Download the Delmar Nurse's Drug Handbook iPhone®/iPod touch® Application

With Delmar Nurse's Drug Handbook iPhone®/iPod touch® application, access detailed information for nearly **800 of the most commonly prescribed drugs** right at your fingertips!

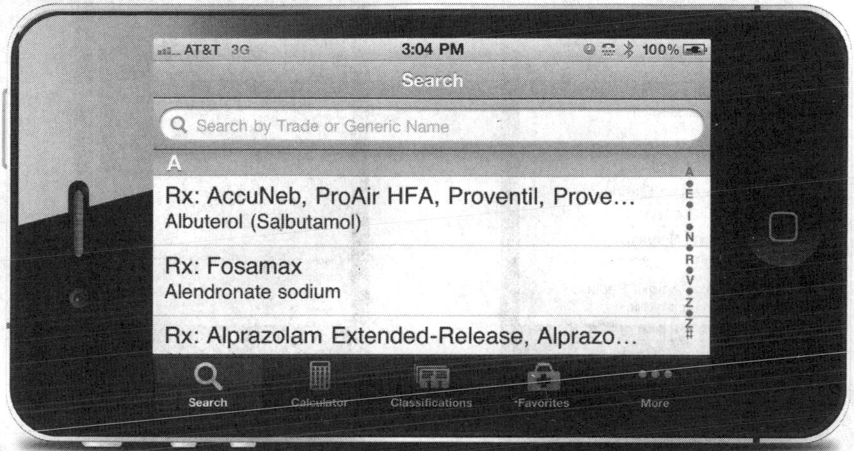

Available on the App Store

FEATURES INCLUDE:

- **Drug search** by trade or generic name
- **Auto-complete** to predict the drug name you seek
- **Search by classification**
- **"Notes" feature** to record your own notes on a specific drug
- **"Favorites" feature** allows uick reference to frequently-cessed drugs
- **"Pinch to zoom" feature** allows for quick enlargement of text using a familiar iPhone®/iPod touch® zoom method
- **Dosage calculators** for solids, liquids, IV drugs and pediatric drugs, plus an IV rate calculator are included
- **Link to individual drugs that comprise a combination drug** for additional drug information

source code:13M-HC0235

2013 NURSE'S DRUG HANDBOOK WEBSITE:

www.cengage.com/community/nursesdrughandbook

ACCESS ADDITIONAL RESOURCES: New FDA-approved drugs Drug administration guidelines • Expanded color photo quick reference guide • Appendices of more resource information

app at
obi

With Delmar Nurse's Drug Handbook iPhone®/iPod touch® "Lite" application, access detailed information for **50 of the most commonly prescribed drugs** right at your fingertips for ***FREE!***

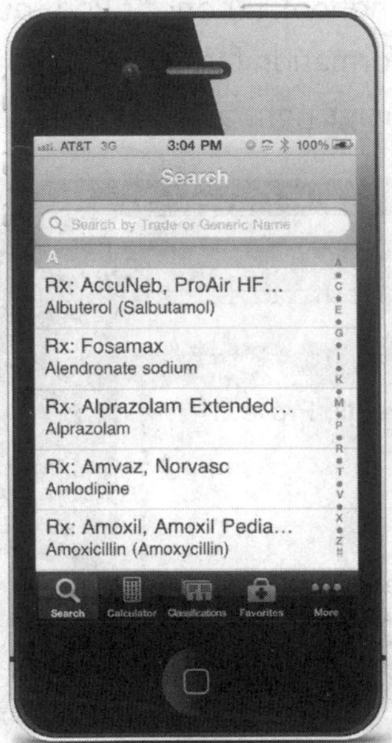

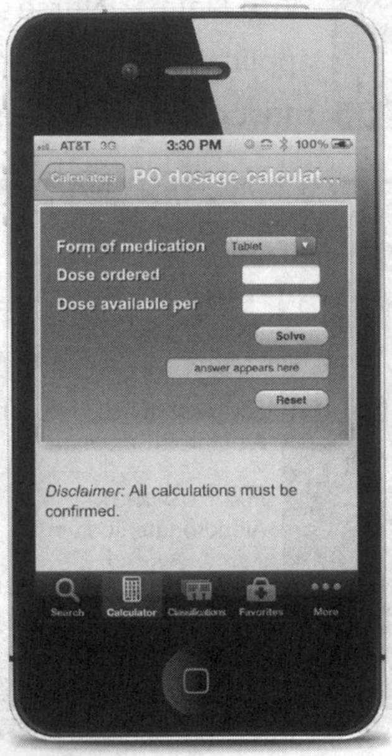

Available on the App Store

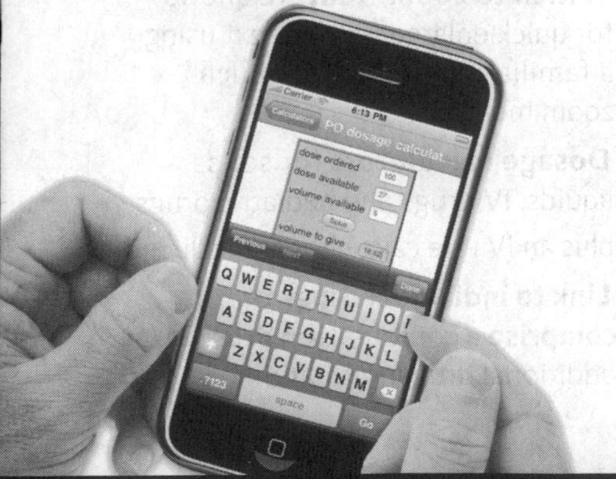

FEATURES INCLUDE:

- **Drug search** by trade or generic name
- **Auto-complete** to predict the drug name you seek
- **Tabbed browsing** to find the information you need fast
- **"Notes" feature** to record your own notes on a specific drug
- **"Favorites" feature** allows quick reference to frequently-accessed drugs
- **Dosage calculators** for solids, liquids, IV drugs and pediatric drugs, plus an I rate calculator are included

2013 NURSE'S DRUG HANDBOOK WEBS

www.cengage.com/community/nursesdrughan

ACCESS ADDITIONAL RESOURCES: New FDA-approve Drug administration guidelines • Expanded color pho reference guide • Appendices of more resource info

Get the free mobile app at http://gettag.mobi

2013 EDITION

DELMAR NURSE'S DRUG HANDBOOK

The information standard for prescription drugs and nursing implications for over 20 years

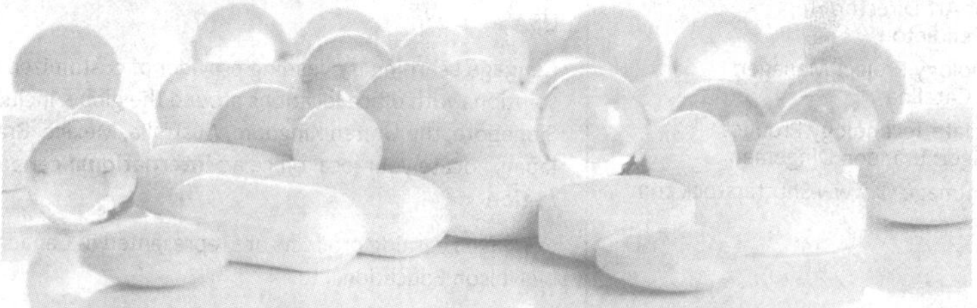

GEORGE R. SPRATTO, PHD
Dean Emeritus and Professor
School of Pharmacy
West Virginia University
Morgantown, West Virginia

ADRIENNE L. WOODS, MSN, FNP-BC
Nurse Practitioner
President AF6E LO34 National Representative NVAC
Department of Veterans Affairs Medical and Regional Office Center
Wilmington, Delaware

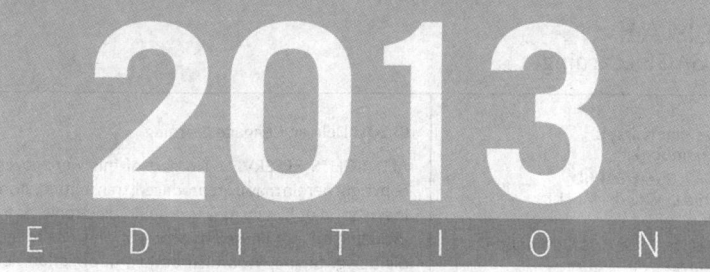

DELMAR
CENGAGE Learning™

2013 Delmar Nurse's Drug Handbook™

George R. Spratto, PhD
Adrienne L. Woods, MSN, FNP-BC

Vice President, Careers & Computing: Dave Garza

Director of Learning Solutions: Matthew Kane

Executive Editor: Maureen Rosener

Managing Editor: Marah Bellegarde

Senior Product Manager: Debra Myette-Flis

Editorial Assistant: Samantha Miller

Vice President, Marketing: Jennifer Ann Baker

Marketing Director: Wendy E. Mapstone

Senior Marketing Manager: Michele McTighe

Marketing Coordinator: Scott A. Chrysler

Production Manager: Andrew Crouth

Content Project Manager: Brooke Greenhouse

Senior Art Director: Jack Pendleton

Technology Project Manager: Chris Catalina

Associate Technology Product Manager: Brandon Dingeman

Cover image © www.Shutterstock.com

Library of Congress Control Number: 2012937927

ISBN-13: 978-1-133-28028-6

ISBN-10: 1-133-28028-5

Delmar
5 Maxwell Drive
Clifton Park, NY 12065-2919
USA

Cengage Learning is a leading provider of customized learning solutions with office locations around the globe, including Singapore, the United Kingdom, Australia, Mexico, Brazil, and Japan. Locate your local office at: **international.cengage.com/region**

Cengage Learning products are represented in Canada by Nelson Education, Ltd.

To learn more about Delmar, visit **www.cengage.com/delmar**
Purchase any of our products at your local college store or at our preferred online store **www.cengagebrain.com**

Printed in the United States of America
4 5 6 7 16 15 14 13

Table of Contents

Notice to the Reader

The monographs in this edition of the *Delmar Nurse's Drug Handbook*™ are the work of two distinguished authors: George R. Spratto, PhD, Dean Emeritus and Professor of Pharmacology of the School of Pharmacy at West Virginia University, Morgantown, West Virginia, and Adrienne L. Woods, MSN, FNP-BC, Nurse Practitioner, President AF6E L0342 and National Representative NVAC, Department of Veterans Affairs Medical and Regional Office Center, Wilmington, Delaware.

The publisher and the authors do not warrant or guarantee any of the products described herein or perform any independent analysis in connection with any of the product information contained herein. The publisher and the authors do not assume and expressly disclaim any obligation to obtain and include information other than that provided by the manufacturer.

The reader is expressly warned to consider and adopt all safety precautions that might be indicated by the activities described herein and to avoid all potential hazards. By following the instructions contained herein, the reader willingly assumes all risks in connection with such instructions.

The publisher and the authors make no representations or warranties of any kind, including but not limited to the warranties of fitness for a particular purpose or merchantability nor are any such representations implied with respect to the material set forth herein, and the publisher and the authors take no responsibility with respect to such material. The publisher and the authors shall not be liable for any special, consequential, or exemplary damages resulting, in whole or in part, from the reader's use of, or reliance upon, this material.

The authors and publisher have made a conscientious effort to ensure that the drug information and recommended dosages in this book and companion web site are accurate and in accord with accepted standards at the time of publication. However, pharmacology and therapeutics are rapidly changing sciences, so readers are advised, before administering any drug, to check the package insert provided by the manufacturer for the recommended dose, for any contraindications for administration, and for any added warnings and precautions. This recommendation is especially important for new, infrequently used, or highly toxic drugs.

Preface

The *2013 Delmar Nurse's Drug Handbook* is a trusted resource used by nursing students, practicing nurses, and other health care professionals. Each annual edition provides updates affecting thousands of bits of information and introduces monographs of drugs recently approved by the FDA and marketed by the drug manufacturers. Drug information changes rapidly, including the development of new drugs, new uses for established drugs, revised and new administration routes (dosage forms), newly identified side effects and drug interactions, and changes in dosing and use recommendations based on feedback from health care professionals, researchers, and consumers. Nurses and other health care professionals depend on this handbook to provide the latest information on drug therapy, guidelines for monitoring efficacy of therapy, and recommendations for teaching the client and family about important aspects of the drug therapy. These uses are critically important to minimize errors in drug therapy.

ORGANIZATION OF CONTENT

Chapter 1 contains individual drug monographs in alphabetical order by generic name. Newly marketed drugs are also included in Chapter 1. The purpose and meaning of each of the components of a monograph are described under "Using the Drug Monographs." See also the "Quick Reference Guide to a Drug Monograph" on page xvi.

Chapter 2 includes general information on important therapeutic or chemical classes of drugs. The classes are listed alphabetically. Consult the Table of Contents for a listing of the therapeutic/chemical classes included in Chapter 2. Each class begins with a list of drugs for which a monograph appears in Chapter 1 as well as the 2013 Delmar Nurse's Drug Handbook Website (www.cengage.com/community/nursesdrughandbook). The information provided in the class applies to all drugs listed for the class. For complete knowledge of a specific drug, consult the class information in Chapter 2, as well as the appropriate monograph in Chapter 1.

The **Color Photo Quick Reference Guide** is a color insert that provides rapid identification of 98 most-commonly prescribed drugs. Products shown in the guide are identified by a camera icon in the drug name area of the related monograph in Chapter 1. Actual-sized tablets and capsules, with their strengths listed, are organized alphabetically by generic name. Each product is also labeled with its trade name and the name of the manufacturer.

The **Appendices** provide additional information to assist in administering drugs and monitoring drug therapy. A complete listing of the appendices is provided in the Table of Contents. Appendices are revised annually, as appropriate, to reflect the latest available information.

The FDA has added a boxed warning to prescribing information for numerous drugs whose side effects can be toxic or life-threatening and in some cases have resulted in death. In this handbook, these "Black Box Warnings" are indicated by a black box icon ■ following the drug name and by the black box icon and highlighted content in the "Special Concerns" portion of the monograph.

Two indexes are found in the back of the handbook. The **IV Index** lists IV drugs by generic name and trade name. The **General Index** is extensively cross-referenced: each generic drug name entry includes the major trade name(s) entry in parentheses and each trade name entry is followed by the generic drug name in parentheses. This is helpful when you or the client can only remember one name of the drug prescribed (especially by another provider). Each page of the general index contains a key identifying boldface as the generic drug name, italics as the therapeutic drug class, regular type as the trade name, and capitals as the name of combination drugs.

USING THE DRUG MONOGRAPHS

The following components are described in the order in which they appear in the monographs. All components may not appear in each monograph but are represented where appropriate and when information is available. Refer also to the "Quick Reference Guide to a Drug Monograph," with explanatory notes for the purpose and use of each component.

Drug Name: The generic drug name is the first item in the name block (in color at the beginning of each monograph). One or more icons may follow the drug name:

■ Black box to indicate that the FDA has issued a boxed warning about potentially dangerous or life-threatening side effects

Ear to indicate that sound-alike drug names may be linked to medication errors

Camera to indicate that the oral form of a drug is shown in the Visual Identification Guide

IV to indicate that the drug can also be given IV

Phonetic Pronunciation: Guide for generic name to assist in mastering the pronunciation of often complex names.

Classification: Defines the type of drug or the class under which the drug is listed. A classification or descriptor is provided for each drug name in Chapter 1. If the drug class is new and/or only a few drugs are available in the class at the time of printing the handbook, the classification will not appear in Chapter 2. It will be added at a later date as more drugs in the class reach the market.

Pregnancy Category: Lists the FDA pregnancy category (A, B, C, D, or X) assigned to the drug (pregnancy categories are defined in Appendix 4).

Trade Name: Trade names are identified as OTC (over-the-counter, no prescription required) or Rx (prescription required). If numerous dosage forms of the drug are available, the trade names are preceded by identifying the dosage form. Trade names available only in Canada are identified by a maple leaf icon ✤.

Controlled Substance: If the drug is controlled by the U.S. Federal Controlled Substances Act, the schedule in which the drug is placed (C-I, C-II, C-III, C-IV, C-V) follows the trade name listing. See Appendix 3 for a listing of controlled substances in both the United States and Canada.

Combination Drug: This heading at the top of the name block indicates that the drug is a combination of two or more drugs in the same product. An extensive list of combination drugs is found in Appendix 8, List of Combination Drugs.

The following components may appear in the body of a drug monograph.

Cross Reference: "See also…" directs the reader to the classification entry in Chapter 2 that matches the classification of the drug being reviewed or to another related drug in Chapter 1. General information about the drugs in the class is provided in Chapter 2.

General Statement: This appears in a few drug monographs but is more common in the class entries in Chapter 2. Information about the drug class and/or anything specific or unusual about a group of drugs is presented. Information may also be presented about the disease(s), condition(s) for which the drugs are indicated, or drug therapy for the disease.

Uses: Approved therapeutic uses for the drug are listed. Some investigational uses are also listed for selected drugs.

Content: For combination drugs, provides the generic name and amount of each drug in the combination product.

Action/Pharmacokinetics: The action portion describes the proposed mechanism(s) by which a drug achieves its therapeutic effect. Not all mechanisms of action are known, and some are self-evident, as when a hormone is administered as a replacement. The pharmacokinetics portion lists critical information, if known, about the rate of drug absorption (including, when known, the percent bioavailable), distribution, time for peak plasma levels or peak effect, minimum effective serum or plasma level, biological half-life, duration of action, mechanism for metabolism, and excretion route(s). Metabolism and excretion routes may be important for clients with systemic liver disease, kidney disease, or both.

Many drugs bind to plasma proteins. If a client is prescribed two or more drugs that bind to plasma proteins, there is the potential for altered effects (either increased or decreased) because of competition for binding sites. It may be necessary to change the dose of one or more of the drugs to improve the therapeutic action. The percent of the drug bound to plasma proteins is included when known.

The half-life (the time required for half the drug to be excreted or removed from the blood, serum, or plasma—t½) is important in determining how often a drug is to be administered and how long the client is to be assessed for side effects. Therapeutic levels indicate the desired concentration, in serum or plasma, for the drug to exert its beneficial effect and are helpful in predicting the onset of side effects or the lack of effect. Drug therapy is often monitored in this manner (e.g., antibiotics, theophylline, phenytoin, amiodarone).

Contraindications: Disease states or conditions in which the drug should not be used are noted. The safe use of many of the newer pharmacologic agents during pregnancy, lactation, or childhood has not been fully established. As a general rule, the use of drugs during pregnancy is contraindicated unless the benefits of drug therapy are determined to far outweigh the potential risks.

Special Concerns: Numerous drugs have life-threatening or dangerous adverse effects that may lead to organ/system damage and possibly death. The FDA provides boxed warnings with the prescribing information for these drugs to alert health care professionals to the potential for serious side effects. A black box icon ■ and highlighted content in this section of the monograph draw attention to the warning information. This section also covers considerations for use with pediatric, geriatric, pregnant, or lactating clients. Situations and disease states when the drug should be used with caution are also listed.

Side Effects: Undesired or bothersome effects the client may experience while taking a particular agent are described. The most common side effects (shown in color) are listed first for quick reference, followed by a complete list of side effects organized by the body organ or system affected. Nearly all potential side effects are listed. In any given clinical situation, however, a client may experience no side effects, one or two side effects, or several, side effects. If potentially life-threatening, the side effect is displayed in ***bold italic*** type.

Overdose Management: When appropriate, this section provides a list of the symptoms observed following an overdose (Symptoms) as well as treatment approaches and/or antidotes for the overdose (Treatment).

Drug Interactions: Alphabetical listing of drugs and herbals that may interact with the drug under discussion. The study of drug interactions is an important area of pharmacology that changes constantly. Because of the significant increase in the use of herbal products, interactions of medications with herbals are included in this section if known or suspected. These interactions are designated by the icon H. The listing of drug/drug and drug/herbal interactions is far from complete; therefore, listings in this handbook are to be considered only as general cautionary guidelines.

Drug interactions may result from a number of different mechanisms: (1) additive or inhibitory effects; (2) increased or decreased metabolism of the drug; (3) increased or decreased rate of elimination; (4) decreased absorption from the GI tract; and (5) competition for or displacement from receptor sites or plasma protein binding sites. Drug interactions may manifest themselves in a variety of ways; however, an attempt has been made throughout the handbook to describe these interactions whenever possible as an increase (↑) or a decrease (↓) in the effect of the drug, and a reason for the change and, in some cases, monitoring cautions. It is important to realize that any side effects that accompany the administration of a particular agent may be increased as a result of a drug or herbal interaction.

Laboratory Test Considerations: The manner by which a drug may affect laboratory test values is presented. Some of the effects are caused by the therapeutic or toxic effects of the drugs; others result from interference with the testing method itself. The laboratory considerations are described as increased (↑) or false positive (+) values and as decreased (↓) or false negative (-) values. Also included, when available, are drug-induced changes in blood or urine levels of endogenous substances (e.g., glucose, electrolytes, and so on).

How Supplied: The various dosage forms available for the drug and amounts of the drug in each of the dosage forms are presented. Such information is important as one dosage form may be more appropriate for a client than another. This information also allows the user to ensure the appropriate dosage form and strength is being administered.

Dosage: The dosage form and route of administration (in color) is followed by the disease state or condition (in italics) and the recommended dosage. Both adult and pediatric doses are given, when available. The listed dosage is to be considered as a general guideline; the exact amount of the drug to be given is determined by the provider. However, one should question orders when dosages differ markedly from the accepted norm.

Nursing Implications: The guidelines provided in this section are designed to help the practitioner in applying the nursing process to pharmacotherapeutics to ensure safe practice and to minimize medication errors. When applicable, this section begins with an ear icon denoting that either the generic and/or trade name(s) of the drug being discussed sound similar to one or more other drugs. Caution must be exercised to ensure that the correct drug is being used as many drug names do sound similar. In each monograph the following sections are provided when applicable.

- *Implementation/Administration/Storage*: Guidelines for preparing medications for administration, administering the medication, things to be aware of during administration and storage and disposal of the medication. Guidelines for administration by IV route are indicated by an icon **IV**. A feature with COMPATIBILITY and INCOMPATIBILITY icons, found under the IV icon when appropriate, lists compatibilities and incompatibilities for that drug when administered by the IV route.
- *Assessment*: Guidelines for monitoring/assessing the client before, during, and after prescribed drug therapy.
- *Interventions*: Additional guidelines for specific nursing actions related to the drug being administered.
- *Client/Family Teaching*: Guidelines to promote education, active participation, understanding, and adherence to drug therapy by the client, family, and/or care givers. Precautions, including side effects related to the drug therapy are also noted for communication to the client/family/care giver.
- *Outcomes/Evaluate*: Desired outcomes of the drug therapy and client response. These will help determine the effectiveness and positive therapeutic outcome of the prescribed drug therapy.

Notes on Assessment and Administration. The following tasks are critical in assessing the client for drug therapy and for planning the interventions needed to undertake the therapy:

- Gather relevant physical data and client history
- Assess specific physiologic functions likely to be affected by the drug therapy
- Determine specific laboratory tests needed to monitor the course of the drug therapy
- Identify sensitivities/interactions and conditions that may preclude a particular drug therapy
- Document specific indications for therapy and describe symptom characteristics related to this condition
- Know the physiologic, pharmacologic, and psychologic effects of the drug and how these may affect the client and impact the nursing process and client response

- Know side effects that can arise as a result of drug therapy and be prepared with appropriate nursing interventions, reporting, and documentation
- Monitor the client for side effects and document/report them to the provider. Severe side effects generally require dosage modification or discontinuation of the drug
- Ensure client safety when receiving drug therapy
- Determine all other drugs/herbals/agents taken by the client

When taking the nursing history, place emphasis on the client's ability to read and to follow directions. Language barriers must be identified and appropriate written translations should be provided to promote understanding and adherence to the drug therapy. In addition, client lifestyle, culture, income, availability of health insurance, medications, and access to transportation are important factors that may affect adherence with therapy and follow-up care. Appendix 13 discusses cultural aspects of medication therapy.

The assessment should include the potential for the client being/becoming pregnant, and if a mother is breastfeeding her infant.

The age and orientation level of the client, whether learned from personal observation or from discussion with close friends or family members can be critical in determining potential relationships between drug therapy and/or drug interactions.

Including these factors in the nursing assessment will assist all members of the health care team to determine the type of pharmacotherapy, drug delivery system, and monitoring and follow-up plan best suited to a particular client to promote the highest level of adherence and desired results.

Notes on Client/Family Teaching: Specific understandable information for the client is provided for each drug. Client/family teaching assists the client/family to recognize side effects and avoid potentially dangerous situations, and alleviates anxiety associated with starting and maintaining drug therapy.

Details on administration are included to enhance client understanding and adherence. Side effects that require medical intervention are included, as are recommendations for minimizing the side effects for certain medications (e.g., take medication with food to decrease GI upset, or take at bedtime to minimize daytime sedative effects).

The proper education of clients is one of the most challenging aspects of nursing. The instructions must be tailored to the needs, awareness, and sophistication of each client. For example, clients who take medication to lower blood pressure should assume responsibility for taking their own blood pressure or having it taken and recorded for provider review. Promote use of pill box to help compliance.

Clients should carry identification listing the drugs currently prescribed and consumed. They should know what they are taking and why, and develop a mechanism to remind themselves to take their medication as prescribed. Clients should always carry this drug list with them whenever they go for a checkup or seek medical care, and it should be updated by providers at each visit. The drug list may also be shared with the pharmacist if there is a question concerning drugs prescribed, if the client is considering taking an over-the-counter medication, if the client has to change pharmacies, or if the client patronizes more than one pharmacy.

The records, especially subjective reports as well as pulse or blood pressure readings, should be shared with the health care provider to ensure accurate evaluation of the response to the prescribed drug therapy. This may also alert the provider to any drug/food/herbal consumption by the client that they did not prescribe, were not aware of, or that may interfere with (i.e., potentiate or antagonize) the current pharmacologic regimen. The provider may also encourage the client to call with any questions or concerns about the drug therapy to discourage stopping therapy or self-medicating.

Remember: The components described previously are covered for all drugs or drug classes. When drugs are presented as a group (as in Chapter 2), the information for each component is given only once for the group. Check each component for information relevant to all drugs covered in the class. Note that many of the drug monographs in Chapter 1 are cross-referenced to the general information in Chapter 2 or to another drug appearing in Chapter 1. Critical information or information relevant to a specific drug is provided in the individual drug monograph in Chapter 1 under appropriate headings, such as Additional Contraindications or Additional Side Effects. These are **in addition to** and **not instead of** the entry in Chapter 2, which is referenced and must be consulted.

2013 NURSE'S DRUG HANDBOOK ONLINE WEBSITE

Additional content on website includes:

- A FREE iPhone®/iPod® touch "lite version" application with 50 drug monographs
- A "full version" iPhone®/iPod® touch application with nearly 800 monographs
- Full monographs of new drugs added to the 2013 edition
- Bonus drug monographs that include information on addtional drugs
- Expanded color photo quick reference guide
- Drug adminstration guidelines
- Appendices

Enjoy the benefits of the 2013 Delmar Nurse's Drug Handbook Website absolutely free! With your purchase of the *2013 Delmar Nurse's Drug Handbook*, you are entitled to access the website at www.cengage.com/community/nursesdrughandbook

Acknowledgments

We would like to extend our thanks and appreciation to the Delmar Cengage Learning team who works so diligently to ensure that the manuscript process flows smoothly and to keep us on the appropriate time schedule. Team members include Matthew Kane, Director of Learning Solutions; Maureen Rosener, Executive Editor; Deb Myette-Flis, Senior Product Manager; Brooke Greenhouse, Content Project Manager; Jack Pendleton, Senior Art Director; Mary Colleen Liburdi, Senior Product Manager, Digital Solutions Group; Chris Catalina, Technology Project Manager; and Brandon Dingeman, Associate Technology Product Manager.

George Spratto extends greatest appreciation and love to his wife, Lynne, as well as son Chris and his family (daughter-in-law Mary Alice and grandchildren Patrick and Victoria Santopietro) and Gregg and his family (daughter-in-law Kim and grandchildren Alexandra and Dominic), each of whom make the work of this project worthwhile by their unfailing love, support, and encouragement. Special thanks to Dr. Marie Abate and Dr. Matthew Blommel of the West Virginia Center for Drug and Health Information, West Virginia University, who assisted in researching information on new and existing drugs.

Adrienne Woods would like to extend her appreciation to her colleagues and friends at the VA and AFGE. To her husband, Howard, who always finds time and energy to keep it all together. She thanks him for all his patience, caring, love, and understanding. To her children, Katy and Nate, she extends thanks for enduring hectic schedules, missed games, visits, and for understanding the complexities of her work. Finally, to her friends, Cindy and Maryann, for all their support, help, and encouragement during very stressful times.

Quick Reference Guide to a Drug Monograph

IV

1 **Diazepam**

2 (dye-**AYZ**-eh-pam)

3 **Classification(s):** Antianxiety drug, benzodiazepine

4 **Pregnancy Category: D**

5 **Rx:** Diastat AcuDial, Diazepam Intensol, Valium, **C-IV** 6

Rx: Apo-Diazepam, Diazemuls, Valium Roche Oral.

7 SEE ALSO ***TRANQUILIZERS/ANTIMANIC DRUGS/HYPNOTICS***.

8 **INDICATIONS/USES**

PO: (1) Management of anxiety disorders or for short-term relief of symptoms of anxiety. (2) Adjunct therapy in convulsive disorders; effectiveness as sole therapy has not been proven. (3) Adjunct for relief of skeletal muscle spasm caused by reflex spasm to local pathology (e.g., inflammation of muscles or joints or secondary to trauma). Also, spasticity due to upper motor neuron disorders (e.g., cerebral palsy, paraplegia). Athetosis, stiff-man syndrome. (4) Acute alcohol withdrawal for symptomatic relief of acute agitation, tremor, impending or acute delirum tremens, and hallucinosis.

1 **GENERIC NAME OF DRUG**

One or more icons may be found here: black box (adverse effects warning), camera (photo of dosage form), ear (sound-alike drug), IV (drug can be given IV).

2 **PHONETIC PRONUNCIATION**

A phonetic pronunciation of the generic name is provided.

3 **CLASSIFICATION**

Defines the type of drug or the class under which the drug is listed.

4 **PREGNANCY CATEGORY**

Assigned by the FDA. Defined in Appendix 4.

5 **TRADE NAMES**

Names by which a drug is marketed. If numerous forms of the drug are available, the trade names are identified by dosage form. **Rx** denotes prescription drugs. **OTC** denotes over-the-counter, non-prescription drugs. Trade names unique in Canada are indicated by a maple leaf.

6 **CONTROLLED SUBSTANCES**

If the drug is controlled by the U.S. Federal Controlled Substances Act, the schedule in which the drug is placed follows the trade name listing. Controlled substance schedules are placed after Rx drugs (e.g., **C-II**). See Appendix 3.

7 **CROSS REFERENCE (for selected drugs)**

"See also …" directs the reader to the classification entry in Chapter 2 or to other parts of Chapter 1 that give a complete profile or additional information for the drug.

8 **APPROVED THERAPEUTIC USES**

Some investigational uses are also listed for selected drugs.

9 **ACTION/KINETICS**

Action

Reduces anxiety by increasing or facilitating the inhibitory neurotransmitter activity of GABA. The skeletal muscle relaxant effect may be due to enhancement of GABA-mediated presynaptic inhibition at the spinal level as well as in the brain stem reticular formation.

Pharmacokinetics

Onset: PO, 30–60 min; **IM,** 15–30 min; **IV,**
10 more rapid. **Peak plasma levels: PO,** 0.5–2 hr;
IM, 0.5–1.5; **IV,** 0.25 hr. **Duration:** 3 hr. **t½:** 11
20–50 hr. Metabolized in the liver to the active metabolites desmethyldiazepam, oxazepam, and temazepam. Diazepam and metabolites are excreted through the urine. **Plasma protein binding:** 12
97–99%.

13 **CONTRAINDICATIONS**

Lactation.

14 **SPECIAL CONCERNS**

(1) Tablets are for treatment of HIV-1 infection in combination with appropriate antiretroviral agents when therapy is warranted. (2) Resistant virus emerges rapidly when delavirdine is given as monotherapy. Always give in combination with appropriate antiretroviral therapy.

- Use with caution in impaired hepatic function.
- Use with combination therapy as resistant viruses emerge with monotherapy.
- Safety and efficacy in combination with other antiretroviral drugs not determined in HIV-1-infected clients less than 16 years of age.

15 **SIDE EFFECTS**

Most Common

Rash, maculopapular rash, N&V, diarrhea, headache, fatigue, pruritus.

Body as a whole: Headache, fatigue, asthenia, allergic reaction, angioedema, chest pain, chills, general or local edema, fever, flu syndrome, leth-

9 **ACTION/KINETICS**

The mechanism of action is stated when known. **Pharmacokinetics:** Critical information about the rate of drug absorption, bioavailability, distribution, time for peak plasma levels or peak effect, minimum effective serum or plasma level, duration of action, metabolism, and excretion route(s). Metabolism and excretions routes may be important for clients with systemic liver disease, kidney disease, or both.

10 **MAXIMUM PLASMA LEVELS**

Achieved at therapeutic doses or at steady state.

11 **BIOLOGICAL HALF-LIFE**

The time required for half the drug to be excreted or removed from the blood, serum, or plasma. This information is important in determining dosing intervals.

12 **PLASMA PROTEIN BINDING**

The extent to which a drug is bound to plasma protein, when applicable.

13 **CONTRAINDICATIONS**

Lists disease states or conditions in which the drug should not be used.

14 **SPECIAL CONCERNS**

When appropriate, the FDA Black Box Warning is included. Considerations for use with caution in pediatric, geriatric, pregnant, or lactating clients, and in unique situations or disease states.

15 **SIDE EFFECTS**

The most common side effects are listed in color first for quick reference, followed by the complete list of side effects organized by body organ or system affected. If potentially life-threatening, the side effect is bold-italic.

LABORATORY TEST CONSIDERATIONS

16 ↑ AST, ALT, GGT, alkaline phosphatase, bilirubin, uric acid, serum amylase, lipase.

17 **OVERDOSE MANAGEMENT**

Symptoms: Pancreatitis, peripheral neuropathy, diarrhea, hyperuricemia, hepatic dysfunction. *Treatment:* There are no antidotes; treatment should be symptomatic. There may be some clearance using hemodialysis.

18 **DRUG INTERACTIONS**

Digoxin / ↑ Digoxin bioavailability

19 H *Evening primrose oil* / Potential for ↑ antiplatelet effect

H *Feverfew* / Potential for ↑ antiplatelet effect

H *Garlic* / Potential for ↑ antiplatelet effect

H *Ginger* / Potential for ↑ antiplatelet effect

H *Ginkgo biloba* / Potential for ↑ antiplatelet effect

H *Ginseng* / Potential for ↑ antiplatelet effect

H *Grapeseed extract* / Potential for ↑ antiplatelet effect

Warfarin / ↑ Risk of major bleeding

20 **HOW SUPPLIED**

Tablets: 25 mg, 50 mg, 75 mg.

21 **DOSAGE**

TABLETS

Adjunct in prophylaxis of thromboembolism after cardiac valve replacement.

Adults: 75–100 mg 4 times per day as an adjunct to warfarin therapy. Do not give aspirin concomitantly.

16 **LABORATORY TEST CONSIDERATIONS**

The manner by which the drug may affect laboratory test values is presented as increased values (↑) or false positive values (+) or decreased values (↓) or false negative values (–). Also included, when available, are drug-induced changes in blood or urine levels of endogenous substances.

17 **OVERDOSE MANAGEMENT**

Symptoms observed following an overdose or toxic reaction and treatment approaches and/or antidotes for the overdose.

18 **DRUG INTERACTIONS**

Alphabetical listing of drugs and herbals that may interact with the drug: ↑ (increase) effect, ↓ (decrease) effect, → leading to. Monitoring information may also be presented.

19 **HERBALS**

Known or suspected drug interactions with herbal products.

20 **HOW SUPPLIED**

Dosage forms and amounts of the drug in each of the dosage forms. One dosage form may be more appropriate for a client than another. This information also allows the user to ensure the appropriate dosage form and strength is being administered.

21 **DOSAGE**

The dosage form (in color) and/or route of administration is followed by the disease state or condition (in italics) and the recommended dosage.

22 **NURSING IMPLICATIONS**

23 ℞ Do not confuse Avelox with Asacol (mesalamine, an anti-inflammatory drug).

24 **IMPLEMENTATION/ADMINISTRATION/STORAGE**

1. Avoid high humidity when storing tablets. Not for IM, SC, intrathecal, or intraperitoneal use.
2. Store tablets from 15–30°C (59–86°F) avoiding high humidity and the ophthalmic solution from 2–25°C (36–77°F).

25 3. **IV** No dosage adjustment needed when switching from IV to PO dosing.

4. Give only by IV infusion over 60 min through a Y-type IV infusion set. Avoid rapid or bolus IV infusion. If Y-type or piggyback method used, temporarily discontinue administration of other solutions during moxifloxacin IV administration.
5. The premix containers are for single use only; discard any unused portion.
6. Store IV solution from 15–30°C (59–86°F); do not refrigerate.

26 7. COMPATIBILITY 0.9% NaCl, D5W, D10W, LR.

8. INCOMPATIBILITY Administer separately; flush line before and after moxifloxacin infusion with a compatible solution.

27 **ASSESSMENT**

1. Note onset, location, characteristics of S&S, clinical presentation, and culture results. List drugs prescribed to ensure none interact.

28 **CLIENT/FAMILY TEACHING**

1. Drug is administered every 2–3 weeks IV to inhibit/control rapid cell division of abnormal cells. Anticipate premedication with other agents to prevent hypersensitivity reactions.
2. Anticipate hair loss; should regrow. Avoid crowds and those with infections during therapy.

29 **INTERVENTIONS**

For induction and stimulation of labor and/or oxytocin challenge test:

1. Before initiating therapy, inform client of rationale for using oxytocic agents and reassure that this procedure is not unusual. Explain

30 **OUTCOMES/EVALUATE**

- Induction of labor with effective uterine contractions
- ↑ Uterine tone with ↓ postpartum bleeding

22 **NURSING IMPLICATIONS**

Guidelines to help the practitioner in applying the nursing process to pharmacotherapeutics to ensure safe practice and patient safety.

23 **SOUND ALIKE WARNINGS**

Drug names that sound alike are listed for which caution must be exercised to ensure the correct drug has been chosen.

24 **IMPLEMENTATION/ADMINISTRATION/STORAGE**

Guidelines for preparing medications for administration, administering the medication, and proper storage and disposal of the medication.

25 **GUIDELINES FOR ADMINISTRATION BY IV**

26 **COMPATIBILITY AND INCOMPATIBILITY**

Compatibility and Incompatibility drug-related information is included for IV drug administration.

27 **ASSESSMENT**

Guidelines for monitoring/assessing before, during, and after prescribed drug therapy, including labs and tests indicated.

28 **CLIENT/FAMILY TEACHING**

Guidelines to promote education, active participation, understanding, and adherence to drug therapy by the client and/or family members. Precautions about drug therapy are also noted for communication to the client/family.

29 **INTERVENTIONS (for selected drugs)**

Guidelines for specific nursing actions and approaches related to the drug being administered.

30 **OUTCOMES/EVALUATE**

Desired outcome(s) of the drug therapy and client response.

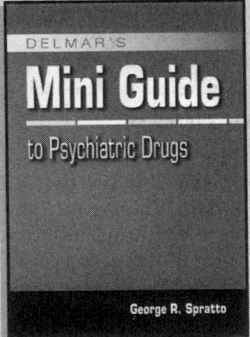

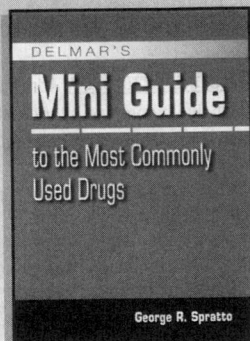

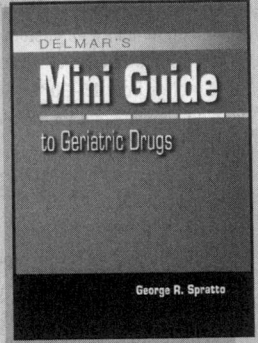

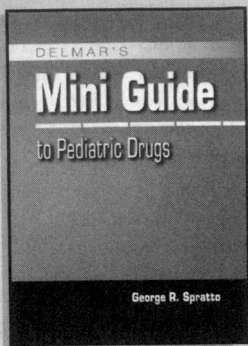

A

chapter 1

A–Z Listing of Drugs

A

Abacavir sulfate

(uh-**BACK**-ah-veer)

Classification(s): Antiviral, nucleoside reverse transcriptase inhibitor

Pregnancy Category: C

RX: Ziagen.

SEE ALSO ***ANTIVIRAL DRUGS***.

INDICATIONS/USES

Treat HIV-1 infection in combination with other antiretroviral drugs (e.g., lamivudine and zidovudine). Do not add as a single agent when antiretroviral regimens are changed due to loss of virologic response.

ACTION/KINETICS

Action

Synthetic nucleoside analog. Converted intracellularly to the active carbovir triphosphate, which inhibits the activity of HIV-1 reverse transcriptase by competing with the natural substrate deoxyguanosine-5'-triphosphate and by incorporation into viral DNA. Prevents the formation of the 5'- to 3'-phosphodiester linkage essential for DNA chain elongation; thus, viral DNA growth is terminated. Cross resistance in vitro has been seen to lamivudine, didanosine, and zalcitabine.

Pharmacokinetics

Rapidly and extensively absorbed after PO use. Bioavailability of the tablet is about 80%. Oral solution and tablets may be used interchangeably. Not significantly metabolized by cytochrome P450 enzymes, but it is metabolized by alcohol dehydrogenase in the liver and excreted in both the urine and feces. **Plasma protein binding:** About 50%.

CONTRAINDICATIONS

Hypersensitivity to abacavir or any component of the product. Lactation. The safety, efficacy, and pharmacokinetic properties have not been determined in clients with moderate or severe hepatic impairment; do not use abacavir in these clients. Reintroduction to clients with a prior history of a hypersensitivity reaction to abacavir.

SPECIAL CONCERNS

(1) **Hypersensitivity reactions.** Serious and sometimes fatal hypersensitivity reactions have been associated with abacavir therapy (see *Side Effects*). Hypersensitivity to abacavir is a multi-organ clinical syndrome usually characterized by a sign or symptom in two or more of the following groups:

- Constitutional, including achiness, fatigue, or generalized malaise
- Fever
- GI, including abdominal pain, diarrhea, nausea, or vomiting
- Rash
- Respiratory, including cough, dyspnea, or pharyngitis

Discontinue as soon as hypersensitivity reaction is suspected. (2) Clients who carry the HLA-B*5701 allele are at high risk for experiencing a hypersensitivity reaction to abacavir. Prior to initiating therapy with abacavir, screening for the HLA-B*5701 allele is recommended; this approach has been found to decrease the risk of hypersensitivity reaction. Screening is also recommended prior to reinitiating abacavir in clients of unknown HLA-B*5701 status who have previously tolerated abacavir. HLA-B*5701-negative clients may develop a suspected hypersensitivity reaction to abacavir; however, this occurs significantly less frequently than in HLA-B*5701–positive clients. (3) Regardless of HLA-B*5701 status, permanently discontinue if hypersensitivity cannot be ruled out, even when other diagnoses are possible. (4) Following a hypersensitivity reaction to abacavir, never re-

A

start abacavir or any abacavir-containing product because more severe symptoms can occur within hours and may include life-threatening hypotension and death. (5) Reintroduction of abacavir or any other abacavir-containing product, even in clients who have no identified history or unrecognized symptoms of hypersensitivity to abacavir therapy, can result in serious or fatal hypersensitivity reactions. Such reactions can occur within hours. (6) **Lactic acidosis and severe hepatomegaly**. Lactic acidosis and severe hepatomegaly with steatosis, including fatal cases, have been reported with the use of nucleoside analogs alone or in combination, including abacavir and other antiretroviral drugs. ■

- **Cross-resistance is possible between abacavir and other nucleoside reverse transcriptase inhibitors.**
- **There is an increased risk of MI.**
- **Use with caution in the elderly.**

SIDE EFFECTS

Most Common

N&V, malaise/fatigue, dreams/sleep disorders, headache, migraine, abdominal pain/gastritis, diarrhea, fever/chills, fatigue, malaise, drug hypersensitivity.

Hypersensitivity: See Black Box Warning. Also, abnormal chest x-ray findings (predominantly infiltrates, which can be localized), edema, lethargy, myolysis, paresthesia, adult respiratory distress syndrome, ***anaphylaxis, death***, hypotension, ***liver failure***, renal failure, ***respiratory failure***, lymphadenopathy, mucous membrane lesions (including conjunctivitis, mouth ulceration), maculopapular/urticarial rash, erythema multiforme. **GI:** N&V, diarrhea, abdominal pain, gastritis, loss of appetite, ***pancreatitis, severe hepatomegaly with steatosis (may be fatal)***. **CNS:** Dreams, sleep disorders, headache, migraine, depressive disorders, dizziness, anxiety, worsening of pre-existing depression. **CV:** ***MI***. **Respiratory:** Bronchitis, viral respiratory infections, pneumonia (in children). **Musculoskeletal:** Musculoskeletal pain. **Dermatologic:** Rash, ***Stevens-Johnson syndrome, and toxic epidermal necrolysis, especially in combination with drugs known to cause these effects***. **GU:** Renal signs/symptoms. **Hematologic:** Neutropenia, anemia, thrombocytopenia, leukopenia. **Body as a whole:** Fatigue, malaise, skin rashes, fever, chills, ear/nose/throat infections, non-site specific pain. Redistribution/accumulation of body fat, including central obesity, dorsocervical fat enlargement (buffalo hump), peripheral/facial wasting, breast enlargement, and cushinoid appearance. **Miscellaneous**: Lactic acidosis, immune reconstitution syndrome.

LABORATORY TEST CONSIDERATIONS

Abnormal LFTs. ↑ ALT, AST, CPK, GGT, creatinine. Hypertriglyceridemia, hyperamylasemia, hyperglycemia.

DRUG INTERACTIONS

Ethanol / ↓ Excretion of abacavir → ↑ abacavir AUC and t½

Methadone / ↑ Methadone clearance; may need to ↑ dose in some clients

HOW SUPPLIED

Oral Solution: 20 mg/mL; *Tablets:* 300 mg.

DOSAGE

ORAL SOLUTION; TABLETS

Treat HIV-1 infection.

Adults: 300 mg twice a day or 600 mg once a day with other antiretroviral drugs. **Pediatric, 3 months to 16 years:** 8 mg/kg twice a day, not to exceed 300 mg twice a day, in combination with other antiretroviral drugs. Use the following doses in hepatic impairment: **Child-Pugh score 7–9:** 200 mg twice a day. To enable dose reduction, use abacavir oral solution, 10 mL twice a day. Do not use in those with a Child-Pugh score of 10–15.

NURSING IMPLICATIONS

IMPLEMENTATION/ADMINISTRATION/STORAGE

1. Give with or without food.
2. Do not restart after hypersensitivity reaction. More severe symptoms will occur within hours; may include life-threatening hypotension or death.
3. Store tablets and oral solution from 20–25°C (68–77°F). Do not freeze oral solution; it may be refrigerated.

ASSESSMENT

1. List reasons for therapy, assess for changes in HIV presentation and S&S of opportunistic infections during therapy; note other agents trialed.
2. Observe for hypersensitivity reactions, even if alternative diagnosis possible. Once experienced, never resume therapy with abacavir. If discontinued and no hypersensitivity reactions, may reintroduce cautiously if medical care readily accessible.
3. Several products contain abacavir. Before starting abacavir, review medical history for prior exposure to any abacavir-containing product to avoid reintroduction in a client with a history of hypersensitivity to abacavir.
4. Drug has been associated with an ↑ risk of MI.
5. Screen blood for gene variation HLA-B*5701; report hypersensitivity reactions to the Abacavir Hypersensitivity Registry at 1-800-270-0425 Monday–Friday 8 a.m. to 6 p.m.
6. Get electrolytes, CD_4, CPK, renal and LFTs; assess for liver enlargement, steatosis, lactic acidosis (↑ lactate levels), opportunistic infections. Lactic acidosis and hepatomegaly has been noted with steatosis (including fatal cases); monitor closely.

CLIENT/FAMILY TEACHING

1. Take with or without food and with other antiretroviral agents twice daily as directed. Also, continue all other HIV medications as prescribed.
2. Measure prescribed dose of solution using dosing spoon or dosing syringe.
3. Review guide accompanying product; report any S&S of allergic reactions (fever, severe fatigue, skin rash, N&V, palpitations, diarrhea, or abdominal pain) and stop drug.
4. Does not prevent or cure disease; works to lower viral count.
5. If allergic reaction experienced, never restart—may be fatal.
6. Report if profound weakness/tiredness, feeling cold, dizzy, or light-headed, pain/tingling in hands/feet or muscle/joint pain occurs.
7. Practice safe sex; drug does not prevent disease transmission.
8. Use reliable birth control; do not breast-feed. Redistribution/accumulation of body fat may occur.
9. Keep all F/U to assess response, labs, and for adverse SE.

OUTCOMES/EVALUATE

- Suppression of HIV RNA
- Increase in CD4 counts

IV

Abatacept

(ah-**BAY**-tah-sept)

Classification(s): Immunomodulator

Pregnancy Category: C

RX: Orencia.

INDICATIONS/USES

(1) Reduce signs and symptoms, slow progression of structural damage, and improve physical function in adults with moderate to severe rheumatoid arthritis. Used alone or with other disease-modifying antirheumatic drugs other than tumor necrosis factor antagonists. (2) Reduce signs and symptoms in children 6 years of age and older with moderately to severely active polyarticular juvenile idiopathic arthritis. May be used as monotherapy or with methotrexate.

ACTION/KINETICS

Action

Inhibits T-lymphocyte activation; activated T-lymphocytes are implicated in the pathogenesis of rheumatoid arthritis. Decreases serum levels of soluble interleukin-2 receptor, interleukin-6, rheumatoid factor, C-reactive protein, metalloproteinase-3, and tumor necrosis factor-al (relationship of these biological markers to rheumatoid arthritis is not known).

Pharmacokinetics

Steady state, adults: By day 60 at doses of 10 mg/kg. **t½, terminal:** 8–25 days in rheumatoid arthritis clients. Is a trend toward highe clearance with increasing baseline body weight.

CONTRAINDICATIONS

Hypersensitivity to abatacept or any of its components. Use with TNF antagonists (due to increased incidence of infections) or ana' ra. Use of live vaccines concurrently with abat pt or within 3 months of its discontinuation. Lactation.

A

SPECIAL CONCERNS

- **Concomitant use of abatacept and tissue necrosis factor (TNF) antagonists result in more infections (including serious infections) compared with use of TNF antagonists alone.**
- **Use with caution in clients with a history of recurrent infections, underlying conditions that may predispose these clients to infections, or chronic, latent, or localized infections.**
- **Use with caution in COPD clients as side effects are more frequent in this group, as well as exacerbation of their COPD.**
- **A higher rate of infections may occur in abatacept-treated clients as well as clients 65 years of age and older.**
- **The possibility exists that the drug may affect host defenses against infections and malignancies because T cells mediate cellular immune responses.**
- **Use with caution in the elderly.**
- **Safety and efficacy not established in children less than 6 years of age.**

SIDE EFFECTS

Most Common

Adults: Headache, URTI, nasopharyngitis, nausea, infections (pneumonia, bronchitis).
Children: Nasopharyngitis, URTI, abdominal pain, cough, diarrhea, headache, nausea, pyrexia.
Infections: URTI, bronchitis, herpes zoster, pneumonia, localized infection, sinusitis, influenza, rhinitis, herpes simplex, cellulitis, diverticulitis, acute pyelonephritis, UTI. **GI:** Nausea, dyspepsia, abdominal pain, diarrhea. **CNS:** Headache, dizziness. **CV:** Hypertension. **Respiratory:** Cough, nasopharyngitis, worsening of COPD in COPD clients, dyspnea, rhonchi, pneumonia. **Malignancies:** Lung cancer, lymphoma, myelodysplastic syndrome, acute lymphocytic leukemia in children, melanoma; cancer of the skin, breast, bile duct, bladder, cervix, endometrium, ovary, prostate, kidney, thyroid, and uterus. **Acute infusion reaction:** Dizziness, headache, hypertension, hypotension, increased BP, dyspnea, nausea, flushing, urticaria, cough, hypersensitivity, pruritus, rash, wheezing. **Hypersensitivity reactions:** Dyspnea, hypotension, urticaria, ***anaphylaxis***, anaphylactoid reactions. **Miscellaneous:** Back pain, pain in extremity, rash, UTI, pyrexia, immunogenicity.

LABORATORY TEST CONSIDERATIONS

Glucose dehydrogenase pyrroloquinoline quinone-based monitoring systems may react with the maltose found in abatacept, resulting in falsely elevated blood glucose readings on the day of infusion.

DRUG INTERACTIONS

Anakinra / Concomitant use is not recommended as there is insufficient experience to assess safety and efficacy
Tissue necrosis factor (TNF) antagonists / ↑ Risk of serious infections and no significant additional efficacy over use of TNF antagonists alone; do not use together

HOW SUPPLIED

Injection, Lyophilized Powder for Solution: 250 mg; ***Injection Solution:*** 125 mg/mL.

DOSAGE

IV INFUSION

Adults, moderate to severe rheumatoid arthritis.

Adults, less than 60 kg: 500 mg. **Adults, 60–100 kg:** 750 mg. **Adults, over 100 kg:** 1,000 mg. Given as a 30 min IV infusion. Give at 2 and 4 weeks after the first infusion and then q 4 weeks thereafter.

Juvenile idiopathic arthritis.

Children, 6–17 years of age, weighing less than 75 kg: 10 mg/kg based on client body weight at each administration; **children, weighing 75 kg or more:** Calculate the dose following the adult dosing regimen. **Maximum dose:** 1,000 mg. Following the initial dose, give at 2 and 4 weeks after the first infusion and then q 4 weeks thereafter.

SC

Adults, moderate to severe rheumatoid arthritis.

Adults: Following a single IV loading dose (see preceding IV dose), give the first 125 mg SC injection within a day followed by 125 mg SC once weekly. *NOTE:* Clients who are unable to receive an IV infusion may initiate weekly SC injections without an IV loading dose.

A

NURSING IMPLICATIONS

IMPLEMENTATION/ADMINISTRATION/STORAGE

1. Clients transitioning from IV abatacept to SC administration should administer the first SC dose instead of the next scheduled IV dose.
2. The 125 mg/mL solution is not intended for IV use.
3. Rotate injection sites. Never give into areas where the skin is tender, bruised, or hard.
4. After proper training in SC injection technique, the client may self-inject if appropriate.
5. Clients using SC administration should be instructed to inject the full amount in the syringe (1 mL), which delivers 125 mg of abatacept.
6. IV Give by IV infusion only. Not for intradermal, subcutaneous, IM, IV bolus, or intra-arterial administration.
7. Use aseptic technique. Reconstitute powder for injection with 10 mL of sterile water for injection, using only the silicone-free disposable syringe provided and an 18- to 21-gauge needle. Do not use vial if the vacuum is not present. Rotate vial with gentle swirling until contents completely dissolve. Avoid prolonged or vigorous agitation. Do not shake. Vent the vial with a needle to dissipate any foam that may be present.
8. If the abatacept powder is accidentally reconstituted using a siliconized syringe, the solution may develop a few translucent particles. Discard any solutions prepared using siliconized syringes.
9. After reconstitution, the concentration in the vial will be 25 mg/mL. The solution should be clear and colorless to pale yellow. Do not use if opaque particles, discoloration, or other foreign particles are present.
10. Reconstituted solution must be further diluted to 100 mL. From a 100 mL infusion bag or bottle, withdraw a volume of 0.9% NaCl injection equal to the volume of the reconstituted solution needed for the client's dose. Slowly add the reconstituted solution into the infusion bag or bottle using the same silicone-free disposable syringe provided with each vial. Mix gently. Do not shake the bag or bottle. The final concentration of abatacept in the bag or bottle will depend on the amount of drug added but will be no more than 10 mg/mL. Immediately discard any unused portion in the vials.
11. Administer with an infusion set and a sterile, nonpyrogenic, low-protein-binding filter (pore size of 0.2–1.2 micrometers). Administer each dose as a 30-min infusion. The infusion of the fully diluted abatacept solution must be completed within 24 hr of reconstitution.
12. In clients with juvenile rheumatoid arthritis, bring all immunizations up-to-date before initiating abatacept therapy.
13. Store unopened vials in refrigerator (2–8°C; 36°–46°F). Protect from light. Infusion of fully diluted abatacept solution must be completed within 24 hr of reconstitution of the abatacept vials. If not used immediately, fully diluted abatacept solution may be stored at room temperature or in refrigerator before use.
14. COMPATIBILITY Reconstitute powder for injection with 10 mL of sterile water for injection; 0.9% NaCl.
15. INCOMPATIBILITY Do not infuse concurrently in same IV line with other agents.

ASSESSMENT

1. List reasons for therapy, other disease modifying antirheumatic drugs (DMARDs) trialed/failed, extent of disease, ROM, level of mobility.
2. Identify all drugs prescribed/OTC to ensure none interact.
3. When switching from TNF therapy to abatacept, monitor closely for S&S of infection.
4. Perform TB test; CXR to ensure no lung disease. Monitor those with COPD closely for worsening of respiratory symptoms. Closely monitor if any new infection occurs during therapy; reduces T cell defenses against infections and malignancies.
5. Monitor BS, CBC, renal and LFTs.

CLIENT/FAMILY TEACHING

1. Used to help slow joint destruction in rheumatoid arthritis when other agents have failed. Given by IV infusion over 30 min at varying times. Ensure ability to complete scheduled therapy.
2. Avoid crowds, sick people, and live vaccinations (up to 3 months after stopping drug) while on therapy.
3. Report lack of response, headaches, runny nose, or dizziness.

4. Advise diabetics: may falsely raise blood sugar readings.
5. Use [illegible]on; avoid activities that require mental [illegible]s until drug effects realized.
6. R[illegible], chills, non-healing wound, burni[illegible]tion, night sweats, Wt loss, [illegible]gh, skin rash, itching, flushing, [illegible]
7. [illegible]ble contraception; stop drug if p[illegible]spected.
8. Kee[illegible]U visits to assess response, labs, and for adverse SE.

OUTCOMES/EVALUATE

- ↓ Progression of joint damage in RA
- Improved physical function/mobility

IV

Abciximab

(ab-**SIX**-ih-mab)

Classification(s): Antiplatelet drug

Pregnancy Category: C

RX: ReoPro.

INDICATIONS/USES

Adjunct to percutaneous coronary intervention (PCI) to prevent cardiac ischemic complications in clients undergoing PCI and in those with unstable angina not responding to conventional therapy when PCI is planned within 24 hr. Used with aspirin and heparin. *Investigational:* Early treatment of acute MI.

ACTION/KINETICS

Action

Binds to a glycoprotein receptor on human platelets, thus inhibiting platelet aggregation by preventing the binding of fibrinogen, von Willebrand factor, and other adhesive molecules to receptor sites on activated platelets.

Pharmacokinetics

$t^{1/2}$, after IV bolus/infusion: 10 min initially and a second phase half-life of about 30 min. **Recovery of platelet function:** About 48 hr, although the drug remains in the circulation bound to platelets for up to 15 days. Following IV infusion, free drug levels in the plasma decrease rapidly for about 6 hr and then decline at a slower rate.

CONTRAINDICATIONS

Due to a potential for drug-induced bleeding, abciximab is contraindicated as follows: History of CVA (within 2 years) or CVA with a significant residual neurologic deficit; active internal bleeding; within 6 weeks of GI or GU bleeding of clinical significance; bleeding diathesis; within 7 days of administration of oral anticoagulants unless the PT is less than 1.2 times control; thrombocytopenia (less than 100,000 cells/μL); within 6 weeks of major surgery or trauma; intracranial neoplasm; arteriovenous malformation or aneurysm; severe uncontrolled hypertension; presumed or documented history of vasculitis; use of IV dextran before PCI or intent to use it during PCI; hypersensitivity to murine proteins.

SPECIAL CONCERNS

- Assess benefits versus the risk of increased bleeding in clients who weigh less than 75 kg, are 65 years of age or older, have a history of GI disease, and are receiving thrombolytics and heparin.
- Also assess benefits versus the risk of increased bleeding in conditions associated with an increased risk of bleeding in the angioplasty setting and which may be additive to that of abciximab: PCI within 12 hr of onset of symptoms for acute MI, PCI lasting more than 70 min, and failed PCI.
- Use with caution during lactation and when abciximab is used with other drugs that affect hemostasis, including thrombolytics, oral anticoagulants, NSAIDs, dipyridamole, and ticlopidine.
- Safety and efficacy not determined in children.

SIDE EFFECTS

Most Common

Back/chest pain, bleeding, hypotension, N&V, headache, bradycardia, puncture site pain, abdominal pain.

Bleeding tendencies: ***Major bleeds, including intracranial hemorrhage.*** Minor bleeding, including spontaneous gross hematuria/hematemesis. Loss of hemoglobin. **CV:** Hypotension, bradycardia, atrial fibrillation/flutter, vascular disorder, pulmonary edema, incomplete or ***complete AV block***, VT, weak pulse, palpitations, nodal arrhythmia, limb embolism, thrombophlebitis, intermittent claudication, pericardial effusion, pseudoaneurysm, AV fistula, ventricular arrhythmia.

GI: N&V, abdominal pain, diarrhea, dry mouth, dyspepsia, enlarged abdomen, ileus, gastroesophageal reflux. **Hematologic**: Thrombocytopenia, anemia/hemolytic anemia, leukocytosis, petechiae. **CNS**: Hypesthesia, confusion, abnormal thinking, agitation, anxiety, dizziness, ***coma, brain ischemia***, insomnia. **Respiratory**: Pleural effusion, pleurisy, pneumonia, rales, bronchitis, bronchospasm, ***PE***, rhonchi. **Musculoskeletal**: Myopathy, cellulitis, myalgia, muscle contraction/pain. **GU**: UTI, urinary retention, abnormal renal function, dysuria, frequent micturition, cystalgia, incontinence, prostatitis. **Dermatologic:** Pruritus, pallor, increased sweating, bullous eruption.
Ophthalmic: Diplopia, abnormal vision. **Miscellaneous**: Pain, peripheral edema, development of human antichimeric antibody, dysphonia, abscess, asthenia, incisional pain, wound abscess, cellulitis, peripheral coldness, injection site pain, diabetes mellitus, hypertonia, inflammation, immunogenicity, hypersensitivity reactions including ***anaphylaxis***.

LABORATORY TEST CONSIDERATIONS

Hyperkalemia.

DRUG INTERACTIONS

Anticoagulants / ↑ Risk of bleeding
H *Bromelain* / Possible ↑ bleeding risk
Dipyridamole / ↑ Risk of bleeding
H *Evening primrose oil* / Possible ↑ antiplatelet effect
H *Feverfew* / Possible ↑ antiplatelet effect
H *Garlic* / Possible ↑ antiplatelet effect
H *Ginger* / Possible ↑ antiplatelet effect
H *Ginkgo biloba* / Possible ↑ antiplatelet effect
H *Ginseng* / Possible ↑ antiplatelet effect
H *Grapeseed extract* / Possible ↑ antiplatelet effect
NSAIDs / ↑ Risk of bleeding
Ticlopidine / ↑ Risk of bleeding

HOW SUPPLIED

Injection: 2 mg/mL.

DOSAGE

IV BOLUS FOLLOWED BY IV INFUSION

Prevention of cardiac ischemic complications with concomitant use of heparin and aspirin.

IV bolus: 0.25 mg/kg 10–60 min before the start of the intervention, followed by **continuous IV infusion:** 0.125 mcg/kg/min (to a maximum of 10 mcg/min) for 12 hr. Those with unstable angina not responding to usual therapy and who require PCI within 24 hr may be given abciximab, 0.25 mg/kg IV bolus, followed by an 18–24 hr IV infusion of 10 mcg/min, ending 1 hr after the PCI.

NURSING IMPLICATIONS

IMPLEMENTATION/ADMINISTRATION/STORAGE

1. **IV** Stop infusion after 12 hr; avoids prolonged platelet receptor blockade effects.
2. Inspect visually for particulate matter prior to administration; do not use if visibly opaque particles noted. Use aseptic procedures.
3. Arterial access site care is important to prevent bleeding. Only the anterior wall of the femoral artery should be punctured. Avoid femoral vein sheath placement unless needed. While the vascular sheath is in place, maintain clients on complete bed rest with the head of the bed 30° or less and the affected limb restrained in a straight position. Medicate clients for back/groin pain as needed.
4. Following sheath removal, apply pressure to the femoral artery for at least 30 min using either manual compression or a mechanical device for hemostasis. Apply a pressure dressing following hemostasis. Maintain the client on bed rest for 6–8 hr after sheath removal or discontinuation of the drug, or 4 hr following discontinuation of heparin, whichever is later. Remove the pressure dressing prior to ambulation.
5. The following conditions may be associated with an increased risk of bleeding and may be additive with the effect of abciximab in the angioplasty setting: PCI within 12 hr of onset of symptoms for acute MI, prolonged PCI (lasting more than 70 min), and failed PCI.
6. Stop continuous infusion with failed PCIs; no evidence it is effective in such situations.
7. Stop abciximab and heparin immediately if serious bleeding occurs not controlled by compression.
8. If symptoms of an allergic reaction or anaphylaxis occur, stop infusion immediately; institute treatment. Have epinephrine, dopamine,

A

theophylline, antihistamines, and corticosteroids for immediate use.

9. For the bolus injection, withdraw the appropriate amount of drug into a syringe. Filter through a sterile, nonpyrogenic, low-protein-binding 0.2- or 5-micrometer filter into syringe; give bolus 10–60 min before procedure.
10. For continuous infusion, withdraw the appropriate amount of drug into a syringe. Inject into a container of sterile 0.9% NSS or D5W. Filter either upon admixture using a sterile, nonpyrogenic, low-protein-binding 0.2- or 5-micrometer filter or upon administration using an inline, sterile, nonpyrogenic low-protein-binding 0.2- or 0.22-micrometer filter. Discard any unused drug at the end of the infusion.
11. Use the following guidelines to minimize the risk of bleeding:
    - When abciximab is started 18–24 hr before PCI, maintain the aPTT between 60 and 85 seconds during the abciximab and heparin infusion period.
    - During PCI, maintain the ACT between 200 and 300 seconds.
    - If anticoagulation is continued in these clients following PCI, maintain the aPTT between 55 and 75 seconds.
    - Check the aPTT or ACT prior to arterial sheath removal. Do not remove the sheath, unless aPTT is 50 seconds or less or ACT is 175 seconds or less.
12. Store vials at 2–8°C (36–46°F); do not freeze or shake vials.
13. COMPATIBILITY Sterile 0.9% NSS or D5W.
14. INCOMPATIBILITY Give through separate IV line with no other medications added to solution. No incompatibilities have been noted with glass bottles or PVC bags or IV sets.

ASSESSMENT

1. Obtain thorough nursing history; note indications/goals of therapy.
2. Determine any history of CVA, bleeding disorders, recent episodes of bleeding, use of anticoagulants, previous abciximab use, trauma, or surgery; precludes therapy.
3. List other agents prescribed/OTC and when last consumed to prevent any bleeding potential.
4. If undergoing PCI, will receive a bolus of abciximab (0.25 mg/kg) 10–60 min before procedure followed by a continuous IV infusion (10 mcg/min) for 12 hr.
5. Insert separate IV lines (avoid noncompressible sites) with saline locks for blood draws. Observe during infusion; anaphylaxis may occur at any time.
6. Administer 325 mg aspirin orally 2 hr before procedure, and prepare heparin bolus and infusion for administration.
7. Observe for any bleeding sites: catheter sites, needle punctures, GI, GU, and retroperitoneal sites. Remove tape/dressings gently.
8. If serious bleeding develops (not controlled with pressure), stop infusions of abciximab and heparin.
9. Complete bed rest while vascular access sheath is in place. Restrain limb straight, and raise HOB no more than 30°. Stop heparin infusion at least 4 hr before sheath removal. Palpate/monitor distal pulses of involved extremity.
10. Apply pressure for 30 min over femoral artery once sheath is removed. When hemostasis evident, apply pressure dressing with sandbag and check frequently for bleeding. Monitor hematoma for enlargement. Enforce bed rest 6–8 hr after infusion completed and sheath removed.
11. Monitor PT, INR, PTT, CBC, VS, and ECG. Check platelet count 2–4 hr after initial bolus and again in 24 hr.

CLIENT/FAMILY TEACHING

1. Review indications, what to expect, clinical management, and anticipated results.
2. Identify risks with therapy, e.g., bleeding from intracranial hemorrhage/stroke, which may be lethal, or bloody urine/vomit; may require blood/platelet transfusions.
3. Report fever, chills, rash, or other adverse side effects and any bleeding or bruising immediately. It may take longer to stop bleeding, and pressure will be applied to bleeding sites to help stop the flow.
4. Drug may cause formation of human antichimeric antibody (HACA), which may cause hypersensitivity reactions when treated with other monoclonal antibodies, low platelets, or diminished response on readministration.

OUTCOMES/EVALUATE

Prevention of abrupt coronary vessel closure with associated ischemic complications during percutaneous coronary intervention (PCI)

Abiraterone acetate

(ay-bir-**AYE**-ter-own)

Classification(s): Antiandrogen.

Pregnancy Category: X

RX: Zytiga.

INDICATIONS/USES

In combination with prednisone to treat metastatic castration—resistant prostate cancer in those who have received prior chemotherapy containing docetaxel.

ACTION/KINETICS

Action

Abiraterone acetate is converted to abiraterone which is an inhibitor of androgen biosynthesis by inhibiting 17-alpha-hydroxylase. This enzyme is present in testicular, adrenal, and prostate tumor tissues and is required for androgen synthesis. Thus, inhibition of the enzyme results in a decrease in androgen levels. Abiraterone may also cause an increased mineralocorticoid production by the adrenal glands.

Pharmacokinetics

T_{max}: 2 hr. Food increases both AUC and C_{max}; taking the drug with meals has the potential to cause increased and highly variable exposure to abiraterone. Abiraterone acetate is an inhibitor of P-glycoprotein. **t½, terminal:** 12 hr. About 88% of the dose is excreted in the feces and 5% in the urine, mainly as unchanged drug. t½ is prolonged to about 18 hr in those with mild hepatic impairment and to about 19 hr in those with moderate hepatic impairment.

CONTRAINDICATIONS

Severe hepatic impairment. Women who are or who may become pregnant. Use in children. Lactation.

SPECIAL CONCERNS

- **Use with caution in those with a history of CV disease and in those whose underlying medical conditions may be compromised by increases in BP, hypokalemia, or fluid retention.**
- **The safety in those with left ventricular ejection fraction less than 50% or New York Heart Association class III or IV heart failure has not been established.**

SIDE EFFECTS

Most Common

Joint swelling/discomfort, arrhythmia, cough, diarrhea, dyspepsia, edema, hot flush, hypertension, hypokalemia, muscle discomfort, nocturia, urinary frequency, URTI, UTI.

GI: Diarrhea, dyspepsia, hepatotoxicity. **CV:** Arrhythmia, hypertension, atrial fibrillation/tachycardia, atrial flutter, bradycardia, complete AV block, conduction disorder, bradyarrhythmias, supraventricular/***ventricular tachycardia***, left ventricular dysfunction, ***cardiogenic shock***, cardiomegaly, cardiomyopathy, decreased ejection fraction, angina pectoris, unstable angina, chest pain/discomfort, ***cardiac failure***. **Musculoskeletal:** Joint swelling/discomfort, muscle discomfort, arthritis, arthralgia, joint stiffness, muscle spasms, musculoskeletal pain/discomfort, myalgia. **Respiratory:** Cough, URTI. **GU:** Nocturia, urinary frequency, UTI, urosepsis. **Dermatologic:** Hot flush. **Metabolic:** Peripheral/pitting/generalized edema, adrenal insufficiency.

LABORATORY TEST CONSIDERATIONS

↑ AST, ALT, triglycerides, total bilirubin, alanine aminotransferase, aspartate aminotransferase. ↓ Phosphorus, potassium.

OVERDOSE MANAGEMENT

Treatment: General supportive measures, including monitoring for arrhythmias and cardiac failure. Assess liver function.

DRUG INTERACTIONS

CYP3A4 inducers or inhibitors / Abiraterone is a substrate of CYP3A4. The effects of strong CYP3A4 inhibitors or inducers on the pharmacokinetics of abiraterone have not been evaluated; avoid coadministration or use with caution. Strong CYP3A4 inhibitors include atazanavir, clarithromycin, indinavir, itraconazole, ketoconazole, nefazodone, nelfinavir, ritonavir, saquinavir, telithromycin, and voriconazole. Strong CYP3A4 inducers include carbamazepine, phenobarbital, phenytoin, rifabutin, rifampin, and rifapentine.

A

Dextromethorphan / ↑ Dextromethorphan C_{max} and AUC R/T inhibition of metabolism by CYP2D6; do not use together with abiraterone/prednisone
Thioridazine / ↑ Thioridazine C_{max} and AUC R/T inhibition of metabolism by CYP2D6; do not use together with abiraterone/prednisone

HOW SUPPLIED

Tablets: 250 mg.

DOSAGE

TABLETS

Castration-resistant prostate cancer.

Adults: 1,000 mg once a day in combination with prednisone, 5 mg twice a day. For moderate hepatic impairment (Child-Pugh class B): 250 mg once a day.

NURSING IMPLICATIONS

IMPLEMENTATION/ADMINISTRATION/STORAGE

1. Interrupt treatment with abiraterone if ALT and/or AST is greater than 5 × ULN or total bilirubin is >3 × ULN. Restart abiraterone at 750 mg once a day following return of liver function tests to the client's baseline or to AST and ALT to 2.5 × ULN or lower and total bilirubin to 1.5 × ULN or lower. If hepatotoxicity recurs at the 750 mg once daily dose, restart at 500 mg once a day following return of LFTs to the client's baseline or to AST and ALT less than or equal to 2.5 × ULN and total bilirubin less than or equal to 1.5 × ULN. Discontinue treatment if hepatotoxicity recurs at the 500 mg once daily dose.
2. Take on an empty stomach. No food should be consumed for at least 2 hr before and for at least 1 hr after abiraterone is taken. Swallow tablets whole with water.
3. Abiraterone may harm a developing fetus. Thus, women who are pregnant or may become pregnant should not handle abiraterone without protection (e.g., gloves).
4. Store from 15–30°C (59–86°F)

ASSESSMENT

1. Note indications for therapy, when chemotherapy (docetaxel) received and other therapies trialed.
2. Identify any history of cardiovascular disease, hypertension, hypokalemia, or fluid retention R/T ACTH drive.
3. Use cautiously with heart failure, recent MI, or ventricular arrhythmia.
4. Assess for S&S of adrenocortical insufficiency, especially if withdrawn from prednisone (given twice a day with abiraterone), have prednisone dose reductions, or experience unusual stress.
5. Monitor BP, K^+, renal and LFTs; reduce dose with dysfunction.

CLIENT/FAMILY TEACHING

1. Do not consume food for at least two hours before the dose of drug is taken and for at least one hour after taking Zytiga. Swallow the tablets whole with water. Food causes increased exposure and may result in adverse reactions.
2. Drug is taken once a day and prednisone is to be taken twice a day as ordered.
3. If also prescribed GnRH agonists, client will need to maintain this treatment during the course of treatment with Zytiga and prednisone.
4. Men who are sexually active with a pregnant woman must use a condom during and for one week after treatment with Zytiga. If sexual partner may become pregnant, a condom and another form of birth control must be used during and for one week after treatment with Zytiga (drug may harm fetus).
5. May experience peripheral edema, hypokalemia, hypertension, and urinary tract infection. Report any dizziness, headache, confusion, pain in legs, swelling of legs or feet, SOB, or chest pain.
6. Keep all F/U to assess response, BP, labs and for adverse SE.

OUTCOMES/EVALUATE

- Treatment of castration-resistant prostate cancer (CRPC)
- Inhibition of malignant cell proliferation

■

AbobotulinumtoxinA (Botulinum toxin Type A)

(a-bo-**BOT**-you-lye-num-**TOX**-in-ay)

Classification(s): Botulinum toxin Type A

Pregnancy Category: C

RX: Dysport.

INDICATIONS/USES

(1) Cervical dystonia in adults to decrease the severity of abnormal head position and neck pain in toxin-naive and previously treated clients. (2) Temporary improvement in the appearance of moderate to severe glabellar lines associated with corrugator and procerus muscle activity in adults younger than 65 years. *Investigational:* (1) Achalasia. (2) Acquired nystagmus. (3) Facial lines and wrinkles. (4) Gustatory sweating (Frey syndrome). (5) Hand dystonia. (6) Tension-type headache. (7) Palmar hyperhidrosis. (8) Sialorrhea (drooling) in adults and children. (9) Spasticity of cerebral palsy.

ACTION/KINETICS

Action

AbobotulinumtoxinA blocks cholinergic transmission at the neuromuscular junction by inhibiting the release of acetylcholine. Impulse transmission is reestablished by the formation of new nerve endings.

Pharmacokinetics

Using available technology, it is not possible to detect abobotulinumtoxinA in the peripheral blood following IM injection at the recommended doses.

CONTRAINDICATIONS

Hypersensitivity to any botulinum toxin preparation or to any components of the product, including cow's milk protein. Infection at the proposed injection site(s). Use in children younger than 18 years of age.

SPECIAL CONCERNS

Spread of toxin effect. Postmarketing reports indicate that the effects of all botulinum toxin products may spread from the area of injection to produce symptoms consistent with botulinum toxin effects. These may include asthenia, generalized muscle weakness, diplopia, ptosis, dysphagia, dysphonia, dysarthria, urinary incontinence, and breathing difficulties. These symptoms have been reported hours to weeks after injection. Swallowing and breathing difficulties can be life-threatening, and there have been reports of death. The risk of symptoms is probably greatest in children treated for spasticity, but symptoms can also occur in adults treated for spasticity and other conditions, particularly in those clients who have underlying conditions that would predispose them to these symptoms. In unapproved uses, including spasticity in children and adults, and in approved indications, cases of spread of effect have been reported at doses comparable with those used to treat cervical dystonia and at lower doses.

- **Use with caution in clients with surgical alterations to the facial anatomy, excessive weakness or atrophy in the target muscle(s), marked facial asymmetry, inflammation at the injection site(s), ptosis, excessive dermatochalasis, deep dermal scarring, thick sebaceous skin, or the inability to substantially lessen glabellar lines by physically spreading them apart.**
- **Exceeding the recommended dose and frequency of administration increases the incidence of eyelid ptosis.**
- **Clients with peripheral motor neuropathic diseases, amyotrophic lateral sclerosis, or neuromuscular junction disorders (e.g., myasthenia gravis, Lambert-Eaton syndrome) may be at increased risk of clinically significant effects, including severe dysphagia and respiratory compromise.**
- **Safety for treating hyperhidrosis has not been established.**
- **Risk to a breast-feeding infant is probably nil.**
- **Elderly clients may have an increased number of ocular side effects.**

SIDE EFFECTS

Most Common

Muscle weakness, dysphagia, dry mouth, dysphonia, eye disorders, fatigue, headache, injection-site discomfort/pain, neck pain, musculoskeletal pain.

Musculoskeletal: Muscular weakness, musculoskeletal pain, neck pain, muscle atrophy, amyotrophy. **CNS:** Headache, dizziness, burning sensation, facial paresis, hypesthesia, vertigo. **GI:** Dysphagia, dry mouth, nausea. **CV:** ↓ HR. **Respiratory:** Dysphonia, dyspnea, cough, sinusitis, bronchitis, pharyngolaryngeal pain, nasopharyngitis, URTI. **Dermatologic:** Contact dermatitis, erythema, excessive granulation tissue. **Injection site:** Discomfort, pain, bruising, erythema, irrita-

A

tion, itching, numbness, stinging, swelling, tenderness, tightness, tingling, warmth. **Ophthalmic:** Blurred vision, diplopia, reduced visual acuity and accommodation, eyelid edema, eyelid ptosis, photophobia. **Body as a whole:** Fatigue, injections, influenza, malaise, hypersensitivity. **Miscellaneous:** Dysphonia, immunogenicity.

LABORATORY TEST CONSIDERATIONS

↑ Mean blood glucose.

OVERDOSE MANAGEMENT

Symptoms: Neuromuscular weakness with a variety of symptoms. Paralysis. *Treatment:* Symptomatic treatment. Respiratory support may be needed where excessive doses cause paralysis of respiratory muscles. Antitoxin against botulinum is available from the Centers for Disease Control and Prevention but the antitoxin will not reverse any botulinum toxin-induced effects already apparent by the time of the antitoxin administration.

DRUG INTERACTIONS

Aminoglycosides (e.g., gentamicin) / Enhanced neuromuscular action → protracted respiratory depression; use together with caution
Anticholinergic drugs (e.g., atropine) / Potentiation of systemic anticholinergic effects (e.g., blurred vision); use together with caution
Cholinesterase inhibitors / Enhanced neuromuscular action → protracted respiratory depression; use together with caution
Magnesium sulfate / Enhanced neuromuscular action → protracted respiratory depression; use together with caution
Muscle relaxants (e.g., metaxalone) / Exaggeration of excessive weakness; use together with caution
Nondepolarizing muscle relaxants (e.g., tubocurarine) / Enhanced neuromuscular activity → protracted respiratory depression; use together with caution
Other botulinum neurotoxins (e.g., botulinum toxin B) / Administration at the same time or within several months of each other → exacerbation of excessive neuromuscular weakness
Quinidine / Enhanced neuromuscular action → protracted respiratory depression; use together with caution

HOW SUPPLIED

Injection, Lyophilized Powder for Solution: 300 units, 500 units.

DOSAGE

IM

Cervical dystonia.

Adults, initial: 500 units IM as a divided dose among affected muscles in clients with or without a history of prior treatment with botulinum toxin. The peak effect occurs between 2 and 4 weeks after injection. **Usual dose:** 250–1,000 units IM q 12 weeks or longer. Make dosage adjustments in 250 unit steps dependent on client response, with retreatment q 12 weeks or longer as needed, based on return of clinical symptoms.

Glabellar lines.

Adults, usual: 50 units IM in 5 equal aliquots of 10 units each. The clinical effect may last up to 4 months. Administer no more frequently than q 3 months.

NURSING IMPLICATIONS

IMPLEMENTATION/ADMINISTRATION/STORAGE

1. Potency units of abobotulinumtoxinA are specific to the preparation and assay method utilized. They are not interchangeable with other preparations of botulinum toxin products.
2. **Use for cervical dystonia.** (a) Reconstitute each 500 unit vial with 1 mL of preservative-free NaCl 0.9% injection to yield a solution of 500 units/mL. Reconstitute each 300 unit vial with 0.6 mL of preservative-free 0.9% NaCl injection to yield a solution equivalent to 250 units/0.5 mL. Swirl gently to dissolve. (b) Administer IM. Limiting the dose injected into the sternocleidomastoid muscle may reduce the occurrence of dysphagia. Simultaneous EMG-guided application may help in locating active muscle not identified by physical exam alone.
3. **Use for glabellar lines.** (a) Reconstitute each 300 unit vial with 2.5 mL preservative-free 0.9% NaCl. The resulting concentration will be 10 units/0.08 mL to be delivered in 5 equally divided aliquots of 0.08 mL each. (b) The 300 unit vial may also be reconstituted with 1.5 mL of preservative-free 0.9% NaCl for a solution of 10 units/0.05 mL to be delivered

in 5 equally divided aliquots of 0.05 mL each. (c) To inject, advance the needle through the skin into the underlying muscle while applying finger pressure on the superior medial orbital rim. Using a 30-gauge needle, inject 10 units into 5 sites, 2 in each corrugator muscle and 1 in the procerus muscle. (d) Take the following steps to reduce the complication of ptosis: Avoid injection near the levator palpebrae superioris, especially in those with larger brow depressor complexes; place injections into the mediator corrugator at least 1 cm above the body supraorbital ridge; ensure the injected volume/dose is accurate; and do not inject closer than 1 cm above the central eyebrow.

4. Store vials from 2–8°C (36–46°F). Protect from light. Administer within 4 hr of reconstitution; during this period, store under refrigeration between 2–8°C (36–46°F). Do not freeze after reconstitution. Discard any remaining solution after injection.
5. Reconstitute with sterile 0.9% NaCl injection only.

ASSESSMENT

1. Note reasons for therapy, age at onset, extent of abnormal head/neck positioning with cervical dystonia or clinical presentation with glabellar lines and other agents/therapies trialed.
2. Assess for any evidence/history of neuropathic, neurologic, or neuromuscular disorders. These clients may be at increased risk of clinically significant effects including severe dysphagia and respiratory compromise from typical doses.
3. For use/administration only by those individuals trained to administer.
4. Advise and monitor carefully for post injection effects (hours to weeks later) which may spread from the area of injection to other body areas to produce symptoms consistent with botulinum toxin effects. Swallowing and breathing difficulties can be life-threatening, and there have been reports of death related to spread of toxin effects.
5. Review associated risk factors to ensure client understanding. Drug contains albumin which may present the remote risk of viral disease transmission.

CLIENT/FAMILY TEACHING

1. Drug is administered IM by a trained provider to treat the abnormal head position and neck pain associated with cervical dystonia or to decrease frown lines between the eyebrows.
2. Do not perform activities that require mental alertness until drug effects realized; may cause dizziness. Resume activity slowly and carefully following administration. May cause loss of strength or general muscle weakness, blurred vision, or drooping eyelids within hours to weeks of drug administration.
3. May experience injection site pain, headaches, neck/muscle pain, eye problems and tiredness; report if persistent.
4. Any S&S of allergic reaction (itching, rash, red itchy welts), wheezing or asthma type symptoms require immediate reporting.
5. Keep all F/U to assess response, need for repeat treatment (after 12 weeks), and for adverse SE.

OUTCOMES/EVALUATE

- Relief of painful muscle spasms/contractures permitting improved posture, movement, and activity
- Smoothing of wrinkle/frown lines

Acarbose

(ah-**KAR**-bohs)

Classification(s): Antidiabetic, oral; alpha-glucosidase inhibitor

Pregnancy Category: B

RX: Precose.

SEE ALSO ***ANTIDIABETIC AGENTS: HYPOGLYCEMIC AGENTS***.

INDICATIONS/USES

(1) Alone as an adjunct to diet to treat type 2 diabetes mellitus in those whose hyperglycemia is not managed by diet alone. (2) With a sulfonylurea, insulin, or metformin when diet plus either acarbose or a sulfonylurea do not control diabetes.

ACTION/KINETICS

Action

Causes a competitive, reversible inhibition of pancreatic alpha-amylase and membrane-bound intestinal alpha-glucosidase hydrolase enzymes. This

A

causes delayed glucose absorption, resulting in a smaller increase in blood glucose following meals. Glycosylated hemoglobin levels are decreased in those with NIDDM. Additive effect with sulfonylureas due to different mechanism of action (the drug does not enhance insulin secretion).

Pharmacokinetics

Approximately 65% of an oral dose of acarbose remains in the GI tract, which is the site of action. **Peak plasma levels of active drug:** About 1 hr. Metabolized in the GI tract by both intestinal bacteria and intestinal enzymes. Acarbose and metabolites that are absorbed are excreted in the urine.

CONTRAINDICATIONS

Diabetic ketoacidosis, cirrhosis, IBD, colonic ulceration, partial intestinal obstruction or predisposition to intestinal obstruction, chronic intestinal diseases associated with marked disorders of digestion or absorption, conditions that may deteriorate as a result of increased gas formation in the intestine. In significant renal dysfunction (serum creatinine >2 mg/dL). Severe, persistent bradycardia. Lactation.

SPECIAL CONCERNS

- **Safety and efficacy have not been determined in children.**
- **Acarbose, alone, does not cause hypoglycemia; however, sulfonylureas and insulin can lower blood glucose sufficiently to cause symptoms or even life-threatening hypoglycemia.**
- **Loss of BG control may occur during stress, such as fever, trauma, infection, and surgery.**

SIDE EFFECTS

Most Common

Flatulence, diarrhea, abdominal pain.

GI: Flatulence, diarrhea, abdominal pain. GI side effects may be severe and may be confused with paralytic ileus. **Miscellaneous**: Skin rash and edema (rare).

LABORATORY TEST CONSIDERATIONS

↑ Serum transaminases (especially long-term use with doses up to 300 mg 3 times/day). Small ↓ in hematocrit. ↓ Serum calcium. Low plasma vitamin B_6 levels.

OVERDOSE MANAGEMENT

Symptoms: Flatulence, diarrhea, abdominal discomfort. *Treatment:* Reduce dose; symptoms will subside.

DRUG INTERACTIONS

Charcoal / ↓ Acarbose effect; do not use together
Digestive enzymes / ↓ Acarbose effect; do not use together
Digoxin / ↓ Serum digoxin levels
Insulin / ↑ Hypoglycemia; possible severe hypoglycemia
Sulfonylureas / ↑ Hypoglycemia; possible severe hypoglycemia

HOW SUPPLIED

Tablets: 25 mg, 50 mg, 100 mg.

DOSAGE

TABLETS

Type 2 diabetes mellitus.

Individualized, depending on effectiveness and tolerance, but not to exceed 100 mg 3 times per day. **Adults, initial:** 25 mg 3 times per day with the first bite of each main meal. Some may benefit from more gradual dose titration by starting with 15 mg once a day and then increasing to 25 mg twice a day. **Maintenance:** Increase dose to 50 mg 3 times per day. Some may benefit from 100 mg 3 times per day. The dosage can be adjusted at 4- to 8-week intervals. **Recommended maximum daily dose:** 50 mg 3 times per day for clients weighing less than 60 kg and 100 mg 3 times per day for those weighing more than 60 kg.

NURSING IMPLICATIONS

IMPLEMENTATION/ADMINISTRATION/STORAGE

1. **Start with low dose; reduces GI side effects and helps determine minimum effective dose.**
2. **If dose missed, take usual dose at start of next main meal.**

ASSESSMENT

1. **List reasons for therapy, age at symptom onset, other agents trialed and outcome.**

A

2. Note any cirrhosis, chronic intestinal diseases, or disorders of digestion/absorption. Avoid if C_{CR} <25 mL/min.
3. Initiate/titrate acarbose based on BS results. Ideally, measure 1 hr postprandial plasma glucose level to determine effective dose.
4. May enhance glycemic control with a sulfonylurea, but may also be used alone.
5. Obtain baseline ht, Wt, CBC, HbA1c, BS, electrolytes, U/A, Ca, renal and LFTs; assess for B_6 deficiency. Also monitor HbA1c and LFTs q 3 months for first year of therapy.

CLIENT/FAMILY TEACHING

1. Take three times daily with first bite of each meal. May be used with insulin or other oral agents. If dose missed and meal completed, then skip dose and take at next meal.
2. Delays digestion of ingested carbohydrates (glucose); used in addition to diet.
3. Caloric restrictions and weight loss, especially in obese, must be continued to control BS and prevent complications of diabetes; continue regular daily exercise, BP and cholesterol control. Complete diabetes education classes to enhance success.
4. Most common side effects are of GI origin (abdominal discomfort, diarrhea, gas); should subside in frequency and intensity with continued use. Report persistent or adverse side effects, including allergic skin rash, yellow skin discoloration, severe abdominal pain, swelling of extremities, or bleeding abnormalities.
5. Monitor glucose (finger sticks), and record to assess response and provider review.
6. Loss of glucose control may result when exposed to stress, such as fever, trauma, infection, or surgery. In this event, temporary insulin therapy may be needed. Do not use candy bars to counteract hypoglycemia; use glucose tablets/gel or lactose. Cane sugar (table sugar) absorption is inhibited by acarbose.
7. Keep all F/U to assess response (weight, FS, BP log), labs, and for adverse SE.

OUTCOMES/EVALUATE

Control of BS with NIDDM; A1c <8

IV

Acetaminophen (APAP, Paracetamol)

(ah-**SEAT**-ah-**MIN**-oh-fen)

Classification(s): Non-narcotic analgesic

Pregnancy Category: B (C if used IV.)

OTC: Capsules: Mapap, Masophen Extra Strength. **Elixir:** Apra Children's, Mapap Children's, Q-Pap Children's, Silapap Children's. **Gelcaps:** Genapap Extra Strength Gelcaps, Mapap Gelcaps, Tylenol Extra Strength Rapid Release Gels. **Oral Liquid:** Apap 500, Mapap Extra Strength, Q-Pap Children's, Silapap Children's, Tylenol Extra Strength, Tylenol Sore Throat Daytime. **Oral Solution:** Ed-Apap Children's, ElixSure Children's Fever Reducer/Pain Reliever, Pain and Fever Relief Children's. **Solution, Oral Concentrate (Drops):** Apap Infant's Drops, Infantaire Drops, Little Fever, Mapap Infant Drops, Pain and Fever Relief Children's Drops, Q-Pap Infants Drops, Silapap Infants, Triaminic Infants' Drops, Triaminic Infants' Fever Reducer/Pain Reliever, Tylenol Infants' Drops. **Suppositories:** Acephen, FeverAll, FeverAll Children's, FeverAll Infants, FeverAll Junior Strength. **Suspension, Oral:** Nortemp Children's, Q-Pap Children's, Triaminic Syrup, Tylenol Children's, Tylenol with Flavor Creator Children's. **Tablets (including Caplets):** Acetaminophen Caplets, Acetaminophen Extra Strength Caplets, Aminofen, Aminofen Max Extra Strength, Anacin Aspirin Free, Apap, Cetafen, Cetafen Extra, Genapap, Mapap Caplets, Mapap Regular Strength, Masophen, Non-Aspirin Extra Strength Caplets, Pain and Fever, Pain Relief Extra Strength Caplets, Pain Reliever, Pain Reliever Extra Strength, Q-Pap, Q-Pap Extra Strength, Tylenol Extra Strength Caplets, Tylenol Extra Strength EZ Tabs, Tylenol Regular Strength Tablets, UN-Aspirin Extra Strength, Valorin. **Tablets, Chewable:** Acetaminophen Children's, Genapap Children's, Mapap Children's, Mapap Junior Strength, Pain and Fever Children's, Tylenol Extra Strength Go Tabs. **Tablets, Chewable/ Dispersible:** Tylenol Children's Meltaways, Tylenol Jr. Meltaways. **Tablets, Extended-Release:** Mapap Arthritis Pain, Tylenol 8 Hour Caplets, Tylenol Arthritis Pain. **Tablets, Oral Disintegrating:** Quick Melts Children's Non-Aspirin, Quick Melts Jr. Strength Non-Aspirin. :

✤ **OTC: Caplets:** Atasol. **Oral Liquid/Syrup:** Atasol, Children's Acetaminophen Elixir Drops, Pediatrix, Tempra, Tempra Children's Syrup. **Oral Solution:** Atasol, Pediatrix. **Oral**

A

Suspension: Tylenol Children's Suspension, Tylenol Infants' Suspension. **Tablets, Chewable:** Children's Chewable Acetaminophen, Tempra, Tylenol Junior Strength Tablets Meltaways. **Tablets:** A.F. Anacin, A.F. Anacin Extra Strength, Apo-Acetaminophen, Atasol, Tylenol Tablets 325 mg, 500 mg.

Acetaminophen, buffered

OTC: Bromo Seltzer Effervescent Granules.

INDICATIONS/USES

PO. (1) **Adults and children at least 12 years of age:** Temporary reduction of fever and relief of minor aches and pains due to backache, the common cold, headache, menstrual cramps, minor arthritis pain, muscular aches, and toothache. (2) **Children, 2–11 years of age:** Temporary reduction of fever and relief of minor aches and pains due to the common cold, flu, headache, sore throat, and toothache. *Investigational:* Prevention of side effects with diphtheria, tetanus toxoids, and pertussis vaccination, including clients at risk for seizures.

Rectal. Temporary reduction of fever and the temporary relief of occasional aches and pains, and headaches. *Investigational:* Prophylaxis to decrease incidence of fever and injection site pain in children receiving diphtheria, tetanus toxoid, and acellular pertussis vaccination.

IV. (1) Reduction of fever. (2) Management of mild to moderate pain and the management of moderate to severe pain with adjunctive opioid analgesics.

ACTION/KINETICS

Action

Decreases fever by (1) a hypothalamic effect leading to sweating and vasodilation and (2) inhibits the effect of pyrogens on the hypothalamic heat-regulating centers. May cause analgesia by inhibiting CNS prostaglandin synthesis; however, due to minimal effects on peripheral prostaglandin synthesis, acetaminophen has no anti-inflammatory or uricosuric effects. Does not cause any anticoagulant effect or ulceration of the GI tract. Antipyretic and analgesic effects are comparable to those of aspirin.

Pharmacokinetics

Immediate-release PO products are absorbed rapidly; **peak plasma levels:** 30–60 min. **t½:** 2–3 hr. **Therapeutic serum levels** (analgesia): 5–20 mcg/mL. Metabolized in the liver and excreted in the urine as glucuronide and sulfate conjugates. Less than 5% is excreted unchanged. The t½ may be increased twofold in those with liver disease. In children, acetaminophen rectal suppositories reach peak levels from 107–288 min; bioavailability is from 30–40%. Following IV administration, the C_{max} occurs at the end of the 15-min infusion. After the same dose, the C_{max} following IV use is 70% higher compared with PO administration.

The pharmacokinetic exposure of acetaminophen injection seen in children and adolescents is similar to adults, but higher in infants and neonates. Dose reductions of 33% in infants 1 month to younger than 2 years of age, and 50% in neonates up to 28 days of age, with a minimum dosing interval of 6 hr, will lead to pharmacokinetic exposure similar to that seen in children 2 years of age and older.

A highly reactive intermediate hydroxylated metabolite normally combines with glutathione. The resulting complex is rendered harmless and is excreted. However, after large doses of acetaminophen, this pathway becomes saturated and glutathione stores are depleted. Concentrations of the reactive intermediate product rise leading to possible hepatotoxicity.

The extended-relief products use a bilayer system that allows the outer layer to release acetaminophen rapidly while the inner layer is designed to release the remainder of the dose more slowly. This allows prolonged relief of symptoms. The buffered product is a mixture of acetaminophen, sodium bicarbonate, and citric acid that effervesces when placed in water. It also has a high sodium content (0.76 grams per ¾ capful). **Plasma protein binding:** Approximately 10–25%.

CONTRAINDICATIONS

Hypersensitivity to acetaminophen or any component of the product. Renal insufficiency, anemia, liver failure. Clients with cardiac or pulmonary disease are more susceptible to acetaminophen toxicity. IV use in those with severe hepatic impairment or severe active liver disease.

A

SPECIAL CONCERNS

- **Serious liver damage (hepatocyte necrosis and apoptosis) from doses not far from labeled doses, especially using high doses and taking more than one product containing acetaminophen and with three or more alcoholic drinks/day.**
- **Use with caution during pregnancy.**
- **Consult MD before use if more than three alcoholic drinks consumed/day.**
- **May decrease ability in infants to produce a full immune response to a vaccine if drug given prophylactically to prevent fever.**
- **Use IV with caution during lactation, alcoholism, chronic malnutrition, severe hypovolemia (e.g., due to dehydration or blood loss), or severe renal impairment (C_{CR} 30 mL/min or less).**
- **Efficacy of IV use not studied in children less than 2 years of age.**

SIDE EFFECTS

Most Common

PO, Rectal. Few when taken in usual therapeutic doses. GI upset in some.
IV. Adults: Headache, insomnia, N&V. **Children:** Agitation, atelectasis, constipation, N&V, pruritus.

PO and Rectal Use. Chronic and even acute toxicity can develop after long symptom-free usage. **CNS:** Dizziness, disorientation, and excitement following high doses; drowsiness, CNS stimulation. **Hematologic**: Methemoglobinemia, ***hemolytic anemia***, neutropenia, thrombocytopenia, pancytopenia, leukopenia. **Hepatic:** Mild ↑ liver enzymes. Liver damage, especially after overdose. Jaundice. Possible liver damage in those who consume three or more alcoholic drinks daily. **Hypersensitivity:** Urticarial and erythematous skin reactions, mucosal lesions, drug fever. **GU:** Renal damage without hepatic damage. **Miscellaneous**: Hypoglycemic coma, glossitis.

IV Use. Adults. CNS: Headache, insomnia, anxiety, fatigue. **GI:** N&V. **CV:** Hyper-/hypotension. **Musculoskeletal:** Muscle spasms, trismus. **Respiratory:** Abnormal breath sounds, dyspnea. **Metabolic/Nutritional:** Peripheral edema, hypokalemia. **Miscellaneous:** Pyrexia, injection-site pain, increased AST. **Children. CNS:** Agitation, headache, insomnia. **GI:** N&V, constipation, abdominal pain, diarrhea. **CV:** Hyper-/hypotension, tachycardia. **Musculoskeletal:** Muscle spasms, pain in extremity. **Respiratory:** Atelectasis, hypoxia, pleural effusion, pulmonary edema, stridor, wheezing. **Metabolic/Nutritional:** Increased hepatic enzymes, hypervolemia, hypoalbuminemia, hypokalemia, hypomagnesemia, hypophosphatemia, peripheral edema. **Dermatologic:** Pruritus, periorbital edema, rash. **Miscellaneous:** Anemia, oliguria, injection-site pain, pyrexia. Hypersensitivity reactions can occur in both adults and children, including symptoms of swelling of the face, mouth, and throat; respiratory distress; urticaria; rash, pruritus, ***anaphylaxis***.

OVERDOSE MANAGEMENT

Symptoms: Are four stages of acetaminophen poisoning. **Stage 1:** Onset may be within a few hours of ingestion and may resolve within 24 hr. Symptoms include abdominal pain, N&V, diaphoresis, anorexia, drowsiness, malaise, pallor. LFTs may be normal. **Stage 2:** Onset is 24–36 hr after acute ingestion. Liver damage develops and is noted by right upper quadrant pain and elevation of ALT, AST, bilirubin, and PT. **Stage 3:** Onset is 72–96 hr after acute ingestion. Hepatotoxicity peaks and is evident by fulminant hepatic failure, encephalopathy, coma, levels of AST and ALT more than 10,000 units/L, and abnormal PT, bilirubin, glucose, lactate, and phosphate. Fatalities caused by hepatic failure may occur 3 to 5 days after acute ingestion. **Stage 4:** Recovery for those who survive stage 3. *Treatment:* The optimal time to draw an acetaminophen level is 4 hr after an acute ingestion or as soon as possible after 4 hr. Initially, induction of emesis, gastric lavage, activated charcoal. Oral *N*-acetylcysteine is said to reduce or prevent hepatic damage by inactivating acetaminophen metabolites, which cause liver toxicity.

DRUG INTERACTIONS

Alcohol, ethyl / Chronic use → ↑ liver toxicity of larger therapeutic doses of acetaminophen
Barbiturates (e.g., phenobarbital) / ↑ Potential hepatotoxicity R/T ↑ liver breakdown of acetaminophen to a reactive metabolite; also, ↓ acetaminophen therapeutic effects
Carbamazepine / ↑ Potential hepatotoxicity R/T ↑ liver breakdown of acetaminophen
Charcoal, activated / ↓ Absorption of acetaminophen when given ASAP after overdose
Diuretics, loop / ↓ Effect R/T ↓ renal prostaglandin excretion and ↓ plasma renin activity

A

Hydantoins (including Phenytoin) / ↑ Potential hepatotoxicity R/T ↑ liver breakdown of acetaminophen to a reactive metabolite; also, ↓ acetaminophen therapeutic effects
Isoniazid / ↑ Potential hepatotoxicity R/T ↑ liver breakdown of acetaminophen
Lamotrigine / ↓ Serum lamotrigine levels → ↓ effect
H ***Milk thistle*** / Helps prevent acetaminophen liver damage
NSAIDs / ↑ Risk of hypertension in women
Oral contraceptives / ↑ Liver breakdown of acetaminophen → ↓ t½
Propranolol / ↑ Effect R/T ↓ liver breakdown
Rifampin / ↑ Hepatotoxicity potential R/T ↑ liver breakdown of acetaminophen
Smoking / Possible ↓ serum acetaminophen levels R/T ↑ hepatic metabolism
Sulfinpyrazone / ↑ Hepatotoxicity potential R/T ↑ liver breakdown of acetaminophen to a reactive metabolite; also, ↓ acetaminophen therapeutic effects
Warfarin / ↑ Warfarin antithrombotic effect in a dose-dependent manner; monitor coagulation parameters 1–2 times a week when starting or stopping acetaminophen (especially if more than 2,275 mg/week are consumed)
Zidovudine / ↓ Zidovudine effect R/T ↑ nonhepatic or renal clearance

HOW SUPPLIED

Acetaminophen. ***Capsules:*** 500 mg; ***Elixir:*** 160 mg/5 mL; ***Gelcaps:*** 500 mg; ***Injection Solution:*** 10 mg/mL; ***Oral Liquid:*** 160 mg/5 mL, 166.6 mg/5 mL, 500 mg/5 mL; ***Oral Solution:*** 160 mg/5 mL; ***Solution, Oral Concentrate:*** 80 mg/mL, 100 mg/mL; ***Suppositories, Rectal:*** 80 mg, 120 mg, 325 mg, 650 mg; ***Suspension, Oral:*** 160 mg/5 mL; ***Tablets (including Caplets):*** 325 mg, 500 mg; ***Tablets, Chewable:*** 80 mg, 160 mg, 500 mg; ***Tablets, Chewable/Dispersible:*** 80 mg, 160 mg; ***Tablets, Extended-Release:*** 650 mg; ***Tablets, Oral Disintegrating:*** 80 mg, 160 mg.
Acetaminophen, buffered: ***Granules, Effervescent:*** 1 or 2 three-quarter capfuls.

DOSAGE

Acetaminophen

CAPSULES; ELIXIR; GELCAPS; ORAL LIQUID; ORAL SOLUTION; SOLUTION, ORAL CONCENTRATE (DROPS); SUSPENSION, ORAL; TABLETS (INCLUDING CAPLETS); TABLETS, CHEWABLE; TABLETS, CHEWABLE/DISPERSIBLE; TABLETS, DISINTEGRATING; TABLETS, EXTENDED-RELEASE; TABLETS, ORAL DISINTEGRATING

Analgesic, antipyretic.

Adults: 325–650 mg q 4–6 hr of immediate-release or 1,300 mg q 6 hr of extended-release; **maximum per 24 hr:** 3 grams. **Children, 12 years of age (96 lbs or more or 43.6 kg or more):** 640 mg q 4–6 hr, not to exceed 5 doses (3.2 grams total) in 24 hr; **11 years of age (72–95 lbs or 32.7–42.3 kg):** 480 mg q 4–6 hr, not to exceed 5 doses (2.4 grams total) in 24 hr; **9–10 years of age (60–71 lbs or 27.3–32.3 kg):** 400 mg q 4–6 hr, not to exceed 5 doses (2 grams total) in 24 hr; **6–8 years of age (48–59 lbs or 21.8–26.8 kg):** 320 mg q 4–6 hr, not to exceed 5 doses (1.6 grams total) in 24 hr; **4–5 years of age (36–47 lbs or 16.4–21.4 kg):** 240 mg q 4 hr, not to exceed 5 doses (1.2 grams total) in 24 hr; **2–3 years of age (24–35 lbs or 10.9–15.9 kg):** 160 mg q 4 hr, not to exceed 5 doses (800 mg total) in 24 hr; **1–2 years of age (18–23 lbs or 8.2–10.5 kg):** 120 mg q 4 hr, not to exceed 5 doses (600 mg total) in 24 hr; **4–11 months of age (12–17 lbs or 5.5–7.7 kg):** 80 mg q 4 hr, not to exceed 5 doses (total of 400 mg) in 24 hr; **0–3 months of age (6–11 lbs or 2.7–5 kg):** 40 mg q 4 hr, not to exceed 5 doses (total of 200 mg) in 24 hr.

Prevention of side effects with diphtheria, tetanus toxoids, and pertussis vaccination, including clients at risk for seizures (investigational).

10–15 mg/kg given with or prior to the vaccination and continued for several doses after vaccination.

JUNIOR STRENGTH CHEWABLE AND DISINTEGRATING TABLETS, 160 MG

Analgesic, antipyretic.

Children, 12 years of age (96 lbs or more or 43.6 kg or more): 640 mg (4 tablets) q 4 hr, up to 5 times per day; **11 years of age (72–95 lbs or 32.7–42.3 kg):** 480 mg (3 tablets) q 4 hr, up to 5 times per day; **9–10 years of age (60–71 lbs or 27.3–32.3 kg):** 400 mg (2.5 tablets) q 4 hr, up to 5 times per day; **6–8 years of age (48–59 lbs or 21.8–26.8 kg):** 320 mg (2 tablets) q 4 hr, up to 5 times per day. *NOTE:* This dosage form is not recommended for children less than 6 years of age.

CHILDREN'S CHEWABLE AND DISINTEGRATING TABLETS, 80 MG

Analgesic, antipyretic.

Children, 11 years of age (72–95 lbs or 32.7–42.3 kg): 480 mg (6 tablets) q 4 hr, up to 5 times per day; **9–10 years of age (60–71 lbs or 27.3–32.3 kg):** 400 mg (5 tablets) q 4 hr, up to 5 times per day; **6–8 years of age (48–59 lbs or 21.8–26.8 kg):** 320 mg (4 tablets) q 4 hr, up to 5 times per day; **4–5 years of age (36–47 lbs or 16.4–21.4 kg):** 240 mg (3 tablets) q 4 hr, up to 5 times per day; **2–3 years of age (24–35 lbs or 10.9–15.9 kg):** 160 mg (2 tablets) q 4 hr, up to 5 times per day. *NOTE:* This dosage form is not recommended for children less than 2 years of age.

CHILDREN'S LIQUID, SOLUTION, OR SUSPENSION, 160 MG/5 ML

Analgesic, antipyretic.

Children, 11 years of age (72–95 lbs or 32.7–42.3 kg): 480 mg (15 mL) q 4 hr, up to 5 times per day; **9–10 years of age (60–71 lbs or 27.3–32.3 kg):** 400 mg (12.5 mL) q 4 hr, up to 5 times per day; **6–8 years of age (48–59 lbs or 21.8–26.8 kg):** 320 mg (10 mL) q 4 hr, up to 5 times per day; **4–5 years of age (36–47 lbs or 16.4–21.4 kg):** 240 mg (7.5 mL) q 4 hr, up to 5 times per day; **2–3 years of age (24–35 lbs or 10.9–15.9 kg):** 160 mg (5 mL) q 4 hr, up to 5 times per day; **1–2 years of age (18–23 lbs or 8.2–10.5 kg):** 120 mg (3.75 mL) q 4 hr, up to 5 times per day; **4–11 months of age (12–17 lbs or 5.5–7.7 kg):** 80 mg (2.5 mL) q 4 hr, up to 5 times per day. *NOTE:* This dosage form is not recommended for children less than 4 months of age.

INFANTS' CONCENTRATED DROPS (80 MG/0.8 ML)

Analgesic, antipyretic.

Children, 2–3 years of age (24–35 lbs or 10.9–15.9 kg): 160 mg (1.6 mL or 2 droppersful) q 4 hr, up to 5 times per day; **1–2 years of age (18–23 lbs or 8.2–10.5 kg):** 120 mg (1.2 mL or 1.5 droppersful) q 4 hr, up to 5 times per day; **4–11 months of age (12–17 lbs or 5.5–7.7 kg):** 80 mg (0.8 mL or 1 dropperful) q 4 hr, up to 5 times per day; **0–3 months of age (6–11 lbs or 2.7–5 kg):** 40 mg (0.4 mL or ½ dropperful) q 4 hr, up to 5 times per day.

SUPPOSITORIES

Analgesic, antipyretic.

Adults and children over 12 years of age: 650 mg (given as two 325 mg suppositories or one 650 mg suppository) q 4–6 hr, not to exceed 3.9 grams per 24 hr. Clients on long-term therapy should not exceed 2.6 grams/day. **Children, 6–12 years of age:** 325 mg q 4–6 hr with no more than 1.95 grams in 24 hr; **3–6 years of age:** 120 mg q 4–6 hr, with no more than 720 mg in 24 hr; **1–3 years of age:** 80 mg q 4 hr, with no more than 480 mg in 24 hr; **3–11 months of age:** 80 mg q 6 hr. Given as needed while symptoms persist. For neonates, may also use a dose of 10–15 mg/kg/dose rectally q 6–8 hr. Some suggest a loading dose of 30 mg/kg/dose rectally.

IV

Analgesic, antipyretic.

Adults, usual: 1,000 mg q 6 hr or 650 mg q 4 hr IV; **maximum:** 1,000 mg as a single dose and 4,000 mg/day. **Children, 13 years and older, 50 kg or more, usual:** See adult dosing; **less than 50 kg, usual:**

A

15 mg/kg q 6 hr or 12.5 mg/kg q 4 hr IV; **maximum:** 15 mg/kg (up to 750 mg) as a single dose and 75 mg/kg (up to 3,750 mg)/day. **Children, 2–12 years, usual:** 15 mg/kg q 6 hr or 12.5 mg/kg q 4 hr; **maximum:** 15 mg/kg as a single dose and 75 mg/kg/day. *NOTE:* The minimum recommended dosing interval for adults and children of all ages is 4 hr.

Acetaminophen Buffered

GRANULES, EFFERVESCENT

Analgesic, antipyretic.

Adult, usual: 1 or 2 three-quarter capfuls are placed into an empty glass; add half a glass of cool water. May be taken while fizzing or after settling. Can be repeated q 4 hr as required or directed by provider.

NURSING IMPLICATIONS

IMPLEMENTATION/ADMINISTRATION/STORAGE

1. The maximum dose is now 3 grams in 24 hr for adults and children older than 12 years of age. A dose of 10 mg/kg has been used in children 2–12 years of age. Even though dosages are presented for children younger than 2 years of age (or less than 24 lbs), a health care provider should be consulted before use. Chronic alcoholics should limit the dose to 2 grams or less per day.
2. For neonates a dose of 10–15 mg/kg/dose PO q 6–8 hr has been recommended. A PO loading dose of 20–25 mg/kg/dose may also be used.
3. If possible use client weight to determine the dose; otherwise, use age.
4. Consult a provider if pain gets worse or lasts for more than 5 days in children or 10 days in adults; if fever lasts for more than 3 days in adults or children; or if swelling is present or new symptoms occur, as these could be signs of a serious condition.
5. Dissolve dispersible tablets in the mouth or chew before swallowing.
6. Shake the elixir, suspension, or concentrated infants' drops well before using.
7. Put orally disintegrating tablets on the tongue and allow to dissolve. Do not chew or swallow the tablet whole.
8. Take ER product with water; do not crush, chew, or dissolve before swallowing.
9. Pediatric products come in a variety of flavors, including bubble gum, cherry, grape, apple, chocolate, or strawberry.
10. Store PO forms from 15–30°C (59–86°F). Avoid high humidity and excessive heat; protect from freezing. Store suppositories from 2–27°C (36–80°F); do not use if imprinted suppository paper is opened or damaged.
11. IV No dose adjustment is needed when converting between PO acetaminophen and acetaminophen injection dosing in adults and adolescents.
12. Longer dosing intervals and a reduced daily dose may be needed in those with severe impaired renal function (C_{CR} of 30 mL/min or less).
13. Administer IV over 15 min; may be given without further dilution.
14. For those requiring acetaminophen, 1,000 mg, administer by inserting a vented IV set through the septum of the 100 mL vial (10 mg/mL in 100 mL vial).
15. Use the following procedure for acetaminophen doses less than 1,000 mg. Withdraw the appropriate dose from an intact sealed vial, and place the measured dose in a separate empty, sterile container (e.g., glass bottle, plastic IV container, syringe) for IV infusion to avoid inadvertent delivery and administration of the total volume of the commercially available container. Place small volume doses for children of up to 60 mL in volume in a syringe, and administer over 15 min using a syringe pump. Monitor the end of the infusion in order to prevent a possible air embolism, especially in cases where the acetaminophen infusion is the primary infusion.
16. Store vials from 20–25°C (68–77°F). Use within 6 hr after the vacuum seal of the vial has been penetrated, or the contents transferred to another container. Do not refrigerate or freeze. Vials are for single use; discard any unused portion.
17. COMPATIBILITY No further dilution; may administer as diluted.
18. INCOMPATIBILITY Do not add other medications to the acetaminophen vial or infusion device. Diazepam and chlorpromazine

are physically incompatible with acetaminophen; thus, give separately.

ASSESSMENT

1. Note reasons for therapy, VS, prescribed form and dosage (weight and age based), and expected outcomes. Review potential adverse SE.
2. Assess for prolonged pain/fever and any conditions that may preclude therapy.
3. With IV therapy, assess for hepatic impairment or active hepatic disease, alcoholism, chronic malnutrition, severe hypovolemia (dehydration or blood loss), or severe renal impairment (C_{cr}, 30 mL/min); precludes therapy.
4. Monitor closely for any hypersensitivity reaction during IV therapy.
5. Rate pain; note type, onset, location, duration, intensity, and triggers.
6. Determine alcohol use: frequency and amount; avoid if more than 3 drinks/day (alcohol induces hepatic cytochromes and is competitive inhibitor of acetaminophen metabolism).
7. Check urine for occult blood and albumin; assess for nephritis.
8. With long-term therapy, use lower daily dose and monitor CBC, renal and LFTs.

CLIENT/FAMILY TEACHING

1. Do not combine products containing acetaminophen, many of which are OTC. Read labels on all OTC products consumed.
2. Review with parents the difference between concentrated dropper dose formulation and teaspoon dose formulation. Shake elixir, suspension, or concentrated infants' drops well before using.
3. Dissolve dispersible tablets in the mouth, or chew before swallowing.
4. Put orally disintegrating tablets on the tongue and allow to dissolve. Do not chew or swallow the tablet whole.
5. Take ER product with water; do not crush, chew, or dissolve before swallowing.
6. Dosage is weight determined; follow guidelines carefully. Use lower total daily amounts with long-term use to prevent cumulative effects.
7. Take as directed with food or milk to decrease GI upset. If diabetic, use sugar-free form of drug.
8. S&S of acute toxicity that require immediate reporting include N&V or abdominal pain. Yellow discoloration of skin and eyes, dark urine, itching, clay-colored stools may also indicate liver toxicity. Bluish coloration of skin/nailbeds or complaints of SOB, weakness, headache, or dizziness are S&S of methemoglobinemia caused by lack of oxygen and require immediate attention. Different stages of toxicity occur over 4–5 days and warrant close medical supervision.
9. Report paleness, weakness, and heartbeat skips; S&S of hemolytic anemia.
10. Consult provider promptly if sore throat is severe, persists for more than 2 days, or is accompanied by fever, headache, N&V, or rash.
11. SOB, fast/weak pulse; cold extremities; unexplained bleeding, bruising, sore throat, fatigue, feeling clammy/sweaty; or low temperatures may be S&S of chronic poisoning; report. Requires close monitoring over a 3–5-day period and treatment to prevent liver failure.
12. Phenacetin, the major active metabolite, may cause urine to become dark brown or wine-colored.
13. Headache and minor pain relievers containing combinations of salicylates, acetaminophen, and caffeine may be no more beneficial than the drug alone.
14. Report any unexplained pain or fever that persists for longer than 3–5 days.
15. Avoid alcohol; may cause toxicity. Not for regular use or high dose with any form of liver disease.
16. Keep all F/U to assess response, labs, and for adverse SE.

OUTCOMES/EVALUATE

- ↓ Fever
- Relief/control of pain
- Control of pain with adjunctive opioid analgesics

Combination Drug

Acetaminophen and Codeine phosphate

(ah-**SEAT**-ah-**MIN**-oh-fen, **KOH**-deen)

Classification(s): Non-narcotic/narcotic analgesic combination

A

Pregnancy Category: C

RX: Cocet, Tylenol with Codeine, Vopac, **C-III**

SEE ALSO ***ACETAMINOPHEN*** AND ***CODEINE PHOSPHATE***.

INDICATIONS/USES

Relief of mild to moderately severe pain.

CONTENT

Each Tylenol with Codeine No. 3 Tablet contains: Acetaminophen (non-narcotic analgesic), 300 mg, and Codeine phosphate (narcotic analgesic), 30 mg.

Each Tylenol with Codeine No. 4 Tablet contains: Acetaminophen, 300 mg, and Codeine phosphate, 60 mg.

Each 5 mL of Tylenol with Codeine Elixir (oral solution) contains: Acetaminophen, 120 mg, and Codeine phosphate, 12 mg.

Each Cocet or Vopac Capsule contains: Acetaminophen, 650 mg, and Codeine phosphate, 30 mg.

ACTION/KINETICS

Action

Acetaminophen may cause analgesia by inhibiting CNS prostaglandin synthesis. The mechanism of morphine is believed to involve decreased permeability of the cell membrane to sodium, which results in diminished transmission of pain impulses and therefore analgesia.

Pharmacokinetics

Both are well absorbed after PO. Acetaminophen, plasma **t½**: 1–4 hr; codeine plasma **t½**: 2.5–3 hr. Acetaminophen is metabolized mainly in the liver and excreted in the urine. Codeine is metabolized in the liver and excreted in the urine.

CONTRAINDICATIONS

Renal insufficiency, anemia. Those with cardiac or pulmonary disease are more susceptible to acetaminophen toxicity. During labor when delivery of a premature infant is expected. Hypersensitivity to any component of the product.

SPECIAL CONCERNS

- **Tablets contain sodium metabisulfite that may cause allergic-type reactions, including anaphylaxis and life-threatening or less severe asthmatic episodes in susceptible individuals.**
- **Use with caution in the elderly, debilitated, in those with severe hepatic or renal impairment, hypothyroidism, Addison's disease, and prostatic hypertrophy or urethral stricture.**
- **Serious liver damage and apoptosis may occur with acetaminophen doses not far beyond labeled dosing. If more than three alcoholic drinks per day are consumed, consult provider before use.**
- **Significant codeine levels may appear in breast milk in those abusing codeine.**
- **Safety and efficacy of the tablets have not been determined in children. Safety and efficacy of the elixir (oral solution) have not been determined in children 3 years of age and younger.**

SIDE EFFECTS

Most Common

Light-headedness, dizziness, sedation, shortness of breath, N&V, respiratory depression (high doses of codeine).

See *Acetaminophen* and *Narcotic Analgesics* for a complete list of possible side effects. Codeine can produce drug dependence of the morphine type and thus has the potential to be abused. Psychological and physical dependence, as well as tolerance, can result upon repeated use.

OVERDOSE MANAGEMENT

SEE ALSO ***ACETAMINOPHEN*** AND ***NARCOTIC ANALGESICS***.

DRUG INTERACTIONS

See also ***Acetaminophen,*** and ***Narcotic Analgesics.***

Anticholinergics / Possible paralytic ileus
CNS Depressants (other narcotic analgesics, antipsychotics, antianxiety drugs, alcohol) / Additive CNS depression

HOW SUPPLIED

See *Content.*

DOSAGE

ELIXIR (ORAL SOLUTION)

Mild to moderately severe pain.

Adults: 15 mL (360 mg acetaminophen and 36 mg codeine phosphate) q 4 hr.
Children, 7–12 years of age: 10 mL (240 mg acetaminophen and 24 mg codeine phosphate) 3–4 times per day.
Children, 3–6 years of age: 5 mL (120 mg acetaminophen and 12 mg codeine phosphate) 3–4 times per day.

A

TABLETS
Mild to moderately severe pain.

Adults, acetaminophen:
200–1,000 mg is the single dose range; maximum daily dose: 4,000 mg.

Adults, codeine: 15–60 mg is the single dose range; maximum daily dose: 360 mg. Doses may be repeated q 4 hr.

TABLETS (VOPAC)
Mild to moderately severe pain.

Adults: ½–2 tablets q 4 hr, up to 6 tablets per day.

NURSING IMPLICATIONS

IMPLEMENTATION/ADMINISTRATION/STORAGE
1. Adult doses of codeine higher than 60 mg do not give commensurate relief of pain, but do prolong analgesia and are associated with a significant increase in the incidence of side effects.
2. Store tablets from 15–30°C (59–86°F). Dispense in a tight, light-resistant container.

ASSESSMENT
1. List reasons for therapy, onset, duration, characteristics of symptoms; rate pain level, list other drugs trialed/outcome. Note baseline mental status and orientation level.
2. Assess for hypothyroidism, CAD, BPH, liver disease, alcoholism, asthma; seizures may preclude therapy or require lower dosage.
3. With cough, determine comorbidities, fever, change in sputum color/amount, leukocytosis, need for CXR/ATX.
4. Monitor CBC, renal and LFTs. If used with severe hepatic or renal disease, monitor serial liver/renal function tests.

CLIENT/FAMILY TEACHING
1. Take as directed with full glass of water. May take with food/milk if GI upset.
2. Do not drive/perform activities that require mental alertness until drug effects realized; may cause dizziness, drowsiness.
3. For constipation, increase fluid and fiber intake to offset.
4. Store away from bedside; out of reach of children. Do not exceed prescribed dose.
5. Do not stop suddenly with prolonged use, may cause withdrawal.
6. Avoid excessive alcohol intake (>3 drinks per day).
7. Report any unusual or sudden onset side effects, especially rash or breathing problems.
8. Keep all F/U visits to assess response and for adverse SE.

OUTCOMES/EVALUATE
Control of pain/cough

IV

Acetylcysteine

(ah-see-till-**SIS**-tay-een)

Classification(s): Mucolytic; Detoxification agent

Pregnancy Category: B

RX: Acetadote.

INDICATIONS/USES
(1) Adjunct in clients with abnormal, viscid, or inspissated mucous secretions in such conditions as chronic emphysema, emphysema with bronchitis, chronic asthmatic bronchitis, tuberculosis, bronchiectasis, primary amyloidosis of lung, acute bronchopulmonary disease (bronchitis, pneumonia, tracheobronchitis). Inhalation solution only. (2) Routine care of clients with tracheostomy, pulmonary complications after thoracic or CV surgery, use during anesthesia, atelectasis due to mucus obstruction, and in posttraumatic chest conditions. (3) Pulmonary complications of cystic fibrosis. (4) Diagnostic bronchial studies, including bronchograms, bronchospirometry, and bronchial wedge catheterization. (5) Antidote in acetaminophen poisoning to reduce or prevent hepatotoxicity. Give as soon as possible after the overdose and definitely within 24 hr of ingestion if acetylcysteine given PO and within 8–10 hr if given IV. *Investigational:* As an ophthalmic solution for dry eye syndrome. As an enema to treat bowel obstruction due to meconium ileus or equivalent. Prevention of contrast media nephrotoxicity.

ACTION/KINETICS
Action
Reduces the viscosity of purulent and nonpurulent pulmonary secretions and facilitates their removal by splitting disulfide bonds. Action increases with increasing pH (peak: pH 7–9). Also reduces liver injury due to acetaminophen over-

dosage by maintaining or restoring glutathione levels or by acting as an alternate substrate for the reactive metabolite of acetaminophen.

Pharmacokinetics

Onset, inhalation: Within 1 min; **by direct instillation:** immediate. **Time to peak effect:** 5–10 min. Excreted in the urine. **t½, terminal, after IV:** 5.6 hr. t½ increases by up to 80% in those with severe liver damage. t½, elimination is longer in newborns (11 hr) than in adults (5.6 hr). **Plasma protein binding:** 83%.

CONTRAINDICATIONS

Sensitivity to drug.

SPECIAL CONCERNS

- **Use with caution during lactation, in the elderly, and in clients with asthma or a history of bronchospasm.**
- **There are no adequate and well controlled studies in children for IV use.**

SIDE EFFECTS

Most Common

After PO use. Bronchial/tracheal irritation, N&V, rash, stomatitis.
After IV use. Urticaria, pruritus, anaphylactoid reaction, immune system disorders.

After PO use. Respiratory: Bronchoconstriction; rarely, **bronchospasm** even in those with asthmatic bronchitis or bronchitis complicating bronchial asthma. Bronchial and tracheal irritation, tightness in chest. **Dermatologic:** Rash, with or without mild fever; urticaria. **GI:** N&V, stomatitis. **Miscellaneous:** Fever, clamminess, drowsiness, rhinorrhea, **hypersensitivity** (rare).

After IV use. Respiratory: Pharyngitis, rhinorrhea, rhonchi, throat tightness, cough, wheezing, stridor, SOB, chest tightness, respiratory distress, **bronchospasm**. **CV:** Tachycardia, hypotension, vascular disorders. **GI:** N&V. **Dermatologic:** Urticaria, facial flushing, pruritus. **Miscellaneous:** Anaphylactoid reaction/***anaphylaxis***, immune system disorders, edema.

DRUG INTERACTIONS

Acetylcysteine is incompatible with antibiotics and should be administered separately.

HOW SUPPLIED

Injection: 20% (200 mg/mL); ***Inhalation Solution:*** 10%; ***Inhalation Solution, Concentrate:*** 20%; ***Oral Solution:*** 10%; ***Oral Solution, Concentrate:*** 20%.

DOSAGE

10% INHALATION SOLUTION, 20% INHALATION SOLUTION CONCENTRATE

Abnormal, viscid, or inspissated mucous secretions: Nebulization with face mask, tracheostomy, mouth piece.

Adults, usual: 3–5 mL of 20% solution or 6–10 mL of 10% solution 3–4 times per day. Alternate dosage: 1–10 mL of the 20% solution or 2–20 mL of the 10% solution given q 2–6 hr.

Abnormal, viscid, or inspissated mucous secretions: Nebulization with tent or croupette.

Adults: Recommended dose is the volume of acetylcysteine, using the 10% or 20% solution that will maintain a very heavy mist in the tent or croupette for the desired period. Up to 300 mL of solution during a single treatment may be needed. It may be desirable to administer for intermittent or continuous prolonged periods (e.g., overnight).

Abnormal, viscid, or inspissated mucous secretions: Direct instillation for routine care of tracheostomy.

Adults: 1–2 mL of 10% or 20% solution q 1–4 hr by instillation into the tracheostomy.

Abnormal, viscid, or inspissated mucous secretions: Direct instillation into percutaneous intratracheal catheter.

Adults: 1–2 mL of the 20% solution or 2–4 mL of the 10% solution q 1–4 hr by a syringe attached to the catheter.

Abnormal, viscid, or inspissated mucous secretions: Instillation to particular segment of bronchopulmonary tree using small plastic catheter into the trachea.

Adults: 2–5 mL of 20% solution instilled into the trachea by means of a syringe connected to a catheter. Insert under local anesthesia and direct vision.

Diagnostic bronchial studies.

Adults: 2–3 doses of 1–2 mL of 20% or 2–4 mL of 10% solution by nebulization or intratracheal instillation before the procedure.

A

IV

Acetaminophen overdosage.

Adults, loading dose: 150 mg/kg in 200 mL of D5W given over 60 minutes; **second dose:** 50 mg/kg in 500 mL of D5W given over 4 hr; **third dose:** 100 mg/kg in 1,000 mL of D5W given over 16 hr. To avoid fluid overload, reduce the volume of D5W in clients weighing less than 50 kg and in those with a restriction on fluid intake.

10% ORAL SOLUTION, 20% ORAL SOLUTION CONCENTRATE

Acetaminophen overdose.

Adults and children, PO, loading dose: 140 mg/kg; **maintenance dose:** 70 mg/kg 4 hr after the loading dose and q 4 hr thereafter for a total of 17 doses.

NURSING IMPLICATIONS

Do not confuse Mucomyst with Mucinex (guaifenesin, an expectorant).

IMPLEMENTATION/ADMINISTRATION/STORAGE

1. Use nonreactive plastic, glass, or stainless steel for administration.
2. For PO use to treat acetaminophen overdosage: Dilute 10% or 20% solution with diet cola or other diet soft drinks to final concentration of 5%. If given via gastric tube or Miller-Abbott tube, water may be used as the diluent. Freshly prepare solutions, and use within 1 hr. Remaining undiluted solutions may be stored in the refrigerator for up to 96 hr.
3. When using the solution for acetaminophen overdosage, empty the stomach promptly by lavage. If there is mixed drug overdosage, activated charcoal may be given. However, if activated charcoal is given, lavage before administering acetylcysteine treatment. If the client vomits within 1 hr of administration, repeat the dose. If the client is persistently unable to retain the PO administered drug, administer by duodenal intubation.
4. For use as a mucolytic, the 10% solution may be used undiluted. Use either water for injection or saline to dilute the 20% solution.
5. May administer via face mask, face tent, oxygen tent, head tent, or by positive-pressure apparatus.
6. Inhalation incompatible with antibiotics; administer separately.
7. Administer with compressed air for nebulization. Hand nebulizers are contraindicated.
8. There may be stickiness of the face after nebulization using a face mask. Remove by washing with water.
9. After prolonged nebulization, dilute the last fourth of the medication with sterile water to prevent drug concentration.
10. An increased volume of liquefied bronchial secretions may result if acetylcholine is administered properly; if cough is inadequate, maintain an open airway by mechanical suction.
11. If encephalopathy caused by hepatic failure becomes evident, discontinue acetylcysteine treatment to avoid further administration of nitrogenous substances.
12. Solution may develop a light purple color; does not affect action.
13. Store unopened vials from 15–30°C (59–86°F). Store open bottles at 2–8°C (36–46°F) and use within 96 hr. Once opened, record time/date to prevent use beyond 96 hr.
14. IV Stability and safety of acetylcysteine not determined when mixed with other drugs.
15. Dose based on weight and over varying administration times (3) to be completed in 21 hr.
16. Adjust the total volume administered for clients less than 40 kg and for those requiring fluid restriction. To avoid fluid overload, reduced the volume of diluent as needed. If volume is not adjusted, fluid overload can occur, potentially resulting in hyponatremia, seizures, and death.
17. Store unopened vials of IV solution from 20–25°C (68–77°F). Reconstituted solution stable for 24 hr at controlled room temperature. Single-dose vials are preservative-free; discard any unused portion.
18. COMPATIBILITY Dilute in D5W, 0.45% NaCl, or water for injection.
19. INCOMPATIBILITY IV acetylcysteine is incompatible with rubber and metals, especially iron, copper, and nickel. Administer separately.

ASSESSMENT

1. Identify reason for therapy: acetaminophen overdosage (IV or PO) or mucolytic (inh). Note

A

pulmonary findings; determine when spasms occur. List conditions likely to cause congestion and wheezing.
2. Note previous approaches (successful and unsuccessful) used to treat symptoms.
3. Determine smoking status. If currently taking antibiotics, do not administer together.
4. With acetaminophen overdosage: document time and amount of ingestion. Administer drug within 8–10 hr following overdose to protect from hepatoxicity and death. May administer IV especially if vomiting; determine any asthma history as may trigger hypersensitivity reaction. Monitor closely for any reactions during infusion.
5. Wash face following nebulization treatments; may cause face to become sticky.
6. As a mucolytic: check airway patency, baseline lung sounds, and effectiveness of cough. If increased volume of liquefied secretions noted and cough inadequate to clear, position to facilitate removal of secretions. If unable to cough up secretions, provide suction. If bronchospasm occurs, stop therapy and report. Have short-acting bronchodilator (i.e., isoproterenol for HFN) readily available.
7. Monitor VS and I&O. Follow dosing guidelines based on condition being treated. Obtain baseline acetaminophen level/CBC, PT, electrolytes, BS, renal and LFTs. Monitor LFTs and acetaminophen levels with overdose.

CLIENT/FAMILY TEACHING

1. Use as directed; do not exceed prescribed dosage. Medication may turn a light purple color after opening bottle. This is normal and does not alter the safety or effectiveness of the medication.
2. Report changes in sputum color, consistency, characteristics, or new onset fever. If using face mask, a sticky residue may appear on the face; can be easily removed by washing with water. Clear airway by coughing deeply prior to starting nebulizer treatments.
3. Dilute nebulizer solution with sterile water to prevent solution from becoming concentrated and plugging the nebulizer. Do not add other medications or solutions to nebulizer canister unless advised. Wash face after treatment; may feel sticky.
4. Nauseous odor (rotten eggs) when treatment begins will become less noticeable as therapy continues.
5. Avoid any triggers that may stimulate bronchospasm (i.e., cigarette smoke, dust, chemicals, cold air).
6. Report if rash or S&S of allergic reaction, new/worsening wheezing, chest tightness, difficulty breathing, or persistent nausea or vomiting occur.
7. Attend smoking cessation classes and support groups to help stop smoking.
8. Keep all F/U to assess response and for adverse SE.

OUTCOMES/EVALUATE

- Improved airway exchange with ↓ viscosity. Mobilization and expectoration of secretions
- ↓ Acetaminophen levels and associated liver toxicity

IV

Acyclovir (Acycloguanosine)

(ay-**SYE**-kloh-veer, ay-**SYE**-kloh-**GWON**-oh-seen)

Classification(s): Antiviral

Pregnancy Category: B

RX: Zovirax.

Rx: Apo-Acyclovir, Gen-Acyclovir, Nu-Acyclovir.

SEE ALSO ***ANTIVIRAL DRUGS***.

INDICATIONS/USES

PO. (1) Initial and recurrent genital herpes in immunocompromised and nonimmunocompromised clients. (2) Prophylaxis of frequently recurring genital herpes infections in nonimmunocompromised clients. (3) Treatment of chickenpox in children ranging from 2 to 18 years of age. (4) Acute treatment of herpes zoster (shingles).

Parenteral. (1) Mucosal and cutaneous herpes simplex virus types 1 and 2 infections in immunocompromised clients. (2) Shingles in immunocompromised clients. (3) Herpes simplex encephalitis. (4) Neonatal herpes simplex infections.

Topical. (1) To decrease healing time and duration of viral shedding in initial herpes genitalis. (2) Limited non-life-threatening mucocutaneous

HSV infections in immunocompromised clients. No beneficial effect in recurrent herpes genitalis or in herpes labialis in nonimmunocompromised clients. (3) Recurrent herpes labialis in adults and children 12 years and older. *Investigational:* Cytomegalovirus and HSV infection following bone marrow or renal transplantation; herpes simplex ocular infections; herpes simplex proctitis; herpes simplex labialis; herpes simplex whitlow; herpes zoster encephalitis; disseminated primary eczema herpeticum; herpes simplex-associated erythema multiforme; infectious mononucleosis; and varicella pneumonia.

ACTION/KINETICS

Action

Converted by HSV-infected cells to acyclovir triphosphate, which interferes with HSV DNA polymerase, thereby inhibiting DNA replication.

Pharmacokinetics

Systemic absorption is slow from the GI tract (although therapeutic levels are reached) and following topical administration. Food does not affect absorption. **Peak levels after PO:** 1.5–2 hr. Widely distributed in tissues and body fluids. The half-life and total body clearance depend on renal function. **t½, PO, C_{CR} >80 mL/min/1.73 m^2:** 2.5 hr. Metabolites and unchanged drug (up to 85%) are excreted through the kidneys. Reduce dosage in clients with impaired renal function.

CONTRAINDICATIONS

Hypersensitivity to formulation. Use of the cream or ointment in the eyes, nose, or mouth. Use to prevent recurrent HSV infections.

SPECIAL CONCERNS

- Use with caution during lactation or with concomitant intrathecal methotrexate or interferon.
- Higher plasma levels in geriatric clients cause a higher incidence of side effects (especially N&V, dizziness, and CNS effects); reduced dosage in geriatric clients with renal impairment may be necessary.
- Safety and efficacy of PO form not established in children 2 years or less or of the cream or ointment in children 12 years and younger.
- Prolonged or repeated doses in immunocompromised clients may result in emergence of resistant viruses.
- Use of oral acyclovir does not eliminate latent HSV and is not a cure.

SIDE EFFECTS

Most Common

IV: N&V, inflammation/phlebitis at injection site, itching, rash, hives, increased BUN or creatinine.
PO: N&V, headache, diarrhea, malaise.
Topical: Mild pain with transient burning/stinging, pruritus.

- **After PO or parenteral use**

GI: Diarrhea, GI distress, N&V, sore throat, taste of drug, constipation, abdominal pain, flatulence. **CNS:** Aggressive behavior, agitation, ataxia, coma, confusion, delirium, dizziness, encephalopathy, hallucinations, paresthesia, psychosis, ***seizure***, somnolence, tremors, headache. **Hematologic:** Leukocytoclastic vasculitis, leukopenia, lymphadenopathy. **Hepatic:** Elevated LFTs, hepatitis, hyperbilirubinemia, jaundice. **Renal:** ***Fatal renal failure, fatal thrombotic thrombocytopenic purpura or hemolytic uremic syndrome in immunocompromised clients***, increased BUN or creatinine, hematuria. **Dermatologic:** Alopecia, erythema multiforme, photosensitive rash, pruritus, rash, ***Stevens-Johnson syndrome, toxic epidermal necrolysis***, urticaria. **Hematologic:** Anemia. **Musculoskeletal:** Myalgia. **Ophthalmologic:** Visual abnormalities. **Miscellaneous:** Anaphylaxis, ***angioedema***, fever, pain, peripheral edema.

- **Additional symptoms after parenteral use**

At injection site: Inflammation/phlebitis at site, itching, rash, hives. **CV:** Hypotension. **CNS:** Anorexia. Encephalopathic changes, including lethargy, obtundation, tremors, agitation, confusion, hallucination, ***seizures, coma***, jitters, headache. **Hematologic:** Hematuria, neutropenia, thrombocytopenia, thrombocytosis, leukocytosis, neutrophilia, ***DIC***, hemolysis. **Dermatologic:** Tissue necrosis following infusion into extravascular tissues. **Miscellaneous:** Elevated transaminases.

- **Additional symptoms after PO use**

CNS: Decreased consciousness, malaise. **Hematologic:** Thrombocytopenia.

- **After topical use**

Cream: Dry lips/skin, desquamation, cracked lips, pruritus, skin flakiness, stinging/burning on skin. Also, ***angioedema, anaphylaxis***, contact dermatitis, eczema, inflammation at application site.

OVERDOSE MANAGEMENT

Symptoms: Precipitation in renal tubules may occur when the solubility (2.5 mg/mL) in the intratubular fluid is exceeded. **After parenteral use:** Overdose has resulted with bolus injections, inappropriately high doses, and in those whose fluid and electrolyte balance was not properly monitored. Increased BUN and serum creatinine, followed by ***renal failure.*** **After PO use:** Agitation, ***coma, seizures***, lethargy. *Treatment:* Hemodialysis (a 6 hr hemodialysis results in a 60% decrease in plasma acyclovir levels); peritoneal dialysis is less effective.

DRUG INTERACTIONS

Cimetidine / ↑ Acyclovir peak plasma levels and AUC; not clinically important in those with normal renal function
Hydantoins / ↓ Hydantoin plasma levels
Interferon / ↑ Or synergistic antiviral effects
Ketoconazole / ↑ Or synergistic antiviral effects
Mycophenolate mofetil / ↑ Acyclovir AUC, peak concentration, and time to reach maximum concentration; ↓ acyclovir $t^{1/2}$ and renal clearance
Probenecid / ↑ Bioavailability and half-life of acyclovir → ↑ effect
Theophyllines / ↑ Theophylline plasma levels; monitor plasma levels and side effects
Valproic acid / ↓ Valproic acid plasma levels
Zidovudine / Severe lethargy and drowsiness

HOW SUPPLIED

Capsules: 200 mg; ***Cream:*** 5%; ***Injection:*** 50 mg/mL; ***Powder for Injection:*** 500 mg/vial; ***Suspension:*** 200 mg/5 mL; ***Tablets:*** 400 mg, 800 mg.

DOSAGE

CAPSULES; SUSPENSION; TABLETS

Initial, genital herpes.

200 mg q 4 hr 5 times per day for 10 days.

Chronic suppressive therapy for recurrent genital herpes.

400 mg twice a day, 200 mg 3 times per day, or 200 mg 5 times per day for up to 12 months.

Intermittent therapy for genital herpes.

200 mg q 4 hr 5 times per day for 5 days. Start therapy at the first symptom/sign of recurrence.

Herpes zoster, acute treatment.

800 mg q 4 hr 5 times per day for 7–10 days.

Chickenpox.

Adults and children over 40 kg: 800 mg 4 times per day for 5 days. **Children, 2 years and older, 40 kg or less:** 20 mg/kg (of the suspension) 4 times per day for 5 days. A single dose should not exceed 800 mg. Begin therapy at the earliest sign/symptom.

IV INFUSION

Mucosal and cutaneous herpes simplex in immunocompromised clients.

Adults: 5 mg/kg infused at a constant rate over 1 hr, q 8 hr (15 mg/kg/day) for 7 days. **Children less than 12 years of age:** 10 mg/kg infused at a constant rate over 1 hr q 8 hr for 7 days.

Varicella-zoster infections (shingles) in immunocompromised clients.

Adults: 10 mg/kg infused at a constant rate over 1 hr q 8 hr for 7 days.

Children less than 12 years of age: 20 mg/kg infused at a constant rate over at least 1 hr q 8 hr for 7 days.

Herpes simplex encephalitis.

Adults: 10 mg/kg infused at a constant rate over at least 1 hr q 8 hr for 10 days.

Children less than 12 years of age and greater than 3 months of age: 20 mg/kg infused at a constant rate over at least 1 hr q 8 hr for 10 days.

Neonatal herpes simplex virus (HSV) infections.

Children, birth-3 months: 10 mg/kg infused at a constant rate over 1 hr q 8 hr for 10 days. Doses as high as 15 mg/kg or 20 mg/kg infused at a constant rate over 1 hr q 8 hr have also been used.

CREAM, 5%

Recurrent herpes labialis.

Adults and children 12 years and older: Apply 5 times per day for 4 days.

NURSING IMPLICATIONS

Do not confuse Zovirax with Zyvox (an antibiotic).

IMPLEMENTATION/ADMINISTRATION/STORAGE

1. **Do not exceed recommended dosage, frequency, or length of treatment. Adjust dosage based on estimated C_{CR}.**

2. Store ointment in dry place at room temperature.
3. Adjust both PO and parenteral dose and/or dosing interval in acute or chronic renal impairment.
4. May use suspension to treat varicella zoster infections.
5. IV Prepare IV solution by dissolving contents of the 500- or 1,000-mg vial in 10 or 20 mL sterile water for injection, respectively (final concentration of 50 mg/mL). Infusion concentrations of 7 mg/mL or lower are recommended; thus, the calculated dose must be added to an appropriate IV solution at the correct volume. Reconstituted solution should be used within 12 hr.
6. Administer infusion over 1 hr to prevent renal tubular damage; do not administer by rapid or bolus IV, IM, or SC injections.
7. Accompany IV infusion by hydration (3 L/day) to prevent precipitation in renal tubules (crystalluria).
8. If refrigerated, reconstituted solution may show a precipitate, which dissolves at room temperature.
9. COMPATIBILITY D5W, 0.9% NaCl, dextrose/saline combinations, or LR.
10. INCOMPATIBILITY Avoid bacteriostatic water containing benzyl alcohol or parabens; causes precipitate. Avoid biologic or colloidal fluids (e.g., blood products, protein solutions).

ASSESSMENT

1. List reasons for therapy; assess skin lesions noting location, size, distribution, and number. Monitor neurologic status with neuro involvement.
2. With chickenpox or herpes zoster, institute appropriate precautions for all susceptible individuals (i.e., pregnant women, immunocompromised clients, and those who have not had chickenpox [may check titer if unknown]).
3. Monitor CBC, electrolytes, renal and LFTs closely, especially with IV therapy and if immunocompromised.

CLIENT/FAMILY TEACHING

1. Drug is not a cure; used only to help manage symptoms. Virus may remain latent for lifetime or may emerge periodically to cause S&S as it lies dormant in the ganglia. Drug will not prevent disease transmission to others or prevent reinfection. Most effective when started at first S&S of outbreak.
2. Take oral with or without food unless GI upset; then take with food. Take exactly as prescribed. Shake oral suspension well and use calibrated cup, syringe, or dropper to ensure correct dosage.
3. Do not cover cold sores with a bandage or dressing. Apply cream to lesions, washing hands with soap and water after each application. Report any burning, stinging, itching, and rash when applying.
4. Cream dose form is not to be used for genital herpes. Complete all exams/tests to rule out presence of other STDs. Return if lesions recur.
5. Wash area with soap and water 3–4 times per day and dry well. Adequately cover all lesions with topical acyclovir as ordered; do not exceed dosage, frequency of application, or treatment time. Avoid any contact near eyes; herpetic transmission to eye may contribute to blindness.
6. Apply ointment with a finger cot or rubber glove to prevent transmission of infection to other body sites. Wash hands before and after application. Apply enough ointment to adequately cover all lesions every 3 hr (6 times per day) for 7 days; (a ½-inch ribbon of ointment should cover about 4 square inches). Wear loose-fitting clothing and cotton underwear.
7. Use condoms for sexual intercourse to prevent reinfections while undergoing treatment. Abstain during acute outbreaks (lesions present), and use condoms at all other times.
8. Total dose and dosage schedule differ depending on whether the infection is initial or chronic and whether intermittent therapy regimen is being used. Follow prescribed dosage guidelines, dosage combinations (i.e., with zidovudine), and duration of treatment. With recurrent episodes of genital herpes, start therapy at the first S&S or recurrence; may not be effective if started more than 6 hr after onset of S&S of recurrence.
9. Consume 2–3 L/day of fluids, especially during parenteral therapy; prevents renal toxicity/crystalluria.

A

10. Females need annual Pap test; increased risk of cervical cancer may be associated with genital herpes.
11. Do not exceed dosage or share medications. With shingles, take tablets as directed, cover any open draining lesions to prevent disease transmission, avoid contact with children who have not had chickenpox, and pregnant women as fetuses may be vulnerable to the disease.
12. Keep all F/U to assess response, labs, and for adverse SE.

OUTCOMES/EVALUATE

- Less severe and less frequent herpes outbreaks
- Crusting and healing of herpetic lesions
- ↓ Pain with shingles outbreak

■

Adalimumab

(**ay**-dah-**LIM**-you-mab)

Classification(s): Immunomodulator

Pregnancy Category: B

RX: Humira.

INDICATIONS/USES

(1) Reduce signs and symptoms of rheumatoid arthritis, including major clinical response, inhibiting the progression of structural damage, and improving physical function in adults with moderate to severe rheumatoid arthritis. May be used alone or in combination with methotrexate or other disease-modifying antirheumatic drugs. (2) Reduce signs and symptoms of active ankylosing spondylitis in adults. (3) Treatment of adults with moderate to severe chronic plaque psoriasis who are candidates for systemic therapy or phototherapy and when other systemic therapies are medically less appropriate. Give only to those who will be closely monitored and have regular follow-up visits with a health care provider. (4) Reduce signs and symptoms and inducing and maintaining clinical remission in adults with moderate to severe active Crohn's disease who have had an inadequate response to conventional therapy. Also, for those who have lost response to or are intolerant to infliximab. (5) Reduce signs and symptoms of moderate to severe active polyarticular juvenile idiopathic arthritis in clients 4 years of age and older. Can be used alone or in combination with methotrexate. (6) Reduce signs and symptoms, inhibiting the progression of structural damage, and improving physical function in adults with active psoriatic arthritis. Used alone or with nonbiologic disease-modifying antirheumatic drugs.

ACTION/KINETICS

Action

Tissue necrosis factor (TNF) is a naturally occurring cytokine involved in normal inflammatory and immune responses. TNF plays an important role in the pathologic inflammation and joint destruction in rheumatoid arthritis. Adalimumab binds specifically to TNF-alpha and blocks its interaction with p55 and p75 cell surface TNF receptors. This results in a rapid decrease in levels of the acute phase reactants of inflammation and erythrocyte sedimentation rate and serum cytokines.

Pharmacokinetics

Maximum serum levels: 131 hr following a single SC injection of 40 mg (absolute bioavailability is 64%). **Adults, mean steady-state trough levels:** About 5 mcg/mL (without methotrexate) or 8–9 mcg/mL (with methotrexate) after 40 mg every other week. **Children, mean steady-state trough levels:** 6.8 mcg/mL (without methotrexate) or 10.9 mcg/mL (with methotrexate) after 20 mg every other week in those less than 30 kg. **$t^{1/2}$, terminal:** 2 weeks. Clearance is lower in clients 40 to 75 years of age and older. Methotrexate reduces adalimumab apparent clearance.

CONTRAINDICATIONS

Hypersensitivity to adalimumab or components of the product. Administration of live vaccines. Use in active infections, including chronic or localized infections. Lactation.

SPECIAL CONCERNS

■ **Serious infections.** (1) Clients treated with adalimumab are at increased risk for developing serious infections that may lead to hospitalization or death. Most clients who developed these infections were taking concomitant immunosuppressants, such as methotrexate or corticosteroids. (2) Discontinue adalimumab if a client develops a serious infection or sepsis. Reported infections include the following: (a) Active tuberculosis (TB), including reactivation of latent TB. Clients with TB frequently have presented with disseminated or extrapulmonary disease. Test clients for latent TB before adalimumab use and during therapy. Initiate treatment for latent infection prior to adalimumab use. (b) Invasive fungal infections, including histoplasmosis, coccidioidomycosis, candidiasis, aspergillosis, blastomycosis, and pneumocystosis. Clients with histoplasmosis or other invasive fungal infections may present with disseminated, rather than localized disease. Antigen and antibody testing for histoplasmosis may be negative in some clients with active infection. Consider empiric antifungal therapy in clients at risk for invasive fungal infections who develop severe systemic illness. (c) Bacterial, viral, and other infections caused by opportunistic pathogens. (3) Carefully consider the risks and benefits of treatment with adalimumab prior to initiating therapy in clients with chronic or recurrent infection. (4) Closely monitor clients for the development of S&S of infection during and after treatment with adalimumab, including the possible development of TB in clients who tested negative for latent TB infection prior to initiating therapy. **Malignancy.** Lymphoma and other malignancies, some fatal, have been reported in children and adolescents treated with tumor necrosis factor (TNF) blockers, of which adalimumab is a member. Postmarketing cases of hepatosplenic T-cell lymphoma, a rare type of T-cell lymphoma, have been reported in clients treated with TNF blockers, including adalimumab. These cases have had a very aggressive disease course and have been fatal. The majority of reported TNF blocker cases occurred in clients with Crohn's disease or ulcerative colitis, and the majority were in adolescent and young adult males. Almost all these clients had received treatment with azathioprine or 6-mercaptopurine concomitantly with a TNF blocker at or prior to diagnosis. It is uncertain whether the occurrence of hepatosplenic T-cell lymphoma is related to use of a TNF blocker or a TNF blocker in combination with these other immunosuppressants. ■

- **Use with caution in the elderly, in those with preexisting or recent-onset CNS demyelinating disorders, in those with active infections or a history of recurrent infection, in underlying conditions that may predispose to infections, in those with heart failure, or in those who have resided in regions where tuberculosis and histoplasmosis are endemic.**
- **Simultaneous use with other TNF-blocking drugs is discouraged.**
- **Safety and efficacy not determined in children other than for juvenile idiopathic arthritis.**
- **The frequency of serious infection and malignancy is higher for those 65 years of age and older; use with caution in this population.**

SIDE EFFECTS

Most Common

Adults: Injection site reactions (erythema and/or itching, ***hemorrhage***, pain, swelling), headache, sinusitis, URTI, rash, nausea, UTI, accidental injury. **Children:** Injection site pain reaction.

Body as a whole: Serious infections (including opportunistic infections) and ***sepsis***, especially in those also receiving immunosuppressants. Fever, lymphomas, adenoma, flu syndrome, immunosuppression, new or reactivation of tuberculosis (miliary, lymphatic, peritoneal, pulmonary), lupus-like syndrome (due to development of autoantibodies), prosthetic and postsurgical infections. Fungal infections, including aspergillosis, candidiasis, coccidioidomycosis, listeriosis, pneumocytosis. Cancers, including breast, skin, GI, urogenital, colon-rectum, uterine-cervical, prostate, melanoma, gallbladder-bile ducts. Reactivation of hepatitis B virus. New onset or exacerbation of demyelinating diseases, including multiple sclerosis and Guillain-Barré syndrome. **Hypersensitivity:** Rash, ***anaphylaxis***, fixed and/or nonspecific drug reaction, urticaria, angioneurotic edema. **Injection site:** Erythema, itching, hemorrhage, pain, swelling, clinical flare reaction, rash. **GI:** N&V, abdominal pain, cholecystitis, cholelithiasis, esophagitis, gastroenteritis, GI disorder, diverticulitis, ***pancreatitis, GI hemorrhage, hepatic necrosis, large bowel perforations*** (including perforations associated with diverticulitis and appendiceal perforations associated with appendicitis). **Respiratory:** Pneumonia, URTI, bronchitis, sinusitis, flu syndrome, asthma, ***bronchospasm***, dyspnea, lung disorder, decreased lung function, pleural effusion, interstitial lung disease (including pulmonary fibrosis). **CNS:** Confusion, headache, multiple sclerosis, paresthesia, ***subdural hematoma***, tremor. **CV:** Hypertension, arrhythmia, atrial fibrillation, CV disorder, chest pain,

A

CHF (new onset or worsening), coronary artery disorder, ***MI***, ***cardiac arrest***, hypertensive encephalopathy, palpitation, pericardial effusion, pericarditis, syncope, tachycardia, vascular disorder, leg thrombosis, cutaneous vasculitis. **Hematologic:** Agranulocytosis including ***aplastic anemia***, granulocytopenia, leukopenia, lymphoma-like reaction, pancytopenia, polycythemia, thrombocytopenia. **GU:** UTI, hematuria, pyelonephritis, cystitis, kidney calculus, menstrual disorder. **Dermatologic:** Erysipelas, cellulitis, herpes zoster, cutaneous vasculitis, erythema multiforme, new or worsening psoriasis (including pustular and palmoplantar), ***Stevens Johnson syndrome***. **Musculoskeletal:** Arthritis, arthralgia, bone disorder, bone fracture (not spontaneous), bone necrosis, joint disorder, muscle cramps, myasthenia, pain in extremities, pyogenic (septic) arthritis, synovitis, tendon disorder. **Metabolic:** Dehydration, abnormal healing, peripheral edema, ketosis, paraproteinemia. **Miscellaneous:** Accidental injury, back pain, pelvic pain, thorax pain, parathyroid disorder, cataract, immunogenicity, ***systemic vasculitis***.

Side effects observed in children, 4–17 years of age with juvenile idiopathic arthritis: Injection site pain/ reaction, neutropenia, streptococcal pharyngitis, increased aminotransferases (ALT, AST), herpes zoster, myositis, metrorrhagia, appendicitis, herpes simplex, pneumonia, UTI, granuloma annulare (rare), hypersensitivity reactions (localized allergic hypersensitivity reactions, allergic rash), mild to moderate increased creatine phosphokinase, development of autoantibodies.

LABORATORY TEST CONSIDERATIONS

↑ ALT (more common), AST, alkaline phosphatase. Hypercholesterolemia, hyperlipidemia, hematuria.

OVERDOSE MANAGEMENT

Treatment: In case of overdose, monitor for signs and symptoms of side effects. Begin appropriate symptomatic treatment immediately.

DRUG INTERACTIONS

Abatacept / ↑ Risk of infection; coadministration not recommended; if used together, monitor for infection

Anakinra / Coadministration with anakinra → increased risk of serious infections, neutropenia, pancytopenia (including aplastic anemia) and hypersensitivity reactions (including anaphylaxis); do not use together

Immunosuppressants / Possible development of malignancies and/or infection

Methotrexate / ↓ Adalimumab clearance after single and multiple dosing; dosage adjustment not needed

Rituximab / ↑ Rate of serious infections if rituximab use followed by a TNF blocker; use together not recommended

Tocilizumab / ↑ Rate of infection may occur; do not use together

HOW SUPPLIED

Injection Solution: 20 mg/0.4 mL, 40 mg/0.8 mL.

DOSAGE

SC

Rheumatoid arthritis, psoriatic arthritis, ankylosing spondylitis.

Adults: 40 mg every other week SC. Rheumatoid arthritis clients not taking methotrexate concomitantly may benefit more by increasing the dosing frequency to 40 mg every week.

Juvenile idiopathic arthritis.

Children, 4–17 years, 15 kg (33 lbs) to <30 kg (66 lbs): 20 mg every other week (use 20 mg prefilled syringe); **30 kg (66 lbs) or greater:** 40 mg every other week (use adalimumab pen or 40 mg prefilled syringe). Limited data are available for use in children weighing less than 15 kg.

Crohn's disease.

Adults, initial: 160 mg on day 1 (given as four 40 mg injections in 1 day or two 40 mg injections per day for 2 consecutive days) followed by 80 mg 2 weeks later (i.e., day 15). **Maintenance:** Two weeks later (i.e., day 29) begin a maintenance dose of 40 mg every other week.

Plaque psoriasis.

Adults, initial: 80 mg; **then** 40 mg every other week starting 1 week after the initial dose.

NURSING IMPLICATIONS

IMPLEMENTATION/ADMINISTRATION/STORAGE

1. During treatment, aminosalicylates, analgesics, corticosteroids, immunomodulatory drugs (e.g., 6-mercaptopurine and azathioprine), methotrexate, NSAIDs, salicylates, and other disease-modifying antirheumatic drugs may be continued.
2. Syringe needle cover is made of latex; if sensitive to latex, do not handle the product.
3. May increase the risk of reactivation of hepatitis B virus (HBV) in those who are chronic carriers of the virus. If HBV is reactivated, stop adalimumab and begin effective antiviral therapy with appropriate supportive therapy.
4. Discard unused portions remaining in the vial/syringe; no preservative in product.
5. Refrigerate at 2–8°C (36–46°F). Do not freeze.
6. Protect vial/prefilled syringe from exposure to light. Store in original carton until administered.

ASSESSMENT

1. Note reasons for therapy, joints affected, presenting symptoms, extent of disease, ROM, level of mobility, other agents trialed/failed.
2. Assess carefully for evidence of chronic/local infections, and initiate complete diagnostic workup with any new onset infection. Look for latent tuberculosis infection with a tuberculin skin test. Begin treatment of latent TB prior to adalimumab therapy. Discontinue if a serious infection develops.
3. Discontinue in confirmed significant hematologic abnormalities.
4. Use cautiously in elderly and those with preexisting or recent-onset CNS demyelinating disorders, recurrent infections or those who have resided in regions endemic with TB or histoplasmosis.
5. Observe client perform first injection after instruction, and monitor injection site for reactions. Administer subcutaneous at 45° angle into abdomen or upper thighs, rotating sites.
6. Caution that hepatosplenic T-cell lymphoma (HSTCL), a rare type of T-cell lymphoma, has been reported with use of TNF blockers including adalimumab.
7. Monitor VS, ROM, for S&S of infection, CPK, LFT, and CBC.

CLIENT/FAMILY TEACHING

1. Used to preserve joint structure and stability. Methotrexate, glucocorticoids, salicylates, NSAIDs, analgesics, and other prescribed antirheumatic drugs may be continued during treatment.
2. May self-administer drug after proper training in injection technique. Review procedures for storage (refrigerate in original container), reconstitution, inspection, withdrawal, administration, site rotation, and disposal of syringes. Use the prefilled syringes or pen to inject the full amount in the syringe (0.8 mL), which provides the full 40 mg dose. When using the pediatric prefilled syringe (clients 15 to <30 kg), inject the full amount in the syringe (0.4 mL), which provides the full 20 mg dose.
3. Prepare selected site with alcohol, pinch skin, and administer following enclosed guidelines. Use calendar stickers provided to prompt dosing schedule.
4. Always rotate sites for self-injection, which include the thigh, abdomen, or upper arm. Give new injections at least 1 inch from the old site and never into areas where the skin is tender, bruised, red, or hard. Do not rub, and avoid injection within 2 inches of umbilicus.
5. May experience rash, pain, or swelling at injection site. A cool, moist compress should relieve. If no relief or S&S worsen, report.
6. Any evidence of dizziness, infection, numbness or tingling, weakness of legs or vision problems as well as facial swelling, chest pain, increased cough, fever, SOB, flu-like symptoms, rash, or joint pains require medical evaluation.
7. Drug may make one more likely to get infections or make any infection that you may have worse.
8. Serious infections, including TB (tuberculosis) and infections caused by viruses, fungi, or bacteria, may occur with this therapy; report immediately—may be fatal.
9. Avoid immunizations with live vaccines.
10. Review risks of therapy related to lymphoma, and some types of cancer. Report bumps/open sores that do not heal or lupus-like reactions (chest discomfort/pain that does not go away, SOB, joint pain, rash on cheeks or arms that gets worse in the sun).

11. When travelling, store in a cool carrier with an ice pack.
12. If sensitive to latex, do not handle the needle cover of the syringe. Keep all F/U to evaluate response to therapy and for any adverse SE.

OUTCOMES/EVALUATE

- ↓ Joint pain/swelling; delayed structural damage with RA
- Improvement in S&S of rheumatoid/juvenile/psoriatic arthritis, ankylosing spondylitis
- ↓ Skin severity with chronic plaque psoriasis
- Symptom improvement with Crohn's disease

Adefovir dipivoxil

(ah-**DEH**-foh-veer)

Classification(s): Antiviral
Pregnancy Category: C
RX: Hepsera.

SEE ALSO ***ANTIVIRAL DRUGS***.

INDICATIONS/USES

Chronic hepatitis B in adults and children 12 years of age and older with evidence of active viral replication and evidence of persistent increases of ALT or AST or histologically active disease.

ACTION/KINETICS

Action

A prodrug that is phosphorylated to the active metabolite, adefovir diphosphate, by cellular kinases. Adefovir diphosphate inhibits HBV DNA polymerase (reverse transcriptase) by competing with the natural substrate deoxyadenosine triphosphate. This causes DNA chain termination after being incorporated into viral DNA. Resistance and cross-resistance may develop.

Pharmacokinetics

Approximate bioavailability is 59%. **Peak plasma level:** 18.4 ng/mL after 0.6–4 hr (median = 1.75 hr). May be taken without regard for food. **t½, terminal:** About 7.5 hr. Modify dose in those with renal impairment. Excreted in the urine. **Plasma protein binding:** 4% or less.

CONTRAINDICATIONS

Hypersensitivity to any of the product components. Use in children less than 12 years of age. Lactation (if used during lactation, there is a potential risk of toxicity for the infant, such as nephrotoxicity).

SPECIAL CONCERNS

■ (1) **Hepatitis.** Severe acute exacerbations of hepatitis have been reported in those who have discontinued anti-hepatitis B therapy, including use of adefovir dipivoxil. Closely monitor hepatic function with both clinical and laboratory follow-up for at least several months in clients who discontinue anti-hepatitis B therapy. If appropriate, resumption of anti-hepatitis B therapy may be warranted. (2) **Nephrotoxicity.** In clients at risk of or having underlying renal dysfunction, chronic use of adefovir dipivoxil may result in nephrotoxicity. Closely monitor renal function in these clients; they may require dosage adjustment. (3) **HIV resistance**. HIV resistance may emerge in chronic hepatitis B clients with unrecognized or untreated HIV infection treated with anti-hepatitis B therapies that may have activity against HIV (e.g., adefovir). (4) **Lactic acidosis and severe hepatomegaly.** Lactic acidosis and severe hepatomegaly with steatosis, including fatal cases, have been reported with the use of nucleoside analogs alone or in combination with other antiretrovirals. ■

- Use with caution in the elderly due to a greater frequency of decreased renal or cardiac function as a result of concomitant disease or other drug therapy.
- Possible exacerbations of hepatitis after discontinuing treatment.
- Safety and efficacy not determined in children.

SIDE EFFECTS

Most Common

Asthenia, headache, abdominal pain, nausea, flatulence, diarrhea, dyspepsia.

Hepatic: Severe acute exacerbation of hepatitis in clients who have discontinued anti-hepatitis B therapy. ***Severe hepatomegaly with steatosis, hepatic failure***, abnormal liver function. **CNS:** Headache. **GI:** N&V, flatulence, diarrhea, dyspepsia, abdominal pain. **GU:** Nephrotoxicity (including renal failure, renal insufficiency), Fanconi syndrome, proximal renal tubulopathy, renal failure. **Musculoskeletal:** Myopathy, osteomalacia. **Respiratory:** Increased cough, pharyngitis, sinusitis. **Dermatologic:** Pruritus, rash. **Miscellaneous:** Lactic acidosis, asthenia, headache, fever, HIV resistance, hypophosphatemia.

Side effects in pre- and post-liver transplantation clients. GI: Abdominal pain, diarrhea, flatulence, N&V. **GU:** Renal failure, ↑ creatinine, renal insufficiency. **Dermatologic:** Pruritus, rash. **Respiratory:** Increased cough, pharyngitis, sinusitis. **Hepatic:** Abnormal liver function, hepatic failure, ↑ AST and ALT. **Body as a whole:** Asthenia, fever. **Miscellaneous:** Headache, resistance (resulting in viral load rebound, worsening of hepatitis B, and possible death).

LABORATORY TEST CONSIDERATIONS

↑ ALT, AST, creatine kinase, amylase, serum creatinine. ↓ Serum phosphorus. Glycosuria, hematuria.

OVERDOSE MANAGEMENT

Symptoms: GI side effects. *Treatment:* Monitor for evidence of toxicity. Provide standard supportive treatment as needed. Hemodialysis will remove a portion of the dose.

DRUG INTERACTIONS

Aminoglycosides / ↑ Risk of nephrotoxicity
Cyclosporine / ↑ Risk of nephrotoxicity
Drugs that reduce renal function or compete for active tubular secretion / ↑ Serum levels of adefovir or coadministered drugs
Ibuprofen / ↑ C_{max}, AUC, and urinary recovery of adefovir
NSAIDs / ↑ Risk of nephrotoxicity
Tacrolimus / ↑ Risk of nephrotoxicity
Vancomycin / ↑ Risk of nephrotoxicity

HOW SUPPLIED

Tablets: 10 mg.

DOSAGE

TABLETS

Chronic hepatitis B.

Adults and children, 12 years of age and older: 10 mg (maximum) once daily without regard to food. Adjust dose as follows in clients with impaired renal function: **C_{CR} 30–49 mL/min:** 10 mg q 48 hr; **C_{CR} 10–29 mL/min:** 10 mg q 72 hr; **hemodialysis clients:** 10 mg q 7 days following dialysis.

NURSING IMPLICATIONS

IMPLEMENTATION/ADMINISTRATION/STORAGE

Store in original container from 15–30°C (59–86°F).

ASSESSMENT

1. Note onset, characteristics of S&S, and contacts. Assess HIV risks/test results.
2. List drugs prescribed/consumed to ensure none interact.
3. Check HIV status before starting therapy if exposure possible.
4. Resistance in those with lamivudine-resistant HBV may occur, use adefovir dipivoxil combined with lamivudine; do not use adefovir monotherapy. To reduce risk of resistance in those receiving adefovir monotherapy, may modify treatment if serum HBV DNA levels remain above 1,000 copies/mL with continued treatment.
5. To monitor fetal outcomes of pregnant women exposed to adefovir, call the established antiviral pregnancy register at 1-800-258-4263.
6. Obtain baseline viral load, renal and LFTs, BS, CK, amylase, and U/A; monitor for liver/renal failure and reduce dose with renal dysfunction—may result in nephrotoxicity. Lactic acidosis and hepatomegaly with steatosis (including fatal cases) may also occur; assess lactate levels.

CLIENT/FAMILY TEACHING

1. Take as directed once daily with or without food. If dose is missed, take as soon as remembered on that day. Do not take more than 1 dose of adefovir in a day, and do not take 2 doses at the same time to catch up.
2. Review enclosed patient literature before starting therapy and with each refill. Do not stop suddenly; severe acute exacerbation of hepatitis may occur.
3. May experience weakness, headaches, and GI upset. Report appetite loss, light-colored BMs, yellowing of skin/eyes, dark-colored urine, cold feeling in arms and legs, difficulty breathing, persistent dizziness/lightheadedness, fast/irregular heartbeat, stomach pain with N&V, unexplained drowsiness, or unusual muscle pain.
4. Does not cure disease but controls it; does not prevent transmission; safe behaviors must continue to be practiced. Do not share nee-

A

dles or injection equipment, personal items that have blood or body fluids on them (e.g., toothbrushes, razor blades). Practice safe sex using condoms or dental dams.

5. Keep all F/U to assess response, labs, and for adverse SE.

OUTCOMES/EVALUATE

↓ Viral replication in hepatitis B; improved LFTs

IV

Adenosine

(ah-**DEN**-oh-seen)

Classification(s): Antiarrhythmic

Pregnancy Category: C

RX: Adenocard, Adenoscan.

SEE ALSO ***ANTIARRHYTHMIC DRUGS***.

INDICATIONS/USES

(1) **Adenocard:** Conversion to sinus rhythm of PSVT, including that associated with accessory bypass tracts (Wolff-Parkinson-White syndrome). If clinically advisable, try appropriate vagal maneuvers (e.g., Valsalva maneuver) prior to use. *Investigational:* With thallium-201 tomography in noninvasive assessment of clients with suspected CAD who cannot exercise adequately prior to being stress-tested. Adenosine is not effective in converting rhythms other than PSVT. (2) **Adenoscan:** Adjunct to thallium-201 myocardial perfusion scintigraphy in clients unable to exercise adequately. For details on dosing, see package insert.

ACTION/KINETICS

Action

Found naturally in all cells of the body. A potent vasodilator in most vascular beds, except in renal afferent aretrioles and hepatic veins where it causes vasoconstriction. Thought to exert its pharmacological effects by activation of purine receptors (cell-surface A_1 and A_2 adenosine receptors). Mechanism for relaxation of vascular beds thought to be by inhibition of the slow inward calcium current reducing calcium uptake and activation of adenylate cyclase through A_2 receptors in smooth muscle cells. Adenosine may also decrease vascular tone by modulating sympathetic neurotransmission.

Pharmacokinetics

Onset, after IV: 34 sec. **t½:** Less than 10 sec (taken up by erythrocytes and vascular endothelial cells). **Duration:** 1–2 min. Exogenous adenosine becomes part of the body pool. Intracellular adenosine is rapidly metabolized via phosphorylation to adenosine monophosphate by adenosine kinase or via deamination to inosine by adenosine deaminase.

CONTRAINDICATIONS

Known hypersensitivity to adenosine. Second- or third-degree AV block (except in clients with a functioning artificial pacemaker), sick sinus syndrome (SSS) or symptomatic bradycardia (except in clients with a functioning artificial pacemaker), atrial flutter, atrial fibrillation, ventricular tachycardia. History of MI or cerebral hemorrhage. Bronchoconstriction or bronchospasm (e.g., asthma). Use in those who develop high-level block on one dose of adenosine additional doses.

SPECIAL CONCERNS

- **At time of conversion to normal sinus rhythm, new rhythms (PVC, PACs, sinus bradycardia, skipped beats, varying degrees of AV block, sinus tachycardia) lasting a few seconds may occur.**
- **Use with caution in the elderly due to diminished cardiac function, nodal dysfunction, concomitant disease, or drug therapy that may alter hemodynamic function and produce severe bradycardia and AV block.**
- **Use with caution in obstructive lung disease not associated with bronchoconstriction (e.g., bronchitis, emphysema).**
- **Safety and efficacy as a diagnostic agent not determined in clients less than 18 years of age.**

SIDE EFFECTS

Most Common

Facial flushing, shortness of breath/dyspnea, chest pressure, headache, lightheadedness, nausea.

CV: Short-lasting first-, second-, or ***third-degree AV block; cardiac arrest***, atrial premature contractions, atrial fibrillation, premature ventricular contractions, ***sustained ventricular tachycardia*** (requiring resuscitation), bradycardia, hypertension (systolic BP >200 mm Hg), hypotension (may be significant), palpitations, chest pain/discomfort, nonfatal MI, prolonged asystole, ***torsades de pointes***, sinus bradycardia, sinus tachycardia, sinus exit block, sinus pause, T-wave changes, skipped beats, varying degrees of AV nodal block, SA nodal block, ST segment depression, nonfatal MI, transient increase in BP, ***ventricular arrhythmia, ventricular fibrillation*** (rare). **CNS:** Lightheadedness, dizziness, numbness, headache, apprehension, paresthesia, drowsiness, emotional instability, tremors, nervousness, loss of consciousness and seizure activity (including generalized ***tonic-clonic seizures***). **Dermatologic:** Facial flushing, sweating. **Musculoskeletal:** Tingling/heaviness in arms, neck/back pain, back discomfort, lower/upper extremity discomfort. **GI:** N&V, metallic taste, tightness in throat, dry mouth, GI/tongue discomfort. **Respiratory:** SOB or dyspnea, urge to breathe deeply, chest pressure or discomfort, cough, hyperventilation, nasal congestion, bronchoconstriction in asthmatics, ***bronchospasm, respiratory arrest***. **GU:** Urinary urgency, vaginal pressure. **Ophthalmic:** Blurred vision. **Otic:** Ear discomfort. **Body as a whole:** Burning sensation, weakness, scotomas. **Miscellaneous:** Pressure in head, pressure in groin, discomfort in throat, neck, or jaw, injection site reaction.

OVERDOSE MANAGEMENT

Symptoms: Due to a short half-life (<10 sec), side effects are usually rapidly self-limiting when the infusion is stopped. *Treatment:* If side effects are prolonged, individualize treatment toward the specific side effect. Caffeine and theophylline are antagonists of adenosine.

DRUG INTERACTIONS

ACE inhibitors (e.g., captopril) / Potential additive or synergistic depressant effects on the SA and AV nodes; use together with caution

H ***Aloe; Buckthorn bark/berry; Cascara sagrada bark; Rhubarb root; Senna pod and leaf*** / Possible ↑ adenosine effect

Antiarrhythmic drugs (e.g., quinidine) / Potential additive or synergistic depressant effects on the SA and AV nodes; use together with caution

Beta-adrenergic blocking agents (e.g., propranolol) / Potential additive or synergistic depressant effects on the SA and AV nodes; use together with caution

Caffeine / Competitively antagonizes adenosine effect; larger doses of adenosine may be needed

Calcium channel blocking drugs (e.g., verapamil) / Potential additive or synergistic depressant effects on the SA and AV nodes; use together with caution. Also, possible ventricular fibrillation (rare)

Carbamazepine / ↑ AV block (higher degrees of heart block); closely monitor cardiac function

Digoxin / Potential additive or synergistic depressant effects on the SA and AV nodes; use together with caution. Also, possible ventricular fibrillation (rare)

Dipyridamole / Potentiates adenosine effect; possibly use smaller adenosine doses

Smoking (nicotine) / ↑ CV effects of adenosine; lower doses may be needed

Theophylline / Competitively antagonizes adenosine effect; larger doses of adenosine may be needed

HOW SUPPLIED

Injection: 3 mg/mL.

DOSAGE

Adenocard

IV BOLUS (ONLY), RAPID

Paroxysmal supraventricular tachycardia.

Adults and children 50 kg or more, initial: 6 mg over 1–2 sec. If the first dose does not reverse the PSVT within 1–2 min, 12 mg should be given as a rapid IV bolus. The 12-mg dose may be repeated a second time, if necessary. Doses greater than 12 mg are not recommended. **Children, less than 50 kg, initial:** 0.05–0.1 mg/kg as a rapid IV bolus given either centrally or peripherally; follow by a saline flush. If conversion of PSVT does not occur within 1–2 min, additional bolus injections can be given at increasing doses of 0.05–0.1 mg/kg. Continue this until sinus rhythm is established or a maximum single dose of 0.3 mg/kg is given. **Maximum dose, children:** 0.3 mg/kg as a single dose, up to 12 mg. Doses greater than 12 mg are not recommended.

Adenoscan

IV INFUSION

Stress testing diagnostic aid.

Adults, usual: 140 mcg/kg/min infused for 6 min (total dose of 0.84 mg/kg). The required dose of thallium-201 should be injected at the midpoint of the adenosine infusion (i.e., after the first 3 min of adenosine).

NURSING IMPLICATIONS

IMPLEMENTATION/ADMINISTRATION/STORAGE

1. **IV Can be stored at room temperature; crystallization may result if refrigerated. If crystals form, dissolve by warming to room temperature. Solution must be clear when administered.**
2. **Discard any unused portion; contains no preservatives.**
3. **When used for conversion of sinus rhythm, administer directly into a vein over 1–2 sec. If given into IV line, introduce in most proximal line.**
4. **Whenever possible, withhold drugs that might inhibit or increase the effect of adenosine for at least 5 half-lives prior to the use of adenosine.**
5. **Store from 15–30°C (59–86°F); do not refrigerate, as crystallization may occur.**
6. **COMPATIBILITY Administer undiluted, and follow with rapid saline flush (20 mL) to ensure delivery to systemic circulation.**
7. **INCOMPATIBILITY Avoid coadministration with other drugs.**

ASSESSMENT

1. **Note reasons for therapy, onset of symptoms, ECG confirmation of arrhythmia.**
2. **Monitor ECG continuously for evidence of varying degrees of AV block and increased arrhythmias, asystole during conversion to sinus rhythm, usually only transient due to short half-life of adenosine.**
3. **Monitor BP during therapy and pulse (q 15–30 sec). Report complaints of numbness, tingling in the arms, blurred vision, or apprehensiveness; may be indication to discontinue therapy.**
4. **Document chest pressure, SOB, heaviness of the arms, palpitations, or dyspnea. Note any history of MI/CVA; drug contraindicated; may cause bronchoconstriction with asthma; assess respiratory status closely.**

CLIENT/FAMILY TEACHING

1. **Drug helps restore heart to a normal, slower rhythm when given IV.**
2. **Avoid caffeine; report if prescribed theophylline, digoxin, or dipyridamole.**
3. **Facial flushing is common temporary side effect of therapy. Report chest pain, numbness/tingling, increased SOB, or other adverse side effects.**
4. **Change positions slowly to prevent any sudden drop in BP.**

OUTCOMES/EVALUATE

Conversion of PSVT to NSR

Aflibercept

Classification(s): Selective vascular endothelial growth factor antagonist

Pregnancy Category: C

RX: Eylea.

INDICATIONS/USES

Treatment of neovascular (wet) age-related macular degeneration.

ACTION/KINETICS

Action

By binding to receptors, vascular endothelial growth factor A can act as mitogenic, chemotactic, and vascular permeability factors for endothelial cells. This results in neovascularization and vascular permeability. Aflibercept is an inhibitor of vascular endothelial growth factor A thus preventing the effects on endothelial cells.

Pharmacokinetics

After intravitreal injection, small amounts are found in the plasma.

CONTRAINDICATIONS

Known hypersensitivity to aflibercept or any components of the product. Ocular or periocular infections. Active intraocular inflammation. Lactation.

SPECIAL CONCERNS

Safety and efficacy not established in children.

SIDE EFFECTS

Most Common

Conjunctival hemorrhage, eye pain, cataract, vitreous detachment, vitreous floaters, increased intraocular pressure.

A

Ophthalmic: Conjunctival hemorrhage, eye pain, cataract, vitreous detachment, vitreous floaters, increased intraocular pressure, conjunctival hyperemia, corneal edema/erosion, detachment of the retinal pigment epithelium, eyelid edema, foreign body sensation in the eyes, injection site hemorrhage/pain, increased lacrimation, tear of retinal pigment epithelium, vision blurred, retinal detachment/tear, endophthalmitis. **CV:** Potential risk of arterial thromboembolic events, including, nonfatal stroke, nonfatal MI, ***vascular death*** (including those of unknown cause). **Miscellaneous:** Hypersensitivity, immunogenicity.

HOW SUPPLIED

Injection Solution, Intravitreal: 40 mg/mL.

DOSAGE

INTRAVITREAL INJECTION ONLY.

Neovascular (wet) age-related macular degeneration.

Adults: 2 mg (0.05 mL) by intravitreal injection q 4 weeks for the first 12 weeks, followed by 2 mg (0.05 mL) once q 8 weeks.

NURSING IMPLICATIONS

IMPLEMENTATION/ADMINISTRATION/STORAGE

1. Give adequate anesthesia and a topical broad-spectrum antibiotic before the injection.
2. Each vial is to be used for the treatment of a single eye. If the contralateral eye requires treatment, use a new vial. Change the sterile field, syringe, gloves, drapes, eyelid speculum, filter, and injection needles before injection into the other eye.
3. Administer the intravitreal injection using a 30 gauge × ½-inch injection needle under controlled aseptic conditions (i.e., surgical hand disinfection and use of sterile gloves, sterile drape, and sterile eyelid speculum, or equivalent).
4. Store from 2–8°C (36–46°F). Do not freeze; protect from light. Store in original container until time of use. Discard any unused product.

ASSESSMENT

1. Note reasons for therapy, clinical presentation, visual acuity, other agents trialed and outcome.
2. Injection is performed by trained provider under aseptic conditions. Adequate anesthesia and a topical broad-spectrum antibiotic should be given prior to the injection.
3. Immediately after injection monitor for elevations of IOP (check for perfusion of the optic nerve head or tonometry).
4. Assess for and report eye pain, redness, light sensitivity or blurred vision (S&S of endophthalmitis or retinal detachment).

CLIENT/FAMILY TEACHING

1. Drug is administered by a trained individual into the eye once anesthetized.
2. Do not drive or operate equipment after injection; may experience visual disturbances.
3. Report if the eye becomes red, sensitive to light, painful, or develops a change in vision, and seek immediate care from an ophthalmologist due to risk of developing endophthalmitis or retinal detachment.
4. Keep all F/U to assess vision and IOP, for adverse SE, and need for additional therapy.

OUTCOMES/EVALUATE

- ↓ IOP
- Maintenance of vision

Albuterol (Salbutamol)

(al-**BYOU**-ter-ohl)

Classification(s): Sympathomimetic

Pregnancy Category: C

RX: AccuNeb, ProAir HFA, Proventil, Proventil HFA, Ventolin HFA, VoSpire ER.

✤ **Rx:** Airomir, Gen-Salbutamol Respirator Solution, Gen-Salbutamol Sterinebs P.F., ratio-Salbutamol HFA.

SEE ALSO ***SYMPATHOMIMETIC DRUGS.***

INDICATIONS/USES

Inhalation: (1) Prophylaxis and relief of bronchospasm in reversible obstructive airway disease in clients 4 years of age and older. (2) Acute attacks of bronchospasm (inhalation solution) including for children 2 years of age and older. (3) Prophylaxis of exercise-induced bronchospasm in clients 4 years of age and older.

Syrup: Relief of bronchospasm in adults and children 2 years and older with reversible obstructive airway disease.

Tablets and Extended-Release Tablets: Relief of bronchospasm in adults and children 6 years and older with reversible obstructive airway disease.

Investigational: Asthma, using the metered–dose inhaler, in children 4 years of age and younger. Nebulized albuterol as an adjunct (with treatments that promote potassium excretion) to treat moderate to severe serious acute hyperkalemia.

ACTION/KINETICS

Action

Stimulates beta-2 receptors of the bronchi, leading to bronchodilation. Also stimulates beta-1 receptors but activity is less. Causes less tachycardia and is longer-acting than isoproterenol. Has minimal beta-1 activity. Available as an inhaler that contains no chlorofluorocarbons (Proventil HFA).

Pharmacokinetics

Onset, PO: 15–30 min; **inhalation,** within 5–7 min. **Peak effect, PO:** 2–3 hr; **inhalation,** 60–90 min (after 2 inhalations). **Duration, PO:** 6–12 hr (extended-release); **inhalation,** 3–6 hr. Metabolites and unchanged drug excreted in urine and feces.

CONTRAINDICATIONS

Aerosol for prevention of exercise-induced bronchospasm and tablets are not recommended for children less than 12 years of age. Use during lactation.

SPECIAL CONCERNS

■ Long-acting beta-2 agonists may increase the risk of asthma-related death. Data from a large placebo-controlled U.S. study that compared the safety of salmeterol or placebo added to usual asthma therapy showed an increase in asthma-related deaths in clients receiving salmeterol. This finding is considered a class effect of long-acting beta-2 agonists. All long-acting beta-2 agonists are contraindicated in clients with asthma without the use of a long-term asthma control medication. Currently available data are inadequate to determine whether current use of inhaled corticosteroids or other long-term asthma control drugs mitigates the increased risk of asthma-related death from long-acting beta-2 adrenergic agonists.

Once asthma control is achieved and maintained, assess the client at regular intervals and step down therapy (e.g., discontinue long-acting beta-2 agonists) if possible without loss of asthma control and maintain the client on a long-term asthma control medication, such as an inhaled corticosteroid. Do not use long-acting beta-2 agonists for clients whose asthma is adequately controlled on low- or medium-dose inhaled corticosteroids.

Children and adolescents:

Available data from controlled clinical trials suggest that long-acting beta-2 agonists increase the risk of asthma-related hospitalization in children and adolescents. For children and adolescents with asthma, who require addition of a long-acting beta-2 agonist to an inhaled corticosteroid, a fixed-dose combination product containing both an inhaled corticosteroid and a long-acting beta-2 agonist should ordinarily be used to ensure adherence with both drugs. In cases where use of a separate long-term asthma control medication (e.g., inhaled corticosteroid) and a long-acting beta-2 agonist is clinically indicated, appropriate steps must be taken to ensure adherence with both treatment components. If adherence cannot be ensured, a fixed-dose combination product containing both an inhaled corticosteroid and a long-acting beta-2 agonist is recommended. ■

- **Use with caution in CV disorders, including coronary insufficiency, ischemic heart disease, coronary artery disease, cardiac arrhythmias, CHF, and hypertension.**
- **Due to the potential of additive effects, do not use 2 or more beta-adrenergic aerosol bronchodilators simultaneously.**
- **AccuNeb has not been studied for treating acute bronchospasms.**
- **PO use may delay preterm labor.**
- **Use not established for use of the aerosol and inhalation powder in children less than 4 years of age and the solution for inhalation in children less than 2 years of age.**
- **Safety and efficacy not established for the syrup in children less than 2 years of age and for tablets and extended-release tablets in children less than 6 years of age.**

ADDITIONAL SIDE EFFECTS

Most Common

Headache, hyperactivity, hyperkinesia, shakiness/nervousness, tension, tremor, bronchitis, URTI, rhinitis, dry throat, pharyngitis, N&V, palpitations/tachycardia, bronchospasm.

GI: N&V, dry mouth, heartburn/GI distress, dyspepsia, appetite loss or stimulation, epigastric pain, stomachache, bad or unusual taste, teeth discoloration. **CNS:** Hyperkinesia, excitement, hyperactivity, nervousness, tension, tremor, dizziness, vertigo, weakness, drowsiness, restlessness, headache, insomnia, malaise, emotional lability, light-headedness, nightmares, disturbed sleep, aggressive behavior, irritability, migraine, shakiness/nervousness, tension. **Respiratory:** Cough, wheezing, dyspnea, asthma, bronchospasm, dry throat, rhinitis, pharyngitis, throat irritation, bronchitis, URTI, lung disorder, epistaxis, hoarseness (especially in children), nasal/sinus congestion, increase in sputum, wheezing, paradoxical bronchospasm (rare). Increased risk of ***asthma-related death***. **CV:** Palpitations, tachycardia, BP changes, hypertension, tight chest, chest pain/discomfort, angina. **Musculoskeletal:** Back pain, muscle cramps, musculoskeletal pain. **Hypersensitivity** (may be immediate): Urticaria, ***angioedema***, rash, ***bronchospasm***. Rarely, erythema multiforme and ***Stevens-Johnson syndrome*** following use of syrup in children. **Metabolic:** Aggravation of pre-existing diabetes mellitus and ketoacidosis (large IV doses), hypokalemia (transient). **Dermatologic:** Flushing, sweating, pallor. **Body as a whole:** Flu syndrome, malaise, fatigue, viral infection. **Ophthalmic:** Conjunctivitis, dilated pupils. **Miscellaneous:** Change in smell, difficult urination, voice changes, ***oropharyngeal edema***.

OVERDOSE MANAGEMENT

SEE ALSO ***SYMPATHOMIMETIC DRUGS.***

Symptoms: Seizures, anginal pain, hypertension, hypokalemia, tachycardia (rate may increase to 200 beats/min).

ADDITIONAL DRUG INTERACTIONS

H *Fir needle oil; Pine needle oil* / ↑ Risk of bronchospasm

HOW SUPPLIED

Inhalation Aerosol: 90 mcg/actuation; ***Inhalation Solution:*** 0.021% (0.63 mg as sulfate/3 mL), 0.042% (1.25 mg as sulfate/3 mL), 0.083% (2.5 mg as sulfate/3 mL), 0.5% (5 mg as sulfate/mL); ***Syrup:*** 2 mg as sulfate/5 mL; ***Tablets:*** 2 mg as sulfate, 4 mg as sulfate; ***Tablets, Extended-Release:*** 4 mg as sulfate, 8 mg as sulfate.

DOSAGE

INHALATION AEROSOL (METERED-DOSE INHALER)

Asthma, bronchospasm.

Metered-dose inhaler. Adults and children over 4 years of age (12 and over for Proventil), usual: 180 mcg (2 inhalations) q 4–6 hr. In some clients 1 inhalation (90 mcg) q 4 hr may be sufficient. More frequent administration or use of a larger number of inhalations is not recommended. **Maintenance (Proventil only):** 180 mcg (2 inhalations) 4 times per day.

Prophylaxis of exercise-induced bronchospasm.

Adults and children over 4 years of age (12 and over for Proventil): 180 mcg (2 inhalations) 15–30 min before exercise.

INHALATION SOLUTION (NEBULIZER)

Asthma, bronchospasm.

Adults and children over 12 years of age: 2.5 mg 3–4 times per day by nebulization; up to 5 mg q 4–8 hr has been used. To administer 2.5 mg, dilute 0.5 mL of the 0.5% solution with 2.5 mL sterile NSS and deliver over 5–15 min or give 3 mL of 0.083% (1 unit-dose vial) and deliver over 5–15 min. **Children, 2–12 years of age (15 kg or over), initial:** 0.1–0.15 mg/kg (about 2.5 mg) (1 Unit-dose vial) 3–4 times per day by nebulization. Deliver over 5–15 min. **Children weighing 10–15 kg who require less than the 2.5 mg dose:** 0.1–0.15 mg/kg (about 1.25 mg) 3–4 times per day. Use the 0.5% inhalation solution. Give over 5–15 min.

ACCUNEB

Relief and prophylaxis of bronchospasms.

Initial, children 2–12 years: 1.25 mg or 0.63 mg given 3–4 times per day, as needed, by nebulization. Do not give

A

more frequently. Administer over about 5–15 min. Children, 6–12 years of age, with more severe asthma (baseline FEV_1 less than 60% predicted), who weigh more than 40 kg, or those 11–12 years of age may achieve a better initial response with the 1.25 mg dose. Titrate dosing to the desired clinical response.

SYRUP

Bronchospasm.

Adults and children over 14 years of age, usual initial: 2–4 mg (5–10 mL) 3–4 times per day. Use a dosage above 4 mg 4 times per day only when the client fails to respond; the dosage should be increased cautiously stepwise up to a maximum of 8 mg 4 times per day (i.e., 32 mg total/day), as tolerated. In geriatric clients and those sensitive to beta-adrenergic stimulation, restrict initial dose to 2 mg (5 mL) 3 or 4 times per day; adjust individually thereafter. **Children, over 6–12 years, initial:** 2 mg (5 mL) 3–4 times per day; **then** increase cautiously stepwise as necessary to a maximum of 24 mg/day in divided doses. **Children, 2–6 years, initial:** 0.1 mg/kg 3 times per day, not to exceed 2 mg (5 mL) 3 times per day; **then** increase stepwise as necessary up to 0.2 mg/kg 3 times per day, not to exceed 4 mg (10 mL) 3 times per day (i.e., 12 mg total). **Neonates (investigational):** 0.1–0.3 mg/kg q 6–8 hr.

TABLETS

Bronchospasm.

Adults and children over 12 years of age, initial: 2 or 4 mg 3–4 times per day; **then** increase dose stepwise cautiously as needed up to a maximum of 8 mg 4 times per day (i.e., 32 mg/day total), as tolerated. In geriatric clients or those sensitive to beta-agonists, start with 2 mg 3–4 times per day; increase dose gradually, if needed, to a maximum of 8 mg 3–4 times per day, not to exceed 32 mg/day in adults and children over 12 years of age. **Children, 6–12 years of age, usual, initial:** 2 mg 3–4 times per day; **then**, if necessary, increase the dose in a stepwise fashion to a maximum of 24 mg/day in divided doses.

EXTENDED-RELEASE TABLETS (VOSPIRE ER)

Bronchodilation.

Adults and children over 12 years of age: 8 mg q 12 hr; in some clients (e.g., low adult body weight), 4 mg q 12 hr may be sufficient initially and then increased to 8 mg q 12 hr, depending on the response. The dose can be increased stepwise and cautiously (under provider supervision) to a maximum of 32 mg/day in divided doses q 12 hr. **Children, 6–12 years of age:** 4 mg q 12 hr. The dose can be increased stepwise and cautiously (under provider supervision) to a maximum of 24 mg/day in divided doses q 12 hr.

NURSING IMPLICATIONS

Do not confuse albuterol with atenolol (a beta-blocker); Ventolin with Benylin (an expectorant); or Volmax with Flomax (an alpha-adrenergic blocker).

IMPLEMENTATION/ADMINISTRATION/STORAGE

1. The aerosol and inhalation powder are indicated for children 4 years and older (12 years and older for Proventil); the solution for inhalation and syrup are indicated for children 2 years and older. Tablets, including extended-release, are for use in children 6 years of age and over.
2. Clients maintained on the tablets or syrup may be switched to the extended-release tablets. For example, the administration of one 4 mg extended-release tablet q 12 hr is comparable to one 2 mg tablet q 6 hr.
3. To prepare the 0.5% inhalation solution for administration, dilute the appropriate volume in sterile normal saline solution to a total volume of 3 mL before administration by nebulization. To administer albuterol, 2.5 mg, dilute 0.5 mL of the 0.5% inhalation solution with 2.5 mL sterile normal saline solution. *NOTE:* Albuterol, 0.083% inhalation solution requires no dilution before administration by nebulization.

4. If a previously effective regimen does not provide the usual response, reevaluate the client as it is possible corticosteroids may be required.
5. When given by nebulization, use either a face mask or mouthpiece. Use compressed air or oxygen with a gas flow of 6–10 L/min; a single treatment lasts from 5 to 15 min.
6. When given by IPPB, the inspiratory pressure should be from 10 to 20 cm water, with the duration of treatment ranging from 5 to 20 min depending on the client and instrument control.
7. The MDI may also be administered on a mechanical ventilator through an adapter.
8. Take extended-release tablets whole with the aid of liquids; do not chew or crush. The outer coating of Volmax Extended-Release Tablets is not absorbed and is excreted in the feces; empty outer coating may be seen in the stool.
9. Contents of the MDI container are under pressure. Do not store near heat or open flames, and do not puncture the container.
10. Proventil HFA and Ventolin HFA contain hydrofluoroalkane as the propellant rather than chlorofluorocarbons.
11. AccuNeb, either 0.63 mg/3 mL or 1.25 mg/3 mL is intended for relief of bronchospasm in children 2–12 years of age with asthma. AccuNeb has not been studied in the setting of acute attacks of bronchospasms.
12. Store Volmax tablets refrigerated at 2–8°C (36–46°F).
13. Albuterol inhalation solution may be used with cromolyn solution, budesonide inhalant suspension, or ipratropium solution for nebulization.
14. Store the inhalation solution, 0.5%, from 2–25°C (36–77°F). Store the inhalation solution, 0.083%, under refrigeration from 2–8°C (36–46°F); may be held at room temperature for up to 2 weeks before use. Store the HFA inhalation aerosol (canisters) from 15–25°C (59–77°F); store canisters with mouthpiece down. For optimum results, bring the canister to room temperature before use. Shake well before using.

ASSESSMENT

1. Note characteristics of S&S: onset, duration, frequency, any precipitating factors, and obtain history; assess ECG and CNS status. Avoid use with cardiac tachyarrhythmias.
2. List any convulsive disorders, hyperthyroidism, diabetes, CAD or HTN, and assess closely.
3. Document PFTs, CXR, oxygen sats, and lung sounds. Monitor pulmonary status (i.e., breath sounds, VS, peak flow/ABGs).
4. Determine if able to self-administer medication. Assess environmental/home issues and note anxiety; may contribute to air hunger.
5. List drugs prescribed; beta-blockers may induce severe bronchospasms, digoxin levels may decrease, and diuretic effects (↓ K) may be aggravated by albuterol.
6. Observe for allergic responses, and monitor for renal dysfunction.

CLIENT/FAMILY TEACHING

1. Take as directed; do not exceed prescribed dose and do not chew or crush capsules.
2. Maintain calm, reassuring approach. Do not leave client/child unattended if acutely short of breath; should improve 30–60 min after therapy. Report if persists and accompanied by chest pain, diaphoresis, or dizziness.
3. Ensure comfortable administering therapy, and have provider review technique to ensure correct administration procedure.
4. Practice how to inhale through nose and exhale with pursed lips or diaphragmatic breathing; prolongs expiration and keeps the airways open longer, thus reducing the work of breathing. May experience a bad taste in mouth after therapy.
5. With new inhaler (or if not used for 2 weeks), prime with 4 sprays prior to use. To use: shake inhaler several times and uncap mouthpiece. Breathe out fully. Hold the inhaler 1 to 2 inches in front of your open mouth, or attach a spacer to the inhaler and place the spacer in your mouth, above your tongue and past your teeth to prevent drug from depositing on tongue/throat. Take a deep, slow breath as you push down on the canister. Hold your breath for 10 seconds; then exhale slowly. If more than one puff ordered, wait for at least 1 full minute after each puff; then repeat the procedure. Avoid exhaling into mouthpiece to avoid moisture accumulation. Rinse mouth and clean inhaler after use. Keep mouthpiece capped to avoid getting dirt inside it.

6. Keep the plastic actuator clean to prevent blockage and medication buildup. If it becomes blocked (little or no medication coming out of the mouthpiece), remove by washing the actuator.
7. A spacer used with the MDI may enhance drug dispersion. Maintain fluid intake of 2,000 mL/day. Always thoroughly rinse mouth and equipment with water following each use/dose to prevent oral fungal infections.
8. When using inhalers, do not use other albuterol inhalation medication unless specifically prescribed. If a steroid (Vanceril) inhaler is also prescribed, use this 20–30 min after albuterol to permit better lung penetration.
9. Establish dosing regimens that fit lifestyle, i.e., 1–2 puffs q 6 hr or 4 puffs 4 times per day; usual dosing is q 4–6 hr with an as-needed order, or before exercise. Check peak flows; call if requiring more puffs more frequently than prescribed or if drug dose used previously does not provide relief. Report lack of response, chest pain, dizziness, weakness, heart palpitations, significant drop in peak flow readings, changes in sputum color/amount.
10. Use caution, may cause dizziness/drowsiness. Keep record of pulse and BP for provider review. Overuse of inhalers may cause cardiac-related adverse side effects.
11. To check inhaler content, place in glass of water: full inhalers sink, empty inhalers float, and half-full inhalers are partially submerged. If metered for a certain number of sprays, i.e., 200, then discard when number is reached. Check to ensure you do not run out of medication.
12. If using albuterol via nebulizer, do not dilute AccuNeb and the 0.083% solution before use; the 0.5% solution requires dilution with sterile normal saline solution prior to use.
13. Do not add or mix drugs with solutions in a nebulizer unless specifically ordered by provider.
14. Keep all F/U to evaluate response to therapy and for adverse SE.

OUTCOMES/EVALUATE

- Improved breathing patterns/airway exchange
- Prevention/treatment of reversible bronchospasm R/T asthma or obstructive pulmonary diseases (inhalation solution)
- Prevention of exercise-induced bronchospasm (aerosol)

■ IV

Aldesleukin (Interleukin-2: IL-2)

(al-des-**LOO**-kin)

Classification(s): Antineoplastic, miscellaneous

Pregnancy Category: C

RX: Proleukin.

SEE ALSO ***ANTINEOPLASTIC AGENTS.***

INDICATIONS/USES

(1) Metastatic renal cell carcinoma in adults 18 years of age and older. (2) Metastatic melanoma in adults. *Investigational:* In combination with highly active antiretroviral therapy to treat HIV clients. In combination for treatment of cutaneous T cell lymphoma.

ACTION/KINETICS

Action

Aldesleukin possesses the biologic activity of human native IL-2, even though it is not identical. The drug produces several immunologic effects including (1) activation of cellular immunity with profound lymphocytosis, (2) eosinophilia and thrombocytopenia, (3) production of cytokines (including tissue necrosis factor, IL-2, gamma interferon), and (4) inhibition of tumor growth. The exact antitumor effect is not known.

Pharmacokinetics

High plasma levels reached after a short IV infusion; rapidly distributed to the extravascular, extracellular space. Rapidly cleared from the circulation by both glomerular filtration and peritubular extraction; metabolized in the kidneys with little or no active form excreted through the urine. **t½, distribution:** 13 min; **t½, elimination:** 85 min.

CONTRAINDICATIONS

Hypersensitivity to IL-2 or any components of the product. Abnormal thallium stress test or pulmonary function tests. Organ allografts. Use in either men or women not practicing effective contraception. Lactation.

Retreatment is contraindicated in those who have experienced the following during a previous

A

course of therapy: Sustained ventricular tachycardia; uncontrolled or unresponsive cardiac rhythm disturbances; recurrent chest pain with ECG changes that are consistent with angina or MI; intubation required for more than 72 hr; pericardial tamponade; renal dysfunction requiring dialysis for more than 72 hr; coma or toxic psychosis lasting more than 48 hr; seizures that are repetitive or difficult to control; ischemia or perforation of the bowel; and GI bleeding requiring surgery.

SPECIAL CONCERNS

(1) **Capillary leak syndrome**. Use has been associated with capillary leak syndrome (CLS). CLS results in hypotension and reduced organ perfusion that may result in death (see *Side Effects*). Restrict therapy to clients with normal cardiac and pulmonary function as defined by thallium stress testing and formal pulmonary function testing. Use extreme caution in those with normal thallium stress tests and pulmonary function tests who have a history of prior cardiac or pulmonary disease. (2) Withhold use in those who develop moderate to severe lethargy or somnolence; continued use may result in coma. (3) CLS may be associated with cardiac arrhythmias (supraventricular and ventricular), angina, MI, respiratory insufficiency requiring intubation, GI bleeding or infarction, renal insufficiency, edema, and mental status changes. (4) Aldesleukin treatment is associated with impaired neutrophil function (reduced chemotaxis) and with an increased risk of disseminated infection, including sepsis and bacterial endocarditis. Adequately treat pre-existing bacteria prior to initiation of therapy.

- Symptoms may worsen in unrecognized or untreated CNS metastases.
- Use of nephrotoxic or hepatotoxic drugs may further increase toxicity to the kidney and liver caused by aldesleukin.
- May increase the risk of allograft rejection in transplant clients.
- Safety and efficacy not established in children less than 18 years of age.

SIDE EFFECTS

Most Common

Fever, chills, rigors, GI side effects, hypotension, sinus tachycardia, mental status changes, pruritus/erythema, N&V, diarrhea, pulmonary congestion/dyspnea, oliguria/anuria, anemia/thrombocytopenia.

Side effects are frequent, often serious, and sometimes fatal. The frequency and severity of side effects are usually dose-related and schedule-dependent. Incidence of side effects is greater in PS 1 clients than in PS 0 clients. The side effects listed have an incidence of 1% or greater. **Capillary leak syndrome (CLS):** Results from extravasation of plasma proteins and fluid into the extracellular space with loss of vascular tone. This results in a drop in mean arterial BP within 2–12 hr after the start of treatment and reduced organ perfusion that may be severe and result in death. CLS causes hypotension, hypoperfusion, and extravasation that leads to edema and effusion. ***CLS may be associated with supraventricular and ventricular arrhythmias, MI***, angina, respiratory insufficiency requiring intubation, GI bleeding or infarction, renal insufficiency, and changes in mental status. **CV:** Hypotension (sometimes requiring vasopressor therapy), sinus tachycardia, ***arrhythmias (atrial, junctional, supraventricular, ventricular)***, bradycardia, PVCs, PACs, myocardial ischemia, ***MI, cardiac arrest, CHF***, myocarditis, endocarditis, gangrene, ***stroke, pericardial effusion, thrombosis***. **Respiratory:** Pulmonary congestion/edema, dyspnea, ***respiratory failure***, tachypnea, pleural effusion, wheezing, apnea, pneumothorax, hemoptysis. **GI:** N&V, diarrhea, stomatitis, anorexia, ***GI bleeding*** (sometimes requiring surgery), dyspepsia, constipation, ***intestinal perforation***, intestinal ileus, pancreatitis. **CNS:** Changes in mental status (may be an early indication of bacteremia or early bacterial sepsis), dizziness, sensory dysfunction, disorders of special senses (speech, taste, vision), syncope, motor dysfunction, ***coma, seizure***. **GU:** Oliguria or anuria, proteinuria, hematuria, dysuria, impaired renal function requiring dialysis, urinary retention/frequency. **Hepatic:** Jaundice, ascites, hepatomegaly. **Hematologic:** Anemia, thrombocytopenia, leukopenia, coagulation disorders, leukocytosis, eosinophilia. **Dermatologic:** Pruritus, erythema, rash, dry skin, exfoliative dermatitis, purpura, petechiae, urticaria, alopecia. **Musculoskeletal:** Arthralgia, myalgia, arthritis, muscle spasm. **Electrolyte and other disturbances:** Hypomagnesemia, acidosis, hypocalcemia/-kalemia, hypophosphatemia, hyperuricemia, hypoalbuminemia/-proteinemia, hypona-

A

tremia, hyperkalemia, alkalosis, hypo-/hyperglycemia, hypocholesterolemia, hypercalcemia, hypernatremia/-phosphatemia. **Miscellaneous:** Fever, chills, pain (abdominal, chest, back), fatigue, malaise, weakness, edema, infection (including the injection site, urinary tract, catheter tip, phlebitis, sepsis), weight gain/loss, headache, conjunctivitis, reactions at the injection site, allergic reactions, hypothyroidism.

LABORATORY TEST CONSIDERATIONS

↑ BUN, bilirubin, serum creatinine, transaminase, alkaline phosphatase. See also *Electrolyte and other disturbances* under *Side Effects*.

OVERDOSE MANAGEMENT

Symptoms: See *Side Effects*. Exceeding the recommended dose may cause a more rapid onset of toxicity. *Treatment:* Side effects will usually reverse if the drug is stopped, especially because the serum half-life is short. Continuing toxicity is treated symptomatically. Life-threatening side effects have been treated by the IV administration of dexamethasone (which may result in loss of the therapeutic effectiveness of aldesleukin).

DRUG INTERACTIONS

Aminoglycosides / ↑ Risk of kidney toxicity
Antihypertensives / Potentiate hypotension due to aldesleukin
Asparaginase / ↑ Risk of hepatic toxicity
Cardiotoxic agents / ↑ Risk of cardiac toxicity
Corticosteroids / Concomitant use may ↓ antitumor effectiveness of aldesleukin (although corticosteroids ↓ aldesleukin side effects)
Cytotoxic chemotherapy / ↑ Risk of myelotoxicity
Doxorubicin / ↑ Risk of cardiac toxicity
Hepatotoxic drugs / ↑ Risk of liver toxicity
Indinavir / ↑ Indinavir plasma levels R/T ↓ liver breakdown
Indomethacin / ↑ Risk of kidney toxicity
Methotrexate / ↑ Risk of hepatic toxicity
Myelotoxic agents / ↑ Risk of myelotoxicity
Nephrotoxic agents / ↑ Risk of kidney toxicity
Psychotropic drugs (e.g., analgesics, antiemetics, narcotics, sedatives, tranquilizers) / Possible alteration of CNS function

HOW SUPPLIED

Powder for Injection, Lyophilized: 22 million international units/vial (18 million international units/mL or 1.1 mg/mL when reconstituted).

DOSAGE

IV INFUSION, INTERMITTENT

Metastatic renal cell carcinoma in adults and metastatic melanoma in adults.

Each course of treatment consists of two 5-day treatment cycles separated by a rest period. **Adults:** 600,000 international units/kg (0.037 mg/kg) given q 8 hr by a 15-min IV infusion for a maximum of 14 doses. Following 9 days of rest, repeat schedule for another 14 doses, for a maximum of 28 doses per course as tolerated. *NOTE:* Due to toxicity, clients may not be able to receive all 28 doses (median number of doses given is 20 during the first course of therapy for renal cell carcinoma and 18 during the first course of therapy for metastatic melanoma).

Retreatment for metastatic renal cell carcinoma and metastatic melanoma.

Evaluate for a response about 4 weeks after completion of a course of therapy and again just prior to the start of the next treatment course. Give additional courses only if there is evidence of some tumor shrinkage following the last course and retreatment is not contraindicated (see preceding *Contraindications*). Separate each treatment course by at least 7 weeks from the date of hospital discharge.

NURSING IMPLICATIONS

IMPLEMENTATION/ADMINISTRATION/STORAGE

1. **IV Undertake dose modification for toxicity by withholding/interrupting dose rather than reducing dose to be given.**
2. **Decisions to stop, hold, or restart therapy must be made after a global assessment of the client. *Permanently discontinue* therapy for the following toxicities:**
   - **CV: Sustained VT (greater than or equal to 5 beats), uncontrolled/unresponsive cardiac rhythm disturbances, recurrent chest pain with ECG changes indicating angina or MI, cardiac tamponade**
   - **Pulmonary: Intubation >72 hr**
   - **Renal failure requiring dialysis >72 hr**

- CNS: Coma or toxic psychosis lasting >48 hr; repetitive/difficult to control seizures
- GI: Bowel ischemia/perforation, GI bleeding requiring surgery

3. Consult product information for withheld and subsequent doses of aldesleukin, as well as guidelines for discontinuing therapy.
4. Reconstitute vials aseptically with 1.2 mL sterile water; each mL will contain 18 million international units (1.1 mg) of aldesleukin.
5. During reconstitution, direct sterile water at the side of the vial. Swirl contents gently to avoid foaming. *Do not shake vial.* Solutions should be clear and colorless to slightly yellow.
6. The vial is for single use only; discard any unused portion. Not for use with transplants; risk of allograft rejection.
7. Reconstituted drug may be diluted in 50 mL of D5W and infused over 15 min.
8. Use plastic bags for more consistent drug delivery. Do NOT use in-line filters.
9. After reconstitution, drug stable for 48 hr if stored at room temperature or 2–8°C (36–46°F). Administer within 48 hr of reconstitution; bring solution to room temperature before infusing. Do not freeze.
10. Undiluted drug stable for 5 days if refrigerated in 1-mL B-D syringes.
11. COMPATIBILITY D5W, sterile water, glass, PVC (preferred), or polypropylene syringes.
12. INCOMPATIBILITY Due to increased aggregation, do not reconstitute or dilute using bacteriostatic water or 0.9% NaCl injection. Do not mix with albumin or other drugs.

ASSESSMENT

1. Note diagnosis of metastatic melanoma or renal cell carcinoma, treatments, and any liver/renal dysfunction; cardiac, pulmonary, or CNS impairment.
2. Screen with a thallium stress test to document normal ejection fraction and unimpaired wall motion. If minor abnormalities in wall motion noted, a stress echocardiogram may help to exclude significant CAD.
3. Assess for any S&S of infection. Obtain cultures to R/O any potential sources. Pre-existing bacterial infections must be treated prior to initiation of therapy, as intensive treatment may cause impaired neutrophil function and an increased risk of disseminated infection leading to sepsis and bacterial endocarditis.
4. All those with indwelling central lines should receive antibiotic prophylaxis against *Saccharomyces aureus.*
5. Give premedications (e.g., NSAIDs, meperidine, H_2 antagonists) as ordered before starting infusion and for 12 hr after final aldesleukin dose. Initiate in a closely monitored environment where VS and I&O are assessed often.
6. Assess cardiac function daily by clinical examination and assessment of VS. Those with chest pain, murmurs, gallops, irregular rhythm, or palpitations should be further assessed with an ECG and CPKs. If ischemia or CHF evident, get a repeat thallium or cardiolyte stress test.
7. Perform daily CV evaluations to identify early S&S of drug toxicity. Monitor for symptoms of CLS characterized by hypotension and hypoperfusion, altered mental status, and decreased urine output. Mental status changes are usually transient but should be evaluated carefully. Hold drug in those developing moderate to severe lethargy or somnolence; continued administration may result in coma. Alterations in urinary output may signal renal toxicity. Monitor for dehydration, liver, or renal failure. Stop infusion and transport to ICU for intubation and dialysis if progressive toxicity evident.
8. Obtain baseline PFTs with ABGs. Determine the following baseline parameters prior to therapy and daily during drug use: CBC, blood chemistries, CPK, renal and LFTs, and CXRs.

CLIENT/FAMILY TEACHING

1. Report any persistent chest/abdominal pain/discomfort, unusual bruising or bleeding, fatigue, confusion, or ↑ SOB.
2. Review dosing schedules and list of drug side effects; note those (SOB, palpitations, blood in sputum, confusion, chest pain, or impaired vision) requiring immediate intervention.
3. Practice reliable contraception.
4. Avoid any OTC drugs unless specifically ordered.

OUTCOMES/EVALUATE

Disease regression with evidence of ↓ tumor size and spread

A

Alemtuzumab

IV

(**ah**-lem-**TOOZ**-uh-mab)

Classification(s): Monoclonal antibody

Pregnancy Category: C

RX: Campath.

INDICATIONS/USES

As a single agent to treat B-cell chronic lymphocytic leukemia. *Investigational:* Treat rheumatoid arthritis; multiple sclerosis.

ACTION/KINETICS

Action

Recombinant DNA-derived humanized monoclonal antibody. Binds to CD52, a nonmodulating antigen, that is present on the surface B and T lymphocytes, a majority of monocytes, macrophages, NK cells, and a subpopulation of granulocytes. Probably acts by by antibody-dependent cellular-mediated lysis of leukemic cells following cell surface binding.

Pharmacokinetics

t½, mean: 11 hr (range: 2–32 hr) after the first 30 mg dose and 6 days (range: 1–14 days) after the last 30 mg dose.

CONTRAINDICATIONS

Active systemic infections, underlying immunodeficiency (e.g., seropositive for HIV), or known Type I hypersensitivity or anaphylactic reaction to alemtuzumab or any of its components. Immunization of clients who have recently received the drug. Lactation.

SPECIAL CONCERNS

■ Administer under the supervision of a health care provider experienced in the use of antineoplastic therapy. (1) **Cytopenias.** Serious, including fatal, pancytopenia/marrow hypoplasia, autoimmune idiopathic thrombocytopenia, and autoimmune hemolytic anemia have occurred. Single doses of alemtuzumab of >30 mg or cumulative doses >90 mg/week increase the incidence of pancytopenia. (2) **Infusion reactions.** Alemtuzumab administration can result in serious, including fatal, infusion reactions. Carefully monitor clients during infusions, and withhold alemtuzumab for grade 3 or 4 infusion reactions. Gradually escalate the recommended dose at the initiation of therapy and after interruption of therapy for 7 days or more. (3) **Infections.** Serious, including fatal, bacterial, viral, fungal, and protozoan infections can occur in clients receiving alemtuzumab. Administer prophylaxis against (see *Implementation/Administration/Storage*) *Pneumocystis jiroveci* pneumonia and herpes virus infections. ■

- **Due to immunosuppression by the drug, do not immunize with live viral vaccines in clients who have recently received alemtuzumab.**
- **Safety and efficacy not determined in children.**

SIDE EFFECTS

Most Common

Cytopenias (anemia, lymphopenia, neutropenia, thrombocytopenia), N&V, abdominal pain, infections (CMV infection, CMV viremia, others), infusion reaction (rigors, dyspnea, hypotension, pyrexia, rash, tachycardia, urticaria), anxiety, insomnia.

Infusion-reaction: Hypotension, rigors, drug-related fever, N&V, SOB, bronchospasm, chills, rash, fatigue, urticaria, dyspnea, pruritus, headache, diarrhea, syncope, pulmonary infiltrates, acute cardiac insufficiency, angioedema, ***acute respiratory distress syndrome, respiratory arrest***, cardiac arrhythmias, ***MI, and cardiac arrest, anaphylactoid shock, fatal infusion reactions***. **GI:** N&V, diarrhea, stomatitis, ulcerative stomatitis, mucositis, abdominal pain, dyspepsia, constipation. **CNS:** Headache, dysesthesias, dizziness, insomnia, anxiety, depression, tremor, somnolence, chronic inflammatory demyelinating polyradiculoneuropathy, Guillain-Barré syndrome, optic neuropathy. **CV:** Hypotension, tachycardia, SVT, hypertension, decreased ejection fraction (in those previously treated with cardiotoxic drugs), dysrhythmias, ***cardiomyopathy***. **Hematologic:** ***Myelosuppression*** (may be prolonged), anemia, thrombocytopenia, neutropenia, profound lymphopenia, bone marrow aplasia, hypoplasia, ***severe/fatal autoimmune anemia***, ***aplastic anemia***, hemolytic anemia, pure red cell aplasia, purpura, pancytopenia, purpura. **Respiratory:** Dyspnea, cough, bronchitis, pneumonitis, pneumonia, pharyngitis, bronchospasm, rhinitis, epistaxis. **Musculoskeletal:** Musculoskeletal pain, myalgias, back/chest pain. **Dermatologic:** Rash (including maculopapular, erythematous), erythema, urticaria, pruritus, increased sweating. **Infections:** Opportunistic bacterial, viral, fungal, and protozoan infections, including CMV infection, CMV viremia (may be fatal), Epstein Barr virus, Goodpasture's syndrome, ***sepsis,*** febrile neutropenia. **Body as a whole:** Rigors, fever, fatigue, anorexia, chills, asthenia, edema, peripheral edema, malaise. **Miscellaneous:** Grave's disease, progressive multifocal leukoencephalopathy, serum sickness, tumor lysis syndrome, herpes simplex, moniliasis, temperature change sensation, immunogenicity.

LABORATORY TEST CONSIDERATIONS

Interference with diagnostic serum tests that use antibodies.

OVERDOSE MANAGEMENT

Symptoms: Bone marrow aplasia, infections, severe infusion reactions. *Treatment:* No known specific antidote. Discontinue the drug, and provide supportive therapy.

HOW SUPPLIED

Solution for Injection, Concentrate: 30 mg/mL.

DOSAGE

IV ONLY

B-cell chronic lymphocytic leukemia.

Adults, initial: 3 mg/day given as a 2 hr infusion. When the 3 mg dose is tolerated (Grade 2 or less infusion-related toxicities), escalate the dose to 10 mg and continue as tolerated. When the 10 mg dose is tolerated (i.e., infusion reactions of grade 2 or less); then gradually escalate to the maximum recommended single dose of 30 mg IV. Escalation can usually be attained in 3–7 days. **Maintenance:** 30 mg/day IV 3 times per week on alternate days (e.g., Monday, Wednesday, Friday). Single doses greater than 30 mg or weekly doses greater than 90 mg are associated with an increased incidence of pancytopenia. The total duration of therapy, including dose escalation is 12 weeks.

NURSING IMPLICATIONS

IMPLEMENTATION/ADMINISTRATION/STORAGE

1. **IV** Administer as an IV infusion over 2 hr. Do not give as IV push/bolus.
2. Alemtuzumab is a cytotoxic agent. Follow safe handling procedures when preparing, dispensing, and administering the drug. Using aseptic technique, withdraw correct amount of drug from ampule into syringe. To prepare the 3 mg dose, withdraw 0.1 mL into a 1 mL syringe calibrated in increments of 0.1 mL. To prepare the 10 mg dose, withdraw 0.33 mL into a 1 mL syringe calibrated in increments of 0.1 mL. To prepare the 30 mg dose, withdraw 1 mL in either a 1 or 3 mL syringe calibrated in 0.1 mL increments. Inject into 100 mL sterile 0.9% NaCl or D5W. Gently invert bag to mix the solution. Discard syringe. Use within 8 hr after dilution. Discard any unused portion after withdrawal of the dose.
3. Do not use if particulate matter is present or solution discolored. Do not shake prior to use.
4. To minimize infusion-related effects, premedicate 30 min prior to first dose, at dose escalations, and as needed. Premedication consists of diphenhydramine, 50 mg, and acetaminophen, 500–1,000 mg, prior to the first infusion and with each dose escalation. In those who experience severe infusion reactions, hydrocortisone sodium succinate may be added to the pretreatment regimen prior to subsequent doses at a dose of 200 mg IV. Institute appropriate medical management (e.g., epinephrine, meperidine, steroids) for infusion reactions as needed.
5. Gradually escalate to the recommended dose at the initiation of therapy and after interruption of therapy for 7 or more days. Temporarily interrupt the infusion or decrease the rate if severe reactions occurs (e.g., hypotension, hypertension, SOB, rash). Symptoms may be treated with hydrocortisone sodium succinate, diphenhydramine, acetaminophen, bronchodilators, oxygen, and/or IV fluids. Monitor client until symptoms resolve completely.
6. Give trimethoprim/sulfamethoxazole DS twice a day 3 times per week to prevent *Pneumocystis jiroveci* pneumonia. Give famciclovir (or equivalent) 250 mg twice a day as herpetic prophylaxis. Continue prophylaxis for 2 months after completion of therapy or until $CD4^+$ count is 200 or more cells/microliter (whichever occurs later).
7. Discontinue during serious infection, serious hematologic toxicity, or other serious toxicity,

A

until problem resolved. Permanently discontinue if autoimmune anemia or thrombocytopenia occurs. If severe neutropenia or thrombocytopenia occurs, use the following dose modification and reinitiation therapy protocol:

- For first occurrence of ANC <250/mcL and/or platelet count 25,000/mcL or less, withhold therapy. When ANC is 500/mcL or more and platelet count is 50,000/mcL or more, resume therapy at the same dose. If delay between dosing is 7 days or more, start therapy at 3 mg and escalate to 10 mg and then 30 mg as tolerated.
- For second occurrence of ANC <250/mcL and/or platelet count 25,000/mcL or less, withhold therapy. When ANC is 500/mcL or more and platelet count is 50,000/mcL or more, resume therapy at 10 mg. If dosing delay is 7 days or more, initiate therapy at 3 mg and escalate to 10 mg only.
- For a third incidence of ANC <250/mcL and/or platelet count 25,000/mcL or less, stop therapy permanently.
- If there is a first occurrence of ↓ ANC and/or platelet count of 50% or less of baseline value in those who started therapy with a baseline ANC of 500/mcL or less and/or a baseline platelet count of 25,000/mcL or less, withhold therapy. When ANC and platelet counts return to baseline value(s), resume therapy. If the dosing delay is 7 days or more, start therapy at 3 mg and escalate to 10 mg and then to 30 mg as tolerated. If there is a second occurrence, withhold therapy and resume therapy at 10 mg upon return to baseline values. For a third occurrence, discontinue alemtuzumab therapy.

8. Alemtuzumab contains no preservative; use within 8 hr of dilution. Store diluted solutions at room temperature or refrigerate. Protect from light. Prior to dilution, store ampule at 2–8°C (36–46°F). Do not freeze. Discard if ampule has been frozen. Protect from direct sunlight.
9. COMPATIBILITY 0.9% NaCl or D5W; alemtuzumab is compatible with polyvinylchloride bags and PVC or polyethylene-lined PVC administration sets.
10. INCOMPATIBILITY Do not add any drugs or simultaneously infuse any other drug through the same IV line.

ASSESSMENT

1. Note reasons for therapy (B-cell CLL), disease characteristics, physical condition; list fludarabine failure/other alkylating agents used.
2. Premedicate with diphenhydramine 50 mg and acetaminophen 650 mg 30 min before infusion, at dose escalations, and as indicated. Hydrocortisone 200 mg may help decrease infusion-related events.
3. Give *P. jiroveci* pneumonia (PCP) prophylaxis with trimethoprim/sulfamethoxazole double-strength twice daily 3 times/wk. Administer famciclovir 250 mg twice daily or equivalent for herpetic prophylaxis. Continue PCP and herpes viral prophylaxis for at least 2 months after completion of alemtuzumab or until the CD4+ count is at least 200 cells/mcL, whichever occurs later.
4. Assess for infusion reactions and for evidence of infections, especially CMV infection. Monitor VS and assess skin, urine, and lungs frequently. Follow infection prophylaxis under administration. Drug is extremely toxic; requires close observation.
5. Monitor CBCs and platelets at weekly intervals during therapy and more frequently if worsening anemia, neutropenia, or thrombocytopenia noted. Assess CD4 counts after treatment until recovery to at least 200 cells/mcL. Follow guidelines under administration for dosing/resuming therapy if ANC depressed or CD4 count <200 cells/mcL.

CLIENT/FAMILY TEACHING

1. Used to treat CLL in those who have failed to respond to fludarabine and other alkylating agents.
2. Once maintenance dose of 30 mg has been reached, drug is given 3 times per week (over 2 hr) on alternating days for up to 12 weeks. If the ANC or platelets drop, the dose may be modified.
3. May cause drowsiness/dizziness; avoid activities requiring mental alertness or coordination until drug effects realized.
4. Report any sign of infection, fever, chills, unusual bruising/bleeding, chest pain, diarrhea, fainting, hives/rash, mouth sores, persistent

N&V, sore throat, ↑ SOB, or difficulty breathing; drug is highly toxic.

5. Avoid live viral vaccines during therapy R/T drug-induced immunosuppression.
6. Women of childbearing age and men of reproductive potential should practice reliable contraception during treatment and for a minimum of 6 months after therapy. Consider egg/sperm harvesting prior to therapy.
7. Keep all F/U to assess response, labs, and for adverse SE.

OUTCOMES/EVALUATE

Control of malignant cell proliferation in B-cell CLL

Alendronate sodium

(ay-**LEN**-droh-nayt)

Classification(s): Bone growth regulator, bisphosphonate

Pregnancy Category: C

RX: Fosamax.

🍁 **Rx:** CO Alendronate, Gen-Alendronate, Novo-Alendronate, PMS-Alendronate, ratio-Alendronate, Sandoz Alendronate.

INDICATIONS/USES

Daily dosing: (1) Prevent osteoporosis in women who are at risk of developing osteoporosis and to maintain bone mass and reduce the risk of future fracture. (2) Treat osteoporosis in postmenopausal women to increase bone mass and reduce the incidence of fractures, including those of the hip and spine. Has been used in combination with estrogen/progestin replacement therapy. (3) Increase bone mass in men with osteoporosis. (4) Treatment of glucocorticoid-induced osteoporosis in men and women receiving daily dosage equivalent to prednisone 7.5 mg or greater and who have low bone mineral density. Used with adequate amounts of calcium and vitamin D. (5) Paget's disease of bone in men and women with alkaline phosphatase at least two times the upper limit of normal, for those who are symptomatic, or those at risk for future complications from the disease. *Investigational:* Osteogenesis imperfecta in adults, adolescents, and children. Postoperative knee arthroplasty.

Weekly dosing: Treatment or prevention of postmenopausal osteoporosis in women or osteoporosis in men.

ACTION/KINETICS

Action

Binds to bone hydroxyapatite and inhibits osteoclast activity, thereby preventing bone resorption. Appears to reduce fracture risk and reverse the progression of osteoporosis. Does not inhibit bone mineralization.

Pharmacokinetics

Well absorbed orally and initially distributed to soft tissues, but then quickly redistributed to bone. Food and beverages (e.g., coffee, orange juice) decreases absorption. Not metabolized; excreted through the urine. Somewhat great accumulation in those with impaired renal function. **t½, terminal:** Believed to be more than 10 years, due to slow release from the skeleton.

CONTRAINDICATIONS

Hypersensitivity to the drug or any component of the product. In hypocalcemia. Severe renal insufficiency (C_{CR} less than 35 mL/min). Use of hormone replacement therapy with alendronate for osteoporosis in postmenopausal women. Use of the PO solution in clients at increased risk of aspiration. In those with esophagus abnormalities that delay esophageal emptying (e.g., stricture or achalasia). Inability to stand or sit upright for at least 30 min.

SPECIAL CONCERNS

- Use with caution in those with upper GI problems (e.g., dysphagia, symptomatic esophageal diseases, gastritis, duodenitis, or ulcers).
- Safety and efficacy have not been determined in children.
- Some elderly clients may be more sensitive to the drug effects.
- Rarely, visual and auditory hallucinations when switched from daily to weekly use.
- Use with caution during lactation.

SIDE EFFECTS

Most Common

Abdominal pain, dyspepsia, nausea, constipation, diarrhea.

GI: Flatulence, acid regurgitation, esophageal ulcer, dysphagia, esophagitis, esophageal erosions/ulcers, esophageal strictures/perforation (rare),

A

oropharyngeal ulceration, abdominal pain/distention, gastritis, melena, constipation, diarrhea, dyspepsia, N&V, gastric/duodenal ulcers, local irritation of upper GI mucosa. **CNS:** Headache. **Musculoskeletal:** Bone/muscle/joint/skeletal pain, leg/muscle cramps, osteonecrosis of the jaw. **Dermatologic:** Rash (may be severe and with complications), photosensitivity, erythema (rare). **Ophthalmic:** Glaucoma, uveitis. **Body as a whole:** Accidental injury, edema, flu-like symptoms, hypersensitivity reactions (e.g., urticaria, angioedema). **Miscellaneous:** Pain, taste perversion, accidental injury.

LABORATORY TEST CONSIDERATIONS

↓ Serum calcium and phosphate.

OVERDOSE MANAGEMENT

Symptoms: Hypocalcemia, hypophosphatemia, upset stomach, heartburn, esophagitis, gastritis, ulcer. *Treatment:* Consider giving milk or antacids to bind the drug. Dialysis is not beneficial.

DRUG INTERACTIONS

Antacids / ↓ Absorption of alendronate
Aspirin / ↑ Risk of GI side effects with alendronate doses >10 mg/day
Calcium supplements / ↓ Absorption of alendronate
Naproxen / ↑ Risk of drug-induced gastric ulcers
Ranitidine / ↑ Bioavailability of alendronate (significance not known)

HOW SUPPLIED

Oral Solution: 70 mg as base (0.93 mg/mL); *Tablets:* 5 mg, 10 mg, 35 mg, 40 mg, 70 mg.

DOSAGE

ORAL SOLUTION; TABLETS

Prevention of osteoporosis in postmenopausal women.

One 35 mg tablet once weekly or one 5 mg tablet once daily.

Treatment of osteoporosis in postmenopausal women.

One 70 mg tablet once weekly, 1 bottle of 70 mg oral solution once weekly, or one 10 mg tablet once daily.

Osteoporosis in men.

One 70 mg tablet once weekly, 1 bottle of 70 mg oral solution once weekly, or one 10 mg tablet once daily.

Glucocorticoid-induced osteoporosis.

One 5 mg tablet once daily for men and women. For postmenopausal women not receiving estrogen, the recommended dose is one 10 mg tablet daily. Also give clients adequate amounts of calcium and vitamin D.

Paget's disease of the bone.

40 mg once daily for 6 months for both men and women. Retreatment for Paget's disease may be considered following a 6-month posttreatment evaluation in clients who have relapsed, based on increases in serum alkaline phosphatase. Retreatment may also be appropriate for those who failed to normalize serum alkaline phosphatase.

Osteogenesis imperfecta in adults Investigational.

10 mg once daily.

Postoperative knee arthroplasty (Investigational).

10 mg once daily beginning after knee arthroplasty.

NURSING IMPLICATIONS

Do not confuse Fosamax (alendronate) a bisphosphonate with Flomax (tamsulosin) an alpha-adrenergic blocking drug.

IMPLEMENTATION/ADMINISTRATION/STORAGE

1. **To facilitate stomach delivery and reduce esophagus irritation, do not lie down for at least 30 min following administration.**
2. **Due to possible interference with absorption, at least 30 min should elapse before taking antacids or calcium supplements.**
3. **Hypocalcemia must be corrected before beginning alendronate therapy.**
4. **If dietary intake is insufficient, give supplemental calcium and vitamin D when used for glucocorticoid-induced osteoporosis or Paget's disease. A product called Fosamax Plus D containing alendronate sodium 70 mg and vitamin D_3, 2,800 international units, is available to treat osteoporosis in postmenopausal women and to increase bone mass in men with osteoporosis.**
5. **No dosage adjustment needed for the elderly.**

6. Store tablets and oral solution in a tight container from 15–30°C (59–86°F). Do not freeze oral solution.

ASSESSMENT

1. Note reasons for therapy: osteoporosis prevention/treatment in postmenopausal women, steroid-induced osteoporosis, or Paget's disease. Note symptoms, onset, physical changes.
2. Note any history of GI problems (i.e., gastritis, dysphagia, duodenitis, or ulcers). Assess for any S&S of esophageal reaction (e.g., dysphagia, retrosternal pain, new/worsening reflux); precludes therapy.
3. Document bone mineral density (BMD) studies before starting therapy and after 6–12 months of treatment especially with glucocorticoid-induced disease and osteoporosis.
4. Assess for fractures; manage client to prevent further injury and loss of function.
5. With Paget's disease, monitor baseline S&S, assess for bone pain, changes in vision and hearing, headaches and skull size changes. Check alkaline phosphatase levels.
6. Obtain baseline BMD, VS, height, calcium, phosphate, electrolytes, renal and LFTs; correct any calcium or vitamin D deficiencies, and monitor periodically.

CLIENT/FAMILY TEACHING

1. Osteoporosis usually occurs after age 40 and is a systemic skeletal disease characterized by low bone mass due to a higher amount of bone resorbed than formed; may be induced by chronic steroid therapy at any age.
2. Take as prescribed. Benefit seen only when each tablet is taken with 6–8 oz of plain water first thing in the morning at least 30 min before the first food, beverage, or medication of the day. Do not lie down after taking drug. Taking with juice or coffee will markedly reduce absorption. Do not take at bedtime or before arising for the day.
3. Once-weekly therapy may enhance compliance. If taking alendronate once weekly and a dose is missed, take dose the next morning, and then resume taking 1 dose a week as originally scheduled on chosen day. Do not take 2 doses on the same day to catch up.
4. Do not chew, crush, or suck on tablets; take whole. If using oral solution, swallow entire contents of bottle and then drink at least 6 oz of water and remain standing or sitting for at least 30 min. Do not take aspirin or aspirin-containing products unless approved by provider.
5. Consume well balanced diet. If dietary intake is inadequate or levels low, take calcium with vitamin D supplements.
6. Things that can help prevent/inhibit progression of osteoporosis: take 1,500 mg/day of calcium and 800 international units of vitamin D/day supplements; regular daily weight-bearing exercises; cessation of cigarette smoking and reduction of excessive alcohol consumption.
7. Stop drug and report if swallowing difficulty, pain behind breastbone or new/worsening heartburn occurs.
8. Report blurred vision, eye pain, and notify provider prior to dental surgery.
9. Keep all F/U visits to evaluate response to therapy, BMD, and for adverse SE.

OUTCOMES/EVALUATE

- Prevention/decreased progression of osteoporosis in postmenopausal women (at risk)
- Increased bone mass in men with osteoporosis
- Treatment of glucocorticoid-induced osteoporosis
- Inhibition of kyphosis and pain R/T bone fracture or deformity
- ↓ Serum alkaline phosphatase levels with Paget's disease with ↓ disease progression

IV

Alfentanil hydrochloride

(al-**FEN**-tah-nil)

Classification(s): Narcotic analgesic

Pregnancy Category: C

RX: Alfentanil hydrochloride, **C-II**

SEE ALSO ***NARCOTIC ANALGESICS***.

INDICATIONS/USES

(1) **Continuous infusion:** As an analgesic with nitrous oxide/oxygen to maintain general anesthesia. (2) **Incremental doses:** Adjunct with barbiturate/nitrous oxide/oxygen to maintain general anesthesia. (3) **Anesthetic induction:** As primary agent when ET intubation and mechanical ventilation are necessary. (4) Analgesic component for monitored anesthesia care.

A

ACTION/KINETICS

Onset: Immediate. **t½:** 1–2 hr (after IV use).

CONTRAINDICATIONS

Use during labor and in children less than 12 years of age.

SPECIAL CONCERNS

Use with caution during lactation.

SIDE EFFECTS

Most Common

N&V, hyper-/hypotension, arrhythmias, tachycardia, chest wall rigidity.

See *Narcotic Analgesics*. Bradycardia, postoperative confusion, blurred vision, hypercapnia, shivering, injection-site pain/reaction, and ***asystole***. Neonates with respiratory distress syndrome have manifested hypotension with doses of 20 mcg/kg.

ADDITIONAL DRUG INTERACTIONS

Fluconazole / ↑ Alfentanil plasma levels due to ↓ liver breakdown

H *Indian snakeroot* / Potentiation of alfentanil effects

H *Kava kava* / Potentiation of alfentanil effects

HOW SUPPLIED

Injection: 0.5 mg/mL.

DOSAGE

Individualize dosage and titrate to desired effect according to body weight, physical status, underlying disease states, use of other drugs, and type and duration of surgical procedure and anesthesia.

IV

Induction of anesthesia—spontaneously breathing/assisted ventilation.

Initial for induction: 8–20 mcg/kg; give slowly over 3 min; **maintenance:** 3–5 mcg/kg q 5–20 min or 0.5–1 mcg/kg/min. **Total dose:** 8–40 mcg/kg.

Assisted or controlled ventilation: Incremental induction to attenuate response to laryngoscopy and intubation.

Initial for induction: 20–50 mcg/kg given slowly over 3 min; **maintenance:** 5–15 mcg/kg q 5–20 min. **Total dose:** Up to 75 mcg/kg.

Assisted or controlled ventilation: Continuous infusion to provide attenuation of response to intubation and incision.

Initial for induction: 50–75 mcg/kg given slowly over 2 min; **maintenance:** 0.5–3 mcg/kg/min. Average infusion rate: 1–1.5 mcg/kg/min. **Total dose:** Dependent on duration of procedure. With nitrous oxide/oxygen in general surgery, give 0.5–3 mcg/kg/min alfentanil. Following the anesthetic induction dose, reduce the infusion rate requirements by 30–50% for the first hour of maintenance. *NOTE:* (1) Vital sign changes that indicate the response to surgical stress or lightening of anesthesia may be controlled by increasing the rate to a maximum of 4 mcg/kg/min alfentanil or giving bolus doses of 7 mcg/kg. If changes are not controlled after 3 bolus doses given over 5 min, a barbiturate, vasodilator, and/or inhalation agent should be used. Always adjust infusion rates downward in absence of above signs until there is some response to surgical stimulation.

(2) Rather than an increase in infusion rate, give 7 mcg/kg alfentanil bolus doses or a potent inhalation agent in response to signs of anesthesia lightening within the last 15 min of surgery. Discontinue infusion at least 10–15 min prior to the end of surgery.

Assisted or controlled ventilation: Anesthetic induction.

Initial for induction: 130–245 mcg/kg given slowly over 3 min; **maintenance:** 0.5–1.5 mcg/kg/min or general anesthetic. At these doses, expect truncal rigidity; use a muscle relaxant. **Total dose:** Dependent on duration of procedure. *NOTE:* Reduce concentration of inhalation agents by 30–50% for the initial hour.

Assisted or controlled ventilation: Monitored anesthesia care, for sedated and responsive spontaneously breathing clients.

Initial for induction: 3–8 mcg/kg; **maintenance:** 3–5 mcg/kg every 5–20 min (or 0.25–1 mcg/kg/min, up to a total dose of 3–40 mcg/kg). Infusions may be continued until the end of the procedure.

NURSING IMPLICATIONS

Do not confuse fentanyl with alfentanil or sufentanil (opioid analgesic).

IMPLEMENTATION/ADMINISTRATION/STORAGE

1. IV Individualize drug dosage for each client and for each use:
   - Reduce dosage for elderly or debilitated clients.
   - For those who are more than 20% above IBW, base dosage on lean body weight.
   - Individualize selection of preanesthetic medication.
2. Neuromuscular-blocking drugs should be compatible with client condition.
3. Use a tuberculin-type syringe to ensure accuracy when giving small volumes of drug.
4. Direct IV administration over 1½–3 min. For continuous IV administration dilute 20 mL of alfentanil in 230 mL diluent to provide a solution of 40 mcg/mL.
5. Discontinue infusion 10–15 min prior to the end of surgery.
6. Protect from light. Store at room temperature from 15–25°C (59–77°F).
7. COMPATIBILITY NSS, D5/NSS, RL solution, or D5W.
8. INCOMPATIBILITY Administer separately.

ASSESSMENT

1. Qualified personnel and adequate facilities are essential for the management of intraoperative and postoperative respiratory depression in clients given anesthetic (induction) doses. Drug is individualized and titrated according to physical condition, body weight, underlying pathology, other drugs used, and type and duration of procedure.
2. Note any history of drug hypersensitivity reactions. Those with chronic opioid use may become tolerant to alfentanil.
3. Obtain baseline weight and VS.
4. Report any muscular rigidity before giving next dose.
5. Assess respiratory and CV status continuously during therapy; note oxygen saturations.

CLIENT/FAMILY TEACHING

1. May experience dizziness, drowsiness, and orthostatic hypotension; change positions slowly and call for assistance to prevent falls.
2. Avoid alcohol or any CNS depressants for at least 24 hr following drug administration.

OUTCOMES/EVALUATE

- Induction/maintenance of anesthesia
- Facilitation of intubation and mechanical ventilation

Alfuzosin hydrochloride

(al-fue-**ZO**-sin)

Classification(s): Treat benign prostatic hypertrophy (alpha-1 receptor antagonist)

Pregnancy Category: B

RX: Uroxatral.

INDICATIONS/USES

Signs and symptoms of benign prostatic hyperplasia.

ACTION/KINETICS

Action

Selective antagonist of postsynaptic alpha-1 adrenergic receptors located in various areas of the prostate. Blockade of these receptors causes relaxation of smooth muscle in the bladder neck and prostate, resulting in an improvement in urine flow and a reduction in symptoms of BPH.

Pharmacokinetics

About 49% is bioavailable after PO dosing in the fed state. **Maximum levels:** 8 hr after multiple dosing. Absorption is 50% lower under fasting conditions; thus, take immediately following a meal. Extensively metabolized by the liver principally by CYP3A4, with only 11% excreted unchanged in the urine. Metabolites and unchanged drug are excreted in the feces (69%) and urine (24%). **t½, elimination:** 10 hr. C_{max} and AUC are increased by 50% in those with mild to severe renal impairment. Plasma levels are increased with moderate to severe hepatic impairment. **Plasma protein binding:** 82–90%.

A

CONTRAINDICATIONS

Hypersensitivity to alfuzosin or any component of the product. Use with moderate to severe hepatic impairment. Concomitant use with itraconazole, ketoconazole, ritonavir, other alpha-adrenergic blockers, or another potent inhibitor of CYP3A4. Treatment of hypertension. Use in children or in women.

SPECIAL CONCERNS

- **Postural hypotension, with or without symptoms, may develop within a few hours of taking alfuzosin. Thus, use with caution in clients with symptomatic hypotension or who have had a hypotensive response to other drugs.**
- **Marked hypotension (especially postural hypotension) and syncope with sudden loss of consciousness may occur with the first few doses or after therapy is interrupted for more than a few doses, if dosage is increased rapidly, or if another antihypertensive drug is introduced.**
- **Use with caution in severe renal insufficiency.**

SIDE EFFECTS

Most Common

Dizziness, headache, fatigue, URTI.

CV: Hypotension/postural hypotension (with or without dizziness), syncope, tachycardia. **CNS:** Dizziness, drowsiness, headache. **GI:** Abdominal discomfort/pain, dyspepsia, constipation, nausea. **Respiratory:** URTI, bronchitis, cold symptoms, ***bronchospasm***, sinusitis, pharyngitis, rhinitis. **Body as a whole:** Fatigue, malaise, pain, rash. **Miscellaneous:** Impotence, chest pain, priapism, intraoperative floppy iris syndrome.

OVERDOSE MANAGEMENT

Symptoms: Hypotension. *Treatment:* Restoration of BP and normalization of HR by keeping client supine. If this is inadequate, consider IV fluids. If needed, vasopressors can be given. Monitor renal function; support as needed. Dialysis may not be effective.

DRUG INTERACTIONS

Atenolol / ↑ Risk of significant ↓ in mean BP and mean HR

Beta-adrenergic blockers / Enhanced acute postural hypotension

Diltiazem / ↑ Alfuzosin plasma levels R/T inhibition of CYP3A4 metabolizing enzyme; monitor BP

Cimetidine / ↑ Alfuzosin C_{max} and AUC

Clarithromycin / ↑ Alfuzosin plasma levels R/T inhibition of CYP3A4 metabolizing enzyme; do not use together

Erythromycin / ↑ Alfuzosin plasma levels R/T inhibition of CYP3A4 metabolizing enzyme; monitor BP

Itraconazole / ↑ Alfuzosin plasma levels R/T inhibition of CYP3A4 metabolizing enzyme; do not use together

Ketoconazole / ↑ Alfuzosin plasma levels R/T inhibition of CYP3A4 metabolizing enzyme; do not use together

Ritonavir / ↑ Alfuzosin plasma levels R/T inhibition of CYP3A4 metabolizing enzyme; do not use together

Verapamil / ↑ Alfuzosin plasma levels R/T inhibition of CYP3A4 metabolizing enzyme; monitor BP

HOW SUPPLIED

Tablets, Extended-Release: 10 mg.

DOSAGE

TABLETS, EXTENDED-RELEASE

Benign prostatic hyperplasia.

10 mg daily immediately after the same meal each day.

NURSING IMPLICATIONS

Ⓢ Do not confuse Uroxatral with either Oxytrol (an anticholinergic) or Roxanol (an opioid analgesic).

IMPLEMENTATION/ADMINISTRATION/STORAGE

1. **Do not chew/crush tablets.**
2. **Discontinue if symptoms of angina pectoris newly appear or worsen.**
3. **Store between 15–30°C (59–86°F). Protect from light and moisture.**

ASSESSMENT

1. **Note reasons for therapy, characteristics of S&S. List other drugs used for BPH and outcome.**
2. **Note drugs currently prescribed to ensure none interact. Check for CAD and any QT prolongation.**
3. **Document DRE and PSA to R/O prostatic pathology. Assess for any urinary symptoms.**
4. **Monitor BP, renal and LFTs; note any dysfunction.**

A

CLIENT/FAMILY TEACHING

1. Take as directed after the same meal each day with a full glass of water.
2. Do not chew, break, or crush extended release tablets.
3. Avoid tasks that require mental alertness until drug effects realized; may experience dizziness, drowsiness, and headaches.
4. May experience drop in BP with sudden change in position; change positions slowly and use caution. Alert older clients/family of fall risk.
5. Report chest pain, dizziness, fainting, prolonged or painful erection, or lack of improvement of urinary S&S.
6. Avoid OTC cough, cold, or allergy meds without provider approval.
7. Advise eye provider prior to any surgery.
8. Keep all F/U to assess response and for adverse SE.

OUTCOMES/EVALUATE

Improved urine stream; ↓ nocturia/frequency/hesitancy

Aliskiren hemifumarate

(a-lis-**KYE**-ren)

Classification(s): Direct renin inhibitor

Pregnancy Category: C ((first trimester)); **D** ((second and third trimester))

RX: Tekturna.

INDICATIONS/USES

Treatment of hypertension alone or with other antihypertensive drugs.

ACTION/KINETICS

Action

Renin cleaves angiotensinogen to form angiotensin I (inactive); angiotensin I is converted to the active angiotensin II by angiotensin-converting enzyme (ACE) and non-ACE pathways. Angiotensin II is a powerful vasoconstrictor. It also promotes aldosterone secretion and sodium reabsorption. Together these effects increase BP. Aliskiren is a direct renin inhibitor, decreasing plasma renin activity and inhibiting the conversion of angiotensinogen to angiotensin I.

Pharmacokinetics

Poorly absorbed; bioavailability is about 2.5%. **t½, accumulation:** 24 hr. **Peak plasma levels:** 1–3 hr. **Steady-state blood levels:** 7–8 days. High-fat meals significantly decrease absorption from the GI tract. Metabolized by CYP3A4. About 25% excreted in the urine unchanged.

CONTRAINDICATIONS

Lactation.

SPECIAL CONCERNS

Use in pregnancy. When used in pregnancy during the second and third trimesters, drugs that act on the renin-angiotensin system can cause injury and even death to the developing fetus. When pregnancy is detected, discontinue aliskiren as soon as possible.

- Use with caution in impaired renal function.
- Safety and efficacy not determined in children.

SIDE EFFECTS

Most Common

Diarrhea, abdominal pain, dyspepsia, gastroesophageal reflux, rash.

GI: Diarrhea, abdominal pain, dyspepsia, gastroesophageal reflux. **CNS:** Dizziness, headache, ***seizures*** (rare). **CV:** Hypotension. **Respiratory:** Increased cough, nasopharyngitis, URTI. **Musculoskeletal:** Back pain. **Body as whole:** ***Angioedema*** of the face, extremities, lips, tongue, glottis, and/or larynx; rash, gout, fatigue. **Miscellaneous:** Renal stones.

LABORATORY TEST CONSIDERATIONS

↑ Creatine kinase, serum K, BUN, serum creatinine, serum uric acid. Small ↓ H&H.

OVERDOSE MANAGEMENT

Symptoms: Hypotension (most likely). *Treatment:* Initiate supportive treatment.

DRUG INTERACTIONS

ACE inhibitors / ↑ Risk of elevated serum potassium in diabetics; monitor electrolytes and renal function if used together

Atorvastatin / ↑ Aliskiren plasma levels → ↑ pharmacologic/toxic effects; monitor clinical response and adjust dose if needed

Cyclosporine / ↑ Aliskiren plasma levels → ↑ pharmacologic/toxic effects; do not use together

A

Furosemide / ↓ Furosemide AUC and C_{max} 30% and 50% respectively → ↓ efficacy; monitor diuretic response and adjust furosemide dose if needed
Hydrochlorothiazide / Additive ↑ in serum uric acid levels; use together with caution especially in those at risk for hyperuricemia
Irbesartan / ↓ Aliskiren C_{max} up to 50% after multiple dosing → ↓ effect; monitor BP
Ketoconazole / ↑ Aliskiren plasma levels → ↑ pharmacologic/toxic effects; monitor clinical response and adjust dose if needed
Potassium-containing salt substitutes / ↑ Serum potassium; use together with caution and monitor electrolytes
Potassium-sparing diuretics (e.g., spironolactone) / ↑ Serum potassium; use together with caution and monitor electrolytes
Potassium supplements / ↑ Serum potassium; use together with caution and monitor electrolytes

HOW SUPPLIED

Tablets: 150 mg, 300 mg.

DOSAGE

TABLETS

Hypertension.

Initial: 150 mg once daily. The daily dose may be increased to 300 mg in those whose BP is not adequately controlled. Doses above 300 mg are not more effective but do increase the incidence of diarrhea.

NURSING IMPLICATIONS

IMPLEMENTATION/ADMINISTRATION/STORAGE

1. May be given with other antihypertensives, most commonly diuretics and an angiotensin receptor blocker (e.g., valsartan). It is not known if additive effects occur when taken with ACE inhibitors or beta-blockers.
2. The antihypertensive effect is usually reached within 2 weeks.
3. If angioedema occurs, promptly discontinue aliskiren and provide appropriate therapy and monitoring until complete and sustained resolution of the symptoms has occurred.
4. Store from 15–30°C (59–86°F). Protect from moisture.

ASSESSMENT

1. Note reasons for therapy, presenting symptoms, other agents trialed, outcome.
2. List drugs prescribed to ensure none interact.
3. Record ECG, VS, and weight. Determine if pregnant.
4. Monitor CBC, electrolytes, renal and LFTs. Reduce dose or avoid use with impaired renal function.

CLIENT/FAMILY TEACHING

1. For BP lowering, take at the same time each day. High-fat meals substantially decrease absorption.
2. Use caution, may cause low BP effects and dizziness. Consume adequate fluids; excessive perspiration, diarrhea, or vomiting can lead to fall in BP.
3. Maintain healthy diet, limit intake of caffeine, and avoid alcohol, salt substitutes, potassium supplements, or high Na^+ and high K^+ foods. Lose/control weight, exercise daily, and do not smoke to help control BP.
4. Practice reliable contraception. Stop drug and report if pregnancy suspected; may cause fetal harm.
5. Immediately report/seek help if swelling of the eyes, face, extremities, lips, or tongue, difficulty in breathing/swallowing noted.
6. Any persistent dry cough, flu-like symptoms, rash, fatigue, SOB, diarrhea, or unusual side effects should be reported immediately.
7. Keep all F/U to assess response, review BP log, labs, and for adverse SE.

OUTCOMES/EVALUATE

↓ BP; hypertension control

IV

Allopurinol

(al-oh-**PYOUR**-ih-nohl)

Classification(s): Antigout drug

Pregnancy Category: C

RX: Aloprim for Injection, Zyloprim.

Rx: Apo-Allopurinol.

INDICATIONS/USES

IV: Management of clients with leukemia, lymphoma, and solid tumor malignancies in whom cancer chemotherapy causes elevations of serum and urinary uric acid levels and who cannot tolerate PO therapy.

PO: (1) Primary or secondary gout (acute attacks, tophi, joint destruction, nephropathy, uric acid lithiasis). (2) Clients with leukemia, lymphoma, or other malignancies in whom drug therapy causes elevations of serum and urinary uric acid. (3) Recurrent calcium oxalate calculi where daily uric acid excretion exceeds 800 mg/day in males and 750 mg/day in females.

Investigational: (1) Mixed with methylcellulose as a mouthwash to prevent stomatitis following fluorouracil administration. (2) Prevent ischemic reperfusion tissue damage. (3) Reduce the incidence of perioperative mortality and postoperative arrhythmias in coronary artery bypass surgery. (4) Reduce rates of *Helicobacter pylori*–induced duodenal ulcers and treatment of hematemesis from NSAID-induced erosive esophagitis. (5) Ex vivo preservation and function of organs for liver and kidney transplantation by supplementing preservation solutions with allopurinol. (6) To reduce rejection episodes in adult cadaver renal transplant recipients by adding low-dose allopurinol on alternate days to a triple immunosuppressive regimen of azathioprine/cyclosporine/prednisolone. (7) Alleviate pain due to acute pancreatitis (rectal use). (8) Treatment of American cutaneous leishmaniasis and against *Trypanosoma cruzi*. (9) Treat Chagas' disease. (10) As an alternative in epileptic seizures refractory to standard therapy.

ACTION/KINETICS

Action

Allopurinol and its major metabolite, oxipurinol, are potent inhibitors of xanthine oxidase, an enzyme involved in the synthesis of uric acid. The drug decreases uric acid production by inhibiting the biochemical reactions immediately preceding uric acid formation. Also, allopurinol increases reutilization of xanthine and hypoxanthine for synthesis of nucleotide and nucleic acid by acting on the enzyme hypoxanthine-guanine phosphoribosyltransferase. The resultant increases in nucleotides cause a negative feedback to inhibit synthesis of purines and a decrease in uric acid levels (usually within 2–3 days).

Pharmacokinetics

About 90% absorbed from the GI tract. **Peak plasma levels, after PO:** 1.5 hr for allopurinol and 4.5 hr for oxipurinol. **Onset, after PO:** 2–3 days. **t½, after PO** (allopurinol); 1–2 hr; **t½** (oxipurinol): about 15 hr. **Peak serum levels after PO, allopurinol:** 2–3 mcg/mL; **oxipurinol:** 5–6.5 mcg/mL (up to 50 mcg/mL in clients with impaired renal function). **Maximum therapeutic effect, after PO:** 1–3 weeks. Well absorbed from GI tract, metabolized in liver, excreted in urine and feces (20%).

CONTRAINDICATIONS

Hypersensitivity to drug. Clients with idiopathic hemochromatosis or relatives of clients suffering from this condition. Children except as an adjunct in treatment of neoplastic disease. Severe skin reactions on previous exposure. To treat asymptomatic hyperuricemia.

SPECIAL CONCERNS

- **Use with caution during lactation and in clients with liver or renal disease.**
- **Acute gout attacks may occur during early stages of use; give maintenance doses of colchicine.**
- **In children use has been limited to rare inborn errors of purine metabolism or hyperuricemia as a result of malignancy or cancer therapy.**

SIDE EFFECTS

Most Common

Skin rash, maculopapular rash, nausea, diarrhea, increased attacks of acute gout.

Dermatologic: Rash, maculopapular rash, purpura, vesicular bullous dermatitis, exfoliative dermatitis, eczematoid dermatitis, pruritus, urticaria, alopecia, onycholysis, lichen planus, furunculosis, facial edema, sweating, skin edema. **Hypersensitivity:** Fever, chills, leukopenia, eosinophilia, arthralgia, skin rash, pruritus, N&V, nephritis, mild leukocytosis/leukopenia; exfoliative, urticarial, and purpuric lesions; ***toxic epidermal necrolysis***, ***Stevens-Johnson syndrome***, and/or generalized vasculitis, ***irreversible hepatotoxicity, death (rare)***. Hypersensitivity reactions may be increased in those with impaired renal function. **GI:** N&V, diarrhea, intermittent abdominal pain, gastritis, dyspepsia, ***hemorrhagic pancreatitis***, GI bleeding, stomatitis, salivary gland swelling, tongue edema, anorexia, taste loss/perversion. **Hepatic:** Hepatomegaly, cholestatic jaundice, ***hepatic necrosis, liver failure***, jaundice, granulomatous hepatitis. **CNS:** Headache, peripheral neuropathy, neuritis, paresthesia, somnolence, confusion, dizziness, vertigo, foot drop, depression, amnesia,

A

asthenia, insomnia. **Hematologic:** Thrombocytopenia, ***aplastic anemia***, agranulocytosis, eosinophilic fibrohistiocytic lesion of bone marrow, ***pancytopenia***, anemia, hemolytic anemia, reticulocytosis, lymphadenopathy, lymphocytosis. **CV:** Necrotizing angiitis, vasculitis, pericarditis, peripheral vascular disease, thrombophlebitis, bradycardia, vasodilation. **GU:** Renal failure/insufficiency, uremia, nephritis, impotence, primary hematuria, decreased libido, male infertility, male gynecomastia. **Respiratory:** Epistaxis, bronchospasm, asthma, pharyngitis, rhinitis. **Musculoskeletal:** Myalgia, myopathy, arthralgias. **Ophthalmic:** Cataracts, macular retinitis, iritis, conjunctivitis, amblyopia. **Miscellaneous:** Ecchymosis, fever, malaise.

LABORATORY TEST CONSIDERATIONS

↑ ALT, AST, alkaline phosphatase. ↓ Serum glucose, prothrombin. Hyperbilirubinemia, hypercalcemia, hyperlipidemia, albuminuria.

DRUG INTERACTIONS

ACE inhibitors / ↑ Risk of hypersensitivity reactions
Al salts / ↓ Allopurinol effect
Amoxicillin/Ampicillin / ↑ Rate of drug-induced skin rashes
Anticoagulants, oral / ↑ Anticoagulant effect R/T ↓ liver breakdown; may not occur with warfarin, however
Azathioprine / ↑ Azathioprine effect R/T ↓ liver breakdown; ↓ azathioprine dose by ⅓–¼
Chlorpropamide / ↑ Plasma t½ of chlorpropamide R/T competition for excretion in renal tubules; ↑ risk of hypoglycemia
Cyclophosphamide / ↑ Risk of bleeding or infection due to ↑ drug myelosuppressive effects
Cyclosporine / ↑ Cyclosporine levels
Iron preparations / Allopurinol ↑ hepatic iron concentrations
Mercaptopurine / ↑ Mercaptopurine effects and toxicity R/T ↓ liver breakdown; ↓ mercaptopurine dose by ⅓–¼
Theophylline / Allopurinol ↑ plasma drug levels → possible toxicity
Thiazide diuretics / Possible ↑ risk of hypersensitivity reactions to allopurinol
Thiopurines, oral / ↑ Pharmacologic and toxic effects of thiopurines
Uricosuric agents / ↓ Effect of oxipurinol R/T ↑ rate of excretion

HOW SUPPLIED

Injection: 500 mg/30 mL; ***Tablets:*** 100 mg, 300 mg.

DOSAGE

IV INFUSION

Lower serum uric acid in leukemia, lymphoma, or solid malignancies.

Adults: 200–400 mg/m^2/day, to a maximum of 600 mg/day. **Children, initial:** 200 mg/m^2/day.

TABLETS

Gout/hyperuricemia.

Adults: 200–300 mg/day for mild gout and 400–600 mg/day for moderately severe tophaceous gout, not to exceed 800 mg/day. Minimum effective dose: 100–200 mg/day. Give in divided doses if dosage requirements exceed 300 mg/day. To reduce the possibility of flare-up of acute gouty attacks, start with 100 mg daily and increase at weekly intervals by 100 mg until a serum uric acid level of 6 mg/dL or less is reached without exceeding the maximal recommended dose.

Prevention of uric acid nephropathy during vigorous treatment of neoplasms.

Adults, usual: 600–800 mg/day for 2–3 days (with high fluid intake).

Recurrent calcium oxalate stones.

Usual: 200–300 mg/day in single or divided doses. Adjust dose up or down depending on the 24 hr urinary urate determination. Clients may also benefit from dietary changes, such as reduction of animal protein, sodium, refined sugars, oxalate-rich foods, and excessive calcium intake, as well as an increase in oral fluids and dietary fiber.

Children, hyperuricemia associated with malignancy.

Children, 6–10 years of age: 300 mg/day either as a single dose or 100 mg 3 times per day. Alternative dosage: 1 mg/kg/day divided q 6 hr to a maximum of 600 mg/day. For either dosage regimen, evaluate response after 48 hr; adjust dosage if necessary according to serum uric acid levels. **Children,**

under 6 years of age, usual:
150 mg/day in three divided doses. Alternative dosage: 1 mg/kg/day divided q 6 hr, to a maximum of 600 mg/day. For either dosage regimen, evaluate response after 48 hr and adjust dose according to serum uric acid levels.

To ameliorate granulocyte suppressant effect of fluorouracil.
600 mg/day.

Reduce perioperative mortality and postoperative arrhythmias in coronary artery bypass surgery.
300 mg 12 hr and 1 hr before surgery.

Reduce relapse rates of H. pylori*-induced duodenal ulcers; treat hematemesis from NSAID-induced erosive gastritis.*
50 mg 4 times per day.

Alleviate pain due to acute pancreatitis.
50 mg 4 times per day.

Treat American cutaneous leishmaniasis and T. cruzi.
20 mg/kg for 15 days.

Treat Chagas' disease.
600–900 mg/day for 60 days.

Alternative to treat epileptic seizures refractory to standard therapy.
300 mg/day, except use 150 mg/day in those less than 20 kg.

MOUTHWASH

Prevent fluorouracil-induced stomatitis.
5 mg/mL to 16 mg/mL in methylcellulose in adults receiving fluorouracil as monotherapy or in combination with other antineoplastic drugs.

NURSING IMPLICATIONS

Do not confuse allopurinol with apresoline (an antihypertensive) or Zyloprim with ZORprin (aspirin).

IMPLEMENTATION/ADMINISTRATION/STORAGE

1. Individualize use for each client. The maximum dose should not exceed 800 mg/day but may differ depending on use.
2. Keep urine slightly alkaline to prevent uric acid stone formation.
3. Transfer from colchicine, uricosuric agents, and/or anti-inflammatory agents to allopurinol should be made gradually by decreasing the dosage of one and increasing the dosage of allopurinol until a normal serum uric acid level achieved.
4. Reduce PO dose as follows in impaired renal function: C_{CR} 10–20 mL/min: 200 mg/day; C_{CR} <10 mL/min: do not exceed 100 mg/day; C_{CR} <3 mL/min: Interval between doses may also need to be lengthened. Do not reuse in those who develop a severe reaction.
5. Normal serum urate levels are usually reached in 1–3 weeks. The ULN is about 7 mg/mL for men and postmenopausal women and 6 mg/mL for premenopausal women. Using the appropriate dosage and, in some clients, using uricosuric drugs concurrently, it is possible to reduce serum uric acid levels to as low as 2 to 3 mg/mL indefinitely.
6. Store from 15–25°C (59–77°F) in a dry place protected from light.
7. **IV** For either adults or children, give daily dose as a single infusion or in equally divided infusions at 6-, 8-, or 12-hr intervals at concentration not to exceed 6 mg/mL.
8. Whenever possible, administer 24–48 hr before start of chemotherapy known to cause tumor cell lysis (including corticosteroids).
9. Dissolve contents of each 30 mL vial with 25 mL of sterile water for injection. Then dilute to the desired concentration with 0.9% NaCl or D5W injection); administer over 30–60 min.
10. Store reconstituted solution at 20–25°C (68–77°F); begin administration within 10 hr after reconstitution.
11. Do not refrigerate either the reconstituted and/or diluted product.
12. COMPATIBILITY Sterile water, D5W, NSS.
13. INCOMPATIBILITY Sodium bicarbonate-containing solutions; administer separately.

ASSESSMENT

1. Take complete drug history; list drugs prescribed that may interact unfavorably.
2. Note reasons for therapy, type, onset of S&S, any previous allopurinol use. List location, severity, and frequency of gout attacks; joint size, swelling, color, deformity, pain and x-ray joint to assess for destruction.
3. If female and of childbearing age, or if nursing, avoid allopurinol.
4. Assess for idiopathic hemochromatosis; precludes therapy.

A

5. Any skin rash or allergic reaction warrants stopping therapy; may be severe and fatal.
6. May need to take colchicine with allopurinol for acute flare, especially during first 6 weeks of therapy.
7. Monitor CBC, uric acid, liver and renal function studies. Reduce dose with renal dysfunction.

CLIENT/FAMILY TEACHING

1. Take with food or immediately after meals to lessen gastric irritation. Consume at least 2 L of fluid/day to prevent stone formation.
2. When used IV, ensure sufficient fluid intake to yield a daily urinary output of at least 2 L in adults; maintain neutral, or preferably, a slightly alkaline urine (pH >7)
3. May cause drowsiness; use caution while driving or performing tasks requiring mental alertness.
4. Monitor weight with N&V or other signs of gastric irritation; report persistent weight loss/gain.
5. Report if rash or flu-like symptoms develop. Skin rashes may start after months of therapy; stop therapy/report to determine if drug-related.
6. Do not take iron salts; high iron concentrations may occur in liver.
7. Avoid excessive intake of vitamin C; may cause kidney stones.
8. Avoid caffeine and excessive intake of alcohol; decreases allopurinol effect and increases uric acid concentrations.
9. Keep food diary to identify any triggers; may avoid foods high in purine, which include sardines, roe, salmon, scallops, anchovies, organ meats (impact questionable).
10. Gouty attacks may not end for 2 to 6 weeks after beginning therapy; take as prescribed and continue to take NSAID or colchicine during acute attacks.
11. Minimize exposure to UV light due to increased risk of cataracts; report vision changes.
12. Keep F/U visits to evaluate serum/urinary uric acid levels, response to therapy, and adverse SE.

OUTCOMES/EVALUATE

- ↓ Uric acid levels (6 mg/dL)/frequency of gout attacks
- ↓ Joint pain and inflammation
- ↓ Recurrent calcium oxalate renal calculi
- ↓ Hyperuricemia R/T chemo for cancer treatment
- Prevention of fluorouracil-induced stomatitis/granulocyte suppression (unlabeled)

Almotriptan maleate

(**AL**-moh-**trip**-tin)

Classification(s): Antimigraine drug (serotonin 5-HT_1 receptor agonist)

Pregnancy Category: C

RX: Axert.

INDICATIONS/USES

Acute treatment of migraine, with and without aura, in adults and children, 12 years and older (use when untreated headache lasts 4 or more hours). Use only where there is a clear diagnosis of migraine.

ACTION/KINETICS

Action

As an agonist, binds to 5-HT_{1D}, 5-HT_{1B}, and 5-HT_{1F} receptors on the extracerebral, intracranial blood vessels that become dilated during a migraine headache, as well as on nerve terminals in the trigeminal system. Activation of these receptors causes cranial vessel vasoconstriction, inhibition of neuropeptide release, and reduced transmission in trigeminal nerve pathways.

Pharmacokinetics

Well absorbed after PO use; **onset:** 30 min; **peak plasma levels:** 1–3 hr. **t½, mean:** 3–4 hr. Metabolized in the liver; metabolites and unchanged drug (40%) are excreted mainly in the urine. **Plasma protein binding:** Approximately 35%.

CONTRAINDICATIONS

Use to prevent migraine or in management of hemiplegic or basilar migraine. Use in those with ischemic heart disease (angina pectoris, history of MI, documented silent ischemia) or who have symptoms or findings consistent with ischemic heart disease, coronary artery vasospasm (including Prinzmetal's variant angina), or other significant underlying CV disease. Use when unrecognized coronary artery disease is predicted by presence of risk factors such as hypertension, hypercholesterolemia, smoking, diabetes, strong family history of CAD, females with surgical or physiologic menopause, or males over 40 years of age unless a CV evaluation shows individual is reasonably free of CAD or ischemic myocardial disease. Use in uncontrolled hypertension, within 24 hr of treatment with another 5-HT_1 agonist or an ergotamine-containing or ergot-type medication (e.g., dihydroergotamine, methysergide). Use in children less than 18 years of age.

SPECIAL CONCERNS

- **Use with caution during lactation and in diseases that may alter the absorption, metabolism, or excretion of the drug, such as impaired hepatic or renal function.**
- **Safety and efficacy not determined for cluster headaches (present in an older, predominantly male population).**
- **Use caution with dose selection in the elderly.**
- **Safety not established for treating more than 4 headaches in a 30-day period.**

SIDE EFFECTS

Most Common

Drowsiness, dry mouth, headache, nausea, paresthesia, dizziness.

CV: ***Acute MI, disturbances of cardiac rhythm, death, cerebral hemorrhage, subarachnoid hemorrhage, stroke, hypertensive crisis, ventricular fibrillation***, peripheral vascular ischemia, transient myocardial ischemia, ***ventricular tachycardia***, coronary artery vasospasm, vasodilation, palpitations, ***colonic ischemia*** (with abdominal pain and bloody diarrhea). **CNS:** Somnolence, drowsiness, dizziness, headache, tremor, vertigo, anxiety, hypesthesia, restlessness, CNS stimulation, insomnia, shakiness. **GI:** N&V, dry mouth, abdominal cramps or pain, diarrhea, dyspepsia. **Body as a whole:** Paresthesia, asthenia, chills, back pain, chest pain, neck pain, fatigue, rigid neck. **Musculoskeletal:** Myalgia, muscular weakness. **Respiratory:** Pharyngitis, rhinitis, dyspnea, laryngismus, sinusitis, bronchitis, epistaxis. **Dermatologic:** Diaphoresis, dermatitis, erythema, pruritus, rash. **Ophthalmic:** Conjunctivitis, eye irritation. **Miscellaneous:** Ear pain, hyperacusis, taste alteration, dysmenorrhea. Sensations of tightness, pain, and heaviness in the precordium, throat, neck, and jaw.

LABORATORY TEST CONSIDERATIONS

↑ Serum creatine phosphokinase. Hyperglycemia.

DRUG INTERACTIONS

Clarithromycin / Possible ↑ almotriptan levels R/T inhibition of CYP3A4
Dihydroergotamine / Possible additive vasospastic effects; do not use within 24 hr of each other
Erythromycin / Possible ↑ almotriptan levels
Itraconazole / Possible ↑ almotriptan AUC and plasma levels R/T inhibition of CYP3A4
Ketoconazole / Possible ↑ almotriptan levels R/T inhibition of CYP3A4
MAOIs / ↓ Almotriptan clearance
Methysergide / Possible additive vasospastic effects; do not use within 24 hr of each other
Nefazodone / Possible ↑ almotriptan levels R/T inhibition of CYP3A4
Nelfinavir / Possible ↑ almotriptan levels R/T inhibition of CYP3A4
Ritonavir / Possible ↑ almotriptan levels R/T inhibition of CYP3A4
Selective serotonin reuptake inhibitors / Rarely, weakness, hyperreflexia, and incoordination
Troleandomycin / Possible ↑ almotriptan levels R/T inhibition of CYP3A4
Verapamil / ↑ Plasma levels of almotriptan

HOW SUPPLIED

Tablets: 6.25 mg, 12.5 mg.

DOSAGE

TABLETS

Migraine headache.

Adults and children, 12 to 17 years: Single dose of either 6.25 or 12.5 mg (more effective). Choice of dose is on an individual basis. If the headache returns, dose may be repeated after 2 hr, but give no more than 2 doses in a 24 hr period. **Maximum daily dose:** 25 mg. In either hepatic or renal impairment, do not exceed a daily dose of 12.5 mg over a 24 hr period; use an initial dose of 6.25 mg.

NURSING IMPLICATIONS

Do not confuse almotriptan with alvimopan (drug for postoperative ileus). Do not confuse Axert with Antivert (antiemetic/antimotion sickness).

A

IMPLEMENTATION/ADMINISTRATION/STORAGE

1. If first dose does not produce response, reconsider diagnosis of migraine before giving a second dose.
2. Safety of treating an average of more than 4 headaches in a 30-day period has not been studied.
3. For those with hepatic or renal impairment or concomitant use with CYP3A4 inhibitors, do not exceed a maximum daily dose of 12.5 mg and a starting dose of 6.25 mg.
4. Store from 15–30°C (59–86°F).

ASSESSMENT

1. Review symptom characteristics listing location, type, intensity, duration, triggers; ensure not hemiplegic or basilar migraine type of headaches. Have neurologist evaluate if unclear.
2. Note drugs currently prescribed to ensure none interact. List those taken within the past 24 hr and ensure no other serotonin agonist or ergotamine derivatives prescribed.
3. Avoid in those with ischemic heart disease (angina pectoris, history of myocardial infarction, or documented silent ischemia) or stroke/TIA, or PVD.
4. Obtain ECG immediately following the first dose in those with CAD risk factors or the potential for CAD.
5. Assess for uncontrolled HTN and cardiac risk factors. Obtain ECG, BP, renal and LFTs; use lowest dose with dysfunction.

CLIENT/FAMILY TEACHING

1. Take only as directed for migraine headaches; do not share medications with another person regardless of symptoms. Use only to treat actual migraine attack; does not prevent or reduce the number of attacks.
2. Drug acts to shrink swollen blood vessels surrounding the brain that cause migraine headaches. Keep a headache diary, and identify factors/foods/events that surround/trigger migraine headaches. Lie down in a quiet, dark room to facilitate desired effects.
3. Take as soon as symptoms of migraine appear. If effective and headache returns, may repeat dose in 2 hr unless otherwise instructed due to renal dysfunction. Do not exceed 2 tablets in 24 hr.
4. Use caution if driving or performing activities that require mental alertness; may cause dizziness or drowsiness.
5. Store away from heat, light, and moisture; store in a safe place.
6. Avoid known migraine triggers, i.e., chocolate, cheese, citrus fruit, caffeine, alcohol, missing sleep or meals, etc.
7. Report unusual side effects, chest pain/heaviness, new onset jaw, throat or neck pain, intolerance, or lack of response.
8. Not for use during pregnancy; practice reliable contraception.
9. Avoid prolonged sun exposure and use sunscreen when exposed.
10. Keep all F/U to evaluate response and for adverse SE.

OUTCOMES/EVALUATE

Resolution of migraine headaches

Alprazolam

(al-**PRAYZ**-oh-lam)

Classification(s): Antianxiety drug, benzodiazepine

Pregnancy Category: D

RX: Alprazolam Extended-Release, Alprazolam Intensol, Niravam, Xanax, Xanax XR, **C-IV**

Rx: Apo-Alpraz, Apo-Alpraz TS, Gen-Alprazolam, Xanax TS.

SEE ALSO ***TRANQUILIZERS/ANTIMANIC DRUGS/HYPNOTICS***.

INDICATIONS/USES

Immediate-Release Tablets, Orally Disintegrating Tablets and Intensol: (1) Anxiety. (2) Anxiety associated with depression with or without agoraphobia.

Immediate- and Extended-Release Tablets, Orally Disintegrating Tablets: Panic disorder with or without agoraphobia. *Investigational:* Agoraphobia with social phobia, depression, PMS.

ACTION/KINETICS

Action

Reduces anxiety by increasing or facilitating the inhibitory neurotransmitter activity of GABA. The skeletal muscle relaxant effect may be due to enhancement of GABA-mediated presynaptic in-

A

hibition at the spinal level as well as in the brain stem reticular formation.

Pharmacokinetics

Onset: Intermediate. **Peak plasma levels: PO,** 8–37 ng/mL after 1–2 hr. **t½:** 12–15 hr. Sublingual absorption is as rapid as PO use; completeness of absorption is comparable. Metabolized to alpha-hydroxyalprazolam, an active metabolite. **t½:** 12–15 hr. Excreted in urine. **Plasma protein binding:** 80%.

CONTRAINDICATIONS

Use with fluconazole, itraconazole, ketoconazole, posaconazole, or voriconazole. Acute narrow-angle glaucoma.

SIDE EFFECTS

Most Common

Drowsiness, ataxia, confusion.
See *Tranquilizers, Antimanic Drugs,* and *Hypnotics* for a complete list of possible side effects.

ADDITIONAL DRUG INTERACTIONS

Azole antifungal drugs, clarithromycin, erythromycin, protease inhibitors, or SSRIs decrease the metabolism of alprazolam. Decrease the dose of alprazolam by 50–75%.

H ***Possible lethargy and disorientation when combined with kava kava.***

HOW SUPPLIED

Oral Solution (Intensol): 1 mg/mL; *Tablets, Extended-Release:* 0.5 mg, 1 mg, 2 mg, 3 mg; *Tablets, Immediate-Release:* 0.25 mg, 0.5 mg, 1 mg, 2 mg; *Tablets, Oral Disintegrating:* 0.25 mg, 0.5 mg, 1 mg, 2 mg.

DOSAGE

ORAL SOLUTION; TABLETS, IMMEDIATE-RELEASE; TABLETS, ORAL DISINTEGRATING

Anxiety disorders.

Adults, initial: 0.25–0.5 mg 3 times per day; **then** titrate to needs of client at intervals of 3–4 days in increments of no more than 1 mg/day, with total daily dosage not to exceed 4 mg. **In elderly or debilitated, initial:** 0.25 mg 2–3 times per day; **then** adjust dosage to needs of client.

TABLETS, EXTENDED-RELEASE; TABLETS, IMMEDIATE-RELEASE; TABLETS, ORAL DISINTEGRATING

Panic disorders (use Niravam, Xanax, Xanax XR).

Immediate-Release Tablets, Oral Disintegrating Tablets: Adults, initial: 0.5 mg 3 times per day; increase dose as needed, every 3–4 days in increments of no more than 1 mg/day up to a maximum of 10 mg/day (mean dose: 5–6 mg/day). **Extended-Release Tablets: Adults, initial:** 0.5 mg–1 mg once daily. **Total daily dose:** 3–6 mg/day.

Agoraphobia with social phobia (Investigational).

Adults: 2–8 mg/day.

Premenstrual syndrome (Investigational).

0.25 mg 3 times per day.

NURSING IMPLICATIONS

Do not confuse alprazolam with lorazepam (antianxiety drug) or Xanax with Zantac (H-2 receptor blocker).

IMPLEMENTATION/ADMINISTRATION/STORAGE

1. Reduce dosage in elderly and debilitated clients. Starting dose of immediate-release and Intensol is 0.25 mg, given 2 or 3 times per day. Increase dose gradually if needed. For extended-release tablets, begin with 0.5 mg once a day; gradually increase if needed and tolerated.
2. To switch therapy from immediate-release to extended-release tablets, start with a once-daily dose of the extended-release product equal to the total daily dose of the immediate-release tablets.
3. Avoid abrupt discontinuation due to the possibility of withdrawal. When discontinuing therapy or decreasing the daily dose, reduce dosage gradually. It is recommended the daily dose be decreased by no more than 0.5 mg q 3 days; some clients may require an even slower dosage reduction. If significant withdrawal symptoms develop, reinstitute the previous dosing schedule and try a less rapid discontinuation schedule.
4. Store from 15–30°C (59–86°F) protected from moisture.

A

ASSESSMENT

1. Note reasons for therapy, describe symptoms and clinical presentation, other agents trialed, and outcome.
2. Note any pulmonary disease, severe depression or suicide ideations; assess response closely.
3. With anxiety, evaluate/compare before and after therapy initiated for mood, behavior, subjective reports, drowsiness, and dizziness.
4. Assess need for counselling and/or assisted care. With prolonged use physical/psychological dependence may occur; do not stop suddenly.
5. Have flumazenil available in the event of overdose, and follow dosing guidelines.
6. Monitor CBC, liver and renal function (to avoid accumulation of drug) during prolonged therapy; may cause neutropenia and decreased Hct.

CLIENT/FAMILY TEACHING

1. Do not chew, crush, or break the extended-release tablet.
2. Immediate-release and extended-release tablets are interchangeable on a daily mg-to-mg basis. Immediate-release tablets may be administered sublingually if difficulty swallowing tablets.
3. Mix Intensol oral solution with liquids or semi-solid foods such as water, juices, soda, or soda-like beverages, applesauce, and puddings. Use the calibrated dropper provided. Draw up the required amount, squeeze the dropper contents into the liquid or semi-solid food, and stir gently for a few seconds. Do not prepare and store doses for future use.
4. Just before giving orally disintegrating tablets, remove the tablet from the bottle with dry hands. Immediately place the tablet on top of the tongue where it will disintegrate and be swallowed with saliva. Giving with a liquid is not necessary. If only one-half of a scored tablet is used, discard the unused portion of the tablet immediately as it may not remain stable. Discard any cotton included in the bottle, and reseal the bottle tightly to prevent introduction of moisture that may cause tablet disintegration.
5. May take tablets with milk or food to decrease GI upset.
6. Include extra fluids and bulk in the diet to minimize constipation.
7. Avoid activities that require mental alertness, until tolerance is assessed; may cause drowsiness or impair judgment, thinking, or reflexes. Rise slowly to prevent light-headedness or fainting.
8. Seek appropriate psychological therapy as prolonged use may cause dependence. Provider will gradually taper dose (e.g., no more than 0.5 mg every 3 days) when therapy no longer indicated. Report withdrawal symptoms (e.g., increased anxiety, tremor, palpitations, muscle or abdominal cramps, sweating). If significant withdrawal symptoms develop, they may reinstitute previous dosing schedule and determine need for in-house detoxification or a less rapid tapering regimen once stabilized as MI or death may occur in severe cases.
9. Use support devices as needed, especially at night; elderly tend to become confused. Store drug away from bedside to prevent overdose.
10. Avoid smoking, alcohol consumption, or any other CNS depressants without provider approval. Keep all F/U to evaluate response and adverse SE.

OUTCOMES/EVALUATE

- Positive behaviors with phobias
- ↓ Anxiety/restlessness; ↓ panic attacks
- Treatment of irritable bowel syndrome, depression, PMS (unlabeled)

IV

Alteplase, recombinant

(**AL**-teh-playz)

Classification(s): Thrombolytic, tissue plasminogen activator

Pregnancy Category: C

RX: Activase, Cathflo Activase.

🍁 **Rx:** Activase rt-PA.

INDICATIONS/USES

Activase. (1) Improvement of ventricular function following AMI, including reducing the incidence of CHF and decreasing mortality. (2) Acute ischemic stroke, after intracranial hemorrhage has been excluded by CT scan or other diagnostic imaging.

A

(3) Acute pulmonary embolism (confirm diagnosis by pulmonary angiography or noninvasive procedures as lung scanning).

Cathflo Activase. Restoration of function to central venous access devices that have become occluded by a blood clot or thrombus.

Investigational: Unstable angina pectoris.

ACTION/KINETICS

Action

Alteplase, a tissue plasminogen activator, binds to fibrin in a thrombus, causing a conversion of plasminogen to plasmin. This conversion results in local fibrinolysis and a decrease in circulating fibrinogen.

Pharmacokinetics

Within 10 min following termination of an infusion, 80% of the alteplase has been cleared from the plasma by the liver. The enzyme activity of alteplase is 580,000 international units/mg. **t½, initial:** 4 min; **final:** 35 min (elimination phase).

CONTRAINDICATIONS

When used for AMI or pulmonary embolism: Active internal bleeding, history of CVA, within 2 months of intracranial or intraspinal surgery or trauma, intracranial neoplasm, AV malformation or aneurysm, bleeding diathesis, severe uncontrolled hypertension.

When used for acute ischemic stroke: Symptoms of intracranial hemorrhage on pretreatment evaluation, suspected subarachnoid hemorrhage, recent intracranial surgery or serious head trauma, recent previous stroke, history of intracranial hemorrhage, uncontrolled hypertension (above 185 mm Hg systolic or above 110 Hg diastolic) at time of treatment, active internal bleeding, seizure at onset of stroke, intracranial neoplasm, AV malformation or aneurysm, bleeding diathesis.

SPECIAL CONCERNS

- **Use with caution in the presence of recent GI or GU bleeding (within 10 days), subacute bacterial endocarditis, acute pericarditis, significant liver dysfunction, concomitant use of oral anticoagulants, diabetic hemorrhagic retinopathy, septic thrombophlebitis or occluded arteriovenous cannula (at infected site), lactation, mitral stenosis with atrial fibrillation.**
- **Since fibrin will be lysed during therapy, give careful attention to potential bleeding sites such as sites of catheter insertion and needle puncture sites.**
- **Use with caution within 10 days of major surgery (e.g., obstetrics, coronary artery bypass) and in clients over 75 years of age.**
- **Safety and efficacy not established in children.**
- **Doses greater than 150 mg have been associated with an increase in intracranial bleeding.**
- **Use Cathflo Activase with caution in presence of suspected infection in a catheter.**

SIDE EFFECTS

Most Common

GU bleeding, ecchymosis, strokes, N&V, fever, hypotension.

Bleeding tendencies: ***Internal bleeding*** (including the GI and GU tracts and intracranial or retroperitoneal site). Superficial bleeding (e.g., gums, sites of recent surgery, venous cutdowns, arterial punctures). Ecchymosis, epistaxis. **CV:** Bradycardia, hypotension, ***cardiogenic shock***, arrhythmias, ***heart failure, cardiac arrest/tamponade, myocardial rupture***, recurrent ischemia, reinfarction, mitral regurgitation, pericardial effusion, pericarditis, venous thrombosis and embolism, ***electromechanical dissociation***, cholesterol embolism. **Allergic:** Rash, ***laryngeal edema, orolingual angioedema, anaphylaxis.*** **GI:** N&V. **Miscellaneous:** Fever, urticaria, pulmonary edema, cerebral edema. **Due to accelerated infusion:** ***Strokes, hemorrhagic stroke***, nonfatal stroke. Incidence increases with age.

OVERDOSE MANAGEMENT

Symptoms: Bleeding disorders. *Treatment:* Discontinue therapy immediately as well as any concomitant heparin therapy.

DRUG INTERACTIONS

Abciximab / ↑ Risk of bleeding
Aspirin / ↑ Risk of bleeding
Dipyridamole / ↑ Risk of bleeding
Heparin / ↑ Risk of bleeding, especially at arterial puncture sites
Nitroglycerin / ↓ Alteplase concentrations → ↓ thrombolytic effect
Vitamin K antagonists / ↑ Risk of bleeding

HOW SUPPLIED

Powder for Injection: 50 mg, 100 mg; *Single-patient vial (Cathflo Activase):* 2 mg.

A

DOSAGE

IV INFUSION ONLY

Acute myocardial infarction (AMI), accelerated infusion.

Weight >67 kg: 100 mg as a 15 mg IV bolus, followed by 50 mg infused over the next 30 min and then 35 mg infused over the next 60 min. **Weight <67 kg:** 15 mg IV bolus, followed by 0.75 mg/kg infused over the next 30 min (not to exceed 50 mg) and then 0.50 mg/kg infused over the next 60 min (not to exceed 35 mg). The safety and efficacy of this regimen have only been evaluated using heparin and aspirin concomitantly.

AMI, 3 hr infusion.

100 mg total dose subdivided as follows: 60 mg (34.8 million international units) the first hour with 6–10 mg given in a bolus over the first 1–2 min and the remaining 50–54 mg given over the first hour; 20 mg (11.6 million international units) over the second hour and 20 mg (11.6 million international units) given over the third hour. **Clients less than 65 kg:** 1.25 mg/kg given over 3 hr, with 60% given the first hour with 6–10% given by direct IV injection within the first 1–2 min; 20% is given the second hour and 20% during the third hour. Doses of 150 mg have caused an increase in intracranial bleeding.

Pulmonary embolism.

100 mg over 2 hr; heparin therapy should be instituted near the end of or right after the alteplase infusion when the partial thromboplastin or thrombin time returns to twice that of normal or less.

Acute ischemic stroke.

0.9 mg/kg (maximum of 90 mg) infused over 60 min with 10% of the total dose given as an initial IV bolus over 1 min. Doses greater than 0.9 mg/kg may cause an increased incidence of intracranial hemorrhage. Use with aspirin and heparin during the first 24 hr after onset of symptoms has not been investigated.

Restoration of function to central venous access device.

2 mg in 2 mL of solution for clients weighing 30 kg or more; for those weighing between 10 and 30 kg, use a dose of 1 mg/mL solution equivalent to 110% of the volume of the catheter's internal lumen but not more than 2 mg. A second dose may be instilled if the catheter is not functioning 120 min after the first dose.

NURSING IMPLICATIONS

IMPLEMENTATION/ADMINISTRATION/STORAGE

1. **IV** Initiate alteplase therapy as soon as possible after onset of symptoms of acute MI and within 3 hr after the onset of stroke symptoms.
2. For acute MI, nearly 90% of clients also receive heparin concomitantly with alteplase and either aspirin or dipyridamole during or after heparin therapy.
3. Reconstitute with only sterile water for injection without preservatives immediately prior to use. The reconstituted preparation contains 1 mg/mL and is a colorless to pale yellow transparent solution.
4. Using an 18-gauge needle, direct the stream of sterile water into the lyophilized cake. Leave product undisturbed for several minutes to allow dissipation of any large bubbles.
5. If necessary, the reconstituted solution may be further diluted immediately prior to use in an equal volume of 0.9% NaCl injection or D5W injection to yield a concentration of 0.5 mg/mL. Dilute by gentle swirling or slow inversion.
6. Either glass bottles or PVC bags may be used for administration.
7. Stable for up to 8 hr following reconstitution or dilution; stability will not be affected by light.
8. Do not use 50 mg vials if vacuum is not present (100-mg vials do not contain a vacuum). Reconstitute 50 mg vials with a large-bore needle (e.g., 18 gauge) directing stream of sterile water into lyophilized cake. For the

100-mg vial, use provided transfer device for reconstitution.

9. Use infusion device for administration. Anticipate 3 lines for access (1-alteplase; 1-heparin and other drugs such as lidocaine; 1-blood drawing and transfusions).
10. Store lyophilized alteplase at room temperatures not to exceed 30°C (86°F) or under refrigeration between 2–8°C (36–46°F).
11. Have emergency drugs (especially aminocaproic acid) and resuscitative equipment available.
12. COMPATIBILITY Sterile water, D5W, 0.9% NaCl.
13. INCOMPATIBILITY Do not add any other medications to the infusion or line.

ASSESSMENT

1. Note reasons for therapy, any history of hypertension, internal bleeding, PUD, or recent surgery.
2. Document onset/characteristics of chest pain and/or stroke symptoms; note deficits and monitor.
3. Assess/document overall physical condition; note CV and neurologic findings, weight, and ECG. Obtain drug history. List those currently taking; note any anticoagulants/antiplatelets.
4. Carefully review/follow instructions for drug reconstitution. Review contraindications before initiating therapy and document if accelerated or 3 hr infusion is prescribed.
5. Observe in a closely monitored environment; obtain VS, review and document monitor strips. Anticipate and assess for reperfusion reactions such as:
   - Reperfusion arrhythmias usually of short duration; may include accelerated idioventricular rhythm and sinus bradycardia.
   - Reduction of chest pain
   - Return of the elevated ST segment to near baseline levels
   - Smaller Q waves
6. Check all access sites for any evidence of bleeding. During IV therapy, arterial sticks require 30 min of manual pressure followed by application of a pressure dressing. In event of any uncontrolled bleeding, terminate alteplase and heparin infusions and report; have protamine available.
7. Monitor neuro status; document findings every 15–30 min during infusion. During treatment of stroke, note CT or MRI results.
8. During treatment for pulmonary embolism, ensure that the PTT/PT is no more than twice that of normal before heparin therapy is added.
9. Keep on bed rest; observe for S&S of abnormal bleeding (hematuria, hematemesis, melena, CVA, cardiac tamponade, ↑ HR, ↓ BP).
10. Monitor appropriate postinfusion labs (cardiac marker, platelets, H&H, PTT, ECG) as directed. Obtain baseline hematologic parameters, type and cross, coagulation times, cardiac marker panel, renal and LFTs.

CLIENT/FAMILY TEACHING

1. Review goals of therapy and inherent risks during acute coronary artery occlusion and/or stroke.
2. To be effective, therapy should be instituted within 3 hr of stroke and 4–6 hr of MI S&S.
3. Report any chest pain, SOB, bleeding, N&V, heart palpitations or other adverse effects. Call for assistance prior to getting out of bed to prevent injury.
4. Encourage family members to learn CPR.

OUTCOMES/EVALUATE

- Lysis of thrombi with reperfusion of ischemic cardiac and/or cerebral tissue or PE
- ↓ Infarct size with restoration of coronary perfusion and improved ventricular function (↑ CO, ↓ incidence of CHF, ↓ mortality)
- Restoration of function to central venous access devices that have become occluded by a blood clot or thrombus (Cathflo Activase)

Amantadine hydrochloride

(ah-**MAN**-tah-deen)

Classification(s): Antiviral, antiparkinson drug

Pregnancy Category: C

RX: Symmetrel.

✤ **Rx:** Endantadine, Gen-Amantadine.

SEE ALSO ***ANTIVIRAL DRUGS***.

A

INDICATIONS/USES

(1) Prophylaxis of influenza A viral infections when early vaccination is not feasible or if vaccine is contraindicated or not available. (2) Treatment of uncomplicated respiratory tract infection caused by influenza A virus strains, especially if given early in the illness. It is not known if amantadine will prevent development of influenza A virus pneumonitis or other complications in high-risk clients. (3) Symptomatic treatment of idiopathic parkinsonism and parkinsonism syndrome resulting from encephalitis, carbon monoxide intoxication, or cerebral arteriosclerosis. For parkinsonism, is usually used concomitantly with other agents, such as levodopa and anticholinergic agents. (4) Drug-induced extrapyramidal reactions. *NOTE:* The H1N1 virus is resistant to amantadine.

Amantadine is recommended for prophylaxis in the following situations:

- High-risk clients vaccinated after flu outbreak has begun; may take up to 2 weeks for immunity.
- Unvaccinated caretakers of high-risk clients during peak flu activity.
- High-risk clients who are expected to have inadequate antibody response to flu vaccine (e.g., HIV).
- High-risk clients who should not be vaccinated or those who wish to avoid the flu.

ACTION/KINETICS

Action

For parkinsonism, the mechanism is unknown, but amantadine may (1) enhance cellular concentrations of dopamine by increasing the release or decreasing reuptake of dopamine into presynaptic neurons, (2) stimulate the dopamine receptor itself, or (3) drive the postsynaptic dopaminergic system to a more dopamine sensitive state. The drug decreases extrapyramidal symptoms, including akinesia, rigidity, tremors, excessive salivation, gait disturbances, and total functional disability. As an antiviral, amantadine may prevent the release of infectious viral nucleic acid into the host cell by interfering with the function of the transmembrane domain of the viral M2 protein. It may also prevent virus assembly during virus replication. The drug reduces symptoms (70–90% effective) of viral infections if given within 24–48 hr after onset of illness.

Pharmacokinetics

Well absorbed from GI tract. **Peak blood levels:** 4 hr. **Onset:** 48 hr. **Mean peak serum concentration:** 0.22 mcg/mL after 1.5–8 hr. **t½:** Approximately 17 hr; elimination half-life increases two- to threefold when C_{CR} <40 mL/min/1.73 m^2. Renal clearance is reduced and plasma levels increased in otherwise healthy clients, aged 65 years and older. Primarily excreted unchanged in urine. Acidification of the urine may increase the elimination of the drug.

CONTRAINDICATIONS

Hypersensitivity to drug. Use in those with untreated angle closure glaucoma. Lactation.

SPECIAL CONCERNS

- **Use with caution in clients with liver and renal disease, history of epilepsy (possible increased seizure activity), CHF (possible worsening of CHF), peripheral edema, orthostatic hypotension, recurrent eczematoid dermatitis, psychosis or severe psychoneurosis, in clients taking CNS stimulant drugs, and in those exposed to rubella.**
- **Abrupt withdrawal in Parkinson's clients may cause a parkinsonian crisis (e.g., symptoms of delirium, agitation, delusions, hallucinations, paranoid reaction, stupor, anxiety, depression, slurred speech).**
- **Safe use in newborn infants and children less than 1 year not established.**

SIDE EFFECTS

Most Common

Nausea, dizziness, lightheadedness, insomnia.

CNS: Dizziness, lightheadedness, insomnia, depression, anxiety, irritability, hallucinations, confusion, ataxia, headache, somnolence, nervousness, abnormal dreams, agitation, psychosis, slurred speech, euphoria, abnormal thinking, amnesia, hyperkinesia, ***convulsion, suicidal attempt/ideation, suicide***, coma, stupor, delirium, hypokinesia, hypertonia, delusions, aggressive behavior, paranoid reaction, manic reaction, gait abnormalities, paresthesia, EEG changes, tremor. **GI:** Nausea, anorexia, dry mouth, constipation, diarrhea, vomiting, dysphagia. **CV:** Orthostatic hypotension, CHF, hypertension, ***cardiac arrest***, arrhythmias (including ***malignant arrhythmias***), hypotension, tachycardia. **Dermatologic:** Livedo reticularis, skin rash, eczematoid dermatitis, pruritus, diaphoresis. **Respiratory:** Dyspnea, dry nose,

A

acute respiratory failure, pulmonary edema, tachypnea. **GU:** Urinary retention, decreased libido. **Hematologic:** Leukopenia, neutropenia, leukocytosis. **Ophthalmic:** Visual disturbance (including punctate subepithelial or other corneal opacity), corneal edema, decreased visual acuity, photophobia, optic nerve palsy, oculogyric episodes, mydriasis, keratitis. **Body as a whole:** Fatigue, peripheral edema. **Miscellaneous:** ***Neuroleptic malignant syndrome***, allergic reactions (including anaphylactic reactions, edema, fever).

LABORATORY TEST CONSIDERATIONS

↑ CPK, BUN, serum creatinine, alkaline phosphatase, LDH, bilirubin, GGT, AST, ALT.

OVERDOSE MANAGEMENT

Symptoms: Arrhythmia, tachycardia, hypertension, pulmonary edema, respiratory distress, renal dysfunction. CNS effects include insomnia, anxiety, aggressive behavior, hypertonia, hyperkinesia, tremor, confusion, disorientation, depersonalization, fear, delirium, hallucinations, psychotic reactions, lethargy, somnolence, ***coma, seizures***, hyperthermia. *Treatment:*

- Gastric lavage or induction of emesis followed by supportive measures.
- Ensure that client is well hydrated; give IV fluids if necessary.
- To treat CNS toxicity: Slow IV physostigmine, 1–2 mg given q 1–2 hr in adults or 0.5 mg at 5–10-min intervals (maximum of 2 mg/hr) in children.
- Sedatives and anticonvulsants may be given if needed; antiarrhythmics and vasopressors may also be required. Force fluids and if necessary, give IV.
- Administration of urine acidifying drugs may increase the elimination of amantadine.
- Monitor BP, pulse, respiration, and temperature. Monitor blood electrolytes, urine pH, and urinary output.
- Exercise care if giving adrenergic drugs, such as isoproterenol, since the dopaminergic activity of amantatinde may induce malignant arrhythmias.

DRUG INTERACTIONS

Acidic drugs / ↑ Elimination of amantadine
Anticholinergics / Additive anticholinergic effects (including hallucinations, confusion), especially with trihexyphenidyl and benztropine; consider ↓ anticholinergic drug dose
H ***Belladonna leaf/root*** / ↑ Anticholinergic effect
CNS stimulants / May ↑ CNS and psychic effects of amantadine; use together cautiously
H ***Henbane leaf*** / ↑ Anticholinergic effects
Hydrochlorothiazide/triamterene combination / ↓ Urinary excretion of amantadine → ↑ amantadine plasma levels
Levodopa / Effects potentiated by amantadine
H ***Pheasant's eye herb*** / ↑ Amantadine effect
Quinidine/Quinine / ↓ Renal amantadine clearance
H ***Scopolia root*** / ↑ Amantadine effect
Thiazide diuretics / ↑ Plasma amantadine levels
Thioridazine / Worsening of tremors in the elderly with Parkinson's disease
Triamterene / ↑ Plasma amantadine levels
Trimethoprim/Sulfamethoxazole / ↓ Amantadine renal clearance → ↑ plasma levels

HOW SUPPLIED

Capsules: 100 mg; ***Syrup:*** 50 mg/5mL; ***Tablets:*** 100 mg.

DOSAGE

CAPSULES; SYRUP; TABLETS

Prophylaxis and treatment of uncomplicated influenza A viral illness.

Adults, 13–64 years: 200 mg/day as a single or 100 mg twice daily (may be used in those who develop CNS effects to once daily dosage as side effects may be less with this regimen). A 100 mg daily dose has been used as prophylaxis in healthy adults who are not at high risk for flu-related complications, but this dose is not as effective as the 200 mg daily dose for prophylaxis. **Adults, over 65 years:** 100 mg once daily. **Children, 1–9 years:** 4.4–8.8 mg/kg/day up to a maximum of 150 mg/day in one or two divided doses (use syrup); **9–12 years:** 100 mg twice daily. Continue daily dosage for at least 10 days following a known exposure. Treat influenza A virus illness as soon as possible, preferably within 24–48 hr after onset of symptoms; continue treatment for 24–48 hr after signs and symptoms disappear.

A

Parkinsonism.

Use as sole agent, usual: 100 mg twice a day, up to 400 mg/day in divided doses, if necessary. **Use with other antiparkinson drugs (e.g., levodopa):** 100 mg 1–2 times per day.

Drug-induced extrapyramidal symptoms.

100 mg twice daily; up to 300 mg/day in divided doses may be required in some. Reduce dose in impaired renal function.

NURSING IMPLICATIONS

Do not confuse amantadine with memantine (Alzheimer's drug).

IMPLEMENTATION/ADMINISTRATION/STORAGE

1. Protect capsules from moisture.
2. Dispense in a tight container with a child-resistant closure.
3. Decrease dose in renal impairment as follows: **C_{CR} 30–50 mL/min:** 200 mg the first day and 100 mg/day thereafter; **C_{CR} 15–29 mL/min:** 200 mg the first day and 100 mg on alternate days thereafter; **C_{CR} less than 15 mL/min or in hemodialysis clients:** 200 mg q 7 days.
4. Reduce dose to 100 mg/day for persons with active seizure disorders R/T increased risk of seizure frequency with 200 mg daily dose.
5. Reduce dose in clients age 65 or older. Dose may need to be reduced in clients with CHF, peripheral edema, orthostatic hypotension, or impaired renal function.
6. Store from 15–30°C (59–86°F); protect tablets/capsules from moisture.

ASSESSMENT

1. List reasons for therapy: influenza prophylaxis, Parkinson's disease or drug-induced extrapyramidal reactions.
2. Note evidence of seizures, CHF, and renal insufficiency.
3. With seizure disorder, reduce dosage to prevent breakthrough seizures. With an increase in seizure activity, take precautions and reduce dosage to 100 mg/day to prevent loss of seizure control.
4. With Parkinson's disease, following loss of drug effectiveness, benefits may be regained by increasing dosage or discontinuing the drug for several weeks and then reinstituting.
5. Assess for NMS (neuroleptic malignant syndrome) with dose reductions or withdrawal of amantadine therapy.
6. Monitor VS, I&O; observe clients with renal impairment for crystalluria, oliguria, and increased BUN or creatinine levels and reduce dose; ensure adequate hydration. Avoid with liver failure.

CLIENT/FAMILY TEACHING

1. To prevent insomnia, give last dose several hours before bedtime.
2. Do not drive or work where alertness is important until drug effects realized; can affect vision, concentration, and coordination. Rise slowly from prone position; low BP may occur. Lie down if dizzy/weak to relieve symptoms.
3. Report diffuse patchy discoloration or skin mottling. Discoloration lessens when legs elevated; usually fades completely within weeks after stopping drug.
4. With flu protection, report if S&S do not improve or worsen. Report any exposure to rubella; drug may increase disease susceptibility.
5. Susceptible individuals (elderly, immunocompromised) should avoid crowds during flu season, receive annual flu shot and the pneumonia vaccine.
6. Report any psychologic changes such as confusion, mental status changes, nervousness, depression, or suicide ideations.
7. Avoid alcohol or any other unprescribed OTC products.
8. Clients with parkinsonism: do not stop drug abruptly; may take up to 2 weeks to notice any improvement.
9. With seizure disorders, report any early S&S of seizure activity; dosage may require adjustment.
10. Report if any new or increased gambling urges, increased sexual urges, or other intense urges experienced during therapy.
11. Keep all F/U to assess response and for adverse SE.

OUTCOMES/EVALUATE

- ↓ Drug-induced extrapyramidal S&S
- Improved motor control; ↓ tremor
- Influenza A prophylaxis; ↓ spread of infection to high-risk individuals during outbreaks

IV

Amifostine

(**am**-ih-**FOS**-teen)

Classification(s): Cytoprotective drug

Pregnancy Category: C

RX: Ethyol.

INDICATIONS/USES

(1) To decrease cumulative renal toxicity due to repeated use of cisplatin in clients with advanced ovarian cancer or in those with non-small-cell lung cancer. (2) Reduce incidence of moderate-to-severe xerostomia in those undergoing postoperative radiation treatment for head and neck cancer, where the radiation port includes a significant part of the parotid glands. *Investigational:* Prevent or reduce cisplatin-induced neurotoxicity and cyclophosphamide-induced granulocytopenia. Prevent or reduce toxicity of radiation therapy to other areas. Reduce toxicity of paclitaxel.

ACTION/KINETICS

Action

Amifostine, an organic thiophosphate prodrug, is dephosphorylated by alkaline phosphatase in tissue to the active free thiol metabolite. The thiol metabolite reduces the toxic effects of cisplatin. The ability to protect normal tissues differentially is due to the higher capillary alkaline phosphatase activity, higher pH, and better vascularity of normal tissues compared with tumor tissue. This results in a more rapid generation of the active thiol metabolite as well as greater uptake into tissues. The higher levels of the thiol metabolite in normal tissues bind to, and thus detoxify, reactive metabolites of cisplatin; the thiol metabolite can also scavenge free radicals that may be generated in tissues exposed to cisplatin.

Pharmacokinetics

Rapidly cleared from the plasma. **t½, distribution:** less than 1 min; **t½, elimination:** about 8 min. The thiol metabolite is further broken down to a disulfide metabolite that is less active.

CONTRAINDICATIONS

Hypersensitivity to aminothiol compounds or mannitol. Use in hypotensive or dehydrated clients, in those on antihypertensive therapy that cannot be terminated for 24 hr, and in clients receiving chemotherapy for malignancies that are potentially curable (e.g., certain malignancies of germ cell origin). Use in clients receiving definitive radiotherapy, except during a clinical trial. Lactation.

SPECIAL CONCERNS

- **Safety not determined in clients over 70 years of age or in those with pre-existing CV or cerebrovascular conditions, such as ischemic heart disease, arrhythmias, CHF, or history of stroke or transient ischemic attacks.**
- **Use with caution in clients where N&V or hypotension may be more likely to have serious consequences.**
- **Safety and efficacy not determined in children.**

SIDE EFFECTS

Most Common

N&V, skin rashes, feeling of warmth, chills, fever, dizziness.

CV: Transient decrease in BP. Hypotension associated with ***apnea***, dyspnea, hypoxia, tachycardia, bradycardia, extrasystoles, chest pain, myocardial ischemia, and convulsions; also, rarely atrial fibrillation/flutter, SVT. **GI:** Severe N&V. **CNS:** Dizziness, somnolence; rarely, reversible loss of consciousness or seizures. **Hypersensitivity:** Mild skin rash, fever, chills, dyspnea, urticaria, rigors, cutaneous eruptions, erythema multiforme, toxoderma; rarely, ***Stevens-Johnson syndrome***, ***toxic epidermal necrolysis***, ***anaphylaxis*** (hypoxia, ***laryngeal edema***, chest tightness, ***cardiac arrest***). **Miscellaneous:** Flushing or feeling of warmth, chills or feeling of coldness, hiccoughs, fever, sneezing, hypocalcemia.

DRUG INTERACTIONS

Amifostine may cause hypotension in clients receiving antihypertensive drugs or other drugs that may potentiate hypotension.

HOW SUPPLIED

Injection, Lyophilized Powder for Solution: 500 mg (anhydrous).

DOSAGE

IV INFUSION

Decrease cumulative renal toxicity with chemotherapy.

Initial: 910 mg/m² given once daily as a 15 min IV infusion, starting within 30 min prior to cisplatin chemotherapy.

Reduce dry mouth in postoperative radiation treatment for head and neck cancer.

200 mg/m^2 given once daily as a 3 min IV infusion, starting 15 to 30 min before standard fraction radiation therapy.

NOTE: Select dosage carefully in the elderly due to greater frequency of hepatic, renal, or cardiac function and of concomitant disease or other drug therapy.

NURSING IMPLICATIONS

IMPLEMENTATION/ADMINISTRATION/STORAGE

1. IV The 15 min infusion is better tolerated than longer duration infusions.
2. Adequately hydrate clients prior to amifostine infusion, and keep them supine during administration; monitor BP every 5 min.
3. Stop infusion if systolic BP decreases significantly from recommended baseline values. Place the client in either the Trendelenburg or supine position, and give a normal saline solution using a separate IV line. If BP returns to normal within 5 min and the client has no symptoms, the infusion may be restarted so the full dose of amifostine can be given. If the full dose of amifostine cannot be given, the dose for subsequent cycles should be 740 mg/m^2.
4. Prior to and in conjunction with amifostine, antiemetic medication, including dexamethasone 20 mg IV and a serotonin 5HT$_3$ receptor antagonist should be given. Additional antiemetics may be needed based on the chemotherapy drugs given concomitantly.
5. Reconstituted solution contains 500 mg amifostine/10 mL and is stable for 5 hr at room temperature (25°C; 77°F) or up to 24 hr under refrigeration (2–8°C; 36–46°F).
6. COMPATIBILITY To reconstitute, add 9.5 mL of 0.9% NaCl injection (other solutions not recommended).
7. INCOMPATIBILITY Do not mix with other fluids or other meds.

ASSESSMENT

1. Note type of malignancy, onset, duration of symptoms, other agents trialed, anticipated dose, and duration of cisplatin therapy.
2. List drugs currently prescribed; ensure none interact.
3. Hydrate well and ensure not hypotensive. Monitor VS, I&O and keep supine during 15 min infusion, checking BP every 5 min.
4. Review/follow manufacturer's guidelines for interrupting infusion due to decreased SBP and suggested dose for drug readmission.
5. Give an antiemetic, including dexamethasone (20 mg IV) and a serotonin 5HT$_3$ receptor antagonist, prior to and with amifostine. Monitor for before, during and after infusion for cutaneous reactions.
6. Obtain baseline VS, calcium, renal and LFTs; monitor throughout therapy. Those at risk of hypocalcemia (e.g., nephrotic syndrome) or after multiple doses; give calcium supplements.

CLIENT/FAMILY TEACHING

1. Given to protect kidneys during repeated cisplastin therapy or to offset severe dry mouth effects (xerostomia) in those undergoing radiation with head and neck cancer.
2. Stop BP medications 24 hr prior to therapy; ensure well hydrated and that BP at designated level.
3. Chills, flushing, dizziness, somnolence, hiccoughs, and sneezing may occur. Report anxiety, sweating, N&V, rapid heartbeat, SOB or difficulty breathing, swelling of the throat, or rash/itching.
4. Stay supine during infusion. Report any reactions.

OUTCOMES/EVALUATE

- ↓ Renal toxicity with cisplatin chemotherapy
- Reduction of xerostomia from XRT of head and neck cancer

■ IV

Amikacin sulfate

(am-ih-**KAY**-sin)

Classification(s): Antibiotic, aminoglycoside

Pregnancy Category: D

RX: Amikin.

SEE ALSO ***ANTI-INFECTIVE DRUGS*** AND ***AMINOGLYCOSIDES***.

INDICATIONS/USES

(1) Short-term treatment of gram-negative bacterial infections including *Pseudomonas, Escherichia coli, Proteus, Providencia, Klebsiella, Enterobacter,*

Serratia, and *Acinetobacter.* (2) For infections due to gentamicin- or tobramycin-resistant strains of *Providencia rettgeri, P. stuartii, Serratia marcescens,* and *Pseudomonas aeruginosa.* Infections include bacterial septicemia (including neonatal sepsis); serious infections of the respiratory tract, bones, joints, skin, soft tissue, and CNS (including meningitis); intra-abdominal infections (including peritonitis); burns; postoperative infections (including postvascular surgery). Also, serious complicated and recurrent infections of the urinary tract. (3) May be used as initial therapy in certain situations in the treatment of known or suspected staphylococcal disease. *Investigational:* Intrathecal or intraventricular use. As part of multiple drug regimen for *Mycobacterium avium* complex (commonly seen in AIDS clients).

ACTION/KINETICS

Action

Its spectrum is somewhat broader than that of other aminoglycosides, including *Serratia* and *Acinetobacter* species, as well as certain staphylococci and streptococci. Effective against both penicillinase- and non-penicillinase-producing organisms.

Pharmacokinetics

Peak therapeutic serum levels: IM, 16–32 mcg/mL. **t½:** 2–3 hr. Toxic serum levels: >35 mcg/mL (peak measured after 1 hr) and >10 mcg/mL (trough measured before next dose).

CONTRAINDICATIONS

Concurrent use of nephrotoxic agents or diuretics.

SPECIAL CONCERNS

See *Aminoglycosides.*

- **Use with caution in premature infants and neonates.**
- **Neurotoxicity and nephrotoxicity may occur.**

SIDE EFFECTS

Most Common

Arthralgia, oliguria, hearing loss/deafness, loss of balance, apnea, acute muscle paralysis.

See *Aminoglycosides* for a complete list of possible side effects.

ADDITIONAL DRUG INTERACTIONS

Cidofovir / ↑ Risk of nephrotoxicity

Foscarnet / ↑ Risk of nephrotoxicity

HOW SUPPLIED

Injection: 250 mg/mL; *Pediatric Injection:* 50 mg/mL.

DOSAGE

IM (PREFERRED); IV

Infections.

Adults, children, and older infants: 15 mg/kg/day in two to three equally divided doses q 8–12 hr for 7–10 days; **maximum daily dose:** 15 mg/kg.

Uncomplicated urinary tract infections (UTIs).

250 mg twice a day; **newborns:** loading dose of 10 mg/kg followed by 7.5 mg/kg q 12 hr.

Use in neonates.

Initial: Loading dose of 10 mg/kg; **then** 7.5 mg/kg q 12 hr. Lower doses may be safer during the first 2 weeks of life.

Intrathecal or intraventricular use.

8 mg/24 hr.

As part of multiple drug regimen for M. avium *complex.*

15 mg/kg/day IV in divided doses q 8–12 hr.

In clients with impaired renal function.

Normal loading dose of 7.5 mg/kg; **then** monitor administration by serum level of amikacin (35 mcg/mL maximum) or creatinine clearance rates. Duration of treatment: **Usual:** 7–10 days.

NURSING IMPLICATIONS

IMPLEMENTATION/ADMINISTRATION/STORAGE

1. **IV Add 500 mg vial to 200 mL of sterile diluent (NSS or D5W).**
2. **Administer over 30- to 60-min period for adults.**
3. **Administer to infants in prescribed fluid amount over 1–2 hr.**
4. **Store colorless liquid no longer than 2 years at room temperature.**
5. **Potency not affected if solution turns light yellow.**
6. **COMPATIBILITY D5W, NSS, LR, or dextrose/saline solutions.**
7. **INCOMPATIBILITY Flush between use.**

A

ASSESSMENT

1. Note reasons for therapy, location, onset, characteristics of S&S; C&S results.
2. Obtain audiometric assessment with high doses or prolonged use. Note vestibular dysfunction (ataxia, vertigo, N&V); monitor for 8th CN impairment R/T elevated peak drug levels, and stop drug if new onset hearing loss or tinnitus occur.
3. Assess weight, hydration status, C&S, U/A, CBC, renal and LFTs; reduce dose with renal dysfunction (assess for nephrotoxicity).

CLIENT/FAMILY TEACHING

1. Drug is administered parenterally (IV or IM) to treat susceptible infections.
2. Report lack of response; adverse side effects. Consume 2–3 liters per day of fluids to ensure hydration.
3. Report alterations in hearing, vision, ambulation, S&S of superinfection (black, furry tongue; loose, foul-smelling stools, vaginal itching).
4. Keep all F/U to assess response, labs, for adverse SE.

OUTCOMES/EVALUATE

- Resolution of infection
- Therapeutic drug levels (peak <35 mcg/mL; trough >10 mcg/mL)

■ IV

Amiodarone hydrochloride

(am-ee-**OH**-dah-rohn)

Classification(s): Antiarrhythmic, class III

Pregnancy Category: D

RX: Cordarone, Nexterone, Pacerone.

✦ **Rx:** Cordarone I.V., Gen-Amiodarone, Novo-Amiodarone, ratio-Amiodarone, Rhoxal-Amiodarone.

SEE ALSO ***ANTIARRHYTHMIC DRUGS***.

INDICATIONS/USES

PO and IV: Use should be reserved for life-threatening ventricular arrhythmias unresponsive to other therapy, such as recurrent ventricular fibrillation and recurrent, hemodynamically unstable ventricular tachycardia. During or after treatment with amiodarone injection, clients may be transferred to PO amiodarone therapy. Reserve IV use for acute treatment until the client's ventricular arrhythmias are stabilized (usually 48–96 hr); may be given IV for longer periods if needed. *Investigational:* Conversion of atrial fibrillation and maintenance of sinus rhythm, supraventricular tachycardia, IV for AV nodal reentry tachycardia.

ACTION/KINETICS

Action

Blocks sodium channels at rapid pacing frequencies, causing an increase in the duration of the myocardial cell action potential and refractory period, as well as alpha- and beta-adrenergic blockade. The drug decreases sinus rate, increases PR and QT intervals, results in development of U waves, and changes T-wave contour. After IV use, amiodarone relaxes vascular smooth muscle, reduces peripheral vascular resistance (afterload), and increases cardiac index slightly. No significant changes are seen in left ventricular ejection fraction after PO use.

Pharmacokinetics

Absorption is slow and variable, but food increases the rate and extent of absorption. **Maximum plasma levels:** 3–7 hr after a single dose. **Onset:** Several days up to 1–3 weeks. Drug may accumulate in the liver, lung, spleen, and adipose tissue. **Therapeutic serum levels:** 0.5–2.5 mcg/mL. **t½, biphasic, initial:** 2.5–10 days; **final t½:** 26–107 days. Effects may persist for several weeks or months after therapy is terminated. **Therapeutic serum levels:** 0.5–2.5 mcg/mL; **toxic serum levels:** >2.5 mcg/mL. Neither amiodarone nor its major metabolite, desethylamiodarone, is dialyzable. Excreted primarily through the bile. **Plasma protein binding:** 96%.

CONTRAINDICATIONS

Known hypersensitivity to the drug or any of its components, including iodine. Marked sinus bradycardia due to severe sinus node dysfunction, second- or third-degree AV block unless a functioning pacemaker is available, cardiogenic shock, and when bradycardia has caused syncope except when used with a pacemaker. Lactation. Use in children is not recommended.

SPECIAL CONCERNS

■ (1) Amiodarone is intended for use only in clients with the indicated life-threatening arrhythmias, because its use is accompanied by substantial toxicity. (2) Amiodarone has several potentially fatal toxicities, the most important of which is pulmonary toxicity (hypersensitivity pneumonitis or interstitial/alveolar pneumonitis) that has resulted in clinically manifest disease rates as high as 10–17% in some series of clients with ventricular arrhythmias given doses around 400 mg/day, and as abnormal diffusion capacity without symptoms in a much higher percentage of clients. Pulmonary toxicity has been fatal approximately 10% of the time. (3) Liver injury is common with amiodarone, but is usually mild and evidenced only by abnormal liver enzymes. Overt liver disease can occur, however, and has been fatal in a few cases. Like other antiarrhythmics, amiodarone can exacerbate the arrhythmia, e.g., by making the arrhythmia less well tolerated or more difficult to reverse. This has occurred in 2–5% of clients in various series, and significant heart block or sinus bradycardia has been seen in 2–5%. All of these events should be manageable in the proper clinical setting in most cases. Although the frequency of such proarrhythmic events does not appear greater with amiodarone than with many other agents used in this population, the effects are prolonged when they occur. (4) Even in clients at high risk of arrhythmic death, in whom the toxicity of amoidarone is an acceptable risk, amiodarone poses major management problems that could be life-threatening in a population at risk of sudden death, so that every effort should be made to utilize alternative agents first. (5) The difficulty of using amiodarone effectively and safely itself poses a significant risk to clients. Clients with the indicated arrhythmias must be hospitalized while the loading dose of amiodarone is given, and a response generally requires at least 1 week, usually 2 or more. Because absorption and elimination are variable, maintenance-dose selection is difficult, and it is not unusual to require dosage decrease or discontinuation of treatment. (6) The time at which a previously controlled life-threatening arrhythmia will recur after discontinuation or dose adjustment is unpredictable, ranging from weeks to months. The client is obviously at great risk during this time and may need prolonged hospitalization. Attempts to substitute other antiarrhythmic agents when amiodarone must be stopped will be made difficult by the gradually, but unpredictably, changing amiodarone body burden. A similar problem exists when amiodarone is not effective; it still poses the risk of an interaction with whatever subsequent treatment is tried. ■

- **Although not recommended for use in children, minimize the potential for the drug to leach out di-(2-ethylhexyl)phthalate (DEHP, a plasticizer) from IV tubing during administration to children (DEHP may alter development of the male reproductive tract when given in high amounts).**
- **Benzyl alcohol, found in some products, may cause a fatal "gasping syndrome" in premature infants.**
- **Geriatric clients may be more sensitive, especially in thyroid dysfunction.**
- **Carefully monitor the IV product in geriatric clients and in those with severe left ventricular dysfunction.**
- **Those on amiodarone undergoing general anesthesia may be more sensitive to the myocardial depressant and conduction effects of halogenated inhalation anesthetics.**
- **May cause fatal hepatocellular necrosis after administration of a much higher loading dose and at a rate much faster than the product's labeling.**
- **Use with caution with drugs that may cause hypokalemia and/or hypomagnesemia.**

SIDE EFFECTS

Most Common

After PO use: CHF, cardiac arrhythmias, malaise, fatigue, tremor, involuntary movements, poor coordination, peripheral neuropathy, paresthesias, photosensitivity, N&V, constipation, anorexia, pulmonary inflammation.

After IV use: Hypotension, bradycardia, AV block, CHF, ***ventricular tachycardia***, nausea, fever, injection site reactions, abnormal LFTs, heart arrest.

Adverse reactions, some potentially fatal, are common with doses greater than 400 mg/day. **Respiratory:** Pulmonary infiltrates or ***fibrosis***, interstitial/alveolar pneumonitis, hypersensitivity pneumonitis, alveolitis, pulmonary inflammation or ***fibrosis, ARDS (after both PO and parenteral use)***, lung edema, cough and progressive dyspnea, respiratory distress/***failure***, ***respiratory failure,***

A

bronchiolitis obliterans organizing pneumonia, bronchospasm, hemoptysis, hypoxia, pleuritis, ***possibly fatal respiratory disorders***, wheezing. Oral use may cause a clinical syndrome of cough and progressive dyspnea accompanied by functional, radiographic, gallium scan, and pathologic data indicating ***pulmonary toxicity***. **CV:** ***Worsening of arrhythmias, paroxysmal ventricular tachycardia***, proarrhythmias, symptomatic bradycardia, sinus arrest, SA node dysfunction, AV block, ***asystole***, ***CHF***, edema, hypotension (especially with IV use), venous thrombosis, phlebitis, thrombophlebitis, ***ventricular tachycardia***, vasculitis, ***cardiac conduction abnormalities, coagulation abnormalities, cardiac arrest (after IV use), cardiogenic shock***. IV use may result in atrial fibrillation, nodal arrhythmia, prolonged QT interval, sinus bradycardia, ***pulseless electrical activity***, ***ventricular fibrillation, electromechanical dissociation***, ***heart arrest***. **Hepatic:** Abnormal LFTs, overt liver disease, nonspecific hepatic disorders, cholestatic hepatitis, cirrhosis, hepatitis, steatohepatitis (with cumulative doses), ***fatal hepatocellular necrosis***, ***hepatic failure***. **CNS:** Malaise, tremor, lack of coordination, fatigue, ataxia, paresthesias, peripheral neuropathy, abnormal involuntary movements, sleep disturbances, dizziness, insomnia, headache, decreased libido, abnormal gait, hallucinations, confusion, disorientation, delirium, pseudotumor cerebri. **Hematologic:** ***Hemolytic anemia, aplastic anemia***, thrombocytopenia, neutropenia, pancytopenia, agranulocytosis, granuloma. **GI:** N&V, constipation, diarrhea, anorexia, abdominal pain, abnormal taste and smell, abnormal salivation, ***pancreatitis***. **Hepatic:** Cholestatic jaundice, cirrhosis, hepatitis. **Musculoskeletal:** Myopathy, muscle weakness, rhabdomyolysis. **Ophthalmologic:** Ophthalmic abnormalities, including optic neuropathy and/or optic neuritis (may progress to permanent blindness). Papilledema, corneal degeneration, photosensitivity, eye discomfort, scotoma, lens opacities, macular degeneration. Corneal microdeposits (asymptomatic) in clients on therapy for 6 months or more, photophobia, dry eyes, visual disturbances, blurred vision, halos. **Dermatologic:** Photosensitivity, pruritus, flushing, solar dermatitis, blue discoloration of skin, rash, alopecia, spontaneous ecchymosis, erythema, erythema multiforme, exfoliative dermatitis, pigment changes, flushing, skin sloughing, angioedema, skin cancer, ***Stevens-Johnson syndrome***, ***fatal toxic epidermal necrolysis***. **GU:** Epididymitis, impotence, renal impairment/insufficiency, acute renal failure. **At injection site:** Cellulitis, edema, erythema, necrosis, pain, phlebitis, pigment changes, skin sloughing, thrombophlebitis, venous thrombosis. **Miscellaneous:** Hypothyroidism or hyperthyroidism, thyroid nodules/tumors, fever, syndrome of inappropriate ADH secretion, necrosis.

IV use may cause abnormal kidney function, pain, ***Stevens-Johnson syndrome, ventricular fibrillation,*** thrombocytopenia, vomiting, respiratory syndrome, ***fatal "gasping syndrome" in neonates following IV use of benzyl alcohol-containing solutions, anaphylactic/anaphylactoid reactions***, and ***shock***.

LABORATORY TEST CONSIDERATIONS

↑ AST, ALT, GGT. Alteration of thyroid function tests (↑ serum T_4, ↓ serum T_3), abnormal LFTs, abnormal kidney function.

OVERDOSE MANAGEMENT

Symptoms: Bradycardia, hypotension, ***disorders of cardiac rhythm, cardiogenic shock***, AV block, hepatoxicity. *Treatment:* Institute supportive treatment. Monitor cardiac rhythm and BP. Use a beta-adrenergic agonist or pacemaker to treat bradycardia; treat hypotension due to insufficient tissue perfusion with a vasopressor or positive inotropic agents. Cholestyramine may hasten the reversal of side effects by increasing elimination. Drug is not dialyzable.

DRUG INTERACTIONS

Anesthetics, volatile / ↑ Sensitivity to the myocardial depressant and conduction effects of halogenated inhalation anesthetics

Atazanavir / Significant ↑ amiodarone levels → ↑ risk of amiodarone toxicity

Azole antifungals (e.g., itraconazole) / ↑ Risk of life-threatening cardiac arrhythmias, including torsades de pointes

Beta-adrenergic blocking agents (e.g., propranolol) / ↑ Bradycardia and hypotension R/T ↓ beta-blocker metabolism

Calcium channel blockers (e.g., diltiazem, verapamil) / ↑ Risk of inhibition of AV conduction and ↓ myocardial conduction; AV block with verapamil or diltiazem or hypotension with any calcium channel blockers

A

Cholestyramine / ↑ Elimination of amiodarone → ↓ serum levels and half-life
Cimetidine / ↑ Serum levels of amiodarone
Cyclosporine / ↑ Cyclosporine plasma levels → elevated creatinine levels (even with ↓ cyclosporine doses)
Dextromethorphan / Chronic use of PO amiodarone (>2 weeks) impairs dextromethorphan metabolism
Digoxin / ↑ Serum digoxin levels by 70% after 1 day → toxicity; reduce digoxin dose by 50% or discontinue
Disopyramide / ↑ QT prolongation → possible arrhythmias; also, ↑ disopyramide plasma levels; reduce disopyramide dose
Fentanyl / Possibility of hypotension, bradycardia, ↓ CO
Flecainide / ↑ Plasma flecainide levels → toxicity; reduce flecainide dose
Fluoroquinolones (e.g., sparfloxacin) / ↑ Risk of life-threatening cardiac arrhythmias, including torsade de pointes R/T prolongation of the QT-interval
Grapefruit juice / ↑ AUC by 50% and peak plasma amiodarone levels by 84% R/T inhibition of CYP3A4 metabolism of amiodarone; stop using grapefruit juice when starting amiodarone therapy
HMG-CoA reductase inhibitors (e.g., rosuvastatin, simvastatin) ↑ Risk of myopathy and rhabdomyolysis
Hydantoins (e.g., phenytoin) / ↑ Hydantoin levels after >2 weeks amiodarone use → toxicity; also, ↓ amiodarone serum levels
Indinavir / ↑ Plasma levels of amiodarone due to ↓ breakdown by liver → ↑ risk of toxicity
Iohexol (contrast media) / ↑ QTc in clients taking amiodarone and undergoing cardiac catheterization
Lidocaine / Sinus bradycardia after PO amiodarone; seizures R/T ↑ lidocaine levels with concomitant IV amiodarone
Macrolide antibiotics (e.g., azithromycin) / ↑ Risk of life-threatening cardiac arrhythmias, including torsades de pointes
Methotrexate / Chronic use of PO amiodarone (>2 weeks) ↓ methotrexate metabolism → toxicity
Nelfinavir / ↑ Amiodarone levels → ↑ risk of amiodarone toxicity
Procainamide / ↑ Serum procainamide levels → toxicity; reduce procainamide dose
Pyridoxine / ↑ Amiodarone-induced photosensitivity
Quinidine / ↑ Quinidine toxicity, including fatal cardiac arrhythmias; reduce quinidine dose
Rifampin / ↓ Serum levels of amiodarone and its active metabolite due to ↑ liver breakdown → ↓ therapeutic effect
Ritonavir / ↑ Levels of amiodarone → ↑ risk of amiodarone toxicity
H ***St. John's wort*** / ↓ Amiodarone levels R/T ↑ metabolism by CYP3A4
Theophylline / ↑ Serum theophylline levels → toxicity (effects may not be seen for 1 week and may last for a prolonged period after amiodarone is discontinued)
Thioridazine / ↑ Risk of life-threatening cardiac arrhythmias, including torsades de pointes
Vardenafil / ↑ Risk of life-threatening cardiac arrhythmias, including torsades de pointes
Warfarin / ↑ PT; ↓ warfarin dose by 30–50%. Effect may persist for months after amiodarone discontinuation
Ziprasidone / ↑ Risk of life-threatening cardiac arrhythmias, including torsades de pointes

HOW SUPPLIED

Injection: 1.5 mg/mL (premixed single-dose), 1.8 mg/mL (premixed single-dose), 50 mg/mL, 150 mg/3 mL, 450 mg/9 mL, 900 mg/18 mL; ***Tablets:*** 100 mg, 200 mg, 400 mg.

DOSAGE

Due to the drug's side effects, unusual pharmacokinetic properties, and difficult dosing schedule, administer amiodarone in a hospital only by physicians trained in treating life-threatening arrhythmias. Loading doses are required to ensure a reasonable onset of action.

IV INFUSION

Life-threatening ventricular arrhythmias (e.g., ventricular fibrillation or hemodynamically unstable ventricular tachycardia).

Loading dose, first rapid: 150 mg over the first 10 minutes (15 mg/min). **Then, slow loading dose:** 360 mg over the next 6 hr (1 mg/min). **Maintenance dose:** 540 mg over the remaining 18 hr (0.5 mg/min). After the first 24 hr, continue maintenance infusion rate

A

of 0.5 mg/min (720 mg/24 hr). This may be continued with monitoring for 2 to 3 weeks.

Once arrhythmias have been suppressed, the client may be switched to PO amiodarone. The following is intended only as a guideline for PO amiodarone dosage after IV infusion. **IV infusion less than 1 week:** Initial daily dose of PO amiodarone, 800–1,600 mg. **IV infusion from 1 to 3 weeks:** Initial daily dose of PO amiodarone, 600–800 mg. **IV infusion longer than 3 weeks:** Initial daily dose of PO amiodarone, 400 mg.

TABLETS

Life-threatening ventricular arrhythmias (e.g., ventricular fibrillation or hemodynamically unstable ventricular tachycardia).

Loading dose: 800–1,600 mg/day for 1–3 weeks (or until initial response occurs); **then**, reduce dose to 600–800 mg/day for 1 month. **Maintenance dose:** 400 mg/day (as low as 200 mg/day or as high as 600 mg/day may be needed in some clients). Give in divided doses with meals for total daily doses of 1,000 mg or higher or when GI intolerance occurs.

NURSING IMPLICATIONS

IMPLEMENTATION/ADMINISTRATION/STORAGE

1. Correct K^+ or Mg^{++} deficiencies before therapy since antiarrhythmics may be ineffective or arrhythmogenic with hypokalemia.
2. When initiating therapy, gradually discontinue other antiarrhythmic drugs.
3. To minimize side effects, determine lowest effective dose; if side effects occur, reduce dose.
4. If dosage adjustments required, monitor client for extended time frame R/T long and variable half-life of drug and the difficulty in predicting time needed to achieve new steady-state plasma drug level.
5. Administer daily PO doses of 1,000 mg or more in divided doses with meals.
6. If additional antiarrhythmic therapy required, initial dose of such drugs should be about one-half usual recommended dose.
7. Review labeling for PO formulation, especially safety and efficacy, before switching route of administration from IV or PO.
8. IV For first rapid loading dose, add 3 mL amiodarone IV (150 mg) to 100 mL D5W for concentration of 1.5 mg/mL; infuse at rate of 100 mL/10 min. For slower loading dose, add 18 mL amiodarone IV (900 mg) to 500 mL of D5W for concentration of 1.8 mg/mL.
9. IV concentrations of amiodarone greater than 3 mg/mL in D5W cause high incidence of peripheral vein phlebitis; concentrations of 2.5 mg/mL or less are not as irritating. For infusions greater than 1 hr, the IV concentration should not exceed 2 mg/mL unless central venous catheter used.
10. Cordarone IV has been found to leach out plasticizers, such as DEHP, which can adversely affect male reproductive tract development in fetuses, infants, and toddlers. Cordarone IV is not indicated to treat arrhythmias in pediatric clients.
11. Store the injection at room temperature protected from light.
12. COMPATIBILITY Amiodarone-D5W; Nexterone-D5W or saline
13. INCOMPATIBILITY Amiodarone IV in D5W is incompatible with aminophylline, cefamandole nafate, cefazolin sodium, mezlocillin sodium, heparin sodium, and sodium bicarbonate as is Nexterone in D5Wor saline. Because amiodarone adsorbs to PVC, IV infusions exceeding 2 hr must be given in glass or polyolefin bottles containing D5W. Nexterone does not contain polysorbate 80 or benzyl alcohol, thus allowing it to be administered in polyvinyl chloride, polyolefin, or glass containers.

ASSESSMENT

1. Note indications for therapy; used only for life-threatening arrhythmias. List other agents prescribed and other antiarrhythmic drugs to ensure none interact.
2. Assess quality of respirations and breath sounds; note cardiac status, ECG, and CV findings. Monitor for hepatic and pulmonary toxicity.
3. Note baseline CXR, PFTs, VS and perfusion (skin temperature, color), and monitor during therapy. Document ABGs; assess for circulatory impairment and hypotension.

4. Assess vision before and during therapy.
5. During administration, observe for increased PR and QRS intervals, increased arrhythmias, and HR <60 bpm. Obtain ECG, document rhythm strips; note EPS findings and BP.
6. Reduce dosages of digoxin, warfarin, quinidine, procainamide, and phenytoin if administered with amiodarone.
7. Monitor thyroid studies (drug inhibits conversion of T_4 to T_3). May require replacement therapy with prolonged use.
8. Obtain ECG, CBC, electrolytes (especially K^+ and Mg^{++}), CXR, renal and LFTs. Monitor LFTs assessing for toxicity and thyroid function regularly during therapy.

CLIENT/FAMILY TEACHING

1. Drug is used to control heartbeat irregularities; take as directed. Avoid grapefruit juice.
2. Report if crystals develop on skin, producing bluish color, so dosage can be adjusted.
3. Avoid direct exposure to sunlight. Wear protective clothing, sunglasses, and a sunscreen if exposed.
4. Report side effects. Some may not appear for several weeks up to a year after therapy and may persist; especially any abnormal swelling, bleeding, or bruising.
5. Painful breathing, wheezing, fever, coughing, or SOB are S&S of pulmonary problems; requires prompt attention.
6. Report CNS S&S such as tremor, lack of coordination, numbness, and dizziness (neurotoxicity).
7. Complaints of headaches, depression, or insomnia as well as any change in behavior such as decreased interest in personal appearance or apparent hallucinations may require evaluation and a change in therapy.
8. Have periodic eye exams; small yellow-brown granular corneal deposits may develop during prolonged therapy. Visual changes require prompt eye evaluation.
9. Requires lab studies and close medical evaluation; drug is highly toxic and may stay in system for many months after stopping.
10. Practice reliable contraception.
11. Health care professionals who dispense amiodarone tablets are required to provide medication guides to clients to review; these should not be used as substitutes for counseling regarding the risks and benefits of the drug.
12. Keep all F/U to assess response, labs, for adverse SE.

OUTCOMES/EVALUATE

- Termination/control of arrhythmias
- Serum drug levels within therapeutic range (0.5–2.5 mcg/mL)

Amitriptyline hydrochloride

(ah-me-**TRIP**-tih-leen)

Classification(s): Antidepressant, tricyclic

Pregnancy Category: C

✤ **Rx:** Apo-Amitriptyline.

SEE ALSO ***ANTIDEPRESSANTS, TRICYCLIC.***

INDICATIONS/USES

(1) Relief of symptoms of depression, including depression accompanied by anxiety and insomnia. (2) Chronic pain due to cancer or other pain syndromes. (3) Prophylaxis of cluster and migraine headaches. *Investigational:* Pathologic laughing and crying secondary to forebrain disease, bulimia nervosa, antiulcer agent, enuresis. Adjunct analgesic for phantom limb pain, migraine, chronic tension headaches, diabetic neuropathy, tic douloureux, cancer pain, peripheral neuropathy with pain, postherpetic neuralgia, arthritic pain. Dermatologic disorders (chronic urticaria and angioedema, nocturnal pruritus in atopic eczema).

ACTION/KINETICS

Action

Amitriptyline is metabolized to an active metabolite, nortriptyline. Has significant anticholinergic and sedative effects with moderate orthostatic hypotension. Very high ability to block serotonin uptake and moderate activity with respect to norepinephrine uptake.

Pharmacokinetics

Peak plasma levels: 2–4 hr. Significant first-pass effect. Metabolized to nortriptyline. **Effective plasma levels of amitriptyline and nortriptyline:** Approximately 110–250 ng/mL. **Time to reach steady state:** 4–10 days. **t½:** 31–46 hr. Up to 1 month may be required for beneficial effects to be manifested.

A

CONTRAINDICATIONS

Use in children less than 12 years old.

SPECIAL CONCERNS

■ Antidepressants increase the risk of suicidal thinking and behavior (suicidality) in short-term studies in children, adolescents, and young adults with major depressive disorders and other psychiatric disorders. Anyone considering the use of amitriptyline or any other antidepressant in a child, adolescent, or young adult must balance this risk with the clinical need. Clients who are started on therapy should be observed closely for clinical worsening, suicidality, or unusual changes in behavior. Families and caregivers should be advised of the need for close observation and communication with the prescriber. Amitriptyline is not approved for use in pediatric clients. Analysis of short-term (4–16 weeks) placebo-controlled trials in children and adolescents with major depressive disorder, obsessive-compulsive disorder, or other psychiatric disorders have revealed a greater risk of adverse reactions representing suicidal thinking or behavior during the first few months of treatment in those receiving antidepressants. The average risk of such reactions in such clients receiving antidepressants was 4%, twice the placebo risk of 2%. No suicides occurred in these trials. ■

SIDE EFFECTS

Most Common

Sedation, dry mouth, blurred vision, constipation, mydriasis, urinary retention, disturbance of accommodation.

See *Antidepressants, Tricyclic* for a complete list of possible side effects. Possible limb reduction anomalies.

ADDITIONAL DRUG INTERACTIONS

Guanethidine and similar drugs / Antihypertensive effect may be blocked

H ***St. John's wort*** / ↓ Blood levels of amitriptyline and its metabolite

Smoking / ↓ Amitriptyline levels R/T ↑ hepatic metabolism; possible ↓ efficacy

Valproic acid / ↑ Amitriptyline levels

HOW SUPPLIED

Tablets: 10 mg, 25 mg, 50 mg, 75 mg, 100 mg, 150 mg.

DOSAGE

TABLETS

Antidepressant.

Adults (outpatients): 75 mg/day in divided doses; may be increased to 150 mg/day. *Alternate dosage:* **Initial,** 50–100 mg at bedtime; **then** increase by 25–50 mg, if necessary, up to 150 mg/day. **Hospitalized clients: initial,** 100 mg/day; may be increased to 200–300 mg/day. **Maintenance: usual,** 40–100 mg/day (may be given as a single dose at bedtime). **Adolescent and geriatric:** 10 mg 3 times per day and 20 mg at bedtime up to a maximum of 100 mg/day.

Chronic pain.

50–100 mg/day.

Analgesic adjunct.

75–300 mg/day.

Dermatologic disorders.

10–50 mg/day.

NURSING IMPLICATIONS

Do not confuse amitriptyline with nortriptyline (also a tricyclic antidepressant).

IMPLEMENTATION/ADMINISTRATION/STORAGE

1. Initiate dosage increases late in afternoon or bedtime.
2. Sedative effects may be manifested before antidepressant effects.
3. When satisfactory improvement is noted, reduce the dose to the lowest effective amount. Continue 3 or more months to lessen the possibility of relapse.

ASSESSMENT

1. Note indications, onset, characteristics/extent of S&S. With depression, assess for suicidal ideations; with pain, identify levels and locations; list other agents trialed, outcome.
2. Assess I&O, weights, VS, ECG, and bowel elimination patterns.
3. Monitor mental status, CBC, electrolytes, BS, renal and LFTs.

CLIENT/FAMILY TEACHING

1. Take with food; minimizes gastric upset; tablets may be crushed. Could take up to 6 weeks to see desired effects.
2. Do not drive or operate hazardous machinery until drug effects realized; causes high degree of sedation. Rise slowly from lying to sitting position to reduce low BP drug effects.
3. Take dose right after food or fluid and in late afternoon or at bedtime if sedative effects are a problem. Report increased appetite may cause some weight gain. Do not stop taking drug abruptly without provider approval.
4. Report if blurred vision, sore throat, fever, increased heart rate, impaired coordination, difficult urination, excessive sedation, or seizures occur.
5. Wear sunscreen; avoid prolonged sun exposure.
6. Urine may appear blue-green in color; harmless. May experience dry mouth. Report urinary retention or constipation; increase fluids/bulk in diet to offset.
7. Encourage regular dental care; oral dryness can increase risk for dental caries.
8. Beneficial antidepressant effects may not be noted for 4 to 6 weeks but side effects may be noted earlier. Report any suicide ideations or abnormal behaviors.
9. Elderly clients may be at increased risk for falls; start low doses, use precautions, and observe closely.
10. Avoid intake of alcohol or other CNS depressants. Keep F/U visits to evaluate response and adverse SE.

OUTCOMES/EVALUATE

- ↓ Symptoms of depression
- Chronic pain control with migraine, tension headache, phantom limb pain, tic douloureux, diabetic neuropathy, peripheral neuropathy, cancer or arthritis
- ↓ Panic attacks; control of eating disorders (unlabeled uses)
- Relief of insomnia/itching

Amlodipine

(am-**LOH**-dih-peen)

Classification(s): Calcium channel blocker

Pregnancy Category: C

RX: Amvaz, Norvasc.

SEE ALSO ***CALCIUM CHANNEL BLOCKING AGENTS.***

INDICATIONS/USES

(1) Hypertension alone or in combination with other antihypertensives. (2) Chronic stable angina alone or in combination with other antianginal drugs. (3) Vasospastic (Prinzmetal's or variant) angina alone or in combination with other antianginal drugs.

ACTION/KINETICS

Action

Inhibits influx of calcium through the cell membrane, resulting in a depression of automaticity and conduction velocity in cardiac muscle. Decreases SA and AV conduction and prolongs AV node effective and functional refractory periods. Slight decrease in HR. Possible slight decrease in myocardial contractility. CO is increased; moderate decrease in peripheral vascular resistance.

Pharmacokinetics

Peak plasma levels: 6–12 hr. **t½, elimination:** 30–50 hr. 90% metabolized in the liver to inactive metabolites; 10% excreted unchanged in the urine. **Plasma protein binding:** About 93%.

CONTRAINDICATIONS

Use with grapefruit juice.

SPECIAL CONCERNS

- Use with caution in clients with CHF and in those with impaired hepatic function or reduced hepatic blood flow.
- Safety and efficacy not determined in children.

SIDE EFFECTS

Most Common

Edema, palpitations, dizziness/light-headedness, headache, fatigue/lethargy, flushing.

CNS: Headache, fatigue, lethargy, somnolence, dizziness, light-headedness, sleep disturbances, depression, amnesia, psychosis, hallucinations, paresthesia, asthenia, insomnia, abnormal dreams, malaise, anxiety, tremor, hand tremor, hypoesthesia, vertigo, depersonalization, migraine, apathy, agitation, amnesia. **GI:** Nausea, abdominal discomfort, cramps, dyspepsia, diarrhea, constipation, vomiting, dry mouth, thirst, flatulence, dysphagia, loose stools. **CV:** Peripheral edema, palpi-

A

tations, hypotension, syncope, bradycardia, unspecified arrhythmias, tachycardia, ventricular extrasystoles, peripheral ischemia, ***cardiac failure***, pulse irregularity, increased risk of MI. **Dermatologic:** Dermatitis, rash, pruritus, urticaria, photosensitivity, petechiae, ecchymosis, purpura, bruising, hematoma, cold/clammy skin, skin discoloration, dry skin. **Musculoskeletal:** Muscle cramps, pain, or inflammation; joint stiffness or pain, arthritis, twitching, ataxia, hypertonia. **GU:** Polyuria, dysuria, urinary frequency, nocturia, sexual difficulties. **Respiratory:** Nasal or chest congestion, sinusitis, rhinitis, SOB, dyspnea, wheezing, cough, chest pain. **Ophthalmic:** Diplopia, abnormal vision, conjunctivitis, eye pain, abnormal visual accommodation, xerophthalmia. **Miscellaneous:** Tinnitus, flushing, sweating, weight gain, epistaxis, anorexia, increased appetite, taste perversion, parosmia.

ADDITIONAL DRUG INTERACTIONS

Diltiazem / ↑ Plasma levels of amlodipine → further ↓ BP
Grapefruit juice / ↑ Plasma amlodipine levels
Indinavir + Ritonavir / ↑ Amlodipine AUC R/T inhibition of CYP3A4 metabolism of amlodipine

HOW SUPPLIED

Tablets: 2.5 mg, 5 mg, 10 mg.

DOSAGE

TABLETS

Hypertension.

Adults, usual, individualized: 5 mg/day, up to a maximum of 10 mg/day. Titrate the dose over 7–14 days. Adjust dose to client needs.

Chronic stable or vasospastic angina.

Adults: 5–10 mg, using the lower dose for elderly clients and those with hepatic insufficiency. Most clients require 10 mg.

NURSING IMPLICATIONS

Ⓢ Do not confuse amlodipine with amiloride (a diuretic) or Norvasc with Navane (an antipsychotic).

IMPLEMENTATION/ADMINISTRATION/STORAGE

1. Food does not affect bioavailability of amlodipine.
2. Elderly clients, small/fragile clients, or those with hepatic insufficiency may be started on 2.5 mg/day. May also use this dose when adding amlodipine with other antihypertensive therapy.
3. Can be given safely with ACEI, beta-blockers, nitrates (long-acting), nitroglycerin (sublingual), or thiazides.
4. Store from 25–30°C (59–86°F).

ASSESSMENT

1. Note reasons for therapy, history of CAD or CHF, angina. Monitor carefully with angina as CCBs may cause increase in frequency/intensity of pain with severe CAD initially and with dose increase.
2. Review list of drugs prescribed to prevent interactions.
3. Monitor HR, BP, ECG, CBC, renal and LFTs. Reduce dose in elderly clients, those with liver dysfunction, or severe heart failure.

CLIENT/FAMILY TEACHING

1. Take once daily as directed; do not stop suddenly as that may precipitate chest pain/MI.
2. May take with/without meals; food helps decrease stomach upset. Avoid grapefruit juice; increases drug concentrations.
3. May experience light-headedness, dizziness, or drowsiness. Avoid activities that require mental alertness until drug effects realized.
4. Report S&S of chest pain, SOB, dizziness, swelling of extremities, irregular pulse, or altered vision immediately. Keep record of daily BP and pulse.
5. Change positions slowly to prevent sudden drop in BP. Avoid OTC cold preparations and CNS depressants during therapy.
6. To help control BP: maintain healthy diet and limit intake of caffeine; avoid alcohol, salt substitutes, or high Na and high K foods; perform regular exercise, maintain weight, and stop smoking.
7. Keep all F/U to assess response and adverse SE.

OUTCOMES/EVALUATE

- Desired BP control
- ↓ Frequency/intensity of angina

Combination Drug

Amlodipine besylate and Benazepril hydrochloride

(am-**LOH**-dih-peen, beh-**NAYZ**-eh-prill)

Classification(s): Antihypertensive
Pregnancy Category: D
RX: Lotrel.

SEE ALSO ***AMLODIPINE*** AND ***BENAZEPRIL HYDROCHLORIDE.***

INDICATIONS/USES

Hypertension (not indicated for initial therapy).

CONTENT

Amlodipine besylate (*calcium channel blocker*), 2.5 mg, 5 mg, or 10 mg with benazepril hydrochloride (*ACE inhibitor*), 10 mg, 20 mg, or 40 mg with the following available combinations: 2.5/10 mg, 5/10 mg, 5/20 mg, 5/40 mg, 10/20 mg, and 10/40 mg.

ACTION/KINETICS

Action

Benazepril (and its active metabolite benazeprilat) inhibit angiotensin-converting enzyme resulting in decreased plasma angiotensin II, which leads to decreased vasopressor activity and decreased aldosterone secretion. Amlodipine inhibits the transmembrane influx of calcium ions into vascular smooth muscle and cardiac muscle, resulting in a depression of automaticity and conduction velocity. There is a reduction of both supine and standing BP, with no compensatory tachycardia.

Pharmacokinetics

Absorption of either drug is not affected by food. **Peak plasma levels, amlodipine:** 6–12 hr; **benazepril and benazeprilat:** 0.5–2 hr and 1.5–4 hr, respectively. Amlodipine is metabolized in the liver and excreted through the urine. Benazepril and metabolites are excreted through the urine. **t½, elimination, amlodipine:** 2 days; **benazeprilat:** 10–11 hr.

CONTRAINDICATIONS

Hypersensitivity to benazepril, to any other ACE inhibitor, or to amlodipine. Lactation.

SPECIAL CONCERNS

When used in pregnancy during the second and third trimesters, ACE inhibitors can cause injury and even death to the developing fetus. When pregnancy is detected, discontinue the ACE inhibitor as soon as possible.

- **Use with caution in clients with severe aortic stenosis and in severe renal or hepatic disease.**
- **Possible excessive hypotension in clients with CHF, with or without associated renal insufficiency.**
- **Safety and efficacy have not been determined in children.**

SIDE EFFECTS

Most Common

Cough, hypotension, edema (dependent, ***angioedema***, facial edema), headache, dizziness.

See *Amlodipine* and *Benazepril hydrochloride* for a complete list of possible side effects.

LABORATORY TEST CONSIDERATIONS

↑ Serum creatinine (especially in those with renal insufficiency, those pretreated with a diuretic, and those with renal artery stenosis). ↑ Serum bilirubin, uric acid.

DRUG INTERACTIONS

See ***Amlodipine*** and ***Benazepril hydrochloride***.

HOW SUPPLIED

See *Content*.

DOSAGE

CAPSULES

Hypertension.

One 2.5/10, 5/10, 5/20, 5/40, 10/20, or 10/40 capsule daily. For the small, elderly, frail, or hepatically impaired, initial amlodipine dose is 2.5 mg.

NURSING IMPLICATIONS

IMPLEMENTATION/ADMINISTRATION/STORAGE

1. **To minimize dose-independent hazards, it is usually appropriate to begin Lotrel therapy only after a client has:**
   - **Failed to achieve the desired antihypertensive effect with one or the other monotherapy, or**

A

- Demonstrated inability to achieve adequate antihypertensive effect with amlodipine therapy without developing edema.

2. Store from 15–30°C (59–86°F).

ASSESSMENT

1. List reasons for therapy, other agents trialed, outcome.
2. Check drugs prescribed to ensure none interact.
3. Note risk factors, CAD, CHF, if renal artery stenosis; assess for pregnancy.
4. Monitor VS, ECG, CBC, K^+, renal and LFTs.

CLIENT/FAMILY TEACHING

1. Lotrel is a combination of two drugs in one capsule to better control BP. Take capsule at the same time each day.
2. If swelling of extremities/face, cough, SOB, dizziness, abdominal pain, dark urine, yellowing of skin, persistent sore throat occur, stop drug and report.
3. Lie or sit down if experiencing dizziness or lightheadedness when standing.
4. Poor fluid intake, excessive perspiration, diarrhea, or vomiting can lead to excessive fall in BP resulting in lightheadedness or fainting. Consume adequate fluids during therapy.
5. Use reliable contraception; stop drug/report if pregnant.
6. Review importance of lifestyle changes on BP: weight control, regular exercise, smoking cessation, and moderate intake of alcohol and salt.
7. Record BP and weight log for provider review; report significant changes.
8. Keep all F/U to assess response, labs, and adverse SE.

OUTCOMES/EVALUATE

Control of BP

Amoxicillin (Amoxycillin)

(ah-mox-ih-**SILL**-in)

Classification(s): Antibiotic, penicillin

Pregnancy Category: B

RX: Amoxil, Amoxil Pediatric Drops, DisperMox, Moxatag, Trimox.

🍁 **Rx:** Apo-Amoxi, Gen-Amoxicillin, Novamoxin, Nu-Amoxi.

SEE ALSO ***ANTI-INFECTIVE DRUGS*** AND ***PENICILLINS***.

INDICATIONS/USES

1. Ear, nose, and throat infections due to *Streptococcus* species (alpha- and beta-lactamase-negative only), *S. pneumoniae, Staphylococcus* species, or *Haemophilus influenzae.*
2. GU infections due to *Escherichia coli, Proteus mirabilis,* or *Enterococcus faecalis.*
3. Skin and skin structure infections due to *Streptococcus* species (alpha- and beta-hemolytic strains only), *Staphylococcus* species, or *E. coli.*
4. Lower respiratory tract infections due to *Streptococcus* species (alpha- and beta-hemolytic strains only), *S. pneumoniae, Staphylococcus* species, or *H. haemophilus.*
5. Acute uncomplicated (anogenital and urethral) gonococcal infections due to *Neisseria gonorrhoeae* in males and females.
6. In combination with amoxicillin/lansoprazole (dual therapy) or amoxicillin/lansoprazole/clarithromycin (triple therapy) to treat duodenal ulcers due to *Helicobacter pylori.* Eradication of *H. pylori* has been shown to reduce the risk of duodenal ulcer recurrence.
7. Postexposure prophylaxis following confirmed or suspected exposure to *Bacillus anthracis.*
8. Extended-release tablets (Moxatag) to treat tonsillitis and/or pharyngitis secondary to *Streptococcus pyogenes* in adults and children 12 years of age and older.

ACTION/KINETICS

Action

Semisynthetic broad-spectrum penicillin closely related to ampicillin. Binds to penicillin-binding proteins (PBP-1 and PBP-3) in the cytoplasmic membranes of bacteria, thus inhibiting cell wall synthesis. Cell division and growth are inhibited. Destroyed by penicillinase, acid stable, and better absorbed than ampicillin.

Pharmacokinetics

From 50–80% of a PO dose is absorbed from the GI tract. **Peak serum levels, PO:** 4–11 mcg/mL after 1–2 hr. **t½:** 60 min. Mostly excreted unchanged in urine.

A

ADDITIONAL CONTRAINDICATIONS

Use of the 875 mg tablet in clients with a GFR less than 30 mL/min.

SPECIAL CONCERNS

- Safe use during pregnancy not established.
- Effectiveness of oral contraceptives may be decreased.

SIDE EFFECTS

Most Common

Hypersensitivity, N&V, gastritis, stomatitis. See *Penicillins* for a complete list of potential side effects.

HOW SUPPLIED

Capsules: 250 mg, 500 mg; *Powder for Oral Suspension:* 50 mg/mL, 125 mg/5 mL, 200 mg/5 mL, 250 mg/5 mL (all strengths are after reconstitution); *Tablets:* 500 mg, 875 mg; *Tablets, Chewable:* 125 mg, 200 mg, 250 mg, 400 mg; *Tablets, Extended-Release:* 775 mg; *Tablets for Oral Suspension:* 200 mg, 400 mg, 600 mg.

DOSAGE

CAPSULES; ORAL SUSPENSION; TABLETS; TABLETS, CHEWABLE

Susceptible infections of ear, nose, throat, GU tract, skin, and soft tissues. Mild to moderate infections.

Adults and children 40 kg or more, usual, mild to moderate infections: 250 mg q 8 hr or 500 mg q 12 hr; **severe infections:** 500 mg q 8 hr or 875 mg q 12 hr. **Children 3 months and older and less than 40 kg, mild to moderate infections:** 20 mg/kg/day in divided doses q 8 hr or 25 mg/kg/day in divided doses q 12 hr; **severe infections:** 40 mg/kg/day in divided doses q 8 hr or 45 mg/kg/day in divided doses q 12 hr. For children, do not exceed the maximum adult dose.

Infections of the lower respiratory tract.

Adults and children 40 kg and over, mild/moderate/severe infections: 500 mg q 8 hr or 875 mg q 12 hr. **Children 3 months and older and under 40 kg, mild/moderate/severe infections:** 40 mg/kg/day in divided doses q 8 hr or 45 mg/kg/day in divided doses q 12 hr.

Gonococcal infections, uncomplicated urethral, endocervical, or rectal infections in males and females.

Adults: 3 grams as a single PO dose. **Children, over 2 years (prepubertal):** 50 mg/kg amoxicillin combined with 25 mg/kg probenecid as a single dose.

Eradicate H. pylori *infections to reduce risk of duodenal ulcer recurrence.*

The following regimens may be used. (1) **Dual Therapy (amoxicillin/lansoprazole), adults:** Amoxicillin, 1,000 mg and lansoprazole, 30 mg, each given 3 times per day (q 8 hr) for 14 days. (2) **Triple Therapy (amoxicillin/clarithromycin/lansoprazole), adults:** Amoxicillin, 1,000 mg, clarithromycin, 500 mg, and lansoprazole, 30 mg, each given 2 times per day (q 12 hr) for 14 days.

Anthrax (postexposure prophylaxis following confirmed or suspected exposure to Bacillus anthracis*).*

Adults: 500 mg PO 3 times per day. **Children, less than 9 years of age:** 80 mg/kg/day PO divided into 2–3 doses. Continue prophylaxis until exposure has been excluded. If exposure is confirmed and vaccine is available, continue prophylaxis for 4 weeks and until 3 doses of vaccine have been given or for 30–60 days if vaccine is unavailable.

TABLETS, EXTENDED-RELEASE

Tonsillitis and/or pharyngitis secondary to S. pyogenes.

Adults and children 12 years and older: 775 mg (1 extended-release tablet) daily for 10 days taken within 1 hr of finishing a meal. Ensure completion of the 10-day course of therapy.

NURSING IMPLICATIONS

IMPLEMENTATION/ADMINISTRATION/STORAGE

1. Child's dose should not exceed maximum adult dose.

A

2. Clients with GFR of 10–30 mL/min should receive 250 or 500 mg q 12 hr, depending on severity of infection. Those with GFR <10 mL/min should receive 250 or 500 mg q 24 hr, depending on infection severity. Those on hemodialysis should receive 250 or 500 mg q 24 hr, depending on infection severity; should receive an additional dose both during and at end of dialysis.
3. The recommended upper dose of amoxicillin in neonates and infants 12 weeks of age and younger is 30 mg/kg/day divided every 12 hours.
4. Dry powder stable at room temperature for 18–30 months; reconstituted suspension stable 1 week at room temperature and 2 weeks at 2–8°C (36–46°F).
5. Discard any unused portion of the reconstituted suspension after 14 days. Refrigeration is preferable, but not required.

ASSESSMENT

1. List reasons for therapy; C&S results. Note onset, symptoms, severity, location, other associated factors. Monitor and assess clinical response during therapy.
2. Some forms may contain phenylalanine; assess for phenylketonuria.
3. Note previous reactions to penicillins, cephalosporins, or other antibiotics.
4. Infections caused by *S. pyogenes* require 10 days of treatment to prevent acute rheumatic fever.
5. With gonorrhea treatment, obtain serologic test for syphilis at the time of treatment, and repeat this test after 3 months.
6. Obtain/monitor VS, CBC, cultures, renal and LFTs. Avoid or reduce dose with renal dysfunction.

CLIENT/FAMILY TEACHING

1. Capsules, chewable tablets, and oral suspension may be taken without regard to meals except Moxatag; take with meals.
2. Take entire prescription; don't stop if feeling better; creates antibiotic resistance. Works best on empty stomach but may be taken with food if GI upset.
3. For school-age child, space evenly over 24 hr period; give before school, upon arrival home, and at bedtime.
4. Chewable tablets available for children; may be taken with food.
5. If using tablet for oral suspension (DisperMox), mix 1 tablet in about 10 mL of water. Drink entire mixture, rinse with small amount of water, and drink contents to ensure entire dose is taken. Do not chew or swallow tablets.
6. Place drops directly on child's tongue to swallow. May add to formula, milk, fruit juice, water, ginger ale, or cold drinks; must take immediately and consume completely.
7. Ensure adequate hydration; consume 2–3 L/day of fluids.
8. Use additional form of birth control during therapy if taking oral contraceptives.
9. Report any difficulty breathing, increased bruising/bleeding, sore throat, rash, diarrhea, worsening of symptoms, or lack of response.
10. Keep all F/U to assess response, cultures, and adverse SE.

OUTCOMES/EVALUATE

- Resolution of infection; symptomatic improvement
- Therapeutic peak serum drug levels (4–11 mcg/mL)

Combination Drug

Amoxicillin and Potassium clavulanate

(ah-mox-ih-**SILL**-in, poh-**TASS**-ee-um klav-you-**LAN**-ayt)

Classification(s): Antibiotic, penicillin

Pregnancy Category: B

RX: Amoclan, Augmentin, Augmentin ES-600, Augmentin XR.

🍁 **Rx:** Apo-Amoxi-Clav, Clavulin, ratio-Aclavulanate.

SEE ALSO ***ANTI-INFECTIVE DRUGS*** AND ***PENICILLINS***.

INDICATIONS/USES

Amoxicillin/Clavulanate Potassium Oral Suspension (Amoclan, Augmentin), Tablets (Augmentin), and Chewable Tablets (Augmentin). For beta-lactamase-producing strains of the following organisms: (1) Lower respiratory tract infections, otitis media, and sinusitis caused by *Haemophilus influenzae* and *Moraxella catarrhalis*. (2) Skin and skin structure infections caused by

Staphylococcus aureus, Escherichia coli, and *Klebsiella* species. (3) UTI caused by *E. coli, Klebsiella* species, and *Enterobacter* species.

Amoxicillin/Clavulanate Potassium Oral Suspension (Augmentin ES-600). Recurrent or persistent acute otitis media in pediatric clients due to *Streptococcus pneumoniae* (penicillin MICs less than or equal to 2 mcg/mL), *H. influenzae* (including beta-lactamase-producing strains), or *M. catarrhalis* (including beta-lactamase-producing strains) characterized by the following risk factors: Antibiotic exposure for acute otitis media within the preceding 3 months and **either** 2 years of age or younger or day-care attendance. Do not use Augmentin ES-600 to treat acute otitis media due to *S. pneumoniae* with penicillin MIC at least 4 mcg/mL.

Amoxicillin/Clavulanate Potassium Extended-Release Tablets (Augmentin XR). Community-acquired pneumonia or acute bacterial sinusitis due to confirmed or suspected beta-lactamase-producing pathogens, including *H. influenzae, M. catarrhalis, Haemophilus parainfluenzae, Klebsiella pneumoniae,* methicillin-susceptible *S. aureus,* or *S. pneumoniae* with reduced susceptibility to penicillin. Do not use to treat *S. pneumoniae* with penicillin MIC of 4 mcg/mL or more.

NOTE: Mixed infections caused by ampicillin-susceptible organisms and beta-lactamase-producing organisms susceptible to amoxicillin/clavulanate should not require an additional antibiotic.

CONTENT

Powder for Oral Suspension: '125' Powder for Oral Suspension: 125 mg amoxicillin and 31.25 mg potassium clavulanate/5 mL. *'200' Powder for Oral Suspension:* 200 mg amoxicillin and 28.5 mg potassium clavulanate/5 mL. *'400' Powder for Oral Suspension:* 400 mg amoxicillin and 57 mg potassium clavulanate/5 mL; *Augmentin ES-600:* 600 mg amoxicillin and 42.9 mg clavulanic acid/5 mL. All strengths are after reconstitution.

Tablets: '250' Tablet: 250 mg amoxicillin and 125 mg potassium clavulanate. *'500' Tablet:* 500 mg amoxicillin and 125 mg potassium clavulanate. *'875' Tablet:* 875 mg amoxicillin and 125 mg potassium clavulanate. *'200' Chewable Tablet:* 200 mg amoxicillin and 28.5 mg potassium clavulanate. *'400' Chewable Tablet:* 400 mg amoxicillin and 57 mg potassium clavulanate.

Tablets, Extended-Release: 1,000 mg amoxicillin and 62.5 mg potassium clavulanate.

ACTION/KINETICS

Action

For details, see *Amoxicillin*. Potassium clavulanate inactivates lactamase enzymes, which are responsible for resistance to penicillins. Effective against microorganisms that have manifested resistance to amoxicillin.

Pharmacokinetics

For potassium clavulanate: **Peak serum levels:** 1–2 hr. **t½:** 1 hr.

CONTRAINDICATIONS

Use in those with a history of amoxicillin/clavulanate potassium-associated cholestatic jaundice or hepatic dysfunction. Use of Augmentin XR in severe renal impairment (C_{CR} less than 30 mL/min) and in hemodialysis clients.

SPECIAL CONCERNS

- **The effect of oral contraceptives may be decreased.**
- **Use with caution in hepatic dysfunction.**
- **Safety and efficacy of Augmentin XR not established in children less than 16 years of age.**

SIDE EFFECTS

Most Common

Hypersensitivity, N&V, gastritis, stomatitis.

See *Amoxicillin* and *Penicillins* for a complete list of possible side effects.

HOW SUPPLIED

See *Content.*

DOSAGE

Augmentin

ORAL SUSPENSION (STANDARD); TABLETS; TABLETS, CHEWABLE

Susceptible infections.

Adults, usual and children over 40 kg: One 500 mg tablet q 12 hr or one 250 mg tablet q 8 hr. For more severe infections or infections of the respiratory tract, give one 875 mg tablet q 12 hr or one 500 mg tablet q 8 hr. Adults unable to take tablets can be given the 125 mg/5 mL or the 250 mg/5 mL suspension in place of the 500 mg tablet or the 200 mg/5 mL or 400 mg/5 mL suspension can be given in place of the 875 mg tablet. **Children less than 3**

months old: 30 mg/kg/day amoxicillin in divided doses q 12 hr. Use of the 125 mg/5 mL suspension is recommended. **Children over 3 months old:** 200 mg/5 mL or 400 mg/5 mL q 12 hr. Or, 125 mg/5 mL or 250 mg/5 mL q 8 hr for otitis media, sinusitis, lower respiratory tract infections, or severe infections. For less severe infections the dose is 25 mg/kg/day (200 mg/5 mL or 400 mg/5 mL q 12 hr) or 20 mg/kg/day (125 mg/5 mL or 250 mg/5 mL q 8 hr).

Recurrent or persistent acute otitis media, sinusitis, lower respiratory tract infections, severe infections in children 3 months and older.

45 mg/kg/day of amoxicillin in divided doses q 12 hr or 40 mg/kg/day amoxicillin in divided doses q 8 hr. For less severe infections, use 25 mg/kg/day in divided doses q 12 hr or 20 mg/kg/day in divided doses q 8 hr.

Respiratory tract and severe infections.

Adults: One 875-mg tablet q 12 hr or one 500-mg tablet q 8 hr.

Augmentin ES-600

ORAL SUSPENSION

Recurrent or persistent acute otitis media in children.

Children, 3 months and older: 90 mg/kg/day amoxicillin in divided doses q 12 hr for 10 days. Experience is not available for pediatric clients weighing more than 40 kg or for adults.

Augmentin XR

TABLETS, EXTENDED-RELEASE

Acute bacterial sinusitis.

Adults: 2 tablets (2 grams amoxicillin) q 12 hr for 10 days. Do not use extended-release tablets in children less than 16 years of age.

Community-acquired pneumonia.

Adults: 2 tablets (2 grams amoxicillin) q 12 hr for 7–10 days. Do not use the extended-release tablets in children less than 16 years of age.

NURSING IMPLICATIONS

IMPLEMENTATION/ADMINISTRATION/STORAGE

1. Both 250 mg and 500 mg tablets contain 125 mg clavulanic acid; therefore, two 250 mg tablets are not the same as one 500 mg tablet. The 250 mg tablet and the 250 mg chewable tablet do not contain the same amount of potassium clavulanate and are thus not interchangeable. The 250 mg tablet should not be used until children are over 40 kg.
2. Two Augmentin 500 mg tablets are not equivalent to one Augmentin XR tablet, because Augmentin XR contains 62.5 mg clavulanic acid while each Augmentin 500 mg tablet contains 125 mg clavulanic acid. The XR tablet provides an extended time course of plasma amoxicillin levels compared with the immediate-release tablets.
3. Amoxicillin/Clavulanate potassium ES-600 suspension, 600 mg/5 mL, does not contain the same amount of clavulanic acid (as the potassium salt) as any of the other amoxicillin/clavulanate potassium suspensions. Therefore, do not substitute the ES-600 for other dosage forms as they are not interchangeable.
4. Pediatric formulations are available in fruit flavors for oral suspension and chewable tablets. These formulations allow twice-daily dosing—more convenient than 3 times daily dosing, and incidence of diarrhea is significantly reduced.
5. The 200 and 400 mg suspensions and chewable tablets contain aspartame; do not use with phenylketonuria.
6. For adults who have difficulty swallowing, do not give the ES-600 suspension in place of the 500 or 875 mg tablets

ASSESSMENT

1. List reasons for therapy; C&S results. Note onset, symptoms, severity, location, other associated factors. Assess clinical response during therapy.
2. Note previous reactions to penicillins, cephalosporins, or other antibiotics.
3. Avoid with C_{CR} less than 30 mL/min and in hemodialysis patients.

4. Monitor VS, cultures, CBC, renal and LFTs. May need to reduce dose with severe liver/renal dysfunction.

CLIENT/FAMILY TEACHING

1. Take as directed; complete entire prescription.
2. May take without regard for meals; absorption of potassium clavulanate enhanced if taken just before a meal. To lessen stomach upset, take with food.
3. Do not chew or crush; swallow tablets whole. Consume increased fluids to ensure adequate hydration.
4. Report side effects, i.e., rash, persistent diarrhea, lack of response, worsening of symptoms after 48–72 hr.
5. Refrigerate reconstituted suspension; discard after 10 days.
6. With oral contraceptives, use additional contraception during treatment.
7. Keep all F/U visits to assess response and adverse SE.

OUTCOMES/EVALUATE

Resolution of infection; symptomatic improvement

Amphetamine mixtures

(am-**FET**-ah-meen)

Classification(s): CNS stimulant

Pregnancy Category: C

RX: Adderall, Adderall XR, Amphetamine Salt Combo, **C-II**

SEE ALSO ***AMPHETAMINES AND DERIVATIVES***.

INDICATIONS/USES

(1) As a part of a total treatment program (including psychological, educational, social aspects) to stabilize adults and children 3 years and older with attention deficit/hyperactivity disorder (ADHD). Use with the following symptoms: Moderate to severe distractibility, short attention span, hyperactivity, emotional lability, and impulsivity. Learning disability and abnormal EEG may or may not be present; a diagnosis of CNS dysfunction may or may not be warranted. (2) Narcolepsy in adults and children over 6 years of age (use tablets).

ACTION/KINETICS

Action

Thought to act on the cerebral cortex and reticular activating system by releasing norepinephrine from central adrenergic neurons. Adderall or Adderall XR contain equal amounts of dextroamphetamine sulfate, dextroamphetamine saccharate, amphetamine sulfate, and amphetamine aspartate monohydrate in each dosage form.

Pharmacokinetics

Completely absorbed in 3 hr. **Peak effects:** 2–3 hr. **Duration:** 4–24 hr. **Therapeutic blood levels:** 5–10 mcg/dL. **t½, if urine pH is 5.6 or less:** 7–8 hr; **t½, if urine pH is alkaline:** 18.6–33.6 hr. For every one unit increase in urinary pH, there is an average 7 hr increase in plasma t½. Metabolized in the liver and excreted in urine.

ADDITIONAL CONTRAINDICATIONS

Fatalities have occurred following concurrent use of MAOIs (e.g., isocarboxazid, phenelzine, selegiline, tranylcypromine, rasagiline) and amphetamine. At least 2 weeks should elapse between the use of any MAOI and any CNS stimulant, including amphetamine.

CONTRAINDICATIONS

Use in children less than 3 years of age for attention deficit disorders, in children less than 6 years of age for narcolepsy, or in children or adults with a structural cardiac abnormality due to the possibility of sudden death. Use as an appetite suppressant.

SPECIAL CONCERNS

Amphetamines have a high potential for abuse. Administration of amphetamines for prolonged periods of time may lead to drug dependence and must be avoided. Particular attention should be paid to the possibility of subjects obtaining amphetamines for nontherapeutic use or distribution to others, and the drugs should be prescribed or dispensed sparingly.

- Extended-release amphetamine has not been studied in children less than 6 years of age.
- NOTE: Adderall XR has been removed from the Canadian market due to concerns about sudden deaths, heart-related deaths, and strokes in children and adults taking recommended doses.

SIDE EFFECTS

Most Common

Decreased appetite, upset stomach, insomnia, increased anxiety, irritability.

See *Amphetamine and Derivatives* for a complete list of possible side effects.

HOW SUPPLIED

Capsules, Extended-Release: 5 mg, 10 mg, 15 mg, 20 mg, 25 mg, 30 mg; ***Tablets:*** 5 mg, 7.5 mg, 10 mg, 12.5 mg, 15 mg, 20 mg, 30 mg.

DOSAGE

CAPSULES, EXTENDED-RELEASE

Attention deficit/hyperactivity disorder.

Adults and children 6 years and older, initial: 10 mg once daily in the morning if starting treatment for the first time or switching from another medication. Daily dosage may be increased in increments of 10 mg at weekly intervals. **Maximum dose:** 30 mg/day.

TABLETS

Attention deficit/hyperactivity disorder.

Adults and children 6 years and older, initial: 5 mg once or twice a day. Daily dosage may be increased in increments of 5 mg at weekly intervals until optimum response is reached. **Maximum dose:** 40 mg/day. **Children, 3–5 years of age, initial:** 2.5 mg/day. Daily dosage may be increased in increments of 2.5 mg at weekly intervals until optimum response is reached.

Narcolepsy.

Adults and children age 12 and older, initial: 10 mg/day. Daily dosage may be increased in increments of 10 mg at weekly intervals until optimum response is reached. If bothersome side effects occur (e.g., anorexia, insomnia), reduce the dose. **Usual dose range:** 5–60 mg/day in divided doses, depending on client response. *NOTE:* Narcolepsy rarely occurs in children less than 12 years of age. If it does occur, dextroamphetamine sulfate may be used, starting with a dose of 5 mg/day and increasing in increments of 5 mg at weekly intervals until optimum response is reached.

NURSING IMPLICATIONS

IMPLEMENTATION/ADMINISTRATION/STORAGE

1. Administer the lowest effective dose; determine dosage individually. Avoid late evening doses to prevent insomnia.
2. Take extended-release capsules whole or sprinkle contents on applesauce. If applesauce used, take immediately (do not store). Do not chew applesauce sprinkled with amphetamine beads.
3. Take extended-release capsules and tablets upon awakening. For tablets, give additional doses (1 or 2) at intervals of 4–6 hr. Avoid afternoon doses R/T possibility of insomnia.
4. Clients taking divided doses of immediate-release amphetamine (e.g., twice a day) may be switched to amphetamine extended-release at the same total daily dose taken once a day. Titrate at weekly intervals to appropriate dosage levels.
5. When possible, interrupt therapy occasionally to determine the need for continued therapy.
6. Store from 15–30°C (59–86°F) in light-resistant containers.

ASSESSMENT

1. Document symptom type, onset, pretreatment findings, and/or educational testing results. Note clinical presentation.
2. Review CNS/neurologic/cardiac status before starting therapy.
3. Determine if pregnant. Note any evidence of psychiatric disorders, seizures, thyroid disease, tics, alcohol or drug problems.
4. Monitor ht/Wt, HR, BP, ECG; assess CBC, chemistry profile, TSH, urinalysis, and ECG.

CLIENT/FAMILY TEACHING

1. For attention deficit disorders (ADD) or narcolepsy, give the first dose on awakening with additional one or two doses given at intervals of 4–6 hr. Give the last dose 6 hr before bedtime. Extended-release product administered once daily upon awakening. The correct dose must be given at the right time; never give doses more than 2 hours late, unless told otherwise by the provider. Never double doses. It

is safer for a child to skip a dose than inadvertantly be given two doses.

2. Take with water; do not take with milk, juice, or antacids. Fruit juices and vitamin C intake may decrease drug absorption.
3. Extended-release capsules may be taken whole or the capsule opened and the contents sprinkled on applesauce. If sprinkled on applesauce, consume immediately, without chewing. Do not divide the dose of a single capsule.
4. May impair reactions; use care with activities such as driving or activities that requires alertness until drug effects realized. After stimulant effects have worn off, drowsiness, trembling, unusual tiredness or weakness, or mental depression may occur.
5. Report changes in mood or affect, including S&S of impaired thinking. Also report headaches, extremity weakness or chest pain/SOB immediately.
6. Do not use caffeine/caffeine-containing products. Avoid OTC preparations containing caffeine or other stimulants.
7. Keep weight records; report excessive loss. Store safely; has potential for abuse.
8. Drink 2.5 L/day; increase intake of high-fiber foods/fruits to decrease constipation.
9. Chew sugarless gum/candies and rinse mouth frequently with nonalcoholic mouth rinses for dry mouth.
10. Children receiving amphetamines may have growth retarded. Drug should periodically be discontinued (i.e., during the summer) by provider to allow growth to proceed normally and to evaluate need for continued drug therapy.
11. Keep all F/U to assess response, dose adequacy, and for adverse SE.

OUTCOMES/EVALUATE

- Improved attention span/concentration/grades
- ↓ Episodes of narcolepsy

IV

Amphotericin B desoxycholate

(am-foe-**TER**-ih-sin)

Classification(s): Antibiotic, antifungal

Pregnancy Category: B

SEE ALSO ***ANTI-INFECTIVE DRUGS.***

INDICATIONS/USES

Drug is toxic; used mainly for clients with progressive and potentially fatal fungal infections. **Parenteral:** (1) Systemic, potentially fatal life-threatening invasive fungal infections, including aspergillosis; cryptococcosis; North American blastomycosis; systemic candidiasis; coccidiodomycosis; histoplasmosis; sporotrichosis; zygomycosis including mucormycosis caused by susceptible species of the genera *Mucor, Rhizopus,* and *Absidia* species. (2) Infections due to susceptible species of *Conidiobolus* and *Basidiobolus.*
(3) Secondary therapy to treat American mucocutaneous leishmaniasis. *Investigational:* Prophylaxis of fungal infection in bone marrow transplantation; treatment of primary amoebic meningoencephalitis due to *Naegleria fowleri;* subconjunctival or intravitreal injection in ocular aspergillosis; chemoprophylaxis for low dose IV, intranasal, or nebulized administration in immunocompromised clients at risk of aspergillosis; intrathecally in severe meningitis unresponsive to IV therapy; intra-articularly or IM for coccidioidal arthritis.

ACTION/KINETICS

Action

Binds to sterols in the cell membrane causing a change in membrane permeability leading to leakage of a variety of intracellular components. Fungistatic or fungicidal depending on the level of drug in body fluids and susceptibility of the fungus. Can also bind to cholesterol in the mammalian cell leading to cytotoxicity.

Pharmacokinetics

Peak plasma levels: 0.5–2 mcg/mL. **t½, initial:** 24 hr; **second phase:** 15 days. Slowly excreted (weeks to months) by the kidneys. Kinetics differ in adults and children. **Plasma protein binding:** >90%.

CONTRAINDICATIONS

Hypersensitivity to drug unless the condition is life-threatening and amenable only to amphotericin B therapy. Use to treat noninvasive forms of fungal disease such as oral thrush, vaginal candidiasis, and esophageal candidiasis in clients with normal neutrophil counts. Lactation. Avoid rapid IV infusion due to possible hypotension, hypokalemia, arrhythmias, and shock.

A

SPECIAL CONCERNS

■ (1) Use primarily for treatment of clients with progressive and potentially fatal fungal infections. It should not be used to treat noninvasive forms of fungal disease such as oral thrush, vaginal candidiasis, and esophageal candidiasis in clients with normal neutrophil counts. (2) Exercise caution to prevent inadvertent overdose with amphotericin B. Verify the product name and dosage if dose exceeds 1.5 mg/kg. ■

- **The bone marrow depressant effects may result in increased incidence of microbial infection, delayed healing, and gingival bleeding.**
- **Although used in children, safety and efficacy have not been determined.**
- **Use with caution in clients receiving leukocyte transfusions; separate administration of each as much as possible.**
- **Use with caution in reduced renal function.**

SIDE EFFECTS

Most Common

Hypotension, headache, epigastric pain, normocytic anemia, muscle/joint pain, tachypnea.

GI: Anorexia, N&V, diarrhea, dyspepsia, cramping, epigastric pain, acute liver failure, hepatitis, melena, jaundice, hemorrhagic gastroenteritis. **CNS:** Headache, ***convulsions,*** vertigo (transient), peripheral neuropathy, encephalopathy, leukoencephalopathy, other neurologic symptoms. **CV:** Hypotension, ***cardiac arrest, cardiac failure, ventricular fibrillation***, arrhythmias, hypertension. **Respiratory:** Tachypnea, ***shock***, pulmonary edema, hypersensitivity pneumonitis, dyspnea. **Dermatologic:** Rash especially maculopapular, flushing, pruritus. **Hematologic:** Normochromic anemia, normocytic anemia (most common), ***agranulocytosis***, coagulation defects, thrombocytopenia, leukopenia, eosinophilia, leukocytosis. **GU:** Decreased renal function, azotemia, hyposthenuria, renal tubular acidosis, nephrocalcinosis, acute renal failure, anuria, oliguria. **Allergic:** Bronchospasm, wheezing, ***anaphylactoid*** and other allergic reactions. **Infusion reactions:** Fever, shaking, chills, hypotension, anorexia, N&V, headache, tachypnea all within 1–3 hr after starting an IV infusion. Extravasation may cause chemical irritation. **Ophthalmic:** Visual impairment, diplopia. **Ophthalmic:** Visual impairment, diplopia. **Otic:** Tinnitus, hearing loss. **Miscellaneous:** Fever (with chills, shaking) occurring within 15 to 20 min after starting treatment, malaise, weight loss, pain at injection site (with or without phlebitis or thrombophlebitis), generalized pain (including muscle and joint pain), ***anaphylaxis.***

LABORATORY TEST CONSIDERATIONS

↑ AST, ALT, GGT, LDH, alkaline phosphatase, serum creatinine, BUN, bilirubin. Hypomagnesemia, hyperkalemia, hypokalemia, hypercalcemia, hypocalcemia, acidosis, hypoglycemia, hyperglycemia, hyperamylasemia, hyperuricemia, hypophosphatemia. Abnormal serum electrolytes, liver function, renal function.

OVERDOSE MANAGEMENT

Symptoms: Cardiopulmonary arrest. *Treatment:* Discontinue therapy, monitor clinical status, and provide supportive therapy.

DRUG INTERACTIONS

Aminoglycosides / Additive nephrotoxicity and/or ototoxicity

Antineoplastic drugs / ↑ Risk for renal toxicity, bronchospasm, and hypotension

Azole antifungals / ↑ Risk of fungal resistance to amphotericin B; administer with caution, especially in immunocompromised clients

Corticosteroids, Corticotropin / ↑ Risk of hypokalemia → cardiac dysfunction; do use together unless needed to control side effects

Cyclosporine / ↑ Risk of renal toxicity

Digitalis glycosides / ↑ Risk of hypokalemia → ↑ incidence of digitalis toxicity

Flucytosine / ↑ Risk of flucytosine toxicity due to ↑ cellular uptake or ↓ renal excretion

Foscarnet / ↑ Risk of renal toxicity due to additive or synergistic effects; if used together, use aggressive hydration and close monitoring

Leukocyte transfusions / Acute pulmonary toxicity; do not coadminister

Nephrotoxic drugs (e.g., aminoglycosides, pentamidine) / ↑ Risk of nephrotoxicity; use caution if used together

Skeletal muscle relaxants, surgical (e.g., succinylcholine, d-tubocurarine) / ↑ Muscle relaxation due to amphotericin B-induced hypokalemia; monitor serum K levels closely

Thiazides / ↑ Electrolyte depletion, especially potassium; monitor levels

Zidovudine / Possible ↑ risk of myelotoxicity and nephrotoxicity

HOW SUPPLIED

Powder for Injection: 50 mg (as desoxycholate).

DOSAGE

IV

Test dose by slow IV infusion.

Single dose: 1 mg in 20 mL of D5W injection should be infused over 20 to 30 min to determine tolerance. Record client's temperature, pulse, respiration, and BP q 30 min for 2–4 hr.

Life-threatening fungal infections.

Adults, initial: 0.25 mg/kg/day in those with good cardio-renal function and a well-tolerated test dose. In those with severe and rapidly progressing fungal infections, therapy may be initiated with a daily dose of 0.3 mg/kg body weight. In clients with impaired cardio-renal function or a severe reaction to the test dose, initiate therapy with a smaller daily doses (e.g., 5–10 mg). **Maintenance:** Depending on the cardio-renal status, the dose may be increased gradually by 5–10 mg/day to a final daily dosage of 0.5–0.7 mg/kg. For clients with a C_{CR} <10 mL/min, the dosage should be 0.5–0.7 mg/kg q 24–48 hr. **Maximum dose:** 1.5 mg/kg/day. The total daily dose may range up to 1 mg/kg/day or up to 1.5 mg/kg/day when given on alternate days. *NOTE:* Amphotericin overdoses may cause cardiorespiratory arrest.

Dosage for treatment of the following infections:**Aspergillosis:** Amphotericin B IV has been given for up to 11 months with a total dose up to 3.6 grams.

Rhinocerebral phycomycosis: A cumulative dose of at least 3 grams is recommended. Although a total dose of 3–4 grams will infrequently cause permanent renal impairment, this is a reasonable minimum if there is clinical evidence of invasion of deep tissue.

Sporotrichosis: Dosage has ranged up to 9 months with a total dose of 2.5 grams.

Adults receiving continuous renal replacement therapy.

Adults: 0.5–1 mg/kg IV q 24 hr for clients receiving continuous venovenous hemofiltration, continuous venovenous hemodialysis, or continuous venovenous hemodiafiltration. *NOTE:* This dosage assumes ultrafiltration and dialysis flow rates of 1–2 liters/hr.

Adults receiving intermittent hemodialysis.

Adults: 0.5–1 mg/kg IV q 24 hr given after the dialysis session. This recommendation assumes the client is receiving standard intermittent hemodialysis 3 times/week and completes the full dialysis session.

NURSING IMPLICATIONS

Do not confuse amphotericin B desoxycholate with amphotericin B lipid-based.

IMPLEMENTATION/ADMINISTRATION/STORAGE

1. **IV** Client tolerance varies greatly. Thus, individualize dosage based on client clinical status, including site and severity of infection, etiologic agent, and cardio-renal function. Give a test dose prior to administration.
2. Infusion reactions (see *Side Effects*) are common 1–3 hr after starting an IV infusion. These reactions are usually more severe with the first few doses but usually diminish with subsequent doses.
3. The following approaches may decrease severe side effects:
   - Give aspirin, acetaminophen, antihistamines, and antiemetics before infusion and maintain sodium balance.
   - Give on alternate days to decrease anorexia and phlebitis.
   - Small doses of IV corticosteroids before infusion may decrease febrile reactions; keep steroid administration to a minimum.
   - Adding a small amount of heparin (500–2,000 units) to infusion, removing the needle after infusion, rotating the infusion sites, giving through a large central vein, and using a pediatric scalp-vein may

A

decrease the incidence of thrombophlebitis.
- Meperidine, 25–50 mg IV, may decrease duration of shaking, chills, and fever that may occur.
- Hydration and sodium repletion prior to administration may reduce the risk of nephrotoxicity.

4. Separate leukocyte transfusions as far as possible from administration of IV amphotericin. Monitor pulmonary function.
5. *Preparation of amphotericin B desoxycholate:* To obtain initial concentration of 5 mg/mL, rapidly inject 10 mL sterile water (without a bacteriostatic agent) directly into lyophilized cake, using a sterile 20-gauge needle. Shake vial immediately until colloidal solution clear. To obtain infusion solution of 0.1 mg/mL, further dilute 1:50 with D5W with a pH of 4.2 or above.
6. Determine pH of each container of dextrose injection before use (pH usually >4.2). If pH <4.2, add 1 or 2 mL of buffer to dextrose injection before used to dilute concentrated amphotericin B solution. Preferred buffer is dibasic sodium phosphate (anhydrous), 1.59 grams; monobasic sodium phosphate (anhydrous), 0.96 gram; and water for injection which is diluted to 100 mL. Sterilize buffer before adding to dextrose injection. Sterilize either by filtration through a bacterial retentive stone, mat, or membrane or by autoclaving for 30 min at 15 lb pressure and 121°C (249.8°F).
7. Strict aseptic technique must be used in preparation; contains no bacteriostatic agent.
8. Do not use the initial concentrate or the infusion solution if there is any precipitation of foreign matter in either solution.
9. If given through an existing IV line, flush with D5W prior to and after infusion. Do not use initial concentrate if any precipitate is present. An inline filter may be used for IV infusion; however, the mean pore diameter of the filter should not be less than 1 micron in order to ensure passage of the antibiotic dispersion.
10. Administer by slow IV infusion given over a period of 2–6 hr. Rapid IV administration may cause hypotension, hypokalemia, arrhythmias, and shock.
11. Protect from light during administration. Loss of drug activity during administration is likely negligible if the solution is exposed for 8 hr or less.
12. Initiate therapy in the most distal veins. When administered peripherally, changing sites with each dose may decrease phlebitis.
13. If therapy is interrupted for 7 days or more, resume therapy starting with the lowest dosage level (e.g., 0.25 mg/kg body weight) and increase gradually (see *Dosage*).
14. Before reconstitution, vials should be refrigerated and protected from light. After reconstitution concentrate may be stored in the dark at room temperature for 24 hr or under refrigeration for 1 week with minimal loss of potency and clarity. Discard any unused solution. Use diluted solutions promptly after preparation. Protect from light during administration.
15. COMPATIBILITY Sterile water, D5W.
16. INCOMPATIBILITY DO NOT dilute or reconstitute with saline solution or mix with other drugs or electrolytes.

ASSESSMENT

1. Note indications for therapy, clinical presentation, any allergy to amphotericin B, adverse effects, or hypersensitivity reactions. Drug is toxic, not for use with non-invasive forms of fungal disease with normal neutrophil counts.
2. Obtain cultures and/or histologic studies prior to systemic therapy.
3. Note mental status and age.
4. Describe characteristics of any severe systemic infections/lesions requiring therapy. Different organisms require different lengths of treatment, i.e., sporotrichosis may require 9 months of IV therapy, whereas topical lesions may require only 2–4 weeks.
5. Ensure correct drug form prepared for administration; IV form in D5W only.
6. Note results of 1-mg test dose (1 mg in 20 mL D5W over 20–30 min).
7. Premedicate with antipyretics, antihistamines, corticosteroids, and/or antiemetic drugs to reduce side effects. Rashes, fevers, and chills may occur.
8. Infuse slowly, monitor VS every 15–30 min during first dose; interrupt infusion for adverse effects. Monitor pulmonary function.
9. Monitor I&O; report change in output; cloudy urine. Hydration and sodium repletion prior to

administration may reduce the risk of nephrotoxicity.

10. Weigh twice weekly; assess for malnutrition/dehydration.
11. List drugs prescribed; ensure none interact unfavorably.
12. Anticipate hypokalemia with digoxin therapy. Observe for toxicity and muscle weakness, and monitor digoxin and potassium levels.
13. With impaired cardio-renal function, interruption of therapy for 7 days or more, or severe reactions to test dose, start therapy with lower daily doses.
14. Monitor VS, ECG, CBC, K^+, Mg^{++}, renal and LFTs, and cultures during therapy. Stop therapy; report any adverse effects. Monitor for bleeding.

CLIENT/FAMILY TEACHING

1. GI effects reduced by antihistamine or antiemetic drug before therapy and taking drug before mealtime. Try small frequent meals if diarrhea occurs.
2. Report anorexia, N&V, headache, rashes, fever, chills or other adverse effects.
3. Consume 2.5 L/day of fluids to prevent toxic kidney effects. Report decrease in I&O, extreme weight loss.
4. Therapy usually requires long-term treatments (6–11 weeks) to ensure adequate response and to prevent relapse.
5. Report neurologic S&S such as ringing in ears, blurred vision, or dizziness as well as fever, chills, difficulty breathing or swallowing, or malaise.
6. Keep all F/U to assess response, labs, for adverse SE.

OUTCOMES/EVALUATE

- Resolution of fungal infection
- Reduction in number of skin lesions
- Symptomatic improvement

IV

Amphotericin B lipid-based

Classification(s): Antibiotic, antifungal

Pregnancy Category: B

RX: Abelcet, AmBisome.

SEE ALSO ***ANTI-INFECTIVE DRUGS*** AND ***AMPHOTERICIN B DESOXYCHOLATE.***

INDICATIONS/USES

Drug is toxic; use mainly for clients with progressive and potentially fatal fungal infections. Lipid products decrease the severe renal toxicity of amphotericin B and are indicated for use in clients with renal impairment when amphotericin B can not or should not be used.

(1) **Abelcet:** Systemic invasive fungal infections in those refractory to conventional amphotericin B desoxycholate therapy. Is used in adults, children, and the elderly. *Investigational:* (a) Prophylaxis of fungal infections in those with bone marrow transplantation. (b) Treatment of primary amoebic meningoencephalitis due to *Naegleria fowler.* (c) Subconjunctival or intravitreal injection in ocular aspergillosis. (d) Chemoprophylaxis by low-dose IV, intranasal, or nebulized administration in immunocompromised clients at risk of aspergillosis. (e) Intra-articularly or IM for coccidioidal arthritis. (f) Empiric treatment of fungal infections. (g) Treatment of visceral leishmaniasis.

(2) **AmBisome:** Treatment of infections due to *Aspergillus, Candida,* or *Cryptococcus* in those refractory to conventional amphotericin B desoxycholate or when renal impairment or unacceptable toxicity precludes use; empirical treatment in febrile, neutropenic clients with presumed fungal infection; cryptococcal meningitis in HIV-infected clients; visceral leishmaniasis. *Investigational:* See (a) to (e) above.

ACTION/KINETICS

Action

See *Amphotericin B desoxycholate.*

Pharmacokinetics

Lipid-based products increase the circulation time and alter the biodistribution of amphotericin. Since lipid-based drugs stay in the circulation longer, they can localize and attain higher concentrations in areas with increased capillary permeability (e.g., inflammation, infection, solid tumors). Importantly, the two amphotericin lipid-based products have different physical and chemical properties that affect their use, pharmacokinetic properties, and side effects. Each of the products has a long terminal t½ and varies depending on the product (mean t½ about 100–153 hr hr for AmBisome and about 173.4 hr for Abelcet).

A

CONTRAINDICATIONS

See *Amphotericin B desoxycholate.*

SPECIAL CONCERNS

> Use primarily for progressive and potentially fatal fungal infections. Not used to treat noninvasive fungal disease, including oral thrush, vaginal candidiasis, and esophageal candidiasis in clients with normal neutrophil counts.

- Use with caution in impaired renal function.
- Carefully monitor elderly clients.
- Amphotericin B liposome (Ambisome) is significantly less toxic than amphotericin B desoxycholate; however, side effects may still occur.

SIDE EFFECTS

Most Common

Chills, fever, hypotension, tachycardia, N&V, dyspnea.

- **Common to all products**

CV: Hypotension, hypertension, ***cardiac arrest***, chest pain, tachycardia. **GI:** N&V, diarrhea, abdominal pain, ***GI hemorrhage***. **CNS:** Headache, anxiety, confusion, insomnia, leukoencephalopathy. **Respiratory:** ***Respiratory failure***, dyspnea, respiratory disorder, hypoxia, increased cough, epistaxis, lung disorder, pleural effusion, rhinitis. **Hematologic:** Thrombocytopenia, anemia, leukopenia. **Dermatologic:** Rash, pruritus, sweating. **GU:** Hematuria, kidney failure. **Infusion reactions:** Fever, shaking, chills, rigors, hypotension, anorexia, N&V, headache, tachypnea. **Body as a whole:** Chills, rigors, fever, infection, pain, asthenia. **Miscellaneous:** ***Multiple organ failure, sepsis, anaphylactic reaction***, back pain.

- **Reported for Abelcet**

CV: ***Cardiac failure, MI, cardiomyopathy, CVA***, thrombophlebitis, arrhythmias, including ***ventricular fibrillation***. **GI:** Melena, dyspepsia, cramping, epigastric pain. **CNS:** Convulsions, peripheral neuropathy, transient vertigo, encephalopathy, extrapyramidal syndrome, and other neurologic symptoms. **Hematologic:** Coagulation defects, leukocytosis, eosinophilia. **GU:** Oliguria, decreased renal function, kidney failure, anuria, renal tubular acidosis, impotence, dysuria. **Respiratory:** Bronchospasm, wheezing, asthma, pulmonary edema, hemoptysis, ***pulmonary embolus***, tachypnea, pleural effusion. **Hepatic:** Hepatitis, jaundice, ***acute liver failure***, veno-occlusive liver disease, hepatomegaly, cholangitis, cholecystitis. **Dermatologic:** Maculopapular rash, exfoliative dermatitis, erythema multiforme. **Musculoskeletal:** Myasthenia, bone pain, muscle pain, joint pain. **Hypersensitivity:** Asthma, bronchospasm, wheezing, ***anaphylactoid*** and other allergic reactions. **Ophthalmic:** Visual impairment, diplopia. **Otic:** Deafness, tinnitus, hearing loss. **Miscellaneous:** Malaise, weight loss, reaction at injection site (including inflammation, shock, weight loss) thrombophlebitis, anorexia, acidosis.

- **Reported for AmBisome**

CV: Arrhythmia, atrial fibrillation, bradycardia, cardiomegaly, ***hemorrhage***, postural hypotension, valvular heart disease, vascular disorder, flushing, veno-occlusive disease, phlebitis, vasodilation. **GI:** Anorexia, constipation, enlarged abdomen, dry mouth/nose, dyspepsia, dysphagia, eructation, fecal incontinence, flatulence, ***GI hemorrhage***, hemorrhoids, gum/oral hemorrhage, hematemesis, ileus, mucositis, rectal disorder, stomatitis, ulcerative stomatitis. **Hepatic:** Hepatocellular damage, hepatomegaly, venoocclusive liver disease. **CNS:** Agitation, ***coma, convulsions***, cough, depression, dysesthesia, dizziness, hallucinations, nervousness, paresthesia, somnolence, abnormal thinking, tremor. **Hematologic:** Coagulation disorder, ecchymosis, fluid overload, petechia, agranulocytosis. **GU:** Abnormal renal function, acute renal failure, dysuria, nephrotoxicity, toxic nephropathy, urinary incontinence, vaginal hemorrhage, hemorrhagic cystitis. **Respiratory:** Asthma, atelectasis, bronchospasm, hemoptysis, hiccough, hyperventilation, flu-like symptoms, lung edema, pharyngitis, pneumonia, respiratory insufficiency, sinusitis, cyanosis, hypoventilation, pulmonary edema. **Dermatologic:** Alopecia, dry skin, herpes simplex, inflammation at injection site, maculopapular rash, purpura, skin discoloration, skin disorder/ulcer, urticaria, vesiculobullous rash. **Musculoskeletal:** Arthralgia, bone pain, dystonia, myalgia, neck pain, rigors. **Ophthalmic:** Conjunctivitis, dry eyes, eye hemorrhage. **Metabolic:** Edema, peripheral edema, facial edema, acidosis, respiratory alkalosis. **Miscellaneous:** Enlarged abdomen, cellulitis, cell-mediated immunological reaction, graft-versus-host disease, malaise, chest pain/tightness, angioedema, erythema, blood product transfusion reaction.

LABORATORY TEST CONSIDERATIONS

Common to all products

↑ ALT, AST, creatinine, BUN, alkaline phosphatase. Hyperbilirubinemia, hypokalemia, hypomagnesemia, hyperglycemia, hypernatremia, hypocalcemia, hypervolemia. Abnormal liver function tests.

For Abelcet

Hyperkalemia, hypercalcemia, ↑ LDH, hyperamylasemia, hypoglycemia, hyperuricemia, hypophosphatemia.

For AmBisome

↑ Amylase, LDH, NPN. ↑ or ↓ Prothrombin. Hyperchloremia, hyperkalemia, hypermagnesemia, hyperphosphatemia, hyponatremia, hypophosphatemia, hypoproteinemia. Abnormal LFTs.

OVERDOSE MANAGEMENT

SEE ALSO ***AMPHOTERICIN B DESOXYCHOLATE.***

DRUG INTERACTIONS

See *Amphotericin B desoxycholate.*

HOW SUPPLIED

Abelcet. *Suspension for Injection (as lipid complex):* 100 mg/20 mL.
AmBisome. *Powder for Injection (as liposomal):* 50 mg.

DOSAGE

Abelcet

IV

Systemic fungal infections.

Adults and children: 5 mg/kg/day prepared as a 1 mg/mL infusion and given at a rate of 2.5 mg/kg/hr. For children and those with CV disease, dilute the drug to a final concentration of 2 mg/mL. If the infusion exceeds 2 hr, mix the contents by shaking the infusion bag. Do not use an in-line filter.

AmBisome

IV

Empirical fungal infections.

Adults and children: 3 mg/kg/day using a controlled infusion device over about 2 hr. Can reduce infusion time to 60 min if well tolerated or increase if client is uncomfortable.

Infections due to Aspergillus, Candida, Cryptococcus.

Adults and children; 3–5 mg/kg/day prepared as a 1–2 mg/mL infusion and given initially over 2 hr. Can reduce infusion time to 60 min if well tolerated or increase if client is uncomfortable. For infants and small children, infusion concentrations of 0.2–0.5 mg/mL may be better. A micron or more in-line filter may be used.

Cryptococcal meningitis in human immunodeficiency virus (HIV).

Adults and children: 6 mg/kg/day using a controlled infusion device over 2 hr. Can reduce infusion time to 60 min if well tolerated or increase if client is uncomfortable.

Leishmaniasis.

Adults and children, immunocompetent clients: 3 mg/kg/day on days 1 through 5, 14, and 21; repeat course may be given if parasite is not eradicated. **Adults and children, immunosuppressed clients:** 4 mg/kg/day on days 1 through 5, 10, 17, 24, 31, and 38 to immunosuppressed clients; if parasite is not eradicated or relapse occurs, seek expert advice regarding further therapy.

NURSING IMPLICATIONS

Do not confuse amphotericin B lipid-based with amphotericin B desoxycholate.

IMPLEMENTATION/ADMINISTRATION/STORAGE

1. **IV Acute reactions, including fever and chills, may occur 1–2 hr after beginning an IV infusion. These reactions are more common with the first few doses and usually decrease with subsequent doses. Infusion reactions may be reduced by pretreatment with antihistamines and corticosteroids or by reducing the rate of infusion and prompt administration of antihistamines and corticosteroids.**
2. **The following approaches may decrease severe side effects:**
   - **Give aspirin, acetaminophen, antihistamines, and antiemetics before infusion and maintain sodium balance.**
   - **Give on alternate days to decrease anorexia and phlebitis.**
   - **Small doses of IV corticosteroids before infusion may decrease febrile reactions.**

A

- Adding small amount of heparin (500–2,000 units) to infusion, removing the needle after infusion, rotating the infusion sites, giving through a large central vein, and using a pediatric scalp-vein may decrease incidence of thrombophlebitis.
- Meperidine, 25–50 mg IV, may decrease duration of shaking, chills, and fever that may occur.

3. *Preparation of amphotericin B lipid complex (Abelcet):* Shake vial gently until there is no yellow sediment at the bottom. Withdraw appropriate dose from the required number of vials into one or more sterile syringes using an 18-gauge needle. Remove needle from each syringe filled with liposomal amphotericin B, and replace with a 5-micron filter needle. Each filter needle may be used to filter the contents of up to four 100 mg vials. Insert filter needle of the syringe into an IV bag containing D5W and empty syringe contents into the bag. The infusion concentration should be 1 mg/mL. For pediatric clients and those with CV disease, the drug may be diluted with D5W to a final infusion concentration of 2 mg/mL. Shake the bag until the contents are mixed thoroughly. Do not use the admixture if there is any evidence of foreign matter. Vials are for single use; discard any unused material.
4. *Administration of amphotericin B lipid complex (Abelcet):* Before infusion, shake the bag until the contents are mixed thoroughly. Administer at a rate of 2.5 mg/kg/hr. Do not use an in-line filter. If C_{CR} is <10 mL/min, give 5 mg/kg q 24–36 hr. If the infusion exceeds 2 hr, mix the contents by shaking the infusion bag q 2 hr. Flush an existing IV line with D5W injection before infusing amphotericin B lipid complex; or use a separate line.
5. *Preparation of liposomal amphotericin B (AmBisome):* Add 12 mL of sterile water for injection to each vial to yield 4 mg/mL. Immediately shake vial vigorously for 30 sec to completely disperse drug until a yellow, translucent suspension is formed. Visually inspect the vial for particulate matter; continue shaking until completely dispersed. After calculating dose of reconstituted drug, withdraw appropriate amount into a sterile syringe. Attach 5 micron filter provided and inject syringe contents through the filter needle into an appropriate volume of D5W for final concentration of 1–2 mg/mL. Use only one filter needle/vial. Lower concentrations of 0.2–0.5 mg/mL may be more appropriate for infants and small children. Discard partially used vials.
6. *Administration of liposomal amphotericin B (AmBisome):* Administer using a controlled infusion device over about 120 min. An in-line membrane filter of at least 1 micron mean pore diameter may be used. If given through an existing IV line, flush with D5W injection prior to and following the infusion; otherwise, give via a separate line. C_{CR} is <10 mL/min, give 3 mg/kg q 24 hr. Give a dose of 3–5 mg/kg/day IV for clients receiving continuous venovenous hemofiltration, continuous venovenous hemodialysis, or continuous venovenous hemodiafiltration; this assumes ultrafiltration and dialysis flow rates of 1–2 L/hr. Also, a dose of 3–5 mg/kg IV q 24 hr is given after the dialysis session; assumes the client is receiving standard intermittent hemodialysis 3 times/week and completes the full dialysis session.
7. Strict aseptic technique must be used in preparation; contains no bacteriostatic agent. Do not use initial concentrate if any precipitate is present.
8. Protect from light during administration. Loss of drug activity during administration is likely negligible if the solution is exposed for <8 hr.
9. Initiate therapy in the most distal veins. When administered peripherally, changing sites with each dose may decrease phlebitis.
10. *Storage/stability of amphotericin B lipid complex (Abelcet):* Prior to admixture store at 2–8°C (36–46°F). Protect from exposure to light; do not freeze. Keep in the carton until used. Admixture may be stored for up to 48 hr at 2–8°C (36–46°F) and an additional 6 hr at room temperature.
11. *Storage/stability of liposomal amphotericin B (AmBisome):* Store unopened vials at 2–8°C (36–46°F), without freezing. Keep product in the carton until used. Store reconstituted product concentrate at 2–8°C (36–46°F) for up to 24 hr. Do not freeze. Use within 6 hr of diluted with D5W. Discard any unused drug.
12. COMPATIBILITY Sterile water, D5W.

A

13. INCOMPATIBILITY Do not dilute or reconstitute with saline solution or mix with other drugs or electrolytes. Use of a bacteriostatic agent (e.g., benzyl alcohol) may cause precipitation. If given through an existing IV line, flush with D5W before and after infusion.

ASSESSMENT

1. Check for any allergy to amphotericin, adverse effects, hypersensitivity reactions. If hypersensitivity reactions occur, immediately discontinue the infusion.
2. Assess mental status; note age and reasons for therapy.
3. Document and describe characteristics of systemic infections requiring therapy. Different organisms require different lengths of treatment time.
4. List drugs prescribed; ensure none interact unfavorably.
5. Ensure correct form prepared for administration.
6. Premedicate with antipyretics, antihistamines, corticosteroids, and/or antiemetic drugs to reduce side effects. Rashes, fevers, and chills may occur.
7. Infuse slowly until response identified. May increase infusion time if well tolerated or decrease if not tolerated according to manufacturer's guidelines and orders. Monitor VS every 15–30 min during first dose; interrupt infusion for adverse effects.
8. Monitor I&O; report change in output, cloudy urine. Weigh twice weekly; assess for malnutrition/dehydration.
9. Identify and protect those who are severely immunocompromised.
10. Assess for hypokalemia with digoxin therapy; and hyponatremia with this therapy. Observe for toxicity/muscle weakness and monitor K^+, Na^+, Mg^{++}, and digoxin levels.
11. Monitor CBC, electrolytes, Mg^{++}, renal and LFTs, and cultures during therapy. Stop therapy/report any adverse effects. Monitor for bleeding, progressive liver and kidney dysfunction. The lipid form is generally used with kidney impairment.

CLIENT/FAMILY TEACHING

1. Reduce GI effects with an antihistamine or antiemetic before drug therapy; administer before mealtime. Try small frequent meals if diarrhea occurs.
2. Report any anorexia, N&V, headache, rashes, fever, or chills.
3. Consume ↑ fluids as directed to prevent dehydration and further toxic kidney effects. Report any changes in I&O and extreme weight loss.
4. Therapy usually requires long-term treatments to ensure adequate response (eradication of organism) and prevent relapse.
5. Report neurologic symptoms such as ringing in ears, blurred vision, or dizziness as well as fever, chills, difficulty breathing or swallowing, or malaise.
6. Fever reaction may diminish with prolonged therapy; muscle pain/aches may be R/T low potassium.
7. Report any bleeding, bruising, or soft-tissue swelling as well as vertigo or hearing loss.
8. Keep all F/U to assess response, labs, and adverse SE.

OUTCOMES/EVALUATE

- Resolution of fungal infection
- Eradication of parasites
- Symptomatic improvement

IV

Ampicillin oral

(am-pih-**SILL**-in)

Classification(s): Antibiotic, penicillin

Pregnancy Category: B

RX: Principen.

♣ **Rx:** Novo-Ampicillin.

Ampicillin sodium, parenteral

Pregnancy Category: B

RX: Ampicillin sodium.

SEE ALSO ***ANTI-INFECTIVE DRUGS*** AND ***PENICILLINS***.

INDICATIONS/USES

(1) Respiratory tract infections due to non-penicillinase-producing *Haemophilus influenzae,* penicillinase (injection only) and non-penicillinase-producing staphylococci, and streptococci, including *Streptococcus pneumoniae.*

(2) GI infections due to *Shigella, Salmonella typhosa* and other salmonella, *Escherichia coli, Proteus mirabilis,* and enterococci.

A

(3) GU infections due to *E. coli, P. mirabilis, Shigella, S. typhosa* and other salmonella, enterococci, and non-penicillinase-producing *Neisseria gonorrhoeae.*

(4) Use of the injection only for bacterial meningitis due to *Neisseria meningitides, E. coli, Listeria monocytogenes,* and Group B streptococci. Addition of an aminoglycoside may enhance effectiveness against gram-negative bacteria.

(5) Use of the injection only for septicemia and endocarditis due to *Streptococcus* species, penicillin G susceptible staphylococci, enterococci, *E. coli, P. mirabilis,* and *Salmonella.* Addition of an aminoglycoside may enhance effectiveness when treating streptococcal endocarditis.

ACTION/KINETICS

Action

Synthetic, broad-spectrum antibiotic suitable for gram-negative bacteria. Acid resistant, destroyed by penicillinase.

Pharmacokinetics

Absorbed more slowly than other penicillins. From 30 to 60% of PO dose absorbed from GI tract. **Peak serum levels; PO:** 1.8–2.9 mcg/mL after 2 hr; **IM,** 4.5–7 mcg/mL. **t½:** 80 min-range 50–110 min. Partially inactivated in liver; 25–85% excreted unchanged in urine.

SIDE EFFECTS

Most Common

Hypersensitivity, N&V, gastritis, stomatitis.

See *Penicillins* for a complete list of potential side effects.

ADDITIONAL DRUG INTERACTIONS

Allopurinol / ↑ Skin rashes

Oral contraceptives / ↓ Effect of ampicillin

HOW SUPPLIED

Ampicillin oral. *Capsules (trihydrate):* 250 mg, 500 mg; *Powder for Oral Suspension (trihydrate):* 125 mg/5 mL, 250 mg/5 mL.

Ampicillin sodium, parenteral. *Injection, Powder for Solution:* 250 mg, 500 mg, 1 gram, 2 grams, 10 grams.

DOSAGE

AMPICILLIN ORAL: CAPSULES, ORAL SUSPENSION; AMPICILLIN SODIUM: IM, IV

Respiratory tract and soft-tissue infections.

PO, 20 kg or more: 250 mg q 6 hr; **less than 20 kg:** 50 mg/kg/day in equally divided doses q 6–8 hr. **IV, IM, 40 kg or more:** 250–500 mg q 6 hr; **less than 40 kg:** 25–50 mg/kg/day in equally divided doses q 6–8 hr.

GI and GU infections, other than N. gonorrhoeae.

Adults/children, more than 20 kg: 500 mg PO q 6 hr. Use larger doses, if needed, for severe or chronic infections. **Children, less than 20 kg:** 100 mg/kg/day q 6 hr.

Bacterial meningitis.

Adults and children: 150–200 mg/kg/day in divided doses q 3 to 4 hr. Initially give IV drip, followed by IM q 3 to 4 hr.

Septicemia.

Adults and children: 150–200 mg/kg/day, IV for first 3 days, then IM q 3–4 hr.

Enterococcal endocarditis.

12 grams/day IV either continuously or in equally divided doses q 4 hr plus 1 mg/kg gentamicin, IM or IV, q 8 hr for 4–6 weeks.

Bacterial endocarditis prophylaxis (dental, oral, or upper respiratory tract procedures).

Clients at moderate risk or those unable to take PO medications: **Adults, IM, IV:** 2 grams 30 min prior to procedure; **children:** 50 mg/kg, 30 min prior to procedure. Clients at high risk: **Adults, IM, IV:** 2 grams ampicillin plus gentamicin, 1.5 mg/kg, given 30 min before procedure followed in 6 hr by ampicillin, 1 gram IM or IV, or amoxicillin, 1 gram PO. **Children, IM, IV:** Ampicillin, 50 mg/kg, plus gentamicin, 1.5 mg/kg, 30 min prior to procedure followed in 6 hr by ampicillin, 25 mg/kg IM or IV, or amoxicillin, 25 mg/kg PO.

N. gonorrhoeae *infections.*

PO: Single dose of 3.5 grams given together with probenecid, 1 gram. **Parenteral, Adults/children over 40 kg:** 500 mg IV or IM q 6 hr. **Children, less than 40 kg:** 50 mg/kg/day IV or IM in equally divided doses q 6 to 8 hr.

A

Urethritis in males caused by N. gonorrhoeae.

Parenteral, males over 40 kg: Two 500 mg doses IV or IM at an interval of 8 to 12 hr. Repeat treatment if necessary. In complicated gonorrheal urethritis, prolonged and intensive therapy is recommended.

Prophylaxis for neonatal Group B streptococcal disease.

If culture is positive or risk factors are present, give 2 grams IV during labor; **then,** 1 gram IV q 4 hr until delivery.

In preterm, premature rupture of membranes in Group B negative women, give 2 grams ampicillin IV q 6 hr plus erythromycin, 250 mg IV, q 8 hr for 48 hr; **then,** amoxicillin, 250 mg plus erythromycin base, 333 mg, q 8 hr PO for 5 days.

NURSING IMPLICATIONS

Do not confuse ampicillin with amoxicillin (another penicillin product).

IMPLEMENTATION/ADMINISTRATION/STORAGE

1. Reconstituted PO solution stable for 7 days at room temperature, not exceeding 25°C (77°F); 14 days refrigerated.
2. For IM use, dilute only with sterile or bacteriostatic water for injection.
3. If the C_{CR} <10 mL/min, dosing interval should be increased to 12 hr.
4. IV After reconstitution for IM or direct IV administration, solution **must be used within the hour to prevent loss of potency.**
5. For IVPB, ampicillin may be reconstituted with NaCl injection.
6. Once reconstituted (50 mL), give IV slowly over at least 10–15 min.
7. For IV, check compatibility and length of time drug retains potency in a particular solution.
8. COMPATIBILITY For reconstitution: sterile water; for infusion: D5W, NSS, D5/0.45% NaCl, LR.
9. INCOMPATIBILITY Flush well between infusions.

ASSESSMENT

1. List characteristics of S&S. Identify onset, severity, location, other associated factors.
2. Note history of sensitivity/reactions to this or related drugs.
3. IM route may be painful; rotate/document sites.
4. Monitor urinary output and serum K⁺ levels, especially in elderly. Monitor CBC, cultures, renal and LFTs.

CLIENT/FAMILY TEACHING

1. Take 1 hr before or 2 hr after meals; food may interfere with absorption.
2. Ampicillin chewable tablets should not be swallowed whole. Refrigerate liquid oral preparations; discard any unrefrigerated preparations more than 7 days old.
3. Review method for administration/storage. Consume fluids; ensure adequate hydration.
4. Take for prescribed number of days even if symptoms subside. Report adverse effects or if S&S do not improve/worsen during therapy.
5. Do not save pills for future use or share with family members/friends who have similar symptoms.
6. May decrease effectiveness of oral contraceptives; use additional form of contraception during therapy.
7. Review importance of prophylaxis before invasive procedures in those with valve replacement or history of rheumatic heart disease.
8. Report SOB and any *ampicillin rashes*; a dull, red, itchy, flat, or raised rash occurs more often with this drug than with other penicillins; usually benign. If late skin rash develops with symptoms of fever, fatigue, sore throat, generalized lymph node swelling, and enlarged spleen, a heterophil antibody test may be ordered to rule out mononucleosis.
9. Keep all F/U to assess response and for adverse SE.

OUTCOMES/EVALUATE

- Resolution of infection; symptomatic improvement
- Negative culture reports
- Endocarditis prophylaxis

Combination Drug

IV

Ampicillin sodium and Sulbactam sodium

(am-pih-**SILL**-in, sull-**BACK**-tam)

Classification(s): Antibiotic, penicillin

A

Pregnancy Category: B

RX: Unasyn.

SEE ALSO ***ANTI-INFECTIVE DRUGS*** AND ***PENICILLINS***.

INDICATIONS/USES

Infections caused by beta-lactamase-producing strains of the following: (1) Skin and skin structure infections caused by *Staphylococcus aureus, Escherichia coli, Klebsiella* species (including *K. pneumoniae*), *Proteus mirabilis, Bacteroides fragilis, Enterobacter* species, and *Acinetobacter calcoaceticus.* (2) Intra-abdominal infections caused by *E. coli, Klebsiella* species (including *K. pneumoniae*), and *Bacteroides* (including *B. fragilis)* and *Enterobacter.* (3) Gynecologic infections caused by *E. coli* and *Bacteroides* (including *B. fragilis). NOTE:* Mixed infections caused by ampicillin-susceptible organisms and beta-lactamase-producing organisms are susceptible to this product; thus, additional antibiotics do not have to be used.

CONTENT

Injection, Powder for Solution: 1 gram ampicillin sodium/0.5 gram sulbactam sodium, 2 grams ampicillin sodium/1 gram sulbactam sodium, or 10 grams ampicillin sodium/5 grams sulbactam sodium.

ACTION/KINETICS

Action

For details, see *Ampicillin oral.* Sulbactam is present in this product because it irreversibly inhibits beta-lactamases, thus ensuring activity of ampicillin against beta-lactamase-producing microorganisms. Thus, sulbactam broadens the antibiotic spectrum of ampicillin to those bacteria normally resistant to it.

Pharmacokinetics

Peak serum levels, after IV infusion: 15 min. **t½, both drugs:** about 1 hr. From 75–85% of both drugs are excreted unchanged in the urine within 8 hr after administration.

SPECIAL CONCERNS

Safety and efficacy in children 1 year of age and older not established for intra-abdominal infections or for IM administration.

SIDE EFFECTS

Most Common

Hypersensitivity, N&V, gastritis, stomatitis.

See *Penicillins* for a complete list of potential side effects. **At site of injection:** Pain and thrombophlebitis. **GI:** Diarrhea, N&V, flatulence, abdominal distention, glossitis. **CNS:** Fatigue, malaise, headache. **GU:** Dysuria, urinary retention. **Miscellaneous:** Itching, chest pain, edema, facial swelling, erythema, chills, tightness in throat, epistaxis, substernal pain, mucosal bleeding, candidiasis.

LABORATORY TEST CONSIDERATIONS

↑ AST, ALT, alkaline phosphatase, LDH, creatinine, BUN; also, ↑ basophils, eosinophils, lymphocytes, monocytes, platelets. ↓ Serum albumin and total proteins, H&H, RBCs, WBCs, and platelets. Presence of RBCs and hyaline casts in urine.

OVERDOSE MANAGEMENT

Symptoms: Neurologic symptoms, including ***convulsions.*** *Treatment:* Both ampicillin and sulbactam may be removed by hemodialysis.

HOW SUPPLIED

See *Content.*

DOSAGE

IM; IV

All infections.

Adults: 1 gram ampicillin/0.5 gram sulbactam to 2 grams ampicillin/1 gram sulbactam q 6 hr, not to exceed 4 grams sulbactam daily. Doses must be decreased in renal impairment. **Children, over 40 kg:** Use adult doses; total sulbactam dose should not exceed 4 grams/day. **Children, one year and older but less than 40 kg:** 300 mg/kg/day (200 mg ampicillin/100 mg sulbactam) in divided doses q 6 hr.

In clients with impaired renal function, use the following dosage guide: **C_{CR} greater than or equal to 30 mL/min/1.73 m^2:** 1.5–3 grams (ampicillin with sulbactam) q 6–8 hr; **15–29 mL/min/1.73 m^2:** 1.5–3 grams (ampicillin with sulbactam) q 12 hr;

5–14 mL/min/1.73 m²: 1.5–3 grams (ampicillin with sulbactam) q 24 hr.

NURSING IMPLICATIONS

IMPLEMENTATION/ADMINISTRATION/STORAGE

1. For IM use: reconstitute with sterile water for injection or 0.5% or 2% lidocaine HCl injection.
2. Must use solutions for IM administration within 1 hr of preparation.
3. IV After reconstitution, solutions should stand so that any foaming will dissipate; inspect vial to ensure dissolution.
4. Give by slow injection over 10–15 min or, if mixed with 50–100 mL of diluent listed below, over 15–30 min.
5. Store at or below 30°C (86°F) prior to reconstitution.
6. COMPATIBILITY D5W, D5W/0.45% NaCl, 10% invert sugar, RL, 0.9% NaCl, M/6 sodium lactate injection, reconstitute with sterile water for injection.
7. INCOMPATIBILITY Flush between drugs, and if aminoglycosides are also prescribed, administer each separately (1 hr apart) because ampicillin will inactivate aminoglycosides.

ASSESSMENT

1. List reason for therapy, type, onset, characteristics of S&S and culture results.
2. Note sensitivity/reactions to this drug or related drugs.
3. During first 30 min of IV therapy, monitor closely for S&S of hypersensitivity reactions.
4. Ensure adequately hydrated. Assess for diarrhea and S&S of superinfection.
5. Monitor VS, CBC, cultures, renal and LFTs. With impaired renal function, reduce dose or frequency of administration.

CLIENT/FAMILY TEACHING

1. Administered parenterally to treat infections.
2. IM injections painful; expect some discomfort. Report if S&S worsen, diarrhea, vaginal itching occurs or symptoms do not improve.
3. Consume 2–3 L/day of fluids to ensure hydration.
4. Use additional form of birth control if using hormone contraceptive pills.
5. Report any adverse effects including skin rash; if accompanied by fatigue, sore throat and enlarged spleen and lymph nodes (a heterophil antibody test may be ordered to rule out mononucleosis).
6. Keep all F/U to assess response, labs, and for adverse SE.

OUTCOMES/EVALUATE

- Resolution of infection
- Symptomatic improvement

Anagrelide hydrochloride

(an-**AG**-greh-lyd)

Classification(s): Antiplatelet drug

Pregnancy Category: C

RX: Agrylin.

INDICATIONS/USES

Reduce elevated platelet count and the risk of thrombosis in thrombocythemia, secondary to myeloproliferative disorders; also to reduce associated symptoms, including thrombo-hemorrhagic events.

ACTION/KINETICS

Action

May act to reduce platelets by decreasing megakaryocyte hypermaturation; possible disruption in the postmitotic phase of megakaryocyte development and a reduction in megakaryocyte size and ploidy. Does not cause significant changes in white cell counts or coagulation parameters. Inhibits platelet aggregation at higher doses than needed to reduce platelet count.

Pharmacokinetics

Peak plasma levels: 5 ng/mL at 1 hr. **t½:** 1.3 hr; **terminal t½:** About 3 days. Maximum drug levels and total drug exposure in clients 7–14 years old were about one-half the values in clients 16–86 years old. Food modestly (14%) reduces bioavailability but increased total exposure by 20%. Extensively metabolized in liver and excreted in urine and feces.

CONTRAINDICATIONS

Lactation. Severe hepatic impairment.

A

SPECIAL CONCERNS

- **Use with caution in known or suspected heart disease and in impaired renal function.**
- **Serum levels may increase 8-fold in those with moderate hepatic impairment; use lower doses in these clients. Use with caution in severe hepatic impairment (Child-Pugh score from 10 to 15).**
- **Safety and efficacy not determined in those less than 16 years of age.**

SIDE EFFECTS

Most Common

Palpitations, headache, asthenia, dizziness, diarrhea, nausea, abdominal pain, dyspnea, flatulence, edema.

CV: CHF, palpitations, chest pain, tachycardia, arrhythmias, angina pectoris, postural hypotension, hypertension, CVD, vasodilation, migraine, syncope, ***MI, cardiomyopathy, CHB, fibrillation, CVA, pericarditis, hemorrhage, heart failure, pericardial effusion, thrombosis***, cardiomegaly, AF. **GI:** Diarrhea, abdominal pain, pancreatitis, gastric/duodenal ulcers, N&V, flatulence, anorexia, dyspepsia, constipation, GI distress, ***GI hemorrhage***, gastritis, melena, aphthous stomatitis, eructation. **Respiratory:** Rhinitis, pharyngitis, cough, epistaxis, respiratory disease, sinusitis, pneumonia, bronchitis, asthma, pulmonary infiltrate, ***pulmonary fibrosis, pulmonary hypertension, pleural effusion***, pulmonary infiltrates, dyspnea. **CNS:** Headache, ***seizures***, dizziness, paresthesia, depression, somnolence, confusion, insomnia, nervousness, amnesia, migraine, asthenia. **Musculoskeletal:** Arthralgia, myalgia, leg cramps. **Dermatologic:** Pruritus, skin disease, alopecia, rash, urticaria. **Hematologic:** Anemia, thrombocytopenia, ecchymosis, lymphadenoma, lymphadenopathy. **GU:** Dysuria, hematuria. **Body as a whole:** Fever, flu symptoms, chills, photosensitivity, dehydration, malaise, asthenia, edema, peripheral edema, pain. **Ophthalmic:** Amblyopia, abnormal vision, visual field abnormality, diplopia. **Miscellaneous:** Back/chest pain, tinnitus.

LABORATORY TEST CONSIDERATIONS

↑ Liver enzymes.

OVERDOSE MANAGEMENT

Symptoms: Thrombocytopenia. *Treatment:* Close clinical monitoring. Decrease or stop dose until platelet count returns to the normal range.

DRUG INTERACTIONS

Amrinone / Exacerbation of amrinone effects
Aspirin / Less inhibition (slight) of platelet aggregation when given with single 1 mg doses of anagrelide compared with aspirin alone
Cilostazol / Exacerbation of effects
CYP1A2 inhibitors (e.g., theophylline) / Limited inhibition of CYP1A2 by anagrelide; potential for interaction with other products sharing the same clearance mechanism
H ***Evening primrose oil*** / Potential for ↑ antiplatelet effect
H ***Feverfew*** / Potential for ↑ antiplatelet effect
H ***Garlic*** / Potential for ↑ antiplatelet effect
H ***Ginger*** / Potential for ↑ antiplatelet effect
H ***Ginkgo biloba*** / Potential for ↑ antiplatelet effect
H ***Ginseng*** / Potential for ↑ antiplatelet effect
H ***Grapeseed extract*** / Potential for ↑ antiplatelet effect
Milrinone / Exacerbation of effects

HOW SUPPLIED

Capsules: 0.5 mg, 1 mg.

DOSAGE

CAPSULES

Thrombocythemia.

Adults, initial: 0.5 mg 4 times per day or 1 mg twice a day. Maintain for 1 week or more. **Children, initial:** 0.5 mg per day. **Then,** in both children and adults adjust to lowest effective dose to maintain platelet count less than 600,000/mcL and ideally to the normal range. Do not increase the dose by more than 0.5 mg/day in any 1 week. Maintenance dose is not expected to be different between adults and children. **Maximum dose:** 10 mg/day or 2.5 mg in single dose. Most respond at a dose of 1.5 to 3 mg/day. In those with moderate hepatic impairment (Child-Pugh score from 7 to 9), start with 0.5 mg/day and maintain for a minimum of 1 week with careful monitoring of CV effects. Do not exceed a dosage increment of more than 0.5 mg/day in any 1 week.

A

NURSING IMPLICATIONS

IMPLEMENTATION/ADMINISTRATION/STORAGE

1. Initiate under close medical supervision.
2. Platelet count usually responds within 7–14 days. The time to complete response (i.e., platelet count less than or equal to 600,000/mcL) ranged from 4–12 weeks.
3. Store from 15–30°C (59–86°F).

ASSESSMENT

1. List etiology, onset, duration of thrombocythemia.
2. Note any CAD, liver or renal dysfunction; document CV assessment, monitor closely.
3. Determine if pregnant. Monitor VS, CBC, renal and LFTs frequently during lowering of platelet; check platelets every 2 days during first week and then weekly thereafter until stabilized. Monitor for adverse CV effects if used with moderate hepatic impairment (at lower dosage).

CLIENT/FAMILY TEACHING

1. Take as directed. Used to lower platelet counts; increases usually occur within 4 days after therapy stopped.
2. Practice reliable contraception; may cause fetal harm.
3. Report palpitations, fever/chills, SOB, dizziness, chest/abdominal pain, or unusual bruising/bleeding. Report if GI upset severe and persistent.
4. Avoid alcohol intake with oral solution; may increase side effects related to propylene glycol content.
5. Keep all F/U to monitor labs/assess response and for adverse SE.

OUTCOMES/EVALUATE

- Reduction in platelet counts; (maintain <600,000/mcL)
- ↓ Risk of thrombosis

Anakinra

(**an**-ah-**KIN**-rah)

Classification(s): Antiarthritic drug

Pregnancy Category: B

RX: Kineret.

INDICATIONS/USES

Decrease signs and symptoms and slow the progression of structural damage in moderate-to-severe active rheumatoid arthritis in clients 18 and older who have failed 1 or more disease modifying antirheumatic drugs (DMARD). Can be used alone or with DMARDs (except tissue necrosis factor blocking drugs).

ACTION/KINETICS

Action

Interleukin-1 (IL-1) production is induced by inflammation. IL-1 degrades cartilage due to its induction of the rapid loss of proteoglycans, as well as stimulation of bone resorption. Anakinra blocks the biologic activity of IL-1 by competitively inhibiting IL-1 binding to the interleukin-1 type I receptor found in many tissues and organs. Thus, symptoms of rheumatoid arthritis improve.

Pharmacokinetics

Is 95% bioavailable after a 70 mg bolus injection. **Maximum plasma levels:** 3–7 hr. **t½, terminal:** 4–6 hr. Plasma clearance decreased 70–75% in those with severe or end-stage renal disease.

CONTRAINDICATIONS

Known hypersensitivity to *Escherichia coli*–derived proteins, anakinra, or any component of the product. Use of live vaccines concurrently with anakinra.

SPECIAL CONCERNS

- Associated with an increased incidence of serious infections (especially when used with etanercept).
- Safety and efficacy not determined in immunosuppressed clients, in those with chronic infections, when used with blocking agents, or with use for juvenile rheumatoid arthritis.
- Vaccination may not be effective in those receiving anti-anakinra antibodies.
- Use with caution during lactation, in treating geriatric clients, in those with impaired renal function, in those with pre-existing or recent-onset demyelinating disorders, and in those with heart failure.
- Safety and efficacy in clients with juvenile rheumatoid arthritis not determined.
- The elderly may be more sensitive to the drug effects.

A

SIDE EFFECTS

Most Common

Injection site reaction, worsening of RA, URTI, headache, nausea, diarrhea, sinusitis, arthralgia, flu-like symptoms, abdominal pain.

Injection site reactions: Erythema, ecchymosis, inflammation, pain. **CNS:** Headache. **GI:** Nausea, diarrhea, abdominal pain. **Hematologic:** Neutropenia (especially when combined with TNF-blocking drugs). **Musculoskeletal:** Worsening of RA, bone and joint infections, arthralgia. **Respiratory:** Sinusitis, URTI. **Body as a whole:** Increased incidence of serious infections (especially in those with asthma), including cellulitis, pneumonia, bone and joint infections, bacterial pneumonia. Flu-like symptoms, malignancies, immunosuppression, immunogenicity. Rarely, hypersensitivity reactions.

LABORATORY TEST CONSIDERATIONS

↓ Total WBC, platelets, and absolute neutrophil blood counts. Small ↑ mean eosinophil differential percentage. Possible development of anti-anakinra antibodies after 12 months of use.

DRUG INTERACTIONS

Use with adalimumab may result in hypersensitivity reactions, hematologic events, and serious infections.

HOW SUPPLIED

Injection, Single-Use: 100 mg/0.67 mL.

DOSAGE

SC

Rheumatoid arthritis.

100 mg/day SC.

NURSING IMPLICATIONS

IMPLEMENTATION/ADMINISTRATION/STORAGE

1. Give at approximately the same time every day.
2. Before administration, visually inspect for particulate matter or discoloration; do not use prefilled syringes if particulates or discoloration are observed.
3. Give only one dose/day (i.e., entire contents of 1 prefilled glass syringe). Discard any unused portion; no preservative in product.
4. Store in refrigerator at 2–8°C (36–46°F); do not freeze or shake. Protect from light.

ASSESSMENT

1. Note reasons for therapy, onset, extent and characteristics of disease, other agents trialed/failed; rate pain level. Assess joints, (e.g., number of tender or swollen joints, pain, disability), evaluate degree of function; note improvements/loss of mobility.
2. List drugs taking; ensure none interact. Do not administer with TNF blocking agents or to those with juvenile RA.
3. Assess for any evidence of infection before and during therapy; stop drug and report if evident.
4. Monitor CBC, renal and LFTs. Check neutrophil count (ANC) before therapy, then monthly for 3 mo, and then quarterly during the first year of therapy.

CLIENT/FAMILY TEACHING

1. Review drug insert/guidelines. Perform self-injection after instruction. Inject anakinra daily, at same time each day, into the tissues as ordered.
2. Drug comes in single dose syringe and requires refrigeration. Check expiration date, protect from light, heat, and do **not** shake or freeze.
3. The needle cover on the prefilled syringe contains dry natural rubber (a derivative of latex). Do not handle if sensitive to latex.
4. Store syringes safely out of reach; place used needles and syringes in container and dispose of as directed. Do not reuse or share needles.
5. Injection site reactions may occur; usually lasting 1–2 weeks. Rotate sites; report any pain, inflammation, bruising at sites.
6. Avoid immunizations with live vaccines.
7. Stop drug and report if any infection suspected. Drug highly toxic; has been associated with increased incidence of serious infections.
8. Keep all F/U to assess response, labs (q 1 month × 3 months, then q 3 months for CBC) for adverse SE and rheumatologist evaluation.

OUTCOMES/EVALUATE

Control of RA progression; ↓ joint pain; ↓ bone erosion in those unresponsive to 1 or more DMARDs, ↑ mobility

IV

Antihemophilic factor (AHF, Factor VIII)

(an-tie-hee-moh-**FILL**-ick)

Classification(s): Antihemophilic agent

Pregnancy Category: C

RX: Advate, Alphanate, Helixate FS, Hemofil M, Koate-DVI, Kogenate FS, Monoclate-P, Recombinate, ReFacto, Xyntha.

INDICATIONS/USES

(1) Control of bleeding in clients suffering from hemophilia A (Factor VIII deficiency and acquired Factor VIII inhibitors). These products temporarily replace the missing clotting factor in order to correct or prevent bleeding episodes or to perform surgery. AHF is safe and effective for use in children of all ages, including neonates. *NOTE:* Not effective in controlling bleeding due to von Willebrand's disease. (2) Perioperative management of hemophilic clients. (3) ReFacto only: Short-term prophylaxis to decrease frequency of spontaneous bleeding episodes. (4) Kogenate FS: Routine prophylaxis to reduce the frequency of bleeding episodes and the risk of joint damage in children with hemophilia A with no pre-existing joint damage.

ACTION/KINETICS

Action

Plasma protein (Factor VIII) accelerates the conversion of Factor X to activated Factor X, which converts prothrombin to thrombin. Thrombin then converts fibrinogen to fibrin, resulting in clot formation. Since Factor VIII activity is greatly reduced in clients with hemophilia A, replacement therapy is required. *NOTE:* The potency and purity of preparations vary, but each lot is standardized. Details on the package should be noted.

Pharmacokinetics

t½: 10–18 hr. One AHF unit is the activity found in 1 mL of normal pooled human plasma. *NOTE:* ReFacto is albumin free, which reduces the risk of viral transmission.

CONTRAINDICATIONS

Use of monoclonal antibody-derived AHF in clients hypersensitive to bovine, hamster, or mouse protein or to murine or porcine factor.

SPECIAL CONCERNS

- **Since AHF is prepared from human plasma, there is a risk of transmitting hepatitis or AIDS. However, the products are carefully prepared and tested.**
- **Koate-DVI has not been studied in children and limited studies have been conducted with Alphanate. However, consult the package insert of each product to determine whether it should be given to children.**
- **Use with caution during lactation.**

SIDE EFFECTS

Most Common

Chills, N&V, irritation at injection site, drowsiness, headache.

CNS: Headache, somnolence, drowsiness, dizziness, jittery feeling, depersonalization. **CV:** Increased bleeding tendency, vasodilatation, hot flushes, angina pectoris, tachycardia, chest discomfort, mild hypotension, acute hemolytic anemia, hyperfibrinogenemia. **GI:** N&V, constipation, stomachache, diarrhea, anorexia, taste changes, gastroenteritis, abdominal pain, dysgeusia. **Dermatologic:** Rash, flushing of face, acne, increased perspiration, pruritus, urticaria. **Musculoskeletal:** Myalgia, muscle weakness, joint swelling. **Respiratory:** Nose bleeds, rhinitis, dyspnea, coughing. **Hematologic:** Forearm bleeding following venipuncture, anemia, infected hematoma, forehead bruises, permanent venous access catheter complications. **Ophthalmic:** Blurred vision, eye disorder, abnormal vision. **Otic:** Serous otitis media. **Hypersensitivity:** Nausea, fever, hives, chills, urticaria, wheezing, hypotension, chest tightness, stinging at infusion site, hypotension, ***anaphylaxis***. **Body as a whole:** Fever, chills, rigors, asthenia, lethargy, fatigue. **Miscellaneous:** Irritation at injection site, sore throat, cold feet; tingling in arm, ear, and face; adenopathy, cold sensation, finger pain. Antibodies may form to the mouse protein found in AHF derived from monoclonal antibodies. Approximately 10–20% of clients develop inhibitors to Factor VIII, which leads to a significantly decreased response. Antihemophilic factor contains traces of blood group A and B isohemagglutins. These may cause ***intravascular hemolysis*** in clients with types A, B, or AB blood. ***Both hepatitis and AIDS may be transmitted from AHF prepared from human plasma.***

A

LABORATORY TEST CONSIDERATIONS

↑ Aminotransferase, bilirubin, CPK. ↓ Hematocrit, coagulation factor VIII.

HOW SUPPLIED

Powder for Injection: Injection, Lyophilized Powder for Solution (Human): 250 units AHF, 500 units AHF, 1,000 units AHF, 1,500 units AHF, 3,000 AHF; Injection, Lyophilized Powder for Solution (Recombinant): 250 units AHF, 500 units AHF, 1,000 units AHF, 2,000 units AHF; Injection, Lyophilized Powder for Solution: As labeled (greater than or equal to 5 units AHF human/mg total protein); Injection, Powder for Solution (Recombinant): 250 units AHF, 500 units AHF, 1,000 units AHF, 1,500 units AHF, 2,000 units AHF, 3,000 units AHF; Injection Powder for Solution: As labeled (2 to 20 units AHF human/mg total protein).

DOSAGE

IV ONLY

Hemophilia A.

Individualized, depending on severity of bleeding, degree of deficiency, body weight, the presence of inhibitors of Factor VIII, and the level of Factor VIII desired. *NOTE:* AHF levels may rise 2% to 2.5% for every unit of AHF per kilogram administered. The following formula provides a guide for dosage calculation: Expected Factor VIII increase (in % of normal): AHF/international units administered × 2 divided by body weight (in kg). Dosages given are only guidelines. Also, AHF/IU required = body weight (kg) × desired Factor VIII increased (% normal) × 0.5.

Mild hemorrhage.

Minor episodes usually subside with a single infusion of 10 international units/kg if a level of 20% to 30% of normal is obtained. Dosage should not be repeated until further bleeding occurs.

Minor surgery, moderate hemorrhage.

AHF levels should be raised to 30–50% of normal. **Initial:** 15–25 international units/kg; **maintenance, if necessary:** 10–15 international units/kg q 8–12 hr.

Severe hemorrhage involving vital organs (CNS, retropharyngeal, retroperitoneal spaces, iliopsoas sheath).

Increase AHF levels to 80–100% of normal. **Initial:** 40–50 international units/kg; **maintenance:** 20–25 international units/kg q 8–12 hr.

Major surgery.

Raise AHF levels to 80–100% of normal. Administer 1 hr before surgery; check Factor VIII level before surgery. Repeat injections may be given q 6–12 hr. AHF levels should be maintained at 30% or more of normal for a healing period of at least 10–14 days.

Dental extraction.

Factor VIII level should be increased to 60–80% immediately before the procedure. A single infusion plus PO antifibrinolytic therapy within 1 hr is sufficient in about 70% of cases.

ReFacto

IV

Prevent or reduce frequency of spontaneous bleeding episodes.

Give two or more times a week; dosing three times a week may result in a lower bleeding risk than dosing two times a week. In children, shorter dosage intervals or higher doses may be needed.

NURSING IMPLICATIONS

IMPLEMENTATION/ADMINISTRATION/STORAGE

1. IV Factor VIII concentrates may be given on a regular schedule to prevent bleeding.
2. The efficacy of these products can be reduced due to incorrect diagnosis, inappropriate dosage, method of administration, and biological differences in individual clients. Also, ill effects may occur.
3. AHF is labile inactivated within 10 min at 56°C and within 3 hr at 49°C. Store vials at 2–8°C (36–46°F). Check expiration date. **Do not freeze.**
4. Generally do not store products stabilized with sucrose (e.g., Helixate FS) at room temperature. Refrigerate at all times from 2–8°C (36–46°F). However, Kogenate FS may be stored at room temperature for up to 3

A

months, although it is still recommended that it be refrigerated. Do not return products stored at room temperature to refrigeration.

5. Warm concentrate and diluent to room temperature before reconstitution.
6. Place one needle in the concentrate to act as an airway and then aseptically with a syringe and needle add the diluent to the concentrate.
7. Gently agitate/roll vial containing diluent and concentrate to dissolve the drug. **Do not shake vigorously.**
8. Administer within 3 hr of reconstitution to avoid incubation if contamination occurs with mixing.
9. Do not refrigerate after reconstitution; active ingredient may precipitate out.
10. Keep reconstituted drug at room temperature during infusion; at lower temperature, precipitation of active ingredients may occur.
11. Administer at rate of 2 mL/min, although rates up to 10 mL/min can be used if necessary. If pulse rate increases significantly, reduce rate or discontinue administration.
12. There are a large number of products available. It is important to note the actual AHF units, which are indicated on the vial.
13. Give ReFacto 2 or more times a week for short-term prophylaxis to prevent or reduce the frequency of spontaneous musculoskeletal hemorrhage in those with hemophilia A. In children, shorter dosage intervals or higher doses may be necessary.
14. Store from 2–8°C (35–46°F) except for Hyate: C. Do not freeze.
15. COMPATIBILITY Mix with provided diluent.
16. INCOMPATIBILITY Administer separately.

ASSESSMENT

1. Note reasons for therapy and blood type. Clients with A, B, and AB are more prone to hemolytic reactions. Identification of clotting defect as factor VIII deficiency is essential before administering AHF.
2. Identify recent trauma or injury; assess joints/muscles and body carefully.
3. List drugs prescribed; ensure none interact unfavorably.
4. Document baseline VS; monitor HR before and q 5–15 min during infusion. If tachycardia and hypotension occur, slow IV (symptoms should resolve) and report.
5. May premedicate (usually diphenhydramine) to reduce allergic S&S.
6. Should only be administered in a center with specially trained personnel familiar with drug therapy and labs equipped to monitor factor levels.
7. To control spontaneous bleeding, 5% of normal Factor VIII must be present. For moderate bleeding or prior to surgery, 30–50% must be present and for severe bleeding associated with trauma or major surgery, 80–100% of the normal Factor VIII level must be present.
8. Give the first dose 1 hr before surgery, and the second dose (half of the first dose) 5–8 hr after surgery. Maintain Factor VIII levels at 30% of normal for 10–14 days postoperatively as prescribed.
9. Slow infusion and report if headaches, flushing, numbness, back/joint pain, visual disturbances, or chest constriction occur.
10. The general rule is that 1 unit of AHF activity per kg will increase the circulating AHF level by 2%.
11. Document I&O; assess urine for quantity, color, occult blood.
12. May develop Factor VIII inhibitors, which lead to decreased drug response. Note baseline hematologic parameters and Factor VIII levels. Monitor VS, H&H, coagulation studies, and factor levels before and during therapy; obtain Coombs' test during therapy. (When indicated, monitor Factor VIII activity levels by one-stage clotting assay to confirm adequate Factor VIII levels have been achieved and are maintained.)

CLIENT/FAMILY TEACHING

1. Review method for storing/administering AHF at home.
2. If product prepared from human plasma, identify rare but associated potential risks, such as HIV and certain viral infections (e.g., parovirus B19, hepatitis A) as these may seriously affect seronegative pregnant or immunocompromised individuals. Heat treated or monoclonal antibody preparations may decrease risk.
3. Avoid any drugs/OTC agents that may alter clotting (i.e., ASA, NSAIDs).

A

4. **Increase knowledge level concerning disease process and hereditary transmission. Identify areas necessary to ensure compliance. Report lack of clinical response to Factor VIII replacement therapy; may be a manifestation of an inhibitor. Identify need for genetic counselling.**
5. **Reinforce safety measures related to sports, work, risk taking, and sexual activity. Report any unusual bleeding, rash, joint pain, loss of appetite, N&V, or unusual tiredness. Ensure adequate supply of agent for anticipated treatment when traveling; advise provider before traveling.**
6. **Report any S&S of hypersensitivity/anaphylaxis during therapy: generalized itching or rash with itching, drop in BP, chest tightness, and wheezing.**
7. **Identify local support groups that may assist to understand and cope with this disease.**
8. **Keep all F/U to assess response, labs, and for adverse SE.**

OUTCOMES/EVALUATE

- **Prevention/control of bleeding with hemophilia A**
- **Promotion of normal clotting mechanisms**
- **Coagulation times and Factor VIII levels within desired range**

Apomorphine hydrochloride

(ey-poe-**MOR**-feen)

Classification(s): Antiparkinson drug (dopamine receptor agonist)

Pregnancy Category: C

RX: Apokyn.

INDICATIONS/USES

Acute, intermittent treatment of acute hypomobility, "off" episodes ("end-of-dose wearing off" and unpredictable "on/off" episodes) associated with advanced Parkinson's disease. Used as an adjunct to other drugs.

ACTION/KINETICS

Action

Apomorphine is a dopamine receptor agonist. The precise mechanism to treat Parkinson's is not known but may involve stimulation of postsynaptic dopamine D_2 receptors in the caudate-putamen in the brain. *NOTE*: If apomorphine is used with carbidopa/levodopa, the levodopa pharmacokinetics are not changed; however, motor response differences are significant. Also, the threshold levodopa concentration required to improve motor response was reduced significantly if used with apomorphine, leading to an increased duration of action.

Pharmacokinetics

Rapidly absorbed; **time to peak levels after SC:** 10–60 min. **Mean t½, terminal:** About 40 min. Cytochrome P450 enzymes appear to play a minor role in the metabolism of apomorphine.

CONTRAINDICATIONS

Use in those with hypersensitivity to the drug or sodium metabisulfite. IV use. Use with $5HT_3$ antagonists (e.g., alosetron, dolasetron, granisetron, ondansetron, palonosetron) due to the possibility of severe hypotension and loss of consciousness. Lactation.

SPECIAL CONCERNS

- **Use with caution in those with hypokalemia, hypomagnesemia, bradycardia, concomitant use with other drugs that prolong the QTc interval, genetic predisposition to prolongation of the QT interval, known CV and cerebrovascular disease, or in those with mild to moderate hepatic or renal impairment.**
- **Safety and efficacy not determined in children.**
- **Serious side-effects (including those that may be life-threatening) are more common in geriatric clients.**

SIDE EFFECTS

Most Common

N&V, postural hypotension, yawning, dyskinesias, somnolence, dizziness, edema, hallucinations, chest pain, increased sweating, flushing, pallor, rhinorrhea.

GI: N&V, constipation, diarrhea. **CV:** Chest pain/pressure, QT prolongation and potential for proarrhythmic effects, postural hypotension, CHF, angina, ***MI, cardiac arrest and/or sudden death***. **CNS:** Somnolence, dizziness, insomnia, hallucinations, confusion, headache, depression, anxiety, falling asleep during activities of daily living. **Musculoskeletal:** Dyskinesia or exacerbation of existing dyskinesia, arthralgia, limb/back pain, spontaneous hypomobility. **GU:** Prolonged, painful erections; UTI. **Respiratory:** Rhinorrhea, pneumonia, dyspnea. **Body as a whole:** Edema, swelling of extremities, increased sweating, flushing, pallor, fatigue, weakness, dehydration, increased risk of falls. **Injection site reactions:** Bruising, granuloma, pruritus. **Miscellaneous:** Yawning, worsening of Parkinson's disease. Rarely, motivation for apomorphine abuse or a psychosexual reaction (including increased libido, priapism, atypical sexual behavior, heightened libido).

DRUG INTERACTIONS

$5HT_3$ antagonists (e.g., alosetron, dolasetron, granisetron, ondansetron, palomosetron) / Profound hypotension and loss of consciousness; do not use apomorphine with any of these drugs
Antihypertensive drugs / ↑ Possibility of hypotension, MI, serious pneumonia, serious falls, bone/joint injuries
Butyrophenones / ↓ Effect of apomorphine R/T dopamine antagonist effect of butyrophenone
Metoclopramide / ↓ Effect of apomorphine R/T dopamine antagonist effect of metoclopramide
Phenothiazines / ↓ Effect of apomorphine R/T dopamine antagonist effect of phenothiazine
Thioxanthines / ↓ Effect of apomorphine R/T dopamine antagonist effect of thioxanthine
Vasodilators / ↑ Possibility of hypotension, MI, serious pneumonia, serious falls, bone/joint injuries

HOW SUPPLIED

Injection: 10 mg/mL.

DOSAGE

SC ONLY

Parkinson's disease.

Always express the dose of apomorphine in mL to avoid confusion. Doses greater than 0.6 mL (6 mg) are not recommended. Titrate the dose on the basis of effectiveness and tolerance starting at 0.2 mL (2 mg) and up to a maximum recommended dose of 0.6 mL (6 mg). Give clients in an "off" state a 0.2 mL (2 mg) test dose in a setting where BP can be closely monitored. Check both supine and standing BP predose and at 20, 40, and 60 min post dose. Those who develop clinically significant orthostatic hypotension to the test are not candidates for treatment with apopmorphine. If the client tolerates the 0.2 mL (2 mg) dose and responds, the starting dose is 0.2 mL (2 mg) used on an as needed basis to treat existing "off" episodes. If needed, the dose can be increased in 0.1 mL (1 mg) increments every few days on an outpatient basis.

For those who tolerate the test dose of 0.2 mL (2 mg) but achieve no response, give a dose of 0.4 mL (4 mg) at the next "off" period, but no sooner than 2 hr after the initial test dose of 0.2 mL (2 mg). Check both supine and standing BP predose and at 20, 40, and 60 min post dose. If the client tolerates a test dose of 0.4 mL (4 mg), the starting dose should be 0.3 mL (3 mg) used on an as needed basis to treat existing "off" episodes. If necessary, increase the dose in 0.1 mL (1 mg) increments every few days on an outpatient basis. If a client does not tolerate a test dose of 0.4 mL (4 mg), give a test dose of 0.3 mL (3 mg) during a separate "off" period, no sooner than 2 hr after the test dose of 0.4 mL (4 mg). Check both supine and standing BP predose and at 20, 40, and 60 min post dose. If the client tolerates the 0.3 mL (3 mg) dose, the starting dose should be 0.2 mL (2 mg) used on an as needed basis to treat existing "off" episodes. If needed, and the 0.2 mL (2 mg) dose is tolerated, the dose can be increased to 0.3 mL (3 mg) after a few days. In such a client, the dose should ordinarily not be increased to 0.4 mL (4 mg) on an out-patient basis.

Most clients respond to 0.3 mL to 0.6 mL (3 to 6 mg). There is no evidence that doses greater than 0.6 mL (6 mg) give an increased effect, and such doses are not recommended. The average frequency of dosing is 3 times per day. There is limited experience with single doses greater than 0.6 mL (6 mg), dosing more than 5 times per day, or with total daily doses greater than 2 mL (20 mg).

If a single dose of apomorphine is ineffective for a particular "off" period, do

A

not give a second dose for that "off" episode. The safety and efficacy of a second dose for a single "off" episode has not been systematically studied.

Clients who have an interruption in therapy of more than a week should be restarted on a 0.2 mL (2 mg) dose and gradually titrated to effect.

NURSING IMPLICATIONS

IMPLEMENTATION/ADMINISTRATION/STORAGE

1. *To avoid confusion, always express the dose in mL; do not give doses greater than 0.6 mL (6 mg).*
2. Clients and caregivers must be given detailed instructions in the preparation and administration of apomorphine. Pay particular attention to correct use of dosing pen.
3. Give apomorphine with an antiemetic (usually trimethobenzamide, 300 mg 3 times per day PO). Start trimethobenzamide 3 days before the initial dose of apomorphine; continue at least during the first 2 months of therapy. DO NOT use $5HT_3$ antagonist antiemetics (e.g., dolasetron, granisetron, ondansetron, palonosetron).
4. For clients with mild to moderate renal impairment, reduce testing dose and subsequently the starting dose to 0.1 mL (1 mg).
5. Use caution in clients with mild to moderate hepatic impairment due to the increased C_{max} and AUC in these people.
6. Store from 15–30°C (59–86°F).

ASSESSMENT

1. Identify frequency of hypomotility episodes (wearing off/end of dose) with advanced Parkinson's disease.
2. List all drugs prescribed/consumed; ensure none interact unfavorably. Drug contains sodium metabisulfite; assess for sensitivity. Any $5HT_3$ antagonist (ondansetron, etc.) should not be used with this drug due to serious adverse effects.
3. Document test dose and response noting supine and standing BP prior to and 20, 40, and 60 min after each test dose; monitor for S&S of orthostatic hypotension, especially during dose escalation.
4. Advise of risks and monitor for melanoma.
5. Establish when client experiencing an "off" episode. May induce "off" state by withholding client's antiparkinson agents overnight. Dose should be titrated according to response and tolerance.
6. Ensure that premedications administered: antiemetic (i.e., trimethobenzamide hydrochloride 300 mg orally 3 times daily) beginning 3 days prior to initiation of apomorphine; continue for the first 2 months of therapy or until tolerance to nausea and vomiting develops.
7. Assess mental status and neurologic evaluations. Continually reassess for drowsiness or sleepiness.
8. Monitor BP, ECG, renal and LFTs. Reduce dose with renal impairment.

CLIENT/FAMILY TEACHING

1. Used to treat loss of control of body movements during a hypomobility phase with advanced Parkinson's disease. Does not prevent these occurrences but helps to improve them once they occur.
2. Dose determined by provider by performing test dose during "off" period.
3. Drug administered just under the skin by a needle. May administer once careful instruction and observation are given by provider. Drug is dosed in milliliters; do not confuse with milligrams; may overdose. Dose on the dosing pen device is expressed in terms of mL. All directions and dosages will be written out to ensure correct dosing.
4. Read/review patient information sheet that comes with each new refill for any changes and new information. Call provider to clarify dosage and answer questions.
5. The prefilled glass cartridges used in the injector pen may be set to administer a certain dose. If the cartridge contains only a partial dose, you can still set the device for the full dose, but you will need to "re-arm" the device and dial in the correct amount of the remaining dose in order to administer the correct amount. Keep a record of how many doses you have delivered for each cartridge to prevent situation from recurring; share with provider.
6. Wash hands, prep site, and rotate injection sites (stomach, upper arms, or upper legs) each time; report any adverse site reactions. Use ice before and after injection at site to re-

duce chances of swelling, redness, pain, itching, bruising, or soreness.
7. Drug may cause dizziness, fainting, or suddenly falling asleep during activities or drowsiness. Avoid activities that require mental alertness; report if persistent/evident.
8. Change positions slowly to prevent sudden drop in BP resulting in dizziness or fainting.
9. Do not change dose without provider approval. Do not use drug if cloudy, green, or contains particles; should be clear and colorless; if not, return for a replacement.
10. Avoid consuming alcohol and any other CNS depressants.
11. May experience worsening of symptoms, depression, headaches, yawning, runny nose and swelling of hands, arms, legs, and feet; report if persistent/bothersome. May also cause hallucinations (unreal visions, sounds, or sensations) or other manifestations of psychotic-like behavior; report if evident.
12. Report chest pain, SOB, fast heartbeats, severe N&V immediately.
13. Store drug in a safe place at room temperature away from children.
14. Intense urges to gamble, sexual urges, other intense urges, and the inability to control these urges have been reported; contact provider if any new or increased urges experienced.
15. Keep all F/U to assess response, review log of drug dose/usage, and for adverse SE. Provider will monitor for excessive use (e.g., use out of proportion to motor signs).

OUTCOMES/EVALUATE

Improvement in mobility and body control during hypomobility phase with advanced Parkinson's disease

Aprepitant

(ah-**PREH**-pih-tant)

Classification(s): Antiemetic

Pregnancy Category: B

RX: Emend.

INDICATIONS/USES

(1) Antiemetic in combination with other antiemetics to prevent acute and delayed N&V associated with initial and repeat courses of highly emetogenic cancer chemotherapy, including high-dose cisplatin. (2) Antiemetic in combination with other antiemetic agents to prevent N&V associated with initial and repeat courses of moderately emetogenic cancer chemotherapy. (3) Prevention of postoperative N&V. Has not been studied for treatment of N&V.

ACTION/KINETICS

Action

A selective, high-affinity antagonist of human substance P/neurokinin 1 (NK_1) receptors in the brain. It augments the antiemetic action of ondansetron and dexamethasone and inhibits both the acute and delayed phases of cisplatin-induced emesis.

Pharmacokinetics

Absolute bioavailability is about 60–65%. **Peak plasma levels**: 4 hr after a 125 mg dose. The AUC is higher in geriatric and Hispanic clients; the t½ is lower in women compared with men. Undergoes extensive metabolism primarily by CYP3A4 with minor metabolism by CYP1A2 and CYP2C19. Excreted in both the urine and feces. **t½, terminal:** 9–13 hr. **Plasma protein binding:** More than 95%.

CONTRAINDICATIONS

Use with astemizole, cisapride, pimozide, or terfenadine (inhibition of CYP3A4 could cause elevated plasma levels of these drugs). Hypersensitivity to any component of the product. Chronic continuous use to prevent N&V. Lactation.

SPECIAL CONCERNS

- Has not been studied for treatment of established N&V.
- Use with caution in clients receiving concomitant drugs that are primarily metabolized via CYP3A4 as aprepitant inhibits this enzyme system, resulting in elevated plasma levels of these drugs and possible toxicity.
- Use with caution in severe hepatic insufficiency.
- Safety and efficacy not determined in children.

SIDE EFFECTS

Most Common

When used with highly emetogenic chemotherapy: Asthenia/fatigue, anorexia, constipation, diarrhea, N&V, hiccoughs, dehydration, dizziness, headache.

A

When used with moderately emetogenic chemotherapy: Fatigue, headache, constipation, dyspepsia, nausea, stomatitis, neutropenia, alopecia. **CNS:** Headache, dizziness, insomnia, anxiety disorder, confusion, depression, peripheral neuropathy, tremor, taste disturbance, hypesthesia, disorientation, dysarthria, sensory disturbance. **GI:** N&V, constipation, diarrhea, anorexia, heartburn, abdominal pain (including upper), gastritis, stomatitis, epigastric discomfort, acid reflux, deglutition disorder, dry mouth, dysgeusia, dyspepsia, dysphagia, eructation, flatulence, increased salivation, obstipation, abnormal bowel sounds, stomach discomfort, perforating duodenal ulcer, enterocolitis. **CV:** ***DVT***, flushing, hypertension, hypotension, ***MI***, palpitations, ***pulmonary embolism***, tachycardia, sinus tachycardia, syncope, bradycardia, hot flush, ***operative hemorrhage***. **Dermatologic:** Alopecia, acne, diaphoresis, rash, pruritus, urticaria, hematoma. **Respiratory:** Hiccoughs, pharynolaryngeal pain, cough, dyspnea, lower or upper RTI, nasal secretion, pharyngitis, pneumonitis, impaired respiratory function, vocal disturbance, dyspnea, hypoxia, respiratory depression, wheezing, pneumonia. **Hematologic:** Neutropenia, anemia, febrile neutropenia, thrombocytopenia. **GU:** Dysuria, pelvic pain, UTI, impaired renal function. **Musculoskeletal:** Arthralgia, back pain, muscular weakness, musculoskeletal pain, myalgia. **Metabolic/Nutritional:** Dehydration, decreased appetite, diabetes mellitus, edema, weight loss. **Ophthalmic:** Conjunctivitis, miosis, decreased visual acuity. **Otic:** Tinnitus. **Body as a whole:** Asthenia, fatigue, malaise, rigors, pain, pyrexia/fever, hypothermia. **Miscellaneous:** Mucous membrane disorder, mucosal inflammation, candidiasis, herpes simplex, malignant neoplasm, non-small-cell lung carcinoma, postoperative infection, wound dehiscence, neutropenic sepsis, ***septic shock***.

LABORATORY TEST CONSIDERATIONS

↑ Alkaline phosphatase, AST, ALT, BUN, serum creatinine, leukocytes, blood bilirubin, blood/urine glucose. ↓ Hemoglobin, WBCs, blood albumin, blood potassium. Erythrocyturia, hyperglycemia, hyponatremia, hypokalemia, hypovolemia, leukocyturia, proteinuria.

DRUG INTERACTIONS

Alprazolam / ↑ Alprazolam plasma levels R/T inhibition of CYP3A4
Carbamazepine / ↓ Aprepitant plasma levels R/T increased metabolism by CYP3A4
Clarithromycin / ↑ Aprepitant plasma levels R/T inhibition of CYP3A4; use together with caution
Dexamethasone / ↑ Dexamethasone AUC, peak levels, and t½ R/T inhibition of CYP3A4; reduce dexamethasone dose by 50%
Diltiazem / ↑ Aprepitant plasma levels R/T inhibition of CYP3A4; use together with caution
Docetaxel / ↑ Docetaxel plasma levels R/T inhibition of CYP3A4
Etoposide / ↑ Etoposide plasma levels R/T inhibition of CYP3A4
Ifosfamide / ↑ Ifosfamide plasma levels R/T inhibition of CYP3A4
Imatinib / ↑ Imatinib plasma levels R/T inhibition of CYP3A4
Irinotecan / ↑ Irinotecan plasma levels R/T inhibition of CYP3A4
Itraconazole / ↑ Aprepitant plasma levels R/T inhibition of CYP3A4; use together with caution
Ketoconazole / ↑ Aprepitant plasma levels R/T inhibition of CYP3A4; use together with caution
Methylprednisolone / ↑ Methylprednisolone AUC, peak levels, and t½ R/T inhibition of CYP3A4; reduce IV methylprednisolone dose by 25% and PO dose by 50%
Midazolam / ↑ Midazolam AUC, peak plasma levels, and t½ R/T inhibition of CYP3A4; dosage adjustment of IV midazolam may be needed
Nefazodone / ↑ Aprepitant plasma levels R/T inhibition of CYP3A4; use together with caution
Nelfinavir / ↑ Aprepitant plasma levels R/T inhibition of CYP3A4; use together with caution
Oral contraceptives / ↓ Oral contraceptive effectiveness during and for 28 days after the last dose of aprepitant; use alternative or backup contraceptive methods during treatment and for 1 month after the last dose
Paclitaxel / ↑ Paclitaxel plasma levels R/T inhibition of CYP3A4
Paroxetine / ↓ AUC and C_{max} of both drugs
Phenytoin / ↓ Aprepitant plasma levels R/T increased metabolism by CYP3A4; also, ↓ phenytoin plasma levels R/T induction of CYP2C9
Pimozide / ↑ Pimozide plasma levels R/T inhibition of CYP3A4; do not use together
Rifampin / ↓ Aprepitant plasma levels R/T increased metabolism by CYP3A4
Ritonavir / ↑ Aprepitant plasma levels R/T inhibition of CYP3A4; use together with caution

Tolbutamide / ↓ Tolbutamide plasma levels R/T induction of CYP2C9
Triazolam / ↑ Triazolam plasma levels R/T inhibition of CYP3A4
Troleandomycin / ↑ Aprepitant plasma levels R/T inhibition of CYP3A4; use together with caution
Vinblastine / ↑ Vinblastine plasma levels R/T inhibition of CYP3A4
Vincristine / ↑ Vincristine plasma levels R/T inhibition of CYP3A4
Vinorelbine / ↑ Vinorelbine plasma levels R/T inhibition of CYP3A4
Warfarin / ↓ Warfarin plasma levels R/T induction of CYP2C9; closely monitor INR especially 7–10 days after beginning aprepitant

HOW SUPPLIED

Capsules: 40 mg, 80 mg, 125 mg.

DOSAGE

CAPSULES

Antiemetic, highly emetogenic cancer chemotherapy.

Day 1: Aprepitant, 125 mg, 1 hr prior to chemotherapy; dexamethasone, 12 mg PO 30 min prior to chemotherapy; and, ondansetron, 32 mg IV 30 min prior to chemotherapy. **Days 2 and 3:** Aprepitant, 80 mg and dexamethasone, 8 mg PO in the morning. **Day 4:** Only dexamethasone, 8 mg PO, in the morning.

Antiemetic, moderately emetogenic cancer chemotherapy.

Day 1: Aprepitant, 125 mg, 1 hr prior to chemotherapy; dexamethasone, 12 mg PO, 30 min prior to chemotherapy; and, ondansetron, 8 mg PO 30–60 min prior to chemotherapy followed by a second 8 mg capsule 8 hr after the first dose. Dexamethasone, 12 mg PO, 30 min prior to chemotherapy. **Days 2 and 3:** Only aprepitant, 80 mg, in the morning.

Prevention of postoperative nausea and vomiting.

40 mg within 3 hr prior to induction of anesthesia.

NURSING IMPLICATIONS

IMPLEMENTATION/ADMINISTRATION/STORAGE

1. The PO dexamethasone doses should be reduced approximately 50% when coadministered with aprepitant. The IV methylprednisolone dose should be reduced approximately 25% and the PO methylprednisolone dose reduced by approximateley 50% when coadministered with aprepitant.
2. Store bottles and blisters from 20–25°C (68–77°F). Keep the desiccant in the original bottle.

ASSESSMENT

1. Identify type of malignancy and chemotherapy prescribed; note other agents trialed/outcome. Give with other antiemetics and corticosteroid.
2. With post-op N&V prevention, give within 3 h prior to induction of anesthesia. Ensure adequately hydrated, assess GI S&S before and after therapy.
3. List drugs prescribed; ensure none interact.
4. Assess mental status. Monitor CBC, renal and LFTs during therapy.

CLIENT/FAMILY TEACHING

1. Take as directed: first dose 1 hour before start of chemotherapy with other antiemetics and a corticosteroid. Will need to use an additional antiemetic drug for breakthrough vomiting. This drug is part of a regimen that has been found to help alleviate N&V associated with prescribed chemotherapy. Will take a lower dose on days 2 and 3 following the chemotherapy with or without food.
2. Consume plenty of fluids to ensure adequate hydration.
3. Practice reliable nonhormonal contraception.
4. Report adverse effects or lack of response. Use caution when performing tasks that require mental alertness; may cause dizziness and drowsiness especially in higher doses.
5. May require medication to relieve headaches and constipation; report if evident or persistent. Avoid all OTC preparations or herbals without provider approval.
6. Keep all F/U to assess response, labs, and adverse SE.

A

OUTCOMES/EVALUATE

- Prevention/control of chemotherapy-induced N&V
- Prevention of postoperative nausea and vomiting

IV

Argatroban

(are-**GAT**-roh-ban)

Classification(s): Anticoagulant, thrombin inhibitor

Pregnancy Category: B

RX: Argatroban.

INDICATIONS/USES

(1) As an anticoagulant for prophylaxis or treatment in heparin-induced thrombocytopenia (HIT) or heparin-induced thrombosis-thrombocytopenia syndrome (HITTS). (2) Anticoagulant in those with or at risk for heparin-induced thrombocytopenia or heparin-induced thrombosis-thrombocytopenia in those undergoing percutaneous coronary intervention.

ACTION/KINETICS

Action

A synthetic, direct thrombin inhibitor derived from L-arginine. Reversibly binds to the thrombin active site and does not require antithrombin III for antithrombotic activity. Acts by inhibiting thrombin-catalyzed or induced reactions, including fibrin formation; activation of coagulation Factors V, VIII, and XIII; protein C; and platelet aggregation. Inhibits both free and clot-associated thrombin. The small molecule provides the needed anticoagulant effect without worsening hypercoagulable states. Has little or no effect on trypsin, Factor Xa, plasmin, and kallikrein. Does not interact with heparin-induced antibodies. Coadministration with warfarin produces a combined effect on INR, but coadministration exerts no additional effect on vitamin-K-dependent factor Xa activity.

Pharmacokinetics

Distributes mainly in the extracellular fluid. Steady state reached, by IV infusion, in 1–3 hr and is continued until infusion is stopped. Metabolized in the liver by CYP3A4/5. **t½, terminal:** 39–51 min. Excreted in the feces, primarily through biliary excretion. Clearance is decreased in seriously ill children **Plasma protein binding:** 54%.

CONTRAINDICATIONS

Overt major bleeding, hypersensitivity to the product or any of its components. Use with heparin in heparin-induced thrombocytopenia. Lactation.

SPECIAL CONCERNS

- Use with extreme caution in hepatic disease (use lower doses) and in disease states and circumstances with an increased danger of hemorrhage, including severe hypertension, immediately following lumbar puncture, spinal anesthesia, major surgery (especially the brain, spinal cord, or eye), congenital or acquired bleeding disorders, and GI lesions (e.g., ulcerations).
- Hemorrhage can occur at any site in the body.
- Safety and efficacy not determined in children less than 18 years of age, although the drug has been used in seriously ill children.

SIDE EFFECTS

Most Common

Chest pain, hypotension, N&V, headache, major/minor bleeding episodes.

Bleeding: ***Major hemorrhagic events,*** including GI, GU/hematuria, decreased H&H, ***multisystem hemorrhage*** and DIC, limb and below the knee amputation stump, ***intracranial bleeding/hemorrhage***, ***retroperitoneal hemorrhage.*** Minor hemorrhagic events, including GI (including hematemesis), GU/hematuria, groin, hemoptysis, brachial, coronary artery bypass graft, access site, hemoptysis. ***Intracranial bleeding*** in clients with acute MI started on argatroban and streptokinase. **Allergic:** Airway reactions (coughing, dyspnea), rash, bullous eruption, vasodilation. **CNS:** Headache. **GI:** Diarrhea, N&V, GERD, abdominal pain, ***GI hemorrhage.*** **CV:** Hypotension, aortic stenosis, ***cardiac arrest, VT, MI, coronary thrombosis, myocardial ischemia, coronary occlusion, arterial thrombosis***, cerebrovascular/vascular disorder, bradycardia, angina pectoris, atrial fibrillation. **Respiratory:** Dyspnea, pneumonia, coughing, lung edema. **GU:** UTI, abnormal renal function. **Body as a whole:** Fever, pain, infection, allergic reactions, ***sepsis.*** **Miscellaneous:** Back/chest pain.

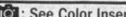

LABORATORY TEST CONSIDERATIONS

↓ H&H. Coadministration of argatroban and warfarin produces a combined effect on laboratory measurement of INR. However, concurrent therapy exerts no additional effect on vitamin-K-dependent Factor Xa activity, compared with warfarin monotherapy.

OVERDOSE MANAGEMENT

Symptoms: Major/minor bleeding events. *Treatment:* Discontinue argatroban or decrease infusion dose. Anticoagulation parameters usually return to baseline within 2–4 hr after discontinuing the drug. Reversal may take longer in hepatic impairment. No specific antidote is available. Provide symptomatic and supportive therapy.

DRUG INTERACTIONS

Alteplase / ↑ Risk of bleeding
Clopidogrel / ↑ Risk of bleeding
Epifibatide / Safety and efficacy of use together not established
Heparin / Prolongation of PT and INR; use together contraindicated in HIT
NSAIDs / ↑ Risk of bleeding
Salicylates / ↑ Risk of bleeding
Streptokinase / ↑ Risk of bleeding
Tirofiban / Safety and efficacy of use together not established
Warfarin / Prolongation of PT and INR; use together contraindicated in HIT

HOW SUPPLIED

Injection, Solution Concentrate: 100 mg/mL.

DOSAGE

IV INFUSION

Heparin-induced thrombocytopenia (HIT) or heparin-induced thrombocytopenia and thrombosis syndrome (HITTS).

Adults, initial, without hepatic impairment: 2 mcg/kg/min as a continuous IV infusion. The infusion rate depends on body weight (see package insert). After the initial dose, adjust dose as clinically indicated, not to exceed 10 mcg/kg/min, until the steady state aPTT is 1.5–3 times initial baseline value, not to exceed 100 seconds. Steady-state levels usually reached within 1–3 hr following initiation of argatroban. Adjustment of dose may be necessary to attain the target aPTT. Check aPTT 2 hr after initiation of therapy to confirm that the aPTT is within the desired therapeutic range.

Percutaneous coronary intervention in HIT/HITTS.

Adults, initial: Start a continuous infusion at 25 mcg/kg/min and a bolus of 350 mcg/kg given via a large bore IV line over 3–5 min. Check activated clotting time (ACT) 5–10 min after the bolus dose is completed. If the ACT is less than 300 sec, give an additional IV bolus dose of 150 mcg/kg, increase the infusion dose to 30 mcg/kg/min, and check the ACT 5–10 min later.

If the ACT is greater than 450 seconds, decrease the infusion rate to 15 mcg/kg/min and check the ACT 5–10 min later. Once an ACT between 300 and 450 sec has been reached, continue this infusion for the duration of the procedure. In the event of dissection, impending abrupt closure, thrombus formation during the procedure, or inability to achieve or maintain ACT over 300 sec, give additional bolus doses of 150 mcg/kg and increase the infusion dose to 40 mcg/kg/min. Check ACT after each additional bolus or change in infusion rate. If anticoagulation is needed after the procedure, argatroban may be continued but at a lower infusion dose (see preceding dose for HIT/HITTS). *NOTE:* Do not use high doses in PCI clients with clinically significant hepatic disease or AST/ALT levels of 3 or more times ULN.

Initial doses are lower for seriously ill children compared with adults with healthy hepatic function.

Impaired hepatic function (for all uses).

Adults, initial, moderate hepatic impairment: 0.5 mcg/kg/min, based on about a 4-fold decrease in argatroban clearance compared with normal hepatic function.

NURSING IMPLICATIONS

IMPLEMENTATION/ADMINISTRATION/STORAGE

1. **IV Discontinue all parenteral anticoagulants before giving argatroban.**

2. If argatroban is begun after cessation of heparin, allow sufficient time for effects of heparin on aPTT to decrease before starting argatroban therapy.
3. To prepare IV infusion: Dilute in 0.9% NaCl, D5W, or LR injection to a final concentration of 1 mg/mL. Dilute each 2.5 mL vial 100-fold by mixing with 250 mL of diluent.
4. Mix reconstituted solution by repeated inversion of the diluent bag for 1 min. After preparation, solution may be briefly hazy R/T formation of microprecipitates; dissolves rapidly upon mixing.
5. If prepared correctly, pH of IV solution is 3.2–7.5.
6. Use of argatroban and warfarin results in prolongation of INR beyond that caused by warfarin alone. If used together, a loading dose of warfarin should not be used. Initiate therapy using the expected daily dose of warfarin. Measure INR daily if argatroban and warfarin are given together. Generally, with doses of argatroban of 2 mcg/kg/min or less, argatroban can be discontinued when the INR is greater than 4 on combined therapy. After argatroban is discontinued, repeat INR measurement in 4–6 hr. If the repeat INR is below the desired range, resume argatroban infusion and repeat the procedure daily until the desired therapeutic range on warfarin alone is reached.
7. For doses of argatroban greater than 2 mcg/kg/min, the relationship of INR on warfarin alone to the INR of both drugs given together is less predictable. Thus, temporarily reduce dose of argatroban to 2 mcg/kg/min. Repeat INR on argatroban and warfarin 4–6 hr after reducing argatroban dose and follow process outlined previously for giving argatroban at doses of 2 mcg/kg/min or less.
8. Argatroban is a clear, colorless to pale yellow, slightly viscous solution. Discard vial if the solution is cloudy or an insoluble precipitate is observed.
9. Store vials in original cartons protected from light from 15–30°C (59–86°F); do not freeze. Prepared solutions stable at 15–30°C (59–85°F) for 24 hr at ambient indoor light. Prepared solutions are stable for 48 hr or less when stored at 2–8°C (36–46°F) in the dark. Do not expose prepared solutions to direct sunlight.
10. COMPATIBILITY 0.9% NaCl, D5W, or LR.
11. INCOMPATIBILITY Do not mix argatroban with other drugs or infusions.

ASSESSMENT

1. Note reasons for therapy: thrombosis prophylaxis or treatment (HIT or during PCI). List all drugs prescribed/consumed; ensure none interact.
2. Review history; note conditions that may preclude drug therapy. Note active bleeding sites/disorders. Stop heparin therapy.
3. Observe closely for evidence of abnormal/hidden bleeding or adverse effects. Perform routine vascular checks.
4. Obtain and monitor weight, INR (when used with warfarin), PT/PTT (with heparin-before, during, and 2 hr after therapy), CBC, and LFTs. Lower dosage with liver dysfunction.

CLIENT/FAMILY TEACHING

1. Review goals of therapy and potential bleeding risks.
2. Report unusual oozing or bleeding sites and wet bandages or bedding.
3. Use soft-bristled toothbrush, electric razor, and avoid IM shots.
4. Report any bleeding or unusual bruising, coughing, difficulty breathing, skin rash, or adverse reaction.
5. Encourage family members to learn CPR.

OUTCOMES/EVALUATE

- Inhibition/treatment of thrombus formation with HIT
- ↓ Risk of HIT during PCI

Aripiprazole

(**ah**-rih-**PIP**-rah-zohl)

Classification(s): Antipsychotic

Pregnancy Category: C

RX: Abilify, Abilify Discmelt.

INDICATIONS/USES

PO. (1) Acute and maintenance treatment of schizophrenia in adults and adolescents 13–17 years of age. (2) Monotherapy in adults and children 10–17 years of age for acute and maintenance treatment of manic and mixed episodes with bipolar I disorder with or without psychotic features. (3) Adjunctive therapy to either lithium or valproate in adults and children 10–17 years of age for acute treatment of manic and mixed episodes associated with bipolar I disorder. (4) Adjunctive treatment to antidepressants for major depressive disorders in adults. (5) Treatment of irritability associated with autistic disorder in children. *Investigational:* Restless legs syndrome, cocaine dependence, Tourette's syndrome in children and adolescents.

IM only. Acute treatment of agitation associated with schizophrenia or bipolar disorder (manic or mixed) in adults.

ACTION/KINETICS

Action

Mechanism not known with certainty but likely due to high affinity for dopamine D_2 (partial agonist) and D_3 receptors as well as 5-HT_{1A} (partial agonist) and antagonist activity at 5-HT_{2A} receptors. The drug has moderate affinity for dopamine D_4, serotonin 5-HT_7, serotonin 5-HT_{2C}, alpha-1 adrenergic, and histamine H_1 receptors. Increased C_{max} in severe renal impairment and in women. Low incidence of sedation and orthostatic hypotension, low to no effect to cause anticholinergic effects, and no effect to cause extrapyramidal symptoms. Is a low incidence of weight gain. Metabolized in the liver by CYP3A4 and CYP 2D6. Clearance decreases (20%) in clients 65 years and older.

Pharmacokinetics

Well absorbed (87% bioavailable). **Peak plasma levels:** 3–5 hr. A high-fat meal will delay the $T_{max.}$ **t½, elimination:** 75 hr for extensive metabolizers and 146 hr for poor metabolizers. Metabolized by CYP2D6 and CYP3A4 enzymes in the liver. Excreted through both the feces (about 55%) and urine (about 25%). Clearance is decreased in the elderly. **Plasma protein binding:** >99%.

CONTRAINDICATIONS

Lactation. Use in those with dementia-related psychosis. Use of alcohol.

SPECIAL CONCERNS

(1) **Increased mortality in elderly clients with dementia-related psychosis.** Elderly clients with dementia-related psychosis treated with atypical antipsychotic drugs are at an increased risk of death, compared with placebo. Analyses of placebo-controlled trials (modal duration, 10 weeks), largely in clients taking atypical antipsychotic drugs, revealed a risk of death in the drug-treated clients of between 1.6 to 1.7 times the death in placebo-treated clients. Over the course of a typical 10-week controlled trial, the rate of death in drug-treated clients was about 4.5% compared with a rate of about 2.6% in the placebo group. Although the causes of death were varied, most of the deaths appeared to be either cardiovascular (e.g., heart failure, sudden death) or infections (e.g., pneumonia) in nature. Observational studies suggest that, similar to atypical antipsychotic drugs, treatment with conventional antipsychotic drugs may increase mortality. The extent to which the findings of increased mortality in observational studies may be attributed to the antipsychotic drug as opposed to some characteristic(s) of the clients is not clear. Aripiprazole is not approved for the treatment of clients with dementia-related psychosis.
(2) **Suicidality and antidepressant drugs.** Antidepressants increased the risk of suicidal thinking and behavior (suicidality) in children, adolescents, and young adults in short-term studies of major depressive disorder and other psychiatric disorders. Anyone considering the use of adjunctive aripiprazole or any other antidepressant in a child, adolescent, or young adult must balance this risk with the clinical need. Short-term studies did not show an increase in the risk of suicidality with antidepressants compared with placebo in adults older than 24 years of age; there was a reduction in the risk with antidepressants compared with placebo in adults 65 years of age and older. Depression and certain other psychiatric disorders are themselves associated with increases in the risk of suicide. Appropriately monitor clients of all ages who are started on antidepressant therapy, and closely observe them for clinical worsening, suicidality, or unusual changes in behavior. Advise families and caregivers of the need for close observation and communication with the prescriber. Aripiprazole is not approved for use in children with depression.

A

- Use with caution in history of MI, ischemic heart disease, heart failure, conduction abnormalities, cerebrovascular disease, or conditions that predispose to hypotension (e.g., dehydration, hypovolemia, antihypertensive drug treatment).
- Use with caution in conditions that may contribute to an increase in body temperature and in those at risk for aspiration pneumonia.
- There is an increased risk of hyperglycemia and diabetes.
- May cause weight gain in young clients.
- Elderly clients with dementia-related psychosis show a higher incidence of stroke, TIAs, and death.
- Safety and efficacy in psychosis associated with dementia, in psychosis associated with Alzheimer's disease, or in children and adolescents have not been evaluated.
- Long-term efficacy has not been established.

SIDE EFFECTS

Most Common

Headache, agitation, anxiety, akathisia, insomnia, asthenia, dyspepsia, pharyngitis, myalgia, tardive dystonia, constipation, N&V, drowsiness/sedation/somnolence, accidental injury, weight gain.

Neuroleptic Malignant Syndrome: Hyperpyrexia, muscle rigidity, altered mental status, autonomic instability, rhabdomyolysis, acute renal failure. **CNS:** Headache, agitation, insomnia, akathisia, depersonalization, drowsiness/sedation, somnolence, dysphoria, anxiety, lightheadedness, tardive dystonia, extrapyramidal symptoms, confusion, depression, abnormal/bizarre dreams, abnormal gait, hostility, hypersomnia, nervousness, hallucinations, akinesia, amnesia, apathy, ataxia, delirium, dysarthria, dyskinesia, dystonia, hyperactivity, hyperkinesia, hyperreflexia, hypesthesia, hyperesthesia, hypokinesia, impaired concentration/memory, migraine, neuropathy, obsessive thought, panic attack, paresthesia, psychosis, manic reaction, suicide attempt/thought, stupor, tardive dyskinesia, vertigo, euphoria, incoordination, slowed thinking, blunted affect, decreased consciousness, decreased reflexes. **GI:** N&V, dyspepsia, constipation, salivation, abdominal discomfort/pain, abdominal distention/enlargement, anorexia, increased appetite, bloating, colitis, diarrhea, dry mouth, duodenal ulcer, dyspepsia, dysphagia, eructation, fecal impaction, fecal incontinence, flatulence, gastritis, gastroenteritis, gastroesophageal reflux, gingivitis, glossitis, ***GI hemorrhage***, hemorrhoids, hiccough, increased sputum, intestinal obstruction, mouth ulceration, pancreatitis, peptic ulcer, periodontal abscess, polydipsia, ***rectal hemorrhage,*** stomatitis, altered taste, tooth caries, esophageal ulcer/esophagitis, gum hemorrhage, hematemesis, melena, esophageal dysmotility and aspiration, cheilitis, oral moniliasis. **Hepatic:** Cholecystitis, cholelithiasis, hepatitis, hepatomegaly. **CV:** Hypertension, bradycardia, hypotension, tachycardia, angina pectoris, premature atrial contractions, atrial fibrillation/flutter, AV block, ***cardiac arrest***, ***CVA***, CHF, extrasystoles, ***MI***, myocardial ischemia, palpitation, phlebitis, prolonged QTc interval, ***pulmonary embolus***, ***hemorrhage***, ***intracranial hemorrhage***, vasodilation, thrombophlebitis (including deep), cardiomegaly, cerebral ischemia, vasovagal reaction, shortened QT interval. **GU:** Amenorrhea, anorgasmia, cystitis, dysmenorrhea, dysuria, ejaculation disorders, gynecomastia, hematuria, impotence, urinary incontinence, mastalgia, acute renal failure, urinary frequency, kidney calculus, urgency increased, urinary retention, uterine/vaginal hemorrhage, increased/decreased libido, menorrhagia, nocturia, polyuria, priapism, vaginal moniliasis, cervicitis, urinary burning, urolithiasis, vaginitis. **Musculoskeletal:** Myalgia, arthralgia, joint pain, arthritis, back pain, bone pain, bradykinesia, bursitis, muscle weakness, myoclonus, myopathy, cogwheel rigidity, muscle cramps, hypertonia, jaw pain/tightness, neck pain/rigidity, restless leg, pelvic pain, arthrosis, spasm, tenosynovitis, rhabdomyolysis, rheumatoid arthritis, tendonitis. **Respiratory:** Pharyngitis, rhinitis, increased cough, asthma, dry nasal passages, dyspnea, epistaxis, pneumonia, aspiration pneumonia, chest pain/tightness, apnea, hemoptysis, hypoxia, laryngitis, pulmonary edema, ***respiratory failure***, throat tight, throat pain, buccoglossal syndrome, URTI. **Dermatologic:** Ecchymosis, acne, alopecia, eczema, pallor, photosensitivity, pruritus, psoriasis, rash, vesiculobullous rash, seborrhea, urticaria, dermatitis (including exfoliative dermatitis), maculopapular skin reactions, dry skin, skin ulcer. **Hematologic:** Anemia, hypochromic anemia, leukocytosis, leukorrhea, iron deficiency anemia, leukopenia, eosinophilia, lymphadenopathy, macrocytic anemia, thrombocythemia, thrombocytopenia. **Metabolic:** Peripheral edema, cyanosis, diabetes mellitus, edema, facial/tongue edema, gout, goiter, hyper-/hypothyroidism. **Ophthalmic:**

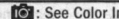

Blurred vision, conjunctivitis, eye hemorrhage, blepharitis, cataracts, dry eyes, diplopia, eye pain, oculogyric crisis, photophobia, amblyopia, increased lacrimation, increased blinking. **Otic:** Tinnitus, ear pain, otitis media/externa, deafness. **Body as a whole:** Asthenia, malaise, weight gain/loss, obesity, allergic reaction, accidental injury, dehydration, diaphoresis, fever, flu syndrome, chills. **Miscellaneous:** Heat stroke, head heaviness, Mendelson syndrome, dental pain.

LABORATORY TEST CONSIDERATIONS

↑ CPK, AST, ALT, BUN, alkaline phosphatase, creatinine, LDH. Albuminuria, glycosuria, hypercholesterolemia, hyper-/hypoglycemia, hyper-/hypokalemia, hyperlipemia, hyponatremia, bilirubinemia, hyperuricemia.

DRUG INTERACTIONS

Alcohol / Possible dystonic reactions
Antihypertensive drugs / Possible enhanced orthostatic hypotension R/T blockade of alpha-adrenergic receptors
Carbamazepine / ↑ Aripiprazole clearance → ↓ blood levels R/T induction of CYP3A4 enzymes; double the aripiprazole dose
Clarithromycin / ↓ Aripiprazole metabolism → ↑ blood levels R/T inhibition of CYP3A4 enzymes; reduce aripiprazole to one-half the usual dose
CNS depressants / Possible enhanced CNS depression, especially impaired motor skills
Famotidine / ↓ Aripiprazole absorption → ↓ C_{max} and AUC
Fluoxetine / ↓ Aripiprazole metabolism → ↑ blood levels R/T inhibition of CYP2D6 enzymes; reduce aripiprazole dose to at least one-half the usual dose
Ketoconazole / ↓ Aripiprazole metabolism → ↑ blood levels R/T inhibition of CYP3A4 enzymes; reduce aripiprazole to one-half the usual dose
Paroxetine / ↓ Aripiprazole metabolism → ↑ blood levels R/T inhibition of CYP2D6 enzymes; reduce aripiprazole to one-half the usual dose
Quinidine / ↓ Aripiprazole metabolism → ↑ blood levels R/T inhibition of CYP2D6 enzymes; reduce aripiprazole to one-half the usual dose
Valproate / ↓ Aripiprazole C_{max} and AUC by 25%

HOW SUPPLIED

Injection Solution: 7.5 mg/mL; ***Oral Solution:*** 1 mg/mL; ***Tablets:*** 2 mg, 5 mg, 10 mg, 15 mg, 20 mg, 30 mg; ***Tablets, Orally Disintegrating (Discmelt):*** 10 mg, 15 mg.

DOSAGE

ORAL SOLUTION; TABLETS; TABLETS, ORALLY DISINTEGRATING

Schizophrenia, adults.

Initial and target dose: 10 or 15 mg/day given on a once-a-day schedule using the tablet formulation. **Maintenance dose range:** 10–30 mg/day (doses higher than 10 or 15 mg/day were not more effective). Do not make dosage increases before 2 weeks, the time required to reach steady state. Maintenance dosing has been used for periods up to 6 months. Periodically assess to determine the need for maintenance treatment.

Schizophrenia, adolescents, 13 to 17 years of age.

Initial: 2 mg/day using the tablet formulation. Usually titrated to 5 mg after 2 days and to the target dose of 10 mg/day after 2 additional days. Give subsequent dose increases in 5 mg increments. A 30 mg/day dose is not more effective than a 10 mg/day dose. Can be given without regard to meals. **Maintenance:** 10–30 mg/day. The 30 mg/day dose was not shown to be more effective than the 10 mg/day dose. Those responding can be continued beyond the acute response; use the lowest dose needed to maintain remission. Periodically assess to determine the need for maintenance treatment.

Bipolar disorder.

Adults, acute treatment, initial and target dose: 15 mg as monotherapy or as adjunctive therapy with lithium or valproate given once a day without regard to meals. The dose may be increased to 30 mg/day based on clinical response. Doses above 30 mg/day have not been evaluated. **Maintenance:** May be used for up to 6 weeks; data are not available to support treatment beyond 6 weeks. **Children, 10–17 years of age, acute treatment, initial:** 2 mg/day using the tablet formulation; titrate to 5 mg/day after 2 days and to the target dose of 10 mg/day after 2 additional days when used as monotherapy or as adjunctive therapy. Make subsequent dose increases in increments of 5 mg/day. **Maintenance:** 10 or 30 mg/day. Responding adults and children, 10–17 years, can be continued beyond the acute response but at the lowest dose needed to maintain remission. Periodically assess to determine the need for maintenance therapy.

Adjunct to antidepressants for major depressive disorder.

Adults, initial: 2–5 mg/day in those already taking an antidepressant. Adjust dosage of up to 5 mg/day gradually, at intervals of no less than 1 week; doses up to 15 mg/day have been used. Long-term efficacy has not been determined; periodically assess to determine the need for maintenance treatment. Efficacy has not been determined for adjunctive treatment of major depressive disorder in children.

Irritability in children associated with autistic disorder.

Children, 6–17 years of age, initial: 2 mg/day. Dosage should be increased to 5 mg/day, with subsequent increases to 10 or 15 mg/day, if needed. Dosage adjustments of up to 5 mg/day should occur gradually, at intervals of no less than 1 week. **Dosage range:** 5–15 mg/day; individualize dosage based on tolerability and response. **Maintenance:** No data exist on how long treatment should continue.

INJECTION (IM ONLY)

Agitation associated with schizophrenia or bipolar mania.

Adults, initial: 9.75 mg; **dose range:** 5.25–15 mg. If agitation persists following the initial dose, cumulative doses up to 30 mg/day may be given. The safety of total daily doses greater than 30 mg or injections given more frequently than q 2 hr have not been adequately evaluated. If ongoing therapy is indicated, PO aripiprazole in a dose range from 10–30 mg/day should replace the injection as soon as possible. The injection has not been evaluated in children.

NURSING IMPLICATIONS

Do not confuse aripiprazole with lansoprazole (proton pump inhibitor).

IMPLEMENTATION/ADMINISTRATION/STORAGE

1. If switching from other antipsychotics, minimize period of overlapping antipsychotic administration.
2. Oral solution can be given on a mg-per-mg basis in place of the 5, 10, 15, or 20 mg tablet strengths. Clients receiving 30 mg tablets should receive 25 mg of the solution.
3. The dosing for the orally disintegrating tablets is the same as for the oral tablets.
4. To administer the injection, draw up the required volume of solution as follows: 0.7 mL for the 5.25 mg dose, 1.3 mL for the 9.75 mg dose, and 2 mL for the 15 mg dose. Inject slowly deep in the muscle mass. Discard any unused portion.
5. Do not give the injection IV or SC.
6. Opened bottles of solution can be used for up to 6 months after opening if refrigerated.
7. Reduce the dose of aripiprazole to one-half the usual dose if given with CYP3A4 inhibitors (e.g., clarithromycin, ketoconazole). When the CYP3A4 inhibitor is withdrawn, increase the dose of aripiprazole.
8. Reduce the dose of aripiprazole to at least one-half the usual dose if given with potential CYP2D6 inhibitors (e.g., fluoxetine, paroxetine, quinidine). When the CYP2D6 inhibitor is withdrawn, increase the dose of aripiprazole.
9. Double the dose of aripiprazole if given with a potential CYP3A4 inducers (e.g., carbamazepine). Base additional increases in dose based on clinical evaluation. When the CYP3A4 inducer is withdrawn, reduce the dose of aripiprazole to 10 or 15 mg.
10. Protect the injection from light by storing in the original container. Keep in carton until time of use.
11. Store the injection, tablets, and oral solution between 15–30°C (59–86°F).

A

ASSESSMENT

1. Identify behaviors/conditions requiring management, other agents trialed and outcome. Note clinical presentation and behavioral manifestations.
2. List drugs prescribed; ensure no interactions or dosage adjustments needed.
3. Assess mental status, evidence/history of CAD, hypo-/hypertension. Use cautiously with CAD, seizure history, or conditions that lower seizure threshold, e.g., Alzheimer's dementia. Use caution; has caused fatal heart attack and stroke in older adults with dementia-related conditions.
4. Aripiprazole has been given for up to 26 weeks, although it can be used for longer-term efficacy; ensure clients assessed regularly by a psychiatrist to determine need for maintenance therapy.
   - DSM III/IV-TR criteria for schizophrenia: delusions, conceptual disorganization, hallucinatory behavior, excitement, grandiosity, suspiciousness/persecution, and hostility.
   - PANSS (Positive and Negative Syndrome Scale) should include 7+ symptoms of schizophrenia: blunted affect, emotional withdrawal, poor rapport, passive apathetic withdrawal, difficulty with abstract thinking, lack of spontaneity/flow of conversation, stereotypical thinking).
5. Monitor VS, weights, ECG, I&O, lipid panel, BS, electrolytes, CPK, renal and LFTs, and for evidence of diabetes.

CLIENT/FAMILY TEACHING

1. Take with or without food once daily with a full glass of water.
2. Do not split or open blister for orally disintegrating tablet until ready to take.
3. Place these tablets on the tongue—disintegration occurs rapidly in saliva so it may be taken without water. Do not split the tablet.
4. With diabetes, each mL of Abilify oral solution contains 400 mg of sucrose and 200 mg of fructose. Use tablets and check blood sugar often to ensure control.
5. Avoid activities that require mental alertness until drug effects realized; may impair judgment, thinking, or motor skills.
6. Change positions slowly; prevents sudden drop in BP. Hot tubs, hot showers, or baths mhot showersay aggravate dizziness.
7. May alter temperature regulation. Avoid alcohol, CNS depressants, OTC agents, strenuous exercise, overheating, or dehydration.
8. May cause esophogeal dysmotility—may result in aspiration; use caution.
9. Do not add any medications or OTC agents without provider approval due to the potential for strong drug interactions.
10. Immediately report any S&S of NMS (neuroleptic malignant syndrome): increased temperature, muscle rigidity, irregular heart rate/BP, arrhythmias or severe diaphoresis.
11. Report any movements that become involuntary, slow, repetitive, rhythmical (tardive dyskinesia) in select or groups of muscles; may become irreversible.
12. Practice reliable contraception, report if pregnancy suspected.
13. Prescriptions will be for small amounts to prevent overdose and for the smallest dose and shortest duration of treatment needed. Report any suicide ideations. Psychiatric therapy and evaluation should be regular and ongoing.
14. Keep all F/U to assess response, labs, BP, weight, and for adverse SE.

OUTCOMES/EVALUATE

- Improvement in PANSS and DSM III/IV-TR schizophrenia criteria
- Improved behavioral and emotional presentation
- ↓ Delusions/suspiciousness and hostility

Armodafinil

(ar-moe-**DAF**-in-il)

Classification(s): Analeptic

Pregnancy Category: C

RX: Nuvigil, **C-IV**

INDICATIONS/USES

(1) Improve wakefulness in clients with excessive sleepiness associated with narcolepsy. (2) Improve wakefulness in clients with excessive sleepiness associated with obstructive sleep apnea-hypopnea syndrome (OSA). May be used with continuous positive airway pressure (CPAP). (3) Improve

A

wakefulness in those with excessive sleepiness associated with shift-work sleep disorder (SWSD).

ACTION/KINETICS

Action

Precise mechanism is unknown. The drug has wake-promoting effects similar to amphetamine or methylphenidate, although the pharmacology is not identical to that of sympathomimetic amines. Modafinil, a similar drug, produces psychoactive and euphoric effects, as well as alterations in mood, perception, thinking, and feelings. *NOTE:* Armodafinil is the R isomer of racemic modafinil.

Pharmacokinetics

Readily absorbed after PO use. **Peak plasma levels:** About 2 hr in the fasted state. **Apparent steady state:** Reached within 7 days. Time to reach T_{max} may be delayed from 2–4 hr in the fed state. Metabolized by liver enzymes, including CYP3A4 and CYP3A5. **t½, terminal:** About 15 hr. 80% excreted in the urine. Clearance may be reduced in geriatric clients. **Plasma protein binding:** Approximately 60%, mainly to albumin.

CONTRAINDICATIONS

Hypersensitivity to armodafinil or modafinil or any component of the product. Use not recommended in those with a history of left ventricular hypertrophy or with mitral valve prolapse who have experienced mitral valve prolapse syndrome when previously receiving CNS stimulants. Not approved for use in children.

SPECIAL CONCERNS

- **Use with caution in those with a history of psychosis, depression, mania; in those with a recent history of MI or unstable angina; and during lactation.**
- **The abuse potential is likely to be similar to that of modafinil.**

SIDE EFFECTS

Most Common

Headache, nausea, dry mouth, insomnia, dizziness, anxiety, diarrhea.

GI: Nausea, diarrhea, dry mouth, dyspepsia, upper abdominal pain, constipation, loose stools, vomiting. **CNS:** Headache, dizziness, insomnia, anxiety, fatigue, depression, agitation, depressed mood, disturbance in attention, migraine, nervousness, parestheisa, tremor. Persistent sleepiness, mania, delusions, hallucinations, ***suicidal ideations***. **CV:** Palpitations, increased HR, small increases in mean systolic and diastolic BP and pulse rate. **Dermatologic:** Rash, including ***Stevens-Johnson syndrome;*** contact dermatitis, hyperhidrosis. **Metabolic/Nutritional:** Anorexia, decreased appetite. **Body as a whole:** Fatigue, angioedema, ***anaphylactoid reactions***, multiorgan hypersensitivity reactions. **Miscellaneous:** Dyspnea, flu-like illness, pain, polyuria, pyrexia, seasonal allergy, thirst.

LABORATORY TEST CONSIDERATIONS

↑ GGT, alkaline phosphatase.

OVERDOSE MANAGEMENT

Symptoms: Similar to modafinil, including excitation, agitation, insomnia, slight or moderate increase in hemodynamic parameters. *Treatment:* No specific antidote exists. Provide supportive treatment, including CV monitoring. If there are no contraindications, consider gastric lavage.

DRUG INTERACTIONS

Alcohol / Avoid concomitant use
Carbamazepine / Possible ↓ armodafinil levels R/T ↑ metabolism by CYP3A4/5
Clomipramine / ↑ Clomipramine levels R/T inhibition of CYP2C19
Contraceptives, steroidal / Possible ↓ efficacy of steroidal contraceptives during and for 1 month after armodafinil co-administration; use of alternative methods of contraception recommended
Cyclosporine / ↓ Cyclosporine levels; monitor levels and adjust dose
Diazepam / ↑ Diazepam levels R/T ↓ metabolism by CYP2C19
Erythromycin / Possible ↑ armodafinil levels R/T ↓ metabolism by CYP3A4/5
Ethinyl estradiol / ↓ Systemic exposure to ethinyl estradiol; dose adjustment may be needed
Ketoconazole / Possible ↑ armodafinil levels R/T ↓ metabolism by CYP3A4/5
MAOIs / Use caution when using together
Midazolam / ↓ Midazolam levels R/T ↑ metabolism by CYP3A4/5
Omeprazole / ↑ Omeprazole levels R/T inhibition of CYP2C19
Phenobarbital / Possible ↓ armodafinil levels R/T ↑ metabolism by CYP3A4/5
Phenytoin / ↑ Phenytoin levels R/T inhibition of CYP2C19; dose reduction may be needed

Propranolol / ↑ Propranolol levels R/T inhibition of CYP2C19; dose reduction may be needed
Rifampin / Possible ↓ armodafinil levels R/T ↑ metabolism by CYP3A4/5
Triazolam / ↓ Triazolam levels R/T ↑ metabolism by CYP3A4/5
Warfarin / Possible interaction; monitor PT and INR more frequently

HOW SUPPLIED

Tablets: 50 mg, 150 mg, 250 mg.

DOSAGE

TABLETS

Narcolepsy, obstructive sleep apnea-hypopnea syndrome.

150 or 250 mg as a single dose in the morning; in obstructive sleep apnea-hypopnea syndrome, doses up to 250 mg/day, given as a single dose, have been well tolerated. However, there is no evidence that the 250 mg/day dose confers additional benefit over the 150 mg/day dose.

Shift-work sleep disorder.

150 mg/day given about 1 hr before the start of the client's work shift.

NURSING IMPLICATIONS

IMPLEMENTATION/ADMINISTRATION/STORAGE

1. The efficacy for more than 12 weeks has not been evaluated.
2. Periodically reevaluate long-term usefulness in each client.
3. Reduce dose in those with severely impaired hepatic function.
4. Store from 20–25°C (68–77°F).

ASSESSMENT

1. Note onset, characteristics of sleepiness episodes and etiology (OSA, narcolepsy, shift work sleep disorder). Identify how often it interferes with normal functioning/work, any associated problems/accidents.
2. List drugs prescribed to ensure none interact or require dosage adjustments.
3. Assess for any evidence or history of mental health issues; may aggravate. Observe for S&S of abuse (e.g., drug-seeking behaviors, increased usage).
4. Discontinue at the first sign of severe rash.
5. Do not use with LVH, MVP, recent MI, ischemic ECG changes, chest pain, or arrhythmias.
6. Obtain ECG, monitor BP and LFTs; reduce dose with liver dysfunction and in the elderly.

CLIENT/FAMILY TEACHING

1. May take with or without food in the morning unless otherwise directed.
2. Drug is used to promote wakefulness. It can cause psychoactive and euphoric effects similar to those with other controlled substances as well as depression.
3. May alter judgment, thinking, motor skills, and cause dizziness. Do not engage in activities that require mental alertness, until drug effects realized.
4. With narcolepsy and obstructive sleep apnea, take as a single dose in the a.m. With shift work sleep disorder, drug should be taken approximately 1 hour prior to the start of the work shift.
5. Use additional protection to avoid pregnancy.
6. Avoid alcohol; do not take any OTC agents unless approved.
7. Immediately report any blisters, hives, mouth sores, peeling skin, rash, trouble swallowing or breathing. Stop drug and report any unusual rash or chest pain.
8. Keep all F/U to assess response, labs, for adverse SE.

OUTCOMES/EVALUATE

- ↑ Daytime wakefulness with narcolepsy
- Improved wakefulness with SWSD and OSA

IV

Asparaginase

(ah-**SPAIR**-ah-jin-ays)

Classification(s): Antineoplastic, miscellaneous

Pregnancy Category: C

RX: Elspar.

🍁 **Rx:** Kidrolase.

SEE ALSO *ANTINEOPLASTIC AGENTS*.

INDICATIONS/USES

Acute lymphocytic leukemia (ALL) in children; mostly used in combination with other drugs in the induction of remissions of the disease. Not to be used as the sole induction agent unless combi-

A

nation therapy is deemed inappropriate. Not recommended for maintenance therapy.

ACTION/KINETICS

Action

Neoplastic cells are unable to synthesize sufficient asparagine, an amino acid, to meet their metabolic needs. The supply of asparagine is further decreased by the enzyme asparaginase, which breaks down asparagine to aspartic acid and ammonia. Asparaginase interferes with synthesis of DNA, RNA, and protein and is cell-cycle specific for the G_1 phase of cell division.

Pharmacokinetics

Time to peak plasma levels, after IM: 14–24 hr. **t½, after IV:** 8–30 hr; **after IM:** 39–49 hr. Accumulates in plasma and tissue, and a small amount (1%) appears in CSF. Excretion is unknown. More toxic in adults than in children.

CONTRAINDICATIONS

Previous anaphylactic reactions to asparaginase. Pancreatitis (acute hemorrhagic pancreatitis has been fatal in some instances when asparaginase has been given) or a history of pancreatitis. Lactation.

SPECIAL CONCERNS

■ It is recommended that asparaginase be administered to clients only in a hospital setting under the supervision of a physician who is qualified by training and experience to administer cancer chemotherapeutic agents, because of the possibility of severe reactions, including anaphylaxis and sudden death. The physician must be prepared to treat anaphylaxis at each administration of the drug. In the treatment of each client, the physician must weigh carefully the possibility of achieving therapeutic benefit versus the risk of toxicity. ■

- **Use with caution in presence of liver dysfunction.**
- **Due to the possibility of an increased risk of hypersensitivity, institute retreatment with great care.**

SIDE EFFECTS

Most Common

N&V (may be severe), anorexia, abdominal cramps, swelling at injection site, headache, malaise, drowsiness.

GI: N&V, anorexia, abdominal cramps, ***pancreatitis (sometimes fulminant)***, ***acute hemorrhagic pancreatitis***. **CNS:** Depression, somnolence, drowsiness, coma, confusion, fatigue, malaise, agitation, mild to severe hallucinations, headache, irritability, Parkinson-like syndrome with tremor and a progressive increase in muscle tone (rare). **Hematologic:** Marked leukopenia, bone marrow depression (rare). Depression of clotting factors (Factors V, VII, VIII, IX); rarely, ***intracranial hemorrhage and fatal bleeding***. **Hypersensitivity:** Skin rashes, urticaria, arthralgia, respiratory distress, ***acute anaphylaxis, death***. **Renal:** Azotemia, proteinuria (rare), acute renal shutdown, ***fatal renal insufficiency***. **Hepatic:** Hepatotoxicity, fatty changes in the liver. **Miscellaneous:** Hyperglycemia with glucosuria and polyuria. Marked hypoalbuminemia associated with peripheral edema, malabsorption syndrome, ***fatal hyperthermia***, chills, fever, mild weight loss, uric acid nephropathy.

LABORATORY TEST CONSIDERATIONS

↑ Blood ammonia, BUN, glucose, serum uric acid, AST, ALT, alkaline phosphatase, bilirubin (direct and indirect). ↓ Serum albumin, cholesterol (total and esters), plasma fibrinogen, circulating lymphoblasts. ↑ or ↓ Total lipids. Interference with interpretation of thyroid function tests.

DRUG INTERACTIONS

Methotrexate / Asparaginase ↓ effect of methotrexate; do not use methotrexate with or following asparaginase

Prednisone / Even though used with asparaginase, may cause ↑ toxicity

Vincristine / Even though used with asparaginase, may cause ↑ toxicity; ↑ hyperglycemic effect

HOW SUPPLIED

Powder for Injection, Lyophilized: 10,000 international units.

DOSAGE

IM; IV

Regimen I for acute lymphocytic leukemia (ALL) in children.

Prednisone: 40 mg/m²/day PO in three divided doses for 15 days, followed by tapering of dosage as follows: 20 mg/m²/day for 2 days, 10 mg/m²/day for 2 days, 5 mg/m²/day for 2 days,

2.5 mg/m²/day for 2 days, and then discontinue. Vincristine sulfate: 2 mg/m² IV once weekly on days 1, 8, and 15. The maximum single dose should not exceed 2 mg. Asparaginase: 1,000 international units/kg/day IV for 10 successive days beginning on day 22.

Regimen II for ALL in children.

Prednisone: 40 mg/m²/day PO in three divided doses for 28 days with the total daily dose to the nearest 2.5 mg; then, discontinue gradually over 14 days. Vincristine sulfate: 1.5 mg/m² IV weekly for four doses on days 1, 8, 15, and 22. The maximum single dose should not exceed 2 mg. Asparaginase: 6,000 international units/m² IM on days 4, 7, 10, 13, 16, 19, 22, 25, and 28. When remission is obtained with either regimen, appropriate maintenance therapy should be instituted. Do not use asparaginase for maintenance therapy.

When used as the sole agent for induction.

Adults and children: 200 international units/kg/day IV for 28 days.

NURSING IMPLICATIONS

Do not confuse asparaginase with pegaspargase (antineoplastic drug).

IMPLEMENTATION/ADMINISTRATION/STORAGE

1. Give intradermal skin test (0.1 mL of a 20 international units/mL solution) at least 1 hr before initial administration of drug and when 1 week or more has elapsed between treatments. Observe for at least 1 hr for wheal/erythema that indicates a positive reaction. A negative skin test reaction does not preclude possibility of an allergic reaction.
2. A desensitization procedure, with increasing amounts of asparaginase may be carried out in those hypersensitive to the drug (1 international unit, then double dose q 10 min until total dose for day or reaction occurs).
3. Due to the unpredictability of side effects, initiate treatment only in hospitalized clients.
4. To prevent uric acid nephropathy, give allopurinol, increase fluid intake, and alkalinize the urine.
5. Do not use asparaginase as sole induction agent unless combined regimen is not possible due to toxicity or because client is refractory.
6. For IM use, reconstitute by adding 2 mL NaCl injection to the 10,000-unit vial. Use within 8 hr and only if clear. Give no more than 2 mL at a single injection site.
7. Handle the drug with care; is a contact irritant.
8. Have emergency equipment readily available during each administration; a severe hypersensitivity reaction is more likely to occur with this drug.
9. Store both the lyophilized product and reconstituted solution at 2–8°C (36–46°F). Discard reconstituted solution after 8 hr (sooner if cloudy).
10. IV Follow IV administration guidelines carefully.
11. For IV use: reconstitute the 10,000-unit vial with either 5 mL sterile water or NaCl injection. Give solution by direct IV administration within 8 hr following reconstitution. For infusion, dilute solutions with NaCl injection or D5W. Infuse through the side arm of an already running infusion of sodium chloride injection or D5W over at least 30 min and within 8 hr of reconstitution only if solution is clear.
12. A very small number of gelatinous fiber-like particles may develop on standing. Filtration through a 5.0 micron filter during administration will remove the particles with no resultant loss in potency.
13. COMPATIBILITY Reconstitute with sterile water or NaCl; infuse D5W, saline solutions.
14. INCOMPATIBILITY Flush after infusion; administer separately.

ASSESSMENT

1. Note reasons for therapy, leukemia history, baseline labs and VS. May cause mild lymphocyte suppression. Nadir: 7–10 days; recovery 14 days.
2. Determine intradermal skin test performed initially and after a 1 week or more interval between doses. (Repeated doses/course of therapy increase hypersensitivity reactions.)
3. Increase fluids and add allopurinol to reduce uric acid levels from tumor necrosis.
4. Expect to administer antiemetic prior to drug therapy. Give vincristine and prednisone be-

A

5. Asparaginase administration 9–10 days before or within 24 hr after methotrexate (MTX) may reduce the GI and hematologic effects of MTX.
6. Weigh weekly, monitor I&O; assess for any evidence of renal failure. Alkalinization of the urine and allopurinol therapy may help prevent urate stone formation.
7. Observe for peripheral edema R/T hypoalbuminemia triggered by asparaginase.
8. Monitor for hyperglycemia, glycosuria, and polyuria, all of which may be precipitated by asparaginase. Have IV fluids and regular insulin available; stop therapy.
9. Assess cardiopulmonary function; document ECG and CXR q 2 weeks.
10. Monitor neurologic status, renal and LFTs, CBC, uric acid, glucose, amylase, and lipase levels; check for S&S of pancreatitis/allergic reactions.

CLIENT/FAMILY TEACHING

1. Used with other drugs to treat acute lymphocytic leukemia (ALL). Report stomach pain, appetite/weight loss, and N&V: S&S of pancreatitis.
2. Report any sudden increase in SOB, coughing, feet swelling, frequent urination, increased thirst, or fever. Consume 2–3 L/day of fluids to prevent dehydration.
3. May cause drowsiness, even several weeks after administration; do not drive a car or operate hazardous machinery.
4. Report shakiness or unusual body movements; a Parkinson-like condition may be precipitated by drug. Report any evidence of rash, hives, breathing problems, fever, chills, sore throat, or other S&S of infection.
5. Skin tests may be used before starting therapy.
6. Follow guidelines for supplemental therapies to protect the kidneys from excessive uric acid (e.g., increased fluid intake, allopurinol, urinary alkalinizing agents).
7. Avoid live immunizations and contact with child who has recently taken poliovirus vaccine. Avoid crowds, especially during flu season. Consider pneumococcal vaccine and annual flu/H1N1 shot.
8. Practice reliable contraception; drug is teratogenic.
9. Do not take any aspirin-containing compounds, NSAIDs, or alcohol; may cause GI bleeding.
10. Keep all F/U to assess response, labs, and for adverse SE.

OUTCOMES/EVALUATE

- Improved hematologic parameters
- Inhibition of malignant cell proliferation

Aspirin (Acetylsalicylic acid, ASA)

(ah-**SEE**-till-sal-ih-**SILL**-ick **AH**-sid)

Classification(s): Nonsteroidal anti-inflammatory drug, analgesic, antipyretic

Pregnancy Category: C

OTC: Caplets/Tablets: Arthritis Foundation Pain Reliever, AspirLow, Empirin, Genprin, Genuine Bayer Aspirin Caplets and Tablets, Maximum Bayer Aspirin Caplets and Tablets, Norwich Extra Strength, Norwich Regular Strength. **Tablets, Chewable:** Aspirin Low Dose, Bayer Children's Aspirin, Miniprin Low Dose, St. Joseph Adult Chewable Aspirin. **Tablets, Coated/Enteric-Coated:** Bayer Advanced Aspirin, Ecotrin Adult Low Strength, Ecotrin Caplets and Tablets, Ecotrin Low Strength, Ecotrin Maximum Strength Caplets and Tablets, Extra Strength Bayer Enteric 500 Aspirin, ½ Halfprin, Halfprin 81, Heartline, Regular Strength Bayer Enteric Coated Caplets. **Tablets, Extended-Release:** Bayer Low Adult Strength, Extended Release Bayer 8-Hour Caplets.

RX: Easprin, ZORprin.

🍁 **OTC:** Asaphen, Asaphen E.C., Entrophen.

Aspirin, buffered

Pregnancy Category: C

OTC: Caplets: Extra Strength Bayer Plus Caplets. **Caplets/Tablets:** Arthritis Pain Formula, Bayer Buffered Aspirin, Buffered Aspirin, Bufferin Extra Strength, Buffex, Cama Arthritis Pain Reliever, Tri-Buffered Bufferin Caplets and Tablets. **Tablets, Coated:** Adprin-B, Ascriptin, Bufferin, Extra-Strength Adprin-B. **Tablets, Effervescent:** Alka-Seltzer Extra

A

Strength with Aspirin, Alka-Seltzer with Aspirin, Alka-Seltzer with Aspirin (Flavored).

SEE ALSO ***NONSTEROIDAL ANTI-INFLAMMATORY DRUGS.***

INDICATIONS/USES

Analgesic: (1) Pain from integumentary structures, myalgias, neuralgias, arthralgias, headache, dysmenorrhea, and similar types of pain. (2) Gout. (3) May be effective in less severe postoperative and postpartum pain; pain secondary to trauma and cancer.

Antipyretic, Anti-Inflammatory: Arthritis, osteoarthritis, SLE, acute rheumatic fever, gout, and many other conditions. Mucocutaneous lymph node syndrome (Kawasaki disease).

Cardiovascular: Despite the increased risk of GI bleeding, low-dose aspirin should be used for the following CV events:

1. Reduce risk of death and nonfatal stroke in those who have had an ischemic stroke or TIA; also combined with dipyridamole for this purpose.
2. Reduce risk of vascular mortality with suspected acute MI.
3. Reduce the combined risk of recurrent MI and death after an MI or unstable angina.
4. Reduce risk of MI and sudden death in chronic stable angina.
5. Pre-existing need for aspirin following coronary artery bypass grafting, PTCA, or carotid endarterectomy.
6. Used with ticlopidine as adjunctive therapy to reduce development of subacute stent thrombosis.
7. *Investigational:* Reduce risk of heart problems in healthy adults with a small risk of heart attack and no history of CV disease. Includes men over 40 years of age, postmenopausal women, and younger people with risk factors including, smoking, diabetes, hypertension, and high cholesterol.

Chronic use to prevent cataract formation; low doses to prevent toxemia of pregnancy; in pregnant women with inadequate uteroplacental blood flow. Reduce colon cancer mortality (low doses). Low doses of aspirin and warfarin to reduce risk of a second heart attack. In addition to treatment for CV risk factors, may reduce risk of dying from heart attack or stroke significantly.

ACTION/KINETICS

Action

Exhibits antipyretic, anti-inflammatory, and analgesic effects. The antipyretic effect is due to an action on the hypothalamus, resulting in heat loss by vasodilation of peripheral blood vessels and promoting sweating. The anti-inflammatory effects are probably mediated through inhibition of cyclo-oxygenase, which results in a decrease in prostaglandin (implicated in the inflammatory response) synthesis and other mediators of the pain response. The mechanism of action for the analgesic effects of aspirin is not known fully but is partly attributable to improvement of the inflammatory condition. Aspirin also produces inhibition of platelet aggregation by decreasing the synthesis of endoperoxides and thromboxanes—substances that mediate platelet aggregation. Large doses of aspirin (5 grams/day or more) increase uric acid secretion, while low doses (2 grams/day or less) decrease uric acid secretion. However, aspirin antagonizes drugs used to treat gout.

Pharmacokinetics

Rapidly absorbed after PO administration. Is hydrolyzed to the active salicylic acid. **Blood levels for arthritis and rheumatic disease:** Maintain 150–300 mcg/mL. **Blood levels for analgesic and antipyretic:** 25–50 mcg/mL. **Blood levels for acute rheumatic fever:** 150–300 mcg/mL. Tinnitus occurs at serum levels above 200 mcg/mL and serious toxicity above 400 mcg/mL. **t½:** Aspirin, 15–20 min; salicylic acid, 2–20 hr, depending on the dose. Salicylic acid and metabolites are excreted by the kidney. The bioavailability of enteric-coated salicylate products may be poor. The addition of antacids (buffered aspirin) may decrease GI irritation and increase the dissolution and absorption of such products. **Plasma protein binding:** As active salicylic acid, 70–90%.

CONTRAINDICATIONS

Hypersensitivity to salicylates. Clients with asthma, hay fever, or nasal polyps have a higher incidence of hypersensitivity reactions. Severe anemia, history of blood coagulation defects, in conjunction with anticoagulant therapy. Salicylates can cause congestive failure when taken in the large doses used for rheumatic diseases. Vitamin K deficiency; 1 week before and after surgery. In pregnancy, especially the last trimester as the drug may cause problems in the newborn child or complica-

A

tions during delivery. In children or teenagers with chickenpox or flu due to possibility of development of Reye's syndrome.

Controlled-release aspirin is not recommended for use as an antipyretic or short-term analgesic because adequate blood levels may not be reached. Also, controlled-release products are not recommended for children less than 12 years of age and in children with fever accompanied by dehydration.

SPECIAL CONCERNS

Do not use in children or teenagers with chickenpox or flu symptoms due to the possibility of Reye's syndrome, a rare but serious illness.

- **Use with caution during lactation and in the presence of gastric or peptic ulcers, in mild diabetes, erosive gastritis, bleeding tendencies, in cardiac disease, and in liver or kidney disease.**
- **There is increased potential for stomach bleeding with aspirin in the following: age 60 years and older, prior ulcers or bleeding, taking an anticoagulant when taking more than one product containing an NSAID, with moderate amounts of alcohol, or when taken for longer than directed.**
- **Aspirin products now carry the following labeling: "It is especially important not to use aspirin during the last 3 months of pregnancy unless specifically directed to do so by a doctor because it may cause problems in the newborn child or complications during delivery."**

SIDE EFFECTS

Most Common

Dyspepsia, nausea, epigastric discomfort. The toxic effects of the salicylates are dose-related.

GI: Dyspepsia, heartburn, anorexia, nausea, occult blood loss, epigastric discomfort, ***massive GI bleeding, potentiation of peptic ulcer.*** Possible stomach bleeding in those who ingest three or more alcoholic drinks/day. **Allergic: *Bronchospasm, asthma-like symptoms, anaphylaxis,*** skin rashes, angioedema, urticaria, rhinitis, nasal polyps. **Hematologic:** Prolongation of bleeding time, thrombocytopenia, leukopenia, purpura, shortened erythrocyte survival time, decreased plasma iron levels. **Miscellaneous:** Thirst, fever, dimness of vision.

NOTE: Use of aspirin in children and teenagers with flu or chickenpox may result in the development of Reye's syndrome. Also, dehydrated, febrile children are more prone to salicylate intoxication.

OVERDOSE MANAGEMENT

Symptoms: **Symptoms of Mild Salicylate Toxicity (Salicylism):** At serum levels between 150 and 200 mcg/mL. **GI:** N&V, diarrhea, thirst. **CNS:** Tinnitus (most common), dizziness, difficulty in hearing, mental confusion, lassitude. **Miscellaneous:** Flushing, sweating, tachycardia. Symptoms of salicylism may be observed with doses used for inflammatory disease or rheumatic fever. **Symptoms of Severe Salicylate Poisoning:** At serum levels over 400 mcg/mL. **CNS:** Excitement, confusion, disorientation, irritability, hallucinations, lethargy, stupor, ***coma, respiratory failure, seizures.*** **Metabolic:** Respiratory alkalosis (initially), respiratory acidosis and metabolic acidosis, dehydration. **GI:** N&V. **Hematologic:** Platelet dysfunction, hypoprothrombinemia, increased capillary fragility. **Miscellaneous: *Hyperthermia, hemorrhage, CV collapse, renal failure,*** hyperventilation, pulmonary edema, tetany, hypoglycemia (late). *Treatment: Mild Toxicity:*

1. If the client has had repeated administration of large doses of salicylates, document and report evidence of hyperventilation or complaints of auditory or visual disturbances (symptoms of salicylism).
2. Severe salicylate poisoning, whether due to overdose or accumulation, will have an exaggerated effect on the CNS and the metabolic system:
   - Clients may develop a salicylate jag characterized by garrulous behavior. They may act as if they were inebriated.
   - Convulsions and coma may follow.
3. When working with febrile children or the elderly who have been treated with aspirin, maintain adequate fluid intake. These clients are more susceptible to salicylate intoxication if they are dehydrated.
4. The following treatment approaches may be considered for treatment of *acute salicylate toxicity:*
   - Initially induce vomiting or perform gastric lavage followed by activated charcoal (most effective if given within 2 hr of ingestion).
   - Monitor salicylate levels and acid-base and fluid and electrolyte balance. If required, administer IV solutions of dex-

A

trose, saline, potassium, and sodium bicarbonate as well as vitamin K.

- Seizures may be treated with diazepam.
- Treat hyperthermia if present.
- Alkaline diuresis will enhance renal excretion. Hemodialysis is effective but should be reserved for severe poisonings.
- If necessary, administer oxygen and artificial ventilation.

DRUG INTERACTIONS

ACE inhibitors / ↓ Effect of ACE inhibitors possibly due to prostaglandin inhibition; also, significantly higher mortality rate using doses of aspirin of at least 325 mg/day
Acetazolamide / ↑ CNS toxicity of salicylates; also, ↑ excretion of salicylic acid in alkaline urine
Alcohol, ethyl / ↑ Chance of GI bleeding caused by salicylates
Alteplase, recombinant / ↑ Risk of bleeding
Aminosalicylate / Possible ↑ effect of PAS due to ↓ excretion by kidney or ↓ plasma protein binding
Ammonium chloride / ↑ Effect of salicylates by ↑ renal tubular reabsorption
Antacids / ↓ Salicylate levels in plasma due to ↑ rate of renal excretion
Anticoagulants, oral / ↑ Effect of anticoagulant by ↓ plasma protein binding and plasma prothrombin
Antirheumatics / Both are ulcerogenic and may cause ↑ GI bleeding
Ascorbic acid / ↑ Effect of salicylates by ↑ renal tubular reabsorption
Beta-adrenergic blocking agents / Salicylates ↓ action of beta-blockers, possibly due to prostaglandin inhibition
Charcoal, activated / ↓ Absorption of salicylates from GI tract
Clopidogrel / ↑ Risk of life-threatening or major bleeding events in high-risk clients with recent ischemic stroke or transient ischemic attacks
Corticosteroids / Both are ulcerogenic; also, corticosteroids may ↓ blood salicylate levels by ↑ breakdown by liver and ↑ excretion
Dipyridamole / Additive anticoagulant effects
H ***Feverfew*** / Possible ↑ antiplatelet effect
Furosemide / ↑ Risk of salicylate toxicity due to ↓ renal excretion; also, salicylates may ↓ effect of furosemide in clients with impaired renal function or cirrhosis with ascites
H ***Garlic*** / Possible ↑ antiplatelet effect
H ***Ginkgo biloba*** / Possible ↑ effect on platelet aggregation → bleeding episodes
H ***Ginseng*** / Possible ↓ effect on platelet aggregation
Griseofulvin / ↓ Salicylate levels
Heparin / Inhibition of platelet adhesiveness by aspirin may result in bleeding tendencies
Hypoglycemics, oral / ↑ Hypoglycemia R/T ↓ plasma protein binding and ↓ excretion
Ibuprofen / Cardioprotective effects of low dose aspirin may be negated or ↓ with concomitant ibuprofen use
Indomethacin / Both are ulcerogenic → ↑ GI bleeding
Insulin / Salicylates ↑ hypoglycemic effect of insulin
Methionine / ↑ Effect of salicylates by ↑ renal tubular reabsorption
Methotrexate / ↑ Methotrexate effect by ↓ plasma protein binding; also, salicylates block drugs' renal excretion
Nitroglycerin / Combination may result in unexpected hypotension
Nizatidine / ↑ Serum levels of salicylates
NSAIDs / Additive ulcerogenic effects; also, aspirin may ↓ serum levels of NSAIDs
Phenytoin / ↑ Phenytoin effect by ↓ plasma protein binding
Probenecid / Salicylates inhibit uricosuric activity of probenecid
Sodium bicarbonate / ↓ Effect of salicylates by ↑ rate of excretion
Spironolactone / Aspirin ↓ diuretic drug effect
Sulfinpyrazone / Salicylates inhibit uricosuric drug activity
Sulfonamides / ↑ Sulfonamides effect R/T displacement from plasma proteins
Valproic acid / ↑ Valproic effect R/T ↓ plasma protein binding

HOW SUPPLIED

Aspirin. ***Suppositories:*** 120 mg, 200 mg, 300 mg, 600 mg; ***Tablets:*** 325 mg, 500 mg; ***Tablets, Chewable:*** 81 mg; ***Tablets, Coated/Enteric-Coated:*** 81 mg, 165 mg, 325 mg, 500 mg, 650 mg, 975 mg; ***Tablets, Delayed-Release:*** 81 mg; ***Tablets, Extended-Release:*** 650 mg, 800 mg.
Aspirin, Buffered. ***Caplets:*** 325 mg; ***Tablets:*** 325 mg, 500 mg; ***Tablets, Coated:*** 325 mg, 500 mg; ***Tablets, Effervescent:*** 325 mg, 500 mg.

A

DOSAGE

CAPLETS; SUPPOSITORIES; TABLETS; TABLETS, CHEWABLE; TABLETS, COATED; TABLETS, DELAYED-RELEASE; TABLETS, EFFERVESCENT; TABLETS, ENTERIC-COATED

Analgesic, antipyretic.

Adults: 325–500 mg q 3 hr, 325–600 mg q 4 hr, or 650–1,000 mg q 6 hr. As an alternative, the adult chewable tablet (81 mg each) may be used in doses of 4–8 tablets q 4 hr as needed. **Pediatric:** 65 mg/kg/day (alternate dose: 1.5 grams/m²/day) in divided doses q 4–6 hr, not to exceed 3.6 grams/day. Alternatively, the following dosage regimen can be used: **Pediatric, 2–3 years:** 162 mg q 4 hr as needed; **4–5 years:** 243 mg q 4 hr as needed; **6–8 years:** 320–325 mg q 4 hr as needed; **9–10 years:** 405 mg q 4 hr as needed; **11 years:** 486 mg q 4 hr as needed; **12–14 years:** 648 mg q 4 hr.

Arthritis, rheumatic diseases.

Adults: 3.2–6 grams/day in divided doses.

Juvenile rheumatoid arthritis.

60–110 mg/kg/day (alternate dose: 3 grams/m²/day) in divided doses q 6–8 hr. When initiating therapy at 60 mg/kg/day, dose may be increased by 20 mg/kg/day after 5–7 days and by 10 mg/kg/day after another 5–7 days.

Acute rheumatic fever.

Adults, initial: 5–8 grams/day. **Pediatric, initial:** 100 mg/kg/day (3 grams/m²/day) for 2 weeks; **then,** decrease to 75 mg/kg/day for 4–6 weeks.

Reduce risk of death and nonfatal stroke following ischemic stroke or transient ischemic attack (TIA).

50–325 mg/day.

Reduce risk of vascular mortality in suspected acute myocardial infarction (MI).

Initial: 160–162.5 mg, **then** daily for 30 days. Consider subsequent prophylactic therapy.

Reduce combined risk of recurrent MI and death in those with a previous MI or unstable angina or to reduce risk of MI and sudden death in those with chronic stable angina.

75–325 mg/day.

Pre-existing need for aspirin following coronary artery bypass grafting, percutaneous transluminal coronary angioplasty (PTCA), carotid endarterectomy.

Dosage varies by procedure.

Kawasaki disease.

Adults: 80–180 mg/kg/day during the febrile period. After the fever resolves, the dose may be adjusted to 10 mg/kg/day.

NOTE: Aspirin Regimen Bayer 81 mg with Calcium contains 250 mg calcium carbonate (10% of RDA) and 81 mg of acetylsalicylic acid for individuals who require aspirin to prevent recurrent heart attacks and strokes.

NURSING IMPLICATIONS

IMPLEMENTATION/ADMINISTRATION/STORAGE

1. Enteric-coated tablets or buffered tablets are better tolerated by some.
2. Take with full glass of water to prevent lodging in the esophagus.
3. Have epinephrine available to counteract hypersensitivity reactions should they occur. Asthma caused by hypersensitivity reaction to salicylates may be refractory to epinephrine, so antihistamines should also be available for parenteral and PO use.

ASSESSMENT

1. Take complete drug history; note any hypersensitivity. If salicylates not tolerated well in the past may suddenly have an allergic or anaphylactoid reaction.
2. For pain, rate and determine the type, location, and pattern of pain, if unusual, or if recurring and triggers/relievers. Note effectiveness of aspirin if previously used for pain and dose used.
3. Identify any asthma, hay fever, ulcer disease or nasal polyps. Note history of peptic ulcers or bleeding disorders, and get PT/INR with prolonged use.

4. Note age; avoid drug if under the age of 12. Assess for chickenpox or the flu; precludes therapy.
5. Determine if diagnostic tests scheduled. Drug causes irreversible platelet effects. Anticipate 4–7 days for body to replace these once drug is discontinued; hence no salicylates 1 week prior to procedure.
6. Review drugs currently prescribed/OTC for drug interactions.
7. The therapeutic serum level of salicylate is 150–300 mcg/mL for adult and juvenile rheumatoid arthritis and acute rheumatic fever. Reassure that higher dosage is needed for anti-inflammatory effects as long as liver and renal function intact.
8. Test stool and urine for blood; monitor renal, LFTs and CBC routinely during high-dose and chronic therapy. PT/INR with prolonged use. Avoid use with severe liver and renal dysfunction.

CLIENT/FAMILY TEACHING

1. Take as directed. To reduce gastric irritation or lodging in the esophagus, administer with meals, milk, a full glass of water, or crackers and remain upright for at least 20–30 min. Avoid antacids within 1 to 2 hr after ingestion of enteric-coated tablets. Sodium bicarbonate may decrease serum level of aspirin, reducing its effectiveness.
2. Do not take if product is off-color or has a strange odor. Note expiration date.
3. Report toxic effects: ringing in the ears, difficulty hearing, dizziness or fainting spells, unusual increase in sweating, severe abdominal pain, or mental confusion.
4. Potentiates effects of antidiabetic drugs. Monitor FS and report low sugars. Avoid high alcohol ingestion; may cause GI bleeding.
5. When administering for antipyretic effect, follow temperature administration parameters:
   - Obtain temperature 1 hr after administering to assess outcome.
   - With marked diaphoresis, dry client, change linens, provide fluids, prevent chilling, avoid dehydration.
6. Cardiac clients on large doses should report symptoms of CHF (e.g., ↑ SOB, ↑ swelling of extremities). Limit use of effervescent or buffered aspirin preparations.
7. Tell dentist and other HCPs you are taking salicylates.
8. Before purchasing other OTC preparations, read labels for salicylate content and advise provider noting quantity used per day.
9. Salicylates should be administered to children only upon specific medical order R/T ↑ risk of Reye's syndrome. Dehydrated children who have a fever are especially susceptible to aspirin intoxication from even small doses.
10. Report gastric irritation/pain; may be S&S of hypersensitivity or toxicity. If child refuses medication or vomits, notify provider.
11. Report unusual bruising or bleeding. Large doses may increase PT and should be avoided. Aspirin and NSAIDs may interfere with blood-clotting mechanisms (antiplatelet effects) and are usually discontinued 1 week before surgery to prevent increased risk of bleeding.
12. If also taking NSAID, i.e., ibuprofen for pain, take at least 8 hours before or 30 minutes after you take the aspirin.
13. Avoid indiscriminate use; store appropriately.
14. Keep all F/U to assess response and for adverse SE.

OUTCOMES/EVALUATE

- Relief of pain/discomfort; Improved joint mobility/function
- ↓ Fever; ↓ Vascular mortality
- ↓ Inflammation
- Prophylaxis of MI/TIA

Atazanavir sulfate

(ah-**tah**-zah-**NAH**-veer)

Classification(s): Antiretroviral agent, protease inhibitor
Pregnancy Category: B
RX: Reyataz.

INDICATIONS/USES

In combination with other antiretroviral drugs for HIV-1 infections in adults and children, 6 to less than 18 years of age.

ACTION/KINETICS

Action

Atazanavir is an azapeptide HIV-1 protease inhibitor that selectively inhibits the virus-specific pro-

A

cessing of viral Gag and Gag-Pol polyproteins in HIV-1 infected cells, thus preventing formation of mature virions. Resistance to the drug has been observed.

Pharmacokinetics

Readily absorbed; $\mathbf{T_{max}}$: 2.5 hr (average). Food enhances bioavailability and reduces pharmacokinetic variability. Steady state is reached between 4 and 8 days. Is extensively metabolized by CYP3A. Metabolites and unchanged drug are excreted in the feces (79%) and urine (13%). **t½, elimination:** 7 hr at steady-state after a 400 mg/day dose with a light meal. t½ increases in clients with impaired hepatic function. **Plasma protein binding:** 86%.

CONTRAINDICATIONS

Previously demonstrated hypersensitivity to any components of the product. Use in clients with severe hepatic insufficiency (Child-Pugh C). Use with drugs that are highly dependent on CYP3A or UGT1A1 for clearance and for which increased plasma levels are associated with serious and/or life-threatening events (e.g., alfuzosin, cisapride, dihydroergotamine, ergonovine, ergotamine, indinavir, irinotecan, lovastatin, methylergonovine, PO administered midazolam, rifampin, sildenafil when dosed as Revatio, St. John's wort, simvastatin, triazolam). Lactation. Use in pediatric clients less than 3 months of age due to the possibility of kernicterus.

SPECIAL CONCERNS

- **Concentration- and dose-dependent prolongation of the PR interval in ECGs has been observed. Use with caution in pre-existing conduction system disease (e.g., marked first-degree AV block or second- or third-degree AV block).**
- **Use with caution when used with drugs that may prolong the PR interval (e.g., beta-blockers, digoxin, verapamil).**
- **Use with caution in clients with moderate hepatic impairment and in the elderly.**
- **Cross-resistance among protease inhibitors has been observed.**
- **Safety and efficacy not determined for children 3 months to younger than 4 years of age. Do not use in children less than 3 months.**

SIDE EFFECTS

Most Common

Adults: N&V, jaundice/scleral icterus, myalgia, rash (all grades), headache, fever, abdominal pain, diarrhea, hyperbilirubinemia.

Children: Cough, fever, rash, jaundice/scleral icterus, diarrhea, vomiting, headache, rhinorrhea, asymptomatic second-degree AV block, hyperbilirubinemia.

Many side effects occur when atazanavir is combined with other antiviral drugs. **CNS:** Headache, depression, dizziness, insomnia, peripheral neurologic symptoms, abnormal dreams/gait, agitation, amnesia, anxiety, confusion, convulsions, decreased libido, emotional lability, hallucinations, hostility, hyperkinesia, hypesthesia, increased reflexes, nervousness, psychosis, sleep disorder, somnolence, ***suicide attempt***, twitch. **GI:** N&V, scleral icterus, jaundice, abdominal pain, diarrhea, acholia, anorexia, aphthous stomatitis, colitis, constipation, dental pain, dyspepsia, enlarged abdomen, esophageal ulcer, esophagitis, flatulence, gastritis, gastroenteritis, GI disorder, increased appetite, mouth ulcer, ***pancreatitis***, peptic ulcer. **Hepatic:** Hepatitis, jaundice, hepatomegaly, hepatosplenomegaly, liver damage, liver fatty deposit, cholecystitis, cholelithiasis, cholestasis, abnormal hepatic function. **Metabolic:** New-onset diabetes mellitus, exacerbation of pre-existing diabetes mellitus, hyperglycemia, diabetic ketoacidosis, ***lactic acidosis syndrome (when used with nucleoside analogs,*** especially in pregnant women), dehydration, dyslipidemia, gout, lipohypertrophy, obesity, weight decrease/gain. Redistribution/accumulation of body fat, including central obesity, dorsocervical fat enlargement (buffalo hump), peripheral/facial wasting, breast enlargement, cushingoid appearance. **CV:** Increased bleeding, including spontaneous skin hematomas and hemarthrosis in hemophilia type A and B; prolongation of PR interval, asymptomatic second-degree AV block in children, left bundle branch block, ***second-degree or third-degree AV block, QTc prolongation. Heart arrest***, heart block, hypertension, myocarditis, palpitation, syncope, vasodilation. **GU:** Abnormal urine, amenorrhea, crystalluria, decreased male fertility, gynecomastia, hematuria, impotence, kidney calculus/failure/pain, menstrual disorder, oliguria, pelvic pain, polyuria, proteinuria, urinary frequency, UTI, nephrolithiasis. **Musculoskeletal:** Bone/extremity pain, muscle atrophy, myalgia, myasthenia, myopathy, arthralgia. **Respiratory:** Dyspnea, hiccough, hypoxia, increased cough, rhinorrhea. **Dermatologic:** Rash (all grades), alopecia, cellulitis, dermatophytosis, dry skin, eczema, nail disorder, pruritus, seborrhea, urticaria, vesiculobullous rash, ecchymosis, purpura, sweating, maculopapular rash. **Otic:** Otitis, tinnitus. **Body as a whole:** Fatigue, fever, lipodystrophy, pain, allergic reaction, angioedema, asthenia, burning sensation, edema, heat sensitivity, infection, malaise, pallor, peripheral edema. **Miscellaneous:** Photosensitivity, taste perversion, back/chest pain, dysplasia, substernal chest pain, immune reconstitution syndrome (inflammatory response to indolent or residual opportunistic infections), hyperbilirubinemia.

LABORATORY TEST CONSIDERATIONS

↑ ALT, AST, total bilirubin, amylase, glucose, lipase, creatine kinase, total cholesterol, HDL-C, LDL-C, triglycerides. ↓ Hemoglobin, neutrophils, platelets.

OVERDOSE MANAGEMENT

Symptoms: Jaundice, PR interval prolongation. *Treatment:* General supportive measures, including monitoring of VS and ECG. Emesis or gastric lavage. Activated charcoal. Dialysis is unlikely to be beneficial.

DRUG INTERACTIONS

1. Concurrent administration of atazanavir and drugs primarily metabolized by CYP3A, CYP2C8, or UTT1A1 may result in increased plasma levels of the other drug that may increase or prolong both therapeutic and side effects.
2. Concurrent administration of drugs that induce CYP3A may decrease atazanavir plasma levels and decrease its therapeutic effect. Concurrent administration of atazanavir and drugs that inhibit CYP3A may increase atazanavir plasma levels.
3. An additive effect may result between atazanavir and drugs that prolong the PR interval (e.g., beta-blockers, other than atenolol; digoxin; verapamil).

Alfuzosin / ↑ Alfuzosin levels → ↑ risk of hypotension; do not use together

Antacids and buffered drugs / ↓ Atazanavir plasma levels; give atazanavir 2 hr before or 1 hr after these medications

Antiarrhythmics (e.g., amiodarone, bepridil, systemic lidocaine, quinidine) / Possible serious/life-threatening side effects; monitor therapeutic levels of the antiarrhythmic if given together

Antidepressants, tricyclic (e.g., amitriptyline) / Possible serious/life-threatening side effects; monitor tricyclic levels

Aripiprazole / ↑ Plasma aripiprazole levels → ↑ pharmacologic and toxic effects; monitor and adjust aripiprazole dose as needed

Bosentan / ↓ Atazanavir plasma levels when bosentan given without ritonavir; use without ritonavir not recommended; also ↑ bosentan plasma levels → ↑ pharmacologic/toxic effects (See ***Implementation Administration/Storage)***

Benzodiazepines (e.g., midazolam, triazolam) / With PO midazolam/triazolam: Potential for serious/life-threatening events, such as prolonged or increased sedation or respiratory depression; do not use together; use IV midazolam with caution

Calcium channel blockers (e.g., amlodipine, diltiazem, felodipine, nicardipine, nifedipene, verapamil) / Possible prolongation of PR interval; dose reduction may be needed (e.g., 50% for diltiazem); monitor ECG

Carbamazepine / ↑ Carbamazepine levels → ↑ risk of toxicity; ↓ atazanavir levels → treatment failure

H ***Cat's claw*** / ↑ Atazanavir levels → ↑ risk of toxicity; do not use together

Cisapride / Serious and/or life-threatening effects, such as cardiac arrhythmias; do not use together

Clarithromycin / ↑ Clarithromycin levels → QTc prolongation; consider a 50% dose reduction; also, significant ↓ in the active 14-OH clarithromycin; consider alternative therapy except for ***Mycobacterium avium*** complex

Colchicine / Do not give combination to those with hepatic or renal impairment

Corticosteroids (e.g., fluticasone, prednisone) / ↑ Corticosteroid plasma levels; monitor for signs of adrenal insufficiency; consider alternatives to fluticasone for long-term use

Delavirdine / ↑ Plasma atazanavir levels → ↑ pharmacologic effects; also, ↓ plasma levels and effects of delavirdine; dose reduction of atazanavir and dose increase of delavirdine may be needed

Didanosine, buffered formulation / ↓ Atazanavir levels; take atazanavir 2 hr before or 1 hr after buffered didanosine

Didanosine, enteric-coated / ↓ Didanosine levels when taken with food; give atazanavir and didanosine at different times

Digoxin / Possible additive effect on PR interval prolongation; use together with caution

A

Dronedarone / ↑ Plasma dronedarone levels → ↑ pharmacologic/toxic effects; do not use together
Efavirenz / ↓ Atazanavir plasma levels and clinical efficacy in treatment-naive clients; do not give atazanavir/efavirenz in treatment-experienced clients
Eletriptan / ↑ Plasma eletriptan levels → ↑ pharmacologic/toxic effects; do not use eletriptan within 72 hr of atazanavir
Eplerenone / ↑ Eplerenone plasma levels → ↑ pharmacologic/toxic effects; monitor closely and adjust eplerenone dose as needed
Ergot derivatives (e.g., dihydroergotamine, ergonovine, ergotamine, methylergonovine) / Potential for serious/life-threatening acute ergot toxicity (e.g., peripheral vasospasm, ischemia of the extremities); do not use together
Erlotinib / ↑ Plasma erlotinib levels → ↑ pharmacologic/toxic effects; monitor for side effects and adjust erlotinib dose as needed
Erythromycin / ↑ Plasma erythromycin levels → ↑ risk of sudden death from cardiac causes; do not use together
Eszopiclone / ↑ Plasma eszopiclone levels → ↑ pharmacologic/toxic effects; monitor and consider ↓ eszopiclone dose
Everolimus / ↑ Everolimus plasma levels → ↑ pharmacologic/toxic effects; monitor response and adjust everolimus dose as needed
Famotidine / Significant ↓ atazanavir plasma levels → possible loss of therapeutic effect and resistance
Fluoxetine / ↑ Fluoxetine plasma levels → possible fluoxetine toxicity; also, possible ↑ atazanavir plasma levels; closely monitor for side effects, including serotonin syndrome; dosage reduction of one or both may be needed
H ***Garlic*** / ↓ Atazanavir plasma levels → ↓ pharmacologic effect; avoid garlic ingestion
Grapefruit juice / ↑ Atazanavir plasma levels → ↑ pharmacologic effect; if used together, closely monitor and adjust atazanavir dose as needed
H_2 receptor antagonists / ↓ Atazanavir plasma levels → ↓ therapeutic effect and resistance; give atazanavir as far apart as possible from H_2-receptor antagonists
HMG-CoA reductase inhibitors (e.g., atorvastatin, lovastatin, rosuvastatin, simvastatin) / ↑ HMG-CoA reductase inhibitor serum levels → ↑ toxicity, including rhabdomyolysis; coadministration with lovastatin or simvastatin contraindicated; start with lowest dose of atorvastatin or rosuvastatin with careful monitoring
Iloperidone / ↑ Plasma iloperidone levels → ↑ pharmacologic effects; ↓ iloperidone dose by ½
Immunosuppressants (e.g., cyclosporine, sirolimus, tacrolimus) / ↑ Immunosuppressant plasma levels; monitor therapeutic levels carefully
Indinavir / Both associated with indirect hyperbilirubinemia; do not use together
Irinotecan / ↑ Irinotecan toxicity R/T ↓ metabolism; do not use together
Itraconazole / Use with caution with atazanavir/ritonavir due to possible ↑ in atazanavir AUC and C_{max}
Ixabepilone / Elevated ixabepilone plasma levels; do not use together
Ketoconazole / Use with caution with atazanavir/ritonavir due to possible ↑ in atazanavir AUC and C_{max}
Maraviroc / ↑ Maraviroc plasma levels → ↑ pharmacologic effects; monitor and adjust maraviroc dose as needed
Muscarinic receptor antagonists (e.g., darifenacin, fesoterodine, solifenacin, tolterodine) / ↑ Muscarinic receptor antagonist plasma levels; if atazanavir coadministered, to not exceed the following doses: darifenacin 7.5 mg/day; fesoterodine 4 mg/day; solifenacin 5 mg/day; tolterodine 2 mg/day
Narcotic analgesics (e.g., buprenorphine, fentanyl, sufentanil) / Possible ↑ narcotic plasma levels and t½; closely monitor respiratory function during and after stopping the narcotic; do not give atazanavir without ritonavir if using buprenorphine
Nevirapine / ↓ Atazanavir exposure and ↑ nevirapine exposure; do not use together
Nilotinib / ↑ Nilotinib plasma levels → ↑ pharmacologic effects; do not use together
Oral contraceptives (ethinyl estradiol, norethindrone, norgestimate) / Levels of hormones may be altered; consider nonhormonal contraception
PDE5 inhibitors (e.g., sildenafil, tadalafil, vardenafil) / ↑ PDE5 inhibitor side effects, including hypotension, visual changes, and priapism; use with caution at reduced doses (sildenafil 25 mg q 48 hr; tadalafil 10 mg q 72 hr; vardenafil up to 2.5 mg q 72 hr); do not use atazanavir and sildenafil to treat pulmonary arterial hypertension
Pimozide / ↑ Pimozide serum levels → serious and/or life-threatening reactions, such as cardiac arrhythmias; do not use together
Protease inhibitors (e.g., amprenavir, darunavir, fosamprenavir, indinavir, nelfinavir, saquinavir, ti-

pranavir) / ↑ Levels of protease inhibitor; do not use together
Proton pump inhibitors (e.g., omeprazole) / Significant ↓ in atazanavir levels → ↓ therapeutic effect and possible resistance; give proton pump inhibitors 12 hr before the atazanavir dose
Quetiapine / ↑ Quetiapine plasma levels → ↑ pharmacologic/toxic effects; use together with caution and monitor; adjust quetiapine dose as needed
Raltegravir / ↑ Raltegravir plasma levels → ↑ pharmacologic/toxic effects; closely monitor and adjust raltegravir dose as needed
Ranolazine / ↑ Risk of dose-related prolongation of the QTc interval, torsades de pointes–type arrhythmias, and sudden death; do not use together
Rifabutin / ↑ Rifabutin levels; reduce dose up to 75% (i.e., 150 mg q other day or 3 times a week)
Rifampin / ↓ Atazanavir plasma levels and AUC by 90% → loss of therapeutic effect and resistance; do not use together
Risperidone / ↑ Risperidone plasma levels → ↑ pharmacologic/toxic effects; closely monitor and adjust risperidone dose as needed
Ritonavir / Decrease the dose of atazanavir to 300 mg once daily with 100 mg ritonavir
Romidepsin / ↑ Romidepsin plasma levels → ↑ pharmacologic/toxic effects, including QT prolongation; if used together, monitor ECG and adjust romidepsin dose as needed
Salmeterol / ↑ Salmeterol levels → ↑ risk of CV events, including QT prolongation, palpitations, and sinus tachycardia; do not use together
H *St. John's wort* / ↓ Atazanavir plasma levels → ↓ effect R/T possible ↑ metabolism by CYP3A4 enzymes; do not use together
Temsirolimus / ↑ Temsirolimus plasma levels → ↑ pharmacologic/toxic effects; monitor response and adjust temsirolimus dose as needed
Tenofovir / ↓ Atazanavir AUC and C_{max}; do not give atazanavir and tenofovir without ritonavir; also, atazanavir ↑ tenofovir levels; monitor for tenofovir side effects; dose as atazanavir 300 mg, ritonavir 100 mg and tenofovir 300 mg
Tetracyclines (e.g., minocycline) / ↓ Atazanavir levels → ↓ therapeutic effect; closely monitor atazanavir levels and adjust atazanavir dose as needed
Trazodone (with or without ritonavir) / Significant ↑ plasma trazodone levels → ↑ risk of toxicity; use with caution and ↓ trazodone dose
Tyrosine kinase inhibitors (e.g., dasatinib, lapatinib, pazopanib, sorafenib, sunitinib) / ↑ Tyrosine kinase inhibitor plasma levels → ↑ pharmacologic/toxic effects; if used together, monitor closely and adjust kinase inhibitor dose as needed
Vasopressor receptor antagonists (e.g., conivaptan, tolvaptan) / ↑ Vasopressor receptor antagonist plasma levels → ↑ pharmacologic effects; do not use together
Voriconazole / Do not use with atazanavir/ritonavir R/T ↑ atazanavir levels
Warfarin / Possible serious and/or life-threatening bleeding; monitor INR

HOW SUPPLIED

Capsules: 100 mg, 150 mg, 200 mg, 300 mg (all as the sulfate).

DOSAGE

CAPSULES

Human immunodeficiency virus-1 (HIV-1) infections, treatment-naive adults and children.

Adults, antiretroviral-naive clients, usual: 300 mg atazanavir with 100 mg ritonavir, once daily, as a single dose with food. For those unable to tolerate ritonavir, give atazanavir, 400 mg (without ritonavir) once daily with food. Consider a dose reduction to 300 mg of atazanavir for those with moderate hepatic insufficiency (Child-Pugh, class B). **Children, 6 to younger than 18 years of age, 15 to <25 kg (33 to <55 lbs):** Atazanavir, 150 mg and ritonavir, 80 mg; **25 to <32 kg (55 to <70 lbs):** Atazanavir, 200 mg and ritonavir, 100 mg; **32 to <39 kg (70 to <86 lbs):** Atazanavir, 250 mg and ritonavir, 100 mg; **39 kg or greater (86 or more lbs):** Atazanavir, 300 mg and ritonavir, 100 mg. For children at least 13 years of age and weighing at least 39 kg who are unable to tolerate ritonavir, give atazanavir, 400 mg (without ritonavir) once daily with food.

HIV-1 infections, treatment-experienced adults and children.

Adults, antiretroviral-experienced clients, usual: 300 mg atazanavir plus 100 mg ritonavir both once daily with food. **Children, 6 to younger than 18**

years of age, 25 to <32 kg (55 to <70 lbs): Atazanavir, 200 mg and ritonavir, 100 mg; **32 to <39 kg (70 to <86 lbs):** Atazanavir, 250 mg and ritonavir, 100 mg; **39 kg or greater (86 lbs or more):** Atazanavir, 300 mg and ritonavir, 100 mg. *NOTE:* Data are insufficient to recommend dosing of treatment-experienced children weighing less than 25 kg.

NURSING IMPLICATIONS

IMPLEMENTATION/ADMINISTRATION/STORAGE

1. PO dosage depends on treatment history of the client and use of other coadministered drugs.
2. Dosage for children, 6 to younger than 18 years, is based on body weight and should not exceed the recommended adult dose.
3. Data are insufficient to recommend doses of atazanavir for the following: Clients less than 6 years of age; without ritonavir in those younger than 13 years of age; and, treatment-experienced children with body weight less than 25 kg.
4. Atazanavir without ritonavir is not recommended for treatment-experienced clients with prior virologic failure.
5. Safety and efficacy of atazanavir with ritonavir in doses greater than 100 mg once daily have not been determined. Use of higher ritonavir doses is not recommended as they may alter the safety profile of atazanavir (e.g., cardiac effects, hyperbilirubinemia).
6. In *treatment-naive* or *treatment-experienced* clients, coadministration of atazanavir with didanosine buffered or enteric-coated should be given with food 2 hr before or 1hr after didanosine.
7. In *treatment-naive* clients who receive efavirenz and atazanavir, the recommended dose of atazanavir is 400 mg with ritonavir 100 mg, all as a single dose with food. Give efavirenz, 600 mg once daily on an empty stomach preferably at bedtime. Do not coadminister atazanavir and efavirenz without ritonavir.
8. Dosing recommendations for atazanavir and efavirenz have not been determined in *treatment-experienced* clients. Do not give atazanavir with efavirenz in treatment-experienced clients, because of decreased atazanavir exposure.
9. In *treatment-naive* clients requiring tenofovir disoproxil fumarate, give atazanavir 300 mg, with ritonavir, 100 mg, and tenofovir, 300 mg (all as a single daily dose with food). Atazanavir should not be given with tenofovir without ritonavir.
10. In clients who require famotidine, give atazanavir 300 mg with ritonavir 100 mg both once daily at the same time with food; do not exceed a dose of 40 mg of famotidine twice daily in *therapy-naive* clients or 20 mg twice daily of famotidine in *therapy-experienced* clients. Give atazanavir/ritonavir at least 2 hr before up to 10 hr after the dose of famotidine.
11. In *treatment-naive* clients who require a proton pump inhibitor, do not exceed a 20 mg dose equivalent to omeprazole. Give about 12 hr prior to atazanavir 300 mg and ritonavir 100 mg. Do not use proton pump inhibitors in treatment-experienced clients receiving atazanavir.
12. *Treatment-naive* clients with end-stage renal disease managed with hemodialysis should receive atazanavir 300 mg with ritonavir 100 mg. Do not give atazanavir to *treatment-experienced* clients with end-stage renal disease managed with hemodialysis.
13. For clients with moderate hepatic impairment (Child-Pugh class B) who have not experienced virologic failure, reduce dose of atazanavir to 300 mg daily. Atazanavir/ritonavir has not been studied in those with hepatic failure and such use is not recommended.
14. In those receiving atazanavir/ritonavir for at least 10 days, start bosentan at 62.5 mg once a day or every other day based on tolerability. In those on bosentan, discontinue bosentan at least 36 hr before starting atazanavir/ritonavir. At least 10 days after starting atazanavir/ritonavir, resume bosentan at 62.5 mg once daily or every other day based on individual tolerability.
15. In pregnancy, recommended is atazanavir 300 mg once daily and ritonavir 100 mg both once daily. Do not give atazanavir without ritonavir to this group. For treatment-experienced pregnant women during the second or third trimester, atazanavir 400 mg with ritona-

vir 100 mg each once daily is recommended when atazanavir is coadministered with either an H_2 receptor antagonist or tenofovir.

16. Store from 15–30°C (59–86°F).

ASSESSMENT

1. Note disease onset, characteristics of S&S, other agents trialed, outcome. Determine if first time treatment or if received previously.
2. List drugs prescribed; ensure none interact.
3. Monitor ECG at baseline and periodically thereafter; assess for prolonged PR interval.
4. Monitor women for at least 2 months postdelivery because atazanavir exposure increases during this time; this may make clients more susceptible to side effects.
5. Check glucose, lipids, and LFTs; reduce dose with dysfunction. Monitor CD4+ cell count and HIV RNA load. Assess for S&S of lactic acidosis. Observe for any new onset diabetes.

CLIENT/FAMILY TEACHING

1. Take with food or snack to increase absorption and effectiveness and with other antiretroviral therapy (always used in combination therapy). Take as directed, do not skip or double doses. Take once daily, at about the same time each day; swallow capsules whole. Do not crush, chew, or open capsules.
2. Do not take any unprescribed or OTC meds/herbals without provider consent. Avoid garlic ingestion, St. John's wort, and erectile dysfunction-type drugs; may cause adverse SE.
3. If taking antacids or didanosine chewable/dispersible buffered tablets, take atazanavir 2 hr before or 1 hr after these medicines.
4. Report dizziness/lightheadedness, palpitations (pounding in the chest), as ECG may be needed (may prolong PR interval). Also report persistent nausea or vomiting, profound weakness or tiredness, unexpected stomach discomfort, trouble breathing, or yellowing of the skin or eyes (may cause bilirubin elevations).
5. Drug may cause changes in body fat distribution/accumulation.
6. Does not prevent disease transmission or STDs; use protection.
7. Caution HIV-infected mother that breast-feeding could cause HIV infection in the baby. Caution may be more susceptible to side effects for 2 months postdelivery as atazanavir exposure increases during this time.
8. Keep all F/U to evaluate response, labs, and adverse SE.

OUTCOMES/EVALUATE

- Management of HIV infection
- ↓ HIVRNA

Atenolol

(ah-**TEN**-oh-lohl)

Classification(s): Beta-adrenergic blocking agent

Pregnancy Category: C

RX: Tenormin.

✤ **Rx:** Apo-Atenol, CO Atenolol, Gen-Atenolol, Novo-Atenol, PMS-Atenolol, RAN-Atenolol, ratio-Atenolol, Sandoz Atenolol.

SEE ALSO ***BETA-ADRENERGIC BLOCKING AGENTS***.

INDICATIONS/USES

(1) Hypertension (either alone or with other antihypertensives such as thiazide diuretics). (2) Long-term treatment of angina pectoris due to coronary atherosclerosis. (3) To reduce CV mortality in definite or suspected acute MI in hemodynamically stable clients. Initiate treatment as soon as the client's clinical condition allows. *Investigational:* Prophylaxis of migraine.

ACTION/KINETICS

Action

Combines reversibly with beta-adrenergic receptors to block the response to sympathetic nerve impulses, circulating catecholamines, or adrenergic drugs. Predominantly beta-1 blocking activity. Has no membrane-stabilizing activity or intrinsic sympathomimetic activity.

Pharmacokinetics

Low lipid solubility. **Peak blood levels:** 2–4 hr. **t½:** 6–9 hr. 50% eliminated unchanged in the feces. Geriatric clients have a higher plasma level than younger clients and a total clearance value of about 50% less.

SPECIAL CONCERNS

Advise clients with coronary heart disease who are being treated with atenolol against abrupt discontinuation of therapy. Severe exacerbation of angina and the occurrence of MI and ventricular arrhythmias have been re-

A

ported in clients with angina following abrupt discontinuation of therapy with beta-blockers. The last 2 complications may occur with or without preceding exacerbation of the angina pectoris. As with other beta-blockers, when discontinuation of atenolol is planned, observe the client carefully and advise the client to limit physical activity to a minimum. If the angina worsens or acute coronary insufficiency develops, it is recommended that atenolol be promptly reinstituted, at least temporarily. Because coronary artery disease is common and may be unrecognized, it may be prudent not to discontinue atenolol therapy abruptly, even in clients treated only for hypertension. ■

Dosage not established in children.

SIDE EFFECTS

Most Common

Dizziness, fatigue, nausea, bradycardia, hypotension, vertigo.

See *Beta-Adrenergic Blocking Agents* for a complete list of possible side effects.

HOW SUPPLIED

Tablets: 25 mg, 50 mg, 100 mg.

DOSAGE

TABLETS

Hypertension.

Adults, initial: 50 mg/day, either alone or with diuretics; an initial dose of 25 mg/day should be used in the elderly. If response is inadequate, 100 mg/day in adults. Doses higher than 100 mg/day will not produce further beneficial effects. Maximum effects usually seen within 1–2 weeks. May be used with thiazide-type diuretics, hydralazine, prazosin, and alpha-methyldopa. **Children, usual (investigational):** 0.5–1 mg/kg/day divided once or twice daily, up to a maximum of 2 mg/kg/day, up to 100 mg daily.

Angina.

Initial: 50 mg/day; if maximum response is not seen in 1 week, increase dose to 100 mg/day (some clients require 200 mg/day).

Prophylaxis of migraine (Investigational).

100 mg/day for 6–12 weeks.

NURSING IMPLICATIONS

Do not confuse atenolol with albuterol (sympathomimetic) or with timolol (beta-blocker). Do not confuse Tenormin with Tenoretic (atenolol plus chlorthalidone).

IMPLEMENTATION/ADMINISTRATION/STORAGE

1. Adjust dosage in cases of renal failure to a maximum of 50 mg/day if C_{CR} is 15–35 mL/min/1.73 m^2 and to a maximum of 25 mg/day if C_{CR} is less than 15 mL/min/1.73 m^2.
2. With hemodialysis, give 25 or 50 mg in the hospital after each dialysis, under hospital supervision, since significant decreases in BP may occur.
3. Atenolol is used in addition to standard coronary care unit therapy.
4. Beta-blockers that are effective in the post-infarction setting may be continued for 1 to 3 years provided there are no contraindications.
5. Control of angina pectoris for 24 hr to achieve an immediate maximum effect. The maximum early effect on exercise tolerance occurs with doses of 50 to 100 mg; however, at these doses, the effect at 24 hr is attenuated, averaging about 50–75% of that observed with 200 mg given once daily.
6. Store from 25–25°C (68–77°F).

ASSESSMENT

1. Identify reasons for therapy, type, onset, and characteristics of S&S; list agents trialed and those prescribed to ensure none interact.
2. Note history of diabetes, pulmonary disease, or cardiac failure; monitor closely.
3. Assess VS, ECG, weight, lung sounds, TSH, renal and LFTs; reduce dose with dysfunction.

CLIENT/FAMILY TEACHING

1. Take at same time each day. May take with food if GI upset occurs.
2. Use caution while driving or performing tasks requiring mental alertness; may cause drowsiness. Dizziness, light-headedness, or fainting may occur, and alcohol, hot weather, exercise, or fever may increase effects. Avoid sudden position changes to prevent sudden drop in BP.

3. May mask symptoms of low blood sugar in those with diabetes. Monitor FS closely; may need to alter insulin dose while taking drug.
4. A beta-blocker drug lowers BP and heart rate, controls angina, and may decrease mortality from recurrent MI. Do not stop suddenly; sharp chest pain, irregular heartbeat, and sometimes heart attack may occur.
5. Report any difficulty breathing; swelling of extremities; irregular heartbeat, altered mood, or depression.
6. Sensitivity to cold may occur due to reduced blood flow to feet and hands. This may cause one to feel chilled and more sensitive to the cold. Dress warmly in cold weather, and use care when out in the cold for long periods of time.
7. To help control BP: maintain healthy diet, and limit intake of caffeine; avoid alcohol, salt substitutes, or high Na and high K foods; perform regular exercise; maintain weight; and stop smoking. Keep log of HR and BP at different times during the day for provider review.
8. Practice reliable contraception, and report if pregnancy suspected.
9. If erectile dysfunction occurs/persists, report so therapy can be adjusted/changed.
10. Monitor/record HR and BP, and report any marked changes.
11. Report any significant changes in mood or depression, swelling of feet or hands, or heart palpitations.
12. Keep all F/U to assess response and adverse SE.

OUTCOMES/EVALUATE

- ↓ BP; ↓ HR
- ↓ Frequency of anginal attacks
- Prevention of repeat infarction

Atomoxetine HCl

(**AT**-oh-mox-eh-teen)

Classification(s): Drug for attention-deficit/hyperactivity disorder

Pregnancy Category: C

RX: Strattera.

INDICATIONS/USES

Treatment of attention-deficit/hyperactivity disorder (ADHD) in adults and children. Used for both inattentive type and hyperactive-impulsive type of disorders. *Investigational:* Nocturnal enuresis, binge eating disorder, obesity.

ACTION/KINETICS

Action

Mechanism not known but thought to be related to selective inhibition of presynaptic norepinephrine transport, thus increasing levels of norepinephrine in nerve synapses.

Pharmacokinetics

Rapidly absorbed after PO use with absolute bioavailability of 63% in extensive metabolizers and 94% in poor metabolizers. High-fat meals decrease the rate of absorption; in children and adolescents, administration with food results in a 9% lower C_{max}. **Maximum plasma levels:** 1–2 hr. Metabolized by the CYP2D6 pathway. Those with reduced activity of this pathway (about 7% of Caucasians and 2% of African Americans) have higher plasma levels. **t½, extensive metabolizers:** About 5.2 hr; **t½, poor metabolizers:** 21.6 hr. Greater than 80% excreted in the urine and 17% in the feces. **Plasma protein binding:** About 98%.

CONTRAINDICATIONS

Hypersensitivity to atomoxetine or other product constituents. Use with a monoamine oxidase inhibitor (MAOI) or within 2 weeks after discontinuing an MAOI. Use in narrow angle glaucoma due to ↑ risk of mydriasis. Pheochromocytoma or a history of pheochromocytoma.

SPECIAL CONCERNS

Suicidal ideation in children and adolescent. (1) Atomoxetine increased the risk of suicidal ideation in short-term studies in children or adolescents with ADHD. Anyone considering the use of atomoxetine in a child or adolescent must balance this risk with the clinical need. Comorbidities occurring with ADHD may be associated with an increase in the risk of suicidal ideation and/or behavior. Closely monitor clients who are started on therapy for suicidality (suicidal thinking and behavior), clinical worsening, or unusual changes in behavior. Advise families and caregivers of the need for close observation and communication with the prescribing health care provider. Atomoxetine is approved for ADHD in children and adults. Atomoxetine is not approved for major depressive disorder. (2) Pooled analyses of short-term (6- to -18 week), placebo-controlled trials of atomoxetine in children and adolescents (12 trials involving more than 2,200 clients, including 11 trials in ADHD and 1 trial in enuresis) have revealed a greater risk of suicidal ideation early during treatment in those receiving atomoxetine compared with placebo. The average risk of suicidal ideation in children and adolescents receiving atomoxetine was 0.4% compared with none in placebo-treated clients. No suicides occurred in these trials. ■

- **Safety and efficacy not determined in children younger than 6 years of age. Efficacy not evaluated systematically beyond 9 weeks of use and safety beyond 1 year of use.**
- **Use with caution in hypertension, tachycardia, cerebrovascular or CV disease, or with pressor agents due to drug-induced increases in BP and HR.**
- **Use with caution in any condition that predisposes to hypotension and during lactation.**
- **Discontinue if jaundice or lab evidence of liver injury occurs.**
- **Use with caution during lactation; observe for constipation, dyspepsia, or upper abdominal pain in the infant.**

SIDE EFFECTS

Most Common

Adults: Dry mouth, nausea, insomnia, decreased appetite, hot flush, constipation, erectile dysfunction, fatigue, urinary hesitation/retention, abdominal pain, dysmenorrhea, dizziness.

Children/Adolescents: Headache, abdominal pain/discomfort, decreased appetite, somnolence, N&V, fatigue, irritability, dizziness.

CNS: Aggression, headache, somnolence, irritability, dizziness, mood swings, feeling jittery, agitation, akathisia, anxiety, hostility, paresthesia, sinus headache, abnormal dreams, sleep disorder, insomnia and/or middle insomnia, sedation, depression (includes depressed mood, depressive symptoms, dysphoria, major depression), tremor, hypomania, impulsivity, mania, panic attacks, crying, tearfulness, nervousness, early morning awakening, hypoesthesia, sensory disturbances, ***seizures***. ↑ ***Risk of suicidal ideation*** in children and adolescents. Emergent of new psychotic or manic symptoms (e.g., delusions, hallucinations, mania) in children and adolescents with no prior history of such. Appearance or worsening of aggressive behavior or hostility especially in children and adolescents during beginning of treatment. **GI:** N&V, abdominal pain/discomfort (including upper abdominal pain), dyspepsia, anorexia, diarrhea, dry mouth, flatulence, constipation, viral gastroenteritis, severe liver injury (rare). **CV:** Postural hypotension, increased BP & HR, sinus tachycardia, tachycardia, syncope, palpitations, hot flushes, QT prolongation, peripheral vascular instability and/or Raynaud phenomenon (new onset or worsening of pre-existing). Elevated BP and tachyarrhythmias in those with pheochromocytoma. ***Sudden death in children with structural cardiac abnormalities or other serious heart problems. Sudden death, stroke, and MI in adults.*** **Hypersensitivity:** ***Angioneurotic edema,*** urticaria, rash, ***anaphylactic reactions.*** **Respiratory:** Cough, rhinorrhea, sore throat, sinusitis, nasal/sinus congestion, nasopharyngitis, URTI, pharyngolaryngeal pain. **Dermatologic:** Rash, dermatitis, flushing, pruritus, increased sweating, peripheral coldness. **GU:** Urinary retention/hesitation (in adolescents and children), dysuria, ejaculatory failure and/or ejaculation disorder, impotence, difficulty in micturition, dysmenorrhea, delayed menses, irregular menstruation, abnormal orgasm, prostatitis, erectile disturbance/dysfunction, priapism (rare). **Ophthalmic:** Mydriasis, conjunctivitis. **Metabolic/Nutritional:** Weight loss, decreased appetite. **Body as a whole:** Fatigue and/or lethargy, feeling abnormal, pyrexia, rigors, chills, flu, arthralgia, myalgia, slower growth and weight gain in children. **Miscellaneous:** Ear infection, chest/back pain, decreased libido, paresthesias, pelvic pain in men, excoriation.

OVERDOSE MANAGEMENT

Symptoms: Agitation, abnormal behavior, dizziness, GI symptoms, tremor, hyperactivity, somnolence, mydriasis, tachycardia, dry mouth, ↑ BP. Less commonly, QT prolongation and mental changes (e.g., disorientation, hallucinations). *Treatment:* Establish an airway. Monitor cardiac and vital signs. Provide symptomatic and supportive care. Gastric lavage (if performed soon after ingestion). Repeated activated charcoal may prevent systemic absorption. Dialysis is not likely to be beneficial.

DRUG INTERACTIONS

Possible additive effect with other drugs that prolong the QT interval. The following drugs may prolong the QT interval and ↑ risk of life-threatening arrhythmias, including torsades de pointes: Amiodarone, arsenic trioxide, bretylium, chlorpromazine, cisapride, disopyramide, dofetilide, dolasetron, droperidol, gatifloxacin, halofantrine, levomethadyl, mefloquine, mesoridazine, moxifloxacin, pentamidine, pimozide, probucol, procainamide, quinidine, sotalol, sparfloxacin, thioridazine, ziprasidone.

Albuterol / Potentiation of CV effects (e.g., ↑ HR & BP) of albuterol; use together with caution

Fluoxetine / ↑ Atomoxetine AUC and C_{max}; dosage reduction may be necessary

MAOIs / Possible serious, and sometimes fatal, reactions, including hyperthermia, rigidity, myoclonus, autonomic instability, extreme agitation, delirium, and coma; also neuroleptic malignant syndrome. Do not give atomoxetine within 2 weeks after discontinuing an MAOI, and do not start treatment with an MAOI within 2 weeks after discontinuing atomoxetine

Midazolam / ↑ Midazolam AUC; no dose adjustment needed

Paroxetine / ↑ Atomoxetine AUC and C_{max}; dosage reduction may be necessary

Pressor drugs (e.g., dopamine, dobutamine) / Possible combined effects on BP; give with caution

Quinidine / ↑ Atomoxetine AUC and C_{max}; dosage reduction may be necessary

HOW SUPPLIED

Capsules: 10 mg, 18 mg, 25 mg, 40 mg, 60 mg, 80 mg, 100 mg.

DOSAGE

CAPSULES

Attention-deficit hyperactivity disorder (ADHD).

Adults and children/adolescents over 70 kg, initial: Total daily dose of 40 mg. May increase after a minimum of 3 days to a target total daily dose of about 80 mg/day given either as a single dose in the a.m. or as evenly divided doses in the morning and late afternoon/early evening. After 2–4 weeks, dose may be increased to a maximum of 100 mg/day in those who have not achieved an optimal response. **Children and adolescents up to 70 kg, initial:** Total daily dose of 0.5 mg/kg. May be increased after a minimum of 3 days to a target total daily dose of about 1.2 mg/kg given either as a single dose in the a.m. or as evenly divided doses in the morning and late afternoon/early evening. No additional benefit is noted for doses higher than 1.4 mg/kg/day. Do not exceed a maximum daily dose of 1.4 mg/kg or 100 mg, whichever is less.

NURSING IMPLICATIONS

IMPLEMENTATION/ADMINISTRATION/STORAGE

1. Take with or without food. Administer as a single daily dose in the morning or as evenly divided doses in the morning and the late afternoon/early evening.
2. The safety of single doses more than 120 mg and total daily doses of 150 mg has not been evaluated.
3. Periodically evaluate the long-term usefulness for each client.
4. Atomoxetine may be discontinued without the dose being tapered.
5. For moderate hepatic insufficiency (Child-Pugh Class B), reduce initial and target doses to 50% of the normal dose. For severe hepatic insufficiency (Child-Pugh Class C), reduce initial and target doses to 25% of the normal dose.
6. **For children and adolescents up to 70 kg:** who have been given strong CYP2D6 inhibitors (e.g., fluoxetine, quinidine, or paroxetine) or in those known to be CYP2D6 poor metabolizers, initiate dosage at 0.5 mg/kg/day and only increase to the usual target dose of 1.2 mg/kg/day if symptoms fail to improve after 4 weeks and initial dose is well tolerated. **Those over 70 kg:** who have been given strong CYP2D6 inhibitors (see above) or who are CYP2D6 poor metabolizers: Initiate dosage at 40 mg/day and only increase to the usual target dose of 80 mg/day if symptoms fail to improve after 4 weeks and the initial dose is well tolerated.

A

7. Store at controlled room temperature between 15–30°C (59–86°F).

ASSESSMENT

1. Note age at diagnosis of ADHD, chronicity/severity and type of symptoms, social/academic, or occupational impairment. Ensure no psychosis, environmental triggers, or undiagnosed psychiatric disorders.
2. Complete history, physical exam, list DSM IV-TR characteristics. Perform LFTs if itchy skin, dark urine, jaundice, tenderness in the right-upper abdominal quadrant, or unexplained flu-like symptoms.
3. Monitor VS, ht, and Wt; may impair growth and weight gain during long-term therapy; may need to interrupt therapy (summer) in children who are not growing or gaining weight satisfactorily.
4. List drugs prescribed to ensure none interact (e.g., Prozac, Paxil, quinidine).
5. May increase HR and BP; assess CNS/neurologic/cardiac status and ECG prior to starting therapy. Use cautiously with HTN.
6. Monitor ECG, CBC, chemistry profile, TSH, urinalysis, renal and LFTs; adjust dosage with dysfunction. Drug metabolized by cytochrome P450 pathway (CYP2D6).

CLIENT/FAMILY TEACHING

1. Take with or without food. If dose missed, take as soon as possible but do not take more than the prescribed total daily dose in any 24-hr period.
2. Do not open capsules. If any eye contact with capsule contents, flush eyes immediately with water and report. Wash hands and any other objects that may have become contaminated with contents.
3. Use caution driving or operating machinery until drug effects realized.
4. Do not take any other prescribed, OTC, herbal, or dietary supplements without provider approval. Albuterol therapy may increase BP and heart rate.
5. May experience emotional upset, abdominal pain, GI upset, dry mouth; should subside with continued therapy. Report significant weight loss/loss of appetite, yellow discoloration of skin or eyes, anxiety, agitation, panic attacks, insomnia, irritability, hostility, aggressiveness, suicidal thoughts, or other unusual changes in behavior to HCP.
6. Do not use caffeine/caffeine-containing products. Avoid OTC preparations containing caffeine or other stimulants.
7. Swelling of lips, face, rash, and itching are S&S of allergic reaction and require immediate treatment.
8. May inhibit sexual functioning and cause urinary retention/hesitancy; report if bothersome. May experience erection (priapism) >4 hr; report if evident.
9. Record weight and report excessive loss. Children may experience growth retardation, so drug should periodically be discontinued (i.e., during the summer) by provider to allow growth to proceed normally and to evaluate the need for continued drug therapy.
10. Keep all F/U to assess response, dose adequacy, and for adverse SE.

OUTCOMES/EVALUATE

- Ability to sit quietly and concentrate
- ↓ Hyperactivity/impulsive behaviors

Atorvastatin calcium

(ah-**TORE**-vah-**stah**-tin)

Classification(s): Antihyperlipidemic, HMG-CoA reductase inhibitor

Pregnancy Category: X

RX: Lipitor.

SEE ALSO ***ANTIHYPERLIPIDEMIC AGENTS—HMG-COA REDUCTASE INHIBITORS.***

INDICATIONS/USES

1. Heterozygous familial and nonfamilial hypercholesterolemia and mixed dyslipidemia. Adjunct to diet to decrease elevated total and LDL cholesterol, apo-B, and triglyceride levels and to increase HDL cholesterol in primary hypercholesterolemia (including heterozygous familial and nonfamilial) and mixed dyslipidemia (including Fredrickson type IIa and IIb).
2. Homozygous familial hypercholesterolemia. Adjunct to other lipid-lowering treatments (e.g., LDL apheresis), or if other treatments are not available, to reduce total and LDL cholesterol.

3. Primary dysbetalipoproteinemia (Fredrickson type III) in those who do not respond adequately to diet.
4. Hypertriglyceridemia. Adjunct to diet to treat elevated serum triglyceride levels (Fredrickson type IV).
5. Heterozygous familial hypercholesterolemia in children 10–17 years of age. Adjunct to diet to reduce total and LDL cholesterol and apo-B levels in boys and postmenarchal girls 10–17 years of age with heterozygous familial hypercholesterolemia; used after a trial of diet therapy if the following are present: (a) LDL cholesterol remains 190 mg/dL or higher or (b) LDL remains 160 mg/dL or higher and there is a positive family history of premature CVD or two or more other CVD risk factors are present.
6. Clinically evident coronary heart disease. Reduce the risk of nonfatal MI, fatal and nonfatal stroke, revascularization procedures, hospitalization for CHF, and angina in clients with clinically evident coronary heart disease.
7. Prevention of cardiovascular disease. Reduce the risk of MI and stroke and the risk for revascularization procedures and angina in adults without clinically evident coronary heart disease but with multiple risk factors for coronary heart disease, including age, smoking, hypertension, low HDL-C, or a family history of early coronary heart disease.
8. Reduce the risk of stroke and MI in type 2 diabetics who show no evidence of coronary heart disease but with other risk factors, including retinopathy, albuminuria, smoking, or hypertension.

NOTE: Use lipid-altering drugs, in addition to a diet restricted in saturated fat and cholesterol, only when the response to diet and other nonpharmacological measures has been inadequate.

ACTION/KINETICS

Action

Competitively inhibits HMG-CoA reductase; this enzyme catalyzes the early rate-limiting step in the synthesis of cholesterol. Thus, plasma levels of LDL and total cholesterol are markedly decreased while Apo-B and triglycerides are decreased to a lesser extent. Also, HDL is increased.

Pharmacokinetics

Absolute bioavailability is about 14%. Undergoes first-pass metabolism by CYP3A4 enzymes in the liver to active metabolites. **Time to peak effect:** 1–2 hr. **t½:** 14 hr. Plasma levels are not affected by renal disease, but they are markedly increased with chronic alcoholic liver disease. Decreases in LDL cholesterol range from 35–40% (10 mg/day) to 50–60% (80 mg/day). Less than 2% excreted in the urine. **Plasma protein binding:** More than 98%.

CONTRAINDICATIONS

Active liver disease or unexplained persistently high liver transaminases. Pregnancy, lactation.

SPECIAL CONCERNS

- **Elderly clients are at an increased risk of myopathy.**
- **Safety and efficacy not determined in children less than 18 years of age.**

SIDE EFFECTS

Most Common

Headache, asthenia, abdominal pain/cramps, infection, diarrhea, sinusitis, myalgia, arthralgia, back pain, rash, flu syndrome, accidental trauma.

See also *Antihyperlipidemic Agents—HMG-CoA Reductase Inhibitors* for a complete list of possible side effects. **GI:** Altered LFTs (usually within the first 3 months of therapy), diarrhea, abdominal pain/cramps, flatulence, dyspepsia, constipation, dry mouth, dysgeusia, gastroenteritis/gastritis, N&V. **CNS:** Headache, asthenia, paresthesia, insomnia, depression, dizziness. **CV:** Angina pectoris, hypertension. **Musculoskeletal:** Myalgia, arthralgia, back pain, arthritis, leg pain, ***rhabdomyolysis with acute renal failure secondary to myoglobinuria***. **Respiratory:** Sinusitis, bronchitis, pharyngitis, rhinitis, dyspnea. **Dermatologic:** Rash, alopecia, eczema, pruritus. **Miscellaneous:** Infection, allergy, influenza, accidental trauma, flu syndrome, allergy/hypersensitivity, peripheral edema, chest pain, edema/swelling, UTI.

LABORATORY TEST CONSIDERATIONS

CPK (due to myalgia).

ADDITIONAL DRUG INTERACTIONS

Amiodarone / ↑ Risk of myopathy R/T ↓ atorvastatin metabolism by CYP3A4; if amiodarone use necessary, use the lowest possible dose

A

Antacids / ↓ Atorvastatin levels by 35%; LDL-C reduction not affected
Bosentan / Possible ↑ metabolism of atorvastatin → ↓ therapeutic effect
Carbamazepine / Possible ↑ metabolism of atorvastatin → ↓ therapeutic effect
Cholestyramine/Colistipol / ↓ Atorvastatin GI tract absorption R/T / binding to bile acid sequestrant
Cilostazole / Possible ↓ metabolism of atorvastatin → ↑ risk of toxicity (e.g., myopathy); monitor closely and adjust dosage if necessary
Cyclosporine / ↑ Risk of myopathy and rhabdomyolysis R/T ↓ atorvastatin metabolism by CYP3A4
Delavirdine / Possible ↓ metabolism of atorvastatin → ↑ risk of toxicity (e.g., myopathy)
Digoxin / ↑ Digoxin levels R/T ↑ digoxin absorption; monitor digoxin levels and adjust dosage as necessary
Diltiazem / Possible ↓ metabolism of atorvastatin → ↑ risk of toxicity (e.g., myopathy)
Efavirenz / Either ↓ metabolism of atorvastatin → ↑ risk of toxicity (e.g., myopathy) or possible induction of CYP3A4 → ↓ atorvastatin plasma levels
Erythromycin / ↑ Risk of myopathy and rhabdomyolysis R/T ↓ atorvastatin metabolism by CYP3A4
Grapefruit juice (1 qt daily) / ↑ Atorvastatin plasma levels → ↑ risk of myopathy; avoid concurrent use
Hydantoins (e.g., phenytoin) / ↓ Atorvastatin plasma levels R/T ↑ metabolism
Imatinib / Possible ↓ metabolism of atorvastatin → ↑ risk of toxicity (e.g., myopathy)
Itraconazole / ↑ Risk of myopathy and rhabdomyolysis R/T ↓ atorvastatin metabolism by CYP3A4
Midazolam / Possible ↓ midazolam metabolism → ↑ and prolonged effects
Nefazodone / ↑ Risk of myopathy and rhabdomyolysis R/T ↓ atorvastatin metabolism by CYP3A4
Nevirapine / Either ↓ metabolism of atorvastatin → ↑ risk of toxicity (e.g., myopathy) or possible induction of CYP3A4 → ↓ atorvastatin plasma levels
Oral contraceptives / ↑ Plasma levels of norethindrone and ethinyl estradiol
Quinine / Possible ↓ metabolism of atorvastatin → ↑ risk of toxicity (e.g., myopathy)
Rifamycins (e.g., rifampin) / Possible ↓ atorvastatin plasma levels
Ritonavir / ↑ Risk of myopathy and rhabdomyolysis R/T ↓ atorvastatin metabolism by CYP3A4
Saquinavir / ↑ Risk of myopathy and rhabdomyolysis R/T ↓ atorvastatin metabolism by CYP3A4
H ***St. John's wort*** / Possible ↑ metabolism of atorvastatin → ↓ therapeutic effect
Telithromycin / Possible ↓ metabolism of atorvastatin → ↑ risk of toxicity (e.g., myopathy)
Verapamil / Possible ↓ metabolism of atorvastatin → ↑ risk of toxicity (e.g., myopathy); if use necessary, decrease atorvastatin dose and monitor; atorvastatin may also ↑ verapamil levels

HOW SUPPLIED

Tablets: 10 mg, 20 mg, 40 mg, 80 mg.

DOSAGE

TABLETS

Hypercholesterolemia (heterozygous familial and nonfamilial) and mixed dyslipidemia (Fredrickson types IIa and IIb).
Initial: 10 or 20 mg once daily (40 mg/day for those who require more than a 45% reduction in LDL cholesterol); **then** a dose range of 10–80 mg once daily may be used. Individualize therapy according to goal of therapy and response.

Homozygous familial hypercholesterolemia.
Initial: 10–80 mg/day. Used as an adjunct to other lipid-lowering treatments (e.g., LDL apheresis) or if such treatments are unavailable.

Heterozygous familial hypercholesterolemia in children 10–17 years of age.
Initial: 10 mg/day; **then** individualize dosage to a maximum of 20 mg/day. Adjust dosage at 4-week or more intervals. Individualize dosage based on recommended goal of therapy.

Prophylaxis of cardiovascular disease.
Adults: 10 mg/day.

NURSING IMPLICATIONS

IMPLEMENTATION/ADMINISTRATION/STORAGE

1. **Place client on a standard cholesterol-lowering diet before giving atorvastatin (except with CAD); continue during treatment.**

2. Give as single dose at any time of the day, with or without food.
3. Up to 10 ounces of grapefruit juice may be consumed daily if on doses of 10, 20, or 40 mg atorvastatin.
4. Determine lipid levels within 2–4 weeks; adjust dosage accordingly.
5. For additive effect, may be used in combination with a bile acid binding resin. Do not use atorvastatin with fibrates (e.g., gemfibrozil).
6. Store tablets from 20–25°C (68–77°F).

ASSESSMENT

1. Note reasons for therapy, other comorbidities, lab/cath results, onset, duration of disease, other agents/measures trialed.
2. Review dietary habits, weight, and exercise patterns; identify lifestyle changes needed.
3. Hold drug with any severe conditions (acute infection, hypotension, major surgery, trauma, and uncontrolled seizures) to ensure no acute renal failure R/T rhabdomyolysis.
4. Obtain baseline lipid profile, CPK, and LFTs. Monitor at 4 and 12 weeks after starting therapy and with any dosage change, then semiannually thereafter. If ALT or AST exceed 3 times the normal level, reduce dose or withdraw drug. Assess need for liver biopsy if elevations continue after stopping therapy.

CLIENT/FAMILY TEACHING

1. Helps to lower blood cholesterol and fat levels, which have been proven to promote CAD.
2. Take at same time each day with or without food; avoid grapefruit juice, as it causes increased drug concentrations.
3. Continue dietary restrictions of saturated fat and cholesterol and alcohol, regular exercise, and weight loss is the overall goal of lowering cholesterol levels. See dietitian for additional dietary recommendations. Read all food labels.
4. Do not add other drugs or OTC agents without provider approval. Reduce or avoid alcohol consumption due to risk of liver damage/problems.
5. Report any unexplained muscle pain, weakness, or tenderness, especially if accompanied by fever or malaise. Any new onset dark urine, fatigue, flu-like symptoms, pain under the right rib cage, persistent nausea, or yellowing of skin or eyes requires reporting; stop drug until cleared.
6. Practice reliable birth control; may cause fetal damage.
7. Report for F/U to assess response, labs, and for adverse SE.

OUTCOMES/EVALUATE

- ↓ LDL, VLDL, triglycerides, apo-B
- ↓ Total cholesterol ↑ HDL

IV

Atropine sulfate

(**AH**-troh-peen)

Classification(s): Cholinergic blocking drug

Pregnancy Category: C

RX: Atropair, AtroPen, Atropine Care, Atropine Sulfate Ophthalmic, Isopto Atropine, Sal-Tropine.

SEE ALSO ***CHOLINERGIC BLOCKING AGENTS***.

INDICATIONS/USES

PO: (1) Adjunct in peptic ulcer treatment. (2) Relieve pylorospasm, small intestine hypertonicity, and colon hypermotility. (3) Relax biliary and ureteral colic spasm and bronchial spasms. (4) Decrease tone of the detrusor muscle of the urinary bladder in treating urinary tract disorders.
(5) Preanesthetic to control salivation and bronchial secretions. (6) Control rhinorrhea of acute rhinitis or hay fever. (7) Has been used for parkinsonism but more effective drugs are available.

Parenteral: (1) Restore cardiac rate and arterial pressure during anesthesia when vagal stimulation, due to intra-abdominal surgical traction, causes a sudden decrease in pulse rate and cardiac action.
(2) Decrease degree of AV heart block when increased vagal tone is a major factor in the conduction defect (e.g., due to digitalis). (3) Overcome severe bradycardia and syncope due to hyperactive carotid sinus reflex. (4) Relax upper GI tract and colon during hypertonic radiography. (5) Antidote (with external cardiac massage) for CV collapse from toxicity due to cholinergic drugs, pilocarpine, physostigmine, or isofluorophate.
(6) Treat anticholinesterase poisoning from organophosphates; antidote for mushroom poisoning due to muscarine. (7) Poisoning by susceptible organophosphorus nerve agents having cholinesterase activity; also, poisoning due to organophosphorus or carbamate insecticides. (8) Control the crying and laughing episodes in clients with

A

brain lesions. (9) Treat closed head injuries that cause acetylcholine to be released or be present in CSF, which causes abnormal EEG patterns, stupor, and neurological symptoms. (10) Relieve hypertonicity of uterine muscle. (11) As a preanesthetic or in dentistry to decrease secretions.

Ophthalmic: Cycloplegic refraction or pupillary dilation in acute inflammatory conditions of the iris and uveal tract. *Investigational:* Treatment of uveitis in children.

ACTION/KINETICS

Action

Blocks acetylcholine effects on postganglionic cholinergic receptors in smooth muscle, cardiac muscle, exocrine glands, urinary bladder, and the AV and SA nodes in the heart. Ophthalmologically, blocks acetylcholine effects on the sphincter muscle of the iris and the accommodative muscle of the ciliary body. This results in dilation of the pupil (mydriasis) and paralysis of the muscles required to accommodate for close vision (cycloplegia).

Pharmacokinetics

Ophthalmic, peak effect: *Mydriasis,* 30–40 min; *cycloplegia,* 1–3 hr. **Ophthalmic, recovery:** *Mydriasis,* 7–10 days; *cycloplegia,* 6–12 days. **PO, duration:** 4–6 hr. **t½:** 2.5 hr. Metabolized by the liver although 30–50% is excreted through the kidneys unchanged.

ADDITIONAL CONTRAINDICATIONS

Ophthalmic use: Infants less than 3 months of age, primary glaucoma or a tendency toward glaucoma, adhesions between the iris and the lens, geriatric clients and others where undiagnosed glaucoma or excessive pressure in the eye may be present, in children who have had a previous severe systemic reaction to atropine.

SPECIAL CONCERNS

- Use with caution in infants, small children, geriatric clients, diabetes, hypo- or hyperthyroidism, narrow anterior chamber angle, individuals with Down syndrome. Excessive use in children may cause systemic toxic symptoms.
- Some ophthalmic products contain sulfites, which may cause allergic reactions, including hives, itching, wheezing, and anaphylaxis.
- Use ophthalmic products with caution during lactation.

SIDE EFFECTS

Most Common

Systemic use: Dry mouth, urinary hesitancy, headache, flushing, constipation, heartburn, N&V.

Ophthalmic use: Blurred vision, stinging, increased intraocular pressure.

See *Cholinergic Blocking Agents* for a complete list of possible side effects. **Ophthalmic:** Blurred vision, stinging, burning, increased intraocular pressure, contact dermatitis, irritation, photophobia, eczematoid dermatitis, conjunctivitis, follicular conjunctivitis, blepharoconjunctivitis, vascular congestion, exudate, hyperemia, edema, eczematoid dermatitis.

OVERDOSE MANAGEMENT

Treatment: Ocular Overdose: Eyes should be flushed with water or normal saline. A topical miotic may be necessary.

HOW SUPPLIED

Autoinjector: 0.25 mg, 0.5 mg/0.7 mL, 1 mg/0.7 mL, 2 mg/0.7 mL; ***Injection:*** 0.05 mg/mL, 0.1 mg/mL, 0.3 mg/mL, 0.4 mg/mL, 0.5 mg/mL, 0.8 mg/mL, 1 mg/mL; ***Ophthalmic Ointment:*** 1%; ***Ophthalmic Solution:*** 1%; ***Tablets:*** 0.4 mg.

DOSAGE

TABLETS

Anticholinergic or antispasmodic.

Adults: 0.4–0.6 mg q 4–6 hr. **Pediatric, over 40.8 kg (90 lbs):** same as adult; **29.5–40.8 kg (65–90 lbs):** 0.4 mg q 4–6 hr; **18.1–29.5 kg (40–65 lbs):** 0.3 mg q 4–6 hr; **10.9–18.1 kg (24–40 lbs):** 0.2 mg q 4–6 hr; **7.3–10.9 kg (16–24 lbs):** 0.15 mg q 4–6 hr; **3.2–7.3 kg (7–16 lbs):** 0.1 mg q 4–6 hr.

Prophylaxis of respiratory tract secretions and excess salivation during anesthesia.

Adults: 2 mg.

Parkinsonism.

Adults: 0.1–0.25 mg 4 times per day.

IM; IV; SC

Anticholinergic (e.g., for surgery).

Adults, IM, IV, SC: 0.4–0.6 mg (average 0.5 mg). Is used as an antisialogogue; inject IM prior to induction of anesthesia. **Children, SC:** 0.01 mg/kg,

A

not to exceed 0.4 mg (or 0.3 mg/m^2) repeated q 4–6 hr as needed. **Infants:** 0.04 mg/kg for those <5 kg or 0.03 mg/kg for those >5 kg repeated q 4–6 hr as needed.

Treatment of toxicity from cholinesterase inhibitors.

Adults, IV, initial: 2–4 mg; **then,** 2 mg repeated q 5–10 min until muscarinic symptoms disappear and signs of atropine toxicity begin to appear. **Pediatric, IM, IV, initial:** 1 mg; **then,** 0.5–1 mg q 5–10 min until muscarinic symptoms disappear and signs of atropine toxicity appear.

Treatment of mushroom poisoning due to muscarine.

Adults, IM, IV: 1–2 mg q hr until respiratory effects decrease.

Treatment of anticholinesterase poisoning.

Adults, IM, IV, Initial: >2–3 mg; repeat until signs of atropine intoxication appear. In 'rapid' type of mushroom poisoning, give sufficient doses to control parasympathomimetic signs before coma and CV collapse occur.

Bradyarrhythmias.

Adults: 0.4–1 mg IV q 1–2 hr as needed; up to a maximum of 2 mg may be needed. **Children:** 0.01–0.03 mg/kg IV.

Prophylaxis of respiratory tract secretions, excessive salivation, succinylcholine- or surgical procedure-induced arrhythmias.

Pediatric, up to 3 kg, SC: 0.1 mg; **7–9 kg:** 0.2 mg; **12–16 kg:** 0.3 mg; **20–27 kg:** 0.4 mg; **32 kg:** 0.5 mg: **41 kg:** 0.6 mg.

ATROPEN

Organophosphorus or carbamate poisoning.

Adults and children weighing more than 90 lbs (and generally over 10 years of age): 2 mg. **Children weighing 40–90 lbs (generally 4–10 years of age):** 1 mg. **Children weighing 15–40 lbs (generally 6 months-4 years of age):** 0.5 mg.

OPHTHALMIC SOLUTION

Mydriasis/cycloplegia.

Adults: 1–2 gtt of the 1% solution into the eye(s) 3 times/day or as directed by health care provider.

Uveitis in children (investigational).

Children: 1–2 gtt of the 0.5% solution into the eye(s) 1–3 times per day.

OPHTHALMIC OINTMENT

Mydriasis/cycloplegia.

Adults: Instill a small amount into the conjunctival sac once or twice a day, or as directed by health care provider.

NURSING IMPLICATIONS

IMPLEMENTATION/ADMINISTRATION/STORAGE

1. After instillation of ophthalmic ointment, compress lacrimal sac by digital pressure for 1–3 min to decrease systemic effects.
2. Have physostigmine available in the event of overdose.
3. Use the AtroPen Auto-injector as soon as symptoms of organophosphorus or carbamate poisoning appear. In moderate to severe poisoning, use of more than 1 AtroPen may be required until atropinization (e.g., flushing, mydriasis, tachycardia, dry mouth and nose) is achieved.
4. Do not use more than 3 AtroPen injections unless under supervision of trained medical provider.
5. In severe poisonings due to organophosphorus nerve agents or carbamate insecticides, it may be desirable to give an anticonvulsant (e.g., diazepam) concomitantly if seizures are suspected in an unconscious client (since classic tonic-clonic jerking may not be seen). Administration of a cholinesterase reactivator (e.g., pralidoxime chloride) may be helpful.
6. See package insert for AtroPen to determine number of AtroPen auto-injectors to use based on symptoms observed.
7. Administer AtroPen as follows:
   - Snap grooved end of the plastic sleeve down and over the yellow safety cap. Remove AtroPen from plastic sleeve. Do not put fingers on the green tip.
   - Firmly grasp AtroPen with the green tip pointed down.
   - Pull off the yellow safety cap with the other hand.
   - Aim and firmly jab the green tip straight down (a 90° angle) against the outer thigh. The AtroPen device will activate and deliver the drug. It is permissible to inject

through clothing, but be sure pockets at the injection site are empty. Very thin clients and small children should also be injected into the thigh, but before giving the injection, bunch up the thigh to provide a thicker area for injection.

- Hold auto-injector firmly in place for at least 10 sec to allow injection to finish.
- Remove AtroPen and massage injection site for several seconds. If the needle is not visible, check to be sure the yellow safety cap has been removed; repeat the preceding steps but press harder.

8. Store AtroPen auto-injector from 15–30°C (59–86°F). Do not freeze, and protect from light.
9. Store ophthalmic ointment or solution from 15–30°C (59–86°F). Use solution only if imprinted neckband is intact. Use ointment only if bottom ridge of tube cap is not exposed.
10. IV May give by direct IV undiluted or may dilute in up to 10 mL sterile water and administer at 0.6–1 mg over 1 min.
11. Do not add to any existing IV solution. May give through three-way stop cock, Y connection, or injection port.
12. Dose is dependent on condition being treated and age of recipient. See drug insert.
13. Store unopened at room temperature 15–30°C (59–86°F) in airtight, light-resistant container.
14. COMPATIBILITY Sterile water.
15. INCOMPATIBILITY Administer separately.

ASSESSMENT

1. Note reasons for therapy, onset, characteristics of S&S. Review underlying presentation/history and update regularly.
2. Check for glaucoma before ophthalmic administration; may precipitate an acute crisis.
3. Perform abdominal assessment, and monitor bowel sounds.
4. Obtain VS, I&O, and ECG; monitor CV status during IV therapy.

CLIENT/FAMILY TEACHING

1. Review indications for drug use, frequency of use, and route of administration.
2. When used in the eye, vision will be temporarily impaired. Close work, operating machinery, or driving a car should be avoided until drug effects have worn off.
3. Do not blink excessively; wait 5 min before instilling other drops. Stop eye drops, and report if eye pain, conjunctivitis, rapid pulse/palpitations, or dizziness occurs.
4. Do not touch dropper tip to any surface as this may contaminate the solution.
5. Drug impairs heat regulation; avoid strenuous activity in hot environments; wear sunglasses.
6. Males with enlarged prostate may experience urinary retention and hesitancy; void before use.
7. Increase fluids and add bulk to diet to ensure hydration and diminish constipating effects.
8. Drug inhibits salivation; use sugarless candies and gums to decrease dry mouth symptoms.
9. Use caution, may experience dizziness, confusion, or visual problems. Report all adverse side effects.
10. Ensure client understands the indications for and use of the auto-injector, including symptoms of poisoning and preparation and use of the auto-injector. Once auto-injector (AtroPen) is used outside of a medical facility, medical attention must be sought immediately.
11. Keep all F/U to assess response and for adverse SE.

OUTCOMES/EVALUATE

- ↑ HR
- Desired pupillary dilatation
- ↓ GI activity; ↓ Salivation
- Reversal of muscarinic effects of anticholinesterase agents

IV

Azacitidine

(ay-za-**SYE**-ti-deen)

Classification(s): Antineoplastic (DNA demethylation agent)

Pregnancy Category: D

RX: Vidaza.

INDICATIONS/USES

Myelodysplastic syndrome with the following subtypes: (a) refractory anemia or refractory anemia with ringed sideroblasts (if accompanied by neutropenia or thrombocytopenia or requiring transfusions), (b) refractory anemia with excess blasts, (c) refractory anemia with excess blasts in transformation, and (d) chronic myelomonocytic leukemia. *Investigational:* Refractory acute lymphocytic leukemia; refractory acute myelogenous leukemia.

ACTION/KINETICS

Action

Antineoplastic effect due to hypomethylation of DNA and by direct cytotoxicity on abnormal hematopoietic cells in the bone marrow. The cytotoxic effects cause death of rapidly dividing cells, including cancer cells that are no longer responsive to normal growth control mechanisms. Nonproliferating cells are relatively insensitive to azacitidine.

Pharmacokinetics

Rapidly absorbed after SC administration. **Peak plasma levels:** 30 min. Bioavailability is 89%. Metabolized by the liver. **t½, mean, after SC administration:** 41 min. Probably metabolized in the liver. Excreted in the urine; **elimination t½:** About 4 hr after either IV or SC use.

CONTRAINDICATIONS

Known hypersensitivity to azacitidine or mannitol. Use in advanced malignant hepatic tumors. Lactation.

SPECIAL CONCERNS

- **Use caution with dose selection in geriatric clients.**
- **Safety and efficacy have not been determined in clients with renal or hepatic impairment or in children.**

SIDE EFFECTS

Most Common

N&V, anemia, thrombocytopenia, pyrexia, leukopenia, diarrhea, fatigue, injection site erythema, constipation, neutropenia, ecchymosis. Also, hypokalemia, petechiae, rigors, weakness (after IV).
GI: N&V, diarrhea, constipation, anorexia, abdominal distension/tenderness/pain (including upper abdominal pain), gingival bleeding, oral mucosal petechiae, stomatitis, dyspepsia, hemorrhoids, loose stools, dysphagia, tongue ulceration, ***mouth hemorrhage***, diverticulitis, ***GI hemorrhage***, mouth hemorrhage, melena, perirectal abscess. **Hepatic:** Cholecystectomy, cholecystitis, ***hepaticcoma.*** **CNS:** Headache, dizziness, anxiety, decreased appetite, depression, confusion, insomnia, syncope, hypoesthesia, ***convulsions,intracranial/cerebral hemorrhage.*** **CV:** Cardiac murmur, tachycardia, hypo-/hypertension, atrial fibrillation, ***congestive cardiac failure***, ***cardiac failure***, ***CHF***, ***cardiorespiratory arrest***, ***congestive cardiomyopathy***, orthostatic hypotension. **Respiratory:** Cough, dyspnea, pharyngitis, pharyngolaryngeal pain, epistaxis, nasopharyngitis, exertional dyspnea, URTI, productive cough, lung crackles, rhinorrhea, rhinitis, rales, pneumonia, wheezing, decreased breath sounds, pleural effusion, rhonchi, postnasal drip, sinusitis, atelectasis, exacerbated dyspnea, hemoptysis, lung infiltration, nasal congestion, pneumonitis, productive cough, respiratory distress. **Dermatologic:** Erythema, pallor, skin lesion, rash, petechiae, pruritus, ecchymosis, increased sweating, night sweats, urticaria, cellulitis, skin nodule, dry skin, pyoderma gangrenosum, pruritic rash, skin induration. **Hematologic:** Anemia, neutropenia, thrombocytopenia, leukopenia, febrile neutropenia, ecchymosis, petechiae, lymphadenopathy, hematoma, postprocedural hemorrhage, aggravated anemia, agranulocytosis, bone marrow depression/failure, pancytopenia, splenomegaly. **Injection site:** Erythema, pain, bruising, injection-site reaction, hematoma, induration, rash, pruritus, swelling, granuloma, pigmentation changes, catheter site reactions (hemorrhage, infection, erythema). **Musculoskeletal:** Arthralgia, pain in limb, myalgia, muscle cramps, aggravated bone pain, muscle weakness, neck pain. **Metabolic:** Peripheral swelling/edema, decreased weight, pitting edema, hypokalemia. **GU:** Dysuria, UTI, renal failure, renal tubular acidosis, hematuria, loin pain. **Infections:** Abscess limb, bacterial infection, blastomycosis, *Klebsiella* sepsis, streptococcal pharyngitis, injection-site infection, *Klebsiella* pneumonia, ***neutropenic sepsis***, staphylococcal bacteremia/infection, ***sepsis***, ***septic shock***, toxoplasmosis. **Ophthalmic:** Eye hemorrhage. **Body as a whole:** Pyrexia, fatigue, weakness, rigors, aggravated fatigue, lethargy, malaise, weight loss, dehydration, pitting edema, peripheral edema/swelling, general physical health deterioration, systemic inflammatory response syndrome. **Miscellaneous:** Back/chest/chest wall pain, pain, herpes simplex, cellulitis, transfusion reaction, postprocedural pain, ***anaphylactic shock***, hypersensitivity, leukemia cutis.

LABORATORY TEST CONSIDERATIONS

↑ Serum creatinine, hypokalemia.

A

DRUG INTERACTIONS

Etoposide in combination with azacitidine → renal tubular acidosis

HOW SUPPLIED

Powder for Injection, Lyophilized: 100 mg.

DOSAGE

SC, IV

Myelodysplastic syndrome.

First treatment cycle: For all clients, regardless of baseline hematology values: 75 mg/m^2 SC or IV daily for 7 days. Premedicate clients for N&V.

Subsequent treatment cycles: 75 mg/m^2 every 4 weeks. The dose may be increased to 100 mg/m^2 if no beneficial effect is seen after 2 treatment cycles and if no toxicity other than N&V has occurred. Four treatment cycles are recommended. Complete or partial response may require more than 4 cycles as long as beneficial effects are observed. *NOTE:* Reduced doses may be necessary in those with impaired renal function.

NURSING IMPLICATIONS

IMPLEMENTATION/ADMINISTRATION/STORAGE

1. Premedicate for N&V.
2. Treat for a minimum of 4 cycles; however, complete or partial response may require more than 4 treatment cycles. Treatment may continue as long as client continues to benefit.
3. Take care with dosage selection in the elderly.
4. Use the following guidelines to adjust the dose based on hematology lab values. For clients with baseline (start of treatment) WBC greater than or equal to 3×10^9/L, ANC greater than or equal to 1.5×10^9/L, and platelets greater than or equal to 75×10^9/L, adjust the dose as follows, based on nadir counts, for any given cycle: (a) If ANC is less than 0.5×10^9/L and platelets are less than 25×10^9/L, give 50% of the dose in the next course; (b) if ANC is between 0.5 and 1.5×10^9/L and platelets are 25 to 50×10^9/L, give 67% of the dose in the next course; (c) if ANC is greater than 1.5×10^9/L and platelets are greater than 50×10^9/L, give 100% of the dose in the next course.
5. For clients with baseline counts of WBC less than 3×10^9/L, ANC less than 1.5×10^9/L, or platelets less than 75×10^9/L, base dosage adjustments on nadir counts and bone marrow biopsy cellularity at the time of the nadir unless there is clear improvement in differentiation at the time of the next cycle, in which case the dose of the current treatment should be continued. Check the package insert for the correct dosage adjustments.
6. If unexplained reductions in serum bicarbonate levels to <20 mEq/L occur, reduce dosage by 50% on next course.
7. If unexplained elevations of BUN or serum creatinine occur, delay next cycle until values return to normal or baseline and reduce dose by 50% on next treatment course.
8. For SC use, reconstitute aseptically with 4 mL sterile water for injection. Inject diluent slowly into vial. Vigorously shake or roll the vial until a uniform suspension occurs. Reconstituted suspension will be cloudy and will contain 25 mg/mL azacitidine.
9. Divide doses greater than 4 mL into 2 syringes. Inject into separate sites. Rotate sites for each injection (thigh, abdomen, or upper arm). Give new injections at least 1 inch from an old site and never into areas where the site is tender, bruised, red, or hard.
10. For immediate SC administration, the product may be held at room temperature for up to 1 hr but must be given within 1 hr after reconstitution. Doses greater than 4 mL should be divided equally into 2 syringes.
11. For delayed SC administration, reconstituted drug may be kept in the vial or drawn into a syringe. Doses greater than 4 mL should be divided equally into 2 syringes. Refrigerate immediately; the product may be held under refrigeration for up to 8 hr. After removal from the refrigerator, allow the suspension to equilibrate to room temperature for up to 30 min before administration.
12. To provide a homogeneous suspension, resuspend the contents by inverting the syringe 2 to 3 times and gently rolling the syringe between the palms for 30 sec immediately prior to administration.

13. Rotate SC sites for each injection (thigh, abdomen, upper arm). Give new injections at least 1 inch from an old site and never into areas where the site is tender, bruised, red, or hard.
14. Azacitidine is a cytotoxic drug; exercise caution when handling and preparing azacitidine. If reconstituted drug comes into contact with the skin, wash with soap and water immediately and thoroughly. If the drug comes into contact with mucous membranes, flush thoroughly with water.
15. IV For IV administration, reconstitute the appropriate number of vials to achieve the desired dose. Reconstitute each vial with 10 mL of sterile water for injection. Shake or roll the vial vigorously until all solids are dissolved. The concentration of the resulting solution will be 10 mg/mL.
16. The solution should be clear. Inspect visually for particulate matter and discoloration before administration.
17. Withdraw the required amount of solution to deliver the correct dose, and inject into a 50 to 100 mL infusion bag of either sodium chloride 0.9% NaCl or Ringer's lactate injection.
18. Administer the total IV dose over 10–40 min. Administration must be complete within 1 hr of reconstitution.
19. Store unreconstituted vials from 15–30°C (59–86°F). The reconstituted product may be held at room temperature for up to 1 hr but must be administered within 1 hr after reconstitution.
20. Discard unused portions of each vial properly. Do not save any unused drug for later use.
21. COMPATIBILITY 0.9% NaCl; Ringer's lactate.
22. INCOMPATIBILITY D5W solutions, hetastarch 6% in sodium chloride 0.9% injection, or solutions that contain bicarbonate. These solutions increase the degradation rate of azacitidine.

ASSESSMENT

1. Note disease onset, subtype, other agents trialed and outcome.
2. Do not use in those with hypersensitivity to azacitidine or mannitol or with advanced malignant hepatic tumors.
3. Review and follow administration guidelines carefully.
4. Monitor renal function closely, especially in the elderly. Renal tubular acidosis (serum bicarbonate <20 mEq/L) in association with alkaline urine and hypokalemia (K^+ <3 mEq/L) may be fatal. Report any changes in renal function, delay next cycle until values return to normal or baseline, and reduce dose 50% on the next treatment course; excreted primarily by the kidneys.
5. Obtain baseline CBC, renal and LFTs; monitor prior to each cycle. Review drug literature for dosage adjustments (delay or reduction of dose), based on hematologic response calculated on nadir counts (ANC, platelets), and bone marrow biopsy cellularity at time of nadir.

CLIENT/FAMILY TEACHING

1. Used to treat resistant types of leukemia; usually administered subcutaneously, once a day for 7 days and repeated every 4 weeks as long as benefit evident.
2. Drug therapy can be very toxic, so blood tests must be performed before and after each treatment cycle and therapy adjusted or discontinued based on these lab results.
3. May cause dizziness, fainting, or lightheadedness; avoid activities that require mental alertness until drug effects realized.
4. Males and females should both practice reliable contraception; drug may cause fetal harm. Men should not father a child while taking azacitidine.
5. Identify candidates for egg or sperm harvesting; drug may cause infertility.
6. Report changes in urine output/color, skin or stool color changes, fever, sore throat, severe muscle aches, abnormal bruising/bleeding or any other adverse effects.
7. Keep all F/U to assess response, labs, and for adverse SE.

OUTCOMES/EVALUATE

Improved hematologic parameters; inhibition of malignant cell proliferation

IV

Azathioprine

(ay-zah-**THIGH**-oh-preen)

Classification(s): Immunosuppressant

Pregnancy Category: D

A

RX: Azasan, Imuran.

Rx: Apo-Azathioprine, Gen-Azathioprine, ratio-Azathioprine.

INDICATIONS/USES

(1) As an adjunct to prevent rejection in renal homotransplantation. (2) In adult clients meeting criteria for classic or definite rheumatoid arthritis as defined by the American Rheumatism Association. Restrict use to clients with severe, active, and erosive disease that is not responsive to conventional therapy. *Investigational:* Chronic ulcerative colitis, generalized myasthenia gravis, to control the progression of Behçet's syndrome (especially eye disease), Crohn's disease (low doses).

ACTION/KINETICS

Action

Antimetabolite that is quickly split to form mercaptopurine. To be effective, must be given during the induction period of the antibody response. The precise mechanism in depressing the immune response is unknown, but it suppresses cell-mediated hypersensitivities and alters antibody production. Inhibits synthesis of DNA, RNA, and proteins and may interfere with meiosis and cellular metabolism. The mechanism for its effect on autoimmune diseases is not known. The anuric client manifests increased effectiveness and toxicity (up to twofold).

Pharmacokinetics

Readily absorbed from the GI tract. **Onset:** 6–8 weeks for rheumatoid arthritis. **t½:** 3 hr.

CONTRAINDICATIONS

Treatment of rheumatoid arthritis in pregnancy or in clients previously treated with alkylating agents. Pregnancy and lactation.

SPECIAL CONCERNS

Chronic immunosuppression with azathioprine increases the risk of neoplasia. Physicians using this drug should be familiar with this risk as well as with the mutagenic potential to both men and women and with possible hematologic toxicities.

- **Hematologic toxicity is dose-related and may occur late in the course of therapy; may be more severe in renal transplant clients undergoing rejection.**
- **Although used in children, safety and efficacy not established.**

SIDE EFFECTS

Most Common

GI toxicity (severe N&V, diarrhea), fever, rash, malaise, myalgias, leukopenia.

Hematologic: Leukopenia, thrombocytopenia, macrocytic anemia, ***severe bone marrow depression***, selective erythrocyte aplasia. **GI:** N&V, diarrhea, abdominal pain, steatorrhea. **CNS:** Fever, malaise. **Miscellaneous:** ***Increased risk of carcinoma***, severe infections (fungal, viral, bacterial, and protozoal), and ***hepatotoxicity*** are major side effects. Also, skin rashes, alopecia, myalgias, increase in liver enzymes, hypotension, negative nitrogen balance.

OVERDOSE MANAGEMENT

Symptoms: Large doses may result in ***bone marrow hypoplasia***, bleeding, infection, and death. *Treatment:* Approximately 45% can be removed from the body following 8 hr of hemodialysis.

DRUG INTERACTIONS

ACE inhibitors / ↑ Risk of severe leukopenia
Allopurinol / ↑ Azathioprine effects R/T ↓ liver breakdown
Anticoagulants / ↓ Anticoagulant effect
Balsalazide / ↑ Rate of leukopenia in Crohn's disease clients R/T inhibition of thiopurine-metabolizing enzyme
Corticosteroids / Possible muscle wasting after prolonged therapy
Cyclosporine / ↑ Plasma cyclosporine levels
H ***Echinacea*** / Do not give with azathioprine
Mercaptopurine / Possibility of profound myelosuppression and severe sepsis; do not use together
Mesalamine / ↑ Rate of leukopenia in Crohn's disease clients R/T inhibition of thiopurine-metabolizing enzyme
Methotrexate / ↑ Plasma levels of the active metabolite, 6-mercaptopurine
Sulfasalazine / ↑ Rate of leukopenia in Crohn's disease clients R/T inhibition of thiopurine-metabolizing enzyme
Tubocurarine / ↓ Tubocurarine (and other nondepolarizing neuromuscular blocking agents) effects

HOW SUPPLIED

Powder for Injection: 100 mg (as sodium); ***Tablets:*** 25 mg, 50 mg, 75 mg, 100 mg.

A

DOSAGE

IV; TABLETS

Use in renal homotransplantation.

Adults and children, initial: 3–5 mg/kg (120 mg/m^2), 1–3 days before or on the day of transplantation; **maintenance:** 1–3 mg/kg (45 mg/m^2) daily.

Rheumatoid arthritis.

Adults and children, tablets, initial: 1 mg/kg (50–100 mg); **then,** increase dose by 0.5 mg/kg/day after 6–8 weeks and thereafter q 4 weeks, up to maximum of 2.5 mg/kg/day; **maintenance:** lowest effective dose. Dosage should be reduced in clients with renal dysfunction.

Myasthenia gravis.

2–3 mg/kg/day. However, side effects occur in more than 35% of clients.

To control progression of Behçet's syndrome.

2.5 mg/kg/day.

Crohn's disease.

75–100 mg/day.

NURSING IMPLICATIONS

Do not confuse Imuran with Imdur (an antianginal drug).

IMPLEMENTATION/ADMINISTRATION/STORAGE

1. For rheumatoid arthritis, a therapeutic response may not be observed for 6–8 weeks.
2. May be discontinued abruptly, but delayed effects are possible.
3. When used with allopurinol, reduce dose of azathioprine by 25–33% of the usual dose.
4. IV Reconstitute drug (100 mg) with 10 mL of sterile water for injection and use within 24 hr. Infusion time ranges from 5 min to 8 hr.
5. COMPATIBILITY Sterile saline or dextrose.
6. INCOMPATIBILITY Administer separately.

ASSESSMENT

1. Note reasons for therapy; include preassessment data. Check for drug interactions.
2. With RA assess joint for functional level: ROM, swelling, erythema, temperature, stiffness, and active synovitis.
3. With transplant procedures, protect from visitors or staff who may carry infectious organisms. Assess for and aggressively treat fungal, viral, bacterial, and protozoal infections–may be fatal.
4. Assess I&O and weigh daily. Report decreases in urine volume, C_{CR}, oliguria or symptoms of kidney transplant rejection.
5. Review increased risk of neoplasia following therapy with azathioprine.
6. May check TPMT level (one person in every 300 lacks TPMT). TPMT is an enzyme that helps remove thiopurine drugs, such as azathioprine, from the body when they are present above therapeutic levels. Individuals with no TPMT enzyme can become severely ill if treated with normal doses of thiopurine drugs, because toxic levels of the drug accumulate.
7. Monitor CBC (weekly during the first month, twice monthly for the second and third months of treatment, then monthly), uric acid, renal and LFTs. Observe for S&S bleeding abnormalities or hepatic dysfunction. Stop drug/report if jaundiced or abnormal LFTs.

CLIENT/FAMILY TEACHING

1. If GI upset occurs, give in divided doses or take with food.
2. Take only as directed, and do not skip or stop drug without approval; increase fluid intake.
3. Practice reliable contraception during and for 4 months following therapy.
4. Report bruising, bleeding, S&S of infection, fever, rash, abdominal pain, yellow eyes or skin, itching, and/or clay-colored stools.
5. Must take this medication for life to prevent transplant rejection.
6. Avoid crowds or contact with anyone who has taken oral poliovirus vaccine recently or persons with active infections.
7. When used for RA, improvement in joint pain, swelling, and stiffness may take 6–12 weeks. Continue other medications and therapies as prescribed for symptom control. Should be considered refractory if no beneficial effect is noted after 12 weeks.
8. Report any S&S of transplant rejection (e.g., localized redness, tenderness and swelling in the area of the transplant, decreased transplant organ function).

A

9. Practice reliable contraception during and for four months following therapy to prevent adverse fetal effects.
10. Keep all F/U to assess response, labs and for adverse SE.

OUTCOMES/EVALUATE

- Prevention of organ transplant rejection
- Suppression of cell-mediated immunity
- With RA ↓ joint pain and inflammation with improved mobility

Azilsartan medoxomil

(ay-zil-**SAR**-tan me-**DOX**-oh-mil)

Classification(s): Angiotensin II receptor antagonist

Pregnancy Category: D

RX: Edarbi.

SEE ALSO ***ANGIOTENSIN II RECEPTOR BLOCKING AGENTS.***

INDICATIONS/USES

Hypertension alone or in combination with other antihypertensive drugs.

ACTION/KINETICS

Action

Azilsartan is a selective AT_1 subtype angiotensin II receptor antagonist. Angiotensin II, formed from angiotensin I, is the primary pressor agent of the renin-angiotensin system. Azilsartan blocks the vasoconstrictor and aldosterone-secreting effects of angiotensin II by selectively blocking the binding of angiotensin II to the AT_1 receptor in various tissues, including vascular smooth muscle and the adrenal gland.

Pharmacokinetics

Azilsartan medoxomil is a prodrug that is hydrolyzed to the active azilsartan in the GI tract during absorption. Absolute bioavailability is about 60%. **Peak plasma levels:** 1.5–3 hr. Food does not affect bioavailability. Steady-state achieved within 5 days. Azilsartan is metabolized to two primary inactive compounds by CYP2C9. About 55% excreted in the feces and 42% in the urine. **t½, elimination:** 11 hr. **Plasma protein binding:** >99%.

CONTRAINDICATIONS

Lactation.

SPECIAL CONCERNS

■ Avoid use in pregnancy. When pregnancy is detected, discontinue azilsartan as soon as possible. Drugs that act directly on the renin-angiotensin system can cause injury and death to the developing fetus. ■

- Abnormally high serum creatinine values are more likely to be reported for clients age 75 and older.
- Safety and efficacy not determined in children less than 18 years of age.

SIDE EFFECTS

Most Common

Diarrhea, excessive hypotension.

GI: Diarrhea, nausea. **CV:** Excessive hypotension (especially in those with an activated renin-angiotensin system), orthostatic hypotension. **CNS:** Dizziness, postural dizziness. **Musculoskeletal:** Muscle spasms. **Respiratory:** Cough. **Body as a whole:** Asthenia, fatigue.

LABORATORY TEST CONSIDERATIONS

Reversible ↑ serum creatinine (increase larger when given with chlorthalidone or hydrochlorothiazide). ↓ Hemoglobin, hematocrit, RBCs. ↓ Platelet and WBCs (infrequent).

OVERDOSE MANAGEMENT

Treatment: Supportive therapy dictated by client's clinical status. Azilsartan is not dialyzable.

DRUG INTERACTIONS

Antihypertensive effects of azilsartan may be ↑ by NSAIDs, including selective COX-2 inhibitors.

HOW SUPPLIED

Tablets: 40 mg, 80 mg.

DOSAGE

TABLETS

Hypertension.

Adults, usual: 80 mg once a day. If BP is not controlled with azilsartan alone, additional BP reduction can be achieved by adding other antihypertensive drugs. *NOTE:* Consider a starting dose of azilsartan of 40 mg in those taking high doses of diuretics.

NURSING IMPLICATIONS

IMPLEMENTATION/ADMINISTRATION/STORAGE

1. Correct volume or salt depletion before giving azilsartan medoxomil.
2. No initial dose adjustment is recommended for the elderly, in those with mild-to-severe renal impairment, end-stage renal disease, or mild-to-moderate hepatic dysfunction (not studied in those with severe hepatic impairment).
3. Store from 15–30°C (59–86°F). Protect from moisture and light. Dispense and store in the original container.

ASSESSMENT

1. Note disease onset, reasons for therapy, characteristics of S&S, risk factors, all medical conditions, other agents trialed, outcome. List drugs prescribed to ensure none interact.
2. Ensure client is well hydrated.
3. Assess renal function in severe heart failure, renal artery stenosis, or volume depletion to prevent progression of renal dysfunction.
4. Monitor BP and electrolytes; ensure females of child bearing age are not pregnant.

CLIENT/FAMILY TEACHING

1. May take with or without food. Continue all other prescribed BP medications.
2. Change positions slowly and avoid dehydration to prevent sudden drop in BP and dizziness. Consume plenty of fluids to ensure adequate hydration. May experience low BP with severe salt or volume depletion.
3. Practice reliable contraception; report if pregnancy suspected as drug may cause fetal death.
4. Continue low-fat, low-sodium diet, regular exercise, weight loss, smoking and alcohol cessation, and stress weight reduction to regain BP control.
5. Report any unusual side effects or swelling of face, lips, or tongue.
6. Keep all F/U to assess response, review log of BP readings, and for adverse SE.

OUTCOMES/EVALUATE

Control of hypertension

IV

Azithromycin

(ah-**zith**-roh-**MY**-sin)

Classification(s): Antibiotic, macrolide

Pregnancy Category: B

RX: AzaSite Ophthalmic Solution, Azithromycin 3-Day Dose Pack, Azithromycin 5-Day Dose Pack, Zithromax, Zithromax Tri-Pak, Zithromax Z-Pak, Zmax.

🍁 **Rx:** CO Azithromycin, Z-Pak.

SEE ALSO ***ANTI-INFECTIVE DRUGS***.

INDICATIONS/USES

Adults, Oral:

1. Acute bacterial sinusitis due to *Haemophilus influenzae, Moraxella catarrhalis,* or *Streptococcus pneumoniae.*
2. Acute bacterial exacerbations of COPD due to *H. influenzae, M. catarrhalis,* or *S. pneumoniae.*
3. Community-acquired pneumonia (CAP) of mild severity due to *H. influenzae, Chlamydia pneumoniae, Mycoplasma pneumoniae,* or *S. pneumoniae.*
4. In men with genital ulcer disease due to *Haemophilus ducreyi* (chancroid). The efficacy in women has not been established.
5. As an alternative to first-line therapy for pharyngitis/tonsillitis due to *Streptococcus pyogenes* in those who cannot use first-line therapy.
6. Alone or with rifabutin to prevent disseminated *Mycobacterium avium* complex (MAC) disease in those with advanced HIV infection.
7. In combination with ethambutol to treat disseminated MAC infections in those with advanced HIV infection.
8. Treatment of uncomplicated skin/skin structure infections due to *Staphyloccus aureus, S. pyogenes,* or *Streptococcus agalactiae.* Abscesses usually require surgical draining.
9. Treatment of urethritis/cervicitis due to *Chlamydia trachomatis* or *Neisseria gonorrhoeae.* Azithromycin should not be relied on to treat gonorrhea or syphilis at the recommended dose.

NOTE: Zmax is approved only for the treatment of acute bacterial sinusitis and CAP.

Adults, IV:

1. Required initial IV therapy in CAP due to *S. pneumoniae, C. pneumoniae, Mycoplasma pneumoniae, S. pneumoniae, H. influenzae, M. catarrhalis, Legionella pneumophila,* and *Staphylococcus aureus.*

A

2. Initial IV therapy in pelvic inflammatory disease (PID) due to *C. trachomatis, N. gonorrhoeae,* or *Mycoplasma hominis.* If anaerobic organisms are suspected of contributing to the infection, an antimicrobial with anaerobic activity may be added to the regimen. Follow IV therapy with the PO route as needed.

Children, Oral:

1. Acute otitis media due to *H. influenzae, M. catarrhalis,* or *S. pneumoniae* in children over 6 months of age.
2. Acute bacterial sinusitis in children 6 months and older due to *H. influenzae, M. catarrhalis,* or *S. pneumoniae.*
3. CAP due to *C. pneumoniae, H. influenzae, M. pneumoniae,* or *S. pneumoniae* in children over 6 months of age who can take PO therapy. Do not use in children with pneumonia who are judged to be inappropriate for PO therapy.
4. Pharyngitis/tonsillitis due to *S. pyogenes* in children over 2 years of age who cannot use first-line therapy. Penicillin IM is the usual drug of choice to treat *S. pyogenes* infections and for prophylaxis of rheumatic fever. Azithromycin is often effective to eradicate susceptible strains of *S. pyogenes* from the nasopharynx; perform susceptibility tests when clients are treated with azithromycin.

Ophthalmic: Bacterial conjunctivitis due to coryneform group G, *H. influenzae, S. aureus, Streptococcus mitis* group, and *S. pneumoniae.*

Investigational:

1. Treatment of cholera in adults.
2. In combination with atovaquone to treat babesiosis.
3. Chlamydial infections due to *C. trachomatis.*
4. In children 45 kg or more who have chlamydial infections but are younger than 8 years of age. Also used in children 8 years of age and older.
5. Second-line therapy for early Lyme disease in those intolerant of or who should not take first-line therapy (e.g., amoxicillin, cefuroxime axetil, or doxycycline).
6. Granuloma inguinale due to *Klebsiella granulomatis.*
7. Prophylaxis after a sexual assault.

ACTION/KINETICS

Action

A macrolide antibiotic derived from erythromycin. Acts by binding to the P site of the 50S ribosomal subunit and may inhibit RNA-dependent protein synthesis by stimulating the dissociation of peptidyl t-RNA from ribosomes.

Pharmacokinetics

Rapidly absorbed and distributed widely throughout the body. Food increases the absorption of azithromycin. **Time to reach maximum concentration:** 2–2.5 hr (about 5 hr for ER PO suspension). **C_{max}:** 0.5 mcg/mL after a single 500 mg dose. **t½, terminal elimination:** 68 hr. A loading dose will achieve steady-state levels more quickly. Mainly excreted unchanged through the bile with a small amount (about 6%) excreted unchanged in the urine. The ophthalmic solution is formulated in a system that enhances retention time of the drug on the surface of the eye, allowing for administration of fewer drops for effective treatment. **Plasma protein binding:** 51% at 0.02 mcg/mL.

CONTRAINDICATIONS

Hypersensitivity to azithromycin, any macrolide antibiotic, erythromycin, or a ketolide antibiotic (e.g., telithromycin). In clients who are not eligible for outpatient PO therapy (e.g., known or suspected bacteremia, immunodeficiency, functional asplenia, nosocomially acquired infections, geriatric or debilitated clients). Use with pimozide. IV use in children less than 16 years of age.

SPECIAL CONCERNS

- **Use with caution in clients with impaired hepatic or renal function and during lactation.**
- **Possible cardiac arrhythmias and torsades de pointes development if used in those at increased risk for prolonged cardiac repolarization.**
- **May aggravate the weakness due to myasthenia gravis.**
- **Local IV site reactions have been reported with IV administration.**
- **An additive effect with other drugs that prolong the QT interval cannot be excluded.**
- **Safety and efficacy in children less than 6 months of age not determined for acute otitis media, acute bacterial sinusitis, or CAP or for pharyngitis/tonsillitis in children less than 2 years of age. Safety and efficacy not determined**

of IV azithromycin in children or adolescents less than 16 years of age. Safety and efficacy of extended-release PO suspension not determined in children less than 6 months of age for CAP or in children of any age for acute bacterial sinusitis. Azithromycin PO suspension, 1 gram single dose, not approved for children.

SIDE EFFECTS

Most Common

Adults: Abdominal pain/discomfort, diarrhea/loose stools, N&V, application site reaction, local inflammation, pain at injection site, pruritus, rash, vaginitis.

Children: Abdominal pain/discomfort, diarrhea/loose stools, N&V, rash.

Adults. GI: N&V, diarrhea/loose stools, abdominal pain/discomfort, abnormal taste, taste perversion, anorexia, stomatitis, constipation, dyspepsia, flatulence, gastritis, melena, mucositis, oral moniliasis, ***pancreatitis***, pseudomembranous colitis. **Hepatic:** Cholestatic jaundice, impaired hepatic function, hepatitis symptoms. **CNS:** Headache, asthenia, dizziness, fatigue, malaise, nervousness, somnolence, vertigo, agitation, ***seizures***. **CV:** Chest pain, palpitations, QT prolongation, ***torsades de pointes***, ventricular tachycardia. **Dermatologic:** Pruritus, rash, urticaria. **GU:** Vaginitis, interstitial nephritis, monilia. **Hypersensitivity:** Angioedema, bronchospasm, photosensitivity, ***anaphylaxis***, erythema multiforme, skin reactions, allergic reactions, ***Stevens-Johnson syndrome*** (rare), ***toxic epidermal necrolysis*** (rare). **Hematologic:** Leukopenia, neutropenia. **Injection-site reactions:** Pain at injection site, local inflammation, application site reaction. **Miscellaneous:** Hearing loss, bronchospasm.

Children. GI: Diarrhea/loose stools, abdominal pain/discomfort, N&V, abnormal taste, anorexia, constipation, dyspepsia, enteritis, flatulence, gastritis, oral moniliasis, ***pancreatitis***, pseudomembranous colitis. **Hepatic:** Cholestatic jaundice, impaired hepatic function, hepatic symptoms, jaundice. **CNS:** Headache, agitation, asthenia, dizziness, fatigue, hyperkinesia, insomnia, malaise, nervousness, somnolence, vertigo, ***seizures***. **CV:** Chest pain, QT prolongation, ***torsade de pointes***, ventricular tachycardia. **Dermatologic:** Rash, eczema, fungal dermatitis, pruritus, sweating, urticaria, vesiculobullous rash. **GU:** Interstitial nephritis, vaginitis. **Respiratory:** Increased cough, pharyngitis, pleural effusions, rhinitis. **Hypersensitivity:** ***Anaphylaxis***, angioedema, erythema multiforme, skin reactions, allergic reactions, ***Stevens-Johnson syndrome*** (rare), ***toxic epidermal necrolysis*** (rare). **Hematologic:** Anemia, leukopenia. **Miscellaneous:** Conjunctivitis, facial edema, fever, fungal infection, hearing loss, pain.

Postmarketing. GI: Oral candidiasis, tongue discoloration (rare). **Hepatic:** Cholestatic jaundice, ***hepatic necrosis*** (rare), ***hepatic failure***. **CNS:** Aggressive reaction, anxiety, hyperactivity, paresthesia, syncope. **CV:** Arrhythmias, hypotension, syncope. **GU:** Acute renal failure. **Hematologic:** Thrombocytopenia. **Otic:** Hearing disturbances, including deafness and/or tinnitus. **Miscellaneous:** Taste loss and smell perversion and/or loss (rare), arthralgia, edema.

LABORATORY TEST CONSIDERATIONS

↑ Alkaline phosphatase, ALT, AST, basophils, bilirubin, BUN, eosinophils, GGT, LDH, lymphocytes, monocytes, neutrophils, phosphate, serum CPK, serum creatinine. ↓ Bicarbonate, blood glucose, hematocrit, hemoglobin, lymphocytes, neutrophils. ↑ or ↓ Platelet count, potassium.

OVERDOSE MANAGEMENT

Symptoms: Abdominal pain, diarrhea, N&V, reversible hearing loss. *Treatment:* Supportive measures. Hemodialysis and peritoneal dialysis are not very effective.

DRUG INTERACTIONS

Al- and Mg-containing antacids / ↓ Azithromycin absorption; do not use simultaneously

Amiodarone / Possible additive or synergistic increase in QTc interval → life-threatening cardiac arrhythmias, including torsades de pointes

Benzodiazepines (e.g., alprazolam, diazepam, midazolam, triazolam) / Possible ↓ metabolism of certain benzodiazepines → ↑ CNS depression and prolonged sedation

Bretylium / Possible additive or synergistic increase in QTc interval → life-threatening cardiac arrhythmias, including torsades de pointes

Cyclosporine / ↑ Serum cyclosporine levels R/T ↓ metabolism → ↑ risk of nephrotoxicity and neurotoxicity

Digoxin / Possible ↑ digoxin levels → toxicity (may persist for several weeks); monitor digoxin levels and adjust dose if needed

A

Disopyramide / Possible additive or synergistic increase in QTc interval → life-threatening cardiac arrhythmias, including torsades de pointes
Dofetilide / Possible additive or synergistic increase in QTc interval → life-threatening cardiac arrhythmias, including torsades de pointes
Ergot derivatives (e.g., dihydroergotamine, ergotamine) / Possible acute ergotism (e.g., peripheral ischemia)
HMG-CoA reductase inhibitors / ↑ HMG-CoA reductase levels → ↑ risk of severe myopathy/rhabdomyolysis
Levofloxacin / Possible prolongation in QTc interval → life-threatening cardiac arrhythmias, including torsades de pointes; do not use together
Moxifloxacin / Possible prolongation in QTc interval → life-threatening cardiac arrhythmias, including torsades de pointes; use together with caution
Phenytoin / ↑ Serum phenytoin levels R/T ↓ metabolism
Pimozide / ↑ Pimozide plasma levels → cardiotoxicity; do not use together
Procainamide / Possible additive or synergistic increase in QTc interval → life-threatening cardiac arrhythmias, including torsades de pointes
Quinidine / Possible additive or synergistic increase in QTc interval → life-threatening cardiac arrhythmias, including torsades de pointes
Ranolazine / ↑ Ranolazine plasma levels → cardiotoxicity; do not use together
Sotalol / Possible additive or synergistic increase in QTc interval → life-threatening cardiac arrhythmias, including torsades de pointes
Sparfloxacin / Possible prolongation in QTc interval → life-threatening cardiac arrhythmias, including torsades de pointes; do not use together
Theophyllines (e.g., aminophylline, theophylline) / Possible ↑ theophylline levels → toxicity; monitor theophylline levels
Valproic acid / Possible ↑ valproic acid serum levels → toxicity
Warfarin / ↑ Anticoagulant effect → possible hemorrhage; monitor and adjust warfarin dose if necessary

HOW SUPPLIED

Ophthalmic Solution: 1%; ***Powder for Injection, Lyophilized:*** 500 mg in 10 mL vials; ***Powder for Oral Suspension:*** 100 mg/5 mL (when reconstituted), 167 mg/5 mL (extended-release microspheres), 200 mg/5 mL (when reconstituted), 1 gram/packet; ***Tablets:*** 250 mg, 500 mg, 600 mg; ***Tri-Pak:*** 3–500 mg tablets; ***Z-Pak:*** 6–250 mg tablets.

DOSAGE

ORAL SUSPENSION; TABLETS

Acute bacterial sinusitis.

Adults: 500 mg once daily for 3 days or a single 2-gram dose of Zmax.

Mild to moderate acute bacterial exacerbations of COPD.

Adults: 500 mg/day for 3 days or 500 mg as a single dose on the first day followed by 250 mg once a day on days 2 through 5.

Mild CAP, second-line therapy for pharyngitis/tonsillitis; uncomplicated skin and skin structure infections.

Adults and children over 16 years of age: 500 mg as a single dose on day 1 followed by 250 mg once daily on days 2–5 for a total dose of 1.5 grams. For CAP, a single 2-gram dose of Zmax may be given.

Genital ulcer disease (chancroid) in men.

A single 1-gram dose.

Prevention of disseminated MAC infections.

1,200 mg once weekly; may be combined with rifabutin.

Treatment of disseminated MAC infections.

600 mg/day in combination with ethambutol, 15 mg/kg. Other effective antibacterial drugs may be added to the regimen.

Nongonococcal urethritis and cervicitis due to C. trachomatis *or genital ulcer disease due to* H. ducreyi.

1 gram given as a single dose.

Gonococcal urethritis/cervicitis due to N. gonorrhoeae.

2 grams given as a single dose.

Chlamydial infections caused by C. trachomatis.

1 gram given as a single dose.

Granuloma inguinale due to K. granulomatis.

1 gram PO once a week for at least 3 weeks and until all lesions have healed completely.

A

ORAL SUSPENSION

Acute otitis media in children 6 months and older.

Children, 6 months and older: 30 mg/kg given as a single dose or 10 mg/kg once daily for 3 days. Or, 10 mg/kg as a single dose on the first day, followed by 5 mg/kg on days 2–5.

Acute bacterial sinusitis in children 6 months and older.

10 mg/kg once daily for 3 days.

CAP in children 6 months and older.

10 mg/kg as a single dose on the first day followed by 5 mg/kg on days 2–5.

Pharyngitis/tonsillitis in children.

Children: 12 mg/kg once daily for 5 days, not to exceed 500 mg/day.

Chlamydial infections in children caused by C. *trachomatis.*

Children 45 kg or more and less than 8 years of age; or over 8 years of age: 1 gram given as a single dose.

IV

CAP.

Adults: 500 mg IV as a single daily dose for at least 2 days followed by a single daily dose of 500 mg PO to complete a 7- to 10-day course of therapy. Switching to PO therapy is at the discretion of the provider and according to clinical response.

Pelvic inflammatory disease.

Adults: 500 mg IV as a single daily dose for 1 or 2 days followed by a single daily dose of 250 mg PO to complete a 7-day course of therapy. Switching to PO therapy is at the discretion of the provider and according to clinical response.

OPHTHALMIC SOLUTION

Bacterial conjunctivitis.

Initial: 1 drop in the affected eye(s) 2 times per day, 8–12 hr apart for the first 2 days; **then** 1 drop in the affected eye(s) once daily for the next 5 days.

NURSING IMPLICATIONS

Do not confuse azithromycin with erythromycin (both antibiotics).

IMPLEMENTATION/ADMINISTRATION/STORAGE

1. Tablets and oral suspension can be taken with or without food; however, there is increased tolerability when tablets are taken with food (can be taken with milk). Zmax should be taken at least 1 hr prior to or 2 hr after a meal.
2. The safety of redosing azithromycin in children who vomit after a 30 mg/kg as a single dose has not been determined.
3. If a client vomits within 5 minutes after dosing with Zmax, consider additional antibiotic treatment since there will be minimal absorption. If a client vomits between 5 and 60 min after dosing, consider alternative therapy.
4. To prepare the single 1-gram packet, thoroughly mix the entire contents of the packet with about 60 mL of water. Drink the entire contents immediately; add an additional 60 mL of water, mix, and drink to ensure complete consumption of dosage. The packet is not for pediatric use.
5. To prepare the 2-gram dose bottle, reconstitute with 60 mL water. Shake well before dispensing. Consume the suspension within 12 hr.
6. **IV** Prepare the initial solution by adding 4.8 mL sterile water for injection to the 500 mg vial; shake the vial until all of the drug is dissolved. It is recommended that a standard 5 mL (nonautomated) syringe be used to ensure the exact amount of 4.8 mL is delivered. Each mL of reconstituted solution contains 100 mg azithromycin. To obtain a concentration range of 1–2 mg/mL, transfer 5 mL of the 100 mg/mL solution to any of the compatible solutions.
7. Infuse IV at a rate of 1 mg/mL over 3 hr or 2 mg/mL over 1 hr; do not give as a bolus or IM.
8. Reconstituted solution for injection is stable for 24 hr if stored below 30°C (86°F) or for 7 days refrigerated at 5°C (41°F).
9. Store unopened bottle of ophthalmic solution from 2–8°C (36–46°F). Once bottle is opened, store from 2–25°C (36–77°F) for up to 14 days; discard after 14 days.
10. COMPATIBILITY 0.9% or 0.45% NaCl, D5W, RL solution, D5/0.45% NaCl with 20 mEq KCl, D5/RL solution, D5/0.3% NaCl, D5/0.45% NaCl, Normosol-M in D5%, or Normosol-R in D5%.

11. INCOMPATIBILITY Do not add other IV substances, additive, or drugs to azithromycin injection or infuse simultaneously through the same IV line.

ASSESSMENT

1. Note history of sensitivity to erythromycins (derivative of this drug) and any previous therapy.
2. List reasons for therapy, onset/characteristics of symptoms, culture results, other agents/remedies trialed.
3. Assess for prolonged QT interval; note ECG, and culture results.
4. List drugs prescribed; may cause an increase in concentrations of certain drugs (digoxin, carbamazepine, cyclosporine, Dilantin).
5. Assess for skin rash during therapy; stop therapy and report to prevent development of severe skin disorder.
6. Test those sexually active for gonorrhea and syphilis at time of diagnosis. Ensure appropriate drug therapy instituted if necessary.
7. Obtain CBC, liver/renal function studies and cultures when warranted.

CLIENT/FAMILY TEACHING

1. Tablets may be taken with food or milk to improve tolerability. Take with a full glass of water 1 hr before or 2–3 hr after a meal. (Food decreases absorption).
2. With suspension, shake well and use dosing spoon, dosing syringe, or medicine cup to ensure correct dose. The 1 g packets can be taken with or without food after constitution.
3. Finish all medication prescribed unless otherwise directed.
4. May cause drowsiness or dizziness; use caution.
5. Avoid ingesting Al- or Mg-containing antacids simultaneously with azithromycin. Take 2 hr before or after.
6. Notify provider if N&V or diarrhea is excessive or debilitating. Report lack of response/unusual side effects if skin rash, hives, itching, or shortness of breath occur.
7. With eye drops, wash hands, do not allow dropper to touch eye. Tilt head back looking up, pull lower eyelid down, and instill prescribed number of drops. Close eye for 1–2 min, apply gentle pressure to bridge of nose for 1–3 min. Do not rub eye or touch top of dropper bottle to eye, fingers, or other surface. If more than 1 topical eye drug is used, give at least 5 min apart administering the ointment last. May experience temporary stinging or burning; report if bothersome or if eye/eyelid inflammation noted. If wearing contact lens, remove before instilling eye drops; may be reinserted 15 min after drug therapy.
8. Avoid sun exposure, and use protection when outside.
9. With STDs, encourage sexual partner to seek medical evaluation and testing/treatment to prevent reinfections. Use condoms during intercourse throughout therapy.
10. Keep all F/U visits to assess response, labs, and adverse SE.

OUTCOMES/EVALUATE

- Resolution of S&S of infection
- Negative cultures

B

Bacitracin intramuscular

(bass-ih-**TRAY**-sin)

Classification(s): Antibiotic, miscellaneous

Pregnancy Category: C

RX: Baci-IM.

Bacitracin ointment

Pregnancy Category: C

RX: Baciguent.

Bacitracin ophthalmic ointment

Pregnancy Category: C

SEE ALSO ***ANTI-INFECTIVE DRUGS***.

INDICATIONS/USES

Parenteral: Limited to the treatment of staphylococcal-induced pneumonia or empyema in infants.

Topical Ointment: Aid to prevent infection in minor cuts, scrapes, burns, and wounds.

Ophthalmic Ointment: Superficial ocular infections of the conjunctiva or cornea (e.g., conjunctivitis, keratitis, keratoconjunctivitis, corneal ulcers, blepharitis, blepharoconjunctivitis, acute meibomianitis, and dacryocystitis) involving species of *Staphylococcus, S. aureus, Streptococcus, S. pneumoniae, S. pyogenes, Corynebacterium, Neisseria, N. gonorrhoeae,* and beta-hemolytic streptococci. Do not use topical antibiotics in deep-seated ocular infections or in those that are likely to become systemic.

ACTION/KINETICS

Action

Interferes with synthesis of cell wall, preventing incorporation of amino acids and nucleotides. Is bactericidal, bacteriostatic, and active against protoplasts. Not absorbed from the GI tract. When given parenterally, drug is well distributed in pleural and ascitic fluids. High nephrotoxicity. Systemic use is restricted to infants (see *Indications/Uses*). Carefully evaluate renal function prior to, and daily, during use.

Pharmacokinetics

Peak plasma levels: IM, 0.2–2 mcg/mL after 2 hr. From 10–40% is excreted in the urine after IM administration.

CONTRAINDICATIONS

Hypersensitivity or toxic reaction to bacitracin. Pregnancy. Epithelial herpes simplex keratitis, vaccinia, varicella, mycobacterial eye infections, fungal diseases of the eye. Concomitant use of nephrotoxic drugs.

SPECIAL CONCERNS

Renal failure. IM use may cause renal failure due to tubular and glomerular necrosis. Restrict use to infants with staphylococcal pneumonia and empyema due to susceptible organisms. Use only where laboratory facilities are adequate and constant supervision is possible. Carefully determine renal function prior to, and daily, during therapy. Do not exceed the recommended daily dose, and maintain fluid intake and urinary output at proper levels to avoid renal toxicity. If renal toxicity occurs, discontinue the drug. Avoid the concurrent use of other nephrotoxic drugs, especially streptomycin, kanamycin, polymyxin B, colistin, and neomycin.

- **Ophthalmic ointments may retard corneal epithelial healing.**
- **Prolonged or repeated use may result in bacterial or fungal overgrowth of nonsusceptible organisms leading to a secondary infection.**
- **Use topical ointment with caution during pregnancy.**

SIDE EFFECTS

Most Common

After IM use: N&V, skin rashes, pain at injection site.

After topical use: Skin rashes.

After ophthalmic use: Transient burning, stinging, itching, irritation.

• IM

N&V, skin rashes, pain at injection site, albuminuria, cylindruria, azotemia. ***Nephrotoxicity due to tubular and glomerular necrosis, renal failure.***

• Topical

Allergic contact dermatitis, skin rashes, superinfection.

• Ophthalmic

Transient burning, stinging, itching, irritation, inflammation, angioneurotic edema, urticaria, vesicular and maculopapular dermatitis.

DRUG INTERACTIONS

Aminoglycosides / Additive nephrotoxicity and neuromuscular blocking activity

Anesthetics / ↑ Neuromuscular blockade → possible muscle paralysis

Neuromuscular blocking agents / Additive neuromuscular blockade → possible muscle paralysis

HOW SUPPLIED

Bacitracin intramuscular. *Powder for Injection:* 50,000 units/vial.

Bacitracin ointment: 500 units/gram.

Bacitracin ophthalmic ointment: 500 units/gram.

DOSAGE

IM ONLY

Staphylococcal-induced pneumonia or empyema in infants.

Infants, 2.5 kg and below: 900 units/kg/day in 2–3 divided doses; **infants over 2.5 kg:** 1,000 units/kg/day in 2–3 divided doses.

TOPICAL OINTMENT

Prophylaxis of topical infections.

Apply small amount equal to the surface area of a fingertip 1–3 times per day after cleaning affected area. Do not use for more than 1 week.

OPHTHALMIC OINTMENT

Acute ophthalmic infections.

Apply ½-inch in lower conjunctival sac q 3–4 hr until improvement occurs. Reduce treatment before the drug is discontinued.

Mild to moderate ophthalmic infections.

Apply ½-inch 2–3 times per day.

NURSING IMPLICATIONS

Do not confuse bacitracin with Bactroban (topical anti-infective).

IMPLEMENTATION/ADMINISTRATION/STORAGE

1. When used IM, maintain adequate fluid intake: PO or parenterally.
2. Give IM in upper outer quadrant of buttocks; alternate sites, avoid multiple injections to same region R/T transient pain after injection.
3. For IM use: dissolve in NaCl injection containing 2% procaine HCl. Ensure bacitracin concentration is not <5,000 units/mL or >10,000 units/mL. Do not use diluents containing parabens. Reconstitution of 50,000 unit vial with 9.8 mL of diluent results in concentration of 5,000 units/mL.
4. Refrigerate unreconstituted drug at 2–8°C (36–46°F). Solutions stable for 1 week if stored the same as the unreconstituted drug.
5. Do not mix with glycerin or other polyalcohols that cause drug to deteriorate.
6. When used topically: may cover affected area with sterile bandage.
7. Administration and dosage varies for individual ophthalmic products; refer to individual manufacturer information.

ASSESSMENT

1. Note reasons for therapy, onset, characteristics of S&S, clinical presentation, culture results.
2. List experiences with this type of infection (especially ocular), agents used, and outcome.
3. Recurrent ophthalmic infections should be cultured and carefully assessed by ophthalmologist.
4. Do not administer with topical or systemic nephrotoxic drug.
5. Test urine pH daily; pH should be kept at 6 or greater; decreases renal irritation. Have $NaHCO_3$ or other alkali available if pH <6.
6. Monitor renal function studies; maintain adequate I&O with parenteral therapy.

CLIENT/FAMILY TEACHING

1. Review type of therapy, frequency, how to administer and site preparation. Wash hands before and after applying.
2. Apply topically as directed. Cleanse area thoroughly before applying bacitracin as wet dressing or ointment.
3. Do not use topical ointment near eyes, nose, mouth, or mucous membranes.
4. With eye ointment place a ribbon inside eyelid and close eyes; lightly press the inner corner of the eye for 60 seconds. Avoid contact of tube with the eye and wash hands before/after application.
5. Report lack of response, rash, fever, stinging, itching, changes in vision, or unusual side effects.
6. Keep all F/U to assess response, labs, and adverse SE.

OUTCOMES/EVALUATE

- Resolution of infection
- Restoration of skin integrity

Baclofen

(**BAK**-low-fen)

Classification(s): Skeletal muscle relaxant, centrally-acting

Pregnancy Category: C

RX: Gablofen, Kemstro, Lioresal, Lioresal Intrathecal.

Rx: Apo-Baclofen, Gen-Baclofen, PMS-Baclofen, ratio-Baclofen.

SEE ALSO ***SKELETAL MUSCLE RELAXANTS, CENTRALLY ACTING***.

INDICATIONS/USES

PO. Multiple sclerosis (flexor spasms, pain, clonus, and muscular rigidity) and diseases and injuries of the spinal cord associated with spasticity. Not effective for the treatment of cerebral palsy, stroke, parkinsonism, or rheumatic disorders. *Investigational:* Trigeminal neuralgia, tardive dyskinesia, intractable hiccoughs.

Intrathecal. Severe spasticity of spinal cord of cerebral origin in clients unresponsive to PO baclofen therapy or who have intolerable CNS side effects.

Investigational: Trigeminal neuralgia; intractable hiccoughs; reduce choreiform movements in Huntington's chorea; reduce rigidity in parkinsonism; reduce spasticity in cerebral lesions, cerebral palsy, or rheumatic disorders; reduce spasticity in CV stroke; acquired periodic alternating nystagmus; acquired pendular nystagmus; reduce number of gastroesophageal reflux episodes; Tourette's syndrome in children; prophylaxis of migraine, neuropathic pain; reduce spasticity in children with cerebral palsy.

ACTION/KINETICS

Action

Related chemically to GABA, an inhibitory neurotransmitter. May act by combining with the $GABA_B$ receptor subtype. It increases threshold for excitation of primary afferent nerves and decreases the release of excitatory amino acids from presynaptic sites. May also act at certain brain sites. Has CNS depressant effects.

Pharmacokinetics

After PO use, baclofen is rapidly and extensively absorbed. **Peak serum levels,** PO: 2–3 hr. **Therapeutic serum levels:** 80–400 ng/mL. **t½, PO:** 3–4 hr. **Onset after intrathecal bolus:** 30–60 min; **peak effect after intrathecal bolus:** 4 hr; **duration after intrathecal bolus:** 4–8 hr. **t½ after bolus lumbar injection of 50 or 100 mcg:** 1.5 hr over the first 4 hr. **Onset after intrathecal continuous infusion:** 6–8 hr; **peak effect after intrathecal continuous infusion:** 24–48 hr. 70–80% is eliminated unchanged by the kidney.

CONTRAINDICATIONS

Hypersensitivity. PO to treat rheumatic disorders, spasm resulting from Parkinson's disease, stroke, cerebral palsy. Intrathecal product for IV, IM, SC, or epidural use.

SPECIAL CONCERNS

■ Abrupt withdrawal after intrathecal use may result in high fever, altered mental status, exaggerated rebound spasticity, and muscle rigidity; rarely advances to rhabdomyolysis, multiple organ system failure, and death. Those at greatest risk include those with communication difficulties, history of baclofen withdrawal, or injuries at level of T-6 or above. ■

- **Use during lactation only if potential benefit outweighs the potential risk.**
- **Safety of PO product for children under 12 years and of the intrathecal product for children under 4 years not established.**
- **Use with caution in impaired renal function, in autonomic dysreflexia and where spasticity is used to sustain an upright posture and balance in locomotion; in psychotic disorders, schizophrenia, or confusional states (worsening of these conditions has occurred after PO use).**
- **Geriatric clients may be at higher risk for developing CNS toxicity, including mental depression, confusion, hallucinations, and significant sedation.**
- **Due to serious, life-threatening side effects after intrathecal use, physicians must be trained and educated in chronic intrathecal infusion therapy.**

SIDE EFFECTS

Most Common

After PO use: Drowsiness, hypotension, dizziness, headache, insomnia, fatigue, confusion, nausea, constipation, urinary frequency.

After intrathecal use: Hypotonia, somnolence, dizziness, convulsions, constipation, N&V, headache, paresthesia.

• PO

CNS: Drowsiness, dizziness, lightheadedness, weakness, lethargy, fatigue, confusion, headaches, insomnia, euphoria, excitement, depression, paresthesia, muscle pain, coordination disorder, tremor, rigidity, dystonia, ataxia, strabismus, dysarthria, slurred speech, ***seizures*** (rare). Hallucinations following abrupt withdrawal. **CV:** Hypotension, chest pain, syncope (rare), palpitations. **GI:** N&V, constipation, dry mouth, anorexia, taste disorder, abdominal pain, diarrhea. **GU:** Urinary

B

frequency, enuresis, urinary retention, dysuria, impotence, inability to ejaculate, nocturia, hematuria (rare). **Dermatologic:** Rash, pruritus, excessive perspiration. **Respiratory:** Nasal congestion, dyspnea (rare). **Ophthalmic:** Nystagmus, miosis, mydriasis, diplopia, blurred vision. **Miscellaneous:** Ankle edema, weight gain, weakness.

- **Intrathecal**

Spasticity of spinal origin. **CNS:** Dizziness, somnolence, paresthesia, headache, ***convulsion,*** confusion, speech disorder, coma, ***death,*** insomnia, anxiety, depression, abnormal tremor, thinking, agitation, hallucinations. **GI:** N&V, constipation, dry mouth, diarrhea, anorexia, increased salivation. **GU:** Urinary retention, impotence, urinary incontinence, urinary frequency, impaired urination. **CV:** Hypotension, hypertension. **Miscellaneous:** Accidental injury, asthenia, amblyopia, pain, peripheral edema, dyspnea, hypoventilation, fever, urticaria, anorexia, diplopia, dysautonomia, hypertonia, back pain, pruritus, asthenia, chills, pneumonia.

LABORATORY TEST CONSIDERATIONS

↑ AST, alkaline phosphatase, blood glucose.

OVERDOSE MANAGEMENT

Symptoms: Symptoms after PO use include vomiting, drowsiness, muscular hypotonia, muscle twitching, accommodation disorders, respiratory depression, seizures, coma. Symptoms after intrathecal use include drowsiness, dizziness, lightheadedness, somnolence, respiratory depression, rostral progression of hypotonia, ***seizures, loss of consciousness leading to coma (for up to 24 hr).*** *Treatment:* After PO use:

- Induce vomiting (only if the client is alert and conscious) followed by gastric lavage.
- If the client is not alert and conscious, undertake only gastric lavage making sure the airway is secured with a cuffed ET tube.
- Maintain an adequate airway.
- Atropine may be used to improve HR, BP, ventilation, and core body temperature. *Treatment:* After intrathecal use:
- Remove residual solution from the pump as soon as possible.
- Intubate the client who has respiratory depression until the drug is eliminated.
- IV physostigmine (total dose of 1–2 mg given over 5–10 min) may be tried, with caution.
- Can withdraw 30–60 mL of CSF to decrease baclofen levels (provided that lumbar puncture is not contraindicated).

DRUG INTERACTIONS

CNS depressants / Additive CNS depression
MAOIs / ↑ CNS depression and hypotension
Tricyclic antidepressants / Muscle hypotonia

HOW SUPPLIED

Injection Solution, Intrathecal: 0.05 mg/mL, 0.5 mg/mL, 2 mg/ mL; ***Kit (Intrathecal):*** 0.05 mg/mL, 0.5 mg/mL, 2 mg/mL; ***Tablets:*** 10 mg, 20 mg; ***Tablets, Oral Disintegrating:*** 10 mg, 20 mg.

DOSAGE

TABLETS; TABLETS, ORAL DISINTEGRATING

Muscle relaxant, spasticity.

Adults, initial: 5 mg 3 times per day for 3 days; **then,** 10 mg 3 times per day for 3 days, 15 mg 3 times per day for 3 days, and 20 mg 3 times per day for 3 days. Additional increases in dose may be required but do not exceed 20 mg 4 times per day. **Children (treatment of spasticity), initial:** 10–15 mg/kg/day in 3 divided doses. Titrate to a maximum of 40 mg/day if less than 8 years of age and to a maximum of 80 mg/day if more than 8 years of age.

Trigeminal neuralgia.

50–60 mg/day.

Tardive dyskinesia.

40 mg/day used in combination with neuroleptics.

INTRATHECAL

Initial screening bolus for severe spasticity of spinal cord of cerebral origin.

50 mcg/mL given into the intrathecal space by barbotage over a period of not less than 1 min. The client is observed for 4–8 hr for a positive response consisting of a decrease in muscle tone, frequency, and/or severity of muscle spasms. If the response is not adequate, a second bolus dose of 75 mcg/1.5 mL, 24 hr after the first bolus dose, can be given with the client observed for 4–8

hr. If the response is still inadequate, a final bolus screening dose of 100 mcg/ 2 mL can be given 24 hr later.

Postimplant dose titration for severe spasticity of spinal cord of cerebral origin.

To determine the initial daily dose of baclofen following the implant for intrathecal use, double the screening dose that gave a positive response and give over a 24-hr period. However, if the effectiveness of the bolus dose lasted for more than 12 hr, the daily dose should be the same as the screening dose but delivered over a period of 24 hr. After the first 24 hr, the dose can be increased slowly by 10–30% increments only once each 24 hr until the desired effect is reached.

Maintenance therapy for severe spasticity of the spinal cord of cerebral origin.

The maintenance dose may need to be adjusted during the first few months of intrathecal therapy. The daily dose may be increased by 10% to no more than 40% daily. If side effects occur, the daily dose may be decreased by 10–20%. Daily doses for long-term continuous infusion have ranged from 12 to 1,500 mcg (usual maintenance is 300–800 mcg/day). Use the lowest dose producing optimal control.

Reduce spasticity of cerebral palsy in children.

25, 50, or 100 mcg. *NOTE:* Intrathecal doses are in micrograms.

NURSING IMPLICATIONS

IMPLEMENTATION/ADMINISTRATION/STORAGE

1. If no beneficial effects noted, withdraw drug slowly.
2. Check manufacturer's manual for specific instructions/precautions for programming implantable intrathecal infusion pump and refilling reservoir.
3. Prior to intrathecal pump implantation, clients must show positive response to a bolus dose of baclofen in screening trial.
4. If no significant clinical response to increases in daily dose given intrathecally, check pump for proper function and catheter for patency.
5. During long-term intrathecal treatment, approximately 10% of clients become tolerant to increasing doses. If this occurs, a drug "holiday" consisting of a gradual decrease of intrathecal baclofen over a 2-week period can be considered. Alternate methods to treat spasticity must be undertaken. After a few days, sensitivity may return. To avoid possible side effects or overdose, discontinue alternative medication slowly.
6. Filling of the reservoir for intrathecal use must be performed by fully trained/qualified personnel. Refill intervals must be carefully calculated to avoid reservoir depletion.
7. Use extreme caution when filling an FDA-approved implantable pump equipped with an injection port (i.e., that allows direct access to the intrathecal catheter). Direct injection into the catheter through the access port may result in a life-threatening overdose of baclofen.
8. For screening purposes, intrathecal baclofen, either 10 mg/20 mL or 10 mg/5 mL, must be diluted with sterile preservative-free NaCl for injection, to a concentration of 50 mcg/mL for bolus administration. For maintenance, baclofen must be diluted with sterile preservative-free NaCl for injection USP for clients who require concentrations other than 500 mcg/mL (i.e., the 10 mg/20 mL product) or 2,000 mcg/mL (i.e., the 10 mg/5 mL product).

ASSESSMENT

1. List reasons and goals for therapy, other agents trialed, pre-treatment findings.
2. With epilepsy assess for clinical S&S of disease. Obtain EEG at regular intervals; assess for reduced seizure control.
3. Must closely monitor clients in fully equipped/staffed facility during both the intrathecal screening phase and dose-titration period following intrathecal implant. Resuscitative equipment should be readily available.
4. Ensure free from S&S of infection. Systemic infection may alter response to screening trials, (during pump implantation) lead to surgical complications, and interfere with pump dosing rate.
5. Assess for level of useful spasticity (e.g., to aid in transfers or to maintain posture) as rigidity is important for gait in some clients.

B

6. In those who require hypertonicity to stand upright, to maintain balance when walking, or to increase functionality, baclofen may be contraindicated; interferes with this coping mechanism.
7. Report evidence of hypersensitivity reaction.
8. If no improvement within 6–8 weeks, drug should be withdrawn gradually.
9. For clients with an intrathecal pump:
   - Calculate pump refill interval to prevent empty reservoir and return of severe spasticity.
   - Access pump reservoir percutaneously. Refill/program by one specifically trained in this procedure.
   - When filling pumps with injection ports permitting direct access to the catheter, use care as an injection directly into the catheter can cause lethal overdose. In this event, immediately remove any residual drug from the pump and follow guidelines for *Treatment* under *Overdose Management*.
   - When dose requirements suddenly escalate, assess for catheter kinks or dislodgement.
   - When programming for increased dosage, e.g., at bedtime, the flow rate should be programmed to change 2 hr before desired effect.
10. Obtain initial renal and LFTs and monitor for dysfunction; assess for diabetes. Monitor BP, blood sugar, weight, renal and LFTs, CK, urine output.

CLIENT/FAMILY TEACHING

1. Take orally with meals/snack to avoid gastric irritation. Report if GI S&S are severe/persistent.
2. To prevent constipation, increase fluids and roughage in diet.
3. Dizziness/drowsiness may occur; use caution. May take several weeks of therapy before improvement occurs.
4. Monitor/record weight/I&O; note frequency/amount of each voiding; report any swelling (edema).
5. May alter insulin requirements.
6. Report impotence; change of drug/dosage may be required. Do not stop abruptly; must be tapered off over 1–2 weeks otherwise may experience hallucinations/seizures.
7. Avoid OTC agents, antihistamines, cough remedies, CNS depressants, and alcohol use.
8. Avoid sudden position changes to prevent sudden drop in BP.
9. With the intrathecal pump:
   - Once screening trials completed, "baclofen pump" will be surgically placed in the abdominal wall and attached to an implanted lumbar intrathecal catheter. Proper postop site care, and S&S of infection that require immediate reporting will be reviewed.
   - Maintain log identifying when spasms are greatest; facilitates proper pump programming to ensure optimal control of spasticity and discomfort.
   - Identify symptoms requiring immediate medical intervention.
   - Report as scheduled (usually monthly with maintenance) to ensure proper reservoir drug levels and prevent loss of effect or air entering the reservoir.
   - Drowsiness, dizziness, and lower extremity weakness may occur; report if persistent/progressive; dose may require adjustment.
   - Those refractory to increasing doses may require hospitalization for "drug holiday"; consists of *gradual reduction* of intrathecal baclofen over a 2-week period and alternative therapy with other agents. Sensitivity to baclofen usually returns after several days and may be resumed intrathecally at the initial continuous dose.
10. Keep all F/U to assess response, for loss of control, and adverse SE.

OUTCOMES/EVALUATE

- Improved muscle tone and involuntary movements; ↓ muscle spasticity and pain
- ↓ Painful/disabling symptoms permitting ↑ functioning level

Balsalazide disodium

(bal-**SAL**-ah-zide)

Classification(s): Ulcerative colitis drug

Pregnancy Category: B

RX: Colazal.

INDICATIONS/USES

Treatment of mild to moderately active ulcerative colitis, including children 5 years of age and older.

ACTION/KINETICS

Action

Delivered intact to the colon where it is cleaved by bacteria to release equimolar amounts of mesalamine, the active portion of the molecule. Exact mechanism unknown but the drug may act locally to diminish inflammation by blocking production of arachidonic acid metabolites in the colon.

Pharmacokinetics

Designed to be delivered to the colon as an intact prodrug. Absorption is low and variable. Metabolites and parent drug are mainly excreted in the feces. **Plasma protein binding:** 99%.

CONTRAINDICATIONS

Hypersensitivity to salicylates, components of balsalazide capsules, or balsalazide metabolites.

SPECIAL CONCERNS

- Ulcerative colitis symptoms may worsen in some.
- Use with caution with known renal dysfunction, history of renal disease, or during lactation.
- Prolonged gastric retention of balsalazide capsules possible with pyloric stenosis.
- Safety and efficacy not determined in children less than 5 years of age.

SIDE EFFECTS

Most Common

Adults: Headache, abdominal pain, N&V, diarrhea, arthralgia, respiratory tract infection.
Children: Headache, upper abdominal pain, abdominal pain, vomiting, diarrhea, nasopharyngitis, pyrexia, ulcerative colitis.

GI: N&V, diarrhea, abdominal pain, rectal bleeding, flatulence, dyspepsia, frequent stools, dry mouth, constipation, cramps, bowel irregularity, aggravated ulcerative colitis, enlarged abdomen, diarrhea with blood, diverticulosis, epigastric pain, eructation, fecal incontinence, abnormal feces, gastroenteritis, giardiasis, glossitis, hemorrhoids, melena, benign neoplasm, pancreatitis, ulcerative stomatitis, tenesmus, tongue discoloration. **Hepatic:** Hepatic toxicity, jaundice, cholestatic jaundice, cirrhosis, hepatocellular damage, abnormal liver function, ***liver necrosis, liver failure***. **CNS:** Headache, insomnia, dizziness, aphasia, dysphonia, abnormal gait, hypertonia, hypoesthesia, paresis, generalized spasm, tremor, anxiety, depression, nervousness, somnolence. **CV:** Bradycardia, DVT, hypertension, leg ulcer, palpitations, pericarditis. **Respiratory:** Respiratory infection, rhinitis, pharyngitis, coughing, sinusitis, bronchospasm, dyspnea, hemoptysis. **Dermatologic:** Alopecia, angioedema, dermatitis, dry skin, erythema nodosum, erythematous rash, pruritus, pruritus ani, psoriasis, skin ulceration. **Hematologic:** Anemia, eosinophilia, granulocytopenia, leukocytosis, leukopenia, lymphadenopathy, lymphoma-like disorder, lymphopenia, ***hemorrhage,*** thrombocytopenia. **GU:** Menstrual disorder, UTI, hematuria, interstitial nephritis, micturition frequency, polyuria, pyuria. **Musculoskeletal:** Myalgia, arthritis, back pain, pain, arthritis, arthropathy, leg stiffness. **Ophthalmic:** Conjunctivitis, iritis, abnormal vision. **Otic:** Earache/infection, tinnitus. **Body as a whole:** Fatigue, fever, myalgia, flu-like disorder, viral infection, asthenia, chills, edema, hot flushes, malaise. **Miscellaneous:** Epistaxis, abnormal hepatic function, abscess, infection, moniliasis, weight increase/decrease, parosmia, taste perversion, chest pain.

LABORATORY TEST CONSIDERATIONS

↑ Bilirubin, AST, ALT, amylase, GGT, creatine phosphokinase, LDH, alkaline phosphatase, plasma fibrinogen. ↓ Immunoglobulins. Hypocalcemia, hypokalemia, hypoproteinemia. Increased/decreased prothrombin.

DRUG INTERACTIONS

The use of PO antibiotics might interfere with the release of mesalamine in the colon.

HOW SUPPLIED

Capsules: 750 mg.

DOSAGE

CAPSULES

Ulcerative colitis.

Adults: Three 750 mg capsules 3 times per day (total daily dose of 6.75 grams) for 8 weeks. Some require treatment for 12 weeks or less. Safety and efficacy beyond 12 weeks have not been determined. **Children, 5–17 years of age:** Either three 750 mg capsules 3 times per day (total daily dose of 6.75 grams) for up to 8 weeks or 1 capsule (750 mg) three times daily (total daily dose of 2.25 grams) for up to 8 weeks. Use in children for more than 8 weeks has not been evaluated.

B

NURSING IMPLICATIONS

IMPLEMENTATION/ADMINISTRATION/STORAGE

Store from 15–30°C (59–86°F).

ASSESSMENT

1. Note onset, character/frequency of stools and rectal bleeding. Assess abdomen for bowel sounds, distension, pain/tenderness and overall functional status.
2. List other agents trialed, outcome. Note history of pyloric stenosis.
3. Monitor CBC, renal and LFTs; assess for liver dysfunction/toxicity.

CLIENT/FAMILY TEACHING

1. Take as directed (3 capsules 3 times per day) to control bowel movements.
2. Alternatively, the drug may be given by carefully opening the capsule and sprinkling the contents on applesauce. The entire drug/applesauce mixture should be swallowed immediately; the contents may be chewed.
3. Practice reliable contraception; avoid drug if breast-feeding.
4. May experience headaches, N&V, diarrhea, abdominal pain and fatigue; report if persistent. Report if S&S do not improve or worsen; course of therapy is usually 8 to 12 weeks.
5. Report prolonged abdominal pain, skin rash/hives, breathing problems, yellowing of eyes/skin; may cause liver toxicity.
6. Keep all F/U to assess response, for labs/colon studies, and adverse SE.

OUTCOMES/EVALUATE

- Control of abnormal/frequent liquid stools with ulcerative colitis
- ↓ Diarrhea/abdominal pain with ulcerative colitis

■ IV

Basiliximab

(**bah**-zih-**LIX**-ih-mab)

Classification(s): Immunosuppressant
Pregnancy Category: B
RX: Simulect.

INDICATIONS/USES

Prophylaxis of acute organ rejection in renal transplantation, including children. Used as part of an immunosuppressive regimen that includes cyclosporine and corticosteroids in adults and children.

ACTION/KINETICS

Action

An interleukin-2 (IL-2) receptor antagonist which is a monoclonal antibody produced by recombinant DNA technology. Acts as an immunosuppressant by binding to and blocking the IL-2 receptor alpha–chain which is selectively expressed on the surface of activated T-lymphocytes. This competitively inhibits IL-2-mediated activation of lymphocytes which is a critical pathway in the cellular immune response involved in allograft rejection.

Pharmacokinetics

To be effective, serum levels must exceed 0.2 mcg/mL. At the recommended dosing regimen, the mean duration of basiliximab saturation of IL-2Rα was 36 days. **t½, terminal, adults and adolescents:** 7.2 days; **t½, terminal, children:** 11.5 days.

CONTRAINDICATIONS

Lactation.

SPECIAL CONCERNS

■ Should be prescribed only by physicians experienced in immunosuppressive therapy and management of organ transplant clients. Have complete information available for follow-up. Manage clients in facilities equipped and staffed with adequate lab and supportive medical resources. ■

- Increased risk to develop opportunistic infections and lymphoproliferative disorders.
- Possible severe acute hypersensitivity reactions within 24 hr with both first and subsequent doses.

SIDE EFFECTS

Most Common (greater than 10%)

Headache, tremor, insomnia, acne, N&V, constipation, diarrhea, abdominal pain, dyspepsia, dyspnea, URTI, anemia, pain, peripheral edema, fever, viral infection, hypertension, UTI.

B

The incidence of side effects following basiliximab is no greater than placebo groups; however, 99% of clients in both groups reported side effects. Those with an incidence of 3% or greater are listed. **GI:** Constipation, N&V, diarrhea, abdominal pain, dyspepsia, moniliasis, enlarged abdomen, flatulence, GI disorder, gastroenteritis, GI hemorrhage, gum hyperplasia, melena, esophagitis, ulcerative stomatitis. **CNS:** Headache, tremor, dizziness, insomnia, hypoesthesia, neuropathy, paresthesia, agitation, anxiety, depression. **CV:** Angina pectoris, cardiac failure, chest pain, abnormal heart sounds, aggravated hypertension, hypotension, arrhythmia, atrial fibrillation, tachycardia, vascular disorder. **GU:** Dysuria, UTI, impotence, genital edema, bladder disorder, hematuria, frequent micturition, oliguria, abnormal renal function, renal tubular necrosis, ureteral disorder, urinary retention. **Respiratory:** Dyspnea, URTI, coughing, rhinitis, pharyngitis, bronchitis, bronchospasm, abnormal chest sounds, pneumonia, pulmonary disorder, pulmonary edema, sinusitis. **Dermatologic:** Surgical wound complications, acne, cysts, herpes simplex, herpes zoster, hypertrichosis, pruritus, rash, skin disorder, skin ulceration. **Musculoskeletal:** Leg pain, back pain, arthralgia, arthropathy, bone fracture, cramps, hernia, myalgia. **Hematologic:** Hematoma, anemia, ***hemorrhage,*** purpura, thrombocytopenia, thrombosis, polycythemia. **Metabolic:** Acidosis, weight increase, dehydration, diabetes mellitus, fluid overload. **Ophthalmic:** Cataract, conjunctivitis, abnormal vision. **Miscellaneous:** Pain, peripheral edema, fever, viral infection, leg edema, asthenia, accidental trauma, chest pain, increased drug level, facial edema, fatigue, infection, malaise, generalized edema, rigors, ***sepsis, hypersensitivity reactions (including anaphylaxis).***

LABORATORY TEST CONSIDERATIONS

↑ NPN, glucocorticoids. Albuminuria, hyper-/hypokalemia, hyper-/hypoglycemia, hyperuricemia, hypophosphatemia, hyper-/hypocalcemia, hyperlipemia, hypercholesterolemia, hypoproteinemia, hypomagnesemia.

DRUG INTERACTIONS

H *Do not give echinacea with basiliximab.*

HOW SUPPLIED

Powder for Injection: 10 mg, 20 mg.

DOSAGE

IV BOLUS; IV INFUSION, CENTRAL OR PERIPHERAL ONLY

Prevent kidney transplant rejection.

Adults: Two 20-mg doses; give the first 20 mg within 2 hr prior to transplant surgery and the second 20 mg dose 4 days after transplantation. **Children, <35 kg:** Two doses of 10 mg each. **Children, 35 kg and higher:** Two doses of 20 mg each. Space the doses as in adults. Withhold the second dose if complications occur (e.g., severe hypersensitivity).

NURSING IMPLICATIONS

IMPLEMENTATION/ADMINISTRATION/STORAGE

1. **IV** To reconstitute: Add 5 mL of sterile water for injection to powder vial (20 mg/5 mL). Do not shake solution; invert bag gently to avoid foaming.
2. After reconstitution, solution should be colorless and clear to opalescent. If particulate matter present or solution colored, do not use.
3. Use reconstituted solution immediately. If not used immediately, store at 2–8°C (36–46°F) for 24 hr or at room temperature for 4 hr. Discard if not used within 24 hr.
4. Reconstituted solution is isotonic. May be given as bolus injection or diluted to a volume of 50 mL with NSS or D5W and infused through a central or peripheral IV over 20–30 min.
5. COMPATIBILITY Sterile water, NSS or D5W.
6. INCOMPATIBILITY Do not add/infuse other drugs simultaneously through same IV line.

ASSESSMENT

1. Note reasons for transplant, other therapies trialed, outcome. Used in conjunction with cyclosporine and corticosteroids to prevent organ rejection.
2. Given as 2 doses: infuse the first dose 2 hr prior to transplant surgery, give the 2nd dose 4 days after transplantation.
3. Have medications available for treatment of hypersensitivity reactions. Withhold second dose if hypersensitivity reactions occur.

4. Assess carefully for evidence of infection. Monitor labs/serum drug levels: CBC, metabolic/lipid panel, and renal function.

CLIENT/FAMILY TEACHING

1. Used to prevent transplant rejection; must comply with treatments to ensure success.
2. Report any fever, chills, fatigue, or sore throat; usually precedes more serious infection. S&S of infections and transplant rejection including fever, pain, and UTIs and require medical intervention.
3. Taken with cyclosporine and steroids. May increase risk of opportunistic infections and lymphoproliferative disorders.
4. Avoid vaccinations for 2 weeks following last dose. Avoid crowds and persons with known infections.
5. Practice reliable contraception during therapy, and for 2 months after the completion of therapy. Do not breast-feed infant during therapy.
6. Keep all F/U to assess for rejection, labs, and adverse SE.

OUTCOMES/EVALUATE

- Prophylaxis of renal transplant rejection
- Serum drug levels of >0.2 mcg/mL

BCG, Intravesical

Classification(s): Antineoplastic, miscellaneous

Pregnancy Category: C

RX: TheraCys, Tice BCG.

INDICATIONS/USES

(1) Treatment and prophylaxis of carcinoma in situ (CIS) of the urinary bladder. (2) Prophylaxis of primary or recurrent stage Ta and/or T1 papillary tumors after transurethral resection. Not recommended for stage TaG1 papillary tumors, unless they are judged to be at high risk of tumor recurrence. *Investigational:* Local control of accessible tumor. *NOTE:* Not to be used as vaccines to prevent cancer.

ACTION/KINETICS

Action

BCG promotes a local acute inflammatory and subacute granulomatous reaction with macrophage and lymphocyte infiltration in the urothelium and lamina propria of the urinary bladder. Precise mechanism is unknown but the anti-tumor effect seems to be T-lymphocyte dependent.

CONTRAINDICATIONS

Immunosuppressed clients with congenital or acquired immune deficiencies, whether due to concurrent disease (e.g., AIDS, leukemia, lymphoma), cancer therapy (e.g., cytotoxic drugs, radiation), or immunosuppressive therapy (e.g., corticosteroids) due to the possibility of a systemic BCG infection. A positive Mantoux test by itself is not a contraindication to use of the drug but an assessment must be made regarding whether the client has signs, symptoms, and/or a chest x-ray consistent with active or latent tuberculosis that requires treatment. Use within 14 days following biopsy, TUR, or traumatic catheterization. Use with active TB. Use with concurrent infections or with an actively bleeding mucosa. SC or IV use. Lactation. **TheraCys:** Use with current symptoms or a previous history of systemic BCG reaction. Use with a bacterial UTI until resolution of the infection.

SPECIAL CONCERNS

■ (1) BCG contains live, attenuated mycobacteria. Because of the risk for transmission, it should be prepared, handled, and disposed of as a biohazardous material. (2) BCG infections have been reported in health care workers, primarily from exposure resulting from accidental needle sticks or skin penetrations during preparation of BCG for administration. Nosocomial infections have been reported in clients, including immunosuppressed clients, receiving parenteral drugs that were prepared in areas in which BCG was reconstituted. BCG live is capable of dissemination when administered by the intravesical route. Serious infections, including fatal infections, have been reported in clients receiving intravesical BCG live. ■

- BCG infection of aneurysms and prosthetic devices (including arterial grafts, cardiac devices, and artificial joints) is possible, although risk is small.
- Administer with extreme caution to those at high risk for HIV infection and only after careful evaluation of risk/benefit.
- Small bladder capacity has been associated with increased risk of severe local reactions.

- **Carefully consider use of TheraCys in those who may require mandatory immunosuppression (e.g., awaiting an organ transplant, myasthenia gravis).**
- **BCG live is not a vaccine to prevent cancer.**
- **BCG vaccine, not Tice BCG, is used to prevent TB.**
- **Safety and efficacy not established in children; do not use TheraCys in children.**

SIDE EFFECTS

Most Common

Dysuria, urinary urgency/frequency, nocturia, urinary incontinence, UTI, fever, flu-like symptoms, abdominal pain, local pain.

Side effects common to both products. GU: Bladder inflammation/irritability, including symptoms of transient fever, hematuria, urinary frequency, dysuria, granulomatous prostatitis, epididymoorchitis, renal abscess. **Hypersensitivity:** Flu-like symptoms, including malaise, fever, chills. **Ophthalmic:** Uveitis, conjunctivitis, iritis, keratitis, granulomatous choreoretinitis. **Systemic BCG Reaction:** Fever of 39.5°C (103.1°F) for 12 hr or fever at least 38.5°C (101.3°F) for at least 48 hr; pneumonitis; hepatitis; organ dysfunction outside the GU tract with granulomatous inflammation on biopsy; classical signs of sepsis, including circulatory collapse, acute respiratory distress, and disseminated intravascular coagulation. **Body as a whole:** Serious infections, including ***disseminated sepsis including death;*** infections of the eye, lung, liver, bone, bone marrow, kidney, regional lymph nodes, peritoneum, prostate, GU tract.

TheraCys. GU: Dysuria, urinary frequency, hematuria, cystitis, UTI, urinary urgency, genital pain, renal toxicity, urinary incontinence, bladder cramps/pain, contracted bladder, tissue in urine, ureteral obstruction, symptomatic granulomatous prostatitis, epididymo-orchitis, renal abscess. **GI:** N&V, anorexia, diarrhea, abdominal pain, constipation, liver involvement. **CV:** Cardiac side effects, coagulopathy. **CNS:** Dizziness, headache. **Musculoskeletal:** Arthralgia, myalgia, flank pain. **Dermatologic:** Skin rash. **Hematologic:** Anemia, leukopenia, thrombocytopenia. **Body as a whole:** Malaise, fever, chills, fatigue. **Miscellaneous:** Local/systemic infection, pulmonary infection.

Tice BCG. GU: Dysuria, urinary frequency, hematuria, urinary urgency, bladder cramps/pain, nocturia, cystitis, genital inflammation/abscess, urinary debris, urinary incontinence, UTI, hemorrhagic cystitis, contracted bladder, epididymitis, prostatitis, orchitis, pyuria, urethritis, urinary obstruction. **GI:** N&V, anorexia, weight loss, abdominal pain, diarrhea, hepatic granuloma, hepatitis. **CNS:** Headache, dizziness. **CV:** Coagulopathy, cardiac side effects. **Musculoskeletal:** Arthritis, myalgia, arthralgia. **Respiratory:** Pneumonitis. **Dermatologic:** Diaphoresis, rash. **Hematologic:** Anemia, leukopenia, thrombocytopenia. **Body as a whole:** Flu-like syndrome, fever, malaise, fatigue, chills, rigors, allergy. **Miscellaneous:** Cardiac, respiratory, or neurologic symptoms; pain, ***BCG sepsis.***

LABORATORY TEST CONSIDERATIONS

May cause tuberculin sensitivity → false + tuberculin reaction.

DRUG INTERACTIONS

Antibiotic therapy / Interference with development of immune response to BCG; do not use together

Antituberculosis drugs / Interference with development of immune response to BCG; do not use together

Bone marrow depressants / Interference with development of immune response to BCG; do not use together

Immunosuppressants / Interference with development of immune response to BCG; do not use together

Radiation / Interference with development of immune response to BCG; do not use together

HOW SUPPLIED

Injection, Lyophilized Powder for Suspension: **TheraCys:** 10.5 +/− 8.7 × 10^8 CFU when resuspended (equivalent to about 81 mg dry weight); **Tice BCG:** 1 to 8 × 10^8 CFU (equivalent to about 50 mg wet weight).

DOSAGE

TheraCys

INTRAVESICALLY ONLY

Carcinoma in situ of the urinary bladder, Stage Ta and/or T1 papillary tumors.

Instill 81 mg BCG (dry weight) into the bladder once a week for 6 weeks. Follow with maintenance therapy, consisting of 1 dose given at 3, 6, 12, 18, and 24 months after initial treatment. *NOTE:* Begin treatment 7 to 14 days after biopsy or transurethral resection.

B

TICE BCG
INTRAVESICALLY ONLY
Carcinoma of the urinary bladder, stage Ta and/or T1 papillary tumors.
One vial (about 50 mg) suspended in 50 mL preservative-free saline and instilled into the bladder once a week for 6 weeks. Schedule may be repeated once if tumor remission has not been achieved. Thereafter, intravesical Tice BCG should continue to be given at about monthly intervals for at least 6 to 12 months. Retain in bladder for 2 hr and then void in a seated position to avoid splashing of urine. *NOTE:* Allow 7–14 days to elapse after bladder biopsy before giving Tice BCG.

NURSING IMPLICATIONS

IMPLEMENTATION/ADMINISTRATION/STORAGE

1. Product contains viable attenuated mycobacteria. Handle as biohazardous substance; use aseptic technique. If cannot be prepared in biocontainment hood, the person preparing product should wear gloves, mask, and gown to avoid inadvertent exposure to broken skin or inhalation of BCG organisms. Product should not be handled by individuals with an immunologic deficiency.
2. Reconstitute using aseptic technique and dilute immediately before use. Any delay between reconstitution and administration must not exceed 2 hr.
3. For *TheraCys:* Should not be handled by those wtih an immunologic deficiency. Do not remove rubber stopper from the vial. Reconstitute contents of 1 vial with 3 mL of diluent provided. Shake gently until a fine, even suspension results. Avoid foaming. Withdraw the entire contents (about 3 mL) of the reconstituted material into the syringe. Further dilute in an additional 50 mL of sterile, preservative-free saline provided to a final volume of 53 mL.
4. Administration of *TheraCys:* Insert a urethral catheter into the bladder under aseptic conditions; drain the bladder. Then instill 53 mL of TheraCys suspension slowly by gravity; withdraw the catheter. The client retains the suspension for as long as possible for a total of up to 2 hr. During the first 15 min following instillation, the client lies prone. Thereafter, the client is allowed to be up. At the end of 2 hr, the client should void in a seated position for safety reasons. Following BCG treatment, clients should increase fluid intake in order to flush the bladder.
5. For *TICE BCG:* Draw 1 mL of sterile preservative-free 0.9% NaCl (temperature of 4–25°C, 39.2–77°F) into a small (e.g., 3 mL) syringe. Add to 1 vial of TICE BCG to resuspend. Gently swirl vial until a homogenous suspension obtained. Avoid forceful agitation that may cause clumping of the mycobacterium. Dispense cloudy BCG suspension into the top end of a catheter-tip syringe containing 49 mL of sterile, preservative-free 0.9% NaCl, bringing the total volume to 50 mL. Gently rotate syringe. Do not filter contents. Avoid exposing Tice BCG to direct sunlight. Avoid bacteriostatic solutions.
6. Administration of *Tice BCG:* Clients should not drink fluids for 4 hr before treatment and should empty their bladder prior to Tice BCG administration. The reconstituted Tice BCG is instilled into the bladder by gravity flow via the catheter. The plunger should not be depressed to force the fluid. Retain in the bladder for 2 hr followed by voiding. If unable to retain the suspension for 2 hr, the client can void sooner. While Tice BCG is in bladder, reposition the client from left side to right side as well as lying on the back and the abdomen. Change these positions every 15 min to maximize bladder surface exposure of the drug.
7. Postpone intravesical instillation of BCG live during treatment with antibiotics as antimicrobial therapy may interfere with the efficacy of BCG live.
8. After usage, place all equipment and materials used for product instillation into the bladder into plastic bags (usually red) labeled "Infectious Waste" and dispose of properly as biohazardous waste.
9. Disinfect urine voided for 6 hr after instillation with equal volume of 5% sodium hypochlorite solution; (undiluted household bleach) allow to stand for 15 min before flushing.
10. Do not use antituberculosis drugs to prevent or treat the local, irritant effects of BCG live.

B

11. Store intact *Tice BCG* vials from 2–8°C (36–46°F). Keep the reconstituted product refrigerated, protected from exposure to direct sunlight, and used within 2 hr. The product contains live bacteria and should be protected from direct sunlight. Do not use after the expiration date printed on the label.
12. Store *TheraCys* and the accompanying diluent from 2–8°C (36–46°F). Do not use after the expiration date. Never expose the freeze-dried product to direct or indirect sunlight. Minimize exposure to artificial light.

ASSESSMENT

1. Note symptom onset, labs, cysto/TUR, and staging results.
2. Avoid BCG in immunocompromised individuals. BCG contains live, attenuated mycobacteria, there is risk of transmission.
3. Handle and mix carefully away from other parenteral drugs; drug contamination may occur. Follow administration guidelines carefully. Discard if not used within 2 hr of reconstitution.
4. Dispose of all equipment used to administer product according to institutional guidelines for hazardous waste.
5. May result in tuberculin skin reactivity; determine PPD (purified protein derivative) testing before treatment initiated.

CLIENT/FAMILY TEACHING

1. Used to treat bladder cancer. Contains a viable mycobacteria and should be handled as a biohazard; can make others ill.
2. Given once a week into the bladder for 6 weeks by provider (initially). Maintenance therapy with TheraCys is given at 3, 6, 12, 18, and 24 months after initial treatment. Tice BCG if indicated will be given monthly.
3. Do not drink fluids for 4 hr before treatment. Empty bladder prior to instillation.
4. Once reconstituted, the suspension is instilled into the bladder slowly by gravity flow, by the catheter within 2 hr or preparing. Do not force the flow.
5. Those mixing the agent should wear gloves and eye protection and avoid contact of BCG with broken skin to prevent BCG infection.
6. Retain in the bladder for 2 hr before voiding. Increase fluid intake in order to flush bladder following BCG treatment.
7. Sit on toilet seat and void to prevent splashing. Disinfect urine for up to 6 hr after instillation with equal volumes of bleach; wait 15 min before flushing to ensure deactivation of bacteria.
8. Report increase in symptoms associated with blood in the urine, rash, fever/chills, increased frequency/urgency, painful urination, or flu-like symptoms.
9. Any development of cough after BCG treatment requires immediate reporting; may signal a toxic systemic infection.
10. Keep all F/U to assess response, labs/cystograms, and adverse SE.

OUTCOMES/EVALUATE

Control/resolution of bladder cancer

Beclomethasone dipropionate

(be-kloh-**METH**-ah-zohn)

Classification(s): Glucocorticoid

Pregnancy Category: C

RX: Aerosol Inhaler: QVAR. **Aerosol Spray:** Beconase AQ.

✱ **Rx: Nasal Aerosol or Spray:** Apo-Beclomethasone, Gen-Beclo AQ, ratio-Beclomethasone AQ, Rivanase AQ. **Topical:** Propaderm.

SEE ALSO ***CORTICOSTEROIDS***.

INDICATIONS/USES

Nasal Aerosol Spray (Beconase AQ): (1) Prevent recurrence of nasal polyps following surgical removal. (2) Relief of symptoms of seasonal or perennial allergic and nonallergic (vasomotor) rhinitis. Relief may take up to 2 weeks.

Respiratory Aerosol Inhaler (QVAR): (1) Maintenance treatment of asthma as a prophylaxis in clients 5 years and older. (2) For asthmatics who require systemic corticosteroids when adding an inhalation product, the drug may reduce or eliminate the need for systemic corticosteroids.

ACTION/KINETICS

Pharmacokinetics

t½, after intranasal: 0.5 hr. **t½, after inhalation:** 2.8 hr; 44% is bioavailable. Rapidly inactivated by the liver, resulting in few systemic effects. Excret-

B

ed in the feces (about 60%) and urine (12%). **Plasma protein binding:** 87%.

CONTRAINDICATIONS

Status asthmaticus, acute episodes of asthma, hypersensitivity to drug or aerosol ingredients.

SPECIAL CONCERNS

- **Safe use during lactation and in children under 5 years of age not established.**
- **Use with caution, if at all, in active or quiescent tuberculosis infections of the respiratory tract, or in untreated fungal, bacterial, or systemic viral infections, or ocular herpes simplex.**

SIDE EFFECTS

Most Common

Beconase AQ: Mild nasopharyngeal irritation, nasal stuffiness, epistaxis, rhinorrhea, sneezing, watery eyes.

QVAR. Pharyngitis, headache, dyspepsia, coughing, nasal congestion, viral infection, URTI, sinusitis.

Beconase AQ. Respiratory: Mild nasopharyngeal irritation, epistaxis, nasal stuffiness/congestion, rhinorrhea, sneezing, nasal dryness, nasal irritation, throat dryness/irritation. Rarely, ulceration of the nasal mucosa and nasal septum perforation or localized *Candida albicans* infections of the nose and pharynx. **CNS:** Headache, lightheadedness. **GI:** Nausea. **Hypersensitivity:** ***Angioedema***, urticaria, ***bronchospasm***, rash, wheezing. **Ophthalmic:** Cataracts, glaucoma, increased intraocular pressure (all rare); watery eyes. **Body as a whole:** Viral infection, flu-like syndrome, pain, fever, rigors. **Miscellaneous:** Loss of taste/smell, unpleasant taste/smell, growth suppression, infection, hypercorticism.

QVAR. Respiratory: Pharyngitis, coughing, URTI, rhinitis, sinusitis, nasal congestion, dysphonia, sneezing, chest congestion, bronchitis, increased asthma symptoms, respiratory disorder, ***bronchospasm*** (rare). **CNS:** Headache, migraine, insomnia, depression. **GI:** Dyspepsia, nausea, diarrhea, ***rectal hemorrhage***. **CV:** Tachycardia, chest pain. **Dermatologic:** Eczema, pruritus, rash, skin discoloration. **GU:** Dysmenorrhea, UTI. **Musculoskeletal:** Back pain, arthralgia. **Hypersensitivity:** Urticaria, ***angioedema***. **Ophthalmic:** Lacrimation. **Otic:** Earache. **Body as a whole:** Viral infection, flu-like syndrome, pain, fever, fatigue, rigors. **Miscellaneous:** Taste alteration, lymphadenopathy.

HOW SUPPLIED

Nasal Spray (Beconase AQ): 0.042% (42 mcg/actuation); ***Respiratory Aerosol Inhaler (QVAR):*** 40 mcg/inh, 80 mcg/inh.

DOSAGE

Beconase AQ

NASAL SPRAY

Allergic or nonallergic rhinitis, prophylaxis of nasal polyps.

Adults and children 12 years or older: 1 or 2 (42 to 84 mcg) nasal inhalations in each nostril twice a day (total dose: 168–336 mcg/day). **Children 6–11 years of age:** Start with 1 nasal inhalation in each nostril twice a day (168 mcg). Those not responding adequately or those with more severe symptoms may use 2 sprays in each nostril twice a day (336 mcg/day). **Maximum daily dose:** 2 sprays in each nostril twice a day (336 mcg/day). **Maintenance:** Once adequate control is achieved, decrease dose to 1 spray in each nostril twice a day.

QVAR

RESPIRATORY AEROSOL INHALER

Asthma, chronic.

Adults and adolescents: If previous therapy was bronchodilators alone, start with 40–80 mcg twice a day. The highest recommended dose is 320 mcg twice a day. If previous therapy was inhaled corticosteroids, start with 40–160 mcg twice a day. The highest recommended dose is 320 mcg twice a day. **Children, 5–11 years of age:** If previous therapy was bronchodilators alone or if previous therapy was inhaled corticosteroids, start with 40 mcg twice a day. The highest recommended dose is 80 mcg twice a day.

NURSING IMPLICATIONS

IMPLEMENTATION/ADMINISTRATION/STORAGE

1. **For nasal use, symptoms usually improve in a few days but relief may not be seen in some for up to 2 weeks. Do not continue therapy beyond 3 weeks if symptoms do not improve. For nasal polyps, treatment may be required**

for several weeks or more before a beneficial result assessed. Recurrence of nasal polyps can occur after stopping treatment.

2. With excessive nasal mucus secretion or edema of the nasal mucosa, the intranasal spray may not reach the site of action. In such cases, use a topical or oral nasal vasoconstrictor/decongestant during the first 2–3 days of beclomethasone intranasal therapy.
3. Improvement usually observed within 1–4 weeks after beginning therapy. Consider tapering to lowest effective dose once desired effect is reached.
4. To prevent explosion of contents under pressure, do not store or use near heat or open flame, or throw into a fire or incinerator. Keep secure from children.
5. If canister is cold, therapeutic effect may be decreased. Shake well before using.
6. Once canister removed from moisture-protected package, use within 6 months.
7. If on systemic steroids, transfer to beclomethasone may be difficult because recovery from impaired adrenal function may be slow.
8. Store the intranasal spray from 15–30°C (59–86°F).

ASSESSMENT

1. Identify reasons for therapy, onset, and characteristics of S&S, other agents trialed, outcome.
2. Note any sensitivity to corticosteroids. If changing from systemic to inhaled or intranasal dosing, observe closely for adrenal insufficiency.
3. Document allergy and congestion history, presenting symptoms, mucosa presentation, PFTs, ENT, and pulmonary findings.

CLIENT/FAMILY TEACHING

1. Use regularly as prescribed to ensure desired effect.
2. With nasal spray, activate new sprayer by pushing down on the pump 6 times. If pump has not been used for 7 days or more, must prime again. Insert tip into one nostril while pressing closed the other nostril. Slowly inhale while pushing down pump. Aim toward the outer eye and not the inside of nose to decrease nasal irritation while inhaling. Shake and repeat steps in the other nostril. Wash cap and tip of activator in warm water and allow to air dry.
3. Review use, care, and storage of inhaler. Rinse out mouth and wash mouthpiece, spacer, sprayer; dry after each use.
4. A spacer may facilitate oral administration. Review video/instruction to ensure proper use.
5. To administer with oral inhaler:
   - Shake metal canister thoroughly immediately prior to use.
   - Exhale as completely as possible.
   - Place spacer/mouthpiece into the mouth and tighten lips around it.
   - Inhale fully through the mouth while pressing the metal canister down with forefinger.
   - Hold breath as long as possible.
   - Remove spacer/mouthpiece.
   - Exhale slowly.
   - A minimum of 60 sec must elapse between inhalations.
   - Rinse mouth with water and expectorate after use.
6. To use nasal inhaler:
   - Using a finger from your other hand, press against the opposite nostril to close it off. Alternate for other nostril.
   - Breathe gently through the open nostril and squeeze the spray container. If using more than 1 inhalation, wait for 1 to 2 minutes between sprays.
   - After using the medicine, rinse the tip of the spray unit in hot water and dry with a clean tissue to prevent contamination.
7. Not to be used for acute asthma attacks but used regularly to prevent attacks.
8. Follow prescribed therapy; may take 1–4 weeks for any improvement to be realized.
9. To check inhaler content, place in a glass of water: full inhalers sink, empty inhalers float, and half-full inhalers are partially submerged. Discard aerosol cannister when labeled doses completed.
10. Report signs of adrenal insufficiency (i.e., muscular pain, lassitude, and depression) even if respiratory function has improved. S&S such as hypotension and weight loss are indications that the dosage of systemic steroid should be boosted temporarily, and then withdrawn more gradually.
11. More than 1 mg in adults or more than 0.5 mg in children may precipitate hypothalamic-pituitary axis depression, resulting in

adrenal insufficiency. Do not overuse inhaler or exceed prescribed dosage.

12. Report any symptoms of localized oral infections as well as cough, dry mouth, facial swelling, rash, sore throat or mouth, worsening asthma symptoms (increasing need for bronchodilator).
13. Gargling and rinsing after treatments, rinsing of the spacer and/or administration port may help prevent infections. May require antifungal meds and possibly discontinuation of drug if oral infections occur. Report any nasal, oral or pharyngeal irritation.
14. If also receiving bronchodilators by inhalation (i.e., albuterol), use the bronchodilator first to open the airways and then use beclomethasone. (Increases penetration of steroid.)
15. For those receiving systemic steroid therapy, initiate beclomethasone therapy VERY slowly, withdrawing the systemic steroids as ordered. The benefit of inhaled steroids is a much lower dose, since it goes to target organ and does not require weaning. Once systemic steroid is withdrawn, keep supply of PO glucocorticoids and take immediately if subjected to unusual stress.
16. Carry ID with diagnosis, treatment, and possible need for systemic glucocorticoids, in the event of exposure to unusual stress.
17. Identify/practice relaxation techniques during stressful situations. Avoid triggers.
18. Keep all F/U to assess response and for adverse SE.

OUTCOMES/EVALUATE

- Maintenance control of asthma S&S (↓ wheezing, dyspnea)
- Relief of rhinitis
- Prophylaxis of nasal polyp recurrence

■ IV

Belatacept

(bel-**AT**-ah-sept)

Classification(s): Immunosuppressive.

Pregnancy Category: C

RX: Nulojix.

INDICATIONS/USES

Prophylaxis of organ rejection in adults receiving a kidney transplant. Use in combination with basiliximab induction, mycophenolate mofetil, and corticosteroids.

ACTION/KINETICS

Action

Belatacept binds to CD80 and CD86 on antigen-presenting cells, thus blocking CD28-mediated costimulation of T lymphocytes. In vitro, belatacept inhibits T lymphocyte proliferation and the production of cytokines, interleukin-2, interferon-gamma, interleukin-4, and TNF-alpha. Activated T lymphocytes are the predominant mediators of immunologic rejection.

Pharmacokinetics

Mean serum levels reached steady state by week 8 in the initial phase following transplantation and by month 6 during the maintenance phase. **t½, terminal:** 8.2–9.8 (depending on the use). In kidney transplant clients, there is a trend toward higher clearance with increasing body weight.

CONTRAINDICATIONS

Transplant clients who are Epstein-Barr virus seronegative or with unknown Epstein-Barr virus serostatus. Lactation.

SPECIAL CONCERNS

■ **Posttransplant lymphoproliferative disorder, other malignancies and serious infections.** (1) Increased risk for developing posttransplant lymphoproliferative disorder, predominantly involving the CNS. Recipients without immunity to Epstein-Barr virus are at particularly increased risk; therefore, use in Epstein-Barr virus seropositive clients only. Do not use belatacept on transplant recipients who are Epstein-Barr virus seronegative or with unknown Epstein-Barr serostatus. (2) Only health care providers experienced in immunosuppressive therapy and management of kidney transplant clients should prescribe belatacept. Manage clients receiving the drug in facilities equipped and staffed with adequate laboratory and supportive medical resources. The health care provider responsible for maintenance therapy should have complete information requisite for the followup of the client. (3) Increased susceptibility to infection and the possible development of malignancies

may result from immunosuppression.
(4) Use in liver transplant clients is not recommended because of an increased risk of graft loss and death.

- **Avoid the use of live vaccines during belatacept treatment, including but not limited to intranasal influenza, measles, mumps, rubella, oral polio, bacille Calmette-Guérin (BCG), yellow fever, varicella, and TY21a typhoid vaccines.**
- **Safety and efficacy not determined in children less than 18 years of age. Is increased potential in children for autoimmunity.**

SIDE EFFECTS

Most Common

Anemia, constipation, cough, diarrhea, graft dysfunction, headache, hyper–/hypokalemia, hypertension, leukopenia, N&V, peripheral edema, pyrexia, UTI.

CNS: Headache, anxiety, dizziness, insomnia, tremor, posttransplant lymphoproliferative disorder, JC virus–associated progressive multifocal leukoencephalopathy. **GI:** N&V, abdominal pain, upper abdominal pain, constipation, diarrhea, stomatitis (including aphthous stomatitis). **CV:** Hyper–/hypotension, atrial fibrillation, hematoma, lymphocele. **GU:** UTI, dysuria, hematuria, renal impairment (including acute renal failure), hydronephrosis, renal artery stenosis, urinary incontinence, renal tubular necrosis, chronic allograft nephropathy, polyma virus–associated nephropathy. **Respiratory:** Cough, bronchitis, dyspnea, nasopharyngitis, URTI. **Dermatologic:** Acne, alopecia, hyperhidrosis, nonmelanoma skin cancer. **Musculoskeletal:** Arthralgia, back pain, musculoskeletal pain. **Hematologic:** Anemia, leukopenia, neutropenia. **Infections:** CMV infection; bacterial, mycobacterial, viral, and fungal infections; herpes infections; tuberculosis; CNS infections. **Metabolic:** New onset diabetes mellitus. **Body as a whole:** Peripheral edema, pyrexia, influenza, malignancies, Guillain–Barré syndrome. **Miscellaneous:** Graft dysfunction, graft complications (including arteriovenous fistula thrombosis, wound dehiscence), infusion reactions (including hypotension and hypertension).

LABORATORY TEST CONSIDERATIONS

Dyslipidemia, proteinuria, hypercholesterolemia, hyperglycemia, hyper-/hypokalemia, hyperuricemia, hypocalcemia, hypomagnesemia, hypophosphatemia.

DRUG INTERACTIONS

Mycophenolate mofetil / ↑ Mycophenolic acid AUC and C_{max} levels; coadminister with caution and monitor clinical response
Vaccines / Vaccinations may be less effective; avoid live vaccines (See ***Special Concerns***).

HOW SUPPLIED

Injection, Lyophilized Powder for Solution: 250 mg.

DOSAGE

IV INFUSION

Prophylaxis of organ rejection following kidney transplantation.

Adults, usual, initial phase. Day 1 (day of transplantation, prior to transplantation) and day 5 (about 96 hr after day 1 dose): 10 mg/kg by IV infusion. **End of week 2 and week 4 after transplantation:** 10 mg/kg by IV infusion. **End of week 8 and week 12 after transplantation:** 10 mg/kg by IV infusion. **Maintenance phase:** End of week 16 after transplantation and q 4 weeks (+/- 3 days) thereafter: 5 mg/kg. **Maximum doses:** 10 mg/kg/dose for initial phase and 5 mg/kg/dose for maintenance phase. *NOTE:* Base the total IV infusion dose on the actual body weight at the time of transplantation; do not modify dosage during therapy unless there is a change in body weight of greater than 10%.

NURSING IMPLICATIONS

IMPLEMENTATION/ADMINISTRATION/STORAGE

1. **IV Prophylaxis for cytomegalovirus is recommended for at least 3 months after transplantation. Prophylaxis for *Pneumocystis jiroveci* is recommended after transplantation.**
2. **Preparation for administration:**
   - **Calculate the number of 250 mg vials required for the total infusion dose.**

B

- Reconstitute the contents of each vial with 10.5 mL of sterile water for injection, 0.9% NaCl, or D5W using the silicone-free disposable syringe provided with each vial and an 18- to 21-gauge needle.
- Remove the flip top from the vial and wipe the vial top with an alcohol swab. Insert the syringe needle into the vial through the center of the rubber stopper and direct the stream of diluent to the glass wall of the vial.
- To minimize foam formation, rotate the vial and invert with gentle swirling until the contents are completely dissolved. Avoid prolonged or vigorous agitation. Do not shake.
- The concentration of the reconstituted solution is 25 mg/mL belatacept. The solution should be clear to slightly opalescent and colorless to pale yellow. Do not use if opaque particles, discoloration, or other foreign particles are present.
- If the belatacept powder is accidentally reconstituted using a different syringe than the one provided, the solution may develop a few translucent particles. Discard any solution prepared using siliconized syringes.
- Transfer the reconstituted solution from the vial to the infusion bag or bottle immediately. Calculate the total volume of the reconstituted belatacept 25 mg/mL solution needed to provide the total infusion dose.
- If belatacept was reconstituted with sterile water for injection, further dilute with either 0.9% NaCl or D5W. If belatacept was reconstituted with 0.9% NaCl or D5W, further dilute with the same solution used for reconstitution.
- From the appropriate size infusion container, withdraw a volume of infusion fluid that is equal to the volume of the reconstituted belatacept solution needed to provide the prescribed dose.
- With the same silicon-free disposable syringe used for reconstitution, withdraw the required amount of belatacept solution from the vial; inject it into the infusion container, and gently rotate the infusion container to ensure mixing.
- The final belatacept concentration in the infusion container should range from 2 to 10 mg/mL. Typically, an infusion volume of 100 mL will be appropriate for most clients and doses, but the total infusion volumes ranging from 50 to 250 mL have been used.
- Any unused solution remaining in the vials must be discarded.

3. Administer the entire infusion over a period of 30 min with an infusion set and a sterile, nonpyrogenic, low-protein binding filter (with a pore size of 0.2 to 1.2 mcm).
4. Infusion must be completed within 24 hr of reconstitution of the lyophilized powder. A maximum of 4 hr of the total 24 hr can be at room temperature and room light.
5. Store vials from 2–8°C (36–46°F). Protect from light; store in original package until use.
6. COMPATIBILITY D5W or 0.9% NaCl.
7. INCOMPATIBILITY Do not infuse concomitantly in the same IV line with other drugs.

ASSESSMENT

1. Note date/type of transplant, other procedures trialed/agents used and outcome. Used in combination with basiliximab induction, mycophenolate mofetil, and corticosteroids.
2. Drug is contraindicated in transplant recipients who are Epstein-Barr virus (EBV) seronegative or with unknown EBV serostatus due to the risk of post-transplant lymphoproliferative disorder (PTLD), predominantly involving the central nervous system (CNS).
3. Monitor VS, BS, CBC, renal and LFTs.

CLIENT/FAMILY TEACHING

1. Drug is administered IV to prevent kidney transplant rejection. Medications to prevent infections will also be prescribed (CMV and *Pneumocystis jiroveci*).
2. With increased immunosuppression the susceptibility to infection and the risk of lymphoproliferative disease and other malignancies may be increased. Report any new/unusual side effects or fever/infections. Avoid live vaccines, crowds, and contact with persons with contagious disease or infection. Vaccinations may be less effective
3. With those at ↑ risk of skin cancer, limit sun and UV exposure; wear protective clothing and sunscreen.
4. Practice reliable form of contraception and report if pregnancy suspected.

5. Report any mood changes, unusual behaviors, changes in walking or talking, or visual changes, as well as decreased strength or weakness on one side of body.
6. Keep all F/U to assess response, labs, and for adverse SE.

OUTCOMES/EVALUATE

Prevent kidney transplant rejection

IV

Belimumab

(bee-**LIM**-you-mab)

Classification(s): Immunosuppressive (monoclonal antibody).

Pregnancy Category: C

RX: Benlysta.

INDICATIONS/USES

Treatment of adults with active, autoantibody positive, systemic lupus erythematosus who are receiving standard therapy.

ACTION/KINETICS

Action

Belimumab is a specific inhibitor that blocks the binding of soluble BLyS, a B-cell survival factor, to its receptors on B cells. The drug does not bind directly to B cells, but by binding to BLyS, belimumab inibits the survival of B cells, including autoreactive B cells, and reduces the differentiation of B cells into immunoglobulin-producing plasma cells.

Pharmacokinetics

t½, distribution: 1.75 days; **t½, terminal:** 19.4 days. Response rates for the primary end point were lower for Black clients.

CONTRAINDICATIONS

Anaphylactic reaction to belimumab. Lactation.

SPECIAL CONCERNS

- Use with caution in Black clients and in those with chronic infections.
- Safety and efficacy not established in children.

SIDE EFFECTS

Most Common

Bronchitis, depression, diarrhea, insomnia, migraine, nasopharyngitis, nausea, pain in extremity, pharyngitis, pyrexia.

CNS: Insomnia, depression (may be serious), migraine. **GI:** Nausea, diarrhea, viral gastroenteritis. **Respiratory:** Nasopharyngitis, bronchitis, pharyngitis. **Musculoskeletal:** Pain in extremity. **GU:** Cystitis, lupus nephritis. **Dermatologic:** Nonmelanoma skin cancers. **Hematologic:** Leukopenia. **Infusion reactions:** Bradycardia, headache, hypotension, myalgia, rash, skin reactions, urticaria. **Hypersensitivity:** Hypotension, ***angioedema***, urticaria, rash, pruritus, dyspnea, ***anaphylaxis***. **Body as a whole:** Pyrexia, infections (including bronchitis, cellulitis, influenza, nasopharyngitis, pneumonia, sinusitis, URI, URTI), hypersensitivity reactions. **Miscellaneous:** Infusion reactions, malignancies, immunogenicity, ***death (including those due to infection, CV disease, and suicide)***. *NOTE:* It may not be possible to distinguish between an infusion reaction and a hypersensitivity reaction.

HOW SUPPLIED

Injection, Lyophilized Powder for Solution: 120 mg, 400 mg.

DOSAGE

IV INFUSION

Systemic lupus erythematosus in adults.

Adults, usual: 10 mg/kg at 2–week intervals for the first 3 doses, and at 4–week intervals thereafter. *NOTE:* Consider giving premedication for prevention of infusion and hypersensitivity reactions.

NURSING IMPLICATIONS

IMPLEMENTATION/ADMINISTRATION/STORAGE

1. IV Should be administered by health professionals prepared to manage infusion/hypersensitivity reactions.
2. Preparation for administration:
   - Remove from the refrigerator and allow to stand 10–15 min for the vial to reach room temperature.
   - Reconstitute the 120-mg vial with 1.5 mL sterile water for injection. Reconstitute the 400-mg vial with 4.8 mL sterile water for injection.
   - Direct the stream of water toward the side of the vial to minimize foaming. Gently swirl the vial for 60 sec.

B

- Allow the vial to sit at room temperature during reconstitution, gently swirling the vial for 60 sec every 5 min until the powder is dissolved. Do not shake. Reconstitution is generally complete within 10–15 min after the sterile water has been added; however, it may take up to 30 min.
- The reconstituted solution will have a concentration of belimumab of 80 mg/mL.
- If a mechanical reconstitution device is used to reconstitute belimumab, it should not exceed 500 rpm; do not swirl the vial for longer than 30 min.
- Once reconstitution is complete, the solution should be opalescent, colorless to pale yellow, and without particles. However, small bubbles may occur and are acceptable.
- Only dilute belimumab in NaCl 0.9% injection. Dilute the reconstituted drug to 250 mL in 0.9% NaCl injection for IV infusion.
- From a 250 mL infusion bag or bottle of normal saline, withdraw and discard a volume equal to the volume of the reconstituted belimumab solution required for the client's dose. Then, add the required volume of the reconstituted belimumab solution into the infusion bag or bottle. Gently invert the bag or bottle to mix the solution.

3. For IV infusion only; do not administer by IV push or bolus.
4. Administer over 1 hr period. If the client develops an infusion reaction, the infusion rate may be slowed or interrupted. Discontinue immediately if the client experiences a serious hypersensitivity reaction.
5. To monitor maternal-fetal outcomes of pregnant women exposed to belimumab, a pregnancy registry has been established. To enroll clients, health care professionals and pregnant women are encouraged to call 1-877-681-6296.
6. Store vials from 2–8°C (36–46°F) protected from light and heat; store in the original container until use. If not used immediately, the reconstituted solution should be stored, protected from direct sunlight from 2–8°C (36–46°F). Solutions diluted in normal saline may be stored from 2–8°C (36–46°F) or at room temperature. Discard any unused solution. The total time from reconstitution to completion of the infusion should be no longer than 8 hr.
7. COMPATIBILITY 0.9% NaCl.
8. INCOMPATIBILITY Dextrose IV solutions. Do not infuse concomitantly in the same IV line with other agents.

ASSESSMENT

1. Note indications for therapy, age at onset of SLE, clinical presentation, other agents trialed and outcome.
2. Monitor closely for the development of infusion and/or hypersensitivity reactions during therapy. Assess carefully those who develop a new infection while undergoing treatment.
3. Determine any history of CAD, infections, any mental health issues or suicide attempts.
4. Review risks associated with therapy: severe infections, increased mortality, malignancy, hypersensitivity reactions, depression.
5. Monitor VS, CBC, renal and LFTs.

CLIENT/FAMILY TEACHING

1. Drug is given as IV infusion (over 1 hr) by provider to help control effects of SLE.
2. After infusion, client will be evaluated for any hypersensitivity and adverse side effects.
3. Avoid persons with infections and report any high fevers, chills, sore throat, painful urination or other symptoms. Avoid live vaccines during therapy.
4. Report any depression or changes in mood or affect.
5. Practice reliable contraception. Report if pregnancy occurs and enroll in the Benlysta (belimumab) Pregnancy Registry by calling 1-877-681-6296.
6. Review risks associated with therapy such as allergic reactions, cancer from immune system suppression, depression, or severe infections and report immediately if evident.
7. Keep all F/U visits to assess response, labs and adverse SE.

OUTCOMES/EVALUATE

Control of lupus symptoms

Benazepril hydrochloride

(beh-**NAYZ**-eh-prill)

Classification(s): Antihypertensive, ACE inhibitor

Pregnancy Category: D (Category C for first trimester and Category D for second and third trimesters.)

RX: Lotensin.

SEE ALSO ***ANGIOTENSIN-CONVERTING ENZYME INHIBITORS.***

INDICATIONS/USES

Hypertension, alone or in combination with other antihypertensives, especially thiazides. *Investigational:* Nondiabetic nephropathy. Heart failure, post MI, high coronary disease risk, diabetes, chronic kidney disease, and recurrent stroke prevention.

ACTION/KINETICS

Action

Benazepril (and its active metabolite benazeprilat) inhibit angiotensin-converting enzyme resulting in decreased plasma angiotensin II, which leads to decreased vasopressor activity and decreased aldosterone secretion (which contributes to sodium and fluid retention). Increased prostaglandin synthesis may also contribute to the antihypertensive action. Both supine and standing BPs are reduced with mild-to-moderate hypertension with an increased cardiac output and no compensatory tachycardia. Also an antihypertensive effect in clients with low-renin hypertension.

Pharmacokinetics

Food does not affect the extent of absorption. Almost completely converted to the active benazeprilat, which has greater ACE inhibitor activity. Is about 37% or more bioavailable. Food slows absorption. **Onset:** 1 hr. **Peak effect:** 2–4 hr. **Duration:** 24 hr. **Peak plasma levels, benazepril:** 30–60 min. **Peak plasma levels, benazeprilat:** 1–2 hr if fasting and 2–4 hr if not fasting. **t½, benazeprilat:** 10–11 hr. **Peak reduction in BP:** 2–4 hr after dosing. **Peak effect with chronic therapy:** 1–2 weeks. About 20% benazeprilat excreted through the urine and 11–12% excreted in the bile. **Plasma protein binding:** About 96.7% for benazepril and about 95.3% for benazeprilat.

CONTRAINDICATIONS

Hypersensitivity to benazepril or any other ACE inhibitor. Use not advised for children less than 6 years of age or in children with a glomerular filtration rate <30 mL.

SPECIAL CONCERNS

Use during pregnancy. When used during pregnancy, ACE inhibitors can cause injury and even death to the developing fetus. When pregnancy is detected, discontinue the ACE inhibitor as soon as possible.

- **May cause a profound drop in BP following the first dose.**
- **Use with caution during lactation.**
- **Safety and efficacy not determined in children.**

SIDE EFFECTS

Most Common

Headache, dizziness, fatigue, somnolence/drowsiness, nausea, cough, postural dizziness.

CNS: Headache, dizziness, anxiety, insomnia, drowsiness, nervousness. **GI:** N&V, constipation, gastritis, melena, pancreatitis, small bowel angioedema. **CV:** Symptomatic hypotension, postural hypotension/dizziness, syncope, angina pectoris, palpitations, peripheral edema, ECG changes. **Dermatologic:** Flushing, photosensitivity, pruritus, rash, diaphoresis, alopecia, dermatitis, pemphigus/pemphigoid, ***Stevens-Johnson syndrome***. **GU:** Decreased libido, impotence, UTI. **Respiratory:** Cough, asthma, bronchitis, dyspnea, sinusitis, bronchospasm. **Musculoskeletal:** Paresthesias, arthralgia, arthritis, asthenia, myalgia. **Hematologic:** Thrombocytopenia, hemolytic anemia, leukopenia, anemia, agranulocytosis, neutropenia. **Body as a whole:** Fatigue, asthenia, infection, ***anaphylactoid reactions***. **Miscellaneous:** ***Angioedema***, which may be associated with involvement of the tongue, glottis, or larynx, hypertonia.

LABORATORY TEST CONSIDERATIONS

↑ Serum creatinine, BUN, serum potassium, uric acid, blood glucose. ↓ Hemoglobin. ECG changes. Proteinuria, hyponatremia.

OVERDOSE MANAGEMENT

Symptoms: Hypotension (most common). *Treatment:* Supportive treatment. Volume expansion with an IV infusion of normal saline is the treatment of choice to restore BP. Only slightly dialyzable; consider dialysis, however, in an overdose in those with severely impaired renal function.

DRUG INTERACTIONS

Diuretics / Excessive ↓ in BP

B

Lithium / ↑ Serum lithium levels with ↑ risk of lithium toxicity
Potassium-sparing diuretics, potassium supplements / ↑ Risk of hyperkalemia

HOW SUPPLIED

Tablets: 5 mg, 10 mg, 20 mg, 40 mg.

DOSAGE

TABLETS

Hypertension in clients not receiving a diuretic.

Adults, initial: 10 mg once daily; **maintenance:** 20–40 mg/day given as a single dose or in two equally divided doses. Total daily doses greater than 80 mg have not been evaluated. **Children, 6 years and older, initial:** 0.2 mg/kg once daily as monotherapy. Doses between 0.1 mg/kg and 0.6 mg/kg once daily have been studied. Doses above 0.6 mg/kg (in excess of 40 mg daily) have not been studied.

Hypertension in clients receiving a diuretic.

Adults: Discontinue the diuretic 2–3 days before starting benazepril therapy. If BP is not controlled, resume diuretic therapy. If the diuretic cannot be discontinued, **initial dose of benazepril:** 5 mg/day.

Heart failure (investigational).

Adults, initial: 10 mg/day; increase at monthly intervals with a maintenance dose usually between 20 and 40 mg/day. Evaluate for potential hypotension within 2 weeks of any change in dose.

Nondiabetic nephropathy (investigational).

Adults: 10–20 mg/day. Less common doses of 1.25–5 mg/day have also been used.

Prevention of recurrent stroke (investigational).

Adults: 10 mg/day in combination with a diuretic and increased at monthly intervals with a maintenance dose usually between 20 and 40 mg/day. Evaluate for potential hypotension within 2 weeks of any change in dosage.

NURSING IMPLICATIONS

Ⓢ Do not confuse Lotensin with lovastatin (antihyperlipidemic).

IMPLEMENTATION/ADMINISTRATION/STORAGE

1. Base dosage adjustment on measuring peak (2–6 hr after dosing) and trough responses. Increase dose or give divided doses if once-daily dosing doesn't provide adequate trough response. Several weeks may be required to reach maximal effects.
2. Coadministration with potassium supplements, potassium salt substitutes, or potassium-sparing diuretics can lead to increases of serum potassium.
3. In impaired renal function (C_{CR} <30 mL/min/1.73 m^2), start with 5 mg/day; **maintenance**: titrate dose upward until BP is controlled or to a maximum total daily dose of 40 mg.
4. For children who cannot swallow tablets or for whom the calculated dosage does not correspond to the available tablet strength, a suspension can be made. To prepare 150 mL of a 2 mg/mL suspension: Add 75 mL Ora-Plus oral suspending vehicle to an amber polyethylene terephthalate bottle containing 15 benazepril 20 mg tablets; shake for at least 2 minutes. Allow suspension to stand for a minimum of 1 hr. After the standing time, shake suspension for a minimum of 1 additional minute. Add 75 mL Ora-Sweet oral syrup to the bottle and shake suspension to disperse. Refrigerate from 2–8°C (36–46°F) for up to 30 days in the polyethylene bottle with a child-resistant screw-cap closure. Shake suspension before each use.
5. Do not store tablets above 30°C (86°F); protect tablets from moisture.

ASSESSMENT

1. Note previous experience with this class of drugs; list other agents trialed.
2. Review diet, weight loss, exercise, and lifestyle changes necessary to control BP. Ensure not pregnant.
3. Monitor BP, CBC, electrolytes, renal (especially in geriatric clients) and LFTs. Check urine for protein.

CLIENT/FAMILY TEACHING

1. Take as directed. May take with or without food. Do not chew or crush; swallow tablets whole.

2. May be dizzy, faint, or lightheaded during first few days of therapy; use caution. Change positions slowly to prevent sudden drop in BP.
3. Avoid concomitant administration of potassium-sparing diuretics/supplements/salt substitutes; may lead to increased K^+ levels.
4. Consume adequate fluids to prevent dehydration and BP drop.
5. Report headache, fatigue, dizziness, drowsiness, mouth sores, rash, sore throat, swelling of hands/feet, chest pain and cough.
6. Avoid prolonged sun exposure, wear sunscreen and protective clothing if exposed to avoid photosensitivity reaction.
7. Use birth control; report if pregnancy suspected.
8. Avoid OTC products without provider approval.
9. Keep all F/U to assess response, BP log, labs, and for adverse SE.

OUTCOMES/EVALUATE

Desired BP control

IV

Bendamustine hydrochloride

(**BEN**-da-mus-teen **HY**-droe-**KLOR**-ide)

Classification(s): Antineoplastic, alkylating agent

Pregnancy Category: D

RX: Treanda.

INDICATIONS/USES

(1) Treatment of chronic lymphocytic leukemia. (2) Treatment of indolent B-cell non-Hodgkin's lymphoma that has progressed during or within 6 months of treatment with rituximab or a rituximab-containing regimen.

ACTION/KINETICS

Action

The drug dissociates into electrophilic alkyl groups. These groups form covalent bonds with electron-rich nucleophilic moieties. The covalent linkage can lead to cell death via several pathways but the exact mechanism of action is unknown.

Pharmacokinetics

Bendamustine is not likely to displace or be displaced by highly protein-bound drugs. The drug distributes freely in human RBCs. Primarily metabolized in the liver by CYP1A2 to two active metabolites. The drug does not induce drug metabolizing enzymes. About 90% excreted in the feces. **t½, intermediate of parent compound:** 40 min. **Plasma protein binding:** 94–96%.

CONTRAINDICATIONS

Known hypersensitivity to bendamustine or mannitol. Use in clients with a C_{CR} <40 mL/min or in those with moderate or severe impaired hepatic function (AST or ALT 2.5–10 × ULN and total bilirubin 1.5–3 × ULN). Lactation.

SPECIAL CONCERNS

- Use with caution in those with mild or moderate impaired renal function or with mild impaired hepatic function.
- Safety and efficacy not established in children.

SIDE EFFECTS

Most Common

When used for chronic lymphocytic leukemia: Pyrexia, N&V, diarrhea, rash, asthenia, fatigue, malaise, weakness, constipation, cough, dry mouth, headache, mucosal inflammation, stomatitis, somnolence.

When used for non-Hodgkin's lymphoma: N&V, fatigue, diarrhea, pyrexia, constipation, febrile neutropenia, pneumonia, hypokalemia, dehydration, stomatitis, abdominal pain, headache, chills, dizziness, insomnia, rash, cough, dyspnea, back pain, anorexia, decreased weight.

When used for acute lymphocytic leukemia. GI: N&V, diarrhea, constipation, dry mouth, stomatitis. **CNS:** Headache, somnolence. **CV:** Worsening of hypertension (hypertensive crisis possible). **Dermatologic:** Rash, pruritus, toxic skin reactions, bullous exanthema. **Respiratory:** Cough, nasopharyngitis. **Hematologic:** Myelosuppression, including neutropenia and febrile neutropenia, anemia, thrombocytopenia, leukopenia, lymphopenia. **Infections:** Pneumonia, ***sepsis***, death. **Infusion reactions:** Chills, fever, pruritus, rash, ***anaphylaxis and anaphylactoid reactions*** (rare). **Body as a whole:** Asthenia, chills, fatigue, malaise, pyrexia, weakness, mucosal inflammation, hypersensitivity, weight loss, herpes simplex.

Tumor lysis syndrome (including acute renal failure and ***death***).

When used for non-Hodgkin's lymphoma. GI: N&V, diarrhea, constipation, stomatitis, abdominal pain, dyspepsia, GERD, dry mouth, oral candidiasis, abdominal distension, upper abdominal pain, dysgeusia/taste disorder. **CNS:** Headache, dizziness, insomnia, anxiety, depression. **CV:** Tachycardia, hypotension, ***cardiac failure***. **Dermatologic:** Rash, pruritus, dry skin, hypertrichosis, night sweats, skin reactions, erythema, dermatitis, skin necrosis, toxic skin reactions, bullous exanthema, ***Stevens-Johnson syndrome*** (when given with allopurinol), ***toxic epidermal necrolysis*** (when given with allopurinol). **Respiratory:** Cough, dyspnea, URTI, sinusitis, pneumonia (including atypical pneumonia), pharyngolaryngeal pain, nasopharyngitis, nasal congestion, wheezing, pulmonary fibrosis. **Hematologic:** Febrile neutropenia, myelosuppression, hemolysis. **Musculoskeletal:** Back pain, arthralgia, bone pain, pain in extremity, chest pain. **GU:** UTI, acute renal failure. **Metabolic/Nutritional:** Anorexia, decreased weight, decreased appetite, dehydration, peripheral edema, hypokalemia. **Infusion reactions:** Chills, fever, pruritus, rash, ***anaphylaxis and anaphylactoid reactions*** (rare). **Body as a whole:** Fatigue, chills, pyrexia, asthenia, pain, hypersensitivity, infections, ***sepsis***. **Miscellaneous:** Infusion-site reaction (pruritus, irritation, pain, swelling), catheter-site pain, herpes zoster. myelodysplastic syndrome, tumor lysis syndrome.

NOTE: The drug may also cause impaired spermatogenesis, azoospermia, and total germinal aplasia in men. Also, malignancies, including myelodysplastic syndrome, myeloproliferative disorders, acute myeloid leukemia, bronchial carcinoma.

LABORATORY TEST CONSIDERATIONS

↑ AST, ALT, bilirubin. ↓ Hemoglobin, leukocytes, lymphocytes, neutrophils, platelets. Changes in creatinine levels. Hyperuricemia.

OVERDOSE MANAGEMENT

Symptoms: ECG changes. Possibly ataxia, ***seizures***, respiratory distress, sedation, tremor. *Treatment:* No known specific antidote. Provide general supportive measures, including monitoring of hematologic parameters and ECGs.

DRUG INTERACTIONS

Ciprofloxacin / ↑ Bendamustine plasma levels and ↓ plasma levels of its active metabolites; coadminister with caution
Fluvoxamine / ↑ Bendamustine plasma levels and ↓ plasma levels of its active metabolites; coadminister with caution
Omeprazole / ↓ Bendamustine plasma levels and ↑ plasma levels of its active metabolites; coadminister with caution
Smoking / ↓ Bendamustine plasma levels and ↑ plasma levels of its active metabolites R/T CYP1A2 induction

HOW SUPPLIED

Injection, Lyophilized Powder for Solution: 25 mg, 100 mg.

DOSAGE

IV INFUSION

Chronic lymphocytic leukemia.

Adults, usual: 100 mg/m² given by IV infusion over 30 min on days 1 and 2 of a 28-day cycle, up to 6 cycles. Delay administration in the event of grade 4 hematologic toxicity or clinically significant grade 2 or higher nonhematologic toxicity (see *Implementation/Administration/Storage*).

Non-Hodgkin's lymphoma.

Adults, usual: 120 mg/m² IV on days 1 and 2 of a 21-day cycle, up to 8 cycles. Delay administration in the event of grade 4 hematologic toxicity or clinically significant grade 2 or higher nonhematologic toxicity. Once nonhematologic toxicity has recovered to grade 1 or lower and/or the blood cell counts have improved (ANC 1×10^9/L or higher, platelet count of 75×10^9/L or higher), the drug can be reinitiated at the discretion of the health care provider. Dose reduction may be needed (see *Implementation/Administration/Storage*).

NURSING IMPLICATIONS

IMPLEMENTATION/ADMINISTRATION/STORAGE

1. **IV Consider measures to prevent severe infusion reactions, including antihistamines, an-**

B

tipyretics, and corticosteroids, in subsequent cycles who have previously manifested grade 1 or 2 infusion reactions. Infusion reactions are more likely in the second and subsequent cycles. Consider discontinuing the drug in those with grade 3 or 4 infusion reactions.

2. For clients at high risk, consider using allopurinol the first few weeks to prevent tumor lysis syndrome.
3. When used for **chronic lymphocytic leukemia**, delay administration in the event of grade 4 hematologic toxicity or clinically significant grade 2 or higher nonhematologic toxicity. Reinitiate therapy, at the discretion of the provider, once the nonhematologic toxicity has recovered to grade 1 or less and/or the blood cell counts have improved (ANC: 1×10^9/L or higher, platelets: 75×10^9/L).
4. For grade 3 or higher hematologic toxicity when used for **chronic lymphocytic leukemia**, reduce the dose to 50 mg/m^2 on days 1 and 2 of each cycle; if grade 3 or higher hematologic toxicity recurs on a dose of 50 mg/m^2, reduce the dose to 25 mg/m^2 on days 1 and 2 of each cycle.
5. For clinically significant nonhematologic toxicity when used for **chronic lymphocytic leukemia**, grade 3 or higher, reduce the dose to 50 mg/m^2 on days 1 and 2 of each cycle. Reescalation of the dose in subsequent cycles may occur at the discretion of the health care provider.
6. Adjust dosage as follows when used for **non-Hodgkin's lymphoma.** For grade 4 or higher hematologic toxicity or grade 3 or higher nonhematologic toxicity, reduce the dose to 90 mg/m^2 IV if the current dose is 120 mg/m^2 IV and to 60 mg/m^2 IV if the current dose is 90 mg/m^2 IV.
7. Aseptically reconstitute each vial as follows: For the 2 mg vial, add 5 mL of only sterile water for injection; for the 100 mg vial, add 20 mL of only sterile water for injection. This yields a clear, colorless to pale yellow solution, with a bendamustine concentration of 5 mg/mL. The lyophilized powder should dissolve completely in 5 min. If particulate matter is observed, do not use the reconstituted product.
8. Reconstituted solution must be further diluted before administration. Aseptically withdraw the volume needed for the required dose (based on the 5 mg/mL concentration) and transfer within 30 min of reconstitution to a 500 mL infusion bag of NaCl 0.9% solution. As an alternative, a 500 mL infusion bag of dextrose 2.5%/NaCl 0.45% injection may be used. After transferring, thoroughly mix the contents of the infusion bag. The admixture should be clear and colorless to slightly yellow. The resulting final concentration in the infusion bag should be within 0.2–0.6 mg/mL.
9. Bendamustine contains no antimicrobial preservative. Thus, prepare the admixture as close as possible to the time of administration. The final admixture is stable for 24 hr under refrigeration and 3 hr at room temperature. Administration must be completed within this period.
10. Exercise care in handling and preparing bendamustine solutions. Use gloves and safety glasses to avoid exposure in the case of breakage of the vial or accidental spillage. If bendamustine solution contacts the skin, immediately wash the skin thoroughly with soap and water. If the drug contacts mucous membranes, flush thoroughly with water.
11. Prior to reconstitution store vials up to 30°C (86°F). Retain in the original package until time of use; protect from light.
12. COMPATIBILITY Sterile water, NaCl 0.9%, dextrose 2.5%/NaCl 0.45%.
13. INCOMPATIBILITY Compatibility with other diluents has not been determined.

ASSESSMENT

1. Note reasons for therapy: chronic lymphocytic leukemia (CLL) or unresponsive non-Hodgkin's lymphoma (NHL), other agents trialed, outcome.
2. May use allopurinol to reduce tumor lysis effects. Closely assess those with any skin reactions.
3. Initiate measures to prevent severe infusion reactions, including antihistamines and corticosteroids, in subsequent cycles for those who have previously experienced minor infusion reactions; do not retreat with severe reactions.
4. Obtain VS, ECG, CBC, uric acid, renal and LFTs; monitor during therapy. Do not use if C_{CR} <40 mL/min or with moderate-severe hepatic impairment.

B

CLIENT/FAMILY TEACHING

1. Drug is given IV on days 1 and 2 of a 21- or 28-day cycle for up to 6–8 cycles for CLL/NHL.
2. Avoid driving or operating dangerous machinery until drug effects realized; may cause tiredness.
3. May experience N&V, diarrhea, mild rash or itching during treatment.
4. Report SOB, significant fatigue, bleeding, fever, or other S&S of infection.
5. Consider sperm/egg harvesting; potential risk to reproductive capacities. Men and women should practice reliable contraception during and for 3 months after therapy stopped.
6. Keep all F/U to assess response, labs and for adverse SE.

OUTCOMES/EVALUATE

Inhibition of malignant cell proliferation

IV

Benztropine mesylate

(**BENS**-troh-peen)

Classification(s): Antiparkinsonian drug, cholinergic blocking drug

Pregnancy Category: C

RX: Cogentin.

✱ **Rx:** Apo-Benztropine.

SEE ALSO ***CHOLINERGIC BLOCKING AGENTS.***

INDICATIONS/USES

(1) Adjunct to treat parkinsonism (all types). (2) Reduce severity of extrapyramidal effects in phenothiazine or other antipsychotic drug therapy (not effective in tardive dyskinesia).

ACTION/KINETICS

Action

Synthetic anticholinergic possessing antihistamine and local anesthetic properties.

Pharmacokinetics

Onset, PO: 1–2 hr; **IM, IV:** Within a few minutes. Effects are cumulative; long-acting (24 hr). **Full effects:** 2–3 days. Low incidence of side effects.

CONTRAINDICATIONS

Use in children under 3 years of age or in those with tardive dyskinesia.

SPECIAL CONCERNS

- Safe use during pregnancy not established.
- Geriatric or emaciated clients cannot tolerate large doses.
- Use with caution in children over 3 years of age.
- Use with caution in those with a tendency to tachycardia or with prostatic hypertrophy.
- Certain drug-induced extrapyramidal symptoms may not respond to benztropine.

SIDE EFFECTS

Most Common

Headache, blurred vision, constipation, mydriasis, dizziness, dry mouth, tachycardia, urinary retention, nausea.

See *Cholinergic Blocking Agents* for a complete list of possible side effects. Also, sudden, uncontrolled somnolence, weakness, inability to move particular muscle groups (especially with large doses), mental confusion, excitement, visual hallucinations, toxic psychosis if used with phenothiazines, tardive dyskinesia.

ADDITIONAL DRUG INTERACTIONS

Possible paralytic ileus, hyperthermia, or heat stroke if used with tricyclic antidepressants.

HOW SUPPLIED

Injection Solution: 1 mg/mL; ***Tablets:*** 0.5 mg, 1 mg, 2 mg.

DOSAGE

TABLETS

Parkinsonism.

Adults: 1–2 mg/day (range: 0.5–6.5 mg/day).

Idiopathic parkinsonism.

Adults, initial: 0.5–1 mg/day, increased gradually to 4–6 mg/day, if necessary.

Postencephalitic parkinsonism.

Adults: 2 mg/day in one or more doses.

Drug-induced extrapyramidal effects.

Adults: 1–4 mg 1–2 times per day.

IM; IV (RARELY)

Acute dystonic reactions.

Adults, initial: 1–2 mg; **then,** 1–2 mg PO twice a day usually prevents recurrence. Clients can rarely tolerate full dosage.

B

NURSING IMPLICATIONS

IMPLEMENTATION/ADMINISTRATION/STORAGE

1. When used as replacement for or supplement to other antiparkinsonism drugs, substitute or add gradually.
2. For difficulty swallowing tablets, may crush tablets and mix with a small amount of food or liquid.
3. Some may benefit by taking entire dose at bedtime while others are best treated by taking divided doses, 2–4 times per day.
4. Initiate therapy with low dose (e.g., 0.5 mg) and increase in increments of 0.5 mg at 5–6-day intervals. Do not exceed 6 mg/day.
5. IV May give IV undiluted at a rate of 1 mg over 1 min, separately.
6. COMPATIBILITY Give undiluted; may flush line with D5W or NSS.
7. INCOMPATIBILITY Give separately.

ASSESSMENT

1. List symptoms, onset, other agents trialed, outcome.
2. Note if phenothiazines or TCAs are being used; may cause paralytic ileus.
3. Elderly require lower dosage. Monitor mental status and assess for depression or mood changes.
4. Monitor I&O. Assess for urinary retention and bowel sounds; especially with limited mobility.
5. Inspect skin at regular intervals for evidence of skin changes.
6. Observe for extrapyramidal symptoms, i.e., drooling, muscle spasms, shuffling gait, muscle rigidity, and pill rolling.
7. If excitation or vomiting occurs, withdraw drug temporarily and resume at lower dose.
8. Assess for tolerance, tardive dyskinesia with prolonged therapy, may require dosage/drug change.

CLIENT/FAMILY TEACHING

1. Review goals of therapy (control of parkinsonian symptoms, i.e., improved gait and balance and less rigidity and involuntary movements; control of extrapyramidal symptoms, i.e., less drooling, muscle spasms, shuffling gait, or pill rolling).
2. With once-a-day dosing take at bedtime to minimize side effects; if taking more often take after meals.
3. Use caution when performing tasks that require mental alertness; drug has a sedative effect and may also cause drop in BP with sudden changes in position.
4. It usually takes 2–3 days for drug to exert desired effect. Take as ordered unless side effects occur; these usually subside with continued drug use.
5. Vision may appear blurry during the first 2 to 3 wks of treatment. Wearing sunglasses outdoors will help to minimize photophobia effects. With long term therapy have periodic eye exams to monitor for glaucoma.
6. Avoid strenuous activity and increased heat exposure. Plan rest periods during the day; ability to tolerate heat will be reduced and heatstroke may occur.
7. Increase fluid intake to minimize dry mouth and constipation effects.
8. Report any difficulty in voiding or inadequate emptying of the bladder.
9. Avoid alcohol, OTC agents, and other CNS depressants.
10. Do not stop drug abruptly; requires gradual reduction in dose over 1 week to prevent withdrawal symptoms.
11. Keep all F/U to assess response and for adverse SE.

OUTCOMES/EVALUATE

- ↓ Involuntary movements and rigidity with improved gait and balance
- Control of extrapyramidal side effects of antipsychotic agents

---

Betamethasone

(bay-tah-**METH**-ah-zohn)

Classification(s): Glucocorticoid

Pregnancy Category: C

RX: Celestone.

Betamethasone dipropionate

RX: Topical: Augmented Betamethasone Dipropionate, Diprolene, Diprolene AF.

✦ **Rx: Topical:** Diprolene Glycol, ratio-Topilene, ratio-Topisone, Taro-Sone.

B

Betamethasone sodium phosphate and Betamethasone acetate

RX: Celestone Soluspan.

Rx: Betaject.

Betamethasone valerate

RX: Topical: Beta-Val, Ectosone Regular, Luxiq, Psorion Cream, Valisone, Valisone Reduced Strength.

Rx: Topical: Betaderm, Prevex B, ratio-Ectosone.

SEE ALSO ***CORTICOSTEROIDS***.

ADDITIONAL USES

(1) Prevention of respiratory distress syndrome in premature infants. (2) Betamethasone dipropionate cream, lotion, and ointment can be used to treat atopic dermatitis in children younger than 12 years of age.

ACTION/KINETICS

Action

Causes low degree of sodium and water retention, as well as potassium depletion.

Pharmacokinetics

The injectable form contains both rapid-acting and repository forms of betamethasone (mixture of betamethasone sodium phosphate and betamethasone acetate). Long-acting. **t½:** over 300 min.

CONTRAINDICATIONS

Replacement therapy in any acute or chronic adrenal cortical insufficiency due to weak sodium-retaining effects.

SPECIAL CONCERNS

Safe use during pregnancy and lactation not established.

HOW SUPPLIED

Betamethasone. ***Syrup:*** 0.6 mg/5 mL.
Betamethasone dipropionate. ***Cream:*** 0.05%; ***Gel:*** 0.05%; ***Lotion:*** 0.05%; ***Ointment:*** 0.05%.
Betamethasone sodium phosphate and betamethasone acetate. ***Injection:*** 3 mg/mL each of sodium phosphate and of acetate.
Betamethasone valerate. ***Cream:*** 0.01%, 0.05%, 0.1%; ***Foam:*** 0.12%; ***Lotion:*** 0.1%; ***Ointment:*** 0.1%.

DOSAGE

Betamethasone

SYRUP

All uses.

Initial: 0.6–7.2 mg/day; individualize dosage.

Betamethasone sodium phosphate and betamethasone acetate

IM

All uses.

Initial: 0.5–9 mg/day (dose ranges are ⅓–½ the PO dose given q 12 hr.) In life-threatening situations, dosages exceeding the usual dose may be acceptable; may be in multiple doses.

INTRA-ARTICULAR; INTRABURSAL; INTRALESIONAL

Bursitis, peritendinitis, tenosynovitis.

1 mL intrabursally.

Rheumatoid arthritis and osteoarthritis.

0.25–2 mL intra-articularly, depending on size of the joint (1–2 mL for very large joints; 1 mL for large joints; 0.5–1 mL for medium joints; and, 0.25–0.5 mL for small joints).

Foot disorders, bursitis.

0.25–0.5 mL under heloma durum or heloma molle; 0.5 mL under calcaneal spur or over hallux rigidus or digiti quinti varus.

Tenosynovitis or periostitis of cuboid.

0.5 mL.

Acute gouty arthritis.

0.5–1 mL.

INTRADERMAL

Dermatologic conditions.

0.2 mL/cm^2, not to exceed 1 mL/week.

Betamethasone dipropionate, betamethasone valerate

CREAM; FOAM; GEL; LOTION; OINTMENT; TOPICAL SPRAY

Dermatological conditions.

Apply sparingly to affected areas and rub in lightly.

B

NURSING IMPLICATIONS

IMPLEMENTATION/ADMINISTRATION/STORAGE

1. Avoid injection into deltoid; SC tissue atrophy may occur.
2. Intralesional use indicated for keloids; localized hypertrophic, infiltrated, inflammatory lesions of lichen planus, psoriatic plaques, granuloma annulare, and lichen simplex chronicus; discoid lupus erythematosus; necrobiosis lipoidica diabeticorum; alopecia areata.

ASSESSMENT

1. List reasons for therapy, type, onset, location, characteristics of S&S and clinical presentation.
2. List agents trialed; outcome. With joints, assess ROM, swelling, erythema and pain level.
3. Monitor uric acid level with gout.

CLIENT/FAMILY TEACHING

1. Review appropriate method for administration and frequency of use. Wash hands before and after application.
2. Report S&S of infection, i.e., increased fever, any redness, odor, or purulent wound drainage. Avoid exposure to those with contagious diseases.
3. Cover lesions to avoid sunburn.
4. Do not overuse joint after injection; may further injure joint.
5. Record weight; report sudden weight gain (>5 lbs/week), swelling of limbs, blood in stools, severe abdominal pain, bruising or lack of response.
6. Keep all F/U to assess response and for adverse SE.

OUTCOMES/EVALUATE

- ↓ Pain/inflammation; ↑ mobility
- Prevention of respiratory distress syndrome in premature infants
- Improved skin integrity; healing of lesions

Betaxolol hydrochloride

(beh-**TAX**-oh-lohl)

Classification(s): Beta-adrenergic blocking agent

Pregnancy Category: C

RX: Betoptic S, Kerlone.

SEE ALSO ***BETA-ADRENERGIC BLOCKING AGENTS.***

INDICATIONS/USES

PO: Hypertension, alone or with other antihypertensive agents (especially thiazide diuretics).

Ophthalmic: (1) Ocular hypertension. (2) Chronic open-angle glaucoma, alone or in combination with other antiglaucoma drugs.

ACTION/KINETICS

Action

Inhibits beta-1-adrenergic receptors (beta-2 receptors inhibited at high doses). Has some membrane stabilizing activity but no intrinsic sympathomimetic activity. Low lipid solubility. Reduces the production of aqueous humor, thus reducing IOP. No effect on pupil size or accommodation.

Pharmacokinetics

t½: 14–22 hr. Metabolized in the liver with most excreted through the urine; about 15% is excreted unchanged.

ADDITIONAL CONTRAINDICATIONS

Avoid use of calcium antagonists in impaired cardiac function.

SPECIAL CONCERNS

- Use with caution during lactation.
- Use catecholamine-depleting drugs with caution.
- Calcium antagonists may be used with betaxolol when heart function is normal; do not use together in those with impaired cardiac function.
- Safety and efficacy not determined in children.
- Elderly are at greater risk of developing bradycardia; start on a lower dose (e.g., 5 mg).
- Clearance of betaxolol is decreased in those with impaired renal function.

SIDE EFFECTS

Most Common

After ophthalmic use: Brief discomfort, tearing, headaches.

See *Beta-Adrenergic Blocking Agents* for a complete list of side effects.

HOW SUPPLIED

Ophthalmic Solution: 0.5%; ***Ophthalmic Suspension:*** 0.25%; ***Tablets:*** 10 mg, 20 mg.

DOSAGE

TABLETS

Hypertension.

Initial: 10 mg once daily either alone or with a diuretic. If desired effect is not reached, may increase dose to 20 mg; doses higher than 20 mg will not increase the therapeutic effect but doses of 40 mg are well tolerated. If monotherapy does not result in the desired effect, a diuretic or another antihypertensive (e.g., chlorthalidone, hydrochlorothiazide, nifedipine have been used) may be added. In geriatric clients or in those with impaired renal function, the initial dose should be 5 mg/day. If the desired effect is not achieved with 5 mg/day in those with impaired renal function, the dose may be increased by 5 mg/day increments q 2 weeks up to a maximum of 20 mg.

OPHTHALMIC SOLUTION; SUSPENSION

Ocular hypertension; chronic open-angle glaucoma.

Adults, usual: 1–2 gtt twice a day. If used to replace another drug, continue the drug being used and add 1 gtt of betaxolol twice a day. Discontinue the previous drug the following day. If transferring from several antiglaucoma drugs being used together, adjust one drug at a time at intervals of not less than 1 week. The agents being used can be continued and add 1 gtt betaxolol twice a day. The next day another agent should be discontinued. The remaining antiglaucoma drug dosage can be decreased or discontinued depending on client response.

NURSING IMPLICATIONS

IMPLEMENTATION/ADMINISTRATION/STORAGE

1. Full antihypertensive effect usually observed within 7 to 14 days.
2. As PO dose increases, HR decreases.
3. Discontinue PO therapy gradually over 2-week period.
4. Shake ophthalmic suspension well before use.
5. Store tablets from 15–25°C (59–77°F). Store ophthalmic products at room temperature; not to exceed 30°C (86°F).

ASSESSMENT

1. Note reasons for therapy, frequency/characteristics of symptoms, other agents trialed.
2. With glaucoma check eye exam and pressures.
3. Monitor lung sounds, weight, VS, ECG, renal and LFTs; reduce dose with dysfunction.

CLIENT/FAMILY TEACHING

1. Review appropriate method/indications for therapy; take/use as directed. Do not stop suddenly.
2. Use caution, may cause dizziness or drowsiness. Change positions slowly; prevents sudden drop in BP.
3. With eye therapy may have burning or stinging with initial instillation. With eye drops, wash hands, do not allow dropper to touch eye. Tilt head back; looking up, pull lower eyelid down and instill prescribed number of drops. Close eye for 1 to 2 min, apply gentle pressure to bridge of nose for 1 to 3 min. Do not rub eye or touch top of dropper bottle to eye, fingers, or other surface.
4. Wear sunglasses, avoid sun exposure; may cause photophobia.
5. Report SOB, wheezes, confusion, rash, unusual bruising/bleeding, slow pulse, cold hands/feet.
6. Do not stop suddenly with prolonged therapy, may cause ↓ BP, ↓ HR, anxiety, angina, MI.
7. May mask S&S of hypoglycemia, and cause increased cold sensitivity.
8. Avoid OTC agents without approval.
9. With HTN, monitor BP and HR and record.
10. Keep all F/U to assess response, labs and for adverse SE.

OUTCOMES/EVALUATE

- ↓ BP (PO)
- ↓ Intraocular pressure (ophthalmic)

■ IV

Bevacizumab

(bev-ah-**CIZ**-yoo-mab)

Classification(s): Antineoplastic, monoclonal antibody

Pregnancy Category: C

RX: Avastin.

INDICATIONS/USES

(1) With IV 5-fluorouracil-based chemotherapy for first- or second-line treatment of metastatic carcinoma of the colon or rectum. (2) With paclitaxel to treat clients who have not received chemotherapy for metastatic human epidermal growth factor receptor 2-negative breast cancer. (3) With carboplatin and paclitaxel for first-line treatment of unresectable, locally advanced, recurrent or metastatic nonsquamous, non-small-cell lung cancer. (4) Monotherapy to treat glioblastoma with progressive disease following previous therapy. (5) With interferon alfa to treat metastatic renal cell carcinoma. *Investigational:* With erlotinib to treat metastatic renal cell carcinoma.

ACTION/KINETICS

Action

Bevacizumab is a recombinant, humanized, monoclonal IgG_1 antibody that binds to and inhibits the biologic activity of human vascular endothelial growth factor (VEGF). Binding of bevacizumab to VEGF prevents the interaction of VEGF to its receptor on the surface of endothelial cells. It is believed this results in reduction of microvascular growth and inhibition of metastatic disease progression.

Pharmacokinetics

t½: About 20 days. **Time to reach steady state:** 100 days. Clearance varies by body weight and gender, as well as by tumor burden.

CONTRAINDICATIONS

Use within 28 days following major surgery. Lactation.

SPECIAL CONCERNS

(1) **GI perforations.** The incidence of GI perforations, some fatal, in bevacizumab-treated clients ranges from 0.3% to 2.4%. Discontinue bevacizumab in clients with GI perforation. (2) **Surgery and wound healing complications.** The incidence of wound healing and surgical complications, including serious and fatal complications, is increased in bevacizumab-treated clients. Discontinue bevacizumab in clients with wound dehiscence. The appropriate interval between termination of bevacizumab and subsequent elective surgery required to reduce the risks of impaired wound healing/wound dehiscence has not been determined. Discontinue at least 28 days prior to elective surgery. Do not initiate bevacizumab for at least 28 days after surgery and until the surgical wound is fully healed. (3) **Hemorrhage.** Severe or fatal hemorrhage, including hemoptysis, GI bleeding, CNS hemorrhage, epistaxis, and vaginal bleeding, occurred up to 5-fold more frequently in clients receiving bevacizumab. Do not administer bevacizumab to clients with serious hemorrhage or recent hemoptysis.

- Safety in clients with clinically significant CV disease not adequately evaluated.
- There is the potential for immunogenicity.
- Use with caution in clients with known hypersensitivity to bevacizumab or any component of the drug product.
- Higher incidence of severe side effects in the elderly.
- There is an increased risk of serious arterial thromboembolic events, including CVA, cerebral infarction, MI, TIAs, angina, and fatal arterial thrombotic events in those receiving bevacizumab plus chemotherapy; risk factors include history of arterial thromboembolism before drug exposure and age 65 years and older.
- Safety and efficacy not evaluated in children.

SIDE EFFECTS

Most Common

Back pain, dry skin, URTI, asthenia, dyspnea, epistaxis, exfoliative dermatitis, headache, hypertension, lacrimation disorder, rectal hemorrhage, rhinitis, taste alteration, N&V, abdominal pain, anorexia, diarrhea, stomatitis.

Most serious: ***CHF, GI perforation, surgery and wound healing complications, serious and nonserious hemorrhagic events, arterial/venous thromboembolic events, thromboembolism, hypertensive crises, nephrotic syndrome, non-GI fistula formation*** (tracheoesophageal, bronchopleural, biliary, vagina, bladder). **Infusion reaction:** Hypertension, ***hypertensive crisis*** associated with neurologic signs and symptoms, wheezing, oxygen desaturation, ***grade 3 hypersensitivity,*** chest pain, headaches, rigors, diaphoresis. **GI:** Diarrhea, abdominal pain, anorexia, constipation, N&V, stomatitis, dyspepsia, flatulence, ***GI/large/small intestine hemorrhage,*** dry mouth, colitis, ileus, anastomotic ulceration, ***gastric ulcer hem-***

B

orrhage, intestinal necrosis, mesenteric venous occlusion, intestinal obstruction, fistula formation, gingival bleeding/pain, gingivitis, GERD, minor gum bleeding, mouth ulceration, tooth abscess, gastritis. **CV:** Hypertension, ***DVT, intra-abdominal thrombosis, MI, CVA, fatal arterial thrombotic events (e.g., cerebral infarction), thromboembolism, aneurysm,*** TIAs, CHF, angina, syncope, hypotension, cerebrovascular ischemia, traumatic hematoma. **Hematologic:** Leukopenia, neutropenia (with infection), febrile neutropenia, thrombocytopenia, pancytopenia. **CNS:** Dizziness, headache, confusion, abnormal gait, sensory neuropathy, ***CNS hemorrhage*.** **Respiratory:** Dyspnea, epistaxis, rhinitis, URTI, voice alteration, pneumonitis/pulmonary infiltrates, hemoptysis, nasal septum perforation, dysphonia, ***respiratory tract hemorrhage, pulmonary embolism/hypertension*.** **Dermatologic:** Alopecia, rash, dry skin, exfoliative dermatitis, nail disorder, skin discoloration, skin ulcer, desquamation. **Musculoskeletal:** Back/bone pain, myalgia. **GU:** Proteinuria, vaginal hemorrhage, urinary frequency/urgency, ureteral stricture, renal thrombotic microangiopathy. **Ophthalmic:** Lacrimation disorder, blurred vision. **Otic:** Tinnitus, deafness. **Body as a whole:** Asthenia, pain, weight loss, fatigue, weakness, dehydration, infection (with or without neutropenia), ***non-GI fistula formation*** (e.g., tracheoesophageal, bronchopleural, biliary, vaginal, renal, bladder). **Miscellaneous:** Taste disorder, polyserositis, impaired fertility, immunogenicity, reversible posterior leukoencephalopathy syndrome (headache, seizure, lethargy, confusion, blindness, visual and neurologic disturbances, mild to severe hypertension).

NOTE: Also listed previously are side effects when bevacizumab is used with other antineoplastic drugs.

LABORATORY TEST CONSIDERATIONS

Proteinuria, hypokalemia, bilirubinemia, albuminuria, hyponatremia.

DRUG INTERACTIONS

Bevacizumab with paclitaxel and carboplatin → significant ↓ paclitaxel exposure after 4 cycles of treatment

HOW SUPPLIED

Injection Solution, Concentrate: 25 mg/mL.

DOSAGE

IV INFUSION; IV INJECTION

Metastatic colon or rectal carcinoma.

Adults: 5 or 10 mg/kg once every 14 days in combination with IV 5-fluorouracil (5-FU). The recommended dose of bevacizumab when used in combination with IV 5-FU/leucovorin/oxaliplatin is 10 mg/kg. The recommended dose of bevacizumab when used in combination with bolus irinotecan/5-FU/leucovorin is 5 mg/kg. Give until disease progression is detected.

Metastatic HER2-negative breast cancer.

Adults: 10 mg/kg as an IV infusion every 14 days in combination with paclitaxel.

Non-squamous non-small-cell lung cancer.

Adults: 15 mg/kg as an IV infusion every 3 weeks in combination with carboplatin and paclitaxel.

Glioblastoma.

Adults: 10 mg/kg, as monotherapy, as an IV infusion q 2 weeks.

Metastatic renal cell carcinoma.

Adults: 10 mg/kg as an IV injection q 14 days in combination with interferon alfa.

NURSING IMPLICATIONS

IMPLEMENTATION/ADMINISTRATION/STORAGE

1. **IV** To prepare: Withdraw necessary amount of drug for a dose of 5 mg/kg; dilute in total volume of 100 mL 0.9% NaCl injection. Discard any unused portion; product contains no preservatives. Use aseptic technique.
2. Give only as IV infusion; do **not** give as IV push or bolus.
3. If first infusion (given over 90 min) is well tolerated, the second infusion may be given over 60 min. If the 60-min infusion is well tolerated, all subsequent infusions may be given over 30 min.
4. There are no dose reduction recommendations. If needed, discontinue or temporarily suspend bevacizumab therapy.
5. Permanently discontinue bevacizumab in those who develop GI perforation (fistula formation in the GI tract, intra-abdominal ab-

scess), fistula formation involving an internal organ, wound dehiscence and wound healing complications requiring medical intervention, serious hemorrhage (i.e., requiring medical intervention), nephrotic syndrome, a severe arterial thromboembolic event, hypertensive crisis, or hypertensive encephalopathy. Discontinue bevacizumab and begin treatment of hypertension, if present, in clients developing reversible posterior leukoencephalopathy.

6. Discontinue temporarily in those with evidence of moderate to severe proteinuria pending further evaluation and with severe infusion reactions, and with severe hypertension not controlled with medical management.
7. Suspend bevacizumab at least 28 days before elective surgery. Do not resume bevacizumab until surgical incision is fully healed (at least 28 days).
8. Refrigerate bevacizumab vials from 2–8°C (36–46°F). Diluted solutions for infusion may be stored at the same temperature as vials for up to 8 hr. Protect
9. COMPATIBILITY 0.9% NaCl.
10. INCOMPATIBILITY Dextrose solutions.

ASSESSMENT

1. Note reasons for therapy, disease onset, physical condition, extent of illness. Document clinical presentation and mental/cognitive status.
2. Drug impairs wound healing, may cause dehiscence and/or GI perforation and hemorrhage; monitor for abdominal pain, constipation, and vomiting. Assess wound/surgical site; discontinue drug with any complications.
3. Monitor BP weekly to ensure no drug-induced HTN. Stop if hypertensive crisis occurs.
4. Assess during infusion for evidence of reaction; interrupt infusion and treat symptoms.
5. Document cardio-pulmonary status; assess for ventricular dysfunction. Drug may induce/worsen CHF; stop infusion, monitor carefully.
6. Monitor those over 65 years for increased incidence of adverse effects.
7. Wait at least 28 days after major surgery ensuring that the incision is fully healed, to initiate therapy. Drug half-life is 20 days. If surgery planned in future, stop therapy at least 1 month before.
8. Assess for proteinuria; monitor serial urines for worsening proteinuria. Assess 24 hr urine; with 2+ protein readings, hold drug to prevent nephrotoxicity. Stop drug permanently with evidence of nephrotic syndrome.

CLIENT/FAMILY TEACHING

1. Used in combo therapy to treat cancer that has spread in the colon or rectum or for other cancers—some of which were unresponsive to other therapy; extremely powerful—can cause many side effects.
2. With any surgery, drug will impair wound healing and may also cause GI bleeding.
3. Monitor/record BP readings and urine dip tests for protein.
4. Practice barrier contraception; drug will harm fetus.
5. Once therapy stopped, drug may stay in system for up to a month or more.
6. Report constipation, abdominal pains, calf pain, SOB, chest pain, swelling of the face, lips, eyes, or tongue, wheezing, infusion site reactions, rash, opening of wound, bleeding, or any unusual side effects immediately.
7. Keep all F/U to prevent adverse outcome, monitor BP, and drug effects.

OUTCOMES/EVALUATE

- Inhibition of malignant cell proliferation
- Prevention of serious drug side effects

Bicalutamide

(**buy**-kah-**LOO**-tah-myd)

Classification(s): Antineoplastic, antiandrogen

Pregnancy Category: X

RX: Casodex.

SEE ALSO ***ANTINEOPLASTIC AGENTS.***

INDICATIONS/USES

Treatment of stage D2 metastatic prostate cancer in combination with a leutinizing hormone-releasing hormone analog.

ACTION/KINETICS

Action

Nonsteroidal antiandrogen that competitively inhibits the action of androgens by binding to cytosolic androgen receptors in target tissues. The drug increases bone mineral density and reduces fat accumulation when used as monotherapy.

B

Pharmacokinetics

Well absorbed after PO; food does not affect the rate or amount absorbed. Metabolized in the liver, and both parent drug and metabolites are eliminated in the urine and feces. **t½:** 5.8 days. **Mean steady-state concentration in prostatic cancer:** 8.9 mcg/mL. **Plasma protein binding:** 96%.

CONTRAINDICATIONS

Hypersensitivity to the drug or any components of the tablet. Pregnancy. Use in women.

SPECIAL CONCERNS

- **Use with caution with moderate to severe hepatic impairment and during lactation.**
- **Safety and efficacy not established in children.**

SIDE EFFECTS

Most Common

Hot flashes, generalized pain, back pain, asthenia, pelvic pain, constipation, nausea, diarrhea, dyspnea, infection, peripheral edema, nocturia, hematuria, abdominal pain, anemia, dizziness.

GI: Constipation, N&V, abdominal pain, diarrhea, anorexia, dyspepsia, ***rectal hemorrhage***, dry mouth, melena, flatulence, dysphagia, GI disorder, periodontal abscess, GI carcinoma, hepatotoxicity (e.g., ***hepatitis***). **CNS:** Dizziness, paresthesia, insomnia, anxiety, headache, depression, decreased libido, hypertonia, confusion, neuropathy, insomnia, somnolence, nervousness, paresthesia. **GU:** Gynecomastia, breast pain, nocturia, hematuria, UTI, impotence, urinary incontinence/frequency, impaired urination, dysuria, urinary retention/urgency, hydronephrosis, urinary tract disorder, inhibition of spermatogenesis. **CV:** Hot flashes (most common), hypertension, angina pectoris, CHF, ***MI, cardiac arrest,*** coronary artery disorder, syncope. **Metabolic:** Peripheral edema, hyperglycemia, weight loss or gain, dehydration, gout, edema. **Musculoskeletal:** Myasthenia, arthritis, myalgia, back/bone pain, leg cramps, pathologic fracture. **Respiratory:** Dyspnea, increased cough, pharyngitis, bronchitis, pneumonia, rhinitis, lung disorder, asthma, epistaxis, sinusitis, interstitial pneumonitis, ***pulmonary fibrosis***. **Dermatologic:** Rash, sweating, dry skin, pruritus, alopecia, herpes zoster, skin carcinoma, skin disorder. **Hematologic:** Anemia, hypochromic and iron deficiency anemia. **Hypersensitivity:** ***Angioneurotic edema***, urticaria. **Body as a whole:** General pain, asthenia, pelvic/abdominal/chest pain, flu syndrome, edema, neoplasm, fever, neck pain, chills, infection, ***sepsis.*** **Miscellaneous:** Bone pain, hernia, cyst, specified cataract, diabetes mellitus.

LABORATORY TEST CONSIDERATIONS

↑ Alkaline phosphatase, creatinine, AST, ALT, bilirubin, BUN, liver enzyme tests. ↓ Hemoglobin, white cell count, glucose tolerance (manifested as diabetes or loss of glycemic control in those with pre-existing diabetes).

DRUG INTERACTIONS

Bicalutamide may displace coumarin anticoagulants from their protein-binding sites, resulting in an increased anticoagulant effect.

HOW SUPPLIED

Tablets: 50 mg.

DOSAGE

TABLETS

Prostatic carcinoma.

Adults: 50 mg (1 tablet) once daily (morning or evening at the same time) in combination with an LHRH analog with or without food.

NURSING IMPLICATIONS

IMPLEMENTATION/ADMINISTRATION/STORAGE

1. Take at same time daily.
2. Start at same time as LHRH analog.

ASSESSMENT

1. Note reasons for therapy, onset/duration of symptoms, staging results, and other agents/therapies trialed.
2. If on warfarin, monitor PT/INR; can displace from protein binding sites.
3. Monitor renal and LFTs, CBC, PSA. Check ALT/AST at regular intervals for the first 4 mo, and periodically thereafter. If ALT/AST increase 2 times normal or jaundice develops, stop drug.

CLIENT/FAMILY TEACHING

1. Used to treat prostate cancer by blocking hormone release.
2. Males should take at same time each day; used with LHRH analog (i.e., goserelin implant or leuprolide depot).

3. Use caution until drug effects realized; may cause drowsiness.
4. Side effects requiring immediate attention: hemorrhage, urinary retention, yellow skin, fracture, respiratory distress, persistent/severe N&V/diarrhea. Also report abdominal pain, dark urine, RUQ tenderness, fatigue, "flu-like" symptoms, and loss of appetite.
5. May experience hot flashes, breast enlargement and pain; drug-related hair loss should regrow following therapy.
6. Keep F/U to assess response, labs, and for adverse SE.

OUTCOMES/EVALUATE

↓ PSA; inhibition of prostate cancer growth

Bisoprolol fumarate

(**BUY**-soh-**proh**-lol)

Classification(s): Beta-adrenergic blocking agent

Pregnancy Category: C

RX: Zebeta.

✱ Rx: Monocor.

SEE ALSO ***BETA-ADRENERGIC BLOCKING AGENTS.***

INDICATIONS/USES

Hypertension alone or in combination with other antihypertensive agents. *Investigational:* Angina pectoris, SVTs, PVCs.

ACTION/KINETICS

Action

Inhibits beta-1-adrenergic receptors and, at higher doses, beta-2 receptors. No intrinsic sympathomimetic activity and no membrane-stabilizing activity.

Pharmacokinetics

$t_{1/2}$: 9–12 hr. Over 90% of PO dose is absorbed. Approximately 50% is excreted unchanged through the urine and the remainder as inactive metabolites; a small amount (less than 2%) is excreted through the feces.

SPECIAL CONCERNS

- Due to selectivity for beta-1 receptors, use with caution in clients with bronchospastic disease who do not respond to, or who cannot tolerate, other antihypertensive therapy.
- Use with caution during lactation.
- Safety and efficacy not determined in children.

SIDE EFFECTS

Most Common

Dizziness, fatigue, headache, diarrhea, rhinitis, URTI, cough, peripheral edema.

See *Beta-Adrenergic Blocking Agents* for a complete list of possible side effects.

HOW SUPPLIED

Tablets: 5 mg, 10 mg.

DOSAGE

TABLETS

Antihypertensive.

Dose must be individualized. **Adults, initial:** 5 mg once daily (in some, 2.5 mg/day may be appropriate). **Maintenance:** If the 5 mg dose is inadequate, the dose may be increased to 10 mg/day and then, if needed, to 20 mg once daily. In impaired renal (C_{CR} <40 mL/min) or hepatic function (hepatitis or cirrhosis), initially give 2.5 mg with caution in titrating the dose upward.

NURSING IMPLICATIONS

Do not confuse bisoprolol with bitolterol (a sympathomimetic drug). Also, do not confuse Zebeta with DiaBeta (an oral hypoglycemic).

IMPLEMENTATION/ADMINISTRATION/STORAGE

1. Food does not affect bioavailability; may give without regard to meals.
2. Bisoprolol is not dialyzable; dose adjustments not required if undergoing hemodialysis.
3. Dosage adjustment not necessary in the elderly.
4. Store from 20–25°C (68–77°F); protect from moisture.

ASSESSMENT

1. Note reasons for therapy, previous agents used, outcome.
2. Once baseline parameters determined, monitor BP in both arms while lying, sitting, and standing. Assess for lower extremity edema and JVD.
3. Determine bronchospastic disease, heart failure, PVD; may preclude therapy.

B

4. Check ECG and CXR. Assess heart/lung sounds and note any arrhythmias.
5. Monitor CBC, glucose, electrolytes, renal and LFTs; reduce dose with dysfunction.

CLIENT/FAMILY TEACHING

1. Take as directed at same time with/without food.
2. Use caution; may cause dizziness/drowsiness. Change positions slowly to avoid sudden drop in low BP.
3. Avoid OTC drugs without approval.
4. With diabetes, monitor FS closely. Report weakness or fatigue; drug does block tachycardia but does not block dizziness and sweating as signs of hypoglycemia.
5. Report any breathing difficulty, or S&S of congestive heart failure or excessive bradycardia.
6. Keep log of BP and pulse for provider review. Do not stop drug suddenly after prolonged use, especially with coronary artery disease.
7. Report if impotence or decreased libido occur.
8. Keep all F/U to assess response, BP/HR, and for adverse SE.

OUTCOMES/EVALUATE

- ↓ BP
- Relief of angina (unlabeled use)
- Stable cardiac rhythm

Combination Drug

Bisoprolol fumarate and Hydrochlorothiazide

(**BUY**-soh-**proh**-lol, **hy**-droh-klor-oh-**THIGH**-ah-zyd)

Classification(s): Antihypertensive

Pregnancy Category: C

RX: Ziac.

SEE ALSO ***BISOPROLOL FUMARATE*** AND ***HYDROCHLOROTHIAZIDE***.

INDICATIONS/USES

First-line therapy for management of mild to moderate hypertension.

CONTENT

Ziac-2.5 mg/6.25 mg: Biosprolol fumarate *(beta-adrenergic blocking agent)*, 2.5 mg and hydrochlorothiazide *(thiazide diuretic)*, 6.25 mg. *Ziac-5 mg/6.25 mg*: Bisoprolol fumarate, 5 mg and hydrochlorothiazide, 6.25 mg. *Ziac-10 mg/6.25 mg:* Bisoprolol fumarate, 10 mg and hydrochlorothiazide, 6.25 mg.

ACTION/KINETICS

Action

Bisoprolol is a beta-1 selective adrenergic blocking drug with no significant membrane stabilizing or intrinsic sympathomimetic action. At higher doses, it also inhibits beta-2 adrenergic receptors located in bronchial and vascular musculature. Hydrochlorothiazide is a diuretic that increases excretion of sodium and chloride in approximately equal amounts. The antihypertensive effects are additive.

Pharmacokinetics

Both drugs are well absorbed; absorption is not affected whether the drug is taken with or without food. The bioavailability of bisoprolol is about 80% while the bioavailability of hydrochlorothiazide is 65–75%. **Peak plasma levels, bisoprolol:** 3 hr; **hydrochlorothiazide:** 2.5 hr. **t½, elimination, bisoprolol:** 7–15 hr; **hydrochlorothiazide:** 4–10 hr. About 50% of bisoprolol is excreted unchanged in the urine. Hydrochlorothiazide is excreted mainly in the urine. **Plasma protein binding:** About 30% of bisoprolol and 40–68% of hydrochlorothiazide are bound to plasma proteins.

CONTRAINDICATIONS

Use in cardiogenic shock, overt cardiac failure, second- or third-degree heart block, marked sinus bradycardia, anuria, hypersensitivity to either drug or to other sulfonamide-derived drugs. Lactation.

SPECIAL CONCERNS

- **Continued depression of the myocardium with beta-blockers may precipitate heart failure.**
- **Use with caution in peripheral vascular disease, in bronchospastic disease, and in those who do not respond to or tolerate other antihypertensive treatment.**
- **Safety and efficacy not determined in children.**

SIDE EFFECTS

Most Common

Cough, fatigue, dizziness, headache, myalgia, diarrhea.

See *Bisoprolol fumarate* and *Hydrochlorothiazide* for a complete list of possible side effects.

LABORATORY TEST CONSIDERATIONS
↑ Uric acid, serum triglycerides.

DRUG INTERACTIONS
See ***Bisoprolol fumarate*** and ***Hydrochlorothiazide***.

HOW SUPPLIED
See *Content.*

DOSAGE

TABLETS
Hypertension.

Initial: One 2.5/6.25 mg tablet once daily; dose may be increased q 14 days to a maximum of two 10/6.25 mg tablets once daily.

NURSING IMPLICATIONS

IMPLEMENTATION/ADMINISTRATION/STORAGE
Store from 20–25°C (68–77°F). Dispense in tight containers.

ASSESSMENT
1. List reasons for therapy, disease onset, other agents trialed, outcome.
2. Assess for sulfonamide sensitivity.
3. Determine any CAD, CHF, or lung disease.
4. Monitor ECG, electrolytes, Mg^{++}, renal and LFTs.

CLIENT/FAMILY TEACHING
1. Ziac is a combination of two drugs (beta blocker and diuretic) in one pill to better control BP.
2. May cause dizziness, use caution operating machinery until drug effects realized.
3. With diabetes, monitor FS closely; may mask low glucose symptoms.
4. Record BP and pulse; report any difficulty breathing, low heart rate, swelling of extremities or adverse effects.
5. Ensure adequate fluid intake to prevent dehydration.
6. Avoid exposure to UV light (sunlight, tanning booths) and use sunscreen when exposed to ↓ photosensitivity reaction.
7. Report if impotence or decreased libido experienced.
8. Keep all F/U to assess response, BP log, and for adverse SE.

OUTCOMES/EVALUATE
Control of BP

IV

Bivalirudin

(**by**-val-ih-**ROO**-din)

Classification(s): Anticoagulant, thrombin inhibitor

Pregnancy Category: B

RX: Angiomax.

SEE ALSO ***ANTICOAGULANTS.***

INDICATIONS/USES
(1) As an anticoagulant with aspirin in clients with unstable angina undergoing percutaneous transluminal coronary angioplasty (PTCA). (2) As an anticoagulant in those undergoing percutaneous coronary intervention. (3) Use for clients with, or at risk of, heparin-induced thrombocytopenia or heparin-induced thrombocytopenia and thrombosis syndrome who are undergoing percutaneous coronary intervention. *NOTE:* Aspirin is intended to be used concomitantly for all indications.

ACTION/KINETICS

Action
Direct-acting thrombin inhibitor by binding to both the catalytic site and to the anion-binding exosite of circulating and clot-bound thrombin. Binding to thrombin is reversible. When bound to thrombin, all effects of thrombin are inhibited, including activation of platelets, cleavage of fibrinogen, and activation of the positive amplification reactions of thrombin. Advantages over heparin include activity against clot-bound thrombin, more predictable anticoagulation, and no inhibition by components of the platelet release reaction.

Pharmacokinetics
t½, after IV: 25 min. t½ is increased in clients with renal impairment. Metabolized in the liver with about 20% excreted unchanged in the urine.

CONTRAINDICATIONS
Use in active major bleeding, cerebral aneurysm, intracranial hemorrhage. IM use.

B

SPECIAL CONCERNS

- Reduce dose in moderate to severe impaired renal function.
- Increased risk of hemorrhage with GI ulceration or hepatic disease.
- Hypertension may increase risk of cerebral hemorrhage.
- Use with caution following recent surgery or trauma and during lactation.
- Use with caution when bivalirudin is used as the antithrombin during brachytherapy procedures due to an increased risk of thrombus formation.
- Safety and efficacy not established when used with glycoprotein IIb/IIIa inhibitors, in clients with unstable angina who are not undergoing PTCA, in those with other acute coronary syndromes, or in children.
- Elderly clients may experience more bleeding events than younger clients.

SIDE EFFECTS

Most Common

N&V, back pain, pain, hypotension, hypertension, headache, pelvic pain, injection-site pain, insomnia, anxiety, bradycardia, abdominal pain, dyspepsia, fever, urinary retention, nervousness.

Bleeding: Major side effect is bleeding with possibility (infrequent) of ***major hemorrhage***, including ***fatal bleeding***, ***intracranial hemorrhage*** and ***retroperitoneal hemorrhage***. Most bleeding occurs at the site of arterial puncture; however, hemorrhage can occur at any site. **CV:** Hypo-/hypertension, bradycardia, syncope, vascular anomaly, angina pectoris, ***thrombus formation during PCI with and without intracoronary brachytherapy (may be fatal), ventricular fibrillation***. **GI:** N&V, dyspepsia, abdominal pain, dyspepsia. **CNS:** Headache, insomnia, anxiety, nervousness, cerebral ischemia, confusion, facial paralysis. **Dermatologic:** Hematoma, pain at injection site. **GU:** Urinary retention, kidney failure, oliguria. **Miscellaneous:** Back/pelvic/chest pain, injection site pain, fever, lung edema, infection, hypersensitivity/allergic reactions, ***sepsis***.

LABORATORY TEST CONSIDERATIONS

Prolongation of aPTT, activated clotting time, thrombin time, and PT.

OVERDOSE MANAGEMENT

Symptoms: Possible bleeding episodes. *Treatment:* Discontinue the drug and monitor closely for signs of bleed. No known antidote. Bivalirudin is hemodialyzable.

DRUG INTERACTIONS

Coadministration of bivalirudin with heparin, warfarin, thrombolytics, or GPIIb/IIIa inhibitors was associated with an increased risk of major bleeding events.

HOW SUPPLIED

Powder for Injection, Lyophilized: 250 mg/vial.

DOSAGE

IV ONLY

Percutaneous coronary intervention or percutaneous transluminal coronary angioplasty.

Adults: IV bolus dose of 0.75 mg/kg followed by an infusion of 1.75 mg/kg/hr for the duration of the PCI procedure. Five minutes after the bolus dose has been given, an activated clotting time should be performed and an additional bolus of 0.3 mg/kg should be given if needed. Continuation of the bivalirudin infusion following PCI for up to 4 hr postprocedure is optional. After 4 hr, an additional IV infusion may be initiated at a rate of 0.2 mg/kg/hr for up to 20 hr if needed. Use with aspirin (300–325 mg/day).

Clients with moderate renal impairment (C_{CR} of 30–59 mL/min) should receive 1.75 mg/kg/hr. If the C_{CR} is <30 mL/min, reduce the infusion rate to 1 mg/kg/hr. If the client is on hemodialysis, reduce the infusion to 0.25 mg/kg/hr. No reduction in the bolus dose is needed.

Heparin-induced thrombocytopenia or heparin-induced thrombocytopenia and thrombosis syndrome.

Adults: IV bolus of 0.75 mg/kg followed by a continuous infusion at a rate of 1.75 mg/kg/hr for the duration of the procedure.

NURSING IMPLICATIONS

IMPLEMENTATION/ADMINISTRATION/STORAGE

1. **IV Initiate just prior to PTCA.**

2. To reconstitute: Add 5 mL sterile water to each 250 mg vial; gently swirl until material dissolved. Each reconstituted vial is further diluted in 50 mL of D5W or 0.9% NaCl for final concentration of 5 mg/mL.
3. Adjust dose according to client weight.
4. If the low-rate infusion (i.e., 0.2 mg/kg/hr) is needed, reconstitute the 250 mg vial with 5 mL of sterile water and further dilute in 500 mL of D5W or 0.9% NaCl for a final concentration of 0.5 mg/mL.
5. Do not use if preparation contains particulate matter.
6. Do not freeze reconstituted or diluted drug.
7. Store reconstituted drug at 2–8°C (36–46°F) for up to 24 hr. Diluted drug (0.5–5 mg/mL) stable at room temperature for up to 24 hr.
8. COMPATIBILITY Sterile water, D5W, 0.9% NaCl.
9. INCOMPATIBILITY The following drugs resulted in haze formation, microparticulate formation, or gross precipitation: Alteplase, amiodarone HCl, amphotericin B, chlorpromazine HCl, diazepam, prochlorperazine edisylate, reteplase, streptokinase, and vancomycin HCl. Do not give in the same IV line with bivalirudin. Do not mix with any other medications before administration.

ASSESSMENT

1. Note reasons for/method of therapy: (bolus/infusion).
2. List history of cerebral aneurysm, intracranial hemorrhage, recent GI bleed or surgery. Assess carefully for any bleeding or hemorrhage at all access sites.
3. Monitor cardiac/neurologic status during therapy; report deficits.
4. Monitor weight, VS, ECG, CBC, bleeding parameters, renal and LFTs; reduce dose/infusion rate with renal dysfunction.

CLIENT/FAMILY TEACHING

1. Review procedure, and reasons for therapy during PTCA.
2. Report adverse effects or unusual bruising/bleeding, back pain, headache, nausea, or pain at the injection site. New onset SOB, chest pain, or edema warrant evaluation. Avoid aspirin or drugs used to treat swelling or pain (NSAIDs).
3. Incorporate lifestyle changes related to smoking cessation, alcohol reduction, diet and exercise into daily routine.
4. Avoid jostling or activities that may cause injury. Use electric razor, soft toothbrush, and nightlight to prevent injury.
5. Encourage family members to learn CPR.

OUTCOMES/EVALUATE

Anticoagulation during angioplasty

IV

Bleomycin sulfate (BLM)

(blee-oh-**MY**-sin)

Classification(s): Antineoplastic, antibiotic

Pregnancy Category: D

SEE ALSO ***ANTINEOPLASTIC AGENTS.***

INDICATIONS/USES

Palliative treatment of cancers listed, either used alone or in combination. (1) Squamous cell carcinoma of the head and neck, including mouth, tongue, tonsil, nasopharynx, oropharynx, sinus, palate, lip, buccal mucosa, gingiva, epiglottis, skin, and larynx. Carcinoma of the penis, cervix, and vulva. (2) Lymphomas, including Hodgkin's and non-Hodgkin's either alone or with other antineoplastic drugs. (3) Testicular carcinoma, including embryonal cell, choriocarcinoma, and teratocarcinoma either alone or with other antineoplastic drugs. (4) Sclerosing agent to prevent or treat malignant pleural effusions associated with cancer. *Investigational:* Malignant peritoneal effusion, malignant pericardial effusion, warts (intralesional use). Also, treatment of mycosis fungoides; osteosarcoma; AIDS-related Kaposi sarcoma. In children for palliative treatment of lymphomas; testicular carcinoma; germ cell tumors; sclerosis of pleural effusions.

ACTION/KINETICS

Action

Mixture of cytotoxic glycopeptide antibiotics that likely inhibit DNA synthesis with less inhibition of RNA and protein synthesis. Causes single- and, to a lesser extent, double-stranded DNA breaks. In vitro studies indicate bleomycin causes cell cycle arrest in G2 and in mitoris. Relatively low bone marrow depressant activity; localizes in cer-

B

tain tissues. Is an important component of some combination regimens.

Pharmacokinetics

Rapidly absorbed afer IM, SC, IP, or intrapleural administration; **peak plasma levels:** 30–60 min. Bioavailability is 100% and 70% after IM and SC administration, respectively and is 45% following both IP and intrapleural use, compared with IV administration. **Peak plasma levels** (after 4–5 days of therapy): 50 ng/mL. Metabolized by many body tissues. **t½, elimination, after IV bolus:** 1–2 hr. Excreted mainly in the urine. Renal insufficiency markedly alters elimination; in clients with a C_{CR} <35 mL/min, the plasma or serum t½ elimination increases exponentially as the C_{CR} decreases. Children less than 3 years of age have a higher total body clearance than adults following IV bolus administration.

CONTRAINDICATIONS

Hypersensitivity or idiosyncratic reactions to bleomycin. Lactation. Renal or pulmonary diseases. Pregnancy.

SPECIAL CONCERNS

(1) It is recommended that bleomycin be administered under the supervision of a qualified physician experienced in the use of cancer chemotherapeutic drugs. Appropriate management of therapy and complications is possible only when adequate diagnostic and treatment facilities are readily available. (2) **Pulmonary fibrosis.** Pulmonary fibrosis is the most severe toxicity associated with bleomycin. The more frequent presentation is pneumonitis that may progress to fibrosis. Its occurrence is higher in geriatric clients and in those receiving >400 units total dose, but toxicity has occurred in young clients and in those treated with low doses. (3) **Idiosyncratic reaction.** A severe idiosyncratic reaction consisting of hypotension, mental confusion, fever, chills, and wheezing has been reported in about 1% of lymphoma clients treated with bleomycin.

- **Pulmonary toxicity may occur at lower doses when used in combination with other antineoplastic drugs.**
- **Use great caution if giving total doses greater than 400 units.**
- **Use with extreme caution in significantly impaired renal function.**
- **Safety and efficacy not determined in children.**

SIDE EFFECTS

Most Common

Pneumonitis, fever, chills, photosensitivity, N&V, weight loss, erythema, skin rash, darkening/thickening of skin, striae, vesiculation, skin tenderness, swollen fingers, changes in fingernails/toenails, colored bumps on fingertips/elbows/palms.

Pulmonary: Pneumonitis, ***pulmonary fibrosis,*** especially in older clients, acute chest pain syndrome, pain after intrapleural administration. **Hypersensitivity/Idiosyncratic reactions:** Hypotension, fever, chills, mental confusion, and wheezing in about 1% of lymphoma clients. **Integumentary and mucous membranes:** Erythema, rash, striae, vesiculation, hyperpigmentation, skin tenderness, hyperkeratosis, alopecia, pruritus, stomatitis, skin toxicity, darkening/thickening of skin, swollen fingers, changes in fingernails/toenails, colored bumps on fingertips/elbows/palms, scleroderma-like skin changes. **GI:** N&V, anorexia, weight loss. **Body as a whole:** Chills, fever, vomiting, anorexia, weight loss that may persist long after termination of the drug, phlebitis, malaise, photosensitivity. **Miscellaneous:** Renal and hepatic toxicity, pain at tumor site.

NOTE: Use of bleomycin in combination with other antineoplastics may result in vascular toxicities, including cerebral arteritis, ***CVA, MI,*** thrombotic microangiopathy, Raynaud phenomenon, hypotension.

DRUG INTERACTIONS

Cisplatin / ↓ Bleomycin elimination → ↑ toxicity R/T cisplatin-induced renal dysfunction; use together with caution and monitor renal function
Digoxin / ↓ Digoxin levels; monitor for signs of ↓ pharmacologic effect
Oxygen / ↑ Risk for pulmonary toxicity
Phenytoin / ↓ Phenytoin levels; monitor phenytoin levels and adjust dose if necessary

HOW SUPPLIED

Powder for Injection: 15 units, 30 units.

DOSAGE

IM; IV; SC

Squamous cell carcinoma, testicular carcinoma.

0.25–0.5 units/kg (10–20 units/m²) IV, IM, or SC once or twice a week.

Lymphoma, Hodgkin's or non-Hodgkin's disease.

Adults, initial: Due to the possibility of anaphylaxis, give 2 units or less for the first two doses; if no acute reaction occurs, follow the regular dosage schedule. **Maintenance:** 0.25–0.5 units/kg (10–20 units/m^2) IV, IM, or SC once or twice weekly. After a 50% response, give 1 unit/day or 5 units/week IM or IV.

INTRAPLEURAL INJECTION

Malignant pleural effusion.

Adults: 60 units given as a single bolus dose by a thoracostomy tube following drainage of excess pleural fluid and confirmation of complete lung expansion.

NURSING IMPLICATIONS

IMPLEMENTATION/ADMINISTRATION/STORAGE

1. For IM or SC use: Reconstitute drug with 1–5 mL (15-unit vial) or 2–10 mL (30-unit vial) 0.9% NaCl injection, sterile water for injection, or bacteriostatic water for injection.
2. For intrapleural use: Dissolve 60 units in 50–100 mL of 0.9% NaCl injection and give through a thoracostomy tube following drainage of excess pleural fluid and confirmation of complete lung expansion. Drainage from chest tube should be as minimal as possible before instillation of bleomycin. Clamp thoracostomy tube after instillation. Move from supine to left and right lateral positions several times during the next 4 hr, followed by removal of the clamp to reestablish suction.
3. Hodgkin's disease and testicular tumors should respond within 2 weeks; squamous cell cancers require at least 3 weeks.
4. Bleomycin in NaCl is stable for 24 hr at room temperature (14 days if refrigerated).
5. If extravasation occurs, phlebitis may result. If signs or symptoms of extravasation occur, stop the infusion immediately. If possible, withdraw 3–5 mL of blood to remove some of the drug. Remove the infusion needle. Delineate the infiltrated area on the skin with a felt-tip marker. Elevate for 48 hr above the heart level using a sling or stockinette dressing with a window for observation. Avoid pressure or friction; do not rub the area. After 48 hr, the client should use the extremity normally to promote full range of motion.
6. Adjust the dose as follows in impaired renal function: C_{CR}, 50 mL/min or >: Give 100% of the dose; C_{CR}, 40–50 mL/min: 70% of the dose; C_{CR}, 30–40 mL/min: 60% of the dose; C_{CR}, 20–30 mL/min: 55% of the dose; C_{CR}, 10–20 mL/min: 45% of the dose; C_{CR}, 5–10 mL/min: 40% of the dose.
7. **IV** For IV use: Reconstitute contents of 15- or 30-unit vial with 5 or 10 mL, respectively, of 0.9% NaCl injection. Administer IV slowly over 10 min. The sterile powder is stable if stored from 2–8°C (36–46°F).
8. COMPATIBILITY 0.9% NaCl.
9. INCOMPATIBILITY Do not reconstitute with D5W or other dextrose-containing solutions.

ASSESSMENT

1. Note reason for therapy, onset, symptom characteristics, method of administration, other agents/therapies trialed.
2. Assess/monitor for basilar crackles, cough, dyspnea, and tachypnea; dose-related symptoms of pulmonary toxicity.
3. Document total cumulative dose; risk of pulmonary toxicity significantly increased with dosing beyond 400 units.
4. Obtain CXR every 1 to 2 weeks during therapy to monitor for pulmonary toxicity. If changes noted stop therapy until changes are decided if drug related. Ensure DLCO (diffusion capacity for carbon monoxide) determined before starting therapy and then monthly during treatment. Stop therapy if DLCO falls below 30% to 35% of pretreatment value.
5. Note and avoid adhesive on the skin; drug accumulates in keratin and may discolor epithelium.
6. Clients with lymphoma may initially receive two test doses of 2 units each to assess for idiosyncratic response.
7. Follow institutional and NIH procedures for handling, administration, and disposal of anticancer drugs. Wear appropriate protective equipment when preparing and administering bleomycin. Avoid exposure by direct contact of the skin, mucous membranes, and eyes.
8. If accidental skin or mucous membrane contact occurs, wash thoroughly with soap and water. If accidental eye contact occurs, imme-

diately institute standard irrigation techniques.

9. May cause mild granulocyte suppression. Nadir: 10 days; recovery: 14 days.
10. Obtain baseline CXR, VS, CBC, LFTs, and PFTs. If receiving digoxin or dilantin, monitor levels.

CLIENT/FAMILY TEACHING

1. Administered IV or IM in the management of certain neoplastic conditions.
2. Report S&S of idiosyncratic reaction (hypoxia, fever, chills, confusion); *may occur with lymphoma.*
3. Fever 3–6 hr after treatment is common; may use acetaminophen. Avoid aspirin or ibuprofen type of analgesics—may cause bleeding. Use soft bristled toothbrush and electric razor.
4. Avoid live vaccinations during therapy.
5. Practice safe, reliable contraception. Do not breast-feed during therapy.
6. Report abnormal mouth/skin rashes, hives, or side effects; may lose hair but should regrow once therapy completed. Chest pain, difficulty breathing/SOB, fever, chills, all require reporting.
7. Persistent nausea, vomiting, or appetite loss as well as worsening general body weakness, skin/nail changes require reporting.
8. Smoking may aggravate pulmonary symptoms. Report changes in breathing or increased coughing.
9. Keep all F/U to assess response, labs, x-rays, breathing tests, and for adverse SE.

OUTCOMES/EVALUATE

- ↓ Tumor size/spread
- Prevention/control of malignant pleural effusion

Boceprevir

(boe-**SE**-pre-vir)

Classification(s): Antiviral drug
Pregnancy Category: X
RX: Victrelis.

INDICATIONS/USES

Treatment of chronic hepatitis C virus genotype 1 infection, in combination with peginterferon alfa and ribavirin in adults (18 years and older) with compensated liver disease, including cirrhosis, who are previously untreated or who have failed previous interferon and ribavirin therapy.

ACTION/KINETICS

Action

Boceprevir is a direct-acting antiviral drug that inhibits a protease that is required for the proteolytic cleavage of the HCV encoded polyprotein into mature forms of certain proteins. The drug covalently binds to the NS3 protease active site serine through and alpha-ketoamide functional group to inhibit viral replication in HCV-infected cells.

Pharmacokinetics

T_{max}: 2 hr. Steady state achieved after about 1 day of 3-times daily dosing. Should be administered with food which enhances exposure up to 54% of the 800 mg 3 times/day dosing schedule. Is metabolized in the liver; excreted in both the feces (8%) and urine (3%). **t½, plasma:** About 3.4 hr. **Plasma protein binding:** About 75%.

CONTRAINDICATIONS

Pregnant women and men whose female partners are pregnant. Coadministration with drugs that are highly dependent on CYP3A4/5 for clearance, including alfuzosin, drospirenone, ergot derivatives (e.g., dihydroergotamine, ergonovine, ergotamine, methylergonovine), cisapride, lovastatin, midazolam (oral), phosphodiesterase 5 enzyme inhibitors (e.g., sildenafil, tadalafil when used to treat pulmonary arterial hypertension), pimozide, simvastatin, and triazolam. Coadministration with CYP3A4/5 inducers, including anticonvulsants (e.g., carbamazepine, phenobarbital, phenytoin), rifampin, and St. John's wort. Lactation.

SPECIAL CONCERNS

- Safety and efficacy not established for use of boceprevir alone or with peginterferon alfa and ribavirin to treat chronic hepatitis C genotype 1 infection in clients coinfected with HIV and HCV or hepatitis B virus and HCV, or in liver or other organ transplant recipients.
- Use caution when administering and monitoring in the elderly due to greater frequency of decreased hepatic function, other diseases, and other drug therapy.
- Safety and efficacy not determined in children.

SIDE EFFECTS

Most Common

Anemia, chills, fatigue, diarrhea, dysgeusia, headache, insomnia, irritability, nausea.

Side effects listed include those when boceprevir is combined with peginterferon alfa and ribavirin. Also see *Side Effects* for *Peginterferon alfa–2a* and *2b,* and *Ribavirin.* **GI:** N&V, dysgeusia, diarrhea, dry mouth. **CNS:** Headache, dizziness, insomnia, irritability. **CV:** Thromboembolic events. **Dermatologic:** Alopecia, dry skin, rash. **Musculoskeletal:** Arthralgia. **Respiratory:** Exertional dyspnea. **Hematologic:** Anemia, neutropenia. **Body as a whole:** Fatigue, asthenia, chills. **Miscellaneous:** Decreased appetite.

LABORATORY TEST CONSIDERATIONS

↓ Hemoglobin, neutrophils, platelets.

DRUG INTERACTIONS

Alpha-1 adrenoreceptor antagonists (e.g., alfuzosin) / ↑ Alfuzosin levels → ↑ pharmacologic/toxic (e.g., hypotension) effects; coadministration with alfuzosin contraindicated
Antiarrhythmic agents (e.g., amiodarone, bepridil, flecainide, propafenone, quinidine) / ↑ Antiarrhythmic agent levels → ↑ risk of serious and/or life–threatening side effects; use together with caution; monitor levels
Antidepressants (e.g., desipramine, trazodone) / ↑ Plasma levels of desipramine and trazodone → ↑ risk of side effects (e.g., hypotension, syncope); use together with caution and consider a lower dose of antidepressant
Benzodiazepines (e.g., alprazolam, midazolam, triazolam) / ↑ Risk of prolonged sedation or respiratory depression; coadministration with PO midazolam or triazolam contraindicated; monitor for respiratory depression and/or prolonged sedation if used with alprazolam and IV midazolam
Bosentan / ↑ Bosentan concentrations; coadminister with caution and monitor
Calcium channel blockers, dihydropyridine type (e.g., felodipine, nifedipine, nicardipine) / ↑ Concentration of dihydropyridine calcium channel blocker; use together with caution and monitor
Carbamazepine / ↓ Boceprevir concentrations → ↓ virologic response; coadministration contraindicated
Cisapride / ↑ Risk of cardiac arrhythmias; coadministration contraindicated
Clarithromycin / ↑ Clarithromycin levels; coadministration contraindicated
Colchicine / Clinically important ↑ colchicine levels; fatal colchicine toxicity seen with other strong CYP3A4 inhibitors; do not coadminister in those with hepatic/renal impairment. See ***Implementation/Administration/Storage*** boceprevir/colchicine dosing recommendations
Contraceptives, hormonal (e.g., drospirenone, ethinyl estradiol) / ↑ Risk of hypokalemia if given with drospirenone; coadministration contraindicated; ↓ ethinyl estradiol levels → ↓ contraceptive effectiveness; use two alternative contraceptive treatment methods during ribavirin treatment
Corticosteroids, systemic / ↓ Boceprevir levels → ↓ effect; if coadministration necessary, use with caution; also inhaled corticosteroid levels may be ↑. Avoid coadministration especially for extended durations
Digoxin / ↑ Digoxin serum levels; start digoxin therapy with the lowest dose with careful titration and monitoring
Ergot derivatives (e.g., dihydroergotamine, ergonovine, ergotamine, methylergonovine) / ↑ Risk of acute ergot toxicity (i.e., peripheral vasospasm and ischemia of extremities); coadministration contraindicated
HMG–CoA reductase inhibitors (e.g., atorvastatin, lovastatin, simvastatin) / ↑ Risk of myopathy, including rhabdomyolysis; do not exceed a max dose of atorvastatin 20 mg daily; coadministration with lovastatin or simvastatin contraindicated
Immunosuppressants (e.g., cyclosporine, sirolimus, tacrolimus) / Significant ↑ immunosuppressant plasma levels; closely monitor immunosuppressant blood levels
Itraconazole / ↑ Levels of both boceprevir and itraconazole; do not exceed a dose of itraconazole, 200 mg
Ketoconazole / ↑ Levels of both boceprevir and ketoconazole; do not exceed a dose of ketoconazole, 200 mg
Narcotic analgesics (e.g., buprenorphine, methadone) / Plasma levels of buprenorphine or morphine may be ↑ or ↓; closely monitor clinical response and adjust dose of narcotic as needed
Nonnucleoside reverse transcriptase inhibitors (e.g., efavirenz) / ↓ Boceprevir tough levels → loss of therapeutic effect; avoid coadministration
Phenobarbital / ↓ Boceprevir concentrations → ↓ virologic response; coadministration contraindicated
Phenytoin / ↓ Boceprevir concentrations → ↓ virologic response; coadministration contraindicated

B

Pimozide / ↑ Risk of cardiac arrhythmias; coadministration contraindicated
Posaconazole / ↑ Levels of both boceprevir and posaconazole
Protease inhibitors (e.g., ribavirin) / ↓ Boceprevir levels; effect on protease inhibitor levels unknown
Rifamycins (rifabutin, rifampin) / ↓ Boceprevir levels and ↑ rifabutin levels; coadministration with rifampin contraindicated while coadministration with rifabutin is not recommended
Salmeterol / ↑ Risk of salmeterol CV effects; coadministration not recommended
Sildenafil / ↑ Risk of visual abnormalities, hypotension, prolonged erection, and syncope when used to treat pulmonary arterial hypertension; coadministration contraindicated; when used to treat erectile dysfunction, use with caution and monitor for side effects - do not exceed a dose of 25 mg q 48 hr.
H ***St. John's wort*** / ↓ Boceprevir levels → ↓ virologic response; coadministration contraindicated
Tadalafil / ↑ Risk of visual abnormalities, hypotension, prolonged erection, and syncope when used to treat pulmonary arterial hypertension; coadministration contraindicated; when used to treat erectile dysfunction, use with caution and monitor for side effects - do not exceed a dose of 10 mg q 72 hr
Vardenafil / When used to treat erectile dysfunction, use with caution and monitor for side effects - do not exceed a dose of 2.5 mg q 24 hr
Voraconazole / ↑ Levels of both boceprevir and voraconazole
Warfarin / ↑ or ↓ Warfarin concentrations; monitor INR and adjust warfarin dose as needed

HOW SUPPLIED

Capsules: 200 mg.

DOSAGE

CAPSULES

Chronic hepatitis C.

Adults (18 years and older), usual: 800 mg (4 × 200 mg capsules) 3 times a day (q 7–9 hr) after 4 weeks of peginterferon alfa and ribavirin treatment. **Duration of treatment:** 44 weeks for clients with cirrhosis. For clients without cirrhosis: (1) Previously untreated clients, undectable HCV–RNA at both week 8 and week 24 or treatment: Complete 3-drug (boceprevir, ribavirin, peginterferon alfa) regimens at treatment week 28. (2) Previously untreated clients, detectable HCV-RNA at week 8 but not week 24: Continue all 3 drugs and finish through treatment week 36; **then,** administer peginterferon alfa and ribavirin and finish through treatment week 48. (3) Previous partial responders or relapsers, undetectable HCV-RNA at both week 8 and week 24: Complete 3 drug regimen at treatment week 36. (4) Previous partial responders or relapsers, detectable HCV–RNA at week 8 but not week 24: Continue all 3 drugs and finish through treatment week 26; **then,** administer peginterferon alfa and ribavirin and finish through treatment week 48.

NURSING IMPLICATIONS

IMPLEMENTATION/ADMINISTRATION/STORAGE

1. Discontinuation of therapy is recommended in all clients with HCV-RNA levels of 100 units/mL or higher at treatment week 12 or confirmed detectable HCV-RNA levels at treatment week 24.
2. If a dose is missed and it is less than 2 hr before the next dose is due, skip the missed dose. If a dose is missed and it is 2 or more hr before the next dose is due, take the missed dose with food and resume the normal dosing schedule.
3. Dose reduction of boceprevir is not recommended. If a client has a serious side effect potentially related to peginterferon alfa and/or ribavirin, reduce the dose of or discontinue peginterferon alfa and/or ribavirin.
4. Administer with food or a light meal/snack. Administer concurrently with peginterferon alfa and ribavirin.
5. Store from 2–8°C (36–46°F). Avoid exposure to excessive heat. May be stored at room temperature for 3 months.

ASSESSMENT

1. Note disease onset, HCV genotype (1), if previously treated with interferon and ribavirin and failed therapy, or untreated with compensated liver disease.
2. List drugs prescribed to ensure none interact.

3. Confirm not pregnant and partners of males taking therapy use reliable contraception due to effects on fetus.
4. Monitor VS, HCV-RNA levels and CBC at weeks 4, 8, 12, and 24, and at the end of treatment.

CLIENT/FAMILY TEACHING

1. Take with interferon and ribavirin as directed; do not take alone.
2. Total daily dose of boceprevir is packaged into a single bottle containing 12 capsules; generally advised to take 4 capsules 3 times daily with food.
3. May experience fatigue, headaches, nausea, and taste changes; report if persistent or bothersome.
4. Females must use two forms of contraception during and for 6 months following therapy, Additionally, client will require a pregnancy test monthly during therapy and for 6 months following therapy. If pregnancy occurs, contact the Ribavirin Pregnancy Registry by calling 1-800-593-2214 for tracking outcome effects. Males receiving therapy must use reliable contraception as should female partners of childbearing age due to teratogenic fetal effects.
5. Review risks and S&S as anemia and neutropenia may be increased when boceprevir is administered with peginterferon alfa and ribavirin.
6. Keep all F/U to assess response, for labs (4, 8, 12 weeks) to determine continuation of therapy, and adverse SE.

OUTCOMES/EVALUATE

Inhibition of HCV replication

IV

Bortezomib

(bor-**TEZ**-oh-mib)

Classification(s): Antineoplastic, proteasome inhibitor

Pregnancy Category: D

RX: Velcade.

SEE ALSO ***ANTINEOPLASTIC AGENTS***.

INDICATIONS/USES

(1) Multiple myeloma. (2) Mantle cell lymphoma in those who have received at least one prior therapy. *Investigational:* Myelomatous pleural effusion.

ACTION/KINETICS

Action

A reversible inhibitor of the chymotrypsin-like activity of the 26S proteasome (large protein that degrades ubiquitinated proteins) in mammalian cells. The ubiquitin-proteasome pathway plays an essential role in regulating the intracellular concentration of specific proteins, thus maintaining homeostasis within cells. Inhibition of the 26S proteasome affects multiple signaling cascades within the cell. This disruption of normal homeostasis can lead to cell death. Bortezomib causes a delay in tumor growth in multiple myeloma clients.

Pharmacokinetics

Primarily metabolized mainly by CYP3A4, 2C19, and 1A2 with CYP2D6 and 2C9 playing a minor role; the major metabolic pathway is deboronation. **t½, elimination:** 40–193 hr after the 1 mg/m^2 dose and 76–108 hr after the 1.3 mg/m^2 dose. The elderly have higher AUC and C_{max} than those younger than 65 years of age. **Plasma protein binding:** Average of 83% over the concentration range of 100 to 1,000 ng/mL.

CONTRAINDICATIONS

Hypersensitivity to the drug, boron, or mannitol. Lactation.

SPECIAL CONCERNS

- Use with caution and closely monitor in impaired hepatic and renal function.
- Elderly may manifest greater sensitivity to the drug.
- Safety and efficacy not determined in children.

SIDE EFFECTS

Most Common

Asthenic conditions, dizziness, lightheadedness, peripheral neuropathy, hypotension, N&V, anorexia, diarrhea, constipation, malaise, weakness, blurred vision, cough, insomnia, pyrexia, psychiatric disorders, thrombocytopenia, dysesthesia, paresthesia, anemia, headache, injection site irritation.

GI: N&V, abdominal pain (including upper), diarrhea, decreased appetite, anorexia, constipation, dyspepsia, dysgeusia, ascites, dysphagia, fecal impaction, stomatitis, ***hemorrhagic gastritis/duo-***

B

denitis, GI hemorrhage, hematemesis, paralytic ileus, small/large intestine obstruction, paralytic intestinal obstruction, large intestine obstruction/perforation, stomatitis, melena, ***acute pancreatitis,*** gastroenteritis, gastroesophageal reflux, hematemesis, paralytic ileus, oral mucosal petechiae, peritonitis, oral candidiasis, ischemic colitis. **Hepatic:** Hepatitis, cholestasis, ***hepatic hemorrhage***, portal vein thrombosis, ***acute liver failure***. **CNS:** Asthenic conditions (fatigue, malaise, weakness), peripheral neuropathy (both sensory and motor, including symptoms of burning sensation, hyperesthesia, hypesthesia, paresthesia, discomfort, neuropathic pain, weakness), dysesthesia, cranial palsy, headache, insomnia, dizziness (including vertigo), anxiety, ataxia, coma, dizziness, agitation, lightheadedness, confusion, psychiatric disorders, ***suicidal ideation,*** dysarthria, dysautonomia, encephalopathy, ***generalized tonic-clonic seizures,*** mental status change, motor dysfunction, neuralgia, paralysis, postherpetic neuralgia, spinal cord compression, psychotic disorder, vertigo. **CV:** Hypotension, aggravated atrial fibrillation/flutter, hypertension, atrial flutter, angina pectoris, atrial fibrillation, bradycardia, cardiac amyloidosis, ***cardiac arrest, CHF, GI and intracerebral hemorrhage, CVA, MI, pulmonary embolism, DIC, complete AV block, hemorrhagic stroke,*** DVT, myocardial ischemia, pericardial effusion, pericarditis, peripheral embolism, subdural hematoma, phlebitis, ***pulmonary embolism***, pulmonary edema/hypertension, sinus arrest, ***torsades de pointes,*** TIA, ventricular tachycardia, subdural hematoma, cardiac tamponade, pulmonary hypertension (in the absence of left heart failure or significant pulmonary disease); acute development of or exacerbation of CHF and/or new onset of decreased left ventricular ejection fraction. **Hematologic:** Thrombocytopenia, anemia, neutropenia, ***disseminated intravascular coagulation***, leukopenia, lymphopenia. **Hypersensitivity: *Anaphylaxis,*** angioedema, drug hypersensitivity, immune complex-mediated hypersensitivity, ***toxic epidermal necrolysis***. **Musculoskeletal:** Arthralgia, back/bone pain, muscle cramps, myalgia, pain in extremity, skeletal fracture. **Respiratory:** Dyspnea, bronchitis, URTI, lower RTI, lung infections, cough, pneumonia, nasopharyngitis, ***acute respiratory distress syndrome,*** interstitial pneumonia, lung infiltration, aspiration pneumonia, atelectasis, worsening COPD, exertional dyspnea, epistaxis, hemoptysis, hypoxia, lung infiltration, pleural effusion, pneumonitis, respiratory distress, sinusitis, ***laryngeal edema, respiratory failure,*** exacerbated chronic obstructive airways disease, acute diffuse infiltrative pulmonary disease (rare). **GU:** Renal calculus, bilateral hydronephrosis, bladder spasm, hematuria, urinary incontinence, urinary retention, acute/chronic renal failure, proliferative glomerular nephritis, hemorrhagic cystitis, UTI. **Dermatologic:** Pruritus, rash, urticaria, leukocytoclastic vasculitis, ***toxic epidermal necrolysis***. **Ophthalmic:** Blurred vision, conjunctival infection, diplopia, eye irritation, ophthalmic herpes. **Otic:** Impaired hearing, bilateral deafness. **Metabolic:** Hypo-/hyperglycemia, dehydration. **Injection site:** Injection site irritation/erythema/pain, phlebitis, catheter-related complication/infection. **Body as a whole:** Fatigue, malaise, weakness, peripheral/lower limb edema, herpes zoster, herpes virus infection, pyrexia, rigors, ***septic shock,*** toxoplasmosis, reactivation of herpes virus infection, tumor lysis syndrome. **Miscellaneous:** Pain in limb, edema in lower limb/face, bacteremia, aspergillosis, listeriosis, herpes meningoencephalitis. Rarely, reversible posterior leukoencephalopathy syndrome, including symptoms of seizures, hypertension, headache, lethargy, confusion, blindness, and other visual/neurological symptoms.

LABORATORY TEST CONSIDERATIONS

↑ Liver enzymes. Hyperbilirubinemia, hyper-/hypokalemia, hyper-/hyponatremia, hyperuricemia, hyper-/hypocalcemia.

OVERDOSE MANAGEMENT

Symptoms: Acute onset of symptomatic hypotension and thrombocytopenia with possible fatal outcomes. *Treatment:* There is no specific antidote. Monitor vital signs and give appropriate supportive care.

DRUG INTERACTIONS

Antihypertensives / Possible potentiation of hypotension; adjust antihypertensive dose as needed
Cyclosporine / ↑ Neurotoxicity of cyclosporine; monitor closely
CYP3A4 inhibitors or inducers / Closely monitor for toxicity or reduced efficacy when bortezomib is coadministered with drugs that are inducers or inhibitors of cytochrome CYP3A4

CYP2A19 substrates / Inhibition of 2C19 isoenzyme activity → ↑ exposure to drugs that are substrates for this isoenzyme
Hypoglycemics, oral / Possible hypo- or hyperglycemia; monitor blood glucose levels closely
Ketoconazole / ↑ Bortezomib AUC by 35%; closely monitor and adjust dose as needed
Melphalan & Prednisolone / ↑ Bortezomib AUC by 17%; not likely to be clinically relevant
Ritonavir / ↑ Bortezomib plasma levels → ↑ possible toxicity R/T inhibition of metabolism; monitor closely

HOW SUPPLIED

Injection, Lyophilized Powder for Solution: 3.5 mg.

DOSAGE

IV BOLUS

Multiple myeloma, previously untreated.

Adults: Bortezomib, 1.3 mg/m^2/dose, given as a 3- to 5-second IV bolus injection in combination with melphalan, 9 mg/m^2/dose, and PO prednisone, 60 mg/m^2/dose, for nine 6-week treatments. In cycles (one cycle is 6 weeks in length) 1 through 4, bortezomib is given twice weekly (days 1, 4, 8, 11, 22, 25, 29, and 32). In cycles 5 through 9, bortezomib is given once a week (days 1, 8, 22, and 29). Note there are rest periods during weeks 3 and 6 for all nine cycles. At least 72 hr should elapse between consecutive doses. For all nine cycles, melphalan and prednisone are given on days 1 through 4 of week 1. *NOTE:* The amount of bortezomib in one vial (3.5 mg) may exceed the usual single dose needed. To prevent overdose, use caution in calculating the dose.

Multiple myeloma, relapsed.

See dosing for *Mantle cell lymphoma.*

Mantle cell lymphoma.

Adults: Bortezomib, 1.3 mg/m^2/dose given as a 3- to 5-second IV bolus twice a week for 2 weeks (days 1, 4, 8, and 11) followed by a 10-day rest period (days 12 to 21). For extended therapy of more than 8 cycles, give bortezomib on the standard schedule or on a maintenance schedule of once a week for 4 weeks (days 1, 8, 15, and 22) followed by a 13-day rest period (days 23 to 35). At least 72 hr should elapse between consecutive doses.

NURSING IMPLICATIONS

IMPLEMENTATION/ADMINISTRATION/STORAGE

1. **IV** Give under the supervision of a provider experienced in the use of antineoplastic therapy.
2. To prevent dehydration, give with fluid and electrolytes.
3. Before beginning any cycle of therapy with bortezomib in combination with melphalan and prednisone, the platelet count should be 70×10^9/L or more and the absolute neutrophil count (ANC) should be 1×10^9/L or more; nonhematological toxicities should have resolved to grade 1 or baseline.
4. Bortezomib is metabolized by CYP3A4, 2C19, and 1A2; thus, monitor clients receiving bortezomib together with potent CYP3A4 inhibitors or inducers.
5. Withhold at the onset of any grade 3 nonhematological or grade 4 hematological toxicity, excluding neuropathy. May restart therapy once toxic symptoms have resolved but at a 25% reduced dose (i.e., 1.3 mg/m^2/dose reduced to 1 mg/m^2/dose; 1 mg/m^2/dose reduced to 0.7 mg/m^2/dose).
6. The following are dose modifications for bortezomib-related neuropathic pain and/or peripheral sensory neuropathy:
   - Grade 1 (paresthesias and/or loss of reflexes) without pain or loss of function: No action required.
   - Grade 1 with pain or grade 2 (interference with function but not with activities of daily living): Reduce dose to 1 mg/m^2.
   - Grade 2 with pain or grade 3 (interference with activities of daily living): Withhold therapy until toxicity resolves. When toxicity resolves, reinitiate with a reduced bortezomib dose of 0.7 mg/m^2 and change treatment schedule to once weekly.
   - Grade 4 (sensory neuropathy that is disabling or motor neuropathy that is life-threatening or leads to paralysis): Discontinue bortezomib.

B

7. The following are dose modifications during cycles of combination bortezomib, melphalan, and prednisone therapy:
   - Hematological toxicity during a cycle: If prolonged grade 4 neutropenia or thrombocytopenia, or thrombocytopenia with bleeding is observed in previous cycle, consider the reduction of the melphalan dose by 25% in the next cycle.
   - If platelet count is 30×10^9/L or less or ANC is 0.75×10^9/L or less on bortezomib dosing day (other than day 1), withhold the bortezomib dose.
   - If several bortezomib doses in consecutive cycles are withheld due to toxicity, the bortezomib dose should be reduced by 1 dose level (from 1.3 mg/m^2 to 1 mg/m^2, or from 1 mg/m^2 to 0.7 mg/m^2).
   - Grade 3 or greater nonhematological toxicities, withhold bortezomib therapy until symptoms of the toxicity have resolved to grade 1 or baseline. Then, bortezomib may be reinitiated with 1 dose level reduction (from 1.3 mg/m^2 to 1 mg/m^2, or from 1 mg/m^2 to 0.7 mg/m^2). For bortezomib-related neuropathic pain and/or peripheral neuropathy, hold or modify bortezomib as directed.
8. The following are dose modifications for bortezomib starting dosage in hepatic impairment. **Mild:** Bilirubin level of $1 \times$ ULN or less and AST >ULN or bilirubin level of >1 to $1.5 \times$ ULN and any AST level: No modification of starting dose. **Moderate:** Bilirubin level of >1.5 to 3 ULN and any AST level: Reduce starting bortezomib dose to 0.7 mg/m^2 in the first cycle. Consider dose escalation to 1 mg/m^2 or further dose reduction to 0.5 mg/m^2 in subsequent cycles based on client tolerance. **Severe:** Bilirubin level $>3 \times$ ULN and any AST level: See dosage modification for moderate hepatic impairment.
9. For treatment beyond 8 cycles, doses may continue to be given on a 3-week cycle or given once weekly on days 1, 8, 15, and 22, followed by a 13-day rest period (days 23–35).
10. Dosage adjustments are not needed for clients with renal insufficiency. However, since dialysis may decrease bortezomib levels, give after the dialysis procedure.
11. Reconstitute each vial with 3.5 mL of NaCl injection, resulting in a final concentration of 1 mg/mL of bortezomib. The reconstituted drug should be a clear and colorless solution.
12. Use caution during handling and preparation. Use gloves and other protective clothing to prevent skin contact.
13. Store unopened vials at controlled room temperature from 15–30°C (59–86°F) protected from light.
14. When reconstituted, drug may be stored from 15–30°C (59–86°F). Give within 8 hr of reconstitution. May store reconstituted drug in original/syringe prior to administration. Product may be stored up to 8 hr in a syringe; however, the total storage time for the reconstituted drug must not exceed 8 hr when exposed to normal indoor lighting.
15. COMPATIBILITY 0.9% NaCl.
16. INCOMPATIBILITY Administer separately.

ASSESSMENT

1. Note reasons for therapy, other therapy trialed and dates administered, and documented progression of multiple/mantle cell myeloma after those therapies.
2. Carefully assess nutritional status, hydration level to prevent adverse effects; ensure well hydrated. Monitor VS: with HTN may require dosage adjustment for BP meds, increased fluid intake and steroids to manage hypotensive effects.
3. Before therapy, may need to administer drugs for diarrhea and nausea as therapy may cause N&V, diarrhea, and/or constipation.
4. Assess for history/presence of peripheral neuropathy (e.g., burning sensation, hyperesthesia, paresthesia, discomfort, neuropathic pain). If new or worsening symptoms, stop drug and report as dose and schedule require adjustment.
5. Monitor BP, renal and LFTs, Ca^{++}, uric acid, electrolytes and CBC.

CLIENT/FAMILY TEACHING

1. Drug administered IV in treatment cycles; used to prevent progression of cancerous cells.
2. Avoid activities that require mental alertness until drug effects realized; may cause dizziness, faintness, lightheadedness, fatigue, and blurred vision.

3. Consume plenty of fluids to prevent dehydration; may have vomiting and diarrhea with therapy.
4. Report any new onset S&S /adverse SE especially worsening neuropathy: burning sensation, numbness, pins and needles sensation, loss of sensation, or discomfort in any extremity. Also report dizziness, fainting, fever, lightheadedness, nerve pain, persistent vomiting or diarrhea, or other S&S of infection.
5. Practice reliable contraception and do not breast-feed during therapy.
6. Keep all F/U to assess response, labs, and adverse SE.

OUTCOMES/EVALUATE

- Inhibition of malignant cell proliferation
- Treatment of multiple myeloma or mantle cell lymphoma in those who have received at least 1 other prior therapy

Bosentan

(boh-**SEN**-tan)

Classification(s): Vasodilator, endothelin receptor antagonist

Pregnancy Category: X

RX: Tracleer.

INDICATIONS/USES

To improve exercise ability and decrease the rate of worsening in pulmonary arterial hypertension (WHO group 1). *Investigational:* Prevention of digital ulcers in systemic sclerosis. *NOTE:* Because of potential liver injury and to decrease the chance as much as possible for fetal exposure, bosentan may be prescribed only through the Tracleer Access Program.

ACTION/KINETICS

Action

Endothelin-1 (ET-1) is a neurohormone whose effects are mediated by binding to ET_A and ET_B receptors in the endothelium and smooth muscle. ET-1 levels are increased in plasma and lung tissue of clients with pulmonary arterial hypertension. Bosentan is a specific and competitive antagonist at endothelin receptor types ET_A and ET_B, thus improving pulmonary arterial hypertension.

Pharmacokinetics

Absolute bioavailability is about 50% and is unaffected by food. **Maximum plasma levels:** 3–5 hr. Metabolized in the liver by CYP3A4 and CYP2C9 and possibly CYP2C19 to 3 metabolites, 1 of which is active. Steady state reached in 3–5 days. Excreted in the bile. **t½, terminal:** About 5 hr. **Plasma protein binding:** More than 98%.

CONTRAINDICATIONS

Use in moderate or severe liver abnormalities or elevated aminotransferases >3 times ULN. Pregnancy or those who may become pregnant. Use with cyclosporine A or glyburide. Hypersensitivity to bosentan or any component of the medication. Lactation.

SPECIAL CONCERNS

(1) **Distribution program.** Because of the risk of liver injury and birth defects, bosentan is available only through a special restricted distribution program called the Tracleer Access Program (TAP), by calling 1-800-228-3546. Only prescribers and pharmacies registered with TAP may prescribe and distribute bosentan. In addition, bosentan may be dispensed only to clients who are enrolled in and meet all conditions of TAP. (2) **Liver injury.** Bosentan causes at least a 3-fold upper limit of normal (ULN) elevation of liver aminotransferases (ALT and AST) in approximately 11% of clients, accompanied by elevated bilirubin in a small number of cases. Because these changes are a marker for potential serious liver injury, serum aminotransferase levels must be measured prior to initiation of treatment and then monthly. In the postmarketing period, in the setting of close monitoring, rare cases of unexplained hepatic cirrhosis were reported after prolonged (more than 12 months) therapy with bosentan in clients with multiple comorbidities and drug therapies. There have also been reports of liver failure. The contribution of bosentan in these cases could not be excluded. (3) In at least 1 case, the initial presentation of liver injury (after more than 20 months of treatment) included pronounced elevations in aminotransferases and bilirubin levels accompanied by nonspecific symptoms, all of which resolved slowly over time after discontinuation of bosentan.

This case reinforces the importance of strict adherence to the monthly monitoring schedule for the duration of treatment and the treatment algorithm, which includes stopping bosentan if a rise of aminotransferase accompanied by signs or symptoms of liver dysfunction occurs. (4) Elevations in aminotransferases require close attention. Avoid using bosentan in clients with elevated aminotransferases (greater than 3 times ULN) at baseline because monitoring liver injury may be more difficult. Stop treatment if liver aminotransferase elevations are accompanied by clinical symptoms of liver injury (e.g., abdominal pain, fever, jaundice, nausea, unusual lethargy or fatigue, vomiting) or increases in bilirubin greater than or equal to 2 times the ULN. There is no experience with the reintroduction of bosentan in these circumstances.
(5) **Pregnancy:** Bosentan is likely to cause major birth defects if used by pregnant women based on animal data. Pregnancy must be excluded before the start of treatment with bosentan. Throughout treatment and for 1 month after stopping bosentan, women of child-bearing potential must use 2 reliable methods of contraception unless the client has a tubal sterilization or Copper T 380A intrauterine device (IUD) or levonorgestrel 20 mcg/day intrauterine system (IUS) inserted, in which case no other contraception is needed. Hormonal contraceptives, including oral, injectable, transdermal, and implantable contraceptives, should not be used as the sole means of contraception because these may not be effective in clients receiving bosentan. Obtain monthly pregnancy tests. ■

- **Use with caution in mildly impaired liver function and in the elderly.**
- **Safety and efficacy not determined in children.**

SIDE EFFECTS

Most Common

Respiratory tract infection, headache, nasopharyngitis, flushing, abnormal hepatic function, hypotension, palpitations, dyspepsia, edema.

CV: Hypotension, palpitations, edema, syncope, lower limb edema, CHF, pulmonary hypertension. **GI:** Dyspepsia. **Hepatic:** Abnormal hepatic function, hepatotoxicity, jaundice, ***liver failure***, unexplained hepatic cirrhosis. **CNS:** Headache, fatigue. **Dermatologic:** Flushing, pruritus, rash. **Respiratory:** Nasopharyngitis, respiratory tract infection, sinusitis. **Musculoskeletal:** Arthralgia, chest pain. **GU:** Decreased sperm counts. **Hematologic:** Anemia requiring transfusion, leukopenia, neutropenia, thrombocytopenia. **Metabolic:** Edema/fluid retention, lower limb edema. **Miscellaneous:** Hypersensitivity, angioneurotic edema.

LABORATORY TEST CONSIDERATIONS

↑ Liver transferases (AST, ALT). Dose-related ↓ H & H.

DRUG INTERACTIONS

Clarithromycin / ↑ Risk of bosentan hepatotoxicity; closely monitor; if interaction suspected, stop both drugs
Contraceptives, hormonal (oral, injectable, implantation, transdermal) / Possible contraceptive failure R/T ↑ liver metabolism of hormones by CYP3A4; clients should use additional methods of contraception
Cyclosporine A / ↑ Bosentan trough levels by about 30-fold and steady-state levels by 3–4 fold; ↓ Cyclosporine A levels by about 50%; **Do not give together.**
Glyburide / ↓ Glyburide levels by about 40% and bosentan levels by about 30%. Also, ↑ risk of elevated liver aminotransferases. **Do not give together.**
Ketoconazole / ↑ Bosentan levels by about 2-fold; possible ↑ bosentan effects
Rifampin / ↑ Bosentan trough levels after the first concomitant dose and ↓ bosentan trough levels at steady state; measure liver function q week for the first 4 weeks of concurrent use
Ritonavir-containing regimens / Coadministration may ↑ bosentan trough levels; adjust dosage
Sildenafil / ↓ Sildenafil levels and $t^{1/2}$ R/T ↑ metabolism by CYP3A4 → ↓ pharmacologic effect; also, ↑ bosentan levels → ↑ pharmacologic/toxic effects; closely monitor
Simvastatin (and other statins, including atorvastatin and lovastatin) / ↓ Plasma simvastatin and other statin levels by about 50% R/T ↑ hepatic metabolism by CYP3A4; monitor statin levels and adjust statin dose accordingly
Tacrolimus / Possible significant ↑ bosentan plasma levels; use together with caution

Warfarin / ↓ S-warfarin and R-warfarin levels 29% and 38% respectively; monitor coagulation parameters and adjust dose as needed

HOW SUPPLIED

Tablets: 62.5 mg, 125 mg.

DOSAGE

TABLETS

Pulmonary arterial hypertension.

Initial: 62.5 mg twice a day for 4 weeks. **Then,** increase to maintenance dose of 125 mg twice a day. In those with a body weight less than 40 kg and who are over 12 years of age, the recommended initial and maintenance doses are 62.5 mg twice a day.

NURSING IMPLICATIONS

IMPLEMENTATION/ADMINISTRATION/STORAGE

1. Use the following guidelines for dosage adjustment and monitoring in clients who develop aminotransferase abnormalities:
   - If ALT/AST levels are >3 and 5 or less times ULN, confirm by another aminotransferase test. If confirmed, reduced the dose to 62.5 mg daily or interrupt treatment and monitor aminotransferase levels at least every 2 weeks. If levels return to pretreatment values, continue or reintroduce the treatment as appropriate.
   - If ALT/AST levels are >5 and 8 or less times ULN, confirm by another aminotransferase test. If confirmed, stop treatment and monitor aminotransferase levels at least every 2 weeks. Once levels return to pretreatment values, consider reintroduction.
   - If ALT/AST levels are >8 times ULN, stop treatment and do not consider bosentan reintroduction. There is no experience with the reintroduction of bosentan in these circumstances.
2. If bosentan is reintroduced, begin again with the starting dose. Check aminotransferase levels within 3 days and thereafter.
3. If aminotransferase levels are accompanied by N&V, fever, abdominal pain, jaundice, unusual lethargy, fatigue (i.e., symptoms of liver injury) or increases in bilirubin 2 or more times ULN, stop drug.
4. To avoid potential for clinical deterioration after abrupt discontinuation, reduce dose gradually (i.e., 62.5 mg twice a day for 3–7 days).
5. Discontinue bosentan use at least 36 hr prior to initiation of ritonavir. After at least 10 days following the initiation of ritonavir, resume bosentan at 62.5 mg once daily or every other day based on individual tolerability.
6. Store from 15–30°C (59–86°F).

ASSESSMENT

1. Note reasons for therapy, other agents trialed, when diagnosed, and PAH (WHO Group I); and NYHA functional class II-IV of pulmonary artery hypertension (PAH) symptoms.
2. List drugs currently prescribed to ensure none interact adversely; drug is highly protein bound.
3. Ensure not pregnant; perform pregnancy test on all females of childbearing potential.
4. Document baseline disease state activity (e.g., exercise capacity, walking distance); reassess regularly.
5. After initial labs, monitor LFTs and pregnancy tests monthly; H&H after 1 and 3 months and then q 3 months to assess for any deficiencies. CXR, ABGs, and PFTs as indicated.

CLIENT/FAMILY TEACHING

1. Drug is used to improve exercise ability and to decrease the rate of clinical worsening with PAH.
2. Review bosentan medication guide for safe drug administration. Take twice a day, with or without food, as directed; increase dosage after 4 weeks upon provider recommendation.
3. Drug has two significant concerns: potential for serious liver damage and fetal damage. It is only administered through the Tracleer Access Program (TAP) at 1-866-228-3546. All adverse drug reactions/pregnancy should also be reported directly to this number by the provider.
4. Drug is not a cure but may improve clinical symptoms of disease. Report all side effects and any changes in breathing or exercise tolerance (exercise capacity, walking distance).
5. Practice reliable contraception; use an additional form of contraception with the hormonal form as drug will cause major birth defects.

6. Stop drug and report new onset abdominal pain, fatigue, fever, nausea, unusual lethargy, vomiting, or yellow skin discoloration.
7. Continue all other therapies prescribed by pulmonologist.
8. Keep all F/U to assess response, monthly labs, and for adverse SE.

OUTCOMES/EVALUATE

- Improved exercise tolerance
- ↓ Pulmonary artery pressure

Botulinum toxin, Type B (RimabotulinumtoxinB)

(**bot**-you-**LIE**-num **TOX**-in)

Classification(s): Botulinum toxin

Pregnancy Category: C

RX: Myobloc.

INDICATIONS/USES

Treatment of cervical dystonia to reduce the severity of abnormal head position and neck pain.

ACTION/KINETICS

Action

The product is a sterile liquid formulation of a purified neurotoxin derived from fermentation of *Clostridium botulinum* type B. It acts to produce flaccid paralysis by inhibiting acetylcholine release at the neuromuscular junction. *NOTE:* Myobloc, formerly called botulinum toxin type B is now called rimabotulinumtoxinB.

SPECIAL CONCERNS

- Use with caution in those with peripheral motor neuropathic diseases (e.g., amyotropic lateral sclerosis, motor neuropathy) or neuromuscular junctional disorders (e.g., myasthenia gravis, Lambert-Eaton syndrome).
- The product contains albumin; there is an extremely remote risk for transmission of viral diseases or Creutzfeldt-Jakob disease.
- The effect of giving different botulinum neurotoxin serotypes at the same time or within less than 4 months of each other is unknown; neuromuscular paralysis may be potentiated by coadministration or overlapping administration of different botulinum toxin serotypes.
- Use with caution during lactation.
- Safety and efficacy not determined in children.

SIDE EFFECTS

Most Common

Dry mouth, dysphagia, dyspepsia, pain at the injection site.

GI: N&V, GI disorder, glossitis, stomatitis, tooth disorder. **CNS:** Dizziness, neck pain related to cervical dystonia, headache, torticollis, pain related to cervical dystonia or torticollis, migraine, anxiety, tremor, hyperesthesia, somnolence, confusion. **Respiratory:** Increased cough, rhinitis, dyspnea, lung disorder, pneumonia. **Musculoskeletal:** Arthralgia, back pain, myasthenia, arthritis, joint disorder. **GU:** UTI, cystitis, vaginal moniliasis. **Dermatologic:** Pruritus, ecchymosis. **Ophthalmic:** Amblyopia, abnormal vision. **Otic:** Otitis media, tinnitus. **Body as a whole:** Infection, pain, flu syndrome, accidental injury, fever, chills, malaise, viral infection. **Miscellaneous:** Injection site pain, peripheral edema, hypercholesterolemia, taste perversion, allergic reaction, chest pain, hernia, abscess, cyst, neoplasm, vasodilation.

DRUG INTERACTIONS

Effect of botulinum toxin may be potentiated by aminoglycosides or any other drug that interferes with neuromuscular transmission (e.g., curare-like drugs).

HOW SUPPLIED

Injection, Suspension: 5,000 units/mL.

DOSAGE

INJECTION

Cervical dystonia.

Clients with a history of tolerating botulinum toxin, initial: 2,500–5,000 units divided among the affected muscles. **Clients without a history of tolerating botulinum toxin:** Use a lower initial dose. Individualize subsequent dosing based on individual client response.

NURSING IMPLICATIONS

Do not confuse Botulinum Toxin, Type B with Botulinum Toxin, Type A. Do not confuse onabotulinumtoxinA (Botulinum Toxin Type A) with rimabotulinumtoxinB (Botulinum Toxin Type B).

IMPLEMENTATION/ADMINISTRATION/STORAGE

1. Duration of effect in those responding to the toxin is between 12 and 16 weeks at doses of 5,000 units or 10,000 units.
2. Administration of the toxin should only be by physicians familiar with and experienced in assessing and managing clients with cervical dystonia.
3. Units of biological activity of botulinum toxin, type B cannot be compared or converted into units of any other botulinum toxin.
4. If a client ingests drug or is accidentally overdosed, monitor for up to several weeks for S&S of systemic weakness or paralysis.
5. Increased incidence of dysphagia with increased dose in the sternocleidomastoid muscle.
6. Incidence of dry mouth may increase when toxin is used in the splenius capitis, trapezius, and sternocleidomastoid muscles.
7. Store under refrigeration at 2–8°C (36–46°F) for up to 21 months. Do not freeze or shake.
8. After dilution with normal saline, use within 4 hr; product does not contain a preservative.

ASSESSMENT

1. Note reasons for therapy, level of pain, extent of abnormal head/neck positioning, and other agents/therapies trialed.
2. Assess for any evidence/history of neuropathic, neurologic, or neuromuscular disorders.
3. For use/administration only by those individuals trained to administer.
4. Monitor carefully for post-injection effects (hours to weeks later) which may spread from the area of injection to other body areas to produce symptoms consistent with botulinum toxin effects.
5. Do not use within 4 months of any other botulinum toxin serotype.
6. Review associated risk factors to ensure client understanding. Drug contains albumin which may present the remote risk of disease transmission of CJD.

CLIENT/FAMILY TEACHING

1. Used to release abnormal muscle spasms/contractures permitting more controlled movements, mobility, and freedom.
2. The clostridium bacteria (B) that makes the toxin is not being injected directly; a sterilized by-product of the bacteria is utilized. May experience a slight sting with injections and dryness of mouth.
3. Do not perform activities that require mental alertness until drug effects realized, may experience dizziness, anxiety, confusion. Resume activity slowly and carefully following administration.
4. Report any swallowing problems, SOB, respiratory disorders/infections, injection site abnormalities, facial drooping, or weakness.
5. With cervical dystonia, should see improvement within the first 2 wk following treatment, and max improvement about 6 wk following treatment. Beneficial effects may last 3 to 4 months before retreatment is needed.
6. Immediately seek medical assistance if swallowing, speech, or breathing problems develop.
7. Practice reliable contraception.
8. An antitoxin is available in the event of significant overdose or misinjection. Contact Elan Pharmaceuticals at 1-888-638-7605 from 9 am to 7 pm EST Mon to Fri., after hours at Elan's Global Safety Surveillance 1-877-352-6477 or the CDC at 1-800-CDC-INFO (1-800-232-4636) or 1-404-639-2888 nights and weekends. The antitoxin would need to be administered within 20 hr of overdosage.
9. Keep all F/U to assess response and for adverse SE.

OUTCOMES/EVALUATE

Relief of painful neck spasms/contractures with cervical dystonia

IV

Brentuximab vedotin

(bren-**TUX**-ih-mab)

Classification(s): Antineoplastic agent: Antibody-drug conjugate

Pregnancy Category: D

RX: Adcetris.

INDICATIONS/USES

(1) Treatment of Hodgkin's lymphoma after failure of autologous stem cell transplant or after failure of at least 2 prior multiagent chemotherapy

regimens in clients who are not autologous stem cell transplant candidates. (2) Treatment of clients with systemic anaplastic large cell lymphoma after failure of at least 1 prior multiagent chemotherapy regimen.

ACTION/KINETICS

Action

Brentuximab vedotin is an antibody-drug conjugate where the antibody is an immunoglobulin (IgG1) that is directed against CD30. The small molecule, monomethyl auristatin E (MMAE) is a microtubule disrupting agent. MMAE is covalently bound to the antibody via a linker. It is believed the anticancer action of brentuximab is due to the binding of the antibody-drug conjugate to CD30-expressing cells, followed by internalization of the antibody-drug conjugate-CD30 complex. This results in the release of MMAE via proteolytic cleavage; binding of MMAE to tubulin disrupts the microtubule network within the cell, subsequently inducting cell cycle arrest and apoptotic death of the cells.

Pharmacokinetics

Steady state of the antibody–drug conjugate: 21 days with every 3 week dosing. **Time to maximum concentration of MMAE:** 1–3 days. Only a small amount of the MMAE released from brentuximab is metabolized by CYP3A4/5. **t½, terminal, antibody drug conjugate:** About 4–6 days. MMAE is excreted in both the feces and urine, mostly unchanged. **Plasma protein binding:** MMAE: 68–82%.

CONTRAINDICATIONS

Lactation.

SPECIAL CONCERNS

Safety and efficacy not determined in children or in the elderly.

SIDE EFFECTS

Most Common

Neutropenia, peripheral sensory neuropathy, fatigue, N&V, anemia, URTI, diarrhea, pyrexia, thrombocytopenia, rash, abdominal pain, cough. **CNS:** Peripheal sensory neuropathy, headache, peripheral motor neuropathy, anxiety, dizziness, insomnia. **GI:** N&V, diarrhea, abdominal pain, constipation. **CV:** Supraventricular arrhythmia. **Dermatologic:** Rash, pruritus, alopecia, night sweats, dry skin, ***Stevens-Johnson syndrome***. **Hematologic:** Anemia, neutropenia, thrombocytopenia, lymphadenopathy. **Musculoskeletal:** Arthralgia, back pain, muscle spasms, myalgia, pain in extremity. **Respiratory:** URTI, cough, dyspnea, oropharyngeal pain, pneumonitis, pneumothorax, ***pulmonary embolism***. **GU:** Pyelonephritis, UTI. **Metabolic/Nutritional:** Decreased appetite, peripheral edema, weight decreased. **Infusion reactions:** Chills, nausea, dyspnea, pruritus, cough, pyrexia, ***anaphylaxis***. **Body as a whole:** Fatigue, pyrexia, chills, pain, ***septic shock***. **Miscellaneous:** Tumor lysis syndrome, immunogenicity.

OVERDOSE MANAGEMENT

Symptoms: Neutropenia. Also, see *Side Effects*. *Treatment:* No known antidote. Closely monitor for side effects, especially neutropenia. Administer supportive treatment.

DRUG INTERACTIONS

CYP3A4 inducers (e.g., rifampin) / ↓ Brentuximab exposure; administer together with caution and closely monitor for side effects
CYP3A4 inhibitors (e.g., ketoconazole) / ↑ Brentuximab exposure; use together with caution and closely monitor for side effects

HOW SUPPLIED

Injection, Lyophilized Powder for Solution: 50 mg.

DOSAGE

IV INFUSION ONLY

Hodgkin's lymphoma; Systemic anaplastic large cell lymphoma.

Adults, usual: 1.8 mg/kg as an IV infusion over 30 min q 3 weeks. Continue treatment with a maximum of 16 cycles, disease progression, or unacceptable toxicity. *NOTE:* The dose for clients who weigh more than 100 kg should be calculated for 100 kg.

NURSING IMPLICATIONS

IMPLEMENTATION/ADMINISTRATION/STORAGE

1. IV To reconstitute, calculate the dose (mg) and number of vials of brentuximab needed. Reconstitute each 50 mg vial with 10.5 mL of sterile water for injection to yield a single-use solution containing 5 mg/mL. Direct the stream toward the wall of the vial and not di-

rectly at the cake or powder. Gently swirl the vial to aid dissolution; do not shake.

2. For dilution, calculate the required volume of the 5 mg/mL reconstituted solution needed and withdraw this amount from the vials. Immediately add the reconstituted solution to an infusion bag containing a minimum volume of 100 mL to achieve a final concentration of 0.4 to 1.8 mg/mL. Brentuximab can be diluted into 0.9% NaCl injection, D5W injection, or Ringer's lactate injection. Gently invert the bag to mix the solution.
3. Administer as an IV infusion over 30 min. Do not administer as an IV push or bolus.
4. If an infusion reaction occurs, interrupt the infusion and institute appropriate medical management. If anaphylaxis occurs, immediately and permanently discontinue administration of brentuximab.
5. Clients who have experienced a prior infusion reaction should be premedicated for subsequent infusions. Premedication may include acetaminophen, an antihistamine, and a corticosteroid.
6. Manage peripheral neuropathy using a combination of dosage delay and reduction of dose to 1.2 mg/kg. For new or worsening grade 2 or 3 neuropathy, hold the dose until neuropathy improves to grade 1 or baseline and then restart at 1.2 mg/kg. Discontinue brentuximab for grade 4 peripheral neuropathy.
7. Manage neutropenia by dosage delays and reductions. Hold the dose for grade 3 or 4 neutropenia until resolution to baseline or grade 2 or lower. Consider growth factor support for subsequent cycles in those who experience grade 3 or 4 neutropenia. In clients with recurrent grade 4 neutropenia despite the use of growth factors, discontinue or reduce the brentuximab dose to 1.2 mg/kg.
8. Store vials from 2–8°C (36–46°F) in the original carton to protect from light. Reconstituted solution and/or diluted solution for infusion may be stored from 2–8°C (36–46°F) and used within 24 hr of reconstitution. Do not freeze. Discard any unused portion left in the vial.
9. COMPATIBILITY 0.9% NaCl, D5W, Ringer's lactate.
10. INCOMPATIBILITY Do not mix with or administer as an infusion with any other drug.

ASSESSMENT

1. Note indications for therapy, if autologous stem cell transplant (ASCT), or prior multi-agent chemotherapy regimens and outcome.
2. Assess for S&S of neuropathy, such as paresthesia, hypo-/hyperesthesia, a burning sensation, pain or weakness. May require a delay, dosage change, or discontinuation if new or worsening peripheral neuropathy experienced.
3. If prior infusion-related reaction occurred, premedicate for subsequent infusions (may use acetaminophen, corticosteroid and an antihistamine).
4. Monitor for infusion reaction or tumor lysis syndrome. May also require a delay, dosage change, or discontinuation of therapy.
5. Monitor VS, CBC (prior to each dose and more often with dysfunction), renal and LFTs.

CLIENT/FAMILY TEACHING

1. Drug is given IV by infusion over 30 minutes every 3 weeks generally until a max of 16 cycles, disease progression, or unacceptable toxicity occurs.
2. Dosing is based on labs which will be evaluated prior to therapy to assess for neutropenia and need for dose reduction or delay in therapy.
3. Report any S&S of peripheral neuropathy (burning sensation, paresthesia, pain) requires dosage adjustments.
4. May experience neutropenia, anemia, peripheral sensory neuropathy, fatigue, nausea, pyrexia, rash, diarrhea, and pain from therapy; report if evident.
5. Practice reliable contraception.
6. Keep all F/U to assess response, labs and for adverse SE.

OUTCOMES/EVALUATE

Inhibition of malignant cell proliferation

Budesonide

(byou-**DES**-oh-nyd)

Classification(s): Glucocorticoid

Pregnancy Category: C

RX: Capsules: Entocort EC. **Inhalation:** Pulmicort Flexhaler, Pulmicort Respules. **Intranasal**: Rhinocort Aqua.

✤ **Rx:** Entocort, Gen-Budesonide AQ, Pulmicort Nebuamp, Rhinocort Turbuhaler.

SEE ALSO ***CORTICOSTEROIDS***.

INDICATIONS/USES

(1) **Entocort EC:** Treatment and maintenance (up to 3 months) of clinical remission of mild-to-moderate active Crohn's disease involving the ileum and/or ascending colon. (2) **Pulmicort Flexhaler:** Prophylaxis and maintenance treatment of asthma in clients 6 years and older, including those requiring PO corticosteroid therapy for asthma. (3) **Pulmicort Respules:** Prophylaxis of and maintenance treatment of asthma in children and infants 6 months to 8 years. (4) **Rhinocort Aqua:** Treat symptoms of seasonal or perennial allergic rhinitis in adults and children 6 years of age and older.

ACTION/KINETICS

Action

Exerts a direct local anti-inflammatory effect with minimal systemic effects when used intranasally.

Pharmacokinetics

Entocort EC capsules contain micronized budesonide which has been coated to prevent release in the stomach. Budesonide is released in the intestine resulting in decreased inflammation by a local action. When taken PO, not absorbed into the body. Exceeding the recommended dose may result in suppression of hypothalamic-pituitary-adrenal function. About 34% bioavailable (doubled by compromised liver function). **Onset, nasal spray:** 10 hr. **t½:** 2–3 hr. Rapidly metabolized by CYP3A liver enzymes. Excreted through both urine and feces. **Plasma protein binding:** 85–90% over a concentration range of 1–100 ng/mL.

CONTRAINDICATIONS

Hypersensitivity to the drug. Untreated localized nasal mucosa infections. Lactation. Use in children less than 6 years of age or for acute or life-threatening asthma attacks, including status asthmaticus. Use in those who have had recent nasal septal ulcers, recurrent epistaxis, or nasal surgery/trauma until healing has occurred.

SPECIAL CONCERNS

- Use with caution in clients already on alternate-day corticosteroids (e.g., prednisone); in clients with active or quiescent tuberculosis infections of the respiratory tract, or in untreated fungal, bacterial infections or systemic viral infections; or ocular herpes simplex.
- Use with caution in clients with recent nasal septal ulcers, recurrent epistaxis, nasal surgery, or trauma.
- Use with caution during lactation.
- Avoid exposure to chickenpox or measles.
- Safety and efficacy of intranasal steroids not determined in children less than 6 years of age.

SIDE EFFECTS

Most Common

Inhalation Powder: Headache, URTI, flu-like symptoms, sinusitis, pharyngitis, back pain/pain, bronchospasm, cough, epistaxis.
Inhalation Suspension: URTI, rhinitis, nasal congestion, otitis media/ear infection, epistaxis.
Oral: Headache, tremor, rash, acne, fainting.

Respiratory: Nasopharyngeal irritation, nasal irritation, pharyngitis, increased cough, hoarseness, nasal pain, burning, stinging, dryness, epistaxis, bloody mucus, rebound congestion, ***bronchial asthma,*** occasional sneezing attacks (especially in children), rhinorrhea, reduced sense of smell, throat discomfort/burning/itching/swelling/pain, throat dryness/irritation, ulceration of the nasal mucosa, nasal septum perforation, sore throat, dyspnea, localized infections of nose and pharynx with *Candida albicans*, wheezing (rare). **CNS:** Lightheadedness, headache, nervousness. **GI:** Nausea, loss of sense of taste, bad taste in mouth, dry mouth, dyspepsia. **CV:** Palpitations. **Dermatologic:** Rash, pruritus, alopecia, contact dermatitis (rare). **Musculoskeletal:** Arthralgia, myalgia. **Hypersensitivity, immediate and delayed:** Angioedema, ***bronchospasm,*** rash, urticaria. **Ophthalmic:** Watery eyes; cataracts, glaucoma, increased IOP (all rare). **Miscellaneous:** Moniliasis, facial edema, herpes simplex, loss of taste/smell, infection, hypercorticism, reduction in growth velocity in children.

OVERDOSE MANAGEMENT

Symptoms: Symptoms of hypercorticism, including menstrual irregularities, acneiform lesions, and cushingoid features (all are rarely seen, however). *Treatment:* Discontinue the drug slowly using procedures that are acceptable for discontinuing oral corticosteroids.

B

DRUG INTERACTIONS

Cimetidine / Slight ↓ in budesonide clearance and an ↑ in its oral bioavailability; also, ↓ metabolism of budesonide by CYP3A4 liver enzymes → ↑ systemic levels of budesonide
Clarithromycin / ↓ Metabolism of budesonide by CYP3A4 liver enzymes → ↑ systemic levels of budesonide
Erythromycin / ↓ Metabolism of budesonide by CYP3A4 liver enzymes → ↑ systemic levels of budesonide
Grapefruit juice / ↑ Systemic levels of budesonide 2-fold
Itraconazole / ↓ Metabolism of budesonide by CYP3A4 liver enzymes → ↑ systemic levels of budesonide
Ketoconazole / ↑ Systemic levels of budesonide more than sevenfold R/T ↓ metabolism by CYP3A4 liver enzymes
Ritonavir / ↓ Metabolism of budesonide by CYP3A4 liver enzymes → ↑ systemic levels of budesonide

HOW SUPPLIED

Capsules, Enteric Coated (Entocort EC): 3 mg; ***Inhalation Powder (Flexhaler):*** 90 mcg/inh, 180 mcg/inh; ***Inhalation Suspension (Respules):*** 0.25 mg/mL, 0.5 mg/mL, 0.5 mg/2 mL, 1 mg/mL, 1 mg/2 mL; ***Nasal Spray Suspension (Rhinocort Aqua):*** 32 mcg/actuation.

DOSAGE

CAPSULES

Crohn's disease.

Adults: 9 mg once daily in the a.m. for up to 8 weeks. If the disease recurs, another 8-week course may be given. Once symptoms are controlled, give 6 mg once daily for maintenance of clinical remission for up to 3 months. If symptom control is still maintained at 3 months, attempt to taper to complete cessation.

PULMICORT RESPULES

Prophylaxis and maintenance treatment of asthma.

Children 12 months to 8 years old: If previous therapy was bronchodilators alone: 0.5 mg total daily dose given either once or twice daily in divided doses (maximum daily dose: 0.5 mg). If previous therapy was inhaled corticosteroids: 0.5 mg total daily dose given either once or twice daily in divided doses (maximum daily dose: 1 mg). If previous therapy was oral corticosteroids: 1 mg total daily dose given either as 0.5 mg twice a day or 1 mg daily (maximum daily dose: 1 mg).

NASAL SPRAY (RHINOCORT AQUA)

Seasonal and perennial allergic rhinitis.

Adults and children 12 years and older, initial: 64 mcg/day (1 spray per nostril) once daily. **Maximum:** 256 mcg/day (4 sprays per nostril) once daily. **Children, 6–11 years of age, initial:** 64 mcg/day (1 spray per nostril) once daily. **Maximum:** 128 mcg/day (2 sprays per nostril) once daily. An improvement in nasal symptoms may be seen within 10 hr of the first dose. Maximum benefit seen in 2 weeks. After the maximum effect is obtained, reduce the maintenance dose to the smallest amount required to control symptoms.

NURSING IMPLICATIONS

IMPLEMENTATION/ADMINISTRATION/STORAGE

1. Clients with Crohn's disease involving ileum/ascending colon have been switched from PO prednisolone to budesonide with no S&S of adrenal insufficiency. Begin tapering of prednisolone with initiation of budesonide.
2. In the presence of excessive nasal mucosa secretions or edema of the nasal mucosa, the drug may not reach the site of intended action. In such cases, use a nasal vasoconstrictor during the first 2–3 days of therapy.
3. Pulmicort Respules may be used in children as young as 12 months. In symptomatic children not responding to nonsteroidal therapy, a starting dose of 0.25 mg using Respules may be tried.
4. Administer Pulmicort Respules using a jet nebulizer connected to an air compressor with an adequate air flow, equipped with a mouthpiece or suitable face mask. Ultrasonic nebulizers are not suitable. Do not administer with other nebulizable medications.

5. Once the desired clinical effect is achieved using Respules, consider tapering to the lowest effective dose.
6. For those not responding adequately when using the Respules, consider giving the total daily dose as a divided dose if a once-daily dosing schedule was followed.
7. Store Pulmicort Respules from 20–25°C (68–77°F). Store Respules upright, protected from light. When an envelope has been opened, the shelf life of the unused Respules is 2 weeks, when protected. After opening the aluminum foil envelope, return the unused Respules to the aluminum foil envelop to protect from light. Use opened Respules promptly; gently shake using a circular motion before use. Do not freeze.
8. Store Entocort EC capsules from 15–30°C (59–86°F) in a tightly closed container.
9. Store Rhinocort Aqua from 20–25°C (68–77°F) with valve up. Protect from light. Shake gently before use. Do not spray in the eyes. Do not freeze. Discard after 120 sprays following initial priming.

ASSESSMENT

1. Note reasons for therapy, onset/characteristics of S&S, other agents trialed/outcome.
2. List drugs prescribed; ensure none interact unfavorably.
3. Assess VS, nasal integrity, PFTs, and lung sounds. Periodically assess S&S during therapy to ensure desired response and/or if dosage requires adjustment.
4. Monitor growth rate in children and bone mineral density (BMD) in those at risk for decreased bone mineral content.
5. Assess for glaucoma or cataracts in those experiencing changes in vision or with history of increased IOP, glaucoma, and/or cataracts.
6. If changing from systemic to inhaled or intranasal dosing, observe closely for adrenal insufficiency.
7. With oral budesonide, monitor moderate to severe liver disease clients for increased S&S of hypercorticisim. Dose reduction may be required.

CLIENT/FAMILY TEACHING

1. Review method/frequency for administration of prescribed agent. Review video/instruction for proper inhalation guidelines and have client return demonstrate proper use.
2. Take oral capsules whole; do not chew, crush, or break. Take once daily in the a.m.; avoid grapefruit juice. Can be taken without regard to meals; take with food if GI upset occurs.
3. With inhalers: rinse mouth (with water and spit out; especially children) and equipment thoroughly after each use to prevent oral fungal infections. Shake canister well before administering. Store valve down and away from areas of high humidity. Discard inhaler when the red mark appears at bottom of indicator window.
4. With nebulizer do not mix with other nebulizer medications unless advised. Review how to prepare, use, and clean equipment. Use immediately upon opening solution and discard any unused solution. Rinse (child's) mouth and wash face after each treatment.
5. Drug is an asthma controller and not to be used to treat acute asthma attacks. Rescue inhalers (bronchodilator) must be used to obtain rapid relief of asthma symptoms.
6. Do not stop medication once symptoms controlled; continued daily use is required.
7. Prior to using nasal form, clear nasal passages of secretions. If nasal passages are blocked, use decongestant first unless <2 y.o. Report if sores or injuries in nasal passages; may prevent or slow proper healing.
8. Gently shake nasal spray container and prime the pump by actuating 8 times. If not used for 2 consecutive days, reprime with 1 spray or until a fine mist appears. If not used for more than 14 days, rinse the applicator and reprime with 2 sprays or until a fine mist appears.
9. Report persistent sneezing, nasal irritation, or nosebleed. Discard bottle when labeled number of sprays have been used, even if bottle is not completely empty.
10. With oral powder for inhalation: Once aluminum pouch opened, use/discard within 6 months. Store respules upright protected from light; gently shake before use, discard open envelopes after 2 weeks.
11. Avoid individuals with chickenpox, measles, or communicable diseases.
12. Report persistent sore throat/mouth, cough, dry mouth, facial swelling, rash, or worsening asthma symptoms (i.e., increasing need for bronchodilator). Symptoms of hoarseness may

be evident; should subside upon completion of therapy.

13. Drug is a steroid; chronic use in excessive amounts may lead to adverse systemic reactions. Do not suddenly stop taking if therapy has been >1 month. If therapy needs to be stopped after prolonged use, should be slowly withdrawn to prevent adrenal insufficiency.
14. S&S of adrenal insufficiency include: nausea, fatigue, dizziness, hypotension, depression, abdominal, joint, or muscle pain. Immediately report if S&S occur.
15. Maximum benefit usually not seen for 3–7 days, although a decrease in symptoms can be seen within 24 hr.
16. Identify triggers/avoid irritants to control symptoms.
17. Report chest pain, lower extremity swelling, severe headaches, respiratory infections, or increased bruising/bleeding.
18. Keep all F/U visits to assess response and for any adverse SE.

OUTCOMES/EVALUATE

- Relief of seasonal and perennial allergic rhinitis, nasal congestion/allergic manifestations
- Asthma prophylaxis
- Crohn's disease remission (Entocort)

IV

Bumetanide

(byou-**MET**-ah-nyd)

Classification(s): Diuretic, loop

Pregnancy Category: C

✦ **Rx:** Burinex.

SEE ALSO ***DIURETICS, LOOP***.

INDICATIONS/USES

Edema associated with CHF and hepatic and renal disease, including the nephrotic syndrome. Especially useful in clients refractory to other diuretics. *Investigational:* PO to treatment of adult nocturia.

ACTION/KINETICS

Action

Inhibits reabsorption of both sodium and chloride in the proximal tubule and the ascending loop of Henle. Possible activity in the proximal tubule to promote phosphate excretion.

Pharmacokinetics

Onset, PO: 30–60 min. **Peak effect, PO:** 1–2 hr. **Duration, PO:** 4–6 hr (dose-dependent). **Onset, IV:** Several minutes. **Peak effect, IV:** 15–30 min. **Duration, IV:** 3.5–4 hr. **t½:** 1–1.5 hr. The t½ decreases from 6 hr at birth to 2.4 hr at one month of age. Metabolized in the liver although 45% excreted unchanged in the urine.

CONTRAINDICATIONS

Anuria. Hepatic coma or severe electrolyte depletion until condition improved/corrected. Hypersensitivity to drug. Lactation.

SPECIAL CONCERNS

Bumetanide is a potent diuretic that, if given in excess amounts, can lead to a profound diuresis with water and electrolyte depletion. Therefore, careful medical supervision is required and dose and dosage schedule have to be adjusted to the individual client's needs.

- SLE may be activated or made worse.
- Clients allergic to sulfonamides may show cross sensitivity to bumetanide.
- Sudden changes in electrolyte balance may cause hepatic encephalopathy and coma in clients with hepatic cirrhosis and ascites.
- Use caution with dose selection in the elderly. Geriatric clients may be more sensitive to the hypotensive and electrolyte effects and are at greater risk for developing thromboembolic problems and circulatory collapse.
- Safety and efficacy in children under 18 not established.

SIDE EFFECTS

Most Common

Dizziness, hypotension, headache, nausea, muscle cramps, encephalopathy in those with pre-existing liver disease.

Electrolyte and fluid changes: Excess water loss, ***dehydration,*** electrolyte depletion including hypokalemia, hypochloremia, hyponatremia, hypovolemia, thromboembolism, ***circulatory collapse.*** **Otic:** Tinnitus, reversible and irreversible hearing impairment, deafness, vertigo (with a sense of fullness in the ears). **CV:** ***Reduction in blood volume may cause circulatory collapse and vascular thrombosis and embolism, especially in geriatric clients.*** Hypotension, ECG changes, chest pain.

B

CNS: Asterixis, encephalopathy in those with preexisting liver disease, vertigo, headache, dizziness. **GI:** Upset stomach, dry mouth, N&V, diarrhea, GI pain. **GU:** Premature ejaculation, difficulty maintaining erection, renal failure. **Musculoskeletal:** Arthritic pain, weakness, muscle cramps, fatigue. **Hematologic:** Agranulocytosis, thrombocytopenia. **Allergic:** Pruritus, urticaria, rashes. **Miscellaneous:** Sweating, hyperventilation, rash, nipple tenderness, photosensitivity, pain following parenteral use.

LABORATORY TEST CONSIDERATIONS

Alterations in LDH, AST, ALT, alkaline phosphatase, creatinine clearance, total serum bilirubin, serum proteins, cholesterol. Changes in hemoglobin, PT, hematocrit, WBCs, platelet and differential counts, phosphorus, carbon dioxide content, bicarbonate, and calcium. ↑ Urinary glucose and protein, serum creatinine. Also, hyperuricemia, hypochloremia, hypokalemia, azotemia, hyponatremia, hyperglycemia.

OVERDOSE MANAGEMENT

Symptoms: Profound loss of water, electrolyte depletion, dehydration, decreased blood volume, ***circulatory collapse (possibility of vascular thrombosis and embolism).*** Symptoms of electrolyte depletion include: Anorexia, cramps, weakness, dizziness, vomiting, and mental confusion. *Treatment:* Replace electrolyte and fluid losses and monitor urinary and serum electrolyte levels. Emesis or gastric lavage. Oxygen or artificial respiration may be necessary. General supportive measures.

HOW SUPPLIED

Injection: 0.25 mg/mL; ***Tablets:*** 0.5 mg, 1 mg, 2 mg.

DOSAGE

TABLETS

Edema.

Adults: 0.5–2 mg once daily; if response is inadequate, a second or third dose may be given at 4–5 hr intervals up to a maximum of 10 mg/day. For continued control of edema, an intermittent dosage schedule is recommended, whereby bumetanide is given on alternate days for 3 or 4 days with rest periods of 1–2 days in between. *Investigational:* **Infants and children >6 months of age, usual:** 0.015–0.1 mg/kg/dose given daily or every other day; **maximum dose:** 10 mg/day. **Neonates and infants 6 months of age and younger, usual:** 0.01–0.05 mg/kg/dose given daily or every other day. Maximal diuretic effect has been reported at 0.04 mg/kg/dose, with greater efficacy at lower doses. *NOTE:* In critically ill neonates, bumetanide may displace bilirubin. Drug elimination is slower in neonates with respiratory disorders.

IM; IV

Edema.

Adults, initial: 0.5–1 mg; if response is inadequate, a second or third dose may be given at 2–3-hr intervals up to a maximum of 10 mg/day. Initiate PO dosing as soon as possible. *Investigational:* **Infants and children >6 months of age, usual:** 0.015–0.1 mg/kg/dose given IM or IV daily or every other day. **Maximum dose:** 10 mg/day. **Neonates and infants 6 months of age and younger:** 0.01–0.05 mg/kg/dose IM or IV daily or every other day. Maximal diuretic effect has been reported at 0.04 mg/kg/dose, with greater efficacy at lower doses. *NOTE:* In critically ill neonates, bumetanide may displace bilirubin. Drug elimination is slower in neonates with respiratory disorders.

NURSING IMPLICATIONS

IMPLEMENTATION/ADMINISTRATION/STORAGE

1. Recommended PO schedule is on alternate days or for 3–4 days with a 1- to 2-day rest period in between.
2. Bumetanide, at a 1:40 ratio of bumetanide: furosemide, may be ordered if allergic to furosemide.
3. In clients with hepatic cirrhosis and ascites, sudden alterations of electrolyte balance may precipitate hepatic encephalopathy and coma. Initiate treatment in such clients in the hospital with small doses with careful monitoring. Supplemental potassium and/or spironolac-

tone may prevent hypokalemia and metabolic alkalosis in these clients.

4. Reserve IV or IM for those in whom PO use is not practical or absorption from the GI tract is impaired.
5. Whether used PO or parenterally, keep dosage to a minimum in those with hepatic failure; if necessary, increase dosage very carefully.
6. Freshly prepare solutions and use within 24 hr.
7. Store injection and tablets from 15–30°C (59–86°F); protect from light.
8. IV In severe chronic renal insufficiency, a continuous infusion (12 mg over 12 hr) may be more effective and cause fewer side effects than intermittent bolus therapy.
9. Prepare solutions fresh for IM or IV; use within 24 hr.
10. Administer IV solutions slowly over 1–2 min.
11. COMPATIBILITY D5W, 0.9% NaCl, or LR in both glass and plasticized polyvinyl chloride containers.
12. INCOMPATIBILITY Fenoldopam mesylate, midazolam HCl.

ASSESSMENT

1. List reasons for therapy, other agents trialed, and pretreatment findings.
2. Note sulfonamide allergy; may have cross sensitivity.
3. Review history; note any hearing impairment, lupus, or thromboembolic events. Assess hearing; check for ototoxicity, especially if receiving other ototoxic drugs.
4. *NOTE:* 1 mg of bumetanide is equivalent to 40 mg of furosemide.
5. Record VS. Rapid diuresis may cause dehydration and circulatory collapse (especially in elderly). Hypotension may occur when administered with antihypertensives.
6. Monitor electrolytes, I&O, Ca^{++}, uric acid, CBC, renal and LFTs; assess for ↓ K^+.

CLIENT/FAMILY TEACHING

1. May take with food to reduce GI upset. Take early in day to prevent nighttime voidings. With alternate-day therapy, keep written record/calendar to ensure proper therapy and no overdosage.
2. Do not perform activities that require mental alertness until drug effects realized. Change positions slowly to prevent sudden drop in BP causing dizziness.
3. Review dietary requirements, e.g., ↓ sodium and ↑ potassium; see dietitian PRN. Ensure adequate fluids intake to prevent dehydration. Record weights; report any sudden weight gain (>3 lbs/day or 5 lbs/week), swelling in the hands or feet, bleeding, weakness, hearing loss, cramps, nausea, or dizziness.
4. Consume necessary fluids to prevent dehydration unless fluid restrictions apply.
5. Avoid prolonged sun exposure, use sunscreen/protective clothing to prevent photosensitivity reaction.
6. With diabetes, monitor FS closely; may cause loss of glycemic control.
7. Keep all F/U to asses response, labs, and for adverse SE.

OUTCOMES/EVALUATE

↓ Peripheral and sacral edema; enhanced diuresis

IV

Buprenorphine hydrochloride

(byou-pren-**OR**-feen)

Classification(s): Narcotic agonist/antagonist

Pregnancy Category: C

RX: Butrans, Subutex, **C-III**

SEE ALSO ***NARCOTIC ANALGESICS***.

INDICATIONS/USES

Injection: Moderate-to-severe pain.

Tablets, sublingual: Treat opioid dependence.

Transdermal Patch: Moderate to severe chronic pain in those who require round-the-clock therapy for an extended period of time.

ACTION/KINETICS

Action

Semisynthetic opiate possessing both narcotic agonist and antagonist activity. Partial agonist at the mu-opioid receptor and an antagonist at the kappa-opioid receptor. A 0.3 mg parenteral dose is equivalent to 10 mg morphine in respiratory depressant and analgesic effects.

Pharmacokinetics

IM, onset: 15 min; **Peak effect:** 1 hr; **Duration:** 6 hr. **t½:** 2–3 hr. May also be given IV with shorter onset and peak effect. Is about equipotent with naloxone as a narcotic antagonist.

B

CONTRAINDICATIONS

Lactation. Use of the patch to treat postoperative pain. Use of the tablets in children less than 16 years of age.

SPECIAL CONCERNS

- **Use with caution in clients with compromised respiratory function, in the elderly or debilitated, CNS depression or coma, toxic psychoses, acute alcoholism, delirium tremens, kyphoscoliosis, in head injuries, in impairment of liver or renal function, Addison's disease, prostatic hypertrophy, biliary tract dysfunction, urethral stricture, myxedema, and hypothyroidism.**
- **If physically dependent on narcotics, administration may result in precipitation of a withdrawal syndrome.**
- **Use may obscure diagnosis or clinical course in acute abdominal conditions.**
- **Safety and efficacy of the tablets not established in children less than 16 years of age.**
- **Use of the injection in children less than 2 years of age not established.**

SIDE EFFECTS

Most Common

Following use of injection: Hypotension, sedation, dizziness, vertigo, sweating, N&V, miosis, hypoventilation.
Following use of tablets: Headache, insomnia, N&V, abdominal pain, constipation, pain, infection, chills, rhinitis, sweating, asthenia, vasodilation, withdrawal syndrome.

- **Injection**

CNS: Sedation, dizziness, vertigo, dreaming, psychosis, weakness, fatigue, nervousness, confusion, headache, euphoria, slurred speech, depression, paresthesia, malaise, depersonalization, tremors, hallucinations, coma, dysphoria, agitation, seizures. **GI:** N&V, constipation, dyspepsia, loss of appetite, flatulence, dry mouth, cytolytic hepatitis and hepatitis with jaundice in addicts, diarrhea. **Ophthalmic:** Miosis, blurred/double vision, conjunctivitis, visual abnormalities, amblyopia (rare). **CV:** Hypotension, bradycardia, hypertension, tachycardia, Wenckebach block. **Respiratory:** Decreased respiratory rate (especially after IV use), cyanosis, dyspnea, apnea (rare). **Dermatologic:** Sweating, rash, pruritus, flushing/warmth, injection site reaction, pallor, urticaria (rare). **Miscellaneous:** Urinary retention, chills, tinnitus, acute and chronic hypersensitivity.

- **Tablets**

CNS: Headache, insomnia. **GI:** N&V, abdominal pain, constipation, diarrhea. **Body as a whole:** Asthenia, chills, infection, pain, vasodilation, sweating. **Miscellaneous:** Back pain, withdrawal syndrome, rhinitis.

DRUG INTERACTIONS

Barbiturate anesthetics / ↑ Respiratory and CNS depression of buprenorphine
Benzodiazepines / Coma and death possible with concomitant IV use of both drugs by addicts
CNS depressants (alcohol, benzodiazepines, general anesthetics, narcotic analgesics, phenothiazines, sedative/hypnotics, tranquilizers) / Additive CNS depression
CYP3A4 inducers (carbamazepine, phenobarbital, phenytoin, rifampin) / Possible increased clearance of buprenorphine; monitor carefully
CYP3A4 inhibitors (azole antifungals, macrolide antibiotics, protease inhibitors) / Use caution; specific data not available

HOW SUPPLIED

Injection: Equivalent to 0.3 mg/mL buprenorphine; ***Tablets, Sublingual:*** 2 mg, 8 mg; ***Transdermal Patch:*** 5 mcg/hr, 10 mcg/hr, 20 mcg/hr.

DOSAGE

IM; SLOW IV

Analgesia.

Clients over 13 years of age: 0.3 mg (1 mL) given over 2 min q 6 hr; repeat once (up to 0.3 mg) if needed, 30–60 min after initial dose. **Children, 2–12 years of age:** 2–6 mcg/kg q 4–6 hr. Do not give single doses greater than 6 mcg/kg.

TABLETS, SUBLINGUAL

Opioid dependence.

Adults: 12–16 mg given as a single daily dose.

TRANSDERMAL PATCH

Moderate to severe chronic pain in those requiring round-the-clock analgesia.

Adults, initial: 5 mcg/hr; do not increase dose until client has been exposed to previous dose for 72 hr. Each patch is designed to be worn for 7 days.

B

NURSING IMPLICATIONS

Do not confuse Buprenex with Bumex (diuretic) or Buprenex with Butrans. Do not confuse buprenorphine with bupropion (an antidepressant).

IMPLEMENTATION/ADMINISTRATION/STORAGE

1. Not all children may clear buprenorphine faster than adults. Thus, fixed interval or "round the clock" dosing should not be undertaken until proper interdose interval has been established.
2. Some pediatric clients may not need to be remedicated with the injection for 6–8 hr.
3. When using injection, have naloxone to reverse drug-induced respiratory depression.
4. Avoid storing injection in excessive heat and light. Do not freeze.
5. Place sublingual tablets under the tongue until dissolved. For doses requiring more than 2 tablets, place all tablets under the tongue at once. If client cannot fit more than 2 tablets comfortably, place 2 tablets at a time under the tongue until dissolved. Swallowing tablets whole will reduce bioavailability.
6. Clients must undergo induction of therapy. Prior to induction, determine type of opioid dependence, time since last opioid use, and degree/level of opioid dependence.
7. An adequate maintenance dose, titrated to clinical effect, should be achieved as rapidly as possible to prevent opioid withdrawal syndrome. In one induction regimen, clients received buprenorphine, 8 mg on day 1 and 16 mg on day 2. From day 3 onward, they received buprenorphine/naloxone tablets at the same buprenorphine dose as on day 2. Induction was achieved in 3 or 4 days.
8. In those taking heroin or other short-acting opioids, give buprenorphine during the initiation of induction at least 4 hr after the individual last used opioids (or when the first signs of withdrawal appear).
9. Preferred medication for maintenance treatment is buprenorphine/naloxone.
10. As part of the comprehensive treatment plan, the decision should be made to discontinue buprenorphine (or buprenorphine/naloxone) therapy after a period of maintenance or brief stabilization. Taper buprenorphine dose at the end of treatment.
11. IV May be administered undiluted IV, over 3–5 min.
12. COMPATIBILITY Isotonic saline, RL solution, and D5W/0.9% NaCl. May be mixed with solutions containing haloperidol, glycopyrrolate, scopolamine hydrobromide, hydroxyzine chloride, or droperidol.
13. INCOMPATIBILITY Do not mix with solutions containing diazepam or lorazepam.

ASSESSMENT

1. Note reasons for therapy, characteristics of S&S, intensity/pain level. Monitor VS and level of consciousness.
2. For induction therapy, document type of opioid dependence (e.g., long-, short-acting), time since last opioid use, and degree/level of opioid dependence prior to starting SL tablets.
3. Observe for 2 hr and assess need for additional dosing. Monitor for respiratory depression; if evident reestablish adequate ventilation with mechanical assistance.
4. Assess for liver or renal dysfunction, diseases of the biliary tract, or BPH. Report head injuries immediately; precludes therapy.
5. If receiving narcotics, observe for withdrawal symptoms.
6. Providers must meet certain qualifications and have registered/notified Health and Human Services of their intent to prescribe buprenorphine and buprenorphine/naloxone fixed combination in the treatment of opiate dependence.
7. Obtain LFT prior to starting therapy and monitor periodically during therapy.

CLIENT/FAMILY TEACHING

1. Take tablets once daily by placing under the tongue until dissolved. If dose requires more than 2 tablets, place all tablets under the tongue and allow to dissolve. If unable to fit more than 2 tablets under the tongue at one time, then place 2 tablets under the tongue at a time and repeat until entire dose has been taken. Swallowing tablets reduces effectiveness.
2. Avoid activities that require mental alertness. May cause drowsiness, dizziness, low BP effects. Lie or sit down if dizziness or lightheadedness evident when standing.

3. Cough and deep breathe every 2 hr to prevent lung collapse especially when used for post-op pain.
4. Avoid alcohol. Report any CNS changes, adverse effects, or allergic S&S.
5. With opioid dependence, follow therapy guidelines. Stay in recovery program to ensure freedom from dependence. Advise other emergency providers of therapy and opioid dependence to ensure appropriate care rendered.

OUTCOMES/EVALUATE

- Relief of pain (IV)
- Treatment of opioid dependence (oral)

Bupropion hydrobromide

(byou-**PROH**-pee-on)

Classification(s): Antidepressant

Pregnancy Category: C

RX: Aplenzin.

Bupropion hydrochloride

(byou-**PROH**-pee-on)

Classification(s): Antidepressant, miscellaneous; smoking deterrent (Zyban)

Pregnancy Category: C

RX: Budeprion SR, Budeprion XL, Wellbutrin, Wellbutrin SR, Wellbutrin XL, Zyban.

✱ **Rx:** ratio-Bupropion SR, Sandoz Bupropion SR.

INDICATIONS/USES

Bupropion hydrobromide. Treatment of major depressive disorder.

Bupropion hydrochloride. (1) Treatment of major depressive disorder (immediate-release and extended-release). (2) Major depressive episodes in those with a history of seasonal affective disorder (Wellbutrin XL only). (3) Aid to stop smoking (Zyban only); may be combined with a nicotine transdermal system. *Investigational:* Bupropion: Attention deficit hyperactivity disorder in children and adolescents. Attention deficit disorder in adults. Bupropion SR: Neuropathic pain, enhancement of weight loss.

ACTION/KINETICS

Action

Mechanism of action is not known; the drug does not inhibit MAO and it only weakly blocks neuronal uptake of epinephrine, serotonin, and dopamine. However, its action is believed to be mediated by noradrenergic and/or dopaminergic mechanisms. Exerts moderate anticholinergic and sedative effects, but only slight orthostatic hypotension.

Pharmacokinetics

Peak plasma levels, Immediate-Release: 2 hr; **Wellbutrin SR and Zyban:** 3 hr; **Wellbutrin XL:** 5 hr. **t½, terminal, immediate-release:** 8–24 hr. **t½, terminal, Zyban:** 21 hr. **Time to steady state:** Within 8 days. Significantly metabolized by a first-pass effect. Metabolized primarily to hydroxybupropion by CYP2B6. Both bupropion and hydroxybupropion may inhibit CYP2D6. During chronic use the plasma levels of two active metabolites may be higher than bupropion. Excreted through both the urine (87%) and the feces (10%). Zyban is a sustained-release formulation. **Plasma protein binding:** 84% at concentrations up to 200 mcg/mL.

CONTRAINDICATIONS

Hypersensitivity to bupropion or any ingredients. Seizure disorders; presence or history of bulimia or anorexia nervosa due to the higher incidence of seizures in such clients. Concomitant use of an MAOI. Use in clients undergoing abrupt discontinuation of alcohol and sedatives, including benzodiazepines. Use in clients who have shown an allergic response to bupropion or other components of the various products. Wellbutrin, Wellbutrin SR, Wellbutrin XL, and Zyban all contain bupropion; do not use together. Lactation.

SPECIAL CONCERNS

(1) Antidepressants increased the risk of suicidal thinking and behavior (suicidality) in short-term studies in children, adolescents, and young adults with major depressive disorder and other psychiatric disorders compared with placebo. Anyone considering the use of bupropion or other antidepressants in a child, adolescent, or young adult must balance this risk with the clinical need. Short-term studies did not show an increase in the risk of suicidality with antidepressants compared with

placebo in adults older than 24 years of age; there was no reduction in risk with antidepressants compared with placebo in adults 65 years of age and older. Depression and certain other psychiatric disorders are themselves associated with increases in suicide risk. Appropriately monitor clients of all ages who are started on antidepressant therapy and closely observe them for clinical worsening, suicidality, or unusual changes in behavior. Advise families and caregivers of the need for close observation and communication with the prescriber. Bupropion is not approved for use in children. (2) Although Zyban is not indicated for the treatment of depression, it contains the same active ingredient as the antidepressant bupropion medications Wellbutrin, Wellbutrin SR, and Wellbutrin XL.

- **Use with extreme caution in clients with cranial trauma, with drugs that lower the seizure threshold (e.g., alcohol use; addiction to opiates, cocaine, or stimulants; use of OTC stimulants and anorectics, antipsychotics, other antidepressants, theophylline, systemic steroids; diabetes treated with oral hypoglycemics or insulin); and, situations that might cause seizures (e.g., abrupt cessation of a benzodiazepine, CNS tumor, severe hepatic cirrhosis).**
- **Adults and children with major depressive disease may show worsening of their depression and/or the emergence of suicidal ideation and behavior or unusual changes in behavior, whether or not they are taking antidepressants.**
- **Use with extreme caution in severe hepatic cirrhosis (do not exceed 150 mg every other day). Use with caution and in lower doses in clients with liver or kidney disease and in those with a recent history of MI or unstable heart disease.**
- **Hypersensitivity reactions are possible characterized by pruritus, urticaria, angioedema, dyspnea and, rarely, erythema multiforme, Stevens-Johnson syndrome, and anaphylaxis.**
- **Safety and efficacy have not been established in clients less than 18 years of age.**

SIDE EFFECTS

Most Common

Immediate-Release. Agitation, dizziness, headache/migraine, insomnia, sedation, tremor, excessive sweating, anorexia, dry mouth, constipation, N&V, weight gain/loss, blurred vision, tachycardia.

Extended-Release (SR). Headache, insomnia, dry mouth, nausea, pharyngitis, constipation, dizziness, agitation.

Extended-Release (XL). Headache, insomnia, dry mouth, nausea, nasopharyngitis, URTI, constipation.

Zyban. Dry mouth, insomnia, dizziness, nausea, rhinitis.

Listed are side effects for IR, SR, and XL forms with an incidence of 0.1% or greater. **Immediate-Release (IR). CNS:** Agitation, dizziness, headache/migraine, tremor, sedation, insomnia, confusion, akinesia/bradykinesia, hostility, impaired sleep quality, sensory disturbance, anxiety, decreased/increased libido, disturbed concentration, akathisia, delusions, euphoria, pseudoparkinsonism, ***seizures,*** ataxia/incoordination, depression, dyskinesia, dystonia, hallucinations, mania/hypomania, myoclonus, depersonalization, dysarthria, dysphoria, formal thought disorder, frigidity, memory impairment, mood instability, paranoia, psychosis, vertigo. **GI:** Dry mouth, constipation, weight loss/gain, N&V, anorexia, diarrhea, increased appetite, dyspepsia, increased salivation, stomatitis, bruxism, dysphagia, gum irritation, oral edema, thirst disturbance, toothache, liver damage, jaundice. **CV:** Tachycardia, cardiac arrhythmias, hypertension, palpitations, hypotension, syncope, chest pain, ECG abnormalities (premature beats, nonspecific ST-T changes). **Dermatologic:** Excessive sweating, rashes (including nonspecific), pruritus, cutaneous temperature disturbance, alopecia, dry skin, photosensitivity. **GU:** Menstrual complaints, impotence, urinary frequency/retention, decreased sexual function, nocturia, painful erection, retarded ejaculation, testicular swelling, UTI, vaginal irritation, gynecomastia. **Musculoskeletal:** Arthritis, muscle spasms. **Respiratory:** URT complaints, shortness of breath, dyspnea, bronchitis. **Hypersensitivity:** Angioedema, dyspnea, pruritus, urticaria, anaphylactoid/anaphylactic reactions, erythema multiforme (rare), ***Stevens-Johnson syndrome*** (rare), delayed hypersensitivity (arthralgia, myalgia, fever, rash). **Ophthalmic:** Blurred vision, mydriasis, visual disturbance. **Otic:** Auditory disturbance. **Body as a whole:** Fatigue, fever, chills, edema, flu symptoms, nonspecific pain. **Miscellaneous:** Gustatory disturbance.

B

Extended-Release (SR). CNS: Headache, insomnia, dizziness, anxiety, agitation, tremor, nervousness, somnolence, irritability, migraine, CNS stimulation, decreased memory, paresthesia, somnolence, abnormal coordination, confusion, decreased libido, decreased memory, depersonalization, dysphoria, emotional lability, hostility, hyperkinesia, hypertonia, hypesthesia, ***suicidal ideation***, vertigo, psychosis, mania. **GI:** Dry mouth, nausea, constipation, abdominal pain, anorexia, diarrhea, vomiting, dysphagia, bruxism, gastric reflux, gingivitis, glossitis, increased salivation, mouth ulcers, stomatitis, thirst, abnormal liver function, jaundice. **CV:** Palpitation, flushing, hot flashes, postural hypotension, stroke, tachycardia, vasodilation. **Dermatologic:** Sweating, rash, pruritus, urticaria, photosensitivity, ecchymosis. **GU:** Urinary frequency/urgency, UTI, ***vaginal hemorrhage,*** impotence, polyuria, prostate disorder. **Musculoskeletal:** Myalgia, arthralgia, twitch, arthritis, chest pain, leg cramps, musculoskeletal chest pain. **Respiratory:** Pharyngitis, sinusitis, increased cough. **Hypersensitivity: *Angioedema,*** dyspnea, pruritus, urticaria, anaphylactoid/anaphylactic reactions, erythema multiforme (rare), ***Stevens-Johnson syndrome*** (rare), delayed hypersensitivity (arthralgia, myalgia, fever, rash). **Ophthalmic:** Amblyopia, abnormal accommodation, dry eye. **Otic:** Tinnitus. **Body as a whole:** Asthenia, infection, pain, fever, chills, facial edema, edema, increased weight, peripheral edema. **Miscellaneous:** Taste perversion, syndrome of inappropriate antidiuretic hormone.

Extended-Release (XL). CNS: Headache, insomnia, anxiety, dizziness, abnormal dreams, feeling jittery, tremor, agitation, irritability, migraine, psychosis, mania. **GI:** Dry mouth, nausea, constipation, flatulence, decreased appetite, abdominal pain, diarrhea, dyspepsia, upper abdominal pain, viral gastroenteritis. **CV:** Hypertension, palpitations. **Dermatologic:** Rash, hyperhidrosis, photosensitivity. **GU:** Dysmenorrhea. **Musculoskeletal:** Myalgia, extremity pain, arthralgia, back/neck pain. **Respiratory:** Nasopharyngitis, URTI, sinusitis, cough, nasal congestion, pharyngolaryngeal pain, sinus congestion. **Hypersensitivity: *Angioedema,*** dyspnea, pruritus, urticaria, ***anaphylactoid/anaphylactic reactions,*** erythema multiforme (rare), ***Stevens-Johnson syndrome*** (rare), delayed hypersensitivity (arthralgia, myalgia, fever, rash). **Otic:** Tinnitus. **Body as a whole:** Fatigue, influenza. *NOTE:* Side effects for bupropion hydrobromide extended-release are similar to bupropion hydrochloride extended-release.

Zyban. CNS: Insomnia, dizziness, disturbed concentration, anxiety, abnormal dreams, nervousness, tremor, somnolence, tremor, abnormal thinking, dysphoria. **GI:** Dry mouth, nausea, constipation, diarrhea, abdominal pain, anorexia, mouth ulcer, thirst, increased appetite. **CV:** Palpitations, hypertension, hot flashes. **Dermatologic:** Rash, pruritus, dry skin, urticaria, photosensitivity. **Musculoskeletal:** Arthralgia, myalgia, chest/neck pain. **Respiratory:** Rhinitis, increased cough, pharyngitis, epistaxis, sinusitis, bronchitis, dyspnea. **Hypersensitivity: *Angioedema,*** dyspnea, pruritus, urticaria, anaphylactoid/anaphylactic reactions, erythema multiforme (rare), ***Stevens-Johnson syndrome*** (rare), delayed hypersensitivity (arthralgia, myalgia, fever, rash). **Otic:** Tinnitus. **Miscellaneous:** Taste perversion, accidental injury, facial edema, allergic reaction.

OVERDOSE MANAGEMENT

Symptoms: ***Seizures,*** ECG changes (conduction disturbances, arrhythmia), hallucinations, loss of consciousness, sinus tachycardia, coma, fever, hypotension, muscle rigidity, rhabdomyolysis, ***respiratory failure***, stupor. Large doses may cause multiple ***uncontrolled seizures***, bradycardia, ***cardiac failure, cardiac arrest prior to death.*** Consider the possibility of multiple-drug involvement. *Treatment:* Client should be hospitalized. Ensure an adequate airway, oxygenation, and ventilation. Monitor cardiac rhythm and vital signs. Monitor EEG for first 48 hr. Use general supportive and symptomatic measures. Do not induce emesis. Gastric lavage with a large-bore orogastric tube with appropriate airway protection, if needed, may be used if undertaken soon after ingestion or in symptomatic clients. Give activated charcoal. Seizures may be treated with IV benzodiazepines and other supportive procedures.

DRUG INTERACTIONS

Alcohol / ↓ Seizure threshold; may precipitate seizures

Amantadine / ↑ Risk of adverse effects, including psychotic reactions and neurotoxicity; use small initial/gradual increases of bupropion

Antiarrhythmics, type 1C / ↑ Antiarrhythmic side effects R/T ↓ liver metabolism by CYP2D6 isoenzymes

Antidepressants / ↓ Seizure threshold → ↑ risk of seizures; use together with extreme caution
Antipsychotics (haloperidol, risperidone, thioridazine) / ↓ Seizure threshold → ↑ risk of seizures; use together with extreme caution; also, ↑ antiarrhythmic side effects R/T ↓ liver metabolism by CYP2D6 isoenzymes
Beta blockers / ↑ Beta blocker side effect R/T ↓ liver metabolism by CYP2D6 isoenzymes
Carbamazepine / ↑ Bupropion metabolism → ↓ plasma levels
Cimetidine / ↓ Bupropion metabolism by CYP2B6 → ↑ pharmacologic/toxic effects
Clopidogrel / ↑ Bupropion AUC and peak plasma levels and ↓ bupropion clearance/AUC of hydroxyl metabolite R/T ↓ metabolism by CYP2B6 hydroxylation
Corticosteroids, systemic / ↓ Seizure threshold → ↑ risk of seizures; use together with extreme caution
Cyclosporine / ↓ Cyclosporine levels; increase dose
Fluoxetine / Panic symptoms/psychotic reactions
Guanfacine / ↑ Risk of bupropion toxicity
Levodopa / ↑ Risk of side effects, including neurotoxicity; use small initial/small gradual dose increases of bupropion
Linezolid / ↑ Risk of hypertensive crisis
MAOIs / ↑ Acute toxicity to bupropion, especially with phenelzine; allow at least 14 days between discontinuation of an MAOI and initiation of bupropion
Metoprolol / ↑ Metoprolol side effects R/T ↓ liver metabolism
Nicotine replacement / Possible severe hypertension; monitor BP
Phenobarbital / ↑ Bupropion metabolism by CYP2B6 → ↓ plasma levels
Phenytoin / ↑ Bupropion metabolism by CYP2B6 → ↓ plasma levels
Rifampin / ↓ Bupropion plasma levels → ↓ therapeutic effect
Ritonavir / ↓ Bupropion plasma levels → ↓ therapeutic effect
Selective serotonin-reuptake inhibitors / ↓ Seizure threshold → ↑ risk of seizures; use together with extreme caution; also, ↑ SSRI side effects R/T ↓ liver metabolism by CYP2D6 isoenzymes (consider dose reduction)
Tamoxifen / ↓ Levels of active metabolite of tamoxifen → ↓ effect; do not use together
Theophylline / ↓ Seizure threshold → ↑ risk of seizures; use together with extreme caution
Ticlopidine / ↑ Bupropion AUC and peak plasma levels and ↓ bupropion clearance/AUC of hydroxyl metabolite R/T ↓ metabolism by CYP2B6 hydroxylation
Tricyclic antidepressants (TCAs) / ↑ TCA side effects R/T ↓ liver metabolism by CYP2D6 isoenzymes (consider dose reduction)
Warfarin / Altered PT or INR with possible hemorrhagic or thrombotic complications

HOW SUPPLIED

Bupropion hydrobromide. *Tablets, Extended-Release:* 174 mg, 348 mg, 522 mg.
Bupropion hydrochloride. *Tablets, Extended-Release 12-hr (Budeprion SR, Wellbutrin SR):* 100 mg, 150 mg, 200 mg; *Tablets, Extended-Release 24-hr (Budeprion XL and Wellbutrin XL):* 150 mg, 300 mg; *Tablets, Extended-Release (Zyban):* 150 mg; *Tablets, Immediate-Release:* 75 mg, 100 mg.

DOSAGE

Bupropion hydrobromide (Aplenzin)

TABLETS, EXTENDED-RELEASE

Major depressive disorder.

Adults, initial: 174 mg/day (equivalent to 150 mg/day of bupropion hydrochloride) given as a single dose in the morning. If the 174 mg dose is tolerated, an increase to 348 mg/day given once daily can be made as early as day 4 of dosing. There should be an interval of at least 24 hr between successive doses. An increase in dose to the maximum of 522 mg/day, given as a single dose, may be considered for those in whom no clinical improvement is noted after several weeks at 348 mg/day. **Usual dose:** 348 mg/day (equivalent to 300 mg/day of bupropion hydrochloride); **maximum dose:** 522 mg/day. It is not known whether the dose needed for maintenance treatment is identical to the dose needed to achieve an initial response. Periodically assess to determine the need for maintenance treatment and the appropriate dose for such treatment. However, acute episodes of depression require several months or longer of sustained therapy.

Bupropion hydrochloride

TABLETS, IMMEDIATE-RELEASE

Major depressive disorder.

Adults, initial: 100 mg in the a.m. and p.m. for the first 3 days; **then,** 100 mg 3 times per day, given in the morning, midday, and in the evening (6 hr should elapse between doses). If no response is observed after 4 weeks or more, the dose may be increased to a maximum of 450 mg/day with individual doses not to exceed 150 mg. **Maintenance:** Lowest dose to control depression. Several months of treatment may be necessary. Discontinue in those who do not demonstrate an adequate response after an appropriate treatment period using 450 mg/day.

Attention deficit hyperactivity disorder in children and adolescents.

Children and adolescents, initial: Up to 3 mg/kg/day or 150 mg/day; **maximum dose:** Up to 6 mg/kg/day or 300 mg/day. Do not exceed a single dose of 150 mg. Usually dose is divided and given twice a day for children and three times a day for adolescents.

TABLETS, EXTENDED-RELEASE (SR AND XL)

Major depressive disorder.

Adults, initial: 150 mg once daily in the a.m. using either the SR or XL form. If 150 mg is tolerated, increase to 300 mg/day once daily (XL form) or 150 mg twice a day (SR form) as early as day 4 of dosing. Allow 8 or more hr between successive doses. Do not exceed a daily dose of 400 mg given as 200 mg twice a day using the SR form or do not exceed a daily dose of 450 mg using the XL form in clients where no clinical improvement was noted after several weeks of 300 mg/day. **Maintenance:** Periodically assess to determine the need for maintenance treatment and the appropriate dose for such treatment, although acute episodes of depression require several months or longer of sustained therapy. It is not known whether the dose needed for maintenance treatment is identical to the dose needed to achieve an initial response.

Attention deficit hyperactivity disorder in children and adolescents.

Children and adolescents, initial: Up to 3 mg/kg/day or 150 mg/day; **maximum dose:** Up to 6 mg/kg/day or 300 mg/day. Do not exceed a single dose of 150 mg. Usually dose is divided and given twice a day for children and three times a day for adolescents.

TABLETS, EXTENDED-RELEASE (XL)

Seasonal affective disorder.

Initial: 150 mg/day as a single dose in the morning generally started in the autumn prior to the onset of depressive symptoms; **maintenance/maximum dose:** if the 150 mg initial dose is well tolerated, increase the dose to the 300 mg/day dose (given in the morning) after 1 week. Reduce the dose to 150 mg/day if the 300 mg/day dose is not tolerated. There should be an interval of at least 24 hr between successive doses. It is not known whether the dose needed for maintenance treatment is identical to the dose needed to achieve an initial response. Continue treatment through the winter season and taper and discontinue in early spring. For those taking 300 mg/day during the autumn-winter seasons, taper the dose to 150 mg/day for 2 weeks prior to discontinuation. Clients whose seasonal depressive episodes are infrequent or not associated with significant impairment should generally not be treated prophylactically.

Zyban

TABLETS, EXTENDED-RELEASE

Smoking deterrent.

Initial: 150 mg/day for the first 3 days; **then,** 150 mg twice a day for 7–12 weeks (up to 6 months). Do not exceed doses of 300 mg/day. Eight hours or more should elapse between successive doses. *NOTE:* Clients should continue to receive counseling and support throughout treatment and for a period of time thereafter.

NURSING IMPLICATIONS

Do not confuse bupropion with buspirone (antianxiety agent) or buprenorphine (narcotic analgesic). Do not confuse the SR product (intended for twice-daily dosing) with the XL product (intended for once-daily dosing).

IMPLEMENTATION/ADMINISTRATION/STORAGE

1. The risk of seizures may be minimized by using the following guidelines: For Bupropion IR: Do not exceed a total daily dose of 450 mg. The daily dose is given 3 times per day with at least 6 hr between successive doses, with each single dose not to exceed 150 mg. The rate of dose increase is very gradual. For Wellbutrin SR: Do not exceed a total daily dose of 400 mg. The daily dose is given twice daily. The rate of dose increase is gradual. No single dose should exceed 200 mg. For Bupropion XL: Do not exceed a total daily dose of 450 mg. The rate of dose increase is gradual. For Zyban: Do not exceed a total daily dose of 300 mg. The recommended daily dose for most clients is 300 mg/day given as 150 mg twice a day. No single dose should exceed 150 mg.
2. Total daily doses of the immediate- and sustained-release tablets can be converted milligram-for-milligram to a once-daily dose of the extended-release formulation.
3. Several months of therapy may be necessary to control acute depression.
4. With severe hepatic cirrhosis, do not exceed a dose of 75 mg of immediate-release product once daily; do not exceed 100 mg every day or 150 mg every other day for SR and 150 mg every other day for XL. For Zyban, give 150 mg every other day in clients with severe hepatic cirrhosis.
5. Reduce the dose and/or frequency of bupropion in clients with impaired renal function.
6. Initiate Zyban treatment while client is still smoking since about 1 week of treatment is needed to reach steady-state blood levels. A "target quit date," usually in the second week, should be set. Continue treatment for 7 to 12 weeks. Dose tapering is not required when discontinuing Zyban treatment.
7. If significant progress has not been made by week 7 of treatment with Zyban, it is not likely client will stop smoking during this attempt. Thus, discontinue treatment.
8. Zyban may be combined with a nicotine transdermal system for smoking cessation.
9. When switching clients from the hydrochloride product to the hydrobromide product, give the equivalent total daily dose when possible. For example, bupropion hydrobromide, 522 mg, is equivalent to bupropion hydrochloride, 450 mg; bupropion hydrobromide, 348 mg, is equivalent to bupropion hydrochloride, 300 mg; and, bupropion hydrobromide, 174 mg, is equivalent to bupropion hydrochloride, 150 mg. Those who are being treated with bupropion hydrochloride tablets at 300 mg/day (e.g., 100 mg 3 times a day) may be switched to bupropion hydrobromide 348 mg once a day. Those who are currently treated with bupropion hydrochloride tablets at 300 mg/day (e.g., 150 mg twice a day) may be switched to bupropion hydrobromide, 348 mg once a day.
10. Store immediate-release tablets at 15–25°C (59–77°F); sustained release (SR) and Zyban at 20–25°C (68–77°F); and extended-release (XL) at 15–30°C (59–86°F). Protect immediate release from light and moisture. Dispense sustained release in a tight, light-resistant container.

ASSESSMENT

1. List reasons for therapy, presenting behaviors, duration of symptoms, other agents/therapies trialed.
2. Note history of seizures, recent MI, head trauma, CNS tumor, bulimia, anorexia nervosa; precludes therapy.
3. Determine if client is of childbearing age or lactating.
4. Assess mental stability and potential for compliance. Fewer side effects (no CV effects, drug interactions, sedation, and weight gain) with bupropion than other antidepressants.
5. With tobacco abuse, ensure ready to quit; note numbers of cigarettes smoked per day, nicotine content, triggers, other failures, and date desired to quit so that treatment can be started 1 week prior.
6. Monitor response to therapy and need for dosage adjustment.

7. Monitor lung sounds, weight, ECG, BP—especially if on nicotine replacement, renal and LFTs; reduce dose with renal/liver dysfunction.

CLIENT/FAMILY TEACHING

1. Take as directed for condition treated. Do not take Zyban with Wellbutrin and do not break, crush, or chew sustained-release products. If dose is missed, do not take extra dose to catch up: increases seizure risk. Avoid taking at bedtime to minimize insomnia effects.
2. The extended-release (XL) tablets are to be taken once daily with at least 24 hr between doses to minimize risk of seizures. Medication in the XL tablet is contained in a plastic shell that slowly releases the medication over 24 hr and is then expelled in the stool. Swallow tablets whole; do not chew, divide, or crush.
3. May experience changes in taste perception; may result in appetite/weight loss. Record weights; report changes. May take with food if GI upset.
4. May cause menstrual irregularities and impotence. Report changes in urinary output. May cause dry mouth; try frequent sips of water, suck on ice chips or sugarless hard candy, or chew sugarless gum if occurs.
5. Beneficial drug effects for depression may not be evident for up to 30 days. Continue and do not be discouraged by delayed response. Do not stop abruptly with prolonged therapy.
6. Dizziness may occur. Do not arise from lying position suddenly. If dizziness occurs during the day, sit until it subsides. May cause drowsiness, hyperactivity, GI upset, diarrhea, constipation, dry mouth. Avoid activities that require mental alertness until effects realized.
7. Report mood swings, anxiety, change in personality, hostility or aggressiveness, impulsivity, insomnia, irritability, panic attacks, or suicidal thoughts immediately and other adverse side effects.
8. Avoid OTC agents without approval and minimize, or completely avoid, consumption of alcoholic beverages; increases seizure risk.
9. May increase sensitivity to sunlight; wear protective clothing and sunscreen and avoid prolonged exposure. Notify provider if pregnancy planned or suspected.
10. With sustained-released formulation for smoking cessation, will be started at a low dose for twice-a-day consumption. Take last dose 4 to 6 hr before bedtime to prevent insomnia. May be used with nicotine patch if needed. Start therapy while still smoking–takes about 1 week to achieve desired drug level; should stop smoking by week 2. A formal smoking cessation program will enhance positive response rates.
11. For prevention of seasonal major depressive episodes, will start therapy in the autumn prior to the onset of depressive symptoms and continue through the winter; taper and discontinue in early spring as directed.
12. Keep all F/U to assess response and for adverse SE.

OUTCOMES/EVALUATE

- Improvement in S&S of depression such as ↓ fatigue, improved eating and sleeping patterns, and ↑ socialization
- Successful nicotine/smoking cessation
- Treatment of neuropathic pain; SAD; weight loss (bupropion SR); treatment of ADHD (unlabeled)

Buspirone hydrochloride

(byou-**SPYE**-rohn)

Classification(s): Antianxiety drug, nonbenzodiazepine

Pregnancy Category: B

RX: BuSpar.

✤ **Rx:** Apo-Buspirone, CO Buspirone, Gen-Buspirone, PMS-Buspirone, ratio-Buspirone.

INDICATIONS/USES

(1) Management of anxiety disorders. (2) Short-term relief of symptoms of anxiety. *Investigational:* Adjunct in treating withdrawal from heroin.

ACTION/KINETICS

Action

The mechanism of action is unknown. Not chemically related to the benzodiazepines; no anticonvulsant, muscle relaxant properties, or significant sedation seen. Binds to serotonin ($5\text{-}HT_{1A}$) and dopamine (D_2) receptors in the CNS; is possible that dopamine-mediated neurologic disorders may occur. These include dystonia, Parkinson-like symptoms, akathisia, and tardive dyskinesia.

Pharmacokinetics

Peak plasma levels: 1–6 ng/mL 40–90 min after a single PO dose of 20 mg. Bioavailability is increased when given with food. **t½:** 2–3 hr. Rapidly absorbed with extensive first-pass metabolism; active and inactive metabolites excreted in the urine and through the feces. **Plasma protein binding:** About 86%.

CONTRAINDICATIONS

Psychoses, severe liver or kidney impairment, lactation. Not usually indicated for treatment of anxiety and tension due to stress of everyday living.

SPECIAL CONCERNS

A decrease in dose may be necessary in geriatric clients due to age-related impaired renal function.

SIDE EFFECTS

Most Common

Dizziness, drowsiness, nausea, headache, nervousness, lightheadedness, excitement.

Side effects listed have an incidence of 0.1% or more. **CNS:** Dizziness, drowsiness, headache, nervousness, insomnia, lightheadedness, decreased concentration, excitement, anger/hostility, confusion, numbness, depression, tremor, incoordination, paresthesia, dream disturbances, depersonalization, dysphoria, noise intolerance, euphoria, akathisia, fearfulness, loss of interest, dissociative reaction, hallucinations, involuntary movements, slowed reaction times, ***suicidal ideation, seizures.*** **GI:** N&V, dry mouth, abdominal/gastric distress, diarrhea, constipation, flatulence, anorexia, increased appetite, salivation, irritable colon, rectal bleeding. **CV:** Tachycardia/palpitations, nonspecific chest pain, syncope, hypotension, hypertension. **Dermatologic:** Skin rash, edema, pruritus, flushing, easy bruising, hair loss, dry skin, facial, edema, blisters. **GU:** Increased or decreased libido, urinary frequency, urinary hesitancy, menstrual irregularity, spotting, dysuria. **Musculoskeletal:** Aches/pains, muscle cramps, muscle spasms, rigid/stiff muscles, arthralgia. **Respiratory:** Hyperventilation, SOB, chest congestion, sore throat, nasal congestion. **Ophthalmic:** Blurred vision, redness and itching of eye, conjunctivitis. **Body as a whole:** Fatigue, weakness, sweating/clamminess, weight gain/loss, fever, malaise. **Miscellaneous:** Tinnitus, altered taste, altered smell, roaring sensation in the head.

LABORATORY TEST CONSIDERATIONS

↑ ALT, AST.

OVERDOSE MANAGEMENT

Symptoms: Dizziness, drowsiness, N&V, gastric distress, miosis. *Treatment:* Immediate gastric lavage; general symptomatic and supportive measures. Monitor respiration, pulse, and BP.

DRUG INTERACTIONS

Alcohol / Avoid concomitant use
Carbamazepine / ↓ Plasma buspirone levels R/T induction of metabolism by CYP3A4 liver enzymes
Cimetidine / ↑ Buspirone C_{max} and T_{max} but minimal effects on AUC
Clarithromycin / ↑ Plasma buspirone levels R/T inhibition of metabolism by CYP3A4 liver enzymes
Dexamethasone / ↓ Plasma buspirone levels R/T induction of metabolism by CYP3A4 liver enzymes
Diazepam / Possible dizziness, headache, and nausea
Diltiazem / ↑ Plasma buspirone levels R/T inhibition of metabolism by CYP3A4 liver enzymes
Erythromycin / ↑ Plasma buspirone levels R/T inhibition of metabolism by CYP3A4 liver enzymes
Fluoxetine / ↓ Buspirone effects
Fluvoxamine / ↑ Plasma buspirone levels R/T inhibition of metabolism by CYP3A4 liver enzymes
Grapefruit juice / ↑ Plasma levels of buspirone → excess sedation
Haloperidol / Possible ↑ haloperidol levels
Itraconazole / ↑ Plasma buspirone levels R/T inhibition of metabolism by CYP3A4 liver enzymes
Ketoconazole / ↑ Plasma buspirone levels R/T inhibition of metabolism by CYP3A4 liver enzymes
MAOIs / ↑ BP; do not use together
Nefazodone / Possible lightheadedness, asthenia, dizzinesss, and somnolence; use a lower dose (2.5 mg/day) of buspirone
Phenobarbital / ↓ Plasma buspirone levels R/T induction of metabolism by CYP3A4 liver enzymes
Phenytoin / ↓ Plasma buspirone levels R/T induction of metabolism by CYP3A4 liver enzymes
Rifabutin / ↓ Plasma buspirone levels R/T induction of metabolism by CYP3A4 liver enzymes
Rifampin / ↓ Plasma buspirone levels R/T induction of metabolism by CYP3A4 liver enzymes
Ritonavir / ↑ Plasma buspirone levels R/T inhibition of metabolism by CYP3A4 liver enzymes

Verapamil / ↑ Plasma buspirone levels R/T inhibition of metabolism by CYP3A4 liver enzymes

HOW SUPPLIED

Tablets: 5 mg, 7.5 mg, 15 mg, 30 mg.

DOSAGE

TABLETS

Anxiety disorders, short-term relief of anxiety.

Adults: 7.5 mg 2 times per day (i.e., 15 mg daily). May increase dose in increments of 5 mg/day q 2–3 days to achieve optimum effects; do not exceed a total daily dose of 60 mg. Divided doses of 20 to 30 mg/day have been commonly used.

NURSING IMPLICATIONS

Do not confuse buspirone with bupropion (antidepressant, smoking deterrent).

IMPLEMENTATION/ADMINISTRATION/STORAGE

1. No cross-tolerance with other sedative-hypnotic drugs, including benzodiazepines.
2. Will not block the withdrawal syndrome, which may occur following cessation of sedative-hypnotics. Withdraw clients on chronic sedative-hypnotic therapy gradually prior to beginning buspirone therapy.
3. To date, no potential for abuse, tolerance, or either physical/psychologic dependence.
4. Up to 2 weeks may be required before beneficial antianxiety effects manifested.

ASSESSMENT

1. List reasons for therapy, causative factor/event triggering disorder, other agents trialed; note pretreatment findings.
2. Determine support systems; encourage active family involvement in treatment plan.
3. Assess for recent benzodiazepine therapy; drug may be less effective.
4. Document mental status and note age; good agent to use in elderly clients because of less CNS suppression.
5. Evaluate for history of drug abuse; observe for signs of misuse/abuse.
6. Takes several weeks for effect; use another agent to supplement for acute symptoms. Monitor LFTs.

CLIENT/FAMILY TEACHING

1. Take dose consistently either always with or without food; food increases bioavailability. Separate buspirone dosage by 6–8 hr from ingestion of grapefruit juice.
2. May take with food or snack to decrease nausea, a common side effect; report if persistent/severe.
3. Use caution when operating a motor vehicle or performing tasks that require mental alertness; may cause drowsiness/dizziness.
4. Avoid OTC agents, CNS depressants, and alcohol.
5. Do not stop suddenly; withdrawal symptoms such as N&V, dry mouth, nasal congestion, or sore throat may occur.
6. Report weakness, restlessness, nervousness, headaches, feelings of depression, or lack of desired response.
7. Report involuntary, repetitive movements of the face or neck muscles (Parkinson's-like symptoms), or suicide ideations immediately.
8. Keep all F/U to assess response, therapy, and for adverse SE.

OUTCOMES/EVALUATE

Relief of agitated depressive S&S; ↓ anxiety

■ IV

Busulfan

(byou-**SUL**-fan)

Classification(s): Antineoplastic, alkylating
Pregnancy Category: D
RX: Busulfex, Myleran.

SEE ALSO ***ANTINEOPLASTIC AGENTS*** AND ***ALKYLATING AGENTS***.

INDICATIONS/USES

Injection: With cyclophosphamide as a conditioning treatment prior to allogeneic hematopoietic progenitor cell transplantation for chronic myelogenous leukemia (CML).

Tablets: Palliative treatment of CML (granulocytic, myelocytic, myeloid). Less effective in individuals with CML who lack the Philadelphia (Ph_1) chromosome. Not effective in individuals where the disease is in the "blastic" phase. *Investigational:* Other myeloproliferative disorders, including severe thrombocytosis and polycythemia vera, myelofibrosis; bone marrow transplantation.

ACTION/KINETICS

Action

Is an alkylating agent. Busulfan hydrolyzes to release methylsulfonate groups that produce reactive carbonium ions; these ions can alkylate DNA. DNA damage is thought to be responsible for the cytotoxicity of busulfan. Leukocyte count drops during the second or third week; thus, weekly laboratory tests are mandatory. Resistance may develop; thought to be due to the altered transport into the cell and/or increased intracellular inactivation.

Pharmacokinetics

Rapidly and completely absorbed from the GI tract; appears in serum 0.6–2 hr after PO administration. **t½, elimination:** About 2.6 hr. Extensively metabolized by conjugation with glutathione and excreted in the urine. Clearance is more rapid in children than in adults. Increased appetite and sense of well-being may occur a few days after therapy is started. Sometimes administered with allopurinol to prevent symptoms of clinical gout. **Plasma protein binding:** 32% and 47% bound to plasma proteins and RBCs, respectively.

CONTRAINDICATIONS

Use of tablets unless a diagnosis of CML has been adequately established. Hypersensitivity to busulfan or any component of the product. Lactation.

SPECIAL CONCERNS

(1) Busulfan is a potent cytotoxic drug. Do not use unless a diagnosis of chronic myelogenous leukemia has been adequately established and the responsible healthcare provider is knowledgeable in assessing response to chemotherapy. (2) Busulfan can induce severe bone marrow hypoplasia. Reduce or discontinue the dosage immediately at the first sign of any unusual depression of bone marrow function as reflected by an abnormal decrease in any of the formed elements of the blood. Perform a bone marrow examination if the bone marrow status is uncertain. (3) Malignant tumors and acute leukemias have been reported in clients who have received busulfan therapy, and this drug may be a human carcinogen. The World Health Organization has concluded that there is a causal relationship between busulfan exposure and the development of secondary malignancies. Four cases of acute leukemia occurred among 243 clients treated with busulfan as adjuvant chemotherapy following surgical resection of bronchogenic carcinoma. All 4 cases were from a subgroup of 19 of these 243 clients who developed pancytopenia while taking busuflan 5 to 8 years before leukemia became clinically apparent. These findings suggest that busulfan is leukemogenic, although its mode of action is uncertain.

- **Avoid use of live vaccines to immunocompromised clients.**
- **Safety and efficacy of the injection not established in children.**

SIDE EFFECTS

Most Common

Profound myelosuppression, N&V, stomatitis (mucositis), diarrhea, anorexia, abdominal pain, insomnia, anxiety, fever, headache.

Hematologic: ***Pancytopenia, severe bone marrow hypoplasia,*** anemia, leukopenia, thrombocytopenia, ***aplastic anemia.*** **GI:** N&V, stomatitis (mucositits), esophagitis, anorexia, diarrhea, abdominal pain/enlargement, ileus, dyspepsia, constipation, dry mouth, rectal disorder/discomfort, hematemesis, pancreatitis. **Hepatic**: Jaundice, hepatomegaly, ***hepatotoxicity,*** centrilobular sinusoidal fibrosis, hepatocellular atrophy/necrosis, ***hepatic venoocclusive disease.*** **CNS:** Insomnia, anxiety, dizziness, depression, confusion, lethargy, hallucinations, delirium, encephalopathy, agitation, seizures, somnolence, ***cerebral hemorrhage/coma.*** **Respiratory:** ***Bronchopulmonary dysplasia with interstitial pulmonary fibrosis.*** Rhinitis, lung disorder, cough, epistaxis, dyspnea, pharyngitis, hiccough, asthma, alveolar hemorrhage, hemoptysis, pleural effusion, sinusitis, atelectasis, hypoxia, pneumonitis. **CV:** Tachycardia, hypertension, thrombosis, vasodilation (flushing, hot flashes), hypotension, arrhythmia, cardiomegaly, atrial fibrillation, abnormal ECG, heart block, left-sided heart failure, pericardial effusion, ventricular extrasystoles, ***third-degree heart block,*** endocardial fibrosis. ***Cardiac tamponade in children with thalessemia.*** **Ophthalmologic:** Cataracts after prolonged use, corneal thining, lens changes. **Dermatologic:** Hyperpigmentation, especially in clients with a dark complexion. Rash, pruritus, alopecia, vesicular rash, vesiculobullous rash, maculopapular rash, acne, exfoliative derma-

B

titis, erythema nodosum, increased local cutaneous reaction after radiotherapy. **Metabolic:** Syndrome resembling adrenal insufficiency, including symptoms of weakness, severe fatigue, weight loss, anorexia, N&V, and melanoderma (especially after prolonged use). Also, hyperuricemia/uricosuria in clients with CML. **GU:** Oliguria, hematuria, dysuria, hemorrhagic cystitis. **Miscellaneous:** Cellular dysplasia in various organs, including lymph nodes, pancreas, thyroid, adrenal glands, bone marrow, and liver. Also, fever, edema, headache, asthenia, infection, ***sepsis***, chills, pain, allergic reaction, chest/back pain, myalgia, inflammation at injection site, arthralgia, pneumonia, ear disorder. Malignant tumors and acute leukemias are possible.

LABORATORY TEST CONSIDERATIONS

↑ AST, alkaline phosphatase, creatinine. Hyperbilirubinemia, hyperglycemia, hypocalcemia, hypokalemia, hypomagnesemia, hypophosphatemia, hyponatremia, hyperuricemia, hyperuricosuria.

OVERDOSE MANAGEMENT

Symptoms: Bone marrow toxicity, CNS stimulation with ***convulsions and death on the first day.*** *Treatment:* If ingestion is recent, gastric lavage or induction of vomiting followed by activated charcoal. Hematologic status must be monitored.

DRUG INTERACTIONS

Acetaminophen / ↓ Busulfan clearance
Cyclophosphamide / Cardiac tamponade in clients with thalessemia (rare), but possibly fatal in those receiving high doses of both drugs
Cytotoxic drugs / Additive pulmonary toxicity
Itraconazole / ↓ Busulfan clearance up to 25%
Metronidazole / ↑ Trough plasma busulfan levels → ↑ risk of toxicity; do not use together
Myelosuppressive drugs / Additive myelosuppression
Phenytoin / ↑ Busulfan clearance by 15% or more R/T induction of glutathione-S-transferase
Thioguanine / ↑ Risk of esophageal varices with abnormal LFTs; use with caution in long-term continuous therapy

HOW SUPPLIED

Injection: 6 mg/mL; *Tablets:* 2 mg.

DOSAGE

IV VIA A CENTRAL VENOUS CATHETER

With cyclophosphamide prior to allogeneic hematopoietic progenitor cell transplantation.

Adults: 0.8 mg/kg of IBW or actual body weight (whichever is lower) of busulfan q 6 hr for 4 days (i.e., total of 16 doses). For obese or severely obese clients, calculate the dose of busulfan based on adjusted IBW. For cyclophosphamide, 60 mg/kg given on each of 2 days as a 1 hr infusion beginning on BMT day minus 3, 6 hr following the 16th busulfan dose.

TABLETS

Chronic myelocytic leukemia (CML).

Adults or children, remission induction, usual dose: 4–8 mg/day (about 60 mcg/kg or 1.8 mg/m^2 per day) until leukocyte count falls below 15,000/mcL; then, withdraw drug. **Maintenance, when leukocyte reaches about 50,000/mcL:** Resume treatment with induction dosage. When remission is less than 3 months, consider 1–3 mg/day that may keep client under control and prevent rapid relapse.

NURSING IMPLICATIONS

Do not confuse Alkeran (melphalan), Leukeran (chlorambucil), and Myleran (busulfan), each of which is an antineoplastic.

IMPLEMENTATION/ADMINISTRATION/STORAGE

1. **IV Do not administer without supervision and facilities for weekly CBCs.**
2. **Premedicate all clients with phenytoin since busulfan crosses the blood brain barrier and induces seizures.**
3. **Give antiemetics prior to the first dose of busulfan; continue on a fixed schedule through busulfan administration.**
4. **Prepare under biologic hood with proper attire: gloves, gown, and mask.**
5. **Busulfan is given via central catheter as a 2 hr infusion (using an infusion pump) q 6 hr for 4 consecutive days. Cyclophosphamide is given IV as a 1 hr infusion each day for 2 days beginning 6 hr following the 16th busulfan dose.**

B

6. Dilute busulfan prior to use with either 0.9% NaCl injection or D5W. The diluent quantity should be 10 times the volume of busulfan, ensuring the final concentration is about 0.5 mg/mL or more. To prepare final solution for infusion, add 9.3 mL of busulfan to 93 mL of diluent. Always add busulfan to diluent, not diluent to busulfan. Mix thoroughly by inverting several times.
7. Diluted busulfan stable at room temperature for up to 8 hr; infusion must be completed by that time. Busulfan diluted in 0.9% NaCl is stable for up to 12 hr if refrigerated; infusion must be completed by that time.
8. Do not infuse rapidly or at the same time with any other IV solution of unknown compatibility.
9. *NOTE:* Consult the package insert for information on blood sample collection for AUC determination, instructions for drug administration and blood sample collection for therapeutic drug monitoring, and preparation for IV administration.
10. Exercise caution in handling and preparing busulfan solutions as skin reactions may occur with accidental exposure. Use a vertical laminar flow safety hood; wear gloves and protective clothing.
11. COMPATIBILITY 0.9% NaCl injection or D5W.
12. INCOMPATIBILITY Administer separately.

ASSESSMENT

1. Note history of disease, previous experience with drug therapy, any noted resistance. Use with extreme caution in those with prior radiation or chemotherapy.
2. In clients with CML note presence of Philadelphia (Ph_1) chromosome. Document when disease in "blastic" phase as drug is not effective.
3. Monitor VS and I&O. Give plenty of fluids and allopurinol to decrease uric acid levels with resultant nephropathy.
4. Assess CXR/lung sounds; may experience pulmonary fibrosis up to 4–6 months following therapy.
5. May require premedication with IV dilantin to decrease risk of seizures seen with IV infusions. Also start antiemetics before treatment on a regular schedule during IV therapy.
6. Assess for S&S of local or systemic infection or bleeding. Advise of risk of malignant tumor occurrence during therapy.
7. Withhold drug when the total leukocyte count is less than 15,000/mm^3. During remission, may resume when monthly WBC reaches 50,000/mm^3. May cause moderate to severe granulocyte suppression. Busulfan-induced bone marrow suppression may be prolonged. WBC may continue to drop for 2 to 3 weeks after therapy is discontinued and may take up to 2 months to recover. Monitor appropriate weekly hematologic profiles. Nadir: 21 days; recovery: 42–56 days.
8. Monitor renal and LFTs; CBC/platelets weekly during therapy and for 2 weeks after stopping therapy.

CLIENT/FAMILY TEACHING

1. Take at the same time each day. May take on an empty stomach if N&V occur. Extra fluid intake may be required to prevent dehydration.
2. Report early symptoms of sore throat, infection, easy bruising/bleeding; expect weekly CBC studies.
3. Avoid live vaccines, persons infected, or those who have recently taken live virus vaccine, and all OTC agents without approval.
4. Practice reliable contraception. Drug has been associated with ovarian failure, including failure to achieve puberty in females. Consider egg/sperm harvesting as indicated.
5. Report skin rash immediately; may cause increased pigmentation, hair loss.
6. Allopurinol may be prescribed to decrease urate crystal formation.
7. Increased cough and visual difficulties may be S&S of toxicity; report increased weight loss, fatigue, loss of appetite, blurred vision, weakness.
8. Ensure awareness of increased risk of secondary malignancy with therapy.
9. Keep all F/U to assess response, labs, and for adverse SE.

OUTCOMES/EVALUATE

- Maintenance of leukocytes at 20,000/mm^3
- Absence of blasts on peripheral blood smear; ↓ spleen size

B

Combination Drug

Butalbital, Acetaminophen, and Caffeine

(byoo-**TAL**-bi-tall, ah-**SEAT**-ah-**MIN**-oh-fen, **KAF**-een)

Classification(s): Barbiturate/Nonnarcotic analgesic/Stimulant combination drug

Pregnancy Category: C

RX: Esgic, Fioricet, Margesic, Repan, Triad.

SEE ALSO *ACETAMINOPHEN*.

INDICATIONS/USES

Treatment of tension headaches or mild migraine headaches.

CONTENT

Each capsule or tablet contains: Butalbital (barbiturate), 50 mg; acetaminophen (nonnarcotic analgesic), 325 mg; and, caffeine (CNS stimulant), 40 mg.

ACTION/KINETICS

Action

The role of each component in the relief of tension headaches is not completely understood.

Pharmacokinetics

Butalbital is well absorbed from the GI tract. It is excreted primarily in the urine as unchanged drug and metabolites. **t½, plasma:** About 35 hr. Acetaminophen is rapidly absorbed from the GI tract. **t½, plasma:** 1.25–3 hr (may be increased by liver damage or overdosage). Acetaminophen is metabolized by the liver and excreted in the urine as unchanged drug and metabolites. Caffeine is also rapidly absorbed. **t½, plasma:** About 3 hr. It is metabolized by the liver and excreted, mostly as metabolites, in the urine.

CONTRAINDICATIONS

Hypersensitivity to any component of the product. Porphyria. Since butalbital is habit-forming and potentially abused, extended use is not recommended.

SPECIAL CONCERNS

- **Use with caution in the elderly, debilitated, in severe renal or hepatic impairment, or acute abdominal conditions.**
- **Use during pregnancy only when clearly needed.**
- **Safety and efficacy not established in children 12 years of age and less.**

SIDE EFFECTS

Most Common

Drowsiness, lightheadedness, dizziness, sedation, shortness of breath, N&V, abdominal pain, intoxicated feeling.

CNS: Headache, drowsiness, lightheadedness, dizziness, sedation, intoxicated feeling, shaky feeling, tingling, agitation, fainting, heavy eyelids, high energy, hot spells, numbness, sluggishness, dependence, irritability, ***seizures***. Mental confusion, excitement, or depression due to intolerance (especially in the elderly or debilitated). **GI:** N&V, abdominal pain, dry mouth, difficulty swallowing, heartburn, flatulence, constipation. **CV:** Tachycardia, cardiac stimulation. **Musculoskeletal:** Leg pain, muscle fatigue. **Hematologic:** Thrombocytopenia, ***agranulocytosis.*** **Respiratory:** Nasal congestion, SOB. **Otic:** Earache, tinnitus. **GU:** Diuresis, nephrotoxicity. **Dermatologic:** Pruritus, rash, erythema multiforme, ***toxic epidermal necrolysis.*** **Body as a whole:** Hyperhidrosis, fatigue, euphoria, allergic reactions, tremor, fever. **Miscellaneous:** Hyperglycemia.

OVERDOSE MANAGEMENT

Symptoms: **Symptoms due to butalbital:** Drowsiness, confusion, coma, respiratory depression, hypotension, ***hypovolemic shock***. **Symptoms due to acetaminophen:** Potentially fatal ***hepatic necrosis, renal tubular necrosis, hypoglycemic coma***, thrombocytopenia, N&V, diaphoresis, general malaise. *NOTE:* Clinical and laboratory evidence of hepatic toxicity may not be apparent until 48–72 hr after ingestion. **Symptoms due to caffeine:** Insomnia, restlessness, tremor, delirium, tachycardia, extrasystoles. *Treatment:* Overdose is potentially fatal. Immediate treatment includes:

- Induction of vomiting.
- Gastric lavage. A cuffed endotracheal tube should be inserted prior to gastric lavage if the client is unconscious.
- Oral activated charcoal (1 gram/kg) should follow gastric emptying. Follow the first dose of charcoal with an appropriate cathartic. If repeated doses are needed, give consideration to giving the cathartic with alternate charcoal doses.

- Treat hypotension with fluids as it is likely due to hypovolemia. Avoid pressors.
- Maintain adequate pulmonary ventilation.
- If renal function is normal, forced diuresis may help in the elimination of butalbital.
- Alkalinization of the urine increases renal excretion of some barbiturates.
- In severe cases of intoxication, peritoneal dialysis or hemodialysis may be considered.
- If hypoprothrombinemia occurs R/T acetaminophen, give IV vitamin K.
- If the dose of acetaminophen exceeded 140 mg/kg, give acetylcysteine asap. Obtain acetaminophen serum levels, since levels 4 or more hours after ingestion help predict toxicity. Do not wait for acetaminophen assay results before initiating treatment. Obtain hepatic enzyme levels initially and at 24 hr intervals.
- Treat methemoglobinemia over 30% with IV methylene blue.

DRUG INTERACTIONS

See also ***Acetaminophen***.

CNS depressants (other narcotic analgesics, general anesthetics, alcohol, anti-anxiety drug, sedative-hypnotics) / Additive CNS depression
MAOIs / ↑ Butalbital effects

HOW SUPPLIED

See *Content*.

DOSAGE

TABLETS

Tension headache or mild migraine headache.

Adults: 1 or 2 tablets q 4 hr, not to exceed 6 tablets a day.

NURSING IMPLICATIONS

IMPLEMENTATION/ADMINISTRATION/STORAGE

1. Since butalbital is habit-forming, it should be taken only for as long as prescribed, in the amounts prescribed, and no more frequently than prescribed.
2. Store from 15–30°C (59–86°F). Dispense in a tight, light-resistant container.

ASSESSMENT

1. Note reasons for therapy, characteristics of headaches, other agents trialed, outcome; document response 1 hr after administering.
2. Assess renal and LFTs; avoid with porphyria, use sparingly in the elderly or debilitated and those with acute abdominal problems.

CLIENT/FAMILY TEACHING

1. Take as directed with a full glass of water.
2. Do not perform activities that require mental alertness until drug effects realized; may cause dizziness/drowsiness.
3. Avoid alcohol and CNS drugs with this therapy. Store safely away from bedside and out of reach of children to prevent OD which may be fatal.
4. May cause dependence; do not stop suddenly without provider supervision.
5. Practice reliable contraception. Consider additional nonhormonal form of contraception during therapy.
6. Keep all F/U to assess response and for adverse SE.

OUTCOMES/EVALUATE

Control of tension headaches

Butenafine hydrochloride

(byou-**TEN**-ah-feen)

Classification(s): Antifungal

Pregnancy Category: B

OTC: Lotrimin Ultra.

RX: Mentax.

SEE ALSO ***ANTI-INFECTIVE DRUGS***.

INDICATIONS/USES

OTC: (1) Superficial dermatophytoses. (2) Athlete's foot between toes, jock itch, ringworm, and the accompanying itching, burning, cracking, and scaling that usually accompanies these conditions.

Rx: (1) Treat interdigital tinea pedis (athlete's foot), tinea corporis (ringworm), and tinea cruris (jock itch) due to *Epidermophyton floccosum, Trichophyton mentagrophytes, T. rubrum,* or *T. tonsurans.* (2) Treatment of tinea (pityriasis) versicolor due to *Malassezia fufur.*

ACTION/KINETICS

Action

Acts by inhibiting epoxidation of squalene, thus blocking the synthesis of ergosterol, an essential component of fungal cell membranes. Depending on the concentration and the fungal species, the drug may be fungicidal.

Pharmacokinetics

Although applied topically, some of the drug is absorbed into the general circulation.

CONTRAINDICATIONS

Known or suspected sensitivity to butenafine or any component of the product. Ophthalmic, oral, or intravaginal use.

SPECIAL CONCERNS

- Use with caution during lactation and in clients sensitive to allylamine antifungal drugs (drugs may be cross-reactive).
- Safety and efficacy not determined in children less than 12 years of age.

SIDE EFFECTS

Most Common

Burning, stinging, itching.

Dermatologic: Contact dermatitis, burning, stinging, worsening of the condition, erythema, irritation, itching.

HOW SUPPLIED

OTC or Rx. Cream: 1%.

DOSAGE

CREAM (1%)

Tinea versicolor, tinea corporis, tinea cruris.

Apply the cream to cover the affected area and immediate surrounding skin once daily for 2 weeks.

Interdigital tinea pedis.

Apply twice a day for 7 days or once daily for 4 weeks.

NURSING IMPLICATIONS

IMPLEMENTATION/ADMINISTRATION/STORAGE

1. For external use only; not for ophthalmic, PO, or intravaginal use.
2. Store the drug at 5–30°C (41–86°F).

ASSESSMENT

1. Note reasons for therapy, onset, location, duration, characteristics of S&S, culture/skin scraping results.
2. Describe clinical presentation. List other agents trialed and results.

CLIENT/FAMILY TEACHING

1. Review method for site preparation and application of cream. Ensure treatment area is dry; apply a thin film of cream to cover affected area(s) and the surrounding skin areas. Gently massage into skin; wash hands before and after applying.
2. After bathing, dry feet thoroughly/carefully between each toe before applying; avoid occlusive dressings.
3. Avoid contact with the eyes, nose, mouth, other mucous membranes. If eye contact, wash with large amounts of cool water.
4. Nursing mothers should not apply butenafine to the breast.
5. Do not stop therapy when condition shows improvement; continue for full prescribed time (usually 2–4 wk). May experience some local stinging, burning, itching, and redness; report if bothersome or persistent.
6. Stop therapy and report any increased swelling, itching, burning, blistering, drainage, irritation, or lack of improvement.
7. Keep all F/U to assess response and for adverse SE.

OUTCOMES/EVALUATE

Resolution of fungal infection

Butoconazole nitrate

(byou-toe-**KON**-ah-zohl)

Classification(s): Antifungal

Pregnancy Category: C

OTC: Femstat 3, Mycelex-3.

RX: Gynazole-1.

INDICATIONS/USES

Vulvovaginal fungal infections caused by *Candida albicans.*

ACTION/KINETICS

Action

By permeating chitin in the fungal cell wall, butoconazole increases membrane permeability to intracellular substances, leading to reduced osmotic resistance and viability of the fungus.

Pharmacokinetics

Approximately 1.7% of drug is absorbed following vaginal administration. **t½:** 21–24 hr.

B

CONTRAINDICATIONS
Use during first trimester of pregnancy.

SPECIAL CONCERNS
- Use with caution during lactation.
- Pediatric dosage not established.

SIDE EFFECTS
Most Common
See *Side Effects*.

GU: Vaginal burning, vulvar burning or itching, discharge; soreness, swelling, and itching of the fingers.

HOW SUPPLIED
Vaginal Cream: 2%.

DOSAGE
VAGINAL CREAM
Vulvovaginal infections.

One applicatorful of Gynazole-1 intravaginally once (remains in vaginal vault for approximately 4 days). Or, one applicatorful a day of Mycelex-3, preferably at bedtime, for 3 consecutive days.

NURSING IMPLICATIONS
IMPLEMENTATION/ADMINISTRATION/STORAGE
1. During pregnancy, use of a vaginal applicator may be contraindicated.
2. If no response, repeat studies to confirm the diagnosis before reinstituting antifungal therapy.
3. Not to be stored above 40°C (104°F).

ASSESSMENT
1. List onset, characteristics of S&S, clinical presentation and any other contributing factors.
2. Determine if pregnant.
3. Assess vault, obtain cultures, labs as indicated.

CLIENT/FAMILY TEACHING
1. Review technique; insert cream high into the vagina. S&S of vulvovaginal candidiasis usually take 3 days to resolve (6 days if pregnant).
2. Use as prescribed and continue during menstrual cycle, with OCs, and antibiotic therapy.
3. Report irritation, burning, head or body aches, rash, vaginal swelling or discharge, light sensitivity, or lack of desired response.
4. Use sanitary napkins to prevent soiling and staining of undergarments, clothing, bedding. Avoid using tampons during treatment.
5. To prevent reinfection, partner should use a condom during intercourse and receive treatment if symptomatic.
6. If having recurrent vaginal infections, exposed to HIV, consult provider to determine the cause of symptoms. If symptoms return within 2 months, R/O pregnancy or serious underlying medical cause (e.g., diabetes, HIV infection). Keep all F/U to assess response.

OUTCOMES/EVALUATE
Eradication of fungal infection; symptomatic improvement

IV

Butorphanol tartrate
(byou-**TOR**-fah-nohl)

Classification(s): Narcotic agonist/antagonist

Pregnancy Category: C

RX: Butorphanol tartrate, **C-IV**

SEE ALSO ***NARCOTIC ANALGESICS***.

INDICATIONS/USES
Nasal: Treatment of migraine headaches.

Parenteral: (1) Preoperative or preanesthetic medication. (2) To supplement balanced anesthesia. (3) Pain during labor.

Parenteral and nasal: Moderate-to-severe pain, especially after surgery.

ACTION/KINETICS
Action
Has both narcotic agonist and antagonist properties. Analgesic potency may be up to 3.5 to 7 times that of morphine, 30–40 times that of meperidine, and 20 times that of pentazocine. The antagonist activity is about 30 times that of pentazocine and 1/40 that of naloxone. A parenteral dose of 2–3 mg produces analgesia and respiratory depression approximately equal to that of 10 mg morphine or 80 mg meperidine. Butorphanol appears to have a ceiling effect at 30–60 mcg/kg in the degree of respiratory depression produced. Overdosage responds to naloxone. After IV use,

CV effects include increased PA pressure, PCWP, LVED pressure, systemic arterial pressure, PVR, and increased cardiac work load.

Pharmacokinetics

Onset, IM: 10–15 min; **IV:** rapid; **nasal:** within 15 min. **Duration, IM, IV:** 3–4 hr; **nasal:** 4–5 hr. **Peak analgesia, IM, IV:** 30–60 min; **nasal:** 1–2 hr. **t½, IM:** 2.1–8.8 hr; **nasal:** 2.9–9.2 hr. The t½ is increased up to 25% in clients over 65 years of age. Metabolized in the liver and excreted by both the kidney (70–80%) and feces (about 15%). **t½** is increased in the elderly and in those with decreased C_{CR}. *NOTE:* 1 mg of tartrate salt is equal to 0.68 mg base.

CONTRAINDICATIONS

Hypersensitivity to butorphanol or any component of the product. Use of the nasal form during labor or delivery. Children less than 18 years of age.

SPECIAL CONCERNS

- Use with extreme caution in clients with AMI, ventricular dysfunction, and coronary insufficiency (morphine or meperidine are preferred).
- Use with caution and in low dosage in clients with respiratory depression, severely limited respiratory reserve, bronchial asthma, obstructive respiratory conditions, or cyanosis.
- Use in clients physically dependent on narcotics will result in precipitation of a withdrawal syndrome.
- Geriatric clients may be more sensitive to side effects, especially dizziness.
- Safe use during pregnancy, during labor for premature infants, or in children under 18 years not established.

SIDE EFFECTS

Most Common

After nasal use: Nasal congestion, insomnia.

After parenteral use: Somnolence, dizziness, N&V.

See *Narcotic Analgesics* for a complete list of possible side effects. May elevate CSF pressure.

ADDITIONAL DRUG INTERACTIONS

Barbiturate anesthetics / Possible ↑ respiratory and CNS depression of butorphanol

Sumatriptan / Transient ↑ BP if used with butorphanol spray to treat migraine

HOW SUPPLIED

Injection: 1 mg/mL, 2 mg/mL; ***Nasal Spray:*** 10 mg/mL.

DOSAGE

IM

Analgesia.

Adults, usual: 2 mg q 3–4 hr, as necessary; **range:** 1–4 mg q 3–4 hr as necessary in clients who will be able to remain recumbent. Single doses should not exceed 4 mg.

Preoperative/preanesthetic.

Adults: 2 mg 60–90 min before surgery. Individualize dosage.

Labor.

Adults: 1–2 mg if at full term in early labor. May be repeated after 4 hr.

IV

Analgesia.

Adults, usual: 1 mg q 3–4 hr; **range:** 0.5–2 mg q 3–4 hr. **Not recommended for use in children.**

Balanced anesthesia.

Adults: 2 mg just before induction or 0.5–1 mg in increments during anesthesia. The increment may be up to 0.06 mg/kg, depending on drugs previously given. Total dose range: <4 mg to >12.5 mg.

Labor.

Adults: 1–2 mg if at full term in early labor. May be repeated after 4 hr.

NASAL SPRAY

Analgesia.

Adults: 1 spray (1 mg) in one nostril. If pain relief is not reached within 60–90 min, an additional 1 mg may be given. The two-dose sequence may be repeated in 3–4 hr if necessary. In severe pain, 2 mg (1 spray in each nostril) may be given initially followed in 3–4 hr by additional 2 mg doses if needed in those who will be able to remain recumbent.

Geriatric clients, initial: 1 mg; allow 90–120 min to elapse before deciding if a second 1 mg dose is needed.

NURSING IMPLICATIONS

IMPLEMENTATION/ADMINISTRATION/STORAGE

1. For parenteral use in geriatric clients, initially use one-half the usual dose at twice the usual interval. Subsequent doses and intervals are based on response.
2. For those with hepatic or renal impairment, increase the initial dosage interval to 6–8 hr. Determine subsequent doses based on client response.
3. Have naloxone available for treatment of overdose.
4. Store nasal product below 30°C (86°F).
5. IV If administered by direct IV infusion, may give undiluted at a rate of 2 mg or less over 3–5 min.
6. COMPATIBILITY Give directly undiluted.
7. INCOMPATIBILITY Administer separately.

ASSESSMENT

1. Note if narcotic dependent; antagonist property of drug may precipitate acute withdrawal symptoms.
2. List reasons for therapy, characteristics of S&S; rate pain level.
3. Monitor VS, I&O, CNS status and auscultate heart and lungs, before and during therapy.
4. With CV problems, morphine may be a preferred drug to use.
5. Give geriatric clients one-half usual dose at twice the usual interval. Have naloxone readily available.
6. With renal/hepatic impairment, increase initial dosage interval to 6–8 hr with subsequent intervals determined by client response.

CLIENT/FAMILY TEACHING

1. Review how to use nasal spray: prime pump prior to initial use (7 to 8 strokes or until fine mist appears) or reprime (1 or 2 strokes) if unit has not been used for 48 hr or longer. Butorphanol may be aerosolized during priming process; aim pump sprayer away from self, other people, and animals.
2. Clear nasal passages, insert spray tip into 1 nostril, pointing tip toward back of the nose away from the septum while holding the other nostril closed and sniff gently. Pump spray unit firmly and quickly while gently sniffing with mouth closed; remove unit from nose, tilt head backward, and continue sniffing gently for a few more seconds.
3. One bottle will deliver 14 to 15 doses if no repriming needed; with intermittent use requiring repriming before each dose, one bottle may deliver only 8 to 10 doses.
4. To properly dispose of used spray units: unscrew cap, rinse bottle, and place parts in waste container.
5. May cause dizziness/drowsiness; use caution while performing activities that require mental alertness until effect realized.
6. Cough and deep breathe every 2 hours following surgery to prevent atelectasis (lung collapse).
7. Drug is habit-forming when used for extended time. Withdrawal S&S may include, N&V, fever, restlessness, lightheadedness, loss of appetite, abdominal cramps. Store appropriately.
8. Avoid alcohol or any CNS depressants.
9. Keep all F/U to assess response and for adverse SE.

OUTCOMES/EVALUATE

- Relief of pain
- Termination of migraine headache

C

IV

C1 Inhibitor, Human

Classification(s): Protein C1 inhibitor

Pregnancy Category: C

RX: Cinryze.

INDICATIONS/USES

Routine prophylaxis against angioedema attacks in adults and adolescents with hereditary angioedema.

C

ACTION/KINETICS

Action

C1 inhibitor is a normal component of human blood. The primary function is to regulate the activation of the complement and intrinsic coagulation pathway; C1 inhibitor also regulates the fibrolytic system. Clients with hereditary angioedema have low levels of endogenous or functional C1 inhibitor. It is believed that increased vascular permeability and the clinical manifestation of hereditary angioedema attacks are primarily mediated through contact system activation. By increasing C1 inhibitor activity, the contact system activation is suppressed.

Pharmacokinetics

T_{max} following a single dose: 3.8 hr. **t½ following a single dose:** 56 hr. One unit is equal to the mean C1 inhibitor concentration of 1 mL of normal human plasma.

CONTRAINDICATIONS

Life-threatening immediate hypersensitivity reactions, including anaphylaxis to the product.

SPECIAL CONCERNS

- **Made from human blood; thus, it may carry a risk of transmitting infectious agents (e.g., viruses and, theoretically, the Creutzfeldt-Jacob agent).**
- **Use with caution during lactation.**
- **Safety and efficacy not determined in neonates, infants, or children.**

SIDE EFFECTS

Most Common

Headache, rash, sinusitis, URTI, abdominal pain, N&V, muscle spasms, pain, diarrhea, subsequent hereditary angioedema attack.

GI: N&V, abdominal pain, diarrhea. **Respiratory:** Sinusitis, URTI, bronchitis, viral URTI. **Dermatologic:** Rash, pruritus. **CNS:** Headache. **CV:** Noncatheter-related foreign body embolus, thrombotic events, ***stroke***. **Hypersensitivity:** Hives, urticaria, tightness of chest, wheezing, hypotension, ***anaphylaxis***. **Musculoskeletal:** Muscle spasms, back pain, limb injury, pain in extremity. **Miscellaneous:** Preeclampsia resulting in emergency C-section, exacerbation of hereditary angioedema attacks.

HOW SUPPLIED

Injection, Lyophilized Powder for Solution: 500 units.

DOSAGE

IV INFUSION

Prevent angioedema attacks in adults/adolescents with hereditary angioedema.

Adults and adolescents: 1,000 units q 3 or 4 days.

NURSING IMPLICATIONS

IMPLEMENTATION/ADMINISTRATION/STORAGE

1. **IV Prepare the injection for administration as follows:**
   - **Bring the C1 inhibitor and sterile water for injection to room temperature if refrigerated.**
   - **Remove the caps from the C1 inhibitor and diluent vials.**
   - **Cleanse stoppers with germicidal solution and allow them to dry prior to use.**
   - **Remove the protective covering from one end of the double-ended transfer needle and insert exposed needle through the center of the diluent vial stopper.**
   - **Remove the protective covering from the other end of the double-ended transfer needle. Invert diluent vial containing 5 mL of sterile water for injection over the upright and slightly angled C1 inhibitor vial. Then, rapidly insert the free end of the needle through the C1 inhibitor vial stopper at its center. The vacuum in the vial will draw in the diluent. If there is no vacuum in the C1 inhibitor vial, do not use the product.**
   - **Disconnect the two vials by removing the needle from the C1 inhibitor vial stopper and discard the diluent vial, as well as the transfer needle, directly into the sharps container.**
   - **Gently swirl the C1 inhibitor vial until all powder is dissolved. Ensure that the C1 inhibitor is completely dissolved.**
2. **One vial of reconstituted C1 inhibitor contains 5 mL at a concentration of 100 units/mL. Reconstitute two vials for 1 dose.**
3. **Administer at an initial infusion rate of 1 mL/min (i.e., for 10 mL, a total of 10 min). If tolerated, administer at a maintenance infusion rate of 1 mL/min (i.e., 10 min for the 1,000 unit dose).**
4. **Administer the dose as follows:**

- Administer at room temperature within 3 hr after reconstitution.
- Attach the filter needle to a sterile, disposable syringe and draw back the plunger to admit air into the syringe.
- Insert the filter needle into the vial of reconstituted C1 inhibitor.
- Inject air into the vial and then withdraw the reconstituted C1 inhibitor into the syringe. Repeat this with a second vial of C1 inhibitor to achieve the complete dose.
- Remove and discard the filter needle in a hard-walled sharps container for proper disposal. Filter needles are intended to filter the contents of a single dose (2 vials) of C1 inhibitor only.
- Attach a suitable needle or infusion set with a winged adapter, and inject IV.
- Dispose of all unused solution, the empty vials, and the used needles and syringes in an appropriate container.

5. Any vial that has been entered should be used promptly. Discard partially used vials according to biohazard procedures.
6. C1 inhibitor is stable for 1 year when stored from 2–25°C (36–77°F). Do not freeze. Store vials in their original containers to protect from light.
7. COMPATIBILITY Sterile water.
8. INCOMPATIBILITY Do not mix C1 inhibitor with any other materials.

ASSESSMENT

1. Note indications for therapy, frequency of occurrence, and when diagnosed with hereditary angioedema (HAE).
2. Discuss risks; drug made from human blood, may carry a risk of transmitting infectious agents, such as viruses, including the Creutzfeldt-Jakob (CJD) agent.
3. Assess for any history of blood clots and review potential. Increased risk of thrombosis with higher doses.
4. All infections that may have been transmitted by Cinryze should be reported to Lev Pharmaceuticals, Inc (877-945-1000) 8 am to 7 pm EST.

CLIENT/FAMILY TEACHING

1. Cinryze is an injectable medicine that is used to help prevent swelling and/or painful attacks in those with hereditary angioedema (HAE). It contains C1 esterase inhibitor protein which is thought to be deficient or not functioning correctly with this condition.
2. Provider will determine ability to take this drug and will provide instruction before you can administer. The "instructions for use" leaflet that accompanies this drug provides step-by-step instruction for preparation and injection of this product. Two vials will be prepared for one dose (record lot number of vials injecting for each dose). Drug must be dissolved before injection into your vein.
3. Protect vial from light and use within 3 hr of reconstitution.
4. If traveling plan accordingly to ensure that you take adequate drug supply for routine prevention.
5. May experience URI, sinusitis, rash, and headache with therapy.
6. S&S of hypersensitivity reactions may include hives, itching, chest tightness, wheezing, drop in BP and/or anaphylaxis experienced during or after injection of Cinryze. Report as epinephrine should be administered immediately.
7. Report if pregnancy suspected or planned; do not breast-feed without provider approval.
8. Keep all F/U to assess response, technique and for adverse SE.

OUTCOMES/EVALUATE

Prophylaxis against hereditary angioedema (HAE) attacks

Calcium carbonate

(**KAL**-see-um **KAR**-bon-ayt)

Classification(s): Calcium salt

OTC: Capsules: Calci-Mix. **Gum:** Chooz, Surpass, Surpass Extra Strength. **Powder, Oral:** TUMS Quik Pak. **Suspension:** Calcium Carbonate. **Tablets:** Cal-Carb Forte, Calcium-600, Caltrate 600, Nephro-Calci, Os-Cal 500, Oysco 500, Oyst-Cal 500, Oyster Shell Calcium. **Tablets, Chewable:** Alka-Mints, Antacid Tablets, Cal-Carb Forte, Calci-Chew, Calcium Antacid Extra Strength, Cal-Gest, Dicarbosil, Equilet, Maalox Antacid Barrier Maximum Strength, Maalox Children's, Mylanta Children's, Os-Cal 500, Pepto Children's, Rolaids Extra Strength Softchews, Trial Antacid, Tums Calcium for Life Bone Health, Tums

Calcium for Life PMS, Tums E-X, Tums Kids, Tums Smooth Dissolve, Tums Ultra.
✤ **OTC:** Apo-Cal, Calcite 500, Calcium 500.

SEE ALSO ***CALCIUM SALTS***.

C

INDICATIONS/USES

(1) As an antacid for relief of acid indigestion, heartburn, sour stomach, and upset stomach. (2) Daily source of calcium for prevention of calcium deficiency. (3) Calcium supplement to treat osteoporosis, osteomalacia, rickets, and latent tetany. *Investigational:* Daily to help reduce typical premenstrual syndrome symptoms, including bloating, cramps, fatigue, and moodiness.

SPECIAL CONCERNS

Dosage for calcium supplementation not established in children.

SIDE EFFECTS

Most Common

Constipation, headache, mild hypercalcemia (anorexia, N&V).
See *Calcium Salts* for a complete list of possible side effects.

ADDITIONAL DRUG INTERACTIONS

Omeprazole / ↓ fractional calcium absorption in fasting elderly women

HOW SUPPLIED

Capsules: 1,250 mg (500 mg elemental Ca^{++}); ***Gum:*** 300 mg (120 mg elemental Ca^{++}), 450 mg (180 mg elemental Ca^{++}), 500 mg (200 mg elemental Ca^{++}); ***Powder, Oral:*** 1,000 mg; ***Suspension:*** 1,250 mg (500 mg elemental Ca^{++})/5 mL; ***Tablets:*** 500 mg (200 mg elemental Ca^{++}), 600 mg (240 mg elemental Ca^{++}), 648–650 mg (260 mg elemental Ca^{++}), 1,250 mg (500 mg elemental Ca^{++}), 1,500 mg (600 mg elemental Ca^{++}); ***Tablets, Chewable:*** 400 mg (160 mg elemental Ca^{++}), 420 mg (168 mg elemental Ca^{++}), 500 mg (200 mg elemental Ca^{++}), 750 mg (300 mg elemental Ca^{++}), 850 mg (340 mg elemental Ca^{++}), 1,000 mg (400 mg elemental Ca^{++}), 1,177 mg (470.8 mg elemental Ca^{++}), 1,250 mg (500 mg elemental Ca^{++}).

DOSAGE

CAPSULES; TABLETS; TABLETS, CHEWABLE

Antacid.

Adults and children 12 years and older: Swallow or chew 2–4 tablets as symptoms occur. Repeat hourly if symptoms return or as directed by provider.

Calcium supplementation.

Adults: 500–2,000 mg 2–4 times a day. Administer 1,500 mg for men older than 65 years of age and for postmenopausal women not taking estrogen replacement therapy. For Cali-Mix, take one capsule daily as directed; capsules may be swallowed whole or pulled apart and mixed with food and drink.

GUM

Antacid.

Adults and children 12 years and older: Chew 1–2 pieces (calcium carbonate 500–1,000 mg) q 2–4 hr.

Calcium supplementation.

Adults: Chew 1–2 pieces after each meal.

SUSPENSION

Calcium supplementation.

Adults: 5 mL (1,250 mg) 2–3 times a day with meals or as directed by provider.

NURSING IMPLICATIONS

IMPLEMENTATION/ADMINISTRATION/STORAGE

1. **Do not use the maximum dosage for more than 2 weeks, except under the supervision of a health care provider.**
2. **Protect the PO suspension from freezing.**
3. **Store from 15–30°C (59–86°F).**

ASSESSMENT

1. **Note reasons for therapy, age, physical condition, DEXA scan results.**
2. **Maintain serum calcium levels at 9–10.4 mg/dL (4.5–5.2 mEq/L); do not allow levels to exceed 12 mg/dL.**
3. **Get calcium level before therapy, monitor during therapy; ensure normal renal function.**

CLIENT/FAMILY TEACHING

1. **Take with or following meals to enhance absorption. Take with a large glass of water.**
2. **With gum, do not exceed 17 pieces per day of 450 mg strength or 26 pieces per day of the 300 mg strength. Do not take maximum dose for more than 2 weeks.**

3. Ensure adequate vitamin D supplementation, weight-bearing exercises, and reductions in cigarette smoking and excessive alcohol consumption.
4. Keep all F/U to assess response, labs and for adverse SE.

OUTCOMES/EVALUATE

- Desired serum calcium levels
- ↓ Gastric upset/acidity

IV

Calcium chloride

(**KAL**-see-um **KLOH**-ryd)

Classification(s): Calcium salt

Pregnancy Category: C

SEE ALSO *CALCIUM SALTS*.

INDICATIONS/USES

(1) Mild hypocalcemia due to neonatal tetany, tetany due to parathyroid deficiency or vitamin D deficiency, and alkalosis. (2) Prophylaxis of hypocalcemia during exchange transfusions. (3) Intestinal malabsorption. (4) Treat effects of serious hyperkalemia as measured by ECG. (5) Cardiac resuscitation after open heart surgery when epinephrine fails to improve weak or ineffective myocardial contractions. (6) Adjunct to treat insect bites or stings to relieve muscle cramping. (7) Depression due to Mg^{++} overdosage. (8) Acute symptoms of lead colic. (9) Rickets, osteomalacia. (10) Reverse symptoms of verapamil overdosage.

CONTRAINDICATIONS

Use to treat hypocalcemia of renal insufficiency. IM or SC use.

SPECIAL CONCERNS

Use usually restricted in children due to significant irritation and possible tissue necrosis and sloughing caused by IV calcium chloride.

SIDE EFFECTS

Most Common

Peripheral vasodilation with moderate decreases in BP.

See *Calcium Salts* for a complete list of possible side effects. If given IM or SC, extravasation can cause severe necrosis, sloughing, or abscess formation.

HOW SUPPLIED

Injection: 100 mg /mL.

DOSAGE

IV ONLY

Hypocalcemia, replenish electrolytes.

Adults: 0.5–1 gram q 1–3 days (given at a rate not to exceed 13.6–27.3 mg/min). **Pediatric:** 25 mg/kg (0.2 mL/kg up to 1–10 mL/kg) given slowly.

Mg^{++} intoxication.

Adults: 0.5 gram promptly; observe for recovery before other doses given.

Cardiac resuscitation.

Adults: 0.5–1 gram IV or 0.2–0.8 gram injected into the ventricular cavity as a single dose. **Pediatric:** 0.2 mL/kg.

Hyperkalemia.

Sufficient amount to return ECG to normal.

NOTE: The preparation contains 27.2% calcium and 272 mg calcium/gram (13.6 mEq/gram).

NURSING IMPLICATIONS

IMPLEMENTATION/ADMINISTRATION/STORAGE

1. Never administer IM or SC.
2. IV May give undiluted IV push.
3. COMPATIBILITY D5W, NSS, D10W, and various combinations; D5/LR.
4. INCOMPATIBILITY Administer separately.

ASSESSMENT

1. Note reasons for therapy, clinical presentation, serum Ca^{++}, K^{+} levels, other agents trialed.
2. If IV infiltration occurs, stop IV administration at once. Local infiltration of the affected area with 1% procaine hydrochloride, to which hyaluronidase may be added, will often reduce venospasm and dilute the calcium remaining in the tissues locally. Local application of heat may also be helpful.
3. Monitor ECG, VS, electrolytes, Mg^{++}, during therapy; ensure normal renal function.

CLIENT/FAMILY TEACHING

1. Administered in health care setting. Rapid injection may cause a tingling sensation, a cal-

C

cium taste, a sense of oppression or "heat wave."
2. Injections of calcium chloride are accompanied by peripheral vasodilation as well as a local "burning" sensation; may experience a fall in BP.
3. Report any adverse effects, rash, or pain at infusion site.

C

OUTCOMES/EVALUATE

- Desired serum calcium levels
- ↓ Mg^{++} and potassium levels

IV

Calcium gluconate

(**KAL**-see-um **GLUE**-koh-nayt)

Classification(s): Calcium salt

Pregnancy Category: C

OTC: Cal-G.

RX: Calcium gluconate.

SEE ALSO ***CALCIUM SALTS***.

INDICATIONS/USES

PO: Dietary calcium supplement. **IV Injection:** (1) Adjunct treatment of rickets, osteomalacia, lead colic, and magnesium sulfate overdosage. (2) Relieve muscle cramping following black widow spider bites. (3) Decrease capillary permeability in allergic conditions, nonthrombocytopenic purpura and exudative dermatoses, such as dermatitis herpetiformis and for pruritus of eruptions due to certain drugs. (4) In hyperkalemia, may aid to antagonize the cardiac toxicity as long as the client is not receiving digitalis therapy. (5) Treat conditions arising from calcium deficiencies, such as hypocalcemic tetany, hypocalcemia related to hypoparathyroidism, and hypocalcemia due to rapid growth or pregnancy.

CONTRAINDICATIONS

IM, intramyocardial, or SC use due to severe tissue necrosis, sloughing, and abscess formation.

SIDE EFFECTS

Most Common

After PO use: Constipation, headache, mild hypercalcemia (anorexia, N&V).
After rapid IV use: Vasodilation, decreased BP, syncope, cardiac arrhythmias.

See *Calcium Salts* for a complete list of possible side effects.

HOW SUPPLIED

OTC: Capsules: 500 mg, 700 mg; ***Powder for Oral Suspension:*** 1,040 mg (equivalent to 346.7 mg elemental Ca^{++}/15 mL); ***Tablets:*** 500 mg (equivalent to 45 mg elemental Ca^{++}), 555.6 mg (equivalent to 50 mg elemental Ca^{++}), 648–650 mg (equivalent to 58.5–60 mg elemental Ca^{++}), 972–975 mg (equivalent to 87.75–90 mg elemental Ca^{++}); ***Tablets, Chewable:*** 650 mg; ***Rx:*** Injection 10%: 9.3 mg/mL (equivalent to 0.465 mEq/mL).

DOSAGE

CAPSULES; POWDER FOR ORAL SUSPENSION; TABLETS; TABLETS, CHEWABLE

Dietary supplement.

Adults, capsules and tablets: 500–8,000 mg/day (as calcium gluconate) in divided doses, preferably 1–2 hr after meals. **Powder:** 3 Tablespoons/day with food or liquid.

IV ONLY

All uses.

Individualize dosage, depending on client needs. **Adults, usual:** 0.5–2 grams IV (5–20 mL of the 10% solution). **Children, usual:** 0.2–0.5 gram IV (2–5 mL of the 10% solution). **Infants, usual:** Not more than 0.2 gram IV (not more than 2 mL of the 10% solution).

NURSING IMPLICATIONS

IMPLEMENTATION/ADMINISTRATION/STORAGE

1. Store PO dosage forms at room temperature; do not expose to excessive heat or moisture.
2. IV If precipitate noted in syringe, do not use.
3. If crystallization noted in vials or ampules, heat to 60–80°C (140–176°F) in a water bath for 15–30 min with occasional shaking; this may dissolve the precipitate. Allow to cool to room temperature. The injection must be clear at the time of use; do not use if precipitate remains.
4. Do not reconstitute or mix ceftriaxone with a calcium-containing product, such as Ringer's

or Hartmann's solution or parenteral nutrition containing calcium, because a particulate can form.

5. Do not give ceftriaxone and IV calcium-containing products, including parenteral nutrition, to anyone by the same or different infusion lines or sites within 48 hr of each other. Cases of fatal reactions with ceftriaxone-calcium precipitates in lungs and kidneys in neonates have been reported.
6. IV rate should not exceed 0.5–2 mL/min.
7. Must be given slowly; give by slow IV injection or by IV infusion. Inject through a small needle into a large vein in order to avoid too rapid an increase in serum calcium and extravasation of calcium solution into the surrounding tissue (can cause necrosis). May also be given by intermittent infusion at a rate not to exceed 200 mg/min.
8. Since tetracycline antibiotics bind with calcium rendering them inactive, do not give together.
9. Store the IV solution from 15–30°C (59–86°F); do not freeze.
10. COMPATIBILITY D5W, D10W, D20W, D5/0.9% NaCl, NSS, D5/LR, LR.
11. INCOMPATIBILITY Ceftriaxone, tetracycline antibiotics.

ASSESSMENT

1. Note reasons for therapy, other agents trialed, desired levels/outcome.
2. Avoid rapid IV infusion and use with ceftriaxone, tetracycline, and digitalized clients.
3. Monitor VS, and Ca^{++} levels closely with renal function impairment and/or if large doses of vitamin D are used.

CLIENT/FAMILY TEACHING

1. Take capsules or tablets with food and liquid, preferably 1–2 hr after meals. Take oral powder with food or liquid.
2. May experience N&V, decreased appetite, increased thirst, constipation, dry mouth, or increased urination; report if persistent.
3. Calcium can decrease the effects of many other medicines by binding to them or by changing the acidity of the stomach or the urine. Do not take together and ensure provider is aware of all drugs prescribed.
4. Keep all F/U to assess response, labs, and for adverse SE.

OUTCOMES/EVALUATE

- Restoration of serum calcium levels
- ↓ Mg^{++}/potassium levels

Calfactant

(kal-**FAK**-tant)

Classification(s): Lung surfactant

Pregnancy Category: C

RX: Infasurf.

INDICATIONS/USES

Prevention and treatment of respiratory distress syndrome in premature infants.

ACTION/KINETICS

Action

Lung surfactant that contains phospholipids, neutral lipids, and hydrophobic surfactant-associated proteins B and C from calf lungs. Calfactant modifies alveolar surface tension thus stabilizing alveoli. Adsorbs rapidly to the surface of the air: liquid interface and modifies surface tension similarly to natural lung surfactant. Treatment often rapidly improves oxygenation and lung compliance.

SPECIAL CONCERNS

- For endotracheal use only.
- Possible increased proportion of clients with both intraventricular hemorrhage and periventricular leukomalacia. These conditions were not associated with increased mortality.

SIDE EFFECTS

Most Common

Cyanosis, airway obstruction, bradycardia, reflux of surfactant into the endotracheal tube, requirement for manual ventilation.

Respiratory: Cyanosis, airway obstruction, reflux of surfactant into the endotracheal tube, requirement for manual ventilation, apnea, reintubation, periventricular leukomalacia, pulmonary air leaks, pulmonary interstitial emphysema, ***pulmonary hemorrhage***. **CV:** Bradycardia, ***intraventricular hemorrhage***, patent ductus arteriosus, ***intracranial hemorrhage***. **GI:** ***Necrotizing enterocolitis.*** **Body as a whole:** ***Sepsis.***

HOW SUPPLIED

Suspension, Intratracheal: 35 mg phospholipids/mL and 0.65 mg proteins.

DOSAGE

SUSPENSION, INTRATRACHEAL

Prophylaxis of respiratory distress syndrome at birth.

Instill 3 mL/kg of birth weight as soon as possible after birth. Give as 2 doses of 1.5 mL/kg each. Care and stabilization of the premature infant born with hypoxemia or bradycardia should precede calfactant therapy.

Treatment of respiratory distress syndrome within 72 hr of birth.

Instill 3 mL/kg of birth weight, given as 2 doses of 1.5 mL/kg. Repeat doses of 3 mL/kg of birth weight may be given, up to a total of 3 doses 12 hr apart.

NURSING IMPLICATIONS

IMPLEMENTATION/ADMINISTRATION/STORAGE

1. Begin calfactant prophylaxis as soon as possible, within 30 minutes after birth.
2. Give only through an endotracheal tube. Draw dose into syringe from single-dose vial using 20-gauge or larger needle. Avoid excessive foaming. Give under supervision of clinician experienced in acute care of newborns requiring intubation.
3. Does not require reconstitution. Do not dilute, sonicate, or shake. Gently swirl/agitate vial for redispersion. Visible flecks in suspension, foaming at the surface are normal. Drug does not have to be warmed before administration.
4. If administered through side-port adapter into the endotracheal tube (ET), two qualified and experienced in the care of high-risk infants should facilitate the dosing: one to instill calfactant while the other monitors and positions infant. After each aliquot is instilled, position infant on the right or left side to facilitate distribution.
5. Calfactant also can be administered through a 5 French feeding catheter inserted into the ET with the tip above the carina. Do not instill into the main stem bronchus. Attach catheter to syringe. Fill with medication and discard any excess through catheter to ensure the total dose to be given remains in syringe. Instill the total dose in 4 equal aliquots with the catheter removed between each of the instillations and active mechanical ventilation resumed for 30 sec to 2 min. Administer each of the aliquots in 1 of 4 different positions (e.g., prone, supine, right, left lateral) to facilitate even distribution of the surfactant. Continue procedure until the total dose is achieved.
6. Avoid suctioning client for 1 hr after administration unless airway obstruction is present.
7. Unopened, unused vials warmed to room temperature may be returned to refrigerator within 24 hr for future use. Avoid repeated warming to room temperature.
8. Refrigerate 2–8°C (36–46°F); protect from light.
9. Vials for single use only; discard any unused drug after opening.

ASSESSMENT

1. Note condition requiring therapy, oxygen saturation, placement of ET tube.
2. Assess for reflux, airway obstruction, cyanosis, bradycardia; stop drug and take appropriate measures to alleviate. Resume dosing once infant is stabilized.
3. Give only under direct supervision of one trained to use in environment with emergency equipment/personnel readily available. Instill through adaptor to ET tube during inspiration while the ventilator cycles 20–30 breaths per each dose (1.5 mL/kg × 2 doses). Have re-intubation supplies and suction readily available.
4. Assess lungs sounds carefully for changes esp. moist rales; adjust oxygen therapy and ventilatory support in response to changes in respiratory status. Reposition infant between each dose.
5. Monitor oxygen and carbon dioxide levels. If oxygen saturation decreases or bradycardia develops, discontinue administration until infant stabilized.

CLIENT/FAMILY TEACHING

1. Drug used to treat/prevent respiratory distress syndrome in newborn and in those under 29 weeks at high risk.
2. Reassure parents infant will be carefully monitored; breathing apparatus may be required to

stay intact for the next week or more while infant continues to improve.

3. Adverse effects may occur; address as they arise. Include family in care, visits, updates, decisions.

OUTCOMES/EVALUATE

Prophylaxis/management of respiratory distress syndrome

Candesartan cilexetil

(**kan**-deh-**SAR**-tan)

Classification(s): Antihypertensive, angiotensin II receptor blocker

Pregnancy Category: C (first trimester); **D** (second and third trimesters)

RX: Atacand.

SEE ALSO ***ANGIOTENSIN II RECEPTOR ANTAGONISTS*** AND ***ANTIHYPERTENSIVE DRUGS***.

INDICATIONS/USES

(1) Treat hypertension alone or in combination with other antihypertensive drugs in adults and children, 1 to younger than 17 years of age. (2) To reduce risk of death and reduce hospitalizations from heart failure (NYHA class II–IV and ejection fraction less than or equal to 40%). There is added benefit when used with an ACE inhibitor. *Investigational:* Prophylaxis of migraine headaches in adults.

ACTION/KINETICS

Pharmacokinetics

Is about 15% bioavailable. Is rapidly and completely bioactivated to candesartan by ester hydrolysis during absorption from the GI tract. Food does not affect bioavailability. Effect somewhat less in Blacks. **t½, elimination:** 9 hr. Excreted mainly unchanged in the urine (33%) and feces (67%). **Plasma protein binding:** More than 99%.

ADDITIONAL CONTRAINDICATIONS

Use in children with a GFR <30 mL/min.

SPECIAL CONCERNS

Use in pregnancy. When used in pregnancy during the second and third trimesters, drugs that act directly on the renin-angiotensin system may cause injury or death to the developing fetus. When pregnancy is detected, discontinue candesartan as soon as possible.

SIDE EFFECTS

Most Common

URTI, dizziness, pain, rhinitis, pharyngitis.

GI: N&V, abdominal pain, diarrhea, dyspepsia, gastroenteritis. **CNS:** Headache, dizziness, paresthesia, vertigo, anxiety, depression, somnolence. **CV:** Tachycardia, palpitation; rarely, angina pectoris, MI. **Respiratory:** URTI, pharyngitis, rhinitis, bronchitis, coughing, dyspnea, sinusitis, epistaxis. **GU:** Impaired renal function, hematuria. **Dermatologic:** Rash, increased sweating. **Body as a whole:** Fatigue, asthenia, fever, peripheral edema. **Miscellaneous:** Back/chest pain, pain, arthralgia, myalgia, ***angioedema***.

LABORATORY TEST CONSIDERATIONS

↑ Creatine phosphatase. Albuminuria, hyperglycemia, triglyceridemia, uricemia.

ADDITIONAL DRUG INTERACTIONS

When used with lithium, serum lithium levels may be increased; monitor carefully.

HOW SUPPLIED

Tablets: 4 mg, 8 mg, 16 mg, 32 mg.

DOSAGE

TABLETS

Hypertension, monotherapy.

Dose individualized. **Adults, usual initial:** 16 mg once daily for monotherapy in those not volume depleted. Can be given once or twice daily in doses from 8 to 32 mg. If BP is not controlled, a diuretic can be added. Most antihypertensive effect is present within 2 weeks; maximal BP reduction obtained within 4–6 weeks. **Children, age 6–less than 17 years:** For those weighing less than 50 kg, dose range is 2–16 mg/day. For those weighing more than 50 kg, the dose range is 4–32 mg/day. **Children, age 1–younger than 6 years, initial:** 0.2 mg/kg (of an PO suspension); **usual:** 0.05–0.4 mg/kg/day. *NOTE:* Children less than 1 year of age must not receive candesartan for hypertension.

Heart failure.

Adults, initial: 4 mg once daily. Target dose is 32 mg once daily; achieve by doubling the dose at approximately 2-week intervals, as tolerated.

NURSING IMPLICATIONS

IMPLEMENTATION/ADMINISTRATION/STORAGE

1. Most effect is noted within 2 weeks and maximum BP reduction in 4 to 6 weeks.
2. Consider a lower starting dose in those with possible depletion of intravascular volume (e.g., after a diuretic).
3. May give with or without food.
4. If BP not controlled by candesartan alone, may add diuretic.
5. May be given with other antihypertensive drugs.
6. No initial dosage adjustment is required for clients with mildly impaired renal or hepatic function. In moderate hepatic impairment, consider initiating at a lower dose.
7. Check the package insert for instructions on preparation of an oral suspension for use in children.
8. Store tablets from 15–30°C (59–86°F). Store the PO suspension at room temperature (i.e., below 30°C, 86°F); do not freeze.

ASSESSMENT

1. Note HTN onset/duration, other agents trialed, outcome.
2. With heart disease note NYHA and ejection fraction.
3. Ensure adequate hydration, especially with diuretic therapy in renal dysfunction.
4. Assess VS, electrolytes, renal and LFTs. Monitor elderly and those with renal dysfunction closely for desired response/adverse side effects.

CLIENT/FAMILY TEACHING

1. Take as directed with or without food; ensure adequate fluid intake.
2. Change positions slowly to prevent sudden drop in BP effects.
3. Practice barrier birth control; report if pregnancy suspected.
4. With heart failure, keep daily record of weights and BP; report Wt increases of >2 lb/day or 5 lb/week.
5. Continue lifestyle modifications, i.e., diet, regular exercise, stress reduction, no smoking, moderate alcohol intake to ensure BP control.
6. Keep all F/U to assess response, labs, BP, and for adverse SE.

OUTCOMES/EVALUATE

- ↓ BP ↓hospitalizations & mortality with CHF
- Migraine prophylaxis (unlabeled)

■ ©

Capecitabine

(cap-**SITE**-ah-bean)

Classification(s): Antineoplastic, antimetabolite

Pregnancy Category: D

RX: Xeloda.

SEE ALSO ***ANTINEOPLASTIC AGENTS***.

INDICATIONS/USES

(1) Single agent for adjuvant treatment for Duke stage C colon cancer in clients who have undergone complete resection of the primary tumor when treatment with fluoropyrimidine therapy alone is preferred. Combination chemotherapy improves disease-free survival compared with 5-fluorouracil/leucovorin. (2) First-line therapy for metastatic colorectal cancer when treatment with fluoropyrimidine therapy alone is preferred. (3) In combination with docetaxel to treat metastatic breast cancer in those for whom anthracycline therapy has failed. (4) Metastatic breast cancer in those resistant to both paclitaxel and an anthracycline-containing chemotherapy regimen or resistant to paclitaxel and for whom further anthracycline therapy is not indicated (e.g., those who have received cumulative doses of 400 mg/m^2 of doxorubicin or doxorubicin equivalents). *Investigational:* Adjuvant treatment of pancreatic cancer.

ACTION/KINETICS

Action

An oral prodrug of 5'-deoxy-5-fluorouridine (5'DFUR) that is converted to 5-fluorouracil (5-FU). 5-FU is metabolized to 5-fluoro-2-deoxyuridine monophosphate (FdUMP) and 5-fluorouridine triphosphate (FUTP) which cause cell injury in 2 ways. First, FdUMP and the folate cofactor, N^{5-10}-methylenetetrahydrofolate, bind to thymidylate synthase to form a ternary complex which inhibits the formation of thymidylate from uracil. Thymidylate is essential for the synthesis of DNA so a deficiency inhibits cell division. Secondly, nuclear transcriptional enzymes can mistakenly incorporate FUTP in place of uridine triphosphate during RNA synthesis; this interferes with RNA processing and protein synthesis.

Pharmacokinetics

Readily absorbed from the GI tract. **Peak blood levels, capecitabine:** 1.5 hr; **peak blood levels, 5-FU:** 2 hr. Food reduces the rate and extent of absorption. **t½, capecitabine and 5-FU:** 45 min. Metabolites excreted in the urine. Food reduces the rate and extent of absorption; however, drug is given with food since safety and efficacy data are based on administration with food.

CONTRAINDICATIONS

Use in cancer clients with severe renal impairment (C_{CR} less than 30 mL/min). Hypersensitivity to capecitabine or 5-fluorouracil. Dihydropyrimidine dehydrogenase deficiency. Lactation.

SPECIAL CONCERNS

Warfarin interaction. Frequently monitor the anticoagulant response (INR or PT) of clients receiving concomitant capecitabine and oral coumarin-derivative anticoagulant therapy in order to adjust the anticoagulant dose accordingly. A clinically important capecitabine-warfarin drug interaction was demonstrated in a clinical pharmacology trial. Altered coagulation parameters and/or bleeding, including death, have been reported in clients taking capecitabine concomitantly with coumarin-derivative anticoagulants such as warfarin and phenprocoumon. Postmarketing reports have shown clinically significant increases in PT and INR in clients who were stabilized on anticoagulants at the time capecitabine was introduced. These events occurred within several days and up to several months after initiating capecitabine therapy and, in a few cases, within 1 month after stopping capecitabine. These events occurred in clients with and without liver metastases. Age older than 60 years and diagnosis of cancer independently predispose clients to an increased risk of coagulopathy.

- **Use with caution in impaired renal function and in the elderly.**
- **Clients 80 years or older may experience a greater incidence of side effects.**
- **Monitor clients carefully with severe diarrhea.**
- **Discontinue drug if nursing.**
- **When combined with docetaxel, more frequent side effects occur, including N&V and fatigue.**
- **Safety and efficacy not determined in children less than 18 years of age.**

SIDE EFFECTS

Most Common

Hand-and-foot syndrome, diarrhea, N&V, stomatitis, abdominal pain, fatigue, lethargy, asthenia, dizziness, dermatitis, headache, alopecia, erythema, rash, anorexia, constipation, dysgeusia, dyspepsia, upper abdominal pain, pyrexia, conjunctivitis, peripheral sensory neuropathy.

GI: Diarrhea (may be severe), N&V, stomatitis, abdominal pain, anorexia, upper abdominal pain, constipation, dyspepsia, intestinal obstruction, rectal bleeding, GI motility disorder, ileus, oral discomfort, taste disturbance, upper GI inflammatory disorders, ***GI hemorrhage***, esophagitis, gastritis, colitis, duodenitis, hematemesis, ***necrotizing enterocolitis***, oral/GI/esophageal candidiasis, gastroenteritis. **CV:** Cardiotoxicity (***MI***, angina, dysrhythmias, ECG changes, ***cardiogenic shock***, ***sudden death***), angina pectoris, ***cardiomyopathy***, hypo-/hypertension, venous phlebitis, thrombophlebitis, DVT, lymphedema, venous thrombosis, ***pulmonary embolism***, ***CVA***. **Hematologic:** Neutropenia (grade 3 or 4), thrombocytopenia, decreased hemoglobin, anemia (grade 3 or 4), lymphopenia, coagulation disorder, IT, pancytopenia, ***sepsis***. **Dermatologic:** Hand-and-foot syndrome, alopecia, erythema, rash, dermatitis, nail disorder, increased sweating, photosensitivity, skin discoloration, radiation recall syndrome. **Neurological:** Paresthesia, fatigue, headache, dizziness, insomnia. **CNS:** Dizziness, headache, ataxia, depression, insomnia, mood alteration, encephalopathy, decreased level/loss of consciousness, confusion. **Metabolic:** Anorexia, dehydration, cachexia, hypertriglyceridemia. **Respiratory:** Dyspnea, cough, epistaxis, pharyngeal disorder, sore throat, ***bronchospasm***, respiratory distress, URTI, bronchitis, pneumonia, bronchopneumonia, laryngitis. **Musculoskeletal:** Myalgia, arthralgia, back pain, pain in limb, bone pain, joint stiffness. **GU:** Nocturia, UTI. **Hepatic:** Hepatic fibrosis, cholestatic hepatitis, hepatitis. **Ophthalmic:** Conjunctivitis, eye irritation, abnormal vision. **Body as a whole:**

Pyrexia, asthenia, fatigue, edema, lethargy, viral infection, dehydration. **Miscellaneous:** Hyperbilirubinemia (grade 3 or 4), chest pain, drug hypersensitivity, decreased appetite.

LABORATORY TEST CONSIDERATIONS

↑ ALT, bilirubin. ↓ Hemoglobin, lymphocytes, neutrophils, granulocytes, platelets. ↑ or ↓ Calcium.

OVERDOSE MANAGEMENT

Symptoms: N&V, diarrhea, GI irritation and bleeding, bone marrow suppression. *Treatment:* Supportive medical interventions, dose interruption, adjust dose. Dialysis may be of some benefit in removing 5'-deoxy-5-fluorouridine (a metabolite).

DRUG INTERACTIONS

Antacids / ↑ Capecitabine levels
Anticoagulants / Altered coagulation parameters and/or bleeding have been reported in clients taking coumarin-derivative anticoagulants (i.e., warfarin); monitor PT/INR closely; adjust anticoagulant dose accordingly
Leucovorin / ↑ 5-FU levels → ↑ toxicity; deaths from severe enterocolitis, diarrhea, and dehydration seen in elderly clients receiving both drugs
Phenytoin / ↑ Phenytoin levels R/T inhibition of CYP2C9; phenytoin dose may need to be ↓

HOW SUPPLIED

Tablets: 150 mg, 500 mg.

DOSAGE

TABLETS

Colorectal cancer, metastatic breast cancer.

For all indications: 1,250 mg/m^2 twice daily (for a total of 2,500 mg/m^2/day). Each dose should be taken about 12 hours apart at the end of a meal for 2 weeks. Follow by a 1-week rest period (i.e., give as 3-week cycles). Reduce the dose to 75% of the starting dose (i.e., 950 mg/m^2 twice daily) in clients with moderate renal impairment (C_{CR}, 30–50 mL/min). Interrupt and/or reduce dose if toxicity occurs; readjust according to adverse effects. *NOTE:* Check the package insert carefully to determine the dose reduction schedule when capecitabine is combined with docetaxel or recommended dose modification if capecitabine is used alone and there is toxicity.

NURSING IMPLICATIONS

Ⓢ Do not confuse Xeloda with Xenical (antiobesity drug).

IMPLEMENTATION/ADMINISTRATION/STORAGE

1. Recommended treatment duration is 6 months (8 3-week cycles) when used as single-agent treatment of metastatic colorectal cancer where entire primary tumor removed and in whom fluoropyrimidine therapy alone is preferred.
2. Follow manufacturer's insert for recommended dosages R/T BSA, for dose reduction when used with docetaxel, and for adjustment of starting dose in those with impaired hepatic/renal function.
3. If dose was reduced due to toxicity, do not increase at a later time.

ASSESSMENT

1. Note reasons for therapy: first line for metastatic colorectal, combo for metastatic breast cancer or resistant metastatic breast cancer, assess physical condition. List other agents/therapies trialed/failed.
2. Assess for CAD, any sensitivity to 5-FU, organ metastasis especially to liver, renal dysfunction. Give cautiously with impaired liver/renal function, assess for coagulation problems in elderly.
3. Monitor PT if taking both capecitabine and oral coumarin therapy; adjust anticoagulant dose accordingly—bleeding can be life threatening and occur up to 30 days after therapy completed.
4. Monitor VS, weight, CBC, INR/PT, renal and LFTs.

CLIENT/FAMILY TEACHING

1. Used to manage progression of cancer. Take within 30 min after meals and twice/day with water. Take for 14 days, rest for 7 days in a 3-week cycle. Ensure adequate fluid intake.
2. Review package for administration guidelines; expect dose adjustments during therapy.
3. Mild diarrhea may be treated with OTC antidiarrheals (i.e., loperamide).

4. May experience nausea/vomiting, diarrhea, mouth ulcers, and painful, swollen joints. Stop therapy immediately and report:
   - Grade 2 diarrhea (>4–6 stools/day or at night)
   - Grade 2 nausea (loss of appetite; ↓ food intake)
   - Grade 2 vomiting (2–5 times per day)
   - Grade 2 stomatitis (painful, red ulcers in mouth/tongue)
   - Grade 2 hand-and-foot syndrome (red swollen hands/feet)
   - Temperature over 100.5° for infection evidence or chills or other S&S of an infection
5. Practice reliable birth control, may harm fetus; do not breast-feed.
6. Keep all F/U to assess response, labs, and for adverse SE.

OUTCOMES/EVALUATE

- ↓ Tumor size/spread
- Treatment of resistant metastatic breast cancer alone or in combination with docetaxel; colorectal cancer
- Adjuvant to pancreatic cancer treatment (unlabeled)

Capsaicin

(kap-**SAY**-ih-sin)

Classification(s): Analgesic, topical

OTC: Axsain, Capsin, Capzasin-HP, Capzasin-P, Icy Hot PM, No Pain-HP, Pain Doctor, Pain-X, R-Gel, Rid-a-Pain-HP, Zostrix, Zostrix Diabetic Foot Pain, Zostrix Maximum Strength, Zostrix-HP.

RX: Qutenza.

✱ **Rx:** Capsaicin HP.

INDICATIONS/USES

OTC. (1) Temporary relief of minor aches and pains of muscles and joints associated with backache, strains, sprains, arthritis, rheumatoid arthritis and osteoarthritis. (2) Treatment of neuralgias (provider should be consulted). *Investigational:* Possible use in psoriasis, vitiligo, intractable pruritus, postmastectomy and postamputation neuroma (i.e., phantom limb syndrome), vulvar vestibulitis, apocrine chromhidrosis, and reflex sympathetic dystrophy. **Rx.** Management of neuropathic pain associated with postherpetic neuralgia.

ACTION/KINETICS

Action

Derived from natural sources. **OTC:** May act to deplete and prevent the reaccumulation of substance P, thought to be the main mediator of pain impulses from the periphery to the CNS. **Rx:** Capsaicin is an antagonist for the transient receptor potential vanilloid 1 receptor (TRPV1), which is expressed on nociceptive nerve fibers in the skin. Topical use of capsaicin causes an initial enhanced stimulation of the TRPV1-expressing cutaneous nociceptors that may cause painful sensations. However, this is followed by pain relief thought to be mediated by a reduction in TRPV1-expressing nociceptive nerve endings. Over several months of use, there may be gradual reemergence of painful neuropathy thought to be caused by TRPV1 nerve fiber reinnervation of the treated area.

Pharmacokinetics

Very little systemic absorption of capsaicin.

CONTRAINDICATIONS

Application around or to the face or scalp or to wounds or damaged/irritated skin.

SPECIAL CONCERNS

- For external use only.
- Aerolization of capsaicin can occur upon rapid removal of Rx capsaicin patches. Inhalation of airborne capsaicin can cause coughing or sneezing.
- Increases in BP can occur with the Rx product, especially in those with unstable or poorly controlled hypertension or a recent history of CV or cerebrovascular events.
- Mothers using the Rx product should not breastfeed on the day of capsaicin treatment.
- Consult a healthcare provider before using OTC capsaicin in children less than 18 years of age.
- Safety and efficacy of the Rx product not determined in children less than 18 years of age.

SIDE EFFECTS

Most Common

OTC: Burning, stinging.

Rx: Application site erythema/pain/papules/pruritus, nausea.

OTC. Dermatologic (at application site): Transient burning, stinging, erythema. **Respiratory:** Cough, respiratory tract irritation. **Miscellaneous:** Hypersensitivity reaction.

Rx. Dermatologic (at application site): Erythema, pain, papules, pruritus, edema, dryness, swelling. Application site anesthesia, bruising, dermatitis, excoriation, exfoliation, hyperesthesia, inflammation, paresthesia, urticaria, warmth. **Respiratory:** Nasopharyngitis, sinusitis, bronchitis, cough throat irritation. **GI:** N&V, dysgeusia. **CV:** Hypertension. **CNS:** Burning sensation, dizziness, headache, hyperesthesia, hypoesthesia, peripiheral sensory neuropathy. **Miscellaneous:** Abnormal skin odor, peripheral edema.

DRUG INTERACTIONS

Topical use of capsaicin may cause or worsen coughing associated with ACE inhibitors and vice versa.

HOW SUPPLIED

OTC. Cream: 0.025%, 0.035%, 0.075%, 0.1%, 0.25%; ***OTC. Gel:*** 0.025%, 0.05%; ***OTC. Lotion:*** 0.025%, 0.075%; ***OTC. Patch:*** 0.025%; ***Rx. Patch:*** 8%; ***OTC. Roll-on:*** 0.075%.

DOSAGE

OTC: CREAM; GEL; LOTION; PATCH; ROLL-ON

Muscle/joint pain.

Adults: Apply a thin film to affected area no more than 3–4 times per day.

RX: PATCH

Neuropathic pain.

Adults: Apply a single, 60-minute application of up to 4 patches. May repeat q 3 months, as determined by return of pain; do not use more frequently than q 3 months.

NURSING IMPLICATIONS

IMPLEMENTATION/ADMINISTRATION/STORAGE

1. The Rx product is only to be administered by physicians or other health care providers under close supervision of physicians. Consult the package insert for the detailed instructions on how to prepare and administer the product.
2. The prescription product contains capsaicin capable of producing severe irritation of eyes, skin, respiratory tract, and mucous membranes. The product is not to be prescribed to clients for self-administration. Use only on dry, intact skin.
3. May pretreat area with a topical anesthetic. Apply topical anesthetic to the entire treatment area and surrounding 1 to 2 cm, keeping the local anesthetic in place until the skin is anesthetized and prior to application of the Rx patch. Remove the topical anesthetic with a dry wipe. If skin not intended to be treated with capsaicin comes in contact with the Rx product, apply cleansing gel for 1 min and wipe off with dry gauze. Do not use latex gloves, use only nitrile gloves when handling this product and when cleansing capsaicin from the skin.
4. After the gel has been removed, wash the area with soap and water.
5. Refer to the manufacturer's prescribing information for application, removal, and disposal directions.
6. To ensure capsaicin maintains contact with the treatment area, a dressing, such as rolled gauze, may be used.
7. Do not to touch the patch or treatment area.
8. For the OTC product, do not apply heat to the treated area immediately before or after application as this may increase the burning sensation.
9. Store the OTC and Rx products from 15–30°C (59–86°F). Keep the Rx product in the sealed pouch until immediately before use.

ASSESSMENT

1. Note indications and type of therapy, area requiring treatment, characteristics of S&S, pain level, other agents trialed, outcome.
2. OTC takes 1–2 weeks for arthritis pain relief, 2–4 weeks for general neuropathies, 4–6 weeks with head and neck neuralgias.
3. Apply to dry, intact, skin after washing and patting dry. With prescription patch may need to apply topical anesthetic prior to applying patch.
4. Monitor BP with patch therapy and periodically assess skin integrity, location, and intensity of pain.

CLIENT/FAMILY TEACHING

1. The Rx patch will only be administered by a provider no more often than every 3 months. A single 60-min application of up to 4 patches may be applied and may be repeated every 3 months or as warranted by the return of pain. Cover lightly with dressing.
2. Transient erythema and burning sensation may occur. Do not touch the patch; if accidently do touch the patch, it may burn and/or sting. The treated area may be sensitive to heat for a few days following treatment.
3. May monitor BP; small increases in BP may occur during and shortly after treatment.
4. Report if irritation of the eyes or airways occurs, or if any of adverse effects become severe.
5. Drug is for external use only. Avoid eyes, mouth, groin area, and broken/irritated skin. Expect transient burning/stinging. Rub medication well into designated area until none noted on skin surface.
6. Use care when handling contact lenses after application.
7. Wash hands before and immediately after application. If treatment is to hands, leave medication on for at least 30 min before washing or apply cotton gloves to protect hands from contaminating other body parts. May use a tongue blade or a small foam paint brush to apply, or wear a glove to prevent contamination of eyes, mouth etc. Foam applicator is best method to apply to prevent hand contamination. Then store in a plastic bag after administration to facilitate reapplication. Flush area with water if it gets into eyes and wash with warm soapy water if it contacts other sensitive body parts.
8. Do not bandage area tightly. Burning sensation increases with heat, sweating, bathing in warm water, clothing contact, and increased humidity.
9. Regular use of OTC topical (3–4 times per day) is required for desired response and helps decrease the intensity and frequency of burning; drug interferes with substance P (pain neurotransmitter). Must use regularly to obtain desired results.
10. Report if condition worsens, if symptoms persist >3 weeks, or if clears then recurs within a few days.
11. Do not use with a heating pad: accentuates burning sensation.
12. Keep all F/U to assess response and for adverse SE.

OUTCOMES/EVALUATE

Relief/reduction of pain R/T: PHN, diabetic neuropathy, RA, and/or osteoarthritis

Captopril

(**KAP**-toe-prill)

Classification(s): Antihypertensive, ACE inhibitor

Pregnancy Category: C (first trimester); **D** (second and third trimesters)

RX: Capoten.

✤ **Rx:** Apo-Capto, Gen-Captopril, PMS-Captopril.

SEE ALSO ***ANGIOTENSIN-CONVERTING ENZYME (ACE) INHIBITORS.***

INDICATIONS/USES

(1) Antihypertensive, alone or in combination with other antihypertensive drugs, especially thiazide diuretics. May be used as initial therapy for those with normal renal function. *NOTE:* In clients with impaired renal function, especially those with collagen vascular disease, reserve captopril for hypertensive clients who have either developed unacceptable side effects on other drugs or have failed to respond satisfactorily to drug combinations. (2) In combination with diuretics and digitalis to treat CHF. (3) To improve survival following MI in clinically stable clients with LV dysfunction manifested as an ejection fraction of 40% or less; to reduce the incidence of overt heart failure and subsequent hospitalization for CHF in these clients. *Investigational:* Pediatric hypertension, Raynaud's syndrome.

ACTION/KINETICS

Action

Inhibits angiotensin-converting enzyme resulting in decreased plasma angiotensin II, which leads to decreased vasopressor activity and decreased aldosterone secretion.

Pharmacokinetics

Bioavailability is 75% or less. **Onset:** 30 min or less. **Peak serum levels:** 30–90 min; presence of food decreases absorption by 30–40%. **Time to peak effect:** 60–90 min. **Duration:** 6–10 hr (dose related). **t½, normal renal function, elimination:** 2 hr; **t½, impaired renal function:** 3.5–32 hr. More than 95% of absorbed dose excreted in urine (40–50% unchanged). **Plasma protein binding:** 25–30%.

C

CONTRAINDICATIONS

Use with a history of angioedema related to previous ACE inhibitor use.

SPECIAL CONCERNS

■ **Pregnancy.** When used in pregnancy during the second and third trimesters, ACE inhibitors can cause injury and even death to the developing fetus. When pregnancy is detected, captopril should be discontinued as soon as possible. ■

- **Use with caution in impaired renal function and during lactation.**
- **Use with caution in obstruction in the outflow tract of the left ventricle (e.g., aortic stenosis, hypertrophic cardiomyopathy).**
- **May cause a profound drop in BP following the first dose or if used with diuretics.**
- **Use in children only if other antihypertensive therapy has proven ineffective in controlling BP.**

SIDE EFFECTS

Most Common

Angina pectoris, tachycardia, flushing, pruritus, rash, dysgeusia, chronic cough.

GI: Dysgeusia, dyspepsia, pancreatitis, glossitis. **Hepatic:** Jaundice, cholestasis, hepatitis (including rarely necrosis). **CNS:** Ataxia, confusion, depression, nervousness, somnolence, drowsiness. **CV:** Hypotension (may be profound after the first dose), angina, CHF, ***MI, cardiac arrest, CVA***, chest pain, orthostatic hypotension/effects, palpitations, rhythm disturbances, syncope, tachycardia, vasculitis, cerebrovascular insufficiency, transient decrease in BP when used to treat heart failure. **Dermatologic:** Rash (usually maculopapular) with pruritus and occasionally fever, eosinophilia, and arthralgia. Erythema multiforme, exfoliative dermatitis, flushing, pemphigus/pemphigoid, photosensitivity, bullous pemphigus, ***Stevens-Johnson syndrome***. **GU:** Impotence, oliguria, proteinuria, renal insufficiency, renal failure, nephrotic syndrome, polyuria, urinary frequency, gynecomastia. **Respiratory: *Bronchospasm***, chronic cough, asthma, rhinitis. **Musculoskeletal:** Myalgia, arthralgia, myasthenia. **Hematologic:** Anemia, agranulocytosis, neutropenia, pancytopenia, thrombocytopenia. **Ophthalmic:** Blurred vision. **Body as a whole:** Asthenia, fever, angioedema, symptomatic hyponatremia, ***anaphylactoid reactions***. **Miscellaneous:** Decrease/loss of taste perception with weight loss (reversible), eosinophilic pneumonitis

LABORATORY TEST CONSIDERATIONS

False + test for urine acetone. ↑ BUN and serum creatinine after long-term use. Hyperkalemia, hyponatremia.

OVERDOSE MANAGEMENT

Symptoms: Hypotension with SBP of <80 mm Hg a possibility. *Treatment:* Volume expansion with NSS (IV) is the treatment of choice to restore BP. Captopril may be removed by hemodialysis.

ADDITIONAL DRUG INTERACTIONS

Allopurinol / ↑ Risk of hypersensitivity
Indomethacin / ↓ 24 hr antihypertensive effects of captopril
Iron salts / ↓ Captopril blood levels; separate administration by at least 2 hr
Probenecid / ↑ Captopril blood levels R/T ↓ renal excretion

HOW SUPPLIED

Tablets: 12.5 mg, 25 mg, 50 mg, 100 mg.

DOSAGE

TABLETS

Hypertension.

Adults, initial: 25 mg 2–3 times per day. If unsatisfactory response after 1–2 weeks, increase to 50 mg 2–3 times per day; if still unsatisfactory after another 1–2 weeks, the dose may be increased to 100 mg 2–3 times per day and then, if necessary, to 150 mg 2–3 times per day (while continuing the diuretic). **Maximum dose:** 450 mg/day. If BP is not satisfactorily controlled after 1–2 weeks at 50 mg 3 times/day (and the client is not already taking a diuretic), a modest dose of a thiazide diuretic (e.g., hydrochlorothiazide, 25 mg/day) should be added. The diuretic dose may be increased at 1- to 2-week intervals until its highest usual antihypertensive dose is reached.

Accelerated or malignant hypertension.

For clients with severe hypertension (e.g., accelerated or malignant hypertension), when temporary discontinuation of current antihypertensive therapy is not practical or desirable, or if prompt titration to more normotensive BP is indicated, the diuretic should be continued but other current antihypertensive therapy discontinued and captopril dosage promptly begun at 25 mg 2–3 times/day; close medical supervision is necessary.

Heart failure.

Adults, initial: 25 mg 3 times per day; **then,** if necessary, increase dose to 50 mg 3 times per day and evaluate response. Delay further increases for at least 2 weeks to determine if a satisfactory response has been attained. **Maintenance:** 50–100 mg 3 times per day for most clients. Do not exceed 450 mg/day. *NOTE:* For adults, give an initial dose of 6.25–12.5 mg (0.15 mg/kg 3 times per day in children) 2–3 times per day to clients who are sodium- and water-depleted due to diuretics, who will continue to be on diuretic therapy, and who have renal impairment.

Left ventricular dysfunction after MI.

Adults: Therapy may be started as early as 3 days after the MI. **Initial dose:** 6.25 mg; **then,** begin 12.5 mg 3 times per day and increase to 25 mg 3 times per day over the next several days. The target dose is 50 mg 3 times per day over the next several weeks. Other treatments for MI may be used concomitantly (e.g., aspirin, beta blockers, thrombolytic drugs).

Pediatric hypertension (investigational).

Infants, 20 days of age and younger: 0.01–0.05 mg/kg q 8–12 hr. **Infants, 30 days to <6 months of age, initial:** 0.01–0.5 mg/kg 2–3 times/day, followed by upward titration, if needed. **Children, >6 months of age, initial:** 0.3–0.5 mg/kg 2–3 times/day, followed by upward titration, if needed; **maximum dose:** 6 mg/kg/day, up to 450 mg/day.

Raynaud phenomenon (investigational).

Adults, initial: 12.5 mg twice a day, titrated gradually up to 25 mg 3 times a day.

C

NURSING IMPLICATIONS

IMPLEMENTATION/ADMINISTRATION/STORAGE

1. Individualize dose. Give 1 hr before or 2 hr after meals.
2. Discontinue previous antihypertensive medication 1 week before starting captopril, if possible.
3. If needed by the client's clinical condition, the daily dose may be increased q 24 hr or less under continuous medical supervision until a satisfactory BP response is obtained or the maximum dose of captopril is reached. Addition of a more potent diuretic (e.g., furosemide) may also be indicated.
4. For all uses, reduce dose in clients with renal impairment. Reduce initial daily dose and use smaller increments for titration, which should be slow (i.e., 1- to 2-week intervals). When concomitant diuretic therapy is needed in those with severe renal impairment, use a loop diuretic (e.g., furosemide), rather than a thiazide diuretic.
5. Tablets can be used to prepare a solution of captopril if desired.
6. Do from 15–30°C (59–86°F); protect from moisture.

ASSESSMENT

1. Note disease onset, other medical conditions/agents trialed, outcome.
2. Document ACE intolerance. Assess ability to understand/comply with therapy.
3. Note ejection fraction (at or below 40%) in stable, post-MI clients. Usually very effective with heart failure, diabetes, arthritis.
4. Observe for drop in BP within 3 hr of initial dose if on diuretic therapy and low-salt diet. If BP falls rapidly, place supine; have saline infusion available.
5. Note if diuretics or nitrates prescribed; may act synergistically causing more pronounced response. Withhold potassium-sparing diuret-

ics; hyperkalemia may result—may occur several months after spironolactone and captopril therapy.

6. Monitor VS, K^+, CBC, renal and LFTs, reduce dose with renal dysfunction. Check for proteinuria monthly for 9 months during therapy, CBC every 2 weeks for first 3 months of therapy.

C

CLIENT/FAMILY TEACHING

1. Take 1 hr before meals, on empty stomach; food interferes with drug absorption.
2. Report fever, skin rash, sore throat, mouth sores, fast/irregular heartbeat, chest pain, cough.
3. Use caution with activities that require mental alertness. May develop dizziness, fainting, lightheadedness (lie down until passes); usually disappear once body adjusts. Avoid sudden changes in position, activities/exercise in hot weather; prevent dizziness/fainting. Consume plenty of fluids; prevent dehydration.
4. Loss of taste may be experienced first 2–3 months; report if persists/interferes with nutrition/weight.
5. With heart failure, weigh self and keep record of daily weights. Notify provider if rapid weight gain (e.g., 5 lb in 1 wk) is noted or if edema or shortness of breath worsen.
6. Carry ID and medication list. Call with questions concerning symptoms/effects of therapy; do not stop taking abruptly.
7. Continue activities to assist with BP/heart failure control: diet, weight control, regular/progressive exercise program, smoking cessation, and moderate intake of alcohol and salt.
8. If insulin-dependent may experience hypoglycemia; monitor FS closely.
9. Avoid prolonged sun exposure, wear sunscreen and protective clothing if exposed to avoid photosensitivity reaction. Avoid OTC agents without approval.
10. Practice reliable contraception; report if pregnancy suspected.
11. Keep all F/U to assess BP, electrolytes/urine protein, and for adverse SE.

OUTCOMES/EVALUATE

- ↓ BP
- Improved S&S CHF (↓ preload, ↓ afterload)
- Improved mortality post-MI

Carbamazepine

(kar-bah-**MAYZ**-eh-peen)

Classification(s): Anticonvulsant, miscellaneous

Pregnancy Category: D

RX: Carbatrol, Epitol, Equetro, Tegretol, Tegretol XR.

Rx: Apo-Carbamazepine, Gen-Carbamazepine CR, PMS-Carbamazepine, Sandoz Carbamazepine, Taro-Carbamazepine.

SEE ALSO ***ANTICONVULSANTS***.

INDICATIONS/USES

(1) Partial seizures with complex symptoms (psychomotor, temporal lobe). (2) Generalized tonic-clonic seizures. (3) Mixed seizure patterns that include the previously mentioned seizures, or other partial or generalized seizures. Carbamazepine is often a drug of choice. *NOTE:* Absence seizures do not appear to be helped by carbamazepine.

(4) Pain associated with trigeminal neuralgia and glossopharyngeal neuralgia (all products except Equetro). The drug is not a simple analgesic; do not use for relief of trivial aches or pains.

(5) Acute manic and mixed episodes associated with bipolar I disorder (use Equetro only). *Investigational:* Restless leg syndrome, alternative to benzodiazepines to treat alcohol withdrawal, alternative or adjunct to treat certain symptoms associated with borderline personality disorder, adjunct to treat schizophrenia, treat postherpetic neuralgia.

NOTE: Prescribe only after a critical benefit-to-risk assessment has been made in clients with a history of cardiac conduction disturbance, including second- and third-degree AV heart block; cardiac, hepatic, or renal damage; adverse hematologic or hypersensitivity reaction to other drugs, including reactions to other anticonvulsant or interrupted courses of therapy with carbamazepine.

ACTION/KINETICS

Action

Chemically similar to the cyclic antidepressants. Also manifests antimanic, antineuralgic, antidiuretic, anticholinergic, antiarrhythmic, and antipsychotic effects. The anticonvulsant action is not known but may involve depressing activity in the nucleus ventralis anterior of the thalamus, resulting in a reduction of polysynaptic responses and blocking posttetanic potentiation. Due to the potentially serious blood dyscrasias, undertake a benefit-to-risk evaluation before the drug is instituted.

Pharmacokinetics

The suspension is absorbed somewhat faster than tablets and ER tablets. Bioavailability of ER tablets is 89% compared with the suspension. A high fat meal increases the rate of absorption of a single 400 mg dose. **Peak serum levels:** 4–5 hr. **t½ (serum):** 12–17 hr with repeated doses. **Therapeutic serum levels:** 4–12 mcg/mL for both adults and children. Metabolized in the liver by the CYP3A4 isozyme to the active 10,11-epoxide. **t½, initial:** 25–65 hr but is reduced to 12–17 hr (35–40 hr for ER capsules) because the drug induces its own metabolism. The pharmacokinetic parameters are similar in children and adults; however, there is poor correlation between plasma levels of carbamazepine and the carbamazepine dose in children. Metabolized mainly by CYP3A4 to active and inactive metabolites that are excreted through the feces (28%) and urine (72%). **Plasma protein binding:** About 75%.

CONTRAINDICATIONS

History of bone marrow depression, coadministration with nefazodone, acute intermittent porphyria. Hypersensitivity to drug or tricyclic antidepressants. Concomitant use of MAOIs; discontinue MAOIs for a minimum of 14 days or longer if possible. Lactation. Use for relief of general aches and pains. Use in those with a history of hepatic porphyria (e.g., acute intermittent porphyria, porphyria cutanea tarda, variegate porphyria).

SPECIAL CONCERNS

(1) Aplastic anemia and agranulocytosis have been reported in association with the use of carbamazepine. The risk of developing these reactions is 5-8 times greater than in the general population; however, the overall risk of these reactions in the untreated general population is low, approximately 6 clients per 1 million per year for agranulocytosis and 2 clients per 1 million per year for aplastic anemia. (2) Although reports of transient or persistent decreased platelet or WBC counts are not uncommon in association with the use of carbamazepine, data are not available to estimate accurately their incidence or outcome. However, the vast majority of the cases of leukopenia have not progressed to the more serious conditions of aplastic anemia or agranulocytosis. (3) Because of the very low incidence of these two conditions, the vast majority of minor hematologic changes observed in monitoring clients on carbamazepine are unlikely to signal the occurrence of either abnormality. However, obtain complete pretreatment hematological testing as a baseline. If a client exhibits low or decreased WBC or platelet counts during the course of treatment, monitor closely. Consider discontinuation of the drug if any evidence of significant bone marrow depression develops.

- Use with caution in glaucoma/increased intraocular pressure and in hepatic, renal, CV disease, and a history of hematologic reaction.
- Use with caution in clients with mixed seizure disorder, including atypical absence seizures (carbamazepine is not effective and may be associated with an increased frequency of generalized convulsions).
- Use in geriatric clients may cause an increased incidence of confusion, agitation, AV heart block, syndrome of inappropriate antidiuretic hormone, and bradycardia.
- If taking MAOIs, discontinue for 14 days before taking carbamazepine.
- Clients with a history of adverse hematologic reaction to any drug may be particularly at risk.

SIDE EFFECTS

Most Common

Dizziness, drowsiness, unsteadiness, headache, N&V, ataxia, somnolence, rash, diarrhea, dyspepsia, infection, pain.

GI: N&V, diarrhea, constipation, gastric distress, dyspepsia, abdominal pain, anorexia, glossitis, stomatitis, dry mouth, and pharynx. **Hepatic:** Abnormal LFTs, cholestatic/hepatocellular jaundice, hepatitis, acute intermittent porphyria, ***hepatic failure***. **Hematologic:** ***Aplastic anemia***, leukopenia, eosinophilia, thrombocytopenia, ***agranulocytosis***, leukocytosis, pancytopenia, ***bone marrow depression***. **CNS:** Dizziness, ataxia, drowsiness, unsteadiness, disturbances of coordination, somnolence, headache, fatigue, confusion or agitation (especially in the elderly), speech disturbances, visual hallucinations, depression with agitation, talk-

C

ativeness, hyperacusis, abnormal involuntary movements, activation of latent psychosis, ***suicide attempts and increased suicidality***, behavioral changes in children. **CV:** CHF, aggravation of hypertension, hypotension, syncope and collapse, edema, recurrence of or primary thrombophlebitis, aggravation of CAD, paralysis and other symptoms of cerebral arterial insufficiency, thromboembolism, ***arrhythmias (including second- and third-degree AV block).*** **GU:** Urinary frequency, acute urinary retention, oliguria with hypertension, impotence, renal failure, azotemia, albuminuria, glycosuria, increased BUN, microscopic deposits in urine. **Pulmonary:** Pulmonary hypersensitivity characterized by fever, dyspnea, pneumonitis, or pneumonia. **Dermatologic:** Pruritus, urticaria, photosensitivity, exfoliative dermatitis, erythematous rashes, alterations in pigmentation, alopecia, sweating, purpura, ***toxic epidermal necrolysis*** (Lyell's syndrome), ***Stevens-Johnson syndrome***, aggravation of disseminated lupus erythematosus, alopecia, erythema nodosum/multiforme. **Ophthalmic:** Nystagmus, double/blurred vision, oculomotor disturbances, conjunctivitis; scattered, punctuate cortical lens opacities. **Miscellaneous:** Peripheral neuritis, infection, pain, paresthesias, tinnitus, fever, chills, joint/muscle aches and leg cramps, adenopathy/lymphadenopathy, SIADH, frank water intoxication with hyponatremia and confusion, multiorgan hypersensitivity reactions.

Equetro Only. CNS: Headache, dizziness, somnolence, asthenia, amnesia, manic depressive reaction, anxiety, depression, ataxia, insomnia, depersonalization, manic reaction, nervousness, extrapyramidal symptoms, ***suicide attempt***. **GI:** Nausea, dyspepsia, diarrhea, constipation, abnormal LFTs. **Dermatologic:** Rash, pruritus, alopecia. **Respiratory:** Bronchitis, pharyngitis, rhinitis, sinusitis. **GU:** UTI. **Hematologic:** Leukopenia, lymphadenopathy. **Ophthalmic:** diplopia. **Otic:** Ear pain. **Body as a whole:** Infections (bacterial, fungal, viral), pain, peripheral edema. **Miscellaneous:** Accidental injury, back/chest pain, allergic reactions, photosensitivity reaction.

LABORATORY TEST CONSIDERATIONS

↓ Calcium, thyroid function tests. Interference with some pregnancy tests. Hyponatremia.

OVERDOSE MANAGEMENT

Symptoms: First appear after 1 to 3 hours. Neuromuscular disturbances are the most common. **Pulmonary:** Irregular breathing, ***respiratory depression.*** **CV:** Tachycardia, hypo- or hypertension, conduction disorders, ***shock.*** **CNS:** Seizures (especially in small children), impaired consciousness (deep coma possible), motor restlessness, muscle twitching or tremors, athetoid movements, ataxia, drowsiness, dizziness, nystagmus, mydriasis, psychomotor disturbances, hyperreflexia followed by hyporeflexia, opisthotonos, dysmetria, dizziness, EEG may show dysrhythmias. **GI:** N&V. **GU:** Anuria, oliguria, urinary retention. *Treatment:* Stomach should be irrigated completely even if more than 4 hr has elapsed following drug ingestion, especially if alcohol has been ingested. Activated charcoal, 50–100 grams initially, using a NGT (dose of 12.5 or more grams/hr until client is symptom free). Diazepam or phenobarbital may be used to treat seizures (although they may aggravate respiratory depression, hypotension, and coma). Respiration, ECG, BP, body temperature, pupillary reflexes, and kidney and bladder function should be monitored for several days. If significant bone marrow depression occurs, discontinue and determine daily CBC, platelet, and reticulocyte counts. Perform bone marrow aspiration and trephine biopsy immediately and repeat often enough to monitor recovery.

DRUG INTERACTIONS

Acetaminophen / ↑ Acetaminophen breakdown → ↓ effect and ↑ risk of hepatotoxicity

Azetazolamide / ↑ Carbamazepine plasma levels; adjust dose of carbamazepine as needed

Anticoagulants (e.g., *warfarin*) / Carbamazepine may ↑ metabolism of anticoagulants → ↓ hypoprothrombinemic effect; monitor PT times

Antimalarials (e.g., *chloroquine, mefloquine*) / Possible antagonism of the activity of carbamazepine; adjust carbamazepine dose as needed

Antipsychotics (e.g., *aripiprazole, clozapine, haloperidol, olanzapine, quetiapine, risperidone, ziprasidone*) / ↓ Antipsychotic plasma levels; also, ↑ effects of carbamazepine when given with haloperidol or quetiapine

Azole, antifungal drugs (e.g., *itraconazole, ketoconazole, voriconazole*) / ↑ Plasma carbamazepine levels; closely monitor carbamazepine levels; also, possible ↓ serum itraconazole and voraconazole levels

Barbiturates (e.g., phenobarbital) / ↓ Plasma carbamazepine levels → ↓ effectiveness; adjust their doses if needed
Benzodiazepines (e.g., alprazolam, clonazepam, diazepam, lorazepam, midazolam, triazolam) / ↓ Effect of benzodiazepines; monitor client response
Bupropion / ↓ Bupropion effect R/T ↑ liver breakdown by CYP3A4 enzymes
Buspirone / ↓Buspirone plasma levels; monitor client response
Charcoal / ↓ Carbamazepine effect R/T ↓ GI tract absorption
Cimetidine / ↑ Carbamazepine plasma levels → possible toxicity R/T ↓ liver breakdown
Cisplatin / ↓ Carbamazepine plasma levels; monitor levels
Clomipramine / ↑ Clomipramine plasma levels
Clozapine / ↓ Effects of clozapine
Cyclosporine / ↓ Cyclosporine effect R/T ↑ liver breakdown; monitor cyclosporine levels and observe for signs of rejection or toxicity
Dalfopristin / ↑ Carbamazepine plasma levels → possible toxicity
Danazol / ↑ Carbamazepine effect → possible toxicity R/T ↓ liver breakdown; avoid coadministration if possible
Delavirdine / ↑ Carbamazepine plasma levels (monitor carbamazepine levels closely); possible loss of virologic response and possible resistance to delavirdine or to nonnucleoside reverse transcriptase inhibitors
Diltiazem / ↑ Carbamazepine effect → possible toxicity R/T ↓ liver breakdown; monitor carbamazepine levels
Doxorubicin / ↓ Carbamazepine plasma levels; monitor carbamazepine levels
Doxycycline / ↓ Doxycycline t½ and serum levels R/T ↑ liver breakdown
Erythromycin / ↑ Carbamazepine effect R/T ↓ liver breakdown
Felbamate / Possible ↓ serum levels of either drug → ↓ efficacy
Felodipine / ↓ Felodipine effect
Fluoxetine / ↑ Carbamazepine levels → possible toxicity
Fluvoxamine / ↑ Carbamazepine levels → possible toxicity
Glucocorticoids (e.g., dexamethasone, hydrocortisone) / ↓ Glucocorticoid plasma levels
Grapefruit juice / ↑ Peak levels of carbamazepine; do not give together
Haloperidol / ↓ Haloperidol effect R/T ↑ liver breakdown; also, ↑ carbamazepine effects
HMG-CoA reductase inhibitors (e.g., atorvastatin, simvastatin) / ↓ Plasma levels of certain HMG-CoA reductase inhibitors → ↓ effect resulting in hypercholesterolemia; monitor closely
Hydantoins / Both ↑ and ↓ plasma hydantoin levels; also, ↓ plasma carbamazepine levels
Isoniazid / ↑ Carbamazepine effect R/T ↓ liver breakdown; also, carbamazepine may ↑ risk of drug-induced hepatotoxicity
Itraconazole / ↓ Itraconazole plasma levels
Lamotrigine / ↓ Lamotrigine effect; also, ↑ levels of active metabolite of carbamazepine
Levetiracetam / ↑ Risk of carbamazepine toxicity
Levothyroxine / ↓ Levothyroxine plasma levels; monitor TSH
Lithium / ↑ CNS toxicity; monitor lithium serum levels and adjust dose accordingly
Loratidine / ↑ Carbamazepine plasma levels; closely monitor carbamazepine levels
Macrolide antibiotics (e.g., clarithromycin, erythromycin, troleandomycin) / ↑ Carbamazepine effect R/T ↓ liver breakdown; avoid coadministration if possible
MAOIs / Do not use together; discontinue MAOI at least 14 days before giving carbamazepine
Melatonin / ↑ Melatonin bioavailability
Methadone / ↓ Methadone effects, possible ↑ methadone dose
Methylphenidate / ↓ Blood levels of methylphenidate
Mirtazapine / ↓ Mirtazapine plasma levels; monitor client response
Muscle relaxants, nondepolarizing (e.g., atracurium) / Resistance to or reversal of the neuromuscular blocking effects; ↑ muscle relaxant dose as needed
Nefazodone / ↑ Serum carbamazepine levels and ↓ nefazodone levels may result; coadministration is contraindicated
Niacin (e.g., niacinamide, niotinamide) / ↑ Carbamazepine plasma levels; monitor carbamazepine levels and adjust dose if needed
Olanzapine / ↓ Plasma olanzapine levels
Oral and other hormonal contraceptives / Breakthrough bleeding and unintended pregnancies possible; reliability of oral contraceptive may be adversely affected
Oxcarbazepine / ↓ Oxcarbazepine plasma levels

C

Phenobarbital / ↓ Carbamazepine effect R/T ↑ liver breakdown
Phenytoin / ↓ Carbamazepine effect R/T ↑ liver breakdown; also, phenytoin levels may ↑ or ↓; monitor levels of both drugs
Praziquantel / ↓ Praziquantel serum levels → possible treatment failures; ↑ praziquantel dose if needed
Primidone / ↓ Carbamazepine effect R/T ↑ liver breakdown; also, either ↑ or ↓ primidone levels; monitor levels of both drugs; adjust doses if needed
Probenecid / ↑ Carbamazepine metabolism by CYP3A4 and CYP2C8
Protease inhibitors (e.g., amprenavir, indinavir) / ↑ Plasma carbamazepine levels → ↑ risk of toxicity; also, ↓ plasma protease inhibitor levels → treatment failure
Quinine / ↑ Carbamazepine plasma levels; monitor and adjust carbamazepine dose
Quinupristin / ↑ Carbamazepine plasma levels; monitor carbamazepine levels
Rifampin / ↓ Carbamazepine plasma levels R/T ↑ metabolism; monitor carbamazepine levels
Selective serotonin reuptake inhibitors (e.g., citalopram, fluoxetine, fluvoxamine, sertraline) / ↑ Carbamazepine levels → toxicity; possible ↓ plasma levels of SSRIs; closely monitor client response and adjust dose if needed
Sertraline / ↓ Sertraline effect R/T ↑ liver breakdown
Simvastatin / ↓ Simvastatin levels
Succinimides (e.g., ethosuximide, methsuximide, phensuximide) / ↓ Carbamazepine and succinimide levels
Theophyllines / Either ↓ or ↑ theophylline levels; possible ↓ carbamazepine levels; monitor levels of both drugs and adjust doses if needed
Thyroxine/Triiodothyronine / ↑ Elimination of thyroid hormone R/T ↑ liver breakdown
Tiagabine / ↓ Plasma tiagabine levels
Ticlopidine / ↑ Carbamazepine effect R/T ↓ liver breakdown
Topiramate / ↓ Topiramate levels → ↓ effects
Tramadol / ↓Tramadol plasma levels
Trazodone / ↓ Trazodone plasma levels
Tricyclic antidepressants (amitriptyline, desipramine, imipramine, nortriptyline) / ↓ TCA levels and TCA effects R/T ↑ liver breakdown; ↑ carbamazepine levels; monitor levels of both drugs and adjust dose if needed
Valproic acid / ↓ Valproic acid effect R/T ↑ liver breakdown; ↑ carbamazepine plasma levels; monitor for seizure activity for 1 month after starting or stopping either drug
Vasopressin / ↑ Vasopressin effect
Verapamil / ↑ Carbamazepine plasma levels → ↑ effect R/T ↓ liver breakdown; may need to ↓ carbamazepine dose by 40–50%
Voriconazole / ↓ Voriconazole levels; do not give together
Warfarin sodium / ↓ Anticoagulant effect R/T ↑ liver breakdown
Zileuton / ↑ Carbamazepine plasma levels
Ziprasidone / ↓ Plasma ziprasidone levels
Zonisamide / ↓ Zonisamide plasma levels

HOW SUPPLIED

Capsules, Extended-Release: 100 mg, 200 mg, 300 mg; ***Oral Suspension:*** 100 mg/5 mL; ***Tablets:*** 200 mg; ***Tablets, Chewable:*** 100 mg, 200 mg; ***Tablets, Extended-Release:*** 100 mg, 200 mg, 400 mg.

DOSAGE

CAPSULES, EXTENDED-RELEASE; ORAL SUSPENSION; TABLETS; TABLETS, CHEWABLE; TABLETS, EXTENDED-RELEASE

Epilepsy (except Carbatrol).

Adults and children over 12 years old. Initial dose: 200 mg 2 times per day if using tablets or extended-release products or 100 mg (5 mL) 4 times per day of the suspension. **Titration:** For tablets or suspension, increase at weekly intervals of no more than 200 mg/day using a 3- or 4-times per day regimen. For extended-release formulations, increase at weekly intervals of no more than 200 mg/day using a 2 times per day regimen. **Maintenance:** For all formulations, adjust to minimum effective dose, usually 800–1,200 mg/day. **Maximum daily dose, all formulations:** Adults (rarely) up to 1,600 mg/day; 16 years of age and older up to 1,200 mg/day; 12 to 15 years of age up to 1,000 mg/day.

Children 6–12 years of age. Initial dose: 100 mg 2 times per day if using tablets or extended-release formulations or 50 mg (2.5 mL) 4 times per day of the suspension. **Titration:** For tablets or suspension, increase at weekly intervals of no more than 100 mg/day using a 3- or 4-times per day regimen. For extended-release formulations, increase at weekly intervals of no more than 100 mg/day using a 2 times per day regimen. **Maintenance:** For all formulations, adjust to minimum effective dose, usually 400–800 mg/day. **Maximum daily dose:** For tablets or suspension, 1,000 mg/day; for capsules, 35 mg/kg/day.

Children younger than 6 years old, initial dose: 10–20 mg/kg/day in 2 to 3 divided doses if using tablets and 10–20 mg/kg/day in 4 divided doses if using the suspension. **Titration:** For tablets or suspension, increase weekly to achieve optimal clinical response given 3–4 times per day. **Maintenance:** For all formulations, usually optimal responses are achieved at daily doses less than 35 mg/kg. **Maximum daily dose:** For all formulations, 35 mg/kg/day.

Anticonvulsant (Carbatrol only).

Adults and children older than 12 years of age, initial: 200 mg twice daily. Increase at weekly intervals by adding up to 200 mg/day until optimal response is reached. Dosage generally should not exceed 1,000 mg/day in children 12 to 15 years of age and 1,200 mg/day in clients older than 15 years of age. However, doses up to 1,600 mg/day have been used in adults. **Maintenance:** Usually 800–1,200 mg/day.

Children younger than 12 years of age: Optimal clinical response is reached at daily doses below 35 mg/kg. Children taking total daily doses of immediate-release carbamazepine, 400 mg or greater, may be converted to the same total daily dose of carbamazepine ER capsules, using a twice-daily regimen.

Trigeminal neuralgia (except Carbatrol).

Initial, first day: 100 mg 2 times per day for tablets and extended-release tablets, 200 mg once daily for extended-release capsules, or 50 mg (2.5 mL) 4 times per day for the suspension. **Titration:** For tablets and extended-release formulations, may increase by up to 200 mg/day using 100 mg increments q 12 hr as needed. **Maintenance:** Usually 400–800 mg/day. Attempt discontinuation of drug at least 1 time every 3 months. **Maximum daily dose:** For all formulations, 1,200 mg/day. At least once every 3 months, attempts should be made to reduce the dose to the minimum effective level or even to discontinue the drug.

Trigeminal neuralgia (Carbatrol only).

Initial, first day: 1 200 mg capsule. Daily dose may be increased by up to 200 mg/day q 12 hr only as needed to achieve freedom from pain. Do not exceed 1,200 mg/day. **Maintenance:** Usually 400–800 mg daily. Some clients require as little as 200 mg daily, while others require as much as 1,200 mg daily. At least once every 3 months, attempts should be made to reduce the dose to the minimum effective level or even to discontinue the drug.

Postherpetic neuralgia.

Initial: 100 mg at bedtime. Increase by 100 mg every 3 days until dosage is 200 mg 2 times/day, response is adequate, or blood level of the drug is 6–12 mcg/mL.

Bipolar I disorder (Equetro only).

Adults, initial: 200 mg two times per day. **Titration:** Adjust in 200 mg daily increments to achieve optimum clinical response. **Maintenance:** Doses greater than 1,600 mg/day have not been studied.

NURSING IMPLICATIONS

Do not confuse Tegretol with Tequin (an antibacterial), Toprol-XL (beta-adrenergic blocker), or Topamax (anticonvulsant/antimigraine).

IMPLEMENTATION/ADMINISTRATION/STORAGE

1. To convert from tablets to suspension: give same number of milligrams/day in smaller, more frequent doses (e.g., tablets 2 times per day to suspension 3 times per day).

C

2. Convert from conventional tablets to extended-release capsules: give the same total daily milligram dose of extended-release drug.
3. Convert from conventional tablets to extended-release tablets: give same total daily milligram dose of extended-release drug.
4. When adding carbamazepine to existing anticonvulsant therapy, add gradually while other anticonvulsants are maintained or gradually decreased, except phenytoin, which may have to be increased.
5. Do not administer for minimum of 2 weeks after MAOI drugs.
6. Protect tablets from moisture.
7. Start therapy gradually; use lowest dose to minimize adverse reactions. A given dose of suspension will produce higher peak levels than same dose given as the tablet; thus, start with low doses in children 6–12 y.o. (i.e., 2.5 mL 4 times per day), increase slowly to avoid unwanted side effects.
8. If must discontinue R/T side effects, abrupt withdrawal may lead to seizures or status epilepticus.
9. Do not store chewable tablets, or tablets above 30°C (86°F). Protect from light and moisture.
10. Store ER capsules or tablets from 15–30°C (59–86°F). Protect capsules from moisture and light and protect tablets from moisture.
11. Do not store suspension above 30°C (86°F). Do not administer suspension simultaneously with other liquid medicinal agents or diluents.

ASSESSMENT

1. List reason for therapy: with seizures, describe type, onset, frequency, characteristics. With trigeminal neuralgia list characteristics of symptoms and with bipolar disorder note mental status and clinical presentation. Assess mental status and for psychosis; may activate symptoms.
2. List all drugs prescribed/consumed; ensure none interact adversely.
3. At first S&S of blood dyscrasia, stop drug.
4. Obtain eye exams; assess for opacities, ↑ IOPs.
5. Obtain EEG during therapy. Use seizure precautions with quick withdrawal; may precipitate status epilepticus.
6. During dosage adjustment, monitor VS, I&O for evidence of fluid retention, renal failure, or CV complications.
7. Carefully monitor high-risk clients taking Equetro for bipolar disorder R/T possibility of suicide attempts.
8. Clients of Asian descent should be tested for presence of (human leukocyte antigen) HLA-B*1502, a genetic blood test, before starting therapy in order to identify a significantly increased risk of serious skin reactions, including toxic epidermal necrosis (TEN) and Stevens-Johnson syndrome.
9. Obtain baseline and periodic eye examinations, including slit-lamp, funduscopy, and tonometry.
10. Monitor CBC, renal and LFTs; assess for dysfunction. With high doses, get weekly CBC first 3 months, then monthly: assess extent of bone marrow depression. Monitor carbamazepine serum levels. Obtain high-resolution HLA-B*1502 typing for those genetically at risk.

CLIENT/FAMILY TEACHING

1. Take each dose with food (except extended-release capsules unless GI upset) to ↓ GI upset. Coating for extended-release tablet is not absorbed; may be noticeable in stool. With extended-release tablet, inspect each tablet for chips or cracks in the outer coating, do not take a damaged tablet. Avoid grapefruit juice/products during therapy.
2. Extended-release capsules may be opened and beads sprinkled over a teaspoon of applesauce or other similar food products. Do not crush/chew capsules or contents. May take with/without meals.
3. Shake suspension well before dose; measure prescribed dose using dosing cup, dosing spoon, or dosing syringe. Do not administer carbamazepine suspension simultaneously with other liquid medications or mix with other diluents.
4. Use caution operating car or other dangerous machinery; may interfere with vision/coordination.
5. Withhold drug and report if any of the following symptoms occur:
   - Fever, sore throat, mouth ulcers, easy bruising/bleeding (early S&S bone marrow depression).

- appetite loss, confusion, persistent nausea or headache, rash, small purple spots under the skin, swollen glands, or yellowing of eyes or skin.
- Urinary frequency, retention, reduced output, sexual impotence.
- CHF, fainting, collapse, swelling, blood clot, or cyanosis.
- coordination problems, difficulty with concentration, excessive drowsiness or fatigue, or speech or language problems develop.
- Loss of symptom control.
- Increased depression or suicide ideations.

6. With prolonged therapy do not stop drug suddenly, should be slowly withdrawn over a period of several weeks unless severe adverse side effects.
7. Report skin eruptions, pigmentation changes, other adverse side effects.
8. Avoid excessive sunlight; wear protective clothing/sunscreen to prevent photosensitivity reactions.
9. If using combination oral contraceptive use additional nonhormonal form of contraception because carbamazepine may cause a reduction in effectiveness of combination oral contraceptives; do not breast-feed.
10. Avoid OTC agents, CNS depressants, and alcohol.
11. Keep all F/U to assesses response, labs, for early blood/organ dysfunction, adverse SE.

OUTCOMES/EVALUATE

- Control of refractory seizures
- ↓ Pain with trigeminal neuralgia
- ↓ Depression/mania with bipolar disorder
- Therapeutic serum drug levels (4–12 mcg/mL)

Carbidopa

(**KAR**-bih-doh-pah)

Classification(s): Antiparkinson drug
Pregnancy Category: C
RX: Lodosyn.

Carbidopa/Levodopa

(**KAR**-bih-doh-pah, **LEE**-voh-doh-pah)

RX: Parcopa, Sinemet CR, Sinemet-10/100, -25/100, or -25/250.

✱ **Rx:** Apo-Levocarb, Novo-Levocarbidopa, Nu-Levocarb.

SEE ALSO *LEVODOPA*.

INDICATIONS/USES

(1) Parkinsonism (idiopathic, postencephalitic, following injury to the nervous system due to carbon monoxide and manganese intoxication). Not effective in drug-induced extrapyramidal symptoms. (2) Carbidopa alone is used in clients who require individual titration of carbidopa and levodopa. (3) Carbidopa is used with levodopa to permit use of lower doses of levodopa to reduce N&V. Clients with markedly irregular "on-off" responses to levodopa have not shown benefit from adding carbidopa. *Investigational:* To reduce peripheral metabolism of L-5–hydroxytryptophan when used for postanoxic intention myoclonus. **Warning:** Discontinue levodopa at least 8 hr before carbidopa/levodopa therapy is initiated.

CONTENT

NOTE: Carbidopa amount in each tablet indicated first followed by levodopa amount.

Carbidopa/Levodopa Orally Disintegrating Tablets: 10 mg/100 mg; 25 mg/100 mg; and 25 mg/250 mg. **Carbidopa/Levodopa Sustained-/Extended-Release Tablets:** 25 mg/100 mg or 50 mg/200 mg. **Carbidopa/Levodopa Tablets:** 10/100; 25/100; and 25/250.

ACTION/KINETICS

Action

Carbidopa inhibits peripheral, but not central, decarboxylation of levodopa because it does not cross the blood-brain barrier. Since peripheral decarboxylation is inhibited, more levodopa is available for transport to the brain, where it will be converted to dopamine, thus relieving the symptoms of parkinsonism. Both plasma levels and plasma $t^{1/2}$ of dopamine are increased. Carbidopa and levodopa are given together (e.g., Sinemet). However, *the dosage of levodopa must be reduced by up to 75–80% when combined with carbidopa.* This decreases the incidence of levodopa-induced side effects. *NOTE:* Pyridoxine will not reverse the action of carbidopa/levodopa.

Pharmacokinetics

$t^{1/2}$, carbidopa: 1–2 hr; when given with levodopa, the $t^{1/2}$ of levodopa increases from 1 hr to 2 hr (may be as high as 15 hr in some clients). About

30% carbidopa is excreted unchanged in the urine.

CONTRAINDICATIONS

Use in suspicious, undiagnosed skin lesions, or a history of melanoma. Narrow-angle glaucoma. Use with nonselective MAOIs. Use of carbidopa in children less than 18 years of age. Lactation.

SPECIAL CONCERNS

■ When carbidopa and levodopa are used together, start with no more than 20–25% of the previous daily dose of levodopa. At least 8 hr should elapse between the last dose of levodopa and the first dose of carbidopa/levodopa. ■

- **Use during pregnancy only if benefits outweigh risks.**
- **Use with caution in chronic wide-angle glaucoma, to those with severe CV or pulmonary disease, bronchial asthma; and renal, hepatic, or endocrine disease. Also, use with care in those with a history of MI who have residual atrial, nodal, or ventricular arrhythmias.**
- **Lower doses may be necessary in the elderly due to age-related decreases in peripheral dopa decarboxylase.**
- **Stop MAOIs 2 weeks before therapy.**
- **Safety and efficacy not determined in children less than 18 years.**

SIDE EFFECTS

Most Common

Choreiform or dystonic movements, anorexia, N&V with or without abdominal pain, dry mouth, dysphagia, dysgeusia, sialorrhea, headache, dizziness.

See *Levodopa* for a complete list of possible side effects. Because more levodopa reaches the brain, dyskinesias may occur at lower doses with carbidopa/levodopa than with levodopa alone. Also, there is increased risk of involuntary movements and mental disturbances. Clients abruptly withdrawn from levodopa may experience ***neuroleptic malignant-like syndrome*** (may be life-threatening) including symptoms of muscular rigidity, involuntary movements, altered consciousness, changes in mental status, autonomic dysfunction, tachycardia, tachypnea, sweating, hyper-/hypotension, increased creatine phosphokinase/serum myoglobin, leukocytosis, and myoglobinuria.

LABORATORY TEST CONSIDERATIONS

↑ Alkaline phosphatase, ALT, AST, lactic dehydrogenase, bilirubin. ↓ Creatinine, BUN, and uric acid. Abnormal Coombs' test. False negative test with use of glucose oxidase method to test for glucosuria.

DRUG INTERACTIONS

Antihypertensive drugs / Symptomatic postural hypotension with carbidopa alone or when used with levodopa
Butyrophenones / ↓ Levodopa effect R/T butyrophenones being dopamine D_2 receptor antagonists
Iron salts / Possible ↓ availability of carbidopa and levodopa
Isoniazid / ↓ Levodopa effect R/T isoniazid being a dopamine D_2 receptor antagonist
Metoclopramide / Possible ↑ bioavailability of levodopa R/T ↑ gastric emptying; also, possible adverse effect on disease control R/T metoclopramide being a dopamine receptor antagonist
Phenothiazines / ↓ Levodopa effect R/T phenothiazine being a dopamine D_2 receptor antagonist
Risperidone / ↓ Levodopa effect R/T risperidone being a dopamine D_2 receptor antagonist
Selegiline / Possible severe orthostatic hypotension
Tricyclic antidepressants / Hypertension and dyskinesia

HOW SUPPLIED

Carbidopa. *Tablets:* 25 mg.
Carbidopa/Levodopa: See *Content.*

DOSAGE

CARBIDOPA/LEVODOPA TABLETS, ORALLY DISINTEGRATING

Parkinsonism, clients not receiving levodopa.

Initial: 1 tablet of 10 mg carbidopa/100 mg levodopa 3–4 times per day or 25 mg carbidopa/100 mg levodopa 3 times per day; **then,** increase by 1 tablet q 1–2 days until a total of 8 tablets/day is taken. If additional levodopa is required, substitute 1 tablet of 25 mg carbidopa/250 mg levodopa 3–4 times per day

Parkinsonism, clients receiving levodopa.

Initial: Carbidopa/levodopa dosage should be about 25% of prior levodopa dosage (levodopa dosage is discontinued 8 hr before carbidopa/levodopa is initiated); **then,** adjust dosage as required. Suggested starting dose is 1 tablet of 25 mg carbidopa/250 mg levodopa 3–4 times per day for clients taking more than 1,500 mg levodopa or 25 mg carbidopa/100 mg levodopa for clients taking less than 1,500 mg levodopa

TABLETS, SUSTAINED RELEASE (SINEMET CR)

Parkinsonism, clients not receiving levodopa.

1 tablet twice a day at intervals of not less than 6 hr. Depending on the response, dosage may be increased or decreased. Usual dose is 2–8 tablets per day in divided doses at intervals of 4–8 hr during waking hours (if divided doses are not equal, the smaller dose should be given at the end of the day)

Parkinsonism, clients receiving levodopa.

1 tablet twice a day. Carbidopa is available alone for clients requiring additional carbidopa (i.e., inadequate reduction in N&V); in such clients, carbidopa may be given at a dose of 25 mg with the first daily dose of carbidopa/levodopa. If necessary, additional carbidopa, at doses of 12.5 or 25 mg, may be given with each dose of carbidopa/levodopa

CARBIDOPA TABLETS

Clients receiving carbidopa/levodopa who require additional carbidopa.

In clients taking 10 mg carbidopa/100 mg levodopa, 25 mg carbidopa may be given with the first dose each day. Additional doses of 12.5 or 25 mg may be given during the day with each dose. If the client is taking 25 mg carbidopa/250 mg levodopa, a dose of 25 mg carbidopa may be given with any dose, as needed. The maximum daily dose of carbidopa is 200 mg

NURSING IMPLICATIONS

IMPLEMENTATION/ADMINISTRATION/STORAGE

1. Individualize dosage.
2. Assess for drug interactions.
3. Do not administer carbidopa/levodopa with levodopa. Allow at least 8 hr to elapse between the last dose of levodopa and the first dose of carbidopa/levodopa.
4. Giving sustained-release form of carbidopa/levodopa with food results in increased levodopa availability by 50% and increased peak levodopa levels by 25%.
5. Do not crush/chew sustained-release form of Sinemet; may administer as whole or half tablets.
6. Allow at least 3 days to elapse between dosage adjustments of sustained-release product.
7. When carbidopa is used as supplement to carbidopa/levodopa, 1 tablet of carbidopa may be added or omitted per day.
8. Other antiparkinson drugs may be continued with use of carbidopa/levodopa; however, the dose of other antiparkinson drugs may need to be adjusted.
9. If general anesthesia necessary, continue as long as PO fluids and other medication are allowed. Resume when able to take PO medication.
10. Store at room temperature in light-resistant containers.

ASSESSMENT

1. Note reasons for therapy. Document motor function, reflexes, gait, strength of grip, amount of tremor, agents prescribed.
2. Observe extent of tremors, noting muscle weakness, muscle rigidity, difficulty walking, or changing directions. During dosage adjustment, involuntary movement may require dosage reduction.
3. Determine usual sleep patterns; assess mental status.
4. Note CV disease, cardiac arrhythmias, COPD.
5. List drugs prescribed. Elderly may require reduced dosage. May take multivitamin with pyridoxine without losing symptom control.
6. Obtain ECG, VS, respiratory assessment; determine level of bladder function. Monitor BP supine/standing for postural hypotension.
7. Assess need for drug "holiday" periodically based on decreased drug response. Ensure regular neurologic F/U.

CLIENT/FAMILY TEACHING

1. Food may alter availability but may take with food to lessen GI upset. Do not crush or chew

C

sustained-release form of Sinemet. May take as whole or half tablets.
2. Use caution with activities; may cause drowsiness; change positions slowly to prevent ↓ BP effects.
3. Report side effects as dose may need to be reduced or temporarily discontinued. May be asked to tolerate certain side effects because of overall benefits gained with therapy.
4. With improvement, which may take several weeks to a month, may resume normal activity gradually; with increased activity, other medical conditions must be considered.
5. Do not stop abruptly. When changing medication, one drug should be withdrawn slowly and the other started in small doses under supervision. To facilitate adjustment, take last dose of levodopa at bedtime; start carbidopa/levodopa upon arising.
6. May discolor/darken urine/sweat.
7. Muscle/eyelid twitching may indicate toxicity; report immediately.
8. Keep all F/U to assess response and for adverse SE.

OUTCOMES/EVALUATE

Control of parkinsonian symptoms (e.g., improvement in motor function, physical mobility, reflexes, gait, strength of grip, and amount of tremor)

■ IV

Carboplatin

(**KAR**-boh-plah-tin)

Classification(s): Antineoplastic, alkylating

Pregnancy Category: D

RX: Paraplatin.

Rx: Paraplatin-AQ.

SEE ALSO ***ANTINEOPLASTIC AGENTS*** AND ***ALKYLATING AGENTS***.

INDICATIONS/USES

(1) Initial treatment of advanced ovarian cancer in combination with other chemotherapeutic agents. (2) Palliative treatment of recurrent ovarian cancer either initially or previously treated with chemotherapy, including cisplatin. *Investigational:* In combination with other chemotherapeutic drugs to treat small cell and non-small-cell lung carcinoma; advanced or recurrent squamous cell tumors of the head and neck; seminoma of testicular cancer.

ACTION/KINETICS

Action

Related to cisplatin. Acts by producing interstrand DNA cross-links; thought to be cell-cycle nonspecific.

Pharmacokinetics

t½, initial: 1.1–2 hr; **postdistribution:** 2.6–5.9 hr. Eliminated unchanged in the urine at a rate related to C_{CR}. **Plasma protein binding:** Not bound to plasma proteins, although platinum from carboplatin is irreversibly bound to plasma protein with a slow half-life (5 days).

ADDITIONAL CONTRAINDICATIONS

History of severe allergy to mannitol or platinum compounds (including cisplatin). Severe bone marrow depression, significant bleeding, lactation.

SPECIAL CONCERNS

■ (1) Give under the supervision of a qualified physician experienced in the use of cancer chemotherapeutic drugs. Appropriate management of therapy and complications is possible only when adequate treatment facilities are readily available. (2) Bone marrow depression is dose-related and may be severe, causing infection or bleeding. Anemia may be cumulative and require blood transfusions. (3) Vomiting is a frequent side effect due to the drug. (4) Anaphylaxis may occur within minutes of giving the drug. Symptoms may be alleviated by epinephrine, corticosteroids, and antihistamines. ■

Safety and efficacy not determined in children.

SIDE EFFECTS

Most Common

Thrombocytopenia, neutropenia, anemia, central neurotoxicity, peripheral neuropathies, ototoxicity, electrolyte (magnesium, calcium, potassium, sodium) loss, N&V, alopecia, pain, asthenia, allergic reactions.

See *Antineoplastic Agents* for a complete list of possible side effects. ***Bone marrow suppression may be severe.*** Vomiting. **Neurologic:** Central neurotoxicity, peripheral neuropathies (more common in ages 65 and over), ototoxicity. **GU:** Nephrotoxicity (including increased BUN and serum creatinine) especially when used with aminoglycosides. **Electrolytes:** Loss of Ca^{++}, Mg^{++}, K^{+}, Na^{+}. **Allergic:** Rash, urticaria, pruritus, erythema; ***bronchospasm*** and hypotension (rare). **Miscellaneous:** Pain, alopecia, asthenia. CV, respiratory, mucosal side effects, ***anaphylaxis***.

LABORATORY TEST CONSIDERATIONS

↑ Alkaline phosphatase, AST, total bilirubin. Abnormal LFTs.

OVERDOSE MANAGEMENT

Symptoms: Bone marrow suppression, hepatic toxicity. *Treatment:* Monitor bone marrow and LFTs. Treat symptomatically.

DRUG INTERACTIONS

Al / Precipitate formation and loss of potency R/T reaction with Al (e.g., needles, IV administration sets)
Phenytoin / ↓ Serum phenytoin levels → loss of therapeutic effect
Warfarin / ↑ Anticoagulant effect of warfarin; monitor coagulation parameters

HOW SUPPLIED

Injection: 10 mg/mL; ***Injection, Lyophilized Powder for Solution:*** 50 mg, 150 mg, 450 mg; ***Powder for Injection:*** 50 mg, 150 mg, 450 mg, 600 mg.

DOSAGE

IV

Ovarian cancer, as a single agent.

360 mg/m^2 q 4 weeks on day 1. Lower doses are recommended in clients with low C_{CR}.

In combination with cyclophosphamide.

Carboplatin, 300 mg/m^2 plus cyclophosphamide, 600 mg/m^2, both on day 1 q 4 weeks for 6 cycles.

NURSING IMPLICATIONS

Do not confuse carboplatin with cisplatin (also an antineoplastic drug).

IMPLEMENTATION/ADMINISTRATION/STORAGE

1. **IV Do not repeat single intermittent doses of carboplatin until neutrophil count is at least 2,000/mm^3 and platelet count is 100,000/mm^3.**
2. **May escalate dose by no more than 125% of starting dose if platelet count is greater than 100,000/mm^3 and neutrophil count is greater than 2,000/mm^3. If platelet count is less than 50,000/mm^3 and neutrophil count is less than 500/mm^3, subsequent doses should be 75% of the prior dose.**
3. **With impaired kidney function, adjust dose: C_{CR} of 41–59 mL/min, 250 mg/m^2 on day 1; C_{CR} of 16–40 mL/min, 200 mg/m^2 on day 1. No recommended dose if the C_{CR} is less than 15 mL/min.**
4. **Cisplatin is easily confused with carboplatin. Store separately; post signs in storage areas warning of the name mix-ups. Do not refer to as "platinum."**
5. **Do not use with needles or IV sets containing aluminum.**
6. **Just before use, reconstitute with either sterile water, D5W, or NaCl injection to final concentration of 10 mg/mL. May further dilute to concentrations as low as 0.5 mg/mL with D5W or NaCl injection. Administered by infusion lasting 15 min or longer.**
7. **Reconstituted solutions stable for 8 hr at room temperature. Discard after 8 hr; no antibacterial preservative in the formulation, although vials are multidose.**
8. **Store unopened vials at room temperature, protected from light.**
9. COMPATIBILITY **D5W or 0.9% NaCl.**
10. INCOMPATIBILITY **Administer separately.**

ASSESSMENT

1. **List reasons for therapy, other agents trialed, outcome.**
2. **Check for any allergic reactions to mannitol or platinum compounds. With hypersensitivity reaction, which may occur within minutes of administration, have epinephrine, corticosteroids, and antihistamines available to alleviate symptoms**
3. **Note any evidence of kidney impairment; reduce dose with dysfunction. The Calvert formula calculates the carboplatin dose in mg as follows: Total dose (mg) = (target AUC) × (GFR + 25).**
4. **Assess neurologic disorders to determine if those occurring at a later date are drug related or exacerbations of a prior condition. Monitor for ototoxicity, peripheral neuropathy, visual disturbances.**
5. **Premedicate with antiemetics; vomiting frequent side effect.**

C

6. Assess for S&S of infection or bleeding. Report if noted and be prepared to treat appropriately (e.g., IV antibiotics, colony stimulating factors, transfusions).
7. With kidney impairment, initially give 1–2 L of fluids slowly. Use diuretics if overhydrated. Check for drug-induced anemia; adjust dose.
8. Drug dose based on CBC and C_{CR}; reduce dose with impaired liver/renal function, hold for platelet counts <100,000/mm^3. Ensure dose adjusted based on lowest posttreatment platelet or neutrophil value following manufacturer's guidelines.
9. Monitor electrolytes, C_{CR}, renal and LFTs, CBC, platelet counts before each treatment course. Platelet nadir: day 21; back to baseline by day 28.

CLIENT/FAMILY TEACHING

1. Use to treat advanced ovarian cancer. N&V may be experienced; report if pretreatment antiemetic ineffective.
2. Report hearing/vision problems, numbness, tingling, skin rash, hives, itching, redness, numbness, tingling, burning, or pain in the hands and feet.
3. Maintain adequate fluid intake using fluids with electrolytes; may see decrease in K+, Ca^{++}.
4. Avoid live vaccines, crowds, and those with known infections.
5. Report fever, chills, sore throat, bleeding, fatigue, breathing problems, mouth sores; may indicate bone marrow depression, can be severe with therapy.
6. May cause hair loss, but reversible once therapy stopped.
7. Avoid pregnancy; practice reliable birth control.
8. Keep all F/U to assess response, labs, and for adverse SE.

OUTCOMES/EVALUATE

↓ Size and spread of tumor; stabilization of malignant process

Carisoprodol

(kar-eye-so-**PROH**-dohl)

Classification(s): Skeletal muscle relaxant, centrally-acting

Pregnancy Category: C

RX: Soma.

SEE ALSO ***SKELETAL MUSCLE RELAXANTS, CENTRALLY-ACTING***.

INDICATIONS/USES

As an adjunct to rest, PT, and other measures to treat skeletal muscle disorders including bursitis, low back disorders, contusions, fibrositis, spondylitis, sprains, and muscle strains.

ACTION/KINETICS

Action

Does not directly relax skeletal muscles. Sedative effects may be responsible for muscle relaxation.

Pharmacokinetics

Onset: 30 min. **Duration:** 4–6 hr. **Peak serum levels:** 4–7 mcg/mL. **t½:** 8 hr. Metabolized in the liver and excreted in urine.

CONTRAINDICATIONS

Acute intermittent porphyria. Hypersensitivity to carisoprodol or meprobamate. Not recommended for use in children under 12 years of age.

SPECIAL CONCERNS

- Use with caution during lactation, in impaired liver or kidney function, and in addiction-prone individuals.
- Idiosyncratic reactions may occur rarely within minutes or hours after the first dose.
- May cause GI upset and sedation in infants.

SIDE EFFECTS

Most Common

Dizziness, drowsiness, N&V, headache, tachycardia.

CNS: Ataxia, dizziness, drowsiness, excitement, tremor, syncope, vertigo, insomnia, irritability, agitation, headache, depressive reactions. **GI:** N&V, epigastric distress, hiccoughs. **CV:** Flushing of face, postural hypotension, tachycardia. **Allergic or idiosyncratic reactions (usually after the first to fourth dose):** Pruritus, skin rashes, erythema multiforme, eosinophilia, fixed drug eruptions. Symptoms of severe reactions include fever, dizziness, ***angioneurotic edema***, asthmatic symptoms, "smarting" of the eyes, weakness, hypotension, ***anaphylaxis***.

OVERDOSE MANAGEMENT

Symptoms: Stupor, coma, ***shock, respiratory depression, and rarely, death***. The effects of overdosage of carisoprodol and alcohol or other CNS depressants or psychotropic drugs can be additive even if one of the drugs has been ingested at the usual recommended dose. *Treatment:* Supportive measures. Remove any remaining drug from the stomach. Institute supportive measures. If respiration and BP become compromised, provide respiratory assistance, CNS stimulants, and pressor agents cautiously as indicated. Diuresis, osmotic diuresis, peritoneal dialysis, hemodialysis. Monitor urinary output to avoid overhydration. Observe client for possible relapse due to incomplete gastric emptying and delayed absorption.

DRUG INTERACTIONS

Alcohol / Additive CNS depressant effects
Antidepressants, tricyclic / ↑ Carisoprodol effect
Barbiturates / Possible ↑ carisoprodol effect, followed by inhibition of carisoprodol
Chlorcyclizine / ↓ Carisoprodol effect
CNS depressants / Additive CNS depression
MAOIs / ↑ Carisoprodol effect R/T ↓ liver breakdown
Phenobarbital / ↓ Carisoprodol effect R/T ↑ liver breakdown
Phenothiazines / Additive CNS depressant effects
Psychotropic drugs / Additive CNS depressant effects

HOW SUPPLIED

Tablets: 250 mg, 350 mg.

DOSAGE

TABLETS

Skeletal muscle disorders.

Adults: 350 mg 3–4 times per day (take last dose at bedtime).

NURSING IMPLICATIONS

IMPLEMENTATION/ADMINISTRATION/STORAGE

Store from 15–30°C (59–86°F). Dispense in tight, light-resistant, well-closed containers.

ASSESSMENT

1. List reasons for therapy, onset, contributing factors, characteristics of S&S. Record extent of skeletal muscular disorders noting baseline ROM, stiffness, level of discomfort.
2. Review drugs prescribed to ensure no interactions.
3. Monitor for S&S of idiosyncratic response: agitation, ataxia, disorientation, dizziness, euphoria, extreme weakness, impaired verbal communication, transient quadriplegia, and vision disturbances. These may appear within minutes or hours of first dose and usually subside over several hours. Withhold drug and report if these reactions occur.
4. Note sensitivity to meprobamate or carisoprodol; assess carefully as potential for addictive behavior precludes therapy.
5. Monitor VS, renal and LFTs; assess for dysfunction and use with caution.

CLIENT/FAMILY TEACHING

1. Take with food if GI upset. If unable to swallow tablets, mix with syrup, chocolate, or a jelly mixture.
2. Used to help relax certain muscles to relieve stiffness, pain, discomfort caused by strains, sprains, or other muscular injury. Report adverse side effects, especially gait disturbance, hiccoughs, palpitations or tremors.
3. Take last dose at bedtime. May cause dizziness, drowsiness; use caution when driving or undertaking tasks requiring mental alertness. Report if severe; may necessitate drug withdrawal.
4. Avoid OTC agents and alcohol.
5. Use judiciously; psychologic dependence may occur.
6. Keep all F/U to assess response, need for PT referrals, and for adverse SE.

OUTCOMES/EVALUATE

Improvement in skeletal muscle pain and spasticity; ↑ ROM

IV

Carmustine (BCNU)

(kar-**MUS**-teen)

Classification(s): Antineoplastic, alkylating

Pregnancy Category: D

RX: BiCNU, Gliadel.

SEE ALSO ***ANTINEOPLASTIC AGENTS*** AND ***ALKYLATING AGENTS***.

C

INDICATIONS/USES

Injection: (1) Alone or in combination with other antineoplastic agents for palliative treatment of primary (e.g., brain stem glioma, astrocytoma, glioblastoma, ependymoma, medulloblastoma) and metastatic brain tumors. (2) Multiple myeloma (in combination with prednisone). (3) Advanced Hodgkin's disease and non-Hodgkin's lymphomas (not drug of choice) in those who relapse or who fail to respond to primary therapy. *Investigational:* Malignant melanoma.

Wafer: (1) Adjunct to surgery and radiation in newly diagnosed high-grade malignant glioma. (2) To prolong survival in recurrent glioblastoma multiforme as an adjunct to surgery.

ACTION/KINETICS

Action

Alkylates DNA and RNA, as well as inhibits several enzymes by carbamoylation of amino acids in proteins. Cell-cycle nonspecific. Not cross-resistant with other alkylating agents.

Pharmacokinetics

Rapidly cleared from plasma and metabolized. Crosses blood-brain barrier (concentration in CSF at least 50% greater than in plasma). **t½:** 15–30 min. Thirty percent excreted in urine after 24 hr, 60–70% after 96 hr. Wafers are biodegradable in the brain when implanted into the cavity after tumor resection. Released carmustine diffuses into the surrounding brain tissue.

CONTRAINDICATIONS

Lactation.

SPECIAL CONCERNS

(1) Bone marrow depression is the major toxic side effect. Monitor CBCs weekly for at least 6 weeks after a dose. Do not give repeat doses more frequently than q 6 weeks. Safety and effectiveness not established in children. Bone marrow toxicity is cumulative; adjust dose based on nadir blood counts from prior dose. (2) Thrombocytopenia and leukopenia may contribute to bleeding and overwhelming infections in an already compromised client. (3) Pulmonary toxicity (can be fatal) is dose-related. Those receiving >1,400 mg/m^2 cumulative dose are at a higher risk. Other risk factors include history of lung disease and treatment duration. Delayed onset pulmonary fibrosis can occur years after treatment (can result in death), particularly in those treated in childhood.

SIDE EFFECTS

Most Common

Headache, hemiplegia, convulsions, confusion, brain edema, aphasia, depression, somnolence, speech disorder, amnesia, alopecia, N&V, constipation, abnormal healing, asthenia, UTI, infection, fever, pain, rash.

See *Antineoplastic Agents* for a complete list of possible side effects. **GI:** N&V within 2 hr after administration, lasting 4–6 hr; hepatic toxicity. **CNS:** Seizures, brain edema, intracranial infection, obstructive hydrocephalus. **GU:** Renal failure, azotemia, decrease in kidney size. **Hepatic:** Reversible increases in alkaline phosphatase, bilirubin, and transaminase. **Miscellaneous:** Rapid IV administration may produce transitory intense flushing of skin and conjunctiva (onset: after 2 hr; duration: 4 hr). ***Pulmonary fibrosis***, ocular toxicity including retinal hemorrhage. The wafer may cause healing abnormalities including wound dehiscence, delayed wound healing, cerebrospinal fluid leak, and subdural, subgaleal, or wound effusions.

DRUG INTERACTIONS

Cimetidine / Additive bone marrow suppression
Digoxin / ↓ Serum digoxin levels → ↓ effect
Mitomycin / Corneal and conjunctival epithelial damage
Phenytoin / ↓ Serum phenytoin levels → ↓ effect

HOW SUPPLIED

Powder for Injection, Lyophilized: 100 mg; *Wafer Implant:* 7.7 mg.

DOSAGE

IV

In previously untreated clients.

150–200 mg/m^2 q 6 weeks as a single dose. Alternate dosing schedule: 75–100 mg/m^2 on 2 successive days q 6 weeks. Reduce subsequent dosage if platelet levels are less than 100,000/mm^3 and leukocyte levels are less than 4,000/mm^3.

WAFER IMPLANT

Recurrent glioblastoma multiforme.

8 wafers placed in the resection cavity if size and shape of the cavity allow. If this is not possible, use the maximum number of wafers allowed.

NURSING IMPLICATIONS

IMPLEMENTATION/ADMINISTRATION/STORAGE

1. Slight overlap of wafer in cavity is acceptable. May use wafer broken in half; discard wafers broken into more than two pieces.
2. To secure wafers against cavity surface, oxidized regenerated cellulose may be placed over the wafers.
3. Irrigate resection cavity after wafer placement; dura should be closed in watertight fashion.
4. Unopened foil pouches of wafers may be kept at ambient room temperature for a maximum of 6 hr. Store at or below –20°C (–4°F).
5. IV Discard vials in which powder has become an oily liquid.
6. Reconstitute powder with absolute ethyl alcohol (provided); then add sterile water. For injection, dilutions stable for 24 hr when stored as noted in #13.
7. Stock solutions diluted to 500 mL with D5W are stable for 48 hr when stored as noted in #13.
8. Administer IV over 1–2 hr; faster injection may produce intense pain and burning at injection site.
9. Check for extravasation if burning/pain at injection site; discomfort may be from alcohol diluent. If no extravasation but burning experienced, reduce rate of flow.
10. Slow rate of infusion; report intense flushing of skin, redness of conjunctiva.
11. Skin contact with reconstituted carmustine may result in hyperpigmentation (transient); wash the skin/mucosa thoroughly with soap and water.
12. *Do not use vial for multiple doses;* no preservatives.
13. Store unopened vials at 2–8°C (36–46°F); protect from light. Store diluted solutions at 4°C (39°F); protect from light.
14. COMPATIBILITY D5W.
15. INCOMPATIBILITY Administer separately.

ASSESSMENT

1. Note reasons for therapy, onset, extent of disease, other agents trialed.
2. Document/monitor pulmonary, oral, ophthalmic exams.
3. Get baseline PFTs and frequent PFTs during therapy. Those with a baseline <70% of predicted forced vital capacity (FVC) or carbon monoxide diffusing capacity (DLCO) are at particular risk.
4. Delayed onset pulmonary fibrosis has occurred up to 17 yr after treatment and has been reported in clients who received injectable carmustine in childhood and early adolescence.
5. Thrombocytopenia and leukopenia may contribute to bleeding, overwhelming infections in already compromised client; monitor closely.
6. Obtain baseline renal and LFTs. Monitor uric acid, CBC up to 6 weeks after drug dose; delayed bone marrow toxicity may develop. Drug causes granulocyte and bone marrow suppression. Nadir: 21 days; recovery: 35–42 days. Do not give repeat doses more frequently than q 6 weeks. Bone marrow toxicity cumulative; adjust dose based on nadir blood counts from prior dose.

CLIENT/FAMILY TEACHING

1. Used as an adjunct to surgery and radiation in those newly diagnosed high-grade malignant glioma and as an adjunct in those with recurrent glioblastoma multiforme (wafer). Given IV with or without other agents for brain tumors, in multiple myeloma with prednisone and secondary therapy with Hodgkin's disease, and non-Hodgkin's lymphoma with relapse.
2. Drugs (antiemetic) administered before IV therapy should help with N&V.
3. Take temperature daily. Report S&S fever/infection; increased SOB, abnormal bruising/bleeding. Consume adequate fluids; prevent dehydration.
4. Avoid live vaccines. Use soft-bristled toothbrush, electric razor; avoid aspirin/NSAIDs, may cause bleeding.
5. Avoid smoking; enhances pulmonary toxicity. This can be fatal and is dose-related; may occur many years after therapy.
6. May experience hair loss. Report if mouth sores develop; a special mouthwash or anesthetic can be prescribed. Avoid rough, hot/

hard foods or citrus products to prevent oral irritation.

7. Severe flushing after IV dose should subside in 2–4 hr; may also experience N&V 2 hr after infusion.
8. Practice reliable contraception; do not breastfeed.
9. With wafers: remnants of implanted wafers may be observed on brain imaging scans or during later operations even though all components are extensively degraded.
10. Keep all F/U to assess response, labs, and for adverse SE.

OUTCOMES/EVALUATE

↓ Size/spread of metastatic process

Carvedilol

(kar-**VAY**-dih-lol)

Classification(s): Alpha-beta adrenergic blocking agent

Pregnancy Category: C

RX: Coreg, Coreg CR.

🍁 **Rx:** Apo-Carvedilol, PMS-Carvedilol, RAN-Carvedilol, ratio-Carvedilol.

SEE ALSO ***ALPHA-1 AND BETA-ADRENERGIC BLOCKING AGENTS.***

INDICATIONS/USES

(1) Essential hypertension used either alone or in combination with other antihypertensive drugs, especially thiazide diuretics. (2) Mild to severe heart failure of ischemic or cardiomyopathic origin; used with diuretics, ACE inhibitors, and digitalis to increase survival and reduce risk of hospitalization. (3) Reduce CV mortality in clinically stable clients who have survived an acute MI and have a left ventricular ejection fraction of 40% or less (with or without symptomatic heart failure). *Investigational:* Chronic, stable angina pectoris; idiopathic cardiomyopathy.

ACTION/KINETICS

Action

Has both alpha- and beta-adrenergic blocking activity. Decreases cardiac output, reduces exercise- or isoproterenol-induced tachycardia, reduces reflex orthostatic hypotension, causes vasodilation, and reduces peripheral vascular resistance. BP is lowered more in the standing than in the supine position. Significantly lowers plasma renin activity when given for at least 4 weeks.

Pharmacokinetics

Significant beta-blocking activity occurs within 60 min, while alpha-blocking action is observed within 30 min. Rapidly absorbed after PO administration; significant first-pass effect. **Terminal t½:** 7–10 hr. Food delays absorption rate. Plasma levels average 50% higher in geriatric compared with younger clients. Extensively metabolized in the liver mainly by CYP2D6 and CYP2C9; metabolites excreted primarily via the bile into the feces. **Plasma protein binding:** Over 98%.

CONTRAINDICATIONS

Clients with NYHA Class IV decompensated cardiac failure requiring the use of IV inotropic therapy (wean from IV therapy before starting carvedilol), bronchial asthma or related bronchospastic conditions, second- or third-degree AV block, SSS or severe bradycardia (unless a permanent pacemaker is in place), cardiogenic shock, drug hypersensitivity. Impaired hepatic function. Lactation.

SPECIAL CONCERNS

- **Use with caution in hypertensive clients with CHF controlled with digitalis, diuretics, or an ACE inhibitor.**
- **Use with caution in PVD, in surgical procedures using anesthetic agents that depress myocardial function, in diabetics receiving insulin or oral hypoglycemic drugs, in those subject to spontaneous hypoglycemia, or in thyrotoxicosis.**
- **Worsening cardiac failure or fluid retention may occur during up-titration of carvedilol.**
- **Signs of hyperthyroidism or hypoglycemia, especially tachycardia, may be masked.**
- **Abrupt withdrawal may cause severe exacerbation of angina and the occurrence of MI and ventricular arrhythmias; discontinue over 1–2 weeks.**
- **Clients with a history of severe anaphylactic reaction to a variety of allergens may be more reactive to repeated challenge while taking beta-blockers.**
- **Safety and efficacy not established in children less than 18 years of age.**

SIDE EFFECTS

Most Common

Dizziness, headache, N&V, diarrhea, URTI, fatigue, pain, bradycardia, hypotension, weight increase, hyperglycemia, increased cough, SOB.

CV: Bradycardia, postural hypotension, AV block (may be complete), BBB, cerebrovascular disorder, extrasystoles, hyper-/hypotension, palpitations, peripheral ischemia, syncope, angina, aggravated angina, ***cardiac failure***, ***CVA***, myocardial ischemia, tachycardia, CV disorder, fluid overload, peripheral vascular disorder, precipitation/worsening of symptoms of arterial insufficiency, chest pain in Prinzmetal variant angina. **CNS:** Dizziness, headache, somnolence, insomnia, ataxia, nervousness, hypesthesia, paresthesia, vertigo, depression, aggravated depression, nervousness, migraine, neuralgia, paresis, amnesia, confusion, sleep disorder, impaired concentration, abnormal thinking, paranoia, convulsions, emotional lability, hypokinesia, paroniria, ***convulsions***. **Body as a whole:** Fatigue, viral infection, rash, allergy, asthenia, malaise, pain, injury, fever, infection, flu syndrome, dependent/peripheral edema, generalized edema, somnolence, sweating, ***sudden death***. **GI:** Diarrhea, abdominal/GI pain, N&V, flatulence, dry mouth, anorexia, dyspepsia, melena, periodontitis, increased hepatic enzymes, hepatotoxicity, ***GI hemorrhage***. **Respiratory:** Rhinitis, pharyngitis, sinusitis, bronchitis, dyspnea, ***asthma***, ***bronchospasm***, pulmonary edema, respiratory disorder/alkalosis, dyspnea, URTI, coughing, rales, interstitial pneumonitis. **GU:** UTI, albuminuria, hematuria, frequency of micturition, abnormal renal function, impotence, renal insufficiency, kidney failure, urinary incontinence in women. **Dermatologic:** Pruritus, erythematous rash, erythema multiforme, ***Stevens-Johnson syndrome***, ***toxic epidermal necrolysis***, alopecia, maculopapular rash, psoriaform rash, photosensitivity reaction, exfoliative dermatitis, increased sweating. **Metabolic:** Hypertriglyceridemia, hypercholesterolemia, hyper-/hypoglycemia, hypo-/hypervolemia, hyperuricemia, weight gain/loss, gout, dehydration, glycosuria, hyponatremia, hypo-/hyperkalemia, diabetes mellitus, worsening of hyperglycemia in diabetes. **Hematologic:** Thrombocytopenia, anemia, leukopenia, pancytopenia, purpura, atypical lymphocytes, ***aplastic anemia (rare)***. **Musculoskeletal:** Back pain, arthralgia, myalgia, arthritis, muscle cramps, hypotonia. **Otic:** Decreased hearing, tinnitus. **Miscellaneous:** Hot flushes, leg cramps, abnormal/blurred vision, decreased hearing, decreased libido in men, ***anaphylactoid reaction***.

LABORATORY TEST CONSIDERATIONS

↑ ALT, AST, BUN, NPN, alkaline phosphatase, GGT, creatinine. ↓ HDL, prothrombin. Bilirubinemia.

OVERDOSE MANAGEMENT

Symptoms: Severe hypotension, bradycardia, cardiac insufficiency, ***cardiogenic shock***, ***cardiac arrest***, ***generalized seizures***, respiratory problems, bronchospasms, vomiting, lapse of consciousness. *Treatment:* Place client in a supine position, monitor carefully, and treat under intensive care conditions. Continue treatment for a sufficient period consistent with the 7- to 10-hr drug half-life:

- For gastric lavage or induced emesis shortly after ingestion.
- For excessive bradycardia, atropine, 2 mg IV. If bradycardia is resistant to therapy, use pacemaker therapy.
- To support cardiovascular function, give glucagon, 5–10 mg IV rapidly over 30 sec, followed by a continuous infusion of 5 mg/hr. Sympathomimetics (dobutamine, isoproterenol, epinephrine) may be given.
- For peripheral vasodilation, give epinephrine or norepinephrine with continuous monitoring of circulatory conditions.
- For bronchospasm, give beta sympathomimetics as aerosol or IV or use aminophylline IVPB.
- With seizures, give diazepam or clonazepam slowly IV.

DRUG INTERACTIONS

Antidiabetic agents / ↑ Hypoglycemic effects R/T beta blockade

Calcium channel blocking agents (e.g., diltiazem, verapamil) / ↑ Risk of conduction disturbances (rarely with hemodynamic compromise); monitor ECG and BP

Catecholamine-depleting drugs / Possible hypotension/severe bradycardia

Cimetidine / ↑ Carvedilol AUC by about 30%; no change in C_{max}

Clonidine / Potentiation of BP- and heart-rate-lowering effects; when stopping both carvedilol and clonidine, discontinue clonidine first (discontinue carvedilol several days later by gradually decreasing dose)

Cyclosporine / ↑ Cyclosporine levels R/T ↓ liver breakdown; monitor cyclosporine levels closely

C

Digoxin / ↑ Digoxin levels by about 15%; monitor digoxin when initiating, adjusting, or discontinue carvedilol
Diphenhydramine / ↑ Carvedilol plasma levels and CV effects R/T inhibition of metabolism
Disopyramide / ↓ Disopyramide clearance → sinus bradycardia and hypotension; monitor carefully
Hydroxychloroquine / ↑ Plasma and CV effects of carvedilol R/T inhibition of metabolism; monitor clients
Insulin / ↑ Glucose-lowering effect of insulin; monitor blood glucose
MAOIs / Monitor for signs of hypotension or severe bradycardia
Oral hypoglycemics / ↑ Glucose-lowering effect of oral hypoglycemics; monitor blood glucose
Propafenone / ↑ Blood levels of the R(+) enantiomer of carvedilol
Quinidine / ↑ Blood levels of the R(+) enantiomer of carvedilol
Rifampin / ↓ Plasma carvedilol AUC and C_{max} by about 70%
Salicylates / ↓BP-lowering effects of carvedilol; ↓ beneficial effects of carvedilol on LVEF in those with chronic heart failure
Selective serotonin reuptake inhibitors (e.g., fluoxetine, paroxetine) / Inhibition of carvedilol metabolism → excessive bradycardia; monitor cardiac function if used together

HOW SUPPLIED

Capsules, Extended-Release: 10 mg, 20 mg, 40 mg, 80 mg (all as the phosphate); ***Tablets, Immediate-Release:*** 3.125 mg, 6.25 mg, 12.5 mg, 25 mg.

DOSAGE

TABLETS, IMMEDIATE-RELEASE

Essential hypertension.

Initial: 6.25 mg 2 times per day. If tolerated, using standing systolic pressure measured about 1 hr after dosing, maintain dose for 7–14 days. **Then** increase to 12.5 mg 2 times per day, if necessary, based on trough BP, using standing systolic pressure 2 hr after dosing. Maintain this dose for 7–14 days; adjust upward to 25 mg 2 times per day if necessary and tolerated. Do not exceed 50 mg/day.

Congestive heart failure.

Individualize dose and closely monitor. **Initial:** 3.125 mg 2 times per day for 2 weeks. If tolerated, increase to 6.25 mg 2 times per day. Double dose every 2 weeks to the highest tolerated level, up to a maximum of 25 mg 2 times per day in those weighing less than 85 kg and 50 mg 2 times per day in those weighing over 85 kg. Reduce dose in those experiencing bradycardia (HR <55 beats/min).

Left ventricular dysfunction following myocardial infarction (MI).

Individualize dose and monitor during up-titration. **Initial:** 6.25 mg 2 times per day; increase after 3–10 days, based on tolerability, to 12.5 mg 2 times per day. Increase again to a target dose of 25 mg 2 times per day. A lower starting dose (3.125 mg 2 times per day) may be used due to low BP, HR, or fluid retention. The dosing regimen does not need to be altered in those who received an IV or PO beta-blocker during the acute phase of the MI.

Angina pectoris.

25–50 mg 2 times per day.

Idiopathic cardiomyopathy.

6.25–25 mg 2 times per day.

CAPSULES, EXTENDED-RELEASE

Essential hypertension.

Initial: 20 mg once daily. If this dose is tolerated, using standing systolic pressure measured about 1 hr after dosing, maintain this dose for 7–14 days; **then** increase to 40 mg once daily if needed, based on trough BP; maintain this dose for 7–14 days. Dose can then be adjusted upward to 80 mg once daily if tolerated and needed. Do not exceed a total daily dose of 80 mg.

Congestive heart failure.

Initial: 10 mg once daily for 2 weeks. Those who tolerate this dose may have their dose increased to 20, 40, or 80 mg over successive intervals of at least 2 weeks. Maintain clients on lower doses if higher doses are not tolerated.

Left ventricular dysfunction following MI.

Initial: 20 mg once daily; increase after 3–10 days, based on tolerability, to 40 mg once daily and then again to the target dose of 80 mg once daily. A dose of 10 mg once daily may be used and/or the rate of up-titration may be slowed if indicated (i.e., due to low BP or HR or fluid retention). Treatment may be started as an inpatient or outpatient and should be initiated after the client is hemodynamically stable and fluid retention has been minimized. The recommended dosing regimen need not be altered in those who received treatment with an IV or PO beta-blocker during the acute phase of the MI.

NURSING IMPLICATIONS

Do not confuse carvedilol with captopril (ACE inhibitor) or carteolol (beta-blocker).

IMPLEMENTATION/ADMINISTRATION/STORAGE

1. Full antihypertensive effect seen within 7–14 days.
2. Clients controlled with immediate-release (IR) carvedilol alone or in combination with other medications, can be switched to extended-release (ER) capsules based on the total daily dose as follows: If the total daily dose of IR capsules is 6.25 mg, give 10 mg once daily of the ER capsules; if the total daily dose of IR is 12.5 mg, give 20 mg once daily of the ER form; if the total daily dose of IR is 25 mg, give 40 mg once daily of the ER form; and, if the total daily dose of IR is 50 mg, give 80 mg once daily of the ER form. Individualize dosage, and carefully monitor during titration.
3. Addition of a diuretic can produce additive effects and exaggerate orthostatic effect.
4. Treat fluid retention with increased dose of diuretics, whether or not heart failure symptoms have worsened.
5. Episodes of dizziness or fluid retention during initiation of therapy can usually be managed by discontinuing drug; does not preclude subsequent successful titration of or a favorable response to the drug.
6. Reduce dose if bradycardia (HR less than 55 beats/min) occurs.
7. Store both IR and ER forms from 15–30°C (59–86°F). Dispense in a tight, light-resistant container.

ASSESSMENT

1. List reasons for therapy, type/onset of symptoms, other agents trialed, outcome.
2. Note history/evidence of bronchospastic conditions, asthma, advanced AV block, severe bradycardia; drug contraindicated.
3. Obtain VS, I&O, weight, ECG, CBC, BNP, lipids, uric acid, renal and LFTs and monitor. Assess lung sounds, check for edema. Note ejection fraction/stress test/cath results.

CLIENT/FAMILY TEACHING

1. Take as prescribed with food to reduce orthostatic effects; slows absorption/decreases low BP effects.
2. Take the extended-release form once daily in the morning with food. Swallow as a whole capsule; do not crush, chew, or divide doses.
3. Extended-release capsules may be opened and the beads sprinkled over a spoonful of cold applesauce. Consume the mixture immediately in its entirety. Do not store applesauce-drug mixture for future use.
4. Avoid activities that require mental acuity until drug effects realized, may cause dizziness or fatigue. To prevent ↓ BP, sit or lie until symptoms subside, rise slowly from a sitting or lying position, and avoid sudden position changes. Adding a diuretic may aggravate low BP drug effects.
5. R/T beta-blocking activity (especially with ischemic heart disease) may cause arrhythmias; do not stop therapy abruptly; therapy should be weaned over 3 weeks.
6. Decreased tearing may be noted by contact lens wearers.
7. Avoid OTC agents. Separate alcohol consumption, including ethanol-containing prescription and OTC medicines, by at least 2 hr.
8. Review lifestyle changes (e.g., weight control, regular exercise, smoking cessation, moderate intake of alcohol and salt) to enhance therapy with BP control.
9. Report low heart rate, dark urine, fainting or persistent dizziness when arising from a sitting or lying position, fatigue, increasing shortness of breath, persistent anorexia, itching, right upper quadrant tenderness, swelling

of feet or ankles, unexplained flu-like symptoms, or weight gain >5 lb/week or 2 lb/day.

10. Keep all F/U to assess response (bring record of weight, BP, pulse) and for adverse SE. Dosing adjustments made every 7–14 days based on standing SBP measured 1 hr after dosing.

C

OUTCOMES/EVALUATE

- Reduction of BP
- ↓ Progression of CHF ↓ Mortality
- Angina pectoris (unlabeled)

Cefaclor

(**SEF**-ah-klor)

Classification(s): Cephalosporin, second generation

Pregnancy Category: B

RX: Ceclor, Raniclor.

🍁 **Rx:** Apo-Cefaclor.

SEE ALSO ***ANTI-INFECTIVES*** AND ***CEPHALOSPORINS***.

INDICATIONS/USES

Capsules, Chewable Tablets, Oral Suspension: (1) Otitis media due to *Streptococcus pneumoniae, Hemophilus influenzae, Streptococcus pyogenes,* and staphylococci. (2) Pharyngitis and tonsillitis caused by *S. pyogenes.* (3) Lower respiratory tract infections (including pneumonia) due to *S. pneumoniae, H. influenzae,* and *S. pyogenes.* (4) UTIs (including pyelonephritis and cystitis) caused by *Escherichia coli, Proteus mirabilis, Klebsiella* species, and coagulase-negative staphylococci.

Extended-Release Tablets: (1) Uncomplicated skin and skin structure infections due to *Staphylococcus aureus* (methicillin-susceptible). (2) Pharyngitis and tonsillitis due to *S. pyogenes.* (3) Acute bacterial exacerbation of chronic bronchitis due to *H. influenzae* (non-beta-lactamase-producing strains only), *Moraxella catarrhalis* (including beta-lactamase-producing strains), and *S. pneumoniae.* (4) Secondary bacterial infections of acute bronchitis due to *H. influenzae* (non-beta-lactamase-producing strains only), *M. catarrhalis* (including beta-lactamase-producing strains), and *S. pneumoniae.*

ACTION/KINETICS

Pharmacokinetics

Peak serum levels: 5–15 mcg/mL after 1 hr. **$t_{1/2}$: PO,** 36–54 min. Well absorbed from GI tract. From 60 to 85% excreted in urine within 8 hr.

SPECIAL CONCERNS

Safety in infants less than 1 month of age not established.

SIDE EFFECTS

Most Common

N&V, diarrhea, abdominal pain, GI upset, headache, yeast infection of the mouth or vagina.

See *Cephalosporins* for a complete list of possible side effects. Also, cholestatic jaundice, lymphocytosis.

DRUG INTERACTIONS

↓ Plasma levels of cefaclor extended-release tablets when used with antacids; take cefaclor 2 hr before or after the antacid

HOW SUPPLIED

Capsules: 250 mg, 500 mg; ***Powder for Oral Suspension:*** 125 mg/5 mL, 187 mg/5 mL, 250 mg/5 mL, 375 mg/5 mL; ***Tablets, Chewable:*** 125 mg, 187 mg, 250 mg, 375 mg; ***Tablets, Extended-Release:*** 250 mg.

DOSAGE

CAPSULES; ORAL SUSPENSION; TABLETS, CHEWABLE

All uses.

Adults, usual: 250 mg q 8 hr. May double dose in more severe infections or those caused by less susceptible organisms. Do not exceed 4 grams/day. **Children:** 20 mg/kg/day in divided doses q 8 hr. May double dose in more serious infections, otitis media, or for infections caused by less susceptible organisms. For otitis media and pharyngitis, the total daily dose may be divided and given q 12 hr. Do not exceed a total dose of 2 grams/day.

TABLETS, EXTENDED-RELEASE

Uncomplicated skin and skin structure infections.

Adults, 16 years of age and older: 375 mg q 12 hr for 7 to 10 days. **Total daily dose:** 750 mg.

Pharyngitis or tonsillitis.
Adults, 16 years of age and older: 375 mg q 12 hr for 10 days. **Total daily dose:** 750 mg.
Acute bacterial exacerbation of chronic bronchitis or secondary bacterial infection of acute bronchitis.
Adults, 16 years of age and older: 500 mg q 12 hr for 7 days. **Total daily dose:** 1,000 mg.

NURSING IMPLICATIONS

IMPLEMENTATION/ADMINISTRATION/STORAGE

1. Continue administration for a minimum of 48–72 hr after fever abates or after evidence of bacterial eradication has been obtained. For beta-hemolytic streptococcal infections, continue treatment for at least 10 days as a prophylaxis for rheumatic fever or glomerulonephritis.
2. 500 mg twice a day of cefaclor extended-release tablets is clinically equivalent to 250 mg 3 times a day of cefaclor immediate-release as a capsule. 500 mg twice a day of cefaclor extended-release tablets is *not* equivalent to 500 mg 3 times a day of other cefaclor formulations.
3. Refrigerate suspension after reconstitution; discard after 2 weeks.
4. The total daily dose for otitis media and pharyngitis can be divided and given q 12 hr.
5. Store capsules, chewable tablets, and extended-release tablets from 15–30°C (59–86°F). Refrigerate suspension after reconstitution; discard after 14 days.

ASSESSMENT

1. List type, onset, characteristics of S&S, clinical presentation, other agents trialed, C&S results.
2. Note any penicillin allergy; cross-sensitivity may occur.
3. Monitor VS, CBC, renal function, and C&S as needed. Use caution with elderly and renal dysfunction.

CLIENT/FAMILY TEACHING

1. Take as directed; do not stop when feeling better. Review how to store drug; may keep suspension refrigerated up to 14 days; shake well before using.
2. Do not cut, chew, or crush tablets. Food does not affect capsule absorption. Consume adequate fluids to prevent dehydration. Take the extended-release tablets with meals (i.e., within 1 hr of eating).
3. Report any rash, severe abdominal pain, bloody diarrhea, or lack of improvement after 48–72 hr. With new onset wheezing seek immediate help.
4. Keep all F/U to assess response, labs, and for adverse SE.

OUTCOMES/EVALUATE

Resolution of infection; symptomatic improvement

Cefadroxil monohydrate

(sef-ah-**DROX**-ill)

Classification(s): Cephalosporin, first generation

Pregnancy Category: B

🍁 **Rx:** Apo-Cefadroxil.

SEE ALSO ***ANTI-INFECTIVES*** AND ***CEPHALOSPORINS.***

INDICATIONS/USES

(1) UTIs caused by *Escherichia coli, Proteus mirabilis,* and *Klebsiella* species. (2) Skin and skin structure infections due to staphylococci or streptococci. (3) Pharyngitis or tonsillitis due to *Streptococcus pyogenes* (group A beta-hemolytic streptococci).

ACTION/KINETICS

Pharmacokinetics

Peak serum levels: PO, 15–33 mcg/mL after 90 min. **t½: PO,** 78–96 min. 90% excreted unchanged in urine within 24 hr.

SPECIAL CONCERNS

- Determine C_{CR} in clients with renal impairment.
- Safe use in children not established.

SIDE EFFECTS

Most Common

Diarrhea, N&V, redness/swelling of skin, skin rash/itching, vaginal inflammation, colitis.

See *Cephalosporins* for a complete list of possible side effects.

HOW SUPPLIED

Capsules: 500 mg; ***Powder for Oral Suspension:*** 125 mg/5 mL, 250 mg/5 mL, 500 mg/5 mL; ***Tablets:*** 1 gram.

DOSAGE

CAPSULES; ORAL SUSPENSION; TABLETS

Pharyngitis, tonsillitis.

Adults: 1 gram/day in single or two divided doses for 10 days. **Children:** 30 mg/kg/day in single or two divided doses q 12 hr (for beta-hemolytic streptococcal infection, give dose for 10 or more days).

Skin and skin structure infections.

Adults: 1 gram/day in single or two divided doses. **Children:** 30 mg/kg/day in divided doses q 12 hr.

Urinary tract infections (UTIs).

Adults: 1 or 2 grams/day in single or two divided doses for uncomplicated lower UTI (e.g., cystitis). For all other UTIs, the usual dose is 2 grams/day in two divided doses. **Children:** 30 mg/kg/day in divided doses q 12 hr.

For clients with C_{CR} rates below 50 mL/min.

Initial: 1 gram; **maintenance,** 500 mg at following dosage intervals: q 36 hr for C_{CR} rates of 0–10 mL/min; q 24 hr for C_{CR} rates of 10–25 mL/min; q 12 hr for C_{CR} rates of 25–50 mL/min.

NURSING IMPLICATIONS

IMPLEMENTATION/ADMINISTRATION/STORAGE

1. Give without regard to meals. Food may decrease GI side effects.
2. Shake suspension well before using.
3. For beta-hemolytic streptococcal infections, treat for 10 days.
4. Refrigerate reconstituted suspension; discard any unused portion after 14 days.
5. Store tablets and capsules from 15–30°C (59–86°F).

ASSESSMENT

1. List reasons for therapy, type/onset of symptoms, clinical presentation, and culture results.
2. Note any penicillin allergy.
3. Monitor VS, CBC, renal function, and C&S as indicated.

CLIENT/FAMILY TEACHING

1. Complete script as directed with/without food.
2. Refrigerate suspension, shake well before using; discard after 14 days.
3. Report any rash, prolonged fever, diarrhea, worsening of condition, lack of response after 72 hr.
4. Keep all F/U to assess response, labs, and adverse SE.

OUTCOMES/EVALUATE

- Symptomatic improvement
- Negative culture reports

Cefdinir

(**SEF**-dih-near)

Classification(s): Cephalosporin, third generation

Pregnancy Category: B

RX: Omnicef.

SEE ALSO ***CEPHALOSPORINS***.

INDICATIONS/USES

Adults and adolescents:

1. Community-acquired pneumonia or acute exacerbations of chronic bronchitis due to *Haemophilus influenzae* (including beta-lactamase producing strains), *Haemophilus parainfluenzae* (including beta-lactamase producing strains), *Streptococcus pneumoniae* (penicillin-susceptible strains only), and *Moraxella catarrhalis* (including beta-lactamase producing strains).
2. Acute maxillary sinusitis due to *H. influenzae* (including beta-lactamase producing strains), *S. pneumoniae* (penicillin-susceptible strains only), and *M. catarrhalis* (including beta-lactamase producing strains).
3. Uncomplicated skin and skin structure infections due to *Staphylococcus aureus* (including beta-lactamase producing strains) and *Streptococcus pyogenes.*
4. Pharyngitis/tonsillitis due to *S. pyogenes.*

Children (6 months through 12 years):

1. Acute bacterial otitis media due to *H. influenzae* (including beta-lactamase producing strains), *S. pneumoniae* (penicillin-susceptible strains only), and *M. catarrhalis* (including beta-lactamase producing strains).
2. Pharyngitis/tonsillitis due to *S. pyogenes*. Acute maxillary sinusitis.
3. Uncomplicated skin and skin structure infections due to *S. aureus* (including beta-lactamase producing strains) and *S. pyogenes*. *NOTE:* The suspension is approved for use for all infections in children previously indicated.

ACTION/KINETICS

Action

Interferes with the final step in cell wall formation (inhibition of mucopeptide biosynthesis), resulting in unstable cell membranes that undergo lysis. Also, cell division and growth are inhibited.

Pharmacokinetics

Maximum plasma levels: 2–4 hr. **t½, elimination:** 1.7 hr. Excreted through the urine.

CONTRAINDICATIONS

Allergy to cephalosporins.

SPECIAL CONCERNS

- Reduce dose in compromised renal function.
- Safety and efficacy not determined in infants less than 6 months of age.
- Not studied for the prevention of rheumatic fever following *S. pyrogenes* pharyngitis/tonsillitis.

SIDE EFFECTS

Most Common

Diarrhea, N&V, vaginal moniliasis/vaginitis, headache, abdominal pain, rash (children).

See *Cephalosporins* for a complete list of possible side effects.

DRUG INTERACTIONS

Antacids, Al- or Mg⁺⁺-containing / ↓ Cefdinir absorption → ↓ plasma levels

Probenecid / ↑ Plasma cefdinir levels → ↑ effect

HOW SUPPLIED

Capsules: 300 mg; *Oral Suspension:* 125 mg/5 mL, 250 mg/5 mL.

DOSAGE

CAPSULES

Community-acquired pneumonia, uncomplicated skin and skin structure infections.

Adults and adolescents age 13 and older: 300 mg q 12 hr for 10 days.

Acute exacerbations of chronic bronchitis, acute maxillary sinusitis, or pharyngitis/tonsillitis.

Adults and adolescents age 13 and older: 300 mg q 12 hr for 5–10 days or 600 mg q 24 hr for 10 days for acute exacerbations of chronic bronchitis or pharyngitis/tonsillitis. Alternatively, 300 mg twice a day for 5 days for acute exacerbations of chronic bronchitis.

ORAL SUSPENSION

Acute bacterial otitis media or pharyngitis/tonsillitis.

Children, 6 months through 12 years: 7 mg/kg q 12 hr for 5–10 days or 14 mg/kg q 24 hr for 10 days.

Uncomplicated skin and skin structure infections.

Children, 6 months through 12 years: 7 mg/kg q 12 hr for 10 days.

Acute maxillary sinusitis.

Children, 6 months through 12 years: 7 mg/kg q 12 hr or 14 mg/kg q 24 hr for 10 days.

NURSING IMPLICATIONS

IMPLEMENTATION/ADMINISTRATION/STORAGE

1. For adults with C_{CR} <30 mL/min, give 300 mg once daily. For children with a C_{CR} of <30 mL/1.73 m^2, give 7 mg/kg (less than or equal to 300 mg) once daily.
2. Once daily dosing (600 mg) in adults and adolescents may be used for acute maxillary sinusitis, acute exacerbations of chronic bronchitis, or pharyngitis/tonsillitis.
3. For children, ages 6 months through 12 years, the total daily dose for all infections is 14 mg/kg, up to a maximum of 600 mg/day. Except for skin infections, once-daily dosing for 10 days is as effective as twice-daily dosing.
4. The dosage of oral suspension for children is:

- **9 kg (20 lb):** 2.5 mL q 12 hr or 5 mL q 24 hr of 125 mg/5 mL formulation.
- **18 kg (40 lb):** 5 mL q 12 hr or 10 mL q 24 hr of 125 mg/5 mL formulation; or, 2.5 mL q 12 hr or 5 mL q 24 hr of 250 mg/5 mL formulation.
- **27 kg (60 lb):** 7.5 mL q 12 hr or 15 mL q 24 hr of 125 mg/5 mL formulation; or, 3.75 mL q 12 hr or 7.5 mL q 24 hr of 250 mg/5 mL formulation.
- **36 kg (80 lb):** 10 mL q 12 hr or 20 mL q 24 hr of 125 mg/5 mL formulation; or, 5 mL q 12 hr or 10 mL q 24 hr of 250 mg/5 mL formulation.
- **Greater than or equal to 43 kg (95 lb):** 12 mL q 12 hr or 24 mL q 24 hr of 125 mg/5 mL formulation; or, 6 mL q 12 hr or 12 mL q 24 hr of 250 mg/5 mL formulation.

5. Hemodialysis removes cefdinir from the body. In those on chronic hemodialysis, the recommended initial dose is 300 mg or 7 mg/kg every other day. At the end of each hemodialysis session, 300 mg or 7 mg/kg should be given followed by 300 mg or 7 mg/kg every other day.
6. Store capsules/powder for suspension from 15–30°C (59–86°F). After mixing, store suspension at room temperature (25°C, 77°F). Discard any unused suspension after 10 days.

ASSESSMENT

1. Note reasons for therapy, onset, characteristics of S&S, clinical presentation, culture results.
2. Check for cephalosporin/PCN allergy.
3. Report severe diarrhea, or abdominal pain/cramping.
4. Monitor VS, cultures, CBC/liver/renal function; if C_{CR} <30 mL/min, reduce dose.

CLIENT/FAMILY TEACHING

1. Take without regard to food.
2. Iron supplements, multivitamins with iron, antacids with Mg^{++} and aluminum interfere with drug absorption; if needed, take either 2 hr before or 2 hr after dose.
3. Oral suspension contains 2.86 grams of sucrose per teaspoon; use capsules with diabetes. Add 38 mL water to 60 mL bottle or 63 mL water to 100 mL bottle, mix well; discard solution after 10 days. Shake well before each use.
4. May give suspension in iron fortified infant formula without losing potency.
5. Stop drug and report if skin rash, hives, itching, or shortness of breath occurs. Report S&S of superinfection: black furry tongue, white patches in mouth, foul-smelling stools, vaginal itching or discharge.
6. Report if diarrhea persistent, exceeds 4 episodes/day, accompanied by abdominal pain, blood or pus in stool. Consume adequate fluids to prevent dehydation.
7. Stools may be discolored red; should subside.
8. Report worsening of condition after 72 hr. Keep F/U to assess response and for adverse SE.

OUTCOMES/EVALUATE

Resolution of infection

IV

Cefepime hydrochloride

(**SEF**-eh-pim)

Classification(s): Cephalosporin, third generation

Pregnancy Category: B

RX: Cefepime hydrochlorite.

SEE ALSO ***CEPHALOSPORINS*** AND ***ANTI-INFECTIVES***.

INDICATIONS/USES

Adults: (1) Uncomplicated and complicated UTIs (including pyelonephritis) caused by *Escherichia coli* or *Klebsiella pneumoniae;* when the infection is severe or caused by *E. coli, K. pneumoniae,* or *Proteus mirabilis;* when the infection is mild to moderate, including infections associated with concurrent bacteremia with these microorganisms.

(2) Uncomplicated skin and skin structure infections caused by *Staphylococcus aureus* (methicillin-susceptible strains only) or *Streptococcus pyogenes.*

(3) Moderate to severe pneumonia due to *Streptococcus pneumoniae,* including cases associated with concurrent bacteremia, *Pseudomonas aeruginosa, K. pneumoniae,* or *Enterobacter* species.

(4) Monotherapy for empiric treatment of febrile neutropenia in those at high risk for infection.

(5) In combination with metronidazole in complicated intra-abdominal infections due to *E. coli,* viridans group streptococci, *P. aeruginosa, K. pneumoniae, Enterobacter* species, or *Bacteroides fragilis.*

Children, 2 months to 16 years: Treatment of complicated and uncomplicated UTIs including pyelonephritis, uncomplicated skin and skin structure infections, pneumonia, and as empiric therapy for febrile neutropenic clients.

ACTION/KINETICS

Action

Antibacterial activity against both gram-negative and gram-positive pathogens, including those resistant to other beta-lactam antibiotics. High affinity for the multiple penicillin-binding proteins that are essential for cell wall synthesis.

Pharmacokinetics

Peak serum levels, after IV: 78 mcg/mL. **t½, terminal:** 2 hr. About 85% of the drug is excreted unchanged in the urine.

CONTRAINDICATIONS

Use after a hypersensitivity reaction to cefepime, cephalosporins, pencillins, or any other beta-lactam antibiotics.

SPECIAL CONCERNS

- **Increased risk of serious side effects in clients with renal insufficiency, including encephalopathy, myoclonus, seizures, and renal failure.**
- **Use with caution during lactation.**
- **Safety and efficacy not determined in children <12 years.**

SIDE EFFECTS

Most Common

Rash, phlebitis, pain, inflammation at injection site, headache, nausea, dizziness, vaginal moniliasis.

See *Cephalosporins* for a complete list of possible side effects.

LABORATORY TEST CONSIDERATIONS

↑ ALT, AST, alkaline phosphatase, BUN, creatinine, potassium, total bilirubin. ↓ Hematocrit, neutrophils, platelets, WBCs. ↑ or ↓ Calcium, phosphorus. Positive Coombs' test. Abnormal PTT, PT.

DRUG INTERACTIONS

Aminoglycosides / ↑ Risk of nephrotoxicity and ototoxicity

Furosemide / ↑ Risk of nephrotoxicity

HOW SUPPLIED

Injection Solution: 1 gram/50 mL; 2 grams/50 mL; ***Powder for Injection:*** 500 mg, 1 gram, 2 grams.

DOSAGE

IM; IV

Mild to moderate uncomplicated or complicated urinary tract infections (UTIs), including pyelonephritis, due to E. coli, K. pneumoniae, *or* P. mirabilis.

Adults: 0.5–1 gram IV or IM (for *E. coli* infections) q 12 hr for 7–10 days.

Severe uncomplicated or complicated UTIs, including pyelonephritis, due to E. coli *or* K. pneumoniae.

Adults: 2 grams IV q 12 hr for 10 days.

Moderate to severe pneumonia due to S. pneumoniae, P. aeruginosa, K. pneumoniae, *or* Enterobacter *species.*

Adults: 1–2 grams IV q 12 hr for 10 days.

Moderate to severe uncomplicated skin and skin structure infections due to S. aureus *or* S. pyogenes.

Adults: 2 grams IV q 12 hr for 10 days.

Febrile neutropenia.

2 grams IV q 8 hr for 7 days, or until resolution of neutropenia.

With metronidazole in complicated intra-abdominal infections due to E. coli, P. aeruginosa, K. pneumoniae, B. fragilis, Enterobacter *species, or viridans group streptococci.*

Adults: 2 grams IV q 12 hr for 7–10 days

Infections in children 2 months to 16 years.

Up to 40 kg: 50 mg/kg q 12 hr (q 8 hr for febrile neutropenia) for same durations as adult dosage. Do not exceed adult dose.

NURSING IMPLICATIONS

IMPLEMENTATION/ADMINISTRATION/STORAGE

1. **For IM use: Reconstitute with 0.9% NaCl, D5W, 0.5% or 1% lidocaine HCl, sterile water**

or bacteriostatic water for injection with parabens or benzyl alcohol.

2. Adjust dose/frequency (see package insert) for impaired renal function (C_{CR} <60 mL/min).
3. IV For IV use: Reconstitute the 1 or 2 gram 100 mL bottle with 50 or 100 mL of compatible solutions and administer over 30 min.
4. Protect reconstituted drug from light; store at room temperature 20–25°C (68–77°F) for 24 hr or refrigerate at 2–8°C (36–46°F) for 7 days.
5. COMPATIBILITY 0.9% NaCl, 5% or 10% dextrose injection, M/6 sodium lactate injection, D5W/0.9% NaCl injection, D5W/RL, or Normosol-R or Normosol-M in D5W injection.
6. INCOMPATIBILITY Ampicillin (greater than 40 mg/mL), aminophylline, gentamicin, metronidazole, netilmicin sulfate, tobramycin, or vancomycin.

ASSESSMENT

1. Note reasons for therapy, onset, characteristics of S&S. List agents trialed; outcome.
2. Check for any sensitivity to penicillin, cephalosporins, or other antibiotics.
3. Assess mental and cognitive status; stop drug and report if S&S of encephalopathy occur: change in consciousness including confusion, hallucinations, stupor, coma and/or seizures.
4. List other agents prescribed; aminoglycosides and furosemide may increase risk of nephrotoxicity/ototoxicity.
5. Obtain baseline cultures, CBC, renal and LFTs. Reduce dose with renal dysfunction.

CLIENT/FAMILY TEACHING

1. Drug administered parenterally. Must have regular dosing to maintain therapeutic blood levels.
2. Pain and inflammation may occur at infusion site; may see rash.
3. Report adverse side effects, lack of response, changes in neurological status (changes in level of consciousness, including confusion, hallucinations, stupor, and coma), seizures, increase in bruising or bleeding, prolonged/persistent diarrhea as overgrowth of colon flora may have occurred; may require additional therapy.
4. Keep all F/U to assess response, labs, and adverse SE.

OUTCOMES/EVALUATE

Symptomatic improvement with resolution of infective organism

Cefixime oral

(seh-**FIX**-eem)

Classification(s): Cephalosporin, third generation

Pregnancy Category: B

RX: Suprax.

SEE ALSO ***ANTI-INFECTIVES*** AND ***CEPHALOSPORINS***.

INDICATIONS/USES

1. Uncomplicated UTIs caused by *Escherichia coli* and *Proteus mirabilis*.
2. Otitis media due to *Haemophilus influenzae* (beta-lactamase positive and negative strains), *Moraxella catarrhalis,* and *Streptococcus pyogenes*.
3. Pharyngitis and tonsillitis caused by *S. pyogenes*.
4. Acute bronchitis and acute exacerbations of chronic bronchitis caused by *S. pneumoniae* and *H. influenzae* (beta-lactamase positive and negative strains).
5. Uncomplicated cervical or urethral gonorrhea due to *Neisseria gonorrhoeae* (both penicillinase- and non-penicillinase-producing strains).

ACTION/KINETICS

Pharmacokinetics

Stable in the presence of beta-lactamase enzymes. **Peak serum levels:** 2–6 hr. **t½:** Averages 3–4 hr. About 50% excreted unchanged in the urine and approximately 10% in the bile.

SPECIAL CONCERNS

Safe use in infants less than 6 months old not established.

SIDE EFFECTS

Most Common

N&V, diarrhea/loose stools, abdominal pain, dyspepsia, flatulence.

See *Cephalosporins* for a complete list of possible side effects. Also, **GI:** Flatulence. **Hepatic:** Elevated alkaline phosphatase levels. **Renal:** Transient increases in BUN or creatinine.

ADDITIONAL LABORATORY TEST CONSIDERATIONS

False + test for ketones using nitroprusside test.

HOW SUPPLIED

Powder for Oral Suspension: 100 mg/5 mL, 200 mg/5 mL.

DOSAGE

ORAL SUSPENSION

All uses.

Adults: Either 400 mg once daily (recommended) or 200 mg q 12 hr. **Children:** Either 8 mg/kg once daily or 4 mg/kg q 12 hr. Give the adult dose to children >50 kg or >12 years of age.

NOTE: For clients on renal dialysis or in whom C_{CR} is 21–60 mL/min, the dose should be 75% of the standard dose (i.e., 300 mg/day). If the C_{CR} < 20 mL/min or continuous ambulatory peritoneal dialysis, the dose should be 50% of the standard dose (i.e., 200 mg/day).

Uncomplicated gonorrhea.

1 400 mg tablet daily.

NURSING IMPLICATIONS

IMPLEMENTATION/ADMINISTRATION/STORAGE

1. Continue therapy for at least 10 days when treating *S. pyogenes.*
2. Use the following pediatric doses if using the 100 mg/5 mL suspension: **6.25 kg:** For a daily dose of 50 mg, give 2.5 mL; **12.5 kg:** For a daily dose of 100 mg, give 5 mL; **18.75 kg:** For a daily dose of 150 mg, give 7.5 mL; **25 kg:** For a daily dose of 200 mg, give 10 mL; **31.25 kg:** For a daily dose of 250 mg, give 12.5 mL; **37.5 kg:** For a daily dose of 300 mg, give 15 mL.
3. Use the following pediatric dose if using the 200 mg/5 mL suspension: **6.25 kg:** For a daily dose of 50 mg, give 1.25 mL; **12.5 kg:** For a daily dose of 100 mg, give 2.5 mL; **18.75 kg:** For a daily dose of 150 mg, give 3.75 mL; **25 kg:** For a daily dose of 200 mg, give 5 mL; **31.25 kg:** For a daily dose of 250 mg, give 6.25 mL; **37.5 kg:** For a daily dose of 300 mg, give 7.5 mL.
4. Once reconstituted, keep suspension at room temperature or under refrigeration; discard after 14 days.
5. Prior to reconstitution, store powder from 20–25°C (68–77°F).

ASSESSMENT

1. List onset, S&S, clinical findings, source of infection, culture results.
2. Note any prior sensitivity to cephalosporins or penicillins.
3. Use suspension in children and when treating otitis media.
4. Monitor VS, CBC, PT, and renal function; reduce dose with dysfunction.

CLIENT/FAMILY TEACHING

1. Take as directed at same time each day; complete entire prescription. Food may ↓ GI upset; report persistent adverse side effects, especially diarrhea.
2. Shake well before use; store suspension at room temperature; discard after 14 days.
3. May alter results of urine glucose and ketone testing; do finger sticks for more accurate results.
4. Report any rash, hives, itching, or shortness of breath, severe abdominal pain, bloody diarrhea, or lack of improvement after 48–72 hr.
5. Keep all F/U to assess response, labs and adverse SE.

OUTCOMES/EVALUATE

Resolution of infection; symptomatic improvement

IV

Cefotaxime sodium

(sef-oh-**TAX**-eem)

Classification(s): Cephalosporin, third generation

Pregnancy Category: B

RX: Claforan.

SEE ALSO ***ANTI-INFECTIVES*** AND ***CEPHALOSPORINS***.

INDICATIONS/USES

1. Lower respiratory tract infections, including pneumonia, due to *Streptococcus pneumoniae, Streptococcus pyogenes* (group A strepto-

cocci) and other streptococci (excluding enterococci), *Staphylococcus aureus* (penicillinase and nonpenicillinase producing), *Eschericia coli, Klebsiella* species, *Haemophilus influenzae* (including ampicillin-resistant strains), *Haemophilus parainfluenzae, Proteus mirabilis, Serratia marcescens, Enterobacter* species, and indole-positive *Proteus* and *Pseudomonas* species (including *P. aeruginosa*).

2. GU infections due to *Enterococcus* species, *Staphylococcus epidermidis, S. aureus* (penicillinase and nonpenicillinase producing), *Citrobacter* species, *Enterobacter* species, *E. coli, Klebsiella* species, *P. mirabilis, Proteus vulgaris, Providencia stuartii, Morganella morganii, Providencia rettgeri, S. marcescens,* and *Pseudomonas* species (including *P. aeruginosa*).
3. Uncomplicated gonorrhea (cervical/urethral, rectal) due to *Neisseria gonorrhoeae,* including penicillinase-producing strains.
4. Gynecologic infections, including PID, endometritis, and pelvic cellulitis due to *S. epidermidis, Streptococcus* species, *Enterococcus* species, *Enterobacter* species, *Klebsiella* species, *E. coli, P. mirabilis, Bacteroides* species (including *Bacteroides fragilis), Clostridium* species, anaerobic cocci (including *Peptostreptococcus* species and *Peptococcus* species), and *Fusobacterium* species (including *F. nucleatum).* Cefotaxime has no activity against *Chlamydia trachomatis.*
5. Bacteremia/septicemia due to *E. coli, Klebsiella* species, and *S. marcescens, S. aureus,* and *Streptococcus* species (including *S. pneumoniae*).
6. Skin and skin structure infections due to *S. aureus* (penicillinase and nonpenicillinase producing), *S. epidermidis, S. pyogenes* (group A streptococci) and other streptococci, *Enterococcus* species, *Acinetobacter* species, *E. coli, Citrobacter* species (including *C. freundii), Enterobacter* species, *Klebsiella* species, *P. mirabilis, P. vulgaris, M. morganii, P. rettgeri, Pseudomonas* species, *S. marcescens, Bacteroides* species, anaerobic cocci (including *Peptostreptococcus* species, and *Peptococcus* species).
7. Intra-abdominal infections, including peritonitis due to *Streptococcus* species, *E. coli, Klebsiella* species, *Bacteroides* species, anaerobic cocci (including *Peptostreptococcus* species and *Peptococcus* species), *P. mirabilis,* and *Clostridium* species.
8. Bone and joint infections due to *S. aureus* (penicillinase-/non-penicillinase-producing strains), *Streptococcus* species (including *S. pyogenes*), *Pseudomonas* species (including *P. aeruginosa*), and *P. mirabilis.*
9. CNS infections (e.g., meningitis, ventriculitis) due to *Neisseria meningitis, H. influenzae, S. pneumoniae, K. pneumoniae,* and *E. coli.*
10. Reduce incidence of certain infections in clients undergoing cesarean section, both intraoperatively (after clamping the umbilical cord) and postoperatively. The IV route is preferable for clients with severe or life-threatening infections; for clients after surgery; or for those manifesting malnutrition, trauma, malignancy, heart failure, or diabetes, especially if shock is present or possible.
11. Preoperatively to reduce the incidence of certain infections in clients undergoing surgical procedures (e.g., abdominal or vaginal hysterectomy, GI and GU tract surgery) that may be classified as contaminated or potentially contaminated.
12. In certain cases of confirmed or suspected gram-positive or gram-negative sepsis or in those with other serious infections in which the causative organism has not been identified; may be used together with an aminoglycoside. It is possible that nephrotoxicity may be potentiated if cefotaxime is used together with an aminoglycoside.

ACTION/KINETICS

Pharmacokinetics

$t^{1/2}$: 1 hr. **Peak serum levels after 1 gram IV:** 42–102 mcg/mL. 60% excreted unchanged in the urine.

SIDE EFFECTS

Most Common

Injection site inflammation after IV, rash, pruritus, N&V, fever, diarrhea, colitis.

See *Cephalosporins* for a complete list of possible side effects. Also, possibility of erythema multiforme, ***Stevens-Johnson syndrome***, and ***toxic epidermal necrolysis***.

HOW SUPPLIED

Injection: 1 gram, 2 grams; ***Powder for Injection:*** 500 mg, 1 gram, 2 grams, 10 grams.

DOSAGE

IM; IV

Uncomplicated infections.

Adults: 1 gram q 12 hr IM or IV.

Moderate to severe infections.

Adults: 1–2 grams q 8 hr IM or IV.

Septicemia and other infections requiring higher doses.

Adults: 2 grams q 6–8 hr IV; daily dose ranges from 6–8 grams.

Life-threatening infections.

Adults: 2 grams q 4 hr IV, not to exceed 12 grams/day.

Gonorrhea.

Adult males, IM: Single dose of 1 gram for rectal gonorrhea. **Adult IM:** Single dose of 0.5 gram for rectal gonorrhea in females or gonococcoal urethritis/cervicitis in males and females. For disseminated gonogoccal infections give 1 gram IV q 8 hr.

Disseminated gonococcal infection and gonococcal scalp abscesses in newborns.

25 mg/kg IV or IM q 12 hr for 7 days, with a duration of 10 to 14 days if meningitis is documented.

Perioperative prophylaxis.

Adults: 1 gram IM or IV 30–90 min prior to surgery.

Cesarean section.

IV: 1 gram as soon as the umbilical cord is clamped; **then,** give 1 gram IM or IV 6 and 12 hr after the first dose.

Use in children.

Pediatric, 0–1 week: 50 mg/kg q 12 hr IV; **1–4 weeks:** 50 mg/kg q 8 hr IV; **1 month–12 years (<50 kg):** 50–180 mg/kg/day in 4 to 6 divided doses either IM or IV. Higher doses may be used for more severe or serious infections, including meningitis. *NOTE:* Use adult dose in children 50 kg or over.

Use in impaired renal function.

If C_{CR} <20 mL/min/1.73 m^2, reduce dose by 50%. If only serum creatinine is available, use the following formulas to calculate C_{CR}:

- Males: Weight (kg) × (140 – age) / 72 × serum creatinine (mg/dL).
- Females: 0.85 × male value.

NURSING IMPLICATIONS

Do not confuse cefotaxime (Claforan) with cefoxitin (Mefoxin), also a cephalosporin.

IMPLEMENTATION/ADMINISTRATION/STORAGE

1. Do not exceed a maximum daily dose of 12 grams.
2. The premixed injection is intended for IV administration after thawing. Reconstituted powder for injection may be given IM or IV.
3. Continue for a minimum of 48–72 hr after the client defervesces or after evidence of bacterial eradication has been determined. Continue therapy for a minimum of 10 days for group A beta-hemolytic streptococcal infections to minimize risk of rheumatic fever/glomerulonephritis.
4. For IM: Reconstitute with sterile/bacteriostatic water for injection. Inject deeply into large muscle. Divide doses of 2 grams and administer into different sites.
5. **IV** Use IV route for those with bacteremia, bacterial septicemia, peritonitis, meningitis, or other severe/life-threatening infections. Also use IV for those who may be poor risks due to lowered resistance as a result of debilitating conditions, such as malnutrition, trauma, surgery, diabetes, heart failure, or malignancy, especially if shock present/impending. Stop other IV solutions during therapy.
6. Cefotaxime sterile powder for injection may be reconstituted in 50 or 100 mL D5W or 0.9% NaCl in the ADD-Vantage diluent container.
7. Add recommended amount of diluent, shake to dissolve. Do not administer if particles are present or solution discolored. The normal solution color ranges from light yellow to amber.
8. For intermittent IV administration, mix 1 or 2 grams cefotaxime with 10 mL sterile water for injection; administer over 3–5 min; do not give over period of less than 3 minutes. For

administration by infusion, dilute in 50–100 mL of solution; infuse over 30 min.

9. After reconstitution, drug remains stable for 24 hr at room temperature, 5 days refrigerated, and 13 weeks frozen. Thaw frozen samples at room temperature before use. Do not refreeze; discard unused portions.
10. Store dry cefotaxime below 30°C (86°F); protect from excess heat/light to prevent darkening.
11. COMPATIBILITY 0.9% NaCl, D5W; for continous IV infusion may add to: D5 or 10%/W, D5/NSS, D5/0.45% NaCl, D5/0.2% NaCl, LR solution, Sodium Lactate Injection (M/6); 10% Invert Sugar Injection, 8.5% Travasol (Amino Acid) Injection without Electrolytes. May administer through the DUPLEX Drug Delivery System which comes self contained.
12. INCOMPATIBILITY Aminoglycosides (give separately); maximally stable at pH of 5–7; do not prepare with diluents having pH >7.5 (e.g., $NaHCO_3$ injection).

ASSESSMENT

1. Note reasons for therapy, onset, characteristics of S&S; assess for PCN/ATX sensitivity.
2. With joint infections, assess ROM/freedom of movement.
3. With gynecologic infections, determine extent of infection, duration, S&S.
4. Monitor labs/review culture results for organism resistance; reduce dose with renal dysfunction.

CLIENT/FAMILY TEACHING

1. Drug given parenterally. Report adverse side effects/lack of response.
2. Review appropriate technique/frequency for administration, proper storage. Inspect site for pain/redness; IM may cause thrombophlebitis.
3. Record I&O; report decrease in urinary output/persistent diarrhea.
4. Keep all F/U to assess response, labs, adverse SE.

OUTCOMES/EVALUATE

- Resolution of infection; symptomatic improvement
- Negative culture reports

IV

Cefoxitin sodium

(seh-**FOX**-ih-tin)

Classification(s): Cephalosporin, second generation

Pregnancy Category: B

SEE ALSO ***ANTI-INFECTIVES*** AND ***CEPHALOSPORINS***.

INDICATIONS/USES

1. Lower respiratory tract infections (pneumonia and lung abscess) due to *Streptococcus pneumoniae,* other streptococci (excluding enterococci such as *Streptococcus faecalis*), *Staphylococcus aureus* (including penicillinase-producing strains), *Escherichia coli, Klebsiella* species, *Haemophilus influenzae,* and *Bacteroides* species.
2. UTIs due to *E. coli, Klebsiella* species, *Proteus mirabilis, Morganella morganii, Proteus vulgaris,* and *Providencia* species (including *P. rettgeri).*
3. Intra-abdominal infections (peritonitis and intra-abdominal abscess) due to *E. coli, Klebsiella* species, *Bacteroides* species (including *B. fragilis),* and *Clostridium* species.
4. Gynecological infections (endometritis, pelvic cellulitis, PID) due to *E. coli, N. gonorrhoeae* (including penicillinase-producing strains), *Bacteroides* species (including *B. fragilis* group), *Clostridium* species, *P. niger, Peptostreptococcus* species, and *Streptococcus agalactiae.* Cefoxitin has no activity against *Chlamydia trachomatis.*
5. Septicemia due to *S. pneumoniae, S. aureus* (including penicillinase-producing strains), *E. coli, Klebsiella* species, and *Bacteroides* species (including *B. fragilis*).
6. Bone/joint infections due to *S. aureus* (including penicillinase-producing strains).
7. Skin/skin structure infections due to *S. aureus* (including penicillinase-producing strains), *Staphylococcus epidermidis* (excluding enterococci, especially *S. faecalis), E. coli, P. mirabilis, Klebsiella* species, *Bacteroides* species (including the *B. fragilis* group), *Clostridium* species, *P. niger* species, and *Peptostreptococcus* species.

8. Perioperative prophylaxis, including vaginal hysterectomy, GI surgery, TURP, prosthetic arthroplasty, and C-section.
9. Infections due to *Chlamydia trachomatis.* *NOTE:* Many gram-negative infections resistant to certain cephalosporins and penicillins respond to cefoxitin.

ACTION/KINETICS

Action

Broad-spectrum cephalosporin that is penicillinase- and cephalosporinase-resistant and is stable in the presence of beta-lactamases.

Pharmacokinetics

Peak serum level after 1 gram IV: 110 mcg/mL. **t½:** 40–60 min; 85% of drug excreted unchanged in urine after 6 hr.

SIDE EFFECTS

Most Common

N&V, diarrhea, thrombophlebitis.

See *Cephalosporins* for a complete list of possible side effects. Higher doses have caused increased incidence of eosinophilia and increased AST levels in children over 3 months of age.

ADDITIONAL LABORATORY TEST CONSIDERATIONS

High concentrations may interfere with the measurement of creatinine by the Jaffe method.

HOW SUPPLIED

Powder for Injection: 1 gram, 2 grams, 10 grams.

DOSAGE

IM; IV

Uncomplicated infections (cutaneous, pneumonia, urinary tract).

Adults, IV: 1 gram q 6–8 hr. **Daily dosage:** 3 to 4 grams.

Moderately severe or severe infections.

Adults, IV: 1 gram q 4 hr or 2 grams q 6–8 hr. **Daily dosage:** 6 to 8 grams.

Infections requiring higher dosage (e.g., gas gangrene).

Adults, IV: 2 grams q 4 hr or 3 grams q 6 hr. **Daily dosage:** 12 grams.

Gonorrhea.

Adults, IV: 2 grams IM with 1 gram probenecid PO.

Prophylaxis in surgery.

Adults, IV: 2 grams 30–60 min before surgery followed by 2 grams q 6 hr after first dose for 24 hr only (72 hr for prosthetic arthroplasty).

Cesarean section, prophylaxis.

IV: 2 grams as soon as the umbilical cord is clamped or a 3-dose regimen consisting of 2 grams given IV as soon as the umbilical cord is clamped followed by 2 grams 4 and 8 hr after the initial dose.

Transurethral resection of the prostate (TURP), prophylaxis.

1 gram before surgery; **then,** 1 gram q 8 hr for up to 5 days.

Impaired renal function.

Adults, initial: 1–2 grams. Then, use the following as a guide: **Mild impairment (30–50 mL/min C_{CR}):** 1–2 grams q 8–12 hr. **Moderate impairment (10–29 mL/min C_{CR}):** 1–2 grams q 12–24 hr. **Severe impairment (5–9 mL/min C_{CR}):** 0.5–1 gram q 12–24 hr. **Essentially no function (<5 mL/min C_{CR}):** 0.5–1 gram q 24–48 hr.

Use in children for infections.

Children over 3 months: 80–160 mg/kg/day divided into 4 to 6 equal doses. Use the higher doses for more severe or serious infections, not to exceed 12 grams/day.

Use in children for prophylaxis.

Children over 3 months: 30–40 mg/kg q 6 hr or at the times designated for adults.

NURSING IMPLICATIONS

Do not confuse cefoxitin with cefotaxime (Claforan), also a cephalosporin.

IMPLEMENTATION/ADMINISTRATION/STORAGE

1. Maintain therapy at least 10 days for group A beta-hemolytic streptococcal infections in order to minimize the risk of rheumatic fever or glomerulonephritis.
2. For IM injections, reconstitute each gram with 2 mL sterile water or 2 mL 0.5% lidocaine HCl

(without epinephrine) to reduce pain at injection site.

3. When used for prophylactic use in surgery, give 30 to 60 minutes before the surgery. Stop prophylactic administration within 24 hr since continuing use increases the risk of side effects but, in the majority of cases, does not reduce the incidence of subsequent infection.
4. **IV** The IV route is preferable for those with bacteremia, bacterial septicemia, other severe or life-threatening infections or for those who may be poor risks because of lowered resistance resulting from debilitating conditions, including malnutrition, trauma, surgery, diabetes, heart failure, or malignancy, especially if shock is present or impending.
5. For IV: Reconstitute 1 gram with 10 or more mL of sterile water and 2 grams with 10–20 mL. The 10 gram vial may be reconstituted with 43 or 93 mL sterile water or other compatible solutions (see below and package insert).
6. For intermittent IV: give 1 or 2 grams in 10 mL sterile water over 3 to 5 min. For continuous IV administration (e.g., for higher doses), add solution to 50–100 mL of compatible solution and give over 15–30 min.
7. For higher doses, cefoxitin solutions may be added to an IV bottle containing D5W injection, 0.9% NaCl injection, or 5% dextrose/0.9% NaCl injection. Butterfly or scalp vein-type needles are preferred for this type of infusion.
8. Store premixed products (for IV use only) at less than −20°C (−4°F). Will maintain potency after thawing for 24 hr at room temperature; 21 days if refrigerated. Discard any unused thawed solutions; do not refreeze.
9. Store dry powder below 30°C (86°F). The dry powder solutions darken depending on storage conditions; potency is unaffected.
10. COMPATIBILITY D5W or D10W, NSS, D5W/0.9% NaCl, or D5W/0.02% or 0.45% NaCl, lactated Ringers, D5/LR, 5% $NaHCO_3$, M/6 sodium lactate, Mannitol 5% and 10%.
11. INCOMPATIBILITY Do not mix or add to aminoglycoside solutions (e.g., gentamicin sulfate, tobramycin sulfate, amikacin sulfate) because of potential interaction. May administer separately. Do not use solutions containing benzyl alcohol in infants.

ASSESSMENT

1. Note reasons for therapy, characteristics of S&S, clinical presentation, culture results. Assess for PCN/ATX sensitivity.
2. Assess infusion site for pain/redness; may cause thrombophlebitis.
3. Monitor I&O, CBC, for coagulation abnormality, liver and renal function, and culture results; reduce dose with renal dysfunction.

CLIENT/FAMILY TEACHING

1. Drug is administered parenterally. Report any adverse effects, significant diarrhea, reduction in urinary output, rash, abnormal bruising/bleeding, persistent fever, breathing difficulty, wheezing, or lack of response.
2. Review appropriate technique/frequency for administration, proper storage. Inspect site for pain/redness.
3. Keep all F/U to assess response, labs, and adverse SE.

OUTCOMES/EVALUATE

- Resolution of infection
- Surgical infection prophylaxis

Cefpodoxime proxetil

(sef-poh-**DOX**-eem)

Classification(s): Cephalosporin, third generation

Pregnancy Category: B

RX: Vantin.

SEE ALSO ***ANTI-INFECTIVES*** AND ***CEPHALOSPORINS***.

INDICATIONS/USES

1. Acute, community-acquired pneumonia due to *Streptococcus pneumoniae* or *Hemophilus influenzae* (including non-beta-lactamase-producing strains).
2. Acute bacterial exacerbation of chronic bronchitis caused by *S. pneumoniae,* non-beta-lactamase-producing *H. influenzae,* or *Moraxella catarrhalis.*
3. Acute otitis media caused by *S. pneumoniae* (excluding penicillin-resistant strains), *Streptococcus pyogenes, H. influenzae* (including beta-lactamase-producing strains), and *M. catarrhalis* (including beta-lactamase-producing strains).

4. Pharyngitis or tonsillitis due to *S. pyogenes.*
5. Acute, uncomplicated urethral and cervical gonorrhea caused by *Neisseria gonorrhoeae* (including penicillinase-producing strains).
6. Acute, uncomplicated anorectal infections in women due to *N. gonorrhoeae* (including penicillinase-producing strains).
7. Uncomplicated skin and skin structure infections due to *Staphylococcus aureus* (including penicillinase-producing strains) or *S. pyogenes.* Abscesses should be surgically drained.
8. Uncomplicated UTIs (cystitis) due to *Escherichia coli, Klebsiella pneumoniae, Proteus mirabilis,* or *Staphylococcus saprophyticus.*
9. Mild-to-moderate acute maxillary sinusitis due to *H. influenzae* (including beta-lactamase-producing strains), *S. pneumoniae,* and *M. catarrhalis.*

ACTION/KINETICS

Pharmacokinetics

t½, after PO: 2–3 hr. From 29 to 33% is excreted unchanged in the urine.

SIDE EFFECTS

Most Common

N&V, diarrhea, anorexia, headache, yeast infection of the mouth or vagina.

See *Cephalosporins* for a complete list of possible side effects.

DRUG INTERACTIONS

Antacids / ↓ Cefpodoxime plasma levels; take cefpodoxime 2 hr before or after the antacid
H_2 antagonists / ↓ Cefpodoxime plasma levels

HOW SUPPLIED

Tablets, Film-Coated: 100 mg, 200 mg; ***Oral Suspension:*** 125 mg/5 mL (after reconstitution).

DOSAGE

TABLETS, FILM-COATED

Acute community-acquired pneumonia.

Adults and children 12 years and over: 200 mg q 12 hr for 14 days.

Acute bacterial exacerbations of chronic bronchitis.

Adults and children 12 years and over: 200 mg q 12 hr for 10 days. Use the tablets.

Uncomplicated gonorrhea (men and women) and rectal gonococcal infections (women).

Adults and children 12 years and over: Single dose of 200 mg.

Skin and skin structure infections.

Adults and children 12 years and over: 400 mg q 12 hr for 7–14 days.

Pharyngitis, tonsillitis.

Adults and children 12 years and over: 100 mg q 12 hr for 5–10 days.
Children, 2 months through 12 years: 5 mg/kg (maximum of 100 mg/dose) q 12 hr (maximum daily dose: 200 mg) for 5–10 days.

Uncomplicated urinary tract infections (UTIs).

Adults and children 12 years and over: 100 mg q 12 hr for 7 days.

Acute otitis media.

Children, 2 months through 12 years: 5 mg/kg (maximum of 200 mg/dose) q 12 hr for 5 days.

Acute maxillary sinusitis.

Adults and children 12 years and older: 200 mg q 12 hr for 10 days. **Children, 2 months through 12 years:** 5 mg/kg (maximum of 200 mg/dose) q 12 hr for 10 days.

NURSING IMPLICATIONS

IMPLEMENTATION/ADMINISTRATION/STORAGE

1. In severe renal impairment (C_{CR} <30 mL/min), increase dosing interval to q 24 hr. If on hemodialysis, use dosage frequency of 3 times/week after hemodialysis. Adjustment not required with cirrhosis.
2. May use the following formula to estimate C_{CR} (mL/min): **males:** weight (kg) × (140 − age)/72 × serum creatinine (mg/dL); **females:** 0.85 × male value.
3. Store tablets from 20–25°C (68–77°F).

ASSESSMENT

1. List onset, source/characteristics of infection; obtain baseline cultures.
2. Note any reactions to cephalosporins/penicillins; cross-sensitivity can occur.
3. Monitor VS and I&O; evaluate persistent diarrhea for other causes, such as *Clostridium difficile.*
4. Discontinue therapy/report if seizures occur.

5. Note renal dysfunction; alter dosage/frequency if evident. Obtain serologic test for syphilis with gonorrhea treatment.

CLIENT/FAMILY TEACHING

1. Take tablets with food to enhance absorption. Complete entire prescription.
2. Report lack of response, adverse effects, rash, persistent N&V, diarrhea; drug or dosage may require adjustment. Consume adequate fluids to prevent dehydration.
3. If receiving treatment for gonorrhea, have partner tested and treated; use barrier contraception to prevent reinfections. Drug is not effective against syphilis; all partners should be tested so that appropriate treatment may be provided.
4. Keep all F/U to assess response, labs, and for adverse SE.

OUTCOMES/EVALUATE

- Resolution of infection
- Symptomatic improvement

Cefprozil

(**SEF**-proh-zill)

Classification(s): Cephalosporin, second generation

Pregnancy Category: B

SEE ALSO ***ANTI-INFECTIVE DRUGS*** AND ***CEPHALOSPORINS***.

INDICATIONS/USES

1. Pharyngitis and tonsillitis due to *Streptococcus pyogenes*.
2. Acute bacterial sinusitis due to *Streptococcus pneumoniae, Staphylococcus aureus, Haemophilus influenzae* (including beta-lactamase-producing strains), and *Moraxella catarrhalis* (including beta-lactamase-producing strains).
3. Otitis media caused by *S. pneumoniae, H. influenzae* (including beta-lactamase-producing strains), and *M. catarrhalis* (including beta-lactamase-producing strains). *NOTE:* Eradication rates are somewhat lower in treating otitis media due to beta-lactamase-producing strains.
4. Uncomplicated skin and skin structure infections due to *S. aureus* (including penicillinase-producing strains) and *S. pyogenes*. Abscesses usually require surgical drainage.
5. Secondary bacterial infection of acute bronchitis and acute bacterial exacerbation of chronic bronchitis due to *S. pneumoniae, H. influenzae* (including beta-lactamase positive and negative strains), and *M. catarrhalis* (including beta-lactamase-producing strains).

ACTION/KINETICS

Pharmacokinetics

t½, after PO: 78 min. Sixty percent is recovered in the urine unchanged.

SIDE EFFECTS

Most Common

N&V, diarrhea, abdominal pain, yeast infection of mouth or vagina.

See *Cephalosporins* for a complete list of possible side effects.

ADDITIONAL DRUG INTERACTIONS

↓ Effectiveness of oral contraceptives.

HOW SUPPLIED

Powder for Oral Suspension: 125 mg/5 mL after reconstitution, 250 mg/5 mL after reconstitution; ***Tablets:*** 250 mg, 500 mg.

DOSAGE

ORAL SUSPENSION; TABLETS

Pharyngitis, tonsillitis.

Adults and children over 13 years: 500 mg q 24 hr for at least 10 days (for *S. pyogenes* infections, give 10 or more days). **Children, 2–12 years:** 7.5 mg/kg q 12 hr for at least 10 days (for *S. pyogenes* infections, give 10 or more days).

Acute sinusitis.

Adults and children over 13 years: 250 mg q 12 hr or 500 mg q 12 hr for 10 days. Use the higher dose for moderate to severe infections. **Children, 6 months–12 years:** 7.5 mg/kg q 12 hr or 15 mg/kg q 12 hr for 10 days. Use the higher dose for moderate to severe infections.

Secondary bacterial infections of acute bronchitis and acute bacterial exacerbation of chronic bronchitis.

Adults and children over 13 years: 500 mg q 12 hr for 10 days.

Uncomplicated skin and skin structure infections.

Adults and children over 13 years: Either 250 mg q 12 hr, 500 mg q 24 hr, or 500 mg q 12 hr (all for a duration of 10 days). **Children, 2–12 years:** 20 mg/kg q 24 hr for 10 days.

Otitis media.

Infants and children 6 months–12 years: 15 mg/kg q 12 hr for 10 days.

NURSING IMPLICATIONS

IMPLEMENTATION/ADMINISTRATION/STORAGE

1. With impaired renal function (C_{CR} of 0–30 mL/min), give 50% of usual dose at standard intervals.
2. To enhance adherence, a suspension is available in a bubble-gum flavor for children.
3. Store powder for oral suspension (before reconstitution) and tablets from 15–30°C (59–77°F). After reconstitution, refrigerate suspension; discard any unused portion after 14 days.

ASSESSMENT

1. Note reasons for therapy, characteristics of S&S, clinical presentation and culture results. List any PCN/antibiotic sensitivity and assess for any reactions.
2. Reduce dose with impaired renal function; monitor I&O and VS.

CLIENT/FAMILY TEACHING

1. Take as directed with/without food; food decreases stomach upset. Complete entire prescription, do not stop if feeling better. Refrigerate suspension and shake well before using; discard after 14 days.
2. Report rash, hives, diarrhea, nausea, vomiting, breathing difficulty/wheezing, or muscle or joint pain. If temperature does not decrease and symptoms do not improve advise provider.
3. Avoid alcohol while taking medication.
4. Keep all F/U to assess response, labs, and for adverse SE.

OUTCOMES/EVALUATE

- Symptomatic improvement
- Resolution of infection

IV

Ceftaroline fosamil monoacetate

(sef-**TAR**-oh-leen)

Classification(s): Cephalosporin

Pregnancy Category: B

RX: Teflaro.

SEE ALSO ***CEPHALOSPORINS.***

INDICATIONS/USES

(1) Acute bacterial skin and skin structure infections due to *Staphylococcus aureus* (including methicillin-susceptible and methicillin-resistant isolates), *Streptococcus pyogenes, Streptococcus agalactiae, Escherichia coli, Klebsiella pneumoniae,* and *Klebsiella oxytoca.* (2) Community-acquired pneumonia due to *Streptococcus pneumoniae* (including cases with concurrent bacteremia), *S. aureus* (methicillin-susceptible), *Haemophilus influenzae, Klebsiella pneumoniae, Klebsiella oxytoca,* and *E. coli.*

ACTION/KINETICS

Action

The bactericidal action is due to binding to essential penicillin-binding proteins (e.g., affinity for PBP2 for *S. aureus* and PBP2x for *S. pneumoniae).* Cross resistance may occur, although isolates resistant to other cephalosporins may be susceptible to ceftaroline.

Pharmacokinetics

t½: 2.7 hr after multiple 600 mg doses given q 12 hr. Ceftaroline fosamil is converted to bioactive ceftaroline in the plasma. The drug is not a substrate for CYP450 enzymes. Ceftaroline and metabolites are excreted primarily by the kidneys (88%) with smaller amounts excreted in the feces (6%). **Plasma protein binding:** 20%.

CONTRAINDICATIONS

Known serious hypersensitivity to ceftaroline or other cephalosporins.

SPECIAL CONCERNS

- Use with caution in clients with known hypersensitivity to beta-lactam antibiotics.
- Dosage adjustment (see *Implementation/Administration/Storage*) is required with moderate or

severe renal impairment and in end-stage renal disease clients, including those on dialysis.
- Use care in dose selection in the elderly due to possible changes in renal function.
- Use with caution during lactation.
- Safety and efficacy not established in children.

C

SIDE EFFECTS

Most Common

Diarrhea, nausea, rash.

GI: Diarrhea (including *Clostridium difficile*-associated diarrhea/colitis), N&V, constipation, abdominal pain, hepatitis. **CNS:** Dizziness, ***seizures***. **CV:** Phlebitis, bradycardia, palpitations. **Dermatologic:** Rash, urticaria. **GU:** Renal failure. **Hematologic:** Anemia, drug-induced hemolytic anemia, eosinophilia, neutropenia, thrombocytopenia. **Hypersensitivity:** Skin reactions, ***anaphylaxis, anaphylactoid reactions***. **Body as a whole:** Pyrexia.

LABORATORY TEST CONSIDERATIONS

Seroconversion from a negative to a positive Coombs' test. ↑ ALT, AST. Hypokalemia, hyperkalemia, hyperglycemia.

OVERDOSE MANAGEMENT

Treatment: Hemodialysis will remove ceftaroline fosamil.

HOW SUPPLIED

Injection, Powder for Solution: 400 mg, 600 mg.

DOSAGE

IV

Acute bacterial skin and skin structure infection.

Adults: 600 mg q 12 hr for 5–14 days.

Community-acquired bacterial pneumonia.

Adults: 600 mg q 12 hr for 5–7 days.

NURSING IMPLICATIONS

IMPLEMENTATION/ADMINISTRATION/STORAGE

1. IV Doses in the elderly should be based on renal function.
2. The following are dosage recommendations for impaired renal function:
   - C_{CR} >50 mL/min: No dosage adjustment necessary.
   - C_{CR} >30 to <50 mL/min: 400 mg IV q 12 hr.
   - C_{CR} > or equal to 15 to <30 mL/min: 300 mg IV q 12 hr.
   - End-stage renal disease (including hemodialysis): 200 mg IV q 12 hr. Give after hemodialysis on hemodialysis days.
3. To prepare for administration, reconstitute the contents of the ceftaroline fosamil vial with 20 mL sterile water for injection. The approximate ceftaroline fosamil concentration will be 20 mg/mL for the 400 mg strength and 30 mg/mL for the 600 mg strength. Reconstitution time is less than 2 min. Mix gently to reconstitute; ensure complete dissolution.
4. The color of the reconstituted solution ranges from clear to light to dark yellow, depending on the concentration and storage conditions.
5. The reconstituted solution must be further diluted in at least 250 mL before infusion. Appropriate infusion solutions include D5W injection, NaCl 0.9% injection, dextrose 2.5% and sodium chloride 0.45% injection, or lactated Ringer's injection.
6. Administer IV over 1 hr.
7. Store vials from 2–8°C (36–46°F). Use the reconstituted solution in the infusion bag within 6 hr when stored at room temperature, or within 24 hr when stored under refrigeration.
8. COMPATIBILITY D5W, 0.9% NaCl, D2.5%/0.45% NaCl, RL injection.
9. INCOMPATIBILITY Not established. Do not mix with or physically add to solutions containing other drugs.

ASSESSMENT

1. Note reasons for therapy, characteristics of S&S, clinical presentation, and culture results. List any PCN/ATX sensitivity and monitor during therapy.
2. Assess infusion site for pain/redness, and monitor for adverse SE.
3. Obtain VS and baseline culture results, monitor renal function studies; reduce dose/frequency with impaired renal function.

CLIENT/FAMILY TEACHING

1. Drug is administered parenterally. Review appropriate technique/frequency for administration, and proper storage. Inspect site for pain/redness.
2. Must have regular dosing to maintain therapeutic blood levels.

3. Report any adverse effects, significant diarrhea, reduction in urinary output, rash, abnormal bruising/bleeding, breathing difficulty, or lack of response.
4. Prolonged/persistent diarrhea as overgrowth of colon flora may have occurred; may occur several weeks/months after therapy, and require treatment.
5. Use caution during lactation.
6. Keep all F/U to assess response, labs, and adverse SE.

OUTCOMES/EVALUATE

- Resolution of S&S of infection
- Negative culture reports

IV

Ceftazidime

(sef-**TAY**-zih-deem)

Classification(s): Cephalosporin, third generation

Pregnancy Category: B

RX: Fortaz, Tazicef, Tazidime.

SEE ALSO ***ANTI-INFECTIVE DRUGS*** AND ***CEPHALOSPORINS***.

INDICATIONS/USES

1. Lower respiratory tract infections (including pneumonia) due to *Pseudomonas aeruginosa* and other *Pseudomonas* species, *Haemophilus influenzae* (including ampicillin-resistant strains), *Klebsiella* species, *Enterobacter* species, *Proteus mirabilis, Escherichia coli, Serratia* species, *Citrobacter* species, *Streptococcus pneumoniae, Staphylococcus aureus* (methicillin-susceptible strains).
2. Skin and skin structure infections due to *P. aeruginosa, Klebsiella* species, *E. coli, Proteus* species (including *P. mirabilis* and indole-positive *Proteus*), *Enterobacter* species, *Serratia* species, *S. aureus* (methicillin-susceptible strains), *S. pyogenes* (group A beta-hemolytic streptococci).
3. UTIs, both complicated and uncomplicated, due to *P. aeruginosa, Enterobacter* species, *Proteus* species (including *P. mirabilis* and indole-positive *Proteus*), *Klebsiella* species, and *E. coli*.
4. Bacterial septicemia due to *P. aeruginosa, Klebsiella* species, *H. influenzae, E. coli, Serratia* species, *S. pneumoniae, S. aureus* (methicillin-susceptible strains).
5. Bone and joint infections due to *P. aeruginosa, Klebsiella* species, *Enterobacter* species, *S. aureus* (methicillin-susceptible strains).
6. Gynecologic infections, including endometritis, pelvic cellulitis, and other infections of the female genital tract, due to *E. coli*.
7. Intra-abdominal infections, including peritonitis, due to *E. coli, Klebsiella* species, *S. aureus* (methicillin-susceptible strains); polymicrobial infections due to aerobic and anaerobic organisms and *Bacteroides* species (many strains of *B. fragilis* are resistant).
8. CNS infections, including meningitis, due to *H. influenzae* and *Neisseria meningitidis* (limited effect against *P. aeruginosa* and *S. pneumoniae*).

NOTE: May be used with aminoglycosides, vancomycin, and clindamycin in severe, life-threatening infections and in the immunocompromised client. Dosage depends on the severity of the infection and the client's condition.

ACTION/KINETICS

Pharmacokinetics

Only for IM or IV use. **t½:** 114–120 min. From 80 to 90% is excreted unchanged in the urine.

SPECIAL CONCERNS

- **Possible resistance when used to treat *Pseudomonas aeruginosa* infections.**
- **Use a sodium carbonate formulation if indicated for children less than 12 years.**

SIDE EFFECTS

Most Common

N&V, diarrhea, yeast infection of the mouth or vagina, abdominal pain, stomach cramps, colitis, thrombophlebitis.

See *Cephalosporins* for a complete list of possible side effects. Also, hyperbilirubinemia, jaundice, renal impairment, urticaria, pain at injection site, ***anaphylaxis, severe allergic reactions (e.g., cardiopulmonary arrest)***. Myoclonia and coma in clients with renal insufficiency.

HOW SUPPLIED

Injection: 1 gram, 2 grams; ***Powder for Injection:*** 500 mg, 1 gram, 2 grams, 6 grams.

C

DOSAGE

IM; IV

Usual recommended dosage.

Adults, IM, IV: 1 gram q 8–12 hr.

Urinary tract infections (UTIs), uncomplicated.

Adults, IM, IV: 0.25 gram q 12 hr.

UTIs, complicated.

Adults, IM, IV: 0.5 gram q 8–12 hr.

Uncomplicated pneumonia, mild skin and skin structure infections.

Adults, IM, IV: 0.5–1 gram q 8 hr.

Bone and joint infections.

Adults, IV: 2 grams q 12 hr.

Serious gynecologic or intra-abdominal infections, meningitis, severe or life-threatening infections (especially in immunocompromised clients).

Adults, IV: 2 grams q 8 hr.

Pseudomonal lung infections in cystic fibrosis clients with normal renal function.

IV: 30–50 mg/kg q 8 hr, not to exceed 6 grams/day.

Use in neonates, infants, and children.

Neonates, 0–4 weeks, IV: 30 mg/kg q 12 hr, not to exceed the adult dose. **Infants and children, 1 month–12 years, IV:** 30–50 mg/kg q 8 hr not to exceed 6 grams/day.

NURSING IMPLICATIONS

IMPLEMENTATION/ADMINISTRATION/STORAGE

1. Reduce dose in clients with a GFR <50 mL/min. An initial loading dose of 1 gram may be given. The following doses are recommended: C_{CR} 31–50 mL/min: 1 gram q 12 hr; C_{CR} 16–30 mL/min: 1 gram q 24 hr; C_{CR} 6–15 mL/min: 0.5 gram q 24 hr; C_{CR} <5 mL/min: 0.5 gram q 48 hr.
2. For dialysis clients, give a loading dose of 1 gram, followed by 1 gram after each hemodialysis period. In clients undergoing intraperitoneal dialysis and continuous ambulatory peritoneal dialysis, give loading dose of 1 gram, followed by 0.5 gram q 24 hr. In addition to IV use, ceftazidime can be incorporated in the dialysis fluid at a concentration of 250 mg for 2 L of dialysis fluid.
3. For IM: Reconstitute in sterile water or bacteriostatic water for injection, or 0.5% or 1% lidocaine HCl injection.
4. If IM, use large muscle mass and inject deeply.
5. IV The IV route is preferred with bacterial septicemia, peritonitis, bacterial meningitis, or other severe/life-threatening infections. Use IV route if poor risks R/T malnutrition, surgery, diabetes, trauma, heart failure, malignancy, or shock present/imminent.
6. For direct IV: Reconstitute 1 gram in 10 mL sterile water for injection; give over 3–5 min.
7. For intermittent administration, further dilute in 50–100 mL of compatible solution and administer over 30–60 min. For IV infusion: The 1- or 2-gram infusion pack is reconstituted with 100 mL sterile water for injection (or a compatible IV solution).
8. A sodium carbonate formulation should be used for children <12 years old.
9. COMPATIBILITY 0.9% NaCl, RL, D5 or D10W, D5W/0.225%, 0.45%, or 0.9% NaCl.
10. INCOMPATIBILITY Do not add ceftazidime to solutions containing aminoglycosides. Less stable with $NaHCO_3$ so should not be used for reconstitution. Give separately.

ASSESSMENT

1. Note reasons for therapy, characteristics of S&S, clinical presentation, and culture results. List any PCN/ATX sensitivity and monitor therapy.
2. Obtain CBC, renal function studies; reduce dose with dysfunction.

CLIENT/FAMILY TEACHING

1. Drug is administered parenterally. Report lack of response, itching, rash, SOB, or diarrhea.
2. Consume adequate fluids to prevent dehydration.
3. Do not drink alcoholic beverages or take alcohol-containing products while taking this medication and for several days after completing therapy.
4. Keep all F/U to assess response, labs, and adverse SE.

OUTCOMES/EVALUATE

- Resolution of infection
- Negative culture reports

Ceftibuten

(sef-ti-**BYOO**-tin)

Classification(s): Cephalosporin, third generation

Pregnancy Category: B

RX: Cedax.

SEE ALSO ***ANTI-INFECTIVES*** AND ***CEPHALOSPORINS***.

INDICATIONS/USES

(1) Acute bacterial exacerbations of chronic bronchitis due to *Haemophilus influenzae* (including beta-lactamase-producing strains), *Moraxella catarrhalis* (including beta-lactamase-producing strains), and penicillin-susceptible strains of *Streptococcus pneumoniae.* (2) Acute bacterial otitis media due to *H. influenzae* (including beta-lactamase-producing strains), *M. catarrhalis* (including beta-lactamase-producing strains), or *Staphylococcus pyogenes.* (3) Pharyngitis and tonsillitis due to *S. pyogenes.*

ACTION/KINETICS

Pharmacokinetics

Resistant to beta-lactamase. Is well absorbed from the GI tract. Food delays the time to peak serum concentration, lowers the peak concentration, and decreases the total amount of drug absorbed. **Peak serum levels:** 2 to 3 hours. **t½:** 144 min. 56% excreted in the urine unchanged.

SPECIAL CONCERNS

Although ceftibuten has been approved for pharyngitis or tonsillitis, only penicillin has been shown to be effective in preventing rheumatic fever.

SIDE EFFECTS

Most Common

Diarrhea, N&V, abdominal pain, dizziness, headache.

See *Cephalosporins* for a complete list of possible side effects. Usually well tolerated.

HOW SUPPLIED

Capsules: 400 mg; ***Powder for Oral Suspension:*** 90 mg/5mL (after reconstitution), 180 mg/5 mL (after reconstitution).

DOSAGE

CAPSULES; ORAL SUSPENSION

All uses.

Adults and children over 12 years: 400 mg once daily for 10 days. The maximum daily dose is 400 mg. Adjust the dose in clients with a creatinine clearance (C_{CR}) <50 mL/min as follows. If the C_{CR} is between 30 and 49 mL/min, the recommended dose is 4.5 mg/kg or 200 mg once daily. If the C_{CR} is between 5 and 29 mL/min, the recommended dose is 2.25 mg/kg or 100 mg once daily. In clients undergoing hemodialysis 2 or 3 times per week, a single 400 mg dose of ceftibuten capsules or a single dose of 9 mg/kg (maximum of 400 mg) of PO suspension can be given at the end of each hemodialysis session.

Pharyngitis, tonsillitis, acute bacterial otitis media.

Children: 9 mg/kg, up to a maximum of 400 mg daily, for a total of 10 days. Give children over 45 kg the maximum daily dose of 400 mg.

NURSING IMPLICATIONS

Do not confuse Cedax with Ceptaz or Cefzil (also cephalosporins).

IMPLEMENTATION/ADMINISTRATION/STORAGE

1. **Follow directions for mixing ceftibuten suspension carefully, depending on the final concentration and the bottle size. First, tap bottle to loosen powder; then add the appropriate amount of water in two portions. Shake well after each portion.**
2. **Suspension may be kept for 14 days under refrigeration. Keep container tightly closed, shake well before each use. Discard any unused drug after 14 days.**
3. **The dosage of the oral suspension in children is as follows:**
   - **10 kg (22 lb): 5 mL daily of the 90 mg/ 5 mL formulation.**
   - **20 kg (44 lb): 10 mL daily of the 90 mg/ 5 mL formulation.**
   - **40 kg (88 lb): 20 mL daily of the 90 mg/ 5 mL formulation.**

4. Store capsules and the powder for oral suspension before reconstitution from 2–25°C (36–77°F). Once reconstituted, the oral suspension is stable for 14 days from 2–8°C (36–46°F).

C

ASSESSMENT

1. Note reasons for therapy, characteristics of S&S; note any PCN/ATX sensitivity.
2. Review conditions requiring treatment; drug is only approved for chronic bronchitis, bacterial otitis media, pharyngitis, tonsillitis, based on the infective organisms.
3. Monitor VS, cultures, and renal function studies; reduce dose with dysfunction.

CLIENT/FAMILY TEACHING

1. Suspension must be consumed on an empty stomach, at least 2 hr before or 1 hr after a meal. Refrigerate suspension, shake well before use, and discard after 14 days.
2. May take tablets with food or milk to avoid GI upset.
3. Complete entire prescription; do not stop despite feeling better.
4. Report lack of response, adverse effects or persistent diarrhea. Note: suspension contains 1 gram sucrose per teaspoon.
5. Return for F/U (e.g., ear check, throat culture, x-ray) to assess response.

OUTCOMES/EVALUATE

- Resolution of underlying infection
- Symptomatic improvement

IV

Ceftizoxime sodium

(sef-tih-**ZOX**-eem)

Classification(s): Cephalosporin, third generation

Pregnancy Category: B

RX: Cefizox.

SEE ALSO ***ANTI-INFECTIVES*** AND ***CEPHALOSPORINS***.

INDICATIONS/USES

1. Lower respiratory tract infections due to *Streptococcus* species (including *S. pneumoniae,* but excluding enterococci), *Klebsiella* species, *Proteus mirabilis, Escherichia coli, Haemophilus influenzae* (including ampicillin-resistant strains), *Staphylococcus aureus* (penicillinase-/non-penicillinase-producing), *Serratia* species, *Enterobacter* species, and *Bacteroides* species.
2. UTIs due to *S. aureus* (penicillinase-/non-penicillinase-producing), *E. coli, Pseudomonas* species (including *P. aeruginosa*), *P. mirabilis, Proteus vulgaris, Providencia rettgeri, Morganella morganii, Klebsiella* species, *Serratia* species (including *S. marcescens*), and *Enterobacter* species.
3. Uncomplicated cervical and urethral gonorrhea due to *Neisseria gonorrhoeae.*
4. PID due to *N. gonorrhoeae, E. coli,* or *Streptococcus agalactiae.* Ceftizoxime has no activity against *Chlamydia trachomatis.*
5. Intra-abdominal infections due to *E. coli, S. epidermidis, Streptococcus* species (excluding enterococci), *Enterobacter* species, *Klebsiella* species, *Bacteroides* species (including *B. fragilis*), and anaerobic cocci (including *Peptococcus* and *Peptostreptococcus* species).
6. Septicemia due to *Streptococcus* species (including *S. pneumoniae,* but excluding enterococci), *S. aureus* (penicillinase-/non-penicillinease-producing), *E. coli, Bacteroides* species (including *B. fragilis*), *Klebsiella* species, and *Serratia* species.
7. Skin and skin structure infections due to *S. aureus* (penicillinase-/non-penicillinase-producing), *S. epidermidis, E. coli, Klebsiella* species, *Streptococcus* species (including *S. pyogenes,* but excluding enterococci), *P. mirabilis, Serratia* species, *Enterobacter* species, *Bacteroides* species (including *B. fragilis*), and anaerobic cocci (including *Peptococcus* and *Peptostreptococcus* species).
8. Bone and joint infections due to *S. aureus* penicillinase-/non-penicillinase-producing), *Streptococcus* species (excluding enterococci), *P. mirabilis, Bacteroides* species (including *B. fragilis*), and anaerobic cocci (including *Peptococcus* and *Peptostreptococcus* species).
9. Meningitis due to *H. influenzae* and limited use for *S. pneumoniae.*
10. Infections due to aerobic gram negative and by mixtures of organisms resistant to other cephalosporins, aminoglycosides, or penicillins have responded to ceftizoxime.

ACTION/KINETICS

Pharmacokinetics

t½: Approximately 1–2 hr. **Peak serum levels after 1 gram IV:** 60–87 mcg/mL. Approximately 80% excreted unchanged in the urine.

SIDE EFFECTS

Most Common

Rash, pruritus, fever, injection site pain/burning/cellulitis, diarrhea.

See *Cephalosporins* for a complete list of possible side effects. Also, transient increased levels of eosinophils, AST, ALT, and CPK have been seen in children over 6 months of age.

HOW SUPPLIED

Injection: 1 gram/50 mL, 2 grams/50 mL; *Powder for Injection:* 0.5 gram, 1 gram, 2 grams, 10 grams.

DOSAGE

IM; IV

Uncomplicated urinary tract infections (UTIs).

Adults: 0.5 gram IM or IV q 12 hr.

Severe or resistant infections.

Adults: 1 gram q 8 hr or 2 grams q 8–12 hr IM or IV.

Life-threatening infections.

Adults: 3–4 grams q 8 hr IV. Doses of 2 grams IV q 4 hr have been given.

Pelvic inflammatory disease (PID).

2 grams q 8 hr IV (doses up to 2 grams q 4 hr have been used).

Infections at other sites.

Adults: 1 gram q 8–12 hr IM or IV.

Uncomplicated gonorrhea.

Adults: 1 gram as a single dose.

Bacterial septicemia.

Initial: 6–12 grams/day IV in those with normal renal function; **then,** gradually reduce the dose according to clinical response and lab findings.

IM

Use in children.

Pediatric, over 6 months: 50 mg/kg q 6–8 hr up to 200 mg/kg/day (not to exceed the maximum adult dose).

Impaired renal function.

Initial, IM, IV: 0.5–1 gram; **then,** use the following dosing schedule: **Mild impairment** (C_{CR} 50–79 mL/min): 0.5 gram q 8 hr; 0.75–1.5 grams q 8 hr for life-threatening infections. **Moderate to severe impairment** (C_{CR} 5–49 mL/min): 0.25–0.5 gram q 12 hr; 0.5–1 gram q 12 hr for life-threatening infections. **Dialysis clients** (C_{CR} <4 mL/min): 0.5 gram q 48 hr or 0.25 gram q 24 hr; 0.5–1 gram q 48 hr or 0.5 gram q 24 hr for life-threatening infections.

NURSING IMPLICATIONS

Do not confuse Cefizox with Ceptaz or Cedax (also cephalosporins).

IMPLEMENTATION/ADMINISTRATION/STORAGE

1. For IM doses of 2 grams, divide dose equally; give in different large muscle masses.
2. IV IV route may be preferred with bacterial septicemia, intra-abdominal abscess, peritonitis, other severe/life-threatening infections.
3. For direct IV: Reconstitute 1 gram in 10 mL sterile water; give slowly over 3–5 min.
4. Because UTIs R/T *P. aeruginosa* are so serious and because many strains of *Pseudomonas* are only moderately susceptible to ceftizoxime, use higher doses. Institute other therapy if response not prompt.
5. For intermittent administration/continuous infusion: Dilute reconstituted solution in 50–100 mL in one of the compatible solutions described in package insert.
6. For piggyback vials: Reconstitute with 50–100 mL of any of recommended IV solutions (see package insert). Shake well; administer as a single dose with primary IV fluids over 30 min.
7. A solution of 1 gram ceftizoxime in 13 mL sterile water for injection is isotonic.
8. Reconstituted solutions stable at room temperature for 8 hr and 48 hr if refrigerated.
9. For frozen solutions, thaw container at room temperature. After thawing, solution stable for 24 hr at room temperature or for 10 days if refrigerated. Do not refreeze or introduce additives into the solution.

10. Store unreconstituted drug, protected from excessive light, from 15–30°C (59–86°F) in the original package until used.
11. COMPATIBILITY D5W, 0.9% NaCl.
12. INCOMPATIBILITY Aminoglycosides; may give separately.

C

ASSESSMENT

1. Note reasons for therapy, characteristics of S&S, clinical presentation, and culture results. Assess for PCN/antibiotic sensitivity and monitor during therapy.
2. Avoid concomitant administration of other cephalosporins and aminoglycosides.
3. Monitor VS, CBC, and renal function; reduce dose with dysfunction.

CLIENT/FAMILY TEACHING

1. Drug is administered parenterally. Report lack of response, rash, itching, diarrhea, breathing problems, or other adverse side effects.
2. Consume enough fluids to prevent dehydration.
3. Avoid ingesting alcohol.
4. Keep all F/U to assess response, labs, and adverse SE.

OUTCOMES/EVALUATE

- Negative culture reports
- Resolution of S&S of infection

IV

Ceftriaxone sodium

(sef-try-**AX**-ohn)

Classification(s): Cephalosporin, third generation

Pregnancy Category: B

RX: Rocephin.

SEE ALSO *ANTI-INFECTIVES* AND *CEPHALOSPORINS*.

INDICATIONS/USES

1. Lower respiratory tract infections due to *Streptococcus pneumoniae, Staphylococcus aureus, Haemophilus influenzae, Haemophilus parainfluenzae, Klebsiella pneumonia, Serratia marcescens, Escherichia coli, Enterobacter aerogenes,* and *Proteus mirabilis.*
2. Skin and skin structure infections due to *S. aureus, Staphylococcus epidermidis, Streptococcus pyogenes,* Viridins group streptococci, *E. coli, Enterobacter cloacae, Klebsiella oxytoca, K. pneumoniae, P. mirabilis, Pseudomonas aeruginosa, Morganella morganii, Serratia marcescens, Acinetobacter calcoaceticus, Bacteroides fragilis, Peptostreptococcus* species.
3. UTIs (complicated and uncomplicated) due to *E. coli, P. mirabilis, P. vulgaris, M. morganii,* and *K. pneumoniae.*
4. Uncomplicated cervical/urethral and rectal gonorrhea due to *Neisseria gonorrhoeae,* including penicillinase-/non-penicillinase-producing strains. Pharyngeal gonorrhea due to non-penicillinase-producing strains of *N. gonorrhoeae.*
5. PID due to *N. gonorrhoeae.* Ceftriaxone has no activity against *Chlamydia trachomatis.*
6. Bacterial septicemia due to *S. aureus, S. pneumoniae, E. coli, H. influenzae,* and *K. pneumoniae.*
7. Bone and joint infections due to *S. aureus, S. pneumoniae, E. coli, P. mirabilis, K. pneumoniae,* and *Enterobacter* species.
8. Intra-abdominal infections due to *E. coli, K. pneumoniae, B. fragilis, Clostridium* species (most strains of *C. difficile* are resistant), and *Peptostreptococcus* species.
9. Meningitis due to *H. influenzae, N. meningitidis,* and *S. pneumoniae.* Possibly effective against *Staphylococcus epidermidis* and *E. coli.*
10. Single preoperative doses may decrease the incidence of postoperative infections following vaginal or abdominal hysterectomy or in coronary artery bypass surgery.
11. Acute bacterial otitis media due to *S. pneumoniae, H. influenzae* (including beta-lactamase-producing strains), and *Moraxella catarrhalis* (including beta-lactamase-producing strains).

Investigational: Neurologic complications, arthritis, and carditis associated with Lyme disease in clients refractory to penicillin G.

ACTION/KINETICS

Pharmacokinetics

t½: Approximately 6–8 hr. **Serum levels after 1 gram IV:** 151 mcg/mL. One-third to two-thirds excreted unchanged in the urine. **Plasma protein binding:** Significant.

SIDE EFFECTS

Most Common

Diarrhea, rash, eosinophilia, nausea, pain/induration/tenderness/warmth at injection site.
See *Cephalosporins* for a complete list of possible side effects. Also, increase in serum creatinine, presence of casts in the urine, alteration of PTs (rare).

HOW SUPPLIED

Injection: 1 gram/50 mL, 2 grams/50 mL (both strengths as base); ***Powder for Injection:*** 250 mg, 500 mg, 1 gram, 2 grams, 10 grams (all strengths as base).

DOSAGE

IM; IV

General infections.

Adults, usual: 1–2 grams/day in single or divided doses q 12 hr depending on the type and severity of infection, not to exceed 4 grams/day. Maintain therapy for 4–14 days, depending on the infection. **Pediatric, serious infections:** *Other than meningitis:* 50–75 mg/kg/day not to exceed total daily dose of 2 grams given in divided doses q 12 hr.

Meningitis.

Pediatric: 100 mg/kg/day, not to exceed total daily dose of 4 grams given once daily or in equally divided doses q 12 hr for 7–14 days.

Skin and skin structure infections and serious infections other than meningitis.

Pediatric: 50–75 mg/kg once daily or in equally divided doses q 12 hr. Do not exceed a daily dose of 2 grams.

Preoperative for prophylaxis of infection in surgery.

1 gram 30–120 min prior to surgery.

Uncomplicated gonorrhea.

Adults, IM: 125 mg as a single dose plus doxycycline, 100 mg twice a day for 7 days or azithromycin, 1 gram, as a single PO dose. Or, a single dose of ceftriaxone 250 mg IM.

Disseminated gonococcal infection.

Adults: 1 gram IM or IV q 24 hr.

Gonococcal meningitis or endocarditis.

Adults: 1–2 grams IV q 12 hr for 10–14 days (meningitis) or 4 weeks (endocarditis).

Gonococcal conjunctivitis.

Adults and children over 20 kg: 1 gram given as a single IM dose.

Haemophilus ducreyi *infection.*

250 mg IM as a single dose.

Acute pelvic inflammatory disease (PID).

250 mg IM plus doxycycline or tetracycline.

Lyme disease in those refractory to penicillin G.

IV: 2 grams/day for 14–28 days.

Acute bacterial otitis media.

IM: Single dose of 50 mg/kg, not to exceed 1 gram.

NOTE: Dosage adjustment is not required for renal or hepatic impairment; however, monitor blood levels

NURSING IMPLICATIONS

IMPLEMENTATION/ADMINISTRATION/STORAGE

1. Give IM injections deep into the body of a large muscle.
2. IV IV infusions should contain concentrations of 10–40 mg/mL. Reconstitute 500 mg in 4.8 mL of sterile water, NSS, or D5W. Then further dilute in 50–100 mL D5W or NSS and infuse over 30 min.
3. Stability of solutions for IM or IV use varies depending on the diluent used; check package insert carefully.
4. Maintain dosage for at least 2 days after symptoms have disappeared (usual course is 4–14 days, although complicated infections may require longer therapy).
5. Continue dosage for at least 10 days when treating *S. pyogenes* infections.
6. COMPATIBILITY D5W or NSS.
7. INCOMPATIBILITY Do not mix drug with other antibiotics. Avoid calcium-containing IV solution or diluents containing calcium to reconstitute. Incompatible with fluconazole, aminoglycosides, and vancomycin admixtures; may give separately after flushing line.

C

ASSESSMENT

1. Note reasons for therapy, characteristics of S&S, clinical presentation, and culture results. List any PCN/antibiotic sensitivity and monitor during therapy.
2. Assess for GI disease, especially colitis; use drug cautiously, report any bruising/bleeding, diarrhea.
3. Monitor renal and LFTs, coagulation studies. May use vitamin K (10 mg/week) prophylactically if bleeding occurs or impaired synthesis of vitamin K.

CLIENT/FAMILY TEACHING

1. Drug is administered parenterally.
2. Report lack of response, injection site pain, abnormal bruising/bleeding, persistent diarrhea, breathing difficulty, or other adverse side effects.
3. Consume adequate fluids to prevent dehydration.
4. Keep all F/U to assess response, labs, adverse SE.

OUTCOMES/EVALUATE

- Resolution of S&S of infection
- Negative culture reports

IV

Cefuroxime axetil

(sef-your-**OX**-eem)

Classification(s): Cephalosporin, second generation

Pregnancy Category: B

RX: Ceftin.

✱ **Rx:** Apo-Cefuroxime, ratio-Cefuroxime.

Cefuroxime sodium

Pregnancy Category: B

RX: Zinacef.

SEE ALSO *ANTI-INFECTIVES* AND *CEPHALOSPORINS*.

INDICATIONS/USES

PO (axetil), Suspension (Children, 3 months–12 years).

1. Pharyngitis or tonsillitis due to *S. pyogenes* (group A beta-hemolytic streptococci).
2. Acute bacterial otitis media due to *S. pneumoniae, H. influenzae* (including beta-lactamase-producing strains), *M. catarrhalis* (including beta-lactamase-producing strains), or *S. pyogenes*.
3. Impetigo due to *S. aureus* (including beta-lactamase-producing strains) and *Streptococcus pyogenes*.

PO (axetil), Tablets.

1. Pharyngitis or tonsillitis due to *S. pyogenes* (group A beta-hemolytic streptococci).
2. Acute bacterial otitis media due to *S. pneumoniae, H. influenzae* (including beta-lactamase-producing strains), *M. catarrhalis* (including beta-lactamase-producing strains), or *S. pyogenes*.
3. Acute bacterial maxillary sinusitis due to *S. pneumoniae* or *H. influenzae* (non-beta-lactamase-producing strains only).
4. Acute bacterial exacerbations of chronic bronchitis and secondary bacterial infections of acute bronchitis due to *S. pneumoniae, H. influenzae* (beta-lactamase-negative strains) or *H. parainfluenzae* (beta-lactamase-negative strains).
5. Uncomplicated UTIs due to *E. coli* or *K. pneumoniae*.
6. Uncomplicated skin and skin structure infections due to *S. aureus* (including beta-lactamase-producing strains) or *S. pyogenes*.
7. Uncomplicated urethral and endocervial gonorrhea due to penicillinase-producing and non-penicillinase-producing strains of *N. gonorrhoeae* and uncomplicated rectal gonorrhea in females due to non-penicillinase-producing strains of *N. gonorrheae*.
8. Early Lyme disease due to *Borrelia burgdorferi*.

IM, IV (sodium).

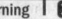

1. Lower respiratory tract infections, including pneumonia, due to *S. pneumoniae, H. influenzae* (including ampicillin-resistant strains), *Klebsiella* species, *S. aureus* (penicillinase-/non-penicillinase-producing), *S. pyogenes, E. coli*.
2. UTIs due to *E. coli* or *Klebsiella* species.
3. Skin and skin structure infections due to *S. aureus* (penicillinase-/non-penicillinase-producing), *S. pyogenes, E. coli, Klebsiella* species, and *Enterobacter* species.
4. Septicemia due to *S. aureus* (penicillinase-/non-penicillinase-producing), *S. pneumoniae, E. coli, H. influenzae* (including ampi-

cillin-resistant strains), and *Klebsiella* species.
5. Meningitis due to *S. pneumoniae, H. influenzae* (including ampicillin-resistant strains), *N. meningitidis* and *S. aureus* (penicillinase-/non-penicillinase-producing strains).
6. Uncomplicated and disseminated gonococcal infections due to *N. gonorrhoeae* (penicillinase-/non-penicillinase-producing strains) in males and females.
7. Bone/joint infections due to *S. aureus* (penicillinase-/non-penicillinase-producing strains).
8. Mixed skin and skin structure infections.
9. Preoperative prophylaxis in clients undergoing surgical procedures (e.g., vaginal hysterectomy) classified as clean-contaminated or potentially contaminated.

ACTION/KINETICS

Pharmacokinetics

Cefuroxime axetil is used PO, whereas cefuroxime sodium is used either IM or IV. **IM, IV: t½, 80 min. Peak serum levels after 1.5 grams IV:** 100 mcg/mL. 66–100% is excreted unchanged in the urine. t½ will be prolonged in clients with renal failure.

SIDE EFFECTS

Most Common

Diarrhea/loose stools, N&V, abdominal pain.

See *Cephalosporins* for a complete list of possible side effects. Also, decrease in H&H.

DRUG INTERACTIONS

H_2 antagonists ↓ cefuroxime plasma levels

ADDITIONAL DRUG INTERACTIONS

↓ Effectiveness of oral contraceptives.

ADDITIONAL LABORATORY TEST CONSIDERATIONS

False/negative reaction in the ferricyanide test for blood glucose.

HOW SUPPLIED

Cefuroxime axetil. ***Powder for Oral Suspension:*** 125 mg/5 mL, 250 mg/5 mL (both when reconstituted); ***Tablets:*** 125 mg, 250 mg, 500 mg. **Cefuroxime sodium.** ***Injection:*** 750 mg/50 mL, 1.5 grams/50 mL; ***Powder for Injection:*** 750 mg, 1.5 grams, 7.5 grams.

DOSAGE

Cefuroxime axetil

SUSPENSION

Pharyngitis, tonsillitis.

Children, 3 months to 12 years: 20 mg/kg/day in 2 divided doses, not to exceed 500 mg total dose/day, for 10 days.

Acute otitis media, impetigo, acute bacterial maxillary sinusitis.

Children, 3 months to 12 years: 30 mg/kg/day in 2 divided doses, not to exceed 1,000 mg total dose/day, for 10 days.

TABLETS

Pharyngitis, tonsillitis.

Adults and children over 13 years: 250 mg q 12 hr for 10 days.

Acute bacterial exacerbations of chronic bronchitis and secondary bacterial infections of acute bronchitis, uncomplicated skin and skin structure infections.

Adults and children over 13 years: 250 or 500 mg q 12 hr for 10 days (5–10 days for secondary bacterial infections of acute bronchitis).

Uncomplicated urinary tract infections (UTIs).

Adults and children over 13 years: 250 mg q 12 hr for 7–10 days.

Acute otitis media.

Children: 250 mg twice a day for 10 days.

Uncomplicated gonorrhea.

Adults and children over 13 years: 1,000 mg as a single dose.

Early Lyme disease.

Adults and children over 13 years of age: 500 mg/day for 20 days.

Acute bacterial maxillary sinusitis.

Adults and children who can swallow tablets whole: 250 mg q 12 hr for 10 days.

Cefuroxime Sodium

IM; IV

Uncomplicated infections, including urinary tract, uncomplicated pneumonia, disseminated gonococcal, skin and skin structure.

Adults: 750 mg q 8 hr. **Pediatric, over 3 months:** 50–100 mg/kg/day in equally divided doses q 6–8 hr (not to exceed adult dose for severe infections).

C

Severe or complicated infections; bone and joint infections.

Adults: 1.5 grams q 8 hr. **Pediatric, over 3 months:** *Bone and joint infections,* **IV:** 150 mg/kg/day in equally divided doses q 8 hr (not to exceed adult dose).

Life-threatening infections or those due to less susceptible organisms.

Adults: 1.5 grams q 6 hr.

Bacterial meningitis.

Adults: Up to 3 grams q 8 hr. **Pediatric, over 3 months, initial, IV:** 200–240 mg/kg/day in divided doses q 6–8 hr; **then,** after clinical improvement, 100 mg/kg/day.

Gonorrhea (uncomplicated).

1.5 grams as a single IM dose given at two different sites together with 1 gram PO probenecid.

Prophylaxis in surgery.

Adults, IV: 1.5 grams 30–60 min before surgery; if procedure is of long duration, **IM, IV:** 0.75 gram q 8 hr.

Open heart surgery, prophylaxis.

IV: 1.5 grams when anesthesia is initiated; **then,** 1.5 grams q 12 hr for a total of 6 grams.

NOTE: Reduce the dose in impaired renal function as follows: C_{CR} over 20 mL/min: 0.75–1.5 grams q 8 hr; C_{CR}, 10–20 mL/min: 0.75 gram q 12 hr; C_{CR}, less than 10 mL/min: 0.75 gram q 24 hr.

NURSING IMPLICATIONS

© Do not confuse cefuroxime with deferoxamine (an iron chelator).

IMPLEMENTATION/ADMINISTRATION/STORAGE

1. Cefuroxime axetil for PO use is available in tablet and suspension forms. Swallow tablets whole, do not crush; crushed tablet has a strong, bitter, persistent taste. Tablets may be taken without regard for food; however, the suspension must be taken with food. Protect tablets from excessive moisture.
2. To reconstitute suspension, loosen powder by shaking the bottle. Add appropriate amount of water (depending on bottle size). Invert bottle and shake vigorously. Shake before each use. Store reconstituted suspension either at room temperature or refrigerate. Discard any unused portion after 10 days.
3. Tablet and suspension are not bioequivalent; not substitutable on a mg-per-mg basis.
4. For IM use, constitute each 750 mg vial with 3 mL sterile water for injection. Shake gently to disperse. Inject deep into a large muscle mass.
5. Store tablets from 15–30°C (59–86°F). Protect unit-dose packs from excessive moisture. Before reconstitution store the dry powder for the oral suspension from 2–25°C (36–77°F). After reconstitution store the suspension either in a refrigerator or at room temperature; discard after 10 days.
6. **IV** Use IV route for severe/life-threatening infections such as septicemia, or in poor-risk clients, especially in presence of shock.
7. Continue treatment for a minimum of 48 to 72 hr after client is asymptomatic or after evidence of bacterial eradication has been obtained. Treat and continue therapy for a minimum of 10 days for *Streptococcus pyogenes* infections in order to minimize the risk of rheumatic fever or glomerulonephritis.
8. For direct IV, reconstitute 750 mg in 8 mL sterile water; give over 3–5 min. For intermittent IV, further dilute in 100 mL of dextrose or saline solution; infuse over 30 min.
9. Reconstitute the 1.5 gram vial with 16 mL sterile water for injection. Withdraw completely the solution for injection. Reconstitute the 7.5-gram pharmacy bulk vial with 77 mL sterile water for injection; each 8 mL of the resulting solution contains 750 mg cefuroxime sodium.
10. For direct intermittent IV administration, slowly inject drug over 3 to 5 min, or give in tubing of other IV solutions. For intermittent IV infusion with a Y-type setup, may give dose in the tubing through which client is receiving other medications; however, during drug infusion, stop other solutions. For continuous IV infusion, the drug may be added to compatible solutions. Prior to reconstitution, protect drug from light. The powder and reconstituted drug may darken without affecting potency.

11. COMPATIBILITY 0.9% NaCl, D5W or D10W, D5/0.45% or 0.9% NaCl, and M/6 sodium lactate injection.
12. INCOMPATIBILITY Aminoglycoside solutions; if both required, flush line and give separately.

ASSESSMENT

1. Note reasons for therapy, characteristics of S&S, culture results, baseline assessments. List any PCN/antibiotic sensitivity.
2. Assess for anemia, renal dysfunction. Reduce dose with impaired renal function.

CLIENT/FAMILY TEACHING

1. Swallow tablets whole; do not chew or crush as crushed tablet has a strong, bitter, persistent taste. Tablets may be taken without regard for food; the suspension must be taken with food. Store suspension at room temperature or refrigerate. Discard after 10 days. Protect tablets from excessive moisture.
2. Crushed tablets have a distinctive bitter taste even when hidden in foods. If intolerable, report so alternative drug therapy may be instituted.
3. Report lack of response, severe abdominal pain, persistent diarrhea, SOB, wheezing, or S&S of anemia (SOB, dizziness, pale skin, etc.) immediately.
4. Ensure adequate fluid intake to prevent dehydration.
5. Keep all F/U to assess response and for adverse SE.

OUTCOMES/EVALUATE

- Resolution of S&S of infection
- Surgical infection prophylaxis

Celecoxib

(**sell**-ah-**KOX**-ihb)

Classification(s): Nonsteroidal anti-inflammatory drug, COX-2 inhibitor

Pregnancy Category: C

RX: Celebrex.

SEE ALSO ***NONSTEROIDAL ANTI-INFLAMMATORY DRUGS.***

INDICATIONS/USES

(1) Relief of signs and symptoms of osteoarthritis and rheumatoid arthritis in adults. (2) Relief of signs and symptoms of juvenile rheumatoid arthritis in clients 2 years of age and older. (3) Relief of signs and symptoms of ankylosing spondylitis. (4) Management of acute pain in adults. (5) Primary dysmenorrhea. (6) Reduce the number of adenomatous colorectal polyps in familial adenomatous polyposis, as an adjunct to usual care (e.g., endoscopic surveillance, surgery).

ACTION/KINETICS

Action

Inhibits prostaglandin synthesis, primarily by inhibiting cyclo-oxygenase-2 (COX-2), thus decreasing inflammation. Does not inhibit the cyclo-oxygenase-1 (COX-1) isoenzyme. Does not affect platelet aggregation; renal effects similar to other NSAIDs. Causes fewer GI complications, such as bleeding and perforation, compared with other NSAIDs.

Pharmacokinetics

Peak plasma levels: 3 hr. **t½, terminal:** 11 hr when fasting; low solubility prolongs absorption. Metabolized in the liver to inactive compounds; excreted in the urine (27%) and feces (57%). Blacks show a 40% increase in the total amount absorbed compared with Caucasians. **Plasma protein binding:** About 97%.

CONTRAINDICATIONS

Use in severe renal impairment or in those with severe hepatic impairment, in those who have shown an allergic reaction to sulfonamides, or in those who have experienced asthma, urticaria, or allergic-type reactions after taking aspirin or other NSAIDs. Use in late pregnancy (may cause premature closure of ductus arteriosus). Lactation.

SPECIAL CONCERNS

(1) **Cardiovascular risk:** Celecoxib may cause an increased risk of serious CV thrombotic events, MI, and stroke, which can be fatal. All NSAIDs may have a similar risk. This risk may increase with duration of use. Clients with CV disease or risk factors for CV disease may be at higher risk. (2) Celecoxib is contraindicated for the treatment of perioperative pain in the setting of coronary artery bypass graft. (3) **GI risk:** NSAIDs, including celecox-

ib, cause an increased risk of serious GI adverse effects, including bleeding, ulceration, and perforation of the stomach or intestines, which can be fatal. These reactions can occur at any time during use and without warning symptoms. Elderly clients are at higher risk for serious GI events.

- **Use with caution in pre-existing asthma, with drugs known to inhibit CYP2C9 in the liver, or when initiating the drug in significant dehydration.**
- **Use with extreme caution in those with a prior history of ulcer disease or GI bleeding. Increased risk of ulceration and bleeding if used with NSAIDs.**
- **Increased risk of serious renal effects in geriatric clients.**
- **Possible serious CV side effects.**
- **Even short-term use may lead to an increased risk of death and recurrent MI in clients with prior MI.**
- **Safety and efficacy not determined in clients less than 18 years of age.**

SIDE EFFECTS

Most Common

Abdominal pain/cramps, diarrhea, nausea, dyspepsia/indigestion, URTI.

Listed are side effects with a frequency of 0.1% or greater. **GI:** Dyspepsia, diarrhea, abdominal pain, N&V, dry mouth, flatulence, constipation, GI bleeding/ulceration, ***GI hemorrhage***, diverticulitis, dysphagia, eructation, esophagitis, gastritis, gastroenteritis, GERD, hemorrhoids, hiatal hernia, melena, stomatitis, tooth disorder, abnormal hepatic function. **CNS:** Headache, dizziness, insomnia, anorexia, anxiety, depression, nervousness, somnolence, hypertonia, hypoesthesia, migraine, neuropathy, paresthesia, vertigo, increased appetite. **CV:** Aggravated hypertension, angina pectoris, CAD, ***MI***, palpitation, tachycardia, thrombocythemia, thrombotic events, CHF-related adverse effects. **Respiratory:** URTI, sinusitis, pharyngitis, rhinitis, bronchitis, bronchospasm, coughing, dyspnea, laryngitis, pneumonia. **Dermatologic:** Rash, ecchymosis, alopecia, dermatitis, nail disorder, photosensitivity, pruritus, erythematous/maculopapular rash, skin disorder, dry skin, increased sweating, urticaria. **Body as a whole:** Accidental injury, back/chest pain, peripheral edema, aggravated allergy, allergic reaction, asthenia, fluid retention, generalized edema, fatigue, fever, hot flushes, flu-like symptoms, pain/peripheral pain, weight increase. **Musculoskeletal:** Arthralgia, arthrosis, bone disorder, accidental fracture, myalgia, stiff neck, synovitis, tendinitis. **Infections:** Bacterial/fungal, or viral infection; herpes simplex/zoster, soft-tissue infection, moniliasis, genital moniliasis, otitis media. **GU:** Cystitis, dysuria, frequent urination, renal calculus, urinary incontinence, UTI, breast fibroadenosis/neoplasm/pain, dysmenorrhea, menstrual disorder, vaginal hemorrhage, vaginitis, prostatic disorder. **Ophthalmic:** Glaucoma, blurred vision, cataract, conjunctivitis, eye pain. **Otic:** Deafness, ear abnormality, earache, tinnitus. **Miscellaneous:** Tenesmus, facial edema, leg cramps, diabetes mellitus, epistaxis, anemia, taste perversion.

LABORATORY TEST CONSIDERATIONS

↑ ALT, AST, BUN, CPK, NPN, creatinine, alkaline phosphatase. Hypercholesterolemia, hyperglycemia, hypokalemia, albuminuria, hematuria.

DRUG INTERACTIONS

ACE Inhibitors / ↓ Antihypertensive effect
Antacids, Al- and Mg-containing / ↓ Celecoxib absorption
Aspirin / ↑ Risk of GI ulceration
Fluconazole / ↑ Plasma celecoxib levels
Furosemide / ↓ Natriuretic drug effect
Lithium / ↑ Plasma lithium levels
Thiazide diuretics / ↓ Natriuretic drug effects
Warfarin / Possible ↑ PT with bleeding, especially in the elderly

HOW SUPPLIED

Capsules: 50 mg, 100 mg, 200 mg, 400 mg.

DOSAGE

CAPSULES

Osteoarthritis.

Adults: 100 mg twice a day or 200 mg as a single dose.

Rheumatoid arthritis.

Adults: 100–200 mg twice a day.

Juvenile rheumatoid arthritis.

Children 2 years and older weighing 10–25 kg: 50 mg twice a day. **Children 2 years of age and older weighing more than 25 kg:** 100 mg twice a day.

Ankylosing spondylitis.
200 mg daily either as a single dose or divided into 2 doses. If no effect is seen after 6 weeks, a trial of 400 mg/day may be beneficial. If no effect is seen after 6 weeks on 400 mg/day, a response is not likely; give consideration to alternate treatments.

Acute pain or primary dysmenorrhea.
Day 1, Initial: 400 mg; **then,** an additional 200 mg, if needed on day 1. On subsequent days, 200 mg 2 times per day, as needed.

Familial adenomatous polyposis.
Usual: 400 mg twice a day with food. Continue usual medical care (e.g., endoscopic surveillance, surgery).

NURSING IMPLICATIONS

Do not confuse Celebrex with Cerebyx (an anticonvulsant) or with Celexa (an antidepressant).

IMPLEMENTATION/ADMINISTRATION/STORAGE

1. The maximum daily dose should be 800 mg in adults and 200 mg in children.
2. For elderly clients less than 50 kg, start therapy at the lowest recommended dose.
3. Reduce daily dose by about 50% in clients with moderate impaired hepatic function (Child-Pugh class B).
4. Consider a starting dose at half the lowest recommended dose in those who are poor metabolizers of CYP2C9. Consider using alternate management in juvenile rheumatoid arthritis clients who are poor metabolizers.
5. For those unable to swallow capsules, the contents of a celecoxib capsule can be added to a level teaspoon of applesauce; ingest immediately with water. The applesauce-celecoxib mixture is stable for up to 6 hr when refrigerated.
6. Store from 15–30°C (59–86°F).

ASSESSMENT

1. Note reasons for therapy, onset, characteristics of disease, ROM, deformity/loss of function, pain level, other agents trialed, outcome. Assess clinical response during therapy.
2. Determine any GI bleed/ulcer history, sulfonamide allergy, aspirin, other NSAID-induced asthma, urticaria, allergic-type reactions.
3. List drugs prescribed; ensure none interact.
4. This class of drugs has been associated with increased risk of heart attacks/stroke (those with CV disease or risk factors for CV disease may be at higher risk); monitor for S&S and advise client.
5. Monitor for GI bleeding, ulceration, and perforation of the stomach or intestines, which can be fatal. Elderly clients are at higher risk for serious GI events.
6. Assess for liver/renal dysfunction; reduce dose. Monitor BP, CBC, electrolytes, renal and LFTs.

CLIENT/FAMILY TEACHING

1. Take with food; decreases stomach upset. Higher doses (e.g., 400 mg twice a day) should be given with food to improve absorption.
2. Avoid alcohol; may aggravate liver function.
3. Report any S&S of liver toxicity (e.g., fatigue, flu-like symptoms, jaundice, lethargy, nausea, pruritus, right upper quadrant tenderness).
4. Seek lowest effective dose. Take as directed, at same time daily. May take several days before desired effect.
5. Do not take aspirin/aspirin-containing products without consent.
6. Report unusual/persistent side effects, including dyspepsia, chest or abdominal pain, weakness, SOB, dizziness, changes in stool/skin color, unusual weight gain or rashes, slurred speech, or problems with vision or balance if occurs.
7. Avoid during pregnancy; use reliable contraception and do not breast-feed.
8. Keep F/U to assess response and for adverse SE.

OUTCOMES/EVALUATE

- Relief of joint pain/inflammation; improved mobility
- ↓ Adenomatous colorectal polyps in familial adenomatous polyposis

Cephalexin

(sef-ah-**LEX**-in)

Classification(s): Cephalosporin, first generation

Pregnancy Category: B

RX: Keflex.

🍁 **Rx:** Apo-Cephalex, Novo-Lexin, Nu-Cephalex.

SEE ALSO ***ANTI-INFECTIVES*** AND ***CEPHALOSPORINS***.

C

INDICATIONS/USES

(1) Respiratory tract infections due to *Streptococcus pneumoniae* and *Streptococcus pyogenes*. (2) GU infections (including acute prostatitis due to *Escherichia coli, Proteus mirabilis,* or *Klebsiella pneumoniae*). (3) Bone infections caused by *P. mirabilis* or *Staphylococcus aureus*. (4) Skin and skin structure infections due to *S. aureus* and/or *S. pyogenes*. (5) Otitis media due to *S. pneumoniae, Haemophilus influenzae, S. pyogenes,* and *Moraxella catarrhalis*.

ACTION/KINETICS

Action

Interferes with the final step in cell wall formation (inhibition of mucopeptide biosynthesis), resulting in unstable cell membranes that undergo lysis. Also, cell division and growth are inhibited.

Pharmacokinetics

Peak serum levels: PO, 9–39 mcg/mL after 1 hr. **t½, PO:** 50–80 min. Absorption delayed in children. The HCl monohydrate does not require conversion in the stomach before absorption. Ninety percent of drug excreted unchanged in urine within 8 hr. **Plasma protein binding:** About 10%.

SIDE EFFECTS

Most Common

Diarrhea, N&V, abdominal pain, dizziness, skin rash, fever, vaginitis.

See *Cephalosporins* for a complete list of potential side effects. Also, nephrotoxicity, cholestatic jaundice.

HOW SUPPLIED

Capsules: 250 mg, 333 mg, 500 mg, 750 mg; ***Powder for Oral Suspension:*** 125 mg/5 mL (after reconstitution), 250 mg/5 mL (after reconstitution); ***Tablets:*** 250 mg, 500 mg; ***Tablets for Oral Suspension:*** 125 mg, 250 mg.

DOSAGE

CAPSULES; ORAL SUSPENSION (FROM POWDER OR TABLETS); TABLETS

General infections.

Adults, usual: 250 mg q 6 hr up to 4 grams/day in divided doses. **Pediatric:** 25–50 mg/kg/day in four equally divided doses.

Infections of skin and skin structures, streptococcal pharyngitis, uncomplicated cystitis, over 15 years of age.

Adults: 500 mg q 12 hr. Large doses may be needed for severe infections or for less susceptible organisms. Continue therapy for cystitis for 7–14 days. For streptococcal pharyngitis **in children over 1 year** and for skin and skin structure infections, the total daily dose should be divided and given q 12 hr. In severe infections, the dose should be doubled.

Otitis media.

Pediatric: 75–100 mg/kg/day in four divided doses.

NURSING IMPLICATIONS

IMPLEMENTATION/ADMINISTRATION/STORAGE

1. Refrigerate suspension after reconstitution; discard after 14 days.
2. If total daily dose is more than 4 grams, use parenteral drugs.
3. Continue for at least 10 days for beta-hemolytic streptococcal infections.
4. May reduce dosage with impaired renal function; or increase for severe infections. Drug action can be prolonged by concurrent use of probenecid.
5. The tablets for oral suspension are used to prepare individual 5 mL doses.
6. Store capsules, powder for oral suspension, and tablets from 20–25°C (68–77°F).

ASSESSMENT

1. Note reasons for therapy, severity of infection, characteristics of S&S, culture results.
2. Monitor cultures, CBC, renal and LFTs; may require reduced dose with renal dysfunction.

CLIENT/FAMILY TEACHING

1. Take as directed/complete prescription; may take with meals for GI upset. Shake the reconstituted suspension well. Refrigerate suspension; discard after 14 days.
2. Consume 2–3 L/day of fluids to prevent dehydration.
3. Report persistent fever, diarrhea, yellow discoloration of the skin/eyes, N&V, skin rash, hives, muscle or joint pain or lack of response. Report S&S of superinfection: black "furry" tongue, white patches in mouth, foulsmelling stools, vaginal itching or discharge.
4. Keep F/U to assess response and for adverse SE.

OUTCOMES/EVALUATE

- Resolution of infection
- Symptomatic improvement

Certolizumab pegol

(**SER**-toe-**LIZ**-oo-mab peg-**OL**)

Classification(s): Immunomodulator

Pregnancy Category: B

RX: Cimzia.

INDICATIONS/USES

(1) Reduce the signs and symptoms of Crohn's disease and maintain clinical response in adults with moderate to severe active disease who have had inadequate response to conventional therapy. (2) Treatment of adults with moderate to severely active rheumatoid arthritis; often used with methotrexate.

ACTION/KINETICS

Action

Certolizumab is a tissue necrosis factor blocker (TNF). It binds to TNF-alpha, a key proinflammatory cytokine with a central role in the inflammatory process. It selectively neutralizes TNF-alpha but does not neutralize TNF-beta. Thus, the drug relieves the inflammation of Crohn's disease.

Pharmacokinetics

Peak plasma levels after SC: 54–171 hr. Bioavailability is about 80% after SC use. **t½, terminal:** 14 days. Pegylation delays the metabolism and elimination of the drug. It is believed that once cleaved from the Fab fragment, the polyethylene glycol moiety is excreted mainly in the urine with no further metabolism. Pharmacokinetic exposure is inversely related to body weight; however no additional beneficial benefit would be expected from a weight-adjusted dosage regimen.

CONTRAINDICATIONS

Initiation of therapy in active infections, including chronic or localized infections. Use in combination with biological disease modifying antirheumatic drugs or other tumor necrosis factor-blocker therapy. Coadministration with live or attenuated vaccines. Lactation.

SPECIAL CONCERNS

Serious infection. (1) Clients treated with certolizumab are at an increased risk for developing serious infections that may lead to hospitalization or death. Most clients who developed these infections were taking concomitant immunosuppressants such as methotrexate or corticosteroids. (2) Discontinue certolizumab if a client develops a serious infection or sepsis. (3) Reported infections include: (a) Active tuberculosis, including reactivation of latent tuberculosis. Clients with tuberculosis have frequently presented with disseminated or extrapulmonary disease. Test clients for latent tuberculosis before certolizumab use and during therapy. Initiate treatment for latent infections prior to certolizumab use. (b) Invasive fungal infections, including histoplasmosis, coccidioidomycosis, candidiasis, aspergillosis, blastomycosis, and pneumocystosis. Clients with histoplasmosis or other invasive fungal infections may present with disseminated, rather than localized disease. Antigen and antibody testing for histoplasmosis may be negative in some clients with active infection. Consider empiric antifungal therapy in clients at risk for invasive fungal infections who develop severe systemic illness. (c) Bacterial, viral, and other infections caused by opportunistic pathogens. (4) Carefully consider the risks and benefits of treatment with certolizumab prior to initiating therapy in clients with chronic or recurrent infection. (5) Closely monitor clients for the development of signs and symptoms of infection during and after treatment with certolizumab, including the possible development of tuberculosis in clients who tested negative for latent tuberculosis infection prior to initiating therapy. (6) **Malignancy.** Lymphoma and other malignancies, some fatal, have been reported in children and adolescent clients treated with tumor necrosis factor (TNF) blockers, of which certolizumab is a member. (7) Certolizumab is not indicated for use in children.

- **Use caution when considering use in those with a history of recurrent infection, concomitant immunosuppressive therapy, or underlying conditions that may predispose the client to infection, or in those who have resided in areas where TB and histoplasmosis are endemic.**
- **Use with caution in pre-existing or recent-onset CNS demyelinating disorders; in those who have ongoing or a history of significant hematologic abnormalities; in those who have heart failure; or, in the elderly.**
- **Safety and efficacy not established in children or in those with immunosuppression.**

SIDE EFFECTS

Most Common

Infections (commonly TB, pneumonia), URTI, UTI, rash, arthralgia, abdominal pain, diarrhea, pyrexia, urticaria.

CNS: Anxiety, bipolar disorder, headache, ***suicide attempt, seizure disorders***, peripheral neuropathy, new onset or exacerbation of demyelinating disease. **GI:** Abdominal pain, diarrhea, intestinal obstruction, hepatitis. **CV:** Worsening or new cases of CHF, angina pectoris, arrhythmias, atrial fibrillation, ***cardiac failure***, hypertensive heart disease, hypertension, ***MI***, myocardial ischemia, pericardial effusion, pericarditis, ***stroke***, thrombophlebitis, TIA, vasculitis. **Respiratory:** URTI, lower RTI, pneumonia, acute bronchitis, nasopharyngitis, pharyngitis. **GU:** UTI, pyelonephritis, menstrual disorder, nephrotic syndrome, renal failure. **Musculoskeletal:** Arthralgia, pain in extremities, back pain. **Dermatologic:** Rash, erythema nodosum, dermatitis, urticaria, alopecia totalis, erythema multiforme, new or worsening psoriasis, ***Stevens-Johnson syndrome, toxic epidermal necrolysis***. **Hematologic:** Leukopenia, thrombocytopenia, anemia, lymphadenopathy, thrombophilia; pancytopenia (rare), including aplastic anemia. **Ophthalmic:** Retinal hemorrhage, uveitis, optic neuritis. **Infections:** Viral (including herpes), bacterial, fungal, protozoal infections possible in all organ systems; ***sepsis, opportunistic infections*** (most frequently TB, histoplasmosis, aspergillosis, candidiasis, coccidioidomycosis, listeriosis, pneumocystosis), tuberculosis (pulmonary and disseminated), reactivation of hepatitis B virus, cellulitis. **Hypersensitivity:** Angioedema, allergic dermatitis, postural dizziness, dyspnea, hot flush, hypotension, injection-site reactions, rash, serum sickness, urticaria, malaise, pyrexia, syncope, vasovagal syncope. **Body as a whole:** Fatigue, pyrexia; malignancies, including lymphoma (including Hodgkin's and non-Hodgkin's lymphoma); acute and chronic leukemia, immunosuppression, peripheral edema, bleeding, new onset or exacerbation of demyelinating disease, development of autoantibodies (including, rarely, a lupus-like syndrome).

LABORATORY TEST CONSIDERATIONS

Erroneous ↑ aPTT.

DRUG INTERACTIONS

Abatacept / Possible ↑ risk of serious infections; do not use together

Anakinra / Possible ↑ risk of serious infections; do not use together

Natalizumab / Possible ↑ risk of serious infections; do not use together

Rituximab / Possible ↑ risk of serious infections; do not use together

Vaccines, live / Contraindicated with certolizumab use

HOW SUPPLIED

Injection, Lyophilized Powder for Solution: 200 mg; ***Injection Solution:*** 200 mg/mL.

DOSAGE

SC

Crohn's disease.

Adults, initial: 400 mg, given as two SC injections of 200 mg simultaneously, initially and at weeks 2 and 4. **Maintenance:** In those who obtain a clinical response, give 400 mg q 4 weeks.

Rheumatoid arthritis.

Adults, initial: 400 mg, given as 2 SC injections of 200 mg, and at weeks 2 and 4; **then,** 200 mg every other week.

Maintenance: Consider 400 mg q 4 weeks.

NURSING IMPLICATIONS

IMPLEMENTATION/ADMINISTRATION/STORAGE

1. Prior to beginning therapy, evaluate all clients for active and latent tuberculosis infection. Consider the possibility of undetected latent TB in those who have immigrated from or traveled to countries with a high prevalence of TB or had close contact with a person with active TB.
2. May be used as monotherapy or with nonbiological disease-modifying antirheumatic drugs. For example, some clients are also taking methotrexate with certolizumab, 200 mg every other week. However, do not use certolizumab with biological disease-modifying antirheumatic drugs or other tumor necrosis factor blocker drugs.
3. Bring to room temperature before reconstituting in order to facilitate dissolution. Reconstitute 2 200 mg vials for each dose. Using aseptic technique, reconstitute each lyophilized vial with 1 mL of sterile water for injection using a syringe with a 20-gauge needle. Gently swirl each vial without shaking so that all the lyophilized powder comes into contact with the diluent. Leave the vials undisturbed to fully reconstitute; this may take as long as 30 min. The reconstituted certolizumab has a concentration of about 200 mg/mL. Once reconstituted, certolizumab is a clear to opalescent, colorless to pale yellow liquid, essentially free from particulate matter.
4. Prior to administration, reconstituted drug should be at room temperature. Using a new 20-gauge needle for each vial, withdraw the reconstituted solution into a separate syringe for each vial (i.e., 2 syringes each containing 1 mL of certolizumab 200 mg). Switch each 20-gauge needle to a 23-gauge needle and inject the full contents of each syringe SC into separate sites on the abdomen or thigh.
5. Rotate injection sites and do not give injections into areas where the skin is tender, bruised, red, or hard. When a 400 mg dose is needed, given as 2 SC injections of 200 mg each; give at separate sites in the thigh or abdomen.
6. Refrigerate the intact carton from 2–8°C (36–46°F). Do not freeze. Do not separate contents of the carton before use. Protect the solution from light.
7. Do not leave reconstituted drug at room temperature for more than 2 hr prior to administration.
8. If prefilled syringes are used, the full amount (1 mL) in the syringe is to be injected.
9. Once reconstituted, the drug can be stored in the vials for up to 24 hr from 2–8°C (36–46°F). Do not freeze the reconstituted drug. Discard any unused portions of the drug as the product does not contain preservatives.

ASSESSMENT

1. Note reasons for therapy: Crohn's disease or rheumatoid arthritis, other agents trialed, outcome.
2. Assess carefully for any S&S of an infection, such as a fever, cough, flu-like symptoms. Check for any open cuts or sores on body.
3. With RA evaluate joints for swelling, nodularity, ROM/mobility, pain, warmth.
4. Determine any evidence of diabetes, HIV, HBV, any type of cancer, seizures, numbness or tingling, or disease that affects the nervous system such as multiple sclerosis, heart failure, tuberculosis (TB), or if have been in close contact with someone with TB, or have had hepatitis B; precludes drug therapy.
5. Test for TB before starting therapy; monitor closely for S&S of TB during treatment.
6. List drugs prescribed to ensure none interact; avoid use with anakinra.
7. Review risk of lymphoma and other malignancies while receiving treatment.
8. Monitor VS, ECG, and CBC during therapy.

CLIENT/FAMILY TEACHING

1. Drug is used to help control S&S of Crohn's disease and rheumatoid arthritis (RA). Given as two separate injections (200 mg each) under the skin in abdomen or upper thigh, and at weeks 2 and 4, then with RA 200 mg every other week. If clinical response, recommended maintenance regimen is 400 mg every 4 weeks.
2. Cimzia affects your immune system; can lower ability of the immune system to fight infections. Some have not survived severe infections during therapy.

3. **Report any S&S of URI, UTI, or joint pains (e.g., fever, cough, non-healing wounds, SOB).**
4. **Avoid immunizations with live vaccines.**
5. **Practice reliable contraception.**
6. **Keep all F/U to assess response, labs, adverse SE.**

OUTCOMES/EVALUATE

- **Control of S&S of Crohn's disease e.g., ↓ abdominal pain, diarrhea, vomiting, fever, and weight loss**
- **Improvement in S&S of rheumatoid arthritis e.g., ↓ swelling, pain, and ↑ROM**

Cetirizine hydrochloride

(seh-**TIH**-rah-zeen)

Classification(s): Antihistamine, second generation, piperazine

Pregnancy Category: B

OTC: All Day Allergy Children's, Zyrtec Allergy, Zyrtec Children's Allergy, Zyrtec Children's Hives Relief, Zyrtec Hives Relief.

Rx: Apo-Cetirizine, Reactine.

SEE ALSO ***ANTIHISTAMINES.***

INDICATIONS/USES

(1) Relief of itching due to urticaria in adults and children. The drug will not prevent hives or an allergic skin reaction from occurring. (2) Temporary relief of runny nose, sneezing, itching of the nose or throat and/or itchy, watery eyes due to hay fever and upper respiratory allergies in adults and children. *Investigational:* Decrease the initial wheal response and pruritus associated with mosquito bites. Improve asthma symptom scores in clients with allergy-related asthma.

ACTION/KINETICS

Action

Potent H_1-receptor antagonist. Mild bronchodilator that protects against histamine-induced bronchospasm; low to negligible anticholinergic and sedative activity. No antiemetic activity.

Pharmacokinetics

Rapidly absorbed after PO administration. Food delays the time to peak serum levels but does not decrease the total amount of drug absorbed. Poorly penetrates the CNS, but high levels are distributed to the skin. **t½:** 8.3 hr (longer in elderly clients and in those with impaired liver or renal function). Excreted mostly unchanged (95%) in the urine; 10% is excreted in the feces.

CONTRAINDICATIONS

Lactation. In those hypersensitive to hydroxyzine. Use of antihistamines in children less than 2 years of age; studies are continuing for use in children, age 2–11 years.

SPECIAL CONCERNS

- **Due to possible sedation, use with caution where mental alertness is required.**
- **Consult a provider before using the syrup in children 4 years and younger and before using the tablets in children 6 years and younger.**

SIDE EFFECTS

Most Common

Somnolence, dry mouth, fatigue, pharyngitis, dizziness.

See *Antihistamines* for complete list of possible side effects. Also, possible aggressive reactions and ***convulsions.***

OVERDOSE MANAGEMENT

Symptoms: Somnolence. *Treatment:* Symptomatic and supportive. Dialysis is not effective in removing the drug from the body.

DRUG INTERACTIONS

Ritonavir ↑ AUC, elimination t½, and volume of distribution of cetirizine

HOW SUPPLIED

Capsules, Liquid-Filled: 10 mg; ***Syrup:*** 1 mg/mL; ***Tablets:*** 5 mg, 10 mg; ***Tablets, Chewable:*** 5 mg, 10 mg; ***Tablets, Oral Disintegrating:*** 10 mg.

DOSAGE

CAPSULES, LIQUID-FILLED; SYRUP; TABLETS; TABLETS, CHEWABLE; TABLETS, ORAL DISINTEGRATING

Urticaria, upper respiratory allergies, hay fever.

Adults and children, 6 years and older: 5–10 mg (5–10 mL of the syrup) once daily, depending on the severity of symptoms, not to exceed 10 mL (10 mg) in 24 hr. **Children, 2–young-**

er than 6 years of age: 2.5 mg (2.5 mL of the syrup) once daily. The dose can be increased to a maximum of 5 mg once daily or 2.5 mg q 12 hr of the syrup. **Elderly, 65 years of age and older:** 5 mL (5 mg) once daily. **Maximum dose:** 10 mg/day for adults and children 6 years and older and 5 mg/day (5 mL/day of the syrup) for children, aged 2–6 years of age.

Bronchial asthma.

Adults and children 12 years and older: 10–20 mg/day.

NURSING IMPLICATIONS

Do not confuse Zyrtec with Zyprexa (olanzapine, an antipsychotic) or Zyrtec with Zantac (ranitidine, an H_2-receptor blocker). Do not confuse Zyrtec with Zyrtec-D 12 Hour (contains pseudoephedrine hydrochloride with cetirizine).

IMPLEMENTATION/ADMINISTRATION/STORAGE

1. Consult a provider before using in clients with impaired renal and/or hepatic function; dosage adjustment should be considered.
2. Store capsules, syrup, and tablets from 20–25°C (68–77°F).

ASSESSMENT

1. Note onset, clinical presentation, and characteristics of allergic symptoms (e.g., rhinitis, nasal congestion, sneezing, itching, watery eyes); identify triggers.
2. Assess for hypersensitivity to hydroxyzine. Check lung sounds and respiratory status; note any increase in secretions, wheezing, breathing rate.
3. List other drugs prescribed; drug is highly protein bound. Monitor for adverse drug interactions.
4. Assess VS, I&O, renal and LFTs; assess for dysfunction.

CLIENT/FAMILY TEACHING

1. May take with or without food; can vary time of administration based on need. Food will decrease stomach upset. Syrup available for pediatric dosing.
2. Use caution when performing activities that require mental alertness until drug effects realized; may cause drowsiness/sedation. Stop drug and report persistent dizziness or excessive drowsiness.
3. May cause dry mouth, fatigue; report adverse effects that prevent taking medications. Increase fluid intake to thin secretions.
4. Avoid alcohol/CNS depressants, and other OTC antihistamines.
5. Stop drug and report any behavioral changes, aggressiveness, or evidence of seizures.
6. Do not take cetirizine for at least 4 days before allergy skin testing scheduled.
7. Review allergens that trigger symptoms, e.g., ragweed, dust mites, molds, animal dander, etc., and how to control/avoid contact.
8. Keep all F/U to assess response and for adverse SE.

OUTCOMES/EVALUATE

- ↓ Itching with idiopathic urticaria
- Relief of runny nose, sneezing, itching of nose/throat, watery eyes R/T hay fever

Combination Drug

Cetirizine hydrochloride and Pseudoephedrine hydrochloride

(seh-**TIH**-rah-zeen, soo-doh-eh-**FED**-rin)

Classification(s): Antihistamine/Decongestant

Pregnancy Category: C

OTC: Zyrtec-D 12 Hour.

SEE ALSO ***CETIRIZINE HYDROCHLORIDE*** AND ***PSEUDOEPHEDRINE HYDROCHLORIDE.***

INDICATIONS/USES

Relief of nasal and non-nasal symptoms associated with seasonal or perennial allergic rhinitis in adults and children 12 years of age and older.

CONTENT

Cetirizine (antihistamine): 5 mg in an immediate-release layer and *pseudoephedrine (decongestant):* 120 mg in an extended-release layer.

ACTION/KINETICS

Action

Cetirizine, an antihistamine, selectively inhibits histamine H_1-receptors. Pseudoephedrine, a sympathomimetic amine, produces direct stimulation of both alpha- and beta-adrenergic receptors, as well as indirect stimulation through release of norepinephrine from storage sites, resulting in a decongestant effect on the nasal mucosa.

C

Pharmacokinetics

Mean peak plasma levels, cetirizine: 2.2 hr; **pseudoephedrine:** 4.4 hr. Food has no significant effect on amount of cetirizine absorption but T_{max} was delayed 1.8 hr and C_{max} was decreased by 30%. About 55–75% of pseudoephedrine is excreted unchanged in the urine and the remainder metabolized in the liver. Moderate renal impairment and chronic liver disease increase the t½ and decrease the clearance of cetirizine. The elimination t½ and apparent total body clearance of cetirizine may be decreased in geriatric clients.

CONTRAINDICATIONS

Due to the pseudoephedrine component, use in narrow-angle glaucoma or urinary retention and in those taking MAOI therapy or within 14 days of stopping such therapy. Also, use in severe hypertension, severe coronary artery disease, or in those who have shown hypersensitivity or idiosyncrasy to product components, to adrenergic drugs, or to other drugs of similar chemical structure. Use with alcohol or other CNS depressants due to additive decreased alertness and impaired CNS performance. Use during lactation is not recommended. Use of decongestants and antihistamines are not recommended for use in children less than 12 years of age.

SPECIAL CONCERNS

- **Use with caution in those with hypertension, diabetes mellitus, ischemic heart disease, increased intraocular pressure, hyperthyroidism, renal impairment, or prostatic hypertrophy.**
- **Use with caution with other sympathomimetic amines; the combined CV effects may be harmful.**

SIDE EFFECTS

Most Common

Insomnia, dry mouth, fatigue, somnolence, pharyngitis, epistaxis, accidental injury, dizziness.
See *Cetirizine hydrochloride* and *Pseudoephedrine hydrochloride*, for the complete list of possible side effects.

DOSAGE

TABLETS

Seasonal or allergic rhinitis.

Adults and children, 12 years and older: One tablet 2 times per day.

NURSING IMPLICATIONS

Ⓢ Do not confuse Zyrtec-D 12 Hour with Zyrtec (contains only cetirizine hydrochloride).

IMPLEMENTATION/ADMINISTRATION/STORAGE

Give a lower initial dose (1 tablet/day) with decreased renal function (C_{CR} 11–31 mL/min), those on hemodialysis (C_{CR} <7 mL/min), and with hepatic impairment.

ASSESSMENT

1. **Note reasons for therapy, characteristics of allergic S&S (e.g., rhinitis, nasal congestion, sneezing, itching, watery eyes); identify triggers. Identify other agents trialed, triggers/seasons if known.**
2. **List drugs prescribed to ensure none interact.**
3. **Assess for hypersensitivity to hydroxyzine. Check lung sounds and respiratory status; note any increase in secretions, wheezing, breathing rate.**
4. **Note any CAD, HTN, BPH or other conditions that may preclude therapy.**
5. **Monitor VS, renal and LFTS; reduce dose with dysfunction.**

CLIENT/FAMILY TEACHING

1. **May be taken with or without food.**
2. **Swallow tablets whole; do not break or chew tablets.**
3. **Avoid alcohol and CNS depressants.**
4. **Do not share drugs; avoid in child <12 y.o.**
5. **May experience dizziness and drowsiness; do not perform activities that require mental alertness until drug effects realized.**
6. **Use sugarless candy or gum, ice chips, or a saliva substitute for dry mouth effects.**
7. **Keep all F/U to assess response and for adverse SE.**

OUTCOMES/EVALUATE

Relief of seasonal allergy symptoms and congestion

■ IV

Cetuximab

(seh-**TUX**-ih-mab)

Classification(s): Antineoplastic, monoclonal antibody

Pregnancy Category: C

RX: Erbitux.

INDICATIONS/USES

(1) Alone to treat epidermal growth factor receptor-expressing metastatic colorectal cancer after failure of both irinotecan- and oxaliplatin-based treatments. (2) Alone to treat epidermal growth factor receptor-expressing metastatic colorectal cancer in those intolerant to irinotecan-based regimens. (3) In combination with irinotecan to treat epidermal growth factor receptor (EGFR)-expressing, metastatic colorectal carcinoma in those who are refractory to irinotecan-based chemotherapy. (4) In combination with radiation for the initial treatment of locally or regionally advanced squamous cell carcinoma of the head and neck.
(5) Alone to treat recurrent or metastatic squamous cell carcinoma of the head and neck when prior platinum-based therapy has failed.

ACTION/KINETICS

Action

Cetuximab is a recombinant, human/mouse chimeric monoclonal antibody that binds specifically to the extracellular domain of the human epidermal growth factor receptor (EGFR) on normal and tumor cells; it competitively inhibits the binding of epidermal growth factor and other ligands (e.g., transforming growth factor-alpha). Binding of cetuximab to the EGFR blocks phosphorylation and activation of receptor-associated kinases; this results in inhibition of cell growth, induction of apoptosis, and decreased matrix metalloproteinase and vascular endothelial growth factor production. Over-expression of EGFR is noted in many human cancers, including the colon and rectum. Thus, cetuximab inhibits growth and survival of tumor cells that over-express the EGFR. Addition of irinotecan or irinotecan plus 5-fluorouracil increases the antitumor effects.

Pharmacokinetics

Steady state is reached by the third weekly infusion. **t½, terminal:** 112 hr (range: 63 to 230 hr). **Mean steady state t½:** 114 hr.

CONTRAINDICATIONS

Use during lactation and for 60 days following the last dose of cetuximab.

SPECIAL CONCERNS

(1) **Infusion reactions.** Severe infusion reactions occurred with the administration of cetuximab in approximately 3% of clients in clinical trials, with fatal outcomes reported in less than 1 in 1,000. Immediately interrupt and permanently discontinue cetuximab infusion for serious infusion reactions. (2) **Cardiopulmonary arrest.** Cardiopulmonary arrest and/or sudden death occurred in 2% of 208 clients with squamous cell carcinoma of the head and neck treated with radiation therapy and cetuximab. Closely monitor serum electrolytes, including serum magnesium, potassium, and calcium, during and after cetuximab administration.

- **Use with caution in clients with known hypersensitivity to cetuximab, murine proteins, or any component of the product.**
- **Safety and efficacy not established in children.**

SIDE EFFECTS

Most Common

Acneform rash, dry skin, mucositis, leukopenia, radiation dermatitis, nail changes, abdominal pain, anorexia, xerostomia, dysphagia, asthenia, malaise, N&V, constipation, diarrhea, fever, headache, dehydration, weight loss, pharyngitis, dyspnea, infection without neutropenia.

Side effects include those for all uses of cetuximab. **GI:** Diarrhea, N&V, xerostomia, abdominal pain, anorexia, constipation, mucositis, stomatitis, dyspepsia, dysphagia. **CV:** ***Cardiopulmonary arrest.*** **Dermatologic:** Acneform rash (including acne, dry skin, exfoliative dermatitis, maculopapular rash, pustular rash, or rash), alopecia, skin disorder, pruritus, increased hair growth, nail changes, desquamation, radiation dermatitis, photosensitivity. **CNS:** Headache, insomnia, depression, confusion, anxiety. **Respiratory:** Dyspnea, pharyngitis, increased cough, ***interstitial lung disease, pulmonary embolus***, SOB. **Hematologic:** Leukopenia, anemia. **Musculoskeletal:** Back/bone pain. **Metabolic:** Weight loss, peripheral edema, dehydration. **Infusion reactions:** Bronchospasm, pyrexia, chills, rigors, stridor, hoarseness, dyspnea, ***bronchospasm***, angioedema, urticaria, hyper-/hypotension, ***cardiac arrest.*** **Body as a whole:** Asthenia/malaise, chills, rigors, fatigue, fever, pain, infections, hypersensitivity reactions, dehydration, peripheral edema, infection without neutropenia, ***sepsis***, electrolyte abnormalities (hypomagnesemia, hypocalcemia, hypokalemia). **Miscellaneous:** Application site reaction, conjunctivitis, renal failure, immunogenicity.

C

LABORATORY TEST CONSIDERATIONS

Hypomagnesemia (may be severe).

HOW SUPPLIED

Injection: 2 mg/mL.

DOSAGE

IV INFUSION

Metastatic colorectal carcinoma.

Initial, either alone or withirinotecan: 400 mg/m^2 given as a 120 min IV infusion (maximum infusion rate, 10 mg/min). **Maintenance, either alone or with irinotecan:** 250 mg/m^2 weekly infused over 60 minutes (maximum infusion rate, 10 mg/min) until disease progression or unacceptable side effects occur.

With radiation therapy for locally or regionally advanced squamous cell cancer of the head and neck.

Initial loading dose: 400 mg/m^2 given as a 120 min IV infusion (maximum infusion rate 10 mg/min) 1 week prior to initiation of a course of radiation therapy. **Weekly maintenance dose (all other infusions):** 250 mg/m^2 infused over 60 min (maximum infusion rate 10 mg/min) for the duration of radiation therapy (6–7 weeks). Complete cetuximab administration 1 hr before radiation therapy.

Monotherapy to treat recurrent or metastatic squamous cell carcinoma of the head and neck.

Initial: 400 mg/m^2 as a 120 min infusion (maximum infusion rate: 10 mg/min). **Maintenance:** 250 mg/m^2 infused per week over 60 min (maximum infusion rate: 10 mg/min) until disease progression or unacceptable toxicity.

NURSING IMPLICATIONS

IMPLEMENTATION/ADMINISTRATION/STORAGE

1. **IV** Do not give as IV push or bolus; give as a 60 or 120 min (depending on whether given alone or with other therapy) IV infusion using an infusion pump or syringe pump. Do not exceed an infusion rate of 10 mg/min.
2. Premedicate with an H_1-histamine antagonist (e.g., 50 mg diphenhydramine IV 30–60 min before the first dose). For subsequent cetuximab doses, base premedication on clinical judgment and presence and/or severity of prior infusion reactions.
3. Give using a low protein-binding 0.22 micrometer in-line filter. The solution should be clear and colorless but may contain a small amount of easily visible, white, amorphous cetuximab particles. Do not shake or dilute.
4. Reduce the infusion rate by 50% for NCI Common Toxicity Criteria grade 1 or 2 and nonserious NCI Common Toxicity Criteria 3 to 4 infusion reactions. Immediately discontinue (permanently) for serious infusion reactions requiring medical intervention and/or hospitalization.
5. If a client experiences severe acneform rash (NCI Common Toxicity Criteria grade 3 or 4, adjust treatment according to the following guidelines:
   - **First occurrence of acneform rash:** Delay infusion 1–2 weeks. If improvement, continue at 250 mg/m^2; if no improvement, discontinue cetuximab.
   - **Second occurrence of acneform rash:** Delay infusion 1–2 weeks. If improvement, reduce dose to 200 mg/m^2; if no improvement, discontinue cetuximab.
   - **Third occurrence of acneform rash:** Delay infusion 1–2 weeks; If improvement, reduce dose to 150 mg/m^2; if no improvement, discontinue cetuximab.
   - **Fourth occurrence of acneform rash:** Discontinue cetuximab.
6. Refrigerate vials from 2–8°C (36–46°F). Increased particulate formation may occur at temperatures at/below 0°C (32°F).
7. Product contains no preservatives. Preparations in infusion containers are chemically and physically stable for up to 12 hr at 2–8°C (36–46°F) and up to 8 hr from 20–25°C (68–77°F). Discard any remaining solution in the infusion container after 8 hr at controlled room temperature or after 12 hr of refrigeration. Discard any unused portion of the vial.

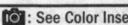

8. COMPATIBILITY NSS to flush; do not dilute.
9. INCOMPATIBILITY Administer separately.

ASSESSMENT

1. Note disease onset, reasons for therapy: combination therapy for immunohistochemical evidence of positive EGFR expression, or irinotecan-based refractory/intolerance for EGFR expressing colorectal cancer.
2. Only to be prescribed by those experienced in this therapy. Follow guidelines for dose modifications, for infusion reactions, dermatologic and related disorder toxicities as directed.
3. Premedicate with an H_1-histamine antagonist (e.g., 50 mg diphenhydramine IV 30–60 min before the first dose).
4. Monitor during and for 1 hr following each infusion for S&S of infusion reaction (e.g., bronchospasm, hives, hoarseness, hypotension, stridor).
5. Closely monitor serum electrolytes, including calcium, magnesium, and potassium, during and after therapy to prevent cardiopulmonary arrest. After initial dose, therapy usually administered once a week. Assess/monitor CBC, CXR, renal and LFTs, VS/I&O, worsening of pulmonary status, skin infections/reactions, infusion reactions.

CLIENT/FAMILY TEACHING

1. Drug used to treat colorectal cancers; may cause a variety of adverse reactions. All must be reported immediately so that dosage/therapy can be adjusted/stopped.
2. Any unusual events should be immediately reported as therapy may be fatal. SOB, wheezing, skin reactions, rash, itching, nail disorders, diarrhea, dehydration, chest pain require immediate attention.
3. Use precautions if sunlight exposed; may cause skin reactions; use hats, sunscreen, clothes to cover extremities during and for 2 months following therapy.
4. Practice reliable contraception (males and females) during and 6 mo following therapy; drug is toxic to developing fetus and may cause loss of pregnancy.
5. Keep all F/U so that any potential problems can be addressed, labs monitored, and therapy stopped or adjusted as needed. Any severe toxicities to this therapy should render one ineligible for another course.

OUTCOMES/EVALUATE

- Inhibition of metastatic colorectal carcinoma (EGFR) in those refractory to irinotecan-based chemotherapy as single agent
- Single-agent treatment of recurrent or metastatic squamous cell carcinoma of the head and neck where prior platinum-based therapy failed

Chlorambucil (CHL)

(klor-**AM**-byou-sill)

Classification(s): Antineoplastic, alkylating

Pregnancy Category: D

RX: Leukeran.

SEE ALSO ***ALKYLATING AGENTS*** AND ***ANTINEOPLASTIC AGENTS***.

INDICATIONS/USES

In adults for palliative treatment of chronic lymphocytic leukemia, malignant lymphomas (including lymphosarcoma), giant follicular lymphomas, and Hodgkin's disease. *Investigational:* (1) Ovarian and testicular carcinoma, non-Hodgkin's lymphoma, Waldenström macroglobulinemia, polycythemia vera. (2) Has been used safely and effectively in children with chronic lymphocytic leukemia, lymphomas, and nephrotic syndrome.

ACTION/KINETICS

Action

Cell-cycle nonspecific; cytotoxic to nonproliferating cells and has immunosuppressant activity. Forms an unstable ethylenimmonium ion that binds (alkylates) with intracellular substances such as nucleic acids. The cytotoxic effect is due to cross-linking of strands of DNA and RNA and inhibition of protein synthesis.

Pharmacokinetics

Rapidly and completely absorbed from the GI tract. **Peak plasma levels:** 1 hr. **t½, terminal:** 1.5 hr. Extensively metabolized by the liver; at least one metabolite is active. Fifteen to 60% is excreted through the urine 24 hr after drug administration; 40% is bound to tissues, including fat. **Plasma protein binding:** 99%, specifically to albumin.

CONTRAINDICATIONS

Resistance to the drug, hypersensitivity. Lactation.

SPECIAL CONCERNS

Chlorambucil can severely suppress bone marrow function. Chlorambucil is carcinogenic in humans. Chlorambucil may be both mutagenic and teratogenic in humans. Chlorambucil produces human infertility.

- May be cross-hypersensitivity with other alkylating agents.
- Although used in children, safety and efficacy not established.

SIDE EFFECTS

Most Common

Bone marrow suppression, N&V, changes in menses.

GI: N&V, diarrhea, oral ulceration (all infrequently). **Hepatic:** Hepatotoxicity with jaundice. **Pulmonary:** ***Pulmonary fibrosis***, bronchopulmonary dysplasia. **CNS:** Children with nephrotic syndrome and those receiving high doses have an increased risk of seizures. Tremors, confusion, agitation, ataxia, hallucinations. **Musculoskeletal:** Muscle twitching, myoclonia, flaccid paresis. **GU:** Impaired fertility in males and females. **Hematologic:** Lymphopenia, leukemia. **Hypersensitivity:** Skin rash progressing to erythema multiforme, ***toxic epidermal necrolysis, Stevens-Johnson syndrome***. Urticaria, angioedema. **Miscellaneous:** Keratitis, drug fever, sterile cystitis, interstitial pneumonia, peripheral neuropathy, secondary malignancies. Cross-sensitivity (skin rashes) may occur with other alkylating agents.

LABORATORY TEST CONSIDERATIONS

↑ Uric acid levels in serum and urine.

OVERDOSE MANAGEMENT

Symptoms: Pancytopenia (reversible), ataxia, agitated behavior, ***clonic-tonic seizures***. *Treatment:* General supportive measures. Monitor blood profiles carefully; blood transfusions may be required. Not dialyzable.

HOW SUPPLIED

Tablets: 2 mg.

DOSAGE

TABLETS

Chronic lymphocytic leukemia or lymphomas.

Individualized according to response of client. **Adults, initial:** 0.1–0.2 mg/kg (or 4–10 mg) daily in single or divided doses for 3–6 weeks. Those with Hodgkin's disease usually require 0.2 mg/kg/day while those with other lymphomas or chronic lymphocytic leukemia usually require only 0.1 mg/kg/day. When lymphocytic infiltration of the bone marrow occurs or when the bone marrow is hypoplastic, do not exceed a daily dose of 0.1 mg/kg (i.e., about 6 mg/day for the average client). **Maintenance:** 0.03–0.1 mg/kg/day (2–4 mg/day) depending on blood counts.

Pulse dosage for chronic lymphocytic leukemia.

Adults, initial: 0.4 mg/kg as a single dose; **then,** repeat this dose biweekly or monthly increasing by 0.1 mg/kg until either toxicity or lymphocytosis is observed.

Children: Chronic lymphocytic leukemia (investigational).

Children, remission induction: 0.1–0.2 mg/kg/day (4–10 mg/day) for 3–6 weeks. As an alternative, 4.5 mg/m^2/day may be given. **Maintenance:** 0.03–0.1 mg/kg/day. Doses of 2–4 mg are typical. Pulse dosage may also be used, initially with a single dose of 0.4 mg/kg. Doses are then given at biweekly or monthly intervals, increasing by 0.1 mg/kg increments until lymphocytosis or toxicity occurs. Subsequent doses are modified to cause mild hematologic toxicity.

Children: Hodgkin's disease, non-Hodgkin lymphoma, Nephrotic syndrome (all investigational).

Children. Hodgkin's disease: 0.2 mg/kg/day. **Non-Hodgkin's lymphoma:** 0.1 mg/kg/day. **Nephrotic syndrome:** 0.1–0.2 mg/kg/day for 5–15 weeks given in combination with prednisone.

NURSING IMPLICATIONS

Do not confuse Alkeran (melphalan), Leukeran (chlorambucil), and Myleran (busulfan), each of which is an antineoplastic.

IMPLEMENTATION/ADMINISTRATION/STORAGE

1. The drug is cytotoxic; thus, follow safe handling procedures when preparing, administering, or dispensing chlorambucil. depending on client response and must be decreased as soon as there is an abrupt fall in WBCs.
2. Dosage must be carefully controlled
3. Short courses of treatment are safer than continuous maintenance therapy. Continuous therapy may give the appearance of 'maintenance' in those who are actually in remission and thus have no need for the drug.
4. Dosage adjustment may be necessary in those with more severe renal impairment according to the following: C_{CR} 50 mL/min or more: Give 100% of usual dose; C_{CR} 10–50 mL/min: Give 75% of the usual dose; C_{CR} <10 mL/min: Give 50% of the usual dose; Hemodialysis or Peritoneal dialysis: Give 50% of the usual dose with no supplemental dosing needed.
5. Store at 15–25°C (59–77°F) in a dry place.

ASSESSMENT

1. List reasons for therapy, noting pretreatment lab and physical assessment findings (weight, spleen size, VS, and extent of disease). List other agents trialed/outcome.
2. Note any recent XRT, chemotherapy, seizure disorder, or if pregnant.
3. Document total cumulative dose. Monitor for S&S of infection. If WBC drops use caution and if platelet drops assess for evidence of bleeding.
4. Caution drug has carcinogenic properties, generally not for use with conditions other than chronic lymphatic leukemia or malignant lymphomas.
5. Monitor CXR, PFTs, CBC, liver and renal function studies, uric acid levels; adjust dose with renal dysfunction. Drug may cause severe granulocyte and lymphocyte suppression. Nadir: 21 days; recovery: 42–56 days.

CLIENT/FAMILY TEACHING

1. Take 1 hr before breakfast, 2 hr after the evening meal or at bedtime to reduce N&V. Take antiemetics as prescribed.
2. Will not receive a full dosage before 4 wk after a full course of radiation therapy or chemotherapy because of bone marrow vulnerability to damage.
3. Consume 2–3 L/day of fluids to prevent dehydration and decrease urate crystals; may be prescribed allopurinol to control.
4. Report side effects: bruising, bleeding, stomach/joint pains, breathing difficulty, seizures, altered gait, fever, sore throat, chills or S&S of infection. Skin rash may result from cross-sensitivity with other alkylating agents.
5. May lose hair; avoid vaccinations and crowds and persons with infections during therapy.
6. Drug is carcinogenic and may also be mutagenic and teratogenic; practice reliable birth control. Advise men that therapy may temporarily or permanently impair their fertility. Evaluate need for sperm/egg harvesting.
7. Keep all F/U to assess response, labs, and for adverse SE.

OUTCOMES/EVALUATE

- Positive tumor response evidenced by ↓ tumor size/spread; suppression of malignant cell proliferation
- Immunosuppressant activity

IV

Chloramphenicol sodium succinate

(klor-am-**FEN**-ih-kohl)

Classification(s): Antibiotic, chloramphenicol

Pregnancy Category: D

SEE ALSO ***ANTI-INFECTIVES.***

INDICATIONS/USES

Use only for serious infections for which less potentially dangerous drugs are ineffective or contraindicated. Chloramphenicol is indicated for the following serious infections. **Systemic:** (1) Acute infections due to *Salmonella typhi*. Not recommended for routine treatment of the typhoid carrier state. (2) Serious infections caused by *Salmonella, Rickettsia, Chlamydia,* and lymphogranuloma-psittacosis group. (3) Meningitis due to *Haemophilus influenzae.* (4) Various gram-negative bacteria causing bacteremia, meningitis, or other serious gram-negative infections. (5) Cystic fibrosis regimens. (6) Susceptible organisms that have been shown to be resistant to all other appropriate antimicrobial drugs.

NOTE: Chloromycetin is no longer approved for ophthalmic or otic use.

C

ACTION/KINETICS

Action

Interferes with or inhibits protein synthesis in bacteria by interfering with the transfer of activated amino acids from soluble RNA to ribosomes. Mostly bacteriostatic.

Pharmacokinetics

Highest levels are found in the liver and kidney and lowest levels in the brain and CSF. Levels are also found in pleural and ascitic fluids, saliva, milk, and in the aqueous and vitreous humors. Transport across the placental barrier occurs with somewhat lower levels in cord blood of neonates than in maternal blood. Metabolized in the liver; 75–90% excreted in urine within 24 hr, as parent drug (8–12%) and inactive metabolites.

CONTRAINDICATIONS

History of previous hypersensitivity or toxic effect. Use to treat trivial infections or where not indicated. Use to prevent bacterial infections. Lactation. Use with other drugs that may depress bone marrow.

SPECIAL CONCERNS

(1) Serious and fatal blood dyscrasias (aplastic anemia, hypoplastic anemia, thrombocytopenia, and granulocytopenia) are known to occur after the administration of chloramphenicol. In addition, there have been reports of aplastic anemia attributed to chloramphenicol that later terminated in leukemia. Blood dyscrasias have occurred after both short-term and prolonged therapy with this drug. Chloramphenicol must not be used when less potentially dangerous agents will be effective. It must not be used in the treatment of trivial infections or where it is not indicated, as in colds, influenza, infections of the throat; or as a prophylactic agent to prevent bacterial infections. (2) It is essential that adequate blood studies be made during treatment with the drug. While blood studies may detect early peripheral blood changes, such as leukopenia, reticulocytopenia, or granulocytopenia, before they become irreversible, such studies cannot be relied on to detect bone marrow depression prior to development of aplastic anemia. To facilitate appropriate studies and observation during therapy, it is desirable that clients be hospitalized.

- Use with caution in clients with intermittent porphyria or G6PD deficiency.
- Avoid repeated courses of treatment, if possible.
- Excessive blood levels may occur in clients with impaired hepatic or renal function; adjust dosage accordingly or, determine blood levels at appropriate intervals.
- To avoid Gray syndrome, use with caution and in reduced doses in premature and full-term infants.

SIDE EFFECTS

Most Common

Headache, N&V, diarrhea.

Hematologic (most serious): ***Aplastic anemia (may end in leukemia), hypoplastic anemia***, thrombocytopenia, granulocytopenia, ***hemolytic anemia***, pancytopenia, hemoglobinuria (paroxysmal nocturnal), leukopenia, decreased reticulocytes. *Hematologic studies should be undertaken before and every 2 days during therapy.* **GI:** N&V, diarrhea, glossitis, stomatitis, unpleasant taste, enterocolitis, pruritus ani. **Allergic:** Fever, angioedema, macular and vesicular rashes, urticaria, hemorrhages of the skin, intestine, bladder, mouth; ***anaphylaxis***. **CNS:** Headache, delirium, confusion, mild depression. **Neurologic:** Optic and peripheral neuritis usually after long-term use. **Body as a whole:** Superinfection.

NOTE: Premature infants and neonates should be observed closely, since the drug accumulates in the bloodstream and the infant is thus subject to greater hazards of toxicity (including the Gray syndrome).

DRUG INTERACTIONS

Anticoagulants, oral / ↑ Anticoagulant effect R/T ↓ liver breakdown

Antidiabetics, oral (e.g., sulfonylureas) / ↑ Hypoglycemic effect R/T ↓ liver breakdown

Barbiturates / ↑ Barbiturate effect R/T ↓ liver breakdown; also, ↓ serum chloramphenicol levels

Bone marrow depressants / ↑ Bone marrow depression; do not use together

Cyclophosphamide / Delayed or ↓ activation of cyclophosphamide

Iron preparations / ↑ Serum levels of iron

Penicillins / Either ↑ or ↓ effect when combined to treat certain microorganisms

Phenytoin (and other hydantoins) / ↑ Phenytoin effect R/T ↓ liver breakdown; also, chloramphenicol levels may be ↑ or ↓

Rifampin / ↓ Chloramphenicol effect R/T ↑ liver breakdown
Tacrolimus / ↑ Tacrolimus blood levels R/T ↓ liver breakdown
Vitamin B_{12} / ↓ Vitamin B_{12} response when treating pernicious anemia

HOW SUPPLIED

Powder for Injection: 100 mg/mL when reconstituted.

DOSAGE

IV ONLY

Serious infections.

Adults: 50 mg/kg/day in four equally divided doses q 6 hr. Can be increased to 100 mg/kg/day in severe infections, but dosage should be reduced as soon as possible. **Infants and children:** 50 mg/kg/day in divided doses q 6 hr. Severe infections (e.g., bacteremia, meningitis) may require doses up to 100 mg/kg/day; however, reduce the dose to 50 mg/kg/day as soon as possible. **Infants and children with suspected immature metabolic function:** 25 mg/kg/day. Carefully follow blood levels. **Neonates, usual:** 25 mg/kg/day in divided doses q 6 hr. Increased dosage should be given as determined by severity of the infection but only to maintain blood levels within a therapeutically effective range. After the first 2 weeks of life, full-term neonates may receive up to a total of 50 mg/kg/day in divided doses at 6 hr intervals. *NOTE:* Carefully follow dosage for premature and newborn infants less than 2 weeks of age because blood levels differ significantly from those of other age groups.

NURSING IMPLICATIONS

IMPLEMENTATION/ADMINISTRATION/STORAGE

1. IV Administer IV as a 10% solution over at least a 60 sec interval by reconstituting 1 gram in 10 mL of water for injection or D5W.
2. Change clients started on IV chloramphenicol to the PO form of another appropriate antibiotic as soon as practical.
3. Store from 15–25°C (59–77°F).
4. COMPATIBILITY Water for injection or D5W.
5. INCOMPATIBILITY Administer separately.

ASSESSMENT

1. Note hypersensitivity/previous reaction to other agents. Assess for acute intermittent porphyria or G6PD deficiency.
2. List reasons/type of therapy, symptom characteristics, culture results, other agents prescribed. If receiving drugs that cause bone marrow depression, do not use chloramphenicol.
3. If nursing, transmission of drug to breast milk can result in infant also receiving drug; infants have underdeveloped capacity to metabolize chloramphenicol.
4. If taking oral hypoglycemic agents, may need insulin during therapy.
5. Note drugs that enhance chloramphenicol; monitor closely for evidence of severe toxicity. Avoid repeated courses of therapy; drug is highly toxic.
6. Monitor for any of the following and report:
   - *Bone marrow depression* characterized by weakness, fatigue, sore throat, bleeding.
   - *Optic neuritis* characterized by reduced visual acuity bilaterally.
   - *Peripheral neuritis* characterized by pain/sensation disturbance.
   - Development of *Gray syndrome* in premature and newborn infants, characterized by rapid respiration, failure to feed, abdominal distention with/without vomiting, loose green stools, progressive cyanosis, vasomotor collapse.
7. Assess for toxic and irritative effects, such as N&V, unpleasant taste, diarrhea, perineal irritation following PO administration. Differentiation of drug-induced diarrhea from that caused by a superinfection is critical and may be accomplished by assessment and analysis of all presenting symptoms.
8. Arrange for frequent observation and hematologic studies (CBC, platelets, reticulocytes, iron q 2 days during therapy) to detect for early S&S bone marrow depression; may develop weeks to months after therapy.
9. Monitor VS, I&O, CBC, renal and LFTs; reduce dose with impaired renal and in newborn infants with immature metabolic functions to

avoid Gray syndrome toxicity. Obtain weekly serum levels.

CLIENT/FAMILY TEACHING

1. Given IV at regularly spaced intervals *around the clock;* a bitter taste may be experienced; should subside after several minutes.
2. Avoid alcohol during therapy.
3. Do not take salicylates (aspirin) or NSAIDs (Advil, Motrin).
4. Report adverse side effects, unusual bruising/bleeding, sore throat, fatigue or lack or response and in infants: failure to feed, abdominal distention, drowsiness, blue or gray skin color, or breathing problems.
5. Keep all F/U to assess response, labs, for adverse SE.

OUTCOMES/EVALUATE

- Resolution of infection
- Therapeutic drug level 10 to 20 mcg/mL (peak)

Chlordiazepoxide

(klor-dye-**AYZ**-eh-**POX**-eyed)

Classification(s): Antianxiety drug, benzodiazepine

Pregnancy Category: D

RX: Librium, **C-IV**

✦ **Rx:** Apo-Chlordiazepoxide.

SEE ALSO ***TRANQUILIZERS/ANTIMANIC DRUGS/HYPNOTICS.***

INDICATIONS/USES

PO: (1) Anxiety disorders or for short-term relief of anxiety symptoms. (2) Acute withdrawal symptoms in chronic alcoholics. (3) Preoperatively to reduce anxiety and apprehension.

ACTION/KINETICS

Pharmacokinetics

Onset: PO, 30–60 min. **Peak plasma levels (PO):** 0.5–4 hr. **Duration:** $t^{1/2}$**:** 5–30 hr. Is metabolized to four active metabolites: desmethylchlordiazepoxide, desmethyldiazepam, oxazepam, and demoxepam. Has less anticonvulsant activity and is less potent than diazepam. About 96% protein bound.

SIDE EFFECTS

Most Common

Drowsiness, ataxia, confusion, headache, blurred vision, nausea, constipation.

See *Tranquilizers, Antimanic Drugs, Hypnotics* for a complete list of possible side effects. Also, jaundice, acute hepatic necrosis, hepatic dysfunction.

LABORATORY TEST CONSIDERATIONS

↑ 17-Hydroxycorticosteroids, 17-ketosteroids, alkaline phosphatase, bilirubin, serum transaminase, porphobilinogen. ↓ PT (clients on coumarin).

HOW SUPPLIED

Capsules: 5 mg, 10 mg, 25 mg.

DOSAGE

CAPSULES

Mild to moderate anxiety.

Adults: 5 or 10 mg 3 to 4 times per day. **Children, initial:** 5 mg 2 to 4 times per day; may be increased in some children to 10 mg 2 to 3 times per day. Not recommended for children less than 6 years old. **Elderly clients or those with debilitating disease:** 5 mg 2 to 4 times per day.

Severe anxiety.

Adults: 20 or 25 mg 3 to 4 times per day. For elderly clients or those with debilitating disease give 5 mg 2 to 4 times per day.

Acute alcohol withdrawal.

50–100 mg; repeat as needed (up to 300 mg/day). Reduce dose to maintenance levels.

Preoperative apprehension and anxiety.

5–10 mg 3 or 4 times per day on days preceding surgery.

NURSING IMPLICATIONS

IMPLEMENTATION/ADMINISTRATION/STORAGE

Store capsules from 15–30°C (59–86°F).

ASSESSMENT

1. Note reasons for therapy, pretreatment symptoms, mental status, motor responses.
2. Maintain quiet, supervised environment; keep recumbent for 3 hr following parenteral administration.

3. Assess VS, CBC, renal and LFTs to R/O impairment.

CLIENT/FAMILY TEACHING

1. May take with food as directed; do not double doses if dose forgotten.
2. Consume extra fluids and bulk; minimizes constipating effects.
3. Use caution, may cause dizziness/drowsiness and sedation.
4. Do not stop drug suddenly after prolonged use, taper off over a week.
5. Avoid all OTC agents, alcohol, and any other CNS depressants.
6. Practice reliable contraception; increased risk of congenital malformations especially in first trimester.
7. Keep all F/U to assess response, labs (CBC, LFTs), and adverse SE.

OUTCOMES/EVALUATE

- ↓ Tremors; ↓ anxiety; sedation
- Termination of panic attacks
- ↓ Alcohol withdrawal symptoms

Chlorpheniramine maleate

(klor-fen-**EAR**-ah-meen)

Classification(s): Antihistamine, first generation, alkylamine

Pregnancy Category: B

OTC: Syrup: Aller-Chlor. **Tablets, Chewable:** Chlo-Amine. **Tablets:** Aller-Chlor, Allergy, Allergy Relief, Allergy-Time. **Tablets, Extended-Release:** Chlor-Trimeton Allergy 8 Hour and 12 Hour.

RX: Caplets: ED-CHLOR-TAN. **Capsules, Extended-Release/Sustained-Release:** Chlorpheniramine maleate, ODALL AR. **Oral Suspension:** Pediox-S, TanaHist PD.

SEE ALSO ***ANTIHISTAMINES***.

INDICATIONS/USES

Allergic rhinitis, including sneezing; itchy, watery eyes; itchy throat, and runny nose due to hay fever and other upper respiratory allergies.

ACTION/KINETICS

Action

Moderate anticholinergic and low sedative activity; no antiemetic activity.

Pharmacokinetics

Onset: 15–30 min. **t½:** 21–27 hr. **Time to peak effect:** 6 hr. **Duration:** 3–6 hr.

ADDITIONAL CONTRAINDICATIONS

Use in children 4 years of age or younger, although some recommend not to use in children less than 6 years of age.

SPECIAL CONCERNS

Geriatric clients may be more sensitive to the adult dose.

SIDE EFFECTS

Most Common

Constipation, diarrhea, dizziness, drowsiness, dry mouth/nose/throat, headache, anorexia, N&V, anxiety, insomnia, GI upset, asthenia.

See *Antihistamines* for a complete list of possible side effects.

HOW SUPPLIED

Caplets: 8 mg (as tannate); ***Capsules, Extended-Release/Sustained-Release:*** 8 mg, 12 mg; ***Oral Suspension:*** 2 mg/5 mL, 4 mg/5 mL; ***Syrup:*** 2 mg/5 mL; ***Tablets:*** 4 mg; ***Tablets, Chewable:*** 2 mg; ***Tablets, Extended-Release:*** 8 mg, 12 mg, 16 mg.

DOSAGE

CAPLETS

Allergic rhinitis.

Adults and children 12 years and older: 8 mg q 12 hr, up to 16–24 mg/day. **Children, 6–12 years of age:** Consult a provider.

CAPSULES, EXTENDED-RELEASE; CAPSULES, SUSTAINED-RELEASE

Allergic rhinitis.

Adults and children over 12 years: 8 or 12 mg q 12 hr, up to 16 or 24 mg/day. **Children, 6–12 years:** 8 mg at bedtime or during the day as indicated. For ODALL AR, give 12 mg once daily, up to 24 mg in 24 hr, to those age 12 and over.

C

ORAL SUSPENSION

Allergic rhinitis.

Children, over 12 years of age: 4–8 mg q 12 hr. **Children, 6–12 years of age:** 2–4 mg q 12 hr; **children, less than 2 years of age:** As directed by provider.

SYRUP; TABLETS; TABLETS, CHEWABLE

Allergic rhinitis.

Adults and children over 12 years: 4 mg q 4–6 hr, not to exceed 24 mg in 24 hr. **Pediatric, 6–12 years:** 2 mg (break 4 mg tablets in half) q 4–6 hr, not to exceed 12 mg in 24 hr. **2–6 years:** Not to be used.

TABLETS, EXTENDED-RELEASE

Allergic rhinitis.

Adults and children over 12 years: 8 mg q 8–12 hr or 12 mg q 12 hr, not to exceed 24 mg in 24 hr.

NURSING IMPLICATIONS

IMPLEMENTATION/ADMINISTRATION/STORAGE

ODALL AR contains 2 mg chlorpheniramine maleate, immediate release, and 10 mg chlorpheniramine maleate, sustained release.

ASSESSMENT

1. Note indications for therapy, other agents trialed and outcome. Attempt to identify triggers/causative agents.
2. Perform/document ENT findings; note any drainage in pharynx, pressure with sinus palpation, condition of turbinates, and any headaches. Assess lung sounds and document findings.
3. Monitor VS and caution that may alter skin testing results; stop 4 days before testing.

CLIENT/FAMILY TEACHING

1. Take as directed with a full glass of water. Food delays absorption but use if GI upset.
2. Report any mental status changes, adverse effects, or lack of response. May cause dizziness/drowsiness; use caution.
3. Avoid alcohol in any form and CNS depressants.
4. Anticipate dry mouth and use appropriate remedies.
5. Avoid excessive/prolonged sun exposure; may cause sensitivity reaction. Wear protective clothing and sunscreens until tolerance determined.
6. If scheduled for skin testing, do not take drug for at least 4 days before skin testing.
7. Keep all F/U to assess response, triggers, for adverse SE.

OUTCOMES/EVALUATE

↓ Nasal congestion and allergic manifestations

Cholestyramine resin

(koh-less-**TEER**-ah-meen)

Classification(s): Antihyperlipidemic, bile acid sequestrant

Pregnancy Category: B

RX: Cholestyramine Light, Prevalite, Questran, Questran Light.

Rx: PMS-Cholestyramine.

INDICATIONS/USES

(1) Adjunct to reduce elevated serum cholesterol in primary hypercholesterolemia in those who do not respond adequately to diet. Not indicated for those in whom hypertriglyceridemia is the abnormality of most concern. (2) Pruritus associated with partial biliary obstruction. *Investigational:* Diarrhea, *Clostridium difficile* (binds to the toxin), digitalis toxicity, adjunct to treat hyperthyroidism, hyperoxaluria.

ACTION/KINETICS

Action

Binds sodium cholate (bile salts) in the intestine; thus, the principal precursor of cholesterol is not absorbed due to formation of an insoluble complex, which is excreted in the feces. Decreases cholesterol and LDL and either has no effect or increases triglycerides, VLDL, and HDL. Also, itching is relieved as a result of removing irritating bile salts. The antidiarrheal effect results from the binding and removal of bile acids.

Pharmacokinetics

Onset, to reduce plasma cholesterol: Within 24–48 hr, but levels may continue to fall for 1 yr; **to relieve pruritus:** 1–3 weeks; **relief of diarrhea associated with bile acids:** 24 hr. Cholesterol levels return to pretreatment levels 2–4 weeks after discontinuance. Fat-soluble vitamins (A, D, K) and possibly folic acid may have to be administered IM during long-term therapy because cholestyramine binds these vitamins in the intestine.

CONTRAINDICATIONS

Complete obstruction or atresia of bile duct.

SPECIAL CONCERNS

- **Elderly may be more likely to manifest adverse GI and nutritional effects.**
- **Exercise caution in clients with phenylketonuria as Prevalite contains 14.1 mg phenylalanine per 5.5-gram dose.**
- **Use during pregnancy only if benefits outweigh risks.**
- **Use with caution during lactation and in children (long-term effects and efficacy in decreasing cholesterol levels in pediatric clients not known).**

SIDE EFFECTS

Most Common

Constipation (may be severe), aggravation of hemorrhoids, abdominal pain, bloating, vomiting, diarrhea, weight loss, flatulence, infection.

GI: Constipation (may be severe), N&V, diarrhea, heartburn, GI bleeding, anorexia, flatulence, belching, abdominal distention/pain or cramping, bloating, loose stools, indigestion, aggravation or bleeding of hemorrhoids, rectal bleeding or pain, blood in stools, bleeding duodenal ulcer, peptic ulceration, ulcer attack, GI irritation, dysphagia, dyspepsia, dental bleeding, dental caries, erosion of tooth enamel, tooth discoloration, hiccoughs, eructation, sour taste, ***pancreatitis***, diverticulitis, cholecystitis, cholelithiasis, ***intestinal obstruction*** (rare). Fecal impaction in elderly clients. Large doses may cause steatorrhea. **CNS:** Migraine/sinus headaches, dizziness, anxiety, vertigo, insomnia, fatigue, lightheadedness, syncope, drowsiness, femoral nerve pain, paresthesia. **CV:** Chest pain, angina, syncope, shortness of breath. **Hypersensitivity:** Urticaria, dermatitis, asthma, wheezing, rash. **Hematologic:** Increased PT, ecchymosis, anemia. **Musculoskeletal:** Muscle or joint pain, aches and pains in the extremities, arthritis, backache, arthritis, osteoporosis, swelling of hands/feet. **Dermatologic:** Rash, irritation of the skin, tongue, and perianal area. **GU:** Hematuria, dysuria, burnt odor to urine, diuresis. **Ophthalmic:** Uveitis. **Otic:** Tinnitus. **Body as a whole:** Edema, weakness, weight loss/gain. **Miscellaneous:** Bleeding tendencies (due to hypoprothrombinemia). Deficiencies of vitamins A and D. Uveitis, swollen glands, increased libido; hyperchloremic acidosis in children.

LABORATORY TEST CONSIDERATIONS

Liver function abnormalities.

OVERDOSE MANAGEMENT

Symptoms: GI tract obstruction.

DRUG INTERACTIONS

Anticoagulants, PO / ↓ Anticoagulant effect R/T ↓ GI tract absorption
Aspirin / ↓ Aspirin absorption from GI tract
Clindamycin / ↓ Clindamycin absorption from GI tract
Clofibrate / ↓ Clofibrate absorption from GI tract
Corticosteroids / ↓ Corticosteroid serum levels R/T ↓ GI absorption
Digoxin / ↓ Digitalis effect R/T ↓ GI tract absorption
Doxepin / ↓ Doxepin serum levels R/T ↓ GI absorption
Estrogens/Progestins / ↓ Estrogen/progestin serum levels R/T ↓ GI absorption
Furosemide / ↓ Furosemide absorption from GI tract
Gemfibrozil / ↓ Gemfibrozil bioavailability
Glipizide / ↓ Serum glipizide levels
HMG-CoA reductase inhibitors / ↓ HMG-CoA reductase inhibitor serum levels R/T ↓ GI absorption
Hydrocortisone / ↓ Hydrocortisone effect R/T ↓ GI tract absorption
Imipramine / ↓ Imipramine absorption from GI tract
Iopanoic acid / Results in abnormal cholecystography
Lovastatin / Effects may be additive
Methyldopa / ↓ Methyldopa absorption from GI tract
Mycophenolate / ↓ Mycophenolate AUC by about 40%
Nicotinic acid / ↓ Nicotinic acid absorption from GI tract
NSAIDs / ↓ NSAID serum levels R/T ↓ GI absorption
Penicillin G / ↓ Penicillin G effect R/T ↓ GI tract absorption
Phenobarbital / ↓ Phenobarbital serum levels R/T ↓ GI absorption

C

Phenytoin / ↓ Phenytoin absorption from GI tract
Phosphate supplements / ↓ Phosphate absorption from GI tract
Piroxicam / ↑ Piroxicam elimination
Propranolol / ↓ Propranolol effect R/T ↓ GI tract absorption
Tetracyclines / ↓ Tetracycline effects R/T ↓ GI tract absorption
Thiazide diuretics / ↓ Thiazide effects R/T ↓ GI tract absorption
Thyroid hormones, Thyroxine / ↓ Thyroid effects R/T ↓ GI tract absorption
Tolbutamide / ↓ Tolbutamide absorption from GI tract
Troglitazone / ↓ Troglitazone absorption from the GI tract
Ursodiol / ↓ Ursodiol effects R/T ↓ GI tract absorption
Valproic acid / ↓ Valproic acid serum levels R/T ↓ GI absorption
Verapamil, sustained-release / ↓ Verapamil, sustained-release AUC and C_{max} by about 11% and 31% respectively
Vitamins A, D, E, K / Malabsorption of fat-soluble vitamins
Vitamin C / ↑ Vitamin C absorption
NOTE: These drug interactions may also be observed with colestipol.

HOW SUPPLIED

Powder for Suspension: 4 grams/5.5 grams powder, 4 grams/5.7 grams powder, 4 grams/6.4 grams powder, 4 grams/9 grams powder.

DOSAGE

POWDER

Hypercholesterolemia; pruritus due to biliary obstruction.

Adults, initial: 4 grams 1–2 times per day, usually at mealtime. Dose is individualized. For Prevalite, give 1 packet or 1 level scoopful (5.5 grams Prevalite: 4 grams anhydrous cholestyramine). **Maintenance:** 2–4 packets or scoopfuls/day (8–16 grams anhydrous cholestyramine resin) mixed with 60–180 mL water or noncarbonated beverage. The recommended dosing schedule is 2 times per day but it can be given in one to six doses per day. Maximum daily dose: 6 packets or scoopfuls (equivalent to 24 grams cholestyramine). **Children, usual:** 240 mg/kg/day of anhydrous cholestyramine resin in 2–3 divided doses, normally not to exceed 8 grams/day; base dose titration on response and tolerance. When calculating pediatric doses, note the following content of anhydrous cholestyramine resin: 80 mg in 110 mg Prevalite, 44.4 mg in 100 mg of Questran powder, and 62.7 mg in 100 mg of Questran Light.

NURSING IMPLICATIONS

Do not confuse cholestyramine with colestipol.

IMPLEMENTATION/ADMINISTRATION/STORAGE

1. Always mix powder with 60–180 mL water or noncarbonated beverage before administering; resin may cause esophageal irritation or blockage. Highly liquid soups or pulpy fruits such as applesauce or crushed pineapple may be used. Do not take in dry form.
2. After placing contents of 1 packet of resin on the surface of 4–6 oz of fluid, allow it to stand without stirring for 2 min, occasionally twirling the glass, and then stir slowly (to prevent foaming) to form a suspension.
3. Avoid inhaling powder; may be irritating to mucous membranes.
4. Cholestyramine may interfere with the absorption of other drugs taken orally; thus, take other drug(s) 1 hr before or 4–6 hr after cholestyramine dosing.
5. In clients with pre-existing constipation, the initial dose should be 1 packet or 1 scoop once daily for 5–7 days, increasing to two times daily with monitoring of constipation and of serum lipoproteins, at least twice, 4–6 weeks apart.
6. Store powder from 15–30°C (59–86°F).

ASSESSMENT

1. List reasons for therapy (hypercholesterolemia, pruritus, diarrhea), symptom type/onset, other agents trialed.
2. Note onset of pruritus, bile acid level with cholestasis.
3. Assess skin and eyes for evidence of jaundice or bile deposits.
4. Vitamins A, D, E, K, and folic acid will need to be administered in a water-miscible form dur-

ing long-term therapy. Assess nutritional status and diet.

5. Monitor CBC, lipid profile, renal and LFTs.

CLIENT/FAMILY TEACHING

1. Other prescribed medications should be taken at least 1 hr before or 4–6 hr after taking drug. These drugs interfere with the absorption and desired effects of other medications.
2. Do not take drug in dry form; always sprinkle powder on surface of liquid (preferably milk, water or juice) and let stand a few min, then stir and drink. Avoid carbonated beverages as these cause too much foaming. Add extra fluid to bottom of glass and swirl to ensure entire dose consumed. Take before meals and at bedtime. Powder also can be mixed with highly fluid soups or pulpy fruits with high moisture content (e.g., applesauce, crushed pineapple).
3. Avoid sipping or holding the resin suspension in the mouth for prolonged periods; may lead to tooth surface changes resulting in discoloration, erosion of enamel, or decay.
4. Review constipating effects of drug and ways to control: daily exercise, fluid intake of 2.5–3 L/day, increased intake of citrus fruits, fruit juices, and high-fiber foods; also, a stool softener may help. If constipation persists, a change in dosage or drug may be indicated.
5. Clients with high cholesterol levels should follow dietary restrictions of fat and cholesterol as well as risk factor reduction such as smoking cessation, alcohol reduction, weight loss, and regular exercise.
6. Report tarry stools or abnormal bleeding as supplemental vitamin K (10 mg/week) may be necessary. CBC, PT, and renal function tests should be done routinely.
7. Itching (pruritus) may subside 1–3 weeks after taking the drug but may return after the medication is discontinued. Cornstarch or tepid oatmeal baths may also alleviate symptoms. Report any unusual bruising/bleeding or intolerable side effects.
8. Keep all F/U to assess response, labs, and for adverse SE.

OUTCOMES/EVALUATE

- Control of pruritus
- ↓ Serum cholesterol/TG levels
- ↓ Diarrheal stools
- ↓ Bile acid levels

Choriogonadotropin alfa

(**KOR**-ee-oh-goh-**nah**-dah-**troh**-pin **AL**-fah)

Classification(s): Ovarian stimulant

Pregnancy Category: X

RX: Ovidrel.

INDICATIONS/USES

(1) Induction of final follicular maturation and early luteinization in infertile women who have undergone pituitary desensitization and who have been pretreated appropriately with FSH as part of an assisted reproductive technology program (e.g., in vitro fertilization and embryo transfer). (2) For the induction of ovulation and pregnancy in anovulatory infertile clients where the cause of infertility is functional and not due to primary ovarian failure.

ACTION/KINETICS

Action

The physicochemical, biologic, and immunologic effects of recombinant choriogonadotropin (hCG) are comparable to those of hCG derived from placental and human pregnancy urine. hCG stimulates late follicular maturation and resumption of oocyte meiosis and initiates rupture of the preovulatory ovarian follicle. Choriogonadotropin alfa binds to the LH/hCG receptor of the granulosa and theca cells of the ovary and initiates its effects in the absence of an endogenous LH surge. Choriogonadotropin alfa is given when sufficient follicular development has occurred following FSH treatment for ovulation induction.

Pharmacokinetics

Maximum serum levels: 12–24 hr. **$t^{1/2}$, distribution, initial:** About 4.5 hr; **$t^{1/2}$ terminal:** About 29 hr.

CONTRAINDICATIONS

Hypersensitivity to hCG products and their components; primary ovarian failure; uncontrolled thyroid or adrenal dysfunction; uncontrolled organic intracranial lesions (e.g., pituitary tumor); abnormal uterine bleeding of undetermined origin; ovarian cyst or enlargement of undetermined origin; sex-hormone-dependent tumors of the reproductive tract and accessory organs; pregnancy.

SPECIAL CONCERNS

- **Ovarian enlargement, ovarian hyperstimulation syndrome, or multiple births may occur.**
- **Use with caution during lactation.**

C

SIDE EFFECTS

Most Common

When used for assisted reproductive technology: Injection site pain/bruising, abdominal pain, N&V, GI system disorder, post-operative pain. **When used for induction of ovulation:** Injection site pain/bruising/inflammation, ovarian cyst/hyperstimulation, abdominal pain.

Ovarian enlargement: Abdominal distention/pain. **Ovarian hyperstimulation syndrome:** Increase in vascular permeability resulting in rapid accumulation of fluid in the peritoneal cavity, thorax, and potentially the pericardium. Early warning signs include severe pelvic pain, N&V, weight gain. Symptoms include abdominal pain/distention, N&V, diarrhea, severe ovarian enlargement, weight gain, dsypnea, oliguria. Also, hypovolemia, hemoconcentration, electrolyte imbalances, ascites, hemoperitoneum, pleural effusions, hydrothorax, ***acute pulmonary distress, thromboembolism***.

Side effects when used for assisted reproductive technology: GI: GI system disorder, abdominal pain, N&V, flatulence, diarrhea, hiccough. **GU:** Ectopic pregnancy, intermenstrual bleeding, breast pain, vaginal hemorrhage, cervical lesion, ovarian hyperstimulation, leukorrhea, uterine disorders, vaginitis, vaginal discomfort, UTI, urinary incontinence, dysuria, albuminuria, genital moniliasis, genital herpes, cervical carcinoma. **CNS:** Dizziness, headache, paresthesias, emotional lability, insomnia. **Respiratory:** URTI, cough. **CV:** Cardiac arrhythmias, heart murmur. **At injection site:** Pain/bruising. **Miscellaneous:** Body/back pain, fever, hot flashes, malaise, leukocytosis.

Side effects when used for induction of ovulation. At injection site: Pain, bruising, inflammation. **GU:** Ovarian cyst, ovarian hyperstimulation, breast pain. **GI:** Abdominal pain, GI system disorders, flatulence, abdominal enlargement. **Respiratory:** URTI, pharyngitis. **Miscellaneous:** Hyperglycemia, pruritus.

Side effects in pregnancies resulting from HCG therapy. Spontaneous abortion, ectopic pregnancy, premature labor, postpartum fever, congenital abnormalities.

HOW SUPPLIED

Prefilled Syringes, Single-Dose: 250 mcg/0.5 mL.

DOSAGE

SC

Infertile women undergoing assisted reproductive technology; Induction of ovulation in infertile women.

250 mcg 1 day following the last dose of FSH. Do not give until adequate follicular development is confirmed by serum estradiol and vaginal ultrasonography. Withhold when there is an excessive ovarian response as indicated by clinically significant ovarian enlargement or excessive estradiol production.

NURSING IMPLICATIONS

IMPLEMENTATION/ADMINISTRATION/STORAGE

1. Give as single SC injection following reconstitution with 1 mL sterile water for injection. Use immediately after reconstitution.
2. Discard any unused reconstituted drug.
3. Vials for reconstitution may be stored refrigerated or at room temperature. Protect from light.
4. Store prefilled syringes at 2–8°C before dispensing to clients; syringes may then be stored at temperatures not exceeding 25°C for up to 30 days.

ASSESSMENT

1. List reasons for therapy: induction of ovulation or for in vitro fertilization program, symptom onset, clinical presentation.
2. Document thorough gynecologic exam, pelvic anatomy, and endocrinologic evaluation. Ensure not pregnant and note partners fertility.
3. Note any drug sensitivity. Ensure FSH treatment for ovulation induction.
4. Assess for any pituitary or sex hormone dependent tumors; uncontrolled thyroid or adrenal dysfunction or abnormal uterine bleeding as these preclude therapy.
5. Obtain estradiol levels and vaginal ultrasound to assess follicular development. If levels too high or follicles significantly enlarged, hold therapy.

CLIENT/FAMILY TEACHING

1. Review reasons for therapy and anticipated results.
2. Follow self administration guideline pamphlet once initial injection done in office. May cause pain at injection site.
3. Record basal body temperature to determine if ovulation has occurred. Record daily weights. Report edema, which is common.
4. If ovulation determined (slight ↓ temperature then sharp ↑ for ovulation) attempt intercourse 3 days before and every other day until after ovulation.
5. Delayed menses, excessive menstrual bleeding, pain in the lower abdomen, weakness/fatigue are S&S of ectopic pregnancy; report immediately.
6. Be prepared, may experience multiple births.
7. Therapy requires long-term commitment.
8. Report headache, SOB, easy fatigue, restlessness; if increasingly irritable, depressed, and changes in attention to physical appearance occur, may have to stop drug.
9. Some pregnancies may result in abortion or birth defects.
10. Keep all F/U to assess response, labs, ultrasound, and adverse SE.

OUTCOMES/EVALUATE

Ovulation with desired pregnancy

Ciclesonide

(sye-**KLES**-oh-nide)

Classification(s): Glucocorticoid

Pregnancy Category: C

RX: Alvesco, Omnaris.

SEE ALSO ***CORTICOSTEROIDS***.

INDICATIONS/USES

Alvesco, Inhalation Aerosol: Prophylaxis and treatment of asthma in adults and adolescents 12 years and older. **Omnaris, Intranasal Suspension:** (1) Treatment of nasal symptoms associated with perennial allergic rhinitis in adults and adolescents, 12 years and older. (2) Treatment of nasal symptoms associated with seasonal allergic rhinitis in adults and children 6 years of age and older.

ACTION/KINETICS

Action

Precise mechanism unknown. Corticosteroids have a wide range of effects on multiple cell types and various mediators involved in allergic inflammation. The effect on adrenal function is not known.

Pharmacokinetics

Ciclesonide is a prodrug that is enzymatically hydrolyzed (by esterases in the nasal mucosa) to the active metabolite, des-ciclesonide, after inhalation. A small amount is absorbed systemically. Is metabolized in the liver mainly by CYP3A4 and to a lesser extent by CYP2D6. Most excreted in the feces (60%) with small amounts (20% or less) excreted in the urine. **Plasma protein binding:** 99%.

CONTRAINDICATIONS

Hypersensitivity to the drug or any component of the product. Use following recent nasal septal ulcers, recurrent epistaxis, or nasal surgery or trauma until healing has occurred.

SPECIAL CONCERNS

- Use with caution during lactation.
- Safety and efficacy not determined in children less than 12 years.

SIDE EFFECTS

Most Common

Inhalation Aerosol (Alvesco): Headache, nasopharyngitis, sinusitis, pharyngolaryngeal pain, URTI, arthralgia, nasal congestion.
Intranasal Spray (Omnaris): Headache, nasopharyngitis, epistaxis.

CNS: Headache. **Respiratory:** Nasopharyngitis, epistaxis, nasal discomfort/congestion, sinusitis, pharyngolaryngeal pain, URTI, wheezing, *Candida albicans* infections of the nose and pharynx, nasal septum perforation (rare). **Musculoskeletal:** Arthralgia, pain in the back and extremities. **Hypersensitivity:** Immediate and delayed hypersensitivity reactions, including angioedema, bronchospasm, rash, urticaria. **Ophthalmic:** Rarely, cataracts, glaucoma, increased IOP. **Otic:** Ear pain. **Miscellaneous:** Reduction in growth velocity in children.

DRUG INTERACTIONS

Cimetidine / Inhibition of metabolism by CYP3A4 → ↑ systemic exposure to ciclesonide

C

Clarithromycin / Inhibition of metabolism by CYP3A4 → ↑ systemic exposure to ciclesonide
Erythromycin / Inhibition of metabolism by CYP3A4 → ↑ systemic exposure to ciclesonide
Itraconazole / Inhibition of metabolism by CYP3A4 → ↑ systemic exposure to ciclesonide
Ketoconazole / Inhibition of metabolism by CYP3A4 → ↑ systemic exposure to ciclesonide
Ritonavir / Inhibition of metabolism by CYP3A4 → ↑ systemic exposure to ciclesonide

HOW SUPPLIED

Inhalation Aerosol (Alvesco): 80 mcg/actuation, 160 mcg/actuation; ***Intranasal Spray Suspension (Omnaris):*** 50 mcg/actuation.

DOSAGE

INHALATION AEROSOL (ALVESCO)

Treatment and prophylaxis of asthma.

Adults and children, 12 years and older. Use in those who receive bronchodilators alone, initial: 80 mcg twice a day; for those who do not respond to the initial dose after 4 weeks, higher doses may provide better asthma control. After asthma stability has been achieved, use the lowest effective dose. **Maximum dose:** 160 mcg twice a day. **Use in those who receive inhaled corticosteroids, initial:** 80 mcg twice a day (see above for dosage adjustment). **Maintenance:** 320 mcg twice a day. **Use in those who receive oral corticosteroids, initial:** 320 mcg twice a day. **Maximum dose:** 320 mcg twice a day. Reduce prednisone gradually, no sooner than 2.5 mg/day on a weekly basis beginning after 1 week or more of ciclesonide therapy.

NASAL SPRAY (OMNARIS)

Perennial allergic rhinitis.

Adults and adolescents, 12 years and older: 200 mcg (i.e., two sprays of 50 mcg/spray) in each nostril once daily. Do not exceed this dose.

Seasonal allergic rhinitis.

Adults and children, 6 years and older: 200 mcg/day given as 2 sprays (50 mcg/spray) in each nostril once daily. **Maximum daily dose:** 200 mcg.

NURSING IMPLICATIONS

IMPLEMENTATION/ADMINISTRATION/STORAGE

1. If used in geriatric clients, start at the low end of the dosing range.
2. Store from 15–30°C (59–86°F). Do not freeze.

ASSESSMENT

1. List reasons for therapy, onset, characteristics of S&S, triggers, other agents trialed, outcome.
2. Examine for evidence of nasal septal ulcers, trauma or recent surgery; note turbinate findings.
3. Assess heart and lungs. Determine if immunocompromised or actively infected. Note any recent systemic steroid therapy use and amount.
4. Perform lung assessment and document findings; note PFT results.
5. Assess closely with change in vision, history of glaucoma or cataracts.
6. Monitor growth rate in children and bone mineral density (BMD) in those at risk for decreased bone mineral content.

CLIENT/FAMILY TEACHING

1. Prior to initial use, gently shake the intranasal spray (Alvesco); prime the pump by actuating 8 times. If the spray is not used for 4 consecutive days, gently shake and reprime with 1 spray or until a fine mist appears. Do not spray onto the nasal septum.
2. Before using the inhalation solution (Omnaris), prime the actuator 3 times prior to using the first dose from a new canister or when the inhaler has not been used for more than 10 days.
3. The inhalation canister should be at room temperature when used. Do not puncture and do not use near heat or open flame.
4. The inhalation product provides 120 metered sprays after initial priming. Discard spray bottle either after 120 sprays following initial priming or after 4 months. Do not use for acute asthma attack. Monitor peak flow and report abnormal readings.
5. Shake gently before each use. Do not spray in the eyes.
6. Use adequate humidity, especially during winter months when dry heat may aggravate mu-

cosa. Report any nasal bleeding, sores, or irritation.

7. Identify/avoid triggers that aggravate symptoms (dust, pollen, smoke, chemicals, pets). Report any visual changes.
8. Keep all F/U to assess response and for adverse SE.

OUTCOMES/EVALUATE

- ↓ Symptoms of seasonal and allergic rhinitis (nasal)
- Control of asthma symptoms S&S (oral inhaler)

Ciclopirox olamine

(sye-kloh-**PEER**-ox)

Classification(s): Antifungal

Pregnancy Category: B

RX: Ciclodan, CNL8 Nail Kit, Loprox, Penlac Nail Lacquer.

INDICATIONS/USES

Loprox. (1) *Cream and Suspension:* Tinea pedis, tinea cruris, and tinea corporis due to *Trichophyton rubrum, T. mentagrophytes, Epidermophyton floccosum,* and *Microsporum canis.* Candidiasis (moniliasis) due to *Candida albicans. Tinea versicolor* due to *Malassezia furfur.* (2) *Gel:* Interdigital tinea pedis and tinea corporis due to *T. rubrum, T. mentagrophytes,* or *E. floccosum.* Topical treatment of seborrheic dermatitis of the scalp. (3) *Shampoo:* Topical treatment of seborrheic dermatitis of the scalp. **Penlac Nail Lacquer:** As part of total program for the topical treatment in immunocompetent clients with mild to moderate onychomycosis, due to *T. rubrum,* of the fingernails and toenails without lunula involvement. Use only on nails and immediately adjacent skin.

ACTION/KINETICS

Action

At lower concentrations the drug blocks the transport of amino acids into the cell, whereas at higher concentrations the cell membrane of the fungus is altered so that intracellular material leaks out. May also inhibit synthesis of RNA, DNA, and protein in growing fungal cells.

Pharmacokinetics

A small amount of drug is absorbed through the skin; it also penetrates to the sebaceous glands and dermis as well as into the hair.

CONTRAINDICATIONS

Ophthalmic, oral, or intravaginal use. Concomitant use of the topical solution and systemic antifungal drugs for onychomycosis.

SPECIAL CONCERNS

- Use with caution during lacatation.
- Safety and efficacy not established in children under 10 years of age.

SIDE EFFECTS

Most Common

See individual formulations below.

- **Cream**

Pruritus at site of application, worsening of the signs and symptoms, burning.

- **Gel**

Skin burning sensation upon application, contact dermatitis, pruritus, dry skin, acne, rash, alopecia, pain upon application, eye pain, facial edema.

- **Shampoo**

Increased itching, burning, erythema, itching, seborrhea, rash, headache, ventricular tachycardia, skin disorder.

- **Topical Suspension**

Pruritus, burning.

- **Penlac Topical Solution**

Periungual erythema, erythema of the proximal nail fold, nail disorders (shape change, irritation, ingrown toenail, discoloration), application site reactions, burning of the skin, mild rash.

HOW SUPPLIED

Cream: 0.77%; ***Gel:*** 0.77%; ***Lotion:*** 0.77%; ***Shampoo:*** 1%; ***Solution, Topical:*** 8%; ***Topical Suspension:*** 0.77%.

DOSAGE

Loprox

CREAM; GEL; LOTION; TOPICAL SUSPENSION

Dermatologic conditions.

Massage gently into the affected area and surrounding skin morning and evening. If there is no improvement after 4 weeks, re-evaluate diagnosis.

C

SHAMPOO

Seborrheic dermatitis of scalp in adults.

Wet hair and apply about 5 mL to scalp; up to 10 mL can be used on long hair. Lather and leave on hair for 3 min. Rinse. Repeat twice/week for 4 weeks with a minimum of 3 days between applications.

CNL8 Nail Kit, Penlac

TOPICAL SOLUTION

Mild to moderate onychomycosis of the nails.

Apply once daily preferably at bedtime or 8 hr before washing to all affected nails using the applicator brush provided. Apply evenly over the entire nail plate and 5 mm of surrounding skin.

NURSING IMPLICATIONS

IMPLEMENTATION/ADMINISTRATION/STORAGE

Protect from light.

ASSESSMENT

1. List onset/characteristics of S&S, clinical presentation.
2. Describe lesion presentation, obtain scrapings; confirms diagnosis.
3. Weigh risk of removing unattached, infected nail before prescribing with insulin-dependent diabetes/diabetic neuropathy.

CLIENT/FAMILY TEACHING

1. Cleanse skin with soap/water; dry thoroughly. Massage cream into affected area and surrounding skin (may use glove) twice a day; wash hands before/after therapy.
2. Avoid occlusive dressings/wrappings; adult incontinence pads/diapers are occlusive.
3. Even if symptoms have improved, use for the full course.
4. Change shoes and socks at least once daily. Shoes should be well-fitted and ventilated.
5. Report any blistering, burning, itching, oozing, redness, swelling, adverse side effects.
6. When using solution, apply to nail bed, surround skin, under nail plate surface when free of nail bed. Do not remove; apply daily over the previous coat and remove with alcohol every 7 days. Up to 48 weeks may be needed, along with weekly nail trimmings and monthly professional removal of the unattached, infected nail.
7. For Penlac, avoid skin contact other than skin immediately surrounding the treated nail(s).
8. Do not use nail polish or other nail cosmetics on treated nails.
9. Do not use near heat or open flame because the product is flammable.
10. Keep all F/U to assess response and for adverse SE.

OUTCOMES/EVALUATE

- Resolution of fungal infection; wound healing
- Symptomatic improvement

■ IV

Cidofovir

(sih-**DOF**-oh-veer)

Classification(s): Antiviral

Pregnancy Category: C

RX: Vistide.

SEE ALSO ***ANTIVIRAL DRUGS.***

INDICATIONS/USES

CMV retinitis in clients with AIDS.

ACTION/KINETICS

Action

A nucleotide analog that suppresses CMV replication by selective inhibition of viral DNA synthesis. The drug inhibits CMV DNA polymerase by cidofovir diphosphate, the active intracellular metabolite. Must be administered with probenecid. There may be cross resistance with ganciclovir and foscarnet.

Pharmacokinetics

Must be given with probenecid as renal tubular secretion contributes to excretion of cidofovir. **Plasma protein binding:** <6%.

CONTRAINDICATIONS

Direct intraocular injection (may be associated with iritis, ocular hypotony, and permanent impaired vision). History of severe hypersensitivity to probenecid or other sulfa-containing drugs. In clients with a serum creatinine greater than 1.5 mg/dL, a calculated C_{CR} of 55 mL/min or less, or a urine protein of 100 mg/dL or more (equivalent to 2+ proteinuria or more). Use with other nephrotoxic drugs (discontinue 7 or more days prior to starting cidofovir therapy). Lactation.

SPECIAL CONCERNS

(1) Renal impairment is the major toxicity of cidofovir. Cases of acute renal failure resulting in dialysis or contributing to death have occurred with as few as 1 or 2 doses of cidofovir. To minimize possible nephrotoxicity, IV prehydration with normal saline and administration of probenecid must be used with each cidofovir infusion. Monitor renal function (serum creatinine and urine protein) within 48 hr prior to each dose of cidofovir and modify the dose or changes in renal function as appropriate. Cidofovir is contraindicated in clients who are receiving other nephrotoxic agents. (2) Neutropenia has been observed in association with cidofovir. Monitor neutrophil counts during cidofovir therapy. (3) Cidofovir is indicated only for treating CMV retinitis in clients with acquired AIDS. (4) In animal studies, cidofovir was carcinogenic, teratogenic, and caused hypospermia.

- **Increased risk of ocular hypotony in those with pre-existing diabetes.**
- **Use caution in clients with risk factors for nephrotoxicity.**
- **Safety and efficacy not determined for children or for treatment of other CMV infections, including pneumonitis, gastroenteritis, congenital or neonatal CMV disease; also for CMV disease in non-HIV-infected clients.**

SIDE EFFECTS

Most Common

Proteinuria, neutropenia, asthenia, decreased IOP, decreased serum bicarbonate, fever, infection, elevated creatinine, pneumonia, dyspnea, N&V, rash, alopecia, diarrhea, pain, anemia, anorexia, chills, increased cough, oral moniliasis.

GU: Nephrotoxicity, Fanconi syndrome and decreases in serum bicarbonate associated with renal tubular damage, hematuria, urinary incontinence, UTI, ***acute renal failure***, dysuria, glycosuria, kidney stone, mastitis, metrorrhagia, nocturia, polyuria, prostatic disorder, toxic nephropathy, urethritis, urinary casts, urinary retention. **GI:** N&V, diarrhea, anorexia, abdominal pain, colitis, constipation, tongue discoloration, dyspepsia, dysphagia, flatulence, gastritis, hepatomegaly, hepatitis, abnormal LFTs, melena, oral candidiasis, oral moniliasis, rectal disorder, stomatitis, aphthous stomatitis, mouth ulceration, dry mouth, cholangitis, esophagitis, gingivitis, fecal incontinence, ***GI hemorrhage***, gingivitis, hepatitis, hepatosplenomegaly, jaundice, liver damage, ***liver necrosis***, pancreatitis, proctitis, tooth caries. **CNS:** Headache, amnesia, agitation, confusion, ***convulsions***, depression, dizziness, abnormal gait, hallucinations, insomnia, neuropathy, paresthesia, migraine, somnolence, abnormal dreams, acute brain syndrome, anxiety, agitation, ataxia, cerebrovascular disorder, delirium, dementia, drug dependence, encephalopathy, facial paralysis, hemiplegia, hyperesthesia, hypertonia, hypotony, incoordination, increased libido, myoclonus, nervousness, personality disorder, speech disorder, tremor, twitching, vertigo. **CV:** Hypotension, postural hypotension, vasodilation, pallor, syncope, tachycardia, vasodilation, CHF, ***cardiomyopathy, shock***, migraine, CV disorder, hypertension, peripheral vascular disorder, phlebitis, edema. **Hematologic:** Neutropenia, thrombocytopenia, anemia, hypochromic anemia, leukocytosis, leukopenia, lymphadenopathy, lymphoma-like reaction, pancytopenia, splenic disorder, splenomegaly, thrombocytopenic purpura. **Respiratory:** Pneumonia, asthma, bronchitis, increased cough, dyspnea, hiccough, increased sputum, lung disorder, pharyngitis, pneumonia, rhinitis, sinusitis, epistaxis, hemoptysis, hyperventilation, hypoxia, ***larynx edema***, pneumothorax. **Dermatologic:** Alopecia, rash, acne, skin discoloration, pruritus, pallor, dry skin, herpes simplex, pruritus, sweating, urticaria, ***angioedema***, eczema, exfoliative dermatitis, furunculosis, nail disorder, seborrhea, skin disorder, skin hypertrophy, skin ulcer. **Musculoskeletal:** Arthralgia, myasthenia, myalgia, arthrosis, bone necrosis, bone pain, joint disorder, leg cramps, pathological fracture. **Metabolic:** Edema, metabolic acidosis, dehydration, weight loss/gain, cachexia, peripheral edema, hypoglycemic reaction, respiratory alkalosis, thirst. **Ophthalmic:** Ocular hypotony, amblyopia, conjunctivitis, eye disorder, iritis, retinal detachment, uveitis, decreased IOP (may cause abnormal vision), blindness, cataract, corneal lesion, corneal opacity, diplopia, dry eyes, eye pain, keratitis, miosis, refraction disorder, retinal disorder/detachment, visual field defect. **Otic:** Ear disorder, ear pain, hearing loss, hyperacusis, otitis externa, otitis media, tinnitus. **Body as a whole:** Allergic reactions, asthenia, malaise, fever, infections, pain, chills, flu-like syndrome, photosensitivity, hypothermia, *sarcoma, sepsis*. **Miscellaneous:** Facial edema, back/chest/neck pain, taste perversion, accidental injury, adrenal cortical insufficiency, AIDS, cellulitis, cryptococcosis, cyst, ***death***, injection site reaction, mucous membrane disorder, catheter blocked.

C

LABORATORY TEST CONSIDERATIONS

↑ Creatinine, alkaline phosphatase, BUN, lactic dehydrogenase, ALT, AST. ↓ Serum bicarbonate, creatinine clearance. Proteinuria, hematuria, glycosuria, hypercalcemia, hyperglycemia, hyperkalemia, hyperlipidemia, hypocalcemia, hypoglycemia, hypokalemia, hypomagnesemia, hyponatremia, hypophosphatemia, hypoproteinemia, respiratory alkalosis.

DRUG INTERACTIONS

Amikacin / ↑ Risk of nephrotoxicity; do not use together
Amphotericin B / ↑ Risk of nephrotoxicity; do not use together
Aminoglycosides, IV (amikacin, gentamicin, tobramycin) / ↑ Risk of nephrotoxicity; do not use together
Foscarnet / ↑ Risk of nephrotoxicity; do not use together
Gentamicin / ↑ Risk of nephrotoxicity; do not use together
NSAIDs / ↑ Risk of nephrotoxicity; do not use together
Pentamidine, IV / ↑ Risk of nephrotoxicity; do not use together
Tenofovir / ↑ Risk of nephrotoxicity; do not use together
Tobramycin / ↑ Risk of nephrotoxicity; do not use together
Vancomycin / ↑ Risk of nephrotoxicity; do not use together
Zidovudine / ↓ Zidovudine clearance R/T concomitant probenecid administration to prevent nephrotoxicity; temporarily discontinue or decrease zidovudine dose by 50% on day of cidofovir administration only

HOW SUPPLIED

Injection: 75 mg/mL.

DOSAGE

IV INFUSION

Cytomegalovirus (CMV) retinitis.

Induction: 5 mg/kg given once weekly for 2 consecutive weeks as an IV infusion at a constant rate over 1 hr. **Maintenance:** 5 mg/kg given once q 2 weeks as an IV infusion at a constant rate over 1 hr. Do not exceed the recommended dosage, frequency, or infusion rate.

NURSING IMPLICATIONS

IMPLEMENTATION/ADMINISTRATION/STORAGE

1. IV A full course of probenecid and IV saline prehydration must be done with each dose of cidofovir. For probenecid, give 2 grams 3 hr prior to the cidofovir dose and give 1 gram at 2 hr and again at 8 hr after completion of the 1 hr cidofovir infusion (i.e., total of 4 grams probenecid).
2. Give 1 L of 0.9% normal saline solution; infuse the saline solution over a 1 to 2 hr period immediately before cidofovir. Those who can tolerate the additional fluid load should receive a second liter. If given, start the second liter of saline at the start of the cidofovir infusion or immediately afterward; infuse over a 1 to 3 hr period.
3. Use probenecid after a meal or with an antiemetic to decrease nausea.
4. Nephrotoxic drugs must be discontinued 7 or more days before starting cidofovir therapy.
5. Prior to administration, dilute cidofovir in 100 mL of 0.9% NaCl solution; administer over 1 hr.
6. Consider possible viral resistance for those who show a poor clinical response or experience recurrent retinitis progression during therapy.
7. Serum creatinine may not provide an accurate picture of the client's underlying renal status. Thus, use the Cockcroft-Gault formula to estimate more accurately creatinine clearance. Calculate C_{CR} (mL/min) according to the following formula:
   - Males: Weight (kg) × (140 – age)/72 × serum creatinine (mg/dL) = C_{CR}
   - Females: 0.85 × male value
8. If serum creatinine increases by 0.3 to 0.4 mg/dL, reduce the dose of cidofovir from 5 to 3 mg/kg. Discontinue cidofovir if the serum creatinine increases by 0.5 mg/dL or more or if there is development of 3+ or more proteinuria.

9. Since cidofovir is mutagenic, use adequate precautions, including use of appropriate safety equipment, for the preparation, administration, and disposal of cidofovir. If cidofovir contacts the skin, wash membranes and flush thoroughly with water.
10. Store the injection from 20–25°C (36–46°F). Store admixtures at 2–8°C (36–46°F) for no more than 24 hr. Bring to room temperature prior to use. Discard partially used vials.
11. COMPATIBILITY 0.9% NaCl.
12. INCOMPATIBILITY Do not mix with other meds or solutions.

ASSESSMENT

1. List reasons for therapy, onset, duration, symptom characteristics.
2. Note sensitivity to probenecid or sulfa drugs; review ophthalmic exam.
3. Monitor IOP, visual acuity, and ocular symptoms. Assess for progression of CMV retinitis.
4. Consider viral resistance if poor clinical response or recurrent retinitis progression during therapy.
5. Identify other medical conditions/those at risk for nephrotoxicity. To minimize potential for nephrotoxicity follow administration guidelines:
   - Initiate therapy only if serum creatinine is less than or equal to 1.5 mg/dL.
   - Monitor serum creatinine and urine protein within 48 hr prior to each dose; modify/discontinue dose based on renal function.
   - Prehydrate with at least 1L IV of NSS and ensure adequate fluid volume status and follow with 1L NSS if tolerated.
   - Coadminister PO probenecid, 4 grams total, with each cidofovir dose; 2 grams given 3 hr prior to the cidofovir dose and 1 gram given 2 hr and again at 8 hr after completion of the cidofovir infusion.
   - Avoid concomitant nephrotoxic drugs at least 7 days before initiating cidofovir.
   - Neutropenia may occur. Monitor neutrophil counts during therapy.
6. Monitor CBC, renal function (serum creatinine and urine protein), LFTs, and BMP.

CLIENT/FAMILY TEACHING

1. Not a cure but controls symptoms. Retinitis may progress as well as other CMV symptoms; must have regular medical/eye exams.
2. Stop zidovudine or decrease dose by 50% on cidofovir days; probenecid inhibits zidovudine clearance.
3. Report any change/decrease in urinary output; may cause renal toxicity.
4. Complete a full course of probenecid with each dose (2 grams 3 hr before and 1 gram 2 hr and 8 hr after completing infusion). Take after meals or use antiemetics to decrease nausea.
5. Women should use reliable contraception during and for 1 month following therapy. Men should practice barrier contraception during and for 3 months following therapy. Infertility may result; identify if candidate for sperm/egg harvesting.
6. Drug causes tumors (e.g., mammary adenocarcinomas) in rats; considered a potential carcinogen in humans. May also impair renal function.
7. Keep all F/U to assess response, labs, and for adverse SE.

OUTCOMES/EVALUATE

Control of symptoms of CMV retinitis with HIV

Cilostazol

(sih-**LESS**-tah-zohl)

Classification(s): Antiplatelet drug

Pregnancy Category: C

RX: Pletal.

INDICATIONS/USES

Reduce symptoms of intermittent claudication, as indicated by an increased walking distance.

ACTION/KINETICS

Action

Inhibits cellular phosphodiesterase (PDE), especially PDE III. Cilostazol and several metabolites inhibit cyclic AMP PDE III. Suppression of this isoenzyme causes increased levels of cyclic AMP resulting in vasodilation and inhibition of platelet aggregation. Inhibits platelet aggregation caused by thrombin, ADP, collagen, arachidonic acid, epinephrine, and shear stress.

Pharmacokinetics

High fat meals significantly increase absorption. Extensively metabolized by the liver mainly by

CYP3A4 and to a less extent by CYP2C19. Two of the metabolites are active. Primarily excreted through the urine (74%) with the rest in the feces. **t½, elimination:** 11–13 hr. **Plasma protein binding:** 95–98%.

C

CONTRAINDICATIONS

Use with CHF of any severity. Use in those with hemostatic disorders or active pathologic bleeding, such as bleeding peptic ulcer and intracranial bleeding. Known or suspected hypersensitivity to any component of the product. Concurrent use of grapefruit juice. Lactation.

SPECIAL CONCERNS

■ Cilostazol and several of its metabolites are phosphodiesterase III inhibitors. Such compounds have caused decreased survival in those with class III-IV CHF. Contraindicated in clients with CHF of any severity. ■

Safety and efficacy not determined in children.

SIDE EFFECTS

Most Common

Headache, diarrhea, abnormal stools, rhinitis, infection, dizziness, peripheral edema, pharyngitis, dyspepsia, nausea, palpitations, tachycardia, vertigo, abdominal pain, flatulence, back pain, myalgia, increased cough.

GI: Abnormal stool, diarrhea, dyspepsia, flatulence, N&V, abdominal pain, anorexia, colitis, duodenal ulcer, duodenitis, ***esophageal/GI/rectal hemorrhage***, esophagitis, gastritis, gastroenteritis, gum hemorrhage, hematemesis, melena, peptic ulcer, periodontal abscess, ***rectal hemorrhage***, stomach ulcer, tongue edema. **Hepatic:** Hepatic dysfunction/abnormal LFTs, cholelithiasis, jaundice. **CNS:** Headache, dizziness, vertigo, anxiety, insomnia, neuralgia, subdural hematoma pain, ***cerebral/intracranial hemorrhage***. **CV:** Palpitation, tachycardia, hypertension, angina pectoris, atrial fibrillation/flutter, cerebral infarct/ischemia, CHF, ***heart arrest, hemorrhage***, hypotension, MI, myocardial ischemia, nodal arrhythmia, postural hypotension, supraventricular tachycardia, syncope, varicose veins, vasodilation, ventricular extrasystole or ***ventricular tachycardia***, subacute thrombosis, ***CVA, torsades de pointes, QTc prolongation***. **Respiratory:** Rhinitis, pharyngitis, increased cough, dyspnea, bronchitis, asthma, epistaxis, hemoptysis, pneumonia, sinusitis, interstitial pneumonia, ***pulmonary hemorrhage***. **Musculoskeletal:** Back pain, myalgia, leg cramps, arthritis, arthralgia, bone pain, bursitis, neck rigidity. **Dermatologic:** Rash, dry skin, furunculosis, skin hypertrophy, urticaria, subcutaneous hemorrhage, pruritus, skin eruptions, dermatitis medicamentosa, extradural hematoma, subdural hematoma pain, ***Stevens-Johnson syndrome***. **GU:** Hematuria, UTI, cystitis, urinary frequency, vaginal hemorrhage, vaginitis. **Hematologic:** Anemia, ecchymosis, iron deficiency anemia, polycythemia, purpura, agranulocytosis, bleeding tendency, granulocytopenia, leukopenia, thrombocytopenia or leukopenia progressing to agranulocytosis when cilostazol not immediately discontinued. **Metabolic/Nutritional:** Generalized edema, diabetes mellitus, gout, peripheral/facial/generalized edema. **Ophthalmic:** Amblyopia, blindness, conjunctivitis, diplopia, eye hemorrhage, retinal hemorrhage. **Otic:** Tinnitus, ear pain. **Body as a whole:** Infection, hypesthesia, paresthesia, flu syndrome, asthenia, chills, fever, hot flashes, malaise. **Miscellaneous:** Pelvic/chest pain, ***retroperitoneal hemorrhage***.

LABORATORY TEST CONSIDERATIONS

↑ GGT, creatinine, blood glucose, uric acid, BUN, serum urea. ↓ Platelets, WBCs. Albuminuria, hyperlipemia, hyperuricemia.

OVERDOSE MANAGEMENT

Symptoms: Excessive pharmacologic effects, including severe headache, diarrhea, hypotension, tachycardia, possible cardiac arrhythmias. *Treatment:* Observe client carefully and provide symptomatic treatment. Since drug is highly protein bound, it is unlikely to be removed by hemodialysis or peritoneal dialysis.

DRUG INTERACTIONS

Clopidogrel / Possible additive effects on bleeding time; monitor bleeding times if used together

Diltiazem / ↑ Cilostazol levels R/T inhibition of liver metabolizing enzymes; consider dose reduction of cilostazol

Erythromycin / ↑ Cilostazol levels R/T inhibition of liver metabolizing enzymes; consider dose reduction of cilostazol

Grapefruit juice / ↑ Cilostazol levels R/T inhibition of liver metabolizing enzymes

Itraconazole / ↑ Cilostazol levels R/T inhibition of liver metabolizing enzymes; consider dose reduction of cilostazol
Ketoconazole / ↑ Cilostazol levels R/T inhibition of liver metabolizing enzymes; consider dose reduction of cilostazol
Lovastatin / ↓ Cilostazol C_{max} and AUC by 15%; ↑ lovastatin AUC by about 70%
Macrolide antibiotics / ↑ Cilostazol levels R/T inhibition of liver metabolizing enzymes; consider dose reduction of cilostazol
Omeprazole / ↑ Cilostazol levels R/T inhibition of liver metabolizing enzymes; consider dose reduction of cilostazol

HOW SUPPLIED

Tablets: 50 mg, 100 mg.

DOSAGE

TABLETS

Intermittent claudication.

100 mg twice a day taken 30 min or more before or 2 hr after breakfast and dinner. Consider a dose of 50 mg twice a day during coadministration of CYP3A4 inhibitors, including diltiazem, erythromycin, itraconazole, or ketoconazole and during coadministration of CYP2C19 inhibitors such as omeprazole.

NURSING IMPLICATIONS

Do not confuse Pletal with Plavix (also an antiplatelet drug).

IMPLEMENTATION/ADMINISTRATION/STORAGE

1. **Clients may respond as early as 2–4 weeks after beginning therapy but treatment for up to 12 weeks may be needed.**
2. **The dosage of cilostazol may be reduced or discontinued without platelet hyperaggregability.**
3. **Store from 15–30°C (59–86°F).**

ASSESSMENT

1. **Note onset/characteristics of symptoms; contributing factors. Measure distance walked before pain elicited.**
2. **List drugs currently prescribed to ensure none interact. Identify any S&S bleeding, CV disease or CHF (↓ survival with class III to IV CHF).**
3. **Perform/document ABIs.**
4. **Assess extent/amount/duration of nicotine use; nicotine constricts blood vessels.**
5. **Monitor CBC, and for liver/renal dysfunction.**

CLIENT/FAMILY TEACHING

1. **Take 30 min before or 2 hr after meals. Avoid grapefruit juice.**
2. **Read patient insert carefully before starting therapy; each time renewed.**
3. **Use caution, may experience headaches, GI upset, dizziness, or runny nose; report if bothersome. Report any unusual bleeding, skin rash, or diarrhea.**
4. **Do not smoke; enroll in formal smoking cessation program.**
5. **Continue to walk past the point of severe pain before resting, then resume walking to improve symptoms and distance able to walk before pain recurs.**
6. **Avoid becoming pregnant due to potential hazard to the fetus.**
7. **Beneficial effects may be seen in 2 to 4 weeks; up to 12 weeks may be needed before evident.**
8. **Keep all F/U to assess response, ABIs, and adverse SE.**

OUTCOMES/EVALUATE

- **Increased walking distance without pain**
- **↓ S&S intermittent claudication**

IV

Cimetidine

(sye-**MET**-ih-deen)

Classification(s): Histamine H_2-receptor blocking drug

Pregnancy Category: B

OTC: Acid Reducer 200, Tagamet HB 200.

RX: Tagamet.

♣ **Rx:** Apo-Cimetidine, Gen-Cimetidine, Nu-Cimet.

SEE ALSO ***HISTAMINE H_2-ANTAGONISTS***.

INDICATIONS/USES

Rx. (1) Short-term treatment and maintenance therapy for duodenal ulcers. (2) Short-term (6 weeks) treatment of benign gastric ulcers (in rare cases, healing has occurred). (3) Treatment of gastric acid hypersecretory states (Zollinger-Ellison syndrome, systemic mastocytosis). (4) GERD, including erosive esophagitis. (5) Prophylaxis of UGI bleeding in critically ill hospitalized clients (IV only). *Investigational:* As part of a multidrug regimen to eradicate *Helicobacter pylori* in the treatment of peptic ulcer; in the perioperative setting to suppress gastric acid secretion, prevent stress ulcers, and prevent aspiration pneumonitis; in combination with histamine H_1-antagonists to treat certain types of urticaria; treat cutaneous warts (conflicting data). IV only: Prevent paclitaxel hypersensitivity and reduce incidence of GI hemorrhage associated with stress-related ulcers.

OTC. (1) Relief of heartburn associated with acid indigestion and sour stomach. (2) Prevent heartburn associated with acid indigestion and sour stomach caused by certain foods and beverages.

ACTION/KINETICS

Action

Reduces postprandial daytime and nighttime gastric acid secretion by about 50–80%. May increase gastromucosal defense and healing in acid-related disorders (e.g., stress-induced ulcers) by increasing production of gastric mucus, increasing mucosal secretion of bicarbonate and gastric mucosal blood flow as well as increasing endogenous mucosal synthesis of prostaglandins. It also inhibits cytochrome P-450 and P-448, which will affect metabolism of drugs. Also possesses antiandrogenic activity and will increase prolactin levels following an IV bolus injection.

Pharmacokinetics

Well absorbed from GI tract. **Peak plasma level, PO:** 45–90 min. **Time to peak effect, after PO:** 1–2 hr. **Peak plasma levels, after PO use:** 0.7–3.2 mcg/mL (after a 300 mg dose); **after IV:** 3.5–7.5 mcg/mL. **Duration, nocturnal:** 6–8 hr; **basal:** 4–5 hr. **t½:** 2 hr, longer in presence of renal impairment. After PO use, most metabolized in liver; after parenteral use, about 75% of drug excreted unchanged in the urine. **Plasma protein binding:** 13–25%.

CONTRAINDICATIONS

Children under 12, lactation. Cirrhosis, impaired liver and renal function.

SPECIAL CONCERNS

Confusion is more likely to occur in the elderly with impaired renal or hepatic function.

SIDE EFFECTS

Most Common

Headache, dizziness, diarrhea, gynecomastia, arthralgia.

GI: Diarrhea, pancreatitis (rare), hepatitis, hepatic fibrosis. **CNS:** Dizziness, sleepiness, headache, confusion, delirium, hallucinations, double vision, dysarthria, ataxia. Severely ill clients may manifest agitation, anxiety, depression, disorientation, hallucinations, mental confusion, and psychosis. **CV:** Hypotension and arrhythmias following rapid IV administration. **Hematologic:** Agranulocytosis, thrombocytopenia, ***hemolytic or aplastic anemia***, granulocytopenia. **GU:** Impotence (high doses for prolonged periods of time), gynecomastia (long-term treatment). **Dermatologic:** Exfoliative dermatitis, erythroderma, erythema multiforme. **Musculoskeletal:** Arthralgia, reversible worsening of joint symptoms with pre-existing arthritis (including gouty arthritis). **Miscellaneous:** Hypersensitivity reactions, pain at injection site, myalgia, rash, cutaneous vasculitis, peripheral neuropathy, galactorrhea, alopecia, bronchoconstriction.

DRUG INTERACTIONS

Acyclovir / ↑ Acyclovir peak plasma level and AUC; not clinically important in those with normal renal function

Antacids / ↓ Effect of cimetidine R/T ↓ GI tract absorption

Anticholinergics / ↓ Effect of cimetidine R/T ↓ GI tract absorption

Benzodiazepines / ↑ Benzodiazepine effects R/T ↓ liver breakdown

Beta-adrenergic blocking drugs / ↑ Beta-adrenergic effects R/T ↓ liver breakdown

Caffeine / ↑ Caffeine effect R/T ↓ liver breakdown

Calcium channel blockers / ↑ Calcium channel blocker effects R/T ↓ liver breakdown

Carbamazepine / ↑ Carbamazepine effect R/T ↓ liver breakdown

Carmustine / Additive bone marrow depression

Chloroquine / ↑ Chloroquine effects R/T ↓ liver breakdown

Chlorpromazine / ↓ Chlorpromazine effect R/T ↓ GI tract absorption

Cyanocobalamin / ↓ Cyanocobalamin absorption

Digoxin / ↓ Serum digoxin levels

Escitalopram / ↑ Escitalopram AUC and t½

Flecainide / ↑ Flecainide effect
Fluconazole / ↓ Fluconazole effect R/T ↓ GI tract absorption
Fluorouracil / ↑ Serum fluorouracil levels following chronic cimetidine use
Indomethacin / ↓ Indomethacin effect R/T ↓ GI tract absorption
Iron salts / ↓ Iron salt effects R/T ↓ GI tract absorption
Ketoconazole / ↓ Ketoconazole effect R/T ↓ GI tract absorption
Labetalol / ↑ Labetalol effect R/T ↓ liver breakdown
Lidocaine / ↑ Lidocaine effect R/T ↓ liver breakdown
Metoclopramide / ↓ Cimetidine effect R/T ↓ GI tract absorption
Metoprolol / ↑ Metoprolol effect R/T ↓ liver breakdown
Metronidazole / ↑ Metronidazole effect R/T ↓ liver breakdown
Moricizine / ↑ Moricizine effect R/T ↓ liver breakdown
Narcotics / Possible ↑ toxic effects (respiratory depression) of narcotics
Pentoxifylline / ↑ Pentoxifylline effect R/T ↓ liver breakdown
Phenytoin / ↑ Phenytoin effect R/T ↓ liver breakdown
Procainamide / ↑ Procainamide effect R/T ↓ kidney excretion
Propafenone / ↑ Propafenone effect R/T ↓ liver breakdown
Propranolol / ↑ Propranolol effect R/T ↓ liver breakdown
Quinidine / ↑ Quinidine effect R/T ↓ liver breakdown
Quinine / ↑ Quinine effect R/T ↓ liver breakdown
Saquinavir / ↑ Saquinavir AUC and peak plasma levels R/T inhibition of CYP3A4 liver enzymes
Sildenafil / ↑ Sildenafil effect R/T ↓ liver breakdown
Succinylcholine / ↑ Neuromuscular blockade → respiratory depression and extended apnea
Sulfonylureas / ↑ Sulfonylurea effects R/T ↓ liver breakdown
Tacrine / ↑ Tacrine effect R/T ↓ liver breakdown
Tetracyclines / ↓ Tetracycline effects R/T ↓ GI tract absorption
Theophyllines / ↑ Theophylline effects R/T ↓ liver breakdown
Tocainide / ↓ Tocainide effect
Triamterene / ↑ Triamterene effect R/T ↓ liver breakdown
Tricyclic antidepressants / ↑ TCA effects R/T ↓ liver breakdown
Valacyclovir / ↑ Valacyclovir peak plasma level and AUC; not clinically important in those with normal renal function
Valproic acid / ↑ Valproic acid effect R/T ↓ liver breakdown
Warfarin / ↑ Anticoagulant effects R/T ↓ liver breakdown; do not use together

HOW SUPPLIED

Injection: 150 mg/mL; ***Injection, Premixed:*** 6 mg/mL; ***Liquid Oral Solution:*** 300 mg/5 mL; ***Tablets:*** 200 mg (OTC or Rx), 300 mg, 400 mg, 800 mg.

C

DOSAGE

ORAL SOLUTION; TABLETS (RX)

Duodenal ulcers, short-term treatment.

Adults: 800 mg at bedtime. Alternate dosage: 300 mg 4 times per day with meals and at bedtime for 4–6 weeks (administer with antacids, staggering the dose of antacids) or 400 mg 2 times per day (in the morning and evening). **Maintenance:** 400 mg at bedtime.

Active benign gastric ulcers.

Adults: 800 mg at bedtime (preferred regimen) or 300 mg 4 times per day with meals and at bedtime for no more than 8 weeks.

Pathologic hypersecretory conditions.

Adults: 300 mg 4 times per day with meals and at bedtime up to a maximum of 2,400 mg/day for as long as needed. Individualize dosage. If needed, give 300 mg doses more often.

Erosive gastroesophageal reflux disease.

Adults: 800 mg 2 times per day or 400 mg 4 times per day for 12 weeks. Use beyond 12 weeks has not been determined.

Prophylaxis of aspiration pneumonitis.

Adults: 400–600 mg 60–90 min before anesthesia.

C

TABLETS (OTC)

Heartburn, acid indigestion, sour stomach (OTC only).

200 mg, as symptoms present, up to 2 times per day. Take tablets with water. Do not take maximum dose for more than 2 weeks continuously unless directed by provider.

IM; IV; IV INFUSION

Hospitalized clients with pathologic hypersecretory conditions or intractable ulcers or those unable to take PO medication.

Adults: 300 mg IM or IV q 6–8 hr. If an increased dose is necessary, administer 300 mg more frequently than q 6–8 hr, not to exceed 2,400 mg per day. Give concomitant antacids as needed for pain relief.

Prophylaxis of upper GI bleeding.

Adults: 50 mg/hr by continuous IV infusion. If C_{CR} <30 mL/min, use one-half the recommended dose. Treatment beyond 7 days has not been studied.

Prophylaxis of aspiration pneumonitis.

Adults: 300 mg IV 60–90 min before induction of anesthetia.

NURSING IMPLICATIONS

Ⓢ Do not confuse Tagamet (Rx product) with Tagamet HB 200 (OTC product).

IMPLEMENTATION/ADMINISTRATION/STORAGE

1. If antacids used, stagger dose with that of cimetidine; antacids (but not food) decrease absorption.
2. Administer PO medication with meals and with a snack at bedtime.
3. In renal dysfunction, a dose of 300 mg PO or IV q 12 hr may be necessary. The dose may be given, with caution, q 8 hr if needed.
4. For IM use, give undiluted.
5. IV For IV injections, dilute in 0.9% NaCl (or other compatible solution) to a total volume of 20 mL. Inject over at least 2 min.
6. For intermittent IV infusion, dilute 300 mg in at least 50 mL of D5W or other compatible solution and infuse over 15–20 min.
7. For continuous IV infusion, give loading dose of 150 mg (by intermittent IV infusion); then, administer 37.5 mg/hr (900 mg/day) in compatible solutions. Stable for 24 hr at room temperature if mixed with these diluents.
8. May be diluted in 100–1,000 mL; if the volume for a 24 hr infusion is less than 250 mL, use a pump.
9. Do not expose premixed single-dose product to excessive heat; store at 15–30°C (59–86°F).
10. COMPATIBILITY 0.9% NaCl, D5W or D10W, 5% $NaHCO_3$ injection, RL, or standard TPN solutions.
11. INCOMPATIBILITY Stop other drugs while administering and do not add drugs or additives to mixtures; flush lines before and after therapy.

ASSESSMENT

1. Note reasons for therapy, type/onset of S&S, anticipated length of therapy.
2. Assess location, characteristics, extent of abdominal pain; note blood in emesis, stool, or gastric aspirate. Report loss of bowel sounds, absence of BM/gas, crampy pain or distension. Maintain gastric pH above 5 to enhance mucosal healing.
3. Note general client condition. Those receiving radiation therapy or myelosuppressive drugs may have additional side effects.
4. List drugs prescribed; ensure none interact.
5. Monitor VS, I&O. Review radiologic/endoscopic findings; check for *H. pylori*.
6. Monitor CBC, electrolytes, B_{12} level, renal and LFTs, especially in elderly, severely ill, with renal impairment; most susceptible to confusion.

CLIENT/FAMILY TEACHING

1. Take with meals/snack at bedtime. Avoid antacids 1 hr before or after dose; establish regular schedule.
2. Take as prescribed even if symptoms disappear.
3. Review dietary modifications, especially if being treated for GI problems; consult dietitian.
4. Do not perform tasks that require mental alertness until effects realized.
5. Report any breast swelling/discharge/pain or impotence.
6. Report if abdominal pain, bloody stools, or other S&S of reactivated ulcer evident.
7. Avoid alcohol, caffeine, spicy or tomato-based foods, mints, NSAIDs, aspirin-containing products; may enhance GI irritation.

8. Do not smoke after the last dose of cimetidine to ensure optimal suppression of nocturnal gastric acid secretion. Attend smoking cessation program if unable to quit.
9. Report new S&S of confusion, mood swings; more common with elderly.
10. Note increased susceptibility to infections. Report if diarrhea develops, maintain adequate hydration, monitor frequency/severity.
11. Report skin rashes/changes, adverse effects, lack of response. May alter response to skin tests with allergenic extracts; stop drug 48–72 hr prior to testing.
12. Keep all F/U to assess response, labs, for adverse SE.

OUTCOMES/EVALUATE

- ↓ Abdominal pain; ulcer healing
- Control of acid hypersecretion
- Prophylaxis of GI bleeding

IV

Ciprofloxacin hydrochloride

(sip-row-**FLOX**-ah-sin)

Classification(s): Antibiotic, fluoroquinolone

Pregnancy Category: C

RX: Cetraxal Otic, Ciloxan Ophthalmic, Cipro, Cipro I.V., Cipro XR, Proquin XR.

✱ **Rx:** Apo-Ciproflox, Cipro XL, CO Ciprofloxacin, Gen-Ciprofloxacin, PMS-Ciprofloxacin, RAN-Ciprofloxacin, ratio-Ciprofloxacin, Sandoz Ciprofloxacin, Taro-Ciprofloxacin.

SEE ALSO ***FLUOROQUINOLONES***.

INDICATIONS/USES

Adults: Immediate Release (IR) Tablets and Oral Suspension.

1. Acute sinusitis due to *Haemophilus influenzae, Streptococcus pneumoniae* (penicillin-sensitive), or *Moraxella catarrhalis.*
2. Acute uncomplicated cystitis in women due to *Escherichia coli* or *Staphylococcus saprophyticus.*
3. Chronic bacterial prostatitis due to *E. coli* or *Proteus mirabilis.*
4. UTIs due to *E. coli, Klebsiella pneumoniae, Enterobacter cloacae, Serratia marcescens, P. mirabilis, Providencia rettgeri, Morganella morganii, Citrobacter diversus, Citrobacter freundii, Pseudomonas aeruginosa, Staphylococcus epidermidis* (methicillin-sensitive), *S. saprophyticus,* or *Enterococcus faecalis.*
5. Bone and joint infections due to *E. cloacae, S. marcescens,* or *P. aeruginosa.*
6. With metronidazole for complicated intra-abdominal infections due to *E. coli, P. aeruginosa, P. mirabilis, K. pneumoniae,* or *Bacteroides fragilis.*
7. Infectious diarrhea due to *E. coli* (enterotoxigenic strains), *Campylobacter jejuni, Shigella boydii, Shigella dysenteriae, Shigella flexneri,* or *Shigella sonnei.*
8. Lower respiratory tract infections due to *E. coli, K. pneumoniae, E. cloacae, P. mirabilis, P. aeruginosa, H. influenzae, Haemophilus parainfluenzae,* or *S. pneumoniae* (methicillin-susceptible). Not a drug of first choice to treat presumed or confirmed pneumonia secondary to *S. pneumoniae.*
9. Acute exacerbations of chronic bronchitis due to *M. catarrhalis.*
10. Skin and skin structure infections due to *E. coli, K. pneumoniae, E. cloacae, P. mirabilis, Proteus vulgaris, P. stuartii, M. morganii, C. freundii, P. aeruginosa, Staphylococcus aureus* (methicillin-susceptible), *S. epidermidis* (methicillin-sensitive), or *Streptococcus pyogenes.*
11. Typhoid fever (enteric fever) due to *Salmonella typhi.* Efficacy in eradicating the chronic typhoid carrier state has not been demonstrated.
12. Uncomplicated cervical and urethral gonorrhea due to *Neisseria gonorrhoeae.*

Adults and Children: Immediate-Release (IR) Tablets, IV, and Oral Suspension. Reduce the incidence or progression of disease following exposure to aerosolized *Bacillus anthracis.*

Children, 1–17 years of age: Immediate-Release (IR) Tablets, IV, and Oral Suspension. Complicated UTIs and pyelonephritis due to *E. coli* (not the first drug of choice due to increased incidence of side effects).

Cipro XR (Extended-Release Tablets) Only. (1) Uncomplicated UTIs (acute cystitis) due to *E. coli, P. mirabilis, E. faecalis,* or *S. saprophyticus.* (2) Complicated UTIs due to *E. coli, P. aeruginosa, E. faecalis, P. mirabilis,* or *K. pneumoniae.* (3)

Acute uncomplicated pyelonephritis due to *E. coli*. *NOTE:* Ciprofloxacin ER and immediate-release tablets are not interchangeable.

Proquin XR (Extended-Release Tablets) Only. Uncomplicated UTIs (acute cystitis) due to *E. coli* and *K. pneumoniae*. *NOTE:* Proquin XR is not interchangeable with other ciprofloxacin ER or immediate-release oral formulations.

Investigational, PO forms:

1. Traveler's diarrhea.
2. Cystic fibrosis in children (for periods of 10 days to 6 months).
3. Gastroenteritis in children.
4. Atypical mycobacterial infections when used with ciprofloxacin as part of combination therapy.
5. Multi-drug resistant tuberculosis.
6. Alternative regimen for tularemia in adults and children.
7. Prophylaxis of anthrax in adults.
8. Plague in adults and children.
9. Mycobacterial diseases.
10. Disseminated gonorrhea (alternative regimen).
11. Chancroid.
12. Granuloma inguinale.
13. Infective endocarditis in adults, adolescents, and children.
14. As monotherapy for urologic surgical procedures or in combination with metronidazole or clindamycin for abdominal or vaginal hysterectomies, cesarean sections, and colorectal surgical procedures in clients with a beta-lactam allergy.

Adults: IV.

1. Acute sinusitis due to *H. influenzae, S. pneumoniae* (penicillin-sensitive), or *M. catarrhalis*.
2. Chronic bacterial prostatitis due to *E. coli* or *P. mirabilis*.
3. UTIs due to *E. coli* (including cases with secondary bacteremia), *K. pneumoniae* (subspecies *pneumoniae*), *E. cloacae, S. marcescens, P. mirabilis, P. rettgeri, M. morganii, C. diversus, C. freundii, P. aeruginosa, S. epidermidis* (methicillin-susceptible), *S. saprophyticus,* or *E. faecalis*.
4. Bone and joint infections due to *E. cloacae, S. marcescens,* or *P. aeruginosa*.
5. With metronidazole for complicated intra-abdominal infections due to *E. coli, P. aeruginosa, P. mirabilis, K. pneumoniae,* or *B. fragilis*.
6. Lower respiratory tract infections due to *E. coli, K. pneumoniae* (subspecies *pneumoniae*), *E. cloacae, P. mirabilis, P. aeruginosa, H. influenzae, H. parainfluenzae,* or *S. pneumoniae* (penicillin–susceptible). *NOTE:* Not the first drug of choice to treat presumed or confirmed pneumonia secondary to *S. pneumoniae*.
7. Acute exacerbations of chronic bronchitis due to *M. catarrhalis*.
8. Nosocomial pneumonia due to *H. influenzae* or *K. pneumoniae*.
9. With piperacillin sodium as empirical therapy for febrile neutropenic clients.
10. Skin and skin structure infections due to *E. coli, K. pneumoniae* (subspecies *pneumoniae*), *E. cloacae, P. mirabilis, P. vulgaris, P. stuartii, M. morganii, C. freundii, P. aeruginosa, S. aureus* (methicillin-susceptible), *S. epidermidis,* or *S. pyogenes*.

Investigational, IV: (1) Multi-drug resistant tuberculosis. (2) Alternative regimen for tularemia in adults and children. (3) Alternative regimen for cutaneous, oropharyngeal, and GI anthrax. (4) Alternative regimen for the plague in adults and children. (5) Cystic fibrosis in children for periods of 10 days to 6 months without documented side effects or intolerance. (6) Alternative regimen for disseminated gonorrhea. (7) Prophylaxis of anthrax in adults. (8) Infective endocarditis in adults, adolescents, and children. (9) As monotherapy for urologic surgical procedures or in combination with metronidazole or clindamycin for abdominal or vaginal hysterectomy's, cesarean sections, and colorectal surgical procedures in clients with a beta-lactam allergy.

Ocular Infections. Superficial ocular infections involving the conjunctiva or cornea, including conjunctivitis, keratitis, keratoconjunctivitis, corneal ulcers, blepharitis, blepharoconjunctivitis, acute meibomianitis, and dacryocystitis.

Ophthalmic Ointment. Bacterial conjunctivitis due to *S. aureus, S. epidermidis, S. pneumoniae, Streptococcus* (viridans group), and *H. influenzae*.

Ophthalmic Solution. (1) Corneal ulcers due to *P. aeruginosa, S. marcescens, S. aureus, S. epidermidis, S. pneumoniae,* and *Streptococcus* (viridans group). (2) Conjunctivitis due to *H. influenzae, S. aureus, S. epidermidis,* and *S. pneumoniae*.

Otic Solution. Acute otitis externa due to susceptible isolates of *P. aeruginosa* or *S. aureus.*

ACTION/KINETICS

Action

Interferes with DNA gyrase and topoisomerase IV. DNA gyrase is an enzyme needed for replication, transcription, and repair of bacterial DNA. Topoisomerase IV plays a key role in the partitioning of chromosomal DNA during bacterial cell division. Effective against both gram-positive and gram-negative organisms.

Pharmacokinetics

Rapidly and well absorbed following PO administration. Food delays absorption of the drug. **Maximum serum levels:** 2–4 mcg/mL 1–2 hr after dosing. **t½:** 4 hr for PO use and 5–6 hr for IV use. Avoid peak serum levels above 5 mcg/mL. About 40–50% of a PO dose and 50–70% of an IV dose are excreted unchanged in the urine.

CONTRAINDICATIONS

Hypersensitivity to quinolones. Use in children. Lactation. Ophthalmic use in the presence of dendritic keratitis, varicella, vaccinia, and mycobacterial and fungal eye infections and after removal of foreign bodies from the cornea.

SPECIAL CONCERNS

Tendonitis and tendon rupture: Fluoroquinolones, including ciprofloxacin hydrochloride, are associated with an increased risk of tendinitis and tendon rupture in all ages. This risk is further increased in older clients (usually older than 60 years of age), in clients taking corticosteroid drugs, and in clients with kidney, heart, or lung transplants. **Myasthenia gravis:** Fluoroquinolones, including ciprofloxacin, may exacerbate muscle weakness in persons with myasthenia gravis. Avoid ciprofloxacin in clients with known history of myasthenia gravis.

Possible antibiotic resistance when used to treat *P. aeruginosa* infections.

ADDITIONAL SIDE EFFECTS

Most Common

After systemic use: Headache, N&V, diarrhea, restlessness, rash.
After ophthalmic use: Irritation, burning, stinging, itching, inflammation.
After otic use: Ear pruritus, application site pain, headache.
See also *Side Effects* for *Fluoroquinolones.* **GI:** N&V, abdominal pain/discomfort, diarrhea, dry/painful mouth, dyspepsia, heartburn, constipation, flatulence, pseudomembranous colitis, oral candidiasis, ***intestinal perforation***, anorexia, GI bleeding, bad taste in mouth. **CNS:** Headache, dizziness, fatigue, lethargy, malaise, drowsiness, restlessness, insomnia, nightmares, hallucinations, tremor, light-headedness, irritability, confusion, ataxia, mania, weakness, psychotic reactions, depression, depersonalization, seizures. **GU:** Nephritis, hematuria, cylindruria, renal failure, urinary retention, polyuria, vaginitis, urethral bleeding, acidosis, renal calculi, interstitial nephritis, vaginal candidiasis. **Skin:** Urticaria, photosensitivity, hypersensitivity, flushing, erythema nodosum, cutaneous candidiasis, hyperpigmentation, rash, paresthesia, edema (of lips, neck, face, conjunctivae, hands), ***angioedema***, ***toxic epidermal necrolysis***, exfoliative dermatitis, ***Stevens-Johnson syndrome***. **Ophthalmic:** Blurred or disturbed/double vision, eye pain, nystagmus. **CV:** Hypertension, syncope, angina pectoris, palpitations, atrial flutter, ***MI***, ***cerebral thrombosis***, ventricular ectopy, ***cardiopulmonary arrest***, postural hypotension. **Respiratory:** Dyspnea, ***bronchospasm***, ***pulmonary embolism***, ***edema of larynx or lungs***, hemoptysis, hiccoughs, epistaxis. **Hematologic:** Eosinophilia, pancytopenia, leukopenia, anemia, leukocytosis, ***agranulocytosis***, bleeding diathesis. **Miscellaneous:** Superinfections; fever; chills; tinnitus; joint pain/stiffness; back/neck/chest pain; gout flare-up; flushing; worsening of myasthenia gravis; ***hepatic necrosis***; cholestatic jaundice; hearing loss, dysphasia.

After ophthalmic use. Irritation, burning, itching, ***angioneurotic edema***, urticaria, maculopapular/vesicular dermatitis, crusting of lid margins, conjunctival hyperemia, bad taste in mouth, corneal staining, keratitis, keratopathy, allergic reactions, photophobia, decreased vision, tearing, lid edema. Also, a white, crystalline precipitate in the superficial part of corneal defect (onset within 1–7 days after initiating therapy; lasts about 2 weeks and does not affect continued use of the medication).

After otic use. Ear pruritus, fungal ear superinfection, application site pain, headache.

C

LABORATORY TEST CONSIDERATIONS

↑ ALT, AST, alkaline phosphatase, serum bilirubin, LDH, serum creatinine, BUN, GGT, amylase, uric acid, blood monocytes, potassium, PT, triglycerides, cholesterol. ↓ H&H. Either ↑ or ↓ blood glucose, platelets.

ADDITIONAL DRUG INTERACTIONS

Azlocillin / ↓ Ciprofloxacin excretion → possible ↑ effect
Caffeine / ↓ Caffeine excretion → ↑ pharmacologic effects
Calcium acetate / ↓ Relative ciprofloxacin bioavailability R/T ↓ absorption
Cyclosporine / ↑ Nephrotoxic effects
Foscarnet / ↑ Seizure potential
Hydantoins / ↓ Phenytoin levels
Sevelamer / ↓ Relative ciprofloxacin bioavailability R/T ↓ absorption
Tizanidine / ↑ Tizanidine AUC/peak plasma levels R/T inhibition of CYP1A2 metabolism
Theophylline / Do not take with ciprofloxacin

HOW SUPPLIED

Injection Solution Concentrate: 10 mg/mL (1%); ***Injection Solution:*** 2 mg/mL (0.2%) in D5W; ***Microcapsules for Oral Suspension:*** 250 mg/5 mL (5%), 500 mg/5 mL (10%) (both when reconstituted); ***Ophthalmic Ointment:*** 3.33 mg/gram (equivalent to 3 mg base); ***Ophthalmic Solution:*** 3.5 mg/mL (equivalent to 3 mg base); ***Otic Solution:*** 0.2%; ***Tablets:*** 100 mg, 250 mg, 500 mg, 750 mg; ***Tablets, Extended-Release:*** 500 mg, 1,000 mg.

DOSAGE

ORAL SUSPENSION; TABLETS, IMMEDIATE-RELEASE

Mild to moderate acute sinusitis.

Adults: 500 mg q 12 hr for 10 days.

Mild to moderate chronic bacterial prostatitis.

Adults: 500 mg q 12 hr for 28 days.

Urinary tract infections.

Adults. Acute, uncomplicated infections: 250 mg q 12 hr for 3 days. **Mild to moderate infections:** 250 mg q 12 hr for 7–14 days. **Severe/complicated infections:** 500 mg q 12 hr for 7–14 days.

Bone and joint infections.

Adults, mild to moderate infections: 500 mg q 12 hr for 4 to 6 weeks; **severe/complicated infections:** 750 mg q 12 hr for 4 to 6 weeks.

Intra-abdominal infections, complicated.

Adults: 500 mg q 12 hr for 7–14 days with metronidazole.

Infectious diarrhea, mild to severe.

Adults: 500 mg q 12 hr for 5–7 days.

Skin and skin structures or lower respiratory tract infections.

Adults, mild to moderate infections: 500 mg q 12 hr for 7–14 days; **severe/complicated infections:** 750 mg q 12 hr for 7–14 days.

Typhoid fever, mild to moderate.

Adults: 500 mg q 12 hr for 10 days.

Inhalational anthrax (postexposure).

Adults: 500 mg q 12 hr for 60 days. **Children:** 15 mg/kg/dose (maximum), not to exceed 500 mg/dose, q 12 hr for 60 days. Begin treatment as soon as possible after suspected or confirmed exposure.

Urethral or cervical gonococcal infections, uncomplicated.

Adults: 250 mg as a single dose.

Complicated urinary tract infections or pyelonephritis in children 1–17 years of age.

10–20 mg/kg (maximum, 750 mg per dose) q 12 hr for 10–21 days. **Maximum dose:** 750 mg/dose, not to be exceeded even in children weighing more than 51 kg.

TABLETS, EXTENDED-RELEASE (ER)

Complicated UTIs or acute uncomplicated pyelonephritis.

Adults: 1,000 mg q 24 hr (i.e., once daily) for 7–14 days.

Uncomplicated UTIs (acute cystitis).

Adults: 500 mg q 24 hr (i.e., once daily) for 3 days.

PROQUIN XR

Uncomplicated UTIs (acute cystitis).

500 mg once a day for 3 days with a main meal of the day (preferably the evening meal).

IV INFUSION

Acute sinusitis, mild to moderate.

Adults: 400 mg q 12 hr for 10 days.

Chronic bacterial prostatitis, mild to moderate.

Adults: 400 mg q 12 hr for 28 days.

UTIs.

Adults, mild to moderate infections: 200 mg q 12 hr for 7–14 days; **severe/complicated infections:** 400 mg q 12 hr for 7–14 days.

Bone and joint infections.

Adults, mild to moderate infections: 400 mg q 12 hr for 4–6 weeks; **severe/complicated infections:** 400 mg q 8 hr for 4–6 weeks.

Intra-abdominal infections, complicated.

Adults: 400 mg q 12 hr for 7–14 days with metronidazole.

Skin and skin structures or lower respiratory tract infections.

Adults. Mild to moderate infections: 400 mg q 12 hr for 7–14 days. **Severe/complicated infections:** 400 mg q 8 hr for 7–14 days.

Nosocomial pneumonia, mild to severe.

Adults: 400 mg q 8 hr for 10–14 days.

Febrile neutropenic clients, empirical therapy, severe.

Adults: Ciprofloxacin, 400 mg q 8 hr, with piperacillin, 50 mg/kg q 4 hr, not to exceed 24 grams/day, each for 7–14 days.

Inhalational anthrax, postexposure.

Adults: 400 mg q 12 hr for 60 days. **Children:** 10 mg/kg q 12 hr, not to exceed 400 mg/day, for 60 days. Begin treatment as soon as possible after suspected or confirmed exposure.

Disseminated gonococcal infections (alternate regimen).

Adults, initial: 400 mg IV q 12 hr for 24–48 hr after improvement begins; **then**, 500 mg PO twice a day for 7 days.

Complicated urinary tract infections or pyelonephritis in children, 1–17 years of age.

6–10 mg/kg q 8 hr for 10–21 days. **Maximum dose:** 400 mg/dose, not to be exceeded even in children weighing more than 51 kg.

OPHTHALMIC OINTMENT

Bacterial conjunctivitis.

Adults and children, 2 years and older, initial: Apply ½ in. ribbon to conjunctival sac 3 times per day for the first 2 days; **then**, ½ in. ribbon twice a day for the next 5 days.

OPHTHALMIC SOLUTION

Corneal ulcers.

Adults and children, 1 year and older, first day, initial: 2 gtt into the affected eye q 15 min for the first 6 hr; **then**, 2 gtt into the affected eye q 30 min for the remainder of the first day. **Second day:** 2 gtt into the affected eye hourly. **Third-fourteenth day:** 2 gtt into the affected eye q 4 hr. If corneal reepithelialization has not occurred after 14 days, treatment may be continued.

Bacterial conjunctivitis.

Adults and children, 1 year and older, initial: 1–2 gtt into the conjunctival sac q 2 hr while awake for 2 days; **then**, 1 or 2 gtt q 4 hr while awake for the next 5 days.

OTIC SOLUTION

Otitis externa.

Adults and children, 1 year and older: Instill the contents of 1 single-use container (0.25 mL) into the affected ear twice a day, about 12 hr apart, for 7 days.

NURSING IMPLICATIONS

IMPLEMENTATION/ADMINISTRATION/STORAGE

1. Dose must be reduced in adults with severely impaired renal function (i.e., <50 mL/min). If the C_{CR} is 30–50 mL/min, the dose of immediate-release tablets and suspension should be 250–500 mg q 12 hr; if the C_{CR} is 5–29 mL/min, the dose of immediate-release tablets and suspension should be 250–500 mg q 18 hr. For IV use, give 200–400 mg q 18–24 hr if the C_{CR} is 5–29 mL/min. If the client is on hemodialysis or peritoneal dialysis, the dose of immediate-release and suspension should be 250–500 mg q 24 hr after dialysis. No dosage adjustment is needed for those with uncompli-

cated UTIs receiving ciprofloxacin ER, 500 mg or Proquin XR with mild to moderate impaired renal function. In those with complicated UTIs and acute uncomplicated pyelonephritis and who have a C_{CR} <30 mL/min, reduce the dose of ciprofloxacin from 1,000 to 500 mg a day.

C

2. Five mL of ciprofloxacin, 5% PO suspension equals ciprofloxacin, 250 mg; 5 mL of ciprofloxacin, 10% PO suspension equals ciprofloxacin, 500 mg.
3. Due to physical characteristics, do not give the PO suspension through feeding tubes.
4. Although food delays drug absorption, it may be taken with or without meals; however, coadministration with dairy products alone or with calcium-fortified products should be avoided due to decreased absorption. A minimum of 2 hr between substantial calcium intake (>80 mg) and dosing with ciprofloxacin ER is recommended.
5. Ciprofloxacin ER, ciprofloxacin immediate release, and Proquin XR are not interchangeable. Give Proquin XR once daily for 3 days with a main meal of the day (preferably the evening meal). Give Proquin XR at least 4 hr before or 2 hr after antacids containing magnesium or aluminum, sucralfate, Videx (didanosine) chewable/buffered tablets or pediatric powder, metal cations such as iron, and multivitamin products containing zinc. Never split, crush, or chew Proquin XR.
6. Clients whose therapy began with IV ciprofloxacin for UTIs may be switched to extended-release ciprofloxacin at the discretion of the health care provider when clinically indicated.
7. Clients on theophylline or probenecid require close observation and potential medication adjustments.
8. Do not administer to children.
9. Following instillation of ophthalmic solution, apply light finger pressure to lacrimal sac for 1 min. Safety and efficacy of the ophthalmic ointment has not been established in children younger than 2 years of age. Safety and efficacy of the ophthalmic solution has not been established in children younger than 1 year of age.
10. Store immediate-release tablets below 30°C (86°F). Store extended-release tablets from 15–30°C (59–86°F). Prior to reconstitution, store oral suspension below 25°C (77°F); after reconstitution, store below 30°C (86°F) for 14 days protected from freezing.
11. Store ophthalmic ointment from 2–25°C (36–77°F) and ophthalmic solution from 2–30°C (36–86°F). Protect from light.
12. **IV** Reconstitute IV solution, using appropriate diluents (see below in 13), to a final concentration of 1–2 mg/mL and give over 60 min. The solutions in flexible containers do not require dilution.
13. Ciprofloxacin injection, 1% (10 mg/mL), when diluted with the following IV solutions to concentrations of 0.5–2 mg/mL is stable for up to 14 days at room temperature or refrigerated: NaCl 0.9% injection, D5W injection, sterile water for injection, D10W for injection, D5 and NaCl 0.225% for injection, D5 and NaCl 0.45% for injection, or Ringer's lactate for injection.
14. Administer by IV infusion over 60 min by direct infusion or through a Y-type IV infusion set (may already be in place). Slow infusion of a dilute solution into a larger vein will minimize client discomfort and decrease the risk of vein irritation.
15. If the Y-type or the piggyback method of administration is used, it is recommended that the administration of any other drug be temporarily discontinued during infusion of ciprofloxacin.
16. The IV dose must be adjusted in adults with impaired renal function as follows: If the C_{CR} is >30 mL/min, give the usual dose; if the C_{CR} is 5–29 mL/min, the dose is 200–400 mg q 18–24 hr.
17. If started on IV ciprofloxacin, may be switched to tablets or suspension when clinically indicated. Equivalent dosing regimens are as follows:
    - 250 mg tablet q 12 hr = 200 mg IV q 12 hr.
    - 500 mg tablet q 12 hr = 400 mg IV q 12 hr.
    - 750 mg tablet q 12 hr = 400 mg IV q 8 hr.
18. Store vials for IV use from 5–30°C (41–86°F) and flexible containers from 5–25°C (41–77°F). Protect from light, excessive heat, and freezing.
19. COMPATIBILITY 0.9% NaCl, D5W, 10% dextrose, DIOW, D5/0.225% NaCl, D5/0.45% NaCl, or LR.

20. INCOMPATIBILITY Incompatible with aminophylline, amoxicillin sodium, amoxicillin sodium/potassium clavulanate, clindamycin, and mezlocillin.

ASSESSMENT

1. Note reasons for therapy; onset, characteristics of S&S, culture results.
2. Not for systemic use in children under 18, as irreversible collagen destruction has occurred.
3. Monitor in the elderly; more susceptible to tendon and QT interval effects.
4. Note medications currently prescribed. Fatal reactions have been reported with concurrent administration of IV ciprofloxacin and theophylline. Drug inhibits hepatic CYP1A2 enzyme pathway; coadministration with drugs such as theophylline, methylxanthines, tizanidine could result in adverse effects.
5. Monitor VS, cultures, CBC, renal and LFTs; adjust dose with renal dysfunction.

CLIENT/FAMILY TEACHING

1. XR tablets may be taken with meals that include milk; however, avoid with dairy products alone or with calcium-fortified products because of decreased absorption. A 2 hr window between substantial calcium intake (more than 800 mg) and dosing with XR tablets is recommended. With oral suspension, shake vigorously for 15 sec before measuring dose.
2. Swallow XR tablets whole; do not split, crush, or chew. XR and IR tablets are not interchangeable.
3. Take 2 hr before or 6 hr after Mg/Al antacids, sucralfate, didanosine chewable/buffered tablets, pediatric powder for oral solution, or other products containing calcium, iron, or zinc.
4. May cause dizziness; use caution in any activity that requires mental alertness or coordination.
5. Drink 2–3 L per day of fluids to keep the urine acidic and reduce risk of crystalluria.
6. Minimize caffeine intake: ciprofloxacin may cause caffeine to accumulate in the body, resulting in exaggerated caffeine effects. Avoid OTC meds, and notify of any prescribed meds before taking drug.
7. Complete entire prescription to ensure desired results and to ensure bacteria does not become resistant to the antibiotic.
8. Use caution; avoid sun exposure; direct or artificial sunlight may cause photosensitivity reaction. Wear protective clothing and sunscreen if exposed.
9. Report any persistent joint/tendon pain (especially knee) or GI symptoms such as diarrhea, vomiting, or abdominal pain. Stop therapy, report and refrain from exercise if pain, tenderness, or rupture of tendon occurs or nerve problems, e.g., burning, pain, tingling, numbness, and/or weakness develops (peripheral neuropathy).
10. With eye drops: wash hands, tilt head back, and look up. Pull lower eyelid down, and instill prescribed number of drops. Close eye for 1–2 min, and apply gentle pressure to bridge of nose for 3–5 min. Do not rub eye. Do not allow dropper to touch eye. Avoid contact lenses with any S&S bacterial conjunctivitis.
11. With eye ointment: wash hands, do not touch eye with tube or tip. Tilt head back looking up, and pull lower eyelid down to form pocket. Place prescribed dose of ointment into pocket. Look downward before closing eye, and do not rub eye.
12. If using more than 1 topical ophthalmic drug, administer the drugs at least 5 min apart, administering ointment last. Temporary blurred vision, eye pain, or eye discomfort may occur; report if persistent or bothersome.
13. With ear drops: warm container in hands for at least 1 min prior to use. Lie down with affected ear up, and place contents of 1 container into the ear; stay in this position for at least 1 min.
14. Keep F/U to assess response, labs, adverse SE, or intolerance.

OUTCOMES/EVALUATE

- Resolution of infection with symptomatic improvement; ↓ fever, ↓ WBCs, ↑ appetite
- Treatment of corneal ulcers (solution only), conjunctivitis and/or external otitis
- Negative culture reports
- ↓ Incidence/progression of disease following exposure to aerosolized *Bacillus anthracis* (anthrax)

IV

Cisatracurium besylate

(sis-ah-trah-**KYOU**-ree-um)

Classification(s): Neuromuscular blocking drug

Pregnancy Category: B

RX: Nimbex.

SEE ALSO ***NEUROMUSCULAR BLOCKING AGENTS***.

C

INDICATIONS/USES

Neuromuscular blocking agent for in- and out-patients as an adjunct to general anesthesia, to facilitate tracheal intubation, and to cause skeletal muscle relaxation during surgery or mechanical ventilation in the intensive care unit.

ACTION/KINETICS

Action

Nondepolarizing neuromuscular blocking agent that binds competitively to cholinergic receptors on the motor end-plate, resulting in antagonism of the action of acetylcholine and therefore neuromuscular blockade. The neuromuscular blocking potency of cisatracurium is about three times greater than that for atracurium.

Pharmacokinetics

Intermediate onset and duration. **Time to maximum blockade:** 2 min. **Time to recovery:** Approximately 55 min. Continuous infusion for up to 3 hr may be undertaken without tachyphylaxis or cumulative neuromuscular blockade. The time required for recovery following successive maintenance doses does not change with the number of doses given, provided that partial recovery is allowed to occur between doses. Onset, duration, and recovery are faster in children. About 95% of a dose is excreted as metabolites and unchanged drug (10%) in the urine and 4% is eliminated through the feces. Laudanosine, a major biologically active metabolite with no neuromuscular activity, may cause transient hypotension and cerebral excitatory effects (in high doses).

CONTRAINDICATIONS

Hypersensitivity to cisatracurium or other bisbenzylisoquinolinium agents or hypersensitivity to benzyl alcohol. Use for rapid-sequence ET intubation due to its intermediate onset of action.

SPECIAL CONCERNS

- **Since the drug has no effect on consciousness, pain threshold, or cerebration, do not undertake administration before unconsciousness.**
- **May cause a profound effect in those with myasthenia gravis or the myasthenic syndrome.**
- **Burn clients may require higher doses.**
- **Onset time is faster (about 1 min) and recovery is slower (by about 1 min) in impaired hepatic function.**
- **The time to maximum blockage is about 1 min slower in geriatric clients and in those with impaired renal function.**
- **Use with caution during lactation.**
- **Safety and efficacy not determined in children less than 2 years of age.**

SIDE EFFECTS

Most Common

Bradycardia, hypotension, flushing, ***bronchospasm***, rash.

See *Neuromuscular Blocking Agents* for a complete list of possible side effects.

OVERDOSE MANAGEMENT

Symptoms: Neuromuscular blockade beyond the time needed for surgery and anesthesia. *Treatment:* Maintain a patent airway and control ventilation until recovery of normal function is ensured. Once recovery begins, facilitate the process by using neostigmine or edrophonium with an anticholinergic drug. Do not give these antidotes when complete blockade is evident.

DRUG INTERACTIONS

Aminoglycosides / ↑ Cisatracurium effect
Bacitracin / ↑ Cisatracurium effect
Carbamazepine / Resistance to neuromuscular blockage → slightly shorter duration.
Clindamycin / ↑ Cisatracurium effect
Colistin, sodium colistimethate / ↑ Cisatracurium effect
Enflurane/nitrous oxide/oxygen / ↑ Cisatracurium duration
Isoflurane/nitrous oxide/oxygen / ↑ Cisatracurium duration
Lincomycin / ↑ Cisatracurium effect
Lithium / ↑ Cisatracurium effect
Local anesthetics / ↑ Cisatracurium effect
Mg^{++} salts / ↑ Cisatracurium effect
Phenobarbital / Resistance to neuromuscular blockade → slightly shorter duration
Polymyxins / ↑ Cisatracurium effect
Procainamide / ↑ Cisatracurium effect
Quinidine / ↑ Cisatracurium effect
Succinylcholine / Time to onset of maximum block of cisatracurium is about 2 min faster
Tetracyclines / ↑ Cisatracurium effect

HOW SUPPLIED

Injection: 2 mg/mL, 10 mg/mL.

DOSAGE

IV BOLUS

Neuromuscular blockade.

Adults, initial: Depending on the desired time to intubation and the anticipated length of surgery, either 0.15 or 0.2 mg/kg is used. These doses are components of a propofol/nitrous oxide/oxygen induction-intubation technique. **Maintenance during prolonged surgery:** 0.03 mg/kg given 40–50 min following an initial dose of 0.15 mg/kg and 50–60 min following an initial dose of 0.2 mg/kg.

Children, 2–12 years of age: 0.1 mg/kg over 5–10 sec during either halothane or opioid anesthesia. When given during stable opioid/nitrous oxide/oxygen anesthesia, 0.1 mg/kg produces maximum effects in about 2.8 min and a clinically effective blockade for 28 min.

IV INFUSION

Neuromuscular blockade during extended surgery or in the intensive care unit (ICU).

In the OR or ICU, following an initial bolus dose, a diluted solution can be given by continuous infusion to both adults and children over 2 years of age. The rate is dependent on the response of the client determined by peripheral nerve stimulation. An infusion rate of 3 mcg/kg/min can be used to counteract rapid spontaneous recovery of neuromuscular blockade. Thereafter, an infusion rate of 1–2 mcg/kg/min is usually adequate to maintain blockade. Reduce infusion rate by 30–40% when given during stable isoflurane or enflurane anesthesia.

NURSING IMPLICATIONS

IMPLEMENTATION/ADMINISTRATION/STORAGE

1. IV Due to slower times of onset in geriatric clients and those with impaired renal function, extend interval between drug administration and intubation.
2. Spontaneous recovery following infusion will proceed at a rate comparable to that following administration of a bolus dose.
3. The 10 mL multiple-dose vial contains benzyl alcohol, which has been associated with neurological and other complications that are sometimes fatal in neonates
4. Cisatracurium diluted in D5W, 0.9% NaCl, or D5/0.9% NaCl may be refrigerated or stored at room temperature for 24 hr without significant loss of potency. Dilutions to 0.1 or 0.2 mg/mL in DW5/RL may be refrigerated for 24 hr. Refrigerate vials at 2–8°C (36–46°F) and protect from light. Once removed from the refrigerator, use vials within 21 days, even if rerefrigerated.
5. COMPATIBILITY D5W, 0.9% NaCl, D5/0.9% NaCl, sufentanil, alfentanil HCl, fentanyl, midazolam HCl, and droperidol.
6. INCOMPATIBILITY Propofol or ketorolac for Y-site administration. Due to chemical instability, do not dilute in RL or alkaline solutions with a pH greater than 8.5 (e.g., barbiturate solutions).

ASSESSMENT

1. List reasons for therapy, other agents trialed, anticipated duration of therapy.
2. Note hypersensitivity to benzyl alcohol or note any neuromuscular disorders.
3. Administered only by those trained in giving neuromuscular blocking agents.
4. Client requires constant monitoring and ventilatory support.
5. Those with burns, hemiparesis, or paraparesis may have resistance to cisatracurium.
6. Medicate with analgesics for pain, agents for anxiety based on assessed need.
7. Utilize a peripheral nerve stimulator to evaluate response to therapy, to ensure partial recovery between doses.
8. Have antagonists (e.g., neostigmine) readily available. Do not use when complete blockade present.
9. Prevent overdosage during infusions by frequent evaluations with a peripheral nerve stimulator to document antagonism of neuromuscular blockade and recovery of muscle function and strength.

10. Document/monitor VS, neurologic and respiratory assessments, ABGs, electrolytes, and other labs as condition indicates.

CLIENT/FAMILY TEACHING

1. During drug administration you will be able to see and hear things around you but you will be completely unable to move or breathe on your own. A machine will perform breathing for you while medicated.
2. This will resolve once the medication is discontinued. Medications will be given for anxiety and pain as needed.
3. Eye drops and patches to protect corneas during prolonged therapy may be used as blink reflex suppressed.
4. Passive range-of-motion exercises may be performed to prevent loss of function and contractures with prolonged therapy.

OUTCOMES/EVALUATE

- Facilitation of ET intubation
- Skeletal muscle relaxation

IV

Cisplatin (CDDP)

(sis-**PLAH**-tin)

Classification(s): Antineoplastic, alkylating
Pregnancy Category: D

RX: Cisplatin.

SEE ALSO ***ANTINEOPLASTIC AGENTS***.

INDICATIONS/USES

Palliative therapy. (1) Combination therapy for metastatic testicular tumors or for metastatic ovarian tumors (e.g., with cyclophosphamide) in those who have received appropriate surgical or radiotherapeutic procedures. (2) Single agent in metastatic ovarian tumors as secondary therapy in those refractive to standard therapy who have not previously received cisplatin. (3) Single agent in transitional cell bladder cancer that is no longer amenable to surgery or radiotherapy. *Investigational:* Adjuvant therapy for non-small-cell lung cancer.

ACTION/KINETICS

Action

Binds to DNA and causes production of intrastrand cross-links and formation of DNA adducts. The drug is cell-cycle nonspecific.

Pharmacokinetics

t½, plasma: 20–30 min. **Terminal t½, blood cells:** 36–47 days. Incomplete urinary excretion (only 35–51% after 5 days). Concentrates in liver, kidneys, and large and small intestines, with low penetration of CNS. About 10–40% excreted in the urine within 24 hr. **Plasma protein binding:** More than 90%.

ADDITIONAL CONTRAINDICATIONS

Lactation. Pre-existing renal impairment, myelosuppression, impaired hearing, history of allergic reactions to platinum-containing compounds.

SPECIAL CONCERNS

(1) Administer under the supervision of a qualified physician experienced in the use of cancer chemotherapy. Appropriate management of therapy and complications is possible only when adequate diagnostic and treatment facilities are readily available. (2) Cumulative renal toxicity is severe. Other major dose-related toxicities are myelosuppression and N&V. (3) Ototoxicity, which may be more pronounced in children, is manifested by tinnitus or loss of high frequency hearing; occasionally deafness is significant. (4) Anaphylactic-type reactions have occurred. Facial edema, bronchoconstriction, tachycardia, and hypotension may occur within minutes of cisplatin administration. Epinephrine, corticosteroids, and antihistamines have been effectively used to alleviate symptoms. (5) Exercise caution to prevent inadvertent cisplatin overdose. Doses >100 mg/m^2/cycle once every 3 to 4 weeks are rarely used. Take care to avoid inadvertent cisplatin overdose due to confusion with carboplatin or prescribing practices that fail to differentiate daily doses from total dose per cycle.

- The elderly may be more susceptible to drug-related nephrotoxicity, myelosuppression, or infectious complications.
- Safety and efficacy not determined in children.

ADDITIONAL SIDE EFFECTS

Most Common

Renal toxicity, ototoxicity, myelosuppression, N&V, diarrhea.

Renal: Severe cumulative renal toxicity, including renal tubular damage and renal insufficiency.

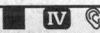

CNS: Seizures, peripheral neuropathies, dorsal column myelopathy, Lhermitte's sign, autonomic neuropathy, paresthesias. Neurotoxicity may occur 4–7 months after prolonged therapy. **GI:** N&V, anorexia, diarrhea, loss of taste, hiccoughs. **CV:** Cardiac abnormalities, MI, CVA, thrombotic microangiopathy, cerebral arteritis. **Hematologic:** Myelosuppression, including anemia and hemolytic anemia, leukopenia, thrombocytopenia. **Electrolytes:** Low levels of calcium, Mg^{++}, potassium, phosphate, and sodium. **Musculoskeletal:** Muscle cramps, including localized, painful, involuntary skeletal muscle contractions (sudden onset and short duration) with high cumulative doses. **GU:** Renal insufficiency, renal tubular damage. **Dermatologic:** Alopecia, rash, local soft tissue toxicity (rare). **Otic:** Ototoxicity characterized by tinnitus, especially in children; high frequency hearing loss, vestibular toxicity. **Ophthalmologic:** Papilledema, cerebral blindness, optic neuritis. High doses have resulted in blurred vision and altered color perception. **Metabolic:** Tetany due to hypomagnesemia and hypocalcemia. **Hypersensitivity reaction:** ***Anaphylactic reactions***, facial edema, wheezing, tachycardia, hypotension. **Body as a whole:** Asthenia, malaise. **Miscellaneous:** Hepatotoxicity, ADH syndrome.

LABORATORY TEST CONSIDERATIONS

↑ Plasma iron levels, serum amylase, liver enzymes, bilirubin. Nephrotoxicity results in ↑ serum uric acid, BUN, and creatinine and ↓ C_{CR}. Hypomagnesemia, hypocalcemia, hyponatremia, hypokalemia, hypophosphatemia, hyperuricemia.

OVERDOSE MANAGEMENT

Symptoms: Liver and kidney failure, deafness, ocular toxicity (including retinal detachment), significant myelosuppression, intractable N&V, neuritis, death. *Treatment:* General supportive measures

ADDITIONAL DRUG INTERACTIONS

Aminoglycosides / Cumulative nephrotoxicity
Anticonvulsants / Anticonvulsant plasma levels may become subtherapeutic
Loop diuretics / Additive ototoxicity
Phenytoin / ↓ Phenytoin effect R/T ↓ plasma levels

HOW SUPPLIED

Injection: 1 mg/mL.

DOSAGE

IV INFUSION ONLY

Metastatic testicular tumors.

Adults: 20 mg/m²/day for 5 days per cycle in combination with other chemotherapeutic drugs.

Metastatic ovarian tumors.

Adults: Cisplatin: 75–100 mg/m² once every 4 weeks per cycle. Cyclophosphamide: 600 mg/m² once every 4 weeks on day 1. Administer cisplatin and cyclophosphamide sequentially.

Advanced bladder cancer.

Adults: 50–70 mg/m² per cycle once q 3–4 weeks, depending on prior radiation or chemotherapy. For those heavily pretreated, give an initial dose of 50 mg/m²/cycle repeated q 4 weeks. *NOTE:* Repeat courses should not be administered until (1) serum creatinine is below 1.5 mg/dL and/or the BUN is below 25 mg/dL; (2) platelets are equal to or greater than 100,000/mm³ and leukocyte count is equal to or greater than 4,000/mm³; and (3) auditory activity is within the normal range.

NURSING IMPLICATIONS

Do not confuse cisplatin with carboplatin (also an antineoplastic drug).

IMPLEMENTATION/ADMINISTRATION/STORAGE

1. **IV** Before administration, hydrate with 1–2 L of IV fluid over a period of 8–12 hr.
2. Add dosage recommended from vial to 2 L of D5W in one-half or one-third NSS containing 37.5 grams mannitol. (Do not just dilute cisplatin in D5W.) Infuse over a period of 6–8 hr. Furosemide may be used instead of mannitol. Maintain adequate hydration, urinary output for 24 hr following infusion.
3. If diluted solution is not to be used within 6 hours, protect solution from light.
4. Cisplatin has been confused with carboplatin. Place signs/label warnings to prevent name mix-ups. Do not refer to as "platinum."
5. Have emergency equipment available for anaphylactic reaction.

6. Aluminum reacts with cisplatin; avoid using equipment with aluminum as a black precipitate will form and loss of potency occurs.
7. COMPATIBILITY D5W, D5% in ½ to ⅓ normal saline.
8. INCOMPATIBILITY Administer separately.

C

ASSESSMENT

1. List reasons for therapy, onset, and characteristics of symptoms. Identify previous cancer treatments (XRT, chemotherapy).
2. Obtain audiometry testing before and after therapy to ensure hearing has not been affected; get ECG during induction therapy to assess for myocarditis or focal irritability.
3. Hydrate well (1–2 L fluid over 8–12 hr) prior to initial dose; give parenteral antiemetic at least 30 min before therapy and regularly during therapy. Hydrate to prevent urate deposits; monitor I&O during and for 24 hr after treatment.
4. *During therapy monitor for:*
   - Facial edema, bronchoconstriction, tachycardia, and shock.
   - Tremors that may progress to seizures due to hypomagnesemia.
   - Tetany, confusion, or signs of hypocalcemia associated with hypomagnesemia; monitor Ca^{++}/Mg^{++} levels.
   - Bone marrow suppression (↑ bruising/bleeding).
   - Irritation and extravasation at IV site.
5. Obtain baseline CBC, uric acid, electrolytes, Ca^{++}, Mg^{++}, renal and LFTs. May cause severe cumulative renal toxicity; additional cisplatin doses should not be administered until renal function returned to baseline and usually not more frequently than every 3–4 weeks. Assess for mild granulocyte suppression. Nadir: 14 days; recovery: 21 days.

CLIENT/FAMILY TEACHING

1. Review reasons and frequency for therapy; administered parenterally.
2. Report ringing in ears, difficulty hearing, pain at injection site, abnormal bruising/bleeding, N&V, edema of lower extremities, decreased urination, numbness, tingling, swelling, or joint pain.
3. Avoid alcohol and salicylates; may increase gastric bleeding. Avoid vaccinations.
4. Use reliable birth control; may cause infertility. Identify candidates for egg/sperm harvesting.
5. Keep all F/U to assess response, labs, and for adverse SE.

OUTCOMES/EVALUATE

↓ Tumor size; suppression of malignant cell proliferation

■ ©

Citalopram hydrobromide

(sigh-**TAL**-oh-pram)

Classification(s): Antidepressant, selective serotonin reuptake inhibitor

Pregnancy Category: C

RX: Celexa.

✱ **Rx:** Apo-Citalopram, CO Citalopram, Gen-Citalopram, PMS-Citalopram, RAN-Citalopram, ratio-Citalopram, Sandoz Citalopram.

SEE ALSO ***ANTIDEPRESSANTS.***

INDICATIONS/USES

Treatment of depression in those with DSM-III and DSM III-R category of major depressive disorder. *Investigational:* Panic disorder, premenstrual dysphoric disorder (intermittent use), posttraumatic stress disorder, generalized anxiety disorder, obsessive-compulsive disorder.

ACTION/KINETICS

Action

Significant effect to inhibit reuptake of serotonin into CNS neurons, resulting in increased levels of serotonin in synapses. Has minimal effects on reuptake of norepinephrine and dopamine. Minimal to no anticholinergic, sedative, or orthostatic hypotensive effects.

Pharmacokinetics

Is about 80% bioavailable. **Peak plasma levels:** 120–150 nmol/L after about 4 hr. **t½, terminal:** 33 hr. Half-life and AUC are increased in geriatric clients. **Steady state plasma levels:** About 1 week. Metabolized in the liver and excreted in the urine (20%) and feces (65%). **Plasma protein binding:** About 80%.

CONTRAINDICATIONS

Use with MAOIs or with alcohol. Lactation.

SPECIAL CONCERNS

> Suicidality in children, adolescents, and young adults. Antidepressants increased the risk compared with placebo of suicidal thinking and behavior (suicidality) in short-term studies in children, adolescents and young adults with major depressive disorders and other psychiatric disorders. Anyone considering the use of citalopram or any other antidepressant in a child, adolescent, or young adult must balance this risk with the clinical need. Closely observe clients who are started on therapy for clinical worsening, suicidality, or unusual changes in behavior. Advise families and caregivers of the need for close observation and communication with the health care provider. Citalopram is not approved for use in pediatric clients. The average risk of adverse reactions representing suicidal thinking or behavior (suicidality) during the first few months of treatment in those receiving antidepressants was 4%, twice the placebo risk of 2%. No suicides occurred in these trials.

- **Use with caution in severe renal impairment (dosage adjustment not necessary), a history of seizure disorders, or in diseases or conditions that produce altered metabolism or hemodynamic responses.**
- **Safety and efficacy not determined in children.**
- **Complications can develop immediately on delivery of the neonate and may require prolonged hospitalization, respiratory support, and tube feeding.**

SIDE EFFECTS

Most Common

Somnolence, insomnia, nausea, excessive sweating, dry mouth, tremor, loose stools/diarrhea.
CNS: Activation of mania/hypomania, dizziness, insomnia, agitation, somnolence, anorexia, paresthesia, migraine, hyperkinesia, vertigo, hypertonia, extrapyramidal disorder, neuralgia, dystonia, abnormal gait, hypesthesia, ataxia, aggravated depression, ***suicide ideation/attempt***, confusion, aggressive reaction, drug dependence, depersonalization, hallucinations, euphoria, psychotic depression, delusions, paranoid reaction, emotional lability, panic reaction, psychosis. **GI:** N&V, dry mouth, diarrhea, dyspepsia, abdominal pain, increased salivation, flatulence, gastritis, gastroenteritis, stomatitis, eructation, hemorrhoids, dysphagia, teeth grinding, gingivitis, esophagitis. **CV:** Tachycardia, postural hypotension, hypertension, bradycardia, edema of extremities, angina pectoris, extrasystoles, ***cardiac failure, MI, CVA***, flushing, myocardial ischemia. **Musculoskeletal:** Arthralgia, myalgia, arthritis, muscle weakness, skeletal pain, leg cramps, involuntary muscle contraction. **Hematologic:** Purpura, anemia, leukocytosis, lymphadenopathy. **Metabolic/Nutritional:** Decreased/increased weight, thirst. **GU:** Ejaculation disorder, impotence, dysmenorrhea, decreased/increased libido, amenorrhea, galactorrhea, breast pain/enlargement, ***vaginal hemorrhage***, polyuria, frequent micturition, urinary incontinence/retention, dysuria. **Respiratory:** Coughing, epistaxis, bronchitis, dyspnea, pneumonia. **Dermatologic:** Rash, pruritus, photosensitivity reaction, urticaria, acne, skin discoloration, eczema, dermatitis, dry skin, psoriasis. **Ophthalmic:** Abnormal accommodation, conjunctivitis, eye pain. **Body as a whole:** Asthenia, fatigue, fever. **Miscellaneous:** Hyponatremia, increased sweating, yawning, hot flushes, rigors, alcohol intolerance, syncope, flu-like symptoms, taste perversion, tinnitus.

LABORATORY TEST CONSIDERATIONS

↑ Hepatic enzymes, alkaline phosphatase. Abnormal glucose tolerance.

OVERDOSE MANAGEMENT

Symptoms: Dizziness, sweating, N&V, tremor, somnolence, sinus tachycardia. Rarely, amnesia, confusion, coma, convulsions, hyperventilation, cyanosis, rhabdomyolysis, ECG changes (including QTc prolongation, nodal rhythm, ventricular arrhythmias). *Treatment:* Establish and maintain an airway. Gastric lavage with use of activated charcoal. Monitor cardiac and vital signs. General symptomatic and supportive care.

DRUG INTERACTIONS

See also ***Drug Interactions*** for ***Selective Serotonin Reuptake Inhibitors.***

Azole antifungals / ↑ Citalopram levels
Beta-blockers / ↑ Beta-blocker effect; reduce initial beta blocker dose
Carbamazepine / ↓ Citalopram levels; ↑ carbamazepine levels
Imipramine / ↑ Drug metabolite (desimpramine) by 50%

Lithium / Possible ↑ serotonergic citalopram effects
Macrolide antibiotics (e.g., erythromycin) / ↑ Citalopram levels
MAOIs / Possible serious and sometimes fatal reactions, including hyperthermia, rigidity, myoclonus, autonomic instability, mental status changes (extreme agitation, delirium, coma); do not use together

HOW SUPPLIED

Oral Solution: 10 mg/5 mL; *Tablets:* 10 mg, 20 mg, 40 mg; *Tablets, Orally Disintegrating:* 10 mg, 20 mg, 40 mg.

DOSAGE

ORAL SOLUTION; TABLETS; TABLETS, ORALLY DISINTEGRATING

Depression.

Adults, initial: 20 mg once daily in a.m. or p.m. with or without food. Increase dose in increments of 20 mg at intervals of no less than 1 week. Doses greater than 40 mg/day are not recommended. For the elderly or those with hepatic impairment, 20 mg/day is recommended; titrate to 40 mg/day only for nonresponders. Initial treatment is continued for 6 or 8 weeks. **Maintenance:** Up to 24 weeks following 6 or 8 weeks of initial treatment. Periodically re-evaluate the long-term usefulness of the drug if used for extended periods.

Panic disorder.

20–30 mg/day.

NURSING IMPLICATIONS

Do not confuse Celexa with Cerebyx (an anticonvulsant) or with Celebrex (nonsteroidal anti-inflammatory drug).

IMPLEMENTATION/ADMINISTRATION/STORAGE

1. Allow at least 14 days to elapse between discontinuation of an MAOI and initiation of citalopram or vice versa.
2. A gradual reduction in dose, rather than abrupt cessation, is recommended whenever possible. Resume a previously prescribed dose if intolerable symptoms occur following a decrease in dose or upon discontinuation of treatment.
3. Dosage adjustment is not needed in clients with mild to moderate renal impairment.
4. Store from 15–30°C (59–86°F).

ASSESSMENT

1. Note reasons for therapy, onset/characteristics of S&S, any events/triggers, and other agents trialed/outcome.
2. List other drugs prescribed; ensure none interact. Avoid use within 14 days before or after MAOI use.
3. If discontinued, monitor for the following symptoms: Dysphoric mood, irritability, agitation, dizziness, sensory disturbances, anxiety, confusion, headache, lethargy, emotional lability, or hypomania. If intolerable symptoms occur following decrease in dose or discontinuation of the drug, consider resuming the previously prescribed dose. Subsequently the dose may be decreased but at a more gradual rate.
4. Document behaviors and clinical presentation.
5. Monitor weight, ECG, VS, electrolytes, renal and LFTs. Note any liver/renal dysfunction, or seizure disorder; reduce dose with dysfunction.

CLIENT/FAMILY TEACHING

1. Take as directed, once daily, with or without food.
2. Use caution operating machines or cars until drug effects known. May impair judgment, thinking, motor skills, or cause drowsiness.
3. Avoid alcohol or other CNS depressants. Do not take aspirin or aspirin-containing products, NSAIDs, ginkgo biloba, or any other medication or herbal product that can affect coagulation.
4. Monitor and report any changes in personality, mood swings, anxiety, agitation, ↑ panic attacks, insomnia, irritability, hostility, aggressiveness, impulsivity, or suicidal thoughts/behaviors.
5. May see improvement in 1–4 weeks; children should be seen weekly during initiation of therapy. Do not stop suddenly unless instructed.
6. Report if excessive drowsiness, diarrhea, tremors, nausea, diarrhea, nervousness, changes in sexual function, rash, hives, or itching occur.

7. **May increase sensitivity to sunlight; wear sunscreen, protective clothing, and avoid prolonged exposures.**
8. **Report pregnancy, intent to become pregnant, or breast-feeding to provider. If using, taper off during last trimester.**
9. **Keep all F/U to assess response, dose, labs, and for adverse SE.**

OUTCOMES/EVALUATE

- Relief/control of major depression/panic attacks
- Control PTSD/OCD (unlabeled)

Clarithromycin

(klah-**rith**-roh-**MY**-sin)

Classification(s): Antibiotic, macrolide

Pregnancy Category: C

RX: Biaxin, Biaxin XL.

✤ **Rx:** Apo-Clarithromycin, Biaxin BID.

SEE ALSO ***ANTI-INFECTIVES***.

INDICATIONS/USES

Oral Suspension, Tablets. Mild to moderate infections caused by susceptible strains of the following.

1. Pharyngitis/tonsillitis in adults or children due to *Streptococcus pyogenes*. Efficacy in prevention of rheumatic fever is not available.
2. Acute maxillary sinusitis in adults or children due to *Streptococcus pneumoniae, Haemophilus influenzae,* and *Moraxella catarrhalis.* The active metabolite, 14-OH clarithromycin, has significant activity (twice the parent compound) against *H. influenzae.*
3. Acute bacterial exacerbation of chronic bronchitis in adults due to *S. pneumoniae, H. influenzae, H. parainfluenzae, M. catarrhalis.*
4. Community-acquired pneumonia in adults or children due to *Mycoplasma pneumoniae, S. pneumoniae, Chlamydia pneumoniae* (TWAR strain), or *H. influenzae* (adults only).
5. Acute otitis media in children due to *H. influenzae, M. catarrhalis,* or *S. pneumoniae.*
6. Uncomplicated skin and skin structure infections in adults or children due to *Staphylococcus aureus* or *S. pyogenes.* Abscesses usually require surgical drainage.
7. Disseminated mycobacterial infections in adults or children due to *Mycobacterium avium* (commonly seen in AIDS clients) and *M. intracellulare.* Prevention of disseminated *M. avium* complex in adults or children with advanced HIV.
8. Dual therapy to treat *Helicobacter pylori;* clarithromycin in combination with omeprazole.
9. Triple therapy to treat *Helicobacter pylori;* clarithromycin in combination with lansoprazole or omeprazole, and amoxicillin. To treat *H. pylori* infection and duodenal ulcer disease (active or 5-year history of duodenal ulcer) to eradicate *H. pylori.*

Investigational: Treatment of early Lyme disease.

Extended-Release Tablets. Mild to moderate infections in adults of the following:

1. Acute maxillary sinusitis due to *H. influenzae, M. catarrhalis,* or *S. pneumoniae.*
2. Acute bacterial exacerbation of chronic bronchitis due to *H. influenzae, H. parainfluenzae, M. catarrhalis,* or *S. pneumoniae.*
3. Community-acquired pneumonia due to *H. influenzae, H. parainfluenzae, M. catarrhalis, S. pneumoniae, C. pneumoniae* (TWAR), or *M. pneumoniae.*

ACTION/KINETICS

Action

Macrolide antibiotic that acts by binding to the 50S ribosomal subunit of susceptible organisms, thus interfering with or inhibiting microbial protein synthesis. Nucleic acid synthesis is not affected.

Pharmacokinetics

Rapidly absorbed from the GI tract although food slightly delays the onset of absorption and the formation of the active metabolite but does not affect the extent of the bioavailability (50–55% for tablets). **Peak serum levels:** 2–3 hr for tablets, about 3 hr for the suspension, and 5–8 hr for extended-release tablets. **Steady-state peak serum levels:** 1–2 mcg/mL within 2–3 days after 250 mg q 12 hr and 2–3 mcg/mL after 500 mg q 8–12 hr. Clarithromycin and 14-OH clarithromycin (active metabolite) are readily distributed to body tissues and fluids. **t½, elimination:** 3–7 hr (depending on the dose) for clarithromycin and 5–9 hr for 14-OH clarithromycin. Up to 20–30% of a dose of tablets and 40% of a dose of the suspension are excreted unchanged in the urine. **Plasma protein binding:** 40–70%.

CONTRAINDICATIONS

C

Hypersensitivity to clarithromycin, other macrolide antibiotics, or erythromycin. Use in pregnancy unless no alternative therapy is appropriate. Use in those taking cisapride, pimozide, ergotamine, or dihydroergotamine. Use with ranitidine bismuth citrate in those with a history of acute porphyria or in those with a C_{CR} <25 mL/min.

SPECIAL CONCERNS

- **Use with caution in severe renal impairment with or without concomitant hepatic impairment and during lactation.**
- **Safety and efficacy not determined in children less than 6 months of age.**
- **Safety has not been determined in MAC clients less than 20 months of age.**
- **Use with caution during lactation.**

SIDE EFFECTS

Most Common

Adults: Diarrhea/loose stools, abdominal pain/discomfort, N&V, dyspepsia, flatulence, abnormal taste/taste perversion, headache.

Children: Diarrhea, vomiting, abdominal pain, rash, and headache.

GI: N&V, abnormal taste, taste perversion, taste loss, abdominal pain/discomfort, diarrhea/loose stools, *Clostridium difficile*–associated diarrhea, flatulence, dyspepsia, anorexia, oral moniliasis, ***pancreatitis***, glossitis, stomatitis, tongue/tooth discoloration. **Hepatic:** Impaired hepatic function, hepatocellular and/or cholestatic hepatitis (with or without jaundice), ***hepatic failure***. **CV:** QT prolongation, ***torsades de pointes***, ventricular arrhythmias/tachycardia. **CNS:** Headache, agitation, asthenia, ***convulsions***, dizziness, insomnia, vertigo, anxiety, behavioral changes, confusion, depersonalization, disorientation, hallucinations, manic behavior, nightmares, psychosis, tremor. **Dermatologic:** Rash, urticaria. **GU:** Interstitial nephritis. **Hematologic:** Leukopenia, neutropenia, thrombocytopenia. **Hypersensitivity:** Urticaria, mild skin eruptions and, rarely, ***anaphylaxis***, ***Stevens-Johnson syndrome***, and ***toxic epidermal necrolysis***. **Otic:** Hearing loss, tinnitus. **Miscellaneous:** Alterations of smell, hypoglycemia, superinfection.

LABORATORY TEST CONSIDERATIONS

↑ ALT, AST, liver enzymes, GGT, alkaline phosphatase, LDH, total bilirubin, BUN, serum creatinine, PT. ↓ Hemoglobin, platelet count, WBC count.

OVERDOSE MANAGEMENT

Symptoms: Abdominal pain, diarrhea, nausea, vomiting, reversible hearing loss. *Treatment:* Supportive measures. Hemodialysis and peritoneal dialysis are not particularly effective.

DRUG INTERACTIONS

NOTE: (1) Clarithromycin is a substrate and inhibitor of CYP3A enzymes. Coadministration of clarithromycin and a drug primarily metabolized by CHP3A may cause increases in drug levels → ↑ pharmacologic/toxic effects. Consider dosage adjustments when possible.
(2) A possible additive effect of clarithromycin with other drugs that prolong the QT interval may occur. The following drugs may prolong the QT interval and ↑ the risk of life-threatening cardiac arrhythmias, including torsades de pointes: Amiodarone, arsenic trioxide, bretylium, chlorpromazine, cisapride, disopyramide, dofetilide, dolasetron, droperidol, gatifloxacin, halofantrine, levomethadyl, mefloquine, mesoridazine, moxifloxacin, pentamidine, pimozide, probucol, procainamide, quinidine, sotalol, sparfloxacin, tacrolimus, thioridazine, and ziprasidone.

Alfentanil / ↑ Alfentanil pharmacologic effects

Amiodarone / Additive or synergistic ↑ in QT interval → ↑ risk of life-threatening cardiac arrhythmias, including torsades de pointes

Benzodiazepines (e.g., alprazolam, diazepam, midazolam, triazolam) / ↑ Plasma levels of certain benzodiazepines → ↑ CNS depression and prolonged sedation

Bretylium / Additive or synergistic ↑ in QT interval → ↑ risk of life-threatening cardiac arrhythmias, including torsades de pointes

Bromocriptine / ↑ Bromocriptine serum levels → ↑ pharmacologic/toxic effects

Buspirone / ↑ Buspirone levels → ↑ risk of pharmacologic/toxic effects

Calcium channel blockers / ↑ Risk of hypotension or shock requiring hospitalization in elderly clients

Carbamazepine / ↑ Carbamazepine levels → ↑ toxicity; do not use together

Cilostazol / ↑ Cilostazol levels → ↑ risk of pharmacologic/toxic effects
Cimetidine / ↓ Clarithromycin antimicrobial effect
Cisapride / ↑ Cisapride levels → QT prolongation, ventricular tachycardia, ventricular fibrillation, and torsades de pointes R/T inhibition of cisapride metabolism; do not use together
Clopidogrel / ↓ Clopidogrel antiplatelet effect; monitor platelet function; adjust clopidogrel dose as needed
Colchicine / Severe colchicine intoxication R/T inhibition of metabolism by CYP3A4; death has resulted; do not use together
Conivaptan / ↑ Conivaptan plasma levels → ↑ risk of toxic effects; do not use together
Cyclosporine ↑ Cyclosporine levels → ↑ risk of nephrotoxicity and neurotoxicity; monitor cyclosporine levels and serum creatinine, and adjust dose as needed
Digoxin / ↑ Digoxin levels R/T ↓ digoxin metabolism by the gut flora; monitor digoxin levels, and adjust dose as needed
Diltiazem / Possible ↑ clarithromycin plasma levels → ↑ risk of cardiotoxicity; do not use together
Disopyramide / Additive or synergistic ↑ in QT interval → ↑ risk of life-threatening cardiac arrhythmias, including torsades de pointes
Dofetilidei / Additive or synergistic ↑ in QT interval → ↑ risk of life-threatening cardiac arrhythmias, including torsades de pointes
Eletriptan / ↑ Eletriptan plasma levels →↑ pharmacologic/toxic effects; do not take eletriptan within 72 hr of potent CYP3A4 inhibitors (e.g., clarithromycin)
Eplerenone / ↑ Eplerenone plasma levels → ↑ risk of hyperkalemia and serious, sometime fatal, arrhythmias; do not use together
Ergot alkaloids (e.g., dihydroergotamine, ergotamine) / Acute drug toxicity, including severe peripheral vasospasm and dysesthesia; use together contraindicated
Esomeprazole / ↑ Levels of omeprazole, clarithromycin, and 14-OH-clarithromycin
Fluconazole / ↑ Clarithromycin mean steady-state minimum plasma levels and AUC
Grapefruit juice / May inhibit the metabolism of clarithromycin → ↑ plasma levels; do not use together
HMG-CoA reductase inhibitors (e.g., atorvastatin, lovastatin, simvastatin) / ↑ Risk of severe myopathy or rhabdomyolysis
Lansoprazole / ↑ Levels of omeprazole, clarithromycin, and 14-OH-clarithromycin
Lapatinib / ↑ Lapatinib plasma levels → ↑ toxicity; if use together cannot be avoided, ↓ lapatinib dose to 500 mg/day
Levofloxacin / Prolongation of QT interval → ↑ risk of life-threatening cardiac arrhythmias, including torsades de pointes; do not use together
Methylprednisolone / ↑ Methylprednisolone pharmacologic/toxic effects
Moxifloxacin / Prolongation of QT interval → ↑ risk of life-threatening cardiac arrhythmias, including torsades de pointes; use together with caution
Omeprazole / ↑ Levels of omeprazole, clarithromycin, and 14-OH-clarithromycin
Phenytoin / ↑ Phenytoin serum levels
Pimozide / ↑ Risk of sudden death R/T cardiac effects; use together contraindicated
Procainamide / Additive or synergistic ↑ in QT interval → ↑ risk of life-threatening cardiac arrhythmias, including torsades de pointes
Quetiapine / ↑ Quetiapine plasma levels → ↑ pharmacologic/toxic effects
Quinidine / Additive or synergistic ↑ in QT interval → ↑ risk of life-threatening cardiac arrhythmias, including torsades de pointes
Ranolazine / ↑ Ranolazine plasma levels with cardiotoxicity; use together contraindicated
Repaglinide / ↑ Repaglinide levels likely R/T ↓ liver metabolism → ↑ pharmacologic/toxic effects; monitor blood glucose levels and adjust repaglinide dose as needed
Rifabutin, Rifampin / ↓ Clarithromycin effect and ↑ frequency of GI and rifamycin side effects
Ritonavir / ↑ Clarithromycin AUC by 77% and ↓ 14-OH-clarithromycin AUC by 100%; if C_{CR} is 30–60 mL/min, ↓ clarithromycin dose by 50% and if C_{CR} is <30 mL/min, ↓ clarithromycin dose by 75%
Sildenafil / ↑ Sildenafil plasma levels → ↑ risk of side effects; consider lower dose of sildenafil
Sotalol / Additive or synergistic ↑ in QT interval → ↑ risk of life-threatening cardiac arrhythmias, including torsades de pointes
Sparfloxacin / Prolongation of QT interval → ↑ risk of life-threatening cardiac arrhythmias, including torsades de pointes; use together contraindicated

Tacrolimus / ↑ Tacrolimus levels → ↑ risk of toxicity (e.g., nephrotoxicity); monitor tacrolimus levels and adjust dose as needed
Theophyllines (e.g., aminophylline, theophylline) / ↑ Theophylline levels → ↑ risk of toxicity
Valproic acid / ↑ Valproic acid serum levels → toxicity
Verapamil / ↑ Plasma levels of both drugs; ↑ risk of cardiotoxicity
Vinorelbine / ↑ Vinorelbine toxicity R/T inhibition of CYP3A4
Warfarin / ↑ Warfarin anticoagulant effect → possible hemorrhage; monitor anticoagulant parameters and adjust warfarin dose as needed
Zidovudine (AZT) / Either ↑ or ↓ levels of zidovudine

HOW SUPPLIED

Granules for Oral Suspension (after reconstitution): 125 mg/5 mL, 250 mg/5 mL; ***Tablets:*** 250 mg, 500 mg; ***Tablets, Extended-Release:*** 500 mg.

DOSAGE

ORAL SUSPENSION; TABLETS

Pharyngitis, tonsillitis.

Adults: 250 mg q 12 hr for 10 days.

Acute maxillary sinusitis.

Adults: 500 mg q 12 hr for 14 days.

Acute exacerbation of chronic bronchitis due to H. parainfluenzae *or* H. influenzae.

Adults: 500 mg q 12 hr for 7–14 days for *H. influenzae* and 7 days for *H. parainfluenzae.*

Acute exacerbation of chronic bronchitis due to M. catarrhalis *or* S. pneumoniae.

Adults: 250 mg q 12 hr for 7–14 days.

Community-acquired pneumonia due to S. pneumoniae, M. pneumoniae, H. influenzae, *or* C. pneumoniae.

Adults: 250 mg q 12 hr for 7–14 days (7 days for *H. influenzae).*

Uncomplicated skin and skin structure infections.

Adults: 250 mg q 12 hr for 7–14 days.

Disseminated M. avium *complex or prophylaxis of* M. avium *complex.*

Adults: 500 mg twice a day; **children:** 7.5 mg/kg twice a day up to 500 mg twice a day.

Active duodenal ulcers associated with H. pylori *infection.*

The following drug regimens are used:

Triple Therapy: Clarithromycin, 500 mg twice a day; amoxicillin, 1,000 mg twice a day; and *either* lansoprazole, 30 mg twice a day *or* omeprazole, 20 mg twice a day, each for 10–14 days. Take each drug with meals. In clients with an ulcer present at the time therapy begins, give omeprazole, 20 mg once daily, for an additional 18 days.

Dual Therapy: Clarithromycin, 500 mg three times per day and omeprazole, 40 mg once daily in the morning each for 14 days. Give omeprazole, 20 mg once daily, for an additional 14 days for ulcer healing and symptom relief.

Use in children.

For all uses, the usual daily dose for children is 15 mg/kg q 12 hr for 10 days. See *Implementation/Administration/Storage.*

TABLETS, EXTENDED-RELEASE

Acute maxillary sinusitis.

Adults: 1,000 mg once daily for 14 days.

Acute exacerbation of chronic bronchitis or community-acquired pneumonia due to susceptible organisms.

Adults: 1,000 mg once daily for 7 days.

NURSING IMPLICATIONS

IMPLEMENTATION/ADMINISTRATION/STORAGE

1. Usual dose for children is 15 mg/kg/day divided q 12 hr for 10 days. Use the following guidelines: **9 kg:** 62.5 mg q 12 hr; **17 kg:** 125 mg q 12 hr; **25 kg:** 187.5 mg q 12 hr; **33 kg:** 250 mg q 12 hr.
2. Tablets and granules may be given with or without food; both tablets and suspension can be given with milk. Give ER tablets with food. Food delays both the onset of absorption and the formation of 14-OH-clarithromycin (the active metabolite).
3. Give without dosage adjustment in hepatic impairment if there is normal renal function. If severe renal impairment (C_{CR} 30 mL/min)

with/without hepatic impairment, halve the dose or double the dosing interval.

4. Shake reconstituted suspension well before each use; use within 14 days and do not refrigerate. After mixing store at 15–30°C (59–86°F).
5. Store tablets and granules at controlled room temperature in a well-closed container. Protect 250 mg tablets from light. Store ER tablets from 20–25°C (68–77°F).

ASSESSMENT

1. Document onset, severity, characteristics of S&S and culture results.
2. Note sensitivity to erythromycin or any of the macrolide antibiotics.
3. List drugs currently prescribed to prevent any interactions.
4. Avoid use with pimozide and with ranitidine bismuth citrate in those with a history of acute porphyria.
5. Obtain baseline cultures/sensitivity; monitor CBC, renal and LFTs. Reduce dose with renal dysfunction.

CLIENT/FAMILY TEACHING

1. May take with/without meals. Food may decrease chance of stomach upset but delays onset of absorption. Shake suspension well before therapy, use dosing spoon, and store at room temperature. Do not refrigerate suspension and discard unused suspension after 14 days.
2. Do not chew, break, or crush extended-release tablets; take XL tablets with food. Take all tablets with a full glass of water.
3. Drug may cause a bitter taste. Take with sufficient amount of water. Avoid taking with grapefruit juice. Contains FD&C Yellow No. 5 (tartrazine); may cause allergic reaction if sensitive.
4. Report any severe abdominal pain or persistent or bloody diarrhea; an antibiotic-associated colitis may be precipitated by *C. difficile* and require alternative management.
5. Complete entire prescription to prevent resistance; ensure adequate hydration.
6. Practice reliable contraception; may cause fetal harm.
7. Do not take any other medications without first clearing with provider; may interact.
8. Keep all F/U to assess response, labs/cultures, and for adverse SE.

OUTCOMES/EVALUATE

- Resolution of infection
- Symptomatic improvement; ulcer treatment
- Negative F/U cultures

IV

Clindamycin hydrochloride

(klin-dah-**MY**-sin)

Classification(s): Antibiotic, lincosamide

Pregnancy Category: B

RX: Cleocin.

✤ **Rx:** Apo-Clindamycin, Dalacin C, Gen-Clindamycin, ratio-Clindamycin, Taro-Clindamycin.

Clindamycin palmitate hydrochloride

Pregnancy Category: B

RX: Cleocin Pediatric.

✤ **Rx:** Dalacin C Flavored Granules.

Clindamycin phosphate

Pregnancy Category: B

RX: Foam, Gel, Lotion, Pledget, Topical Solution: Cleocin T, Clindagel, ClindaMax, Clindets, Evoclin, PledgaClin. **Injection**: Cleocin Phosphate. **Injection Solution, Concentrate**: Cleocin Phosphate. **Vaginal Cream**: Cleocin, ClindaMax, Clindesse. **Vaginal Suppositories**: Cleocin.

✤ **Rx:** Clinda-T, Dalacin C Phosphate Sterile Solution, Dalacin T Topical Solution, Dalacin Vaginal Cream.

SEE ALSO *ANTI-INFECTIVES*.

INDICATIONS/USES

Should not be used for trivial infections.

Clindamycin hydrochloride and palmitate hydrochloride. Systemic.

1. *Anaerobes:* Serious respiratory tract infections (e.g., empyema, lung abscess, anaerobic pneumonitis).
2. Serious skin and soft-tissue infections, septicemia, intra-abdominal infections (e.g., peritonitis, intra-abdominal abscess), infections of the female pelvis and genital tract (e.g.,

PID, endometritis, nongonococcal tubo-ovarian abscess, pelvic cellulitis, postsurgical vaginal cuff infection).

3. *Streptococci/staphylococci:* Serious respiratory tract infections, serious skin and soft-tissue infections.
4. *Pneumonococcus:* Serious respiratory tract infections.
5. Serious infections caused by susceptible strains of streptococci, pneumococci, staphylococci, and anaerobic bacteria. Reserve use for those allergic to penicillin or in those in whom penicillin is inappropriate. Before selecting clindamycin consider the type of infection and the appropriateness of less toxic alternatives (e.g., erythromycin) due to the risk of antibiotic-associated pseudomembranous colitis.

Investigational: Alternative to sulfonamides in combination with pyrimethamine in the acute treatment of CNS toxoplasmosis in AIDS clients. Treatment of *Chlamydia trachomatis* infections in women. Bacterial vaginosis due to *Gardnerella vaginalis* (may be an alternative to metronidazole).

Clindamycin phosphate (parenteral). Indicated to treat serious infections due to susceptible anaerobic bacteria.

1. Acute hematogenous osteomyelitis due to *S. aureus* and as adjunctive therapy in the surgical treatment of chronic bone and joint infections due to susceptible organisms.
2. Gynecological infections, including endometritis, nongonococcal tubo-ovarian abscess, pelvic cellulitis, and postsurgical vaginal cuff infection due to susceptible anaerobes.
3. Intra-abdominal infections, including peritonitis and intra-abdominal abscess due to susceptible anaerobic organisms.
4. Lower respiratory tract infections, including pneumonia, empyema, and lung abscess due to anaerobes, *Streptococcus pneumoniae,* other streptococci (except *Enterococcus faecalis*), and *S. aureus.*
5. Septicemia due to S. aureus, streptococci (except *E. faecalis,*) and susceptible anaerobes.
6. To treat serious infections due to susceptible strains of streptococci, pneumococci, and staphylococci.
7. Skin and skin structure infections due to *Staphylococcus pyogenes, S. aureus,* and anaerobes.

Investigational: As an alternative to sulfonamides in combination with pyrimethamine in acute treatment of CNS toxoplasmosis in AIDS clients.

Topical.

1. Inflammatory acne vulgaris.
2. Vaginally to treat bacterial vaginosis (*Haemophilus* vaginitis, *Gardnerella* vaginitis, nonspecific vaginitis, *Corynebacterium* vaginitis, or anaerobic vaginosis). Treatment of rosacea (lotion used).

ACTION/KINETICS

Action

Suppresses protein synthesis by microorganisms by binding to ribosomes (50S subunit) and preventing protein synthesis. Is both bacteriostatic and bactericidal. Possible cross resistance with lincomycin.

Pharmacokinetics

Rapidly absorbed after PO administration. Does not diffuse adequately into CSF to be used to treat meningitis. Is 90% bioavailable. **Mean peak serum concentration: PO,** 2.5 mcg/mL; **IM,** 9 mcg/mL for adults and 6 mcg/mL for children; **IV,** 11.9 mcg/mL for adults and 10 mcg/mL for children. Widely distributed in body fluids and tissues, including bones. **t½:** 2.4 hr (in the elderly t½ is about 4 hr). In serious infections the rate of IV administration is adjusted to maintain appropriate serum drug concentrations: 4–6 mcg/mL. Over 90% metabolized in the liver. About 10% excreted unchanged in the urine.

CONTRAINDICATIONS

Hypersensitivity to either clindamycin or lincomycin. Use in treating viral and minor bacterial infections or in clients with a history of regional enteritis, nonbacterial infections (e.g., most URTIs), ulcerative colitis, meningitis, or antibiotic-associated colitis. Lactation.

SPECIAL CONCERNS

■ (1) Pseudomembranous colitis has been reported with nearly all antibacterial agents, including lincosamides, and may range in severity from mild to life-threatening. Therefore, it is important to consider this diagnosis in clients who present with diarrhea subsequent to the administration of antibacterial agents. (2) Because lincosamide therapy has been associated with severe colitis, which may end fatally, it should be reserved for serious infections for which less toxic antimicrobial agents are inappropriate. It should not be used in clients with nonbacterial infections such as most upper respiratory tract infections. Treatment with antibacterial agents alters the normal flora of the colon and may permit overgrowth of clostridia. Studies indicate that a toxin produced by *Clostridium difficile* is one primary cause of antibiotic-associated colitis. (3) After the diagnosis of pseudomembranous colitis has been established, initiate therapeutic measures. Mild cases of pseudomembranous colitis usually respond to drug discontinuation alone. In moderate to severe cases, consider management with fluids and electrolytes, protein supplementation, and treatment with an antibacterial drug clinically effective against *C. difficile* colitis. (4) Diarrhea, colitis, and pseudomembranous colitis have begun up to several weeks following cessation of therapy with lincosamides. ■

- **Use with caution in clients with GI, impaired liver or renal function, or a history of allergy or asthma.**
- **Use topical gel, lotion, or suspension with caution in atopic individuals.**
- **Due to the potential for diarrhea, bloody diarrhea, and pseudomembranous colitis, other drugs may be more appropriate to treat acne.**
- **Safety and efficacy of topical products not established in children less than 12 years old. Safety and efficacy of systemic products not established in children younger than 1 month of age.**

SIDE EFFECTS

Most Common

After systemic use: Diarrhea, pseudomembranous colitis, tinnitis, N&V, skin rashes.
After topical use: Dry skin, burning, itching, erythema, peeling, oily skin.

GI: N&V, diarrhea, ***pseudomembranous colitis*** (more frequent after PO use), abdominal pain, esophagitis, unpleasant or metallic taste (after high IV doses), glossitis, stomatitis. **CV:** Hypotension, thrombophlebitis; ***rarely, cardiopulmonary arrest after too rapid IV use.*** **Allergic:** Morbilliform rash (most common), skin rashes, urticaria, erythema multiforme, ***anaphylaxis***, ***Stevens-Johnson-like syndrome***, maculopapular rash, ***angioneurotic edema***. **Hematologic:** Leukopenia, neutropenia, thrombocytopenia, transient eosinophilia, ***agranulocytosis***. **Dermatologic:** Exfoliative and vesiculobullous dermatitis, pruritus, skin rashes, urticaria. **Hepatic:** Jaundice, abnormal LFTs. **GU:** Renal dysfunction (azotemia, oliguria, proteinuria), vaginitis. **Hypersensitivity reactions:** Maculopapular rash, urticaria, angioneurotic edema, serum sickness, ***anaphylaxis;*** rarely, erythema multiforme, some resembling Stevens-Johnson syndrome. **Miscellaneous:** Superinfection, tinnitus, polyarthritis, sore throat, fatigue, urinary frequency, headache; sterile abscesses, pain, and induration after IV use.

Following IV use: Thrombophlebitis, erythema, pain, swelling.

Following IM use: Pain, induration, sterile abscesses.

Following topical use: Erythema, irritation, dryness, peeling, itching, burning, oiliness of skin, pruritus.

Following vaginal use: Cervicitis, vaginitis, vulvar irritation/moniliasis, urticaria, rash, trichomonal vaginitis, vulvovaginal disorder, vulvovaginitis, body moniliasis.

NOTE: The injection contains benzyl alcohol, which has been associated with ***a fatal "gasping syndrome"*** in infants.

LABORATORY TEST CONSIDERATIONS

↓ Levels of AST, ALT, NPN, alkaline phosphatase, bilirubin, BSP retention, and ↓ platelet count.

DRUG INTERACTIONS

Antiperistaltic antidiarrheals (opiates, Lomotil) / ↑ Diarrhea R/T ↓ toxin removal from colon
Ciprofloxacin HCl / Additive antibacterial activity
Cyclosporine / ↓ Cyclosporine levels
Erythromycin / Cross-interference → ↓ effect of both drugs; do not give together
Kaolin/Pectin (e.g., Kaopectate) / ↓ Effect R/T ↓ GI tract absorption
Neuromuscular blocking agents (pancuronium, tubocurarine) / ↑ Effect of blocking agents → profound and severe respiratory depression

HOW SUPPLIED

Clindamycin hydrochloride. ***Capsules:*** 75 mg, 150 mg, 300 mg.

Clindamycin palmitate hydrochloride. *Granules for Oral Solution:* 75 mg/5 mL.
Clindamycin phosphate. *Cream:* 2%; *Foam:* 1%; *Gel:* 1%; *Injection:* 300 mg, 600 mg, 900 mg; *Injection Solution, Concentrate:* 150 mg/mL; *Lotion:* 1%; *Pledget:* 1%.; *Topical Solution:* 1%; *Topical Suspension:* 1%; *Vaginal Cream:* 2%; *Vaginal Suppositories:* 100 mg (as the base).

DOSAGE

CAPSULES (CLINDAMYCIN HYDROCHLORIDE); ORAL SOLUTION (CLINDAMYCIN PALMITATE HYDROCHLORIDE)

Serious and severe infections.

Clindamycin hydrochloride. Adults, serious infections: 150–300 mg q 6 hr; **more severe infections:** 300–450 mg q 6 hr. **Pediatric, serious infections:** 8–16 mg/kg per day divided into three or four equal doses; **more serious infections**: 16–20 mg//kg per day divided into 3 or 4 equal doses.

Clindamycin palmitate hydrochloride. Pediatric, serious infections: 8–12 mg/kg per day divided into three or four equal doses; **severe infections:** 13–16 mg/kg per day divided into 3 or 4 equal doses; **more severe infections:** 17–25 mg/kg per day divided into 3 or 4 equal doses. **Children less than 10 kg:** Minimum recommended dose is 37.5 mg 3 times per day.

IM; IV (CLINDAMYCIN PHOSPHATE)

Serious infections due to aerobic gram-positive cocci and more susceptible anaerobes.

Adults: 600–1,200 mg per day in 2–4 equal doses. **Pediatric, over 1 month to 16 years:** 20–40 mg/kg per day in 3 or 4 equal doses. Use the higher doses for more severe infections. As an alternative to dosing by body weight, children may be dosed on body surface area using a dose of 350 mg/m^2 per day for serious infections and 450 mg/m^2 per day for more severe infections. **Neonates, less than 1 month of age:** 15–20 mg/kg per day in 3 or 4 equal doses. The lower dose may be more appropriate for small premature infants.

More severe infections due to B. fragilis, Peptococcus, *or* Clostridium *(other than* C. perfringens*).*

Adults: 1,200–2,700 mg/day in 2–4 equal doses. May have to be increased in more serious infections. The maximum daily dose for adults should not exceed 4.8 grams IV. Single IM doses of 600 mg are not recommended. The maximum dose for children, at least 1 month of age is 40 mg/kg per day or 450 mg/m^2 per day.

Life-threatening infections due to aerobes or anaerobes.

Adults: 4.8 grams per day IV.

Acute pelvic inflammatory disease.

IV: 900 mg q 8 hr plus gentamicin loading dose of 2 mg/kg IV or IM; **then,** gentamicin, 1.5 mg/kg q 8 hr IV or IM. Therapy may be discontinued 24 hr after client improves. After discharge from the hospital, continue with doxycycline PO, 100 mg 2 times per day for 10–14 days. Alternatively, give clindamycin, PO, 450 mg 4 times per day for 14 days.

CREAM; LOTION; PLEDGET; TOPICAL GEL; TOPICAL SOLUTION; TOPICAL SUSPENSION (ALL ARE CLINDAMYCIN PHOSPHATE)

Inflammatory acne vulgaris.

Apply thin film once (Clindagel) or twice daily to affected areas. One or more pledgets may also be used.

VAGINAL CREAM (2%)

Bacterial vaginosis.

One applicatorful (5 grams containing about 100 mg clindamycin phosphate), preferably at bedtime, for 3 or 7 days (nonpregnant women) or 7 (pregnant women) consecutive days. Cleocin and ClindaMax creams can be used to treat pregnant women during the second and third trimesters. For Clindesse, use a single applicatorful (5 grams containing 100 mg clindamycin phosphate) given once intravaginally at any time of the day.

VAGINAL SUPPOSITORIES (CLINDAMYCIN PHOSPHATE)

Bacterial vaginosis.

One suppository (100 mg) intravaginally/day, preferably at bedtime, for 3 days.

FOAM (CLINDAMYCIN PHOSPHATE)

Acne vulgaris.

Apply once daily to the affected area. Dispense the foam into the cap of the can or onto a cool surface; apply foam with fingertips.

NURSING IMPLICATIONS

IMPLEMENTATION/ADMINISTRATION/STORAGE

1. For anaerobic infections, use parenteral form initially; may be followed by PO therapy.
2. For beta-hemolytic streptococci infections, continue treatment for at least 10 days.
3. If significant diarrhea occurs, discontinue clindamycin.
4. Coadministration of food does not affect the absorption of clindamycin.
5. Reduce dosage in severe renal impairment.
6. Single IM injections greater than 600 mg are not advisable. Inject deeply into muscle to prevent induration, pain, and sterile abscesses.
7. Do not refrigerate reconstituted solution; may become thickened and difficult to pour.
8. Store PO dosage forms from 20–25°C (68–77°F).
9. Shake lotion well just before using.
10. IV Give parenteral clindamycin only to hospitalized clients.
11. Infuse over at least 10–60 min; do not inject IV undiluted as a bolus.
12. Dilute IV injections to maximum concentration of 18 mg/mL, with no more than 1,200 mg administered in 1 hr.
13. Administer IV over a period of 20–60 min, depending on dose and desired therapeutic serum concentration.
14. The phosphate is stable in NSS, D5W, and RL solution in both glass or PVC containers at concentrations of 6, 9, and 12 mg/mL for 8 weeks frozen, 32 days refrigerated, or 16 days at room temperature.
15. Parenteral therapy may be changed to PO therapy when the condition warrants or at the discretion of the health care provider.
16. Store vials from 20–25°C (68–77°F).
17. COMPATIBILITY D5W, 0.9% NaCl, D5/0.9% or 0.45% NaCl, LR.
18. INCOMPATIBILITY Administer separately.

ASSESSMENT

1. List reasons for therapy, onset, characteristics of S&S; note culture results.
2. Auscultate lungs; assess extent of respiratory tract infections.
3. Describe skin/soft-tissue infections; note complaints indicative of PID or intra-abdominal infections.
4. With IV therapy, observe for hypotension; keep in bed for 30 min following infusion. Bitter taste may be evident.
5. Observe for drug interactions caused by concurrent administration of neuromuscular blocking agents. Be alert to hypotension, bronchospasms, cardiac disturbances, hyperthermia, respiratory depression.
6. Observe closely for:
   - Skin rash; frequently reported
   - Renal/hepatic impairment; newborns for organ dysfunction
   - GI disturbances, such as abdominal pain, diarrhea, anorexia, N&V, bloody/tarry stools, excessive flatulence.
7. Monitor organ system function when used in children up to 16 years of age.
8. Monitor CBC, C&S, renal and LFTs; note any history of liver/renal disease, allergies, or GI problems.

CLIENT/FAMILY TEACHING

1. Take oral medication with a full glass of water to prevent esophageal ulceration. May be taken with or without food.
2. Report side effects such as persistent vomiting, diarrhea, fever, abdominal pain, cramping or with topical any excessive drying or increased irritation.
3. Pseudomembranous colitis may occur 2–9 days or several weeks after initiation of therapy. Fluids, electrolytes, protein supplements, systemic corticosteroids, and oral antibiotics may be needed. Do not use antiperistaltic agents if diarrhea occurs; these can prolong or aggravate condition. Kaolin will reduce ab-

sorption of antibiotic; if prescribed, take 3 hr before drug.

4. With vaginal creams:
   - Review how to fill and administer applicator; applicator is disposable, do not reuse. With bacterial vaginosis, partner treatment not generally needed.
   - The vaginal cream contains mineral oil, and vaginal suppository contains an oil-type base which may weaken latex or rubber products, such as condoms or vaginal contraceptive diaphragms; avoid for 72 hr following treatment.
   - Do not engage in intercourse when using the vaginal cream; may enhance irritation.
5. With vaginal suppositories, review how to load and administer with applicator and how to clean for reuse; suppository may also be inserted directly using fingers.
6. Do not use any acne or topical mercury preparations containing a peeling agent in affected area; severe irritation may occur. Wait 30 min after shaving to apply.
7. Avoid contact of the gel, lotion, or topical suspension with the eyes; alcohol base will cause burning and irritation. Use caution: solution is flammable so avoid smoking or using near flame. In case of accidental contact with eyes, abraded skin, or mucous membranes, wash with copious amounts of cool tap water. To apply, wash area with soap and water, rinse, and pat dry. Gently rub into affected area as directed.
8. With pledget, remove from foil just before use. Do not use if seal is broken and discard pledget after each use.
9. Apply the foam once daily to affected area(s) after washing the skin with mild soap and allowing it to dry fully. Use enough to cover the entire affected area. To use the foam:
   - Do not dispense directly onto the hands or face because the foam will begin to melt on contact with warm skin.
   - Remove the clear cap. Align the black mark with the nozzle of the activator.
   - Hold the can at an upright angle and press firmly to dispense. Dispense enough to cover the affected area into the cap or onto a cool surface. If the can is warm or the foam is runny, run the can under cold water.
   - Pick up small amounts of the foam with the fingertips and gently massage into the affected area until the foam disappears.
   - Use with caution around the mouth area.
10. Keep all F/U to assess response, labs, adverse SE.

OUTCOMES/EVALUATE

- Resolution of infection
- Clearing of skin lesions
- Therapeutic drug levels with IV therapy (4–6 mcg/mL)

Clobazam

(**KLOE**-ba-zam)

Classification(s): Anticonvulsant, benzodiazepine

Pregnancy Category: C

RX: Onfi, **C-IV**

SEE ALSO *ANTICONVULSANTS.*

INDICATIONS/USES

Adjunctive treatment of seizures associated with Lennox-Gastaut syndrome in adults and children 2 years and older.

ACTION/KINETICS

Action

Exact mechanism unknown. Action thought to involve potentiation of gamma-aminobutyric acid (GABA)-ergic neurotransmission as a result of binding at the benzodiazepine site of the $GABA_A$ receptor.

Pharmacokinetics

Rapidly and extensively absorbed. $\mathbf{T_{max}}$: 0.5–4 hr after single or multiple doses. Relative bioavailability: About 100%. Food does not affect absorption. Extensively metabolized in the liver primarily by CYP3A4 and to a lesser extent by CYP2C19 and CYP2B6 mainly to to the active N-desmethylclobazam. N-desmethylclobazam is further metabolized mainly by CYP2C19; there are both rapid and poor CYP2C19 metabolizers. Excreted in both the urine (82%) and feces (11%). **t½, elimination:** 36–42 hr clobazam and 71–82 hr for N-desmethylclobazam. Clearance is lower in the elderly.

SPECIAL CONCERNS

- **Clobazam may be abused similarly as other benzodiazepines.**
- **Physical dependence to clobazam may develop, even using recommended doses. This risk increases in those with a history of alcohol or drug abuse.**
- **Withdrawal symptoms occur following abrupt discontinuation of clobazam. Symptoms include headache, insomnia, irritability, palpitations, diarrhea, psychosis, hallucinations, behavioral disorders, tremor, anxiety, and convulsions. The higher the dose of clobazam being taken, the more severe the withdrawal symptoms.**
- **Elevated clobazam levels are possible in breast-feeding infants.**
- **Safety and efficacy not determined in children younger than 2 years of age.**

SIDE EFFECTS

Most Common

Lethargy, somnolence, sedation, ataxia, aggression, fatigue, insomnia, URTI, pyrexia, UTI.

CNS: Lethargy, somnolence, ataxia, insomnia, aggression, drooling, dysarthria, irritability, psychomotor hyperactivity, sedation, somnolence, agitation, anxiety, apathy, confusional state, delirium, delusion, depression, hallucination, ***suicidal behavior and ideation***. **GI:** Vomiting, dysphagia, constipation, abdominal distention. **Respiratory:** URTI, bronchitis, cough, pneumonia, aspiration, respiratory depression. **Dermatologic:** Rash, ***Stevens-Johnson syndrome, toxic epidermal necrolysis***, urticaria. **GU:** UTI. **Musculoskeletal:** Muscle spasms. **Hematologic:** Anemia, eosinophilia, leukopenia, thrombocytopenia. **Metabolic/Nutritional:** Weight decreased/increased. **Ophthalmic:** Diplopia, blurred vision. **Body as a whole:** Fatigue, pyrexia.

LABORATORY TEST CONSIDERATIONS

↑ Liver enzymes.

OVERDOSE MANAGEMENT

Symptoms: CNS depression, including drowsiness, confusion, lethargy, ataxia, respiratory depression, hypotension and, rarely coma or death. Risk of coma/death increases if other CNS depressants, including alcohol, were used. *Treatment:*

- Gastric lavage and/or administration of activated charcoal.
- IV fluid replenishment.
- Early control of airway.
- Monitor level of consciousness and vital signs.
- Treat hypotension by replenishment with plasma substitutes and, if necessary, sympathomimetic drugs.
- General supportive measures.
- Use of flumazenil in clients with epilepsy is not recommended.

DRUG INTERACTIONS

CNS depressants (e.g., alcohol, opioids, tricyclic antidepressants) / ↑ CNS depressant effects; alcohol ↑ maximum plasma exposure to clobazam by about 50% - avoid concomitant use

CYP2C19 inhibitors (e.g., fluconazole, fluvoxamine, omeprazole, ticlopidine) / ↑ Exposure to the active N-desmethylclobazam; dosage adjustment may be needed

CYP2D6 substrates (e.g., dextromethorphan) / ↑ Exposure to CYP2D6 substrates; lower doses of substrates may be needed

CYP3A4 substrates (e.g., midazolam, some hormonal contraceptives) / ↓ Exposure to CYP3A4 substrates; dosage adjustments generally not needed; hormonal contraceptive efficacy may be ↓—use additional nonhormonal contraception

Ketoconaozle / Significant ↑ clobazam levels R/T inhibition of CYP3A4; no significant changes in AUC and C_{max} of N-desmethylclobazam

HOW SUPPLIED

Tablets: 5 mg, 10 mg, 20 mg.

DOSAGE

TABLETS

Lennox-Gastaut seizures.

Adults and children, 2 years and older, initial: 5 mg/day for clients weighing 30 kg or less and 10 mg/day for clients weighing 30 kg or more; **starting on Day 7:** 10 mg/day for clients weighing 30 kg or less and 20 mg/day for clients weighing 30 kg or more; **starting Day 14:** 20 mg/day for clients weighing 30 kg or less and 40 mg/day for clients weighing 30 kg or more. Dosage escalation should not proceed more rapidly than weekly because serum levels of clobazam and its active metabolite, require 5 to 9 days, respectively to reach steady state. **Elderly:** 5 mg/day. **Maximum dose:** 20 mg/day for those weighing 30 kg or less or 40 mg/day for those weighing more than 30 kg. Plasma levels are generally higher in the elderly; thus proceed slowly with dose escalation. Titrate according to weight, but to half the dose listed for adults and children. If necessary, and based on clinical response, an additional titration to the maximum dose (20 or 40 mg/day, depending on weight), may be started on day 21.

NURSING IMPLICATIONS

IMPLEMENTATION/ADMINISTRATION/STORAGE

1. To provide information regarding the effects of in utero exposure to clobazam, pregnant clients should enroll in the North American Antiepileptic Drug Pregnancy Registry. Enroll by calling 1-888-233-2334. Only clients themselves or their caretakers may register. Information on the registry may be found on the website at: http://www.aedpregnancyregistry.org.
2. Dosing recommendations for mild to moderate hepatic impairment (Child-Pugh score 5 to 9). **Initial dose:** 5 mg/day. Titrate according to weight using half the dose recommended under *Dosage.* If necessary and based on clinical response, an additional titration to the maximum dosage (20 or 40 mg/day), depending on the weight group, may be started on day 21. **Maximum dose:** 20 mg/day for those weighing 30 kg or less or 40 mg/day for those weighing more than 30 kg.
3. Dosing recommendations for CYP2C19 poor metabolizers: **Initial dose:** 5 mg/day. Dose titration should proceed slowly according to weight, but to half the dose recommended under *Dosage.* If necessary and based on clinical response, an additional titration to the maximum dosage (20 or 40 mg/day), depending on weight, may be started on day 21. **Maximum dose:** 20 mg/day for those weighing 30 kg or less or 40 mg/day for those weighing more than 30 kg.
4. Withdraw clobazam gradually. Taper by decreasing the total daily dosage by 5 to 10 mg/day on a weekly basis until discontinued.
5. Administer in divided doses twice a day; the 5 mg dose can be given as a single daily dose.
6. Store from 20–25°C (68–77°F).

ASSESSMENT

1. Note age of seizure onset, characteristics of seizures and type, clinical presentation and behaviors, other agents trialed and outcome.
2. Assess for history of substance abuse. The predisposition may contribute to habituation and dependence (may occur at prescribed dose levels).
3. Monitor for the emergence or worsening of depression, suicidal thoughts or behavior, and/or any unusual changes in mood or behavior.
4. Check VS, emotional status and LFTs; reduce dose with dysfunction.

CLIENT/FAMILY TEACHING

1. May be taken without regard to timing of meals.
2. Tablets can be administered whole or crushed and mixed in applesauce.
3. Avoid activities that require mental alertness until drug effects realized; may impair judgement, thinking, or motor skills.
4. Report any development or worsening of symptoms of depression, unusual changes in mood or behavior, suicidal thoughts, behavior, or thoughts of self-harm immediately.
5. Do not stop abruptly; may increase seizure risk.
6. Practice reliable contraception during therapy and for one month following therapy. If pregnancy occurs enroll in the NAAED Pregnancy Registry at 1-888-233-2334.
7. Avoid alcohol and other CNS depressants.
8. Store drug safely and out of reach; may be abused and cause dependence.
9. Keep all F/U to assess response, labs, and adverse SE.

OUTCOMES/EVALUATE

Control of seizures

Clobetasol propionate

(kloh-**BAY**-tah-sohl)

Classification(s): Glucocorticoid

Pregnancy Category: C

RX: Clobevate Gel, Clobex, Cormax, Embeline, Olux, Olux-E, Temovate, Temovate Emollient.
✦ **Rx:** Dermovate, Gen-Clobetasol Cream/Ointment, Gen-Clobetasol Scalp Application, ratio-Clobetasol, Taro-Clobetasol.

SEE ALSO ***CORTICOSTEROIDS***.

INDICATIONS/USES

(1) Relief of inflammatory and pruritic dermatoses of the skin and scalp, including eczema, atopic dermatitis, contact dermatitis, seborrhea. (2) **Foam:** Short-term treatment of inflammatory and pruritic manifestations of moderate to severe corticosteroid responsive scalp dermatoses and for short-term topical treatment of mild to moderate plaque-type psoriasis of non-scalp regions, excluding the face and intertriginous areas. (3) **Lotion:** Also used for moderate to severe plaque psoriasis if lesions occupy less than 10% of body surface area. (4) **Shampoo:** Moderate to severe scalp psoriasis in those 18 years and older. (5) **Solution:** Short-term treatment of inflammatory and pruritic manifestations of moderate to severe corticosteroid responsive scalp dermatoses. (6) **Spray:** Moderate to severe plaque psoriasis affecting up to 20% of body surface area in clients 18 years of age and older.

ACTION/KINETICS

Action

Has anti-inflammatory, antipruritic, and vasoconstrictive effects.

CONTRAINDICATIONS

Use in children less than 12 years old, use for more than 2 weeks, to treat rosacea or perioral dermatitis, and use on face, groin, axillae.

SPECIAL CONCERNS

- **May suppress hypothalamic-pituitary-adrenal (HPA) axis at doses as low as 2 grams/day.**
- **Use with caution during lactation.**

SIDE EFFECTS

Most Common

Burning, cracking/fissuring of skin, irritation, itching, numbness of fingers, reddened skin, skin atrophy, stinging.

Dermatologic: Burning sensation, itching, stinging, irritation, dryness, pruritus, erythema, folliculitis, hypertrichosis, acneform eruptions, hypopigmentation, perioral dermatitis, allergic contact dermatitis, skin maceration, reddened skin, secondary infection, striae, milaria, cracking and fissuring of the skin, skin atrophy, numbness of fingers, telangiectasia. **Miscellaneous:** Cushing's syndrome.

HOW SUPPLIED

Cream: 0.05%; ***Foam:*** 0.05%; ***Gel:*** 0.05%; ***Lotion:*** 0.05%; ***Ointment:*** 0.05%; ***Shampoo:*** 0.05%; ***Solution for Scalp Application:*** 0.05%; ***Spray:*** 0.05%.

DOSAGE

CREAM; FOAM; GEL; LOTION; OINTMENT

Dermatoses.

Apply thin layer to affected skin or scalp twice a day, once in the morning and once in the evening. Rub in gently and completely. Use no more than 50 grams per week.

FOAM

Mild to moderate plaque-type psoriasis of non-scalp regions, moderate to severe scalp dermatoses.

Apply a small amount to the affected area twice a day, morning and evening.

LOTION

Plaque psoriasis.

Apply to lesions 2 times per day with no more than 50 grams given in 1 week. May be used for up to 4 weeks.

SHAMPOO

Moderate to severe scalp psoriasis.

Apply a thin film to the affected areas of the scalp daily for no more than 4 weeks; apply to a dry scalp and leave on for 15 min before lathering and rinsing. Do not use more than 50 mL of the shampoo per week.

SOLUTION FOR SCALP APPLICATION

Scalp dermatoses.

Apply to affected scalp areas twice a day, morning and evening. Do not exceed a total weekly dosage of 50 mL. Not to be used with occlusive dressings.

SPRAY

Moderate to severe plaque psoriasis.

Adults 18 years and older: Up to 50 grams/week. Limit treatment beyond 2 weeks to localized moderate to severe lesions that have not improved sufficiently.

NURSING IMPLICATIONS

IMPLEMENTATION/ADMINISTRATION/STORAGE

1. Do not use occlusive dressings.
2. Do not refrigerate.
3. Do not use the gel on the face, groin, or axillae.

ASSESSMENT

1. Note onset, location, and characteristics of S&S (photo) as well as clinical presentation; note agents trialed/outcome.
2. Drug is a potent corticosteroid for short-term use; assess for S&S of HPA axis suppression-may use ACTH stimulation test, a.m. cortisol, and urinary free cortisol test.

CLIENT/FAMILY TEACHING

1. Apply thin layer to affected area; gently rub in. Review type of product prescribed and use as directed; externally; avoid eye contact.
2. Wash hands before/after application. Do not cover, wrap, or bandage treatment area; may increase absorption/cause skin to shrink (atrophy).
3. Report failure to heal, may indicate contact dermatitis from agent. Also if skin infections, may need antifungal/antibacterial agent as well as any severe burning, stinging, swelling, or numbness.
4. Do not use continuously for more than 2 weeks.
5. Keep all F/U to assess response and for adverse SE.

OUTCOMES/EVALUATE

Relief/healing of inflamed/pruritic skin manifestations

Clonazepam

(kloh-**NAY**-zeh-pam)

Classification(s): Anticonvulsant, miscellaneous

RX: Klonopin, Klonopin Wafers, **C-IV**

Rx: Apo-Clonazepam, CO Clonazepam, Gen-Clonazepam, PMS-Clonazepam, ratio-Clonazepam, Rivotril.

SEE ALSO ***ANTICONVULSANTS***.

INDICATIONS/USES

(1) Alone or as an adjunct to treat absence seizures (petit mal variant) including Lennox-Gastaut syndrome. (2) Alone or as an adjunct to treat akinetic and myoclonic seizures. (3) Some effectiveness in absence seizures resistant to succinimide therapy. (4) Panic disorder with or without agoraphobia, as defined by DSM-IV. *Investigational:* Parkinsonian (hypokinetic) dysarthria, acute manic episodes of bipolar affective disorder, leg movements (periodic) during sleep, adjunct in treating schizophrenia, neuralgias (deafferentation pain syndrome), multifocal tic disorders.

ACTION/KINETICS

Action

Benzodiazepine derivative that increases presynaptic inhibition and suppresses the spread of seizure activity.

Pharmacokinetics

Peak plasma levels: 1–2 hr. **t½:** 18–60 hr. **Therapeutic serum levels:** 20–80 ng/mL. Metabolized almost completely in the liver to inactive metabolites, which are excreted in the urine. Even though a benzodiazepine, clonazepam is used mainly as an anticonvulsant. However, contraindications, side effects, and so forth are similar to those for diazepam. **Plasma protein binding:** 50–85%.

CONTRAINDICATIONS

Sensitivity to benzodiazepines. Severe liver disease, acute narrow-angle glaucoma. Pregnancy.

SPECIAL CONCERNS

- Effects on lactation not known.
- Safety and efficacy not evaluated for panic disorder in clients less than 18 years of age.

SIDE EFFECTS

Most Common

Drowsiness, dizziness, fatigue, asthenia, dry mouth, diarrhea, GI upset, changes in appetite.

See *Diazepam* for a complete list of potential side effects. Also, in clients in whom different types of seizure disorders exist, clonazepam may elicit or precipitate ***grand mal seizures***.

DRUG INTERACTIONS

CNS depressants / Potentiation of clonazepam CNS depressant effect

Phenobarbital / ↓ Clonazepam effect R/T ↑ liver breakdown
Phenytoin / ↓ Clonazepam effect R/T ↑ liver breakdown
Valproic acid / ↑ Chance of absence seizures

HOW SUPPLIED

Tablets: 0.5 mg, 1 mg, 2 mg; ***Tablets, Oral Disintegrating (also called Wafers):*** 0.125 mg, 0.25 mg, 0.5 mg, 1 mg, 2 mg.

DOSAGE

TABLETS; TABLETS, ORAL DISINTEGRATING (ALSO CALLED WAFERS)

Seizure disorders.

Adults, initial: 0.5 mg 3 times per day; do not exceed this dose. Increase by 0.5–1 mg/day q 3 days until seizures are under control or side effects become excessive; **maximum:** 20 mg/day. In those over 65 years, start on low doses and closely observe. **Pediatric up to 10 years or 30 kg:** 0.01–0.03 mg/kg/day in two to three divided doses up to a maximum of 0.05 mg/kg/day. Increase by increments of no more than 0.25–0.5 mg q 3 days until seizures are under control or maintenance of 0.1–0.2 mg/kg is attained.

Panic disorder.

Adults, initial: 0.25 mg twice a day. Can increase to the target dose by 1 mg/day after 3 days. Some may benefit from doses up to 4 mg/day (increase dose in increments of 0.125–0.25 mg twice a day every 3 days), although incidence of side effects may increase. To reduce somnolence, give 1 dose at bedtime. Discontinue treatment gradually with a decrease of 0.125 mg q 3 days until the drug is completely withdrawn.

Parkinsonian dysarthria (investigational).

Adults: 0.25–0.5 mg/day.

Acute manic episodes of bipolar affective disorder (investigational).

Adults: 0.75–16 mg/day.

Periodic leg movements during sleep (investigational).

Adults: 0.5–2 mg nightly.

Adjunct to treat schizophrenia (investigational).

Adults: 0.5–2 mg/day.

Neuralgias (investigational).

Adults: 2–4 mg/day.

Multifocal tic disorders (investigational).

Adults: 1.5–12 mg/day.

NURSING IMPLICATIONS

Do not confuse clonazepam with diazepam (an antianxiety drug) or Klonopin with clonidine (an antihypertensive).

IMPLEMENTATION/ADMINISTRATION/STORAGE

1. About one-third of clients show some loss of anticonvulsant activity within 3 months; dosage adjustment may reestablish effectiveness.
2. Adding clonazepam to existing anticonvulsant therapy may increase depressant effects.
3. Divide daily dose in three equal doses; if doses cannot be divided equally, give largest dose at bedtime.
4. With panic disorder, discontinue treatment gradually with a decrease of 0.125 mg twice a day every 3 days until drug is completely withdrawn. Re-evaluate long-term usefulness periodically.
5. Store from 15–30°C (59–86°F); protect from moisture.

ASSESSMENT

1. Note reasons for therapy, onset/cause of S&S, other agents prescribed, outcome. With seizure disorder, note onset, frequency, characteristics of seizures, other agents trialed.
2. Assess mental status and behavioral presentation; monitor clinical response.
3. Monitor CBC, renal and LFTs, with prolonged therapy.

CLIENT/FAMILY TEACHING

1. Take with water and swallow whole. May take with food if GI upset occurs. Do not crush, chew, or break tablet.
2. Give orally disintegrating tablet with water as follows: After opening the pouch, peel back foil on the blister. Do not push tablet through foil. Immediately upon opening the blister, using dry hands, remove tablet and place in the mouth. Tablet disintegration occurs rapidly in saliva, so it can be swallowed easily with or without water.

3. Take as directed; report any loss of seizure control or adverse side effects.
4. Assess drug effects before performing activities that require mental alertness. May cause drowsiness or impair judgment, thinking, or reflexes.
5. Report oversedation, increased depression, lack of attentiveness, or any other adverse SE.
6. Do not stop suddenly after long-term use; taper to prevent seizure and withdrawal S&S.
7. Report if pregnancy suspected; if taking during pregnancy, enroll in the NAAED Pregnancy Registry. Call 1-888-233-2334 (Mon.–Fri.) to enroll. Information on this registry can also be found at the website http://www.aedpregnancyregistry.org/
8. Avoid alcohol and any other CNS depressants. Keep all F/U to assess response, labs, and for adverse SE.

OUTCOMES/EVALUATE

- ↓ Number and frequency of seizures
- Control of panic disorder
- Therapeutic drug levels 20–80 ng/mL

Clonidine hydrochloride

(**KLOH**-nih-deen)

Classification(s): Antihypertensive, centrally-acting

Pregnancy Category: C

RX: Catapres, Catapres-TTS-1, -TTS-2, and -TTS-3, Jenloga, Kapvay, Nexiclon XR.

✤ **Rx:** Apo-Clonidine, Dixarit.

SEE ALSO ***ANTIHYPERTENSIVE AGENTS***.

INDICATIONS/USES

Oral. (1) Hypertension (immediate release and modified release only). (2) Attention deficit hyperactivity disorder in children as monotherapy and as adjunctive therapy to stimulant medications (extended release only). *Investigational:* Alcohol withdrawal syndrome, atrial fibrillation, attention deficit hyperactivity disorder (immediate release), constitutional growth delay in children, diabetic diarrhea, diagnosis of pheochromocytoma, Gilles de la Tourette syndrome, growth hormone stimulation test, hot flashes, hyperhidrosis, hypertensive urgencies (diastolic BP >120 mm Hg), opiate detoxification, methadone/opiate withdrawal, postherpetic neuralgia, prevention of migraine headache (adults, adolescents, children), psychosis in schizophrenic clients, restless leg syndrome, smoking cessation, Tourette syndrome (adults, adolescents, children), ulcerative colitis.

Transdermal: Alone or with a diuretic or other antihypertensives to treat mild to moderate hypertension. *Investigational:* Attention deficit hyperactivity disorder in adolescents and children, cyclosporine-associated nephrotoxicity, diabetic diarrhea, hot flashes, hyperhidrosis, postherpetic neuralgia, prevention of migraine (adults, adolescents, children), smoking cessation, ulcerative colitis.

Epidural: With opiates for severe pain in cancer clients not relieved by opiate analgesics alone. Most effective for neuropathic pain than for somatic or visceral pain. *Investigational:* Postanesthetic shivering, postherpetic neuralgia, prevention of migraine in children/adolescents.

ACTION/KINETICS

Action

Is a centrally-acting alpha-2 adrenergic agonist that stimulates alpha-2 adrenergic receptors in the brain stem. This results in reduced sympathetic outflow from the CNS and decreased peripheral resistance, renal vascular resistance, HR and BP. Plasma renin levels are decreased and there is excretion of aldosterone and catecholamines. Peripheral venous pressure remains unchanged. Few orthostatic effects. Although NaCl excretion is markedly decreased, potassium excretion remains unchanged. Tolerance to the drug may develop. Clonidine stimulates growth hormone release in both children and adults acutely but does not cause chronic elevation of growth hormone with long-term use. The mechanism for use in attention deficit hyperactivity disorder is not known. Epidural use causes analgesia at presynaptic and postjunctional alpha-2-adrenergic receptors in the spinal cord due to prevention of pain signal transmission to the brain. Epidural clonidine is not antagonized by narcotic antagonists.

Pharmacokinetics

Food has no effect on absorption of immediate- or extended-release products. **Hypertensive effect. Onset, PO:** 30–60 min after an immediate-release dose; **maximum effect:** 2–4 hr. **Onset,**

transdermal: 2–3 days. **Peak plasma levels, immediate-release:** 3–5 hr; **modified-release:** 4–7 hr; **transdermal:** 2–3 days. **Duration, PO:** 12–24 hr; **transdermal:** 7 days (with system in place). **t ½, immediate-release or extended-release:** 12–16 hr; **modified-release**: 13 hr. Systemic bioavailability of extended-release product is about 89% that following immediate-release clonidine. The t½ of immediate-release tablets increases up to 41 hr in those with severe renal impairment. Approximately 50% excreted unchanged in the urine; 20% excreted through the feces. **Epidural: t½, distribution,** 19 min; **elimination:** 22 hr. After epidural, it rapidly distributes to the CNS. **Plasma protein binding:** 20–40% following epidural use.

CONTRAINDICATIONS

Known hypersensitivity to clonidine. Epidurally if presence of an injection site infection, clients on anticoagulant therapy, in bleeding diathesis, administration above the C4 dermatome, in those with severe CV disease, in those hemodynamically unstable. Use of the injection for obstetric, postpartum, or perioperative pain. Use of modified-release tablets during lactation.

SPECIAL CONCERNS

(1) The 500 mcg/mL injection should be diluted in an appropriate solution prior to use. (2) Epidural clonidine is not recommended for obstetrical, postpartum, or perioperative pain management. The risk of hemodynamic instability, especially hypotension and bradycardia, from epidural clonidine may be unacceptable in these clients. However, in a rare obstetrical, postpartum, or perioperative client, potential benefits may outweigh the possible risks.

- Use the immediate-release tablets, extended-release products, and transdermal products with caution during lactation.
- Use with caution in those with severe coronary insufficiency, conduction disturbances, recent MI, cerebrovascular disease, or chronic renal failure.
- Safety and efficacy of immediate-release tablets or transdermal system not established in children less than 12 years of age and use of modified-release tablets not established in children less than 18 years of age. Clonidine ER has not been studied in children less than 6 years of age with attention deficit hyperactivity disorder.
- A decreased dosage may be necessary in geriatric clients due to age-related decreases in renal function; geriatric clients may also be more sensitive to the hypotensive and CNS adverse effects.
- In clients who develop skin sensitivity to transdermal clonidine, continued use of the transdermal product or substitution of PO therapy may cause a generalized skin rash.
- Sudden withdrawal of immediate-release tablets may cause agitation, headache, nervousness, and tremor accompanied or followed by a rapid rise in BP and elevated plasma catecholamine levels. Sudden withdrawal of modified-release tablets may cause anxiety, brief lightheadedness, flushing, headache, nausea, tachycardia, tightness in chest, or warm feeling; rebound hypertension was not noted.
- For children, restrict epidural use to severe intractable pain from malignancy that is unresponsive to epidural or spinal opiates or other analgesic approaches.

SIDE EFFECTS

Most Common

Epidural: Hypotension, postural hypotension, bradycardia, dry mouth, N&V, somnolence, dizziness, confusion, fever, anxiety, rebound hypertension.
Extended-Release Tablets: Constipation, dry mouth, ear pain, emotional disorder, fatigue, increased body temperature, insomnia, irritability, nasal congestion, nightmares, somnolence, throat pain, URTI.
Immediate-Release Tablets: Dry mouth, drowsiness, dizziness, sedation, constipation.
Modified-Release Tablets: Dry mouth, fatigue, dizziness, headache, somnolence.
Transdermal Products: Dry mouth, drowsiness, erythema, pruritus, contact dermatitis.

Epidural. CV: Hypotension (may be severe), postural hypotension, bradycardia, AV block (greater than first degree), tachycardia, rebound hypertension, palpitations, syncope, Raynaud phenomenon, CHF, sinus node arrest, functional bradycardia. **CNS:** Sedation, somnolence, dizziness, confusion, anxiety, hallucination, hyperesthesia, nervousness, agitation, mental depression, insomnia, vivid dreams/nightmares, restlessness, delirium, headache. **GI:** Dry mouth, N&V, constipation,

C

anorexia, hepatitis, parotitis, ileus and pseudo obstruction, abdominal pain, abnormal LFTs. **Dermatologic:** Sweating, skin ulcer, rash, pruritus, hives, angioneurotic edema, urticaria, alopecia. **Respiratory:** Ventilatory abnormalities, dyspnea, hypoventilation, dryness of nasal mucosa. **Musculoskeletal:** Muscle/joint pain, leg cramps, chest pain. **GU:** UTI, decreased sexual activity, impotence, decreased libido, nocturia, micturition difficulty, urinary retention, gynecomastia. **Withdrawal symptoms:** After abrupt cessation: Agitation, headache, nervousness, tremor, increase in BP; rarely, hypertensive encephalopathy, ***CVA, death***. **Ophthalmic:** Dry eyes, burning of the eyes, blurred vision. **Otic:** Tinnitus. **Body as a whole:** Infection, asthenia, pain, fever, malaise, fatigue, weakness, pallor, weight gain. **Miscellaneous:** Infection at catheter site, thrombocytopenia (rare), increased sensitivity to alcohol, weakly positive Coombs' test.

Extended-Release Tablets. CNS: Headache, emotional disorder, insomnia, irritability, nightmares, somnolence, abnormal sleep-related event, aggression, dizziness, emotional disorder, sleep terror, tremor, anxiety. **GI:** Upper abdominal pain, dry mouth, constipation, diarrhea, GI viral, nausea, thirst, decreased appetite, viral gastroenteritis. **CV:** Bradycardia, increased HR, BP changes. **GU:** Enuresis, pollakiuria. **Respiratory:** URTI, lower respiratory tract infection, asthma, nasal congestion, nasopharyngitis, throat pain, epistaxis, rhinorrhea. **Ophthalmic:** Tearfulness. **Otic:** Ear pain, acute otitis media. **Body as a whole:** Fatigue, increased body temperature, flu-like illness, rash. **Miscellaneous:** Pain in extremity.

Immediate-Release Tablets. CNS: Drowsiness, sedation, dizziness, agitation, anxiety, delirium, delusional perception, headache, insomnia, mental depression, nervousness, behavioral changes, paresthesia, restlessness, sleep disorder, visual and auditory hallucinations, vivid dreams/nightmares. **GI:** Dry mouth, constipation, abdominal pain, anorexia, N&V, parotitis, salivary gland pain, pseudo-obstruction, including colonic pseudo-obstruction. **Hepatic:** Hepatitis, mild transient abnormalities in LFTs. **CV:** CHF, bradycardia, ECG abnormalities (e.g., sinus node arrest, functional bradycardia, high-degree AV block, arrhythmias), orthostatic symptoms, palpitations, Raynaud phenomenon, sinus bradycardia and AV block (both with and without use of concomitant digitalis), syncope, tachycardia. **Dermatologic:** Alopecia, angioneurotic edema, hives, pruritus, skin pallor/rashes, sweating, urticaria. **GU:** Decreased sexual activity, difficulty in urination, erectile dysfunction, gynecomastia, loss of libido, nocturia, urinary retention. **Musculoskeletal:** Muscle/joint pain, leg cramps, weakness. **Metabolic:** Weight gain. **Ophthalmic:** Accommodation disorder, blurred vision, burning/dryness of eyes, decreased lacrimation. **Body as a whole:** Fatigue, fever, infection, malaise, pain. **Miscellaneous:** Increased sensitivity to alcohol, chest pain, pallor, tinnitus, hyperesthesia, thrombocytopenia, withdrawal syndrome, dryness of nasal mucosa. *NOTE*: When used for ADHD in children, can cause serious side effects, including bradycardia, hypotension, and respiratory depression.

Modified-Release Tablets. CNS: Fatigue, dizziness, insomnia, headache, somnolence. **GI:** Dry mouth, nausea.

Transdermal products. Dermatologic: Erythema, pruritus, contact dermatitis, localized vesiculation, localized hypo-/hyperpigmentation, edema, excoriation, burning, papulas, throbbing, blanching, generalized macular rash, urticaria, angioedema of the face/tongue, angioneurotic edema, localized or generalized rash, hives, urticaria, alopecia. **GI:** Dry mouth, dry throat, constipation, N&V, change in taste, anorexia. **CNS:** Drowsiness, headache, sedation, insomnia, dizziness, nervousness, delirium, mental depression, visual/auditory hallucinations, localized numbness, vivid dreams/nightmares, restlessness, anxiety, agitation, irritability. **CV:** CHF, ***CVA***, electrocardiographic abnormalities (e.g., bradycardia, sick sinus syndrome disturbances, arrhythmias), chest pain, orthostatic symptoms, syncope, increase in BP, sinus bradycardia, AV block (with and without concomitant digitalis use), Raynaud phenomenon, tachycardia, palpitations. **Musculoskeletal:** Muscle/joint pain, leg cramps. **GU:** Impotence/sexual dysfunction, difficult micturition, loss of libido, decreased sexual activity. **Metabolic:** Gynecomastia or breast enlargement, weight gain. **Ophthalmic:** Blurred vision, burning/dryness of eyes. **Body as a whole:** Fatigue, lethargy, fever, malaise, weakness, pallor. **Miscellaneous:** Withdrawal syndrome.

NOTE: Rebound hypertension may be manifested if clonidine is withdrawn abruptly.

LABORATORY TEST CONSIDERATIONS

Transient ↑ blood glucose, serum phosphatase, and serum CPK. Weakly + Coombs' test. Electrolyte imbalance.

OVERDOSE MANAGEMENT

Symptoms: Hypertension (may develop early) followed by hypotension, bradycardia, respiratory and CNS depression (may be higher in children), hypothermia, drowsiness, decreased or absent reflexes, weakness, irritability, miosis. Large overdoses may cause reversible cardiac conduction defects or dysrhythmias, apnea, coma, and ***seizures***. Signs and symptoms of overdose may occur within 30–120 min after exposure. *NOTE:* As little as 0.1 mg may cause signs of toxicity in children. *Treatment:* Maintain respiration; perform gastric lavage followed by activated charcoal. Mg sulfate may be used to hasten the rate of transport through the GI tract. Supportive care includes atropine for bradycardia, IV fluids or vasopressor drugs for hypotension, and vasodilators for hypertension. Naloxone may be useful as an adjunct to manage clonidine-induced respiratory depression, hypotension, and/or coma. Monitor BP. Dialysis is not likely to enhance clonidine elimination.

DRUG INTERACTIONS

Anesthetics, local / Epidural clonidine may prolong duration of action of epidural local anesthetics, including both motor and sensory blockade
Beta-adrenergic blocking agents (e.g., atenolol) / Attenuation or reversal of antihypertensive effect; potentially life-threatening ↑ BP. Also, possible additive effects (e.g., bradycardia, AV block) if used with agents known to affect sinus node function or AV nodal conduction. If clonidine discontinued in those receiving a beta-blocker, withdraw the beta-blocker several days before gradual discontinuation of clonidine
Calcium channel blockers (e.g., verapamil) / Possible additive bradycardia and AV block; use together with caution; monitor HR and BP and adjust dose of either agent as needed
CNS depressants (e.g., alcohol, barbiturates) / ↑ CNS depressant effect; monitor and adjust CNS depressant dose as needed
Cyclosporine / Possible ↑ cyclosporine pharmacologic/toxic effects; monitor cyclosporine levels; may need to ↓ cyclosporine dose or stop clonidine
Digitalis / ↑ Risk for additive bradycardia and AV block; use together with caution and monitor HR
Levodopa / ↓ Levodopa effect; monitor and adjust levodopa dose as needed
Methylphenidate / Possible serious side effects, including death in those with an underlying CV condition
Mirtazapine / Loss of BP control by clonidine R/T antagonism of alpha-2 adrenergic receptors
Narcotic analgesics / Possible potentiation of clonidine's hypotensive effects
Prazosin / ↓ Clonidine antihypertensive effect; monitor and adjust clonidine dose as needed
Tizanidine / Possible additive hypotensive effects; avoid coadministration
Tricyclic antidepressants (e.g., amitriptyline) / Blocks antihypertensive effect and possible life-threatening ↑ BP may occur

HOW SUPPLIED

Film, Extended Release, Transdermal: Catapres-TTS-1: 2.5 mg clonidine (surface area 3.5 cm^2), with 0.1 mg released daily; Catapres-TTS-2: 5 mg clonidine (surface area 7 cm^2), with 0.2 mg released daily; and Catapres-TTS-3: 7.5 mg clonidine (surface area 10.5 cm^2), with 0.3 mg released daily.

Clonidine (generic): 3.57 mg clonidine (surface area 10.8 cm^2), with 0.1 mg released daily; Clonidine (generic): 7.34 mg clonidine (surface area 21.6 cm^2, with 0.2 mg released daily; Clonidine (generic): 11.02 mg clonidine (surface area 32.4 cm^2, with 0.3 mg released daily; ***Injection (Duraclon):*** 100 mcg/mL, 500 mcg/mL; ***Suspension, Extended-Release (Nexiclon XR):*** 0.09 mg/mL; ***Tablets:*** 0.1 mg, 0.2 mg, 0.3 mg; ***Tablets, Extended-Release (Kapvay):*** 0.1 mg, 0.2 mg; ***Tablets, Modified-Release (Jenloga):*** 0.1 mg.

DOSAGE

FILM, EXTENDED-RELEASE, TRANSDERMAL

Hypertension.

Adults and children 12 years and older, initial: Use 0.1-mg system; **then,** if after 1–2 weeks adequate control has not been achieved, can use another 0.1-mg system or a larger system. An in-

C

crease in dose more than 2 clonidine 0.3 mg transdermal systems is usually not associated with additional effectiveness. Titrate dosage according to individual requirements. The antihypertensive effect may not be seen for 2–3 days. Thus, when substituting the transdermal product for the PO product or for other antihypertensive medications, gradually decrease the prior drug dosage. The system should be changed q 7 days.

Attention deficit hyperactivity disorder (investigational).

Children: 0.2–0.3 mg/day. The higher dose may be needed to maintain clinical response.

Hot flashes (investigational).

Adults: 0.1 mg patch q 7 days.

Hyperhidrosis (investigational).

Adults: 0.2 mg patch for 14 days, although documentation is insufficient.

Facilitate cessation of smoking (investigational).

Adults: 0.1–0.2 mg/day for 3–10 weeks. Begin initial dose up to 3 days before the quit date (usually 0.1 mg/day), increasing by 0.1 mg q 7 days, if needed.

Ulcerative colitis (investigational).

Adults: 15 mg/week for up to 8 weeks.

EPIDURAL INFUSION

Severe pain in cancer clients.

Adults, initial: 30 mcg/hr by continuous epidural infusion. Dose may then be titrated up or down, depending on pain relief and side effects. Experience with doses above 40 mcg/hr is limited. **Children, initial:** 0.5 mcg/kg/hr by continuous epidural infusion. Adjust dose cautiously depending on response.

Postanesthetic shivering (investigational).

Adults: 3 mcg/kg **IV** as a single dose. Single doses of 2 mcg/kg or 150 mcg IV have also been used. Give at induction of anesthesia, end of surgery, or upon return of laryngeal reflexes and spontaneous breathing.

Postherpetic neuralgia (investigational).

Adults: 20 mL repetitive paravertebral block injections of clonidine, 150 mcg/mL, and bupivacaine, 0.5%, have been used.

SUSPENSION, EXTENDED-RELEASE; TABLETS, IMMEDIATE-RELEASE, EXTENDED-RELEASE, OR MODIFIED-RELEASE

Hypertension

Adults, initial: 0.1 mg twice a day of immediate release, 0.1 mg at bedtime of modified release, or 0.17 mg (2 mL) once daily of the suspension; **then,** increase by 0.1 mg/day (0.09 mg [1 mL] of the suspension) at weekly intervals until desired response is attained. **Maintenance, immediate-release or modified-release:** 0.2–0.6 mg/day in divided doses or 0.17 mg (2 mL)–0.52 mg (6 mL) once daily of the suspension; **modified-release:** doses higher than 0.3 mg twice a day have not been evaluated and thus are not recommended. **Maximum dose:** 2.4 mg/day of immediate-release or 0.52 mg (6 mL)/day of the suspension. Tolerance necessitates increased dosage or concomitant administration of a diuretic. Gradual increase of dosage after initiation minimizes side effects. **Children, 12 years and older, initial:** 0.1 mg twice a day (morning and bedtime) of the immediate-release; increments of 0.1 mg/day may be made at weekly intervals, if needed, until the desired effect is reached. **Usual dose:** 0.2–0.6 mg/day given in divided doses; **maximum dose:** 2.4 mg/day.

Attention deficit hyperactivity disorder using extended-release product.

Children, 6 years and older, initial: 0.1 mg of the extended-release product at bedtime; adjust dosage in increments of 0.1 mg/day at weekly intervals until the desired response is reached. **Maximum dose:** 0.4 mg/day. The dosing schedule should be as follows: If the dose is 0.1 mg/day, give at bedtime; if the dose is 0.2 mg/day, give 0.1 mg in the morning and 0.1 mg at bedtime; if the dose is 0.3 mg/day, give 0.1 mg in the morning and 0.2 mg at bedtime; and, if the dose is 0.4 mg/day, give 0.2 mg in the morning and 0.2 mg at bedtime. *NOTE:* Efficacy has not been determined for long-term use exceeding 5 weeks; thus, periodically reevaluate the need for continued therapy.

Attention deficit hyperactivity disorder using immediate-release tablets (investigational).

Children, initial: 0.05 mg/day with increases of 0.05 mg q 3–7 days to a maximum dose of 0.3–0.4 mg/day. Daily doses have been given 3–4 times/day. Dose titration should be undertaken over several weeks to 0.15–0.3 mg/day in 3–4 divided doses.

Alcohol withdrawal (investigational).

Adults, initial: Up to 0.3 mg. Decrease dose as alcohol withdrawal symptoms subside.

Diabetic diarrhea (investigational).

Adults: 0.1 mg q 12 hr titrated to 0.5 or 0.6 mg q 12 hr over the following 3 days; follow by maintenance dosing up to 24 months.

Diagnosis of pheochromocytoma (investigational).

Adults: Single oral dose of 0.3 mg or 0.3 mg/70 kg.

Growth hormone stimulation test (investigational).

Adults and children: 200 mcg or 0.15 mg/m^2 orally.

Hot flashes (investigational).

Adults: 0.05–0.4 mg twice a day.

Hyperhidrosis (investigational).

Adults: 0.3–0.6 mg/day for several months. Doses of 3.5 mg/day for several weeks have also been investigated.

Methadone withdrawal (investigational).

Adults: 0.2 mg 3–4 times/day. Individualize dosage to each client. Usually, clonidine can be discontinued in 2–3 weeks.

Opiate withdrawal (investigational).

Adults, clonidine monotherapy: 0.1 mg 3 times/day titrated to withdrawal symptoms. **Clonidine adjunctive therapy with naltrexone:** Titrate dose for both drugs to specific client needs.

Postherpetic neuralgia (investigational).

Adults: 0.2 mg/day orally.

Restless leg syndrome (investigational).

Adults: 0.1–0.3 mg/day, up to 0.9 mg/day have shown improvement. Titrate PO doses to client needs. Recommended is 0.5 mg given 2 hr before onset of symptoms for 2–3 weeks.

Smoking cessation (investigational).

Adults: 0.15–0.75 mg/day for 3–10 weeks. Initial dosing should begin up to 3 days before the quit date and is usually 0.1 mg PO twice a day, increasing by 0.1 mg weekly if needed.

Tourette syndrome in adults (investigational).

Adults, adolescents, children: 0.0025–0.015 mg/kg/day for 6 weeks to 3 months.

Ulcerative colitis (investigational).

Adults: 0.3 mg 3 times/day for 6 weeks.

NURSING IMPLICATIONS

Do not confuse Catapres with Cataflam (a nonsteroidal anti-inflammatory drug) or with Combipres (combination antihypertensive drug). Do not confuse clonidine with Klonopin (an anticonvulsant).

IMPLEMENTATION/ADMINISTRATION/STORAGE

1. Divide daily PO doses above 0.1 mg and take in the morning and at bedtime. Taking the higher dose at bedtime may minimize transient dry mouth and drowsiness.
2. The elderly may benefit from lower initial doses.
3. Although modified-release clonidine is dosed twice a day, it is not to be used interchangeably with the immediate-release tablets, which are also dosed twice a day. Also, the extended-release clonidine products are not to be used interchangeably with the immediate-release formulation.
4. May take 2–3 days to achieve effective blood levels using transdermal system. Therefore, reduce any prior drug dosage gradually.

5. For impaired renal function, adjust the dose according to degree of impairment and uptitrate slowly. Monitor to prevent excessive BP lowering or bradycardia.
6. With severe hypertension may require other antihypertensive drug therapy in addition to transdermal clonidine.
7. Continue use up until 4 hr before surgery and resume as soon as possible after.
8. Remove the transdermal system before attempting defibrillation or cardioversion due to the potential for altered electrical conductivity which may increase the risk of arcing.
9. If drug is to be discontinued, do so gradually over a period of 2–4 days to avoid withdrawal symptoms. When the extended-release tablet is to be discontinued, taper the total daily dose in decrements of no more than 0.1 mg q 3–7 days.
10. If the drug is to be discontinued in clients receiving a beta-blocker and clonidine concurrently, withdraw the beta-blocker several days before the gradual discontinuation of clonidine.
11. To prepare the drug for epidural use, dilute the 500 mcg/mL strength in NaCl, 0.9% to a final concentration of 100 mcg/mL. Further dilute according to instructions provided to obtain the proper concentration and volume needed.
12. Do not use preservative when given epidurally.
13. Store immediate-release tablets from 15–30°C (59–86°F) and the modified-release and extended-release tablets from 20–25°C (68–77°F). Store transdermal patches below 30°C (86°F). Store injection at 25°C; discard any unused portion of the injection.

ASSESSMENT

1. Identify reasons for therapy, onset, type of symptoms, clinical presentation, and any previous treatments.
2. Note occupation; drug may interfere with the ability to work.
3. List drugs currently prescribed to prevent any interactions. With propranolol, observe for a paradoxical hypertensive response. With tolazoline or TCA, be aware that these may block the antihypertensive action of clonidine; clonidine dosage may need to be increased. If clonidine therapy is discontinued in those receiving a beta-blocker, withdraw beta-blocker several days before gradual discontinuation of clonidine.
4. Tolerance may develop with long-term use; an increased dose or addition of diuretic may improve response.
5. May be used alone or as adjunctive therapy to a psychostimulant for treatment of ADHD.
6. Note evidence of alcohol, drug, or nicotine addiction. These agents usually work well in this group of clients (especially the once-a-week patch).
7. Monitor BP closely. BP decreases occur within 30–60 min after administration and may persist for 8 hr. Note any fluctuations to determine whether to use clonidine alone or concomitantly with a diuretic. A stable BP reduces orthostatic effects with postural changes.
8. Patch (transdermal) may take 2–3 days to exert effects and therefore oral therapy may be needed during this time. Assess skin sites for rash or itching and change sites weekly.
9. Epidural therapy—implantable epidural catheters with ↑ risk of catheter-related infections. Any fevers should include evaluation for catheter-related infection such as meningitis or epidural abscess.
10. Obtain ECG, CBC, renal and LFTs; reduce dose with severe renal dysfunction. Promote periodic eye exams.

CLIENT/FAMILY TEACHING

1. With transdermal system, apply patch to hairless area of skin, such as upper arm or torso, then apply the adhesive overlay to ensure adhesion of patch. Change system q 7 days; use different site with each application.
2. If taken PO, take last dose (the higher of the two if unequal) of the day at bedtime to ensure overnight control of BP. Keep a log of BP and HR.
3. Extended-release tablets are to be swallowed whole; do not crush, cut, or chew. Extended-release tablets may be taken with or without food. Not to be used interchangeably with the immediate-release formulation.
4. Do not engage in activities that require mental alertness, such as operating machinery or driving a car; may cause drowsiness, dizziness, lightheadedness, or blurred vision.

5. Do not change regimen or stop drug abruptly. May experience nervousness, agitation, headache, tremor followed by a rapid rise in BP.
6. Record weight daily, in the morning, in clothing of the same weight, to determine if there is edema caused by sodium retention. Any fluid retention should disappear after 3–4 days. Change positions slowly to prevent sudden drop in BP and associated dizziness.
7. Clonidine may reduce the effect of levodopa; report any increase in the S&S of Parkinson's disease previously controlled with levodopa.
8. Advise women using modified-release tablets not to breast-feed.
9. Report any depression (may be precipitated by drug), especially with history of mental depression.
10. Avoid alcohol and any sedatives without approval.
11. Drug may may cause dryness of eyes; use caution if wearing contact lenses.
12. Keep all F/U to assess response and for adverse SE.

OUTCOMES/EVALUATE

- ↓ BP
- In combination with opiates for epidural use for relief of cancer pain
- Treatment of ADHD in children (extended-release only)
- ↓ Menopausal flushing; postherpetic neuralgia; diagnosis of pheochromocytoma; control of withdrawal symptoms (unlabeled)

Clopidogrel bisulfate

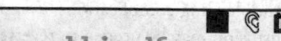

(kloh-**PID**-oh-grel)

Classification(s): Antiplatelet drug

Pregnancy Category: B

RX: Plavix.

INDICATIONS/USES

(1) Non-ST-segment elevation acute coronary syndrome (unstable angina/non-ST-elevation MI), including those who are to be managed medically and those who are to be managed with coronary revascularization. Clopidogrel decreases the rate of a combined end point of CV death, MI, or stroke, as well as the rate of a combined end point of CV death, MI, stroke, or refractory ischemia. (2) To reduce the rate of death from any cause and the rate of a combined end point of death, reinfarction, or stroke in those with ST-segment elevation acute MI. (3) To reduce the rate of a combined end point of new ischemic stroke (fatal or not), new MI (fatal or not), and other vascular death in those with a recent MI, recent stroke, or established peripheral arterial disease. *Investigational:* As a loading dose with aspirin to prevent cardiac side effects in those undergoing coronary stent implantation. Treatment of arterial ischemic stroke in children. Antiplatelet therapy in children with a cardiac condition and at risk for arterial thrombosis (i.e., a systemic to pulmonary artery shunt or another cardiac condition with a risk for arterial thrombosis, including a stent replacement).

ACTION/KINETICS

Action

Must be metabolized mainly by CYP2C19 to produce the active metabolite. Inhibits platelet aggregation by inhibiting binding of adenosine diphosphate (ADP) to its platelet receptor ($P2Y_{12}$) and subsequent ADP-mediative activation of glycoprotein GPIIb/IIIa complex. Effect on receptors is irreversible; thus, platelets are affected for the remainder of their lifespan (about 7–10 days). Also inhibits platelet aggregation caused by agonists other than ADP by blocking amplification of platelet activation by released ADP.

Pharmacokinetics

Rapidly absorbed from GI tract; food does not affect bioavailability. **Peak plasma levels:** About 1 hr. **Steady-state:** 3–7 days. Platelet aggregation and bleeding time return to baseline values gradually (about 5 days) after treatment is discontinued. Extensively metabolized in liver; about 50% excreted in urine and 46% in feces. **t½, elimination:** 8 hr.

CONTRAINDICATIONS

Hypersensitivity to the drug or any component of the product. Active pathological bleeding such as peptic ulcer or intracranial hemorrhage. Avoid concomitant use of clopidogrel and drugs that inhibit CYP2C19 activity (e.g., omeprazole). Lactation.

SPECIAL CONCERNS

Diminished effectiveness in poor metabolizers. The effectiveness of clopidogrel is dependent on its activation to an active metabolite by the cytochrome P450 (CYP-450) system, principally CYP2C19. Poor metabolizers treated with clopidogrel at recommended doses exhibit higher cardiovascular event rates following acute coronary syndrome or percutaneous coronary intervention than clients with normal CYP2C19 function. Tests are available to identify a client's CYP2C19 genotype and can be used as an aid in determining therapeutic strategy. Consider alternative treatment or treatment strategies in clients identified as CYP2C19 poor metabolizers. ■

- **Use with caution in those at risk of increased bleeding from trauma, surgery, or other pathological conditions; also, in severe impaired renal or hepatic function.**
- **Moderate to severe renal impairment lowers (25%) inhibition of ADP-induced platelet aggregation.**
- **Safety and efficacy not determined in children.**

SIDE EFFECTS

Most Common

Skin/appendage disorders, headache, URTI, chest pain, flu-like symptoms.

CV: Edema, hyper-/hypotension, syncope, palpitations, atrial fibrillation, ***intracranial hemorrhage, major/life-threatening bleeding, major noncerebral bleeding, hemorrhagic stroke, retroperitoneal hemorrhage, hemorrhage of operative wound, cardiac failure, pulmonary hemorrhage, GI and retroperitoneal hemorrhage***, ocular hemorrhage with significant loss of vision. **GI:** Abdominal pain, dyspepsia, diarrhea, constipation, N&V, taste disorders, colitis (including lymphocytic or ulcerative), ***pancreatitis***, stomatitis, ***hemorrhage***, ulcers (peptic, gastric, duodenal), GI bleeding, ***perforated hemorrhagic gastritis, hemorrhagic upper GI ulcer, perforated gastric ulcer***. **Hepatic:** Infectious hepatitis, fatty liver, noninfectious hepatitis, ***acute liver failure***. **CNS:** Headache, dizziness, depression, hypoesthesia, neuralgia, paresthesia, vertigo, anxiety, insomnia, confusion, hallucinations. **Body as a whole:** Chest pain, accidental injury, flu-like symptoms, pain, fatigue, asthenia, fever, allergic reactions, ischemic necrosis, generalized edema, leg cramps, gout. **Respiratory:** URTI, epistaxis, dyspnea, rhinitis, bronchitis, coughing, pneumonia, sinusitis, hemothorax, bronchospasm, interstitial pneumonitis, respiratory tract bleeding. **Hematologic:** Purpura/bruises, ***thrombotic thrombocytopenic purpura*** (rare), epistaxis, hematoma, anemia, hemarthrosis, hemoptysis, thrombocytopenia, agranulocytosis, ***aplastic anemia, pancytopenia***, hypochromic anemia, neutropenia, ***agranulocytosis***, granulocytopenia, leukemia, leukopenia, allergic purpura. **Musculoskeletal:** Arthralgia, back pain, arthritis, arthrosis, myalgia, musculoskeletal bleeding. **Dermatologic:** Disorders of skin/appendages, rash, pruritus, eczema, hematoma, skin ulceration, bullous eruption, erythematous rash, maculopapular rash, urticaria, ***angioedema***, erythema multiforme, lichen planus, skin bleeding, ***Stevens-Johnson syndrome, toxic epidermal necrolysis***. **GU:** UTI, cystitis, menorrhagia, abnormal renal function, ***acute renal failure***, hematuria, glomerulopathy. **Hypersensitivity:** ***Angioedema***, bronchospasm, serum sickness, ***anaphylactoid reactions***. **Ophthalmic:** Cataract, conjunctivitis; conjunctival, ocular, and retinal bleeding. **Miscellaneous:** Hernia, fever, cardiovasculitis.

LABORATORY TEST CONSIDERATIONS

Hypercholesterolemia, hematuria, bilirubinemia, hyperuricemia. ↑ Hepatic enzymes, creatinine, NPN. ↓ Platelets, neutrophils. Prolonged bleeding time. Abnormal creatinine levels, abnormal LFTs.

OVERDOSE MANAGEMENT

Symptoms: Prolonged bleeding time and subsequent bleeding complications. *Treatment:* Platelet transfusion may be needed to reverse the effects of clopidogrel if a quick reversal is required.

DRUG INTERACTIONS

Aspirin / ↑ Risk of life-threatening or major bleeding events (e.g., intracranial and GI hemorrhage) in high-risk clients with recent ischemic stroke or TIAs; avoid concomitant use in these clients

Atorvastatin / Inhibition of clopidogrel effects on platelet function R/T inhibition of metabolic conversion (by CYP2C19) of the prodrug clopidogrel to the active drug

Bupropion / ↑ Bupropion AUC and peak plasma levels R/T inhibition of metabolism by CYP2B6 hydroxylation of bupropion; ↑ bupropion pharmacologic and toxicologic effects

Cimetidine / ↓ Pharmacologic effect of clopidogrel R/T inhibition of CYP2C19 → ↓ clopidogrel

metabolism to the active metabolite; avoid concurrent use
Esomeprazole / ↓ Pharmacologic effect of clopidogrel R/T inhibition of CYP2C19 → ↓ clopidogrel metabolism to the active metabolite; avoid concurrent use
Etravirine / ↓ Pharmacologic effect of clopidogrel R/T inhibition of CYP2C19 → ↓ clopidogrel metabolism to the active metabolite; avoid concurrent use
H ***Evening primrose oil*** / Potential for ↑ antiplatelet effect
Felbamate / ↓ Pharmacologic effect of clopidogrel R/T inhibition of CYP2C19 → ↓ clopidogrel metabolism to the active metabolite; avoid concurrent use
H ***Feverfew*** / Potential for ↑ antiplatelet effect
Fluconazole / ↓ Pharmacologic effect of clopidogrel R/T inhibition of CYP2C19 → ↓ clopidogrel metabolism to the active metabolite; avoid concurrent use
Fluoxetine / ↓ Pharmacologic effect of clopidogrel R/T inhibition of CYP2C19 → ↓ clopidogrel metabolism to the active metabolite; avoid concurrent use
Fluvoxamine / ↓ Pharmacologic effect of clopidogrel R/T inhibition of CYP2C19 → ↓ clopidogrel metabolism to the active metabolite; avoid concurrent use
H ***Garlic*** / Potential for ↑ antiplatelet effect
H ***Ginger*** / Potential for ↑ antiplatelet effect
H ***Ginkgo biloba*** / Potential for ↑ antiplatelet effect
H ***Grapeseed extract*** / Potential for ↑ antiplatelet effect
Ketoconazole / ↓ Pharmacologic effect of clopidogrel R/T inhibition of CYP2C19 → ↓ clopidogrel metabolism to the active metabolite; avoid concurrent use
Macrolide antibiotics (e.g., erythromycin, telithromycin) / Inhibition of antiplatelet effect of clopidogrel; monitor platelet function and adjust clopidogrel dose as needed
NSAIDs (e.g., naproxen) / ↑ Risk of occult blood loss; use together with caution
Omeprazole / ↓ Pharmacologic effect of clopidogrel R/T inhibition of CYP2C19 → ↓ clopidogrel metabolism to the active metabolite; avoid concurrent use
Proton pump inhibitors (e.g., esomeprazole, omeprazole) / Significantly ↑ risk of major CV events (pantoprazole may not alter clopidogrel's effects); use together with caution
Rifamycins (e.g., rifampin) / ↑ Clopidogrel antiplatelet effect; monitor platelet function when starting, stopping, or changing the rifamycin dose; adjust clopidogrel dose as needed
Simvastatin / Inhibition of clopidogrel effects on platelet function R/T inhibition of metabolic conversion (by CYP2C19) of the prodrug clopidogrel to the active drug
Ticlopidine / ↓ Pharmacologic effect of clopidogrel R/T inhibition of CYP2C19 → ↓ clopidogrel metabolism to the active metabolite; avoid concurrent use
Voriconazole / ↓ Pharmacologic effect of clopidogrel R/T inhibition of CYP2C19 → ↓ clopidogrel metabolism to the active metabolite; avoid concurrent use
Warfarin / Clopidogrel prolongs bleeding time → ↑ risk of major bleeding; use together with caution

HOW SUPPLIED

Tablets: 75 mg, 300 mg.

DOSAGE

TABLETS

Acute coronary syndrome, non-ST elevation myocardial infarction.

Adults, initial: Single 300 mg loading dose; **then,** 75 mg once daily. Initiate and continue aspirin (75–325 mg once daily). Many clients also receive heparin acutely.

Acute coronary syndrome, ST-elevation MI.

Usual: 75 mg once daily, given with aspirin, 75–325 mg/day. Given with or without thrombolytics. Clopidogrel may be initiated with or without a loading dose of 300 mg.

Recent MI, stroke, or established peripheral arterial disease.

Adults: 75 mg once daily.

Loading dose regimen in those undergoing coronary stent placement (investigational).

Adults, loading dose: 150–600 mg; **then,** 75 or 100 mg/day. Loading doses have been given from 3–24 hr before the procedure or within 24 hr after the procedure.

Arterial ischemic stroke in children (investigational).

Children, 1 month and older: 1 mg/kg/day (up to 75 mg). *NOTE:* The risk of intracranial bleeding is increased when given concomitantly with aspirin.

Cardiac condition at risk for arterial thrombosis in children (investigational).

Children, 24 months of age and younger: 0.2 mg/kg/day.

C

NURSING IMPLICATIONS

Do not confuse Plavix with Pletal (also an antiplatelet drug) or Paxil (antidepressant).

IMPLEMENTATION/ADMINISTRATION/STORAGE

1. Dosage adjustment not necessary for geriatric clients, those with impaired hepatic function, or those with renal disease (experience limited in those with moderate and severe renal impairment).
2. Clients with polymorphisms in CYP2C19 have a significantly reduced response to clopidogrel and an increased risk for death, MI, or stroke. Although higher doses of clopidogrel (600 mg loading dose followed by 150 mg once/day), an appropriate dose regimen for this population has not been established.
3. If necessary, discontinue clopidogrel 5 days before surgery.
4. Avoid lapses in therapy. If clopidogrel must be discontinued temporarily, restart as soon as possible. Premature discontinuation may increase the risk of CV events.
5. Store from 15–30°C (59–86°F).

ASSESSMENT

1. Note atherosclerotic event (MI, stroke), CABG, stent (note type), or established peripheral arterial disease requiring therapy; monitor during therapy for any S&S of progression of CVA, PVD, or MI.
2. Assess for fever or any active bleeding as with ulcers or intracranial bleeding; precludes therapy.
3. List all drugs prescribed/consumed especially OTC (i.e., NSAIDs, ASA, herbals).
4. Monitor renal and LFTs, platelets, CBC and for bleeding, unusual bruising, or TTP.

CLIENT/FAMILY TEACHING

1. Take exactly as directed; may take without regard to food. Food will lessen chance of stomach upset.
2. May cause dizziness, assess drug response.
3. Avoid OTC agents especially aspirin, aspirin-containing products, or NSAIDs, unless prescribed.
4. Be prepared, it may take longer than usual to stop bleeding and one may bruise and bleed much easier. Report any unusual or prolonged bruising or bleeding, fever or chills; advise all providers of prescribed therapy.
5. Those found to be CYP2C19 poor metabolizers may have to take larger doses to attain same desired effects.
6. Stop drug 5–7 days prior to elective surgery. Ensure provider notified before any dental procedures.
7. Keep all F/U to assess response, labs, and for adverse SE.

OUTCOMES/EVALUATE

- Inhibition of platelet aggregation
- Reduction of atherosclerotic events (e.g., MI, stroke, vascular death) with atherosclerosis
- Treatment of acute coronary syndrome

Clorazepate dipotassium

(klor-**AYZ**-eh-payt)

Classification(s): Antianxiety drug, benzodiazepine; anticonvulsant, miscellaneous

Pregnancy Category: D

RX: Tranxene T-tab, **C-IV**

Rx: Apo-Clorazepate.

SEE ALSO ***TRANQUILIZERS/ANTIMANIC DRUGS/HYPNOTICS***.

INDICATIONS/USES

(1) Anxiety disorders or short-term relief of symptoms of anxiety. (2) Symptomatic relief of acute alcohol withdrawal. (3) Adjunct to treat partial seizures.

ACTION/KINETICS

Pharmacokinetics

Peak plasma levels: 1–2 hr. **t½:** 40–50 hr. Hydrolyzed in the stomach to desmethyldiazepam, the active metabolite. Oxazepam is also an active metabolite. Also metabolized in the liver. **t½, desmethyldiazepam:** 30–100 hr; **t½, oxazepam:** 5–15 hr. **Time to peak plasma levels:** 0.5–2 hr. Slowly excreted by the kidneys. **Plasma protein binding:** 97–98%.

ADDITIONAL CONTRAINDICATIONS

Depressed clients, lactation.

SPECIAL CONCERNS

Use with caution with impaired renal or hepatic function.

SIDE EFFECTS

Most Common

Drowsiness, dizziness, fatigue, dry mouth, stomach upset, constipation, blurred vision, headache. See *Tranquilizers/Antimanic Drugs/Hypnotics* for a complete list of possible side effects.

HOW SUPPLIED

Tablets, Immediate-Release: 3.75 mg, 7.5 mg, 15 mg.

DOSAGE

TABLETS, IMMEDIATE-RELEASE

Anxiety.

Initial: 30 mg/day in divided doses; gradually adjust dose to 15–60 mg/day. **Alternative.** Single daily dosage: **Adult, initial,** 15 mg at bedtime; subsequent dosage adjustment may be needed. **Elderly or debilitated clients, initial:** 7.5–15 mg/day.

Acute alcohol withdrawal.

Day 1, initial: 30 mg; **then,** 30–60 mg in divided doses; **day 2:** 45–90 mg in divided doses; **day 3:** 22.5–45 mg in divided doses; **day 4:** 15–30 mg in divided doses. Thereafter, reduce to 7.5–15 mg/day and discontinue as soon as possible. Maximum daily dose: 90 mg.

Partial seizures.

Adults and children over 12 years, initial: 7.5 mg 3 times/day; increase no more than 7.5 mg/week to maximum of 90 mg/day. **Children (9–12 years), initial, maximum:** 7.5 mg twice a day; increase by no more than 7.5 mg/week to maximum of 60 mg/day. Not recommended for children under 9 years of age.

NURSING IMPLICATIONS

IMPLEMENTATION/ADMINISTRATION/STORAGE

Store at controlled room temperature from 15-30°C (59-86°F). Protect from moisture and light.

ASSESSMENT

1. Note reasons for therapy, symptom characteristics/behavioral presentation, any evidence of depression.
2. With excessive alcohol intake, determine timing of last drink.
3. Monitor CBC, renal and LFTs; assess for dysfunction especially with prolonged therapy.

CLIENT/FAMILY TEACHING

1. Take as directed; do not alter prescribed dose. Do not crush, chew, divide, or break tablets. Do not take with food unless GI upset occurs.
2. Avoid activities requiring mental alertness until drug effects realized; drowsiness may occur initially and with dosage increases.
3. May use sugarless gum or candy to control dry mouth symptoms.
4. Avoid alcohol and any other CNS depressants.
5. Report increased depression or behavioral changes.
6. Drug may be habit forming, do not stop suddenly after prolonged therapy—may trigger withdrawal S&S. Provider will regularly assess response and need to continue therapy.
7. With seizure disorder take other meds as prescribed; report loss of seizure control.
8. With anxiety issues identify alternative ways to control; ensure stress reduction training and counselling as indicated.
9. Keep all F/U to assess response, labs, and for adverse SE.

OUTCOMES/EVALUATE

- ↓ Anxiety and tension
- ↓ S&S of alcohol withdrawal
- Control of seizures

Clotrimazole

(kloh-**TRY**-mah-zohl)

Classification(s): Antifungal

Pregnancy Category: C (systemic B (topical/vaginal use)

OTC: Topical Cream, Lotion, S... n (all 1%): Cruex, Desenex, Fungi C... tensive, Lotrimin AF. **Vaginal Cream:** ...-Lotrimin-3 and -7, Mycelex-7. **Vaginal ...positories:** Gyne-Lotrimin 3. **Vaginal ...m and Vaginal Suppositories:** Gyne-Lot... 3, Mycelex-7.
RX: Oral Troche: Mycel... **Topical Cream, Lotion, Solution:** Lotri...
✦ OTC: Canesten To...al/Vaginal, Clotrimaderm.

SEE ALSO ***ANTI-INFE...IVES.***

INDICATIONS/USES

Broad-spectrum antifungal.

Oral troche (Rx): (1) Oropharyngeal candidiasis. (2) Reduce incidence of oropharyngeal candidiasis in clients who are immunocompromised due to chemotherapy, radiotherapy, or steroid therapy used for leukemia, solid tumors, or kidney transplant.

Topical OTC products: Tinea pedis, tinea cruris, and tinea corporis due to *T. rubrum, T. mentagrophytes, E. floccosum,* and *M. canis.* Relieves itching, burning, cracking, and discomfort.

Topical Rx products: Candidiasis due to *C. albicans* and tinea versicolor due to *M. furfur.* **Vaginal products:** Vulvovaginal candidiasis.

ACTION/KINETICS

Action

Depending on concentration, may be fungistatic or fungicidal. Acts by inhibiting the biosynthesis of sterols, resulting in damage to the cell wall and subsequent loss of essential intracellular elements due to altered permeability. May also inhibit oxidative and peroxidative enzyme activity and inhibit the biosynthesis of triglycerides and phospholipids by fungi. When used for *Candida albicans,* the drug inhibits transformation of blastophores into the invasive mycelial form.

Pharmacokinetics

Well absorbed from the GI tract and metabolized in the liver to inactive compounds that are excreted through the feces. **Duration:** Up to 3 hr. Minimally absorbed when used topically or vaginally.

CONTRAINDICATIONS

Hypersensitivity. First trimester of pregnancy. Topically in children less than 2 years of age. Use around the eyes.

SPECIAL CONCERNS

- Use with caution during lactation.
- Safety and efficacy for PO use in children younger than age 3 or for topical use in children younger than age 2 not determined.
- For topical use, supervise children under age 12.

SIDE EFFECTS

Most Common

Topical use on skin: Irritation, rash, stinging, burning, pruritus.
Topical use in vagina: Vaginal irritation, itching, burning.
Use of troche: N&V.

Skin: Irritation including rash, stinging, pruritus, urticaria, erythema, burning, peeling, blistering, edema, general skin irritation. **Vaginal:** Lower abdominal cramps; urinary frequency; bloating; vaginal irritation, itching or burning; dyspareunia. **Hepatic:** Abnormal liver function tests. **GI:** N&V following use of troche.

HOW SUPPLIED

Oral Troche: 10 mg; ***Topical Cream:*** 1%; ***Topical Lotion:*** 1%; ***Topical Solution/Spray Solution:*** 1%; ***Vaginal Cream:*** 1%, 2%; ***Vaginal Suppositories:*** 200 mg; ***Combination/Twin Packs, Suppositories/Cream:*** 100 mg/1%, 200 mg/1%.

DOSAGE

TOPICAL CREAM; LOTION; SOLUTION

OTC for Tinea pedis/corporis.

Apply a thin layer over the affected area(s) morning and evening for 4 weeks. If no improvement, consult provider.

OTC for Tinea cruris.

Apply a thin layer over the affected area morning and evening for 2 weeks. If no improvement, consult provider.

OTC cream for vaginal yeast infections.

Apply to affected areas morning and evening for 7 consecutive days or as needed.

Rx for candidiasis and tinea versicolor.

Massage into affected skin and surrounding areas twice a day (in morning and evening). Diagnosis should be reevaluated if no improvement occurs in 4 weeks.

TROCHE

Treatment of oropharyngeal candidiasis.

One troche (10 mg) 5 times per day for 14 consecutive days.

Prophylaxis of oropharyngeal candidiasis.

One troche 3 times per day for duration of chemotherapy or until maintenance doses of steroids are instituted.

VAGINAL CREAM

Vulvovaginal candidiasis.

Insert 1 full applicator at bedtime for 3–7 consecutive days.

VAGINAL SUPPOSITORIES

Vulvovaginal candidiasis.

Insert 1 suppository (200 mg) at bedtime for 3 consecutive days.

NURSING IMPLICATIONS

IMPLEMENTATION/ADMINISTRATION/STORAGE

1. Do not allow topical products to come in contact with the eyes.
2. Slowly dissolve the troche in the mouth.
3. Store topical products from 20–25°C (68–77°F). Store Mycelex-7 vaginal cream at 2–30°C (36–86°F). Do not store Mycelex-7 100 mg vaginal troche above 35°C (95°F); store the 500 mg vaginal troche below 30°C (86°F).

ASSESSMENT

1. Note location, onset, and characteristics of S&S. List other agents/therapies trialed and outcome.
2. Describe clinical presentation. Document skin scraping/culture results.
3. Monitor LFTs periodically during prolonged therapy with oral troches, especially with hepatic dysfunction.

CLIENT/FAMILY TEACHING

1. Review goals of therapy/appropriate method for administration. Wash hands before/after treatments. Unless otherwise directed, apply only after cleaning the affected area.
2. For lotions, creams, solutions: Shake lotion well before use. With cream, lotion, or solutions, massage cream or lotion thoroughly into affected area and surrounding skin as prescribed.
3. Avoid contact with eyes; if occurs, flush immediately and thoroughly with water.
4. Report any adverse side effects N&V abdominal pain, or S&S of increased irritation (redness, itching, burning, blistering, swelling, oozing); suggests possible sensitization.
5. Avoid use of occlusive dressings/wraps and sources of infection or reinfection.
6. For oral troche: slowly dissolve (over 15–30 min) troche in mouth and retain saliva as long as possible before swallowing. Do not chew or swallow troche.
7. With vaginal infections, do not engage in intercourse; or, to prevent reinfection or pain, have partner wear a condom. Avoid contact with eyes.
8. Cream may also be applied to irritated area(s) of vulva to relieve external vaginal itching.
9. Vaginal cream may reduce effectiveness of vaginal spermicides and may damage condoms and diaphragms, causing them to fail. Use another method of birth control while using vaginal cream. Avoid using tampons while treating infection.
10. To prevent staining of clothes, use sanitary napkin with vaginal tablets or cream.
11. If exposed to HIV and recurrent vaginal yeast infections occur, seek prompt medical care to determine cause of symptoms.
12. Keep all F/U to assess response and for adverse SE.

OUTCOMES/EVALUATE

- Eradication of fungal infection
- Symptomatic improvement

Combination Drug

Clotrimazole and Betamethasone dipropionate

(kloh-**TRY**-mah-zohl, bay-tah-**METH**-ah-zohn)

Classification(s): Topical antifungal/corticosteroid

Pregnancy Category: C

RX: Lotrisone.

SEE ALSO ***CLOTRIMAZOLE*** AND ***BETAMETHASONE DIPROPIONATE***.

C

INDICATIONS/USES

Topical treatment of symptomatic inflammatory tinea pedis, tinea cruris, and tinea corporis due to *Epidermophyton floccosum, Trichophyton mentagrophytes,* and *T. rubrum.*

CONTENT

Each gram of lotion contains: Clotrimazole (antifungal), 10 mg, and Betamethasone dipropionate (corticosteroid), 0.643 mg (equivalent to 0.5 mg betamethasone).

ACTION/KINETICS

Action

Clotrimazole inhibits the biosynthesis of sterols, resulting in cell wall damage and subsequent loss of essential intracellular elements due to altered permeability. May also inhibit oxidative and peroxidative enzyme activity and inhibit the biosynthesis of triglycerides and phospholipids by fungi. The anti-inflammatory effect of betamethasone results from inhibition of prostaglandin synthesis. The drug also inhibits accumulation of macrophages and leukocytes at sites of inflammation and inhibits phagocytosis and lysosomal enzyme release.

Pharmacokinetics

Skin penetration and systemic absorption of clotrimazole have not been studied. Betamethasone is absorbed after topical use, the extent of which depends on the vehicle, integrity of the epidermal barrier, and use of occlusive dressings.

CONTRAINDICATIONS

Use in clients less than 17 years of age and in those who are sensitive to clotrimazole, betamethasone, other corticosteroids or imidazoles, or to any component of the product. Use for diaper dermatitis is not recommended.

SPECIAL CONCERNS

- **Systemic absorption can cause reversible hypothalamic-pituitary-adrenal axis suppression with possible glucocorticoid insufficiency after treatment is withdrawn.**
- **Children may be more susceptible to systemic toxicity (e.g., Cushing's syndrome, linear growth retardation, delayed weight gain, intracranial hypertension) from equivalent doses due to their large skin surface to body mass ratios.**
- **Use with caution during lactation.**

SIDE EFFECTS

Most Common

Use of the Lotion: Burning/dry skin, stinging.

Dermatologic: Itching, irritation, dryness, folliculitis, hypertrichosis, acneiform eruptions, hypopigmentation, perioral dermatitis, allergic contact dermatitis, maceration of the skin, secondary infection, skin atrophy, striae, milaria, erythema, stinging, blistering, peeling, edema, pruritus, urticaria, general skin irritation, paresthesia, rash, burning or dry skin.

HOW SUPPLIED

See *Content.*

DOSAGE

LOTION

Symptomatic inflammatory tinea pedis, tinea cruris, and tinea corporis.

Adults and children over 17 years of age: Gently massage sufficient lotion into the affected skin areas twice a day, in the morning and evening.

NURSING IMPLICATIONS

IMPLEMENTATION/ADMINISTRATION/STORAGE

1. **Do not use the lotion longer than 2 weeks when treating tinea corporis or tinea cruris and amounts greater than 45 mL of the lotion should not be used.**
2. **When treating tinea corporis or tinea cruris, review the diagnosis if no improvement is seen after 1 week.**
3. **Do not use the lotion for longer than 4 weeks when treating tinea pedis.**
4. **When treating tinea pedis, review the diagnosis if no improvement is seen after 2 weeks.**
5. **Do not use the lotion with occlusive dressings.**
6. **Do not use the lotion for more than 2 weeks in the groin area. Loose-fitting clothing should be worn.**
7. **Shake the lotion well before each use.**
8. **Store the lotion from 15–30°C (59–86°F).**

ASSESSMENT

1. **Note onset, location, and characteristics of skin condition.**
2. **Describe clinical presentation and do skin scraping if lesion not definitive.**

CLIENT/FAMILY TEACHING

1. Lotion contains a combination of a steroid and an antifungal used to treat the inflammation and infection. Use as directed for the time directed—2 weeks for tinea cruris and tinea corporis; 4 weeks for tinea pedis.
2. Do not take Lotrisone lotion internally and keep away from eyes. Wash hands before and after each use.
3. Wash and completely dry skin in the affected area. Gently rub the medicine into the affected and surrounding areas until evenly distributed. If in the groin area, use only for 2 weeks and apply sparingly; wear loose-fitting clothing.
4. Wash clothes separately with tinea corporis (ringworm) to prevent contamination of others.
5. Report any blistering, burning, dry skin, hives, infection, itching, peeling, reddened skin, skin eruptions, and rash.
6. Avoid occlusive coverings/bandages unless ordered.
7. Keep all F/U to assess response and for adverse SE.

OUTCOMES/EVALUATE

- Healing/clearing of lesions
- Resolution of fungal infection

Clozapine

(**KLOH**-zah-peen)

Classification(s): Antipsychotic

Pregnancy Category: B

RX: Clozaril, FazaClo.

✱ **Rx:** Apo-Clozapine, Gen-Clozapine.

INDICATIONS/USES

(1) Severely ill schizophrenic clients who do not respond adequately to conventional antipsychotic therapy, either because of ineffectiveness or intolerable side effects from other drugs. May be effective in chronic refractory schizophrenia. Due to the possibility of agranulocytosis and seizures associated with clozapine, use the drug only in those who have failed to respond adequately to other treatment regimens. (2) Recurrent suicidal behavior in schizophrenia or schizoaffective disorders in clients who are at chronic risk of re-experiencing suicidal behavior. (3) Tetanus. *Investigational:* Acute manic and/or mixed episodes associated with bipolar disorder, psychosis/agitation in dementia or Alzheimer's disease, psychosis in Parkinson's disease.

ACTION/KINETICS

Action

High receptor affinity for dopamine D_4 receptors thus interfering with the binding of dopamine. Also blocks D_1, D_2, D_3, and D_5 receptors; more active at limbic than at striatal dopamine receptors. Thus, is relatively free from extrapyramidal side effects and does not induce catalepsy. Also acts as an antagonist at adrenergic, cholinergic, histaminergic, and serotonergic receptors. Increases the amount of time spent in REM sleep. Causes a high incidence of sedation, anticholinergic effects, orthostatic hypotension, and weight gain. It does not cause extrapyramidal symptoms.

Pharmacokinetics

Is 27–47% bioavailable; food does not affect the bioavailability of clozapine. **Peak plasma levels:** 2.5 hr. **Mean C_{max} at steady state:** 319 ng/mL. **t½:** 12 hr at steady state. Metabolized in the liver to inactive compounds by CYP1A2, 2D6, and 3A4. Excreted through the urine (50%) and feces (30%). **Plasma protein binding:** About 97%.

CONTRAINDICATIONS

Hypersensitivity to the drug or any component of the product. Myeloproliferative disorders. Uncontrolled epilepsy. Use in those with a history of clozapine-induced agranulocytosis or severe granulocytopenia; use with other agents known to suppress bone marrow function. Use with other agents having a known potential to cause agranulocytosis or otherwise suppress bone marrow function. Severe CNS depression or coma due to any cause, including use of CNS depressants. Due to the possibility of development of agranulocytosis and seizures, avoid continued use in clients failing to respond. Lactation.

SPECIAL CONCERNS

(1) **Agranulocytosis**. Because of a significant risk of agranulocytosis, a potentially life-threatening adverse reaction, reserve clozapine for use in (a) the treatment of severely ill clients with schizophrenia who fail to show an acceptable response to adequate courses of standard antipsychotic drug treatment or

(b) for reducing the risk of recurrent suicidal behavior in clients with schizophrenia or schizoaffective disorder who are judged to be at risk of re-experiencing suicidal behavior. (2) Clients being treated with clozapine must have a baseline white blood cell (WBC) and differential count before initiation of treatment, as well as regular WBC counts during treatment and for at least 4 weeks after discontinuation of treatment. (3) Clozapine is available only through a distribution system that ensures monitoring of WBC counts according to the following schedule prior to delivery of the next supply of medication. (4) **Seizures.** Seizures have been associated with the use of clozapine. Dose appears to be an important predictor of seizure, with a greater likelihood at higher clozapine doses. Use caution when administering clozapine to clients who have a history of seizures or other predisposing factors. Advise clients not to engage in any activity in which sudden loss of consciousness could cause serious risk to themselves or others. (5) **Myocarditis**. Analysis of postmarketing safety databases suggest that clozapine is associated with an increased risk of fatal myocarditis, especially during, but not limited to, the first month of therapy. In clients in whom myocarditis is suspected, discontinue clozapine treatment promptly. (6) **Orthostatic hypotension**, with or without syncope, can occur with clozapine treatment. Rarely, collapse can be profound and be accompanied by respiratory and/or cardiac arrest. Orthostatic hypotension is more likely to occur during initial titration in association with rapid dose escalation. In clients who have had even a brief interval off clozapine (2 or more days since the last dose), start treatment with 12.5 mg once or twice daily. (7) Because collapse, respiratory arrest, and cardiac arrest during initial treatment have occurred in clients who were being administered benzodiazepines or other psychotropic drugs, caution is advised when clozapine is initiated in clients taking a benzodiazepine or any other psychotropic drug. (8) Elderly clients with dementia-related psychosis treated with atypical antipsychotic drugs are at an increased risk of death compared with placebo. Analyses revealed a risk of death in the drug-treated clients of between 1.6 and 1.7 times that seen in placebo-treated clients. Over the course of a typical 10-week controlled trial, the rate of death in drug-treated clients was about 4.5% compared with a rate of about 2.6% in the placebo group. Although the causes of death were varied, most of the deaths appeared to be either cardiovascular (e.g., heart failure, sudden death) or infectious (e.g., pneumonia) in nature. (9) Clozapine is not approved for the treatment of clients with dementia-related psychosis. ■

- **Use with caution in clients with known CV disease, prostatic hypertrophy, narrow-angle glaucoma, hepatic or renal disease.**
- **Increased incidence of cardiomyopathy.**
- **Increased mortality in the elderly with dementia-related psychosis.**
- **Safety and efficacy not determined in children.**

SIDE EFFECTS

Most Common

Drowsiness, sedation/somnolence, dizziness, vertigo, tachycardia, headache, tremor, syncope, salivation, constipation, dyspepsia, hypotension.

CNS: Drowsiness, sedation/somnolence, dizziness, vertigo, headache, syncope, tremor, hypokinesia, restlessness, agitation, akathisia, akinesia, confusion, ***convulsions***, insomnia, anxiety, ataxia, depression, hyperkinesia, lethargy, slurred speech, weakness, pseudoparkinsonism, amnesia, delirium, abnormal/bizarre/increased dreams, dysarthria, hallucinations, increased/decreased/loss of libido, psychosis, aphasia, altered EEG tracings, delusions, amentia, mild catalepsy, poor coordination, epileptiform movements, histrionic/involuntary movements, irritability, impaired memory, shakiness, stuttering, tics, nightmares, sleep disturbance, ***status epilepticus, suicide***. **GI:** Salivation, constipation, dyspepsia, dry mouth, N&V, gastroesophageal reflux, abdominal discomfort/pain, weight gain/loss, diarrhea, anorexia, increased appetite, dysphagia, eructation, fecal impaction, gastroenteritis, hematemesis, intestinal obstruction, rectal hemorrhage, paralytic ileus, GI distress, bitter taste, gastric ulcer, abnormal stools, dry throat, throat pain/discomfort, numb/sore tongue, ***acute pancreatitis***. **Hepatic:** Impaired liver function, cholelithiasis, hepatitis, jaundice, cholestasis. **CV:** Tachycardia, hypotension with or without syncope, hypertension, ECG changes, angina pectoris, ***myocarditis***, ***cardiomyopathy***, premature atrial contractions, atrial fibrillation/flutter, bradycardia, CHF, ***MI***, phlebitis, ***pulmonary embolus***, T-wave flattening/inversion, thrombophlebitis (including deep), twitch, arrhythmias, DVT, ST-depression, ischemic changes, pericardial effusions, pericarditis, petechiae, PVCs, vasculitis, cardiac abnormality, ***ventricular fibrillation***. **Hematologic:** Leukopenia, ***agranulocytosis***, eosinophilia, anemia, leukocytosis, thrombocythemia, thrombocytopenia, increased erythrocyte sed rate, granulocytopenia, neutropenia. **Dermatologic:** Rash, dermatitis, diaphoresis, ecchymosis, eczema, erythema, photosensitivity, urticaria, erythema multiforme, hot flashes, ***Stevens-Johnson syndrome***. **GU:** Ejaculation disorders, urinary frequency, increased urinary urgency, urinary retention, dysmenorrhea, priapism, impotence, mastalgia, acute interstitial nephritis, vaginal infection/itch, urinary abnormalities, incontinence. **Respiratory:** Dyspnea, nasal congestion, aspiration, increased cough, epistaxis, hyperventilation, pneumonia, bronchopneumonia, bronchitis, laryngitis, pleural effusion, pneumonia-like symptoms, rhinorrhea, sneezing, wheezing, ***pulmonary embolism***. **Musculoskeletal:** Rigidity, arthralgia/joint/leg pain, muscle weakness, muscle rigidity, myalgia, myoclonus, back/chest pain, neck pain/rigidity, rhabdomyolysis. **Neuroleptic malignant syndrome: *Hyperpyrexia***, muscle rigidity, altered mental status, irregular pulse or BP, tachycardia, diaphoresis, cardiac dysrhythmias. **Metabolic:** Hyperglycemia, diabetes mellitus. **Ophthalmic:** Visual disturbances, conjunctivitis, glaucoma, periorbital edema, eyelid disorder, bloodshot eyes. **Otic:** Ear disorder. **Body as a whole:** Fatigue, chills, fever, allergic/hypersensitivity reaction, cyanosis, edema, transient temperature elevations, hypothermia, numbness, ***sepsis, sudden death***. **Miscellaneous:** Parotid swelling.

LABORATORY TEST CONSIDERATIONS

↑ CPK, hematocrit, hemoglobin. ↓ WBCs. Hyperglycemia, hyperprolactinemia, hyperuricemia, hyponatremia.

OVERDOSE MANAGEMENT

Symptoms: Drowsiness, delirium, tachycardia, ***respiratory depression***, hypotension, hypersalivation, ***seizures, coma***. *Treatment:* Establish airway; maintain with adequate oxygenation and ventilation. Give activated charcoal and sorbitol. Monitor cardiac status and VS. General supportive measures.

DRUG INTERACTIONS

NOTE: Use contraindicated with drugs having a well-known potential to cause agranulocytosis or suppress bone marrow function.

Anticholinergic drugs / Additive anticholinergic effects

Antihypertensive drugs / Additive hypotensive effects

Benzodiazepines / Possible orthostatic hypotension, collapse, respiratory arrest, and cardiac arrest possible with certain benzodiazepines; use together with caution

Caffeine / ↑ Caffeine plasma levels → ↑ side effects; avoid caffeine if an interaction is noted

Citalopram / ↑ Clozapine plasma levels → ↑ pharmacologic/toxic effects; adjust dose as needed

CYP1A2 inducers (e.g., carbamazepine, omeprazole, rifampin) / May ↓ clozapine serum levels

CYP 1A2 inhibitors (e.g., fluvoxamine) / May ↑ clozapine plasma levels; dose reduction may be needed

CYP3A4 inhibitors (e.g., ketoconazole) / Possible ↑ clozapine plasma levels

Digoxin / ↑ Digoxin effect R/T ↓ plasma protein binding

Epinephrine / Clozapine may reverse effects when given for hypotension

Fluoxetine / ↑ Clozapine plasma levels → ↑ pharmacologic/toxic effects; adjust dose as needed

Fluvoxamine / ↑ Clozapine plasma levels → ↑ pharmacologic/toxic effects; adjust dose as needed

Phenobarbital / ↓ Clozapine levels R/T ↑ liver breakdown

Risperidone / Chronic use together may ↓ risperidone clearance; also, ↑ pharmacologic/toxic effects of clozapine; adjust dose as needed

Ritonavir / ↑ Clozapine serum levels → ↑ pharmacologic/toxic effects

Sertraline / ↑ Clozapine plasma levels → ↑ pharmacologic/toxic effects; adjust dose as needed

Smoking / ↓ Clozapine levels R/T ↑ hepatic metabolism by CYP1A2

H ***St. John's wort*** / Possible ↓ clozapine levels R/T ↑ metabolism

Warfarin / ↑ Warfarin effect R/T ↓ plasma protein binding

HOW SUPPLIED

Tablets: 12.5 mg, 25 mg, 50 mg, 100 mg, 200 mg; ***Tablets, Oral Disintegrating:*** 12.5 mg, 25 mg, 100 mg, 150 mg, 200 mg.

C

DOSAGE

TABLETS; TABLETS, ORAL DISINTEGRATING

Treatment-resistant schizophrenia.

Adults, initial: 12.5 mg 1–2 times per day; **then,** if drug tolerated, the dose can be increased by 25–50 mg/day to a dose of 300–450 mg/day at the end of 2 weeks. Subsequent dosage increments should occur no more often than once or twice a week in increments not to exceed 100 mg. **Usual maintenance dose:** 300–600 mg/day (although doses up to 900 mg/day may be required in some clients). Total daily dose should not exceed 900 mg due to a risk of agranulocytosis and seizures. Continue responding clients on the lowest level needed to maintain remission. If treatment must be discontinued, a gradual reduction in dose over a 1–2 week period is recommended. If abrupt discontinuation is required (i.e., leukopenia), carefully observe the client for recurrence of psychotic symptoms and symptoms related to cholinergic rebound (i.e., headache, N&V, diarrhea). *NOTE:* Consult manufacturer's clozapine guidelines based on WBC and ANC for treatment alterations, including reinitiation of treatment.

Recurrent suicidal behavior.

Follow the dosage and administration recommendations for schizophrenia. **Mean daily dose:** 300 mg; **range:** 12.5–900 mg. A course of treatment for at least 2 years is recommended in order to maintain the reduction of risk for suicidal behavior. After 2 years, reassess risk of suicidal behavior.

NURSING IMPLICATIONS

Do not confuse Clozaril with Clinoril (a NSAID).

IMPLEMENTATION/ADMINISTRATION/STORAGE

1. Clozapine is available through independent "Clozaril treatment systems" based on a plan developed by physicians and pharmacists to ensure safe use of the drug with respect to weekly CBC monitoring, data reporting, and drug dispensing. Prescriptions are limited to 1-week supplies, and drug may only be dispensed following receipt, by the pharmacist, of weekly WBC test results that fall within the established limits. All weekly blood test results must be reported by participating pharmacists to the Clozaril National Registry (1-800-448-5938).
2. If drug is effective, seek lowest maintenance doses possible to maintain remission.
3. If termination of therapy is planned, gradually reduce dose over a 1–2 week period. If cessation of therapy is abrupt due to toxicity, observe client carefully for recurrence of psychotic symptoms.
4. Clozapine therapy may be initiated immediately upon discontinuation of other antipsychotic medication; however, a 24 hr "washout period" is desirable.
5. When restarting clients who have had even a brief interval off of clozapine (i.e., 2 days or more since the last dose), treatment should be reinitiated with 12.5 mg once or twice daily. If this dose is well tolerated, it may be possible to titrate clients back to a therapeutic dose more quickly than is recommended for initial treatment. However, any client who has previously experienced respiratory or cardiac arrest with initial dosing, but was then able to be titrated successfully to a therapeutic dose should be retitrated with extreme caution, even after 24 hr of discontinuation.
6. Clients discontinued for WBC counts below 2,000/mm^3 or an ANC below 1,000/mm^3 must not be restarted on clozapine.
7. Store orally disintegrating tablets, protected from moisture, from 15–30°C (59–86°F). Store tablets below 30°C (86°F).

ASSESSMENT

1. List reasons for therapy; assess behavioral manifestations. Identify other therapies trialed and outcome; due to adverse side effects should only be used in those who have failed to respond adequately to other treatment regimens.

2. Note seizure disorder, enlarged prostate, C or glaucoma.
3. Check baseline VS and ECG; report any irregular pulse, tachycardia, hyperpyrexia, or hypotension. Monitor S&S closely; may cause myocarditis/cardiomyopathy.
4. Follow manufacturer's guidelines for clients reinitiated on clozapine starting at lower dose. Ensure adequate time to respond to a dose before increasing to higher dose.
5. Monitor for S&S of hyperglycemia and diabetes mellitus; may aggravate control.
6. Assess risks vs benefits of therapy with family/client. Periodically reassess to determine continued need for therapy.
7. Monitor BS, CBC, and LFTs. Monitor and report WBCs once weekly for the first 6 months of therapy, then every 2 weeks if stable.
8. Only available through a distribution system that ensures monitoring and uses the following therapy guidelines based on WBC and ANC:
   - Do not begin treatment if WBC is <3,500/mm^3 or there is a history of myeloproliferative disorder or previous clozapine-induced agranulocytosis or granulocytopenia.
   - If WBC is <3,500/mm^3 or >3,500/mm^3 with a substantial drop from baseline, or presence of immature forms following initiation of treatment, repeat WBC and differential counts. S&S of infection include lethargy, weakness, fever, and sore throat.
   - If WBC is 3,000/mm^3 to 3,500/mm^3 on subsequent counts and ANC is >1,500/mm^3, perform twice weekly WBC and differential counts.
   - If WBC is <3,000/mm^3 or ANC is <1,500/mm^3, interrupt therapy and monitor for flu-like symptoms or orther symptoms of infection. Perform WBC count and differential daily. May resume therapy if no signs of infection develop, WBC count is >3,000/mm^3 and ANC is >1,500/mm^3. However, continue twice weekly WBC and differential counts until WBC returns to >3,500/mm^3 and then monitor WBC weekly for 6 months.
   - If WBC is <2,000/mm^3 or ANC is <1,000/mm^3, monitor WBC count and differential daily. Consider bone marrow aspiration to determine granulopoetic status. If granulopoiesis is deficient, consider protective isolation. If infection develops, perform cultures and begin antibiotics. Do not rechallenge with clozapine because agranulocytosis may develop with a shorter latency.

CLIENT/FAMILY TEACHING

1. Dru… script… only be provided in 1 or 2 week … Ensure r…d on lab results and monitoring. … rupted the… …ments met to provide uninter-
2. Do not push o… disintegrating tablet through foil. Just …r to use, peel foil from the blister and gen… …emove orally disintegrating tablet. Immediately place tablet in mouth, allow to disintegra… …nd swallow with saliva. No water is needed. De…oy half tablets. Contains phenylalanine.
3. Take as directed; do not stop abruptly. Used only when conventional therapies fail due to risk of adverse side effects.
4. Report symptoms of lethargy, weakness, chest pain, involuntary body or facial movements, fever, sore throat, malaise, mucous membrane ulceration, S&S of infection, or other adverse effects. Also any muscle rigidity, pounding in the chest, rapid or difficult breathing, rapid or irregular heartbeat, unexplained shortness of breath, unquenchable thirst, or weight gain should be reported to health care provider.
5. Rinse mouth frequently; perform regular oral care to minimize potential for candidiasis. With diabetes monitor FS frequently and report loss of blood sugar control.
6. Use caution and avoid driving or other hazardous activity due to possibility of seizures and drowsiness.
7. Because of (orthostatic) drop in BP, use care when rising from a lying or sitting position. Avoid hot showers or baths, strenuous exercise in hot/humid weather.
8. Report if pregnancy occurs or client desires to become pregnant. Do not breast-feed.
9. Avoid other prescription drugs (sedatives), OTC drugs, or alcohol.
10. Report any changes in mental status, mood, or personality.
11. Stress importance of weekly WBC to assess for agranulocytosis. These are reported to a national registry (Clozaril Patient Management System at 1-800-448-5938) and must be

completed before prescriptions will be iss and filled.

12. Keep all F/U to assess response, lab adverse SE.

OUTCOMES/EVALUATE

- Improved behavior patterns with ↓ agitation, ↓ hyperactivity, ↓ delusions, and hallucinations
- Improved coping behaviors, thought patterns

Codeine phosphate

(**KOH**-deen)

Classification(s): Narcotic analgesic, **C-II**

Pregnancy Category: C

Codeine sulfate

Classification(s): Narcotic analgesic, **C-II**

Pregnancy Category: C

SEE ALSO ***NARCOTIC ANALGESICS.***

INDICATIONS/USES

(1) Relief of mild to moderate pain. (2) In combination with aspirin or acetaminophen to enhance analgesia. (3) Antitussive, often in combination with other respiratory drugs to treat cough.

ACTION/KINETICS

Action

Produces less respiratory depression and N&V than morphine. Moderately habit-forming and constipating. Dosages over 60 mg often cause restlessness and excitement and irritate the cough center. In lower doses it is a potent antitussive and is an ingredient in many cough syrups.

Pharmacokinetics

Onset, PO: 10–30 min. **Peak effect:** 30–60 min. **Duration, PO:** 4–6 hr. **t½, elimination:** 2.5–3 hr. Metabolized in the liver and excreted in the urine. Codeine is two-thirds as effective PO as parenterally. Codeine phosphate may be given as an oral solution or by injection.

CONTRAINDICATIONS

Premature infants or during labor when delivery of a premature infant is expected.

SPECIAL CONCERNS

- Use with caution and reduce the initial dose in clients with seizure disorders, acute abdominal conditions, renal or hepatic disease, fever, Addison's disease, hypothyroidism, prostatic hypertrophy, ulcerative colitis, urethral stricture, following recent GI or GU tract surgery, and in the young, geriatric, or debilitated clients.
- May increase the duration of labor.
- Nursing mothers who are ultrarapid metabolizers of codeine may have abnormally high levels of morphine in their breast milk that can cause serious, even fatal, side effects (increased tiredness, difficulty breathing, limpness, difficulty breast-feeding) in nursing infants.
- Administer to infants and small children only with great caution and in carefully monitored dosage. Safety and efficacy not established in newborns.

SIDE EFFECTS

Most Common

Orthostatic hypotension, tachycardia, anxiety, dizziness, lethargy, mood changes, sedation, sweating, biliary tract spasm, constipation, dry mouth, N&V, urinary hesitancy/retention, skin rash, miosis, visual disturbances.

See *Narcotic Analgesics*, for a complete list of possible side effects.

ADDITIONAL DRUG INTERACTIONS

Combination with chlordiazepoxide may induce coma.

HOW SUPPLIED

Codeine phosphate. ***Injection:*** 15 mg/mL, 30 mg/mL; ***Oral Solution:*** 15 mg/5 mL. **Codeine sulfate.** ***Tablets:*** 15 mg, 30 mg, 60 mg.

DOSAGE

Codeine Phosphate/Sulfate

ORAL SOLUTION; TABLETS

Analgesia.

Adults: 15–60 mg q 4–6 hr, not to exceed 360 mg/day. **Pediatric, over 1 year:** 0.5 mg/kg or 15 mg/m^2 q 4–6 hr, up to a maximum of 60 mg/dose.

Antitussive.

Adults: 10–20 mg q 4–6 hr, not to exceed 120 mg/day. **Pediatric, 2–6 years:**

2.5–5 mg q 4–6 hr, not to exceed 30 mg/day; **6–12 years:** 5–10 mg q 4–6 hr, not to exceed 60 mg/day.

IM, SC

Analgesic.

Adults: 30 mg SC or IM q 4 hr as needed. **Usual dose range:** 15–60 mg. **Children:** 500 micrograms/kg or 15 mg/m^2 SC or IM q 4 hr as needed.

NURSING IMPLICATIONS

IMPLEMENTATION/ADMINISTRATION/STORAGE

1. Adjust the dose depending on the severity of the pain and client response. Occasionally, it may be necessary to exceed the usual recommended dosage in cases of more severe pain or in those clients who have become more tolerant to the analgesic effect of narcotics.
2. Codeine is incompatible with soluble barbiturates.
3. Store oral solution and tablets from 15–30°C (59–86°F); protect from moisture. Store injection below 40°C (104°F); protect from light and freezing.

ASSESSMENT

1. List reasons for therapy, onset, location, characteristics of S&S, other agents trialed, outcome.
2. Assess for conditions that may warrant lowered dose or cautious use. With pain, rate pain level. With cough document lung sounds and cough characteristics. Identify name, dose, form, and route prescribed. With prolonged use may experience dependence/tolerance.
3. Monitor renal and LFTs; reduce dose with dysfunction.

CLIENT/FAMILY TEACHING

1. Take as directed; acetaminophen and aspirin act synergistically with codeine and are usually given together. May take with food or milk to decrease GI upset.
2. Increase intake of fluids, fruits, and fiber to decrease constipation.
3. Avoid activities that require mental alertness; may cause dizziness/drowsiness. Report altered mental patterns.
4. If taking codeine syrups to suppress coughs, do not overuse. If productive coughing is suppressed, may cause additional congestion.
5. May be habit forming. Avoid sudden position changes to prevent sudden drop in BP.
6. Avoid alcohol/CNS depressants. May cause coma if taken with chlordiazepoxide-derivatives.
7. Keep all F/U to assess response and for adverse SE.

OUTCOMES/EVALUATE

- Relief of pain
- Control of coughing with improved sleeping patterns

Colchicine

(**KOHL**-chih-seen)

Classification(s): Antigout drug

Pregnancy Category: C

RX: Colchicine Tablets, Colcrys.

INDICATIONS/USES

(1) Prophylaxis and treatment of acute attacks of gout. Often effective in aborting an attack when taken at the first sign of symptoms. (2) Treatment of familial Mediterranean fever in adults and children 4 years and older (Colcrys only). *Investigational:* Adjunct in the treatment of primary amyloidosis; Behçet's syndrome; primary biliary or hepatic cirrhosis; pericarditis in adults/children/adolescents; scleroderma; Sweet syndrome; sarcoid arthritis; acute inflammatory calcific tendonitis; arthritis associated with erythema nodosum; leukemia; adenocarcinoma of the GI tract; mycosis fungoides; intraurethral condyloma acuminata in men (topically).

ACTION/KINETICS

Action

May reduce the crystal-induced inflammation by reducing lactic acid production by leukocytes (resulting in a decreased deposition of sodium urate), by inhibiting leukocyte migration, and by reducing phagocytosis. May also inhibit the synthesis of kinins and leukotrienes. Although pain is reduced, colchicine is not an analgesic or a uricosuric.

Pharmacokinetics

Rapidly absorbed after PO use. **Onset, PO:** 12 hr. **Time to peak levels, PO:** 0.5–2 hr. **t½, plasma:** About 20 min; **t½, leukocytes:** 60 hr. High levels found in the liver, kidney, and spleen. Metabolized in the liver and mainly excreted in the feces with 10–20% excreted unchanged through the urine.

C

CONTRAINDICATIONS

Hypersensitivity to colchicine. Blood dyscrasias. Serious GI, hepatic, cardiac, or renal disorders. Use with P-glycoprotein or strong CYP3A4 inhibitors (includes all protease inhibitors, except fosamprenavir) in those with renal or hepatic impairment (Colcrys only). Use in presence of combined renal and hepatic disease.

SPECIAL CONCERNS

- **Use with caution during pregnancy and lactation.**
- **Has been approved to treat Mediterranean fever in children 4 years and older; safety and efficacy not determined in children to treat gout (which is rare in children).**
- **Life-threatening and fatal drug interactions reported in those treated with colchicine with P-gp and CYP3A4 inhibitors.**
- **Geriatric clients may be at greater risk of developing cumulative toxicity.**
- **Use with extreme caution for elderly, debilitated clients, especially in the presence of chronic renal, hepatic, GI, or CV disease.**
- **May impair fertility.**
- **Fatal overdoses, both accidental and intentional, have occurred in both adults and children.**

SIDE EFFECTS

Most Common

N&V, diarrhea (may be severe), pharyngolaryngeal pain, abdominal pain/cramps, dermatoses.

The drug is toxic; thus clients must be carefully monitored. **GI:** N&V, diarrhea, abdominal cramps/pain/discomfort, lactose intolerance, liver dysfunction. **CNS:** Neuropathy, headache, sensory motor neuropathy. **CV:** Disseminated intravascular coagulation, thrombophlebitis at injection site (rare). **Hematologic:** Bone marrow depression, ***aplastic anemia***, ***agranulocytosis***, leukopenia, granulocytopenia, pancytopenia, thrombocytopenia. **Respiratory:** Pharyngolaryngeal pain, respiratory thoracic mediastinal disorders. **Musculoskeletal:** Myopathy, rhabdomyolysis, muscle pain/weakness, myotonia. **Dermatologic:** Purpura, alopecia, dermatoses, rash (including maculopapular). **GU:** Azoospermia (reversible), oligospermia. **Body as a whole:** Hypersensitivity reactions, fatigue. **Miscellaneous:** Peripheral neuritis; injury to cells in the renal, hepatic, circulatory, and central nervous systems. *NOTE:* If such symptoms appear, discontinue drug at once and wait at least 48 hr before reinstating drug therapy.

LABORATORY TEST CONSIDERATIONS

Alters liver function tests. ↑ Alkaline phosphatase, ALT, AST. ↓ Thrombocyte values. False + for hemoglobin or RBCs in urine.

OVERDOSE MANAGEMENT

Symptoms: **Acute Intoxication:** Onset usually delayed for several hr or more after ingestion of an acute overdose. N&V, abdominal pain, and diarrhea occur first. Diarrhea may be bloody due to hemorrhagic gastroenteritis. Burning sensation of the throat, stomach, and skin may occur. Extensive vascular damage may result in shock. Hematuria and oliguria may indicate kidney damage. May be marked muscular weakness and ascending paralysis of the CNS. Client usually remains conscious. Delirium and convulsions may occur. ***Death*** due to respiratory arrest may result. *NOTE:* Death may occur with low doses but others survive after having taken much higher doses. *Treatment:* **Acute Intoxication:** Begin with gastric lavage and measures to prevent shock. Hemodialysis and peritoneal dialysis are helpful. Provide symptomatic support, including atropine and morphine for relief of abdominal pain and artificial respiration with oxygen to combat respiratory distress. There is no known antidote.

DRUG INTERACTIONS

Acidifying agents / Inhibit colchicine action; avoid coadministration

Alkalinizing agents / Potentiate colchicine action; avoid coadministration

Aprepitant / ↑ Colchicine plasma levels R/T inhibition of CYP3A4 metabolism → ↑ risk of myopathy; use together with caution

Atazanavir / ↑ Colchicine plasma levels R/T inhibition of CYP3A4 metabolism → ↑ risk of life-threatening/fatal drug interactions; use together contraindicated in those with renal/hepatic impairment

Clarithromycin / ↑ Colchicine plasma levels R/T inhibition of CYP3A4 metabolism → ↑ risk of life-threatening/fatal drug interactions; use together contraindicated in those with renal/hepatic impairment
CNS depressants / Clients may be more sensitive to CNS depressant effects; monitor and adjust depressant dose as needed
Cyclosporine / ↑ Risk of myopathy or rhabdomyolysis; monitor; also possible life-threatening and fatal drug interaction R/T inhibition of colchicine metabolism by P-glycoprotein; use together is contraindicated in those with renal/hepatic impairment
Digoxin / ↑ Risk of myopathy or rhabdomyolysis; if coadministration cannot be avoided, monitor for unexplained muscle weakness/pain/tenderness
Diltiazem / ↑ Colchicine plasma levels R/T inhibition of CYP3A4 metabolism → ↑ risk of myopathy; use together with caution
Erythromycin / ↑ Colchicine plasma levels R/T inhibition of CYP3A4 metabolism → ↑ risk of myopathy; use together with caution
Fibric acids (e.g., fenofibrate, gemfibrozil) / ↑ Risk of myopathy or rhabdomyolysis; if coadministration cannot be avoided, monitor for unexplained muscle weakness/pain/tenderness
Fluconazole / ↑ Colchicine plasma levels R/T inhibition of CYP3A4 metabolism → ↑ risk of myopathy; use together with caution
Fosamprenavir / ↑ Colchicine plasma levels R/T inhibition of CYP3A4 metabolism → ↑ risk of myopathy; use together with caution
HMG Co-A reductase inhibitors (e.g., atorvastatin, fluvastatin, pravastatin, simvastatin) / ↑ Risk of myopathy or rhabdomyolysis; if coadministration cannot be avoided, monitor for unexplained muscle weakness/pain/tenderness
Indinavir / ↑ Colchicine plasma levels R/T inhibition of CYP3A4 metabolism → ↑ risk of life-threatening/fatal drug interactions; use together contraindicated in those with renal/hepatic impairment
Itraconazole / ↑ Colchicine plasma levels R/T inhibition of CYP3A4 metabolism → ↑ risk of life-threatening/fatal drug interactions; use together contraindicated in those with renal/hepatic impairment
Ketoconazole / ↑ Colchicine plasma levels R/T inhibition of CYP3A4 metabolism → ↑ risk of life-threatening/fatal drug interactions; use together contraindicated in those with renal/hepatic impairment
Macrolide antibiotics / Severe colchicine toxicity (sometimes leading to death) R/T inhibition of metabolism by CYP3A4
Nefazodone / ↑ Colchicine plasma levels R/T inhibition of CYP3A4 metabolism → ↑ risk of life-threatening/fatal drug interactions; use together contraindicated in those with renal/hepatic impairment
Nelfinavir / ↑ Colchicine plasma levels R/T inhibition of CYP3A4 metabolism → ↑ risk of life-threatening/fatal drug interactions; use together contraindicated in those with renal/hepatic impairment
Ranolazine / Possible life-threatening and fatal drug interaction R/T inhibition of colchicine metabolism by P-glycoprotein; use together is contraindicated in those with renal/hepatic impairment
Ritonavir / ↑ Colchicine plasma levels R/T inhibition of CYP3A4 metabolism → ↑ risk of life-threatening/fatal drug interactions; use together contraindicated in those with renal/hepatic impairment
Saquinavir / ↑ Colchicine plasma levels R/T inhibition of CYP3A4 metabolism → ↑ risk of life-threatening/fatal drug interactions; use together contraindicated in those with renal/hepatic impairment
Sympathomimetic agents / Enhanced by colchicine; monitor and adjust sympathomimetic dose as needed
Telithromycin / ↑ Colchicine plasma levels R/T inhibition of CYP3A4 metabolism → ↑ risk of life-threatening/fatal drug interactions; use together contraindicated in those with renal/hepatic impairment
Verapamil / ↑ Colchicine plasma levels R/T inhibition of CYP3A4 metabolism → ↑ risk of myopathy; use together with caution
Vitamin B_{12} / Colchicine may interfere with gut absorption
Voriconazole / ↑ Colchicine plasma levels R/T inhibition of CYP3A4 metabolism → ↑ risk of life-threatening/fatal drug interactions; use together contraindicated in those with renal/hepatic impairment

HOW SUPPLIED

Tablets: 0.6 mg.

DOSAGE

Colchicine (generic)

TABLETS

Prophylaxis of gout flares.

Adults, usual: 0.6 mg once or twice a day. **Less than 1 attack/year:** 0.6 mg/day for 3 or 4 days a week. **More than 1 attack/year:** 0.6 mg daily; severe cases may require 2–3 0.6 mg tablets/day. **Surgical clients:** 0.6 mg 3 times/day for 3 days before and 3 days after surgery.

Treatment of gout flares.

Adults, usual, initial: 1.2 mg at the first sign of an attack, followed by 0.6 mg 1 hr later. **Maximum dose:** 1.8 mg over a 1 hr period. **Alternative dose: Initial,** 0.6–1.2 mg at the first sign of a flare, followed by 0.6 mg q hr or 1.2 mg q 2 hr until pain is relieved or until diarrhea occurs. After the initial dose, it may be sufficient to take 0.6 mg q 2–3 hr. **Total amount usually required:** 4–8 mg. Articular pain and swelling usually relieved within 12 hr and usually gone in 24–48 hr. *NOTE:* If also taking colchicine for prophylaxis of gout flares, wait 12 hr after taking the last dose for treatment of the flare; then, resume the prophylaxis dose.

Behçet's syndrome (investigational).

Adults: 1–2 mg/day in divided doses (e.g., 0.5 or 0.6 mg 3 times/day) used as primary or adjunctive therapy. Treatment is for a prolonged period.

Pericarditis in adults and children (investigational).

Acute pericarditis, adults, initial: Loading dose from 1–2 mg/day; **maintenance:** 0.5–1 mg/day for at least 3 months. **Recurrent pericarditis, adults, initial:** Loading dose from 1–3 mg/day; **maintenance:** 0.5–2 mg/day for at least 6 months. **Pericarditis, adolescents/children, initial:** Loading dose from 0.5–1.5 mg/day; **maintenance:** 0.25–2 mg/day up to several months.

Colcrys only.

TABLETS

Familial Mediterranean fever.

Adults and children, 13 years and older, usual: 1.2–2.4 mg/day in 1 or 2 divided doses. Increase dose as needed in increments of 0.3 mg/day to a maximum recommended daily dose to control the disease and as tolerated. If intolerable side effects occur decrease the dose in increments of 0.3 mg. **Children, 6–12 years or age:** 0.9–1.8 mg/day in 1 or 2 divided doses; **4–6 years of age:** 0.3–1.8 mg/day in 1 or 2 divided doses. If needed, increase in increments of 0.3 mg/day to a maximum daily dose to control disease and as tolerated. If intolerable side effects occur, decrease the dose in increments of 0.3 mg/day.

NURSING IMPLICATIONS

IMPLEMENTATION/ADMINISTRATION/STORAGE

1. If ACTH is given to treat an attack of gouty arthritis, give colchicine in doses of at least 1 mg/day; continue colchicine for a few days after ACTH is withdrawn.
2. An interval of 3 days between colchicine courses is recommended to minimize cumulative toxicity.
3. Treatment of gout flares with prophylactic colchicine is not recommended for those with mild to severe (C_{CR} <30–80 mL/min) renal impairment.
4. The dose may need to be reduced or interrupted in those with normal renal and hepatic function if treatment with a P-gp or CYP3A4 inhibitor is required.
5. Dosage adjustment may be necessary when treating clients for familial Mediterranean fever and who have mild to severe renal impairment. For those with severe renal impairment, start with 0.3 mg/day of colchicine; monitor before increasing dose.
6. In geriatric clients, base dosing on renal function.
7. Store below 30°C (86°F).

ASSESSMENT

1. List symptom onset and characteristics; any other attacks, frequency, and any preventive therapy prescribed.
2. Note age and general physical condition.
3. Identify joint involvement, noting pain, swelling, and degree of mobility; may need to aspirate joint for definitive diagnosis.
4. Monitor CBC, joint x-ray, uric acid levels, B_{12}, renal and LFTs.

CLIENT/FAMILY TEACHING

1. Drug seems to alter body's response to deposited uric acid crystals. This leads to less swelling and less pain. Take as prescribed; at the first sign of joint pain or other symptom of impending gout attack. The maximum dose is 10 tablets or 4–8 mg in 24 hr; do not exceed. It usually takes 12–48 hr for relief of symptoms; wait 3 days before starting second course to prevent cumulative toxicity.
2. Stop drug and report if N&V, or diarrhea develops; these are signs of toxicity. With severe diarrhea, medication (paregoric) may be needed.
3. Acute episodes may be precipitated by aspirin, alcohol, or foods high in purine; avoid.
4. Report evidence of liver dysfunction (yellow discoloration of eyes, skin, or stool).
5. Females should avoid pregnancy.
6. Drug will not prevent the progression of this disease; it only controls symptoms when taken regularly.
7. Consume 3–3.5 L/day of fluids to enhance crystal excretion.
8. NSAIDs may help with pain and inflammation; use as prescribed. Report any unusual bruising/bleeding, weakness, numbness or tingling, fatigue, rash, sore throat, or fever; bone marrow depression may occur.
9. Keep all F/U to assess response, labs, and for adverse SE.

OUTCOMES/EVALUATE

- ↓ Joint pain/swelling/destruction
- Termination of acute gout attacks
- Relief of pain

Colestipol hydrochloride

(koh-**LESS**-tih-poll)

Classification(s): Antihyperlipidemic, bile acid sequestrant

Pregnancy Category: B

RX: Colestid.

INDICATIONS/USES

As adjunctive therapy to diet to reduce elevated serum total and LDL cholesterol in those with primary hypercholesterolemia (elevated LDL, cholesterol) who do not respond adequately to diet. *Investigational:* Digitalis toxicity; hyperoxaluria; diarrhea due to bile acids; adjunctive treatment for hyperthyroidism; relief of pruritus associated with partial biliary obstruction (including primary biliary cirrhosis and various other forms of bile stasis); binds to the toxin produced by *Clostridium difficile*.

ACTION/KINETICS

Action

An anion exchange resin that binds bile acids in the intestine, forming an insoluble complex excreted in the feces. The loss of bile acids results in increased oxidation of cholesterol to bile acids and a decrease in LDL and serum cholesterol. Does not affect (or may increase) triglycerides or HDL and may increase VLDL.

Pharmacokinetics

Not absorbed from the GI tract. **Onset:** 1–2 days; **maximum effect:** 1 month. Return to pretreatment cholesterol levels after discontinuance of therapy: 1 month.

CONTRAINDICATIONS

Complete obstruction or atresia of bile duct.

SPECIAL CONCERNS

- Children may be more likely to develop hyperchloremic acidosis although dosage has not been established.
- Use during pregnancy only if benefits outweigh risks.
- Clients over 60 years may be at greater risk of GI side effects and adverse nutritional effects.
- Use with caution during lactation and in children.

C

SIDE EFFECTS

Most Common

Constipation (may be severe), N&V, anorexia, flatulence, abdominal distention/cramping, bloating, heartburn, anorexia, headache, dizziness, drowsiness, sour taste in mouth.

GI: Constipation (may be severe and accompanied by fecal impaction), N&V, diarrhea, heartburn, GI bleeding, anorexia, flatulence, steatorrhea, abdominal distention/cramping/pain, bloating, loose stools, indigestion, rectal bleeding/pain, blood in stools, hemorrhoidal aggravated/bleeding, ***bleeding duodenal ulcer, peptic ulceration***, ulcer attack, GI irritation, dysphagia, dental bleeding/caries, hiccoughs, sour taste, pancreatitis, diverticulitis, cholecystitis, cholelithiasis, calcified material in biliary tree and gallbladder. **CV:** Chest pain, angina, tachycardia (rare). **CNS:** Migraine or sinus headache, anxiety, vertigo, dizziness, lightheadedness, insomnia, tinnitus, syncope, drowsiness, femoral nerve pain, paresthesia, increased libido. **Hematologic:** Ecchymosis, anemia, bleeding tendencies due to hypoprothrombinemia. **Allergic:** Urticaria, dermatitis, asthma, wheezing, rash. **Musculoskeletal:** Backache, muscle/joint pain, arthritis, osteoporosis, aches and pains in extremities, swelling of hands/feet. **Dermatologic:** Rash, dermatitis, urticaria (rare). **GU:** Hematuria, burnt odor to urine, dysuria, diuresis. **Body as a whole:** Fatigue, edema, weakness, weight loss/gain. **Miscellaneous:** Uveitis, swollen glands, SOB, hyperchloremic acidosis in children.

LABORATORY TEST CONSIDERATIONS

Transient and modest ↑ ALT, AST, alkaline phosphatase.

DRUG INTERACTIONS

See ***Cholestyramine***. Also, colestipol ↓ bioavailability of diltiazem if colestipol is given with, 1 hr before, or 4 hr after diltiazem.

HOW SUPPLIED

Granules: 5 grams/7.5 grams; *Granules for Oral Suspension:* 5 gram packets; *Tablets:* 1 gram.

DOSAGE

GRANULES; GRANULES FOR ORAL SUSPENSION

Antihyperlipidemic.

Adults, initial: 5 grams once or twice daily with a daily increment of 5 grams at 1- or 2-month intervals. **Range:** 5–30 grams/day (1–6 packets or level scoopfuls) given once daily or in divided doses.

TABLETS

Antihyperlipidemic.

Adults, initial: 2 grams 1–2 times per day. Dose can be increased by 2 grams, once or twice daily, at 1–2-month intervals. **Total dose:** 2–16 grams/day given once or in divided doses.

NURSING IMPLICATIONS

Do not confuse colestipol with cholestyramine.

IMPLEMENTATION/ADMINISTRATION/STORAGE

1. If compliance is good and side effects acceptable but desired effect is not obtained with 2–16 grams/day using tablets, consider combined therapy or alternative treatment.
2. In those with pre-existing constipation, the starting dose of tablets should be 2 grams once daily and the starting dose of granules is 1 packet or 1 scoop once daily for 5–7 days, increasing to twice daily with monitoring of constipation and of serum lipoproteins, at least twice, 4–6 weeks apart.
3. Granules available in an orange-flavored product.
4. Store granules or tablets from 20–25°C (68–77°F).

ASSESSMENT

1. Note reasons for therapy, other agents trialed, outcome.
2. Assess family history, for CAD, risk factors, dietary patterns, and exercise regimes.
3. Because it sequesters bile acids, colestipol may interfere with normal fat absorption; may reduce absorption of folic acid and fat-soluble vitamins such as A, D, and K.
4. Monitor lipid panel, LFTs, and electrolytes.

CLIENT/FAMILY TEACHING

1. Take 30 min before meals, preferably with the evening meal, since cholesterol synthesis is increased during the evening hours. Take only 1 tablet at a time and swallow whole with plenty of fluids. Caution not to crush, chew, or cut tablet. Report if any tablets get stuck after swallowing or cause a choking sensation. Take other drugs 1 hr before or 4 hr after to reduce interference with absorption.

2. Never take dose in dry form; avoid inhaling powder. Always mix (1 packet or 1 level scoop) granules with 90 mL or more of fruit juice, milk, water, carbonated beverages, applesauce, soup, cereal, or pulpy fruit before administering to disguise unpalatable taste and to prevent resin from causing esophageal irritation or blockage.
3. Rinse glass with a small amount of fluid and swallow to ensure the total amount of the drug is taken.
4. Tablets should be swallowed whole one at a time (i.e., they should not be cut, crushed, or chewed); may be taken with plenty of water or other fluids.
5. Consume adequate amounts of fluids, fruits, and fiber to diminish constipating drug effects. Report unusual bruising/bleeding or adverse effects.
6. Continue to follow dietary restrictions of fat and cholesterol, regular exercise program, smoking cessation, and weight reduction in the overall goal of cholesterol reduction.
7. Serum cholesterol level will return to pretreatment levels within 1 month if drug is discontinued.
8. Keep all F/U to assess response, labs, and for adverse SE.

OUTCOMES/EVALUATE

↓ LDL-cholesterol levels

Combination Drug

Conjugated estrogens and Medroxyprogesterone acetate

(**KON**-jyou-**gay**-ted **ES**-troh-jens, meh-**drox**-see-proh-**JESS**-ter-ohn)

Classification(s): Sex hormones

Pregnancy Category: X

RX: Premphase, PremPro.

✱ **Rx:** Premplus.

SEE ALSO ***ESTROGENS CONJUGATED*** AND ***MEDROXYPROGESTERONE ACETATE.***

INDICATIONS/USES

(1) Moderate to severe vasomotor symptoms associated with menopause in women with an intact uterus. (2) Vulvular and vaginal atrophy.

CONTENT

PremPro: Each tablet contains: Conjugated estrogens/Medroxyprogesterone, 0.3/1.5 mg, 0.45 mg/1.5 mg, 0.625 mg/2.5 mg, 0.625 mg/5 mg. *Premphase:* Two tablet types: One containing conjugated estrogens, 0.625 mg (14 tabs), and one containing conjugated estrogens, 0.625 mg, and medroxyprogesterone acetate, 5 mg (14 tabs).

ACTION/KINETICS

Action

Estrogens combine with receptors in the cytoplasm of cells, resulting in an increase in protein synthesis. During menopause, estrogens are used as replacement therapy. Medroxyprogesterone acetate reduces endometrial hyperplasia and may decrease the number of estrogen receptors.

Pharmacokinetics

Estrogens are metabolized in the liver and excreted mainly in the urine. **Medroxyprogesterone acetate, maximum levels:** 1–2 hr. **$t^{1/2}$, after PO:** 2–3 hr for first 6 hr; then, 8–9 hr.

CONTRAINDICATIONS

Known or suspected pregnancy, including use for missed abortion or as a diagnostic test for pregnancy. Known or suspected cancer of the breast or estrogen-dependent neoplasia. Undiagnosed abnormal genital bleeding. Active or past history of thrombophlebitis, thromboembolic disease, or stroke. Liver dysfunction or disease. Lactation.

SPECIAL CONCERNS

Estrogens reportedly increase the risk of endometrial carcinoma in postmenopausal women. Do not use estrogens during pregnancy. Use of progestins during the first 4 weeks of pregnancy is not recommended.

- Use with caution in conditions aggravated by fluid retention, including asthma, epilepsy, migraine, and cardiac or renal dysfunction.
- Estrogens may cause significant increases in plasma triglycerides that may cause pancreatitis and other complications in clients with familial defects of lipoprotein metabolism.

C

SIDE EFFECTS

Most Common

Abdominal/back pain, headache, nausea, infection, depression, breast pain.

See *Estrogens* and *Progesterone and Progestins*, for a complete list of possible side effects.

DRUG INTERACTIONS

See individual drug entries.

HOW SUPPLIED

See *Content.*

DOSAGE

TABLETS

Vasomotor symptoms due to menopause, vulvar and vaginal atrophy, prevention of osteoporosis.

PremPro: One 0.625/2.5 mg tablet once daily. *Premphase:* One 0.625 mg conjugated estrogen tablet once daily on days 1 to 14 and one 0.625/5 mg tablet once daily on days 15 to 28.

NURSING IMPLICATIONS

IMPLEMENTATION/ADMINISTRATION/STORAGE

PremPro, 0.3 mg/1.5 mg, is approved for moderate to severe symptoms associated with menopause while the 0.45/1.5 mg product is approved for the prevention of postmenopausal osteoporosis.

ASSESSMENT

1. List reasons for therapy (hormone replacement for significant menopausal symptoms), onset, duration, and characteristics of S&S, anticipated length of therapy.
2. Note history or experience with replacement therapy. Do not give for cardiac protection; give for postmenopausal symptom control only.
3. Document Pap smear and breast, abdominal, and pelvic exams completed before starting and annually thereafter with prolonged therapy.
4. Evaluate for active or past conditions that may preclude drug therapy: liver dysfunction, hyperlipidemia, thrombophlebitis, thromboembolic disorders, cancer of the breast or estrogen-dependent neoplasia, or any undiagnosed abnormal vaginal bleeding (AVB). Monitor closely during use.
5. Monitor BP, lipid panel, TSH, BS, and LFTs.

CLIENT/FAMILY TEACHING

1. Take tablet at the same time every day as directed from the dispensing dial.
2. May be taken without regard to meals; take with food if GI upset occurs.
3. Do not take tablets out of sequence and when dispensing dial is empty, begin a new cycle of tablets the next day.
4. Keep tablets in provided plastic dispensing device until dose is needed.
5. When used for treating vasomotor symptoms or vulval and vaginal atrophy, reevaluate every 3–6 months.
6. Report any pain, swelling, redness, or warmth in calves; sudden severe headache, visual disturbances, weakness or numbness of arms or legs, signs of liver dysfunction (e.g., dark urine, jaundice) or signs of depression.
7. Should not be used to prevent osteoporosis. Nonhormonal modalities that help prevent osteoporosis include 1,500 mg/day of calcium, vitamin D supplementation, and exercise and therapies such as bisphosphonates for fracture prevention. Diagnostic procedures should be undertaken to rule out malignancy in the event of persistent or recurring abnormal vaginal bleeding (AVB).
8. Have regular mammograms and pelvic exams with Pap smear. Perform regular BSE.
9. Use may increase risk of endometrial cancer or other carcinomas.
10. Keep all F/U to assess response, need for continued therapy, adverse SE.

OUTCOMES/EVALUATE

Control/reduction of menopausal S&S

Cortisone acetate

(**KOR**-tih-zohn)

Classification(s): Glucocorticoid

Pregnancy Category: D

SEE ALSO ***CORTICOSTEROIDS***.

C

ADDITIONAL USES

(1) Replacement therapy in chronic cortical insufficiency. (2) Short-term (due to strong mineralocorticoid effect) for inflammatory or allergic disorders.

ACTION/KINETICS

Action

Possesses both glucocorticoid and mineralocorticoid activity.

Pharmacokinetics

Short-acting. **t½, plasma:** 30 min; **t½, biologic:** 8–12 hr.

SPECIAL CONCERNS

Use during pregnancy only if benefits outweigh risks.

SIDE EFFECTS

Most Common

Insomnia, N&V, GI upset, fatigue, dizziness, muscle weakness, joint pain, increased hunger/thirst, problems with diabetes control.

See *Corticosteroids* for a complete list of possible side effects.

HOW SUPPLIED

Tablets: 25 mg.

DOSAGE

TABLETS

Initial or during crisis.

25–300 mg/day. Decrease gradually to lowest effective dose.

Anti-inflammatory.

25–150 mg/day, depending on severity of the disease.

Acute rheumatic fever.

200 mg twice a day on day 1, thereafter, 200 mg/day.

Addison's disease.

Maintenance: 0.5–0.75 mg/kg/day.

NURSING IMPLICATIONS

IMPLEMENTATION/ADMINISTRATION/STORAGE

1. Single course of therapy should not exceed 6 weeks. Rest periods of 2–3 weeks are indicated between treatments.
2. If cortisone is to be discontinued after more than a few days of therapy, it should be withdrawn gradually.
3. It may be necessary to increase the dose during periods of stress.
4. Store from 15–30°C (59–86°F). Protect from light and moisture.

ASSESSMENT

1. Note reasons for therapy: crisis or anti-inflammatory, rheumatic fever, or Addison's disease.
2. Identify levels, characteristics of S&S and previous experience with this drug.
3. Assess for HPA suppression with long term therapy. Monitor BP, BS, electrolytes, and LFT.

CLIENT/FAMILY TEACHING

1. Drug reduces swelling and decreases the body's immune response. Do not take if you have serious bacterial, viral, fungal infection; reduces ability to fight infection
2. Take in the a.m. with milk or food to minimize GI upset.
3. Review correct dosage, length of therapy, rest periods, F/U labs and visit schedules. Do not stop suddenly with long-term therapy; wean as directed.
4. Avoid receiving live virus vaccine during therapy.
5. With long term therapy, have annual eye exams. Obtain BP, blood glucose, and electrolytes checked at least every 6 months. Report persistent weight gain.
6. Keep all F/U to assess response, labs, and for adverse SE.

OUTCOMES/EVALUATE

- Replacement with adrenal cortex insufficiency
- Relief of allergic manifestations; inflammatory conditions
- Normal plasma cortisol levels (138–635 nmol/L at 8 a.m.)

Crizotinib

(kriz-**OH**-tih-nib)

Classification(s): Tyrosine kinase inhibitor

Pregnancy Category: D

RX: Xalkori.

C

INDICATIONS/USES

Treatment of locally advanced or metastatic non-small cell lung cancer that is anaplastic lymphoma kinase-positive as detected by a Food and Drug Administration-approved test.

ACTION/KINETICS

Action

Crizotinib is a tyrosine kinase inhibitor. The drug demonstrated concentration-dependent inhibition of anaplastic lymphoma kinase leading to antitumor activity. May prolong the QT interval.

Pharmacokinetics

Mean absolute bioavailability: 43% (range of 32–66%). A high fat meal reduces AUC and C_{max}. **Peak levels:** 4–6 hr. Steady state reached within 15 days and remains stable. Metabolized predominantly by CYP3A4/5. Metabolites and parent drug excreted in both the feces and urine. **t½, terminal:** 42 hr. Hepatic impairment is likely to increase plasma levels. Both AUC and C_{max} are higher in Asian clients. **Plasma protein binding:** 91%.

CONTRAINDICATIONS

Lactation.

SPECIAL CONCERNS

- **Use with caution in severe renal impairment or end-stage renal disease and in those with impaired hepatic function.**
- **Safety and efficacy not established in children.**

SIDE EFFECTS

Most Common

Vision disorder, N&V, diarrhea, edema, constipation.

GI: N&V, diarrhea, constipation, abdominal discomfort/pain/tenderness, dyspepsia, dysphagia, epigastric discomfort/pain/burning, esophagitis, esophageal obstruction/pain/spasm/ulcer, GERD, odynophagia, reflux esophagitis, mouth ulceration, glossodynia, glossitis, cheilitis, mucosal inflammation, oropharyngeal pain/discomfort, oral pain, stomatitis. **CNS:** Dizziness, dysgeusia, headache, insomnia, burning sensation, dysesthesia, hyperesthesia, hypoesthesia, neuralgia, paresthesia, peripheral neuropathy, peripheral motor/sensory neuropathy. **CV:** Bradycardia, QT interval prolongation, disseminated intravascular coagulopathy. **Musculoskeletal:** Arthralgia, back pain, chest pain/discomfort, musculoskeletal chest pain. ***Respiratory:*** Pneumonia, cough, hypoxia, acute respiratory distress syndrome, dyspnea, ***pneumonitis***, empyema, nasopharyngitis, rhinitis, pharyngitis, URTI, ***pulmonary hemorrhage, pulmonary embolism***. **GU:** Complex renal cysts. **Hematologic:** Neutropenia, thrombocytopenia, lymphopenia. **Ophthalmic:** Diplopia, photopsia, photophobia, blurred vision, visual field defect, visual impairment, vitreous floaters, visual brightness, decreased visual acuity. **Body as a whole:** Edema/peripheral edema, localized edema, fatigue, fever, rash, ***septic shock***. **Miscellaneous:** Decreased appetite

LABORATORY TEST CONSIDERATIONS

↑ ALT, AST.

DRUG INTERACTIONS

(1) An additive effect of crizotinib with other drugs that prolong the QT interval cannot be excluded. The following drugs may prolong the QT interval and increase the risk of life-threatening cardiac arrhythmias, including torsades de pointes: Amiodarone, arsenic trioxide, bretylium, chlorpromazine, cisapride, disopyramide, dofetilide, dolasetron, droperidol, gatifloxacin, halofantrine, levomethadyl, mefloquine, mesoridazine, moxifloxacin, pentamidine, pimozide, probucol, procainamide, quinidine, sotalol, tacrolimus, thioridazine, and ziprasidone.
(2) Crizotinib is an inhibitor of P-glycoprotein (in vitro); therefore, crizotinib may ↑ plasma levels of coadministered P-gp drugs.
(3) Crizotinib is metabolized mainly by the CYP3A enzyme system. Thus, substances known to inhibit these enzymes may ↓ metabolism or ↑ bioavailability of crizotinib. Drugs known to induce these enzyme systems may result in an ↑ metabolism of crizotinib or ↓ bioavailability. Monitor blood levels and appropriate dosage adjustments when such drugs are used together.

Alfentanil / ↑ Alfentanil plasma levels R/T inhibition of CYP3A enzymes → ↑ pharmacologic/toxic effects; avoid coadministration
Antacids / ↑ Gastric pH may ↓ crizotinib solubility and ↓ bioavailability
Aprepitant / ↑ Crizotinib plasma levels → ↑ pharmacologic/toxic effects; coadminister with caution
Atazanavir / ↑ Crizotinib plasma levels R/T inhibition of metabolism by CYP3A enzymes → ↑

pharmacologic/toxic effects; avoid coadministration
Carbamazepine / ↓ Crizotinib plasma levels R/T ↑ metabolism by CYP3A enzymes; avoid coadministration
Clarithromycin / ↑ Crizotinib plasma levels R/T inhibition of metabolism by CYP3A enzymes → ↑ pharmacologic/toxic effects; avoid coadministration
Cyclosporine / ↑ Cyclosporine plasma levels R/T inhibition of CYP3A enzymes → ↑ pharmacologic/toxic effects; avoid coadministration
Dihydroergotamine / ↑ Dihydroergotamine plasma levels R/T inhibition of CYP3A enzymes → ↑ pharmacologic/toxic effects; avoid coadministration
Drugs that prolong the QT interval / See (1) at the beginning of this section.
Diltiazem / ↑ Crizotinib plasma levels → ↑ pharmacologic/toxic effects; coadminister with caution
Ergotamine / ↑ Ergotamine plasma levels R/T inhibition of CYP3A enzymes → ↑ pharmacologic/toxic effects; avoid coadministration
Erythromycin / ↑ Crizotinib plasma levels → ↑ pharmacologic/toxic effects; coadminister with caution
Fentanyl / ↑ Fentanyl plasma levels R/T inhibition of CYP3A enzymes → ↑ pharmacologic/toxic effects; avoid coadministration
Fluconazole / ↑ Crizotinib plasma levels → ↑ pharmacologic/toxic effects; coadminister with caution
Fosamprenavir / ↑ Crizotinib plasma levels → ↑ pharmacologic/toxic effects; coadminister with caution
Grapefruit/Grapefruit juice / ↑ Crizotinib plasma levels → ↑ risk of side effects; avoid coadministration
H_2 blockers (e.g., cimetidine) / ↑ Gastric pH may ↓ crizotinib solubility and ↓ bioavailability
Indinavir / ↑ Crizotinib plasma levels R/T inhibition of metabolism by CYP3A enzymes → ↑ pharmacologic/toxic effects; avoid coadministration
Itraconazole / ↑ Crizotinib plasma levels R/T inhibition of metabolism by CYP3A enzymes → ↑ pharmacologic/toxic effects; avoid coadministration
Ketoconazole / ↑ Crizotinib plasma levels R/T inhibition of metabolism by CYP3A enzymes → ↑ pharmacologic/toxic effects; avoid coadministration
Nefazodone / ↑ Crizotinib plasma levels R/T inhibition of metabolism by CYP3A enzymes → ↑ pharmacologic/toxic effects; avoid coadministration
Nelfinavir / ↑ Crizotinib plasma levels R/T inhibition of metabolism by CYP3A enzymes → ↑ pharmacologic/toxic effects; avoid coadministration
Phenobarbital / ↓ Crizotinib plasma levels R/T ↑ metabolism by CYP3A enzymes; avoid coadministration
Phenytoin / ↓ Crizotinib plasma levels R/T ↑ metabolism by CYP3A enzymes; avoid coadministration
Pimozide / ↑ Pimozide plasma levels R/T inhibition of CYP3A enzymes → ↑ pharmacologic/toxic effects; avoid coadministration
Proton pump inhibitors (e.g., omeprazole) / ↑ Gastric pH may ↓ crizotinib solubility and ↓ bioavailability
Quinidine / ↑ Quinidine plasma levels R/T inhibition of CYP3A enzymes → ↑ pharmacologic/toxic effects; avoid coadministration
Rifabutin/Rifampin / ↓ Crizotinib plasma levels R/T ↑ metabolism by CYP3A enzymes; avoid coadministration
Ritonavir / ↑ Crizotinib plasma levels R/T inhibition of metabolism by CYP3A enzymes → ↑ pharmacologic/toxic effects; avoid coadministration
Saquinavir / ↑ Crizotinib plasma levels R/T inhibition of metabolism by CYP3A enzymes → ↑ pharmacologic/toxic effects; avoid coadministration
Sirolimus / ↑ Sirolimus plasma levels R/T inhibition of CYP3A enzymes → ↑ pharmacologic/toxic effects; avoid coadministration
H ***St. John's wort*** / ↓ Crizotinib plasma levels R/T ↑ metabolism by CYP3A enzymes; avoid coadministration
Tacrolimus / ↑ Tacrolimus plasma levels R/T inhibition of CYP3A enzymes → ↑ pharmacologic/toxic effects; avoid coadministration
Telithromycin / ↑ Crizotinib plasma levels R/T inhibition of metabolism by CYP3A enzymes → ↑ pharmacologic/toxic effects; avoid coadministration
Verapamil / ↑ Crizotinib plasma levels → ↑ pharmacologic/toxic effects; coadminister with caution

Voriconazole / ↑ Crizotinib plasma levels R/T inhibition of metabolism by CYP3A enzymes → ↑ pharmacologic/toxic effects; avoid coadministration

C

HOW SUPPLIED

Capsules: 200 mg, 250 mg.

DOSAGE

CAPSULES

Non-small-cell cancer.

Adults, usual: 250 mg twice a day. If dose reduction is needed, reduce the dose to 200 mg twice a day. If further dose reduction is necessary, reduce the dose to 250 mg once a day, based on individual safety and tolerance. **Duration:** Continue treatment as long as the client is deriving clinical benefit from therapy.

NURSING IMPLICATIONS

IMPLEMENTATION/ADMINISTRATION/STORAGE

1. If a dose is missed, take as soon as the client remembers unless it is less than 6 hr until the next dose, in which case the missed dose should not be taken. Clients should not take 2 doses at the same time to make up for a missed dose.
2. No dosage adjustment is needed for clients with mild (C_{CR} 60–80 mL/min) and moderate (C_{CR} 30–60 mL/min) renal impairment.
3. Use the following crizotinib dosage adjustment for hematologic toxicities (except lymphopenia unless associated with clinical events as opportunistic infections): (a) For Grade 3 National Cancer Institute (NCI) Common Terminology Criteria for Adverse Events (CTCAE), withhold crizotinib until recovery to grade 2 or less; then, resume at the same dose schedule. (b) For Grade 3 NCI, CTCAE, withhold crizotinib until recovery to grade 2 or less; then, resume at 200 mg twice a day.
4. Use the following crizotinib dosage adjustment for nonhematologic toxicities using CTCAE: (a) For Grade 3 or 4 ALT or AST elevation with grade 1 or less total bilirubin, withhold crizotinib until recovery to grade 1 or less or baseline; then, resume at 200 mg twice a day. In case of recurrence, withhold until recovery to grade 1 or less; then resume at 250 mg once a day. Permanently discontinue if further grade 3 or 4 recurrence. (b) For grade 2, 3, or 4 ALT or AST elevation with concurrent grade 2, 3, or 4 total bilirubin elevation (in the absence of cholestasis or hemolysis), permanently discontinue crizotinib. (c) For any grade pneumonitis not attributable to non–small cell lung cancer, other pulmonary disease, or radiation effect, permanently discontinue crizotinib. (d) For Grade 3 QTc prolongation, withhold crizotinib until recovery to grade 1 or less; then, resume at 200 mg twice a day. (e) For Grade 4 QTc prolongation, permanently discontinue crizotinib.
5. Store from 15–30°C (59–86°F).

ASSESSMENT

1. Drug indicated for advanced or metastatic non–small cell lung cancer that is anaplastic lymphoma kinase-positive. Note detection of ALK-positive NSCLC using an FDA-approved test (necessary for selection of patients for treatment with crizotinib).
2. List drugs prescribed to ensure none interact.
3. Assess for congenital long QT syndrome; precludes therapy. Obtain ECG to assess for QT prolongation and monitor electrolytes in those with CHF, bradyarrhythmias, electrolyte abnormalities and in those taking drugs known to prolong QT interval.
4. Monitor for pulmonary symptoms indicative of pneumonitis. Check for other causes of pneumonitis, and permanently discontinue in those diagnosed with treatment-related pneumonitis.
5. Obtain eye exam if vision disorders occur, particularly in those who experience photopsia or new or increased vitreous floaters.
6. Monitor VS, ECG, CBC, and LFTs; follow labs and dosing guidelines closely and withhold, decrease dose or discontinue based on ALT/AST levels and hematologic parameters.

CLIENT/FAMILY TEACHING

1. Take crizotinib as directed with or without food. Swallow capsules whole, do not crush, dissolve or open capsules. Avoid grapefruit and grapefruit juice during therapy.
2. Use caution with activities that require mental alertness until drug effects realized; may experience dizziness, visual disturbances and fatigue.

3. **Report any flashes or floaters to provider. Visual changes (e.g., perceived flashes of light, blurry vision, light sensitivity, floaters) were commonly reported and usually began during the first 2 weeks of therapy.**
4. **Most common GI side effects include nausea, vomiting, diarrhea and constipation; report if bothersome or persistent so anti-emetics, antidiarrheals or laxatives can be ordered.**
5. **Report S&S of liver dysfunction: weakness, fatigue, N&V, anorexia, RUQ pain, dark urine, yellowing of skin/eyes, itching, or easy bruising/bleeding.**
6. **Advise provider if abnormal heartbeats, feeling dizzy, or faintness occur; may be S&S related to QT prolongation and require ECG evaluation.**
7. **Any SOB, difficulty breathing, cough with or without mucus and fever may signal pneumonitis; report immediately.**
8. **Males and females should practice reliable contraception during and for 90 days following therapy; report if pregnancy suspected—may cause fetal harm. Do not breast feed during therapy.**
9. **Keep all F/U to assess response, labs, ECG, and for adverse SE.**

OUTCOMES/EVALUATE

Inhibition of continued progression of ALK-positive metastatic non-small cell lung cancer

Cromolyn sodium (Sodium cromoglycate)

(**CROH**-moh-lin)

Classification(s): Antiasthmatic drug; antiallergic drug

Pregnancy Category: B

OTC: Nasalcrom.

RX: Crolom, Cromolyn Sodium Ophthalmic Solution, Gastrocrom, Intal.

✤ **Rx:** Apo-Cromolyn Nasal Spray/Sterules, Nalcrom, Opticrom.

INDICATIONS/USES

Oral Inhalation Aerosol/Solution (Rx): (1) Management of bronchial asthma. (2) Prophylaxis of acute bronchospasms induced by exercise, toluene diisocyanate, known allergens, or environmental pollutants.

Nasal (OTC): Prophylaxis and treatment of allergic rhinitis, including children 2 years and older, due to airborne pollens from trees, grasses, or ragweed and by mold, animals, and dust.

PO (Rx): Mastocytosis (improves symptoms including diarrhea, flushing, headaches, vomiting, urticaria, nausea, abdominal pain, and itching).

Ophthalmic (Rx): Vernal keratoconjunctivitis, vernal conjunctivitis, and vernal keratitis.

Investigational: PO to treat food allergies and mucosal and serosal eosinophilic gastroenteritis. As alternative therapy in refractory forms of chronic urticaria/angioedema.

ACTION/KINETICS

Action

Considered a mast cell stabilizer that acts locally to inhibit the degranulation of sensitized mast cells that occurs after exposure to certain antigens. Prevents the release of histamine, slow-reacting substance of anaphylaxis, and other endogenous substances causing hypersensitivity reactions. When effective, reduces the number and intensity of asthmatic attacks as well as decreasing allergic reactions in the eye. No antihistaminic, anti-inflammatory, or bronchodilator effects and has no role in terminating an acute attack of asthma.

Pharmacokinetics

After inhalation, some drug is absorbed systemically. **t½:** 81 min; from lungs: 60 min. About 50% excreted unchanged through the urine and 50% through the bile. When used in the eye, approximately 0.03% is absorbed. **Onset, ophthalmic:** Several days. **Onset, nasal:** Less than 1 week. **Time to peak effect, nasal:** Up to 4 weeks.

CONTRAINDICATIONS

Hypersensitivity. Acute attacks and status asthmaticus. For mastocytosis in premature infants.

SPECIAL CONCERNS

- **Due to the propellants in the aerosol, use with caution in CAD or cardiac arrhythmias.**
- **Use with caution for long periods of time, in the presence of renal or hepatic disease, during pregnancy, and during lactation.**
- **Safety and efficacy not established for the aerosol in children under 5 years, for the nebulizer in children under 2 years, and for the ophthalmic solution in children under 4 years.**

- **Reserve use in children under 2 years old for severe disease in which potential benefits clearly outweigh potential risks.**

SIDE EFFECTS

Most Common

After PO/aerosol use: ***Bronchospasm*** (maybe severe), cough, nasal congestion, pharyngeal irritation, wheezing.

After ophthalmic use: Transient ocular stinging or burning after instillation

Following nebulization (oral solution): Sneezing, wheezing, nasal itching, cough, nose bleeds, burning, nasal congestion, nausea, drowsiness, serum sickness, stomach ache.

Following aerosol: Lacrimation, swollen parotid gland, dysuria, urinary frequency, dizziness, headache, rash, urticaria, ***angioedema***, joint swelling and pain, nausea, dry or irritated throat, bad taste, cough, wheezing, substernal burning, myopathy (rare).

Following nasal solution: Burning, stinging, irritation of nose; sneezing, nosebleeds, headache, bad taste in mouth, postnasal drip, rash.

Following ophthalmic use: Ocular stinging/burning following instillation; conjunctival injection, watery/itchy eyes, dryness around the eye, puffy eyes, eye irritation, styes. Rarely, immediate hypersensitivity reactions, including dyspnea, edema, and rash.

Following PO use (oral concentrate): GI: Diarrhea, abdominal pain, constipation, dyspepsia, dysphagia, eosphagospasm, flatulence, glossitis, N&V, stomatitis. **CNS:** Headache, irritability, anxiety, behavior change, convulsions, depression, dizziness, hallucinations, hypoesthesia, insomnia, lethargy, migraine, nervousness, paresthesia, postprandial lightheadedness, psychosis. **CV:** Palpitations, PVCs, tachycardia. **Dermatologic:** Flushing, rash, ***angioedema***, urticaria, skin burning, skin erythema, photosensitivity, pruritus. **GU:** Dysuria, urinary frequency. **Respiratory:** Dyspnea, pharyngitis. **Hematologic:** Neutropenia, pancytopenia, polycythemia. **Musculoskeletal:** Arthralgia, myalgia, stiffness and weakness in legs, chest pain. **Otic:** Tinnitus. **Body as a whole:** Fatigue, edema. **Miscellaneous:** Altered liver function test, unpleasant taste, lupus erythematosus syndrome, hypersensitivity (rare).

HOW SUPPLIED

OTC. *Nasal Solution:* 40 mg/mL (5.2 mg/inh). **Rx.** *Aerosol Spray:* 800 mcg/actuation; *Ophthalmic Solution:* 4%; *Oral Concentrate:* 100 mg/5 mL; *Solution for Inhalation:* 20 mg/2 mL.

DOSAGE

SOLUTION FOR INHALATION

Prophylaxis of bronchial asthma.

Adults and children over 2 years old: 20 mg (1 vial) inhaled 4 times per day at regular intervals.

Prophylaxis of exercise-induced bronchospasm.

Inhale 20 mg (1 vial) of the nebulizer solution no more than 1 hr (the shorter the interval between the dose and exercise, the better the effect) before anticipated exercise. Repeat as required for protection during prolonged exercise.

AEROSOL SPRAY (INTAL)

Management of bronchial asthma.

Adults and children 5 years and older, initial: 2 metered sprays inhaled 4 times per day at regular intervals. Do not exceed this dose.

Prophylaxis of acute bronchospasm.

Inhalation of 2 metered dose sprays 10–15 min (but not more than 60 min) before exposure to precipitating factor.

NASAL SOLUTION (NASALCROM: OTC)

Allergic rhinitis.

Adults and children 2 years and older: 1 spray in each nostril 3–4 times/day at regular intervals q 4–6 hr. May be used up to 6 times/day if needed. Maximum effect may not be seen for 1–2 weeks. Use every day while in contact with the allergen, preferably before contact with the cause of the allergy. For best results, use up to 1 week before contact.

ORAL CONCENTRATE

Mastocytosis.

Adults and children 13 years and older: 200 mg (i.e., 2 ampules) 4 times per day 30 min before meals and at bedtime. **Pediatric, 2–12 years:** 100 mg (i.e., 1 ampule) 4 times per day 30 min before meals and at bedtime. If relief is not seen within 2–3 weeks, dose may be increased, but should not exceed

40 mg/kg/day. **Maintenance:** Reduce dose to minimum amount to maintain client with minimum symptoms.

OPHTHALMIC SOLUTION

Vernal keratoconjunctivitis, vernal conjunctivitis, vernal keratitis.

Adults and children, 4 years and older: 1–2 gtt in each eye 4–6 times per day at regular intervals. 1 gtt contains 1.6 mg cromolyn sodium. Treatment may be required for up to 6 weeks. If needed, corticosteroids may be used concomitantly with cromolyn sodium ophthalmic solution.

NURSING IMPLICATIONS

IMPLEMENTATION/ADMINISTRATION/STORAGE

1. Continue corticosteroid dosage when initiating PO cromolyn therapy. If improvement occurs, taper the steroid dosage slowly. May have to reinstitute steroids if cromolyn inhalation is impaired, in times of stress, or in adrenocortical insufficiency.
2. Cromolyn should be added to existing treatment regimens for bronchial asthma (e.g., bronchodilators). When a clinical response to cromolyn is noted and asthma is under good control, attempts may be made to decrease gradually concomitant drug use.
3. Products for inhalation must not be used for injection.
4. Safety and stability of oral inhalation products have not been established if mixed with other drugs in a nebulizer.
5. Store oral concentrate and ophthalmic solution from 15–30°C (59–86°F) protected from light; store ampules in foil pouch until ready to use. Store aerosol, solution for inhalation, and nasal solution from 20–25°C (68–77°F) protected from light; store ampules in foil pouch until ready to use.

ASSESSMENT

Note reasons for therapy, onset, characteristics of S&S, triggers, other agents trialed, PFTs, CXR, and pulmonary assessment findings.

CLIENT/FAMILY TEACHING

1. Institute only after acute episode is over, when airway is clear and able to inhale adequately. Acts to inhibit acute reaction by preventing histamine release.
2. Report any adverse effects or loss of response. Remember to rinse/dry all equipment thoroughly and to rinse mouth after each treatment.
3. Directions for using aerosol:
   - Remove cap from mouthpiece and shake the inhaler with canister in place for 5–10 seconds.
   - Breathe out to the end of a normal breath. Place mouthpiece into mouth, use a chamber, or position mouthpiece 2–3 finger widths from open mouth.
   - Slightly tilt head back. Breathe in through mouth slowly for 3–5 sec and press the top of the canister at the same time.
   - Remove inhaler from mouth and hold breath for about 10 sec; allow at least 1 min between inhalations.
4. Directions for using nebulizer solution:
   - Assemble the face mask or mouthpiece and connect the tubing from the port to the compressor unit.
   - Sit in an upright and comfortable position. Put the mask over your nose and mouth, making sure it fits properly to prevent mist from going into the eyes. If a mouthpiece is used, place it into your mouth.
   - Turn on compressor and take slow, deep breaths. If possible, hold breath for 10 sec before slowly exhaling. Continue until medication chamber is empty.
5. Do not swallow nebulizer solution as it is poorly absorbed. When using nebulizer solution, do not mix different types of medications without provider permission.
6. Directions for using nasal spray/solution:
   - Blow nose before using spray.
   - Hold pump with thumb at bottom and nozzle between fingers. When using for the first time, prime the pump by initially spraying 5 times into the air until a fine mist appears.
   - Insert nozzle into nostril, spray upward while breathing through the nose. Repeat in other nostril.
   - Wipe nozzle to remove debris; cleanse.
   - If the pump has not been used for 2 weeks, spray 2 times into the air before using again.

- Consult provider if used continuously for more than 12 weeks.

7. Directions for PO use:
   - Take at least 30 min before meals.
   - Break open ampule and squeeze contents into a glass of water. Do not mix with fruit juice, milk, or foods.
   - Stir solution and drink all of the liquid.
8. Continue prescribed medications; may take up to 4 weeks for frequency of asthmatic attacks to decrease.
9. With exposure induced bronchoconstriction, use inhaler within 10–15 min prior to precipitating agent (i.e., exercise, antigen, environmental pollutants) for best results.
10. Use a peak expiratory flow meter to monitor asthma control; establish level to seek medical assistance.
11. Do not discontinue inhalation or nasal medication abruptly. Rapid withdrawal of the drug may precipitate an asthmatic attack, and concomitant corticosteroid therapy may require adjustment.
12. Report any increase in wheezing or coughing after inhalation or stinging effect after nasal instillation, joint pain, severe wheezing, difficulty breathing, chills, sweating, or chest pain; may indicate eosinophilic pneumonia.
13. With eye drops, wash hands, review method for instillation. Do not wear soft contact lenses during therapy; wait for several hours after therapy is discontinued. May experience slight burning or stinging upon instillation.
14. Keep all F/U to assess response and for adverse SE.

OUTCOMES/EVALUATE

- ↓ Frequency of asthmatic attacks
- Prevention of exposure-induced bronchoconstriction
- Control of symptoms of mastocytosis (↓ diarrhea, N&V, headache, flushing, and abdominal pain)
- Relief of nasal allergic manifestations

Cyanocobalamin (Vitamin B_{12})

(sye-**an**-oh-koh-**BAL**-ah-min)

Classification(s): Vitamin B_{12}

Pregnancy Category: A (**C** in doses that exceed the RDA)

OTC: Lozenges, Tablets: Twelve Resin-K. **Sublingual Spray Solution:** Rapid B-12 Energy.

RX: Nasal Spray: CaloMist, Nascobal.

Cyanocobalamin crystalline

Pregnancy Category: C

INDICATIONS/USES

Oral Cyanocobalamin (OTC). Nutritional vitamin B_{12} deficiency. (These products are not for the treatment of pernicious anemia.)

Cyanocobalamin Nasal Spray (Rx). Nutritional vitamin B_{12} deficiency. **CaloMist:** Maintenance of vitamin B_{12} concentrations after normalization with IM vitamin B_{12} therapy in those with vitamin B_{12} deficiency who have no nervous system involvement. **Nascobal:** (1) Maintenance of hematologic status in those who are in remission following IM vitamin B_{12} therapy and who have no nervous system involvement. (2) As a supplement for other vitamin B_{12} deficiencies, including the following: (a) Dietary deficiency of vitamin B_{12} in strict vegetarians (isolated vitamin B_{12} deficiency is rare); (b) Malabsorption of vitamin B_{12} due to structural or functional damage to the stomach where intrinsic factor is secreted or to the ileum where intrinsic factor facilitates vitamin B_{12} absorption, including HIV infection, AIDS, Crohn's disease, tropical sprue, nontropical sprue (idiopathic steatorrhea, gluten-induced enteropathy); (c) Inadequate secretion of intrinsic factor due to lesions that destroy the gastric mucosa (e.g., ingestion of corrosives, extensive neoplasia) and conditions associated with a variable degree of gastric atrophy (e.g., multiple sclerosis, HIV infection, AIDS, certain endocrine disorders, iron deficiency, subtotal gastrectomy); (d) Competition for vitamin B_{12} by intestinal parasites or bacteria; and, (e) Inadequate use of vitamin B_{12} (i.e., if antimetabolites for the vitamin are used to treat neoplasms).

Cyanocobalamin Crystalline Parenteral: (1) Vitamin B_{12} deficiency due to malabsorption syndrome as seen in pernicious anemia, GI pathology, dysfunction, or surgery. (2) Fish tapeworm infestation, malignancy of pancreas or bowel, gluten enteropathy, small bowel overgrowth of bacteria, sprue, accompanying folic acid deficiency, or total or partial gastrectomy. *NOTE:* Gel can be used in clients with HIV, AIDS, multiple sclerosis, or Crohn's disease.

ACTION/KINETICS

Action

Required for hematopoiesis, cell reproduction, nucleoprotein and myelin synthesis. Plasma vitamin B_{12} levels: 150–750 pg/mL. Following absorption, vitamin B_{12} is carried by plasma proteins to the liver where it is stored until required for various metabolic functions.

Pharmacokinetics

Bioavailability is about 25% after PO use. Rapidly absorbed following IM or SC administration. **t½:** 6 days (400 days in the liver). **Time to peak levels, after intranasal:** 1–2 hr. Bioavailability is 8.9%. Most vitamin B_{12} is reabsorbed from the GI tract. Unbound vitamin B_{12} is excreted in the urine if the binding capacity of plasma proteins and the liver are saturated.

CONTRAINDICATIONS

Hypersensitivity to cobalt or any component of the product, Leber's disease.

SPECIAL CONCERNS

- Use with caution in clients with gout and during lactation. For the elderly, start at the low end of the dosage range.
- Those with severe megaloblastic anemia treated intensely with vitamin B_{12} may develop hypokalemia and sudden death.
- Folic acid is **not** a substitute for vitamin B_{12}.
- A blunted or impeded therapeutic response to vitamin B_{12} may be caused by infection, uremia, bone marrow suppressants (e.g., chloramphenicol), and concurrent iron or folic acid deficiency.
- Doses of vitamin B_{12} exceeding 10 mcg/day may cause a hematologic response in those with folate deficiency. Indiscriminate use may mask the true diagnosis.
- Vitamin B_{12} deficiency may mask signs of polycythemia vera.
- Safety and efficacy of CaloMist not determined in children.

SIDE EFFECTS

Most Common

After intranasal use: N&V, glossitis, headache, rhinitis.

After parenteral use: Itching, diarrhea, pain at injection site.

- **Following intranasal use**

CaloMist. Respiratory: Nasopharyngitis, rhinorrhea, bronchitis, nasal discomfort, asthma, cough, epistaxis, pharyngolaryngeal pain, postnasal drip, sinus headache, sinusitis. **CNS:** Dizziness, headache, hypersomia. **Dermatologic:** Rash. **Musculoskeletal:** Arthralgia, back pain. **Body as a whole:** Flu-like illness, malaise, pain, pyrexia. **Miscellaneous:** Procedural pain, scab, tooth abscess.

Nascobal. GI: Glossitis, nausea. **CNS:** Headache, asthenia, paresthesia. **Respiratory:** Rhinitis. **Miscellaneous:** Infection. NOTE: Benzyl alcohol, which is present in certain products, may cause ***fatal "gasping syndrome"*** in premature infants.

- **Following parenteral use**

Allergic: Urticaria, itching, transitory exanthema, ***anaphylaxis, shock, death***. **CV:** ***Peripheral vascular thrombosis***, CHF, ***pulmonary edema***. **Hypersensitivity:** Allergic reactions (e.g., angioedema, angioedema-like reaction), ***anaphylactic shock, death***. However, vitamin B_{12} is essentially nontoxic in humans. **Miscellaneous:** Polycythemia vera, optic nerve atrophy in clients with hereditary optic nerve atrophy, diarrhea, hypokalemia, body feels swollen, pain at injection site.

LABORATORY TEST CONSIDERATIONS

Antibiotics, methotrexate, or pyrimethamine invalidate folic acid and vitamin B_{12} diagnostic blood assays.

DRUG INTERACTIONS

Alcohol / ↓ Vitamin B_{12} absorption
Aminosalicylic acid / ↓ Vitamin B_{12} effect. Also, abnormal Schilling test and symptoms of vitamin B_{12} deficiency
Chloramphenicol / ↓ Response to vitamin B_{12} in pernicious anemia
Cholestyramine / ↓ Vitamin B_{12} absorption
Cimetidine / ↓ Digestion and release of vitamin B_{12}; ↓ absorption of cyanocobalamin
Colchicine / ↓ Vitamin B_{12} absorption
Neomycin / ↓ Vitamin B_{12} absorption
Para-aminosalicylic acid / ↓ Vitamin B_{12} absorption
Potassium, timed-release / ↓ Vitamin B_{12} absorption

C

HOW SUPPLIED

Cyanocobalamin (OTC). ***Lozenges:*** 50 mcg, 100 mcg, 250 mcg, 500 mcg; ***Sublingual Spray Solution:*** 200 mcg/spray; ***Tablets:*** 100 mcg, 500 mcg, 1,000 mcg, 1,000 mcg (on resin); ***Tablets, Sublingual:*** 1,000 mcg, 2500 mcg.
Cyanocobalamin (Rx). ***Nasal Gel (Nascobal):*** 500 mcg/0.1 mL (500 mcg/actuation); ***Nasal Spray (CaloMist):*** 25 mcg/0.1 mL.
Cyanocobalamin crystalline (Rx). ***Injection:*** 100 mcg/mL, 1,000 mcg/mL.

DOSAGE

Cyanocobalamin (OTC)

LOZENGES; SUBLINGUAL SPRAY SOLUTION; TABLETS; TABLETS SUBLINGUAL

Vitamin B_{12} deficiency.

Dosage varies. See individual product package inserts. The RDA for adults is 2 mcg/day.

CaloMist (Rx)

NASAL SPRAY

Maintenance of vitamin B_{12} levels after normalization with IM vitamin B_{12} therapy in vitamin B_{12} deficiency.

Initial: 1 spray (25 mcg) in each nostril once daily (total daily dose is 50 mcg). Increase the dose to one spray in each nostril twice a day (total daily dose of 100 mcg) for those with an inadequate response to once daily dosing.

Nascobal (Rx)

NASAL GEL

Maintenance of hematologic status in those who are in remission following IM vitamin B_{12} therapy.

One spray (500 mcg) in 1 nostril once a week at least 1 hr before or after ingestion of hot foods or liquids. Monitor serum B_{12} levels periodically to assess adequacy of therapy.

Cyanocobalamin crystalline

IM, SC (DEEP)

Addisonian pernicious anemia.

Adults: 100 mcg/day for 6–7 days; **then,** if improvement noted along with a reticulocyte response, give 100 mcg every other day for seven doses and then 100 mcg q 3–4 days for 2–3 weeks. **Maintenance, IM:** 100 mcg once a month for life. Give folic acid if necessary.

Vitamin B_{12} deficiency.

Adults: 30 mcg daily for 5–10 days; **then,** 100–200 mcg/month. Doses up to 1,000 mcg have been recommended. **Pediatric, for hematologic signs:** 10–50 mcg/day for 5–10 days followed by 100–250 mcg/dose q 2–4 weeks. **Pediatric, for neurologic signs:** 100 mcg/day for 10–15 days; **then,** 1–2 times/week for several months (can possibly be tapered to 250–1,000 mcg/month by 1 year).

Diagnosis of vitamin B_{12} deficiency.

Adults: 1 mcg/day IM for 10 days plus low dietary folic acid and vitamin B_{12}. Loading dose for the Schilling test is 1,000 mcg given IM.

NURSING IMPLICATIONS

IMPLEMENTATION/ADMINISTRATION/STORAGE

1. With pernicious anemia, the drug cannot be administered PO.
2. Clients should be in hematologic remission before use of the nasal gel.
3. The dose of CaloMist and other intranasal drugs should be separated by several hours; monitor vitamin B_{12} levels due to the potential for erratic absorption.
4. Clients with chronic nasal symptoms or significant nasal pathology are not ideal candidates for intranasal vitamin B_{12} therapy.
5. Protect the intranasal spray from light and from freezing. Store from 15–30°C (59–86°F).
6. Protect cyanocobalamin crystalline injection from light and from freezing.

ASSESSMENT

1. Note reasons for therapy, onset, characteristics of S&S and levels.
2. Check if allergic to cobalt. Obtain dietary history. Assess peripheral pulses, check for neuropathy.
3. Note if prescribed chloramphenicol; antagonizes hematopoietic response to vitamin B_{12}.

4. With pernicious anemia and malabsorption syndromes give parenterally and administer intrinsic factor simultaneously.
5. Hypokalemia and thrombocytosis may occur upon conversion of severe megaloblastic to normal erythropoiesis with vitamin B_{12} therapy. Monitor serum potassium levels and platelet count during therapy.
6. Monitor VS, CBC, reticulocyte, potassium, folate, iron, and B_{12} levels if being treated for megaloblastic anemia.

CLIENT/FAMILY TEACHING

1. With pernicious anemia, *must* take vitamin B_{12} replacement for life. May take orally daily or monthly shots.
2. When repository vitamin B_{12} used, provides drug for 4 weeks.
3. The stinging, burning sensation after injection is transitory.
4. If vitamin B_{12} therapy is the result of dietary deficiency, identify foods (such as meats, especially liver, fermented cheeses, egg yolks, and seafood) high in B_{12} and review diet.
5. Avoid alcohol; interferes with drug absorption.
6. Report any symptoms of urticaria, itching, and evidence of anaphylaxis immediately.
7. If diarrhea occurs, record frequency, quantity, and consistency of stools; may require a drug change.
8. When using CaloMist nasal spray, prime pump before the first time used. Place the nozzle between the first and second finger with the thumb on the bottom of the bottle. Pump the unit firmly and quickly; repeat this priming an additional 6 times for a total of 7 sprays. If 5 or more days elapse since last use, reprime the pump with two repriming sprays.
9. When using Nascobal nasal spray, prime the pump before the first time used. Remove the clear plastic cover and the plastic safety clip from the pump. To prime the pump, place the nozzle between the first and second fingers with the thumb on the bottom of the bottle. Pump unit firmly and quickly until the first appearance of spray; then, prime an additional 2 times. Unit is now ready for use.
10. Use the intranasal gel at least 1 hr before or 1 hr after ingestion of hot foods or liquids.
11. Keep all F/U to assess response, labs, and for adverse SE.

OUTCOMES/EVALUATE

- Relief of fatigue/improved functioning level
- Plasma vitamin B_{12} levels of 350–750 pg/mL

Cyclobenzaprine hydrochloride

(sye-kloh-**BENZ**-ah-preen)

Classification(s): Skeletal muscle relaxant, centrally-acting

Pregnancy Category: B

RX: Amrix, Fexmid, Flexeril.

✤ **Rx:** Apo-Cyclobenzaprine, Gen-Cyclobenzaprine, PMS-Cyclobenzaprine, ratio-Cyclobenzaprine.

SEE ALSO ***SKELETAL MUSCLE RELAXANTS, CENTRALLY-ACTING***.

INDICATIONS/USES

Adjunct to rest and physical therapy for relief of muscle spasms associated with acute and/or painful musculoskeletal conditions. *Investigational:* Management of fibromyalgia.

ACTION/KINETICS

Action

Thought to inhibit reflexes by reducing tonic somatic motor activity. Does not interfere with muscle function. Related to the tricyclic antidepressants; possesses both sedative and anticholinergic properties.

Pharmacokinetics

Tablets are from 33–55% bioavailable. **Onset:** 1 hr. **Time to peak plasma levels:** About 8 hr. **Therapeutic plasma levels:** 20–30 ng/mL. Food increases the C_{max} and AUC. **Duration:** 12–24 hr. **t½, elimination:** About 18 hr for tablets and 32 hr for capsules. Metabolized mainly by CYP3A4 and CYP1A2. Inactive metabolites are excreted in the urine. **Plasma protein binding:** Highly bound.

CONTRAINDICATIONS

Hypersensitivity. Arrhythmias, heart block or conduction disturbances, CHF, or during acute recovery phase of MI. Hyperthyroidism. Concomitant use of MAOIs or within 14 days of their discontinuation; hyperpyretic crisis seizures and death may result if used together. Treatment of spastic diseases or cerebral palsy. Moderate to severe hepatic impairment.

SPECIAL CONCERNS

C

- **Safety in children under age 15 has not established.**
- **Due to atropine-like effects, use with caution where cholinergic blockade is not desired (e.g., history of urinary retention, angle-closure glaucoma, increased intraocular pressure).**
- **Geriatric clients may be more sensitive to cholinergic blockade.**
- **Use with caution in mild hepatic impairment and during lactation.**

SIDE EFFECTS

Most Common

Drowsiness, dizziness, dry mouth, confusion, nausea, constipation, dyspepsia, unpleasant taste, headache, fatigue.

Since cyclobenzaprine resembles tricyclic antidepressants, side effects to these drugs should also be noted. **GI:** Dry mouth, N&V, constipation, dyspepsia, unpleasant taste, anorexia, diarrhea, GI pain, gastritis, thirst, flatulence, ageusia, dysgeusia, paralytic ileus, discoloration/edema of tongue, stomatitis, parotid swelling, dry throat, unpleasant taste. **Hepatic:** Abnormal liver function; rarely, cholestasis, hepatitis, jaundice. **CNS:** Drowsiness, dizziness, fatigue, asthenia, blurred vision, nervousness, headache, somnolence, fatigue/tiredness, disturbance in attention, ***convulsions***, ataxia, vertigo, dysarthria, paresthesia, hypertonia, tremors, malaise, abnormal gait, delusions, Bell's palsy, alteration in EEG patterns, extrapyramidal symptoms. Psychiatric symptoms include: Confusion, insomnia, disorientation, depressed mood, abnormal sensations, anxiety, agitation, abnormal thinking or dreaming, excitement, hallucinations, psychosis. **CV:** Tachycardia, syncope, ***arrhythmias***, vasodilation, palpitations, hypotension, edema, chest pain, hypertension, MI, heart block, stroke. **GU:** Urinary frequency or retention, impaired urination, dilation of urinary tract, impotence, decreased or increased libido, testicular swelling, gynecomastia, breast enlargement, galactorrhea. **Dermatologic:** Sweating, skin rashes, pruritus, photosensitivity, alopecia, acne. **Musculoskeletal:** Muscle twitching, weakness, myalgia. **Hematologic:** Purpura, bone marrow depression, leukopenia, eosinophilia, thrombocytopenia. **Hepatic:** Abnormal liver function, hepatitis, jaundice, cholestasis. **Ophthalmic:** Diplopia, blurred vision. **Hypersensitivity:** ***Anaphylaxis***, angioedema, pruritus, facial edema, urticaria, rash. **Body as a whole:** Local weakness, malaise, sweating. **Miscellaneous:** Tinnitus, peripheral neuropathy, increase and decrease of blood sugar, weight gain or loss, inappropriate ADH syndrome, dyspnea.

OVERDOSE MANAGEMENT

Symptoms: Temporary confusion, dizziness, disturbed concentration, transient visual hallucinations, agitation, hyperactive reflexes, muscle rigidity, vomiting, ***hyperpyrexia.*** Also, drowsiness, hypothermia, tachycardia, hypertension, nausea, slurred speech, tremor, ***cardiac arrhythmias such as bundle branch block, ECG evidence of impaired conduction***, CHF, dilated pupils, ***seizures, severe hypotension, cardiac arrest, neuroleptic malignant syndrome***, chest pain, stupor, ***coma***, paradoxical diaphoresis, ECG changes. *Treatment:* In addition to the treatment outlined for skeletal muscle relaxants, physostigmine salicylate, 1–3 mg IV may be used to reverse symptoms of severe cholinergic blockade; however, profound bradycardia and asystole may occur.

DRUG INTERACTIONS

NOTE: Because of the similarity of cyclobenzaprine to tricyclic antidepressants, the drug interactions for tricyclics should also be consulted.

Anticholinergics / Additive anticholinergic side effects
CNS depressants / Additive depressant effects
Guanethidine / Cyclobenzaprine may block effect of guanethidine and similar drugs
MAOIs / Hyperpyretic crisis seizures and death are possible; do not use together or within 14 days of their discontinuation
Tramadol / ↑ Seizure risk
Tricyclic antidepressants / Additive side effects

HOW SUPPLIED

Capsules, Extended-Release: 15 mg, 30 mg; ***Tablets:*** 5 mg, 7.5 mg, 10 mg.

DOSAGE

CAPSULES, EXTENDED-RELEASE

Skeletal muscle disorders.

Adults: 15 mg once daily. Some may require 30 mg/day given once daily or 15 mg 2 times per day.

TABLETS

Skeletal muscle disorders.

Adults: 5 mg 3 times per day. Depending on client response, may be increased to either 7.5 or 10 mg 3 times per day. Doses of 5 mg produce less sedation.

NURSING IMPLICATIONS

Do not confuse cyclobenzaprine with cyproheptadine (an antihistamine).

IMPLEMENTATION/ADMINISTRATION/STORAGE

1. Use only for 2–3 weeks.
2. If taking an MAOI, do not administer cyclobenzaprine for at least 2 weeks after discontinuing.
3. Store from 15–30°C (59–86°F).

ASSESSMENT

1. List reasons for therapy, extent of acute or painful musculoskeletal condition, DTRs, ROM, degree of stiffness, and evidence of weakness. Review RICE (rest, ice, compression, and elevation) with acute injury to reduce swelling and recovery time.
2. Note any hypersensitivity or spastic diseases.
3. Check for evidence of cardiac arrhythmias; note history of MI.
4. With injury/fall, assess need for x-rays.
5. Obtain ECG, CBC, and LFTs.

CLIENT/FAMILY TEACHING

1. Take as directed; at about the same times each day. Moist heat, gentle stretching, and PT may help during the recovery phase; do not rush. Avoid lifting or exercising too soon; may damage muscles further.
2. Due to drug-induced drowsiness, dizziness, and/or blurred vision, observe caution if performing activities that require mental alertness. Rise slowly from a sitting or standing position to avoid injury.
3. Report any unusual fatigue, sore throat, fever, easy bruising/bleeding; S&S of blood dyscrasia. Nausea or abdominal pain, itchy skin, or evidence of yellow sclera or skin; S&S of hepatic toxicity. Blurred vision, dizziness, tachycardia, constipation, or urinary retention should be reported.
4. Take frequent sips of water, suck on ice chips/sugarless hard candy, or chew sugarless gum for dry mouth symptoms. Avoid alcohol during therapy.
5. Keep all F/U to assess response, and adverse SE.

OUTCOMES/EVALUATE

- ↑ ROM
- Relief of musculoskeletal spasms/pain

IV

Cyclosporine

(sye-kloh-**SPOR**-een)

Classification(s): Immunosuppressant

Pregnancy Category: C

RX: Gengraf, Neoral, Restasis, Sandimmune.

✤ **Rx:** Sandimmune IV, Sandoz Cyclosporine.

INDICATIONS/USES

(1) Prophylaxis of rejection in kidney, liver, and heart allogeneic transplants. Sandimmune is always to be taken with adrenal corticosteroids while Neoral or Gengraf have been used in combination with azathioprine and corticosteroids. (2) **Sandimmune:** Treatment of chronic rejection in clients previously treated with other immunosuppressants. Sandimmune has been used in children as young as 6 months with no unusual side effects. (3) **Neoral or Gengraf:** Severe, active rheumatoid arthritis, which has not responded to methotrexate alone. Neoral and Gengraf may be used with methotrexate in RA clients who do not respond adequately to methotrexate alone. (4) **Neoral or Gengraf:** Adult, nonimmunocompromised clients with severe (i.e., extensive and/or disabling) recalcitrant, plaque psoriasis who have failed to respond to at least 1 systemic therapy (e.g., PUVA, retinoids, methotrexate) or in those for whom other systemic therapies are contraindicated or cannot be tolerated. (5) **Restasis:** Increase tear production where tear production is presumed to be suppressed due to ocular inflammation associated with keratoconjunctivitis sicca.

ACTION/KINETICS

Action

Thought to act by inhibiting the immunocompetent lymphocytes in the G_0 or G_1 phase of the cell cycle. T-lymphocytes are specifically inhibited; both the T-helper cell and the T-suppressor cell may be affected. Also inhibits interleukin 2 or

T-cell growth factor production and release. Absorption from the GI tract is incomplete and variable. Children often require larger PO doses than adults, which may be due to the smaller absorptive surface area of their intestines.

C

Pharmacokinetics

Peak plasma levels: 3.5 hr. Food may both delay and impair drug absorption. **t½:** Approximately 19 hr for adults and 7 hr in children. Metabolized by the liver; inactive metabolites are excreted mainly through the bile. Neoral immediately forms a microemulsion in an aqueous environment. This product has better bioequivalency; thus, Sandimmune and Neoral are not bioequivalent and cannot be used interchangeably without medical supervision. **Time to peak blood levels:** 1.5–2 hr. Food decreases the amount of drug absorbed.

CONTRAINDICATIONS

Hypersensitivity to cyclosporine or polyoxyethylated castor oil. Lactation. Use of potassium-sparing diuretics. Neoral in psoriasis or rheumatoid arthritis with abnormal renal function, uncontrolled hypertension, or malignancies. Neoral together with PUVA or UVB in psoriasis. Use in psoriasis if client is taking other immunosuppressive drugs or radiation therapy. Use of the ophthalmic emulsion with active ocular infections. Administration of the ophthalmic emulsion in those wearing contact lenses.

SPECIAL CONCERNS

■ (1) Only physicians experienced in immunosuppression therapy and management of organ transplant clients should prescribe cyclosporine. Manage clients in facilities equipped and staffed with adequate lab and supportive medical resources. The physician responsible for maintenance therapy should have complete information necessary for client follow-up. (2) Give Sandimmune with adrenal corticosteroids but not with other immunosuppressants as there is increased susceptibility to infection and possible development of lymphoma from immunosuppression. (3) Neoral and Gengraf may increase susceptibility to infection and the development of neoplasia. In kidney, liver, and heart transplant clients, Gengraf and Neoral may be given with other immunosuppressive agents. Increased susceptibility to infection and possible development of lymphoma and other neoplasms may result from the increase in the degree of immunosuppression in transplant clients. (4) Oral absorption during chronic Sandimmune use is erratic. Monitor cyclosporine blood levels during PO therapy at repeated intervals, and make dosage adjustments to avoid toxicity or possible organ rejection. This is especially important in liver transplants. (5) Sandimmune capsules and oral solution have decreased bioavailability compared with Neoral capsules, Neoral oral solution, Gengraf capsules, and Gengraf oral solution. Gengraf and Neoral are not bioequivalent to Sandimmune and cannot be used interchangeably without physician approval. For a given trough concentration, cyclosporine exposure will be greater with Neoral and Gengraf than with Sandimmune. If a client receiving exceptionally high doses of Sandimmune is converted to Neoral or Gengraf, exercise particular caution. Monitor cyclosporine blood levels in transplant and rheumatoid arthritis clients taking Gengraf and Neoral to minimize possible organ rejection due to high concentrations. Make dose adjustments in transplant clients to minimize possible organ rejection due to low concentrations. Comparison of blood concentrations in the published literature with blood concentrations obtained using current assays must be done with detailed knowledge of the assays used. (6) Psoriasis clients previously treated with PUVA and to a lesser extent, methotrexate or other immunosuppressants, UVB, coal tar, or radiation therapy are at increased risk of developing skin malignancies when taking Neoral or Gengraf. (7) In recommended doses cyclosporine can cause systemic hypertension and nephrotoxicity. Risk increases with increasing dose and duration of cyclosporine therapy. Renal dysfunction, including structural kidney damage, is a potential consequence of therapy; monitor renal function during therapy. ■

- **Use with caution with impaired renal or hepatic function.**
- **Clients with malabsorption may not achieve therapeutic levels following PO use.**
- **Use the ophthalmic product with caution during lactation.**

- **Safety and efficacy have not been established in children.**

SIDE EFFECTS

Most Common

After systemic use: Renal dysfunction, hypertension, hirsutism, tremor, gum hyperplasia, diarrhea, paresthesia, seizures, acne, N&V.
After ophthalmic use: Ocular burning.

Systemic use. GI: N&V, diarrhea, gum hyperplasia, anorexia, gastritis, hiccoughs, peptic ulcer, abdominal discomfort, UGI bleeding, pancreatitis, constipation, mouth sores, swallowing difficulty. **Hematologic:** Leukopenia, lymphoma, thrombocytopenia, anemia, microangiopathic hemolytic anemia syndrome. **Allergic:** ***Anaphylaxis (rare).*** **CV:** Hypertension, edema, chest pain, cramps, ***MI*** (rare). **CNS:** Headache, tremor, confusion, fever, ***seizures***, anxiety, depression, weakness, lethargy, ataxia. **GU:** Renal dysfunction, glomerular capillary thrombosis, nephrotoxicity. **Dermatologic:** Acne, hirsutism, brittle fingernails, hair breaking, pruritus. **Miscellaneous:** Hepatotoxicity, flushing, paresthesia, sinusitis, gynecomastia, conjunctivitis, hearing loss, tinnitus, muscle pain, infections (including fungal, viral), *Pneumocystis carinii* pneumonia, hematuria, blurred vision, weight loss, joint pain, night sweats, tingling, tremor, hypomagnesemia in some clients with seizures, infectious complications, increased risk of cancer. **Ophthalmic use.** Ocular burning, conjunctival hyperemia, discharge, epiphora, eye pain, foreign body sensation, pruritus, stinging, visual blurring.

LABORATORY TEST CONSIDERATIONS

↑ Serum creatinine, potassium, BUN, total bilirubin, alkaline phosphatase. Possibly ↑ cholesterol, LDL, and apolipoprotein B. Hyperglycemia/hyperkalemia/hyperuricemia.

OVERDOSE MANAGEMENT

Symptoms: Transient hepatotoxicity and nephrotoxicity. *Treatment:* Induction of vomiting (up to 2 hr after ingestion). General supportive measures.

DRUG INTERACTIONS

Allopurinol / ↑ Cyclosporine levels
Aminoglycosides / ↑ Risk of nephrotoxicity
Amiodarone / ↑ Cyclosporine blood levels → ↑ risk of nephrotoxicity
Amphotericin B / ↑ Risk of nephrotoxicity
Androgens / ↑ Cyclosporine blood levels → possible nephrotoxicity
Azathioprine / ↑ Immunosuppression R/T suppression of lymphocytes → possible infection and malignancy
Bosentan / ↑ Bosentan trough levels → ↑ risk of toxicity; ↓ cyclosporine plasma levels
Bromocriptine / ↑ Cyclosporine plasma level R/T ↓ liver breakdown
Bupropion / Possible ↓ cyclosporine levels; ↑ cyclosporine dose
Calcium channel blockers / ↑ Cyclosporine plasma levels R/T ↓ liver breakdown; ↑ risk of toxicity
Carbamazepine / ↓ Cyclosporine plasma level R/T ↑ liver breakdown
Carvedilol / ↑ Cyclosporine blood levels → possible nephrotoxicity and neurotoxicity
Chloramphenicol / ↑ Cyclosporine blood levels in renal transplant clients
Cimetidine / ↑ Risk of nephrotoxicity
Clarithromycin / ↑ Cyclosporine plasma levels R/T ↓ liver breakdown; ↑ risk of nephro-/neurotoxicity
Clindamycin / ↓ Cyclosporine serum levels
CMV-IVIG / ↑ Risk of reversible acute kidney failure
Colchicine / Severe side effects, including GI, hepatic, renal, and neuromuscular toxicity; ↑ Risk of nephrotoxicity
Corticosteroids / ↑ Immunosuppression R/T suppression of lymphocytes → possible infection and malignancy
Cyclophosphamide / ↑ Immunosuppression R/T suppression of lymphocytes → possible infection and malignancy
Danazol / ↑ Cyclosporine plasma levels R/T ↓ liver breakdown
Diclofenac / ↑ Risk of nephrotoxicity; also, doubling of diclofenac blood levels
Digoxin / ↑ Digoxin levels R/T ↓ clearance; also, ↓ volume of distribution of digoxin → toxicity
Diltiazem / ↑ Cyclosporine plasma levels R/T ↓ liver breakdown → possible nephrotoxicity
H ***Echinacea*** / Do not give with cyclosporine
Erythromycin / ↑ Cyclosporine plasma levels R/T ↓ liver breakdown and ↓ biliary excretion → possible nephrotoxicity
Etoposide / ↓ Etoposide renal clearance → increased toxicity

Fluconazole / ↑ Cyclosporine plasma levels R/T ↓ gut and liver metabolism → possible nephrotoxicity
Fluoroquinolones / ↑ Cyclosporine toxicity possible
Foscarnet / ↑ Risk of renal failure
Ganciclovir / Additive nephrotoxicity and myelosuppression
Grapefruit juice / ↑ Cyclosporine blood levels due to ↓ liver breakdown
Griseofulvin / ↓ Cyclosporine levels → ↓ effect
HIV protease inhibitors / ↑ Cyclosporine plasma levels R/T ↓ liver breakdown → toxicity
Imipenem-cilastatin / ↑ CNS effects of both drugs
Isoniazid / ↓ Cyclosporine plasma levels R/T ↑ liver breakdown
Itraconazole / ↑ Plasma levels of cyclosporine R/T ↓ liver breakdown
Ketoconazole / ↑ Cyclosporine plasma levels R/T ↓ breakdown by gut and liver metabolism → possible nephrotoxicity
Lovastatin / ↑ Risk of myopathy and rhabdomyolysis R/T↓ cyclosporine breakdown
Melphalan / ↑ Risk of nephrotoxicity
Methotrexate / ↑ Methotrexate plasma levels and AUC perhaps R/T ↓ metabolism
Methylphenidate / Possible ↑ cyclosporine levels; ↓ cyclosporine dose
Methylprednisolone / ↑ Cyclosporine blood levels R/T ↓ liver breakdown → toxicity
Metoclopramide / ↑ Cyclosporine plasma levels R/T ↓ liver breakdown → toxicity
Micafungin / ↑ Cyclosporine single-dose whole-blood levels and ↓ cyclosporine PO clearance after single-dose and steady-state administration of micafungin
Mycophenolate / Possible ↑ Mycophenolate side effects if cyclosporine discontinued
Naproxen / ↑ Risk of nephrotoxicity
Nephrotoxic drugs / Additive nephrotoxicity
Nicardipine / ↑ Cyclosporine plasma levels R/T ↓ liver breakdown → possible nephrotoxicity
Nifedipine / ↑ Risk of gingival hyperplasia
Octreotide / ↓ Cyclosporine plasma levels R/T ↑ liver breakdown
Oral contraceptives / ↑ Cyclosporine plasma levels R/T ↓ liver breakdown; possible severe hepatotoxicity
Orlistat / Possible ↓ cyclosporine blood levels R/T ↓ absorption
Phenobarbital / ↓ Cyclosporine plasma levels R/T ↑ liver breakdown
Phenytoin / ↓ Cyclosporine plasma levels R/T ↑ liver breakdown
Probucol / ↓ Cyclosporine bioavailability → ↓ clinical effect
H ***Quercetin (in apples, berries, ginkgo, grapefruit, onions, red wine, and tea)*** / ↑ Cyclosporine bioavailability, AUC, and peak levels
Quinupristin/Dalfopristin / ↑ Cyclosporine blood levels
Ranitidine / ↑ Risk of nephrotoxicity
Repaglinide / ↑ Repaglinide peak serum levels R/T inhibition of hepatic metabolism
Rifabutin/Rifampin / ↓ Cyclosporine plasma levels R/T ↑ liver breakdown
Saquinavir / ↑ Cyclosporine blood levels
Simvastatin / ↑ Risk of myopathy and rhabdomyolysis R/T ↓ cyclosporine breakdown
H ***St. John's wort*** / Possible induction of liver enzymes → ↓ cyclosporine effect
Sulfamethoxazole and/or trimethoprim / ↑ Risk of nephrotoxicity; also, ↓ cyclosporine serum levels → possible organ rejection
Sulindac / ↑ Risk of nephrotoxicity
Tacrolimus / ↑ Risk of nephrotoxicity
Vancomycin / ↑ Risk of nephrotoxicity
Verapamil / ↑ Immunosuppression

HOW SUPPLIED

Capsules, Soft Gelatin: 25 mg, 50 mg, 100 mg; ***Capsules, Soft Gelatin for Microemulsion:*** 25 mg, 100 mg; ***Injection:*** 50 mg/mL; ***Ophthalmic Emulsion:*** 0.05%; ***Oral Solution:*** 100 mg/mL.

DOSAGE

CAPSULES; ORAL SOLUTION

Allogeneic transplants.

Adults and children, initial: A single 15 mg/kg dose given 4–12 hr before transplantation; there is a trend to use lower initial doses of 10–14 mg/kg/day. The dose should be continued postoperatively for 1–2 weeks followed by 5% decrease in dose per week to maintenance dose of 5–10 mg/kg/day (some have used a dose of 3 mg/kg/day successfully). Compared with Sandimmune, lower maintenance doses of Neoral may be sufficient.

If converting from Sandimmune to Neoral, start with a 1:1 conversion. Then, adjust the Neoral dose to reach the pre-conversion cyclosporine blood trough levels. Until this level is reached, monitor the cyclosporine trough level q 4–7 days.

Rheumatoid arthritis (Neoral only).

Initial: 1.25 mg/kg twice a day PO. Salicylates, NSAIDs, and PO corticosteroids may be continued. If sufficient beneficial effect is not seen and the client is tolerating the medication, the dose may be increased by 0.5–0.75 mg/kg/day after 8 weeks and again after 12 weeks to a maximum dose of 4 mg/kg/day. If no benefit is seen after 16 weeks, discontinue therapy. If Neoral is combined with methotrexate, the same initial dose and dose range of Neoral can be used.

Psoriasis (Neoral only).

Initial: 1.25 mg/kg twice a day PO. Maintain this dose for 4 weeks if tolerated. If significant improvement is not seen, increase the dose at 2-week intervals. Based on client response, make dose increases of about 0.5 mg/kg/day to a maximum of 4 mg/kg/day. Discontinue treatment if beneficial effects cannot be achieved after 6 weeks at 4 mg/kg/day. Once beneficial effects are seen, decrease the dose (doses less than 2.5 mg/kg/day may be effective). To control side effects, make dose decreases by 25–50% at any time.

IV (ONLY IN CLIENTS UNABLE TO TAKE PO MEDICATION)

Allogeneic transplants.

Adults: 5–6 mg/kg/day 4–12 hr prior to transplantation and postoperatively until client can be switched to PO dosage. *NOTE:* Steroid therapy must be used concomitantly.

Investigational uses.

Oral doses ranging from 1 to 10 mg/kg/day.

OPHTHALMIC SOLUTION

Keratoconjunctivitis sicca.

1 gtt twice a day in each eye about 12 hr apart.

NURSING IMPLICATIONS

Do not confuse cyclosporine with cyclophosphamide (an antineoplastic) or with cycloserine (an antineoplastic).

IMPLEMENTATION/ADMINISTRATION/STORAGE

1. Sandimmune and Neoral are not bioequivalent and should not be used interchangeably without the supervision of someone experienced in immunosuppressive therapy. Conversion from Neoral to Sandimmune using a 1:1 ratio (mg/kg/day) may result in lower cyclosporine blood levels.
2. Sandimmune capsules and oral solution are bioequivalent. Neoral capsules and oral solution are bioequivalent.
3. May dilute the PO solution with milk, chocolate milk, orange, or apple juice immediately before administering. Dilute Neoral, preferably, with orange or apple juice; grapefruit juice affects metabolism of cyclosporine and is not to be used. After removal of the protective cover, transfer the solution, using the dosing syringe supplied, to a glass of diluent. Stir well and drink at once. Do not allow diluted solution to stand before drinking. Use a glass container (not plastic). Rinse the glass with more diluent and swallow to ensure the total dose is taken. Do not store PO solutions in the refrigerator; contents should be used within 2 months after being opened.
4. At temperatures less than 20°C (68°F), Neoral solution may gel; light flocculation or the formation of a light sediment may also occur. This will not affect product performance or dosing using the syringe provided. Allow to warm to room temperature to reverse such changes.
5. Due to variable absorption of the PO solution, monitor blood levels.
6. Clients with malabsorption from the GI tract may not achieve appropriate blood levels.
7. The ophthalmic emulsion can be used with artificial tears; allow a 15 min interval between use of products.
8. IV Reserve the injection for those unable to take the soft gelatin capsules or oral solution.
9. Dilute IV concentrate 1 mL (50 mg) in 20–100 mL 0.9% NaCl or D5W injection; give infusion slowly over 2–6 hr. Do not refrigerate

C

once cyclosporine has been added to an IV solution.
10. Following addition to an IV solution, shake vigorously to disperse the drug.
11. Protect IV solution from light.
12. The polyoxyethylated castor oil found in the concentrate for IV infusion may cause phthalate stripping from PVC.
13. Due to possibility of anaphylaxis, monitor clients receiving IV cyclosporine closely for 30 min at the start of therapy. Have epinephrine (1:1,000) for anaphylaxis.
14. COMPATIBILITY D5W, 0.9% NaCl.
15. INCOMPATIBILITY Administer separately.

ASSESSMENT

1. Note reasons for therapy, clinical presentation, any previous treatments. List drugs prescribed and any potential interactions. Anticipate concomitant administration of adrenal corticosteroids.
2. Differentiate nephrotoxicity from rejection using criteria provided by the manufacturer.
3. Monitor VS, CBC, cyclosporine levels, renal and LFTs. Drug may increase BP, K^+, lipid, and uric acid levels.

CLIENT/FAMILY TEACHING

1. Review importance of following the written guidelines for medication therapy explicitly. Drug must be taken throughout one's lifetime to prevent transplant rejection.
2. Because this drug is so important in preventing rejection, a written list of all possible drug side effects and those that need to be reported will be provided. Do not change brands or switch to another dose form of cyclosporine without provider approval.
3. Taking the drug with food may reduce nausea and GI upset. If PO form is unpalatable, mix with milk or orange juice in a glass container to minimize container adherence. Measure dose accurately and take immediately after mixing.
4. Do not take with grapefruit juice due to biometabolic concerns.
5. Do not stop abruptly; must be discontinued gradually.
6. Record BP, I&O, weights daily. Report any changes or persistent diarrhea and N&V.
7. Avoid crowds and persons with infectious illnesses. Review risk of lymphoproliferative disorders and other malignancies.
8. May increase skin cancer risk; avoid unnecessary exposure to UV light (sunlight, tanning booths) and use sunscreen and protective clothing if exposed.
9. Practice additional reliable nonhormonal contraception (e.g., diaphragm, condom) while taking cyclosporine
10. Use nystatin swish and swallow to prevent development of thrush; perform regular oral care and routine dental exams.
11. May develop acne and hairiness; dermatology referral may be needed.
12. Yellow discoloration of eyes, skin, or stools; fever; S&S of hepatotoxicity require reporting.
13. Report increased fatigue, malaise, unexplained bleeding or bruising, or blood in urine.
14. If using the eye emulsion, wash hands and invert vial a few times to obtain a uniform, white, opaque emulsion. Do not allow tip of dropper bottle to touch eye, eyelid, fingers, or any other surface. Tilt head back; looking up, pull lower eyelid down to form pocket. Instill 1 drop in the pocket, looking downward before closing eye. Compress lacrimal sac for 2 to 3 min. Do not rub eyes.
15. Discard ophthalmic emulsion vial immediately after each use. Do not save vial or contents for future use. May be used simultaneously with artificial tears but allow 15 min between use of products.
16. If contact lenses are worn, remove them prior to using the drug. Lenses may be reinserted 15 min after therapy.
17. Keep all F/U to assess response, labs, and for adverse SE.

OUTCOMES/EVALUATE

- Prevention of organ rejection with kidney, liver, and heart allogeneic transplants
- Treatment of chronic rejection in those previously treated with other immunosuppressive agents
- Cyclosporine trough levels (100–200 ng/mL)
- ↑ Tear production (ocular inflammation R/T keratoconjunctivitis sicca)

IV

Cytomegalovirus immune globulin intravenous, human (CMV-IGIV)

(**sigh**-toh-**meg**-ah-lo-**VIGH**-rus im-**MYOUN GLOB**-you-lin)

Classification(s): Immune globulin

Pregnancy Category: C

RX: CytoGam.

INDICATIONS/USES

(1) Attenuation of primary cytomegalovirus (CMV) disease for kidney transplant recipients who are seronegative for CMV and who receive a kidney from a CMV seropositive donor. (2) With ganciclovir to prevent CMV in clients undergoing liver, lung, pancreas, and heart transplants from CMV-seropositive donors to CMV-seronegative recipients. *NOTE:* There is a 50% decrease in primary CMV disease in renal transplant clients given this product. *Investigational:* Prevention or attenuation of primary CMV disease in immunosuppressed clients of organ transplants (e.g., bone marrow, liver). Also to prevent CMV disease or CMV pneumonia in immunocompromised clients.

ACTION/KINETICS

Action

Obtained from pooled adult human plasma that has been selected for high titers of antibody for CMV. Is purified. When reconstituted, each mL contains 50 mg of immunoglobulin that is primarily IgG with trace amounts of IgA and IgM; albumin is also present. In individuals exposed to CMV, the immune globulin can increase the relevant antibodies to levels that prevent or reduce the incidence of serious CMV disease.

CONTRAINDICATIONS

Use in clients with a history of a prior severe reaction to this product or other human immunoglobulin preparations.

SPECIAL CONCERNS

- **Individuals with selective immunoglobulin (Ig) A deficiency may develop antibodies to IgA and could develop anaphylactic reactions to subsequent administration of blood products that contain IgA.**
- **Use with caution in pre-existing renal insufficiency and in those at an increased risk of developing renal insufficiency (including, but not limited to those with diabetes mellitus, age over 65 years, volume depletion, paraproteinemia, sepsis, and in those receiving known nephrotoxic drugs).**

SIDE EFFECTS

Most Common

During infusion: Nausea, backache, flushing.
At site of injection: Muscle stiffness, pain, tenderness.
Other side effects: Flushing, chills, muscle cramps, fever, N&V, SOB.

Side effects often due to the rate of infusion; adhere closely to the infusion schedule. **GI:** N&V. **Body as a whole:** Flushing, chills, fever. **Respiratory:** SOB. **Musculoskeletal:** Muscle cramps, back pain, backache. **Respiratory:** Wheezing. Hypotension and allergic reactions such as ***angioneurotic edema*** and ***anaphylactic shock*** are possible but have not been observed. **Site of injection:** Muscle stiffness, pain, tenderness.

OVERDOSE MANAGEMENT

Symptoms: Major effects would be those related to volume overload. Also possible are anaphylaxis and a drop in BP. *Treatment:* Stop infusion immediately and have epinephrine and diphenhydramine available for treatment of acute allergic symptoms.

DRUG INTERACTIONS

The antibodies present in this product may interfere with the immune response to live virus vaccines, including measles, mumps, and rubella. Thus, such vaccinations should be deferred until at least 3 months after administration of CMV immune globulin or revaccination may be required.

HOW SUPPLIED

Solution for Injection: 50 ± 10 mg/mL.

DOSAGE

IV

Prevention of rejection of kidney transplants.

The maximum total dose/infusion is 150 mg/kg given according to the following schedule:

C

- Within 72 hr of transplant: 150 mg/kg.
- 2, 4, 6, and 8 weeks after transplant: 100 mg/kg.
- 12 and 16 weeks after transplant: 50 mg/kg.

The rate of infusion for the initial dose is 15 mg/kg per hr. If no side effects occur after 30 min, the rate may be increased to 30 mg/kg per hr. If no side effects occur after a subsequent 30 min period, the dose may be increased to 60 mg/kg per hr at a volume not to exceed 7.5 mL per hr. **This rate of infusion must not be exceeded.** For subsequent doses, the rate of infusion is 15 mg/kg per hr for 15 min. If no side effects occur, increase the rate to 30 mg/kg per hr for 15 min and then increase to a maximum rate of 60 mg/kg per hr at a volume not to exceed 7.5 mL per hr. **This rate of infusion must not be exceeded.**

Prevent rejection in liver, pancreas, lung, or heart transplants.

The maximum recommended total dose per infusion is 150 mg/kg, given according to the following schedule:

- Within 72 hr of transplant: 150 mg/kg
- 2, 4, 6, and 8 weeks after transplant: 150 mg/kg
- 12 and 16 weeks after transplant: 100 mg/kg.

Initially, give IV at 15 mg/kg per hr. If no side effects occur after 30 min, the rate may be increased to 30 mg/kg per hr. If no side effects occur after a subsequent 30 min, the infusion may be increased to 60 mg/kg per hr (do not exceed a volume of 70 mL per hr) or the rate of 15 mg/kg per hr. For subsequent doses, administer at 15 mg/kg per hr for 15 min. If no side effects occur, increase to 30 mg/kg per hr for 15 min and then increase to a maximum rate of 60 mg/kg per hr with a volume not to exceed 70 mL per hr. **This rate of infusion must not be exceeded.** Monitor the client closely during each rate change.

NURSING IMPLICATIONS

IMPLEMENTATION/ADMINISTRATION/STORAGE

1. **IV** The reconstituted solution should be colorless and translucent. Do not use solution if turbid.
2. After removing tab portion of the vial cap, the rubber stopper is cleaned with 70% alcohol or equivalent. Reconstitute the lyophilized powder with 50 mL of sterile water for injection using a double-ended transfer needle or large syringe. When using a double-ended transfer needle, insert one end first into the vial of water. The lyophilized powder is supplied in an evacuated vial; thus, the water should transfer by suction. To avoid foaming, do not shake vial. After water is transferred into the evacuated vial, release the residual vacuum to hasten dissolution. Rotate container gently to wet all the undissolved powder. Allow 30 min for complete dissolution of the powder.
3. This product does not contain a preservative. After reconstitution, enter vial only once; begin the infusion within 6 hr of entering vial and complete within 12 hr.
4. Administer drug through a separate IV line using a constant infusion pump. If not possible, the drug may be "piggybacked" into a pre-existing line that contains either NaCl or one of the following dextrose solutions (with or without NaCl added): 2.5%, 5%, 10%, or 20% dextrose in water. If used with a pre-existing line, do not dilute drug more than 1:2 with any solutions. See *Dosage* for administration guidelines.
5. If minor side effects occur, slow or temporarily interrupt the infusion.
6. Store from 2–8°C (35.6–46.4°F); use within 6 hr after entering the vial and complete within 12 hr of entering the vial.
7. COMPATIBILITY NaCl or one of the following dextrose solutions (with or without NaCl added): 2.5%, 5%, 10%, or 20% dextrose in water.
8. INCOMPATIBILITY Administer through separate line. Gamunex is incompatible with saline; may dilute with D5W if indicated.

ASSESSMENT

1. Document indications for therapy, with transplant note type, location, and date.

2. List any previous experience with human immunoglobulin preparations.
3. Note any IgA deficiency; these clients may experience anaphylactic reactions with subsequent exposures to IgA products. Assess transplant before therapy.
4. Follow infusion dosing schedules carefully and assess closely during each rate change. Monitor VS continuously; if side effects develop (fever, chills, flushing, nausea, back pain), or BP drops, slow/stop infusion and report.
5. Made from human plasma and may contain infectious agents (e.g., viruses) that can cause disease.
6. Have epinephrine available in the event of an acute anaphylactic reaction.
7. Monitor CBC, electrolytes, renal and LFTs.

CLIENT/FAMILY TEACHING

1. Used to help prevent infection by cytomegalovirus in people who receive an organ transplant. If seronegative for CMV and receives a seropositive donor kidney, CMV disease may develop.
2. Drug has been associated with the development of kidney problems, sometimes resulting in kidney failure and/or death. Report decreased urination, sudden weight gain, fluid retention/swelling, or shortness of breath; signs of kidney problems.
3. Rarely, aseptic meningitis syndrome (AMS) has been associated with these products. Immediately report severe headache, neck stiffness, drowsiness, fever, eye sensitivity to light, painful eye movements, nausea or vomiting. Stopping therapy has resulted in resolution of AMS without any lasting problems.
4. Avoid vaccinations for at least 3 months following therapy; may require revaccination. Antibodies in suspension may interfere with immune response to live virus vaccines.
5. In order to prevent transmission of infectious agents/hepatitis virus from one client to another, sterile disposable syringes and needles should be used; do not reuse.
6. Identify support groups that may assist to cope with chronic disease condition.
7. Keep all F/U to assess response, labs, and for adverse SE.

OUTCOMES/EVALUATE

- CMV prophylaxis in renal transplant recipients
- Improved kidney function

D

D

Dabigatran etexilate

(dah-bye-**GAT**-ran)

Classification(s): Anticoagulant, thrombin inhibitor

Pregnancy Category: C

RX: Pradaxa.

INDICATIONS/USES

Reduce the risk of stroke and systemic embolism in nonvalvular atrial fibrillation.

ACTION/KINETICS

Action

Dabigatran is a direct thrombin inhibitor. Because thrombin enables the conversion of fibrinogen to fibrin during coagulation, inhibition of thrombin prevents the development of a thrombus. Free and clot-bound thrombin and thrombin-induced platelet aggregation are inhibited by the drug.

Pharmacokinetics

Dabigatran etexilate mesylate is absorbed as dabigatran etexilate ester. The ester is then hydrolyzed forming dabigatran, which is the active form. Absolute bioavailability is 3–7%. **Maximal plasma levels:** 1 hr in the fasted state. Administration with a high-fat meal delays the time to C_{max} by about 2 hr. The drug may be given with or without food. Metabolized in the liver and after PO use 86% excreted in the feces and 7% in the urine. **t½:** 12–17 hr.

CONTRAINDICATIONS

Serious hypersensitivity (anaphylactoid reaction/shock) to dabigatran. Active pathological bleeding.

D

SPECIAL CONCERNS

- **Consider the risks of bleeding and stroke if using dabigatran in labor and delivery.**
- **Use with caution during lactation.**
- **The risk of bleeding and stroke increase with age but the risk-benefit is favorable in the elderly (as well as all age groups).**
- **Safety and efficacy not determined in children.**

SIDE EFFECTS

Most Common

Bleeding, dyspepsia, nausea, upper abdominal pain, diarrhea.

CV: Bleeding, including intraocular, ***intracranial***, intraspinal, intramuscular, retroperitoneal, intra-articular, pericardial. ***Intracranial hemorrhage***, including ***hemorrhagic stroke***; subarachnoid and subdural bleeds. **GI:** Dyspepsia, nausea, upper abdominal pain, ***GI hemorrhage***, diarrhea, abdominal pain/discomfort, epigastric discomfort, GERD, esophagitis, erosive gastritis, hemorrhagic gastritis, hemorrhagic erosive gastritis, GI ulcer. **Hypersensitivity:** Urticaria, rash, pruritus, allergic edema, ***anaphylactic reaction, anaphylactic shock***.

OVERDOSE MANAGEMENT

Symptoms: Hemorrhagic complications. *Treatment:* There is no antidote available. Initiate appropriate support. Discontinue dabigatran use. Investigate the source of bleeding. Maintain adequate diuresis. The drug is dialyzable (can remove about 60% over 2 hr). Consider surgical hemostasis or the transfusion of fresh frozen plasma or RBCs. If thrombocytopenia is present, consider giving platelet concentrates. Measurement of activated partial thromboplastic time may help guide therapy.

DRUG INTERACTIONS

Amiodarone / Amiodarone, single dose of 600 mg, ↑ dabigatran AUC and C_{max} 58% and 50%, respectively; ↑ exposure mitigated by a 65% ↑ in dabigatran renal clearance; ↑ renal clearance may persist after amiodarone discontinued due to long amiodarone t½

Clopidogrel / ↑ Dabigatran AUC and C_{max} 30% and 40%, respectively, after a loading dose of clopidogrel, 300 to 600 mg; coadministration did not further prolong capillary bleeding times compared with clopidogrel monotherapy; also, ↑ risk of severe bleeding; monitor for S&S of blood loss; discontinue dabigatran in those with active pathologic bleeding

Fibrinolytic therapy (e.g., alteplase) / ↑ Risk of severe bleeding; monitor for S&S of blood loss (↓ hemoglobin, hypotension); discontinue dabigatran in those with active pathologic bleeding

Heparin / ↑ Risk of severe bleeding; monitor for S&S of blood loss (↓ hemoglobin, hypotension); discontinue dabigatran in those with active pathologic bleeding

Ketoconazole / Multiple dose ketoconazole ↑ dabigatran AUC and C_{max} 153% and 149%, respectively

NSAIDs, chronic use (e.g., ibuprofen) / ↑ Risk of severe bleeding; monitor for S&S of blood loss (↓ hemoglobin, hypotension); discontinue dabigatran in those with active pathologic bleeding

Quinidine / ↑ Dabigatran AUC and C_{max} 53% and 56%, respectively

Rifamycins (e.g., rifampin) / ↓ Dabigatran exposure → ↓ efficacy; avoid coadministration

Verapamil / Possible ↑ dabigatran AUC and C_{max}; depends on the verapamil formulation and time of administration

HOW SUPPLIED

Capsules: 75 mg, 150 mg.

DOSAGE

CAPSULES

Stroke/Systemic embolism prevention.

Adults, usual: 150 mg twice a day. If a dose is not taken at the scheduled time, take as soon as possible on the same day. Skip the missed dose if it cannot be taken at least 6 hr before the next scheduled dose. Do not double the dose to make up for a missed dose. Adjust the dose as follows in impaired renal function: **C_{CR} 15–30 mL/min:** 75 mg twice a day; **C_{CR} <15 mL/min or dialysis:** Dosing recommendations not provided.

NURSING IMPLICATIONS

IMPLEMENTATION/ADMINISTRATION/STORAGE

1. **When converting from warfarin to dabigatran, discontinue warfarin and begin dabigatran when the INR is below 2.**

2. When converting from dabigatran to warfarin, adjust the starting time of warfarin based on C_{CR} as follows; For C_{CR} >50 mL/min, start warfarin 3 days before discontinuing dabigatran; for C_{CR} from 31 to 50 mL/min, start warfarin 2 days before discontinuing dabigatran; for C_{CR} from 15 to 30 mL/min, start warfarin 1 day before discontinuing dabigatran; and, for C_{CR} <15 mL/min, no recommendation can be made for dosing.
3. For clients receiving a parenteral anticoagulant, begin dabigatran 0–2 hr before the time that the next dose of the parenteral drug was to have been given or at the time of discontinuation of a continuously administered parenteral drug (e.g., IV unfractionated heparin).
4. For clients currently taking dabigatran, wait 12 hr (if the C_{CR} is 30 mL/min or more) or 24 hr (if the C_{CR} is less than 30 mL/min) after the last dose of dabigatran before starting treatment with a parenteral anticoagulant.
5. If possible, discontinue dabigatran 1–2 days (if C_{CR} is 50 mL/min or more) or 3–5 days (if C_{CR} is <50 mL/min) before invasive or surgical procedures because of the increased risk of bleeding. Consider longer times for those undergoing major surgery, spinal puncture, or placement of a spinal or epidural catheter or port, in whom a complete hemostasis may be required.
6. Store from 15–30°C (59–86°F). Once opened, contents of the bottle must be used within 30 days. Store in the original package to protect from moisture.

ASSESSMENT

1. Note indications for therapy, characteristics of S&S, onset of AF, other agents trialed, outcome.
2. Review list of drugs prescribed to ensure none interact; avoid use with rifampin derivatives.
3. Stop drug therapy 1 to 2 days (C_{CR} 50 mL/min or more) or 3 to 5 days (C_{CR} less than 50 mL/min) before invasive or surgical procedures. Consider longer times for those undergoing major surgery, spinal puncture, or placement of a spinal or epidural catheter or port.
4. If emergency surgery necessary, a bleeding risk can be assessed by the ecarin clotting time (ECT). This test is a better marker of the anticoagulant activity of dabigatran than activated partial thromboplastin time (aPTT). If ECT not available, the aPTT test provides an approximation of Pradaxa anticoagulant activity.
5. Monitor ECG, CBC, INR, PTT and renal function; reduce dose (75 mg twice daily) if C_{CR} 15–30 mL/min.

CLIENT/FAMILY TEACHING

1. Drug is a blood thinner used to reduce the risk of clots forming in body.
2. Swallow capsules whole; do not break, chew, or empty capsule contents. Doing so can result in increased concentrations.
3. If regular dose is missed, take as soon as possible on the same day. If unable to take at least 6 hr before the next regular dose, then it should be skipped. Do not double up dose of Pradaxa to make up for a missed dose.
4. Take with or without food.
5. May experience GI upset, stomach pain, nausea, heartburn, and bloating; report if bothersome or evidence of any unusual bruising, bleeding or bloody secretions/stools.
6. May cause severe bleeding; do not undergo any surgery or dental procedures without provider approval and do not interrupt therapy without approval.
7. Avoid all OTC and prescribed drugs unless medically cleared.
8. Store safely out of child's reach.
9. Practice reliable contraception; long-term effects not known.
10. Keep all F/U to assess response, ECG, labs, adverse SE.

OUTCOMES/EVALUATE

↓ Risk of stroke and systemic embolism with nonvalvular atrial fibrillation

IV

Dacarbazine (DTIC, Imidazole carboxamide)

(dah-**KAR**-bah-zeen)

Classification(s): Antineoplastic, alkylating

Pregnancy Category: C

RX: DTIC-Dome.

SEE ALSO ***ANTINEOPLASTIC AGENTS*** AND ***ALKYLATING AGENTS***.

D

INDICATIONS/USES

(1) Metastatic malignant melanoma. (2) Hodgkin's disease (second-line therapy with other agents). *Investigational:* In combination with cyclophosphamide and vincristine for malignant pheochromocytoma. In combination with other drugs to treat advanced metastatic soft-tissue sarcoma. Alone or in combination with other drugs to manage Kaposi's sarcoma.

ACTION/KINETICS

Action

Exact mechanism of action unknown. May act by three ways: (1) Alkylation by an activated carbonium ion; (2) Antimetabolite to inhibit DNA and RNA synthesis; or (3) Alkylation by combining with protein sulfhydryl groups. Is cell-cycle nonspecific.

Pharmacokinetics

t½, biphasic, initial: 19 min; **terminal:** 5 hr. The t½ is increased to 55 min and 7.2 hr in those with renal and hepatic dysfunction. Probably localizes in liver. Limited amounts (14% of plasma level) enter CSF. Approximately 40% of drug excreted in urine unchanged within 6 hr. Secreted through the kidney tubules rather than filtered through the glomeruli.

CONTRAINDICATIONS

Hypersensitivity to dacarbazine. Lactation.

SPECIAL CONCERNS

■ (1) Administer under the supervision of a qualified physician experienced in the use of cancer chemotherapeutic drugs. (2) Hemopoietic depression is the most common toxic effect. (3) Hepatic necrosis has been reported. (4) The drug is carcinogenic and teratogenic when used in animals. (5) In treating each client, the physician must carefully weigh the possibility of achieving therapeutic benefit against the risk of toxicity. ■

Dosage not established in children.

ADDITIONAL SIDE EFFECTS

Most Common

Leukopenia, thrombocytopenia, anorexia, N&V.

Hematologic: Hemopoietic depression, especially ***leukopenia and thrombocytopenia, which may cause death***. **GI**: N&V (more than 90% of clients within 1 hr after initial administration, which persists for 12–48 hr), anorexia, diarrhea. **Dermatologic**: Erythematous and urticarial rashes, photosensitivity reactions, alopecia, facial flushing, paresthesia. **Miscellaneous**: Flu-like syndrome, including fever, myalgia, and malaise.

Hepatotoxicity (***accompanied by hepatic vein thrombosis and hepatocellular necrosis resulting in death***), hypersensitivity, facial paresthesia, ***anaphylaxis***.

LABORATORY TEST CONSIDERATIONS

↑ AST, ALT, and other enzymes.

OVERDOSE MANAGEMENT

Treatment: Monitor blood cell counts; supportive treatment.

HOW SUPPLIED

Powder for Injection: 100 mg, 200 mg.

DOSAGE

IV ONLY

Malignant melanoma.

2–4.5 mg/kg/day for 10 days; may be repeated at 4-week intervals; or

250 mg/m²/day for 5 days; may be repeated at 3-week intervals.

Hodgkin's disease.

150 mg/m²/day for 5 days in combination with other drugs, and repeated q 4 weeks; or, 375 mg/m² on day 1, with other drugs and repeated q 15 days.

NURSING IMPLICATIONS

IMPLEMENTATION/ADMINISTRATION/STORAGE

1. **IV Avoid extravasation due to the possibility of tissue damage and severe pain.**
2. **Reconstitute under a biologic hood with sterile water for injection: 9.9 mL for the 100 mg vials and 19.7 mL for the 200 mg vials for a final concentration of 10 mg/mL with a pH of 3–4. May give by IV push over 1 min period. May further dilute with 50–250 mL D5W or NaCl injection and given over 30 min.**
3. **Stop infusion immediately with infiltration, and apply ice for 24 to 48 hr.**
4. **Protect dry vials from light and store at 2–8°C (36–46°F).**
5. **Reconstituted solutions stable for up to 72 hr at 4°C (39°F) or for 8 hr at 20°C (68°F). More dilute solutions for IV infusions are sta-**

ble for 24 hr when stored at 2–8°C (36–46°F).

6. Do not use solution that has turned pink.
7. COMPATIBILITY D5W or 0.9% NaCl.
8. INCOMPATIBILITY Administer separately.

ASSESSMENT

1. Note disease onset, staging, other agents trialed.
2. Monitor I&O; ascertain how fluid status is to be handled (fast for 4–6 hr before treatment to reduce emesis or have fluids up to 1 hr before administration to minimize).
3. To reduce GI adverse reactions, restrict food intake for 4 to 6 h prior to treatment if possible.
4. Give antiemetic before and throughout therapy. Have agents available for palliation of vomiting. Assess IV site closely for any evidence of extravasation.
5. Assess for S&S of bacterial, viral, or fungal infection.
6. Monitor client and CBC closely for bone marrow depression, liver or renal toxicity, or hypersensitivity reaction (hepatic necrosis has occurred). Anticipate mild granulocyte toxicity. Nadir: 10 days; recovery: 21 days.

CLIENT/FAMILY TEACHING

1. Used to treat cancer of the lymph system, malignant melanoma (a type of skin cancer) and other types. It interferes with the growth of cancer cells, and destroys them. The growth of normal body cells may also be affected; hence other effects can occur.
2. To minimize GI effects, antiemetics, fasting, and limited fluid intake (4–6 hr preceding treatment) may be ordered. After the first 1–2 days of therapy, vomiting should cease as tolerance develops.
3. Report any unusual bruising/bleeding or flu-like symptoms (fever, aches, fatigue) that may occur. Usually occurs 1 week after treatment and may persist for 1–3 weeks. Acetaminophen may relieve symptoms. Avoid OTC agents including aspirin and NSAIDs.
4. Avoid prolonged exposure to sun or UV light and wear protective clothing; photosensitivity reaction may occur for up to 2 days following therapy.
5. Prepare for hair loss; report any blurred vision or numbness.
6. Practice contraception during and for several months following therapy.
7. Some effects may not occur for months or years after the medicine is used.
8. Keep all F/U to assess response, labs, and for adverse SE.

OUTCOMES/EVALUATE

↓ Tumor size/spread with suppression of malignant cell proliferation

Dalfampridine (4-Aminopyridine)

(dal-**FAM**-prih-deen)

Classification(s): Potassium channel blocker.

Pregnancy Category: C

RX: Ampyra.

INDICATIONS/USES

Improve walking in clients with multiple sclerosis.

ACTION/KINETICS

Action

Mechanism is not fully known. Dalfampridine is a broad-spectrum potassium channel blocker. It may increase conduction of action potentials in demyelinated axons through inhibition of potassium channels.

Pharmacokinetics

Rapidly and completely absorbed from the GI tract. Relative bioavailability is 96%. **Peak plasma levels:** 3–4 hr. May be taken with or without food. Metabolized in the liver mainly by CYP2E1 and parent drug and metabolites excreted in the urine (90.3%). **t½, elimination:** 5.2–6.5 hr. Severely impaired renal function significantly affects the terminal t½. **Plasma protein binding:** Largely unbound.

CONTRAINDICATIONS

Moderate to severe impaired renal function. History of seizures. Use with other forms of 4-aminopyridine. Lactation.

SPECIAL CONCERNS

- Dalfampridine is excreted mainly by the kidneys; because the elderly are more likely to have decreased renal function, know the estimated C_{CR} in these clients.

- Safety and efficacy not determined in children less than 18 years of age.

SIDE EFFECTS

Most Common

UTI, insomnia, asthenia, dizziness, headache, back pain, nausea.

Most side effects listed are those with an incidence of 2% or more. **CNS:** Headache, insomnia, balance disorder, dizziness, confusion, MS relapse, paresthesia, increased incidence of ***seizures.*** **GI:** Nausea, constipation, dyspepsia. **Respiratory:** Nasopharyngitis, pharyngolaryngeal pain. **Musculoskeletal:** Back pain. **GU:** UTI. **Body as a whole:** Asthenia.

HOW SUPPLIED

Tablets, Extended-Release: 10 mg.

DOSAGE

TABLETS, EXTENDED-RELEASE

Multiple sclerosis.

Adults: 10 mg twice a day; **maximum dose:** 20 mg/day.

NURSING IMPLICATIONS

IMPLEMENTATION/ADMINISTRATION/STORAGE

1. The risk of seizures is increased with increasing exposure to dalfampridine. An estimated C_{CR} should be known before beginning dalfampridine therapy.
2. Store from 15–30°C (59–86°F).

ASSESSMENT

1. Note indications for therapy, disease onset, walking speed/distance, degree of gait disorder, and other agents trialed.
2. Determine any seizure disorder; precludes therapy. If seizure occurs during therapy, do not restart drug.
3. Monitor gait, walking speed/distance, and renal function studies (C_{CR}); avoid with dysfunction.

CLIENT/FAMILY TEACHING

1. Take tablets whole; do not divide, crush, chew, or dissolve.
2. May be taken with or without food. Take with food if GI upset.
3. Take doses about 12 hr apart, and do not double up if dose missed. Drug is released slowly over time. If tablet broken, may cause the medicine to be released too fast. This raises chance of seizure occurrence.
4. Stop drug and do not restart therapy if seizure experienced.
5. Avoid all OTC and prescribed drugs without provider approval.
6. May experience headaches, dizziness, insomnia, constipation, back pain, weakness, balance problems, and urinary tract infections. Keep provider advised of all adverse SE.
7. Keep all F/U to assess response, labs, and adverse SE.

OUTCOMES/EVALUATE

Improvement in walking with MS

Dalteparin sodium

(**DAL**-tih-**pair**-in)

Classification(s): Anticoagulant, low molecular weight heparin

Pregnancy Category: B

RX: Fragmin.

SEE ALSO ***HEPARINS, LOW MOLECULAR WEIGHT.***

INDICATIONS/USES

(1) Prevent deep vein thrombosis (DVT) in clients undergoing hip replacement or abdominal surgery who are at risk for thromboembolic complications (i.e., pulmonary embolism). High risk includes obesity, general anesthesia more than 30 min, malignancy, history of DVT or pulmonary embolism, age 40 and over. (2) Prevent DVT in those who are at risk for thromboembolic complications (which may lead to pulmonary embolism) due to severely restricted mobility during acute illness. (3) Prevent ischemic complications due to blood clot formation in life-threatening unstable angina and non-Q-wave MI in clients coadministered aspirin. (4) Extended treatment of symptomatic venous thromboembolism (proximal deep vein thrombosis and/or pulmonary embolism) to reduce the occurrence of venous thromboembolism in clients with cancer. *Investigational:* Primary venous thromboembolism prophylaxis in cancer clients; venous thromboembolism prophylaxis in cancer clients with central venous catheters; in general surgery; or in gynecologic surgery.

ACTION/KINETICS

Pharmacokinetics

About 87% bioavailable. **Peak plasma levels:** 4 hr. **t½, SC:** 3–5 hr. t½ increased in those with chronic renal insufficiency requiring hemodialysis.

ADDITIONAL CONTRAINDICATIONS

IM administration.

SPECIAL CONCERNS

See also *Heparins, Low Molecular Weight*.

(1) **Spinal/epidural hematomas.** When neuraxial anesthesia (spinal/epidural anesthesia) or spinal puncture is employed, those who are anticoagulated or scheduled to be anticoagulated with low molecular weight heparins or heparinoids for prevention of thromboembolic complications are at risk of developing a spinal or epidural hematoma that can result in long-term or permanent paralysis. The risk is increased using indwelling epidural catheters for administering analgesics; the concomitant use of drugs affecting hemastasis, such as NSAIDs, platelet inhibitors, or other anticoagulants; a history of traumatic or repeated epidural or spinal puncture; or a history of spinal deformity, spinal injury, or spinal surgery. (2) Frequently monitor clients for signs and symptoms of neurological impairment. If neurological compromise is noted, urgent treatment is necessary. (3) Consider the potential benefits versus risk before neuraxial intervention in clients anticoagulated or scheduled to be anticoagulated for thromboprophylaxis.

- **The multiple dose vial contains benzyl alcohol that has been associated with a fatal "gasping syndrome" in premature infants.**
- **Use with caution in severe hepatic or renal impairment.**

SIDE EFFECTS

Most Common

Hematomas (injection site, wound), significant bleeding, pruritus/rash, hematuria, allergic reaction, fever, injection site reactions.

CV: Significant bleeding (fatal/nonfatal) from any tissue or organ, hematoma at injection site, wound hematoma, spinal or epidural hematoma, reoperation due to bleeding, postoperational transfusions. **Hematologic:** Thrombocytopenia. **Hypersensitivity:** Allergic reactions, including pruritus, rash, fever, injection site reaction, bullous eruption, maculopapular rash, vesiculobullous rash, bullous eruption, skin necrosis (rare), ***anaphylaxis***. ***Dermatologic:*** Alopecia. **Miscellaneous:** Pain at injection site, hematuria. *NOTE:* Hemorrhagic complications may present as, but not limited to, any of the following: headache; paralysis; paresthesias; chest, abdomen, join, muscle, or other pain; dizziness; shortness of breath or difficulty breathing or swallowing; swelling; weakness; hypotension; shock; coma.

HOW SUPPLIED

Injection: 2,500 international units/0.2 mL (16 mg/0.2 mL); 5,000 international units/0.2 mL (32 mg/0.2 mL); 7,500 international units/0.3 mL (48 mg/0.3 mL); 10,000 international units/0.4 mL or 1 mL (64 mg/0.4mL or 64 mg/1 mL); 12,500 units/0.5 mL (80 mg/0.5 mL); 15,000 units/0.6 mL (96 mg/0.6 mL); 18,000 units/0.72 mL (115.2 mg/0.72 mL); 95,000 units/3.8 mL (160 mg/mL); 95,000 international units/9.5 mL (64 mg/mL).

DOSAGE

SC ONLY

Prevention of deep vein thrombosis (DVT) in abdominal surgery.

Adults: 2,500 international units each day starting 1–2 hr prior to surgery and repeated once daily for 5–10 days postoperatively. **High-risk clients:** 5,000 international units the night before surgery and repeated once daily for 5–10 days postoperatively. **In malignancy:** 2,500 international units 1–2 hr before surgery followed by 2,500 international units 12 hr later and 5,000 international units once daily for 5–10 days postoperatively.

Prevention of DVT following hip replacement surgery.

Adults, preoperative start, day of surgery: 2,500 international units within 2 hr before surgery with a second dose of 2,500 international units 4–8 hr after surgery (or later if hemostasis has not been achieved). This is followed by 5,000 units once daily postoperatively, usually for 5–10 days (up to 14 days was well tolerated). **Adults, preoperative start, evening before surgery:** 5,000 units 10–14 hr before surgery. This is followed by 5,000 units 4–8 hr after surgery (or later if hemostasis has not been achieved). Then, give 5,000 units once daily postoperatively, usually for 5–10 days (up to 14 days was well tolerated). **Adults, postoperative start:** 2,500 units 4–8 hr after surgery (or later if hemostasis has not been achieved). This is followed by 5,000 units once daily postoperatively, usually for 5–10 days (up to 14 days was well tolerated).

Severely restricted mobility during acute illness.

Adults: 5,000 international units once daily for up to 12 to 14 days.

Prevent ischemic complications in unstable angina/non-Q-wave MI.

Adults: 120 international units/kg, not to exceed 10,000 international units q 12 hr with concurrent PO aspirin (75–165 mg/day). Continue treatment until client is clinically stabilized (usually 5–8 days).

Venous thromboembolism in clients with cancer.

First 30 days of treatment: 200 units/kg total body weight once daily, not to exceed 18,000 units per day. **Months 2–6:** Approximately 150 units/kg once daily, not to exceed 18,000 units per day. Safety and efficacy beyond 6 months have not been determined.

Thrombocytopenia in clients with cancer and acute symptomatic venous thromboembolism.

Platelet counts between 50,000 and 100,000/mm^3: Reduce the daily dose by 2,500 units until platelet count recovers to at least 100,000/mm^3. **Platelets less than 50,000/mm^3:** Discontinue dalteparin until platelet count recovers above 50,000/mm^3.

NURSING IMPLICATIONS

IMPLEMENTATION/ADMINISTRATION/STORAGE

1. In clients in extended treatment of symptomatic venous thromboembolism and who have severe impaired renal function (C_{CR} <30 mL/min), monitor for anti-factor Xa levels. Target anti-factor Xa range is 0.5–1.5 units/mL. When monitoring anti-factor Xa in these clients, perform sampling 4–6 hr after dalteparin dosing and only after the client has received 3–4 doses.
2. Available in single-dose prefilled syringes affixed with a 27-gauge × ½-inch needle. Consult the package insert for instructions for using the prefilled single-dose syringes preassembled with needle-guard devices.
3. Before withdrawing drug, inspect vial for particulate matter or discoloration.
4. Do not mix with other infusions or injections unless compatibility data known.
5. To ensure delivery of full dose, do not expel air bubble from prefilled syringe before injection.
6. Store drug at controlled room temperature of 20–25°C (68–77°F). After the first penetration of rubber stopper, may store multidose vials at room temperature for up to 2 weeks. Discard any unused drug after 2 weeks.

ASSESSMENT

1. Note reasons for therapy, any evidence of active major bleeding, bleeding disorders, or thrombocytopenia.
2. List sensitivity to heparin or pork products.
3. Identify criteria for inclusion or if at risk for DVT (i.e., over 40, obese, prolonged general anesthesia, additional risk factors).
4. Monitor anticoagulant using anti-factor Xa in those with severe renal dysfunction, if abnormal coagulation parameters, or if bleeding occurs.
5. Monitor CBC with platelets, urinalysis, chemistry, renal function, and FOB during therapy.

CLIENT/FAMILY TEACHING

1. Review reasons for therapy and administration technique. Used to prevent blood clot development after major surgery.
2. Give by deep SC injection while sitting or lying down. May give in a U-shape area around the navel, the upper outer side of the thigh, or the upper outer quadrangle of the buttock. Change/rotate the injection site daily.
3. If the area around the navel or thigh is used, a fold of skin must be lifted, using the thumb and forefinger, while giving the injection.

4. Insert the entire length of the needle at a 45–90° angle.
5. Avoid OTC aspirin-containing products. Use electric razor and soft toothbrush to prevent tissue trauma.
6. Report any unusual bruising/bleeding or hemorrhage. Therapy may last for 5–10 days.
7. Keep all F/U to assess response, labs, and for adverse SE.

OUTCOMES/EVALUATE

Post-operative DVT prophylaxis

Danazol

(**DAN**-ah-zohl)

Classification(s): Androgen, synthetic

Pregnancy Category: X

✤ **Rx:** Cyclomen.

INDICATIONS/USES

(1) Endometriosis amenable to hormonal management in clients who cannot tolerate or who have not responded to other drug therapy. (2) Fibrocystic breast disease. (3) Hereditary angioedema in males and females. *Investigational:* Gynecomastia, menorrhagia, precocious puberty, idiopathic immune thrombocytopenia, lupus-associated thrombocytopenia, and autoimmune hemolytic anemia.

ACTION/KINETICS

Action

Inhibits the release of gonadotropins (FSH and LH) by the anterior pituitary; thus, inhibits synthesis of sex steroids and competitively inhibits binding of steroids to their cytoplasmic receptors in target tissues. In women this action arrests ovarian function, induces amenorrhea, and causes atrophy of normal and ectopic endometrial tissue. Has weak androgenic effects.

Pharmacokinetics

Onset, fibrocystic disease: 4 weeks. **Time to peak effect, amenorrhea and anovulation:** 6–8 weeks; **fibrocystic disease:** 2–3 months to eliminate breast pain and tenderness and 4–6 months for elimination of nodules. **t½:** 4.5 hr. **Duration:** Ovulation and cyclic bleeding usually resume 60–90 days after cessation of therapy.

CONTRAINDICATIONS

Undiagnosed genital bleeding; markedly impaired hepatic, renal, and cardiac function; porphyria; pregnancy and lactation.

SPECIAL CONCERNS

(1) Use contraindicated in pregnancy. A sensitive test (e.g., beta subunit test, if available) capable of determining early pregnancy is recommended immediately prior to starting therapy. Also, a nonhormonal method of contraception should be used during therapy. If the client becomes pregnant while taking danazol, discontinue the drug and advise the client of the potential risk to the fetus.
(2) Thromboembolism, thrombotic and thrombophlebitic events, including sagittal sinus thrombosis and life-threatening or fatal strokes have been reported. (3) Experience with long-term danazol therapy is limited. Long-term use has resulted in peliosis hepatitis and benign adenoma; these may be silent until complicated by acute, potentially life-threatening intra-abdominal hemorrhage. Attempt to determine the lowest dose that will provide adequate protection. (4) Drug has been associated with several cases of benign intracranial hypertension. Early signs include papilledema, headache, N&V, and visual disturbances. Screen clients with these symptoms for papilledema and, if present, advise client to discontinue the drug immediately and refer to a neurologist for further diagnosis and care.

- Use with caution in children treated for hereditary angioedema due to the possibility of virilization in females and precocious sexual development in males.
- Use with caution in conditions aggravated by fluid retention (e.g., epilepsy, migraine, cardiac, or renal dysfunction).
- Elderly may have an increased risk of prostatic hypertrophy or prostatic carcinoma.

SIDE EFFECTS

Most Common

Headache, dizziness, fatigue, appetite changes, GI upset, anxiety, bloating, vaginal dryness, mood changes, hot flashes.

Androgenic: Acne, edema, mild hirsutism, seborrhea, decrease in breast size, oily hair/skin, weight

D

gain, deepening of voice and hair growth, clitoral hypertrophy, testicular atrophy. **Estrogen deficiency:** Flushing, sweating, vaginitis, vaginal dryness/irritation, decreased breast size, nervousness, changes in emotions, hot flashes. **GU**: Menstrual disturbances (e.g., spotting), alteration of the timing cycle, amenorrhea (may be persistent), abnormalities in semen volume, viscosity, sperm count, and motility with long-term use. **GI**: N&V, constipation, gastroenteritis, GI upset. **Hepatic**: Jaundice, dysfunction, peliosis hepatitis and benign hepatic adenoma (***intra-abdominal hemorrhage possible***) with long-term use. **CV**: ***Thromboembolism***, thrombotic and thrombophlebitic events including sagittal sinus thrombosis and ***life-threatening or fatal strokes***. **CNS**: Fatigue, tremor, headache, dizziness, mood changes, sleep problems, paresthesia of extremities, anxiety, depression, appetite changes, pseudotumor cerebri. **Musculoskeletal**: Muscle cramps or spasms, joint swelling or lock-up, pain in back, legs, or neck. **Miscellaneous**: Allergic reactions (skin rashes and rarely nasal congestion), hematuria, increased BP, chills, pelvic pain, carpal tunnel syndrome, hair loss, change in libido.

LABORATORY TEST CONSIDERATIONS

↓ HDL and ↑ LDL (temporary but may be severe). Interference with lab determinations of testosterone, androstenedione, and dehydroepiandrosterone.

DRUG INTERACTIONS

Carbamazepine / ↑ Carbamazepine levels
Cyclosporine / ↑ Cyclosporine blood levels → possible nephrotoxicity
Insulin / ↑ Insulin requirements
Warfarin / ↑ PT in warfarin-stabilized clients

HOW SUPPLIED

Capsules: 50 mg, 100 mg, 200 mg.

DOSAGE

CAPSULES

Endometriosis.

400 mg twice a day (moderate to severe) or 100–200 mg twice a day (mild) for 3–6 months (up to 9 months may be required in some clients). Begin therapy during menses, if possible, to be sure that client is not pregnant.

Fibrocystic breast disease.

50–200 mg twice a day beginning on day 2 of menses. Begin therapy during menses to ensure client is not pregnant.

Hereditary angioedema.

Initial: 200 mg 2–3 times per day; after desired response, decrease dosage by 50% (or less) at 1–3-month intervals. Treat subsequent attacks by doses up to 200 mg/day. No more than 800 mg/day should be given to adults.

NURSING IMPLICATIONS

Do not confuse Danazol with Dantrium (a skeletal muscle relaxant).

IMPLEMENTATION/ADMINISTRATION/STORAGE

Breast pain and tenderness in fibrocystic disease are usually relieved within 30 days and eliminated in 2–3 months; elimination of nodularity requires 4–6 months of uninterrupted therapy. Treatment may be reinstituted if symptoms recur (50% have recurring symptoms within 6 months).

ASSESSMENT

1. Note reasons for therapy. Assess reports of endometrial pain, breast pain, tenderness, and the presence of any nodules. Perform regular breast exams. Exclude breast carcinoma before initiating therapy for fibrocystic disease.
2. Determine any undiagnosed vaginal bleeding; note onset, frequency, extent, and precipitating factors.
3. CTS may develop due to drug-induced edema with compression of median nerve.
4. Assess for early signs of intracranial hypertension (e.g., headache, nausea, vomiting, visual disturbances).
5. Identify factors that trigger angioedema (e.g., C-1 inhibitor deficiency).
6. Obtain baseline CBC, renal and LFTs; determine if pregnant.

CLIENT/FAMILY TEACHING

1. Take with meals to ↓ GI upset.
2. Virilization may occur with drug therapy (e.g., abnormal hair growth, acne, reduced breast size, increased skin oiliness, enlarged clitoris, voice deepening); report so dosage can be adjusted to prevent voice damage. These side

effects usually disappear once drug is discontinued; ovulation will resume in 60–90 days.

3. Wear cotton underwear, and pay careful attention to hygiene to diminish danazol-induced vaginitis.
4. Practice nonhormonal birth control as ovulation may not be suppressed until after 6–8 weeks of therapy; continue breast self-exams and report changes.
5. Clients with a history of epilepsy, migraines, and cardiac or renal dysfunction may develop fluid retention; stop drug and report. Report any early S&S of intracranial hypertension (e.g., headache, nausea, vomiting, visual disturbances).
6. With cystic breast disease, pain and discomfort usually resolve in 2–3 months while nodules take 4–6 months. Endometriosis may recur once the drug is stopped.
7. With long-term therapy, advise peliosis hepatitis and benign hepatic adenoma have occurred as have thrombotic events.
8. Keep all F/U to assess response, labs, and for adverse SE.

OUTCOMES/EVALUATE

- ↓ Endometrial pain (3–6 months)
- ↓ Breast pain (2–3 months)
- Relief angioedema attack (hereditary)

IV

Daptomycin

(**DAP**-toe-my-sin)

Classification(s): Antibiotic, cyclic lipopeptide

Pregnancy Category: B

RX: Cubicin.

INDICATIONS/USES

(1) Treatment of complicated skin and skin structure infections due to the following susceptible strains of gram positive organisms: *Staphylococcus aureus* (including methicillin-resistant strains), *Streptococcus pyogenes, Streptococcus agalactiae, Streptococcus dysgalactiae* subspecies *equisimilis,* and *Enterococcus faecalis* (vancomycin-susceptible strains only). Combination therapy may be used if the documented or presumed pathogens include gram-negative or anaerobic organisms. (2) Treatment of *Staphylococcus aureus* bacteremia, including right-sided infective endocarditis caused by methicillin–susceptible and methicillin–resistant isolates. Combination therapy may be used if the documented or presumed pathogens include gram-negative or anaerobic organisms.

ACTION/KINETICS

Action

Daptomycin is a cyclic lipopeptide that binds to bacterial membranes and causes a rapid depolarization of membrane potential. The loss of membrane potential leads to inhibition of protein, DNA, and RNA synthesis, leading to bacterial cell death. Daptomycin exhibits rapid, concentration-dependent bactericidal activity against gram-positive organisms.

Pharmacokinetics

Steady-state levels are achieved by the third daily dose. It is reversibly bound to human plasma proteins (primarily serum albumin). **t½:** About 8 hr. Site of metabolism of the drug has not been determined. Excreted primarily by the kidney. **Plasma protein binding:** 90–93%.

CONTRAINDICATIONS

Hypersensitivity to daptomycin. Treatment of pneumonia.

SPECIAL CONCERNS

- Dosage adjustment is necessary in clients with severe renal insufficiency (C_{CR} <30 mL/min).
- Mild to life-threatening pseudomembranous colitis may develop.
- To decrease the risk of rhabdomyolysis, temporarily suspend HMG-CoA reductase inhibitors in clients receiving daptomycin.
- Clearance is decreased in clients older than 65 years; this group may experience more side effects.
- Use with caution during lactation.
- Safety and efficacy not determined in children less than 18 years.

SIDE EFFECTS

Most Common

Constipation, N&V, headache, insomnia, diarrhea, rash, injection site reactions.

Side effects listed are for all uses. **GI:** Constipation, N&V, diarrhea, loose stools, dyspepsia, abdominal pain, ***pseudomembranous colitis***, superinfections, abdominal distention, flatulence, stomatitis, dry mouth, epigastric discomfort, gingival pain, oral hypesthesia, jaundice, oral candidiasis,

C. difficile–associated diarrhea. ***GI hemorrhage***. **CNS:** Headache, insomnia, dizziness, anxiety, confusion, vertigo, mental status change, paresthesia, dyskinesia, hallucinations, peripheral neuropathy. **Dermatologic:** Rash (heat, vesicular), pruritus, eczema, increased sweating, ***Stevens-Johnson syndrome***, vesiculobullous rash with or without membrane involvement. **CV:** Hyper-/hypotension, ***cardiac failure/arrest***, supraventricular arrhythmia, atrial fibrillation/flutter. **GU:** Renal failure (including acute), UTI, vaginal candidiasis, proteinuria, impaired renal function, fungal UTI. **Hematologic:** Anemia, leukocytosis, thrombocythemia, thrombocytopenia, thrombocytosis, eosinophilia, lymphadenopathy. **Respiratory:** Dyspnea, cough, sore throat, pneumonia, pharyngolaryngeal pain, pleural effusion, eosinophilic pneumonia. **Musculoskeletal:** Limb/back pain, arthralgia, chest pain, myalgia, muscle cramps/pain/weakness, pain in extremity, osteomyelitis, myopathy, rhabdomyolysis. **Metabolic:** Hypo-/hyperglycemia, hypokalemia, hypomagnesemia, electrolyte disturbance. **Ophthalmic:** Eye irritation, blurred vision. **Otic:** Tinnitus. **Hypersensitivity:** Difficulty swallowing, hives, pruritus, pulmonary eosinophilia, SOB, truncal erythema, ***anaphylaxis***. **Body as a whole:** Injection site reactions (including erythema), fever, edema (including peripheral edema), cellulitis, *Candida* infections, superinfection, fungemia, bacteremia, ***sepsis***, fatigue, weakness, asthenia, rigors, discomfort, jitteriness, flushing. **Miscellaneous:** Decreased appetite, taste disturbance, *S. aureus* bacteremia/endocarditis.

LABORATORY TEST CONSIDERATIONS

↑ CPK, ALT, AST, INR ratio, myoglobin, serum LDH, alkaline phosphatase, phosphorus, serum bicarbonate, alanine aminotransferase, aspartate aminotransferase. Prolonged PT. Abnormal LFTs.

OVERDOSE MANAGEMENT

Treatment: Provide supportive care with maintenance of GFR. Daptomycin is slowly cleared by hemodialysis or by peritoneal dialysis. The use of high-flux dialysis membranes during 4 hr of hemodialysis may increase the percentage of dose removed compared with low-flux membranes.

DRUG INTERACTIONS

HMG-CoA reductase inhibitors / ↑ Risk of rhabdomyolysis; temporarily suspend HMG-CoA reductase inhibitor; monitor CPK levels weekly and more frequently in those receiving recent, prior, or concomitant HMG-CoA reductase therapy

Tobramycin / ↑ Daptomycin C_{max} and AUC; ↓ tobramycin C_{max} and AUC; use caution if given together

HOW SUPPLIED

Injection, Lyophilized Powder for Solution: 500 mg.

DOSAGE

IV INFUSION

Complicated skin and skin structure infections.

Adults, usual: 4 mg/kg once every 24 hr for 7–14 days. Administer by IV injection over 2 min or by infusion over 30 min period. Do not dose more frequently than once a day. For clients with C_{CR} < 30 mL/min (including hemodialysis or CAPD), give 4 mg/kg q 48 hr.

Bacteremia due to Staphylococcus aureus, *including right-sided endocarditis caused by methicillin-susceptible or methicillin-resistant strains.*

Adults, usual: 6 mg/kg q 24 hr for a minimum of 2–6 weeks. Administer by IV injection over 2 min or by infusion over 30 min period. For clients with a C_{CR} of 30 mL/min or less, give 6 mg/kg once q 48 hr.

NURSING IMPLICATIONS

IMPLEMENTATION/ADMINISTRATION/STORAGE

1. **IV** To reduce development of drug-resistant bacteria and maintain effectiveness of daptomycin, use drug only to treat/prevent infections that are proven/strongly suspected to be caused by susceptible organisms.
2. Reconstitute the 500 mg vial with 10 mL of 0.9% NaCl injection. The product contains no preservative or bacteriostatic agent.
3. For IV injection over 2 min, give the appropriate volume of the reconstituted daptomycin solution, which has a concentration of 50 mg/mL. For IV infusion over 30 min, the appropriate volume of the reconstituted solution (i.e., concentration of 50 mg/mL) should be further diluted using aseptic technique into

a 50 mL IV infusion bag containing NaCl, 0.9% injection.

4. A dose of 4–6 mg/kg IV q 48 hr is recommended for clients receiving continuous venovenous hemofiltration, continuous venovenous hemodialysis, or continuous venovenous hemodiafiltration. This recommendation assumes ultrafiltration and dialysis flow rates of 1–2 liters/hr.
5. For critically ill clients receiving continuous renal replacement therapy who have severe infections, give consideration to decreasing the dosing interval to 4–6 mg/kg IV q 24 hr or 8 mg/kg IV q 48 hr.
6. The dose for clients receiving intermittent hemodialysis is 4–6 mg/kg IV q 48–72 hr. This assumes the client is receiving standard intermittent dialysis 3 times/week and completes the full dialysis session.
7. Reconstituted solution stable in vial for 12 hr at room temperature, up to 48 hr if refrigerated at 2–8°C (36–46°F). The diluted solution is stable in the infusion bag for 12 hr at room temperature or 48 hr if refrigerated. The combined time (vial and infusion bag) should not exceed 12 hr at room temperature and 48 hr if refrigerated.
8. Vials are for single use only.
9. Store original packages refrigerated at 2–8°C (36–46°F). Avoid excessive heat.
10. COMPATIBILITY 0.9% NaCl, LR.
11. INCOMPATIBILITY Dextrose-containing diluents. Do not add additives or other medications to daptomycin single-use vials or infuse simultaneously through the same IV line. If the same IV line is used for sequential infusion of several different drugs, flush line with compatible infusion solution before and after infusion with daptomycin. Do not use in conjunction with ReadyMED elastomeric infusion pumps.

ASSESSMENT

1. Note reasons for therapy, onset, characteristics of S&S, other agents trialed, culture results, outcome.
2. Assess regularly for any GI, CNS, musculoskeletal, and adverse body effects. Monitor for S&S of myopathy or neuropathy.
3. List drugs prescribed; hold statins during therapy, monitor anticoagulant activity for several days after starting daptomycin if receiving warfarin.
4. Monitor VS, CBC, renal and LFTs; reduce dose with renal dysfunction. Check CPK levels weekly.

CLIENT/FAMILY TEACHING

1. Drug is prepared and administered by IV infusion.
2. Report immediately any muscle pain/weakness, infusion site pain or reactions, abnormal sensations in the legs or arms (e.g., pain, numbness), breathlessness, cough, fever, or lack of improvement.
3. Report if severe diarrhea, rash, or infection is evident. Black, furry tongue, foul-smelling stools, vaginal itching/discharge, white patches in mouth may indicate superinfection.

OUTCOMES/EVALUATE

Resolution of infection; healing/clearing of skin lesions

IV

Darbepoetin alfa

(**DAR**-beh-**poh**-eh-tin **AL**-fah)

Classification(s): Erythropoietin, human recombinant

Pregnancy Category: C

RX: Aranesp.

INDICATIONS/USES

(1) Anemia associated with chronic kidney disease, including those on or not on dialysis. (2) Treat anemia in nonmyeloid malignancies in which anemia is caused by the effect of coadministered chemotherapy, and upon initiation, there is a minimum of two additional months of planned chemotherapy. *Investigational:* Anemia associated with malignancy.

ACTION/KINETICS

Action

Production of endogenous erythropoietin is decreased in those with chronic renal failure, and a deficiency in erythropoietin is the causative factor. Darbepoetin alfa, produced by recombinant DNA technology, stimulates erythropoiesis-stimulating protein. Darbepoetin interacts with progenitor stem cells to increase RBC production. Usually takes 2–6 weeks to see increased hemoglobin levels.

Pharmacokinetics

Darbepoetin has about a 3-fold longer terminal **t½** when given IV or SC than does epoetin alfa. **Distribution**, **t½, after IV:** About 1.4 hr (distribution) and about 21 hr (terminal). **Distribution, t½, after SC:** 49 hr. Bioavailability after SC is about 37% in adults and about 54% in children. **Peak levels after SC:** 48 hr. **t½, terminal after IV:** 21 hr, which is about 3 times higher than for epoetin alfa; **t½, terminal after SC:** 74 hr. With once weekly dosing, steady-state serum levels are reached in 4 weeks.

CONTRAINDICATIONS

Hypersensitivity to darbepoetin alfa or any component of the product. Uncontrolled hypertension, red cell aplasia that begins after treatment with darbepoetin alfa or other erythropoietin protein drugs.

SPECIAL CONCERNS

Erythropoiesis-stimulating agents (ESAs) increase the risk of death, myocardial infarction, stroke, venous thromboembolism, thrombosis of vascular access, and tumor progression or recurrence. **Chronic kidney disease.** (1) In controlled trials, clients experienced greater risks for death, serious adverse CV reactions, and stroke when administered erythropoiesis-stimulating agents (ESAs) to target a hemoglobin level of greater than 11 grams/dL. (2) No trial has identified a hemoglobin target level, darbepoetin alfa dose, or dosing strategy that does not increase these risks. (3) Use the lowest darbepoetin alfa dose sufficient to reduce the need for red blood cell transfusions. **Cancer.** (1) ESAs shortened overall survival and/or increased the risk of tumor progression or recurrence in clinical studies of clients with breast, non-small-cell lung, head and neck, lymphoid, and cervical cancers. (2) Because of these risks, prescribers and hospitals must enroll in and comply with the ESA APPRISE Oncology Program to prescribe and/or dispense darbepoetin to clients with cancer. To enroll in the ESA APPRISE Oncology Program, visit www.esa-apprise.com or call 1-866-284-8089 for further assistance. (3) To decrease these risks, as well as the risk of serious CV and thromboembolic reactions, use the lowest dose to avoid RBC transfusions. (4) Use ESAs only for anemia from myelosuppressive chemotherapy. (5) ESAs are not indicated for clients receiving myelosuppressive chemotherapy when the anticipated outcome is cure. (6) Discontinue following the completion of a chemotherapy course.

- **Product is formulated with two different excipients (one containing polysorbate 80 and the other containing albumin); there is a remote risk for transmission of viral diseases with the albumin product.**
- **There is the potential for immunogenicity to develop resulting in pure red cell aplasia and severe anemia, especially in those with chronic renal failure receiving the drug SC.**
- **Possible increased mortality and/or increased risk of tumor progression or recurrence.**
- **Clients on dialysis may require adjustments in their dialysis prescriptions after beginning darbepoetin alfa therapy. They may require increased anticoagulation with heparin to prevent clotting of the extracorporeal circuit during hemodialysis.**
- **Use with caution during lactation.**
- **Safety and efficacy not determined in children, in children with cancer, or in clients with underlying hematologic diseases (e.g., hemolytic anemia, sickle cell anemia, thalassemia, porphyria).**

SIDE EFFECTS

Most Common

Adults: Hypertension, hypotension, muscle spasm, ***cardiac arrhythmias/death,*** headache, fatigue, abdominal pain, diarrhea, constipation, N&V, arthralgia, limb pain, myalgia, cough, dyspnea, URTI, infection, peripheral edema, fever, dehydration.
Children: Cough, fever, headache, hypertension, hypotension, injection site pain, rash, seizures, URTI.

CV: Hypertension, vascular access thrombosis, ***access hemorrhage***, ***pulmonary emboli***, ***arterial and venous thromboembolic reactions***, AV graft thrombosis, thrombophlebitis (deep and/or superficial), thrombosis, CHF, ***cardiac arrhythmia/death***, ***cardiac arrest***, ***acute MI***, ***stroke***, hemodialysis graft occlusion, TIA, angina pectoris, cardiac chest pain, hypertensive encephalopathy, procedural hypotension, vascular access complications. **CNS:** ***Seizures***, headache, dizziness. **GI:** Diarrhea, N&V, abdominal pain, constipation, ***GI hemorrhage***. **Hematologic:** Pure red cell aplasia, severe anemia, compromised erythropoietic response. **Musculoskeletal:** Muscle spasm, myalgia, arthralgia, limb/back pain. **Dermatologic:** Pruritus, erythema, rash. **Respiratory:** URTI, dyspnea, cough, bronchitis, pneumonia, ***pulmonary embolism***. **Hypersensitivity:** Skin rash, urticaria, allergic reaction, bronchospasm, angioedema, ***anaphylaxis***. **Body as a whole:** ***Sepsis***, infection (includes abscess, bacteremia, peritonitis, pneumonia), fever, fatigue, flu-like symptoms, asthenia, edema, dehydration, ***death***. **Miscellaneous:** Chest pain, peripheral edema, injection site pain, fluid overload, access infection, immunogenicity.

NOTE: Increasing hemoglobin levels to more than 11 grams/dL in men or women may cause increased thrombotic vascular events (e.g., pulmonary emboli, thrombophlebitis, thrombosis in cancer clients) and mortality. Also, there is increased mortality and/or tumor progression in cancer clients.

OVERDOSE MANAGEMENT

Symptoms: Increases in hemoglobin greater than about 1 gram/dL during any 2-week period may cause an increased incidence of cardiac arrest, seizures, stroke, exacerbations of hypertension, CHF, vascular thrombosis, ischemia/infarction, acute MI, and fluid overload/edema. *Treatment:* In the event of polycythemia, temporarily withhold darbepoetin alfa. If clinically indicated, undertake phlebotomy. Reduce the dose in those with an excessive hematopoietic response.

HOW SUPPLIED

Solution for Injection: **Single-dose vials:** 25 mcg/mL, 40 mcg/mL, 60 mcg/mL, 100 mcg/mL, 150 mcg/0.75 mL, 200 mcg/mL, 300 mcg/mL. **Single-dose prefilled syringes:** 25 mcg/0.42 mL, 40 mcg/0.4 mL, 60 mcg/0.3 mL, 100 mcg/0.5 mL, 150 mcg/0.3 mL, 200 mcg/0. 4 mL, 300 mcg/0.6 mL, 500 mcg/mL.

DOSAGE

IV; SC

Anemia associated with chronic kidney disease on dialysis.

Adults, initial: 0.45 mcg/kg IV or SC once weekly or 0.75 mcg/kg once q 2 weeks as appropriate. If the hemoglobin level approaches or exceeds 11 grams/dL, reduce or interrupt the dose and use the lowest dose sufficient to reduce the need for RBC transfusions. If the hemoglobin rises rapidly (e.g., more than 1 gram/dL in any 2-week period), reduce the dose by 25% or more as needed to reduce rapid responses. For those who do not respond adequately, if the hemoglobin has not increased by more than 1 gram/dL after 4 weeks of therapy, increase the dose by 25%. Do not increase the dose more frequently than once q 4 weeks. Decreases in dose can occur more frequently. Avoid frequent dose adjustments.

When converting from epoetin alfa to darbepoetin alfa, estimate the starting weekly dose of darbepoetin alfa on the basis of the weekly dose of epoetin alfa at the time of substitution (see package insert for initial dosages). Titrate dose to maintain target hemoglobin. Due to a longer darbepoetin alfa half-life, give less frequently than epoetin alfa (e.g., give darbepoetin alfa once a week if epoetin alfa was given 2–3 times per week and give darbepoetin alfa once every 2 weeks if epoetin alfa was given once per week). Maintain the route of administration (i.e., either IV or SC).

Anemia associated with chronic kidney disease not on dialysis.

Adults, initial: 0.45 mcg/kg IV or SC given once at 4-week intervals as appropriate. If the hemoglobin level exceeds 10 grams/dL, reduce or interrupt the dose. If the hemoglobin rises rapidly (e.g., more than 1 gram/dL in any 2-week period), reduce the dose by 25% or more as needed to reduce rapid responses. For those who do not respond adequately, if the hemoglobin has not increased by more than 1 gram/dL after 4 weeks of therapy, increase the dose by 25%. Do not increase the dose more frequently than once q 4 weeks. Decreases in dose can occur more frequently. Avoid frequent dose adjustments.

Children, 1 year and older: The starting weekly dose should be estimated based on the weekly epoetin alfa dosage at the time of substitution. See package insert for specific information.

Anemia in cancer clients receiving chemotherapy.

Adults, initial: 2.25 mcg/kg weekly SC or 500 mcg q 3 weeks SC until completion of a chemotherapy course. The following are dosage adjustments in clients on cancer chemotherapy: (1) If the hemoglobin increases by more than 1 gram/dL in a 2-week period or if the hemoglobin reaches a level needed to avoid RBC transfusion, reduce the dose by 40% whether on the weekly schedule or the every 3-week schedule. (2) If hemoglobin exceeds a level needed to avoid RBC transfusion, withhold the dose until hemoglobin approaches a level where RBC transfusion may be required. Reinitiate at a dose 40% below the previous dose whether on the weekly schedule or every 3-week schedule. (3) If hemoglobin increases by less than 1 gram/dL and remains less than10 grams/dL after 6 weeks of therapy, increase the dose to 4.5 mcg/kg/week of on the weekly schedule. No dosage adjustment is necessary if on the every 3-week schedule. (4) If there is no response as measured by hemoglobin levels or if RBC transfusions are still required after 8 weeks of therapy and following completion of a chemotherapy course, discontinue darbepoetin alfa therapy whether on the weekly or every 3-week schedule.

NURSING IMPLICATIONS

IMPLEMENTATION/ADMINISTRATION/STORAGE

1. IV For those who respond to darbepoetin with a rapid increase in hemoglobin (e.g., >1 gram/dL in any 2-week period), reduce dose due to side effects as a result of an excessive rate of rise of hemoglobin.
2. Those with CRF not yet requiring dialysis may require lower maintenance doses of darbepoetin alfa than those receiving dialysis.
3. Therapy causes an increase in RBCs and a decrease in plasma volume, which could decrease dialysis efficiency.
4. When preparing injection, do not shake; vigorous shaking may denature the drug. Do not leave vials, prefilled syringes, or prefilled SureClick autoinjectors exposed to bright light. Store in their cartons until use.
5. Visually inspect vials; do not use if there is particulate matter and/or discoloration.
6. Do not shake or dilute the vials or prefilled syringes. Do not use vials or prefilled syringes that have been shaken.
7. Both prefilled syringes and autoinjectors are supplied with a 27-gauge, ½-inch needle. Each prefilled syringe is equipped with an "UltraSafe" needle guard that is manually activated to cover the needle during disposal. The needle cover of the prefilled syringe contains dry natural rubber (a derivative of latex), which may cause an allergic reaction in sensitive individuals.
8. Prefilled syringes: Following administration from the prefilled syringe, activate the "UltraSafe" needle guard. Place hands behind the needle, grasp the guard with one hand, and slide the guard forward until the needle is completely covered and the guard clicks into place. If an audible click is not heard, the needle guard may not be activated completely.
9. Autoinjectors: The prefilled "SureClick" autoinjector is designed to deliver the full dose. The completion of the injection is determined by an audible click. Removal of the autoinjector from the injection site automatically extends a needle cover. Only use autoinjectors for those who require the full dose. If the required dose is not available in an autoinjector, prefilled syringes or vials should be used to give the required dose. Autoinjectors are for SC administration only.
10. Discard any unused portion; drug is packaged in single-use vials and contains no preservative. Do not pool unused portions, and do not reenter the vial.
11. Store at 2–8°C (36–46°F). Do not freeze; protect from light.

12. After removing the vials, prefilled syringes, or autoinjectors from the cartons, keep them covered to protect from room light until administration.
13. COMPATIBILITY Do not dilute product.
14. INCOMPATIBILITY Do not give with any other drug solutions.

ASSESSMENT

1. List reasons for therapy, other agents trialed, outcome, and if epoetin alfa conversion.
2. Note baseline neurologic status; assess for seizure history, uncontrolled HTN, other medical conditions that may preclude therapy.
3. Drug dose and therapy by trained individuals only under closely monitored conditions.
4. Assess for any neurologic S&S during first few months of therapy.
5. Since ESAs (erythropoiesis-stimulating agents) increase risk of tumor progression or recurrence, providers and hospitals must enroll in and comply with the ESA APPRISE Oncology Program to prescribe and/or dispense darbepoetin alfa to those with cancer. To enroll in the ESA APPRISE Oncology Program, may visit www.esa-apprise.com or call 1-866-284-8089 for further assistance. Review product literature for administration guidelines carefully. Follow dosing guidelines based on Hb levels (maintain around 10 to 11 g/dL) to ensure no adverse SE.
6. Obtain baseline iron panel, ferritin or transferrin saturation, H&H, and BP. Monitor weekly until stabilized or until dosage change. Add supplemental iron therapy if serum ferritin <100 mcg/L or iron saturation <20%.

CLIENT/FAMILY TEACHING

1. Drug stimulates bone marrow to produce red blood cells. Supplemental iron/vitamins may be used to enhance drug effects. Stop drug once chemotherapy completed.
2. Review how to store, prepare, and administer dose, and how/where to dispose of used equipment and supplies. The needle cover on the prefilled syringe contains dry natural rubber (a derivative of latex), which should not be handled by persons allergic to latex.
3. Administer as directed once a week; do not increase/skip dose. Do not shake vial or prefilled syringe; inactivates drug. Keep refrigerated.
4. Review increased risks of mortality, serious CV reactions, thromboembolic reactions, stroke, and tumor progression with this therapy.
5. Follow prescribed dietary and dialysis recommendations; schedule activities to permit rest periods. Monitor BP and record. May experience seizures and brain dysfunction with chronic renal failure if BP is not controlled.
6. Do not perform any tasks that require mental alertness until drug effects realized.
7. Review list of drug side effects; practice reliable contraception. Immediately report any hives, persistent GI effects (e.g., nausea, vomiting, diarrhea), SOB, palpitations, rash, severe headache, S&S infection (e.g., fever, chills), swelling of eyes, mouth, or throat or swelling of feet/ankles.
8. Report any new-onset neurologic symptoms or change in seizure frequency.
9. Keep all F/U to assess response, VS, weekly labs, adverse SE. Dose based on weekly hemoglobin levels.

OUTCOMES/EVALUATE

- ↑ RBC production in anemia from CRF/chemotherapy
- Reduction of RBC transfusions

Darifenacin hydrobromide

(dar-ih-**FEN**-ah-sin)

Classification(s): Cholinergic blocking drug

Pregnancy Category: C

RX: Enablex.

INDICATIONS/USES

Overactive bladder with symptoms of urge urinary incontinence, urgency, and frequency.

ACTION/KINETICS

Action

Darifenacin is a competitive muscarinic receptor antagonist. Muscarinic receptors play an important role in contractions of the urinary bladder smooth muscle and stimulation of salivary secretion. Has a greater affinity for the M_3 receptor than for other known muscarinic receptors. By blocking muscarinic receptors, activity of the bladder is reduced.

D

Pharmacokinetics

Oral bioavailability in extensive metabolizers is about 15% and 19% for the 7.5 and 15 mg tablets, respectively. **Peak plasma levels:** About 7 hr after multiple doses. **Steady-state plasma levels:** 6 days. Extensively metabolized by the liver by CYP2D6 and CYP3A4. **t½, elimination:** 13–19 hr. Excreted in both the urine (60%) and feces (40%). Clearance decreases with age. **Plasma protein binding:** About 98%.

CONTRAINDICATIONS

Use with severe hepatic impairment (Child-Pugh scores of 10–15), urinary retention, gastric retention, or uncontrolled narrow-angle glaucoma and in those who are at risk for these conditions. Hypersensitivity to the drug or components.

SPECIAL CONCERNS

- **Use with caution in clients being treated for narrow-angle glaucoma, in those with GI obstructive disorders, in those with clinically significant bladder outflow obstruction, and during lactation.**
- **Safety and efficacy not determined in children.**

SIDE EFFECTS

Most Common

Constipation, dry mouth, dyspepsia, nausea, headache, UTI, flu syndrome.

GI: Dry mouth, constipation, N&V, dyspepsia, abdominal pain, diarrhea. **CNS:** Headache, asthenia, dizziness. **CV:** Hypertension. **GU:** UTI, acute urinary retention, urinary tract disorder, vaginitis. **Musculoskeletal:** Arthralgia, back pain. **Respiratory:** Bronchitis, pharyngitis, rhinitis, sinusitis. **Dermatologic:** Dry skin, pruritus, rash. **Ophthalmic:** Dry eyes, blurred vision, abnormal vision. **Body as a whole:** Flu syndrome, heat prostration (when used in a hot environment), pain, weight gain. **Miscellaneous:** Accidental injury.

OVERDOSE MANAGEMENT

Symptoms: Severe antimuscarinic effects. *Treatment:* Symptomatic and supportive. In the event of overdosage, monitor ECG.

DRUG INTERACTIONS

Anticholinergic drugs / Additive anticholinergic side effects

Clarithromycin / ↑ Darifenacin levels R/T inhibition of metabolism by CYP3A4; do not exceed 7.5 mg darifenacin/day

Desipramine / Possible ↑ desipramine C_{max} and AUC R/T ↓ metabolism by CYP2D6

Diltiazem / ↑ Darifenacin levels R/T inhibition of metabolism by CYP3A4

Erythromycin / ↑ Darifenacin levels R/T inhibition of metabolism by CYP3A4

Flecainide / Possible ↑ flecainide C_{max} and AUC R/T ↓ metabolism by CYP2D6

Fluoconazole / ↑ Darifenacin levels R/T inhibition of metabolism by CYP3A4

Imipramine / Possible ↑ imipramine C_{max} and AUC R/T ↓ metabolism by CYP2D6

Itraconazole / ↑ Darifenacin levels R/T inhibition of metabolism by CYP3A4; do not exceed 7.5 mg darifenacin/day

Ketoconazole / ↑ Darifenacin levels R/T inhibition of metabolism by CYP3A4; do not exceed 7.5 mg darifenacin/day

Nefazodone / ↑ Darifenacin levels R/T inhibition of metabolism by CYP3A4; do not exceed 7.5 mg darifenacin/day

Nelfinavir / ↑ Darifenacin levels R/T inhibition of metabolism by CYP3A4; do not exceed 7.5 mg darifenacin/day

Ritonavir / ↑ Darifenacin levels R/T inhibition of metabolism by CYP3A4; do not exceed 7.5 mg darifenacin/day

Thioridazine / Possible ↑ thioridazine C_{max} and AUC R/T ↓ metabolism by CYP2D6

Verapamil / ↑ Darifenacin levels R/T inhibition of metabolism by CYP3A4

HOW SUPPLIED

Tablets, Extended-Release: 7.5 mg, 15 mg.

DOSAGE

TABLETS, EXTENDED-RELEASE

Overactive bladder.

Initial: 7.5 mg once daily. Based on individual response, dose may be increased to 15 mg once daily as early as 2 weeks after starting therapy. For clients with moderate hepatic impairment (Child-Pugh scores of 7–9), do not exceed a daily dose of 7.5 mg.

NURSING IMPLICATIONS

IMPLEMENTATION/ADMINISTRATION/STORAGE

1. Do not exceed a daily dose of 7.5 mg if given with potent CYP3A4 inhibitors, such as clarithromycin, itraconazole, ketoconazole, nefazodone, nelfinavir, or ritonavir.
2. Store from 15–30°C (59–86°F); protect from light.

ASSESSMENT

1. Note reasons for therapy, onset/characterictics (degree of urgency, frequency, incontinence), other agents trialed, outcome.
2. List other drugs prescribed to ensure none interact. Note any glaucoma, and rule out UTI, obstruction, stones, etc. prior to starting therapy.
3. Review voiding patterns; assess abdomen to ensure no urinary retention or gastric motility problems. Identify nonpharmacologic therapies trialed first (i.e., Kegal exercises, estrogen rings, weights, etc.). Stop therapy if any evidence of severe abdominal pain, sudden eye pain, or urinary retention.
4. Assess BP, renal and LFTs; do not exceed 7.5 mg dose with liver impairment.

CLIENT/FAMILY TEACHING

1. Take with liquid, with/without food once daily.
2. Swallow whole; do not chew, divide, or crush tablets.
3. Use caution until drug effects realized; may cause dizziness or blurred vision.
4. Keep a voiding diary noting frequency and triggers; note any changes in voiding patterns after starting therapy.
5. May experience dry mouth, constipation, urinary retention. Avoid exercise in hot weather; sweating may be decreased, heat prostration may occur.
6. Immediately report any adverse side effects especially inability to pass urine, severe abdominal pain, or sudden eye pain.
7. May cause pupils to dilate, resulting in intolerance to bright lights or sunlight; wear dark glasses if evident.
8. Keep all F/U to assess response and need for dosage adjustment, labs, and for adverse SE.

OUTCOMES/EVALUATE

↓ Urinary symptoms R/T frequency, urgency and/or incontinence

Darunavir ethanolate

(dar-**UE**-na-vir)

Classification(s): Antiviral drug, antiretroviral protease inhibitor

Pregnancy Category: B (Category C per manufacturer's prescribing information)

RX: Prezista.

SEE ALSO ***ANTIVIRAL DRUGS***.

INDICATIONS/USES

Treatment of HIV infection in adults and children, 6 years and older, coadministered with ritonavir, and other antiretroviral drugs.

ACTION/KINETICS

Action

Inhibits HIV-1 protease. Selectively inhibits the cleavage of HIV encoded Gag-Pol polyproteins in infected cells, thus preventing the formation of mature virus particles. Darunavir is primarily metabolized by CYP3A; ritonavir is given because it inhibits CYP3A, thus increasing plasma levels of darunavir. Ritonavir, 100 mg twice daily, given with darunavir, 600 mg, results in about a 14-fold increase in systemic exposure to darunavir. The information for ritonavir should also be consulted.

Pharmacokinetics

Absolute bioavailability of darunavir, 600 mg alone, and after coadministration with ritonavir, 100 mg, twice daily is 37% and 82%, respectively. **Time to maximum levels:** 2.5–4 hr when taken with ritonavir. Food increases the C_{max} and AUC of darunavir by about 30% when given with ritonavir. Metabolized by CYP3A; unchanged drug and metabolites are excreted in the feces (about 80%) and urine (about 14%). **t½, terminal:** About 15 hr when combined with ritonavir. *NOTE:* Darunavir/ritonavir combination is an inhibitor of the P-glycoprotein transporters. **Plasma protein binding:** 95%.

CONTRAINDICATIONS

Known hypersensitivity to any component of the product. Use in severely impaired hepatic function. Coadministration with drugs that are highly dependent on CP3A for clearance and for which increased plasma levels may result in serious and/or life-threatening events (see *Drug Interactions*). Use of phosphodiesterase type 5 inhibitors (e.g., sildenafil) to treat pulmonary arterial hypertension due to increased risk for sildenafil side effects (e.g., visual disturbances, hypotension, prolonged erection, syncope). Use in children less than 3 years old. Lactation.

SPECIAL CONCERNS

- Use with caution in those with a known sulfonamide allergy since darunavir contains a sulfonamide moiety.
- Use with caution in impaired hepatic function and in the elderly.
- Those with pre-existing impaired liver function, including chronic active hepatitis B or C coinfection, have an increased risk for abnormal liver function, including severe hepatic side effects.
- During the initial phase of treatment, those responding to antiretrovial therapy may develop an inflammatory response to indolent or residual opportunistic infections (e.g., *Mycobacterium avium* complex, cytomegalovirus, *Pneumocystis jiroveci* pneumonia, tuberculosis) that may require further evaluation and treatment.
- Cross resistance with other protease inhibitors has been observed.
- Safety and efficacy not determined in children aged 3 to younger than 6 years.

SIDE EFFECTS

Most Common

Diarrhea, headache, nasopharyngitis, N&V, abdominal pain, rash, constipation.

Included are side effects that might occur when darunavir is combined with ritonavir. **GI:** Abdominal pain/distension, diarrhea, constipation, dry mouth, dyspepsia, flatulence, N&V, ***acute pancreatitis***. **Hepatic:** Acute hepatitis, cytolytic hepatitis, hepatotoxicity, hyperbilirubinemia. **CNS:** Headache, abnormal dreams, altered mood, anxiety, confusion, disorientation, hypesthesia, irritability, impaired memory, nightmares, paresthesia, peripheral neuropathy, somnolence, vertigo. **CV:** Hypertension, ***MI***, tachycardia, TIAs. Increased bleeding, including spontaneous skin hematomas and hemarthrosis in hemophilia type A and B clients. **Dermatologic:** Rash, pruritus, urticaria, angioedema, allergic dermatitis, alopecia, dermatitis medicamentosa, eczema, hyperhidrosis, liopatrophy, maculopapular rash, night sweats, skin inflammation, toxic skin eruption. Severe skin rash, including erythema multiforme, ***toxic epidermal necrolysis***, ***Stevens-Johnson syndrome***. Severe skin rashes accompanied by fever, general malaise, fatigue, muscle/joint aches, blisters, oral lesions, conjunctivitis, hepatitis, and/or eosinophilia. **Musculoskeletal:** Arthralgia, myalgia, osteopenia, osteonecrosis, osteoporosis, rhabdomyolysis (with coadministration with HMG-CoA reductase inhibitors), pain in extremity. **Respiratory:** Cough, dyspnea, hiccough. **GU:** Acute renal failure, gynecomastia, nephrolithiasis, polyuria, renal insufficiency. **Metabolic:** Anorexia, decreased appetite, obesity, peripheral edema, polydipsia. New onset diabetes mellitus or exacerbation of pre-existing diabetes mellitus and hyperglycemia. **Hematologic:** Increased bleeding, including spontaneous skin hematomas and hemarthrosis in those with hemophilia type A and B. **Body as a whole:** Asthenia, fatigue, hypersensitivity; redistribution/accumulation of body fat, including central obesity, dorsocervical fat enlargement, peripheral wasting, facial wasting, breast enlargement, pyrexia, rigors, and "cushingoid appearance." **Miscellaneous:** Folliculitis, hyperthermia, decreased susceptibility, immune reconstitution syndrome, possible resistance and cross-resistance among protease inhibitors.

LABORATORY TEST CONSIDERATIONS

↑ ALT, AST, alkaline phosphatase, gammaglutamyltransferase, pancreatic amylase, pancreatic lipase, total cholesterol, LDL, PTT, plasma prothrombin. ↓ Bicarbonate, platelet count, total absolute neutrophil count, lymphocytes, WBCs. Hyperbilirubinemia, hypertriglyceridemia, hyper-/hypoglycemia, hyper-/hyponatremia, hyperuricemia, hypoalbuminemia, hypocalcemia, hypercholesterolemia, hyperlipidemia.

OVERDOSE MANAGEMENT

Treatment: No specific antidote available. Treatment consists of general supportive measures, including monitoring of vital signs and clinical status of the client. Unabsorbed drug may be removed by gastric lavage or administration of activated charcoal. Dialysis is unlikely to be of benefit due to darunavir being highly protein bound.

DRUG INTERACTIONS

NOTE: Drug interactions are based on coadministration of darunavir and ritonavir. Darunavir and ritonavir are inhibitors of CYP3A and CYP2D6; use together with drugs that are primarily metabolized by these enzymes may result in increased plasma levels of such drugs, which could increase or prolong their therapeutic and side effects.

Alpha-1 adrenergic receptor antagonists (e.g., alfuzosin) / Possible serious and/or life-threatening side effects, as hypotension; do not use together
Amiodarone / ↑ Amiodarone concentrations; use together with caution and monitor therapeutic levels
Bepridil / ↑ Bepridil concentrations; use together with caution and monitor therapeutic levels
Beta-adrenergic blockers (e.g., metoprolol, timolol) / Possible dose ↓ may be needed; use together with caution
Buprenorphine / ↑ Buprenorphine plasma levels and t½ → ↑ risk of side effects, especially respiratory depression; monitor respiratory function closely
Carbamazepine / Significant ↓ darunavir levels → loss of therapeutic effect; carbamazepine levels may ↑; consider alternative drugs
Cisapride / Possible serious and/or life-threatening reactions, as cardiac arrhythmias; do not use together
Clarithromycin / ↑ Clarithromycin levels; if C_{CR} is 30–60 mL/min, decrease clarithromycin dose by 50%, and if C_{CR} is <30 mL/min decrease clarithromycin dose by 75%
Colchicine / ↑ Plasma colchicine levels → ↑ risk of life-threatening and fatal colchicine toxicity; use together contraindicated in those with renal/hepatic impairment; in normal renal function, do not exceed a dose of 0.3 mg colchicine twice a day; monitor closely
Cyclosporine / ↑ Cyclosporine levels; monitor levels
Desipramine / Possible ↑ desipramine plasma levels; use together with caution and at lower desipramine doses
Dexamethasone / ↓ Darunavir levels → ↓ therapeutic effect R/T ↑ metabolism by CYP3A → loss of darunavir therapeutic effect
Dextromethorphan / ↑ Dextromethorphan plasma levels; monitor for dextromethorphan side effects and adjust dose if needed
Didanosine / Give didanosine on an empty stomach 1 hr before or 2 hr after darunavir/ritonavir (which are given with food)
Digoxin / Significant ↑ serum digoxin levels; monitor digoxin levels closely and use lowest possible dose; use digoxin serum levels to gauge dose
Dihydroergotamine / ↑ Darunavir levels → ↑ risk of serious and/or life-threatening side effects (e.g., peripheral vasospasm, ischemia of extremities); do not use together
Dronedarone / ↑ Dronedarone plasma levels and pharmacologic effect; do not use together
Efavirenz / ↓ Darunavir AUC and C_{min}; ↑ efavirenz AUC and C_{min}; monitor response and use together with caution
Ergonovine / ↑ Darunavir levels → ↑ risk of serious and/or life-threatening side effects (e.g., peripheral vasospasm, ischemia of extremities); do not use together
Ergotamine / ↑ Darunavir levels → ↑ risk of serious and/or life-threatening side effects (e.g., peripheral vasospasm, ischemia of extremities); do not use together
Felodipine / ↑ Felodipine levels; use together with caution and monitor
Fentanyl / ↑ Fentanyl plasma levels and t½ → ↑ risk of side effects, especially respiratory depression; monitor respiratory function closely
Flecainide / ↑ Flecainide concentrations; use together with caution and monitor therapeutic levels
Fluticasone propionate (inhaled) / ↑ Fluticasone levels; consider an alternative to fluticasone especially for long-term use
HMG-CoA reductase inhibitors (e.g., atorvastatin, lovastatin, pravastatin, rosuvastatin, simvastatin) / ↑ Risk of myopathy (including rhabdomyolysis); start with the lowest HMG-CoA reductase inhibitor dose; coadministration with lovastatin or simvastatin contraindicated
Iloperidone / ↑ Iloperidone plasma levels and pharmacologic effect; reduce iloperidone dose by one-half when given with darunavir
Indinavir / Appropriate dose of indinavir with darunavir/ritonavir not established
Itraconazole / ↑ Darunavir and ↑ itraconazole levels; if used together, do not exceed a daily dose of itraconazole of 200 mg
Ketoconazole / ↑ Darunavir and ↑ ketoconazole levels; if used together, do not exceed a daily dose of ketoconazole of 200 mg
Lidocaine / ↑ Lidocaine concentrations; use together with caution and monitor therapeutic levels
Lopinavir/Ritonavir / ↓ Darunavir AUC → ↓ efficacy; also, ↑ lopinavir levels; do not coadminister

D

lopinavir/ritonavir and darunavir with or without ritonavir
Maraviroc / ↑ Plasma maraviroc levels; if used together, decrease maraviroc dose to 150 mg twice a day
Methadone / Monitor for possible abstinence syndrome; may need to ↑ methadone dose
Methylergonovine / ↑ Darunavir levels → ↑ risk of serious and/or life-threatening side effects (e.g., peripheral vasospasm, ischemia of extremities); do not use together
Midazolam / ↑ Midazolam levels → ↑ risk of serious and/or life-threatening side effects, such as prolonged or increased sedation or respiratory depression; do not use together; consider ↓ midazolam dose
Nevirapine / ↓ Darunavir levels → ↓ efficacy; also, possible ↑ nevirapine levels; use together with caution; monitor response and adjust dose as needed
Nicardipine / ↑ Nicardipine levels; use together with caution and monitor
Nifedipine / ↑ Nifedipine levels; use together with caution and monitor
Omeprazole / Possible ↓ omeprazole plasma levels → ↓ efficacy; may need to ↑ omeprazole dose
Oral Contraceptives (e.g., ethinyl estradiol, norethindrone) / ↓ Ethinyl estradiol levels R/T ↑ metabolism by ritonavir; use alternative or additional contraceptive measures
Phenobarbital / Significant ↓ darunavir or phenobarbital levels → loss of therapeutic effect; monitor phenobarbital levels and adjust dose as needed
Phenytoin / Significant ↓ darunavir or phenytoin levels → loss of therapeutic effect; monitor phenytoin levels and adjust dose as needed
Pimozide / ↑ Darunavir levels → ↑ risk of serious and/or life-threatening side effects (e.g., cardiac arrhythmias); do not use together
Propafenone / ↑ Propafenone concentrations; use together with caution and monitor therapeutic levels
Quetiapine / ↑ Plasma quetiapine levels → ↑ pharmacologic and side effects; use together with caution and closely monitor; adjust quetiapine dose as needed
Quinidine / ↑ Quinidine concentrations; use together with caution and monitor therapeutic levels
Rifamycins (e.g., rifabutin, rifampin) / Significant ↓ darunavir levels → loss of therapeutic effect; also, rifabutin + ritonavir → ↑ ritonavir levels. When the three drugs are used together, give rifabutin 150 mg once every other day
Risperidone / Possible dose ↓ of risperidone; monitor clinical response
Saquinavir / ↓ Darunavir AUC by about 25%; do not use together with or without ritonavir
Selective serotonin reuptake inhibitors (e.g., paroxetine, sertraline) / Carefully titrate SSRI dose based on antidepressant response
Sildenafil / Use together with caution; do not exceed sildenafil dose of 25 mg within 48 hr; use together contraindicated to treat pulmonary arterial hypertension
Sirolimus / ↑ Sirolimus levels; monitor levels
H ***St. John's wort*** / Significant ↓ darunavir levels → loss of therapeutic effect; do not use together
Tacrolimus / ↑ Tacrolimus levels; monitor levels
Tadalafil / Use together with caution; do not exceed tadalafil dose of 10 mg within 72 hr
Tenofovir / ↑ AUC of tenofovir by 22%; not clinically significant
Thioridazine / Possible dose ↓ of thioridazine; monitor clinical response
Trazodone / ↑ Trazodone levels; possible nausea, dizziness, hypotension, syncope; use together with caution; consider a lower dose of trazodone
Triazolam / ↑ Darunavir levels → ↑ risk of serious and/or life-threatening side effects, such as prolonged or increased sedation or respiratory depression; do not use together
Vardenafil / Use together with caution; do not exceed vardenafil dose of 2.5 mg within 72 hr
Voraconazole / ↓ Voraconazole AUC about 39% when given with ritonavir, 100 mg twice a day; do not give together unless benefit/risk ratio justifies use
Warfarin / Possible ↓ warfarin levels; monitor INR frequently

HOW SUPPLIED

Tablets: 75 mg, 150 mg, 400 mg, 600 mg.

DOSAGE

TABLETS

Human immunodeficiency virus (HIV) infection.

Adults, treatment-naive: 800 mg (two 400 mg tablets) with ritonavir, 100 mg, once daily with food. **Adults, treatment-experienced:** 600 mg twice daily taken with ritonavir, 100 mg, twice daily with food in those with no darunavir resistance-associated substitutions. With one or more darunavir resistance-associated substitution, the dose is 600 mg darunavir twice daily with ritonavir 100 mg twice daily and food. **Children, 6 years of age and older, 20 kg or greater to <30 kg (44 lbs or greater to <66 lbs):** darunavir, 375 mg and ritonavir, 50 mg twice daily with food; **30 kg or greater to <40 kg (66 lbs or greater to <88 lbs):** darunavir, 450 mg and ritonavir, 60 mg twice daily with food; **40 kg or greater (88 lbs or greater):** darunavir, 600 mg and ritonavir, 100 mg twice daily with food. **Maximum dose:** Darunavir, 600 mg and ritonavir, 100 mg twice daily with food. *NOTE:* Children must be at least 20 kg (44 lbs) in order to initiate therapy.

NURSING IMPLICATIONS

IMPLEMENTATION/ADMINISTRATION/STORAGE

1. Failure to coadminister darunavir with ritonavir and food will result in decreased darunavir plasma levels that are not high enough to achieve the desired antiviral effect. Also, some drug interactions may be altered.
2. **Missed doses, once daily doses.** (a) If clients taking darunavir once daily miss a dose of darunavir or ritonavir by more than 12 hours, the client should wait and take the next dose of darunavir/ritonavir at the regularly scheduled time. (b) If the client misses a dose of darunavir or ritonavir by less than 12 hr, the client should take darunavir/ritonavir immediately and then take the next dose of darunavir/ritonavir at the regularly scheduled time. (c) If a dose of darunavir or ritonavir is skipped, the client should not double the next dose. The client should not take more or less than the prescribed dose of darunavir or ritonavir.
3. **Missed doses, twice daily doses.** (a) If the client misses a dose of darunavir or ritonavir by more than 6 hr, the client should wait and take the next dose of darunavir/ritonavir at the regularly scheduled time. (b) If the client misses a dose of darunavir or ritonavir by less than 6 hr, the client should take darunavir/ritonavir immediately and then take the next dose of darunavir/ritonavir at the regularly scheduled time. (c) If a dose of darunavir or ritonavir is skipped, the client should not double the next dose. The client should not take more or less than the prescribed dose darunavir or ritonavir at any one time.
4. Do not use once daily dosing in children or treatment-experienced adults.
5. Store tablets from 15–30°C (59–86°F).

ASSESSMENT

1. Note treatment history, onset, when available, genotypic or phenotypic testing results; may aid in determining darunavir susceptibility.
2. Assess for any sulfa allergy; precludes therapy.
3. Interrupt or discontinue therapy if there is evidence of new or worsening impaired liver function, such as elevation of liver enzymes and/or symptoms including anorexia, dark urine, fatigue, hepatomegaly, jaundice, liver tenderness, or nausea.
4. To monitor maternal-fetal outcomes of pregnant women exposed to darunavir, an antiretroviral pregnancy register has been established. To register clients, call 1-800-258-4263.
5. List drugs prescribed/consumed to ensure none interact unfavorably.
6. Diabetes may aggravate control; may also cause diabetes. With hemophilia may cause increased bleeding; monitor closely.
7. Drug is coadministered with 100 mg ritonavir and with other antiretroviral agents.
8. Has not been used in treatment-naive adults or pediatric clients.
9. Monitor renal and LFTs closely especially with dysfunction.

CLIENT/FAMILY TEACHING

1. Drug must be coadministered with ritonavir and food to work effectively. Swallow tablets whole with water or milk. Follow guidelines for missed doses.
2. If a child is not able to swallow a tablet, use of darunavir may not be appropriate.
3. Prezista is not a cure for HIV infection. May continue to develop opportunistic infections and other complications associated with HIV disease.
4. Use reliable contraception. With birth control pills, use alternate contraceptive measures during therapy because hormonal levels may

decrease. Use a condom or other barrier method to lower the chance of sexual contact with any body fluids such as semen, vaginal secretions, or blood. Never reuse or share needles.

5. May experience a redistribution or accumulation of body fat in the upper back and neck, breast, and around the back, chest, and stomach area. Loss of fat from the legs, arms, and face may also occur.
6. Diarrhea, nausea, headaches, cold symptoms may occur; report if bothersome or persistent.
7. Report all drugs prescribed, and avoid OTC or herbal products, including St. John's wort.
8. Drug interacts with many drugs; review pamphlet for list of drugs to avoid.
9. Store medications safely, do not share with others and keep out of the reach of children.
10. Keep all F/U to assess response, labs, and for adverse SE.

OUTCOMES/EVALUATE

- Decreases in HIV RNA
- ↑ CD4 cells

■ IV ©

Daunorubicin hydrochloride (DNR)

(daw-noh-**ROO**-bih-sin)

Classification(s): Antineoplastic, antibiotic

Pregnancy Category: D

RX: Cerubidine.

Daunorubicin citrate liposomal

Pregnancy Category: D

RX: DaunoXome.

SEE ALSO ***ANTINEOPLASTIC AGENTS***.

INDICATIONS/USES

Daunorubicin HCl: (1) In combination with other drugs (e.g., cytarabine) for remission induction in acute nonlymphocytic leukemia (erythroid, monocytic, myelogenous) in adults. (2) Remission induction in acute lymphocytic leukemia in children and adults (increased effectiveness when combined with prednisone and vincristine).

Daunorubicin liposomal: First-line cytotoxic therapy for advanced HIV-associated Kaposi's sarcoma. *Investigational:* Ewing's sarcoma, chronic myelocytic leukemia, neuroblastoma, non-Hodgkin's lymphomas, Wilms' tumor.

ACTION/KINETICS

Action

Anthracycline antibiotic. The liposomal product contains an aqueous solution of the citrate salt of daunorubicin encapsulated within lipid vesicles, which are composed of a lipid bilayer of distearoylphosphatidylcholine and cholesterol. Acts by a number of possible mechanisms. Forms complexes with DNA by intercalation between base pairs. It inhibits topoisomerase II activity by stabilizing the DNA-topoisomerase II complex, preventing the religation portion of the ligation-religation reaction that topoisomerase II catalyzes. Single-strand and double-strand DNA breaks result. Daunorubicin may also inhibit polymerase activity, affect regulation of gene expression, and produce free radical damage to DNA.

Pharmacokinetics

Rapidly cleared from the plasma. The liposomal preparation helps protect daunorubicin from chemical and enzymatic breakdown; also, it minimizes protein binding and decreases uptake by normal tissues. Is released from the liposomal preparation over time and improves selectivity for solid tumors. Metabolized to the active daunorubicinol. About 40% of the drug in the plasma is present as daunorubicinol within 30 min and 60% in 4 hr after dosage. **t½:** daunorubicin (nonliposomal product), 18.5 hr; daunorubinicol, 27 hr. **t½, elimination:** 4.4 hr for liposomal form. Drug rapidly taken up by heart, kidneys, lung, liver, and spleen. Chiefly excreted in bile (40%) and active form in urine (25%). Does not pass blood-brain barrier.

CONTRAINDICATIONS

Lactation. Hypersensitivity to previous doses. IM or SC use. Use in those who have previously received the maximum cumulative dose of either daunorubicin or doxorubicin.

SPECIAL CONCERNS

■ (1) Give daunorubicin hydrochloride into a rapidly flowing IV infusion. Do not give IM or SC; severe local tissue necrosis will result if extravasation occurs. (2) Myocardial toxicity, in its most severe form, as potentially fatal CHF, may occur when the total cumulative dose exceeds 400–550 mg/m^2 in adults, 300 mg/m^2 in children over 2 years of age or 10 mg/kg in children less than 2 years of age. May occur during therapy or several months or years after therapy. (3) It is recommended that daunorubicin be administered only by physicians experienced in leukemia chemotherapy and in facilities with lab and supportive resources adequate to monitor drug tolerance and protect and maintain a client compromised by drug toxicity. (4) The physician and institution must be capable of responding rapidly and completely to severe hemorrhagic conditions or overwhelming infection. (5) Severe myelosuppression occurs when using therapeutic doses; may lead to infection or hemorrhage. (6) Reduce dose in clients with impaired hepatic or renal function. (7) A triad of back pain, flushing, and chest tightness has been reported in clients treated with liposomal daunorubicin. This triad usually occurs during the first 5 min of the infusion, subsides with interruption of the infusion, and generally does not recur if the infusion is then resumed at a slower rate.

- **Use with caution in pre-existing heart disease or bone marrow depression.**
- **Cardiotoxicity may be more frequent in children (and at lower doses) and in the elderly. Use caution in the elderly who have inadequate bone marrow reserves due to old age.**

SIDE EFFECTS

Most Common

Daunorubicin hydrochloride: N&V, alopecia, mucositis, rash.
Daunorubicin citrate liposomal: N&V, fatigue, headache, fever, diarrhea, rigors, cough, dyspnea, rhinitis, neuropathy, abdominal pain, anorexia, back pain, allergic reactions.

Myocardial toxicity: ***Potentially fatal CHF***, (especially if total dosage exceeds 400–550 mg/m^2 for adults, 300 mg/m^2 for children more than 2 years of age, and 10 mg/kg for children less than 2 years of age.) Mucositis (3–7 days after administration), red-colored urine, hyperuricemia. Severe tissue necrosis if extravasation occurs. Cross-resistance with doxorubicin (produced by similar microorganism) and vinca alkaloids. Hyperuricemia may occur due to lysis of leukemic cells; give allopurinol as a precaution, before starting antileukemic therapy.

For daunorubicin hydrochloride. GI: Acute N&V, mucositis, diarrhea, abdominal pain. **Dermatologic:** Alopecia (reversible), rash, contact dermatitis, urticaria. **At injection site due to extravasation:** Tissue necrosis, severe cellulitis, thrombophlebitis, painful induration. **Miscellaneous:** Anaphylaxis (rare), fever, chills, hyperuricemia.

For daunorubicin citrate liposomal. CNS: Fatigue, headache, neuropathy, malaise, dizziness, depression, insomnia, amnesia, anxiety, ataxia, confusion, ***seizures***, emotional lability, abnormal gait, hallucinations, hyperkinesia, hypertonia, meningitis, somnolence, abnormal thinking, tremors. **GI:** Nausea, diarrhea, anorexia, abdominal pain, vomiting, stomatitis, constipation, increased appetite, dysphagia, ***GI hemorrhage***, gastritis, gingival bleeding, hemorrhoids, hepatomegaly, melena, dry mouth, tooth caries. **Hematologic:** Myelosuppression, especially of the granulocytic series. Neutropenia. **CV:** Cardiomyopathy associated with a decrease in left ventricular ejection fraction (especially in clients who have received prior anthracyclines or who have pre-existing cardiac disease). Also, hot flushes, hypertension, palpitation, syncope, tachycardia, angina pectoris, atrial fibrillation, ***cardiac arrest***, hot flashes, ***MI***, pericardial effusion, pericardial tamponade, pulmonary hypertension, sinus tachycardia, SVT, ventricular extrasystoles. **Respiratory:** Cough, dyspnea, rhinitis, sinusitis, hemoptysis, hiccoughs, pulmonary infiltration, increased sputum. **Musculoskeletal:** Rigors, back pain, myalgia, arthralgia. **Dermatologic:** Alopecia, pruritus, folliculitis, seborrhea, dry skin. **GU:** Dysuria, nocturia, polyuria. **Ophthalmic:** Abnormal vision, conjunctivitis, eye pain. **Otic:** Deafness, ear pain, tinnitus. **Miscellaneous:** Fever, allergic reactions, sweating, chest pain, edema, taste perversion, tenesmus, flu-like symptoms, opportunistic infections/illnesses, inflammation at injection site, lymphadenopathy, splenomegaly, dehydration, thirst. Back pain, flushing, and chest tightness have been reported within the first 5 min of the infusion.

LABORATORY TEST CONSIDERATIONS

Hyperuricemia secondary to rapid lysis of leukemic cells.

D

OVERDOSE MANAGEMENT

Symptoms: Granulocytopenia, fatigue, N&V. Also, extension of side effects. *Treatment:* Supportive care; maintain glomerular filtration. Slowly cleared from the body by both hemodialysis and peritoneal dialysis.

DRUG INTERACTIONS

Cyclophosphamide / ↑ Risk of cardiotoxicity
Methotrexate / Impaired liver function → ↑ risk of toxicity
Myelosuppressive drugs / Reduce dose of daunorubicin

HOW SUPPLIED

Daunorubicin HCl. ***Injection:*** 5 mg/mL; ***Powder for Injection, Lyophilized:*** 20 mg/10 mL, 50 mg/20 mL.
Daunorubicin Citrate Liposomal. ***Injection:*** 2 mg/mL.

DOSAGE

IV INFUSION OF DAUNORUBICIN HCl

Acute nonlymphocytic leukemia.

Adults, less than 60 years old: Daunorubicin, 45 mg/m^2/day on days 1, 2, and 3 of the first course and days 1 and 2 of additional courses; cytosine arabinoside (Ara-C), 100 mg/m^2/day, by IV infusion, for 7 days during first course and for 5 days during any additional courses of treatment. **Adults, 60 years and older:** Daunorubicin, 30 mg/m^2/day on days 1, 2, and 3 of the first course and days 1 and 2 of additional courses. Use the same dose of cytosine arabinoside as for adults less than 60 years old. Up to three courses may be required.

Acute lymphocytic leukemia, adults.

Adults: Daunorubicin, 45 mg/m^2, IV, on days 1, 2, and 3; vincristine, 2 mg IV, on days 1, 8, and 15; prednisone, PO, 40 mg/m^2/day for days 1–22 and then taper between days 22 and 29; and, l-asparaginase, IV, 500 international units/kg/day on days 22–32.

Acute lymphocytic leukemia, children.

Children: Daunorubicin, 25 mg/m^2, and vincristine, 1.5 mg/m^2, each IV, on day 1 every week with prednisone, 40 mg/m^2, PO, daily. Usually 4 courses will induce remission. If after 4 courses the client is in partial remission, an additional 1 or, if needed, 2 courses may be given to obtain a complete remission. *NOTE:* Calculate the dose on the basis of milligrams per kilogram if the child is less than 2 years of age or if the body surface is less than 0.5 m^2.

IV INFUSION OF DAUNORUBICIN CITRATE LIPOSOMAL

Advanced human immunodeficiency virus (HIV)-associated Kaposi's sarcoma.

40 mg/m^2 given over 1 hr. Dose is repeated q 2 weeks. This regimen is continued until there is progression of the disease or other complications of HIV disease or until other intercurrent complications preclude continued therapy. Reduce dosage for renal or hepatic disease. Recommended dose for liposomal product: three-fourths of normal dose if serum bilirubin is 1.2 to 3 mg/dL; one-half of normal dose if serum bilirubin is less than 3 mg/dL and serum creatinine is greater than 3 mg/dL.

NURSING IMPLICATIONS

Ⓢ Do not confuse daunorubicin with doxorubicin (also an antineoplastic).

IMPLEMENTATION/ADMINISTRATION/STORAGE

1. **IV Do not start therapy in clients with preexisting drug-induced bone marrow suppression unless the benefit from such treatment warrants the risk.**
2. **Reduce the dose as follows in impaired hepatic or renal function. Reduce the dose by 25% if serum bilirubin is 1.2–3 mg; reduce the dose by 50% if serum bilirubin is greater than 3 mg or if serum creatinine is greater than 3 mg.**
3. **Dilute the hydrochloride in vial with 4 mL sterile water for injection USP. Agitate gently until dissolved (solution contains 5 mg daunorubicin/mL). Withdraw desired dose into syringe containing 10–15 mL isotonic saline.**
4. **Inject into tubing of rapidly flowing D5W or NSS IV and administer over 3–5 min. May further dilute in 50 mL of D5W or NSS and in-**

fuse over 10–15 min (or in 100 mL of solution and infuse over 30–45 min).

5. Give into a rapidly flowing IV infusion. *Never administer IM or SC, as severe local tissue necrosis will result.*
6. Extravasation may cause severe local tissue necrosis.
7. Reconstituted solution stable for 24 hr at room temperature; 48 hr refrigerated. Protect from sunlight.
8. Dilute the liposomal product 1:1 with D5W dextrose injection before use. Do not use an in-line filter.
9. Store unopened vials of the hydrochloride from 2–8°C (36–46°F). Store prepared solution for infusion at room temperature (15–30°C, 59–86°F) for 24 hr or less. Discard unused portion; protect from light.
10. Refrigerate liposomal product at 2–8°C (36–46°F). Do not store the reconstituted solution for longer than 6 hr; do not freeze; protect from light.
11. COMPATIBILITY HCL product with D5W or NSS; liposomal product 1:1 with D5W.
12. INCOMPATIBILITY Do not mix with other drugs or heparin.

ASSESSMENT

1. Note reasons for therapy, ensure adequate hydration; medicate 1 hr before therapy with antiemetic and again 6–8 hr after therapy to decrease N&V. Assess hydration status.
2. Assess during and following therapy for myocardial toxicity: changes in baseline ECG, edema, dyspnea, and cyanosis. A 30% decrease in QRS voltage and reduction in the systolic ejection fraction may be early signals of cardiomyopathy. Clients with a cardiac history who receive doses above 50 mg/m^2 are more susceptible to CHF.
3. Follow appropriate guidelines for dose adjustment in liver dysfunction (e.g., bilirubin 1.2–3.0 mg, give 75% of dose; bilirubin greater than 3.0 mg, give 50% of dose) and renal dysfunction.
4. Drug may precipitate hyperuricemia; may use allopurinol.
5. Review risk of secondary leukemias with combo therapy.
6. Ensure CBC done prior to starting therapy and before each dose. Withhold therapy if ANC <750 cells/mm^3. Monitor for S&S of infection.
7. Monitor VS, CBC, renal and LFTs; drug may cause severe granulocyte and platelet toxicity. Allow bone marrow recovery before subsequent treatments. Nadir: 10 days; recovery: 21–28 days.

CLIENT/FAMILY TEACHING

1. Drug is used parenterally to treat leukemia and lymphoma.
2. Report S&S of cardiac toxicity (i.e., increased SOB/fatigue, and swelling of hands/feet).
3. Report back pain, flushing, breathing problems, chest pain during infusion, S&S of infection, or if mouth ulcers or pain interferes with eating. N&V usually controlled with antiemetics.
4. Urine may appear red for several days following therapy; this is not blood. Consume 1.5–2 L/day of fluids. Record I&O and report alterations.
5. Avoid alcohol, NSAIDs, aspirin, and foods high in purines.
6. Practice contraception during and for at least 1 month after therapy. Consider sperm/egg harvesting as needed.
7. Avoid crowds and those with active infections. Avoid vaccinations during therapy.
8. Anticipate hair loss; should grow back about 5 weeks later.
9. Report any unusual bruising/bleeding; use soft toothbrush and electric razor, and avoid contact sports or excessive jostling.
10. Keep all F/U to assess response, labs, ECGs, and adverse SE.

OUTCOMES/EVALUATE

- Suppression of malignant cell proliferation
- Treatment HIV-associated Kaposi's sarcoma

IV

Decitabine

(de-**SIT**-a-been)

Classification(s): DNA demethylation agent

Pregnancy Category: D

RX: Dacogen.

INDICATIONS/USES

Treatment of myelodysplastic syndromes, including previously treated and untreated, *de novo* and secondary myelodysplastic syndromes. *Investigational:* Acute myelogenous leukemia, chronic myelogenous leukemia.

ACTION/KINETICS

Action

Antineoplastic effects occur after phosphorylation and direct incorporation of the drug into DNA and inhibition of DNA methyltransferase, causing hypomethylation of DNA and cellular differentiation or apoptosis. In rapidly dividing cells, the cytotoxicity of decitabine may be due to the formation of covalent adducts between DNA methyltransferase and decitabine incorporated into DNA. Nonproliferating cells are relatively insensitive to the drug.

Pharmacokinetics

t½, terminal: 0.62 hr after a 15 mg/m^2 dose. Exact route of metabolism and excretion not known in humans. One pathway for elimination may be deamination by cytidine deaminase found in the liver (mainly), granulocytes, intestinal epithelium, and whole blood. **Plasma protein binding:** Negligible (less than 1%).

CONTRAINDICATIONS

Hypersensitivity to decitabine or any component of the product. Use in men if trying to father a child while receiving treatment and for 2 months afterwards (decitabine alters DNA synthesis and can cause fetal harm). Lactation.

SPECIAL CONCERNS

- **Use caution with renal or hepatic dysfunction.**
- **Safety and efficacy not determined in children.**

SIDE EFFECTS

Most Common

Anemia, fatigue, constipation, cough, dyspnea, diarrhea, fatigue, hyperglycemia, nausea, neutropenia, petechiae, pyrexia, thrombocytopenia, headache, insomnia, pallor.

GI: Constipation, diarrhea, N&V, anorexia, decreased appetite, abdominal pain (including upper)/distention, dyspepsia, oral mucosa petechiae, stomatitis, ascites, gingival bleeding, hemorrhoids, loose stools, tongue ulceration, dysphagia, GERD, glossodynia, lip ulceration, oral soft-tissue disorder, upper abdominal pain, oral pain, tooth abscess, toothache, gingival pain, hemoptysis, cholecystitis, peridiverticular abscess, upper ***GI hemorrhage***. **CNS:** Headache, insomnia, dizziness, confusion, anxiety, hypesthesia, depression, ***intracranial hemorrhage***, changes in mental status. **CV:** Hypo-/hypertension, tachycardia, ***CHF***, ***MI***, cardiac murmur, ***cardiorespiratory arrest***, atrial fibrillation, ***intracranial hemorrhage, cardiac myopathy***, supraventricular tachycardia. **Dermatologic:** Petechiae, pallor, ecchymosis, rash, erythema, cellulitis, pruritus, skin lesions, alopecia, face swelling, urticaria, cellulitis, contusion, dry skin, night sweats, skin lesion. **GU:** UTI, dysuria, urinary frequency, renal failure, urethral hemorrhage, Sweet's syndrome. **Respiratory:** Cough, pneumonia, pharyngitis, lung crackles, hypoxia, decreased breath sounds, rales, postnasal drip, pulmonary edema, sinusitis, URTI, epistaxis, pharyngolaryngeal pain, sinus congestion, pleural effusion, abnormal breath sounds, bronchopulmonary aspergillosis, lung infiltration, pseudomonal lung infection, pulmonary mass, ***pulmonary embolism, respiratory arrest***, respiratory tract infection. **Musculoskeletal:** Rigors, arthralgia, pain in limb, back pain, chest wall pain, musculoskeletal discomfort/pain, myalgia, muscle spasms/weakness, bone pain. **Hematologic:** Neutropenia, thrombocytopenia, anemia, febrile neutropenia, leukopenia, lymphadenopathy, hematoma, thrombocythemia, splenomegaly, myelosuppression, ***pancytopenia***. **Metabolic:** Edema (including peripheral), dehydration. **At administration site:** Catheter-related infection/hemorrhage, catheter-site erythema/pain, injection site swelling. **Ophthalmic:** Blurred vision. **Otic:** Ear pain. **Body as a whole:** Pyrexia, fatigue, lethargy, malaise, pain, tenderness, chills, abrasion, intermittent pyrexia, mucosal inflammation, hypersensitivity (including ***anaphylaxis***), ***sepsis***. **Miscellaneous:** Falls, central line infection, *Mycobacterium avium* complex infection, candidal infection, oral candidiasis, chest discomfort, crepitations, bacteremia, transfusion reaction, staphylococcal infection, fungal infection, postprocedural hemorrhage/pain.

LABORATORY TEST CONSIDERATIONS

↑ AST, blood alkaline phosphatase, blood lactate dehydrogenase, blood urea. ↓ Albumin, blood bilirubin, blood chloride, total protein. ↑ or ↓ Blood bicarbonate. Hyperbilirubinemia, hyper-/hypokalemia, hypoalbuminemia, hyperglycemia, hypomagnesemia, hyponatremia. Abnormal LFTs.

OVERDOSE MANAGEMENT

Symptoms: Increased myelosuppression, including prolonged neutropenia and thrombocytopenia. *Treatment:* No known antidote. Provide supportive measures.

HOW SUPPLIED

Powder for Injection Solution, Lyophilized: 50 mg.

DOSAGE

CONTINUOUS IV INFUSION

Myelodysplastic syndromes.

First treatment cycle: 15 mg/m^2 given by continuous IV infusion over 3 hr, repeated q 8 hr for 3 days. Repeat the preceding cycle every 6 weeks. **Alternative dosage:** 20 mg/m^2 by continuous IV infusion over 1 hr, repeated daily for 5 days. Repeat cycle q 4 weeks. For both treatment regimens, it is recommended that clients be treated for a minimum of 4 cycles; a complete or partial response may take longer than 4 cycles. Treatment may be continued as long as beneficial effects are obtained.

Acute myelogenous leukemia (investigational) or chronic myelogenous leukemia, acute phase or blast phase (investigational).

15 mg/m^2 IV once a day on days 1 to 5 and 8 to 12 of each cycle; repeat cycles q 6 weeks. Infuse over 1 hr.

Chronic myelogenous leukemia, chronic phase (investigational).

10 mg/m^2 IV once a day on days 1 to 5 and 8 to 12 of each cycle; repeat cycles q 6 weeks. Infuse over 1 hr.

NURSING IMPLICATIONS

IMPLEMENTATION/ADMINISTRATION/STORAGE

1. IV Aseptically reconstitute with 10 mL sterile water for injection; after reconstitution, product contains approximately 5 mg/mL at a pH of 6.7–7.3. Immediately after reconstitution, further dilute with 0.9% NaCl injection, D5W, or Ringer's lactate injection to a final concentration of 0.1–1 mg/mL. Unless used within 15 min of reconstitution, the diluted solution must be prepared using cold (2–8°C, 36–46°F) infusion fluids and stored from 2–8°C (36–46°F) for up to a maximum of 7 hr until administration.
2. **Dosage adjustment: Hematological toxicities after 15 mg/m^2:** If hematologic recovery (ANC at least 1,000/mcL and platelets at least 50,000/mcL) from a previous decitabine treatment cycle requires more than 6 weeks, the next cycle should be delayed and dosing reduced temporarily by the following: (a) For recovery requiring more than 6 weeks but less than 8 weeks, delay decitabine dosing for up to 2 weeks and reduce the dose temporarily to 11 mg/m^2 q 8 hr (33 mg/m^2/day, 99 mg/m^2/cycle) upon restarting therapy; then maintain or increase dose in subsequent cycles, as clinically indicated. (b) For recovery requiring more than 8 but less than 10 weeks, assess the client for disease progression (by bone marrow aspirates). In the absence of progression, the decitabine dose should be delayed up to 2 more weeks and the dose reduced to 11 mg/m^2 q 8 hr (33 mg/m^2/day, 99 mg/m^2/cycle) upon restarting therapy; then maintain or increase dose in subsequent cycles, as clinically indicated.
3. **Dosage adjustment: Nonhematologic toxicities after 15 mg/m^2 or 20 mg/m^2:** If any of the following nonhematologic toxicities are present, do not start decitabine treatment until the toxicity is resolved: serum creatinine at least 2 mg/dL; ALT, total bilirubin at least 2 times ULN; and active or uncontrolled infection.
4. **Dosage adjustment: Hematologic toxicities after 20 mg/m^2:** If myelosuppression is present, delay subsequent treatment cycles until there is hematologic recovery (ANC at least 1,000/mcL and platelets at least 50,000/mcL).
5. Store from 15–30°C (59–86°F).
6. COMPATIBILITY 0.9% NaCl, D5W, or Ringer's lactate.
7. INCOMPATIBILITY Administer separately.

ASSESSMENT

1. Note onset of myelodysplastic syndrome (MDS), if previously treated and with what, or if untreated; note hematologic status (myeloblasts, plt, H/H) and physical condition of client.

2. List drugs prescribed; no data on interactions at this time.
3. Assess infusion site for erythema or phlebitis. Give antiemetics before starting each infusion, after labs drawn. Cycles will be continued as long as client benefits.
4. Monitor VS, CBC (with platelets), renal and LFTs. Determine if pregnant—drug will cause fetal damage.

D

CLIENT/FAMILY TEACHING

1. Drug is administered by IV infusion over 3 hr every 8 hr for 3 days, then every 6 weeks for at least 4 cycles.
2. Labs will be drawn before each infusion to assess for toxicity.
3. May experience fatigue, fever, nausea, cough, constipation, diarrhea, bruising, and elevated blood sugars. Will be given medication before treatments to prevent N&V; report if other S&S persistent or bothersome.
4. Practice reliable contraception. Report if pregnancy suspected. Men should not father a child while receiving decitabine treatment and for 2 months after therapy is terminated.
5. Keep all F/U to assess response, labs, and for adverse SE.

OUTCOMES/EVALUATE

- Inhibition of MDS with <5% myeloblasts and Hb >11 g/dL
- Hematologic recovery

Delavirdine mesylate

(deh-lah-**VIR**-deen)

Classification(s): Antiviral, non-nucleoside reverse transcriptase inhibitor

Pregnancy Category: C

RX: Rescriptor.

SEE ALSO ***ANTIVIRAL DRUGS***.

INDICATIONS/USES

Treatment of HIV-1 infections in combination with at least 2 other active antiretroviral agents when therapy is warranted.

ACTION/KINETICS

Action

Non-nucleoside reverse transcriptase inhibitor that binds directly to reverse transcriptase and blocks RNA-dependent and DNA-dependent DNA polymerase activities. Effect is additive if used with other antiviral drugs. Delavirdine may confer cross-resistance to other non-nucleoside reverse transcriptase inhibitors when used alone or in combination.

Pharmacokinetics

Rapidly absorbed. **Peak plasma levels:** About 1 hr. Median area under the curve is about 30% higher in females than males. Converted to inactive metabolites by both CYP3A and CYP2D6. Excreted in urine and feces. It inhibits its own metabolism. **t½, plasma:** 2–11 hr. Resistance to the drug develops; also cross-resistance may develop to other non-nucleoside reverse transcriptase inhibitors. **Plasma protein binding:** About 98%.

CONTRAINDICATIONS

Hypersensitivity to delavirdine or any component of the product. Use with drugs that are highly dependent on CYP3A for clearance and for which increased plasma levels are associated with serious or life-threatening events; drugs include alprazolam, cisapride, dihydroergotamine, ergonovine, ergotamine, methylergonovine, midazolam, pimozide, and triazolam. Lactation.

SPECIAL CONCERNS

■ (1) Delavirdine tablets are for treatment of HIV-1 infection in combination with appropriate antiretroviral agents when therapy is warranted. The indication is based on surrogate marker changes in clinical studies. Clinical benefit was not demonstrated for delavirdine based on survival or incidence of AIDS-defining clinical events in a completed trial comparing delavirdine plus didanosine with didanosine monotherapy. (2) Resistant virus emerges rapidly when delavirdine is given as monotherapy. Therefore, always give in combination with appropriate antiretroviral therapy. ■

- Use with caution in impaired hepatic function.
- Use with combination therapy as resistant viruses emerge with monotherapy.
- Use caution when dosing elderly clients.
- Safety and efficacy in combination with other antiretroviral drugs not determined in HIV-1-infected clients less than 16 years of age.

SIDE EFFECTS

Most Common

Rash, maculopapular rash, N&V, diarrhea, headache, fatigue, pruritus.

Body as a whole: Headache, fatigue, abscess, asthenia, allergic reaction, angioedema, chest pain, chills, general or local edema, fever, flu syndrome, infection (including viral), lethargy, malaise, neck rigidity, general or local pain, trauma. Fat redistribution or accumulation of body fat, including central obesity, dorsocervical fat enlargement (buffalo hump), peripheral wasting, facial wasting, breast enlargement, and "cushingoid appearance." **GI:** N&V, diarrhea, anorexia, aphthous stomatitis, bloody stool, colitis, constipation, appetite decreased or increased, diarrhea (*Clostridium difficile*), duodenitis, dry mouth, diverticulitis, dyspepsia, dysphagia, fecal incontinence, flatulence, enteritis (at all levels), eructation, esophagitis, gastritis, gagging, gastroenteritis, gastroesophageal reflux, GI bleeding or disorder, gingivitis, gum hemorrhage, hiccoughs, increased saliva, increased thirst, mouth ulcer, abdominal cramps/distention/pain (local or generalized), lip edema, oral/enteric moniliasis, ***pancreatitis***, rectal disorder, sialadenitis, stomatitis, mouth/tongue inflammation/ulcers, tongue edema, tooth abscess/ache. **Hepatic:** Hepatomegaly, hepatitis (nonspecific), jaundice, impaired hepatic function, ***hepatic failure***. **CV:** Bradycardia, migraine, pallor, palpitation, postural hypotension, syncope, tachycardia, vasodilation, abnormal cardiac rate/rhythm, cardiac insufficiency, cardiomyopathy, hypertension, vascular disorder. **CNS:** Headache, abnormal coordination, agitation, amnesia, anxiety, change in dreams, cognitive impairment, confusion, decreased libido, depression, disorientation, dizziness, emotional lability, euphoria, hallucinations, hyperesthesia, hyperreflexia, hypertonia, hypesthesia, impaired coordination, insomnia, mania, nervousness, neuropathy, nightmares, paralysis, paranoia, paresthesia, restlessness, sleep cycle disorder, somnolence, tingling, tremor, vertigo, weakness. **Dermatologic:** Skin rashes, maculopapular rash, pruritus, angioedema, dermal leukocytoblastic vasculitis, dermatitis, dry/moist desquamation, ulceration, diaphoresis, discolored skin, dry skin, erythema, erythema multiforme, folliculitis, fungal dermatitis, alopecia, herpes simplex/zoster, nail disorder, petechial rash, seborrhea, skin disorder, skin hypertrophy, skin nodule, ***Stevens-Johnson syndrome***, urticaria, vesiculobullous rash, vesiculation, wart, sebaceous/epidermal cyst. **GU:** Breast enlargement, amenorrhea, kidney calculi, chromaturia, epididymitis, hematuria, hemospermia, impotence, impaired urination, kidney pain, metrorrhagia, nocturia, polyuria, proteinuria, testicular pain, UTI, vaginal moniliasis, acute kidney failure. **Musculoskeletal:** Back pain, neck rigidity, arthritis or arthralgia of single or multiple joints, rhabdomyolysis, bone disorder or pain, leg cramps, muscle weakness, myalgia, tendon disorder, tenosynovitis, tetany, muscle cramps, flank pain. **Respiratory:** URTI, bronchitis, chest congestion, cough, dyspnea, epistaxis, laryngismus, pharyngitis, pneumonia, rhinitis, sinusitis. **Hematologic:** Anemia, adenopathy, bruises, ecchymosis, eosinophilia, granulocytosis, hemolytic anemia, leukopenia, neutropenia, pancytopenia, petechiae, purpura, spleen disorder, thrombocytopenia. **Ophthalmic:** Nystagmus, blepharitis, blurred vision, conjunctivitis, diplopia, dry eyes, photophobia. **Otic:** Tinnitus, ear pain, otitis media. **Miscellaneous:** Alcohol intolerance, peripheral edema, weight increase or decrease, parosmia, taste perversion, *Mycobacterium tuberculosis* infection.

LABORATORY TEST CONSIDERATIONS

↑ ALT, AST, APTT, bilirubin, GGT, lipase, serum alkaline phosphatase, serum amylase, serum creatinine phosphatase, serum creatine, serum creatinine. Bilirubinemia, hyperglycemia, hyperkalemia, hypertriglyceridemia, hyperuricemia, hypocalcemia, hyponatremia, hypophosphatemia. Prolonged PTT.

DRUG INTERACTIONS

NOTE: Delavirdine is an inhibitor of CYP3A isoform and to a lesser extent CYP2C9, CYP2D6, and CYP2C19. Coadministration of delavirdine and drugs metabolized mainly by CYP3A may result in ↑ plasma levels of the coadministered drug → ↑ or prolonged therapeutic and side effects.

Amprenavir / Possible ↑ amprenavir plasma levels

Antacids / ↓ Delavirdine absorption; separate doses by 1 hr

Benzodiazepines (e.g., alprazolam, midazolam, triazolam) / Possible serious/life-threatening drug side effects such as prolonged or ↑ sedation or respiratory depression R/T ↓ metabolism

Calcium channel blockers, dihydropyridine-type / Possible serious or life-threatening drug side effects R/T ↓ metabolism
Carbamazepine / Possible loss of virologic response or resistance to delavirdine or other non-nucleoside reverse transcriptase inhibitors R/T ↓ delavirdine plasma levels R/T ↑ metabolism
Cisapride / Potential for serious/life-threatening reactions, such as cardiac arrhythmias; also, ↑ plasma cisapride levels; use together contraindicated
Clarithromycin / ↑ Delavirdine plasma levels R/T ↑ absorption; also, ↑ plasma clarithromycin levels
Dapsone / Possible serious or life-threatening drug side effects of dapsone R/T ↑ plasma dapsone levels R/T ↓ metabolism
Didanosine / ↓ Absorption of both drugs; separate administration by at least 1 hr
Ergot derivatives (e.g., dihydroergotamine, ergonovine, ergotamine, methylergonovine) / Possible serious or life-threatening ergot side effects, such as acute ergot toxicity characterized by peripheral vasospasm and ischemia of the extremities and other tissues
Fluoxetine / ↑ Trough levels of delavirdine by 50%
HMG-CoA reductase inhibitors (e.g., lovastatin, simvastatin) / Potential for serious side effects, such as myopathy, including rhabdomyolysis
H_2-receptors antagonists / Possible ↓ absorption of delavirdine R/T ↑ gastric pH
Indinavir / ↑ Indinavir levels R/T ↓ metabolism; possible serious side effects (reduce indinavir dose to 600 mg 3 times per day)
Ketoconazole / ↑ Trough levels of delavirdine by 50%
Phenobarbital / Possible loss of virologic response or resistance to delavirdine or other non-nucleoside reverse transcriptase inhibitors R/T ↓ delavirdine plasma levels R/T ↑ metabolism
Phenytoin / Possible loss of virologic response or resistance to delavirdine or other non-nucleoside reverse transcriptase inhibitors R/T ↓ delavirdine plasma levels R/T ↑ metabolism
Pimozide / Potential for serious/life-threatening reactions, such as cardiac arrhythmias; use together contraindicated
Quinidine / Possible serious or life-threatening drug side effects R/T ↓ metabolism
Rifabutin, Rifampin / ↓ Delavirdine levels R/T ↑ hepatic metabolism; also, possible ↑ rifabutin plasma levels; possible loss of virologic response or resistance to delavirdine or other non-nucleoside reverse transcriptase inhibitors
H ***St. John's wort*** / Possible loss of virologic response or resistance to delavirdine or other non-nucleoside reverse transcriptase inhibitors R/T ↑ CYP3A4 metabolism
Saquinavir / ↑ Saquinavir levels R/T ↓ metabolism; possible serious side effects. Also, possible ↓ delavirdine AUC; monitor ALT/AST levels closely
Sildenafil / ↑ Sildenafil levels (do not exceed a single 25 mg dose of sildenafil in a 48-hr period)
Warfarin / ↑ Warfarin levels → possible serious or life-threatening warfarin side effects R/T ↓ metabolism

HOW SUPPLIED

Tablets: 100 mg, 200 mg.

DOSAGE

TABLETS

Human immunodeficiency virus (HIV)-1 infection.

Adults and children, 16 years and older: 400 mg 3 times per day in combination with other antiretroviral therapy.

NURSING IMPLICATIONS

IMPLEMENTATION/ADMINISTRATION/STORAGE

1. Give with or without food.
2. In achlorhydria, take with an acidic beverage (e.g., cranberry or orange juice).
3. The 200 mg tablets are about ⅓ smaller than the 100 mg tablets.
4. An Antiretroviral Pregnancy Registry has been established to monitor maternal-fetal outcomes of pregnant women exposed to delavirdine and other antiretroviral drugs. Register clients by calling 1-800-258-4263.
5. Store from 20–25°C (68–77°F). Protect from high humidity.

ASSESSMENT

1. Note disease onset/exposure times, likelihood of transmission, disease characteristics such as stage of infection, viral load.
2. List drugs prescribed. Assess lifestyle and potential to resume risky behaviors.
3. Monitor CBC, LFTs, viral load, CD4 counts.

CLIENT/FAMILY TEACHING

1. **Take as directed, with or without food. Take didanosine or antacids 1 hr before or 1 hr after drug ingestion. Always take with other antiretroviral therapy.**
2. **The 100 mg tablets may be dispersed with water prior to consumption. To prepare, add four 100 mg tablets to at least 3 ounces of water and allow to stand for a few minutes. Stir until a uniform dispersion occurs and consume promptly. Rinse glass and swallow to ensure entire dose is taken. Do not disperse the 200 mg tablets with water, as they are not readily dispersible.**
3. **In achlorhydria (lack of stomach acid production), take with an acidic beverage (e.g., cranberry or orange juice).**
4. **Drug does not cure HIV infection but only slows virus replication; may continue to have HIV-related illnesses.**
5. **Rash on upper body and arms may require interruption of therapy. Report especially if accompanied by fever, blistering, myalgia, eye or mouth lesions.**
6. **Avoid OTC agents without approval.**
7. **Continue barrier contraception; does not reduce risk of transmission.**
8. **If prescribed Viagra (sildenafil), do not exceed 25 mg in a 48 hr period due to risk of adverse effects such as drop in BP, vision changes and sustained painful erection (priapism).**
9. **Keep all F/U to assess response, labs, and adverse SE.**

OUTCOMES/EVALUATE

Post-exposure prophylaxis HIV; ↓ viral load

IV

Denileukin diftitox

(den-ih-**LOO**-kin **DIF**-tih-tox)

Classification(s): Antineoplastic, miscellaneous

Pregnancy Category: C

RX: Ontak.

INDICATIONS/USES

Treatment of persistent or recurrent cutaneous T-cell lymphoma whose malignant cells express the CD25 component of the IL-2 receptor. *Investigational:* Treatment of chronic lymphocytic leukemia refractory to fludarabine; non-Hodgkin's lymphoma.

ACTION/KINETICS

Action

A recombinant DNA-derived cytotoxic protein designed to direct the cytocidal action of diphtheria toxin to cells that express the IL-2 receptor. The human IL-2 receptor consists of 3 forms: low (CD25), intermediate (CD122/CD132), and high affinity (CD25/CD122/CD132). The high affinity form is usually found only on activated T-lymphocytes, activated B-lymphocytes, and activated macrophages. Malignant cells expressing 1 or more of the subunits of the IL-2 receptor are found in certain leukemias and lymphomas, including cutaneous T-cell lymphoma. It is believed denileukin interacts with the high affinity IL-2 receptor on the cell surface leading to inhibition of cellular protein synthesis and cell death within hours.

Pharmacokinetics

t½, distribution: About 2–5 min; **t½, terminal:** About 70–80 min. Metabolized by proteolytic degradation. Development of antibodies significantly impacts clearance rates.

CONTRAINDICATIONS

Hypersensitivity to denileukin, diphtheria toxin, interleukin-2, or excipients in the product.

SPECIAL CONCERNS

The following adverse reactions have been reported: (1) Serious and fatal infusion reactions. Administer denileukin diftitox in a facility equipped and staffed for cardiopulmonary resuscitation. Immediately stop and permanently discontinue denileukin diftitox for serious infusion reactions. (2) Capillary leak syndrome resulting in death. Monitor weight, edema, BP, and serum albumin levels prior to and during denileukin diftitox treatment. (3) Loss of visual acuity and color vision.

- **Pre-existing low serum albumin levels may predict and predispose clients to the vascular leak syndrome.**
- **Wait about 4 hr after a dose to breast-feed; this should limit the exposure of the infant to the drug.**
- **Safety and efficacy not determined in children or in cutaneous T-cell lymphoma whose malignant**

cells do *not* express the CD25 component of the IL-2 receptor.

SIDE EFFECTS

Most Common

Cough, diarrhea, dyspnea, fatigue, headache, N&V, peripheral edema, pruritus, pyrexia, rigors, capillary leak syndrome, infusion reactions, visual changes.

Up to 5% of side effects are severe or life-threatening. **Hypersensitivity**: Hypotension, back pain, dyspnea, vasodilation, rash, chest pain/tightness, tachycardia, dysphagia or laryngismus, syncope, allergic reaction, ***anaphylaxis***. **Capillary leak syndrome:** Hypotension, edema, hypoalbuminemia, ***death***. **GI**: N&V, anorexia, diarrhea, dysgeusia, constipation, dyspepsia, dysphagia, pancreatitis. **CNS**: Dizziness, headache, paresthesia, nervousness, confusion, insomnia. **CV**: Hypo-/hypertension, vasodilation, tachycardia, thrombotic events, arrhythmia. **Dermatologic:** Acute or delayed onset rash (generalized maculopapular, petechial, vesicular bullous, urticarial, or eczematous), pruritus, sweating. **GU**: Hematuria, albuminuria, pyuria, acute renal insufficiency, microscopic hematuria. **Hematologic:** Anemia, thrombocytopenia, leukopenia. **Metabolic:** Peripheral edema, weight decrease, dehydration (due to GI events). **Respiratory:** Dyspnea, increased cough, URTI, pharyngitis, rhinitis, lung disorder. **Musculoskeletal:** Myalgia, arthralgia, back pain. **Ophthalmic:** Loss of visual acuity, usually with loss of color vision, with or without retinal pigment mottling. **Body as a whole:** Chills, fever, fatigue, asthenia, rigors, infection, pain, headache, flu-like syndrome. **Miscellaneous:** Chest pain, injection site reaction, infectious complications (decreased lymphocyte counts), hyper-/hypothyroidism, immunogenicity.

LABORATORY TEST CONSIDERATIONS

↑ Creatinine, ALT, AST. Hypoalbuminemia, hypocalcemia, hypokalemia.

HOW SUPPLIED

Injection Solution, Concentrate: 150 mcg/mL.

DOSAGE

IV ONLY

Cutaneous T-cell lymphoma.

For each treatment cycle, give 9 or 18 mcg/kg/day by IV infusion over 30–60 min for 5 consecutive days q 21 days for 8 cycles. Premedicate with an antihistamine and acetaminophen before each denileukin diftitox infusion.

NURSING IMPLICATIONS

IMPLEMENTATION/ADMINISTRATION/STORAGE

1. **IV If side effects occur during IV infusion, stop/reduce rate, depending on reaction severity. Withhold administration if serum albumin levels are less than 3 grams/dL.**
2. **Optimal duration of therapy has not been determined.**
3. **Prepare and hold diluted denileukin in plastic syringes or soft plastic IV bags (adsorption will occur if glass containers are used).**
4. **Concentration must be 15 or more mcg/mL during all steps in the preparation of the solution for IV infusion. Ensure by withdrawing calculated dose from the vial(s) and injecting it into an empty IV infusion bag. For each 1 mL of denileukin removed from the vial(s), no more than 9 mL of sterile saline without preservative should be added to the IV bag.**
5. **Store frozen at −10°C (14°F) or lower. Bring to room temperature before preparing dose. May thaw vials in refrigerator for 24 hr or less or at room temperature for 1–2 hr. Do not heat. Administer prepared solutions within 6 hr. Do not refreeze.**
6. **Mix solution in the vial by gently swirling (do not shake vigorously). After thawing, a haze may be visible, which should clear when solution reaches room temperature. Do not use unless clear, colorless, and without visible particulate matter.**
7. **Infuse over 30–60 min using a syringe pump or IV infusion bag. Do not administer as a bolus injection or through an in-line filter.**
8. **Administer prepared solution within 6 hr, using a syringe pump or IV infusion bag.**
9. **Discard any unused portion immediately.**
10. COMPATIBILITY **0.9% NaCl.**
11. INCOMPATIBILITY **Do not physically mix with other drugs or administer through an in-line filter.**

ASSESSMENT

1. **Note disease onset, other agents trialed, outcome.**

2. Assess albumin levels; delay administration until levels are >3 grams/dL. Low albumin levels may predispose to vascular leak syndrome.
3. Premedicate with an antihistamine and acetaminophen prior to each infusion.
4. Manage hypersensitivity reactions as follows:
   - Interrupt/decrease rate of infusion, depending on severity of reaction.
   - IV antihistamines, corticosteroids, and epinephrine may be required.
   - Have resuscitative equipment readily available.
5. Monitor VS, weight, for edema, or S&S of infection during therapy.
6. Test malignant cells for CD25 expression prior to starting therapy. Obtain CBC, electrolytes, albumin, renal and LFTs prior to starting therapy and weekly during therapy.

CLIENT/FAMILY TEACHING

1. Used to treat cutaneous T-cell lymphoma, a rare type of cancer that affects certain WBCs and causes lesions to develop on the skin.
2. Monitor weight daily; report any significant gain/loss.
3. Report adverse effects, any S&S of infection, anemia, or unusual bruising/bleeding. Avoid alcohol, aspirin products, or ibuprofen.
4. Practice reliable contraception during and for several months following therapy.
5. Back pain, chest pain, dizziness or faintness, difficulty swallowing, fast or irregular heartbeat, fever or chills, infection, rash, SOB, swelling of face, feet, or lower legs, warmth and flushing of skin may be experienced.
6. Report any visual changes e.g., loss of acuity or color vision.
7. Keep all F/U to assess response, labs, and adverse SE.

OUTCOMES/EVALUATE

Inhibition of malignant cell proliferation; ↓ tumor burden

Denosumab

(den-**OH**-sue-mab)

Classification(s): Monoclonal antibody for osteoporosis.

Pregnancy Category: C

RX: Prolia, Xgeva.

INDICATIONS/USES

(1) **Prolia only:** Treatment of osteoporosis in postmenopausal women at high risk for fracture; defined as a history of osteoporotic fracture, or multiple risk factors for fracture, or those who have failed or are intolerant to other available osteoporosis therapies. (2) **Xgeva only:** Prevention of skeletal-related events in clients with bone metastases from solid tumors.

ACTION/KINETICS

Action

Binds to receptor activator of nuclear factor kappa-B ligand (RANKL), a transmembrane or soluble protein essential for the formation, function, and survival of osteoclasts (cells responsible for bone resorption). Denosumab prevents RANKL from activating its receptor on the surface of osteoclasts and their precursors. Prevention of the interaction with the receptor inhibits osteoclast formation, function, and survival, thus decreasing bone resorption and increasing bone mass and strength in both cortical and trabecular bone.

Pharmacokinetics

Prolia. Time to C_{max}: 10 days. Serum levels then decline over a period of 4–5 months. **t½, mean:** 25.4 days. **Xgeva.** Is 62% bioavailable. **Steady-state:** Achieved in 6 months. **t½, mean:** 28 days.

CONTRAINDICATIONS

Hypocalcemia. Use in children. Lactation.

SPECIAL CONCERNS

It is important to distinguish the dosing and use differences between Prolia and Xgeva.

SIDE EFFECTS

Most Common

Prolia: Back pain, pain in the extremities, musculoskeletal pain, hypercholesterolemia, cystitis.
Xgeva: Fatigue, asthenia, hypophosphatemia, nausea.

Prolia. Musculoskeletal: Back pain, pain in the extremities, musculoskeletal pain, bone pain, myalgia, spinal osteoarthritis, osteonecrosis of the jaw, suppression of bone remodeling, atypical fractures, delayed fracture healing. **GI:** Constipation, upper abdominal pain, flatulence, GERD, ***pancreatitis***. **CNS:** Vertigo, sciatica, insomnia. **CV:** Angina pectoris, atrial fibrillation, endocarditis. **Respiratory:** URTI, pneumonia, pharyngitis. **GU:** Cystitis, breast cancer. **Dermatologic:** Rash, pruritus, dermatitis, eczema. **Hematologic:** Anemia. **Metabolic:** Hypercholesterolemia, hypocalcemia (may be severe). **Body as a whole:** Asthenia, peripheral edema, herpes zoster, ***infections*** (may be serious; includes UTI; abdomen; ear; and, skin, including erysipelas and cellulitis), new malignancies (e.g., breast, reproductive, GI). **Miscellaneous:** Immunogenicity.

D

Xgeva. Musculoskeletal: Osteonecrosis of the jaw. **GI:** Nausea, diarrhea. **CNS:** Headache. **Respiratory:** Dyspnea, cough. **Metabolic:** Hypocalcemia, hypophosphatemia. **Body as a whole:** Fatigue, asthenia.

LABORATORY TEST CONSIDERATIONS

Hypocalcemia, hypercholesterolemia, hypophosphatemia (Xgeva).

HOW SUPPLIED

Injection Solution: 60 mg/mL (Prolia), 70 mg/mL (Xgeva).

DOSAGE

SC

Osteoporosis in postmenopausal women (Prolia only).

Adults, usual: 60 mg once q 6 months. If an injection is missed, give it as soon as the client is available; thereafter, schedule injections q 6 months from the date of the last injection. *NOTE:* All clients should receive 1,000 mg calcium/day and at least 400 units vitamin D/day.

Bone metastases from solid tumors (Xgeva only).

Adults: 120 mg q 4 weeks. Administer with calcium and vitamin D as needed to treat or prevent hypocalcemia.

NURSING IMPLICATIONS

IMPLEMENTATION/ADMINISTRATION/STORAGE

1. Pre-existing hypocalcemia must be corrected prior to beginning denosumab therapy.
2. Consider the benefit to risk when giving denosumab to those with severe renal impairment (C_{CR} <30 mL/min) or dialysis as they may be at greater risk of developing hypocalcemia.
3. Prior to administration, may be removed from the refrigerator and brought to room temperature in the original container. Takes 15–30 min. Do not warm denosumab any other way. Avoid vigorous shaking.
4. Administer by SC injection in the upper arm, upper thigh, or abdomen.
5. Use a 27-gauge needle to withdraw and inject the dose.
6. Women who become pregnant during denosumab therapy are encouraged to enroll in the manufacturer's Pregnancy Surveillance Program. Clients or their provider should call 1-800-772-6436 to enroll.
7. Store in the refrigerator (2–8°C; 36–46°F) in the original carton. Do not freeze. Once removed from the refrigerator, do not expose to temperatures above 25°C (77°F). Must be used within 14 days; if not, discard. Protect from direct light and heat.

ASSESSMENT

1. Note indications for therapy, age at onset, dexa scan confirmation or fracture history, other agents trialed and outcome.
2. Obtain dental exam prior to starting therapy. Observe for osteonecrosis of jaw, which has been associated with tooth extraction and/or local infection with delayed healing and usually with prolonged therapy.
3. Identify any skin rashes/changes or disorders noted with therapy.
4. Determine any hypocalcemia, thyroid/parathyroid surgery, malabsorption syndrome, or renal disorders. Monitor cholesterol, calcium, phosphorus, and magnesium levels.

CLIENT/FAMILY TEACHING

1. Administered by HCP via injection just under the skin once every 6 months in the upper arm, the upper thigh, or the abdomen for fracture prevention with osteoporosis.
2. Take calcium 1,000 mg and vitamin D 400 international units daily with this therapy.
3. Those sensitive to latex should not handle the gray needle cap on the single-use prefilled syringe.
4. Report any S&S of infection: fever, chills, severe abdominal pain, red swollen skin surfaces, or painful frequent urination. Also, any S&S of hypocalcemia (paresthesias or muscle stiffness, twitching, spasms, or cramps) requires reporting.

5. May experience back, muscle or extremity pain; report if persistent or bothersome.
6. Practice daily, careful oral hygiene with regular brushing and flossing. Report any pain or dental problems immediately. Ensure dentist is aware of drug therapy.
7. Not for use during pregnancy. If pregnancy occurs, report to Amgen's Pregnancy Surveillance Program, or call 1-800-772-6436 (1-800-77-AMGEN).
8. Keep all F/U to assess response, labs, and adverse SE.

OUTCOMES/EVALUATE

↓ Incidence of vertebral, nonvertebral, and hip fractures in high-risk post-menopausal women with osteoporosis

Desipramine hydrochloride

(dess-**IP**-rah-meen)

Classification(s): Antidepressant, tricyclic

Pregnancy Category: C

RX: Norpramin.

🍁 **Rx:** Apo-Desipramine, Novo-Desipramine, Nu-Desipramine, PMS-Desipramine, ratio-Desipramine.

SEE ALSO ***ANTIDEPRESSANTS, TRICYCLIC.***

INDICATIONS/USES

Treatment of depression. *Investigational:* Bulimia nervosa, panic disorder, premenstrual symptoms, facilitation of cocaine withdrawal, chronic urticaria and angioedema, nocturnal pruritus in atopic eczema.

ACTION/KINETICS

Action

Significant norepinephrine uptake blocking activity and moderate serotonin uptake blocking activity. Slight anticholinergic, sedative, and orthostatic hypotensive effects.

Pharmacokinetics

Well absorbed. **Peak plasma levels:** 2–4 hr. **Effective plasma levels:** 125–300 ng/mL. **t½:** 12–24 hr. **Time to reach steady state:** 2–11 days. Response usually seen within the first week. Significant first-pass effect. **Plasma protein binding:** >90%.

CONTRAINDICATIONS

Use in children less than 12 years of age. Tricyclic antidepressant and MAOI combined use.

SPECIAL CONCERNS

(1) Antidepressants increase the risk of suicidal thinking and behavior (suicidality) in short-term studies in children, adolescents, and young adults with major depressive disorders and other psychiatric disorders compared with placebo. Anyone considering the use of desipramine or any other antidepressant in a child, adolescent, or young adult must balance this risk with the clinical need. (2) Short-term studies did not show an increase in the risk of suicidality with antidepressants compared with placebo in adults older than 24 years of age; there was a reduction in risk with antidepressants compared with placebo in adults 65 years of age and older. (3) Depression and certain other psychiatric disorders are themselves associated with increases in the risk of suicide. Closely observe and appropriately monitor clients of all ages who are started on antidepressant therapy for clinical worsening, suicidality, or unusual changes in behavior. Advise families and caregivers of the need for close observation and communication with the prescribing health care provider. Desipramine is not approved for use in children.

- Use with caution with seizure disorders or other predisposing factors to seizures (e.g., brain damage, alcoholism, concomitant drugs known to lower the seizure threshold).
- Due to anticholinergic effects, use with caution with a history of urinary retention, narrow-angle glaucoma, or increased IOP.
- Use with extreme caution in CV disorders due to possible conduction defects, arrhythmias, CHF, sinus tachycardia, MI, strokes, and tachycardia.
- Schizophrenic or paranoid clients may show worsening of psychosis.
- Safe use during pregnancy not established.
- Safety and efficacy not established in children.

SIDE EFFECTS

Most Common

Dizziness, drowsiness, dry mouth, taste alteration, photosensitivity, tremors, constipation, decreased libido, blurred vision.

See *Antidepressants, Tricyclic* for a complete list of possible side effects. Also, bad taste in mouth, hypertension during surgery, mania, or hypomania. Impending toxicity from high doses is prolongation of the QRS or QT intervals on ECG, as well as drowsiness, dizziness, and postural hypotension.

D

HOW SUPPLIED

Tablets: 10 mg, 25 mg, 50 mg, 75 mg, 100 mg, 150 mg.

DOSAGE

TABLETS

Antidepressant.

Initial: 100–200 mg per day in single or divided doses. **Maximum daily dose:** 300 mg in severely ill clients. **Maintenance:** 50–100 mg given once per day. **Geriatric and adolescent clients:** 25–100 mg per day in single or divided doses up to a maximum of 150 mg per day.

NURSING IMPLICATIONS

Do not confuse desipramine with diphenhydramine (an antihistamine), imipramine, clomipramine, nortriptyline; or Norpramin with Normodyne (labetalol, an antihypertensive).

IMPLEMENTATION/ADMINISTRATION/STORAGE

1. Initiate in hospital setting for those requiring 300 mg/day.
2. Lower doses are recommended for outpatients compared with hospitalized clients. Also lower doses are recommended for adolescents and the elderly.
3. Give maintenance doses for at least 2 months following satisfactory response.
4. Store from 15–30°C (59–86°F). Protect from excessive heat.

ASSESSMENT

1. Note reasons for therapy, onset, characteristics of S&S, other agents trialed, outcome.
2. Assess mental status; note any suicide behaviors.
3. Obtain ECG; prolongation of the QRS or QT and PR interval may occur.
4. Check for CAD, thyroid disease, seizure disorders, glaucoma, or BPH. Monitor BP, HR, weight, lipid panel, BS, renal and LFTs. Initiate at lower doses in elderly, adolescents, and with dysfunction

CLIENT/FAMILY TEACHING

1. Take as directed; may take 4–6 weeks to note desired effects.
2. Take single daily dose or any dosage increases at bedtime; reduce daytime sedation. Report lack of desired response/adverse side effects.
3. Use caution; drowsiness, dizziness, or drop in BP may occur. May require dosage reduction.
4. Avoid prolonged sun exposure and use precautions when exposed. Increase fluid intake to prevent dehydration.
5. Keep log of BP, HR, and weight for provider review.
6. Avoid alcohol and all OTC drugs without approval. Do not stop drug suddenly; with prolonged therapy may experience headaches, nausea and malaise.
7. Advise males of possible sexual dysfunction and difficult urination.
8. Store safely out of child's reach. Report any increased depression, behavior changes, or suicide ideations immediately.
9. Keep all F/U to assess response, VS, depression scores, and adverse SE.

OUTCOMES/EVALUATE

- ↓ Depression; ↑ self-worth
- Relief of neurogenic pain
- Therapeutic levels (125–300 ng/mL)

Desirudin

(**DEH**-sih-rue-din)

Classification(s): Antithrombin drug

Pregnancy Category: C

RX: Iprivask.

INDICATIONS/USES

Prophylaxis of DVT that may lead to pulmonary embolism in clients undergoing elective hip replacement surgery.

ACTION/KINETICS

Action

A specific inhibitor of free-circulating and clot-bound human thrombin. Desirudin prolongs the clotting time of human plasma by increasing aPTT. One molecule of desirudin binds to 1 molecule of thrombin, thereby blocking the thrombogenic activity of thrombin. As a result, all thrombin-dependent coagulation assays are affected. Thrombin time may exceed 200 seconds, even at low plasma desirudin levels; thus, this test is unsuitable for routine monitoring of desirudin therapy. At therapeutic serum levels, the drug has no effect on factors IXa, Xa, kallikrein, plasmin, tissue plasminogen activator, or activated protein.

Pharmacokinetics

Absorption is complete. **Maximum plasma levels:** 1–3 hr. Primarily metabolized and eliminated by the kidney with about 40–50% excreted unchanged. **t½, elimination:** 2–3 hr after SC use. **Plasma protein binding:** >99%.

CONTRAINDICATIONS

IM use. Known hypersensitivity to natural or recombinant hirudins and in those with active bleeding and/or irreversible coagulation disorders.

SPECIAL CONCERNS

(1) **Spinal/Epidural Hematomas.** When neuraxial anesthesia (epidural/spinal anesthesia) or spinal puncture is employed, clients anticoagulated or scheduled to be anticoagulated with selective thrombin inhibitors, such as desirudin, may be at risk of developing an epidural or spinal hematoma, which can result in long-term or permanent paralysis. (2) The risk of the preceding events may be increased by the use of indwelling spinal catheters for administration of analgesia or by the concomitant use of drugs affecting hemostasis, such as NSAIDs, platelet inhibitors, or other anticoagulants. Likewise with such agents, the risk appears to be increased by traumatic or repeated epidural or spinal puncture. (3) Frequently monitor clients for signs and symptoms of neurological impairment. If neurological compromise is noted, urgent treatment is required. (4) The physician should consider the potential benefit versus risk before neuraxial intervention, in clients anticoagulated or to be anticoagulated for thromboprophylaxis.

- **Use with caution in clients with increased risks of hemorrhage, including those with recent major surgery, organ biopsy, or puncture of a noncompressible vessel within the last month; also, a history of hemorrhagic stroke, intracranial or intraocular bleeding including diabetic retinopathy, recent ischemic stroke, severe uncontrolled hypertension, bacterial endocarditis, congenital or acquired hemostatic disorder (e.g., hemophilia, liver disease), or a history of GI or pulmonary bleeding within the past 3 months.**
- **Use with caution in clients with renal impairment, especially in those with moderate and severe renal impairment (C_{CR} less than 60 mL/min/1.74 m^2 body surface area) and in those with impaired liver function. See *Implementation/Administration/Storage* for adjustments to dosage in renal insufficiency.**
- **Risk of side effects may be greater in elderly clients.**
- **Use with caution during lactation.**
- **Safety and efficacy not determined in children.**

SIDE EFFECTS

Most Common

Hemorrhage, injection site mass, wound secretion, anemia, deep thrombophlebitis, nausea.

Hemorrhagic events: Hematomas; ***hemorrhages, including retroperitoneal, intracranial, intraocular, intraspinal, or in a major prosthetic joint.*** **CV:** Deep thrombophlebitis, thrombosis, hypotension, CV disorder. **GI:** N&V. **Body as a whole:** Wound secretion, fever, impaired healing. **Miscellaneous:** Injection site mass, anemia, leg edema, decreased hemoglobin, hematuria, dizziness, epistaxis, leg pain, hematemesis, hypersensitivity reactions, including ***anaphylaxis***.

OVERDOSE MANAGEMENT

Symptoms: Hemorrhagic complications, excessively high aPTT values. *Treatment:* Discontinue desirudin therapy. Effects of desirudin are partially reversed by using thrombin-rich plasma concentrates. aPTT levels can be decreased by IV administration of 0.3 mcg/kg of desmopressin. Institute emergency procedures as appropriate.

DRUG INTERACTIONS

Abciximab / Use with caution with desirudin
Alteplase / ↑ Risk of bleeding
Anticoagulants (heparin, low molecular weight heparins) / Prolongation of aPTT; do not use together
Aspirin / Use with caution with desirudin
Clopidogrel / Use with caution with desirudin
Dextran / ↑ Risk of bleeding

Dipyridamole / Use with caution with desirudin
Glucocorticoids / ↑ Risk of bleeding
Ketorolac / Use with caution with desirudin
NSAIDs / Use with caution with desirudin
Salicylates / Use with caution with desirudin
Streptokinase / ↑ Risk of bleeding
Sulfinpyrazone / Use with caution with desirudin
Ticlopidine / Use with caution with desirudin

D

HOW SUPPLIED

Powder for Injection, Lyophilized: 15 mg.

DOSAGE

SC

Prophylaxis of deep vein thrombosis (DVT) during hip replacement surgery.

Adults: 15 mg q 12 hr with the initial dose given up to 5–15 min before surgery, but after induction of regional block anesthesia (if used). May be given up to 12 days (average is 9–12 days).

NURSING IMPLICATIONS

IMPLEMENTATION/ADMINISTRATION/STORAGE

1. Reduce dosage with renal insufficiency as follows:
   - **Moderate insufficiency.** If C_{CR} is between 31 and 60 mL/min/1.73 m^2, begin therapy at 5 mg SC q 12 hr. Monitor aPTT and serum creatinine at least daily. If aPTT exceeds 2 times control, (a) interrupt therapy until the value returns to <2 times control and (b) resume therapy at a reduced dose guided by the initial degree of aPTT abnormality.
   - **Severe insufficiency.** If C_{CR} <31 mL/min/1.73 m^2, begin therapy at 1.7 mg SC q 12 hr. Monitor aPTT and serum creatinine at least daily. If aPTT exceeds 2 times control, (a) interrupt therapy until the value returns to <2 times control and (b) consider further dose reductions guided by the initial degree of aPTT abnormality.
2. Reconstitute each vial under sterile conditions with 0.5 mL of provided diluent (mannitol, 3%, in water for injection). Shake gently until drug is fully reconstituted.
3. Once reconstituted, each 0.5 mL contains 15.75 mg of desirudin.
4. Use the reconstituted solution immediately, although stable for up to 24 hr when stored at room temperature and protected from light. Discard any unused solution. Do not mix with other injections, solvents, or infusions.
5. To administer SC, use a 26- or 27-gauge ½-inch needle. Withdraw the entire reconstituted solution (15.75 mg/0.5 mL) into the syringe, and inject the total volume (will deliver 15 mg).
6. Desirudin cannot be used interchangeably with other hirudins as they differ in their manufacturing process and specific biological activity.
7. Do not use any vial that is discolored or that has particles in it.
8. Store unopened vials from 15–30°C (59–86°F); protect from light.

ASSESSMENT

1. With elective THR, administer initial dose 5–15 min before surgery but after induction of regional block anesthesia if used. Given every 12 hr SC for 9–12 days following surgery. If epidural/spinal anesthesia or spinal puncture employed assess carefully for epidural or spinal hematoma, which can result in long-term or permanent paralysis.
2. Assess for any recent surgery or bleeding episodes, bleeding or coagulation disorders, or other conditions that may preclude therapy.
3. With epidural catheter, immediately report any (neuro impairment) midline back pain, numbness or weakness in lower extremities, bowel and/or bladder dysfunction.
4. Monitor CBC, aPTT, renal and LFTs. Decrease dosage with impaired renal function.

CLIENT/FAMILY TEACHING

1. Drug is used to prevent the development of blood clots in the legs or lungs after elective hip replacement surgery.
2. To administer (after instruction), wash hands, lie down and grasp a fold of skin on the abdomen between the thumb and forefinger. Insert the entire length of the needle straight in; use a ½-inch, 26- to 27-gauge needle to minimize tissue trauma. Hold the skin fold throughout the injection. Do not rub or massage area after administration; rotate sites with each injection. Alternate between the left and right anterolateral and posterolateral abdominal walls.

3. Avoid OTC aspirin-containing products. Use electric razor, soft-bristle toothbrush to prevent tissue trauma.
4. Report any unusual chest pain, SOB, bruising/bleeding, acute SOB, itching, rash, or swelling of extremities.
5. Keep all F/U to assess response, labs, adverse SE.

OUTCOMES/EVALUATE

Postoperative DVT prophylaxis

Desloratadine

(**des**-lor-**AT**-ah-deen)

Classification(s): Antihistamine, second generation, piperidine

Pregnancy Category: C

RX: Clarinex, Clarinex Reditabs.

SEE ALSO ***ANTIHISTAMINES (H_1 BLOCKERS)***.

INDICATIONS/USES

(1) Relief of nasal and nonnasal symptoms of seasonal allergic rhinitis in adults and children 6 years and older. (2) Relief of nasal and nonnasal symptoms of perennial allergic rhinitis in adults and children 6 years and older. (3) Symptomatic relief of chronic idiopathic pruritus and reduction in the number and size of hives in adults and children 6 years and older.

ACTION/KINETICS

Action

Desloratadine, a major metabolite of loratadine, is a long-acting selective histamine H_1-receptor antagonist. Low to no anticholinergic or sedative activity.

Pharmacokinetics

Maximum plasma levels: About 3 hr. Neither food nor grapefruit juice affects bioavailability. Metabolized to 3-hydroxydesloratadine, which is also active. There are both slow and normal metabolizers of desloratadine; people of African descent have a higher frequency of slow metabolism. **t½, elimination:** 27 hr. Reduce dose in clients with renal or hepatic impairment.

CONTRAINDICATIONS

Lactation. Use in children less than 4 years of age.

SPECIAL CONCERNS

Use with caution in elderly clients.

SIDE EFFECTS

Most Common

Dizziness, drowsiness/somnolence, headache, fatigue, pharyngitis, myalgia, dry mouth/nose/throat.

See also *Antihistamines* (H_1-blockers) for a complete list of possible side effects. **CNS**: Fatigue, drowsiness/somnolence, headache, dizziness. **GI**: Dry mouth, nausea, dyspepsia. **Miscellaneous**: Pharyngitis, myalgia, dysmenorrhea, tachycardia, dry nose/throat, rarely hypersensitivity reactions (e.g., rash, pruritus, urticaria, edema, dyspnea, ***anaphylaxis***).

LABORATORY TEST CONSIDERATIONS

↑ Liver enzymes, bilirubin.

HOW SUPPLIED

Syrup: 2.5 mg/5 mL; ***Tablets:*** 5 mg; ***Tablets, Rapidly Disintegrating:*** 2.5 mg, 5 mg.

DOSAGE

SYRUP; TABLETS; TABLETS, RAPIDLY DISINTEGRATING

Perennial/seasonal allergic rhinitis; chronic idiopathic urticaria.

Adults and children over 12 years: 5 mg once daily (10 mL of the syrup). **Children, 6–11 years:** 2.5 mg once daily (5 mL of the syrup). **Children, 4–6 years:** Consult provider. In adults with liver or renal impairment, start with 5 mg every other day.

NURSING IMPLICATIONS

IMPLEMENTATION/ADMINISTRATION/STORAGE

1. Protect syrup from light.
2. Protect tablets from excessive moisture.
3. Store tablets, syrup, and disintegrating tablets from 15–30°C (59–86°F).

ASSESSMENT

1. Note reasons for therapy, onset, characteristics of S&S, time of year, triggers if known, clinical presentation. List other agents trialed/outcome.

2. Assess lung sounds, renal and LFTs; reduce dose/frequency with dysfunction.

CLIENT/FAMILY TEACHING

1. May be taken without regard to meals; take with food if GI upset. Use calibrated measuring device for syrup.
2. With dry hands, place the rapidly disintegrating tablet on the tongue immediately after opening the blister. Do not push the tablet through the foil backing. Peel back the foil backing, and remove the tablet (disintegrates rapidly); give with or without water.
3. Do not increase dose or dosing frequency as effectiveness is not increased and sleepiness may occur.
4. Avoid activities that require mental alertness until drug effects realized; may cause drowsiness.
5. Avoid alcohol and CNS depressants.
6. May cause dry mouth; use sips of water, sugar-free gum or ice chips to offset.
7. If allergy skin testing planned, do not take drug for at least 4 days before testing.
8. Keep a diary and attempt to identify triggers.
9. Keep all F/U visits; report unusual/persistent side effects, lack of response, or worsening of symptoms.

OUTCOMES/EVALUATE

- Control of S&S of seasonal/allergic rhinitis
- Relief from idiopathic urticaria
- ↓ Number and size of hives

IV

Desmopressin acetate

(des-moh-**PRESS**-in)

Classification(s): Antidiuretic hormone, synthetic

Pregnancy Category: B

RX: DDAVP, Stimate.

Rx: Apo-Desmopressin, DDAVP Rhinyle Nasal Solution, Minirin, Novo-Desmopressin, Octostim Injection/Spray.

INDICATIONS/USES

Injection. (1) As antidiuretic replacement therapy to manage central (cranial) diabetes insipidus. (2) Manage temporary polyuria and polydipsia following head trauma or surgery in the pituitary region. (3) Hemophilia A clients with factor VIII coagulant activity more than 5%. (4) Maintain hemostasis in clients with hemophilia A during surgical procedures and postoperatively when given 30 min prior to the scheduled procedure. (5) Stop bleeding in hemophilia A clients with episodes of spontaneous or trauma-induced injuries, such as hemarthroses, IM hematomas, or mucosal bleeding. (6) Mild to moderate classic von Willebrand's disease (type I) with factor VIII levels more than 5%. (7) Maintain hemostasis in clients with mild to moderate von Willebrand's disease during surgical procedures and postoperatively when given 30 min prior to the scheduled procedure. (8) Stop bleeding in mild to moderate von Willebrand's clients with episodes of spontaneous or trauma-induced injuries, such as hemarthroses, IM hematomas, or mucosal bleeding.

Intranasal Spray. DDAVP only: (1) Antidiuretic replacement therapy to manage central cranial diabetes insipidus. (2) Manage temporary polyuria and polydipsia following head trauma or surgery in the pituitary region. *NOTE:* Is ineffective to treat nephrogenic diabetes insipidus. **Stimate only:** (1) Hemophilia A with factor VIII coagulant activity levels more than 5%. (2) To stop bleeding in clients with hemophilia A with episodes of spontaneous or trauma-induced injuries, such as hemarthroses, IM hematomas, or mucosal bleeding. (3) Mild to moderate classic von Willebrand's disease (type I) with factor VIII levels more than 5%. (4) To stop bleeding in clients with mild to moderate von Willebrand's disease with episodes of spontaneous or trauma-induced injuries, such as hemarthroses, IM hematomas, mucosal bleeding, or menorrhagia. *Investigational:* Treat chronic autonomic failure (e.g., nocturnal polyuria, overnight weight loss, morning postural hypotension).

Oral (Tablets). (1) Management of central diabetes insipidus. (2) Management of temporary polyuria and polydipsia following head trauma or surgery in the pituitary region. (3) Management of primary nocturnal enuresis. (4) Alone or as an adjunct to behavioral conditioning or other nonpharmacologic intervention.

ACTION/KINETICS

Action

A synthetic analog of arginine vasopressin, which possesses antidiuretic activity but is devoid of vasopressor and oxytocic effects. Acts to increase absorption of water in the kidney by increasing permeability of cells in the collecting ducts. The drug usually will allow resumption of a more normal lifestyle, with a decrease in urinary frequency and nocturia.

Pharmacokinetics

Bioavailability of tablets is about 5% compared with intranasal desmopressin and about 0.16% compared with IV use. **Onset:** 1 hr. **Time to peak levels, intranasal:** 40–45 min; **time to peak levels, PO:** 45 min. **Maximum effect, after PO:** 4–7 hr. **Duration:** 8–20 hr. **t½, plasma:** 1.5–2.5 hr (3.3–3.5 hr after intranasal use). **t½, terminal:** 3 hr in healthy clients and 9 hr in clients with severely impaired renal function. Effect ceases abruptly. Desmopressin also increases factor VIII levels (**onset:** 30 min; **peak:** 1.5–2 hr) and von Willebrand's factor activity. Excreted through the urine.

CONTRAINDICATIONS

Hypersensitivity to desmopressin or any components of the products. Moderate to severe impaired renal function (C_{CR} below 50 mL/min). Hyponatremia or a history of hyponatremia. Use to treat von Willebrand's disease (type IIB) because platelet aggregation may be induced. Parenteral administration for DI in infants under 3 months and intranasal administration in infants less than 11 months to treat hemophilia A or von Willebrand's disease.

SPECIAL CONCERNS

- **Use with caution and with restricted fluid intake in infants due to an increased risk of hyponatremia and water intoxication.**
- **Possible greater risk of developing hyponatremia and water intoxication in the elderly.**
- **Use with caution with coronary artery insufficiency and/or hypertensive CV disease due to possible rise in BP.**
- **Use cautiously with other pressor agents.**
- **Use with caution in those with habitual or psychogenic polydipsia who may be more likely to drink excessive amounts of water leading to increased risk of hyponatremia.**
- **Use with caution in conditions associated with fluid and electrolyte imbalance (e.g., cystic fibrosis, heart failure, renal disorders) as these clients are more prone to hyponatremia.**
- **Use with caution during lactation.**
- **Safety and efficacy not determined in children less than 12 years of age (parenteral) or less than 2 months of age (intranasal) with DI.**

SIDE EFFECTS

Most Common

See below.

The following side effects may be seen with any of the dosage forms. **Metabolic:** Hyponatremia that includes symptoms of headache, N&V, decreased serum sodium, weight gain, restlessness, fatigue, lethargy, disorientation, depressed reflexes, loss of appetite, irritability, muscle weakness/spasms/cramps, hallucinations, decreased consciousness, confusion, ***seizure***, coma, ***respiratory arrest***. **Hypersensitivity:** Severe allergic reactions (rare), ***anaphylaxis*** after intranasal or IV use (rare).

Intranasal. CNS: Headache, agitation, dizziness, insomnia, somnolence. **GI:** N&V, mild abdominal cramps, abdominal pain, dyspepsia, GI disorder. **CV:** Palpitations, tachycardia. **Respiratory:** Nasal congestion, rhinitis, nosebleed, sore throat, cough, URTI, epistaxis, nostril pain, changes in nasal mucosa (scarring, edema). **Dermatologic:** Flushing. **GU:** Balanitis. **Ophthalmic:** Itchy or light-sensitive eyes, conjunctivitis, eye edema, lacrimation disorder. **Body as a whole:** Chills, edema, asthenia, pain, warm feeling. **Miscellaneous:** Chest pain.

Parenteral GI: Abdominal cramps (mild), nausea. **CNS:** Headache (transient). **CV:** Slight elevation or transient decrease in BP and a compensatory increase in HR; acute CV thrombosis or acute MI in those predisposed to thrombus formation. **Dermatologic:** Facial flushing. **GU:** Vulval pain. **At injection site:** Local burning pain, erythema, swelling. **Miscellaneous:** Vulval pain.

Tablets. CNS: Headache (when used for nocturnal enuresis), abnormal thinking. **Miscellaneous:** Diarrhea, edema weight gain.

LABORATORY TEST CONSIDERATIONS

↑ AST (transient) after PO use.

OVERDOSE MANAGEMENT

Symptoms: Continuing headache, confusion, drowsiness, problems with passing urine, rapid weight gain due to fluid retention. *Treatment:* Reduce dose, decrease frequency of administration, or withdraw the drug, depending on the severity of the condition. No known specific antidote.

Observe client and provide appropriate symptomatic therapy.

DRUG INTERACTIONS

Carbamazepine / ↑ Risk of water intoxication with hyponatremia; use together with caution
Chlorpromazine / ↑ Risk of water intoxication with hyponatremia; use together with caution
Imipramine / Possible hyponatremic convulsions
Lamotrigine / ↑ Risk of water intoxication with hyponatremia; use together with caution
NSAIDs (e.g., naproxen) / ↑ Risk of water intoxication with hyponatremia; use together with caution
Opiate analgesics (e.g., methadone) / ↑ Risk of water intoxication with hyponatremia; use together with caution
Oxybutynin / Possible hyponatremic convulsions
Pressor drugs / Use large nasal or parenteral doses (0.3 mcg/kg) of desmopressin with caution with other pressor drugs
Selective serotonin reuptake inhibitors / ↑ Risk of water intoxication with hyponatremia; use together with caution
Tricyclic antidepressants / ↑ Risk of water intoxication with hyponatremia; use together with caution

HOW SUPPLIED

Injection: 4 mcg/mL; ***Intranasal Solution, Spray:*** 0.1 mg/mL, 1.5 mg/mL; ***Tablets:*** 0.1 mg, 0.2 mg.

DOSAGE

INJECTION: DIRECT IV, SC

Central diabetes insipidus.

Individualize dose and adjust according to pattern of response. Estimate response by adequate duration of sleep and adequate, not excessive, water turnover. Observe fluid intake. **Adults:** 0.5–1 mL/day (2–4 mcg/day), usually in two divided doses. **Maximum daily dose:** 4 mcg. The morning and evening doses should be separately adjusted for an adequate diurnal rhythm of water turnover. If switching from intranasal to IV, the comparable IV antidiuretic dose is about 1/10 the intranasal dose.

Hemophilia A, von Willebrand's disease (type I).

Adults and children weighing more than 10 kg: 0.3 mcg/kg diluted in 50 mL 0.9% NaCl injection infused IV over 15–30 min; dose may be repeated, if necessary. **Children, weighing 10 kg or less, IV:** 0.3 mcg/kg diluted in 10 mL of 0.9% NaCl injection and given over 15–30 min; repeat if necessary. Monitor BP and pulse during infusion. If used preoperatively, administer 30 min prior to the scheduled procedure. Observe fluid intake.

INTRANASAL SOLUTION, SPRAY

Central diabetes insipidus.

DDAVP only. Dosage must be determined for each individual client and adjusted, based on the diurnal pattern of response. **Adults, usual:** 0.1–0.4 mL/day, either as a single dose or divided into two to three doses (usual: 0.2 mL/day in two divided doses). Adjust morning and evening doses separately for an adequate diurnal rhythm of water turnover. **Children, 3 months to 12 years:** 0.05–0.3 mL/day, either as a single dose or two divided doses. About 1/3 to 1/4 of children can be controlled by a single daily dose. Fluid restriction should be observed.

Hemophilia A and type I von Willebrand's disease.

Stimate only. In clients weighing 50 kg or more: One spray per nostril (total dose of 300 mcg), using nasal insufflation. **In clients weighing less than 50 kg:** Given as a single spray of 150 mcg. The drug is to be given 2 hr prior to minor surgery in the same doses as described above. Before the initial therapeutic administration, establish that there is an appropriate change in the coagulation profile following a test dose of intranasal desmopressin.

TABLETS

Central cranial diabetes insipidus.

Adults and children, initial: 0.05 mg (i.e., one-half of the 0.1 mg tablet) twice a day; adjust individually to optimum therapeutic dose and adjust each dose for an adequate diurnal rhythm of water turnover. Total daily dose should be increased or decreased (range 0.1–1.2 mg divided 2–3 times per day) as needed to obtain adequate antidiuresis. For most clients, the optimal dose was 0.1–0.8 mg/day. Observe fluid restriction. Careful restriction of fluid intake in children is required to prevent hyponatremia and water intoxication.

Primary nocturnal enuresis.

Children 6 years and older, initial: 0.2 mg at bedtime. May be increased to 0.6 mg, depending on client response. Fluid restriction should be observed and fluid intake limited to a minimum from 1 hr before administration until the next morning or at least 8 hr after administration. Those on previous intranasal desmopressin therapy can begin tablet therapy the night following (24 hr) the last intranasal dose. *NOTE:* Interrupt therapy during acute intercurrent illness characterized by fluid and/or electrolyte imbalance (e.g., systemic infections, fever, recurrent vomiting, diarrhea) or under conditions of extremely hot weather, during vigorous exercise, or other conditions associated with increased water intake.

NURSING IMPLICATIONS

IMPLEMENTATION/ADMINISTRATION/STORAGE

1. When used for central diabetes insipidus, estimate response by two parameters: adequate duration of sleep and adequate, not excessive, water turnover.
2. Measure the dosage exactly because the drug is potent.
3. Only use intranasal desmopressin in those where PO tablet administration is not feasible.
4. The intranasal route may be compromised by nasal congestion and blockage, nasal discharge, atrophy of nasal mucosa, or severe atrophic rhinitis. Intranasal administration may be inappropriate if there is an impaired level of consciousness.
5. Use an alternative route of administration, other than intranasal, following cranial surgical procedures (e.g., transsphenoidal hypophysectomy).
6. The DDAVP nasal spray pump can deliver only 0.1 mL (10 mcg) doses or multiples of 0.1 mL. If doses other than these are needed, the rhinal tube delivery system should be used.
7. The DDAVP spray pump must be primed prior to the first use. To prime the pump, press down 4 times. The bottle will deliver 0.1 mL. Discard after 50 sprays since the amount delivered per spray may be substantially less than 10 mcg desmopressin.
8. Using the DDAVP rhinal tube, desmopressin is delivered into the nose through a soft, flexible plastic rhinal tube with four graduation marks: 0.2, 0.15, 0.1, and 0.05 mL. The 0.05-level is not designated by number. Cleanse and dry tube appropriately.
9. Stimate nasal spray pump can only deliver 0.1 mL (150 mcg) or multiples of 0.1 mL. If doses other than these are needed, desmopressin acetate injection may be used. The pump must be primed prior to the first use by pressing down four times. Discard the bottle after 25 (150 mcg per dose) doses since the amount delivered thereafter may be much less than 150 mcg.
10. If used for hemophilia A or von Willebrand's disease, do not use it more often than q 2 days as tachyphylaxis may occur.
11. To determine the renal concentration capacity in adults, the urine voided within 1 hr after drug administration is discarded; the two subsequent urines collected within 8 hr are saved and tested for osmolality. In children, osmolality is measured on urine voided during 3-5 hr after drug administration. Advise to drink only small amounts of fluid during the test day.
12. Store DDAVP nasal spray upright from 20–25°C (68–77°F). Store DDAVP rhinal tube and Stimate in the refrigerator from 2–8°C (36–46° F). When traveling, the product will be stable for up to 3 weeks when stored at room temperature.
13. Store tablets from 20–25°C (68–77°F). Avoid exposure to excessive heat or light.
14. IV Determine the necessity for repeat administration or use of any blood products for hemostasis by lab response, as well as the clinical condition of the client.
15. A lessening of response may occur with repeated administration given more frequently than q 48 hr.

16. Follow the package insert carefully to prepare for IV use.
17. Store from 2–8°C (36–46°F).
18. COMPATIBILITY 0.9% NaCl.
19. INCOMPATIBILITY Administer separately.

ASSESSMENT

1. Note reasons for therapy and clinical presentation.
2. Observe for early S&S of water intoxication (drowsiness, headache, and vomiting, excessive fluid consumption, weight gain, and/or seizures). Adjust fluid intake to avoid water intoxication and hyponatremia; use diuretic for excessive retention.
3. With hemophilia or von Willebrand's disease (type I), monitor BP and HR closely during IV therapy. Do coagulation testing before administration. These may include factor VIII coagulant activity, factor VIII antigen, ristocetin cofactor, activated PTT, and skin bleeding time. If factor VIII coagulant activity is less than 5% of normal, do not rely on desmopressin.
4. With neurogenic DI, monitor urine osmolarity and volume; weigh daily; assess for edema/dehydration.
5. With enuresis monitor duration of sleep. The amount of sleep, together with the client's daily I&O, provide parameters to estimate the clinical response to drug therapy.
6. Monitor BP, CBC, calcium, blood sugar, electrolytes, and factor levels.

CLIENT/FAMILY TEACHING

1. Drug is a synthetic analogue of vasopressin and an antidiuretic hormone. It may be used to maintain bleeding or for antidiuretic replacement therapy in the management of central (cranial) diabetes insipidus and for the management of the temporary polyuria and polydipsia following head trauma or surgery in the pituitary region.
2. If intranasal solution is prescribed, administer after instruction using the special catheter provided. Insert tip of catheter into nose, and blow on the other end of the catheter to deliver the medication deep into the nasal cavity. (A syringe filled with air may be used in children and comatose persons; rinse after use.)
3. The *Stimate* nasal spray pump accurately delivers 25 doses of 150 mcg per spray. Any solution remaining after 25 sprays should be discarded since the amount left may contain less than 150 mcg of drug. Do not transfer any remaining solution to another bottle. For first use, prime pump by pressing down 4 times. Then place the spray nozzle in the nostril and press spray pump once. If a 300 mcg dose is prescribed, then spray once in each nostril. Frequently inspect nasal mucosa to ensure mucosa intact.
4. DDAVP nasal spray can deliver 50 doses. Discard any solution remaining after the 50 doses since remaining amount may be substantially less than prescribed.
5. Review recommendations concerning fluid intake. Measure I&O and keep an accurate record of fluid status. Report any symptoms of water intoxication and swelling.
6. Notify provider at the earliest signs of trouble, such as ↓ urinary output, headaches, or severe nasal congestion, which may be mistaken for an URI.
7. Interrupt during acute intercurrent illness characterized by fluid and/or electrolyte imbalance (fevers, diarrhea, or vomiting) or in extremely hot weather, vigorous exercise, or other conditions associated with increased water intake.
8. Avoid alcohol in any form.
9. Tolerance may develop over time, and response may be diminished.
10. Keep all F/U to assess response, labs, and adverse SE.

OUTCOMES/EVALUATE

- Prevention of hemorrhage
- Control of nocturnal enuresis
- Desired antidiuretic effects (↓ urine volume, ↑ urine osmolarity, and relief of polydipsia) with DI

Desvenlafaxine succinate

(des-**VEN**-la-**FAX**-een **SUX**-ih-nate)

Classification(s): Antidepressant, serotonin and norepinephrine reuptake inhibitor.

Pregnancy Category: C

RX: Pristiq.

INDICATIONS/USES

Treatment of major depressive disorder.

ACTION/KINETICS

Action

Desvenlafaxine is a potent serotonin and norepinephrine reuptake inhibitor, thus increasing the levels of these neurotransmitters in the CNS. No anticholinergic, sedative, or orthostatic hypotensive effects.

Pharmacokinetics

Absolute bioavailability is about 80%. **Peak plasma levels:** About 7.5 hr. Steady-state plasma levels are reached in about 4–5 days with once daily dosing. Maximal drug concentration was increased in the fed state. Primarily metabolized by CYP3A4. **$t^{1/2}$, mean terminal:** 11.1 hr; mean terminal $t^{1/2}$ is increased to 13.5, 15.5, and 17.6 hr in mild, moderate, and severe renal impairment. Unchanged drug (about 45%) and metabolites are excreted in the urine. **Plasma protein binding:** 30% (is independent of drug concentration).

CONTRAINDICATIONS

Hypersensitivity to desvenlafaxine, venlafaxine, or any component of the product. Use in clients taking MAOIs. Only give during lactation if benefits outweigh any possible risk.

SPECIAL CONCERNS

Suicidality and antidepressant drugs. Antidepressants increased the risk compared with placebo of suicidal thinking and behavior (suicidality) in children, adolescents, and young adults in short-term studies of major depressive disorder and other psychiatric disorders. Anyone considering the use of desvenlafaxine or any other antidepressant in a child, adolescent, or young adult must balance this risk with the clinical need. Short-term studies did not show an increase in the risk of suicidality with antidepressants compared with placebo in adults beyond 24 years of age; there was a reduction in risk with antidepressants compared with placebo in adults 65 years of age and older. Depression and certain other psychiatric disorders are associated with increases in the risk of suicide. Monitor clients of all ages who are started on antidepressant therapy appropriately, and observe closely for clinical worsening, suicidality, or unusual changes in behavior. Advise families and caregivers of the need for close observation and communication with the prescriber. Desvenlafaxine is not approved for use in children.

- **Neonates exposed to serotonin and norepinephrine reuptake inhibitors during the third trimester may develop complications requiring prolonged hospitalization, respiratory support, and tube feeding.**
- **Clinical worsening of depression and/or emergence of suicidal ideation and behavior may occur.**
- **Use with caution in pre-existing hypertension or other conditions that might be compromised by increases in BP, in those with a family history of mania or hypomania, or in those with CV, cerebrovascular, or lipid metabolism disorders.**
- **The elderly may be more sensitive to the effects of the drug.**
- **Safety and efficacy not determined in children.**

SIDE EFFECTS

Most Common

Anxiety, constipation, diarrhea, dry mouth, decreased appetite, dizziness, hyperhidrosis, insomnia, nausea, somnolence, disorders of male sexual function.

CNS: Dizziness, headache, mania/hypomania activation, anxiety, insomnia, somnolence, abnormal dreams, irritability, nervousness, paresthesia, tremor, disturbed attention, jitteriness, ***seizures***, depersonalization, extrapyramidal disorder. Worsening of depression and/or emergence of ***suicidal ideation and suicidality*** or unusual changes in behavior. **GI:** N&V, diarrhea, constipation, dry mouth, dysgeusia, decreased appetite. **Serotonin syndrome/Neuroleptic malignant syndrome:** Hyperthermia, labile BP, tachycardia, diarrhea, N&V, agitation, coma, hallucinations, hyperreflexia, incoordination. **CV:** Elevated BP, palpitations, tachycardia, sustained hypertension, increased risk of bleeding, orthostatic hypotension, syncope, coronary occlusion, ***MI***, myocardial ischemia, ECG changes. **Respiratory:** Rarely, interstitial lung disease and eosinophilic pneumonia, epistaxis. **Dermatologic:** Hyperhidrosis, rash, hot flush. **GU:** Disorders of male sexual function (including delayed ejaculation, ejaculation disorder/failure, erectile dysfunction, decreased libido, abnormal orgasm, sexual dysfunction), urinary hesitation, anorgasmia (both men and women). **Ophthalmic:** Mydriasis, blurred vision. **Otic:** Tinnitus. **Body as a whole:** Fatigue, asthenia, chills, de-

D

creased weight. **Miscellaneous:** Yawning, hypersensitivity. *NOTE:* Abrupt discontinuation, dose reduction, or tapering of treatment can lead to the following reactions: Abnormal dreams, anxiety, diarrhea, dizziness, fatigue, headache, hyperhidrosis, insomnia, irritability, nausea.

D

LABORATORY TEST CONSIDERATIONS

↑ Blood prolactin. Dose-related ↑ fasting serum total cholesterol, LDL, cholesterol, and triglycerides (fasting). Hyponatremia, proteinuria. Abnormal LFT.

OVERDOSE MANAGEMENT

Symptoms: Changes in the level of consciousness (somnolence to coma), mydriasis, seizures, tachycardia, vomiting, ECG changes (e.g., prolongation of QT interval, BBB, QRS prolongation), sinus and ventricular tachycardia, bradycardia, hypotension, rhabdomyolysis, vertigo, ***liver necrosis, serotonin syndrome, death.*** *Treatment:* The following measures can be employed:

- Ensure an adequate airway, oxygenation, and ventilation.
- Monitor cardiac rhythm and vital signs.
- General supportive and symptomatic care.
- Gastric lavage with a large-bore orogastric tube with appropriate airway protection, if needed, and performed soon after ingestion or in symptomatic individuals.
- Administer activated charcoal. *NOTE:* Induction of emesis is not recommended. Also, forced diuresis, hemoperfusion, and exchange transfusion are unlikely to be beneficial.

DRUG INTERACTIONS

Aspirin / ↑ Risk of GI bleeding
CNS drugs (including alcohol) / Use together with caution; avoid consumption of alcohol
Desipramine / ↑ Desipramine C_{max} and AUC
Ketoconazole / ↑ Desvenlafaxine AUC and C_{max} R/T inhibition of CYP3A4
Linezolid / Possible life-threatening serotonin syndrome (see ***Side Effects***); do not use together
Lithium / Serotonin syndrome may occur
MAOIs (e.g., phenelzine, selegiline) / Possible serious and sometimes fatal reactions, including hyperthermia, rigidity, myoclonus, autonomic instability, mental status changes, delirium, coma; do not use together
Metoclopramide / Possible life-threatening serotonin syndrome (see ***Side Effects***); do not use together
Midazolam / ↓ Midazolam C_{max} and AUC R/T midazolam is a substrate for CYP3A4
NSAIDs / ↑ Risk of GI bleeding
Serotonergic drugs (e.g., SSRIs, other SNRI, triptans) / Possible life-threatening serotonin syndrome (see ***Side Effects***); do not use together
H ***St. John's wort*** / Serotonin syndrome may occur
Tramadol / Possible life-threatening serotonin syndrome (see ***Side Effects***); do not use together
Trazodone / Possible life-threatening serotonin syndrome (see ***Side Effects***); do not use together
Tricyclic antidepressants (TCAs) / ↑ Levels of TCAs
Triptans (e.g., sumatriptan) / Possible life-threatening serotonin syndrome (see ***Side Effects***); do not use together
Tryptophan / Do not use together
Warfarin / ↑ Bleeding; monitor when desvenlafaxine is initiated or discontinued

HOW SUPPLIED

Tablets, Extended-Release: 50 mg, 100 mg.

DOSAGE

TABLETS, EXTENDED-RELEASE

Major depressive disorder.

Adults, initial: 50 mg once daily at about the same time each day, with or without food. Acute episodes of major depressive disorder require several months or longer of therapy. Periodically reassess to determine the need for continued treatment.

NURSING IMPLICATIONS

IMPLEMENTATION/ADMINISTRATION/STORAGE

1. **When discontinuing the drug, use a gradual reduction in dose by giving desvenlafaxine, 50 mg, less frequently rather than abrupt cessation of the drug. If intolerable symptoms occur following a decrease in dose or discontinuation of the drug, consider resuming the previously prescribed dose.**
2. **Carefully consider tapering desvenlafaxine dosage during the third trimester of pregnancy.**

3. Use the following dosage guidelines for renal impairment: Administer 50 mg/day if the 24 hr C_{CR} is 30 to 50 mL/min; administer 50 mg every other day if the C_{CR} is less than 30 mL/min or the client is in end-stage renal disease. Do not give supplemental doses after dialysis.
4. No adjustment of the starting dose is required for those with impaired hepatic function. However, do not give more than 100 mg/day.
5. At least 14 days must elapse between discontinuation of an MAOI and initiation of therapy with desvenlafaxine. Also, at least 7 days must elapse after stopping desvenlafaxine and initiating an MAOI.
6. Store from 15–30°C (59–86°F).

ASSESSMENT

1. List reasons for therapy, onset, characteristics of S&S, mental status, clinical presentation. Note other agents trialed, outcome.
2. List agents prescribed to ensure none interact.
3. May cause increased bleeding with certain agents (ASA, NSAIDS, and warfarin), sustained hypertension; monitor HR and BP regularly. Use cautiously with narrow angle glaucoma.
4. Prior to beginning treatment with an antidepressant, adequately screen clients with depressive symptoms to determine if they are at risk for bipolar disorder—may cause a mixed/manic episode.
5. Monitor VS, weight, CBC, lipid panel, renal and LFTs; reduce dose with renal dysfunction.

CLIENT/FAMILY TEACHING

1. Do not chew, crush, divide, or dissolve extended-release tablets; swallow whole with fluids. Take at approximately the same time each day. May notice an inert matrix tablet in stool; this is normal and not worrisome.
2. Do not perform activities that require mental alertness until drug effects realized; may cause dizziness or drowsiness. Avoid alcohol and any unprescribed or OTC preparations. The use of aspirin, NSAIDs, warfarin, or other drugs affecting coagulation may cause increased risk of bleeding.
3. When discontinuing therapy, gradually reduce the dose; do not stop suddenly.
4. Report any rash, hives, difficulty breathing or other allergic manifestations immediately. May experience anxiety, palpitations, headaches, and constipation; report if persistent or intolerable.
5. Use reliable contraception. Notify provider if pregnant or intend to become pregnant while taking drug.
6. Any suicide ideations or abnormal behaviors should be reported. Due to the possibility of suicide, high-risk clients should be observed closely during initial therapy. Prescriptions should be written for the smallest quantity to reduce the risk of overdose. Family should supervise medication administration with severely depressed clients and report increased agitation, akathisia (psychomotor restlessness), anxiety, change in mood, change in personality, hostility or aggressiveness, impulsivity, insomnia, irritability, panic attacks, suicidal thoughts or behavior immediately.
7. Keep all F/U to assess response, labs, BP/HR, and for adverse SE.

OUTCOMES/EVALUATE

- Improvement in S&S of depression
- Control of anxiety/panic disorder

Dexamethasone

(dex-ah-**METH**-ah-zohn)

Classification(s): Glucocorticoid

Pregnancy Category: C

RX: Ophthalmic: Maxidex Ophthalmic, Ozurdex Intravitreal Implant. **Oral:** Baycadron, Dexamethasone Intensol, DexPak 13 Day TaperPak, DexPak 6 Day TaperPak, DexPak Jr. 10 Day TaperPak, DexPak TaperPak, Zema-Pak 10 Day, Zema-Pak 13 Day. **Topical Spray:** Aeroseb-Dex.

✤ **Rx:** Apo-Dexamethasone, PMS-Dexamethasone, ratio-Dexamethasone.

SEE ALSO ***CORTICOSTEROIDS***.

ADDITIONAL USES

Systemic. (1) In acute allergic disorders, PO dexamethasone may be combined with dexamethasone sodium phosphate injection and used for 6 days. (2) Test for adrenal cortical hyperfunction. (3) Cerebral edema due to brain tumor, craniotomy, or head injury. *Investigational:* Diagnosis of depression. Antiemetic in cisplatin-induced vomiting. Prophylaxis or treatment of acute mountain sickness. Decrease hearing loss in bacterial meningitis. Hirsutism.

Ophthalmic Solution/Suspension. (1) Treat corneal injury due to chemical, radiation, or thermal burns, or penetration of foreign bodies. (2) Inflammatory conditions of the palpebral and bulbar conjunctiva, cornea, and anterior segment of the globe, including allergic conjunctivitis, acne rosacea, superficial punctate keratitis, cyclitis, herpes zoster keratitis, iritis, and selected infective conjunctivitis when the risks of steroid use are expected to obtain decreased edema and inflammation.

Ophthalmic Implant. Treatment of macular edema following branch retinal vein occlusion or central retinal vein occlusion.

ACTION/KINETICS

Action

Long-acting. Low degree of sodium and water retention. Diuresis may ensue when transferred from other corticosteroids to dexamethasone.

Pharmacokinetics

t½: 110–210 min.

CONTRAINDICATIONS

Use for replacement therapy in adrenal cortical insufficiency.

SPECIAL CONCERNS

Use during pregnancy only if benefits outweigh risks.

SIDE EFFECTS

Most Common

Dizziness, nausea, indigestion, increased appetite, weight gain, weakness, sleep disturbances.

See *Corticosteroids* for a complete list of possible side effects.

ADDITIONAL DRUG INTERACTIONS

Aprepitant / ↑ Dexamethasone AUC, peak levels, and t½ R/T inhibition of metabolism of CYP3A4 first pass and systemic metabolism

Ephedrine / ↓ Dexamethasone effect R/T ↑ liver breakdown

Oral Contraceptives / ↓ Effect of oral contraceptives R/T ↑ liver breakdown

Smoking / Antagonism of the suppressive effects of dexamethasone on adrenal cortical secretion

HOW SUPPLIED

Aerosol, Topical: 0.01%; ***Elixir:*** 0.5 mg/5 mL; ***Intravitreal Implant:*** 0.7 mg; ***Ophthalmic Solution:*** 0.1% (as sodium phosphate); ***Ophthalmic Suspension:*** 0.1%; ***Oral Solution:*** 0.5 mg/0.5 mL; ***Oral Solution, Concentrated:*** 1 mg/mL; ***Tablets:*** 0.25 mg, 0.5 mg, 0.75 mg, 1 mg, 1.5 mg, 2 mg, 4 mg, 6 mg.

DOSAGE

ELIXIR; ORAL SOLUTION; TABLETS

Most uses.

Individualize dose based on disease and client response. **Adults, initial:** 0.75–9 mg/day; **maintenance:** gradually reduce to minimum effective dose that maintains an adequate clinical response (0.5–3 mg/day). **Children, initial:** 0.02–0.3 mg/kg per day in 3 or 4 divided doses (0.6–9 mg/m^2 body surface area per day).

Acute allergic disorders or acute worsening of chronic allergic disorders.

Dosage regimen combines parenteral and PO therapy (0.75 mg tablets and dexamethsone sodium phosphate injection, 4 mg/mL). **Day 1:** Dexamethasone sodium phosphate injection, 4 or 8 mg IM. **Day 2 and 3:** Four 0.75 mg tablets in 2 divided doses. **Day 4:** Two 0.75 mg tablets in 2 divided doses. **Days 5 and 6:** One 0.75 mg tablet. **Day 7:** No treatment. **Day 8:** Follow-up visit to provider.

Palliative management of recurrent or inoperable brain tumors.

2 mg 2 or 3 times per day for maintenance therapy.

Suppression test for Cushing's syndrome.

For greatest accuracy, 0.5 mg q 6 hr for 48 hr. Collect 24 hr urine to determine 17-hydroxycorticosteroid excretion. Alternatively, 1 mg at 11 p.m. with blood withdrawn at 8 a.m. for blood cortisol determination.

Test to distinguish Cushing's syndrome because of adrenocorticotropic hormone (ACTH) excess from Cushing's syndrome due to other causes.

2 mg q 6 hr for 48 hr. Collect 24 hr urine to determine 17-hydroxycorticosteroid excretion.

AEROSOL, TOPICAL

Apply sparingly as a light film to affected area 2–3 times per day.

OPHTHALMIC SOLUTION

Corneal injury, ophthalmic inflammation.

Initial: Instill 1–2 gtt into the conjunctival sac q hr during the day and q 2 hr during the night. When a favorable response is reached, reduce dose to 1 qtt q 4 hr. Further reduction in dose to 1 qtt 3–4 times per day may control symptoms. Treatment may be required from a few days to several weeks, depending on the response. Relapses usually respond to retreatment.

OPHTHALMIC SUSPENSION

Corneal injury, ophthalmic inflammation.

Instill 1 or 2 drops in the conjunctival sac(s). In mild disease, use up to 4 to 6 times per day. Drops may be used hourly in severe disease; taper to discontinuation as inflammation subsides.

INTRAVITREAL IMPLANT

Macular edema.

One implant is inserted carefully following the instructions provided by the manufacturer. Each applicator can be used only for the treatment of a single eye. If the contralateral eye requires treatment, a new applicator must be used. Also, the sterile field, syringe, gloves, drapes, and eyelid speculum should be changed before the implant is administered to the contralateral eye.

NURSING IMPLICATIONS

IMPLEMENTATION/ADMINISTRATION/STORAGE

1. For maintenance therapy, decrease the initial PO dose in small decrements at appropriate time intervals until the lowest dose that maintains an adequate response is reached.
2. If the drug is to be discontinued after more than a few days of treatment, it usually should be withdrawn gradually. If, after long-term therapy, the drug is to be discontinued, withdraw gradually rather than abruptly.
3. During times of stress, it may be necessary to increase the dose temporarily.
4. Store tablets and oral solution from 20–25°C (68–77°F). Do not freeze oral solution, and do not use if it contains a precipitate. Store the elixir at controlled room temperature; avoid freezing.
5. Carry out the intravitreal injection procedure under controlled aseptic conditions that includes use of sterile gloves, a sterile drape, and a sterile eyelid speculum. Adequate anesthesia and a broad-spectrum antibiotic are recommended to be given before the injection by trained provider.
6. Carefully follow the instructions provided for instillation of the implant.
7. Store ophthalmic solution and the intravitreal implant from 15–30°C (59–86°F) and the ophthalmic suspension upright from 8–27°C (46–80°F).

ASSESSMENT

1. Note reasons for therapy, characteristics of S&S, onset/contact, other agents trialed, outcome.
2. Describe clinical presentation; assess for any evidence of infection. Assess for bone and muscle weakness with prolonged therapy.
3. After intravitreal injection, monitor for elevation in IOP and endophthalmitis. This may consist of a check for perfusion of the optic nerve head immediately after injection, tonometry within 30 min following the injection, and biomicroscopy between 2 and 7 days.
4. Monitor BP, weight, mental status, serum glucose, electrolyes, thyroid function; IOP with eye therapy.

CLIENT/FAMILY TEACHING

1. Drug is a steroid used to treat a variety of conditions but mainly for anti-inflammatory effects in disorders of many organ systems.
2. Use exactly as directed; do not exceed dose and do not stop abruptly or may result in symptoms of corticosteroid withdrawal syndrome, including muscle/joint pain, and malaise.
3. May take with food to decrease GI upset. Monitor weight with long-term therapy.
4. Mix the Intensol with liquid or semi-solid foods such as water, juices, soda or soda-like beverages, applesauce, and puddings. Use the calibrated dropper provided to introduce the drug into the liquid or semi-solid food. Stir gently for a few seconds. Consume the entire

amount of the liquid or food immediately. Do not store for future use.
5. Review S&S of infection; fever, swelling, and redness may be masked in infection.
6. With eye injection, report if eye becomes red, light sensitive, painful, or vision change; may experience temporary visual blurring after intravitreal injection. Do not drive or use machines until this has resolved.
7. Report adverse effects, lack/loss of response, worsening of symptoms, excessive thirst, and urinary frequency.
8. Avoid immunizations, those with active infections, and exposure to chickenpox or measles during therapy; report if exposed.
9. Keep all F/U to assess response, labs, and adverse SE.

OUTCOMES/EVALUATE

- Status of adrenal cortical function
- ↓ Symptoms of allergic response
- ↓ Cerebral edema
- Treatment of macular edema

IV

Dexamethasone sodium phosphate

Classification(s): Glucocorticoid

Pregnancy Category: C

RX: Ophthalmic/Topical: Decadron Phosphate. **Injection:** Cortastat, Dalalone, Decadron Phosphate, Decaject, Dexasone.

🍁 **Rx:** PMS-Dexamethasone Injection.

SEE ALSO ***CORTICOSTEROIDS***.

ADDITIONAL USES

Systemic: For IV or IM use in emergency situations when dexamethasone cannot be given PO.

Intranasal: Nasal polyps, allergic or inflammatory nasal conditions.

Ophthalmic: Ophthalmic inflammatory conditions (See *Dexamethasone*).

Otic: Inflammatory conditions of the external auditory meatus, such as allergic otitis externa and selected purulent and nonpurulent infective otitis external when the risks of steroid use are expected to obtain decreased edema and inflammation.

ACTION/KINETICS

Pharmacokinetics

Rapid onset and short duration of action.

CONTRAINDICATIONS

Acute infections, persistent positive sputum cultures of *Candida albicans.* Lactation.

SPECIAL CONCERNS

- Use during pregnancy only if benefits outweigh risks.
- Safety and efficacy of the otic solution not determined in children.

SIDE EFFECTS

Most Common

Following ophthalmic use: Increased intraocular pressure, eye pain, blurred vision, dry eye, eye inflammation, abnormal sensation in eye, glaucoma, tearing, conjunctival hemorrhage, cataracts. **Following otic use:** Rarely, stinging and burning. **Following topical use:** Burning, itching, irritation, erythema, dryness.

See *Corticosteroids* for a complete list of possible side effects.

HOW SUPPLIED

Cream: 0.1%; ***Injection:*** 4 mg/mL, 10 mg/mL, 20 mg/mL, 24 mg/mL; ***Ophthalmic Ointment:*** 0.05%; ***Ophthalmic Solution:*** 0.1%; ***Otic Solution:*** 0.1% (as phosphate).

DOSAGE

IM; IV

Most uses.

Range: 0.5–9 mg/day (1/3 to 1/2 the PO dose q 12 hr).

Cerebral edema.

Adults, initial: 10 mg IV; **then,** 4 mg IM q 6 hr until maximum effect is obtained (usually within 12–24 hr). Switch to PO therapy (1–3 mg 3 times per day) as soon as feasible and then slowly withdraw over 5–7 days.

Shock, unresponsive.

Initial: Either 1–6 mg/kg IV or 40 mg IV; **then,** repeat IV dose q 2–6 hr as long as necessary.

INTRA-ARTICULAR; INTRALESIONAL; SOFT-TISSUE INJECTIONS

0.4–6 mg, depending on the site (e.g., small joints: 0.8–1 mg; large joints:

2–4 mg; soft-tissue infiltration: 2–6 mg; ganglia: 1–2 mg; bursae: 2–3 mg; tendon sheaths: 0.4–1 mg).

OPHTHALMIC OINTMENT

Instill a small amount of the ointment into the conjunctival sac 3–4 times per day. As response is obtained, reduce the number of applications.

OPHTHALMIC SOLUTION

Initial: Instill 1–2 gtt into the conjunctival sac q hr during day and q 2 hr at night until response is obtained. After favorable response, reduce to 1 gtt q 4 hr and later 1 gtt 3–4 times per day.

OTIC SOLUTION

Otic inflammatory conditions.

Initial: 3 or 4 qtt 2 or 3 times daily directly into the aural canal. Reduce dose when a favorable response is obtained. Duration of treatment may extend from a few days to several weeks. Relapses usually respond to retreatment.

TOPICAL CREAM

Apply sparingly to affected areas and rub in.

NURSING IMPLICATIONS

IMPLEMENTATION/ADMINISTRATION/STORAGE

1. The ophthalmic ointment is useful when an eye pad is used and for situations when prolonged contact of dexamethasone with ocular tissues is required.
2. If preferred, the aural canal may be packed with a gauze wick saturated with the solution. Keep the wick moist with the solution, and remove from the ear after 12–24 hr. Repeat treatment as often as needed.
3. IV For IV administration may give undiluted over 1 min. Do not use preparation containing lidocaine IV.
4. COMPATIBILITY D5W, 0.9% NaCl.
5. INCOMPATIBILITY Administer separately.

ASSESSMENT

1. Note reasons for therapy, clinical presentation, onset, characteristics of S&S, any triggers, other agents trialed, outcome.
2. With joint pain describe ROM, pain, erythema and x-rays as indicated.
3. With prolonged use monitor thyroid function, cholesterol, BS, and potassium.

CLIENT/FAMILY TEACHING

1. Provide appropriate method/frequency for administration; use as directed.
2. Review procedure for ear, eye or skin application to ensure compliance.
3. Keep all F/U to assess response and for adverse SE.

OUTCOMES/EVALUATE

- ↓ Pain/swelling
- Relief of allergic manifestations
- Suppression of inflammatory response; enhanced tissue perfusion

Dexlansoprazole

(**DEX**-lan-**SOE**-pra-zole)

Classification(s): Proton pump inhibitor.

Pregnancy Category: B

RX: Dexilant.

NOTE: The manufacturer has changed the trade name from Kapidex to Dexilant to avoid confusion with products with similar names..

SEE ALSO ***PROTON PUMP INHIBITORS.***

INDICATIONS/USES

(1) Healing of all grades of erosive esophagitis for up to 8 weeks. (2) Maintain healing of erosive esophagitis for up to 6 months. (3) Treatment for 4 weeks of heartburn associated with nonerosive gastroesophageal reflux disease (GERD) in adults.

ACTION/KINETICS

Action

Suppresses gastric acid secretion by specific inhibition of the (H^+, K^+)-ATPase in the gastric parietal cell. By a specific action on the proton pump, the drug blocks the final step of acid production. Effect is dose-related and inhibits both basal and stimulated acid secretion regardless of the stimulus. Serum gastrin increases.

Pharmacokinetics

Peak plasma levels: 1–2 hr (first peak) and 4–5 hr (second peak). **t½, elimination:** 1–2 hr. Metabolized in the liver by CYP3A4 and CYP2C19. Excreted in both the urine (about 51%) and feces. AUC is about 2 times greater in those with moderate hepatic impairment. t½, elimination is increased in the elderly and AUC is increased in women; however, no dosage adjustment is needed in either group. Systemic exposure of dexlansoprazole is usually higher in intermediate and poor metabolizers of CYP2C19. **Plasma protein binding:** 96.1–98.8%.

CONTRAINDICATIONS

Known hypersensitivity to any component of the product. Lactation.

SPECIAL CONCERNS

- **Symptomatic response does not preclude the presence of gastric malignancy.**
- **Greater sensitivity in the elderly cannot be ruled out.**
- **Safety and efficacy not determined in children less than 18 years of age.**

SIDE EFFECTS

Most Common

Diarrhea, abdominal pain, N&V, URTI, flatulence.

GI: Diarrhea, abdominal pain/discomfort, N&V, flatulence, abdominal tenderness, abnormal feces, altered taste, anal discomfort, Barrett's esophagus, bezoar, abnormal bowel sounds, breath odor, microscopic colitis, colonic polyp, constipation, dry mouth, duodenitis, dyspepsia, dysphagia, enteritis, eructation, esophagitis, gastric polyp, gastritis, gastroenteritis, GERD, GI disorder, GI hypermotility disorders, ***GI*** ulcers/***perforation,*** hematemesis, hematochezia, hemorrhoids, impaired gastric emptying, irritable bowel syndrome, mucus stools, oral mucosal blistering, painful defecation, proctitis, oral paresthesia, ***rectal hemorrhage.*** **Hepatic:** Biliary colic, cholelithiasis, hepatomegaly. **CNS:** Convulsion, dizziness, headache, migraine, impaired memory, paresthesia, psychomotor hyperactivity, tremor, trigeminal neuralgia, abnormal dreams, anxiety, depression, insomnia, libido changes, vertigo. **CV:** Angina, arrhythmia, bradycardia, chest pain, edema, ***MI***, palpitation, tachycardia, ***DVT***, hot flush, hypertension, leukocytoclastic vasculitis. **Musculoskeletal:** Arthralgia, arthritis, muscle cramps, musculoskeletal pain, myalgia, falls, fractures, joint sprains, greater risk for osteoporosis-related fractures of the hip, wrist, or spine. **GU:** Dysuria, micturition urgency, dysmenorrhea, dyspareunia, menorrhagia, menstrual disorder, vulvovaginal infection. **Respiratory:** URTI, aspiration, asthma, bronchitis, cough, dyspnea, hiccoughs, hyperventilation, respiratory tract congestion, sore throat, throat tightness, nasopharyngitis, pharyngitis, pharyngeal edema, sinusitis. **Dermatologic:** Acne, dermatitis, erythema, pruritus, rash, skin lesion, urticaria, generalized rash, ***Stevens-Johnson syndrome, toxic epidermal necrolysis.*** **Hematologic:** Anemia, lymphadenopathy. **Metabolic/Endocrine:** Appetite changes, goiter, facial/oral edema. **Ophthalmic:** Eye irritation/swelling, blurred vision. **Otic:** Ear pain, tinnitus. **Body as a whole:** Asthenia, chest pain, chills, feeling abnormal, inflammation, influenza, mucosal inflammation, nodule, pain, pyrexia, sunburn, weight increased. **Miscellaneous:** Hypersensitivity including ***anaphylaxis***, *Candida* infections, oral herpes, viral infection, procedural pain.

LABORATORY TEST CONSIDERATIONS

↑ALP, ALT, AST, blood creatinine, blood gastrin, blood glucose, blood potassium, total protein, weight. ↓ Platelet count. ↑ or ↓ Bilirubin. Abnormal LFTs. Hypercalcemia, hypokalemia.

OVERDOSE MANAGEMENT

Treatment: Treatment should be supportive and symptomatic. Drug is extensively protein bound and is not readily dialyzable.

DRUG INTERACTIONS

NOTE: Since gastric acid secretion is inhibited, dexlansoprazole may interfere with the absorption of drugs where gastric pH is an important determinant of bioavailability (see below).

Ampicillin esters / ↓ Absorption of ampicillin R/T ↓ gastric pH
Atazanavir / ↓ Serum atazanavir levels R/T inhibition of gastric secretion, which is needed for atazanavir absorption → loss of therapeutic effect; do not use together
Clarithromycin / Serum levels of both drugs may be ↑
Digoxin / ↑ Digoxin serum levels
Indinavir / ↓ Serum indinavir levels R/T inhibition of gastric secretion, which is needed for atazanavir absorption → loss of therapeutic effect; do not use together
Iron salts / ↓ Absorption of iron salts R/T ↓ gastric pH
Itraconazole / ↓ Absorption of itraconazole R/T ↓ gastric pH

Ketoconazole / ↓ Absorption of ketoconazole R/T ↓ gastric pH
Nelfinavir / ↓ Serum nelfinavir levels R/T inhibition of gastric secretion, which is needed for atazanavir absorption → loss of therapeutic effect; do not use together
Tacrolimus / ↑ Whole blood tacrolimus levels especially in transplant clients who are intermediate or poor metabolizers of CYP2C19 → ↑ pharmacologic/toxic effects
Warfarin / Possible ↑ INR and PT→ abnormal bleeding and death; monitor INR and PT

HOW SUPPLIED

Capsules, Delayed-Release: 30 mg, 60 mg.

DOSAGE

CAPSULES, DELAYED-RELEASE

Healing of erosive esophagitis.

Adults, over 18 years of age: 60 mg once a day for up to 8 weeks.

Maintain healing of erosive esophagitis.

Adults, over 18 years of age: 30 mg once a day. *NOTE:* Studies did not extend for use beyond 6 months.

Symptomatic nonerosive gastroesophageal reflux disease (GERD).

Adults, over 18 years of age: 30 mg once a day for 4 weeks.

NURSING IMPLICATIONS

IMPLEMENTATION/ADMINISTRATION/STORAGE

1. Can be taken without regard to food.
2. Consider a maximum dose of 30 mg a day for those with moderate hepatic impairment (Child-Pugh Class B). No dosage adjustment is needed for mild hepatic impairment (Child-Pugh Class A). Studies not conducted in those with Child-Pugh Class C hepatic impairment.
3. No dosage adjustment is needed for the elderly, for gender, or for those with renal impairment.
4. Store from 15–30°C (59–86°F).

ASSESSMENT

1. List reasons for therapy, type, onset, and characteristics of symptoms. List other agents prescribed; ensure no interaction. Altered pH may interfere with antiviral effects.
2. Record abdominal assessments, radiographic/endoscopic and *Helicobacter pylori* findings.
3. Monitor CBC and LFTs; reduce dose with liver dysfunction.

CLIENT/FAMILY TEACHING

1. May take with or without food. Swallow capsules whole.
2. If swallowing problems, may open capsules and sprinkle contents on 1 tablespoon of applesauce; swallow immediately.
3. Report any persistent gas, diarrhea, stomach pain, common cold, symptoms, and vomiting.
4. Keep all F/U to assess response and for adverse SE.

OUTCOMES/EVALUATE

Suppression of gastric acid secretion

IV

Dexmedetomidine hydrochloride

(dex-**med**-ih-**TOM**-ih-deen)

Classification(s): Sedative-hypnotic, nonbenzodiazepine

Pregnancy Category: C

RX: Precedex.

INDICATIONS/USES

(1) ICU sedation. For sedation in initially intubated and mechanically ventilated clients for treatment in an intensive care setting. (2) Procedural sedation. Sedation of nonintubated clients prior to and/or during surgical and other procedures. *Investigational:* (a) Treat postanesthetic shivering in adults, adolescents, and children. (b) Adjunct to epidural or spinal anesthesia. (c) Benzodiazepine withdrawal in adults and children. (d) Cyclic vomiting syndrome in children. (e) Sedation during awake craniotomy. (f) As an adjunct to regional or general anesthesia. (g) As a bridge to ICU sedation and analgesia. (h) As a supplement to regional block in clients undergoing carotid endarterectomy. (i) In selected clients with CHF. (j) To control agitation while receiving noninvasive ventilatory support, such as mask or continuous bilevel positive airway pressure.

D

ACTION/KINETICS

Action

An alpha-2-adrenoceptor agonist with sedative effects. No evidence of respiratory depression when given at recommended doses.

Pharmacokinetics

Rapidly distributed; **t½:** About 6 min. Almost completely metabolized in the liver primarily by CYP2D6; excreted in the urine and feces. **t½, terminal:** About 2 hr. Possibility of accumulation of metabolites with long-term infusions in clients with impaired renal function. **Plasma protein binding:** Average of 94%.

CONTRAINDICATIONS

Use for infusions lasting over 24 hr, during labor and delivery (including cesarean section deliveries), or in pediatric patients under 18 years of age.

SPECIAL CONCERNS

- Consider dose reduction in geriatric and hypovolemic clients due to a higher incidence of hypotension and bradycardia.
- Use with caution in advanced heart block, severe ventricular dysfunction, or during lactation.
- Hypotension may be more pronounced in clients with hypovolemia, diabetes mellitus, chronic hypertension, or in the elderly.
- If chronically given and then abruptly discontinued, withdrawal symptoms (e.g., nervousness, agitation, headaches, increase in BP, elevated catecholamine levels in the plasma) may occur.
- Use beyond 24 hr has been associated with tolerance and tachyphylaxis and a dose-related increase in side effects.

SIDE EFFECTS

Most Common

Bradycardia, dry mouth, hypotension, hypertension, respiratory depression, nausea.

CV: Hypotension, hypertension (transient), diastolic/systolic hypertension, bradycardia, atrial fibrillation, tachycardia, sinus tachycardia, sinus arrest, arrhythmia, AV block, BP fluctuation, ***cardiac arrest***, extrasystoles, heart block, heart disorder, ***MI***, supraventricular tachycardia, tachycardia, T wave inversion, ventricular arrhythmia, ventricular tachycardia. **GI:** N&V, dry mouth, constipation, abdominal pain, diarrhea. **Hepatic:** Abnormal hepatic function. **CNS:** Agitation, anxiety, confusion, ***convulsion***, delirium, dizziness, hallucination, headache, illusion, neuralgia, neuritis, speech disorder. **Respiratory:** Depressed respiration, atelectasis, bradypnea, hypoxia, pleural effusion, pulmonary edema, hypoxia, wheezing, apnea, bronchospasm, dyspnea, hypercapnia, hypoventilation, pulmonary congestion, ***ARDS, respiratory failure***. **GU:** Oliguria, decreased urine output, acute renal failure. **Metabolic:** Acidosis, hypovolemia, peripheral edema, respiratory acidosis, thirst. **Ophthalmic:** Abnormal vision, photopsia. **Body as a whole:** Anemia, chills, hypertermia, pyrexia, increased sweating, light anesthesia, pain, rigors. **Miscellaneous:** ***Postprocedural hemorrhage, hemorrhage.***

LABORATORY TEST CONSIDERATIONS

↑ AST, ALT, GGT, alkaline phosphatase, serum urea nitrogen. Hyper-/hypoglycemia, hypocalcemia, hyperbilirubinemia, hyperkalemia.

DRUG INTERACTIONS

Possible enhanced CNS depression when given with anesthetics, hypnotics, narcotics, or sedatives. Consider dosage reduction.

HOW SUPPLIED

Injection, Solution Concentrate: 100 mcg/mL.

DOSAGE

IV INFUSION

Intensive care unit sedation.

Adults, loading dose: Up to 1 mcg/kg over 10 min, followed by a maintenance infusion of 0.2–0.7 mcg/kg/hr. Adjust rate to achieve desired level of sedation. *NOTE:* For clients being converted from alternate sedative therapy, a loading dose may not be needed.

Procedural sedation.

Adults, loading dose: 1 mcg/kg over 10 min, including fiberoptic intubation clients. For less invasive procedures (e.g., ophthalmic surgery), a loading infusion of 0.5 mcg/kg given over 10 min may be appropriate. **Maintenance:** Initiate at 0.6 mcg/kg/hr and titrate to achieve the desired effect with doses ranging from 0.2–1 mcg/kg/hr. Adjust the rate of infusion to achieve the targeted level of sedation. For awake fiberoptic intubation, give 0.7 mcg/kg/hr until the endotracheal tube is secured.

For the elderly, use a loading dose of 0.5 mcg/kg over 10 min; for maintenance, consider a dose reduction.

NURSING IMPLICATIONS

IMPLEMENTATION/ADMINISTRATION/STORAGE

1. IV Administer using a controlled infusion device.
2. Has been infused continuously in mechanically ventilated clients prior to extubation, during extubation, and postextubation. It is not necessary to discontinue the drug prior to extubation.
3. Individualize dosage and titrate to the desired response.
4. Reduce the dose in impaired renal or hepatic function and in the elderly. Consider reduction of the dose if given with anesthetics, sedatives, opioids, or hypnotics.
5. To prepare the infusion, withdraw 2 mL and add to 48 mL of 0.9% NaCl injection (i.e., total of 50 mL). Shake gently to mix. Ampules and vials are intended for single use only. The concentration will be 4 mcg/mL prior to administration.
6. Administer by continuous IV infusion using a controlled infusion device, not to exceed 24 hr.
7. May adsorb to some types of natural rubber; use administration components made with synthetic or coated natural rubber gaskets.
8. Store from 15–30°C (59–86°F).
9. COMPATIBILITY LR, D5W, 0.9% NaCl, 20% mannitol, as well as a large number of drugs. (See package insert for the comprehensive list.)
10. INCOMPATIBILITY Do not coadminister with blood or plasma; amphotericin B or diazepam through same IV catheter.

ASSESSMENT

1. Note reasons for and goals of therapy, length of use (up to 24 hr). May also be used before, during and after extubation.
2. Use with caution in the elderly, with HTN, DM, or CAD.
3. Give in a continuously monitored environment. Client may develop cardiac arrhythmias, heart block, ↓ BP, significant bradycardia and sinus arrest, GI upset, respiratory distress. Ensure not hypovolemic; note if diabetic.
4. Monitor ECG, VS, renal and LFTs; reduce dose with dysfunction.

CLIENT/FAMILY TEACHING

1. Drug is used to sedate before surgery and during procedures. Do not attempt to get up or walk without assistance.
2. Not for use during labor and delivery.
3. May awaken when stimulated; may experience arrhythmia, burning at injection site, change in mental status, and respiratory suppression. Therefore, drug is only administered in a carefully monitored environment by trained personnel where client can be closely monitored and attended.

OUTCOMES/EVALUATE

Desired sedation; control of intubated clients being mechanically ventilated

Dexmethylphenidate hydrochloride

(dex-**meth**-il-**FEN**-ah-dayt)

Classification(s): CNS stimulant

Pregnancy Category: C

RX: Focalin, Focalin XR, **C-II**

INDICATIONS/USES

As part of a total program to treat attention deficit hyperactivity disorder in children 6 years of age and older. Effectiveness of use for more than 6 weeks using tablets or for more than 7 weeks using extended-release capsules has not been studied.

ACTION/KINETICS

Action

Precise mechanism to treat attention deficit disorder is not known. Drug is thought to block reuptake of norepinephrine and dopamine into the presynaptic neuron and increase the release of these neurotransmitters into the extraneuronal space.

Pharmacokinetics

Immediate-release tablets: Rapidly absorbed; **maximum levels after fasting:** 1–1.5 hr. Food delays the time to maximum levels. Metabolized in the liver; 90% excreted through the urine. **t½, elimination:** About 2.2 hr. **Extended-release**

capsules: Produce a bimodal concentration-time profile about 4 hr apart. The initial release is similar to immediate-release tablets. High-fat meals cause a longer lag time until absorption begins and variable delays until the first peak concentration, the time until the interpeak minimum, and the time until the second peak. The drug is metabolized in the liver and excreted mainly in the urine.

CONTRAINDICATIONS

Hypersensitivity to dexmethylphenidate or any component of the product. Clients with marked anxiety, tension, and agitation. Those with glaucoma, motor tics, or with a family history or diagnosis of Tourette's syndrome; during treatment with MAOIs or within a minimum of 14 days following discontinuation of an MAOI (hypertensive crisis may result). Use to treat severe depression or to prevent or treat normal fatigue states.

SPECIAL CONCERNS

■ (1) **Drug dependence.** Give dexmethylphenidate cautiously to clients with a history of drug dependence or alcoholism. (2) Long-term, abusive use may lead to marked tolerance and psychological dependence with varying degrees of abnormal behavior. (3) Frank psychotic episodes can occur, especially with parenteral abuse. (4) Careful supervision is required during drug withdrawal from abusive use because severe depression may occur. (5) Withdrawal following long-term therapy may unmask symptoms of the underlying disorder that may require follow-up. ■

- **In psychotic children, worsening of symptoms of behavior disturbance and thought disorder may occur.**
- **Use with caution during lactation and in medical conditions that might be compromised by increases in BP or HR (e.g., pre-existing hypertension, heart failure, recent MI, hyperthyroidism).**
- **Use in geriatric clients is considered high risk.**
- **Safety and efficacy not determined in children less than 6 years of age.**

SIDE EFFECTS

Most Common

Immediate-Release (Tablets): Abdominal pain, nausea, anorexia, fever, nervousness, anxiety, irritability, insomnia, weight loss, tachycardia, motor/vocal tics.

Extended-Release (Capsules): Headache, dyspepsia, decreased appetite, anxiety, dry mouth, pharyngolaryngeal pain, feeling jittery, dizziness.

CNS: Nervousness, insomnia, dizziness, drowsiness, anxiety, irritability, dyskinesia, headache, motor/vocal tics, feeling jittery, mood swings, Tourette's syndrome (rare), toxic psychosis (rare), transient depressed mood, lowering of seizure threshold in those with a history of seizures or with prior EEG abnormalities, treatment emergent psychotic or manic symptoms, aggressive behavior or hostility. Worsening of symptoms of behavioral disturbances and thought disorder in those with a pre-existing psychotic condition. **GI:** Abdominal pain, anorexia/decreased appetite, nausea, dyspepsia, dry mouth. **CV:** Tachycardia, angina, arrhythmia, palpitations, increased or decreased pulse/BP, cerebral arteritis or occlusion, ***sudden death, stroke, or MI in those with structural cardiac abnormalities or other serious heart problems.*** **Dermatologic:** Skin rash, scalp hair loss. **Hematologic:** Anemia, leukopenia. **Hypersensitivity:** Arthralgia, erythema multiforme with histopathological findings of necrotizing vasculitis, exfoliative dermatitis, fever, skin rash, thrombocytopenic purpura, urticaria. **Ophthalmic:** Difficulties with accommodation and blurring of vision. **Body as a whole:** Fever, weight loss (during prolonged therapy). **Miscellaneous:** Temporary slowing of growth rate in consistently medicated children, ***neuroleptic malignant syndrome*** (rare).

LABORATORY TEST CONSIDERATIONS

↑ Urinary excretion of epinephrine. Abnormal liver function (ranging from ↑ transaminase levels to hepatic coma).

OVERDOSE MANAGEMENT

Symptoms: Agitation, cardiac arrhythmias, confusion, convulsions (may be followed by coma), delirium, dry mucous membranes, euphoria, flushing, hallucinations, headache, hyperpyrexia, hyperreflexia, hypertension, muscle twitching, mydriasis, palpitations, sweating, tachycardia, tremors, vomiting. *Treatment:* Appropriate supportive measures. Protect against self-injury and external stimuli. Gastric lavage (control agitation and seizures before gastric lavage). Administration of activated charcoal and a cathartic. Maintain adequate circulation and respiratory exchange. External cooling procedures to treat hyperpyrexia. Effect of peritoneal dialysis not established. *NOTE:* There is an extended-release (i.e., long-acting) form of dexmethylphenidate.

DRUG INTERACTIONS

Anesthetics, halogenated / Possible sudden ↑ BP during surgery; dexmethylphenidate contraindicated on the day of planned surgery using halogenated anesthetics

Antacids / Possible alteration of the release of dexmethylphenidate from the extended-release capsule

Antihypertensives / ↓ Effect of antihypertensives

Clonidine / Possible serious side effects

Gastric acid suppressants / Possible alteration of the release of dexmethylphenidate from the extended-release capsule

MAOIs (e.g., isocarboxazid, phenelzine, selegiline) / Possible hypertensive crisis, hyperthermia, convulsions, coma; do not use together or within 14 days following discontinuation of MAO therapy

Phenobarbital / ↑ Effect of phenobarbital R/T ↓ metabolism; possibly ↓ phenobarbital dose

Phenytoin / ↑ Effect of phenytoin R/T ↓ metabolism; possibly ↓ phenytoin dose

Pressor drugs (dopamine, epinephrine, phenylephrine) / Due to possible effects on BP, use cautiously with pressor drugs

Primidone / ↑ Effect of primidone R/T ↓ metabolism; possibly ↓ primidone dose

Selective serotonin reuptake inhibitors (e.g., fluoxetine) / ↑ Effect of SSRIs R/T ↓ metabolism → possible serotonin syndrome; use together with caution

Tricyclic antidepressants (e.g., clomipramine, desipramine, imipramine) / ↑ TCA effect R/T ↓ metabolism; consider possible dosage adjustment

Warfarin / ↓ Metabolism of warfarin; monitor coagulation times when starting or stopping therapy with possible dosage adjustment

HOW SUPPLIED

Capsules, Extended-Release: 5 mg, 10 mg, 15 mg, 20 mg, 30 mg, 40 mg; ***Tablets, Immediate-Release:*** 2.5 mg, 5 mg, 10 mg.

DOSAGE

CAPSULES, EXTENDED-RELEASE

Attention deficit hyperactivity disorder.

Adults, initial, those not currently taking racemic methylphenidate or those not currently on other stimulants: 10 mg/day. Adjust dosage in 10 mg/day increments at weekly intervals to a maximum of 40 mg/day. **Children, 6 years and older, those not currently taking racemic methylphenidate or those not currently on other stimulants:** 5 mg/day. Adjust dosage in 5 mg/day increments at weekly intervals to a maximum of 30 mg/day. Observe both adults and children for a sufficient period of time at a given dose to ensure that a maximum benefit has been reached before a dose increase is considered. Periodically assess need for the drug.

TABLETS, IMMEDIATE-RELEASE

Attention deficit hyperactivity disorder.

Adults and children 6 years and older, initial, those not currently taking racemic methylphenidate or those who are on other stimulants: 2.5 mg twice a day (i.e., total of 5 mg/day). Adjust dosage in 2.5 to 5 mg increments at weekly intervals to a maximum of 20 mg/day (i.e., 10 mg twice a day). Observe both adults and children for a sufficient period of time at a given dose to ensure that a maximum benefit has been reached before a dose increase is considered. Periodically assess need for the drug.

NURSING IMPLICATIONS

IMPLEMENTATION/ADMINISTRATION/STORAGE

1. Give immediate-release tablets twice a day at least 4 hr apart, with/without food. Give extended-release capsules once a day in the morning.
2. Clients currently taking the immediate-release product may be switched to the same daily dose of the extended-release product.
3. The recommended starting dose of dexmethylphenidate immediate- or extended-release products is one-half the dose of racemic methylphenidate.
4. If extended treatment deemed necessary, evaluate long-term usefulness with periods off drug to assess ability to function without medication.

D

5. If paradoxical aggravation of symptoms or other side effects occur, decrease/discontinue drug.
6. Discontinue drug if improvement is not seen after appropriate dosage adjustment over a 1-month period.
7. Withdrawal after use may cause severe depression.
8. Withdrawal from chronic therapeutic use may unmask symptoms of underlying disorder.
9. Store from 15–30°C (59–86°F). Protect from light and moisture.

ASSESSMENT

1. Note reasons for therapy, symptom characteristics, other agents trialed, outcome. List other drugs prescribed that may interact unfavorably.
2. Assess for family history of Tourette's syndrome, evidence of glaucoma, tics, or depression; may preclude therapy.
3. Ensure psychologic evaluations show no evidence of psychotic disorder or severe stress/anxiety reaction.
4. Assess for possible growth suppression. Monitor height and weight especially with long-term therapy and provide periodic "drug holiday" to determine need for continued therapy.
5. Obtain baseline VS, ht, Wt, LFTs, CBC, CNS evaluation, ECG, and monitor.

CLIENT/FAMILY TEACHING

1. Drug thought to work by restoring the balance of certain natural substances (neurotransmitters) in the brain. It helps increase ability to pay attention, stay focused on an activity, and control-related behavior problems. Used in conjunction with psychological, educational, and social interventions/therapy.
2. Take before/with breakfast and lunch to avoid interference with sleep. For immediate-release tablets, take twice daily at least 4 hr apart, with or without food. Take extended-release capsules once daily in the morning.
3. Take extended-release capsules whole or by sprinkling the contents on a small amount of applesauce. Do not crush, chew, or divide capsules. Consume the mixture with applesauce immediately; do not store for future use.
4. Store safely out of reach, may cause tolerance and psychological dependence. Alert school or day care provider of use and administration guidelines.
5. Do NOT stop suddenly with long-term therapy; reduce dose with supervised direction.
6. Use caution when driving or operating hazardous machinery; may mask fatigue and/or cause physical incoordination, dizziness, drowsiness.
7. Record weight twice a week; weight loss may occur.
8. Report any overt changes in client mood or attention span. Any adverse S&S as well as skin rashes, fever, or joint pains should be reported immediately. Also any visual changes, appetite loss, nervousness, or difficulty sleeping as well as unusual or unexplained symptoms or feelings should be reported.
9. Therapy may be interrupted periodically ("drug holiday") to assess behavior and to determine if it is still necessary in those responsive to therapy and in some to permit normal growth.
10. Keep all F/U to assess response and for adverse SE.

OUTCOMES/EVALUATE

Ability to sit quietly and concentrate

Dextroamphetamine sulfate

(dex-troh-am-**FET**-ah-meen)

Classification(s): CNS stimulant

Pregnancy Category: C

RX: Dexedrine Spansules, Dextrostat, ProCentra, **C-II**

SEE ALSO ***AMPHETAMINES AND DERIVATIVES.***

INDICATIONS/USES

(1) As part of a total treatment program for attention deficit disorders with hyperactivity in adults and children 3 to 16 years of age. (2) Narcolepsy. *Investigational:* Treatment of cocaine dependence; autism.

ACTION/KINETICS

Action

Stronger CNS effects and weaker peripheral action than amphetamine; thus, dextroamphetamine manifests fewer undesirable CV effects.

Pharmacokinetics
After PO, completely absorbed in 3 hr. **Duration: PO,** 4–24 hr; **t½, adults:** 10–12 hr; **children:** 6–8 hr. Excreted in urine. Acidification will increase excretion, while alkalinization will decrease it.

ADDITIONAL CONTRAINDICATIONS
Lactation. Use for obesity. Not recommended for use in children less than 3 years of age. Use with MAOIs.

SPECIAL CONCERNS
(1) Amphetamines have a high potential for abuse. Administration of amphetamines for prolonged periods of time may lead to drug dependence and must be avoided. Pay particular attention to the possibility of subjects obtaining amphetamines for nontherapeutic use or distribution to others; prescribe and dispense the drugs sparingly. (2) Misuse of amphetamines may cause sudden death and serious CV adverse reactions.

- **Higher rates of serious CV events and sudden death are seen with amphetamine compared with methylphenidate in both children and adults, with more events seen in adults rather than children.**
- **Use not recommended of extended-release capsules for attention deficit disorders in children less than 6 years of age and the tablets for attention deficit disorders in children less than 3 years of age.**
- **Dosage for narcolepsy not determined in children less than 6 years of age.**

SIDE EFFECTS
Most Common
Nausea, GI upset, cramps, anorexia, diarrhea, constipation, dry mouth, headache, nervousness, dizziness, insomnia, irritability, restlessness.

See *Amphetamines and Derivatives* for a complete list of possible side effects.

HOW SUPPLIED
Capsules, Extended-Release: 5 mg, 10 mg, 15 mg; ***Oral Solution:*** 5 mg/5 mL; ***Tablets:*** 5 mg, 10 mg.

DOSAGE
CAPSULES, EXTENDED-RELEASE; ORAL SOLUTION; TABLETS
Attention deficit disorders in adults and children.

Adults, initial: 5 mg once or twice a day. Daily dose may be increased in increments of 5 mg at weekly intervals until the optimum response is achieved. Only rarely, will a dose greater than 40 mg/day be needed. **Children, 6 years and older, initial:** 5 mg once or twice daily initially; increase in increments of 5 mg/day at weekly intervals until optimum response reached. Dosage will rarely exceed 40 mg/day. **Children, 3–5 years, initial:** 2.5 mg/day initially; increase in increments of 2.5 mg/day at weekly intervals until optimum response reached. When appropriate, use the extended-release capsules for once daily dosing. For all clients, interrupt dosage occasionally to determine continued need.

Narcolepsy.

Adults and children, 12 years and older, initial: 10 mg/day. Daily dose may be increased in increments of 5 mg at weekly intervals until optimal response is reached. **Children, 6–12 years of age, initial:** 5 mg/day; increase in increments of 5 mg at weekly intervals until optimum effect is reached. With all clients, if bothersome side effects occur (e.g., anorexia, insomnia), reduce the dose.

NURSING IMPLICATIONS
IMPLEMENTATION/ADMINISTRATION/STORAGE
1. **Use the lowest effective dose; adjust dosage individually.**
2. **Avoid late evening doses, especially with sustained-release capsules, due to the possibility of insomnia.**
3. **Sustained-release capsules may be used for once-a-day dosing in attention deficit disorders and narcolepsy.**
4. **When tablets are used for ADD or narcolepsy, give first dose upon awakening with one or two additional doses given at intervals of 4–6 hr. Give the last dose 6 hr before bedtime.**
5. **If receiving a MAOI, wait 14 days after stopping before initiating dextroamphetamine.**
6. **Where possible, interrupt drug administration occasionally to determine the need for continued therapy.**

7. Store from 15–30°C (59–86°F); dispense in a tight, light- and child-resistant container.

ASSESSMENT

1. Note reasons for therapy, characteristics of S&S, testing results, other agents trialed, outcome.
2. Products contain FD&C Yellow No. 5 (tartrazine).
3. Monitor HR and BP; assess for the appearance or worsening of aggressive behavior or hostility.
4. Obtain baseline labs, ECG, vital signs, ht and Wt; monitor during therapy.

CLIENT/FAMILY TEACHING

1. Do not crush or chew SR tablets.
2. With tablets, give the first dose upon awakening; give additional doses (1 or 2) at intervals of 4–6 hr. Take last dose at least 6 hr before bedtime to ensure adequate rest.
3. Avoid activities that require alertness until drug effects realized. May experience fatigue as drug starts to wear off.
4. Stress importance of good oral hygiene to prevent or treat dry mouth and changes in breath odor.
5. Check weight weekly to ensure no significant loss. In children check height and growth rate and record. Eat regular meals with snacks to prevent weight loss. Avoid caffeine or caffeinated drinks such as sodas, coffee, tea, and chocolate.
6. Report increased agitation, dizziness, and palpitations; use caution when performing tasks that require physical coordination or mental alertness.
7. Do not stop suddenly after prolonged use; drug may cause psychological dependence. Reduce dose gradually to prevent acute withdrawal effects or severe depression.
8. Keep all F/U to assess response and for adverse SE.

OUTCOMES/EVALUATE

- Improved attention span and concentration levels
- ↓ Daytime sleeping

Dextromethorphan hydrobromide

(dex-troh-meth-**OR**-fan)

Classification(s): Antitussive, nonnarcotic

Pregnancy Category: C

OTC: Freezer Pops: PediaCare Children's Long-Acting Cough. **Gelcaps:** DexAlone, Robitussin Cough Gels. **Liquid/Oral Solution:** Buckley's Cough Mixture, Creo-Terpin, Robitussin Maximum Strength Cough, Simply Cough, Vicks 44 Cough Relief. **Lozenges:** Hold DM, Scot-Tussin DM Cough Chasers, Sucrets DM Cough Formula, Sucrets DM Cough Suppressant, Trocal. **Oral Suspension, Extended-Release:** Delsym. **Solution, Oral:** Children's PediaCare Long-Acting Cough. **Solution, Oral Concentrate:** Little Colds Cough Formula, PediaCare Infants' Long-Acting Cough. **Strips, Orally Disintegrating:** TheraFlu Thin Strips Long Acting Cough, Triaminic Thin Strips Long Acting Cough. **Syrup:** Creomulsion Adult Formula, Creomulsion for Children, ElixSure Children's Cough, Robitussin Pediatric Cough, Silphen DM, Triaminic Long Acting Cough.

RX: Suspension: AeroTuss 12.

🍁 **OTC:** Balminil DM, Balminil DM Children, Koffex DM, Robitussin Children's, Robitussin DM Cough Gels.

INDICATIONS/USES

Temporary relief of cough due to minor throat and bronchial irritation, including the common cold or inhaled irritants.

ACTION/KINETICS

Action

Selectively depresses the cough center in the medulla. Dextromethorphan 15–30 mg is equal to 8–15 mg codeine as an antitussive. Does not produce physical dependence or respiratory depression.

Pharmacokinetics

Rapidly absorbed from GI tract. **Onset:** 15–30 min. **Duration:** 3–6 hr. Metabolized in the liver and both unchanged drug and metabolites are excreted in the urine. The sustained liquid contains dextromethorphan plistirex equivalent to 30 mg dextromethorphan hydrobromide per 5 mL.

CONTRAINDICATIONS

Persistent or chronic cough or when cough is accompanied by excessive secretions. Use during first trimester of pregnancy unless directed otherwise by physician. Use in children less than 4 years of age is not recommended. Use with MAOIs.

SPECIAL CONCERNS

- Use with caution in clients with nausea, vomiting, high fever, rash, or persistent headache.
- Abuse can lead to brain damage, seizures, loss of consciousness, irregular heartbeat, and death.
- Some products contain tartrazine, which may cause an allergic reaction in some clients, especially in those allergic to aspirin.
- Not known if dextromethorphan is excreted in breast milk.

SIDE EFFECTS

Most Common

Dizziness, drowsiness, GI disturbances.

CNS: Dizziness, drowsiness. **GI:** N&V, stomach pain. **Respiratory:** May slow rate or breathing.

OVERDOSE MANAGEMENT

Symptoms: **Adults:** Dysphoria, slurred speech, ataxia, altered sensory perception. **Children:** Ataxia, ***convulsions, respiratory depression.*** *Treatment:* Treat symptoms and provide support.

DRUG INTERACTIONS

Grapefruit juice / ↑ Bioavailability of dextromethorphan
MAOIs / May cause hyperpyrexia, abnormal muscle movement, hypotension, coma, and death; avoid concomitant use for 2 weeks after stopping MAOI
Quinidine / ↑ Plasma dextromethorphan levels R/T quinidine ↓ liver metabolism by CYP2D6
Silbutramine / Accumulation of brain serotonin → serotonin syndrome (myoclonus, hyperreflexia, confusion, disorientation, agitation, hypomania, rigidity, tremor, sweating, shivering, seizures, coma, hypertension)

HOW SUPPLIED

Freezer pops: 7.5 mg/25 mL (per pop); ***Gelcaps:*** 15 mg, 30 mg; ***Liquid:*** 3.33 mg/5 mL, 5 mg/5 mL, 10 mg/5 mL, 12.5 mg/5 mL, 15 mg/5 mL; ***Lozenges:*** 5 mg, 7.5 mg, 10 mg; ***Oral Suspension, Extended-Release:*** 30 mg/5 mL; ***Solution, Oral:*** 7.5 mg/5 mL; ***Solution, Oral Concentrate:*** 3.75 mg/0.8 mL, 7.5 mg/mL; ***Strips, Orally Disintegrating:*** 7.5 mg, 15 mg; ***Suspension, Oral:*** 30 mg/5 mL; ***Syrup:*** 5 mg/5 mL, 7.5 mg/5 mL, 10 mg/5 mL, 20 mg/15 mL.

DOSAGE

NOTE: The use of dextromethorphan is generally not recommended for use in children less than 4 years of age. However, dosage is provided for children, aged 2 and higher.

FREEZER POPS

Antitussive.

Children, 6 to <12 years old: 2 freezer pops (50 mL as liquid), if needed, repeat dose q 6–8 hr, up to 8 freezer pops per day (i.e., four doses per day or 200 mL per day). **Children, 2 to <6 years of age:** One freezer pop (25 mL as liquid); if needed, repeat dose q 6–8 hr, up to 4 freezer pops per day (i.e., four doses in 24 hr).

GELCAPS

Antitussive.

Adults and children 12 years and older: 30 mg q 6–8 hr, not to exceed 120 mg per 24 hr. Do not use in children less than 12 years old.

LOZENGES

Antitussive.

Adults and children 12 years and older: 5–15 mg q 1–4 hr, up to 120 mg/day. **Children, 6 to <12 years of age:** 5–10 mg q 1–4 hr, not to exceed 60 mg/day. Do not give to children under 6 years of age unless directed by provider.

LIQUID; SYRUP

Antitussive.

Adults and children 12 years and older: 10–20 mg q 4 hr or 30 mg q 6–8 hr, not to exceed 120 mg per day. **Children, 6 to <12 years of age:** 15 mg q 6–8 hr, up to 60 mg per day. **Children, 2 to <6 years of age:** 7.5 mg q 6–8 hr, up to 30 mg per day.

ORAL SUSPENSION, EXTENDED-RELEASE

Antitussive.

Adults and children 12 years and older: 60 mg q 12 hr, up to 120 mg per day. **Children, 6 to <12 years of age:** 30 mg q 12 hr, up to 60 mg per day. **Children, 2 to <6 years of age:** 15 mg q 12 hr, up to 30 mg per day.

D

STRIPS, ORALLY DISINTEGRATING
Antitussive.

Adults and children, age 12 and older: 30 mg q 6–8 hr, up to 120 mg per day. **Children, 6 to <12 years of age:** 15 mg q 6–8 hr, up to 60 mg per day.

SOLUTION, ORAL
Antitussive.

Children, 6 to < 12 years of age: 15 mg (10 mL) q 6–8 hr, up to 60 mg per day. **Children, 2 to <6 years of age:** 7.5 mg (5 mL) q 6–8 hr, up to 30 mg per day.

NURSING IMPLICATIONS

IMPLEMENTATION/ADMINISTRATION/STORAGE
1. Increasing the dose of dextromethorphan will not increase its effectiveness but will increase the duration of action.
2. Do not give lozenges to children under 6 years of age.

ASSESSMENT
1. Note duration of cough. If persists beyond several weeks, stop drug and reassess cause. Document lung sounds, sputum characteristics, C&S results and any triggers. List drugs prescribed to ensure none interact.
2. Determine presence of nausea, vomiting, persistent headaches, or a high fever.
3. If pregnant, determine trimester; contraindicated in first trimester.
4. Assess VS, ENT, lung sounds; determine need for CXR/sinus films.

CLIENT/FAMILY TEACHING
1. Take exactly as directed, and do not exceed dosing schedule or prescribed amount.
2. Avoid tasks that require mental alertness until drug effects realized.
3. Practice cough and deep breathing several times per hour to enhance lung expansion.
4. Avoid alcohol in any form.
5. Store freezer pops safely out of reach of children.
6. Add humidity to environment. Increase fluid intake to decrease thickness of secretions.
7. Cigarette smoke, dust, and chemical fumes are irritants that may aggravate condition.
8. Symptoms that persist for more than a week require medical intervention; record/report onset, triggers, characteristics of secretions, fever/chills, medications, and response to therapy.
9. Keep all F/U to assess response and adverse SE.

OUTCOMES/EVALUATE
Control of cough with improved sleep patterns

IV

Diazepam
(dye-**AYZ**-eh-pam)

Classification(s): Antianxiety drug, benzodiazepine

Pregnancy Category: D

RX: Diastat AcuDial, Diazepam Intensol, Valium, **C-IV**

Rx: Apo-Diazepam, Diazemuls, Valium Roche Oral.

SEE ALSO ***TRANQUILIZERS/ANTIMANIC DRUGS/HYPNOTICS.***

INDICATIONS/USES
PO: (1) Management of anxiety disorders or for short-term relief of symptoms of anxiety. (2) Adjunct therapy in convulsive disorders; effectiveness as sole therapy has not been proven. (3) Adjunct for relief of skeletal muscle spasm caused by reflex spasm to local pathology (e.g., inflammation of muscles or joints or secondary to trauma). Also, spasticity due to upper motor neuron disorders (e.g., cerebral palsy, paraplegia). Athetosis, stiff-man syndrome. (4) Acute alcohol withdrawal for symptomatic relief of acute agitation, tremor, impending or acute delirum tremens, and hallucinosis.

Parenteral: (1) Adjunct therapy in status epilepticus and severe recurrent convulsive seizures. (2) IV prior to cardioversion for relief of anxiety and tension and to decrease client's recall. (3) Relief of anxiety and tension in those undergoing surgical procedures. As an adjunct prior to endoscopic or surgical procedures if apprehension, anxiety, or acute stress reactions are present; also, to diminish client recall of the procedures. (4) Treatment of tetanus. (5) Adjunct for the relief of skeletal muscle spasm due to reflex spasm caused by local pathology (e.g., inflammation of muscles or joints, secondary to trauma). Also, spasticity due to upper motor neuron disorders (e.g., cerebral palsy, paraplegia); athetosis; stiff-man syndrome. (6) Symptomatic relief of acute agitation, tremor, impending or acute delirium tremens, and hallucinosis.

Rectal gel: Management of selective refractory clients with epilepsy who are stable on regimens of anticonvulsant drugs and who require intermittent diazepam to control increased seizure activity.

ACTION/KINETICS

Action

Reduces anxiety by increasing or facilitating the inhibitory neurotransmitter activity of GABA. The skeletal muscle relaxant effect may be due to enhancement of GABA-mediated presynaptic inhibition at the spinal level as well as in the brain stem reticular formation.

Pharmacokinetics

Onset: PO, 30–60 min; **IM,** 15–30 min; **IV,** more rapid. **Peak plasma levels: PO,** 0.5–2 hr; **IM,** 0.5–1.5; **IV,** 0.25 hr. **Duration:** 3 hr. **t½:** 20–50 hr. Metabolized in the liver to the active metabolites desmethyldiazepam, oxazepam, and temazepam. Diazepam and metabolites are excreted through the urine. **Plasma protein binding:** 97–99%.

ADDITIONAL CONTRAINDICATIONS

Narrow-angle glaucoma, children under 6 months, lactation, and parenterally in children under 12 years.

SPECIAL CONCERNS

- When used as an adjunct for seizure disorders, diazepam may increase the frequency or severity of clonic-tonic seizures; an increased dose of anticonvulsant medication is necessary.
- Safety and efficacy of parenteral diazepam not determined in neonates less than 30 days of age. Prolonged CNS depression has been observed in neonates, probably due to inability to biotransform diazepam into inactive metabolites.
- Use IV diazepam with extreme caution in the elderly, in very ill clients, and in those with limited pulmonary reserve as apnea or cardiac arrest may occur.
- Due to the long t½, the drug can accumulate in the elderly and cause excessive sedation, thus increasing the risk of falls and fractures.
- Tonic status epilepticus may be precipitated when IV diazepam is used for petit mal status or petit mal variant status.

SIDE EFFECTS

Most Common

Drowsiness (transient), ataxia, confusion.

See *Tranquilizers/Antimanic Drugs/Hypnotics* for a complete list of possible side effects.

ADDITIONAL DRUG INTERACTIONS

1. Diazepam potentiates antihypertensive effects of thiazides and other diuretics.
2. Diazepam potentiates muscle relaxant effects of d-tubocurarine and gallamine.

Fluoxetine / ↑ Diazepam half-life
Isoniazid / ↑ Diazepam half-life
Ranitidine / ↓ GI absorption of diazepam
Smoking / Possible ↑ Diazepam hepatic metabolism → ↓ response

HOW SUPPLIED

Injection: 5 mg/mL; ***Oral Solution:*** 1 mg/mL; ***Rectal Gel:*** 2.5 mg, 10 mg, 20 mg; ***Solution, Intensol:*** 5 mg/mL; ***Tablets:*** 2 mg, 5 mg, 10 mg.

DOSAGE

ORAL SOLUTION; SOLUTION, INTENSOL; TABLETS

Management and relief of anxiety disorders.

Adults: 2–10 mg 2 to 4 times per day. **Children, initial:** 1–2.5 mg 3–4 times per day; **then,** increase gradually as needed and tolerated. Not to be used in children less than 6 months of age. **Elderly clients or in presence of debilitating disease, initial:** 2–2.5 mg 1 or 2 times per day; **then,** increase gradually as needed and tolerated.

Adjunct in convulsive disorders.

Adults: 2–10 mg 2–4 times per day. **Elderly or debilitated clients, initial:** 2–2.5 mg 1 or 2 times per day; **then,** increase dose gradually as needed and tolerated. Limit dose to the smallest effective amount to preclude development of ataxia or oversedation. **Children at least 6 months of age, initial:** 1–2.5 mg 3 or 4 times per day; **then,** increase dose gradually as needed and tolerated.

Adjunct in skeletal muscle spasms.

Adults: 2–10 mg 3 or 4 times per day. **Children:** 0.12–0.8 mg/kg per 24 hr divided 3 to 4 times per day.

Acute alcohol withdrawal.

10 mg 3 or 4 times per day during the first 24 hr; reduce to 5 mg 3 or 4 times per day, as needed.

IM; IV

Status epilepticus or severe recurrent convulsive seizures.

Adults, initial: 5–10 mg IV (preferred); **then**, may be repeated at 10–15 min intervals up to a maximum of 30 mg, if needed. May repeat therapy in 2–4 hr. Use with extreme caution in chronic lung disease or unstable cardiovascular status. **Children, at least 5 years of age:** 1 mg q 2–5 min IV (preferred) up to a maximum of 10 mg. Repeat in 2–4 hr if needed. **Infants older than 30 days of age and younger than 5 years of age:** 0.2–0.5 mg by slow IV q 2–5 min up to a maximum of 5 mg. May be repeated in 2–4 hr if needed.

Cardioversion.

Adults: 5–15 mg IV, 5–10 min prior to procedure.

Moderate anxiety disorders and symptoms of anxiety.

Adults: 2–5 mg IM or IV. Repeat in 3–4 hr if needed.

Severe anxiety disorders and symptoms of anxiety.

Adults: 5–10 mg IM or IV. Repeat in 3–4 hr if needed.

Preoperative medication.

Adults: 10 mg IM before surgery. If atropine, scopolamine, or other premedications are desired, use separate syringes.

Endoscopic procedures.

Adults, IV: Titrate dosage to desired sedative response (e.g., slurring of speech). Give slowly and just prior to procedure. Reduce narcotic dosage by at least one-third; in some cases, narcotics may be omitted. **Usual:** 10 mg or less; up to 20 mg may be used, especially when concomitant narcotics are omitted. **Adults, IM:** 5–10 mg 30 min prior to procedure if IV route cannot be used.

Tetanus.

Children, 5 years and older: 5–10 mg given q 3–4 hr, if needed. **Infants older than 30 days of age:** 1–2 mg IM or slowly IV given q 3–4 hr as needed.

Muscle spasms.

Adults, initial: 5–10 mg IM or IV; **then,** 5–10 mg in 3–4 hr if needed. Tetanus may require larger doses.

Sedation or muscle relaxation in children.

0.04–0.2 mg/kg per dose q 2–4 hr up to a maximum of 0.6 mg/kg within an 8 hr period.

Acute alcohol withdrawal.

Adults, initial: 10 mg IM or IV; **then,** 5–10 mg in 3–4 hr if needed.

RECTAL GEL

Convulsive disorders.

Depending on age dose ranges from 0.2–0.5 mg/kg; calculate the recommended dose by rounding up to the next available unit dose. If needed, a second dose may be given 4–12 hr after the first dose. Do not treat more than 5 episodes per month or more than 1 episode q 5 days. **Adults and children 12 years and older:** 0.2 mg/kg. In the elderly or debilitated, adjust dose downward to reduce ataxia or oversedation. **Children, 6–11 years of age:** 0.3 mg/kg; **children, 2–5 years of age:** 0.5 mg/kg.

NURSING IMPLICATIONS

Do not confuse diazepam with clonazepam (an anticonvulsant).

IMPLEMENTATION/ADMINISTRATION/STORAGE

1. Mix Intensol solution with beverages such as water, soda, and juices or soft foods such as applesauce or puddings. Use only the calibrated dropper provided to withdraw drug; once withdrawn and mixed, use immediately.
2. Except for the deltoid muscle, absorption from IM sites is slow, erratic, and painful and not generally recommended.
3. The rectal delivery system includes a plastic applicator with a flexible, molded tip available in two lengths. The Diastat AcuDial 2.5 mg and 10 mg syringes are available with a

4.4 cm tip and the Diastat AcuDial 20 mg syringe is available with a 6 cm tip.

4. Store the rectal gel from 15–30°C (59–86°F).
5. IV IV route is preferred in the convulsing client; EEG monitoring of seizure may be helpful.
6. IV diazepam will control seizures promptly; however, many clients experience a return to seizure activity (probably due to the short duration of IV diazepam). Be prepared to readminister.
7. Diazepam is not recommended for maintenance of seizure control. Consider other agents for long-term control.
8. In children, EEG monitoring of seizures may be helpful.
9. Parenteral administration may cause bradycardia, respiratory/cardiac arrest; have emergency equipment/drugs available.
10. To reduce IV site reactions, give diazepam slowly (5 mg/min); avoid small veins or intraarterial administration. For pediatric use, give IV solution slowly over a 3 min period.
11. Due to the possibility of precipitation and instability, do not infuse diazepam. Do not mix or dilute with other solutions or drugs in the syringe or infusion container.
12. Store injection at room temperature protected from light. Do not use if solution is darker than slightly yellow or contains a precipitate.
13. COMPATIBILITY Give solution separately followed by saline flush; not recommended for dilution due to chance of precipitation.
14. INCOMPATIBILITY Diazepam interacts with plastic; putting into plastic containers or administration sets will decrease drug availability.

ASSESSMENT

1. Identify reasons for therapy, onset, characteristics of S&S, other agents prescribed/trialed.
2. Assess emotional status; note any depression or drug abuse. Avoid concurrent use with CNS depressants. Reduce drug gradually to avoid withdrawal S&S (e.g., anxiety, tremors, anorexia, insomnia, weakness, headache, N&V).
3. Avoid use with glaucoma (narrow angle).
4. Review anxiety level; identify contributing factors. Note behavioral presentation, skeletal conditions and/or seizure history.
5. Elderly clients, very ill clients, those with limited pulmonary reserve may experience adverse reactions more quickly than others; use lower dose with these groups.
6. Monitor VS, CBC, renal and LFTs.

CLIENT/FAMILY TEACHING

1. Drug acts by slowing down the nervous system. Review why prescribed, dose, form, frequency, and desired outcome.
2. May take without regard to meals; take with food if GI upset.
3. With solution, if using calibrated dropper, add solution to a liquid (e.g., juice, water, soda) or semisolid food (e.g., applesauce, pudding); stir for a few seconds; then immediately take (give) entire mixture. Do not prepare mixtures ahead of time and store.
4. Inspect prefilled syringes with rectal gel for cracks frequently. Cracks can cause leakage of the drug and may not get sufficient medication to control seizures. Review administration procedure prior to use.
5. May cause dizziness/drowsiness, impair judgement and reflexes; avoid activities that require mental alertness until drug effects realized.
6. Take as directed; do not double doses. Seek alternative methods for anxiety control (e.g., stress reduction, counseling).
7. Avoid alcohol and other CNS depressants. Report if pregnancy suspected; practice reliable birth control.
8. Smoking may increase drug metabolism; thus requiring higher dose than nonsmoker.
9. Prolonged use may cause dependence. Do not stop drug abruptly.
10. Keep all F/U to assess response and for adverse SE.

OUTCOMES/EVALUATE

- ↓ Anxiety/tension episodes
- Relief alcohol withdrawal S&S
- Control of status epilepticus
- Relief of muscle spasms

Diclofenac epolamine

(dye-**KLOH**-fen-ack)

Classification(s): Nonsteroidal anti-inflammatory drug

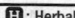

Pregnancy Category: C

RX: Patch, Topical: Flector.

Diclofenac potassium

(dye-**KLOH**-fen-ack)

Pregnancy Category: C

RX: Cambia, Cataflam, Zipsor.

♣ **Rx:** Apo-Diclo Rapide, Novo-Difenac-K, Voltaren Rapide.

Diclofenac sodium

Pregnancy Category: C (**Pennsaid:** C prior to 30 weeks gestation; D starting at 30 weeks gestation. **Solaraze:** B and **Voltaren:** C.)

RX: Gel: Solaraze, Voltaren. **Ophthalmic**: Voltaren. **Solution, Topical**: Pennsaid. **Tablets, Delayed- or Extended-Release**: Voltaren, Voltaren-XR.

♣ **Rx:** Apo-Diclo, Apo-Diclo SR, Novo-Difenac, Nu-Diclo, Nu-Diclo-SR, PMS-Diclofenac, PMS-Diclofenac SR, Sandoz Diclofenac, Sandoz Diclofenac Rapide, Sandoz Diclofenac SR, Voltaren Ophtha.

SEE ALSO ***NONSTEROIDAL ANTI-INFLAMMATORY DRUGS***.

INDICATIONS/USES

Diclofenac epolamine. Transdermal Patch: Topical treatment of acute pain due to minor strains, sprains, and contusions.

Diclofenac potassium. Capsules, Oral Solution, Tablets, Immediate-Release: (1) Acute and chronic treatment of signs and symptoms of rheumatoid arthritis and osteoarthritis. (2) Ankylosing spondylitis. (3) Mild-to-moderate pain in adults. (4) Primary dysmenorrhea. Use immediate-release when prompt relief is desired. (5) Acute treatment of migraine attacks with or without aura in adults (Oral Solution). Safety and efficacy of the oral solution has not been determined for cluster headaches.

Diclofenac sodium. Tablets, Delayed-Release or Extended-Release: (1) Signs and symptoms of rheumatoid arthritis and osteoarthritis. (2) Acute or long-term use for ankylosing spondylitis (Delayed-Release). *Investigational:* Mild-to-moderate pain, juvenile rheumatoid arthritis, acute painful shoulder, sunburn.

Ophthalmic: (1) Postoperative inflammation following cataract removal. (2) Temporary relief of pain and photophobia in those undergoing corneal refractive surgery.

Topical Gel: (1) **Solaraze only:** Actinic keratoses. (2) **Voltaren only:** Relief of the pain of osteoarthritis of joints amenable to topical treatment (e.g., knees and joints of the hand).

Topical Solution (Pennsaid): Relief of the pain of osteoarthritis of only the knee(s).

ACTION/KINETICS

Action

Diclofenac has anti-inflammatory, analgesic, and antipyretic activity. Anti-inflammatory effect is due to inhibition of the enzyme cyclo-oxygenase. Inhibition of cyclo-oxygenase results in decreased prostaglandin synthesis. Prostaglandin will cause inflammation. Effective in reducing joint swelling, pain, and morning stiffness and increases mobility in those with inflammatory disease.

Pharmacokinetics

Available as the epolamine (transdermal patch), potassium (immediate-release), and sodium (delayed-release) salts. *Transdermal patch.* **Peak plasma levels:** 10–20 hr. **t½, plasma:** About 12 hr. Excreted through both the bile and urine. *Immediate-release product.* Is 50–60% bioavailable. **Onset:** 30 min. **Peak plasma levels:** 1 hr. **Duration:** 8 hr. *Delayed-release product.* **Peak plasma levels:** 2–3 hr. **t½:** 1–2 hr. For all dosage forms, food will affect the rate, but not the amount, absorbed from the GI tract. Metabolized in the liver and excreted by the kidneys. **Plasma protein binding:** Greater than 99%.

CONTRAINDICATIONS

- Use to treat perioperative pain following coronary artery bypass graft surgery.
- Use in those who have experienced asthma, urticaria, or allergic reactions after taking aspirin or other NSAIDs. Use with advanced kidney disease.
- Wearers of soft contact lenses.
- Use of the gel in those with hypersensitivity to benzyl alcohol, polyethylene glycol monomethyl ether 350, or hyaluronate sodium.
- Use of the gel in children.
- Use of the oral solution for prophylaxis of migraine.
- Use of the patch with advanced renal disease or application to nonintact or damaged skin re-

sulting from any cause (e.g., exudative dermatitis, eczema, infected lesion, burns, wounds).

- Coadministration of oral NSAIDs and topical diclofenac unless benefits outweigh risks.
- Use not recommended during lactation, although the topical products are considered as a low-risk alternative if an NSAID is needed during lactation.

SPECIAL CONCERNS

(1) NSAIDs may cause an increased risk of serious CV thrombotic events, MI, and stroke, which can be fatal. This risk may increase with duration of use. Clients with CV disease or risk factors for CV disease may be at greater risk. (2) Diclofenac epolamine, potassium, or sodium are contraindicated to treat perioperative pain in the setting of coronary artery bypass graft surgery. (3) NSAIDs cause an increased risk of serious GI side effects including bleeding, ulceration, and perforation of the stomach or intestines, which can be fatal. These events can occur at any time during use and without warning symptoms. Elderly clients are at greater risk for serious GI events.

- **Starting therapy with maximum doses is likely to increase the frequency of side effects in those at increased risk due to renal or hepatic disease, low body weight (less than 60 kg), advanced age, known ulcer diathesis, or known hypersensitivity to NSAIDs.**
- **Use with caution, if at all, during lactation.**
- **Use with caution in those with hypertension, fluid retention, heart failure, history of ulcer disease, or GI bleeding.**
- **Use during late pregnancy may cause premature closure of the ductus arteriosus. Drug may also inhibit uterine contractions and delay parturition.**
- **Safety and efficacy not determined in children.**
- **When used ophthalmically, may cause increased bleeding of ocular tissues in conjunction with ocular surgery. Healing may be slowed or delayed.**

SIDE EFFECTS

Most Common

After PO use: Headache, dizziness, abdominal pain/cramps, nausea, diarrhea, constipation, dyspepsia/indigestion.

After topical use: Application-site reactions (acne, dryness, erythema, induration, paresthesia, pruritus, urticaria, vasodilation, vesicles).

See *Nonsteroidal Anti-Inflammatory Drugs* for a complete list of possible side effects. Also, onset of new hypertension or worsening of pre-existing hypertension, fluid retention/edema, serious GI side effects, hepatotoxicity, renal toxicity, serious skin reactions, anemia, inhibition of platelet aggregation, hypersensitivity reactions.

Following ophthalmic use: Ophthalmic: Keratitis, increased IOP, ocular allergy, N&V, anterior chamber reaction, viral infections, transient burning/stinging on administration. When used with soft contact lenses, may cause ocular irritation, including redness/burning. **GI:** N&V.

Following topical use of the gel (Solaraze, Voltaren): Dermatologic: Application-site reactions (e.g., skin carcinoma, hypertonia, skin hypertrophy, lacrimation disorder, maculopapular rash, purpuric rash, vasodilation, dermatitis, dryness, irritation, papules, paresthesia, pruritus, vesicles), acne, alopecia, contact dermatitis, dry skin, edema, exfoliation, hyperesthesia, pain, paresthesia, photosensitivity reaction, pruritus, rash, seborrhea, skin ulcer, urticaria, vesiculobullous rash. **GI:** Abdominal pain, constipation, diarrhea, dyspepsia. **CV:** Hypertension. **CNS:** Asthenia, headache, hypokinesia. **GU:** Hematuria. **Metabolic:** ↑ ALT and AST, ↑ creatinine and creatine phosphokinase, hypercholesterolemia, hyperglycemia. **Musculoskeletal:** Arthralgia, arthrosis, back pain, myalgia, neck pain. **Respiratory:** Asthma, dyspnea, pharyngitis, pneumonia, rhinitis, sinusitis. **Ophthalmic:** Conjunctivitis, eye pain. **Body as a whole:** Flu syndrome, infection, pain. **Miscellaneous:** Accidental injury, allergic reaction, chest pain.

Following topical use of the solution (Pennsaid): Dermatologic: Rash, eczema, dry skin, ecchymosis, paresthesia at application site, pruritus, contact dermatitis (including with vesicles), skin discoloration, urticaria, vesicles. **CNS:** Depression, dizziness, drowsiness, headache, **GI:** Dyspepsia, abdominal pain, diarrhea, flatulence, nausea, constipation, decreased appetite, diarrhea, dry mouth, gastroenteritis, mouth ulceration, halitosis, ulcerative stomatitis, ***rectal hemorrhage.*** **CV:** CV disorder, palpitation. **Respiratory:** Asthma, dyspnea, laryngismus, laryngitis, pharyngitis, sinusitis. **Musculoskeletal:** Back pain, leg cramps, myalgia, neck rigidity. **Metabolic:** ↑ Creatinine, edema. **Ophthalmic:** Abnormal vision, blurred vision, cataract, eye disorder/pain. **Otic:** Ear pain. **Body as a whole:** Edema, infection, paresthesia, asthenia, lethargy, allergic reaction, body odor, pain. **Miscellaneous:** Accidental injury, taste perversion, chest pain, facial edema.

Following transdermal use (Flector): Dermatologic: Skin reactions at site of treatment, including burning, dermatitis, pruritus. Application-site dryness, atrophy, discoloration, edema, erythema, hyperhidrosis, irritation, itching, vesicles, abnormal sensation. **CNS:** Headache, paresthesia, somnolence, dizziness, hyperkinesia, hypoesthesia. **GI:** Dysgeusia, dyspepsia, N&V, constipation, diarrhea, dry mouth, gastritis, upper abdominal pain.

LABORATORY TEST CONSIDERATIONS

↑ AST, ALT.

DRUG INTERACTIONS

ACE inhibitors (e.g., enalapril) / Possible ↓ ACE inhibitor antihypertensive effect; also, ↑ risk nephrotoxicity
Acetaminophen / ↑ Risk of hepatotoxicity; use together with caution
Alcohol / ↑ Risk of GI bleeding; use together with caution
Aminoglycosides (e.g., amikacin, gentamicin) / Possible ↑ plasma aminoglycoside levels → ↑ risk of acute renal insufficiency; avoid concomitant use but if not possible, ↓ aminoglycoside dose before starting NSAID
Antibiotics (selective ones) / ↑ Risk of hepatoxicity; use together with caution
Anticoagulants (e.g., heparin, warfarin) / ↑ Risk of GI bleeding; monitor closely for signs of bleeding
Antiepileptic drugs / ↑ Risk of hepatotoxicity; use together with caution
Antiplatelet drugs (e.g., clopidogrel) / ↑ Risk of bleeding; use together with caution and monitor closely for signs of bleeding
Azole antifungals (e.g., fluconazole, voriconazole) / Possible ↑ diclofenac plasma levels → ↑ pharmacologic and side effects; adjust diclofenac dose as needed
Bisphosphonates (e.g., alendronate) / ↑ Risk of gastric ulceration; monitor closely
Corticosteroids (e.g., prednisone) / ↑ Risk of GI bleeding; use together with caution
Cyclosporine / ↑ Nephrotoxicity of both drugs; use together with caution
Diuretics (e.g., loop diuretics including furosemide, thiazides) / Possible ↓ natriuretic effect of the diuretic R/T inhibition of renal prostaglandin synthesis; observe for signs of renal failure
H ***Hibiscus sabdariffa*** / ↓ Urinary excretion of diclofenac → ↑ concentrations and ↑ risk of side effects; avoid beverages made from ***H. sabdariffa***
Lithium / ↑ Lithium plasma levels R/T ↓ renal lithium clearance → lithium toxicity
Methotrexate / Enhanced methotrexate toxicity; coadminister with caution
Quinolone (e.g., levofloxacin) / ↑ Risk of CNS stimulation and seizures due to quinolones; also ↑ quinolone plasma levels; use together with caution
Salicylates (e.g., aspirin) / Possible ↑ risk of side effects R/T ↓ diclofenac protein binding
Serotonin-norepinephrine reuptake inhibitors (e.g., venlafaxine) or selective serotonin reuptake inhibitors (e.g., citalopram, fluoxetine) / ↑ Risk of upper GI bleeding; use together with caution
Smoking / ↑ Risk of GI bleeding; use diclofenac in smokers with caution
Tenofovir / ↑ Risk of tenofovir pharmacologic/toxic (e.g., nephrotoxicity) effects; use together with caution
Triamterene / Possible sudden onset of nephrotoxicity

HOW SUPPLIED

Diclofenac epolamine. ***Topical patch:*** 180 mg/patch (1.3%).
Diclofenac potassium. ***Capsules:*** 25 mg; ***Powder for Solution, Oral:*** 50 mg; ***Tablets, Immediate-Release:*** 50 mg.
Diclofenac sodium. ***Gel, Topical:*** 1%, 3%; ***Ophthalmic Solution:*** 0.1%; ***Tablets, Delayed-Release:*** 25 mg, 50 mg, 75 mg; ***Tablets, Extended-Release:*** 100 mg; ***Topical Solution:*** 1.5%.

DOSAGE

Diclofenac epolamine

TRANSDERMAL PATCH (FLECTOR)

Acute pain due to minor strains, sprains, contusions.

Adults: Apply 1 patch to the most painful area twice a day. Change patch once every 12 hr. Remove patch if irritation occurs. Do not apply to damaged or nonintact skin or wear when bathing or showering. Avoid eye contact. Use the lowest effective dose for the shortest duration depending on client needs.

Diclofenac potassium

CAPSULES; ORAL SOLUTION; TABLETS, IMMEDIATE-RELEASE

Rheumatoid arthritis.

Adults: 150–200 mg/day in divided doses given as 50 mg 3 or 4 times per day. Do not exceed 225 mg/day.

Osteoarthritis.

Adults: 100–150 mg/day in divided doses given as 50 mg 2 or 3 times per day. Doses greater than 200 mg/day have not been evaluated.

Ankylosing spondylitis.

Adults: 50 mg 2 times per day; **range:** 100–125 mg/day. Doses greater than 125 mg/day have not been evaluated.

Analgesia, primary dysmenorrhea.

Adults, initial: 50 mg 3 times per day of immediate-release tablets or 25 mg 4 times per day of capsules. In some, an initial dose of 100 mg followed by 50 mg doses may achieve better results. After the first day, when the recommended dose may be 200 mg, the total daily dose should usually not exceed 150 mg.

Migraine, acute treatment.

Adults: Give 50 mg (1 packet of the Powder for Solution reconstituted).

Diclofenac sodium

DELAYED-RELEASE TABLETS

Ankylosing spondylitis, acute or chronic.

100–125 mg/day, given as 25 mg 4 times per day, with an extra 25 mg at bedtime, if necessary.

Osteoarthritis.

100–150 mg/day (e.g., 50 mg 2 or 3 times per day or 75 mg 2 times per day).

Rheumatoid arthritis.

150–200 mg/day in divided doses (50 mg 3 or 4 times per day or 75 mg 2 times per day).

EXTENDED-RELEASE TABLETS

Rheumatoid arthritis.

Extended-Release Tablets. Adults: 100 mg/day. If this dose is ineffective, the dose may be increased to 100 mg 2 times per day if the benefits outweigh potential increased side effects.

Osteoarthritis.

Delayed-Release Tablets. Adults: Extended-Release Tablets. Adults: 100 mg/day.

OPHTHALMIC SOLUTION, 0.1%

Following cataract surgery.

1 gtt in the affected eye 4 times per day beginning 24 hr after cataract surgery and for 2 weeks thereafter.

Corneal refractive surgery.

1–2 gtt within 1 hr prior to surgery; then, apply 1–2 gtt within 15 min of surgery and continue 4 times per day for up to 3 days.

TOPICAL GEL, 3% (SOLARAZE)

Actinic keratoses.

Adults, usual: Apply 0.5 gram gel for each 5 cm × 5 cm lesion site 2 times per day for 60–90 days. *NOTE:* The safety of concomitant use of sunscreens, cosmetics, or other topical medications is not known.

TOPICAL GEL, 1% (VOLTAREN)

Osteoarthritis.

Adults, lower extremities (e.g., knees, ankles, feet): Apply 4 grams of the gel to the affected area 4 times per day. Gently massage into the skin ensuring application to the entire area. Do not apply more than 16 grams per day to any single joint of the lower extremities. **Adults, upper extremities (e.g., elbows, hands, wrists):** Apply 2 grams of the gel to the affected area 4 times per day. Gently massage into the skin ensuring application to the entire area. Do not apply more than 8 grams per day to any single joint of the upper extremities. Concomitant use of the gel with oral NSAIDs has not been studied and may increase NSAID side effects.

NOTE: The total daily dose should not exceed 32 grams of the gel over all affected joints. Also, do not use sunscreens, cosmetics, lotions, moisturizers, insect repellants, or other topical medications on the same skin sites.

TOPICAL SOLUTION 1.5% (PENNSAID)
Osteoarthritis.
Adults: Apply 40 drops/knee four times a day.

NURSING IMPLICATIONS

Do not confuse Cataflam with Catapres (an antihypertensive).

IMPLEMENTATION/ADMINISTRATION/STORAGE

1. The lowest dose should be individualized for each client.
2. Diclofenac potassium is the form for management of acute pain and primary dysmenorrhea when a prompt onset of pain relief is desired; diclofenac potassium is absorbed earlier than diclofenac sodium.
3. In those weighing less than 60 kg (132 lbs) or where the severity of the disease, concomitant medications, or other diseases warrant, reduce the maximum recommended total dose of diclofenac potassium.
4. The various dosage forms are not necessarily bioequivalent even if the milligram strength is the same.
5. Up to 3 weeks may be required for beneficial effects to be realized when used for rheumatoid arthritis or osteoarthritis.
6. Do not store diclofenac potassium or sodium above 30°C (86°F); protect from moisture.
7. Store ophthalmic solution from 15–30°C (59–86°F).
8. Protect ophthalmic solution from light; dispense in original, unopened container.
9. Store the patch from 15–30°C (59–86°F). Keep the envelopes sealed at all times when not in use. Discard unused patches 3 months after opening the envelope.
10. Store the gel and topical solution from 15–30°C (59–86°F). Protect the gel from heat and avoid freezing.

ASSESSMENT

1. Note reasons for therapy, symptom characteristics, other agents trialed/failed.
2. Assess for redness, infection, pain, vision changes with eye therapy.
3. With arthritis, assess joints for inflammation, deformity, erosion, ROM, loss of function; rate pain level.
4. Assess skin integrity; do not apply to damaged or nonintact skin (Flector) or to open wounds. Avoid contact with eyes and mucous membranes. (Pennsaid; Voltaren gel)
5. Ensure drug administered in high enough doses for anti-inflammatory effect when needed and in low doses for an analgesic effect.
6. Assess for CV disease or risk factors; NSAIDs may cause an increased risk of serious CV thrombotic events, MI, and stroke, which can be fatal.
7. Monitor VS, elecytrolytes, CBC, renal and LFTs; stop with liver dysfunction. Monitor for bleeding, and perform FOB with long-term therapy.

CLIENT/FAMILY TEACHING

1. Take with meals, a full glass of water or milk if GI upset occurs; remain upright for 30 min after taking drug to reduce esophageal irritation. Do not crush or chew delayed-release tablets.
2. To reconstitute the powder for oral solution, empty the contents of 1 packet into a cup containing 1–2 ounces of water. Mix well and drink immediately; giving with food may decrease effectiveness.
3. May cause dizziness or drowsiness; avoid activities that require mental alertness until drug effects realized.
4. Administration of Pennsaid Topical Solution: (a) Apply to clean, dry skin. To avoid spillage, dispense 10 drops at a time either directly onto the knee or first onto the hand and then onto the knee. Spread evenly around the front, back, and side of the knee. Repeat this procedure until 40 drops have been applied; the knee is to be completely covered with solution. Repeat the procedure if the other knee is to be treated. Do not apply more or less than the recommended dose. (b) Wash and dry hands after use. Avoid bathing/showering for at least 30 min after application. (c) Do not apply to open wounds. (d) Avoid contact with eyes and mucous membranes. (e) Do not apply external heat and/or occlusive dressings to treated knees. Avoid wearing clothing over the treated knee(s) until the treated knee is dry. (f) Protect treated knee(s) from sunlight. Wait until treated knee(s) dry before applying sunscreen, insect repellant, lotion, moisturizer, cosmetics, or other topical products.

5. Administration of Solaraze Topical Gel: Smooth onto the affected area gently. Ensure enough gel is applied to cover each lesion adequately. Do not apply to open skin wounds, infections, or exfoliative dermatitis. Avoid contact with eyes.
6. Administration of Voltaren Topical Gel: (a) Gently massage into the skin; be sure the application covers the entire affected area. The entire foot includes the sole, top of the foot, and the toes. The entire hand includes the palm, back of the hands, and the fingers. (b) Measure the proper amount using the dosing cards supplied in the product carton. Use one dosing card for each application. (c) Apply the gel within the oblong area of the dosing card up to the 2 or 4 gram line (2 grams each for elbow, wrist, or hand, and 4 grams for each knee, ankle, or foot). (d) The dosing card can be used to apply the gel. (e) Avoid bathing/showering for at least 1 hr after application. (f) Wash hands after use, unless hands are the joint being treated. If the gel is used to treat the hand(s), wait at least 1 hr after application before washing. (g) Do not apply to open wounds. Avoid contact with eyes and mucous membranes. (h) Do not apply external heat or occlusive dressings to treated joints. (i) Avoid exposure of treated joint(s) to sunlight. (j) Avoid wearing clothing or gloves for at least 10 min after application.
7. Consult provider before using any other topical agents (e.g., astringents, cosmetics, medicated soaps) on treated skin.
8. With the patch, do not wear when bathing or showering. Wash hands after applying, handling, or removing the patch. Avoid contact with the eyes. If eye contact occurs, immediately wash out the eye with water or saline and contact provider if irritation persists for more than 1 hr.
9. If patch begins to peel off, the edges may be taped down. When disposing of the patch, fold so that the adhesive side sticks to itself. Safely discard where children and pets cannot access.
10. For eye drops, wash hands and do not allow dropper to touch eye. Tilt head back, look up and pull lower eyelid down, instilling prescribed number of drops. Close eye for 2 to 3 min, and apply gentle pressure to bridge of nose for 1 to 2 min. Do not rub eye. If more than 1 topical eye drug being used, give at least 5 min apart, administering ointment last. Do not wear contact lenses during therapy unless hydrogel soft contact lens during first 3 days after refractive surgery.
11. Limit intake of sodium, monitor BP, weights; report any swelling or unusual weight gain.
12. Monitor BS levels closely with diabetes; may alter response to antidiabetic agents.
13. Avoid alcohol, OTC products, and prolonged sun exposure without protection.
14. Maintain adequate fluid intake (2 L/day).
15. Avoid use late in pregnancy; may cause premature closure of the ductus arteriosus.
16. Report changes in stools, ringing in ears, stomach pain, unusual bruising/bleeding; seek help with chest pain, SOB, or weakness on one side of body.
17. Keep all F/U to assess response, labs, and adverse SE.

OUTCOMES/EVALUATE

- Relief of joint pain/inflammation with improved mobility
- ↓ Eye inflammation
- Clearing of AK

Dicyclomine hydrochloride

(dye-**SYE**-kloh-meen)

Classification(s): Cholinergic blocking drug

Pregnancy Category: C

RX: Bentyl, Byclomine.

🍁 **Rx:** Bentylol.

SEE ALSO ***CHOLINERGIC BLOCKING AGENTS***.

INDICATIONS/USES

IM, PO: Treatment of functional bowel/irritable bowel syndrome, including irritable colon, spastic colon, mucous colitis.

ACTION/KINETICS

Action

Prevents acetylcholine from combining with postganglionic parasympathetic nerve receptors (muscarinic) resulting in decreased vagal impulses to the GI tract. Results in a decrease in GI motility.

Pharmacokinetics

The IM injection is about twice as bioavailable as PO dosage forms. **t½, initial:** 1.8 hr; **secondary:** 9–10 hr.

ADDITIONAL CONTRAINDICATIONS

Use for peptic ulcer.

SPECIAL CONCERNS

Lower doses may be needed in elderly clients due to confusion, agitation, excitement, or drowsiness.

SIDE EFFECTS

Most Common

Dry mouth, N&V, constipation, urinary hesitancy/retention, headache, blurred vision.

See *Cholinergic Blocking Agents* for a complete list of possible side effects. Also, brief euphoria, slight dizziness, feeling of abdominal distention. **Use of the syrup in infants less than 3 months of age:** ***Seizures***, syncope, respiratory symptoms, fluctuations in pulse rate, ***asphyxia***, muscular hypotonia, ***coma***.

HOW SUPPLIED

Capsules: 10 mg, 20 mg; *Injection:* 10 mg/mL; *Syrup:* 10 mg/5 mL; *Tablets:* 20 mg.

DOSAGE

CAPSULES; SYRUP; TABLETS

Functional bowel/irritable bowel syndrome.

Individualize dosage. **Adults, initial:** 80 mg/day in 4 equally divided doses; depending on client response during the first week of therapy, increase the dose to 160 mg/day (the only PO effective dose). If efficacy is not achieved within 2 weeks or side effects mandate doses below 80 mg/day, discontinue the drug.

IM ONLY

Functional bowel/irritable bowel syndrome.

Adults: 80 mg/day in 4 equally divided doses. **Not for IV use.** Begin PO therapy as soon as possible; do use the IM form longer than 1 or 2 days.

NURSING IMPLICATIONS

Do not confuse dicyclomine with doxycycline (an antibiotic); do not confuse Bentyl with Benadryl (an antihistamine) or Aventyl (an antidepressant).

IMPLEMENTATION/ADMINISTRATION/STORAGE

1. Aspirate the syringe before injecting to avoid intravascular injection (may cause thrombosis).
2. Inspect the parenteral product visually for particulate matter and discoloration.
3. Can be administered to clients with glaucoma with caution.
4. Store PO forms from 15–30°C (59–86°F). Protect from light, freezing, and moisture. Store the injection below 30°C (86°F); protect from freezing.

ASSESSMENT

1. List reasons for therapy, symptom characteristics, any triggers, other agents trialed, outcome.
2. Determine presence/history PUD, obstructive uropathy/GI disease, hepatic or renal disease or myocardial ischemia; may preclude therapy.
3. Assess abdomen, review renal and LFTs, UGI, endoscopy/colonoscopy findings.

CLIENT/FAMILY TEACHING

1. Take 30 min before meals and at bedtime.
2. Use caution with activities requiring mental alertness; may cause drowsiness, blurred vision.
3. Elderly should report eye pain to provider and undergo testing for glaucoma; use lubricating solutions with contact lens.
4. Consume adequate fluids to prevent dehydration/constipation; may use sugarless candy/gum for dry mouth. Avoid direct sunlight and heat extremes as well as overheating and strenuous activity during hot conditions; heatstroke may occur.
5. Any fever warrants noting due to decreased ability to sweat; report marked changes in bowel or bladder habits.
6. Report any confusion, disorientation, swallowing difficulty, short-term memory loss, hallucinations, gait disturbance, coma, euphoria, ↓ anxiety, fatigue, insomnia, agitation, and inappropriate affect.
7. Keep all F/U to assess response and for adverse SE.

OUTCOMES/EVALUATE

- Restoration of normal bowel function/GI motility

- Relief of GI spasms/pain

Didanosine (ddI, dideoxyinosine)

(die-**DAN**-oh-seen)

Classification(s): Antiviral, nucleoside reverse transcriptase inhibitor

Pregnancy Category: B

RX: Videx, Videx EC.

SEE ALSO ***ANTIVIRAL AGENTS***.

INDICATIONS/USES

Adults and children over 2 weeks of age to treat HIV-1 infections in combination with other antiretroviral drugs.

ACTION/KINETICS

Action

A nucleoside analog of deoxyadenosine. After entering the cell, it is converted to the active dideoxyadenosine triphosphate (ddATP) by cellular enzymes. Due to the chemical structure of ddATP, its incorporation into viral DNA leads to chain termination and therefore inhibition of viral replication. ddATP also inhibits viral replication by interfering with the HIV-RNA-dependent DNA polymerase by competing with the natural nucleoside triphosphate for binding to the active site of the enzyme. Didanosine has shown in vitro antiviral activity in a variety of HIV-infected T-cell and monocyte/macrophage cell cultures.

Pharmacokinetics

Rapidly absorbed. Is broken down quickly at acidic pH; therefore, PO products contain buffering agents to increase the pH of the stomach. Food decreases the rate of absorption. Oral availability differs between adults (about 42%) and children (about 25%). **Peak plasma levels:** 0.25–1.5 hr. **t½, elimination:** 1.5 hr for adults and 0.8 hr for children. Metabolized in the liver and excreted mainly through the urine. Videx EC capsules contain enteric-coated beadlets, which protect against stomach acid degradation; the drug is absorbed from the small intestine.

CONTRAINDICATIONS

Hypersensitivity to any component of the products. Lactation.

SPECIAL CONCERNS

(1) **Pancreatitis.** Fatal and nonfatal pancreatitis has occurred during therapy with didanosine used alone or in combination regimens in both treatment-naive and treatment-experienced clients, regardless of the degree of immunosuppression. Suspend didanosine in those suspected of pancreatitis; discontinue in those with confirmed pancreatitis. (2) **Lactic acidosis and severe hepatomegaly.** Lactic acidosis and severe hepatomegaly with steatosis, including fatal cases, have been reported with the use of nucleoside analogs alone or in combination, including didanosine and other antiretrovirals. (3) Fatal lactic acidosis has been reported in pregnant women who received the combination of didanosine and stavudine with other antiretroviral drugs. Use the combination of didanosine and stavudine with caution during pregnancy; the combination is recommended only if the potential benefit clearly outweighs the potential risk.

- **Use with caution in renal and hepatic impairment and in those on sodium-restricted diets.**
- **Discontinue in clients with confirmed pancreatitis.**
- **Use the combination of didanosine and ribavirin with caution due to increased exposure to the active metabolite of didanosine that may cause fatal hepatic failure, peripheral neuropathy, pancreatitis, and symptomatic hyperlactatemia or lactic acidosis.**
- **Opportunistic infections and other complications of HIV infection may continue to develop; thus, keep clients under close observation.**
- **High rate of virologic failure and emergence of nucleoside reverse transcriptase inhibitor resistance-associated mutations.**
- **Increased risk for MI.**
- **Clients 65 years and older have a higher frequency of pancreatitis. Use care in dose selection in this population.**

SIDE EFFECTS

Most Common

Diarrhea, N&V, headache, peripheral neurologic symptoms/neuropathy, abdominal pain, rash, pruritus, pancreatitis.

Commonly pancreatitis (fatal or nonfatal) and peripheral neuropathy (manifested by distal numbness, tingling, or pain in the feet or hands). Lactic acidosis (may be fatal), including pregnant women also receiving stavudine along with other antiretroviral drugs. Hepatotoxicity (may be fatal) used alone or in combination. Neuropathy occurs more frequently in clients with a history of neuropathy or neurotoxic drug therapy.

D

In adults. GI: Diarrhea, abdominal pain, N&V, anorexia, dyspepsia, dry mouth, ileus, colitis, constipation, eructation, flatulence, gastroenteritis, ***GI hemorrhage***, oral moniliasis, stomatitis, mouth sores, sialadenitis, ***stomach ulcer /hemorrhage***, melena, oral thrush, liver abnormalities, parotid gland enlargement, ***pancreatitis***. **Hepatic:** ***Severe hepatomegaly with steatosis, liver failure,*** hepatitis, liver abnormalities, ***noncirrhotic portal hypertension***. **CNS:** Headache, ***tonic-clonic seizures***, abnormal thinking, anxiety, nervousness, twitching, confusion, depression, acute brain syndrome, amnesia, aphasia, ataxia, dizziness, hyperesthesia, hypertonia, incoordination, ***intracranial hemorrhage***, paralysis, paranoid reaction, peripheral neuropathy, psychosis, insomnia, sleep disorders, speech disorders, tremor. **Hematologic:** Leukopenia, granulocytopenia, thrombocytopenia, anemia, microcytic anemia, ***hemorrhage***, ecchymosis, petechiae. **Dermatologic**: Rash, pruritus, herpes simplex, skin disorder, sweating, eczema, impetigo, excoriation, erythema. **Musculoskeletal**: Asthenia, myopathy, arthralgia, arthritis, myalgia (with or without increases in creatine phosphokinase), muscle atrophy, decreased strength, hemiparesis, neck rigidity, joint disorder, leg cramps, ***rhabdomyolysis, including acute renal failure*** and hemodialysis. **CV:** Chest pain, hypertension, hypotension, migraine, palpitation, peripheral vascular disorder, syncope, vasodilation, arrhythmias, ***MI***. **Metabolic:** Diabetes mellitus, hypo-/hyperglycemia, symptomatic hyperlactatemia, ***lactic acidosis***. **Respiratory**: Pneumonia, dyspnea, asthma, bronchitis, increased cough, rhinitis, rhinorrhea, epistaxis, laryngitis, decreased lung function, pharyngitis, hypoventilation, sinusitis, rhonchi, rales, congestion, interstitial pneumonia, respiratory disorders. **Ophthalmic:** Blurred vision, conjunctivitis, diplopia, dry eyes, glaucoma, retinitis, photophobia, strabismus, optic neuritis, retinal changes, retinal depigmentation. **Otic:** Ear disorder, otitis (externa and media), ear pain. **GU:** Impotency, kidney calculus, kidney failure, abnormal kidney function, nocturia, urinary frequency, vaginal hemorrhage. **Body as a whole:** Chills, fever, asthenia, pain, infection, allergic reaction, pain, abscess, cellulitis, cyst, dehydration, malaise, flu syndrome, numbness of hands and feet, weight loss, alopecia, ***anaphylaxis***. **Miscellaneous:** Peripheral edema, sarcoma, hernia, hypokalemia, lymphoma-like reaction, immune reconstitution syndrome. Fat redistribution, including central obesity, dorsocervical fat enlargement, peripheral wasting, facial wasting, breast enlargement, "cushinoid" appearance.

In children. GI: Diarrhea, N&V, liver abnormalities, abdominal pain, stomatitis, mouth sores, pancreatitis, anorexia, increase in appetite, constipation, oral thrush, melena, dry mouth, ***pancreatitis, liver failure***. **CNS**: Headache, nervousness, insomnia, dizziness, poor coordination, lethargy, neurologic symptoms, ***seizures***. **Hematologic**: Ecchymosis, ***hemorrhage***, petechiae, leukopenia, granulocytopenia, thrombocytopenia, anemia. **Dermatologic**: Rash, pruritus, skin disorder, eczema, sweating, impetigo, excoriation, erythema. **Musculoskeletal:** Arthritis, myalgia, muscle atrophy, decreased strength. **Body as a whole:** Chills, fever, asthenia, pain, malaise, failure to thrive, weight loss, flu syndrome, alopecia, dehydration, lactic acidosis. **CV:** Vasodilation, arrhythmia. **Respiratory:** Cough, rhinitis, dyspnea, asthma, rhinorrhea, epistaxis, pharyngitis, hypoventilation, sinusitis, rhonchi, rales, congestion, pneumonia. **Ophthalmic:** Photophobia, strabismus, visual impairment, optic neuritis, retinal changes. **Otic:** Ear pain, otitis. **Miscellaneous:** Urinary frequency, diabetes mellitus, diabetes insipidus, liver abnormalities.

LABORATORY TEST CONSIDERATIONS

↑ AST, ALT, GGT, alkaline phosphatase, bilirubin, uric acid, serum amylase, lipase.

OVERDOSE MANAGEMENT

Symptoms: Pancreatitis, peripheral neuropathy, diarrhea, hyperuricemia, hepatic dysfunction. *Treatment:* There are no antidotes; treatment should be symptomatic. There may be some clearance using hemodialysis.

DRUG INTERACTIONS

NOTE: (a) Didanosine formulations either contain buffers or are mixed with antacids before use; thus, interactions may occur with drugs whose absorption can be affected by the level of acidity in the stomach and with drugs that interact with antacids containing magnesium, calcium, or aluminum. (b) Coadministration of didanosine with drugs that are known to cause pancreatitis may ↑ the risk of this toxicity.

Allopurinol / ↑ Didanosine levels; coadministration not recommended
Antacids, Mg⁺⁺ or Al-containing / ↑ Risk of side effects R/T antacid components; use powder for the PO solution with caution
Antifungal drugs (azoles: itraconazole, ketoconazole) / ↓ Absorption of azole antifungals → ↓ therapeutic effect; give azoles 2 or more hr before didanosine
Antiretroviral drugs (delavirdine, indinavir) / Significantly ↓ levels delavirdine or indinavir; give delavirdine or indinavir 1 hr before didanosine
Fluoroquinolone antibiotics (e.g., ciprofloxacin) / ↓ Quinolone levels R/T ↓ absorption due to antacid; give the fluoroquinolone 2 hr or more before or 6 hr after didanosine
Ganciclovir / ↑ Didanosine levels when given 2 hr prior to ganciclovir; ↓ ganciclovir levels when given 2 hr prior to didanosine; monitor for didanosine toxicity and adjust dose as needed
Methadone / ↓ Didanosine AUC and C_{max}; do not give methadone with didanosine powder for oral solution due to ↓ didanosine levels; if coadministration is necessary, use the delayed-release capsule
Nelfinavir / Possible ↑ nelfinavir levels; give nelfinavir with a light meal 1 hr after didanosine
Neurotoxic drugs / ↑ Risk of neuropathy; use together with caution, if at all
Pentamidine (IV) / ↑ Risk of pancreatitis
Ranitidine / ↓ Ranitidine absorption R/T gastric pH change caused by buffering agents in didanosine
Ribavirin / ↑ Risk of fatal hepatic failure, peripheral neuropathy, pancreatitis, symptomatic hyperlactatemia, or lactic acidosis; use together contraindicated
Stavudine / ↑ Risk of fatal lactic acidosis including in pregnant women, especially when combined with other drugs; also, ↑ risk of peripheral neuropathy
Stavudine with or without hydroxyurea / ↑ Risk of pancreatitis and liver function abnormalities; avoid the combination of didanosine and hydroxyurea
Tenofovir / ↑ Didanosine toxicity (lactic acidosis, pancreatitis, peripheral neuropathy) and poor therapeutic outcomes (↓ virologic response, ↓ CD4+ T-cell counts); adjust dosage (see ***Implementation/Administration/Storage***).
Tetracyclines / ↓ Tetracycline absorption R/T gastric pH changes caused by buffering agents in didanosine
Valganciclovir / ↑ Didanosine plasma levels

HOW SUPPLIED

Didanosine. *Powder for Oral Solution:* 2 grams, 4 grams.
Didanosine Delayed-Release. *Capsules, Delayed-Release (Enteric-Coated Beadlets):* 125 mg, 200 mg, 250 mg, 400 mg.

DOSAGE

CAPSULE, DELAYED-RELEASE (ENTERIC-COATED BEADLETS); POWDER FOR ORAL SOLUTION

Human immunodeficiency virus (HIV) infection.

Delayed-Release Capsule. Adults, over 60 kg: 400 mg once a day. **Adults, 25 kg to less than 60 kg:** 250 mg once a day. **Adults, 20 kg to less than 25 kg:** 200 mg once a day. **Powder for oral solution. Adults, 60 kg or greater:** 200 mg twice a day (preferred) or 400 mg once a day. **Adults, less than 60 kg:** 125 mg twice a day (preferred) or 250 mg once a day.

Children: Delayed-Release Capsule. See Adult dosing. **Powder for oral solution. Children, older than 8 months:** 120 mg/m^2 twice a day. **Children, 2 weeks to 8 months:** 100 mg/m^2 twice a day.

Children, off-label dosing: Treatment naive (3–21 years): 240 mg/m^2/day. **Older than 8 months:** 90–150 mg/m^2 twice a day. **Neonates/infants, 2 weeks–younger than 3 months:** 50 mg/m^2 twice a day.

For adults with impaired renal function, the following dosage regimens are used: (1) **Weight 60 kg or more, C_{CR} 60 mL or more/min:** 400 mg once a day using delayed-release capsules or 200 mg twice a day using the powder for oral suspension. (2) **Weight 60 kg**

D

or less, C_{CR} 60 mL or more/min: 250 mg once a day using delayed-release capsules or 125 mg twice a day using the powder for oral suspension. (3) **Weight 60 kg or more, C_{CR} 30–59 mL/min:** 200 mg once a day using delayed-release capsules or 200 mg once a day or 100 mg twice a day using the powder for oral suspension. (4) **Weight, 60 kg or less, C_{CR} 30–59 mL/min, <60 kg:** 125 mg once a day using delayed-release capsules or 150 mg once a day or 75 mg twice a day using the powder for oral suspension. (5) **Weight, 60 kg or more, C_{CR} 10–29 mL/min:** 125 mg once a day using the delayed-release capsules or 150 mg once a day using the powder for oral suspension. (6) **Weight, 60 kg or less, C_{CR} 10–29 mL/min:** 125 mg once a day using the delayed-release capsules or 100 mg once a day using the powder for oral suspension. (7) **Weight, 60 kg or more, C_{CR} <10 mL/min:** 125 mg once a day using the delayed-release capsules or 100 mg once a day using the powder for oral suspension. (8) **Weight, 60 kg or less, C_{CR} <10 mL/min:** 75 mg once a day using the powder for oral suspension. Do not use enteric-coated capsules in these clients.

NOTE: For clients requiring continuous ambulatory peritoneal dialysis or hemodialysis, follow dosing recommendation for clients with a C_{CR} <10 mL/min. It is not necessary to give a supplemental dose of didanosine following hemodialysis.

For children with impaired renal function, clearance of didanosine may be altered. Thus, consider dose reduction and/or an increase in the interval between doses.

NURSING IMPLICATIONS

IMPLEMENTATION/ADMINISTRATION/STORAGE

1. Twice daily dosing may be more effective than once daily dosing.
2. Administer all formulations 30 min before or 1 hr after meals.
3. When taken with tenofovir, reduce dose of didanosine as follows: For adults weighing at least 60 kg with a C_{CR} of >60 mL/min, reduce didanosine dose to 250 mg once daily; for adults weighing less than 60 kg with a C_{CR} of at least 60 mL/min, reduce the didanosine dose to 200 mg. The dose of didanosine to be given with tenofovir in those with a C_{CR} <60 mL/min has not been established.
4. May take didanosine pediatric powder for oral solution and tenofovir together in the fasted state. Or, if tenofovir is taken with food, take didanosine on an empty stomach (at least 30 min before or 2 hr after food).
5. May take didanosine delayed-release capsules with tenofovir together with a light meal (400 kcal or less; 20% fat or less) or in the fasted state.
6. To reduce GI side effects, do not give more than 4 capsules at each dose.
7. Clients treated with didanosine in combination with stavudine, with or without hydroxyurea, may be at increased risk for pancreatitis and liver function abnormalities. Also, those treated with didanosine with stavudine may be at increased risk for peripheral neuropathy.
8. To prepare the pediatric powder for oral solution, reconstitute with purified water to an initial concentration of 20 mg/mL by adding 100 or 200 mL of purified water to the didanosine 2 gram or 4 gram powder, respectively. Then, immediately mix 1 part of the 20 mg/mL initial solution with 1 part Maximum Strength Mylanta liquid for a final dispensing concentration of didanosine, 10 mg/mL. This mixture is stable for 30 days under refrigeration. The admixture must be thoroughly shaken prior to each use.
9. To monitor maternal-fetal outcomes of pregnant women exposed to didanosine, an Antiretroviral Pregnancy Register has been established. Enroll clients by calling 1-800-258-4263.
10. Store delayed-release capsules and the bottles of powder from 15–30°C (59–86°F). The didanosine admixture may be stored up to 30 days from 2–8°C (36–46°F). Discard any unused portion after 30 days.

ASSESSMENT

1. Note all experiences with zidovudine therapy; list reasons for transfer to didanosine. List drugs prescribed to ensure none interact.
2. Assess for S&S of lactic acidosis and hepatomegaly. Pregnant women receiving the combination of didanosine and stavudine with other antiretroviral agents have experienced fatal lactic acidosis; monitor closely.
3. Reduce dose with liver and renal impairment. Note baseline VS and weight. Monitor for S&S pancreatitis; withhold if pancreatitis is suspected and discontinue drug with confirmed pancreatitis. Assess for diarrhea with the oral solution.
4. Monitor CBC, CD_4 counts/viral load, uric acid, renal and LFTs; reduce dose with renal dysfunction.

CLIENT/FAMILY TEACHING

1. Used with other drugs to treat HIV infections. Follow dosing guidelines carefully; review drug administration insert. Food decreases the rate of drug absorption by 50%; take 30 min before or 2 hr after meals.
2. Do not swallow tablets whole. Tablets may be chewed or crushed thoroughly before taking or dispersed in at least 1 oz of drinking water (stir thoroughly and drink immediately).
3. Chewable/dispersible buffered tablets contain 73 mg phenylalanine per 2-tablet dose.
4. The pediatric powder for oral suspension is first mixed with purified water for concentration of 20 mg/mL, and then mixed with antacid to obtain final concentration of 10 mg/mL.
5. Report any symptoms of neuropathy (numbness, burning, or tingling in the hands or feet); drug should be discontinued until symptoms subside. May tolerate a reduced dose once these S&S are resolved.
6. Report any abdominal pain and N&V immediately; may be clinical signs of pancreatitis. Stop drug and report; resume only after pancreatitis has been ruled out.
7. With salt-restricted diets, sodium content is higher in the single-dose packet than the 2-tablet dose. Each single-dose packet of buffered powder for oral solution contains 1,380 mg sodium and each 2-tablet dose contains 529 mg sodium.
8. Increase fluid intake; report S&S of diarrhea or hyperuricemia (joint pains).
9. Any changes in vision should be evaluated by an ophthalmologist. Get retinal exams every 6 months to rule out depigmentation with children.
10. Avoid alcohol and any other drugs that may exacerbate toxicity of didanosine.
11. Drug is not a cure, but alleviates the symptoms of HIV infections; may continue to acquire opportunistic infections. *Does not* reduce the risk of transmission of HIV to others through sexual contact or blood contamination; use appropriate precautions/protection.
12. Identify local support groups that may assist client/family to understand and cope with disease.
13. Keep all F/U to assess response, labs, and adverse SE.

OUTCOMES/EVALUATE

- ↓ HIV RNA Replication
- Treatment of HIV infection

Diflunisal

(dye-**FLEW**-nih-sal)

Classification(s): Nonsteroidal anti-inflammatory drug

Pregnancy Category: C

✤ **Rx:** Apo-Diflunisal.

SEE ALSO ***NONSTEROIDAL ANTI-INFLAMMATORY DRUGS.***

INDICATIONS/USES

(1) Acute or long-term use for mild to moderate pain. (2) Acute or long-term use for symptomatic treatment of rheumatoid arthritis or osteoarthritis.

ACTION/KINETICS

Action

Has analgesic, anti-inflammatory, and antipyretic effects. Salicylic acid derivative, although not metabolized to salicylic acid. Mechanism not known; may be an inhibitor of prostaglandin synthetase.

Pharmacokinetics

Rapidly and completely absorbed. **Onset:** 20 min (analgesic, antipyretic). **Peak plasma levels:** 2–3 hr. **Peak effect:** 2–3 hr. **Duration:** 4–6 hr. **t½:**

8–12 hr. Metabolites excreted in urine. **Plasma protein binding:** 99%.

CONTRAINDICATIONS

Hypersensitivity to diflunisal, aspirin, or other anti-inflammatory drugs. Acute asthmatic attacks, urticaria, or rhinitis precipitated by aspirin. Advanced renal disease. During lactation and in children less than 12 years of age.

SPECIAL CONCERNS

■ (1) **Cardiovascular risk.** NSAIDs may cause an increased risk of serious CV thrombotic reactions, MI, and stroke, which can be fatal. This risk may increase with duration of use. Clients with CV disease or risk factors for CV disease may be at greater risk. (2) Diflunisal is contraindicated for the treatment of perioperative pain in the setting of coronary artery bypass graft surgery. (3) **GI risk.** NSAIDs cause an increased risk of serious GI adverse reactions, including bleeding, ulceration, and perforation of the stomach or intestines, which can be fatal. These reactions can occur at any time during use and without warning symptoms. Elderly clients are at greater risk for serious GI reactions. ■

- Use with extreme caution in presence of ulcers or in clients with a history thereof, GI bleeding, in clients with hypertension, compromised cardiac function, or in conditions leading to fluid retention.
- Use with caution in only first two trimesters of pregnancy.
- Geriatric clients may be at greater risk of GI toxicity.
- Use of diflunisal may be associated with Reye's syndrome.

SIDE EFFECTS

Most Common

Headache, rash, nausea, dyspepsia, GI pain, diarrhea, fatigue, tiredness, tinnitus.

GI: N&V, dyspepsia, GI pain and bleeding, diarrhea, constipation, flatulence, peptic ulcer, eructation, anorexia, gastritis, GI inflammation, ulceration, stomatitis, ***perforation of the stomach/small intestine/large intestine.*** **Hepatic:** Cholestasis, hepatitis, jaundice. **CNS:** Headache, fatigue, fever, malaise, tiredness, dizziness, somnolence, insomnia, nervousness, confusion, depression, disorientation, vertigo, hallucinations, lightheadedness, paresthesias. **Dermatologic:** Rashes, pruritus, sweating, ***Stevens-Johnson syndrome, toxic epidermal necrolysis***, exfoliative dermatitis, dry mucous membranes, erythema multiforme, photosensitivity, urticaria. **CV:** Palpitations, syncope, edema, hypertension (new or worsening of existing), ***serious thrombotic events, MI, stroke.*** **GU:** Dysuria, hematuria, interstitial nephritis, proteinuria, impaired renal function including renal failure, nephrotic syndrome (rare), renal papillary necrosis. **Hematologic:** Agranulocytosis, hemolytic anemia, thrombocytopenia, anemia. **Hypersensitivity:** ***Acute anaphylaxis with bronchospasm***, angioedema, flushing, hypersensitivity syndrome, hypersensitivity vasculitis. **Ophthalmic:** Transient visual disturbances including blurred vision. **Otic:** Tinnitus, hearing loss (rare). **Miscellaneous:** Asthenia, chest pain, ***anaphylaxis***, dyspnea, muscle cramps, fluid retention, edema, ***fulminant necrotizing fascititis.***

LABORATORY TEST CONSIDERATIONS

↑ ALT, AST. Abnormal LFTs.

OVERDOSE MANAGEMENT

Symptoms: Drowsiness, N&V, diarrhea, tachycardia, sweating, tinnitus, hyperventilation, stupor, disorientation, diminished urine output, ***coma, cardiorespiratory arrest.*** *Treatment:* Supportive measures to treat symptoms. To empty the stomach perform gastric lavage. Hemodialysis may not be effective since the drug is significantly bound to plasma protein.

DRUG INTERACTIONS

Acetaminophen / ↑ Acetaminophen levels
ACE Inhibitors / ↓ Antihypertensive effect; in those with renal dysfunction → further renal function deterioration
Angiotensin II antagonists / ↓ Antihypertensive effect; in those with renal dysfunction → further renal function deterioration
Antacids / ↓ Diflunisal levels
Anticoagulants / ↑ PT
Aspirin / Potential for ↑ side effects R/T ↓ diflunisal plasma protein binding
Cyclosporine / ↑ Cyclosporine toxicity possibly R/T ↓ synthesis of renal prostacyclin; use together with caution
Furosemide / ↓ Furosemide hyperuricemic effect

Hydrochlorothiazide / ↑ Hydrochlorothiazide levels and ↓ hyperuricemic effect
Indomethacin / ↓ Indomethacin renal clearance → ↑ plasma levels
Lithium / ↑ Lithium levels; monitor for lithium toxicity
Methotrexate / ↑ Methotrexate toxicity
Naproxen / ↓ Urinary naproxen and metabolite excretion
NSAIDs / ↑ Chance of GI toxicity with little or no ↑ efficacy
Probenecid / ↑ Probenecid pharmacologic and toxic effects
Sulindac / ↓ Plasma levels of the active sulindac metabolite by one-third
Thiazide diuretics / ↓ Natriuertic and hyperuricemic effects

HOW SUPPLIED

Tablets: 500 mg.

DOSAGE

TABLETS

Mild to moderate pain.

Adults, initial: 1,000 mg; **then,** 500 mg q 12 hr. Some may require 500 mg q 8 hr. A lower dosage may be appropriate for some (e.g., 500 mg initially followed by 250 mg q 8 hr).

Rheumatoid arthritis, osteoarthritis.

Adults: 250–1,000 mg/day in 2 divided doses. Dose may be increased or decreased depending on client response. Maintenance doses greater than 1,500 mg/day are not recommended.

NURSING IMPLICATIONS

IMPLEMENTATION/ADMINISTRATION/STORAGE

1. Maximum relief occurs in 2–3 weeks when used for pain/swelling of arthritis. Serum salicylate levels are not used as a guide to dosage or toxicity; drug is not hydrolyzed to salicylic acid.
2. Store from 20–25°C (68–77°F).

ASSESSMENT

1. Note reasons for therapy, characteristics of S&S. Assess for hypersensitivity to salicylates, other NSAIDs.
2. With arthritis, assess joints for inflammation, deformity, erosion, ROM, loss of function. Rate pain levels.
3. Determine PUD, HTN, cardiac dysfunction, asthma, CV disease or risk factors. List drugs prescribed to ensure none interact.
4. Check for pregnancy; avoid drug/use with extreme caution during first two trimesters.
5. Give in high enough doses for anti-inflammatory effects when needed; use lower dose for analgesic effects. Reduce dose by half in those over 65 years old.
6. Monitor BP, CBC, renal and LFTs; reduce dose with dysfunction, and assess for bleeding.

INTERVENTIONS

1. Note reasons for therapy, characteristics of S&S. Assess for hypersensitivity to salicylates, other NSAIDs. List drugs prescribed to ensure none interact.
2. With arthritis, assess joints for inflammation, deformity, erosion, ROM, loss of function. Rate pain levels.
3. Determine history of ulcers, HTN, cardiac dysfunction, asthma, CV disease or risk factors. Advise may cause increased risk of serious CV thrombotic events, MI, and stroke, which increases with prolonged use and heart disease.
4. Check for pregnancy; avoid drug/use with extreme caution during first two trimesters.
5. Give in high enough doses for anti-inflammatory effects when needed; use lower dose for analgesic effects. Reduce dose by half in those over 65 years old.
6. Monitor BP, CBC, renal and LFTs; reduce dose with dysfunction and assess for bleeding.

CLIENT/FAMILY TEACHING

1. May give with water, milk, or meals to reduce gastric irritation. Do not crush or chew tablets.
2. Report adverse effects, unusual bruising/bleeding, or lack of response; may inhibit platelets, which is reversible with drug discontinuation. Do not give with acetaminophen or aspirin.
3. May cause dizziness or drowsiness; use care when operating machinery or driving.
4. Report stool color changes or diarrhea; can cause electrolyte imbalance or GI bleed.
5. Must take on a regular basis to sustain anti-inflammatory effect.
6. NSAIDs may cause an increased risk of serious CV thrombotic events, MI, and stroke,

which can be fatal. Drug can precipitate Reye's syndrome.

7. **Pregnant women should avoid use late in pregnancy.**
8. **Keep all F/U to assess response, labs, and for adverse SE. Drug dose needs to be adjusted according to age, condition, and changes in disease activity.**

D

OUTCOMES/EVALUATE

↓ Pain/inflammation; ↑ joint mobility

IV

Digoxin

(dih-**JOX**-in)

Classification(s): Cardiac glycoside

Pregnancy Category: A

RX: Digoxin, Digoxin Injection Pediatric.

🍁 **Rx:** Apo-Digoxin, Digoxin Injection C.S.D., Digoxin Pediatric Injection C.S.D., PMS-Digoxin.

INDICATIONS/USES

(1) CHF, including that due to venous congestion, edema, dyspnea, orthopnea, and cardiac arrhythmia. May be drug of choice for CHF because of rapid onset, relatively short duration, and ability to be administered PO or IV. (2) Control of rapid ventricular contraction rate in clients with atrial fibrillation or flutter. (3) Slow HR in sinus tachycardia due to CHF. (4) SVT. (5) Prophylaxis and treatment of recurrent paroxysmal atrial tachycardia with paroxysmal AV junctional rhythm. (6) Cardiogenic shock (value not established).

ACTION/KINETICS

Action

Increases the force and velocity of myocardial contraction (positive inotropic effect) by increasing the refractory period of the AV node and increasing total peripheral resistance. This effect is due to inhibition of sodium/potassium-ATPase in the sarcolemmal membrane, which alters excitation-contraction coupling. Inhibiting sodium/potassium-ATPase results in increased calcium influx and increased release of free calcium ions within the myocardial cells, which then potentiate the contractility of cardiac muscle fibers. Digoxin also decreases HR, decreases the rate of conduction, and increases the refractory period of the AV node due to an increase in parasympathetic tone and a decrease in sympathetic tone. Clinical effects are not seen until steady-state plasma levels are reached. The initial dose of digoxin is larger (loading dose) and is traditionally referred to as the *digitalizing dose;* subsequent doses are referred to as *maintenance doses.*

Pharmacokinetics

Onset, PO: 0.5–2 hr; **time to peak effect:** 2–6 hr. **Duration:** Over 24 hr. **Onset, IV:** 5–30 min; **time to peak effect:** 1–4 hr. **Duration:** 6 days. **$t^{1/2}$:** 30–40 hr. **Therapeutic serum level:** 0.5–2.0 ng/mL. Serum levels above 2.5 ng/mL indicate toxicity. 50–70% is excreted unchanged by the kidneys. Bioavailability depends on the dosage form: Tablets (60–80%) and elixir (70–85%). Thus, changing dosage forms may require dosage adjustments. **Plasma protein binding:** 20–25%.

CONTRAINDICATIONS

Ventricular fibrillation or tachycardia (unless congestive failure supervenes after protracted episode not due to digitalis), in presence of digoxin toxicity, hypersensitivity to cardiac glycosides, beriberi heart disease, certain cases of hypersensitive, carotid sinus syndrome.

SPECIAL CONCERNS

- **Use with caution in clients with ischemic heart disease, acute myocarditis, hypertrophic subaortic stenosis, hypoxic or myxedemic states, Adams-Stokes or carotid sinus syndromes, cardiac amyloidosis, or cyanotic heart and lung disease, including emphysema and partial heart block.**
- **Also use with caution and at reduced dosage in elderly, debilitated clients, pregnant women and nursing mothers, and newborn, term, or premature infants who have immature renal and hepatic function and in reduced renal and/or hepatic function.**
- **Those with carditis associated with rheumatic fever or viral myocarditis are especially sensitive to digoxin-induced disturbances in rhythm.**
- **Electric pacemakers may sensitize the myocardium to cardiac glycosides.**
- **The $t^{1/2}$ of digoxin is prolonged in the elderly; anticipate smaller doses.**
- **Be especially alert to cardiac arrhythmias in children. This sign of toxicity occurs more frequently in children than in adults.**

SIDE EFFECTS

Most Common

Tachycardia, headache, dizziness, mental disturbances, N&V, diarrhea, anorexia, blurred or yellow vision.

Digoxin is extremely toxic and has caused ***death*** even in clients who have received the drug for long periods of time. There is a narrow margin of safety between an effective therapeutic dose and a toxic dose. Overdosage caused by the cumulative effects of the drug is a constant danger in therapy. Digoxin toxicity is characterized by a wide variety of symptoms, which are hard to differentiate from those of the cardiac disease itself. One of the most serious side effects of digoxin is hypokalemia. This may lead to cardiac arrhythmias, muscle weakness, hypotension, and respiratory distress. Other agents causing hypokalemia reinforce this effect and increase the chance of digitalis toxicity. Such reactions may occur in clients who have been on digoxin maintenance for a long time. **CV:** Changes in the rate, rhythm, and irritability of the heart and the mechanism of the heartbeat. Extrasystoles, bigeminal pulse, coupled rhythm, ectopic beat, and other forms of arrhythmias have been noted. ***Death most often results from ventricular fibrillation***. Discontinue digoxin in adults when pulse rate falls below 60 beats/min. All cardiac changes are best detected by the ECG, which is also most useful in clients suffering from intoxication. ***Acute hemorrhage***. **GI:** Anorexia, N&V, excessive salivation, epigastric distress, abdominal pain, diarrhea, bowel necrosis. Clients on digoxin therapy may experience two vomiting stages. The first is an early sign of toxicity and is a direct effect of digoxin on the GI tract. Late vomiting indicates stimulation of the vomiting center of the brain, which occurs after the heart muscle has been saturated with digoxin. **CNS:** Headaches, fatigue, lassitude, irritability, malaise, muscle weakness, insomnia, stupor. Psychotomimetic effects (especially in elderly or arteriosclerotic clients or neonates) including disorientation, confusion, depression, aphasia, delirium, hallucinations, and, rarely, ***convulsions***. **Neuromuscular:** Neurologic pain involving the lower third of the face and lumbar areas, paresthesia. **Visual disturbances:** Blurred vision, flickering dots, white halos, borders around dark objects, diplopia, amblyopia, color perception changes. **Hypersensitivity: (5–7 days after starting therapy):** Skin reactions (urticaria, fever, pruritus, facial and ***angioneurotic edema***). **Miscellaneous:** Chest pain, coldness of extremities.

LABORATORY TEST CONSIDERATIONS

May ↓ PT. Alters tests for 17-ketosteroids and 17-hydroxycorticosteroids.

OVERDOSE MANAGEMENT

Symptoms: **Adults:** The relationship of digoxin levels to symptoms of toxicity varies significantly from client to client; thus, it is not possible to identify digoxin levels that would define toxicity accurately. **Toxicity: GI:** Anorexia, N&V, diarrhea, abdominal discomfort, or pain. **CNS:** Blurred, yellow, or green vision and halo effect; headache, weakness, drowsiness, mental depression, apathy, restlessness, disorientation, confusion, ***seizures***, EEG abnormalities, delirium, hallucinations, neuralgia, psychosis. **CV:** VT, unifocal or ***multiform PVCs*** (especially in bigeminal or trigeminal patterns), paroxysmal/nonparoxysmal nodal rhythms, AV dissociation, accelerated junctional rhythm, excessive slowing of the pulse, ***AV block (may proceed to complete block)***, atrial fibrillation, ***ventricular fibrillation (most common cause of death)***. **Children:** Visual disturbances, headache, weakness, apathy, and psychosis occur but may be difficult to recognize. **CV:** Conduction disturbances, supraventricular tachyarrhythmias (e.g., ***AV block***), atrial tachycardia with or without block, nodal tachycardia, unifocal or multiform ventricular premature contractions, ***ventricular tachycardia***, sinus bradycardia (especially in infants).

Treatment: In Adults:

- Discontinue drug; admit to ICU for continuous ECG monitoring.
- If serum potassium is below normal, KCl should be administered in divided PO doses totaling 3–6 grams (40–80 mEq). Potassium should not be used when severe or complete heart block is due to digoxin and not related to tachycardia.
- *Atropine:* A dose of 0.01 mg/kg IV to treat severe sinus bradycardia or slow ventricular rate due to secondary AV block.
- *Cholestyramine, colestipol, activated charcoal:* To bind digitalis in the intestine, thus preventing enterohepatic recirculation.
- *Digoxin immune FAB:* See drug entry. Given in approximate equimolar quantities as digoxin, it

reverses S&S of toxicity, often with improvement within 30 min.

- *Lidocaine:* A dose of 1 mg/kg given over 5 min followed by an infusion of 15–50 mcg/kg/min to maintain normal cardiac rhythm.
- *Phenytoin:* For atrial or ventricular arrhythmias unresponsive to potassium, can give a dose of 0.5 mg/kg at a rate not exceeding 50 mg/min (given at 1–2 hr intervals). The maximum dose should not exceed 10 mg/kg/day.
- *Countershock:* A direct-current countershock can be used *only as a last resort.* If required, initiate at low voltage levels.

In Children: Give potassium in divided doses totaling 1–1.5 mEq/kg (if correction of arrhythmia is urgent, a dose of 0.5 mEq/kg/hr can be used) with careful monitoring of the ECG. The potassium IV solution should be diluted to avoid local irritation although IV fluid overload must be avoided.

Digoxin immune FAB may also be used. Digoxin is not removed effectively by dialysis, by exchange transfusion, or during cardiopulmonary bypass as most of the drug is found in tissues rather than the circulating blood.

DRUG INTERACTIONS

The following drugs increase serum digoxin levels, leading to possible toxicity: Aminoglycosides, amiodarone, anticholinergics, atorvastatin, benzodiazepines, captopril, clarithromycin, diltiazem, dipyridamole, erythromycin, esmolol, flecainide, hydroxychloroquine, ibuprofen, indomethacin, itraconazole, nifedipine, quinidine, quinine, telmisartan, tetracyclines, tolbutamide, verapamil.

Albuterol / ↑ Digoxin binding to skeletal muscle

H ***Aloe*** / Potential for ↑ digoxin effect R/T aloe-induced hypokalemia

Amiloride / ↓ Digoxin inotropic effects

Aminoglycosides / ↓ Digoxin effect R/T ↓ GI tract absorption

Aminosalicylic acid / ↓ Digoxin effect R/T ↓ GI tract absorption

Amphotericin B / ↑ K^+ depletion caused by digoxin; ↑ risk of digitalis toxicity

Antacids / ↓ Digoxin effect R/T ↓ GI tract absorption

Beta blockers / Complete heart block possible

H ***Buckthorn bark/berry*** / Potential for ↑ digoxin effect R/T to buckthorn-induced hypokalemia

Calcium preparations / Cardiac arrhythmias following parenteral calcium

H ***Cascara sagrada bark*** / Potential for ↑ digoxin effect R/T to cascara-induced hypokalemia

Chlorthalidone / ↑ K^+ and Mg^{++} loss with ↑ chance of digitalis toxicity

Cholestyramine / Binds digoxin in the intestine and ↓ its absorption

Colestipol / Binds digoxin in the intestine and ↓ its absorption

Disopyramide / May alter effect of digoxin

H ***Ephedra*** / ↑ Chance of cardiac arrhythmias

Ephedrine / ↑ Chance of cardiac arrhythmias

Epinephrine / ↑ Chance of cardiac arrhythmias

Ethacrynic acid / ↑ K^+ and Mg^{++} loss with ↑ chance of digitalis toxicity

Fluoxetine / Possible ↑ serum digoxin levels

Furosemide / ↑ K^+ and Mg^{++} loss with ↑ chance of digoxin toxicity

H ***German chamomile flower*** / Potential for ↑ digoxin effect R/T to chamomile-induced hypokalemia

H ***Ginseng*** / ↑ Digoxin levels

Glucose infusions / Large infusions of glucose may cause ↓ K^+ and ↑ chance of digoxin toxicity

Grapefruit juice / ↑ Digoxin bioavailability; do not take digoxin with grapefruit juice

H ***Hawthorn*** / Potentiation of digoxin effect

Hypoglycemic drugs / ↓ Effect of digitalis glycosides R/T ↑ liver breakdown

H ***Iceland moss*** / Potential for ↑ digoxin effect R/T to iceland moss-induced hypokalemia

H ***Indian snakeroot*** / ↑ Risk of bradycardia

H ***Ivy leaf*** / Potential for ↑ digoxin effect R/T to ivy leaf-induced hypokalemia

Levothyroxine / ↓ Serum levels and therapeutic digoxin effect

H ***Licorice*** / Potential for ↑ digoxin effect R/T to licorice-induced hypokalemia

H ***Marshmallow root*** / Potential for ↑ digoxin effect R/T to marshmallow root-induced hypokalemia

Methimazole / ↑ Chance of toxic effects of digitalis

Metoclopramide / ↓ Digoxin effect R/T ↓ GI tract absorption

Muscle relaxants, nondepolarizing / ↑ Risk of cardiac arrhythmias

Penicillamine / ↓ Serum digoxin levels

Propranolol / Potentiates digitalis-induced bradycardia

H ***Rhubarb root*** / Potential for ↑ digoxin effect R/T to rhubarb root-induced hypokalemia

H *St. John's wort* / ↓ Digoxin plasma levels R/T ↑ renal excretion
H *Sarsaparilla root* / Potential for ↑ absorption of digoxin
H *Senna pod/leaf* / Potential for ↑ digoxin effect R/T to senna-induced hypokalemia
Spironolactone / Either ↑ or ↓ toxic effects of digoxin
Succinylcholine / ↑ Chance of cardiac arrhythmias
Sulfasalazine / ↓ Digoxin effect R/T ↓ GI tract absorption
Sympathomimetics / ↑ Chance of cardiac arrhythmias
Thiazides / ↑ K^+ and Mg^{++} loss with ↑ chance of digoxin toxicity
Thioamines / ↑ Effect and toxicity of digoxin
Thyroid / ↓ Digoxin effect
Triamterene / ↑ Digoxin effects

HOW SUPPLIED

Elixir, Pediatric: 0.05 mg/mL; *Injection:* 0.1 mg/mL (pediatric), 0.25 mg/mL; *Tablets:* 0.125 mg, 0.25 mg.

DOSAGE

ELIXIR; TABLETS

Digitalization: Rapid.

Adults: A total of 0.75–1.25 mg divided into two or more doses each given at 6–8-hr intervals.

Digitalization: Slow.

Adults: 0.125–0.5 mg/day for 7 days. **Pediatric.** (Digitalizing dose is divided into two or more doses and given at 6–8-hr intervals.) **Children, 10 years and older, rapid or slow:** Same as adult dose. **5–10 years:** 0.02–0.035 mg/kg. **2–5 years:** 0.03–0.05 mg/kg. **1 month–2 years:** 0.035–0.06 mg/kg. **Premature and newborn infants to 1 month:** 0.02–0.035 mg/kg.

Maintenance.

Adults: 0.125–0.5 mg/day. **Pediatric:** One-fifth to one-third the total digitalizing dose daily. *NOTE:* An alternate regimen (referred to as the "small-dose" method) is 0.017 mg/kg/day. This dose causes less toxicity.

IV

Digitalization.

Adults: Same as tablets. **Maintenance:** 0.125–0.5 mg/day in divided doses or as a single dose. **Pediatric:** Same as tablets.

NURSING IMPLICATIONS

IMPLEMENTATION/ADMINISTRATION/STORAGE

1. Due to decreased renal clearance in the elderly, daily doses should not exceed 0.125 mg except when treating atrial arrhythmias.
2. Measure liquids precisely using calibrated dropper/syringe.
3. Obtain written parameters for high/low pulse rates, at which cardiac glycosides are to be held; changes in rate or rhythm may indicate toxicity.
4. Differences in bioavailability have been noted between products; monitor when changing from one product to another.
5. If switching from tablets or elixir to the parenteral route, expect reduction in dosage; absorption is much higher with the parenteral form.
6. Protect from light.
7. IV Give IV injections over 5 min (or longer) either undiluted or diluted fourfold or greater with sterile water for injection.
8. COMPATIBILITY 0.9% NaCl, or D5W.
9. INCOMPATIBILITY Administer separately.

ASSESSMENT

1. List type, onset, characteristics of S&S. If administered for heart failure, note causes; ensure failure not solely related to diastolic dysfunction—drug's positive inotropic effect may increase cardiac outflow obstruction with hypertrophic cardiomyopathy.
2. List drugs prescribed that would adversely interact with digoxin and monitor; diuretics may increase toxicity.
3. Assess for hyper-/hypothyroidism; hypothyroid sensitive to glycosides, while hyperthyroid may require a higher dose of drug.
4. Obtain ECG; note rhythm/rate. Check apical pulse for 1 full min before administering. Identify when to withhold dose i.e., HR <60 bpm in adult, <70 bpm in child, or <90 bpm in infant.

5. Document cardiopulmonary findings; note presence of S3, JVD, HJR, displaced PMI, HR above 100 bpm, rales, peripheral edema, DOE, PND, and echo, MUGA, cardiac catheterization findings. Note NYHA Classification.
6. Observe S&S of toxicity (N&V, abdominal pain, anorexia, confusion, visual disturbances, bradycardia, ECG changes, arrhythmias, headache, seizure). With elderly, rate of drug elimination is slower.
7. Calculate doses based upon lean (ideal) body weight. Consider differences in bioavailability between digoxin injection, tablets, and oral solution when changing from one dosage form to another.
8. Monitor closely during digitalization:
   - Observe for bradycardia/arrhythmias, count apical rate for at least 1 min before administering drug. Obtain written parameters to hold drug (e.g., HR <60 bpm adults; <70 child; <90 infant) for drug administration.
   - Anticipate more than once daily dosing in most children (up to age 10) R/T higher metabolic activity.
   - With coworker simultaneously take apical and radial pulse for 1 min; report pulse deficit (e.g., the wrist rate is less than the apical rate); may indicate adverse drug reaction.
   - Monitor weights and I&O; check for edema. Adequate intake will help prevent cumulative toxic drug effects.
   - If taking non-potassium-sparing diuretics as well as digoxin, will need potassium supplements. Provide the most palatable preparation available. (Liquid potassium preparations usually bitter.)
   - If gastric distress experienced, use antacid. Antacids containing Al or Mg^{++} and kaolin/pectin mixtures should be given 6 hr before or 6 hr after dose of cardiac glycoside to prevent decreased therapeutic effects.
   - When given to newborns, use monitor to identify early evidence of toxicity: excessive slowing of sinus rate, sinoatrial arrest, prolonged PR interval.
   - Monitor digoxin levels periodically, assess for S&S of toxicity; draw serum levels just before the next scheduled dose or 6–8 hr after last dose.
   - Use caution; digoxin withdrawal may worsen heart failure.
9. Have available digoxin antibodies (digoxin-immune Fab) for severe overdose toxicity.
10. Monitor I&O, VS, CBC, electrolytes, Ca^{++}, Mg^{++}, BNP, TSH, renal and LFTs. Reduce dose with renal dysfunction. Monitor digoxin levels.

CLIENT/FAMILY TEACHING

1. Take at the same time each day; after meals to lessen gastric irritation. Do not take with grapefruit juice.
2. Maintain written record of pulse rates and weights; review guidelines for withholding medication and reporting abnormal pulse rates. Report weight gains of >2 lb/day or >5 lb/week.
3. Do not change brands; different preparations have variations in bioavailability and may cause toxicity or loss of effect.
4. Follow directions carefully for taking medication. If one dose is accidentally missed, do not double up on the next dose.
5. Report adverse effects or toxic drug symptoms: Anorexia, N&V, abdominal pain and diarrhea are often early symptoms due to the toxic effects on the GI tract and brain. Disorientation, agitation, visual disturbances, changes in color perception, irregular heartbeat, and hallucinations may also occur.
6. Maintain a sodium-restricted diet. Read labels and review foods low in sodium; consult dietitian for assistance in food selection, meal planning, and preparation.
7. Consult provider before taking any other medications, whether prescribed or OTC, because drug interactions occur frequently with cardiac glycosides.
8. Report persistent cough, difficulty breathing, or extremity swelling (S&S of CHF).
9. Identify community health agencies to assist in maintaining health.
10. Keep all F/U to assess response, labs, ECG, and adverse SE.

OUTCOMES/EVALUATE

- Stable cardiac rate and rhythm, ↓ severity of S&S of CHF, improved CO, improved activity tolerance
- Serum drug levels within therapeutic range (e.g., digoxin 0.5–2.0 ng/mL)

IV

Digoxin immune fab (Ovine)

Classification(s): Antidote for digoxin poisoning

Pregnancy Category: C

RX: Digibind, DigiFab.

INDICATIONS/USES

Life-threatening digoxin toxicity or overdosage. Symptoms of toxicity include severe sinus bradycardia, second- or third-degree heart block, which does not respond to atropine, ventricular tachycardia, and ventricular fibrillation.

NOTE: Cardiac arrest can be expected if a healthy adult ingests more than 10 mg digoxin or a healthy child ingests more than 4 mg. Also, use DigiFab to treat steady-state serum concentrations of digoxin greater than 10 ng/mL in adults or 4 ng/mL in children. Use digoxin immune Fab for life-threatening toxicity including severe ventricular arrhythmias (e.g., ventricular tachycardia or fibrillation), progressive bradycardia, and second- or third-degree heart block not responsive to atropine, serum potassium levels exceeding 5 mEq/L (Digibind) or 5.5 mEq/L in adults or 6 mEq/L in children (DigiFab) with rapidly progressing signs and symptoms of digoxin toxicity.

ACTION/KINETICS

Action

Digoxin immune Fab are antibodies that bind to digoxin making them unavailable to bind at their site of action. In cases of digoxin toxicity, the antibodies bind to digoxin and the complex is excreted through the kidneys. As serum levels of digoxin decrease, digoxin bound to tissue is released into the serum to maintain equilibrium and this is then bound and excreted. The net result is a decrease in both tissue and serum digoxin.

Pharmacokinetics

Onset: Less than 1 min. Improvement in signs of toxicity occurs within 30 min. **t½:** 15–20 hr (after IV administration). Each vial contains either 38 mg or 40 mg of pure digoxin immune Fab, which will bind approximately 0.5 mg digoxin.

CONTRAINDICATIONS

Use for mild cases of digitalis toxicity.

SPECIAL CONCERNS

- Use with caution during lactation.
- Use in infants only if benefits outweigh risks.
- Clients sensitive to products of sheep origin may also be sensitive to digoxin immune Fab. Skin testing may be appropriate for high-risk clients.

SIDE EFFECTS

Most Common

Hypokalemia.

CV: Worsening of CHF or low CO, atrial fibrillation (all due to withdrawal of the effects of digoxin). **Miscellaneous:** Hypokalemia. Rarely, hypersensitivity reactions occur, including fever and ***anaphylaxis***.

HOW SUPPLIED

Digibind. *Powder for Injection, Lyophilized:* 38 mg/vial (each vial will bind about 0.5 mg digoxin).

DigiFab. *Powder for Injection, Lyophilized:* 40 mg/vial (each vial will bind about 0.5 mg digoxin).

DOSAGE

IV

Dosage depends on the serum digoxin concentration. A large dose has a faster onset, but there is an increased risk of allergic or febrile reactions. The package insert should be carefully consulted.

Acute ingestion of an unknown amount of digoxin.

Adults and children: Twenty vials (760 mg Digibind or 800 mg DigiFab). In small children, monitor the amount of overload.

Toxicity during chronic therapy.

Adults: Six vials (228 mg of Digibind or 240 mg DigiFab) is usually enough to reverse most cases of toxicity. **Children, <20 kg:** A single vial (38 mg Digibind or 40 mg DigiFab) should be sufficient.

NURSING IMPLICATIONS

IMPLEMENTATION/ADMINISTRATION/STORAGE

1. IV Dose of antidote estimated based on ingested digoxin differs significantly from that calculated based on the serum digoxin levels.

Errors in amount of antidote required may result from inaccurate estimates of amount of digoxin ingested or absorbed from non-steady-state serum digoxin concentrations. Also, inaccurate serum digoxin level measurements are a possible source of error.

2. Dosage calculations are based on a steady-state volume of distribution of about 5 L/kg for digoxin (0.5 L/kg for digitoxin) to convert serum digitalis levels to the amount of digitalis in the body. Many clients, however, need higher doses for complete neutralization. Round the doses up to the next whole vial.
3. **Dosage for acute ingestion of unknown amount:** Twenty vials (760 mg Digibind or 800 mg DigiFab) are adequate to treat most life-threatening ingestion for both adults and children. In small children, monitor for volume overload. In general, a large dose of digoxin immune Fab has a faster onset, but may increase the risk of a febrile reaction. One approach used is to administer 10 vials and observe client response; then, if clinically indicated, an additional 10 vials may be given.
4. **Dosage for toxicity during chronic therapy:** For adults, 6 vials (228 mg Digibind or 240 mg DigiFab) are usually adequate to reverse most toxicity. In infants and small children (20 kg or less), a single vial usually should suffice.
5. Failure of the client to respond to digoxin immune Fab may indicate the possibility that symptoms may not be due to digitalis toxicity.
6. To calculate dose (in number of vials) of antidote for acute ingestion of a known amount of digitalis, divide the total digitalis body load (in mg) by 0.5 (i.e., amount of digitalis bound/vial). The total body load (mg) will be about equal to the amount ingested in mg for digoxin capsules or digitoxin; or, the amount ingested in milligrams multiplied by 0.8 (to account for incomplete absorption) for digoxin tablets.
7. To estimate number of vials for adults when a steady-state serum digoxin level is known, multiply the serum digoxin concentration in ng/mL times the weight in kg and divide by 100.
8. Because infants and small children may require much smaller dosages, reconstituted the 38 mg vial of Digibind, as directed, and administer with a tuberculin syringe. For very small doses, dilute the reconstituted vial with 34 mL of sterile isotonic saline to achieve a 1 mg/mL concentration.
9. Reconstitute lyophilized material with 4 mL of sterile water for injection to give a concentration of 10 mg/mL (DigiFab) or 9.5 mg/mL (Digibind). If small doses required (e.g., in infants), Digibind or DigiFab can be further diluted (34 mL sterile isotonic saline when using Digibind or 36 mL sterile isotonic saline for DigiFab) for a concentration of 1 mg/mL.
10. Administer over a 30 min period. May use bolus injection if immediate danger of cardiac arrest. However, there is an increased incidence of infusion-related reactions. If infusion-rate-related reactions occur, stop the infusion and restart at a slower rate. Infuse Digibind through a 0.22 micron membrane filter to ensure no undissolved particles are administered.
11. Use reconstituted antibody immediately. May store up to 4 hr at 2–8°C (36–46°F). Unreconstituted vials of Digibind can be stored up to 30°C (86°F) for a total of 30 days. Do not freeze DigiFab.
12. If acute digoxin ingestion results in severe symptoms and serum concentration is not known, 800 mg (20 vials) of digoxin immune Fab may be given. Monitor for volume overload in small children.
13. COMPATIBILITY 0.9% NaCl.
14. INCOMPATIBILITY Do not mix with other drugs or solutions.

ASSESSMENT

1. Determine if for acute ingestion of unknown amount or toxicity during chronic therapy; list amount, time of drug ingestion if known, and serum digoxin level.
2. If previous reaction suspected or high-risk client, perform skin testing: Prepare a 10 mL solution (0.1 mL of drug in 9.9 mL NSS). Administer 0.1 mL intradermally or perform a scratch test by placing 1 drop of solution on the skin and making a scratch through the drop with a sterile needle; assess site in 20 min. **Do not** use if reaction is positive: urticarial wheal with erythematous surrounding skin.
3. **Do not** administer with known allergy to sheep proteins.

4. Wait several days for redigitalization to ensure complete elimination of Digibind. Levels will take 5–7 days to stabilize following treatment, although improvement in S&S of toxicity should be evident in 30 min.
5. Monitor VS, ECG, K^+ and digoxin levels. Assess for electrolyte imbalance; note hypokalemia, and any evidence of CHF.

CLIENT/FAMILY TEACHING

1. Drug is used to reverse the effects of too high a concentration of digoxin in the body.
2. Should take effect in a couple of hours but digoxin levels will not show changes until about 2 days later.
3. Report any chest pain, dizziness, breathing difficulty or other adverse SE.

OUTCOMES/EVALUATE

- Resolution of digoxin toxicity
- Controlled cardiac rhythm

IV

Diltiazem hydrochloride

(dill-**TIE**-ah-zem)

Classification(s): Calcium channel blocker

Pregnancy Category: C

RX: Capsule, Extended-Release: Cardizem CD, Cartia XT, Dilt-CD, Diltia XT, Diltiazem HCl Extended Release, Dilt-XR, Taztia XT, Tiazac. **Injection:** Diltiazem Injection. **Powder for Injection:** Cardizem. **Tablets, Extended-Release:** Cardizem LA, Diltzac, Matzim LA. **Tablets, Immediate-Release:** Cardizem.

✱ **Rx:** Apo-Diltiaz, Apo-Diltiaz CD, Apo-Diltiaz Injectable, Apo-Diltiaz SR, Gen-Diltiazem, Gen-Diltiazem CD, Novo-Diltazem SR, Novo-Diltiazem, Novo-Diltiazem CD, Nu-Diltiaz, Nu-Diltiaz-CD, ratio-Diltiazem CD, Sandoz Diltiazem CD.

SEE ALSO ***CALCIUM CHANNEL BLOCKING AGENTS***.

INDICATIONS/USES

PO: (1) Chronic stable angina (use extended-release tablets). (2) Chronic stable angina and angina due to coronary artery spasm (use extended-release capsules and immediate-release tablets). (3) Hypertension as monotherapy or in combination with other antihypertensives (use extended-release capsules and tablets).

Investigational: As a 2% gel, cream, or ointment to reduce pain/bleeding and promote healing of anal fissures.

Parenteral: (1) Temporary control of rapid ventricular rate in atrial fibrillation or flutter. Do not use with atrial fibrillation or atrial flutter associated with an accessory bypass tract such as in Wolff-Parkinson-White syndrome or short PR syndrome. (2) Rapid conversion of paroxysmal SVT to sinus rhythm (including AV nodal re-entrant tachycardias and reciprocating tachycardias associated with an extranodal accessory pathway such as Wolff-Parkinson-White syndrome or short PR syndrome).

ACTION/KINETICS

Action

Inhibits influx of calcium through the cell membrane, resulting in a depression of automaticity and conduction velocity in cardiac muscle. Decreases SA and AV conduction and prolongs AV node effective and functional refractory periods. Also decreases myocardial contractility and peripheral vascular resistance. Slight decrease in HR.

Pharmacokinetics

Tablets, Immediate-Release: Onset, 30–60 min; **time to peak plasma levels:** 2–4 hr; **t½, elimination:** about 3–4.5 hr (5–8 hr with high and repetitive doses); **duration:** 4–8 hr. **Extended-Release Capsules/Tablets: Onset,** 2–3 hr; **time to peak plasma levels:** 10–14 hr; **t½, elimination:** 4–9.5 hr; **duration:** 12 hr. **IV, t½, elimination:** About 3.4 hr. **Therapeutic serum levels:** 0.05–0.2 mcg/mL. Metabolized in the liver to desacetyldiltiazem, which manifests 25–50% of the activity of diltiazem. Excreted through both the bile and urine. **Plasma protein binding:** 70–80%.

CONTRAINDICATIONS

Hypotension or cardiogenic shock. Second- or third-degree AV block and sick sinus syndrome except in presence of a functioning ventricular pacemaker. Acute MI, pulmonary congestion. IV diltiazem with IV beta-blockers. Atrial fibrillation or atrial flutter associated with an accessory bypass tract (e.g., as in W-P-W syndrome or PR syndrome). Ventricular tachycardia. Use of Cardizem LyoJect Syringe in newborns (due to presence of benzyl alcohol). Lactation.

D

SPECIAL CONCERNS

- Safety and efficacy in children not determined.
- The t½ may be increased in geriatric clients.
- Use with caution in hepatic disease and in CHF.
- Abrupt withdrawal may cause an increase in the frequency and duration of chest pain.
- Use with beta blockers or digitalis is usually well tolerated, although the effects of coadministration cannot be predicted (especially in clients with left ventricular dysfunction or cardiac conduction abnormalities).

SIDE EFFECTS

Most Common

AV block, bradycardia, edema, dizziness/lightheadedness, headache, pain, dyspnea, rhinitis, infection.

CV: AV block, bradycardia, CHF, hypotension, syncope, palpitations, peripheral edema, ***arrhythmias***, angina, tachycardia, ***abnormal ECG***, ***ventricular extrasystoles***. **GI:** N&V, diarrhea, constipation, anorexia, abdominal discomfort, cramps, dry mouth, dysgeusia. **CNS:** Weakness, nervousness, dizziness, lightheadedness, headache, depression, psychoses, hallucinations, disturbances in sleep, somnolence, insomnia, amnesia, abnormal dreams. **Dermatologic:** Rashes, dermatitis, pruritus, urticaria, erythema multiforme, ***Stevens-Johnson syndrome***. **Miscellaneous:** Photosensitivity, joint pain/stiffness, flushing, nasal/chest congestion, dyspnea, SOB, nocturia/polyuria, sexual difficulties, weight gain, paresthesia, tinnitus, tremor, asthenia, gynecomastia, gingival hyperplasia, petechiae, ecchymosis, purpura, bruising, hematoma, leukopenia, double vision, epistaxis, eye irritation, thirst, alopecia, ***bundle branch block***, abnormal gait, hyperglycemia.

LABORATORY TEST CONSIDERATIONS

↑ Alkaline phosphatase, CPK, LDH, AST, ALT.

ADDITIONAL DRUG INTERACTIONS

Amiodarone / Possible cardiotoxicity with bradycardia and ↓ CO
Amlodipine / ↑ Amlodipine levels possibly R/T ↓ liver metabolism
Anesthetics / ↑ Risk of depression of cardiac contractility, conductivity, and automaticity as well as vascular dilation
Buspirone / ↑ Buspirone effects
Carbamazepine / ↑ Diltiazem effect R/T ↓ liver breakdown
Cimetidine / ↑ Diltiazem bioavailability
Colestipol / ↓ Diltiazem bioavailability when colestipol given 1 hr before or 4 hr after diltiazem R/T ↓ diltiazem absorption
Cyclosporine / ↑ Cyclosporine effect → possible renal toxicity
Digoxin / Possible ↑ digoxin levels
HMG-CoA reductase inhibitors / ↑ HMG-CoA reductase inhibitors levels
Imipramine / ↑ Serum levels
Indinavir + Ritonavir / ↑ Diltiazem AUC R/T ↓ CYP 3A metabolism of diltiazem
Lithium / ↑ Risk of neurotoxicity
Methylprednisolone / ↑ Pharmacologic and toxicologic effects of methylprednisolone
Moricizine / ↑ Moricizine levels and ↓ diltiazem levels
Quinidine / ↑ Therapeutic and toxic effects of quinidine
Ranitidine / ↑ Diltiazem bioavailability
Sirolimus / ↑ Sirolimus levels
Tacrolimus / ↑ Tacrolimus levels → ↑ toxicity
Theophyllines / ↑ Risk of pharmacologic and toxicologic theophylline effects

HOW SUPPLIED

Capsules, Extended-Release: 60 mg, 90 mg, 120 mg, 180 mg, 240 mg, 300 mg, 360 mg, 420 mg; ***Injection:*** 5 mg/mL; ***Powder for Injection:*** 25 mg; ***Tablets, Extended-Release:*** 120 mg, 180 mg, 240 mg, 300 mg, 360 mg, 420 mg; ***Tablets, Immediate-Release:*** 30 mg, 60 mg, 90 mg, 120 mg.

DOSAGE

CAPSULES, EXTENDED-RELEASE

Angina.

Cardizem CD and Cartia XT: Adults, initial: 120 or 180 mg once daily. Up to 480 mg/day may be required. Dosage adjustments should be carried out over a 7–14-day period.

Dilacor XR and Diltia XT: Adults, initial: 120 mg once daily; **then,** dose may be titrated, depending on the needs of the client, up to 480 mg once daily. Titration may be carried out over a 7–14-day period.

Tiazac: Adults, initial: 120–180 once daily. Some may respond to higher doses up to 540 mg once daily. When necessary, carry out titration over 7–14 days.

Hypertension.

Cardizem CD and Cartia XT: Adults, initial: 180–240 mg once daily. Some respond to lower doses. Maximum antihypertensive effect usually reached within 14 days. Usual range is 240–360 mg once daily.

Dilacor XR and Diltia XT: Adults, initial: 180–240 mg once daily. Clients 60 years and older may respond to a lower dose of 120 mg. Usual range is 180–480 mg once daily. The dose may be increased to 540 mg/day with little or no increased risk of side effects. May be used alone or in combination with other antihypertensive drugs, such as diuretics

Tiazac: Adults, initial: 120–240 mg once daily. Maximum effect usually reached by 14 days of therapy; thus, schedule dosage adjustments accordingly. Usual range is 120–540 mg once daily. May be used alone or with other antihypertensive drugs.

TABLETS, EXTENDED-RELEASE

Hypertension.

Individualize dose. **Adults, initial, monotherapy:** 180–240 mg once daily; some may respond to lower doses. May be titrated to a maximum dose of 540 mg/day. Schedule dosage adjustments accordingly as maximum effect usually seen within 14 days.

Angina.

Individualize dose. **Adults, initial:** 180 mg once daily; **then,** may increase dose at intervals of 7–14 days if adequate response not obtained. Doses above 360 mg appear not to have any additional benefit.

TABLETS, IMMEDIATE-RELEASE

Exertional angina pectoris due to atherosclerotic coronary artery disease or angina pectoris at rest due to coronary artery spasm.

Individualize dose. **Adults, initial:** 30 mg 4 times per day before meals and at bedtime; **then,** increase gradually to total daily dose of 180–360 mg (given in three to four divided doses). Increments may be made q 1–2 days until the optimum response is attained.

IV BOLUS

Atrial fibrillation/flutter; paroxysmal supraventricular tachycardia.

Adults, initial: 0.25 mg/kg (average 20 mg) given over 2 min; **then,** if response is inadequate, a second dose may be given after 15 min. The second bolus dose is 0.35 mg/kg (average 25 mg) given over 2 min. Subsequent doses should be individualized. Some clients may respond to an initial dose of 0.15 mg/kg (duration of action may be shorter).

IV, CONTINUOUS INFUSION

Atrial fibrillation/flutter.

Adults, initial: For continuous reduction of HR (up to 24 hr) for those with atrial fibrillation/flutter, begin an IV infusion immediately after an IV bolus dose of 20 mg (0.25 mg/kg) or 25 mg (0.35 mg/kg). Initial infusion rate is 10 mg/hr; may be increased in 5 mg increments to 15 mg/hr. Infusion longer than 24 hr at a dose of 15 mg/hr is not recommended.

NURSING IMPLICATIONS

Do not confuse Cardizem with Cardene (also a calcium channel blocker). Do not confuse Cartia-XT with Cartia (an enteric-coated aspirin tablet).

IMPLEMENTATION/ADMINISTRATION/STORAGE

1. Sublingual nitroglycerin may be taken concomitantly for acute angina. Diltiazem may also be taken together with long-acting nitrates.
2. Clients treated with diltiazem alone or in combination with other medications may be switched safely to once daily extended-release diltiazem capsules or tablets at the nearest equivalent total daily dose. However, subsequent titration to a higher or lower dose may be necessary and should be initiated if needed.
3. Use with beta blockers or digitalis is usually well tolerated, but the combined effects can-

not be predicted, especially with cardiac conduction abnormalities or LV dysfunction.

4. Store from 15–30°C (59–86°F). Avoid excessive humidity.
5. IV May administer direct IV over 2 min or as infusion (see *Dosage*).
6. Infusion may be maintained for up to 24 hr; beyond 24 hr is not recommended.
7. Refrigerate the injection at 2–8°C (36–46°F). May be stored at room temperature for 1 month; then, discard remaining solution.
8. Store Cardizem LyoJect and Cardizem Monovial at room temperature (15–20°C; 59–86°F). Do not freeze. Reconstituted drug is stable for 24 hr at controlled room temperature. Discard any unused portion of Cardizem LyoJect.
9. COMPATIBILITY NSS, D5W, or D5/0.45% NaCl.
10. INCOMPATIBILITY Give separately.

ASSESSMENT

1. Note reasons for therapy, onset, and characteristics of S&S, other drugs trialed and outcome.
2. List meds prescribed to ensure none interact.
3. Review history and assess for edema or CHF; review ECG for AV block.
4. Drug half-life may be prolonged in elderly; monitor closely.
5. Monitor BP & HR, ECG, Wt, CBC, renal and LFTs; may need to reduce dose with dysfunction.

CLIENT/FAMILY TEACHING

1. Take extended-release capsules at same time each day. Do not open, chew, or crush; swallow whole.
2. Tiazac extended-release capsules may also be given by opening the capsule and sprinkling the contents on a spoonful of applesauce. Swallow the applesauce immediately without chewing; follow with a glass of cool water to ensure complete swallowing of the capsule contents.
3. Drug does not cure high BP or angina, just controls it; continue taking even when BP is not elevated or angina symptoms are not present.
4. Use caution; may cause drowsiness/dizziness. Keep record of BP and HR for review.
5. Rise slowly from a lying to a sitting and standing position; may cause ↓ BP. Report frequent dizzy episodes when arising, slow heart rate, persistent fatigue, any other unusual or persistent/bothersome side effects including headaches, constipation, unusual tiredness, or weakness.
6. Continue carrying short-acting nitrites (nitroglycerin) at all times; use as directed. Report changes in frequency or severity of chest pain or need for sublingual nitroglycerin increases.
7. Avoid prolonged sun exposure; use precaution if exposed to prevent photosensitivity reaction.
8. Continue diet (low-fat/low Na^+), regular exercise, weight loss/control, and decreased caffeine; stop tobacco and alcohol. Reduce fluid and salt intake to control swelling.
9. Keep all F/U to assess response and for adverse SE.

OUTCOMES/EVALUATE

- ↓ Frequency and intensity of vasospastic anginal attacks
- ↓ BP; stable cardiac rhythm

IV

Dimenhydrinate

(dye-men-**HY**-drih-nayt)

Classification(s): Cholinergic blocking drug, antiemetic

Pregnancy Category: B

OTC: Liquid: Children's Dramamine, Dramamine. **Tablets:** Dramamine, Triptone. **Tablets, Chewable:** Dramamine.

RX: Injection: Dramanate, Dymenate. **Liquid:** Dramamine.

Rx: Tablets, Chewable: Apo-Dimenhydrinate, Gravol.

SEE ALSO ***ANTIHISTAMINES*** AND ***ANTIEMETICS***.

INDICATIONS/USES

Prophylaxis and treatment of N&V, dizziness, or vertigo due to motion sickness.

ACTION/KINETICS

Action

Contains both diphenhydramine and chlorotheophylline. Antiemetic mechanism not known, but it does depress labyrinthine and vestibular function. May mask ototoxicity due to aminoglycosides. Possesses anticholinergic activity.

Pharmacokinetics

Duration: 3–6 hr.

CONTRAINDICATIONS

Neonates. Hypersensitivity to dimenhydrinate or any component of the product. Lactation. Use in children less than 2 years of age unless directed by provider.

SPECIAL CONCERNS

- **Use with caution in conditions that might be aggravated by anticholinergic therapy (e.g., prostatic hypertrophy, stenosing peptic ulcer, pyloroduodenal obstruction, bladder neck obstruction, narrow angle glaucoma, bronchial asthma, cardiac arrhythmias).**
- **Geriatric clients may be more sensitive to the usual adult dose.**
- **Some products contain benzyl alcohol, which has been associated with a fatal "gasping" syndrome in premature infants.**

SIDE EFFECTS

Most Common

Drowsiness, confusion (especially in children), headache, dizziness, blurred vision, diplopia.

CNS: Drowsiness, confusion, nervousness, restlessness, headache, insomnia (especially in children), tingling, heaviness and weakness of hands, vertigo, dizziness, lassitude, excitation. **GI:** N&V, diarrhea, epigastric distress, constipation, anorexia. **CV:** Palpitations, hypotension, tachycardia. **Ophthalmic:** Blurred vision, diplopia. **Respiratory:** Nasal stuffiness, tightness of chest, wheezing, thickening of bronchial secretions, dryness of mouth, nose, throat. **Dermatologic:** Photosensitivity, urticaria, drug rash. **Miscellaneous:** ***Anaphylaxis***, hemolytic anemia, difficult or painful urination.

OVERDOSE MANAGEMENT

Symptoms: Drowsiness (usual). Also ***convulsions***, coma, ***respiratory depression*** following massive doses. *Treatment:* No specific antidote known. Treat respiratory depression using mechanically assisted respiration and administer oxygen. Treat convulsions with diazepam. Give phenobarbital (5–6 mg/kg) to control convulsions in children.

DRUG INTERACTIONS

Alcohol / Additive CNS depressant effect

Antibiotics / Use caution when given with certain antibiotics that may cause ototoxicity as dimenhydrinate may mask ototoxic symptoms → irreversible damage

CNS depressants / Additive CNS depressant effect

HOW SUPPLIED

OTC. *Liquid:* 12.5 mg/4 mL; *Tablets:* 50 mg; *Tablets, Chewable:* 50 mg.
Rx. *Injection:* 50 mg/mL.

DOSAGE

LIQUID; TABLETS; TABLETS, CHEWABLE

Motion sickness.

Adults: 50–100 mg q 4 hr, not to exceed 400 mg/day. **Pediatric, 6–12 years:** 25–50 mg q 6–8 hr, not to exceed 150 mg/day; **2–6 years:** 12.5–25 mg q 6–8 hr, not to exceed 75 mg/day. Use in children less than 2 years of age only on advice of a provider.

IM

Motion sickness.

Adults: 50 mg as required. **Pediatric, 4 years and older:** 1.25 mg/kg (37.5 mg/m^2) 4 times per day, not to exceed 300 mg/day.

IV

Motion sickness.

Adults: 50 mg in 10 mL sodium chloride injection given over 2 min; may be repeated q 4 hr as needed.

NURSING IMPLICATIONS

Do not confuse dimenhydrinate with diphenhydramine (also an antihistamine).

IMPLEMENTATION/ADMINISTRATION/STORAGE

1. **IV Dilute 50 mg in 10 mL of NSS and administer slowly over 2 min.**
2. **Adjust pediatric dosage per BSA.**
3. COMPATIBILITY **Dilute in NSS; compatible with most solutions.**
4. INCOMPATIBILITY **Administer separately.**

ASSESSMENT

1. **List reasons for therapy, onset and characteristics of S&S. Note other agents trialed and outcome.**
2. **Assess for vestibular damage when administered with antihistamines.**
3. **Evaluate need for further neurologic workup.**

CLIENT/FAMILY TEACHING

1. Take at least 30 min before departure; may repeat before meals and upon retiring for motion sickness prevention.
2. Avoid activities that require mental alertness until effects realized. Avoid alcohol and any other CNS depressants.
3. Report N&V to provider if being used as antiemetic.
4. Take frequent sips of water and sugarless gum for dry mouth S&S; increase fluids and bulk in diet to relieve constipation.
5. May alter skin testing results; wait 72 hr after use.
6. Keep all F/U to assess response and for adverse SE.

OUTCOMES/EVALUATE

- Prevention of N&V R/T motion sickness
- Control of vertigo

Dinoprostone (PGE_2)

(**die**-noh-**PROS**-tohn)

Classification(s): Abortifacient

Pregnancy Category: C

RX: Cervidil, Prepidil Gel, Prostin E_2.

INDICATIONS/USES

(1) Ripening of an unfavorable cervix in pregnant women at or near term with a medical or obstetric need for induction of labor. (2) Evacuation of uterus in the management of missed abortion or intrauterine fetal death up to 28 weeks gestational age. (3) Management of nonmetastatic gestational trophoblastic disease (benign hydatidiform mole). (4) Termination of pregnancy from 12–20 weeks calculated from the first day of the last normal menstrual period.

ACTION/KINETICS

Action

Interacts with prostaglandin receptor to produce changes in the consistency, dilation, and effacement of the cervix. May also stimulate the smooth muscle of the GI tract, causing vomiting and diarrhea.

Pharmacokinetics

Extensively metabolized in the lungs on first pass through the pulmonary circulation. Metabolites are excreted through the kidneys. **t½:** 2.5–5 min.

CONTRAINDICATIONS

Use when oxytocic drugs are contraindicated or when prolonged uterine contractions are inappropriate (e.g., history of cesarean section or major uterine surgery), presence of cephalopelvic disproportion, history of difficult labor and/or traumatic delivery, grand multiparae with six or more previous term pregnancies, non-vertex presentation, hyperactive or hypertonic uterine patterns, fetal distress where delivery is not imminent, obstetric emergencies when surgical intervention may be favored. Also, use is contraindicated in ruptured membranes, hypersensitivity to prostaglandins or constituents of the gel, placenta previa or unexplained vaginal bleeding during current pregnancy, or when vaginal delivery is contraindicated (e.g., vasa previa or active herpes genitalis). Use in conjunction with oxytocic agents.

SPECIAL CONCERNS

- **Uterine rupture is possible when high-tone uterine contractions are sustained.**
- **Use with caution in clients with asthma or a history thereof; hypotension or hypertension; cardiovascular, renal, or hepatic disease; anemia; jaundice; diabetes; epilepsy; a compromised (scarred) uterus; glaucoma or increased intraocular pressure.**
- **Use dinoprostone suppositories with caution in presence of cervicitis, infected endocervical lesions, or acute vaginitis.**

SIDE EFFECTS

Most Common

N&V, diarrhea, headache, chills/shivering.

GI: N&V, diarrhea. **CV:** Arrhythmias, chest pain/tightness, **MI** (in those with a history of CV disease), transient diastolic BP decreases of >20 mm Hg. **CNS:** Headache, flushing, anxiety, tension, hot flashes, paresthesia, syncope, dizziness, weakness. **GU:** Endometritis, uterine rupture, uterine/vaginal pain, vaginitis, vulvitis, vaginismus, breast tenderness, urine retention. **Respiratory:** Coughing, dyspnea, wheezing, pharyngitis, laryngitis. **Musculoskeletal:** Joint inflammation, arthralgia, myalgia, stiff neck, backache, muscle cramp/pain, leg cramps. **Dermatologic:** Skin discoloration, rash. **Ophthalmic:** Eye pain, blurred vision. **Body as a whole:** Chills, shivering, tremor, dehydration, diaphoresis, fever. **Miscellaneous:** Hearing impairment.

OVERDOSE MANAGEMENT

Symptoms: Uterine hypercontractility, uterine hypertonus. *Treatment:* Symptoms may be relieved by changing maternal position, giving oxygen to the mother, or the use of beta-adrenergic drugs to treat hyperstimulation.

DRUG INTERACTIONS

Dinoprostone may ↑ action of other oxytocics.

HOW SUPPLIED

Vaginal Gel/Jelly: 0.5 mg/3 grams; ***Vaginal Insert, Controlled-Release:*** 10 mg (releases 0.3 mg/hr); ***Vaginal Suppositories:*** 20 mg.

DOSAGE

GEL

All uses.

Initial: 0.5 mg. If there is no cervical/uterine response, repeat doses of 0.5 mg may be given q 6 hr. The maximum cumulative dose for 24 hr is 1.5 mg dinoprostone.

VAGINAL INSERT

All uses.

One insert (10 mg), designed to release approximately 0.3 mg dinoprostone/hr over a 12 hr period. The insert should be removed upon onset of active labor or 12 hr after insertion.

VAGINAL SUPPOSITORIES

All uses.

20 mg repeated every 3–5 hr; dose adjusted according to client response.

NURSING IMPLICATIONS

IMPLEMENTATION/ADMINISTRATION/STORAGE

1. Bring gel to room temperature just prior to administration.
2. Avoid contact with the skin; wash hands thoroughly with soap and water after administration.
3. Gel is intended for endocervical placement; do not administer above level of the internal os. The degree of cervical effacement will regulate shielded catheter size to be used (20 mm catheter for no effacement and 10 mm catheter for 50% effacement).
4. Administer gel by sterile technique; introduce just below level of the internal os.
5. Keep supine for at least 15–30 min after administration.
6. If desired response obtained from the initial dose, the recommended interval before giving oxytocin is 6–12 hr. A dosing interval of at least 30 min is recommended following removal of vaginal insert.
7. The insert is placed transversely in the posterior fornix of the vagina immediately after removal from the foil package. Insertion does not require sterile conditions. Do not use insert without its retrieval system.
8. Insert may be placed in the vagina with a minimal amount of water-miscible lubricant. Prevent excess contact or coating with the lubricant, thus preventing optimal swelling and release of the drug.
9. The gel has a shelf life of 24 months when stored under refrigeration at 2–8°C (36–46°F). Store the insert in a freezer between −20 to −10°C (−4 to −14°F). When stored in a freezer, the insert is stable for up to 3 years.

ASSESSMENT

1. Note reasons for therapy and maternal condition. List calculated and ultrasound-derived due date; note fetopelvic relationships.
2. Check cervix for degree of effacement (shortening of cervical canal) to determine size of shielded endocervical catheter needed.
3. Prevent skin contact with this drug; use latex gloves and thoroughly wash hands with soap and water after insertion.
4. Note system used, time of insertion, and dosing intervals. Insert must be removed with retrieval system after 12 hr or with onset of labor. Wait at least 6 to 12 hr after administration of gel before using IV oxytocin, (dosing interval of at least 30 min recommended after removal of insert).
5. Monitor uterine contractions, fetal heart tones, cervical dilation and effacement by visual physical assessment, auscultation, and electronic fetal monitor.
6. Continuous monitoring of uterine activity and fetal status should be undertaken especially

with history of hypertonic uterine contractility or tetanic uterine contractions. Monitor for uterine rupture with sustained high-tone myometrial contractions.

7. Monitor VS during therapy reporting any increase in temperature and/or changes in BP.
8. Assess closely for adverse reactions including nausea, vomiting, or diarrhea. Monitor for hypersensitivity reactions such as bronchospasms, cardiac arrhythmias, or seizures.

D

CLIENT/FAMILY TEACHING

1. Review reasons for therapy and anticipated outcome.
2. Gel may produce increased vaginal warmth and uterine contractions; report if pain from contractions severe so analgesics may be considered.
3. Must remain supine for 30 min after gel insertion.
4. Avoid douches, tampons, intercourse, and tub baths for at least 2 weeks.
5. Monitor temperature (late afternoon) for a few days after discharge; report any new onset fever, bleeding, cramps/pain or foul-smelling discharge.
6. Report immediately any nausea, vomiting, difficulty breathing, chest pain, or headache.
7. Pretreatment or concurrent use of antiemetic and antidiarrheal drugs help decrease the incidence of GI effects.

OUTCOMES/EVALUATE

- Desired cervical presentation to facilitate induction of labor (gel)
- Evacuation of uterus (termination of pregnancy) with suppository

IV

Diphenhydramine hydrochloride

(dye-fen-**HY**-drah-meen)

Classification(s): Antihistamine, second generation, ethanolamine

Pregnancy Category: B

OTC: Anti-Allergy/Anti-Cough.
Capsules or Capsules, Soft Gel: Banophen, Benadryl Allergy Kapseals, Benadryl Dye-Free Allergy Liqui Gels, Diphenhist, Genahist. **Elixir:** Banophen Allergy, Siladryl. **Liquid, Oral:** Allermax, Altaryl Children's Allergy, Banophen Allergy, Banophen Children's Allergy, Benadryl Children's Allergy, Benadryl Children's Dye-Free Allergy, Diphen AF, Genahist, O-dryl, Scot-Tussin Allergy Relief Formula Clear, Siladryl. **Lotion, Topical:** DERMA-PAX. **Oral Solution:** Children's PediaCare Nighttime Cough, Diphenhist. **Strips, Oral Disintegrating:** Benadryl Allergy Quick Dissolve Strips, TheraFlu Thin Strips Multi-Symptom, Triaminic Children's Allergy, Triaminic Thin Strips Cough & Runny Nose, Triaminic Thin Strips Multi-Symptoms. **Syrup:** Hydramine Cough, Silphen Cough. **Tablets:** AllerMax Caplets Maximum Strength, Banophen Caplets, Benadryl Allergy Ultratabs, Diphenist Captabs, Genahist. **Tablets, Chewable:** Benadryl Allergy. **Tablets, Oral Disintegrating:** Children's Benadryl Allergy Fastmelt.
Sleep Aids. Capsules: Compoz Gel Caps, Dormin, Maximum Strength Sleepinal Capsules and Soft Gels, Maximum Strength Unisom SleepGels. **Tablets:** 40 Winks, Dormin, Maximum Strength Nytol, Midol PM, Miles Nervine, Nighttime Sleep Aid, Nytol, Simply Sleep, Sleepwell 2-nite, Snooze Fast, Sominex, Twilite. **Tablets, Orally Disintegrating:** Unisom SleepMelts.

RX: Injection: Benadryl. **Syrup:** Tusstat.

SEE ALSO *ANTIHISTAMINES, ANTIEMETICS,* AND *ANTIPARKINSON AGENTS*.

INDICATIONS/USES

(1) Hypersensitivity reactions (type I), including perennial and seasonal allergic rhinitis, vasomotor rhinitis and sneezing caused by the common cold, allergic conjunctivitis caused by inhalant allergens and foods, mild uncomplicated allergic skin manifestations of urticaria and angioedema, amelioration of allergic reactions to blood or plasma, dermatographism, adjunctive anaphylactic therapy, uncomplicated allergic conditions of the immediated type. (2) Motion sickness (injection only). (3) Parkinsonism (postencephalitic, arteriosclerotic, idiopathic, drug/chemical induced). (4) Nighttime sleep aid. (5) Antitussive (syrup only).

ACTION/KINETICS

Action

High sedative, anticholinergic, and antiemetic effects.

CONTRAINDICATIONS
Use in children 6 years of age and younger. Use of oral OTC diphenhydramine products with other products containing diphenhydramine, including topical products.

SPECIAL CONCERNS
Increased risk of cognitive decline in the elderly.

SIDE EFFECTS
Most Common
Drowsiness, constipation, diarrhea, dizziness, dry mouth/nose/throat, headache, anorexia, N&V, anxiety, GI upset, asthenia.
See *Antihistamines* for a complete list of possible side effects.

ADDITIONAL DRUG INTERACTIONS
Diphenhydramine ↑ effects of metoprolol.

HOW SUPPLIED
OTC. ***Capsules:*** 25 mg, 50 mg; ***Capsules, Soft Gel:*** 25 mg; ***Elixir:*** 12.5 mg/5 mL; ***Liquid:*** 12.5 mg/5 mL; ***Lotion, Topical:*** 0.5%.; ***Oral Solution:*** 12.5 mg/5 mL; ***Strips, Orally Disintegrating:*** 12.5 mg, 25 mg; ***Syrup:*** 12.5 mg/5 mL; ***Tablets:*** 25 mg, 50 mg; ***Tablets, Chewable:*** 12.5 mg; ***Tablets, Oral Disintegrating:*** 12.5 mg, 25 mg.
Rx. ***Injection:*** 50 mg/mL; ***Syrup:*** 12.5 mg/5 mL.

DOSAGE

CAPSULES; CAPSULES, SOFT GEL; ELIXIR; LIQUID; ORAL SOLUTION; SYRUP; TABLETS; TABLETS, CHEWABLE; TABLETS, ORAL DISINTEGRATING
Hypersensitivity reactions, motion sickness, parkinsonism.

Adults: 25–50 mg PO 3–4 times per day, not to exceed 300 mg/day; **pediatric, 6–12 years:** 12.5–25 mg PO 3–4 times per day, not to exceed 150 mg/day.

Sleep aid.

Adults and children over 12 years: 50 mg at bedtime.

LIQUID, ORAL
Antitussive.

Adults and children 12 years of age and older: 25–50 mg q 4 hr, not to exceed 300 mg in 24 hr. **Children, 6–12 years of age:** 12.5–25 mg q 4 hr, not to exceed 150 mg in 24 hr. **Children, 6 years and younger:** Do not use without consulting provider.

ORAL SOLUTION
Antitussive.

Children, 6 to <12 years of age: 12.5 mg (5 mL) q 4 hr, up to 75 mg (30 mL)/day. **Children, less than 6 years of age:** Do not use without consulting a provider.

STRIPS, ORALLY DISINTEGRATING
Antiallergic.

Adults: Take one q 4 to 6 hr, up to 6 doses/day.

SYRUP
Antitussive.

Adults: 25 mg q 4 hr, not to exceed 150 mg/day; **pediatric, 6–12 years:** 12.5 mg q 4 hr, not to exceed 75 mg/day; **pediatric, 2–6 years:** do not use without consulting provider although dosage of 6.25 mg q 4 hr, not to exceed 25 mg in 24 hr, has been recommended.

IM (DEEP); IV
Hypersensitivity reactions, motion sickness, parkinsonism.

Adults: 10–50 mg up to 100 mg if needed (not to exceed 400 mg/day); **pediatric, 6 years and older:** 1.25 mg/kg (or 37.5 mg/m^2) 4 times per day, not to exceed a total of 300 mg/day divided into 4 doses given IV at a rate not exceeding 25 mg/min or deep IM.

NURSING IMPLICATIONS

Do not confuse diphenhydramine with desipramine (an antidepressant) or with dimenhydrinate (also an antihistamine).

IMPLEMENTATION/ADMINISTRATION/STORAGE
1. With motion sickness, give full prophylactic dose 30 min prior to travel and 1–2 hr before exposures that precipitate sickness.
2. Take similar doses with meals and at bedtime.
3. Do not use more than 2 weeks to treat insomnia.

4. Store liquid and syrup from 15–30°C (59–86°F).
5. IV For IV, may give undiluted.
6. For adults or children, do not exceed an IV rate of 25 mg/min.
7. Protect the injection from freezing and light.
8. COMPATIBILITY D5W, D10W, 0.45% and 0.9% NaCl, dextrose and saline combinations, RL.
9. INCOMPATIBILITY Administer separately.

ASSESSMENT

1. Note reasons for therapy, onset, S&S of characteristics, other agents trialed, triggers, outcome.
2. List drugs prescribed to ensure none interact.
3. Ensure catheter patency with IV therapy; intradermal or subcutaneous administration may cause tissue necrosis.
4. Note any sleep apnea, recent asthma attack; precludes therapy.
5. Assess for liver dysfunction; requires dose reduction.

CLIENT/FAMILY TEACHING

1. Allow orally disintegrating tablets to dissolve in mouth before swallowing. Use caution if using orally-disintegrating tablet or chewable tablet with phenylketonuria (contains phenylalanine).
2. Consume small amount of water or juice after taking chewable tablet or orally-disintegrating tablet.
3. With liquid, oral solution, elixir, or syrup use dosing syringe, dosing spoon, or dosing cup to measure and ensure correct dose.
4. May cause drowsiness; use caution performing activities that require mental alertness until drug effects realized.
5. Take 30 min before travel to prevent motion sickness. Take 30 min before bedtime when used for sleeping.
6. Use sun protection; may cause photosensitivity reaction.
7. Use sugarless gum/candy to diminish dry mouth effects.
8. Avoid alcohol and any other CNS depressants unless prescribed.
9. Report any persistent dizziness, excessive drowsiness, chest tightness, unexplained SOB or difficulty breathing, difficulty voiding, unusual tiredness or weakness, bleeding or unusual bruising, fast or irregular heartbeat, excitability, confusion, or changes in thinking or behavior.
10. Stop therapy 72 to 96 hr before skin testing performed.
11. May require different antihistamine to offset tolerance if it occurs.
12. Keep all F/U to assess response and for adverse SE.

OUTCOMES/EVALUATE

- ↓ Allergic manifestations
- Relief of nausea/insomnia
- Relief of dyskinesias/extrapyramidal symptoms with parkinsonism

Combination Drug

Diphenoxylate hydrochloride with Atropine sulfate

(dye-fen-**OX**-ih-layt, **AH**-troh-peen)

Classification(s): Antidiarrheal

Pregnancy Category: C

RX: Logen, Lomanate, Lomotil, Lonox, **C-V**

SEE ALSO ***CHOLINERGIC BLOCKING AGENTS***.

INDICATIONS/USES

(1) Symptomatic treatment of chronic and functional diarrhea. (2) Diarrhea associated with gastroenteritis, irritable bowel, regional enteritis, malabsorption syndrome, ulcerative colitis, acute infections, food poisoning, postgastrectomy, and drug-induced. Therapeutic results for control of acute diarrhea are inconsistent. (3) Control of intestinal passage time in clients with ileostomies and colostomies.

CONTENT

Each tablet or 5 mL of oral solution contains: Diphenoxylate HCl (*Antidiarrheal*), 2.5 mg and Atropine sulfate (*Anticholinergic*), 0.025 mg.

ACTION/KINETICS

Action

Chemically related to the narcotic analgesic drug meperidine but without the analgesic properties. Inhibits GI motility and has a constipating effect. May aggravate diarrhea due to organisms that penetrate the intestinal mucosa (e.g., *Escherichia coli, Salmonella, Shigella*) or in antibiotic-induced pseudomembranous colitis. High doses over prolonged periods may cause euphoria and physical dependence. The product also contains small amounts of atropine sulfate, which will prevent abuse by deliberate overdosage.

Pharmacokinetics

Onset: 45–60 min. **t½, diphenoxylate:** 2.5 hr; **diphenoxylic acid:** 12–24 hr. **Duration:** 2–4 hr. Metabolized in the liver to the active diphenoxylic acid and excreted through the urine.

CONTRAINDICATIONS

Obstructive jaundice, liver disease, diarrhea associated with pseudomembranous enterocolitis after antibiotic therapy or enterotoxin-producing bacteria, children under the age of 4.

SPECIAL CONCERNS

- **Use with caution during lactation, when anticholinergics may be contraindicated, and in advanced hepatic-renal disease or abnormal renal functions.**
- **Children (especially those with Down syndrome) are susceptible to atropine toxicity.**
- **Children and geriatric clients may be more sensitive to the respiratory depressant effects of diphenoxylate.**
- **Dehydration, especially in young children, may cause a delayed diphenoxylate toxicity.**

SIDE EFFECTS

Most Common

Dizziness, drowsiness, dry mouth, bloating, anorexia.

GI: N&V, dry mouth, anorexia, abdominal discomfort, bloating, paralytic ileus, megacolon. **Allergic:** Pruritus, ***angioneurotic edema***, swelling of gums. **CNS:** Dizziness, drowsiness, malaise, restlessness, headache, depression, numbness of extremities, ***respiratory depression, coma.*** **Dermatologic:** Dry skin and mucous membranes, flushing. **Miscellaneous:** Anorexia, tachycardia, urinary retention, hyperthermia.

OVERDOSE MANAGEMENT

Symptoms: Dry skin and mucous membranes, flushing, ***hyperthermia***, mydriasis, restlessness, tachycardia followed by miosis, lethargy, hypotonic reflexes, nystagmus, ***coma, severe (and possibly fatal) respiratory depression.*** *Treatment:* Gastric lavage, induce vomiting, establish a patent airway, and assist respiration. Activated charcoal (100 grams) given as a slurry. IV administration of a narcotic antagonist. Administration may be repeated after 10–15 min. Observe client and readminister antagonist if respiratory depression returns.

DRUG INTERACTIONS

Alcohol / Additive CNS depression
Antianxiety agents / Additive CNS depression
Barbiturates / Additive CNS depression
MAOIs / ↑ Chance of hypertensive crisis
Narcotics / ↑ Effect of narcotics

HOW SUPPLIED

See Content.

DOSAGE

Diphenoxylate

ORAL SOLUTION; TABLETS

Diarrhea (various causes); control of intestinal passage time in ileostomies and colostomies.

Adults, initial: 2.5–5 mg (of diphenoxylate) 3–4 times per day; **maintenance:** 2.5 mg 2–3 times per day. **Pediatric, 2–3 years:** 0.75–1.5 mg 4 times per day; **3–4 years:** 1–1.5 mg 4 times per day; **4–5 years:** 1–2 mg 4 times per day; **5–6 years:** 1.25–2.25 mg 4 times per day; **6–9 years;** 1.25–2.5 mg 4 times per day; **9–12 years:** 1.75–2.5 mg 4 times per day. Maintain dosage at initial levels until symptoms are under control; then reduce to maintenance levels.

NURSING IMPLICATIONS

Do not confuse Lomotil with Lamisil (terbinafine, an antifungal), lamivudine (an antiviral), Ludiomil (maprotiline, an antidepressant), or labetalol (an adrenergic blocking agent).

IMPLEMENTATION/ADMINISTRATION/STORAGE

1. **For liquid preparations, use only plastic dropper supplied by manufacturer to measure dosage.**
2. **If clinical improvement not evident after 10 days with a maximum dose of 20 mg/day, further use will not likely control symptoms.**

ASSESSMENT

1. List reasons for therapy, onset/frequency of stools, unusual foods/exposures, and other agents trialed.
2. Note fluid and electrolyte status. Dehydration occurs rapidly in young children: may cause delayed toxicity. Correct before therapy.
3. Review culture reports to determine if drug is appropriate if not effective after 24–36 hr.
4. Assess GI function, for abdominal distension and toxic megacolon.
5. Note mental status, assess for any hepatic or renal dysfunction.

CLIENT/FAMILY TEACHING

1. Used to control diarrhea. Take as prescribed; do not exceed dosage.
2. May cause dizziness or drowsiness; use caution with activities requiring mental alertness.
3. Avoid ETOH and CNS depressants; may aggravate drug effects.
4. Store in child-resistant container out of reach of child; may cause fatal respiratory depression.
5. Avoid in child with Down syndrome; signs of atropinism may occur.
6. Report if fever and palpitations occur or when diarrhea persists or becomes malodorous or bloody.
7. Keep all F/U to assess response and for adverse SE.

OUTCOMES/EVALUATE

Relief of diarrhea

Dipyridamole

(dye-peer-**ID**-ah-mohl)

Classification(s): Anticoagulant, platelet adhesion inhibitor

Pregnancy Category: B

RX: Persantine.

✱ **Rx:** Apo-Dipyridamole-FC.

INDICATIONS/USES

As an adjunct to coumarin anticoagulants in preventing post-operative thromboembolic complications of cardiac valve replacement. *Investigational:* Use with aspirin to prevent myocardial reinfarction and reduction of post-MI mortality (combination therapy does not appear to be any more beneficial than use of aspirin alone).

ACTION/KINETICS

Action

In higher doses may act by several mechanisms, including inhibition of red blood cell uptake of adenosine, itself an inhibitor of platelet reactivity; inhibition of platelet phosphodiesterase, which leads to accumulation of cAMP within platelets; direct stimulation of release of prostacyclin or prostaglandin D_2; and/or inhibition of thromboxane A_2 formation. Dipyridamole prolongs platelet survival time in clients with valvular heart disease and has maintained platelet count in open heart surgery. Also causes coronary vasodilation, which may be due to inhibition of adenosine deaminase in the blood, thus allowing accumulation of adenosine, which is a potent vasodilator. Vasodilation may also be caused by delaying the hydrolysis of cyclic 3',5'-adenosine monophosphate as a result of inhibition of the enzyme phosphodiesterase.

Pharmacokinetics

Incompletely absorbed from the GI tract. **Peak plasma levels, after PO:** 75 min. **t½, after PO: initial,** 40 min; **terminal,** 10–12 hr. Metabolized in the liver and mainly excreted in the bile. **Plasma protein binding:** Significant.

SPECIAL CONCERNS

- Use with caution in hypotension (can cause peripheral vasodilation) and during lactation.
- Safety and efficacy not determined in children less than 12 years of age.

SIDE EFFECTS

Most Common

Dizziness, abdominal distress, headache, rash.

GI: Abdominal distress, diarrhea, vomiting, liver dysfunction (rare). **CNS:** Dizziness, headache. **CV:** Angina pectoris. **Dermatologic:** Rash, flushing, pruritus.

OVERDOSE MANAGEMENT

Symptoms: Hypotension of short duration. *Treatment:* Use of a vasopressor may be beneficial. Due to the high percentage of protein binding of dipyridamole, dialysis is not likely to be beneficial.

DRUG INTERACTIONS

Digoxin / ↑ Digoxin bioavailability

H ***Evening primrose oil*** / Potential for ↑ antiplatelet effect
H ***Feverfew*** / Potential for ↑ antiplatelet effect
H ***Garlic*** / Potential for ↑ antiplatelet effect
H ***Ginger*** / Potential for ↑ antiplatelet effect
H ***Ginkgo biloba*** / Potential for ↑ antiplatelet effect
H ***Ginseng*** / Potential for ↑ antiplatelet effect
H ***Grapeseed extract*** / Potential for ↑ antiplatelet effect
Warfarin / ↑ Risk of major bleeding

HOW SUPPLIED

Tablets: 25 mg, 50 mg, 75 mg.

DOSAGE

TABLETS

Adjunct in prophylaxis of thromboembolism after cardiac valve replacement.

Adults: 75–100 mg 4 times per day as an adjunct to warfarin therapy. Do not give aspirin concomitantly.

NURSING IMPLICATIONS

ASSESSMENT

1. Note reasons for therapy, type, onset, characteristics of S&S.
2. List drugs currently prescribed to ensure none interact unfavorably.
3. Assess mental status, skin color, cardiopulmonary findings.
4. Monitor VS, ECG, CBC, PT, PTT, INR.

CLIENT/FAMILY TEACHING

1. Drug helps prevent clots by inhibiting platelet stickiness; may also decrease frequency of chest pain and increase exercise tolerance. May take several months of therapy before effects evident.
2. Try small frequent meals if nausea or gastric distress experienced.
3. Avoid alcohol and tobacco due to hypotensive vasoconstrictive effects; avoid use of any unprescribed drugs including aspirin without approval.
4. May cause dizziness and lightheadedness; avoid activities that require mental alertness until drug effects realized.
5. Report any rash or hives, unusual bruising or bleeding, difficulty breathing, persistent dizziness when arising from a sitting or lying position, fainting, yellowing of the skin or eyes.
6. Keep all F/U to assess response, labs, adverse SE.

OUTCOMES/EVALUATE

Prevention of thromboembolism

Disulfiram

(dye-**SUL**-fih-ram)

Classification(s): Treatment of alcoholism

Pregnancy Category: C

RX: Antabuse.

INDICATIONS/USES

Aid to manage selected chronic alcoholics who wish to remain in a state of enforced sobriety so that supportive and psychotherapeutic treatment may be undertaken advantageously.

ACTION/KINETICS

Action

Produces severe hypersensitivity to alcohol. Inhibits liver enzymes that participate in the normal degradation of alcohol. This results in accumulation of acetaldehyde in the blood. High levels of acetaldehyde produce a series of symptoms referred to as the disulfiram-alcohol reaction or syndrome. The specific symptoms are listed under *Side Effects.*

Pharmacokinetics

The symptoms vary individually, are dose-dependent with respect to both alcohol and disulfiram, and persist for periods ranging from 30 min to several hours. Slowly absorbed from the GI tract. **Maximum plasma levels:** 8–10 hr for disulfiram and metabolites. **Onset:** May be delayed up to 12 hr because disulfiram is initially localized in fat stores. Mainly excreted in the urine although the carbon disulfide metabolite is excreted in the breath. A single dose of disulfiram may be effective for 1–2 weeks.

CONTRAINDICATIONS

Alcohol intoxication. Severe myocardial or occlusive coronary disease, psychoses, hypersensitivity to disulfiram or other thiuram derivatives used in pesticides and rubber vulcanization, clients receiving or who have recently received metronidazole, paraldehyde, alcohol, or alcohol-containing preparations (e.g., cough syrups, tonics). If client is exposed to ethylene dibromide (possible toxicity). Lactation.

SPECIAL CONCERNS

■ Never give to anyone in a state of alcohol intoxication or without the client's full knowledge. Instruct the client's relatives accordingly. ■

- **Use in pregnancy only if benefits outweigh risks.**
- **Use with caution in narcotic addicts or clients with diabetes mellitus, goiter, cerebral damage, epilepsy, psychosis, hypothyroidism, hepatic cirrhosis or insufficiency, or nephritis (acute or chronic).**
- **Do not expose clients to ethylene dibromide or its vapors; a toxic interaction may occur.**
- **Safety and efficacy not determined in children.**

SIDE EFFECTS

In the absence of alcohol. CNS: Drowsiness, fatigue, headache, psychotic reactions. **Neurologic:** Peripheral neuropathy, peripheral neuritis, polyneuritis, optic neuritis. **GI:** Metallic or garlic-like aftertaste (usually during the first 2 weeks of therapy), hepatotoxicity, cholestatic and fulminant hepatitis, ***hepatic failure***. **Dermatologic:** Skin eruptions (occasional), acneiform eruptions, allergic dermatitis. **Miscellaneous:** Impotence.

In the presence of alcohol. CV: Flushing, chest pain, palpitations, tachycardia, hypotension, syncope, arrhythmias, ***CV collapse, MI, acute CHF***. **CNS:** Throbbing headaches, vertigo, weakness, uneasiness, confusion, unconsciousness, ***seizures, death***. **GI:** Nausea, severe vomiting, thirst. **Respiratory:** Respiratory difficulties, dyspnea, hyperventilation, ***respiratory depression***. **Miscellaneous:** Throbbing in head and neck, sweating. In the event of an Antabuse-alcohol interaction, measures should be undertaken to maintain BP and treat shock. Oxygen, antihistamines, ephedrine, and/or vitamin C may also be used.

DRUG INTERACTIONS

Alcohol / Severe alcohol intolerance reactions (e.g., flushing, increased respiration, pulse rate, and CO); avoid alcohol in all forms
Anticoagulants, oral / ↑ Anticoagulant effects by ↑ hypoprothrombinemia
Barbiturates / ↑ Barbiturate effects R/T ↓ liver breakdown
Caffeine / ↑ CV and CNS stimulant effects of caffeine
Chlordiazepoxide, diazepam / ↑ Chlordiazepoxide/diazepam effects R/T ↓ plasma clearance
Chlorzoxazone / Inhibition of chlorzoxazone metabolism; ↓ chlorzoxazone dose
Cocaine / ↑ CV side effects of cocaine
Hydantoins / ↑ Serum hydantoin levels → ↑ pharmacologic and toxic effects
Isoniazid / ↑ Isoniazid side effects (e.g., unsteady gait, changes in behavior)
Metronidazole / Acute toxic psychosis or confusional state; do not use together
Paraldehyde / Antabuse-like effects
Phenytoin / ↑ Phenytoin effects R/T ↓ liver breakdown
Theophyllines / ↓ Theophylline metabolism → toxic effects
Tricyclic antidepressants / ↑ Risk of acute organic brain syndrome
Warfarin / ↑ Anticoagulant effect of warfarin

HOW SUPPLIED

Tablets: 250 mg, 500 mg.

DOSAGE

TABLETS

Prevent further ingestion of alcohol in chronic alcoholics.

Adults, initial (after alcohol-free interval of 12–48 hr): 500 mg/day for 1–2 weeks; **maintenance: usual,** 250 mg/day (range: 120–500 mg/day). Do not exceed 500 mg/day. Maintenance may be needed for months or years.

NURSING IMPLICATIONS

IMPLEMENTATION/ADMINISTRATION/STORAGE

1. **Disulfiram is usually taken in the morning; however, if a sedative effect is noted, it can be taken at bedtime or a decrease in dose can be implemented.**
2. **The test reaction has been largely abandoned. Do not administer to a client over 50 years of age.**
3. **Store tablets from 15–30°C (59–86°F).**

ASSESSMENT

1. **Note reasons for therapy, other agents/therapies trialed, living situation, client's mental**

status/level of understanding. Identify length of time with disease.
2. Perform baseline and follow-up LFTs (10–14 days) to detect any hepatic dysfunction. Perform CBC, chemistry, renal and LFTs every 6 months during therapy.

CLIENT/FAMILY TEACHING

1. Drug is used in those alcoholics who want enforced sobriety so that supportive and psychotherapeutic treatment may be administered.
2. May crush tablets or mix with liquid.
3. Never give without client's knowledge. Ingesting 30 mL of 100-proof alcohol (e.g., one shot) may cause severe symptoms (within 15 min; lasting several hours) and possibly death. Avoid alcohol in any form, in foods, sauces, or other medications, such as cough syrups or tonics; avoid vinegar, paregoric, skin products, linaments, or lotions containing alcohol. Read all labels before consuming.
4. 1 (or even 2) weeks after last dose of disulfiram, ingestion of alcohol may produce unpleasant symptoms. Prolonged administration of disulfiram does not produce tolerance; the longer on therapy, the more sensitive one becomes to alcohol.
5. CNS side effects should lessen with continued therapy. May feel tired, experience drowsiness, headaches, and develop a metallic or garlic-like taste; should subside after 2 weeks of therapy.
6. May have occasional impotence, usually transient; report.
7. Report if skin eruptions occur; an antihistamine may be prescribed.
8. Carry card stating "taking disulfiram" and describing symptoms and treatment if a disulfiram reaction occurs. Include provider/contact person, and phone number.
9. Attend local support group meetings, e.g., Alcoholics Anonymous and Al-Anon, to gain the support, structure, referral, and encouragement to obtain an alcohol-free life.

OUTCOMES/EVALUATE

Freedom from alcohol and its effects; sobriety

Divalproex sodium

(dye-**VAL**-proh-ex)

Pregnancy Category: D

RX: Depakote.

✦ **Rx:** Apo-Divalproex, Epival, Nu-Divalproex.

SEE ALSO ***VALPROIC ACID*** FOR ALL INFORMATION FOR THIS PRODUCT.

ADDITIONAL USES

Extended-Release Tablets: Treatment of acute manic or mixed episodes associated with bipolar disorder, with or without psychotic features.

LABORATORY TEST CONSIDERATIONS

False + for ketonuria. Altered thyroid function tests.

HOW SUPPLIED

Capsules, Enteric-Coated: 125 mg; ***Tablets, Enteric-Coated:*** 125 mg, 250 mg, 500 mg; ***Tablets, Extended-Release:*** 500 mg.

IV

Dobutamine hydrochloride

(doh-**BYOU**-tah-meen)

Classification(s): Sympathomimetic, direct-acting

Pregnancy Category: B

RX: Dobutamine Hydrochloride, Dobutamine Hydrochloride in 5% Dextrose.

SEE ALSO ***SYMPATHOMIMETIC DRUGS***.

INDICATIONS/USES

When parenteral therapy is needed for inotropic support in the short-term treatment of cardiac decompensation in adults secondary to depressed contractility resulting from organic heart disease or cardiac surgical procedures. Experience does not extend beyond 48 hr of use. In clients with atrial fibrillation with rapid ventricular response, use a digitalis preparation before starting dobutamine therapy. *Investigational:* Congenital heart disease in children undergoing diagnostic cardiac catheterization.

ACTION/KINETICS

Action

Directly stimulates beta-1 receptors (in the heart), increasing cardiac function, CO, and SV, with minor effects on HR. Decreases afterload reduction although SBP and pulse pressure may remain unchanged or increased (due to increased CO). Also decreases elevated ventricular filling pressure and helps AV node conduction. It does not cause the release of norepinephrine. In children, dobutamine-induced increases in CO and systemic pressure are generally seen in any given client at lower infusion rates than those that cause significant tachycardia.

D

Pharmacokinetics

Onset: 1–2 min. **Peak effect:** Up to 10 min. **t½:** 2 min. **Therapeutic plasma levels:** 40–190 ng/mL. Metabolized by the liver and excreted in urine.

CONTRAINDICATIONS

Idiopathic hypertrophic subaortic stenosis. Previous hypersensitivity to dobutamine. Solutions containing dextrose in clients with known allergy to corn or corn products.

SPECIAL CONCERNS

- Safe use after AMI not established.
- May precipitate or exacerbate ventricular ectopic activity (but rarely causes ventricular tachycardia).
- Dobutamine is less effective than dopamine in premature neonates in raising systemic BP without causing undue tachycardia.
- Use with caution during lactation.

SIDE EFFECTS

Most Common

Marked increase in HR, BP, ventricular ectopic activity; premature ventricular beats, hypotension, nausea, headache, SOB.

CV: Marked increase in HR, BP, and ***ventricular ectopic activity***, precipitous drop in BP, premature ventricular beats, anginal pain, palpitations. **Hypersensitivity:** Skin rash, pruritus of the scalp, fever, eosinophilia, ***bronchospasm***. **Infusion site reactions:** Inadvertant infiltration, phlebitis, cutaneous necrosis, local inflammation. **Miscellaneous:** Nausea, headache, nonspecific chest pain, SOB, fever.

LABORATORY TEST CONSIDERATIONS

Thrombocytopenia. Mild ↓ serum potassium.

OVERDOSE MANAGEMENT

Symptoms: Excessive alteration of BP, anorexia, N&V, tremor, anxiety, palpitations, headache, SOB, anginal and nonspecific chest pain, hypertension, hypotension, tachyarrhythmias, ***myocardial ischemia, ventricular fibrillation or tachycardia.*** *Treatment:* Reduce the rate of administration or discontinue temporarily until the condition stabilizes. Establish an airway, ensuring oxygenation and ventilation. Initiate resuscitative measures immediately. Treat severe ventricular tachyarrhythmias with propranolol or lidocaine.

DRUG INTERACTIONS

Beta-blocking drugs / Possible ineffectiveness of dobutamine
Desflurane / Potential death associated with cardiac ischemia; drug interaction not proven
Halogenated hydrocarbon anesthetics / Possible sensitization of the myocardium → serious arrhythmias; use together with extreme caution
Methyldopa / ↑ Pressor response → hypertension; monitor BP closely
Nitroprusside / ↑ CO and ↓ pulmonary wedge pressure
Oxytocics (e.g., ergonovine, oxytocin) / Possible severe persistent hypertension
Tricyclic antidepressants / Possible potentiation of the pressor response; use together with caution

HOW SUPPLIED

Injection Solution, Concentrate: 12.5 mg/mL; ***Injection Solution in 5% Dextrose:*** 250 mg/250 mL (1 mg/mL), 500 mg/500 mL (1 mg/mL), 500 mg/250 mL (2 mg/mL), 1,000 mg/250 mL (4 mg/mL).

DOSAGE

IV INFUSION

Treatment of cardiac decompensation.

Adults, initial: 0.5–1 mcg/kg/min as a continuous infusion. **Usual dose:** 2.5–10 mcg/kg/min (up to a maximum of 40 mcg/kg/min) as a continuous infusion. For the elderly start at the low end of the dosage range. Rate of administration and duration of therapy depend on response of client, as determined by HR, presence of ectopic activity, BP, and urine flow and, when possible, measurement of central venous or pulmonary wedge and cardiac output. Adjust duration of therapy according to client response, as determined by the parameters listed above.

Children with congenital heart disease undergoing diagnostic cardiac catheterization.

Children: 2 and 7.75 mcg/kg/min infused for 10 min. *NOTE:* This dosage is investigational.

NURSING IMPLICATIONS

Do not confuse dobutamine with dopamine (also a sympathomimetic).

IMPLEMENTATION/ADMINISTRATION/STORAGE

1. IV When conventional vials are used, reconstituted dobutamine must be further diluted in an IV container at the time of administration. Dilute 20 mL of dobutamine in at least 50 mL of diluent, and dilute 40 mL of dobutamine in at least 100 mL of diluent. IV solutions should be used within 24 hr.
2. Do not administer solutions containing dextrose through the same administration set as blood as this may result in pseudoagglutination or hemolysis.
3. Inspect parenteral products visually for particulate matter and discoloration prior to administration, whenever solution and container permit. Do not administer unless solution is clear and seal is intact.
4. Administer by IV infusion. A calibrated electronic infusion device is recommended for controlling the rate of flow in mL/hr or drops/min.
5. Excess administration of potassium-free solutions may cause significant hypokalemia.
6. Fluid overload may occur resulting in dilution of serum electrolyte concentrations, overhydration, congested states, or pulmonary edema.
7. Concentrations of up to 5,000 mcg/mL have been given (i.e., 250 mg/50 mL). Determine the final volume given by the fluid requirements of the client.
8. The Pediatric Advanced Life Support guidelines and the American Academy of Pediatrics recommend the following formula for preparation of the infusion: 6 × (desired dose [mcg/kg/min]/desired rate [mL/hr] × Wt (kg) = mg drug/100 mL fluid. Dobutamine in 5% Dextrose Injection may be inappropriate for the dosage requirements in children weighing less than 30 kg.
9. Dobutamine hydrochloride in D5W injection may exhibit a pink color that, if present, will increase with time. There is no significant loss of potency.
10. Store from 15–30°C (59–86°F). Avoid excessive heat and protect from freezing.
11. COMPATIBILITY D5W, D5/0.45% NaCl, D5/0.9% NaCl, D10W, Isolyte M with D5W injection, RL, D5/RL, Normosol-M in D5W, 20% mannitol in water for injection, 0.9% NaCl, and sodium lactate injection. Also compatible when given through same tubing with dopamine, lidocaine, tobramycin, verapamil, nitroprusside, KCl, and protamine sulfate.
12. INCOMPATIBILITY Because of potential physical incompatibilities, advised not to mix with other drugs in the same solution. Do not add dobutamine to sodium bicarbonate 5% injection or to any other strongly alkaline solution. Also, do not use dobutamine in conjunction with other agents or diluents containing both sodium bisulfite and ethanol.

ASSESSMENT

1. Note reasons for therapy; ensure hydrated prior to infusion. Administered in a monitored environment; assess for increased ectopy with dose titration.
2. Ensure patency and placement of IV catheter to ↓ risk of extravasation and phlebitis.
3. During acute use:
   - Monitor CVP to assess vascular volume and cardiac pumping efficiency. Normal range 5–10 cm water (1–7 mm Hg). Elevated CVP may indicate disruption of CO, as in pump failure or pulmonary edema; low CVP may indicate hypovolemia.
   - Monitor PAWP to assess the pressures in the left atrium and ventricle and to measure the efficiency of CO; usual range is 6–12 mm Hg.
   - Assess ECG and BP continuously during drug administration; review written parameters for SBP and titrate infusion. Drug increases AV node conduction causing those with AFib to develop rapid ventricular rate; have digoxin available to give in this event.
   - Record I&O; monitor glucose in diabetics; more insulin may be needed.
4. Monitor VS, ECG, serum K^+, electrolytes, renal function, cardiac output, pulmonary capillary

wedge pressure, central venous pressure, and urinary output during infusion.

CLIENT/FAMILY TEACHING

1. Drug is administered IV to improve cardiac function, thus increasing BP and improving urine output.
2. Report any chest pain, increased SOB, headaches, or IV site pain.

OUTCOMES/EVALUATE

- ↑ CO; ↑ urine output
- SBP >90 mm Hg

■ IV ©

Docetaxel

(doh-seh-**TAX**-ell)

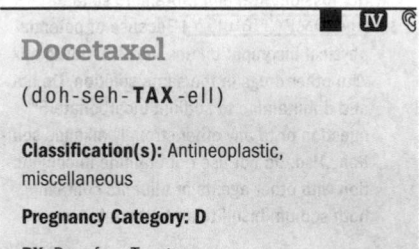

Classification(s): Antineoplastic, miscellaneous

Pregnancy Category: D

RX: Docefrez, Taxotere.

SEE ALSO ***ANTINEOPLASTIC AGENTS***.

INDICATIONS/USES

(1) Locally advanced or metastatic breast cancer after failure of prior chemotherapy. (2) In combination with doxorubicin and cyclophosphamide for the adjuvant treatment of operable node-positive breast cancer. (3) As a single agent to treat locally advanced or metastatic non-small-cell lung cancer after failure of prior platinum-based chemotherapy. (4) With cisplatin for first-line treatment of unresectable locally advanced or metastatic non-small-cell lung cancer in clients who have not received prior chemotherapy. (5) With prednisone to treat androgen-independent (hormone-refactory) advanced metastatic prostate cancer. (6) With cisplatin and 5-fluorouracil to treat advanced gastric adenocarcinoma, including adenocarcinoma of the gastroesophageal junction, in those who have not previously received chemotherapy for advanced disease. (7) With cisplatin and fluorouracil for induction of treatment of inoperable locally advanced squamous cell carcinoma of the head and neck. *Investigational:* Ovarian cancer, urothelial cancer, small cell lung cancer, esophageal cancer.

ACTION/KINETICS

Action

Effect is due to disruption of the microtubular network in cells that is required for mitotic and interphase cellular functions. Thus, mitosis is inhibited.

Pharmacokinetics

t½, 3 phases: 4 min, 36 min, and 11.1 hr. Metabolized in the liver, and metabolites and small amounts of unchanged drug are excreted through both the feces (75%) and urine (6%). **Plasma protein binding:** About 94%.

CONTRAINDICATIONS

Severe hypersensitivity to docetaxel or to other drugs formulated with polysorbate 80. Use in those with neutrophil counts less than 1,500 cells/mm^3, in those with bilirubin greater than the upper limit of normal (ULN), or in those with AST or ALT greater than 1.5 times the ULN. Lactation.

SPECIAL CONCERNS

■ (1) Give docetaxel under the supervision of a qualified health care provider experienced in the use of antineoplastic drugs. Appropriate management of complications is possible only when adequate diagnostic and treatment facilities are readily available. (2) The incidence of treatment-related mortality is increased in clients with abnormal liver function, in those receiving higher doses, and in clients with non-small-cell lung cancer and a history of prior treatment with platinum-based chemotherapy who receive docetaxel as a single agent at a dose of 100 mg/m^2. (3) **Hepatic function impairment**. In general, do not give to clients with bilirubin greater than the upper limit of normal (ULN) or to those with AST and/or ALT over 1.5 × ULN concomitant with alkaline phosphatase over 2.5 × ULN. Those with elevations of bilirubin or abnormalities of transaminase concurrent with alkaline phosphatase are at increased risk for developing grade 4 neutropenia, febrile neutropenia, infections, severe thrombocytopenia, severe stomatitis, severe skin toxicity, and toxic death. Those with isolated elevations of transaminases greater than 1.5 × ULN also had a higher rate of febrile neutropenia grade 4 but did not have an increased incidence of toxic death. Obtain and review bilirubin, AST or ALT, and alkaline phosphatase values before each cycle of docetaxel therapy. (4) **Neutropenia**. Do not give to those with a neutrophil count less than 1,500 cells/mm^3. In order to monitor the occurrence of neutropenia, which may be severe and result in infection, perform frequent blood cell counts on all clients receiving docetaxel. (5) **Hypersensitivity**. Severe hypersensitivity reactions, characterized by general rash/erythema, hypotension and/or bronchospasm or, very rarely, fatal anaphylaxis, have been reported in clients who received the recommended 3-day dexamethasone premedication. Hypersensitivity reactions require immediate discontinuation of the docetaxel infusion and administration of appropriate therapy. Do not give docetaxel to clients who have a history of severe hypersensitivity reactions to docetaxel or other drugs formulated with polysorbate 80. (6) **Fluid retention.** Severe fluid retention is a possibility despite use of 3-day dexamethasone premedication regimen. Fluid retention was characterized by one or more of the following reactions: poorly tolerated peripheral edema, generalized edema, pleural effusion requiring urgent drainage, dyspnea at rest, cardiac tamponade, or pronounced abdominal distention (due to ascites).

- **The incidence of treatment-related mortality is increased in clients with abnormal liver function and in those receiving higher doses.**
- **Select doses carefully in the elderly; side effects may be more common.**
- **Safety and efficacy not determined in children less than 16 years of age.**

SIDE EFFECTS

Most Common

Neutropenia, leukopenia, asthenia, fatigue, neurosensory effects, alopecia, nail changes, N&V, diarrhea, stomatitis, anemia, hypersensitivity reactions, fluid retention, myalgia, fever, infections, skin toxicity, constipation.

Hematologic: Neutropenia (virtually in 100% of clients given 100 mg/m^2). Leukopenia, thrombocytopenia, anemia, febrile neutropenia, acute myeloid leukemia. **GI:** N&V, diarrhea (may be severe), stomatitis (may be severe), pharyngitis, anorexia (may be severe/life-threatening), abdominal pain, colitis, constipation, duodenal ulcer, esophagitis, dysphagia, odynophagia, GI pain/cramps, heartburn, ***GI perforation, GI hemorrhage/bleeding***, intestinal obstruction, ileus, ischemic colitis, neutropenic enterocolitis, taste perversion, duodenal ulcer, impaired hepatic function, ***hepatitis***. **CNS:** Confusion, dizziness, lethargy, motor/sensory neuropathy, loss of consciousness (rare), ***seizures*** (rare). **CV:** Fluid retention (even with premedication), hypotension, atrial fibrillation, ***DVT***, ECG abnormalities, cardiac arrhythmias, thrombophlebitis, CHF, ***pulmonary embolism, heart failure***, syncope, tachycardia, sinus tachycardia, atrial flutter, dysrhythmia, unstable angina, vasodilation, pulmonary edema, myocardial ischemia, ***MI***, cardiac left ventricular function, hypertension (rare). **Respiratory:** Dyspnea, cough, epistaxis, pleural effusion, interstitial pneumonia, ***acute pulmonary edema, ARDS***, pulmonary fibrosis, radiation pneumonitis (in those also receiving radiotherapy). **Dermatologic:** Reversible cutaneous reactions characterized by a rash, including localized eruptions on the hands, feet, arms, face, or thorax, and usually associated with pruritus. Localized erythema of the extremities with edema followed by desquamation. Nail changes, alopecia, itching, dry skin, cutaneous lupus erythematosus (rare), bullous eruption (e.g., erythema multiforme), ***Stevens-Johnson syndrome, toxic epidermal necrolysis***. **Hypersensitivity:** Flushing, localized skin reactions, back pain, chest tightness, chills, drug fever, dyspnea, rash (with or without pruritus). Severe hypersensitivity reactions characterized by hypotension, bronchospasm, or generalized rash/erythema, ***anaphylactic shock***. **Musculoskeletal:** Myalgia, arthralgia. **GU:** Amenorrhea, impaired renal function. **Neurologic:** Paresthesia, dysesthesia, pain in those with anthracycline-resistant breast cancer, paresthesia, dysestheisa, pain. Distal extremity weakness. **Reactions at infusion site:** Hyperpigmentation, inflammation, redness or dryness of the skin, phlebitis, extravasation, mild swelling of the vein. **Ophthalmic:** Conjunctivitis, lacrimation disorder (tearing), flashes, flashing lights, scotomata. **Otic:** Altered hearing, hearing loss. **Metabolic:** Fluid retention, peripheral edema, weight gain/loss. **Body as a whole:** Infections, asthenia, fatigue, lymphedema, dehydration (due to GI reactions), bleeding episodes. **Miscellaneous:** ***Septic/nonseptic death, treat-***

ment-related death, fever (including in absence of infections), diffuse pain, chest pain, renal insufficiency, syncope, allergy, cancer pain.

LABORATORY TEST CONSIDERATIONS

↑ ALT, AST, alkaline phosphatase.

D

OVERDOSE MANAGEMENT

Symptoms: Bone marrow suppression, peripheral neurotoxicity, mucositis. *Treatment:* No known antidote. Keep client in a specialized unit to monitor vital functions. Give therapeutic G-CSF as soon as possible after overdose discovered. Treat symptomatically.

DRUG INTERACTIONS

Clarithromycin / Substantial ↑ docetaxel levels
Itraconazole / ↑ Docetaxel levels → ↑ risk of toxicity (e.g., neutropenia); coadminister with caution and ↓ dose as needed
Ketoconazole / ↑ Docetaxel levels → ↑ risk of toxicity (e.g., neutropenia); coadminister with caution and ↓ dose as needed
Nefazodone / Substantial ↑ docetaxel levels
Nelfinavir / Substantial ↑ docetaxel levels

HOW SUPPLIED

Injection Solution, Concentrate: 10 mg/mL, 20 mg/mL, 80 mg/4 mL.

DOSAGE

IV

Breast cancer.

60–100 mg/m^2 given IV over 1 hr q 3 weeks. Reduce the dose to 75 mg/m^2 or discontinue therapy in those who are dosed initially at 100 mg/m^2 and who experience febrile neutropenia, neutrophils less than 500/mm^3 for more than 1 week, severe or cumulative cutaneous reactions, or severe peripheral neuropathy. If these reactions continue, either decrease the dosage from 75 to 55 mg/m^2 or discontinue treatment. Those who are dosed at 60 mg/m^2 and do not experience these symptoms may tolerate higher doses. Discontinue treatment in those who develop greater than grade 3 peripheral neuropathy.

Combination therapy with doxorubicin and cyclophosphamide for breast cancer.

Docetaxel, 75 mg/m^2 given as a 1hr IV infusion after doxorubicin, 50 mg/m^2, and cyclophosphamide, 500 mg/m^2, every 3 weeks for 6 treatment cycles. Give when the neutrophil count is 1,500 cells/mm^3 or more. Prophylactic granulocyte colony-stimulating factor may be given to reduce the risk of hematological toxicities. Those who experience febrile neutropenia should receive granulocyte colony-stimulating factor in all subsequent cycles. Clients who continue to experience febrile neutropenia should remain on granulocyte colony-stimulating factor and have their docetaxel dose decreased to 60 mg/m^2. Those who experience grade 3 or 4 stomatitis, severe or cumulative cutaneous reactions, or moderate neurosensory signs and/or symptoms should have their docetaxel dose reduced to 60 mg/m^2. If the client continues to experience these reactions at 60 mg/m^2, discontinue treatment.

Non-small-cell lung cancer, after failure of prior platinum-based chemotherapy.

75 mg/m^2 IV over 1 hr q 3 weeks. Withhold treatment until toxicity is resolved for those who experience either febrile neutropenia, neutrophils less than 500/mm^3 for more than 1 week, severe or cumulative cutaneous reactions, or severe peripheral neuropathy. Resume at 55 mg/m^2. Discontinue entirely if clients develop grade 3 or greater peripheral neuropathy.

Non-small-cell lung cancer, chemotherapy naive clients.

75 mg/m^2 IV over 1 hr immediately followed by cisplatin, 75 mg/m^2 over 30–60 min q 3 weeks. In those whose nadir of platelet count during the previous course of therapy is less than 25,000 cells/mm^3, in those who experience febrile neutropenia, and in clients with serious nonhematologic toxicities, reduce the docetaxel dosage in subse-

quent cycles to 65 mg/m^2. If the client requires a further dose reduction, a dose of 50 mg/m^2 is recommended.

Metastatic prostate cancer.

75 mg/m^2 by IV infusion over 1 hr q 3 weeks with PO prednisone, 5 mg, twice a day continuously. For androgen-dependent metastatic prostate cancer, give dexamethasone 8 mg PO at 12 hr, 3 hr, and 1 hr before the docetaxel infusion. Reduce the dose of docetaxel from 75 mg/m^2 to 60 mg/m^2 if febrile neutropenia, neutrophils less than 500/mm^3 for more than 1 week, severe or cumulative cutaneous reactions, or moderate neurosensory signs and/or symptoms occur during docetaxel therapy. If the client continues to experience these reactions at 60 mg/m^2, discontinue the drug.

Gastric adenocarcinoma.

75 mg/m^2 as a 1 hr IV infusion, followed by cisplatin, 75 mg/m^2, as a 1 to 3 hr IV infusion (both on day 1), followed by fluorouracil, 750 mg/m^2/day given as a 24 hr continuous IV infusion for 5 days (start at the end of the cisplatin infusion). Repeat treatment q 3 weeks. Clients must receive premedication with antiemetics and appropriate hydration for cisplatin administration. *NOTE:* See information under *Head and Neck Cancer* below for dose reduction guidelines in the event of toxicities.

Head and neck cancer.

75 mg/m^2 as a 1 hr IV infusion, followed by cisplatin, 75 mg/m^2 IV over 1 hour both on day 1; follow with fluorouracil, 750 mg/m^2 as a continuous IV infusion for 5 days. Give this regimen q 3 weeks for 4 cycles. Following chemotherapy, clients should receive radiotherapy. Clients must receive premedication with antiemetics and appropriate hydration (prior to and after cisplatin administration). Prophylactic antibiotics are also often given.

Granulocyte colony-stimulating factor has been given during the second and/or subsequent cycles in the event of febrile neutropenia, documented infection with neutropenia, or neutropenia lasting longer than 7 days. If these symptoms occur despite granulocyte colony-stimulating factor use, reduce the dose of docetaxel to 60 mg/m^2. If subsequent episodes of complicated neutropenia occur, reduce the docetaxel dose to 45 mg/m^2.

In cases of grade 4 thrombocytopenia, reduce the docetaxel dose to 60 mg/m^2. Do not retreat clients with subsequent cycles of docetaxel until neutrophils recover to a level more than 1,500 cells/mm^3 and platelets recover to a level of more than 100,000/mm^3. Discontinue treatment if these toxicities persist.

The recommended dose modifications for diarrhea, stomatitis, and/or mucositis are as follows: (1) Diarrhea grade 3: Reduce the fluorouracil dose by 20% after the first episode. Reduce the docetaxel dose by 20% after the second episode. (2) Diarrhea, grade 4: Reduce the docetaxel and fluorouracil doses by 20% after the first episode. Discontinue treatment after the second episode. (3) Stomatitis/mucositis, grade 3: Reduce the fluorouracil dose by 20% after the first episode. For the second episode, discontinue fluorouracil only, at all subsequent cycles. For the third episode, reduce the docetaxel dose by 20%. (4) Stomatitis/mucositis, grade 4: Discontinue fluorouracil only, at all subsequent cycles, at the first episode. Reduce the docetaxel dose by 20% at the second episode.

NURSING IMPLICATIONS

Do not confuse Taxotere with Taxol (also an antineoplastic).

IMPLEMENTATION/ADMINISTRATION/STORAGE

1. **IV Premedicate clients with oral corticosteroids, such as dexamethasone, 16 mg/day (e.g., 8 mg twice a day) for 3 days starting 1 day prior to docetaxel in order to reduce the incidence and severity of fluid retention and hypersensitivity reactions.**

2. Check package insert for cisplatin and fluorouracil dose modifications and delays.
3. A one-vial formulation, rather than the original two-vial product is available to treat various types of cancer. The new one-vial formulation eliminates the need for dilution and can be added directly to the infusion solution. One-vial formulation is available in both 20 and 80 mg strengths.
4. Withdraw the required amount of docetaxel using a calibrated syringe. Inject into a 250 mL infusion bag or bottle of either 0.9% NaCl injection or D5W to produce a final concentration of 0.3–0.9 mg/mL; administer as a 1 hr infusion. If doses greater than 240 mg are required, use more solution so that the concentration to be infused does not exceed 0.9 mg/mL.
5. Protect drug from light; refrigerate at 2–8°C (36–46°F). The premixed solution is stable for 8 hr. Do not store in PVC bags.
6. COMPATIBILITY 0.9% NaCl injection or D5W.
7. INCOMPATIBILITY Do not mix with other drugs or solutions.

ASSESSMENT

1. List reasons for therapy, disease onset, previous agents used, outcome.
2. Note previous experience with this drug. If previous hypersensitivity, do not rechallenge. Premedication helps prevent hypersensitivity reactions and reduce adverse side effects.
3. Premedicate with oral corticosteroids to reduce incidence and severity of fluid retention and hypersensitivity reactions. Assess for rash, joint and muscle pains, numbness/tingling, and abnormal bruising or bleeding.
4. List other drugs prescribed; ensure none interact. Advise of increased mortality with liver dysfunction.
5. Monitor CBC, LFTs. Drug causes bone marrow suppression. Do not give if AST or ALT above 1.5 ULN, alkaline phosphatase above 2.5 ULN or neutrophil count <1,500/mm^3; Nadir: 8 days. Check bilirubin, ALT, AST, and alkaline phosphatase prior to each cycle.

CLIENT/FAMILY TEACHING

1. Used to treat resistant cancers and can cause a drop in WBCs and altered liver function, which must be monitored closely to prevent any severe reactions.
2. Drug will be prepared and administered in a monitored setting; pretreatment corticosteroid (e.g., dexamethasone) will be given to reduce adverse treatment SE.
3. May experience a rash 1 week after treatment; should subside.
4. Report adverse effects including infection, fever; sore throat, unusual bruising/bleeding; swelling in feet, hands, or legs; fever, chills, or S&S of infection; chest tightness, difficulty breathing, or unexplained SOB. Muscle or joint pain; numbness, tingling, or burning sensation in hands or feet; rapid, unexplained weight gain, rash, hives, or any other sign of allergic reaction; severe or persistent diarrhea or vomiting; or sores in mouth require intervention.
5. Hair loss may occur but is usually reversible after therapy completed.
6. Color changes to fingernails or toenails may occur and, in extreme cases, the nails may fall off. They will usually grow back after therapy completed.
7. Women of childbearing age should avoid pregnancy during therapy.
8. Avoid crowds and people with contagious diseases.
9. Keep all F/U to assess response, labs, and adverse SE.

OUTCOMES/EVALUATE

Control of metastatic proliferation

Docusate calcium (Dioctyl calcium sulfosuccinate)

(**DOCK**-you-sayt)

Classification(s): Laxative, emollient

Pregnancy Category: C

OTC: DC Softgels, Pro-Cal-Sof, Sulfolax Calcium, Surfak Liquigels, Surfak Stool Softener.

✱ **OTC:** ratio-Docusate Calcium.

Docusate sodium (Dioctyl sodium sulfosuccinate)

Pregnancy Category: C

OTC: Colace, D.O.S., Dioctyn Softgels, Docu, Docusol Mini-Enema, D-S-S, Dulcolax Stool Softener, Ex-Lax Stool Softener, Gena Soft, Non-Habit Forming Stool Softener, Phillips Liqui-Gels, Silace Stool Softener, Sof-lax.

✦ **OTC:** ratio-Docusate Sodium, Selax, Soflax.

SEE ALSO ***LAXATIVES***.

INDICATIONS/USES

(1) To lessen strain of defecation in persons with hernia or CV diseases or other diseases in which straining at stool should be avoided. (2) Megacolon or bedridden clients. (3) Constipation associated with dry, hard stools. *NOTE:* The microemulsion formulation is indicated for relief of occasional constipation in children over the age of 3 years.

ACTION/KINETICS

Action

Acts by lowering the surface tension of the feces and promoting penetration by water and fat, thus increasing the softness of the fecal mass. Not absorbed systemically and does not seem to interfere with the absorption of nutrients.

Pharmacokinetics

A microenema formulation is available for clients aged 3 and older. **Onset:** 12–72 hr.

CONTRAINDICATIONS

Nausea, vomiting, abdominal pain, and intestinal obstruction.

SIDE EFFECTS

Most Common

Diarrhea, N&V, perianal irritation, flatulence, cramps.

See *Laxatives* for a complete list of possible side effects.

DRUG INTERACTIONS

Docusate may ↑ absorption of mineral oil from the GI tract

HOW SUPPLIED

Docusate calcium. ***Capsules:*** 50 mg, 240 mg; ***Capsules, Softgel:*** 240 mg.

Docusate sodium. ***Capsules:*** 50 mg, 100 mg, 250 mg; ***Capsules, Soft Gel:*** 50 mg, 100 mg, 250 mg; ***Mini-Enema:*** 283 mg.; ***Oral Liquid:*** 10 mg/mL; ***Syrup:*** 20 mg/5 mL, 50 mg/15 mL, 60 mg/15 mL, 100 mg/30 mL; ***Tablets:*** 100 mg.

DOSAGE

Docusate Calcium

CAPSULES; CAPSULES, SOFT GEL

Laxative.

Adults: 240 mg/day until bowel movements are normal; **pediatric, over 6 years:** 50–150 mg/day.

Docusate Sodium

CAPSULES; CAPSULES, SOFT GEL; ORAL LIQUID; SYRUP; TABLETS

Laxative.

Adults and children over 12 years: 50–500 mg, depending on the product; **6–12 years:** 40–120 mg, depending on the product; **3–6 years:** 20–60 mg; **pediatric, under 3 years:** 10–40 mg.

MINI-ENEMA

Laxative.

Children, over 12 years of age: 1 to 3 units/day; **6–12 years of age:** 1 unit/day.

NURSING IMPLICATIONS

Several OTC products use the brand name Dulcolax. Bisacodyl is one product and docusate sodium is in another. There is also a liquid formulation that contains magnesium hydroxide that is also sold as Dulcolax.

ASSESSMENT

1. Note reasons for therapy, onset, causes, other agents prescribed.
2. Assess activity levels, diet, water intake, exercise routines. Have client identify habits and BM frequency.
3. Document bowel sounds, abdominal distension, and characteristics of any stool produced.
4. When used in enemas, add 50–100 mg (5–10 mL) to a retention or flushing enema.

CLIENT/FAMILY TEACHING

1. May give oral solutions with milk or juices to help mask bitter taste.
2. Swallow tablets whole; do not chew. Drink a glass of water with each dose.
3. Because docusate salts are minimally absorbed, it may require 1–3 days to soften fecal matter.
4. Do not use mineral oil while taking this drug.

5. **With enema therapy, lubricate enema tip prior to insertion with a few drops of water or product.**
6. **Review other methods to stimulate regular bowel evacuation: attempt to evacuate bowels at same time each day, drink 6 to 8 full glasses of water/day, eat a high-fiber diet, exercise daily, and respond to urge for BM as soon as possible.**
7. **Report any nausea, vomiting, abdominal cramping, rectal bleeding, or diarrhea.**
8. **Keep all F/U to assess response and for adverse SE.**

OUTCOMES/EVALUATE
Elimination of a soft, formed stool; ↓ straining

Dofetilide

(doh-**FET**-ih-lyd)

Classification(s): Antiarrhythmic

Pregnancy Category: C

RX: Tikosyn.

SEE ALSO ***ANTIARRHYTHMIC DRUGS***.

INDICATIONS/USES

(1) Conversion of atrial fibrillation or atrial flutter to normal sinus rhythm. Not shown to be effective in clients with paroxysmal atrial fibrillation. (2) Maintenance of normal sinus rhythm in clients with atrial fibrillation/atrial flutter of more than 1 week duration and who have been converted to normal sinus rhythm. Reserve for those in whom atrial fibrillation/atrial flutter is highly symptomatic due to life-threatening ventricular arrhythmias. *NOTE:* Available only to hospitals and prescribers who receive dosing and treatment initiation education through the *Tikosyn in Pharmacy System* (phone: 1-877-845-6796 or www.tikosyn.com). *Investigational:* Ventricular arrhythmias.

ACTION/KINETICS

Action

Acts by blocking the cardiac ion channel carrying the rapid component of the delayed rectifier potassium currents. Blocks only I_{Kr} with no significant block of other repolarizing potassium currents (e.g., I_{Ks}, I_{K1}). No effect on sodium channels or adrenergic receptors. Dofetilide increases the monophasic action potential duration due to delayed repolarization.

Pharmacokinetics

Maximum plasma levels: 2–3 hr during fasting. Steady state plasma levels reached in 2–3 days. Metabolized in the liver and excreted in the urine. **t½, terminal:** About 10 hr. Women have lower oral clearances than men.

CONTRAINDICATIONS

Congenital or acquired long QT syndromes, in those with a baseline QT interval greater than 440 msec (500 msec in clients with ventricular conduction abnormalities), severe renal impairment (C_{CR} less than 20 mL/min). Concomitant use of verapamil, cimetidine, trimethoprim (alone or with sulfamethoxazole), ketoconazole, prochlorperazine, megestrol. Lactation.

SPECIAL CONCERNS

■ (1) To minimize risk of induced arrhythmia, place clients started or restarted on dofetilide in a facility that can provide calculations on creatinine clearance, continuous ECG monitoring, and cardiac resuscitation for a minimum of 3 days. (2) Dofetilide is available only to hospitals and prescribers who have received appropriate dofetilide dosing and treatment initiation education. ■

- **There is a greater risk of dofetilide-induced torsades de pointes (type of ventricular tachycardia) in female clients than in male clients.**
- **Use with caution in severe hepatic impairment.**
- **Use with drugs that prolong the QT interval has not been studied with dofetilide use; therefore, do not use bepridil, certain macrolide antibiotics, phenothiazines, or TCAs with dofetilide.**
- **Safety and efficacy not determined in children less than 18 years of age.**

SIDE EFFECTS

Most Common

Headache, chest pain, dizziness, ventricular tachycardia/arrhythmias, respiratory tract infection, dyspnea, nausea, flu syndrome, insomnia.
CV: Ventricular arrhythmias (especially TdP type ventricular tachycardia), ***torsades de pointes***, angina pectoris, atrial fibrillation, hypertension, palpitation, supraventricular tachycardia, ventricular tachycardia, bradycardia, cerebral ischemia, ***CVA***, ***MI***, ***heart arrest***, ***ventricular fibrillation***, AV

block, bundle branch block, heart block. **CNS:** Headache, dizziness, insomnia, anxiety, paresthesia. **GI:** Nausea, diarrhea, abdominal pain. **Respiratory:** Respiratory tract infection, dyspnea, increased cough. **Miscellaneous:** Chest pain, flu syndrome, accidental injury, back pain, rash, arthralgia, asthenia, pain, peripheral edema, sweating, UTI, angioedema, edema, facial paralysis, flaccid paralysis, liver damage, paralysis, ***sudden death***, syncope.

OVERDOSE MANAGEMENT

Symptoms: Excessive prolongation of QT interval. *Treatment:* Symptomatic and supportive. Initiate cardiac monitoring. Can use charcoal slur but is effective only when given within 15 min of dofetilide. To treat TdP or overdose, may give isoproterenol infusion, with or without cardiac pacing. IV Mg sulfate may be useful to manage TdP. Monitor until QT interval returns to normal.

DRUG INTERACTIONS

Amiloride / Possible ↑ dofetilide levels
Amiodarone / Possible ↑ dofetilide levels
Cannabinoids / Possible ↑ dofetilide levels
Cimetidine / ↑ Risk of arrhythmia (TdP) R/T ↓ liver metabolism of dofetilide
Digoxin / ↑ Risk of torsades de pointes
Diltiazem / Possible ↑ dofetilide levels
Grapefruit juice / Possible ↑ dofetilide levels
Ketoconazole / ↑ Risk of arrhythmia (TdP) R/T ↓ liver metabolism of dofetilide
Macrolide antibiotics / Possible ↑ dofetilide levels
Megestrol / Possible ↑ dofetilide levels → arrhythmias
Metformin / Possible ↑ dofetilide levels
Nefazadone / Possible ↑ dofetilide levels
Norfloxacin / Possible ↑ dofetilide levels
Potassium-depleting diuretics / Hypokalemia or hypomagnesemia may occur, → ↑ potential for torsades de pointes
Prochlorperazine / Possible ↑ dofetilide levels → arrhythmias
Quinine / Possible ↑ dofetilide levels
Triamterene / Possible ↑ dofetilide levels
Trimethoprim or Trimethoprim/Sulfamethoxazole / ↑ Risk of arrhythmias (TdP) R/T ↓ liver metabolism of dofetilide
Verapamil / Possible ↑ dofetilide levels → arrhythmias
Zafirlukast / Possible ↑ dofetilide levels

HOW SUPPLIED

Capsules: 125 mcg, 250 mcg, 500 mcg.

DOSAGE

CAPSULES

Conversion of atrial fibrillation/flutter; maintenance of normal sinus rhythm.

The dosing for dofetilide must be undertaken using the following steps:

- **Step 1:** Before giving the first dose, determine the QTc using an average of 5–10 beats. If the QTc is greater than 440 msec (500 msec in those with ventricular conduction abnormalities), dofetilide is contraindicated. Also, do not use if the heart rate <60 bpm. Those with heart rates <50 bpm have not been studied.
- **Step 2:** Before giving the first dose, calculate the C_{CR} using the following formulas: *Males:* (Weight [kg] × [140 − age])/(72 × serum creatinine [mg/dL]) *Females:* 0.84 × male value
- **Step 3:** Determine starting dose of dofetilide as follows: **C_{CR} >60 mL/min:** 500 mcg 2 times per day; **C_{CR} 40–60 mL/min:** 250 mcg 2 times per day; **C_{CR} 20 to <40 mL/min:** 125 mcg 2 times per day; **C_{CR} < 20 mL/min:** DO NOT USE DOFETILIDE; CONTRAINDICATED IN THESE CLIENTS. The maximum daily dose is 500 mcg 2 times per day.
- **Step 4:** Give adjusted dose based on C_{CR} and begin continuous ECG monitoring.
- **Step 5:** At 2–3 hr after giving the first dofetilide dose, determine the QTc. If the QTc has increased by >15% compared with the baseline established in Step 1 or if the QTc is 500 msec (550 msec in those with ventricular conduction abnormalities), adjust subsequent dosing as follows: If the starting dose based on C_{CR} is 500 mcg 2 times per day, the adjusted dose (for QTc prolongation) is 250 mcg twice/day. If the starting dose is 250 mcg twice a day, the adjusted dose (for QTc prolongation) is 125 mcg 2 times per day. If the starting dose is 125 mcg twice a day,

the adjusted dose (for QTc prolongation) is 125 mcg once daily.

- **Step 6:** At 2–3 hr after each subsequent dose of dofetilide, determine QTc for in-hospital doses 2 through 5. No further down titration of dofetilide based on QTc is recommended. Discontinue if at any time after the second dose of dofetilide, the QTc is greater than 500 msec (550 msec in those with ventricular conduction abnormalities).
- **Step 7:** Continuously monitor by ECG for a minimum of 3 days or for a minimum of 12 hr after electrical or pharmacologic conversion to normal sinus rhythm, whichever time is greater. Do not discharge within 12 hr of electrical or pharmacological conversion to normal sinus rhythm.

D

NURSING IMPLICATIONS

IMPLEMENTATION/ADMINISTRATION/STORAGE

1. Therapy must be started (and, if necessary, reinitiated) in a setting where continuous ECG monitoring and personnel trained in the management of serious ventricular arrhthymias are available for a minimum of 3 days.
2. Do not discharge clients within 12 hr of electrical or pharmacologic conversion to normal sinus rhythm.
3. Prior to electrical or pharmacologic cardioversion, anticoagulate clients with atrial fibrillation according to usual medical practices. Anticoagulants may be continued after cardioversion. Correct hypokalemia before starting dofetilide therapy.
4. Re-evaluate renal function q 3 months or as warranted. Discontinue dofetilide if the QTc is >500 msec (550 msec in those with ventricular conduction abnormalities) and monitor carefully until QTc returns to baseline levels. If renal function decreases, adjust dose as directed under *Dosage*.
5. The highest dose of 500 mcg twice a day is the most effective. However, the risk of torsades de pointes is increased. Thus, a lower dose may be used. If at any time the lower dose is increased, the client must be hospitalized for 3 days. Previous tolerance of higher doses does not eliminate the need for hospitalization.
6. Do not consider electrical conversion if the client does not convert to normal sinus rhythm within 24 hr after starting dofetilide.
7. Withdraw previous antiarrhythmic drug therapy before starting dofetilide therapy; during withdrawal, carefully monitor for a minimum of 3 plasma half-lives. Do not initiate dofetilide following amiodarone therapy until amiodarone plasma levels are less than 0.3 mcg/mL or until amiodarone has been withdrawn for 3 or more months.
8. Protect capsules from moisture and humidity. Dispense in tight containers.

ASSESSMENT

1. Identify arrhythmia and duration. Note S&S associated with arrhythmia. Monitor ECG rhythm continuously for at least 3 days after starting therapy for evidence of prolonged QT interval; requires reduction in dose or stopping therapy.
2. Note drugs prescribed; ensure none interact. Do not give within 3 months of amiodarone therapy unless level is below 0.3 mcg/mL. Avoid use of drugs that prolong QT interval.
3. Drug is available only through the Tikosyn Dosing Program with provider education.
4. Ensure QTc interval and K^+ have been determined before initiating therapy and periodically (at least every 3 mo) during treatment. Check QTc interval 2 to 3 hr after first dose, and note change from baseline QTc interval. Notify provider if increased more than 15% or is greater than 500 msec.
5. Monitor ECG, VS, electrolytes, renal and LFTs; avoid use with dysfunction. Dose is based on C_{CR}. Low K^+ and Mg^{++} can increase risk of torsades de pointes.

CLIENT/FAMILY TEACHING

1. Take exactly as prescribed without regard to food or meals; avoid grapefruit juice.
2. Do not double the next dose if dose missed. Take next dose at usual time.
3. Report any change in prescriptions or OTC/supplement use. Inform all providers if hospitalized or prescribed a new medication for any condition. Do not take any interacting drugs for at least 2 days after stopping dofetilide; allow drug to get out of system.

4. Avoid OTC Tagamet, may use Zantac, Pepcid, Axid, and Prevacid for acid indigestion or ulcer therapy.
5. Report adverse effects including dizziness, weakness, diarrhea, excessive sweating, vomiting, or loss of thirst/appetite to provider immediately.
6. Read the package insert prior to use. Drug adherence is imperative with this therapy. Must report as scheduled for ECG evaluation and report any adverse effects to ensure no serious drug-related complications. Keep record of BP and HR for provider review.
7. Keep all F/U to assess response, labs, and for adverse SE.

OUTCOMES/EVALUATE

- Conversion of atrial fibrillation/flutter to NSR
- Maintenance of NSR once converted

IV

Dolasetron mesylate

(dohl-**AH**-seh-tron)

Classification(s): Antinauseant, serotonin 5-HT_3 antagonist

Pregnancy Category: B

RX: Anzemet.

INDICATIONS/USES

PO: Prevention of N&V associated with emetogenic cancer chemotherapy (initially and repeat courses) in adults and children 2 years and older. **PO, IV:** Prevention of postoperative N&V in adults and children 2 years and older. *Investigational:* Radiotherapy-induced N&V.

ACTION/KINETICS

Action

Selective serotonin 5-HT_3 antagonist that prevents N&V by inhibiting released serotonin from combining with receptors on vagal efferents that initiate vomiting reflex. May also cause acute, usually reversible, PR and QTc prolongation and QRS widening, perhaps due to blockade of sodium channels by active metabolite of dolasetron.

Pharmacokinetics

Well absorbed from GI tract. Metabolized to active hydrodolasetron. **Peak plasma levels:** 1 hr; **t½:** 8.1 hr. Food does not affect bioavailability. Hydrodolasetron is excreted through urine and feces. Is eliminated more quickly in children than in adults.

CONTRAINDICATIONS

IV use in adults and children to prevent N&V associated with initial and repeat courses of emetogenic cancer chemotherapy due to dose-dependent QT prolongation.

SPECIAL CONCERNS

- Use with caution during lactation.
- Use with caution in those who have or may develop prolongation of cardiac conduction intervals, including QTc (e.g., in hypokalemia or hypomagnesemia, taking diuretics with potential for electrolyte abnormalities, in congenital QT syndrome, taking anti-arrhythmic drugs or other drugs that lead to QT prolongation, and cumulative high dose anthracycline therapy).
- Safety and efficacy not determined in children less than 2 years of age.

SIDE EFFECTS

Most Common

Headache, diarrhea, fatigue, drowsiness, dizziness, bradycardia, hypotension, hypertension, abdominal pain, fever, pain.

Chemotherapy clients. Headache, fatigue, diarrhea, bradycardia, dizziness, pain, tachycardia, dyspepsia, chills, shivering. **Postoperative clients.** Headache, hypotension, dizziness, fever, pruritus, oliguria, hypertension, tachycardia. **Chemotherapy or postoperative clients. CV:** Hypotension, edema, peripheral edema, peripheral ischemia, thrombophlebitis, phlebitis. **GI:** Constipation, dyspepsia, abdominal pain, anorexia, pancreatitis, taste perversion. **CNS:** Flushing, vertigo, paresthesia, tremor, ataxia, twitching, agitation, sleep disorder, depersonalization, confusion, anxiety, abnormal dreaming. **Dermatologic:** Rash, increased sweating. **Hematologic:** Hematuria, epistaxis, anemia, purpura, hematoma, thrombocytopenia. **Hypersensitivity**: Rarely, ***anaphylaxis***, facial edema, urticaria. **Musculoskeletal:** Myalgia, arthralgia. **Respiratory:** Dyspnea, bronchospasm. **GU:** Dysuria, polyuria, acute renal failure. **Ophthalmic:** Abnormal vision, photophobia. **Miscellaneous:** Tinnitus.

LABORATORY TEST CONSIDERATIONS

↑ PTT, AST, ALT, alkaline phosphatase. Prolonged prothrombin time.

DRUG INTERACTIONS

Atenolol / ↓ Hydrodolasetron clearance (by about 27%) when dolasetron given IV
Cimetidine / ↑ Hydrodolasetron levels after given with cimetidine for 7 days
Rifamycins / ↓ Dolasetron levels
Ziprasidone / ↑ Risk of life-threatening cardiac arrhythmias, including torsades de pointes; do not give together

HOW SUPPLIED

Injection: 20 mg/mL; ***Tablets:*** 50 mg, 100 mg.

DOSAGE

TABLETS

Prevention of cancer chemotherapy-induced nausea and vomiting (N&V).

Adults: 100 mg within 1 hr before chemotherapy; **maximum**: 100 mg/dose. **Children, 2 to 16 years, usual:** 1.8 mg/kg within 1 hr before chemotherapy, up to a maximum of 100 mg/dose.

Prevention of postoperative N&V.

Adults: 100 mg within 2 hr before surgery; **maximum:** 100 mg/dose. **Children, 2 to 16 years:** 1.2 mg/kg within 2 hr before surgery, up to a maximum of 100 mg/dose.

IV

Prevention or treatment of postoperative N&V.

Adults: 12.5 mg given as a single dose; **maximum**: 12.5 mg/dose. **Children, 2 to 16 years:** 0.35 mg/kg, up to a maximum of 12.5 mg/dose. Alternative pediatric dose: 1.2 mg/kg, up to 100 mg, within 2 hr before surgery. For adults and children, give about 15 min before cessation of anesthesia or as soon as nausea and vomiting presents.

NURSING IMPLICATIONS

Ⓢ Do not confuse Anzemet with Avandamet (combination drug oral hypoglycemic).

IMPLEMENTATION/ADMINISTRATION/STORAGE

1. For children, injection may be mixed with apple or apple-grape juice and used for oral dosing. When injection is used PO, recommended dose for prevention of cancer chemotherapy N&V is 1.8 mg/kg (up to a maximum of 100 mg) and dose for prevention of postoperative N&V is 1.2 mg/kg (up to a maximum of 100 mg). Diluted injection may be kept up to 2 hr at room temperature before use; do not use beyond 2 hr.
2. Store capsules from 20–25°C (68–77°F); protect from light.
3. IV Injection can be safely infused as rapidly as 100 mg/30 seconds. May also be diluted to 50 mL with compatible solutions. Dilutions are given over 15 min. Diluted product is stable for 24 hr at room temperature and 48 hr if refrigerated.
4. Flush infusion line before and after administration of dolasetron.
5. Inspect visually for particulate matter and discoloration before using.
6. Store injection from 15–30°C (59–86°F); protect from light.
7. COMPATIBILITY 0.9% NaCl, D5W, D5/0.45% NaCl, D5/RL, RL, and 10% mannitol injection.
8. INCOMPATIBILITY Do not mix with any other drugs. Flush infusion line before and after administration.

ASSESSMENT

1. Note reasons for therapy: N&V R/T chemotherapy or postoperatively. List drugs prescribed; ensure none interact.
2. Give 1 hr before chemotherapy or 2 hr before surgery to gain desired effect. Assess bowel sounds and abdomen. May experience headache.
3. With children, calculate appropriate dose (cancer chemotherapy or postop N&V); may administer orally with apple or apple-grape juice.
4. Assess ECG closely in the elderly and in those with CHF, bradycardia, and renal impairment.
5. Monitor CBC, K^+, Mg^{++}, ECG and fluid status. Assess ECG for prolonged QT intervals.

CLIENT/FAMILY TEACHING

1. May take tablets without regard to food. Drug also given parenterally to prevent N&V with chemo/surgery.
2. May mix injection in apple juice for oral administration just before dosing. Discard mixture after 2 hr.
3. Drug may cause serious cardiac arrhythmias, such as QT prolongation or heart block. Re-

port changes in heart rate, light-headedness, or if syncopal episode (fainting) experienced.
4. May experience headaches as well as some N&V but incidence should be reduced.
5. Keep all F/U to assess response and adverse SE.

OUTCOMES/EVALUATE

Inhibition of chemotherapy induced/postop N&V

Donepezil hydrochloride

(dohn-**EP**-eh-zil)

Classification(s): Treatment of Alzheimer's disease

Pregnancy Category: C

RX: Aricept, Aricept 23, Aricept ODT.

INDICATIONS/USES

Treatment of mild to severe dementia of the Alzheimer's type. Is combined with memantine (Namenda) to lower the decline of mental and physical function in Alzheimer's disease. *Investigational:* Vascular dementia; improve memory in multiple sclerosis clients; post-stroke aphasia.

ACTION/KINETICS

Action

A decrease in cholinergic function may be the cause of Alzheimer's disease. Donepezil, a cholinesterase inhibitor, exerts its effect by enhancing cholinergic function by increasing levels of acetylcholine through reversible inhibition of acetylcholinesterase. No evidence that the drug alters the course of the underlying dementing process.

Pharmacokinetics

Well absorbed from the GI tract; is 100% bioavailable. **Peak plasma levels:** 3–4 hr; steady state reached in 15 days. Food does not affect the rate or extent of absorption. **t½, elimination:** 70 hr. Metabolized in the liver, and both unchanged drug and metabolites are excreted in the urine and feces. **Plasma protein binding:** 96%.

CONTRAINDICATIONS

Hypersensitivity to piperidine derivatives.

SPECIAL CONCERNS

- Use with caution with a history of asthma or obstructive pulmonary disease.
- Safety and efficacy not determined in children.

SIDE EFFECTS

Most Common

Anorexia, diarrhea, fatigue, insomnia, muscle cramps, N&V, dizziness, headache, ecchymosis.

NOTE: Side effects with an incidence of 1% or greater are listed. **GI:** N&V, diarrhea, anorexia, fecal incontinence, GI bleeding (especially those at risk of developing ulcers), bloating, epigastric pain, abdominal pain, constipation, dyspepsia, gastroenteritis. **CNS:** Insomnia, dizziness, depression, confusion, abnormal dreams, somnolence, abnormal crying, aggression/hostility, aphasia, ataxia, delusions, increased libido, irritability, nervousness, paresthesia, restlessness, tremor, emotional lability, hallucinations, personality disorder, abnormal gait, anxiety, ***seizures***. **CV:** Hypertension, vasodilation, atrial fibrillation, hot flashes, hypotension, heart block, bradycardia, ***hemorrhage***, syncope, ecchymosis, ECG abnormalities, ***heart failure***. **Body as a whole:** Headache, pain (in various locations), fever, asthenia, infection, accident, fatigue, influenza, fungal infection, chest/back pain, edema, peripheral edema, toothache. **Hematologic:** Anemia. **Musculoskeletal:** Muscle cramps, arthritis, bone fracture. **Dermatologic:** Diaphoresis, urticaria, pruritus, eczema, rash, skin ulcer. **GU:** Urinary incontinence, nocturia, frequent urination, cystitis, hematuria, UTI. **Respiratory:** Dyspnea, sore throat, bronchitis, increased cough, pharyngitis, pneumonia. **Ophthalmic:** Cataract, eye irritation, blurred vision. **Miscellaneous:** Dehydration, ecchymosis, weight loss.

LABORATORY TEST CONSIDERATIONS

↑ CPK, alkaline phosphatase, ALT, AST, LDH. Hyperlipemia, glycosuria.

OVERDOSE MANAGEMENT

Symptoms: Cholinergic crisis characterized by severe N&V, salivation, sweating, bradycardia, hypotension, respiratory depression, collapse, convulsions, increased muscle weakness (may cause death if respiratory muscles are involved). *Treatment:* Atropine sulfate at an initial dose of 1–2 mg IV with subsequent doses based on the response. General supportive measures.

D

DRUG INTERACTIONS

Anticholinergic drugs / The cholinesterase inhibitor activity of donepezil interferes with the activity of anticholinergics
Bethanechol / Synergistic effect
Carbamazepine / ↑ Donepezil elimination R/T induction of CYP3A4 and CYP2D6
Dexamethasone / ↑ Donepezil elimination R/T induction of CYP3A4 and CYP2D6
Ketoconazole / ↑ Peak plasma levels of donepezil R/T ↓ breakdown by liver
NSAIDs / ↑ Gastric acid secretion due to donepezil → ↑ risk of active or occult GI bleeding
Phenobarbital / ↑ Donepezil elimination R/T induction of CYP3A4 and CYP2D6
Quinidine / ↑ Peak plasma levels of donepezil R/T ↓ breakdown by liver
Rifampin / ↑ Donepezil elimination R/T induction of CYP3A4 and CYP2D6
Succinylcholine / ↑ Muscle relaxant effect

HOW SUPPLIED

Tablets: 5 mg, 10 mg, 23 mg; ***Tablets, Oral Disintegrating:*** 5 mg, 10 mg.

DOSAGE

TABLETS; TABLETS, ORAL DISINTEGRATING

Mild to moderate Alzheimer's disease.

Initial: 5 or 10 mg once daily. Use of a 10-mg dose did not provide a clinical effect greater than the 5-mg dose; however, in some clients, 10 mg daily may be superior. Do not increase the dose to 10 mg until clients have been on a daily dose of 5 mg for 4 to 6 weeks.

Severe Alzheimer's disease.

10 mg given once daily. Do not achieve a dose of 10 mg until clients have been on a daily dose of 5 mg for 4–6 weeks. *NOTE:* Donepezil 23 is now marketed. It can be used in clients with moderate to severe Alzheimer's disease who have been on 5 mg once daily initially for 4–6 weeks; then 10 mg once a day for 3 months; then 23 mg once a day. The 23 mg dose is associated with a higher incidence of side effects (N&V, diarrhea, anorexia).

NURSING IMPLICATIONS

Ⓢ Do not confuse Aricept with Aciphex (a proton pump inhibitor).

IMPLEMENTATION/ADMINISTRATION/STORAGE

1. Donepezil orally disintegrating tablets are bioequivalent to donepezil tablets.
2. Store at controlled room temperatures from 15–30°C (59–86°F).

ASSESSMENT

1. Note onset/duration, characteristics of S&S, other agents trialed, outcome.
2. Describe cognitive function, mental status and ADL performance as well as MME (mini mental exam) or similar such scores before and then periodically during therapy to assess clinical response.
3. Note any history of ulcers, asthma, or COPD.
4. Monitor for symptoms of active or occult GI bleeding.
5. Assess Wt, ECG, HR, and labs (renal and LFTs, CBC).

CLIENT/FAMILY TEACHING

1. Take in the evening, just prior to bedtime. May take with or without food.
2. Place the oral disintegrating tablet on the tongue; after the tablet dissolves, drink water.
3. May cause dizziness or drowsiness; avoid activities that require mental alertness until drug effects realized.
4. Drug does not cure disease but helps alleviate symptoms or slow physical and mental progression of disease, especially when used with memantine. May take up to 3 weeks to notice any effects.
5. Report adverse effects including irregular pulse or dizzy/fainting spells, lack of response, worsening of symptoms. May aggravate asthma and other breathing problems and increase risk of seizures.
6. Report persistent diarrhea, N&V, inability to sleep, depression, fainting, or loss of appetite with weight loss.
7. Ensure caregiver is aware of outside programs available for socialization, stimulation, and activity. Advise all providers that drug is prescribed; especially before anesthesia use.
8. Keep all F/U to assess response and adverse SE.

OUTCOMES/EVALUATE

Improved cognitive functioning with Alzheimer's-type dementia.

IV

Dopamine hydrochloride

(**DOH**-pah-meen)

Classification(s): Sympathomimetic, direct-acting and indirect-acting

Pregnancy Category: C

RX: Dopamine hydrochloride.

SEE ALSO ***SYMPATHOMIMETIC DRUGS***.

INDICATIONS/USES

(1) Hypotension due to inadequate cardiac output (use low to moderate doses of dopamine). (2) To increase cardiac output (use low or moderate doses of dopamine). (3) Poor perfusion of vital organs, including the kidney. Coadministration of dopamine and diuretics may produce an additive or potentiating effect. (4) Correction of hemodynamic imbalances present in the shock syndrome due to MI, trauma, endotoxic septicemia, open heart surgery, renal failure, and chronic cardiac decompensation as in refractory congestive failure. *Investigational:* Chronic obstructive pulmonary disease, CHF, respiratory distress syndrome in infants.

ACTION/KINETICS

Action

Dopamine is the immediate precursor of epinephrine in the body. Exogenously administered, it causes positive chronotropic and inotropic effects on the myocardium resulting in an increase in HR and cardiac contractility. This is accomplished directly by exerting an agonist effect on beta receptors and indirectly by causing release of norepinephrine from storage sites in sympathetic nerve endings. Exerts little effect on DBP and induces fewer arrhythmias than are seen with isoproterenol.

Pharmacokinetics

Onset: 5 min after IV. **Duration:** <10 min (MAOIs increase duration to 1 hr). **t½, plasma:** 2 min. Does not cross the blood-brain barrier. Metabolized in liver by MAO and catechol-O–methyltransferase; 80% excreted in urine. About 25% is taken up into adrenergic nerve terminals where it is hydroxylated to form norepinephrine. **t½, elimination, children:** 5–11 min.

ADDITIONAL CONTRAINDICATIONS

Pheochromocytoma, uncorrected tachycardia, ventricular fibrillation, or arrhythmias. Possible contraindication in those with known allergy to corn or corn products.

SPECIAL CONCERNS

Antidote for peripheral ischemia: To prevent sloughing and necrosis in ischemic areas, the area should be infiltrated as soon as possible with 10 to 15 mL of saline solution containing phentolamine 5 to 10 mg, an adrenergic blocking agent. Pediatric dosage of phentolamine should be 0.1 to 0.2 mg/kg up to a maximum of 10 mg per dose. A syringe with a fine hypodermic needle should be used, and the solution liberally infiltrated throughout the ischemic area. Sympathetic blockade with phentolamine causes immediate and conspicuous local hyperemic changes if the area is infiltrated within 12 hr. Therefore, phentolamine should be given as soon as possible after the extravasation is noted.

- **Use with caution during lactation.**
- **Possible dosage adjustment in clients with a history of occlusive vascular disease. Closely monitor.**
- **Use solutions containing dextrose with caution in those with known subclinical or overt diabetes mellitus.**
- **Safety and efficacy not established in children, although dopamine has been used in children.**

SIDE EFFECTS

Most Common

Tachycardia, anginal pain, palpitations, dyspnea, N&V, headache, anxiety, hypertension, hypotension.

CV: Ectopic heartbeats, tachycardia, anginal pain, palpitations, vasoconstriction, hypo-/hypertension, abnormal cardiac conduction, bradycardia, widened QRS complex, ventricular arrhythmia (at very high doses). **CNS:** Headache, anxiety. **GI:** N&V. **Dermatologic:** Piloerection. **Respiratory:** Dyspnea. **Metabolic:** Azotemia. **Due to injection:** Febrile response, infection, venous thrombosis, phlebitis extending from injection site, extravasation, hypervolemia. **Miscellaneous:** Azotemia; gangrene of the extremities, especially if given for long periods or in those with occlusive vascular disease receiving low doses of dopamine; peripheral cyanosis. Extravasation may result in necrosis and sloughing of surrounding tissue.

LABORATORY TEST CONSIDERATIONS

Suppression of pituitary secretion of TSH, growth hormone, and prolactin.

OVERDOSE MANAGEMENT

Symptoms: Extravasation. Overdose may cause excessive BP elevation. *Treatment:* To prevent sloughing and necrosis if extravasation occurs, infiltrate as soon as possible with 10–15 mL of 0.9% NaCl solution containing 5–10 mg phentolamine using a syringe with a fine needle. Infiltrate liberally throughout the ischemic area. For overdosage, reduce the rate of administration or discontinue temporarily until condition has stabilized.

ADDITIONAL DRUG INTERACTIONS

Alpha- or beta-adrenergic blocking drugs / Antagonism of dopamine effects
Anesthetics, halogenated hydrocarbon / Sensitization of myocardium to dopamine → serious arrhythmias; use together with extreme caution
Diuretics (e.g., furosemide) / Additive or potentiating effect on urine flow
Ergonovine / Possible severe hypertension
Haloperidol / Suppression of dopaminergic renal and mesenteric vasodilation induced with low dose dopamine infusion
Hydantoins (e.g., phenytoin) / Possible profound hypotension and possibly cardiac arrest; use together with extreme caution, if at all
MAOIs / ↑ Pressor response to dopamine by 6 to 20 fold → hypertensive crisis and possible cardiac arrest; avoid concomitant use
Methyldopa / Possible ↑ pressor response → hypertension; monitor BP closely
Oxytocic drugs (e.g., ergonovine, oxytocin) / Possible severe persistent hypertension
Phenothiazines / Suppression of dopaminergic renal and mesenteric vasodilation induced with low dose dopamine infusion
Tricyclic antidepressants (e.g., amitriptyline) / Possible potentiation of dopamine pressor response; use together with caution

HOW SUPPLIED

Injection Solution, Concentrate: 40 mg/mL, 80 mg/mL, 160 mg/mL; ***Injection Solution in 5% Dextrose:*** 200 mg/250 mL (0.8 mg/mL), 400 mg/500 mL (0.8 mg/mL), 400 mg/250 mL (1.6 mg/mL), 800 mg/500 mL (1.6 mg/mL), 800 mg/250 mL (3.2 mg/mL).

DOSAGE

IV INFUSION

Hypotension; low cardiac output; poor perfusion of vital organs; shock.

Adults, initial: 2–5 mcg/kg/min in those who are likely to respond to modest increments of heart force and renal perfusion. For the elderly, start at the low end of the dosage range. In more seriously ill clients, begin with 5 mcg/kg/min. **Usual dose:** <20 mcg/kg/min in more than 50% of clients. In severely ill clients, increase the dose gradually, using 5 to 10 mcg/kg/min increments, up to 20 to 50 mcg/kg/min as needed. If doses in excess of 50 mcg/kg/min are needed, check urine output frequently. Consider reducing the dopamine dose if urine flow begins to decrease in the absence of hypotension. *NOTE:* Clients who have been treated with MAOIs within 2–3 weeks prior to the use of dopamine should receive initial doses of dopamine not greater than one-tenth of the usual dose. Also, identify and correct hypovolemia, hypercapnia, and acidosis before or concurrently with dopamine administration. **Children:** Dosing is similar, on a mcg/kg/min basis, to that used in adults.

NURSING IMPLICATIONS

Do not confuse dopamine with dobutamine (also a sympathomimetic).

IMPLEMENTATION/ADMINISTRATION/STORAGE

1. **IV Dopamine is a potent drug. It must be diluted before use; see package insert.**
2. **For conventional vials, transfer the contents of 1 or more vials by aseptic technique to either 250 or 500 mL of a sterile compatible IV solution.**

3. Infuse into a large vein (e.g., veins of the antecubital fossa) when possible to prevent possibility of extravasation into adjacent tissue. Extravasation may cause necrosis and tissue sloughing. Use less suitable infusion sites only when larger veins are unavailable and the client's condition requires immediate attention. Switch to a more suitable site as soon as possible; continuously monitor the infusion site for free flow. Do not use the umbilical artery.
4. Adjust the dose of dopamine according to the client's response, especially with respect to diminution of established urine flow rate, increasing tachycardia, or development of new dysrhythmias (i.e., as indices for decreasing or temporarily suspending dosage).
5. If a disproportionate rise in diastolic pressure (i.e., a marked decrease in pulse pressure) is seen, decrease the infusion rate and observe carefully for further evidence of predominant vasoconstrictor activity, unless such an effect is desired.
6. Treatment of all clients requires constant evaluation of therapy, including blood volume, augmentation of cardiac contractility, urine flow, CO, BP, and distribution of peripheral perfusion.
7. Administer using an electronic infusion device. Control the rate of infusion to avoid inadvertant administration of a bolus of the drug.
8. Do not use if solution is darker than slightly yellow or discolored in any way. Do not give unless solution is clear and the container is undamaged. Discard any unused portion.
9. Do not administer dextrose solutions without electrolytes simultaneously with blood through the same infusion set because of the possibility that pseudoagglutination of red cells may occur.
10. Dopamine is stable for a minimum of 24 hr after dilution in the sterile IV solutions recommended. However, dilution should be made just prior to administration.
11. Hypoxia, hypercapnia, and acidosis may reduce the effectiveness and/or increase the incidence of side effects of dopamine. Correct these conditions prior to or concurrently with dopamine administration.
12. If hypotension occurs during administration, rapidly increase infusion rate until adequate BP is reached. If hypotension persists, discontinue dopamine and use a more potent vasoconstrictor (e.g., norepinephrine).
13. When discontinuing, gradually decrease dose while expanding blood volume with IV fluids, because sudden cessation may cause marked hypotension.
14. Some products contain sodium metabisulfite that may cause allergic reactions, including anaphylaxis and life-threatening or less severe asthmatic symptoms in susceptible people.
15. If an increased number of ectopic beats occurs, reduce the dose, if possible.
16. IV administration can cause fluid and/or solute overload resulting in dilution of serum electrolyte concentrations, overhydration, congested states, or pulmonary edema.
17. Excess administration of potassium-free solutions may cause significant hypokalemia.
18. Store vials from 15–30°C (59–86°F) and premixed single-use containers from 20–25°C (68–77°F). Brief exposure of premixed single-use containers up to 40°C (104°F) does not affect the product adversely. However, avoid excessive heat. Protect from freezing.
19. COMPATIBILITY 0.9% NaCl, D5W, D5/0.9% NaCl, D5/0.45% NaCl, D5/RL, sodium lactate (⅙ molar), and RL.
20. INCOMPATIBILITY Alteplase, amphotericin B; sodium bicarbonate or other alkaline IV solutions as dopamine is inactivated in alkaline media. Avoid contact with oxidizing agents or iron salts.

ASSESSMENT

1. Note reasons for therapy; ensure adequate hydration prior to infusion.
2. List drugs prescribed to ensure none interact.
3. Note significant changes in VS, ECG, deterioration of peripheral pulses, and/or cold, mottled extremities. Assess urine output, cardiac output, CVP, PCWP, and BP during dopamine infusion. Determine any hypovolemia and correct prior to dopamine infusion.
   - Monitor VS, I&O, and ECG; titrate infusion to maintain SBP as ordered.
   - Record CVP and PCWP. Report ectopy, palpitations, anginal pain, or vasoconstriction.
4. Those with history of occlusive vascular disease (e.g., atherosclerosis, arterial embolism, Raynaud disease, cold injury, diabetic endarteritis, Buerger's disease) require close moni-

toring for any changes in skin color or temperature of extremities.

5. Monitor VS, ECG, TSH, growth hormone, and prolactin levels during infusion; dopamine suppresses pituitary secretion.

CLIENT/FAMILY TEACHING

1. Drug is administered IV to improve cardiac function thus increasing BP and improving urine output.
2. Report any chest pain, increased SOB, headaches, discomfort at IV site, or numbness, tingling or burning of extremities.

OUTCOMES/EVALUATE

- SBP >90; ↑ urine output
- Improved organ perfusion

D

Dornase alfa recombinant

(**DOR**-nace **AL**-fah)

Classification(s): Treatment of cystic fibrosis

Pregnancy Category: B

RX: Pulmozyme.

INDICATIONS/USES

In cystic fibrosis (CF) clients in conjunction with standard therapy to decrease the frequency of respiratory infections that require parenteral antibiotics and to improve pulmonary function.

ACTION/KINETICS

Action

This drug is a highly purified solution of genetically engineered recombinant human deoxyribonuclease I (rhDNase), an enzyme that selectively cleaves DNA. The amino acid sequence is identical to that of the native human enzyme. Cystic fibrosis (CF) clients have viscous purulent secretions in the airways that contribute to reduced pulmonary function and worsening of infection. These secretions contain high concentrations of extracellular DNA released by degenerating leukocytes that accumulate as a result of infection. Dornase alfa hydrolyzes the DNA in sputum of CF clients, thereby reducing sputum viscoelasticity and reducing infections.

CONTRAINDICATIONS

Known sensitivity to dornase alfa or products from Chinese hamster ovary cells.

SPECIAL CONCERNS

- Safety and efficacy of daily use not demonstrated in clients with forced vital capacity (FVC) of less than 40% of predicted, or for longer than 12 months.
- Consider use in children less than 5 years of age only if there is the potential for benefit in pulmonary function or if there is risk of respiratory tract infection.
- Use with caution during lactation.

SIDE EFFECTS

Most Common

Pharyngitis, chest pain, rash, voice alteration, conjunctivitis, laryngitis.

Respiratory: Pharyngitis, voice alteration, laryngitis, ***apnea***, bronchiectasis, bronchitis, change in sputum, cough increase, dyspnea, hemoptysis, lung function decrease, nasal polyps, pneumonia, pneumothorax, rhinitis, sinusitis, sputum increase, wheezing. **Body as a whole:** Abdominal pain, asthenia, fever, flu syndrome, malaise, ***sepsis***, weight loss. **GI:** Dyspepsia, intestinal obstruction, gallbladder disease, liver disease, pancreatic disease. **Dermatologic:** Rash, urticaria. **Miscellaneous:** Chest pain, conjunctivitis, diabetes mellitus, hypoxia, development of serum antibodies to dornase alfa.

HOW SUPPLIED

Solution for Inhalation: 1 mg/mL.

DOSAGE

SOLUTION FOR INHALATION

Cystic fibrosis.

Adults and children, 5 years and older: One 2.5 mg (2.5 mL) single-dose ampule inhaled once daily using a recommended nebulizer (see *Implementation/Administration/Storage*). Some clients may benefit from twice-daily dosing.

NURSING IMPLICATIONS

IMPLEMENTATION/ADMINISTRATION/STORAGE

1. Use only with a recommended nebulizer. Approved nebulizers include the Hudson T Updraft II nebulizer with Pulmo-Aide compressor; Marquest Acorn II nebulizer with a Pulmo-Aide compressor; Pari LC Jet+ nebulizer with the

Pari Proneb compressor; Pari Baby nebulizer with the Pari Proneb compressor; Durable Sidestream nebulizer with the Mobilaire compressor; or, the Durable Sidestream nebulizer with the Porta-Neb compressor. *NOTE:* Those who are unable to inhale or exhale orally throughout the entire nebulization period may use the Pari Baby nebulizer.
2. Clients who use the Sidestream nebulizer with the Mobilaire compressor should turn the compressor control knob fully to the right and then turn on the compressor. At this setting the needle on the pressure gauge should vibrate between 35 and 45 psi (highest pressure output).
3. Do not dilute.
4. Refrigerate when transported, and do not expose to room temperature for more than 24 hr.
5. Discard if cloudy or discolored.
6. Product does not contain a preservative; thus, once opened, entire ampule must be used or discarded.
7. Must be stored in the refrigerator from 2–8°C (36–46°F) in the protective foil pouch and protected from strong light.
8. **Do not mix with other drugs in the nebulizer.** Mixing could lead to adverse physicochemical or functional changes in dornase alfa.

ASSESSMENT
1. Note age of CF symptom onset, therapies trialed, and outcome.
2. Drug is produced by genetically engineered Chinese hamster ovary cells; assess for sensitivity.
3. Monitor VS, PFTs, respiratory patterns, and lung sounds.
4. Note characteristics of cough and sputum. Assess ability to clear secretions; determine need for assistance with coughing, positioning (semi-Fowler's or sitting upright) and suctioning. Perform chest physiotherapy (percussion and postural drainage) regularly and hydration to liquefy secretions and replace fluids.

CLIENT/FAMILY TEACHING
1. Drug is administered by inhalation of an aerosol mist generated by a compressed air-driven nebulizer system; review dose, frequency, and method for inhalation. Ensure familiarity with use, care, and storage of equipment and drug. Rinse equipment and mouth after each use. Drug works to reduce sputum viscoelasticity.
2. Must be administered on a daily schedule to obtain full benefits, which may not be apparent for months. Must continue standard therapies for CF, e.g., chest PT, antibiotics, bronchodilators, oral and inhaled corticosteroids, enzyme supplements, vitamins, and analgesics during therapy.
3. May cause sore throat, hoarseness, or voice alterations; report if persistent or bothersome.
4. Avoid contact with those with infections. Report symptoms that require immediate medical intervention: Severe rashes, itching, respiratory distress, fever. Have family members learn CPR.
5. Identify support groups that may assist to cope with this disease. Benefits of treatment may not be apparent for months.

OUTCOMES/EVALUATE
- ↓ Respiratory tract infectious exacerbations; ↓ sputum viscosity with cystic fibrosis
- Improved PFTs

Doxazosin mesylate

(dox-**AYZ**-oh-sin)

Classification(s): Antihypertensive, peripherally-acting

Pregnancy Category: B

RX: Cardura, Cardura XL.

🍁 **Rx:** Apo-Doxazosin, Cardura-1, -2, -4, Gen-Doxazosin.

SEE ALSO ***ALPHA-1-ADRENERGIC BLOCKING AGENTS.***

INDICATIONS/USES
(1) Hypertension, alone or in combination with diuretics, calcium channel blockers, ACE inhibitors, or beta blockers. (2) BPH, both urinary outflow obstruction and obstructive and irritative symptoms. May be used in BPH clients whether hypertensive or normotensive. Cardura XL is used only for BPH.

ACTION/KINETICS
Action
Blocks the alpha-1 (postjunctional) adrenergic receptors resulting in a decrease in systemic vascular resistance and a corresponding decrease in BP.

Pharmacokinetics

About 65% bioavailable. **Peak plasma levels:** 2–3 hr. **Peak effect:** 2–6 hr. First-pass metabolism; metabolized in the liver to active and inactive metabolites, which are excreted through the feces (about 63%) and urine (about 9%). **t½:** 22 hr. **Plasma protein binding:** 98%.

D

CONTRAINDICATIONS

Clients allergic to prazosin or terazosin.

SPECIAL CONCERNS

- **Use with caution during lactation, in impaired hepatic function, or in those taking drugs known to influence hepatic metabolism.**
- **Safety and efficacy not demonstrated in children.**
- **Due to the possible severe hypotension, do not use the 2, 4, or 8 mg tablets for initial therapy.**

SIDE EFFECTS

Most Common

Dizziness, somnolence, headache, edema, fatigue/malaise, N&V, asthenia.

CV: Palpitations, chest pain, postural hypotension/hypotension, arrhythmia, angina pectoris, syncope, tachycardia, peripheral ischemia, bradycardia, ***MI, CVA.*** **CNS:** Dizziness, headache, somnolence, nervousness, depression, paresthesia, insomnia, ataxia, hypertonia, hypesthesia, agitation, paresis, tremor, twitching, confusion, migraine, kinetic disorders, impaired concentration, paroniria, amnesia, emotional lability, abnormal thinking, depersonalization, hypesthesia. **GI:** N&V, diarrhea, constipation, flatulence, dyspepsia, increased appetite, anorexia, fecal incontinence, gastroenteritis, aggravated vomiting, hepatitis, cholestatic hepatitis. **Musculoskeletal:** Arthritis, joint disorder, muscle pain, arthralgia, myalgia, muscle weakness. **Respiratory:** Pharyngitis, rhinitis, dyspnea, epistaxis, sinusitis, bronchitis, cold/flu symptoms, increased cough, bronchospasm. **GU:** Decreased libido/sexual dysfunction, polyuria, incontinence, breast pain, renal calculus, priapism, gynecomastia, hematuria, micturition disorder/frequency, nocturia. **Dermatologic:** Pruritus, rash, flushing, sweating, alopecia, lichen planus, dry skin, eczema, urticaria. **Hematologic:** Lymphadenopathy, purpura, leukopenia, thrombocytopenia. **Ophthalmic:** Abnormal vision, conjunctivitis, reddened sclera, eye pain, photophobia, abnormal lacrimation. **Otic:** Tinnitus, earache. **Body as a whole:** Fatigue/malaise, edema, weight gain/loss, pain, fever, rigors, infection, pallor, hot flushes, gout, allergic reaction. **Miscellaneous:** Facial edema, thirst, taste perversion, parosmia.

OVERDOSE MANAGEMENT

Symptoms: Hypotension. *Treatment:* IV fluids.

HOW SUPPLIED

Tablets: 1 mg, 2 mg, 4 mg, 8 mg; ***Tablets, Extended-Release:*** 4 mg, 8 mg.

DOSAGE

TABLETS

Hypertension.

Adults: initial, 1 mg once daily at bedtime; **then,** depending on the response (client's standing BP both 2–6 hr and 24 hr after a dose), the dose may be increased to 2 mg/day, and then 4 mg, 8 mg, and 16 mg (maximum), if needed to control BP.

Benign prostatic hyperplasia.

Initial: 1 mg once daily in the morning or evening. **Maintenance:** Depending on the urodynamics and symptoms, dose may be increased to 2 mg daily and then 4 or 8 mg once daily (maximum recommended dose). The recommended titration interval is 1–2 weeks.

TABLETS, EXTENDED-RELEASE

Benign prostatic hyperplasia.

Initial: 4 mg once daily with breakfast. Depending on the response and tolerability, the dose may be increased to 8 mg, the maximum recommended dose. Titrate at intervals of 3–4 weeks. If administration is discontinued for several days, restart therapy using the 4 mg daily dose.

NURSING IMPLICATIONS

Do not confuse Cardura with Ridaura (gold-containing anti-inflammatory), Cardene (Ca channel blocker), or with Coumadin (warfarin, an anticoagulant).

IMPLEMENTATION/ADMINISTRATION/STORAGE

1. **To minimize the possibility of severe hypotension, limit initial dosage to 1 mg/day.**

2. Increasing the dose higher than 4 mg/day increases the possibility of severe syncope, postural dizziness, vertigo, and postural hypotension.
3. If switching from immediate-release to extended-release tablets, start therapy with 4 mg once daily. Before starting therapy with extended-release tablets, the final evening dose of the immediate-release tablets should not be taken.
4. Store from 15–30°C (59–86°F).

ASSESSMENT

1. Note reasons for therapy, onset and characteristics of S&S, other agents trialed/outcome.
2. List drugs prescribed to ensure none interact especially therapy for ED.
3. Assess supine and standing BP at 2 to 6 hr and 24 hr after dosing.
4. With BPH, score severity and symptoms.
5. Document changes in urinary symptoms, such as dribbling, frequency, hesitancy, nocturia, volume, weak stream.
6. Monitor BP, I&O, Wt, ECG, CBC, renal and LFTs.

CLIENT/FAMILY TEACHING

1. Take once daily; do not stop abruptly. May take first dose at bedtime to minimize side effects. Swallow ER tablets whole; do not chew, divide, cut, or crush them. May take ER tablets with breakfast.
2. Driving and hazardous tasks should be avoided for 24 hr after first dose until effects realized; use caution, may experience dizziness and fainting.
3. Rise slowly to a sitting position before attempting to stand to prevent ↓ BP. This may occur 2–6 hr after a dose.
4. Record BP and weight; note swelling of hands/feet. Dosage may be increased every 2 weeks for high BP and every 1 to 2 weeks for prostate enlargement. Report any sustained erections.
5. Continue diet, exercise, weight control, to assist in BP control as well as salt and ETOH restrictions, and smoking cessation.
6. Keep all F/U to assess response and for adverse SE.

OUTCOMES/EVALUATE

- ↓ BP
- ↓ S&S of BPH/nocturia

Doxepin hydrochloride

(**DOX**-eh-pin)

Classification(s): Antidepressant, tricyclic

Pregnancy Category: C

RX: Prudoxin Cream 5%, Silenor, Sinequan, Zonalon.

✦ **Rx:** Apo-Doxepin.

SEE ALSO ***ANTIDEPRESSANTS, TRICYCLIC.***

INDICATIONS/USES

PO. (1) Psychoneurotic clients with depression or anxiety. (2) Depression or anxiety due to alcoholism (do not give concomitantly with alcohol). (3) Psychotic depressive disorders with associated anxiety, including involutional depression and manic-depressive disorders. (4) Depression or anxiety associated with organic disease. (5) Insomnia characterized by difficulty with sleep maintenance (Silenor only). *NOTE:* The symptoms of psychoneurosis that are most responsive include anxiety, tension, depression, somatic symptoms and concerns, sleep disturbances, guilt, lack of energy, fear, apprehension, and worry.

Topical. Dermatologic disorders including chronic urticaria, angioedema, atopic dermatitis, lichen simplex chronicus in adults, and nocturnal pruritus due to atopic eczema.

ACTION/KINETICS

Action

Metabolized to the active metabolite, desmethyldoxepin. Moderate anticholinergic effects and orthostatic hypotension; high sedative effects.

Pharmacokinetics

Peak plasma levels: 2–4 hr. **Therapeutic plasma levels of both doxepin and desmethyldoxepin:** 100–200 ng/mL. **Time to reach steady state:** 2–8 days. **t½:** 8–24 hr. Significant first-pass effect. Metabolized in the liver; desmethyldoxepin is an active metabolite.

CONTRAINDICATIONS

Use in children less than 12 years of age. Glaucoma or a tendency for urinary retention. Use with or immediately after MAOIs.

SPECIAL CONCERNS

Antidepressants increase the risk of suicidal thinking and behavior (suicidality) in short-term studies in children, adolescents, and young adults with major depressive disorders and other psychiatric disorders. Anyone considering the use of doxepin or any other antidepressant in a child, adolescent, or young adult must balance this risk with the clinical need. Clients who are started on therapy should be observed closely for clinical worsening, suicidality, or unusual changes in behavior. Families and caregivers should be advised of the need for close observation and communication with the prescriber. Doxepine is not approved for use in pediatric clients. Analysis of short-term (4–16 weeks) placebo-controlled trials in children and adolescents with major depressive disorder, obsessive-compulsive disorder, or other psychiatric disorders have revealed a greater risk of adverse reactions representing suicidal thinking or behavior during the first few months of treatment in those receiving antidepressants. The average risk of such reactions in such clients receiving antidepressants was 4%, twice the placebo risk of 2%. No suicides occurred in these trials.

- **Use with caution with a history of urinary retention, narrow-angle glaucoma, or increased IOP.**
- **Hyperthyroid clients may manifest CV toxicity, including arrhythmias.**
- **Safety not determined in pregnancy.**
- **Possible cross sensitivity to amoxapine.**
- **Use with caution during lactation.**

SIDE EFFECTS

Most Common

Drowsiness, dry mouth, blurred vision, constipation, urinary retention, sweating, tachycardia, weight gain/loss, orthostatic hypotension.

See also *Antidepressants, Tricyclic* for a complete list of possible side effects.

- **After systemic use**

Sedation, decreased libido, extrapyramidal symptoms, dermatitis, pruritus, fatigue, weight gain, edema, paresthesia, breast engorgement, insomnia, tremor, chills, tinnitus, hypomania/mania, and photophobia.

- **After topical use**

Burning, stinging, drowsiness, dry mouth.

HOW SUPPLIED

Capsules: 10 mg, 25 mg, 50 mg, 75 mg, 100 mg, 150 mg; ***Cream:*** 5%; ***Oral Concentrate:*** 10 mg/mL; ***Tablets:*** 3 mg, 6 mg.

DOSAGE

CAPSULES; ORAL CONCENTRATE

Antidepressant, mild to moderate anxiety or depression.

Adults, initial: 25 mg 3 times per day (up to 150 mg can be given at bedtime); **then,** adjust dosage to individual response (usual optimum dosage: 75–150 mg/day). **Geriatric clients, initially:** 25–50 mg/day; dose can be increased as needed and tolerated.

More severe anxiety or depression.

Initial: 50 mg 3 times per day; **then,** gradually increase to 300 mg per day, if needed. Additional effects rarely obtained using doses over 300 mg/day. Although the optimal antidepressant effects may take 2 to 3 weeks, the antianxiety effect is evident rapidly.

Mild symptomatology or emotional symptoms associated with organic disease.

25–50 mg/day.

CREAM, 5%

Dermatological disorders.

Apply thin film 4 times per day with at least a 3–4 hr interval between applications.

TABLETS

Insomnia characterized by difficulty with sleep maintenance.

Adults: 6 mg within 30 min of bedtime. A lower dose of 3 mg may be used in some clients, if clinically indicated (e.g., geriatric clients).

NURSING IMPLICATIONS

Do not confuse doxepin with Doxapram (an analeptic), doxycycline (antibiotic), or doxazosin (antiadrenergic drug). Do not confuse Sinequan with saquinavir (antiviral) or with Singulair (an antiasthmatic).

IMPLEMENTATION/ADMINISTRATION/STORAGE

1. **Dilute oral concentrate with 4 oz water, milk, or orange, grapefruit, tomato, prune, or pine-**

apple juice just before ingestion. Do not mix concentrate with carbonated beverages or grape juice.

2. For clients on methadone maintenance, concentrate can be mixed with methadone syrup and lemonade, orange juice, water, or sugar water (but not with grape juice).
3. Do not prepare or store bulk dilutions.
4. The antianxiety effect is manifested rapidly; however, it may take 2 to 3 weeks to observe optimum antidepressant effect.
5. The oral concentrate should not be used to treat anxiety.

ASSESSMENT

1. Note type, onset, characteristics of S&S, mental status, and clinical presentation. List other therapy trialed, outcome.
2. Assess depression/anxiety and identify any contributing factors. List all drugs prescribed to ensure none interact.
3. With insomnia, identify sleep patterns.
4. Monitor BP, Wt, CBC, renal and LFTs.

CLIENT/FAMILY TEACHING

1. Take at bedtime to minimize sedative effects. Beneficial antidepressant effects may take up to 3 weeks, whereas antianxiety effects occur more rapidly.
2. Do not perform activities that require mental alertness until drug effects realized; may experience drowsiness/dizziness (should subside after several weeks of therapy). Change positions slowly to prevent sudden drop in BP.
3. Avoid alcohol and any other CNS depressants. Do not stop drug abruptly.
4. Use sunscreen and avoid prolonged sun exposure until tolerance determined to prevent photosensitivity reaction.
5. Keep all F/U to assess response, counselling, and for adverse SE.

OUTCOMES/EVALUATE

- ↓ S&S of anxiety/depression
- Improved sleeping patterns
- Control of neurogenic pain
- Relief of nocturnal pruritus

IV

Doxorubicin hydrochloride, conventional (ADR)

(dox-oh-**ROO**-bih-sin)

Classification(s): Antineoplastic, antibiotic

Pregnancy Category: D

RX: Adriamycin PFS, Adriamycin RDF.

Doxorubicin hydrochloride, liposomal

Pregnancy Category: D

RX: Doxil.

🍁 **Rx:** Caelyx.

SEE ALSO ***ANTINEOPLASTIC AGENTS.***

INDICATIONS/USES

Conventional doxorubicin: To produce regression in the following disseminated cancers: Acute lymphoblastic leukemia, acute myeloblastic leukemia, Wilms' tumor, soft-tissue and osteogenic sarcomas, neuroblastoma; cancer of the breast, ovaries, lungs, bladder, stomach, and thyroid; Hodgkin's disease, malignant lymphoma, and bronchogenic carcinoma (in which the small-cell histologic type is the most responsive compared with other cell types). *Investigational:* Refractory multiple myeloma; endometrial, islet cell, and lung cancers; AIDS-related Kaposi's sarcoma.

Liposomal doxorubicin: (1) AIDS-related Kaposi's sarcoma in clients where the disease has progressed on prior combination therapy or in those who are intolerant of such therapy. (2) Metastatic ovarian cancer in women who have failed or relapsed after cisplatin- or paclitaxel-based chemotherapy. (3) In combination with bortezomib to treat multiple myeloma in those who have not previously received bortezomib and have received at least one prior therapy. *Investigational:* Refractory metastatic breast cancer.

ACTION/KINETICS

Action

Antineoplastic activity may be due to nucleotide base intercalation and cell membrane lipid-binding activity. Intercalation inhibits nucleotide replication and action of DNA and RNA polymerases.

The interaction of doxorubicin with topoisomerase II to form DNA-cleavable complexes is thought to be an important mechanism for the drugs cytocidal activity. Cells treated with doxorubicin appear to manifest characteristic morphologic changes associated with apoptosis or programmed cell death. Apoptosis may be an integral component of the cellular mechanism of action related to therapeutic effects, toxicity, or both.

The liposomal product is produced with surface-bound methoxypolyethylene in order to protect liposomes from detection by mononuclear phagocytes and to increase blood circulation time. It is believed the liposomes are able to penetrate altered and often compromised vasculature of tumors.

Pharmacokinetics

Conventional product is rapidly distributed to body tissues. Conventional doxorubicin is significantly bound to tissue and plasma proteins whereas the liposomal product is confined mostly to the vascular fluid and does not bind to plasma proteins. Metabolized in the liver to the active doxorubicinol as well as inactive metabolites, which are excreted mainly through the bile. **t½, doxorubicin, conventional: triphasic:** 12 min (distributive), 3.3 hr, and about 20–48 hr (terminal). **t½, liposomal:** About 55 hr. **Plasma protein binding:** About 75%.

CONTRAINDICATIONS

History of hypersensitivity to conventional or liposomal doxorubicin or their components. Malignant melanoma, cancer of the kidney, large bowel carcinoma, brain tumors and metastases to the CNS (not responsive to doxorubicin therapy). Initiation of therapy in those with marked myelosuppression induced by previous treatment with other drugs or with radiotherapy. Use in pre-existing heart disease. Previous treatment with complete cumulative doses of doxorubicin, daunorubicin, idarubicin, or other anthracyclines and anthracenes. Lactation. Depressed bone marrow or cardiac disease. IM or SC use.

SPECIAL CONCERNS

■ **Doxorubicin, Conventional.** (1) Severe local tissue necrosis will occur if there is extravasation during administration. On IV administration of doxorubicin, extravasation may occur with or without an accompanying burning or stinging sensation, even if blood returns well on aspiration of the infusion needle. If any signs of extravasation have occurred, the injection or infusion should be immediately terminated and restarted in another vein. If extravasation is suspected, intermittent application of ice to the site for 15 minutes 4 times daily for 3 days may be useful. The benefit of local administration of drugs has not been clearly established. Because of the progressive nature of extravasation reactions, close observation and plastic surgery consultation is recommended. Blistering, ulceration, or persistent pain are indications for wide excision surgery, followed by split-thickness skin grafting. (2) Doxorubicin must not be given by the IM or SC route. (3) Myocardial toxicity manifested in its most severe form by potentially fatal congestive heart failure may occur during therapy or months to years after termination of therapy. The probability of developing impaired myocardial function based on a combined index of signs, symptoms, and decline in left ventricular ejection fraction(LVEF) is estimated to be 1%–2% at a total cumulative dose of 300 mg/m², 3%–5% at a dose of 400 mg/m², 5%–8% at a dose of 450 mg/m², and 6%–20% at 500 mg/m². The risk of developing CHF increases rapidly with increasing total cumulative doses of doxorubicin in excess of 450 mg/m². This toxicity may occur at lower cumulative doses in those with prior mediastinal irradiation or on concurrent cyclophosphamide therapy or with pre-existing heart disease. Pediatric clients are at increased risk for developing delayed cardiotoxicity. (4) Reduce the dose in those with impaired hepatic function. (5) Severe myelosuppression may occur. (6) Give only under the supervision of a physician who is experienced in the use of cancer chemotherapeutic drugs.

Doxorubicin, Liposomal. (1) **Cardiotoxicity.** The use of liposomal doxorubicin may lead to cardiac toxicity. Myocardial damage may lead to CHF and may occur as the total cumulative dose of doxorubicin (conventional or liposomal) approaches 550 mg/m². Cardiac toxicity also may occur at lower cumulative doses in clients with mediastinal irradiation or who concurrent cardiotoxic agents. (2) **Infu-**

sion reactions. Acute infusion-related reactions, sometimes reversible upon terminating or slowing infusions, occurred in up to 10% of clients. Serious and sometimes fatal allergic/ anaphylactoid-like reactions have been reported. Medications/emergency equipment to treat such reactions should be available for immediate use. Administer liposomal doxorubicin at an initial rate of 1 mg/min to minimize the risk of infusion reactions. (3) Severe myelosuppression may occur. (4) Reduce the dose in those with impaired hepatic function. (5) Accidental substitution of liposomal doxorubicin for conventional doxorubicin has resulted in severe side effects. Do not substitute liposomal doxorubicin for conventional doxorubicin on a mg-per-mg basis. ■

- **Use with caution in necrotizing colitis.**
- **Liposomal doxorubicin may potentiate the toxicity of other anticancer therapies, such as exacerbation of cyclophosphamide-induced hemorrhagic cystitis, enhancement of hepatotoxicity of 6-mercaptopurine, and radiation-induced toxicity to the liver, mucosae, myocardium, and skin.**
- **Safety and efficacy of the liposomal product not established in children.**

SIDE EFFECTS

Most Common

Conventional: N&V, diarrhea, anorexia, alopecia, rash, hoarseness, red color to urine/sweat/ tears, opportunistic infections (candidiasis, cytomegalovirus, herpes simplex, ***Pneumocystis carinii*** pneumonia, mycobacterium avium).
Liposomal: Palmar-plantar skin eruptions, neutropenia, thrombocytopenia, anemia, asthenia, alopecia, rash, abdominal pain, anorexia, N&V, constipation, diarrhea, dyspepsia, stomatitis, dyspnea, pharyngitis, fever, fatigue, mucous membrane disorder, pain/back pain, infection.

See also *Antineoplastic Agents* for a complete list of potential side effects. Side effects listed are for both conventional and liposomal products. **CV:** Potentially fatal ***CHF, including acute left ventricular failure; cardiac arrest***, deep thrombophlebitis, hypotension, tachycardia, vasodilation, chest pain, bundle branch block, palpitation, thrombophlebitis, thrombosis, ventricular arrhythmia. **Infusion reactions** (liposomal product): Flushing, fever, SOB, facial swelling, headache, chills, chest/back pain, tightness in chest and throat, hypotension, tachycardia, pruritus, rash, cyanosis, syncope, ***bronchospasm, asthma, apnea, anaphylaxis***. **Neurologic:** Peripheral neurotoxicity (e.g., local-regional sensory or motor disturbances), ***seizures***, coma. **CNS:** Dizziness, headache, depression, somnolence, neuralgia, paresthesia, dysesthesia. **GI**: N&V, abdominal pain, mucositis (stomatitis, esophagitis—may cause ulceration), anorexia, diarrhea, dyspepsia, dysphagia, esophagitis, ileus, mouth ulceration, oral moniliasis, rectal bleeding, hepatitis. ***Ulceration and necrosis of the colon***. **Dermatologic**: Reversible complete alopecia, rash, acne, dry skin, itching, exfoliative dermatitis, fungal dermatitis, furunculosis, herpes simplex, herpes zoster, maculopapular rash, pruritus, skin discoloration, vesiculobullous rash, hyperpigmentation of nail beds and dermal creases (especially in children), onycholysis, recall of skin reaction to prior radiotherapy, palmar-plantar erythrodysesthesia (swelling, pain, erythema, and desquamation of the skin on the hands and feet). Severe cellulitis, vesication, and tissue necrosis if the drug is extravasated. Erythematous streaking along the vein next to injection site. Burning or stinging indicative of perivenous infiltration. **Respiratory:** Increased cough, dyspnea, pharyngitis, epistaxis, pneumonia, rhinitis, sinusitis, ***pulmonary embolism*** (rare). ***GU:*** Hematuria, UTI, vaginal moniliasis. **Hypersensitivity**: Fever, chills, urticaria, cross-sensitivity with lincomycin, ***anaphylaxis***. **Hematologic**: Myelosuppression, neutropenia, anemia, thrombocytopenia, ecchymosis, secondary acute myeloid leukemia with or without a preleukemic phase. **Ophthalmic**: Conjunctivitis, lacrimation, dry eyes. **Body as a whole:** Asthenia, infection, chills, dehydration, taste perversion, muscle spasms, weight loss, cryptococcosis, moniliasis, ***sepsis***, mucous membrane disorder.

LABORATORY TEST CONSIDERATIONS

↑ Alkaline phosphatase, ALT. Hyperbilirubinemia, hypercalcemia, hypokalemia, hyponatremia.

OVERDOSE MANAGEMENT

Symptoms: Mucositis, leukopenia, thrombocytopenia, pancytopenia. Increased risk of ***cardiomyopathy*** and subsequent ***CHF*** with chronic overdosage. *Treatment:* If the client is myelosuppressed, hospitalization, antibiotics, and platelet and granulocyte transfusions may be necessary. Treat symptoms of mucositis. Treat doxorubicin-induced CHF with digitalis preparations, diuretics, after load reducers (such as angiotensin I converting enzyme [ACE] inhibitors), low salt diet, and bed rest.

DRUG INTERACTIONS

Actinomycin-D / Acute "recall" pneumonitis in pediatric clients
Ciprofloxacin/other quinolones / Liposomal doxorubicin ↓ PO absorption of quinolones
Cyclophosphamide / ↑ Risk of hemorrhagic cystitis; also, potentiation of cardiotoxicity due to both drugs
Cyclosporine / ↑ Doxorubicin levels R/T ↓ metabolism → more profound and prolonged hematologic toxicity
Digoxin / ↓ Digoxin plasma levels R/T ↓ absorption
6-Mercaptopurine / ↑ Risk of hemorrhagic cystitis
Paclitaxel / ↓ Doxorubicin clearance → more profound neutropenic and stomatitis episodes
Phenobarbital / ↑ Elimination of doxorubicin R/T ↑ metabolism
Phenytoin / Possible ↓ phenytoin levels; monitor phenytoin levels and adjust dose if necessary
Progesterone / More pronounced doxorubicin-induced neutropenia and thrombocytopenia
Radiation / ↑ Radiation-induced toxicity to the myocardium, mucosa, skin, and liver
Streptozocin / Possible inhibition of doxorubicin hepatic metabolism; also, ↑ neutropenia and thrombocytopenia
Verapamil / Possible ↑ initial peak doxorubicin levels in the heart → ↑ incidence and severity of degenerative changes in cardiac muscle resulting in shorter survival
Zidovudine / ↓ Antiviral activity of zidovudine

HOW SUPPLIED

Conventional. ***Injection:*** 2 mg/mL; ***Powder for Injection, Lyophilized:*** 10 mg, 20 mg, 50 mg, 150 mg.
Liposomal. ***Injection, Suspension, Liposomal Concentrate:*** 20 mg/ 10 mL (2 mg/mL), 50 mg/ 30 mL (1.67 mg/mL).

DOSAGE

Conventional Doxorubicin

IV ONLY

Various cancers (see Indications/Uses).

Adults, highly individualized: 60–75 mg/m² as a single injection q 21 days. Use the lower dose for clients with inadequate marrow reserves due to old age, prior therapy, or neoplastic marrow infiltration. The most common dosage when used with other chemotherapeutic agents is 40–60 mg/m² given as a single IV injection q 21 to 28 days.

Liposomal Doxorubicin

IV ONLY

Acquired-immune-deficiency-syndrome-related Kaposi's sarcoma.

Adults: 20 mg/m² over 30 min once q 3 weeks, as long as the client responds satisfactorily and tolerates the drug. Use an initial rate of 1 mg/min to minimize the risk of infusion-related reactions. If no infusion-related side effects occur, increase the infusion rate to complete administration of the drug over 1 hr. For clients with hepatic dysfunction, use the same dosing schedule as conventional doxorubicin.

Metastatic ovarian carcinoma.

Adults: 50 mg/m² at an initial rate of 1 mg/min. If no adverse effects occur, increase the rate of infusion to complete administration in 1 hr. Give q 4 weeks as long as the client does not progress, shows no signs of cardiotoxicity, and continues to tolerate the drug. A minimum of 4 courses is recommended.

Multiple myeloma.

Give bortezomib at a dose of 1.3 mg/m² as an IV bolus on days 1, 4, 8, and 11 every 3 weeks. Administer liposomal doxorubicin at a dose of 30 mg/m² as a 1 hr IV infusion on day 4 following bortezomib. With the first liposomal doxorubicin dose, infuse at an initial rate of 1 mg/min to minimize infusion reactions. If no infusion reactions occur, increase the infusion rate to complete drug administration over 1 hr. Clients may be treated for up to 8 cycles, until disease progression or the occurrence of unacceptable side effects.

NURSING IMPLICATIONS

Do not confuse doxorubicin with daunorubicin (also an antineoplastic). Also, do not confuse Adriamycin with Aredia (bone growth regulator).

IMPLEMENTATION/ADMINISTRATION/STORAGE

1. IV Use reduced dosage of both conventional and liposomal doxorubicin in clients with hepatic dysfunction, depending on serum bilirubin level. If bilirubin is 1.2–3 mg/100 mL, give 50% of usual dose; if it is greater than 3 mg/100 mL, give 25% of usual dose.
2. Initiate while hospitalized. Give by slow IV into the tubing of a running NaCl or D5W infusion attached to a butterfly needle inserted into a large vein. Avoid veins over joints or in extremities with compromised venous or lymphatic drainage. Although infusion rate depends on vein size, do not administer in less than 3 to 5 min. Local erythematous streaking along the vein and facial flushing may be signs of too rapid an administration. Perivenous infiltration may be manifested by burning or stinging; immediately terminate the infusion and restart in another vein.
3. Do not substitute liposomal doxorubicin for conventional doxorubicin hydrochloride on a mg to mg basis. Accidental substitution has resulted in severe adverse reactions.
4. Reconstitute conventional drug with NaCl injection to give a final concentration of 2 mg/mL (e.g., dilute 10 mg vial with 5 mL, 20 mg vial with 10 mL, the 50 mg vial with 25 mL, and the 150 mg vial with 75 mL of 0.9% NaCl) and administer over 3–5 min. After adding the NaCl injection, shake the vial to dissolve the contents. The reconstituted solution is stable for 7 days at room temperature and 15 days if stored at 2–8°C (36–46°F). Protect from exposure to sunlight; discard any unused solution from the 10 mg, 20 mg, or 50 mg single-dose vials. Discard any unused solution from the multiple-dose vial beyond the recommended storage times.
5. The liposomal product is diluted, up to 90 mg, in 250 mL of D5W prior to administration. Dosages higher than 90 mg should be diluted in 500 mL of D5W prior to administration. Aseptic technique must be strictly followed as the product has no preservative or bacteriostatic agent. The product is a translucent, red liposomal dispersion. Do not use in-line filters. If the powder or solution comes in contact with the skin or mucous membranes, wash with soap and water thoroughly.
6. **Do not** administer SC or IM because severe necrosis of tissue may result. To minimize danger of extravasation, inject as directed. Monitor carefully; stinging, burning, or edema may indicate extravasation. Stop infusion, and change sites to avoid tissue necrosis.
7. Be prepared with an injectable corticosteroid for local infiltration and flood site with NSS. Examine area frequently for ulceration, which may necessitate early wide excision followed by plastic surgery.
8. Do not give liposomal product as a bolus injection or as undiluted solution. Rapid infusion may increase risk of infusion-related events. Have emergency equipment and medication available for immediate use in the event of serious, life-threatening symptoms.
9. Check package insert carefully for recommended dosage modifications for liposomal doxorubicin in clients with palmar-plantar erythrodysesthesia, hematologic toxicity, or stomatitis.
10. The functional properties of the liposomal product may differ significantly from the conventional product.
11. Store conventional doxorubicin powder from 15–30°C (59–86°F) protected from light. Store conventional doxorubicin solution from 2–8°C (36–46°F) protected from light.
12. Store unopened vials of the liposomal product from 2–8°C (36–46°F). Refrigerate diluted liposomal doxorubicin at 2–8°C (36–46°F), and administer within 24 hr. Short-term freezing (less than 1 month) should not affect liposomal product.
13. COMPATIBILITY Conventional drug with NaCl; liposomal product with D5W.
14. INCOMPATIBILITY Do not mix conventional doxorubicin with heparin or fluorouracil; a precipitate may form. Mixing with aminophylline or 5-FU will result in a change from red to blue-purple indicating decomposition. Do not mix liposomal doxorubicin with other drugs, and do not use with any diluent other than D5W. Liposomal doxorubicin is a translucent, red, liposomal dispersion.

ASSESSMENT

1. Note reasons for therapy, onset, characteristics of S&S; list other agents/therapies trialed.

2. Observe for cardiac arrhythmias, ST segment depression, sinus tachycardia, and/or respiratory difficulties indicative of cardiac toxicity. Have dexrazoxane available to prevent drug-induced cardiomyopathy. Monitor for late-onset (up to 6 mo) CHF.
3. Administer antiemetics 30–45 min before therapy and ATC as needed.
4. Monitor VS and I&O; encourage fluid intake of 2–3 L/day. Anticipate allopurinol administration and alkalinization of urine to decrease urate stone formation.
5. Assess radionuclide left ventricular ejection fraction. Monitor ECG and systolic EF as the maximum cumulative lifetime dose approaches.
6. Hospitalize during at least the first phase of treatment.
7. Monitor CBC, uric acid, potassium, calcium, phosphate, renal and LFTs; drug may cause granulocyte toxicity. Nadir: 10–14 days; recovery: 21 days.

CLIENT/FAMILY TEACHING

1. If medication reactivates previous radiotherapy damage, such as erythema, edema, and desquamation, should resolve after 7 days.
2. Consume 2–3 L/day of fluids. Avoid foods with citric acid, hot or rough textures.
3. Report mouth ulcers; inflammation may occur 5–10 days after dose and last for 3–7 days. A special mouth rinse may help control symptoms.
4. May experience increased tearing; avoid rubbing eyes.
5. Urine will turn red-brown for 1–2 days; this is not blood.
6. Nail beds may become discolored.
7. Any hair loss should grow back 2–3 months after therapy.
8. Report any flu-like symptoms; causes severe myelosuppression. Avoid vaccinations.
9. Practice contraception during and for 4 mo after therapy.
10. Keep all F/U to assess response, ECGs/heart function, labs, and for adverse SE.

OUTCOMES/EVALUATE

Inhibition of malignant cell proliferation

IV

Doxycycline anhydrous

(dox-ih-**SYE**-kleen)

Classification(s): Antibiotic, tetracycline

Pregnancy Category: D

RX: Alodox Convenience Kit, NutriDox, Oracea.

Doxycycline calcium

Pregnancy Category: D

RX: Vibramycin.

Doxycycline hyclate

Pregnancy Category: D

RX: Atridox, Doryx, Doxy 100 and 200, Periostat, Vibramycin, Vibra-Tabs.

Rx: Apo-Doxy, Apo-Doxy-Tabs, Doxycin, Nu-Doxycycline.

Doxycycline monohydrate

Pregnancy Category: D

RX: Adoxa, Monodox, Vibramycin.

SEE ALSO *ANTI-INFECTIVES* AND *TETRACYCLINES*.

INDICATIONS/USES

Doxycycline calcium, doxycycline hyclate, and doxycycline monohydrate.

1. Gram-negative organisms, including *Haemophilus ducreyi* (chancroid), *Francisella tularensis* (tularemia), *Yersenia pestis* (plague), *Bartonella bacilliformis* (bartonellosis), *Campylobacter fetus* (fetus infections), *Vibrio cholerae* (cholera), *Brucella* species (with streptomycin) to treat brucellosis, *Calymmatobacterium granulomatis* (granuloma inguinale).
2. *Rickettsiae* (e.g., Rocky Mountain spotted fever, typhus fever and the typhus group, Q fever, rickettsialpox, tick fevers).
3. *Mycoplasma pneumoniae* (e.g., respiratory tract infections).
4. *Chlamydia trachomatis* (e.g., lymphogranuloma venereum, trachoma, inclusion conjunctivitis, uncomplicated urethral, endocervical, or rectal infections).
5. *Chlamydia psittaci* (psittacosis).
6. *Borellia recurrentis* (e.g., relapsing fever).
7. *Ureaplasma urealyticum* (e.g., nongonococcal urethritis).

8. For the following infections following susceptibility testing as resistance has been documented: *Escherichia coli, Enterobacter aerogenes, Acinetobacter* species, *Haemophilus influenzae* (e.g., respiratory tract infections), *Klebsiella* species (e.g., upper and lower respiratory and urinary tract infections), *Streptococcus pneumoniae* (e.g., upper respiratory tract infections), *S. pyogenes* (including skin and skin structure infections), *S. pneumoniae, Mycoplasma pneumoniae* (Eaton agent), *Staphylococcus aureus, Bacteroides,* and *Shigella* species.
9. Alternative therapy for the following infections when penicillin is contraindicated: Uncomplicated gonorrhea due to *Neisseria gonorrhoeae,* syphilis due to *Treponema pallidum,* yaws due to *Treponema pertenue,* listeriosis due to *Listeria monocytogenes,* anthrax due to *Bacillus anthracis,* Vincent's infection due to *Fusobacterium fusiforme,* actinomycosis due to *Actinomyces israelii,* and infections due to *Clostridium* species.
10. Adjunct to amebicides for acute intestinal amebiasis due to *Entamoeba histolytica.*
11. Adjunctive therapy for severe acne.
12. Reduce incidence or progression of anthrax (including inhalational anthrax) following exposure to aerosolized *Bacillus anthracis.*
13. Prophylaxis of malaria due to *Plasmodium falciparum* in short-term travelers (less than 4 months) to areas with chloroquine and/or pyrimethamine-sulfadoxine resistant strains.
14. *Investigational:* Lyme disease, syphilis, pelvic inflammatory disease, epididymitis due to gonococcal or chlamydial infection, sexual assault prophylaxis.

Doxycycline hyclate. (1) Trachoma (infectious agent not always eliminated). (2) Inclusion conjunctivitis (may also be combined with topical drugs). (3) Acute epididymo-orchitis due to *Chlamydia trachomatis.*

Doxycycline monohydrate. Treatment of only inflammatory lesions (papules and pustules) or rosacea in adults.

Dental: (1) Atridox injection for chronic adult periodontitis for a gain in clinical attachment, reduction in probing depth, and reduction in bleeding on probing. (2) Periostat as an adjunct to scaling and root planing to promote attachment level gain and reduce pocket depth in adult periodontitis. (3) Oraxyl as an adjunct to scaling and root planing to promote attachment level gain and reduce pocket depth in those with adult periodontitis.

NOTE: Do not use for streptococcal disease unless organism is susceptible. Tetracyclines are not the drugs of choice to treat any type of staphylococcal infection.

ACTION/KINETICS

Action

Inhibits protein synthesis by binding to the ribosomal 30S subunit. Blocks binding of aminoacyl transfer RNA to the messenger RNA complex, thus inhibiting protein synthesis and cell growth. Cell wall synthesis is not inhibited.

Pharmacokinetics

More slowly absorbed, and thus more persistent, than other tetracyclines. 90–100% absorbed. Preferred for clients with impaired renal function for treating infections outside the urinary tract. Time to maximum levels: 2 hr for hyclate and 2.6 hr for monohydrate each after a 200 mg PO dose. **t½, serum:** 18–22 hr; 40% excreted unchanged in urine. High lipid solubility. **Plasma protein binding:** From 80–95%.

CONTRAINDICATIONS

Prophylaxis of malaria in pregnant individuals and in children less than 8 years old. Use during pregnancy (may stunt fetal growth) and in children up to 8 years of age (tetracycline may cause permanent discoloration of the teeth). Lactation.

SPECIAL CONCERNS

Safety for IV use in children less than 8 years of age not established.

SIDE EFFECTS

Most Common

Anorexia, N&V, diarrhea, dizziness, headache, rashes.

See *Tetracyclines* for complete listing of possible side effects.

ADDITIONAL DRUG INTERACTIONS

Barbiturates, carbamazepine, phenytoin / ↓ Doxycycline effect R/T ↑ liver breakdown

Methotrexate / Possible GI and hematologic toxicity after high doses of methotrexate

D

HOW SUPPLIED

Doxycycline anhydrous. *Capsules:* 40 mg (30 mg immediate-release and 10 mg delayed-release); 75 mg; *Powder for Oral Suspension:* 25 mg/5 mL (after reconstitution); *Tablets:* 20 mg (equivalent to 23 mg doxycycline hyclate).
Doxycycline calcium. *Syrup:* 50 mg/5 mL.
Doxycycline hyclate. *Capsules:* 20 mg, 50 mg, 100 mg; *Capsules, Coated Pellets:* 75 mg, 100 mg; *Gel:* 10%; *Powder for Injection, Lyophilized:* 100 mg, 200 mg; *Tablets:* 20 mg, 100 mg; *Tablets, Delayed-Release:* 75 mg, 100 mg, 150 mg, 500 mg.
Doxycycline monohydrate. *Capsules:* 50 mg, 100 mg, 150 mg; *Powder for Oral Suspension:* 25 mg/5 mL (after reconstitution); *Tablets:* 50 mg, 75 mg, 100 mg, 150 mg.

DOSAGE

CAPSULES; CAPSULE, ENTERIC-COATED; IV; ORAL SUSPENSION; SYRUP; TABLETS; TABLETS, DELAYED-RELEASE

Infections.

Adult: First day, 100 mg q 12 hr; **maintenance:** 100 mg/day. For more severe infections (e.g., chronic UTIs), give 100 mg q 12 hr. **Children, over 8 years (45 kg or less): First day,** 4.4 mg/kg in 2 doses; **then,** 2.2–4.4 mg/kg/day in divided doses depending on severity of infection. Children over 45 kg should receive the adult dose.

Uncomplicated gonorrhea in adults (except anorectal infections in men).

Adults: 100 mg twice a day for at least 7 days. Alternatively, 300 mg immediately followed in 1 hr with 300 mg. Give with plenty of water.

Nongonococcal urethritis due to C. trachomatis *or* U. urealyticum.

100 mg PO twice a day for 7 days.

Syphilis, early.

100 mg PO twice a day for 2 weeks (except Doryx). When using Doryx: Give 300 mg/day in divided PO doses for 10 days.

Syphilis, more than 1 year duration.

100 mg PO 2 times per day for 4 weeks (except Adoxa, Doryx, Monodox).

Uncomplicated urethral, endocervical or rectal infections in adults due to C. trachomatis.

100 mg PO twice a day for at least 7 days.

Acute epididymo-orchitis due to N. gonorrhoeae *or* C. trachomatis.

100 mg PO twice a day for at least 10 days.

Pelvic inflammatory disease.

100 mg PO or IV q 12 hr *plus* cefotetan, 2 grams IV, q 12 hr *or* cefoxitin, 2 grams IV, q 6 hr. May discontinue parenteral therapy after 24 hr; continue PO therapy with doxycycline for 14 days.

Epididymitis likely due to gonococcal or chlamydial infection.

100 mg twice a day for 10 days *plus* a single dose of ceftriaxone, 250 mg IM.

Sexual assault prophylaxis.

100 mg twice a day for 7 days plus ceftriaxone and metronidazole.

Prophylaxis of malaria.

Adults: 100 mg PO once daily (except Doryx); **children, over 8 years of age:** 2 mg/kg/day up to 100 mg/day. Begin 1–2 days before travel to endemic area, and continue during travel and for 4 weeks after returning.

Anthrax, inhalation, post-exposure.

Adults and children weighing 45 kg or more: 100 mg q 12 hr for 60 days. **Children, less than 45 kg:** 2.2 mg/kg q 12 hr for 60 days.

Lyme disease.

Tick bite from endemic area: 200 mg once. **Early Lyme disease:** 100 mg twice a day for 14–21 days. **Carditis (first degree AV block):** 100 mg twice a day for 14–21 days. **Facial nerve paralysis:** 100 mg twice a day for 14–21 days. **Arthritis:** 100 mg twice a day for 30–60 days.

Oracea

TABLETS

Inflammatory lesions of rosacea.

40 mg once daily in the morning on an empty stomach, preferably at least 1 hr

before or 2 hr after meals. Oracea contains 30 mg immediate release and 10 mg delayed release anhydrous doxycycline.

Oraxyl

CAPSULES

Adjunct to promote attachment and level gain and to reduce pocket depth in adult periodontitis.

One capsule (20 mg) twice a day, up to 9 months.

Periostat

TABLETS

Adjunct to promote attachment and level gain and to reduce pocket depth in adult periodontitis.

20 mg twice a day following scaling and planing. May be used for up to 9 months. Do not exceed recommended dose.

Atridox

INJECTION

Chronic adult periodontitis.

After preparing the injection (see package insert), keeping the tip near the base of the pocket, express the drug into the pocket until the formulation reaches the top of the gingival margin. Cover the pocket containing doxycycline with either Coe-Pak periodontal dressing or Octyldent dental adhesive.

IV INFUSION ONLY

Infections.

Adults: 200 mg IV on day 1 given in 1 or 2 infusions; **then,** 100–200 mg, depending on severity of condition (give 200 mg in 1 or 2 infusions). **Children, over 8 years of age, up to 45 kg:** 4.4 mg/kg on day 1 in 1 or 2 infusions; **then,** 2.2–4.4 mg/kg given as 1 or 2 infusions, depending on severity of the infection. **Children, over 45 kg:** Use adult dose.

GEL, 10%

Reduce bacteria due to periodontal disease.

Apply to affected area; gel conforms to shape of the periodontal pocket and solidifies. It releases doxycycline for about 7 days.

NURSING IMPLICATIONS

Do not confuse doxycycline with dicyclomine (an anticholinergic/antispasmodic) or doxepin (TCA).

IMPLEMENTATION/ADMINISTRATION/STORAGE

1. When used for streptococcal infections, continue therapy for 10 days.
2. Malaria prophylaxis can begin 1–2 days before travel begins, during travel, and for 4 weeks after leaving the malarial area.
3. The powder for suspension expires 12 months from date of issue.
4. Reconstituted PO solution is stable for 2 weeks when refrigerated.
5. IV Avoid rapid administration. Duration of IV infusion may vary with the dose; usually from 1–4 hr. A recommended minimum infusion time for 100 mg of a 0.5 mg/mL solution is 1 hr. Switch to oral therapy as soon as possible.
6. Continue therapy for at least 24–48 hr after symptoms and fever have subsided.
7. Follow directions on vial for dilution. Concentrations should be no lower than 0.1 mg/mL and no higher than 1.0 mg/mL.
8. During infusion protect solution from light.
9. When diluted with NaCl injection, D5W, Ringer's injection, 10% invert sugar in water, Normosol-M in D5W, Normosol-R in D5W, Plasma-Lyte 56 in D5W, or Plasma-Lyte 148 in D5W, infusion of the solution (about 1 mg/mL) or lower concentrations (not less than 0.1 mg/mL) must be completed within 12 hr after reconstitution to ensure adequate stability.
10. Administer solutions diluted with RL or D5/RL within 6 hr.
11. Reconstituted solutions (0.1–1 mg/mL) may be stored up to 72 hr prior to start of the infusion, if refrigerated and protected from sun or artificial light.
12. COMPATIBILITY 0.9 % NaCl, D5W, D5/RL, RL.
13. INCOMPATIBILITY Administer separately.

ASSESSMENT

1. Note reasons for therapy, onset, characteristics of S&S, culture results clinical presentation and other agents trialed.
2. Check for any allergic/hypersensitivity reactions; note expiration date as expired tetracycline products are nephrotoxic.

3. Monitor VS, cultures, CBC, renal and LFTs.

CLIENT/FAMILY TEACHING

1. May take with food; take caps with full glass of water to prevent esophageal ulceration and remain upright for 45 min. With syrup or oral suspension measure and give prescribed dose using dosing spoon/syringe, or medicine cup.
2. Take either 2 hr before or 2 hr after antacids containing aluminum, calcium, or magnesium, preparations containing iron or zinc, or dairy products (e.g., milk, cheese, ice cream).
3. May cause dizziness, light-headedness, or blurred vision; use caution while performing activities that require mental alertness until drug effects realized.
4. Discard any unused doxycycline by the expiration date noted on the label.
5. Take entire prescription; do not stop if symptoms subside. Stop drug and report if skin rash, hives, itching, SOB, headache, or blurred vision occur.
6. Avoid direct exposure to sunlight and wear protective clothing and sunscreens when exposed to prevent photosensitivity.
7. For malaria prophylaxis take daily, beginning 1 to 2 days prior to arrival in malaria-infected area, while in the malaria-infected area, and for 28 days after leaving the malaria-infected area. Drug is not 100% effective; protective clothing, insect repellents, and bed nets are also needed to help prevent malaria.
8. Women taking oral contraceptives should use nonhormonal forms of contraception during treatment. Drug may make birth control pills less effective. With STDs advise that partner be tested and treated. Use condoms until medically cleared.
9. Not for use in children under 8 y.o. or during the last half of pregnancy due to the potential for permanent tooth discoloration during tooth development stages.
10. With Periostat:
    - Will take daily for up to 9 months to help treat periodontitis
    - Dose is too small to treat infections–do not use for that purpose
    - Used q 12 hr so allow at least 1 hr prior to or 2 hr after meals
11. With subgingival injection: avoid any mechanical oral hygiene procedure (e.g., tooth-brushing, flossing) on any treated areas for 7 days after application.
12. Keep all F/U visits to assess response, cultures, or for adverse SE.

OUTCOMES/EVALUATE

- Resolution of infection
- Promote gum attachment, and reduce pocket depth
- Prophylaxis of malaria caused by *Plasmodium falciparum*/anthrax (including inhalational anthrax)/severe acne

Dronedarone

(**DROE**-**NEH**-dah-rone)

Classification(s): Antiarrhythmic agent.

Pregnancy Category: X

RX: Multaq.

INDICATIONS/USES

Reduce the risk of CV hospitalization in clients with paroxysmal or persistent atrial fibrillation or atrial flutter, with a recent episode of atrial fibrillation/atrial flutter and associated with CV risk factors (i.e., >70 years of age, hypertension, diabetes, prior CVA, left atrial diameter 50 mm or more or left ventricular ejection fraction less than 40%), who are in sinus rhythm or who will be cardioverted.

ACTION/KINETICS

Action

Mechanism is unknown. Has antiarrhythmic properties belonging to all four Vaughan-William classes; the contribution of each of these activities to the clinical effect is not known.

Pharmacokinetics

Peak plasma levels: 3–6 hr. **Steady state**: 4–8 days after repeated administration of 400 mg twice a day. Bioavailability is increased by food; absolute bioavailability of about 4% but increases to about 15% when given with a high-fat meal. Extensively metabolized by CYP3A. Most excreted in the feces (84%) with a small amount excreted in the urine (6%). **t½, elimination:** 13–19 hr.

CONTRAINDICATIONS

NYHA class IV heart failure or NYHA class II or III heart failure with a recent decompensation requiring hospitalization or referral to a specialized heart failure clinic. Second- or third-degree heart AV block or sick sinus syndrome (except when used in conjunction with a functioning pacemaker); bradycardia less than 50 beats/min; concomitant use of strong CYP3A inhibitors (e.g., clarithromycin, cyclosporine, itraconazole, ketoconazole, nefazodone, ritonavir, telithromycin, voriconazole); concomitant use of drugs or herbal products that prolong the QT interval and might increase the risk of torsades de pointes (e.g., phenothiazines, antipsychotics, tricyclic antidepressants, certain oral macrolide antibiotics, class I and III antiarrhythmics); QTc Bazett interval 500 milliseconds or more or PR interval more than 280 milliseconds; severe hepatic impairment; pregnancy; lactation.

SPECIAL CONCERNS

■ (1) Dronedarone is contraindicated in clients with New York Heart Association (NYHA) class IV heart failure or NYHA class II to III heart failure with a recent decompensation requiring hospitalization or referral to a specialized heart failure clinic. (2) In a placebo-controlled study in clients with severe heart failure requiring recent hospitalization or referral to a specialized heart failure clinic for worsening symptoms, clients given dronedarone had a greater than 2-fold increase in mortality. Do not give such clients dronedarone. ■

Safety and efficacy not established in children less than 18 years of age.

SIDE EFFECTS

Most Common

Diarrhea, asthenia, nausea, rashes.

GI: Diarrhea, N&V, abdominal pain, dyspeptic signs and symptoms, dysgeusia. **CV:** Bradycardia, QT prolongation. **Dermatologic:** Rashes, including generalized, macular, maculopapular, erythematous; pruritus, eczema, dermatitis, allergic dermatitis. **Body as a whole:** Asthenia, photosensitivity reactions.

LABORATORY TEST CONSIDERATIONS

↑ Serum creatinine levels; reaches a plateau in 7 days (use the increased value as a new baseline).

OVERDOSE MANAGEMENT

Treatment: Monitor cardiac rhythm and BP. Provide supportive treatment based on symptoms. There is no specific antidote.

DRUG INTERACTIONS

NOTE: It is possible an additive effect can occur with other drugs that prolong the QT interval.

Amiodarone / Potential risk of torsades-de-pointes-type ventricular tachycardia; use together contraindicated

Beta-blockers (metoprolol, propranolol) / ↑ Frequency of bradycardia; possible ↑ dronedarone exposure; give lower initial beta-blocker dosage and ↑ only after ECG verification of good tolerance

Calcium channel blockers (e.g., diltiazem, verapamil) / Possible ↑ dronedarone and calcium channel blocker exposure; give lower initial calcium channel blocker dosage and ↑ only after ECG verification of good tolerance

Carbamazepine / Possible ↓ dronedarone exposure; use together contraindicated

Cyclosporine / Possible ↑ dronedarone exposure R/T inhibition of CYP3A

Digoxin / Potentiation of the electrophysiologic effects of dronedarone; ↓ digoxin dose by 50%; monitor serum levels and observe for toxicity

Disopyramide / Potential risk of torsades-de-pointes-type ventricular tachycardia; use together contraindicated

Dofetilide / Potential risk of torsades-de-pointes-type ventricular tachycardia; use together contraindicated

Flecainide / Potential risk of torsades-de-pointes-type ventricular tachycardia; use together contraindicated

Itraconazole / Possible ↑ dronedarone exposure R/T inhibition of CYP3A

Ketoconazole / Possible ↑ dronedarone exposure R/T inhibition of CYP3A

Macrolide antibiotics (e.g., clarithromycin, telithromycin) / Possible ↑ dronedarone exposure R/T inhibition of CYP3A

Midazolam / Possible ↑ plasma levels of midazolam; dosage adjustment may be needed

Nefazodone / Possible ↑ dronedarone exposure R/T inhibition of CYP3A

Phenobarbital / Possible ↓ dronedarone exposure; use together contraindicated

Phenothiazine antipsychotics (e.g., chlorpromazine, thioridazine) / Potential risk of torsades-de-pointes-type ventricular tachycardia; use together contraindicated

Pimozide / Possible ↑ plasma levels of pimozide; dosage adjustment may be needed

Propafenone / Potential risk of torsades-de-pointes-type ventricular tachycardia; use together contraindicated
Quinidine / Potential risk of torsades-de-pointes-type ventricular tachycardia; use together contraindicated
Rifampin / Possible ↓ dronedarone exposure; use together contraindicated
Ritonavir / Possible ↑ dronedarone exposure R/T inhibition of CYP3A
Selective serotonin reuptake inhibitors (fluoxetine) / Possible ↑ plasma levels of SSRIs; dosage adjustment may be needed
Simvastatin / ↑ Simvastatin exposure
Sirolimus / Possible ↑ plasma levels of sirolimus; dosage adjustment may be needed
Sotalol / Potential risk of torsades-de-pointes-type VT; use together contraindicated
H ***St. John's wort*** / Possible ↓ dronedarone exposure; use together contraindicated
Tacrolimus / Possible ↑ plasma levels of tacrolimus; dosage adjustment may be needed
Tricyclic antidepressants (e.g., amitriptyline) / Potential risk of torsades-de-pointes-type ventricular tachycardia; use together contraindicated; also possible ↑ TCA exposure
Voriconazole / Possible ↑ dronedarone exposure R/T inhibition of CYP3A
Warfarin / Possible ↑ S-warfarin exposure; monitor INR

HOW SUPPLIED

Tablets: 400 mg.

DOSAGE

TABLETS

Paroxysmal or persistent atrial fibrillation or atrial flutter.

Adults, usual: 400 mg twice a day with the morning and evening meals.
NOTE: Treatment with class I or III antiarrhythmics (e.g., amiodarone, disopyramide, dofetilide, flecainide, propafenone, quinidine, or sotalol) or drugs that are strong inhibitors of CYP3A4 (e.g., ketoconazole) must be discontinued before taking dronedarone.

NURSING IMPLICATIONS

IMPLEMENTATION/ADMINISTRATION/STORAGE

1. Potassium levels should be within the normal range prior to dronedarone administration and maintained in the normal range during administration.
2. Premenopausal women who have not undergone a hysterectomy or oophorectomy must use effective contraception while using dronedarone.
3. Store from 15–30°C (59–86°F).

ASSESSMENT

1. Note reasons for therapy, frequency of hospitalizations, other agents trialed and outcome.
2. List drugs prescribed to ensure none interact.
3. Identify CV risk factors (i.e., >70 years old, hypertension, prior CVA, diabetes, left atrial diameter at least 50 mm or LVEF less than 40%).
4. Determine if heart failure develops or worsens. Assess for development of liver injury.
5. Obtain ECG, assess rhythm, note NYHA class, assess for CHF, QT prolongation, heart block;
6. Note last hospitalization, treatments and any referrals to heart failure clinics.
7. Monitor ECG, BP, K^+, Mg^{++}, renal and LFTs.

CLIENT/FAMILY TEACHING

1. Take each dose twice a day with food; avoid grapefruit juice.
2. Report any S&S of worsening heart failure such as rapid weight gain (>3 lb/day or >5 lb/week), swelling of feet or legs, ↑ shortness of breath.
3. May experience N&V, stomach pain, diarrhea, fatigue or skin changes; report if persistent or bothersome.
4. Practice reliable contraception and avoid pregnancy during therapy.
5. Record HR, BP and weight for provider review.
6. Keep all F/U to assess response, labs, ECG, and for adverse SE.

OUTCOMES/EVALUATE

↓ Risk of hospitalization with paroxysmal AFib/flutter

Duloxetine hydrochloride

(doo-**LOX**-eh-teen)

Classification(s): Antidepressant, selective serotonin and norepinephrine reuptake inhibitor

Pregnancy Category: C (D if used during the second half of pregnancy)

RX: Cymbalta.

INDICATIONS/USES

(1) Acute and maintenance treatment of major depressive disorder. (2) Management of neuropathic pain associated with diabetic peripheral neuropathy. (3) Acute treatment of generalized anxiety disorder. (4) Management of fibromyalgia. (5) Management of chronic musculoskeletal pain. *Investigational:* Stress urinary incontinence.

ACTION/KINETICS

Action

Mechanism is unknown. Antidepressant and pain inhibitory effect believed to be related to potentiation of serotonergic and noradrenergic activity in the CNS. Potent inhibitor of neuronal reuptake of serotonin and norepinephrine. Slight anticholinergic, orthostatic hypotensive, and sedative effects.

Pharmacokinetics

Well absorbed after PO administration. **Maximum plasma levels:** 6 hr (there is a 2-hr lag until absorption begins). Food delays the time to peak levels from 6 to 10 hr. There is a 3-hr delay in absorption and a one-third increase in apparent clearance after an evening dose compared with a morning dose. **Time to steady state:** 3 days. Undergoes extensive metabolism by the liver isoenzymes, CYP2D6 and CYP1A2. **t½, elimination:** About 12 hr (range: 8–17 hr) hr. Excreted in both the urine (70%) and feces (20%). **Plasma protein binding:** More than 90%.

CONTRAINDICATIONS

Use in end-stage renal disease or severe renal impairment (C_{CR} less than 30 mL/min), any hepatic insufficiency, chronic liver disease, substantial alcohol use, uncontrolled narrow-angle glaucoma, or concomitant use in those taking MAOIs. Lactation.

SPECIAL CONCERNS

(1) **Suicidality and antidepressant drugs.** Antidepressants increased the risk compared with placebo of suicidal thinking and behavior (suicidality) in children, adolescents, and young adults in short-term studies of major depressive disorder and other psychiatric disorders. Anyone considering the use of duloxetine or other antidepressants in a child, adolescent, or young adult must balance this risk with the clinical need. Short-term studies did not show an increase in the risk of suicidality with antidepressants compared with placebo in adults older than 24 years of age; there was a reduction in the risk with antidepressants compared with placebo in adults 65 years of age and older. (2) Depression and certain other psychiatric disorders are themselves associated with increases in the risk of suicide. Appropriately monitor clients of all ages who are started on antidepressant therapy and closely observe clients for clinical worsening, suicidality, or unusual changes in behavior. Advise families and caregivers of the need for close observation and communication with the prescribing health care provider. (3) Duloxetine is not approved for use in children.

- **Adults and children may experience worsening of depression and/or the emergence of suicidal ideation and behavior or unusual changes in behavior, whether or not they are taking antidepressants.**
- **Use with caution in clients with a history of mania, seizure disorder, with controlled narrow-angle glaucoma, and in the elderly.**
- **Use with caution in conditions that may slow gastric emptying (e.g., diabetes) as in extremely acidic conditions; duloxetine, unprotected by the enteric coating, may undergo hydrolysis to form naphthol. Drugs that raise the GI pH may lead to an earlier release of duloxetine.**
- **Safety and efficacy not determined in children and adolescents.**
- **Use during labor and delivery only if the potential benefit justifies the potential risk to the fetus.**

SIDE EFFECTS

Most Common

N&V, somnolence, dizziness, headache, constipation, dry mouth, fatigue, insomnia, decreased appetite, increased sweating, agitation.

Listed are side effects with an incidence of 1% or greater, those identified post-marketing, and those that are life-threatening. **CNS:** Headache, dizziness, fatigue, insomnia, somnolence, asthenia, agitation, tremor, abnormal dreams/nightmares, paresthesia, migraine, anxiety, lethargy, hypesthe-

D

sia, sleep disorder, activation of mania/hypomania, dysgeusia, aggression, anger (especially early in treatment or when treatment discontinued), extrapyramidal disorder, hallucinations, restless legs syndrome, trismus, ***seizures*** (upon treatment discontinuation). **Serotonin syndrome/Neuroleptic malignant-like reaction:** Agitation, coma, hallucinations, hyperthermia, labile BP, tachycardia, hyperreflexia, incoordination, diarrhea, N&V, ***death***. **CV:** Hot flush, palpitations, orthostatic hypotension, syncope; increased risk of bleeding events, including ecchymoses, hematomas, epistaxis, and petechiae to ***hemorrhages*** (especially when used with NSAIDs, warfarin, or other anticoagulants); increased BP and/or HR, ***hypertensive crisis***, supraventricular arrhythmia. **GI:** N&V, dry mouth, constipation, diarrhea, decreased appetite, anorexia, dyspepsia, loose stools, dysgeusia, viral gastroenteritis, abdominal discomfort/pain/tenderness, flatulence, ***hepatic failure***. **GU:** Ejaculation dysfunction/failure/delayed, erectile dysfunction, decreased/loss of libido, abnormal orgasm, anorgasmia, penis disorder, UTI, pollakiuria, urinary hesitancy/retention, gynecologic bleeding. **Dermatologic:** Hyperhidrosis, flushing, rash, pruritus, erythema multiforme, urticaria, ***Stevens-Johnson syndrome***, serious skin reactions. **Musculoskeletal:** Muscle cramps, myalgia, muscle spasms, musculoskeletal pain. **Respiratory**: Nasopharyngitis, cough, influenza, oropharyngeal pain, pharyngolaryngeal pain, URTI, yawning. **Ophthalmic:** Blurred vision, increased risk of mydriasis, glaucoma. **Otic:** Tinnitus after treatment discontinued. **Body as a whole:** Asthenia, chills, rigors, decreased/increased appetite, pyrexia, influenza, seasonal allergy, weight decreased/increased, dehydration, thirst, ***anaphylaxis***, angioneurotic edema, hypersensitivity. **Miscellaneous:** Decreased glycemic control in diabetics, vertigo, yawning.

LABORATORY TEST CONSIDERATIONS

Slight ↑ AST, ALT, CPK, alkaline phosphatase. ↑ WBCs, blood cholesterol, blood creatinine. Hyponatremia, hyperglycemia.

OVERDOSE MANAGEMENT

Symptoms: Serotonin syndrome, somnolence, coma, hyper-/hypotension, syncope, tachycardia, ***seizures***, vomiting, ***death*** (rare and usually with mixed drugs). *Treatment:* Treat serotonin syndrome with cyproheptadine and/or temperature control. Ensure an adequate airway, oxygenation, and ventilation; monitor cardiac rhythm and vital signs. Do not induce vomiting. Gastric lavage with a large-bore orogastric tube with appropriate airway protection, if needed, may be performed soon after ingestion or in symptomatic clients. Activated charcoal may limit duloxetine absorption from the GI tract. Consider the possibility of multiple drug involvement.

DRUG INTERACTIONS

Alcohol (heavy use) / Liver injury manifested by ↑ ALT and total bilirubin; do not use in clients with heavy alcohol use
Antiarrhythmics, type 1C (e.g., flecainide, propafenone) / ↑ Antiarrhythmic plasma levels R/T inhibition of CYP2D6; give together with caution
Aspirin / ↑ Risk of bleeding events (e.g., ecchymoses, hematomas, epistaxis, petechiae, life-threatening hemorrhages)
Beta-adrenergic blockers (e.g., carvedilol, metoprolol, propranolol) / Excessive beta blockade (e.g., bradycardia); possible inhibition of CYP2D6 metabolism of certain beta blockers; monitor cardiac function
Cimetidine / ↑ Duloxetine AUC, C_{max}, and t½ R/T inhibition of the CYP1A2 isoenzyme
Ciprofloxacin / ↑ Duloxetine AUC, C_{max}, and t½ R/T inhibition of the CYP1A2 isoenzyme
CNS drugs (e.g., narcotic analgesics) / Use together with caution
Cyclobenzaprine / Possible serotonin syndrome (e.g., agitation, altered consciousness, ataxia, myoclonus, overactive reflexes, shivering); do not use together
Fluoxetine / ↑ Duloxetine levels R/T inhibition of CYP2D6 isoenzyme
Fluvoxamine / ↑ Duloxetine AUC, C_{max}, and t½ R/T inhibition of the CYP1A2 isoenzyme
Linezolid / Possible serotonin syndrome, including agitation, altered consciousness, ataxia, myoclonus, overactive reflexes, shivering; allow at least 2 weeks between stopping linezolid and starting duloxetine
Lithium / Possible serotonin syndrome (e.g., agitation, altered consciousness, ataxia, myoclonus, overactive reflexes, shivering); do not use together
Methylene blue / ↑ Risk of neurologic symptoms, including serotonin syndrome; do not use together

NSAIDs (e.g., naproxen) / ↑ Risk of bleeding events (e.g., ecchymoses, hematomas, epistaxis, petechiae, life-threatening hemorrhages)
Paroxetine / ↑ Duloxetine levels R/T inhibition of CYP2D6 isoenzyme
Phenelzine / ↑ Risk of serious side effects, including hyperthermia, rigidity, myoclonus, autonomic instability, mental status changes, and death, R/T ↑ levels of serotonin and norepinephrine. Do not use with an MAOI or within at least 14 days of discontinuing an MAOI; allow 5 days after stopping duloxetine before starting an MAO
Phenothiazines (e.g., thioridazine) / Both are metabolized by CYP2D6 → ↑ levels of phenothiazine → life-threatening arrhythmias and sudden death; do not use together
Phenytoin / ↑ Levels of phenytoin R/T displacement from plasma protein binding sites
Quinidine / ↑ Duloxetine levels R/T inhibition of CYP2D6 isoenzyme
Quinolone antibiotics / ↑ Duloxetine AUC, C_{max}, and t½ R/T inhibition of the CYP1A2 isoenzyme
Rasagiline / ↑ Risk of serious side effects, including hyperthermia, rigidity, myoclonus, autonomic instability, mental status changes, and death, R/T ↑ levels of serotonin and norepinephrine. Do not use with an MAOI or within at least 14 days of discontinuing an MAOI; allow 5 days after stopping duloxetine before starting an MAOI
Selective norepinephrine reuptake inhibitors / Possible serotonin syndrome (e.g., agitation, altered consciousness, ataxia, myoclonus, overactive reflexes, shivering); do not use together
Selective serotonin reuptake inhibitors / Possible serotonin syndrome (e.g., agitation, altered consciousness, ataxia, myoclonus, overactive reflexes, shivering); do not use together
Selegiline / ↑ Risk of serious side effects, including hyperthermia, rigidity, myoclonus, autonomic instability, mental status changes, and death, R/T ↑ levels of serotonin and norepinephrine. Do not use with an MAOI or within at least 14 days of discontinuing an MAOI; allow 5 days after stopping duloxetine before starting an MAOI
H ***St. John's wort*** / ↑ Sedative-hypnotic effects; also possible serotonin syndrome; do not use together
Sympathomimetics (e.g., amphetamine, dextroamphetamine, phentermine) / ↑ Sensitivity to sympathomimetic effects and ↑ risk of serotonin syndrome; if coadministration cannot be avoided, monitor for ↑ CNS effects; adjust therapy as needed
Terbinafine / ↑ Duloxetine levels R/T inhibition of CYP2D6 isoenzyme
Theophylline / ↑ Theophylline AUC; not expected to be clinically significant; monitor clinical response
Thioridazine / Both are metabolized by CYP2D6 → ↑ risk of serious arrhythmias and sudden death; do not use together
Tramadol / Possible serotonin syndrome (e.g., agitation, altered consciousness, ataxia, myoclonus, overactive reflexes, shivering); do not use together
Tricyclic antidepressants (e.g., amitriptyline, desipramine, imipramine, nortriptyline) / Both are metabolized by CYP2D6 → ↑ levels of tricyclic antidepressant; approach coadministration with caution; may need to ↓ TCA dose
Triptans (e.g., almotriptan, eletriptan, naratriptan, sumatriptan) / ↑ Risk of serotonin syndrome, including symptoms of agitation, overactive reflexes, ataxia, shivering, myoclonus, altered consciousness; use together with caution
Tryptophan / Possible serotonin syndrome (e.g., agitation, altered consciousness, ataxia, myoclonus, overactive reflexes, shivering); do not use together
Warfarin / ↑ Free levels of warfarin due to displacement from plasma protein binding sites by duloxetine → ↑ bleeding; monitor warfarin therapy

HOW SUPPLIED

Capsules, Delayed-Release: 20 mg, 30 mg, 60 mg.

DOSAGE

CAPSULES, DELAYED-RELEASE

Major depressive disorder.

Adults, initial: 20 mg twice a day to 60 mg/day (given once a day or as 30 mg twice a day). For some, give 30 mg once a day for 1 week to allow adjustment to the medication before increasing to 60 mg once daily. **Maintenance:** 40 mg/day, given as 20 mg twice a day to 60 mg/day, given once a day or as 30 mg twice a day. Although 120 mg/day is effective, there is no evidence that dosages more than 60 mg/day confer any additional benefits. Several months of therapy may be necessary. Periodically evaluate to determine need for maintenance treatment.

Diabetic peripheral neuropathic pain.

Adults, usual: 60 mg/day given once a day without regard to meals. Periodically evaluate to determine need for maintenance treatment.

Generalized anxiety disorder.

Adults, initial: 60 mg once daily without regard to meals. For some, it may be beneficial to start at 30 mg once daily for 1 week to allow adjustment to the drug before increasing to 60 mg once daily. There is no evidence that doses higher than 60 mg daily confer additional benefit. If doses greater than 60 mg are used, increase doses in increments of 30 mg once daily up to a maximum of 120 mg once daily. Periodically evaluate the long-term usefulness of the drug.

Fibromyalgia.

Adults, initial: 30 mg once daily for the first week to allow adjustment to the drug; **then,** 60 mg once a day. Some clients may respond to the initial dose.

Chronic musculoskeletal pain.

Adults, initial: 30 mg/day for 1 week to allow adjustment to the drug; **then,** 60 mg once daily.

Stress urinary incontinence (investigational).

Adults: 80 mg once a day or in 2 divided doses; **range:** 20–120 mg/day for 12 weeks.

NURSING IMPLICATIONS

Ⓢ Do not confuse duloxetine with fluoxetine (also a selective serotonin reuptake inhibitor).

IMPLEMENTATION/ADMINISTRATION/STORAGE

1. Before beginning therapy with duloxetine, screen clients with depressive symptoms carefully to determine if they are at risk for bipolar disorder.
2. Dosage adjustment is not needed for geriatric clients on the basis of age.
3. Treatment for several months or longer may be needed for acute episodes of major depression. Periodically reassess clients to determine need for and appropriate dose for maintenance therapy.
4. Consider a lower starting dose and a gradual increase in dose in those with renal impairment.
5. Abrupt discontinuation may cause withdrawal symptoms, including dizziness, N&V, headache, paresthesia, irritability, nightmares, anxiety, fatigue, hyperhidrosis, and insomnia. Reduce dose gradually rather than abruptly discontinuing the drug.
6. If intolerable symptoms occur following a decrease in dose or upon discontinuing the drug, resume the previously prescribed dose. The provider may continue decreasing the dose but at a more gradual rate.
7. Wait at least 14 days between discontinuing a MAOI and initiating duloxetine. Also, at least 5 days should elapse after stopping duloxetine and starting a MAOI.
8. Consider tapering the dose in the third trimester of pregnancy.
9. Store from 15–30°C (59–86°F).

ASSESSMENT

1. List reasons for therapy, characteristics of S&S, contributing factors, other agents trialed, outcome, and behavioral presentation. Monitor clinical response during therapy.
2. Prior to initiating treatment with an antidepressant, adequately screen clients with depressive symptoms to determine if they are at risk for bipolar disorder.
3. Assess history and use cautiously with seizures, controlled narrow angle glaucoma, history of mania, or drug abuse/dependence, and conditions that may slow gastric emptying.
4. Note electromyogram (EMG) results, extent of neuropathy and any contributing factors.
5. Monitor ECG, BP, Wt, electrolytes, renal and LFTs; avoid use with dysfunction. May cause elevation of liver enzymes; avoid in those that have substantial alcohol use.

CLIENT/FAMILY TEACHING

1. Take as directed without regard to meals. Do not chew, crush, or sprinkle contents, or mix with liquids; swallow whole to protect enteric coating.
2. Avoid activities that require mental alertness until drug effects realized; may impair judgment, thinking, or motor skills, and cause drowsiness or dizziness.
3. Bleeding may be precipitated when used with NSAIDs, aspirin, or warfarin; do not take to-

gether. Avoid other antidepressants unless specifically prescribed.

4. May experience dizziness, N&V, headache, paresthesia, irritability, and nightmares. Do not stop suddenly; reduce dose gradually. Report new onset adverse side effects, especially worsening of depression, inability to sleep, suicide thoughts, anxiety, agitation, hostility, and impulsiveness.
5. Avoid excess alcohol use; may cause severe liver injury.
6. Practice reliable contraception; report if pregnant, desire to become pregnant, or if breastfeeding.
7. Record BP and pulse for provider review.
8. Keep all F/U to assess response, counselling, and adverse SE. May take up to 4 weeks before improvement noted.

OUTCOMES/EVALUATE

- Relief of depression/anxiety
- Control of neuropathic pain R/T diabetic peripheral neuropathy
- ↓ Fibromyalgia symptoms

Dutasteride

(dew-**TAS**-teer-ide)

Classification(s): Androgen hormone inhibitor
Pregnancy Category: X
RX: Avodart.

INDICATIONS/USES

Alone or with tamsulosin to treat symptomatic benign prostatic hypertrophy in men with enlarged prostate to improve symptoms, decrease risk of acute urinary retention, and decrease risk/need for surgery. *Investigational:* Prevention of prostate cancer.

ACTION/KINETICS

Action

Competitively inhibits conversion of testosterone to the active 5 alpha-dihydrotestosterone (DHT) by 5 alpha-reductase. DHT develops and enlarges the prostate gland. Reduces total serum prostate-specific antigen levels by about 40% after 3 months and by 50% after 6–24 months.

Pharmacokinetics

Time to peak serum levels: 2–3 hr. Absolute bioavailability: Averages 60%. **Maximum effect:** Within 1–2 weeks. Metabolized by the CYP3A4 and CYP3A5 isoenzymes. Excreted mainly in the feces. **t½, terminal:** About 5 weeks at steady state. **Steady-state serum level after 0.5 mg for 1 year:** 40 ng/mL. **Plasma protein binding:** Over 99%.

CONTRAINDICATIONS

Pregnancy, women of child-bearing age, all other women, and children. Lactation. Known hypersensitivity to dutasteride or other 5 alpha-reductase inhibitors.

SPECIAL CONCERNS

- Use with caution in liver disease.
- Men should not donate blood until at least 6 months after their last dutasteride dose.

SIDE EFFECTS

Most Common

Impotence, decreased libido, ejaculation disorder, gynecomastia (both breast enlargement and tenderness).

Monotherapy or combination with tamsulosin. GU: Impotence, decreased libido, ejaculation disorder, gynecomastia (both breast enlargement and tenderness). **CNS:** Dizziness. **Hypersensitivity:** Rash, pruritus, urticaria, localized edema, serious skin reactions, angioedema. **CV:** ***Cardiac failure*** (causal relationship to use of dutasteride alone or with tamsulosin not established).

LABORATORY TEST CONSIDERATIONS

↓ PSA levels.

DRUG INTERACTIONS

Calcium channel antagonists (e.g., diltiazem, verapamil) / ↓ Dutasteride clearance R/T inhibition of CYP3A4; use amlodipine as an alternative
CYP3A4 inhibitors (e.g., cimetidine, ciprofloxacin, ketoconazole, ritonavir, troleandomycin) / ↑ Dutasteride levels in presence of potent, chronic CYP3A4 inhibitors; use together with caution
Tamsulosin / Possible ejaculation disorders; however, the combination is indicated for symptomatic BPH

HOW SUPPLIED

Capsules, Softgel: 0.5 mg.

DOSAGE

CAPSULES

Benign prostatic hypertrophy.

Monotherapy: 0.5 mg once a day with or without food. **Combination therapy**

E

with tamsulosin: Dutasteride, 0.5 mg once daily with tamsulosin, 0.4 mg once daily.

Prevention of prostate cancer (investigational).

Adults: 0.5 mg once daily.

NURSING IMPLICATIONS

IMPLEMENTATION/ADMINISTRATION/STORAGE

1. Dutasteride is both a hormonal agent and a teratogen. Follow safe handling procedures when preparing, administering, or dispensing the drug.
2. Dutasteride is absorbed through the skin. Women who are pregnant or who may become pregnant should not handle the drug due to the risk to a developing male fetus. If contact is made with a leaking capsule, wash the contact area immediately with soap and water.
3. Swallow capsules whole. Contact with the capsule contents may cause irritation of the oropharyngeal mucosa.
4. Store between 15–30°C (59–77°F).

ASSESSMENT

1. Note characteristics of S&S, other agents trialed/outcome.
2. List other drugs prescribed to ensure none interact.
3. Assess urinary tract symptoms to R/O other urological diseases; assess for obstructive uropathy with reduced flow or increased residual volume. Note prostate exam findings.
4. Reduces total serum prostate-specific antigen levels by about 40% after 3 months and by 50% after 6–24 months. Obtain baseline/monitor PSA, DRE, and LFTs; assess for liver dysfunction.

CLIENT/FAMILY TEACHING

1. Take as directed once daily. May take with or without food, but swallow capsule whole. Review printed drug guide for updates.
2. Drug causes the prostate to decrease in size and thus decreases urination complaints. Do not stop taking dutasteride when symptoms have improved must continue to achieve results; may take 3–6 months to see results.
3. Ejaculation volume may decrease; this does not appear to affect normal sexual function. Drug-related side effects (impotence, ↓ libido, and ejaculation disorder) may decrease with continued therapy.
4. May experience breast enlargement/tenderness; report if persistent.
5. Women should use caution when handling dutasteride capsules; if contact is made with leaking capsules, wash contact area immediately with soap and water.
6. Women who are pregnant or who may be pregnant should not handle dutasteride capsules due to the possibility of absorption and potential risk to a male fetus.
7. Men treated with dutasteride should not give blood until at least 6 months have passed since the last dose.
8. Keep all F/U to assess response and adverse SE.

OUTCOMES/EVALUATE

Control of S&S of BPH: ↓ nocturia ↑ urinary stream

E

Ecallantide

(ee-**KAL**-lan-tide)

Classification(s): Kallikrein inhibitor
Pregnancy Category: C
RX: Kalbitor.

INDICATIONS/USES

Acute attacks of hereditary angioedema in adults and children 16 years of age and older.

ACTION/KINETICS

Action

The kallikrein-kinin system is a complex proteolytic cascade involved in the initiation of both inflammatory and coagulation pathways. In hereditary angioedema, normal regulation of plasma kallikrein activity and the complement cascade is not present. During attacks, unregulated activity of plasma kallikrein results in excessive bradykinin generation. Bradykinin is a vasodilator that may be responsible for the characteristic hereditary angioedema symptoms of localized swelling, inflammation, and pain. Ecallantide is a potent, selective, reversible inhibitor of plasma kallikrein. Ecallantide binds to plasma kallikrein and blocks its binding site. By directly inhibiting plasma kallikrein, ecallantide reduces formation of bradykinin, thereby decreasing symptoms during acute episodic attacks of hereditary angioedema.

Pharmacokinetics

Maximum plasma levels: 2–3 hr. **t½, elimination:** 2 hr. Excreted in the urine.

CONTRAINDICATIONS

Hypersensitivity to ecallantide.

SPECIAL CONCERNS

Anaphylaxis has been reported after administration of ecallantide. Because of the risk of anaphylaxis, ecallantide should only be administered by a health care provider with appropriate medical support to manage anaphylaxis and hereditary angioedema. Health care providers should be aware of the similarity of symptoms between hypersensitivity reactions and hereditary angioedema, and clients should be monitored closely. Do not administer ecallantide to clients with known hypersensitivity to ecallantide.

- Use with caution during lactation.
- Use caution in dose selection in the elderly, starting at the low end of the dosing range.
- Safety and efficacy not determined in children less than 16 years of age.

SIDE EFFECTS

Most Common

Headache, N&V, fatigue, diarrhea, URTI, injection-site reactions, nasopharyngitis, pruritus, upper abdominal pain.

GI: N&V, diarrhea, upper abdominal pain. **CNS:** Headache. **Dermatologic:** Pruritus. **Respiratory:** Nasopharyngitis, URTI. **Injection site:** Local bruising, erythema, pain, irritation, pruritus, urticaria. **Hypersensitivity:** Chest discomfort, flushing, pharyngeal edema, pruritus, rhinorrhea, sneezing, nasal congestion, throat irritation, urticaria, wheezing, hypotension, rash, ***anaphylaxis***. **Body as a whole:** Fatigue, pyrexia. **Miscellaneous:** Immunogenicity.

HOW SUPPLIED

Injection Solution: 10 mg/mL.

DOSAGE

SC

Hereditary angioedema.

Adults and children, 16 years and older: 30 mg (3 mL) given SC in three 10 mg (1 mL) injections. If the attack persists, an additional dose of 30 mg may be given within a 24 hr period.

NURSING IMPLICATIONS

IMPLEMENTATION/ADMINISTRATION/STORAGE

1. Using aseptic technique, withdraw 1 mL (10 mg) from the vial using a large bore needle. Change the needle on the syringe to a needle suitable for SC injection (27 gauge is recommended).
2. Inject into the skin of the abdomen, thigh, or upper arm.
3. The injection site for each of the injections may be in the same or in different anatomic locations. There is no need for site rotation. However, injection sites should be separated by at least 2 inches away from the anatomical site of attack.
4. Store from 2–8°C (36–46°F). When removed from the refrigerator, store below 30°C (86°F) and use within 14 days or return to the refrigerator until use. Protect vials from light until use.

ASSESSMENT

1. Note indications for therapy (hereditary angioedema—HAE), onset and characteristics of S&S, frequency of occurrence, triggers, other agents trialed and outcome.
2. List medical history, and assess for conditions that may preclude therapy.
3. Assess skin integrity, and ensure not administered into red, hard, or infected skin areas.
4. Serious allergic reactions may occur and can be life-threatening; usually occur within 1 hour after receiving injection, so monitor closely during this time frame.

5. Perform respiratory and cardiac assessments; monitor VS.

CLIENT/FAMILY TEACHING

1. Drug is administered by HCP in a controlled setting, and used to treat an acute attack of a certain immune disease passed down through families (angioedema–HAE).
2. Each dose consists of three injections under the skin. It does not cure disease; only treats the symptoms.
3. Three separate shots will be administered under the skin separated by at least 2 inches (5 cm). An additional three shots may be given in a 24 hr period if the HAE attack continues.
4. After administration, you will remain at facility (approximately 1 hr), and be monitored for any allergic reaction.
5. Any S&S of allergic reaction, such as rash, itching/swelling (especially of the face/tongue/throat), severe dizziness, trouble breathing, or chest pain (similar to condition being treated) requires immediate medical attention, and you should not receive this drug again.
6. May experience redness, bruising, itching, and swelling at the injection site. Nausea, fever, or stuffy nose may also occur; report if persistent or worsens.
7. Practice reliable contraception; report if pregnancy suspected, as benefits should outweigh risks with this therapy.
8. Keep all F/U to assess response and for adverse SE.

OUTCOMES/EVALUATE

- ↓ Swelling, inflammation, and pain with hereditary angioedema
- Control of symptoms of angioedema

Efavirenz

(eh-**FAH**-vih-rehnz)

Classification(s): Antiviral, non-nucleoside reverse transcriptase inhibitor

Pregnancy Category: D (Category C per Briggs' *Drugs in Pregnancy and Lactation*)

RX: Sustiva.

SEE ALSO ***ANTIVIRAL AGENTS***.

INDICATIONS/USES

In combination with other antiretroviral drugs (e.g., protease inhibitor and/or nucleoside analog reverse transcriptase inhibitors) to treat HIV-1 infection.

ACTION/KINETICS

Action

A nonnucleoside reverse transcriptase inhibitor of HIV-1 that acts mainly by noncompetitive inhibition of HIV-1 reverse transcriptase.

Pharmacokinetics

Peak plasma levels: 3–5 hr in HIV clients. **Steady-state plasma levels:** 6–10 days. Metabolized mainly by CYP3A4 and CYP 2B6 to inactive metabolites, which are excreted in the urine (14–34%) and feces (16–61%). Will induce its own metabolism. **t½, terminal:** 52–76 hr after a single dose and 40–55 hr after multiple doses. **Plasma protein binding:** 99.5–99.75%.

CONTRAINDICATIONS

Hypersensitivity (e.g., Stevens-Johnson syndrome, erythema multiforme, toxic skin eruptions) to efavirenz or any component of the product. Use as a single agent to treat HIV (resistant virus emerges rapidly) or added on as a sole agent to a failing regimen. High-fat meals (increase absorption). Use with bepridil, ergot derivatives, midazolam, pimozide, triazolam, or with standard doses of voriconazole. Pregnancy or in those of childbearing age due to increased risk of birth defects. Lactation (to prevent postnatal transmission of HIV infection).

SPECIAL CONCERNS

- Use with caution in impaired hepatic function and in dose selection in the elderly.
- Not studied in children younger than 3 years of age or who weigh less than 13 kg.

SIDE EFFECTS

Most Common

Adults: Rash, N&V, dizziness, headache, insomnia, diarrhea, impaired concentration, dyspepsia, fatigue, abnormal dreams, somnolence, depression, anxiety, nervousness.
Children: Rash, diarrhea/loose stools, fever, cough, dizziness, lightheadedness, fainting, aches/pain/discomfort, N&V, headache.

CNS: Dizziness, headache, insomnia, impaired concentration, depression (may be severe), abnormal dreams, nervousness, somnolence, anxiety, severe depression, abnormal thinking, agitation, amnesia, confusion, depersonalization, euphoria, hallucinations, stupor, ***suicidal ideation***, nonfatal suicide attempts, aggressive behavior, paranoid reactions, manic reactions, abnormal coordination, ataxia, cerebellar coordination and balance disturbances, ***convulsions***, delusions, emotional lability, hypesthesia, neuropathy, neurosis, paranoia, paresthesia, psychosis, ***suicide***, tremor. **Dermatologic:** Rash (including blistering, moist/dry desquamation, ulceration, mucosal involvement, vesiculation, ulceration, fever), mild to moderate maculopapular skin eruptions, pruritus, erythema multiforme, nail disorders, flushing, photoallergic dermatitis, skin discoloration, necrosis requiring surgery, exfoliative dermatitis, ***Stevens-Johnson syndrome, toxic epidermal necrolysis***. **GI:** N&V, anorexia, dyspepsia, diarrhea, abdominal pain, constipation, malabsorption, ***pancreatitis***. **Hepatic:** ***Hepatic failure***, hepatitis. **CV:** Palpitations. **Musculoskeletal:** Arthralgia, myalgia, myopathy. **Respiratory:** Dyspnea. **GU:** Gynecomastia. **Ophthalmic:** Abnormal vision. **Otic:** Tinnitus. **Body as a whole:** Fatigue, asthenia, allergic reactions, pain, redistribution/accumulation of body fat (including central obesity, dorsocervical fat enlargement, peripheral wasting, facial wasting, breast enlargement, "cushingoid" appearance). **Miscellaneous:** Immune reconstitution syndrome, including an inflammatory response to indolent or residual opportunistic infections (such as *Mycobacterium avium* infection, cytomegalovirus, *Pneumocystis jiroveci* pneumonia, or tuberculosis).

NOTE: The following side effects were noted in 10% or more of children, aged 3–16 years: Rash, diarrhea, loose stools, fever, cough, dizziness, lightheadedness, fainting, ache, pain, discomfort, N&V, headache, rash.

LABORATORY TEST CONSIDERATIONS

↑ AST, ALT, GGT, total cholesterol, LDL, serum amylase, glucose, serum triglycerides. ↓ Neutrophils. False + urine cannabinoid tests using the CEDIA DAU Multi-Level THC assay.

OVERDOSE MANAGEMENT

Symptoms: Increased nervous system symptoms. *Treatment:* General supportive measures, including monitoring of vital signs. Activated charcoal may be used to aid removal of unabsorbed drug. Dialysis is not likely to be effective.

DRUG INTERACTIONS

NOTE: Efavirenz coadministered with drugs primarily metabolized by CYP3A4, CYP2C9, and CYP2C19 may result in altered plasma levels of the coadministered drug. Thus, dose adjustments may be necessary.

Amprenavir / ↓ Serum amprenavir levels
Atazanavir / ↓ Atazanavir plasma levels and efficacy; dosage adjustment is necessary; see ***Implementation/Administration/Storage;*** coadministration is not recommended in treatment-experienced clients
Bepridil / Competition for CYP3A4 by efavirenz → possible cardiac arrhythmias, prolonged sedation, or respiratory depression; use together contraindicated
Cabazitaxel / ↓ Cabazitaxel plasma levels and efficacy; do not use together
Calcium channel blockers (diltiazem, felodipine, nicardipine, nifedipine, verapamil) / Possible ↓ plasma levels of the calcium channel blocker; monitor and adjust dosage if necessary
Carbamazepine / ↓ Levels of both drugs; monitor carbamazepine levels and adjust dose if necessary
Cisapride / Competition for CYP3A4 by efavirenz → serious/life-threatening side effects, including cardiac arrhythmias, prolonged or increased sedation, respiratory depression; use together contraindicated
Clarithromycin / ↓ Clarithromycin levels and ↑ levels of metabolite; use alternative therapy such as azithromycin
Ergot derivatives (dihydroergotamine, ergotamine, methylergotamine) / Competition for CYP3A4 by efavirenz → serious/life-threatening side effects, including possible cardiac arrhythmias, prolonged sedation or respiratory depression, acute ergot toxicity; use together contraindicated
HMG-CoA reductase inhibitors (atorvastatin, pravastatin, simvastatin) / ↓ Plasma levels of the HMG-CoA reductase inhibitor; monitor LDL levels
Hormonal contraceptives (e.g., etonogestrel, levonorgestrel, norgestimate) / Significant ↓ of progestin levels; use a reliable barrier contraceptive in addition to the hormonal contraceptive; no effect on ethinyl estradiol levels

Immunosuppressants (e.g., cyclosporine, sirolimus, tacrolimus) / ↓ Levels of immunosuppressants metabolized by CYP3A4; closely monitor immunosuppressant levels for at least 2 weeks when starting/stopping efavirenz
Indinavir / ↓ Indinavir levels R/T enzyme induction; ↑ indinavir dose
Itraconazole / Possible ↓ itraconazole plasma levels
Ixabepilone / ↓ Ixabepilone plasma levels and efficacy; avoid concurrent use
Ketoconazole / Possible ↓ ketoconazole plasma levels
Lopinavir / ↓ Lopinavir plasma levels and efficacy; do not give lopinavir/ritonavir once/day with efavirenz; in treatment-experienced consider a dose increase in lopinavir/ritonavir if used with efavirenz
Maraviroc / ↓ Maraviroc plasma levels and efficacy; dosage adjustment of maraviroc may be needed; concurrent use contraindicated in those with severe renal impairment (C_{CR} <30 mL/min)
Methadone / ↑ Risk of methadone withdrawal symptoms R/T ↑ liver breakdown; ↑ methadone dose as needed
Midazolam / Competition for CYP3A4 by efavirenz → serious/life-threatening side effects, including possible cardiac arrhythmias, prolonged sedation, or respiratory depression; use together contraindicated
Nevirapine / ↓ Efavirenz plasma levels → ↓ efficacy; ↑ risk of side effects; do not use together
Phenobarbital / ↓ Levels of both drugs R/T ↑ metabolism; monitor phenobarbital levels
Phenytoin / ↓ Levels of both drugs R/T ↑ metabolism; monitor phenytoin levels
Pimozide / Competition for CYP3A4 by efavirenz → possible cardiac arrhythmias, prolonged sedation, or respiratory depression; use together contraindicated
Posaconazole / Possible ↓ posaconazole plasma levels
Rifabutin / Possible ↓ rifabutin levels and ↑ clearance of efavirenz; ↑ rifabutin daily dose by 50%
Rifampin / Possible ↓ rifampin levels and ↑ clearance of efavirenz
Ritonavir / ↑ Levels of both drugs; higher frequency of dizziness, nausea, paresthesia, and elevated liver enzymes; monitor liver enzymes
Saquinavir / ↓ Saquinavir AUC and C_{max}; do not use saquinavir as the sole protease inhibitor with efavirenz
Sertraline / Possible ↓ sertraline AUC and C_{max}; possible adjustment of dosage needed
H ***St. John's wort*** / Possible significant ↓ efavirenz levels R/T ↑ hepatic metabolism by CYP3A4 isoenzymes; do not use together; ↑ risk of resistance to efavirenz or other nonnucleoside reverse transcriptase inhibitors
Triazolam / Competition for CYP3A4 by efavirenz → serious/life-threatening side effects, including possible cardiac arrhythmias, prolonged sedation, or respiratory depression; use together is contraindicated
Voraconazole / ↑ Efavirenz plasma levels and significant ↓ voriconazole plasma levels; dosage adjustment is necessary; see ***Implementation/Administration/Storage***
Warfarin / Possible ↑ or ↓ levels of warfarin; monitor coagulation parameters and adjust warfarin dose as needed

HOW SUPPLIED

Capsules: 50 mg, 200 mg; ***Tablets:*** 600 mg.

DOSAGE

CAPSULES; TABLETS

Human immunodeficiency virus-1 infections.

Adults: 600 mg once daily in combination with a protease inhibitor and/or nucleoside analog reverse transcriptase inhibitors. **Children, 3 years and older, 10 to <15 kg (22 to <33 lbs):** 200 mg at bedtime; **15 to <20 kg (33 to <44 lbs):** 250 mg at bedtime; **20 to <25 kg (44 to <55 lbs):** 300 mg at bedtime; **25 to <32.5 kg (55 to <71.5 lbs):** 350 mg at bedtime; **32.5 to <40 kg (71.5 to <88 lbs):** 400 mg at bedtime; **40 kg or more (88 lbs or more):** 600 mg at bedtime. **Maximum dose:** 600 mg/day.

NURSING IMPLICATIONS

IMPLEMENTATION/ADMINISTRATION/STORAGE

1. **Always initiate therapy with 1 or more other new antiretroviral drugs to which client has not been previously exposed.**

2. Initiating efavirenz therapy using a stepwise dosage schedule over a 2-week period reduces the incidence and intensity of neuropsychiatric side effects without affecting virologic efficacy.
3. Should be taken on an empty stomach, preferably at bedtime. Food may lead to an increase in the frequency of side effects.
4. Use bedtime dosing during first 2 to 4 weeks to improve tolerability of nervous system side effects.
5. If coadministered with voraconazole, increase the maintenance dose of voriconazole to 400 mg q 12 hr, and decrease the efavirenz dose to 300 mg once daily using the capsule formulation (one 200 mg and two 50 mg capsules or six 50 mg capsules).
6. If coadministered with atazanavir in treatment-naive clients, the recommended dosage is atazanavir 400 mg, ritonavir 100 mg, and efavirenz 600 mg, each once daily. In treatment-experienced clients, coadministration of efavirenz and atazanavir is not recommended.
7. Appropriate antihistamines and/or corticosteroids may improve tolerability, and prevent or hasten the resolution of rash.
8. To monitor fetal outcomes of pregnant women exposed to efafirenz, an Antiretroviral Pregnancy Registry has been established. To register clients, call 1-800-258-4263.
9. Store from 15–30°C (59–86°F).

ASSESSMENT

1. Note reasons for therapy, date confirmed, other agents trialed, outcome.
2. Determine any history of psychiatric disorders or seizure disorders; may aggravate these conditions. Assess carefully for any evidence of rash, especially during first 2–4 weeks of therapy.
3. May cause false-positive cannabinoid urine test.
4. Monitor lipid profile and LFTs with history of hepatitis B and/or C. Record viral load, CD4 counts during therapy.

CLIENT/FAMILY TEACHING

1. Take as directed and with other antiretroviral agents. Should be taken on an empty stomach, preferably at bedtime.
2. Do not break efavirenz tablets.
3. May cause dizziness, drowsiness, delusions, and impaired concentration. Take at bedtime to increase tolerability; avoid tasks requiring concentration/dexterity until effects realized.
4. Drug does not cure disease but works to reduce viral load.
5. Practice reliable barrier contraception with additional form of birth control; do not breast-feed due to potential for adverse reactions from the drug in breast-feeding infants and transmission of the HIV virus. Practice abstinence or safe sex, and do not share needles. Continue to use contraception for 12 wk after stopping therapy.
6. Most clients will experience a rash. This should resolve after several weeks; report if persistent or extensive. Report if accompanied by fever, blistering, oral lesions, conjunctivitis, swelling, muscle or joint aches, general malaise, or infection such as a sore throat, fever, cough, or respiratory congestion. Therapy that was stopped for blistering rash should not be restarted unless accompanied by steroids or antihistamines.
7. Immediately report if S&S of serious psychiatric adverse reactions occur; i.e., increased depression, or suicide thoughts.
8. May cause false+ urine cannabinoid test results.
9. Avoid alcohol and psychoactive drugs; may alter effects.
10. Keep all F/U to assess response and for adverse SE. Long-term effects and adverse reactions are not known.

OUTCOMES/EVALUATE

- Treatment of HIV-1 infection in combination with other antiretroviral agents
- ↓ HIV-RNA levels; ↑ CD_4 cell counts

Eletriptan hydrobromide

(**EH**-leh-trip-tan)

Classification(s): Antimigraine drug

Pregnancy Category: C

RX: Relpax.

SEE ALSO ***SEROTONIN 5-HT$_1$ RECEPTOR AGONISTS (ANTIMIGRAINE DRUGS)***.

INDICATIONS/USES

Treatment of migraine with or without aura.

ACTION/KINETICS

Action

Binds with high affinity to 5-HT_{1B}, 5-HT_{1D}, and 5-HT_{1F} receptors. It is believed activation of these receptors located on intracranial blood vessels leads to vasoconstriction, which causes relief of migraine headache. The drug may also activate 5-HT_1 receptors on sensory nerve endings in the trigeminal system resulting in inhibition of pro-inflammatory neuropeptide release.

Pharmacokinetics

Well absorbed; **peak plasma levels:** About 1.5 hr. Is approximately 50% bioavailable. A high-fat meal increases AUC and C_{max} by 20–30%. Is metabolized by the CYP3A4 enzyme. The N-demethylated metabolite is active and contributes significantly to the overall effect of eletriptan. **t½, terminal:** 4 hr. The half-life is increased in the elderly. **Plasma protein binding:** About 85%.

CONTRAINDICATIONS

Use for prophylaxis of migraine or use in the management of hemiplegic or basilar migraine. Use in clients with the following: ischemic heart disease (e.g., angina pectoris, history of MI, documented silent ischemia) or in those who have symptoms or findings consistent with ischemic heart disease, coronary artery vasospasm (including Prinzmetal's variant angina), or other significant underlying CV disease. Use in clients with cerebrovascular syndromes (including, but not limited to, strokes of any type as well as transient ischemic attacks), in peripheral vascular disease (including, but not limited to, ischemic bowel disease), in those with uncontrolled hypertension, within 24 hr of treatment with another 5-HT_1 agonist (e.g., dihydroergotamine, methysergide), or in those with severe hepatic impairment.

SPECIAL CONCERNS

- **Safety and efficacy not determined for cluster headache.**
- **Use with caution during lactation.**

SIDE EFFECTS

Most Common

Asthenia, dizziness, nausea, paresthesia, somnolence, headache, chest tightness/pressure/heaviness, dry mouth.

See *Serotonin 5-HT_1 Receptor Agonists (Antimigraine Drugs)* for a complete list of possible side effects. **GI:** Nausea, dry mouth, dyspepsia, dysphagia. **CNS:** Somnolence, dizziness, headache. **Body as a whole:** Paresthesia, flushing/feeling of warmth, asthenia. **Miscellaneous:** Chest tightness, pain or pressure; abdominal pain, discomfort; stomach pain; cramps/pressure.

DRUG INTERACTIONS

Ergot-containing drugs (e.g., dihydroergotamine) / Prolonged vasospastic reactions; do not use within 24 hr of each other

Erythromycin / ↑ Eletriptan C_{max} and AUC R/T ↓ metabolism

Fluoconazole / ↑ Eletriptan C_{max} and AUC R/T ↓ metabolism

Ketoconazole / ↑ Eletriptan C_{max} and AUC R/T ↓ metabolism

SSRIs / Possible weakness, hyperreflexia, and incoordination

Verapamil / ↑ Eletriptan C_{max} and AUC R/T ↓ metabolism

HOW SUPPLIED

Tablets: 24.2 mg eletriptan hydrobromide (equivalent to 20 mg of the base), 48.5 mg eletriptan hydrobromide (equivalent to 40 mg of the base).

DOSAGE

TABLETS

Migraine with or without aura.

Adults: Individualize dose. Usually a single 20 mg or 40 mg dose (greater chance of a response). Maximum single dose: 40 mg; maximum daily dose: 80 mg. If after the initial dose the headache improves and then returns, a repeat dose may be beneficial. If a second dose is required, take at least 2 hr after the initial dose. If the initial dose is ineffective, a second dose may not be beneficial either.

NURSING IMPLICATIONS

IMPLEMENTATION/ADMINISTRATION/STORAGE

1. **Do not use within 72 hr of treatment with clarithromycin, ketoconazole, itraconazole, nefazodone, nelfinavir, ritonavir, and troleandomycin.**
2. **Safety of treating an average of >3 headaches in a 30-day period has not been determined.**

ASSESSMENT

1. Note reasons for therapy, neurologic evaluations, characteristics of S&S (pain location, intensity, duration), and other agents trialed.
2. Assess for CHD, uncontrolled BP, CVA, severe liver problems; precludes drug therapy.
3. Monitor for any S&S of cardiac problems, and assess risk factors.
4. Obtain ECG and LFTs. Note any evidence of increased cholesterol, obesity, smoking, or menopause S&S.

CLIENT/FAMILY TEACHING

1. Drug works by reducing swollen blood vessels around the brain and reducing release of nerve substances that cause migraine headache symptoms.
2. Take as directed; do not exceed prescribed dosage. Read info sheet accompanying product; do not share medications. Take at first sign of migraine; if headache returns, may take a second dose after 2 hr. Lying down in a darkened room after taking medication may help with symptoms. Continue other prophylactic meds as prescribed.
3. May cause fatigue or dizziness; use caution when performing activities requiring mental alertness.
4. Avoid unnecessary exposure to sunlight or tanning lamps; use sunscreen/protective clothing to avoid photosensitivity reactions.
5. Use caution, may experience nausea, dizziness, tiredness, or weakness, as well as pain or pressure in chest/throat. Report any increased SOB, pains, heaviness, or tightness in chest, jaw, or neck.
6. Immediately report any severe chest pain, or chest pain that does not go away, sudden or severe stomach pain, shortness of breath, wheezing, swelling of the eyelids, face, or lips.
7. Do not take if you have used any other type of special headache medicines, or within 24 hr of clarithromycin, itraconazole, ketoconazole, nefazodone, nelfinavir, ritonavir, or troleandomycin. Do not use within 72 hr with drugs that have demonstrated potent CYP3A4 inhibition. Contact provider if unsure; avoid all OTC agents without approval.
8. Avoid alcohol; may aggravate symptoms.
9. Keep all F/U to assess response, labs, and adverse SE.

OUTCOMES/EVALUATE

Relief of migraine headaches

Emtricitabine

(em-trih-**SIGH**-tah-been)

Classification(s): Antiretroviral drug, nucleoside reverse transcriptase inhibitor

Pregnancy Category: B

RX: Emtriva.

SEE ALSO ***ANTIVIRAL DRUGS***.

INDICATIONS/USES

Treatment of HIV-1 infection in adults and children; used in combination with other antiretroviral agents.

ACTION/KINETICS

Action

Emtricitabine is phosphorylated by cellular enzymes to form emtricitabine 5'-triphosphate, which then inhibits the activity of the HIV-1 reverse transcriptase by competing with the natural substrate deoxycytidine 5'-triphosphate. It is also incorporated into nascent viral DNA, which results in chain termination.

Pharmacokinetics

Pharmacokinetic data for children from birth to 3 months of age is similar to those of older infants, children, and adolescents. Rapidly and extensively absorbed; **peak plasma levels:** 1–2 hr. Bioavailability of capsules is 75% and of the oral solution is 80%. May be taken with or without food. Metabolized in the liver and excreted in both the feces (14%) and urine (86%). **t½, plasma:** About 10 hr. **t½, terminal, children:** About 8.9 hr. Is eliminated in the urine by both glomerular filtration and active tubular secretion; thus, there may be competition for elimination with other drugs/compounds that are also renally eliminated. **Plasma protein binding:** < 4%.

CONTRAINDICATIONS

Hypersensitivity to the drug or any components of the product. Lactation.

SPECIAL CONCERNS

(1) Lactic acidosis and severe hepatomegaly with steatosis, including fatal cases, have been reported with the use of nucleoside an-

alogs alone or in combination with other antiretroviral drugs. (2) Emtricitabine is not approved for the treatment of chronic hepatitis B virus (HBV) infection, and the safety and efficacy of emtricitabine have not been established in clients coinfected with HBV and HIV-1. Severe acute exacerbations of hepatitis B have been reported in clients after the discontinuation of emtricitabine. Closely monitor hepatic function with clinical and laboratory follow-up for at least several months in clients who discontinue emtricitabine and are coinfected with HIV-1 and HBV. If appropriate, initiation of anti-HBV therapy may be warranted. ■

- **Use with caution in the elderly.**
- **Safety and efficacy not determined in children less than 3 months of age.**

SIDE EFFECTS

Most Common

Adults: Abdominal pain, abnormal dreams, asthenia, depression, diarrhea, dizziness, fatigue, headache, increased cough, insomnia, nausea, rash, rhinitis.

Children: Infection, hyperpigmentation, increased cough, vomiting, otitis media, rash, rhinitis, diarrhea, fever, pneumonia, gastroenteritis, abdominal pain, anemia.

CNS: Headache, depression, insomnia, depressive disorders, paresthesia, dizziness, neuropathy/peripheral neuritis, abnormal dreams. **GI:** Diarrhea, N&V, abdominal pain, dyspepsia, gastroenteritis. **Metabolic:** Redistribution or accumulation of body fat, including central obesity, dorsocervical fat enlargement (buffalo hump), peripheral/facial wasting, breast enlargement, and "cushingoid" appearance; ***lactic acidosis/severe hepatomegaly with steatosis***. **Musculoskeletal:** Myalgia, arthralgia. **Respiratory:** Rhinitis, increased cough, nasopharyngitis, sinusitis, URTI, otitis media (children), pneumonia. **Dermatologic:** Rash, pruritus, urticaria maculopapular/vesiculobullous/pustular rash, skin discoloration (hyperpigmentation on the palms and/or soles). **Hematologic:** Anemia (children). **Body as a whole:** Asthenia, fatigue, fever, infections, immune reconstitution syndrome (inflammatory response to indolent or residual opportunistic infections, including *Mycobacterium avium*, cytomegalovirus, *Pneumocystis jirovecii*, pneumonia, tuberculosis), ***allergic reactions.***

LABORATORY TEST CONSIDERATIONS

↑ ALT, AST, alkaline phosphatase, bilirubin, creatine kinase, pancreatic amylase, serum amylase, serum lipase, triglycerides, fasting cholesterol. ↓ Neutrophils, hemoglobin. ↑ or ↓ Serum glucose. Glycosuria, hematuria. Possible laboratory abnormalities in children include: ↑ Amylase, ALT, creatine phosphokinase, bilirubin, GGT, and lipase; and, ↓ neutrophils, hemoglobin, and glucose.

OVERDOSE MANAGEMENT

Symptoms: If overdose occurs, monitor for signs of toxicity and begin standard supportive care. *Treatment:* There is no known antidote. Hemodialysis removes about 30% of an emtricitabine dose over a 3 hr period starting within 1.5 hr of emtricitabine dosing.

DRUG INTERACTIONS

1. Emtricitabine is a component of two combination drugs: Atripla (fixed-dose combination of emtricitabine, efavirenz, and tenofovir disproxil fumarate) and Truvada (fixed-dose combination of emtricitabine and tenofovir disoproxil fumarate). **Do not coadminister emtricitabine with Atripla or Truvada.**
2. Due to similarities between emtricitabine and lamivudine, do not coadminister emtricitabine with any other drug containing lamivudine, including lamivudine/zidovudine, abacavir/lamivudine, or abacavir/lamivudine/zidovudine.

HOW SUPPLIED

Capsules: 200 mg; *Oral Solution:* 10 mg/mL.

DOSAGE

CAPSULES; ORAL SOLUTION

Human immunodeficiency virus-1 infection in adults and children.

Adults, 18 years and older: 200 mg of the capsules or 240 mg (24 mL) of the oral solution once daily. **Children, 3 months through 17 years:** For children weighing more than 33 kg who can swallow an intact capsule, one 200 mg capsule once daily. For the oral solution, 6 mg/kg, up to a maximum of

240 mg (24 mL) once daily. **Children, 0–3 months of age:** 3 mg/kg once a day. *NOTE:* May be taken with or without food. See *Implementation/Administration/Storage* for the dosing interval in clients with baseline C_{CR} <50 mL/min.

NURSING IMPLICATIONS

IMPLEMENTATION/ADMINISTRATION/STORAGE

1. Adjust the dose as follows in clients with impaired renal function:
   - C_{CR}, 50 mL/min and greater: 200 mg q 24 hr of the capsule or 240 mg (24 mL) q 24 hr of the oral solution.
   - C_{CR}, 30–49 mL/min: 200 mg q 48 hr of the capsule or 120 mg (12 mL) q 24 hr of the oral solution.
   - C_{CR}, 15–20 mL/min: 200 mg q 72 hr of the capsule or 80 mg (8 mL) q 24 hr of the oral solution.
   - C_{CR}, <15 mL/min and those clients requiring hemodialysis: 200 mg q 96 hr of the capsule and 60 mg (6 mL) of the oral solution q 24 hr. If dosing on the day of dialysis, give after dialysis.
2. There are insufficient data regarding adjustment of emtricitabine dosage in children with renal impairment; however, a dose reduction and/or an increase in the dosing interval similar to adjustments for adults should be considered.
3. An antiretroviral pregnancy registry has been established to monitor fetal outcomes of pregnant women exposed to emtricitabine. To register clients, call 1-800-258-4263.
4. Store capsules from 15–30°C (59–86°F) and the oral solution refrigerated from 2–8°C (36–46°F). Use the oral solution within 3 months if stored from 15–30°C (59–86°F).

ASSESSMENT

1. Note disease onset, characteristics of S&S, other agents trialed, outcome. List drugs prescribed to ensure none interact.
2. Check for hepatitis B; may preclude therapy.
3. Monitor HIV RNA, renal and LFTs; reduce dose based on C_{CR}. Assess for lactic acidosis and liver dysfunction during and for several months following therapy.

CLIENT/FAMILY TEACHING

1. Take as directed with other antiretroviral therapy; always used in combination therapy. Must take for life.
2. Do not take any unprescribed/OTC medications/herbals without provider consent.
3. Drug may cause a redistribution of body fat.
4. Does not prevent disease transmission or STDs; practice safe sex, and use protection. Practice reliable birth control, and report immediately if pregnancy suspected.
5. May continue to experience opportunistic infections. Long-term drug effects are unknown; may cause liver toxicity, and lactic acidosis.
6. Keep all F/U to assess response, labs, and for adverse SE.

OUTCOMES/EVALUATE

↓ HIV RNA

IV

Enalapril maleate

(en-**AL**-ah-prill)

Classification(s): Antihypertensive, ACE inhibitor

Pregnancy Category: D (Category C first trimester; Category D second and third trimesters)

RX: Enalaprilat, Vasotec.

SEE ALSO ***ANGIOTENSIN-CONVERTING ENZYME INHIBITORS***.

INDICATIONS/USES

PO: (1) Alone or in combination with other antihypertensives (especially thiazide diuretics) for the treatment of hypertension. Hypertension in children. (2) In combination with digitalis and diuretic in acute and chronic CHF. (3) Asymptomatic left ventricular dysfunction (ejection fraction less than 35%) in clinically stable asymptomatic clients.

IV: Treatment of hypertension when PO therapy is not practical.

Investigational: Hypertension related to scleroderma renal crisis. Treatment of diabetic nephropathy in normotensive clients. Enalaprilat may be used for hypertensive emergencies (effect is variable).

E

ACTION/KINETICS

Action

Enalapril (and its active metabolite enalaprilat) inhibit angiotensin-converting enzyme resulting in decreased plasma angiotensin II, which leads to decreased vasopressor activity and decreased aldosterone secretion. The parenteral product is enalaprilat injection.

Pharmacokinetics

About 60% bioavailable after PO. Enalapril rapidly converted to the active enalaprilat. **Onset, PO:** 1 hr; **IV:** 15 min. **Time to peak action, PO:** 4–6 hr; **IV:** 1–4 hr. **Duration, PO:** 24 hr or more; **IV:** About 6 hr. **t½, enalapril, PO:** 1.3 hr; **IV:** 15 min. **t½, enalaprilat, PO:** 11.5 hr. Excreted through the urine (half unchanged) and feces; over 90% of enalaprilat is excreted through the urine. *NOTE:* With a GFR of 30 mL/min or less, peak and trough enalaprilat levels increase, time to reach C_{max} increases, and time to steady state may be delayed. **Plasma protein binding:** Approximately 50–60%.

ADDITIONAL CONTRAINDICATIONS

Use of enalapril or enalaprilat with hereditary or idiopathic angioedema. Use in neonates and children with a GFR less than 30 mL/min/1.73 m^2.

SPECIAL CONCERNS

■ When used during the second and third trimesters of pregnancy, ACE inhibitors can cause injury and even death to the developing fetus. When pregnancy is detected, discontinue as soon as possible. ■

- **May cause a profound drop in BP following the first dose.**
- **Use with caution during lactation.**

SIDE EFFECTS

Most Common

Dizziness, headache, hypotension, syncope, chest pain, fatigue, diarrhea, cough.

CV: Palpitations, hypotension, chest pain, angina pectoris, ***CVA, MI***, orthostatic hypotension/effects, disturbances in rhythm, tachycardia, ***cardiac arrest***, atrial fibrillation, tachycardia, bradycardia, Raynaud phenomenon, vasculitis. **GI:** N&V, diarrhea, abdominal pain, alterations in taste, anorexia, dry mouth, constipation, dyspepsia, glossitis, ileus, melena, stomatitis. **Hepatic:** Hepatitis, hepatocellular or cholestatic jaundice, pancreatitis, elevated liver enzymes, ***hepatic failure***. **CNS:** Insomnia, headache, fatigue, dizziness, paresthesias, nervousness, sleepiness, ataxia, confusion, depression, dysesthesia, vertigo, abnormal dreams, sleep disturbances, somnolence, drowsiness. **Respiratory:** Bronchitis, chronic cough, dyspnea, bronchospasm, URTI, pneumonia, pulmonary infiltrates, asthma, rhinorrhea, sore throat, hoarseness, ***pulmonary embolism and infarction, pulmonary edema***. **Renal:** Renal dysfunction, oliguria, UTI, transient increases in creatinine and BUN. **Musculoskeletal:** Arthralgia, arthritis, myalgia, muscle cramps, myositis, flank pain. **Hematologic:** Rarely, neutropenia, agranulocytosis, leukopenia; thrombocytopenia, eosinophilia, bone marrow depression, decreased H&H in hypertensive or CHF clients. Hemolytic anemia, including hemolysis, in clients with G6PD deficiency. **Dermatologic:** Rash, pruritus, alopecia, flushing, erythema multiforme, exfoliative dermatitis, photosensitivity, urticaria, diaphoresis, increased sweating, pemphigoid/pemphigus, ***Stevens-Johnson syndrome***, herpes zoster, ***toxic epidermal necrolysis***. **GU:** Impotence, gynecomastia, oliguria, UTI, renal failure, renal dysfunction. **Ophthalmic:** Blurred vision, conjunctivitis, tearing, dry eyes. **Otic:** Tinnitus, hearing loss. **Body as a whole:** Asthenia, fever, peripiheral edema. **Miscellaneous:** ***Angioedema***, syncope, loss of sense of smell, peripheral neuropathy, anosmia, serositis.

ADDITIONAL DRUG INTERACTIONS

Rifampin may ↓ the effects of enalapril. Do not discontinue without first reporting to the provider.

ADDITIONAL LABORATORY TEST CONSIDERATIONS

↑ BUN and serum creatinine after ↓ BP in those with unilateral or bilateral renal artery stenosis.

HOW SUPPLIED

Injection: 1.25 mg/mL (as enalaprilat); ***Tablets:*** 2.5 mg, 5 mg, 10 mg, 20 mg.

DOSAGE

Enalapril

TABLETS

Hypertension in clients not taking diuretics.

Initial: 5 mg once a day; **then,** adjust dosage according to response (range: 10–40 mg/day in one to two doses). In some clients treated once daily, the antihypertensive effect may decrease toward the end of the dosing interval; if this occurs, consider an increase in dosage or twice daily administration.

Hypertension in clients taking diuretics.

Initial: 2.5 mg. Since hypotension may occur following the initiation of enalapril, the diuretic should be discontinued, if possible, for 2–3 days before initiating enalapril. If BP is not maintained with enalapril alone, diuretic therapy may be resumed.

Hypertension in clients with impaired renal function.

Initial: 5 mg/day if C_{CR} ranges between 30 and 80 mL/min and serum creatinine is less than 3 mg/dL; 2.5 mg/day if C_{CR} is less than 30 mL/min and serum creatinine is more than 3 mg/dL and in dialysis clients on dialysis days.

Hypertension in children.

Initial: 0.08 mg/kg, up to 5 mg, once daily. Adjust dose depending on response. Do not give to neonates and children with a GFR <30 mL/min/1.73 m^2.

Heart failure (adjunct with diuretics and digitalis).

Initial: 2.5 mg 1–2 times per day; **then,** depending on the response, 2.5–20 mg/day in 2 divided doses. Dose should not exceed 40 mg/day. Dosage must be adjusted in clients with renal impairment or hyponatremia.

Heart failure and renal impairment or hyponatremia.

Initial: 2.5 mg/day if serum sodium is less than 130 mEq/L or serum creatinine is more than 1.6 mg/dL. The dose may be increased to 2.5 mg twice a day and then 5 mg twice a day or higher if required; dose is given at intervals of 4 or more days. Maximum daily dose is 40 mg.

Asymptomatic left ventricular dysfunction.

2.5 mg twice a day, titrated as tolerated to the daily dose of 20 mg in divided doses.

Enalaprilat

IV

Hypertension.

1.25 mg over a 5 min period; repeat q 6 hr.

Antihypertensive in clients taking diuretics.

Initial: 0.625 mg over 5 min; if there is an inadequate response after 1 hr, administer another 0.625 mg dose. Thereafter, 1.25 mg q 6 hr.

Hypertension in clients with impaired renal function.

C_{CR} >30 mL/min (serum creatinine up to about 3 mg/mL): 1.25 mg enalaprilat. **C_{CR} <30 mL/min or less (serum creatinine up 3 mg/mL or less):** 0.625 mg initially. If there is an inadequate response after 1 hr, repeat the 0.625 mg dose. Additional doses of 1.25 mg may be given at 6 hr intervals.

Hypertensive emergency.

1.25 mg IV over 5 min q 6 hr; titrate by 1.25 mg increments up to a maximum dose of 5 mg.

NURSING IMPLICATIONS

Do not confuse enalapril with Anafranil (an antidepressant) or with Eldepryl (an antiparkinson drug).

IMPLEMENTATION/ADMINISTRATION/STORAGE

1. To convert from IV to PO therapy in clients on a diuretic, begin with 2.5 mg/day for clients responding to a 0.625 mg IV dose. Thereafter, 2.5 mg/day may be given.
2. Use lower dose if receiving diuretics or impaired renal function.
3. A 1 mg/mL suspension may be prepared for use in children (see instructions in the labeling).
4. Carefully select dosage of all enalapril products in the geriatric client R/T decreased renal function with advancing age.
5. Coadministration of enalapril with potassium supplements, potassium salt substitutes, or potassium-sparing diuretics may lead to increases in serum potassium.
6. **IV** To convert from PO to IV therapy in clients not on a diuretic, use the recommended IV dose (i.e., 1.25 mg every 6 hr). To con-

vert from IV to PO therapy, begin with 5 mg/day.

7. Following IV administration, first dose peak effect may take 4 hr (whether or not on a diuretic). For subsequent doses, the peak effect is usually within 15 min.
8. Give enalaprilat as a slow IV infusion (over 5 min) either alone or diluted up to 50 mL with an appropriate diluent. When used initially for heart failure, observe for at least 2 hr after initial dose and until BP has stabilized for an additional hour. If possible, reduce dose of diuretic.
9. Store below 30°C (86°F).
10. COMPATIBILITY D5W, D5/RL, 0.9% NaCl, D5/0.9% NaCl.
11. INCOMPATIBILITY Administer separately.

ASSESSMENT

1. Note reasons for therapy, presenting symptoms, other agents trialed, outcome.
2. Record ECG, VS, and weight. With CHF, monitor for S&S of worsening failure (e.g., daily weights, evaluation of peripheral edema, shortness of breath).
3. Monitor BP, HR, CBC, electrolytes, renal and LFTs. Reduce dose with impaired renal function/hyponatremia/hyperkalemia.

CLIENT/FAMILY TEACHING

1. For BP lowering, use caution; may cause low BP effects and dizziness. Avoid sudden position changes to prevent drop in BP.
2. To help control BP, maintain healthy diet and limit intake of caffeine, avoid alcohol, salt substitutes, or high Na^+ and high K^+ foods, perform regular exercise, maintain weight, and stop smoking.
3. Report any weight loss that may result from the loss of taste, or rapid weight gain that may result from fluid overload.
4. With heart failure, record daily weights, and notify provider of rapid weight gain (e.g., 5 pounds in 1 week) or if extremity swelling or SOB worsen.
5. Any persistent dry cough, flu-like symptoms, rash, or unusual side effects should be reported immediately. Report pregnancy as soon as noted.
6. Consume adequate fluids to prevent dehydration.
7. Keep all F/U to assess response, BP record, for adverse SE.

OUTCOMES/EVALUATE

- ↓ BP
- ↓ Preload and afterload with CHF

Enfuvirtide

(en-**FYOU**-vir-tide)

Classification(s): Antiretroviral drug, fusion inhibitor

Pregnancy Category: B

RX: Fuzeon.

SEE ALSO ***ANTIVIRAL DRUGS***.

INDICATIONS/USES

In combination with other antiretroviral drugs to treat HIV-1 infection in treatment-experienced clients with evidence of HIV-1 replication despite ongoing antiretroviral therapy.

ACTION/KINETICS

Action

Enfuvirtide is an inhibitor of the fusion of HIV-1 with CD4+ cells. The drug interferes with the entry of HIV-1 into cells by inhibiting the fusion of the viral and cellular membranes.

Pharmacokinetics

Time to peak levels: 3–12 hr. Is about 84% bioavailable. Since the drug is a peptide, it is expected to undergo catabolism into its constituent amino acids with subsequent recycling of the amino acids in the body pool. **t½:** 3.8 hr. Clearance is 20% lower in women than men; no dosage adjustment is necessary, however. Clearance decreases with decreased body weight; no dosage adjustment is necessary. **Plasma protein binding:** About 92% in HIV-infected plasma.

CONTRAINDICATIONS

Hypersensitivity to the drug or any component of the product. Lactation.

SPECIAL CONCERNS

- Theoretically, enfuvirtide use may cause production of anti-enfuvirtide antibodies that cross-react with HIV gp41, resulting in a false + HIV test with an ELISA. A confirmatory Western blot test would be expected to be negative.
- SC injections with the needle-free Biojector 2000 is associated with neuralgia and/or paresthesia lasting up to 6 months when used at sites

where large nerves course close to the skin (e.g., elbow, knee, groin, medial sections of the buttocks).

- Safety and efficacy not determined in children less than 6 years of age.

SIDE EFFECTS

Most Common

Injection site reaction (pain/discomfort, induration, erythema, nodules/cysts, pruritus, ecchymosis), diarrhea, nausea, fatigue, weight loss, sinusitis, abdominal pain, cough, herpes simplex.

Local injection site reactions: Pain, discomfort, induration, erythema, nodules and cysts, pruritus, ecchymosis. **Hypersensitivity:** Rash, fever, N&V, chills, rigors, hypotension, elevated serum liver transaminases, primary immune complex reaction, respiratory distress, glomerulonephritis, Guillain-Barré syndrome. **CNS:** Insomnia, peripheral neuropathy, depression, anxiety, taste disturbance, sixth nerve palsy. **GI:** Diarrhea, nausea, decreased appetite, constipation, anorexia, pancreatitis, upper abdominal pain. **Hematologic:** Thrombocytopenia, neutropenia, fever. **Infections:** Increased rate of bacterial pneumonia, herpes simplex, sinusitis, skin papilloma, influenza. **GU:** Glomerulonephritis, renal failure. **Body as a whole:** Fatigue, decreased weight, asthenia, pruritus. **Miscellaneous:** Cough, myalgia, sinusitis, lymphadenopathy, conjunctivitis, hyperglycemia.

LABORATORY TEST CONSIDERATIONS

↑ Amylase, lipase, ALT, AST, creatine phosphokinase, GGT, triglycerides. ↓ Hemoglobin. Eosinophilia.

HOW SUPPLIED

Powder for Injection, Lyophilized: 108 mg (about 90 mg/mL when reconstituted).

DOSAGE

SC

Human immunodeficiency virus-1 infection.

Adults: 90 mg (1 mL) twice a day SC into the upper arm, anterior thigh, or abdomen. **Children, 6–16 years:** 2 mg/kg twice a day, up to a maximum of 90 mg twice a day SC into the upper arm, anterior thigh, or abdomen. (See *Implementation/Administration/Storage* for specific pediatric dosing guidelines.)

NURSING IMPLICATIONS

IMPLEMENTATION/ADMINISTRATION/STORAGE

1. Pediatric dosing guidelines for enfuvirtide using the 90 mg/mL reconstituted solution are:
   - **11–15.5 kg:** 27 mg/dose (0.3 mL)
   - **15.6–20 kg:** 36 mg/dose (0.4 mL)
   - **20.1–24.5 kg:** 45 mg/dose (0.5 mL)
   - **24.6–29 kg:** 54 mg/dose (0.6 mL)
   - **29.1–33.5 kg:** 63 mg/dose (0.7 mL)
   - **33.6–38 kg:** 72 mg/dose (0.8 mL)
   - **38.1–42.5 kg:** 81 mg/dose (0.9 mL)
   - **42.6 kg or greater:** 90 mg/dose (1 mL)
2. Reconstitute only with 1.1 mL of sterile water for injection.
3. Enfuvirtide contains no preservatives. Once reconstituted, inject immediately or keep refrigerated in original vial; use within 24 hr. Bring refrigerated reconstituted solution to room temperature before injection. Visually inspect vial to ensure that the contents are fully dissolved in solution, and solution is clear, colorless, and without bubbles or particulate matter.
4. Product is for single use only; discard unused portions.
5. Give each injection at a different site from preceding injection site, and only where there is no current injection site reaction from an earlier dose.
6. Do not inject enfuvirtide directly over a blood vessel or into moles, scar tissue, bruises, tattoos, burn sites, near the navel, or where there is an injection site reaction.
7. Store lyophilized powder for injection from 15–30°C (59–86°F). Store reconstituted solution under refrigeration at 2–8°C (36–46°F); use within 24 hr.

ASSESSMENT

1. Note disease onset, characteristics of S&S, other agents trialed, outcome.
2. List drugs prescribed to ensure none interact.
3. Observe injection site for reactions, bruising, hematomas, and nerve pain.
4. Assess lung sounds, and for the development of bacterial pneumonia especially in those with initial low CD4 lymphocyte count, high initial viral load, intravenous drug use, smoking, and a prior history of lung disease.
5. FUZEON use may lead to the production of anti-enfuvirtide antibodies, which cross-react

with HIV gp41. This could result in a false + HIV test with ELISA; in this case a Western blot confirmatory test would be expected to be negative.

CLIENT/FAMILY TEACHING

1. Drug is given subcutaneously by injection twice a day. Injections with the needle-free Biojector 2000 has been associated with neuralgia and/or paresthesia lasting up to 6 months when used near elbow, knee, groin, medial sections of the buttocks. It is taken with other antiretroviral drugs.
2. If given SC, may experience pain and inflammation at injection site. Review how to prepare and inject medication, dispose of needles, rotate sites, and notify provider if redness and swelling at site do not resolve.
3. Do not perform activities that require mental alertness until drug effects realized; may experience dizziness.
4. Report fever, increased SOB, cough, and labored breathing as pneumonia has been reported. Clients developing S&S of hypersensitivity reaction (rash, N&V, fever, chills) should discontinue drug and seek medical evaluation immediately. Do not restart therapy.
5. Practice safe sex and reliable contraception; report if pregnant or plan to become pregnant. Alert provider if planning to breast-feed. Drug is not a cure for HIV; may continue to experience opportunistic infections.
6. Clients may have medication dispensed by their own pharmacist at the pharmacy of their choice (no longer available only through Chronimed, Inc.). May call 1-877-438-9366 Mon–Fri 6 a.m. to 5 p.m. EST or go to www.fuzeon.com for more information. May enroll or call for a wealth of information support.
7. Keep all F/U to assess response, labs, and for adverse SE.

OUTCOMES/EVALUATE

↓ HIV RNA

■ IV ©

Enoxaparin

(ee-**nox**-ah-**PAIR**-in)

Classification(s): Anticoagulant, low molecular weight heparin

Pregnancy Category: B

RX: Lovenox.

Rx: Lovenox HP.

SEE ALSO ***HEPARINS, LOW MOLECULAR WEIGHT.***

INDICATIONS/USES

(1) Prophylaxis of deep vein thrombosis (DVT), which may lead to pulmonary embolism in those undergoing abdominal surgery who are at risk for thromboembolic complications; those undergoing hip replacement surgery during and following hospitalization; clients undergoing knee replacement surgery; and medical clients who are at risk for thromboembolic complications due to severely restricted mobility during acute illness. (2) With warfarin for inpatient treatment of DVT with and without pulmonary embolism; with warfarin for outpatient treatment of DVT without pulmonary embolism. (3) With aspirin to prevent ischemic complications of unstable angina and non-Q-wave MI. Can be used in geriatric clients. (4) Acute ST-segment elevation myocardial infarction in those receiving thrombolysis and being managed medically or with percutaneous coronary intervention (PCI). *Investigational:* Prevention of exercise-induced bronchoconstriction, prophylaxis of venous thromboembolism in cancer clients with central venous catheters, prophylaxis of venous thromboembolism in general or gynecologic surgery.

ACTION/KINETICS

Action

Enhances the inhibition of Factor Xa and thrombin by binding to and accelerating antithrombin II activity. Only slightly affects thrombin and clotting time (i.e., thrombin time or aPTT).

Pharmacokinetics

Bioavailability: 100%. **Maximum activity:** 3–5 hr. **t½, elimination:** 4.5 hr after a single dose and 7 hr after repeated doses. AUC is increased significantly (average of 65%) in those with severe renal impairment (C_{CR} <30 mL/min). Anti-factor Xa exposure is 52% higher in low-weight women (less than 45 kg). Elimination may be delayed in the elderly. **Duration:** 12 hr following a 40 mg dose. Excreted mainly through the urine.

CONTRAINDICATIONS

IM use. Use with prosthetic heart valves due to possible valve thrombosis, especially in pregnant women. Hypersensitivity to enoxaparin, heparin, pork products and in those with active major bleeding; also hypersensitivity to sulfites or benzyl alcohol (multidose vials). History of thrombocytopenia associated with in vitro tests for antiplatelet antibody in the presence of low molecular weight heparins.

SPECIAL CONCERNS

(1) **Spinal/epidural hematomas.** Epidural or spinal hematomas may occur in clients who are anticoagulated with low molecular weight heparins or heparinoids and are receiving neuraxial anesthesia or undergoing spinal puncture. These hematomas may result in long-term or permanent paralysis. Consider these risks when scheduling clients for spinal procedures. (2) Factors that can increase the risk of developing epidural or spinal hematomas in these clients include use of indwelling epidural catheters; concomitant use of other drugs that affect hemostasis, such as NSAIDs, platelet inhibitors, and other anticoagulants; a history of traumatic or repeated epidural or spinal punctures; and a history of spinal deformity or spinal surgery. (3) Monitor clients frequently for signs and symptoms of neurological impairment. If neurological compromise is noted, urgent treatment is necessary. (4) Consider the benefits and risks before neuraxial intervention in clients anticoagulated or to be anticoagulated for thromboprophylaxis.

- **Use with caution during pregnancy.**
- **Use with caution in the elderly as delayed elimination may occur.**
- **The use of enoxaparin has not been studied adequately for thromboprophylaxis or long-term use in those with mechanical prosthetic heart valves.**

SIDE EFFECTS

Most Common

Anemia, dyspnea, edema, fever, peripheral edema, confusion, pruritus/rash, nausea, diarrhea, thrombocytopenia, injection site reactions including hemorrhage.

Hematologic: Thrombocytopenia (with thrombosis), anemia, thrombocythemia, thrombocytosis, hematoma, ***hemorrhage***, hypochromic anemia, ecchymosis, epidural/spinal hematoma when used with spinal/epidural anesthesia or spinal puncture. **Injection site:** Mild local irritation, pain, hematoma, ecchymosis, erythema, hemorrhage, inflammation, nodules, skin necrosis, oozing. **GI:** Nausea, diarrhea. **CNS:** Confusion. **CV:** Atrial fibrillation, ***heart failure***. **Dermatologic:** Pruritus, rash, cutaneous vasculitis, purpura, vesiculobullous rash. **GU:** Hematuria. **Respiratory:** Dyspnea, lung edema, pneumonia. **Miscellaneous:** Fever, pain, edema, peripheral edema, hypersensitivity/allergic reactions.

LABORATORY TEST CONSIDERATIONS

Hyperlipidemia (rare).

HOW SUPPLIED

Injection: 30 mg/0.3 mL, 40 mg/0.4 mL, 60 mg/0.6 mL, 80 mg/0.8 mL, 100 mg/1 mL, 120 mg/0.8 mL, 150 mg/1 mL, 300 mg/3 mL.

DOSAGE

SC ONLY

Prophylaxis of deep vein thrombosis (DVT) in abdominal surgery.

Adults: 40 mg once daily, with the initial dose given 2 hr prior to surgery. Give for 7–10 days, up to 12 days.

Prophylaxis of DVT in hip or knee replacement.

Adults: 30 mg q 12 hr with the initial dose given within 12–24 hr after surgery (providing hemostasis has been established) for 7–10 days (usually), up to 14 days. For hip replacement, a dose of 40 mg once daily may be considered; give 9–15 hr before surgery and continue for 3 weeks.

Prophylaxis of DVT for medical clients during acute illness.

40 mg once daily for 6–11 days (up to 14 days has been well tolerated).

Treatment of DVT with or without pulmonary embolism for outpatients.

1 mg/kg SC q 12 hr.

Treatment of DVT with or without pulmonary embolism for inpatients.

1 mg/kg SC q 12 hr or 1.5 mg/kg SC once daily at the same time each day.

NOTE: For both in- and outpatients, initiate warfarin within 72 hr of enoxaparin. Continue enoxaparin for a minimum of 5 days and until an INR of 2–3 is reached (average duration is 7 days; up to 17 days has been well tolerated).

Acute ST-segment elevation myocardial infarction.

Single IV bolus of 30 mg plus a 1 mg/kg SC dose followed by 1 mg/kg given SC q 12 hr (maximum of 100 mg for the first 2 doses only, followed by 1 mg/kg dosing for the remaining doses). Adjust dosage in those over 75 years of age.

When given with a thrombolytic (fibrin-specific or nonfibrin-specific), give enoxaparin between 15 minutes before and 30 minutes after the start of fibrolytic therapy. All clients should receive aspirin as soon after acute ST-segment elevation MI has been diagnosed and maintained with 75–325 mg aspirin once daily unless contraindicated.

For clients managed with percutaneous coronary intervention, no additional dosing is needed if the last SC injection was given less than 8 hr before balloon inflation. If the last SC injection was given more than 8 hr before balloon inflation, give an IV bolus of enoxaparin of 0.3 mg/kg.

Acute ST-segment elevation myocardial infarction (MI) in those 75 years of age and older (STEMI).

Initial: 0.75 mg/kg SC q 12 hr (maximum of 75 mg for the first 2 doses only) followed by 0.75 mg/kg for the remaining doses. **Do not use an initial IV bolus.**

Prophylaxis of ischemic complications of unstable angina/Non-Q-wave MI.

Usual: 1 mg/kg q 12 hr with PO aspirin (100–325 mg once per day). Use for a minimum of 2 days; usual duration for enoxaparin is 2–8 days, up to 12.5 days.

Prophylaxis of venous thromboembolism in cancer clients with central venous catheters (investigational).

Adults: 40 mg SC once daily; enoxaparin was initiated 2 hr before insertion of the central venous catheter and continued for 6 weeks.

Prophylaxis of venous thromboembolism in general surgery (investigational).

Adults: 40 mg once daily SC with the initial dose given 2 hr before surgery. **Duration, usual:** 7–10 days. For those undergoing high-risk general surgery, including some having undergone major cancer surgery or have previously experienced venous thromboembolism, enoxaparin may be given for up to 28 days after hospital discharge.

Prophylaxis of venous thromboembolism in gynecologic surgery (investigational).

Adults: 40 mg once daily with the initial dose given 2 hr before surgery. For those undergoing major gynecologic surgery who are at high risk for venous thromboembolism, including those with a history of such or who had surgery for cancer, consider continuing enoxaparin for up to 28 days after hospital discharge. *NOTE:* All clients who have major gynecologic surgery should receive thromboprophylaxis at least until hospital discharge.

Thrombosis in children (investigational).

Thrombosis prophylaxis. Children, 2 months and older: 0.5 mg/kg SC q 12 hr; **younger than 2 months of age:** 0.75 mg/kg SC q 12 hr.

Thrombosis treatment. Children, 2 months and older: 1 mg/kg SC q 12 hr; **younger than 2 months of age:** 1.5 mg/kg SC q 12 hr. *NOTE:* Preterm infants younger than 2 months of age may require higher doses to achieve therapeutic anti-factor Xa concentrations; 2 mg/kg SC q 12 hr has been recommended.

NURSING IMPLICATIONS

Do not confuse enoxaparin with enoxacin (a fluoroquinolone antibiotic).

IMPLEMENTATION/ADMINISTRATION/STORAGE

1. Consider adjusting dose for low weight (<45 kg) clients and those with a C_{CR} <30 mL/min.
2. Dosage regimens for clients with severe renal impairment (C_{CR} less than 30 mL/min): (a) DVT prophylaxis in abdominal surgery, hip or knee replacement surgery, or medical clients during acute illness: 30 mg SC once a day. (b) Prophylaxis of ischemic complications of unstable angina and non-Q-wave MI (when used with aspirin), inpatient treatment of

acute DVT with or without pulmonary embolism (when used with warfarin), or outpatient treatment of acute DVT without pulmonary embolism (when given with warfarin): 1 mg/kg once daily. (c) Acute ST-segment elevation MI in clients less than 75 years of age, the dose is 30 mg as a single IV bolus plus a 1 mg/kg SC dose followed by 1 mg/kg given SC once a day. (d) Acute ST-segment elevation MI in clients over 75 years of age, give 1 mg/kg SC once daily (no initial bolus).

3. Use a tuberculin syringe or equivalent to ensure withdrawal of appropriate drug volume.
4. Usually given only by deep SC while lying down; do *not* give IM. Can be used IV (see below).
5. Continue treatment throughout postsurgical period until risk of DVT decreased.
6. Do not mix with other injections/infusions.
7. Discard any unused solution.
8. Do *not* interchange (unit for unit) with unfractionated heparin or other low molecular weight heparins, as they differ in their manufacturing process, molecular weight distribution, anti-Xa and anti-IIa activities, units, and dosage.
9. Injection is clear and colorless to pale yellow; store at 15–30°C (59–86°F). Do not freeze.
10. Do not store the multidose vial for more than 28 days after the first use.
11. IV For IV use, the multidose vial should be used. Give through an IV line. To avoid possible mixture with other drugs, the IV access chosen should be flushed with a sufficient amount of saline or dextrose solution before and following the IV bolus administration (i.e., to clear the port of the drug). For IV use, drug can be mixed with normal saline solution (0.9%) or D5W.
12. Store from 15–30°C (59–86°F). Do not store the multidose vials for more than 28 days after using the first time.
13. COMPATIBILITY 0.9%NaCl or D5W.
14. INCOMPATIBILITY Do not mix or coadminister with other drugs or infusions.

ASSESSMENT

1. Note reasons for therapy, clinical presentation, S&S of pulmonary embolism or DVT for SC versus acute STEMI for IV administration.
2. Assess for a bleeding disorder before giving enoxaparin, unless drug urgently needed.
3. Assess for heparin or pork product sensitivity; may preclude drug therapy.
4. List baseline hematologic parameters, liver function, and coagulation studies. If normal coagulation, monitor platelet counts. Drug may cause significant, nonsymptomatic increases in ALT/AST.
5. Monitor VS; observe for early S&S of bleeding. Any unexplained fall in hematocrit or BP should lead to search for a bleeding site. Those with spinal or epidural anesthesia should have neuro assessments regularly.
6. Assess clients with renal dysfunction and the elderly closely. Drug is extremely expensive; order in small lots. Report any evidence of thromboembolic event.
7. Monitor CBC with platelet count, and stool occult blood tests.

CLIENT/FAMILY TEACHING

1. May self-inject SC once instructed and observed. Lie down during self-administration; use prefilled syringes, and administer at the same time(s) each day.
2. Alternate injections between the left and right anterolateral and posterolateral abdominal wall. Insert entire length of needle into a skin fold held between the thumb and forefinger; hold throughout injection. To minimize bruising, do not rub site.
3. May experience mild discomfort, irritation, hematoma at site. Report unusual weakness, bruising, bleeding, black, bloody, or tarry stools immediately. Practice reliable contraception.
4. Avoid OTC agents that contain aspirin, NSAIDs; take safety precautions to prevent cuts, bruising, or falls (e.g., use electric razor, soft toothbrush, handrails, night-light).
5. Keep all F/U to assess response, and for adverse SE.

OUTCOMES/EVALUATE

- DVT prophylaxis post hip or knee replacement surgery or abdominal surgery
- Thromboembolic occurrence/recurrence prophylaxis
- Prevention of ischemic complications of unstable and non-Q-wave MI when coadministered with aspirin

E

Entacapone

(en-**TAH**-kah-pohn)

Classification(s): Antiparkinson drug

Pregnancy Category: C

RX: Comtan.

E

INDICATIONS/USES

As an adjunct with levodopa/carbidopa to treat idiopathic parkinsonism clients who experience signs and symptoms of end-of-dose "wearing off."

ACTION/KINETICS

Action

A selective and reversible catechol-O-methyltransferase (COMT) inhibitor. COMT eliminates catechols (e.g., dopa, dopamine, norepinephrine, epinephrine) and in the presence of a decarboxylase inhibitor (e.g., carbidopa), COMT becomes the major metabolizing enzyme for DOPA. Thus, in the presence of a COMT inhibitor, levels of dopa and dopamine increase. When entacapone is given with levodopa and carbidopa, plasma levels of levodopa are greater and more sustained than after levodopa/carbidopa alone. This leads to more constant dopaminergic stimulation in the brain resulting in improvement of the signs and symptoms of Parkinson's disease.

Pharmacokinetics

Rapidly absorbed. Almost completely metabolized in the liver with most excreted in the feces. **t½, elimination:** Biphasic 0.4–0.7 hr and 2.4 hr. **Plasma protein binding:** 98%.

CONTRAINDICATIONS

Concomitant use with a nonselective MAOI (e.g., phenelzine, tranylcypromine).

SPECIAL CONCERNS

- **Use with caution during lactation and in clients with biliary obstruction.**
- **At present, there is no potential use in children.**
- **Use with caution with drugs known to be metabolized by COMT (e.g., apomorphine, bitolterol, dobutamine, dopamine, epinephrine, isoetharine, isoproterenol, methyldopa, norepinephrine) due to the possibility of increased HR, arrhythmias, and excessive changes in BP.**

SIDE EFFECTS

Most Common

Dyskinesia, nausea, hyperkinesia, diarrhea, urine discoloration, hypokinesia, dizziness, abdominal pain, constipation, fatigue, aggravation of Parkinson's symptoms.

CNS: Dyskinesia, hyper-/hypokinesia, dizziness, anxiety, somnolence (may be sudden and uncontrolled), agitation, hallucinations, aggravation of Parkinson's symptoms. **GI:** Nausea, diarrhea, abdominal pain, constipation, vomiting, dry mouth, dyspepsia, flatulence, gastritis, GI disorders. **Body as a whole:** Fatigue, asthenia, increased sweating, bacterial infection. **Miscellaneous:** Urine discoloration, back pain, dyspnea, purpura, taste perversion, rhabdomyolysis.

OVERDOSE MANAGEMENT

Symptoms: Abdominal pain, loose stools. *Treatment:* Symptomatic with supportive care. Consider hospitalization. Monitor respiratory and circulatory systems. Review for possible drug interactions.

DRUG INTERACTIONS

Ampicillin / Interference with biliary excretion → ↓ excretion

Apomorphine / Possible ↑ HR, arrhythmias, and excessive BP changes

Bitolterol / Possible ↑ HR, arrhythmias, and excessive BP changes

Chloramphenicol / Interference with biliary excretion → ↓ excretion

Cholestyramine / Interference with biliary excretion → ↓ excretion

Dobutamine / Possible ↑ HR, arrhythmias, and excessive BP changes

Dopamine / Possible ↑ HR, arrhythmias, and excessive BP changes

Epinephrine / Possible ↑ HR, arrhythmias, and excessive BP changes

Erythromycin / Interference with biliary excretion → ↓ excretion

Isoetharine / Possible ↑ HR, arrhythmias, and excessive BP changes

Isoproterenol / Possible ↑ HR, arrhythmias, and excessive BP changes

MAOIs (phenelzine, tranylcypromine) / Significant ↑ levels of catecholamines

Methyldopa / Possible ↑ HR, arrhythmias, and excessive BP changes

Norepinephrine / Possible ↑ HR, arrhythmias, and excessive BP changes
Probenecid / Interference with biliary excretion → ↓ excretion
Rifampicin / Interference with biliary excretion → ↓ excretion

HOW SUPPLIED

Tablets: 200 mg.

DOSAGE

TABLETS

Parkinsonism.

200 mg given concomitantly with each levodopa/carbidopa dose up to a maximum of 8 times per day (i.e., 1,600 mg/day).

NURSING IMPLICATIONS

IMPLEMENTATION/ADMINISTRATION/STORAGE

1. Always give in combination with levodopa/carbidopa; entacapone has no antiparkinson effect by itself.
2. Most clients required a decreased daily levodopa dose (about 25%) if their daily levodopa dose was 800 mg or more, or if they had moderate or severe dyskinesias prior to entacapone treatment.
3. Entacapone can be given with immediate- or sustained-release levodopa/carbidopa formulations.
4. Rapid withdrawal or abrupt reduction in entacapone dose can lead to emergence of S&S of parkinsonism, and could lead to a complex resembling neuroleptic malignant syndrome (hyperpyrexia and confusion).
5. If necessary to discontinue treatment, withdraw clients slowly from entacapone.

ASSESSMENT

1. Note onset of Parkinson's disease, levodopa/carbidopa dosage, and when symptoms occur in dosage cycle. Assess mental status, mood, and involuntary movement/occurrence.
2. List drugs prescribed to ensure none interact. Assess for melanoma regularly.
3. Observe for postural hypotension, increased dyskinesia, and CNS changes (e.g., hallucinations).
4. Determine any evidence of liver or biliary dysfunction. Monitor renal and LFTs, H&H and ferritin levels with prolonged therapy.

CLIENT/FAMILY TEACHING

1. Take as directed with levodopa/carbidopa with or without food. Do not crush or chew tablets.
2. Drug is used to prevent end-of-dose "wearing off" effects of levodopa/carbidopa; alone it has no antiparkinson effect.
3. Never stop abruptly! Report any high fever or rigidity immediately.
4. Do not perform activities that require mental or physical alertness until drug effects realized. Rise slowly from a sitting or lying position to prevent sudden drop in BP or dizziness.
5. May experience loss of consciousness, nausea, diarrhea (may be delayed onset), hallucinations, increase in involuntary movements, altered pulmonary or kidney function. Report if evident.
6. Urine may appear brownish-orange in color.
7. Avoid alcohol during therapy.
8. May experience intense urges while taking one or more of the medications generally used to treat Parkinson's disease, notify provider if experiencing new or increased gambling urges, sexual urges, or other intense urges while taking entacapone.
9. Drug is not for use during pregnancy or breast-feeding. Report if pregnancy suspected or desired.
10. Keep all F/U to assess response, labs, and for adverse SE.

OUTCOMES/EVALUATE

Improved control of Parkinson's disease; (↓ dyskinesia: stiffness, tremor and shuffling; ↑ coordination)

IV

Epinephrine

(ep-ih-**NEF**-rin)

Classification(s): Sympathomimetic, direct-acting

Pregnancy Category: C

OTC: Aerosol: Epinephrine Mist, Primatene Mist.

RX: Injection: EpiPen, EpiPen Jr.

E

Epinephrine hydrochloride

Pregnancy Category: C

OTC: Inhalation Solution (as Racenephrine hydrochloride): S2.

RX: Inhalation/Topical Solution: Adrenalin Chloride. **Injection:** Adrenalin Chloride.

SEE ALSO ***SYMPATHOMIMETIC DRUGS***.

E

INDICATIONS/USES

Inhalation (Rx and OTC): Temporary relief of shortness of breath, tightness of chest, and wheezing due to bronchial asthma. Inhalation of a 1:100 epinephrine solution eases breathing for asthmatics by reducing bronchial muscle spasms. Do not use for asthma until a diagnosis of asthma has been made by a provider.

1:1,000 (1 mg/mL) solution: (1) Relieve respiratory distress due to bronchospasms. (2) Rapid relief of hypersensitivity reactions to drugs and other allergens. (3) Prolong the action of anesthetics used in local and regional anesthesia. (4) Restore cardiac rhythm in cardiac arrest due to various causes, although it is not used in cardiac failure or in hemorrhagic, traumatic, or cardiogenic shock. (5) Hemostatic agent. (6) Treat mucosal congestion of hay fever, rhinitis, and acute sinusitis. (7) Relieve bronchial asthmatic paroxysms. (8) In syncope because of complete heart block or carotid sinus hypersensitivity. (9) Symptomatic relief of serum sickness, urticaria, or angioneurotic edema. (10) Resuscitation in cardiac arrest following anesthetic accidents. (11) Simple (open-angle) glaucoma. (12) Relaxation of uterine musculature and to inhibit uterine contractions.

Injection, 1:1,000 (autoinjector) and 1:2,000 (autoinjector): Emergency treatment of allergic reactions (anaphylaxis) to insect stings or bites, foods, drugs, and other allergens, as well as idiopathic or exercise-induced anaphylaxis. Autoinjectors are for emergency supportive therapy only and are not replacements or substitutes for immediate medical or hospital care.

1:10,000 (0.1 mg/mL) solution. (1) Injection (IV) to treat acute hypersensitivity (anaphylactoid reactions) to drugs, animal serums, and other allergens. (2) In acute asthmatic attacks to relieve bronchospasm not controlled by inhalation or SC administration of other solutions of the drug. (3) Treatment and prophylaxis of cardiac arrest in the absence of ventricular fibrillation and attacks of transitory AV heart block with syncopal seizures (Stokes-Adams syndrome). Not used in cardiac failure or in hemorrhagic, traumatic, or cardiogenic shock. (4) Stimulate the heart in syncope due to complete heart block or carotid sinus sensitivity. (5) Resuscitation in cardiac arrest following anesthetic accidents. (6) Acute attacks of ventricular standstill (use physical measures first). When external cardiac compression and attempts to restore circulation by electrical defibrillation or use of a pacemaker fail, intracardiac puncture, and intramyocardial injection of epinephrine may be effective. *NOTE:* Intracardiac injection is not recommended any longer in Advanced Cardiac Life Support guidelines.

Investigational: (1) Endoscopic injection to manage acute lower GI bleeding. (2) Treat tricyclic antidepressant (and other sodium channel blockers) overdosage, calcium channel blocker overdosage, and beta-adrenergic blocker overdosage. (3) Symptomatic bradycardia or hypotension in those who have failed to respond to atropine or transcutaneous pacing, or if transcutaneous pacing is not available.

ACTION/KINETICS

Action

Causes marked stimulation of alpha, beta-1, and beta-2 receptors, causing sympathomimetic stimulation, pressor effects, cardiac stimulation, bronchodilation, and decongestion. It crosses the placenta but not the blood-brain barrier. **Extreme caution must be taken never to inject 1:100 solution intended for inhalation-injection of this concentration has caused death.**

Pharmacokinetics

SC: Onset, 5–10 min; **duration:** 4–6 hr. **Inhalation: Onset,** 1–5 min; **duration:** 1–3 hr. **IM, Onset:** variable; **duration:** 1–4 hr. **IV, Onset:** Immediate; intense response seen. After IV, drug disappears rapidly from the bloodstream. Ineffective when given PO. Excreted in the urine both unchanged and as metabolites.

ADDITIONAL CONTRAINDICATIONS

Organic heart disease, organic brain damage, hypertension, thyroid disease, local anesthesia of certain areas (e.g., fingers/toes) due to risk of tissue sloughing, labor, cardiac dilation, coronary insufficiency, cerebral arteriosclerosis, difficulty in urination due to enlarged prostate gland. Also, narrow angle glaucoma, non-anaphylactic shock during general anesthesia with halogenated hydrocarbons or cyclopropane. Use if taking a MAOI or for 4 weeks after stopping the MAOI. Inhalation if the client has ever been hospitalized for asthma or if the client is taking prescription medication for asthma. Do not use parenteral epinephrine in obstetrics when maternal BP exceeds 130/80 (increased risk of acceleration of fetal heart rate). Pregnancy and lactation.

SPECIAL CONCERNS

- May cause anoxia in the fetus.
- Administer parenteral epinephrine to infants and children with caution.
- Syncope may occur if epinephrine is given to asthmatic children.
- Administration of the SC injection by the IV route may cause severe or fatal hypertension or cerebrovascular hemorrhage.
- Extravasation may cause tissue necrosis.
- May temporarily increase the rigidity and tremor of parkinsonism.
- Use with caution and in small quantities in the toes, fingers, nose, ears, and genitals or in the presence of peripheral vascular disease as vasoconstriction-induced tissue sloughing may occur.
- Use the injection with caution in geriatric clients and in those with CV disease, hypertension, diabetes, hyperthyroidism, psychoneurotic clients, during pregnancy, and in those with long-standing bronchial asthma and emphysema who have developed degenerative heart disease. This is especially true if using epinephrine autoinjectors.
- Autoinjectors may increase the risk of side effects in children under 30 kg (66 lbs) if using the EpiPen and in children under 15 kg (33 lbs) if using EpiPen Jr. However, epinephrine is essential for treating anaphylaxis.
- May cause potentially serious cardiac arrhythmias in clients not suffering from heart disease and in those with organic heart disease or who are receiving drugs that sensitize the myocardium.

SIDE EFFECTS

Most Common

When used for bronchodilation: Palpitations, tachycardia, PVCs, dizziness/vertigo, nervousness, headache, insomnia, N&V, sweating, anorexia.

When used to treat shock: Anginal pain, tachycardia, palpitations, restlessness, headache, tremor, dizziness, N&V, sweating, anxiety.

See *Sympathomimetic Drugs* for a complete list of possible side effects. **Use of autoinjectors:** Palpitations, tachycardia, sweating, N&V, respiratory difficulty, pallor dizziness, weakness, tremor, headache, apprehension, nervousness, anxiety. **CV:** BP changes, hypertension, chest tightness/pain/discomfort, angina, palpitations, PVCs, arrhythmias, skipped beats, tachycardia. ***A rapid and large increase in BP may cause aortic rupture, cerebral hemorrhage, or angina pectoris.*** **GI:** N&V. **CNS:** Dizziness, vertigo, drowsiness, headache, insomnia, restlessness, shakiness, nervousness, tension, tremor, weakness, anxiety, fear. **GU:** Decreased urine formation, urinary retention, painful urination, direct vasoconstrictive effect on renal circulation after parenteral use. **Respiratory:** Dyspnea, ***pulmonary edema.*** **Dermatologic:** Flushing, pallor, sweating. **Miscellaneous:** Prolonged use or overdose may cause elevated serum lactic acid with severe metabolic acidosis. Anorexia and appetite loss. Skeletal injury. **At injection site:** Bleeding, urticaria, wheal formation, pain. Repeated injections at the same site may cause vascular necrosis from vascular constriction.

Parenteral use: CV: Parenteral use may cause ***cerebral hemorrhage, fatal ventricular fibrillation, cerebral or subarachnoid hemorrhage***, obstruction of central retinal artery, angina in coronary artery disease. **GU:** Direct vasoconstriction on renal circulation. **CNS:** Assaultive behavior, disorientation, hallucinations, hemiplegia, memory impairment, induce or aggravate psychomotor agitation, panic, hallucinations, ***suicidal or homicidal tendencies***, schizophrenic-type behavior, paranoid delusions, syncope in children, temporary rigidity and tremor in those with Parkinson's disease. **Miscellaneous:** Shock, hemorrhage at injection site, urticaria

OVERDOSE MANAGEMENT

Symptoms: **After Inhalation.** Exaggeration of side effects. **CNS:** ***Seizures***, nervousness, headache, tremor, dizziness, fatigue, malaise, insomnia. **GI:** Dry mouth, nausea. **CV:** Anginal pain, hypo-/hypertension, tachycardia (rates up to 200 beats/min), arrhythmias, palpitation, prolongation of QTc interval, ***cardiac arrest, death***. **Metabolic:** Hypokalemia, hyperglycemia, metabolic acidosis.

Musculoskeletal: Muscle cramps.

After Systemic use. CNS: Insomnia, anxiety, nervousness, drowsiness, dizziness, fatigue, malaise, insomnia, ***seizures,*** headache, tremor, delirium, ***coma***. **GI:** N&V. **CV:** Palpitations, tachycardia, transient arrhythmias, bradycardia, extrasystoles, heart block, angina, hypo-/hypertension, significant drop in BP due to peripheral vasodilation. **Musculoskeletal:** Muscle cramps. **Metabolic:** Hyperglycemia and increased insulin levels followed by rebound hypoglycemia; hypokalemia. **Ophthalmic:** Mydriasis. **Body as a whole:** Fever, chills, cold perspiration, collapse, blanching of the skin. *Treatment:* **Inhalation toxicity.** (a) Discontinue the drug; begin supportive measures. (b) Monitor BP and ECG. (c) Judiciously use a cardioselective beta-blocker (e.g., atenolol, metoprolol); note that there is danger of causing an asthmatic attack. (d) Dialysis is not appropriate.

Systemic toxicity. (a) Discontinue the drug or reduce dosage. Begin supportive measures. (b) Gastric lavage or charcoal may be useful following overdosage with PO drug. (c) If pronounced a beta-adrenergic blocker (e.g., propranolol) may be used; note there is danger of aggravating the airway obstruction. (d) Phentolamine may be used to block strong alpha-adrenergic effects. (e) Monitor BP, pulse, respiration, and ECG. (f) If respirations are shallow or cyanosis is present, give artificial respiration. (g) Do not use vasopressors. In CV collapse, maintain BP. (h) Control convulsions by diazepam. (i) Cool applications and dexamethasone (1 mg/kg) given slowly may control pyrexia.

ADDITIONAL DRUG INTERACTIONS

Alpha-adrenergic blocking agents / Antagonism of vasoconstrictor and pressor effects
Antihistamines (e.g., chlorpheniramine, diphenhydramine) / Pressor effects of direct-acting vasopressors potentiated
Beta-adrenergic blocking agents (e.g., propranolol) / Possible hypertension and reflex bradycardia R/T predominance of alpha-receptor effects
Bromocriptine / ↑ Risk of bromocriptine toxicity; closely monitor if coadministration is necessary
Cardiac glycosides (e.g., digoxin) / Possible sensitization of the myocardium to actions of epinephrine
COMT inhibitors (e.g., entacapone, tolcapone) / Inhibition of pathway responsible for normal catecholamine metabolism → excessive sympathetic stimulation
Diuretics / ↓ Vascular response to epinephrine
Ergot alkaloids / Reversal of pressor effects of epinephrine
General anesthetics (halothane, cyclopropane) / ↑ Sensitivity of myocardium to epinephrine → serious arrhythmias; do not use together
Guanethidine / Potentiation of effects of epinephrine; possible reversal of hypotensive effect of guanethidine
Levothyroxine / Potentiation of pressor effects of epinephrine
MAOIs / Appear to be minimal interaction but possible severe headache, hypertension, high fever, and hypertensive crisis; avoid coadministration or within 2 weeks of each other
Methyldopa / Possible ↑ pressor response → hypertension
Nitrites / Antagonism of vasoconstrictor and pressor effects
Oxytocic drugs (e.g., ergonovine) / Possible hypertension
Phenothiazines (e.g., chlorpromazine) / Reversal of epinephrine pressor effects
Quinidine / Possible sensitization of the myocardium to actions of epinephrine
Steroids / Possible potentiation of any hypokalemic effect
Sympathomimetic drugs / Possible additive effects and ↑ toxicity (e.g., serious cardiac arrhythmias) when used with other sympathomimetic drugs; do not use together
Tricyclic antidepressants (e.g., amitriptyline, imipramine) / Possible potentiation of direct-acting vasopressors (e.g., dysrhythmias); use together with caution
Xanthine derivatives (e.g., aminophylline, theophylline) / Possible potentiation of any hypokalemic effect; ↑ toxicity (especially cardiotoxicity)

HOW SUPPLIED

Epinephrine. ***Aerosol (OTC):*** 0.22 mg/spray; ***Injection Solution, Autoinjectors (Rx):*** 1:1,000 (0.15 mg/0.15 mL, 0.3 mg/0.3mL), 1:2,000 (0.15 mg/0.3 mL); ***Injection Solution, Ampules/Prefilled Syringes (Rx):*** 1:1,000 (0.3 mg/0.3 mL). **Epinephrine hydrochloride.** ***Intranasal Solution (Rx):*** 1:1000 (1 mg/mL); ***Inhalation Solution (Racenephrine HCl) (OTC):*** 2.25% (1.125% epinephrine base); ***Injection Solution (Rx):*** 1:1,000

(1 mg/mL), 1:10,000 (0.1 mg/mL); *Topical Solution (Rx):* 1:1,000 (1 mg/mL).

DOSAGE

Epinephrine/Epinephrine hydrochloride

AEROSOL (OTC)

Bronchodilation.

Adults and children 4 years and older: Start with 1 inhalation, and wait at least 1 min. If not relieved, use once more. Do not use again for at least 3 hr. Each inhalation delivers 0.22 mg epinephrine. **Children younger than 4 years of age:** Consult a provider.

INHALATION AEROSOL (RX)

Bronchodilation.

Adults and children 4 years and older, initial: 1–3 inhalations no more often than q 3 hr. **Children less than 4 years of age:** Consult a provider. See *Implementation/Administration/Storage* for specific instructions.

IM; IV; SC; AUTOINJECTORS

Asthma.

Adults, initial: 0.2–1 mg (0.2–1 mL) of the **1:1,000** solution SC (preferred) or IM q 4 hr. Start with a small dose and increase if necessary. Or, 0.1–0.25 mg (1–2.5 mL) of the **1:10,000** solution injected slowly IV. *Investigational (recommendation from the American Heart Association):* For acute severe asthma, give 0.01 mg/kg divided into 3 doses of about 0.3 mg given SC at 30-min intervals. Use the **1:1,000** (1 mg/mL) solution. **Infants and children:** 0.01 mg/kg or (0.3 mg/m^2) SC of the **1:1,000** solution, up to a maximum 0.5 mg repeated q 4 hr as needed. For an infant, 0.05 mg is an adequate initial dose that may be repeated at 20 to 30 min intervals to manage asthma attacks. **Neonates:** 0.01 mg/kg of the **1:1,000** solution given SC.

Anaphylaxis.

Adults: 0.2–1 mg of the **1:1,000** (1 mg/mL) solution SC or IM. Start with a small dose and increase, if required. Repeat q 10–15 min as needed. Or, 0.1–0.25 mg (1–2.5 mL) of the **1:10,000** solution (0.1 mg/mL) given slowly IV; may be repeated q 5–15 min, as needed. **Epinephrine autoinjectors:** 0.3 mg IM or SC into the anterolateral aspect of the thigh, through clothing if necessary. Repeat injection with an additional epinephrine autoinjector if necessary. *Investigational (recommendation from the American Heart Association):* 0.3–0.5 mg IM q 15–20 min as needed using the **1:1,000** (1 mg/mL) solution. If the anaphylaxis is severe with life-threatening symptoms, give epinephrine 0.1 mg by slow IV over 5 min using the **1:10,000** (0.1 mg/mL) solution. If frequent epinephrine administration is anticipated, a continuous IV infusion (1–4 micrograms/min) may be used. For anaphylactic reactions progressing to cardiac arrest, use high-dose epinephrine in a sequence, such as 1–3 mg IV over 3 min, followed by 3–5 mg IV over 3 min, and then 4–10 **micrograms** infusion.

Children: 0.1 mg/kg (or 0.3 mg/m^2) of the **1:1,000** (1 mg/mL) solution, up to a maximum of 0.5 mg given SC; repeat q 15 min for 2 doses and then q 4 hr as needed. Or, 0.3 mg (3 mL) of the **1:10,000** (0.1 mg/mL) solution given slowly IV; repeat q 15 min for 3 or 4 doses, as needed. **Epinephrine autoinjectors:** Base dose on body weight: **15–29 kg:** 0.15 mg; **30 kg or more:** 0.3 mg. Give IM or SC into the anterolateral aspect of the thigh, through clothing if necessary. Repeat injections with an additional epinephrine autoinjector as needed.

Cardiac stimulation.

Adults: 0.1–1 mg (1–10 mL) of the **1:10,000** (0.1 mg/mL) solution repeated q 5 min, if necessary. IV administration using the **1:10,000** solution (0.1 mg/mL) may last only a few minutes; thus, the IV dose may be followed with 0.3 mg (0.3 mL) of the **1:1,000** (1 mg/mL) solution given SC. **Children:** 0.005–0.01 mg/kg

(0.05–0.1 mL) of the **1:10,000** (0.1 mg/mL) solution IV; repeat q 5 min, if necessary. *NOTE:* For both adults and children, epinephrine is given by IV injection and/or, in cardiac arrest, by intracardiac injection into the left ventricular chamber. Intracardiac injection should only be undertaken by personnel well trained in the technique, if there has not been sufficient time to establish an IV route. **Intracardiac injection is no longer recommended in the ACLS guidelines.**

INTRASPINAL

Epinephrine added to anesthetic spinal fluid mixture.

Adults, usual: 0.2–0.4 mg (0.2–0.4 mL) of the **1:1,000** (1 mg/mL) solution added to anesthetic spinal fluid mixture. Epinephrine **1:100,000** (0.01 mg/mL) to **1:20,000** (0.05 mg/mL) is the usual concentration used with local anesthetics. *NOTE:* Intraspinal injection should only be undertaken by trained personnel.

OPHTHALMOLOGIC PRODUCTS

Conjunctival decongestion, control hemorrhage, produce mydriasis, reduce intraocular pressure.

Adults: Use concentrations of 1:10,000 (0.1 mg/mL) to 1:1,000 (1 mg/mL).

NURSING IMPLICATIONS

IMPLEMENTATION/ADMINISTRATION/STORAGE

1. **Medication errors, including deaths, have occurred due to inadvertant administration of the 1:1,000 (1 mg/mL) solution instead of the 1:10,000 (0.1 mg/mL) solution. The 1:1,000 solution must be diluted before administering IV. Use extreme caution.**
2. The following information is for use of the inhalation aerosol (Rx: 1:1,000):
   - Place 10 drops (not more) in the reservoir of the nebulizer.
   - Place the nozzle just inside the partially opened mouth. As the bulb is squeezed once or twice, the client inhales deeply, drawing the vaporized solution into the lungs.
   - Start treatment at the first symptoms.
   - Rinsing the mouth with water immediately after using the nebulizer will help prevent the sensation of dry mouth and throat.
   - When the nebulizer contains any liquid and is not in use, cap the container, and keep in an upright position.
   - Because of oxidation, epinephrine solution, 1:100, will turn pink to brown when exposed to air. Light, heat, alkalis, and certain metals (e.g., copper, iron, zinc) will also promote deterioration.
   - Never use a discolored (pinkish or darker than slightly yellow) inhalation solution or one containing a precipitate.
3. The 1:1,000 injection solution may be given IM or SC (preferred). The 1:10,000 injection solution is given by IV injection or, in cardiac arrest, by intracardiac injection into the left ventricular chamber or via endotracheal tube directly into the bronchial tree.
4. The 1:100 epinephrine inhalation solution is intended only for PO (not nasal) use. Because of the higher concentration of the 1:100 solution, it is not suitable for parenteral use.
5. Seek medical attention immediately if symptoms are not relieved within 20 min, or if they become worse after using the inhalation solution.
6. Excessive use of the inhalation solution may cause nervousness and rapid heartbeat, and possibly adverse cardiac effects.
7. Briskly massage site of SC or IM injection to hasten drug action. Do not expose drug to heat, light, or air as this causes deterioration.
8. Solution should be clear. Do not use the injection if the color is pinkish or darker than slightly yellow, or if it contains a precipitate. Protect from light. Discard unused portion. Epinephrine deteriorates rapidly on exposure to air and light, turning, due to oxidation, to adrenochrome and brown.
9. Accidental injection of the autoinjector into the hands or feet may result in loss of blood flow to the area and should be avoided.
10. Store autoinjectors in the tube provided from 15–30°C (59–86°F); do not refrigerate. Autoinjectors do not contain latex.
11. Store the OTC inhalation solution and parenteral forms from 15–30°C (59–86°F), and the Rx inhalation solution from 15–25°C (59–77°F), protected from light and freezing.

12. **Never administer** 1:100 solution IV; use the 1:10,000 solution.
13. Use a tuberculin syringe to measure. Parenteral doses are small and drug is potent, thus errors in measurement may be disastrous.
14. IV For direct IV administration to adults, the drug must be well diluted as a 1:10,000 solution; inject quantities of 0.05–0.1 mL of solution cautiously, taking about 1 min for each injection; note response (BP and pulse). Dose may be repeated several times if necessary.
15. COMPATIBILITY D5W or NSS.
16. INCOMPATIBILITY Administer separately.

ASSESSMENT

1. List reasons for therapy; describe type/onset of symptoms, anticipated results and method of administration.
2. Assess for sulfite sensitivity. Note cardiopulmonary function.
3. During IV therapy, continuously monitor ECG, BP, and pulse until desired effect achieved. Take VS every 2–5 min until stabilized; once stable, monitor BP q 15–30 min.
4. Note any symptoms of shock such as cold, clammy skin, cyanosis, and loss of consciousness.
5. With inhalation/aerosol therapy, monitor respiratory status during each treatment; stop treatment if bronchospasm worsens. Document PFTs.
6. Check to ensure proper concentration and dosage form are being used, as multiple forms and concentrations are available.

CLIENT/FAMILY TEACHING

1. Take as directed. Review method for administration carefully. When prescribed for anaphylaxis, administer autoinjector immediately, and seek medical care. Check expiration dates.
2. Report any increased restlessness, chest pain, heart fluttering, SOB, lack of response, adverse effects, or insomnia, as dosage adjustment may be necessary. May elevate blood sugar.
3. Limit intake of caffeine (colas, coffee, tea, and chocolate); avoid OTC drugs without approval.
4. Rinse mouth and inhaler after use. If also prescribed steroid inhaler, take bronchodilator first, and wait at least 5 min before administering steroid inhaler so air passages are open and receptive.
5. Nasal application may sting slightly. Nasal OTC products may work initially but with prolonged use exacerbate symptoms.
6. Ophthalmic solution may burn initially, and a brow headache may occur; this should subside. Remove contact lenses; may stain lenses.
7. Use caution when performing activities that require careful vision; ophthalmic solution may diminish visual fields, cause double vision, and alter night vision.
8. Discard any discolored or precipitated solutions.
9. Keep all F/U to assess response, and for adverse SE.

OUTCOMES/EVALUATE

- Restoration of cardiac activity
- ↓ IOP
- Reversal of S&S of anaphylaxis
- Improved airway exchange
- Hemostasis with ocular surgery

IV

Epirubicin hydrochloride

(ep-ee-**ROO**-bih-sin)

Classification(s): Antineoplastic, antibiotic

Pregnancy Category: D

RX: Ellence.

✦ **Rx:** Pharmorubicin PFS.

SEE ALSO ***ANTINEOPLASTIC AGENTS***.

INDICATIONS/USES

Adjunct to treat breast cancer in clients with evidence of axillary node tumor involvement after resection of primary breast cancer. *Investigational:* In combination with cisplatin and 5-fluorouracil to treat advanced esophageal cancer. Also, small-cell lung cancer, non-small-cell lung cancer, Hodgkin's lymphoma, and non-Hodgkin's lymphoma.

ACTION/KINETICS

Action

Cell cycle phase nonspecific anthracycline; has maximum cytotoxic effects on the S and G_2 phases. Precise mechanism of action is not known.

It does form a complex with DNA by intercalation of its planar rings between nucleotide base pairs resulting in inhibition of DNA and RNA synthesis. Intercalation triggers DNA cleavage by topoisomerase II, resulting in cell death. The drug also inhibits DNA helicase activity, which prevents enzymatic separation of double-stranded DNA and interferes with replication and transcription. The drug is also involved in oxidation-reduction reactions by generating cytotoxic free radicals.

Pharmacokinetics

Following IV, it is rapidly and widely distributed; appears to concentrate in RBCs. Extensively and rapidly metabolized by the liver and RBCs. Parent drug and metabolites are excreted through both the feces (main route) and urine. **t½:** Triphasic with half-lives of about 3 min, 2.5 hr, and 33 hr. **Plasma protein binding:** About 77% (not affected by drug concentration).

CONTRAINDICATIONS

Severe hepatic dysfunction; previous anthracycline treatment up to the maximum cumulative dose; severe myocardial insufficiency or recent MI; severe arrhythmias; hypersensitivity to epirubicin, other anthracyclines, or anthracenediones; baseline neutrophil count <1,500 cells/mm^3. Lactation.

SPECIAL CONCERNS

(1) Severe local tissue necrosis will occur if extravasation occurs during administration. It is recommended that epirubicin be slowly administered into the tubing of a freely running IV infusion usually between 3 and 20 minutes depending upon dosage and volume of the infusion solution. If possible, veins over joints or in extremities with compromised venous or lymphatic drainage should be avoided. A burning or stinging sensation may be indicative of perivenous infiltration, and the infusion should be immediately terminated and restarted in another vein. Perivenous infiltration may occur without causing pain. Epirubicin must not be given by the IM or SC route. (2) Myocardial toxicity, manifested in its most severe form by potentially fatal CHF, may occur either during therapy with epirubicin or months or years after termination of therapy. The probability of developing clinically evident CHF is estimated as approximately 0.9% at a cumulative dose of 550 mg/m^2, 1.6% at 700 mg/m^2, and 3.3% at 900 mg/m^2. In the adjuvant treatment of breast cancer, the maximum cumulative dose used in clinical trials was 720 mg/m^2. The risk of developing CHF increases rapidly with increasing total cumulative doses of epirubicin in excess of 900 mg/m^2; this cumulative dose should only be exceeded with extreme caution. Active or dormant CV disease, prior or concomitant radiotherapy to the mediastinal/pericardial area, previous therapy with other anthracyclines or anthracenediones, or concomitant use of other cardiotoxic drugs may increase the risk of cardiac toxicity. Cardiac toxicity with epirubicin may occur at lower cumulative doses whether or not cardiac risk factors are present. (3) Secondary acute myelogenous leukemia (AML) has been reported in clients with breast cancer treated with anthracyclines, including epirubicin. The occurrence of refractory secondary leukemia is more common when such drugs are given in combination with DNA-damaging antineoplastic agents, when clients have been heavily pretreated with cytotoxic drugs, or when doses of anthracyclines have been escalated. The cumulative risk of developing treatment-related AML in 3,844 clients with breast cancer who received adjuvant treatment with epirubicin-containing regimens, was estimated as 0.2% at 3 years and 0.8% at 5 years. (4) Dosage should be reduced in clients with impaired hepatic function. Definitive recommendation regarding use of epirubicin in clients with hepatic dysfunction are not available because clients with hepatic abnormalities were excluded from participation in adjuvant trials. In clients with elevated serum AST or serum total bilirubin concentrations, the following dose reductions were recommended in clinical trials, although few clients experienced hepatic impairment: (a) Bilirubin 1.2 to 3 mg/dL or AST 2 to 4 times ULN, give one-half of the recommended starting dose.
(b) Bilirubin greater than 3 mg/dL or AST greater than 4 times ULN, give one-fourth of the recommended starting dose. (5) Severe myelosuppression may occur. (6) Epirubicin should be administered only under the super-

vision of a physician who is experienced in the use of cancer chemotherapeutic agents.

- Use of epirubicin after previous radiation therapy may cause an inflammatory recall reaction at the site of irradiation.
- When used in combination with other cytotoxic drugs, additive hematologic and GI toxicity may occur.
- Use with caution in women over 70 years of age due to lower plasma clearance.
- Safety and efficacy not determined in children.

SIDE EFFECTS

Most Common

Leukopenia, neutropenia, anemia, thrombocytopenia, amenorrhea, lethargy, N&V, mucositis, alopecia, hot flashes.

GI: N&V, mucositis (oral stomatitis, esophagitis), diarrhea, anorexia, abdominal pain, hyperpigmentation of the oral mucosa. **CV:** CHF, sinus tachycardia, nonspecific ST-T wave changes, asymptomatic decrease in LVEF, PVCs, ***ventricular tachycardia***, bradycardia, AV and bundle branch block, tachyarrhythmias (including PVTs), thrombophlebitis, ***thromboembolism***. **Dermatologic:** Alopecia, local toxicity, rash, itch, skin changes, flushes, skin and nail hyperpigmentation, photosensitivity, hypersensitivity to irradiated skin, urticaria, ***anaphylaxis*** (including symptoms of skin rash, pruritus, fever, chills, and shock), injection site reactions (e.g., venous sclerosis, extravasation causing local pain, severe tissue lesions, and necrosis). **Hematologic:** Leukopenia, neutropenia, anemia, thrombocytopenia, secondary acute myelogenous leukemia (with or without a preleukemic phase), acute lymphoid leukemia, acute myelogenous leukemia. **Endocrine:** Amenorrhea, hot flashes. **Miscellaneous:** Lethargy, infection, febrile neutropenia, fever, conjunctivitis/keratitis, tumor lysis syndrome, injection site reactions (venous sclerosis, local pain, severe tissue lesions, necrosis), hypersensitivity (urticaria, ***anaphylaxis***), inflammatory recall reaction at the site of the irradiation.

OVERDOSE MANAGEMENT

Symptoms: Symptoms are similar to the known toxicity of epirubicin (see *Side Effects*), including delayed CHF. *Treatment:* Supportive treatment, including antibiotic therapy, blood and platelet transfusions, colony-stimulating factors, and intensive care. Observe over time for signs of CHF; provide supportive therapy.

DRUG INTERACTIONS

Cardioactive drugs (e.g., calcium channel blockers) / Possible heart failure; close monitoring required
Cimetidine / ↑ Epirubicin blood levels by 50%; stop cimetidine therapy during use of epirubicin
Cytotoxic drugs / Additive toxicity, especially hematologic and GI effects
Radiation therapy / Possible sensitization of tissues to the cytotoxic action of irradiation

HOW SUPPLIED

Injection Solution: 2 mg/mL; *Injection, Lyophilized Powder for Solution:* 50 mg, 200 mg.

E

DOSAGE

IV INFUSION

Breast cancer with evidence of axillary node tumor.

The following regimens are recommended: (1) epirubicin, 100 mg/m^2; 5-fluorouracil, 500 mg/m^2; and cyclophosphamide, 500 mg/m^2. All drugs are given on day 1 and repeated q 21 days for 6 cycles. Clients given epirubicin, 120 mg/m^2 are also given prophylactic antibiotic therapy with trimethoprim-sulfamethoxazole or a fluoroquinolone. (2) epirubicin, 60 mg/m^2 on days 1 and 8; 5-fluorouracil, 500 mg/m^2 on days 1 and 8 and repeated q 28 days for 6 cycles; and cyclophosphamide, 75 mg/m^2 PO on days 1 to 14.

NURSING IMPLICATIONS

IMPLEMENTATION/ADMINISTRATION/STORAGE

1. IV Epirubicin should only be given under the supervision of a qualified physician experienced in the use of cytotoxic therapy.
2. Make dosage adjustments after the first treatment cycle based on hematologic and nonhematologic toxicity:
   - Reduce day 1 dose in subsequent cycles to 75% of the day 1 dose given in the current cycle in clients experiencing cycle nadir platelet counts <50,000/mm^3, absolute neutrophil counts (ANC) <250/mm^3, neu-

tropenic fever, or Grades 3/4 nonhematologic toxicity. Delay day 1 chemotherapy in subsequent courses of treatment until platelet counts are 100,000/mm^3 or more, ANC is 1,500/mm^3 or more, and nonhematologic toxicities have recovered to Grade 1 or less.
- For clients receiving a divided dose of epirubicin on days 1 and 8, reduce the day 8 dose to 75% of day 1 if platelet counts are 75,000–100,000/mm^3 and ANC is 1,000–1,499/mm^3. Omit the day 8 dose, if day 8 platelet counts are <75,000/mm^3, ANC is < 1,000/mm^3, or Grade 3/4 nonhematologic toxicity has occurred.

3. Consider a lower starting dose (75–90 mg/m^2) for heavily pretreated clients, those with pre-existing bone marrow depression, or in the presence of neoplastic bone marrow infiltration.
4. With elevated serum AST or serum total bilirubin levels, consider the following doses of epirubicin:
   - Bilirubin, 1.2–3 mg/dL, or AST, 2–4 times ULN, give one-half the recommended starting dose.
   - Bilirubin >3 mg/dL or AST >4 times ULN, give one-fourth the recommended starting dose.
5. Consider lower doses of epirubicin with severe renal impairment (serum creatinine >5 mg/dL).
6. Clients given 120 mg/m^2 of epirubicin as part of combination therapy should receive prophylactic antibiotic therapy with a fluoroquinolone or trimethoprim-sulfamethoxazole.
7. Consider prophylactic use of antiemetics to reduce N&V, especially if epirubicin given with other emetogenic drugs.
8. The solution is manufactured preservative-free and as a ready-to-use solution. Give over a 3–5 min period into the tubing of a freely flowing IV infusion. Do not use a direct push injection due to the possibility of extravasation.
9. Wear protective clothing when handling drug, and do not handle if pregnant. Use within 24 hr of first penetration of the rubber stopper.
10. Treat spillage or leakage with dilute sodium hypochlorite (1% available chlorine), preferably by soaking, and then water. Treat accidental contact with the skin immediately by copious lavage with water, or soap and water, or sodium bicarbonate solution; however, do not abrade the skin by using a scrub brush.
11. Store from 2–8°C (36–46°F); do not freeze. Protect from light. Discard any unused drug.
12. Epirubicin can be used in combination with other antitumor drugs; do not, however, mix with other drugs in the same syringe.
13. COMPATIBILITY 0.9% NaCl or D5W.
14. INCOMPATIBILITY Do not mix epirubicin with heparin or fluorouracil due to chemical incompatibility that may cause precipitation. Avoid prolonged contact with any alkaline solution; hydrolysis of the drug will occur.

ASSESSMENT

1. Note disease onset, symptom characteristics, staging, other medical conditions, other agents trialed.
2. Monitor ECG and for anthracyline-induced cardiomyopathy by ECHO or MUGA determination of LVEF during therapy. Note any rhythm changes, S_3, SOB, edema; may experience delayed cardiac toxicity 2–3 months to years after completing therapy. Do not exceed 900 mg/m^2 cumulative dose. May cause inflammatory reaction at previous XRT sites.
3. Assess IV site carefully; drug is a vessicant. Venous sclerosis at injection site or extravasation may occur; may cause pain and tissue necrosis. Give slowly over 3–5 min to prevent facial flushing or erythematous streaking along vein.
4. Give antiemetics 30–60 min before therapy to diminish N&V. Ensure adequate hydration, alkalinization of urine, treatment for tumor lysis syndrome (allopurinol).
5. With 120 mg/m^2 regimen in combination therapy, also give ATX prophylaxis with trimethoprim-sulfamethoxazole or fluoroquinolone.
6. Lower dose with hematologic, renal or liver dysfunction; follow dosing guidelines carefully. Secondary leukemias have occurred.
7. Obtain baseline CBC before and during therapy; renal and LFTs, and reduce dose with dysfunction. WBC nadir 10–14 days; recovery 21 days.

CLIENT/FAMILY TEACHING

1. Therapy usually given once every 3 weeks for 6 cycles for node positive resectable primary

breast cancer. Used in combination with other agents to achieve maximum benefits.
2. May experience N&V, diarrhea, hair loss, inflammation or sores in the oral mucosa; report side effects or complaints.
3. There is a risk of irreversible myocardial damage and treatment-related leukemia; need frequent studies (ECG, ECHO or MUGA scans) and blood work.
4. Report increased SOB, chest pains, lower extremity swelling, vomiting, dehydration, fever, infection or injection site pain after therapy.
5. Urine may be red for several days after therapy; not worrisome.
6. If platelet counts, white count, or nonhematologic toxicities occur, dosage will be reduced with next dose or discontinued if prolonged.
7. Use reliable birth control; men may experience chromosomal sperm damage, and women may develop premature menopause or irreversible amenorrhea. Determine if sperm/egg harvesting indicated.
8. Avoid crowds and persons with known infections and live vaccinations during therapy.
9. Keep all F/U to assess response, labs, and adverse SE.

OUTCOMES/EVALUATE

Control of malignant cell proliferation in breast cancer

IV

Epoetin alfa recombinant

(ee-**POH**-ee-tin)

Classification(s): Erythropoietin, human recombinant

Pregnancy Category: C

RX: Epogen, Procrit.

♣ **Rx:** Eprex.

INDICATIONS/USES

(1) Treatment of anemia associated with chronic kidney disease in adults and children, including clients on dialysis (end-stage renal disease) or adults not on dialysis to decrease the need for RBC transfusion. For clients on dialysis, initiate treatment when the hemoglobin level is <10 grams/dL. For those not on dialysis, consider starting epoetin alfa only when the hemoglobin level is <10 grams/dL, the rate of hemoglobin decline indicates the likelihood of requiring a RBC transfusion, and reducing the risk of alloimmunization and/or other RBC transfusion-related risks is a goal.

(2) Treatment of anemia due to zidovudine administered at 4,200 mg or less per week in HIV-infected clients with endogenous serum erythropoietin levels of 500 milliunits/mL or less.

(3) Treatment of anemia in clients with nonmyeloid malignancies in which anemia is due to the effect of coadministered chemotherapy and upon initiation there is a minimum of 2 additional months of planned chemotherapy.

(4) To reduce the need for allogeneic RBC transfusions in clients with perioperative hemoglobin greater than 10–13 grams/dL who are at high risk of perioperative blood loss from elective, noncardiac, nonvascular surgery.

Investigational: Anemia associated with critically ill clients, CHF, chronic disease (e.g., rheumatoid arthritis), postpartum anemia, sickle cell disease, thalassemia, multiple myeloma, Jehovah's witnesses, radiation treatment, epidermolysis bullosa, porphyria. For athletic enhancement, sexual dysfunction, and transfusional iron overload.

ACTION/KINETICS

Action

Made by recombinant DNA technology; it has the identical amino acid sequence and same biologic effects as endogenous erythropoietin (which is normally synthesized in the kidney and stimulates RBC production). Epoetin alfa will stimulate RBC production and thus elevate or maintain the RBC level, decreasing the need for blood transfusions. The reticulocyte count increases within 10 days of initiating therapy, followed by increases in the RBC count, hemoglobin, and hematocrit, usually within 2–6 weeks.

Pharmacokinetics

Peak serum levels after SC: 5–24 hr. **t½, chronic renal failure:** 4–13 hr (20% longer in those with chronic renal failure compared with healthy subjects); **t½, anemic cancer clients:** 16–67 hr. Distribution volume is 1.5–2 times higher in preterm neonates than in healthy adults; clearance is about 3 times higher in preterm neonates than in healthy adults.

CONTRAINDICATIONS

Uncontrolled hypertension. Pure red cell aplasia that begins after treatment with epoetin alfa or other erythropoietin protein drugs. Hypersensitivity to mammalian cell-derived products or to human albumin. Use in chronic renal failure clients who need severe anemia corrected. To treat anemia in HIV-infected or cancer clients due to factors such as iron or folate deficiencies, hemolysis, or GI bleeding. Anemic clients willing to donate autologous blood. Use from multidose vials that contain benzyl alcohol in neonates, infants, pregnant women, and breast-feeding mothers.

SPECIAL CONCERNS

■ Erythropoiesis-stimulating agents (ESAs) increase the risk of death, myocardial infarction, stroke, venous thromboembolism, thrombosis of vascular access, and tumor progression or recurrence. **Chronic kidney disease.** (1) In controlled trials, clients experienced greater risks for death, serious adverse CV reactions, and stroke when administered ESAs to target a hemoglobin level of greater than 11 grams/dL. (2) No trial has identified a hemoglobin target level, darbepoetin alfa dose, or dosing strategy that does not increase these risks. (3) Use the lowest darbepoetin alfa dose sufficient to reduce the need for red blood cell transfusions. **Cancer.** (1) ESAs shortened overall survival and/or increased the risk of tumor progression or recurrence in clinical studies of clients with breast, non-small-cell lung, head and neck, lymphoid, and cervical cancers. (2) Because of these risks, prescribers and hospitals must enroll in and comply with the ESA APPRISE Oncology Program to prescribe and/or dispense darbepoetin to clients with cancer. To enroll in the ESA APPRISE Oncology Program, visit www.esa-apprise.com or call 1-866-284-8089 for further assistance. (3) To decrease these risks, as well as the risk of serious CV and thromboembolic reactions, use the lowest dose to avoid RBC transfusions. (4) Use ESAs only for anemia from myelosuppressive chemotherapy. (5) ESAs are not indicated for clients receiving myelosuppressive chemotherapy when the anticipated outcome is cure. (6) Discontinue following the completion of a chemotherapy course. **Perisurgery.** Due to increased risk of deep venous thrombosis, DVT prophylaxis is recommended. ■

- **Use with caution in clients with porphyria, during lactation, and pre-existing vascular disease.**
- **Increased anticoagulation with heparin may be required in clients on epoetin alfa undergoing hemodialysis.**
- **Since epoetin alfa contains albumin, there is a remote risk for transmission of viral diseases or Creutzfeldt-Jakob disease.**
- **There is an increased risk of MI, stroke, thromboembolism, and mortality at higher hemoglobin targets (i.e., 13–14 grams/dL) compared with lower targets (9–11.5 grams/dL).**
- **Use of high doses to treat acute ischemic stroke is associated with an increased risk of death.**
- **Some clients treated with epoetin alfa may show a lack or loss of hemoglobin response; causes should be investigated.**
- **Use benzyl alcohol free epoetin alfa with caution during lactation.**
- **Safety and efficacy not established in children less than 1 month of age, in children less than 5 years of age with cancer, or in clients with a history of seizures or underlying hematologic disease (e.g., hypercoagulable disorders, myelodysplastic syndromes, sickle cell anemia).**

SIDE EFFECTS

Most Common

Hypertension, headache, fatigue, N&V, diarrhea, edema, asthenia, respiratory congestion, cough, pyrexia, rash, SOB, insomnia, pruritus, DVT (in surgery clients), hyperkalemia.

All uses. CV: Hypertension. Increased risk for ***death*** and serious CV events when given to target a hemoglobin of more than 12 grams/dL. There is an increased risk of serious arterial and venous thromboembolic reactions, including ***MI,*** stroke, CHF, and hemodialysis graft occlusion. **CNS:** ***Seizures.*** **Dermatologic:** Injection-site reactions, including irritation and pain. **Hematologic:** Pure red cell aplasia, porphyria. **Hypersensitivity:** Angioedema, bronchospasm, skin rash, urticaria, ***anaphylaxis.*** **Miscellaneous:** Absolute or functional iron deficiency. Immunogenicity.

In chronic kidney disease clients (symptoms may be due to the disease). CV: Hypertension (including hypertensive encephalopathy), tachycardia, edema, ***MI***, ***CVA***, TIA, clotted vascular access. Rarely, thromboembolic reactions, including microvascular thrombosis, migratory thrombophlebitis, pulmonary embolus, and thrombosis of the retinal artery and temporal and renal veins. **CNS:** Headache, fatigue, dizziness, ***seizures*.** **GI:** N&V, diarrhea, worsening of porphyria. **Musculoskeletal:** Myalgia, arthralgias, muscle spasm. **Respiratory:** SOB, URTI. **Allergic reactions:** Skin rashes, urticaria, circumoral edema, ***anaphylaxis*.** **Hematologic:** Pure red cell aplasia, severe anemia (with or without cytopenias). **Body as a whole:** Asthenia, edema, pyrexia, erythema. **Miscellaneous:** Hyperkalemia, chest pain, skin reaction at administration site, injection site stinging in dialysis clients, worsening of porphyria.

Children with chronic kidney disease. The pattern of most side effects was similar to adults. The following additional side effects were observed: Abdominal pain, constipation, cough, dialysis access complications (e.g., infections, peritonitis), fever, pharyngitis, URTI.

In zidovudine-treated HIV-infected clients. CNS: Pyrexia, fatigue, headache, dizziness, ***seizures*.** **CV:** Increased risk of thrombotic events. **Respiratory:** Cough, ***pulmonary embolism***, respiratory tract congestion, SOB. **GI:** Diarrhea, nausea. **Dermatologic:** Rash, urticaria, skin reaction at injection site, urticaria. **Body as a whole:** Asthenia, pyrexia.

In cancer clients. CNS: Pyrexia, fatigue, depression, headache, insomnia, dizziness, ***seizures*.** **GI:** Diarrhea, N&V, dysphagia, stomatitis. **CV:** Increased ***thrombotic reactions, thrombosis*.** **Musculoskeletal:** Asthenia, arthralgia, bone pain, myalgia, paresthesia, trunk pain. **Respiratory:** SOB, cough, URTI. **Metabolic:** Hyperglycemia, hypokalemia, weight decrease. **Body as a whole:** Edema, asthenia, rash. **Miscellaneous: *Increased mortality*** and/or tumor progression, leukopenia.

In surgery clients. CNS: Pyrexia, insomnia, headache, dizziness, anxiety. **GI:** N&V, constipation, diarrhea, dyspepsia. **CV:** Hypertension, ***DVT***, edema. **Dermatologic:** Pruritus, reaction/pain at injection site, skin pain, rash. **GU:** UTI. **Body as a whole:** Chills, cough.

LABORATORY TEST CONSIDERATIONS

↑ Platelets, WBCs, BUN, creatinine, phosphorus, potassium in CRF clients (all increases not clinically significant). Hyperkalemia.

OVERDOSE MANAGEMENT

Symptoms: Polycythemia. Symptoms associated with an excessive and/or rapid increase in hemoglobin levels (including CV symptoms). Hypertension (may be severe). *Treatment:* Withhold drug until hematocrit returns to the target range. Phlebotomy may be used to decrease hemoglobin. Reduce dose in those with an excessive hematopoietic response.

HOW SUPPLIED

Injection Solution: 2,000 units/mL, 3,000 units/mL, 4,000 units/mL, 10,000 units/mL, 20,000 units/mL, 40,000 units/mL.

DOSAGE

IV; SC

Anemia caused by chronic kidney disease.

Adults, initial: 500–100 units/kg IV or SC 3 times a week. The IV route is recommended for clients on hemodialysis. Do not increase the dose more frequently than once q 4 weeks. Decreases in dose can occur more frequently. Avoid frequent dose adjustments. When initiating or adjusting therapy, monitor hemoglobin levels at least weekly until stable; then, monitor monthly.

Dosage increase for those who do not respond adequately: If the hemoglobin has not increased by more than 1 gram/dL after 4 weeks of therapy, increase the dose by 25%. For clients who do not respond adequately over a 12-week escalation period, increasing the epoetin alfa dose further will not likely improve the response and may increase risks. Discontinue epoetin alfa if the response does not improve.

Dosage decrease: If the hemoglobin rises rapidly (e.g., more than 1 gram/dL in any 2-week period), reduce the dose of epoetin alfa by 25% or more as needed to reduce rapid progression.

Children, 1 month–16 years of age, dialysis clients only, initial: 50 units/kg IV or SC 3 times a week. The IV route is recommended for clients on hemodialysis. See preceding adult information for dosage adjustment and monitoring.

Children, 3 months–18 years of age, not on dialysis (investigational), initial: 50–250 units/kg 3 times a week. Reduce the dose by 25% if hemoglobin increases more than 1 gram/dL in any 2-week period or hemoglobin reaches a level needed to avoid RBC transfusion.

E

Anemia in zidovudine-treated, human immunodeficiency virus infections.

Adults, initial: 100 units/kg 3 times per week IV or SC. If hemoglobin does not increase after 8 weeks of therapy, increase the epoetin alfa dose by about 50–100 units/kg at 4- to 8-week intervals until hemoglobin reaches a level needed to avoid RBC transfusions or 300 units/kg.

Withhold epoetin alfa if the hemoglobin exceeds 12 grams/dL. Resume therapy at a dose of 25% below the previous dose when hemoglobin declines to less than 11 grams/dL.

Discontinue epoetin alfa if an increase in hemoglobin is not reached at a dosage of 300 units/kg for 8 weeks.

Children, 8 months–17 years of age (investigational), usual dose: 50–400 units/kg 2–3 times a week. If the response is not satisfactory after 8 weeks of therapy, the dose may be increased by 50–100 units/kg per dose 3 times a week. Re-evaluate after 4–8 weeks. Clients are not likely to respond to dosages greater than 300 units/kg 3 times a week.

Anemia in cancer clients on chemotherapy.

Adults, initial: 150 units/kg 3 times a week or 40,000 units per week SC until completion of a chemotherapy course. Initiate epoetin alfa therapy in clients on cancer chemotherapy only if the hemoglobin is less than 10 grams/dL and if there is a minimum of 2 additional months of planned chemotherapy.

Children, 5–18 years of age, initial: 600 units/kg IV weekly until completion of a chemotherapy course. **Maximum dose:** 60,000 units a week. After the initial 4 weeks of epoetin alfa therapy, if hemoglobin increase by less than 1 gram/dL and remains below 10 grams/dL, increase the dose to 900 units/kg, up to a maximum of 60,000 units a week.

If hemoglobin increases by less than 1 gram/dL and remains below 10 grams/dL after the initial 4 weeks of epoetin alfa therapy, increase the dose to 300 units/kg 3 times a week or 60,000 units a week.

Reduce the dose by 25% if hemoglobin increases greater than 1 gram/dL in any 2-week period or hemoglobin reaches a level needed to avoid RBC transfusions. Withhold the dose if hemoglobin exceeds a level needed to avoid RBC transfusion. Reinitiate at a dose 25% below the previous dose when hemoglobin reaches a level needed to avoid RBC transfusion.

If there is no response after 8 weeks of therapy as measured by hemoglobin levels or if RBC transfusions are still required, discontinue epoetin alfa.

Surgery to reduce allogeneic blood transfusions.

Obtain a hemoglobin before surgery to determine that it is more than 10 to less than or equal to 13 grams/dL. **Adults, SC:** 300 units/kg/day for 10 days before surgery, on the day of surgery, and for 4 days after surgery. Alternative: 600 units/kg SC once a week 21, 14, and 7 days before surgery plus a fourth dose on the day of surgery. Iron supplementation is required at the time of epoetin therapy and continuing throughout the course of therapy. DVT prophylaxis is recommended during epoetin alfa therapy.

NURSING IMPLICATIONS

IMPLEMENTATION/ADMINISTRATION/STORAGE

1. ***Do not*** **give with any other drug solutions. At time of SC administration, the drug may be admixed in a syringe with bacteriostatic 0.9% NaCl injection with benzyl alcohol, 0.9%, at a**

1:1 ratio. The benzyl alcohol acts as a local anesthetic that may reduce discomfort at the SC injection site.

2. A hemoglobin rise of more than 1 gram/dL over 2 weeks may contribute to increased mortality, serious CV and thromboembolic events.
3. Absolute or functional iron deficiency may develop.
4. Using aseptic technique, attach a sterile needle to a sterile syringe. Remove the flip top from the vial containing epoetin alfa, and wipe the septum with a disinfectant. Insert the needle into the vial, and withdraw into the syringe an appropriate volume of solution.
5. Do not dilute or give in conjunction with other drug solutions. At the time of SC administration, however, preservative-free epoetin alfa from single-use vials may be mixed in a syringe with bacteriostatic sodium chloride (0.9% injection with benzyl alcohol 0.9%) at a 1:1 ratio using aseptic technique. Admixing is not necessary when using multidose vials as these contain benzyl alcohol.
6. Therapy with epoetin alfa results in an increase in hematocrit and a decrease in plasma volume; this could affect efficiency of dialysis. During hemodialysis, clients may need increased anticoagulation with heparin to prevent clotting of the artificial kidney.
7. IV IV usually given as a bolus 3 times/week. May be given into venous line at end of dialysis procedure to obviate need for additional venous access.
8. The IV route is recommended for those on hemodialysis. For adults with CRF not on dialysis, epoetin alfa may be given IV or SC.
9. During hemodialysis, may require increased anticoagulation with heparin to prevent clotting of artificial kidney.
10. Determine hematocrit twice weekly until stabilized in the target range and the maintenance dose of epoetin alfa has been determined. Do not adjust more often than once a month, unless clinically indicated. After any dosage adjustment, monitor hematocrit twice a week for 2–6 weeks.
11. Individualize hemoglobin target level. If rate of rise of hemoglobin exceeds 1 gram/dL over a 2-week period, interrupt dose and modify rate of rise of hemoglobin. Target hemoglobin levels in those with cancer to avoid RBC transfusions. See *Dosage* for specific information.
12. Do **not** shake; shaking will denature the glycoprotein, making it biologically inactive.
13. Do not use vials showing particulate matter or discoloration.
14. The 1 mL single-dose vial contains no preservative; use only one dose/vial. Do not reenter the vial; discard unused portions.
15. The multidose 1 and 2 mL vials contain preservative. Store from 2–8°C (36–46°F) after initial entry and between doses. Discard 21 days after initial entry.
16. Store single-dose at 2–8°C (36–46°F). Do not freeze or shake. Protect from light. Discard unused portions in single-dose vials.
17. COMPATIBILITY 0.9% NaCl; single dose vials: bacteriostatic NaCl 0.9% injection with benzyl alcohol 0.9% in a 1:1 ratio.
18. INCOMPATIBILITY Administer separately. Do not mix with other drug solutions.

ASSESSMENT

1. Note any sensitivity to mammalian cell-derived products or human albumin.
2. List reasons/conditions requiring therapy, goal Hb, expected duration of therapy. Follow dosing guidelines carefully; initially monitor H&H 2 times weekly in CRF clients and once weekly in zidovudine-treated HIV clients until stabilized and maintenance dose established then at least every 4 weeks.
3. DVT prophylaxis recommended with surgical orthopedic procedures or when ESAs are used for the reduction of allogeneic RBC transfusions in surgical patients.
4. Assess BP; control hypertension. Assess for seizures with any significant hematocrit increases.
5. Review product literature for administration guidelines. Follow dosing guidelines carefully and based on Hb levels to ensure no adverse SE.
6. Those with cancer must sign the patient-health care provider acknowledgment before the start of each treatment course with epoetin alfa and must be provided written acknowledgment of a discussion of the risks of Epogen. Hospital/provider must be enrolled in ESA-APPRISE; to enroll visit www.esa-apprise.com or call 1-866-284-8089 for further assistance.

7. Determine CBC and iron stores. Transferrin saturation should be at least 20%, and serum ferritin should be at least 200 ng/mL. Provide supplemental iron to increase or maintain transferrin to levels required to support stimulation of erythropoiesis by epoetin alfa.
8. Review the potential for increased risk of death, MI, stroke, venous thromboembolism, thrombosis of vascular access, and tumor progression or recurrence with this type of drug therapy.
9. Regularly monitor CBC, renal function studies, I&O, electrolytes, phosphorus, iron, and uric acid levels. Drug dose and therapy by trained and registered individuals only under closely monitored conditions.

CLIENT/FAMILY TEACHING

1. Avoid shaking vial; keep refrigerated. Goal is to achieve lowest level Hb to avoid transfusion. Review medication information sheet with each renewal.
2. Over 95% of clients with CRF manifested significant increases in hematocrit, and nearly all were transfusion-independent within 2 months after beginning therapy; drug does not cure renal disease and desired drug response may take up to 6 weeks.
3. Supplemental iron and vitamins are administered to enhance drug effects; take as directed.
4. Do not perform tasks that require mental alertness until drug effects realized (especially during first 3 months of therapy due to risk of seizures).
5. Report any new-onset neurologic symptoms or change in seizure frequency.
6. Review list of drug side effects; immediately report: hives, intolerable GI effects (e.g., nausea, vomiting, diarrhea), intolerable injection-site reaction, palpitations, rash, severe headache, SOB, swelling of eyes, mouth, or throat or swelling of feet/ankles.
7. Practice reliable contraception during therapy.
8. Must continue to follow prescribed dietary and dialysis recommendations; schedule activities to permit rest periods. Record BP for provider review.
9. May cause tumor progression with some types of cancer. There may be greater risks for death and serious CV events when erythropoiesis-stimulating agents (ESAs) targeted to higher versus lower Hb levels.
10. Keep all F/U to assess response, labs, for dose adjustment, and adverse SE.

OUTCOMES/EVALUATE

- ↑ Hemoglobin (10–12 g/dL)
- Relief of symptoms of anemia R/T CRF, zidovudine therapy with HIV, and nonmyeloid malignancies R/T chemo
- Reduction of RBC transfusions

Eprosartan mesylate

(eh-proh-**SAR**-tan)

Classification(s): Antihypertensive, angiotensin II receptor blocker

Pregnancy Category: C (first trimester); **D** (second and third trimesters)

RX: Teveten.

SEE ALSO ***ANTIHYPERTENSIVE AGENTS***.

INDICATIONS/USES

Hypertension, alone or with other antihypertensives (e.g., diuretics, calcium channel blockers).

ACTION/KINETICS

Action

Acts by blocking the vasoconstrictor and aldosterone-secreting effects of angiotensin II by blocking selectively the binding of angiotensin II to angiotensin II receptors located in the vascular smooth muscle and adrenal gland. BP is thus reduced.

Pharmacokinetics

About 13% bioavailable. **Peak plasma levels:** 1–2 hr. Food delays absorption. **t½, terminal:** 5–9 hr. Excreted mostly unchanged in both the feces (about 90%) and urine (about 7%). **Plasma protein binding:** About 98%.

SPECIAL CONCERNS

■ **Use in pregnancy.** When used in pregnancy during the second and third trimesters, drugs that act directly on the renin-angiotensin system can cause injury and even death to the developing fetus. When pregnancy is detected, eprosartan mesylate tablets should be discontinued as soon as possible. ■

- Symptomatic hypotension may be seen in clients who are volume- and/or salt-depleted (e.g., those taking diuretics).
- Safety and efficacy not determined in children.

SIDE EFFECTS

Most Common

URTI, cough, pharyngitis, rhinitis, UTI, viral infection, arthralgia, abdominal pain, fatigue.

GI: Abdominal pain, diarrhea, dyspepsia, anorexia, constipation, dry mouth, esophagitis, flatulence, gastritis, gastroenteritis, gingivitis, nausea, periodontitis, toothache, vomiting. **CNS:** Depression, headache, dizziness, anxiety, ataxia, insomnia, migraine, neuritis, nervousness, paresthesia, somnolence, tremor, vertigo. **CV:** Angina pectoris, bradycardia, abnormal ECG, extrasystoles, atrial fibrillation, hypotension, tachycardia, palpitations, peripheral ischemia. **Respiratory:** URTI, sinusitis, bronchitis, chest pain, rhinitis, pharyngitis, cough, asthma, epistaxis. **Musculoskeletal:** Arthralgia, myalgia, arthritis, aggravated arthritis, arthrosis, skeletal/back pain, tendonitis. **GU:** UTI, albuminuria, cystitis, hematuria, frequent micturition, polyuria, renal calculus, urinary incontinence. **Metabolic:** Diabetes mellitus, gout. **Body as a whole:** Viral infection, injury, fatigue, alcohol intolerance, asthenia, substernal chest pain, peripheral edema, dependent edema, fever, hot flushes, flu-like symptoms, malaise, rigors, pain, leg cramps, herpes simplex. **Hematologic:** Anemia, purpura, leukopenia, neutropenia, thrombocytopenia. **Dermatologic:** Eczema, furunculosis, pruritus, rash, maculopapular rash, increased sweating. **Ophthalmic:** Conjunctivitis, abnormal vision, xerophthalmia. **Otic:** Otitis external, otitis media, tinnitus.

LABORATORY TEST CONSIDERATIONS

↑ ALT, AST, creatine phosphokinase, BUN, creatinine, alkaline phosphatase. ↓ Hemoglobin. Glycosuria, hypercholesterolemia, hyperglycemia, hyper-/hypokalemia, hyponatremia.

HOW SUPPLIED

Tablets: 400 mg, 600 mg.

DOSAGE

TABLETS

Hypertension.

Adults, initial: 600 mg once daily as monotherapy in clients who are not volume-depleted. Can be given once or twice daily with total daily doses ranging from 400–800 mg. There is limited experience with doses exceeding 800 mg/day.

NURSING IMPLICATIONS

IMPLEMENTATION/ADMINISTRATION/STORAGE

1. If antihypertensive effect using once-daily dosing is inadequate, a twice-a-day regimen at the same total daily dose or an increase in dose may be more effective.
2. Maximum BP reduction may not occur for 2–3 weeks.
3. May be used in combination with thiazide diuretics or calcium channel blockers if additional BP lowering effect is needed.
4. Discontinuing treatment does not lead to a rapid rebound increase in BP.
5. No initial dosage adjustment is needed for the elderly or those with hepatic or renal impairment (maximum dose: 600 mg/day for those with moderate to severe renal impairment).
6. Store from 20–25°C (68–77°F).

ASSESSMENT

1. Note onset, symptoms, other agents trialed/outcome.
2. Correct volume depletion. Monitor BP, CBC, K^+, sodium, microalbumin, renal and LFTs.

CLIENT/FAMILY TEACHING

1. Take as directed once or twice daily with or without food.
2. Continue lifestyle modifications, i.e., maintain healthy diet and limit intake of caffeine, avoid alcohol, salt substitutes, or high Na^+ and high K^+ foods, perform regular exercise, maintain weight, and stop smoking for BP control.
3. Practice reliable birth control. Report if pregnant.
4. Immediately report any lip, tongue, or facial swelling as well as any fever or sore throat. Report any persistent dry cough.
5. Keep a record of BP readings and bring for provider review.
6. Keep all F/U to assess response and for adverse SE.

OUTCOMES/EVALUATE

↓ BP; control of HTN

E

IV

Eptifibatide

(**ep**-tih-**FY**-beh-tide)

Classification(s): Antiplatelet drug, glycoprotein IIb/IIIa inhibitor

Pregnancy Category: B

RX: Integrilin.

E

INDICATIONS/USES

(1) Treatment of acute coronary syndrome (unstable angina or non-Q-wave MI), including those to be managed medically and those undergoing percutaneous coronary intervention. (2) Treatment of those undergoing percutaneous coronary intervention, including those undergoing intracoronary stenting.

ACTION/KINETICS

Action

Reversibly inhibits platelet aggregation by preventing the binding of fibrinogen, von Willebrand's factor, and other adhesive ligands to GP IIb/IIIa.

Pharmacokinetics

Immediately effective after IV use. **t½, elimination:** 2.5 hr. Drug and metabolites are excreted through kidneys.

CONTRAINDICATIONS

History of bleeding diathesis or evidence of active abnormal bleeding within the past 30 days. Severe hypertension (systolic BP >200 mm Hg or diastolic BP >110 mm Hg) inadequately controlled. Major surgery within the past 6 weeks, history of stroke within 30 days or any history of hemorrhagic stroke, current or planned use of another parenteral GP IIb/IIIa inhibitor, platelet count less than 100,000/mm^3, dependency on renal dialysis. Serum creatinine of 2.0 mg/dL or more (for the 180 mcg/kg bolus and the 2 mcg/kg/min infusion) or 4.0 mg/dL or more (for the 135 mcg/kg bolus and the 0.5 mcg/kg/min infusion). Lactation.

SPECIAL CONCERNS

- **Bleeding is the most common complication; there is a greater risk in older clients.**
- **Use with caution when used with drugs that affect hemostasis, including thrombolytics, oral anticoagulants, NSAIDs, dipyridamole, ticlopidine, and clopidogrel.**
- **Use with caution during lactation.**
- **Safety and efficacy not determined in children.**

SIDE EFFECTS

Most Common

Bleeding, hypotension.

CV: ***Major bleeding***, including ***intracranial hemorrhage***, bleeding from the femoral artery access site, and bleeding that leads to decreases in hemoglobin greater than 5 grams/dL. Minor bleeding, including spontaneous gross hematuria, spontaneous hematemesis, or blood loss with a hemoglobin decrease of more than 3 grams/dL. Oropharyngeal (especially gingival), genitourinary, GI, and retroperitoneal bleeding. Hypotension. **Hypersensitivity/allergy:** ***Anaphylaxis***, other allergic S&S.

DRUG INTERACTIONS

Possible additive effects when used with thrombolytics, anticoagulants, or other antiplatelet drugs.

H *Evening primrose oil* / Potential for ↑ antiplatelet effect
H *Feverfew* / Potential for ↑ antiplatelet effect
H *Garlic* / Potential for ↑ antiplatelet effect
H *Ginger* / Potential for ↑ antiplatelet effect
H *Ginkgo biloba* / Potential for ↑ antiplatelet effect
H *Ginseng* / Potential for ↑ antiplatelet effect
H *Grapeseed extract* / Potential for ↑ antiplatelet effect

HOW SUPPLIED

Injection: 0.75 mg/mL, 2 mg/mL.

DOSAGE

IV

Acute coronary syndrome.

Adults, initial: IV bolus of 180 mcg/kg as soon as possible following diagnosis, followed by a continuous infusion of 2 mcg/kg/min until hospital discharge or initiation of coronary artery bypass surgery, up to 72 hr. If the client is to undergo a PCI while receiving eptifibatide, continue the infusion up to hospital discharge, or for up to 18 to 24 hr after the procedure, whichever comes first, allowing up to 96 hr of therapy.

The recommended adult dosage in clients with acute coronary syndrome with an estimated C_{CR} <50 mL/min or a serum creatinine >2 mg/dL (if C_{CR} is not available) is an IV bolus of 180 mcg/kg as soon as possible following diagnosis, immediately followed by a continuous infusion of 1 mcg/kg/min.

Percutaneous coronary intervention.

Adults with normal renal function: IV bolus of 180 mcg/kg given immediately before initiation of PCI followed by a continuous infusion of 2 mcg/kg/min and a second bolus dose of 180 mcg/kg 10 min after the first bolus. This is followed by a continuous infusion until hospital discharge or for up to 18–24 hr, whichever comes first. A minimum of 12 hr of infusion is recommended. Give those weighing more than 121 kg a maximum of 22.6 mg/bolus followed by a maximum infusion rate of 7.5 mg/hr.

Adults, in those with a C_{CR} <50 mL/min or creatinine >2 mg/dL: IV bolus of 180 mcg/kg given immediately before initiation of PCI, immediately followed by a continuous infusion of 1 mcg/kg/min and a second 180 mcg/kg bolus given 10 min after the first. Give those weighing more than 121 kg a maximum of 22.6 mg/bolus followed by a maximum infusion rate of 7.5 mg/hr.

NURSING IMPLICATIONS

IMPLEMENTATION/ADMINISTRATION/STORAGE

1. **IV** If undergoing CABG surgery, discontinue prior to surgery.
2. Aspirin has been used with eptifibatide with the following possible doses: In acute coronary syndrome, aspirin, 160–325 mg initially and daily thereafter; in PCI, aspirin, 160–325 mg 1–24 hr prior to intervention and daily thereafter.
3. The following aspirin and heparin doses are recommended:
   - **Acute coronary syndrome:** Aspirin, 160–325 mg PO initially and daily thereafter. For heparin, achieve a target aPTT of 50–70 sec during medical management of the following: If weight is 70 or more kg, give a 5,000 units heparin bolus followed by infusion of 1,000 units/hr. If the weight is <70 kg, give a 60 units/kg bolus followed by infusion of 12 units/kg/hr. If heparin is initiated prior to PCI, additional boluses during PCI to maintain an ACT target of 200 to 300 seconds. Heparin infusion after the PCI is discouraged.
   - **PCI:** Aspirin, 160–325 mg PO 1 to 24 hr prior to PCI and daily thereafter. For heparin, achieve a target ACT of 200–300 seconds for the following: Heparin, 60 units/kg, as a bolus initially in those not treated with heparin within 6 hr prior to PCI. Give additional boluses during PCI to maintain ACT within target. Do not give heparin infusion after the PCI.
4. Inspect vial for particulate matter or discoloration before use.
5. Withdraw bolus dose from the 10 mL vial and give by IV push over 1–2 min. Immediately following the bolus dose, start continuous infusion. If using an infusion pump, give undiluted directly from the 100 mL vial by spiking the 100 mL vial with a vented infusion set. Center spike within the circle on the stopper top.
6. Store vials at 2–8°C (36–46°F). Protect from light until use. Discard any portion left in the vial.
7. COMPATIBILITY 0.9% NaCl or D5/NSS (may also contain up to 60 mEq/L of KCl). May be given in the same IV line as alteplase, atropine, dobutamine, heparin, lidocaine, meperidine, metoprolol, midazolam, morphine, nitroglycerin, or verapamil.
8. INCOMPATIBILITY Do not give in same line as furosemide.

ASSESSMENT

1. Identify onset, duration, characteristics of S&S.
2. Note conditions that preclude therapy: recent CVA or surgery, platelets <100,000/mm^3, uncontrolled BP, abnormal bleeding or history of bleeding diathesis, hemorrhagic stroke, renal failure, or dialysis.
3. Stop drug prior to CABG surgery.
4. Used in conjunction with aspirin and heparin; review dosing guidelines.

5. Assess femoral artery access site for evidence of bleeding. Stop heparin and eptifibatide therapy if unable to stop bleeding with pressure.
6. Monitor VS, ECG, CBC, bleeding times, renal and LFTs, and also activated clotting time (ACT) in those undergoing PCI.

CLIENT/FAMILY TEACHING

1. Review risks associated with therapy. Drug is a blood thinner given IV and used to prevent clot formation with unstable angina, non-Q-wave MI, and those undergoing PCI including stenting.
2. Bleeding is most common side effect of therapy; usually occurs at graft site but may also occur as GU, GI, oropharyngeal, or retroperitoneal bleeding. Report any unusual bleeding, change in mental status, sudden drop in BP, or other adverse side effects.
3. Encourage family to learn CPR.

OUTCOMES/EVALUATE

- Inhibition of platelet aggregation
- ↓ Death/MI with acute coronary syndrome

IV

Eribulin mesylate

(**er**-ih-**BUE**-lin)

Classification(s): Antineoplastic drug, antimitotic agent.

Pregnancy Category: D

RX: Halaven.

INDICATIONS/USES

Treatment of metastatic breast cancer in those who have previously received at least two chemotherapeutic regimens to treat metastatic disease. Prior therapy should have included an anthracycline and a taxane in either the adjuvant or metastatic setting.

ACTION/KINETICS

Action

Inhibits the growth phase of microtubules without affecting the shortening phase, and sequesters tubulin into nonproductive aggregates. Eribulin exerts its effects via a tubulin-based antimitotic mechanism resulting in G_2/M cell-cycle block, disruption of mitotic spindles, and ultimately, apoptotic cell death after prolonged mitotic blockage.

Pharmacokinetics

t½, elimination: About 40 hr. Eliminated primarily in the feces (82%) unchanged with a small amount eliminated in the urine (9%). Levels are increased in those with moderate renal impairment and mild and moderate hepatic impairment. **Plasma protein binding:** 49–65%.

CONTRAINDICATIONS

Lactation.

SPECIAL CONCERNS

Safety and efficacy not determined in children 18 years and younger.

SIDE EFFECTS

Most Common

Neutropenia, anemia, asthenia, fatigue, alopecia, peripheral neuropathy, nausea, constipation.

CNS: Headache, peripheral neuropathy, paresthesia, depression, dizziness, insomnia. **GI:** Anorexia, constipation, diarrhea, N&V, abdominal pain, dry mouth, dyspepsia, stomatitis, dysgeusia. **CV:** QT prolongation. **Dermatologic:** Alopecia, rash. **Musculoskeletal:** Arthralgia, myalgia, back/bone pain, pain in extremity, muscle spasms, muscular weakness. **Respiratory:** Cough, dyspnea, URTI. **GU:** UTI. **Hematologic:** Anemia, neutropenia, febrile neutropenia. **Ophthalmic:** Increased lacrimation. **Metabolic:** Decreased weight, peripheral edema. **Body as a whole:** Asthenia, fatigue, pyrexia, mucosal inflammation.

LABORATORY TEST CONSIDERATIONS

↑ ALT. Hypokalemia.

DRUG INTERACTIONS

An additive effect of eribulin with other drugs that prolong the QT interval is possible. The following drugs may prolong the QT interval and increase the risk of life-threatening cardiac arrhythmias, including torsades de pointes: Amiodarone, arsenic trioxide, bretylium, chlorpromazine, cisapride, disopyramide, dofetilide, dolasetron, droperidol, gatifloxacin, halofantrine, levomethadyl, mefloquine, mesoridazine, moxifloxacin, pentamidine, pimozide, probucol, procainamide, quinidine, sotalol, sparfloxacin, thioridazine, ziprasidone.

HOW SUPPLIED

Injection Solution: 0.5 mg/mL.

DOSAGE

IV

Metastatic breast cancer.

Adults, usual: 1.4 mg/m^2 over 2–5 min on days 1 and 8 of a 21-day cycle. See *Implementation/Administration/Storage* for dosage adjustments.

NURSING IMPLICATIONS

IMPLEMENTATION/ADMINISTRATION/STORAGE

1. **IV** Do not give eribulin on day 1 or day 8 for any of the following: ANC <1,000/mm^3, platelets <75,000/mm^3, or grade 3 or 4 nonhematological toxicities.
2. The day 8 dose may be delayed for a maximum of 1 week. If toxicities do not resolve or improve to grade 2 severity or less by day 15, omit the dose. If toxicities resolve or improve to grade 2 severity or less by day 15, administer eribulin at a reduced dose and initiate the next cycle no sooner than 2 weeks later. Do not reescalate eribulin dose after it has been reduced.
3. The following are recommended dose reductions for eribulin if the listed toxicities occur: (a) ANC <500/mm^3 for >7 days, ANC <1,000/mm^3 with fever or infection, platelets <25,000/mm^3, platelets <50,000/mm^3 requiring transfusion, nonhematologic grade 3 or 4 toxicities, omission or delay of day 8 eribulin dose in previous cycle for toxicity: Permanently reduce the dose to 1.1 mg/m^2. (b) Occurrence of any event requiring permanent dose reduction while receiving eribulin 1.1 mg/m^2: Permanently reduce the dose to 0.7 mg/m^2. (c) Occurrence of any event requiring permanent dose reduction while receiving eribulin 0.7 mg/m^2: Discontinue eribulin.
4. No dosage adjustment is needed in those with a C_{CR} from 50–80 mL/min. For moderate renal impairment (30–50 mL/min), give 1.1 mg/m^2 IV over 2–5 min on days 1 and 8 of a 21-day cycle.
5. For mild hepatic impairment (Child-Pugh class A), give 1.1 mg/m^2 IV over 2–5 min on days 1 and 8 of a 21-day cycle. For moderate hepatic impairment (Child-Pugh class B), give 0.7 mg/m^2 IV over 2–5 min on days 1 and 8 of a 21-day cycle.
6. To prepare the drug for administration, aseptically withdraw the required amount of eribulin from the single-use vial and administer undiluted or diluted in 100 mL NaCl 0.9% injection.
7. Store vials in the original cartons from 15–30°C (59–86°F). Do not freeze. Store undiluted eribulin in the syringe for up to 4 hr at room temperature or for up to 24 hr if refrigerated. Store dilution eribulin solutions for up to 4 hr at room temperature or for up to 24 hr if refrigerated. Discard unused portions of the vial.
8. COMPATIBILITY 0.9% NaCl.
9. INCOMPATIBILITY Do not dilute in or administer through IV line containing solutions with dextrose. Do not give in the same IV line with other drugs.

ASSESSMENT

1. Document disease progression, indications for therapy and when other regimens were received for metastatic breast cancer with anthracycline and a taxane.
2. Assess for peripheral neuropathy, and monitor closely for S&S of peripheral motor and sensory neuropathy.
3. In those with CHF, bradyarrhythmias, electrolyte abnormalities, or prescribed drugs that may prolong the QT interval, ensure regular ECG monitoring.
4. Obtain Mg^{++}, K^+, CBC prior to each dose; monitor CBC more frequently in those who develop grade 3 or 4 cytopenias. Monitor VS, ECG, U/A, renal and LFTS, and reduce dose with dysfunction.

CLIENT/FAMILY TEACHING

1. Drug is used to treat breast cancer that has spread to other parts of the body in those who have already received certain types of anticancer medicines for this condition.
2. Therapy is administered IV in cycles with each cycle lasting 21 days. An injection will be given 1 time each week for 2 weeks in a row (day 1 and day 8 of a treatment cycle). The frequency and dose will be determined after blood tests have been reviewed.

3. **Report any S&S of infection during therapy such as fever, chills, temperature, cough, or painful urination.**
4. **Drug therapy may cause numbness, tingling, or burning in your hands and feet; report if evident.**
5. **May experience hair loss, N&V, constipation and fatigue; report if persistent or intolerable as well as chest pain or palpitations.**
6. **Practice reliable contraception during therapy; may cause fetal harm.**
7. **Keep all F/U to assess response, labs, ECG, and for adverse SE.**

OUTCOMES/EVALUATE

Inhibition of malignant cell proliferation with previously treated metastatic breast cancer

Erlotinib

(er-**LOE**-tye-nib)

Classification(s): Epidermal growth factor receptor inhibitor

Pregnancy Category: D

RX: Tarceva.

INDICATIONS/USES

(1) As monotherapy for non-small-cell lung cancer (locally advanced or metastatic) after failure of at least 1 prior chemotherapy regimen. (2) As monotherapy for the maintenance treatment of clients with non-small-cell lung cancer (locally advanced or metastatic) whose disease has not progressed after 4 cycles of platinum-based first-line chemotherapy. (3) With gemcitabine for first-line treatment of locally advanced, unresectable, or metastatic pancreatic cancer. *Investigational:* Squamous cell head and neck cancer.

ACTION/KINETICS

Action

Erlotinib inhibits the intracellular phosphorylation of tyrosine kinase associated with the epidermal growth factor receptor. Epidermal growth factor receptors are expressed on the cell surface of both normal and cancer cells. Precise mechanism is not known.

Pharmacokinetics

Bioavailability is about 60%; food increases bioavailability to almost 100%. **Peak plasma levels:** 4 hr. Solubility decreases as pH increases. **t½:** 36 hr. **Time to reach steady-state plasma levels:** 7–8 days. Metabolized predominantly by CYP3A4 and to a lesser extent by CYP1A2. Excreted mainly through the feces (83%) with 8% excreted in the urine. **Plasma protein binding:** About 93%.

CONTRAINDICATIONS

Lactation.

SPECIAL CONCERNS

- **Use with caution in impaired hepatic function; interrupt therapy if total bilirubin levels are more than 3 times the ULN and/or transaminases are more than 5 times the ULN.**
- **Safety and efficacy not determined in children.**

SIDE EFFECTS

Most Common

When used to treat non-small-cell lung cancer: Rash, diarrhea, anorexia, N&V, stomatitis, cough, dyspnea, fatigue, infection, dry skin, pruritus.
When used to treat pancreatic cancer (with gemcitabine): Rash, diarrhea, fatigue, N&V, anorexia, abdominal pain, constipation, depression, weight loss, infection, pyrexia, edema, bone pain, myalgia.

When used to treat non-small-cell lung cancer. Respiratory: Dyspnea, cough, fever, epistaxis, ***interstitial lung disease.*** **CV:** ***MI***, ischemia, ***CVA***. **GI:** Diarrhea, GI bleeding, anorexia, N&V, stomatitis, abdominal pain, gastritis, gastroduodenal ulcers, hematemesis, hematochezia, melena, hemorrhage from possible colitis, GI bleeding, ***GI perforation***, ***hepatic failure***. **Hematologic:** Microangiopathic hemolytic anemia with thrombocytopenia (when used for pancreatic cancer). **Dermatologic:** Rash, acne, dry skin, pruritus, dermatitis acneiform, paronychia; itching, tenderness, and/or burning skin; bullous, hyperpigmentation or dry skin with or without digital skin fissures; brittle/loose nails; bullous, blistering, and exfoliative skin conditions (including ***Stevens-Johnson syndrome, toxic epidermal necrolysis***). **GU:** Hepatorenal syndrome, ***acute renal failure***, renal insufficiency. **Ophthalmic:** Conjunctivitis, keratoconjunctivitis sicca, corneal perforation/ulceration, abnormal eyelash growth, keratitis. **Body as a whole:** Fatigue, infection, dehydration, decreased weight, non-GI bleeding.

When used with gemcitabine to treat pancreatic cancer. GI: N&V, diarrhea, anorexia, abdominal pain, constipation, stomatitis, dyspepsia, flatulence, ileus, pancreatitis, GI bleeding, gastritis, gastroduodenal ulcers, hematemesis, hematochezia, melena, ***hemorrhage from possible colitis, GI perforation, hepatic failure.*** **CNS:** Depression, dizziness, headache, insomnia, anxiety, neuropathy, rigors. **CV:** Syncope, arrhythmias, DVT, ***MI***/ischemia, ***CVA (including cerebral hemorrhage)***. **Dermatologic:** Rash, alopecia; itching, tenderness, and/or burning skin; hyperpigmentation or dry skin with or without digital skin fissures; brittle/loose nails; bullous, blistering, and exfoliative skin conditions (including ***Stevens-Johnson syndrome, toxic epidermal necrolysis***). **Musculoskeletal:** Bone pain, myalgia. **Respiratory:** Dyspnea, cough, epistaxis, ***interstitial lung disease***. **Hematologic:** Hemolytic anemia (including microangiopathic hemolytic anemia with thrombocytopenia). ***GU:*** Hepatorenal syndrome, ***acute renal failure***, renal insufficiency. **GU:** Renal insufficiency. **Ophthalmic:** Conjunctivitis, keratitis, corneal perforation/ulceration, abnormal eyelash growth, keratoconjunctivitis sicca. **Body as a whole:** Fatigue, weight loss, edema, infection, pyrexia, dehydration, non-GI bleeding.

LABORATORY TEST CONSIDERATIONS

↑ INR, ALT, AST, bilirubin.

OVERDOSE MANAGEMENT

Symptoms: Doses of 400 mg daily may cause diarrhea, rash, and elevated liver transaminases. *Treatment:* Withhold erlotinib and begin symptomatic treatment.

DRUG INTERACTIONS

Antacids / ↓ Bioavailability of erlotinib R/T alteration of pH of upper GI tract; separate dose of antacids and erlotinib by several hours

Ciprofloxacin / Possible ↓ erlotinib dose R/T inhibition of CYP3A4 and CYP1A2; consider ↓ erlotinib dosage if side effects occur

Clarithromycin / ↑ Erlotinib levels R/T inhibition of CYP3A4 and CYP1A2; consider ↓ erlotinib dosage if side effects occur

Coumarin derivatives / ↑ Risk of bleeding episodes

CYP3A4 inducers (e.g., carbamazepine, phenobarbital, phenytoin, rifabutin, rifampin, rifapentine, St. John's wort) / Potential ↓ erlotinib AUC by 2/3–4/5 R/T ↑ metabolism by CYP3A4; use alternative drugs. If an alternative is not possible, consider an increase in erlotinib dose at 2-week intervals and monitor client safety

CYP3A4 inhibitors (e.g., atazanavir, clarithromycin, grapefruit/grapefruit juice, indinavir, itraconazole, ketoconazole, nefazodone, nelfinavir, ritonavir, saquinavir, telithromycin, troleandomycin, voriconazole) / ↑ Erlotinib levels R/T inhibition of CYP3A4 and CYP1A2; consider ↓ erlotinib dosage if side effects occur

Grapefruit/Grapefruit juice / ↑ Erlotinib AUC R/T inhibition of CYP3A4 metabolism

H-2 receptor antagonists (e.g., ranitidine) / ↓ Bioavailability of erlotinib R/T alteration of pH of upper GI tract; give erlotinib 10 hr after the H-2 receptor blocker and at least 2 hr before the next H-2 antagonist

Midazolam / ↓ Midazolam levels R/T metabolism by CYP3A4; adjust midazolam dose as needed

NSAIDs / ↑ Risk of bleeding episodes

Proton pump inhibitors (e.g., omeprazole) / ↓ Bioavailability of erlotinib R/T alteration of pH of upper GI; avoid coadministration if possible

Warfarin / ↑ Risk of bleeding episodes both GI and non-GI R/T ↑ INR; monitor for changes in PT or INR

HOW SUPPLIED

Tablets: 25 mg, 100 mg, 150 mg.

DOSAGE

TABLETS

Non-small-cell lung cancer.

Adults: 150 mg once daily taken at least 1 hr before or 2 hr after ingestion of food. Continue treatment until disease progresses or unacceptable toxicity occurs. When reduction of dose is necessary, reduce in 50 mg decrements.

Pancreatic cancer.

Adults: 100 mg per day taken at least 1 hr before or 2 hr after ingestion of food. Taken in combination with gemcitabine. Continue treatment until disease progresses or unacceptable toxicity occurs. When dose reduction is needed, reduce the erlotinib dose in 50 mg decrements.

Squamous cell head and neck cancer (investigational).

Adults: 150 mg/day. Higher doses cause increased toxicity without increased benefit.

NURSING IMPLICATIONS

IMPLEMENTATION/ADMINISTRATION/STORAGE

1. Adjust dosage as follows based on hepatic function: If AST is <3 times the ULN and serum direct bilirubin is <1 mg/dL, no change in initial dose is needed. If AST is 3 or more times the ULN and and serum direct bilirubin is 1–7 mg/dL, reduce the initial dose to 75 mg/day. May gradually increase to labeled dose as tolerated. There is no information if serum direct bilirubin is >7 mg/dL.
2. In those who develop an acute onset of new or progressive pulmonary symptoms (e.g., dyspnea, cough, or fever), interrupt treatment pending diagnostic evaluation. If interstitial lung disease diagnosed, discontinue and institute appropriate treatment.
3. Diarrhea can usually be managed by loperamide. Severe diarrhea unresponsive to loperamide or in those who become dehydrated may require dose reduction or temporary interruption of therapy. Discontinue for GI perforation.
4. Those with severe skin reactions (e.g., severe bullous, blistering, or exfoliative skin conditions) may require dose reduction or temporary interruption of therapy.
5. Interrupt or discontinue therapy in acute/worsening ocular disorders and in those with dehydration who are at risk for renal failure.
6. Smoking reduces erlotinib exposure. Clients should stop smoking. If the client continues to smoke, a cautious increase in the erlotinib dose, not exceeding 300 mg, may be considered. However, efficacy and long-term safety (>14 days) of a higher than the recommended starting dose have not been established in these clients. If the erlotinib dose is increased in smokers, it should be reduced immediately to the indicated starting dose upon cessation of smoking.
7. Store from 15–30°C (59–86°F).

ASSESSMENT

1. Note reasons for therapy, disease onset, other chemotherapy regimen trialed/failed with non-small-cell lung cancer or with gemcitabine for pancreatic cancer. List drugs prescribed to ensure none interact.
2. Assess/monitor pulmonary condition; include PFTs, CXR and CT/MRI findings, bronchoscopy biopsy results. Monitor for dermatologic, GI, ophthalmic, respiratory, and/or general body adverse reactions.
3. Monitor CBC, electrolytes, renal and LFTs; may need to reduce dose or stop therapy with dysfunction, with diarrhea unresponsive to loperamide, with dehydration or if severe skin reactions occur.

CLIENT/FAMILY TEACHING

1. Drug is used to treat non-small-cell lung cancer after at least one other therapy trialed/failed or with gemcitabine for advanced pancreatic cancer.
2. Take once daily at least 1 hour before or 2 hours after food.
3. If the client cannot swallow whole tablets, place the tablet in 100 mL of distilled water (do not crush). Stir until dispersed; drink the mixture immediately. To ensure the entire dose is taken, rinse the inside of the container with another 40 mL of water; drink immediately. The suspension may also be given using an enteral feeding tube.
4. Smoking interferes with absorption; advise to stop smoking during therapy.
5. May cause worsening of lung condition; report any increased SOB, coughing, fever, or sudden change in breathing condition.
6. Report inability to eat, severe diarrhea or vomiting, eye irritation, onset/worsening of SOB or cough.
7. Diarrhea is managed with loperamide. In those with severe diarrhea who are unresponsive to loperamide or who become dehydrated, dose will be reduced or therapy temporarily interrupted until resolved.
8. Practice reliable contraception during and for 2 weeks after completing therapy.
9. Avoid sun exposure, and wear sunscreen and protection if exposed.
10. Keep all F/U to assess response, labs, and for adverse SE.

OUTCOMES/EVALUATE

Inhibition of malignant cell proliferation with non-small-cell lung cancer or pancreatic cancer

Erythromycin base

(eh-**rih**-throw-**MY**-sin)

Classification(s): Antibiotic, macrolide

Pregnancy Category: B (A/T/S, Eryderm 2%, Erymax, Staticin, and T-Stat are C)

RX: Capsules, Delayed-Release (with Enteric-Coated Pellets): Erythromycin. **Gel, Topical:** A/T/S, Emgel, Erygel. **Ointment, Topical:** Akne-Mycin. **Ophthalmic Ointment:** Ilotycin Ophthalmic. **Pledgets, Topical:** Ery Pads. **Solution, Topical:** A/T/S, Eryderm 2%. **Tablets, Delayed-Release (Enteric-Coated):** Ery-Tab, PCE Dispertab. **Tablets, Film-Coated:** Erythromycin Filmtab.

✤ Rx: Capsules: Tablets: Apo-Erythro Base, Apo-Erythro E-C.

SEE ALSO ***ANTI-INFECTIVE AGENTS.***

INDICATIONS/USES

1. Mild to moderate upper respiratory tract infections due to *Streptococcus pyogenes* (group A beta-hemolytic streptococci), *Streptococcus pneumoniae,* and *Haemophilus influenzae* (combined with sulfonamides).
2. Mild-to-moderate lower respiratory tract infections due to *S. pyogenes* (group A beta-hemolytic streptococci) and *S. pneumoniae.* Respiratory tract infections due to *Mycoplasma pneumoniae.*
3. Pertussis (whooping cough) caused by *Bordetella pertussis;* may also be used as prophylaxis of pertussis in exposed individuals.
4. Mild-to-moderate skin and skin structure infections due to *S. pyogenes* and *Staphylococcus aureus* (resistant staphylococci may emerge during treatment). Acne vulgaris.
5. As an adjunct to antitoxin in diphtheria (caused by *Corynebacterium diphtheriae),* to prevent carriers, and to eradicate the organism in carriers.
6. Intestinal amebiasis due to *Entamoeba histolytica* (PO erythromycin only). Extraenteric amebiasis requires treatment with other drugs.
7. As an alternative to penicillin to treat acute pelvic inflammatory disease due to *Neisseria gonorrhoeae* (erythromycin lactobionate IV followed by PO erythromycin).
8. Erythrasma due to *Corynebacterium minutissimum.*
9. *Chlamydia trachomatis* infections causing urogenital infections during pregnancy, conjunctivitis in the newborn, or pneumonia during infancy. Also, uncomplicated chlamydial infections of the urethra, endocervix, or rectum in adults (when tetracyclines are contraindicated or not tolerated).
10. Nongonococcal urethritis caused by *Ureaplasma urealyticum* when tetracyclines are contraindicated or not tolerated (PO erythromycin only).
11. Legionnaires' disease due to *Legionella pneumophila.*
12. PO as an alternative to penicillin (in penicillin-allergic clients) to treat primary syphilis caused by *Treponema pallidum.*
13. Prophylaxis of initial or recurrent attacks of rheumatic fever in clients allergic to penicillin or sulfonamides.
14. Alternative to treat *T. pallidum* in clients allergic to penicillin.
15. Listeriosis.
16. Pneumonia of infancy.

Investigational:

1. Acne vulgaris to decrease population of lipophilic bacteria.
2. Bacillary angiomatosis in immunocompromised clients due to *Bartonella henselae* or *Bartonella quintana.*
3. Enteritis due to *Campylobacter jejuni.*
4. As an alternative to treat erysipelas cellulitis of the extremities not associated with venous catheter or diabetes.
5. Chancroid due to *Haemophilus ducreyi.*
6. As an alternative to doxycycline or trimethoprim-sulfamethoxazole to treat granuloma inguinale due to *Calymmatobacterium granulomatis.*
7. As an alternative to treat nonbullous lesions of ecthyma impetigo.
8. As an alternative to treat inclusion conjunctivitis in adults due to *Chlamydia trachomatis.*
9. As an alternative to treat mild to moderate, uncomplicated, infected wounds of the extremities.
10. Moderate to severe leptospirosis due to *Leptospira* species.
11. Alternative to treat early Lyme disease due to *Borrelia burgorferi.*
12. Genital, inguinal, or anorectal lymphogranuloma venereum.
13. Tick-borne relapsing fever and louse-borne relapsing fever.

14. As an alternative to treat tetanus due to *Clostridium tetani.*
15. Early syphilis (primary or secondary) in nonpregnant clients for whom compliance with therapy and follow-up can be ensured.
16. In combination with neomycin prior to elective colorectal surgery to reduce wound complications.
17. As an alternative to penicillins to treat anthrax, Vincent's gingivitis, erysipeloid, actinomycosis, *Nocardia* infections (with a sulfonamide), *Eikenella corrodens* infections, *Borrelia* infections.

Ophthalmic ointment:

1. Treatment of superficial ocular infections involving the conjunctiva and cornea (e.g., conjunctivitis, keratitis, keratoconjunctivitis, corneal ulcers, blepharitis, blepharoconjunctivitis, acute meibomianitis, and dacryocystitis) due to *S. pneumoniae, S. aureus, S. pyogenes, Corynebacterium* species, *H. influenzae,* and *Bacteroides* infections.
2. Prophylaxis of ophthalmia neonatorum due to *N. gonorrhoeae* and *C. trachomatis.* The efficacy in preventing ophthalmia caused by penicillinase-producing *N. gonorrhoeae* is not established.

Topical gel/solution: Acne vulgaris.

Topical ointment:

1. Prophylaxis of infection in minor skin abrasions; treatment of superficial infections of the skin.
2. Acne vulgaris.

ACTION/KINETICS

Action

Erythromycins are macrolide antibiotics. They inhibit protein synthesis of microorganisms by binding reversibly to a ribosomal subunit (50S), thus interfering with the transmission of genetic information and inhibiting protein synthesis. The drugs are effective only against rapidly multiplying organisms.

Pharmacokinetics

Absorbed from the upper part of the small intestine. Food may reduce antibiotic efficacy. Those for PO use are manufactured in enteric-coated or film-coated forms to prevent destruction by gastric acid. Achieves concentrations in body tissues about 40% of those in the plasma. Diffuses into body tissues: Peritoneal, pleural, ascitic, and amniotic fluids; saliva; through the placental circulation; and across the mucous membrane of the tracheobronchial tree. Diffuses poorly into spinal fluid, although penetration is increased in meningitis. Alkalinization of the urine (to pH 8.5) increases the gram-negative antibacterial action. **Peak serum levels: PO,** 4 hr. **C_{max}:** 0.3–1.9 mcg/mL. **$t^{1/2}$:** 1.5–2 hr, *but prolonged in clients with renal impairment* (e.g., 5 hr in those with anuria). Partially metabolized by the liver and primarily excreted unchanged in bile and urine. Also excreted in breast milk. **Plasma protein binding:** Approximately 70–80%.

CONTRAINDICATIONS

Hypersensitivity to erythromycin; in utero syphilis. Use of topical preparations in the eye or near the nose, mouth, or any mucous membrane. Ophthalmic use in dendritic keratitis, vaccinia, varicella, myobacterial infections of the eye, fungal diseases of the eye. Use with steroid combinations following uncomplicated removal of a corneal foreign body. Concomitant use with cisapride, pimozide. Use during pregnancy only when clearly needed.

SPECIAL CONCERNS

- **Use with caution in liver disease and during lactation.**
- **Use may result in bacterial and fungal overgrowth (i.e., superinfection).**
- **Use of other drugs for acne may result in a cumulative irritant effect.**
- **Use to treat whooping cough in newborns may cause pyloric stenosis.**
- **It is possible that erythromycin does not reach the fetus in adequate concentrations to prevent congenital syphilis. Use an appropriate penicillin regimen.**
- **Use with certain CYP3A inhibitors, such as certain calcium-channel blockers, certain antifungal drugs, and some antidepressants, causes a greater risk of sudden death from cardiac causes.**
- **The elderly, especially those with reduced renal or hepatic function, may be at increased risk to develop erythromycin-induced hearing loss. Also, the elderly may be at increased risk to develop torsades de pointes arrhythmias.**
- **Safety and efficacy of topical products not established in children.**

SIDE EFFECTS

Most Common

After systemic use: Abdominal pain/discomfort, headache, diarrhea/loose stools, increased cough, dyspepsia, N&V, dizziness, rash.

GI: Abdominal discomfort or pain, anorexia, diarrhea or loose stools, dyspepsia, flatulence, GI disorder, N&V, pseudomembranous colitis, hepatotoxicity, *C. difficile*–diarrhea, ***pancreatitis*** (rare). Possibility of hypertrophic pyloric stenosis in infants. **Hepatic:** Impaired hepatic function, symptoms of hepatitis, hepatocellular and/or cholestatic hepatitis with or without jaundice. **CV:** Ventricular arrhythmias, including ***ventricular tachycardia and torsades de pointes in clients with prolonged QT intervals.*** After IV, increase in heart rate and prolongation of QT interval. **Dermatologic:** Pruritus, rash, bullous eruptions, eczema, photosensitivity, mild skin reactions, erythema multiforme; rarely, ***Stevens-Johnson syndrome, toxic epidermal necrolysis.*** **CNS:** Dizziness, headache, insomnia, ***convulsions*** (rare). **Hypersensitivity:** Urticaria, ***anaphylaxis***, **Miscellaneous:** Asthenia, dyspnea, increased cough, nonspecific pain, vaginitis, allergic reaction, superinfection. Reversible hearing loss in those with renal or hepatic insufficiency, in the elderly, and after doses greater than 4 grams/day. Aggravation of weakness in clients with myasthenia gravis.

Following IV use: Venous irritation, thrombophlebitis.

Following IM use: Pain at the injection site, with development of necrosis or sterile abscesses.

Following topical use: Erythema, desquamation, burning sensation, eye irritation, tenderness, dryness, pruritus, oily skin, peeling, itching, contact sensitization, generalized urticaria.

LABORATORY TEST CONSIDERATIONS

↑ Bicarbonate, eosinophils, liver enzymes, platelet count, segmented neutrophils, serum CPK. Interference with fluorometric assay for urinary catecholamines.

OVERDOSE MANAGEMENT

Symptoms: N&V, diarrhea, epigastric distress, acute pancreatitis (mild), hearing loss (with or without tinnitus and vertigo). *Treatment:* Induce vomiting. General supportive measures. Allergic reactions should be controlled with conventional therapy. Hemodialysis and peritoneal dialysis are not particularly effective.

DRUG INTERACTIONS

NOTE: (1) Erythromycin is a substrate and inhibitor of CYP3A. Coadministration of erythromycin and a drug primarily metabolized by CYP3A may be associated with increases in drug levels that could increase or prolong both the therapeutic and side effects of the concomitant drug. Consider dosage adjustments and if possible closely monitor serum levels of such drugs.

(2) An additive effect is possible with other drugs that prolong the QT interval. When used with erythromycin, the following drugs may prolong the QT interval and increase the risk of life-threatening cardiac arrhythmias, including torsades de pointes: Amiodarone, bretylium, chlorpromazine, cisapride, disopyramide, dofetilide, dolasetron, droperidol, gatifloxacin, mefloquine, mesoridazine, moxifloxacin, pentamidine, pimozide, probucol, procainamide, quinidine, sotalol, sparfloxacin, tacrolimus, thioridazine, and ziprasidone.

Alfentanil / ↑ Pharmacological effects of alfentanil

Benzodiazepines (alprazolam, diazepam, midazolam, triazolam) / ↑ Benzodiazepine levels R/T ↓ metabolism → ↑ CNS depressant effects

Bromocriptine / ↑ Bromocriptine levels → ↑ pharmacologic/toxic effects

Buspirone / ↑ Buspirone levels → ↑ pharmacologic/toxic effects

Calcium channel blockers / ↑ Risk of hypotension and shock; may require hospitalization

Carbamazepine / ↑ Carbamazepine effect (and toxicity requiring hospitalization and resuscitation) R/T ↓ liver breakdown

Cilostazol / ↑ Cilostazol levels → ↑ pharmacologic/toxic effects

Clopidogrel / Inhibition of clopidogrel antiplatelet effect; monitor platelet function carefully and adjust dose as needed

Clozapine / ↑ Serum clozapine levels → ↑ pharmacologic/toxic effects

Colchicine / Possible severe colchicine toxicity (may cause death) R/T inhibition of CYP3A4 metabolism of colchicine; coadministration contraindicated

Cyclosporine / ↑ Cyclosporine effect R/T ↓ excretion (possibly with nephrotoxicity and neurotoxicity); monitor cyclosporine levels and adjust dosage as needed

E

Digoxin / ↑ Digoxin levels → toxicity; effects may last for several weeks following erythromycin administration
Diltiazem / ↑ Erythromycin plasma levels R/T ↓ metabolism by CYP3A4 → ↑ risk of cardiotoxicity; avoid coadministration
Eletriptan / ↑ Plasma eletriptan levels → ↑ pharmacologic/toxic effects; do not take eletriptan within 72 hr of a potent CYP3A4 inhibitor
Ergot alkaloids (e.g., dihydroergotamine, ergotamine) / Acute ergotism manifested by peripheral ischemia and dysesthesia
Felodipine / ↑ Felodipine drug levels → ↑ pharmacologic/toxic effects
Fluoroquinolones (e.g., levofloxacin, moxifloxacin, sparfloxacin) / Prolongation of QT interval → ↑ risk of life-threatening arrhythmias, include torsades de pointes; avoid coadministration with levofloxacin and sparfloxacin and use with caution with moxifloxacin
Grapefruit juice / ↑ Erythromycin levels and AUC R/T ↓ metabolism in the small intestine
HMG-CoA reductase inhibitors (e.g., atorvastatin, lovastatin, simvastatin) / ↑ Risk of myopathy or rhabdomyolysis; also ↑ levels of atorvastatin, lovastatin, or simvastatin R/T ↓ liver breakdown
Methylprednisolone / ↑ Methylprednisolone pharmacologic/toxic effects R/T ↓ liver breakdown
Phenytoin / ↑ Serum phenytoin levels
Pimozide / ↑ Pimozide plasma levels → possible cardiotoxicity; coadministration contraindicated
Quetiapine / ↑ Quetiapine AUC, peak plasma levels, and t½ R/T inhibition of metabolism by CYP3A4 → ↑ pharmacologic/toxic effects
Ranolazine / ↑ Ranolazine plasma levels → cardiotoxicity; coadministration contraindicated
Repaglinide / ↑ Plasma repaglinide levels → ↑ pharmacologic/toxic effects; monitor blood glucose levels carefully and adjust dose as needed
Rifabutin, rifampin / ↓ Erythromycin effect; ↑ risk of GI and rifamycin side effects
Sildenafil / ↑ AUC and peak sildenafil levels R/T inhibition of sildenafil first pass metabolism; consider lower dose of sildenafil
Tacrolimus / ↑ Tacrolimus plasma levels → ↑ risk of toxicity; monitor renal function and tacrolimus blood levels; adjust tacrolimus dose as needed
Theophyllines (e.g., aminophylline, theophylline) / ↑ Theophylline effects → toxicity R/T ↓ liver breakdown; ↓ erythromycin levels may also occur
Valproic acid / ↑ Serum valproic acid → valproic acid toxicity
Verapamil / ↑ Plasma levels of both drugs → ↑ risk of cardiotoxicity; closely monitor cardiac function
Vinblastine / ↑ Risk of vinblastine toxicity (constipation, myalgia, neutropenia); coadministration contraindicated
Warfarin / ↑ Warfarin anticoagulant effect → possible hemorrhage; monitor anticoagulant parameters and adjust warfarin dose as needed

HOW SUPPLIED

Capsules, Delayed-Release: 250 mg; ***Gel, Topical:*** 2%; ***Ointment, Topical:*** 2%; ***Ophthalmic Ointment:*** 0.5%; ***Pledgets, Topical:*** 2%; ***Solution, Topical:*** 2%; ***Tablets, Delayed-Release (Enteric-Coated):*** 250 mg, 333 mg, 500 mg; ***Tablets, Film-Coated:*** 250 mg, 500 mga ; ***Tablets, Polymer Coated Particles:*** 333 mg, 500 mg.

DOSAGE

NOTE: Doses are listed as erythromycin base.

CAPSULES, DELAYED-RELEASE; TABLETS, DELAYED-RELEASE; TABLETS, FILM-COATED; TABLETS, POLYMER COATED PARTICLES

Respiratory tract infections due to Mycoplasma pneumoniae.

Adults: 500 mg q 6 hr for 14–21 days (for severe infections). **Children:** 20–50 mg/kg/day in 3 or 4 divided doses for 14–21 days.

Upper respiratory tract infections (URTIs) (mild to moderate) due to S. pyogenes *or* S. pneumoniae.

Adults: 250 mg q 6 hr, or 333 mg q 8 hr, or 500 mg q 12 hr for 10 days or longer, up to a maximum of 4 grams/day. **Children:** 20–50 mg/kg/day in divided doses, not to exceed the adult dose, for 10 days or longer.

URTIs due to H. influenzae.

Erythromycin ethylsuccinate, 50 mg/kg/day for children, plus sulfisoxazole, 150 mg/kg/day, given together for 10 days.

Lower UTRIs (mild to moderate) due to S. pyogenes *or* S. pneumoniae.

250–500 mg 4 times per day (or 20–50 mg/kg/day in divided doses) for 10 days.

Intestinal amebiasis due to Entamoeba histolytica.

Adults: 250 mg of the base (or 400 mg of ethylsuccinate) 4 times per day or 333 mg of the base q 8 hr or 500 mg q 12 hr for 10–14 days; **pediatric:** 30–50 mg/kg/day in divided doses for 10–14 days.

Legionnaires' disease.

1–4 grams/day in divided doses for 10–14 days.

Bordetella pertussis.

500 mg 4 times per day for 10 days (or for children, 40–50 mg/kg/day in divided doses for 5–14 days).

Infections due to Corynebacterium diphtheriae.

500 mg q 6 hr for 14 days (7 days for cutaneous diphtheria and carriers).

Primary syphilis.

30–40 grams (or 48–64 grams of ethylsuccinate) in divided doses over 10–15 days.

Conjunctivitis of the newborn, pneumonia of infancy, urogenital infections during pregnancy due to Chlamydia trachomatis.

Infants: 50 mg/kg/day in four divided doses for 14 (conjunctivitis) to 21 (pneumonia) days or longer. **Adults:** 500 mg 4 times per day or 666 mg q 8 hr for urogenital infections during pregnancy. For women unable to tolerate the preceding regimen, give 250 mg q 6 hr or 333 mg q 8 hr, or 500 mg q 12 hr for 14 days or longer.

Mild to moderate skin and skin structure infections due to S. pyogenes *or* S. aureus.

250–500 mg q 6 hr (or 20–50 mg/kg/day for children, in divided doses—to a maximum of 4 grams/day) for 10 days.

Listeria monocytogenes *infections.*

Adults: 500 mg q 12 hr (or 250 mg q 6 hr), up to maximum of 4 grams/day.

Pelvic inflammatory disease, acute due to N. gonorrhoeae.

Erythromycin lactobionate, 500 mg IV q 6 hr for 3 days; **then,** erythromycin base, 250 mg PO q 6 hr or 333 mg q 8 hr for 7 days.

Prevention of initial rheumatic fever attack; Prophylaxis of recurrent attacks of rheumatic fever.

Prevention of initial attack: 400 mg q 6 hr for 10 days. Prevention of recurrent attacks: 250 mg twice a day of the base or 400 mg of ethylsuccinate given continuously.

Bacterial endocarditis due to alpha-hemolytic streptococcus.

Adults: 1 gram 1–2 hr prior to the procedure; **then,** 500 mg 6 hr after the initial dose. **Pediatric,** 20 mg/kg 2 hr prior to the procedure; **then,** 10 mg/kg 6 hr after the initial dose.

Uncomplicated urethral, endocervical, or rectal infections due to C. trachomatis.

500 mg 4 times per day for 7 days (or 250 mg 4 times per day for 14 days).

Nongonococcal urethritis due to Ureaplasma urealyticum.

Adults: 500 mg 4 times per day, or 666 mg q 8 hr, or 800 mg (as ethylsuccinate) 4 times per day for 7 days or longer. **Children, 45 kg or less:** 50 mg/kg/day in 4 divided doses for 14 days.

Erythrasma due to Corynebacterium minutissimum.

250 mg q 6 hr for 14 days.

OPHTHALMIC OINTMENT (0.5%)

Ophthalmic infections.

Approximately 1 cm of ointment applied directly to the eye(s) up to 6 times/day, depending on the severity of the infection.

Prophylaxis of neonatal gonococcal or chlamydial conjunctivitis.

Approximately 1 cm of ointment instilled into each lower conjunctival sac. Do not flush the ointment from the eye after instillation.

TOPICAL GEL (2%); TOPICAL OINTMENT (2%); TOPICAL PLEDGETS (2%); TOPICAL SOLUTION (2%)

Acne vulgaris.

Clean the affected area thoroughly and pat dry. **Gel:** Apply sparingly and lightly as a thin film to affected area(s) once or twice a day. If there is no improvement after 6–8 weeks, or if the condition gets worse, discontinue treatment. **Ointment:** Apply to affected area in the morning and evening. **Pledgets:** Rub the pad over the affected area(s) twice a day after the skin is thoroughly washed with warm water and soap and patted dry. Use each pledget once and discard. **Solution:** Apply to the affected area(s) in the morning and evening after the skin is thoroughly washed with warm water and soap and patted dry. Use enough solution to thoroughly wet the affected area(s).

INVESTIGATIONAL USES

Diarrhea due to Campylobacter enteritis *or enterocolitis. Chancroid due to* Haemophilus ducreyi.

500 mg 4 times per day for 7 days.

Genital, inguinal, or anorectal infections due to Lymphogranuloma venereum. *Early syphilis due to* Treponema pallidum.

500 mg 4 times per day for 14 days.

Tetanus due to Clostridium tetani.

500 mg q 6 hr for 10 days.

Granuloma inguinale due to Calymmatobacterium granulomatis.

500 mg PO 4 times per day for 21 or more days.

NURSING IMPLICATIONS

(Sound Alike Drug) Do not confuse Eryc with Ery-Tab, both of which are trade names for erythromycin base.

IMPLEMENTATION/ADMINISTRATION/STORAGE

1. Daily dose should not exceed 4 grams.
2. Erythromycin base is inactivated by gastric acids; thus, it is given as enteric-coated tablets or capsules containing enteric-coated pellets.
3. The therapeutic dosage of erythromycin should be given for at least 10 days when treating streptococcal infections of the upper respiratory tract (e.g., tonsillitis, pharyngitis).
4. It is recommended that erythromycin 250 mg twice a day be given for long-term prophylaxis of streptococcal upper respiratory tract infections to prevent recurring attacks of rheumatic fever in those allergic to penicillin and sulfonamides.
5. Prepare topical gel by adding 3 mL of ethyl alcohol to the vial and immediately shaking to dissolve erythromycin. This solution is added to the gel and stirred until it appears homogenous (1–1.5 min). Refrigerate gel.
6. The gel and topical solution are flammable; keep away from heat and flame. Store the gel in the original container and the topical solution in a light-resistant container, tightly closed, from 15–25°C (59–77°F). Store the pledgets from 15–25°C (59–77°F) in a tightly closed jar. Store ointment below 27°C (80°F).
7. Store capsules and tablets below 30°C (86°F). Protect capsules from moisture and excessive heat.

ASSESSMENT

1. List type, onset, characteristics of S&S, clinical presentation, other agents used, outcome.
2. Note allergy to any antibiotics; assess for sensitivity reactions.
3. Avoid if also prescribed digoxin and theophyllines; erythromycins can inhibit cytochrome P-450 and enhance effects of these drugs or cause lethal arrhythmias. Assess for hepatotoxicity and ototoxicity.
4. Obtain cultures, LFTs, CBC, wound documentation, appropriate diagnostic studies.

CLIENT/FAMILY TEACHING

1. Take on an empty stomach; delayed-release forms of base can be taken without regard for meals. Do not administer with or immediately prior to ingestion of fruit juice or other acidic drinks; acidity may decrease drug activity. Consume up to 8 oz of water with each dose, and ensure a fluid intake of 2.5 L/day.
2. May take with food to diminish GI upset; food decreases absorption of most erythromycins. Take as directed and complete entire prescription despite feeling better.
3. Stomach acid destroys erythromycin base; must be administered with enteric coating.

4. Evenly space doses over 24 hr. Swallow whole; do not crush, chew, break, or open. Report any unusual/intolerable side effects or lack of response.
5. If nausea intolerable, report so prescription can be changed to coated tablets; can be taken with meals.
6. Report symptoms of superinfection, i.e., furry tongue, vaginal itching, rectal itching, or diarrhea. Also rash, yellow discoloration of skin or eyes, or irritation of the mouth or tongue should be reported.
7. Drug may increase GI motility with diabetic gastric paresis.
8. With topical use, clean affected area before applying ointment; wash hands before and after therapy. If no improvement in 6–8 weeks or if condition worsens, consult provider.
9. A sterile bandage may be used with the topical ointment. Drying and peeling following topical use may be controlled by reducing the frequency of applications.
10. With eye therapy, wash hands before and after instilling ointment; tilt head backward and gently pull down lower lid to form a pouch. Place prescribed amount of ointment with a sweeping motion inside the lower eyelid. Close eye(s) for 1 to 2 min, and roll the eye around in all directions. May remove excessive ointment around eye with tissue.
11. Avoid contaminating ointment by not touching tip of tube to any surface and replace cap after using. May cause temporary blurring of vision, so avoid activities requiring visual acuity until blurriness clears.
12. If using more than 1 eye product, wait at least 10 min before instilling second drug. Topical and ophthalmic products are for external use only.
13. Report any hearing loss; usually temporary.
14. Keep all F/U to assess response, labs/cultures, and for adverse SE.

OUTCOMES/EVALUATE

- Resolution of infection (negative culture reports, ↓ temperature, ↑ wound healing, ↓ WBCs)
- Desired infection prophylaxis

Erythromycin ethylsuccinate

Classification(s): Antibiotic, macrolide

Pregnancy Category: B

RX: E.E.S. 400 Filmtab, E.E.S. 400 Liquid, E.E.S. Granules, EryPed 200, EryPed 400, EryPed Drops.

✤ **Rx:** Apo-Erythro-ES.

SEE ALSO ***ERYTHROMYCIN BASE***.

INDICATIONS/USES

See *Erythromycin Base* for more specific details on use, including causative organisms.

1. Acute pelvic inflammatory disease.
2. Diphtheria.
3. Erythrasma.
4. *Chlamydia trachomatis* infections.
5. Intestinal amebiasis.
6. Legionnaires' disease.
7. Listeriosis.
8. Lower respiratory tract infections. Mild to moderate upper respiratory tract infections due to *Streptococcus pyogenes, Streptococcus pneumoniae,* or *Haemophilus influenzae* (when used with sulfonamides).
9. Nongonococcal urethritis.
10. Pertussis.
11. Prevention of initial (drug of choice) and recurrent attacks of rheumatic fever.
12. Primary syphilis due to *Treponema pallidum* (is an alternate drug to penicillin).
13. Respiratory tract infections due to *Mycoplasma pneumoniae.*
14. Mild to moderate skin and skin structure infections due to *S. pyogenes* or *Staphylococcus aureus* (resistance may occur during treatment).

ADDITIONAL CONTRAINDICATIONS

Pre-existing liver disease.

HOW SUPPLIED

Powder for Oral Suspension: 100 mg (of the base)/2.5 mL (when reconstituted), 200 mg (of the base)/5 mL (when reconstituted), 400 mg (of the base)/5 mL (when reconstituted); ***Suspension, Oral:*** 200 mg (as the base)/5 mL, 400 mg (as the base)/5 mL; ***Tablets:*** 400 mg.

DOSAGE

NOTE: For adults, 400 mg of erythromycin ethylsuccinate will achieve the same blood levels of erythromycin as 250 mg of the base or stearate forms.

ORAL SUSPENSION; TABLETS

Most uses.

Adults, usual: 400 mg q 6 hr; dose may be increased up to 4 grams/day, according to the severity of the infection. **Children, usual:** For mild to moderate infections, 30–50 mg/kg/day in equally divided doses q 6 hr. For more severe infections, the dose may be doubled. For children, age, weight, and severity of the infection are important factors in determining the appropriate dose. See *Implementation/Administration/Storage* for specific dosing information for children. For adults or children, one-half of the daily dose may be given q 12 hr or one-third of the daily dose q 8 hr.

Intestinal amebiasis.

Adults: 400 mg 4 times per day for 10–14 days. **Children:** 30–50 mg/kg/day in divided doses for 10–14 days.

Legionnaires' disease.

Usual: 1.6–4 grams/day in divided doses. *NOTE:* Optimal doses have not been established.

Pertussis.

Usual: 40–50 mg/kg/day in divided doses for 5–14 days. *NOTE:* Optimal dosage and duration have not been established.

Primary syphilis.

Adults: 48–64 grams given in divided doses over a period of 10–15 days.

Urethritis due to C. trachomatis *or* U. urealyticum.

800 mg 3 times per day for 7 days.

Streptococcal infections.

Give a therapeutic dose of erythromycin ethylsuccinate for at least 10 days. For continuous prophylaxis against recurrent streptococcal infections in those with a history of rheumatic heart disease, the usual dose is 400 mg twice a day.

NURSING IMPLICATIONS

1. Maximum daily dosage is 4 grams/day.
2. The following doses are used in children: **<4.5 kg (<10 lbs):** 30–50 mg/kg/day or 15–25 mg/kg q 12 hr; **4.5–6.8 kg (10–15 lbs):** 200 mg/day; **7.3–11.4 kg (16–25 lbs):** 400 mg/day; **11.8–22.7 kg (26–50 lbs):** 800 mg/day; **23.2–45.5 kg (51–100 lbs):** 1,200 mg/day; **>45.5 kg (>100 lbs):** 1,600 mg/day.
3. For streptococcal infections, a therapeutic dose should be given for at least 10 days.
4. In continuous prophylaxis against recurrences of streptococcal infections in those with a history of rheumatic heart disease, the usual dose is 400 mg twice a day.
5. To prepare the oral suspension of EryPed 200, reconstitute with 2.9 mL of water; for EryPed 400, reconstitute with 2.7 mL of water.
6. Prior to mixing the granules for oral suspension, store below 30°C (86°F). After mixing, refrigerate and use within 10 days.
7. Prior to mixing the powder for oral suspension, store below 30°C (86°F). After reconstitution, store at or below 25°C (77°F); use within 25 days. Refrigeration is not required.
8. Refrigerate the suspension to preserve taste. Refrigeration is not required if used within 14 days.
9. Store tablets below 30°C (86°F).

ASSESSMENT

1. List reasons for therapy, onset/characteristics of S&S, clinical presentation and culture results.
2. Monitor CBC, renal and LFTs; avoid use with severe liver dysfunction.

CLIENT/FAMILY TEACHING

1. Take tablets with a full glass of water 1 hr before or 2 hr after meals. May take with food if GI upset. Complete entire prescription.
2. Shake suspension well before using measure, and administer prescribed dose using dosing spoon, dosing syringe, or medicine cup. Refrigerate after opening.
3. Report any persistent palpitations, SOB, syncope, cyanosis, seizures, hallucinations, rash/hives, bleeding, diarrhea, inability to void, abdominal pain, or signs of superinfection.
4. Avoid exposure to sunlight and use sunscreen, or wear protective clothing to avoid photosensitivity reaction

5. Keep all F/U to assess response, labs/cultures, and adverse SE.

OUTCOMES/EVALUATE

Resolution of infection

IV

Erythromycin lactobionate

Classification(s): Antibiotic, macrolide

Pregnancy Category: B

RX: Erythromycin lactobionate.

SEE ALSO ***ERYTHROMYCIN BASE.***

INDICATIONS/USES

See *Erythromycin Base* for specific information, including causative organisms. *NOTE:* To reduce development of drug-resistant bacteria and maintain the efficacy of erythromycin, use only to treat or prevent infections that are proven or strongly suspected to be due to susceptible bacteria.

1. Acute pelvic inflammatory disease due to *Neisseria gonorrhoeae* in females with a history of sensitivity to penicillin. Use IV erythromycin followed by PO erythromycin.
2. Diphtheria due to *Corynebacterium diphtheriae* to prevent establishment of carriers and to eradicate the organism in carriers.
3. Erythrasma due to *Corynebacterium minutissimum.*
4. Legionnaires' disease due to *Legionella pneumophila.*
5. Mild to moderate lower and upper respiratory tract infections due to *Streptococcus pyrogenes* (group A beta-hemolytic streptococci) or *Streptococcus pneumoniae.*
6. Prevention of initial and recurrent attacks of rheumatic fever.
7. Skin and skin structure infections due to *S. pyogenes* or *Staphylococcus aureus* (resistance may emerge during treatment).
8. Respiratory tract infections due to *Mycoplasma pneumoniae.*
9. Mild to moderate upper respiratory tract infections due to *S. pyogenes* (group A beta-hemolytic streptococci), *S. pneumoniae,* or *Haemophilus influenzae* (when used with sulfonamides).

ADDITIONAL DRUG INTERACTIONS

Do not add drugs to IV solutions of erythromycin lactobionate.

HOW SUPPLIED

Injection, Lyophilized Powder for Solution: 500 mg, 1 gram.

DOSAGE

IV

Most infections.

Adults and children:
15–20 mg/kg/day up to 4 grams/day (maximum) in severe infections.

Acute pelvic inflammatory disease caused by gonorrhea.

Adults: 500 mg IV q 6 hr for 3 days, followed by 500 mg PO q 12 hr, 333 mg PO q 8 hr, or 250 mg PO q 6 hr for 7 days.

Legionnaires' disease.

Adults: 1–4 grams/day in divided doses. Change to PO therapy as soon as possible. *NOTE:* The optimal dosage has not been established.

NURSING IMPLICATIONS

IMPLEMENTATION/ADMINISTRATION/STORAGE

1. IV The maximum recommended dose is 4 grams/day.
2. In the treatment of streptococcal infections of the upper respiratory tract (e.g., tonsillitis, pharyngitis), administer a therapeutic dose for at least 10 days.
3. To prevent recurring attacks of rheumatic fever in those allergic to penicillin and sulfonamides, it is recommended that erythromycin, 250 mg PO twice a day, be given for long-term prophylaxis of streptococcal upper respiratory tract infections.
4. To prepare the initial solution for IV use, add 10 mL of sterile water for injection to the 500 mg vial or 20 mL of sterile water for injection to the 1 gram vial. Use only sterile water for injection, as other diluents may cause precipitation during reconstitution. Do not use diluents containing preservatives or inorganic salts. After reconstitution, each mL contains 50 mg of erythromycin activity.

5. Add the initial dilution to one of the following diluents before administration to give a concentration of 1 gram of erythromycin activity/liter (i.e., 1 mg/mL) for continuous infusion or 1–5 mg/mL for intermittent infusion: NaCl 0.9% injection, Ringer's lactate injection, or Normosol-R.
6. The following solutions may also be used provided they are first buffered with sodium bicarbonate 4% (1 mL/100 mL of solution): D5W injection, D5 and Ringer's lactate injection, D5 and NaCl 0.9% injection. A pH of at least 5.5 is desirable for the final diluted solution of erythromycin.
7. IV erythromycin may be given only by continuous or intermittent IV infusion (at 6 hr intervals). IV push is not acceptable due to the irritating properties of erythromycin.
8. For slow continuous infusion, the final diluted erythromycin solution should be 1 mg/mL (i.e., 1 gram/L).
9. For intermittent infusion, give one-fourth the total daily dose over 20–60 min at intervals no greater than q 6 hr. The final diluted solution is prepared to give a concentration of 1–5 mg/mL. No less than 100 mL of IV diluent should be used. The infusion should be sufficiently slow to minimize pain along the vein.
10. Replace IV erythromycin by PO erythromycin as soon as possible.
11. The initial solution is stable refrigerated for 2 weeks or for 24 hr at room temperature. The final diluted solution of erythromycin should be completely administered within 8 hr as it is not suitable for storage.
12. Store vials from 20–25°C (68–77°F).
13. COMPATIBILITY 0.9 % NaCl, LR or Normosol-R.
14. INCOMPATIBILITY No drug or chemical agent should be added to infusion.

ASSESSMENT

1. Note reasons for therapy, onset, characteristics of S&S and clinical presentation.
2. Assess for hearing deficits.
3. Monitor CBC, cultures, renal and LFTs.

CLIENT/FAMILY TEACHING

1. Drug is administered by injection for severe infections. Will be switched to oral dosing when condition permits.
2. Report any rash, fever, nausea, abdominal pain, diarrhea, or lack of response.

OUTCOMES/EVALUATE

Resolution of infection; negative C&S

Erythromycin stearate

Classification(s): Antibiotic, macrolide

Pregnancy Category: B

RX: Erythrocin Stearate.

✤ **Rx:** Apo-Erythro-S.

SEE ALSO ***ERYTHROMYCIN BASE.***

INDICATIONS/USES

See *Erythromycin Base* for more specific details on use, including causative organisms. *NOTE:* To reduce development of drug-resistant bacteria and maintain the efficacy of erythromycin, use only to treat or prevent infections that are proven or strongly suspected to be due to susceptible bacteria.

1. Acute pelvic inflammatory disease.
2. Diphtheria.
3. Erythrasma.
4. *Chlamydia trachomatis* infections.
5. Intestinal amebiasis.
6. Legionnaires' disease.
7. Listeriosis.
8. Lower and upper respiratory tract infections.
9. Nongonococcal urethritis.
10. Pertussis.
11. Primary syphilis.
12. Prevention of initial and recurrent attacks of rheumatic fever.
13. Skin and skin structure infections. *Investigational:* Primary or secondary early syphilis (*Treponema pallidum)* in those for whom compliance with therapy and follow-up can be ensured. Lymphogranuloma venerum, granuloma inguinale, *Haemophilus ducreyi* (chancroid).

ADDITIONAL SIDE EFFECTS

Causes more allergic reactions (e.g., skin rash and urticaria) than other erythromycins.

HOW SUPPLIED

Tablets, Film-Coated: 250 mg.

DOSAGE

TABLETS, FILM-COATED

Most infections.

Adults: 250 mg q 6 hr or 500 mg q 12 hr; dose may be increased up to 4 grams/day according to the severity of the infection. *NOTE:* Twice-a-day dosing is not recommended when doses are larger than 1 gram/day. **Children:** 30–50 mg/kg/day in equally divided doses. For more severe infections, the dose may be doubled, but should not exceed 4 grams/day. Age, weight, and severity of the infection are important factors in determining the proper dose in children.

Acute pelvic inflammatory disease.

Adults: 500 mg erythromycin for IV injection (e.g., erythromycin lactobionate) q 6 hr for 3 days followed by 500 mg erythromycin for PO use q 12 hr, or 333 mg q 8 hr, or 250 mg q 6 hr for 7 days.

Intestinal amebiasis.

Adults: 500 mg q 12 hr, 333 mg q 8 hr, or 250 mg q 6 hr for 10–14 days. **Children:** 30–50 mg/kg/day in divided doses for 10–14 days.

Legionnaires' disease.

1–4 grams/day in divided doses. *NOTE:* The optimal dosage has not been established.

Nongonococcal urethritis.

Adults: 500 mg PO 4 times per day for at least 7 days.

Pertussis.

Usual: 40–50 mg/kg/day in divided doses for 5–14 days. *NOTE:* The optimal dosage has not been established.

Primary syphilis.

Adults: 30–40 grams in divided doses over a period of 10–15 days.

Adults with uncomplicated urethral, endocervical, or rectal infections due to C. trachomatis *when tetracycline is contraindicated or not tolerated.*

Adults: 500 mg 4 times per day.

Urogenital infections during pregnancy.

Suggested treatment: 500 mg 4 times per day for at least 7 days. For women who cannot tolerate this dose, a decreased dosage of 500 mg q 12 hr or 250 mg 4 times per day should be used for 14 days.

NURSING IMPLICATIONS

IMPLEMENTATION/ADMINISTRATION/STORAGE

1. The maximum daily dose should not exceed 4 grams.
2. The therapeutic dosage of erythromycin should be given for at least 10 days when treating streptococcal infections of the upper respiratory tract (e.g., tonsillitis, pharyngitis).
3. It is recommended that erythromycin 250 mg twice a day be given for long-term prophylaxis of streptococcal upper respiratory tract infections to prevent recurring attacks of rheumatic fever in those allergic to penicillin and sulfonamides.
4. Store tablets below 30°C (86°F).

ASSESSMENT

1. List reasons for therapy, onset, characteristics of S&S, and clinical presentation.
2. Obtain and monitor culture results, CBC, renal and LFTs.

CLIENT/FAMILY TEACHING

1. Take on an empty stomach; food decreases absorption.
2. Report lack of effect or evidence of allergic reaction, i.e., rash or itching. Keep all F/U to assess response, labs, and adverse SE.

OUTCOMES/EVALUATE

Resolution of infection

Escitalopram oxalate

(eh-sye-**TAL**-oh-pram)

Classification(s): Antidepressant, selective serotonin reuptake inhibitor

Pregnancy Category: C

RX: Lexapro.

SEE ALSO ***SELECTIVE SEROTONIN REUPTAKE INHIBITORS.***

E

INDICATIONS/USES

(1) Major depressive disorder, including maintenance, in adults and children, age 12–17 years. (2) Generalized anxiety disorder. *Investigational:* Posttraumatic stress disorder, panic disorder.

ACTION/KINETICS

Action

Inhibits CNS neuronal reuptake of serotonin. Minimal effects on norepinephrine and dopamine reuptake. Little to no anticholinergic or sedative effects; does not cause orthostatic hypotension.

Pharmacokinetics

80% is bioavailable. **Peak plasma levels:** About 5 hr. Absorption is not affected by food. **Steady state:** About 1 week following once-daily dosing. Metabolized in the liver by the CYP3A4 and CYP2C19 isoenzymes. **t½, terminal:** 27–32 hr. About 7% excreted in the urine. **Plasma protein binding:** About 56%.

CONTRAINDICATIONS

Clients taking MAOIs or citalopram (Celexa). Hypersensitivity to the drug or any component of the product. Alcohol use.

SPECIAL CONCERNS

■ **Suicidality and antidepressant drugs.** Antidepressants increased the risk compared with placebo of suicidal thinking and behavior (suicidality) in children, adolescents, and young adults in short-term studies of major depressive disorder and other psychiatric disorders. Anyone considering the use of escitalopram or any other antidepressant in a child, adolescent, or young adult must balance this risk with the clinical need. Short-term studies did not show an increase in the risk of suicidality with antidepressants compared with placebo in adults beyond 24 years of age; there was a reduction in risk with antidepressants compared with placebo in adults 65 years of age and older. Depression and certain other psychiatric disorders are themselves associated with increases in the risk of suicide. Appropriately monitor clients of all ages who are started on antidepressant therapy and closely observe for clinical worsening, suicidality, or unusual changes in behavior. Advise families and caregivers of the need for close observation and communication with the prescriber. Escitalopram is not approved for use in children younger than 12 years of age. ■

- **Do not use escitalopram in combination with an MAOI, within 14 days of discontinuing treatment with an MAOI, or within 14 days after discontinuing escitalopram before starting an MAOI.**
- **Some risk of developing a serotonin syndrome.**
- **Use with caution during lactation; in seizure disorders; in clients with diseases or conditions that produce altered metabolism or hemodynamic responses; in impaired hepatic function; severe renal impairment; and with use of CNS drugs.**
- **Risk of clinical worsening and suicidal ideation/behavior, especially at the beginning of drug therapy and during dosage adjustments.**
- **Safety and efficacy have not been determined in children.**
- **Possible need for prolonged hospitalization, respiratory support, and tube feeding in neonates exposed to escitalopram late in the third trimester.**

SIDE EFFECTS

Most Common

Nausea, dry mouth, increased sweating, dizziness, diarrhea, flu-like symptoms, fatigue, insomnia, somnolence, rhinitis, ejaculation disorder.

CNS: Insomnia, somnolence, dizziness, decreased appetite, activation of mania/hypomania, ***suicide attempts***, paresthesia, light-headedness, migraine, tremor, vertigo, abnormal dreaming, yawning, irritability, impaired concentration, seizures. **GI:** N&V, dry mouth, diarrhea, constipation, indigestion, abdominal pain, flatulence, heartburn, toothache, gastroenteritis, abdominal cramps, gastroesophageal reflux. **CV:** Palpitation, hypertension. **GU:** Ejaculatory delay, decreased libido, impotence, anorgasmia (females), menstrual cramps, UTI, urinary frequency. **Respiratory:** Rhinitis, sinusitis, bronchitis, sinus headache/congestion, coughing, nasal congestion. **Musculoskeletal:** Arthralgia, neck/shoulder pain, muscle cramps, myalgia. **Dermatologic:** Increased sweating. **Body as a whole:** Fatigue, flu-like symptoms, allergy, hot flushes, fever, increased/decreased weight, lethargy. **Miscellaneous:** Pain in limb, chest pain, blurred vision, earache, tinnitus.

DRUG INTERACTIONS

Cimetidine / ↑ Escitalopram AUC and t½ R/T possible inhibition of metabolism

MAOIs / Serious (may be fatal) reactions, including hyperthermia, rigidity, myoclonus, autonomic instability, mental status changes (extreme agitation, delirium, coma)
Metoprolol / ↑ Metoprolol C_{max} and AUC
Omeprazole / ↑ Escitalopram AUC and t½ R/T possible inhibition of metabolism
Sumatriptan / Potential for weakness, hyperreflexia, incoordination

HOW SUPPLIED

Oral Solution: 1 mg (as base)/mL; *Tablets:* 5 mg (as base), 10 mg (as base), 20 mg (as base).

DOSAGE

ORAL SOLUTION; TABLETS

Major depressive illness.

Adults, initial: 10 mg once daily, including the elderly or those with hepatic impairment. Increase dose to 20 mg, if necessary, after a minimum of 1 week. **Maintenance therapy:** 10 or 20 mg/day for up to 36 weeks after an initial 8 weeks of treatment. Periodically reassess to determine the need for maintenance treatment. **Children, 12–17 years, initial:** 10 mg once daily. If the dose is increased to 20 mg, it should occur over a minimum of 3 weeks. See above for maintenance therapy.

Generalized anxiety disorder.

Initial: 10 mg once daily. Dose may be increased to 20 mg once daily after a minimum of 1 week. Efficacy after 8 weeks of treatment has not been determined.

Post-traumatic stress disorder (Investigational).

Initial: 10 mg once daily; may be increased to 20 mg once daily after 4 weeks. May need to continue therapy indefinitely. Tapering may be considered after 6–12 months in those with acute post-traumatic stress syndrome and after 12–24 months in those with chronic post-traumatic stress syndrome. Taper gradually over 2 weeks to 1 month to avoid withdrawal symptoms. In those at risk for relapse, taper over 4–12 weeks.

NURSING IMPLICATIONS

IMPLEMENTATION/ADMINISTRATION/STORAGE

1. For the elderly and those with impaired hepatic function, the recommended dose is 10 mg/day.
2. Give once daily in the morning or evening with or without food.
3. No dosage adjustment is needed for those with mild or moderate impaired renal function.
4. Discontinuing escitalopram may cause symptoms, including dysphoric mood, irritability, agitation, dizziness, sensory disturbances, anxiety, confusion, headache, lethargy, emotional lability, hypomania, or insomnia. A gradual reduction in dose, rather than abrupt cessation, is recommended whenever possible.
5. Store from 15–30°C (59–86°F).

ASSESSMENT

1. List reasons for therapy, onset/characteristics of symptoms, any events/triggers and other agents trialed/outcome.
2. Note other drugs prescribed; ensure none interact. Avoid use within 14 days before/after MAOI use.
3. Determine seizure disorder or any liver, renal, or sexual dysfunction.
4. Document behaviors (mood changes and anxiety levels), cognitive function, and clinical response. Assess closely for any suicide ideations.
5. Monitor ECG, electrolytes, renal and LFTs.

CLIENT/FAMILY TEACHING

1. Take as directed, once daily, with or without food.
2. Drug is an isomer of Celexa and should not be taken with Celexa.
3. Use caution operating machines or cars until drug effects known. May experience insomnia, fatigue, nausea, sweating, and ejaculation disorders. Report unusual bleeding, appetite/wt changes, seizures or S&S of electrolyte imbalances.
4. Avoid alcohol, OTC agents, or CNS depressants.
5. Report any abnormal changes in mood or thinking, especially: agitation, anxiety, hostility or aggressiveness, impulsivity, irritability, panic attacks, suicidal thoughts or behavior.

6. Use reliable birth control; report if pregnancy suspected.
7. May see improvement in 1 to 4 weeks; continue as prescribed. Children will be seen weekly during first 4 weeks of therapy, then regularly thereafter.
8. Keep all F/U to assess response, counselling, and adverse SE.

OUTCOMES/EVALUATE

Relief/control of depression/anxiety

IV

Esmolol hydrochloride

(**EZ**-moh-lohl)

Classification(s): Beta-adrenergic blocking agent

Pregnancy Category: C

RX: Brevibloc.

SEE ALSO ***BETA-ADRENERGIC BLOCKING AGENTS***.

INDICATIONS/USES

(1) Supraventricular tachycardia in those with atrial fibrillation or atrial flutter in perioperative, postoperative, or other emergent situations when short-term control is needed. (2) Noncompensatory sinus tachycardia when rapid heart rate requires intervention. (3) Tachycardia and hypertension during induction and tracheal intubation, during surgery, on emergence from anesthesia, and postoperatively. *Investigational:* Unstable angina.

ACTION/KINETICS

Action

Preferentially inhibits beta-1 receptors. Has no membrane-stabilizing or intrinsic sympathomimetic activity. Decreases HR and AV nodal conduction velocity and increases AV refractory period.

Pharmacokinetics

Rapid onset (<5 min) and a short duration of action. Low lipid solubility. **t½:** 9 min. Rapidly metabolized by esterases in RBCs.

SPECIAL CONCERNS

Dosage not established in children.

SIDE EFFECTS

Most Common

N&V, dizziness, sweating, pain/redness at injection site, headache, confusion, fatigue, hypotension, somnolence, local thrombophlebitis, rash, itchy skin.

See *Beta-Adrenergic Blocking Agents* for a complete list of possible side effects. **Dermatologic:** Inflammation at site of infusion, flushing, pallor, induration, erythema, burning, skin discoloration, edema. **Miscellaneous:** Urinary retention, midscapular pain, asthenia, changes in taste.

ADDITIONAL DRUG INTERACTIONS

Digoxin / ↑ Digoxin levels
Morphine / ↑ Esmolol levels

HOW SUPPLIED

Injection: 10 mg/mL, 250 mg/mL.

DOSAGE

IV INFUSION

Supraventricular tachycardia.

Individualize dosage. The dosing regimen assumes that 3 loading doses (maximum recommended) are infused over 1 min and incremental maintenance doses are required after each loading dose. There should be no fourth loading dose, but the maintenance dose may be increased by 1 more increments. **Dosing regimen:** 500 mcg/kg/min over 1 min; **then,** 50 mcg/kg/min over 4 min. If after 5 min an adequate effect is not achieved, repeat the loading dose (i.e., 500 mcg/kg/min given over 1 min) followed by a maintenance infusion of 100 mcg/kg/min over 4 min. This procedure may be repeated, **if necessary**, increasing the maintenance infusion to 150 mcg/kg/min over 4 min (i.e., elapsed time of 11 to 15 min since the first loading dose). **Then,** omit the loading infusion and give a maintenance dose of 200 mcg/kg/min over 4 min (i.e., over minutes 16 to 20 after the initial loading dose). After 20 min have elapsed since the first loading dose, give maintenance doses titrated to heart rate or other clinical end point. Use of esmolol infusions over a 24 hr period has been well documented; there are limited data with use up to 48 hr. *NOTE:* Loading and maintenance doses after the first loading dose are determined by clinical need.

Responses to esmolol usually occur over a range of 50–200 mcg/kg/min with the average effective dose being 100 mcg/kg/min (doses as low as 25 mcg/kg/min have been effective in some).

After adequate control of HR and a stable clinical status has been achieved in clients with SV, transition to alternative antiarrhythmic agents (e.g., propranolol, digoxin, or verapamil) is warranted. Doses to consider are (a) Propranolol: 10–20 mg q 4–6 hr. (b) Digoxin: 0.125–0.5 mg q 6 hr (either PO or IV). (c) Verapamil: 80 mg q 6 hr. The dosage of esmolol should be reduced as follows: (a) 30 min following the first dose of the alternative drug, reduce the esmolol infusion rate by one-half. (b) Following the second dose of the alternative drug, monitor client response and, if satisfactory control is maintained for the first hr, discontinue esmolol.

Intraoperative and postoperative tachycardia and hypertension.

It is not always advisable to titrate the esmolol dose slowly to a therapeutic effect. Thus, there are 2 dosing options: immediate control and gradual control. **Immediate control (intraoperative tachycardia and hypertension):** 80 mg (about 1 mg/kg) bolus dose over 30 sec followed by 150 mcg/kg/min, if necessary. Adjust the infusion rate as needed, up to 300 mcg/kg/min to maintain the desired HR or BP. **Gradual control (postoperative tachycardia and hypertension):** Initiate treatment with a loading dosage infusion of 500 mcg/kg/min for 1 min followed by a 4-min maintenance infusion of 50 mcg/kg/min. If an adequate effect is not seen within 5 min, repeat the same loading dosage and follow with a maintenance infusion increased to 100 mcg/kg/min. ***NOTE:* Dosage above is given in both milligrams (mg) and micrograms (mcg); do not confuse the two.**

Unstable angina (investigational).

Adults: 2 to 24 mg/min as a continuous infusion.

Children, acute severe hypertension (investigational).

Children, 1–17 years of age, loading dose: 100–500 mcg/kg IV over 1 min; **then,** 25–100 mcg/kg/min by IV infusion. Titrate to individual response. Readminister loading dose or increase maintenance dose by 25–50 mcg/kg/min q 5–10 min as needed to achieve the desired effect. **Maintenance:** 50–500 mcg/kg/min; doses as high as 1,000 mcg/kg/min have been given.

Children, less than 1 year of age, initial: 50 mcg/kg/min by continuous IV infusion. Titrate to the desired BP, increasing by 25–50 mcg/kg/min q 5 min. Rarely titrate above 300 mcg/kg/min due to side effects.

Children, supraventricular tachycardia (investigational).

Children, 1–17 years of age: Same dosage as *"Children, acute severe hypertension."* **Children, less than 1 year of age, initial:** 100 mcg/kg/min by continuous IV infusion; titrate for control of ventricular rate, increasing by 50–100 mcg/kg/min q 5 min.

NURSING IMPLICATIONS

IMPLEMENTATION/ADMINISTRATION/STORAGE

1. IV Infusions may be necessary for 24–48 hr.
2. Not for direct IV push administration.
3. Do not dilute concentrate with sodium bicarbonate.
4. To minimize irritation and thrombophlebitis, do not infuse concentrations greater than 10 mg/mL. If a side effect occurs, the dose may be reduced or discontinued. Do not use butterfly needles.
5. If a local infusion site reaction occurs, use an alternate infusion site; take care to prevent extravasation.

6. Although abrupt cessation of esmolol therapy has not been reported to cause withdrawal effects, care should still be used in abruptly discontinuing infusion of esmolol.
7. Store from 15–30°C (59–86°F). Protect from freezing; avoid excessive heat.
8. COMPATIBILITY Diluted esmolol (concentration of 10 mg/mL) is compatible with D5W, D5/RL, D5/Ringer's injection, D5/0.9% NaCl, D5/0.45% NaCl, 0.45% NaCl, RL, KCl (40 mEq/L) in D5W, and 0.9% NaCl.
9. INCOMPATIBILITY Administer separately.

E

ASSESSMENT

1. Note reasons for therapy, type, onset, characteristics of S&S.
2. Administer in a monitored environment; wean using guidelines.
3. List CP assessments, ECG, VS. Assess for hypotension, bradycardia, heart block, DM, or CHF.
4. May reduce dose with renal or liver dysfunction.

CLIENT/FAMILY TEACHING

1. Drug is administered IV to control cardiac arrhythmias.
2. May cause drowsiness; use caution and change positions slowly to prevent any sudden drop in BP.
3. With diabetes monitor BS closely.
4. Report any itching, SOB, vertigo, syncope, or inability to void.

OUTCOMES/EVALUATE

- Suppression of SVT
- Restoration of stable rhythm

IV

Esomeprazole magnesium

(**es**-oh-**MEP**-rah-zole)

Classification(s): Proton pump inhibitor

Pregnancy Category: B

RX: Nexium.

SEE ALSO ***PROTON PUMP INHIBITORS***.

INDICATIONS/USES

PO only: (1) Healing of erosive esophagitis. Short-term treatment (4–8 weeks) in the healing and symptomatic resolution of diagnostically confirmed erosive esophagitis. An additional 4- to 8-week course may be instituted for those who have not healed. (2) To maintain symptom resolution and healing of erosive esophagitis. (3) Symptomatic GERD. Short-term (4–8 weeks) treatment of heartburn and other symptoms associated with GERD in adults and children, 1 year and older. (4) Reduce occurrence of gastric ulcers associated with continuous NSAID therapy in those at risk for developing gastric ulcers (those 60 years and older and/or documented history of gastric ulcers). (5) *Helicobacter pylori* eradication. In combination with amoxicillin and clarithromycin (Triple Therapy) to treat and eradicate *H. pylori* infection and duodenal ulcer disease (active or history in the past 5 years). Eradication has been shown to reduce the risk of duodenal ulcer recurrence. (6) Long-term treatment of pathological hypersecretory conditions, including Zollinger-Ellison syndrome. *Investigational:* Non-GERD dyspepsia, Barrett esophagus, stress ulcer prophylaxis. Reduction of GI bleeding in clients receiving antiplatelets (e.g., clopidogrel).

IV only: Short-term treatment (up to 10 days) of GERD with erosive esophagitis in adults and children, 1 month to 17 years of age, inclusively as an alternative to PO therapy when therapy with PO esomeprazole is not possible or inappropriate. *Investigational:* Stress ulcer prophylaxis. Prevention of GI bleeding in clients receiving antiplatelets (e.g., clopidogrel).

ACTION/KINETICS

Action

Suppresses the final step in gastric acid production by inhibiting the H^+/K^+-ATPase system at the secretory surface of the gastric parietal cells. This decreases gastric acid secretion. This effect is dose-related and inhibits both basal and stimulated acid secretion regardless of the stimulant.

Pharmacokinetics

Products contain enteric-coated granules. Absorption is rapid but occurs only after the granules leave the stomach. About 90% bioavailable after multiple doses. **Peak plasma levels:** 1.5 hr. Absorption is decreased by food. Extensively metabolized in the liver by the cytochrome P450 enzyme system. **t½, elimination:** 1–1.5 hr. The AUC is increased 2–3 times in those with severe hepatic insufficiency. About 80% excreted as inactive metabolites in the urine with 20% excreted in the feces. **Plasma protein binding:** 97%.

CONTRAINDICATIONS

Known hypersensitivity to any component of the formulation or to any macrolide antibiotic. Lactation.

SPECIAL CONCERNS

- Symptomatic response does not preclude gastric malignancy.
- Safety and efficacy not determined in children except where noted under *Indications/Uses.*

SIDE EFFECTS

Most Common

Headache, flatulence, dyspepsia, nausea, dizziness, diarrhea, stomach pain, constipation, dry mouth, mild focal erythema and pruritus at IV injection site.

GI: Diarrhea, N&V, flatulence, enlarged abdomen, bowel irregularity, aggravated constipation, dyspepsia, dysphagia, epigastric pain, eructation, esophageal disorder, frequent stools, gastroenteritis, GI dysplasia, ***GI hemorrhage***, melena, dry mouth, hiccough, melena, mouth/rectal/tongue disorder, tongue edema, ulcerative stomatitis. **CNS:** Headache, anorexia, apathy, increased appetite, confusion, aggravated depression, dizziness, hypertonia, nervousness, hypoesthesia, insomnia, migraine, paresthesia, sleep disorder, somnolence, tremor, vertigo. **CV:** Hypertension, tachycardia. **Hematologic:** Anemia, hypochromic anemia, cervical lymphoadenopathy, leukocytosis, leukopenia, thrombocytopenia. **Respiratory:** Aggravated asthma, cough, dyspnea, epistaxis, ***laryngeal edema***, pharyngitis, pharynx disorder, rhinitis, sinusitis. **Dermatologic:** Acne, ***angioedema***, dermatitis, flushing, pruritus, pruritus ani, rash, erythematous/maculopapular rash, skin inflammation, increased sweating, urticaria. **Otic:** Earache, tinnitus, otitis media. **Ophthalmic:** Conjunctivitis, abnormal vision, visual field defect. **Musculoskeletal:** Arthralgia, aggravated arthritis, arthropathy, cramps, fibromyalgia syndrome, hernia, polymyalgia rheumatica. **GU:** Dysmenorrhea, menstrual disorder, vaginitis, abnormal urine, cystitis, dysuria, fungal infection, hematuria, impotence, frequent micturition, moniliasis, genital moniliasis, polyuria. **Body as a whole:** Enlarged abdomen, ***allergic reaction***, ***anaphylaxis***, asthenia, back/chest/substernal chest pain, facial/generalized/peripheral/leg edema, hot flushes, fatigue, fever, flu-like symptoms, malaise, pain, rigors. **Miscellaneous:** Goiter, abnormal hepatic function, thirst, weight gain/loss, vitamin B_{12} deficiency, parosmia, taste loss/perversion, mild focal erythema and pruritus at IV injection site.

Postmarketing. CNS: Aggression, agitation, hallucination. **GI:** GI candidiasis, pancreatitis, stomatitis, taste disturbance. **Hepatic:** Hepatic encephalopathy, ***hepatic failure***, hepatitis (with or without jaundice). **Hematologic:** ***Agranulocytosis, pancytopenia***. **Dermatologic:** Alopecia, erythema multiforme, hyperhidrosis, photosensitivity, ***Stevens-Johnson syndrome.*** **Musculoskeletal:** Bone fracture, muscular weakness, myalgia. **GU:** Gynecomastia, interstitial nephritis. **Respiratory:** Bronchospasm. **Ophthalmic:** Blurred vision. **Body as a whole:** ***Anaphylactic reaction***, shock.

LABORATORY TEST CONSIDERATIONS

↑ AST, ALT, GGT, alkaline phosphatase, total bilirubin, serum creatinine, serum gastrin, uric acid, TSH, hemoglobin, platelets, WBC count, potassium, sodium, thyroxine. Glycosuria, hyponatremia, hypoglycemia, hypomagnesemia. Bilirubinemia, hyperuricemia, albuminuria.

DRUG INTERACTIONS

See also ***Proton Pump Inhibitors.***

Esomeprazole may interfere with the absorption of drugs where gastric pH is an important factor in bioavailability (e.g., digoxin, iron salts, ketoconazole).

Benzodiazepines (e.g., diazepam, triazolam) / Oxidative metabolism of the benzodiazepine may be ↓ → ↓ clearance, prolonged t½, and ↑ serum levels; ↓ benzodiazepine dose or ↑ the dosing interval

Cilostazol / Possible ↑ cilostazol plasma levels → ↑ therapeutic and toxic effects; consider cilostazol dosage adjustment

Clarithromycin / ↑ Serum levels of both clarithromycin and esomeprazole

HOW SUPPLIED

Capsules, Delayed-Release: 20 mg, 40 mg; *Injection, Lyophilized Powder for Solution:* 20 mg, 40 mg; *Powder for Suspension, Delayed-Release Oral:* 10 mg, 20 mg, 40 mg.

DOSAGE

CAPSULES, DELAYED-RELEASE; SUSPENSION, DELAYED-RELEASE

Healing of erosive esophagitis.

Adults, initial: 20 or 40 mg once daily for 4–8 weeks; **maintenance:** 20 mg/day. For those who do not heal within 4–8 weeks, consider an additional 4–8 weeks of therapy.

Healing of erosive esophagitis in children, 1-11 years.

Children, <20 kg: 10 mg once daily for 8 weeks. **Children, 20 kg or more:** 10 or 20 mg once daily for 8 weeks.

Maintenance of healing of erosive esophagitis.

20 mg once daily, for up to 6 months.

Symptomatic GERD in adults and children, 1-11 years of age.

Adults: 20 mg once daily for 4 weeks. If symptoms do not resolve completely, consider an additional 4 weeks of therapy. **Children, 1–11 years:** 10 mg once daily for up to 8 weeks.

Short-term treatment of GERD in adolescents, 12-17 years of age.

Children, 12–17 years of age: 20 or 40 mg once daily for up to 8 weeks.

Reduce risk of NSAID-associated gastric ulcers.

Adults: 20 or 40 mg once daily for up to 6 months.

Eradication of H. pylori *to reduce risk of duodenal ulcer recurrence—Triple Therapy.*

Adults: Use the following triple therapy. Esomeprazole, 40 mg once daily for 10 days; amoxicillin, 1,000 mg twice a day for 10 days; and, clarithromycin, 500 mg twice a day for 10 days.

Pathological hypersecretory conditions, including Zollinger-Ellison syndrome.

Adults: 40 mg twice daily; adjust dose to needs of client. Doses up to 240 mg/day have been used.

IV

GERD with erosive esophagitis.

Adults: 20 or 40 mg given once daily by IV injection (no less than 3 minutes) or by IV infusion over 10–30 minutes. **Children, 1–17 years:** 20 mg per day by IV infusion if weight of 55 kg or more; 10 mg once daily by IV infusion is weight is less than 55 kg. **Children, 1 month to <1 year, usual:** 0.5 mg/kg once daily by IV infusion.

NURSING IMPLICATIONS

IMPLEMENTATION/ADMINISTRATION/STORAGE

1. Do not exceed a dose of 20 mg daily in clients with severe hepatic dysfunction (Child-Pugh class C).
2. For clients unable to swallow capsules, add 1 tablespoon of applesauce to an empty bowl. Carefully empty the pellets from the capsule onto the applesauce. Mix the pellets with the applesauce, and swallow immediately. Do not use hot applesauce, and do not chew or crush the pellets. Do not store the pellet/applesauce mixture for future use.
3. For clients with a nasogastric tube in place, open the capsules and empty the intact granules into a 60 mL syringe. Mix with 50 mL of water. Replace the plunger, and shake the syringe vigorously for 15 seconds. Hold the syringe with the tip up, and check for granules remaining in the tip. Attach the syringe to the NG tube, and deliver the contents through the NG tube into the stomach. Flush the NG tube with additional water.
4. Store between 15–30°C (59–86°F) with container tightly closed.
5. IV Discontinue treatment as soon as the client is able to resume therapy with the delayed-release capsule.
6. Safety and efficacy of esomeprazole IV for use for more than 10 days in GERD clients with a history of erosive esophagitis has not been demonstrated. In clients with severe impaired liver function (Child-Pugh class C), do not exceed a dose of 20 mg.
7. **Adults, IV Injection:** For use as an IV injection, reconstitute the freeze-dried powder with 5 mL of 0.9% NaCl injection. Withdraw 5 mL of the reconstituted solution, and give IV over no less than 3 min.
8. **Adults, IV Infusion:** For use by IV infusion over 10–30 min, reconstitute the contents of 1 vial with 5 mL of 0.9% NaCl injection, Ringer's lactate injection or D5W injection; further dilute to a final volume of 50 mL. Give the final

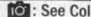

diluted solution as an IV infusion over 10–30 min.

9. **Children, IV infusion, 1–17 years of age, 40 mg vial:** First reconstitute the contents of 1 vial with 5 mL of NaCl 0.9% injection; further dilute to a final volume of 50 mL. The resultant concentration after diluting to a final volume of 50 mL is 0.8 mg/mL. For a 20 mg dose, withdraw 25 mL of the final solution and give as an IV infusion. For a 10 mg dose, withdraw 12.5 mL of the final solution and give as an IV infusion. **Children, IV infusion, 1–17 years of age, 20 mg vial:** First reconstitute the contents of 1 vial with 5 mL of NaCl 0.9% injection; further dilute to a final volume of 50 mL. The resultant concentration after diluting to a final volume of 50 mL is 0.4 mg/mL. For a 20 mg dose, administer the final solution (50 mL) and give as an IV infusion. For a 10 mg dose, withdraw 25 mL of the final solution and give as an IV infusion. **Infants, 1 month to younger than 1 year:** First reconstitute the contents of 1 vial with 5 mL of NaCl 0.9% injection; further dilute to a final volume of 50 mL. The resultant concentration after diluting to a final volume of 50 mL is as follows: 40 mg vial: 0.8 mg/mL and the 20 mg vial: 0.4 mg/mL. Withdraw the appropriate volume for the desired dose (0.5 mg/kg) and give as an IV infusion. For children, only administer by IV infusion over 10–30 min.
10. Store unreconstituted vials from 15–30°C (59–86°F). Protect from light. Store in carton until use.
11. Store the reconstituted IV injection at room temperature up to 30°C (86°F), and give within 12 hr after reconstitution. Store the IV infusion up to 30°C (86°F), and give within 12 hr if diluted with 0.9% NaCl or LR and within 6 hr if diluted with D5W.
12. COMPATIBILITY 0.9% NaCl, LR, or D5W.
13. INCOMPATIBILITY Do not give esomeprazole IV with any other medication through the same IV site and/or tubing. Always flush the IV line with the diluent both prior to and after administration of the drug.

ASSESSMENT

1. List reasons for therapy, type, onset, and characteristics of symptoms. List other agents prescribed; ensure no interaction. Altered pH may interfere with antiviral effects.
2. Determine if pregnant.
3. Drug may interfere with iron absorption and contribute to vitamin B_{12} deficiency in some clients.
4. Record abdominal assessments, pain level, contributing factors, radiographic/endoscopic and *H. pylori* findings.
5. Review potential risks of increased risk for osteoporosis-related fractures of the hip, wrist, or spine.
6. Monitor CBC, Mg^{++}, and LFTs; reduce dose with liver dysfunction.

CLIENT/FAMILY TEACHING

1. Take the delayed-release capsules whole at least 1 hr before meals. If unable to swallow whole, may empty capsule onto 1 tablespoon of applesauce in a cup. Mix pellets into applesauce and swallow immediately, taking care not to chew pellets. The capsule may also be opened and the intact granules emptied into a syringe and delivered through a nasogastric tube.
2. Mix the contents of 10, 20, or 40 mg packet of delayed-release powder for suspension with 15 mL of water; leave 2–3 min to thicken; stir and drink within 30 min. The suspension may also be administered via a nasogastric or gastric tube. To do so, add 15 mL water to a syringe and add contents of the packet. Shake the syringe; leave 2–3 min to thicken. Shake the syringe, and inject through the nasogastric or gastric tube within 30 min. Refill the syringe with 15 mL water; shake and flush any remaining contents from the nasogastric or gastric tube into the stomach.
3. May take antacids.
4. Avoid alcohol and OTC products unless approved.
5. Drug is for short-term use only; it inhibits gastric acid secretion. Side effects of prolonged therapy and suppression of acid secretion alter bacterial colonization and lead to hypochlorhydria and hypergastrinemia, which may lead to an increased risk for gastric tumors.
6. Report if bloody or coffee-ground-like vomit; black, tarry stools; recurrent heartburn/indigestion or abdominal pain occur; increased need for antacid use; or bothersome adverse

reactions (e.g., constipation, gas, headache) are noted.

7. Keep all F/U appointments to assess response, need to continue therapy, and for adverse SE.

OUTCOMES/EVALUATE

- Promotion of ulcer healing; relief of pain; ↓ gastric acid production
- Relief of S&S of GERD
- Eradication of *H. pylori* with designated ATXs

E

Esterified estrogens

(es-**TER**-ih-fyd **ES**-troh-jens)

Classification(s): Estrogen, natural

Pregnancy Category: X

RX: Menest.

SEE ALSO ***ESTROGENS***.

INDICATIONS/USES

(1) Moderate to severe vasomotor symptoms associated with menopause. No evidence that estrogens are effective for nervous symptoms or depression that might occur during menopause; do not use estrogens to treat these conditions. (2) Atrophic vaginitis and kraurosis vulvae due to menopause. (3) Female hypogonadism. (4) Female castration and primary ovarian failure. (5) Inoperable, progressing breast cancer (palliation only) in selected women and men with metastatic disease. (6) Inoperable, progressing, prostate cancer (palliation only).

ACTION/KINETICS

Pharmacokinetics

This product is a mixture of sodium salts of sulfate esters of natural estrogenic substances: 75–85% estrone sodium sulfate and 6–15% equilin sodium sulfate in such proportion that the total of the components is not less than 90% of the total esterified estrogens content. Less potent than estrone.

ADDITIONAL CONTRAINDICATIONS

Pregnancy as use may cause severe harm to the fetus.

SPECIAL CONCERNS

■ See *Estrogens* for Black Box Warnings. ■

SIDE EFFECTS

Most Common

N&V, breakthrough bleeding/spotting, loss of menses or excessively long menses, breast pain, breast enlargement, edema, increased/decreased libido.

See *Estrogens* for a complete list of possible side effects.

HOW SUPPLIED

Tablets: 0.3 mg, 0.625 mg, 1.25 mg, 2.5 mg.

DOSAGE

TABLETS

Moderate to severe vasomotor symptoms.

1.25 mg/day given cyclically (3 weeks on and then 1 week off).

Atrophic vaginitis, kraurosis vulvae.

0.3–1.25 mg or more daily depending on the individual tissue response. Short-term use only. Give cyclically. Reevaluate at 3- to 6- month intervals for tapering or terminating therapy.

Female hypogonadism.

2.5–7.5 mg daily in divided doses for 20 days followed by a 10-day rest period. If bleeding does not occur by the end of this period, repeat the same dosage schedule. The number of courses of therapy to produce bleeding depends on the endometrial responsiveness. If bleeding occurs before the end of the 10-day period, begin with an estrogen-progestin cyclic regimen of 2.5–7.5 mg daily of estrogen in divided doses for 20 days. During the last 5 days of estrogen therapy give a PO progestin. If bleeding occurs before the end of this regimen, discontinue therapy and resume on the 5th day of bleeding.

Female castration, primary ovarian failure.

1.25 mg/day; give cyclically. Adjust dose up or down according to severity of symptoms and client response. For maintenance, adjust dose to lowest level that will provide effective control.

Prostatic cancer, inoperable, progressing.

1.25–2.5 mg 3 times per day given chronically. Judge effectiveness of therapy by symptomatic improvement and phosphatase determinations.

Breast cancer, inoperable, progressing in selected men and women.

10 mg 3 times per day for at least 3 months.

NURSING IMPLICATIONS

IMPLEMENTATION/ADMINISTRATION/STORAGE

1. Given cyclically (3 weeks on, 1 week off) for short-term use only. Use the lowest dose that will control symptoms; discontinue as soon as possible.
2. When used for moderate to severe vasomotor symptoms: If client has not menstruated within the last 2 months or more, cyclic administration is started arbitrarily. If the client is menstruating, start cyclic use on day 5 of bleeding. For short-term use only. Use the lowest dose to control symptoms and discontinue as soon as possible. Reevaluate at 3–6 month intervals for tapering or discontinuation of therapy.
3. When used for atrophic vaginitis, kraurosis vulvae: For short-term use only. Discontinue as soon as possible. Reevaluate at 3–6 month intervals for tapering or stopping therapy.
4. When estrogen is used for a postmenopausal woman with an intact uterus, monitor closely for signs of endometrial cancer; undertake appropriate diagnostic measures to rule out malignancy in the event of persistent or recurring abnormal vaginal bleeding.

ASSESSMENT

1. Note reasons for therapy, type, onset, characteristics of S&S.
2. Review associated hazards of prolonged therapy.
3. Monitor BP, Wt, lipids, and LFTs.

CLIENT/FAMILY TEACHING

1. May take oral tablets as directed at bedtime or mealtime to minimize GI upset or nausea.
2. Report abdominal pain, severe headaches, SOB, chest pain, visual changes, vaginal bleeding/discharge, breast lumps, yellow skin or eyes, dark urine, light-colored stools or swelling of hands and feet.
3. Stop therapy 1 month before planned procedure that may result in prolonged immobilization to reduce risk of blood clot formation.
4. Smoking significantly increases risk of blood clots.
5. Keep all F/U appointments and yearly exams. Will need lipid and liver panel, BP, and body weight monitored; perform BSE regularly. Report unusual side effects or lack of desired response.

OUTCOMES/EVALUATE

- Stimulation of menses
- Relief of postmenopausal S&S
- Suppression of tumor growth/spread

Estradiol gel

(ess-trah-**DYE**-ohl)

Classification(s): Estrogen, semisynthetic

Pregnancy Category: X

RX: Divigel, Elestrin, Estrogel.

SEE ALSO ***ESTROGENS***.

INDICATIONS/USES

(1) Moderate to severe vasomotor symptoms associated with menopause. (2) Moderate to severe symptoms of vulvar and vaginal atrophy associated with menopause (Estrogel only).

SPECIAL CONCERNS

(1) **Endometrial cancer.** Close clinical surveillance of all women taking estrogen is important. Adequate diagnostic measures, including endometrial sampling when indicated, should be undertaken to rule out malignancy in all cases of undiagnosed persistent or recurring abnormal vaginal bleeding. There is no evidence that the use of "natural" estrogens results in a different endometrial risk profile than synthetic estrogens at equivalent estrogenic doses. (2) **CV and other risks.** Estrogens with or without progestins should not be used for the prevention of CV disease or dementia. The Women's Health Initiative (WHI) estrogen alone substudy reported increased risk of stroke and deep vein thrombosis (DVT) in postmenopausal women (50 to 79 years of age) during 6.8 and 7.1 years, respectively of treatment with daily oral conjugated estrogens, 0.625 mg, relative to placebo. (3) The estrogen and progestin WHI substudy reported increased risks of MI, stroke,

invasive breast cancer, pulmonary emboli, and DVT in postmenopausal women (50 to 79 years of age) during 5.6 years of treatment with daily oral conjugated estrogens, 0.625 mg, combined with medroxyprogesterone acetate, 2.5 mg relative to placebo. (4) The WHI Memory Study, a substudy of the WHI, reported an increased risk of developing probable dementia in postmenopausal women 65 years of age and older during 5.2 years of treatment with daily conjugated estrogen, 0.625 mg alone and during 4 years of treatment with daily conjugated estrogens, 0.625 mg combined with medroxyprogesterone acetate, 2.5 mg, relative to placebo. It is unknown whether this finding applies to younger postmenopausal women. (5) Other doses of conjugated estrogens and medroxyprogesterone acetate, and other combinations of estrogens and progestins, were not studied in the WHI and, in the absence of comparable data, these risks should be assumed to be similar. Because of these risks, estrogens with or without progestins should be prescibed at the lowest effective doses and for the shortest duration consistent with treatment goals and risks for the individual woman. ■

SIDE EFFECTS

Most Common

Dizziness, lightheadedness, headache, N&V, GI upset, bloating, weight changes, increased/decreased libido, breast tenderness, edema, redness/irritation at application site.

See *Estrogens* for a complete list of possible side effects.

HOW SUPPLIED

Gel: **Divigel:** 0.1% estradiol in 0.25, 0.5, or 1 gram per single-dose foil packet. **Elestrin:** 0.06% estradiol (0.52 mg/0.87 gram unit dose). **Estrogel:** 0.06% estradiol (0.75 mg/1.25 gram unit dose).

DOSAGE

DIVIGEL

Moderate to severe vasomotor symptoms associated with menopause.

Initial, usual: 0.25 gram. Adjust subsequent doses based on individual client response. Doses of 0.25 gram, 0.5 gram, and 1 gram/day may be used. Each gram of Divigel contains 1 mg of estradiol. Periodically assess.

ELESTRIN

Moderate to severe vasomotor symptoms associated with menopause.

Apply 1 pump per day (0.87 gram/day containing 0.52 mg estradiol) to the upper arm. Adjust subsequent doses based on client response.

ESTROGEL

Moderate to severe vasomotor symptoms and/or moderate to severe symptoms of vulvar and vaginal atrophy associated with menopause.

1.25 grams (containing 0.75 mg estradiol). The lowest effective dose has not been determined. When prescribing solely to treat moderate to severe symptoms of vulvar and vaginal atrophy, consider using a topical vaginal product.

NURSING IMPLICATIONS

IMPLEMENTATION/ADMINISTRATION/STORAGE

1. When estrogen is prescribed for a postmenopausal woman with a uterus, initiate a progestin to reduce the risk of endometrial cancer. A woman without a uterus does not need a progestin.
2. Store from 15–30°C (59–86°F).

ASSESSMENT

1. Note reasons for therapy, age at menopause onset, other therapies trialed, GYN findings.
2. The use of unopposed estrogen in women with intact uteri has been associated with an increased risk of endometrial cancer.
3. Note mental status.
4. Review risks associated with prolonged therapy (dementia, CHD, malignant neoplasms).
5. Monitor BP, Wt, thyroid function, lipids and LFTs.

CLIENT/FAMILY TEACHING

1. Before using pump for the first time, it must be primed. Remove the large pump cover, and fully depress pump twice. After priming, the pump is ready to use. Discard unused gel by thoroughly rinsing down the sink or placing it

in the household trash in a manner that prevents accidental exposure or ingestion by household members or pets.

2. *Estrogel:*
   - Estrogel pump contains enough drug to allow for initial priming of the pump twice and to deliver 64 daily doses. Discard the pump after priming twice and after 64 doses have been used.
   - Apply the gel at the same time each day. Apply daily dose of gel to clean, dry, unbroken skin. Apply after bath, shower, or sauna. Be sure skin is completely dry before applying the gel.
   - Leave as much time as possible between applying the gel and going swimming.
   - To obtain gel from the pump, collect gel into the palm of the hand by pressing the pump firmly and fully with 1 fluid motion without hesitation.
   - Apply the gel to one arm using the hand. Spread the gel as thinly as possible over the entire area on the inside and outside of the arm from wrist to shoulder to cover 750 cm^2 of skin.
   - Always place the cap back on the tip of the pump and the large pump cover over the top of the pump after each use.
   - To reduce the chance that the estradiol will spread to other people, wash hands with soap and water after applying the gel.
   - It is not necessary to massage or rub in the gel. Allow the gel to dry for up to 5 min before dressing.
3. *Divigel:*
   - Apply once daily on the skin of either the right or left upper thigh. The application surface area should be about 5 by 7 inches (about the size of 2 palm prints).
   - The entire contents of a unit dose packet should be applied each day.
   - To avoid potential skin irritation, apply to the right or left upper thigh on alternating days.
   - Do not apply to the face, breasts, or irritated skin, or in or around the vagina.
   - After application, allow the gel to dry before dressing.
   - Do not wash the application site within 1 hr after applying Divigel.
   - Avoid contact of the gel with eyes.
   - Wash hands after each application.
4. Alcohol-based gels are flammable. Avoid fire, flame, or smoking until the gel has dried.
5. When using the tube, apply the gel to one arm using the applicator. Be sure to transfer all of the gel from the applicator to the arm.
6. Report if any of the following occur: abnormal vaginal bleeding, breast lumps, dizziness or fainting, pain in groin or calves, severe abdominal pain or swelling, severe depression, sharp chest pain or sudden shortness of breath, sudden severe headache, vision or speech problems, weakness or numbness of arms or legs, yellowing of skin or eyes.
7. Keep all regular visits for F/U and lab evaluation. Review associated adverse effects of estrogen. Report any rash, adverse side effects, or lack of response.

OUTCOMES/EVALUATE
Relief of menopausal symptoms

Estradiol hemihydrate

(ess-trah-**DYE**-ohl)

Classification(s): Estrogen, semisynthetic

Pregnancy Category: X

RX: Vagifem.

SEE ALSO ***ESTROGENS.***

INDICATIONS/USES

Atrophic vaginitis—effective in relieving vaginal dryness, vaginal and vulvar irritation and itching, painful intercourse, and vaginal bleeding associated with intercourse.

SPECIAL CONCERNS

See *Estrogens* for Black Box Warnings.

SIDE EFFECTS

Most Common

Breakthrough bleeding/spotting, dizziness, lightheadedness, headache, GI upset, bloating, N&V, weight changes, increased/decreased libido, breast tenderness, edema.
See *Estrogens* for a complete list of possible side effects.

HOW SUPPLIED

Vaginal Tablets: 10 mcg, 25 mcg.

E

E

DOSAGE

VAGINAL TABLETS

Atrophic vaginitis.

Initial: 1 tablet, inserted vaginally, once daily for 2 weeks; **maintenance:** 1 tablet, inserted vaginally, twice a week.

NURSING IMPLICATIONS

IMPLEMENTATION/ADMINISTRATION/STORAGE

Attempt to discontinue or taper the drug at 3- to 6-month intervals.

ASSESSMENT

1. List reasons for therapy, age at menopause onset, characteristics of S&S.
2. Review associated hazards of therapy and alternative treatments available.
3. Note mental status, VS, and baseline labs.

CLIENT/FAMILY TEACHING

1. Gently insert the vaginal tablet into the vagina as far as it can comfortably go without force. Use the supplied applicator and insert tablet at the same time each day.
2. Report any pain, odor, increased discharge.
3. Keep all F/U to assess response and adverse SE.

OUTCOMES/EVALUATE

Relief of S&S of atrophic vaginitis

Estradiol topical emulsion

(ess-trah-**DYE**-ohl)

Classification(s): Estrogen, semisynthetic

Pregnancy Category: X

RX: Estrasorb.

SEE ALSO ***ESTROGENS***.

INDICATIONS/USES

Moderate to severe vasomotor symptoms associated with menopause.

SPECIAL CONCERNS

See *Estrogens* for Black Box Warnings.

SIDE EFFECTS

Most Common

Dizziness, lightheadedness, headache, N&V, GI upset, bloating, weight changes, increased/decreased libido, breast tenderness, edema, redness/irritation at application site.

See *Estrogens* for a complete list of possible side effects.

HOW SUPPLIED

Topical Emulsion: 2.5 mg estradiol hemihydrate/gram.

DOSAGE

TOPICAL EMULSION

Moderate to severe vasomotor symptoms.

The single approved dose is 3.48 grams/day (of the product). The lowest effective dose has not been determined. Use the lowest effective dose and for the shortest period of time determined by goals of treatment and risks involved. Periodically reevaluate (e.g., at 3 and 6 months) to determine need for continued treatment.

NURSING IMPLICATIONS

IMPLEMENTATION/ADMINISTRATION/STORAGE

1. When estrogen is prescribed for a women with a uterus, also initiate a progestin to reduce the risk of endometrial cancer. When indicated, rule out malignancy in cases of undiagnosed persistent or recurring abnormal vaginal bleeding.
2. Store at 15–30°C (59–86°F).

ASSESSMENT

1. List reasons for therapy, age at onset, other agents trialed, outcome. Review potential hazards of therapy.
2. Determine if client has undergone GYN exam, understands risks associated with and is a candidate for therapy.
3. Therapy may increase risk of thromboembolism especially with smoking.
4. Review potential risks R/T to prolonged therapy in postmenopausal women. Progestin helps minimize risk of endometrial hyperplasia.

5. Monitor VS, weight, blood sugar, liver and lipid panels.

CLIENT/FAMILY TEACHING

1. Drug is administered topically to relieve S&S of post-menopausal symptoms.
2. The following procedure for application of two-1.74 grams foil-laminated pouches should be followed:
   - Open each pouch individually, and apply in a comfortable sitting position to clean, dry skin on both legs each morning.
   - Cut or tear the first pouch at the notches indicated near the top of the pouch.
   - Apply the emulsion in the pouch to the top of the left thigh; push the entire contents from the bottom through the neck of the pouch.
   - Using one or both hands, rub the emulsion into the entire left thigh and left calf for 3 minutes until thoroughly absorbed. Rub any excess estradiol remaining on both hands on the buttocks.
   - Cut or tear the second pouch at the notches indicated near the top of the pouch. Apply the emulsion in the pouch to the top of the right thigh; push the entire contents from the bottom through the neck of the pouch.
   - Using one or both hands, rub the emulsion into the entire right thigh and right calf for 3 minutes until thoroughly absorbed. Rub any excess estradiol remaining on both hands on the buttocks.
   - To avoid transfer to other persons, allow the application to dry completely before covering with clothing.
   - When application is completed, wash both hands with soap and water to remove any residual estradiol.
3. Report any rash, irritation or skin discoloration at application sites. Do not smoke.
4. Any sudden pain in chest or calves, severe headaches, dizziness, swelling of hands or feet, speech or vision changes, SOB, changes in mental status or abnormal vaginal bleeding, yellow skin or other adverse side effects should be reported immediately.
5. Keep all F/U to assess response and adverse SE.

OUTCOMES/EVALUATE

Relief/control of post menopausal vasomotor symptoms

Estradiol transdermal system

Classification(s): Estrogen, semisynthetic

Pregnancy Category: X

RX: Alora, Climara, Estraderm, Estradiol Transdermal System, Menostar, Vivelle, Vivelle-Dot.

✱ **Rx:** Sandoz Estradiol derm.

SEE ALSO ***ESTROGENS***.

INDICATIONS/USES

(1) Vasomotor symptoms (moderate to severe) associated with menopause (except Menostar). (2) Hypoestrogenism due to hypogonadism, castration, or primary ovarian failure (except Menostar). (3) Vulvar and vaginal atrophy associated with menopause (except Menostar). When prescribing solely for vulvar and vaginal atrophy, consider topical vaginal products. (4) Prevention of postmenopausal osteoporosis. Consider this therapy only for women at significant risk of osteoporosis; carefully consider nonestrogen medications.

ACTION/KINETICS

Action

This transdermal system allows a constant low dose of estradiol to directly reach the systemic circulation. The system overcomes certain problems associated with PO use, including first-pass hepatic metabolism, GI upset, and induction of liver enzymes.

Pharmacokinetics

The system is available in various surface areas, release rates, and total estradiol content (the package insert should be carefully consulted). The patches are made either with a reservoir and a rate-controlling membrane or using a matrix where estradiol is embedded in the adhesive, allowing for a translucent, small, thin patch.

ADDITIONAL CONTRAINDICATIONS

Use with liver dysfunction or disease.

SPECIAL CONCERNS

(1) **Endometrial cancer.** Close clinical surveillance of all women taking estrogen is important. Adequate diagnostic measures, including endometrial sampling when indicated, should be undertaken to rule out malignancy in all cases of undiagnosed persistent or recurring abnormal vaginal bleeding. There is no evidence that the use of "natural" estrogens results in a different endometrial risk profile than synthetic estrogens at equivalent estrogenic doses. (2) **CV and other risks.** Estrogens with or without progestins should not be used for the prevention of CV disease or dementia. The Women's Health Initiative (WHI) estrogen alone substudy reported increased risk of stroke and deep vein thrombosis (DVT) in postmenopausal women (50 to 79 years of age) during 6.8 and 7.1 years, respectively of treatment with daily oral conjugated estrogens, 0.625 mg, relative to placebo. (3) The estrogen and progestin WHI substudy reported increased risks of MI, stroke, invasive breast cancer, pulmonary emboli, and DVT in postmenopausal women (50 to 79 years of age) during 5.6 years of treatment with daily oral conjugated estrogens, 0.625 mg, combined with medroxyprogesterone acetate, 2.5 mg relative to placebo.
(4) The WHI Memory Study, a substudy of the WHI, reorted an increased risk of developing probable dementia in postmenopausal women 65 years of age and older during 5.2 years of treatment with daily conjugated estrogen, 0.625 mg alone and during 4 years of treatment with daily conjugated estrogens, 0.625 mg combined with medroxyprogesterone acetate, 2.5 mg, relative to placebo. It is unknown whether this finding applies to younger postmenopausal women. (5) Other doses of conjugated estrogens and medroxyprogesterone acetate, and other combinations of estrogens and progestins, were not studied in the WHI and, in the absence of comparable data, these risks should be assumed to be similar. Because of these risks, estrogens with or without progestins should be prescibed at the lowest effective doses and for the shortest duration consistent with treatment goals and risks for the individual woman.

SIDE EFFECTS

Most Common

Breakthrough bleeding/spotting, dizziness, lightheadedness, headache, GI upset, bloating, N&V, weight changes, increased/decreased libido, breast tenderness, edema, redness/irritation at site of application.
See *Estrogens* for a complete list of possible side effects.

HOW SUPPLIED

Transdermal System: Release rate: 0.014 mg/24 hr, 0.025 mg/24 hr, 0.0375 mg/24 hr, 0.05 mg/24 hr, 0.06 mg/24 hr, 0.075 mg/24 hr, 0.1 mg/24 hr.

DOSAGE

TRANSDERMAL SYSTEM

Menopausal symptoms, including hypoestrogenism and vulvar/vaginal atrophy.

Initial: To treat vasomotor symptoms, use a system that delivers 0.025 mg estradiol/day. To treat moderate to severe vasomotor symptoms, vulvar and vaginal atrophy associated with menopause, hypoestrogenism caused by hypogonadism, castration, or primary ovarian failure, use a system that delivers 0.025–0.05 mg estradiol/day. Depending on the system selected, apply to the skin once or twice weekly. Do not make dosage adjustments until after the first month of therapy. Try to taper or discontinue at 3- to 6-month intervals but try to discontinue as soon as possible.

Prevention of postmenopausal osteoporosis.

Initial: 0.05 mg/day is the minimum established dosage; initiate as soon as possible after menopause. Adjust dosage to control concurrent menopausal symptoms. In women who are not taking oral estrogens or in women switching from another estradiol transdermal product, start treatment immediately. In women who are currently taking oral estrogens, start treatment 1 week after withdrawal of oral therapy or sooner if symptoms reappear in less than 1 week.

NURSING IMPLICATIONS

IMPLEMENTATION/ADMINISTRATION/STORAGE

1. Therapy may be given continuously to those who do not have an intact uterus. For clients with an intact uterus, give cyclically (3 weeks on, 1 week off). Vivelle may be given continuously or on a cyclic schedule with a progestin.
2. A progestin is given to postmenopausal women with an intact uterus to reduce the risk of endometrial cancer. A woman without a uterus does not require a progestin. Menostar may be used in women both with and without a uterus.
3. Alora, Estraderm, Esclim, Vivelle, and Vivelle-Dot are applied twice a week. Climara and Menostar are applied once a week.
4. Menostar should only be prescribed to postmenopausal women who are at significant risk of osteoporosis. Carefully consider nonestrogen approaches. It is recommended that women who have a uterus and are to be treated with Menostar receive a progestin for 14 days q 6 to 12 months, as well as undergo an endometrial biopsy at yearly intervals or as clinically indicated.
5. Store at 25°C (77°F). Do not store above 30°C (86°F). Do not store unpouched. Apply immediately upon removal from the protective pouch.

ASSESSMENT

1. Note reasons for therapy, age, other agents trialed, outcome. Review potential hazards of therapy. List drugs prescribed to ensure none interact.
2. Ensure client has undergone GYN exam, understands the risks associated with contraception and is a candidate for therapy.
3. Therapy may increase risk of thromboembolism especially with smoking, CVA, and ↑ BP readings. Monitor weight, TSH, blood sugar, and lipid panel.

CLIENT/FAMILY TEACHING

1. If taking oral estrogens, stop tablets and wait 1 week before applying transdermal system.
2. Without a hysterectomy, the system is usually used for 3 weeks, followed by 1 week of rest. May be used continuously in those without an intact uterus.
3. Place system on a clean, dry area of the skin on the trunk of the body (preferably the abdomen). Avoid using areas with excessive amounts of hair. Also may use on the hip or buttock. Do not apply to the breasts or the waistline.
4. Rotate application site; date patch. Allow 1 week intervals between reapplication to same site. Wear only 1 patch at a time.
5. Apply system immediately after the pouch is opened and the protective liner is removed. Firmly press in place with the palm for approximately 10 sec. Ensure good contact, especially around the edges. If system falls off, reapply the same system (except Climara or Menostar) or place a new one and follow the same schedule. If Climara or Menostar falls off, apply a new system for the remainder of the 7-day dosing interval. Continue the original treatment schedule.
6. If forget to apply a patch, apply a new one as soon as possible on the original treatment schedule. Interruption of treatment may increase the likelihood of breakthrough bleeding, spotting, and recurrence of symptoms.
7. Swimming, bathing, or using a sauna while the patch is in place may decrease adhesion of the patch and thus delivery of estradiol.
8. To avoid irritation, slowly and carefully remove the system. If any adhesive remains on the skin after removal of the system, allow the area to dry for 15 min. Then, gently rub the area with an oil-based cream or lotion to remove the adhesive residue.
9. Used patches still contain estradiol. Thus, carefully fold each patch in half so that it sticks to itself before discarding. Discard in household trash such that accidental application or ingestion by children, pets, or others is prevented.
10. Weight gain may occur; report if marked or if extremity swelling noted.
11. Stop smoking; smoking increases risk of blood clots.
12. To help prevent osteoporosis: 1,500 mg/day of calcium, vitamin D supplementation, exercise.
13. Addition of a progestin for 7 or more days may reduce the incidence of endometrial hyperplasia.
14. Report adverse side effects, sudden pain in chest or calves, headaches, speech or vision

changes, SOB, changes in mental status or abnormal vaginal bleeding.

15. Keep all F/U to assess response and for adverse SE.

OUTCOMES/EVALUATE

- Relief of menopausal symptoms
- Therapeutic estrogen levels

IV

Estrogens conjugated, oral (conjugated estrogenic substances)

(**ES**-troh-jens)

Classification(s): Estrogen, natural and synthetic

Pregnancy Category: X

RX: Premarin.

Rx: C.E.S..

Estrogens conjugated, parenteral

Pregnancy Category: X

RX: Premarin Intravenous.

Estrogens conjugated, synthetic (A & B)

Pregnancy Category: X

RX: Cenestin, Enjuvia.

Estrogens conjugated, vaginal

Pregnancy Category: X

RX: Premarin Vaginal Cream.

SEE ALSO ***ESTROGENS*** AND ***ESTERIFIED ESTROGENS***.

INDICATIONS/USES

Conjugated Estrogens, PO: (1) Moderate to severe vasomotor symptoms due to menopause. (2) Moderate to severe symptoms of vulvar and vaginal atrophy associated with menopause. (3) Prophylaxis of postmenopausal osteoporosis. (4) Hypoestrogenism due to hypogonadism, castration, or primary ovarian failure. (5) Palliation of breast cancer in selected women and men with metastatic disease. (6) Palliation only of advanced androgen-dependent prostatic carcinoma.

Conjugated Estrogens, Parenteral: Abnormal bleeding due to imbalance of hormones and in the absence of disease.

Conjugated Estrogens, Synthetic, A & B, PO: (1) Moderate to severe vasomotor symptoms associated with menopause. (2) Moderate to severe vulvar and vaginal atrophy associated with menopause (Synthetic Conjugated Estrogens A). (3) Moderate to severe vaginal dryness and pain with intercourse and symptoms of vulvar and vaginal atrophy associated with menopause (Synthetic Conjugated Estrogens B).

Conjugated Estrogens, Vaginal: Atrophic vaginitis and kraurosis vulvae associated with menopause.

ACTION/KINETICS

Action

Estrogens combine with receptors in the cytoplasm of cells, resulting in an increase in protein synthesis. During menopause, estrogens are used as replacement therapy. These products contain a blend of various estrogenic substances.

Pharmacokinetics

Metabolized in the liver and excreted mainly in the urine.

CONTRAINDICATIONS

Use for prevention of CV disease due to increased risk of MI, stroke, invasive breast cancer, and venous thromboembolism.

SPECIAL CONCERNS

See *Estrogens* for Black Box Warnings. Also, due to the increased risk of MI, stroke, invasive breast cancer, and venous thromboembolism, give for the shortest amount of time consistent with treatment goals.

Use of estrogen replacement therapy for prolonged periods may increase the risk of fatal ovarian cancer and endometrial cancer.

SIDE EFFECTS

Most Common

After PO Use: Abdominal/back pain, asthenia, breast pain, headache, infection, dyspepsia, nausea, arthralgia, pharyngitis, URTI.

See *Estrogens* for a complete list of possible side effects.

HOW SUPPLIED

Estrogens conjugated, oral. *Tablets:* 0.3 mg, 0.45 mg, 0.625 mg, 0.9 mg, 1.25 mg.
Estrogens conjugated, parenteral. *Injection:* 25 mg.
Estrogens conjugated, synthetic A (Cenestin). *Tablets:* 0.3 mg, 0.45 mg, 0.625 mg, 0.9 mg, 1.25 mg.
Estrogens conjugated, synthetic B (Enjuvia). *Tablets:* 0.3 mg, 0.45 mg, 0.625 mg, 0.9 mg, 1.25 mg.
Estrogens conjugated, vaginal. *Cream:* 0.625 mg/gram.

DOSAGE

Estrogens conjugated, oral (Premarin)

TABLETS

Moderate to severe vasomotor symptoms due to menopause, moderate to severe symptoms of vulvar and vaginal atrophy associated with menopause.

Start with the lowest dose. If the client has not menstruated in 2 or more months, begin therapy on any day; if, however, the client is menstruating, begin therapy on day 5 of bleeding.

Prophylaxis of osteoporosis.

0.625 mg/day continuously or cyclically (such as 25 days on, 5 days off). Mainstays of therapy include calcium; exercise and nutrition may be important adjuncts.

Primary ovarian failure, female castration.

1.25 mg/day given cyclically (3 weeks on, 1 week off). **Maintenance:** Adjust dose to lowest effective level.

Hypogonadism in females.

0.3–0.625 mg/day given cyclically (3 weeks on, 1 week off). Adjust dose depending on severity of symptoms and responsiveness of the endometrium. Dose may be gradually titrated upward at 6–12 month intervals as needed to achieve appropriate bone age advancement and eventual epiphyseal closure. Chronic dosing with 0.625 mg is sufficient to induce artificial cyclical menses with sequential progestin administration and to maintain bone density after skeletal maturity has been achieved.

Palliation of mammary carcinoma in men or postmenopausal women.

10 mg 3 times/day for at least 90 days.

Palliation of prostatic carcinoma (advanced androgen-dependent).

1.25–2.5 mg 3 times per day. Effectiveness can be measured by phosphatase determinations and symptomatic improvement.

Estrogens conjugated, parenteral (Premarin Intravenous)

IM; IV

Abnormal bleeding.

25 mg; repeat after 6–12 hr if necessary.

Estrogens conjugated, synthetic A (Cenestin)

TABLETS

Moderate-to-severe vasomotor symptoms due to menopause.

Initial: 0.45 mg daily; **then,** adjust dose based on individual client response. Discontinue as soon as possible. Attempt to discontinue or taper dosage at 3- to 6-month intervals.

Vulvar and vaginal atrophy.

0.3 mg/day.

Estrogens conjugated, synthetic B (Enjuvia)

TABLETS

Moderate-to-severe vasomotor symptoms due to menopause.

Initial: 0.3 mg daily. Adjust dosage based on individual client response. Periodically reassess dosage.

Vaginal dryness/vulvar and vaginal atrophy associated with menopause.

0.3 mg once daily. If to be used solely for treating moderate to severe vaginal dryness and pain during intercourse, consider using topical vaginal products.

Estrogens conjugated, vaginal (Premarin Vaginal Cream)

VAGINAL CREAM

Atrophic vaginitis and kraurosis vulvae associated with menopause.

0.5–2 grams daily for 3 weeks on and 1 week off. Repeat as needed. Attempt to taper the dose or discontinue the medication at 3- to 6-month intervals.

E

NURSING IMPLICATIONS

IMPLEMENTATION/ADMINISTRATION/STORAGE

1. For all uses, except palliation of mammary and prostatic carcinoma, oral conjugated estrogens are best administered cyclically—3 weeks on and 1 week off.
2. When used vaginally, insert the cream high into the vagina (two-thirds the length of the applicator).
3. When estrogen is used for a postmenopausal woman with a uterus, also initiate a progestin to reduce the risk of endometrial cancer. Those without a uterus do not require a progestin.
4. For women who have a uterus, undertake adequate diagnostic measures, such as endometrial sampling, when indicated to rule out malignancy in cases of undiagnosed persistent or recurring abnormal vaginal bleeding.
5. Limit the use of estrogen, alone or with a progestin, to the shortest duration consistent with treatment goals and risks. Evaluate periodically to determine if treatment is still required.
6. IV To reconstitute, first withdraw air from the vial to facilitate introduction of the diluent. Then, introduce the sterile diluent slowly against the side of the vial and agitate gently. Do not shake violently.
7. Administer IV Premarin slowly to prevent flushing.
8. Use reconstituted parenteral solutions within a few hours after mixing if kept at room temperature. Note date and time of reconstitution on the label. If refrigerated, the reconstituted solution is stable for 60 days. Do not use if solution is dark or has a precipitate.
9. IV use is preferred over IM as it induces a more rapid response.
10. Store the parenteral package from 2–8°C (36–46°F).
11. COMPATIBILITY NSS, invert sugar solutions, and dextrose solutions.
12. INCOMPATIBILITY Acid solutions, ascorbic acid solutions, and protein hydrolysates.

ASSESSMENT

1. Indicate reasons for therapy, age, characteristics of S&S, other agents trialed and any family history of blood clots.
2. Review potential risks R/T the development of breast and fatal ovarian cancers with prolonged therapy.
3. List drug prescribed to ensure no interaction or loss of potency (AEDs for seizure disorder, antimicrobials)
4. Obtain baseline breast, abdominal, and pelvic exams with Pap smear before starting therapy and obtain annually.
5. Ensure client understands the risks associated with contraception and is a candidate for therapy. Therapy may increase risk of thromboembolism especially with smoking, CVA, and ↑ BP readings.
6. Ensure females are advised that the use of unopposed estrogen with intact uteri has been associated with an increased risk of ovarian/endometrial cancer.
7. Monitor serum phosphatase levels with prostatic cancer. Monitor weight, TSH, K^+, renal and LFTs, blood sugar, and lipid panel.

CLIENT/FAMILY TEACHING

1. Take tablets cyclically as directed, i.e., 3 weeks on, 1 week off.
2. May take with food to decrease GI upset.
3. Include nonhormonal modalities to help prevent osteoporosis: 1,500 mg/day of calcium, vitamin D supplementation, exercise.
4. Perform breast self-examinations monthly. Spotting may occur first 3 months of therapy.
5. Cenestin is the only plant derived form of estrogen.
6. Review potential risks of prolonged therapy, i.e., ovarian/endometrial cancer, abnormal blood clotting, gallbladder disease, and breast cancer.
7. If no hysterectomy has been performed, a progestin should be added to help prevent cancer. Review hazards related to hormone replacement therapy.
8. Report to provider if pain in groin/calves, chest pain, difficulty breathing or unexplained SOB, abnormal vaginal bleeding, breast

lumps, sudden severe headache, dizziness/fainting, vision or speech problems, weakness or numbness of arms or legs, severe abdominal pain or swelling, yellowing of skin or eyes, severe depression experienced.

9. Stop smoking; smoking and obesity increases risk of blood clots and breakthrough bleeding.
10. Keep F/U visits to monitor therapy and for examinations, including Pap smear at least once a year.

OUTCOMES/EVALUATE

- Control of abnormal uterine bleeding
- Relief of menopausal symptoms
- Treatment of urogenital S&S R/T postmenopausal atrophy of vagina and lower urinary tract

Eszopiclone

(ess-**ZOP**-eye-klone)

Classification(s): Sedative-hypnotic, nonbenzodiazepine

Pregnancy Category: C

RX: Lunesta, **C-IV**

INDICATIONS/USES

Treatment of insomnia (decreases sleep latency and improves sleep maintenance). With newly diagnosed severe obstructive sleep apnea, will improve adherence to therapy if given for the first 14 nights of continuous positive airway pressure (CPAP).

ACTION/KINETICS

Action

Precise mechanism is unknown but may interfere with GABA-receptor complexes at binding domains located close to or allosterically coupled to benzodiazepine receptors.

Pharmacokinetics

Rapidly absorbed; **peak plasma levels:** 1 hr. Extensively metabolized by CYP3A4 and CYP2E1 enzymes; one of the metabolites has hypnotic activity. **t½:** About 6 hr (9 hr in elderly clients). Excreted in the urine (75%); less than 10% is excreted as the parent drug. **Plasma protein binding:** 52–59%.

CONTRAINDICATIONS

Use with alcohol.

SPECIAL CONCERNS

- Use with caution during lactation; in those with diseases that could affect metabolism or hemodynamic responses; in those with compromised respiratory function; and, in those with signs and symptoms of depression.
- Eszopiclone has no established use in labor and delivery.
- Safety and efficacy not demonstrated in children less than 18 years of age.

SIDE EFFECTS

Most Common

Unpleasant taste, headache, dizziness, diarrhea, dry mouth, dyspepsia, nervousness, somnolence.

Listed are side effects with an incidence of 0.1% or greater as well as life-threatening side effects. **CNS:** Headache, somnolence, nervousness, dizziness, depression, anxiety, confusion, hallucinations, abnormal dreams, neuralgia, decreased libido, agitation, apathy, ataxia, emotional lability, hostility, hypertonia, hypesthesia, incoordination, insomnia, impaired memory, neurosis, nystamus, paresthesia, decreased reflexes, difficulty concentrating, abnormal thinking, behavioral changes, vertigo. **GI:** N&V, dry mouth, diarrhea, unpleasant taste, dyspepsia, anorexia, cholelithiasis, increased appetite, melena, mouth ulceration, thirst, ulcerative stomatitis, halitosis. **CV:** Hypertension, migraine, thrombophlebitis. **GU:** Dysmenorrhea, gynecomastia (in men), UTI, amenorrhea, breast engorgement/enlargement/pain, breast neoplasm, cystitis, dysuria, female lactation, hematuria, kidney calculus/pain, mastitis, menorrhagia, metrorrhagia, urinary frequency/incontinence, ***uterine/vaginal hemorrhage***, vaginitis. **Dermatologic:** Rash, pruritus, acne, alopecia, contact dermatitis, dry skin, eczema, skin discoloration, sweating, urticaria. **Musculoskeletal:** Arthrits, bursitis, joint disorder (pain, stiffness, swelling) leg cramps, myasthenia, twitching. **Respiratory:** Asthma, bronchitis, dyspnea, epistaxis, hiccough, laryngitis. **Hematologic:** Anemia, lymphadenopathy. **Hypersensitivity:** ***Angioedema***, dyspnea, N&V, ***throat closing***. **Ophthalmic:** Conjunctivitis, dry eyes. **Otic:** Ear pain, otitis externa, otitis media, tinnitus, vestibular disorder. **Body as a whole:** Allergic reaction, cellulitis, fever, heat stroke, malaise, photosensitivity, accidental injury, pain. **Miscellaneous:** Infection, viral infection, migraine, hypertension, peripheral edema, hypercholesteremia, weight gain/loss, chest pain, facial edema, hernia, neck rigidity, drug dependence.

OVERDOSE MANAGEMENT

Symptoms: Exaggeration of the pharmacologic effects, including impairment of consciousness ranging from somnolence to coma. *Treatment:* General symptomatic and supportive care. Immediate gastric lavage, if appropriate. Give IV fluids as needed. Flumazenil may be useful. Monitor respiration, pulse, BP, hypotension, and CNS depression. The value of dialysis has not been determined.

E

DRUG INTERACTIONS

Clarithromycin / ↑ Eszoplicone levels, C_{max}, and t½ R/T ↓ metabolism by CYP3A4; do not exceed a starting dose of 1 mg when given with potent CYP3A4 inhibitors
CNS depressants, including anticonvulsants, antihistamines / Additive CNS depressant effects
Ethanol / Additive CNS depression; do not use together
Ketoconazole / ↑ Eszoplicone levels, C_{max}, and t½ R/T ↓ metabolism by CYP3A4; do not exceed a starting dose of 1 mg when given with potent CYP3A4 inhibitors
Nefazodone / ↑ Eszoplicone levels, C_{max}, and t½ R/T ↓ metabolism by CYP3A4; do not exceed a starting dose of 1 mg when given with potent CYP3A4 inhibitors
Olanzapine / ↓ Psychomotor function
Rifampin / ↓ Eszopiclone levels R/T ↑ metabolism by CYP3A4
Ritonovir / ↑ Eszoplicone levels, C_{max}, and t½ R/T ↓ metabolism by CYP3A4; do not exceed a starting dose of 1 mg when given with potent CYP3A4 inhibitors

HOW SUPPLIED

Tablets: 1 mg, 2 mg, 3 mg.

DOSAGE

TABLETS

Insomnia.

Individualize dosage. **Adults, initial:** 2 mg immediately before bedtime for most nonelderly clients. May be initiated at or raised to 3 mg if indicated, as 3 mg is more effective for sleep maintenance. **Elderly, initial:** 1 mg immediately before bedtime; dose may be increased to 2 mg if indicated. For the elderly who have difficulty staying asleep, give 2 mg immediately before bedtime. **Severe hepatic impairment, initial:** 1 mg; use with caution in this group.

NURSING IMPLICATIONS

IMPLEMENTATION/ADMINISTRATION/STORAGE

1. Absorption is slowed if taken with or immediately after a heavy, high-fat meal; this results in a reduced effect on sleep latency.
2. Do not exceed a starting dose of 1 mg in clients coadministered eszopiclone with potent CYP3A4 inhibitors (e.g., ketoconazole).
3. A rapid dose decrease or abrupt discontinuation may cause signs and symptoms of withdrawal.
4. Store from 15–30°C (59–86°F).

ASSESSMENT

1. List reasons for therapy: difficulty falling asleep, nocturnal awakening, and/or early morning awakening; other agents trialed, outcome. List drugs prescribed to ensure none interact.
2. Indentify triggers (i.e., napping during daytime, high caffeine intake, depression, or pain).
3. Assess for depression, memory problems, and any dependent behaviors.
4. Monitor renal and LFTs. Anticipate reduced dosage with the elderly and those with impaired liver function.

CLIENT/FAMILY TEACHING

1. Take as directed just before bedtime as drug acts quickly. Do not crush or break tablets, and ensure at least 8 hours before required to be up and active.
2. Take with a full glass of water on an empty stomach. May take with food if GI upset. Avoid high-fat meal as drug may not work
3. Use caution, do not perform activities that require mental alertness until drug effects realized. May experience unpleasant taste, dizziness, drowsiness, lightheadedness, and impaired coordination.
4. Avoid alcohol and OTC meds without provider approval.

5. **Report any unusual or disturbing thoughts or behavior or other adverse side effects or lack of response immediately.**
6. **May experience more sleeping problems after stopping drug for the first one or two nights. With prolonged therapy may experience mild withdrawal symptoms.**
7. **Caution elderly and debilitated that falls may occur with therapy; ensure safe, clear path or help to get up or to use bathroom.**
8. **Do not share medications. Store safely out of reach of children.**
9. **Do not use if nursing or pregnant.**
10. **Keep F/U visits to assess response and for adverse SE.**

OUTCOMES/EVALUATE
Relief of insomnia

Etanercept

(eh-**TAN**-er-sept)

Classification(s): Immunomodulator
Pregnancy Category: B
RX: Enbrel.

INDICATIONS/USES

(1) Reduce S&S, delays structural damage, and improves physical function in moderate to severe active rheumatoid arthritis in adults. May be used alone or in combination with methotrexate.
(2) Reduce signs and symptoms of active ankylosing spondylitis. (3) Reduce signs and symptoms of moderate to severe active polyarticular-course juvenile rheumatoid arthritis in children 2 years and older. (4) Reduce signs and symptoms, inhibiting the progression of structural damage of active arthritis, and improving physical function in those with psoriatic arthritis. Can be used in combination with methotrexate in those who do not respond adequately to methotrexate alone.
(5) Chronic, moderate to severe plaque psoriasis in adults 18 years of age and older who are candidates for systemic therapy or phototherapy.

ACTION/KINETICS

Action

Binds specifically to tumor necrosis factor (TNF) and blocks its interaction with cell surface TNF receptors. TNF is a cytokine that is involved in normal inflammatory and immune responses. Thus, the drug renders TNF biologically inactive. It is possible for etanercept to affect host defenses against infections and malignancies since TNF mediates inflammation and modulates cellular immune responses. It may also reverse CHF by decreasing inflammation in the heart.

Pharmacokinetics

t½: About 102 hr. Individual clients may undergo a two- to five-fold increase in serum levels with repeated dosing. The clearance of etanercept is reduced slightly in children aged 4–8 years.

CONTRAINDICATIONS

Hypersensitivity to etanercept or any component of the product. Sepsis. Use in any chronic or localized active infection. Concurrent administration of live vaccines. Use in clients with Wegener's granulomatosis receiving immunosuppressants or in clients receiving concurrent cyclophosphamide. Lactation.

SPECIAL CONCERNS

(1) **Risk of serious infections.** Clients treated with etanercept are at increased risk for developing serious infections that may lead to hospitalization or death. Most clients who developed these infections were taking concomitant immunosuppressants, such as methotrexate or corticosteroids. Discontinue etanercept if a client develops a serious infection or sepsis. (2) Reported infections include the following: (a) Active tuberculosis (TB), including reactivation of latent TB. Clients with TB have frequently presented with disseminated or extrapulmonary disease. Clients should be tested for latent TB before etanercept use and during therapy. Treatment for latent infection should be initiated prior to etanercept use.
(b) Invasive fungal infections, including histoplasmosis, coccidiodomycosis, candidiasis, aspergillosis, blastomycosis, and pneumocystosis. Clients with histoplasmosis or other invasive fungal infections may present with disseminated, rather than localized, disease. Antigen and antibody testing for histoplasmosis may be negative in some clients with active infection. Consider empiric antifungal therapy in clients at risk for invasive fungal infections who develop severe systemic illness. (c) Bacterial, viral, and other infections caused by

opportunistic pathogens. (3) Carefully consider the risks and benefits of treatment with etanercept prior to initiating therapy in clients with chronic or recurrent infections. (4) Closely monitor clients for the development of signs and symptoms of infection during and after treatment with etanercept, including the possible development of TB in clients who tested negative for latent TB infection before initiating therapy. ■

- **Use with caution in the elderly and in those with a history of recurring infections or with a condition that predisposes to infections (e.g., advanced or poorly controlled diabetes).**
- **Use with caution in those with pre-existing or recent-onset CNS-demyelinating disorders.**
- **Safety and efficacy not determined in those with immunosuppression, chronic infections, in children with plaque psoriasis, or in children less than 2 years of age.**

SIDE EFFECTS

Most Common

Adults: URTI, non-URTI, injection site reaction, infections, headache, nausea, dizziness, rash, abdominal pain, cough, pharyngitis, asthenia, peripheral edema.

Children: Headache, N&V, abdominal pain.

Injection site reactions: Erythema, itching, pain, swelling, injection site bleeding, bruising. **GI:** Abdominal pain, N&V, diarrhea, altered taste sense, mouth ulcer, dyspepsia, dry mouth, cholecystitis, pancreatitis, appendicitis, GI bleeding, autoimmune/noninfectious hepatitis, ***GI hemorrhage, intestinal perforation***. **CNS:** Headache, dizziness, depression, ***stroke, seizures***, paresthesias, normal pressure hydrocephalous, ***seizure, CVA***. Rarely, demyelinating disorders (multiple sclerosis, transverse myelitis, optic neuritis, new onset or exacerbation of seizure disorders). **CV:** ***Heart failure***, chest pain, flushing, ***MI***, myocardial ischemia, cerebral ischemia, DVT, thrombophlebitis, coagulopathy, cutaneous vasculitis, hypertension, hypotension, vasodilation, cutaneous vasculitis, CHF (either new or worsening of existing). **Hematologic:** ***Pancytopenia, including aplastic anemia***; adenopathy, anemia, leukopenia, neutropenia, thrombocytopenia, lymphadenopathy. **Respiratory:** URTI, non-URTI, sinusitis, rhinitis, pharyngitis, cough, pneumonitis, pneumonia, respiratory disorder, dyspnea, interstitial lung disease, worsening of prior lung disorder, pulmonary disease, sarcoidosis, ***pulmonary embolism***. **Ophthalmic:** Ocular inflammation, dry eyes, optic neuritis. **Dermatologic:** Urticaria, pruritus, rash, alopecia, cutaneous vasculitis, subcutaneous nodules, worsening psoriasis, erythema multiforme, ***Stevens-Johnson syndrome, toxic epidermal necrolysis***. **GU:** Membranous glomerulonephropathy, UTI, kidney calculus. **Musculoskeletal:** Bursitis, polymyositis, joint pain, urticaria, SC nodules, transverse myelitis, lupus-like syndrome (including rash consistent with subacute or discoid lupus). **Body as a whole:** Formation of autoimmune antibodies (resulting in a lupus-like syndrome or autoimmune hepatitis), immunogenicity, malignancies (including lymphoma and noncutaneous solid malignancies), asthenia, ***serious infections (including bacterial, viral, fungal, protozoan) and sepsis, hypersensitivity reactions (including angioedema and anaphylaxis)***, generalized pain, fatigue, angioedema, abscess with bacteremia, fever, flu-like symptoms, tuberculosis arthritis. In plaque psoriasis clients treated with etanercept, infections include cellulitis, gastroenteritis, pneumonia, abscess, and osteomyelitis. **Miscellaneous:** Peripheral edema, reactivation of hepatitis B virus, anorexia, weight gain, chest pain.

Side effects noted in juveniles. GI: N&V, gastroenteritis, abdominal pain, esophagitis, gastritis. **CNS:** Depression, headache, personality disorder, ***seizures***. **CV:** Cutaneous vasculitis. **Hematologic:** Coagulopathy, pancytopenia. **GU:** UTI. **Ophthalmic:** Optic neuritis. **Body as a whole:** Group A streptococcal septic shock, type 1 diabetes mellitus, soft-tissue and postoperative wound infection, infections, abscess with bacteremia. **Miscellaneous:** Varicella, cutaneous ulcer, tuberculosis arthritis, ↑ transaminases.

DRUG INTERACTIONS

Anakinra / ↑ Incidence of serious infections compared with use of etanercept alone

Cyclophosphamide / ↑ Incidence of noncutaneous solid malignancies in clients with Wegener's granulomatosis when etanercept added to cyclophosphamide/methotrexate/corticosteroid therapy

Immunosuppressants / Do not use etanercept in those with Wegener's granulomatosis receiving immunosuppressive drugs

Sulfasalazine / Mild ↓ in mean neutrophil counts; clinical significance not known

HOW SUPPLIED

Injection, Lyophilized Powder for Solution: 25 mg; *Injection, Solution:* 25 mg/0.5 mL, 50 mg/mL.

DOSAGE

SC

Moderate to severe active rheumatoid arthritis; psoriatic arthritis; ankylosing spondylitis.

Adults: 50 mg per week given as one SC injection using a 50 mg/mL single-use prefilled syringe, or as two 25 mg injections given either on the same day or 3 or 4 days apart. Doses greater than 50 mg per week are not recommended. Methotrexate, glucocorticoids, salicylates, NSAIDs, or analgesics may be used during treatment.

Children with active polyarticular-course juvenile rheumatoid arthritis.

Children, 2–17 years: 0.8 mg/kg/week (up to a maximum of 50 mg/week). Maximum dose at a single injection site: 25 mg. For children weighing from 31–62 kg, give the total weekly dose as 2 SC injections, either on the same day or 3 or 4 days apart using the multiple-use vial. Give the dose for children weighing less than 31 kg as a single SC injection once weekly using the correct volume from the multiple-use vial. The 25 mg prefilled syringe is not recommended for children weighing less than 31 kg (68 lbs). Glucocorticoids, NSAIDs, or analgesics may be continued during treatment. Concurrent use of methotrexate and higher doses of etanercept have not been studied in children.

Plaque psoriasis in adults.

Adults, initial: 50 mg given twice weekly (3 or 4 days apart) for 3 months; **then,** reduce dose to 50 mg/week. Starting doses of 25 mg or 50 mg per week were also shown to be effective.

NURSING IMPLICATIONS

IMPLEMENTATION/ADMINISTRATION/STORAGE

1. Clients must enroll with the makers of etanercept so that pharmacies can obtain the product.
2. Reconstitute multiple-use vial aseptically with 1 mL of the supplied sterile bacteriostatic water for injection (benzyl alcohol 0.9%) to yield a solution containing 25 mg/mL. The reconstituted solution should be clear and colorless. Withdraw only the dose to be given from the vial into the syringe. Some foam or bubbles may remain in the vial. Do not filter the reconstituted solution during preparation or administration.
3. A vial adapter is provided for use when reconstituting the lyophilized powder. Do not use the vial adapter if multiple doses are going to be withdrawn from the vial. If the vial will be used for multiple doses, use a 25-gauge needle for reconstituting and withdrawing etanercept; apply the supplied "Mixing Date" sticker to the vial and enter the date of reconstitution. Reconstitution with bacteriostatic water for injection, using a 25-gauge needle, yields a preserved multiple-use solution that must be used within 14 days.
4. If using the vial adapter, twist the vial adapter onto the diluent syringe. Place the vial adapter over the etanercept vial, and insert the vial adapter into the vial stopper. Push down on the plunger to inject the diluent into the etanercept vial. Some foaming will occur (which is normal). Swirl the contents gently during dissolution. To avoid excessive foaming, do not shake or agitate vigorously.
5. If using a 25-gauge needle to reconstitute and withdraw etanercept, inject the diluent very slowly into the etanercept vial. Some foaming will occur (which is normal). Swirl the contents gently during dissolution. To avoid excessive foaming, do not shake or agitate vigorously. Generally dissolution takes less than 10 min.
6. Using the multidose vial, withdraw the correct dose of reconstituted solution into the syringe. Remove the syringe from the vial adapter or remove the 25-gauge needle from the syringe. Attach a 27-gauge needle to inject etanercept.
7. Do not mix the contents of 1 vial of etanercept solution with, or transfer into, the contents of another vial of etanercept.
8. Allow the single-use prefilled syringe or the single-use prefilled SureClick autoinjector to come to room temperature (about 15–30

min) before using. Do not remove the needle shield while allowing the prefilled syringe to reach room temperature. Check to determine if the amount of liquid in the prefilled syringe falls between the 2 purple fill level indicator lines on the syringe; do not use that syringe if it does not have the right amount of liquid.

9. Prior to administration, visually inspect the solution for particulate matter and discoloration. Small white particles of protein may be present in the solution; this is not unusual. Do not use the solution if it is discolored or cloudy, or if foreign particulate matter is present.
10. Sites for SC injection include the thigh, abdomen, or upper arm and should be rotated. Never inject into areas where the skin is tender, bruised, red, or hard.
11. Methotrexate, glucocorticoids, salicylates, NSAIDs, or analgesics may be continued during therapy for rheumatoid arthritis.
12. Glucocorticoids, NSAIDs, or analgesics may be continued during treatment for polyarticular juvenile rheumatoid arthritis.
13. Some clients treated, without interruption, for 3 years may be able to reduce the dose or stop concomitant therapy with methotrexate or corticosteroids.
14. The needle cover of the diluent syringe contains latex; do not handle if sensitive to latex.
15. The diluent for multiple-use vials containing lyophilized powder contains benzyl alcohol, which has been associated with a fatal "gasping syndrome" in premature infants.
16. Do not add other medications to solutions containing etanercept, and do not reconstitute with other diluents.
17. Give a 50 mg dose as 1 SC injection using a 50 mg/mL single-use prefilled syringe or a 50 mg single-use prefilled SureClick autoinjector. Also, a 50 mg dose can be given as two 25 mg SC injections using 25 mg single-use prefilled syringes or multiple-use vials. Give the two 25 mg injections either on the same day or 3–4 days apart.
18. The 25 mg prefilled syringe is not recommended for children weighing less than 31 kg (68 lbs). The 50 mg prefilled syringe or SureClick autoinjector may be used for children weighing 63 kg (138 lbs) or more.
19. Store the sterile powder at 2–8°C (36–46°F). Refrigerate etanercept sterile powder (do not freeze). Solutions reconstituted with the diluent provided may be stored for up to 14 days if refrigerated. Do not freeze.
20. Keep single-use prefilled syringes refrigerated at 2–8°C (36–46°F). Do not freeze. Keep prefilled syringes in the original carton to protect from light until the time of use. Do not shake.

ASSESSMENT

1. Note reasons for therapy, joints affected, presenting characteristics, other agents/therapies trialed/failed. Assess baseline ROM, functionality and clinical presentation; monitor.
2. Observe as client performs first injection after instruction.
3. Perform HBV and TB testing prior to starting therapy. Monitor closely if a new infection occurs during treatment; stop if serious infection develops.
4. Certain joints may require individual steroid injections during flares to control pain and enhance mobility.
5. Ensure juvenile clients brought up to date with all immunizations prior to starting etanercept therapy.
6. Review risks associated with this class of drugs as lymphoma and other malignancies, some fatal, have been reported in children and adolescent patients treated with TNF blockers.
7. A pregnancy register is available to monitor outcomes of pregnant women exposed to etanercept. Providers should register clients by calling 1-877-311-8972.
8. Monitor CBC and for S&S of blood dyscrasias.

CLIENT/FAMILY TEACHING

1. Drug consists of a protein injected under the skin. Each tray contains all materials needed for administration. Follow written guidelines for mixing and administering explicitly. May request prefilled syringes and autoinjector to facilitate administration.
2. Review procedures for storage, reconstitution, inspection, withdrawal, administration, site rotation, and disposal of syringes.
3. Always rotate sites for self-injection including the thigh, abdomen, or upper arm. Give new injections at least 1 inch from the old site and never into areas where the skin is tender, bruised, red, or hard.

4. It is recommended that children with juvenile idiopathic arthritis be brought up to date (if possible) with all immunizations prior to initiating etanercept therapy.
5. Terminate temporarily etanercept in clients with significant exposure to varicella virus and consider prophylactic treatment with varicella-zoster immune globulin.
6. Report any abdominal pain, S&S of infection, dizziness, SOB, chest pain, rash, or worsening S&S of heart failure (e.g., shortness of breath, swelling of ankles/feet).
7. If latex-sensitive, beware as needle cover on the prefilled syringe contains dry natural rubber (latex).
8. When traveling must keep refrigerated or carry in cooler.
9. Avoid immunizations with live vaccines.
10. Practice reliable contraception. Do not use if breast-feeding.
11. The manufacturer maintains an active website www.enbrel.com with patient support services and information. Additionally may call 1-888-4ENBREL (1-888-436-2735) with questions and nurse support.
12. Keep all F/U to assess response, labs, and adverse SE.

OUTCOMES/EVALUATE

- ↓ Joint pain/swelling
- Improved ROM
- Delayed structural damage with RA
- ↓ S&S of psoriatic arthritis/ankylosing spondylitis

IV

Ethacrynate sodium

(eth-ah-**KRIH**-nayt)

Classification(s): Diuretic, loop

Pregnancy Category: B

RX: Edecrin Sodium.

Ethacrynic acid

(eth-ah-**KRIH**-nik)

Pregnancy Category: B

RX: Edecrin.

SEE ALSO ***DIURETICS, LOOP***.

INDICATIONS/USES

PO. Edema when a drug with greater diuretic potential than those usually used is needed. (1) Edema associated with CHF, cirrhosis of the liver, and renal disease, including nephrotic syndrome. (2) Short-term management of ascites caused by malignancy, idiopathic edema, and lymphedema. (3) Short-term management of hospitalized children, other than infants, with congenital heart disease or the nephrotic syndrome. **IV.** Treatment of edema when a rapid onset of diuresis is desired (e.g., acute pulmonary edema) or when GI absorption is impaired or PO medication is not practical.

ACTION/KINETICS

Action

Inhibits the reabsorption of sodium and chloride in the loop of Henle; it also decreases reabsorption of sodium and chloride and increases potassium excretion in the distal tubule. Also acts directly on the proximal tubule to enhance excretion of electrolytes. Large quantities of sodium and chloride and smaller amounts of potassium and bicarbonate ion are excreted during diuresis.

Pharmacokinetics

Onset, PO: 30 min; **IV:** Within 5 min. **Peak, PO:** 2 hr; **IV:** 15–30 min. **Duration, PO:** 6–8 hr. **IV:** 2 hr. **t½, after PO:** 60 min. Metabolites are excreted through the urine. Diuresis and electrolyte loss are more pronounced with ethacrynic acid than with thiazide diuretics. Is often effective in clients refractory to other diuretics. Careful monitoring of the diuretic effects is necessary.

CONTRAINDICATIONS

Pregnancy (usually), lactation, use in neonates. Anuria and severe renal damage. SC or IM use due to local pain and irritation. IV use in infants.

SPECIAL CONCERNS

> Potent diuretic; excess amounts can lead to a profound diuresis with water and electrolyte depletion. Careful medical supervision is required; individualize dosage.

- Elderly may be more sensitive to the usual adult dose.
- Use with caution in diabetics and in those with hepatic cirrhosis (who are particularly susceptible to electrolyte imbalance).
- Monitor gout clients carefully.

- **Safety and efficacy of oral use in infants and IV use in children not established.**

SIDE EFFECTS

Most Common

Dizziness, lightheadedness, blurred vision, anorexia, itching, GI upset, headache, weakness, muscle cramps, N&V, hearing difficulty, pain.

Electrolyte imbalance: Hypokalemia, hyponatremia, hypochloremic alkalosis, hypomagnesemia, hypocalcemia. **GI:** Anorexia, N&V, diarrhea (may be sudden, watery, profuse diarrhea), acute pancreatitis, abdominal discomfort/pain, jaundice, ***GI bleeding or hemorrhage***, dysphagia. **Hematologic:** Severe neutropenia, thrombocytopenia, ***agranulocytosis***, rarely Henöch-Schönlein purpura in clients with rheumatic heart disease. **CNS:** Apprehension, confusion, dizziness, lightheadedness, vertigo, headache. **Body as a whole:** Fever, chills, fatigue, malaise, weakness, muscle cramps. **Otic:** Sense of fullness in the ears, tinnitus, irreversible hearing loss. **Miscellaneous:** Hematuria, acute gout, abnormal LFTs in seriously ill clients on multiple drug therapy including ethacrynic acid, blurred vision, rash, local irritation and pain following parenteral use, hyperuricemia/glycemia.

Ethacrynic acid may cause death in critically ill clients refractory to other diuretics. These include (a) clients with severe myocardial disease who also received digitalis and who developed acute hypokalemia with fatal arrhythmias and (b) those with severely decompensated hepatic cirrhosis with ascites, with or without encephalopathy, who had electrolyte imbalances. ***Death is due to intensification of the electrolyte effect.***

OVERDOSE MANAGEMENT

Symptoms: Profound water loss, electrolyte depletion (causes dizziness, weakness, mental confusion, vomiting, anorexia, lethargy, cramps), dehydration, reduction of blood volume, ***circulatory collapse (possibility of vascular thrombosis and embolism).*** *Treatment:* Replace electrolytes and fluid and monitor urine output and serum electrolyte levels. Induce emesis or perform gastric lavage. Artificial respiration and oxygen may be needed. Treat other symptoms.

ADDITIONAL DRUG INTERACTIONS

Carbonic anhydrase inhibitors / Ethacrynic acid may potentiate the effect of carbonic anhydrase inhibitors

Diuretics, other / Additive effect when used with ethacrynic acid

HOW SUPPLIED

Ethacrynate Sodium: ***Powder for Injection:*** 50 mg/vial.
Ethacrynic Acid: ***Tablets:*** 25 mg.

DOSAGE

Ethacrynate Sodium

IV

Diuresis.

Adults: 50 mg (base) (or 0.5–1 mg/kg); may be repeated in 2–4 hr, although only one dose is usually needed. A single 100 mg (maximum) dose IV has been used in critical situations. **Children:** 0.5–1 mg/kg (investigational); may be repeated q 8–12 hr as needed.

Ethacrynic Acid

TABLETS

Diuresis.

Adults, initial: 50–100 mg/day in single or divided doses. Use the smallest dose to produce a gradual weight loss of 1–2 lb/day. **Day 1:** 50 mg once after a meal; **day 2:** 50 mg twice a day after meals (if needed); **day 3:** 100 mg in the morning and 50–100 mg following the afternoon or evening meal, depending on the response to the morning dose. Usually adjust doses in 25–50 mg increments. **Maintenance:** Usually 50–200 mg (up to a maximum of 400 mg) daily may be required in severe, refractory edema. If used with other diuretics, the initial dose should be 25 with increments of 25 mg. **Children, 13 months and older, initial:** 25 mg/day; can increase by 25 mg/day if needed. **Maintenance:** Adjust dose to needs of client. Use contraindicated in infants.

NURSING IMPLICATIONS

IMPLEMENTATION/ADMINISTRATION/STORAGE

1. **Due to local pain and irritation, do not give SC or IM.**

2. Ammonium chloride or arginine chloride may be prescribed for those at a higher risk of developing metabolic acidosis.
3. Salt liberalization usually prevents development of hyponatremia and hypochloremia.
4. Discontinue if increasing electrolyte imbalance, azotemia, and/or oliguria occur during treatment of severe, progressive renal disease.
5. Potassium chloride or potassium-sparing agents (or both) should be given during treatment with ethacrynic acid, especially in clients with cirrhosis or nephrosis and in those taking digitalis.
6. Store tablets and injection from 15–30°C (59–86°F).
7. **IV** Reconstitute by adding 50 mL of D5W or NaCl injection to powder.
8. Administer intermittent IV slowly over a 30 min period, given either directly or through IV tubing. For direct IV, may give at a rate of 10 mg/min.
9. When reconstituted with D5W injection, do not use if the resulting solution is hazy or opalescent. Do not mix solution with whole blood or its derivatives.
10. If a second IV injection is necessary, use a different site to prevent thrombophlebitis.
11. Use reconstituted solutions within 24 hr; discard any unused solution.
12. COMPATIBILITY D5W or normal saline.
13. INCOMPATIBILITY Do not administer drug with other drugs or with blood products.

ASSESSMENT

1. Note reasons for therapy, other agents trialed, outcome.
2. Assess for diabetes or cirrhosis; ensure not anuric.
3. Drug acts on the ascending loop of Henle and on the proximal and distal tubules. Urinary output usually dose dependent and R/T fluid accumulation. Water and electrolyte excretion may be several times that with thiazide diuretics, since drug inhibits reabsorption. Monitor VS, I&O, and weight. Note excessive diuresis or weight loss; electrolyte imbalance may occur quickly.
4. With rapid excessive diuresis, assess for pain in calves, pelvic area, or the chest; rapid hemoconcentration may cause thromboembolic effects.
5. Drug should be withdrawn if severe, watery diarrhea presents. Test for occult blood in urine and stools.
6. Observe for vestibular disturbances. Do not administer concomitantly with any other ototoxic agent. Hearing loss is most common following high or rapid IV dosing.
7. Monitor serum K^+ levels; assess need for supplemental potassium.
8. Since drug has such a profound effect on sodium excretion, dietary salt restriction is not necessary; if sodium is restricted, hyponatremia may result.
9. Monitor BP, I&O, electrolytes, CO_2, CBC, BS, renal and LFTs; avoid with severe liver/renal failure. With prolonged therapy, obtain hearing test.

CLIENT/FAMILY TEACHING

1. Take tablets after meals and early in the day to ensure sleep is not interrupted due to voiding.
2. Change positions slowly to prevent any sudden drop in BP and associated dizziness. Avoid activities that require mental alertness until drug effects realized.
3. Monitor weight, I&O, and BP; report any excessive weight gain, SOB, swelling of hands or feet, adverse effects, or lack of response.
4. Avoid prolonged exposure to sunlight or UV light; wear protective clothing/sunscreen to prevent photosensitivity reaction.
5. Keep all F/U to assess response, labs, and adverse SE.

OUTCOMES/EVALUATE

- Enhanced diuresis
- ↓ Edema (↑ weight loss)
- ↓ Abdominal girth R/T ascites

Ethosuximide

(eth-oh-**SUCKS**-ih-myd)

Classification(s): Anticonvulsant, succinimide

Pregnancy Category: C

RX: Zarontin.

SEE ALSO ***ANTICONVULSANTS***.

INDICATIONS/USES

Absence (petit mal) seizures. May be given concomitantly with other anticonvulsants if other types of epilepsy are manifested with absence seizures.

ACTION/KINETICS

Action

Suppresses the paroxysmal 3-cycle/sec spike and wave activity that is associated with lapses of consciousness seen in absence seizures. Acts by depressing the motor cortex and by raising the threshold of the CNS to convulsive stimuli.

Pharmacokinetics

Rapidly absorbed from the GI tract. **Peak serum levels:** 3–7 hr. **t½, adults:** 60 hr; **t½, children:** 30 hr. Steady serum levels reached in 7–10 days. **Therapeutic serum levels:** 40–100 mcg/mL. Extensively metabolized in the liver. Both inactive metabolites and unchanged drug (25%) are excreted in the urine. Not bound to plasma protein.

CONTRAINDICATIONS

Hypersensitivity to succinimides.

SPECIAL CONCERNS

- **Use with extreme caution in clients with abnormal liver and kidney function.**
- **When used alone in mixed types of epilepsy, may increase the frequency of tonic-clonic seizures.**
- **Safe use during pregnancy not established.**

SIDE EFFECTS

Most Common

Drowsiness, dizziness, blurred vision, GI upset, anorexia, headache, hiccoughs.

CNS: Drowsiness, ataxia, dizziness, headaches, euphoria, lethargy, fatigue, insomnia, irritability, nervousness, dream-like state, hyperactivity. Psychiatric or psychologic aberrations such as mental slowing, hypochondriasis, sleep disturbances, inability to concentrate, depression, night terrors, instability, confusion, aggressiveness. Rarely, auditory hallucinations, paranoid psychosis, increased libido, ***suicidal behavior***. **GI:** N&V, hiccoughs, anorexia, diarrhea, GI upset, weight loss, abdominal/epigastric pain, cramps, constipation. **Hematologic:** Leukopenia, granulocytopenia, eosinophilia, ***agranulocytosis***, pancytopenia with or without bone marrow suppression, monocytosis. **Dermatologic:** Pruritus, urticaria, erythema multiforme, systemic lupus erythematosus, ***Stevens-Johnson syndrome***, pruritic erythematous rashes, skin eruptions, alopecia, hirsutism. **GU:** Urinary frequency, vaginal bleeding, renal damage, microscopic hematuria. **Ophthalmic:** Blurred vision, myopia, photophobia, periorbital edema. **Miscellaneous:** Muscle weakness, hyperemia, hypertrophy of gums, swollen tongue.

OVERDOSE MANAGEMENT

Symptoms: **Acute Overdose:** Confusion, sleepiness, slow shallow respiration, N&V, ***CNS depression with coma and respiratory depression***, hypotension, cyanosis, hyper-/hypothermia, absence of reflexes, unsteadiness, flaccid muscles. **Chronic Overdose:** Ataxia, dizziness, drowsiness, confusion, depression, proteinuria, skin rashes, hangover, irritability, poor judgment, N&V, muscle weakness, periorbital edema, hepatic dysfunction, ***fatal bone marrow aplasia, delayed onset of coma***, nephrosis, hematuria, casts. *Treatment:* General supportive measures. Charcoal hemoperfusion or hemodialysis may be helpful. Forced diuresis and exchange transfusions are ineffective.

DRUG INTERACTIONS

Estrogens, Progestins / ↓ Plasma hormone levels → ↓ effect
Hydantoins / ↑ Hydantoin effect R/T ↓ breakdown by the liver
Isoniazid / ↑ Ethosuximide effects
Phenobarbital/Primidone / Lower levels of phenobarbital and primidone
Valproic acid / Both ↑ and ↓ ethosuximide levels observed

HOW SUPPLIED

Capsules: 250 mg; ***Syrup:*** 250 mg/5 mL.

DOSAGE

CAPSULES; SYRUP

Absence seizures.

Adults and children over 6 years, initial: 250 mg twice a day; the dose may be increased by 250 mg/day at 4–7-day intervals until seizures are controlled or until total daily dose reaches 1.5 grams. Administer doses over 1.5 grams only under the strict supervision of the health care provider. **Children 3–6 years, initial:** 250 mg/day; dosage may be increased by small increments every 4–7 days until control is established or total daily dose reaches 1 gram. The optimal dose for most children is 20 mg/kg/day, which provides plasma levels in the therapeutic range of 40–100 mcg/mL.

NURSING IMPLICATIONS

IMPLEMENTATION/ADMINISTRATION/STORAGE

1. May be given with other anticonvulsants when other forms of epilepsy are present.
2. Store capsules from 15–30°C (59–86°F). Store syrup below 30°C (86°F) protected from freezing and light.

ASSESSMENT

1. Note reasons for therapy, onset, characteristics of seizures, other agents trialed, outcome. List any predisposing factors (e.g., SAH, head trauma, etc.).
2. Assess clinical presentation, mental/emotional status; ensure not pregnant.
3. Any S&S of infection (e.g., sore throat, fever) warrant blood counts. There have been several cases of lupus associated with drug therapy.
4. Monitor ECG, CBC, uric acid, renal and LFTs.

CLIENT/FAMILY TEACHING

1. Take with meals to minimize GI upset. Do not stop abruptly; may increase severity and frequency of seizures. Report any increase in frequency of seizures or unusual side effects.
2. Avoid hazardous activities while on drug therapy. May experience dizziness, drowsiness, confusion, headaches, and blurred vision.
3. Any persistent fever, swollen glands, and bleeding gums may signal a blood dyscrasia and require reporting. Report significant weight loss, rash, joint pain, fever.
4. Avoid alcohol and CNS depressants during therapy.
5. May change urine color to pink, red, or red-brown; not worrisome.
6. Any transient personality changes, hypochondriacal behavior, and aggressiveness, should be reported.
7. Keep all F/U to assess response, labs, and adverse SE.

OUTCOMES/EVALUATE

- ↓ Frequency; ↑ control of seizures
- Therapeutic serum drug levels (40–100 mcg/mL)

Etidronate disodium

(eh-tih-**DROH**-nayt)

Classification(s): Bone growth regulator, bisphosphonate

Pregnancy Category: B

RX: Didronel.

INDICATIONS/USES

PO: (1) Paget's disease (osteitis deformans), especially of the polyostotic type accompanied by pain and increased urine levels of hydroxyproline and serum alkaline phosphatase. In many, the disease process will be suppressed for at last 1 year following cessation of therapy. (2) Prevention and treatment of heterotopic ossification due to spinal cord injury or total hip replacement. Among those who form heterotopic bone, etidronate retards the progression of immature lesions and reduces the severity by at least 50%. *Investigational:* Prevention and treatment of corticosteroid-induced osteoporosis.

ACTION/KINETICS

Action

Slows bone metabolism, thereby decreasing bone resorption, bone turnover, and new bone formation; it also reduces bone vascularization. Renal tubular reabsorption of calcium is not affected.

Pharmacokinetics

Absorption: Dose-dependent; after 24 hr, one-half of absorbed drug is excreted unchanged. Absorption is affected by food or preparations containing divalent ions. **Onset:** 1 month for Paget's disease and within 24 hr for hypercalcemia. The drug remaining in the body is adsorbed to bone, where therapeutic effects for Paget's disease persist 3–12 months after discontinuation of the drug. **Plasma t½:** 6 hr; **bone t½:** Over 90 days. Approximately 50% excreted unchanged in the urine; unabsorbed drug is excreted through the feces.

CONTRAINDICATIONS

Enterocolitis, fracture of long bones, hypercalcemia of hyperparathyroidism. Serum creatinine greater than 5 mg/dL.

SPECIAL CONCERNS

- Use with caution in renal dysfunction, in active UGI problems, and during lactation.

- Safety and efficacy not established in children.

SIDE EFFECTS

Most Common

Diarrhea, nausea, increased or recurrent bone pain at pagetic sites, onset of pain at previously asymptomatic sites.

GI: Nausea, diarrhea, constipation, ulcerative stomatitis, altered taste, loss of taste. **Bones:** Increased incidence of bone fractures and increased or recurrent bone pain. Drug should be discontinued if fracture occurs and not restarted until healing takes place. Onset of pain at previously asymptomatic sites. Osteonecrosis, primarily in the jaw, especially with cancers of the oral cavity. **Allergy:** Angioedema, rash, pruritus, urticaria. **Electrolytes:** Hypophosphatemia, hypomagnesemia. **Miscellaneous:** Metallic taste, chest pain, abnormal hepatic function, fever, fluid overload, dyspnea, convulsions. Symptoms of rachitic syndrome have been reported in children receiving 10 mg or more/kg daily for long periods (up to 1 year) to treat heterotopic ossification or soft-tissue calcification.

LABORATORY TEST CONSIDERATIONS

Hypomagnesemia, hypophosphatemia.

OVERDOSE MANAGEMENT

Symptoms: Following PO ingestion, hypocalcemia may occur. Rapid IV administration may cause renal insufficiency. *Treatment:* Gastric lavage following PO ingestion. Treat hypocalcemia by giving calcium IV.

DRUG INTERACTIONS

Products containing calcium or other multivalent cations ↓ absorption of etidronate

HOW SUPPLIED

Tablets: 200 mg, 400 mg.

DOSAGE

TABLETS

Paget's disease.

Adults, initial: 5–10 mg/kg/day for 6 months or less; or, 11–20 mg/kg for a maximum of 3 months. Reserve doses above 10 mg/kg when lower doses are ineffective, when there is a need for suppression of increased bone turnover, or when a prompt decrease in cardiac output is needed. Do not exceed doses of 20 mg/kg/day. Another course of therapy may be instituted after a rest period of 3 months if there is evidence of active disease process. For most clients, the original dose will be adequate for retreatment. If not, consider increasing the dose within recommended guidelines. Monitor every 3 to 6 months.

Heterotopic ossification due to spinal cord injury.

Adults, usual: 20 mg/kg/day for 2 weeks; **then** 10 mg/kg/day for 10 weeks. Total treatment period is 12 weeks. Treatment should be initiated as soon as possible after the injury, preferably before evidence of heterotopic ossification.

Heterotopic ossification due to total hip replacement.

Adults, initial: 20 mg/kg/day for 1 month preoperatively and 3 months postoperatively for a total treatment duration of 4 months. Retreatment has not been studied.

NURSING IMPLICATIONS

IMPLEMENTATION/ADMINISTRATION/STORAGE

1. Administer PO as a single dose (if GI upset occurs, divide dose) with juice or water 2 hr before meals.
2. There are no indications to date that etidronate will affect mature heterotopic bone.
3. Reduce the dose when decreases in glomerular filtration rate is present.
4. Avoid excessive heat (over 40°C or 104°F) for tablets.

ASSESSMENT

1. Note reasons for therapy, other agents trialed, clinical presentation; rate pain level. List dates of previous treatment with etidronate.
2. Review x-rays/bone density for evidence of bone loss/fracture or pagetic lesions.
3. Determine if pregnant.
4. Assess for evidence of renal dysfunction. Monitor uric acid, alkaline phosphatase, urinary hydroxyproline excretion, electrolytes, Mg^{++},

phosphate, calcium, vitamin D level, PTH, and renal function studies.

CLIENT/FAMILY TEACHING

1. Drug slows accelerated bone turnover (resorption and accretion) in pagetic lesions and, to a lesser extent, in normal bone.
2. Maintain a well-balanced diet with calcium and vitamin D supplementation; see dietitian PRN.
3. Take with a full glass of water. Do not eat for 2 hr after taking medication. Foods high in calcium (e.g., milk, milk products), and vitamins with mineral supplements (e.g., Al, calcium, iron, or Mg^{++}) may decrease absorption. If GI upset with single dose, may divide dose.
4. With jaw pain, obtain periodic dental exams to R/O osteonecrosis of the jaw (ONJ). Any invasive dental procedures, consider discontinuation of bisphosphonate treatment to reduce risk for ONJ.
5. Report any unusual pain, muscle twitching/spasms, diarrhea, headaches, restricted mobility or pain/heat over bone site, and S&S of hypercalcemia, (i.e., lethargy, N&V, anorexia, tremors, and pain).
6. Obtain lab studies as scheduled; with Paget's disease, reduced levels of urinary hydroxyproline excretion and serum alkaline phosphatase indicate a beneficial therapeutic response. Levels usually decrease 1–3 months after initiation of therapy.
7. With hypercalcemia, serum calcium levels show drug response and need for continued therapy. Reduction usually occurs in 2–8 days in hypercalcemia R/T bone metastasis. Therapy may be repeated only after 7 days of rest.
8. Keep all F/U to assess response, labs, radiologic exams, and for adverse SE.

OUTCOMES/EVALUATE

- Suppression of bone resorption
- Reductions in serum alkaline phosphatase and urinary hydroxyproline levels
- ↓ Bone pain with Paget's disease

Etodolac

(ee-toh-**DOH**-lack)

Classification(s): Nonsteroidal anti-inflammatory drug

Pregnancy Category: C

✱ **Rx:** Apo-Etodolac.

SEE ALSO ***NONSTEROIDAL ANTI-INFLAMMATORY DRUGS.***

INDICATIONS/USES

(1) Relief of signs and symptoms of osteoarthritis and rheumatoid arthritis. (2) Juvenile rheumatoid arthritis (use extended-release tablets). (3) Mild to moderate pain.

ACTION/KINETICS

Action

Etodolac is an NSAID in a class called the pyranocarboxylic acids. Anti-inflammatory effect likely due to inhibition of cyclo-oxygenase, which results in decreased prostaglandin synthesis. Effective in reducing joint swelling, pain, and morning stiffness in those with inflammatory disease.

Pharmacokinetics

Over 80% bioavailable. **Time to peak levels:** 1–2 hr. **Onset of analgesic action:** 30 min; **duration:** 4–12 hr. **t½:** 7.3 hr. The drug is metabolized by the liver and metabolites are excreted through the kidneys (72%) and feces (16%). **Plasma protein binding:** More than 99%.

CONTRAINDICATIONS

Clients in whom etodolac, aspirin, or other NSAIDs have caused asthma, rhinitis, urticaria, or other allergic reactions. Use during lactation, during labor and delivery, and in children.

SPECIAL CONCERNS

- Use caution with impaired renal or hepatic function, heart failure, those on diuretics, and in geriatric clients.
- Safety and efficacy not determined in children.

ADDITIONAL SIDE EFFECTS

Most Common

Dizziness, asthenia/malaise, abdominal pain/cramps, diarrhea, nausea, flatulence.

See *Nonsteroidal Anti-Inflammatory Drugs* for a complete listing of side effects. **GI:** Diarrhea, gastritis, thirst, ulcerative stomatitis, anorexia. **CNS:** Nervousness, depression. **CV:** Syncope. **Respiratory:** Asthma. **Dermatologic:** ***Angioedema***, vesiculobullous rash, cutaneous vasculitis with purpura, hyperpigmentation. **Miscellaneous:** Jaundice, hepatitis.

LABORATORY TEST CONSIDERATIONS

False + reaction for urinary bilirubin and for urinary ketones (using the dip-stick method). ↑ Liver enzymes, serum creatinine. ↑ Bleeding time.

OVERDOSE MANAGEMENT

Symptoms: N&V, drowsiness, lethargy, epigastric pain, ***anaphylaxis.*** Rarely, hypertension, acute renal failure, respiratory depression. *Treatment:* Since there are no antidotes, treatment is supportive and symptomatic. If discovered within 4 hr, emesis followed by activated charcoal and an osmotic cathartic may be tried.

ADDITIONAL DRUG INTERACTIONS

Cyclosporine / ↑ Cyclosporine levels R/T ↓ renal excretion; ↑ risk of cyclosporine-induced nephrotoxicity
Digoxin / ↑ Digoxin levels R/T ↓ renal excretion
Lithium / ↑ Lithium levels R/T ↓ renal excretion
Methotrexate / ↑ Methotrexate levels R/T ↓ renal excretion

HOW SUPPLIED

Capsules: 200 mg, 300 mg; *Tablets:* 400 mg, 500 mg; *Tablets, Extended-Release:* 400 mg, 500 mg, 600 mg.

DOSAGE

CAPSULES; TABLETS; TABLETS, EXTENDED-RELEASE

Osteoarthritis, rheumatoid arthritis.

Adults, initial: 300 mg 2–3 times per day, 400 mg 2 times/day, or 500 mg 2 times per day using capsules or tablets. Dose may be adjusted up or down during long-term use, depending on the clinical response. A dose of 600 mg may suffice for chronic administration. In clients who tolerate 1,000 mg/day, the dose may be increased to 1,200 mg/day if a higher level of activity is needed.
Tablets, Extended-Release: 400–1,000 mg given once daily. Doses above 1,200 mg/day have not been evaluated adequately, although the dose may be increased to 1,200 mg/day if needed.

Juvenile rheumatoid arthritis (use extended-release tablets).

Children, 6–16 years of age based on body weight. 20–30 kg: 1–400 mg tablet once daily. **31–45 kg:** 1–600 mg tablet once daily. **46–60 kg:** 2–400 mg tablets once daily. **>60 kg:** 2–500 mg tablets once daily.

Acute pain.

Adults: 200–400 mg q 6–8 hr, up to 1,000 mg/day. In some, the dose may be increased to 1,200 mg/day. Use capsules or tablets.

NOTE: Do not exceed 20 mg/kg in clients weighing 60 kg or less.

NURSING IMPLICATIONS

IMPLEMENTATION/ADMINISTRATION/STORAGE

1. Seek the lowest dose and longest dosing interval for each client.
2. Dosage adjustment is usually not required in clients with mild-to-moderate renal impairment.
3. In chronic conditions, a therapeutic response with extended-release tablets may be seen within 1 week, but most often is seen by 2 weeks.
4. Store capsules and tablets from 15–30°C (59–86°F) in tight, light-resistant containers. Store extended-release tablets from 20–25°C (68–77°F) protected from excessive heat and humidity.

ASSESSMENT

1. Note any previous experience with NSAIDs or acetylsalicylic acid and results.
2. List reasons for therapy (i.e., analgesic or anti-inflammatory); include onset, location, characteristics of symptoms, status of ROM; rate pain level.
3. Determine history of ulcers, heart disease, or cardiac failure. May cause an increased risk of serious CV thrombotic events, MI, and stroke.
4. Note age and weight; if currently prescribed diuretics.
5. With long-term therapy, monitor BP, CBC, chemistry, renal and LFTs. Assess closely for skin rash, ulcers, or bleeding.

CLIENT/FAMILY TEACHING

1. Drug works by reducing hormones that cause inflammation and pain in the body
2. Take with milk or food to decrease GI upset.

3. **May cause dizziness or drowsiness; avoid activities requiring alertness until drug effects realized.**
4. **Report any unusual bruising/bleeding, rash, yellow skin discoloration, dark/tarry stools, or lack of response.**
5. **Stop drug and report, sudden weight gain, loss of BP control, swelling in extremities, blood in stools or urine.**
6. **Avoid alcohol, aspirin, and other NSAIDs.**
7. **Use protection if exposed, and avoid prolonged sun exposure.**
8. **Practice reliable contraception during therapy.**
9. **Keep all F/U to assess response, labs, and adverse SE.**

OUTCOMES/EVALUATE

Control of pain and inflammation with improved joint mobility

Combination Drug

Etonogestrel/Ethinyl estradiol vaginal ring

Classification(s): Contraceptive

Pregnancy Category: X

RX: NuvaRing.

SEE ALSO ***ESTROGENS*** AND ***ORAL CONTRACEPTIVES: ESTROGEN-PROGESTERONE COMBINATIONS.***

INDICATIONS/USES

Prevention of pregnancy.

CONTENT

In each ring: 11.7 mg etonogestrel and 2.7 mg ethinyl estradiol.

ACTION/KINETICS

Action

The product is a nonbiodegradable, flexible, transparent, colorless to almost colorless contraceptive vaginal ring containing a progestin (etonogestrel) and an estrogen (ethinyl estradiol). In the vagina, each ring releases an average of 0.12 mg/day of etonogestrel and 0.015 mg/day of ethinyl estradiol over a 3-week period of use. The primary action is inhibition of ovulation although changes in the cervical mucus (decreasing sperm motility) and the endometrium (reducing possibility of implantation) add to the contraceptive effectiveness.

Pharmacokinetics

Both hormones are rapidly absorbed into the systemic circulation; the bioavailability of etonogestrel is 100%, while the bioavailability of ethinyl estradiol is about 56%. Both hormones are metabolized by the liver cytochrome CYP3A4 isoenzyme. The hormones may be poorly metabolized in women with impaired hepatic function. Both hormones are excreted in the urine, bile, and feces. **Plasma protein binding:** Etonogestrel is about 32% bound to sex hormone-binding globulin and about 66% bound to blood albumin. Ethinyl estradiol is about 98.5% bound to serum albumin.

CONTRAINDICATIONS

See *Estrogens* and *Oral Contraceptives: Estrogen-Progesterone Combinations.*

SPECIAL CONCERNS

See both *Estrogens* and *Progesterone/Progestins* for Black Box Warnings.

SIDE EFFECTS

Most Common

Vaginitis, headache, URTI, vaginal secretion, sinusitis, weight gain, nausea.

Device-related events: Foreign body sensation, coital problems, device expulsion, vaginal discomfort, vaginitis/vaginal secretion, leukorrhea, headache, emotional lability, weight gain. **Serious:** ***Thrombophlebitis, venous thrombosis with or without embolism, arterial thromboembolism, pulmonary embolism, MI, cerebral hemorrhage, cerebral thrombosis, hepatic adenomas***, hypertension, gallbladder disease, benign liver tumors, mesenteric thrombosis, retinal thrombosis. **GI:** Cholestatic jaundice, abdominal pain/cramps, bloating, N&V, colitis, exacerbation or development of gallbladder disease, ***pancreatitis***. **CNS:** Headache (including migraine), exacerbation of chorea, migraine, mood changes (including depression), dizziness, nervousness. **GU:** Amenorrhea, breakthrough bleeding, breast tenderness/enlargement/secretion, breast pain, change in cervical erosion and secretion, change in menstrual flow, decrease in lactation when given immediately postpartum, spotting, temporary infertility after discontinuing treatment, vaginitis (including candidiasis), changes in libido, cystitis-like syndrome, dysmenorrhea, hemolytic uremic syndrome, premenstrual syndrome, impaired renal function. **Dermatologic:** Melasma/chloasma (which may persist), acne, erythema multiforme or nodosum, hirsutism, loss of scalp hair. **Hypersensitivity:** ***Anaphylactic/anaphylactoid reactions***, including ***angioedema***, severe reactions with respiratory and circulatory symptoms, urticaria, allergic rash. **Metabolic:** Increase or decrease in weight or appetite, edema/fluid retention, decreased tolerance to carbohydrates. **Ophthalmic:** Steepening of corneal curvature, intolerance to contact lenses, cataracts, optic neuritis (which may lead to partial or complete loss of vision). **Miscellaneous:** Aggravation of varicose veins, exacerbation of porphyria, exacerbation of systemic lupus erythematosus, Budd-Chiari syndrome, hemorrhagic eruption.

E

LABORATORY TEST CONSIDERATIONS

See *Oral Contraceptives: Estrogen-Progesterone Combinations.*

DRUG INTERACTIONS

See *Estrogens* and *Oral Contraceptives: Estrogen-Progesterone Combinations.*

HOW SUPPLIED

See *Content.*

DOSAGE

VAGINAL RING

Prevention of pregnancy.

One vaginal ring is inserted by the woman in the vagina. Ring remains in place for 3 weeks and is removed for a 1-week break, during which withdrawal bleeding usually occurs. Withdrawal bleeding usually starts 2 to 3 days after removal of the ring; bleeding may not have finished before the next ring is inserted. A new ring is inserted 1 week after the last ring was removed on the same day of the week as it was inserted in the previous cycle, even if menstrual bleeding is not finished.

NURSING IMPLICATIONS

IMPLEMENTATION/ADMINISTRATION/STORAGE

1. If switching from a progestin-only method, insert the first vaginal ring as follows:
   - Any day of the month when switching from a progestin-only tablet; do not skip any days between the last tablet and the first day of vaginal ring use.
   - On the same day as the contraceptive implant removal.
   - On the same day as removal of a progestin-containing IUD.
   - On the day when the next contraceptive injection would be due.

   In all of these situations, advise use of an additional method of contraception for the first 7 days after ring insertion.
2. The client may start using the vaginal ring within the first 5 days following a complete first-trimester abortion. No additional method of contraception is required. If the vaginal ring is not inserted within 5 days and no preceding hormonal contraceptive was used in the past month, count the first day of menses as day 1 and insert the vaginal ring on or prior to day 5 of the cycle, even if menses has not finished.
3. Following delivery or a second-trimester abortion, insert the vaginal ring 4 weeks postpartum in women who are not breast-feeding. A woman who is breast-feeding should not use the vaginal ring until the child is weaned. Initiate use of the vaginal ring 4 weeks after a second-trimester abortion. However, there is an increased risk of thromboembolic disease. If a woman begins using the vaginal ring postpartum and has not yet had a period, it is possible that ovulation and conception has occurred prior to the insertion of the vaginal ring.
4. If the client has not adhered to the prescribed regimen, including that the vaginal contraceptive ring has been out of the vagina for more than 3 hr or the preceding ring-free interval was longer than 1 week, consider the possibility of pregnancy at the time of the first missed period. Discontinue the use of the vaginal ring if pregnancy is confirmed. Rule out pregnancy if the client has adhered to the regimen and misses 2 consecutive periods or if the woman has retained 1 contraceptive vaginal ring for more than 4 weeks.
5. Once dispensed to the user, the vaginal rings can be stored for up to 4 months at 15–30°C (59–86°F). Avoid storing in direct sunlight. When dispensed to the user, place an expira-

tion date on the label. The date should not be more than 4 months from the date of dispensing or the expiration date, whichever comes first.

ASSESSMENT

1. Note reasons for therapy, other agents trialed/outcome.
2. Ensure client has undergone GYN exam, understands contraception and ring use, and is a candidate for therapy.
3. Therapy may increase risk of thromboembolism, especially with smoking, CVA, and ↑ BP readings. Monitor VS, TSH, blood sugar, and lipid panel.

CLIENT/FAMILY TEACHING

1. The flexible ring is placed in the vagina to prevent pregnancy. It is inserted and left in place for 3 weeks.
2. Wash and dry your hands. Remove one contraceptive ring from its foil pouch, but do not throw away the pouch. Save the pouch so you can use it to discard the old contraceptive ring after you remove it.
3. May select the insertion position that is most comfortable (e.g., standing with one leg up, squatting, or lying down). Compress the ring, and insert into the vagina. The exact position of the ring inside the vagina is not critical for activity.
4. Remove the vaginal ring after 3 weeks on the same day of the week as it was inserted, and at about the same time. Remove the ring by hooking the index finger under the forward rim, or by grasping the rim between the index and middle finger or thumb and pulling it out. Place the used ring in the foil pouch, and discard in a waste receptacle out of the reach of children and pets. Do not flush in toilet.
5. Withdrawal bleeding usually starts on day 2 to 3 after removal, but may not have finished before the next ring is inserted. However, it is imperative that the new ring be inserted 1 week after the previous one was removed in order to maintain contraceptive efficacy.
6. It is possible that ovulation and conception may occur before the first use of the vaginal ring. During the first cycle, an additional method of contraception should be used until after the first 7 days of ring use.
7. If no preceding hormonal contraceptive was used in the past month, count the first day of menses as day 1 and insert the vaginal ring on days 2 to 5 of the cycle, even if menses has not finished.
8. If switching from a combination oral contraceptive to the vaginal ring, insert the vaginal ring anytime within 7 days after the last combination oral contraceptive tablet, and no later than the day that a new cycle of tablets would have started. No backup method of contraception is required.
9. If changing from a progestin-only method (minipill, implant, or injection), the woman may switch on any day from the minipill. She should switch from the implant on the day when the next injection would be due. The woman should use an additional barrier contraceptive for the first 7 days.
10. If there has been inadvertent removal, expulsion, or prolonged ring-free intervals during the 3-week use period and is left outside the vagina for less than 3 hr, rinse the ring with cool to lukewarm (not hot) water, and reinsert as soon as possible, at the latest within 3 hr. Contraceptive effectiveness is reduced if the ring has been out of the vagina for more than 3 hours. If the ring is lost, a new vaginal ring should be inserted, and the regimen continued without alteration. Thus, use an additional form of contraception until the ring has been used continuously for 7 days. Consider the possibility of pregnancy if the ring-free interval has been extended beyond 1 week.
11. If the ring is out of the vagina during weeks 1 and 2, reinsert the ring as soon as the woman remembers. A barrier method of contraception should be used until the ring has been used continuously for 7 days. If the ring is out of the vagina for more than 3 hours during week 3, discard that ring. Choose one of the following options: (a) Insert a new ring immediately; inserting a new ring will start the next 3-week period. The woman may not experience withdrawal bleeding from her previous cycle. However, breakthrough spotting or bleeding may occur. (b) Have withdrawal bleeding, and insert a new ring no later than 7 days from the time the previous ring was removed or expelled. Choose this option only if the ring was used continuously for the preceding 7 days. A barrier contraceptive method must be used

until the new ring has been used continuously for 7 days.

12. If the vaginal ring has been left in place for up to 1 extra week, the women will remain protected. Remove the ring, and insert a new ring after a 1-week ring-free interval. Rule out pregnancy if the vaginal ring has been left in place for more than 4 weeks.
13. The vaginal ring does not prevent the spread of HIV or other sexually transmitted diseases.
14. Store away from light/heat.
15. Do not smoke. If you choose to smoke, do not use this type of therapy as the risk of cardiovascular events far outweighs the benefits of therapy.
16. Report any problems related to usage, or suspected pregnancy.
17. Keep all F/U to assess response and for adverse SE.

OUTCOMES/EVALUATE
Desired contraception

Etravirine

(ee-tra-**VIR**-een)

Classification(s): Antiviral, non-nucleoside reverse transcriptase inhibitor

Pregnancy Category: B

RX: Intelence.

SEE ALSO ***ANTIVIRAL DRUGS***.

INDICATIONS/USES

In combination with other antiretroviral drugs to treat HIV-1 infection in antiretroviral treatment-experienced clients who have evidence of viral replication and HIV-1 strains resistant to non-nucleoside reverse transcriptase inhibitors and other antiretroviral drugs.

ACTION/KINETICS

Action

Entravirine binds directly to reverse transcriptase and blocks the RNA- and DNA-dependent DNA polymerase activities by causing a disruption of the enzyme's catalytic site. The drug does not inhibit the human DNA polymerases alpha, beta, or gamma.

Pharmacokinetics

Time to maximum plasma levels: About 2.5–4 hr. Absorption is not affected by drugs that increase gastric pH (e.g., omeprazole, ranitidine). The AUC is decreased by about 50% under fasting conditions; thus, always take etravirine following a meal. Metabolized primarily by CYP3A4, CYP2C9, and CYP2C19. Nearly 94% is excreted in the feces. **t½, terminal elimination:** About 41 hr. **Plasma protein binding:** About 99.9%.

CONTRAINDICATIONS

Lactation.

SPECIAL CONCERNS

- Use caution when selecting the dose for the elderly.
- Safety and efficacy not determined in children.

SIDE EFFECTS

Most Common

Rash (any type), N&V, diarrhea, fatigue, abdominal pain, hypertension, peripheral neuropathy, headache.

GI: Diarrhea, N&V, abdominal pain/distension, anorexia, constipation, dry mouth, flatulence, gastritis, GERD, hematemesis, ***pancreatitis***, retching, stomatitis. **Hepatic:** Cytolytic hepatitis, hepatic steatosis, hepatitis, hepatomegaly, ***hepatic failure***. **CNS:** Peripheral neuropathy, headache, abnormal dreams, amnesia, anxiety, confused state, ***convulsion***, disorientation, hypersomnia, hypesthesia, insomnia, nervousness, nightmares, paresthesia, sleep disorders, sluggishness, somnolence, syncope, tremor, vertigo. **CV:** Hypertension, angina pectoris, atrial fibrillation, ***MI, hemorrhagic stroke***. **Dermatologic:** Mild to moderate rash, dry skin, hyperhidrosis, lipohypertrophy, night sweats, prurigo, pruritus, swelling face, ***Stevens-Johnson syndrome, hypersensitivity reaction, erythema multiforme, toxic epidermal necrolysis***. **Respiratory:** ***Bronchospasm***, exertional dyspnea. **GU:** Gynecomastia, renal failure. **Hematologic:** Anemia, hemolytic anemia. **Metabolic:** Diabetes mellitus, dyslipidemia. **Ophthalmic:** Blurred vision. **Body as a whole:** Fatigue, angioneurotic edema, redistribution/accumulation of body fat (including central obesity, dorsocervical fat enlargement, peripheral wasting, facial wasting, breast enlargement, cushingoid appearance), immune reconstitution syndrome (i.e., inflammatory response to indolent or residual opportunistic infections, such as *Mycobacterium avium* complex, cytomegalovirus, *Pneumocystis jiroveci,* pneumonia, tuberculosis), ***angioneurotic edema.*** **Miscellaneous:** Drug hypersensitivity, acquired lipodystrophy.

LABORATORY TEST CONSIDERATIONS

↑ Pancreatic amylase, lipase, creatinine, total cholesterol, LDL, triglycerides, glucose, ALT, AST. ↓ Hemoglobin, neutrophils, platelets. *NOTE:* ALT and AST abnormalities occur more frequently in clients with hepatitis B and/or hepatitis C.

OVERDOSE MANAGEMENT

Symptoms: Extension of side effects. *Treatment:* General supportive measures, including monitoring of vital signs and observation of the clinical status. Eliminate unabsorbed drug by gastric lavage and/or administration of activated charcoal. Because etravirine is highly bound to plasma proteins, it is unlikely hemodialysis or peritoneal dialysis will remove significant quantities of the drug.

DRUG INTERACTIONS

Because etravirine is a substrate of CYP3A4, CYP2C9, and CYP2C19, coadministration with drugs that induce or inhibit these enzymes may alter the therapeutic effect or side effects of etravirine. Also, etravirine is an inducer of CYP3A4 and inhibitor of CYP2C9 and CYP2C19; thus, coadministration of drugs that are substrates of these enzymes with etravirine may alter the therapeutic effect or side effects of the coadministered drug(s).

Antiarrhythmic drugs (e.g., amiodarone, bepridil, disopyramide, flecainide, systemic lidocaine, mexiletine, propafenone, quinidine) / ↓ Concentrations of antiarrhythmic drugs; use together with caution and monitor drug levels if available

Anticonvulsants (e.g., carbamazepine, phenobarbital, phenytoin) / Significant ↓ in etravirine levels → loss of therapeutic effect R/T induction of CYP450 enzymes

Atazanavir/Ritonavir / Etravirine AUC 100% higher; also, possible significant ↓ in atazanavir minimum plasma levels → loss of atazanavir therapeutic effect; do not use together

Charcoal / ↓ Etravirine absorption → ↓ efficacy and toxicity

Clarithromycin / ↓ Clarithromycin levels but ↑ of the active 14-hydroxyclarithromycin; consider using azithromycin

Darunavir/Ritonavir / Etravirine AUC ↓ by about 37%; no dosage adjustments needed

Delavirdine / ↑ Etravirine levels; do not use together

Dexamethasone (systemic) / ↓ Etravirine levels → loss of therapeutic effect; consider an alternative corticosteroid, especially if used long-term

Diazepam / ↑ Diazepam levels; possibly ↓ diazepam dose

Fluconazole / ↑ Etravirine levels

Fosamprenavir/Ritonavir / Significant ↑ amprenavir levels; do not use together

HMG-CoA reductase inhibitors (e.g., atorvastatin, fluvastatin, lovastatin, simvastatin) / ↓ Lovastatin and simvastatin levels and ↑ fluvastatin levels; possibly adjust dosage levels

Immunosuppressants (cyclosporine, sirolimus, tacrolimus) / Use together with caution R/T plasma levels of immunosuppressant may be affected

Itraconazole / ↑ Etravirine levels; ↓ itraconazole levels; dosage adjustment may be needed

Ketoconazole / ↑ Etravirine levels; ↓ ketoconazole levels; dosage adjustment may be needed

Lopinavir/Ritonavir / Etravirine AUC 85% higher; coadminister with caution

Methadone / Methadone maintenance therapy may have to be adjusted in some clients

Non-nucleoside reverse transcriptase inhibitors (e.g., efavirenz, nevirapine) / Significant ↓ etravirine levels → loss of therapeutic effect; avoid coadministration

PDE-5 inhibitors (e.g., sildenafil, tadalafil, vardenafil) / Dose of sildenafil may need adjustment depending on clinical effect

Posaconazole / ↑ Etravirine levels

Protease inhibitors (atazanavir, fosamprenavir, indinavir, nelfinavir) / Possible significant alteration (↑ or ↓) of plasma levels of protease inhibitor if taken without low-dose ritonavir; do not give etravirine with protease inhibitors without low-dose ritonavir

Rifabutin, Rifampin, or Rifapentine / Significant ↓ etravirine levels → loss of therapeutic effect; do not use together

Ritonavir / Significant ↓ etravirine levels if used with ritonavir, 600 mg twice a day → loss of therapeutic effect; do not use together

Saquinavir/Ritonavir / Etravirine AUC ↓ 33%; no dosage adjustment needed

H ***St. John's wort*** / Significant ↓ etravirine levels → loss of therapeutic effect; do not use together

Tipranavir/Ritonavir / Significant ↓ etravirine levels → loss of therapeutic effect; do not use together
Voriconazole / ↑ Plasma levels of both drugs; dosage adjustment may be needed
Warfarin / Possible ↑ warfarin levels; monitor INR

HOW SUPPLIED

Tablets: 100 mg, 200 mg.

E

DOSAGE

TABLETS

Human immunodeficiency virus-1 infection.

200 mg (2 × 100 mg tablets or 1 × 200 mg tablet) twice a day following a meal. The type of food does not affect exposure to the drug.

NURSING IMPLICATIONS

IMPLEMENTATION/ADMINISTRATION/STORAGE

1. To monitor maternal-fetal outcomes of pregnant women exposed to etravirine, health care providers are encouraged to register clients by calling 1-800-258-4263 at the antiretroviral pregnancy registry Mon.-Fri. 8:30 a.m. to 5:30 p.m. EST.
2. Store from 15–30°C (59–86°F) in the original bottle. Protect from moisture. Do not remove the desiccant pouches.

ASSESSMENT

1. Note onset, disease characteristics such as stage of infection, viral load and other therapies trialed/failed.
2. List all drugs prescribed to prevent interactions.
3. Assess for rashes during therapy; if severe may need to terminate therapy.
4. Determine if also infected with hepatitis virus.
5. Assess lifestyle and potential to resume risky behaviors. Determine if pregnant; report to registry.
6. Monitor CBC, LFTs, viral load, CD_4 counts.

CLIENT/FAMILY TEACHING

1. Take as prescribed following a meal twice daily. Swallow tablets whole with water. Always take drug in combination with other antiretroviral drugs.
2. If unable to swallow tablets, may place the tablets in a glass of water. Once dispersed, stir contents well, and drink immediately. Rinse glass with water several times; completely swallow each rinse to ensure the entire dose is taken.
3. If dose is missed within 6 hours of the time it is usually taken, then may take following a meal as soon as possible, and then take the next dose at the regularly scheduled time. If dose is missed by more than 6 hours of when usually taken, do not take the missed dose, just resume the usual dosing schedule. Take only the dose prescribed, do not increase or decrease dose, or stop therapy without provider approval.
4. Drug is not a cure for HIV infection; may continue to develop opportunistic infections and other complications associated with HIV disease.
5. Does not reduce risk of transmitting HIV through sexual contact, sharing needles, or being exposed to blood. Must continue to practice safe sex, and use latex/polyurethane condoms to reduce chance of sexual contact with any body fluids such as semen, vaginal secretions or blood. Never reuse or share needles.
6. Sustained decreases in viral levels have been associated with a reduced risk of progression to AIDS and death.
7. Avoid other prescription or OTC agents; interacts with many other drugs. Herbal products, including St. John's wort has caused severe and potentially life-threatening rash. Stop therapy if severe rash develops.
8. A redistribution or accumulation of body fat may occur in those receiving antiretroviral therapy; cause and long-term health effects of this are unknown at this time. Report any skin rash or skin changes.
9. Practice reliable contraception as drug effects on fetus may be harmful; monitoring by drug company is requested. (1-800-258-4263)
10. Keep all F/U to assess response, labs, and adverse SE.

OUTCOMES/EVALUATE

- ↓ HIV RNA
- Improved survival rates in those with HIV resistant to non-nucleoside reverse transcriptase inhibitors (NNRTI) and other antiretroviral drugs

Everolimus

(eh-ver-**OH**-lee-mus)

Classification(s): Antineoplastic agent-protein-tyrosine kinase inhibitor

Pregnancy Category: D (Category C for Zortress and Category D for Afinitor)

RX: Afinitor, Zortress.

INDICATIONS/USES

Afinitor only. (1) Advanced renal cell carcinoma after treatment failure with sunitinib or sorafenib. (2) Subependymal giant cell astrocytoma associated with tuberous sclerosis who require therapeutic intervention but are not candidates for curative surgical resection. (3) Progressive neuroendocrine tumors located in the pancreas that are unresectable, locally advanced, or metastatic. **Zortress only.** Prophylaxis of organ rejection in adults at low-moderate immunologic risk receiving a kidney transplant.

ACTION/KINETICS

Action

When used for renal cell carcinoma: The mTOR pathway is dysregulated in several human cancers. Everolimus causes an inhibitory complex formation and inhibition of mTOR kinase activity. The drug also inhibits the expression of hypoxia inducible factor and reduces the expression of vascular endothelial growth factor. Inhibition of mTOR by everolimus has been shown to reduce cell proliferation, angiogenesis, and glucose uptake.

When used for renal transplantation and subependymal giant cell astrocytoma: Everolimus inhibits mTOR; the mTOR pathway is dysregulated in several human cancers. Everolimus binds to an intracellular protein (FKBP12) resulting in an inhibitory complex formation and inhibition of mTOR kinase activity. Inhibition of mTOR reduces cell proliferation, angiogenesis, and glucose uptake.

Pharmacokinetics

Peak levels: 1–2 hr after PO administration; **steady-state:** 2 weeks following once daily dosing. Steady-state is reached in 4 days in kidney transplant clients. High-fat meals decrease C_{max}, delayed T_{max} and reduced AUC; thus, take the drug consistently with or without food. Everolimus is a substrate of CYP3A4 and P-glycoprotein. Excreted mainly in the feces (80%) with a small amount excreted in the urine (5%). **t½, elimination:** About 30 hr. Impaired hepatic function increases AUC. Exposure is higher in Japanese clients than non-Japanese clients, and oral clearance is about 20% higher in black clients than in white clients. Clearance is reduced as age increases. **Plasma protein binding:** 74%.

CONTRAINDICATIONS

Hypersensitivity to everolimus, other rapamycin derivatives, or any component of the product. Hypersensitivity to sirolimus (Zortress only). Concomitant use with strong CYP3A4 inducers (e.g., carbamazepine, dexamethasone, phenytoin, rifabutin, rifampin) or strong CYP3A4 and/or P-glycoprotein inhibitors (e.g., aprepitant, atazanavir, clarithromycin, delavirdine, diltiazem, erythromycin, fluconazole, fosamprenavir, grapefruit juice, indinavir, itraconazole, ketoconazole, nefazodone, nelfinavir, ritonavir, saquinavir, telithromycin, verapamil, voriconazole). Use of live vaccines or close contact with those who have received live vaccines. Use in those with rare hereditary problems of galactose intolerance, Lapp lactase deficiency, or glucose-galactose malabsorption (due to increased risk of diarrhea and malabsorption). Severe hepatic impairment (Child-Pugh class C). Lactation.

SPECIAL CONCERNS

Immunosuppression, renal function, and graft thrombosis (Zortress only). (1) Increased susceptibility to infection and the possible development of malignancies, such as lymphoma and skin cancer, may result from immunosuppression. (2) Only health care providers experienced in immunosuppressive therapy and management of transplant clients should use everolimus. Manage clients receiving the drug in facilities equipped and staffed with adequate laboratory and supportive medical resources. The health care provider responsible for maintenance therapy should have complete information requisite for the follow-up. (3) Increased nephrotoxicity can occur with use of standard doses of cyclosporine in combination with everolimus. Therefore, use reduced doses of cyclosporine in combination with everolimus in order to reduce renal dysfunction. It is important to monitor the cyclosporine and everolimus whole blood trough concentrations. (4) An increased risk of kidney arterial and venous thrombosis, resulting in graft loss, was reported, mostly within the first 30 days post-transplantation. ■

Safety and efficacy in kidney transplant or advanced renal cell carcinoma not established in children younger than 18 years of age. Not studied to treat subependymal giant cell astrocytoma in children younger than 3 years of age.

SIDE EFFECTS

Most Common

Afinitor, when used for advanced renal cell carcinoma: Asthenia, cough, diarrhea, fatigue, infections, stomatitis, abdominal pain, dehydration, dyspnea, pneumonitis.
Afinitor, when used for subependymal giant cell astrocytoma: Otitis media, pyrexia, sinusitis, stomatitis, URTI, convulsions, acneiform dermatitis, diarrhea, sinusitis, pyrexia.
Zortress: Anemia, constipation, hyperlipidemia, hypertension, N&V, peripheral edema, UTI, infections, pyrexia.
NOTE: Only the most common or life-threatening side effects are listed.

Afinitor only when used for advanced renal cell carcinoma. GI: Diarrhea, stomatitis, mouth/tongue ulceration, oral mucositis, abdominal pain, diarrhea, anorexia, dysgeusia, N&V, dry mouth, hemorrhoids, dysphagia, ***pancreatitis***. **CNS:** Headache, insomnia, dizziness, paresthesia. **CV:** Hypertension, tachycardia, CHF. **Respiratory:** Cough, pneumonitis, dyspnea, epistaxis, nasopharyngitis, pneumonia, pneumonitis, bronchitis, sinusitis, rhinorrhea, interstitial lung disease, lung infiltration, pulmonary alveolar hemorrhage, pulmonary toxicity, alveolitis, pharyngolaryngeal pain, pleural effusion, noninfectious pneumonitis, ***respiratory failure***. **Dermatologic:** Rash, dry skin, pruritus, hand-foot syndrome (palmar-plantar erythrodysesthesia syndrome), nail syndrome, erythema, onycholysis, skin lesion, acneiform dermatitis. **GU:** UTI, nephrotoxicity, azoospermia, oligospermia, ***acute renal failure***. **Hematologic:** Anemia, lymphopenia. **Metabolic:** Dehydration, peripheral edema, new onset or exacerbation of pre-existing diabetes mellitus. **Ophthalmic:** Eyelid edema, conjunctivitis. **Hypersensitivity:** Dyspnea, flushing, chest pain, angioedema, respiratory impairment, swelling of the airways or tongue, ***anaphylaxis***. **Body as a whole:** Asthenia, fatigue, mucosal inflammation, pain in extremity, pyrexia, decreased weight, chills, ***infections*** (including aspergillosis, candidiasis, ***sepsis***), ***hemorrhage***. **Miscellaneous:** Chest/jaw pain, impaired/delayed wound healing, lymphomas and other malignancies.

Afinitor only when used for subependymal giant cell astrocytoma. GI: Stomatitis, mouth ulcers, oral mucositis, diarrhea, vomiting, gastroenteritis, gastric infection, abdominal pain, constipation, gastritis, ***pancreatitis***, serious ***hepatitis B reactivation***. **CNS:** ***Convulsions,*** dizziness, headache, personality change, anxiety, somnolence. **CV:** Hypertension. **Respiratory:** Sinusitis, URTI, cough, nasal congestion, allergic rhinitis, pharyngitis, sinusitis, pharyngeal inflammation, abnormal chest x-ray, noninfectious pneumonitis. **GU:** Nephrotoxicity, azoospermia, oligospermia. **Dermatologic:** Dermatitis acneiform, body tinea, dry skin, rash, skin infection, contact dermatitis, acne, pityriasis rosea. **Metabolic:** Peripheral edema, new onset or exacerbation of pre-existing diabetes mellitus. **Hypersensitivity:** Dyspnea, flushing, chest pain, angioedema, respiratory impairment, swelling of the airways or tongue, ***anaphylaxis***. **Ophthalmic:** Ocular hyperemia. **Otic:** Otitis media, otitis externa. **Body as a whole:** Pyrexia, infections, cellulitis, excoriation, pyrexia, fatigue. Miscellaneous: Lymphomas and other malignancies. **Miscellaneous:** Delayed/impaired wound healing.

Zortress only when used for renal transplantation. GI: Constipation, GI disorders, N&V, diarrhea, abdominal pain (including upper), dyspepsia, stomatitis, mouth ulceration, oral mucositis, ***pancreatitis***. **CNS:** Nervous system/psychiatric disorders, headache, insomnia, tremor. **CV:** Hypertension, vascular disorders. **Respiratory:** Noninfectious pneumonitis. **GU:** UTI, dysuria, hematuria, renal/urinary disorders, kidney arterial/venous thrombosis resulting in graft loss, nephrotoxicity, azoospermia, oligospermia. **Hematologic:** Anemia, blood lymphatic system disorders, leukopenia. **Musculoskeletal:** Musculoskeletal/connective tissue disorders, pain in extremity, back pain. **Respiratory:** Respiratory/thoracic/mediastinal disorders, URTI, cough. **Metabolic:** Peripheral edema, dyslipidemia, metabolism/nutrition disorders, new onset or exacerbation of pre-existing diabetes mellitus. **Hypersensi-**

tivity: Dyspnea, flushing, chest pain, ***angioedema***, respiratory impairment, swelling of the airways or tongue, ***anaphylaxis***. **Body as a whole:** Infections (bacterial, viral, fungal), fatigue, pyrexia, ***death***. **Miscellaneous:** Incision-site pain; injury/poisoning/procedural complications, procedural pain, lymphomas and other malignancies, delayed/impaired wound healing.

LABORATORY TEST CONSIDERATIONS

Afinitor used for advanced renal cell carcinoma: ↑ ALT, AST, bilirubin, cholesterol, creatinine, glucose, triglycerides. ↓ Hemoglobin, lymphocytes, neutrophils, platelets, phosphate. Proteinuria.

Afinitor used for subependymal giant cell astrocytoma: ↑ ALT, AST, cholesterol, triglycerides, glucose, creatinine. ↓ WBCs, hemoglobin, glucose, platelets, neutrophils. Proteinuria.

Zortress used for renal transplantation: ↑ Cholesterol, triglycerides, glucose, lipids. ↓ Magnesium, phosphate. ↑ or ↓ Potassium. Proteinuria.

DRUG INTERACTIONS

NOTE: Everolimus is metabolized mainly by the CYP3A enzyme systems. Thus, substances that inhibit these enzymes may decrease metabolism or increase bioavailability of everolimus whereas drugs known to induce these enzymes may increase metabolism of everolimus or decrease bioavailability.

ACE inhibitors (e.g., captopril) / ↑ Risk of angioedema; if interaction suspected, stop one or both drugs
Aprepitant / Significant ↑ everolimus exposure R/T inhibition of metabolism by CYP3A4 or P-glycoprotein (Pgp) → ↑ risk of pharmacologic and side effects; if given together monitor everolimus blood levels and adjust dose as needed
Azole antifungals (e.g., fluconazole, itraconazole, ketoconazole, voriconazole) / Significant ↑ everolimus exposure R/T inhibition of metabolism by CYP3A4; avoid coadministration
Calcium channel blockers (e.g., diltiazem, nicardipine, verapamil) / Significant ↑ everolimus exposure R/T inhibition of metabolism by CYP3A4
Carbamazepine / ↓ Everolimus levels → ↓ effect R/T induction of metabolism by CYP3A4; avoid coadministration
Cyclosporine / ↑ Everolimus levels; monitor everolimus levels; adjust dose as needed
Delaviridine / Significant ↑ everolimus exposure R/T inhibition of metabolism by CYP3A4 or pgp; if coadministration is necessary, monitor everolimus blood levels and adjust the dose as needed
Dexamethasone / ↓ Everolimus levels R/T induction of metabolism by CYP3A4; avoid coadministration
Digoxin / ↑ Everolimus blood levels; use together with caution
Efavirenz / ↓ Everolimus blood levels → ↓ efficacy; monitor everolimus blood levels and adjust dose as needed
Grapefruit juice / Significant ↑ exposure of everolimus; do not give together
Lovastatin / ↑ Risk of side effects, including rhabdomyolysis; coadministration discouraged
Macrolide antibiotics (e.g., clarithromycin, erythromycin, telithromycin) / Significant ↑ everolimus exposure R/T inhibition of metabolism by CYP3A4; avoid coadministration
Nefazodone / Significant ↑ everolimus exposure R/T inhibition of metabolism by CYP3A4 or pgp; avoid coadministration
Nevirapine / ↓ Everolimus blood levels → ↓ efficacy; monitor everolimus blood levels and adjust dose as needed
Protease inhibitors (e.g., atazanavir, fosamprenavir, indinavir, nelfinavir, ritonavir, saquinavir) / Significant ↑ everolimus exposure R/T inhibition of metabolism by CYP3A4; avoid coadministration
Phenobarbital / ↓ Everolimus levels R/T induction of metabolism; avoid coadministration
Phenytoin / ↓ Everolimus levels R/T induction of metabolism; avoid coadministration
Rifabutin/Rifampin/Rifapentine / ↓ Everolimus AUC and C_{max} R/T induction of metabolism; avoid coadministration
Simvastatin / ↑ Risk of side effects, including rhabdomyolysis; coadministration discouraged
H *St. John's wort* / ↓ Everolimus blood levels → ↓ efficacy; if used together, closely monitor everolimus blood levels

HOW SUPPLIED

Tablets (Afinitor): 2.5 mg, 5 mg, 10 mg; *Tablets (Zortress):* 0.25 mg, 0.5 mg, 0.75 mg.

DOSAGE

Afinitor

TABLETS

Advanced renal cell carcinoma.

Adults, usual: 10 mg once a day at the same time every day. Reduce the dose

E

to 5 mg/day in those with moderate hepatic impairment (Child-Pugh Class B). If dose reduction is required due to severe and/or intolerable side effects, a dose of 5 mg/day is suggested. Continue treatment as long as clinical benefit is observed or unacceptable toxicity occurs.

Subependymal giant cell astrocytoma.

Adults and children, 3 years and older, initial: If body surface area (BSA) is 0.5–1.2 m^2, give 2.5 mg once a day; if BSA is 1.3–2.1 m^2, give 5 mg once a day; if BSA is 2.2 m^2 or greater, give 7.5 mg once a day. Dosage adjustments may be needed based on everolimus trough blood levels, tolerability, individual response, and change in concomitant medications. Dosage adjustments may not be needed in moderate hepatic impairment (Child-Pugh class B). Individualize dosing based on therapeutic drug monitoring.

Progressive neuroendocrine tumors in the pancreas.

Adults: 10 mg once daily.

Zortress

TABLETS

Renal transplantation.

Adults, initial: 0.75 mg twice a day in combination with a reduced dose of cyclosporine given as soon as possible after transplantation. Adjust dosage based on everolimus blood levels achieved, tolerability, individual response, change in concomitant medications, and the clinical situation. Dose adjustments can be made at 4–5 day intervals. *NOTE:* Initiate PO prednisone once PO medication is tolerated; steroid doses may be further tapered on an individualized basis depending on clinical status of the client and function of the graft. Give cyclosporine as PO capsules twice a day unless cyclosporine PO solution or IV administration cannot be avoided. Initiate cyclosporine as soon as possible but not later than 48 hr after reperfusion of the graft and the dose adjusted to target levels from day 5 onward.

NURSING IMPLICATIONS

IMPLEMENTATION/ADMINISTRATION/STORAGE

1. To avoid variability, take consistently with or without food. Administer Zortress about 12 hr apart and at the same time as cyclosporine. Swallow tablets whole with a glass of water; do not crush or chew tablets.
2. For those unable to swallow Afinitor tablets, disperse completely in a glass of water (about 30 mL) by gently stirring; drink immediately. Rinse the glass with the same volume of water; completely swallow the rinse to ensure the entire dose is consumed.
3. For clients with moderate hepatic impairment (Child-Pugh class B) and being treated for advanced renal cell carcinoma, reduce the everolimus dose to 5 mg/day. Everolimus has not been evaluated in those with severe hepatic impairment and should not be used in this population. For those being treated following renal transplantation and who have moderate hepatic impairment, reduce the daily dose by one-half of the recommended initial daily dose; monitor blood levels and make further dosage adjustments as necessary.
4. If clients require coadministration with a strong CYP3A4 inducer (see *Contraindications*), consider increasing the everolimus dose from 10 mg/day to 20 mg/day, using 5 mg increments. If the strong CYP3A4 inducer is discontinued, the everolimus dose should be returned to the dose used prior to beginning the strong CYP3A4 inducer.
5. Follow procedures for proper handling and disposal of anticancer drugs.
6. When used for renal transplantation, carefully consult the package insert for appropriate therapeutic drug monitoring.
7. Store from 15–30°C (59–86°F). Protect from light and moisture.

ASSESSMENT

1. Note disease onset, treatment failures with sunitinib or sorafenib, staging and any metastasis with afinitor.
2. If using Zortress, give in combination with basiliximab induction and concurrently with reduced doses of cyclosporine and corticosteroids for the prophylaxis of organ rejection in those receiving a kidney transplant.

3. Cyclosporine should be initiated as soon as possible and no later than 48 hr after reperfusion of the graft; adjust dose to target concentrations from day 5 onward. Reduced doses of cyclosporine should be used in combination with everolimus in order to reduce renal dysfunction. Monitor the cyclosporine and everolimus whole blood trough concentrations.
4. List drugs prescribed to ensure none interact.
5. Attempt to achieve control of blood sugar and lipids prior to starting therapy.
6. Review increased risk of malignancy, serious infections, renal dysfunction, pneumonitis, and blood clots associated with this therapy.
7. Assess for S&S of infection and treat; if systemic fungal infection occurs, must stop therapy and treat. Increased risk of noninfectious pneumonitis; monitor closely.
8. Monitor CBC, glucose, lipid panel, urine protein, renal and LFTs. With transplants monitor cyclosporine and everolimus trough levels.

CLIENT/FAMILY TEACHING

1. Afinitor is used to treat advanced renal cell cancer that has failed other therapy. Zortress is used with other drugs to prevent kidney transplant rejection.
2. Take one tablet once daily at the same time with or without food. Swallow tablet whole with a glass of water; do not chew or crush tablet and avoid eating grapefruit or using grapefruit juice.
3. Report any new or worsening respiratory symptoms as well as any evidence of infections since more susceptible to infections. May need to interrupt therapy; prescribe treatment and then reintroduce at lower dose.
4. Avoid taking live vaccines, and avoid close contact with those who have received live vaccines.
5. Practice reliable contraception during and for 8 weeks following therapy.
6. Mouth sores or ulcers may occur; avoid alcohol- or peroxide-containing mouth washes as they may aggravate.
7. Report any new pain in groin, lower back, side or stomach, dark tea colored or reduced urine output, N&V, or fever.
8. Review risk of developing infections, lymphomas and other malignancies, especially of the skin.
9. Avoid prolonged exposure to sunlight and UV light, and wear protective clothing and sunscreen when exposed.
10. Keep all F/U to assess response, labs, and for adverse SE.

OUTCOMES/EVALUATE

- Inhibition of malignant cell proliferation
- Prevention of organ transplant rejection

Exemestane

(ex-eh-**MESS**-tayn)

Classification(s): Antineoplastic, hormone

Pregnancy Category: D

RX: Aromasin.

SEE ALSO ***ANTINEOPLASTIC AGENTS***.

INDICATIONS/USES

(1) Treatment of advanced breast cancer in postmenopausal women where the disease has progressed following tamoxifen therapy. (2) Adjuvant therapy in menopausal women whose estrogen receptor-positive early breast cancer has progressed despite 2 or 3 years of tamoxifen therapy. Exemestane therapy is intended to complete a total of 5 consecutive years of adjuvant hormonal therapy. *Investigational:* Prevention of prostate cancer.

ACTION/KINETICS

Action

Irreversible, steroidal aromatase inactivator. Acts as a false substrate for the aromatase enzyme, which is the principal enzyme that converts androgens to estrogens. Drug is processed to an intermediate form that binds irreversibly to the active enzyme site causing its inhibition (called "suicide inhibition"). Significantly lowers circulating estrogen levels in postmenopausal women; has no detectable effect on adrenal biosynthesis of corticosteroids or aldosterone.

Pharmacokinetics

Rapidly absorbed. **t½, terminal:** About 24 hr. Metabolized in the liver and metabolites (some are active) excreted in both the urine and feces in equal amounts.

CONTRAINDICATIONS

Premenopausal women.

SPECIAL CONCERNS

Safety and efficacy not established in children.

SIDE EFFECTS

Most Common

Hot flashes, fatigue, pain, N&V, depression, insomnia, anxiety, edema, abdominal pain, anorexia, flu-like symptoms, increased sweating.

GI: N&V, abdominal pain, anorexia, GI upset, constipation, diarrhea, increased appetite, dyspepsia. **CNS:** Depression, insomnia, anxiety, dizziness, headache, hypoesthesia, confusion. **Respiratory:** Dyspnea, coughing, bronchitis, sinusitis, chest pain, URTI, pharyngitis, rhinitis. **Body as a whole:** Fatigue, edema, fever, generalized weakness, paresthesia, asthenia, peripheal edema, leg edema, flu-like symptoms, increased sweating, rash, itching, infection. **Miscellaneous:** Hypertension, hot flashes, pain, pathological fracture, UTI, lymphedema, pain at tumor site, arthralgia, skeletal back pain, alopecia, lymphocytopenia.

LABORATORY TEST CONSIDERATIONS

↑ AST, ALT, alkaline phosphatase, gamma glutamyl transferase. Slight ↑ serum LH and FSH. ↓ Sex hormone binding globulin.

HOW SUPPLIED

Tablets: 25 mg.

DOSAGE

TABLETS

Breast cancer.

25 mg once daily after a meal.

NURSING IMPLICATIONS

IMPLEMENTATION/ADMINISTRATION/STORAGE

Glucocorticoid and mineralocorticoid replacement therapy is not necessary.

ASSESSMENT

1. Note reasons for therapy, disease onset, other therapies trialed; tamoxifen failure date.
2. Drug is not for use in premenopausal women.
3. Treatment should continue until tumor progression is evident.
4. List drugs prescribed; if a potent CYP3A4 inducer such as rifampicin or phenytoin, the recommended dose requires adjustment to 50 mg from 25 mg daily.
5. Continue mammograms/CT to follow disease progression.
6. Monitor VS, CBC, chemistry, renal and LFTs, and BMD.

CLIENT/FAMILY TEACHING

1. Used for the treatment of advanced breast cancer in postmenopausal women whose disease has progressed following tamoxifen therapy or adjuvant treatment of postmenopausal women with estrogen-receptor positive early breast cancer who meet criteria.
2. Take once daily after a meal. Consume adequate fluids to prevent dehydration.
3. Drug will lower estrogen levels; anticipate therapy may be for prolonged period of time. May lower bone density and increase risk for fractures.
4. Androgenic effects may occur i.e., acne, hair loss or hoarseness.
5. Report if GI upset, headaches, depression, chest pain, SOB, fatigue or edema occur or become intolerable.
6. Keep all F/U to assess response and adverse SE.

OUTCOMES/EVALUATE

- Treatment of progressive breast cancer in postmenopausal women following tamoxifen therapy
- Adjuvant therapy in estrogen receptor-positive early breast cancer that meets criteria
- Prevention of prostate cancer (unlabeled)

Exenatide

(ex-**EN**-a-tide)

Classification(s): Antidiabetic, incretin mimetic

Pregnancy Category: C

RX: Byetta.

INDICATIONS/USES

Adjunctive therapy to diet and exercise to improve glycemic control in adults with type 2 diabetes mellitus. *NOTE:* Exenatide is not a substitute for insulin in insulin-dependent clients.

ACTION/KINETICS

Action

Exenatide enhances glucose-dependent insulin secretion by pancreatic beta-cells, suppresses inappropriately elevated glucagon secretion, and slows gastric emptying. Exenatide is an incretin (glucagon-like peptide-1) mimetic agent that mimics the enhancement of glucose-dependent insulin secretion, as well as several other antihyperglycemic actions of incretins. The drug binds and activates known human glucagon-like peptide-1 receptors, leading to an increase in both glucagon-dependent synthesis of insulin and secretion of insulin from pancreatic beta cells in the presence of elevated glucose concentrations. Glycemic control is improved by reducing fasting and postprandial glucose levels.

Pharmacokinetics

Peak plasma levels: 2.1 hr. Eliminated mainly by glomerular filtration and subsequent proteolytic degradation. **t½, terminal:** 2.4 hr. Mean clearance is reduced in end-stage renal disease.

CONTRAINDICATIONS

Hypersensitivity to the product or any of its components. Use with type-1 diabetes or to treat diabetic ketoacidosis. Use in end-stage renal disease or severe renal impairment (C_{CR} <30 mL/min) or in severe GI disease.

SPECIAL CONCERNS

- **Clients may develop anti-exenatide antibodies; antibody titers diminish with time.**
- **Exenatide, by slowing gastric emptying time, may reduce the rate and extent of absorption of oral drugs; thus, use with caution in those receiving oral medications that require rapid GI absorption.**
- **Use with caution in clients with renal transplants and during lactation.**
- **Safety and efficacy not determined in children.**

SIDE EFFECTS

Most Common

N&V, dizziness, headache, jittery feeling, diarrhea, dyspepsia.

Side effects include those when exenatide is used alone or with other hypoglycemics. **Metabolic:** Hypoglycemia (mild to moderate usually). **GI:** N&V, diarrhea, dyspepsia, dysgeusia, decreased appetite, gastroesophageal reflux disease, abdominal distention, abdominal pain, ***acute pancreatitis (including fatal and nonfatal necrotizing and hemorrhagic)***, constipation, eructation, flatulence. **CNS:** Dizziness, jittery feeling, headache, somnolence. **GU:** Altered renal function, including renal impairment, worsened chronic renal failure, and acute renal failure. **Respiratory:** Chronic hypersensitivity pneumonitis. **Hypersensitivity:** ***Angioedema***, generalized pruritus and/or urticaria, macular or papular rash, ***anaphylaxis*** (rare). **Body as a whole:** Asthenia, hyperhidrosis, chills, development of anti-exenatide antibodies, hypersensitivity reactions. **Miscellaneous:** Acute renal failure, chest pain, injection-site reactions.

LABORATORY TEST CONSIDERATIONS

↑ Serum creatinine.

OVERDOSE MANAGEMENT

Symptoms: Hypoglycemia (may be a rapid fall in BG), severe N&V. *Treatment:* Treat hypoglycemia with PO carbohydrate. Initiate appropriate supportive treatment according to the client's clinical signs and symptoms.

DRUG INTERACTIONS

Acetaminophen / ↓ Acetaminophen AUC and C_{max} and ↑ acetaminophen T_{max}; give acetaminophen 1 hr before or 4 hr after exenatide
Antibiotics, oral / Possible ↓ absorption of antibiotics; take the antibiotic at least 1 hr before exenatide injection
Digoxin / ↓ Exenatide C_{max} and delayed T_{max} by about 2.5 hr
Lovastatin / ↓ Lovastatin AUC and C_{max}; T_{max} delayed about 4 hr; monitor and adjust dosage if needed
Oral contraceptives / Possible ↓ absorption of contraceptive; take oral contraceptives at least 1 hr before exenatide injection
Oral hypoglycemics (e.g., meglitinides, sulfonylureas) / ↑ Risk of hypoglycemia; closely monitor blood glucose levels and when exenatide is started or stopped in clients receiving oral hypoglycemics
Warfarin / ↑ INR → ↑ risk of bleeding; monitor PT times

HOW SUPPLIED

Injection Solution: 250 mcg/mL.

DOSAGE

SC

Diabetes mellitus, type 2.

Initial: 5 mcg/dose given 2 times per day at any time within the 60 min period before the morning and evening meals (or before the main meals of the day and about 6 hr between doses). Do not give after a meal. Dose can be increased to 10 mcg twice a day after 1 month.

NURSING IMPLICATIONS

IMPLEMENTATION/ADMINISTRATION/STORAGE

1. Initiation with a 5 mcg dose decreases the incidence and severity of GI side effects.
2. Give the dose SC in the thigh, abdomen, or upper arm.
3. Use caution when escalating the dose from 5 to 10 mcg in those with moderate renal impairment (C_{CR} 30–50 mL/min).
4. When exenatide is added to metformin or thiazolidinedione therapy, the current dose of metformin or thiazolidinedione can be continued as it is unlikely the hypoglycemia will require dosage adjustment. When exenatide is added to sulfonylurea therapy, consider a reduction in dose of the sulfonylurea to reduce the risk of hypoglycemia.
5. Prior to the first use, refrigerate from 2–8°C (36–46°F); after the first use, can be kept at a temperature not to exceed 25°C (77°F). Do not freeze; do not use if the drug has been frozen. Protect from light. Discard the pen 30 days after the first use, even if some drug remains in the pen. Do not share the pen with other clients.

ASSESSMENT

1. Note reasons for therapy, age at disease onset, other agents trialed, outcome. List drugs prescribed to ensure none interact unfavorably.
2. Assess for gastroparesis; drug slows stomach emptying so food passes more slowly through stomach. Determine if timing of other prescribed medications, i.e., birth control pills, antibiotics, should be changed to accommodate these effects.
3. If pancreatitis is suspected, discontinue exenatide. Perform confirmatory tests, and initiate appropriate treatment. Do not resume treatment with exenatide if pancreatitis is confirmed and an alternative etiology for the pancreatitis has not been identified.
4. If kidney dysfunction occurs, reevaluate therapy and do not increase dose.
5. Monitor VS, weight, HbA1c, renal and LFTs; ensure C_{CR} is >30 mL/min.

CLIENT/FAMILY TEACHING

1. Drug is used to help control blood sugars in adults with type 2 diabetes. It is injected twice a day 1 hour before breakfast and dinner by a pen. Do not administer after a meal. Review patient information pamphlet.
2. Generally used with metformin or a sulfonylurea. Drug is injected under the skin into upper leg, stomach, or upper arm. After instruction observe first dose in office to assess client technique. Monitor FS and report any unusual readings. Inject as directed.
3. Also comes in a prefilled pen with 60 doses to allow 30 days of therapy. Pen needles are ordered separately and are to be discarded after each injection.
4. Read directions prior to using pen. Must follow directions in the “new pen setup” section for each new pen before first use. May visit www.byetta.com for tutorial of pen setup.
5. Store pen in original carton, and refrigerate once activated. Thirty days after activating, discard Byetta pen even if not completely empty. Mark with date when pen first used.
6. Liquid in the pen cartridge should be clear, colorless, and free of particles. Report any damaged/broken pens or for further instructions call 1-800-868-1190 or go to www.byetta.com.
7. Follow dietary guidelines, perform regular exercise, weight loss, dietary restrictions, and other lifestyle changes consistent with controlling diabetes.
8. Keep out of reach of children.
9. Report any adverse side effects including injection site reactions, persistently low blood sugars, abdominal pain, changes in urine output, dizziness, N&V. Carry easily digestible carbohydrate (peanut butter crackers) to offset low sugars.
10. Practice reliable contraceptive measures. Do not use if breast-feeding.
11. Keep all F/U visits to assess response, labs, and for dosage adjustment as needed.

OUTCOMES/EVALUATE

Control of blood sugars; HbA1c <8

Ezetimibe

(eh-**ZET**-eh-myb)

Classification(s): Antihyperlipidemic drug

Pregnancy Category: C

RX: Zetia.

INDICATIONS/USES

(1) Primary hypercholesterolemia (heterozygous familial and nonfamilial), either as monotherapy or combination therapy as adjunctive therapy with diet, with HMG-CoA reductase inhibitors to reduce elevated total cholesterol, LDL-C, and Apo B. (2) With atorvastatin or simvastatin to reduce elevated total-C and LDL-C levels in homozygous familial hypercholesterolemia as an adjunct to other lipid-lowering treatments (e.g., LDL apheresis) or if such treatments are unavailable. (3) As adjunctive therapy to diet to reduce elevated sitosterol and campesterol levels in homozygous familial sitosterolemia. (4) With fenofibrate as adjunctive therapy to diet to reduce total cholesterol, LDL-C, Apo B, and non-high-density lipoprotein cholesterol (non-HDL-C) in clients with mixed hyperlipidemia.

ACTION/KINETICS

Action

Acts at the brush border of the small intestine to inhibit the absorption of cholesterol, leading to a decrease in the delivery of cholesterol to the liver. This results in a decrease of hepatic cholesterol stores and an increase in clearance of cholesterol from the blood. This complements the mechanism of action of HMG-CoA reductase inhibitors. Reduces total cholesterol, LDL cholesterol, Apo B, and triglycerides as well as increases HDL cholesterol. Has no effect on the fat-soluble vitamins A, D, and E.

Pharmacokinetics

Peak plasma ezetimibe levels: 4–12 hr. C_{max} is increased by a high-fat meal. Converted to the active exetimibe glucuronide. **t½, parent drug and active metabolite:** 22 hr. After PO administration, is rapidly conjugated to the active phenolic glucuronide in the small intestine and liver. Mainly excreted through the feces with smaller amounts through the urine. **Plasma protein binding:** More than 90% (ezetimibe-glucuronide).

CONTRAINDICATIONS

Use with HMG-CoA reductase inhibitors in pregnant or nursing women and in active liver disease or unexplained persistent elevations in serum transaminases. As monotherapy in moderate to severe hepatic insufficiency. Use during lactation unless the potential benefit outweighs the potential risk to the infant. Use in children under 10 years old.

SPECIAL CONCERNS

If used with HMG-CoA reductase inhibitors or fenofibrate, be aware of contraindications, special concerns, and side effects of these drugs as well.

SIDE EFFECTS

Most Common

Back/abdominal pain, diarrhea, arthralgia, sinusitis, coughing, pharyngitis.

GI: Diarrhea, nausea, abdominal pain. **Hepatic:** Cholelithiasis, hepatitis, cholecystitis, ***pancreatitis***. **CNS:** Headache, dizziness. **Hematologic:** Thrombocytopenia. **Musculoskeletal:** Myalgia, back pain, arthralgia, possible myopathy or rhabdomyolysis. **Respiratory:** URTI, sinusitis, pharyngitis, coughing. **Miscellaneous:** Chest pain, fatigue, viral infection; hypersensitivity reactions, including ***anaphylaxis***, ***angioedema***, rash, urticaria.

LABORATORY TEST CONSIDERATIONS

↑ Liver transaminases greater than or equal to 3 times ULN, CPK.

DRUG INTERACTIONS

Antacids / ↓ Ezetimibe C_{max} after both Mg^{++}- and Ca^{++}-containing antacids; no effect on AUC

Cholestyramine / ↓ Ezetimibe AUC probably R/T ↓ absorption

Cyclosporine / ↑ AUC and C_{max} of total ezetimibe; monitor carefully; possibly ↑ cyclosporine AUC

Fenofibrate/Gemfibrozil / ↑ Total ezetimibe levels; concomitant use not recommended

HOW SUPPLIED

Tablets: 10 mg.

DOSAGE

TABLETS

Primary hypercholesterolemia, homozygous familial hypercholesterolemia, homozygous sitosterolemia, with fenofibrate in mixed hyperlipidemia.

10 mg once daily with or without food.

NURSING IMPLICATIONS

Do not confuse Zetia with Zestril (an antihypertensive).

IMPLEMENTATION/ADMINISTRATION/STORAGE

1. Place client on a standard cholesterol-lowering diet before therapy and for duration of treatment.
2. May be given with a HMG-CoA reductase inhibitor or with fenofibrate for an incremental effect. Dose of both drugs can be given at the same time.
3. Give at least 2 hr before or at least 4 hr after giving a bile sequestrant.
4. Before initiating therapy exclude or, if appropriate, treat secondary causes for dyslipidemia (e.g., diabetes, hypothyroidism, obstructive liver disease, chronic renal failure, drugs that increase LDL-C and decrease HDL-C).
5. Plasma levels are about two-fold higher in geriatric clients.
6. Store from 15–30°C (59–86°F) protected from moisture.

ASSESSMENT

1. Note reasons for therapy: plaque stability or elevated TG/LDL cholesterol in CAD. List other agents trialed, outcome.
2. List all drugs prescribed; ensure none interact unfavorably. Identify cardiac risk factors.
3. Assess level of adherence to weight reduction, exercise, cholesterol-lowering diet, and BP or BS control. Note any alcohol abuse or liver dysfunction.
4. Monitor CBC, lipid panel, CK, renal and LFTs. Schedule LFTs at the beginning of therapy (6 weeks) and if stable, semiannually for the first year of therapy. Special attention should be paid to elevated serum transaminase levels.

CLIENT/FAMILY TEACHING

1. Take daily as directed with or without food. Avoid taking with antacids; reduces drug effect.
2. Drug acts by inhibiting cholesterol absorption in the small intestine. May experience GI upset and muscle and back pains; report if persistent.
3. A low-cholesterol diet must continue to be followed during drug therapy. Consult dietitian for assistance in meal planning and food preparation.
4. Report any S&S of infections, unexplained muscle pain, tenderness/weakness (especially if accompanied by fever or malaise), surgery, trauma, or metabolic disorders.
5. Review importance of following a low-cholesterol diet, regular exercise, low alcohol consumption, and not smoking in the overall plan to reduce serum cholesterol levels and inhibit progression of CAD.
6. Not for use during pregnancy; use barrier contraception.
7. Keep all F/U to assess response, labs, and adverse SE.

OUTCOMES/EVALUATE

↓ Total cholesterol, LDL cholesterol, and triglycerides; ↑ HDL cholesterol

Combination Drug

Ezetimibe and Simvastatin

(eh-**ZET**-eh-myb, **sim**-vah-**STAH**-tin)

Classification(s): Combination antihyperlipidemic drugs

Pregnancy Category: X

RX: Vytorin 10/10, 10/20, 10/40, or 10/80.

SEE ALSO ***EZETIMIBE*** AND ***SIMVASTATIN***.

INDICATIONS/USES

(1) Adjunctive therapy to diet to reduce elevated total-C, LDL-C, Apo B, triglycerides, and non-HDL-C and to increase HDL-C in clients with primary (heterozygous familial or nonfamilial) hyperlipidemia or mixed hyperlipidemia. (2) Reduction of elevated total-C and LDL-C in clients with homozygous familial hypercholesterolemia, as an adjunct to other lipid-lowering treatments (e.g., LDL apheresis) or if such treatments are not available.

CONTENT

All strengths contain ezetimibe, 10 mg with either 10 mg, 20 mg, 40 mg, or 80 mg simvastatin.

ACTION/KINETICS

Action

Ezetimibe reduces blood cholesterol by inhibiting absorption of cholesterol by the small intestine, leading to a decrease of hepatic cholesterol stores and an increased clearance of cholesterol from the blood. Simvastatin decreases cholesterol by inhibiting conversion of HMG-CoA to mevolonate, an early step in the biosynthesis of cholesterol. Also, simvastatin reduces VLDL and triglycerides and increases HDL-C.

Pharmacokinetics

Ezetimibe is absorbed and converted to the active exetimibe-glucuronide. High-fat or nonfat meals have no effect on the extent of absorption. Ezetimibe is metabolized in the small intestine and liver by glucuronide conjugation and excreted in both the feces and urine. Simvastatin undergoes extensive first-pass liver metabolism and is mainly excreted in the bile.

CONTRAINDICATIONS

Use not recommended with moderate or severe hepatic insufficiency. Lactation.

SPECIAL CONCERNS

- **Give to women of childbearing age only when conception is highly unlikely.**
- **Use with caution with niacin.**
- **Possible association between use of ezetimibe/simvastatin and increased incidence of cancer.**
- **Due to increased risk of myopathy, use caution when treating Chinese clients with ezetimibe/simvastatin coadministered with lipid-modifying doses of niacin (1 gram/day or more).**
- **Safety and efficacy for use in children not sufficiently evaluated.**

SIDE EFFECTS

Most Common

Headache, myalgia, URTI, influenza, abdominal pain, diarrhea, arthralgia, back pain, sinusitis, pharyngitis, chest pain, dizziness, fatigue.

See *Ezetimibe* and *Simvastatin* for a complete list of possible side effects.

LABORATORY TEST CONSIDERATIONS

↑ Serum transaminases (>3 × ULN).

DRUG INTERACTIONS

Amiodarone / ↑ Risk of myopathy/rhabdomyolysis; do not use more than Vytorin, 10/20 mg daily

Bile acid sequestrants / Give ezetimibe/simvastatin either 2 hr or more before or 4 hr or more after the bile acid sequestrant

Clarithromycin / ↑ Risk of myopathy/rhabdomyolysis; do not use together

Cyclosporine / ↑ Risk of myopathy/rhabdomyolysis; do not use more than Vytorin, 10/10 mg daily; also, do not start ezetimibe/simvastatin unless the client has already tolerated simvastatin at a dose of 5 mg or higher

Danazol / ↑ Risk of myopathy/rhabdomyolysis; do not use more than Vytorin, 10/10 mg daily; also, do not start ezetimibe/simvastatin unless the client has already tolerated simvastatin at a dose of 5 mg or higher

Diltiazem / Do not exceed ezetimibe/simvastatin 10/40 per day

Erythromycin / ↑ Risk of myopathy/rhabdomyolysis; do not use together

Fibrates / Safety and efficacy of ezetimibe/simvastatin not established do not use together

Gemfibrozil / Use generally not recommended R/T ↑ Risk of myopathy/rhabdomyolysis; if coadministration needed, do not use Vytorin more than 10/10 mg daily

Grapefruit juice (>1 qt daily) / ↑ Risk of myopathy/rhabdomyolysis; do not use together

HIV protease inhibitors / ↑ Risk of myopathy/rhabdomyolysis; do not use together

Itraconazole / ↑ Risk of myopathy/rhabdomyolysis; do not use together

Ketoconazole / ↑ Risk of myopathy/rhabdomyolysis; do not use together

Nefazodone / ↑ Risk of myopathy/rhabdomyolysis; do not use together

Telithromycin / ↑ Risk of myopathy/rhabdomyolysis; do not use together

Verapamil / ↑ Risk of myopathy/rhabdomyolysis; do not use more than Vytorin, 10/20 mg daily

HOW SUPPLIED

See *Content*.

DOSAGE

TABLETS

Primary hypercholesterolemia.

Usual, initial: 10/20 mg/day. Beginning with 10/10 mg/day may be considered for those requiring less aggressive LDL-C reductions. Those requiring a larger LDL-C reduction (>55%) may be started on 10/40 mg/day. After initiation or titration of Vytorin, lipid levels may be analyzed after 2 or more weeks; adjust dosage, if necessary. **Dose range:** 10/10 mg/day through 10/80 mg/day.

Homozygous familial hypercholesterolemia.
10/40 mg/day or 10/80 mg/day, with other lipid-lowering treatments (e.g., LDL apheresis).

NURSING IMPLICATIONS

IMPLEMENTATION/ADMINISTRATION/STORAGE

1. Prior to beginning therapy with Vytorin, secondary causes for dyslipidemia (i.e., diabetes, hypothyroidism, obstructive liver disease, chronic renal failure, and drugs that increase LDL-C and decrease HDL-C) should be excluded or, if appropriate, treated.
2. Place client on a standard cholesterol-lowering diet before giving Vytorin; continue the diet during Vytorin treatment.
3. Individualize Vytorin dose according to baseline LDL-C, recommended goal of therapy, and client's response.
4. No dosage adjustment is needed with mild hepatic insufficiency or mild to moderate renal insufficiency. In severe renal insufficiency, do not begin Vytorin unless client has tolerated treatment with simvastatin, at a dose of 5 mg or higher. Use caution when using Vytorin in these clients; monitor closely.
5. If given with bile acid sequestrants, give Vytorin either 2 hr or more before or 4 hr or more after giving the bile acid sequestrant.
6. Store from 20–25°C (68–77°F). Store in original container until time of use.

ASSESSMENT

1. Note reasons for therapy, family history, risk factors, other agents trialed, outcome. List drugs prescribed to ensure none interact.
2. Assess for seizure history and any muscle problems/disease.
3. Identify any metabolic, endocrine, or electrolyte disorders.
4. Check adherence to cholesterol-lowering diet, weight control, and regular daily exercise.
5. Monitor VS, lipid panel, CK, renal and LFTs; reduce with dysfunction. Monitor lipid levels before starting therapy, 2 weeks after starting therapy or dose changed, and periodically thereafter.

CLIENT/FAMILY TEACHING

1. Take as a single dose in the evening, with or without food. If also prescribed bile sequestrant (e.g., cholestyramine, colestipol, colesevelam), take Vytorin at least 2 hr before or 4 hr after bile subsequent dose.
2. May cause visual changes or drowsiness; avoid activities that require mental alertness until drug effects realized.
3. Avoid grapefruit and grapefruit juice; may increase drug concentrations and adverse effects.
4. Report any new onset muscle pain, weakness, abdominal pain, fever, dark urine, yellowing of skin, or appetite loss. Avoid any OTC or unprescribed drug without approval.
5. Use reliable contraception; do not take if pregnancy suspected.
6. Continue dietary changes of reduced saturated fat intake, increased soluble fiber intake, regular daily exercise, weight control, smoking cessation in overall goal of cholesterol control.
7. Avoid alcohol: may increase risk of liver problems.
8. Keep all F/U to assess response, labs, and for adverse SE.

OUTCOMES/EVALUATE

↓ Total and LDL cholesterol ↑ HDL

Ezogabine

(e-**ZOG**-a-been)

Classification(s): Anticonvulsant, potassium channel opener

Pregnancy Category: C

RX: Potiga.

SEE ALSO ***ANTICONVULSANTS***.

INDICATIONS/USES

Adjunctive treatment of partial onset seizures in clients 18 years and older.

ACTION/KINETICS

Action

The mechanism has not been fully elucidated. The drug enhances transmembrane potassium currents resulting in stabilization of the resting membrane potential and thus reduction of brain excitability. It may also augment gamma-aminobutyric acid-mediated currents.

Pharmacokinetics

Rapidly absorbed. T_{max}: 0.5–2 hr. Absolute oral bioavailability is about 60%. A high fat meal increases C_{max} and delays T_{max}. Extensively metabolized in the liver primarily by UGT1A4 and NAT2. One metabolite, the N-acetyl metabolite, has anticonvulsant activity but it is less potent than ezogabine. Excreted mainly (85%) in the urine; about 14% excreted in the feces. Dosage adjustments are required in those with impaired hepatic and renal function, as well as in the elderly.

CONTRAINDICATIONS

Lactation.

SPECIAL CONCERNS

- **Ezogabine may cause urinary retention; elderly males with symptomatic benign prostatic hypertrophy may be at increased risk for urinary retention.**
- **Safety and efficacy not determined in children younger than 18 years.**

SIDE EFFECTS

Most Common

Dizziness, confusional state, somnolence, tremor, vertigo, abnormal coordination, attention disturbance, impaired memory, aphasia, balance disorder, dysarthria, gait disturbance, diplopia, blurred vision, fatigue, asthenia.

CNS: Dizziness, confusional state, somnolence, tremor, vertigo, abnormal coordination, attention disturbance, impaired memory, aphasia, balance disorder, dysarthria, gait disturbance, amnesia, anxiety, disorientation, dysphasia, paresthesia, psychotic disorder, hallucinations, hypokinesia, coma, encephalopathy, euphoric mood, syncope, ***suicidal behavior***, ideation. **GI:** Nausea, constipation, dyspepsia, dry mouth, dysphagia, increased appetite. **CV:** QT prolongation. **GU:** Hematuria, urinary hesitation, dysuria, chromaturia, urinary retention, nephrolithiasis, renal colic. **Dermatologic:** Alopecia, rash, hyperhidrosis. **Respiratory:** Dyspnea. **Hematologic:** Leukopenia, neutropenia, thrombocytopenia. **Ophthalmic:** Diplopia, blurred vision, nystagmus. **Body as a whole:** Fatigue, asthenia, malaise, influenza, increased weight, peripheral edema, muscle spasms. **Miscellaneous**: Myoclonus.

LABORATORY TEST CONSIDERATIONS

Ezogabine interferes with assays of both serum and urine bilirubin → falsely elevated readings.

OVERDOSE MANAGEMENT

Symptoms: In addition to side effects seen at therapeutic doses, other symptoms include agitation, aggressive behavior, and irritability. *Treatment:* There is no specific antidote. Use standard medical practice for treating overdosage. Ensure adequate airway, oxygenation, and maintain ventilation. Monitor cardiac rhythm and measure vital signs.

DRUG INTERACTIONS

An additive effect of ezogabine with other drugs that prolong the QT interval cannot be excluded. The following drugs may prolong the QT interval and increase the risk of life–threatening cardiac arrhythmias, including torsades de pointes: Amiodarone, arsenic trioxide, bretylium, chlorpromazine, cisapride, disopyramide, dofetilide, dolasetron, droperidol, gatifloxacin, halofantrine, levomethadyl, mefloquine, mesoridazine, moxifloxacin, pentamidine, pimozide, probucol, procainamide, quinidine, sotalol, sparfloxacin, thioridazine, and ziprasidone.

Alcohol / ↑ Exposure to ezogabine → ↑ side effects

Carbamazepine / ↑ Ezogabine clearance; dose ↑ may be necessary when used with carbamazepine

Digoxin / Dose–dependent ↑ in digoxin levels; monitor digoxin levels and adjust dosage as needed

Lamotrigine / ↓ Lamotrigine AUC and ↑ clearance; monitor clinical response

Phenytoin / ↓ Ezogabine AUC and C_{max} and ↑ clearance; consider ↑ ezogabine dose when used with phenytoin

HOW SUPPLIED

Tablets: 50 mg, 200 mg, 300 mg, 400 mg.

DOSAGE

TABLETS

Partial-onset seizures.

Adults, initial: 100 mg 3 times a day. For dose titration, increase dosage gradually at weekly intervals by no more than 50 mg 3 times a day. **Maintenance:** 200–400 mg 3 times a day, based on client response and tolerability. **Maximum dose:** 400 mg 3 times a day. **Elderly, older than 65 years, initial:** 50 mg 3 times a day. For dose titration, increase dosage at weekly intervals by no more than 50 mg 3 times a day. **Maximum dose:** 250 mg 3 times a day.

E

NURSING IMPLICATIONS

IMPLEMENTATION/ADMINISTRATION/STORAGE

1. Adjust the dosage as follows in those with impaired renal function. If C_{CR} is less than 50 mL/min or the client is at end-stage renal disease on dialysis, the initial dose should be 50 mg 3 times a day. For dose titration, increase the dose no more than 50 mg 3 times a day at weekly intervals. Do not exceed the maximum dose of 200 mg 3 times a day.
2. Adjust the dosage as follows in those with impaired hepatic function. If the Child-Pugh score is more than 7–9, give an initial dose of 50 mg 3 times a day. For dosage titration, increase the dosage by no more than 50 mg 3 times a day at weekly intervals. Do not exceed the maximum dose of 250 mg 3 times a day. If the Child-Pugh score is more than 9, give an initial dose of 50 mg 3 times a day. For dosage titration, increase the dosage by no more than 50 mg 3 times a day at weekly intervals. Do not exceed the maximum dose of 200 mg 3 times a day.
3. For discontinuation of therapy, gradually reduce the dose over a period of at least 3 weeks, unless safety concerns require abrupt discontinuation.
4. When discontinuing the drug, withdraw slowly to minimize the potential of increased seizure frequency. Reduce the dose over a period of 3 weeks, unless safety concerns mandate abrupt withdrawal.
5. To provide information on the effects of in utero exposure to ezogabine, health care providers are advised to recommend that pregnant clients taking ezogabine enroll in the North American Antiepileptic Drug Pregnancy Registry. Enroll by calling 1-888-233-2334; clients must enroll themselves. Information on the registry can be found at the website: http://www.aedpregnancyregistry.org.
6. Store from 15–30°C (59–86°F).

ASSESSMENT

1. Note indications for therapy, age at seizure onset, characteristics of seizures, mental status, and other agents trialed.
2. List drugs prescribed to ensure none interact.
3. If drug is discontinued, gradually reduce dose over a period of at least 3 weeks, unless safety concerns require abrupt withdrawal.
4. Note any cardiac history; may prolong QT interval. Assess ECG.
5. Carefully assess any urologic symptoms; may cause urinary retention.
6. May cause hallucinations, psychotic symptoms and confusional states: evaluate closely.
7. Monitor VS, ECG, renal and LFTs; reduce dose with dysfunction.

CLIENT/FAMILY TEACHING

1. Swallow tablets whole. Do not break, crush, dissolve, or chew tablets before swallowing. Give in 3 equally divided doses daily with or without food.
2. Use caution performing activities that require mental alertness; may cause dizziness, drowsiness, double or blurred vision.
3. Notify provider if urinary retention (including urinary hesitation and dysuria), inability to urinate, and/or pain with urination occurs.
4. Do not stop drug suddenly, may cause seizures.
5. Avoid alcohol and OTC agents without approval.
6. Drug may increase risk of suicidal thoughts and behavior; report new onset or worsening of symptoms of depression, unusual changes in mood or behavior, or suicidal thoughts, behavior, or thoughts of self-harm to provider immediately.
7. Practice reliable contraception; if pregnancy occurs report and enroll in North American Antiepileptic Drug Pregnancy Registry by calling 1-888-233-2334.
8. Keep all F/U to assess response, labs and adverse SE.

OUTCOMES/EVALUATE

Control of seizures

F

IV

Factor IX Injection

(**FAK**-tor 9)

Classification(s): Antihemophilic agent.

Pregnancy Category: C

RX: AlphaNine SD, BeneFIX, Mononine.

Factor IX Complex

Classification(s): Antihemophilic agent.

Pregnancy Category: C

RX: Bebulin VH, Profilnine SD.

INDICATIONS/USES

Factor IX Injection: (1) To prevent and control bleeding in clients with factor IX deficiency (hemophilia B/Christmas disease). (2) BeneFIX: To control and prevent bleeding in these clients in surgical settings.

Factor IX Complex: To prevent and control bleeding in clients with factor IX deficiency (hemophilia B/Christmas disease).

ACTION/KINETICS

Action

Factor IX is deficient in hemophilia B and in those with acquired factor IX deficiencies. Administration of factor IX (human or recombinant) increases factor IX plasma levels and can temporarily correct the anticoagulation defect in these clients. Factor IX is activated by factor VII/tissue factor complex in the extrinsic coagulation pathway; also activated by factor XIa in the intrinsic coagulation pathway. Activated factor IX, in combination with activated factor VIII, activates factor X. This ultimately causes conversion of prothrombin to thrombin. Thrombin then converts fibrinogen to fibrin; thus, a clot is formed.

Factor IX complex products are a mixture of vitamin-K-dependent clotting factors found in normal plasma. Administration causes an increase in plasma levels of factor IX and can temporarily correct the coagulation defect of those with factor IX deficiency. Administration of Proplex T also increases plasma factor VII levels and can temporarily correct the coagulation defect of those with factor VII deficiency. Plasma levels of factors II and X will also be increased by Bebulin VH and Proplex T.

Pharmacokinetics

t½: Varies, depending on the product. The mean increase in circulating factor IX after IV infusion is 0.67–1.15 international units/dL rise per international units/kg body weight. One unit is the activity present in 1 mL of pooled normal fresh plasma.

CONTRAINDICATIONS

Hypersensitivity to mouse (Mononine) or hamster (BeneFIX) proteins. Disseminated intravascular coagulation (Proplex T). Signs of fibrinolysis (Factor IX Complex).

SPECIAL CONCERNS

- **Assess benefit versus risk prior to use in liver disease or elective surgery.**
- **Factor IX products may be derived from pooled units of human plasma; although precautions are taken, the risk of viral infections from such products cannot be eliminated completely.**
- **Due to the possibility of thromboembolic complications, use Factor IX injection with caution with liver disease, postoperatively, in neonates, or in those at risk for thromboembolic phenomena or disseminated intravascular coagulation.**
- **Safety during lactation not known.**
- **Safety and efficacy not determined in children less than 16 years of age for AlphaNine SD or Profilnine SD. Safety and efficacy have been evaluated for BeneFIX and Mononine. Use special care using Proplex T in newborns because a higher mortality/morbidity may be associated with hepatitis.**

SIDE EFFECTS

Most Common

Nausea, discomfort at IV site, altered taste, burning sensation in the jaw and skull, allergic rhinitis, lightheadedness, headache.

Side effects may be similar, regardless of the product. **CV:** ***DIC, thrombosis. High doses may cause MI, venous or pulmonary thrombosis***, hypotension, thrombosis. **Symptoms due to rapid infusion:** N&V, headache, fever, chills, tingling,

F

flushing, urticaria, and changes in BP or pulse rate. Most of these side effects disappear when rate of administration is slowed. **Hypersensitivity:** Hives, generalized urticaria, angioedema, chest tightness, dyspnea, wheezing, faintness, hypotension, tachycardia, ***anaphylaxis***. **GI:** N&V, diarrhea, altered taste. **CNS:** Lightheadedness, headache, dizziness, drowsiness. **Respiratory:** Dry cough/sneeze, urge to cough with hypoxemia, lung disorder, tight chest, dyspnea, allergic rhinitis, asthma, ***laryngeal edema***. **Dermatologic:** Flushing, hives, rash, photosensitivity reaction, urticaria. **GU:** Nephrotic syndrome, renal infarct. **At injection site:** Burning, stinging, phlebitis, cellulitis, pain. **Body as a whole:** Chills, fever, lethargy, tingling, shaking. **Ophthalmic:** Visual disturbances. **Miscellaneous:** Cyanosis, burning sensation in jaw and skull, inadequate factor IX recovery, factor IX inhibitor, development.

NOTE: The preparation also contains trace amounts of blood groups A and B and isohemagglutinins, which may cause intravascular hemolysis when administered in large amounts to clients with blood groups A, B, and AB. Although careful screening is undertaken, both hepatitis and AIDS may be transmitted using factor IX concentrates since it is derived from pooled human plasma.

LABORATORY TEST CONSIDERATIONS

↑ ALT, AST, alkaline phosphatase.

DRUG INTERACTIONS

↑ Risk of thrombosis if administered with aminocaproic acid

HOW SUPPLIED

Factor IX Injection. ***Injection, Lyophilized Powder for Solution:*** **AlphaNine SD:** 150 or more units of factor IX (human)/mg protein.*
BeneFIX (units of factor IX, recombinant): 250 units, 500 units, 1,000 units, 2,000 units.*
Mononine (units of factor IX, human): About 500 units, about 1,000 units.*
**NOTE:* Actual factor IX activity in units stated on the label of each vial.
Factor IX Complex. ***Injection, Lyophilized Powder for Solution:*** **Bebulin VH and Profilnine SD:** Factors IX, II, X, and low amounts of VII (human).*
NOTE: Actual factor IX activity in units stated on the label of each vial.

DOSAGE

Factor IX: AlphaNine SD

IV

Minor to major hemorrhages; surgery.

Dosage individualized. One unit approximates the activity of 1 mL of pooled normal human plasma. The following formula may be used as a guide to determine the number of units to be given:

No. of factor IX units required = body weight (kg) × desired increase in factor IX (%) × 1 unit/kg.

For minor hemorrhage (bruises, cuts, scrapes; uncomplicated joint hemorrhage): Bring factor IX levels to 20–30% (factor IX 20–30 units/kg twice a day) until hemorrhage stops and healing has been achieved (1–2 days).

For moderate hemorrhage (nose bleeds, mouth/gum bleeds, dental extractions, hematuria): Bring factor IX levels to 25–50% (factor IX 25–50 units/kg twice a day) until healing has been achieved (average, 2–7 days).

For major hemorrhage (joint/muscle hemorrhages, especially in the large muscles; major trauma, hematuria, intracranial and intraperitoneal bleeding): Bring factor IX levels to 50% for 3–5 days (factor IX 30–50 units/kg twice a day). Following this treatment period, maintain factor IX levels at 20% (factor IX 20 units/kg twice a day) until healing has been achieved. Major hemorrhages may require treatment for up to 10 days.

Surgery: Prior to surgery, bring factor IX levels to 50–100% of normal (factor IX 50–100 units/kg twice a day). For the next 7–10 days, or until healing has been achieved, maintain clients at 50–100% factor IX levels (factor IX 50–100 units/kg twice a day).

Factor IX: BeneFIX

IV

Minor to major hemorrhages; surgery.

Titrate doses using the factor IX activity and pharmacokinetic parameters (e.g., half-life and recovery), as well as the clinical situation. The method of calculating the factor IX dose is shown in the following equation:

No. of factor IX units required = body weight (kg) × desired factor IX increase (% or units/dL) × 1.3 (units/kg per units/dL)

Adults: In previously treated adults, on average 1 unit of BeneFIX/kg body weight increased the circulating activity of factor IX by 0.78 +/- 0.19 (range, 0.39 to 1.2) units/dL.

Children, less than 15 years of age: On average, 1 unit of BeneFIX/kg body weight increased the circulating activity of factor IX by 0.7 +/- 0.2 (range, 0.2–2.1 units/dL; median, 0.6 units/dL per units/kg).

The following is used to guide dosing:

Minor hemorrhages (uncomplicated hemarthroses, superficial muscle or soft tissue): 20–30% (units/dL) circulating factor IX activity required using a dosing interval of 12–24 hr for 1–2 days.

Moderate hemorrhages (IM or soft tissue with dissection, mucous membranes, dental extractions, hematuria): 25–50% (units/dL) circulating factor IX activity required using a dosing interval of 12–24 hr. Treat until bleeding stops and healing begins (about 2–7 days).

Major hemorrhages (pharynx, retropharynx, retroperitoneum, CNS); surgery: 50–100% (units/dL) circulating factor IX activity required using a dosing interval of 12–24 hr for 7–10 days.

Factor IX: Mononine

IV

Minor spontaneous hemorrhage prophylaxis; major trauma or surgery.

Titrate dosage to the client response. As a general guideline, 1 unit of factor IX activity/kg is expected to increase the level of circulating factor IX by 1% (units/dL) of normal. The following formula provides a guide to dosage calculation:

No. of factor IX units required = body weight (kg) × desired factor IX increase (% or units/dL) × 1 unit/kg (units/kg per units/dL)

Adults, prophylaxis of minor spontaneous hemorrhage: 15–25% (or units/dL) factor IX needed for hemostasis. Initial dosing is up to 20–30 units/kg to achieve desired level. Give once and repeat in 24 hr if needed.

Adults, major trauma or surgery: 25–50% (or units/dL) factor IX needed for hemostasis. Initial dosing is up to 75 units/kg to achieve desired level. Give q 18–30 hr, depending on the half-life and measured factor IX levels. Give up to 10 days, depending on nature of condition.

Children: Dosing is based on body weight and generally based on the same guidelines as adults.

NOTE: Doses of Mononine of at least 75 units/kg are well tolerated. In the presence of an inhibitor to factor IX, higher doses may be necessary.

Factor IX Complex: Bebulin VH

IV

Factor IX deficiency (hemophilia B/Christmas disease).

As a general rule, 1 international unit of factor IX activity/kg will increase the plasma level of factor IX by 0.8%. Response will vary from client to client. The following formula can be used as a guide to determine the number of factor IX units required:

body weight (kg) × desired factor IX increase (%) × 1.2

For minor bleeding, a single dose will usually suffice; otherwise, a second dose may be given after 24 hr. More severe hemorrhage will require administration of several doses at approximately 24 hr intervals. For maintenance therapy, usually two-thirds of the initial dose is used.

The following guidelines are to determine Bebulin VH dosing according to bleeding type:

- **Minor bleeding (early hemarthrosis, minor epistaxis, gingival bleeding,**

mild hematuria). Approximate factor IX level: 20% of normal. **Typical initial dose:** 25–30 units/kg. Average treatment duration: 1 day.

- **Moderate bleeding (severe joint bleeding, early hematoma, major open bleeding, minor trauma, minor hemoptysis, hematemesis, melena, major hematuria).** Approximate factor IX level: 40% of normal. **Typical initial dose:** 40–55 units/kg. Average treatment duration: 2 days or until adequate wound healing.
- **Major bleeding (severe hematoma, major trauma, severe hemoptysis, hematemesis, melena).** Approximate factor IX level: 60% or more of normal. **Typical initial dose:** 60–70 units/kg. Average treatment duration: 2 or 3 days or until adequate wound healing. The following guidelines are to determine Bebulin VH dosing to manage surgical procedures. Give the preoperative loading dose 1 hr prior to surgery. Depending on the surgery type, replacement therapy may continue over 1 to several weeks until adequate wound healing has occurred. The average treatment interval will be 12 hr initially; in the later postoperative period 24 hr is usually sufficient.
- **Major surgery.** On day of surgery: Approximate factor IX level: 60% or more. **Dose:** 70–95 units/kg. For initial postoperative period (week 1–2). Approximate factor IX level: 60–20% of normal. **Dose:** 70–35 units/kg. Late postoperative period (week 3 on). Approximately factor IX level: 20% of normal. **Dose:** 35–25 units/kg.
- **Minor surgery.** On day of surgery: Approximate factor IX level: 40–60%. **Dose:** 50–60 units/kg. For initial postoperative period (week 1–2). Approximate factor IX level: 40–20% of normal. **Dose:** 55–25 units/kg. Late postoperative period (week 3 on). Not applicable. For tooth extraction, use the same initial dose as for minor surgery.

NOTE: Prophylactic doses of 20–30 units/kg given once or preferably up to twice a week significantly reduce the frequency of spontaneous hemorrhage. However, prophylactic dosage must be individualized for each client.

Factor IX Complex: Profilnine SD

IV

Factor IX deficiency (hemophilia B/Christmas disease).

The amount of Profilnine SD required will vary from client to client. Monitor factor IX levels frequently during replacement therapy. A 1% increase in factor IX (0.01 unit)/units administered/kg can be expected. The following formula can be used as a guide to determine the number of units to be given:

body weight (kg) × 1 unit/kg × desired increase in plasma factor (%)

Mild to moderate hemorrhages: Usually a single administration will raise plasma factor IX levels to 20–30%. Serious hemorrhages: Raise the factor IX level by 30–50%. Infusions are usually required daily.

Surgery: Usually requires factor IX levels be raised to 30–50% for at least 1 week following the operation.

Dental extractions: Raise factor IX levels to 50% immediately prior to the procedure. Additional factor IX complex may be given if bleeding recurs.

NOTE: Profilnine SD may be given by injection (plastic disposable syringe only) or infusion. Give at room temperature.

NURSING IMPLICATIONS

IMPLEMENTATION/ADMINISTRATION/STORAGE

1. **IV** Follow manufacturer's guidelines carefully for preparation of the product and administration guidelines.
2. Rate of administration varies with the product. As a general guideline, infuse about 100–200 international units/min at a rate of 2–3 mL/min, do not exceed 3 mL/min. If headache, flushing, or changes in pulse rate or BP occur, stop the infusion until symptoms

subside; then resume at a slower rate. Use the factor IX assay for precise monitoring.

3. Do not administer AlphaNine SD at a rate exceeding 10 mL/min. Rapid administration may cause vasomotor reactions.
4. Before reconstitution, warm diluent to room temperature but not above 40°C (104°F).
5. Agitate solution gently until powder dissolved.
6. Administer within 3 hr of reconstitution; avoid incubation in case contamination occurred during preparation. Do not refrigerate after reconstitution; active ingredient may precipitate out.
7. Discard any unused contents of Factor IX into an appropriate safety container. Discard administration equipment after a single use into an appropriate safety container. Do not resterilize components. Due to risk of exposure to viral infection, those who administer factor IX (human) should use appropriate caution when handling the drug.
8. Store products from 2–8°C (36–46°F). Mononine may be stored up to 25°C (77°F) and AlphaNine SD up to 30°C (86°F) for up to 1 month. BeneFIX may be stored up to 25°C (77°F) for up to 6 months. Do not freeze provided diluent.
9. Discard 2 years after date of manufacture or as directed.
10. COMPATIBILITY Sterile water for injection.
11. INCOMPATIBILITY Administer separately.

ASSESSMENT

1. List any previous experience/treatment with factor replacement and outcome.
2. Obtain weight, height, and blood type. Dose must be individualized based on weight, degree of deficiency, product, and severity of bleed. Maintain plasma level at least 20% of normal until hemostasis achieved.
3. Note any S&S of liver disease (i.e., urticaria, fever, pruritus, anorexia, N&V).
4. Assess carefully for abnormal bruising/bleeding, i.e., enlarged joints, restricted joint movement, oral mucosa for gingival bleeding, drop in H&H, increased menses etc.
5. Advise Factor IX (FIX) complex concentrates have been linked with thromboembolic complications.
6. Monitor BP and pulse q 30 min during infusion.
   - Report increased bleeding and joint swelling; use rest, ice, and elevation with affected joints.
   - Reduce flow rate and report if a tingling sensation, headache, flushing, chills, changes in HR or BP, or fever occur.
   - Avoid aminocaproic acid administration; may cause clot formation.
   - Assess for DIC if FIX level is increased above 50% of normal. At 50% or greater, there is an increased risk for the development of a thromboembolic event and/or DIC.
   - Make sure client has received hepatitis A and B vaccines.
   - Monitor I&O; test urine for occult blood. Hemolytic reactions are more pronounced in clients with A, B, and AB type blood.
7. Monitor LFTs, VS, CBC, coagulation, and factor assay levels. Monitor for the development of FIX inhibitors.

CLIENT/FAMILY TEACHING

1. This drug is a type of protein that is normally produced in your body that helps your blood to form clots to prevent you from bleeding out.
2. Product is prepared from human plasma; has been treated but may carry risks (i.e., hepatitis, AIDS) of transmitting infectious diseases. The man-made product does not have these viruses.
3. Avoid contact sports and any activities that may lead to injury or excessive jostling.
4. Use soft-bristled toothbrush and electric razor to prevent unnecessary bleeding.
5. Report any uncontrolled bleeding, joint pain, swelling. May note changes in skin coloring, SOB, chest pains. Report dark urine, poor appetite, tiredness, yellowed complexion, or low-grade fever followed by nausea, vomiting, and stomach pain.
6. Ensure family members are screened and genetically counselled; disease is hereditary.
7. Immediately report any S&S of hypersensitivity reactions (e.g., angioedema, chest tightness, difficulty breathing or unexplained shortness of breath, faintness, hives, rapid heartbeat, wheezing).
8. Avoid OTCs and aspirin-containing products.
9. Identify local support groups that may assist to cope with this disease.

10. Keep all F/U to assess response, labs, adverse SE.

OUTCOMES/EVALUATE

- Prevention of hemorrhage
- Factor levels within desired range

Famciclovir

(fam-**SY**-kloh-veer)

Classification(s): Antiviral

Pregnancy Category: B

RX: Famvir.

SEE ALSO ***ANTIVIRAL AGENTS.***

INDICATIONS/USES

(1) Treatment of acute herpes zoster (shingles). (2) Treatment or suppression of recurrent episodes of genital herpes in immunocompetent clients. (3) Treatment of recurrent mucocutaneous herpes simplex infections in HIV-infected clients. (4) Treatment of recurrent herpes labialis (cold sores) in immunocompetent clients. *Investigational:* Management of initial episodes of herpes genitalis. *NOTE:* The efficacy of famciclovir has not been determined for initial episode genital herpes infection, ophthalmic zoster, disseminated zoster, or in immunocompromised clients with herpes zoster.

ACTION/KINETICS

Action

Undergoes rapid biotransformation to the active compound penciclovir. Inhibits viral DNA synthesis and therefore replication in HSV types 1 (HSV-1) and 2 (HSV-2) and varicella-zoster virus.

Pharmacokinetics

Absolute bioavailability is 77%. **Time to C_{max}:** 0.9 hr after PO use. Food decreased C_{max} but not AUC. **t½, plasma:** 2.3 hr following PO use of famciclovir. Penciclovir, the active metabolite, is further metabolized to inactive compounds that are excreted through the urine. Half-life increased in renal insufficiency.

CONTRAINDICATIONS

Use during lactation. Hypersensitivity to famciclovir, its components, or penciclovir cream. Those with galactose intolerance, a severe lactose deficiency, or glucose-galactose malabsorption.

SPECIAL CONCERNS

Safety and efficacy not determined in children less than 18 years of age.

SIDE EFFECTS

Most Common

Headache, N&V, diarrhea, paresthesia, fatigue, flatulence, pruritus, abdominal pain.

GI: N&V, diarrhea, constipation, anorexia, abdominal pain, dyspepsia, flatulence, jaundice. **CNS:** Headache, dizziness, paresthesia, migraine, somnolence, insomnia, confusion (especially in the elderly), hallucinations. **Body as a whole:** Fatigue, fever, pain, rigors, injury. **Musculoskeletal:** Back pain, arthralgia. **Respiratory:** Pharyngitis, sinusitis, URTI. **Hematologic:** Anemia, leukopenia, neutropenia, thrombocytopenia. **Dermatologic:** Pruritus, rash, urticaria, signs/symptoms/complications of zoster and genital herpes, erythema multiforme. **Miscellaneous:** Dysmenorrhea.

LABORATORY TEST CONSIDERATIONS

↑ AST, ALT, total bilirubin, serum creatinine, amylase, lipase.

DRUG INTERACTIONS

Digoxin / ↑ Digoxin levels
Probenecid / ↑ Penciclovir (active form) levels
Theophylline / ↑ Penciclovir (active form) levels

HOW SUPPLIED

Tablets: 125 mg, 250 mg, 500 mg.

DOSAGE

TABLETS

Herpes zoster infections.

500 mg q 8 hr for 7 days. Initiate as soon as herpes zoster is diagnosed. Dosage reduction is recommended in clients with impaired renal function: For C_{CR} of 40–59 mL/min: 500 mg q 12 hr; C_{CR} of 20–39 mL/min: 500 mg q 24 hr; C_{CR} <20 mL/min: 250 mg q 48 hr. For hemodialysis clients: 250 mg given after each dialysis treatment.

Recurrent genital herpes.

1,000 mg q 12 hr for 1 day. Should be taken at the first sign or symptom. Dosage reduction is as follows for those with impaired renal function: For C_{CR} of 40–59 mL/min: 500 mg q 12 hr for 1 day; C_{CR} of 20–39 mL/min: A single dose of 500 mg; C_{CR} <20 mL/min: A single dose of 250 mg. Hemodialysis clients: A single dose of 250 mg after each dialysis treatment.

Suppression of recurrent genital herpes.

250 mg q 12 hr for up to 1 year (safety and efficacy beyond 1 year have not been established). Dosage reduction is as follows for those with impaired renal function: C_{CR}, over 20–39 mL/min: 125 mg q 12 hr hr; C_{CR} <20 mL/min: 125 mg q 24 hr. Hemodialysis clients: 125 mg after each dialysis treatment.

Recurrent orolabial or genital herpes infection in HIV-infected clients.

500 mg twice a day for 7 days. Dosage reduction is as follows for those with impaired renal function: C_{CR} of 40 mL/min or greater: 500 mg q 12 hr; C_{CR} of 20–39 mL/min: 500 mg q 24 hr; C_{CR} <20 mL/min: 250 mg q 24 hr. Hemodialysis clients: 250 mg after each dialysis treatment.

Recurrent herpes labialis (cold sores).

1,500 mg as a single dose. Initiate therapy at the earliest sign or symptom of a cold sore. Dosage reduction is as follows for those with impaired renal function: C_{CR}, 40–59 mL/min: 750 mg as a single dose; C_{CR}, 20–39 mL/min: 500 mg as a single dose; C_{CR}, <20 mL/min: 250 mg as a single dose. Hemodialysis clients: 250 mg as a single dose following dialysis.

Management of initial episodes of herpes genitalis.

250 mg 3 times per day for 5 days.

NURSING IMPLICATIONS

IMPLEMENTATION/ADMINISTRATION/STORAGE

1. Initiate therapy as soon as herpes zoster is diagnosed and at the first symptoms of genital herpes.
2. Therapy is most useful if started within first 48 hr of rash appearance.
3. Effect is greatest in those over 50 years of age.

ASSESSMENT

1. Note onset of symptoms, location, extent of lesions (dermatones involved), clinical presentation, and duration/frequency of recurrence.
2. Initiate as soon as diagnosis of herpes zoster is confirmed or with first symptoms of genital herpes.
3. Advise that famciclovir contains lactose (esp. for those with rare hereditary problems of galactose intolerance, severe lactase deficiency, or glucose-galactose malabsorption).
4. To monitor maternal fetal outcomes of pregnant women exposed to famciclovir, Novartis Pharmaceutical Corporation (manufacturer), maintains a famciclovir pregnancy registry. Register clients by calling 1-888-669-6682, Mon.–Fri. 8:30 a.m.–5 p.m. EST.
5. Monitor CBC and renal function studies. Anticipate reduced dosage with renal dysfunction; follow dosing guidelines.

CLIENT/FAMILY TEACHING

1. Drug is an antiviral that slows spread and growth of virus so body can fight off infections. Does not prevent transmission of infection to others.
2. May be taken without regard to meals.
3. Review frequency, amount of drug to consume, and duration of therapy depending on condition being treated (e.g., cold sores, recurrent genital herpes, shingles).
4. Side effects often associated with therapy include diarrhea, nausea, headaches, and fatigue; report if intolerable. If dizziness or drowsiness experienced, use caution with activities that require mental alertness.
5. When shingle lesions are open and draining, carrier is extremely contagious and should avoid any exposure or outside contact unless confirmed that the person(s) has had the chickenpox and is not pregnant.
6. For recurrent episodes of genital herpes, initiate therapy at first S&S; may not be effective if started more than 6 hr after onset of S&S of recurrence.
7. Drug is not a cure for genital herpes and does not prevent virus transmission. Use condoms and avoid sexual intercourse when lesions and/or symptoms are present to avoid infect-

F

ing partner. May also be transmitted when lesions not present due to viral shedding.

8. Women should practice reliable contraception during therapy and have yearly Pap smears as cervical cancer is a potential risk.
9. Keep all F/U to assess response and for adverse SE.

OUTCOMES/EVALUATE

Resolution/healing of herpetic lesions

IV

Famotidine

(fah-**MOH**-tih-deen)

Classification(s): Histamine H_2 receptor blocking drug

Pregnancy Category: B

OTC: Pepcid AC, Pepcid AC Maximum Strength, Pepcid AC Maximum Strength EZ Chews.

RX: Pepcid, Pepcid RPD.

🍁 **Rx:** Apo-Famotidine, Gen-Famotidine, Nu-Famotidine.

SEE ALSO ***HISTAMINE H_2 ANTAGONISTS.***

INDICATIONS/USES

PO/Injection, Rx: (1) Treatment, up to 8 weeks, of active duodenal ulcers. Maintenance therapy for duodenal ulcer after active ulcer has healed. (2) Pathologic hypersecretory conditions such as Zollinger-Ellison syndrome or multiple endocrine adenomas. (3) Treatment, up to 6 weeks, of GERD, including ulcerative disease diagnosed by endoscopy or erosive esophagitis. (4) Treatment, up to 8 weeks, of active, benign gastric ulcer. *Investigational:* Prevent aspiration pneumonitis; for prophylaxis of stress ulcers; perioperatively to suppress gastric acid secretion; in combination with histamine H-1 antagonists to treat certain types of urticaria; as part of multidrug therapy to eradicate *Helicobacter pylori;* prevent stomach and upper GI ulcers in those taking low-dose aspirin.

PO, OTC: (1) Relief of heartburn associated with indigestion and sour stomach. (2) Prevent heartburn associated with acid indigestion and sour stomach due to certain foods and beverages.

IV: (1) Some hospitalized clients with pathological hypersecretory conditions or intractable ulcers. (2) Alternative to PO dosage forms for short-term use in those who are unable to take PO medication. *Investigational:* Prevent paclitaxel hypersensitivity; prevent recurrent bleeding after successful endoscopic treatment of bleeding peptic ulcer; reduce incidence of GI hemorrhage associated with stress-related ulcers.

ACTION/KINETICS

Action

Competitive inhibitor of histamine H_2 receptors leading to inhibition of gastric acid secretion. Both basal and nocturnal gastric acid secretion stimulated by food or pentagastrin are inhibited.

Pharmacokinetics

Bioavailability after PO use is 40–45%. **Peak plasma levels:** 1–3 hr. **t½:** 2.5–3.5 hr. **Onset:** 1 hr. **Duration:** 10–12 hr. Does not inhibit the cytochrome P450 system in the liver; thus, drug interactions due to inhibition of liver metabolism are not expected to occur. From 25–30% of a PO dose is eliminated through the kidney unchanged; from 65–70% of an IV dose is excreted through the kidney unchanged. **Plasma protein binding:** From 15–20%.

CONTRAINDICATIONS

Cirrhosis of the liver, impaired renal or hepatic function, lactation.

SPECIAL CONCERNS

- CNS side effects possible in those with moderate to severe renal insufficiency.
- Use of IV famotidine in children younger than 1 year not adequately studied.
- OTC product not for children younger than 12 years unless otherwise directed.

SIDE EFFECTS

Most Common

Headache, dizziness, diarrhea, constipation, N&V, anxiety, confusion.

GI: Constipation, diarrhea, N&V, anorexia, dry mouth, abdominal discomfort. **CNS:** Dizziness, headache, paresthesias, depression, anxiety, confusion, hallucinations, insomnia, fatigue, sleepiness, agitation, ***grand mal seizure***, psychic disturbances. **Skin:** Rash, acne, pruritus, alopecia, urticaria, dry skin, flushing. **CV:** Palpitations. **Musculoskeletal:** Arthralgia, asthenia, musculoskeletal pain. **Hematologic:** Thrombocytopenia. **Miscellaneous:** Fever, orbital edema, conjunctival injection, bronchospasm, tinnitus, taste disorders, decreased libido, impotence, pain at injection site (transient).

DRUG INTERACTIONS

Antacids / ↓ Famotidine absorption from the GI tract

Diazepam / ↓ Diazepam absorption from the GI tract

HOW SUPPLIED

OTC. ***Gelcaps:*** 10 mg; ***Tablets:*** 10 mg, 20 mg; ***Tablets, Chewable:*** 10 mg, 20 mg.

Rx. ***Injection:*** 10 mg/mL; ***Injection (Premix):*** 20 mg/50 mL; ***Powder for Oral Suspension:*** 40 mg/5 mL (when reconstituted); ***Tablets:*** 20 mg, 40 mg; ***Tablets, Oral Disintegrating:*** 20 mg, 40 mg.

DOSAGE

RX: ORAL SUSPENSION; TABLETS; TABLETS, ORAL DISINTEGRATING

Duodenal ulcer, acute therapy.

Adults: 40 mg once daily at bedtime or 20 mg twice a day. Most ulcers heal within 4 weeks, and it is rarely necessary to use the full dosage for 6–8 weeks.

Duodenal ulcer, maintenance therapy.

Adults: 20 mg once daily at bedtime.

Pathological hypersecretory conditions.

Adults, individualized, initial: 20 mg q 6 hr; **then,** adjust dose to response, although doses of up to 160 mg q 6 hr may be required for severe cases of Zollinger-Ellison syndrome. Continue as long as clinically indicated.

Benign gastric ulcers, acute therapy.

Adults: 40 mg once daily at bedtime.

Children: Peptic ulcers.

Children, 1–16 years of age: 0.5 mg/kg/day at bedtime or divided twice a day up to 40 mg/day. Individualize dose based on clinical response and/or gastric/esophogeal pH and endoscopy.

Adults: Gastroesophageal reflux disease (GERD).

Adults: 20 mg twice a day for 6 weeks. For esophagitis with erosions and ulcerations, give 20 or 40 mg twice a day for up to 12 weeks.

Children: GERD with or without esophagitis, including erosions and ulcerations.

Children, 1–16 years of age: 1 mg/kg/day PO divided twice daily, up to 40 mg twice daily.

Infants: GERD.

Children, less than 1 year of age, initial: 0.5 mg/kg/dose of the oral suspension for up to 8 weeks. Give once daily (i.e., 0.5 mg/kg) in children younger than 3 months of age and twice daily (i.e., 0.5 mg/kg twice daily) to children from 3 months to younger than 1 year.

Prophylaxis of upper GI bleeding.

Adults: 20 mg twice a day.

Prophylaxis of stress ulcers.

Adults: 40 mg/day.

IV; IV INFUSION

Hospitalized clients with hypersecretory conditions, duodenal ulcers, gastric ulcers; unable to take PO medication.

Adults: 20 mg IV q 12 hr. **Children, 1–16 years of age:** Individualize. **Initial:** 0.25 mg/kg given over 2 or more minutes or as a 15 min infusion q 12 hr up to 40 mg/day. **Initial, infants less than 1 year of age:** 0.5 mg/kg/dose once daily, for up to 8 weeks in infants younger than 3 months of age and 0.5 mg/kg/dose twice daily, for up to 8 weeks in infants 3 months to younger than 1 year of age. These clients should also receive conservative measures (e.g., thickened feedings).

OTC: GELCAPS; TABLETS; TABLETS, CHEWABLE

Relief and prevention of heartburn, acid indigestion, and sour stomach.

Adults and children over 12 years of age, for prevention: 10 or 20 mg 15–60 min before eating food or drinking a beverage expected to cause symptoms. **Relief (acute therapy):** 10 mg or 20 mg with water. **Maximum dose:** 20 mg/24 hr. Not to be used continuously for more than 2 weeks unless medically prescribed. Do not give OTC product to children less than 12 years of age unless otherwise directed.

F

F

NURSING IMPLICATIONS

IMPLEMENTATION/ADMINISTRATION/STORAGE

1. Use antacids concomitantly if needed.
2. The oral suspension may be substituted for tablets for any use.
3. To prepare the oral suspension, slowly add 46 mL of purified water. Shake vigorously for 5–10 seconds immediately after adding the water and immediately before use.
4. Reduce dose in moderate to severe renal impairment to half the usual dose at the usual dosage interval or the usual dose every 36–48 hr.
5. Store PO Rx forms from 15–30°C (59–86°F). Protect suspension from freezing; discard any unused suspension after 30 days. Store OTC forms from 20–30°C (68–86°F); protect from moisture.
6. **IV** For IV, dilute 2 mL (containing 10 mg/mL) with 0.9% NaCl or other compatible IV solution to a total volume of 5–10 mL; give over at least a 2 min period.
7. For IV infusion, dilute 2 mL (20 mg) with 100 mL of D5W or other compatible IV solution and infuse over 15–30 min. Infuse the premixed solution over 15–30 min.
8. A solution is stable for 7 days at room temperature when added to or diluted with water for injection, 0.9% NaCl, D5W or D10W, RL injection, or 5% $NaHCO_3$ injection.
9. Stable when mixed with various TPN solutions. Length of stability depends on the solution.
10. Store non-premixed injection at 2–8°C (36–46°F). Avoid exposure of premixed injection to excessive heat. If the solution freezes, bring to room temperature, allowing sufficient time to solubilize all the components.
11. COMPATIBILITY Water for injection, 0.9% NaCl, D5W and D10W, LR injection.
12. INCOMPATIBILITY Administer separately.

ASSESSMENT

1. List reasons for therapy, type, onset, characteristics of S&S, other agents trialed.
2. Note location, extent, duration, and type of abdominal pain.
3. Review UGI/endoscopic findings; note modifications trialed with GERD (i.e., staying upright for 3 hr after eating, elevating head of bed on 5-inch blocks, avoiding food triggers/tobacco/ethanol).
4. Check for occult blood in stools/GI secretions; note presence of *H. pylori* antibodies.
5. Assess mental status; history of seizures. List other agents prescribed.
6. If pregnant, list benefits versus risks.
7. Monitor CBC, renal and LFTS; reduce dose with dysfunction and assess for bleeding.

CLIENT/FAMILY TEACHING

1. Drug is used to help heal ulcers or control acid reflux S&S by reducing the amount of stomach acid produced. May take with antacids for pain relief. Drug may cause dizziness, headaches, and anxiety; use caution with activities requiring mental alertness, and report if symptoms persist.
2. Take with food at night; do not smoke after last dose (increases acid production) or if more than one dose daily, take last dose at bedtime.
3. With oral suspension, shake suspension vigorously for 5 to 10 sec before measuring dose; measure and administer prescribed dose using dosing syringe, dosing spoon, or dosing cup.
4. OTC chewable Pepcid AC contains phenylalanine 1.4 mg per tablet.
5. Ensure GERD triggers reviewed/understood. Warn that relief of symptoms does not preclude gastric malignancy.
6. Report any increasing lack of concern for personal appearance, depression, or sleeplessness, diarrhea, constipation, reduction in urinary output, appetite loss, easy bruising, or fatigue. Increase fluids and bulk in diet to prevent constipation.
7. Avoid alcohol, aspirin-containing products, OTC cough and cold products, smoking, and foods that increase GI irritation (i.e., citrus, carbonated drinks, caffeine, black pepper, harsh spices). Smoking causes increased secretion of gastric acid and may aggravate problems.
8. Keep all F/U to assess response labs, need for dosage change, adverse SE.

OUTCOMES/EVALUATE

- ↓ Abdominal pain ↓ S&S GERD
- Prophylaxis of stress ulcers/GI bleeding
- Control of hypersecretion of acid
- Duodenal ulcer healing

Febuxostat

(feb-**UX**-oh-stat)

Classification(s): Antigout drug (xanthine oxidase inhibitor)

Pregnancy Category: C

RX: Uloric.

INDICATIONS/USES

Chronic management of hyperuricemia in gout.

ACTION/KINETICS

Action

As a xanthine oxidase inhibitor, it decreases serum uric acid.

Pharmacokinetics

Absorption is at least 49% after PO use. C_{max}: 1–1.5 hr. Extensively metabolized by CYP1A2, 2C8, and 2C9 as well as UGT1A1, 1A3, 1A9, and 2B7. Excreted through both the urine (49%) and the feces (45%) as both unchanged drug and metabolites. **t½, terminal elimination:** 5–8 hr. C_{max} and AUC are higher in women than in men. **Plasma protein binding:** 99.2% (mainly to albumin).

CONTRAINDICATIONS

Clients being treated with azathioprine, mercaptopurine, or theophylline. Use in clients in whom the rate of urate formation is greatly increased (e.g., malignant disease and its treatment, Lesch-Nyhan syndrome).

SPECIAL CONCERNS

- **Use with caution in severe renal impairment (C_{CR} <30 mL/min), severe hepatic impairment (Child-Pugh class C), and during lactation.**
- **Safety and efficacy not determined in children younger than 18 years of age.**

SIDE EFFECTS

Most Common

Abnormal liver function, arthralgia, nausea, rash.

CNS: Agitation, altered taste, anxiety, balance disorder, depression, fatigue, gait disturbance, Guillain-Barré syndrome, headache, hemiparesis, hypoesthesia, hyposmia, insomnia, irritability, lacunar infarction, lethargy, decreased libido, mental impairment, migraine, nervousness, panic attack, paresthesia, personality change, somnolence, tremor, vertigo. **GI:** Abdominal distention/pain, constipation, dry mouth, dyspepsia, flatulence, frequent stools, gastritis, GERD, GI discomfort, gingival pain, hematemesis, hematochezia, hyperchlorhydria, mouth ulceration, N&V, ***pancreatitis***, peptic ulcer. **Hepatic:** Abnormal liver function, cholelithiasis/cholecystitis, hepatic steatosis, hepatitis, hepatomegaly. **CV:** Angina pectoris, atrial fibrillation/flutter, cardiac murmur, ***CVA***, ***MI***, abnormal ECG, hyper-/hypotension, palpitations, sinus bradycardia, tachycardia, TIAs. **Dermatologic:** Rash, alopecia, ***angioedema***, dermatitis, dermographism, ecchymosis, eczema, hair color changes, abnormal hair growth, hyperhidrosis, peeling skin, petechiae, photosensitivity, pruritus, purpura, skin discoloration/altered pigmentation, skin lesion, abnormal skin odor, urticaria. **Musculoskeletal:** Arthralgia, arthritis, joint stiffness/swelling, muscle spasms/twitching/tightness/weakness, musculoskeletal pain/stiffness, myalgia. **Respiratory:** Bronchitis, cough, dyspnea, epistaxis, nasal dryness, paranasal sinus hypersecretion, pharyngeal edema, respiratory tract congestion, sneezing, throat irritation, URTI. **GU:** Breast pain, erectile dysfunction, gynecomastia, hematuria, incontinence, nephrolithiasis, pollakiuria, renal failure/insufficiency, urgency. **Hematologic:** Anemia, idiopathic thrombocytopenic purpura, leukocytosis/leukopenia, neutropenia, pancytopenia, splenomegaly, thrombocytopenia. **Metabolic/Nutritional:** Anorexia, decreased/increased appetite, dehydration, diabetes mellitus, hypercholesterolemia, hyperglycemia, hyperlipidemia, hypertriglyceridemia, hypokalemia, weight decreased/increased. **Ophthalmic:** Blurred vision. **Otic:** Deafness, tinnitus. **Body as a whole:** Asthenia, edema, abnormal feeling, flushing, hot flush, hypersensitivity, flu-like symptoms, pain, thirst. **Miscellaneous:** Chest pain/discomfort, contusion, herpes zoster, mass.

LABORATORY TEST CONSIDERATIONS

↑ ALT, AST, APTT, alkaline phosphatase, amylase, blood urea, cholesterol, creatine, CPK, creatinine, glucose, LDH, LDL, mean corpuscular volume, potassium, PSA, PT, BUN/creatinine ratio, sodium, TSH, triglycerides. ↓ Bicarbonate, hematocrit, hemoglobin, lymphocyte count, neutrophil count, platelet count, RBC count. ↑ or ↓ Urine output, WBC count. Abnormal coagulation test, EEG. Presence of urinary casts, WBCs and protein in urine.

DRUG INTERACTIONS

Azathioprine / ↑ Plasma levels of azathioprine R/T inhibition of xanthine oxidase → toxicity; do not use together
Mercaptopurine / ↑ Plasma levels of mercaptopurine R/T inhibition of xanthine oxidase → toxicity; do not use together
Theophylline / ↑ Plasma levels of theophylline R/T inhibition of xanthine oxidase → toxicity; do not use together

HOW SUPPLIED

Tablets: 40 mg, 80 mg.

DOSAGE

TABLETS

Chronic management of hyperuricemia in gout.

Adults, initial: 40 mg once a day; **usual:** 40–80 mg once a day. For those who do not achieve a serum uric acid level of <6 mg/dL after 2 weeks with 40 mg, a dose of 80 mg is recommended.

NURSING IMPLICATIONS

IMPLEMENTATION/ADMINISTRATION/STORAGE

1. Gout flares may occur after beginning febuxostat therapy; is due to changing serum uric acid levels resulting in mobilization of urate from tissue deposits. Undertake flare prophylaxis with a nonsteroidal anti-inflammatory drug or colchicine. Prophylaxis may be beneficial for up to 6 months.
2. May be taken without regard to food or antacid use.
3. Store from 15–30°C (59–86°F); protect from light.

ASSESSMENT

1. Note reasons for therapy, frequency of attacks, location, presentation, other agents trialed and outcome. Not for use with malignancy (increased urate formation).
2. Assess for any CAD and monitor for S&S of MI and/or stroke.
3. May start therapy with NSAID or colchicine to diminish gout flare R/T mobilization of urate from tissue deposits.
4. Assess renal function, and obtain LFTs at 2 and 4 months following the start of therapy and periodically thereafter. Check for the target serum uric acid level of <6 mg/dL; may check as early as 2 weeks after starting febuxostat therapy. If not attained may need to increase dose to 80 mg.

CLIENT/FAMILY TEACHING

1. Take once a day without regard to food or antacid use.
2. May take with NSAID or colchicine to prevent gout flares upon starting therapy and with mobilization of urate from the tissues deposits.
3. Review ↑ risks related to gout flares, elevated liver enzymes and cardiovascular events with this therapy.
4. Report any chest pain, shortness of breath, rash, or symptoms suggestive of a stroke.
5. Avoid pregnancy unless benefits outweigh risks.
6. Keep all F/U to assess response, labs, and adverse SE.

OUTCOMES/EVALUATE

- Symptomatic relief of gout pain
- Uric acid level of <6 mg/dL

Felbamate

(**FELL**-bah-mayt)

Classification(s): Anticonvulsant, miscellaneous

Pregnancy Category: C

RX: Felbatol.

SEE ALSO ***ANTICONVULSANTS***.

INDICATIONS/USES

(1) Alone or as part of adjunctive therapy for the treatment of partial seizures with and without generalization in adults with epilepsy. (2) Adjunct in the treatment of partial and generalized seizures associated with Lennox-Gastaut syndrome in children. Used only as second-line therapy. *NOTE:* Due to cases of aplastic anemia, it has been recommended that use of felbamate be discontinued unless, in the judgment of the physician, continued therapy is warranted.

ACTION/KINETICS

Action

Mechanism not known. Felbamate may reduce seizure spread and increase seizure threshold. Has weak inhibitory effects on both GABA and benzodiazepine receptor binding.

Pharmacokinetics

Well absorbed after PO use. **Terminal t½:** 20–23 hr. Trough blood levels are dose dependent. From 40–50% excreted unchanged in the urine. **Plasma protein binding:** 22–25%.

CONTRAINDICATIONS

History of hepatic dysfunction or blood dyscrasia. Hypersensitivity to carbamates.

SPECIAL CONCERNS

(1) Use is associated with a marked increase in the incidence of aplastic anemia. Use only in those whose epilepsy is so severe that the risk of aplastic anemia is deemed acceptable in view of the benefits from its use. Clients should not be placed on or continued on felbamate without consideration of appropriate expert hematologic consultation. (2) Clinical manifestations of aplastic anemia may not be seen until after a client has been on the drug for several months (5-30 weeks); however, the injury to bone marrow stem cells may occur weeks to months earlier, placing clients at risk for developing anemia for a variable and unknown period after drug discontinuation. (3) It is not known whether or not the risk of developing aplastic anemia changes with the duration of exposure, dose, or concomitant use of antiepileptic drugs or other drugs. (4) Aplastic anemia typically develops without premonitory clinical or laboratory signs. The full-blown syndrome presents with signs of infection, bleeding, or anemia. Thus, routine blood testing cannot be reliably used to reduce the incidence of aplastic anemia. It will, in some cases, allow the detection of the hematologic changes before the syndrome is seen clinically. Discontinue felbamate if any evidence of bone marrow depression occurs. (5) Hepatic failure resulting in death has been reported with a marked increase in frequency in those taking felbamate. Thus, only use felbamate in those whose epilepsy is so severe that potential benefits of seizure control outweigh the risk of liver failure. Reliable estimates cannot be made of the incidence of hepatic failure or to identify the factors, if any, that might be used to predict which client is at greater risk. (6) It is not known whether the risk of developing hepatic failure changes with duration of exposure, dosage, or concomitant use of other antiepileptic drugs or other drugs. (7) Avoid use in those with a history of hepatic dysfunction. (8) Clients prescribed felbamate should have liver function tests (AST, ALT, bilirubin) performed before starting therapy and at 1- to 2-week intervals while treatment continues. A client who develops abnormal liver function tests should be immediately withdrawn from the drug.

- **Increased risk of suicidal behavior and ideation.**
- **Use with caution during lactation.**
- **Safety and efficacy not established in children other than those with Lennox-Gastaut syndrome.**

SIDE EFFECTS

Most Common

When used as adjunctive therapy: Headache, N&V, somnolence, anorexia, dizziness, fatigue, dyspepsia, constipation.

When used for Lennox-Gastaut in children: Anorexia, URTI, somnolence, vomiting, fever, insomnia, nervousness, constipation, purpura.

CNS: Insomnia, headache, anxiety, somnolence, dizziness, nervousness, tremor, abnormal gait, depression, paresthesia, ataxia, stupor, abnormal thinking, emotional lability, agitation, psychologic disturbance, aggressive reaction, hallucinations, euphoria, ***suicide attempt***, ***suicidal behavior*** and ideation, migraine. **GI**: Dyspepsia, N&V, constipation, diarrhea, dry mouth, nausea, anorexia, abdominal pain, hiccoughs, esophagitis, increased appetite. **Respiratory**: URTI, rhinitis, sinusitis, pharyngitis, coughing. **CV**: Palpitation, tachycardia, SVT. **Body as a whole:** Fatigue, weight decrease or increase, facial edema, fever, chest pain, pain, asthenia, malaise, flu-like symptoms, ***anaphylaxis***. **Ophthalmologic**: Miosis, diplopia, abnormal vision. **GU**: Urinary incontinence, intramenstrual bleeding, UTI. **Hematologic**: ***Aplastic anemia***, purpura, leukopenia, lymphadenopathy, leukocytosis, thrombocytopenia, granulocytopenia, positive antinuclear factor test, ***agranulocytosis***, qualitative platelet disorder. **Dermatologic**: Acne, rash, pruritus, urticaria, bullous eruption, buccal mucous membrane swelling, ***Stevens-Johnson syndrome***. **Miscellaneous**: Otitis media, ***acute liver failure***, taste perversion, myalgia, photosensitivity, substernal chest pain, dystonia, allergic reaction. *NOTE:* Side effects may differ depending on whether the drug is used as monotherapy or adjunctive therapy in adults or for Lennox-Gastaut syndrome in children.

LABORATORY TEST CONSIDERATIONS

↑ ALT, AST, GGT, LDH, alkaline phosphatase, CPK. Hypophosphatemia, hypokalemia, hyponatremia.

DRUG INTERACTIONS

Carbamazepine / ↓ Carbamazepine steady-state levels and ↑ steady-state carbamazepine epoxide (metabolite) levels. Also, drug → 50% ↑ in felbamate clearance
Methsuximide / ↑ Normethsuxmide levels; decrease methsuximide dose
Phenobarbital / ↑ Phenobarbital levels and ↓ in felbamate levels
Phenytoin / ↑ Phenytoin steady-state drug levels necessitating a 40% decrease in drug dose. Also, drug ↑ felbamate clearance
Valproic acid / ↑ Steady-state valproic acid levels

HOW SUPPLIED

Oral Suspension: 600 mg/5 mL; ***Tablets:*** 400 mg, 600 mg.

DOSAGE

ORAL SUSPENSION/TABLETS

Monotherapy, initial therapy.

Adults over 14 years of age, initial: 1,200 mg per day in divided doses 3–4 times per day. The dose may be increased in 600 mg increments q 2 weeks to 2,400 mg/day based on clinical response and thereafter to 3,600 mg/day, if needed.

Conversion to monotherapy.

Adults: Initiate at 1,200 mg/day in divided doses 3–4 times per day. Reduce dose of concomitant antiepileptic drugs by one-third at initiation of felbamate therapy. At week 2, the felbamate dose should be increased to 2,400 mg/day while reducing the dose of other antiepileptic drugs up to another one-third of the original dose. At week 3, increase the felbamate dose to 3,600 mg/day and continue to decrease the dose of other antiepileptic drugs as indicated by response.

Adjunctive therapy.

Add felbamate at a dose of 1,200 mg/day in divided doses 3–4 times per day while reducing current antiepileptic drugs by 20%. Further decreases of concomitant antiepileptic drugs may be needed to minimize side effects due to drug interactions. The dose of felbamate can be increased by 1,200 mg/day increments at weekly intervals to 3,600 mg/day.

Lennox-Gastaut syndrome in children, aged 2–14 years.

As an adjunct, add felbamate at a dose of 15 mg/kg/day in divided doses 3–4 times per day while decreasing present antiepileptic drugs by 20%. Further decreases in antiepileptic drug dosage may be needed to minimize side effects due to drug interactions. The dose of felbamate may be increased by 15 mg/kg/day increments at weekly intervals to 45 mg/kg/day.

NURSING IMPLICATIONS

IMPLEMENTATION/ADMINISTRATION/STORAGE

1. Shake suspension well before use.
2. Store in a tightly closed container at room temperature away from heat, direct sunlight, or moisture. Keep away from children.
3. Most side effects seen during adjunctive therapy resolve as the dose of concomitant antiepileptic drugs is decreased.
4. For geriatric clients, start at the low end of the dosage range.

ASSESSMENT

1. Note type, location, duration, characteristics of seizures, other agents trialed.
2. Check if monotherapy or adjunctive therapy needed.
3. List drugs prescribed to ensure none interact; assess need for dosage change.
4. Inform of potentially lethal side effects R/T aplastic anemia. Provide written explanation of risks and have consent form signed.

5. Assess clinical presentation and psychologic status; note any depression or mood/behavioral disorders.
6. Monitor CBC, renal and LFTs, and seizure occurrence; reduce dose with renal dysfunction. Assess for any liver dysfunction; obtain LFTS (AST, ALT, bilirubin) before starting therapy, at 1- to 2-week intervals during therapy. Stop therapy immediately if abnormal LFTS occur.

CLIENT/FAMILY TEACHING

1. Take only as prescribed; store appropriately to prevent loss of effectiveness (away from sunlight, heat, and moisture).
2. Take tablet with a full glass of water; do not crush. May be taken with food.
3. Shake bottle well before measuring prescribed dosage.
4. Avoid activities that require mental alertness until drug effects realized. May cause dizziness, drowsiness, or visual problems.
5. Side effects include anorexia, vomiting, insomnia, nausea, and headaches; report if persistent.
6. Report any changes in mental status, depression, suicide thoughts, or loss of seizure control; clinical response determines dosage and need for withdrawal.
7. Do not stop taking; may increase seizure frequency.
8. Seizure control benefit should far outweigh the potential for development of aplastic anemia or severe liver failure; assess risk. A Felbatol "Patient Information/Consent" (informed consent) should be reviewed and signed by client/family prior to starting therapy.
9. Keep all F/U to assess response, labs, adverse SE.

OUTCOMES/EVALUATE

Control of seizures unresponsive to other therapies

Felodipine

(feh-**LOHD**-ih-peen)

Classification(s): Calcium channel blocker

Pregnancy Category: C

✦ **Rx:** Renedil.

SEE ALSO ***CALCIUM CHANNEL BLOCKING AGENTS.***

INDICATIONS/USES

Hypertension, alone or with other antihypertensives. *Investigational:* Raynaud syndrome, CHF.

ACTION/KINETICS

Action

Moderate increase in HR and moderate decrease in peripheral resistance. No effect on the QRS complex, PR interval, or QT interval with no effect to a slight decrease on myocardial contractility.

Pharmacokinetics

Onset after PO: 120–300 min. **Peak plasma levels:** 2.5–5 hr. **t½, elimination:** 11–16 hr. Metabolized in the liver with 70% excreted in the urine and 10% excreted in the feces. **Plasma protein binding:** Over 99%.

CONTRAINDICATIONS

Lactation.

SPECIAL CONCERNS

- Use with caution in clients with CHF or compromised ventricular function, especially if used with a beta-adrenergic blocking agent; also, in impaired hepatic function or reduced hepatic blood flow.
- Possible greater hypotensive effect in geriatric clients due to higher plasma levels.
- Safety and efficacy not determined in children.

SIDE EFFECTS

Most Common

Peripheral edema, asthenia, dizziness, lightheadedness, headache, dyspepsia, constipation, cough, URTI, flushing.

CV: Significant hypotension, syncope, angina pectoris, peripheral edema, palpitations, AV block, ***MI***, ***arrhythmias***, tachycardia. **CNS:** Dizziness, lightheadedness, headache, nervousness, sleepiness, irritability, anxiety, insomnia, paresthesia, depression, amnesia, paranoia, psychosis, hallucinations. **Body as a whole:** Asthenia, flushing, muscle cramps, pain, inflammation, warm feeling, influenza. **GI:** Nausea, abdominal discomfort, cramps, dyspepsia, diarrhea, constipation, vomiting, dry mouth, flatulence. **Dermatologic:** Rash, flushing, dermatitis, urticaria, pruritus. **Respiratory:** Rhinitis, URTI, rhinorrhea, pharyngitis, sinusitis, nasal and chest congestion, SOB, wheezing, dyspnea, cough, bronchitis, sneezing, respiratory infection. **Miscellaneous:** Anemia, gingival hyperplasia, sexual difficulties, epistaxis, back pain, facial edema, erythema, urinary frequency or urgency, dysuria.

ADDITIONAL DRUG INTERACTIONS

Barbiturates / ↓ Effect of felodipine
Carbamazepine / ↓ Felodipine effects
Cimetidine / ↑ Bioavailability of felodipine
Cyclosporine / ↑ Pharmacologic and toxic effects of felodipine; ↑ cyclosporine levels and toxicity
Digoxin / ↑ Digoxin peak levels
Erythromycins / ↑ Erythromycin effects; monitor CV status closely
Fentanyl / Possible severe hypotension or ↑ fluid volume
Grapefruit juice / ↑ Felodipine levels R/T ↓ liver breakdown
Itraconazole / ↑ Felodipine levels
Nelfinavir / Possible leg edema and orthostatic hypotension
Oxcarbazepine / ↓ Felodipine effects
Phenytoin / ↓ Effects of felodipine
Ranitidine / ↑ Felodipine bioavailability

HOW SUPPLIED

Tablets, Extended-Release: 2.5 mg, 5 mg, 10 mg.

DOSAGE

TABLETS, EXTENDED-RELEASE

Hypertension.

Initial: 5 mg once daily (2.5 mg in clients over 65 years of age and in those with impaired liver function); **then:** adjust dose according to response, usually at 2-week intervals with the usual dosage range being 2.5–10 mg once daily. Doses greater than 10 mg increase the rate of peripheral edema and other vasodilatory side effects.

NURSING IMPLICATIONS

IMPLEMENTATION/ADMINISTRATION/STORAGE

1. Bioavailability is not affected by food. It is increased more than twofold when taken with doubly concentrated grapefruit juice as compared with water or orange juice.
2. Store below 30°C (86°F). Protect from light.

ASSESSMENT

1. Note disease onset, other agents used, outcome. Check for history of heart failure or compromised ventricular function. Assess ECG, or for evidence of disease associated organ damage.
2. List drugs currently prescribed to ensure no interactions.
3. During dosage adjustments, monitor BP closely esp. in clients over 65 or with impaired hepatic function. Monitor renal and LFTs.

CLIENT/FAMILY TEACHING

1. Swallow tablets whole; do not chew or crush. Take with food or a light meal. Avoid taking with grapefruit juice.
2. Do not stop abruptly; abrupt withdrawal may increase frequency and duration of chest pain.
3. Avoid activities that require mental alertness until effects are realized.
4. Rise slowly from a lying position, and dangle feet before standing to minimize low BP effects.
5. Drug controls, but does not cure, hypertension or angina. Continue taking as prescribed even when BP is not elevated or angina symptoms are controlled. Report if frequency or severity of chest pain, or need for sublingual nitroglycerin appears to be increasing.
6. Report any headaches, flushing, or extremity swelling. Keep written record of BP and HR for review.
7. Practice frequent oral hygiene to minimize incidence and severity of drug-induced gum swelling.
8. Avoid alcohol and OTC drugs without provider approval.
9. Stress importance of weight control, daily exercise, smoking cessation, stress reduction, and moderation of alcohol/salt intake.
10. Keep all F/U to assess response, labs, adverse SE.

OUTCOMES/EVALUATE

Control of hypertension/angina

Fenofibrate

(**fee**-noh-**FY**-brayt)

Classification(s): Antihyperlipidemic

Pregnancy Category: C

RX: Capsules: Lipofen. **Capsules, Delayed-Release**: Trilipix. **Capsules, Micronized**: Antara, Lofibra. **Tablets**: Fenoglide, Fibricor, Lofibra, Tricor, Triglide.

✤ **Rx: Fenofibrate:** Apo-Fenofibrate, Apo-Feno-Micro, Apo-Feno-Super, Lipidil EZ, Sandoz Fenofibrate. **Fenofibrate Microcoated:** Lipidil Supra. **Fenofibrate Micronized:** Gen-Fenofibrate Micro, PMS-Fenofibrate Micro.

INDICATIONS/USES

(1) Adjunctive therapy to diet to reduce elevated LDL-C, total-C, triglycerides, and Apo B and to increase HDL-C in adults with primary hypercholesterolemia or mixed dyslipidemia (Fredrickson Types IIa and IIb). Use lipid-altering agents in addition to diet when diet and nonpharmacologic interventions have not been effective. (2) Adjunctive therapy to diet to treat adults with hypertriglyceridemia (Fredrickson Types IV and V hyperlipidemia). (3) As an adjunct to diet in combination with a statin to reduce triglycerides and increased HDL-C in those with mixed dyslipidemia and coronary heart disease or a CHD risk equivalent who are on optimal statin therapy to achieve their HDL-C goal. CHD risk equivalents include other forms of atherosclerotic disease (e.g., abdominal aortic aneurysm, peripheral arterial disease, symptomatic carotid artery disease), diabetes, multiple risk factors that confer a 10-year risk for CHD greater than 20%. *Investigational:* Hyperuricemia, hypertriglyceridemia associated with HIV lipodystrophy.

ACTION/KINETICS

Action

Lowers total-C, LDL-C, Apo B, total triglycerides, and triglyceride-rich lipoprotein; also increases HDL and apoproteins Apo AI and Apo AII. Increases lipolysis and elimination of triglyceride-rich particles from plasma by activating lipoprotein lipase and reducing production of apoprotein C III, an inhibitor of lipoprotein lipase activity. The resulting decrease in triglycerides produces an alteration in the size and composition of LDL from small, dense particles to large, buoyant particles; larger particles have a greater affinity for cholesterol receptors and are rapidly catabolized. Fenofibrate also decreases serum uric acid levels in hyperuricemic and healthy individuals by increasing urinary uric acid excretion.

Pharmacokinetics

Well absorbed; micronized and nonmicronized products demonstrate bioequivalence. Absorption is increased when given with food. Rapidly hydrolyzed by esterases to the active fenofibric acid. **Peak plasma levels:** 3–8 hr, depending on the product; **steady-state plasma levels:** within 5–7 days. **t½:** 16–23 hr with once daily dosing. The rate of clearance is greatly reduced in severe renal impairment. Fenofibric acid and an inactive metabolite are excreted mainly through the urine (60%) and feces (25%). **Plasma protein binding:** 99%.

F

CONTRAINDICATIONS

Hypersensitivity to fenofibrate. Hepatic dysfunction (including primary biliary cirrhosis and unexplained, persistent abnormal liver function), severe renal dysfunction, and pre-existing gallbladder disease. Lactation.

SPECIAL CONCERNS

- **Due to similarity to clofibrate and gemfibrozil, side effects, including death, are possible.**
- **Fenofibrate, at a dose equivalent to fenofibric acid 135 mg, does not reduce CHD morbidity and mortality.**
- **Select dosage carefully in the elderly due to possible decreased renal function.**
- **Safety and efficacy not determined in children.**

SIDE EFFECTS

Most Common

Abnormal LFTs, respiratory disorder, abdominal/back pain, headache, nausea, diarrhea, rhinitis, asthenia, flu syndrome, respiratory disorder.

GI: ***Pancreatitis***, cholelithiasis, dyspepsia, N&V, diarrhea, abdominal pain, dry mouth, constipation, flatulence, eructation, hepatitis, cholecystitis, hepatomegaly, gastroenteritis, rectal disorder, esophagitis, gastritis, colitis, tooth disorder, anorexia, GI disorder, duodenal/peptic ulcer, ***rectal hemorrhage***, fatty liver deposit. **CNS:** Headache, decreased libido, dizziness, increased appetite, insomnia, paresthesia, depression, vertigo, anxiety, hypertonia, nervousness, neuralgia, somnolence, migraine. **CV:** Angina pectoris, hyper-/hypotension, vasodilation, coronary artery disorder, abnormal ECG, ventricular extrasystoles, ***MI***, peripheral vascular disorder, extrasystoles, migraine, varicose vein, palpitation, CV/vascular disorder, arrhythmia, phlebitis, tachycardia, atrial fibrillation. **Dermatologic:** Rash, pruritus, eczema, herpes simplex/zoster, urticaria, acne, sweating, contact/fungal dermatitis, alopecia, maculopapular rash, nail/skin disorder, skin ulcer. **Respiratory:** Rhinitis, respiratory disorder, increased cough, sinusitis, allergic pulmonary alveolitis, pharyngitis, bronchitis, dyspnea, asthma, pneumonia, laryngitis. **GU:** Polyuria, vaginitis, prostatic disorder, dysuria, abnormal kidney function, urolithiasis, gynecomastia, unintended pregnancy, vaginal moniliasis, cystitis, urinary frequency. **Hematologic:** Anemia, leukopenia, ecchymosis, eosinophilia, lymphadenopathy, thrombocytopenia (rare), agranulocytosis (rare). **Musculoskeletal:** Myopathy (e.g., muscle tenderness/weakness), myositis, arthralgia, myalgia, myasthenia, rhabdomyolysis, arthritis, arthrosis, tenosynovitis, joint disorder, arthrosis, leg cramps, bursitis. **Hypersensitivity:** Severe skin rashes, urticaria; rarely, ***Stevens-Johnson syndrome and toxic epidermal necrolysis.*** **Ophthalmic:** Eye irritation, blurred/abnormal vision, conjunctivitis, eye floaters, eye disorder, amblyopia, cataract, refraction disorder. **Otic:** Ear pain, otitis media. **Body as a whole:** Infections, pain, headache, asthenia, fatigue, flu syndrome, photosensitivity, malaise, allergic reaction, fever, weight gain/loss. **Miscellaneous:** Back/chest pain, cyst, hernia, accidental injury, diabetes mellitus, gout, edema, peripheral edema, increased appetite.

LABORATORY TEST CONSIDERATIONS

↑ AST, ALT, CPK, creatinine, blood urea, GGT. Initial ↓ hemoglobin, hematocrit, WBCs. Hypoglycemia, hyperuricemia. Abnormal LFTs.

OVERDOSE MANAGEMENT

Treatment: If needed, gastric lavage to increase elimination of unabsorbed drug. Maintain the airway. Do not consider hemodialysis (drug is highly bound to plasma proteins).

DRUG INTERACTIONS

Anticoagulants, oral / Potentiation of coumarin anticoagulants (prolongation of PT/INR); determine PT/INR frequently and dose reduction is advisable
Bile acid sequestrants / ↓ Absorption of fenofibrate R/T binding; give fenofibrate at least 1 hr before to 4–6 hr after a bile acid binding resin
Cyclosporine / ↑ Risk of nephrotoxicity; use lowest effective dose
HMG-CoA reductase inhibitors / ↑ Possibility of rhabdomyolysis, ↑ creatine kinase, and myoglobinuria → acute renal failure; avoid concomitant use unless benefits outweigh risks
Warfarin / Possible significant drug interactions; monitor PT and INR

HOW SUPPLIED

Capsules (Lipofen): 50 mg, 150 mg; ***Capsules, Delayed-Release (Trilipix):*** 45 mg, 135 mg; ***Capsules, Micronized (Antara, Lofibra):*** 43 mg, 67 mg, 130 mg, 134 mg, 200 mg; ***Tablets (Fenoglide, Fibricor, Lofibra, Triglide, Tricor):*** 35 mg, 40 mg, 48 mg, 50 mg, 54 mg, 105 mg, 107 mg, 120 mg, 145 mg, 160 mg.

DOSAGE

CAPSULES; TABLETS

Primary hypercholesterolemia, mixed hyperlipidemia.

Individualize dose depending on client response; adjust, if necessary, following repeat lipid determinations at 4- to 8-week intervals. Dosage will differ depending on the product to be used. **Antara, initial:** 130 mg/day without regard to meals; for renal function impairment or the elderly, give 43 mg/day initially. **Lipofen, initial:** 150 mg/day with meals. In the elderly and in impaired renal function, start with 50 mg/day. **Lofibra capsules, initial:** 200 mg/day with meals; for renal function impairment or the elderly, give 67 mg/day. **Lofibra tablets, initial:** 160 mg/day with meals; for renal function impairment or the elderly, give 54 mg/day. **Tricor, initial:** 145 mg/day without regard to meals; for renal function impairment or the elderly, give 48 mg/day initially. **Triglide, initial:** 160 mg/day without regard to meals; for renal function impairment or the elderly, give 50 mg/day. **Trilipix, initial:** 135 mg/day without regard to meals; for renal function impairment, give 45 mg/day. For the elderly, base dosage on renal function.

Hypertriglyceridemia.

Individualize dosage according to client response, and adjust if necessary follow-

F

ing repeat lipid determinations at 4- to 8-week intervals. Dosage will differ depending on the product to be used. **Antara, initial:** 43–130 mg/day without regard to meals; maximum dosage: 130 mg/day. **Lipofen, initial:** 50–150 mg/day with meals; maximum dosage: 150 mg/day. **Lofibra capsules, initial:** 67–200 mg/day with meals; maximum dosage: 200 mg/day. **Lofibra tablets, initial:** 54–160 mg/day with meals; maximum dosage: 160 mg/day. **Tricor, initial:** 48–145 mg/day without regard to meals; maximum dosage: 145 mg/day. **Triglide, initial:** 50–160 mg/day without regard to meals; maximum dosage: 160 mg/day. **Trilipix, initial:** 45–135 mg/day without regard to meals; maximum dosage: 135 mg/day. *NOTE:* For dosage in impaired renal function or in the elderly, see dosage under primary hypercholesterolemia or mixed hyperlipidemia.

Combination therapy with statin for mixed dyslipidemia.

Trilipix, initial: 135 mg/day.

NURSING IMPLICATIONS

IMPLEMENTATION/ADMINISTRATION/STORAGE

1. Place clients on an appropriate triglyceride-lowering diet before starting fenofibrate, and continue during treatment.
2. Reduce dosage in clients who have severe renal impairment (C_{CR} <50 mL/min); no dosage adjustment is needed for moderate impaired renal function.
3. Withdraw therapy in clients who do not have an adequate response after 2 months with the maximum recommended dosage.
4. If possible, discontinue or change drugs known to worsen hypertriglyceridemia (e.g., beta-blockers, thiazides, estrogens) prior to considering triglyceride-lowering drug therapy.
5. Store from 15–30°C (59–86°F); protect from moisture and light.

ASSESSMENT

1. Note reasons for therapy, other agents trialed, cardiac risk factors.
2. List drugs prescribed to ensure none interact or worsen lipid levels.
3. If an adequate response is not achieved after 2 months of treatment with the max dose, drug is generally withdrawn.
4. May increase cholesterol secretion into the bile, leading to cholelithiasis. If cholelithiasis suspected, assess for gallstones; stop therapy if gallstones present.
5. Regularly monitor BP, BS, lipids, CBC, renal and LFTs (in 4–8 weeks) to find lowest effective dose; if ALT or AST >3 times normal, stop therapy. Reduce dosage with C_{CR} <50 mL/min; avoid <30 mL/min.

CLIENT/FAMILY TEACHING

1. Take as directed with/without meals; except take Lofibra capsules and tablets and Lipofen capsules with food to increase absorption and lipid-lowering effectiveness.
2. Take at the same time each day; never take more than 1 dose of fenofibrate/day.
3. If also prescribed a bile acid resin (e.g., cholestyramine), take fenofibrate 1 hr before or 4–6 hr after the resin.
4. Follow prescribed diet for triglyceride reduction (↑ soluble fiber intake; ↓ saturated fat intake) as well as regular exercise program, weight reduction, BP control, smoking cessation, alcohol and salt reduction.
5. Report skin rash, GI upset, persistent abdominal pain, muscle pain, tenderness, fatigue, GU dysfunction or weakness.
6. Avoid therapy with pregnancy and breast-feeding.
7. Report as scheduled for regular liver tests and triglyceride levels. Drug therapy should be reevaluated after 2 months and if desired lipid reduction not evident with maximum dose therapy then alternative therapy should be sought.
8. Keep all F/U to assess response, labs, and for adverse SE.

OUTCOMES/EVALUATE

- ↓ LDL cholesterol, total cholesterol, triglycerides, apolipoprotein B
- ↑ HDL cholesterol

Fenoprofen calcium

(fen-oh-**PROH**-fen)

Classification(s): Nonsteroidal anti-inflammatory drug

Pregnancy Category: B
RX: Nalfon.

SEE ALSO ***NONSTEROIDAL ANTI-INFLAMMATORY DRUGS.***

INDICATIONS/USES

(1) Relief of S&S of rheumatoid arthritis and osteoarthritis. Is used for treatment of acute flare-ups and exacerbations and for long-term management of these diseases. (2) Mild to moderate pain. *Investigational:* Juvenile rheumatoid arthritis, prophylaxis of migraine, migraine due to menses, sunburn.

F

ACTION/KINETICS

Pharmacokinetics

Peak serum levels: 1–2 hr. **Peak effect:** 2 hr. **Duration:** 4–6 hr. **t½:** 2–3 hr. **Onset, as antiarthritic:** Within 2 days; **maximum effect:** 2–3 weeks. Food (but not antacids) delays absorption and decreases the total amount absorbed. 99% eliminated through the kidneys. **Plasma protein binding:** 99%.

CONTRAINDICATIONS

Use in pregnancy and children less than 12 years of age. Renal dysfunction.

SPECIAL CONCERNS

■ (1) **Cardiovascular risk.** NSAIDs may cause an increased risk of serious CV thrombotic events, MI, and stroke, which can be fatal. This risk may increase with duration of use. Clients with CV disease or risk factors for CV disease may be at greater risk. (2) Fenoprofen is contraindicated for treatment of perioperative pain in the setting of coronary artery bypass graft surgery. (3) **GI risk.** NSAIDs cause an increased risk of serious GI adverse events, including bleeding, ulceration, and perforation of the stomach or intestines, which can be fatal. These events can occur at any time during use and without warning symptoms. Elderly clients are at greater risk for serious GI events. ■

Safety and efficacy not established in children.

SIDE EFFECTS

Most Common

Headache, dizziness, asthenia/malaise, nervousness, somnolence, nausea, constipation, dyspepsia/indigestion, peripheral edema.

See *Nonsteroidal Anti-Inflammatory Drugs* for a complete list of possible side effects. Also, **GU:** Dysuria, hematuria, cystitis, interstitial nephritis, nephrotic syndrome. Overdosage has caused tachycardia and hypotension.

HOW SUPPLIED

Capsules: 200 mg, 300 mg, 400 mg; ***Tablets:*** 600 mg.

DOSAGE

CAPSULES; TABLETS

Rheumatoid arthritis and osteoarthritis.

Adults, usual: 400–600 mg 3–4 times per day, not to exceed a total daily dose of 3,200 mg. Adjust dose according to response of client. 2–3 weeks may be needed for improvement. Those with rheumatoid arthritis seem to require larger doses than do those with osteoarthritis.

Mild to moderate pain.

200 mg q 4–6 hr, as needed.

NURSING IMPLICATIONS

Do not confuse fenoprofen with flurbiprofen (also a NSAID).

IMPLEMENTATION/ADMINISTRATION/STORAGE

1. Those over 70 years of age generally require half the usual adult dose.
2. Lower daily dosage may be needed for those with impaired renal function.
3. Store from 20–25°C (68–77°F).

ASSESSMENT

1. List reasons for therapy, symptom characteristics, other agents trialed, outcome.
2. Assess joints for inflammation, swelling, deformities, mobility; rate pain levels.
3. Obtain periodic ophthalmic, auditory tests with chronic therapy.
4. Determine history of ulcers, heart disease, or cardiac failure.
5. May cause an increased risk of serious CV thrombotic events, MI, and stroke.
6. Monitor BP, CBC, PT/PTT, chemistry panel, renal and LFTs with chronic therapy; avoid with renal dysfunction.

CLIENT/FAMILY TEACHING

1. Take 30 min before or 2 hr after meals; peak blood levels are delayed or diminished if taken with food, but the total amount absorbed is not affected. If GI upset occurs, may be taken with meals or milk.
2. With swallowing problems, tablets can be crushed and contents mixed with applesauce or other similar foods.
3. Report any unusual bruising/bleeding, blood oozing from gums/nose, sore throat, fever, extremity swelling, SOB, or Wt gain. May elevate BP.
4. Avoid smoking, aspirin, alcohol, and OTC agents.
5. Report evidence of liver toxicity, such as yellow skin/eyes, RUQ pain, or a change in the color/consistency of stools.
6. If vomiting or diarrhea occurs, monitor appetite, and weight; report if persistent or if increased headaches, sleepiness, dizziness, SOB, chest pain, nervousness, weakness, or fatigue.
7. Review risk of serious GI reactions, including inflammation, bleeding, ulceration, and perforation of the stomach or intestines, which may be fatal.
8. These drugs may increase the chance of a heart attack or stroke that can lead to death; risk increased with longer use and with heart disease.
9. Keep all F/U to assess response, labs, adverse SE.

OUTCOMES/EVALUATE

↓ Joint pain and inflammation with ↑ mobility

IV

Fentanyl citrate

(**FEN**-tah-nil)

Classification(s): Narcotic analgesic

Pregnancy Category: C

RX: Buccal Film: Onsolis. **Buccal Tablets:** Fentora. **Injection:** Sublimaze. **Lozenge on a Stick:** Actiq, Fentanyl Citrate Transmucosal. **Spray, Intranasal Solution:** Lazanda. **Tablets, Sublingual:** Abstral, **C-II**

SEE ALSO ***NARCOTIC ANALGESICS***.

INDICATIONS/USES

Oral (buccal film or tablet, sublingual tablet, transmucosal lozenge), Nasal Spray: Management of breakthrough cancer pain in those (usually over 18 years of age) with cancer who are already receiving and are tolerant of opioid therapy for their underlying persistent cancer pain. *Investigational:* Management of pain and anxiety in pediatric burn clients undergoing dressing change and tubbing. Reduction of postoperative anxiety and excitement in ambulatory children.

Parenteral: (1) Induction and maintenance of anesthesia of short duration and immediate postoperative (recovery room) period. (2) Opioid analgesic supplement in general or regional anesthesia. (3) Combined with droperidol for preanesthetic medication, induction of anesthesia, or as adjunct in maintenance of general or regional anesthesia. (4) Combined with oxygen for anesthesia in select high-risk clients undergoing open heart surgery or certain complicated orthopedic or neurological procedures. (5) Preoperative medication.

ACTION/KINETICS

Action

Effects similar to those of morphine and meperidine. May have profound effects on respiration.

Pharmacokinetics

IV, onset: Immediate; **IM, onset:** 7–8 min. **Peak effect:** Approximately 30 min for the injection and 20–30 min for transmucosal product. **Duration:** 30–60 min after IV and 1–2 hr after IM. **t½:** 3.65 hr for the injection and 7 hr for transmucosal. When the oral lozenge (transmucosal administration) is sucked, fentanyl citrate is absorbed through the mucosal tissues of the mouth and GI tract. Actiq resembles a lollipop; sucking provides a rapid onset of action. The nasal spray is rapidly absorbed into the bloodstream through mucous membranes. Faster-acting and shorter duration than morphine or meperidine. Metabolized by CYP3A4 enzymes in the liver and excreted in the urine.

CONTRAINDICATIONS

The transmucosal form is contraindicated in children who weigh less than 10 kg, for the treatment of acute or chronic pain (safety for this use not established), and for doses in excess of 15 mcg/kg in children and in excess of 5 mcg/kg (maximum of 400 mcg) in adults. Use outside the hospital setting is contraindicated. Myasthenia gravis and other conditions in which muscle relaxants should not be used. Clients particularly sensitive to respiratory depression. Use during labor. Lactation.

SPECIAL CONCERNS

■ (1) Fentanyl is an opioid agonist and a Schedule II controlled substance with an abuse liability similar to other opioid analgesics. Fentanyl can be abused in a manner similar to other opioid agonists, legal or illicit. This should be considered when prescribing or dispensing fentanyl in situations in which the health care provider or pharmacist is concerned about an increased risk of misuse, abuse, or diversion. (2) Schedule II opioid substances, which include morphine, oxycodone, hydromorphone, oxymorphone, and methadone, have the highest potential for abuse and risk of fatal overdose due to respiratory depression. (3) Serious adverse effects, including deaths, in clients treated with oral transmucosal fentanyl products have been reported. Deaths occurred as a result of improper client selection (e.g., use in opioid nontolerant clients) and/or improper dosing. The substitution of fentanyl buccal soluble film for any other fentanyl product may result in fatal overdose. (4) The fentanyl lozenge, buccal and sublingual tablets, and buccal soluble film are indicated only for the management of breakthrough cancer pain in clients with cancer already receiving and tolerant to opioid therapy for their underlying persistent cancer pain. Clients considered opioid-tolerant are those who are taking oral morphine 60 mg/day or more, transdermal fentanyl 25 mcg/hr or more, oxycodone 30 mg/day or more, oral hydromorphone 8 mg/day or more, or an equianalgesic dose of another opioid for a week or longer.
(5) Because life-threatening respiratory depression could occur at any dose in clients not on long-term opiates, it is contraindicated in the management of acute or postoperative pain, including headache/migraine, dental pain, or use in the emergency department. This product is not indicated for use in opioid-non-tolerant clients, including those using opioids intermittently on an as-needed basis. Deaths have occurred in opioid-non-tolerant clients treated with other fentanyl products. (6) Instruct clients and their caregivers that this drug contains a medicine in an amount that can be fatal to children, in individuals for whom it is not prescribed, and in those who are not opioid tolerant. Keep all units out of the reach of children, and discard opened units properly. (7) This medicine should be used only in the care of opioid-tolerant cancer clients and only by health care providers who are knowledgeable of and skilled in the use of Schedule II opioids to treat cancer pain. (8) **Buccal tablet:** Because of the higher bioavailability of fentanyl in the buccal tablet, when converting clients on a mcg-per-mcg basis from other oral fentanyl products (including the fentanyl lozenge) to the buccal tablet, do not substitute the buccal tablet on a mcg-per-mcg basis. Adjust dosage as appropriate. (9) **Buccal soluble film and sublingual tablet:** When prescribing, do not convert clients on a mcg-per-mcg basis from any other oral transmucosal fentanyl product to fentanyl buccal soluble film or sublingual tablet. Clients beginning treatment with fentanyl buccal soluble film must begin with titration from the 200 mcg dose. Clients beginning treatment with sublingual tablets must begin with titration from the 100 mcg dose.
(10) When dispensing, do not substitute a fentanyl buccal soluble film or sublingual tablet prescription for any other fentanyl product. Substantial differences exist in the pharmacokinetic profile of fentanyl buccal soluble film and sublingual tablets compared with other fentanyl products that result in clinically important differences in the extent of absorption of fentanyl. As a result of these differences, the substitution of fentanyl buccal soluble film or sublingual tablet for any other fentanyl product may result in fatal overdose.
(11) Special care must be used when dosing fentanyl buccal soluble film or sublingual tablet. If the breakthrough pain episode is not relieved, clients should wait at least 2 hours before taking another dose. (12) The concomitant use of fentanyl buccal soluble film with CYP3A4 inhibitors may result in an increase in fentanyl plasma concentrations and may cause potentially fatal respiratory depression. (13) Because of the risk for misuse,

abuse, and overdose, fentanyl buccal soluble film is available only through a restricted distribution program, called the FOCUS Program, and the fentanyl sublingual tablets and nasal spray are available only through a restricted program, required by the Food and Drug Administration, called the Risk Evaluation and Mitigation Strategy (REMS). Under the FOCUS program, only prescribers, pharmacies, and clients registered with the program are able to prescribe, dispense, and receive fentanyl buccal soluble film. To enroll in the FOCUS program, call 1-877-466-7654 or visit http://www.onsolisfocus.com. Under the REMS, health providers who prescribe to outpatients, pharmacies, and distributors must enroll in the program to prescribe, receive, dispense, and distribute fentanyl sublingual tablets, respectively. Further information is available at http://www.abstralrems.com or by calling 1-888-227-8725.

- **Safety and efficacy not determined in children less than 2 years of age.**
- **Use with caution and at reduced dosage in poor-risk clients, children, the elderly, with impaired renal and hepatic function, if used with CYP3A4 inhibitors, and when other CNS depressants are used.**
- **Use of the transmucosal form carries a risk of hypoventilation that may result in death. The respiratory depressant effect of fentanyl may last longer than the analgesic effect. Consider the total dose of all opioid analgesics used before ordering narcotic analgesics during recovery from anesthesia. Use opioids in reduced doses initially (i.e., one-fourth to one-third those usually recommended).**
- **Certain forms of conduction anesthesia, such as spinal anesthesia and some peridural anesthetics, can alter respiration by blocking intercostal nerves. Fentanyl can also alter respiration through other mechanisms.**

SIDE EFFECTS

Most Common

Injection: Bradycardia, circulatory depression, hypotension, dizziness, sweating, N&V, chest wall/muscle rigidity, respiratory depression, blurred vision.
Transmucosal: N&V, anxiety, asthenia, confusion, depression, headache, insomnia, sedation/somnolence, itching, rash, constipation, abnormal vision, conjunctivitis, ear disorder, taste perversion, tinnitus, accidental injury.

See *Narcotic Analgesics* for a complete list of possible side effects. Also, skeletal and thoracic muscle rigidity, especially after rapid IV administration. Bradycardia, ***seizures***, diaphoresis. Transmucosal form may cause ***life-threatening hypoventilation.***

ADDITIONAL DRUG INTERACTIONS

Diazepam / ↑ Risk of CV depression
Droperidol / Hypotension and ↓ pulmonary arterial pressure
Nitrous oxide / ↑ Risk of CV depression
Protease inhibitors / ↑ CNS and respiratory depression
Ritonavir / ↑ Fentanyl effect R/T ↓ liver metabolism

HOW SUPPLIED

Fentanyl Citrate: Note that strengths are in micrograms *not* milligrams. ***Buccal Film, Soluble (Onsolis):*** 200 mcg/film, 400 mcg/film, 600 mcg/film, 800 mcg/film, 1,200 mcg/film; ***Buccal Tablet (Fentora):*** 100 mcg, 200 mcg, 400 mcg, 600 mcg, 800 mcg; ***Injection (Fentanyl):*** 50 mcg/mL (as the base); ***Lozenge on a Stick, Transmucosal (Actiq, Fentanyl Citrate):*** 200 mcg, 400 mcg, 600 mcg, 800 mcg, 1,200 mcg, 1,600 mcg (all as the base); ***Tablets, Sublingual (Abstral):*** 100 mcg, 200 mcg, 300 mcg, 400 mcg, 600 mcg, 800 mcg.

DOSAGE

BUCCAL FILM (ONSOLIS)

Breakthrough cancer pain.

The dose of the buccal soluble film cannot be predicted from the daily maintenance dose of opioid used to manage persistent cancer pain; the dose must be determined by dose titration. Individually titrate fentanyl buccal soluble film to a dose that provides adequate analgesia with tolerable side effects. Fentanyl buccal soluble film is not a generic form of any other oral transmucosal fentanyl product. **Adults, 18 years and older, initial:** One 200 mcg film. When prescribing, do not switch clients on a mcg-per-mcg basis from any other PO transmucosal fentanyl product to the fentanyl film, as they are not equivalent on a mcg-to-mcg basis. From the initial dose, closely follow clients and change the dosage level until a dose is reached that provides adequate analgesia.

If adequate analgesia is not achieved after one 200 mcg fentanyl film, titrate using multiples of the 200 mcg film (for doses of 400, 600, or 800 mcg). Increase the dose by 200 mcg in each subsequent episode until the client reaches a dose that provides adequate analgesia with tolerable side effects. Do not use more than four of the 200 mcg films simultaneously. If multiple films are used, do not place on top of each other; they may be placed on both sides of the mouth.

If adequate pain relief is not achieved after 800 mcg of fentanyl films (i.e., four 200 mcg films), and the client has tolerated the 800 mcg dose, treat the next episode by using one 1,200 mcg film. Do not use doses above 1,200 mcg.

Once adequate pain relief has been achieved with a dose between 200 and 800 mcg of fentanyl buccal soluble film, the client should use or safely rid of all remaining fentanyl 200 mcg buccal soluble films. Those who require fentanyl 1,200 mcg buccal soluble film should dispose of all remaining unused 200 mcg buccal soluble films. The client should then obtain a prescription for fentanyl buccal soluble films of the dose determined by titration (i.e., 200, 400, 600, 800, or 1,200 mcg) to treat subsequent episodes. Once a successful dose has been found, each episode is treated with a single film. Limit to 4 or fewer per day of fentanyl buccal soluble film.

Single doses should be separated by at least 2 hours. Films should only be used once per breakthrough cancer pain episode, i.e., the drug should not be redosed within an episode. During any episode of breakthrough cancer pain, if adequate pain relief is not achieved after the film, the client may use a rescue medication (after 30 minutes) as directed by their health care provider.

NOTE: Only prescribers enrolled in the FOCUS program may prescribe fentanyl buccal soluble film.

BUCCAL TABLETS (FENTORA)

Breakthrough cancer pain.

Titrate to a dose of the buccal tablet that provides adequate analgesia with tolerable side effects. Clients should have only one strength of the buccal tablet available at any one time. Follow clients closely, and change the dosage level until a dose is reached that provides adequate analgesia with tolerable side effects. **Adults, initial:** 100 mcg. Initiate titration using multiples of the fentanyl, 100 mcg buccal tablet. Those needing to titrate above 100 mcg can be instructed to use two 100 mcg tablets (one on each side of the mouth). If this dose is not successful in controlling the breakthrough pain, instruct the client to place two 100 mcg tables on each side of the mouth in the buccal cavity (i.e., total of four 100 mcg tablets).

Once a successful dose has been established, more than 4 breakthrough pain episodes per day, reevaluate the dose of the maintenance (around-the-clock) opioid used for persistent pain. Titrate above 400 mcg by 200 mcg increments; note that using more than 4 tablets simultaneously has not been studied.

Dosing may be repeated once during a single episode of breakthrough pain if pain is not adequately relieved by one dose. Redosing may occur 30 min after the start of administration; use the same dosage strength. Once a successful dose has been established (i.e., an average episode is treated with a single unit), if a client experiences more than 4 breakthrough pain episodes per day, reevaluate the dose of the maintenance (around-the-clock) opioid used for persistent pain.

For clients switching from oral transmucosal fentanyl (i.e., the lozenge) to the buccal tablet, use the following conversion:

- Current PO dose of transmucosal fentanyl: 200 mcg or 400 mcg; the initial buccal tablet dose is 100 mcg.
- Current PO dose of transmucosal fentanyl: 600 mcg or 800 mcg; the initial buccal tablet dose is 200 mcg.
- Current PO dose of transmucosal fentanyl: 1,200 mcg or 1,600 mcg; the initial buccal tablet dose is 400 mcg.

NASAL SPRAY (LAZANDA)

Breakthrough cancer pain.

Individualize dosage; the dose is not predicted from the daily maintenance dose of opioid used to manage persistent cancer pain and must be determined by dose titration. **Adults, initial:** One 100 mcg spray (i.e., 1 spray in one nostril), including those switching from another fentanyl product. If adequate analgesia is reached within 30 min of administration of the 100 mcg single spray, treat subsequent episodes of breakthrough pain with this dose. If adequate analgesia is not reached with the first 100 mcg dose, dose escalate in a stepwise manner over consecutive episodes of breakthrough pain until adequate analgesia with tolerable side effects is achieved. Clients must wait at least 2 hr before treating another episode of breakthrough cancer pain with the nasal spray.

The titration steps are as follows: **100 mcg of nasal spray:** use 1 × 100 mcg spray; **200 mcg of nasal spray:** use 2 × 100 mcg spray (1 in each nostril); **400 mcg of nasal spray:** use 1 × 400 mcg spray; **800 mcg of nasal spray:** use 2 × 400 mcg spray (1 in each nostril).

Limit nasal spray use to four or fewer doses/day. If there is inadequate pain relief after 30 min following dosing of the nasal spray or if a separate episode of breakthrough pain occurs before the next dose of the nasal spray is permitted (i.e., within 2 hr), clients may use a rescue medication as prescribed by the health care provider.

Due to differences in pharmacokinetic properties and client variability, do not switch clients on a mcg-per-mcg basis from any other fentanyl product to the nasal spray as the nasal spray is not equivalent with any other fentanyl product. The nasal spray (Lazanda) is not a generic version of any other fentanyl product.

If the response (i.e., analgesia, side effects) to the titrated nasal spray dose markedly changes, it may be necessary to adjust the dosage to ensure that an appropriate dose is maintained. If more than 4 episodes of breakthrough pain are experienced per day, reevaluate the dose of the long-acting opioid used for persistent underlying cancer pain. If the long-acting opioid or dose of long-acting opioid is changed, reevaluate and retitrate the dose of the nasal spray to be sure the client is taking the appropriate dose.

For clients no longer requiring opioid therapy, consider discontinuing the nasal spray, along with a gradual downward titration of other opioids in order to minimize possible withdrawal symptoms. In clients who continue to take their chronic opioid therapy for persistent pain but no longer require treatment for breakthrough pain, the nasal spray can usually be discontinued immediately.

SUBLINGUAL TABLETS (ABSTRAL)

Breakthrough cancer pain.

Adults, initial: A single 100 mcg tablet. Due to differences in the pharmacokinetic properties and client variability, even those switching from other fentanyl-containing products to fentanyl sublingual tablets must start with the 100 mcg dose. The sublingual tablet is not equivalent on a mcg-per-mcg basis with all other fentanyl products; thus, do not switch clients on a mcg-per-mcg basis from any other fentanyl product. Fentanyl sublingual tablets are not a generic version of any other fentanyl product.

Individually titrate fentanyl sublingual tablets to a dose that provides adequate analgesia with tolerable side effects. If adequate analgesia is reached within 30 min of administration of the 100 mcg tablet, continue to treat subsequent episodes of breakthrough pain with this dose. If adequate analgesia is not reached, the client may use a second fentanyl sublingual tablet after 30 min, as directed by their health care provider. No more than 2 doses of fentanyl sublingual tablets may be taken to treat an episode of breakthrough pain. Clients must wait at least 2 hr before treating another episode of breakthrough pain with fentanyl sublingual tablets.

If adequate analgesia is not reached with the first 100 mcg dose, continue dose escalation in a stepwise fashion over consecutive breakthrough episodes until adequate analgesia with tolerable side effects is reached. Increase the dose by 100 mcg multiples up to 400 mcg as needed. If adequate analgesia is not reached with a 400 mcg dose, the next titration step is 600 mcg. If adequate analgesia is not reached with a 600 mcg dose, the next titration step is 800 mcg. During titration, clients can be instructed to use multiples of 100 mcg tablets and/or 200 mcg tablets for any single dose. Instruct clients not to use more than 4 tablets at one time. If adequate analgesia is not reached 30 min after the use of the sublingual tablet, the client may repeat the same dose of the sublingual tablet. No more than 2 doses of fentanyl sublingual tablets may be used to treat an episode of breakthrough pain. Clients must wait at least 2 hr before treating another episode of breakthrough pain with fentanyl sublingual tablets.

Once an appropriate dose for analgesia has been reached, instruct clients to use only one sublingual tablet per dose of the appropriate strength, Maintain clients on this dose.

If the response (analgesia, side effects) to the titrated dose markedly changes, a dose adjustment may be required to ensure that an appropriate dose is maintained. If the long-acting opioid or dose of long-acting opioid is changed, reevaluate and retitrate the fentanyl sublingual dose as needed to ensure the client is on an appropriate dose. It is imperative that any dose retitration is carefully monitored by a health care provider.

Limit the use of sublingual tablets to treat 4 or fewer episodes of breakthrough pain per day. Rescue medication, as prescribed by a health care provider, can be used if adequate analgesia is not reached after use of fentanyl sublingual tablets.

For clients no longer needing opioid therapy, consider discontinuing sublingual tablets along with a gradual downward titration of other opioid to minimize possible withdrawal effects. In those who continue to take long-term opioid therapy for persistent pain but no longer require treatment for breakthrough pain, fentanyl sublingual tablets can usually be discontinued immediately.

TRANSMUCOSAL (ORAL LOZENGE)

Breakthrough cancer pain.

Individualize according to weight, age, physical status, general condition and medical status, underlying pathology, use of other drugs, type of anesthetic to be used, and the type and length of the surgical procedure. **Adults, initial:** 200 mcg; prescribe 6 units and advise clients to use all units before increasing to a higher dose. For dose titration, follow clients closely and change the dose level until the client achieve a dose that provides adequate analgesia using a single lozenge unit per breakthrough cancer pain episode.

Until the appropriate dose is determined, it may be necessary to use an additional unit during a single episode. Redosing may start 15 min after the previous unit has been completed (30 min after the start of the previous unit). Do not give more than 2 units for each individual breakthrough cancer pain episode while clients are in the titration phase and consuming units that individually may be subtherapeutic.

If treatment of several consecutive breakthrough cancer episodes requires more than 1 fentanyl lozenge per episode, consider an increase in dose to the next higher available strength. At each new dose during titration, 6 units of the titration dose should be prescribed. Evaluate each new dose in the titration period of several episodes of breakthrough cancer pain (usually 1–2 days) to determine whether the dose is adequate with acceptable side effects. Once a successful dose has been determined (i.e., an average episode is treated with a single unit), clients should limit consumption to a maximum of 4 units/day or less. If consumption increases to more than 4 units/day, reevaluate the dose of the long-acting opioid for persistent cancer pain. Dosage adjustment of the lozenge and the maintenance (around-the-clock) opioid analgesic may be needed in some clients to provide adequate relief of breakthrough cancer pain. Gradually titrate downward for discontinuation as it is not known at what dose level the opioid may be discontinued without producing the signs and symptoms of abrupt withdrawal.

IM; IV

Preoperative medication.

Adults: 50–100 mcg IM 30–60 min before surgery.

Adjunct to general anesthesia.

Adults, total low dose: 2 mcg/kg IV for minor, painful surgical procedures and postsurgical relief; **maintenance low dose:** 2 mcg/kg (additional doses are infrequently needed in minor procedures).

Adults, total moderate dose: 2–20 mcg/kg IV, depending on length and depth of anesthesia desired; **maintenance moderate dose:** 2–20 mcg/kg when indicated. Use 25–200 mcg total IV or IM when movement and/or changes in vital signs indicate surgical stress or lightening of anesthesia.

Adults, total high dose: 20–50 mcg/kg for "stress free" anesthesia. Use this dose during open heart surgery and complicated neurosurgical and orthopedic procedures where surgery is prolonged and stress response is detrimental. Use with nitrous oxide/oxygen to reduce the stress response. Postoperative ventilation and observation are required. **Maintenance, high dose:** 20–50 mcg/kg (range: 25 to half the initial loading dose). Individualize dose; administer when vital signs indicate surgical stress and lightening of anesthesia.

As general anesthetic with oxygen and a muscle relaxant.

Adults: 50–100 mcg/kg (up to 150 mcg/kg may be required) with oxygen and a muscle relaxant when attenuation of the responses to surgical stress is very important; used for open heart surgery and other major surgical procedures to protect the myocardium from excess oxygen demand and for complicated neurological and orthopedic procedures.

Adjunct to regional anesthesia.

Adults: 50–100 mcg IM or slowly IV over 1–2 min as required.

Postoperatively, recovery room.

Adults: 50–100 mcg IM q 1–2 hr for control of pain, tachypnea, and emergence delirium.

Children, induction and maintenance of anesthesia.

Children, 2–12 years: 2–3 mcg/kg. Safety and efficacy have not been determined in children less than 2 years of age.

NURSING IMPLICATIONS

IMPLEMENTATION/ADMINISTRATION/STORAGE

1. Individually titrate to a dose that provides adequate analgesia and minimizes side effects.

2. Fentanyl buccal tablets (e.g., Fentora) should only be used to treat breakthrough pain in cancer clients already receiving and tolerant to opioids. They should not be used for any short-term pain, such as headaches or migraines.
3. Fentora cannot be substituted for Actiq.
4. Reduce dose of injection in elderly and debilitated clients and those with renal or hepatic dysfunction. Use the lowest possible fentanyl dose in clients receiving CYP3A4 inhibitors.
5. The fentanyl buccal tablet, transmucosal lozenge, and buccal soluble film are supplied in individually sealed child-resistant blister packages. **The amount of fentanyl contained in each tablet, lozenge, or film can be lethal to a child. Keep out of the reach of children.**
6. Consider lower doses of the transmucosal form with head injury, CV, pulmonary/hepatic disease, or liver dysfunction.
7. When using transmucosal form, monitor at all times by an individual skilled in airway management and resuscitative techniques. Have naloxone available in event of overdose.
8. When discontinuing transmucosal fentanyl, titrate downward gradually; not known at what dose level opioid may be discontinued without causing S&S of withdrawal.
9. The following information applies to the administration of the fentanyl buccal soluble film (Onsolis):
   - Only prescribers enrolled in the FOCUS program may prescribe fentanyl buccal soluble film.
   - Use the tongue to wet the inside of the cheek, or rinse the mouth with water to wet the area for placement of the film.
   - Open the package containing the film immediately prior to use.
   - Place the entire film near the tip of a dry finger with the pink side facing up, and hold in place. Place the pink side of the film against the inside of the cheek. Press and hold the film in place for 5 seconds.
   - The film should stay in place on its own after this period. Liquids may be consumed after 5 minutes.
   - If chewed and swallowed, the film might result in lower peak concentrations and lower bioavailability than when used as directed.
   - The film should not be cut or torn prior to use.
   - The film will dissolve within 15 to 30 minutes after application. The film should not be manipulated with the tongue or finger(s), and eating food should be avoided until the film has dissolved.
10. The following applies to administration of the buccal tablet (Fentora):
    - Separate a single blister unit from the blister card by tearing apart at the perforation.
    - Bend along the line where indicated; peel back the blister backing to expose the tablet. Do not push the tablet through the blister, as this may damage the tablet. Do not store the tablet after it has been removed from the blister package, as the tablet's integrity may be compromised; also this increases the risk of exposure to children.
    - Immediately remove the tablet from the blister unit, and place the entire buccal tablet in the buccal cavity above a rear molar between the upper cheek and gum.
    - Do not attempt to split the tablet. Do not suck, chew or swallow the tablet, as this will lower plasma levels.
    - Leave the buccal tablet between the cheek and gum until it has disintegrated (about 14 to 25 min).
    - If remnants remain after 30 min, they may be swallowed with a glass of water.
11. The following applies to administration of the nasal spray (Lazanda):
    - Prime the device before use by spraying into the pouch (4 sprays total). Hold the nasal spray bottle upright so that the spray goes into the pouch.
    - Look at the counting window as a new unused bottle will show 2 thin red lines in the counting window in the white plastic top on the bottle.
    - Firmly press on the grips and then release. A "click" will be heard and one wide red bar will be seen in the counting window.
    - Keep pressing and releasing the grips 3 more times (for a total of 4 times). Each time the red bar will become smaller until a green bar will be seen in the counting window.

- Remove the tip of the bottle from the pouch; do not seal the pouch and do not discard the pouch.
- When ready to use, remove the protective cap from the tip (if it has been replaced).
- Sit up with the head upright, and hold the nasal spray bottle with the thumb on the bottom of the bottle and the first and middle fingers on the finger grips.
- Insert the nozzle of the bottle of nasal spray a short distance (about ½ inch) into the nose and point toward the bridge of the nose, tilting the bottle slightly.
- Close off the other nostril with one finger.
- Press down firmly on the finger grips until a "click" is heard and the number in the counting window advances by one.
- Note that the fine mist spray is not always felt on the nasal mucosa; clients must rely on the audible click and the advancement of the dose counter to confirm a spray has been administered.
- Stay sitting down for at least 1 min after using the nasal spray. Avoid blowing the nose for at least 30 min after each spray.
- Replace the protective cap, and return the bottle to the child-resistant container after each use.

12. The following applies to administration of the sublingual tablets (Abstral):
    - Place sublingual tablets on the floor of the mouth directly under the tongue immediately after removal from the blister unit.
    - Do not chew, suck, or swallow sublingual tablets.
    - Allow tablets to dissolve completely in the sublingual cavity.
    - Allow clients not to eat or drink anything until the tablet is completely dissolved.
    - In clients who have a dry mouth, water may be used to moisten the buccal mucosa before taking sublingual tablets.
13. The following applies to administration of the transmucosal lozenge (Actiq):
    - Open the blister pack with scissors just prior to use.
    - Place the unit in the mouth between the check and lower gum, moving it from one side to the other using the handle.
    - Client should suck, not chew, the lozenge. If chewed and swallowed, a lower peak level might result.
    - Consume the lozenge over a 15 min period. Longer or shorter consumption times may produce less effect.
    - If signs and symptoms of excessive opioid effects occur before the unit is consumed, remove the drug matrix from the mouth immediately and decrease future doses.
14. The respiratory depressant effect of fentanyl may last longer than the analgesic effect. The total dose of all opioid analgesics must be considered before ordering narcotic analgesics during recovery from anesthesia. Use opioid in reduced doses initially, usually ¼–⅓ those recommended.
15. Store buccal soluble film, buccal tablet, sublingual tablet, and lozenge products from 15–30°C (59–86°F). Protect from freezing and moisture. Do not use if package has been tampered with or opened.
16. **IV** Direct IV infusions may be given, undiluted, over a period of 1–3 min.
17. Protect injection from light; store from 15–25°C (59–77°F).
18. COMPATIBILITY D5W or 0.9% NaCl.
19. INCOMPATIBILITY Administer separately.

ASSESSMENT

1. List reasons for therapy, anticipated time frame, any previous use. Assess characteristics of pain and rate levels.
2. Monitor VS; assess for skeletal, thoracic muscle rigidity and weakness. Respiratory depression may persist. Have opioid antagonist (naloxone) available to reverse drug effects.
3. Available (Abstral, Actiq, Fentora and Lazanda) only through a program called the Transmucosal Immediate Release Fentanyl (TIRF) Risk Evaluation and Mitigation Strategy (REMS) Access program. Requires signed Patient-Prescriber Agreement and participating pharmacy for dispensing (www.TIRFREMSAccess.com or 1-866-822-1483). Onsolis available through the FOCUS program (www.OnsolisFocus.com or call 1-877-466-7654).
4. Note any neurovascular or pulmonary disease. Instruct in C&DB exercises before therapy to ensure compliance.

5. Inquire about children in the home, as dose could be fatal if consumed accidently.
6. Monitor respiratory rate, heart rate, and BP frequently. Assess for signs of misuse, abuse, or addiction.

CLIENT/FAMILY TEACHING

1. These drugs are only for opioid-tolerant persons; generally used with cancer pain. Keep out of child's reach—may be fatal if accidently consumed.
2. Rise slowly; may experience orthostatic hypotension (sudden drop in BP).
3. Do not perform activities that require mental alertness; drug causes dizziness and drowsiness.
4. If prescribed buccal tabs, do not open Fentora blister pack until ready to administer and do not store tablet once it has been removed from the blister package.
5. Fentora tablets should not be sucked, chewed, or swallowed. Place tablets between the cheek and gum, and leave until disintegrated, which usually takes 15–25 min. If any remains after 30 min, may be swallowed with a glass of water.
6. Actiq, Fentora, Abstral, and Lazanda require enrollment in TIRF REMS Access program (an FDA-required program to ensure appropriate use and to mitigate overdose, misuse, and complications of therapy).
7. Use caution, Actiq contains approximately 2 grams of sugar/unit; dry mouth associated with fentanyl use may increase risk of dental decay and diabetes control problems.
8. Place the Actiq unit between the cheek and lower gum. The unit should not be sucked or chewed.
9. Reinforce with child that transmucosal agent is not candy; it is a very potent medication that may be fatal and should not be chewed or swallowed. Place in mouth in-between cheek and lower gum, and ensure that the lozenge is sucked and child is able to comply.
10. With Onsolis, complete the "FOCUS Patient Enrollment Form." May receive counseling from the FOCUS program call center. May also contact at www.OnsolisFocus.com or call 1-877-466-7654.
11. The buccal films should not be cut or torn prior to use, or chewed and swallowed.
12. Onsolis buccal films should be placed on the inside of the cheek (pink side against cheek), and held in place for 5 seconds. Leave film in place until it dissolves—usually within 15–30 minutes after you apply it. Liquids can be consumed after 5 min. Do not manipulate film with the tongue or finger, and eating food should be avoided until the film is dissolved. If additional dose prescribed, place in opposite cheek; do not place on top on other film.
13. Dispose of units remaining from a prescription as soon as they are no longer needed. Drug can cause dependence and has the potential for abuse. Store appropriately. Partially consumed units are a special risk because they are no longer protected by a child-resistant pouch, yet may contain enough drug to be fatal to a child. Use temporary storage bottle provided in the event that a partially consumed unit cannot be disposed of promptly.
14. Avoid alcohol, grapefruit juice, and CNS depressants for at least 24 hr after use.
15. Recall or memory may be suppressed; may not fully recall events surrounding procedure. Advise that procedure was done, answer any questions; reassure that this is normal, and provide written guidelines for F/U for client/family to review.
16. Keep all F/U to assess response, ensure pain controlled and to assess for adverse SE.

OUTCOMES/EVALUATE

- Desired analgesia/relaxation during procedures
- Conscious sedation
- Control of pain in opioid tolerant clients

■

Fentanyl transdermal system

(**FEN**-tah-nil)

Classification(s): Narcotic analgesic

Pregnancy Category: C

RX: Duragesic-12, -25, -50, -75, and -100.

🍁 **Rx:** RAN-Fentanyl Transdermal System.

SEE ALSO ***NARCOTIC ANALGESICS*** AND ***FENTANYL CITRATE***.

INDICATIONS/USES

Management of persistent, moderate to severe chronic pain that requires continuous around-the-clock opioid administration for an extended period of time and cannot be managed by other means, such as opioid combinations, nonsteroidal analgesics, immediate-release opioids, acetaminophen-opioid combinations, or as-needed dosing with short-acting opioids. Use only in clients who are already receiving opioid therapy, who have demonstrated opioid tolerance, and who require a total daily dose at least equivalent to fentanyl transdermal system, 25 mcg/hr. Clients who are opioid tolerant are those who have been taking, for a week or longer, morphine, 60 mg/day or more; oral oxycodone, 30 mg/day or more; oral hydromorphone, 8 mg/day or more; or, an equianalgesic dose of another opioid. Can be used in opioid-tolerant pediatric clients 2 years of age and older.

ACTION/KINETICS

Action

The system provides continuous delivery of fentanyl for up to 72 hr. The amount of fentanyl released from each system each hour depends on the surface area (25 mcg/hr is released from each 10 cm^2). Each system also contains 0.1 mL of alcohol/10 cm^2; the alcohol enhances the rate of drug flux through the copolymer membrane and also increases the permeability of the skin to fentanyl.

Pharmacokinetics

Following application of the system, the skin under the system absorbs fentanyl, resulting in a depot of the drug in the upper skin layers, which is then available to the general circulation. After the system is removed, the residual drug in the skin continues to be absorbed so that serum levels fall 50% in about 17 hr. Metabolized in the liver and excreted mainly in the urine.

CONTRAINDICATIONS

Use for acute or postoperative pain (including outpatient surgeries). To manage mild or intermittent pain that can be managed by acetaminophen-opioid combinations, NSAIDs, or short-acting opioids. Hypersensitivity to fentanyl or adhesives. ICP, impaired consciousness, coma, medical conditions causing hypoventilation. Use during labor and delivery. Use of initial doses exceeding 25 mcg per hr, use in children less than 2 years of age. Lactation.

SPECIAL CONCERNS

Transdermal System. (1) Fentanyl transdermal systems contain a high concentration of the potent Schedule II opioid agonist, fentanyl. Schedule II drugs, which include fentanyl, hydromorphone, methadone, morphine, oxycodone, and oxymorphone, have the highest potential for abuse and associated risk of fatal overdose caused by respiratory depression. Fentanyl can be abused and is subject to criminal diversion. The high content of fentanyl in the patches may be a particular target for abuse and diversion. (2) Fentanyl transdermal system is indicated for the management of persistent, moderate to severe chronic pain (such as that of malignancy) that requires continuous around-the-clock opioid administration for an extended period of time and cannot be managed by other means such as acetaminophen-opioid combinations, nonsteroidal analgesics, opioid combination products, or immediate-release opioids, or as-needed dosing with short-acting opioids. (3) Only use the 50, 75, and 100 mcg/hr dosages in clients who are already on and tolerant to opioid therapy.
(4) Only use fentanyl transdermal system in clients who are already receiving opioid therapy, who have demonstrated opioid tolerance, and who require a total daily dose at least equivalent to fentanyl transdermal system, 25 mcg/hr transdermal system. Clients who are considered opioid tolerant are those who have been taking, for a week or longer, morphine 60 mg/day or more, or oral oxycodone 30 mg/day or more, or oral hydromorphone 8 mg/day or more, or an equianalgesic dose of another opioid. (5) Because serious or life-threatening hypoventilation can occur, the transdermal product is contraindicated: (a) in clients who are not opioid tolerant; (b) in the management of acute pain or in clients who require opioid analgesia for a short period of time; (c) in the management of acute or postoperative pain, including use after outpatient or day surgeries (e.g., tonsillectomies); (d) in the management of mild pain; (e) in the management of intermittent

F

pain responsive to as-needed therapy or non-opioid therapy; or, (f) in doses exceeding 25 mcg/hr at the initiation of opioid therapy. (6) Because the peak fentanyl levels occur between 24 and 72 hr after treatment, be aware that serious or life-threatening hypoventilation may occur, even in opioid-tolerant clients, during the initial application period. (7) The concomitant use of fentanyl transdermal system with potent CYP3A4 inhibitors (e.g., clarithromycin, itraconazole, ketoconazole, nefazodone, nelfinavir, ritonavir, troleandomycin) may result in an increase in fentanyl plasma levels, which could increase or prolong adverse drug reactions and may cause potentially fatal respiratory depression. Carefully monitor clients receiving fentanyl transdermal system and potent CYP3A4 inhibitors for an extended period of time and adjust dosage if warranted. (8) The safety of fentanyl has not been established in children younger than 2 years of age. Only administer to children if they are opioid tolerant and 2 years of age or older. (9) Fentanyl transdermal system is only for use in those who are already tolerant to opioid therapy of comparable potency. Use in non-opioid-tolerant clients may lead to fatal respiratory depression. Overestimating the fentanyl transdermal system dose when converting clients from another opioid medication can result in fatal overdose with the first dose. Because of the 17-hour mean elimination half-life of fentanyl transdermal system, those who are thought to have had a serious adverse reaction, including overdose, will require monitoring and treatment for at least 24 hr. (10) Fentanyl transdermal system can be abused in a manner similar to other opioid agonists, legal or illicit. Consider this risk when giving, prescribing, or dispensing in situations where there is concern about increased risk of misuse, abuse, or diversion. (11) Persons at increased risk for opioid abuse include those with a personal or family history of substance abuse (including drug or alcohol abuse or addiction) or mental illness (e.g., major depression). Assess clients for their clinical risks for opioid abuse or addiction prior to prescribing opioids. Routinely monitor all clients receiving opioids for signs of misuse, abuse, and addiction. Clients at increased risk of opioid abuse may still be appropriately treated with modified-release opioid formulations; however, these clients will require intensive monitoring for signs of misuse, abuse, or addiction. (12) Fentanyl transdermal patches are for transdermal use on intact skin only. Using damaged or cut fentanyl transdermal patches can lead to rapid release of the contents of the patch and absorption of a potentially fatal dose of fentanyl. ■

F

- **Use with caution in clients with brain tumors and bradyarrhythmias, as well as in elderly, cachectic, or debilitated individuals.**
- **Administer to children only if they are opioid tolerant and 2 years of age and older.**

SIDE EFFECTS

Most Common

N&V, anxiety, asthenia, confusion, depression, dizziness, euphoria, hallucinations, headache, nervousness, sedation/somnolence, itching/pruritus, abdominal pain, anorexia, constipation, dry mouth, diarrhea, dyspepsia, urinary retention.

See *Narcotic Analgesics* for a complete list of possible side effects. Also, sustained hypoventilation, amblyopia, blurred vision, accidental injury, back pain, edema, fever, flu syndrome, infection.

HOW SUPPLIED

Transdermal Patch, Extended-Release: 12.5 mcg/hr, 25 mcg/hr, 50 mcg/hr, 75 mcg/hr, 100 mcg/hr.

DOSAGE

TRANSDERMAL SYSTEM

Analgesia.

Individualize dose. Adults, usual initial: 25 mcg per hr unless the client is tolerant to opioids (Duragesic-50, -75, and -100 are intended for use only in clients tolerant to opioids). Initial dose should be based on (1) the daily dose, potency, and characteristics (i.e., pure agonist, mixed agonist/antagonist) of the drug the client has been taking; (2) the reliability of the relative potency estimates used to calculate the dose as estimates vary depending on the route of administration; (3) the degree, if any, of tolerance to narcotics; and (4) the general condition and status of the client. Maintain each client at the lowest dose providing acceptable pain control.

Overestimating the fentanyl dose when converting clients from another opioid drug can result in fatal overdose with the first dose. Because of the mean elimination t½ of 17 hr, clients who are thought to have had a serious side effect, including overdose, will require monitoring and treatment for at least 24 hr.

To convert clients from PO or parenteral opioids to the transdermal system, the following method should be used: (1) the previous 24 hr analgesic requirement should be calculated; (2) convert this amount to the equianalgesic PO morphine dose; (3) find the calculated 24 hr morphine dose and the corresponding transdermal fentanyl dose using the table provided with the product; and (4) initiate treatment using the recommended fentanyl dose.

The majority of clients are adequately maintained on fentanyl transdermal system given q 72 hr. Some may not achieve adequate analgesia with this dosing interval and may require systems to be applied q 48 hr. Consider an increase in the fentanyl dose before changing dosing intervals. Dosing intervals less than q 72 hr are not recommended for children and adolescents.

During the initial application, clients should use short-acting analgesics, as needed, until the analgesic effect of the transdermal system is reached. Thereafter, some clients may still require periodic supplemental doses of other short-acting analgesics for breakthrough pain.

The recommended initial dose of transdermal fentanyl is based upon the daily PO morphine dose and is conservative; 50% of clients are likely to require a dose increase after initial application of fentanyl. The initial dose may be increased after 3 days, based on the daily dose of supplemental opioid analgesics needed by the client in the second or third day of initial application.

It may take up to 6 days after increasing the dose for the client to reach equilibrium on the new dose. Thus, clients should wear a higher dose through 2 applications before any further increase in dosage is made on the basis of the average daily use of a supplemental analgesic. Appropriate dosage increments should be based on the daily dose of supplemental opioid, using the ratio of 45 mg/24 hr of PO morphine to a 12.5 mcg/hr increase in the transdermal fentanyl dose.

NURSING IMPLICATIONS

IMPLEMENTATION/ADMINISTRATION/STORAGE

1. The efficacy of fentanyl, 12 mcg/hr, as the initial dose has not been determined. Also, clients who are not opioid tolerant have manifested hypoventilation and death during use of fentanyl. Thus, use fentanyl only in those who are opioid tolerant.
2. Children converting to fentanyl transdermal with a 25 mcg/hr patch should be opioid tolerant and receiving at least morphine 60 mg/day orally.
3. Elderly, cachectic, or debilitated clients should not be started on fentanyl transdermal system doses higher than 25 mcg/hr unless they are already tolerating an around-the-clock opioid at a dose and potency comparable with fentanyl transdermal system, 25 mcg/hr.
4. Multiple systems may be used if the delivery rate needs to exceed 100 mcg/hr.
5. Do not undertake initial evaluation of the maximum analgesic effect until 24 hr after system applied.
6. If required, a short-acting analgesic may be used for the first 24 hr (i.e., until analgesic efficacy reached with transdermal system).
7. Upon removal of the system, it takes 17 hr or more for the serum levels of fentanyl to fall by 50%. To convert to another opioid, remove the fentanyl system and titrate the dose of the new analgesic based on the client's report of pain until adequate analgesia is reached.

8. If opioid therapy is to be discontinued, a gradual decrease in dose is recommended to minimize S&S of abrupt narcotic withdrawal.
9. Do not store the system above 25°C (77°F).

ASSESSMENT

1. List reasons for therapy, characteristics of pain, previous agents used, outcome. Note all drugs prescribed to ensure none compete/interact.
2. Rate pain level at various times throughout the day to ensure adequate dosing. Determine that dose required is based on conversion guidelines provided by manufacturer.
3. It takes 17 hr or more for fentanyl serum levels to fall by 50% after system removal. Titrate dose of new analgesic based on reports of pain until adequate analgesia reached. If opioids are to be discontinued, titrate downward gradually since it is not known at what dose level the opioid may be discontinued without causing S&S of abrupt withdrawal.
4. Note ↑ ICP or brain tumors; precludes drug therapy. Monitor VS; assess for respiratory depression.
5. Assess for any history of illicit drug use; monitor for compliance and level of pain control.

CLIENT/FAMILY TEACHING

1. Apply system to a nonirritated and nonirradiated fatty, flat surface of the skin, preferably on the upper torso. May clip hair (not shave) from site prior to application.
2. Use only clear water, if needed, to cleanse the site prior to application. Do not use soaps, oils, lotions, alcohol, or other agents that might irritate the skin. Allow skin to dry completely prior to applying the system. If liquid comes in contact with the skin, use clear water only to remove.
3. Remove system from sealed package, and apply immediately by pressing firmly in place (for 10–20 sec) with the palm of the hand. *Never cut or open the system.* Ensure complete contact of system, especially around the edges. Date and time patches, and tape securely to avoid confusion or dislodgment.
4. Keep each system in place for 72 hr; if additional analgesia is required, use breakthrough analgesic and record. A new system can be applied to a different skin site after removal of the previous system.
5. Fold system removed from a skin site so that the adhesive side adheres to itself; double bag and discard as directed after removal. Keep systems out of reach of children/pets.
6. Dispose of any unused systems as soon as they are no longer needed, by removing them from their package and double bagging and discarding.
7. Note time and frequency of short-acting analgesic use for breakthrough pain. Report if use exceeds expected needs; transdermal dosage may require adjustment.
8. Use only as prescribed; do not stop suddenly. Directions for use of fentanyl transdermal must be followed exactly to prevent death or serious side effects associated with overdose.
9. Avoid activities that require mental alertness. Excessive heat may increase absorption and excessive perspiration may alter adhesive stickiness.
10. Drug can cause severe constipation; use stool softeners, dietary fiber, and adequate fluids to control.
11. Report if high fever develops; potential for temperature-dependent increase in fentanyl release from the system that could result in fentanyl overdose.

OUTCOMES/EVALUATE

Desired pain control with chronic conditions.

Ferrous sulfate

(**FAIR**-us **SUL**-fayt)

Classification(s): Antianemic, iron

Pregnancy Category: A

OTC: Enfamil Fer-in-Sol, Feosol, Fer-Iron, FeroSul.

✦ **OTC:** Apo-Ferrous Sulfate, Ferodan.

Ferrous sulfate, dried

OTC: Feosol, Feratab, Slow FE, Slow Release Iron.

INDICATIONS/USES

(1) Prophylaxis and treatment of iron deficiency and iron-deficiency anemias. (2) Dietary supplement for iron. Optimum therapeutic responses are usually noted within 2–4 weeks. *Investigational:* Clients receiving epoetin therapy (failure to

give iron supplements either IV or PO can impair the hematologic response to epoetin).

ACTION/KINETICS

Action

The normal daily iron intake for males is 12–20 mg and for females is 8–15 mg, although only about 10% (1–2 mg) of this iron is absorbed. Sustained-release or enteric-coated products reduce the amount of available iron and absorption from these dosage forms is reduced because iron is transported beyond the duodenum. Iron is absorbed from the duodenum and upper jejunum by an active mechanism through the mucosal cells where it combines with the protein transferrin. Iron is stored in the body as hemosiderin or aggregated ferritin, which is found in reticuloendothelial cells of the liver, spleen, and bone marrow. About two-thirds of total body iron is in the circulating RBCs in hemoglobin. Iron-deficiency anemia can affect muscle metabolism, heat production, and catecholamine metabolism; deficiency has been associated with behavioral or learning problems in children.

Pharmacokinetics

Absorption of iron is enhanced when stored iron is depleted or when erythropoesis occurs at an increased rate. Food decreases iron absorption by up to 50%. The daily loss of iron through urine, sweat, and sloughing of intestinal mucosal cells is 0.5–1 mg in healthy men; in menstruating women, 1–2 mg is the normal daily loss. Least expensive, most effective iron salt for PO therapy. Ferrous sulfate products contain 20% elemental iron, whereas ferrous sulfate dried products contain 30% elemental iron. The exsiccated form is more stable in air.

CONTRAINDICATIONS

Hemosiderosis, hemochromatosis, peptic ulcer, regional enteritis, and ulcerative colitis. Hemolytic anemia, pyridoxine-responsive anemia, and cirrhosis of the liver. Use in those with normal iron balance.

SPECIAL CONCERNS

Accidental overdose of iron-containing products is a leading cause of fatal poisoning in children younger than 6 years of age. Keep products out of reach of children. In case of accidental overdose, call a doctor or poison control center immediately.

- **Allergic reactions may result due to certain products containing tartrazine and some products containing sulfites.**
- **Those with normal iron balance should not take iron chronically.**

SIDE EFFECTS

Most Common

Constipation, gastric irritation, nausea, abdominal cramps, anorexia, diarrhea, dark-colored stools.

GI: Abdominal pain, constipation, gastric irritation, N&V, abdominal cramps, anorexia, diarrhea, dark-colored stools. Soluble iron preparations may temporarily stain the teeth (the enamel is not involved); also, when iron-containing drops are given to infants, the membrane covering the teeth may darken.

LABORATORY TEST CONSIDERATIONS

Iron may affect electrolyte balance determinations.

OVERDOSE MANAGEMENT

Symptoms: Symptoms may occur when at least 20 mg/kg is ingested. Acute poisoning will produce symptoms in the following four stages:

1. Within 6 hours: Abdominal pain, coma, diminished tissue perfusion, dyspnea, fever, hyperglycemia, hypotension, lethargy, leukocytosis, metabolic acidosis, N&V, tarry stools, weak-rapid pulse.
2. If not immediately fatal, symptoms may subside within 12–24 hr.
3. Symptoms return 12–48 hr after ingestion and may include: Anuria, ***convulsions***, ***death***, ***diffuse vascular congestion***, hyperthermia, metabolic acidosis, pulmonary edema, ***shock.***
4. If client survives, in 2–6 weeks after ingestion, pyloric or antral stenosis, hepatic cirrhosis, and CNS damage may occur.

Treatment: Maintain a proper airway, respiration, and circulation. Perform gastric lavage in those who are candidates for GI decontamination. Systemic chelation with deferoxamine may be recommended for those with serum iron levels greater than 350–500 mcg/dL or in those with symptoms of iron toxicity. IM deferoxamine therapy may suffice, but severe poisoning (e.g., shock, coma) may require IV deferoxamine therapy. Specific treatment for shock, convulsions, acidosis, and renal failure may be necessary. Treatment includes usual supportive measures.

DRUG INTERACTIONS

Acetohydroxamic acid (AHA) / Possible ↓ iron absorption R/T chelation by AHA
Antacids, oral / ↓ Iron absorption from GI tract
Ascorbic acid / Ascorbic acid, 200 mg or more, ↑ iron absorption
Calcium salts / ↓ GI absorption of iron; separate administration times
Captopril / Concomitant use within 2 hr may promote formation of inactive captopril disulfide dimer
Cefdinir / ↓ GI cefdinir absorption by up to 80%; give cefdinir 2 hr before or after iron supplements
Chloramphenicol / ↑ Serum iron levels
Cholestyramine / ↓ Iron absorption from GI tract
Digestive enzymes / Serum iron response to PO iron may be ↓ by pancreatic extracts
Fluoroquinolones (e.g., ciprofloxacin) / ↓ Fluoroquinolone absorption from GI tract R/T formation of a ferric ion-quinolone complex; do not use together
Histamine H-2 receptor antagonists (e.g., cimetidine) / ↓ Iron absorption from GI tract
Levodopa / ↓ Levodopa absorption R/T formation of chelates with iron salts
Levothyroxine / ↓ Levothyroxine efficacy → hypothyroidism R/T ↓ absorption; do not use together
Methyldopa / ↓ Methyldopa absorption from GI tract
Mycophenolate mofetil / ↓ GI absorption of mycophenolate R/T formation of a drug-iron complex in the GI tract; avoid simultaneous administration
Pancreatic extracts / ↓ Iron absorption from GI tract
Penicillamine / ↓ Penicillamine absorption from GI tract possibly due to chelation
Proton pump inhibitors / ↓ GI absorption of iron
H ***St. John's wort*** / May ↓ absorption of iron
Tetracyclines / ↓ Absorption of both tetracyclines and iron from GI tract
Thyroid hormone / ↓ Thyroid absorption; do not use together
Trientine / The two drugs inhibit absorption of each other; give at least 2 hr apart
Vitamin E / ↓ Response to iron therapy

HOW SUPPLIED

Ferrous sulfate. ***Capsules, Extended-Release:*** 140 mg (45 mg iron); ***Drops:*** 15 mg iron/mL, 75 mg iron/0.6 mL; ***Elixir:*** 220 mg/5 mL (44 mg iron/5 mL); ***Liquid:*** 300 mg/5 mL (60 mg iron/5 mL); ***Tablets:*** 325 mg (66 mg iron).

Ferrous sulfate, dried. ***Tablets:*** 200 mg (65 mg iron), 300 mg (60 mg iron); ***Tablets, Slow-Release/Extended-Release:*** 142 mg (45 mg iron), 160 mg (50 mg iron).

DOSAGE

Ferrous sulfate
Ferrous sulfate, dried
CAPSULES; DROPS; ELIXIR; LIQUID; TABLETS

Prophylaxis of iron deficiency.

Adults: 60 mg/day given in 1–2 divided doses. **Children:** 1–2 mg/kg/day given in 1–3 divided doses, up to a maximum of 15 mg/day. **Premature infants:** 2 mg/kg/day given in 1–3 divided doses, up to a maximum of 15 mg/day.

Iron replacement therapy in deficiency states.

Adults: 150–300 mg/day given in 3 divided doses; Alternatively, can give 60 mg 2–4 times per day to help lessen GI effects. **Children:** 3–6 mg/kg/day given in 1–3 divided doses. **Premature infants:** 2–4 mg/kg/day given in 1–2 divided doses, up to a maximum of 15 mg/day. Consult a provider if the liquid is being considered for a child. The enteric-coated tablets are not recommended for use in children.

Iron supplementation during last 2 semesters of pregnancy.

15–30 mg/day should be adequate to meet the daily requirement during the last 2 semesters of pregnancy.

NURSING IMPLICATIONS

IMPLEMENTATION/ADMINISTRATION/STORAGE

1. Iron therapy should increase hemoglobin levels by about 1 gram/week.
2. Substitution of one iron salt for another without proper adjustment may result in serious over- or under-dosing.
3. For infants and young children, administer liquid preparations with a dropper. Deposit liquid well back against the cheek.
4. Eggs, milk, coffee, or tea consumed with a meal or 1 hr after may significantly inhibit absorption of dietary iron.

5. Ingestion of calcium and iron supplements with food can decrease iron absorption by one-third; iron absorption is not decreased if calcium carbonate is used and taken between meals.
6. Do not crush or chew sustained-release products.
7. Generally about 4–6 months of iron therapy is needed to reverse uncomplicated iron-deficiency anemias.

ASSESSMENT

1. Identify reasons for therapy noting S&S, clinical presentation, labs, and other related conditions.
2. Take a drug history, including:
   - Antacid use; any drugs used that may interact
   - OTC drugs, i.e., iron compounds or vitamin E use
   - Recent abdominal surgery; currently prescribed drugs
   - Allergy to sulfites or tartrazines (may be present in some products)
3. Note any GI bleeding; tarry stools or bright blood in stool or vomitus.
4. Assess for thalassemia (Mediterranean descent); obtain hemoglobin electrophoresis, as iron administration could be lethal.
5. Note any complaints of fatigue, pallor, poor skin turgor, or change in mental status, especially in the elderly.
6. Assess nutritional status and diet history through questioning and intake if possible.
7. Review pregnancies and menstruation history; note frequency, amounts, and heavy or abnormal bleeding. Pregnancy is an indication for iron prophylactically.
8. Discontinue if 500 mg of iron daily does not cause a 1-gram rise of hemoglobin in 1 month. Note cause (i.e., iron-deficient or megaloblastic anemia) or if further workup/studies needed.
9. Monitor VS, CBC, chemistry profile, stool for occult blood, reticulocytes, serum transferrin, and iron panel results.

CLIENT/FAMILY TEACHING

1. Adhere to prescribed regimen; report any problems immediately. Coated tablets may diminish GI effects such as nausea, constipation or diarrhea, gastric irritation, and abdominal cramps.
2. Review form of iron prescribed (bi- or trivalent), frequency of administration.
3. Take with meals to reduce gastric irritation. Taking with citrus juices enhances iron absorption. Milk products, eggs, and antacids inhibit absorption, so avoid unless taking ferrous lactate. Coffee and tea consumed within 1 hr of meals may inhibit absorption of dietary iron.
4. May cause indigestion, change in stool color (black and tarry or dark green), abdominal cramps, diarrhea, or constipation; may be relieved by changing the medication, dosage, or time of administration.
5. Increase intake of fruit, fiber, and fluids to minimize constipating effects. Eat a well-balanced diet with foods high in iron (i.e., meat proteins, dried fruits) and affordable foods (i.e., raisins; dark green, leafy vegetables, and liver vs apricots or prunes).
6. Will reduce tetracycline absorption. If to receive both, allow at least 2 hr to elapse between doses.
7. Store out of reach of children; overdosage can be fatal.
8. Dilute liquid preparations well with water or fruit juice, and use a straw to minimize teeth staining.
9. Note that the dropper for Fer-In-Sol has two markings: 0.5 mL for a 7.5 mg dose of iron and 1 mL for 15 mg dose of iron.
10. Pregnant women need an iron-rich diet. The American Academy of Pediatrics recommends an iron supplement for infants during their first year of life.
11. Follow administration guidelines for each product to minimize side effects. Do not self-medicate with vitamin, mineral, and iron supplements.
12. Keep all F/U to assess response, labs, adverse SE.

OUTCOMES/EVALUATE

- Resolution of S&S of anemia; if hemoglobin has not increased 1 gram in 4 weeks, then reconfirm diagnosis
- Restoration of serum iron/ferritin levels
- Improvement in exercise tolerance and level of fatigue

Fesoterodine fumarate

(fes-oh-**TER**-oh-deen)

Classification(s): Anticholinergic.

Pregnancy Category: C

RX: Toviaz.

F

INDICATIONS/USES

Treat overactive bladder with symptoms of urge urinary incontinence, urgency, and frequency.

ACTION/KINETICS

Action

Muscarinic receptors are involved in urinary bladder smooth muscle contraction. Inhibition of these receptors by fesoterodine causes the anticholinergic (antimuscarinic) effect.

Pharmacokinetics

Rapidly and extensively hydrolyzed by nonspecific esterases to the active metabolite, 5-hydroxymethyl tolterodine. Bioavailability is about 52%. **Maximum plasma levels:** 5 hr. **t½:** 7.3–8.6 (depending on the dose). The active metabolite is further broken down in the liver. Excreted mostly (70%) through the urine.

CONTRAINDICATIONS

Use in those with severe hepatic impairment. Urinary retention, gastric retention, uncontrolled narrow-angle glaucoma. Known hypersensitivity to the drug or any component of the product. Use during lactation unless the potential benefit outweighs the potential risk to the neonate.

SPECIAL CONCERNS

- Use with caution in clinically significant bladder outlet obstruction (risk of urinary retention), in decreased GI motility (e.g., severe constipation), in narrow-angle glaucoma, and in myasthenia gravis.
- The incidence of antimuscarinic side effects (e.g., constipation, dizziness, dry mouth, dyspepsia, increase in residual urine, UTI) is higher in clients 75 years of age and older.
- Safety and efficacy not determined in children.

SIDE EFFECTS

Most Common

Dry mouth, constipation, UTI, URTI.

GI: Dry mouth, constipation, nausea, upper abdominal pain, dyspepsia, gastroenteritis, diverticulitis, irritable bowel syndrome. **GU:** URTI, dysuria, urinary retention. **CV:** Angina, chest pain, QT prolongation on ECG. **Respiratory:** URTI, cough, dry throat. **Miscellaneous:** Peripheral edema, back pain, dry eyes, insomnia, rash.

OVERDOSE MANAGEMENT

Symptoms: Severe anticholinergic effects. *Treatment:* Symptomatic and supportive treatment. ECG monitoring is recommended.

DRUG INTERACTIONS

Anticholinergic drugs / ↑ Frequency and/or severity of anticholinergic side effects (e.g., constipation, dry mouth, urinary retention); also, anticholinergic drugs may ↓ GI tract absorption due to effects on GI motility

CYP3A4 inducers (e.g., rifampin) / ↓ Fesoterodine C_{max} and AUC by 70% and 75% respectively; dosage adjustment not needed

CYP3A4 inhibitors (e.g., clarithromycin, erythromycin, itraconazole, ketoconazole) / ↑ C_{max} and AUC of fesoterodine active metabolite; do not use fesoterodine doses >4 mg

HOW SUPPLIED

Tablets, Extended-Release: 4 mg, 8 mg.

DOSAGE

TABLETS, EXTENDED-RELEASE

Overactive bladder.

Adults, initial: 4 mg once daily. **Usual dose:** 8 mg once daily based on client response and tolerability. Daily dosage should not exceed 4 mg in those with severe renal insufficiency.

NURSING IMPLICATIONS

IMPLEMENTATION/ADMINISTRATION/STORAGE

1. Do not exceed a dose of 4 mg/day in clients taking potent CYP3A4 inhibitors (e.g., clarithromycin, itraconazole, ketoconazole).
2. Store from 15–30°C (59–86°F); protect from moisture.

ASSESSMENT

1. Note reasons for therapy, onset, occurrence/triggers, frequency, characteristics of S&S.

Describe daily bladder function (use a voiding diary) and R/O infections and stones.

2. List drugs currently prescribed to ensure none interact.
3. Determine evidence of urinary/gastric retention, GI obstructive disorders, or glaucoma.
4. Obtain renal and LFTs; reduce dose with dysfunction. Check urine culture to R/O infection.

CLIENT/FAMILY TEACHING

1. Take with liquid and swallow whole; do not chew, divide, or crush the tablets. May be given with or without food.
2. Drug is used to help reduce the frequency and urgency associated with urination. Not for stress incontinence or UTI; for treatment of overactive bladder.
3. Use caution with activities requiring mental alertness; may cause blurred vision and drowsiness. May also experience headache, dry mouth, constipation, and increased heart rate; report if bothersome.
4. Dry mouth symptoms may be relieved with sugar-free candy/gum, ice/water, or saliva substitute. Avoid alcohol and OTC antihistamines.
5. Decreased sweating may occur; use caution in hot environments and with increased physical activity.
6. Practice reliable contraception.
7. Keep all F/U to assess response and for adverse SE.

OUTCOMES/EVALUATE

↑ Bladder control with ↓ urinary frequency, urgency, or urge incontinence

Fexofenadine hydrochloride

(fex-oh-**FEN**-ah-deen)

Classification(s): Antihistamine, second generation, piperidine

Pregnancy Category: C

OTC: Allegra 12-Hour, Allegra 24-Hour, Children's Allegra 12-Hour Oral Suspension and Tablets, Children's Allegra ODT.

SEE ALSO ***ANTIHISTAMINES***.

INDICATIONS/USES

(1) Seasonal allergic rhinitis, including sneezing; rhinorrhea; itchy nose, throat, or palate; and itchy, watery, and red eyes in adults and children 2 years of age and older. (2) Uncomplicated skin manifestations of chronic idiopathic urticaria in adults and children 2 years of age and older. Significantly reduces pruritus and number of wheals.

ACTION/KINETICS

Action

Fexofenadine, a metabolite of terfenadine, is an H_1-histamine receptor blocker. Low to no sedative or anticholinergic effects.

Pharmacokinetics

Rapidly absorbed. **Onset:** Rapid. **Peak plasma levels:** 2.6 hr. **t½, terminal:** 14.4 hr. Approximately 90% of the drug is excreted through the feces (80%) and urine (10%) unchanged. **Plasma protein binding:** 60–70%.

CONTRAINDICATIONS

Hypersensitivity to fexofenadine or any component of the product.

SPECIAL CONCERNS

- Use with caution during lactation.
- The orally disintegrating tablets contain phenylalanine.

SIDE EFFECTS

Most Common

Headache, dyspepsia, coughing, URTI, viral infection, back pain.

CNS: Drowsiness, fatigue, somnolence, headache, dizziness, insomnia, nervousness, sleep disorders. **GI:** N&V, diarrhea, dyspepsia. **Respiratory:** Coughing, URTI, nasopharyngitis, rhinorrhea. **Musculoskeletal:** Back pain, myalgia. **Dermatologic:** Rash, urticaria, pruritus. **Hypersensitivity:** Angioedema, chest tightness, dyspnea, flushing, ***systemic anaphylaxis***. **Body as a whole:** Fever, pain, viral infection (flu, colds). **Miscellaneous:** Dysmenorrhea, back pain, accidental injury, otitis media, pain in extremity, paroniria.

OVERDOSE MANAGEMENT

Symptoms: Overdosage is infrequent. Symptoms observed are dizziness, drowsiness, and dry mouth. *Treatment:* Use standard measures to remove any unabsorbed drug. Treat symptoms and provide supportive treatment.

DRUG INTERACTIONS

Aluminum- or Magnesium-containing antacids / ↓ Fexofenadine AUC by 41% and C_{max} by 43%
Erythromycin / ↑ Fexofenadine plasma levels; no differences seen in side effects or QTc interval
Grapefruit juice / ↓ Fexofenadine absorption from GI tract
Ketoconazole / ↑ Fexofenadine plasma levels; no differences seen in side effects or QTc interval
Orange juice / ↓ Bioavailability of fexofenadine
Probenecid / ↑ Fexofenadine AUC R/T ↓ renal clearance
Verapamil / ↑ Fexofenadine peak plasma level and AUC R/T inhibiting P-glycoprotein transport

F

HOW SUPPLIED

Oral Suspension: 6 mg/mL; ***Tablets:*** 30 mg, 60 mg, 180 mg; ***Tablets, Oral Disintegrating:*** 30 mg.

DOSAGE

ORAL SUSPENSION; TABLETS; TABLETS, ORAL DISINTEGRATING

Seasonal allergic rhinitis.

Adults and children over 12 years: 60 mg twice a day or 180 mg once daily with water. **Children, 6–11 years:** 30 mg twice a day with water. In children, 2–11 years of age, 30 mg (5 mL) of the suspension may be used twice a day. *NOTE:* **Adults and children over 12 years with decreased renal function, initial:** 60 mg once daily. **Children 2–11 years with decreased renal function, initial:** 30 mg once daily.

Chronic idiopathic urticaria.

Adults and children, 12 years and older: 60 mg tablet twice a day or 180 mg tablet once a day with water. **Children, 6–11 years:** 30 mg tablet twice a day with water. Or, 30 mg (5 mL) of the oral suspension twice a day for children 2–11 years. **Children, 6 months–2 years:** 15 mg (2.5 mL) of the oral suspension twice a day. For clients with decreased renal function, give 60 mg once a day to adults, 30 mg once a day in children 2–11 years of age, and 15 mg once a day to children 6 months to less than 2 years of age.

NURSING IMPLICATIONS

IMPLEMENTATION/ADMINISTRATION/STORAGE

1. Store oral suspension and tablets from 20–25°C (68–77°F).
2. Foil blister packs containing tablets or orally disintegrating tablets should be protected from excessive moisture.

ASSESSMENT

1. Note onset, characteristics of S&S; identify triggers/time of year.
2. List other agents trialed, length of use, outcome.
3. Assess for renal dysfunction; reduce dose.

CLIENT/FAMILY TEACHING

1. Take as directed; take tablets with water. May take with food to decrease GI upset. Avoid taking with fruit juices.
2. Do not remove ODT (oral disintegrating tablet) from original blister package until ready to use. Dissolve ODT on the tongue, then swallow with or without water; do not chew. Take on an empty stomach. ODT contains phenylalanine.
3. Shake oral suspension well before each use.
4. Protect from excessive moisture. Store in a tightly closed container in a cool, dry place.
5. Do not take closely within 15 min of aluminum- or magnesium-containing antacids.
6. Avoid activities that require mental alertness until drug effects realized; report persistent dizziness or drowsiness. May experience headaches, sore throat, nausea, and dysmenorrhea.
7. Avoid alcohol and CNS depressants.
8. With allergy skin testing, do not take for at least 4 days before skin testing.
9. Keep all F/U to assess response and adverse SE. Identify and avoid triggers.

OUTCOMES/EVALUATE

- Control of seasonal allergic rhinitis (i.e., ↓ sneezing, pruritus, nasal congestion, watery/red eyes, itchy eyes/nose)
- Relief of chronic idiopathic urticaria.

Combination Drug

Fexofenadine hydrochloride and Pseudoephedrine hydrochloride

(fex-oh-**FEN**-ah-deen, soo-doh-eh-**FED**-rin)

Classification(s): Antihistamine/Decongestant Combination

Pregnancy Category: C

OTC: Allegra-D 12 Hour, Allegra-D 24 Hour.

SEE ALSO ***FEXOFENADINE HYDROCHLORIDE*** AND ***PSEUDOEPHEDRINE HYDROCHLORIDE.***

INDICATIONS/USES

Relief of symptoms associated with seasonal allergic rhinitis in adults and children, 12 years and older. Symptoms relieved include sneezing, rhinorrhea, itchy nose/palate, itchy throat, itchy/watery/red eyes, nasal congestion.

CONTENT

Each Allegra-D 12 Hour tablet contains: Fexofenadine hydrochloride (*antihistamine*), 60 mg for immediate release and Pseudoephedrine hydrochloride (*decongestant*), 120 mg for extended release.

Each Allegra-D 24 Hour tablet contains: Fexofenadine hydrochloride, 180 mg for immediate release and Pseudoephedrine hydrochloride, 240 mg for extended release.

ACTION/KINETICS

Action

Fexofenadine is an antihistamine with selective histamine H_1-receptor antagonist activity. No sedative or other CNS effects are observed. Pseudoephedrine is a sympathomimetic amine that has decongestant activity on the nasal mucosa. CNS effects are similar to, but less intense than, amphetamines. At recommended PO doses, it has little or no pressor activity in normotensive adults.

Pharmacokinetics

Fexofenadine. Rapidly absorbed. **Peak plasma levels:** 2 hr. High-fat meals decrease bioavailability by 50%. About 5% eliminated by hepatic metabolism. **t½, elimination:** 14.4 hr. Excreted mainly in the feces (80%). **Pseudoephedrine. Peak plasma levels:** 6 hr. Food does not affect extent of absorption. Less than 1% is eliminated by hepatic metabolism. **t½, elimination:** 4–6 hr (dependent on urine pH); mainly excreted unchanged in the urine. **Plasma protein binding:** From 60–70% of fexofenadine bound to plasma proteins. Protein binding of pseudoephedrine is unknown.

CONTRAINDICATIONS

Known hypersensitivity to any of the product components. Use with narrow-angle glaucoma or urinary retention, in those receiving MAOI therapy or within 14 days of stopping such treatment, with severe hypertension, or severe coronary artery disease. Antihistamines and decongestants are not recommended for use in children less than 2 years of age (studies continuing on use in children 2–11 years).

SPECIAL CONCERNS

- **Use with caution in those with hypertension, diabetes mellitus, ischemic heart disease, increased intraocular pressure, hyperthyroidism, renal impairment, or prostatic hypertrophy. Also, use with caution during lactation.**
- **Side effects more likely in the elderly due to sympathomimetic amines.**
- **Use during pregnancy only if benefit justifies the potential risk to the fetus.**
- **Safety and efficacy of fexofenadine not determined in children aged 2–12 years of age; do not use in children less than 2 years of age.**

SIDE EFFECTS

Most Common

Headache, insomnia, nausea, dry mouth, dyspepsia, throat irritation, URTI.

See *Fexofenadine hydrochloride* and *Pseudoephedrine hydrochloride* for a complete list of possible side effects. Also, ***seizures or CV collapse*** with accompanying hypotension may occur.

DRUG INTERACTIONS

Antacids (Al- and Mg⁺⁺-containing) / ↓ Fexofenadine AUC and C_{max}

Erythromycin / ↑ Fexofenadine levels R/T enhanced GI absorption

Ketoconazole / ↑ Fexofenadine levels R/T enhanced GI absorption

MAOIs / Significant ↑ BP

Sympathomimetic amines / ↑ Risk of CNS stimulation with seizures or CV collapse with accompanying hypotension

HOW SUPPLIED

See *Content.*

DOSAGE

TABLETS, EXTENDED-RELEASE 12 HOUR

Seasonal allergic rhinitis.

Adults and children over 12 years: One tablet twice daily given on an empty stomach with water. In clients with decreased renal function, initial dose is one tablet once daily.

TABLETS, EXTENDED-RELEASE 24 HOUR

Seasonal allergic rhinitis.

Adults and children over 12 years: One tablet once daily given on an empty stomach with water. Avoid use of the 24 hr product in clients with renal insufficiency.

NURSING IMPLICATIONS

IMPLEMENTATION/ADMINISTRATION/STORAGE

Store from 20–25°C (68–77°F).

ASSESSMENT

1. List reasons for therapy, clinical presentation/symptoms, triggers, other agents trialed. Note lung sounds and any secretion production.
2. Assess HEENT, note findings. List drugs prescribed to ensure none interact.
3. Determine any narrow-angle glaucoma, urinary retention, MAOI therapy, severe CAD/hypertension; precludes drug therapy.
4. Check renal function; reduce dose or avoid with dysfunction.

CLIENT/FAMILY TEACHING

1. Drug prescribed for the relief of symptoms of seasonal allergic rhinitis.
2. Take on an empty stomach with water. Swallow tablet whole; do not break or chew tablet.
3. Something that resembles the tablet may occasionally be eliminated in the feces; this is the inactive ingredients.
4. If nervousness, dizziness, or sleeplessness occur, stop drug and report.
5. Do not take within 30 min of aluminum- and magnesium-containing antacids.
6. Practice reliable contraception. Avoid other OTC agents.
7. Keep all F/U to assess response and adverse SE.

OUTCOMES/EVALUATE

Prevention of sneezing; runny nose; itching, watery eyes; and other allergic symptoms

Fidaxomicin

(fye-dax-oh-**MYE**-sin)

Classification(s): Antibacterial drug.

Pregnancy Category: B

RX: Dificid.

SEE ALSO ***ANTI-INFECTIVE DRUGS.***

INDICATIONS/USES

Treatment of *Clostridium difficile*-associated diarrhea in adults over 18 years of age. *NOTE:* To reduce the development of drug-resistant bacteria and maintain efficacy, fidaxomicin should be used only to treat infections that are proven or strongly suspected to be caused by *Clostridium difficile.*

ACTION/KINETICS

Action

Fidaxomicin is bactericidal against *C. difficile* in vitro by inhibiting RNA synthesis by RNA polymerases.

Pharmacokinetics

Minimal systemic absorption following PO administration. Metabolized in the liver by CYP enzymes. Fidaxomicin and its active metabolite (OP-1118) are substrates for P-glycoprotein. Mainly excreted (>92%) in the feces. **t½**: 9 hr (fidaxomicin) and 10 hr (OP-1118 metabolite).

CONTRAINDICATIONS

Use for systemic infections (fidaxomicin is only minimally absorbed from the GI tract).

SPECIAL CONCERNS

- Use with caution during lactation.
- Safety and efficacy not determined in children less than 18 years of age.

SIDE EFFECTS

Most Common

N&V, abdominal pain.

GI: N&V, abdominal pain/distention/tenderness, dyspepsia, dysphagia, flatulence, intestinal obstruction, megacolon, ***GI hemorrhage***. **Hematologic:** Anemia, neutropenia. **Metabolic:** Hyperglycemia, metabolic acidosis. **Dermatologic:** Drug eruption, pruritus, rash.

LABORATORY TEST CONSIDERATIONS

↑ Blood alkaline phosphatase, hepatic enzymes. ↓ Blood bicarbonate, platelets.

DRUG INTERACTIONS

↑ Fidaxomicin and OP-1118 (metabolite of fidaxomicin) plasma levels if used with cyclosporine.

HOW SUPPLIED

Tablets, Film-Coated: 200 mg.

DOSAGE

TABLETS, FILM-COATED

Clostridium difficile-*associated diarrhea.*

Adults, 18 years and older: One 200 mg tablet twice a day for 10 days given with or without food.

NURSING IMPLICATIONS

IMPLEMENTATION/ADMINISTRATION/STORAGE

1. Dose adjustment is not required for geriatric clients, although plasma levels are higher in the elderly (but still within the normal range).
2. No dose adjustment is required for those with impaired renal function.
3. Impaired hepatic function is not thought to affect metabolism or excretion of fidaxomicin.

ASSESSMENT

1. List reasons for therapy, onset/characteristics of symptoms (stool volume, quality, odor, etc.) culture results, other agents/remedies trialed, and previous antibiotic use.
2. List drugs prescribed to ensure none interact or aggravate diarrhea.
3. Assess for severe GI upset, N&V, abdominal distension/tenderness; check for bowel sounds and any evidence of obstruction.
4. Obtain CBC, alkaline phosphatase, BS, LFTs and cultures when warranted.

CLIENT/FAMILY TEACHING

1. Make take with or without food. Only indicated to treat *C. difficile*-associated diarrhea (CDAD) and not other types of infections.
2. Take exactly as directed. Do not skip doses or not complete therapy as may limit the effectiveness of treatment as well as increase the likelihood of developing resistance of this bacteria in the future.
3. May experience N&V, abdominal pain and distension; report if persistent or intolerable.
4. Avoid during pregnancy and while nursing unless clearly indicated and benefit outweighs risks.
5. Keep all F/U to assess response and for adverse SE.

OUTCOMES/EVALUATE

Treatment of *C. difficile*-associated diarrhea (CDAD)

IV

Filgrastim

(fill-**GRASS**-tim)

Classification(s): Granulocyte colony-stimulating factor, human

Pregnancy Category: C

RX: Neupogen.

INDICATIONS/USES

(1) **Myelosuppressive chemotherapy.** Decrease the incidence of infection, as manifested by febrile neutropenia, in clients with nonmyeloid malignancies who are receiving myelosuppressive anticancer drugs that are associated with severe neutropenia with fever. (2) **Bone marrow transplant.** Reduce the duration of neutropenia and neutropenia-related clinical sequelae (e.g., febrile neutropenia) in clients with nonmyeloid malignancies undergoing myeloablative chemotherapy followed by bone marrow transplantation. (3) **Severe chronic neutropenia.** Chronic administration to reduce the incidence and duration of sequelae of neutropenia (e.g., fever, infections, oropharyngeal ulcers) in symptomatic clients with congenital neutropenia, cyclic neutropenia, or idiopathic neutropenia. (4) **Peripheral blood progenitor cell collection and therapy.** Mobilization of hematopoietic progenitor cells into the peripheral blood for leukapheresis collection. (5) **Acute myelogenous leukemia.** Reduce the

F

time to neutrophil recovery and the duration of fever following induction or consolidation chemotherapy treatment of adults with acute myelogenous leukemia. *Investigational:* Use in AIDS, aplastic anemia, hairy cell leukemia, myelodysplastic syndrome, zidovudine, and other drug-induced neutropenia.

ACTION/KINETICS

Action

Is a human granulocyte colony stimulating factor (G-CSF) produced by recombinant DNA technology. Endogenous colony-stimulating factors are produced by monocytes, fibroblasts, and other endothelial cells; they act on hematopoietic cells by binding to specific cell surface receptors resulting in stimulating proliferation of neutrophils in the bone marrow. Has minimal effects, either in vivo or in vitro, on the production of other hematopoietic cell types. Filgrastim has an amino acid sequence that is identical to the natural sequence predicted from human DNA sequence analysis, except there is an N-terminal methionine that is required for expression in *Escherichia coli.*

Pharmacokinetics

IV infusion of 20 mcg/kg over 24 hr resulted in a mean serum level of 48 ng/mL, whereas SC administration of 11.5 mcg/kg resulted in a maximum serum level of 49 ng/mL within 2–8 hr. **t½, elimination:** 3.5 hr.

CONTRAINDICATIONS

Hypersensitivity to proteins derived from *E. coli.* The safety and efficacy of filgrastim given simultaneously with cytotoxic chemotherapy has not been determined; thus, filgrastim should not be given 24 hr before to 24 hr after cytotoxic chemotherapy.

SPECIAL CONCERNS

- **Use with caution in any malignancy with myeloid characteristics since the drug may act as a growth factor for any tumor type.**
- **Does not cause any greater incidence of toxicity in children than in adults.**
- **Use with caution during lactation.**
- **Safety and efficacy not determined for the following situations: chronic filgrastim therapy; to treat neutropenia due to other hematopoietic disorders, such as myelodysplastic syndrome; simultaneous use with cytotoxic chemotherapy.**
- **Hypersensitivity reactions usually occur within 30 min after administration and are more frequent in clients receiving the drug IV.**
- **Safety and efficacy not determined in neonates and clients with autoimmune neutropenia of infancy.**

SIDE EFFECTS

Most Common

N&V, skeletal pain, alopecia, diarrhea, neutropenic fever, mucositis, fever, fatigue, anorexia, dyspnea, headache.

NOTE: Hypersensitivity reactions may occur for any use on initial (within 30 min especially with IV use) or subsequent treatment. Hypersensitivity characterized by skin rash, urticaria, facial edema, wheezing, dyspnea, hypotension, tachycardia.

When used for myelosuppressive therapy: Musculoskeletal: Medullary bone pain, skeletal pain. **GI:** N&V, diarrhea, anorexia, stomatitis, constipation, peritonitis, splenic rupture. **Hypersensitivity:** Skin rash, facial edema, wheezing, dyspnea, hypotension, tachycardia. **Hematologic:** Leukocytosis; greater risk of thrombocytopenia and anemia. **Respiratory:** Dyspnea, cough, chest pain, sore throat. **Body as a whole:** Alopecia, neutropenic fever, fever, fatigue, headache, skin rash, mucositis, generalized weakness, unspecified pain. **CV:** Decreased BP (transient), cutaneous vasculitis, hypertension, ***arrhythmias, MI.***

When used for bone marrow transplantation. GI: N&V, stomatitis, peritonitis. **CV:** Hypertension, capillary leak syndrome (rare). **Hematologic:** Decreased platelet counts, anemia, increase in neutrophil count, WBC count greater than 100,000/mm³. **Miscellaneous:** Rash, renal insufficiency, erythema nodosum.

When used for severe chronic neutropenia: Musculoskeletal: Mild to moderate bone pain, musculoskeletal pain, abdominal/flank pain, arthralgia, osteoporosis. **Hematologic:** Thrombocytopenia, epistaxis (associated with thrombocytopenia), anemia, myelodysplasia or myeloid leukemia. **Dermatologic:** Exacerbation of certain skin conditions (e.g., psoriasis), rash, alopecia. **Miscellaneous:** Palpable splenomegaly, hepatomegaly, monosomy, injection site reaction, cutaneous vasculitis, hematuria, proteinuria, cytogenic abnormalities.

When used for peripheral blood progenitor cell collection. Musculoskeletal: Medullary bone pain. **CNS:** Headache. **Hematologic:** Mild to moderate anemia, thrombocytopenia.

When used for acute myeloid leukemia. CV: Petechiae, epistaxis, transfusion reactions, hemorrhagic events (respiratory tract, skin, GI tract, urinary tract, eye), ***hemorrhagic death***. **Hematologic:** Persistent leukemia. **Body as a whole:** Infection.

LABORATORY TEST CONSIDERATIONS

↑ Serum uric acid, LDH, alkaline phosphatase. ↓ Platelet counts (remained within normal limits); early myeloid forms in peripheral blood (e.g., metamyelocytes, myelocytes). Possible cyclic fluctuations of neutrophil counts in those with congenital or idiopathic neutropenia after initiation of filgrastim therapy.

OVERDOSE MANAGEMENT

Symptoms: WBC counts greater than 100,000/mm^3. No adverse clinical effects. *Treatment:* Discontinue filgrastim therapy; results in a 50% decrease in circulating neutrophils within 1–2 days, with a return to pretreatment levels in 1–7 days.

DRUG INTERACTIONS

Drug interactions have not been fully evaluated. Use caution with drugs that potentiate the release of neutrophils (e.g., lithium).

HOW SUPPLIED

Injection: 300 mcg/0.5 mL, 300 mcg/mL.

DOSAGE

IV; SC

Myelosuppressive chemotherapy.

Adults, initial: 5 mcg/kg/day as a single injection, either as an SC bolus, by short IV infusion (15–30 min), or by continuous IV infusion. **Range:** 4–8 mcg/kg/day. The dose may be increased in increments of 5 mcg/kg for each chemotherapy cycle depending on the duration and severity of the absolute neutrophil count (ANC) nadir. The dose should be given daily for up to 2 weeks, until ANC has reached 10,000/mm^3 following the expected chemotherapy-induced neutrophil nadir. Discontinue if the ANC surpasses 10,000/mm^3 after the expected chemotherapy-induced neutrophil nadir. Give no earlier than 24 hr after the administration of cytotoxic chemotherapy. Do not give in the period 24 hr before administration of chemotherapy.

Bone marrow transplantation.

Adults, initial: 10 mcg/kg/day given as an IV infusion of 4 or 24 hr or as a continuous 24 hr SC infusion. Administer the first dose at least 24 hr after cytotoxic chemotherapy and at least 24 hr after bone marrow infusion.

NOTE: During the period of neutrophil recovery, the daily dose should be titrated against the neutrophil response as follows:

- When ANC is greater than 1,000/mm^3 for 3 consecutive days, reduce the dose of filgrastim to 5 mcg/kg/day. If ANC decreases to less than 1,000/mm^3 at any time during the 5 mcg/kg/day dosage, increase filgrastim to 10 mcg/kg/day.
- If ANC remains greater than 1,000/mm^3 for 3 more consecutive days, discontinue filgrastim.
- If ANC decreases to less than 1,000/mm^3, resume filgrastim at 5 mcg/kg/day.

Severe chronic neutropenia.

Congenital neutropenia, initial: 6 mcg/kg twice daily SC every day. **Cyclic or idiopathic neutropenia, initial:** 5 mcg/kg as a single SC injection every day. Adjust the dose based on clinical course and ANC. **Usual dosage:** Congenital neutropenia, 6 mcg/kg/day; cyclic neutropenia, 2.1 mcg/kg/day; idiopathic neutropenia, 1.2 mcg/kg/day. *NOTE:* Chronic daily administration is required to maintain beneficial effect.

Peripheral blood progenitor cell collection.

Adults: 10 mcg/kg/day SC, either as a bolus or a continuous infusion. Consider dosage adjustment for those who develop a WBC count greater than 100,000/mm^3. Filgrastim should be given at least 4 days before the first leukapheresis procedure and continued until the last leukapheresis. *NOTE:* Administration of filgrastim for 6–7 days

F

with leukaphereses on days 5, 6, and 7 was found to be safe and effective.

NURSING IMPLICATIONS

IMPLEMENTATION/ADMINISTRATION/STORAGE

1. For myelosuppressive therapy or bone marrow transplantation, do not give filgrastim 24 hr before to 24 hr after administration of chemotherapy.
2. Discontinuing therapy usually results in a 50% decrease in circulating neutrophils within 1–2 days and return to pretreatment levels in 1–7 days.
3. Do not freeze; store in the refrigerator at 2–8°C (36–46°F). Prior to use, can be at room temperature for a maximum of 24 hr. Discard if left at room temperature more than 24 hr.
4. Solution should be clear and colorless. Do not dilute with saline at any time, as a precipitate may form.
5. Do not shake. Use only one dose from each vial; do not reenter the vial.
6. Compatible with glass, PVC, or plastic syringes.
7. IV May be diluted in D5W. When diluted to concentrations between 5 and 15 mcg/mL, protect from adsorption to plastic materials by adding human albumin to a final concentration of 2 mg/mL. When diluted in D5W or D5W plus human albumin, filgrastim is compatible with glass bottles, polyvinyl chloride, and polyolefin IV bags, and polypropylene syringes.
8. Do not dilute filgrastim to a final concentration of less than 5 mcg/mL at any time.
9. COMPATIBILITY D5W.
10. INCOMPATIBILITY Do not dilute filgrastim with saline or administer with Amphotericin B, cefonicid, cefoperazone, cefotaxime, cefoxitin, ceftizoxime, ceftriaxone, cefuroxime, clindamycin, dactinomycin, etoposide, fluorouracil, furosemide, heparin, mannitol, metronidazole, methylprednisolone, mezlocillin, mitomycin, prochlorperazine, piperacillin, and thiotepa.

ASSESSMENT

1. List reasons for therapy (i.e., chemotherapy-induced neutropenia, myelopsuppressive therapy for bone marrow transplantation, leukapheresis), clinical condition, and expected therapy time frame.
2. Note experience/sensitivity to *E. coli*-derived products.
3. With peripheral blood progenitor cell (PBPC) collection/therapy, obtain neutrophil count after 4 days of filgrastim. Consider dose modification if WBC count greater than 100,000/mm^3.
4. Perform bone marrow and cytogenetic evaluations annually with congenital neutropenia.
5. Clients reporting left upper abdominal and/or shoulder-tip pain should be evaluated for an enlarged spleen or splenic rupture.
6. Note last dose of cytotoxic agent and determine ANC nadir. Do not administer from 24 hr before to 24 hr after cytotoxic chemotherapy.
7. Monitor CBC with platelet counts at least 3 times per wk following marrow transplantation, twice weekly during first 4 wk of filgrastim therapy, and during the 2 wk following any dose adjustment; once stable, obtain once monthly for first year, then at least quarterly thereafter.

CLIENT/FAMILY TEACHING

1. Drug helps bone marrow make new white blood cells to protect you from infection. Taking too much may cause too many WBCs to be produced and taking too little filgrastim may not protect against infections.
2. Rotate injection sites and never inject into tissue that is tender, red, bruised, hard, or that has scars or stretch marks.
3. Review appropriate technique and demonstrate administration of first dose for provider. Review written guidelines concerning dose, administration, drug storage/handling, and discarding syringes.
4. Do not shake vial or prefilled syringe; shaking may damage the filgrastim. Only enter the vial once, then discard.
5. Do not use any filgrastim that is foamy, clouding, discolored, or contains particulate matter. Do not stop suddenly or alter prescribed dosing.
6. Flu-like symptoms (N&V and aching; bone pain) may be side effects of drug therapy. Take at bedtime, with prescribed analgesics.
7. Record temperatures; report bone pain, unusual bruising/bleeding or infection (e.g., fever, chills, rash, sore throat, diarrhea, or redness,

swelling, or pain around a cut or open sore, pain in left upper stomach area or left shoulder-tip area, rash, unexplained SOB, wheezing, fast pulse, swelling around mouth or eyes).

8. Avoid crowds and persons with infectious diseases.
9. Keep F/U visits to assess response, labs, and for adverse SE.

OUTCOMES/EVALUATE

- Prevention of infection
- ↓ Duration of neutropenia
- Improved neutrophil counts
- Mobilization of progenitor cells into peripheral blood

Finasteride

(fin-**AS**-teh-ride)

Classification(s): Androgen hormone inhibitor

Pregnancy Category: X

RX: Propecia, Proscar.

INDICATIONS/USES

(1) Improve symptoms of benign prostatic hyperplasia to reduce risk of acute urinary infection and reduce risk for surgery and prostatectomy (Proscar only). (2) In combination with doxazosin to decrease risk of benign prostatic hypertrophy symptoms from progressing over time. (3) Male pattern baldness (vertex and anterior midscalp) in clients between 18 and 41 years of age (Proscar only). *Investigational:* Prostate cancer; prostate cancer chemoprevention; hirsutism (use with caution, if at all, in women of childbearing age), male chronic pelvic pain syndrome (chronic nonbacterial prostatitis).

ACTION/KINETICS

Action

Is a specific inhibitor of 5-alpha-reductase, the enzyme that converts testosterone to the active 5-alpha-dihydrotestosterone (DHT). Thus, there are significant decreases in serum and tissue DHT levels, resulting in rapid regression of prostate tissue and an increase in urine flow and symptomatic improvement. Also a decrease in scalp DHT levels.

Pharmacokinetics

Well absorbed after PO administration with a bioavailability of 63–65%. **Elimination t½:** 6 hr in clients 45–60 years of age and 8 hr in clients over 70 years of age. Slow accumulation after multiple dosing. Metabolized in the liver and excreted through both the urine and feces.

CONTRAINDICATIONS

Hypersensitivity to finasteride or any excipient in the product. Use in women and in children. Handling of crushed or broken tablets by women who may potentially be pregnant. Lactation.

SPECIAL CONCERNS

Use with caution in clients with impaired liver function.

SIDE EFFECTS

Most Common

Impotence, decreased libido, postural hypotension, dizziness, asthenia, headache, ejaculation disorder.

GU: Impotence, decreased libido, decreased volume of ejaculate, ejaculation disorder. **CNS:** Dizziness, somnolence, headache. **CV:** Postural hypotension, hypotension. **Respiratory:** Rhinitis, dyspnea. **Miscellaneous:** Breast tenderness and enlargement (Propecia only), hypersensitivity reactions (including pruritus, urticaria, skin rash and lip swelling), breast cancer in men, testicular pain, gynecomastia, asthenia, peripheral edema.

LABORATORY TEST CONSIDERATIONS

↓ Serum PSA levels.

DRUG INTERACTIONS

Significant ↑ plasma levels of finasteride when used with terazosin

HOW SUPPLIED

Tablets: 1 mg, 5 mg.

DOSAGE

TABLETS

Benign prostatic hyperplasia.

5 mg per day, with or without meals.

Androgenetic alopecia.

Males: 1 mg once a day with or without meals.

NURSING IMPLICATIONS

IMPLEMENTATION/ADMINISTRATION/STORAGE

1. At least 6–12 months of therapy may be required to determine whether a beneficial response has been achieved for BPH.
2. Daily use for 3 months or longer is necessary to observe beneficial effects for androgenetic alopecia.
3. Continued use is required to sustain beneficial effects for hair growth. Withdrawal leads to reversal of effects within 12 months.
4. Women who are pregnant or may become pregnant should not handle crushed finasteride tablets, as there is potential for drug absorption and subsequent potential risk to the male fetus. When the male's sexual partner is or may become pregnant, exposure of semen to his partner should be avoided or drug use discontinued.
5. Do not adjust dosage in the elderly or in those with impaired renal function.

ASSESSMENT

1. Note reasons for therapy, onset, characteristics of S&S, any family history.
2. Complete history/physical exam. Not for use in females. May obtain pre-treatment scalp photos with hair loss to assess/gauge response.
3. Review urologic exam to rule out other conditions similar to BPH (e.g., prostate cancer, infection, stricture, hypotonic bladder, neurogenic disorders).
4. Schedule regular digital rectal exams to assess prostate gland. With liver impairment, monitor closely.
5. Not all clients show a response to finasteride. With a large residual urinary volume or severely diminished urinary flow, assess for obstructive uropathy; may not be finasteride candidate.
6. Monitor VS, LFTs, and PSA. May cause a decrease in PSA levels (prostate-specific antigen: a blood screening study to detect prostate cancer) even in the presence of prostate cancer.

CLIENT/FAMILY TEACHING

1. The following symptoms of BPH should show improvement with continued drug therapy: hesitancy, feelings of incomplete bladder emptying, interruption of urinary stream, impairment of size and force of urinary stream, and terminal urinary dribbling. May take 6–12 months of continued therapy before a beneficial effect is evident.
2. May lower PSA levels (prostate-specific antigen: a blood screening study to detect prostate cancer) even in the presence of prostate cancer.
3. Interruption of therapy will reverse effects within 12 months; BPH S&S will return as well as hair loss.
4. Use barrier contraception. If partner is pregnant or may become pregnant, avoid exposure to semen. Drug may cause damage to male fetus; stop drug or use a condom.
5. Women who are pregnant or desire to become pregnant should not handle crushed or broken tablets due to potential for fetal harm.
6. For male pattern baldness, take once a day with/without meals. More than prescribed dose will not increase hair growth but may cause adverse symptoms. May take 3 mg or more before any response noted for up to 3 months of therapy. Continued use is required to maintain benefit.
7. Decreased volume of ejaculate may occur but does not interfere with sexual function. Impotence and decreased libido may occur; stopping therapy will result in reversal of effect within 12 mo.
8. Immediately report breast lumps, breast pain, or nipple discharge.
9. Keep all F/U to assess response, labs, prostate exams, and adverse SE. Do not donate blood for up to 1 month after therapy completed/stopped.

OUTCOMES/EVALUATE

- ↓ Size of enlarged prostate gland
- Symptomatic improvement
- Regrowth of hair in male pattern baldness

Fingolimod hydrochloride

(fin-**GOL**-ih-mod **HYE**-droe-**KLOR**-ide)

Classification(s): Immunomodulator to treat multiple sclerosis.

Pregnancy Category: C

RX: Gilenya.

INDICATIONS/USES

Relapsing forms of multiple sclerosis to reduce the frequency of clinical exacerbations and to delay the accumulation of physical disability.

ACTION/KINETICS

Action

The mechanism for use in multiple sclerosis is not known but may involve reduction of lymphocyte migration into the CNS.

Pharmacokinetics

Absolute bioavailability is 93%. **Maximum levels:** 12–16 hr. **Steady-state blood levels:** 1–2 months following once daily use. Food does not affect either C_{max} or AUC. Significantly distributed (86%) to RBCs. Biotransformation occurs by three pathways, including by CYP4F2 with minor roles by CYP2D6, CYP2E1, CYP3A4, and CYP4F12. **t½, terminal:** 6–9 days. About 81% excreted in the urine as inactive metabolites.

CONTRAINDICATIONS

Pregnancy should be avoided. Lactation.

SPECIAL CONCERNS

- **Closely monitor clients with severe hepatic impairment as the risk of side effects is greater.**
- **Can decrease the HR and/or AV conduction especially after the first dose.**
- **Clients with a history of uveitis and those with diabetes mellitus are at an increased risk of macular edema.**
- **Lymphocytes may remain decreased for up to 2 months following the last dose.**
- **Use with caution in clients age 65 years and older**
- **Safety and efficacy not determined in children less than 18 years of age.**

SIDE EFFECTS

Most Common

Back pain, diarrhea, headache, influenza, liver enzyme elevations, cough.

GI: Diarrhea, gastroenteritis. **CNS:** Headache, depression, dizziness, migraine, paresthesia. **CV:** Hypertension, AV block, bradycardia, ***ischemic and hemorrhagic strokes***, peripheral arterial occlusive disease, posterior reversible encephalopathy syndrome. **Respiratory:** Cough, bronchitis, dyspnea, sinusitis. Dose-dependent reductions in FEV-1 and diffusing lung capacity for carbon monoxide. **Dermatologic:** Alopecia, eczema, pruritus. **Musculoskeletal:** Back pain. **Hematologic:** Leukopenia, lymphopenia. **Ophthalmic:** Eye pain, blurred vision, macular edema. **Body as a whole:** Asthenia, influenza viral infections, herpes viral infections, tinea infections, weight loss. **Miscellaneous:** Cutaneous T-cell lymphoproliferative disorders and diffuse B-cell lymphoma (relationship to drug use uncertain).

LABORATORY TEST CONSIDERATIONS

↑ AST, ALT, blood triglycerides, GGT. ↓ Blood lymphocytes counts. ↓ Pulmonary function tests.

DRUG INTERACTIONS

An additive effect of fingolimod with other drugs that prolong the QT interval is possible. The following drugs may prolong the QT interval and increase the risk of life-threatening cardiac arrhythmias, including torsades de pointes: Antiarrhythmic drugs (e.g., amiodarone, bretylium, disopyramide, dofetilide, procainamide, quinidine, sotalol), arsenic trioxide, chlorpromazine, cisapride, dolasetron, droperidol, gatifloxacin, halofantrine, levomethadyl, mefloquine, mesoridazine, moxifloxacin, pentamidine, pimozide, probucol, sparfloxacin, thioridazine, and ziprasidone.

Antiarrhythmics Class Ia (e.g., procainamide, quinidine) and Class III (e.g., amiodarone, sotalol) / Use associated with torsades de pointes in clients with bradycardia; since fingolimod ↓ HR, closely monitor coadministration

Antineoplastic drugs / ↑ Risk of immunosuppression and infection; use caution when switching from long-acting therapies with immune effects

Beta-blockers / ↑ Heart-rate lowering effects; monitor carefully during initiation of therapy

Diltiazem / ↑ Heart-rate lowering effects; monitor carefully during imitation of therapy

Immune modulating therapies / ↑ Risk of immunosuppression and infection; use caution when switching from long-acting therapies with immune effects

Immunosuppressive drugs / ↑ Risk of immunosuppression and infection; use caution when switching from long-acting therapies with immune effects

Ketoconazole (oral) / ↑ Fingolimod and fingolimod phosphate blood levels → ↑ risk of side effects; closely monitor

Vaccines / ↓ Efficacy of vaccinations for up to 2 months after discontinuing fingolimod; avoid live attenuated vaccine administration during this period

HOW SUPPLIED

Capsules: 0.5 mg.

DOSAGE

CAPSULES

Multiple sclerosis.

Adults: 0.5 mg once/day.

NURSING IMPLICATIONS

F

IMPLEMENTATION/ADMINISTRATION/STORAGE

1. Observe clients for 6 hr after the first dose to monitor for S&S of bradycardia.
2. Closely monitor clients with severe hepatic impairment as side effects may be greater.
3. Dose modification is not required in those with renal impairment.
4. If fingolimod therapy is discontinued for more than 2 weeks, the effects on HR and AV conduction may recur upon reintroduction of fingolimod treatment. Use the same precautions as for initial dosing.
5. A pregnancy register has been established to collect information about the effect of fingolimod use during pregnancy. Health care providers or pregnant women may enroll by calling 1-877-598-7237.
6. Store from 15–30°C (59–86°F). Protect from moisture.

ASSESSMENT

1. Note disease onset, frequency of exacerbations, other therapies trialed, and outcome.
2. List drugs prescribed to ensure none interact.
3. Assess for any CAD, heart block, arrhythmia, or infection. Obtain baseline ECG, and observe for S&S of bradycardia for 6 hr after first dose.
4. Determine history of chickenpox; if unknown or antibody-negative, consider VZV vaccination prior to starting fingolimod treatment. Wait 1 month after vaccination to permit full effect of vaccination to occur.
5. Assess pulmonary status and lung sounds. Consider spirometric evaluation of respiratory function, and evaluation of DLCO with reports or evidence of pulmonary problems.
6. Obtain baseline ophthalmologic evaluation, and again 3–4 months after starting treatment. If any visual disturbances reported, have additional an eye exam performed. Monitor VS, CBC, ECG, renal and LFTs; assess for dysfunction.

CLIENT/FAMILY TEACHING

1. Take with or without food once daily as directed. Drug is used to reduce the frequency of exacerbations of relapsing MS.
2. Infections more likely when taking fingolimod; advise provider if S&S of infection. Some vaccines should be avoided during treatment, and for 2 months after completed. Report any fever, chills, body aches or S&S of infection, or new onset or worsening of SOB.
3. Symptoms of hepatic dysfunction (unexplained N&V, RUQ abdominal pain, fatigue, yellow skin discoloration and/or dark urine) require reporting and interruption of therapy.
4. Report any dizziness, drowsiness, slow or irregular heart rate.
5. If changes in visual acuity, light sensitivity, blurriness, shadows, or blind spots in center of vision is experienced, report as eye exam will be required.
6. Practice reliable contraceptive during and for 2 months after stopping treatment; report if pregnancy suspected. Notify the Gilenya Pregnancy Registry at 1-877-598-7237 if you become pregnant during therapy.
7. Drug remains in the blood and continues to have effects, including decreased WBCs, for up to 2 mo following the last dose.
8. Keep all F/U to assess response, labs, and adverse SE.

OUTCOMES/EVALUATE

↓ Frequency of relapsing MS exacerbations

Flecainide acetate

(fleh-**KAY**-nyd)

Classification(s): Antiarrhythmic, Class IC

Pregnancy Category: C

RX: Tambocor.

SEE ALSO ***ANTIARRHYTHMIC DRUGS***.

INDICATIONS/USES

(1) Life-threatening arrhythmias manifested as sustained ventricular tachycardia. (2) Prevention of paroxysmal atrial fibrillation associated with

disabling symptoms and paroxysmal supraventricular tachycardias (PSVT), including atrioventricular nodal reentrant tachycardia, atrioventricular reentrant tachycardia, and other supraventricular tachycardias of unspecified mechanism associated with disabling symptoms in those without structural heart disease.

NOTE: Not recommended in those with less severe ventricular arrhythmias even if clients are symptomatic.

ACTION/KINETICS

Action

The antiarrhythmic effect is due to a local anesthetic action, especially on the His-Purkinje system in the ventricle. Drug decreases single and multiple PVCs and reduces the incidence of ventricular tachycardia.

Pharmacokinetics

Peak plasma levels: 3 hr; **steady state levels:** 3–5 days. **Effective plasma levels:** 0.2–1 mcg/mL (trough levels). **t½:** 20 hr (12–27 hr). Approximately 30% is excreted in urine unchanged. Metabolized by the CYP2D6 isoenzyme system. Impaired renal function decreases rate of elimination of unchanged drug and prolongs the half-life. Food or antacids do not affect absorption. **Plasma protein binding:** 40%.

CONTRAINDICATIONS

Cardiogenic shock, pre-existing second- or third-degree AV block, RBBB when associated with bifascicular block (unless pacemaker is present to maintain cardiac rhythm). Recent MI. Chronic atrial fibrillation. Frequent PVCs and symptomatic nonsustained ventricular arrhythmias. Lactation.

SPECIAL CONCERNS

(1) Flecainide was included in the National Heart Lung and Blood Institutes Cardiac Arrhythmia Suppression Trial. An excessive mortality or nonfatal cardiac arrest rate was seen in those treated with flecainide compared with that seen in those assigned to a carefully matched placebo-control group. The average duration of treatment with flecainide in the study was 10 months. (2) The applicability of this study to other populations is uncertain. However, it is advisable to consider the risks of Class IC agents (including flecainide), coupled with the lack of any evidence of improved survival, generally unacceptable in those without life-threatening ventricular arrhythmias, even if the clients are experiencing unpleasant, but not life-threatening, symptoms or signs. (3) Ventricular tachycardia was noted (0.4%) in clients treated with PO flecainide for paroxysmal atrial fibrillation. Flecainide is not recommended for use in those with chronic atrial fibrillation. Case reports of ventricular proarrhythmic effects in those treated with flecainide for atrial fibrillation/flutter have included increased PVCs, ventricular tachycardia, ventricular fibrillation, and death. (4) As with other Class I drugs, those treated with flecainide for atrial flutter have been reported with a 1:1 atrioventricular conduction due to slowing the atrial rate. A paradoxical increase in the ventricular rate may also occur in those with atrial fibrillation who receive flecainide. Concomitant negative chronotropic therapy, such as digoxin or beta-blockers, may lower the risk of this complication.

- **Use with caution in SSS, in clients with a history of CHF or MI, in disturbances of potassium levels, in clients with permanent pacemakers or temporary pacing electrodes, renal and liver impairment.**
- **The incidence of proarrhythmic effects may be increased in geriatric clients.**
- **Safety and efficacy not established in children less than 18 years of age.**

SIDE EFFECTS

Most Common

Dizziness, lightheadedness, faintness, unsteadiness and near syncope, dyspnea, headache, nausea, fatigue, palpitation, chest pain, asthenia, tremor, constipation, edema, abdominal pain.

CV: ***New or worsened ventricular arrhythmias, increased risk of death in clients with non-life-threatening cardiac arrhythmias***, new or worsened CHF, palpitations, chest pain, sinus bradycardia, sinus pause, sinus arrest, ***ventricular fibrillation, ventricular tachycardia that cannot be resuscitated***, second- or third-degree AV block, nonfatal cardiac arrest, tachycardia, hypertension, hypotension, bradycardia, angina pectoris. **CNS:** Dizziness, faintness, syncope, lightheadedness, neuropathy, unsteadiness and near syncope, headache, fatigue, paresthesia, paresis, hy-

F

poesthesia, insomnia, anxiety, twitching, weakness, neuropathy, malaise, vertigo, depression, ***seizures***, euphoria, confusion, depersonalization, apathy, morbid dreams, speech disorders, stupor, amnesia, weakness, somnolence. **GI:** Nausea, constipation, abdominal pain, vomiting, anorexia, dyspepsia, dry mouth, diarrhea, flatulence, change in taste. **Ophthalmic:** Blurred vision, difficulty in focusing, spots before eyes, diplopia, photophobia, eye pain, nystagmus, eye irritation. **Hematologic:** Leukopenia, thrombocytopenia. **GU:** Decreased libido, impotence, urinary retention, polyuria. **Musculoskeletal:** Asthenia, tremor, ataxia, arthralgia, myalgia. **Dermatologic:** Skin rashes, urticaria, exfoliative dermatitis, pruritus, alopecia. **Miscellaneous:** Edema, dyspnea, fever, fatigue, ***bronchospasm***, flushing, increased sweating, tinnitus, swollen mouth, lips, and tongue.

F

OVERDOSE MANAGEMENT

Symptoms: Lengthening of PR interval; increase in QRS duration, QT interval, and amplitude of T wave; decrease in HR and contractility; conduction disturbances; hypotension; ***respiratory failure*** or ***asystole.*** *Treatment:* Charcoal will remove unabsorbed drug up to 90 min after drug ingestion. Administration of dopamine, dobutamine, or isoproterenol. Artificial respiration. Intra-aortic balloon pumping, transvenous pacing (to correct conduction block). Acidification of the urine may be beneficial, especially in those with an alkaline urine. Due to the long duration of action of the drug, treatment measures may have to be continued for a prolonged period of time.

DRUG INTERACTIONS

Acidifying agents / ↑ Renal excretion of flecainide → ↓ bioavailability
Alkalinizing agents / ↓ Renal excretion of flecainide → ↑ bioavailability
Amiodarone / ↑ Flecainide levels
Cimetidine / ↑ Flecainide levels and half-life
Digoxin / ↑ Digoxin levels
Disopyramide / Additive negative inotropic effects; do not use together unless benefits outweigh risks
Propranolol / Additive negative inotropic effects; also, ↑ levels of both drugs
Ritonavir / Significant ↑ flecainide levels; do not use together
Smoking (Tobacco) / ↑ Plasma clearance of flecainide; dose of flecainide may need to be ↑
Verapamil / Additive negative inotropic effects

HOW SUPPLIED

Tablets: 50 mg, 100 mg, 150 mg.

DOSAGE

TABLETS

Sustained ventricular tachycardia.

Initial: 100 mg q 12 hr; **then,** increase by 50 mg twice/day q 4 days until effective dose reached. **Usual effective dose:** 150 mg q 12 hr, not to exceed 400 mg/day.

Paroxysmal supraventricular tachycardia, paroxysmal atrial fibrillation (PAF).

Initial: 50 mg q 12 hr; **then,** dose may be increased in increments of 50 mg twice/day q 4 days until effective dose reached. Maximum recommended dose for those with paroxysmal supraventricular arrhythmias: 300 mg/day.

NOTE: For PAF clients, increasing the dose from 50 to 100 mg twice a day may increase efficacy without a significant increase in side effects. For clients with a C_{CR} <35 mL/min/1.73 m^2, the starting dose is 100 mg once daily (or 50 mg twice a day). For less severe renal disease, the initial dose may be 100 mg q 12 hr.

NURSING IMPLICATIONS

Do not confuse Tambocor with Pamelor (a tricyclic antidepressant).

IMPLEMENTATION/ADMINISTRATION/STORAGE

1. For most situations, start in a hospital setting (especially in clients with symptomatic CHF, sustained ventricular arrhythmias, compensated clients with significant myocardial dysfunction, or sinus node dysfunction).
2. In renal impairment, increase dose at intervals greater than 4 days. Monitor for adverse toxic effects.
3. Most clients treated successfully had trough plasma levels between 0.2 and 1 mcg/mL. The chance of toxic effects increases if the trough plasma levels exceed 1 mcg/mL.
4. If being transferred to flecainide from another antiarrhythmic, allow at least 2–4 plasma half-lives to elapse for the drug being discontinued before initiating flecainide therapy.
5. Dosing at 8 hr intervals may benefit some.

6. If given with amiodarone, reduce flecainide dose by 50% and monitor closely for side effects.
7. To minimize toxicity, reduce dose once arrhythmia controlled.

ASSESSMENT

1. Note reasons for therapy and physical assessment findings i.e., heart, lungs, JVD, weight. Review history, echocardiograms, ECGs for evidence of CHF, ventricular arrhythmias, sinus node dysfunction, abnormal EF.
2. Monitor VS, ECG, CXR; monitor for labile BP. Assess ECG for increased arrhythmias, RBBB with LAH, or AV block. Pre-existing hypo/hyperkalemia may alter drug effects; correct.
3. Concomitant administration with disopyramide, propranolol, or verapamil will promote negative inotropic (depressant) effects. Avoid with SSS or CHF.
4. Avoid with ventricular arrhythmias following recent MI and chronic atrial fibrillation due to ventricular pro-arrhythmic effects.
5. Check pacing thresholds with pacemakers; adjust before and 1 week following drug therapy.
6. Obtain urinary pH to detect alkalinity or acidity. Alkalinity decreases renal excretion and acidity increases renal excretion, affecting rate of drug elimination.
7. Monitor VS, ECG, electrolytes, renal and LFTs.

CLIENT/FAMILY TEACHING

1. Take at dose and frequency prescribed. Drug controls, but does not cure, abnormal heart rhythm; continue taking as prescribed. Report changes in elimination.
2. Avoid hazardous activities until drug effects realized; may cause dizziness or drowsiness. Change positions slowly from lying to standing to prevent drop in BP. Keep log of BP and HR.
3. Report adverse CNS effects, such as dizziness, visual disturbances, headaches, nausea, depression as well as bruising or increased bleeding tendencies, dyspnea, edema, chest pain.
4. Advise with heart failure, or if taking other medications with negative inotropic effect, to monitor and record weight on a daily basis and report unexplained or rapid weight gain.
5. Keep all F/U to assess response, labs, adverse SE, and need for dosage adjustment.
6. Encourage family/significant other to learn CPR.

OUTCOMES/EVALUATE

- Termination of lethal ventricular arrhythmias; stable cardiac rhythm
- Therapeutic serum (trough) drug levels (0.2–1.0 mcg/mL)

Floxuridine

(flox-**YOUR**-ih-deen)

Classification(s): Antineoplastic, antimetabolite

Pregnancy Category: D

RX: FUDR.

SEE ALSO ***ANTINEOPLASTIC AGENTS***.

INDICATIONS/USES

Intra-arterially as palliative treatment of GI adenocarcinoma metastatic to the liver (especially in clients incurable by surgery or other treatment). Used in clients with disease limited to an area capable of infusion by a single artery. *Investigational:* Tumors of the liver, ovaries, or kidneys.

ACTION/KINETICS

Action

Cell-cycle specific for the S phase of cell division. Rapidly metabolized to fluorouracil. The drug inhibits DNA and RNA synthesis. Crosses blood-brain barrier.

Pharmacokinetics

t½: 5–20 min. From 60 to 80% of fluorouracil is excreted as respiratory CO_2 (8–12 hr); small amount (15%) excreted in urine (1–6 hr).

CONTRAINDICATIONS

If client is at poor risk, including depressed bone marrow function, nutritionally poor, or potentially serious infections. Lactation. Do not use during pregnancy unless benefits clearly outweigh risks.

SPECIAL CONCERNS

(1) It is recommended that floxuridine be given only by or under the supervision of a qualified physician who is experienced in cancer chemotherapy and intra-arterial drug therapy and is well versed in the use of potent antimetabolites. (2) Because of the possibility of severe toxic reactions, all clients should be hospitalized for initiation of the first course of therapy.

SIDE EFFECTS

Most Common

N&V, diarrhea, enteritis, stomatitis, localized erythema, anemia, leukopenia, thrombocytopenia.

CNS: Lethargy, malaise, weakness, acute cerebellar syndrome (may persist after treatment discontinued), headache, disorientation, confusion, euphoria. **GI:** Stomatitis/esophagopharyngitis (may lead to sloughing/ulceration), diarrhea, anorexia, N&V, enteritis, cramps, duodenal ulcer, watery stools, duodenitis, gastritis, glossitis, pharyngitis, intra-/extrahepatic biliary sclerosis, acalculus cholecystitis, GI ulceration/bleeding. **CV:** Myocardial ischemia, angina. **Dermatologic:** Alopecia, dermatitis (often as pruritic maculopapular rash on extremities or trunk), nonspecific skin toxicity, photosensitivity (erythema, increased skin pigmentation), nail changes (e.g., loss of nails), dry skin, fissuring, vein pigmentation. **Hematologic:** Leukopenia, thrombocytopenia, pancytopenia, agranulocytosis, anemia, thrombophlebitis. **Hypersensitivity:** Generalized allergic reactions, anaphylaxis. **Ophthalmic:** Photophobia, lacrimation, decreased vision, nystagmus, diplopia, lacrimal duct stenosis, visual changes. **At catheter site:** Bleeding, occluded/displaced/leaking catheters, embolism, fibromyositis, infection, thrombophlebitis. **Miscellaneous:** Complications of intra-arterial administration are arterial aneurysm, arterial ischemia, arterial thrombosis. Fever, epistaxis.

LABORATORY TEST CONSIDERATIONS

↑ Excretion of 5-hydroxyindoleacetic acid. ↑ Serum transaminase and bilirubin, LDH, alkaline phosphatase. ↓ Plasma albumin.

HOW SUPPLIED

Powder for Injection, Lyophilized: 0.5 gram.

DOSAGE

INTRA-ARTERIAL INFUSION ONLY

Palliation of gastrointestinal adenocarcinoma metastatic to the liver.

0.1–0.6 mg/kg/day by continuous infusion over 24 hr. Infusion is continued as long as a response continues.

NURSING IMPLICATIONS

IMPLEMENTATION/ADMINISTRATION/STORAGE

1. Higher doses (0.4–0.6 mg) are best given by hepatic artery infusion; liver metabolizes drug, reducing possibility of systemic toxicity.
2. Give until adverse effects manifested; resume therapy after effects have subsided. Maintain therapy as long as the response to floxuridine continues.
3. Use infusion pump to overcome pressure in large arteries and to ensure a uniform infusion rate.
4. Reconstitute each vial with 5 mL sterile water to yield a 100 mg/mL concentration. This may be further reconstituted in D5W or NSS and infused intra-arterially.
5. Store reconstituted vials in the refrigerator at 2–8°C (36–46°F) for no longer than 2 weeks.

ASSESSMENT

1. Note reasons for therapy; CT/MRI confirmation of metastasis.
2. Administered via pump as hepatic artery infusion; assess carefully for bleeding at catheter site, S&S of infection, catheter displacement. Should be inserted under fluoroscopy (IA) by trained individual.
3. Monitor CBC, uric acid, creatinine and LFTs. WBC nadir: 1 week; Platelet nadir: 10 days.

CLIENT/FAMILY TEACHING

1. Drug is administered under pressure into an artery. Any dislodgment may cause significant bleeding; report immediately.
2. Report any mouth lesions, diarrhea, intractable vomiting or infections. Consume plenty of fluids to prevent dehydration.
3. Will be premedicated for N&V, report recurrence so that therapy may be re-administered.
4. Males and females should practice reliable contraception during therapy.
5. May cause transient thinning and loss of hair.
6. Keep all F/U to assess response, labs, adverse SE.

OUTCOMES/EVALUATE

Suppression of metastatic processes

Fluconazole

(flew-**KON**-ah-zohl)

Classification(s): Antifungal

Pregnancy Category: C

RX: Diflucan.

✱ **Rx:** Apo-Fluconazole, Apo-Fluconazole-150, Diflucan-150, Gen-Fluconazole, PMS-Fluconazole.

INDICATIONS/USES

(1) Oropharyngeal and esophageal candidiasis. (2) Serious systemic candidal infection (including UTIs, peritonitis, candidemia, disseminated candidiasis, and pneumonia). (3) Cryptococcal meningitis. (4) Vaginal candidiasis and infections due to *Candida*. (5) Decrease the incidence of candidiasis in clients undergoing a bone marrow transplant who receive cytotoxic chemotherapy or radiation therapy. (6) Cryptococcal meningitis and candidal infections in children.

ACTION/KINETICS

Action

Is a highly selective inhibitor of fungal cytochrome P450 and sterol C-14 alpha-demethylation. The loss of normal sterols correlates with accumulation of 14-alpha-methyl sterols in fungi and may be responsible for the fungistatic activity. There is a decrease in cell wall integrity and extrusion of intracellular material, leading to death.

Pharmacokinetics

Bioavailability is 90% after PO use. Apparently does not affect the cytochrome P-450 enzyme in animals or humans. **Peak plasma levels:** 1–2 hr. **Steady-state levels:** 5–10 days after 50–400 mg given once a day. **t½:** 30 hr, which allows for once daily dosing. Penetrates all body fluids at steady state. Not affected by agents that increase gastric pH. Eighty percent of the drug is excreted unchanged by the kidneys. **Plasma protein binding:** 11–12%.

CONTRAINDICATIONS

Hypersensitivity to fluconazole. Lactation.

SPECIAL CONCERNS

- **Use with caution if client is hypersensitive to other azoles.**
- **Use with extreme caution in renal impairment.**
- **Efficacy not determined in children less than 6 months of age.**

SIDE EFFECTS

Most Common

Following single doses: Headache, nausea, abdominal pain, diarrhea.
Following multiple doses: Nausea, headache, skin rash, vomiting, abdominal pain.
Following single doses: GI: Nausea, abdominal pain, diarrhea, dyspepsia, taste perversion. **CNS:** Headache, dizziness. **Miscellaneous:** ***Angioedema*, *anaphylaxis (rare)*.**

Following multiple doses: Side effects are more frequently reported in HIV-infected clients than in non-HIV-infected clients. **GI**: N&V, abdominal pain, diarrhea, ***serious hepatic reactions***. **CNS**: Headache, ***seizures***. **Dermatologic**: Skin rash, exfoliative skin disorders (including ***Stevens-Johnson syndrome***, and ***toxic epidermal necrolysis***), alopecia. **Hematologic**: Leukopenia, thrombocytopenia. **Miscellaneous:** Hypercholesterolemia/triglyceridemia, hypokalemia.

LABORATORY TEST CONSIDERATIONS

↑ AST, serum transaminase (especially if used with isoniazid, oral hypoglycemic agents, phenytoin, rifampin, valproic acid).

DRUG INTERACTIONS

Alfentanil / ↑ Pharmacologic and side effects R/T ↓ liver metabolism by CYP3A4
Benzodiazepines / ↑ And prolonged serum levels R/T inhibition of CYP3A4 → CNS depression and psychomotor impairment
Buspirone / ↑ Buspirone levels R/T ↓ metabolism
Carbamazepine / ↑ Carbamazepine levels R/T ↓ metabolism by CYP3A4
Cimetidine / ↓ Fluconazole AUC and C_{max}
Corticosteroids / ↑ Corticosteroid effects and toxicity R/T ↓ metabolism
Cyclosporine / ↑ Cyclosporine levels in renal transplant clients with or without impaired renal function
Glipizide / ↑ Glipizide levels R/T ↓ liver breakdown
Glyburide / ↑ Glyburide levels R/T ↓ liver breakdown
Haloperidol / ↑ Haloperidol levels → ↑ risk of side effects
HMG-CoA reductase inhibitors / ↑ HMG-CoA reductase inhibitor levels → possible rhabdomyolysis
Hydrochlorothiazide / ↑ Fluconazole levels R/T ↓ renal clearance

Losartan / ↑ Losartan antihypertensive and toxicity R/T ↓ metabolism by CYP2D9
Nateglinide / ↑ Nateglinide levels R/T ↓ metabolism by CYP2C9
Nisoldipine / ↑ Effects/toxicity of nisoldipine levels R/T ↓ metabolism by CYP3A4
Oral contraceptives / Possible ↑ or ↓ ethinyl estradiol and levonorgestrel levels
Phenytoin / ↑ Phenytoin levels
Pimozide / ↑ Pimozide levels R/T inhibition of CYP3A4
Protease inhibitors / Possible ↑ protease inhibitor levels with possible ↑ toxicity
Rifabutin, Rifampin / ↓ Fluconazole levels R/T ↑ liver breakdown; possible uveitis if rifabutin/fluconazole given together
Sirolimus / ↑ Sirolimus levels R/T ↓ gut metabolism
Sulfonamides / ↑ Sulfonamide levels
Sulfonylureas / ↓ Sulfonylurea metabolism → ↑ plasma levels
Tacrolimus / ↑ Tacrolimus levels R/T ↓ gut metabolism; possible nephrotoxicity
Theophylline / ↑ Theophylline levels
Tolbutamide / ↑ Tolbutamide levels R/T ↓ liver breakdown
Tolterodine / ↑ Tolterodine levels; do not give more than 1 mg twice daily of tolterodine when given with azole antifungals
Tricyclic antidepressants / ↑ TCA effects/toxicity R/T ↓ metabolism by CYP2C9
Vinca alkaloids / ↑ Risk of vinca toxicity (constipation, myalgia, neutropenia)
Warfarin / ↑ Warfarin effect → ↑ PT
Zidovudine / ↑ Zidovudine levels
Zolpidem / ↑ Zolpidem effects; possible toxicity

HOW SUPPLIED

Powder for Oral Suspension: 10 mg/mL, 40 mg/mL; ***Tablets:*** 50 mg, 100 mg, 150 mg, 200 mg.

DOSAGE

ORAL SUSPENSION TABLETS

Oropharyngeal or esophageal candidiasis.

Adults, first day: 200 mg; **then,** 100 mg/day for a minimum of 14 days (for oropharyngeal candidiasis) or 21 days (for esophageal candidiasis). Up to 400 mg/day may be required for esophageal candidiasis. **Children, first day:** 6 mg/kg; **then,** 3 mg/kg once daily for a minimum of 14 days (for oropharyngeal candidiasis) or 21 days (for esophageal candidiasis).

Systemic candidiasis (e.g., candidemia, disseminated candidiasis, and pneumonia).

Optimal dosage and duration in adults have not been determined although doses up to 400 mg/day have been used. **Children:** 6–12 mg/kg/day.

Acute cryptococcal meningitis.

Adults, first day: 400 mg; **then,** 200 mg/day (up to 400 mg may be required) for 10 to 12 weeks after CSF culture is negative. **Children, first day:** 12 mg/kg; **then,** 6 mg/kg once daily for 10 to 12 weeks after CSF culture is negative.

Vaginal candidiasis.

150 mg as a single oral dose.

Candidal UTI and peritonitis.

50–200 mg/day.

Maintenance to prevent relapse of cryptococcal meningitis in AIDS clients.

Adults: 200 mg once daily. **Pediatric:** 6 mg/kg once daily.

Prevention of candidiasis in bone marrow transplant.

400 mg once daily. In clients expected to have severe granulocytopenia (less than 500 neutrophils/mm^3), start fluconazole several days before the anticipated onset of neutropenia and continue for 7 days after the neutrophil count rises above 1,000 cells/mm^3. In clients with renal impairment, an initial loading dose of 50–400 mg can be given; then daily dose is based on C_{CR}.

NURSING IMPLICATIONS

IMPLEMENTATION/ADMINISTRATION/STORAGE

1. Daily dose is the same for PO and IV administration. Store tablets below 30°C (86°F).
2. A loading dose of twice the daily dose is recommended for the first day of therapy in order to obtain plasma levels close to the steady state by the second day of therapy.
3. Due to a long half-life, once daily dosing (either IV or PO) is possible.

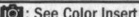

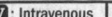

4. To prevent relapse, maintenance therapy is usually required in clients with AIDS, cryptococcal meningitis, or recurrent oropharyngeal candidiasis.
5. Do not give more than 1 mg of tolterodine twice a day when given with azole antifungals.
6. To reconstitute the oral suspension, add 24 mL distilled water or purified water; shake vigorously to suspend powder. Shake oral suspension well before using. Store reconstituted suspension at 5–30°C (41–86°F). Discard any unused drug after 2 weeks. Do not freeze suspension.
7. Store glass bottles from 5–30°C (41–86°F); protect from freezing.

ASSESSMENT

1. Note indications and describe clinical presentation (fungal infection); endoscopic results and/or culture reports. Note sensitivity to azoles or similar drugs.
2. List drugs prescribed to ensure no interactions/dosage adjustments.
3. If HIV infected, may increase risk for side effects and relapse; may need maintenance therapy.
4. Obtain baseline cultures, renal and LFTs. Monitor hematologic, renal, and hepatic status. If abnormal LFTs, monitor closely for development of more serious liver toxicity. Reduce dose with renal dysfunction.

CLIENT/FAMILY TEACHING

1. Review goals of therapy, appropriate method and schedule for administration. Take as directed; complete entire script even if infection has cleared. A single oral dose may be ordered for vaginal yeast infections.
2. Take tablets with a full glass of water without regard to meals; may take with food if GI upset occurs.
3. Shake suspension well before measuring dose using dosing cup, spoon, or syringe. Suspension can be taken without regard to meals but may take with food if GI upset occurs.
4. Consume adequate fluids to prevent dehydration.
5. Report rash, N&V, diarrhea, yellowing of skin, clay-colored stools, dark urine, lack of response, or persistent side effects; may need to be discontinued.
6. Keep all F/U to assess response and adverse SE.

OUTCOMES/EVALUATE

- Elimination of pathogenic fungi
- Candida prophylaxis in transplant recipients
- Resolution of oropharyngeal and esophageal candidiasis and/or vaginal candidiasis

IV

Fludarabine phosphate

(floo-**DAIR**-ah-bean)

Classification(s): Antineoplastic, antimetabolite

Pregnancy Category: D

RX: Fludara, Oforta.

SEE ALSO ***ANTINEOPLASTIC AGENTS.***

INDICATIONS/USES

As a single drug for the treatment of adults with B-cell chronic lymphocytic leukemia whose disease has not responded to or has progressed during treatment with at least one standard alkylating agent-containing regimen. *Investigational (IV):* Hodgkin's lymphoma. Combination therapy to treat primary resistant or relapsing acute myelogenous leukemia, acute lymphoblastic leukemia, and secondary acute myelogenous leukemia.

ACTION/KINETICS

Action

Rapidly dephosphorylated to 2-fluoro-ara-A and then phosphorylated within the cell by the enzyme deoxycytidine kinase to the active 2-fluoro-ara-ATP. Once incorporated in DNA, 2-fluoro-ara-ATP functions as a DNA chain terminator; inhibits DNA polymerase alpha, gamma, and delta; and inhibits ribonucleoside diphosphate reductase. 2-fluoro-ara-ATP also inhibits DNA primase and DNA ligase I.

Pharmacokinetics

Maximum plasma levels after PO use: 1–2 hr. **Absolute bioavailability of 2-fluoro-ara-A after PO:** 50–65%. A high-fat meal does not affect AUC, C_{max}, or terminal **t½**, but the time to reach maximum concentration is delayed from 1.3–2.2 hr. **t½, 2-fluoro-ara-A:** About 20 hr. Approximately 23% of a dose of fludarabine is excreted in the urine as unchanged 2-fluoro-ara-A. **Plasma protein binding:** 19–29% (fludarabine).

CONTRAINDICATIONS

Hypersensitivity to the drug or any component of the product. Use with live vaccines during and after fludarabine treatment. Lactation.

SPECIAL CONCERNS

■ (1) Ensure that fludarabine is administered under the supervision of a qualified health care provider experienced in the use of antineoplastic therapy. (2) Fludarabine can severely suppress bone marrow function. (3) Severe neurologic effects, including blindness, coma, and death, were observed in dose-ranging studies in clients with acute leukemia when fludarabine was administered at high doses. This severe CNS toxicity occurred in 36% of clients treated with doses approximately 4 times greater (96 mg/m^2/day for 5 to 7 days) than the recommended intravenous dose (25 mg/m^2/day). Similar severe CNS toxicity has been rarely (0.2% or less) reported in clients treated at doses in the range of the dose recommended for chronic lymphocytic leukemia (CLL). Periodic neurological assessments are recommended. (4) Instances of life-threatening and sometimes fatal autoimmune hemolytic anemia have been reported after 1 or more cycles of treatment with fludarabine. Clients undergoing treatment with fludarabine should be evaluated and closely monitored for hemolysis. (5) High incidence of fatal pulmonary toxicity was observed in a clinical investigation using fludarabine in combination with pentostatin (deoxycoformycin) for the treatment of refractory CLL. Therefore, the use of fludarabine in combination with pentostatin is not recommended. ■

- **Use with caution in clients with renal insufficiency and in impaired health (impaired bone marrow function, immunodeficiency, or a history of opportunistic infection).**
- **An increased risk of toxicity is possible in geriatric clients, in renal insufficiency, and in bone marrow impairment.**
- **The safety and efficacy of fludarabine not established in children and in previously untreated or nonrefractory chronic lymphocytic leukemia clients.**

SIDE EFFECTS

Most Common

Fever, N&V, infection, chills, malaise, fatigue, anorexia, weakness, serious opportunistic infections, pneumonia, myelosuppression (neutropenia, thrombocytopenia, anemia).

CNS: Agitation, blindness, coma, confusion, objective weakness, peripheral neuropathy, headache, cerebellar syndromes, depression, impaired mentation, paresthesia, sleep disorder, ***seizures, neurotoxicity*** (at high IV doses: delayed blindness, coma, ***death***). **GI:** N&V, anorexia, abdominal pain, diarrhea, stomatitis, GI bleeding, esophagitis, mucositis, constipation, dysphagia. **Hepatic:** Liver failure, cholelithiasis, abnormal LFTs. **CV:** Edema, ***aneurysm***, DVT, phlebitis, TIA, angina, arrhythmia, ***CVA***, CHF, ***MI***, phlebitis, SVT, ***hemorrhage***. **Dermatologic:** Skin rashes, diaphoresis, pruritus, alopecia, seborrhea, erythema multiforme, pemphigus, herpes simplex, increased sweating, ***Stevens-Johnson syndrome, toxic epidermal necrolysis***, worsening or flare-up of pre-existing skin cancer lesions, new onset of skin cancer. **GU:** Hemorrhagic cystitis, dysuria, hematuria, urinary infection, abnormal renal function test, renal failure, urinary hesitancy, proteinuria, UTI. **Hematologic:** Neutropenia, thrombocytopenia, anemia, myelodysplastic syndrome, acute myeloid leukemia. Trilineage bone marrow hypoplasia or aplasia resulting in pancytopenia. Acquired hemophilia, autoimmune thrombocytopenia/thrombocytopenic purpura, Evans syndrome, ***hemolytic anemia*** (including autoimmune). **Respiratory:** Pneumonia, dyspnea, cough, interstitial pulmonary infiltrate, rhinitis, sinusitis, URTI, bronchitis, pharyngitis, allergic pneumonitis, epistaxis, hemoptysis, hypoxia, ***acute respiratory distress syndrome***, respiratory distress, ***pulmonary hemorrhage***, pulmonary fibrosis, ***respiratory failure***. **Musculoskeletal:** Myalgia, osteoporosis, arthralgia, back/chest pain. **Metabolic:** Tumor lysis syndrome (hyperuricemia, hyperphosphatemia, hypocalcemia, metabolic acidosis, hyperkalemia, hematuria, urate crystalluria, renal failure, flank pain), peripheral edema, decreased weight. **Ophthalmic:** Optic neuritis, optic neuropathy, visual disturbances. **Otic:** Hearing loss. **Body as a whole:** Serious, and sometimes fatal, infections, including opportunistic infections and reactivation of latent viral infections (e.g., herpes zoster, Epstein-Barr virus, John Cunningham virus [***progressive multifocal leukoencephalopathy***]). Fever, chills, fatigue, weakness, malaise, pain, flu syndrome, pain, paresthesia, ***anaphylaxis***, dehydration. **Miscellaneous:** ***Progressive multifocal leukoencephalopathy***, transfusion associated graft-versus-host disease after transfusion of nonirradiated blood.

LABORATORY TEST CONSIDERATIONS

↑ LDH. Abnormal renal function test. Proteinuria, hyperglycemia.

OVERDOSE MANAGEMENT

Symptoms: Irreversible CNS toxicity including delayed blindness, ***coma, and death.*** Severe thrombocytopenia and neutropenia. *Treatment:* Discontinue the drug and treat symptoms. Monitor the hematologic profile.

DRUG INTERACTIONS

Digoxin / ↓ Digoxin effects R/T ↓ GI absorption; monitor serum digoxin levels

Pentostatin / ↑ Risk of severe pulmonary toxicity; do not use together

HOW SUPPLIED

Injection Solution (Fludarabine phosphate): 25 mg/mL; *Injection, Lyophilized Cake for Solution (Fludara):* 50 mg; *Tablets (Oforta):* 10 mg.

DOSAGE

IV (FLUDARA)

B-cell chronic lymphocytic leukemia.

Adults, usual: 25 mg/m² daily given over a period of 30 min for 5 consecutive days. Initiate a 5-day course of therapy every 28 days. Dosage may be decreased or delayed based on evidence of hematologic or nonhematologic toxicity. The optimal duration of treatment has not been established. It is recommended that 3 additional cycles of fludarabine be given following achievement of a maximal response; then, discontinue the drug.

Acute myelogenous leukemia in children (investigational).

Children: 10 mg/m² IV over 15 min as a single dose, followed by a continuous IV infusion of 30.5 mg/m²/day for 5 consecutive days. If used in combination with other antineoplastic drugs, give fludarabine, 30 mg/m²/day for 5 days.

Solid tumors in children (investigational).

Children: 9 mg/m² IV bolus as a single dose, followed by a continuous IV infusion of 27 mg/m²/day for 5 days.

TABLETS (OFORTA)

B-cell chronic lymphocytic leukemia.

Adults, usual: 40 mg/m²/day for 5 consecutive days. Each 5-day course of treatment should begin q 28 days. The dose may be decreased or delayed based on evidence of hematologic or nonhematologic toxicity. If neurotoxicity occurs, delay or discontinue the drug. The optimum duration of treatment has not been determined. It is recommended that 3 additional cycles of fludarabine be given following the achievement of a maximual response; the drug should then be discontinued.

NURSING IMPLICATIONS

IMPLEMENTATION/ADMINISTRATION/STORAGE

1. Dose may be decreased or delayed based on presence of hematologic or neurotoxicity.
2. Advanced age, renal insufficiency and bone marrow impairment may predispose to increased fludarabine toxicity. Monitor such clients closely for excessive toxicity and modify dosage accordingly. Reduce the IV and PO dose of fludarabine by 20% in clients with a C_{CR} from 30–70 mL/min/1.73 m². Reduce the PO dose of fludarabine by 50% if the C_{CR} is <30 mL/min/1.73 m²; do not give IV to clients with severe renal impairment.
3. Follow appropriate procedures for handling and disposal of cytotoxic drugs.
4. Store tablets from 15–30°C (59–86°F).
5. IV Reconstitute lyophilized product aseptically with 2 mL of sterile water for injection, USP; the cake should fully dissolve in 15 seconds or less. Each mL of the resulting solution will contain 25 mg fludarabine, 25 mg mannitol, and sodium hydroxide to adjust the pH from 7.2 to 8.2. The reconstituted product or the injection solution may then be diluted in 100 or 125 mL of D5W, or 0.9% NaCl, and given over 30 min.

6. Use reconstituted drug within 8 hr; contains no preservatives. If solution comes in contact with the skin or mucous membranes, wash thoroughly with soap and water. Rinse eyes thoroughly with plain water. Record exposure.
7. Store the product under refrigeration at 2–8°C (36–46°F).
8. COMPATIBILITY D5W, 0.9% NaCl.
9. INCOMPATIBILITY Do not mix with other drugs.

ASSESSMENT

1. Note reasons for therapy, onset, previous agents used/failed.
2. List baseline CNS assessment, bone marrow impairment, and renal dysfunction; high doses may cause toxicity.
3. Assess regularly for anemia, neutropenia, thrombocytopenia, and hemolysis. Monitor those with advanced age, renal impairment, and bone marrow impairment closely for excessive toxicity.
4. Monitor hematologic, renal and LFTs; reduce dose/stop with renal impairment. Causes severe bone marrow suppression; Nadir: 5–25 days.

CLIENT/FAMILY TEACHING

1. Take tablets either on an empty stomach or with food. Swallow tablets whole with water; do not chew, crush, or break them. Avoid any skin or mucous membrane exposure by direct contact or by inhalation. If contact occurs, wash area thoroughly with soap and water or wash out the eyes immediately with water for at least 15 min.
2. Report any evidence of infection (sore throat, fever), abnormal bruising or bleeding, tingling of the hands or feet, persistent N&V, diarrhea, appetite loss, worsening of body weakness, mental confusion, or loss of coordination.
3. Fludarabine is given parenterally to treat resistant leukemia.
4. Use caution may reduce the ability to drive or use machinery.
5. Report flank pain or blood in urine; may precede a tumor lysis syndrome.
6. Practice barrier contraception; evaluate for sperm/egg harvesting. May interfere with menstrual cycle in women and may stop sperm production in men.
7. Do not use with pentostatin; increased incidence of fatal pulmonary toxicity.
8. Avoid live vaccines during and after therapy.
9. Keep all F/U to assess response, labs, for neurotoxicity, autoimmune hemolytic anemia, or other adverse SE.

OUTCOMES/EVALUATE

- Hematologic improvement
- Control of malignant process

■ IV

Flumazenil

(floo-**MAZ**-eh-nill)

Classification(s): Benzodiazepine receptor antagonist

Pregnancy Category: C

RX: Romazicon.

Rx: Anexate.

INDICATIONS/USES

Adults: Complete or partial reversal of the sedative effects of benzodiazepines in cases where general anesthesia has been induced or maintained by benzodiazepines, where sedation has been produced by benzodiazepines for diagnostic and therapeutic procedures, and for the management of benzodiazepine overdosage. **Children, 1–17 years:** Reversal of conscious sedation induced with benzodiazepines. *Investigational:* Hepatic encephalopathy. *NOTE:* Flumazenil is intended as an adjunct to, not a substitute for, proper management of airway, assisted breathing, circulatory access and support, internal decontamination by lavage and charcoal, and adequate clinical evaluation.

ACTION/KINETICS

Action

Antagonizes the effects of benzodiazepines on the CNS by competitively inhibiting their action at the benzodiazepine recognition site on the GABA/benzodiazepine receptor complex. Does not antagonize the CNS effects of ethanol, general anesthetics, barbiturates, or opiates. IV administration antagonizes sedation, impairment of recall, psychomotor impairment, and ventilatory depression caused by benzodiazepines. The duration and degree of reversal of benzodiazepine effects are related to the dose and plasma levels of flumazenil. Generally doses of about 0.1–0.2 mg produce partial antagonism whereas higher doses of 0.4–1 mg usually cause complete antagonism following sedative doses of benzodiazepines.

Pharmacokinetics

Onset of reversal: 1–2 min. **Peak effect:** 6–10 min. The duration of reversal is related to the plasma levels of the benzodiazepine and the dose of flumazenil. **Distribution $t^{1/2}$, initial:** 4–11 min; **terminal $t^{1/2}$:** 40–80 min. Completely metabolized in the liver with 90–95% excreted through the urine and 5–10% excreted in the feces. Hepatic impairment prolongs the half-life of the drug. Ingestion of food results in a 50% increase in clearance of flumazenil.

CONTRAINDICATIONS

Hypersensitivity to flumazenil or benzodiazepines. Use in clients given a benzodiazepine for control of intracranial pressure or status epilepticus. Use in epileptic clients who have been receiving benzodiazepine treatment for a prolonged period. In clients manifesting signs of serious cyclic antidepressant overdose. Use during labor and delivery. To treat benzodiazepine dependence or for the management of protracted benzodiazepine abstinence syndrome. Use until the effects of neuromuscular blockade have been fully reversed.

SPECIAL CONCERNS

The use of flumazenil has been associated with the occurrence of seizures. These are most frequent in clients who have been on benzodiazepines for long-term sedation or in overdose cases where clients are showing signs of serious cyclic antidepressant overdose. Practitioners should individualize the dosage of flumazenil and be prepared to manage seizures.

- **Reversal of benzodiazepine effects may be associated with the onset of seizures in certain high-risk clients (e.g., concurrent major sedative-hypnotic drug withdrawal, recent therapy with repeated doses of parenteral benzodiazepines, myoclonic jerking or seizure activity prior to administration of flumazenil in cases of overdose, and concurrent cyclic antidepressant overdosage).**
- **Use with caution in clients with head injury as the drug may precipitate seizures or alter cerebral blood flow.**
- **Use with caution in clients with alcoholism and other drug dependencies due to the increased frequency of benzodiazepine tolerance and dependence.**
- **May precipitate a withdrawal syndrome if client is dependent on benzodiazepines.**
- **May cause panic attacks in clients with a history of panic disorder.**
- **Use with caution in mixed-drug overdosage as toxic effects (e.g., cardiac dysrhythmias, convulsions) may occur (especially with cyclic antidepressants).**
- **Use with caution in the ICU due to increased risk of unrecognized benzodiazepine dependence; withdrawal symptoms may include convulsions.**
- **Use with caution during lactation.**
- **Safety and efficacy not established in the reversal of conscious sedation in children less than 1 year of age.**

SIDE EFFECTS

Most Common

Sweating, flushing, hot flashes, dizziness, agitation, dry mouth, tremors, palpitations, insomnia, dyspnea, hyperventilation, N&V, abnormal vision, blurred vision, headache, injection site pain.

Deaths have occurred in clients receiving flumazenil, especially in those with serious underlying disease or in those who have ingested large amounts of nonbenzodiazepine drugs (usually cyclic antidepressants) as part of an overdose. Seizures are the most common serious side effect noted. **CNS**: Dizziness, vertigo, ataxia, anxiety, nervousness, tremor, insomnia, abnormal crying, depersonalization, euphoria, increased tears, confusion, depression, dysphoria, paranoia, delirium, difficulty concentrating, ***seizures***, somnolence, stupor, speech disorder (dysphonia, thick tongue), fear, panic attacks in those with a history of panic disorders. **Respiratory:** Dyspnea, hyperventilation, hypoventilation (i.e., resedation, respiratory depression). **GI**: N&V, hiccoughs, dry mouth. **CV**: Sweating, flushing, hot flushes, palpitations, ***arrhythmias (atrial, nodal, ventricular extrasystoles)***, bradycardia, tachycardia, hypertension, chest pain. **At injection site:** Pain, inflammation, thrombophlebitis, rash, skin abnormality. **Body as a whole:** Headache, increased sweating, asthenia, fatigue, malaise, rigors, shivering, hypoesthesia, paresthesia. **Ophthalmologic**: Abnormal vision including visual field defect and diplopia; blurred vision. **Otic**: Transient hearing impairment, tinnitus, hyperacusis. **Miscellaneous:** Withdrawal symptoms following rapid injection in clients with long-term exposure to benzodiazepines.

HOW SUPPLIED

Injection: 0.1 mg/mL.

DOSAGE

IV ONLY

Reversal of conscious sedation.

Adults, initial: 0.2 mg (2 mL) given IV over 15 sec. If the desired level of consciousness is not reached after waiting an additional 45 sec, a second dose of 0.2 mg (2 mL) can be given and repeated at 60 sec intervals, up to a maximum total dose of 1 mg (10 mL). Most clients will respond to doses of 0.6–1 mg. To treat resedation, repeat doses may be given at 20 min intervals; give no more than 1 mg (given as 0.2 mg/min) at any one time and give no more than 3 mg in any 1 hr. **Children, initial:** 0.01 mg/kg (up to 0.2 mg) IV over 15 sec. If the desired level of consciousness is not reached after waiting an additional 45 sec, further injections of 0.01 mg/kg (up to 0.2 mg) can be given and repeated at 60 sec intervals where necessary (up to a maximum of 4 additional times) to a maximum total dose of 0.05 mg/kg or 1 mg, whichever is lower. Individualize the dose based on client response.

Reversal of general anesthesia in adults.

Adults, initial: 0.2 mg (2 mL) IV over 15 sec. If the desired level of consciousness is not obtained after waiting an additional 45 sec, a further dose of 0.2 mg (2 mL) can be given and repeated at 60 sec intervals, where necessary (up to a maximum of 4 times) to a maximum total dose of 1 mg (10 mL). Individual dosage based on client response; most respond to doses from 0.6–1 mg. If resedation occurs, repeated doses may be given at 20 min intervals, as needed. For repeat treatment, no more than 1 mg (given as 0.2 mg/min) should be given at at any one time, and no more than 3 mg should be given in any 1 hr.

Management of suspected benzodiazepine overdose in adults.

Adults, initial: 0.2 mg (2 mL) given IV over 30 sec. If the desired level of consciousness is not obtained after waiting 30 sec, a further dose of 0.3 mg (3 mL) can be given IV over 30 sec. Further doses of 0.5 mg (5 mL) can be given over 30 sec at 1 min intervals up to a total dose of 3 mg (although some clients may require up to 5 mg given slowly as described). If the client has not responded 5 min after receiving a cumulative dose of 5 mg, the major cause of sedation is probably not due to benzodiazepines and additional doses of flumazenil are likely to have no effect. For resedation, repeated doses may be given at 20 min intervals; no more than 1 mg (given as 0.5 mg/min) at any one time and no more than 3 mg in any 1 hr should be administered. *NOTE:* Clients should have a secure airway and IV access before flumazenil administration; they should be wakened gradually.

Hepatic encephalopathy (investigational).

1 mg by IV bolus injection.

NURSING IMPLICATIONS

IMPLEMENTATION/ADMINISTRATION/STORAGE

1. **IV** Must individualize dosage. Give only smallest amount effective. The 1 min wait between individual doses in dose-titration recommended for general uses may be too short for high-risk clients as it takes 6–10 min for any single dose of flumazenil to reach full effects. Slow rate of administration in high-risk clients.
2. Major risk is resedation; duration of effect of a long-acting or a large dose of a short-acting benzodiazepine may exceed that of flumazenil. With resedation, give repeated doses at 20 min intervals as needed.
3. Best given as a series of small injections to allow provider to control reversal of sedation to desired end point and to decrease possibility of side effects.
4. Reduce dose to 40–60% of normal with severe hepatic dysfunction, especially with repeat injections.

5. Give through freely running IV infusion into a large vein to minimize pain at injection site.
6. Doses larger than a total of 3 mg do not reliably produce additional effects.
7. For optimum sterility, keep in the vial until just before use.
8. Before administering, have a secure airway and IV access; awaken clients gradually.
9. Store from 15–30°C (59–86°F).
10. COMPATIBILITY D5W, RL, and NSS.
11. INCOMPATIBILITY Administer separately.

ASSESSMENT

1. List type/time and amount of drug ingested; note any TCA or mixed-drug overdose.
2. Note history of seizure disorder or panic attacks. Drug may cause seizures and respiratory impairment.
3. Assess for evidence of head injury or increased ICP.
4. Note evidence of sedative or benzodiazepine dependence, alcohol abuse, or any recent use; may precipitate withdrawal symptoms.
5. The effects of flumazenil usually wear off before the effects of many benzodiazepines. Observe closely for resedation, depressed respirations, or other benzodiazepine effects up to 2 hr after administration.
   - Intended as an adjunct to, not a substitute for, proper management of the airway, assisted breathing, circulatory access and support, use of lavage and charcoal, and adequate clinical evaluation. Prior to giving flumazenil, proper measures should be undertaken to secure an airway for ventilation and IV access. Be prepared for clients attempting to withdraw ET tubes or IV lines due to confusion and agitation following awakening; awakening should be gradual. Drug should be used with caution in the ICU due to increased risk of unrecognized benzodiazepine dependence; may produce convulsions. Drug is not intended to be used to diagnose benzodiazepine-induced sedation in the ICU. Failure to respond may be masked by metabolic disorders, traumatic injury, or drugs.
   - Use seizure precautions; increased risk for seizures with large overdoses of cyclic antidepressants and with long-term benzodiazepine sedation. Drug-associated convulsions may be treated with benzodiazepines, phenytoin, or barbiturates. (Higher doses of benzodiazepines may be needed.)
   - Do not use until the effects of neuromuscular blockade have been fully reversed.
   - May provoke panic attacks in those with a history of panic disorder.
   - Flumazenil does not consistently reverse amnesia. Therefore, clients may not remember instructions during the postprocedure period; provide written instructions.
6. Check for liver dysfunction; subsequent doses require adjustment.

CLIENT/FAMILY TEACHING

1. Used to reverse sedative effects of benzodiazepines either with sedation for diagnostic or therapeutic procedures, or for management of benzodiazepine overdose.
2. Do not undertake activities requiring complete alertness; do not operate hazardous machinery or motor vehicle until at least 18–24 hr after discharge and until determined that no residual sedative effects of benzodiazepines remain. Memory and judgment may be impaired.
3. Avoid alcohol or nonprescription drugs for 18–24 hr after administration of flumazenil or if the effects of the benzodiazepines persist.

OUTCOMES/EVALUATE

Reversal of benzodiazepine sedative/psychomotor effects

Flunisolide

(flew-**NISS**-oh-lyd)

Classification(s): Glucocorticoid

Pregnancy Category: C

RX: Intranasal: Flunisolide.

✤ **Rx:** Apo-Flunisolide, ratio-Flunisolide.

Flunisolide hemihydrate

Classification(s): Glucocorticoid

Pregnancy Category: C

RX: Aerosol: AeroSpan.

SEE ALSO ***CORTICOSTEROIDS***.

INDICATIONS/USES

Aerosol (AeroSpan): (1) Maintenance treatment of asthma as prophylactic therapy in adults and children, 6 years and older. (2) For those who require systemic corticosteroids where adding flunisolide may reduce or eliminate the need for PO corticosteroids. **Intranasal (Flunisolide):** Relief and management of nasal symptoms of seasonal and perennial allergic rhinitis.

ACTION/KINETICS

Action

Minimal systemic effects with intranasal use.

Pharmacokinetics

Significant first-pass after inhalation; rapidly metabolized by the liver. Several days may be required for full beneficial effects. 50% bioavailable. **t½:** 1–2 hr. Metabolized in the liver and excreted by the feces (50%) and urine (50%).

CONTRAINDICATIONS

Active or quiescent TB, especially of the respiratory tract. Untreated fungal, bacterial, systemic viral infections. Ocular herpes simplex. Use until healing occurs following recent ulceration of nasal septum, nasal surgery, or trauma. Lactation.

SPECIAL CONCERNS

■ (1) Use care when transferring from systemic corticosteroids to flunisolide inhaler due to possibility of death because of adrenal insufficiency. Several months may be needed to restore hypothalamic-pituitary-adrenal function. During this period, clients may exhibit signs and symptoms of adrenal insufficiency when exposed to trauma, surgery, or infections (especially gastroenteritis). (2) Although flunisolide inhaler may provide control of asthmatic symptoms during these episodes, it does not provide the systemic steroid needed for coping with these emergencies. During periods of stress or a severe asthmatic attack, instruct clients who have been withdrawn from systemic steroids to resume systemic steroids (in large doses) immediately and to contact their provider for further instructions. (3) Instruct clients to carry a warning card indicating they may need supplementary systemic steroids during periods of stress or a severe asthmatic attack. (4) To assess the risk of adrenal insufficiency in emergency situations, perform routine tests of adrenal cortical function periodically, including measurement of early morning resting cortisol levels. An early morning resting cortisol level may be accepted as normal if it falls at or near the normal mean level. ■

Safety and efficacy not determined in children less than 6 years of age.

SIDE EFFECTS

Most Common

After use of the aerosol: N&V, diarrhea, flu, sore throat, headache, cold symptoms, nasal congestion, URTI, unpleasant taste.

After use of the solution/spray: Burning, dryness, nasal irritation, sneezing, throat irritation/itching.

See *Corticosteroids* for a complete list of possible side effects. Also, **Respiratory:** Hoarseness, coughing, throat irritation; *Candida* infections of nose, larynx, and pharynx.

● **Intranasal use**

Respiratory: Nasopharyngeal irritation, stinging, burning, dryness; wheezing, epistaxis, nasal stuffiness/congestion, sneezing, throat discomfort (burning, itching, swelling pain), localized infection of the nose and pharynx, nasal septum perforation (rare). **CNS:** Headache. **Ophthalmic:** Watery eyes, cataracts, glaucoma, increased IOP. **GI:** Dry mouth, N&V, temporary or permanent loss of the sense of smell and taste. Systemic corticosteroid effects, especially if recommended dose is exceeded. **Hypersensitivity:** Angioedema, bronchospasm, rash, urticaria. May be immediate or delayed. **Miscellaneous:** Inhibition of wound healing, infection (rare), reduction of growth velocity in children.

HOW SUPPLIED

Flunisolide. ***Solution/Spray (Intranasal):*** 25 mcg/inh.

Flunisolide Hemihydrate. ***Aerosol:*** About 80 mcg flunisolide hemihydrate (78 mcg flunisolide)/actuation.

DOSAGE

Flunisolide

SOLUTION/SPRAY (INTRANASAL)

Seasonal and perennial allergic rhinitis.

Adults: 2 sprays in each nostril twice a day. Dose may be increased to 2 sprays in each nostril 3 times per day. **Maximum dose:** 8 sprays in each nostril daily. **Children, 6–14 years:** 1 spray in each nostril 3 times per day or 2 sprays

F

in each nostril twice a day. **Maximum dose:** 4 sprays in each nostril daily. **Maintenance, adults, children:** Smallest dose necessary to control symptoms. Some clients (approximately 15%) are controlled on 1 spray in each nostril daily.

Flunisolide hemihydrate

AEROSOL (AEROSPAN)

Chronic asthma.

Adults, 12 years of age and older, initial: 160 mcg twice daily, not to exceed 320 mcg twice daily. **Children, 6–11 years of age, initial:** 80 mcg twice daily, not to exceed 160 mcg twice daily.

NURSING IMPLICATIONS

IMPLEMENTATION/ADMINISTRATION/STORAGE

1. When initiating in those receiving systemic corticosteroids, use aerosol concomitantly with the systemic steroid for 1 week. Then, slowly withdraw the systemic corticosteroid over several weeks.
2. The recommended dosage of flunisolide hemihydrate relative to flunisolide is lower due to differences in delivery characteristics between the products. Any client switched from flunisolide to flunisolide hemihydrate should be dosed appropriately, taking into account the recommended dosage; monitor to ensure that the dose of the hemihydate is safe and effective.
3. When flunisolide is used chronically at 2 mg/day for asthma, periodically monitor for effects on the hypothalamic-pituitary-adrenal axis.
4. If nasal congestion is present, use a decongestant before administration to ensure drug reaches site of action.
5. If beneficial effects do not occur within 3 weeks, discontinue therapy. Improvement of symptoms usually is evident within a few days, but may take up to 2 weeks for allergic rhinitis and 1–4 weeks for chronic asthma.
6. Store products from 15–30°C (59–86°F).

ASSESSMENT

1. Note onset, characteristics of S&S, triggers and clinical presentation. List other agents trialed and outcome.
2. Assess for any active or quiescent infections (TB, URI), or ocular herpes simplex.
3. When used chronically, periodically review need to continue or to adjust dosage; monitor children for growth and effects on the HPA axis.

CLIENT/FAMILY TEACHING

1. The effects of drug are not immediate; benefit requires daily use and starts to occur within 1 or 2 days. Full benefit may take 2 to 4 weeks depending on the condition being treated and the dose and route of administration.
2. Do not stop the medication once symptoms have been controlled. Continued daily use is necessary to continue to control symptoms.
3. Before use, prime the nasal spray by pushing down on the pump 5 or 6 times until a fine mist appears. If the pump has not been used for 5 days or more, the spray must be primed again.
4. Review how to administer nasal spray or inhalant. If prescribed a bronchodilator, use that first so steroid can better penetrate mucosa.
5. Clear nasal passages before using nasal spray. Gargle and rinse mouth with water after inhalation to prevent alterations in taste and to maintain adequate oral hygiene. Report any symptoms of irritation or fungal infections.
6. Mild nasal bleeding may occur; this is usually transient.
7. Rinse mouth and inhaler with water after each use to prevent infections.
8. With inhaler (AeroSpan), prime by releasing 2 sprays into air away from face before first use or when inhaler not used for more than 2 weeks. The white ring on opening of the actuator is normal, and the performance of aerosol is not affected by this residue. Do not chew or bite the gray spacer or remove spacer from the purple actuator.
9. With Aerobid, clean inhaler system every few days: remove metal cartridge, rinse plastic inhaler and cap with briskly running warm water and dry thoroughly. Replace the cartridge and cap.
10. Do not puncture the aerosol, store or administer near heat or open flame, or throw container into a fire or incinerator.
11. Keep all F/U to assess response and adverse SE.

F

OUTCOMES/EVALUATE

- Improved airway exchange
- ↓ Allergic manifestations

IV

Fluorouracil (5-Fluorouracil, 5-FU)

(flew-roh-**YOUR**-ah-sill)

Classification(s): Antineoplastic, antimetabolite

Pregnancy Category: X

RX: Adrucil, Carac, Fluoroplex.

SEE ALSO ***ANTINEOPLASTIC AGENTS.***

INDICATIONS/USES

Systemic: (1) Palliative management of certain cancers of the rectum, stomach, colon, pancreas, and breast. (2) In combination with levamisole for Dukes' stage C colon cancer after surgical resection. (3) In combination with leucovorin for metastatic colorectal cancer. *Investigational:* Cancer of the bladder, ovaries, prostate, cervix, endometrium, lung, liver, head, and neck. Also, malignant pleural, peritoneal, and pericardial effusions.

Topical (as solution or cream): (1) Multiple actinic or solar keratoses. (2) Superficial basal cell carcinoma (5% strength) when conventional methods are not practical (e.g., multiple lesion sites). *Investigational:* Condylomata acuminata (1% solution in 70% ethanol or the 5% cream).

ACTION/KINETICS

Action

Pyrimidine antagonist that inhibits the methylation reaction of deoxyuridylic acid to thymidylic acid. Thus, synthesis of DNA and, to a lesser extent, RNA is inhibited. Cell-cycle specific for the S phase of cell division. When used topically, the following response occurs:

- Early inflammation: Erythema for several days (minimal reaction)
- Severe inflammation: Burning, stinging, vesiculation
- Disintegration: Erosion, ulceration, necrosis, pain, crusting, reepithelialization
- Healing: Within 1–2 weeks with some residual erythema and temporary hyperpigmentation

Pharmacokinetics

t½, initial: 5–20 min; **final:** 20 hr. From 60 to 80% eliminated as respiratory CO_2 (8–12 hr); small amount (15%) excreted unchanged in urine (1–6 hr). Highly toxic; initiate use in hospital.

ADDITIONAL CONTRAINDICATIONS

Systemic: Clients in poor nutritional state, with severe bone marrow depression, severe infection, or recent (4-week-old) surgical intervention. Pregnancy or lactation. **Topical:** Use in women who are pregnant or who may become pregnant. Lactation. Use in dihydropyrimidine dehydrogenase enzyme deficiency due to possible cytotoxic activity and other toxicities. Application to mucous membranes due to possible local inflammation and ulceration and miscarriage/birth defects when applied during pregnancy.

SPECIAL CONCERNS

It is recommended that fluorouracil injection be given only by or under the supervision of a qualified physician who is experienced in cancer chemotherapy and who is well versed in the use of potent antimetabolites. Because of the possibility of severe toxic reactions, it is recommended that clients be hospitalized at least during the initial course of therapy.

- **Occlusive dressings may result in increased inflammation in adjacent normal skin when topical products are used.**
- **Use with caution with hepatic or liver dysfunction.**
- **Safety and efficacy of topical products not established in children less than 18 years of age.**

SIDE EFFECTS

Most Common

After systemic use: Diarrhea, heartburn, sores in mouth and on lips, anorexia, N&V, skin rash, itching, weakness, alopecia.

After topical use: Rash, skin/eye irritation, burning, inflammation, itching, pain, tenderness, changes in skin color at application site.

Systemic use. GI: Stomatitis, sores in mouth and on lips, esophagopharyngitis (may lead to sloughing and ulceration), diarrhea, anorexia, N&V, enteritis, cramps, duodenal ulcer, watery stools, duodenitis, gastritis, glossitis, pharyngitis, intra- and extrahepatic biliary sclerosis, acalculus cholecystitis, GI ulceration, bleeding. **CNS:** Lethargy, malaise, weakness, acute cerebellar syndrome (may persist after discontinuation of treatment), headache, disorientation, confusion, euphoria. **CV:** Myocardial ischemia, angina. **Dermatologic:** Alopecia, dermatitis (often as a pruritis maculopapular rash on the extremities or trunk), nonspecific skin toxicity, itching, photosensitivity (erythema, increased skin pigmentation), nail changes (including nail loss), dry skin, fissuring, vein pigmentation. Burning, dryness, edema, erosion, erythema, and pain when used on the face. **Hematologic:** Leukopenia, thrombocytopenia, pancytopenia, ***agranulocytosis***, anemia, thrombophlebitis, low WBC counts. **Ophthalmic:** Photophobia, lacrimation, decreased vision, nystagmus, diplopia, lacrimal duct stenosis, visual changes. **Regional arterial infusion complications:** ***Arterial aneurysm***, arterial ischemia, arterial thrombosis, bleeding at catheter site, catheter blocked/displaced/leaking, ***embolism***, fibromyositis, abscesses, infection at catheter site, thrombophlebitis. **Hypersensitivity:** ***Anaphylaxis***, generalized allergic reactions. **Miscellaneous:** Fever, epistaxis. *NOTE:* Rarely, life-threatening toxicity, including diarrhea, neutropenia, neurotoxicity, and stomatitis may occur with IV use of fluorouracil in those with dihydropyrimidine dehydrogenase enzyme deficiency.

Topical Use. Dermatologic: Local pain, pruritus, itching, urticaria, hyperpigmentation, scarring, skin irritation, inflammation, alopecia, burning at site of application, allergic contact dermatitis, soreness, ulceration, tenderness, suppuration, scaling, crusting, erosions, erythema, swelling, blistering, bullous pemphigoid, discomfort, ichthyosis, suppuration, swelling, telangiectasia, change in skin color at application site. **GI:** Stomatitis, medicinal taste. **CNS:** Insomnia, irritability, headache, emotional upset. **Musculoskeletal:** Muscle soreness. **Respiratory:** URTI, common cold, nasal irritation, sinusitis. **Hematologic:** Leukocytosis, eosinophilia, thrombocytopenia, toxic granulation. **Ophthalmic:** Eye irritation, lacrimation, conjunctival/corneal reaction. **Miscellaneous:** Photosensitivity, hypersensitivity reactions, allergy, herpes simplex.

NOTE: The following side effects are possible when using Carac: **Dermatologic:** Application site reaction, burning, dryness, edema, erosion, erythema, irritation, pain. **Miscellaneous**: Eye irritation, sinusitis, common cold, headache, allergy.

LABORATORY TEST CONSIDERATIONS

↑ Alkaline phosphatase, LDH, serum bilirubin, and serum transaminase. Abnormal lab tests: BSP, prothrombin, total proteins, sed rate, thrombocytopenia.

OVERDOSE MANAGEMENT

Symptoms: N&V, diarrhea, GI ulceration, GI bleeding, thrombocytopenia, ***agranulocytosis***, leukopenia. *Treatment:* Monitor hematologically for at least 4 weeks.

DRUG INTERACTIONS

Leucovorin calcium ↑ toxicity of fluorouracil.

HOW SUPPLIED

Cream, Topical: 0.5%, 1%, 5%; ***Injection:*** 50 mg/mL; ***Solution, Topical:*** 2%, 5%.

DOSAGE

IV

Palliative management of selected carcinomas.

Individualize dosage. Initial: 12 mg/kg/day for 4 days, not to exceed 800 mg/day. If no toxicity seen, administer 6 mg/kg on days 6, 8, 10, and 12. Discontinue therapy on day 12 even if there are no toxic symptoms. **Maintenance:** Repeat dose of first course q 30 days or when toxicity from initial course of therapy is gone; or, give 10–15 mg/kg/week as a single dose. Do not exceed 1 gram/week. **If client is debilitated or is a poor risk:** 6 mg/kg/day for 3 days; if no toxicity, give 3 mg/kg on days 5, 7, and 9 (daily dose should not exceed 400 mg).

Metastatic colorectal cancer.

Leucovorin, **IV,** 200 mg/m^2/day for 5 days followed by fluorouracil, **IV,** 370 mg/m^2/day for 5 days. Repeat q 28 days to maximize response and to prolong survival.

CREAM; TOPICAL SOLUTION

Multiple actinic or solar keratoses.

Apply to cover lesion 2 times per day for 2–6 weeks. Complete healing may not be evident for 1–2 months following cessation of fluorouracil therapy.

F

Superficial basal cell carcinoma.
Apply 5% cream or solution to cover lesion twice a day for 3–6 weeks (up to 10–12 weeks may be required before lesions are obliterated).

NURSING IMPLICATIONS

IMPLEMENTATION/ADMINISTRATION/STORAGE

1. Apply cream or solution with fingertips, nonmetallic applicator, or rubber gloves. Wash hands immediately thereafter.
2. Avoid contact with eyes, nose, and mouth.
3. Limit occlusive dressings to lesions; causes inflammatory reactions in normal skin. Increased absorption is possible through ulcerated or inflamed skin.
4. There is the possibility of increased absorption through inflamed or ulcerated skin.
5. Store 0.5% cream from 20–25°C (68–77°F). Store the 1% cream, 5% cream, and the 2% and 5% solution from 15–30°C (59–86°F).
6. IV Further dilution not needed; solution may be injected directly into the vein with a 25-gauge needle over 1–2 min.
7. Drug can be diluted in D5W or NSS and administered by IV infusion for periods of 30 min–8 hr. This method produces less systemic toxicity than rapid injection.
8. If precipitate forms, resolubilize by heating to 60°C (140°F) with vigorous shaking. Allow to return to room temperature; allow air to settle out before withdrawing and administering medication.
9. Solution may discolor slightly during storage; potency and safety not affected.
10. Store in a cool place (10–27°C, or 50–80°F). Do not freeze. Excessively low temperature causes precipitation. Do not expose the solution to light.
11. COMPATIBILITY D5W or NSS.
12. INCOMPATIBILITY Do not mix with other drugs or IV additives.

ASSESSMENT

1. List reasons for therapy, onset, characteristics of S&S or area requiring treatment, clinical presentation, other agents trialed.
2. Observe for intractable vomiting, stomatitis, diarrhea; early signs of toxicity with injections requiring immediate withdrawal of drug.
3. Hydrate well before and after therapy. Give antiemetics 1 hr before therapy.
4. Protect and supervise ambulation if symptoms of cerebellar dysfunction occur (altered balance, dizziness, or weakness).
5. With topical therapy, biopsy unresponsive lesions (solar keratosis) to confirm diagnosis. Perform follow-up biopsies as indicated in the management of superficial basal cell carcinoma.
6. Reduce dose with toxicity (severe diarrhea, stomatitis, ↓ platelets, ↓ WBC) as directed.
7. Use precautions and strict asepsis when WBC count is below 2,000/mm^3. Check CBC before each injection.
8. Obtain electrolytes and LFTs prior to each treatment for the first three cycles, then prior to every other cycle. Discontinue if WBC and platelet counts are depressed below 3,500/mm^3 and 100,000/mm^3, respectively. Nadir: 10–20 days; recovery: 30 days.

CLIENT/FAMILY TEACHING

1. Infusions usually administered in clinical setting. If administering at home, review how to store, prepare, and administer medication, and how to dispose of used equipment and supplies.
2. Review method for topical application. Do not wear plastic eyeglass frames during facial treatment. Contact may cause severe skin burns. Apply at night when glasses may be removed.
3. With solutions or cream, apply twice daily until ulceration of application site occurs, then discontinue use of solution or cream. Avoid contact with eyes, nose, mouth, and mucous membranes or inflamed skin.
4. To apply Carac, use the following procedure:
   - Apply once a day using fingertips; cover lesions with a thin film.
   - Do not apply near eyes, nostrils, or mouth. Apply 10 min after thoroughly washing, rinsing, and drying the entire area.
   - Wash hands thoroughly immediately after application.
   - Continued treatment up to 4 weeks results in greater lesion reduction. Local irritation is not significantly increased by extending treatment from 2 to 4 weeks; irritation is generally resolved within 2 weeks after stopping treatment.

5. Affected area may appear much worse before healing takes place in 1–2 months. Expect severe red skin areas, and then scaling and peeling of area. If dressing is needed, use only porous gauze; avoid occlusive dressings. May apply moisturizer and sunscreen two hours after application.
6. Drink plenty of fluids (2–3 L/day) during therapy.
7. Report if 4–6 diarrhea stools/day or diarrhea at night, fever, chills, or other signs of infection, persistent vomiting, redness, swelling, and pain of the hands or feet, or sores in the mouth.
8. Practice barrier contraception during systemic therapy.
9. Avoid exposure to sunlight. If exposed, wear protective clothing, sunglasses, and sunscreen.
10. With parenteral therapy, hair loss, skin reactions, and mouth sores may occur but are usually transient.
11. Avoid contact with people who have colds, the flu, or other contagious illnesses; do not receive vaccines that contain live strains of a virus (e.g., live oral polio vaccine) during treatment. Avoid contact with individuals who have recently been vaccinated with a live vaccine.
12. Keep all F/U to assess response, labs/biopsy, adverse SE.

OUTCOMES/EVALUATE

- Control of malignant process
- Reepithelialization of skin lesion

Fluoxetine hydrochloride

(flew-**OX**-eh-teen)

Classification(s): Antidepressant, selective serotonin reuptake inhibitor

Pregnancy Category: B

RX: Prozac, Prozac Pulvules, Prozac Weekly, Sarafem, Selfemra.

✦ **Rx:** Apo-Fluoxetine, CO Fluoxetine, Gen-Fluoxetine, Novo-Fluoxetine, Nu-Fluoxetine, PMS-Fluoxetine, ratio-Fluoxetine, Sandoz Fluoxetine.

SEE ALSO ***SELECTIVE SEROTONIN REUPTAKE INHIBITORS.***

INDICATIONS/USES

Prozac: (1) Major depressive disorder in adults and children 8–18 years of age. (2) Obsessive-compulsive disorders (OCD) in adults and children 8–18 years of age. (3) Long-term treatment of binge-eating and vomiting behaviors in moderate to severe bulimia nervosa. (4) Short-term treatment of panic disorder in adults with or without agoraphobia. (5) With olanzapine for acute treatment of depressive episodes associated with bipolar I disorder in adults. Fluoxetine monotherapy is not indicated for this condition. (6) With olanzapine for short-term treatment of treatment-resistant depression in adults who do not respond to 2 separate trials of different antidepressants of adequate dose and duration. Fluoxetine monotherapy is not indicated for this condition. **Sarafem:** Premenstrual dysphoric disorder. *Investigational:* Posttraumatic stress disorder in adults and children, borderline personality disorder, Raynaud phenomenon.

ACTION/KINETICS

Action

Antidepressant effect likely due to inhibition of CNS neuronal uptake of serotonin and, to a lesser extent. Little to no anticholinergic, sedative, or orthostatic hypotensive effects.

Pharmacokinetics

Metabolized in the liver to norfluoxetine, a metabolite with equal potency to fluoxetine. Norfluoxetine is further metabolized by the liver to inactive metabolites that are excreted by the kidneys. **Time to peak plasma levels:** 6–8 hr. **Peak plasma concentrations:** 15–55 ng/mL. **t½, fluoxetine:** 1–6 days; **t½, norfluoxetine:** 4–16 days. **Time to steady state:** 2–4 weeks. Active drug maintained in the body for weeks after withdrawal. Impaired hepatic function increases the half-life. **Plasma protein binding:** About 94.5%.

CONTRAINDICATIONS

Use of thioridazine with fluoxetine or within a minimum of 5 weeks after fluoxetine has been discontinued.

SPECIAL CONCERNS

(1) Antidepressants increased the risk compared with placebo of suicidal thinking and behavior (suicidality) in short-term studies in children, adolescents, and young adults with

major depressive disorder and other psychiatric disorders. Anyone considering the use of fluoxetine or any other antidepressant in a child, adolescent, or young adults must balance this risk with the clinical need. Short-term studies did not show an increase in the risk of suicidality with antidepressants compared with placebo in adults older than 24 years of age; there was a reduction in risk with antidepressants compared with placebo in adults 65 years of age and older. Depression and certain other psychiatric disorders are themselves associated with increases in the risk of suicide. Appropriately monitor and closely observe clients of all ages who are started on antidepressant therapy for clinical worsening, suicidality, or unusual changes in behavior. Clients who are started on therapy should be observed closely for clinical worsening, suicidality, or unusual changes in behavior. Advise families and caregivers of the need for close observation and communication with the prescribing health provider. (2) Fluoxetine is approved for use in pediatric clients with major depressive disorder and obsessive-compulsive disorder. Sarafem is not approved for use in children. (3) Short-term placebo-controlled trials of 9 antidepressant drugs in children and adolescents with major depressive disorder, obsessive-compulsive disorder, or other psychiatric disorders revealed a greater risk of adverse reactions during the first few months of treatment. The average risk of such reactions in clients receiving antidepressants was 4%, twice the placebo risk of 2%. No suicides occurred in these trials. ■

- **Consider a lower dose or less frequent dosing for those with impaired hepatic function, the elderly, those with concurrent diseases, or those taking multiple medications.**
- **Use in hospitalized clients, for longer than 5–6 weeks for depression, or for more than 13 weeks for OCD; not studied adequately.**

SIDE EFFECTS

Most Common

Insomnia, nausea, somnolence, nervousness, anxiety, tremor, diarrhea/loose stools, anorexia, dry mouth.

A large number of side effects have been reported for this drug. Listed are those with a reported frequency of greater than 1%. **CNS**: Headache, activation of mania or hypomania, insomnia, anxiety, nervousness, dizziness, fatigue, sedation, decreased libido, drowsiness, somnolence, light-headedness, decreased ability to concentrate, tremor, disturbances in sensation, agitation, abnormal dreams. Although less frequent than 1%, ***some clients may experience seizures or attempt suicide***. **GI**: Nausea, diarrhea/loose stools, vomiting, constipation, dry mouth, dyspepsia, anorexia, abdominal pain, flatulence, alteration in taste, gastroenteritis, increased appetite. **CV**: Hot flashes, palpitations. **GU**: Sexual dysfunction, impotence, anorgasmia, frequent urination, UTI, dysmenorrhea. **Respiratory**: URTI, pharyngitis, cough, dyspnea, rhinitis, bronchitis, nasal congestion, sinusitis, sinus headache, yawn. **Skin**: Rash, pruritus, excessive sweating. **Musculoskeletal**: Muscle, joint, limb or back pain. **Miscellaneous**: Flu-like symptoms, asthenia, fever, chest pain, allergy, visual disturbances, blurred vision, weight loss, bacterial or viral infection, chills.

ADDITIONAL DRUG INTERACTIONS

Alprazolam / ↑ Alprazolam levels and ↓ psychomotor performance
Buspirone / ↓ Buspirone effects; worsening of OCD
Carbamazepine / ↑ Carbamazepine levels → toxicity
Clozapine / ↑ Clozapine levels
Cyproheptadine / ↓ or Reversal of fluoxetine effect
Dextromethorphan / Possibility of hallucinations
Diazepam / ↑ Diazepam $t_{1/2}$ → excessive sedation or impaired psychomotor skills
Digoxin / ↓ AUC of digoxin; use together with caution
Haloperidol / ↑ Haloperidol levels
Lithium / ↑ Lithium levels → possible neurotoxicity
Olanzapine / ↑ Olanzapine peak levels
Phenytoin / ↑ Phenytoin levels
Tamoxifen / Concomitant use contraindicated R/T ↓ levels of the active metabolite of tamoxifen → ↓ pharmacologic effect

HOW SUPPLIED

Capsules: 10 mg, 20 mg, 40 mg; ***Capsules, Delayed-Release:*** 90 mg; ***Oral Solution:*** 20 mg/5 mL; ***Tablets:*** 10 mg, 15 mg, 20 mg.

DOSAGE

Prozac

CAPSULES; CAPSULES, DELAYED-RELEASE; ORAL SOLUTION; TABLETS

Major depressive disorder.

Adults, initial: 20 mg/day in the morning. If clinical improvement is not observed after several weeks, the dose may be increased to a maximum of 80 mg/day in two equally divided doses. For weekly dosing for stabilized clients requiring maintenance therapy, can use Prozac Weekly (90 mg delayed release capsule), given 7 days after the last 20 mg dose. If satisfactory response is not maintained, reestablish a daily dosing regimen. **Children, 8–18 years of age, initial:** 10 or 20 mg/day. After 1 week at 10 mg/day, increase the dose to 20 mg/day.

Obsessive compulsive disorder.

Adults, initial: 20 mg/day in the morning. If improvement is not significant after several weeks, the dose may be increased. Full effect may be delayed until 5 weeks of treatment or longer. **Usual dosage range:** 20–60 mg/day; the total daily dosage should not exceed 80 mg. Adjust dose to maintain client on lowest effective dosage. **Adolescents and higher weight children, initial:** 10 mg/day. After 2 weeks, increase the dose to 20 mg/day; additional dose increases may be considered after several more weeks if clinical improvement is insufficient. Recommended dose range: 20–60 mg/day. **Lower weight children, initial:** 10 mg/day. Dosage may be increased after several weeks if there is not sufficient improvement. Dose range: 20–30 mg/day. **Maintenance, adults and children:** Clients have been continued on therapy for an additional 6 months after an initial 13 weeks of treatment, without loss of efficacy. Adjust dose to maintain on lowest effective dose; periodically reassess to determine need for continued treatment.

Moderate to severe bulimia nervosa.

Initial: 60 mg/day given in the morning. May be necessary to titrate up to this dose over several days. **Maintenance:** Therapy has been continued for an additional 52 weeks beyond the initial 8 weeks.

Panic disorder.

Initial: 10 mg/day. After 1 week, increase the dose to 20 mg/day. A dose increase may be considered after several weeks if no improvement is noted. Doses above 60 mg/day have not been evaluated in panic disorders. **Maintenance:** Consider maintenance therapy for responding clients; periodically assess to determine the need for continued treatment.

Raynaud phenomenon.

20–60 mg/day.

With olanzapine for depressive episodes associated with bipolar I disorder; with olanzapine for treatment-resistant depression.

Adults, initial: Fluoxetine, 20 mg and olanzapine, 5 mg once daily in the evening without regard to meals. Adjust dosage depending on efficacy and tolerability within dose ranges of fluoxetine, 20 to 50 mg and olanzapine, 5 to 12.5 mg. Safety of coadministration of fluoxetine, above 75 mg, and olanzapine, above 18 mg, each per day, has not been evaluated. *NOTE:* Symbyax is a fixed-dosed combination of fluoxetine and olanzapine. Fixed-doses include olanzapine/fluoxetine: 3 mg/25 mg, 6 mg/25 mg, 12 mg/25 mg, 6 mg/50 mg, and 12 mg/50 mg.

Posttraumatic stress disorder in adults and children (Investigational).

Adults, initial: 10–20 mg/day. Evaluate for response every 1–2 weeks; increase dose, as needed, for at least an 8-week treatment trial. **Target daily dose:** 20–50 mg/day (20 mg/day in older adults), up to a maximum of 80 mg/day. **Children:** Average target daily dose is 10–20 mg. **Duration of treatment for adults and children:** 6–12 months for acute posttraumatic stress syndrome and 12–24 months for

F

chronic posttraumatic stress syndrome. Discontinuation may be tried after 6–24 months, depending on the type of posttraumatic stress. Taper dose over 2–4 weeks to avoid withdrawal syndrome.

Raynaud phenomenon (Investigational).

Adults: 20–60 mg/day.

Sarafem

CAPSULES

Premenstrual dysphoric disorder.

Initial: 20 mg/day (not to exceed 80 mg/day) given every day of the menstrual cycle or intermittently (starting a daily dose 14 days before anticipated menses onset through the first full day of menses; repeat with each new cycle). Efficacy has been maintained for up to 6 months at doses of 20 mg/day given continuously and up to 3 months at a dose of 20 mg/day given intermittently. Reassess clients to determine continued need for the drug.

NURSING IMPLICATIONS

Do not confuse fluoxetine with duloxetine (another selective serotonin reuptake inhibitor) or with fluvoxamine (another selective serotonin reuptake inhibitor).

IMPLEMENTATION/ADMINISTRATION/STORAGE

1. Doses greater than 20 mg/day may be given once a day (i.e., in the morning) or twice a day (i.e., morning and noon).
2. If doses lower than 20 mg are necessary, the drug may be emptied from the capsule into cranberry, orange, or apple juice; this should not be refrigerated (is stable for 2 weeks). *NOTE:* A liquid preparation (20 mg/5 mL) is also available.
3. The maximum therapeutic effect may not be observed until 4–5 weeks after beginning therapy.
4. If therapy needs to be discontinued, gradually reduce the dose, rather than abrupt discontinuation.
5. Elderly clients, clients taking multiple medications, and those with liver or kidney dysfunction should take lower or less frequent doses.
6. When used for obsessive-compulsive disorders and therapy has been continued for over 6 months, reassess periodically to determine if continued drug therapy is needed.
7. When given with tricyclic antidepressants for major depressive disorder or if fluoxetine has been recently discontinued, the dose of TCA may need to be reduced and plasma levels monitored temporarily.
8. Allow 14 days to elapse between discontinuing an MAOI and starting fluoxetine therapy; also, allow 5 weeks or more to elapse between stopping fluoxetine and starting an MAOI.
9. Do not give thioridazine with fluoxetine or within a minimum of 5 weeks after fluoxetine has been discontinued.
10. Store from 15–30°C (59–86°F). Protect Sarafem from light.

ASSESSMENT

1. Note reasons for therapy, onset, characteristics of S&S, any events/triggers and other agents trialed/outcome. Document behavioral and cognitive functions; assess clinical response.
2. Review drugs currently prescribed to ensure that none interact.
3. Determine if pregnant or lactating.
4. Periodically reassess to determine need for continued therapy. Document mood, behaviors and clinical presentation.
5. Drug has long half-life up to 3 days and its metabolite 16 days.
6. Obtain weight, renal and LFTs; reduce dose with elderly or debilitated, and with hepatic/renal dysfunction.

CLIENT/FAMILY TEACHING

1. Take at the designated times; nervousness and insomnia may occur.
2. May be taken with food to decrease chance of stomach upset.
3. Use caution when driving or performing tasks that require mental alertness; may cause drowsiness/dizziness. Change positions slowly to avoid drop in BP.
4. Report side effects, especially rashes, hives, increased anxiety, loss of appetite, or lack of response. Use reliable birth control during therapy.
5. Usually takes 1 month to note any significant benefits from therapy. Do not become discouraged and discontinue before benefits attained.

6. **Avoid alcohol; do not take any OTC agents without approval. Use sunscreen and avoid prolonged sun exposure.**
7. **Any thoughts of suicide or evidence of increased suicide ideations should be reported immediately. Parents should monitor children carefully for any indications of suicide ideations.**
8. **Keep all F/U to assess response, counselling, and adverse SE.**

OUTCOMES/EVALUATE

- **↓ Symptoms of depression, as evidenced by improved sleeping and eating patterns, ↓ fatigue, and ↑ social involvement and activity**
- **Control of repetitive behavioral manifestations (OCD), bulimia nervosa, panic disorder**
- **↓ PTSD symptoms**

Flutamide

(**FLOO**-tah-myd)

Classification(s): Antineoplastic, hormone

Pregnancy Category: D

✤ **Rx:** Apo-Flutamide, Euflex.

SEE ALSO ***ANTINEOPLASTIC AGENTS***.

INDICATIONS/USES

(1) In combination with leuprolide acetate (i.e., a LHRH agonist) to treat locally confined Stage B_2-C and Stage D_2 prostate cancer. (2) In combination with goserelin acetate depots (Zoladex) to treat locally confined early stage B_2-C prostate cancer before and during radiation therapy. *NOTE:* Other than investigational use for hirsutism in women, flutamide has no indication for women and should not be used in this population. *Investigational:* Treat hirsutism in women.

ACTION/KINETICS

Action

Has antiandrogen effects. Acts either to inhibit uptake of androgen or to inhibit nuclear binding of androgen in target tissues. Thus, the effect of androgen is decreased in androgen-sensitive tissues, such as seen in prostate cancer.

Pharmacokinetics

Rapidly and completely absorbed. **Maximum plasma levels:** 2 hr. Food has no effect on bioavailability. Metabolized to active (alpha-hydroxylated derivative) and inactive metabolites in the liver and mainly excreted in the urine. **t½ of active metabolite:** 6 hr (8 hr in geriatric clients). **Plasma protein binding:** 94–96%.

CONTRAINDICATIONS

Hypersensitivity to flutamide or any component of the product. Use in women or severe hepatic impairment (if baseline serum ALT values exceed twice ULN). Lactation.

SPECIAL CONCERNS

(1) **Hepatic injury**. There have been postmarketing reports of hospitalization and rarely death from liver failure. Evidence of hepatic injury included elevated serum transaminase levels, jaundice, hepatic encephalopathy, and death related to hepatic failure. Hepatic injury was reversible after discontinuation of therapy in some clients. Approximately half of the reported cases occurred within the initial 3 months of treatment with flutamide. (2) Serum transaminase levels should be measured before starting treatment with flutamide. Flutamide is not recommended in clients whose ALT values exceed twice ULN. Serum transaminase levels should then be measured monthly for the first 4 months of therapy, and periodically thereafter. LFTs also should be obtained at the first signs and symptoms suggestive of liver dysfunction (e.g., N&V, abdominal pain, fatigue, anorexia, flu-like symptoms, hyperbilirubinemia, jaundice, right upper quadrant tenderness). If at any time a client has jaundice or their ALT rises above 2 times ULN, flutamide should be immediately discontinued with close follow-up of LFTs until resolution.

- **May cause fetal harm when given to pregnant women.**
- **A metabolite may result in methemoglobinemia, hemolytic anemia, and cholestatic jaundice in those susceptible to aniline toxicity.**

SIDE EFFECTS

Most Common

Hot flashes, loss of libido, impotence, diarrhea, N&V, anorexia, gynecomastia, anemia, edema.

Side effects are listed for treatment with flutamide and LHRH agonist or use with goserelin. **CV**: Hot flashes, hypertension. **GI**: N&V, diarrhea, GI disturbances, anorexia, rectal bleeding, proctitis. **CNS**: Confusion, depression, drowsiness, anxiety, nervousness. **Hematologic**: Anemia, leukopenia, thrombocytopenia, ***hemolytic anemia***, macrocytic anemia, methemoglobinemia, sulfhemoglobinemia. **Hepatic**: Hepatitis, cholestatic jaundice, hepatic encephalopathy, jaundice, ***hepatic necrosis, liver failure***. **Dermatologic**: Rash, injection site irritation, erythema, ulceration, bullous eruptions, photosensitivity, ***epidermal necrolysis***. **Respiratory:** Pulmonary symptoms. **GU:** Gynecomastia, cystitis, hematuria, urine discoloration, loss of libido, impotence, GU symptoms. **Miscellaneous**: Edema, neuromuscular symptoms, malignant breast tumors in male clients.

F

LABORATORY TEST CONSIDERATIONS

↑ AST, ALT, serum creatinine, SGGT, BUN, bilirubin. Urine may be colored amber or yellow-green due to the drug or its metabolites.

OVERDOSE MANAGEMENT

Symptoms: Breast tenderness, gynecomastia, increases in AST. Also possible are ataxia, anorexia, vomiting, decreased respiration, lacrimation, sedation, hypoactivity, and piloerection. *Treatment:* Induce vomiting if client is alert. Frequently monitor VS and observe closely. Drug is not cleared by hemodialysis.

DRUG INTERACTIONS

↑ PT time in clients receiving long-term warfarin; closely monitor PT time and adjust anticoagulant dose if necessary.

HOW SUPPLIED

Capsules: 125 mg.

DOSAGE

CAPSULES

Locally confined stage B_2-C and stage D_2 metastatic cancer of the prostate.

250 mg (2 capsules) 3 times/day q 8 hr for a total daily dose of 750 mg.

Hirsutism in women (investigational).

Use a monotherapy or combination therapy at doses ranging from 125–500 mg/day in 1–2 divided doses.

NURSING IMPLICATIONS

Ⓢ Do not confuse flutamide with remantadine (an antiviral).

IMPLEMENTATION/ADMINISTRATION/STORAGE

1. For stage B_2-C prostatic cancer, start flutamide and the LHRH agonist 8 weeks prior to initiating and continue during radiation therapy.
2. For maximum benefit in stage D_2 metastatic prostatic cancer, start flutamide and the LHRH agonist together and continue until disease progression.
3. Flutamide is a potential teratogen; follow safe handling procedures when preparing, administering, or dispensing flutamide.
4. Store from 15–30°C (59–86°F). Should be dispensed in a child-resistant, tight, light-resistant container.

ASSESSMENT

1. Note reasons for therapy, staging, agents previously used, outcome.
2. Administer with an LHRH agonist (such as leuprolide acetate).
3. Assess methemoglobinemia in those susceptible to aniline toxicity (i.e., G6PD deficiency, hemoglobin M disease, smokers).
4. Monitor CBC, PSA, and LFTs; check liver function prior to therapy, monthly for the first 4 months, and periodically thereafter. Stop therapy (or do not start therapy) if ALT exceeds 2 × ULN or if jaundice develops to prevent acute liver failure.

CLIENT/FAMILY TEACHING

1. Used to treat cancer of the prostate gland; blocks the effect of the male hormone testosterone in the body. Take flutamide and the LHRH agonist (leuprolide) at the same time, which works to lower levels of testosterone produced by the testicles.
2. Drug therapy should not be interrupted or discontinued without consulting provider.
3. Hot flashes, impotence, and diarrhea are all potential side effects of drug therapy; report if persistent or bothersome. Compliance may be a problem if diarrhea experienced. Manage diarrhea by cutting down on dairy products, drinking plenty of fluids, not using laxatives, using antidiarrheal products, and eating smaller, more frequent meals high in dietary fibers.
4. Urine may appear amber or yellow-green.

5. Use caution, photosensitization may occur.
6. Report any N&V, abdominal pain, fatigue, anorexia, flu-like symptoms, right upper quadrant pain/tenderness, loss of appetite, dark yellow or brown urine, and yellowing of the skin or eyes.
7. Sexual problems may be drug induced (impotence, decreased libido, gynecomastia). Counseling may be indicated.
8. Keep all F/U to assess response, labs, adverse SE.

OUTCOMES/EVALUATE

- ↓ Production of testosterone
- ↓ Prostatic tumor size
- Control of metastatic processes

Fluticasone furoate

(flu-**TIH**-kah-sohn)

Classification(s): Glucocorticoid

Pregnancy Category: C

RX: Veramyst.

Fluticasone propionate

(flu-**TIH**-kah-sohn)

Classification(s): Glucocorticoid

Pregnancy Category: C

RX: Cream, Lotion, Ointment: Cutivate. **Aerosol/Powder, Inhalation**: Flovent Diskus, Flovent HFA. **Spray, Intranasal**: Flonase.

🍁 **Rx:** Apo-Fluticasone.

SEE ALSO ***CORTICOSTEROIDS***.

INDICATIONS/USES

Fluticasone furoate. Intranasal (Veramyst): Symptoms of seasonal and perennial allergic rhinitis in clients 2 years of age and older.

Fluticasone propionate. Aerosol, inhalation (Flovent HFA) and Powder, inhalation (Flovent Diskus): Maintenance treatment of asthma as prophylactic therapy in clients 4 years of age and older. Also for those requiring oral corticosteroid therapy. **Intranasal (Flonase Spray):** To manage nasal symptoms of seasonal and perennial allergic and nonallergic rhinitis in adults and children over 4 years of age. **Topical:** (1) Relief of inflammatory and pruritic corticosteroid-responsive dermatoses in adults. (2) Atopic dermatitis in clients as young as 3 months.

ACTION/KINETICS

Action

Anti-inflammatory due to ability to inhibit prostaglandin synthesis. Also inhibits accumulation of macrophages and leukocytes at sites of inflammation as well as to inhibit phagocytosis and lysosomal enzyme release.

Pharmacokinetics

Following intranasal use, a small amount is absorbed into the general circulation. Bioavailability is less than 2%. **Onset:** Approximately 12 hr. **Maximum effect:** May take several days. **$t_{1/2}$:** About 3.1 hr. Absorbed drug is metabolized in the liver by CYP3A4 and excreted in the feces (>95%) and urine (<5%). **Plasma protein binding:** About 91%.

CONTRAINDICATIONS

Use for relief of acute bronchospasm. Use following nasal septal ulcers, nasal surgery, or nasal trauma until healing has occurred. Use of Flovent Rotadisk in those with hypersensitivity to any ingredient, including lactose.

SPECIAL CONCERNS

(1) Use care when transferring from systemic corticosteroids to fluticasone propionate because deaths due to adrenal insufficiency have occurred in those with asthma during and after transfer from systemic corticosteroids to less systemically available inhaled corticosteroids. After withdrawal from systemic corticosteroids, a number of months are required for recovery of hypothalamic-pituitary-adrenal (HPA) function. (2) Clients who have been previously maintained on 20 mg/day or more of prednisone (or its equivalent) may be most susceptible, particularly when their systemic corticosteroids have been almost completely withdrawn. During this period of HPA suppression, clients may exhibit signs and symptoms of adrenal insufficiency when exposed to trauma, surgery, or infections (particularly gastroenteritis) or other conditions associated with severe electrolyte loss. Although fluticasone propionate inhalation may provide control of asthma symptoms during these episodes, in recommended doses it supplies less than normal physiological

amounts of glucocorticoid systemically and does not provide the mineralocorticoid activity that is necessary for coping with these emergencies. (3) During periods of stress or severe asthma attack, clients who have been withdrawn from systemic corticosteroids should be instructed to resume oral corticosteroids (in large doses) immediately and to contact their providers for further instruction. These clients should also be instructed to carry a warning card indicating that they may need supplementary systemic corticosteroids during periods of stress or a severe asthma attack. ■

- **Clients on immunosuppressant drugs, such as corticosteroids, are more susceptible to infections.**
- **Use with caution, if at all, in active or quiescent tuberculosis infections; untreated fungal, bacterial, or systemic viral infections; or ocular herpes simplex.**
- **Use with caution during lactation.**

SIDE EFFECTS

Most Common

Use of Flonase: Headache, pharyngitis, epistaxis, nasal burning/irritation, N&V, asthma symptoms, cough.

Use of Flovent: Throat irritation, URTI, sinusitis/sinus infection, oral candidiasis, headache, fever.

Allergic: Rarely, immediate hypersensitivity reactions or contact dermatitis. Rotadisk blisters contain lactose; ***anaphylaxis*** may occur in those allergic to milk protein. **Respiratory:** Epistaxis, URTI, nasal burning/ulcer, blood in nasal mucus, pharyngitis, cough, asthma symptoms, irritation of nasal mucous membranes, sneezing, runny nose, sinusitis/sinus infection, nasal congestion/dryness, bronchitis, nasal septum excoriation, ***possible severe fatal asthma.*** **CNS:** Headache, dizziness. **Ophthalmic:** Eye disorder, cataracts, glaucoma, increased intraocular pressure. **GI:** N&V, xerostomia, oral candidiasis. **Miscellaneous:** Unpleasant taste, fever, urticaria. High doses have resulted in hypercorticism and adrenal suppression.

DRUG INTERACTIONS

Cimetidine / ↑ Fluticasone plasma levels R/T ↓ liver breakdown by CYP3A4

Clarithromycin / ↑ Fluticasone levels R/T ↓ liver breakdown by CYP3A4

Erythromycin / ↑ Fluticasone levels R/T ↓ liver breakdown by CYP3A4

Itraconazole / ↑ Fluticasone levels R/T ↓ liver breakdown by CYP3A4

Ketoconazole / ↑ Fluticasone levels R/T ↓ liver breakdown by CYP3A4

Ritonavir / ↑ Fluticasone levels R/T ↓ liver breakdown by CYP3A4

HOW SUPPLIED

Fluticasone furoate. ***Intranasal Suspension Spray (Veramyst):*** 27.5 mcg/actuation.

Fluticasone propionate. ***Aerosol, Inhalation Suspension (Flovent HFA):*** 44 mcg/actuation, 110 mcg/actuation, 220 mcg/actuation; ***Cream:*** 0.05%; ***Lotion:*** 0.05%; ***Ointment:*** 0.005%; ***Powder, Inhalation (Flovent Diskus):*** 50 mcg/actuation, 100 mcg/actuation, 250 mcg/actuation; ***Spray, Intranasal (Flonase):*** 50 mcg/actuation.

DOSAGE

Fluticasone furoate (Veramyst)

SPRAY, INTRANASAL SUSPENSION

Seasonal and perennial allergic rhinitis.

Adults and children 12 years and older, initial: 110 mcg once daily given as 2 sprays (27.5 mcg/spray) in each nostril. Titrate to the minimum effective dose to reduce the possibility of side effects. When the maximum benefit has been reached, reduce the dose to 55 mcg (1 spray in each nostril) once daily. **Children, 2–11 years of age, initial:** 55 mcg once daily given as 1 spray (27.5 mcg/spray) in each nostril. Children not responding adequately to the 55 mcg dose may use 110 mcg (2 sprays/nostril) once daily. Once symptoms have been controlled, decrease the dose to 55 mcg daily.

Fluticasone propionate

AEROSOL, INHALATION SUSPENSION (FLOVENT HFA)

Asthma.

Adults and children over 12 years of age, initial: 88 mcg twice a day (maximum: 440 mcg twice a day) if previous therapy was bronchodilators alone;

88–220 mcg twice a day (maximum: 440 mcg twice a day) if previous therapy was inhaled corticosteroids; and 440 mcg twice a day (maximum: 880 mcg twice a day) if previous therapy was oral corticosteroids. Starting doses more than 88 mcg twice daily may be considered for those with poor asthma control or those who have previously required doses of inhaled corticosteroids that are in the higher range for that specific agent. **Children, 4–11 years of age:** 88 mcg twice a day (maximum: 88 mcg twice a day), regardless of prior therapy.

POWDER, INHALATION (FLOVENT DISKUS)

Asthma.

Adults and children over 12 years of age: 100 mcg twice a day (maximum: 500 mcg twice a day) if previous therapy was bronchodilators alone; 100–250 mcg twice a day (maximum: 500 mcg twice a day) if previous therapy was inhaled corticosteroids; 500–1,000 mcg twice a day (maximum: 1,000 mcg twice a day) if previous therapy was oral corticosteroids. **Children, 4–11 years of age:** 50 mcg twice a day (maximum: 100 mcg twice a day) if previous therapy was either bronchodilators alone or inhaled corticosteroids. Starting doses greater than 100 mcg twice a day for adults and children over 12 years of age and starting doses greater than 50 mcg twice a day may be considered for those with poorer asthma control or those who have previously required doses of inhaled corticosteroids that are in the higher range for that specific drug.

Fluticasone propionate

SPRAY, INTRANASAL (FLONASE)

Allergic and nonallergic rhinitis.

Adults, initial: Two sprays (50 mcg each) per nostril once daily (total daily dose: 200 mcg). Or, 100 mcg given twice a day (e.g., 8 a.m. and 8 p.m.) Maximum dose is two sprays (200 mcg) in each nostril once a day. After a few days, may reduce dose to 100 mcg (1 spray/nostril) once daily for maintenance. **Adolescents and children 4 years and older, initial:** 100 mcg (1 spray/nostril once a day). If no response to 100 mcg, may use 200 mcg/day (2 sprays/nostril). Once control achieved, decrease dose to 100 mcg (1 spray/nostril) daily. Do not exceed a dose of 200 mcg/day. The spray is not recommended for children under 4 years of age. *NOTE:* For both adults and children, as needed use may be effective for symptom control in doses not to exceed 200 mcg daily.

CREAM; LOTION; OINTMENT

Dermatoses in adults, atopic dermatitis.

Apply sparingly to affected area 2–4 times daily. For Cutivate Cream, apply a thin film to the affected areas once daily. For Cutivate Lotion, apply a thin film to the affected areas once daily.

NURSING IMPLICATIONS

IMPLEMENTATION/ADMINISTRATION/STORAGE

1. Effectiveness depends on regular use. Individuals will vary with respect to time to onset and degree of relief. Improvement may occur within 24 hr, while maximum benefits may not occur for 1–2 weeks or longer.
2. If taking chronic oral steroids, reduce prednisone no faster than 2.5 mg/day on a weekly basis, beginning after 1 or more weeks of aerosol therapy. After prednisone reduction is complete, decrease fluticasone dosage to the lowest effective dose.
3. Store aerosol canister (Flovent HFA) with nozzle end down; protect from freezing and direct sunlight. For best results, the aerosol canister should be at room temperature before use. Prime the inhaler before using for the first time by releasing 4 test sprays into the air away from the face, shaking well before each spray. If the spray has not been used for more than 7 days or when it has been dropped, prime again by shaking well and releasing 1 spray into the air away from the face.
4. For Flonase, initially prime the pump with 6 actuations before use or after a period of nonuse of 1 week or more.

F

5. Before use of Flonase, shake gently. Discard the Flonase bottle when the labeled number of actuations has been used.
6. Before use of Veramyst, prime for the first time by shaking the container well and release 6 test sprays into the air away from the face. When the product has not been used for more than 30 days or if the cap has been left off the bottle for 5 days or longer, prime the pump again until a fine mist appears. Shake well before each use.
7. Store nasal spray (Flonase) at 4–30°C (39–86°F). Store aerosol (Flovent HFA) and inhalation powder (Flovent Diskus) from 15–30°C (59–86°F) in a dry place. Store the intranasal spray (Veramyst) upright from 15–30°C (59–86°F); do not freeze or refrigerate; discard the nasal device after 120 sprays have been used, even if the container is not empty.

ASSESSMENT

1. List reasons for therapy, onset, characteristics of S&S, other agents trialed, outcome.
2. Document clinical presentation, and assess therapy to note clinical response.
3. If for nasal use, examine for evidence of nasal septal ulcers; note turbinate findings.
4. Determine if immunocompromised or actively infected. Note recent systemic steroid therapy use and amount.
5. Note any evidence of glaucoma or cataracts; risk increased.
6. Assess heart and lungs and for HPA axis effects; note PFTs and CXR findings.

CLIENT/FAMILY TEACHING

1. Review technique for administration. With nasal spray (Flonase), clear nasal passages before using, initially prime the pump with 6 actuations before use or after a period of nonuse of 1 week or more. Shake inhalation and nasal product gently. If more than 1 spray/dose is ordered, administer each spray individually, waiting a few seconds between sprays.
2. Take a drink of water to moisten throat before using inhaler. To use: breathe out fully, hold inhaler 1 to 2 inches in front of mouth or attach a spacer to the inhaler and place the spacer in your mouth (above tongue and past teeth to prevent drug from depositing on tongue/throat). Take a deep, slow breath as you push down on the canister. Hold your breath for 10 seconds; then exhale slowly. If more than one puff ordered, wait for at least 1 full minute after each puff; then repeat the procedure. Avoid exhaling into mouthpiece to avoid moisture accumulation. Keep inhaler capped to avoid dirt getting inside.
3. With inhalers, if others prescribed, use the bronchodilator first so steroid better permeates mucosa. Rinse mouth and inhaler with water after use to prevent infections.
4. Prime Flovent HFA before using for the first time by releasing 4 test sprays into the air away from the face; shake well before each spray. If the inhaler has not been used for more than 7 days or when it has been dropped, prime the inhaler again by shaking well and releasing 1 spray into the air away from the face.
5. With the intranasal suspension spray (Veramyst), prime before using for the first time by shaking the container well and releasing 6 test sprays into the air away from the face. When the drug has not been used for more than 2 weeks or if the cap has been left off the bottle for 5 days or more, prime the pump again until a fine mist appears. Store upright, shake well before each use. Discard after 120 sprays have been used, even though the bottle is not completely empty.
6. Avoid spacer device with the Flovent Diskus. Remember to discard 50 mcg strength 6 weeks after removal and the 100 or 250 mcg strengths 8 weeks after removal from the moisture-protective foil pouch or after all blisters have been used (i.e., when the dose indicator reads 0), whichever comes first.
7. Do not exceed prescribed dose; it may take several days to achieve full benefits. Take at regular intervals to ensure effectiveness.
8. Do not interrupt therapy if side effects evident; notify provider as drug may require slow withdrawal. The dosage should also be slowly reduced if S&S of hypercorticism or adrenal suppression occur, such as depression, lassitude, joint and muscle pain; report if evident, especially when replacing systemic corticosteroids with topical.
9. Use adequate humidity, especially during winter months when dry heat may aggravate mucosa.

10. Avoid persons with active infections. Report exposure to chickenpox or measles. (If not immunized or previously infected with the disease, varicella or immune globulin prophylaxis may be given to high-risk clients on long-term therapy.)
11. Height and weight will be monitored periodically in adolescents to detect any growth suppression.
12. Identify/avoid triggers that aggravate asthma (dust, pollen, smoke, chemicals, pets). Use peak flow meter to help manage asthma.
13. During high stress or acute asthma attack, if previously on systemic corticosteroids, resume oral corticosteroids (in large doses) immediately and contact provider for further instruction. Carry an alert indicating they may need supplementary systemic corticosteroids during periods of stress or a severe asthma attack.
14. With topical products report evidence of infection, lack of healing, or lack of response; do not cover with occlusive dressing (diapers or plastic pants). Do not apply to face, underarms, or groin areas unless specifically directed.
15. Keep all F/U to assess response and adverse SE.

OUTCOMES/EVALUATE

- Control of asthma
- ↓ Symptoms of allergic rhinitis
- Relief of inflammatory and pruritic corticosteroid-responsive dermatoses in adults/atopic dermatitis

Combination Drug

Fluticasone propionate and Salmeterol xinafoate

(flu-**TIH**-kah-sohn, sal-**MET**-er-ole)

Classification(s): Anti-asthmatic combination drug.

Pregnancy Category: C

RX: Advair Diskus, Advair HFA.

SEE ALSO ***FLUTICASONE PROPIONATE*** AND ***SALMETEROL XINAFOATE***.

INDICATIONS/USES

Advair Diskus: (1) Long-term, twice-daily maintenance treatment of asthma in clients 4 years of age and older. (2) Twice-daily maintenance treatment of airflow obstruction in COPD, including chronic bronchitis and/or emphysema. (3) Fluticasone 250 mcg/salmeterol 50 mcg is used to reduce exacerbations of COPD in clients with a history of exacerbations. **Advair HFA:** Long-term, twice-daily maintenance treatment of asthma in clients 12 years of age and older.

CONTENT

Advair Diskus Inhalation Powder: Fluticasone propionate *(corticosteroid),* 100 mcg and Salmeterol *(beta-2 adrenergic agonist),* 50 mcg/actuation; Fluticasone propionate, 250 mcg and Salmeterol, 50 mcg/actuation; Fluticasone propionate, 500 mcg, and Salmeterol, 50 mcg/actuation.

Advair HFA Inhalation Aerosol Spray: Fluticasone propionate *(corticosteroid),* 45 mcg and Salmeterol *(beta-2 adrenergic agonist),* 21 mcg/actuation; Fluticasone propionate, 115 mcg and Salmeterol, 21 mcg/actuation; Fluticasone propionate, 230 mcg, and Salmeterol, 21 mcg/actuation.

ACTION/KINETICS

Action

Fluticasone is an anti-inflammatory corticosteroid. The precise mechanism is unknown, but corticosteroids inhibit multiple cell types (e.g., mast cells, eosinophils, basophils, lymphocytes, macrophages, and neutrophils) and mediator production or secretion (e.g., histamine, eicosanoids, leukotrienes, cytokines) involved in the asthmatic response. Salmeterol is a long-acting beta-2 adrenergic agonist that catalyzes the conversion of ATP to cyclic-AMP. Increased cyclic-AMP levels cause relaxation of bronchial smooth muscle and inhibition of release of mediators of immediate hypersensitivity, especially from mast cells.

Pharmacokinetics

Onset: 30–60 min; **maximum improvement in forced expiratory volume in 1 second (FEV_1):** Within 3 hr; **duration:** 12 hr.

Fluticasone propionate. Peak plasma levels: 1–2 hr. **t½, elimination:** 7.8 hr. Metabolized by CYP3A4 in the liver. Excreted in the feces as parent drug and metabolites.

Salmeterol xinafoate. Peak plasma levels: About 5 min, but plasma levels are low. Extensively metabolized; eliminated mostly in the feces. **Plasma protein binding:** About 91% of fluticasone and 96% of salmeterol.

CONTRAINDICATIONS

Hypersensitivity to any component of the product. Primary treatment of status asthmaticus or other acute episodes of asthma where intensive measures are needed. Use to relieve acute bronchospasm. Do not use Advair Diskus for transferring clients from systemic corticosteroid therapy due to the possibility of deaths due to adrenal insufficiency.

SPECIAL CONCERNS

Long-acting beta-2 adrenergic agonists, such as salmeterol, an active ingredient in fluticasone/salmeterol, may increase the risk of asthma-related death. Data from a large placebo-controlled U.S. study that compared the safety of salmeterol or placebo added to usual asthma therapy showed an increase in asthma-related deaths in clients receiving salmeterol (13 deaths of 13,176 clients treated for 28 weeks on salmeterol versus 3 deaths of 13,179 clients on placebo). Currently available data are inadequate to determine whether concurrent use of inhaled corticosteroids or other long-term asthma control drugs mitigates the increased risk of asthma-related death from long-acting beta-2 adrenergic agents. Available data from controlled clinical trials suggest that long-acting beta-2 adrenergic agents increase the risk of hospitalization in pediatric and adolescent clients.

Therefore, when treating clients with asthma, only prescribe fluticasone/salmeterol for clients not adequately controlled on other asthma-control medications (e.g., inhaled corticosteroids) or whose disease severity clearly warrants initiation of treatment with both an inhaled corticosteroid and long-acting beta-2 adrenergic agent. Once asthma control is achieved and maintained, assess the client at regular intervals and step down therapy (e.g., discontinue fluticasone/salmeterol) if possible without loss of asthma control and maintain the client on a long-term asthma control medication, such as an inhaled corticosteroid. Do not use fluticasone/salmeterol for clients whose asthma is adequately controlled on low or medium dose inhaled corticosteroids.

- **Use with caution in lactation, hepatic disease, and in CV disorders, especially coronary insufficiency, cardiac arrhythmias, and hypertension.**
- **Use with caution, if at all, with active quiescent tuberculosis infections of the respiratory tract; untreated systemic fungal, bacterial, viral, or parasitic infections; or ocular herpes simplex.**
- **Restrict use during labor where the benefits clearly outweigh the risks.**
- **Safety and efficacy have not been shown in children less than 12 years of age.**

SIDE EFFECTS

Most Common

URTI, pharyngitis, headache, URT inflammation, cough, hoarseness/dysphonia, bronchitis, N&V.

See *Fluticasone propionate* and *Salmeterol xinafoate* for a complete list of possible side effects. Also, **Respiratory:** ***Paradoxical bronchospasm, laryngeal spasm***, irritation, swelling of upper airway, stridor, ***choking***. **Immediate Hypersensitivity:** Urticaria, ***angioedema***, rash, ***bronchospasm***. **CV:** Changes in BP and pulse rate. **Hematologic:** Systemic eosinophilia, vasculitis consistent with Churg-Strauss syndrome. **Miscellaneous:** Immunosuppression.

OVERDOSE MANAGEMENT

Symptoms: **Salmeterol:** Excessive beta-adrenergic stimulation and/or occurrence or exaggeration of side effects, including ***seizures***, angina, hypertension/hypotension, tachycardia (rates up to 200 beats/min), arrhythmias, nervousness, headache, tremor, muscle cramps, dry mouth, palpitation, nausea, dizziness, fatigue, malaise, insomnia, hypokalemia, hyperglycemia. Also, prolongation of the QTc interval, which can produce ***arrhythmias***. *Treatment:* **Salmeterol:** Discontinue salmeterol. Institute appropriate supportive therapy based on symptoms. Use a cardioselective beta-receptor blocker but such drugs can cause bronchospasm. Cardiac monitoring is recommended.

DRUG INTERACTIONS

Beta-adrenergic blockers / Block pulmonary effects of salmeterol; also may produce severe bronchospasms

Diuretics (loop or thiazide) / ECG change and/or hypokalemia may be worsened

Ketoconazole / ↑ Fluticasone levels R/T inhibition of metabolism by CYP3A4
MAOIs / Action of salmeterol may be potentiated; administer with extreme caution or within 2 weeks of discontinuation of MAOIs
Ritonavir / ↑ Fluticasone levels R/T inhibition of metabolism by CYP3A4
Tricyclic antidepressants / Action of salmeterol may be potentiated; administer with extreme caution or within 2 weeks of discontinuation of TCAs

HOW SUPPLIED

See *Content*.

DOSAGE

INHALATION POWDER (ADVAIR DISKUS)

Asthma, chronic.

Adults and children 12 years and older: 1 inhalation twice daily (morning and evening) about 12 hr apart. **Maximum dose:** One inhalation of fluticasone 500 mcg/salmeterol 50 mcg twice a day. Recommended starting doses depend on clients' current asthma therapy. Clients not currently on inhaled corticosteroid, whose disease severity warrants treatment with two maintenance therapies, including those on non-corticosteroid maintenance therapy, start with Advair Diskus 100/50 twice daily. For clients on inhaled corticosteroid, dosage depends on the steroid being used; consult the package insert as the dosage varies significantly. **Children, 4–11 years of age who are symptomatic on an inhaled steroid:** 1 inhalation of fluticasone 100 mcg/salmeterol 50 mcg Diskus twice daily (morning and evening), approximately 12 hr apart.

COPD associated with chronic bronchitis and/or emphysema.

Adults: 1 inhalation of fluticasone 250 mcg/salmeterol 50 mcg twice daily (morning and evening) about 12 hr apart (maximum dose). The 250 mcg/50 mcg product is the only strength approved for COPD with chronic bronchitis. If shortness of breath occurs in the period between doses, an inhaled short-acting beta-2 agonist (e.g., formoterol) should be taken for immediate relief.

INHALATION AEROSOL (ADVAIR HFA)

Asthma.

Adults and children over 12 years of age: Two inhalations of fluticasone 230 mcg/salmeterol 21 mcg twice a day (morning and evening about 12 hr apart) every day. The starting dose depends on the client's current asthma therapy. See package insert, as dosage varies over a wide range. For those who do not respond adequately to the initial dose after 2 weeks of therapy, replace the current strength of Advair HFA with a higher strength. **Maximum dosage:** Two inhalations of Advair HFA fluticasone 230 mcg/salmeterol 21 mcg twice a day.

FLUTICASONE/SALMETEROL DISKUS OR HFA

Asthma, clients not currently on inhaled corticosteroids.

Diskus: One inhalation of fluticasone/salmeterol Diskus 100 mcg/50 mcg or 250 mcg/50 mcg twice a day. **HFA:** Two inhalations of fluticasone/salmeterol HFA 45 mcg/21 mcg or 115 mcg/21 mcg twice a day.

NURSING IMPLICATIONS

IMPLEMENTATION/ADMINISTRATION/STORAGE

1. Do not use inhaled, long-acting beta-2 agonists in conjunction with Advair Diskus, including for prevention of exercise-induced bronchospasm.
2. Titrate to the lowest effective strength after adequate asthma stability is achieved. The maximum dose is 1 inhalation of fluticasone/salmeterol Diskus 500 mcg/50 mcg twice a day or 2 inhalations of fluticasone/salmeterol HFA 230 mcg/21 mcg twice a day. Higher doses may cause side effects.
3. More frequent administration than twice daily is not recommended. If symptoms arise be-

tween doses, an inhaled, short-acting beta-2 agonist should be used for immediate relief.

4. Improvement in asthma control can occur within 30 min, but maximum benefits may not be reached for 1 week or longer after beginning treatment.
5. For those who do not respond adequately to the initial dose after 2 weeks of therapy, replacing the current strength of Advair Diskus with a higher strength may provide additional asthma control.
6. Those receiving fluticasone/salmeterol twice a day should not use additional salmeterol or other inhaled, long-acting beta-2 agonists (e.g., formoterol) for prevention of exercise-induced bronchospasms or for any other reason.
7. If a previously effective dosage regimen fails to provide adequate asthma control, reevaluate the therapeutic regimen and consider additional therapeutic options, including replacing the current strength with a higher strength, adding additional inhaled corticosteroid, or initiating oral corticosteroids.
8. Do not use fluticasone/salmeterol to transfer clients from systemic corticosteroid therapy.
9. The Diskus inhalation device is not reusable. Discard 1 month after removal from the moisture-protective foil overwrap pouch or after every blister has been used (i.e., when the dosage indicator reads "0").
10. Store the Diskus product from 20–25°C (68–77°F) in a dry place away from direct heat or sunlight. Store the HFA product from 15–30°C (59–86°F); store with the mouthpiece down.

ASSESSMENT

1. List reasons for therapy, characteristics of S&S, clinical presentation, other agents trialed/outcome.
2. Assess/monitor for conditions that may preclude drug therapy; i.e., seizure disorder, glaucoma, TB, osteoporosis, CV disease, uncontrolled HTN, thyroid disorder, infections, or renal/liver disorder.
3. Determine that ECG, CXR, PFTs completed. Note pulmonary and cardiac findings as well as clinical response to therapy.
4. Long-term use of product may increase risk of some eye problems (e.g., cataracts, glaucoma). Salmeterol ingredient may increase the risk of asthma-related death.
5. Monitor VS, lung sounds, peak flow, renal and LFTs.

CLIENT/FAMILY TEACHING

1. Administer Advair Diskus or Advair HFA by the orally inhaled route only. After inhalation, rinse the mouth with water and spit out without swallowing.
2. Follow the enclosed medication guideline to prepare and use the inhaler correctly. Remove inhaler from the foil pouch, and discard the foil pouch and the drying packet that comes inside the pouch.
3. Prime Advair HFA before using for the first time by releasing 4 test sprays into the air, away from the face. Shake well for 5 seconds before each spray. If the inhaler has not been used for more than 4 weeks or when it has been dropped, prime the inhaler again by shaking well before each spray and releasing 2 test sprays into the air, away from the face. Do not use the purple actuator supplied with Advair HFA with any other product canisters; also, do not use actuators from other canisters with the Advair HFA canister.
4. For best results the HFA inhaler should be at room temperature before use. Shake well for 5 seconds before using. Do not spray into the eyes.
5. The correct amount of medication in each inhalation of Advair HFA cannot be ensured after 120 inhalations (i.e., when the counter reads "000"), even though the canister is not completely empty and will continue to operate. Discard the inhaler when 120 actuations have been used and counter reads "000". Contact pharmacy for refill when counter reads "020". Do not alter the numbers or remove the counter from the metal canister.
6. Inhaler improves lung function and makes breathing easier by reducing airway swelling and irritation and by causing muscle relaxation; combination of steroid and bronchodilator. Do not administer with a spacer device.
7. Drug will not treat an asthma attack that has already begun. Not for use with acute breathing problems.
8. Monitor peak flow readings, and identify when to seek additional medical care.
9. Do not give Advair HFA to child under 12 years; it can affect growth in children. Keep

F/U to assess growth rate of child if using this medication.

10. Long-term use of steroids may lead to bone loss (osteoporosis), especially in smokers, if no regular exercise, if vitamin D or calcium deficient in diet, or if family history of osteoporosis.
11. Can lower the blood cells that help your body fight infections. This can make it easier to get sick. Avoid being near people who are sick or have infections. Avoid exposure to chickenpox or measles, and report if exposed.
12. Keep all F/U to assess response and adverse SE.

OUTCOMES/EVALUATE

- Improved breathing patterns and air exchange
- Asthma control
- Control of COPD associated with chronic bronchitis

Fluvastatin sodium

(flu-vah-**STAH**-tin)

Classification(s): Antihyperlipidemic, HMG-CoA reductase inhibitor

Pregnancy Category: X

RX: Lescol, Lescol XL.

SEE ALSO ***ANTIHYPERLIPIDEMIC AGENTS—HMG-COA REDUCTASE INHIBITORS.***

INDICATIONS/USES

1. Hypercholesterolemia (heterozygous familial and nonfamilial) and mixed dyslipidemia. Reduce elevated total and LDL cholesterol, Apo B, and triglyceride levels and to increase HDL cholesterol in clients with primary hypercholesterolemia (heterozygous familial and nonfamilial) and mixed dyslipidemia (Fredrickson types IIa and IIb) whose response to diet and other nondrug measures has been inadequate. The lipid-lowering effects of fluvastatin are enhanced when it is combined with a bile-acid binding resin or with niacin.
2. Heterozygous familial hypercholesterolemia in children. Adjunct to diet to reduce total and LDL cholesterol and Apo B levels in adolescent boys and girls 10 to 16 years of age who are at least 1 year postmenarche, with heterozygous familial hypercholesterolemia whose response to dietary restriction has not been adequate and the following are present: (a) LDL-C remains at 190 mg/dL or more or (b) LDL-C remains at 160 mg/dL or more and there is a positive family history of premature CV disease or 2 or more other CV disease risk factors present.
3. Atherosclerosis. To slow the progression of coronary atherosclerosis in coronary heart disease as part of a treatment plan to lower total and LDL cholesterol to target levels.
4. Secondary prevention of coronary events. Reduce the risk of undergoing coronary revascularization procedures in those with coronary heart disease.

ACTION/KINETICS

Action

Decreases cholesterol, triglycerides, VLDL, and HDL and increases HDL.

Pharmacokinetics

98% absorbed. **Absolute bioavailability:** 24% for immediate-release (IR) and 29% for extended-release (ER). Undergoes extensive first-pass metabolism by CYP2C9. **Time to peak:** <1 hr for IR and 3 hr for ER. Food decreases the rate, but not the extent of absorption; food increases bioavailability by about 50%. Metabolized in the liver by CYP3A4 and CYP2C9 with 90% excreted through the feces and 5% through the urine. **t½:** Less than 3 hr for IR and about 9 hr for ER. Is potential for drug accumulation with hepatic insufficiency. **Plasma protein binding:** More than 98%.

ADDITIONAL CONTRAINDICATIONS

Lactation.

SPECIAL CONCERNS

Use with caution in clients with severe renal impairment, a history of liver disease, or heavy alcohol consumption.

SIDE EFFECTS

Most Common

Diarrhea, headache, dyspepsia, abdominal pain/cramps, N&V, myalgia, arthralgia, flu syndrome, accidental trauma.

GI: N&V, diarrhea, abdominal pain/cramps, flatulence, dyspepsia, tooth disorder, anorexia, ***pancreatitis.*** **Hepatic:** Cholestatic jaundice, cirrhosis, fatty change in liver, ***hepatic necrosis***, hepatitis (including chronic active hepatitis), hepatoma. **Musculoskeletal:** Myalgia, arthralgia, arthritis, arthropathy, myopathy, rhabdomyolysis. **CNS:** Headache, dizziness, insomnia, depression, paresthesia, vertigo, anxiety, alteration of taste, facial paresis, impairment of extraocular movement, memory loss, peripheral nerve palsy, peripheral neuropathy, psychic disturbances, tremor. **Respiratory:** Sinusitis, bronchitis. **GU:** UTI, erectile dysfunction, gynecomastia, loss of libido. **Dermatologic:** Photosensitivity, changes to hair/nails, skin discoloration, dryness of skin/mucous membranes, skin nodules. **Hematologic:** Anemia, leukopenia, thrombocytopenia. **Ophthalmic:** Ophthalmoplegia, lens opacities. **Miscellaneous:** Accidental trauma, flu syndrome, fatigue, allergy/hypersensitivity.

F

LABORATORY TEST CONSIDERATIONS

↑ Serum transaminases, alkaline phosphatase, GGT, CK. Abnormal thyroid function.

ADDITIONAL DRUG INTERACTIONS

Alcohol / ↑ Fluvastatin absorbed
Cholestyramine, colestipol / ↓ Fluvastatin absorption R/T adsorption to cholestyramine/colestipol; give fluvastatin at least 2 hr after cholestyramine/colestipol
Clopidogrel / Possible interference with clopidogrel platelet inhibition
Diclofenac / ↑ Mean diclofenac C_{max} and AUC
Digoxin / ↑ Digoxin C_{max} and slight ↑ digoxin urinary clearance
Glyburide / ↑ Glyburide C_{max}, AUC, and $t^{1/2}$ and ↑ fluvastatin C_{max} and AUC
Histamine H-2 antagonists (e.g., cimetidine, ranitidine) / Significant ↑ in fluvastatin C_{max} and AUC
HMG-CoA Reductase Inhibitors / Concomitant use not recommended
Omeprazole / Significant ↑ in fluvastatin C_{max} and AUC
Phenytoin / ↑ Fluvastatin C_{max} and AUC; minimal ↑ phenytoin C_{max} and AUC
Rifampin / Possible ↓ fluvastatin levels
Warfarin / ↑ INR → ↑ anticoagulant effect

HOW SUPPLIED

Capsules (Lescol): 20 mg (as the sodium salt), 40 mg (as the sodium salt); ***Tablets, Extended-Release (Lescol XL):*** 80 mg (as the sodium salt).

DOSAGE

CAPSULES; TABLETS, EXTENDED-RELEASE

Hypercholesterolemia and mixed dyslipidemia. Antihyperlipidemic to slow progression of coronary atherosclerosis. Secondary prevention of coronary events.

For those requiring LDL cholesterol reduction of 25% or more, **Adults, initial:** 40 mg as one capsule in the evening or 80 mg as one extended-release tablet any time of day. Or, 80 mg in divided doses using the 40 mg capsule twice a day. For those requiring LDL cholesterol reduction of less than 25%, **Adults, initial:** 20 mg. **Dose range:** 20–80 mg/day. **Children:** 1–20 mg capsule. Adjust dosage at 6-week intervals, up to a maximum daily dose of 40 mg capsules twice a day or 1–80 mg extended-release tablet once a day.

Slow progression of coronary atherosclerosis in coronary heart disease.

40 mg twice a day, initiated shortly after a first percutaneous coronary intervention procedure.

NURSING IMPLICATIONS

IMPLEMENTATION/ADMINISTRATION/STORAGE

1. Place on standard cholesterol-lowering diet before receiving fluvastatin; continue diet during therapy.
2. Lipid-lowering effects on total cholesterol and LDL cholesterol are additive when immediate-release fluvastatin is combined with a bile-acid-binding resin or niacin. Maximum reductions of LDL cholesterol are usually seen within 4 weeks; order periodic lipid determinations during this time, with dosage adjusted accordingly.
3. To avoid fluvastatin binding to a bile-acid binding resin (if given together), give the fluvastatin at bedtime and the resin at least 2 hr before.
4. Dosage adjustment is not necessary in clients with mild to moderate impaired renal function. Use doses above 40 mg with caution in clients with severe impaired renal function.

5. Store from 15–30°C (59–86°F). Dispense in tight containers and protect from light.

ASSESSMENT

1. List reasons for therapy, identify coronary risk factors; attempt to change/modify as many as possible. Note lipid profile.
2. Evaluate on a standard cholesterol-lowering diet before giving fluvastatin unless client has CAD with increased risk factors, HTN with microalbuminuria or diabetes. Continue diet during treatment.
3. Monitor cholesterol, triglycerides, and LFTs prior to starting treatment, 6–8 weeks into therapy, 3 months later, then yearly if stable; 12 weeks after a dose increase.

CLIENT/FAMILY TEACHING

1. Used to lower blood cholesterol and fat levels, which have been proven to promote CAD.
2. May be taken with/without food; usually consumed with evening meal. Swallow ER tablet whole; do not cut, chew, or crush tablet.
3. If also taking a bile acid resin (e.g., cholestyramine), take the resin at least 2 hr before fluvastatin.
4. Practice reliable contraception; report if pregnancy suspected or desired.
5. Must continue risk factor reduction, dietary restrictions of saturated fat and cholesterol, and regular daily exercise in addition to drug therapy in the overall goal of lowering cholesterol levels and CHD risk.
6. Report muscle pain or weakness, especially with fever or severe fatigue. Avoid alcohol consumption.
7. Keep all F/U to assess response, labs, adverse SE.

OUTCOMES/EVALUATE

- ↓ Triglycerides, LDL, and total cholesterol levels
- Slow progression of coronary atherosclerosis in coronary heart disease

Fluvoxamine maleate

(flu-**VOX**-ah-meen)

Classification(s): Antidepressant, selective serotonin reuptake inhibitor

Pregnancy Category: C

RX: Luvox, Luvox CR.

✦ **Rx:** Apo-Fluvoxamine, CO Fluvoxamine, PMS-Fluvoxamine, ratio-Fluvoxamine, Sandoz Fluvoxamine.

SEE ALSO ***SELECTIVE SEROTONIN REUPTAKE INHIBITORS***.

INDICATIONS/USES

Capsules, Extended-Release: (1) Treatment of obsessive compulsive disorder, as defined in DSM-IV. (2) Social anxiety disorder, as defined in DSM-IV. **Tablets:** Obsessive-compulsive disorder (as defined in DSM-III-R) for adults, adolescents, and children. *Investigational:* Depression, panic disorder, bulimia nervosa, social phobia, nocturnal enuresis.

ACTION/KINETICS

Action

Highest effect on blocking uptake of serotonin but minimal to no effect on blocking uptake of norepinephrine. Minimal to no anticholinergic or sedative effects; no orthostatic hypotension.

Pharmacokinetics

About 53% is bioavailable. **Maximum plasma levels:** 3–8 hr. **$t^{1/2}$:** 15.6 hr. **Peak plasma concentration:** 88–546 ng/mL. **Time to reach steady state:** About 7 days. Elderly clients manifest higher mean plasma levels and a decreased clearance. Metabolized in the liver and about 94% excreted through the urine. The extended-release capsule is designed to minimize peak-to-trough fluctuations in plasma levels over a 24 hr period. **Plasma protein binding:** About 80%.

ADDITIONAL CONTRAINDICATIONS

Alcohol ingestion. Use with alosetron, pimozide, thioridazine, or tizanidine.

SPECIAL CONCERNS

Suicidality in children and adolescent. Antidepressants increased the risk of suicidal thinking and behavior (suicidality) in short-term studies in children, adolescents, and young adults with major depressive disorder and other psychiatric disorders. Anyone considering the use of fluvoxamine or any other antidepressant in a child, adolescent, or young adult must balance this risk with the clinical need. Short-term studies did not show an increase in the risk of suicidality with antidepressants compared with placebo in adults older than 24 years of age; there was a reduction in risk with antidepressants compared with placebo in adults 65 years of age and older. Depression and certain other psychiatric disorders are themselves associated with increases in the risk of suicide. Closely observe clients of all ages who are started on therapy for clinical worsening, suicidality, or unusual changes in behavior. Advise families and caregivers of the need for close observation and communication with the prescriber. Fluvoxamine tablets are not approved for use in children, except for clients with OCD. Fluvoxamine extended-release capsules are not approved for use in children.

- **Use with caution in clients with a history of mania, seizure disorders, and liver dysfunction and in those with diseases that could affect hemodynamic responses or metabolism.**
- **Treatment of pregnant women late in the third trimester may result in the neonate having complications requiring prolonged hospitalization, respiratory support, and tube feeding.**

SIDE EFFECTS

Most Common

Nausea, insomnia, somnolence, headache, nervousness, asthenia, dizziness, diarrhea/loose stools, dyspepsia, dry mouth, constipation, URTI.

Side effects listed occur at an incidence of 0.1% or greater. **CNS**: Somnolence, insomnia, nervousness, dizziness, tremor, anxiety, hypertonia, agitation, decreased libido, depression, CNS stimulation, amnesia, apathy, hyperkinesia, hypokinesia, manic reaction, myoclonus, psychoses, fatigue, malaise, agoraphobia, akathisia, ataxia, ***convulsion***, delirium, delusion, depersonalization, drug dependence, dyskinesia, dystonia, emotional lability, euphoria, extrapyramidal syndrome, unsteady gait, hallucinations, hemiplegia, hostility, hypersomnia, hypochondriasis, hypotonia, hysteria, incoordination, increased libido, neuralgia, paralysis, paranoia, phobia, sleep disorders, stupor, twitching, vertigo, activation of mania/hypomania, seizures. **GI**: Nausea, dry mouth, diarrhea/loose stools, constipation, dyspepsia, anorexia, vomiting, flatulence, toothache, tooth caries, dysphagia, colitis, eructation, esophagitis, gastritis, gastroenteritis, ***GI hemorrhage***, GI ulcer, gingivitis, glossitis, hemorrhoids, melena, ***rectal hemorrhage***, stomatitis. **CV**: Palpitations, hypertension, postural hypotension, vasodilation, syncope, tachycardia, angina pectoris, bradycardia, ***cardiomyopathy***, CV disease, cold extremities, conduction delay, ***heart failure, MI***, pallor, irregular pulse, ST segment changes. **Respiratory**: URTI, dyspnea, yawn, increased cough, sinusitis, asthma, bronchitis, epistaxis, hoarseness, hyperventilation. **Body as a whole**: Headache, asthenia, flu syndrome, chills, malaise, edema, weight gain or loss, dehydration, hypercholesterolemia, allergic reaction, neck pain, neck rigidity, photosensitivity, ***suicide attempt***. **Dermatologic**: Excessive sweating, acne, alopecia, dry skin, eczema, exfoliative dermatitis, furunculosis, seborrhea, skin discoloration, urticaria. **Musculoskeletal**: Arthralgia, arthritis, bursitis, generalized muscle spasm, myasthenia, tendinous contracture, tenosynovitis. **GU**: Delayed ejaculation, urinary frequency, impotence, anorgasmia, urinary retention, anuria, breast pain, cystitis, delayed menstruation, dysuria, female lactation, hematuria, menopause, menorrhagia, metrorrhagia, nocturia, polyuria, PMS, urinary incontinence, UTI, urinary urgency, impaired urination, ***vaginal hemorrhage***, vaginitis. **Hematologic**: Anemia, ecchymosis, leukocytosis, lymphadenopathy, thrombocytopenia. **Ophthalmic**: Amblyopia, abnormal accommodation, conjunctivitis, diplopia, dry eyes, eye pain, mydriasis, photophobia, visual field defect. **Otic**: Deafness, ear pain, otitis media. **Miscellaneous**: Taste perversion or loss, parosmia, hypothyroidism, hypercholesterolemia, dehydration.

OVERDOSE MANAGEMENT

Treatment: Establish an airway and maintain respiration as needed. Monitor VS and ECG. Activated charcoal may be as effective as emesis or lavage in removing drug from the GI tract. Since absorption in overdose may be delayed, measures to reduce absorption may be required for up to 24 hr.

ADDITIONAL DRUG INTERACTIONS

Beta-adrenergic blockers / Possible ↑ effects on BP and HR
Buspirone / ↓ Buspirone effects
Carbamazepine / ↑ Risk of carbamazepine toxicity
Clozapine / ↑ Risk of orthostatic hypotension and seizures
Diazepam / ↑ Diazepam effect R/T ↓ clearance
Diltiazem / ↑ Risk of bradycardia

Grapefruit juice / ↑ Fluvoxamine mean AUC and C_{max}
Haloperidol / ↑ Haloperidol levels
Lansoprazole / ↑ Lansoprazole AUC and prolongation of t½ in homozygous and heterozygeous extensive metabolizers R/T inhibition of CYP2C19 metabolism
Lidocaine (IV) / ↓ Lidocaine elimination R/T inhibition of metabolism by CYP1A2; adding erythromycin further ↓ lidocaine elimination R/T inhibition of metabolism by CYP3A4
Lithium / ↑ Risk of seizures
MAO inhibitors / Possible hypertensive crisis; do not take MAOIs within 2 weeks of stopping fluvoxamine and fluvoxamine within 2 weeks of stopping MAOIs
H ***Melatonin*** / ↑ Plasma melatonin levels
Methadone / ↑ Risk of methadone toxicity
Mexiletine / ↓ Mexiletine clearance R/T ↓ metabolism
Midazolam / ↑ Midazolam effect R/T ↓ clearance
Nitroprusside / ↑ Nitroprusside-induced venodilation
Olanzapine / ↑ Olanzapine levels R/T ↓ liver metabolism
Sildenafil / ↑ Sildenafil exposure and t½
Smoking / ↓ Fluvoxamine plasma levels R/T ↑ metabolism by CYP1A2; smokers may need to ↑ dose
Sumatriptan / ↑ Risk of weakness, hyperreflexia, incoordination
Theophylline / ↑ Risk of theophylline toxicity (decrease dose by one-third the usual daily maintenance dose)
Thioridazine / ↑ Thioridazine levels
Tizanidine / ↑ Tizanidine intensity and duration of effects R/T ↓ metabolism by CYP1A2 enzymes
Tolbutamide / ↓ Tolbutamide clearance R/T ↓ metabolism
Triazolam / ↑ Triazolam effect R/T ↓ clearance

HOW SUPPLIED

Capsules, Extended-Release: 100 mg, 150 mg; ***Tablets:*** 25 mg, 50 mg, 100 mg.

DOSAGE

CAPSULES, EXTENDED-RELEASE

Obsessive-compulsive disorder; social anxiety disorder.

Adults, initial: 100 mg as a single dose before bedtime. Titrate in 50 mg increments every week until a maximum therapeutic effect has been reached, but not to exceed 300 mg/day. In geriatric clients and in those with impaired hepatic function, titrate slowly following the initial 100 mg dose. Social anxiety disorder and OCD are chronic conditions; thus, it is reasonable to continue therapy for those clients responding to the drug. Adjust the dosage to maintain the client on the lowest effective dosage; periodically reassess to determine the need for continued treatment.

TABLETS

Obsessive-compulsive disorder.

Adults, initial: 50 mg as a single daily dose at bedtime; **then,** increase the dose in 50 mg increments q 4–7 days, as tolerated, until a maximum benefit is reached, not to exceed 300 mg/day. Give total daily doses greater than 100 mg in 2 divided doses; if doses are unequal, give the larger dose at bedtime. **Children and adolescents, 8 to 17 years, initial:** 25 mg as a single daily dose at bedtime; **then,** increase the dose in 25 mg increments q 4–7 days until a maximum benefit is reached, not to exceed 200 mg/day up to 11 years of age and 300 mg/day up to 17 years of age. Divide total daily doses more than 50 mg into 2 doses; if the 2 divided doses are not equal, give the larger dose at bedtime. The therapeutic effect may be reached in female children with lower doses. **Maintenance:** Although efficacy has not been documented beyond 10 weeks, consider continuation in a responding client since OCD is a chronic condition. Adjust dose to maintain the lowest effective dosage; periodically reassess to determine need for continued treatment.

NURSING IMPLICATIONS

Do not confuse fluoxetine (another SSRI) with fluvoxamine.

IMPLEMENTATION/ADMINISTRATION/STORAGE

1. If total daily dose exceeds 100 mg for adults or 50 mg in children, give in two divided

doses. If the doses are unequal, give the larger dose at bedtime.
2. Initial and incremental doses may need to be lower in geriatric clients and in those with impaired hepatic function.
3. Consider the potential risks and benefits of treating pregnant women during the third trimester with fluvoxamine. Neonates exposed to fluvoxamine late in the third trimester have developed complications requiring prolonged hospitalization, respiratory support, and tube feeding.
4. At least 14 days should elapse between discontinuation of an MAOI and beginning fluvoxamine extended-release capsules. Similarly, at least 14 days should elapse after stopping fluvoxamine extended-release capsules and beginning an MAOI.
5. If terminating therapy, a gradual reduction in dosage should be considered rather than abrupt cessation of the drug.
6. Store extended-release capsules and tablets from 15–30°C (59–86°F); protect from high humidity. Avoid exposure to temperatures above 30°C (86°F).

ASSESSMENT

1. Note reasons for therapy, presenting/reported behavioral manifestations, other agents trialed, outcome.
2. List agents currently prescribed to ensure none interact.
3. Note history of mania, seizure disorders, liver dysfunction.
4. Monitor ECG, CBC, renal and LFTs; reduce dose with dysfunction.

CLIENT/FAMILY TEACHING

1. Take only as directed, usually at bedtime, do not exceed dosage. May initially experience N&V; should subside.
2. May cause dizziness and drowsiness. Do not perform activities that require mental or physical alertness until drug effects realized.
3. Report any rash, hives, or unusual itching or bleeding; increased agitation/irritability or depression, unusual behavioral changes, or suicide ideations.
4. Avoid alcohol and other drugs or herbals without approval. Smoking may reduce drug effectiveness.
5. Practice reliable birth control.
6. Keep all F/U to assess response, dosage/need to continue therapy, adverse SE.

OUTCOMES/EVALUATE

- Reduction in excessive, repetitive behaviors
- ↓ Depression; ↓ social anxiety

IV ©

Folic acid

(**FOH**-lik **AH**-sid)

Classification(s): Vitamin B complex
Pregnancy Category: A
RX: Deplin, Folvite.
🍁 **Rx:** Apo-Folic.

INDICATIONS/USES

Treatment of megaloblastic anemias due to folic acid deficiency (e.g., tropical and nontropical sprue, pregnancy, infancy or childhood, nutritional causes). Diagnosis of folate deficiency.

ACTION/KINETICS

Action

Folic acid (which is converted to tetrahydrofolic acid) is necessary for normal production of RBCs and for synthesis of nucleoproteins. Tetrahydrofolic acid is a cofactor in the biosynthesis of purines and thymidylates of nucleic acids. Megaloblastic and macrocytic anemias in folic acid deficiency are believed to be due to impairment of thymidylate synthesis. Natural sources of folic acid include liver, dried beans, peas, lentils, whole-wheat products, asparagus, beets, broccoli, brussels sprouts, spinach, and oranges.

Pharmacokinetics

Synthetic folic acid is absorbed from the GI tract even if the client suffers from malabsorption syndrome. **Peak plasma levels after an oral dose:** 1 hr. It is stored in the liver.

CONTRAINDICATIONS

Use in aplastic, normocytic, or pernicious anemias (is ineffective). Folic acid injection that contains benzyl alcohol should not be used in neonates or immature infants.

SPECIAL CONCERNS

- **Folic acid doses of 0.1 mg/day or greater may obscure pernicious anemia.**

- **Prolonged folic acid therapy may cause decreased vitamin B_{12} levels.**

SIDE EFFECTS

Most Common

Folic acid is relatively nontoxic in humans.

Allergic: Skin rash, itching, erythema, general malaise, respiratory difficulty due to ***bronchospasm.*** **GI:** Nausea, anorexia, abdominal distention, flatulence, bitter or bad taste (in those taking 15 mg/day for 1 month). **CNS:** In doses of 15 mg daily, altered sleep patterns, irritability, excitement, difficulty in concentration, overactivity, depression, impaired judgment, confusion.

DRUG INTERACTIONS

Aminosalicylic acid / ↓ Serum folate levels
Corticosteroids (chronic use) / ↑ Folic acid requirements
Methotrexate / Folic acid antagonist
Oral contraceptives / ↑ Risk of folate deficiency
Phenytoin / ↑ Seizure frequency; ↓ folic acid levels
Pyrimethamine / ↓ Pyrimethamine effect in toxoplasmosis; also, a folic acid antagonist
Sulfonamides / ↓ Absorption of folic acid
Triamterene / ↓ Utilization of folic acid; folic acid antagonist
Trimethoprim / ↓ Utilization of folic acid; folic acid antagonist

HOW SUPPLIED

Injection: 5,000 mcg/mL; *Tablets:* 400 mcg, 800 mcg, 1,000 mcg; 7.5 mg (as L-methylfolate).

DOSAGE

DEEP SC; IM; IV

Treatment of deficiency.

Adults and children: 250–1,000 mcg/day until a hematologic response occurs.

Diagnosis of folate deficiency.

Adults, IM: 100–200 mcg/day for 10 days plus low dietary folic acid and vitamin B_{12}.

TABLETS

Dietary supplement.

Adults and children: 100 mcg/day (up to 1 mg in pregnancy); may be increased to 500–1,000 mcg if requirements increase.

Treatment of deficiency.

Adults, initial: 250–1,000 mcg/day until a hematologic response occurs; **maintenance:** 400 mcg/day (800 mcg during pregnancy and lactation). **Pediatric, initial:** 250–1,000 mcg/day until a hematologic response occurs. **Maintenance, infants:** 100 mcg/day; **children up to 4 years:** 300 mcg/day; **children 4 years and older:** 400 mcg/day.

NURSING IMPLICATIONS

Do not confuse folic acid with folinic acid (leucovorin calcium).

IMPLEMENTATION/ADMINISTRATION/STORAGE

1. Given PO; if there is severe malabsorption, give either IV or SC.
2. Regardless of age, dosage should never be less than 0.1 mg/day.
3. IV Folic acid will remain stable in solution if the pH is kept above 5.
4. May be administered IM, by direct IV push or added to infusions. When given IV, do not exceed 5 mcg/min.
5. When parenteral forms are used, have drugs and equipment available to treat anaphylactic reactions.
6. COMPATIBILITY Dextrose or 0.9% NaCl; may add to TPN solution.
7. INCOMPATIBILITY Administer separately.

ASSESSMENT

1. Note reasons for therapy, other agents trialed, and outcome.
2. Review drugs prescribed; oral contraceptives, trimethoprim, hydantoins, and alcohol may cause increased body loss of folic acid.
3. Monitor CBC, reticulocytes, MCV, serum folate and B_{12} levels. Assess for pernicious anemia with Shilling test; serum B_{12} levels to prevent permanent neurologic damage.

CLIENT/FAMILY TEACHING

1. Take only as directed. Avoid alcohol.
2. Dietary sources of folic acid include dark green leafy vegetables, beans, fortified breads, and cereals. Prolonged cooking destroys folate in vegetables.
3. Drug may discolor urine a deep yellow.
4. U.S. Public Health Service recommends that all women of childbearing age consume

0.4 mg of folic acid to reduce the risk of neural tube birth defects. Folic acid may prevent the development of spinal canal or brain defects, which occur during the first month of pregnancy.

5. Keep all F/U to assess response, labs, adverse SE.

OUTCOMES/EVALUATE

- Desired hematologic response (↑ retic count in 5 days)
- Reversal of symptoms of folic acid deficiency and megaloblastic anemia
- Prophylaxis of newborn neural tube defects

F

Fondaparinux sodium

(**fon**-dah-**PAIR**-in-uks)

Classification(s): Anticoagulant, antithrombin
Pregnancy Category: B

RX: Arixtra.

INDICATIONS/USES

(1) Prophylaxis of deep vein thrombosis, which may lead to pulmonary embolism, in clients undergoing hip fracture surgery (including extended prophylaxis), hip replacement surgery, knee replacement surgery, or abdominal surgery in those at risk for thromboembolic complications. May be used for up to 60 days in clients undergoing hip fracture surgery. (2) With warfarin to treat acute DVT. (3) With warfarin to treat acute pulmonary embolism when initial therapy is started in the hospital.

ACTION/KINETICS

Action

Antithrombotic action is due to antithrombin III (ATIII)-mediated selective inhibition of Factor Xa. By selectively binding to ATIII, fondaparinux potentiates the innate neutralization of Factor Xa by ATIII. Neutralization of Factor Xa interrupts the blood coagulation cascade and thus inhibits thrombin formation and thrombus development. Does not inactivate thrombin (activated Factor II), has no known effect on platelet function, and does not affect fibrinolytic activity or bleeding time.

Pharmacokinetics

Rapidly and completely absorbed following SC administration; 100% bioavailable. **Maximum levels:** 2 hr. Excreted unchanged in the urine. **t½, elimination:** 17–21 hr. Elimination is prolonged in the elderly, in those with renal impairment, and in those weighing less than 50 kg. Anticoagulant effect may last for 2–4 days after discontinuation in clients with normal renal function and even longer in those with renal impairment. **Plasma protein binding:** Does not significantly bind to plasma proteins or RBCs.

CONTRAINDICATIONS

IM use. In those with severe renal impairment (C_{CR} <30 mL/min) or with body weight <50 kg needing prophylactic therapy and undergoing hip-fracture or knee-replacement surgery (due to increased risk for major bleeding episodes). In those with active major bleeding, bacterial endocarditis, thrombocytopenia associated with a positive in vitro test for antiplatelet antibody in the presence of fondaparinux, or with known sensitivity to fondaparinux.

SPECIAL CONCERNS

(1) When epidural/spinal anesthesia is used, clients anticoagulated or scheduled to be anticoagulated with low molecular weight heparins, heparinoids, or fondaparinux for prevention of thromboembolic complications are at risk of developing an epidural or spinal hematoma that can cause long-term or permanent paralysis. The risk of such events is increased by the use of indwelling epidural catheters for administration of analgesia or by the concomitant use of drugs affecting hemostasis, such as NSAIDs, platelet inhibitors, or other anticoagulants. The risk also seems to be increased by traumatic or repeated epidural or spinal puncture. (2) Frequently monitor clients for signs and symptoms of neurologic impairment. If neurologic compromise is noted, urgent treatment is necessary.
(3) Consider the potential benefit vs risk before neuraxial intervention in clients anticoagulated or to be anticoagulated for thromboprophylaxis. (4) Fondaparinux, like other anticoagulants should be used with extreme caution in conditions with increased risk of hemorrhage, such as congenital or acquired bleeding disorders, active ulcerative and an-

giodysplastic GI disease, hemorrhagic stroke, or shortly after brain, spinal, or ophthalmological surgery, or in those treated concomitantly with platelet inhibitors.

- **The risk of hemorrhage increases with increasing renal impairment.**
- **Use with caution during lactation, in moderate renal impairment (C_{CR} 30–50 mL/min), in the elderly, in those with a history of heparin-induced thrombocytopenia, in those with a bleeding diathesis, uncontrolled arterial hypertension, history of recent GI ulceration, diabetic retinopathy, and hemorrhage.**
- **Use with extreme caution in conditions with increased risk of hemorrhage, including congenital or acquired bleeding disorders, active ulcerative and angiodysplastic GI disease, hemorrhagic stroke, in those treated concomitantly with platelet inhibitors, or shortly after brain, spinal, or ophthalmologic surgery.**
- **Safety and efficacy not determined in children.**

SIDE EFFECTS

Most Common

Bleeding complications (see below), hypotension, confusion, dizziness, insomnia, constipation, headache, N&V, UTI, anemia, purpura, rash, edema, fever.

The most common side effect is ***bleeding complications (hemorrhage)***, which include intracranial, cerebral, retroperitoneal, intra-ocular, pericardial, or spinal bleeding, bleeding in the adrenal gland, or reoperation due to bleeding. **CV:** Edema, hypotension. **GI:** N&V, constipation, diarrhea, dyspepsia, abdominal pain. **CNS:** Insomnia, dizziness, confusion, headache, anxiety. **GU:** UTI, urinary retention. **Dermatologic:** Rash, bullous eruption, pruritus, bruising. **Respiratory:** Coughing, epistaxis. **Hematologic:** Anemia, hematoma, purpura, ***postoperative hemorrhage***. **Miscellaneous:** Thrombocytopenia, injection site bleeding, anemia, fever, increased wound drainage, pain, back/chest/leg pain, abnormal hepatic function.

LABORATORY TEST CONSIDERATIONS

↑ AST, ALT, hepatic enzymes. ↓ Prothrombin. Hypokalemia.

OVERDOSE MANAGEMENT

Symptoms: Hemorrhagic complications. *Treatment:* Discontinue treatment. There is no known antidote. Initiate appropriate therapy. Clearance can increase by 20% during hemodialysis.

DRUG INTERACTIONS

Increased risk of hemorrhage if used with agents that enhance the risk of hemorrhage; discontinue such agents or if coadministration is essential, monitor closely.

HOW SUPPLIED

Injection: 2.5 mg/0.5 mL, 5 mg/0.4 mL, 7.5 mg/0.6 mL, 10 mg/0.8 mL (all in prefilled syringes).

DOSAGE

SC

Prophylaxis of deep vein thrombosis (DVT) in hip fracture, hip or knee replacement surgery.

Adults, initial: 2.5 mg given 6–8 hr after surgery. Administration before 6 hr after surgery has been associated with an increased risk of major bleeding. **Duration:** Give 2.5 mg once daily for 5–9 days (up to 11 days has been tolerated).

Treatment of acute DVT without pulmonary embolism; acute pulmonary embolism.

Adults: 5 mg/day for clients weighing less than 50 kg, 7.5 mg for those weighing 50–100 kg, and 10 mg for those over 100 kg. Continue therapy for at least 5 days and until an INR of 2.0–3.0 is achieved with warfarin sodium.

Abdominal surgery in those at risk for thromboembolic complications.

Adults: 2.5 mg once daily for 5–9 days, with the first dose given 6–8 hr after surgery, once hemostasis has been established. Can be given for up to 10 days.

NURSING IMPLICATIONS

IMPLEMENTATION/ADMINISTRATION/STORAGE

1. **Stop therapy if major bleeding occurs or coagulation indicators change unexpectedly.**
2. **Drug provided in single dose, prefilled syringe affixed with an automatic needle protection system.**
3. **Cannot be used interchangeably (unit for unit) with heparin, low molecular weight heparins,**

or heparinoids; products differ in manufacturing process, anti-Xa and anti-IIa activity, units, and dosage.
4. To avoid loss of drug with the prefilled syringe, do not expel the air bubble from the syringe before injection.
5. Do not mix with other injections or infusions.
6. Give in the fatty tissue, alternating injection sites (i.e., between the left and right anterolateral, or the left and right posterolateral abdominal walls).
7. Store between 15–30°C (59–86°F). Keep out of the reach of children.

F

ASSESSMENT

1. Note condition(s) requiring therapy, onset, estimated duration of therapy. Give initial dose SC 6–8 hr after surgery and then once every 24 hr. When used to treat acute pulmonary embolus or DVT, ensure correct body weight.
2. Assess for conditions that may affect therapy (i.e. age, weight, history of GI ulcerations, diabetic retinopathy, uncontrolled HTN, bleeding diathesis/disorders, hemorrhage, hemorrhagic stroke, or shortly after brain, spinal or eye surgery or in those treated concomitantly with platelet inhibitors). Risk of hemorrhage increases with increasing renal impairment or heparin-induced thrombocytopenia.
3. Do not use interchangeably with heparin, low molecular weight heparins, or heparinoids.
4. Monitor all sites, incisions, orifices for bleeding. Assess mobility and adherence to exercise program.
5. Assess carefully for S&S of neurologic impairment (e.g., midline back pain, numbness or weakness in lower extremities, bowel and/or bladder dysfunction); anticoagulated clients undergoing epidural/spinal anesthesia may sustain a spinal/epidural hematoma that could result in paralysis. Risk increased with postoperative use of indwelling epidural catheters, or concomitant use of other drugs affecting hemostasis such as NSAIDs.
6. The anti-factor Xa activity of fondaparinux can be measured by anti-Xa assay using fondaparinux as the calibrator.
7. Monitor CBC, creatinine, K^+, renal and LFTs, and stool for occult blood.

CLIENT/FAMILY TEACHING

1. Drug is used to prevent the formation of blood clots in those extremities that have compromised functioning due to a surgical procedure. Clots may enter the circulation and be transported to the lung, causing a pulmonary embolus that can be lethal.
2. Review guidelines for SC administration, and demonstrate. Start with proper skin prep, pinching and holding a fold of skin for the injection, injecting the solution, removing the syringe, and discarding into a designated container. The syringe has a retractable needle to prevent punctures. Rotate sites to prevent hardening of the tissues between the right and left anterolateral/posterolateral abdominal wall.
3. Store prefilled syringes and used syringes safely out of reach, and dispose of properly.
4. Report adverse effects as well as extremity pain, chest pain, SOB, S&S bleeding (e.g., black, tarry stools, blood in the urine, dizziness when standing, excessive bruising, nosebleed, paleness).
5. Avoid OTC agents including aspirin, NSAIDs, and other agents without provider approval.
6. Keep all F/U to assess response, labs, adverse SE.

OUTCOMES/EVALUATE

DVT (blood clot) prevention in those undergoing hip fracture repair, hip/knee replacements, or abdominal surgery where mobility is impaired

Formoterol fumarate

(for-**MOH**-tur-all)

Classification(s): Sympathomimetic, direct-acting

Pregnancy Category: C

RX: Foradil Aerolizer, Perforomist.

SEE ALSO ***SYMPATHOMIMETICS.***

INDICATIONS/USES

Inhalation Powder in Capsules only: (1) Long-term, twice-daily (morning and evening) maintenance treatment of asthma and to prevent bronchospasms in adults and children 5 years of age and older who have reversible obstructive airway disease, including nocturnal asthma, who require regular treatment with inhaled, short-acting, beta-2-agonists. Not to be used in those whose asthma can be managed successfully by inhaled corticoste-

roids or other medications along with occasional use of inhaled, short-acting beta-2-agonists.
(2) Acute prevention of exercise-induced bronchospasm in adults and children, 5 years and older, when given on an occasional, as needed, basis.

Inhalation Powder or Inhalation Solution: Long-term, twice-daily (morning and evening) use in the maintenance treatment of bronchoconstriction in those with COPD, including chronic bronchitis and emphysema.

ACTION/KINETICS

Action

Long-acting selective beta-2-agonist. Acts locally in the lung as a bronchodilator. Acts in part by increasing cyclic AMP levels causing relaxation of bronchial smooth muscle and inhibition of release of mediators of immediate hypersensitivity, especially from mast cells.

Pharmacokinetics

When inhaled, is rapidly absorbed into the plasma reaching maximum plasma levels within 5 min and onset of action within 12 min. **Duration:** 12 hr. Metabolized in the liver to inactive metabolites. Excreted in the urine and feces. **t½, terminal:** 10 hr. **Plasma protein binding:** 61–64%.

CONTRAINDICATIONS

Use for those whose asthma can be controlled by occasional use of inhaled, short-acting, beta-2-agonists. Use to treat acute symptoms of asthma or COPD. Use with asthma without use of a long-term asthma control medication.

SPECIAL CONCERNS

(1) Long-acting beta-2-adrenergic agonists may increase the risk of asthma-related death. All long-acting beta-2-agonists are contraindicated in clients with asthma without the use of a long-term asthma control medication. Currently available data are inadequate to determine whether current use of inhaled corticosteroids or other long-term asthma control drugs mitigates the increased risk of asthma-related death from long-acting beta-2-agonists. (2) Once asthma control is achieved and maintained, assess the client at regular intervals and step-down therapy (e.g., discontinue long-acting beta-2-agonist) if possible without loss of asthma control and maintain the client on a long-term asthma control medication, such as an inhaled corticosteroid. Do not use long-acting beta-2-agonists for clients whose asthma is adequately controlled on low- or medium-dose inhaled corticosteroids. (3) **Children and adolescents.** Available data from controlled clinical trials suggest that long-acting beta-2-agonists increase the risk of asthma-related hospitalizations in children and adolescents. For children and adolescents with asthma who require addition of a long-acting beta-2-agonist to an inhaled corticosteroid, a fixed-dose combination product containing both an inhaled corticosteroid and a long-acting beta-2-agonist should ordinarily be used to ensure adherence with both drugs. In cases where use of a separate long-term asthma control medication (e.g., inhaled corticosteroid) and a long-acting beta-2-agonist is clinically indicated, appropriate steps must be taken to ensure adherence with both treatment components. If adherence cannot be ensured, a fixed-dose combination product containing both an inhaled corticosteroid and a long-acting beta-2-agonist is recommended.

- May cause life-threatening, paradoxical bronchospasms.
- Use with extreme caution in clients treated with MAOIs, tricyclic antidepressants, or drugs known to prolong the QTc interval (effect of adrenergic agonists may be prolonged).
- Use with caution during the coadministration of beta-2-agonists with nonpotassium-sparing diuretics (loop or thiazide diuretics) since ECG changes and/or hypokalemia can be acutely worsened by beta-agonists.
- Use with caution in CV disorders (especially coronary insufficiency, ischemic heart disease, coronary artery disease, CHF, cardiac arrhythmias, and hypertension), in convulsive disorders, in thyrotoxicosis, in those unusually responsive to sympathomimetics, and during lactation.
- Safety and efficacy of the inhalation powder not established in children less than 5 years of age; the inhalation solution is not for use in children.

SIDE EFFECTS

Most Common

Viral infection, bronchitis, chest infection/pain, dyspnea, tremor, dizziness, dry mouth, insomnia. See also *Sympathomimetics* for a complete list of possible side effects. Also, **CV:** Hypertension, chest tightness/pain/discomfort, angina, palpitations, PVCs, arrhythmias, skipped beats, tachycardia. Increased pulse rate and BP, hypertension, ECG changes (e.g., flattening of T wave, prolongation of QTc interval, and ST segment depression). **GI:** Dry mouth, diarrhea, N&V. **CNS:** Dizziness, vertigo, insomnia, tremor, headache, shakiness, nervousness, tension, anxiety. **Musculoskeletal:** Back pain, leg/muscle cramps, back pain. **Respiratory:** Worsening of asthma (can be fatal), throat dryness/irritation, pharyngitis, sinusitis, dyspnea, URTI, bronchitis, nasopharyngitis, chest infection, tonsillitis, dysphonia, increased sputum. **Dermatologic:** Pruritus, rash. **Hypersensitivity:** Immediate hypersensitivity reactions, including severe hypotension, rash, urticaria, bronchospasm, ***anaphylaxis***, and angioedema. **Body as a whole:** Viral infection, fever, fatigue, malaise. **Miscellaneous:** Metabolic acidosis.

F

LABORATORY TEST CONSIDERATIONS

Hypokalemia (transient and usually does not require supplementation). Hyperglycemia.

DRUG INTERACTIONS

See also ***Drug Interactions*** for Sympathomimetics. An additive effect of formoterol with other drugs that prolong the QT interval cannot be excluded. The following drugs may prolong the QT interval and increase the risk of life-threatening cardiac arrhythmias, including torsades de pointes: Amiodarone, arsenic trioxide, bretylium, chlorpromazine, cisapride, disopyramide, dofetilide, dolasetron, droperidol, mefloquine, mesoridazine, moxifloxacin, pentamidine, pimozide, procainamide, quinidine, sotalol, tacrolimus, thioridazine, and ziprasidone.

HOW SUPPLIED

Foradil: Powder in Capsules for use in Aerolizer: 12 mcg; ***Perforomist: Inhalation Solution:*** 20 mcg/2 mL.

DOSAGE

Foradil Aerolizer

CAPSULES FOR USE IN AEROLIZER

Maintenance treatment of asthma and to prevent bronchospasm.

Adults and children over 5 years: Inhale contents of one 12 mcg capsule q 12 hr (morning and evening) using the Aerolizer inhaler. Do not exceed 24 mcg/day. If symptoms appear between doses, use an inhaled short-acting beta-2-agonist for immediate relief.

Prevention of exercise-induced bronchospasm.

Adults and children 5 years and older: Inhale contents of one 12 mcg capsule, using the inhaler provided, at least 15 min before exercise. Give on an occasional, as needed, basis. When used intermittently for prevention, protection may last up to 12 hr; do not use additional doses for 12 hr. *NOTE:* Only use the inhalation powder.

Maintenance treatment of chronic obstructive pulmonary disease (COPD).

Adults: Inhale contents of one 12 mcg capsule of the inhalation powder q 12 hr (morning and evening) using the Aerolizer inhaler provided. Do not exceed 24 mcg/day.

Perforomist Inhalation Solution

INHALATION SOLUTION

Maintenance treatment of COPD, including chronic bronchitis and emphysema.

Adults: 20 mcg given twice daily (morning and evening) by nebulization, not to exceed 40 mcg/day.

NURSING IMPLICATIONS

IMPLEMENTATION/ADMINISTRATION/STORAGE

1. Use only with Aerolizer inhaler provided; do not take the inhalation powder orally.
2. Use the inhalation solution with a standard jet nebulizer connected to an air compressor (e.g., Pari–LC Plus nebulizer with a face mask, mouthpiece, or the Proneb Ultra compressor).
3. Can be used together with short-acting beta-2-agonists, inhaled or systemic corticosteroids, and theophylline.
4. If asthma symptoms arise between doses, an inhaled short-acting, beta-2-agonist may be used for immediate relief.
5. If a previously used dose for asthma or COPD does not result in the usual response, seek medical advice immediately; this is often a sign of deteriorating asthma or COPD. Reevaluate therapeutic regimen and consider additional options such as systemic corticosteroids.

6. If taking formoterol in twice-daily doses for asthma, do not take additional doses for exercise-induced bronchospasms.
7. A satisfactory response to formoterol does not eliminate the need for continued treatment with an anti-inflammatory drug.
8. Do not start formoterol therapy in clients with significantly worsening or acutely deteriorating asthma, which may be a life-threatening condition.
9. Formoterol is not a substitute for inhaled or oral corticosteroids.
10. When starting formoterol therapy, instruct clients who have been taking inhaled, short-acting beta-2-agonists on a regular basis (4 times per day) to discontinue the regular use of these drugs, and use only for symptomatic relief of acute asthma symptoms.
11. Do not swallow orally. Store in the blister, and remove immediately before use.
12. Before dispensing, store at 2–8°C (36–46°F). After dispensing, store at 2–25°C (36–77°F). Protect from heat and moisture.

ASSESSMENT

1. List reasons for therapy, symptom characteristics, PFT results, other agents trialed/failed, outcome.
2. Assess for CAD, arrhythmias, heart failure, and HTN.
3. Used only as additional therapy (asthma) in those who are currently taking but are inadequately controlled on a long-term asthma control medication. Once symptoms are controlled, regularly assess client, and step down formoterol therapy as symptoms permit.
4. Document lung sounds, sputum production/characteristics, BP and HR, PFTs, CXR.
5. Monitor VS, serum K^+, and glucose.

CLIENT/FAMILY TEACHING

1. Use only as directed; do not take orally. Not to be used as the only therapy for the treatment of asthma; only used as additional therapy. Demonstrate appropriate method for administration and storage. Review *Patient Use Instructions.*
2. Use the capsules only with the Aerolizer inhaler provided, not by mouth. Do not use Aerolizer inhaler with any other capsules. Do not exceed dosage of 2 capsules per day. Capsules must be punctured by Aerolizer inhaler in order to release powder. Always store capsules in the blister package, and remove from the blister immediately before use.
3. Administer the inhalation solution by the orally inhaled route via a standard jet nebulizer connected to an air compressor. Do not swallow or inject solution; for inhalation use only.
4. Inhalation powder contains lactose, which contains trace amounts of milk protein.
5. If symptoms of asthma arise between doses, an inhaled short-acting, beta-2-agonist may be used for immediate relief. If more than 1 inhaled medication prescribed, use short-acting bronchodilator medication first, if needed, and then use this medicine.
6. If a previously used dose for asthma or COPD does not result in the usual response, seek medical advice immediately as this is often a sign of deteriorating asthma or COPD. Use incentive spirometer to monitor breathing status. Not for use with marked reduction in spirometry readings, or acute worsening of asthma condition.
7. Clients taking formoterol in twice daily doses for asthma should not take additional doses for exercise-induced bronchospasms.
8. With exercise-induced asthma, use 15 min before exercise and do not reuse for at least 12 hr.
9. Do not expose capsules to moisture; handle with dry hands. Do not wet or wash the Aerolizer inhaler; keep dry. Always use the new Aerolizer inhaler with each refill.
10. Do not use Aerolizer inhaler with a spacer, and never exhale into the Aerolizer inhaler.
11. Store capsules as directed, and only pierce once. If gelatin capsule breaks, the screen in the Aerolizer inhaler should retain it. Be aware that it may escape into the mouth or throat after inhalation.
12. May increase the risk of asthma-related death, and may increase the risk of asthma-related hospitalizations in children and adolescents.
13. Practice reliable contraception; report if pregnancy suspected.
14. Report any unusual side effects, loss of control of breathing patterns, or intolerance to therapy.
15. Store the inhalation solution in the foil pouch, and only remove immediately before use. Dis-

F

card the contents of any partially used container.

16. Keep all F/U assess response, prevent deterioration of lung function, adverse SE.

OUTCOMES/EVALUATE

- Improved breathing patterns with asthma
- Maintenance of bronchoconstriction
- Prevention of exercise-induced bronchospasm

Fosamprenavir calcium

(fos-am-**PREN**-ah-veer)

Classification(s): Antiretroviral agent, protease inhibitor

Pregnancy Category: C

RX: Lexiva.

SEE ALSO *ANTIVIRAL AGENTS.*

INDICATIONS/USES

In combination with other antiretroviral drugs to treat HIV-1 infection in adults and children. When initiating therapy with fosamprenavir plus ritonavir in protease-inhibitor experienced clients, consider the following: (a) Studies were unable to reach a definitive conclusion that fosamprenavir plus ritonavir and lopinavir plus ritonavir are clinically equivalent and (b) once-daily administration of fosamprenavir plus ritonavir is not recommended for protease inhibitor-experienced adults or any children.

ACTION/KINETICS

Action

Fosamprenavir is a prodrug of amprenavir, which is a HIV-1 protease inhibitor. Fosamprenavir is rapidly converted to amprenavir and inorganic phosphate by cellular phosphatases in the gut epithelium. Amprenavir binds to the active site of HIV-1 protease, thus preventing the processing of viral Gag and Gag-Pol polyprotein precursors; this results in formation of immature noninfectious viral particles. *NOTE:* Varying degrees of cross-resistance among HIV-1 protease inhibitors have been observed.

Pharmacokinetics

Time to peak amprenavir levels: 1.5–4 hr after a single dose. Food does not affect the C_{max}, T_{max}, or AUC of the tablets. However there is a reduction in the C_{max}, T_{max}, and AUC if the oral suspension is taken with a high-fat meal. Fosamprenavir is almost completely hydrolyzed to amprenavir and inorganic phosphate by the gut epithelium before the drug reaches the systemic circulation. Amprenavir is rapidly and almost completely metabolized in the liver by the CYP3A4 enzyme system. Metabolites are excreted in both the urine (14%) and feces (75%). **Plasma t½, elimination of amprenavir:** About 7.7 hr. Hepatic impairment increases the AUC of amprenavir; thus, dosage adjustment is required (see *Implementation/Administration/Storage*). **Plasma protein binding:** About 90%.

CONTRAINDICATIONS

Clinically significant hypersensitivity (e.g., Stevens-Johnson syndrome) to the drug or any component of the product or to amprenavir. Coadministration with delavirdine, dihydroergotamine, ergotamine, ergonovine, flecainide, lovastatin, methylergonovine, midazolam, pimozide, propafenone, rifampin, simvastatin, St. John's wort, or triazolam. Fosamprenavir with ritonavir coadministered with either flecainide or propafenone; also this combination is not recommended for protease inhibitor experienced adults or children. Use not recommended in those with severe hepatic disease. Lactation.

SPECIAL CONCERNS

- **Select doses carefully in geriatric clients.**
- **Use with caution in those with impaired hepatic function and in those with known sulfonoamide allergy (due to possible cross-sensitivity).**
- **If used with ritonavir at doses higher than recommended, elevations in serum transaminase may occur.**
- **Varying degrees of cross-resistance among protease inhibitors have been noted.**
- **Safety and efficacy not determined in children less than 2 years of age.**

SIDE EFFECTS

Most Common

N&V, diarrhea, abdominal pain, headache, fatigue, rash, redistribution of body fat, symptoms of hyperglycemia.

Side effects include those possible when fosamprenavir is combined with ritonavir. **GI:** Diarrhea, N&V, abdominal pain. Worsening of transaminase elevations in those with hepatitis B or C. **CNS:** Headache, depressive mood disorders, oral paresthesia. **CV:** ***MI.*** **Hematologic:** ***Acute hemolytic anemia***, neutropenia, spontaneous bleeding in hemophilia A and B clients treated with protease inhibitors. **Dermatologic:** Severe or ***life-threatening skin reactions***, including mild or moderate maculopapular rashes, some with pruritus, and ***Stevens-Johnson syndrome***. **GU:** Nephrolithiasis. **Metabolic:** New-onset diabetes mellitus, exacerbation of pre-existing diabetes mellitus, diabetic ketoacidosis, hyperglycemia. Redistribution of body fat, including central obesity, dorsocervical fat enlargement (buffalo hump), peripheral/facial wasting, breast enlargement, and "cushingoid" appearance. **Body as a whole:** Fatigue, angioedema. **Miscellaneous:** Development of opportunistic infections including those due to *Mycobacterium avium* complex, cytomegalovirus, *Pneumocystis carinii,* and tuberculosis. Immune reconstitution syndrome (including an inflammatory response to indolent or residual opportunistic infections such as *M. avium*, cytomegalovirus, *P. jirovecii* pneumonia, and tuberculosis); hypersensitivity reactions.

LABORATORY TEST CONSIDERATIONS

↑ Triglycerides, cholesterol, serum lipase, ALT, AST. ↓ Neutrophils. Hyperglycemia.

OVERDOSE MANAGEMENT

Symptoms: Increased frequency of grade 2/3 ALT elevations and grade 1/2 AST elevations. *Treatment:* Transaminase elevations resolved if the drug is discontinued. There is no known fosamprenavir antidote. If overdosage occurs, monitor the client for evidence of toxicity and use standard supportive treatment as needed.

DRUG INTERACTIONS

Amprenavir, the active form of fosamprenavir, is metabolized by CYP3A4 enzyme system and is an inhibitor (and possible inducer) of CYP3A4. Coadministration of fosamprenavir and drugs that induce CYP3A4 may decrease amprenavir levels and decrease efficacy. Coadministration of amprenavir and drugs that inhibit CYP3A4 may increase amprenavir levels and increase the incidence of side effects. Also, the potential for drug interactions changes when fosamprenavir is given with ritonavir, a potent CYP3A4 inhibitor. Because ritonavir is also a CYP2D6 inhibitor, significant interactions may occur when fosamprenavir plus ritonavir are given with drugs metabolized by CYP2D6.

Amiodarone / Possible serious/life-threatening reactions (e.g., cardiac arrhythmias); give together with caution

Amiodarone plus ritonavir / Possible ↑ amiodarone plasma levels → serious and/or life-threatening reactions, including cardiac arrhythmias when the three are given together

Anticholinergic drugs (e.g., darifenacin, fesoterodine, solifenacin, tolterodine) / Possible ↑ anticholinergic plasma levels → ↑ pharmacologic and side effects; when given with fosamprenavir, do not exceed a daily dose of 7.5 mg darifenacin, 4 mg of fesoterodine, 5 mg solifenacin, or 2 mg tolterodine

Aripiprazole / ↑ Aripiprazole plasma levels → ↑ risk of pharmacologic and side effects; monitor and adjust aripiprazole dose if needed

Benzodiazepines (alprazolam, clorazepate, diazepam, flurazepam, midazolam, triazolam) / ↑ Alprazolam, clorazepate, diazepam and flurazepam levels → ↑ pharmacologic effects; do not use fosamprenavir with midazolam or triazolam R/T possible serious/life-threatening reactions, such as prolonged or increased sedation/respiratory depression

Bepridil plus ritonavir / Possible ↑ bepridil plasma levels → serious and/or life-threatening reactions, including cardiac arrhythmias when the three are given together; use together with caution

Calcium channel blockers (e.g., amlodipine, diltiazem, felodipine, nicardipine, nifedipine, nimodipine, nisoldipine, verapamil) / Possible ↑ levels of CCBs; use together with caution and monitor

Carbamazepine / ↑ Carbamazepine levels → ↑ risk of toxicity; also, ↓ amprenavir plasma levels → ↓ efficacy

Clarithromycin / Possible ↑ amprenavir plasma levels R/T inhibition of CYP3A4; use together with caution

Colchicine / ↑ Colchicine plasma levels → life-threatening and fatal colchicine toxicity; do not use together in those with hepatic or renal impairment. In those with healthy renal and hepatic function, if used together do not exceed a dose of 0.3 mg colchicine twice a day; carefully monitor

Contraceptive hormones (e.g., ethinyl estradiol/norethindrone) / ↓ Fosamprenavir AUC → loss of virologic response; also, alteration of hormone lev-

F

els; use alternative methods of nonhormonal contraceptives
Corticosteroids (e.g., nasal fluticasone, oral prednisone) / Possible inhibition of corticosteroid metabolism by CYP3A4 → ↑ risk of toxicity; do not give fluticasone together with fosamprenavir and ritonavir unless benefits outweigh risks
Cyclosporine / Possible ↑ cyclosporine levels; monitor therapeutic levels of cyclosporine as toxicity may occur; adjust cyclosporine dose as needed
Delavirdine / ↑ Amprenavir levels; possible loss of virologic response and resistance to delavirdine; coadministration is contraindicated
Dexamethasone / Possible loss of virologic response and resistance to fosamprenavir/other protease inhibitors; use together with caution
Dronedarone / ↑ Dronedarone plasma levels → ↑ pharmacologic and toxic effects; do not use together
Efavirenz / ↓ Fosamprenavir levels if given with/without ritonavir; give an additional 100 mg/day of ritonavir; no change in ritonavir dosage needed when efavirenz given with fosamprenavir plus ritonavir twice daily
Efavirenz plus ritonavir / ↑ Amprenavir C_{max} and AUC if fosamprenavir is also given with ritonavir
Eplerenone / ↑ Eplerenone plasma levels → ↑ pharmacologic and toxic effects; monitor closely and adjust eplerenone dose as needed
Ergot derivatives (e.g., dihydroergotamine, ergonovine, ergotamine, methylergonovine) / Do not use together R/T potential for serious/life-threatening reactions, such as acute ergot toxicity (peripheral vasospasm, ischemia of the extremities)
Erythromycin / ↑ Erythromycin plasma levels→ ↑ pharmacologic and toxic effects, such as cardiac arrhythmias; do not use together
Esomeprazole / Possible ↑ esomeprazole plasma levels; monitor for side effects and adjust esomeprazole dose as needed
Eszopiclone / ↑ Eszopiclone plasma levels → ↑ pharmacologic and toxic effects; monitor closely and adjust eszopiclone dose as needed
Everolimus / Possible ↑ plasma levels of mammalian target of rapamycin (mTOR) inhibitors (e.g., everolimus) → ↑ pharmacologic and toxic effects; do not use together
Flecainide plus ritonavir / Possible ↑ plasma levels of flecainide if given with fosamprenavir and ritonavir → serious and/or life-threatening cardiac arrhythmias; do not use together
Fluconazole / Possible ↑ fluconazole side effects; dosage may need to be reduced
H ***Garlic*** / ↓ Amprenavir plasma levels → ↓ pharmacologic effect; do not use together
Grapefruit juice / Possible ↑ amprenavir plasma levels; if grapefruit juice use cannot be avoided, monitor and adjust fosamprenavir dose as needed
Histamine H_2-receptor antagonists (e.g., cimetidine, famotidine, nizatidine, ranitidine) / Possible decreased virologic response and resistance R/T ↓ amprenavir plasma levels; use together with caution
HMG-CoA reductase inhibitors (e.g., atorvastatin, lovastatin, rosuvastatin, I simvastatin) / Possible ↑ serum levels of HMG-CoA reductase inhibitors → ↑ toxicity, including myopathy and rhabdomyolysis; also ↓ amprenavir C_{max} and AUC; avoid concurrent use with lovastatin or simvastatin; use lowest possible doses of atorvastatin or rosuvastatin with monitoring
Indinavir / ↑ Amprenavir levels; possible ↓ indinavir levels
Itraconazole / Possible ↑ itraconazole side effects; dosage reduction may be needed in those receiving >400 mg per day of itraconazole; possible ↑ amprenavir plasma levels → ↑ risk of toxicity; doses higher than 200 mg/day itraconazole not recommended
Ixabepilone / Possible ↑ ixabepilone plasma levels → ↑ pharmacologic and toxic effects; do use together
Ketoconazole / Possible ↑ ketoconazole side effects; may require dosage reduction in those receiving >400 mg per day of ketoconazole; possible ↑ amprenavir plasma levels → ↑ risk of toxicity; doses higher than 200 mg/day ketoconazole not recommended
Lidocaine (systemic) plus ritonavir / Possible ↑ lidocaine plasma levels → serious and/or life-threatening reactions, including cardiac arrhythmias when the three are given together; use together with caution
Lopinavir plus ritonavir / ↓ Amprenavir C_{max} and AUC if also given with ritonavir; ↑ lopinavir C_{max} and AUC; ↑ incidence of side effects
Methadone / Possible ↓ methadone levels—may need to ↑ methadone dose; also, ↓ amprenavir C_{max}, AUC, and C_{min}

Maraviroc / Possible ↑ maraviroc plasma levels → ↑ pharmacologic and toxic effects; monitor and adjust maraviroc dose as needed
Narcotic analgesics (e.g., alfentanil, buprenorphine, fentanyl, sufentanil) / Possible ↑ narcotic analgesic plasma levels and ↑ t½ → ↑ risk of toxicity; monitor respiratory function and adjust dose as needed
Nevirapine / ↓ Amprenavir levels; possible ↑ nevirapine plasma levels; do not give nevirapine and fosamprenavir without ritonavir
Nilotinib / Possible ↑ nilotinib plasma levels → ↑ pharmacologic and toxic effects, such as cardiac arrhythmias; do not use together
Paroxetine / Significant ↓ paroxetine plasma levels when given with fosamprenavir and ritonavir; adjust paroxetine dose on tolerance and efficacy
Phenobarbital / ↓ Efficacy of fosamprenavir R/T ↓ plasma levels; use together with caution
Phenytoin / ↓ Efficacy of fosamprenavir R/T ↓ plasma levels; also, possible ↓ phenytoin plasma levels; monitor phenytoin levels and increase dose as needed; use together with caution
Pimozide / Do not use together; possible serious and/or life-threatening reactions, including cardiac arrhythmias
Propafenone plus ritonavir / Possible ↑ propafenone plasma levels → serious and/or life-threatening reactions, including cardiac arrhythmias when the three are given together; use together is contraindicated
Protein-tyrosine kinase inhibitors (e.g., dasatinib, sorafenib, sunitinib) / ↑ Protein-tyrosine kinase inhibitor → ↑ pharmacologic and toxic effects; monitor response and adjust inhibitor dose as needed
Quetiapine / ↑ Quetiapine plasma levels → ↑ pharmacologic and toxic effects; monitor and adjust quetiapine dose as needed
Quinidine plus ritonavir / Possible serious/life-threatening reactions (e.g., cardiac arrhythmias) when the three are given together; use together with caution
Ranolazine / Possible ↑ Ranolazine plasma levels → ↑ risk of dose-related prolongation of the QTc interval, torsades de pointes-type arrhythmias, and sudden death; do not use together
Rapamycin / Possible ↑ rapamycin levels; monitor therapeutic levels of rapamycin as toxicity may occur; adjust rapamycin dose as needed
Rifabutin / Monitor weekly for neutropenia; reduce rifabutin dose by at least one-half when given with fosamprenavir or three-fourths if given with both fosamprenavir and ritonavir; possible ↑ fosamprenavir AUC and C_{max}
Rifampin / Possible ↓ amprenavir plasma levels → loss of virologic response and resistance to fosamprenavir/other protease inhibitors; coadministration is contraindicated
Saquinavir / ↓ Amprenavir levels; appropriate doses not established
Sildenafil / ↑ Sildenafil plasma levels → ↑ risk of side effects (hypotension, priapism, visual changes); ↓ sildenafil dose to 25 mg q 48 hr and monitor for side effects
H ***St. John's wort*** / Possible loss of virologic response and resistance R/T ↑ fosamprenavir hepatic metabolism by CYP3A4 enzymes → significant ↓ amprenavir levels; do not use together
Tacrolimus / Possible ↑ tacrolimus levels; monitor therapeutic levels of tacrolimus as toxicity may occur; adjust tacrolimus dose as needed
Tadalafil / ↑ Tadalafil plasma levels → ↑ side effects (hypotension, priapism, visual changes); ↓ tadalafil dose to no more than 10 mg q 72 hr
Temsirolimus / Possible ↑ plasma levels of mammalian target of rapamycin (mTOR) inhibitors (e.g., temsirolimus) → ↑ pharmacologic and toxic effects; do not use together
Trazodone / ↑ Trazodone plasma levels → ↑ pharmacologic and side effects when given with fosamprenavir alone or with fosamprenavir and ritonavir; decrease trazodone dose
Tricyclic antidepressants (e.g., amitriptyline, imipramine) / Serious and/or life-threatening reactions possible; monitor TCA plasma levels
Vardenafil / ↑ Vardenafil plasma levels → ↑ side effects; ↓ vardenafil dose to 2.5 mg q 24 hr; if given with fosamprenavir and ritonavir, ↓ vardenafil dose to no more than 2.5 mg q 72 hr
Vasopressin receptor antagonists (e.g., conivaptan, tolvaptan) / ↑ Plasma levels of vasopressin receptor antagonist → ↑ pharmacologic and toxic effects; do not use together
Warfarin / Levels of warfarin may be affected; monitor INR
Zidovudine / Possible ↑ in levels of both amprenavir and zidovudine; monitor for side effects and adjust dose if needed

F

HOW SUPPLIED

Oral Suspension: 50 mg/mL (equivalent to 43 mg/mL amprenavir); ***Tablets:*** 700 mg (equivalent to 600 mg amprenavir).

DOSAGE

ORAL SUSPENSION; TABLETS

Human immunodeficiency virus (HIV) infections, therapy-naive clients.

Adults: Fosamprenavir, 1,400 mg twice a day (without ritonavir); or, fosamprenavir, 1,400 mg once daily plus ritonavir, 200 mg once daily; or, fosamprenavir, 700 mg twice a day plus ritonavir, 100 mg once a day; or, fosamprenavir, 700 mg twice daily plus ritonavir, 100 mg twice daily. **Children, 6 years and older, usual:** fosamprenavir, 30 mg/kg (suspension), twice a day or fosamprenavir, 18 mg/kg (suspension) twice a day plus ritonavir, 3 mg/kg, twice a day. **Maximum dose, children, 6 years and older:** Fosamprenavir, 1,400 mg twice a day or fosamprenavir, 700 mg twice a day plus ritonavir, 100 mg twice a day. **Children, 2–5 years of age, usual:** 30 mg/kg (suspension) twice a day. **Maximum dose, children, 2–5 years:** 1,400 mg twice a day.

HIV infections, protease inhibitor-experienced clients.

Adults: Fosamprenavir, 700 mg twice a day plus ritonavir, 100 mg twice a day. Once daily fosamprenavir and ritonavir is not recommended. **Children, 6 years and older, usual:** Fosamprenavir, 18 mg/kg twice a day plus ritonavir, 3 mg/kg twice a day. **Maximum dose, children, 6 years and older:** Fosamprenavir, 700 mg twice a day plus ritonavir, 100 mg twice a day. **Children, 2–5 years of age:** Data are insufficient to recommend any dosing regimen.

HIV infections, concomitant therapy with efavirenz.

Adults: An additional 100 mg/day (i.e., 300 mg total) of ritonavir is recommended when efavirenz is given with fosamprenavir plus ritonavir once daily. No change in ritonavir dosage is needed when efavirenz is given with fosamprenavir plus ritonavir twice a day.

NURSING IMPLICATIONS

IMPLEMENTATION/ADMINISTRATION/STORAGE

1. When given without ritonavir, the adult regimen of fosamprenavir, 1,400 mg tablets twice a day may be used for children weighing at least 47 kg. When given with ritonavir, the tablets may be used for children weighing at least 39 kg; ritonavir capsules may be used for children weighing at least 33 kg.
2. Use the following guidelines for use of fosamprenavir in clients with hepatic impairment:
   - **For mild hepatic impairment (Child-Pugh score from 5 to 6):** Reduce dosage of fosamprenavir to 700 mg twice daily without ritonavir or 700 mg twice daily plus ritonavir, 100 mg once daily in therapy-naive or protease inhibitor-experienced clients.
   - **For moderate hepatic impairment (Child-Pugh score from 7 to 9):** Use fosamprenavir with caution at reduced dosage of fosamprenavir to 700 mg twice daily (therapy-naive clients) without ritonavir or 450 mg twice daily plus ritonavir, 100 mg once daily in therapy-naive or protease inhibitor-experienced clients.
   - **For severe hepatic impairment (Child-Pugh score from 10 to 15):** Use fosamprenavir with caution at reduced dosage of fosamprenavir to 350 mg twice daily without ritonavir (therapy-naive clients) or 300 mg fosamprenavir twice a day plus ritonavir, 100 mg once a day (therapy-naive or protease inhibitor-experienced clients).
3. Higher than approved dose combinations of fosamprenavir and ritonavir are not recommended due to an increased risk of transaminase elevations.
4. Store tablets from 15–30°C (59–86°F) and the oral suspension from 5–30°C (40–86°F). Shake the suspension vigorously before using; do not freeze.

ASSESSMENT

1. Note disease onset, characteristics of S&S, other agents trialed, outcome. List drugs prescribed to ensure none interact. Identify if protease inhibitor-experienced adults or children.

2. List sulfa allergy; precludes drug therapy.
3. Obtain triglyceride and cholesterol levels before starting therapy, and monitor periodically during therapy. Monitor HIV RNA, CBC, renal and LFTs; reduce dose with liver dysfunction.

CLIENT/FAMILY TEACHING

1. Works by blocking protease, a protein that HIV needs to make more copies of itself.
2. Take tablets as directed with or without food and with other antiretroviral therapy; always used in combination therapy. Do not double or change dose; if dose missed, take when remembered (unless more than 4 hr, then just wait for next dose). Adults should take the oral suspension without food, while children should take the oral suspension with food. If vomiting occurs within 30 min after dosing, redose the fosamprenavir oral suspension.
3. If prescribed oral suspension, shake product vigorously before each use. Refrigeration may improve the taste.
4. Do not take any unprescribed or OTC medications/herbals without approval due to potential for adverse interactions.
5. Report persistent diarrhea, nausea, vomiting, or rash. May experience a change in body fat distribution/accumulation, high cholesterol, increased bleeding in those with hemophilia, high blood sugar levels, and onset or worsening of diabetes.
6. Use nonhormonal contraception; drug may alter hormone levels. Does not prevent disease transmission or STDs; practice safe sex and do not breast-feed.
7. If taking drugs for impotence may be at an increased risk of PDE5 inhibitor-associated adverse reactions, including hypotension, priapism, and visual changes; report if evident.
8. Keep all F/U to assess response, labs, adverse SE. May continue to experience opportunistic infections. Long-term drug effects unknown.

OUTCOMES/EVALUATE

↓ HIV RNA ↑ CD4 cell counts

IV

Fosaprepitant dimeglumine

(**FOS**-ap-**RE**-pih-tant dye-**MEG**-loo-meen)

Classification(s): Antiemetic

Pregnancy Category: B

RX: Emend.

INDICATIONS/USES

In combination with other antiemetic agents to prevent acute and delayed N&V associated with initial and repeat courses of highly and moderately emetogenic cancer chemotherapy, including high-dose cisplatin. *NOTE:* Has not been studied to treat established N&V. Long-term continuous administration is not recommended.

ACTION/KINETICS

Action

Fosaprepitant is a prodrug of aprepitant; thus, its antiemetic effect is due to aprepitant. Aprepitant is a selective high-affinity antagonist of human substance NK_1 receptors. Aprepitant augments the antiemetic activity of the 5-HT_3-receptor antagonist ondansetron and the corticosteroid dexamethasone and inhibits the acute and delayed phases of cisplatin-induced emesis.

Pharmacokinetics

Fosaprepitant is rapidly converted to the active aprepitant in the liver, kidney, lung, and ileum. The mean aprepitant plasma level at 24 hr post-dose was similar between the dose of PO aprepitant, 125 mg PO, and the dose of fosaprepitant, 115 mg IV. Fosaprepitant is rapidly converted to aprepitant in the liver and other tissues. Aprepitant undergoes extensive metabolism primarily by CYP3A4 with minor metabolism by CYP1A2 and CYP2C19. Metabolites are excreted in the urine and feces. **t½, terminal:** 9–13 hr. **Plasma protein binding:** >95%.

CONTRAINDICATIONS

Hypersensitivity to fosaprepitant, aprepitant, polysorbate 80, or any other components of the product. Concurrent use with cisapride or pimozide. Chronic use to prevent N&V (has not been studied and the drug interaction profile may change with chronic continuous use). Lactation.

SPECIAL CONCERNS

- Use with caution in severe hepatic dysfunction (Child-Pugh score higher than 9).
- The elderly may show greater sensitivity to the drug although dosage adjustment is not necessary.

- Use with caution in clients receiving concomitant drugs that are primarily metabolized through CYP3A4.
- Use caution and careful monitoring in clients receiving chemotherapeutic agents (e.g., ifosfamide, vinblastine, vincristine) that are metabolized by CYP3A4.
- Safety and efficacy not determined in children.

SIDE EFFECTS

Most Common

Infusion site pain/induration, headache, asthenia, fatigue, anorexia, diarrhea, N&V, constipation, hiccoughs.

Side effects listed are those for aprepitant and/or the aprepitant regimen. **CNS:** Headache, dizziness, insomnia, anxiety disorder, cognitive disorder, confusion, depression, disorientation, dream abnormality, euphoria, peripheral/sensory neuropathy, somnolence, taste disturbance, tremor, hyperesthesia, hypoesthesia, syncope, dysarthria, sensory disturbance. **GI:** N&V, constipation, diarrhea, hiccoughs, anorexia, dyspepsia, stomatitis, heartburn, abdominal pain (including upper), abdominal distention, gastritis, epigastric discomfort, acid reflux, deglutition disorder, dry mouth, dysgeusia, dysphagia, eructation, flatulence, GERD, obstipation, thirst, increased salivation, abnormal bowel sounds, stomach discomfort, neutropenic colitis, perforating duodenal ulcer, polydipsia, hard feces. **CV:** DVT, flushing/hot flush, hypertension, hypotension, ***MI***, palpitations, tachycardia, bradycardia, CV disorder, operative hemorrhage. **Dermatologic:** Alopecia, acne, diaphoresis, erythema, rash, pruritus, hematoma, wound dehiscence, urticaria, oily skin, photosensitivity, skin lesion. **Respiratory:** Pharyngolaryngeal pain, cough, dyspnea, lower/upper RTI, nasal secretion, pharyngitis, pneumonitis, postnasal drip, ***pulmonary embolism***, respiratory insufficiency, non-small-cell lung carcinoma, hypoxia, respiratory depression, sneezing, throat irritation, wheezing. **GU:** Dysuria, microscopic hematuria, pollakiuria, polyuria, pelvic pain, UTI, impaired renal function. **Musculoskeletal:** Arthralgia, back pain, muscle weakness, musculoskeletal pain, muscle cramps, myalgia, gait disturbance. **Hematologic:** Neutropenia, febrile neutropenia, anemia, thrombocytopenia. **Hypersensitivity:** Flushing, erythema, dyspnea, angioedema, ***anaphylaxis*** (may be immediate). **At infusion site:** Pain, erythema, pruritus, induration, thrombophlebitis. **Ophthalmic:** Conjunctivitis, miosis, decreased visual acuity. **Otic:** Tinnitus. **Body as a whole:** Dehydration, fever, asthenia, fatigue, chills, chest discomfort, edema, malaise, lethargy, rigors, mucous membrane disorder, mucosal inflammation, weight gain/loss, hypothermia, hypovolemia, postoperative infection, ***neutropenic sepsis***. **Miscellaneous:** Decreased appetite, diabetes mellitus, hypokalemia, vocal disturbance, candidiasis, herpes simplex, staphylococcal infection, ***malignant neoplasm***, ***septic shock***.

LABORATORY TEST CONSIDERATIONS

↑ AST, ALT, BUN, serum creatinine, alkaline phosphatase, leukocytes. ↓ Hemoglobin, WBCs, albumin. Hypokalemia, proteinuria, hyperglycemia, hyponatremia, erythrocyturia, leukocyturia, urinary glucose.

DRUG INTERACTIONS

Fosaprepitant is a moderate inhibitor and an inducer of CYP3A4 when given as a 3-day antiemetic dosing regimen. It is also an inducer of CYP2A9.

Benzodiazepines (e.g., alprazolam, midazolam, triazolam) / ↑ Plasma levels of benzodiazepines → ↑ pharmacologic and toxicologic effects; closely monitor for side effects (e.g., CNS depression)

Carbamazepine / Possible ↓ aprepitant plasma levels → ↓ efficacy; use together with caution and monitor

Clarithromycin / Possible ↑ aprepitant plasma levels; use together with caution

Cisapride / ↑ Risk of life-threatening cardiac arrhythmias R/T ↑ cisapride levels due to inhibition of CYP3A4; do not use together

Colchicine / ↑ Colchicine plasma levels → ↑ risk of toxicity; use together with caution

Contraceptives, hormonal / ↓ Efficacy of hormonal contraceptives during and for 28 days after the last dose of aprepitant; use alternative or backup methods of contraception

Dexamethasone / Reduce dose of PO dexamethasone by 50% when given with fosaprepitant followed by aprepitant (125 mg and 80 mg regimen)

Diltiazem / ↑ Plasma levels of both diltiazem and aprepitant; closely monitor the clinical response

Docetaxel / ↑ Docetaxel plasma levels R/T inhibition of CYP3A4; use together with caution

Etoposide / ↑ Etoposide plasma levels R/T inhibition of CYP3A4; use together with caution

Everolimus / ↑ Everolimus plasma levels → ↑ pharmacologic/toxic effects; closely monitor everolimus levels
Fentanyl / ↑ Fentanyl plasma levels → ↑ pharmacologic/toxic effects; closely monitor
Ifosfamide / ↑ Ifosfamide plasma levels R/T inhibition of CYP3A4; use together with caution
Imatinib / ↑ Imatinib plasma levels R/T inhibition of CYP3A4; use together with caution
Irinotecan / ↑ Irinotecan plasma levels R/T inhibition of CYP3A4; use together with caution
Itraconazole / Possible ↑ aprepitant plasma levels; use together with caution
Ketoconazole / Possible ↑ aprepitant plasma levels; use together with caution
Methylprednisolone / Reduce dose of methylprednisolone IV by 25% and the PO dose by 50% when given with fosaprepitant followed by aprepitant (125 mg and 80 mg regimen)
Nefazodone / Possible ↑ aprepitant plasma levels; use together with caution
Nelfinavir / Possible ↑ aprepitant plasma levels; use together with caution
Paclitaxel / ↑ Paclitaxel levels R/T inhibition of CYP3A4; use together with caution
Paroxetine / ↓ AUC and C_{max} of both aprepitant and paroxetine; monitor the clinical response
Phenytoin / Possible ↓ aprepitant plasma levels → ↓ efficacy; use together with caution and monitor
Pimozide / ↑ Risk of life-threatening cardiac arrhythmias R/T ↑ pimozide levels due to inhibition of CYP3A4 do not use together
Ranolazine / ↑ Ranolazine plasma levels → ↑ pharmacologic/toxic effects; closely monitor for QT prolongation; limit the ranolazine dose to 500 mg twice a day
Rifampin / Possible ↓ aprepitant plasma levels → ↓ efficacy; use together with caution and monitor
Ritonavir / Possible ↑ aprepitant plasma levels; use together with caution
Tolbutamide / ↓ Tolbutamide plasma levels R/T induction of metabolism by CYP2C9
Tolvaptan / ↑ Tolvaptan plasma levels → ↑ pharmacologic/toxic effects; avoid coadministration
Troleandomycin / Possible ↑ aprepitant plasma levels; use together with caution
Vinblastine / ↑ Vinblastine plasma levels R/T inhibition of CYP3A4; use together with caution
Vincristine / ↑ Vincristine plasma levels R/T inhibition of CYP3A4; use together with caution
Vinorelbine / ↑ Vinorelbine plasma levels R/T inhibition of CYP3A4; use together with caution
Warfarin / ↓ Warfarin plasma levels R/T induction of metabolism by CYP2C9; monitor INR closely in the 2-week period following initiation of the 3-day antiemetic regimen

HOW SUPPLIED

Injection, Lyophilized Powder for Solution: 115 mg, 150 mg.

DOSAGE

IV

Prevention of chemotherapy-induced nausea and vomiting.

Highly emetogenic cancer chemotherapy. 115 mg injection (3-day dosing regimen using fosaprepitant/aprepitant). Day 1: Fosaprepitant 115 mg IV; dexamethasone 12 mg PO 30 min prior to chemotherapy treatment on day 1 and in the morning on days 2 through 4; and, ondansetron 32 mg IV given 30 min prior to chemotherapy treatment on day 1. *NOTE:* Aprepitant 125 mg PO may be substituted for fosaprepitant 115 mg IV on day 1. **Days 2 and 3:** Aprepitant 80 mg PO and dexamethasone 8 mg PO once a day. **Day 4:** Dexamethasone 8 mg PO once a day.

Highly emetogenic cancer chemotherapy. 150 mg injection (single-dose regimen). Day 1: Fosaprepitant 150 mg IV infused over 20–30 min given 30 min prior to chemotherapy; dexamethasone 12 mg PO given 30 min prior to chemotherapy treatment on day 1 and in the morning on days 2 through 4; ondansetron 32 mg IV given 30 min prior to chemotherapy treatment on day 1. **Days 2 through 4:** Dexamethasone 8 mg PO once a day.

Moderately emetogenic cancer chemotherapy. 115 mg injection (3-day dosing regimen using fosaprepitant/aprepitant). Day 1: Fosaprepitant 115 mg IV 30 min prior to chemotherapy on treatment day 1; dexamethasone 12 mg PO given 30 min prior to chemotherapy treatment on day 1; ondan-

F

setron 8 mg PO twice a day given 30–60 min prior to chemotherapy treatment and 8 hr after the first dose on day 1. *NOTE:* Aprepitant, 125 mg PO, may be substituted for fosaprepitant 115 mg IV on day 1. **Days 2 and 3:** Aprepitant 80 mg PO.

NURSING IMPLICATIONS

IMPLEMENTATION/ADMINISTRATION/STORAGE

1. IV To prepare the injection, aseptically inject 5 mL of NaCl 0.9% for injection into the vial. To prevent foaming, the saline is added to the vial along the vial wall. Swirl the vial gently; avoid shaking and jetting saline into the vial.
2. Aseptically prepare an infusion bag filled with 110 mL (115 mg vial) or 145 mL (150 mg vial) of NaCl 0.9% injection. Aseptically withdraw the entire volume from the vial and transfer it into the infusion bag to yield a total volume of a final concentration of 1 mg/mL. Gently invert the bag 2 to 3 times.
3. Administer as an IV infusion over 15 min for the 115 mg injection and over 20–30 min for the 150 mg injection. Infuse 30 min prior to chemotherapy
4. The reconstituted final drug solution is stable for 24 hr at ambient room temperature at or below 25°C (77°F).
5. Do not mix or reconstitute fosaprepitant injection with solutions for which physical and chemical compatibility have not been established. Fosaprepitant injection may be given with or without food.
6. Store vials from 2–8°C (36–46°F).
7. COMPATIBILITY 0.9% NaCl.
8. INCOMPATIBILITY Any solutions containing divalent cations (e.g., calcium, magnesium), including Ringer's lactate solution and Hartmann's solution.

ASSESSMENT

1. Note reasons for therapy, cytotoxic agents prescribed, other therapy trialed and outcome.
2. List all drugs prescribed to ensure none interact.
3. Depending on chemotherapy prescribed usually given in conjunction with a corticosteroid and a 5-HT_3 antagonist such as ondansetron.
4. Monitor VS, renal and LFTs; adjust dose with dysfunction and with the elderly.

CLIENT/FAMILY TEACHING

1. Drug is used to inhibit N&V induced by cytotoxic chemotherapeutic agents. Usually given as an IV infusion over 15 minutes, 30 minutes prior to chemotherapy on day 1. Injection may be administered with or without food; then a capsule is administered each morning for the 2 days following chemotherapy based on dosing regimens prescribed.
2. Use nonhormonal form of contraception during and for 1 month following the last dose of the 3-day regimen.
3. If prescribed chronic warfarin therapy, may need to have blood tests after each 3-day treatment to check blood clotting and at 7 to 10 days after initiation.
4. Report any adverse SE, skin rash, itching, or lack of desired response.
5. Keep all F/U to assess response, labs, and adverse SE.

OUTCOMES/EVALUATE

Prevention of N&V R/T emetogenic cancer chemotherapy

■ IV

Foscarnet sodium

(fos-**KAR**-net)

Classification(s): Antiviral

Pregnancy Category: C

RX: Foscarnet.

SEE ALSO *ANTIVIRAL AGENTS*.

INDICATIONS/USES

(1) Treatment of CMV retinitis in clients with AIDS. (2) Treatment of acyclovir-resistant HSV infections in immunocompromised clients. (3) With ganciclovir in those who have relapsed after monotherapy with either drug.

ACTION/KINETICS

Action

Inhibits replication of all known herpes viruses by selective inhibition at the pyrophosphate binding site on virus-specific DNA polymerases and reverse transcriptases at levels that do not affect cellular DNA polymerases. Active against herpes simplex virus mutants deficient in thymidine kinase. CMV strains resistant to ganciclovir may be sensitive to foscarnet; viral reactivation of CMV occurs after termination of foscarnet therapy. The latent state of any of the human herpes viruses is not sensitive to foscarnet.

Pharmacokinetics

Believed to accumulate in human bone and has variable penetration into the CSF. **t½, plasma:** About 3 hr. Approximately 80–90% of IV foscarnet is excreted unchanged through the urine.

SPECIAL CONCERNS

(1) Renal impairment is the major toxicity. Continually assess client risk, frequently monitor serum creatinine with dose adjustment for changes in renal function. Ensure adequate hydration when drug is administered. (2) Seizures, related to alterations in plasma minerals and electrolytes, have been associated with foscarnet. Carefully monitor clients for such changes and their potential sequelae. Mineral and electrolyte supplementation may be required. (3) Foscarnet is indicated only for use in immunocompromised clients with CMV retinitis and mucocutaneous acyclovir-resistant HSV infections.

- Use with caution during lactation and in clients with impaired renal function (the effects of the drug have not been determined in clients with a C_{CR} <50 mL/min or serum creatinine >2.8 mg/dL).
- Use with caution with drugs that alter serum calcium levels as foscarnet decreases serum levels of ionized calcium.
- Safety and efficacy not determined in children, for the treatment of other CMV infections such as pneumonitis or gastroenteritis, for congenital or neonatal CMV disease, and in nonimmunocompromised clients.
- Transient changes in electrolytes may increase the risk of cardiac disturbances and seizures.
- Side effects such as renal impairment, electrolyte abnormalities, and seizures may contribute to client death.
- Drug is not a cure for HSV infections, and relapse occurs in most clients.
- Repeated treatment has led to the development of viral resistance.

SIDE EFFECTS

Most Common

Fever, N&V, anemia, diarrhea, abnormal renal function, headache, seizures.

GU: Renal impairment (most common), albuminuria, dysuria, polyuria, urinary retention, urethral disorder, UTIs, ***acute renal failure***, nocturia, hematuria, glomerulonephritis, urinary frequency, toxic nephropathy, nephrosis, urinary incontinence, pyelonephritis, renal tubular disorders, urethral irritation, uremia, perineal pain in women, penile inflammation. **Metabolic/Electrolyte:** Hypocalcemia, hypokalemia, hypomagnesemia, hypophosphatemia, hyponatremia, hyperphosphatemia, hypercalcemia, acidosis, thirst, decreased weight, dehydration, glycosuria, diabetes mellitus, abnormal glucose tolerance, hypochloremia, hypervolemia, hypoproteinemia. **Hematologic:** Anemia (one-third of clients), granulocytopenia, neutropenia, leukopenia, thrombocytopenia, platelet abnormalities, thrombosis, WBC abnormalities, lymphadenopathy, coagulation disorders, decreased coagulation factors, decreased prothrombin, hypochromic anemia, pancytopenia, hemolysis, leukocytosis, cervical lymphadenopathy, lymphopenia. **Body as a whole:** Fever, fatigue, asthenia, pain, infection, rigors, malaise, ***sepsis***, death, back or chest pain, cachexia, flu-like symptoms, edema, bacterial or fungal infections, abscess, moniliasis, leg edema, peripheral edema, hypothermia, syncope, substernal chest pain, ascites, ***malignant hyperpyrexia***, herpes simplex, viral infections, toxoplasmosis. **CNS:** Headache, dizziness, ***seizures (including tonic-clonic)***, tremor, ataxia, dementia, stupor, meningitis, aphasia, abnormal coordination, EEG abnormalities, vertigo, coma, encephalopathy, dyskinesia, extrapyramidal disorders, hemiparesis, paraplegia, speech disorders, tetany, cerebral edema, depression, confusion, anxiety, insomnia, somnolence, amnesia, aggressive reaction, nervousness, agitation, hallucinations, impaired concentration, emotional lability, psychosis, ***suicide attempt***, delirium, sleep disorders, personality disorders. **Peripheral nervous system:** Hypesthesia, neuropathy, sensory disturbances, generalized spasms, abnormal gait, hyperesthesia, hypertonia, hyperkinesia, vocal cord paralysis, hyporeflexia, hyperreflexia, neuralgia, neuritis, peripheral neuropathy. **Musculoskeletal:** Arthralgia, myalgia, involuntary muscle contrac-

F

tions, leg cramps, arthrosis, synovitis, torticollis. **GI:** N&V, diarrhea, anorexia, abdominal pain, dry mouth, dysphagia, dyspepsia, rectal hemorrhage, constipation, melena, flatulence, pancreatitis, ulcerative stomatitis, enteritis, glossitis, enterocolitis, proctitis, stomatitis, tenesmus, pseudomembranous colitis, gastroenteritis, oral leukoplakia, oral hemorrhage, rectal disorders, colitis, duodenal ulcer, hematemesis, paralytic ileus, ulcerative proctitis, tongue ulceration, esophageal ulceration. **Hepatic:** Abnormal hepatic function, cholecystitis, cholelithiasis, hepatitis, hepatosplenomegaly, cholestatic hepatitis, jaundice. **CV:** Hypertension, palpitations, sinus tachycardia, first-degree AV block, nonspecific ST-T segment changes, hypotension, flushing, cerebrovascular disorder, ***cardiomyopathy, cardiac failure, cardiac arrest***, bradycardia, arrhythmias, extrasystole, atrial fibrillation, phlebitis, superficial thrombophlebitis of arm, mesenteric vein thrombophlebitis. **Respiratory:** Cough, dyspnea, pneumonia, sinusitis, rhinitis, pharyngitis, respiratory insufficiency, pulmonary infiltration, ***pulmonary embolism***, pneumothorax, hemoptysis, stridor, bronchospasm, laryngitis, bronchitis, respiratory depression, pleural effusion, ***pulmonary hemorrhage***, pneumonitis. **Ophthalmic:** Visual field defects, nystagmus, periorbital edema, eye pain, conjunctivitis, diplopia, blindness, retinal detachment, mydriasis, photophobia. **Otic:** Deafness, earache, tinnitus, otitis. **Dermatologic:** Increased sweating, rash, skin ulceration, pruritus, seborrhea, erythematous rash, maculopapular rash, facial edema, skin discoloration, acne, alopecia, dermatitis, anal pruritus, genital pruritus, aggravated psoriasis, psoriaform rash, skin disorders, dry skin, urticaria, skin hypertrophy, verruca. **Miscellaneous:** Epistaxis, taste perversions, pain or inflammation at injection site, lymphoma-like disorder, sarcoma, ***malignant lymphoma***, ADH disorders, decreased gonadotropins, gynecomastia.

LABORATORY TEST CONSIDERATIONS

↑ Alkaline phosphatase, AST, ALT, LDH, BUN, CPK, serum creatinine. ↓ C_{CR}. Abnormal x-ray. Abnormal A-G ratio.

OVERDOSE MANAGEMENT

Symptoms: Extensions of the preceding side effects. Of most concern are development of ***seizures***, renal function impairment, paresthesias in limbs or periorally, and electrolyte disturbances especially involving calcium and phosphate. *Treatment:* Monitor the client for S&S of electrolyte imbalance and renal impairment. Symptomatic treatment. Hemodialysis and hydration may be of some benefit.

DRUG INTERACTIONS

Aminoglycosides / ↓ Elimination of foscarnet → ↑ risk of renal impairment
Amphotericin B / ↓ Elimination of foscarnet → ↑ risk of renal impairment
Cidofovir / ↑ Risk of nephrotoxicity
Didanosine / ↓ Elimination of foscarnet → ↑ risk of renal impairment
Ganciclovir / Additive or synergistic effects
Pentamidine, IV / ↓ Elimination of foscarnet → ↑ risk of renal impairment; also, pentamidine causes hypocalcemia
Valganciclovir / Additive or synergistic effects
Zidovudine / ↑ Risk of anemia

HOW SUPPLIED

Injection: 24 mg/mL.

DOSAGE

IV INFUSION

Cytomegalovirus retinitis in acquired immunodeficiency syndrome.

Individualized, initial, normal renal function: Either 60 mg/kg over a minimum of 1 hr q 8 hr or 90 mg/kg q 12 hr for 2–3 weeks, depending on the response. **Maintenance:** 90–120 mg/kg/day (depending on renal function) given as an IV infusion over 2 hr. Start most clients on the 90 mg/kg/day dose; however, consider increasing the dose to 120 mg/kg/day due to progression of retinitis.

Acyclovir-resistant herpes simplex virus infections in immunocompromised clients.

Initial: 40 mg/kg for clients with normal renal function given IV at a constant rate over a minimum of 1 hr q 8 or 12 hr for 2 to 3 weeks or until lesions are healed. **Maintenance:** See dose for CMV retinitis.

NURSING IMPLICATIONS

IMPLEMENTATION/ADMINISTRATION/STORAGE

1. **IV To avoid local irritation, infuse only into veins with adequate blood flow to allow rapid dilution and distribution.**

2. Rate of infusion must be no more than 1 mg/kg/min using controlled IV infusion, either by a central venous line or a peripheral vein. Do not give by rapid or bolus IV injection.
3. If using a central venous catheter for infusion, the standard 24 mg/mL solution may be used without dilution. If peripheral vein catheter is used, dilute the 24 mg/mL solution to 12 mg/mL with D5W or NSS to avoid vein irritation. Use diluted solutions within 24 hr of first entry into sealed bottle.
4. To minimize potential for renal impairment, hydrate during drug administration; establish and maintain diuresis.
5. Adjust dose in renal impairment; use dosing guide.
6. Store drug at room temperature of 15–30°C (59–86°F). Do not freeze. Concentrations of 12 mg/mL in NSS are stable for 30 days at 5°C (41°F).
7. COMPATIBILITY D5W or NSS.
8. INCOMPATIBILITY Do not give any other drug or supplement through the same catheter. Administer separately; a precipitate can result if foscarnet is given at the same time as divalent cations.

ASSESSMENT

1. List reasons for therapy: induction or maintenance of CMV retinitis or acyclovir-resistant HSV clients.
2. Confirm CMV retinitis by indirect ophthalmoscopy reports.
3. Note history of cardiac or neurologic dysfunction.
4. Hydrate to minimize potential for renal impairment; establish and maintain diuresis. Determine C_{CR} 2–3 times per week during induction therapy, and at least once every 1–2 weeks during maintenance therapy, especially in geriatric clients who commonly have decreased GFRs.
5. Observe for possibility of chelation of divalent metal ions, which will alter serum levels of electrolytes.
6. Observe for any seizure activity; use seizure precautions.
7. Follow dilution and administration guidelines carefully. Ideally, product should be prepared daily, under a biologic hood, by the pharmacist. Refer to home infusion program for home therapy.
8. Monitor CBC, electrolytes, minerals, calcium, phosphorus, Mg^{++}, renal and LFTs. Ensure adequately hydrated.

CLIENT/FAMILY TEACHING

1. Foscarnet is not a cure; may continue to experience progression of condition during or following treatment.
2. Report if sore throat, swollen lymph nodes, fatigue, fever and other S&S of infection occur.
3. Consume plenty of fluids and good hygiene to help reduce risk of genital irritation or ulceration.
4. Report any evidence of numbness of the extremities, loss of sensation, or oral tingling as these are symptoms of hypocalcemia. Stop infusion, and notify provider to correct imbalance before resuming the infusion.
5. Keep all F/U for eye exams, response, adverse SE.

OUTCOMES/EVALUATE

- Ophthalmic evidence of successful treatment of CMV retinitis
- Treatment of acyclovir-resistant mucocutaneous HSV infections

Fosinopril sodium

(foh-**SIN**-oh-prill)

Classification(s): Antihypertensive, ACE inhibitor

Pregnancy Category: D (Category C the first trimester and Category D the second and third trimesters)

RX: Monopril.

SEE ALSO ***ANGIOTENSIN-CONVERTING ENZYME INHIBITORS***.

INDICATIONS/USES

(1) Alone or in combination with other antihypertensive agents (especially thiazide diuretics) to treat hypertension. Diabetic hypertensive clients show a reduction in major CV events. (2) Treat CHF as adjunctive therapy when added to conventional therapy, including diuretics with or without digoxin.

ACTION/KINETICS

Action

Fosinopril inhibits angiotensin-converting enzyme resulting in decreased plasma angiotensin II, which leads to decreased vasopressor activity and decreased aldosterone secretion.

Pharmacokinetics

About 36% bioavailable. **Onset:** 1 hr. **Time to peak serum levels:** 3 hr. Metabolized in the liver to the active fosinoprilat. **Peak effect:** 2–6 hr. **t½:** 11.5 hr for fosinoprilat (prolonged in impaired renal function) following IV administration. **t½** is 14 hr in those with CHF. **Duration:** 24 hr. Approximately 50% excreted through the urine and 50% in the feces. In those with end-stage renal disease (C_{CR} <10 mL/min) or hepatic insufficiency (e.g., alcoholic or biliary cirrhosis), the total body clearance is about half of that in clients with healthy renal or hepatic function. Food decreases the rate, but not the extent, of absorption of fosinopril. **Plasma protein binding:** More than 99%.

CONTRAINDICATIONS

Hypersensitivity to any component of the product. Clients with a history of angioedema following previous treatment with an ACE inhibitor. Use during lactation.

SPECIAL CONCERNS

■ When used in pregnancy during the second and third trimesters, ACE inhibitors can cause injury and even death to the developing fetus. When pregnancy is detected, discontinue as soon as possible. ■

May be a profound drop in BP following the first dose.

SIDE EFFECTS

Most Common

Dizziness, headache, hypotension, chest pain, fatigue, diarrhea, URTI.

CV: Orthostatic hypotension, hyper-/hypotension, chest pain, bradycardia, rhythm disturbances, angina pectoris, ***CVA, MI***, palpitations, tachycardia, ***cardiac arrest, hypertensive crisis***, claudication, conduction disorder, ***cerebral infarction, cardiorespiratory arrest, shock***, TIA. **CNS:** Dizziness, confusion, depression, headache, insomnia, sleep disturbances, paresthesias, somnolence, drowsiness, vertigo, memory disturbance, tremor, mood change, numbness, behavior change. **GI:** N&V, constipation, diarrhea, dry mouth, ***pancreatitis***, dysphagia, abdominal distention, flatulence, heartburn, appetite/weight change. **Hepatic:** Hepatitis, hepatomegaly, ***hepatic failure***, hepatocellular or cholestatic jaundice. **Respiratory:** Cough (may be chronic), bronchospasm, dyspnea, pharyngitis, rhinitis, sinusitis, URTI, pleuritic chest pain, tracheobronchitis, abnormal breathing, sinus abnormalities, laryngitis, hoarseness, epistaxis, symptom complex of cough, bronchospasm, and eosinophilia. **Dermatologic:** Diaphoresis, hyperhidrosis, sweating, exfoliative dermatitis, flushing, pemphigus/pemphigoid, photosensitivity, pruritus, rash, urticaria. **GU:** Decreased libido, renal insufficiency, urinary frequency, abnormal urination, kidney pain, sexual dysfunction. **Musculoskeletal:** Arthralgia, arthritis, muscle cramps/ache, myalgia, musculoskeletal pain, swelling/weakness of extremities. **Hematologic:** Anemia, eosinophilia, lymphadenopathy, neutropenia, leukopenia. **Ophthalmic:** Vision disturbance, eye irritation. **Otic:** Tinnitis. **Body as a whole:** Fatigue, ***angioedema***, fever, edema, influenza, cold sensation, pain, syncope, weakness, ***sudden death***. **Miscellaneous:** Taste disturbance, fall, gout, abnormal vocalization.

LABORATORY TEST CONSIDERATIONS

↑ Serum potassium, LDH, alkaline phosphatase. Transient ↓ H&H. False low measurement of serum digoxin levels with DigiTab RIA Kit for Digoxin.

HOW SUPPLIED

Tablets: 10 mg, 20 mg, 40 mg.

DOSAGE

TABLETS

Hypertension.

Initial: 10 mg once daily; **then,** adjust dose depending on BP response at peak (2–6 hr after dosing) and trough (24 hr after dosing) blood levels. **Maintenance:** Usually 20–40 mg/day, although some clients manifest beneficial effects at doses up to 80 mg.

In clients taking diuretics.

Symptomatic hypotension may occur following the initial dose. To reduce this possibility, discontinue diuretic

2–3 days before starting fosinopril. If diuretic cannot be discontinued, use an initial dose of 10 mg fosinopril.

Congestive heart failure.

Initial: 10 mg once daily; **then,** following initial dose, observe the client for at least 2 hr for the presence of hypotension or orthostasis (if either is present, monitor until BP stabilizes). An initial dose of 5 mg is recommended in heart failure with moderate to severe renal failure or in those who have had significant diuresis. Increase the dose over several weeks, not to exceed a maximum of 40 mg daily (usual effective range is 20–40 mg once daily).

NURSING IMPLICATIONS

Do not confuse Monopril with minoxidil (an antihypertensive).

IMPLEMENTATION/ADMINISTRATION/STORAGE

1. If antihypertensive effect decreases at end of dosing interval with once-daily dosing, consider twice a day administration.
2. If also taking a diuretic, discontinue diuretic 2–3 days prior to beginning fosinopril therapy. If BP not controlled, restart diuretic. If the diuretic cannot be discontinued, give an initial dose of 10 mg fosinopril.
3. Fosinopril given with potassium supplements, potassium salt substitutes, or potassium-sparing diuretics can lead to increases of serum potassium. Use together cautiously if at all.
4. Do not adjust the dose of fosinopril in renal insufficiency.
5. Store from 15–30°C (59–86°F). Protect from moisture by keeping bottle tightly closed.

ASSESSMENT

1. Note disease onset, other agents trialed, outcome.
2. With heart failure monitor weights and edema noting any worsening of condition.
3. Monitor BP, CBC, BNP, electrolytes, microalbumin, renal and LFTs.

CLIENT/FAMILY TEACHING

1. Take as directed with or without food. BP control does not exceed 24 hr; take at same time(s) each day.
2. May initially cause dizziness and lightheadedness; use care. Change positions slowly to avoid sudden drop in BP.
3. Avoid dehydration, use caution in hot weather and with increased exercise.
4. Record BP and HR at different times during the day several times per week for provider review.
5. With CHF, keep record of daily weights; report weight gain >2 lb/day or 5 lb/wk or if edema or shortness of breath worsen.
6. Avoid OTC agents without provider approval; salt substitutes containing potassium should be avoided.
7. Avoid exposure to UV light (sunlight, tanning booths), and use sunscreen/protective clothing when exposed to prevent photosensitivity reaction.
8. Use reliable contraception. Stop drug, and report if pregnancy suspected.
9. Report adverse side effects, especially S&S infection, sore throat, swelling of hands and feet, chest pain, SOB, mouth sores, unusual bruising/bleeding, irregular heartbeat, or persistent cough.
10. Continue lifestyle changes aimed at controlling BP; salt/fat restriction, regular exercise, weight reduction, and smoking/alcohol cessation.
11. Keep all F/U to assess response, labs, adverse SE.

OUTCOMES/EVALUATE

Control of BP/CHF

IV

Fosphenytoin sodium

(**FOS**-fen-ih-toyn)

Classification(s): Anticonvulsant, hydantoin

Pregnancy Category: D

RX: Cerebyx.

SEE ALSO ***ANTICONVULSANTS*** AND ***PHENYTOIN***.

INDICATIONS/USES

Short-term parenteral use for the control of generalized convulsive status epilepticus and prophylaxis and treatment of seizures occurring during neurosurgery. It can be substituted, short term, for PO phenytoin when PO administration is not possible.

ACTION/KINETICS

Action

Fosphenytoin is a prodrug of phenytoin; thus, its anticonvulsant effects are due to phenytoin. For every millimole of fosphenytoin administered, 1 mmol of phenytoin is produced. Fosphenytoin is better tolerated at the infusion site than is phenytoin (i.e., pain and burning associated with IV phenytoin is decreased).

F

Pharmacokinetics

t½ plasma, fosphenytoin: 15 min after IV infusion. **Peak plasma levels, after IM:** 30 min; **after IV:** 30–60 min after end of infusion. Typical therapeutic plasma total phenytoin levels are 10–20 mcg/mL (unbound phenytoin levels of 1–2 mcg/mL). Fosphenytoin displaces phenytoin from plasma protein binding sites. The IV infusion rate for fosphenytoin is three times faster than for IV phenytoin. IM use results in systemic phenytoin concentrations that are similar to PO phenytoin, thus allowing interchangeable use. Phenytoin derived from fosphenytoin is extensively metabolized in the liver and excreted in the urine. **Plasma protein binding:** 95–99%.

CONTRAINDICATIONS

Hypersensitivity to fosphenytoin, phenytoin, or other hydantoins. Use in clients with sinus bradycardia, SA block, second- and third-degree AV block, and Adams-Stokes syndrome. Use to treat absence seizures. Use during lactation.

SPECIAL CONCERNS

- **Safety and efficacy of fosphenytoin not determined for longer than 5 days.**
- **Use in children is investigational.**
- **Lower or less frequent dosing in the elderly may be appropriate.**
- **After administration of fosphenytoin to those with renal and/or hepatic dysfunction or in those with hypoalbuminemia, fosphenytoin clearance to phenytoin may be increased without a similar increase in phenytoin clearance, thus increasing the potential for serious side effects.**

SIDE EFFECTS

Most Common

Ataxia, dizziness, headache, nystagmus, paresthesia, pruritus, tinnitus, somnolence.

CNS: Dizziness, nystagmus, ataxia, somnolence, extrapyramidal syndrome, headache, incoordination, stupor, paresthesia, agitation, tremor, brain edema, dysarthria, hypesthesia, decreased reflexes, vertigo, CNS depression, insomnia, mental confusion, motor twitching, nervousness, intracranial hypertension, increased reflexes, speech disorder, abnormal thinking, acute brain syndrome, akathisia, amnesia, aphasia, positive Babinski sign, brain edema, circumoral paresthesia, coma, convulsion, depersonalization, depression, emotional lability, encephalitis, encephalopathy, hemiplegia, hyperesthesia, hyperkinesia, hypokinesis, hypotonia, meningitis, myoclonus, neurosis, paralysis, personality disorder, psychosis, subdural hostility. **GI:** N&V, dry mouth, tongue disorder/edema, diarrhea, constipation, anorexia, dyspepsia, dysphagia, flatulence, gastritis, ***GI hemorrhage***, ileus, increased salivation, abnormal LFTs, tenesmus. **CV:** Hypotension, vasodilation, tachycardia, ***CV collapse***, hypertension, atrial flutter, BBB, ***cardiac arrest***, cardiomegaly, ***cerebral hemorrhage***, cerebral infarct, CHF, migraine, palpitation, postural hypotension, ***pulmonary embolus***, prolonged QT interval, sinus bradycardia, syncope, thrombophlebitis, ventricular extrasystoles, hematoma. **Dermatologic:** Pruritus, ecchymosis, skin rash, contact dermatitis, maculopapular rash, pustular rash, skin discoloration, skin nodule, sweating, urticaria. **Musculoskeletal:** Myasthenia, arthralgia, leg cramps, myalgia, myopathy. **GU:** Dysuria, genital edema, kidney failure, oliguria, polyuria, urethral pain, urinary incontinence/retention, vaginitis, vaginal moniliasis. **Respiratory:** Pneumonia, apnea, aspiration pneumonia, asthma, atelectasis, bronchitis, increased cough, dyspnea, epistaxis, hemoptysis, hyperventilation, hypoxia, pharyngitis, pneumothorax, rhinitis, sinusitis, increased sputum. **Hematologic:** Leukopenia, lymphadenopathy, thrombocytopenia, anemia, cyanosis, hypochromic anemia, leukocytosis, petechia. **Metabolic:** Diabetes insipidus, facial edema, acidosis, alkalosis, dehydration, generalized edema, ketosis. **At injection site:** Inflammation, tenderness, pain, edema, hemorrhage. **Ophthalmic:** Amblyopia, diplopia, conjunctivitis, eye pain, mydriasis, photophobia, visual field defect. **Otic:** Deafness, tinnitus, ear pain, hyperacusis. **Body as a whole:** Asthenia, fever, chills, infection, flu syndrome, malaise, sepsis, ***shock***, accidental injury. **Miscellaneous:** Back/pelvic pain, taste perversion/loss, parosmia, cachexia, cryptococcus, photosensitivity.

LABORATORY TEST CONSIDERATIONS

See *Phenytoin.* Alters LFTs. ↑ blood glucose values, and ↓ PBI values. ↑ Gamma globulins. Phenytoin ↓ immunoglobulins A and G. False + Coombs' test.

OVERDOSE MANAGEMENT

Symptoms: N&V, ***cardiac dysrhythmia or arrest***, hypotension, syncope, hypocalcemia, metabolic acidosis, ***death.*** *Treatment:* See *Phenytoin.*

DRUG INTERACTIONS

See *Phenytoin.*

HOW SUPPLIED

NOTE: Doses of fosphenytoin are expressed as phenytoin sodium equivalents (PE = phenytoin sodium equivalent) to avoid the need to perform molecular weight adjustments when converting between fosphenytoin and phenytoin sodium doses.

Injection Solution, Concentrate: 75 mg/mL (equivalent to phenytoin sodium 50 mg/mL).

DOSAGE

IV

Seizures.

Adults, loading dose: Phenytoin equivalent 15–20 mg/kg given IV at phenytoin equivalent 100–150 mg/min. **Maintenance:** The initial maintenance dose/day is phenytoin sodium equivalent 4–6 mg/kg/day. The loading dose is followed by maintenance doses of either fosphenytoin or phenytoin, either PO or parenterally.

IM; IV

Prevention of seizures during neurosurgery.

Adults, loading dose: 10–20 mg PE/kg given IM or IV at a rate of 100–150 mg PE/min. **Maintenance:** 4–6 mg PE/kg/day.

Status epilepticus in children (investigational).

Loading dose for neonates: PE 15–24 mg/kg. Phenobarbital or a benzodiazepine may be preferable in this age group. **Loading dose for infants and children:** PE 15–20 mg/kg given IV.

Maintenance for seizure disorder in children (investigational).

Infants and children, initial dosage: PE 5 mg/kg IM or IV divided 2–3 times a day. Follow with usual dosage within 24 hr. **Usual dosage: Neonates (30 days of age and younger):** PE 4–8 mg/kg IM or IV divided 2–3 times a day; **6 months–3 years of age:** PE 8–10 mg IM or IV divided 2–3 times a day; **4–6 years of age:** PE 7.5–9 mg/kg IM or IV divided 2–3 times a day; **7–9 years of age:** PE 7–8 mg/kg IM or IV divided 2–3 times a day; **10–16 years of age:** PE 6–7 mg/kg IM or IV divided 2–3 times a day.

F

NURSING IMPLICATIONS

Do not confuse Cerebyx with Celebrex (nonsteroidal anti-inflammatory drug) or with Celexa (an antidepressant).

IMPLEMENTATION/ADMINISTRATION/STORAGE

1. Fosphenytoin can be substituted for PO phenytoin sodium therapy at the same total daily dose. Always prescribe and dispense in phenytoin sodium equivalent units.
2. Phenytoin capsules as Dilantin are approximately 90% bioavailable by the PO route and fosphenytoin (available as Cerebyx) is 100% bioavailable by both the IM and IV routes. Plasma phenytoin may increase modestly when IM or IV fosphenytoin (as Cerebyx) is substituted for PO phenytoin sodium therapy.
3. If rapid phenytoin loading is the primary goal, IV fosphenytoin is preferred because the time to achieve therapeutic plasma levels is greater following IM administration than IV administration.
4. If administration of fosphenytoin does not terminate seizures, consider use of other anticonvulsants and other appropriate measures.
5. Do not use IM fosphenytoin to treat status epilepticus, because therapeutic phenytoin concentrations may not be reached as quickly as with IV administration.
6. Phenytoin levels should be monitored only after conversion to phenytoin is essentially complete about 2 hr after the end of IV infusion and 4 hr after IM injection.

7. Do not abruptly discontinue fosphenytoin, because of the possibility of increased seizure frequency, including status epilepticus. If there is a need to reduce the dose or discontinue the drug, substitute an alternative antiepileptic medication gradually.
8. Do not use vials that develop particulate matter.
9. Do not store at room temperature for more than 48 hr. Store under refrigeration at 2–8°C (36–46°F).
10. IV Prior to IV infusion fosphenytoin must be diluted in D5W or NSS solution to obtain a concentration ranging from 1.5 to 25 mg/PE (phenytoin sodium equivalents)/mL.
11. Due to risk of hypotension, do not administer at a rate greater than 150 PE/min.
12. Because the full antiepileptic effect of phenytoin (given as either fosphenytoin or parenteral phenytoin) is not known immediately, other measures to control status epilepticus (e.g., use of an IV benzodiazepine) will be necessary.
13. COMPATIBILITY D5W or NSS.
14. INCOMPATIBILITY Administer separately.

ASSESSMENT

1. Note type, onset, characteristics of seizures; identify reasons for short-term substitution for oral phenytoin. List other agents trialed, outcome.
2. Fosphenytoin converts to phenytoin and may be administered IV or IM; prescribed and dispensed in PE units.
3. During IV administration, continuously monitor ECG, BP, and respirations.
4. Do not use with bradycardia or heart block; may cause atrial and ventricular conduction depression.
5. Monitor ECG, albumin, CBC, renal and LFTs. The waiting period before ordering laboratory tests for phenytoin plasma levels is 2 hr following IV infusion and 4 hr following IM injection. Periodically measure plasma phenytoin levels in the management of pregnant women.

CLIENT/FAMILY TEACHING

1. Review goals of therapy; drug is for short-term use of seizure control.
2. Report fever, sore throat, bruising/bleeding, rash, jaundice, slurred speech, joint pain, N&V, severe headaches, swollen lymph glands.
3. Use caution with activities that require alertness; may experience dizziness and drowsiness, itching, tingling of groin and face. Presence of REMs, gait and speech impairment may indicate toxicity.
4. If rash appears, stop therapy and report. If mild, therapy may resume once rash has cleared. If rash recurs, do not reuse this class of drugs.
5. Practice reliable contraception; use additional nonhormonal form during therapy and until next menstrual cycle.
6. Avoid alcohol or other CNS drugs.
7. Never suddenly stop drug without reporting; may lead to status epilepticus.
8. Keep all F/U to assess response, labs, adverse SE.

OUTCOMES/EVALUATE

- Control of seizures
- Seizure prophylaxis with surgery
- Short-term substitution for PO phenytoin

Frovatriptan succinate

(**froh**-vah-**TRIP**-tan)

Classification(s): Antimigraine drug

Pregnancy Category: C

RX: Frova.

INDICATIONS/USES

Acute treatment of migraine, with or without aura, in adults. Use only where a clear diagnosis of migraine has been established.

ACTION/KINETICS

Action

Frovatriptan is a selective $5\text{-HT}_{1B/1D}$ receptor agonist, which binds with high affinity to 5-HT_{1B} and 5-HT_{1D} receptors. Believed to act on extracerebral, intracranial arteries to cause constriction and to inhibit excessive dilation of these vessels in migraine.

Pharmacokinetics

From 29.6% (2.5 mg PO) to 17.5% (40 mg PO) bioavailable. **Maximum blood levels:** 2–4 hr. **Time to onset of action:** 2–3 hr. **Time to peak effect:** 2–4 hr. Food has no significant effect on bioavailability but delays the maximum levels by 1 hr. Metabolized in the liver with about ⅓ unchanged drug and metabolites excreted in the urine and ⅔ in the feces. **t½, mean terminal:** 25.7–29.7 hr, depending on the dose. **Plasma protein binding:** About 15%.

CONTRAINDICATIONS

Use for prophylaxis of migraine or use in management of hemiplegic or basilar migraine. Use in those with ischemic heart disease (e.g., angina pectoris, history of MI, documented silent ischemia) or in those who have symptoms or findings consistent with ischemic heart disease, coronary artery vasospasm (including Prinzmetal's variant angina), or other significant underlying CV disease. Use in those with CV syndromes, including (but not limited to) strokes of any type as well as TIAs. Use in those with peripheral vascular disease (including, but not limited to ischemic bowel disease), uncontrolled hypertension, use within 24 hr of treatment with another 5-HT_1 agonist or an ergotamine-containing or ergot-type medication (e.g., dihydroergotamine, methysergide), or in those hypersensitive to frovatriptan or any ingredients of the product. Use in those with documented ischemic or vasospastic CAD or in whom unrecognized CAD is predicted by the presence of risk factors (e.g., hypertension, hypercholesterolemia, smoking, obesity, diabetes, strong history of CAD, females with surgical or physiological menopause, or males over 40 years of age) unless a CV evaluation provides evidence that the client is reasonably free of CAD and ischemic myocardial disease. Use in children less than 18 years of age.

SPECIAL CONCERNS

- **Use with caution during lactation.**
- **Safety and efficacy not established for use in children less than 18 years of age or for cluster headaches (present in an older, predominantly male population).**

SIDE EFFECTS

Most Common

Palpitations, dysesthesia, hypesthesia, insomnia, anxiety, increased sweating, N&V, abdominal pain, diarrhea, sinusitis, rhinitis, abnormal vision, tinnitus, pain.

GI: Dry mouth, dyspepsia, vomiting, abdominal pain, diarrhea, dysphagia, flatulence, constipation, anorexia, esophagospasm, increased salivation. **CNS:** Dizziness, paresthesia, headache, dysesthesia, hypoesthesia, tremor, hyperesthesia, aggravated migraine, vertigo, ataxia, abnormal gait, speech disorder, insomnia, anxiety, confusion, nervousness, agitation, euphoria, impaired concentration, depression, emotional lability, amnesia, abnormal thinking, depersonalization. **CV:** ***Acute MI, life-threatening disturbances of cardiac rhythm, death, cerebral hemorrhage, subarachnoid hemorrhage, stroke, ventricular fibrillation***, coronary artery vasospasm, transient myocardial ischemia, ventricular tachycardia, peripheral vascular ischemia, colonic ischemia (with abdominal pain and bloody diarrhea), hypertension, palpitations, tachycardia, abnormal ECG. **Body as a whole:** Fatigue, flushing, hot or cold sensation, pain, asthenia, rigors, fever, hot flashes, malaise, dehydration, syncope. **Musculoskeletal:** Skeletal pain, involuntary muscle contraction, myalgia, back pain, arthralgia, arthrosis, leg cramps, muscle weakness. **Respiratory:** Sinusitis, rhinitis, pharyngitis, dyspnea, hyperventilation, laryngitis, epistaxis. **Dermatologic:** Increased sweating, pruritis, bullous eruption. **GU:** Frequent micturition, polyuria. **Ophthalmic:** Abnormal vision, eye pain, conjunctivitis, abnormal lacrimation. **Otic:** Tinnitus, earache, hyperacusis. **Miscellaneous:** Chest pain, thirst, taste perversion. Sensations of pain, tightness, pressure, and heaviness in the chest, throat, neck, and jaw.

DRUG INTERACTIONS

Dihydroergotamine / Prolonged vasospastic reaction; do not use within 24 hr of each other
Ergotamine / Frovatriptan maximum levels and AUC ↓ 25%
Methysergide / Prolonged vasospastic reaction; do not use within 24 hr of each other
Oral contraceptives / Frovatriptan maximum levels and AUC ↑ 30%
Propranolol / ↑ Frovatriptan maximum levels and AUC
Selective serotonin reuptake inhibitors / Possible weakness, hyperreflexia, incoordination

HOW SUPPLIED

Tablets: 2.5 mg (as base).

DOSAGE

TABLETS

Migraine headache.

Adults: Single dose of 2.5 mg taken with fluids. If the headache recurs after initial relief, a second tablet (2.5 mg) may be taken provided there is an interval of at least 2 hr between doses. Do not exceed a total daily dose of 3 tablets (7.5 mg).

NURSING IMPLICATIONS

IMPLEMENTATION/ADMINISTRATION/STORAGE

1. If first dose does not produce response, reconsider diagnosis of migraine before giving a second dose. There is no evidence that a second dose is effective in clients who do not respond to a first dose.
2. The safety of treating an average of 4 migraine attacks in a 30-day period has not been determined.
3. Store at controlled room temperature of 15–30°C (59–86°F). Protect from moisture and light.

ASSESSMENT

1. Note reasons for therapy, onset, family history, characteristics of symptoms, location, intensity, duration, and associated symptoms of migraine attack as well as other agents trialed, outcome.
2. Ensure not hemiplegic or basilar type of migraine headaches. Review neurologist reports/findings.
3. List drugs currently prescribed to ensure none interact.
4. Assess for CAD, uncontrolled HTN, circulation problems, IBD, or history of CVA/TIAs. Review risk of severe cardiovascular and cerebrovascular events associated with drug therapy.
5. Obtain ECG; give first dose in the office and assess client for adverse effects.
6. Determine renal and LFTs; evaluate for dysfunction.

CLIENT/FAMILY TEACHING

1. Take as soon as symptoms of migraine headache appears; do not use for other types of headaches. Never share medications with others no matter what the symptoms.
2. If headache returns, may repeat dose in 2 hours; do not exceed 3 tablets (7.5 mg) in 24 hr. Use only during migraine does not prevent or reduce the number of attacks. Continue migraine prophylactic meds as prescribed. Lying down in a quiet, darkened room may help alleviate headache.
3. Use caution if driving or performing activities that require mental alertness; may cause dizziness, fatigue, or drowsiness.
4. Store in a safe place and away from heat, light, and moisture. Do not take within 24 hr of taking any other ergotamine or serotonin receptor agonist type headache medicine.
5. Drug acts to shrink swollen blood vessels surrounding the brain that cause migraine headaches. Keep a headache diary, and identify factors/foods/events that surround migraine headaches.
6. Avoid known triggers, i.e., chocolate, cheese, citrus fruit, caffeine, alcohol, missing sleep/meals, etc.
7. Report any chest pain, SOB, palpitations, rash/itching, heaviness in chest, throat, neck, or jaw or unusual side effects, intolerance, or lack of response.
8. Avoid exposure to sunlight/tanning lamps; use sunscreen/protective clothing to prevent photosensitivity reaction.
9. Keep all F/U to assess response and adverse SE.

OUTCOMES/EVALUATE

Resolution of acute migraine attack

■ IV ℭ 📷

Furosemide

(fur-**OH**-seh-myd)

Classification(s): Diuretic, loop

Pregnancy Category: C

RX: Lasix.

🍁 **Rx:** Apo-Furosemide, Lasix Special.

SEE ALSO ***DIURETICS, LOOP***.

INDICATIONS/USES

IV, PO. Use in adults and children to treat edema associated with CHF, renal disease (including nephrotic syndrome), and hepatic cirrhosis. Is especially useful when a drug with greater diuretic activity is desired. **IV.** Adjunctive therapy in acute pulmonary edema. Indicated when a rapid onset of diuresis is desired. **PO.** Treat hypertension alone or in conjunction with other diuretics *except* ethacrynic acid. *Investigational:* Pediatric hypertension. Dyspnea in cancer clients (nebulized furosemide).

ACTION/KINETICS

Action

Inhibits the reabsorption of sodium and chloride in the proximal and distal tubules as well as the ascending loop of Henle; this results in the excretion of sodium, chloride, and, to a lesser degree, potassium and bicarbonate ions. The resulting urine is more acid. Diuretic action is independent of changes in clients' acid-base balance. Has a slight antihypertensive effect.

Pharmacokinetics

Onset: PO, IM: 30–60 min; **IV:** 5 min. **Peak: PO, IM:** 1–2 hr; **IV:** 20–60 min. **t½:** About 2 hr after PO use. **Duration: PO, IM:** 6–8 hr; **IV:** 2 hr. Metabolized in the liver and excreted through the urine. May be effective for clients resistant to thiazides and for those with reduced GFRs.

CONTRAINDICATIONS

Never use with ethacrynic acid. Anuria, hypersensitivity to drug, severe renal disease associated with azotemia and oliguria, hepatic coma associated with electrolyte depletion. Lactation.

SPECIAL CONCERNS

■ Furosemide is a potent diuretic which, if given in excessive amounts, can lead to profound diuresis with water and electrolyte depletion. Therefore, careful medical attention is required and dose and schedule must be adjusted to the individual client's needs. ■

- **Use with caution in premature infants and neonates due to prolonged half-life; extend the dosing interval.**
- **Geriatric clients may be more sensitive to the usual adult dose.**
- **Allergic reactions may be seen in those hypersensitive to sulfonamides.**

SIDE EFFECTS

Most Common

Jaundice, tinnitus, hearing impairment, hypotension, water/electrolyte depletion, pancreatitis, abdominal pain, dizziness, anemia.

Electrolyte and fluid effects: Fluid and electrolyte depletion leading to dehydration, hypovolemia, thromboembolism. Hypokalemia and hypochloremia may cause metabolic alkalosis. Hyperuricemia, azotemia, hyponatremia. **GI:** Nausea, oral and gastric irritation, abdominal pain, vomiting, anorexia, diarrhea (especially in children) or constipation, cramps, pancreatitis, jaundice, ischemic hepatitis. **Otic:** Tinnitus, hearing impairment (may be reversible or permanent), reversible deafness (usually following rapid IV or IM administration of high doses). **CNS:** Vertigo, headache, dizziness, blurred vision, restlessness, paresthesias, xanthopsia. **CV:** Orthostatic hypotension, thrombophlebitis, chronic aortitis. **Hematologic:** Anemia, thrombocytopenia, neutropenia, leukopenia, ***agranulocytosis***, purpura. ***Rarely, aplastic anemia***. **Allergic:** Rashes, pruritus, urticaria, photosensitivity, exfoliative dermatitis, vasculitis, erythema multiforme. **Miscellaneous:** Interstitial nephritis, fever, weakness, hyperglycemia, glycosuria, exacerbation/aggravation/worsening of SLE, increased perspiration, muscle spasms, urinary bladder spasm, urinary frequency.

Following IV use: Thrombophlebitis, ***cardiac arrest***.

Following IM use: Pain and irritation at injection site, ***cardiac arrest***. Because this drug is resistant to the effects of pressor amines and potentiates the effects of muscle relaxants, it is recommended that the PO drug be discontinued 1 week before surgery and the IV drug 2 days before surgery.

OVERDOSE MANAGEMENT

Symptoms: Profound water loss, electrolyte depletion (manifested by weakness, anorexia, vomiting, lethargy, cramps, mental confusion, dizziness), decreased blood volume, ***circulatory collapse (possibly vascular thrombosis and embolism)***. *Treatment:* Replace fluid and electrolytes. Monitor urine electrolyte output and serum electrolytes. Induce emesis or perform gastric lavage. Oxygen or artificial respiration may be needed. Treat symptoms.

ADDITIONAL DRUG INTERACTIONS

Charcoal / ↓ Absorption of furosemide from GI tract
Clofibrate / Enhanced diuretic effect
Hydantoins / ↓ Diuretic effect of furosemide
Propranolol / ↑ Plasma propranolol levels

HOW SUPPLIED

Injection: 10 mg /mL; *Oral Solution:* 10 mg/mL, 40 mg/5 mL; *Tablets:* 20 mg, 40 mg, 80 mg.

DOSAGE

IM; IV

Edema.

Adults, initial: 20–40 mg given as a single dose IM or slowly IV over 1–2 min; if response inadequate after 2 hr another dose may be given or an increased dose of 20 mg given no sooner than 2 hr after the previous dose until the desired diuretic effect is observed. **Maintenance:** Individualized; a single dose given once or twice daily. **Pediatric, initial:** 1 mg/kg given slowly IM or IV; if response inadequate after 2 hr, increase dose by 1 mg/kg until the desired effect is observed, up to a maximum of 6 mg/kg. Do not exceed a dose of 1 mg/kg/day for premature infants.

F

IV

Acute pulmonary edema.

Adults: 40 mg slowly over 1–2 min; if response inadequate after 1 hr, give 80 mg slowly over 1–2 min. Concomitant oxygen and digitalis may be used.

ORAL SOLUTION; TABLETS

Edema.

Adults, initial: 20–80 mg/day as a single dose. For resistant cases, dosage can be increased by 20–40 mg q 6–8 hr until desired diuretic response is attained. **Maintenance:** Individualized and given once or twice a day. **Maximum daily dose:** Do not exceed 600 mg. **Pediatric, initial:** 2 mg/kg as a single dose; **then** dose can be increased by 1–2 mg/kg q 6–8 hr until desired response is attained (up to 6 mg/kg may be required in children with nephrotic syndrome; maximum dose should not exceed 6 mg/kg). A dose range of 0.5–2 mg/kg twice a day has also been recommended. **Maintenance:** Individualized to the minimum effective level. *NOTE:* Dosing may be most efficient and edema safely mobilized if administered on 2 to 4 consecutive days each week.

Hypertension.

Adults, initial: 40 mg twice a day. Adjust dosage depending on response. If response is unsatisfactory, add other antihypertensive medication(s).

Pediatric hypertension (investigational).

Children: 0.5–2 mg/kg/dose once or twice daily. **Maximum daily dose:** 6 mg/kg. *NOTE:* There are safety concerns with this use.

NURSING IMPLICATIONS

(Sound Alike Drug) Do not confuse Lasix with Lanoxin (a cardiac glycoside), or furosemide with torsemide (diuretic).

IMPLEMENTATION/ADMINISTRATION/STORAGE

1. Give 2–4 consecutive days per week.
2. Food decreases bioavailability of furosemide and ultimately the degree of diuresis.
3. Slight discoloration resulting from light does not affect potency. However, do not dispense discolored tablets or injection.
4. If used with other antihypertensives, reduce dose of other agents by at least 50% when furosemide is added in order to prevent an excessive drop in BP.
5. Store the oral solution and tablets in light-resistant containers at room temperature (15–30°C or 59–86°F). Discard opened oral solution after 60 days; protect from light.
6. In CHF or chronic renal failure, oral and parenteral doses of 2–2.5 grams/day (or higher) are well tolerated.
7. IV Give IV injections slowly over 1–2 min.
8. If high-dose parenteral therapy is prescribed, add furosemide to either NaCl Injection, Lactated Ringer's Injection, or D5W injection after the pH has been adjusted to above 5.5. Do not use if the solution is discolored.
9. Store injection from 15–30°C (59–86°F); protect from light.
10. COMPATIBILITY After pH adjustment, furosemide can be mixed with NaCl injection, RL injection, and D5W and infused at a rate not to exceed 4 mg/min, to prevent ototoxicity.
11. INCOMPATIBILITY Do not mix with solutions with a pH below 5.5. A precipitate may form if mixed with ciprofloxacin, gentamicin, netilmicin, or milrinone in either D5W or NSS.

ASSESSMENT

1. Note reasons for therapy, clinical presentation, other agents trialed, outcome. When more than 40 mg/day is required, give in divided doses, i.e., 40 mg PO twice a day (7 a.m. and 3 p.m.)
2. With renal impairment or if receiving other ototoxic drugs, observe for ototoxicity.

3. Assess closely for signs of vascular thrombosis and embolism, particularly in the elderly. With history of gout, monitor uric acid levels.
4. With rapid diuresis, observe for dehydration and circulatory collapse; monitor BP and pulse.
5. With chronic use, assess for thiamine deficiency. If used with Zaroxolyn, assess for low phosphate levels as well as electrolyte imbalance.
6. Monitor BP, weight, edema, breath sounds, I&O, electrolytes, Mg^{++}, Ca^{++}, uric acid, CO_2; observe for S&S of hypokalemia. Assess for blood dyscrasia and liver damage.

CLIENT/FAMILY TEACHING

1. Take in the morning on an empty stomach to enhance absorption, and avoid interruption of sleep from frequent urination. May take with food or milk if GI upset. Time administration to participate in social activities.
2. Drug may cause BP drop. Change positions slowly from lying to standing. Avoid alcohol, and do not exercise heavily in hot weather.
3. Refrigerate solution. Sorbitol in the solution may result in diarrhea, especially in children.
4. Consult provider before taking excessive aspirin for any reason. Salicylate intoxication occurs at lower levels than normal because of competition at the renal excretory sites.
5. Use sunscreens and protective clothing when sun exposed, to minimize the effects of drug-induced photosensitivity.
6. Management of end stage heart disease requires diligent monitoring, management, and titration on provider and client part; keep all visits and report any changes or adverse effects.
7. Record BP and weights; report any gains of >2 lb per day or >5 lb per week.
8. Supplement diet with vegetables and fruits that are high in potassium (bananas, oranges, peaches, dried dates) if oral supplements are not prescribed. Those on a salt-restricted diet should not increase salt intake; NSAIDs and alpha-blockers may also cause sodium retention. May increase blood glucose levels.
9. Immediately report any muscle pain/weakness/cramps, dizziness, ringing in the ears/hearing loss, sore throat, fever, severe abdominal pain, numbness, or tingling, persistent nausea or vomiting, diarrhea, excessive thirst, unexplained tiredness, drowsiness, feeling of the room spinning, confusion or changes in thinking, increased heart rate, or unexplained joint pain.
10. Keep all F/U visits to assess response, labs, and for adverse SE.

OUTCOMES/EVALUATE

- Enhanced diuresis; ↓ BP
- Resolution of pulmonary edema
- ↓ Edema associated with CHF, hepatic cirrhosis, and renal disease

G

Gabapentin

(**gab**-ah-**PEN**-tin)

Classification(s): Anticonvulsant, miscellaneous

Pregnancy Category: C

RX: Gabarone, Gralise, Neurontin.

✤ **Rx:** Apo-Gabapentin, CO Gabapentin, Gen-Gabapentin, Novo-Gabapentin, PMS-Gabapentin, ratio-Gabapentin.

Gabapentin enacarbil

Pregnancy Category: C

RX: Horizant.

SEE ALSO ***ANTICONVULSANTS***.

INDICATIONS/USES

(1) Treatment of partial seizures with and without secondary generalization in clients 12 years and older. (2) Adjunct to treat partial seizures in children 3–12 years of age. (3) In adults, management of postherpetic neuralgia or pain in the area affected by herpes zoster after treating the disease. (4) **Gralise:** Treatment of postherpetic neuralgia. (5)

Horizant: Treatment of adults with moderate to severe primary restless legs syndrome. *Investigational:* Neuropathic pain, bipolar disorder, prevent migraine, tremors associated with MS. With morphine to treat diabetic neuropathy or postherpetic neuralgia.

ACTION/KINETICS

Action

Anticonvulsant and analgesic mechanisms are not known. Is related chemically to GABA but does not interact with GABA receptors.

Pharmacokinetics

Food has no effect on the rate and extent of absorption; however, as the dose increases, the bioavailability decreases. **t½:** 5–7 hr. Excreted unchanged through the urine. Adjust dosage in those with impaired renal function. Horizant is a prodrug of gabapentin and has a different pharmacokinetic profile. **Plasma protein binding:** Less than 3%.

G

SPECIAL CONCERNS

- Use during lactation only if benefits outweigh risks.
- Plasma clearance is reduced in geriatric clients and in impaired renal function.
- May cause an increased risk of suicidal behavior and ideation.
- Use in children 3–12 years of age is associated with neuropsychiatric side effects (e.g., emotional lability, hostility including aggression, thought disorder including concentration problems and change in school performance, hyperkinesia).
- Safety and efficacy not determined in children less than 3 years of age.

SIDE EFFECTS

Most Common

Dizziness, somnolence, peripheral edema, ataxia, nystagmus, tremor.

Side effects listed are those with an incidence of 0.1% or greater. **CNS:** Most common: Somnolence, ataxia, dizziness, and fatigue. Also, nystagmus, tremor, nervousness, dysarthria, amnesia, depression, abnormal thinking/coordination, twitching, headache, ***convulsions (including the possibility of precipitation of status epilepticus)***, confusion, insomnia, emotional lability, vertigo, hyperkinesia, paresthesia, decreased/increased/absent reflexes, anxiety, hostility, CNS tumors, syncope, abnormal dreaming, aphasia, hyperesthesia, ***intracranial hemorrhage***, hypo-/dystonia, dysesthesia, paresis, hemiplegia, facial paralysis, stupor, cerebellar dysfunction, positive Babinski's sign, decreased position sense, subdural hematoma, apathy, hallucinations, decreased or loss of libido, agitation, depersonalization, euphoria, "doped-up" sensation, ***suicidal tendencies, sudden unexplained deaths***, psychoses. **Neuropsychiatric effects in children:** Emotional lability (behavioral problems), hostility (aggressive behavior), thought disorder (concentration problems and change in school performance), restlessness, hyperactivity. **GI:** Most common are: N&V. Also, dyspepsia, dry mouth and throat, constipation, dental abnormalities, increased appetite, abdominal pain, diarrhea, anorexia, flatulence, gingivitis, glossitis, ***gum hemorrhage***, thirst, stomatitis, taste loss, unusual taste, increased salivation, gastroenteritis, hemorrhoids, bloody stools, fecal incontinence, hepatomegaly. **CV:** Hyper-/hypotension, vasodilation, angina pectoris, peripheral vascular disorder, palpitation, tachycardia, migraine, murmur. **Musculoskeletal:** Myalgia, fracture, tendonitis, arthritis, joint stiffness/swelling, positive Romberg's test. **Respiratory:** Rhinitis, pharyngitis, coughing, pneumonia, epistaxis, dyspnea, apnea. **Dermatologic:** Pruritus, abrasion, rash, acne, alopecia, eczema, dry skin, increased sweating, urticaria, hirsutism, seborrhea, cyst, herpes simplex. **Body as a whole:** Back pain, weight increase/decrease, peripheral edema, asthenia, facial edema, allergy, chills. **GU:** Hematuria, dysuria, frequent urination, cystitis, urinary retention/incontinence, ***vaginal hemorrhage***, amenorrhea, dysmenorrhea, menorrhagia, breast cancer, inability to climax, abnormal ejaculation, impotence. **Hematologic:** Leukopenia, decreased WBCs, purpura, anemia, thrombocytopenia, lymphadenopathy. **Ophthalmic:** Diplopia, amblyopia, abnormal vision, cataract, conjunctivitis, dry eyes, visual field defect, photophobia, bilateral/unilateral ptosis, eye twitching/pain/hemorrhage, hordeolum. **Otic:** Hearing loss, earache, tinnitus, inner ear infection, otitis, ear fullness.

OVERDOSE MANAGEMENT

Symptoms: Double vision, slurred speech, drowsiness, lethargy, diarrhea. *Treatment:* Hemodialysis.

DRUG INTERACTIONS

Alcohol / Intensifies effects of gabapentin

Antacids / ↓ Bioavailability of gabapentin
Cimetidine / ↓ Renal excretion of gabapentin
Hydrocodone / ↑ Gabapentin AUC values and ↓ hydrocodone C_{max} and AUC
Morphine / ↑ Morphine AUC by 44%

HOW SUPPLIED

Gabapentin. *Capsules:* 100 mg, 300 mg, 400 mg; *Oral Solution:* 250 mg/5 mL; *Tablets:* 100 mg, 300 mg, 400 mg, 600 mg, 800 mg.
Gabapentin enacarbil. *Tablets, Extended-Release:* 600 mg.

DOSAGE

Gabapentin
CAPSULES; ORAL SOLUTION; TABLETS

Partial seizures with and without secondary generalization.

Clients 12 years and older: Dose range of 900–1,800 mg/day in three divided doses using 300 or 400 mg capsules or 600 or 800 mg tablets. **Initial dose:** 300 mg 3 times per day; dose may be increased, as needed, up to 1,800 mg/day. Doses up to 2,400 and 3,600 mg/day have been well tolerated for short periods. In clients with a C_{CR} of 30–60 mL/min, the dose is 300 mg twice a day; if the C_{CR} is 15–30 mL/min, the dose is 300 mg/day; if the C_{CR} <15 mL/min, the dose is 300 mg every other day.

Adjunctive therapy for partial seizures in children.

Ages 3–12 years, initial: 10–15 mg/kg/day in 3 divided doses. Attain effective dose by titration over 3 days. Effective dose in clients 5 years and older is 25–35 mg/kg/day and in clients 3 and 4 years of age is 40 mg/kg/day; give in divided doses 3 times per day. May use capsules, oral solution or tablets.

Postherpetic neuralgia.

Adults, initial: Single 300 mg dose on day 1; 600 mg/day on day 2 (divided twice daily); and 900 mg/day on day 3 (divided 3 times daily). Then titrate dose up as needed for pain relief to a daily dose of 1,800 mg (divided 3 times daily). Beneficial effects of dose greater than 1,800 mg/day not determined.

Gabapentin enacarbil
TABLETS, EXTENDED-RELEASE

Restless legs syndrome.

Adults: 600 mg once daily with food at 5:00 p.m.

NURSING IMPLICATIONS

Do not confuse Neurontin with Noroxin (a fluoroquinolone antibiotic).

IMPLEMENTATION/ADMINISTRATION/STORAGE

1. Do not allow 12 hr to pass between any 2 doses using the 3 times per day daily regimen.
2. If gabapentin discontinued or alternate anticonvulsant added to regimen, dose gradually over a 1-week period.
3. The first dose on day 1 may be taken at bedtime to minimize somnolence, dizziness, fatigue, and ataxia.
4. Gralise is intended to swell in the stomach and gradually release gabapentin. It is not interchangeable with other gabapentin products, due to different pharmacokinetic profiles.
5. Horizant is not interchangeable with other gabapentin products.
6. Horizant is not indicated for use in those with a C_{CR} <30 mL/min or in those undergoing hemodialysis.

ASSESSMENT

1. Note reasons for therapy, onset, frequency, characteristics of seizures/symptoms, other agents prescribed, outcome. With chronic pain/neuralgia, rate pain level.
2. List other drugs prescribed to ensure none interact.
3. Note mental and behavioral presentation; assess for depression, agitation or suicide ideations.
4. When drug therapy is discontinued or supplemental therapy added, do so gradually over at least 1 week.
5. Monitor renal and LFTs; reduce dose in elderly and with impaired renal function.

CLIENT/FAMILY TEACHING

1. May be taken with or without food. Do not chew or crush; use half tablets within several days of breaking the scored tablet. May take first dose at bedtime to decrease sedative effects.
2. Do not take antacids at any time while taking gabapentin, or at least stagger 2 hr apart; decreases drug absorption.
3. If having trouble swallowing, may open capsule and mix with applesauce or juice. Mix only one dose at a time just before taking it.
4. May cause dizziness, fatigue, drowsiness, incoordination, and eye twitching. Do not perform any activities that require mental alertness until full drug effects realized.
5. Report any ↑ seizures, visual changes, unusual bruising/bleeding or effects, emotional lability, hostility, thought disorders/abnormal thinking, restlessness/hyperactivity, excessive dizziness/drowsiness, or ↑ swelling in feet or ankles.
6. Report worsening depression S&S, any unusual changes in mood or behavior, or the emergence of suicidal/self-harm thoughts immediately to provider.
7. Avoid alcohol, CNS depressants; do not take any OTC agents without approval.
8. If pregnancy occurs report and enroll in AED Registry @ 1-888-233-2334.
9. Keep all F/U to assess response, labs, and for adverse SE. Do not stop suddenly with prolonged therapy.

OUTCOMES/EVALUATE

- Control of seizure activity
- Relief postherpetic neuralgia/diabetic neuropathy

Galantamine hydrobromide

(gah-**LAN**-tah-meen)

Classification(s): Treatment of Alzheimer's disease

Pregnancy Category: B

RX: Razadyne, Razadyne ER.

INDICATIONS/USES

Treatment of mild to moderate dementia of the Alzheimer's type. *Investigational:* Vascular dementia.

ACTION/KINETICS

Action

The drug is a competitive and reversible inhibitor of acetylcholinesterase. It is believed the drug enhances cholinergic function, which is believed to be impaired in Alzheimer's disease. The drug's effect may lessen as the disease process advances and as fewer cholinergic neurons remain functionally intact. There is no evidence the drug alters the course of the underlying dementing process.

Pharmacokinetics

Well absorbed; absolute bioavailability: 90%. **Time to peak levels, immediate-release:** About 1 hr; **time to peak levels, delayed-release:** 4.5–5 hr. Food does not affect the amount absorbed but does delay the maximum time by 1.5 hr. Metabolized by CYP2D6 and CYP3A4. **t½, terminal:** 7 hr. Mainly excreted in the urine.

CONTRAINDICATIONS

Hypersensitivity to galantamine or any components of the product. Use in those with severe hepatic impairment (Child-Pugh class 10–15) or severe renal impairment or C_{CR} less than 9 mL/min. Lactation, use in children.

SPECIAL CONCERNS

- Use with caution in those with severe asthma, obstructive pulmonary disease, or moderately impaired renal function
- Possible increase in mortality in clients with mild cognitive impairment due to various vascular causes (e.g., MI, stroke, and sudden death).

SIDE EFFECTS

Most Common

Dry mouth, headache, depression, dizziness, insomnia, N&V, fever, malaise, anorexia, diarrhea, weight decrease, dyspepsia, urinary incontinence, UTI, fatigue/lethargy, syncope.

GI: N&V, anorexia, diarrhea, abdominal pain, dyspepsia, constipation, active/occult GI bleeding, PUD, flatulence, gastritis, melena, dysphagia, ***rectal hemorrhage***, dry mouth, increased salivation, diverticulitis, gastroenteritis, hiccough, ***esophageal perforation*** (rare), upper and lower GI bleeding. **CNS:** Dizziness, headache, tremor, depression, insomnia, somnolence, agitation, confusion, anxiety, hallucination, vertigo, hypertonia, aggression, ***convulsions***, paresthesia, ataxia, hypo-/hyperkinesia, apraxia, aphasia, apathy, paroniria, paranoid reaction, increased libido, delirium, suicidal ideation (rare), ***suicide*** (very rare). **CV:** Bradycardia (rarely severe), AV block, syncope, hyper-/hypotension, chest pain, postural hypotension, ***cardiac failure***, palpitation, atrial arrhythmias/fibrillation, prolonged QT, BBB, SVT, VT-wave inversion, ***myocardial ischemia or infarction***, purpura, TIA, ***CVA***. **GU:** UTI, hematuria, urinary retention/hesitancy/difficulty, urinary incontinence, frequent micturition, cystitis, nocturia, renal calculi. **Respiratory:** Rhinitis, URTI, bronchitis, coughing, epistaxis. **Musculoskeletal:** Leg cramps, involuntary muscle contractions. **Hematologic:** Purpura, thrombocytopenia, anemia. **Body as a whole:** Weight decrease, fever, malaise, fatigue/lethargy, anemia, peripheral/dependent edema, asthenia, dehydration (may lead to impaired renal function and renal failure). **Miscellaneous:** Injury, back/chest pain, fall, injury, tinnitus.

LABORATORY TEST CONSIDERATIONS

↑ Alkaline phosphatase. Hyperglycemia, hypokalemia.

OVERDOSE MANAGEMENT

Symptoms: Severe N&V, GI cramping, salivation, lacrimation, urination, defecation, sweating, bradycardia, hypotension, respiratory depression, muscle weakness, fasciculations, ***collapse, convulsions.*** Also, ***increasing muscle weakness that may result in death*** if respiratory muscles are involved. *Treatment:* General supportive measures. IV atropine sulfate at an initial dose of 0.5–1 mg with subsequent doses based on clinical response.

DRUG INTERACTIONS

Amitriptyline / ↓ Galantamine clearance R/T ↓ liver metabolism
Anticholinergic drugs / Possible interference with activity of anticholinergics
Bethanecol / Synergistic effects
Cimetidine / ↑ Galantamine bioavailability
Cholinesterase inhibitors / Synergistic effect
CYP2D6 or CYP3A4 inhibitors / Possible ↑ galantamine AUC
Erythromycin / ↑ Galantamine AUC R/T ↓ liver metabolism
Fluoxetine / ↓ Galantamine clearance R/T ↓ liver metabolism
Fluvoxamine / ↓ Galantamine clearance R/T ↓ liver metabolism
Ketoconazole / ↑ Galantamine AUC R/T ↓ liver metabolism
Neuromuscular blocking drugs / Possible exaggeration of neuromuscular blockade
Nonsteroidal anti-inflammatory drugs / Galantamine ↑ gastric secretion; monitor for symptoms of active or occult GI bleeding
Paroxetine / ↑ Galantamine bioavailability R/T ↓ liver metabolism
Quinidine / ↓ Galantamine clearance R/T ↓ liver metabolism
Succinylcholine-type drugs / Exaggeration of neuromuscular blocking effects

HOW SUPPLIED

Capsules, Extended-Release: 8 mg, 16 mg, 24 mg; *Oral Solution:* 4 mg/mL; *Tablets:* 4 mg, 8 mg, 12 mg.

DOSAGE

CAPSULES, EXTENDED-RELEASE

Dementia of the Alzheimer's type.

Initial: 8 mg/day; increase the dose to the initial maintenance dose of 16 mg/day after a minimum of 4 weeks. Attempt a further increase to 24 mg/day after a minimum of 4 weeks at 16 mg/day. **Dose range:** 16–24 mg/day.

ORAL SOLUTION; TABLETS

Dementia of the Alzheimer's type.

Initial: 4 mg twice a day. After a minimum of 4 weeks if this dose is well tolerated, increase to 8 mg twice a day. Attempt a further increase to 12 mg twice a day only after a minimum of 4 weeks. Although a dosage range of 16–32 mg/day given as twice daily dosing is possible, due to side effects the recommended dose range is 16–24 mg/day given as twice a day dosing.

NURSING IMPLICATIONS

Due to errors confusing Reminyl with Amaryl (glimepiride: an oral hypoglycemic), the manufacturer has changed the name from Reminyl to Razadyne. Also, do not confuse galantamine with glimepiride (an oral antidiabetic agent).

IMPLEMENTATION/ADMINISTRATION/STORAGE

1. Do not exceed a dose of 16 mg/day in those with moderately impaired hepatic function (Child-Pugh class 7–9) or in those with moderate renal function impairment.
2. Store all dosage forms from 15–30°C (59–86°F). Do not freeze the oral solution.

ASSESSMENT

1. Identify onset/duration of behavioral changes, family history, other agents trialed, outcome.
2. Note cognitive functioning, MMSE/Alzheimer's Disease Assessment Scale (ADAS-cog), ability to perform ADLs, clinical presentation, family reports. Monitor mental status, and assess for improvement with therapy.
3. List history of GI bleed, asthma, CAD, COPD, BPH, liver/renal dysfunction. Assess for GI bleeding; may cause ↑ gastric acid secretion and vagotonic effects.
4. Monitor ECG, VS, CBC, renal and LFTs; reduce dose with liver/renal dysfunction.

CLIENT/FAMILY TEACHING

1. Drug does not alter the Alzheimer's process; efficacy of galantamine may lessen over time.
2. Take oral solution or tablets twice daily, with morning and evening meals; take extended-release capsules once in the morning with food.
3. Most side effects occur during periods of increasing dosage. Make dose adjustments no more often than every 4 weeks. Take with food, use prescribed anti-emetics, ensure adequate fluid intake to reduce impact of side effects, especially N&V.
4. If therapy interrupted for several days or longer, must restart at the lowest dose and increase back up to the current dose.
5. Report any irregular, slow pulse, dizzy spells, ↑ abdominal pain, GI bleeding, urinary difficulty, lack of response, worsening of symptoms, persistent N&V or significant weight loss.
6. Keep all F/U to assess response, labs, mental status and functioning, adverse SE.

OUTCOMES/EVALUATE

Improved cognitive functioning with Alzheimer's disease

■ IV

Ganciclovir sodium (DHPG)

(gan-**SYE**-kloh-veer)

Classification(s): Antiviral

Pregnancy Category: C

RX: Cytovene, Vitrasert, Zirgan.

SEE ALSO *ANTIVIRAL AGENTS*.

INDICATIONS/USES

IV (Cytovene): (1) Treatment of CMV retinitis in immunocompromised clients, including those with AIDS. Diagnosis may be confirmed by culture of CMV from the blood, urine, or throat; note that a negative CMV culture does not rule out CMV retinitis. (2) Prevention of CMV disease in transplant clients at risk; duration of treatment depends on duration and degree of immunosuppression.

Intravitreal implant (Vitrasert): CMV retinitis in those with AIDS. *NOTE:* The implant provides localized therapy only to the implanted eye; it does not provide treatment for systemic CMV disease.

Ophthalmic gel (Zirgan): Acute herpetic keratitis (dendritic ulcers).

ACTION/KINETICS

Action

Upon entry into viral cells infected by CMV, ganciclovir is converted to ganciclovir triphosphate by the CMV. Ganciclovir triphosphate inhibits viral DNA synthesis by competitive inhibition of viral DNA polymerases and direct incorporation into viral DNA; this results in eventual termination of viral DNA elongation. Ganciclovir is active against CMV, herpes simplex virus-1 and -2, Epstein-Barr virus, and varicella zoster virus. Use of the intraocular implant causes a significantly slower disease progression than did the use of IV ganciclovir.

Pharmacokinetics

A high-fat meal significantly prolongs the time to peak levels (from 1.8 to 3 hr) as well as a higher C_{max}. **t½, systemic use:** Approximately 2.9 hr. Believed to cross the blood-brain barrier. Most excreted unchanged through the urine. Renal impairment increases the t½ of the drug; make dosage adjustments based on C_{CR}. There is minimal systemic absorption following use of the ophthalmic gel.

CONTRAINDICATIONS

Hypersensitivity to acyclovir or ganciclovir. Lactation when used systemically or if using the intravitreal implant. Use when the absolute neutrophil count is less than 500/mm^3 or the platelet count is less than 25,000/mm^3. Use of the implant with any contraindications for intraocular surgery, such as external infection, severe thrombocytopenia.

SPECIAL CONCERNS

(1) Clinical toxicity includes granulocytopenia, anemia, and thrombocytopenia. In animal studies, the drug was carcinogenic and teratogenic, and caused aspermatogenesis. (2) IV ganciclovir is indicated only to treat cytomegalovirus retinitis in immunocompromised clients and for the prevention of CMV disease in transplant clients at risk for CMV disease. (3) The capsules are indicated only for prevention of CMV disease in clients with advanced HIV infection at risk for CMV disease, for maintenance treatment of CMV retinitis in immunocompromised clients, and for prevention of CMV disease in solid organ transplant recipients. (4) Oral ganciclovir is associated with a risk of more rapid rate of CMV retinitits progression; thus, use as maintenance treatment only in those clients for whom this risk is balanced by the benefit associated with avoiding daily IV infusions.

- Safety and efficacy not established for nonimmunocompromised clients, treatment of other CMV infections (e.g., pneumonitis or colitis), or congenital or neonatal CMV disease.
- Use with caution in impaired renal function, in elderly clients, with pre-existing cytopenias, or with a history of cytopenic reactions to other drugs, chemicals, or irradiation.
- Not a cure for CMV retinitis; progression of the disease may continue in immunocompromised clients.
- Treatment with zidovudine and ganciclovir (e.g., in AIDS clients) will likely not be tolerated and lead to severe granulocytopenia.
- CMV retinitis may be associated with CMV else where in the body. The ganciclovir implant provides only localized therapy limited to the implanted eye.
- Use with caution during lactation if using the ophthalmic gel.
- Use in children only if potential benefits outweigh potential risks, including carcinogenicity and reproductive toxicity. Safety and efficacy of the implant not established in children less than 9 years of age; safety and efficacy of the ophthalmic gel not established in children 2 years of age and less.

SIDE EFFECTS

Most Common

Adults: Diarrhea, fever, rash, leukopenia, anemia, anorexia, vomiting, sweating, infection, neuropathy, chills, sweating, puritus, thrombocyopenia. **Children:** Hypokalemia, abnormal kidney function, sepsis, thrombocytopenia, leukopenia, coagulation disorders, hypertension, pneumonia, immune system disorder.

Systemic use. Hematologic: Granulocytopenia, thrombocytopenia, neutropenia (may be irreversible), eosinophilia, leukopenia, anemia, hemolytic anemia, hemolytic uremic syndrome, hypochromic anemia, bone marrow depression, pancytopenia, ***leukemia, lymphoma***. **CNS:** Ataxia, ***coma***, neuropathy, confusion, abnormal dreams or thoughts, dizziness, headache, paresthesia, psychosis, nervousness, somnolence, tremor, agitation, amnesia, anxiety, depression, euphoria, hypertonia, hypesthesia, insomnia, manic reaction, ***seizures***, trismus, emotional lability, irritability, loss of memory, loss of sense of smell, dysphasia, extrapyramidal reaction, hallucinations. **GI:** N&V, aphthous stomatitis, diarrhea, anorexia, dry mouth, ***GI hemorrhage, pancreatitis, GI perforation***, abdominal pain, flatulence, dyspepsia, constipation, dysphagia, esophagitis, eructation, fecal incontinence, melena, intestinal/mouth ulceration, tongue disorder, splenomegaly. **Hepatic:** Cholestasis, cholelithiasis, cholangitis, hepatitis, ***hepatic failure***. **CV:** Hypertension or hypotension, arrhythmias, phlebitis, deep thrombophlebitis, ***cardiac arrest, intracranial hypertension, MI, stroke***, pericarditis, vasodilation, migraine, cardiac conduction abnormality, peripheral ischemia, ***torsades de pointes***, vasculitis, ventricular tachycardia. **Dermatologic:** Rash, sweating, alopecia, pruritus, urticaria, sweating, acne, dry skin, fixed eruption, herpes simplex, maculopapular rash, skin discoloration, vesiculobullous rash, photosensitivity, phototoxicity, exfoliative dermatitis, ***Stevens-Johnson syndrome***. **GU:** Hematuria, breast pain, kidney failure, abnormal kidney function, urinary frequency, UTI, decreased libido, impotence, infertility, renal tubular disorder, testicular hypotrophy. **At injection site:** Catheter infection, catheter sepsis, inflammation or pain, abscess, edema, hemorrhage, phlebitis. **Musculoskeletal:** Arthralgia, arthritis, bone pain, leg cramps, myalgia, myasthenia, myelopathy, transverse myelitis, abnormal gait, rhabdomyolysis. **Respiratory:** Dyspnea, increased cough, pneumonia, bronchospasm, pulmonary fibrosis. **Metabolic:** Weight loss, acidosis. **Ophthalmologic:** Abnormal vision, amblyopia, blindness, conjunctivitis, dry eyes, eye pain, glaucoma, retinitis, photophobia, cataracts, vitreous disorder, oculomotor nerve paralysis, retinal detachment in CMV retinitis clients. **Otic:** Tinnitus, deafness. **Body as a whole:** Fever, chills, edema, infections, malaise, neuropathy, ***sepsis, multiple organ failure***, asthenia, enlarged abdomen, abscess, back/chest pain, cellulitis, facial edema, neck pain or rigidity. **Miscellaneous:** ***Anaphylaxis***, allergic reaction, taste perversion, congenital anomaly, encephalopathy, facial palsy, ***unexplained death***.

Intravitreal. Implant. Ophthalmic: Vitreous loss, vitreous hemorrhage, cataract formation, retinal detachment, uveitis, endophthalmitis, decrease/loss in visual acuity, lens opacities, macular abnormalities, spikes in intraocular pressure, optic disk/nerve changes, hyphemas. Less frequently: Angle closure glaucoma with anterior chamber swallowing, anterior chamber cell and flare, astigmatism, chemosis, choroidal folds, choroiditis, corneal dellen, cotton wool spots, endophthalmitis gliosis, hemorrhage (other than vitreous), hypotony, keratopathy, microangiopathy, pellet extrusion from scleral wound, phthisis bulbi, retinal hole, retinal tear, retinopathy, sclerosis, severe postoperative inflammation, synechia, vitreous detachment, vitreous traction.

Ophthalmic Gel. Blurred vision, eye irritation, punctate keratitis, conjunctival hyperemia.

LABORATORY TEST CONSIDERATIONS

↑ Serum creatinine, BUN, alkaline phosphatase, CPK, LDH, AST, ALT. ↓ Blood glucose. Abnormal LFT. Hypocalcemia, hypokalemia, hyponatremia. Inappropriate serum ADH.

OVERDOSE MANAGEMENT

Symptoms: **After IV use:** Irreversible pancytopenia, GI symptoms, acute renal failure, persistent bone marrow suppression, reversible neutropenia or granulocytopenia, hepatitis, renal toxicity, seizures. *Treatment:* Hydration, hemodialysis. Consider the use of hematopoietic growth factors.

DRUG INTERACTIONS

Adriamycin / Additive cytotoxicity in rapidly dividing cells
Amphotericin B / Additive cytotoxicity in rapidly dividing cells; also, ↑ serum creatinine levels; additive nephrotoxicity
Antineoplastic drugs / Additive myelosuppression
Cyclosporine / ↑ Serum creatinine levels; additive nephrotoxicity and additive myelosuppression
Cytotoxic drugs / Additive cytotoxicity
Didanosine / ↑ Didanosine AUC R/T ↑ didanosine plasma levels
Flucytosine / Additive cytotoxicity in rapidly dividing cells
Foscarnet / Additive or synergistic effects
Imipenem/Cilastatin combination / Possibility of seizures
Mycophenolate mofetil / ↑ Plasma levels of both drugs in clients with renal impairment
Nephrotoxicity / ↑ Serum creatinine
Pentamidine / Additive cytotoxicity in rapidly dividing cells
Probenecid / ↑ Effect of ganciclovir R/T ↓ renal excretion
Sulfamethoxazole/Trimethoprim combinations / Additive cytotoxicity in rapidly dividing cells
Tacrolimus / Additive myelosuppression
Tenofovir / ↑ Plasma levels of ganciclovir or tenofovir
Vinblastine / Additive cytotoxicity in rapidly dividing cells
Vincristine / Additive cytotoxicity in rapidly dividing cells
Zidovudine / Severe myelosuppression → neutropenia and anemia; if used together, full dosage may not be possible

HOW SUPPLIED

Intravitreal Implant (Vitrasert): 4.5 mg; ***Ophthalmic Gel (Zirgan):*** 0.15%; ***Powder for Injection (Cytovene):*** 500 mg/vial.

DOSAGE

IV INFUSION

Cytomegalovirus (CMV) retinitis.

Induction treatment: 5 mg/kg IV over 1 hr q 12 hr for 14–21 days in clients with normal renal function. **Maintenance, IV:** 5 mg/kg over 1 hr by IV infusion daily for 7 days or 6 mg/kg/day for 5 days each week. Dosage must be reduced in clients with renal impairment.

Prevention of CMV retinitis in those with advanced human immunodeficiency virus (HIV) infection and normal renal function.

1,000 mg 3 times per day with food.

Prophylaxis of CMV disease in transplant clients

Initial dose, IV: 5 mg/kg over 1 hr q 12 hr for 7–14 days in those with normal renal function. **Maintenance:** 5 mg/kg/day on 7 days each week (or 6 mg/kg/day on 5 days each week). The PO prophylactic dose is 1,000 mg 3 times per day with food.

In renal impairment, the following dosages are recommended. **IV. C_{CR} 50–69 mL/min:** Induction dose of 2.5 mg/kg q 12 hr and maintenance dose of 2.5 mg/kg q 24 hr; **C_{CR} 25–49 mL/min:** Induction dose of 2.5 mg/kg q 24 hr and maintenance dose of 1.25 mg/kg q 24 hr; **C_{CR} 10–24 mL/min:** Induction dose of 1.25 mg/kg q 24 hr and maintenance dose of 0.625 mg/kg q 24 hr; **C_{CR} <10 mL/min:** Induction dose of 1.25 mg/kg 3 times per week following hemodialysis and maintenance dose of 0.625 mg/kg 3 times per week following hemodialysis.

INTRAVITREAL IMPLANT

CMV retinitis.

Adults and children, 9 years and older: One implant inserted into each affected eye by intravitreal implantation. The 4.5 mg implant releases the drug over a 5- to 8-month period. Following depletion of the ganciclovir from the implant, it may be removed and replaced.

OPHTHALMIC GEL

Acute herpetic keratitis.

Adults and children, 2 years and older, initial: 1 drop in affected eye 5 times per day (about q 3 hr while awake) until the corneal ulcer heals. **Maintenance:** 1 drop 3 times per day for 7 days.

NURSING IMPLICATIONS

Do not confuse Cytovene with Cytosar (an antineoplastic) or Cytotec (prevents NSAID-induced ulcers).

IMPLEMENTATION/ADMINISTRATION/STORAGE

1. Use caution in handling the implant in order to avoid damage to the polymer coating, which may result in an increased rate of drug release. Handle the implant only by the suture tab. Maintain aseptic technique at all times prior to and during the surgical implantation procedure.
2. Clients should not wear contact lenses if there are signs and symptoms of herpetic retinitis.
3. Store the implant and ophthalmic gel from 15–30°C (59–86°F); protect implant from freezing, excessive heat, and light. Protect gel from freezing.
4. IV Reconstitute by injecting 10 mL sterile water for injection followed by shaking. Discard if particulate matter or discoloration is noted.
5. Parabens is incompatible with ganciclovir; do not use bacteriostatic water for injection for reconstitution.
6. IV infusion concentrations greater than 10 mg/mL are not recommended. Further reconstitute ganciclovir with 100 mL of any of the following solutions: D5W, RL or Ringer's solution, 0.9% NaCl. Infuse over 1 hr. Doses greater than 6 mg/kg infused over 1 hr may result in increased toxicity.
7. Due to high pH (9–11) of reconstituted ganciclovir, do not give IM or SC. Do not give by IV bolus or rapid IV injection.
8. To minimize phlebitis/pain at injection site, give into veins with an adequate blood flow to allow rapid dilution and distribution.
9. Do not exceed 1.25 mg/kg/day in clients undergoing hemodialysis.

G

10. Reconstituted solution stable for 12 hr at room temperature.
11. Follow guidelines for handling and disposal of cytotoxic drugs. Avoid inhalation and contact with skin. Wear latex gloves and safety glasses and mix under a biologic hood.
12. COMPATIBILITY D5W, RL, or Ringer's solution, 0.9% NaCl.
13. INCOMPATIBILITY Do not mix with other IV medications.

ASSESSMENT

1. Note disease onset, other medical conditions, characteristics of S&S, therapies trialed.
2. Confirm CMV retinitis by indirect ophthalmoscopy reports.
3. Assess orientation and mentation levels.
4. Monitor I&O. Ensure adequate hydration before/during IV therapy.
5. May experience pain/phlebitis at infusion site because pH of *diluted* solution is high (pH 9–11). Follow administration guidelines carefully. Avoid skin contact with drug.
6. List drugs prescribed, and review list of drug interactions; some may induce renal failure, have additive toxicity if given during ganciclovir therapy.
7. Review drug-related carcinogenic, teratogenic and aspermatogenesis findings in animal studies.
8. Monitor CBC, CD4+ cell count, renal function studies; reduce dose with impaired renal function. Granulocytopenia and thrombocytopenia are side effects of drug therapy; do not administer if neutrophil count drops below 500 cells/mm^3 or platelet count falls below 25,000/mm^3. Concomitant therapy with zidovudine may increase neutropenia.

CLIENT/FAMILY TEACHING

1. Not a cure; used to control symptoms. Take tablets with food to increase bioavailability. Ensure adequate hydration
2. Do not interrupt drug therapy, unless by provider; a relapse may occur.
3. Report dizziness, S&S of infection, bleeding, seizures, headache, mental status changes, rash, pain at the injection site, nausea, or black, tarry stools.
4. Use protection (sunglasses, clothing/hat, sunscreen) with sun exposure to prevent photosensitivity reaction. Do not wear contact lenses with S&S herpetic keratitis.
5. Have regular eye exams (every 6 weeks) because retinitis may progress to blindness (retinal detachment). Following surgical insertion of the ocular implant, may experience blurred vision in the eye, which clears within 2–4 weeks. Implant can be removed when depleted of drug, usually within 5–8 months, and a new Vitrasert Implant can be inserted. Effect is only on the eye and not elsewhere in the body.
6. Potential complications, include intraocular infection or inflammation, detachment of the retina, and formation of cataract in the natural crystalline lens, following intraocular surgery.
7. In HIV therapy with zidovudine may cause very low WBCs, and with didanosine may cause ↑ serum didanosine concentrations; may not be tolerated.
8. May impair fertility; determine if candidate for sperm/egg harvesting. During and for 90 days following drug therapy, women of childbearing age should use safe contraception and men should practice barrier contraception; inhibits sperm production—may cause temporary or permanent male infertility.
9. Causes tumors in animals, thus considered a potential carcinogen
10. Avoid crowds and persons with known infections. Report any unusual behavior or altered thought processes.
11. Keep all F/U to assess response, frequent labs, q 6 week eye exams, and adverse SE.

OUTCOMES/EVALUATE

- ↓ Progression of CMV retinitis
- CMV prophylaxis with immunocompromised clients
- Prevention of CMV retinitis in those with advanced HIV infection

Gatifloxacin

(**gat**-ih-**FLOX**-ah-sin)

Classification(s): Antibiotic, quinolone

Pregnancy Category: C

RX: Zymar, Zymaxid.

SEE ALSO ***ANTI-INFECTIVE DRUGS*** AND ***FLUOROQUINOLONES***.

INDICATIONS/USES

Ophthalmic. Bacterial conjunctivitis due to susceptible strains of *Corynebacterium propinquum, Staphylococcus aureus, Staphylococcus epidermidis, Streptococcus mitis, Streptococcus oralis, Streptococcus pneumoniae,* or *Haemophilis influenzae.* May be used in clients 1 year of age and older.

ACTION/KINETICS

Pharmacokinetics

Used only ophthalmically.

CONTRAINDICATIONS

Hypersensitivity to any component of the product. Use with epithelial herpes, dendritic keratitis, vaccinia, varicella, mycobacterial infections of the eye, or fungal disease of the ocular structure. Injection subconjunctivally or introduction directly into the anterior chamber of the eye.

SPECIAL CONCERNS

Systemic use may prolong the QTc interval.

SIDE EFFECTS

Most Common

After ophthalmic use: Transient irritation, burning, stinging, itching, inflammation.

Transient irritation, burning, stinging, itching, inflammation, angioneurotic edema, urticaria, vesicular and maculopapular dermatitis.

HOW SUPPLIED

Ophthalmic Solution: 0.3% (3 mg/mL: Zymar), 0.5% (5 mg/mL: Zymaxid).

DOSAGE

OPHTHALMIC SOLUTION (ZYMAR)

Bacterial conjunctivitis.

Days 1 and 2: 1 gtt in affected eye(s) q 2 hr while awake, up to 8 times per day. **Days 3 through 7:** 1 gtt up to 4 times per day while awake.

OPHTHALMIC SOLUTION (ZYMAR OR ZYMAXID)

Bacterial conjunctivitis.

Adults and children, 1 year and older: Days 1 and 2 (Zymar) or Day 1 (Zymaxid): Instill 1 drop in affected eye(s) q 2 hr while awake, up to 8 times per day. **Days 3 through 7 (Zymar) or Days 2 through 7 (Zymaxid):** Instill 1 drop up to 4 times per day while awake.

NURSING IMPLICATIONS

Do not confuse gatifloxacin with gemifloxacin (also a fluoroquinolone antibiotic).

IMPLEMENTATION/ADMINISTRATION/STORAGE

Store ophthalmic solution from 15–25°C (59–77°F). Protect from freezing.

ASSESSMENT

1. Note onset and characteristics of S&S and clinical presentation.
2. Review eye exam; confirm bacterial conjunctivitis.
3. Assess for quinolone sensitivity. Monitor for increased burning, painful stinging, irritation or worsening of symptoms.

CLIENT/FAMILY TEACHING

1. Protect the ophthalmic solution from freezing.
2. When instilling eye drops: wash hands and do not allow dropper to touch eye. Tilt head back; looking up, pull lower eyelid down and instill prescribed number of drops. Close eye for 1 to 2 min; apply gentle pressure to bridge of nose. Do not rub eye.
3. If more than 1 topical eye drug is being used, administer drugs at least 5 min apart.
4. Avoid wearing contacts with bacterial conjunctivitis.
5. Report persistent burning, stinging pain, or irritation.
6. Keep all F/U to assess response and for adverse SE.

OUTCOMES/EVALUATE

Resolution of infection; symptomatic improvement

Gefitinib

(geh-**FIH**-tih-nib)

Classification(s): Antineoplastic, epidermal growth factor receptor inhibitor

Pregnancy Category: D

RX: Iressa.

SEE ALSO ***ANTINEOPLASTIC AGENTS***.

INDICATIONS/USES

Monotherapy for locally advanced or metastatic non-small-cell lung cancer after failure of platinum-based and docetaxel chemotherapies. *NOTE:* The drug should be used only in cancer clients who have already taken the drug; new clients should not be started on the medication, as it does not improve survival. *Investigational:* Treatment of squamous cell head and neck cancer.

ACTION/KINETICS

Action

Mechanism not fully characterized. Gefitinib inhibits intracellular phosphorylation of numerous tyrosine kinases associated with transmembrane cell surface receptors, including the tyrosine kinases associated with epidermal growth factor receptor. Epidermal growth factor receptor is expressed on the cell surface of many normal and cancer cells.

Pharmacokinetics

Slowly absorbed; **peak plasma levels:** 3–7 hr. About 60% bioavailable. Steady-state plasma levels reached within 10 days. Undergoes extensive hepatic metabolism, predominantly by CYP3A4. Cleared mainly by the liver; **t½, elimination:** 48 hr. Excreted mainly by the feces (86%) with a small amount (4%) through the urine. **Plasma protein binding:** 90%.

CONTRAINDICATIONS

Severe hypersensitivity to gefitinib or any component of the product. Lactation.

SPECIAL CONCERNS

- **Pulmonary toxicity (can be fatal) may occur.**
- **Has the potential to inhibit the cardiac action potential repolarization (i.e., QT interval); clinical relevance not known presently.**
- **Use with caution in impaired renal and hepatic function.**
- **Safety and efficacy not determined in children.**

SIDE EFFECTS

Most Common

Diarrhea, rash, acne, dry skin N&V, pruritus, anorexia, asthenia, weight loss.

Pulmonary: ***Interstitial lung disease***, including interstitial pneumonia, pneumonitis, alveolitis, acute onset dyspnea (sometimes associated with cough or low-grade fever). **GI:** Diarrhea, N&V, anorexia, mouth ulceration, pancreatitis (rare). **CV:** Inhibition of cardiac action potential repolarization process (QT interval). **GU:** Impaired renal function. **Dermatologic:** Rash, acne, dry skin, pruritus, vesiculobullous rash; rarely, ***toxic epidermal necrolysis***, erythema multiforme. **Ophthalmic:** Amblyopia, conjunctivitis, eye pain, corneal erosion/ulcer (sometimes with aberrant eyelash growth); very rarely corneal membrane sloughing, ocular ischemia/hemorrhage. **Body as a whole:** Asthenia, weight loss, ***hemorrhage*** (including epistaxis and hematuria). **Miscellaneous:** Peripheral edema. Rarely, allergic reactions, including angioedema and urticaria.

DRUG INTERACTIONS

Cimetidine / ↓ Gefitinib levels R/T ↑ gastric pH → ↓ GI absorption and ↓ efficacy
CYP3A4 inducers (e.g., phenytoin, rifampin) / ↓ Gefitinib levels R/T ↑ liver metabolism; consider a dosage increase
CYP3A4 inhibitors (e.g., itraconazole, ketoconazole) / ↑ Gefitinib levels R/T ↓ liver metabolism; use together with caution
Metoprolol / ↑ Metoprolol levels
Ranitidine / ↓ Gefitinib levels R/T ↑ gastric pH → ↓ GI absorption and ↓ efficacy
Sodium bicarbonate / ↓ Gefitinib levels R/T ↑ gastric pH → ↓ GI absorption and ↓ efficacy
Vinorelbine / Exacerbation of neutropenic effect of vinorelbine
Warfarin / ↑ INR and bleeding events; monitor PT or INR regularly

HOW SUPPLIED

Tablets: 250 mg.

DOSAGE

TABLETS

Non-small-cell lung cancer.

Adults: 250 mg once a day with or without food. Higher doses do not give a better response and may increase toxicity. Continue therapy as long as response is favorable (median duration is about 9 months).

Squamous cell head and neck cancer (investigational).

Adults: 250–500 mg once a day.

NURSING IMPLICATIONS

IMPLEMENTATION/ADMINISTRATION/STORAGE

1. Gefitinib is available only to clients registered in AstraZeneca's restrictive distribution program, the Iressa Access Program. Health care providers must register clients with the program before prescribing gefitinib. To qualify for the program: (a) clients must have been treated with gefitinib prior to September 15, 2005; (b) clients must have been previously benefited from gefitinib, or the client's health care provider believes the client will benefit from further gefitinib therapy; or, (c) the client is enrolled in a clinical trial that was approved by an Institutional Review Board prior to June 17, 2005. Additional information about the Iressa Access Program is available from AstraZeneca at 800-601-8933 (8 a.m. to 6:00 p.m. EST, Mon. through Fri.) or online at http://www.iressa-access.com/
2. Clients with poorly tolerated diarrhea (possibly with dehydration) or skin toxicity may be successfully managed by up to a 14-day drug-free period followed by reinstatement of the 250 mg/day dose.
3. If acute onset or worsening of pulmonary symptoms (e.g., dyspnea, cough, fever) occur, stop gefitinib therapy, evaluate promptly, and begin appropriate treatment. If interstitial lung disease is confirmed, stop therapy and treat appropriately.
4. If new eye symptoms develop (e.g., pain), evaluate and manage appropriately, including stopping gefitinib therapy and removing an aberrant eyelash if present. After symptoms and eye changes resolve, decide on reinitiating the 250 mg/day dose. Eye pain and corneal erosion/ulcer have been reported with gefitinib use.
5. In those receiving a potent CYP3A4 inducer (e.g., phenytoin or rifampin), consider increasing dose to 500 mg/day, provided there are no severe side effects; carefully monitor response and toxicity.
6. Store tablets at room temperature (20–25°C 68–77°F).

ASSESSMENT

1. Note reasons for therapy, other agents trialed, outcome. Should only be used in cancer clients who have already taken the drug; new clients should not be started on this drug as it does not improve survival. List drugs prescribed to ensure none interact.
2. Assess eye findings/symptoms, lungs sounds, CXR and ECG. If pulmonary symptoms (dyspnea, cough, fever) occur, stop drug and determine source of problem and R/O pulmonary toxicity.
3. May temporarily interrupt therapy for eye symptoms, persistent diarrhea and dehydration, or skin reactions.
4. Administered only through the Iressa Access Program; for more information contact AstraZeneca at 1-800-601-8933.
5. Monitor CBC, renal and LFTs; reduce dose with dysfunction.

CLIENT/FAMILY TEACHING

1. Take exactly as directed with or without food.
2. For those unable to swallow tablets whole, place tablet in a half glass of noncarbonated water; do not crush tablet. Stir approximately 10 min until dispersed; drink mixture immediately. To ensure that the entire dose is given, rinse the inside of the container with another half glass of water and drink immediately. The suspension may also be given by a gastric enteral feeding tube.
3. Stop drug and report any persistent diarrhea, increased SOB, N&V, eye problems, or rash.
4. Consume adequate fluids to prevent dehydration. Report any severe or persistent diarrhea, N&V, anorexia, or new onset or worsening of pulmonary symptoms (e.g., shortness of breath, cough).
5. Practice reliable contraception. Avoid pregnancy; may harm fetus.
6. Review side effects related to pulmonary toxicity, which may be lethal.
7. Keep all F/U to assess response, labs, adverse SE.

OUTCOMES/EVALUATE

Inhibition of malignant cell proliferation

IV

Gemcitabine hydrochloride

(jem-**SIGHT**-ah-been)

Classification(s): Antineoplastic, miscellaneous

Pregnancy Category: D

RX: Gemzar.

SEE ALSO ***ANTINEOPLASTIC AGENTS***.

INDICATIONS/USES

(1) In combination with paclitaxel as first-line treatment of metastatic breast cancer after failure of prior anthracycline-containing adjuvant chemotherapy, unless anthracyclines were contraindicated. (2) In combination with cisplatin as first-line treatment of inoperable, locally advanced (stage IIIA or IIIB) or metastatic (stage IV) non-small-cell lung cancer. (3) In combination with carboplatin for advanced ovarian cancer that has relapsed at least 6 months after completion of platinum-based therapy. (4) As first-line treatment of locally advanced (nonresectable stage II or stage III) or metastatic (stage IV) adenocarcinoma of the pancreas. Indicated for those previously treated with 5-fluorouracil. *Investigational:* Biliary cancer, bladder cancer, relapsed or refractory testicular cancer, squamous cell carcinoma of the head and neck.

ACTION/KINETICS

Action

A nucleoside analog that kills cells undergoing DNA synthesis (S-phase) and by blocking the progression of cells through the G1/S-phase boundary. Metabolized within cells by nucleoside kinases to the active gemcitabine diphosphate and triphosphate nucleosides. The diphosphate inhibits ribonucleotide reductase, which is responsible for catalyzing reactions that generate the deoxynucleoside triphosphate for DNA synthesis. Inhibition of the reductase enzyme causes a decrease in the levels of deoxynucleotides. The triphosphate competes with triphosphate nucleosides for incorporation into DNA, resulting in inhibition of DNA synthesis. DNA polymerase is not able to remove the gemcitabine nucleoside and repair the growing DNA strands.

Pharmacokinetics

The metabolite of gemcitabine nucleoside is excreted through the urine. **t½, short infusions:** 42–94 min; **t½, long infusions:** 245–638 min (depends on age and gender). Higher levels are found in women and the elderly due to lower clearance.

CONTRAINDICATIONS

Lactation.

SPECIAL CONCERNS

- Use with caution with pre-existing renal impairment or hepatic insufficiency.
- Safety and efficacy not determined in children.

SIDE EFFECTS

Most Common

N&V, anemia, leukopenia, neutropenia, pain, fever, dyspnea, thrombocytopenia, constipation, diarrhea, ***hemorrhage***, infection, alopecia.

Side effects include those observed with combination therapy. **GI:** N&V, diarrhea, constipation, stomatitis, anorexia, pharyngitis. **CNS:** Somnolence, mild to severe paresthesias, insomnia, neuropathy (motor and sensory). **CV:** Arrhythmia, hypo-/hypertension, CHF, ***MI, CVA***, gangrene, vasculitis. **Hematologic:** Anemia, leukopenia, neutropenia, thrombocytopenia, platelet transfusions. **Respiratory:** Dyspnea, ***bronchospasm***, cough, rhinitis, rarely parenchymal lung toxicity, including ***adult respiratory distress syndrome***, interstitial pneumonitis, ***pulmonary edema***, and ***pulmonary fibrosis***, ***respiratory failure, death*** (rare). **Musculoskeletal:** Myalgia, arthralgia, bone pain. **Dermatologic:** Alopecia, rash, desquamation, macular or finely granular maculopapular pruritic eruptions, pruritus, hair loss (minimal), cellulitis, injection site reactions, bullous skin eruptions. **GU:** Renal failure, hemolytic uremic syndrome. **Body as a whole:** Pain, fever, fatigue, peripheral edema; flu syndrome (including fever), asthenia, chills, sweating, malaise. **Miscellaneous:** ***Hemorrhage, sepsis***, infections, petechiae, anaphylaxis (rare).

LABORATORY TEST CONSIDERATIONS

↑ ALT, AST, alkaline phosphatase, bilirubin, BUN, creatinine, GGT. Proteinuria, hematuria, hyperglycemia, hypocalcemia, hypomagnesemia.

OVERDOSE MANAGEMENT

Symptoms: Myelosuppression, paresthesias, severe rash. *Treatment:* Monitor with appropriate blood counts. Supportive therapy as needed.

DRUG INTERACTIONS

↓ Clearance and ↑ gemcitabine levels when given with paclitaxel.

HOW SUPPLIED

Powder for Injection, Lyophilized: 200 mg, 1 gram, 2 grams.

DOSAGE

IV ONLY

Metastatic breast cancer not responding to anthracycline-containing adjuvant chemotherapy.

Gemcitabine, 1,250 mg/m^2 by IV infusion over 30 min on days 1 and 8 of each 21-day cycle and paclitaxel, 175 mg/m^2 by IV infusion over 3 hr before the administration of gemcitabine on day 1.

Adjust the gemcitabine dosage as follows for hematological toxicity based on granulocyte and platelet counts taken on day 8 of therapy: (a) If the absolute granulocyte count is greater than or equal to 1,200 × 10^6/L and the platelet count is greater than 75,000 × 10^6/L, give 100% of the full dose. (b) If the absolute granulocyte count is between 1,000 and 1,199 × 10^6/L or the platelet count is between 50,000 and 75,000 × 10^6/L, give 75% of the full dose. (c) If the absolute granulocyte count is between 700 and 999 × 10^6/L and the platelet count is greater than or equal to 50,000 × 10^6/L, give 50% of the full dose. (d) If the absolute granulocyte count is less than 700 × 10^6/L or the platelet count is less than 50,000 × 10^6/L, withhold the dose.

Non-small-cell lung cancer.

Two schedules are used. (1) Four-week schedule: Gemcitabine, 1,000 mg/m^2 over 30 min on days 1, 8, and 15 of each 28-day cycle. Give cisplatin, IV, 100 mg/m^2 on day 1 after gemcitabine. (2) Three-week schedule: Gemcitabine, 1,250 mg/m^2 over 30 min on days 1 and 8 of each 21-day cycle. Give cisplatin, IV, 100 mg/m^2 after gemcitabine on day 1. Dosage modifications may be required for hematologic toxicity.

Ovarian cancer.

Adults: Gemcitabine 1,000 mg/m^2 over 30 min on days 1 and 8 of each 21-day cycle plus carboplatin AUC 4 should be given IV on day 1 after gemcitabine administration. Monitor clients prior to each dose; clients should have an absolute granulocyte count of 1,500 × 10^6/L or greater and a platelet count of 100,000 × 10^6/L or greater prior to each cycle.

If marrow suppression is observed on day 8 of therapy within a treatment cycle, use the following dosage modifications: (a) If the absolute granulocyte count is 1,500 × 10^6/L or greater and the platelet count is 100,000 × 10^6/L or greater, give 100% of the full dose; (b) If the absolute granulocyte count is between 1,000 and 1,499 × 10^6/L and/or the platelet count is between 75,000 and 99,999 × 10^6/L, give 50% of the dose. (c) If the absolute granulocyte count is less than 1,000 × 10^6/L and/or the platelet count is less than 75,000 × 10^6/L, withhold the dose.

The dose of gemcitabine should be reduced to 800 mg/m^2 on days 1 and 8 in case of any of the following hematologic toxicities: (a) Absolute granulocyte count less than 500 × 10^6/L for more than 5 days; (b) absolute granulocyte count less than 100 × 10^6/L for more than 3 days; (c) febrile neutropenia; (d) platelets less than 25,000 × 10^6/L; (e) cycle delay of more than 1 week because of toxicity.

Adenocarcinoma of the pancreas.

Adults: 1,000 mg/m^2 given over 30 min once a week for up to 7 weeks (or until toxicity necessitates reducing or holding a dose). This is followed by a 1-week rest period. Subsequent cycles should consist of infusions once a week for 3 consecutive weeks out of 4. Those who complete the entire 7 weeks of initial therapy or a subsequent 3-week cycle at the 1,000 mg/m^2 dose may have the dose for subsequent cycles increased by 25% to 1,250 mg/m^2 provided that the absolute neutrophil count nadir exceeds 1,500 × 10^6/L and the platelet nadir exceeds 100,000 × 10^6/L and if nonhematologic toxicity has not been

G

greater than World Health Organization Grade 1. If clients tolerate a dose of 1,250 mg/m^2 once weekly, the dose for the next cycle can be increased to 1,500 mg/m^2 provided the absolute neutrophil count and platelet nadirs are as defined previously.

The dose should be reduced to 75% of the full dose if the absolute granulocyte count is 500–999 × 10^6/L and the platelet count is 50,000–99,000 × 10^6/L. The dose should be held if the absolute granulocyte count falls below 500 × 10^6/L and the platelet count falls below 50,000 × 10^6/L.

G

NURSING IMPLICATIONS

IMPLEMENTATION/ADMINISTRATION/STORAGE

1. IV To reconstitute drug, use 0.9% NaCl injection without preservatives. The maximum concentration upon reconstitution is 40 mg/mL; greater concentrations may cause incomplete dissolution.
2. Give over 30 min; prolonging infusion time beyond 60 min and more frequent administration than once weekly increases toxicity.
3. To reconstitute, add 5 mL of 0.9% NaCl to the 200 mg vial or 25 mL to the 1-gram vial. Shake to dissolve. This results in a concentration of 40 mg/mL, which may be further diluted, if needed, with 0.9% NaCl to concentrations as low as 0.1 mg/mL.
4. Do not refrigerate reconstituted drug as crystallization may occur. Store diluted product at controlled room temperatures of 20–25°C (68–77°F). Reconstituted solutions are stable at these temperatures for 24 hr.
5. COMPATIBILITY 0.9% NaCl.
6. INCOMPATIBILITY Administer separately.

ASSESSMENT

1. Note disease type/stage, onset, symptoms, organ(s) involved, and other therapies trialed.
2. Assess lung sounds, if pulmonary symptoms (dyspnea, cough, fever) occur, determine source and R/O pulmonary toxicity.
3. Monitor CBC prior to each dose; check CBC, renal and LFTs, K^+, Ca^{++}, and Mg^{++} prior to starting therapy; monitor liver and renal function tests periodically; causes thrombocytopenia and myelosuppression. Nadir: 1 week.

CLIENT/FAMILY TEACHING

1. Anticipate IV therapy once weekly over 30 min for up to 7 weeks; then weekly for 3 out of every 4 weeks.
2. May experience fever and flu-like symptoms as well as a rash involving trunk and extremities.
3. Report any changes in skin, numbness/tingling of hands/feet, infusion site pain, prolonged/uncomfortable swelling, severe constipation/diarrhea, sore mouth/throat, fever >38°C (100.4°F) or shaking chills, unusual bruising/bleeding, vomiting >24 hr after treatment or evidence of blood or pain with voiding.
4. May experience hair loss; avoid live vaccines during therapy.
5. Use reliable birth control during and for several months following therapy; can cause fetal harm.
6. Keep all F/U to assess response, labs, and adverse SE.

OUTCOMES/EVALUATE

Suppression of malignant cell proliferation

Gemfibrozil

(jem-**FIH**-broh-zill)

Classification(s): Antihyperlipidemic, fibric acid derivative

Pregnancy Category: C

RX: Lopid.

Rx: Apo-Gemfibrozil, Gen-Gemfibrozil, PMS-Gemfibrozil.

INDICATIONS/USES

(1) Hypertriglyceridemia (type IV and type V hyperlipidemia) unresponsive to dietary control or in clients who are at risk of pancreatitis and abdominal pain. (2) Reduce risk of coronary heart disease in clients with type IIb hyperlipidemia who have not responded to diet, weight loss, exercise, and other drug therapy.

ACTION/KINETICS

Action

Gemfibrozil, a fibric acid derivative, decreases triglycerides, cholesterol, and VLDL and increases HDL; LDL levels either decrease or do not change. Also, decreases hepatic triglyceride production by inhibiting peripheral lipolysis and decreasing extraction of free fatty acids by the liver. Also, gemfibrozil decreases VLDL synthesis by inhibiting synthesis of VLDL carrier apolipoprotein B, as well as inhibits peripheral lipolysis and decreases hepatic extraction of free fatty acids (thus decreasing hepatic triglyceride production). May be beneficial in inhibiting development of atherosclerosis.

Pharmacokinetics

Well absorbed from the GI tract; absorption maximum if given 30 min before food. **Onset:** 2–5 days. **Peak plasma levels:** 1–2 hr; **t½:** 1.5 hr. Metabolized in the liver with nearly 70% excreted in the urine. **Plasma protein binding:** Highly bound.

CONTRAINDICATIONS

Pre-existing gallbladder disease, primary biliary cirrhosis, hepatic or severe renal dysfunction. Concurrent use with repaglinide. Lactation.

SPECIAL CONCERNS

- **Possible dose reduction in geriatric clients due to age-related decreases in renal function.**
- **Use caution with anticoagulants; dosage of anticoagulant may need to be reduced.**
- **Use with caution with mild to moderate renal impairment.**
- **Safety and efficacy not established in children.**

SIDE EFFECTS

Most Common

Fatigue, vertigo, dyspepsia, eczema, rash, abdominal pain, diarrhea, N&V.

GI: Cholelithiasis (with greater prevalence of gallstones; surgery may be needed), abdominal/epigastric pain, N&V, diarrhea, dyspepsia, constipation, acute appendicitis, colitis, ***pancreatitis***, cholestatic jaundice, hepatoma. **CNS:** Dizziness, headache, fatigue, vertigo, somnolence, paresthesia, hypesthesia, depression, confusion, syncope, peripheral neuritis, ***seizures***. **CV:** Atrial fibrillation, extrasystoles, peripheral vascular disease, ***intracerebral hemorrhage***. **Hematologic:** Anemia, leukopenia, eosinophilia, thrombocytopenia, bone marrow hypoplasia. **Musculoskeletal:** Painful extremities, arthralgia, myalgia, myopathy, myositis, myasthenia, rhabdomyolysis, synovitis. **Allergic:** Urticaria, lupus-like syndrome, ***angioedema***, ***laryngeal edema***, vasculitis, ***anaphylaxis***. **Dermatologic:** Eczema, dermatitis, pruritus, skin rashes, exfoliative dermatitis, alopecia, photosensitivity. **GU:** Impotence, decreased libido/male fertility, impaired renal function, UTI. **Ophthalmic:** Blurred vision, retinal edema, cataracts. **Miscellaneous:** Increased chance of viral and bacterial infections (e.g., cold, cough, UTIs), taste perversion, weight loss.

LABORATORY TEST CONSIDERATIONS

↑ AST, ALT, LDH, CPK, alkaline phosphatase, bilirubin, creatine phosphokinase. Hypokalemia, hyperglycemia. Positive antinuclear antibody. ↓ Hemoglobin, WBCs, hematocrit.

OVERDOSE MANAGEMENT

Symptoms: Abdominal cramping, N&V, diarrhea, abnormal LFTs, ↑ serum creatine phosphokinase, joint and muscle pain. *Treatment:* Initiate symptomatic supportive measures.

DRUG INTERACTIONS

Anticoagulants, oral (e.g., warfarin) / ↑ Anticoagulant effects; monitor for signs of bleeding and PT; adjust dosage

Bexarotene / ↑ Bexarotene plasma levels → ↑ pharmacologic/toxic effects; monitor response and adjust dose if necessary

Colestipol / ↓ Gemfibrozil effect; separate administration times by at least 2 hr

Cyclosporine / ↓ Cyclosporine effect; monitor whole blood cyclosporine levels, and adjust dose if needed

HMG-CoA reductase inhibitors (e.g., lovastatin, rosuvastatin, simvastatin) / ↑ Risk of skeletal muscle toxicity, including rhabdomyolysis, markedly ↑ CPK levels, myositis, and myoglobinuria

Loperamide / ↑ Loperamide plasma levels → ↑ risk of side effects, including respiratory depression; monitor and adjust dose as necessary

Montelukast / ↑ Montelukast plasma levels → ↑ pharmacologic/toxic effects; monitor and adjust montelukast dose as necessary

Pioglitazone / ↑ Pioglitazone AUC R/T inhibition of the CYP2C8 isoenzyme → side effects, including hypoglycemia and peripheral edema; adjust pioglitazone dose as needed

Repaglinide / Significant ↑ repaglinide levels R/T ↓ metabolism by CYP2C8 → severe and protracted hypoglycemia; coadministration contraindicated

Rosiglitazone / ↑ Rosiglitazone AUC R/T inhibition of the CYP2C8 isoenzyme → side effects, including hypoglycemia and peripheral edema; adjust pioglitazone dose as needed
Sulfonylureas / ↑ Hypoglycemic effect; monitor blood glucose levels
Tiagabine / ↑ Tiagabine plasma levels → ↑ pharmacologic/toxic (e.g., confusion, lightheadedness) effects; monitor and adjust tiagabine dose as needed

HOW SUPPLIED

Tablets: 600 mg.

G

DOSAGE

TABLETS

Hypertriglyceridemia, hyperlipidemia, prevention of cardiovascular (CV) disease.

Adults: 600 mg twice a day 30 min before the morning and evening meal. Dosage has not been established in children. Discontinue if significant improvement not observed within 3 months.

NURSING IMPLICATIONS

Do not confuse gemfibrozil with gemifloxacin (a fluoroquinolone antibiotic) or Lopid with Lorabid (a beta-lactam antibiotic) or Levbid.

ASSESSMENT

1. Note reasons for therapy, other agents trialed, outcome, serum HDL and TG levels; identify risk factors.
2. Assess compliance with therapeutic regimens/lifestyle changes (i.e., restriction of fat in diet, blood sugar control, weight reduction, regular exercise, avoidance of alcohol).
3. Monitor CBC, K^+, blood sugars (HbA1c), CPK, LFTs; assess for gallbladder disease, liver/renal dysfunction.

CLIENT/FAMILY TEACHING

1. Take 30 min before meals (twice a day) as directed. Pill is rather large, so use care when swallowing.
2. Use caution when driving/performing dangerous tasks until drug effects realized; may experience dizziness, blurred vision.
3. Continue to follow prescribed dietary guidelines restricting sugar/CHO and fats, avoid tobacco/alcohol, and follow regular exercise program to reduce cardiac risk factors.
4. Report unusual bruising/bleeding. If also on anticoagulant therapy, a reduction in anticoagulant may be necessary.
5. Limit intake of alcohol. Report any muscle pain/cramps, RUQ abdominal pain, or change in stool color or consistency.
6. S&S of gallstones, such as abdominal pain and vomiting should be reported.
7. Keep all F/U to assess response, labs, adverse SE.

OUTCOMES/EVALUATE

↓ Cholesterol and triglyceride levels ↑ HDL

Gemifloxacin mesylate

(gem-ih-**FLOCK**-sah-sin)

Classification(s): Antibiotic, fluoroquinolone

Pregnancy Category: C

RX: Factive.

SEE ALSO ***FLUOROQUINOLONES***.

INDICATIONS/USES

(1) Acute bacterial exacerbation of chronic bronchitis due to *Streptococcus pneumoniae, Haemophilus influenzae, Haemophilus parainfluenzae,* or *Moraxella catarrhalis.* (2) Community-acquired pneumonia (mild to moderate) due to *S. pneumoniae* (including multidrug resistant strains), *H. influenzae, M. catarrhalis, Mycoplasma pneumoniae, Chlamydia pneumoniae,* or *Klebsiella pneumoniae.*

NOTE: To prevent development of drug-resistant bacteria and maintain efficacy, use only to treat infections proven or strongly suspected to be caused by susceptible bacteria.

ACTION/KINETICS

Pharmacokinetics

Rapidly absorbed from the GI tract. **Peak plasma levels:** 0.5–2 hr. About 71% of the drug is bioavailable. Food does not affect absorption. Widely distributed throughout the body after PO administration. A small percentage is metabolized in the liver. Unchanged drug and metabolites are excreted in the feces (about 61%) and urine (about 36%). **t½, elimination:** About 7 hr.

CONTRAINDICATIONS

Hypersensitivity to gemifloxacin, fluoroquinolone antibiotics, or any component of the product. Use in clients with a history of prolongation of the QTc interval, those with uncorrected electrolyte disorders (hypokalemia, hypomagnesemia), in clients taking class IA (e.g., quinidine, procainamide) or class III (e.g., amiodarone, sotalol) antiarrhythmic drugs. Use in those with myasthenia gravis. Lactation.

SPECIAL CONCERNS

(1) Fluoroquinolones, including gemifloxacin, are associated with an increased risk of tendonitis and tendon rupture in all ages. This risk is further increased in clients older than 60; in clients taking corticosteroid drugs; and in clients with kidney, heart, or lung transplants. (2) Fluoroquinolones, including gemifloxacin, may exacerbate muscle weakness in individuals with myasthenia gravis. Avoid gemifloxacin in clients with known history of myasthenia gravis.

- **Use reduced dosage in clients with a C_{CR} <40 mL/min.**
- **Use with caution when given with erythromycin, antipsychotics, and tricyclic antidepressants and in clients with ongoing proarrhythmic conditions (clinically significant bradycardia, acute myocardial ischemia) due to possible prolongation of QTc interval. Possibility of prolongation of the QTc interval increases with increasing doses.**
- **Safety and efficacy not determined in children <18 years old, in pregnancy, or during lactation.**

SIDE EFFECTS

Most Common

Nausea, GI upset, anorexia, diarrhea, drowsiness, dizziness, headache, dry mouth, altered taste, constipation, insomnia.

GI: N&V, diarrhea, GI upset, abdominal pain, taste perversion, anorexia, constipation, dry mouth, dyspepsia, flatulence, gastritis, gastroenteritis, nonspecified GI disorder. **CNS:** Headache, dizziness, insomnia, somnolence/drowsiness, nervousness, vertigo. **Dermatologic:** Rash, dermatitis, pruritus, urticaria, eczema, flushing. **CV:** Prolongation of QT interval. **Hypersensitivity:** ***Anaphylaxis, CV collapse, hypotension/shock, acute respiratory distress, seizures***, loss of consciousness, tingling, ***angioedema***, ***bronchospasm***, shortness of breath, dyspnea, urticaria, itching, serious skin reactions. **Hematologic:** Leukopenia, thrombocythemia, anemia, eosinophilia, granulocytopenia, thrombocytopenia. **Musculoskeletal:** Back pain, leg cramps, myalgia. **Respiratory:** Dyspnea, pharyngitis, pneumonia. **GU:** Genital moniliasis, vaginitis, abnormal urine. **Body as a whole:** Arthralgia, fatigue, fungal infection, moniliasis, asthenia, pain, tremor. **Miscellaneous:** Hot flashes, vision abnormality.

LABORATORY TEST CONSIDERATIONS

↑ ALT, AST, creatine phosphokinase, GGT, potassium, alkaline phosphatase, total bilirubin, BUN, serum creatinine, calcium. ↓ Sodium, albumin, total protein. Hyperglycemia, bilirubinemia.

DRUG INTERACTIONS

Antacids, Al- or Mg^{++}-containing / ↓ Absorption of gemifloxacin from the GI tract
Didanosine (chewable/buffered tablets, pediatric powder for PO solution) / ↓ Absorption of gemifloxacin from the GI tract
Ferrous sulfate or iron-containing products / ↓ Absorption of gemifloxacin from the GI tract
Probenecid / Significant ↑ in gemifloxacin AUC and prolongation of half-life
Sucralfate / ↓ Absorption of gemifloxacin from the GI tract

HOW SUPPLIED

Tablets: 320 mg.

DOSAGE

TABLETS

Acute bacterial exacerbation of chronic bronchitis

Adults: One 320 mg tablet daily for 5 days.

Mild to moderate community-acquired pneumonia.

Adults. Community-acquired pneumonia due to *S. pneumoniae, H. influenzae, M. pneumoniae,* **or** *C. pneumoniae*: One 320 mg tablet daily for 5 days. **Community-acquired pneumonia due to multidrug resistant strains,** *K. pneumoniae,* **or** *M. catarrhalis*: One 320 mg tablet daily for 7 days.

NURSING IMPLICATIONS

Do not confuse gemifloxacin with gatifloxacin (also a fluoroquinolone antibiotic).

IMPLEMENTATION/ADMINISTRATION/STORAGE

1. For both uses, a dose of 160 mg q 24 hr should be used in those with C_{CR} of 40 mL/min or less and in those requiring routine hemodialysis or continuous ambulatory peritoneal dialysis. For C_{CR} >40 mL/min, use usual doses.
2. Store from 15–30°C (59–86°F) protected from light.

ASSESSMENT

1. Note reasons for therapy, characteristics of S&S, other agents trialed/outcome, culture results. Review family history for QT prolongation; avoid with any history.
2. Note drugs prescribed to ensure none interact.
3. Determine sensitivity reactions. Assess for CNS effects such as anxiety, tremors.
4. Review increased risk of tendonitis and tendon rupture in all ages. Risk increased in those older than 60 y.o., in those taking corticosteroids, and with kidney, heart, or lung transplants.
5. Monitor ECG, CBC, LFTs; liver enzymes may become elevated during therapy but should resolve.

CLIENT/FAMILY TEACHING

1. May take without regard to meals. Swallow tablets whole with a full glass of water. Consume eight 8 oz glasses of water daily.
2. Complete entire therapy even if feeling better, to prevent resistance to antibiotic.
3. Allow 3 hr before or 2 hr after dosing if using calcium, iron, sucrafate, multivitamins with zinc, or antacids.
4. Avoid activities that require mental alertness until drug effects realized. May cause dizziness, tremors, and anxiety; report.
5. Use protection when exposed; avoid excessive exposure to sunlight/photosensitivity reaction.
6. Report persistent diarrhea. Consume adequate fluids to prevent dehydration.
7. Stop drug and report any pain, inflammation, or tendon rupture; more pronounced in those over age 60, taking corticosteroids, and with kidney, heart, or lung transplants. Avoid OTC agents without provider approval.
8. Women on hormone therapy, as well as clients under age 40 may experience rash; stop drug if evident and report.
9. May produce prolongation of the QTc interval on an ECG; report cardiac S&S.
10. Keep all F/U to assess response, labs, adverse SE.

OUTCOMES/EVALUATE

Resolution of infection

■ IV

Gentamicin sulfate

(jen-tah-**MY**-sin)

Classification(s): Antibiotic, aminoglycoside

Pregnancy Category: C

RX: Injection: Gentamicin Sulfate, Gentamicin Sulfate in 0.9% Sodium Chloride, Pediatric Gentamicin Sulfate. **Ophthalmic Ointment:** Gentak, Gentamicin Sulfate Ophthalmic. **Ophthalmic Solution:** Gentamicin Ophthalmic.

✤ **Rx:** ratio-Gentamicin.

SEE ALSO *AMINOGLYCOSIDES*.

INDICATIONS/USES

Injection: (1) Serious infections of the conjunctiva or cornea caused by *Pseudomonas aeruginosa, Proteus, Klebsiella, Enterobacter, Serratia, Citrobacter,* and *Staphylococcus.* Infections include bacterial neonatal sepsis, bacterial septicemia, and serious infections of the skin, bone, soft tissue (including burns), urinary tract, GI tract (including peritonitis), and CNS (including meningitis). Should be considered as initial therapy in suspected or confirmed gram-negative infections. (2) In combination with carbenicillin for treating life-threatening infections due to *P. aeruginosa.* (3) In combination with penicillin for treating endocarditis caused by group D streptococci. (4) In combination with penicillin for treating suspected bacterial sepsis or staphylococcal pneumonia in the neonate. (5) Intrathecal administration is used in combination with systemic gentamicin for treating meningitis, ventriculitis, or other serious CNS infections due to *Pseudomonas. Investigational:* Pelvic inflammatory disease.

Ophthalmic: Ophthalmic bacterial infections, including conjunctivitis, keratitis, keratoconjunctivitis, corneal ulcers, blepharitis, blepharoconjunctivitis, acute meibomianitis, and dacryocystitis infections due to *Staphylococcus epidermidis, Streptococcus pyogenes, Streptococcus pneumoniae, Enterobacter aerogenes, Escherichia coli, Haemophilus influenzae, Klebsiella pneumoniae, Neisseria gonorrhoeae, Pseudomonas aeruginosa, Serratia marcescens.*

Topical: (1) Primary skin infections, including impetigo contagiosa, superficial folliculitis, ecthyma, furunculosis, sycosis barbae, and pyoderma gangrenosum. (2) Secondary skin infections, including infectious eczematoid dermatitis, pustular acne, pustular psoriasis, infected seborrheic dermatitis, infected contact dermatitis (including poison ivy), infected excoriations, and bacterial superinfections of fungal or viral infections. (3) Infected skin cysts and certain other skin abscesses when preceded by incision and drainage to permit adequate contact between the antibiotic and the causative bacteria. (4) Other infections, including infected stasis and other skin ulcers, superficial burns, paronychia, infected insect bites and stings, lacerations and abrasions, and wounds from minor surgery.

ACTION/KINETICS

Pharmacokinetics

Therapeutic serum levels: IM, 4–8 mcg/mL. **Toxic serum levels:** >12 mcg/mL (peak) and >2 mcg/mL (trough). Prolonged serum levels above 12 mcg/mL should be avoided. **t½:** 2 hr. Can be used with carbenicillin to treat serious *Pseudomonas* infections; do not mix these drugs in the same flask, as carbenicillin will inactivate gentamicin.

CONTRAINDICATIONS

Ophthalmic use to treat dendritic keratitis, vaccinia, varicella, mycobacterial infections of the eye, fungal diseases of the eye, use with steroids after uncomplicated removal of a corneal foreign body. Concurrent use with nephrotoxic drugs or diuretics. Lactation.

SPECIAL CONCERNS

See Aminoglycosides.

- **Ophthalmic ointments may retard corneal epithelial healing.**
- **Addition of short-term, low-dose gentamicin therapy to antistaphylococcal penicillins or vancomycin to treat *Staphylococcus aureus* bacteremia and native valve endocarditis increases the risk of renal side effects.**
- **Use with caution in premature infants and neonates.**

SIDE EFFECTS

Most Common

After parenteral use: GI upset, diarrhea, anorexia, N&V, tinnitus, dizziness.
After ophthalmic use: Transient irritation, burning, stinging, itching, inflammation, mydriasis, lid itching/swelling.
After topical use: Erythema, pruritus.
See *Aminoglycosides* for a complete list of possible side effects. Also, muscle twitching, numbness, ***seizures***, increased BP, alopecia, purpura, pseudotumor cerebri. Photosensitivity when used topically.

After ophthalmic use: Transient irritation, burning, stinging, itching, inflammation, angioneurotic edema, urticaria, vesicular and maculopapular dermatitis, mydriasis, conjunctival paresthesia, conjunctival hyperemia, nonspecific conjunctivitis, conjunctival epithelial defects, lid itching/swelling, bacterial/fungal corneal ulcers.

After topical use: Erythema, pruritus, photosensitivity; overgrowth of nonsusceptible organisms (superinfection), including fungi.

ADDITIONAL DRUG INTERACTIONS

Carbenicillin / ↑ Effect when used for ***Pseudomonas*** infections
Cidofovir / ↑ Risk of nephrotoxicity
Diuretics / ↑ Risk of ototoxicity
Nephrotoxic drugs / ↑ Risk of toxicity
Ticarcillin / ↑ Effect when used for ***Pseudomonas*** infections

HOW SUPPLIED

Injection: 10 mg/mL, 40 mg/mL; ***Ophthalmic Ointment:*** 3 mg/gram; ***Ophthalmic Solution:*** 3 mg/mL; ***Topical Cream:*** 0.1% (as base); ***Topical Ointment:*** 0.1%; ***Injection in 0.9% Sodium Chloride:*** 0.8 mg/mL, 0.9 mg/mL, 1 mg/mL, 1.2 mg/mL, 1.4 mg/mL, 1.6 mg/mL.

DOSAGE

IM (USUAL); IV

Infections.

Adults with normal renal function: 1 mg/kg q 8 hr, up to 5 mg/kg/day in life-threatening infections; **children:** 2–2.5 mg/kg q 8 hr; **infants and neonates:** 2.5 mg/kg q 8 hr; **premature in-**

fants or neonates less than 1 week of age: 2.5 mg/kg q 12 hr. Therapy may be required for 7–10 days.

Prevention of bacterial endocarditis, dental or respiratory tract procedures.

Adults: 1.5 mg/kg gentamicin (not to exceed 80 mg) plus 1 gram ampicillin, each IM or IV, 30–60 min before the procedure; one additional dose of each can be given 8 hr later (alternative: Penicillin V, 1 gram PO, 6 hr after initial dose).

Prophylaxis of bacterial endocarditis in gastrointestinal or genitourinary tract procedures or surgery.

Adults: 1.5 mg/kg gentamicin (not to exceed 80 mg) plus 2 grams ampicillin, each IM or IV, 30–60 min before procedure; dose should be repeated 8 hr later. **Children:** 2 mg/kg gentamicin plus penicillin G, 30,000 units/kg, or ampicillin, 50 mg/kg in same dosage interval as for adults. Pediatric dosage should not exceed single or 24 hr adult doses. *NOTE:* In clients allergic to penicillin, vancomycin, 1 gram IV given slowly over 1 hr, may be substituted; the dose of vancomycin should be repeated 8–12 hr later. **Adults with impaired renal function**: To calculate interval (hr) between doses, multiply serum creatinine (mg/100 mL) by 8.

IV

Septicemia.

Initially: 1–2 mg/kg infused over 30–60 min; **then,** maintenance doses may be administered.

Pelvic inflammatory disease.

Initial: 2 mg/kg IV; **then,** 1.5 mg/kg 3 times per day plus clindamycin, 500 mg IV 4 times per day. Continue for at least 4 days and at least 48 hr after client improves. Continue clindamycin, 450 mg PO 4 times per day for 10–14 days.

INTRATHECAL

Meningitis.

Use only the intrathecal preparation. Adults, usual: 4–8 mg/day; **children and infants 3 months and older:** 1–2 mg/day

OPHTHALMIC SOLUTION (3 MG/ML)

Ophthalmic bacterial infections.

Initially: 1–2 gtt in conjunctival sac q 4 hr. For severe infections, dose may be increased to 2 gtt once every hour.

OPHTHALMIC OINTMENT (3 MG/GRAM)

Ophthalmic bacterial infections.

Apply a small amount (about ½ inch) to the affected eye 2–3 times a day.

TOPICAL CREAM/OINTMENT (0.1%)

All uses.

Apply 3–4 times per day to affected area. The area may be covered with a sterile bandage.

NURSING IMPLICATIONS

IMPLEMENTATION/ADMINISTRATION/STORAGE

1. When used intrathecally, the usual site is the lumbar area.
2. PO administration of N-acetylcysteine (600 mg twice a day) may lower the incidence of aminoglycoside-induced ototoxicity.
3. Store ophthalmic ointment and solution from 2–30°C (36–86°F).
4. IV For intermittent IV administration, dilute adult dose in 50–200 mL of NSS or D5W and administer over a 30–120 min period; use less volume for infants and children.
5. For parenteral use, the duration of treatment is 7–10 days; a longer course may be required for severe or complicated infections.
6. COMPATIBILITY NSS or D5W.
7. INCOMPATIBILITY Do not mix with other drugs for parenteral use.

ASSESSMENT

1. Note type, onset, characteristics of S&S and clinical presentation.
2. With eye disorders, note baseline ophthalmologic examinations.
3. List drugs prescribed to ensure none interact or potentiate nephrotoxicity.
4. Assess for tinnitus, vertigo, or hearing losses during therapy (auditory or vestibular ototoxicity). Persistently increased gentamicin levels have been associated with 8th CN dysfunction. Monitor levels and ensure adequate hydration. Partial or total irreversible deafness

may continue to develop after drug is stopped.

5. Monitor renal and LFTs, CBC, and appropriate specimens for culture. Reduce dose with renal dysfunction and elevated drug levels.

CLIENT/FAMILY TEACHING

1. Review appropriate method and frequency for administration. Wash hands before and after treatment; prepare site and apply as directed.
2. With topical administration:
   - Remove crusts (of impetigo contagiosa) before applying cream/ointment to permit maximum contact between antibiotic and infection.
   - Wash affected area with soap and water, rinse, and dry thoroughly.
   - Apply cream or ointment gently, and cover with gauze dressing if ordered.
   - Avoid direct exposure to sunlight; photosensitivity reaction may occur.
   - Avoid further contamination of infected skin.
3. With parenteral therapy, report decreased urinary output, hearing changes (e.g., ringing in ears, hearing loss), dizziness, tingling/numbness in hands/feet, growth on tongue, vaginal itch or discharge.
4. Identify symptoms and wound changes that require medical attention; i.e., pain, redness, swelling, increased drainage or odor.
5. With eye therapy, wash hands and do not allow dropper or container tip to touch eye. Tilt head back, looking up; pull lower eyelid down and instill prescribed number of drops. With ointment, pull lower lid downward and insert ½-inch ribbon to sac. Close eye for 1 to 2 min; apply gentle pressure to bridge of nose. Do not rub eye. If more than 1 topical eye drug is being used, administer drugs at least 5 min apart.
6. May experience blurred vision for several min following therapy. Report any visual impairment, vertigo, dizziness, hearing impairment/changes, or worsening of S&S.
7. Avoid prolonged sun exposure; use sunscreen/protective clothing to avoid photosensitivity reaction.
8. Consume adequate fluids to prevent dehydration.
9. Avoid vaccinations during treatment.
10. Practice reliable contraception to prevent pregnancy during parenteral therapy.
11. Keep all F/U to assess response, labs, adverse SE.

OUTCOMES/EVALUATE

- Resolution of infection
- Therapeutic serum drug levels 4–8 mcg/mL; (peak: 4–8 mcg/mL; trough: 2 mcg/mL) with parenteral use.

Glimepiride

(**GLYE**-meh-pye-ride)

Classification(s): Antidiabetic, oral; second generation sulfonylurea

Pregnancy Category: C

RX: Amaryl.

✤ **Rx:** Apo-Glimepiride, CO Glimepiride, ratio-Glimepiride, Sandoz Glimepiride.

SEE ALSO ***ANTIDIABETIC AGENTS: HYPOGLYCEMIC AGENTS***.

INDICATIONS/USES

(1) As an adjunct to diet and exercise to lower blood glucose in non-insulin-dependent diabetes mellitus (type 2 diabetes mellitus) whose hyperglycemia cannot be controlled by diet and exercise alone. (2) In combination with insulin to decrease blood glucose in those whose hyperglycemia cannot be controlled by diet and exercise in combination with an oral hypoglycemic drug. (3) In combination with metformin (Glucophage) if control is not reached with diet, exercise, and either hypoglycemic alone.

ACTION/KINETICS

Action

Lowers blood glucose by stimulating the release of insulin from functioning pancreatic beta cells and by increasing the sensitivity of peripheral tissues to insulin.

Pharmacokinetics

Completely absorbed from the GI tract within 1 hr. **Onset:** 2–3 hr. **t½, serum:** About 9 hr. **Duration:** 24 hr. Completely metabolized in the liver and metabolites are excreted through both the urine and feces.

CONTRAINDICATIONS

Diabetic ketoacidosis with or without coma. Use during lactation.

SPECIAL CONCERNS

- Increased risk of CV mortality compared with diet alone or diet plus insulin.
- Safety and efficacy not determined in children.

SIDE EFFECTS

Most Common

Hypoglycemia, dizziness, weakness, headache, blurred vision, N&V, stomach pain, photosensitivity.

GI: N&V, GI pain, diarrhea, stomach pain, cholestatic jaundice (rare). **CNS:** Dizziness, headache. **Dermatologic:** Pruritus, erythema, urticaria, morbilliform or maculopapular eruptions, photosensitivity. **Hematologic:** Leukopenia, agranulocytosis, thrombocytopenia, hemolytic anemia, ***aplastic anemia***, pancytopenia. **Body as a whole:** Hypoglycemia, weakness. **Miscellaneous:** Hyponatremia, increased release of ADH, changes in accommodation and/or blurred vision.

G

DRUG INTERACTIONS

See *Antidiabetic Agents: Hypoglycemic Agents.*

HOW SUPPLIED

Tablets: 1 mg, 2 mg, 4 mg.

DOSAGE

TABLETS

Non-insulin-dependent diabetes mellitus (type 2 diabetes).

Adults, initial: 1–2 mg once daily, given with breakfast or the first main meal. The initial dose should be 1 mg in those sensitive to hypoglycemic drugs, in those with impaired renal or hepatic function, and in elderly, debilitated, or malnourished clients. The maximum initial dose is 2 mg or less daily. **Maintenance:** 1–4 mg once daily up to a maximum of 8 mg once daily. After a dose of 2 mg is reached, increase the dose in increments of 2 mg or less at 1- to 2-week intervals (determined by the blood glucose response). **When combined with insulin therapy:** 8 mg once daily with the first main meal with low-dose insulin. The fasting glucose level for beginning combination therapy is greater than 150 mg/dL glucose in the plasma or serum. After starting with low-dose insulin, upward adjustments of insulin can be done about weekly as determined by frequent fasting blood glucose determinations.

Type 2 diabetes—transfer from other hypoglycemic agents.

When transferring clients to glimepiride, no transition period is required. However, observe clients closely for 1 to 2 weeks for hypoglycemia when being transferred from longer half-life sulfonylureas (e.g., chlorpropamide) to glimepiride.

NURSING IMPLICATIONS

Do not confuse Amaryl with Reminyl (an anti-Alzheimer's drug). NOTE: The manufacturer has changed the trade name of Reminyl to Razadyne. Also, do not confuse glimepiride with galantamine (a CNS drug for Alzheimer's disease).

IMPLEMENTATION/ADMINISTRATION/STORAGE

1. Dispense tablets in well-closed containers with safety caps.
2. Store tablets at 15–30°C (59–86°F).

ASSESSMENT

1. Note reasons for therapy, if newly diagnosed or transferred therapy, glycemic control, disease characteristics, family history.
2. List other agents trialed, drugs currently taking to ensure none interact. Avoid with G6PD clients—may cause hemolytic anemia.
3. Review risk of increased cardiovascular mortality as compared to treatment with diet and insulin.
4. Assess lifestyle and diet; identify risk factors and changes needed.
5. Monitor VS, Wt, electrolytes, BS, HbA1c, Ca^{++}, Mg^{++}, microalbumin, renal and LFTs; reduce dose with dysfunction.

CLIENT/FAMILY TEACHING

1. Drug stimulates insulin release from pancreas and helps insulin get into the cells where it can work properly to lower blood sugar and help restore the way you use food to make energy.

2. Review dose, frequency for administration and S&S of hypo-/hyperglycemia. Usually taken once a day with first main meal of day.
3. Record finger sticks, include 1 or 2 hr post-meal FS.
4. Continue regular exercise and dietary restrictions, BP and cholesterol control in addition to drug therapy. No alcohol without approval.
5. Report persistent diarrhea, heartburn, N&V, rash, sore throat, or unusual bruising or bleeding.
6. Avoid direct/artificial sun exposure; may cause photosensitivity reaction.
7. Keep all F/U to assess response, teaching reinforcement, labs, BP, eye/foot exams, and for adverse SE.

OUTCOMES/EVALUATE

FBS <100 and HbA1c <8

Glipizide

(**GLIP**-ih-zyd)

Classification(s): Antidiabetic, oral; second-generation sulfonylurea

Pregnancy Category: C

RX: Glipizide Extended-Release, Glucotrol, Glucotrol XL.

SEE ALSO ***ANTIDIABETIC AGENTS: HYPOGLYCEMIC AGENTS.***

INDICATIONS/USES

Adjunct to diet for control of hyperglycemia in clients with type 2 diabetes. Begin therapy when diet alone has been unsuccessful in controlling hyperglycemia.

ACTION/KINETICS

Action

Lowers blood glucose by stimulating the release of insulin from functioning pancreatic beta cells and by increasing the sensitivity of peripheral tissues to insulin. Also has mild diuretic effects.

Pharmacokinetics

Onset: 1–3 hr. **t½:** 2–4 hr. **Duration:** 10–24 hr. Metabolized in liver to inactive metabolites, which are excreted through the kidneys.

SIDE EFFECTS

Most Common

Hypoglycemia, headache, dizziness, hives, skin rash, jaundice.

See *Antidiabetic Agents: Hypoglycemic Agents* for a complete list of possible side effects.

ADDITIONAL DRUG INTERACTIONS

Cimetidine may ↑ glipizide effect R/T ↓ liver breakdown.

HOW SUPPLIED

Tablets, Extended-Release: 2.5 mg, 5 mg, 10 mg; *Tablets, Immediate-Release:* 5 mg, 10 mg.

DOSAGE

TABLETS, IMMEDIATE-RELEASE

Type 2 diabetes.

Adults, initial: 5 mg 30 min before breakfast; **then,** adjust dosage by 2.5–5 mg every few days, depending on the blood glucose response, until adequate control is achieved. **Maintenance:** 15–40 mg/day; divide total daily doses over 15 mg/day. Older clients or those with liver disease should begin with 2.5 mg.

TABLETS, EXTENDED-RELEASE

Type 2 diabetes.

Adults (including geriatric clients), initial: 5 mg with breakfast. Monitor response to therapy by measuring HbA1c at 3-month intervals. Dose can be increased to 10 mg if response is inadequate. **Maintenance:** 5 or 10 mg once daily; some may require 20 mg/day (maximum).

NURSING IMPLICATIONS

Do not confuse glipizide with glyburide (another oral hypoglycemic drug).

IMPLEMENTATION/ADMINISTRATION/STORAGE

1. Some clients are better controlled on once daily dosing, while others are better controlled with divided dosing.
2. Divide maintenance doses greater than 15 mg/day; give before the morning and evening meals. Total daily doses of 30 mg or more may be given safely on twice daily dosing.

G

3. If on immediate-release glipizide, can be safely switched to extended-release tablets once a day at the nearest equivalent total daily dose. Can also be titrated to the appropriate dose of extended-release tablets starting with 5 mg once daily.
4. No transition period needed when transferring to extended-release tablets from other oral antidiabetic drugs. Observe for 1–2 weeks if transferred from long half-life sulfonylureas (e.g., chlorpropamide) to extended-release glipizide due to overlapping effects.
5. When transferring from insulin dose of <20 units/day, insulin may be discontinued abruptly. When transferring from an insulin dose of >20 units/day, reduce insulin dose by 50%; further reduce depending on response. The initial glipizide dose when transferring from insulin is 5 mg/day.
6. Assess lifestyle to ensure that maximal changes in the areas of diet and exercise have been taken before increasing dosage. Once maximum dosage is attained, if renal function is normal, consider adding metformin, pioglitazone, or rosiglitazone for better control.
7. Store immediate-release tablets below 30°C (86°F) and extended-release tablets, protected from moisture and humidity, from 15–30°C (59–86°F).

ASSESSMENT

1. List reasons for therapy, if newly diagnosed or transferred therapy; glycemic control, disease characteristics, family history.
2. List other agents trialed, drugs currently taking to ensure none interact.
3. Assess lifestyle and diet, identify changes needed, identify risk factors.
4. Monitor BP, weight. electrolytes, BS, HbA1c, Ca^{++}, Mg^{++}, U/A, microalbumin, renal and LFTs.

CLIENT/FAMILY TEACHING

1. Helps insulin get into cells where it can work properly to lower blood sugar and help restore the way you use food to make energy.
2. Take 30 min before or with meals (to lessen chance of stomach upset). Do not chew or crush extended-release form (i.e., Glucotrol XL).
3. Report CNS side effects: drowsiness, headache; check finger stick.
4. May have anorexia, constipation, diarrhea, vomiting, stomach pain. Report if severe, record weight, I&O.
5. Report if skin reactions occur. Avoid exposure to direct/artificial light; use sunscreen, sunglasses, protective clothing when outdoors.
6. Assess lifestyle and diet; identify changes needed. Practice barrier contraception
7. Avoid alcohol and OTC agents without approval.
8. Continue prescribed diet, weight loss, and regular exercise program. Record FS, also obtain FS 1–2 hr after eating.
9. Keep all F/U to assess response, labs, teaching reinforcement, BP, eye/foot exams, and for adverse SE.

OUTCOMES/EVALUATE

FBS <100; HbA1c <8

Glyburide

(**GLYE**-byou-ryd)

Classification(s): Antidiabetic, oral; second-generation sulfonylurea

Pregnancy Category: B

RX: Diaβeta, Glynase PresTab.

Rx: Apo-Glyburide, Gen-Glybe, Novo-Glyburide, Nu-Glyburide, PMS-Glyburide, ratio-Glyburide, Sandoz Glyburide.

SEE ALSO ***ANTIDIABETIC AGENTS: HYPOGLYCEMIC AGENTS***.

INDICATIONS/USES

Type 2 diabetes whose hyperglycemia cannot be controlled by diet alone. May be used with metformin when diet and glyburide or diet and metformin alone do not provide adequate control.

ACTION/KINETICS

Action

Lowers blood glucose by stimulating the release of insulin from functioning pancreatic beta cells and by increasing the sensitivity of peripheral tissues to insulin. Has a mild diuretic effect.

Pharmacokinetics

Onset, nonmicronized: 2–4 hr; **micronized:** 1 hr. **t½, nonmicronized:** 10 hr; **micronized:** Approximately 4 hr. **Time to peak levels:** 4 hr. **Duration, nonmicronized:** 16–24 hr; **micronized:**

12–24 hr. Metabolized in liver to weakly active metabolites. Excreted in bile (50%) and through the kidneys (50%). Micronized glyburide (3 mg tablets) produces serum levels that are not bioequivalent to those from nonmicronized glyburide (5 mg tablets).

SIDE EFFECTS

Most Common

Hypoglycemia, nausea, epigastric distress, heartburn, allergic skin reactions, blurred vision.
See *Antidiabetic Agents: Hypoglycemic Agents* for a complete list of possible side effects.

ADDITIONAL DRUG INTERACTIONS

Anticoagulants / Either ↑ or ↓ anticoagulant effect
Ciprofloxacin / Potentiation of hypoglycemic effect

HOW SUPPLIED

Tablets, Micronized: 1.5 mg, 3 mg, 4.5 mg, 6 mg; *Tablets, Nonmicronized:* 1.25 mg, 2.5 mg, 5 mg.

DOSAGE

Diaβeta

TABLETS, NONMICRONIZED

Type 2 diabetes.

Adults, initial: 2.5–5 mg/day given with breakfast (or the first main meal); **then,** increase by 2.5 mg at weekly intervals to achieve the desired response. **Maintenance:** 1.25–20 (maximum) mg/day. Clients sensitive to sulfonylureas should start with 1.25 mg/day.

Glynase Prestab

TABLETS, MICRONIZED

Type 2 diabetes.

Adults, initial: 1.5–3 mg/day given with breakfast (or the first main meal). Those sensitive to sulfonylureas should start with 0.75 mg/day. Increase by no more than 1.5 mg at weekly intervals to achieve the desired response. **Maintenance:** 0.75–12 (maximum) mg/day.

NURSING IMPLICATIONS

Do not confuse glyburide with glipizide (also an oral hypoglycemic) or glyburide with Glucotrol (also an oral hypoglycemic). Do not confuse Diaβeta with Zebeta (a beta-adrenergic blocker).

IMPLEMENTATION/ADMINISTRATION/STORAGE

1. For best results, administer 30 min prior to meals.
2. To avoid hypoglycemic reactions, the initial and maintenance doses should be conservative in the elderly, the debilitated, or in those with impaired hepatic or renal function.
3. Do not exceed 20 mg/day of the nonmicronized product and 12 mg/day of the micronized product.
4. If daily dosage of the nonmicronized product exceeds 15 mg or the micronized product exceeds 6 mg, dividing the dose and giving before the morning and evening meals may be more effective.
5. When transferring from oral hypoglycemics, other than chlorpropamide, no transition and no initial priming dose are required. When transferring from chlorpropamide, use caution for the first 2 weeks due to the long duration of action of chlorpropamide and possible overlapping drug effects.
6. A maintenance dose of 5 mg nonmicronized glyburide or 3 mg of micronized glyburide tablets provides about the same degree of blood glucose control as 250–375 mg chlorpropamide, 250–375 mg tolazamide, 500–750 mg acetohexamide, or 1,000–1,500 mg tolbutamide.
7. Add glyburide tablets gradually to the dosing regimen of those who have not responded to the maximum dose of metformin monotherapy after 4 weeks. Attempt to find the optimal dose of each drug needed to achieve blood glucose control.
8. Use the following guidelines when transferring from insulin to glyburide:
   - Insulin dose <20 units/day, start with 1.5–3 mg/day micronized or 2.5–5 mg/day nonmicronized glyburide. Insulin may be discontinued abruptly.
   - Insulin dose from 20–40 units/day, start with 3 mg/day micronized or 5 mg/day nonmicronized glyburide. Insulin may be discontinued abruptly.
   - Insulin dose >40 units/day, start with 3 mg/day micronized or 5 mg/day nonmicronized glyburide. Reduce insulin dose by 50%; reduce further as determined by re-

sponse. Consider hospitalization during the transition.

9. Store from 15–30°C (59–86°F).

ASSESSMENT

1. Note reasons for therapy, if newly diagnosed or transferred therapy; glycemic control, disease characteristics, family Hx.
2. List other agents trialed, drugs currently taking to ensure none interact.
3. Assess BMI, lifestyle, diet, identify risk factors and changes needed.
4. Monitor BP, electrolytes, BS, HbA1c, Ca^{++}, Mg^{++}, U/A, microalbumin, lipid panel, renal and LFTs.

G

CLIENT/FAMILY TEACHING

1. Works by causing your pancreas to release more insulin into the bloodstream, helps insulin get into the cells to lower blood sugar and help restore the way you use food to make energy. Take as directed with meals.
2. Record finger sticks at various times (i.e., fasting, 1 or 2 hr after meal, bedtime).
3. Continue regular daily exercise, lifestyle changes, BP control, weight loss, and dietary restrictions to control cholesterol and glucose.
4. Report S&S of hypoglycemia (e.g., fatigue, excessive hunger, profuse sweating, numbness of extremities) or if blood glucose is below 60 mg/dL. Report if persistent S&S of hyperglycemia (e.g., excessive thirst, urination, or FS >300).
5. Avoid alcohol, OTC agents without approval. Practice reliable contraception.
6. Report as scheduled for teaching reinforcement, F/U labs, foot/eye exams, and medication response.

OUTCOMES/EVALUATE

- FBS <100
- HbA1c <8

Combination Drug

Glyburide and Metformin hydrochloride

(**GLYE**-byou-ryd, met-**FOR**-min)

Classification(s): Antidiabetic, oral

Pregnancy Category: B

RX: Glucovance.

SEE ALSO ***GLYBURIDE*** AND ***METFORMIN*** AND ***ANTIDIABETIC AGENTS: HYPOGLYCEMIC AGENTS.***

INDICATIONS/USES

(1) As an adjunct to diet and exercise, and as initial therapy, to improve glycemic control in type 2 diabetes in those who cannot be controlled satisfactorily with diet and exercise alone. (2) Second-line therapy when diet, exercise, and initial therapy with a sulfonylurea or metformin do not provide adequate control in those with type 2 diabetes. If additional control is needed, a thiazolidinedione may be added to Glucovance therapy.

CONTENT

Each tablet, glyburide (listed first)/metformin contains: 1.25 mg/250 mg, 2.5 mg/500, 5 mg/500 mg.

ACTION/KINETICS

Action

Glyburide stimulates release of insulin from the pancreas, which is dependent upon functioning pancreatic beta islets. Extrapancreatic effects may also be involved in the long-term effectiveness of glyburide. Metformin decreases hepatic glucose production, decreases intestinal absorption of glucose, and improves insulin sensitivity by increasing peripheral glucose uptake and utilization. Thus the mechanisms are complementary.

Pharmacokinetics

Glyburide is rapidly absorbed; **peak levels:** 4 hr. Food decreases the extent and slightly delays the absorption of metformin. Glyburide is significantly bound to plasma proteins while metformin is negligibly bound. Steady state metformin levels are reached within 24–48 hr. **Glyburide, t½, terminal:** About 10 hr; excreted as metabolites in the bile and urine (about 50% by each route). Metformin is excreted unchanged in the urine; **t½, elimination:** About 17.6 hr.

CONTRAINDICATIONS

Use in renal disease or renal dysfunction (including that due to shock, acute MI, septicemia), CHF requiring pharmacologic treatment, acute or chronic metabolic acidosis (including diabetic ketoacidosis, with or without coma), and known hypersensitivity to glyburide or metformin. Not recommended for use during pregnancy or in children.

SPECIAL CONCERNS

(1) Lactic acidosis is a rare, but serious, metabolic complication that can occur due to metformin accumulation during treatment with Glucovance. When it occurs, it is fatal in approximately 50% of cases. Lactic acidosis may also occur in association with a number of pathophysiologic conditions, including diabetes mellitus, and whenever there is significant tissue hypoperfusion and hypoxemia. (2) Lactic acidosis is characterized by elevated blood lactate levels (>5 mmol/L), decreased blood pH, electrolyte disturbances with an increased anion gap, and an increased lactate/pyruvate ratio. When metformin is implicated as the cause of lactic acidosis, metformin plasma levels >5 micrograms/mL are generally found. (3) The reported incidence of lactic acidosis in those receiving metformin hydrochloride is low (approximately 0.03 cases/1,000 client years, with approximately 0.015 fatal cases/1,000 client years). In more than 20,000 client-years' exposure to metformin in clinical trials, there were no reports of lactic acidosis. Reported cases have occurred primarily in diabetic clients with significant renal insufficiency, including both intrinsic renal disease and renal hypoperfusion, often in the setting of multiple concomitant medical/surgical problems and multiple concomitant medications. (4) Clients with CHF requiring pharmacologic management, in particular those with unstable or acute CHF who are at risk of hypoperfusion and hypoxemia, are at increased risk of lactic acidosis. The risk of lactic acidosis increases with the degree of renal dysfunction and the client's age. The risk of lactic acidosis, therefore, may be significantly decreased by regular monitoring of renal function in clients taking metformin and by use of the minimum effective dose of metformin. (5) In particular, treatment of the elderly should be accompanied by careful monitoring of renal function. Do not initiate glyburide/metformin treatment in clients >80 years of age unless measurement of creatinine clearance demonstrates that renal function is not reduced, because these clients are more susceptible to developing lactic acidosis. In addition, promptly withhold glyburide/metformin in the presence of any condition associated with dehydration, hypoxia, or sepsis. (6) Because impaired hepatic function may significantly limit the ability to clear lactate, generally avoid glyburide/metformin in clients with clinical or laboratory evidence of hepatic disease. (7) Caution clients against excessive alcohol intake, either acute or chronic, when taking glyburide/metformin, because alcohol potentiates the effects of metformin on lactate metabolism. In addition, temporarily discontinue glyburide/metformin prior to any intravascular radiocontrast study and for any surgical procedure. (8) The onset of lactic acidosis often is subtle, and accompanied only by nonspecific symptoms such as malaise, myalgias, respiratory distress, increasing somnolence, and nonspecific abdominal distress. There may be associated hypothermia, hypotension, and resistant bradyarrhythmias with more marked acidosis. The client and the client's provider must be aware of the possible importance of such symptoms. Instruct the client to notify the provider immediately if they occur. Withdraw glyburide/metformin until the situation is clarified. (9) Serum electrolytes, ketones, blood glucose, and if indicated, blood pH, lactate levels, and even blood metformin levels may be useful. Once a client is stabilized on any dose level of glyburide/metformin, GI symptoms, which are common during initiation of therapy with metformin, are unlikely to be drug related. Later occurrence of GI symptoms could be caused by lactic acidosis or other serious disease. (10) Levels of fasting venous plasma lactate above the upper limit of normal but less than 5 mmol/L in clients taking glyburide/metformin do not necessarily indicate impending lactic acidosis and may be explainable by other mechanisms, such as poorly controlled diabetes or obesity, vigorous physical activity, or technical problems in sample handling. (11) Suspect lactic acidosis in any diabetic client with metabolic acidosis lacking evidence of ketoacidosis (ketonuria and ketonemia). (12) Lactic acidosis is a medical emergency that must be treated in a hospital setting. In a

G

client with lactic acidosis taking glyburide/metformin, immediately discontinue the drug and institute general supportive measures promptly. Because metformin is dialyzable (with a clearance of up to 170 mL/min under good hemodynamic conditions), prompt hemodialysis is recommended to correct the acidosis and remove the accumulated metformin. Such management often results in prompt reversal of symptoms and recovery. ■

To avoid the risk of hypoglycemia, generally do not titrate the elderly, debilitated, or malnourished clients to the maximum dose of glyburide/metformin.

SIDE EFFECTS

Most Common

URTI, diarrhea, hypoglycemia, headache, N&V, abdominal pain, dizziness.

See *Glyburide, Metformin*, and *Antidiabetic Agents: Hypoglycemic Agents* for a complete list of possible side effects. Lactic acidosis is a possible severe side effect.

DRUG INTERACTIONS

See ***Glyburide, Metformin***, and ***Antidiabetic Agents; Hypoglycemic Agents*** for a complete list of possible drug interactions.

HOW SUPPLIED

See *Content.*

DOSAGE

TABLETS

Type 2 diabetes, initial therapy.

Individualize dosage. **Initial:** 1.25 mg/250 mg once or twice a day with a meal. In those with baseline HbA1c >9% or an FPG >200 mg/dL, give an initial dose of 1.25 mg/250 mg twice a day with the morning and evening meals. Do not use glyburide/metformin, 5 mg/500 mg, as initial therapy due to the increased risk of hypoglycemia. Make dosage increases in increments of 1.25 mg/250 mg per day every 2 weeks up to the minimum effective dose needed to control blood glucose, not to exceed 20 mg glyburide/2,000 mg metformin daily.

Type 2 diabetes, in previously treated clients (second-line therapy).

Initial: Either 2.5 mg/500 mg or 5 mg/500 mg twice a day with the morning and evening meals. To avoid hypoglycemia, do not exceed the daily doses of glyburide or metformin already being taken. Titrate the daily dose in increments of no more than 5 mg/500 mg, up to the minimum effective dose to achieve adequate blood glucose control or a maximum dose of 20 mg/2,000 mg daily.

NURSING IMPLICATIONS

Do not confuse Glucovance with Glucophage (metformin only).

IMPLEMENTATION/ADMINISTRATION/STORAGE

1. For those previously treated with combination therapy of glyburide (or another sulfonylurea) plus metformin, if switched to glyburide/metformin, do not exceed the daily dose of glyburide (or equivalent dose of another sulfonylurea) and metformin already being taken. Monitor closely for S&S of hypoglycemia.
2. For clients not adequately controlled on glyburide/metformin, a thiazolidinedione can be added to therapy. When a thiazolidinedione is added, the current dose of glyburide/metformin can be continued and the thiazolidinedione added at its recommended starting dose. If additional glycemic control is needed, the dose of the thiazolidinedione can be increased based on its recommended titration schedule. However, the risk of hypoglycemia increases. If hypoglycemia occurs, reduce dose of the glyburide component of glyburide/metformin.
3. In the elderly, the initial and maintenance doses should be conservative due to decreased renal function in this group. Carefully assess renal function before dosage adjustment. For those 80 years and older, do not titrate glyburide/metformin to the maximum dose.
4. To avoid the risk of hypoglycemia, do not titrate debilitated or malnourished clients to the maximum dose.
5. Temporarily discontinue glyburide/metformin in those undergoing radiologic studies involv-

ing intravascular administration of iodinated contrast materials; use of such products may result in acute alteration of renal function.

6. Store up to 25°C (77°F); protect from light.

ASSESSMENT

1. Note reasons for therapy, disease onset, characteristics of S&S, other agents trialed, outcome.
2. List agents prescribed to ensure none interact.
3. Assess for alcohol use; this potentiates the effects of metformin on lactate metabolism.
4. Determine any heart disease, history of MI, stroke, or liver disease.
5. Lactic acidosis can be caused by metformin accumulation during treatment with glyburide/metformin; assess renal function and S&S as can be fatal in some cases.
6. Monitor renal and LFTs; avoid use in elderly, debilitated clients. Stop therapy if creatinine >1.5 males or >1.4 females to prevent acidosis.

CLIENT/FAMILY TEACHING

1. Drug is a combination of two oral hypoglycemic agents (glyburide and metformin) to help control blood sugar.
2. Take with meals as directed. Do not take if meal skipped.
3. May cause drowsiness, dizziness, blurred vision; avoid activities that require mental alertness until drug effects realized.
4. Monitor FS to ensure glucose control. Follow prescribed diabetic diet, exercise, and weight control program.
5. Report symptoms of lactic acidosis: weakness, unexplained sleepiness, slow heart rate, cold feeling, muscle pain, shortness of breath, stomach pain, N&V, feeling lightheaded, fainting.
6. Avoid alcohol: lowers blood sugar and may predispose one to lactic acidosis.
7. May cause photosensitivity; avoid prolonged sun exposure and use protection if exposed.
8. Practice reliable contraception.
9. Any procedure scheduled (x-ray or CT scan) using dye injected into veins, client should temporarily stop taking drug to prevent renal failure.
10. Keep all F/U to assess response, labs, foot/eye exams, and adverse SE.

OUTCOMES/EVALUATE

- HbA1c <8
- Control of BS

Goserelin acetate

(**GO**-seh-rel-in)

Classification(s): Antineoplastic, hormone

Pregnancy Category: X (when used for endometriosis); **D** (when used for breast cancer)

RX: Zoladex.

✤ **Rx:** Zoladex 3.6 mg, Zoladex LA.

SEE ALSO ***ANTINEOPLASTIC AGENTS***.

INDICATIONS/USES

Implant, 3.6 mg or 10.8 mg: Palliative treatment of advanced prostatic carcinoma as an alternative to orchiectomy or estrogen administration when these are either unacceptable to the client or not indicated. **Implant, 3.6 mg only:** (1) Endometriosis, including pain relief and reduction of endometriotic lesions. Use limited to women 18 years and older who have been treated for 6 months. (2) Palliative treatment of advanced breast cancer in pre- and postmenopausal women. (3) For endometrial thinning prior to ablation for dysfunctional uterine bleeding. **Implant, 10.8 mg only:** In combination with flutamide to manage locally confined T2b-T4 (Stage B2 to C) cancer of the prostate. Begin treatment 8 weeks prior to beginning radiation therapy and continue during radiation therapy.

ACTION/KINETICS

Action

Synthetic decapeptide analog of LHRH (or GnRH), which is a potent inhibitor of gonadotropin secretion from the pituitary gland. Initially, there is actually an increase in serum luteinizing hormone and FSH. This is followed by a long-term suppression of pituitary gonadotropins with serum levels of testosterone decreasing to those seen in surgically castrated males. When used for endometriosis, the drug controls the secretion of hormones required for the ovary to synthesize estrogen resulting in plasma estrogen levels seen in menopause.

Pharmacokinetics

Peak serum levels after SC implantation of 3.6 mg: 12–15 days in males and 8–22 days in females. **Mean peak serum levels:** Approximately 2.5 ng/mL. Available as an implant in a preloaded syringe. For the first 8 days of the treatment cycle, the rate of absorption of the 3.6 mg implant is slower than for the remainder of the period. For the 10.8 mg implant, mean levels increase to a peak within the first 24 hr and then decline rapidly until day 4; thereafter, mean levels remain constant until the end of the treatment period. **t½, elimination:** 4.2 hr in males and 2.3 hr in females with normal renal function and 12.1 hr for C_{CR} less than 20 mL/min. Rapidly cleared by a combination of hepatic metabolism and urinary excretion.

G

CONTRAINDICATIONS

Pregnancy, lactation, nondiagnosed vaginal bleeding, hypersensitivity to LHRH or LHRH agonist analogs. Use of the 10.8 mg implant in women.

SPECIAL CONCERNS

- May be initial worsening of the symptoms or occurrence of additional symptoms of prostate or breast cancer.
- Use with caution in males who are at particular risk of developing ureteral obstruction or spinal cord compression.
- Safety and efficacy not determined in children <18 years of age.

SIDE EFFECTS

Most Common

Hot flashes, headache, vaginitis, emotional lability, decreased libido, depression, sweating, acne, breast atrophy, vasodilation, peripheral edema, seborrhea.

In males. GU: Sexual dysfunction, decreased erections, lower urinary tract symptoms, gynecomastia, renal insufficiency, urinary obstruction/retention, UTI, bladder neoplasm, hematuria, impotence, urinary frequency, incontinence, urinary tract disorder, impaired urination. **CV:** CHF, ***CVA, MI, heart failure, pulmonary embolus***, arrhythmia, hypertension, peripheral vascular disorder, chest pain, angina pectoris, cerebral ischemia, varicose veins. **CNS:** Lethargy, dizziness, insomnia, asthenia, anxiety, depression, headache, paresthesia. **GI:** N&V, abdominal pain, diarrhea, constipation, ulcer, anorexia, hematemesis. **Respiratory:** URTI, COPD, increased cough, dyspnea, pneumonia. **Dermatologic:** Hot flashes, pruritus, rash, sweating, herpes simplex. **Metabolic:** Gout, hypercalcemia, weight increase, diabetes mellitus. **Body as a whole:** Anemia, chills, fever, flu syndrome, ***sepsis***, aggravation reaction, hypersensitivity, pain, edema. **Miscellaneous:** Pelvic or bone pain, breast pain, breast swelling or tenderness, abdominal or back pain, peripheral edema, injection site reaction, complications of surgery.

In females. GU: Vaginitis, decreased or increased libido, pelvic symptoms (including pain), dyspareunia, dysmenorrhea, menorrhagia, uterine hemorrhage, vulvovaginitis, urinary frequency, UTI, vaginal bleeding (during the first 2 months) of varying duration and intensity, ovarian hyperstimulation syndrome, ovarian cyst formation. **CV:** ***Hemorrhage***, hypertension, palpitations, migraine, tachycardia, vasodilation. **CNS:** Emotional lability, depression, headache, insomnia, dizziness, nervousness, anxiety, paresthesia, somnolence, abnormal thinking, migraine. **GI:** N&V, abdominal pain, increased appetite, anorexia, constipation, diarrhea, dry mouth, dyspepsia, flatulence. **Musculoskeletal:** Asthenia, back pain, myalgia, hypertonia, arthralgia, joint disorder, decrease of vertebral trabecular bone mineral density. **Dermatologic:** Sweating, acne, seborrhea, hirsutism, pruritus, alopecia, dry skin, ecchymosis, rash, skin discoloration, hair disorders. **Respiratory:** Pharyngitis, bronchitis, increased cough, epistaxis, rhinitis, sinusitis. **Ophthalmic:** Amblyopia, dry eyes. **Body as a whole:** Edema, fever, peripheral edema, hypersensitivity, malaise, fatigue, lethargy, infection, pain, allergic reaction, weight gain, flu syndrome. **Miscellaneous:** Hot flashes, breast atrophy or enlargement, breast pain, tumor flare, application site reaction, voice alterations, chest pain, hypercalcemia, osteoporosis.

LABORATORY TEST CONSIDERATIONS

↑ LDL and HDL cholesterol, triglycerides, AST, ALT. Misleading results of pituitary-gonadotropic and gonadal function tests conducted during treatment.

HOW SUPPLIED

Implant: 3.6 mg, 10.8 mg.

DOSAGE

SC IMPLANT, 3.6 MG

Endometriosis, advanced breast cancer.

3.6 mg q 28 days into the upper abdominal wall using sterile technique under the direction of the provider.

Thinning prior to endometrial ablation for dysfunctional uterine bleeding.

1 or 2 depots (each depot given 4 weeks apart).

SC IMPLANT, 10.8 MG

Advanced prostatic carcinoma.

10.8 mg q 12 weeks into the upper abdominal wall using sterile technique under the direction of the provider.

With flutamide to treat Stage B2-C prostatic carcinoma.

One goserelin 3.6 mg implant followed in 28 days by one 10.8 mg implant. Alternatively, 4 injections of the 3.6 mg depot can be given at 28-day intervals, 2 depots preceding and 2 during radiotherapy.

NURSING IMPLICATIONS

IMPLEMENTATION/ADMINISTRATION/STORAGE

1. Do not remove sterile syringe containing the drug until immediately before use. Examine syringe for damage and to ensure drug is visible in the translucent chamber.
2. Administer drug under physician supervision/orders.
3. Clean the area with an alcohol swab; a topical (i.e., ethyl chloride) or a local anesthetic may be used prior to the injection.
4. To administer, stretch the skin with one hand and grip the needle with the fingers around the barrel of the syringe. Insert needle into the SC fat; do not aspirate. If a large vessel is penetrated, blood will be seen immediately in the syringe; withdraw needle and make injection elsewhere with a new syringe.
5. The direction of the needle is changed so it parallels the abdominal wall. The needle is then pushed in until the barrel hub touches the skin. The plunger is depressed to deliver the drug. The needle is then withdrawn and the area bandaged.
6. To confirm the drug has been delivered, ensure that the tip of the plunger is visible within the tip of the needle.
7. If there is need to remove goserelin surgically, it can be located by ultrasound.
8. Adhere to the 28-day and 12-week schedules as closely as possible.
9. Store at room temperatures not exceeding 25°C (77°F).
10. There is no evidence the drug accumulates with either hepatic and/or renal dysfunction.
11. Duration of treatment for endometriosis is 6 months.
12. Males with ureteral obstruction or spinal cord compression should have appropriate treatment prior to initiating goserelin therapy.

ASSESSMENT

1. Note reasons for therapy, clinical presentation, other agents trialed, outcome.
2. Assess BMD and for osteoporosis. Note any S&S CV disease or loss of glycemic control.
3. During the first month of therapy, assess those at risk carefully for ureteral obstruction or spinal cord compression.
4. List BP, BS; PSA and testosterone levels with prostate cancer, radiologic findings, pain with endometriosis.

CLIENT/FAMILY TEACHING

1. Drug will be implanted into abdomen with a syringe every 28 days to 3 months as prescribed. Be sure not to miss scheduled administration days. The drug pellet is biodegradable and will be absorbed by the body; does not have to be removed.
2. The most common side effects (e.g., hot flashes, decreased erections, and sexual dysfunction) R/T ↓ testosterone levels.
3. Symptoms may grow worse initially as a result of transient increases of testosterone.
4. With palliative treatment of breast cancer or treatment of endometriosis (3.6 mg), menses should stop.
5. May experience increased bone pain, and develop spinal cord compression or ureteral obstruction; usually only temporary but must be reported promptly so that appropriate treatment may be initiated. Report all unusual/adverse side effects.
6. Not for use in women who are likely to become pregnant or who are pregnant. Drug may harm fetus and may impair fertility; identify for

sperm or egg harvesting. Use nonhormonal form of contraception.

7. Clients with prostate cancer who decide against surgery (orchiectomy) for medication therapy must come in regularly for abdominal implants for the rest of their lives.
8. Keep all F/U to assess response, labs, and for adverse SE.
9. Identify appropriate resources and support groups.

OUTCOMES/EVALUATE

- Symptom control; ↑ comfort
- ↓ Tumor size and spread
- ↓ Testosterone levels

G

IV

Granisetron hydrochloride

(gran-**ISS**-eh-tron)

Classification(s): Antiemetic, 5-HT_3 receptor antagonist

Pregnancy Category: B

RX: Granisol, Kytril, Sancuso.

INDICATIONS/USES

IV. (1) Prevention of N&V associated with initial/repeat cancer chemotherapy, including high-dose cisplatin. (2) Prevention/treatment of postoperative nausea and vomiting. *Investigational:* Postanesthetic shivering. **PO.** (1) Prevention of N&V associated with initial/repeat cancer chemotherapy, including high-dose cisplatin. (2) Prevention of N&V associated with radiation, including total body irradiation/fractionated abdominal radiation. **Transdermal Patch.** Prevention of nausea and vomiting in clients receiving moderately and/or highly emetogenic chemotherapy regimens of up to 5 consecutive days' duration.

ACTION/KINETICS

Action

Selective 5-HT_3 (serotonin) receptor antagonist with little or no affinity for other 5-HT, beta-adrenergic, dopamine, or histamine receptors. During chemotherapy-induced vomiting, mucosal enterochromaffin cells release serotonin, which stimulates 5-HT_3 receptors. The stimulation of 5-HT_3 receptors by serotonin causes vagal discharge resulting in vomiting. Granisetron blocks serotonin stimulation and subsequent vomiting.

Pharmacokinetics

In adult cancer clients undergoing chemotherapy, infusion of a single 40 mcg/kg dose over 5 min produced the following data. **Peak plasma level:** 63.8 ng/mL. **Plasma t½, terminal:** 5–9 hr, depending on age and disease state. Metabolized in the liver with unchanged drug (12%) and metabolites excreted through both the urine and feces.

CONTRAINDICATIONS

Known hypersensitivity to the drug.

SPECIAL CONCERNS

- Use with caution during lactation.
- Safety and efficacy not established in children <2 years of age.

SIDE EFFECTS

Most Common

After IV use: Headache, asthenia, constipation, pain, fever, anemia, abdominal pain, constipation, dizziness, bradycardia, somnolence, diarrhea.

After PO use: Headache, constipation, asthenia, diarrhea, abdominal pain, dyspepsia, dizziness, insomnia, N&V, leukopenia, anorexia, fever, anemia.

After IV use. CNS: Headache, somnolence, dizziness, agitation, anxiety, CNS stimulation, insomnia, extrapyramidal syndrome. **GI:** Diarrhea, constipation, taste disorder, abdominal pain. **CV:** Hyper-/hypotension, arrhythmias (e.g., sinus bradycardia, atrial fibrillation, ***AV block***, ventricular ectopy including nonsustained tachycardia, ECG abnormalities). **Allergic:** ***Hypersensitivity reactions (anaphylaxis)***, skin rashes. **Hematologic:** Anemia. **Miscellaneous:** Asthenia, fever, pain.

After PO use. CNS: Headache, dizziness, insomnia, anxiety, somnolence. **GI:** N&V, diarrhea, constipation, abdominal pain, dyspepsia. **CV:** Hyper-/hypotension, angina, atrial fibrillation, syncope (rare). **Hypersensitivity:** Rarely, hypersensitivity reactions; ***severe anaphylaxis***, shortness of breath, urticaria. **Miscellaneous:** Fever, asthenia, leukopenia, decreased appetite, anemia, alopecia, thrombocytopenia.

LABORATORY TEST CONSIDERATIONS

↑ AST, ALT.

DRUG INTERACTIONS

Because granisetron is metabolized by hepatic cytochrome P-450 drug-metabolizing enzymes, agents that induce or inhibit these enzymes may alter the clearance (and thus the half-life) of granisetron.

HOW SUPPLIED

Injection Solution: 0.1 mg/mL, 1 mg/mL; ***Oral Solution:*** 1 mg/5 mL; ***Tablets:*** 1 mg; ***Transdermal Patch:*** 34.3 mg (releases 3.1 mg/24 hr).

DOSAGE

IV

Prevention of chemotherapy-induced nausea and vomiting (N&V).

Adults and children over 2 years of age: 10 mcg/kg within 30 min before initiation of chemotherapy and only on day(s) chemotherapy is given. May be given either undiluted over 30 seconds, or diluted with either 0.9% NaCl or D5W and infused over 5 min.

Prevention and treatment of postoperative N&V.

Adults: 1 mg, undiluted, given over 30 seconds, before induction of anesthesia or immediately before reversal of anesthesia. Treatment of nausea and/or vomiting after surgery is 1 mg, undiluted, given over 30 seconds. Safety and efficacy have not been established in children for this use.

ORAL SOLUTION; TABLETS

Protection from chemotherapy-induced N&V.

Adults: 2 mg (two 1 mg tablets or 10 mL of oral solution) once daily or 1 mg (one 1 mg tablet or 5 mL of oral solution) twice daily. In the 2 mg once daily regime, two 1 mg tablets are given up to 1 hr before chemotherapy. In the 1 mg twice a day regime, the first 1 mg tablet is given up to 1 hr before chemotherapy and the second tablet is given 12 hr after the first. Either regimen is administered only on the day(s) chemotherapy is given. Data are not available for PO use in children.

Protection from radiation-induced (total body irradiation or fractionated abdominal radiation) N&V.

Adults: 2 mg (two 1 mg tablets or 10 mL of oral solution) once daily taken within 1 hr of radiation.

TRANSDERMAL PATCH

Prevention of chemotherapy-induced N&V.

Adults: Apply a single patch to the upper outer arm a minimum of 24 hr before chemotherapy (may be applied up to a maximum of 48 hr before chemotherapy). Remove the patch a minimum of 24 hr after completion of chemotherapy. The patch can be worn for up to 7 days, depending on the duration of the chemotherapy regimen.

NURSING IMPLICATIONS

IMPLEMENTATION/ADMINISTRATION/STORAGE

1. Give drug only on the day chemotherapy is given.
2. Dosage adjustment not necessary for geriatric clients or with impaired renal/hepatic function.
3. Store oral solution and tablets from 15–30°C (59–86°F) protected from light.
4. Store the patch from 15–30°C (59–86°F); store in the original packaging.
5. IV Administer either undiluted over 30 seconds or diluted with NSS or D5W to a total volume of 20 to 50 mL; infuse over 5 minutes. Drug is stable for at least 24 hr when diluted in NSS or D5W and stored at room temperature under normal lighting.
6. Inspect for particulate matter and discoloration before administration.
7. Once multidose vial is penetrated, use within 30 days.
8. Do not freeze vial; protect from light.
9. Store single- and multi-use vials from 15–30°C (59–86°F).
10. COMPATIBILITY D5W or NSS.
11. INCOMPATIBILITY Do not mix in solution with other drugs.

ASSESSMENT

1. Note reasons for therapy: XRT/chemo/postoperative N&V.
2. Drug contains benzyl alcohol.

3. Give drug 30 min before the start of emetogenic cancer chemotherapy.
4. Monitor ECG (QT interval), LFTs, frequency/severity of vomiting, and fluid balance.

CLIENT/FAMILY TEACHING

1. Review the appropriate method/frequency of dosing.
2. May be given IV/orally to ↓ chemotherapy-induced N&V.
3. Take tablets or solution no more than 1 hr before chemotherapy or radiation therapy for greatest protection against nausea and vomiting.
4. Apply the transdermal patch to clean, dry, intact healthy skin on the upper outer arm. Apply the patch immediately after removing from the pouch. Do not apply to skin that is red, irritated, or damaged, and remove patch if rash appears.
5. Do not cut the patch into pieces.
6. Report constipation/diarrhea/rashes/adverse effects. May experience headaches; usually relieved with acetaminophen. Drug may mask an ileus and/or gastric distention.
7. Advise to cover patch application site with clothing to avoid risk of exposure to sunlight; avoid direct exposure for 10 days following removal of patch.
8. Keep all F/U to assess response, labs, adverse SE.

OUTCOMES/EVALUATE

- Prevention of N&V
- Protection from XRT/chemotherapy-induced N&V

Guaifenesin

(gwye-**FEN**-eh-sin)

Classification(s): Expectorant

Pregnancy Category: C

OTC: Granules: Mucinex Mini-Melts Children's, Mucinex Mini-Melts Junior Strength. **Oral Liquid:** Buckley's Chest Congestion, Iophen NR, Mucinex Children's, Naldecon Senior EX, Robitussin, Scot-Tussin Expectorant, Siltussin SA. **Syrup:** Altarussin, Guiatuss. **Tablets:** MucusRelief, Organ-I NR. **Tablets, Extended-Release:** Humabid Maximum Strength, Mucinex, Mucinex Maximum Strength.

RX: Oral Liquid: Diabetic Tussin, Organidin NR. **Tablets:** Liquidbid, Organidin NR.

✦ OTC: Balminil DM, Balminil DM Children, Balminil Expectorant.

INDICATIONS/USES

(1) Dry, nonproductive cough due to colds and minor upper respiratory tract infections when there is mucus in the respiratory tract. (2) To loosen phlegm and thin bronchial secretions.

ACTION/KINETICS

Action

May increase the output of fluid from the respiratory tract by reducing the viscosity and surface tension of respiratory secretions, thereby removing accumulated secretions from the upper and lower airway.

Pharmacokinetics

Readily absorbed from the GI tract. Rapidly metabolized and excreted in the urine. **t½:** 1 hr.

CONTRAINDICATIONS

Chronic cough (e.g., due to smoking, asthma, or emphysema), cough accompanied by excess secretions. Use in children under age 6. Lactation.

SPECIAL CONCERNS

- Persistent cough may indicate a serious infection; thus, the provider should be consulted if cough lasts for more than 1 week, is recurring, or is accompanied by high fever, rash, or persistent headache.
- Taking large quantities of guaifenesin products may increase the risk of drug-induced kidney stones.

SIDE EFFECTS

Most Common

N&V, GI discomfort.

GI: N&V, GI upset/discomfort. **CNS:** Dizziness, headache. **Dermatologic:** Rash, urticaria.

LABORATORY TEST CONSIDERATIONS

↑ Renal urate clearance and thus ↓ serum uric acid levels. ↑ Urinary 5-hydroxyindoleacetic acid and falsely ↑ vanillylmandelic acid test for catechols.

OVERDOSE MANAGEMENT

Symptoms: N&V. *Treatment:* Treat symptomatically.

DRUG INTERACTIONS

Inhibition of platelet adhesiveness by guaifenesin may result in bleeding tendencies.

HOW SUPPLIED

Granules: 50 mg/packet, 100 mg/packet; ***Oral Liquid:*** 100 mg/5 mL, 200 mg/5 mL; ***Syrup:*** 100 mg/5 mL; ***Tablets:*** 200 mg, 400 mg; ***Tablets, Extended-Release:*** 600 mg, 1,200 mg.

DOSAGE

GRANULES

Expectorant.

Children, 12 years and older: 200–400 mg (2 to 4 of the 100 mg/packet strength) q 4 hr, up to 6 doses/day. **Children, 6 to <12 years of age:** 100–200 mg (1 to 2 of the 100 mg/packet strength or 2 to 4 of the 50 mg/packet strength) q 4 hr, up to 6 doses/day. **Children, 2 to <6 years of age:** 50–100 mg (1 to 2 of the 50 mg/packet strength or 1 of the 100 mg/packet strength) q 4hr, up to 6 doses/day. **Children, <2 years of age:** Do not use without physician approval.

ORAL LIQUID; SYRUP; TABLETS

Expectorant.

Adults and children 12 years and older: 200–400 mg q 4 hr, not to exceed 2,400 mg/day; **pediatric, 6–11 years:** 100–200 mg (5 to 10 mL) q 4 hr, not to exceed 1,200 mg/day; **pediatric, 2 to less than 6 years of age:** 50–100 mg (2.5 to 5 mL) q 4 hr, not to exceed 600 mg/day; **pediatric, less than 2 years of age:** Do not use without physician approval.

TABLETS, EXTENDED-RELEASE

Expectorant.

Adults and children 12 years and over: 600–1,200 mg q 12 hr, not to exceed 2,400 mg/day. *NOTE:* The liquid dosage forms may be more suitable for children from 6–12 years of age.

NURSING IMPLICATIONS

Do not confuse Mucinex with Mucomyst (a mucolytic).

IMPLEMENTATION/ADMINISTRATION/STORAGE

Naldecon Senior EX and Mucinex are not recommended for children less than 12 years of age.

ASSESSMENT

1. Note type, frequency, onset, duration, and characteristics of cough and sputum production.
2. List clinical presentation, pulmonary assessment findings, VS, CXR, oxygen saturations.
3. Assess for tobacco/nasal drug use, kidney stones, fever/chills, loss of appetite, or increased fatigue.

CLIENT/FAMILY TEACHING

1. Take only as directed, and do not exceed prescribed dose. Take tablets with a full glass of water.
2. Use dosing spoon, syringe, or cup when giving liquid or syrup to children.
3. If symptoms persist more than 1 week, recur, or are accompanied by a persistent headache, fever, or rash, notify provider.
4. Report any evidence of increased bruising/bleeding, fever, change in secretions, or lack of response.
5. Do not perform activities that require mental alertness; drug may cause drowsiness.
6. Increase fluids to 2.5 L/day to decrease secretion viscosity.
7. Avoid triggers: dust, chemicals, cleansers, cigarette smoke, environmental pollutants, and perfumes.
8. Keep all F/U to assess response, pulmonary findings, adverse SE.

OUTCOMES/EVALUATE

- Control of coughing episodes
- Mobilization of mucus

H

Haloperidol

(hah-low-**PAIR**-ih-dohl)

Classification(s): Antipsychotic

Pregnancy Category: C

Rx: Apo-Haloperidol.

Haloperidol decanoate

Pregnancy Category: C

RX: Haldol Decanoate 100.

Rx: Haloperidol LA.

Haloperidol lactate

Pregnancy Category: C

RX: Haldol.

INDICATIONS/USES

(1) Psychotic disorders including schizophrenia. (The decanoate is used for prolonged therapy in chronic schizophrenia). (2) Severe behavior problems in children (those with combative, explosive hyperexcitability not accounted for by immediate provocation). Use reserved only after failure to respond to psychotherapy or drugs other than antipsychotics. (3) Short-term treatment of hyperactive children who show excessive motor activity with accompanying conduct consisting of impulsivity, poor attention, aggression, mood lability, or poor frustration tolerance. (4) Control of tics and vocal utterances associated with Tourette's syndrome in adults and children. *Investigational:* Intractable hiccoughs, prevention of chemotherapy-induced N&V, obsessive-compulsive disorder.

ACTION/KINETICS

Action

Precise mechanism not known. Competitively blocks dopamine D_2 receptors in the tuberoinfundibular system to cause sedation. Also causes alpha-adrenergic and histamine H_1, and serotonin 5-HT_2 blockade; decreases release of growth hormone, and increases prolactin release by the pituitary. Causes significant extrapyramidal effects, as well as a low incidence of sedation, anticholinergic effects, and orthostatic hypotension. Narrow margin between the therapeutically effective dose and that causing extrapyramidal symptoms. Also has antiemetic effects.

Pharmacokinetics

Is 60–65% bioavailable after PO administration. **Peak plasma levels, PO:** 3–5 hr; **IM:** 20 min; **IM, decanoate:** approximately 6 days. **Therapeutic serum levels:** 3–10 ng/mL. **t½, PO:** About 18 hr; **IM:** 13–36 hr; **IM, decanoate:** 3 weeks; **IV:** approximately 14 hr. Metabolized in liver, slowly excreted in urine and feces. **Plasma protein binding:** 92%.

CONTRAINDICATIONS

Hypersensitivity to the drug or any component of the product. Use in comatose or greatly depressed states because of CNS depression or from any other cause. Use with extreme caution, or not at all, in clients with parkinsonism. Use in children less than 3 years of age. Lactation.

SPECIAL CONCERNS

Increased mortality in elderly clients with dementia-related psychosis. Elderly clients with dementia-related psychosis treated with antipsychotic drugs are at an increased risk of death. Analyses of 17 placebo-controlled trials (modal duration, 10 weeks), largely in clients taking atypical antipsychotic drugs, revealed a risk of death in drug-treated clients of between 1.6 and 1.7 times the risk of death in placebo-treated clients. Over the course of atypical 10-week controlled trial, the rate of death in drug-treated clients was about 4.5% compared with a rate of about 2.6% in the placebo group. Although the causes of death were varied, most of the deaths appeared to be cardiovascular (e.g., heart failure, sudden death) or infectious (e.g., pneumonia) in nature. Observational studies suggest that, similar to atypical antipsychotic drugs, treatment with conventional antipsychotic drugs may increased mortality. The extent to which the findings increased mortality in observational studies may be attributed to the antipsychotic drug as opposed to some characteristic(s) of the clients is not clear. Haloperidol is not approved for the treatment of clients with dementia-related psychosis.

- **Geriatric clients more likely to exhibit orthostatic hypotension, anticholinergic effects, sedation, and extrapyramidal side effects (such as parkinsonism and tardive dyskinesia).**
- **When used for mania in cyclic disorders, a rapid mood swing to depression may occur.**
- **PO dosage not determined in children less than 3 years old; IM dosage not recommended in children.**

SIDE EFFECTS

Most Common

Extrapyramidal symptoms, drowsiness, dizziness, blurred vision, GI upset, anorexia, headache, salivation, dry mouth, sweating, sleep disturbances, restlessness, constipation.

CNS: Extrapyramidal symptoms, agitation, akathisia, anxiety, catatonic-like states, confusion, ***convulsions***, depression, drowsiness, sedation, somnolence, dystonia, euphoria, hallucinations, headache, insomnia, lethargy, increased libido, neuroleptic malignant syndrome, pseudoparkinsonism, psychosis, restlessness, tardive dyskinesia, tardive dystonia, vertigo, transient dyskinetic signs after abrupt withdrawal. **GI:** Anorexia, constipation, diarrhea, dry mouth, dyspepsia, N&V, salivation. **Hepatic:** Jaundice, impaired liver function. **CV:** ECG pattern changes, hyper-/hypotension, prolongation of QTc interval, tachycardia, BP fluctuations, ***torsades de pointes***–type arrhythmias. **Dermatologic:** Acne, alopecia, maculopapular skin reactions, photosensitivity. **Respiratory:** Bronchopneumonia, ***bronchospasm, laryngospasm***, increased respiration depth. **GU:** Breast engorgement, galactorrhea, gynecomastia, impotence, mastalgia, menstrual irregularities, priapism, urinary retention. **Hematologic:** Anemia, leukocytosis, leukopenia, lymphomonocytosis, agranulocytosis (rare). **Musculoskeletal:** Opisthotonos. **Ophthalmic:** Cataracts, oculogyric crisis, blurred vision, visual disturbances, pigmentary retinopathy, lenticular pigmentation. **Miscellaneous:** Diaphoresis, hyperpyrexia, hyperthermia, heatstroke, local tissue reactions, withdrawal syndrome (including transient dyskinetic signs after abrupt withdrawal), limb malformations following maternal use, ***sudden death***. *NOTE:* When used with lithium an encephalopathic syndrome may occur; symptoms include weakness, lethargy, fever, tremulousness, confusion, extrapyramidal symptoms, leukocytosis, and elevated serum enzymes, BUN, and fasting blood sugar.

LABORATORY TEST CONSIDERATIONS

↑ Alkaline phosphatase, bilirubin, serum transaminase; ↓ PT (clients on coumarin), serum cholesterol, RBC count. Hyper-/hypoglycemia, hyponatremia, hyperammonemia.

OVERDOSE MANAGEMENT

Symptoms: CNS depression, hyper-/hypotension, extrapyramidal symptoms (may be severe), agitation, restlessness, fever, hypo-/hyperthermia, ***seizures, cardiac arrhythmias***, changes in the ECG, autonomic reactions, ***coma***. *Treatment:* Treat symptomatically. Antiparkinson drugs, diphenhydramine, or barbiturates can be used to treat extrapyramidal symptoms. Fluid replacement and vasoconstrictors (either norepinephrine or phenylephrine) can be used to treat hypotension. Ventricular arrhythmias can be treated with phenytoin. To treat seizures, use pentobarbital or diazepam. A saline cathartic can be used to hasten the excretion of sustained-release products.

H

DRUG INTERACTIONS

Amphetamine / ↓ Amphetamine effect by ↓ uptake of drug at its site of action

Anticholinergics / ↓ Serum haloperidol levels, worsening schizophrenic symptoms, and tardive dyskinesia; use together with caution

Antidepressants, tricyclic / ↑ TCA effects R/T ↓ liver breakdown

Azole antifungal drugs / ↑ Haloperidol plasma levels → ↑ risk of side effects; adjust haloperidol dosage as needed

Barbiturates / ↓ Effect of haloperidol R/T ↑ liver breakdown

Carbamazepine / ↓ Haloperidol therapeutic effects; adjust dose as needed

Fluoxetine / ↑ Haloperidol levels; possible severe extrapyramidal reactions

H ***Ginkgo biloba*** / ↑ Beneficial effect and decreased extrapyramidal symptoms when used to treat schizophrenia

Guanethidine / ↓ Guanethidine effect by ↓ uptake of drug at site of action

Lithium / Possible encephalopathic syndrome; see ***Side Effects***

Methyldopa / ↑ Toxicity of haloperidol

Phenytoin / ↓ Effect of haloperidol R/T ↑ liver breakdown
Rifamycins / ↓ Haloperidol plasma levels and therapeutic effects; adjust haloperidol dose as needed
Smoking / ↑ Haloperidol clearance → ↓ serum levels

HOW SUPPLIED

Haloperidol. ***Tablets:*** 0.5 mg, 1 mg, 2 mg, 5 mg, 10 mg, 20 mg.
Haloperidol decanoate. ***Injection:*** 50 mg/mL, 100 mg/mL.
Haloperidol lactate. ***Injection:*** 5 mg/mL; ***Oral Concentrate:*** 2 mg/mL.

DOSAGE

Haloperidol, Haloperidol lactate (PO)

ORAL CONCENTRATE; TABLETS

Psychoses.

Adults: 0.5–2 mg 2–3 times per day for moderate symptoms; up to 3–5 mg 2–3 times per day for severe symptoms or chronic or resistant clients. **Maintenance:** Reduce dosage to lowest effective level. Up to 100 mg/day may be required in some, although the safety of prolonged use of high doses has not been demonstrated. **Geriatric or debilitated clients:** 0.5–2 mg 2–3 times per day. **Pediatric, 3–12 years or 15–40 kg:** 0.5 mg/day (25–50 mcg/kg/day) in two to three divided doses; if necessary the daily dose may be increased by 0.5 mg increments q 5–7 days until a therapeutic effect is reached. **Maintenance:** 0.05–0.15 mg/kg/day given in 2–3 divided doses. Upon achieving a satisfactory therapeutic response, reduce the dose to the lowest effective maintenance level.

Behavioral disorders/hyperactivity in children.

Children, 3 to 12 years or 15–40 kg, initial: 0.5 mg/day. If needed, increase the dose in 0.5 mg increments at 5- to 7-day intervals until the therapeutic effect is reached. **Maintenance:** 0.05–0.075 mg/kg/day given in 2–3 divided doses. Upon reaching a satisfactory therapeutic response, reduce the dose to the lowest effective maintenance level. There is little evidence that behavior improvement is further enhanced with doses greater than 6 mg/day.

Tourette's syndrome.

Adults, initial: 0.5–1.5 mg 3 times per day, up to 10 mg daily PO. Adjust dose carefully to obtain the optimum response. **Children, 3 to 12 years or 15–40 kg:** 0.05–0.075 mg/kg/day. Higher doses may be needed for those severely disturbed.

Intractable hiccoughs (investigational).

Adults: 0.5–2 mg 1–3 times per day.

Prevention of chemotherapy-induced nausea and vomiting (investigational).

Adults: 1–2 mg PO a 4–6 hr. Give on a set schedule, not on an as-needed basis.

Haloperidol decanoate

IM

Chronic therapy.

Adults, initial dose, first month: 10–15 times the daily PO dose for those stabilized on low daily PO doses (10 mg/day or less) and in the elderly or debilitated. **Then, monthly maintenance:** 10–15 times the previous daily PO dose (decanoate is not to be given IV). For clients stabilized on higher doses with risk of relapse or those tolerant to oral haloperidol, give 20 times the daily PO dose the first month followed by monthly maintenance doses of 10–15 times the previous daily PO dose. For elderly or debilitated clients, give lower initial doses and more gradual adjustments. *NOTE:* The initial dose should not exceed 100 mg, regardless of the previous oral antipsychotic dose. If the conversion requires more than 100 mg haloperidol decanoate as an initial dose, give that dose in 2 injections (maximum of 100 mg initially followed by the balance in 3–7 days). Upon achieving a satisfactory therapeutic response, reduce the dose gradually to the lowest effective maintenance level.

Haloperidol lactate

IM

Acute psychoses.

Adults and adolescents, initial: 2–5 mg to control moderate to severe acute agitation. Depending on response, may be repeated q 60 min, although q 4–8 hr may be satisfactory. Switch to **PO** therapy as soon as possible.

NURSING IMPLICATIONS

Do not confuse Haldol with Medrol (a corticosteroid).

IMPLEMENTATION/ADMINISTRATION/STORAGE

1. Individualize dosage. Less haloperidol may be needed in children, elderly, debilitated, or those with a history of side effects to neuroleptic drugs. Upon reaching a satisfactory response, reduce dosage gradually to the lowest effective maintenance level.
2. Give the decanoate by deep IM injection using a 21-gauge needle. Do not exceed a volume of 3 mL/site. The recommended interval between doses is monthly or every 4 weeks.
3. Do not give decanoate IV.
4. Replace injectable with PO form asap. For an approximation of the total daily dose needed, determine parenteral dose given during the preceding 24 hr; carefully monitor for the first several days. Give the first PO dose within 12–24 hr after the last parenteral dose.
5. Store tablets from 15–30°C (59–86°F) in a tight, light-resistant container. Store injection from 15–30°C (59–86°F) protected from light and do not freeze.
6. Has been given undiluted at a rate of 5 mg/min or diluted in 30–50 mL D5W and infused over 30 min. (not FDA approved).

ASSESSMENT

1. Note behavior, appearance, response to environment, clinical presentation, characteristics of S&S. Assess for any S&S of parkinsonism and tardive dyskinesias, and monitor for relapse of psychotic symptoms.
2. Use with caution in the elderly; they tend to exhibit toxicity more frequently and problems that may not be resolvable. There is an increased risk of death in those with dementia-related psychosis, so avoid in this group.
3. Assess heart and lungs and for any CAD or lung disorders: may preclude therapy
4. List onset of extrapyramidal symptoms; may be drug induced. Irreversible, involuntary dyskinetic movements may develop.
5. Assess VS, CBC, electrolytes, liver, and renal function; reduce dose in the elderly and with dysfunction.

CLIENT/FAMILY TEACHING

1. Take exactly as prescribed. Do not stop abruptly with long-term therapy.
2. Avoid activities that require mental alertness until drug effects realized; may cause drowsiness and impaired judgment.
3. Avoid alcohol. May use sugarless gum, ice chips, or sips of water for dry mouth effects.
4. Report muscle weakness/stiffness. Change position slowly to avoid sudden drop in BP.
5. Ensure adequate hydration, and avoid strenuous activity during periods of high temperature or humidity.
6. May take up to 6 weeks for full benefits to occur.
7. Sunlight sensitivity may occur; avoid unnecessary exposure to UV light (sunlight, tanning booths), use sunscreen/protective clothing when exposed.
8. Immediately report any new onset involuntary, dyskinetic movements, temperature elevation, muscle rigidity, altered mental status; stop drug.
9. Keep all F/U to assess response, labs, need for continued therapy and adverse SE.

OUTCOMES/EVALUATE

- Improved behavior patterns: ↓ Agitation, hostility, psychosis, delusions
- Control of tics/vocal utterances, intractable hiccoughs
- ↓ Hyperactive behaviors

IV

Heparin sodium injection

(**HEP**-ah-rin)

Classification(s): Anticoagulant, heparin

Pregnancy Category: C

✦ **Rx:** Hepalean, Hepalean-Lok, Heparin LEO.

Heparin sodium and sodium chloride

Pregnancy Category: C

RX: Heparin Sodium and 0.45% Sodium Chloride, Heparin Sodium and 0.9% Sodium Chloride.

Heparin sodium lock flush solution

Pregnancy Category: C

RX: Heparin I.V. Flush, Heparin Lock Flush, Hepflush-10, Hep-Lock, Hep-Lock U/P.

INDICATIONS/USES

(1) Prophylaxis and treatment of venous thrombosis and its extension; pulmonary embolism; peripheral arterial embolism; atrial fibrillation with embolization. (2) Diagnosis and treatment of acute and chronic consumption coagulopathies (disseminated intravascular coagulation). (3) Low-dose regimen for the prevention of post-operative deep venous thrombosis and pulmonary embolism in those undergoing major abdominothoracic surgery or who are at risk of developing thromboembolic disease. (4) Prevention of clotting in arterial and heart surgery, blood transfusions, extracorporeal circulation, dialysis procedures, and blood samples. *Investigational:* (1) Prophylaxis of left ventricular thrombi and cerebrovascular accidents after MI. (2) Continuous infusion for treating MI in unstable angina refractory to conventional treatment. Heparin decreases the number of anginal attacks and silent ischemic episodes and reduces the daily duration of ischemia. (3) Prevention of cerebral thrombosis in the evolving stroke. (4) Adjunct in treating coronary occlusion with acute MI.

Heparin lock flush solution: Maintain patency of indwelling catheters used for intermittent injection or blood sampling. May be used following initial placement of the device in the vein, after each injection of a medication, or after withdrawal of blood for lab tests. Not to be used therapeutically.

ACTION/KINETICS

Action

Anticoagulants do not dissolve previously formed clots, but they do forestall their enlargement and prevent new clots from forming. Heparin potentiates the inhibitory action of antithrombin III on various coagulation factors including factors IIa, IXa, Xa, XIa, and XIIa. This occurs due to the formation of a complex with antithrombin III and causing a conformational change in the antithrombin III molecule. Inhibition of factor Xa results in interference with thrombin generation; thus, the action of thrombin in coagulation is inhibited. Heparin also increases the rate of formation of antithrombin III-thrombin complex, causing inactivation of thrombin and preventing the conversion of fibrinogen to fibrin. By inhibiting the activation of fibrin-stabilizing factor by thrombin, heparin also prevents formation of a stable fibrin clot. Therapeutic doses of heparin prolong thrombin time, whole blood clotting time, activated clotting time, and PTT. Heparin also decreases the levels of triglycerides by releasing lipoprotein lipase from tissues; the resultant hydrolysis of triglycerides causes increased blood levels of free fatty acids.

Pharmacokinetics

Onset: IV, immediate; **deep SC:** 20–60 min. **Peak plasma levels, after SC:** 2–4 hr. **t½:** 30–180 min in healthy persons. t½ increases with dose, severe renal disease, and cirrhosis and in anephric clients and decreases with pulmonary embolism and liver impairment other than cirrhosis. **Metabolism:** Probably by reticuloendothelial system, although up to 50% is excreted unchanged in the urine. Clotting time returns to normal within 2–6 hr.

CONTRAINDICATIONS

Hypersensitivity to heparin. Active bleeding, blood dyscrasias (or other disorders characterized by bleeding tendencies such as hemophilia), clients with frail or weakened blood vessels, purpura, severe thrombocytopenia, liver disease with hypoprothrombinemia, suspected intracranial hemorrhage, suppurative thrombophlebitis, inaccessible ulcerative lesions (especially of the GI tract), open wounds, extensive denudation of the skin, and increased capillary permeability (as in ascorbic acid deficiency). IM use (due to hematoma formation).

Do not administer during surgery of the eye, brain, or spinal cord or during continuous tube drainage of the stomach or small intestine. Use is also contraindicated in subacute endocarditis, shock, threatened abortion, severe hypertension, diverticulitis, colitis, SBE, or hypersensitivity to drug. Premature neonates due to the possibility of a fatal "gasping syndrome." Also, regional anesthesia and lumbar block, vitamin K deficiency, leukemia with bleeding tendencies, open wounds or ulcerations, acute nephritis, or impaired hepatic or renal function. In the presence of drainage tubes in any orifice. Alcoholism.

SPECIAL CONCERNS

- **Use with caution in menstruation, in pregnant women (heparin may cause hypoprothrombinemia in the infant), during lactation, during the postpartum period, and following cerebrovascular accidents.**
- **Geriatric clients may be more susceptible to developing bleeding complications, unusual hair loss, and itching.**
- **Safety and efficacy not determined in newborns; germinal matrix intraventricular hemorrhage occurs more often in low-birth weight infants receiving heparin.**
- **Use heparin lock flush with caution in infants with disease states in which there is an increased risk of hemorrhage. The use of the 100 units/mL product is not advised due to bleeding risk, especially in low birth-weight infants.**
- **Benzyl alcohol, a component in some products as a preservative, may cause a fatal "gasping" syndrome in in premature infants.**
- **Increased resistance is noted frequently in fever, thrombosis, thrombophlebitis, infections with thrombosing tendencies, MI, cancer, and postoperative states.**

SIDE EFFECTS

Most Common

Hemorrhage (see below), chills, fever, urticaria, local irritation, erythema, mild pain, hematoma, thrombocytopenia.

CV: ***Hemorrhage ranging from minor local ecchymoses to major hemorrhagic complications from any organ or tissue. Adrenal hemorrhage*** (causes acute adrenal insufficiency). ***Ovarian (corpus luteum) hemorrhage. Retroperitoneal hemorrhage. Germinal matrix-intraventricular hemorrhage*** in low-birth weight infants. Subacute bacterial endocarditis. Severe hypertension. ***CNS hemorrhage*** during and immediately after spinal tap, spinal anesthesia or major surgery, especially of the brain, spinal cord, or eye. Higher incidence is seen in women over 60 years of age. Hemorrhagic reactions are more likely to occur in prophylactic administration during surgery than in the treatment of thromboembolic disease. White clot syndrome. Vasospastic reactions (6–10 days after starting therapy and last 4–6 hr); affected limb is painful, ischemic, and cyanotic (client may also develop chest pain, elevated BP, arthralgia, or headache). **GI:** Ulcerative lesions, diverticulitis, ulcerative colitis, continuous tube drainage of the stomach or small intestine, liver disease with impaired hemostasis. **GU:** Menstruation, severe renal disease. **Hematologic:** Heparin-induced thrombocytopenia (both early and delayed). Early thrombocytopenia (type I) develops 2–3 days after starting heparin, tends to be mild and is the result of a direct action of heparin on platelets. Delayed thrombocytopenia (type II) develops 7–12 days after either low-dose or full-dose heparin, can have serious consequences, and may reflect presence of an immunoglobulin that induces platelet aggregation. **Hypersensitivity:** Chills, fever, urticaria are the most common. Rarely, asthma, lacrimation, headache, N&V, rhinitis, ***shock, anaphylaxis***. Allergic vasospastic reaction within 6–10 days after initiation of therapy (lasts 4–6 hr) including painful, ischemic, cyanotic limbs. Use a test dose of 1,000 units in clients with a history of asthma or allergic disease. **Miscellaneous:** Hyperkalemia, cutaneous necrosis, osteoporosis (after long-term high doses), delayed transient alopecia, priapism, suppressed aldosterone synthesis. Discontinuance of heparin has resulted in rebound hyperlipemia.

Following IM (not recommended), SC: Local irritation, erythema, mild pain, ulceration, hematoma, and tissue sloughing.

LABORATORY TEST CONSIDERATIONS

↑ AST and ALT. Hyperlipidemia.

OVERDOSE MANAGEMENT

Symptoms: Nosebleeds, hematuria, and tarry stools may be the first sign of overdose. Petechiae formations and easy bruising may precede frank bleeding. *Treatment:* Drug withdrawal is usually sufficient to correct heparin overdosage. Protamine sulfate (1%) solution; each mg of protamine neutralizes about 100 USP heparin units.

DRUG INTERACTIONS

Alteplase, recombinant / ↑ Risk of bleeding, especially at arterial puncture sites
Anticoagulants, oral / Additive ↑ PT
Antihistamines / May partially counteract heparin's anticoagulant action

Aspirin / ↑ Risk of bleeding R/T interference with platelet aggregation
H ***Bromelain*** / ↑ Tendency for bleeding
Cephalosporins / ↑ Risk of bleeding R/T additive coagulopathy effect
H ***Cinchona bark*** / ↑ Anticoagulant effect
Dextran / ↑ Risk of bleeding R/T interference with platelet aggregation
Digitalis / May partially counteract heparin's anticoagulant action
Dipyridamole / ↑ Risk of bleeding R/T interference with platelet aggregation
H ***Feverfew*** / Possible additive antiplatelet effect
H ***Ginger*** / Possible additive antiplatelet effects
H ***Ginkgo biloba*** / ↑ Effect on blood coagulation
H ***Ginseng*** / Potential for ↓ effect on platelet aggregation
H ***Goldenseal*** / Antagonizes action of heparin
Hydroxychloroquine / ↑ Risk of bleeding R/T interference with platelet aggregation
Ibuprofen / ↑ Risk of bleeding R/T interference with platelet aggregation
Indomethacin / ↑ Risk of bleeding R/T interference with platelet aggregation
Insulin / Heparin antagonizes insulin effect
Nicotine / May partially counteract heparin's anticoagulant action
Nitroglycerin / ↓ Effect of heparin
NSAIDs / ↑ Risk of bleeding R/T interference with platelet aggregation
Penicillins / ↑ Risk of bleeding R/T alterations in platelet aggregation
Salicylates / ↑ Risk of bleeding
Smoking / Possible ↑ heparin elimination, ↓ t½; dosage may need to be ↑
Streptokinase / Relative resistance to effects of heparin
Tetracyclines / May partially counteract heparin's anticoagulant action
Ticlopidine / ↑ Risk of bleeding R/T interference with platelet aggregation

HOW SUPPLIED

Heparin sodium injection. ***Injection:*** **Multiple Dose Vials:** 1,000 units/mL, 2,000 units/mL, 2,500 units/mL, 5,000 units/mL, 10,000 units/mL, 20,000 units/mL, 40,000 units/mL. **Single Dose Ampules/Vials:** 1,000 units/mL, 5,000 units/mL, 10,000 units/mL, 20,000 units/mL, 40,000 units/mL. **Unit Dose:** 1,000 units/dose, 2,500 units/dose, 5,000 units/dose, 7,500 units/dose, 10,000 units/dose, 20,000 units/dose.

Heparin sodium and sodium chloride. ***Injection:*** 12,500 units in 250 mL 0.45% NaCl; 25,000 units in 250 and 500 mL 0.45% NaCl; 1,000 units in 500 mL 0.9% NaCl; 2,000 units in 1,000 mL 0.9% NaCl.

Heparin sodium lock flush solution. 1 unit/mL, 10 units/mL, 100 units/mL, 100 units/10 mL.

DOSAGE

NOTE: Adjusted for each client on the basis of laboratory tests. Dosage is adequate when whole blood clotting time is about 2.5 to 3 times control value, or when aPTT is 1.5 to 2 times normal.

DEEP SC

General heparin dosage.

Initial loading dose: 10,000–20,000 units (immediately preceded by an IV loading dose of 5,000 units); **maintenance:** 8,000–10,000 units q 8 hr or 15,000–20,000 units q 12 hr. Use concentrated solution. *NOTE:* Dosage is based on a 68 kg (150 lb) client.

Prophylaxis of postoperative thromboembolism.

5,000 units of concentrated solution 2 hr before surgery and 5,000 units q 8–12 hr thereafter for 7 days or until client is ambulatory, whichever is longer. Administer by deep SC above the ileac crest or abdominal fat layer, arm, or thigh. Reserve use for clients >40 years of age undergoing major surgery. If bleeding occurs during or after surgery, discontinue heparin and neutralize with protamine sulfate.

IV, INTERMITTENT

General heparin dosage.

Initial loading dose: 10,000 units undiluted or in 50–100 mL saline; **then,** 5,000–10,000 units q 4–6 hr undiluted or in 50–100 mL saline. *NOTE:* Dosage is based on a 68 kg (150 lb) client.

IV, CONTINUOUS INFUSION

General heparin dosage.

Initial loading dose: 20,000–40,000 units/day in 1,000 mL saline (preceded initially by 5,000 units IV). *NOTE:* Dosage is based on a 68 kg (150 lb) client.

SPECIAL USES

Use in children.

Use the following as a guideline. **Initial:** 50 units/kg IV bolus. **Maintenance:** 100 units/kg/dose IV drip q 4 hr or 20,000 units/m^2/24 hr continuous IV infusion.

Deep venous thrombosis.

If the PTT is <45 seconds give 5,000 units as a bolus and increase by 250 units/hr. If the PTT is from 45–54 seconds, increase by 150 units/hr. If the PTT is from 55–85 seconds, do not change dosage. If the PTT is 86–110 seconds, stop the infusion for 1 hr and decrease by 150 units/hr. If the PTT is >110 seconds, stop the infusion for 1 hr and decrease by 250 units/hr.

Surgery of heart and blood vessels.

Initial, Not less than 150 units/kg to clients undergoing total body perfusion for open heart surgery. *NOTE:* 300 units/kg may be used for procedures less than 60 min while 400 units/kg is used for procedures lasting more than 60 min. To prevent clotting in the tube system, add heparin to fluids in pump oxygenator.

Extracorporeal renal dialysis.

See instructions on equipment.

Blood transfusion.

Add 400–600 units/100 mL whole blood to prevent coagulation. 7,500 units should be added to 100 mL 0.9% sodium chloride injection; from this dilution, add 6–8 mL/100 mL whole blood. Perform leukocyte counts on heparinized blood within 2 hr of addition of heparin. Do not use heparinized blood for isoagglutinin complement, erythrocyte fragility tests, or platelet counts.

Laboratory samples.

Add 75–150 units/10–20 mL sample of whole blood to prevent coagulation of sample.

Heparin Sodium Lock Flush

HEPARIN LOCK SETS

Prevention of clotting.

To prevent clot formation in a heparin lock set, inject 10–100 units/mL heparin solution through the injection hub in a sufficient quantity to fill the entire set to the needle tip. Replace the solution each time the device is used. Aspirate before administering any solution via the lock in order to confirm patency and location of the needle or catheter tip. If the drug to be given is incompatible with heparin, flush the entire heparin lock set with sterile water or normal saline before and after the medication is given; following the second flush, the heparin lock flush solution may be reinstilled into the set. Consult the manufacturer's instructions for specifics.

Prevent coagulation of laboratory samples.

70–150 units/10 to 20 mL sample to prevent coagulation. When heparin (or sodium chloride) would interfere with or alter the results of blood tests, clear the heparin solution from the device by aspirating and discarding it before withdrawing the blood sample.

NURSING IMPLICATIONS

Do not confuse heparin with low molecular weight heparins (LMWH).

IMPLEMENTATION/ADMINISTRATION/STORAGE

1. **May be given by intermittent IV injection, continuous IV infusion, or deep SC injection. Continuous IV infusion is generally preferred due to the higher chance of bleeding complications with other routes. Do *not* administer IM.**
2. **Administer by deep SC injection to minimize local irritation, hematoma, and tissue sloughing, and to prolong drug action.**
   - **Z-track method: Use any fat roll, but abdominal fat rolls are preferred. Use a ½-in. or ⅝-in. 25- or 27-gauge needle. Grasp skin layer of the fat roll, and lift up. Insert needle at about a 45° angle to the skin's fat layer, and then administer the medication. Not necessary to aspirate to check if needle is in a blood vessel. Rapidly withdraw the needle while releasing the skin.**
   - **"Bunch technique" method: Grasp tissue around injection site, creating a tissue roll of about ½ in. in diameter. Insert needle into tissue roll at a 90° angle to the skin surface and inject medication. Not neces-**

H

sary to aspirate. Withdraw needle rapidly when skin is released.
- Do not administer within 2 in. of umbilicus (R/T increased vascularity of area).

3. Do not massage site. Rotate sites of administration.
4. Inspect products visually for particulate matter and discoloration before administration. Use only if the solution is clear and seal is intact. Do not use if solution contains a precipitate or is discolored or hazy. Do not use if the container is damaged, leaking, or opened.
5. Store heparin sodium lock flush from 15–30°C (59–86°F). For single use only. Discard unused portion after initial use.
6. IV Hospitalize for IV therapy.
7. May be diluted and administered over 4–24 hr with an infusion pump.
8. Protect solutions from freezing.
9. Have protamine sulfate, a heparin antagonist, available should excessive bleeding occur.
10. NaCl, 0.9%, is effective in maintaining patency of peripheral (noncentral) intermittent infusion devices and in reducing medical costs. The following procedure is recommended:
    - Determine patency by aspirating lock.
    - Flush with 2 mL NSS.
    - Administer medication therapy (flush between drugs).
    - Flush with 2 mL NSS.
    - Frequency of flushing to maintain patency when not actively in use varies from every 8 hr to every 24–48 hr.
    - This does *NOT* apply to any central venous access devices. Must use heparin.
11. COMPATIBILITY Dextrose, NSS, or Ringer's solution.
12. INCOMPATIBILITY To prevent incompatibility flush lock with sterile water or NSS before and after administering IV medications.

ASSESSMENT

1. Note reasons for therapy, onset, characteristics and clinical presentation. Identify any bleeding incidents, i.e., bleeding tendencies, family history, or any other incidents of unexplained or active bleeding.
2. Review PMH for conditions that may preclude therapy: alcoholic, chronic GI tract ulcerations, severe renal or liver dysfunction, infections of the endocardium, or PUD, which may be a potential site of bleeding. Note any evidence of intracranial hemorrhage.
3. When heparin given by continuous IV infusion, perform coagulation tests every 4 hr in the early stages. When given by intermittent IV infusion, perform coagulation tests before each dose during early stages and at appropriate intervals thereafter. After deep SC injection, perform coagulation tests 4–6 hr after the injections.
4. Perform test dose (1,000 units SC) on clients with multiple allergies or asthma history.
5. Review drug profile to ensure none interact unfavorably; otherwise, anticipate heparin dosage adjustment.
6. Assess for defects in clotting mechanism or any capillary fragility; obtain baseline coagulation values. PTT values 1½ to 2 times control indicates anticoagulation.
7. Note time frame for therapy (i.e., DVT [initial] 6 months; certain valve replacements-life-time), and desired INR, PT/PTT and record.
8. Assess for defects in clotting mechanism or any capillary fragility; obtain baseline coagulation values. PTT values 1½ to 2 times control indicates anticoagulation.
9. Some studies question the need/benefits of short-term anti-coagulation in hospitalized clients.
10. Monitor CBC with platelets, PT, PTT, renal, and LFTs. Note bleeding precautions at bedside and assess regularly for any evidence of abnormal bleeding.

INTERVENTIONS

For Heparin:

1. Post/advise at bedside "client receiving anticoagulant therapy."
2. Monitor CBC and PTT closely.
3. Question about bleeding (gums, urine, stools, vomit, bruises). If urine discolored, determine cause (i.e., from drug therapy or hematuria). Indanedione-type anticoagulants turn alkaline urine a red-orange color; acidify urine or test for occult blood.
4. Sudden lumbar pain may indicate retroperitoneal hemorrhage.
5. GI dysfunction may indicate intestinal hemorrhage. Test for blood in urine and feces; check H&H to assess for bleeding.
6. Have protamine sulfate for heparin overdose available (generally for every 100 units of

heparin administer 1 mg protamine sulfate IV).

7. Apply pressure to all venipuncture and injection sites to prevent bleeding and hematoma formation.
8. In heparin lock devices, the presence of heparin or NSS may cause lab test interferences.
   - To clear flush solution: aspirate and discard 1 mL of fluid from device before withdrawing blood sample.
   - Inject 1 mL of flush solution into lock after blood samples are drawn.
   - With excessively abnormal results, obtain a repeat sample from another site before altering treatment.
9. With SC administration, do not aspirate or massage; administer in lower abdomen and rotate sites.

For Heparin Lock Flush Solution:

1. Aspirate lock to determine patency. Maintain patency: inject 1 mL of flush solution into device diaphragm after each use (maintains catheter patency for up to 24 hr).
2. If administering a drug incompatible with heparin, flush with 0.9% NaCl solution or sterile water for injection before and immediately after incompatible drug administered. Inject another dose of heparin lock flush solution after the final flush.
3. Observe coagulation times carefully with underlying bleeding disorders; ↑ risk for hemorrhage.
4. The presence of heparin or NSS may cause lab test interferences. To clear flush solution:
   - Aspirate and discard 1 mL of fluid from device before withdrawing blood sample.
   - Inject 1 mL of flush solution into lock after blood samples are drawn.
   - With excessively abnormal results, obtain a repeat sample from another site before initiating treatment.
5. Monitor for allergic reactions due to various biologic sources of heparin.

CLIENT/FAMILY TEACHING

1. Review administration technique. Can only be given parenterally. For SC administration inject in lower abdomen. Do not massage after injection. Rotate sites with each dose.
2. Report signs of active bleeding or any excessive menstrual flow; may need to withhold/reduce dosage.
3. Report alterations in urine function, urine color, or any injury.
4. Use an electric razor for shaving and a soft-bristle toothbrush to decrease gum irritation. Hair loss is generally temporary.
5. Arrange furniture to allow open space for unimpeded ambulation and to diminish chances of bumping into objects that may cause bruising/bleeding. Use a night-light to illuminate trips to the bathroom. Always wear shoes or slippers.
6. Avoid contact sports and any activities where excessive bumping, bruising, or injury may occur.
7. Eat potassium-rich foods (e.g., baked potato, orange juice, bananas, beef, flounder, haddock, sweet potato, turkey, raw tomato). Avoid eating large amounts of vitamin-K food (yellow and dark-green vegetables).
8. Report increased bruising, bleeding of nose, mouth, gums, mucous or oral secretions, tarry stools, GI upset, SOB, chest pain, or difficulty breathing.
9. Avoid alcohol, aspirin, tobacco, and NSAIDs due to increased anticoagulant response.
10. Alert all providers of therapy and wear/carry drug identification.
11. Keep all F/U to assess response, labs, adverse SE.

OUTCOMES/EVALUATE

- PTT: 2–2.5 times the control/normal
- Prevention of thrombus formation
- Clot prophylaxis/treatment
- Indwelling catheter patency

Hyaluronic acid derivatives, dermal

(hie-loo-**RON**-ik)

Classification(s): Physical adjunct

Pregnancy Category: C

RX: Gel or Solution for Injection: Coease, Healon5, Hylaform, Juvederm 24 HV, 30, and 30 HV, Juvederm Ultra, Juvederm Ultra Plus, Perlane, Perlane-L, Restylane, Restylane-L, Shellgel. **Topical Cream, Gel, Lotion, Spray:** Bionect, HyGel, Sodium Hyaluronate.

INDICATIONS/USES

Injection: Mid-to-deep dermal implantation for the correction of moderate to severe facial wrinkles and folds, such as nasolabial folds. **Topical Cream, Gel, Spray:** Dressing and management of partial- to full-thickness dermal ulcers (e.g., pressure sores, venous stasis ulcers, arterial ulcers, diabetic ulcers), wounds (e.g., cuts abrasions, donor sites, postoperative incisions), irritations of the skin, and first- and second-degree burns. The product is intended to cover a wound or burn and protect against abrasions, friction, and desiccation. **Topical Lotion:** Symptoms associated with dry, scaly skin.

ACTION/KINETICS

Action

Hyaluronic acid is a naturally occurring polysaccharide of the glycosamin-oglycan family. It contains repeating disaccharide units of sodium-glucuronate-N-acetyl glucosamine. The exact mechanism of action is not known.

CONTRAINDICATIONS

Injection: Severe allergies manifested by a history of anaphylaxis or history or presence of multiple severe allergies. Use in those with a history of allergies to proteins found in gram-positive bacteria (the product contains trace amounts of gram-positive bacterial proteins). Use in breast augmentation and for implantation into bone, tendon, ligament, muscle, or blood vessels. Implantation into blood vessels (implantation into dermal vessels may cause vascular occlusion, infarction, or embolic phenomena). Use in those with known hypersensitivity to keloid formation or hypertrophic scarring. Use in sites in which an active inflammatory process or infection is present (e.g., cysts, pimples, rash, hives); defer treatment until the inflammation has been controlled. Long-term safety and efficacy have not been determined for use beyond 1 year. **Topical Products:** Known hypersensitivity to the product.

SPECIAL CONCERNS

Injection:

- Use with caution in clients on immunosuppressive therapy.
- Use in those with increased susceptibility to keloid formation and hypertrophic scarring not studied.
- Safety and efficacy not established to treat anatomic regions other than nasolabial folds, or for use in pregnancy, during lactation, and in children under 18 years of age.
- Inflammation at the implant site is possible if laser treatment, chemical peeling, or any other procedure based on active dermal response is used after hyaluronic acid treatment.
- Use for more than 1 year not studied.
- Injection carries a risk of infection.

Topical:

- Prolonged use may cause a sensitization reaction.

SIDE EFFECTS

Most Common

Bruising, itching, pain, redness, swelling, tenderness, acne.

Injection: Dermatologic: Bruising, itching, pain, redness, swelling, tenderness, acne, contact dermatitis, localized superficial necrosis, inflammatory reaction at injection site (including swelling, redness, tenderness, induration, and rarely acneiform papules at the injection site); inflammation at the implant site if laser treatment, chemical peeling, or any other procedure is undertaken. **Hypersensitivity:** Swelling, redness, tenderness, induration, acneiform papules (rare). **CNS:** Depression, headache, migraine, aggravation of depression. **Respiratory:** URTI, sinusitis, bronchitis, pneumonia. **Musculoskeletal:** Arthralgia, osteoporosis. **Miscellaneous:** Inflicted injury, tooth disorder, back pain, allergic reaction, herpes simplex, urinary incontinence, bacterial infection, hypercholesterolemia, necrosis.

DRUG INTERACTIONS

Aspirin / ↑ Bleeding or bruising if used with hyaluronic acid injection

Quaternary ammonium salts / Precipitation of hyaluronic acid in topical products if used together

NSAIDs / ↑ Bleeding or bruising if used with hyaluronic acid injection

HOW SUPPLIED

Gel or Solution for Injection: 5.5 mg/mL (as hylan B), 12 mg/mL, 20 mg/mL, 23 mg/mL, 24 mg/mL; ***Topical Cream, Gel, Spray:*** Each form is 0.2%; ***Topical Lotion:*** 0.1%.

DOSAGE

GEL FOR INJECTION

Facial wrinkles and folds.

Usual: Limit to 1.5 mL per treatment site.

TOPICAL CREAM, GEL, SPRAY

Dermal ulcers, wounds, skin irritation, burns.

Apply a thin layer of the product without extensive rubbing onto the wound surface, 2 or 3 times a day. Cover the lesion area with a sterile gauze pad and, if necessary, with an elastic or compressive bandage.

TOPICAL LOTION

Dry, scaly skin.

Use a liberal amount 2–3 times per day and rub in thoroughly.

NURSING IMPLICATIONS

IMPLEMENTATION/ADMINISTRATION/STORAGE

1. Hyaluronic acid is supplied in a syringe ready for use; never mix with other products prior to injection of the device.
2. If the content of a syringe shows signs of separation and/or appears cloudy, do not use.
3. Do not resterilize hyaluronic acid, as this may damage or alter the product.
4. Hyaluronic acid is packaged for single-client use.
5. Use the following administration procedure when using the injection:
   - Counsel the client and discuss the indication, risks, benefits, and expected responses to treatment. Advise of necessary precautions before beginning the procedure.
   - Assess the need of the client for pain management.
   - Clean the area to be treated with alcohol or other suitable antiseptic solution.
   - Before injecting, press the rod carefully until a small droplet is visible at the tip of the needle.
   - Inject, applying even pressure on the plunger rod while slowly pulling the needle backward.
   - The wrinkle should be lifted and eliminated by the end of the injection.
   - Stop the injection just before the needle is pulled out of the skin, to prevent material from leaking out or ending up too superficially in the skin.
   - Only correct to 100% of the dermal volume effect; do not overcorrect.
   - With cutaneous contour deformities, the best results are seen if the defect can be manually stretched to the point where it is eliminated.
   - When the injection is completed, gently massage the treated site so that it conforms to the contour of the surrounding tissue. If an overcorrection has occurred, massage the area firmly between the fingers or against the underlying superficial bone to obtain optimal results.
6. Administer using a thin gauge needle (30 gauge × ½ in.). The needle is inserted at an approximate angle of 30° parallel to the length of the wrinkle or fold. The bevel of the needle should face upward and the drug injected into the middle of the dermis. For mid-dermis placement, the contour of the needle should be visible but not the color of it.
7. If the product is injected too deep or IM, the duration of action will be shorter. If the product is injected too superficially, visible lumps and/or grayish discoloration may result.
8. If "blanching" is observed (i.e., the overlying skin turns a whitish color), stop the injection immediately and massage the area until it returns to a normal color.
9. The degree and duration of correction depend on the character of the defect treated, the tissue stress at the implant site, the depth of the implant in the tissue, and the injection technique. Markedly indurated defects may be difficult to correct.
10. If the treated area is swollen directly after the injection, an ice pack can be applied on the site for a short period.
11. If further treatment is needed, repeat the same procedure with several punctures of the skin until a satisfactory result is obtained. Additional treatment may be needed to achieve the desired correction. With clients who have localized swelling, the degree of correction is sometimes difficult to judge at the time of treatment. In such cases, a touch-up session may be needed after 1 or 2 weeks.

H

12. Defer use at specific sites in which an active inflammatory process (e.g., skin eruptions such as cysts, pimples, rashes, or hives) or infection are present until the inflammation has been controlled.
13. A mild to moderate injection site reaction may occur; it typically resolves in a few days.
14. Use the following procedure when using the topical cream, gel, or spray: Clean and disinfect the wounds or ulcers before treatment. If there are ulcers of long duration, it may be advisable to clean and/or debride the wound by surgical or enzymatic means prior to treatment.
15. Do not resterilize hyaluronic acid injection; may damage or alter the product.
16. If a sensitization reaction occurs to a topical product, discontinue treatment and follow a suitable therapy.
17. To reduce the risk of cross-infection, each tube of a product should be used by only one client.
18. The injection must be used prior to expiration date. Do not freeze and protect from sunlight. Store at a temperature up to 25°C (77°F); refrigeration is not needed.
19. Store the topical products at room temperature. The cream and gel may be stored for up to 24 months and the spray for up to 36 months.

ASSESSMENT

1. Note indications and conditions for therapy, identify form, dose and method of administration, onset, characteristics of S&S, clinical presentation, other agents trialed/outcome.
2. Determine need for topical or injectable anesthetics to manage pain during and after therapy.
3. Obtain pretreatment photos to document extent of wrinkles and folds if indicated.
4. Ensure no history of multiple allergies or keloid formation.
5. Assess emotional status and ensure ready for procedure; review potential adverse reactions.

CLIENT/FAMILY TEACHING

1. The injection is placed into nasolabial folds to decrease folds and wrinkling.
2. To be administered only by those trained to use this therapy.
3. May experience bruising, itching, pain, redness, swelling, and acne at treatment site. If treated area is swollen directly after the injection, may apply an ice pack on swollen site for short period of time.
4. With topical products, clean and disinfect wound or ulcer and then apply a thin layer onto wound surface 2 or 3 times daily. Cover lesion with a sterile gauze pad and, if needed, with an elastic or compressive bandage. Longstanding ulcers may require debriding by surgical or enzymatic means prior to treatment.
5. Minimize exposure of the treated area to excessive sun, UV lamps, and extreme cold weather until any initial swelling and redness have resolved.
6. Report any adverse effects, including infection, elevated cholesterol levels, or deformity, and keep all F/U to assess response.

OUTCOMES/EVALUATE

- Correction of nasolabial wrinkles and folds
- Treatment of ulcers/wounds

Hydrochlorothiazide

(**hy**-droh-klor-oh-**THIGH**-ah-zyd)

Classification(s): Diuretic, thiazide

Pregnancy Category: B

RX: Ezide, HydroDIURIL, Hydro-Par, Microzide Capsules.

Rx: Apo-Hydro, PMS-Hydrochlorothiazide.

SEE ALSO ***DIURETICS, THIAZIDE.***

INDICATIONS/USES

(1) Hypertension. Used alone or with other drugs used to treat hypertension. (2) Diuretic to treat edema due to CHF, hepatic cirrhosis, or corticosteroid or estrogen therapy. May also be used for edema due to various types of renal dysfunction, including nephrotic syndrome, acute glomerulonephritis, or chronic renal failure. (3) Microzide may be used for once-daily, low-dose treatment for hypertension. *NOTE:* Hydrochlorothiazide is a component of many combination products used to treat hypertension.

ACTION/KINETICS

Action

Promote the excretion of sodium and chloride, and thus water, by the distal renal tubule. Also increases excretion of potassium and to a lesser extent bicarbonate. The antihypertensive activity is thought to be due to direct dilation of the areterioles, as well as to a reduction in the total fluid volume of the body and altered sodium balance.

Pharmacokinetics

Onset: 2 hr. **Peak effect:** 4–6 hr. **Duration:** 6–12 hr. **t½:** 5.6–14.8 hr. Hydrochlorothiazide is not metabolized but is eliminated rapidly by the kidney.

SPECIAL CONCERNS

Geriatric clients may be more sensitive to the usual adult dose.

SIDE EFFECTS

Most Common

Orthostatic hypotension, hypokalemia, weakness, headache, diarrhea, dizziness, gastric upset/irritation/cramping.

See also *Diuretics, Thiazides* for a complete list of possible side effects. Also, **CV:** Allergic myocarditis, hypotension. **Dermatologic:** Alopecia, exfoliative dermatitis, ***toxic epidermal necrolysis***, erythema multiforme, ***Stevens-Johnson syndrome***. **Miscellaneous:** ***Anaphylactic reactions, respiratory distress including pneumonitis and pulmonary edema***, cognitive and neurologic impairment.

HOW SUPPLIED

Capsules: 12.5 mg; *Tablets:* 12.5 mg, 25 mg, 50 mg, 100 mg.

DOSAGE

CAPSULES (INCLUDING MICROZIDE)

Hypertension.

Adults: 12.5 mg (1 capsule) once daily either alone or with other antihypertensives. **Maximum recommended dose:** 50 mg daily.

TABLETS

Hypertension.

Adults, initial: 25 mg/day as a single dose. The dose may be increased to 50 mg/day in one to two daily doses. Doses greater than 50 mg may cause significant reductions in serum potassium. **Children:** 1–2 mg/kg/day in single or 2 divided doses, not to exceed 37.5 mg/day in infants up to 2 years of age or 100 mg/day in children 2–12 years of age. In infants less than 6 months of age, doses up to 3 mg/kg/day in 2 divided doses may be needed.

Diuretic.

Adults, initial: 25–100 mg/day as a single or divided dose. Some clients with edema respond to administration on alternate days or on 3–5 days each week. Intermittent administration, an excessive response, and possible undesirable side effects are minimized. **Children:** 1–2 mg/kg/day in single or 2 divided doses, not to exceed 37.5 mg/day in infants up to 2 years of age or 100 mg/day in children 2–12 years of age. In infants less than 6 months of age, doses up to 3 mg/kg/day in 2 divided doses may be needed.

NURSING IMPLICATIONS

IMPLEMENTATION/ADMINISTRATION/STORAGE

1. Divide daily doses in excess of 100 mg.
2. Give twice a day at 6–12 hr intervals.
3. When used with other antihypertensives, hydrochlorothiazide dose is usually not more than 50 mg.
4. Store from 15–30°C (59–86°F). Protect from light, freezing, and moisture.

ASSESSMENT

1. Note reasons for therapy, disease onset, other agents trialed, outcome.
2. Assess for glucose intolerance and any other conditions that may warrant caution.
3. May take 2 to 3 weeks for desired therapeutic response.
4. Monitor BP, weight, uric acid, renal function, microalbumin, and electrolytes; replace potassium as needed.

CLIENT/FAMILY TEACHING

1. Take in the a.m. to prevent nighttime urinary frequency with 4 oz orange juice or one half a banana. May take with food if GI upset. Consume 2 to 3 L/day of fluids.
2. May cause blurred vision and dizziness; change positions slowly and avoid activities that require mental alertness until drug effects realized.

H

3. **Report swelling of extremities or weight gain of >2 lb/day or 5 lb/week.**
4. **Avoid alcohol, OTC drugs, and prolonged sun exposure; may cause delayed (10–14 days) photosensitivity reaction.**
5. **With diabetes, monitor BS and potassium closely; may cause glucose intolerance.**
6. **Record BP and weight to share with provider. Report persistent GI upset, ↓ urinary output, jaundice, muscle cramps, weakness, nausea, blurred vision, dizziness.**
7. **Keep all F/U to assess response, labs, and adverse SE.**

OUTCOMES/EVALUATE

- ↓ BP
- ↑ Urine output; ↓ edema

H

Combination Drug

Hydrocodone bitartrate and Acetaminophen

(**high**-droh-**KOH**-dohn, ah-**seat**-ah-**MIN**-oh-fen)

Classification(s): Analgesic
Pregnancy Category: C
RX: Anexia 10/660, Anexia 5/500, Anexia 7.5/325, Anexia 7.5/650, Ceta-Plus, Co-Gesic, Dolacet, Duocet, Hycet, Hydrogesic, Hy-Phen, Liquicet, Lorcet Plus, Lorcet-10/650, Lortab 10/500, Lortab 5/500, Lortab 7.5/500, Margesic H, Maxidone, Norco, Norco 5/325, Norco 7.5/325, Stagesic, T-Gesic, Vicodin, Vicodin ES, Vicodin HP, Xodol, Zydone, **C-III**

SEE ALSO ***NARCOTIC ANALGESICS*** AND ***ACETAMINOPHEN***.

INDICATIONS/USES

Relief of moderate to moderately severe pain.

CONTENT

Capsules/Tablets: Several possible combinations of hydrocodone bitartrate (*narcotic analgesic*) and acetaminophen (*nonnarcotic analgesic*)—amount of hydrocodone listed first: 2.5 mg/108 mg, 2.5 mg/325 mg, 2.5 mg/500 mg, 5 mg/300 mg, 5 mg/325 mg, 7.5 mg/300 mg, 7.5 mg/325 mg, 10 mg/325 mg, 5 mg/500 mg, 7.5 mg/325 mg, 7.5 mg/400 mg, 7.5 mg/500 mg, 7.5 mg/650 mg, 7.5 mg/750 mg, 10 mg/300 mg, 10 mg/325 mg, 10 mg/400 mg, 10 mg/500 mg, 10 mg/650 mg, 10 mg/660 mg, 10 mg/750 mg.

Elixir/Oral Solution: Hydrocodone bitartrate, 2.5 mg and acetaminophen, 108 mg/5 mL (oral solution); hydrocodone bitartrate, 2.5 mg and acetaminophen, 167 mg/5 mL (elixir); hydrocodone bitartrate, 10 mg and acetaminophen, 500 mg/15 mL (oral solution).

ACTION/KINETICS

Action

Hydrocodone produces its analgesic activity by an action on the CNS via opiate receptors. The analgesic action of acetaminophen is produced by both peripheral and central mechanisms.

Pharmacokinetics

Hydrocodone, maximum serum levels: About 1.3 hr. **Acetaminophen, t½:** 1.25–3 hr. Both hydrocodone and acetaminophen are metabolized in the liver and excreted through the urine.

CONTRAINDICATIONS

Hypersensitivity to acetaminophen or hydrocodone. Lactation.

SPECIAL CONCERNS

- **Use with caution, if at all, with head injuries as the CSF pressure may be increased further.**
- **Use with caution in geriatric or debilitated clients; in those with impaired hepatic or renal function; in hypothyroidism, Addison's disease, prostatic hypertrophy or urethral stricture, and in clients with pulmonary disease.**
- **Use shortly before delivery may cause respiratory depression in the newborn.**
- **Safety and efficacy have not been determined in children.**

SIDE EFFECTS

Most Common

N&V, urinary retention, light-headedness, dizziness, sedation, mental clouding.

CNS: Light-headedness, dizziness, sedation, drowsiness, mental clouding, lethargy, impaired mental and physical performance, anxiety, fear, dysphoria, psychologic dependence, mood changes. **GI:** N&V. **Respiratory:** Respiratory depression (dose-related), irregular and periodic breathing. **GU:** Ureteral spasm, spasm of vesical sphincters, urinary retention.

OVERDOSE MANAGEMENT

Symptoms: ***Acetaminophen overdose may result in potentially fatal hepatic necrosis.*** Also, renal tubular necrosis, hypoglycemic coma, and thrombocytopenia. Symptoms of hepatotoxic overdose include N&V, diaphoresis, and malaise. Symptoms of hydrocodone overdose include respiratory depression, somnolence progressing to stupor or ***coma***, skeletal muscle flaccidity, cold and clammy skin, bradycardia, and hypotension. ***Severe overdose may cause apnea, circulatory collapse, cardiac arrest, and death.*** *Treatment:* **Acetaminophen:**

- Empty stomach promptly by lavage or induction of emesis.
- Serum acetaminophen levels should be determined as early as possible but no sooner than 4 hr after ingestion.
- Determine liver function initially and at 24 hr intervals.
- The antidote, N-acetylcysteine, should be given within 16 hr of overdose for optimal results.

Hydrocodone:

- Reestablish adequate respiratory exchange with a patent airway and assisted or controlled ventilation.
- Respiratory depression can be reversed by giving naloxone IV.
- Oxygen, IV fluids, vasopressors, and other supportive measures may be instituted as required.

DRUG INTERACTIONS

Anticholinergics / ↑ Risk of paralytic ileus
CNS depressants, including other narcotic analgesics, antianxiety agents, antipsychotics, alcohol / Additive CNS depression
MAOIs / ↑ Effect of either the narcotic or the antidepressant
Tricyclic antidepressants / ↑ Effect of either the narcotic or the antidepressant

HOW SUPPLIED

See *Content.*

DOSAGE

CAPSULES; TABLETS

Analgesia.

For 2.5/500 product: 1 or 2 q 4–6 hr, up to 8 per day. **For 5/500 products:** 1 or 2 q 4–6 hr, up to 8 per day. **For 5/300, 5/325, 7.5/325, 10/325, and 7.5/400 products:** 1 or 2 q 4–6 hr, up to 6 or 12 (lower amounts) per day, depending on the product. **For 7.5/500 and 7.5/650 products:** 1 q 4–6 hr. **For the 7.5/750 product:** 1 q 4–6 hr, up to 5 per day. **For 10/325, 10/400, 10/500, and 10/650 products:** 1 q 4–6 hr, up to 6 per day. **For 10/650, 10/660, and 10/750 products:** 1 q 4–6 hr, up to 5 per day.

ORAL SOLUTION

Analgesia.

Children, 14 years and older: 15 mL q 4–6 hr, up to 120 mL/day; **10–13 years:** 10 mL q 4–6 hr, up to 60 mL/day; **7–9 years:** 7.5 mL q 4–6 hr, up to 45 mL/day; **4–6 years:** 5 mL q 4–6 hr, up to 30 mL/day; **2–3 years:** 3.75 mL q 4–6 hr, up to 22.5 mL/day. *NOTE:* **Dosages are based on a concentration of 2.5 mg hydrocodone bitartrate and 108 mg acetaminophen/5 mL.**

NURSING IMPLICATIONS

Do not confuse Lorcet and Lortab, both of which are a combination of hydrocodone bitartrate and acetaminophen.

ASSESSMENT

1. Note onset, location, and characteristics of S&S, other agents prescribed/therapies trialed, outcome, if pain acute or chronic; rate pain level.
2. Assess for head injury, hypothyroidism, BPH, urethral stricture, Addison's disease, severe pulmonary disease; precludes therapy.
3. Monitor VS, renal and LFTs; avoid with dysfunction.

CLIENT/FAMILY TEACHING

1. Take as directed. May take with food/milk to decrease GI upset.
2. Do not perform activities that require mental alertness; causes dizziness, lethargy, and impaired physical and mental performance.
3. Report evidence of abnormal bruising/bleeding, breathing problems, N&V, constipation, urinary difficulty, excessive sedation or lack of desired pain control.
4. Avoid alcohol and OTC agents or CNS depressants.

5. Store appropriately, away from the bedside and safely out of the reach of children.
6. Drug is for short-term use; may be habit forming.
7. Keep all F/U to assess response and adverse SE.

OUTCOMES/EVALUATE

Desired pain control

IV

Hydrocortisone (Cortisol)

(hy-droh-**KOR**-tih-zohn)

Classification(s): Glucocorticoid

Pregnancy Category: C

OTC: Roll-on Applicator: Maximum Strength Cortaid Faststick. **Topical Cream:** Allercort, Bactine, Cortizone-10, Cortizone-10 External Anal Itch, Cortizone-10 Plus, Dermolate Anti-Itch, Dermtex HC, HydroSkin, Hydro-Tex. **Topical Foam:** Itch-X. **Topical Gel:** Alcortin, Extra Strength CortaGel. **Topical Liquid:** Scalpicin, T/Scalp. **Topical Lotion:** Balneol Convenience Packets, Dermolate Scalp-Itch, HydroSkin. **Topical Ointment:** HydroSkin. **Topical Spray:** Cortaid, Cortizone-10 Quickshot, Dermolate Anti-Itch, Maximum Strength Cortaid, Procort.

RX: Parenteral: Sterile Hydrocortisone Suspension. **Rectal Cream/Gel:** Dermolate Anal-Itch, Proctocort, ProctoCream-HC 2.5%. **Retention Enema (Suspension):** Colocort. **Roll-on:** Cortaid FastStick. **Tablets:** Hydrocortone. **Topical Cream:** Ala-Cort, Alphaderm, Cort-Dome, Cortifair, Dermacort, DermiCort, H_2Cort, Hi-Cor 1.0 and 2.5, Hytone, Nutracort, Penecort, Synacort. **Topical Gel:** Alcortin. **Topical Lotion:** Acticort 100, Ala-Cort, Ala-Scalp, Allercort, Cetacort, Cort-Dome, Delacort, Dermacort, Gly-Cort, Hytone, LactiCare-HC, Lemoderm, Lexocort Forte, My Cort, Nutracort, Pentacort, Rederm, Scalacort DK, S-T Cort. **Topical Ointment:** Allercort, Cortril, Hytone, Lemoderm, Penecort. **Topical Solution:** Emo-Cort Scalp Solution, Penecort, Texacort Scalp Solution.

🍁 **Rx: Topical Lotion:** Emo-Cort, Sarna HC. **Topical Cream:** Emo-Cort. **Topical Ointment:** Cortoderm.

Hydrocortisone acetate

Pregnancy Category: C (topical and dental products)

OTC: Topical Cream: Cortaid, Cortef Feminine Itch, Corticaine, FoilleCort, Gynecort Female Cream, Lanacort 10, Lanacort 5, Maximum Strength Cortaid, Rhulicort. **Topical Lotion:** Cortaid, Rhulicort. **Topical Ointment:** Cortef Acetate, Hydrocortisone Acetate Maximum Strength, Lanacort, Lanacort 5, Maximum Strength Cortaid.

RX: Intrarectal Foam: Cortifoam. **Parenteral:** Hydrocortone Acetate. **Paste:** Orabase-HCA. **Rectal Gel:** Cort-Dome High Potency, Cortenema, Corticaine, Cortifoam. **Topical Cream:** CaldeCORT Light, Carmol-HC, Gynecort, Keratol HC, Lanacort, Pharma-Cort, U-Cort. **Topical Cream/Topical Ointment:** Maximum Strength Hydrocortisone Acetate, U-cort. **Topical Gel:** Novacort. **Topical Lotion:** NuCort.. **Topical Ointment:** Nov-Hydrocort.

🍁 **Rx: Topical Cream:** Hyderm.

Hydrocortisone butyrate

Pregnancy Category: C (topical products)

RX: Topical Cream, Lotion, Ointment, Solution: Locoid, Locoid Lipocream.

Hydrocortisone probutate

Pregnancy Category: C

RX: Topical Cream: Pandel.

Hydrocortisone sodium succinate

Pregnancy Category: C

RX: Parenteral: A-Hydrocort, Solu-Cortef.

Hydrocortisone valerate

Pregnancy Category: C (topical products)

RX: Cream/Topical Ointment: Westcort.

🍁 **Rx:** HydroVal.

SEE ALSO ***CORTICOSTEROIDS***.

INDICATIONS/USES

See *Corticosteroids.*

ACTION/KINETICS

Pharmacokinetics

Short-acting. **t½:** 80–118 min. Topical products are available without a prescription in strengths of 0.5% and 1%.

SIDE EFFECTS

See *Corticosteroids.*

HOW SUPPLIED

Hydrocortisone (Cortisol). ***Cream:*** 0.5%, 1%, 2.5%; ***Enema (Suspension):*** 100 mg/60 mL; ***Foam:*** 1%; ***Gel:*** 1%, 2%; ***Liquid:*** 1%; ***Lotion:*** 0.25%, 0.5%, 1%, 2%, 2.5%; ***Ointment:*** 0.5%, 1%, 2.5%; ***Pad:*** 0.5%, 1%; ***Rectal Cream:*** 2.5%; ***Solution:*** 1%, 2.5%; ***Spray:*** 1%; ***Spray Pump:*** 1%; ***Stick, Roll-On:*** 1%; ***Tablets:*** 5 mg, 10 mg, 20 mg.
Hydrocortisone acetate. ***Cream:*** 0.5%, 1%; ***Foam:*** 10%; ***Gel:*** 2%; ***Injection:*** 25 mg/mL, 50 mg/mL; ***Lotion:*** 2%; ***Ointment:*** 0.5%, 1%; ***Suppositories:*** 10 mg, 25 mg, 30 mg.
Hydrocortisone butyrate. ***Cream:*** 0.1%; ***Lotion:*** 0.1%; ***Ointment:*** 0.1%; ***Solution:*** 0.1%.
Hydrocortisone probutate. ***Cream:*** 0.1%, 1%.
Hydrocortisone sodium succinate. ***Powder for Injection:*** 100 mg, 250 mg, 500 mg, 1 gram.
Hydrocortisone valerate. ***Cream:*** 0.2%; ***Ointment:*** 0.2%.

DOSAGE

Hydrocortisone

TABLETS

20–240 mg/day, depending on disease.

ENEMA

100 mg in retention enema nightly for 21 days (up to 2 months of therapy may be needed; discontinue gradually if therapy exceeds 3 weeks).

CREAM; GEL; LOTION; SOLUTION; SPRAY; TOPICAL OINTMENT

Apply sparingly to affected area and rub in lightly 3–4 times per day.

Hydrocortisone acetate

INTRA-ARTICULAR; INTRALESIONAL; SOFT TISSUE

Large joints: 25 mg (occasionally, 37.5 mg). **Small joints:** 10–25 mg. **Tendon sheaths:** 5–12.5 mg. **Soft tissue infiltration:** 25–50 mg (occasionally 75 mg). **Bursae:** 25–37.5 mg. **Ganglia:** 12.5–25 mg.

INTRARECTAL FOAM

1 applicatorful (90 mg) 1–2 times per day for 2–3 weeks; **then** every second day.

TOPICAL

See *Hydrocortisone.*

Hydrocortisone butyrate

OINTMENT; SOLUTION; TOPICAL CREAM

Apply a thin film to the affected area 2–3 times per day.

Hydrocortisone probutate

TOPICAL CREAM

Apply a thin film to the affected area 1–2 times per day.

Hydrocortisone sodium succinate

IM; IV

Initial: 100–500 mg; **then,** may be repeated at 2-, 4-, and 6-hr intervals depending on response and severity of condition.

Hydrocortisone valerate

OINTMENT; TOPICAL CREAM

See *Hydrocortisone.*

NURSING IMPLICATIONS

Do not confuse hydrocortisone with hydrocodone (a narcotic analgesic). Also, do not confuse Hytone with Vytone (also a topical corticosteroid). Do not confuse HCTZ (hydrochlorothiazide) with HCT (hydrocortisone); spell out all drug names to prevent error and confusion.

IMPLEMENTATION/ADMINISTRATION/STORAGE

1. **IV** Check label of parenteral hydrocortisone because IM and IV preparations are not necessarily interchangeable.
2. Give reconstituted direct IV solution at a rate of 100 mg over 30 sec. Doses larger than 500 mg should be infused over 10 min. Drug may be further diluted in 50–100 mL of dextrose or saline solutions and administered as ordered within 24 hr.

3. COMPATIBILITY Dextrose or saline solutions.
4. INCOMPATIBILITY Administer separately.

ASSESSMENT

1. Note reasons for therapy, conditions requiring treatment, type, location, onset, characteristics of S&S and form/route prescribed. List other agents used and the outcome.
2. Describe clinical presentation; use photographs to document as indicated.
3. Identify any medical conditions that may preclude therapy. Note findings of x-ray, TB skin test, labs, and/or ECG.
4. Assess weight, VS, CBC, BS, chemistry profile, renal and LFTs.

CLIENT/FAMILY TEACHING

1. May take oral medication with food to minimize GI upset.
2. When using topical products, wash area prior to application or shower/bathe first, to increase drug penetration. Use only a small amount and rub into area thoroughly. Do not allow topical product to come in contact with the eyes.
3. Avoid prolonged use of topical products near the genital/rectal areas and eyes, on the face, and in skin creases.
4. For the butyrate topical products, use an occlusive dressing only on advice of the provider if used to treat psoriasis or other deep-seated dermatoses.
5. Do not use probutate products in the diaper area. With the probutate products, do not use tight-fitting diapers or plastic pants (occlusive).
6. No part of the intrarectal foam aerosol container should be inserted into the anus. With the suspension, shake well. Lie on left side with left leg extended and the right leg forward and flexed. Insert applicator tip of the suspension into the rectum pointed toward the navel, and slowly instill medication as directed.
7. Report worsening of condition requiring treatment, any fever, sore throat, muscle aches, slow healing, sudden weight gain, or swelling of extremities.
8. With eye products, use sunglasses—may reduce sensitivity to sunlight.
9. With diabetes, insulin or oral hypoglycemic agent needs may increase.
10. For elderly clients, have BP, blood glucose, and electrolytes monitored at least every 6 months.
11. With prolonged use of oral products, do not stop suddenly. Drug must be weaned/tapered down to prevent adrenal crisis. Cushingoid S&S of adrenal insufficiency include fatigue, dizziness, nausea, lack of appetite, weakness, SOB, joint pain.
12. Avoid alcohol, caffeine, and all OTC agents without approval.
13. Use appropriate prescribed form only as directed; call with questions or problems.
14. Keep all F/U to assess response, labs, adverse SE.

OUTCOMES/EVALUATE

- Replacement of adrenocortical deficiency
- Restoration of skin integrity
- Relief of allergic manifestations
- ↓ Inflammation

IV

Hydromorphone hydrochloride

Classification(s): Narcotic analgesic

Pregnancy Category: C

RX: Dilaudid, Dilaudid-HP, Exalgo, **C-II**

Rx: Dilaudid Sterile Powder, Dilaudid-HP-Plus, Dilaudid-XP, Hydromorph Contin, Hydromorphone HP 10, 20, and 50, Hydromorphone HP Forte, PMS-Hydromorphone.

SEE ALSO ***NARCOTIC ANALGESICS***.

INDICATIONS/USES

PO, Injection, Rectal. Moderate to severe pain (e.g., surgery, cancer, biliary colic, burns, renal colic, MI, bone or soft-tissue trauma). Dilaudid-HP is a concentrated solution intended for those tolerant to narcotics and who require larger than usual doses of opioids to attain adequate pain relief. Exalgo is indicated for managing moderate to severe pain in opioid-tolerant clients requiring continuous around-the-clock opioid analgesia for an extended period of time.

ACTION/KINETICS

Action

Hydromorphone is 7–10 times more analgesic than morphine, with a shorter duration of action.

It manifests less sedation, less vomiting, and less nausea than morphine, although it induces pronounced respiratory depression.

Pharmacokinetics

Onset: 15 min (IM, SC); 30 min (PO). **Peak effect:** 30–60 min. **Duration:** 4–5 hr (immediate release) and 4–5 hr (IM, SC). **t½, elimination:** 2.3 hr (immediate release) and 2.6 hr (IM, SC). Metabolized in the liver and excreted in the urine. Give rectally for prolonged activity. **Plasma protein binding:** 60–80%.

ADDITIONAL CONTRAINDICATIONS

Migraine headaches. Use in children or during labor. Status asthmaticus, obstetrics, respiratory depression in absence of resuscitative equipment. Use as an as-needed analgesic or for the management of acute or postoperative pain. Lactation.

SPECIAL CONCERNS

Hydromorphone Extended-Release Tablets (Exalgo): (1) **Potential for abuse.** Hydromorphone is an opioid agonist and a schedule II controlled substance with an abuse liability similar to other opioid analgesics. Hydromorphone can be abused in a manner similar to other opioid agonists, legal or illicit. These risks should be considered when administering, prescribing, or dispensing hydromorphone in situations where the health care provider is concerned about increased risk of misuse, abuse, or diversion. Schedule II opioid substances, which include hydromorphone, morphine, oxycodone, fentanyl, oxymorphone, and methadone, have the highest potential for abuse and risk of fatal overdose due to respiratory depression. (2) **Proper client selection.** Hydromorphone is an extended-release (ER) formulation of hydromorphone hydrochloride indicated for the management of moderate to severe pain in opioid-tolerant clients when a continuous around-the-clock opioid analgesic is needed for an extended period of time. Clients considered opioid-tolerant are those who are taking at least oral morphine 60 mg/day, oral hydromorphone 8 mg/day, oral oxymorphone 25 mg/day, or an equianalgesic dose of another opioid, for a week or longer. (3) Hydromorphone ER is for use in opioid-tolerant clients only. (4) Fatal respiratory depression could occur in clients who are not opioid tolerant. (5) Accidental consumption of hydromorphone ER, especially in children, can result in a fatal overdose of hydromorphone. (6) Limitations of use: Hydromorphone ER is not indicated for the management of acute or postoperative pain. (7) Hydromorphone ER is not intended for use as an as-needed analgesic. (8) Hydromorphone ER tablets are to be swallowed whole and are not to be broken, chewed, dissolved, crushed, or injected. Taking broken, chewed, dissolved, or crushed hydromorphone ER or its contents leads to rapid release and absorption of a potentially fatal dose of hydromorphone ER.

Hydromorphone Injection: (1) High potency hydromorphone injection is a highly concentrated solution of hydromorphone intended for use in opioid-tolerant clients. Do not confuse HP injection with standard parenteral formulations of injection or other opioids. Overdose and death could result. (2) Schedule II opioid agonists (e.g., hydromorphone, fentanyl, methadone, morphine, oxycodone, oxymorphone) have the highest risk of fatal overdoses because of respiratory depression, as well as the highest potential for abuse. (3) People at increased risk for opioid abuse include those with a personal or family history of substance abuse (including drug or alcohol abuse or addiction) or mental illness (e.g., major depression). Assess clients for clinical risks of opioid abuse or addiction prior to prescribing opioids. Routinely monitor all clients receiving opioids for signs of misuse, abuse, and addiction. Clients at increased risk of opioid abuse may still be appropriately treated with modified-release opioid formulations; however, these clients will require intensive monitoring for signs of misuse, abuse, or addiction. Use Dilaudid-HP with caution in clients with circulatory shock.

SIDE EFFECTS

Most Common

Constipation, N&V, asthenia, headache, infection, sleepiness/sedation/somnolence, itching/pruritus.

See *Narcotic Analgesics* for a complete list of potential side effects. Also, nystagmus.

ADDITIONAL DRUG INTERACTIONS

↑ CNS and respiratory depression when used with protease inhibitors.

HOW SUPPLIED

Injection Solution: 1 mg/mL, 2 mg/mL, 4 mg/mL; *Injection Solution, Concentrate:* 10 mg/mL; *Injection, Lyophilized Powder for Solution:* 250 mg/vial (10 mg/mL after reconstitution); *Liquid, Oral:* 1 mg/mL; *Suppositories:* 3 mg; *Tablets:* 2 mg, 4 mg, 8 mg; *Tablets, Extended-Release (Exalgo):* 8 mg, 12 mg, 16 mg.

DOSAGE

IM; IV; SC

Analgesia using the 1, 2, and 4 mg/mL products.

Adults, initial: 1–2 mg IM or SC q 4–6 hr as needed. For severe pain, 3–4 mg q 4–6 hr. May be given by slow IV over 2–3 min. Those with terminal cancer may be tolerant to opioid analgesics and may require higher doses for adequate analgesia.

Analgesia using the 10 mg/mL (high potency) product.

Give only to those already receiving high doses of opioids. Use this product only if the amount of hydromorphone required can be given accurately. Doses in those with terminal cancer range from 1 to 14 mg SC or IM. Experience with giving the high-potency hydromorphone IV is limited. If IV administration is needed, give slowly over at least 2 to 3 min.

ORAL LIQUID

Analgesia.

Initial: 2.5–10 mg (2.5–10 mL) q 3–6 hr as determined by client need. In some clients, PO dosages higher than usual doses may be needed.

SUPPOSITORIES

Analgesia from moderate to severe pain.

Individualize dosage. **Adults:** 3 mg q 6–8 hr or as directed by provider. In chronic pain, administer doses around-the-clock. A supplemental dose of 5 to 15% of the total daily dose may be given q 2 hr on an as-needed basis. The suppositories may provide a longer duration of relief, which is beneficial during sleeping hours.

TABLETS

Analgesia.

Individualize dosage based on severity of pain, client response, and client size. **Adults, initial:** 2–4 mg q 4–6 hr; for more severe pain, 4 or more mg q 4–6 hr. A gradual increase may be needed if the pain increases in severity, analgesia is not adequate, or tolerance occurs. If pain is exceedingly severe, or if a prompt effect is desired, use parenteral hydromorphone in adequate amounts to control the pain.

TABLETS, EXTENDED-RELEASE (EXALGO)

Analgesia in those opioid-tolerant.

Dose range: 8–64 mg. Initiate the dosing regimen individually for each client. Overestimating the dose of hydromorphone ER when converting from another opioid medication can cause a fatal overdose with the first dose of the ER product. Give ER tablets q 24 hr with or without food. Discontinue all other ER opioids when beginning hydromorphone ER therapy. *Do not begin anyone on hydromorphone ER as the first opioid.* When hydromorphone ER therapy is no longer required, taper doses gradually by 25–50% every 2 or 3 days down to a dose of 8 mg before discontinuing therapy in order to prevent withdrawal symptoms.

NURSING IMPLICATIONS

Do not confuse hydromorphone with morphine (also a narcotic analgesic).

IMPLEMENTATION/ADMINISTRATION/STORAGE

1. **Individualize dosage. Guide dose titration more by the need for analgesia than by the absolute dose of opioid used. Select a dose so that at least 3–4 hr of pain relief may be achieved.**
2. ***Use care when prescribing/dispensing hydromorphone ER 8 mg tablets because 8 mg tablets are also available as hydromorphone immediate-release tablets.***

3. Use lower starting doses in the elderly, in debilitated clients, and in those with impaired hepatic and renal function. Use particular care when using hydromorphone ER tablets.
4. Refrigerate suppositories.
5. Once the total daily dose of hydromorphone has been estimated, divide it into the desired number of doses. Due to individual variation in response to different opioid drugs, only one-half to two-thirds of the estimated hydromorphone dose calculated from equivalence tables should be given for the first few doses. The dose may then be increased as needed.
6. For chronic pain, give the drug around the clock. A supplemental dose of 5–15% of the total daily dose may be given q 2 hr on an as-needed basis.
7. Reduce the dose if excessive side effects are observed early in the dosing interval. If this results in breakthrough pain at the end of the dosing interval, the dosing interval may need to be shortened.
8. Reconstitute the lyophilized sterile powder for injection (i.e., the high-potency product) immediately prior to use with 25 mL sterile water for injection to provide a sterile solution containing 10 mg/mL.
9. If using the 500 mg/50 mL vial (i.e., 10 mg/mL of this single-dose product), do not penetrate the stopper with a syringe. Rather, remove both the aluminum flipseal and rubber stopper in a suitable work area (e.g., under a laminar flow hood). The contents may then be withdrawn for preparation of a single, large-volume parenteral solution. Discard any unused portion.
10. If high-potency hydromorphone is to be substituted for a different opioid analgesic, consult the package insert to determine the appropriate dose of the high-potency hydromorphone.
11. SC injections of high-potency hydromorphone are well accepted when given with a short 30-gauge needle.
12. Store PO and injectable products from 15–30°C (59–86°F); protect from light. Store suppositories in a refrigerator from 2–8°C (36–46°F).
13. **IV** Because the high-potency injection contains 10 mg/mL, a small injection volume can be used than with other formulations. Thus, discomfort from a large volume given IM or SC can be avoided.
14. May be given slowly over at least 2–3 min, depending on the dose. Administer slowly to minimize hypotensive effects and respiratory depression.
15. COMPATIBILITY Dextrose and saline solutions, Ringer's solution, and LR.
16. INCOMPATIBILITY Sodium bicarbonate, thiopental.

ASSESSMENT

1. Note type, location, onset, and characteristics of symptoms. Use a rating scale to rate pain.
2. Assess for respiratory depression; more profound with hydromorphone than with other narcotic analgesics. Encourage to turn, cough, deep breathe or use incentive spirometry every 2 hr to prevent atelectasis.
3. List drugs prescribed to ensure none interact unfavorably. Avoid use with migraine headaches, during labor, or with status asthmaticus.
4. Drug may mask symptoms of acute pathology; assess abdomen carefully.
5. Monitor VS and mental status. Assess bowel function, cognitive functioning, and for fall risk.

CLIENT/FAMILY TEACHING

1. Use exactly as directed at the onset of pain and in the dose prescribed. May take with milk or food to ↓ GI upset.
2. Do not perform activities that require mental alertness or coordination. Change positions slowly to avoid dizziness.
3. Increase intake of fluids and fiber to offset constipating effects; request therapy when needed.
4. Do not stop suddenly with long-term use; drug dependence occurs.
5. Avoid alcohol and any other CNS depressants without approval.
6. Report any unusual or intolerable side effects, difficulty breathing, or loss of pain control.
7. Store away from bedside to prevent accidental overdose.
8. Keep all F/U to assess response and for adverse SE.

OUTCOMES/EVALUATE

Control of pain

Hydroxyzine, Hydroxyzine hydrochloride

(hy-**DROX**-ih-zeen)

Classification(s): Antianxiety drug, nonbenzodiazepine

Pregnancy Category: C

Rx: Apo-Hydroxyzine.

Hydroxyzine pamoate

Pregnancy Category: C

RX: Vistaril.

H

INDICATIONS/USES

IM, PO: (1) Sedation when used as premedication and following general anesthesia. (2) Anxiety and tension associated with psychoneurosis and as an adjunct in organic diseases in which anxiety is manifested. (3) Pruritus due to allergic conditions such as chronic urticaria or atopic or contact dermatoses; also, histamine-mediated pruritus.

ACTION/KINETICS

Action

Action may be due to a suppression of activity in selected key regions of the subcortical areas of the CNS. Manifests anticholinergic, antiemetic, antispasmodic, local anesthetic, antihistaminic, and skeletal relaxant effects. Has mild antiarrhythmic activity and mild analgesic effects. Significant sedative and antiemetic effects and moderate anticholinergic activity.

Pharmacokinetics

Rapidly absorbed. **Onset:** 15–30 min. **t½:** 3 hr. **Duration:** 4–6 hr. Metabolized by the liver and excreted through the urine. The pamoate salt is believed to be converted to the hydrochloride in the stomach.

CONTRAINDICATIONS

Hypersensitivity to hydroxyzine or cetirizine. Pregnancy (especially early) or lactation. Treatment of morning sickness during pregnancy or as sole agent for treatment of psychoses or depression. Use in porphyria. IV, SC, or intra-arterial use.

SPECIAL CONCERNS

Has potent anticholinergic effects and can cause confusion and sedation in the elderly.

SIDE EFFECTS

Most Common

Sedation, drowsiness, tiredness, dizziness, disturbed coordination, drying/thickening of oral and other respiratory secretions, stomach upset.

Low incidence at recommended dosages. **CNS:** Drowsiness, dizziness, sedation, tiredness, sleepiness, confusion, nervousness, irritability, tremor. **GI:** Stomach upset, loss of appetite, nausea, dry mouth. **Respiratory:** Drying and thickening of oral and other respiratory secretions. **Dermatologic:** Urticaria, skin reactions. **Ophthalmic:** Blurred vision, double vision. **Miscellaneous:** Disturbed coordination, involuntary motor activity, hypersensitivity, worsening of porphyria, ECG abnormalities (e.g., alterations in T-waves). Marked discomfort, induration, and even gangrene at site of IM injection.

OVERDOSE MANAGEMENT

Symptoms: Oversedation. *Treatment:* Immediate gastric lavage. General supportive care with monitoring of VS. Control hypotension with IV fluids and either levarterenol, norepinephrine, or metaraminol (do not use epinephrine).

DRUG INTERACTIONS

See ***Drug Interactions*** for ***Tranquilizers***. Additive effects when used with other CNS depressants, including narcotics, nonnarcotic analgesics, and barbiturates.

HOW SUPPLIED

Hydroxyzine. ***Syrup:*** 10 mg/5 mL; ***Tablets:*** 10 mg, 25, mg, 50 mg.
Hydroxyzine hydrochloride. ***Injection:*** 25 mg/mL, 50 mg/mL.
Hydroxyzine pamoate. ***Capsules:*** 25 mg, 50 mg, 100 mg.

DOSAGE

Hydroxyzine Hydrochloride

IM

Sedation.

Adults: 50–100 mg as premedication or following general anesthesia. **Children:** 0.6 mg/kg as premedication or following general anesthesia.

Anxiety and tension.

Adults: 50–100 mg 4 times per day. **Children (investigational):** 0.5–1 mg q 4–6 hr as needed.

Pruritus.

Adults: 25 mg 3–4 times per day. **Children (investigational):** 0.5–1 mg/kg q 4–6 hr as needed.

Hydroxyzine and Hydroxyzine Pamoate

CAPSULES; SYRUP; TABLETS

Sedation.

Adults: 50–100 mg as premedication or following general anesthesia. **Children:** 0.6 mg/kg as premedication or following general anesthesia.

Anxiety and tension.

Adults: 50–100 mg 4 times per day. **Children over 6 years old:** 50–100 mg/day in divided doses. **Children less than 6 years old:** 50 mg/day in divided doses.

Pruritus.

Adults: 25 mg 3–4 times per day. **Children, over 6 years old:** 50–100 mg/day in divided doses. **Children, < 6 years old:** 50 mg/day in divided doses.

NURSING IMPLICATIONS

Do not confuse hydroxyzine with hydralazine (an antihypertensive).

IMPLEMENTATION/ADMINISTRATION/STORAGE

1. Start geriatric clients on low doses and observe closely.
2. Start clients on IM therapy only when indicated; maintain on PO therapy whenever possible.
3. Inject IM only. Make injection into the upper, outer quadrant of the buttocks or the midlateral muscles of the thigh. In children, inject into the midlateral muscles of the thigh. In infants and small children, to minimize sciatic nerve damage, use the periphery of the upper outer quadrant of the gluteal region only when necessary (e.g., burn clients). Do not make IM injections into the lower and mid-third of the upper arm.
4. Shake suspension vigorously until completely resuspended.
5. Store PO dosage forms from 15–30°C (59–86°F). Dispense in tight, light-resistant containers.
6. Store injection below 30°C (86°F); protect from freezing.

ASSESSMENT

1. List reasons for therapy, type, onset, and characteristics of S&S; identify triggers.
2. Note any associated contributing factors (i.e., dehydration, sweating, hives, asthma, urticaria, areas of pruritus and any potential contact).
3. Assess mental status and cognitive functioning; causes sedation.
4. Monitor VS, ECG and clinical presentation/response.

CLIENT/FAMILY TEACHING

1. Take only as directed, do not exceed dosing guidelines. May take with food if GI upset occurs.
2. Wait and evaluate sedative effects of drug before performing tasks that require mental alertness; may cause drowsiness.
3. Careful mouth care with frequent rinsing, sucking hard candy, chewing sugarless gum, and increased fluid intake may relieve S&S of dry mouth.
4. Avoid alcohol, CNS depressants, or any OTC antihistamines.
5. Drug is for short-term use. If scheduled for skin testing, stop drug for at least 4 days before skin testing.
6. Keep all F/U to assess response and for adverse SE.

OUTCOMES/EVALUATE

- ↓ Anxiety and agitation
- Desired sedation
- Control of N&V/chronic urticaria

H

I

Ibandronate sodium

IV

(eye-**BAN**-droh-nayt)

Classification(s): Bone growth regulator, bisphosphonate

Pregnancy Category: C

RX: Boniva.

INDICATIONS/USES

Tablets: Prophylaxis of postmenopausal osteoporosis in women who are at risk of developing osteoporosis and for whom the desired clinical outcome is to maintain bone mass and reduce the risk of fracture. **Injection/Tablets:** Treatment of postmenopausal osteoporosis to increase bone mineral density and reduce the incidence of vertebral fractures. *Investigational:* Prevention and treatment of complications of metastatic bone disease in breast cancer.

ACTION/KINETICS

Action

A bisphosphonate that inhibits osteoclast activity and reduces bone resorption and turnover. In postmenopausal women, the drug reduces the elevated rate of bone turnover, leading to a net gain in bone mass.

Pharmacokinetics

Absorption occurs in the upper GI tract. **Time to maximum plasma levels, after PO:** 0.5–2 hr. Absorption is impaired by food or beverages (other than plain water). After absorption, ibandronate either binds rapidly to bone or is excreted in the urine. Drug not bound to bone is excreted unchanged by the kidney (about 50–60% of the absorbed dose). Unabsorbed drug is excreted unchanged in the feces. **t½, terminal, after 150 mg PO:** 37–157 hr. **Plasma protein binding:** 90.9–99.5%.

CONTRAINDICATIONS

Hypersensitivity to the drug or any component of the product. Abnormalities of the esophagus that delay esophageal emptying (e.g., stricture or achalasia). Uncorrected hypocalcemia. Inability to stand or sit upright for at least 60 min. Severe renal impairment (C_{CR} less than 30 mL/min or serum creatinine >2.3 mg/mL).

SPECIAL CONCERNS

- **Use with caution with aspirin or NSAIDs and during lactation.**
- **Safety and efficacy have not been determined in children.**
- **Greater sensitivity cannot be ruled out in some geriatric clients.**

SIDE EFFECTS

Most Common

Back/arm/leg pain, diarrhea, dyspepsia, abdominal pain, constipation, pain/difficulty swallowing, headache, nausea, rash.

GI: UGI disorders, including dysphagia, esophagitis, esophageal, gastric ulcer, irritation of the mucosa. Dyspepsia, diarrhea, constipation, abdominal pain, pain/difficulty swallowing, tooth disorder, nausea, gastritis, gastroenteritis. **CNS:** Headache, dizziness, depression, insomnia, vertigo, nerve root lesion. **CV:** Hypertension. **Musculoskeletal:** Myalgia, arthralgia, back pain, arthritis, jaw osteonecrosis, localized osteoarthritis; severe and often incapacitating bone, joint and/or muscle pain. **Respiratory:** URTI, bronchitis, nasopharyngitis, pneumonia, pharyngitis. **GU:** UTI, cystitis, decreased renal function, renal failure. **Dermatologic:** Rash. **Injection site:** Redness, swelling. **Hypersensitivity:** Rash, bronchospasm, ***angioedema***, ***anaphylaxis***. **Ophthalmic:** Ocular inflammation, including uveitis and scleritis. **Body as a whole:** Influenza, influenza-like symptoms, asthenia, fatigue, allergic reaction.

LABORATORY TEST CONSIDERATIONS

↓ Alkaline phosphatase. Hypercholesterolemia, hypocalcemia.

OVERDOSE MANAGEMENT

Symptoms: Hypocalcemia/phosphatemia, UGI side effects, including upset stomach, dyspepsia, esophagitis, gastritis, ulcer. *Treatment:* Milk or antacids to bind the drug. Do not induce vomiting due to the risk of esophageal irritation. Keep client fully upright. Dialysis is not beneficial.

DRUG INTERACTIONS

***Antacids containing Ca, Al, Mg**$^{++}$* / ↓ Ibandronate absorption from GI tract
***Foods containing Ca**$^{++}$* / ↓ Ibandronate absorption from GI tract
Iron-containing products / ↓ Ibandronate absorption from GI tract

HOW SUPPLIED

Injection: 1 mg/mL (as base); ***Tablets:*** 150 mg (as base).

DOSAGE

IV ONLY

Treatment of postmenopausal osteoporosis.

Adults: 3 mg q 3 months given over 15–30 seconds.

TABLETS

Treat or prevent postmenopausal osteoporosis.

Adults: 150 mg tablet taken once monthly on the same date each month.

NURSING IMPLICATIONS

IMPLEMENTATION/ADMINISTRATION/STORAGE

1. Therapy must include calcium and vitamin D supplements if dietary intake is inadequate.
2. No dosage adjustment needed with mild or moderate renal impairment (where C_{CR} is equal to or greater than 30 mL/min).
3. IV Do not administer intra-arterially or paravenously due to possible tissue damage.
4. Use the needle provided; prefilled syringes are for single use only.
5. If the IV dose is missed, administer as soon as it can be rescheduled. Thereafter, schedule injections every 3 months from the date of the last injection. Do not give more frequently than every 3 months.
6. Store injection and tablets from 15–30°C (59–86°F). Discard any unused portion of the injection.
7. COMPATIBILITY Use prefilled syringe as a 15–30 second bolus.
8. INCOMPATIBILITY Do not mix the injection with calcium-containing solutions or other IV administered drugs.

ASSESSMENT

1. Note reasons for therapy, risk factors, BMD. List drugs prescribed to ensure none interact.
2. Monitor for S&S of esophageal reaction (e.g., dysphagia, new or worsening heartburn, retrosternal pain); stop drug if evident. Advise periodic dental exams to assess for S&S of osteonecrosis of the jaw.
3. Ensure supplemental calcium and vitamin D with injection and also with oral therapy if dietary intake inadequate.
4. Assess electrolytes, Ca^{++}, vitamin D, renal function; check creatinine prior to each injection and avoid with dysfunction. May cause elevated cholesterol and reduced total alkaline phosphatase.

CLIENT/FAMILY TEACHING

1. Take as directed once daily at least 60 min before the first food or drink (other than water) of the day and before any PO medications containing aluminum, Ca^{++}, or Mg^{++}, including supplements and vitamins.
2. Swallow tablets whole with a full glass of plain water (6–8 oz) while standing or sitting in an upright position. Do not lie down for 60 min after taking the drug. Do not double up or take dose later in the day.
3. Taking the tablets with food, other medications, juices, mineral water, coffee, or any other beverage will reduce drug absorption and its effectiveness.
4. If once-monthly dose is missed, and the next scheduled ibandronate day is more than 7 days away, take one 150 mg tablet in the morning of the date that it is remembered. Return to taking the one 150 mg tablet every month in the morning of the chosen day, according to the original schedule.
5. Do not take two 150 mg tablets during the same week. If the next scheduled ibandronate tablet is only 1–7 days away, wait until the next scheduled ibandronate day to take the tablet. Return to taking one 150 mg tablet every month in the morning of the chosen day, according to the original schedule.
6. Do not chew or suck the tablet due to the possibility of throat ulceration.
7. Review drug insert with each refill. May experience heartburn, swallowing problems, diarrhea, bone pain, ulcers, or chest pain.
8. Eat well-balanced meals, perform regular daily exercise, stop smoking, avoid alcohol consumption; avoid behaviors that add to osteoporosis risk.

9. **Do not take any OTC medications, vitamins, or supplements without approval. Should be prescribed supplemental calcium and vitamin D.**
10. **Practice reliable contraception; report if pregnancy suspected or if planning to breast-feed. Keep all F/U visits to evaluate response, bone mineral density, and for adverse SE.**

OUTCOMES/EVALUATE

↑ Bone mineral density in postmenopausal women; ↓ vertebral fractures

■ IV

Ibritumomab tiuxetan

(ib-rih-**TOO**-moh-mab)

Classification(s): Antineoplastic agent

Pregnancy Category: D

RX: Zevalin.

SEE ALSO ***ANTINEOPLASTIC AGENTS.***

INDICATIONS/USES

Relapsed or refractory low-grade, follicular, or transformed B-cell non-Hodgkin's lymphoma, including the treatment of previously untreated follicular non-Hodgkin's lymphoma in those who achieve a partial or complete response to first-line chemotherapy. Ibritumomab tiuxetan is part of a therapeutic regimen that first includes an infusion of rituximab followed by an injection of ibritumomab tiuxetan. This same regimen is repeated 7–9 days after the first course of therapy.

ACTION/KINETICS

Action

Drug is the immunoconjugate from a stable thiourea covalent bond between the monoclonal antibody, ibritumomab, and the linker-chelator, tiuxetan. The linker-chelator provides a high affinity, conformationally restricted chelation site for either Indium-111 or Yttrium-90. The ibritumomab antibody acts against the CD20 antigen, which is found on the surface of normal and malignant B lymphocytes. The chelate, tiuxetan, which tightly binds In-111 or Y-90 is covalently linked to the amino groups of exposed lysines and arginines contained within the antibody. The beta emission from Y-90 causes cellular damage by forming free radicals in the target and neighboring cells. Administration of ibritumomab tiuxetan results in sustained depletion of B cells. Median serum levels of IgG and IgA remain within the normal range through the period of B-cell depletion. However, median IgM levels drop below normal after treatment but recover to normal values within 6 months after therapy.

Pharmacokinetics

t½ of Y-90: 30 hr. A median of 7.2% of the injected activity is excreted in the urine over 7 days.

CONTRAINDICATIONS

Type I hypersensitivity or anaphylactic reactions to murine proteins or any component of the product, including rituximab, yttrium chloride, or indium chloride. Administration of Y-90 ibritumomab tiuxetan to those with altered biodistribution as determined by imaging with In-111 ibritumomab tiuxetan. Lactation.

Use in clients with 25% or more lymphoma marrow involvement or impaired bone marrow reserve; platelet count <100,000 cells/mm^3; neutrophil count <1,500 cells/mm^3; hypocellular bone marrow (less than or equal to 15% cellularity or marked reduction in bone marrow precursors); or a history of failed stem cell collection.

Receipt of growth factor for 2 weeks prior to ibritumomab tiuxetan therapy and for 2 weeks following completion of the regimen.

Administration of rituximab as an IV push or bolus.

SPECIAL CONCERNS

■ (1) **Fatal infusion reactions.** Deaths have occurred within 24 hr of rituximab infusion, an essential component of the ibritumomab tiuxetan therapeutic regimen. These fatalities were associated with acute respiratory distress syndrome, cardiogenic shock, hypoxia, MI, pulmonary infiltrates, or ventricular fibrillation. About 80% of fatal infusion reactions occurred in association with the first rituximab infusion. Discontinue rituximab, In-111 ibritumomab tiuxetan, and Y-90 ibritumomab tiuxetan infusions in clients who develop severe infusion reactions. (2) **Prolonged and severe cytopenias.** Y-90 ibritumomab tiuxetan administration results in severe and prolonged cytopenias in most clients. Do not administer any further component of the ibritumomab tiuxetan administration regimen to clients with at least 25% lymphoma marrow involvement

and/or impaired bone marrow reserve.
(3) **Severe cutaneous and mucocutaneous reactions.** Severe cutaneous and mucocutaneous reactions, some with fatal outcome, have been reported in association with the ibritumomab tiuxetan therapeutic regimen. Discontinue rituximab, In-111 ibritumomab tiuxetan, and Y-90 ibritumomab tiuxetan infusions in clients experiencing severe cutaneous or mucocutaneous reactions.
(4) **Dosing.** (a) The dose of Y-90 ibritumomab tiuxetan should not exceed 32 mCi (1,184 MBq). (b) Do not administer Y-90 ibritumomab tiuxetan to clients with altered biodistribution as determined by imaging with In-111 ibritumomab tiuxetan. ■

- **Use with caution with drugs that interfere with platelet function or coagulation after the ibritumomab tiuxetan therapeutic regimen; monitor clients carefully who receive such drugs.**
- **Lower doses may be necessary in the elderly.**
- **The therapeutic regimen contains albumin, derived from human blood. There is an extremely remote change for transmission of Creutzfeldt-Jakob disease.**
- **Safety and efficacy not determined in children.**

SIDE EFFECTS

Most Common

Abdominal pain, asthenia, cough, cytopenias (anemia, leukopenia, lymphopenia, neutropenia, thrombocytopenia), diarrhea, fatigue, nasopharyngitis, nausea, pyrexia, thrombocytopenia.

Severe/fatal infusion reactions: Hypotension, angioedema, hypoxia, bronchospasms, urticaria, pulmonary infiltrate, ***ARDS, MI, ventricular fibrillation, cardiogenic shock, death***. **Hematologic:** Prolonged and severe cytopenias (may be accompanied by hemorrhage and severe infection), including thrombocytopenia (most common) and neutropenia; leukopenia, lymphopenia, anemia, ecchymosis, pancytopenia. **CV:** ***Hemorrhage (while thrombocytopenic), including fatal cerebral hemorrhage and severe infections***, hyper-/hypotension, tachycardia. **GI:** N&V, abdominal pain/enlargement, anorexia, diarrhea, throat irritation, constipation, dyspepsia, melena, ***GI hemorrhage***, hematemesis, biliary stent-associated cholangitis. **CNS:** Dizziness, anxiety, headache, insomnia, encephalopathy, ***subdural hematoma***. **Respiratory:** Increased cough, nasopharyngitis, bronchitis, dyspnea, rhinitis, sinusitis, bronchospasm, epistaxis, ***apnea***, lung edema, pharyngolaryngeal pain, ***pulmonary embolus***. **Musculoskeletal:** Arthralgia, myalgia, arthritis. **Dermatologic:** Urticaria, night sweats, petechia, pruritus, rash, flushing, erythema multiforme, ***Stevens-Johnson syndrome, toxic epidermal necrolysis***, bullous dermatitis, exfoliative dermatitis. **Infusion site:** Extravasation, erythema, ulceration. **Infections:** UTI, febrile neutropenia, ***sepsis***, pneumonia, cellulitis, colitis, diarrhea, osteomyelitis, URTI. Serious infections (primarily bacterial), including ***sepsis***, empyema, pneumonia, febrile neutropenia, biliary stent-associated colangitis. Serious infections from 3 months to 4 years after start of treatment, including UTI, bacterial or viral pneumonia, febrile neutropenia, perihilar infiltrate, pericarditis, IV drug-associated viral hepatitis, respiratory disease, ***sepsis***. **Body as a whole:** Development of secondary malignancies (myelodysplastic syndrome and/or acute myelogenous leukemia), possible immunogenicity, allergic reactions (***bronchospasm, angioedema***), peripheral edema, asthenia, fatigue, infection, chills, fever, pain, flu-like illness, back/tumor pain, empyema, ***vaginal hemorrhage***. **Miscellaneous:** Immunogenicity, radiation injury in tissues near areas of lymphomatous involvement within a month of therapy.

DRUG INTERACTIONS

Anticoagulant drugs (e.g., enoxaparin, heparin, warfarin) / Possible ↑ risk of bleeding and hemorrhage as well as cytopenias; avoid coadministration. If coadministration necessary, monitor anticoagulant function and monitor frequently for thrombocytopenia

Antiplatelet drugs (e.g., aspirin, clopidogrel, dipyridamole) / Possible ↑ risk of bleeding and hemorrhage as well as cytopenias; avoid coadministration. If coadministration necessary, monitor anticoagulant function and monitor frequently for thrombocytopenia

Hematopoietic growth factors (e.g., darbepoetin alfa, epoetin alfa, filgrastim, pegfilgrastim) / May ↑ biodistribution pattern by ↑ bone marrow uptake of ibritumomab tiuxetan; reassess biodistribution after correction of underlying factors

HOW SUPPLIED

Injection: 3.2 mg in 2 mL single-use vials.

I

DOSAGE

IV

Non-Hodgkin's lymphoma.

Day 1: Step 1, Give rituximab, 250 mg/m² IV at an initial rate of 50 mg/hr. Do not mix or dilute rituximab with other drugs. If hypersensitivity or infusion-related events do not occur, escalate the infusion rate in 50 mg/hr increments every 30 min to a maximum of 400 mg/hr. Immediately stop the rituximab infusion for serious infusion reactions and discontinue the ibritumomab tiuxetan therapeutic regimen. Temporarily slow or interrupt the rituximab infusion for less severe infusion reactions. If symptoms improve, continue the infusion at ½ the previous rate. **Then,** within 4 hr following completion of the rituximab dose, inject 5 mCi (1.6 mg total antibody dose) IV of In-111 ibritumomab tiuxetan over a 10-min period. Assess biodistribution as follows: First image, 2–24 hr after In-111 ibritumomab tiuxetan; second image, 48–72 hr after In-111 ibritumomab tiuxetan. An optional third image may be taken 90–120 hr after In-111 ibritumomab tiuxetan. If biodistribution is not acceptable, do not proceed. **Day 7, 8, or 9:** Initiate Step 2, 7 to 9 days following Step 1. Give rituximab, 250 mg/m² IV at an initial rate of 100 mg/hr (50 mg/hr if infusion-related events were documented during Step 1). Increase by 100 mg/hr increments at 30-min intervals to a maximum of 400 mg/hr, as tolerated. **Then,** within 4 hr after completion of the rituximab dose, inject IV, Y-90 ibritumomab tiuxetan, over a period of 10 min, 0.4 mCi/kg (14.8 MBq/kg) actual body weight for clients with a platelet count greater than 150,000 cells/mm³ and 0.3 mCi/kg (11.1 MBq/kg) actual body weight for clients with a platelet count of 100,000 to 149,000 cells/mm³. The prescribed, measured, and administered dose of Y-90 ibritumomab tiuxetan must not exceed the maximum allowable dose of 32 mCi (1,184 MBq) regardless of the client's weight. Do not give ibritumomab tiuxetan if platelets are less than 100,000/mm³.

NURSING IMPLICATIONS

IMPLEMENTATION/ADMINISTRATION/STORAGE

1. **IV** The ibritumomab tiuxetan regimen is intended as a single-course of therapy.
2. Due to hypersensitivity reactions, premedicate with acetaminophen 650 mg PO and diphenhydramine 50 mg PO prior to each rituximab infusion.
3. Initiate the ibritumomab tiuxetan therapeutic regimen following recovery of platelet counts to 150,000/mm³ or higher at least 6 weeks, but no more than 12 weeks, following the last dose of first-line chemotherapy.
4. Establish free-flowing IV line prior to Y-90 ibritumomab tiuxetan injection. Monitor carefully for extravasation when giving drug. If any signs of extravasation occur, immediately terminate the infusion and restart in another vein.
5. Reduce the dose of Y-90 ibritumomab tiuxetan to 0.3 mCi/kg (11.1 MBq/kg) for clients with a baseline platelet count between 100,000/mm³ and 149,000/mm³.
6. Monitor clients closely for extravasation during the injection of Y-90 ibritumomab tiuxetan. If any signs or symptoms of extravasation occur, stop infusion immediately and restart in another limb.
7. For product preparation, see manufacturer's product labeling.
8. Two separate kits (distinctly labeled) are to be ordered for the preparation of a single dose each of In-111 ibritumomab tiuxetan and Y-90 ibritumomab tiuxetan. Note that these are both radiopharmaceuticals and must be used only by physicians and other professionals qualified by training in the safe use and handling of such agents.
9. Give In-111 ibritumomab tiuxetan within 12 hr of radiolabeling and give Y-90 ibritumomab tiuxetan within 8 hr of radiolabeling.
10. To administer ibritumomab tiuxetan use a 0.22 micron low-protein-binding in-line filter between the syringe and the infusion port. After injection, flush the line with at least 10 mL of normal saline.

11. Administer Y-90 ibritumomab tiuxetan through a free flowing IV line within 4 hr following completion of rituximab infusion.
12. Changing the ratio of any of the reactants in the radiolabeling process may adversely impact results.
13. Do not use either In-111 ibritumomab tiuxetan or Y-90 ibritumomab tiuxetan in the absence of the rituximab predose.
14. The expected biodistribution is as follows: Activity faintly visible in the blood pool areas (e.g., heart, abdomen, neck, and extremities; moderately high to high update in healthy liver and spleen; moderately low or very low uptake in healthy kidneys, urinary bladders, and healthy (uninvolved) bowel. Delayed imaging may be necessary to confirm GI clearance. Will be focal fixed areas of uptake in the bowel wall (localization to lymphoid aggregates in bowel wall).
15. Tumor uptake may be visualized; however, tumor visualization on the In-111 ibritumomab tiuxetan scan is not required for Y-90 ibritumomab tiuxetan therapy.
16. Altered biodistribution may occur; check package insert for the criteria for altered biodistribution.
17. Store kits from 2–8°C (36–46°F); do not freeze.
18. COMPATIBILITY Use prepared infusions; may flush the line with at least 10 mL of isotonic sodium chloride solution.
19. INCOMPATIBILITY Do not mix or dilute with any other drugs.

ASSESSMENT

1. Note reasons for therapy, other agents trialed, outcome.
2. Premedicate with acetaminophen 650 mg and diphenhydramine 50 mg prior to each infusion of rituximab.
3. Follow administration guidelines and steps carefully. Inject within 4 hr following completion of the rituximab dose. Monitor closely for any evidence of extravasation during therapy.
4. Infusion reactions (ARDS, hypoxia, pulmonary infiltrates, MI, VF, or cardiogenic shock) may occur. Monitor closely and stop infusion as reactions may be fatal. Must only be administered by qualified trained individuals in radiopharmaceuticals.
5. Do not administer Y-90 ibritumomab tiuxetan to those with altered biodistribution as determined by imaging with In-111 ibritumomab tiuxetan.
6. Do not administer the ibritumomab tiuxetan therapeutic regimen to those with at least 25% lymphoma marrow involvement and/or impaired bone marrow reserve.
7. Review risks of secondary malignancy with therapy and risk of transmitting viral infections related to content—albumin, a derivative of human blood.
8. Assess carefully for infections, allergic reactions, skin reactions, and hemorrhage. Drug is radiopharmaceutical; utilize radionuclide precautions (minimize exposure to client and medical staff).
9. Avoid drugs that interfere with platelet function or bleeding times.
10. Monitor platelet and CBC weekly following the ibritumomab tiuxetan therapeutic regimen and continue until levels recover. Monitor platelets and CBC more frequently in those who develop severe cytopenia, are receiving medications that interfere with platelet function or coagulation, or as clinically indicated.

CLIENT/FAMILY TEACHING

1. Used to treat relapsed or refractory non-Hodgkin's lymphoma; consists of two infusions approximately 1 week apart.
2. Elderly may show greater sensitivity to the regimen.
3. Report any evidence of rash, skin eruptions, infection, fatigue, easy bruising or bleeding abnormalities.
4. Use effective contraception during treatment and for 12 months following regimen. Do not breast-feed before and after treatments.
5. Avoid live vaccines during therapy and for 12 months after therapy. Ensure client/family are aware of risks: that myeloid malignancies have occurred with therapy and that infusion reactions may be fatal.
6. Do not consume any drugs that may alter platelet function unless provider prescribed.
7. Keep all F/U to assess response, labs, and for adverse SE.

OUTCOMES/EVALUATE

Inhibition of malignant cell proliferation

Ibuprofen

(eye-byou-**PROH**-fen)

Classification(s): Nonsteroidal anti-inflammatory drug

Pregnancy Category: B (first two trimesters); **D** (third trimester)

OTC: Capsules: Advil Liqui-Gels, Advil Migraine. **Gelcaps**: Motrin IB. **Oral Drops**: Advil Pediatric Drops, Motrin Infants', PediaCare Fever. **Suspension**: Children's Advil, Children's Motrin, PediaCare Fever. **Tablets/Caplets**: Advil, Ibutab, Junior Strength Motrin, Midol Maximum Strength Cramp Formula, Motrin IB, Motrin Migraine Pain (Caplets). **Tablets, Chewable**: Children's Motrin, Junior Strength Motrin.

RX: Tablets: Various generic products.

✤ **Rx:** Apo-Ibuprofen, Apo-Ibuprofen Prescription.

Ibuprofen lysine

RX: NeoProfen.

SEE ALSO ***NONSTEROIDAL ANTI-INFLAMMATORY DRUGS***.

INDICATIONS/USES

Ibuprofen. Rx, Tablets: (1) Analgesic for mild to moderate pain. (2) Primary dysmenorrhea. (3) Relief of signs and symptoms of rheumatoid arthritis or osteoarthritis. **Injection:** (1) Management of mild to moderate pain. (2) Management of moderate to severe pain as an adjunct to opioid analgesics in adults. (3) Reduction of fever in adults.

Ibuprofen. OTC: Liquid-Filled Capsules, Adults: Migraine headaches. **Gelcaps and Tablets, Adults:** (1) Temporary relief of minor aches and pains due to the common cold, headache, toothache, muscular aches, backache, minor pain of arthritis, menstrual cramps. (2) Reduce fever temporarily. **Chewable Tablets, Junior Strength Tablets, Oral Suspension, Oral Drops, Children:** (1) Temporary reduction of fever. (2) Relief of minor aches and pains due to colds, flu, sore throat, headaches, and toothaches. *Investigational:* Prevention of side effects with diphtheria and tetanus toxoids and pertussis (DTP) vaccination. Prevention of side effects with DTP vaccination in those at risk for seizures. Juvenile rheumatoid arthritis.

Ibuprofen lysine. Rx, IV (NeoProfen): To close clinically significant patent ductus arteriosus in infants whose gestational age is 32 weeks or less, weight is 500–1,500 grams, and condition cannot be managed through usual therapy (e.g., diuretics, fluid restriction, respiratory support).

ACTION/KINETICS

Action

Anti-inflammatory effect is likely due to inhibition of cyclo-oxygenase. Inhibition of cyclo-oxygenase results in decreased prostaglandin synthesis. Effective in reducing joint swelling, pain, and morning stiffness, as well as to increase mobility in those with inflammatory disease. Ibuprofen does not alter the course of the disease, however. The antipyretic action occurs by decreasing prostaglandin synthesis in the hypothalamus, resulting in an increase in peripheral blood flow and heat loss, as well as promoting sweating. The mechanism to close patent ductus arteriosus is not known.

Pharmacokinetics

Greater than 80% bioavailable after PO. **Time to peak levels:** 1–2 hr. **Onset:** 30 min for analgesia and approximately 1 week for anti-inflammatory effect. **Peak serum levels:** 1–2 hr. **Duration:** 4–6 hr for analgesia and 1–2 weeks for anti-inflammatory effect. Food delays absorption rate but not total amount of drug absorbed. **$t^{1/2}$:** 1.8–2 hr. 45–79% excreted in the urine. **Plasma protein binding:** 99%.

CONTRAINDICATIONS

Pregnancy, especially during the last trimester (premature closure of ductus arteriosus may occur). Use in clients with the aspirin triad (bronchial asthma, rhinitis, aspirin intolerance). Use to treat perioperative pain in the setting of coronary artery bypass graft surgery. Ibuprofen lysine is contraindicated in preterm infants with a proven or suspected infection not receiving treatment; congenital heart disease needing a patent ductus arteriosus to achieve satisfactory pulmonary or systemic blood flow; thrombocytopenia; in those who are bleeding (especially those with active intracranial hemorrhage or GI bleeding); a coagulation defect, proven or suspected necrotizing enterocolitis, or significant impaired renal function.

SPECIAL CONCERNS

■ (1) **Cardiovascular risk.** NSAIDs may cause an increased risk of serious CV thrombotic events, MI, and stroke, which can be fatal. This risk may increase with duration of use. Clients with CV disease or risk factors for CV disease may be at a greater risk. (2) Ibuprofen is contraindicated for treatment of perioperative pain in the setting of coronary artery bypass graft surgery. (3) **GI risk.** NSAIDs cause an increased risk of serious GI adverse events, including bleeding, ulceration, and perforation of the stomach or intestines, which can be fatal. These events can occur at any time during use and without warning symptoms. Elderly clients are at greater risk for serious GI events. ■

- Individualize dosage by body weight for children less than 12 years of age as safety and efficacy not established.
- May cause stomach bleeding in individuals who consume large amounts of alcohol regularly.
- Blocks the heart-protecting effects of aspirin.
- Ibuprofen chewable tablets may cause stomach bleeding if more than the recommended dose is taken.
- Use with caution in CHF, as fluid retention and edema can occur.
- Use can lead to onset of new hypertension, worsening of pre-existing hypertension, and impairment of the response of antihypertensive therapy (e.g., ACE inhibitors, thiazides, loop diuretics).
- Even short-term use may lead to an increased risk of death and recurrent MI in clients with prior MI.
- Ibuprofen lysine may alter the usual signs of infection. Use the drug with extra care in the presence of controlled infection and in infants at risk of infection. Use with caution in infants with elevated total bilirubin.

SIDE EFFECTS

Most Common

Ibuprofen: Dizziness, rash, nausea, epigastric/GI pain, heartburn.
Ibuprofen lysine: Skin lesion/irritation, ***sepsis***, GI disorders, anemia, ***intraventricular hemorrhage***, impaired renal function, ***apnea***, respiratory failure, RTI.
See also *Nonsteroidal Anti-Inflammatory Drugs* for a complete list of possible side effects.

Ibuprofen: Also, dermatitis (maculopapular type), rash. Hypersensitivity reaction consisting of abdominal pain, fever, headache, ***meningitis***, N&V, abnormal platelet function (returns to normal within 24 hr), signs of liver damage; especially seen in clients with SLE. Renal papillary necrosis, serious skin reactions, including exfoliative dermatitis, ***Stevens-Johnson syndrome***, and ***toxic epidermal necrolysis***.

Ibuprofen lysine: GI: GI disorders, including non-necrotizing enterocolitis, abdominal distention, gastritis, gastroesophageal reflux, ileus, cholestasis, jaundice. **CNS: *Convulsions*. CV: *Cardiac failure***, hypotension, tachycardia. **GU:** UTI, reduced urine output, inguinal hernia. **Hematologic:** Anemia, ***intraventricular hemorrhage*** (all grades), other bleeding disorders, neutropenia, thrombocytopenia. **Metabolic:** Hypernatremia, hypocalcemia, hypo-/hyperglycemia. **GU:** Renal failure, impaired renal function, decreased urine output. **Respiratory:** Apnea, ***respiratory failure***, atelectasis, RTI. **Dermatologic:** Skin lesions/irritation. **Miscellaneous: *Sepsis***, edema, adrenal insufficiency, injection site reactions, feeding problems, various infections.

LABORATORY TEST CONSIDERATIONS

Ibuprofen: Borderline ↑ liver transaminases. **Ibuprofen lysine:** ↑ Blood urea, blood urea increased with hematuria, blood creatinine.

ADDITIONAL DRUG INTERACTIONS

Aspirin / Ibuprofen may ↓ or negate the cardioprotective effects of low-dose aspirin
Furosemide / ↓ Diuretic effect R/T ↓ renal prostaglandin synthesis
H *Ginkgo biloba* / Possible (rare) intracerebral mass bleeding
Lithium / ↑ Plasma lithium levels
Thiazide diuretics / See *Furosemide*

HOW SUPPLIED

Ibuprofen. OTC: Caplets/Capsules: 200 mg; *Oral Drops:* 40 mg/mL; *Suspension:* 100 mg/5 mL; *Tablets:* 100 mg, 200 mg; *Tablets, Chewable:* 50 mg, 100 mg; **Rx:** Injection Solution, Concentrate: 100 mg/mL; *Tablets:* 400 mg, 600 mg, 800 mg.
Ibuprofen lysine. *Injection:* 17.1 mg/mL (equivalent to 10 mg/mL ibuprofen).

DOSAGE

Ibuprofen

RX: TABLETS

Rheumatoid arthritis and osteoarthritis, including flare-ups of chronic disease.

400, 600, or 800 mg 3–4 times per day; adjust dosage according to client response. Individual clients may show a better response to 3,200 mg daily compared with 2,400 mg. However, evaluate the increased clinical benefits of the higher dose to potential increased risk. Full therapeutic response may not be noted for 2 or more weeks.

Mild to moderate pain.

Adults: 400 mg q 4–6 hr, as needed. Doses greater than 400 mg are no more effective than the 400 mg dose.

Primary dysmenorrhea.

Adults: 400 mg q 4 hr, as needed, for the relief of pain. Begin treatment with the earliest onset of pain.

IV: *Management of pain.*

Adults, usual: 400–800 mg q 4–8 hr as necessary, up to a maximum of 3,200 mg/day.

IV: *Reduce fever.*

Adults, usual: 400 mg followed by 400 mg q 4–6 hr or 100–200 mg q 4 hr, as necessary, up to a maximum of 3,200 mg/day.

OTC: CAPSULES

Migraine headaches.

Adults: 400 mg (2 capsules) with a glass of water. If symptoms persist or worsen, contact provider. No more than 2 capsules should be taken in a 24-hr period.

OTC: GELCAPS AND TABLETS

Mild to moderate pain, antipyretic, dysmenorrhea.

Adults: 200 mg (1 gelcap or tablet) q 4–6 hr while symptoms persist. If pain or fever does not respond to 1 gelcap or tablet, 2 gelcaps or tablets (i.e., 400 mg) may be taken, but do not exceed 6 gelcaps or tablets (i.e., 1,200 mg) in 24 hr unless directed by provider.

OTC: CHEWABLE TABLETS (50 MG)

Pain, fever.

Children, 4–5 years of age (36–47 pounds): 150 mg (3 tablets) q 6–8 hr, up to 4 times per day. **Children, 6–8 years of age (48–59 pounds):** 4 tablets (200 mg) q 6–8 hr, up to 4 times per day. **Children, 9–10 years of age (60–71 pounds):** 250 mg (5 tablets) q 6–8 hr, up to 4 times per day. **Children, 11 years of age (72–95 pounds):** 300 mg (6 tablets) q 6–8 hr, up to 4 times per day. Usually use weight to dose; otherwise, use age.

OTC: JUNIOR STRENGTH CHEWABLE TABLETS (100 MG)

Pain, fever.

Children, 6–8 years of age (48–59 pounds): 200 mg (2 tablets) q 6–8 hr, up to 4 times per day. **Children, 9–10 years of age (60–71 pounds):** 250 mg (2.5 tablets) q 6–8 hr, up to 4 times per day. **Children, 11 years of age (72–95 pounds):** 300 mg (3 tablets) q 6–8 hr, up to 4 times per day. Use weight to dose; otherwise use age.

OTC: ORAL DROPS

Antipyretic.

Children, 6–11 months (12–17 pounds): 50 mg (1.25 mL) q 6–8 hr, up to 4 times per day. **Children, 12–23 months (18–23 pounds):** 75 mg (1.875 mL) q 6–8 hr, up to 4 times per day.

OTC: ORAL SUSPENSION

Pain, fever.

Usual dose: 7.5 mg/kg. **Children, 2–3 years of age (24–35 pounds):** 100 mg (5 mL) q 6–8 hr, up to 4 times per day. **Children, 4–5 years of age (36–47 pounds):** 150 mg (7.5 mL) q 6–8 hr, up to 4 times per day. **Children, 6–8 years of age (48–59 pounds):** 200 mg (10 mL) q 6–8 hr, up to 4 times per day. **Children, 9–10 years of age (60–71 pounds):** 250 mg (12.5 mL) q 6–8 hr, up to 4 times per day. **Children, 11 years of age (72–95 pounds):** 300 mg (15 mL) q 6–8 hr, up to 4 times per day.

OTC

Prevention of side effects with DTP vaccination, including those at risk for seizures (investigational).

Dose range: 7–10 mg/kg/dose.

Juvenile rheumatoid arthritis (investigational).

Usual: 30–50 mg/kg/day in divided doses q 6 hr.

Ibuprofen lysine

IV INFUSION

Patent ductus arteriosus.

10 mg/kg by IV infusion over 15 min for one dose and then 5 mg/kg 24 and 48 hr later, with all doses based on birth weight. Administration of the second or third dose to an infant with urinary output <0.6 mL/kg/hr should be delayed until renal function returns to normal.

NURSING IMPLICATIONS

IMPLEMENTATION/ADMINISTRATION/STORAGE

1. Do not use OTC ibuprofen as an antipyretic for more than 3 days or as an analgesic for more than 10 days, unless medically prescribed.
2. Children's Chewable Tablets are for children 4–11 years of age; Junior Strength Tablets are for children 6–11 years of age; Oral Suspension is for children 2–11 years of age; and Oral Drops are for children 6 months to 3 years of age.
3. Do not take more than 3.2 grams/day of prescription products.
4. If GI distress occurs with any product, take with meals or milk.
5. Oral Drops: Consult a provider before giving to children who are less than 6 months of age or weigh less than 24 pounds.
6. Oral Suspension: Consult a provider before giving to children who are less than 2 years of age or weigh less than 24 pounds.
7. Chewable Tablets (50 mg): Consult a provider before giving to children who are less than 4 years of age or weigh less than 36 pounds.
8. Chewable Tablets (100 mg): Consult a provider before giving to children who are less than 6 years of age or weigh less than 48 pounds.
9. Store Capsules, Gelcaps, and Tablets from 20–25°C (68–77°F). Avoid excessive heat greater than 40°C (104°F). Store Oral Suspension and Oral Drops from 15–30°C (59–86°F).
10. IV To reduce the risk of renal side effects, hydrate clients well before administration.
11. Dilute the solution for injection to an appropriate volume with dextrose, saline, or Ringer's lactate. Dilute to a final concentration of 4 mg/mL or less. Prepare for infusion, and administer within 30 min of preparation. Maintain line patency using dextrose or saline.
12. Infuse continuously over a period of no less than 30 min.
13. Administer through the IV port that is nearest the insertion site.
14. After the first withdrawal from the vial, discard any remaining solution because ibuprofen lysine contains no preservative.
15. Administer carefully to avoid extravasation as the product is irritating to tissues.
16. Store the injection from 20–25°C (68–77°F) protected from light. Store vials in the carton until used. Diluted solutions are stable for up to 24 hr at 20–25°C (68–77°F).
17. COMPATIBILITY Dextrose or saline.
18. INCOMPATIBILITY Do not administer in the same IV line with TPN. If necessary, interrupt TPN for 15 min prior to and after drug administration.

ASSESSMENT

1. Note reasons for therapy, onset, location, characteristics of S&S. With pain, rate level; evaluate for effectiveness.
2. Review history for any conditions that may preclude drug therapy, i.e., PUD, lupus, ASA intolerance, heavy alcohol intake, aspirin-sensitive asthma.
3. Determine history of ulcers, heart disease, or cardiac failure. May cause an increased risk of serious CV thrombotic events, MI, and stroke. Also, there is increased risk of serious GI adverse reactions, especially in the elderly, including inflammation, bleeding, ulceration, and perforation of stomach or intestines, which can be fatal.
4. Observe preterm infants for signs of bleeding. Monitor infants' skin and tissue as leaking from infusion can cause irritation.

5. Obtain/monitor VS, CBC, renal and LFTs, x-rays, eye exam prior to initiating long-term therapy.

CLIENT/FAMILY TEACHING

1. Take the dosage prescribed with a snack, milk, antacid, or meals to decrease GI upset.
2. May cause dizziness/drowsiness. Perform activities that require mental alertness with caution.
3. With history of CHF or compromised cardiac function, keep weight records, and report weight gain/swelling (drug causes sodium retention). Seek immediate care if ↑ SOB or trouble breathing, chest pain, weakness in one side of body or extremity, slurred speech, swelling of face or throat.
4. Report any persistent/recurrent GI upset or stomach pain, skin rash/itching, vomiting blood, bloody or black stools, rapid weight gain/swelling, changes in urine output, ↑ joint pain, unusual bruising/bleeding, unexplained tiredness/fatigue, ringing in ears, intestinal flu-like symptoms, yellowing of the skin or eyes, visual changes. Obtain periodic eye exams with chronic therapy.
5. Avoid alcohol, other NSAIDs, corticosteroids, and ASA; bleeding may occur.
6. Keep all F/U visits to assess response, labs, and for adverse SE.

OUTCOMES/EVALUATE

- ↓ Joint pain and ↑ mobility with RA and osteoarthritis
- ↓ Fever, ↓ Inflammation
- ↓ Pain, ↓ Dysmenorrhea
- Relief of migraine headache
- Closure of PDA in premature infants (IV)

Icatibant acetate

(eye-**KAT**-i-bant)

Classification(s): Bradykinin inhibitor.

Pregnancy Category: C

RX: Firazyr.

INDICATIONS/USES

Treatment of acute attacks of hereditary angioedema in adults 18 years and older.

ACTION/KINETICS

Action

Icatibant is a competitive antagonist selective for the bradykinin B2 receptor. Hereditary angioedema is caused by an absence or dysfunction of C1-esterase-inhibitor which is a key regulator of the cascade that leads to bradykinin production. Bradykinin is a vasodilator that is thought to be responsible for the characteristic symptoms of hereditary angioedema, including inflammation and pain. Icatibant inhibits bradykinin from binding to the B2 receptor and thus treats the clinical symptoms of an acute, episodic attack of hereditary angioedema.

Pharmacokinetics

Absolute bioavailability is about 97% after a 30 mg SC dose. Extensively metabolized by proteolytic enzymes to inactive metabolites that are primarily excreted in the urine; less than 10% of a dose is excreted unchanged. After a single 30 mg dose, elderly men and women showed about a 2-fold higher AUC compared with younger men and women. Women show about a 2-fold higher systemic exposure (both AUC and C_{max}) than men.

SPECIAL CONCERNS

- Use only if benefit exceeds the theoretical risk to the client during acute coronary ischemia, unstable angina pectoris, or in the weeks following a stroke.
- Use with caution during lactation.
- Safety and efficacy not established in children less than 18 years of age.

SIDE EFFECTS

Most Common

Injection site reactions.

GI: Nausea. **CNS:** Dizziness, headache. **Dermatologic:** Rash. **At injection site:** Hematoma, burning, erythema, hypoesthesia, irritation, numbness, edema, pain, pressure sensation, pruritus, swelling, urticaria, warmth. **Body as a whole:** Pyrexia.

DRUG INTERACTIONS

As a bradykinin B2 receptor antagonist, icatibant has the potential to attenuate the antihypertensive effect of angiotensin-converting enzyme (ACE) inhibitors. Use together with caution and monitor.

HOW SUPPLIED

Injection Solution: 10 mg/mL.

DOSAGE

SC

Hereditary angioedema.

Adults, usual: 30 mg. Additional doses may be given at intervals of at least 6 hr if response is inadequate or if symptoms recur. **Maximum dose:** 3 doses per 24 hr.

NURSING IMPLICATIONS

IMPLEMENTATION/ADMINISTRATION/STORAGE

1. Administer SC in the abdominal area.
2. Administer over 30 sec.
3. Clients may self-administer the drug upon recognition of symptoms and adequate training under the guidance of a health care provider.
4. Store from 2–25°C (36–77°F).

ASSESSMENT

1. Note indications for therapy (hereditary angioedema-HAE), onset and characteristics of S&S, frequency of occurrence, triggers, other agents trialed and outcome.
2. List medical history, and assess for conditions that may preclude therapy.
3. Assess skin integrity, and ensure not administered into red, hard, or infected skin areas.
4. Perform respiratory and cardiac assessments; monitor renal function and VS.

CLIENT/FAMILY TEACHING

1. Review Patient Information Guide for step-by-step instructions on injection. Administer SC in abdominal area after instruction. Drug does not cure disease; only treats the symptoms. May repeat dose if needed after 6 hr; do not exceed 3 doses in 24 hr.
2. Avoid activities that require mental alertness until drug effects realized; may cause dizziness and drowsiness.
3. May experience fever, increase in liver enzymes, dizziness, and rash. Seek immediate medical care if laryngeal symptoms occur.
4. Keep all F/U to assess response and for adverse SE.

OUTCOMES/EVALUATE

- ↓ Swelling, inflammation, and pain with hereditary angioedema
- Control of symptoms of angioedema

IV

Idarubicin hydrochloride

(eye-dah-**ROOB**-ih-sin)

Classification(s): Antineoplastic, antibiotic

Pregnancy Category: D

RX: Idamycin PFS.

✤ **Rx:** Idamycin.

SEE ALSO *ANTINEOPLASTIC AGENTS*.

INDICATIONS/USES

In combination with other drugs (often cytarabine) to treat acute myelocytic leukemia (AML) in adults, including French-American-British classifications M1–M7. Compared with daunorubicin, idarubicin is more effective in inducing complete remissions in clients with AML.

ACTION/KINETICS

Action

Inhibits nucleic acid synthesis and interacts with the enzyme topoisomerase II. Rapidly taken up into cells due to significant lipid solubility.

Pharmacokinetics

$t^{1/2}$ terminal: 22 hr when used alone and 20 hr when used with cytarabine. Metabolized in the liver to the active idarubicinol, which is excreted through both the bile and urine. **Plasma protein binding:** Idarubicin: 97%; Idarubicinol: 94%.

CONTRAINDICATIONS

Lactation. Pre-existing bone marrow suppression induced by previous drug therapy or radiotherapy (unless benefit outweighs risk). Administration by the IM or SC routes.

SPECIAL CONCERNS

(1) Give idarubicin slowly into a freely flowing IV infusion; never give IM or SC. Severe local tissue necrosis can occur if there is extravasation during administration. (2) The use of idarubicin can cause myocardial toxicity leading to CHF. Cardiac toxicity is more common in those who have received prior anthracyclines

or who have pre-existing heart disease. (3) As is usual with antileukemic agents, severe myelosuppression occurs at therapeutic doses. (4) It is recommended that idarubicin be administered only under the supervision of a physician experienced in leukemia chemotherapy and in facilities with lab and supportive resources adequate to monitor drug tolerance and protect and maintain a client compromised by drug toxicity. The physician and institution must be capable of responding rapidly and completely to severe hemorrhagic conditions or overwhelming infections. (5) Dosage should be reduced in clients with impaired hepatic or renal function. Idarubicin should not be administered if the bilirubin level exceeds 5 mg/dL. ■

- **Skin reactions may occur if the powder is not handled properly.**
- **Clients over age 60 experienced CHF, serious arrhythmias, chest pain, MI, and asymptomatic declines in LVEF more frequently than younger clients.**
- **Safety and efficacy not demonstrated in children.**

SIDE EFFECTS

Most Common

Infection, N&V, alopecia, abdominal cramps, diarrhea, hemorrhage, mucositis, changes in mental status, fever, headache.

GI: N&V, mucositis, diarrhea, abdominal pain/cramps, ***hemorrhage, severe enterocolitis with perforation*****. Hematologic:** ***Severe myelosuppression, hemorrhage*****. Dermatologic:** Alopecia, generalized rash, urticaria, bullous erythrodermatous rash of the palms/soles, hives at injection site. **CNS:** Headache, ***seizures***, altered mental status. **CV:** CHF (may be fatal), ***serious arrhythmias including AF, chest pain, MI, cardiomyopathies***, decreased LV ejection fraction. *NOTE:* Cardiac toxicity more common in clients who received anthracycline drugs previously or who have pre-existing cardiac disease. **Miscellaneous:** Altered hepatic/renal function tests, infection (95% of clients), ***sepsis***, fever, pulmonary allergy, neurologic changes in peripheral nerves.

LABORATORY TEST CONSIDERATIONS

Changes in hepatic/renal function tests (usually transient and occurred in those with sepsis and who were receiving potentially hepatotoxic and nephrotoxic antibiotics and antifungal drugs).

OVERDOSE MANAGEMENT

Symptoms: Severe GI toxicity, myelosuppression. *Treatment:* Supportive treatment including antibiotics and platelet transfusions. Treat mucositis.

HOW SUPPLIED

Injection: 5 mg, 10 mg, 20 mg/vial.

DOSAGE

IV

Induction therapy in adults with acute myelocytic leukemia (AML).

12 mg/m^2/day for 3 days by slow (10–15 min) IV injection in combination with cytarabine, 100 mg/m^2/day given by continuous infusion for 7 days or as a 25 mg/m^2 IV bolus followed by 200 mg/m^2/day for 5 days by continuous infusion. A second course may be given if there is evidence of leukemia after the first course. Delay the second course in those with severe mucositis until recovery occurs; a dosage reduction of 25% is recommended. Consider a dosage reduction in clients with impaired hepatic or renal function; do not give if the bilirubin level is greater than 5 mg/dL.

NURSING IMPLICATIONS

Do not confuse Idamycin (Idarubicin) with Adriamycin (Doxorubicin HCl, also an antibiotic antineoplastic).

IMPLEMENTATION/ADMINISTRATION/STORAGE

1. **IV Reconstitute the 5, 10, and 20 mg vials with 5, 10, and 20 mL, respectively, of 0.9% NaCl injection to give a final concentration of 1 mg/mL. Do not use diluents containing bacteriostatic agents. The reconstituted solution is hypotonic.**
2. **Vial contents under negative pressure. To minimize aerosol formation during reconstitution use care when needle is inserted. Avoid inhalation of any aerosol formed.**
3. **Give slowly into a freely flowing IV infusion of 0.9% NaCl injection or D5W over 10–15 min.**

Attach tubing to a butterfly needle or other suitable device and insert into a large vein.

4. If extravasation suspected/evident, terminate injection or infusion immediately and restart in another vein. Keep extremity elevated and apply intermittent ice packs over area (immediately for ½ hr, then 4 times per day at ½ hr intervals for 3 days).
5. Reconstituted solutions are stable for 7 days if refrigerated and 3 days at room temperature. Discard unused solution.
6. If drug comes in contact with skin, wash area thoroughly with soap and water. Use goggles, gloves, and protective gowns to prepare/administer.
7. Store the preservative free injection from 2–8°C (36–46°F); protect from light. Retain in carton until time of use.
8. COMPATIBILITY 0.9% NaCl or D5W.
9. INCOMPATIBILITY Do not mix IV solution with any other drugs. Precipitation occurs when mixed with heparin. Prolonged contact with any alkaline pH solution will cause drug degradation. Do not use diluents containing bacteriostatic agents. The reconstituted solution is hypotonic.

ASSESSMENT

1. Note disease onset, other agents trialed, outcome. Drug is given in combination with other drugs (often cytarabine) to treat AML in adults.
2. List any pre-existing cardiac disease; assess cardiac status closely. Monitor closely (ECG, CXR, echo and EF evaluation) for any evidence of cardiac toxicity: arrhythmias, CHF, and cardiomyopathy.
3. Give antiemetics 30–45 min before and during therapy to prevent protracted N&V.
4. Note previous radiation therapy or treatment with anthracyclines. Assess infusion site carefully to ensure no extravasation.
5. Reduce dosage by 25% for subsequent courses in those experiencing severe mucositis; delay additional therapy until recovery from mucositis.
6. Monitor ECG (cardiac function), VS, I&O, CBC, platelets, (platelets and WBC nadir 10–14 days; recovery 21 days), uric acid, renal and LFTs (before and during therapy). Reduce dose with impaired hepatic or renal function; hold if bilirubin levels >5 mg/dL.

CLIENT/FAMILY TEACHING

1. Drug administered IV as part of chemo regimen for acute myelocytic leukemia.
2. Nausea and diarrhea are frequent side effects of therapy; take antiemetic 1 hr before therapy.
3. Report any severe abdominal pains, SOB, or chest pain; may cause myocardial toxicity.
4. Consume high fluid intake; keep urine slightly alkaline to prevent the formation of uric acid stones. Those with gout may require therapy.
5. Report S&S of anemia, i.e., dyspnea, fatigue, or faintness. Severe myelosuppression may occur; report any abnormal bruising/bleeding or infection.
6. Hair loss may occur; should regrow once therapy completed.
7. May cause a red coloration of the urine; not worrisome.
8. Use reliable contraception before, during, and for several months after therapy.
9. Avoid all OTC products without provider approval; avoid vaccinia, crowds, and those with infections.
10. Keep all F/U to assess response, labs, tests for cardiac function, and adverse SE.

OUTCOMES/EVALUATE

- Presence of leukemia cells (second course of therapy may be indicated after hematologic recovery)
- Complete remission; improved hematologic parameters

IV

Ifosfamide

(eye-**FOS**-fah-myd)

Classification(s): Antineoplastic, alkylating

Pregnancy Category: D

RX: Ifex.

SEE ALSO ***ANTINEOPLASTIC AGENTS*** AND ***ALKYLATING AGENTS***.

INDICATIONS/USES

(1) As third-line therapy, in combination with other antineoplastic drugs, for germ cell testicular cancer. *Always give with mesna to prevent ifosfamide-induced hemorrhagic cystitis.* (2) Has been used safely and effectively in children to treat bone and soft-tissue carcinomas. *Investigational:* Cancer of

the breast, lung, pancreas, ovary, and stomach. Also for sarcomas, acute leukemias (except AML), malignant lymphomas. Treatment of soft-tissue, Ewing's and osteogenic sarcomas; non-Hodgkin's lymphomas; bladder and cervical carcinoma.

ACTION/KINETICS

Action

Synthetic analog of cyclophosphamide that must be converted in the liver to active metabolites. The alkylated metabolites of ifosfamide then interact with DNA.

Pharmacokinetics

t½, elimination: 7 hr after doses of 1.6–2.4 grams/m^2/day and 15 hr after doses of 3.8–5 grams/m^2/day. Excreted in the urine both as unchanged drug and metabolites.

CONTRAINDICATIONS

Severe bone marrow depression. Hypersensitivity to ifosfamide. Lactation.

SPECIAL CONCERNS

■ (1) Ifosfamide for injection should be administered under the supervision of a qualified physician experienced in the use of cancer chemotherapeutic agents. (2) Urotoxic side effects (especially hemorrhagic cystitis) as well as CNS toxicities such as confusion and coma have been associated with ifosfamide. When they occur, cessation of ifosfamide therapy may be required. (3) Severe myelosuppression has occurred. ■

- **Use with caution in clients with compromised bone marrow reserve and impaired renal function.**
- **May interfere with wound healing.**
- **Although used (investigationally) in children, safety and efficacy not established.**

SIDE EFFECTS

Most Common

Hematuria, alopecia, myelosuppression, hemorrhagic cystitis, dysuria, urinary frequency, metabolic acidosis, somnolence, confusion, depressive psychosis, hallucinations.

GU: ***Hemorrhagic cystitis***, hematuria, dysuria, urinary frequency, renal impairment, renal tubular acidosis, Fanconi syndrome, renal rickets, acute renal failure. **CNS:** Confusion, depressive psychosis, somnolence, hallucinations, polyneuropathy. Less frequently: Dizziness, disorientation, cranial nerve dysfunction, ***seizures, coma***. **GI:** N&V, salivation, diarrhea, stomatitis, anorexia, constipation, liver dysfunction. **CV:** Phlebitis, hyper-/hypotension, coagulopathy, ***cardiotoxicity***. **Dermatologic:** Alopecia (common), dermatitis. **Hematologic:** Myelosuppression (especially when given with other chemotherapeutic drugs), including leukopenia and thrombocytopenia. **Body as a whole:** Infection, allergic reaction, fever of unknown origin, fatigue, malaise. **Miscellaneous:** Metabolic acidosis, pulmonary symptoms, interference with normal wound healing.

LABORATORY TEST CONSIDERATIONS

↑ Liver enzymes, bilirubin, BUN, serum creatinine.

OVERDOSE MANAGEMENT

Symptoms: See *Side Effects*. *Treatment:* General supportive measures.

HOW SUPPLIED

Powder for Injection: 1 gram/single-dose vial, 3 grams/single-dose vial.

DOSAGE

IV INFUSION

Testicular cancer.

Adults: 1.2 grams/m^2/day by IV infusion for 5 consecutive days. Treatment is repeated q 3 weeks or after recovery of hematologic toxicity (platelet counts are at least 100,000/mm^3 and WBCs are at least 4,000/mm^3). Other regimens (investigational) use ifosfamide 2 grams/m^2/day by IV infusion on days 1 through 3. Thus, the total dose is 6 grams/m^2/day by continuous IV infusion over 24 hr in combination with other antineoplastic agents.

Bone and soft-tissue sarcomas in children (investigational).

Children, usual: 1.2–1.8 grams/m^2/day by IV infusion for 5 days; repeat this course q 3–4 weeks. Delay further courses until platelets are at least 100,000 cells/mm^3 and WBC count is at least 4,000 cells/mm^3. Consider dose reduction if severe myelosuppression occurs. Other regimens use ifosfamide 3 grams/m^2/day by IV infusion on days 1 and 2, or doses as high as 5 grams/m^2/day by continuous IV infusion over 24 hr in combination with other antineoplastic agents.

NURSING IMPLICATIONS

IMPLEMENTATION/ADMINISTRATION/STORAGE

1. IV To prevent bladder toxicity, give with at least 2 L/day of PO or IV fluid as well as with mesna.
2. Consider decreasing ifosfamide to 25% of the usual dose if serum AST is greater than 300 units/L or if bilirubin is greater than 3 mg/mL.
3. Dose reduction is necessary in renal impairment as follows: If GFR is >60 mL/min, give 100% of the usual dose; if GFR is 30–60 mL/min, give 75% of the usual dose; if GFR is 10–30 mL/min, give 50% of the usual dose; if GFR is <10 mL/min, do not give ifosfamide.
4. Conventional hemodialysis is 75–100% effective in removing ifosfamide.
5. Ifosfamide is a cytotoxic agent. Follow safe handling procedures when preparing, administering, or dispensing. To reconstitute, add either sterile or bacteriostatic water for injection for a final concentration of 50 mg/mL. Solutions may be further diluted to achieve concentrations from 0.6–20 mg/mL by adding D5W, 0.9% NaCl, RL, or sterile water for injection. Infuse slowly by IV infusion over 30 min.
6. Reconstituted solutions (50 mg/mL) are stable for 1 week at 30°C (86°F) or 3 weeks at 5°C (41°F).
7. Refrigerate dilutions of ifosfamide not prepared with bacteriostatic water for injection; use within 6 hr.
8. COMPATIBILITY D5W, 0.9% NaCl, RL, or sterile water for injection. Compatible at a concentration of 100 mg/mL with bacteriostatic water for injection with benzyl alcohol.
9. INCOMPATIBILITY Administer separately.

ASSESSMENT

1. Note reasons for therapy, other agents/therapies trialed. Anticipate concomitant administration with mesna to minimize hemorrhagic cystitis.
2. Document neurologic status; assess for hallucinations, agitation, confusion, or unusual fatigue; stop infusion if evident.
3. Monitor renal and LFTs, urinalysis, and CBC; immunosuppression may activate latent infections such as herpes. Send urine for analysis prior to each dose of ifosfamide. If hematuria occurs (>10 RBCs per HPF), hold therapy until it clears and adjust dose of mesna as needed.

CLIENT/FAMILY TEACHING

1. Antiemetic may be given before therapy to decrease nausea. Give mesna with or before drug therapy to prevent hemorrhagic cystitis.
2. Consume adequate fluids to prevent dehydration and reduce bladder irritation.
3. Report presence of frothy dark urine, jaundice, or light-colored stools; S&S of hepatotoxicity requiring dosage adjustments. Consume 2–3 L/day of fluids and void frequently to lessen irritation.
4. Hair loss and N&V are frequent side effects of drug therapy.
5. Hyperpigmentation of skin and mucous membranes may occur; report any injury or interference with normal wound healing.
6. Report confusion, hallucinations, or marked drowsiness as dosage may require reduction.
7. Males and females should practice contraceptive measures during and for at least 4 months following treatments. Infertility may result if treatment lasts 6 months.
8. Joint or flank pain may be caused by the increase in uric acid that results from the rapid cytolysis of tumor and RBCs.
9. Report symptoms of neurotoxicity (numbness, tingling). Assess for evidence of infection. Monitor and record temperature daily. Elicit family support in making observations/evaluations and recording.
10. Do not take salicylates or alcohol.
11. Avoid crowds, vaccinations, and persons with known infections.
12. Keep all F/U to assess response, labs, adverse SE.

OUTCOMES/EVALUATE

- ↓ Tumor size and spread
- Desired hematologic parameters

Imatinib mesylate

(eh-**MAT**-eh-nib)

Classification(s): Antineoplastic, miscellaneous

Pregnancy Category: D

RX: Gleevec.

INDICATIONS/USES

(1) Treatment of adults with relapsed or refractory Philadelphia chromosome-positive (Ph+) acute lymphoblastic leukemia. (2) Treatment of adults with aggressive systemic mastocytosis without the D816V c-Kit mutation or with c-Kit mutation status unknown. (3) Treatment of newly diagnosed adults and children with Ph+ chronic myeloid leukemia (CML) in chronic phase; for the treatment of Ph+ CML in blast crisis, accelerated phase, or in chronic phase after failure of interferon alpha therapy; for the treatment of children with Ph+ chronic phase CML whose disease has recurred after stem-cell transplant or who are resistant to interferon alpha therapy. (4) Treatment of adults with unresectable, recurrent, and/or metastatic dermatofibrosarcoma protuberans. (5) Treatment of Kit (CD117) positive unresectable and/or metastatic malignant GI stromal tumors. Also, post-resection of positive GI stromal tumors. (6) Treatment of adults with hypereosinophilic syndrome and/or chronic eosinophilic leukemia who have the FIP1L1-platelet, derived growth factor receptor (PDGFR)α fusion kinase and for those with hypereosinophilic syndrome and/or chronic eosinophilic leukemia who are FIP1L1-PDGFRα fusion kinase negative or unknown. (7) Treatment of adults with myelodysplastic/myeloproliferative diseases associated with platelet-derived growth factor receptor gene rearrangements.

ACTION/KINETICS

Action

Imatinib is a protein-tyrosine kinase inhibitor that inhibits the Bcr-Abl tyrosine kinase which is the abnormal form of tyrosine kinase created by the Philadelphia chromosome abnormality in chronic myeloid leukemia (CML). Imatinib inhibits proliferation and causes apoptosis in Bcr-Abl positive cell lines, as well as fresh leukemic cells from Philadelphia chromosome positive CML. The drug may also inhibit receptor tyrosine kinases for platelet-derived growth factor and stem cell factor, c-Kit; inhibits platelet-derived growth factor and stem cell factor cellular events.

Pharmacokinetics

Well absorbed after PO administration; mean absolute bioavailability is 98%. **Maximum levels:** 2–4 hr. **t½, terminal, imatinib and N-desmethyl derivative (active metabolite):** About 18 and 40 hr, respectively. Metabolized in the liver by the CYP3A4 enzyme with 68% excreted in the feces and 13% in the urine. **Plasma protein binding:** 95%.

CONTRAINDICATIONS

Hypersensitivity to any component of the product. Pregnancy, lactation.

SPECIAL CONCERNS

- **Chance of edema is increased in clients 65 years and older.**
- **Safety and efficacy determined only in children with Ph+ chronic phase CML with recurrence after stem cell transplantation or resistance to interferon-alfa therapy.**
- **There are no data in children younger than 2 years.**

SIDE EFFECTS

Most Common

When used for acute lymphoblastic leukemia: Diarrhea, mild nausea, muscle cramps, myalgia, rash, vomiting, superficial edemas (periorbital or lower limb).
When used for aggressive systemic mastocytosis: Anemia, ascites, diarrhea, dyspnea, fatigue, lower RTI, muscle cramps, nausea, peripheral edema, pruritus, rash.
When used for chronic myeloid leukemia: Diarrhea, edema (periorbital, lower limb), fatigue, muscle cramps, musculoskeletal pain, N&V, abdominal pain, rash.
When used for GI stromal tumors: Abdominal pain, anemia, anorexia, diarrhea, edema, fatigue, myalgia, N&V, rash, superficial edema.

Side effects listed are either those with a frequency of 0.1% or more or those that are potentially serious. **GI:** N&V, diarrhea, abdominal pain/cramping/distention, dyspepsia, constipation, anorexia, heartburn, flatulence, dysgeusia, dry mouth, gastritis, gastroesophageal reflux, ascites, cheilitis, dysphagia, eructation, esophagitis, gastric ulcer, gastroenteritis, hematemesis, melena, mouth ulceration, stomatitis, ***pancreatitis***. ***GI hemorrhage***. **Hepatic:** Liver toxicity, hepatitis, jaundice. **CNS:** Fatigue, headache, dizziness, depression, insomnia, anxiety, lightheadedness, peripheral neuropathy, hypesthesia, paresthesia, decreased libido, impaired memory, migraine, restless legs syndrome, sciatica, somnolence, stupor, tremor, vertigo, ***CNS hemorrhage***. **CV:** Hemorrhage, flushing, CHF, hematoma, hypertension, hypotension, palpitations, peripheral coldness. **Musculoskeletal:** Muscle cramps, musculoskeletal pain, joint pain/swelling, arthralgia, myalgia, bone pain, rigors, chest/back pain, muscle spasms, extremity pain, joint/muscle stiffness. **Respiratory:** Nasopharyngitis, upper RTI, cough, pharyngolaryngeal pain, sinusitis, dyspnea (including exertional), pharyngitis, stomatitis, pneumonia, rhinitis, pulmonary edema, epistaxis, pleural effusion. **Dermatologic:** Skin rash (including exfoliative), night sweats, pruritus, alopecia, desquamation, sweating, dry skin, Raynaud phenomenon, tachycardia, erythema, photosensitivity reaction, bullous eruption, contusion, ecchymosis, exfoliative dermatitis, folliculitis, hypotrichosis, increased bruising tendency, nail disorder, onycholysis, petechiae, psoriasis, purpura, pustular rash, skin hyper-/hypopigmentation, urticaria, ***Stevens-Johnson syndrome***, erythema multiforme. **GU:** Breast enlargement, erectile dysfunction, gynecomastia, hematuria, menorrhagia, irregular menstruation, nipple pain, acute renal failure, renal pain, scrotal edema, sexual dysfunction, increased urinary frequency, UTI. **Hematologic:** Neutropenia, thrombocytopenia, anemia, leukopenia, lymphopenia, granulocytopenia, febrile neutropenia, pancytopenia, bone marrow depression, eosinophilia, lymphadenopathy, thrombocythemia. **Ophthalmic:** Eye edema, periorbital edema, increased lacrimation, blurred vision, conjunctival hemorrhage, conjunctivitis, dry eye, blepharitis, eye irritation, eye pain, macular edema, retinal hemorrhage, scleral hemorrhage. **Otic:** Tinnitus, hearing loss. **Body as a whole:** Fluid retention, superficial/facial edema, anasarca, fever (including in absence of neutropenia), influenza, asthenia, lethargy, malaise, chills, weakness, infection (without neutropenia), pain (including tumor-related), increased/decreased weight, dehydration, gout, ***sepsis***. **Miscellaneous:** Cellulitis, hypothyroidism, increased/decreased appetite, herpes simplex/zoster.

LABORATORY TEST CONSIDERATIONS

↑ AST, ALT, bilirubin, creatinine, alkaline phosphatase, blood creatine phosphokinase, blood lactate dehydrogenase, albumin. ↓ Hemoglobin, neutrophil count, platelets, WBCs. Hypokalemia, hypophosphatemia, hyperglycemia, hyper-/hypocalcemia, hyperuricemia, hyponatremia.

OVERDOSE MANAGEMENT

Treatment: Observe the client; give appropriate supportive treatment.

DRUG INTERACTIONS

Acetaminophen / ↑ Risk of hepatotoxicity
Alfentanil / ↑ Plasma levels of alfentanil R/T ↓ metabolism by CYP3A4
Atazanavir / ↑ Imatinib levels R/T ↓ metabolism by CYP3A4
Benzodiazepines (certain ones) / ↑ Benzodiazepine plasma levels R/T ↓ metabolism by CYP3A4
Calcium channel blockers (dihydropyridine-type) / ↑ Plasma CCB levels R/T ↓ metabolism by CYP3A4
Carbamazepine / ↓ Imatinib levels R/T ↑ metabolism by CYP3A4; avoid coadministration if possible
Clarithromycin / ↑ Imatinib levels R/T ↓ metabolism by CYP3A4
Cyclosporine / ↑ Plasma levels of cyclosporine R/T ↓ metabolism by CYP3A4
Dexamethasone / ↓ Imatinib levels R/T ↑ metabolism by CYP3A4; avoid coadministration if possible
Dihydropyridine / ↑ Plasma levels of dihydropyridine levels R/T ↓ metabolism by CYP3A4
Ergot alkaloids / ↑ Plasma levels of ergot alkaloids R/T ↓ metabolism by CYP3A4
Erythromycin / ↑ Imatinib levels R/T ↓ metabolism by CYP3A4
Ethinyl estradiol / ↑ Ethinyl estradiol levels R/T ↓ metabolism by CYP3A4
Fentanyl / ↑ Plasma levels of fentanyl R/T ↓ metabolism by CYP3A4
Indinavir / ↑ Imatinib levels R/T ↓ metabolism by CYP3A4
Itraconazole / ↑ Imatinib levels R/T ↓ metabolism by CYP3A4
Ketoconazole / ↑ Imatinib levels R/T ↓ metabolism by CYP3A4

Levothyroxine / Symptoms of hypothyroidism and ↑ TSH levels after undergoing thyroidectomy; ↑ levothyroxine dose
Nefazodone / ↑ Imatinib levels R/T ↓ metabolism by CYP3A4
Nelfinavir / ↑ Imatinib levels R/T ↓ metabolism by CYP3A4
Oral contraceptives (e.g., ethinyl estradiol) / ↑ Plasma OC levels R/T ↓ metabolism by CYP3A4
Phenobarbital / ↓ Imatinib levels R/T ↑ metabolism by CYP3A4; avoid coadministration if possible
Phenytoin / ↓ Imatinib levels R/T ↑ metabolism by CYP3A4; avoid coadministration if possible
Pimozide / ↑ Plasma levels of pimozide R/T ↓ metabolism by CYP3A4
Quinidine / ↑ Plasma levels of quinidine R/T ↓ metabolism by CYP3A4
Rifampicin / ↓ Imatinib levels R/T ↑ metabolism
Rifampin / ↓ Imatinib levels R/T ↑ metabolism by CYP3A4; avoid coadministration if possible
Ritonavir / ↑ Imatinib levels R/T ↓ metabolism by CYP3A4
Saquinavir / ↑ Imatinib levels R/T ↓ metabolism by CYP3A4
Simvastatin / ↑ Plasma levels of simvastatin R/T ↓ metabolism by CYP3A4
Sirolimus / ↑ Plasma levels of sirolimus R/T ↓ metabolism by CYP3A4
H ***St. John's wort*** / ↓ Imatinib levels R/T ↑ metabolism by CYP3A4; avoid coadministration if possible
Tacrolimus / ↑ Plasma levels of tacrolimus R/T ↓ metabolism by CYP3A4
Telithromycin / ↑ Imatinib levels R/T ↓ metabolism by CYP3A4
Thyroid hormones (e.g., levothyroxine) / ↑ Levothyroxine clearance → symptoms of hypothyroidism; monitor thyroid function
Triazolobenzodiazepines / ↑ Triazolobenzodiazepine levels
Voriconazole / ↑ Imatinib levels R/T ↓ metabolism by CYP3A4
Warfarin / Possible ↑ warfarin effect R/T ↓ metabolism by CYP2C9 and CYP3A4; use low molecular weight heparins or standard heparin

HOW SUPPLIED

Tablets: 100 mg, 400 mg.

DOSAGE

TABLETS

Acute lymphoblastic leukemia.

Adults: 600 mg/day in those with relapsed/refractory Ph+ acute lymphoblastic leukemia.

Aggressive systemic mastocytosis.

Adults: 400 mg/day in those without the D816V c-kit mutation. For those with aggressive systemic mastocytosis associated with eosinophilia, begin with 100 mg/day. May increase the dose from 100 to 400 mg/day in the absence of adverse side effects if assessment shows an insufficient response to therapy.

Chronic myeloid leukemia (CML) in adults.

Accelerated phase or blast crisis: 600 mg/day. A dose increase from 600 to 800 mg (given as 400 mg twice a day) may be considered in the absence of severe side effects and severe non-leukemia-related neutropenia or thrombocytopenia in the following situations: Disease progression, failure to achieve a satisfactory hematologic response after 3 or more months of treatment, or loss of a previously achieved hematologic response. **Chronic phase:** 400 mg/day. Increases in dose from 400 mg to 600 mg may be considered using the same guidelines as listed earlier for accelerated phase or blast crisis.

CML in chronic phase in children.

Children, newly diagnosed Ph+ CML: 340 mg/m^2/day (not to exceed 600 mg). **Children with Ph+ chronic phase CML recurrent after stem-cell transplant or resistant to interferon alpha:** 260 mg/m^2/day given either once daily or split into two daily doses.

Dermatofibrosarcoma protuberans.

Adults: 800 mg/day.

Gastrointestinal stromal tumors, adjuvant treatment.

Adults, initial: 400 mg/day. The optimal treatment duration is not known.

Malignant GI stromal tumors, unresectable and/or metastatic.

Adults, initial: 400 mg/day. Dose may be increased up to 800 mg/day (given as 400 mg twice a day) in those showing clear signs or symptoms of disease progression at a lower dose and in the absence of severe side effects.

Adjunctive treatment of post-resection of positive GI stromal tumors.

400 mg/day.

Hypereosinophilic syndrome and/or chronic eosinophilic leukemia.

Adults: 400 mg/day. In those with demonstrated FIP1L1-PDGFRα fusion kinase, give a starting dose of 100 mg/day. Dose may be increased from 100 mg/day to 400 mg/day in the absence of side effects if assessments show an insufficient response to therapy.

Myelodysplastic/myeloproliferative diseases.

Adults: 400 mg/day.

NURSING IMPLICATIONS

IMPLEMENTATION/ADMINISTRATION/STORAGE

1. Therapy should be initiated by a health care provider experienced in the treatment of those with hematological malignancies or malignant sarcomas.
2. Give PO with a meal and a large glass of water. Administer doses of 400 mg or 600 mg once daily; give a dose of 800 mg as 400 mg twice a day. For children, give once a day or the daily dose may be split into two (once in the morning and once in the evening).
3. Do not crush tablets. Avoid direct contact of crushed tablets with the skin or mucous membranes.
4. Start with a dose of 400 mg/day in those with mild to moderate impaired hepatic function. Start with a dose of 300 mg/day (i.e., a 25% reduction) in those with severe hepatic impairment.
5. For moderate renal impairment (C_{CR}, 20–39 mL/min), a 50% decrease in the recommended starting dose is suggested (dose not to exceed 400 mg); increase as tolerated. Doses more than 600 mg are not recommended in those with a C_{CR}, 40–59 mL/min. Use with caution in those with severe renal impairment.
6. The use of concomitant strong CYP3A4 inducers (e.g., carbamazepine, dexamethasone, phenobarbital, phenyton, rifampin, St. John's wort) should be avoided. If concomitant use is needed, however, increase the dose of imatinib by at least 50%; carefully monitor clinical response.
7. For daily dosing of 800 mg or more, use the 400 mg tablet to reduce exposure to iron.
8. Continue treatment as long as there is no evidence of disease progression or unacceptable side effects/toxicity.
9. If severe hepatotoxicity or fluid retention occurs, withhold imatinib until event resolved. Treatment can be resumed depending on the initial severity of the event.
10. Use the following guidelines to adjust dose for neutropenia and thrombocytopenia:
    - **For chronic phase CML (starting dose 400 mg), myelodysplastic/myeloproliferative diseases (starting dose 400 mg), or aggressive systemic mastocytosis, hypereosinophilic syndrome/chronic eosinophilic leukemia (starting dose 400 mg), or GI stromal tumors (starting dose 400 mg):** If ANC is $<1 \times 10^9$/L and/or platelets are $<50 \times 10^9$/L, stop imatinib until ANC is 1.5 or more $\times 10^9$/L and platelets are 75 or more $\times 10^9$/L. Resume treatment at the original starting dose of 400 mg. If recurrence of ANC and/or platelets occur at levels indicated above, repeat the previous step and resume imatinib at a reduced dose of 300 mg.
    - **For accelerated phase of CML and blast crisis (starting dose 600 mg) and relapsed or refractory Philadelphia chromosome-positive acute ALL (starting dose 600 mg):** If ANC is $<0.5 \times 10^9$/L and/or platelets are $<10 \times 10^9$/L, check if cytopenia is related to leukemia (marrow aspirate or biopsy). If cytopenia is unrelated to leukemia, reduce dose of imatinib to 400 mg. If cytopenia persists 2 weeks, reduce further to 300 mg. If cytopenia persists 4 weeks and is still unrelated to leukemia, stop imatinib until ANC is 1 or more $\times 10^9$/L and platelets are 20 or more $\times 10^9$/L and then resume treatment at 300 mg.
    - **Aggressive systemic mastocytosis associated with eosinophilia (starting dose 100 mg):** If ANC is $<1 \times 10^9$/L and/or platelets $<50 \times 10^9$/L, stop imatinib until

ANC is 1.5×10^9/L or more and platelets are 75×10^9/L or more. Resume treatment with imatinib at previous dose (i.e., before severe side effects).

- **Hypereosinophilic syndrome/chronic eosinophilic leukemia with FIP1L1-PDGFRα fusion kinase (starting dose 100 mg):** If ANC is $<1 \times 10^9$/L and/or platelets $<50 \times 10^9$/L, stop imatinib until ANC is 1.5×10^9/L or more and platelets are 75×10^9/L or more. Resume treatment with imatinib at previous dose (i.e., before severe side effects).
- **Dermatofibrosarcoma protuberans (starting dose 800 mg):** If ANC is $<1 \times 10^9$/L and/or platelets $<50 \times 10^9$/L, stop imatinib until ANC is 1.5×10^9/L or more and platelets are 75×10^9/L or more. Resume treatment with imatinib at 600 mg. In the event of recurrence of ANC $<1 \times 10^9$/L and/or platelets $<50 \times 10^9$/L, repeat the previous step and resume imatinib at reduced dose of 400 mg.
- **Newly diagnosed pediatric chronic CML (start at dose 340 mg/m²):** If ANC is $<1 \times 10^9$/L and/or platelets $<50 \times 10^9$/L, stop imatinib until ANC is 1.5×10^9/L or more and platelets are 75×10^9/L or more. Resume treatment with imatinib at previous dose (i.e., before serious side effects). In the event of recurrence of ANC $<1 \times 10^9$/L and/or platelets $<50 \times 10^9$/L, repeat the previous step and resume imatinib at reduced dose of 250 mg/m².
- **Children with chronic phase CML recurring after transplant or resistant to interferon (start at dose 260 mg/m²):** If ANC is $<1 \times 10^9$/L and/or platelets $<50 \times 10^9$/L, stop imatinib until ANC is 1.5×10^9/L or more and platelets are 75×10^9/L or more. Resume treatment with imatinib at previous dose (i.e., before severe side effects). In the event of recurrence of ANC $<1 \times 10^9$/L and/or platelets $<50 \times 10^9$/L, repeat the previous step and resume imatinib at reduced dose of 200 mg/m².

11. Use the following guidelines to adjust dose for hepatotoxicity:

- **Adults:** If bilirubin is $>3 \times$ institutional ULN, withhold imatinib until bilirubin levels have returned to $<1.5 \times$ IULN. If liver transaminases are $>5 \times$ IULN, withhold imatinib until transaminase levels have returned to $<2.5 \times$ IULN. Treatment with imatinib may then be continued at a reduced daily dose of 300 mg if the previous dose was 400 mg, 400 mg if the previous dose was 600 mg, or 600 mg if the previous dose was 800 mg.
- **Children:** If bilirubin is $>3 \times$ institutional ULN, withhold imatinib until bilirubin levels have returned to $<1.5 \times$ IULN. If liver transaminases are $>5 \times$ IULN, withhold imatinib until transaminase levels have returned to $<2.5 \times$ IULN. Daily dosages can be reduced under the same circumstances from 260 to 200 mg/m²/day or from 340 to 260 mg/m²/day.

12. Store tablets from 15–30°C (59–86°F); protect from moisture.

ASSESSMENT

1. Note reasons for therapy, disease onset, phase of disease, other therapies trialed/failed, last interferon-alpha therapy.
2. List drugs prescribed to ensure none interact unfavorably.
3. Closely monitor those with hepatic impairment; exposure to imatinib may increase liver dysfunction.
4. Follow administration guidelines carefully; dose is adjusted for various phases of disease, types of disease, as well as altered renal/liver function, neutropenia/thrombocytopenia.
5. Treatment may be continued as long as there is no evidence of progressive disease or unacceptable toxicity.
6. Closely monitor growth of children under treatment. Obtain echocardiogram and serum troponin levels with hypereosinophilic syndrome and/or chronic eosinophilic leukemia and in those with myelodysplastic/myeloproliferative diseases or aggressive systemic mastocytosis associated with high eosinophil levels.
7. Note VS, weight, TSH, CBC, renal and LFTs. Assess for unexpected rapid weight gain (fluid retention/edema) and treat. Perform CBC and platelet counts weekly for first month, biweekly for second month, and periodically thereafter as indicated. Monitor liver function (alkaline phosphatase, bilirubin, transaminases)

prior to therapy, then monthly or as indicated during treatment.

CLIENT/FAMILY TEACHING

1. Take with food and a large glass of water to minimize GI irritation. Avoid grapefruit and grapefruit juice while taking imatinib.
2. Drug is given once daily initially; may be increased to twice daily or temporarily stopped based on lab test results, development of adverse reactions, and response to therapy.
3. If not able to swallow tablets they may be dispersed in a glass of water or apple juice. Place required number of tablets in a glass with appropriate volume of beverage (e.g., 2 oz for 100 mg tablet, 6 oz for 400 mg tablet) and stir with spoon until tablets have disintegrated. Suspension must be swallowed immediately after complete disintegration of the tablets.
4. Do not crush tablets; avoid direct contact of crushed tablets with the skin or mucous membranes. If contact occurs, wash thoroughly.
5. Use caution with activities that require mental alertness; may cause dizziness.
6. Monitor weight; report any significant increases/decreases.
7. Avoid OTC agents especially with acetaminophen unless provider approved.
8. Women of childbearing age should practice reliable contraception and avoid pregnancy during therapy.
9. May experience N&V, diarrhea, swelling of extremities/around the eyes, skin rash, muscle cramps. May also experience increased SOB, changes in urinary output, ↑ bruising/bleeding, and ↓ exercise intolerance; report if evident.
10. Growth retardation has occurred in children and preadolescents during therapy; growth should be monitored closely during treatment.
11. Keep all F/U visits so drug may be adjusted as needed and labs monitored.

OUTCOMES/EVALUATE

- Hematologic stabilization of CML
- Control of malignant cell proliferation with metastatic GI stromal tumors or metastatic dermatofibrosarcoma protuberans (DFSP) as well as other malignancies

Combination Drug

IV

Imipenem-Cilastatin sodium

(em-ee-**PEN**-em, sigh-lah-**STAT**-in)

Classification(s): Antibiotic, carbapenem

Pregnancy Category: C

RX: Primaxin IM, Primaxin IV.

SEE ALSO ***ANTI-INFECTIVE DRUGS***.

INDICATIONS/USES

IM:

1. Lower respiratory tract infections, including pneumonia and bronchitis as an exacerbation of COPD due to *S. pneumoniae* and *H. influenzae*.
2. Intra-abdominal infections including acute gangrenous or perforated appendicitis and appendicitis with peritonitis that are caused by group *Streptococccus,* including *E. faecalis,* streptococcus (viridans group), *E. coli, Klebsiella pneumoniae, P. aeruginosa, Bacteroides* sp., including *B. fragilis, B. distasonis, B. intermedius, B. thetaiotaomicron, Fusobacterium* sp., and *Peptostreptococcus* sp.
3. Skin and skin structure infections, including abscesses, cellulitis, infected skin ulcers, and wound infections due to *S. aureus* (including penicillinase-producing strains), *Streptococcus pyogenes,* group D streptococcus including *E. faecalis, Acinetobacter* sp., including *A. calcoaceticus, Citrobacter* sp., *E. coli, Enterobacter cloacae, K. pneumoniae, P. aeruginosa, Bacteroides* sp., including *B. fragilis.*
4. Gynecologic infections, including postpartum endomyometritis due to group D streptococcus such as *E. faecalis, E. coli., K. pneumoniae, B. intermedius,* and *Peptostreptococcus* sp.

NOTE: IM use is not intended for severe or life-threatening infections, including bacterial sepsis or endocarditis, or in major physiological impairments (e.g., shock).

IV:

1. Lower respiratory tract infections due to *Staphylococcus aureus* (penicillinase-producing), *Escherichia coli, Klebsiella* sp., *Enterobacter* sp., *Haemophilus influenzae, Haemo-*

I

philus parainfluenzae, Acinetobacter sp., and *Serratia marcescens.*

2. Urinary tract infections (complicated and uncomplicated) due to *Enterococcus faecalis, S. aureus* (penicillinase-producing), *E. coli, Klebsiella* sp., *Enterobacter* sp., *Proteus vulgaris, Providencia rettgeri, M. morganii,* and *P. aeruginosa.*
3. Intra-abdominal infections due to *E. faecalis, S. aureus* (penicillinase-producing), *Staphylococcus epidermidis, E. coli, Klebsiella* sp., *Enterobacter* sp., *Proteus* sp., *Morganella morganii, P. aeruginosa, Citrobacter* sp., *Clostridium* sp., *Bacteroides* sp., including *B. fragilis, Fusobacterium* sp., *Peptococcus* sp., *Peptostreptococcus* sp., *Eubacterium* sp., *Propionibacterium* sp., and *Bifidobacterium* sp.
4. Gynecologic infections due to *E. faecalis, S. aureus* (penicillinase-producing), *S. epidermidis, Streptococcus agalactiae* (group B streptococcus), *E. coli, Klebsiella* sp., *Proteus* sp., *Enterobacter* sp., *Bifidobacterium* sp., *Bacteroides* sp., including *B. fragilis, Gardnerella vaginalis, Peptococcus* sp., *Peptostreptococcus* sp., *Propionibacterium* sp.
5. Bacterial septicemia due to *E. faecalis, S. aureus* (penicillinase-producing), *E. coli, Klebsiella* sp., *P. aeruginosa, Serratia* sp., *Enterobacter* sp., *Bacteroides* sp.
6. Bone and joint infections due to *E. faecalis, S. aureus* (penicillinase-producing), *S. epidermidis, Enterobacter* sp., *P. aeruginosa.*
7. Skin and skin structure infections due to *E. faecalis, S. aureus* (penicillinase-producing), *S. epidermidis, E. coli, Klebsiella* sp., *Enterobacter* sp., *P. vulgaris, P. rettgeri, M. morganii, P. aeruginosa, Serratia* sp., *Citrobacter* sp., *Acinetobacter* sp., *Bacteroides* sp., *Fusobacterium* sp., *Peptococcus* sp., and *Peptostreptococcus* sp.
8. Endocarditis due to *S. aureus* (penicillinase-producing).
9. Polymicrobic infections, including those in which *S. pneumoniae* (pneumonia, septicemia), *S. pyogenes* (skin and skin structure), or non-penicillinase-producing *S. aureus* is one of the causative organisms.

CONTENT

The powder for IM injection contains: Imipenem, 500 mg, and cilastatin, 500 mg. The powder for IV injection contains: Imipenem, 250 mg, and cilastatin, 250 mg; or, imipenem, 500 mg, and cilastatin, 500 mg.

ACTION/KINETICS

Action

Inhibits cell wall synthesis. Is bactericidal against a wide range of gram-positive and gram-negative organisms. Stable in the presence of beta-lactamases. Addition of cilastatin prevents the metabolism of imipenem in the kidneys by dehydropeptidase I, thus ensuring high levels of the imipenem in the urinary tract.

Pharmacokinetics

t½, after IV: 1 hr for each component. **Peak plasma levels, after IM:** 10–12 mcg/mL within 2 hr. **Peak plasma levels of imipenem, after 20 min IV infusion:** 14–24 mcg/mL for the 250 mg dose, 21–58 mcg/mL for the 500 mg dose, and 41–83 mcg/mL for the 1 gram dose. Compared with IV administration, imipenem is approximately 75% bioavailable after IM use with cilastatin being 95% bioavailable. **t½, imipenem:** 2–3 hr. About 70% of imipenem and cilastatin is recovered in the urine within 10 hr of administration.

CONTRAINDICATIONS

IM use in clients allergic to local anesthetics of the amide type and use in clients with heart block (due to the use of lidocaine HCl diluent) or severe shock. Use in clients with a C_{CR} of less than or equal to 5 mL/min/1.73 m^2, unless hemodialysis is begun within 48 hr. IV use in children with CNS infections due to the risk of seizures and in children less than 30 kg with impaired renal function.

SPECIAL CONCERNS

- **Due to cross-sensitivity, use with caution in clients with penicillin allergy.**
- **Use with caution in pregnancy and lactation.**
- **Safety and efficacy not determined for IM use in children less than 12 years of age.**

SIDE EFFECTS

Most Common

After IM use: Pain at injection site, nausea, diarrhea, rash, vomiting.

After IV use: Hypotension, phlebitis/thrombophlebitis, pain, erythema at injection site, N&V, diarrhea, fever, seizures, dizziness, rash, pruritus.

GI: Pseudomembranous colitis, nausea, diarrhea, vomiting, abdominal pain, heartburn, increased salivation, ***hemorrhagic colitis***, gastroenteritis, glossitis, pharyngeal pain, tongue papillar hypertrophy, hepatitis, jaundice, staining of the teeth or tongue. **CNS:** Fever, confusion, ***seizures***, dizziness, sleepiness, myoclonus, headache, vertigo, paresthesia, encephalopathy, tremor, psychic disturbances (including hallucinations). **CV:** Hypotension, tachycardia, palpitations. **Dermatologic:** Rash, urticaria, pruritus, flushing, cyanosis, facial edema, erythema multiforme, skin texture changes, hyperhidrosis, angioneurotic edema, ***toxic epidermal necrolysis, Stevens-Johnson syndrome.*** **CV:** Hypotension, palpitations, tachycardia. **Respiratory:** Chest discomfort, dyspnea, hyperventilation. **GU:** Pruritus vulvae, anuria/oliguria, acute renal failure, polyuria, urine discoloration. **Hematologic:** Pancytopenia, bone marrow depression, thrombocytopenia, neutropenia, leukopenia, hemolytic anemia. **Miscellaneous:** Candidiasis, superinfection, tinnitus, polyarthralgia, asthenia, muscle weakness, transient hearing loss in clients with existing hearing impairment, taste perversion, thoracic spine pain. **Children, 3 months and older:** Diarrhea, rash, phlebitis, gastroenteritis, vomiting, IV site irritation, urine discoloration. **Children, newborn to 3 months:** Convulsions, diarrhea, oliguria, anuria, oral candidiasis, rash, tachycardia.

The following side effects may occur at the injection site: Thrombophlebitis, phlebitis, pain, erythema, vein induration, infused vein infection.

LABORATORY TEST CONSIDERATIONS

IM: ↑ AST, ALT, alkaline phosphatase, bilirubin, BUN, creatinine, PT. ↓ Hemoglobin, hematocrit, erythrocytes. ↑ or ↓ WBCs and platelets. Presence of RBCs, WBCs, casts, and bacteria in urine.

IV: ↑ AST, ALT, alkaline phosphatase, bilirubin, LDH, BUN, creatinine, eosinophils, monocytes, lymphocytes, basophils, potassium, chloride. ↓ Neutrophils, hemoglobin, hematocrit. ↑ or ↓ WBCs, platelets. Positive Coombs' test and abnormal PT. Presence of protein, RBCs, WBCs, casts, bilirubin, or urobilinogen in the urine.

DRUG INTERACTIONS

Cyclosporine / ↑ CNS side effects of both drugs
Ganciclovir / ↑ Risk of generalized seizures
Probenecid / ↑ Imipenem levels and half-life; do not use together
Valganciclovir / ↑ Risk of generalized seizures

HOW SUPPLIED

See *Content.*

DOSAGE

IM

Mild to moderate lower respiratory tract, skin and skin structure, or gynecologic infections.

500 or 750 mg q 12 hr depending on severity.

Mild to moderate intra-abdominal infections.

Adults: 750 mg q 12 hr. The total daily dose should not exceed 1.5 grams.

Children: 10–15 mg/kg q 6 hr for all uses.

IV

Fully susceptible gram-positive organisms, gram-negative organisms, anaerobes.

Mild: 250 mg q 6 hr (total daily dose: 1 gram); **moderate:** 500 mg q 6 hr or q 8 hr (total daily dose: 1.5 or 2 grams); **severe/life-threatening:** 500 mg q 6 hr (total daily dose: 2 grams).

Urinary tract infections due to fully susceptible organisms.

Uncomplicated: 250 mg q 6 hr (total daily dose: 1 gram); **complicated:** 500 mg q 6 hr (total daily dose: 2 grams).

Moderately susceptible organisms (especially some strains of P. aeruginosa*).*

Mild: 500 mg q 6 hr (total daily dose: 2 grams); **moderate,** 500 mg q 6 hr to 1 gram q 6 hr (total daily dose: 2 or 3 grams); **severe/life-threatening,** 1 gram q 6 or 8 hr (total daily dose: 3 or 4 grams).

Urinary tract infections due to moderately susceptible organisms.

Uncomplicated: 250 mg q 6 hr (total daily dose: 1 gram); **complicated:** 500 mg q 6 hr (total daily dose: 2 grams).

Pediatric, non-CNS infections.

Children, 3 months of age or older: 15–25 mg/kg/dose q 6 hr, up to a maximum dose of 2 grams/day for treating infections with fully susceptible organisms and up to a maximum of 4 grams/day for infections with moderately susceptible organisms. Doses as high as 90 mg/kg/day have been used in older children with cystic fibrosis. **Children, 3 months of age or less (weighing 1,500 grams or more):** Less than 1 week of age, 25 mg/kg q 12 hr; 1–4 weeks of age, 25 mg/kg q 8 hr; 4 weeks to 3 months of age, 25 mg/kg q 6 hr. Give doses less than or equal to 500 mg by IV infusion over 15 to 20 min; give doses greater than 500 mg by IV infusion over 40 to 60 min. *NOTE*: IV use is not recommended for children with CNS infections due to the risk of seizures and in children <30 kg with impaired renal function as no data are available.

NURSING IMPLICATIONS

IMPLEMENTATION/ADMINISTRATION/STORAGE

1. When used IM, give in large muscle mass (e.g., gluteal muscles or lateral part of the thigh) with a 21-gauge 2-inch needle.
2. Total daily IM doses >1,500 mg/day are not recommended.
3. For IM use, prepare with 1% lidocaine HCl solution without epinephrine. Prepare the 500 mg vial with 2 mL and the 750 mg vial with 3 mL of lidocaine HCl. Use reconstituted IM solutions within 1 hr of preparation.
4. Continue IM use for at least 2 days after S&S of infection are absent. Safety and efficacy not established for use more than 14 days.
5. Reduce dosage with a C_{CR} of 70 mL/min/1.73 m^2 or less. Check package insert for dosage information.
6. IV Reconstitute for IV use by mixing with 100 mL of diluent.
7. Base initial dose on the type and severity of infection. Give doses of 125 mg, 250 mg, and 500 mg by IV infusion over 20–30 min. Give doses of 750 mg or 1 gram by IV infusion over 40–60 min. If nausea develops, decrease infusion rate. Do not exceed more than 50 mg/kg/day or 4 grams/day, whichever is lower as there is no evidence higher doses provide greater efficacy.
8. Reconstituted IV solutions vary from colorless to yellow while reconstituted IM solutions vary from white to light tan in color. Color variations do not affect potency.
9. Most reconstituted IV solutions can be stored at room temperature for 4 hr and, if refrigerated, for 24 hr. The exception is imipenem-cilastatin reconstituted with 0.9% NaCl solution, which is stable at room temperature for 10 hr and, if refrigerated, for 48 hr.
10. COMPATIBILITY 0.9% NaCl or D5W. The following solutions can be used as diluents: 0.9% NaCl, D5W or D10W, D5/0.9% NaCl, D5W with either 0.225% or 0.45% saline solution, D5W with 0.15% KCl solution, or mannitol (2.5%, 5%, or 10%).
11. INCOMPATIBILITY Do not mix with other antibiotics; however, may be administered concomitantly with other antibiotics (e.g., aminoglycosides).

ASSESSMENT

1. Note reasons for therapy, onset, duration, characteristics of S&S, clinical presentation, and culture results.
2. Do not use in clients allergic to local anesthetics of the amide type or with heart block (R/T lidocaine HCl diluent) or severe shock. Use cautiously with penicillin, beta-lactams or cephalosporin allergy. Assess for seizure history. The cilastatin component prevents renal metabolism of imipenem.
3. Avoid IV use in children with CNS infections R/T risk of seizures and in children <30 kg with impaired renal function.
4. Assess IV site for phlebitis, pain, erythema.
5. Monitor renal function; avoid if C_{CR} is less than or equal to 5 mL/min/1.73 m^2, unless hemodialysis is begun within 48 hr. See administration guidelines. Monitor CBC, cultures, renal and LFTs.

CLIENT/FAMILY TEACHING

1. Drug is administered parenterally and used to kill organisms that cause infection. May experience pain at injection site.
2. Report any rash, breathing problems, persistent or delayed watery diarrhea (2–3 months after therapy).
3. Keep all F/U to assess response, labs, and for adverse SE.

OUTCOMES/EVALUATE

- Resolution of infection
- Symptomatic improvement

IV

Immune globulin IV (Human)

(im-**MYOUN GLOH**-byou-lin)

Classification(s): Immune globulin

Pregnancy Category: C

RX: Carimune NF, Flebogamma DIF, Gammagard Liquid, Gammaplex, Gamunex, Iveegam EN, Octagam, Privigen.

✤ **Rx:** Iveegam Immuno.

INDICATIONS/USES

All products (additional uses listed under individual products): Severe combined immunodeficiency and primary immunoglobulin deficiency syndromes, including common variable immunodeficiency, x-linked agammaglobulinemia, severe combined immunodeficiency, and Wiskott-Aldrich syndrome. *Investigational:* Several products are being investigated to treat posttransfusion purpura, Guillain-Barré syndrome, chronic inflammatory demyelinating polyneuropathy (as an alternative to plasma exchange), or multiple sclerosis. **Carimune NF:** (1) Preferable to IM immune globulin to treat those who require an immediate and large increase in intravascular immunoglobulin levels, in those with limited muscle mass, and in those with bleeding tendencies for whom IM injections are contraindicated.
(2) Acute and chronic ITP in adults and children. *Investigational:* Guillain-Barré syndrome, myasthenia gravis, multiple sclerosis, postpoliomyelitis syndrome. **Flebogamma:** Especially useful when rapid replacement of immunoglobulin G (IgG) or the attainment of high serum levels of IgG is needed. **Gamunex:** (1) In idiopathic thrombocytopenic purpura to raise platelet counts rapidly to prevent bleeding or to allow surgery.
(2) Chronic inflammatory demyelinating polyneuropathy to improve neuromuscular disability and impairment and to maintain therapy to prevent relapse. *Investigational:* Myasthenia gravis, postpoliomyelitis syndrome. **Iveegam EN:** Treatment of Kawasaki syndrome. **Octagam:** Primary immune deficient diseases, including congenital agammaglobulinemia and hypogammaglobulinemia, common variable immunodeficiency, Wiskott-Aldrich syndrome, and severe combined immunodeficiencies. **Privigen:** Chronic ITP to raise platelet counts rapidly to prevent bleeding.

ACTION/KINETICS

Action

Derived from a human volunteer pool. Contains the various IgG antibodies normally occurring in humans. The products may also contain traces of IgA and IgM. Plasma in the manufacturing pool has been found nonreactive for hepatitis B antigen. No documented cases of viral transmission. Antibodies present in the products will cause both opsonization and neutralization of microbes and toxins. Reconstituted products may contain sucrose, maltose, protein, and/or small amounts of sodium chloride. Immune globulin IV provides immediate antibody levels. The globulin contains a high level of antibodies directed against CMV. In those who may be exposed to CMV, the globulin can raise the relevant antibodies to levels sufficient to attenuate or reduce the incidence of serious CMV disease.

Pharmacokinetics

The percentage of IgG in the products is over 90%.

CONTRAINDICATIONS

Clients with selective IgA deficiency who have antibodies to IgA (the products contain IgA). Sensitivity to human immune globulin. Use of Privigen with hyperprolinema due to the stabilizer L-proline in the product. Use in those with expanded fluid volumes or where fluid volume may be of concern.

SPECIAL CONCERNS

IGIV (human) products, particularly those containing sucrose, have been associated with renal dysfunction, acute renal failure, osmotic nephrosis, and death. Clients predisposed to acute renal failure include those with any degree of pre-existing renal insufficiency, diabetes mellitus, advanced age (above 65 years of age), volume depletion, sepsis, paraproteinemia, or those receiving known nephrotoxic drugs. Especially in such clients, administer IGIV products at the minimum concentration available and the minimum rate of infusion practical. While these reports of renal dysfunction and acute renal failure have been associated with the use of many of the IGIV products, those containing sucrose as a stabilizer account for a disproportionate share of the total number. Gammagard S/D, Gamimune N, Iveegam, and Venoglobulin-S do not contain sucrose. ■

- The various products are used for different conditions and at different doses; thus, check information carefully, noting especially if they contain sucrose.
- Possible thrombotic events, especially following rapid infusion or high doses.
- Infusing too rapidly may cause flushing and changes in pulse rate and BP; slowing or stopping the infusion usually results in prompt disappearance of signs.
- Antibodies in IGIV products may interfere with responses to live vaccines (e.g., measles, mumps, rubella).
- Safety and efficacy not established in neonates and infants with primary defective antibody synthesis.

I

SIDE EFFECTS

Most Common

Backache, chills, dizziness, fatigue, fever, flushing, headache, increased sweating, leg cramps, muscle aches/pains, N&V, malaise, pain/tenderness at injection site.

CNS: Headache, malaise, feeling of faintness, dizziness. Aseptic meningitis syndrome, including symptoms of severe headache, nuchal rigidity, drowsiness, fever, photophobia, painful eye movements, coma, LOC, ***seizures***, tremor. **GI:** N&V, diarrhea, stomach discomfort, abdominal pain, hepatic dysfunction. **CV:** Tachycardia, BP changes, intravascular hemolysis, thrombotic events, RBC hemolysis, thromboembolism, vascular collapse, hypotension, ***cardiac arrest.*** **GU:** Renal dysfunction, acute renal failure, osmotic nephrosis. **Respiratory:** Dyspnea, bronchospasm, cough, chest tightness, wheezing, epistaxis, apnea, acute respiratory distress syndrome (ARDS), cyanosis, noncardiogenic pulmonary edema (severe respiratory distress, pulmonary edema, hypoxemia, fever). **Musculoskeletal:** Chest, back, or hip pain; leg cramps, arthralgia, myalgia. **Dermatologic:** Skin reactions, ***Stevens-Johnson syndrome***, epidermolysis, erythema multiforme, bullous dermatitis. **Allergic:** Hypersensitivity or ***anaphylactic reactions***. **Hematologic:** Pancytopenia, leukopenia, hemolysis. **Body as a whole:** Fever, hyperpyrexia, fatigue, chills, rigors, flushing, increased sweating. **At injection site:** Pain, tenderness. **Miscellaneous:** Mild erythema following infiltration; burning sensation in the head; tachycardia. Bloodborne viral transmission (low risk).

Agammaglobulinemic and hypogammaglobulinemic clients never having received immunoglobulin therapy or where the time from the last treatment is more than 8 weeks may manifest side effects if the infusion rate exceeds 1 mL/min. Symptoms include flushing of the face, hypotension, tightness in chest, chills, fever, dizziness, diaphoresis, and nausea.

LABORATORY TEST CONSIDERATIONS

↑ BUN, creatinine, serum viscosity, blood conjugated/unconjugated bilirubin, blood total bilirubin. ↓ Hematocrit. Hyperproteinemia, hyponatremia. Negative direct antiglobin test.

DRUG INTERACTIONS

Passive transfer of antibodies may interfere with the immune response to live virus vaccines, such as measles, mumps, and rubella.

HOW SUPPLIED

Injection: Flebogamma DIF (5%: 50 mg/mL; 10%: 100 mg/mL); Octagam (10%; 100 mg/mL); Gammagard Liquid (10%; 100 mg/mL); Gamunex (10%; 100 mg /mL); ***Injection Solution:*** Privigen (10%; 100 mg/mL); Octagam (10%; 100 mg/mL); ***Injection, Freeze-Dried Powder for Solution:*** Iveegam EN (5 grams); ***Injection, Lyophilized Powder for Solution:*** Carimune NF (1 gram, 3 grams, 6 grams, 12 grams).

DOSAGE

NOTE: Due to differences in products, dosage must be listed separately for each product.

Carimune NF

IV ONLY

Immunodeficiency syndrome.

Adults and children: 0.2 gram/kg given once a month by IV infusion. If clinical response is inadequate, the dose may be increased to 0.3 gram/kg or the infusion may be repeated more frequently than once a month. The first infusion in previously untreated agammaglobulinemic or hypogammaglobulinemic clients must be given as a 3% immunoglobulin solution. Start with a flow rate of 10–20 gtt (0.5–1 mL/min). After 15–30 min, the rate of infusion may be further increased to 30–50 gtt (1.5–2.5 mL/min). After the first bottle of 3% solution is given and the client shows good tolerance, subsequent infusions may be given at a higher rate or concentration. Make such increases gradually allowing 15–30 min before each increment. *NOTE:* The first infusion may lead to systemic side effects, some of which may be due to release of proinflammatory cytokines by activated macrophages in immunodeficient recipients. Subsequent administration usually does not cause further side effects.

A maximum safe dose, concentration, and rate of infusion have not been determined in clients with existing or potential impaired renal function. It is recommended, however, that the product should be infused in such clients at a rate less than 2 mg/kg/min.

ITP.

Induction: 0.4 gram/kg on 2–5 consecutive days. If an initial platelet count response in children to the first 2 doses is adequate (30,000–50,000/mcL), therapy may be discontinued after the second day of the 5-day course. **Maintenance, chronic ITP, adults and children:** If after the induction therapy, platelets fall to less than 30,000/mcL and/or the client manifests clinically significant bleeding, 0.4 gram/kg may be given as a single infusion. If an adequate response does not result, the dose may be increased to 0.8–1 gram/kg given as a single infusion.

Flebogamma DIF

IV ONLY

Primary humoral immunodeficiency disorders.

300–600 mg/kg q 3–4 weeks. Dose may be adjusted over time to achieve the desired trough IgG levels and clinical response. Begin the infusion for Flebogamma at a rate of 0.01 mL/kg body weight/min (0.5 mg/kg/min). If during the first 30 min, the client does not experience any discomfort, the rate may be increased gradually to a maximum of 0.1 mL/kg/min (5 mg/kg/min). For those at risk of developing renal dysfunction, infuse at a maximum rate less than 0.06 mL/kg/min (3 mg/kg/min).

Gammagard Liquid (10%)

IV ONLY

Immunodeficiency disease.

Individualize, usual: 300–600 mg/kg q 3–4 weeks, with the first dose given at an initial rate of 0.5 mL/kg/hr (0.8 mg/kg/min) and increased gradually q 30 min to the level the client can tolerate but no more than 5 mL/kg/hr (8.9 mg/kg/min). In clients at risk of renal dysfunction or thrombotic complications, the recommended rate of administration is <2 mL/kg/hr (3.3 mg/kg/min). *NOTE:* Those beginning therapy with IGIV or switching from one IGIV product to another should be started at the lower rates and then advanced to the maximal rate if the client has tolerated several infusions at intermediate rates of infusion.

Gamunex

IV ONLY

ITP.

Adults and children: Total dose of 2 grams/kg divided in two doses of 1 gram/kg (10 mL/kg) given on two consecutive days or into five doses of 0.4 mg/kg given on five consecutive days. If after giving the first of two daily 1 gram/kg doses, an adequate increase in the platelet count is seen at 24 hr, the second dose of 1 gram/kg may be withheld. This high dose regimen should not be given to those with expanded fluid volumes or where fluid volume may be a concern.

Primary humoral Immunodeficiency.

Adults and children: Individualize dose. **Dose range:** 300–600 mg/kg (3–6 mL/kg) q 3–4 weeks. The dose may be adjusted over time to achieve the desired trough levels and clinical response. For those with impaired renal function, reduce the amount infused per unit of time at a rate less than 8 mg/kg/min (0.08 mL/kg/min).

I

Chronic inflammatory demyelinating polyneuropathy.

Adults, initial: Total loading dose of 2 grams/kg (20 mL/kg) given in divided doses over 2–4 consecutive days. May be given as a maintenance infusion of 1 gram/kg (10 mL/kg) administered over 1 day or divided into 2 doses of 0.5 gram/kg (5 mL/kg) given on 2 consecutive days q 3 weeks. *NOTE:* The safety and efficacy not established in children with chronic inflammatory demyelinating purpura.

Iveegam EN

IV ONLY

Immunodeficiency syndromes.

200 mg/kg per month. If the desired response is not obtained, the dose may be increased up to 4-fold or intervals between infusions shortened. Doses up to 800 mg/kg per month were tolerated. The usual rate of administration is 1 mL/min, up to a maximum 2 mL/min for the 5% solution. For clients at risk for developing impaired renal function, reduce the amount infused per unit time at a rate less than 1.5 mg/kg/min (0.03 mL/kg/min).

Kawasaki syndrome.

Initiate within 10 days of onset of the disease. Give either a dose of 400 mg/kg daily for 4 consecutive days or a single dose of 2,000 mg/kg over a 10 hr period. The treatment regimen should also include aspirin, 100 mg/kg each day through the 14th day of illness; then, 3–5 mg/kg each day for a period of 5 weeks.

Octagam

IV ONLY

Immunodeficiency disease.

The frequency and amount of immunoglobulin therapy may vary from client to client. **Adults, usual:** 300–600 mg/kg q 3–4 weeks. Dose may be adjusted over time to achieve the desired trough IgG levels and clinical response. Initially infuse the 5% solution at a rate of 30 mg/kg/hr for the first 30 min; if tolerated, increased to 60 mg/kg/hr for the second 30 min; and if further tolerated, increase to 120 mg/kg/hr for the third 30 min. Thereafter, the infusion can be maintained at a rate up to, but not exceeding, 200 mg/kg/hr. For those with impaired renal function, consider reducing the amount infused per unit of time at a maximum rate less than 0.07 mL/kg (3.3 mg/kg/min or 200 mg/kg/hr). The product should be at room temperature during infusion.

Privigen

IV ONLY

Primary immunodeficiency disease.

200–800 mg/kg given q 3–4 weeks. Adjust doses to achieve the desired serum trough levels and clinical response. The recommended initial infusion rate is 0.5 mg/kg/min (0.005 mL/kg/min). If the infusion is well tolerated, increase the rate gradually to a maximum of 8 mg/kg/min (0.08 mL/kg/min). For those clients at risk of impaired renal function or thrombotic events, administer at the minimum infusion rate practicable.

The following clients may be at risk of developing inflammatory responses on rapid infusion (>4 mg/kg/min or >0.04 mL/kg/min): (1) those who have not received Privigen or another IgG product; (2) those who are switching from another IgG product; and (3) those who have not received IgG in more than 8 weeks. For these clients, start a slow rate of infusion (e.g., 0.5 mg/kg/min or 0.005 mL/kg/min); gradually increase to the maximum rate as tolerated.

Chronic ITP.

1 gram/kg given daily for 2 consecutive days (total dose of 2 grams/kg). The recommended initial infusion rate is 0.5 mg/kg/min (0.005 mL/kg/min). If the infusion is well tolerated, gradually increase the rate to a maximum of 4 mg/kg/min (0.04 mL/kg/min). For those at risk of impaired renal function or thrombotic events, administer at the minimum infusion rate practicable.

NURSING IMPLICATIONS

IMPLEMENTATION/ADMINISTRATION/STORAGE

1. **IV** Check the product information for each product carefully as there are differences in reconstitution procedures, incompatibilities, methods of administration, and rates of infusion.
2. Store Carimune NF at room temperature, not exceeding 30°C (86°F). Do not use after expiration date.
3. Octagam may be stored for 24 months at 2–8°C (36–46°F) or may be stored at temperatures not to exceed 25°C (77°F) for up to 18 months from the date of manufacture. Do not use after expiration date.
4. Store Flebogamma DIF from 2–25°C (36–77°F); do not freeze. Discard after expiration date.
5. Store Gammagard Liquid at 25°C (77°F) for up to 9 months after manufacture or from 2–8°C (36–46°F) for up to 36 months. Should be at room temperature during administration.
6. Follow administration guidelines explicitly and the manufacturer's directions carefully for reconstitution of either the 5% or 10% Gammagard solution. Do not use normal saline as a diluent. If dilution is preferred, use D5W.
7. Administer Gammagard Liquid separate from other drugs or medications. Do not mix with IGIV products from other manufacturers.
8. Do not freeze Gamunex; if frozen do not use. The Gamunex vial is for single use only; it contains no preservative. Open vials should be used promptly. Discard partially used vials.
9. Gamunex should be at room temperature when administered. Infuse using a separate line without mixing with other IV fluids or medications. Flush the infusion before and after administration with D5W.
10. Infuse Gamunex initially at a rate of 0.01 mL/kg/min (1 mg/kg/min) for the first 30 min when used for primary humoral immunodeficiency or ITP. Infuse at a rate of 0.02 mL/kg/min (2 mg/kg/min) if used for chronic inflammatory demyelinating polyneuropathy. For all uses, if well tolerated, the rate may be increased gradually to a maximum of 0.08 mL/kg/min (8 mg/kg/min).
11. Admixture of Octagam with other drugs and IV solutions not evaluated. Administer separately from other drugs; do not mix with IGIVs from other manufacturers.
12. Octagam contains maltose which could interfere with blood and urine glucose tests.
13. Infuse only if the solution is clear and at room temperature. Do not shake the solutions because excessive foaming will occur.
14. Give only IV using a pump to administer; the IM or SC routes have not been evaluated.
15. A rapid decrease in serum IgG level in the first week postinfusion will be observed; this is expected and due to the equilibration of IgG between the plasma and extravascular space.
16. Have epinephrine readily available in the event of an acute anaphylactic reaction.
17. COMPATIBILITY Gamunex may be diluted with D5W if dilution is required. If other medications or IV fluids will be sequentially administered, flush IV line with D5W before and after infusion of immune globulin IV.
18. INCOMPATIBILITY Give by a separate IV line; do not mix with other fluids or medications. Gamunex is incompatible with saline.

ASSESSMENT

1. List reasons for therapy; for passive immunization note date and type of exposure; assess closely for anaphylaxis. Various products are used for different conditions and at different doses; thus, check information carefully.
2. Give within 2 weeks of exposure to hepatitis A, within 6 days after measles exposure, and within 7 days after hepatitis B exposure.
3. Any history of ITP warrants close hematologic monitoring. Monitor CBC, determine if pregnant; requires close observation/management.
4. If S&S of aseptic meningitis syndrome present, conduct neuro exam including CSF studies, to R/O other causes of meningitis.
5. Monitor VS; if hypotension occurs, decrease/interrupt infusion rate until hypotension subsides.
6. Administer in a closely monitored environment away from persons with active infections if immunocompromised.
7. Monitor for S&S of hemolysis and pulmonary reactions. Obtain baseline assessment of blood viscosity in those at risk for hyperviscosity.
8. To reduce the risk of IGIV-associated acute renal failure:

- Ensure adequately hydrated before infusing IGIV. Monitor VS.
- Be especially cautious when giving IGIV to those at increased risk for acute renal failure (renal insufficiency, diabetes mellitus, those over 65 years of age, volume depletion, sepsis, paraproteinemia, or if taking nephrotoxic drugs).
- Do not exceed the recommended dose. For those at risk of acute renal failure, dilute or reconstitute the product so the IGIV concentration is as low and the infusion rate as slow as is practical. Do not exceed infusion rate of 3 mg/kg/min.
- Assess renal function before infusing IGIV and at regular intervals.
- Has been associated with renal dysfunction, acute renal failure, osmotic nephrosis, and death. Products containing sucrose as a stabilizer account for a disproportionate share of the total number of cases of renal dysfunction and acute renal failure. For those at increased risk of developing renal dysfunction, reduce amount of product infused per unit time. Do not exceed recommended dose, and the concentration and infusion rate should be the minimum level practicable.

9. Monitor renal and LFTs, hematologic parameters, IgG levels, and appropriate blood/urine chemistries.

CLIENT/FAMILY TEACHING

1. Immunoglobulin helps to prevent and/or reduce intensity of various infectious diseases. With thrombocytopenia, expect increased platelets and enhanced clotting.
2. Once-monthly therapy is needed to maintain IgG serum levels.
3. Dosage and frequency depend on condition being treated. Drug is administered by IV infusion.
4. Drug may cause N&V, fever, chills, flushing, lightheadedness, respiratory difficulty, and tightness in the chest; report immediately. Also report ↓ urine output, sudden weight gain, fluid retention/swelling, unexplained SOB, fever, severe headache, stiff neck, unexplained drowsiness/fatigue, painful eye movements, sensitivity to bright light, persistent or worsening nausea and vomiting.
5. Close observation and frequent labs are essential with pregnancy to improve chances of a healthy baby and to ensure maternal safety.
6. Advise to vaccinate all at-risk infants as soon after birth as possible and again at 3 mo.
7. For postexposure prophylaxis, give drug as soon after exposure as possible (preferably within 7 days).
8. Warm soaks to injection site and PO acetaminophen may relieve discomfort.
9. Drug is derived from human plasma (except for those engineered genetically); be aware of potential risks.
10. Keep all F/U to assess response, labs, and for adverse SE.

OUTCOMES/EVALUATE

- IgG levels within normal range
- ↑ Antibody titer; passive immunity
- ↑ Platelets; ↓ hemorrhaging

IncobotulinumtoxinA (Botulinum Toxin A)

(in-koe-bot-you-**LYE**-num-**TOX**-in-ay)

Classification(s): Botulinum Toxin Type A

Pregnancy Category: C

RX: Xeomin.

INDICATIONS/USES

(1) Adults with blepharospasm who were previously treated with onobotulinumtoxinA.
(2) Adults with cervical dystonia to decrease the severity of abnormal head position and neck pain in botulinum toxin-naive and previously treated clients. (3) Temporary improvement in the appearance of moderate to severe glabellar lines associated with corrugator and/or procerus muscle activity in adults. *Investigational:* Achalasia; facial lines and wrinkles.

ACTION/KINETICS

Action

IncobotulinumtoxinA blocks cholinergic transmission at the neuromuscular junction by inhibiting the release of acetylcholine. Impulse transmission is reestablished by the formation of new nerve endings.

CONTRAINDICATIONS

Hypersensitivity to botulinum toxin type A or any other botulinum toxin type A product. Infection at the injection site.

SPECIAL CONCERNS

Spread of toxin effect. Postmarketing reports indicate that the effects of all botulinum toxin products may spread from the area of injection to produce symptoms consistent with botulinum toxin effects. These may include asthenia, generalized muscle weakness, diplopia, ptosis, dysphagia, dysphonia, dysarthria, urinary incontinence, and breathing difficulties. These symptoms have been reported hours to weeks after injection. Swallowing and breathing difficulties can be life-threatening, and there have been reports of death. The risk of symptoms is probably greatest in children treated for spasticity, but symptoms can also occur in adults treated for spasticity and other conditions, particularly in those clients who have underlying conditions that would predispose them to these symptoms. In unapproved uses, including spasticity in children and adults, and in approved indications, cases of spread of effect have been reported at doses comparable with those used to treat cervical dystonia and at lower doses.

- The product contains albumin; thus, there is an extremely remote risk for transmission of viral disease or Creutzfeldt-Jakob disease.
- Those with neuromuscular disorders (e.g., peripheral motor neuropathic diseases, amyotrophic lateral sclerosis, neuromuscular junctional disorders) may be at increased risk of clinically significant effects, including severe dysphagia and respiratory compromise from typical doses of incobotulinumtoxinA.
- Use with caution during lactation.
- Safety and efficacy not established in children less than 18 years.

SIDE EFFECTS

Most Common

See *Side Effects*.

For all uses. Spread of toxin effect: Asthenia, blurred vision, breathing difficulties, diplopia, dysarthria, dysphagia, dysphonia, muscle weakness, ptosis, urinary incontinence, ocular effects (e.g., reduced blinking, ectropion) and/or hypersensitivity reactions. **GI:** dysphagia. **Respiratory:** Breathing difficulties. **Ophthalmic:** Reduced blinking may lead to corneal exposure, persistent epithelial defect, and corneal ulceration. Ptosis. **Hypersenstivity:** Serum sickness, urticaria, soft tissue edema, dyspnea, ***anaphylaxis***. **Miscellaneous:** Immunogenicity.

When used for blepharospasm. CNS: Headache. **GI:** Diarrhea, dry mouth. **Respiratory:** Nasopharyngitis, respiratory tract infection, dyspnea. **Ophthalmic:** Eye disorders, eyelid ptosis, dry eye, visual impairment (including blurred vision). **Body as a whole:** Infections and infestations.

When used for cervical dystonia. GI: Dysphagia. **Musculoskeletal:** Muscle weakness, musculoskeletal pain, neck pain. **Respiratory:** Respiratory, thoracic, and mediastinal disorders. **Miscellaneous:** Injection site pain, infections and infestations, asthenia, CNS disorders.

When used for glabellar lines. CNS: Headache. **Musculoskeletal:** Muscle disorder (elevation of eyebrow). **At injection site:** Hematoma, pain, swelling. **Ophthalmic:** Blepharospasm, eye disorders, eyelid edema/ptosis. **Miscellaneous:** Facial pain/paresis (brow ptosis), sensation of pressure.

Postmarketing. GI: Dysphagia, nausea. **Musculoskeletal:** Dysarthria, muscle weakness/spasms, myalgia. **Hypersensitivity:** Allergic dermatitis, localized allergic reactions (e.g., swelling, edema, erythema, pruritus, rash). **At injection site:** Pain, injection site reaction. **Ophthalmic:** Eye swelling/edema. **Miscellaneous:** Herpes zoster.

OVERDOSE MANAGEMENT

Symptoms: Neuromuscular weakness, paralysis of respiratory muscles. *Treatment:* Respiratory support if there is paralysis of respiratory muscles. Symptomatic treatment.

DRUG INTERACTIONS

Aminoglycosides (e.g., gentamicin) / Enhanced neuromuscular action → protracted respiratory depression; use together with caution
Anticholinergic drugs (e.g., atropine) / Potentiation of systemic anticholinergic effects (e.g., blurred vision); use together with caution
Cholinesterase inhibitors / Enhanced neuromuscular action → protracted respiratory depression; use together with caution

Magnesium sulfate / Enhanced neuromuscular action → protracted respiratory depression; use together with caution
Muscle relaxants (e.g., metaxalone) / Exaggeration of excessive weakness; use together with caution
Nondepolarizing muscle relaxants (e.g., tubocurarine) / Enhanced neuromuscular activity → protracted respiratory depression; use together with caution
Other botulinum neurotoxins (e.g., botulinum toxin B) / Administration at the same time or within several months of each other → exacerbation of excessive neuromuscular weakness
Quinidine / Enhanced neuromuscular action → protracted respiratory depression; use together with caution

HOW SUPPLIED

Injection, Lyophilized Powder for Solution: 50 units, 100 units.

DOSAGE

IM ONLY.

Blepharospasm.

Adults, initial: Dose should be the same as the client's previous treatment with onabotulinumtoxinA, though responses differ in individual clients. If the previous dose of onabotulinumtoxinA is not known, give an initial dose of 1.25–2.5 units/injection site. Individualize subsequent dosing based on response. Determine the frequency of repeat treatments by clinical response, but generally should be no more frequent than q 12 weeks.

Cervical dystonia.

Adults, initial: 120 units IM. Determine the frequency of repeat treatments by the clinical response, but generally no more frequently than q 12 weeks.

Glabellar lines.

Adults, initial: 20 units per treatment session divided into 5 equal IM injections of 4 units each. The 5 injection sites are: 2 injections in each corrugator muscle and 1 injection in the procerus muscle. Administer retreatment no more frequently than q 3 months.

NURSING IMPLICATIONS

Do not confuse the three types of botulinum toxin type A products: AbobotulinumtoxinA, IncobotulinumtoxinA, or OnabotulinumtoxinA.

IMPLEMENTATION/ADMINISTRATION/STORAGE

1. Potency units are specific to the preparation and assay method used. They are not interchangeable with other products of botulinum toxin. Thus, units of biological activity of onabotulinumtoxinA cannot be compared with or converted into units of any other botulinum toxin products assessed with any other specific assay method.
2. Reconstitute each vial with sterile, preservative-free 0.9% NaCl injection. Gently inject the appropriate amount of NaCl solution into the vial. If the vacuum does not pull the solvent into the vial, the vial must be discarded. Gently mix by rotating the vial.
3. Product is for IM injection only. If the proposed injection sites are marked with a pen, do not inject through the pen marks; otherwise a permanent tattooing effect may occur.
4. The number of injection sites depends on the size of the muscle to be treated and the volume injected.
5. Inject carefully when administering at sites close to sensitive structures, such as the carotid artery, lung apices, and esophagus. Before injecting, be familiar with the client's anatomy and any anatomic alterations (i.e., due to prior surgical procedures).
6. *For blepharospasm:* Use a sterile needle (26 gauge [0.45 mm diameter], 37 mm length) for superficial muscles. Or, use a sterile needle (22 gauge [0.7 mm diameter], 75 mm length) for injection into deeper muscles.
7. *For cervical dystonia:* Usually injected into the sternocleidomastoid, levator scapulae, splenius capitis, scalenus, and/or trapezius muscle(s). Use a sterile needle (26 gauge [0.45 mm diameter], 37 mm length) for superficial muscles. Or, use a sterile needle (22 gauge [0.7 mm diameter], 75 mm length) for injection into deeper muscles.
8. *For glabellar lines:* The 5 injection sites are 2 injections in each corrugator muscle and 1 injection in the procerus muscle. Use a suitable sterile needle, 30–33 gauge (0.3–0.2 mm diameter), 13 mm length.

9. Store from 20–25°C (68–77°F), or in a refrigerator from 2–8°C (36–46°F), or in a freezer from –20–10°C (–4–14°F) for up to 36 months. Store reconstituted solution in a refrigerator from 2–8°C (36–46°F); administer within 24 hr. Discard any unused solution after 24 hr.

ASSESSMENT

1. Note reasons for therapy: abnormal head position and neck pain, blepharospasm, or glabellar lines, associated characteristics, other agents/therapies trialed.
2. Assess carefully for evidence/history of neuropathic, neurologic, or neuromuscular disorders.
3. For use/administration only by those individuals trained to administer.
4. If proposed injection sites are marked with a pen, the product must not be injected through the pen marks; otherwise, a permanent tattooing effect may occur.
5. Monitor carefully for postinjection effects (hours to weeks later) which may spread from the area of injection to other body areas to produce symptoms consistent with botulinum toxin effects.
6. With eye injections, use caution with those at risk for narrow angle glaucoma; may see decreased blink response and ptosis R/T injection site location.
7. Review associated risk factors to ensure client understanding. Drug contains albumin which may present the remote risk of disease transmission of Creutzfeldt-Jakob disease (CJD).

CLIENT/FAMILY TEACHING

1. Drug has many uses: may be used to relieve abnormal muscle spasms/contractures of the head and neck, eye twitching/tics, and to decrease frown lines.
2. Do not perform activities that require mental alertness until drug effects realized; may cause drowsiness. Resume activity slowly, and carefully following administration.
3. Report any swallowing or breathing problems, SOB, respiratory disorders/infections, injection site abnormalities, facial drooping, weakness.
4. Effects usually last up to 3 months; repeat injections may be required.
5. For cervical dystonia, improvement should occur within the first 2 wk following treatment, and maximum improvement should occur within about 6 wk. Beneficial effects may last 3 months before retreatment is needed.
6. For blepharospasm, improvement should occur within the first 3 days following treatment, and maximum improvement should occur within about 1 to 2 wk. Beneficial effects may last 3 months before retreatment is needed.
7. May cause reduced blinking or ineffective blinking; seek immediate attention if eye pain or irritation occur following treatment.
8. For glabellar lines, improvement should occur within the first 2 days following treatment, and maximum improvement should occur within the first week. Beneficial effects may last 3 to 4 months.
9. Practice reliable contraception.
10. Keep all F/U to assess response and for adverse SE.

OUTCOMES/EVALUATE

- Relief of painful muscle spasms/contractures permitting improved posture, movement, and activity
- Smoothing of wrinkles/frown lines
- Control of eye tic/alignment

Indinavir sulfate

(in-**DIN**-ah-veer)

Classification(s): Antiviral, protease inhibitor
Pregnancy Category: C

RX: Crixivan.

SEE ALSO ***ANTIVIRAL DRUGS***.

INDICATIONS/USES

Treatment of HIV infection in adults in combination with other antiretroviral drugs. *Investigational:* Treatment of HIV infection in children.

ACTION/KINETICS

Action

Binds to active sites on the HIV protease enzyme resulting in inhibition of enzyme activity. Inhibition prevents cleavage of the viral polyproteins resulting in the formation of immature noninfectious viral particles. Varying degrees of cross-resistance have been noted between indinavir and other HIV-protease inhibitors. Also, resistance to indinavir has been noted.

Pharmacokinetics

Rapidly absorbed in fasting clients; **time to peak plasma levels:** Approximately 0.8 hr. Administration with a meal high in calories, fat, and protein results in a significant decrease in the amount absorbed and in the peak plasma concentration. **t½:** 1.8 hr. Metabolized in the liver mostly by CYP3A4 with both parent drug and metabolites excreted through the feces (over 80%) and the urine (<20% unchanged). **Plasma protein binding:** Approximately 60%.

CONTRAINDICATIONS

Hypersensitivity to indinavir or any component of the product. Lactation. Use with alfuzosin, alprazolam, amiodarone, cisapride, dihydroergotamine, ergonovine, ergotamine, methylergonovine, midazolam (oral), pimozide, sildenafil (when used to treat pulmonary arterial hypertension), and triazolam. Mild to moderate liver or kidney disease. Use in HIV-infected pregnant women.

SPECIAL CONCERNS

- **Not a cure for HIV infections; clients may continue to develop opportunistic infections and other complications of HIV disease.**
- **Not been shown to reduce the risk of transmission of HIV through sexual contact or blood contamination.**
- **Hemophiliacs treated for HIV infections with protease inhibitors may manifest spontaneous bleeding episodes.**
- **Drug resistance and cross-resistance with other HIV protease inhibitors have been noted.**
- **Use caution with dose selection in the elderly.**

SIDE EFFECTS

Most Common

Nephrolithiasis/urolithiasis, abdominal pain, N&V, back pain, headache, pruritus, dizziness, diarrhea.

NOTE: Many side effects are the result of combination therapy with other antiretroviral drugs. **GI:** N&V, diarrhea, abdominal pain/distention, acid regurgitation, anorexia, dry mouth, aphthous stomatitis, cheilitis, cholecystitis, cholestasis, constipation, dyspepsia, eructation, flatulence, gastritis, gingivitis, glossodynia, gingival hemorrhage, increased appetite, infectious gastroenteritis, oral paresthesia. **Hepatic:** Jaundice, hepatitis, ***pancreatitis, hepatic failure, impaired liver function, liver cirrhosis***. **CNS:** Headache, insomnia, dizziness, somnolence, agitation, anxiety, bruxism, decreased mental acuity, depression, dream abnormality, dysesthesia, excitement, fasciculation, hypesthesia, nervousness, neuralgia, neurotic disorder, oral paresthesia, peripheral neuropathy, sleep disorder, tremor, vertigo. **CV:** CV disorder, palpitation, ***MI***, angina pectoris, vasculitis, spontaneous bleeding in those with hemophilia A and B treated with protease inhibitors. **Musculoskeletal:** Back/leg pain, arthralgia, myalgia, muscle cramps/weakness, musculoskeletal pain, shoulder pain, stiffness. **Hematologic:** Anemia, lymphadenopathy, spleen disorder, ***acute hemolytic anemia***, spontaneous bleeding in hemophilia A and B. **Respiratory:** Cough, dyspnea, halitosis, SOB, difficulty breathing, pharyngeal hyperemia, pharyngitis, pneumonia, rales, rhonchi, ***respiratory failure***, sinus disorder, sinusitis, URTI. **Dermatologic:** Body odor, pruritus, rash, contact dermatitis, dermatitis, dry skin, flushing, folliculitis, herpes simplex/zoster, night sweats, pruritus, seborrhea, alopecia, hyperpigmentation, ingrown toenails, paronychia, skin disorder/infection, sweating, urticaria, erythema multiforme, ***Stevens-Johnson syndrome***. **GU:** Nephrolithiasis, urolithiasis, dysuria, hematuria, hydronephrosis, nocturia, PMS, proteinuria, renal colic, urinary frequency/abnormality, UTI, urine sediment abnormality, tubulointerstitial nephritis, crystalluria, dysuria, interstitial nephritis, leukocyturia, renal insufficiency, acute renal failure, pyelonephritis with or without bacteremia. **Metabolic:** New-onset diabetes mellitus, exacerbation of pre-existing diabetes mellitus, hyperglycemia. **Ophthalmic:** Accommodation disorder, blurred vision, eye pain/swelling, orbital edema. **Body as a whole:** Asthenia, fatigue, fever, malaise, chills, fever, chest/flank pain, flu-like illness, fungal infection, pain, syncope, hypersensitivity (including, urticaria, vasculitis, ***anaphylaxis)***. **Miscellaneous:** Asymptomatic hyperbilirubinemia, food allergy, taste disorder, immune reconstitution syndrome (when given with other antiretroviral drugs). Redistribution of body fat including central obesity, dorsocervical fat enlargement ("buffalo hump"), peripheral wasting, breast enlargement, and "cushingoid appearance."

LABORATORY TEST CONSIDERATIONS

↑ Serum transaminases (ALT, AST), total serum bilirubin, serum amylase, glucose, creatinine, serum cholesterol, serum triglycerides. ↓ Hemoglobin, platelet count, neutrophils. Hyperbilirubinemia.

OVERDOSE MANAGEMENT

Symptoms: Nephrolithiasis, urolithiasis, flank pain, hematuria, N&V, diarrhea. *Treatment:* It is not known if indinavir is dialyzable by peritoneal or hemodialysis.

DRUG INTERACTIONS

NOTE: Indinavir is an inhibitor of CYP3A4; thus coadministration with drugs primarily metabolized by CYP3A4 may result in increased plasma levels of the other drug which could increase or prolong therapeutic and side effects. Also, indinavir is metabolized by CYP3A4; thus, drugs that induce CYP3A4 could increase the clearance of indinavir, resulting in lower plasma levels of indinavir. Drugs that inhibit CYP3A4 may decrease the clearance of indinavir resulting in increased indinavir plasma levels.

Aldesleukin / ↑ Plasma indinavir levels R/T ↓ liver metabolism → ↑ risk of toxicity

Alfuzosin / ↑ Alfuzosin plasma levels → hypotension; do not use together

Amiodarone / Possible ↑ amiodarone levels R/T ↓ liver metabolism; possible serious and/or life-threatening reactions, such as cardiac arrhythmias; do not use together

Amlodipine / ↑ Amlodipine AUC when given with indinavir and ritonovir R/T ↓ CYP3A metabolism of amlodipine

Aripiprazole / ↑ Aripiprazole plasma levels → ↑ risk of pharmacologic/toxic effects; monitor and adjust aripiprazole dose as needed

Atazanavir / Both drugs associated with indirect (unconjugated) hyperbilirubinemia; do not use together

Azole antifungal drugs (e.g., itraconazole, ketoconazole) / ↑ Indinavir levels → ↑ toxicity; reduce dose of indinavir to 600 mg q 8 hr

Benzodiazepines (e.g., alprazolam, midazolam, triazolam) / Possible severe sedation and respiratory depression; do not use with the three benzodiazepines listed

Bepridil / Use together with caution; monitor therapeutic levels

Bosentan / Start or adjust bosentan dose to 62.5 mg/day or every other day; monitor clinical response

Buspirone / ↑ Buspirone plasma levels → ↑ pharmacologic effects; closely monitor for new onset parkinsonism symptoms if coadministered

Calcium channel blockers (dihydropyridine-type: felodipine, nicardipine, nifedipine) / Use with caution together; monitor

Carbamazepine / ↓ Indinavir levels → ↓ effectiveness; use together with caution

Clarithromycin / ↑ Levels of both indinavir and clarithromycin → ↑ pharmacologic and toxic effects; appropriate doses of combination not determined

Cisapride / ↑ Plasma cisapride levels → ↑ risk for serious and/or life-threatening reactions (e.g., cardiac arrhythmias); do not use together

Colchicine / Do not coadminister to those with hepatic or renal impairment

Conivaptan / ↑ Plasma conivaptan levels → ↑ risk of side effects; do not give together

Corticosteroids, inhaled/nasal (e.g., fluticasone) / ↑ Plasma corticosteroid levels; monitor for signs of adrenal insufficiency

Cyclosporine / ↑ Plasma cyclosporine levels; monitor and adjust cyclosporine dose as needed

Darifenacin / ↑ Plasma darifenacin levels; if given with indinavir, do not exceed a dose of 7.5 mg/day darifenacin

Dasatinib / ↑ Plasma dasatinib levels → ↑ risk of toxicity; avoid coadministration or consider dose reduction of dasatinib

Delavirdine / ↑ Indinavir levels → ↑ pharmacologic and side effects; reduce indinavir dose to 600 mg q 8 hr when given with delavirdine, 400 mg 3 times/day

Didanosine (buffered) / pH Dependent ↓ in absorption; give at least 1 hr apart on an empty stomach

Dronedarone / ↑ Dronedarone plasma levels → ↑ pharmacologic/toxic effects; do not coadminister

Efavirenz / ↓ Indinavir levels R/T ↑ metabolism; optimal dose for coadministration not known

Eletriptan / ↑ Eletriptan plasma levels → ↑ pharmacologic/toxic effects; do not use eletriptan within 72 hr of indinavir

Eplerenone / ↑ Eplerenone plasma levels → ↑ pharmacologic/toxic effects; monitor closely and adjust eplerenone dose as needed

Ergot derivatives (dihydroergotamine, ergonovine, ergotamine, methylergonovine) / ↑ Risk of ergot toxicity (peripheral vasospasm, ischemia of the extremities); do not give together

I

Erlotinib / ↑ Erlotinib plasma levels → ↑ pharmacologic/toxic effects; monitor for side effects and adjust erlotinib dose as needed
Erythromycin / ↑ Plasma erythromycin levels → possible sudden death from cardiac causes; do not coadminister
Eszopiclone / ↑ Plasma eszopiclone levels → ↑ pharmacologic/toxic effects; monitor closely and reduce eszopiclone dose when coadministered with indinavir
Everolimus / ↑ Everolimus plasma levels →↑ pharmacologic/toxic effects; if coadministration necessary, monitor and adjust everolimus dose as needed
Fesoterodine / ↑ Fesoterodine plasma levels; do not exceed; if given with indinavir, do not exceed a dose of 4 mg/day of fesoterodine
Fluoxetine / ↑ Plasma levels of both drugs; closely monitor for side effects, including serotonin syndrome; dosage reduction of either or both drugs may be needed
H ***Garlic*** / ↓ Indinavir plasma levels → ↓ pharmacologic effects; do not use together
Grapefruit juice / Delay of time to reach indinavir peak plasma levels
HMG-CoA reductase inhibitors (e.g., atorvastatin, lovastatin, rosuvastatin, simvastatin) / ↑ Plasma levels of HMG-CoA inhibitor → ↑ risk of myopathy, including rhabdomyolysis; do not use together with lovastatin and simvastatin; use lowest possible dose of atorvastatin or rosuvastatin and monitor for side effects
Iloperidone / ↑ Iloperidone plasma levels →↑ pharmacologic effects; reduce iloperidone dose by one-half when given with indinavir; if indinavir therapy discontinued, increase iloperidone to original dose
Ixabepilone / ↑ Ixabepilone plasma levels → ↑ risk of toxicity; avoid coadministration or consider dose reduction of ixabepilone
Lapatinib / ↑ Plasma lapatinib levels → ↑ risk of toxicity; avoid coadministration or consider dose reduction of lapatinib
Lidocaine (systemic) / Use together with caution; monitor therapeutic levels
Maraviroc / ↑ Maraviroc plasma levels → ↑ pharmacologic/toxic effects; monitor and adjust maraviroc dose as needed
Nelfinavir / ↑ Indinavir concentrations; appropriate dose for coadministration not determined
Nevirapine / ↓ Indinavir levels; monitor levels and adjust dose appropriately
Nilotinib / ↑ Nilotinib plasma levels → ↑ pharmacologic effects; avoid coadministration; if they must be coadministered, consider interrupting nilotinib therapy; consult package labeling for specific recommendations
Opioid analgesics (e.g., buprenorphine, fentanyl, oxycodone) / ↑ Opioid analgesic levels → possible toxicity (severe respiratory depression); monitor and adjust opioid dose as needed
Phenobarbital / ↓ Indinavir levels → ↓ effectiveness; use together with caution
Phenytoin / ↓ Indinavir levels → ↓ effectiveness; use together with caution
Pimozide / ↑ Plasma pimozide levels R/T inhibition of CYP3A4 → ↑ risk of serious and/or life-threatening reactions; do not coadminister
Proton pump inhibitors (e.g., esomeprazole, lansoprazole, omeprazole, pantoprazole) / Possible ↓ antiviral activity of indinavir; monitor and adjust indinavir dose as needed
Quetiapine / ↑ Quetiapine plasma levels → ↑ pharmacologic/toxic effects; monitor and adjust quetiapine dose as needed
Quinidine / ↑ Indinavir levels; use together with caution; monitor therapeutic levels
Ranolazine / ↑ Plasma ranolazine levels → ↑ risk of dose-related prolongation in the QTc interval, torsades de pointes-type arrhythmias, and sudden death; do not use together
Rifabutin / ↑ Rifabutin levels and ↓ indinavir levels; ↓ rifabutin dose by 50% and increase indinavir dose to 1,000 mg q 8 hr
Rifampin / ↓ Levels of indinavir and possible resistance to indinavir or other protease inhibitor; use together is not recommended
Risperidone / ↑ Risperidone plasma levels → ↑ pharmacologic/toxic effects; monitor closely and adjust risperidone dose as needed
Ritonavir / ↑ Ritonavir levels → possible toxicity; ↑ incidence of nephrolithiasis
Romidepsin / ↑ Romidepsin plasma levels → ↑ pharmacologic/toxic effects, including QT prolongation; if coadministration necessary, close clinical lab and ECG monitoring needed
H ***St. John's wort*** / Significant ↓ indinavir levels → loss of virologic response and possible resistance to indinavir R/T ↑ liver metabolism

I

Salmeterol / ↑ Risk of CV side effects, including QT prolongation, palpitations, and sinus tachycardia; do not coadminister
Saquinavir / ↑ Saquinavir levels → ↑ pharmacologic and toxic effects
Sildenafil / ↑ Plasma sildenafil levels → severe and potentially fatal hypotension, visual changes, and priapism; do not coadminister when treating pulmonary arterial hypertension; do not exceed a sildenafil dose of 25 mg in a 48 hr period when treating erectile dysfunction
Sirolimus / ↑ Plasma sirolimus levels; monitor and adjust sirolimus dose as needed
Solifenacin / ↑ Solifenacin plasma levels; if given with indinavir, do not exceed a dose of 5 mg/day of solifenacin
Sorafenib / ↑ Plasma sorafenib levels → ↑ risk of toxicity; avoid coadministration or consider dose reduction of sorafenib
Sunitinib / ↑ Plasma sunitinib levels → ↑ risk of toxicity; avoid coadministration or consider dose reduction of sunitinib
Tacrolimus / ↑ Plasma tacrolimus levels; monitor and adjust tacrolimus dose as needed
Tadalafil / ↑ Plasma tadalafil levels → severe and potentially fatal hypotension, visual changes, and priapism; do not exceed a tadalafil dose of 10 mg in a 72 hr period
Temsirolimus / ↑ Temsirolimus plasma levels →↑ pharmacologic/toxic effects; if coadministration necessary, monitor and adjust temsirolimus dose as needed
Thyroid hormone (e.g., thyroxine) / ↑ or ↓ Serum thyroxin levels → hypo- or hyperthyroidism; monitor thyroid function when indinavir started or stopped; adjust thyroid dose as needed
Tolterodine / ↑ Tolterodine plasma levels; if given with indinavir, do not exceed a dose of 2 mg/day tolterodine
Tolvaptan / ↑ Plasma tolvaptan levels → ↑ risk of side effects; do not give together
Trazodone / ↑ Trazodone levels → ↑ pharmacologic and toxic effects (e.g., dizziness, hypotension, syncope); monitor and adjust trazodone dose as needed
Vardenafil / ↑ Plasma vardenafil levels → severe and potentially fatal hypotension, visual changes, and priapism; do not exceed a vardenafil dose of 2.5 mg in a 24 hr period
Warfarin / ↓ Anticoagulant effect of warfarin; monitor coagulation parameters when indinavir is started or stopped; adjust warfarin dose as needed

HOW SUPPLIED
Capsules: 100 mg, 200 mg, 400 mg.

DOSAGE

CAPSULES
HIV infections.

Adults: 800 mg (two 400 mg capsules) q 8 hr ATC. The dosage is the same whether the drug is used alone or in combination with other retroviral agents (except when noted as follows). **Children, 3–18 years:** Although optimal dosing regimens have not been determined in children, a dose of 500 mg/m^2 (maximum of 800 mg/dose) q 8 hr has been studied.

NURSING IMPLICATIONS

IMPLEMENTATION/ADMINISTRATION/STORAGE
1. Clients should drink at least 1.5 L (about 48 oz) of liquids/24 hr.
2. Modify dosage or dosage schedule when indinivir is taken with the following drugs:
   - **Delavirdine:** Consider reducing dose of indinivir to 600 mg q 8 hr when given with delavirdine, 400 mg 3 times per day.
   - **Didanosine:** If indinavir and didanosine are given together, give at least 1 hr apart on an empty stomach.
   - **Itraconazole:** Reduce dose of indinavir to 600 mg q 8 hr when taken with itraconazole, 200 mg twice a day.
   - **Ketoconazole:** Reduce dose of indinavir to 600 mg q 8 hr when taken with ketoconazole.
   - **Rifabutin:** When taken with rifabutin, reduce the dose of rifabutin to one-half the standard dose and increase the indinavir dose to 1,000 mg q 8 hr.
3. In mild to moderate hepatic insufficiency due to cirrhosis, reduce indinavir dosage to 600 mg q 8 hr.
4. In those with nephrolithiasis or urolithiasis, therapy may have to be interrupted temporarily (1–3 days) or discontinued even with adequate hydration.

5. The optimal dosing regimen for use during pregnancy or in children not established.
6. Capsules are moisture sensitive. Store in original container; keep desiccant in the bottle. Keep tightly closed, protected from moisture and at a room temperature of 15–30°C (59–86°F).

ASSESSMENT

1. Note symptom onset, confirmation of HIV, other agents trialed, outcome.
2. Review list of drugs currently prescribed to ensure none interact.
3. Assess for S&S of nephrolithiasis/urolithiasis (including flank pain with/without hematuria). With asymptomatic severe leukocyturia frequently monitor with U/A.
4. Monitor CD4 count, CBC, viral load, LFTs and blood glucose levels closely; new-onset diabetes or exacerbation of pre-existing diabetes associated with protease inhibitor therapy. Anticipate reduced dosage with impaired liver function; drug is hepatically metabolized.

CLIENT/FAMILY TEACHING

1. Take as prescribed at 8 hr intervals ATC with water 1 hr before or 2 hr after meals for optimal absorption. May be taken with other liquids, such as skim milk, juice, coffee, or tea, or with a light meal (e.g., dry toast with jelly, juice, and coffee with skim milk and sugar; or corn flakes, skim milk, and sugar). Avoid grapefruit juice, foods high in calories, fat, or protein.
2. Drug is not to be used alone but is combined with other antiviral agents.
3. If also taking didanosine, must take on an empty stomach 1 hr apart.
4. The original desiccant must be dispensed with the medication. Store drug in original container, tightly closed, at room temperature away from moisture.
5. If a dose is missed by more than 2 hr, wait and take the next dose at the regularly scheduled time. If a dose is missed by less than 2 hr, take immediately.
6. May cause dizziness or drowsiness; avoid activities that require mental alertness until drug effects realized. With diabetes check BS frequently and report loss of control.
7. To ensure adequate hydration, drink at least 1.5 L of liquids during a 24 hr period. Report any symptoms of kidney stones (e.g., flank pain with or without blood); therapy should be interrupted for 1–3 days.
8. Drug is not a cure for HIV; continue to take precautions with disease transmission; opportunistic infections may occur.
9. Use reliable birth control and barrier protection; drug does not decrease the risk of transmitting disease through sexual contact or blood contamination. Do not breast-feed; could cause HIV infection in the baby.
10. If using Viagra, may experience adverse side effects: drop in BP, visual changes, and prolonged erection requiring medical attention; do not exceed 25 mg in 48 hr.
11. Report severe N&V, diarrhea, fever, chills, personality changes or changes in the color of urine or stool. May cause changes in body fat distribution (e.g., ↑ amount of fat in upper back and neck, breasts, and around the back, chest and stomach area; or loss of fat from arms, legs and face).
12. Keep all F/U to assess response, labs, and for adverse SE.

OUTCOMES/EVALUATE

Interference with progression of HIV infection

■ IV ©

Indomethacin

(in-doh-**METH**-ah-sin)

Classification(s): Nonsteroidal anti-inflammatory drug

Pregnancy Category: C (do not use late in pregnancy due to possible premature closure of ductus arteriosus)

RX: Indocin, Indomethacin Extended-Release, Indomethacin SR.

🍁 **Rx:** Apo-Indomethacin, ratio-Indomethacin.

Indomethacin sodium trihydrate

RX: Indocin IV.

SEE ALSO ***NONSTEROIDAL ANTI-INFLAMMATORY DRUGS***.

INDICATIONS/USES

Not a simple analgesic; use only for the conditions listed. Carefully consider the benefits and risks and other treatment options before deciding to use indomethacin. Use the lowest effective dose for the shortest duration.

PO: (1) Moderate to severe rheumatoid arthritis (including acute flares of chronic disease). (2) Moderate-to-severe osteoarthritis. (3) Moderate-to-severe ankylosing spondylitis. (4) Acute painful shoulder (tendinitis, bursitis). (5) Acute gouty arthritis (Immediate-Release Capsules and Oral Suspension only). *Investigational:* Premature labor.

Rectal: (1) Moderate to severe rheumatoid arthritis, including acute flares of chronic disease. (2) Moderate to severe osteoarthritis. (3) Acute gouty arthritis. (4) Moderate to severe ankylosing spondylitis. (5) Acute painful shoulder (bursitis, tendinitis). *Investigational:* Premature labor.

IV: To close hemodynamically significant patent ductus arteriosus in premature infants weighing between 500 and 1750 grams if, after 48 hr, usual medical management is ineffective.

ACTION/KINETICS

Action

Anti-inflammatory effect is likely due to inhibition of cyclo-oxygenase. Inhibition of cyclo-oxygenase results in decreased prostaglandin synthesis. Effective in reducing joint swelling, pain, and morning stiffness, as well as to increase mobility in those with inflammatory disease. Indomethacin does not alter the course of the disease, however.

Pharmacokinetics

PO. Onset: 30 min for analgesia and up to 1 week for anti-inflammatory effect. Is 98% bioavailable. **Peak plasma levels:** 1–2 hr (2–4 hr for sustained-release). **Peak action for gout:** 24–36 hr; swelling gradually disappears in 3–5 days. **Peak activity for antirheumatic effect:** About 4 weeks. **Duration:** 4–6 hr for analgesia and 1–2 weeks for anti-inflammatory effect. **Therapeutic plasma levels:** 10–18 mcg/mL. **t½:** Approximately 5 hr (up to 6 hr for sustained-release). Metabolized in the liver and excreted in both urine and feces. **Plasma protein binding:** Approximately 90%.

ADDITIONAL CONTRAINDICATIONS

Pregnancy and lactation. PO indomethacin in children under 14 years of age. GI lesions or history of recurrent GI lesions. **IV use:** GI or intracranial bleeding, thrombocytopenia, renal disease, defects of coagulation, necrotizing enterocolitis. **Suppositories:** Recent rectal bleeding, history of proctitis.

SPECIAL CONCERNS

(1) **Cardiovascular risk.** NSAIDs may cause an increased risk of serious CV thrombotic events, MI, and stroke, which can be fatal. This risk may increase with duration of use. Clients with CV disease or risk factors for CV disease may be at a greater risk. (2) Indomethacin is contraindicated for treatment of perioperative pain in the setting of coronary artery bypass graft surgery. (3) **GI risks.** NSAIDs cause an increased risk of serious GI adverse reactions including bleeding, ulceration, and perforation of the stomach or intestines, which can be fatal. These reactions can occur at any time during use and without warning symptoms. Elderly clients are at greater risk for serious GI events.

- Restrict use in children to those unresponsive to or intolerant of other anti-inflammatory agents; efficacy not determined in children less than 14 years of age.
- Elderly are at greater risk of developing CNS side effects, especially confusion.
- Use with caution in clients with history of epilepsy, psychiatric illness, or parkinsonism.
- Use with extreme caution in the presence of existing, controlled infections.

ADDITIONAL SIDE EFFECTS

Most Common

After PO: Headache, dizziness, N&V, diarrhea, constipation, dyspepsia/indigestion, GI distress, tinnitus.

After IV: Renal dysfunction in infants, GI bleeding, elevated serum potassium, fluid retention, hyponatremia, intracranial bleeding, retrolental fibroplasia.

See also *Nonsteroidal Anti-Inflammatory Drugs* for a complete list of possible side effects. Also, reactivation of latent infections may mask signs of infection. More marked CNS manifestations than for other drugs of this group. Aggravation of depression or other psychiatric problems, epilepsy, and parkinsonism.

ADDITIONAL DRUG INTERACTIONS

Captopril / ↓ Captopril effect, probably R/T prostaglandin synthesis inhibition

Diflunisal / ↑ Plasma levels of indomethacin; also, possible fatal GI hemorrhage
Digitalis / Digitalis t½ maybe further prolonged in premature infants
Diuretics (loop, potassium-sparing, thiazide) / May reduce antihypertensive and natriuretic action of diuretics
Furosemide / Indomethacin may blunt natriuretic effect of furosemide
Lisinopril / Possible ↓ lisinopril effect
Losartan / ↓ Antihypertensive effect of losartan
Prazosin / ↓ Antihypertensive drug effects

HOW SUPPLIED

Indomethacin. *Capsules:* 25 mg, 50 mg; *Capsules, Sustained-Release:* 75 mg; *Oral Suspension:* 25 mg/5 mL; *Suppositories:* 50 mg.
Indomethacin sodium trihydrate. *Injection, Lyophilized Powder for Solution:* 1 mg.

I

DOSAGE

Indomethacin

CAPSULES; ORAL SUSPENSION; SUPPOSITORIES

Moderate to severe rheumatoid arthritis (including acute flares), osteoarthritis, or ankylosing spondylitis.

Adults, initial: 25 mg 2–3 times per day; may be increased by 25–50 mg at weekly intervals, according to condition and if tolerated until satisfactory response is obtained. With persistent night pain or morning stiffness, a maximum of 100 mg of the total daily dose can be given at bedtime either PO or rectally. **Maximum daily dosage:** 200 mg. In acute flares of chronic rheumatoid arthritis, the dose may need to be increased by 25–50 mg/day until the acute phase is under control.

Acute gouty arthritis.

Adults, initial: 50 mg 3 times per day until pain is tolerable; **then,** reduce dosage rapidly until drug is withdrawn. Pain relief usually occurs within 2–4 hr, tenderness and heat subside in 24–36 hr, and swelling disappears in 3–4 days. Use only Capsules, Oral Suspension, or Suppositories.

Acute painful shoulder (bursitis/tendinitis).

Adults and children 15 years and older: 75–150 mg/day in 3 to 4 divided doses for 1–2 weeks. Discontinue after signs and symptoms of inflammation have been controlled for several days. Usual course of therapy: 7 to 14 days.

Juvenile rheumatoid arthritis.

Initial: 2 mg/kg/day given in divided doses, up to a maximum of 4 mg/kg/day or 150–200 mg/day, whichever is less. As symptoms subside, reduce the total daily dose to the lowest level required to control symptoms, or discontinue the drug.

CAPSULES, EXTENDED-RELEASE

Moderate to severe rheumatoid arthritis, osteoarthritis, and ankylosing spondylitis.

Adults and children 15 years and older: 75 mg, of which 25 mg is released immediately, 1–2 times per day.

Acute painful shoulder (bursitis, tendinitis).

Adults and children, 15 years and older: 150 mg two times per day. Discontinue after signs and symptoms of inflammation have been controlled for several days. Usual course of therapy: 7 to 14 days.

Indomethacin sodium trihydrate

IV

Closure of patent ductus arteriosus.

A course of therapy is defined as 3 IV doses given 12–24 hr apart. Dose according to age as follows:

Age at first dose, <48 hr: First dose is 0.2 mg/kg; doses two and three are 0.1 mg/kg. **Age at first dose, 2–7 days:** All three doses are 0.2 mg/kg. **Age at first dose, >7 days:** First dose is 0.2 mg/kg; doses two and three are 0.25 mg/kg.

NURSING IMPLICATIONS

Do not confuse Indocin with Minocin (an antibiotic).

IMPLEMENTATION/ADMINISTRATION/STORAGE

1. **If indomethacin is used for pediatric clients 2 years of age or older, monitor closely, including periodic assessment of liver function. If in-**

domethacin is initiated, a suggested starting dose is 2 mg/kg/day, in divided doses. Maximum daily dose should not exceed 4 mg/kg/day or 150–200 mg/day, which is less. As symptoms subside, reduce the dose to the lowest level needed to control symptoms, or discontinue the drug.

2. The ER capsules can be given once a day and can be substituted for the 25 mg capsules 3 times per day. However, significant differences will be noted between the 2 dosage regimens in indomethacin blood levels, especially after 12 hours. The ER capsules can also be substituted for the 50 mg capsules 3 times a day.
3. Do not crush sustained-release form; do not use sustained-release form for acute gouty arthritis.
4. With dysphagia, the capsule contents may be emptied into applesauce, food, or liquid to ensure that client receives the prescribed dose.
5. Use smallest effective dose, based on individual need. Adverse reactions are dose related.
6. Do not use in conjunction with aspirin or other salicylates as such a combination does not produce any greater therapeutic effect and the incidence of GI side effects significantly increases.
7. Capsules: Store from 15–30°C (59–86°F). Protect from light. Dispense in a tight, light-resistant container using a child-resistant container.
8. Extended-Release Capsules: Store from 15–30°C (59–86°F). Protect from moisture.
9. Oral Suspension: Store below 30°C (86°F). Avoid temperatures above 50°C (122°F). Protect from freezing.
10. IV If the ductus arteriosus closes or is significantly reduced in size after 48 hr or more from completion of the first course, no further doses are needed. If the ductus arteriosus reopens, a second course of 1 to 3 doses may be given; separate each dose by 12 to 24 hr.
11. Prepare the IV solution with 1–2 mL of sodium chloride 0.9% or water for injection. All diluents should be preservative free.
12. COMPATIBILITY 0.9% NaCl or water for injection.
13. INCOMPATIBILITY Administer separately.

ASSESSMENT

1. List reasons for therapy, onset, characteristics of S&S, other agents prescribed.
2. Assess involved joint(s), including goniometric measurements, ROM, functional ability, swelling, erosion, erythema, pain level; note x-ray/CT/MRI findings.
3. Note any GI dysfunction and assess for GI bleeding.
4. Check for CV disease or risk factors; may cause an increased risk of serious CV thrombotic events, MI, and stroke, which can be fatal. Risk may increase with length of therapy or existing CV disease.
5. Monitor heart sounds, US, and respiratory status throughout therapy with patent ductus arteriosus.
6. Note BP, U/A, CBC, uric acid, renal and LFTs; avoid with severe renal impairment.

CLIENT/FAMILY TEACHING

1. Take all dosage forms (capsules, oral suspension, SR capsules) with food, milk, or antacids immediately after meals to decrease GI upset. Do not crush or break capsules; may sprinkle capsule contents on food if unable to swallow.
2. Use caution when operating potentially hazardous equipment; may cause drowsiness, lightheadedness and decreased alertness.
3. If serious adverse side effects, withhold drug and report, since many may be serious enough to stop therapy. Seek immediate care with chest pain, SOB, breathing problems, abnormal bruising/bleeding, slurred speech, swelling of the face or throat, bleeding, or weakness in one part or on one side of body.
4. Record weights, especially if N/V occur; report any abdominal pain or diarrhea.
5. Indomethacin masks infections; report any S&S of infection or fever.
6. Avoid alcohol and OTC agents without approval.
7. It will take from 2 to 4 days with gout flare and 2 to 4 weeks with arthritic conditions before significant improvement is evident. Follow prescribed dosing regimen carefully.
8. Keep all F/U to assess response, labs, eye exams, and adverse SE.

OUTCOMES/EVALUATE

- ↓ Pain and inflammation; ↑ joint mobility
- Relief from gout flare
- Therapeutic serum drug levels (10–18 mcg/mL)
- Closure of patent ductus arteriosus (IV)

IV

Infliximab

(in-**FLIX**-ih-mab)

Classification(s): Treatment of Crohn's disease; antiarthritic

Pregnancy Category: B

RX: Remicade.

INDICATIONS/USES

(1) In adults and children to reduce S&S and inducing and maintaining clinical remission of moderate to severe Crohn's disease unresponsive to conventional therapy. (2) Long-term use in adults to reduce the number of draining enterocutaneous fistulas and rectovaginal fistulas and to maintain fistula closure in adults with fistulizing Crohn's disease. (3) With methotrexate to reduce signs and symptoms, inhibiting the progression of structural damage, and improving physical function in clients with moderate-to-severely active rheumatoid arthritis. (4) Reduce S&S in active ankylosing spondylitis. (5) Reduce signs and symptoms of active arthritis in those with psoriatic arthritis to inhibit the progression of structural damage and improve physical function. (6) Reduce signs and symptoms, achieve clinical remission and mucosal healing, and eliminate corticosteroid use in those with moderately to severely active ulcerative colitis who have had an inadequate response to conventional therapy. (7) Treat adults with chronic, severe (i.e., extensive and/or disabling), plaque psoriasis who are candidates for systemic therapy and when other systemic therapies are less appropriate. Only administer to those who will be monitored closely and have regular follow-up visits to their health care provider. *Investigational:* Behçet syndrome uveitis, celiac sprue, suppurative hidradenitis in adults, pyoderma gangrenosum; uveitis in adults, adolescents, and children; Wegener granulomatosis.

ACTION/KINETICS

Action

Chimeric IgG1$_K$ monoclonal antibody produced by a recombinant cell line. Acts by neutralizing the biological activity of TNF-alpha by high-affinity binding to its soluble and transmembrane forms and inhibits TNF-alpha receptor binding. In rheumatoid arthritis, infliximab reduces infiltration of inflammatory cells in inflamed areas of the joint, as well as expression of molecules mediating cellular adhesion. In Crohn's disease, infliximab reduces infiltration of inflammatory cells and TNF-alpha production in inflamed areas of the intestine and reduces the proportion of mononuclear cells from the lamina propria able to express TNF-alpha and interferon.

Pharmacokinetics

t½, terminal: 7.7–9.5 days. No systemic accumulation of drug occurs. Development of antibodies increases infliximab clearance.

CONTRAINDICATIONS

Hypersensitivity to any component of the product or to murine proteins. Lactation. Administration of doses greater than 5 mg/kg to those with moderate to severe heart failure (NYHA Class III/IV). CHF or in those with a clinically important, active infection. Readministration to those who have experienced a severe hypersensitivity reaction to the drug. Concurrent use with live vaccines (e.g., measles, mumps, oral polio) as vaccinations may be less effective.

SPECIAL CONCERNS

(1) **Risk of infections.** Clients treated with infliximab are at increased risk for developing serious infections that may lead to hospitalization or death. Most clients who developed these infections were taking concomitant immunosuppressants such as methotrexate or corticosteroids. Discontinue infliximab if a client develops a serious infection or sepsis. (2) Reported infections include: (a) Active tuberculosis (TB), including reactivation of latent TB. Clients with TB have frequently presented with disseminated or extrapulmonary disease. Test clients for latent TB before infliximab use and during therapy. Initiate treatment for latent infection prior to infliximab use. (b) Invasive fungal infections, including histoplasmosis, coccidiodomycosis, candidiasis, aspergillosis, blastomycosis, and pneumocytosis. Clients with histoplasmosis or other invasive fungal infections may present with disseminated, rather than localized, disease. Antigen and antibody testing for histoplasmosis may be negative in some clients with active infection. Empiric antifungal therapy

should be considered in clients who develop severe systemic illness. (c) Bacterial, viral, and other infections caused by opportunistic pathogens. (3) Carefully consider the risks and benefits of treatment with infliximab prior to initiating therapy in clients with long-term or recurrent infection. (4) Carefully monitor clients for the development of signs and symptoms of infection during and after treatment with infliximab, including the possible development of TB in clients who tested negative for latent TB infection prior to initiating therapy. (5) **Malignancy.** Lymphoma and other malignancies, some fatal, have been reported in children and adolescent clients treated with tumor necrosis factor (TNF) blockers, including infliximab. (6) Postmarketing cases of hepatosplenic T-cell lymphoma, a rare type of T-cell lymphoma, have been reported in clients treated with TNF blockers, including infliximab. These cases had a very aggressive disease course, and have been fatal. All reported infliximab cases have occurred in clients with Crohn's disease or ulcerative colitis, and the majority were in adolescent and young adult males. All of these clients received treatment with azathioprine or 6-mercaptopurine concomitantly with infliximab at or prior to diagnosis.

- **Use with caution in the elderly (due to increased incidence of infections in this group) and in, or pre-existing or recent-onset, CNS demyelinating or seizure disorders. Use caution in clients being treated with infliximab who have ongoing or histories of significant hematologic abnormalities.**
- **Serious infections, including sepsis and death, have occurred in those treated with TNF-blocking agents. Thus, use with caution in clients with a chronic infection or a history of recurrent infection, or in mild heart failure.**
- **May worsen CHF.**
- **Those with Crohn's disease or rheumatoid arthritis, especially those with highly active disease or chronic exposure to immunosuppressant therapies, may be at a higher risk for the development of lymphoma.**
- **Use caution when considering use of infliximab in those with moderate to severe COPD.**
- **Use caution when considering resumption of infliximab following reactivation of hepatitis B.**
- **Safety and efficacy not determined for use in children less than 6 years of age with Crohn's disease; also, safety and efficacy not determined in children with juvenile rheumatoid arthritis, ulcerative colitis, or plaque psoriasis.**

SIDE EFFECTS

Most Common

Adults: URTI, nausea, headache, diarrhea, abdominal pain, pharyngitis, sinusitis, coughing, bronchitis, pain, fatigue, rash, dyspepsia, UTI, arthralgia.

Children (for Crohn's disease): Anemia, blood in stool, flushing, leukopenia, infections (URTI, pharyngitis, abscess, viral), bone fracture, neutropenia, respiratory tract allergic reactions.

Infusion-related, mild to severe (during infusion or within 2 hr post-infusion): Flu-like symptoms, headache, dyspnea, hypotension, transient fever, chills, GI symptoms, skin rashes, anaphylaxis (may occur anytime during infusion). **Hypersensitivity:** Urticaria, dyspnea, hypotension, serum sickness-like reactions (e.g., fever, rash, headache, sore throat, myalgias, polyarthralgias, hand and facial edema, dysphagia), ***layrngeal/pharyngeal edema, severe bronchospasms, anaphylaxis (including laryngeal/pharyngeal edema, severe bronchospasm, seizures)***. **Infections (bacterial, fungal, protozoal, viral):** Pneumonia, sinusitis, pharyngitis, bronchitis, UTIs, cellulitis, infection at CNS venous catheter, abscess, skin ulceration, ***sepsis***, cholecystitis, endophthalmitis, aspergillosis, candidiasis, coccidioidomycosis, furunculosis, histoplasmosis, listeriosis, nocardiosis, cytomegalovirus, pneumocytosis, tuberculosis (disseminated or extrapulmonary) either reactivation or new, invasive fungal infections, other opportunistic infections. **GI:** N&V, diarrhea, abdominal pain, constipation, dyspepsia, flatulence, intestinal obstruction, oral pain, ulcerative stomatitis, toothache, ***GI hemorrhage***, ileus, ***intestinal perforation***, intestinal stenosis, pancreatitis, peritonitis, proctaliga. **Hepatic:** ***Acute liver failure***, jaundice, hepatitis, autoimmune hepatitis, cholestasis, biliary pain, cholecystitis, cholelithiasis, hepatotoxicity, hepatitis B reactivation. **CNS:** Headache, dizziness, paresthesia, vertigo, anxiety, depression, insomnia, optic neuritis, ***seizures***, multiple sclerosis, CNS manifestations of systemic vasculitis, confusion, meningitis, neuritis, peripheral neuropathy, ***suicide attempt***. **Neurologic:** Optic neuritis, seizures, new onset or worsening of CNS demyelinating disorders (as multiple sclerosis, neuropathies, Guillain-Barré syndrome, chronic inflammatory demyelinating polyneuropathy, multifocal motor neuropathy). **CV:** Hypotension, hypertension, tachycardia, ***worsening heart failure (may be fatal)***, arrhythmia, bradycardia, brain infarction, ***cardiac arrest, circulatory failure, MI, pulmonary embolism***, syncope, thrombophlebitis, systemic and cutaneous vasculitis, thrombotic thrombocytopenic purpura, ***pericardial effusion***. **Dermatologic:** Rash, pruritus, acne, alopecia, fungal dermatitis, eczema, erythema, erythema multiforme, erythematous/maculopapular rash, papular rash, dry skin, increased sweating, ulceration, urticaria, ecchymoses, flushing, hematoma, erythema multiforme, new onset and worsening psoriasis (including pustular, primarily palmar/plantar), ***Stevens-Johnson syndrome, toxic epidermal necrolysis.*** **Hematologic:** Leukopenia, neutropenia, thrombocytopenia, anemia, idiopathic thrombocytopenic purpura, lymphadenopathy, thrombotic thrombocytopenic purpura, ***hemolytic anemia, pancytopenia***. **GU:** Dysuria, micturition frequency, UTIs, menstrual irregularity, renal calculus, renal failure, moniliasis. **Musculoskeletal:** Myalgia, back pain, arthralgia, arthritis, intervertebral disk herniation, tendon disorder, transverse myelitis. **Respiratory:** Dyspnea, URTI, pharyngitis, bronchitis, rhinitis, coughing, sinusitis, laryngitis, respiratory tract allergic reaction, ARDS, lower RTI (including pneumonia), pleural effusion, pleurisy, pulmonary edema, ***pulmonary embolism***, respiratory insufficiency, interstitial pneumonitis/fibrosis. **Body as a whole:** Fatigue, fever, pain, chills, peripheral edema, fall, hot flashes, malaise, flu syndrome, dehydration, edema. **Miscellaneous:** Moniliasis, chest pain, abscess, cellulitis, conjunctivitis, diaphragmatic hernia, ***malignancies*** (Hodgkin's and non-Hodgkin's lymphoma, ***hepatosplenic T-cell lymphomas***, acute and chronic leukemia, melanoma, nonmelanoma skin cancers, colorectal, and breast), cellulitis, ***sepsis***, serum sickness, diaphragmatic hernia, lymphoproliferative disorders (including lymphoma), lymphoadenopathy, lupus-like syndrome, surgical/procedural sequelae.

Serious side effects in children include opportunistic infections and TB, malignancies (including hepatosplenic T-cell lymphomas), transient hepatic enzyme abnormalities, lupus-like syndrome, hypersensitivity reactions, and development of autoantibodies.

NOTE: Possible formation of autoimmune antibodies (anti-dsDNA antibodies); development of lupus-like syndrome. Retreatment after an extended treatment-free period may cause delayed, potentially serious side effects. Symptoms include fever, myalgia, polyarthralgia, pruritus, rash and, less frequently, facial or hand edema, dysphagia, urticaria, sore throat, and headache. Use of acetaminophen, antihistamines, corticosteroids, or epinephrine helps the symptoms.

LABORATORY TEST CONSIDERATIONS

↑ ALT, AST.

DRUG INTERACTIONS

Abatacept / Possible ↑ rate of infection; concurrent use not recommended

Anakinra / Possible ↑ risk of neutropenia and serious infections

Azathioprine and 6-Mercaptopurine / Possible hepatosplenic T-cell lymphoma in adolescents and young adults with Crohn's disease; occurs in those treated with infliximab, azathioprine, and 6-mercaptopurine

Etanercept / ↑ Risk of neutropenia

TNF blockers (e.g., adalimumab, certolizumab, etanercept, golimumab) / ↑ Risk of serious infections; avoid coadministration

Tocilizumab / ↑ Risk of serious infections; avoid coadministration

HOW SUPPLIED

Injection, Lyophilized Powder for Solution: 100 mg.

DOSAGE

IV

Moderate to severe Crohn's disease or fistulizing Crohn's disease.

Adults, induction: 5 mg/kg IV at 0, 2, and 6 weeks followed by maintenance of 5 mg/kg q 8 weeks thereafter. If response is lost, consider 10 mg/kg. Those who do not respond by week 14 are not likely to respond with continued dosing; consider discontinuing infliximab. **Children, 6 years and older:** 5 mg/kg IV at 0, 2, and 6 weeks followed by a maintenance regimen of 5 mg/kg q 8 weeks.

Rheumatoid arthritis.

Adults: 3 mg/kg followed by additional similar doses at 2 and 6 weeks; then, q 8 weeks thereafter. If response is incomplete, may adjust the dose up to 10 mg/kg or treat as often as q 4 weeks. *NOTE:* The risk of serious infections is increased at higher doses. Give infliximab in combination with methotrexate.

Ankylosing spondylitis.

Adults: 5 mg/kg by IV infusion, followed by additional similar doses at 2 and 6 weeks after the first infusion. Then, give every 6 weeks thereafter.

Psoriatic arthritis.

Adults, usual: 5 mg/kg by IV infusion, followed by additional similar doses 2 and 6 weeks after the first infusion, and every 8 weeks thereafter. Can be used with or without methotrexate.

Ulcerative colitis, moderate to severe.

Adults, initial, induction: 5 mg/kg at 0, 2, and 6 weeks, followed by a maintenance regimen of 5 mg/kg q 8 weeks thereafter.

Plaque psoriasis.

Adults: 5 mg/kg as an IV infusion followed by additional similar doses at 2 and 6 weeks after the first infusion; then, q 8 weeks thereafter. Infliximab can be used with or without methotrexate.

NURSING IMPLICATIONS

IMPLEMENTATION/ADMINISTRATION/STORAGE

1. IV To prevent and minimize infusion reactions, premedicate with antihistamines (H_1-antihistamines with or without H_2-antihistamines), acetaminophen, and/or corticosteroids. Discontinue treatment in those who experience severe infusion-related reactions.
2. Shortening the dosing interval may work as well (or better) than increasing the dose in those who do not respond to the dosage regimen of 3 mg/kg q 8 weeks for treating arthritis.
3. Do not give more than 5 mg/kg to clients with CHF.
4. Use vials immediately after reconstitution as there is no preservative. Do not reuse or store any unused portion of the infusion solution.
5. Infliximab solution is incompatible with PVC equipment or devices. Prepare only in glass infusion bottles or polypropylene or polyolefin infusion bags. Infuse through polyethylene-lined infusion sets.
6. Calculate total amount of reconstituted solution required. Reconstitute each vial with 10 mL sterile water for injection using a syringe equipped with a 21-gauge or smaller needle. Direct stream of water to the glass wall of the vial. Gently swirl solution by rotating the vial to dissolve contents. Do not shake; some foaming is usual. Allow reconstituted solution to stand for 5 min.
7. The solution should be colorless to light yellow and opalescent; a few translucent particles (protein) may develop. Inspect for particulate matter and discoloration prior to administration. If there are visible opaque particles, discoloration, or other foreign particulates, do not use solution.
8. Dilute reconstituted infliximab dose to a total of 250 mL with 0.9% NaCl injection. Slowly add reconstituted solution to the 250 mL infusion bag/bottle. Mix gently.
9. Administer for 2 or more hours using an in-line, sterile, nonpyrogenic, low protein-binding filter (1.2 mcg or less pore size).
10. Store the lyophilized product at 2–8°C (36–46°F). Do not freeze. Product contains no preservative.
11. COMPATIBILITY Sterile water for injection, 0.9% NaCl.
12. INCOMPATIBILITY Do not infuse concomitantly in the same IV line with other agents.

ASSESSMENT

1. Note disease onset, surgeries, previous treatments trialed. List medical conditions that may preclude therapy. In those with worsening CHF, stop infliximab.
2. List stool frequency and consistency with Crohn's disease. Assess abdomen; note pain levels, mucus production. With fistulas, assess number, size, amount, type of drainage.
3. With arthritis, assess characteristics of involved joint(s), including goniometric mea-

surements, ROM, functional ability, swelling, erythema. Rate pain levels.
4. Do not initiate treatment with active infection; use caution in those with chronic infection or history of recurrent infection.
5. Evaluate for tuberculosis risk factors and latent tuberculosis; drug quadruples risk of TB so test prior to starting therapy.
6. Update immunizations prior to starting infliximab therapy.
7. Consider cessation of therapy when significant infections, hematologic or CNS side effects occur.
8. Evaluate liver enzyme levels in those seropositive for hepatitis B surface antigen before beginning infliximab therapy and during treatment.
9. Monitor VS, renal and LFTs. Malignancy has been observed in some clients receiving this therapy.

CLIENT/FAMILY TEACHING

1. Drug is for short-term therapy. Infusion-related symptoms, i.e., headache, fever, itching, nausea, and pain may be managed with antihistamines, acetaminophen, corticosteroids, and/or epinephrine.
2. With prolonged symptoms and diffuse disease in ulcerative colitis, surgical intervention may improve quality of life and prevent increased mortality.
3. Infliximab may cause dizziness; use caution while driving or performing other tasks requiring alertness, coordination, or physical dexterity.
4. Report any new or worsening symptoms of heart failure (e.g., shortness of breath, swelling of ankles/feet) or infections.
5. Do not receive live vaccines while undergoing infliximab therapy.
6. Keep all F/U visits to assess response, labs, and for adverse SE.

OUTCOMES/EVALUATE

- ↓ Number of draining enterocutaneous fistulas in fistulizing Crohn's disease
- Control of arthritis pain with improved mobility
- ↓ S&S active psoriatic arthritis
- Control severe plaque psoriasis

Insulin aspart

(**IN**-sue-lin **AS**-part)

Classification(s): Insulin, rDNA origin

Pregnancy Category: C

RX: NovoLog, Novolog Mix 70/30.

♣ **Rx:** NovoRapid.

SEE ALSO ***ANTIDIABETIC AGENTS: INSULINS***.

INDICATIONS/USES

Treat diabetes mellitus in adults and children (ages 2–18 years). Due to the short duration of action, use with an intermediate or long-acting insulin. Novolog can be given by continuous SC infusion via an external pump in children between age 4 and 18 years. *NOTE:* Insulin aspart is the only insulin analog approved for use in external pump systems for continuous SC insulin infusion.

ACTION/KINETICS

Action

Rapid-acting. Is homologous with regular human insulin except for a single substitution of the amino acid proline by aspartic acid in position B28. This reduces the tendency of the molecule to form hexamers as with regular human insulin.

Pharmacokinetics

Has a faster absorption, faster onset, and shorter duration than regular human insulin after SC use. **Onset:** 15 min. **Peak:** 2.2 hr. **Duration:** 3–5 hr. **t½:** 90 min (compared with 141 min for regular human insulin). *NOTE:* Novolog Mix 70/30 contains 70% insulin aspart protamine suspension and 30% insulin aspart. **Onset:** 15–20 min. **Peak:** 2.4 hr. **Duration:** 1–24 hr.

SPECIAL CONCERNS

- Use with caution during lactation.
- Safety and efficacy of Novolog 70/30 not established in children.

SIDE EFFECTS

Most Common

Hypoglycemia, hypokalemia, injection site reaction, lipodystrophy, pruritus, rash.

See *Antidiabetic Agents: Insulins* for a complete list of possible side effects.

LABORATORY TEST CONSIDERATIONS

Small, but persistent ↑ in alkaline phosphatase.

DRUG INTERACTIONS

ACE inhibitors / ↑ Blood glucose lowering effect and susceptibility to hypoglycemia

Clonidine / Either potentiate or weaken blood-glucose lowering effect of insulin
Danazol / ↓ Blood glucose lowering effect
Disopyramide / ↑ Blood glucose lowering effect and susceptibility to hypoglycemia
Diuretics / ↓ Blood glucose lowering effect
Fluoxetine / ↑ Blood glucose lowering effect and susceptibility to hypoglycemia
Isoniazid / ↓ Blood glucose lowering effect
Lithium salts / Either potentiate or weaken blood-glucose lowering effect of insulin
MAOIs / ↑ Blood glucose lowering effect and susceptibility to hypoglycemia
Niacin / ↓ Blood glucose lowering effect
Octreotide / ↑ Blood glucose lowering effect and susceptibility to hypoglycemia
Salicylates / ↑ Blood glucose lowering effect and susceptibility to hypoglycemia
Somatropin / ↓ Blood glucose lowering effect
Sulfonamides / ↑ Blood glucose lowering effect and susceptibility to hypoglycemia

HOW SUPPLIED

Injection Solution (Novolog): 100 units/mL; *Injection (NovoLog Mix 70/30):* 100 units/mL (70% insulin aspart protamine suspension and 30% insulin aspart).

DOSAGE

Novolog

SC DAILY INJECTIONS

Diabetes mellitus.

Individualized. **Adults and children, 2 years and older:** The total daily individual insulin dosage requirement is usually between 0.5–1 unit/kg/day. About 50–70% may be provided by insulin aspart and the rest by an intermediate- or long-acting insulin. Clients may require more basal insulin and more total insulin when using insulin aspart compared with regular insulin; additional basal insulin injections may be required.

SC CONTINUOUS INFUSION BY EXTERNAL INFUSION PUMP

Diabetes mellitus.

Adults and children, 4 years and older: Base initial programming of the pump based on the total daily insulin dose of the previous regimen. There is significant interclient variability; however, about 50% of the total dose is usually given as meal-related boluses of NovoLog and the remainder given as a basal infusion.

Novolog 70/30

SC ONLY

Diabetes mellitus.

Adults: Usually used on a twice-daily basis (i.e., before breakfast and dinner); each dose is intended to cover 2 meals or a meal and snack. The absorption rate from SC tissue allows dosing within 15 min of starting a meal. Dosage regimens vary among clients and must be determined by the provider based on the client's metabolic needs, eating habits, and other lifestyle variables.

NURSING IMPLICATIONS

Do not confuse NovoLog or NovoLog Mix 70/30 with Novolin N, Novolin R, Novolin 50/50, or Novolin 70/30, which are various forms of isophane insulin suspension.

IMPLEMENTATION/ADMINISTRATION/STORAGE

1. Administer SC in the abdominal region, buttocks, thigh, or upper arm.
2. Dose requirements may be reduced in those with renal or hepatic impairment.
3. Due to the rapid onset of action and shorter duration than human regular insulin, give within 5–10 min before a meal.
4. Addition of color branding has occurred with insulin products to prevent errors when using or dispensing Novolog and Novolog Mix 70/30.
5. If NovoLog is used with NPH human insulin immediately before injection, there is some attenuation in the peak level of insulin aspart but the time to peak and the total bioavailability are not affected significantly.
6. If NovoLog is mixed with NPH human insulin, draw insulin aspart into the syringe first. Make the injection immediately upon mixing. Do not mix NovoLog 70/30 with any other insulin product.
7. Do not mix insulin aspart with crystalline zinc insulin products.
8. May be infused SC by external infusion pumps. Do not mix with any other insulins or

diluent. Insulin aspart in the pump reservoir should be discarded after at least 48 hr of use or after exposure to temperatures that exceed 37°C (86°F).

9. Visually inspect. Never use if the product contains particulate matter or has become viscous or cloudy. Resuspended NovoLog 70/30 must appear uniformly white and cloudy. Do not use after the expiration date.
10. Store between 2–8°C (36–46°F). Do not freeze and do not use if the product has been frozen. Vials may be kept at room temperature below 30°C (86°F) for up to 28 days but should never be exposed to excessive heat or sunlight.
11. IV use of NovoLog is possible under medical supervision with close monitoring of blood glucose and potassium levels to avoid hypoglycemia and hypokalemia. For IV use, use NovoLog at concentrations from 0.05–1 unit/mL in infusion systems using polypropylene infusion bags. Do not inject NovoLog 70/30 IV.

ASSESSMENT

1. Note onset of diabetes, level of control, other agents used, outcome.
2. Monitor VS, weight, BS, electrolytes, HbA1c, U/A, microalbumin, renal and LFTs. Adjust dosage with impaired hepatic/renal function.

CLIENT/FAMILY TEACHING

1. This insulin is of rapid onset (1–3 hr) and short duration (3–5 hr) and may also be used with an intermediate- or long-acting insulin to maintain glucose control.
2. Due to the fast onset of action, immediately follow the insulin aspart injection by a meal within 10–20 min.
3. Store in the refrigerator; keep from freezing. Store away from heat and direct light.
4. After a cartridge has been inserted into a pen, store the cartridge and pen at room temperature, not in the refrigerator.
5. Monitor BS; adjust dosage with any change in physical activity or usual meal plan. Illness, emotional disturbances, and stress may alter insulin requirements.
6. Continue diet, exercise, and lifestyle changes necessary to enhance blood sugar control. Avoid alcohol.
7. May initially experience local itching, swelling or redness; report if persistent. SOB, wheezing, diffuse rash, ↑ heart rate, and ↓ BP are S&S of shock.
8. Avoid pregnancy; if desired notify provider. Keep out of the reach of children.
9. Keep all F/U to assess diabetes control, BP, weight, LDL levels, foot/eye exams and for adverse SE.

OUTCOMES/EVALUATE

Glycemic control; HbA1c <8

Insulin detemir

(**IN**-sue-lin **DE**-te-meer)

Classification(s): Insulin, rDNA origin

Pregnancy Category: C

RX: Levemir.

SEE ALSO ***ANTIDIABETIC AGENTS: INSULINS.***

INDICATIONS/USES

Once- or twice-daily SC treatment of adult and pediatric clients with type 1 diabetes mellitus or adult clients with type 2 diabetes mellitus who require long-acting insulin to control hyperglycemia.

ACTION/KINETICS

Action

Has a low affinity to IGF-1R relative to human insulin. Binds to insulin receptors and lowers blood glucose by facilitating uptake of glucose into skeletal muscle and fat cells and by inhibiting the output of glucose from the liver. Insulin inhibits lipolysis in the adipocyte, inhibits proteolysis, and enhances protein synthesis.

Pharmacokinetics

Slower, more prolonged, absorption over 24 hr compared with NPH human insulin. Absolute bioavailability: 60%. **Maximum serum levels:** 6–8 hr. **t½, terminal:** 5–7 hr, depending on the dose. **Plasma protein binding:** 98% bound to albumin.

SIDE EFFECTS

Most Common

Hypoglycemia, hypokalemia, injection site reaction, lipodystrophy, pruritus, rash.

See *Antidiabetic Agents: Insulins* for a complete list of possible side effects.

HOW SUPPLIED

Injection: 100 units/mL.

DOSAGE

SC

Type 1 diabetes mellitus in adults and children; Type 2 diabetes mellitus in adults.

Once or twice daily. Determine dose according to blood glucose levels. Individualize according to needs of the client.

NURSING IMPLICATIONS

IMPLEMENTATION/ADMINISTRATION/STORAGE

1. For clients treated once daily, give dose with the evening meal or at bedtime. For clients who require twice-daily dosing, the evening dose can be given with the evening meal, at bedtime, or 12 hr after the morning dose.
2. Administer by SC injection in the thigh, abdominal wall, or upper arm. Rotate injection sites within the same region.
3. Do not dilute or mix with any other insulin preparation.
4. Duration of action varies according to the dose, injection site, blood flow, temperature, and level of physical activity.
5. For those with type 1 or type 2 diabetes who are on basal-bolus treatment, changing the basal insulin to insulin detemir can be undertaken on a unit-to-unit basis. Adjust dose of insulin detemir to achieve glycemic targets. In some clients with type 2 diabetes, more insulin detemir may be needed than neutral protamine (NPH) insulin.
6. For clients receiving only basal insulin, changing the basal insulin to insulin detemir can be undertaken on a unit-to-unit basis.
7. For insulin-naive clients with type 2 diabetes who are not controlled on oral hypoglycemic drugs, start insulin determir at a dose of 0.1–0.2 units/kg once daily in the evening or 10 units once or twice daily. Adjust dose to achieve glycemic targets.
8. Store unused insulin detemir from 2–8°C (36–46°F). Do not freeze. Do not use insulin detemir if it has been frozen.
9. After initial use, store vials in a refrigerator (never a freezer). If refrigeration is not possible, the in-use vial can be kept at room temperature, below 30°C (86°F) for up to 42 days, as long as kept as cool as possible and away from direct heat and light.
10. After initial use, a cartridge or prefilled syringe cartridge may be used for up to 42 days if kept at room temperature, below 30°C (86°F). Do not store in-use cartridges and prefilled syringes in a refrigerator or with the needle in place. Keep away from direct heat and sunlight.

ASSESSMENT

1. Note reasons for therapy, age at onset, height and weight, HbA1c, other agents trialed and outcome.
2. List medications prescribed to ensure none interact.
3. Monitor VS, weight, BUN, creatinine, HbA1c, electrolytes, microalbumin, ECG, and blood sugar.

CLIENT/FAMILY TEACHING

1. Use exactly as directed. Demonstrate appropriate use of cartridge or syringe at visit. Store syringes/cartridges in a safe container until destroyed. If on once daily dosing take with evening meal.
2. May cause drowsiness, dizziness, blurred vision, or lightheadedness. Do not drive, operate machinery, or perform any activities that require mental alertness. Using Insulin Detemir Cartridges alone, with certain other medicines, or with alcohol may lessen ability to drive or perform other potentially dangerous tasks; assess response.
3. Illness, especially N&V, emotional problems, stress, or changes in diet or activity level may cause insulin requirements to change. Even if not eating, you still require insulin. Identify a sick day plan to use in case of illness. When sick, test your blood/urine frequently and call provider as directed. If traveling across time zones, ask about adjustments to your insulin schedule.
4. Proper diet, regular exercise, and regular testing of blood sugar are important for best results when using Insulin Detemir Cartridges. If blood sugar level is higher than it should be and you are taking Insulin Detemir Cartridges according to the directions, check with provider.
5. Carry ID card at all times that says you have diabetes.

6. Do not drink alcohol without approval; may increase risk of high/low blood sugar.
7. Do not exceed the recommended dose, use Insulin Detemir Cartridges more often than prescribed, or change type or dose of insulin without first discussing with provider.
8. An insulin reaction resulting from low blood sugar levels (hypoglycemia) may occur if you take too much insulin, skip a meal, or exercise too much. Signs of hypoglycemia include ↑ heartbeat, headache, chills, sweating, tremor, increased hunger, changes in vision, nervousness, weakness, dizziness, drowsiness, or fainting. Carry glucose tablets or gel to treat low blood sugar. If you do not have a reliable source of glucose available, eat a quick source of sugar such as table sugar, honey, or candy, or drink a glass of orange juice or non-diet soda to quickly raise your blood sugar level; advise provider.
9. Developing a fever or infection, eating significantly more than usual, or missing insulin dose may cause high blood sugar (hyperglycemia). Symptoms of hyperglycemia include thirst, increased urination, confusion, drowsiness, flushing, rapid breathing, and fruity breath odor; report if these S&S occur. If not treated, loss of consciousness, coma, or death may occur.
10. Use with caution in the elderly; may be more sensitive to its effects, especially low blood sugar. Use Cartridges with extreme caution in those under 6 years old.
11. Practice reliable contraception; report if pregnancy occurs. Do not breast-feed.
12. Skin depression, enlargement or thickening, redness, swelling, mild pain, or itching at the injection site may occur. Seek medical attention if any severe side effects occur, i.e., severe allergic reactions (rash; hives, difficulty breathing, chest tightness, swelling of mouth, face, lips, or tongue); changes in vision, chills, dizziness, drowsiness, fainting, very fast heartbeat, fast, shallow breathing, hoarseness, loss of consciousness, seizures, slurred speech, sweet or fruity breath, swelling of arms or legs, tremor, or weakness.
13. May contact www.levemir.com website for additional tools and resources.
14. Keep all F/U to assess response, labs, adverse SE.

OUTCOMES/EVALUATE

- HbA1c <8
- Desired control of blood sugar

Insulin glargine

(**IN**-sue-lin **GLAR**-jeen)

Classification(s): Insulin, rDNA origin

Pregnancy Category: C

RX: Lantus.

SEE ALSO ***ANTIDIABETIC AGENTS: INSULINS.***

INDICATIONS/USES

(1) Once daily treatment of adult and pediatric clients (6 years and older) with type 1 diabetes mellitus. (2) Adults with type 2 diabetes mellitus who require long-acting insulin to control hyperglycemia. Not the insulin of choice for treatment of diabetic acidosis (short-acting IV insulin is preferred).

ACTION/KINETICS

Action

Long-acting recombinant human insulin analog. Differs from human insulin in that the amino acid asparagine at position A21 is replaced by glycine and two arginines are added to the C-terminus of the B-chain. Is designed to have low aqueous solubility at neutral pH; at pH 4, it is completely soluble. After injection into SC tissue, the acidic solution is neutralized, leading to formation of microprecipitates from which small amounts of insulin glargine are slowly released. This allows a relatively constant concentration/time profile over 24 hr with no pronounced peak.

Pharmacokinetics

Potency is about the same as human insulin. **Onset:** 1.1 hr. **Peak:** No pronounced peak; small amounts are released slowly, resulting in relatively constant levels over 24 hr. **Duration:** Prolonged (greater than 24 hr) when compared with NPH human insulin (about 14.5 hr). Metabolized in the liver. Dosage adjustment may be necessary in impaired renal or hepatic function.

CONTRAINDICATIONS

IV use (may cause severe hypoglycemia).

SPECIAL CONCERNS

- Use with caution during lactation.

- The long duration may delay recovery from hypoglycemia.
- Not the drug of choice for diabetic ketoacidosis (use a short-acting IV insulin).
- The rate of absorption may be affected by exercise and other variables.
- Safety and efficacy not determined in children under 6 years old.

ADDITIONAL SIDE EFFECTS

Most Common

Hypoglycemia, hypokalemia, injection site reaction, lipodystrophy, pruritus, rash, allergic reactions.

See *Antidiabetic Agents: Insulins* for a complete list of potential side effects. Also, higher incidence of treatment-emergent injection site pain compared with NPH insulin-treated clients.

DRUG INTERACTIONS

ACE inhibitors / ↑ Blood glucose lowering effect and susceptibility to hypoglycemia
Clonidine / Either potentiates or weakens blood-glucose lowering effect of insulin
Danazol / ↓ Blood glucose lowering effect
Disopyramide / ↑ Blood glucose lowering effect and susceptibility to hypoglycemia
Diuretics / ↓ Blood glucose lowering effect
Fluoxetine / ↑ Blood glucose lowering effect and susceptibility to hypoglycemia
Isoniazid / ↓ Blood glucose lowering effect
Lithium salts / Either potentiate or weaken blood-glucose lowering effect of insulin
MAOIs / ↑ Blood glucose lowering effect and susceptibility to hypoglycemia
Niacin / ↓ Blood glucose lowering effect
Octreotide / ↑ Blood glucose lowering effect and susceptibility to hypoglycemia
Salicylates / ↑ Blood glucose lowering effect and susceptibility to hypoglycemia
Somatropin / ↓ Blood glucose lowering effect
Sulfonamides / ↑ Blood glucose lowering effect and susceptibility to hypoglycemia

HOW SUPPLIED

Injection: 100 units/mL.

DOSAGE

SC

Diabetes mellitus.

Dose individualized. Give once daily at the same time every day (any time of the day is appropriate). **Initial:** Average of 10 units once daily at the same time each day; **then,** adjust according to client need to a total daily dose ranging from 2–100 units.

NURSING IMPLICATIONS

Do not confuse insulin glargine with insulin glulisine. Do not confuse Lantus with Lente insulin (insulin zinc suspension).

IMPLEMENTATION/ADMINISTRATION/STORAGE

1. May be given SC in the abdomen, deltoid, or thigh (there is no difference in absorption between these sites). Rotate sites from one injection to the next.
2. Do not dilute or mix with any other insulin or solution, as the mixture may become cloudy and the properties of either insulin glargine or other insulins may be altered.
3. Use only if the solution is clear and colorless with no visible particles.
4. Syringes must not contain any other medicinal product or residue.
5. If changing from an intermediate- or long-acting insulin to insulin glargine, the amount and timing of the short-acting insulin or fast-acting insulin analog may need to be adjusted.
6. Store unopened product in a refrigerator at 2–8°C (36–46°F). Do not store in the freezer, and do not allow product to freeze. Discard if it has been frozen. If refrigeration is not possible, 10 mL vials/cartridges can be kept unrefrigerated for up to 28 days and 5 mL vials/cartridges can be kept unrefrigerated for up to 14 days, away from direct heat and light, as long as the temperature does not exceed 30°C (86°F).
7. Once the cartridge is placed in an OptiPen One, do not put in the refrigerator.
8. Store from 2–8°C (36–46°F).

ASSESSMENT

1. Note disease onset, level of control, other agents trialed, outcome.
2. List drugs prescribed to ensure none interact.
3. Monitor VS, weight, BS, electrolytes, HbA1c, U/A, microalbumin, renal and LFTs. Adjust dosage with hepatic/renal dysfunction.

CLIENT/FAMILY TEACHING

1. Insulin glargine is usually given once daily at any time of the day for continual blood sugar control. Rotate sites.
2. Use only if clear and colorless with no visible particles. Refrigerate unopened vials; once opened may keep in refrigerator or at room temperature away from direct heat or light <86°F (30°C) and use/discard within 28 days of opening. Once placed in OptiPen One, do not refrigerate.
3. Do not dilute or mix with any other insulin solution. Carry oral glucose tablets in event of hypoglycemia (low blood sugar). Monitor/record FS and assess for hypo-/hyperglycemia S&S.
4. Report any systemic rash, cough, or dizziness. Illness, emotional disturbances, and stress may alter insulin requirements.
5. Continue diet, exercise, and lifestyle changes necessary to enhance blood sugar control. Avoid alcohol.
6. Avoid pregnancy; consult provider if desired.
7. Attend diabetes education classes (with spouse).
8. Keep all F/U to assess diabetes control, BP, weight, LDL levels, foot/eye exams and for adverse SE.

OUTCOMES/EVALUATE

Glycemic control; HbA1c <8

Insulin glulisine

(**IN**-sue-lin glue-**LIH**-seen)

Classification(s): Insulin product, rDNA origin

Pregnancy Category: C

RX: Apidra.

SEE ALSO ***ANTIDIABETIC AGENTS: INSULINS.***

INDICATIONS/USES

Control of hyperglycemia in adults and children, age 4–17 years, with diabetes mellitus. Usually used in regimens that include a longer-acting insulin or basal insulin analog. May also be infused SC by external insulin infusion pumps or IV in a clinical setting.

ACTION/KINETICS

Action

A recombinant insulin analog equipotent to human insulin, i.e., one unit of insulin glulisine has the same glucose-lowering effect as 1 unit of regular insulin when given IV.

Pharmacokinetics

After SC administration, it has a more rapid onset of action and a shorter duration of action than regular human insulin. **Onset:** 15 min. **Peak:** 30–90 min. **Duration:** 1–2.5 hr. **$t^{1/2}$:** 0.7 hr.

SIDE EFFECTS

Most Common

Hypoglycemia, hypokalemia, injection site reaction, lipodystrophy, pruritus, rash.

See *Antidiabetic Agents* for a complete list of possible side effects.

HOW SUPPLIED

Injection: 100 units per mL.

DOSAGE

SC

Diabetes mellitus in adults.

Individualize dosage based on needs of client. Usually used in regimens that include an intermediate- or long-acting insulin. The total daily insulin requirement may vary but is usually between 0.5 and 1 unit/kg/day.

NURSING IMPLICATIONS

Do not confuse insulin glulisine with insulin glargine.

IMPLEMENTATION/ADMINISTRATION/STORAGE

1. Give SC in the abdominal wall, thigh, or deltoid, or by continuous SC infusion in the abdominal wall.
2. Rotate injection sites and infusion sites within an injection area (e.g., abdomen, thigh, deltoid) from one injection to the next.
3. The rate of absorption and thus the onset and duration of action may be affected by the injection site, exercise, and other variables.
4. Insulin requirement may be altered during stress, major illness, or with changes in exercise, meal patterns, or coadministered drugs.
5. Use only if solution is clear and colorless with no particles visible.

6. When given by continuous SC infusion (insulin pump), do not mix insulin glulisine with other insulins or with a diluent. Rotate infusion sites within the same region to reduce the risk of lipodystrophy.
7. Do not mix insulin glulisine with other insulin products other than NPH insulin. If glulisine is mixed with NPH human insulin, draw the glulisine into the syringe first. Make injection immediately after mixing.
8. If OptiClik (the insulin delivery device for glulisine insulin) malfunctions, insulin glulisine may be drawn from the cartridge system into a U-100 syringe and injected.
9. Store unopened glulisine vials in the refrigerator at 2–8°C (36–46°F). Protect from light. Do not store in the freezer or allow to freeze. Discard vial if frozen.
10. Opened vials, whether or not refrigerated, must be used within 28 days. Discard if not used within 28 days. If refrigeration is not possible, the open vial may be kept unrefrigerated for up to 28 days away from direct heat and light as long as the temperature does not exceed 25°C (77°F).
11. Do not refrigerate the opened (in-use) cartridge system inserted in OptiClik but keep below 25°C (77°F) and away from direct heat and light. The opened cartridge must be used within 28 days.
12. Discard infusion sets (e.g., reservoirs, tubing, catheters) and insulin glulisine in the reservoir after no more than 48 hours of use or after exposure to temperatures that exceed 37°C (98.6°F).
13. IV administration is possible but only under strict medical supervision with close monitoring of blood glucose and potassium levels (i.e., to avoid hypoglycemia and hypokalemia).
14. For IV use, insulin glulisine should be used at a concentration of 0.05–1 unit/mL in infusion systems with the infusion fluid being sterile 0.9% NaCl solution, using polyvinyl chloride (Viaflex) infusion bags and PVC tubing (Clearlink system Continu-Flo) with a dedicated infusion line.

ASSESSMENT

1. Note reasons for therapy, age at onset, height and weight, HbA1c, other agents trialed and outcome.
2. Monitor VS, weight, BUN, creatinine, LFTs, HbA1c, electrolytes, microalbumin, ECG, and blood sugar.

CLIENT/FAMILY TEACHING

1. Drug onset of action is quicker than regular human insulin. Take within 15 min before a meal or within 20 min after starting a meal. OptiClik is a reusable pen for the injection of insulin; review enclosed leaflet after demonstration on use if prescribed.
2. Administer subcutaneously into the abdomen, thigh or arm. Rotate injection sites and monitor finger sticks regularly.
3. Refrigerate all vials at or below 77°F (25°C) and away from direct heat and light. Throw vial away 28 days after the first use even if it still contains Apidra.
4. If mixing Apidra with NPH human insulin, draw up the Apidra first and inject mixture right away. Do not mix with any other type of insulin than NPH
5. May also be administered via pump into the abdomen as directed. If using pump, do not mix with any other type of insulin. The infusion set, reservoir with insulin, and infusion site should be changed:
   - every 48 hours or less
   - when unexpected hyperglycemia or ketosis occurs
   - when alarms sound, as specified by your pump manual
   - if the insulin has been exposed to temperatures over 98.6°F (37°C). If the insulin or pump could have absorbed radiant heat, e.g., from sunlight, that would heat the insulin to over 98.6°F (37°C). Dark colored pump cases or sport covers can increase this type of heat. The location where the pump is worn may affect the temperature.
   - if skin reactions at the infusion site may need to change infusion sites more often
6. Continue diet, exercise, and weight control along with insulin to control blood sugar and prevent organ damage.
7. For more information and support go to www.apidra.com.
8. Keep all F/U to assess response, BP control, labs (LDL/HbA1c), and for adverse SE.

OUTCOMES/EVALUATE

Control of diabetes; HbA1c <8

Insulin injection (Regular insulin)

(**IN**-sue-lin)

Classification(s): Insulin product

OTC: Human Insulin: Humulin R, Novolin R.

✤ **Rx: Human Insulin:** Novolinge Toronto.

SEE ALSO ***ANTIDIABETIC AGENTS: INSULINS***.

INDICATIONS/USES

Suitable for treatment of diabetic coma, diabetic acidosis, or other emergency situations. Especially suitable for the client suffering from labile diabetes. During acute phase of diabetic acidosis or for the client in diabetic crisis, client is monitored by serum glucose and serum ketone levels.

ACTION/KINETICS

Action

Rarely administered as the sole agent due to its short duration of action. Injections of 100 units/mL are clear; cloudy, colored solutions should not be used. Available only as 100 units/mL.

Pharmacokinetics

Onset, SC: 30–60 min; **IV:** 10–30 min. **Peak, SC:** 2–5 hr; **IV:** 15–30 min. **Duration, SC:** 8–12 hr; **IV:** 30–60 min. Is compatible with all other insulins.

SIDE EFFECTS

Most Common

Hypoglycemia, hypokalemia, injection site reaction, lipodystrophy, pruritus, rash.

See *Antidiabetic Agents: Insulins* for a complete list of possible side effects.

HOW SUPPLIED

Injection: 100 units/mL.

DOSAGE

SC

Diabetes.

Adults, individualized, usual, initial: 5–10 units; **pediatric:** 2–4 units. Injection is given 15–30 min before meals and at bedtime.

Diabetic ketoacidosis.

Adults: 0.1 unit/kg/hr given by continuous IV infusion.

NURSING IMPLICATIONS

Ⓢ Do not confuse Novolin R with NovoLog or NovoLog 70/30 (both are insulin aspart products).

ASSESSMENT

1. Note reasons for therapy, disease onset, height and weight, HbA1c, other agents trialed and outcome.
2. List medications prescribed to ensure none interact.
3. Monitor VS, weight, HbA1c, microalbumin, renal and LFTs, ECG, and blood sugar.

CLIENT/FAMILY TEACHING

1. Use as directed and monitor FS regularly.
2. Illness, emotional disturbances, and stress may alter insulin requirements.
3. Do not exceed the recommended dose, use more often than prescribed, or change type or dose of insulin without first discussing with provider.
4. An insulin reaction resulting from low blood sugar levels (hypoglycemia) may occur if you take too much insulin, skip a meal, or exercise too much.
5. Developing a fever or infection, eating significantly more than usual, or missing insulin dose may cause high blood sugar (hyperglycemia).
6. Continue diet, exercise, and lifestyle changes necessary to enhance blood sugar control. Avoid alcohol.
7. Keep all F/U to assess response, BP control, LDL levels, foot and eye exams, labs, and for adverse SE.

OUTCOMES/EVALUATE

Control of hyperglycemia; A1C <8

Insulin injection, concentrated

Classification(s): Insulin product

Pregnancy Category: C

RX: Humulin R Regular U-500 (Concentrated).

SEE ALSO ***ANTIDIABETIC AGENTS: INSULINS***.

INDICATIONS/USES

Insulin resistance requiring more than 200 units insulin/day (a large dose may be given SC in a reasonable volume). *NOTE:* Insulin resistance is often self-limiting and after several weeks or months of high dosage, responsiveness may be regained and dosage reduced.

ACTION/KINETICS

Action

Concentrated insulin injection (500 units/mL) is a recombinant DNA product. Response varies among clients. Insulin resistance is frequently self-limiting; responsiveness to insulin may be regained after several weeks or months necessitating dosage reduction. Only given SC.

Pharmacokinetics

Has a duration similar to repository insulin; a single dose lasts for 24 hr.

CONTRAINDICATIONS

IV or IM use due to possible inadvertent overdosage.

SPECIAL CONCERNS

- **Inadvertent overdose may cause irreversible insulin shock.**
- **Use with caution during lactation.**

ADDITIONAL SIDE EFFECTS

Most Common

Hypoglycemia, hypokalemia, injection site reaction, lipodystrophy, pruritus, rash.

See *Antidiabetic Agents: Insulins* for a complete list of possible side effects. Also, deep secondary hypoglycemia 18–24 hr after administration; hypoglycemia may be prolonged and severe.

DRUG INTERACTIONS

Do not use together with PO hypoglycemic agents.

HOW SUPPLIED

Injection: 500 units/mL.

DOSAGE

SC ONLY

Individualized, depending on severity of condition. Clients must be kept under close observation until dosage is established. Some clients may require only 1 dose/day while others may require 2 or 3 injections/day.

NURSING IMPLICATIONS

Do not confuse Humulin R Regular U-500 with Humulin R (Insulin Injection 100 units/mL).

IMPLEMENTATION/ADMINISTRATION/STORAGE

1. Administer only water/clear solutions. Discoloration, turbidity, or unusual viscosity means deterioration or contamination.
2. Use a tuberculin or insulin syringe for accuracy of measurement.
3. Deep secondary hypoglycemia may occur 18–24 hr after administration; monitor closely and have 10–20% dextrose solution available.
4. Some clients who have experienced hypoglycemic reactions after transfer from animal-source insulin to human insulin have reported that the early warning symptoms of hypoglycemia were less pronounced or different from those experienced with their previous insulin.
5. Keep in a cold location, preferably a refrigerator. Do not freeze.

ASSESSMENT

1. Observe closely for S&S of hyper- or hypoglycemia until dosage established. Counsel that this insulin is very concentrated and not to share or use without monitoring FS.
2. Note reasons for therapy, age at onset, height and weight, HbA1c, other agents trialed and outcome.
3. Keep all appointments, especially eye exams and foot exams.
4. Monitor VS, weight, HbA1c, renal and LFTs, microalbumin, ECG, and blood sugar.

CLIENT/FAMILY TEACHING

1. Review technique for self-administration.
2. Be alert for signs of hypoglycemia, which may indicate that responsiveness to insulin has been regained and that a reduction in dosage is warranted.
3. Record FS especially 2 hr after meals to assess response.
4. Continue BP/weight control, diet, and exercise to achieve glycemic control and to prevent complications.
5. Keep all F/U to assess response, labs, and for adverse SE.

OUTCOMES/EVALUATE

- BS and HbA1c within desired range
- Prevention of MI and organ damage

Insulin lispro injection

(**IN**-sue-lin **LYE**-sproh)

Classification(s): Insulin, rDNA origin

Pregnancy Category: B

RX: Humalog, Humalog Mix 50/50, Humalog Mix 75/25.

SEE ALSO ***ANTIDIABETIC AGENTS: INSULINS.***

INDICATIONS/USES

Treatment of diabetes mellitus to control hyperglycemia.

ACTION/KINETICS

Action

Is a rapid-acting human insulin analog created when the amino acids at positions 28 and 29 on the insulin B-chain are reversed. Absorbed faster than regular human insulin. Compared to regular insulin, has a more rapid onset of glucose-lowering activity, an earlier peak for glucose lowering, and a shorter duration of glucose-lowering activity. However, is equipotent to human regular insulin (i.e., one unit of insulin lispro has the same glucose-lowering capacity as one unit of regular insulin). May lower the risk of nocturnal hypoglycemia in clients with type 1 diabetes.

Pharmacokinetics

Onset: 15 min. **Peak effect:** 30–90 min. **t½:** 1 hr. **Duration:** 2–5 hr. *NOTE:* Humalog Mix 75/25 is a mixture of insulin lispro protamine suspension (75%) and insulin lispro injection (25%). It has glucose-lowering effects similar to Humulin 70/30 on a unit for unit basis. **Onset:** 5 min. **Peak:** 7–12 hr. **Duration:** 1–24 hr.

CONTRAINDICATIONS

Use during episodes of hypoglycemia. Hypersensitivity to insulin lispro.

SPECIAL CONCERNS

- Use with caution during lactation.
- Since insulin lispro has a more rapid onset and shorter duration of action than regular insulin, clients with type 1 diabetes also require a longer acting insulin to maintain glucose control.
- Requirements may be decreased in impaired renal or hepatic function.
- Safety and efficacy of Humalog not determined in children less than 12 years of age. Safety and efficacy of Humalog Mix 75/25 not determined in children less than 18 years of age.

SIDE EFFECTS

Most Common

Hypoglycemia, hypokalemia, injection site reaction, lipodystrophy, pruritus, rash, allergic reactions.

See *Antidiabetic Agents: Insulins* for a complete list of possible side effects.

DRUG INTERACTIONS

See ***Antidiabetic Agents: Insulins***.

HOW SUPPLIED

Injection: Humalog: 100 units/mL. Humalog Mix 50/50: 50% insulin lispro protamine suspension and 50% insulin lispro injection. Humalog Mix 75/25: 75% insulin lispro protamine suspension and 25% insulin lispro injection.

DOSAGE

SC

Diabetes mellitus.

Individualized. Adults and children 3 years and older, usual: 0.5–1 unit/kg/day. Insulin lispro should generally be used with an intermediate- or long-acting insulin.

NURSING IMPLICATIONS

Do not confuse Humalog, Humalog Mix 50/50 or Humalog Mix 75/25 with Humulin, Humulin 50/50, or Humulin 70/30 (regular insulin product) or with NovoLog or Novolog Mix 50/50 or 70/30 (another insulin product).

IMPLEMENTATION/ADMINISTRATION/STORAGE

1. Give SC in the abdominal wall, thigh, upper arm, or buttocks. Rotate injection sites within the same region from one injection to the next to reduce the risk of lipodystrophy.
2. Dosage reduction may be required in those with renal or hepatic impairment.
3. When used as a mealtime insulin, give within 15 min before a meal or 15 min of finishing a meal, as compared with human regular insulin, which is best given 30–60 min before a meal.

4. Humalog for SC use should not be mixed with insulin preparations other than NPH insulin. If mixed, draw Humalog into the syringe first. Inject immediately after mixing.
5. Given alone or with Humulin N, insulin lispro causes a more rapid absorption and glucose-lowering effect than human regular insulin.
6. After abdominal administration, insulin lispro levels are higher than those following deltoid or thigh injections. Also, the duration of action following abdominal injection is slighter shorter than deltoid or femoral injection.
7. Do not give insulin lispro mixtures IV.
8. May be given by an external insulin pump. The reservoir syringe, tubing, catheter, cartridge adapter, and insulin should be replaced every 3 days. Rotate infusion sites within the same region to avoid lipodystrophy. Change the Humalog in the reservoir at least every 7 days. Do not expose the insulin in the external pump to a temperature above 37°C (86°F).
9. If an external insulin infusion pump is used, base the initial programming on the total daily insulin dose of the previous regimen. Although there is significant interclient variability, about 50% of the total dose is usually given as meal-related boluses and the remainder given as a basal infusion. Recommended pump systems include the MiniMed, Disetronic, and other equivalent pumps.
10. Do not use diluted or mixed insulins in external infusion pumps.
11. Store in the refrigerator at 2–8°C (36–46°F). Do not freeze. If refrigeration not possible, can store unrefrigerated for up to 28 days, provided it is kept as cool as possible and away from direct heat and light. Do not use if the product has been frozen.
12. Diluted insulin lispro may be used for 28 days when stored at 5°C (41°F) and for 14 days when stored at 30°C (86°F).
13. Do not use if the product is cloudy, contains particulate matter, is thickened, or discolored.

ASSESSMENT

1. Note disease onset, level of control, previous agents trialed, outcome.
2. Monitor VS, weight, BS, CBC, HbA1c, U/A: microalbumin, renal and LFTs.

CLIENT/FAMILY TEACHING

1. Review method for preparation, storage, and administration; rotate sites. Ensure correct concentration and correct dose as prescribed.
2. Prime the disposable insulin-delivery device before each injection.
3. Drug has a more rapid onset of action and a shorter duration of action than regular insulin.
4. Take within 15 min of meals and immediately after mixing, with combined therapy.
5. Monitor/record FS, especially 2 hr PP until response evident. Review S&S of hypoglycemia and appropriate management. Continue BP control, diet, and exercise for disease control.
6. Clients with type 1 diabetes also require a longer-acting insulin preparation for adequate glucose control.
7. Continue diet, exercise and weight control along with insulin to control blood sugar and prevent organ damage.
8. Keep all F/U to assess diabetes control, BP, weight, LDL levels, foot/eye exams and for adverse SE.

OUTCOMES/EVALUATE

- HbA1c <8
- Prevention of MI and end organ disease

IV

Interferon alfa-2b recombinant (rIFN-α2; α-2-interferon; IFN-alpha)

(in-ter-**FEER**-on **AL**-fah)

Classification(s): Antineoplastic, miscellaneous

Pregnancy Category: C; X (for combination therapy of interferon alfa-2b and ribavirin capsules)

RX: Intron A.

INDICATIONS/USES

NOTE: Not all strengths are appropriate for some indications. (1) Hairy cell leukemia in clients over age 18 (in both splenectomized and nonsplenectomized clients). (2) Intralesional use for external genital or perianal warts (*Condylomata acuminata*) in clients 18 years and older. (3) AIDS-related Kaposi's sarcoma in clients over age 18. Response is greater in those without systemic symptoms, who have limited lymphadenopathy, and who have a relatively intact immune system as indicated by total CD4 count. (4) Chronic hepatitis C in clients at least 18 years of age with compensated liver disease and a history of blood or blood product exposure or who are HCV antibody positive. In combination with ribavirin in compensated liver disease previously untreated with alpha interferon therapy or who have relapsed following alpha interferon therapy. (5) Chronic hepatitis B in clients 1 year of age and older with compensated liver disease and HBV replication (clients must be serum HBsAg positive for at least 6 months and have HBV replication with elevated serum ALT). (6) Adjunct therapy to surgical treatment for malignant melanoma in those who are 18 years of age or older who are free of the disease but at a high risk for recurrence within 56 days of surgery. (7) With an anthracycline drug for the initial treatment of clinically aggressive non-Hodgkin's lymphoma in clients 18 years and older. *Investigational:* The drug has been used for a large number of conditions. Treatment of angiomatous disorders; mycosis fungoides; ovarian and cervical carcinoma; renal cell carcinoma; basal and squamous cell skin cancer; bladder tumors (local use for superficial tumors); chronic myelogenous leukemia; cutaneous T-cell lymphoma; non-Hodgkin's lymphoma; multiple myeloma; carcinoid tumor; papillomaviruses; West Nile virus infection.

ACTION/KINETICS

Action

Recombinant product whose activity is expressed as international units, which are determined by comparing the antiviral activity of the recombinant interferon with the activity of the international reference standard of human leukocyte interferon. Interferons bind to specific receptors on the cell surface, resulting in induction of certain enzymes, suppression of cell proliferation, immunomodulating activities (e.g., enhancement of the phagocytic activity of macrophages and augmentation of the specific cytotoxicity of lymphocytes for target cells), and inhibition of virus replication in virus-infected cells.

Pharmacokinetics

Peak serum levels after IM, SC: 18–116 international units/mL after 3–12 hr. **t½, IM, SC:** 2–3 hr. **Peak serum levels after IV infusion:** 135–270 international units/mL at the end of the infusion. **t½, IV:** 2 hr. The main site of metabolism may be the kidney.

CONTRAINDICATIONS

Hypersensitivity to interferon alfa-2b or any components of the products. Use to treat rapidly progressive visceral disease in AIDS-related Kaposi's sarcoma. Use in clients with decompensated liver disease, severe renal dysfunction, autoimmune hepatitis, history of autoimmune disease, or immunosuppressed transplant clients. Use of interferon alfa-2b and ribavirin by women who are pregnant, by men whose female partners are pregnant, or in those with autoimmune hepatitis. Lactation.

SPECIAL CONCERNS

■ Alpha interferons, including interferon alfa-2b recombinant, cause or aggravate fatal or life-threatening neuropsychiatric, autoimmune, ischemic, and infectious disorders. Monitor clients closely with periodic clinical and lab evaluations. Withdraw therapy in clients with persistently severe or worsening S&S of these conditions R/T therapy. In many, but not all, these conditions resolve after stopping interferon alfa-2b therapy. ■

- **Use with caution in clients with a history of unstable angina, CV disease, uncontrolled CHF, COPD, diabetes mellitus prone to ketoacidosis, thrombophlebitis, pulmonary embolism, seizure disorders, moderate renal dysfunction, severe hepatic disease, compromised CNS function, severe myelosuppression, and in the elderly.**
- **Safety and efficacy in those less than age 18 not established, other than to treat chronic hepatitis B (except in children younger than 1 year of age).**

SIDE EFFECTS

Most Common

Musculoskeletal pain/weakness, confusion, depression, dizziness/vertigo, paresthesia, alopecia, rash, pruritus, back pain, chills, dry mouth, fatigue, fever, chills, flu-like symptoms, headache, anemia, myalgia, N&V, anorexia, diarrhea, taste alteration, coughing, asthenia, increased sweating, rigors, leukopenia, neutropenia.

Flu-like symptoms: Fever, headache, fatigue, myalgia, chills. **CV:** Hypo-/hypertension, ***arrhythmias***, tachycardia, syncope, coagulation disorders, chest pain, palpitations, ***stroke***, flushing, atrial fibrillation, bradycardia, cardiomegaly, ***cardiac failure, cardiomyopathy, MI***, extrasystoles, postural hypotension, supraventricular arrhythmias, angina, coronary artery disorder, heart valve disorder, peripheral ischemia, poor peripheral circulation, phlebitis, superficial phlebitis, Raynaud disease, thrombosis, varicose vein. **CNS:** Depression, confusion, somnolence, headache, migraine, dizziness, ataxia, insomnia, irritability, paresthesia, anxiety, nervousness, emotional lability, amnesia, impaired concentration, weakness, tremor, twitching, syncope, abnormal coordination, hypesthesia, aggravated depression, manic depression, manic reaction, aggressive reaction, hypertonia, impaired consciousness, neuropathy, agitation, apathy, aphasia, dysphonia, extrapyramidal disorder, hot flashes, hyper-/hypoesthesia, hypo-/hyperkinesia, neurosis, paresis, paroniria, parosmia, personality disorder, speech disorder, vertigo, obtundation, psychosis, impaired coordination, abnormal dreaming, abnormal gait, abnormal thinking, alcohol intolerance, Bell palsy, delirium, feeling of ebriety, loss of consciousness, neuralgia, neuritis, ***seizures, coma***, polyneuropathy, ***suicide attempt, suicidal ideation, completed suicide.*** **GI:** N&V, diarrhea, stomatitis, weight loss, anorexia, taste loss, flatulence, thirst, dehydration, constipation, dry mouth, dyspepsia, eructation, loose stools, abdominal distention/pain, dysphagia, esophagitis, gastric ulcer, ***GI hemorrhage***, GI mucosal discoloration, gum hyperplasia, gingival bleeding, gingivitis, increased saliva/appetite, melena, oral leukoplakia, rectal bleeding after stool, ***oral/rectal hemorrhage***, ulcerative stomatitis, ascites, gallstones, gastroenteritis, halitosis, abdominal ascites, abdominal distension, colitis, gastritis, hemorrhoids, intestinal disorder, mouth ulceration, mucositis, tongue/tooth disorder, ***pancreatitis***. **Hepatic:** Jaundice, RUQ pain, biliary pain, hepatitis, abnormal hepatic function, ***hepatic encephalopathy/failure***. **Hematologic:** Thrombocytopenia, granulocytopenia, anemia, hypochromic anemia, ***hemolytic anemia***, leukopenia, lymphocytosis, neutropenia, thrombocytopenic purpura, ***aplastic anemia*** (rare). **Musculoskeletal:** Arthralgia, leg cramps, asthenia, arthrosis, arthritis (including rheumatoid), arteritis, muscle pain/weakness, musculoskeletal pain, myalgia, bone disorder, back/bone pain, rigors, carpal tunnel syndrome, hyporeflexia, muscle atrophy, polyarteritis nodosa, spondylitis, tendonitis. **Respiratory:** Pharyngitis, coughing, dyspnea, sinusitis, rhinitis, epistaxis, nasal congestion, dry mouth, ***bronchospasm***, pleural pain/effusion, pneumonia, rhinorrhea, sneezing, wheezing, bronchitis, nonproductive cough, cyanosis, lung fibrosis, asthma, bronchitis, hemoptysis, hypoventilation, laryngitis, orthopnea, pneumonitis, pneumothorax, rales, impaired respiratory function, tonsillitis, tracheitis, URTI, ***pulmonary embolism***. **Dermatologic:** Rash, pruritus, alopecia, urticaria, dry skin, dermatitis, purpura, photosensitivity, acne, nail disorder, facial edema, moniliasis, reaction at injection site (e.g., inflammation, bleeding, pain, itching, burning), abnormal hair texture, cold/clammy skin, cyanosis of the hand, epidermal necrolysis, dermatitis lichenoides, furunculosis, increased hair growth, erythema, melanosis, nonherpetic cold sores, peripheral ischemia, skin depigmentation/discoloration, vitiligo, folliculitis, lipoma, psoriasis, hematoma, cellulitis, eczema, erythema nodosum, maculopapular rash, pallor, erythematous rash, sebaceous cyst, skin nodule, vitiligo. **GU:** Amenorrhea, hematuria, dysuria, impotence, leukorrhea, menorrhagia, dysmenorrhea, menstrual irregularity, urinary frequency, nocturia, polyuria, uterine bleeding, incontinence, pelvic pain, nephrotic syndrome, renal failure, impaired renal function, genital pruritus, cystitis, mastitis, UTI, micturition disorder/frequency, penis disorder, sexual dysfunction, vaginal dryness, scrotal/penile edema. **Endocrine:** Gynecomastia, thyroid disorder, goiter, hyper-/hypothyroidism, aggravation of diabetes mellitus, virilism. **Hypersensitivity reactions:** Urticaria, bronchoconstriction, angioedema, transient rashes, ***anaphylaxis***. **Ophthalmic:** Decrease/loss of vision, blurred vision, retinopathy (including macular edema, retinal artery or vein thrombosis, retinal hemorrhage, and cotton wool spots), optic neuritis, papilledema, conjunctivitis, photophobia, eye pain, diplopia, dry eyes, periorbital edema, lacrimal gland disorder, lacrimation, nystagmus, stye, periorbital edema. **Otic:** Earache, tinnitus, hearing disorder/impairment, labyrinth disorder, otitis media. **Body as a whole:** Pain, increased sweating, malaise, abscess, cachexia, peripheral edema, weakness, ***sepsis***, dehydration, bacterial/fungal/viral/nonspecific infection, parasitic infection, hyper-/hypothermia, allergic reaction, nonspecific inflammation, weight increase. **Miscellaneous:** Decreased libido, herpes zoster/simplex, lymphadenopathy, lymphadenitis, chest pain, hernia, hypercalcemia, substernal chest pain, trichomoniasis, alteration/loss of taste, sarcoidosis (or exacerbation thereof).

NOTE: The most common side effects in children are flu-like symptoms, GI system disorders, N&V, neutropenia, thrombocytopenia.

LABORATORY TEST CONSIDERATIONS

↑ AST, ALT, LDH, BUN, serum urea nitrogen, serum creatinine, alkaline phosphatase. ↓ H&H, granulocytes. Abnormal LFT, bilirubinemia. Hyperglycemia, hypertriglyceridemia.

OVERDOSE MANAGEMENT

Symptoms: Similar to side effects. Reported have been hepatic enzyme abnormalities, renal failure, ***hemorrhage, MI.*** *Treatment:* Consult a Poison Control Center. There is no specific antidote. Hemodialysis and peritoneal dialysis are not effective to treat an overdose.

DRUG INTERACTIONS

Myelosuppressive agents (e.g., zidovudine) / Possible synergistic side effects, such as neutropenia; carefully monitor WBC
Theophyllines / Significant ↓ theophylline clearance (100% ↑ in serum theophylline levels) R/T ↓ liver breakdown

HOW SUPPLIED

Injection, Powder for Solution: 10 million international units/vial, 18 million international units/vial, 50 million international units/vial; ***Injection Solution:*** 3 million international units/vial, 5 million international units/vial, 10 million international units/vial, 18 million international units/vial, 25 million international units/vial.

DOSAGE

IM; SC

Hairy cell leukemia.

2 million international units/m² 3 times per week for up to 6 months. Higher doses are not recommended. If the platelet count is <50,000/mm³, do not administer IM; rather use the SC route. Do not use the 50 million-international unit strength of the powder for injection for treating hairy cell leukemia. If severe side effects occur, reduce the dose by 50% or temporarily discontinue the drug until side effects abate. Discontinue if intolerance persists or recurs following adequate dosage adjustment, or if disease progresses.

AIDS-related Kaposi's sarcoma.

30 million international units/m² 3 times per week SC or IM using only the 50 million international unit vial. Do not use the 18 and 25 million international unit multidose strengths for treatment of AIDS-related Kaposi's sarcoma as concentrations are inappropriate. Using this dose, clients should tolerate an average dose of 110 million international units/week at the end of 12 weeks of therapy and 75 million international units/week at the end of 24 weeks of therapy. Reduce the dose by 50% or withhold if there are severe reactions. Permanently discontinue if severe side effects persist or if they recur in clients receiving a reduced dose.

Chronic hepatitis C.

3 million international units 3 times per week for 16 weeks. At 16 weeks, extend treatment to 18 to 24 months at 3 million international units 3 times per week to improve the sustained response of normalization of ALT. Discontinue therapy if there is no response after 16 weeks.

Chronic hepatitis B.

Adults: 30–35 million international units/week SC or IM, given as either 5 million international units/day or 10 million international units 3 times per week for 16 weeks. If serious side effects occur, the dose may be decreased by 50%. **Children:** 3 million international units/m² 3 times per week for the first week followed by dose escalation to 6 million international units/m² 3 times per week (maximum of 10 million international units 3 times per week) for a total of 16–24 weeks.

Follicular lymphoma.

5 million international units SC 3 times per week for up to 18 months in conjunction with an anthracycline-containing chemotherapy regimen. Consider delaying therapy if either the neutrophil count is less than 1,500/mm³ or platelet

count is less than 75,000/mm^3. Withhold for a neutrophil count <1,000/mm^3 or a platelet count <50,000/mm^3; or, reduce the dose by 50% to 2.5 million international units 3 times per week for a neutrophil count of >1,000/mm^3 but <1,500/mm^3. Reinstitution of the initial dose of 5 million international units 3 times per week may be tolerated after resolution of hematologic toxicity. Discontinue therapy if AST exceeds more than 5 times ULN or serum creatinine is more than 2 mg/dL.

IV INFUSION FOLLOWED BY SC

Malignant melanoma.

Induction dose: 20 million international units/m^2 as an IV infusion on 5 consecutive days per week for 4 weeks. **Maintenance dose:** 10 million international units/m^2 SC 3 times per week for 48 weeks. The solution for injection is not recommended for this use. If side effects develop, especially if granulocytes are >250/mm^3 but < 500/mm^3 or ALT/AST rises to more than 5 to 10 times ULN, temporarily withhold the drug until side effects abate. Restart at 50% of the previous dose. If intolerance persists, granulocytes decrease to less than 250/mm^3, or ALT/AST increases to more than 10 times ULN, discontinue the drug.

INTRALESIONAL

Condylomata acuminata (genital or venereal warts).

1 million international units per lesion for a maximum of 5 lesions in a single course. Inject 3 times a week, on alternate days, for 3 weeks. An additional course may be administered at 12 to 16 weeks. Do **not** use the 18 or 50 million unit powder for injection, the 18 million unit multidose solution for injection, or the multidose pens for this purpose. Administer intralesionally using a tuberculin or similar syringe and a 25- to 30-gauge needle. To reduce side effects, give in the evening with acetaminophen. Maximum response usually occurs within 4–8 weeks. If results are unsatisfactory after 12–16 weeks, a second course may be started.

NURSING IMPLICATIONS

IMPLEMENTATION/ADMINISTRATION/STORAGE

1. Prior to administration, reconstitute drug with provided bacteriostatic water for injection. Consult chart with product package to prepare powder for injection based on use.
2. To enhance the tolerability, administer in the evening when possible. The client may self-administer dose at bedtime.
3. If there are decreases in WBC, granulocyte count, or platelet count, use the following guidelines for dose modification: If the granulocyte count is <750/mm^3, the platelet count is <50,000/mm^3, and/or the WBC is <1,500/mm^3, reduce dose by 50%. If the granulocyte count is <500/mm^3, the platelet count <25,000/mm^3, and/or the WBC is <1,000/mm^3, permanently discontinue the drug. Interferon therapy can be resumed up to 100% of the initial dose when WBC, granulocyte, and/or platelet counts return to normal or baseline values.
4. When used for venereal or genital warts, direct needle at the center of the base of the wart and at an angle almost parallel to the plane of the skin. Take care not to go beneath the lesion too deeply; avoid SC administration. Do not inject too superficially as this will result in possible leakage, infiltrating only the keratinized layer and not the dermal core. Maximum response usually occurs 4–8 weeks after therapy is initiated. If results not satisfactory after 12–16 weeks, a second course of therapy may be undertaken.
5. Although the optimal duration of treatment has not been established, clients have been treated for up to 20 consecutive months.
6. If platelet count is <50,000/mm^3, give SC rather than IM.
7. Use a tuberculin-type syringe with a 25- to 30-gauge needle for intralesion administration. Do not give beneath the lesion too deeply or inject too superficially. As many as five lesions can be treated at one time.
8. Store powder from 2–8°C (36–46°F). The reconstituted solution is stable for 30 days when stored from 2–8°C (36–46°F). The so-

lution for injection is stable at 35°C (95°F) for up to 7 days and at 30°C (86°F) for up to 14 days. The undiluted drug is not stable in syringes due to adhesion to syringe surfaces.

9. IV Although not approved by the FDA, interferon alfa-2b has been given by continuous or intermittent IV infusion as well as ophthalmically and intravaginally.
10. For infusion solutions, after reconstitution, withdraw appropriate dose and inject into a 100 mL bag of 0.9% NaCl solution. The final concentration should be 10 million international units/10 mL or more. Infuse over a 20 min period. Prepare solution immediately prior to use.
11. COMPATIBILITY 0.9% NaCl.
12. INCOMPATIBILITY Administer separately.

ASSESSMENT

1. Note reasons for therapy, clinical presentation, other agents trialed, outcome.
2. Identify if previously untreated, relapsed, or nonresponder with hepatitis C.
3. Assess mental status and note any history or evidence of depression.
4. Monitor VS, weight, CBC, renal and LFTs, path reports, and viral loads.

CLIENT/FAMILY TEACHING

1. Review appropriate method for administration, care, disposal, and safe storage of drug and equipment. Demonstrate proper technique for self-injection at visit.
2. The Multidose Pen can provide between 3 to 12 doses depending upon your prescribed dose. Store multidose pen in the refrigerator.
3. May cause dizziness/confusion or low BP; avoid hazardous tasks until drug effects realized.
4. Most common side effects are flu-like symptoms, such as fever, fatigue, headache, chills, nausea, and loss of appetite; may be minimized by taking at bedtime; use acetaminophen for fever and headache.
5. Consume 2–3 L/day of fluids.
6. Fatigue may be experienced. Report any evidence of neurologic or psychologic disturbances, chest pain, vision problems, and if depression, hallucinations, increased agitation/irritability, or suicide ideations occur.
7. Avoid alcohol and any other unprescribed CNS depressants. Hair loss may occur.
8. Males and females should practice reliable contraception.
9. Keep all F/U to assess response, labs/bone marrow (hairy cell) determinations, and adverse/intolerable SE.

OUTCOMES/EVALUATE

- Improved hematologic response
- ↓ Size/number of genital/venereal warts
- ↓ Viral load

Interferon alfacon-1

(in-ter-**FEER**-on **AL**-fah-kon)

Classification(s): Immunomodulator

Pregnancy Category: C

RX: Infergen.

SEE ALSO *INTERFERON ALFA-2B*.

INDICATIONS/USES

(1) Chronic hepatitis C infections in those 18 years of age or older with compensated liver disease who have anti-HCV (hepatitis C virus) serum antibodies or the presence of HCV RNA. *NOTE:* Viral hepatitis B or autoimmune hepatitis should be ruled out prior to beginning therapy with interferon alfacon-1. (2) In combination with ribavirin to retreat chronic hepatitis C. *NOTE:* Combination therapy is now the standard of care for hepatitis C.

ACTION/KINETICS

Action

Prepared by recombinant technology. Has antiviral, antiproliferative, and immunomodulatory effects, regulation of cell surface major histocompatibility antigen expression, and regulation of cytokine expression.

Pharmacokinetics

Plasma levels after SC administration are too low to measure.

CONTRAINDICATIONS

Hypersensitivity to alpha interferons or to products derived from *E. coli*. Use in autoimmune hepatitis or in decompensated hepatic disease (Child-Pugh score >5). Use of interferon alfacon-1/ribavirin in those with a C_{CR} <59 mL/min.

SPECIAL CONCERNS

(1) **Fatal or life-threatening disorders.** Alpha interferons, including interferon alfacon-1, cause or aggravate fatal or life-threatening neuropsychiatric, autoimmune, ischemic, and infectious disorders. Closely monitor clients with periodic clinical and lab evaluations. Clients with persistently severe or worsening symptoms of these conditions should be withdrawn from therapy. In many, but not all, these conditions resolve after stopping interferon alfacon-1 therapy. (2) **Use with ribavirin.** Ribavirin may cause birth defects and/or death of the fetus. Extreme care must be taken to avoid pregnancy in female clients and in female partners of male clients. Ribavirin causes hemolytic anemia. The anemia associated with ribavirin therapy may result in a worsening of cardiac disease. Ribavirin is genotoxic and mutagenic and should be considered a potential carcinogen.

- **Use with caution during lactation and in pre-existing cardiac disease, in depression, in those with abnormally low peripheral blood cell counts, in those receiving myelosuppressive agents, in the elderly, and in autoimmune disorder.**
- **Discontinue in those developing severe depression, suicidal ideation, or other severe psychiatric disorders.**
- **Safety and efficacy not determined using interferon alfacon-1 alone or with ribavirin to treat chronic HCV infection in liver or other organ transplant recipients or in those coinfected with HIV or HBV.**
- **Safety and efficacy not determined in children less than 18 years of age.**

SIDE EFFECTS

Most Common

Headache, fatigue, fever, myalgia, rigors, arthralgia, increased sweating, arthralgia, depression, body pain, abdominal pain, nausea, back pain, insomnia, nervousness, pharyngitis, URTI, dizziness, diarrhea, anorexia, dyspepsia, injection site erythema, limb pain, cough.

Flu-like symptoms: Headache, fatigue, fever, myalgia, rigors, arthralgia, increased sweating. **Hypersensitivity:** Urticaria, angioedema, bronchoconstriction, ***anaphylaxis***. **CNS:** Headache, insomnia, nervousness, depression, dizziness, anxiety, emotional lability, amnesia, paresthesia, hypesthesia, abnormal thinking, aggressive behavior, hypertonia, decreased libido, agitation, confusion, somnolence, apathy, hyperesthesia, psychosis, homicidal ideation, ***suicidal ideation, suicide attempt, suicide,*** ataxia, ***convulsions***, delusions, abnormal gait, hallucinations, LOC, impaired memory, speech disorder, tremors. **GI:** Abdominal pain, N&V, diarrhea, anorexia, dyspepsia, constipation, flatulence, toothache, hemorrhoids, decreased saliva, gingivitis, ulcerative stomatitis, taste perversion, abdominal distention, GI bleeding, gastritis, ***hemorrhagic/ischemic colitis, pancreatitis***. **Hepatic:** Hepatomegaly, tender liver, ascites, hepatic encephalopathy, jaundice, ***hepatic decompensation***. **CV:** Hyper-/hypotension, tachycardia, supraventricular arrhythmias, chest pain, ***MI***, palpitation, angina pectoris, arrhythmias, ischemic and hemorrhagic CV events, ***cardiomyopathy***. **Hematologic:** Granulocytopenia, thrombocytopenia, leukopenia, ecchymosis, lymphadenopathy, lymphocytosis, anemia, ***aplastic anemia*** (rare). **Respiratory:** Pharyngitis, URTI, cough, sinusitis, rhinitis, respiratory tract/URT congestion, epistaxis, dyspnea, bronchitis, bronchiolitis obliterans, interstitial pneumonitis, pneumonia, pulmonary hypertension, pulmonary infiltrates, sarcoidosis, ***respiratory failure***. **Dermatologic:** Alopecia, pruritus, rash, increased sweating, erythema, dry skin, bruising, pyoderma, gangrenosum, ***toxic epidermal necrolysis***. **Musculoskeletal:** Myalgia, arthralgia, back/limb/neck/skeletal pain, musculoskeletal disorder, arthritis, bone pain, rhabdomyolysis. **GU:** Dysmenorrhea, vaginitis, menstrual disorder, menorrhagia, genital moniliasis, impaired renal function, renal failure. **Metabolic:** Occurrence or aggravation of hyperthyroidism or hypothyroidism, hyperglycemia, diabetes mellitus. **Hypersensitivity:** Bronchoconstriction, urticaria, angioedema, ***anaphylaxis***. **Ophthalmic:** Conjunctivitis, eye pain, decrease or loss of vision, macular edema, retinal artery or vein thrombosis, retinal hemorrhages, cotton wool spots, optic neuritis, papilledema, serious retinal detachment, visual field defect. **Otic:** Tinnitus, earache, otitis, hearing impairment/loss. **At injection site:** Erythema, pain, ecchymosis, necrosis, ulcer, bruising. **Body as a whole**: Fatigue, fever, rigors, body pain, hot flushes, malaise, infection, peripheral edema, peripheral neuropathy, asthenia, dehydration, ***hemorrhage***, sepsis, access pain, non-cardiac chest pain, weight loss, infection, immunogenicity, exacerbation of autoimmune disorders (e.g., autoimmune thrombocytopenia, idiopathic thrombocytopenic purpura, psoriasis, rheumatoid arthritis, thyroiditis, interstitial nephritis, systemic lupus erythematosus).

LABORATORY TEST CONSIDERATIONS

↑ ALT, AST, TSH, triglycerides, serum creatinine. ↓ H&H, ANC, WBC, platelets. Abnormal thyroid tests, abnormal hepatic function. Hyperbilirubinemia.

DRUG INTERACTIONS

Drugs metabolized by cytochrome P450 / Possible changes in therapeutic and/or toxic levels of these drugs

Myelosuppressive drugs / Use caution when given with such drugs

HOW SUPPLIED

Injection Solution: 9 mcg/0.3 mL, 15 mcg/0.5 mL.

I

DOSAGE

SC INJECTION

Chronic hepatitis C infection.

Adults over 18 years of age: 9 mcg SC as a single injection 3 times per week for 24 weeks. At least 48 hr should elapse between doses. Those who tolerate therapy but did not respond or relapsed following discontinuation may be subsequently treated with 15 mcg 3 times per week for up to 48 weeks.

With ribavirin to retreat chronic hepatitis C.

Adults. Interferon alfacon-1: 15 mcg/day SC. **Ribavirin:** 1,000 mg/day for those who weigh <75 kg or 1,200 mg/day for those who weigh 75 kg or more; give PO in 2 divided doses/day for up to 48 weeks.

NURSING IMPLICATIONS

IMPLEMENTATION/ADMINISTRATION/STORAGE

1. Just prior to injection, allow interferon alfacon-1 to reach room temperature. Use only 1 vial per dose; do not re-enter the vial. Discard unused portions. Do not save unused drug for later use.
2. Administer undiluted by SC injection. Do not shake.
3. When interferon alfacon-1 is given in combination, take ribavirin with food.
4. Clients who fail to achieve at least a 2 $\log_{10}$ drop for at least 12 weeks or undetectable HCV RNA at week 24 are highly unlikely to achieve sustained viral response; consider discontinuation of therapy.
5. Withhold dose temporarily or modify the dosage if severe side effects experienced. If side effects do not become tolerable, discontinue therapy.
6. Reduction of dose to 7.5 mcg may be necessary following an intolerable side effect. If side effects continue to occur at reduced dosage, discontinue treatment or reduce dosage further. Decreased efficacy may result from continued treatment at doses less than 7.5 mcg.
7. If serious side effects occur during combination therapy, reduce the dose stepwise from 15 to 9 mcg and from 9 to 6 mcg.
8. Do not give 15 mcg 3 times per week if client has not received or tolerated an initial course of therapy.
9. The following are dose modifications in clients with depression and who are taking interferon alfacon-1 and ribavirin: (a) For mild depression, no change in dosage of either interferon alfacon-1 or ribavirin; evaluate once weekly by office visit and/or phone; (b) For moderate depression, decrease the interferon alfacon-1 dose from 15 to 9 mcg or from 9 to 6 mcg; no change to ribavirin dose; evaluate once weekly with an office visit at least once every other week; (c) For severe depression, discontinue interferon alfacon-1 and ribavirin permanently.
10. The following are dose modifications for clients with hematologic toxicities and who are taking interferon alfacon-1 and ribavirin: (a) If ANC is $<0.75 \times 10^9$/L, reduce interferon alfacon-1 dose from 15 to 9 mcg or from 9 to 6 mcg; maintain ribavirin dose at 1,200 or 1,000 mg; (b) If ANC is $<50 \times 10^9$/L, suspend interferon alfacon-1 and ribavirin treatment until ANC values return to more than 1,000/mm^3; (c) If the platelet count is $<50 \times 10^9$/L, reduce interferon alfacon-1 dose from 15 to 9 mcg or from 9 to 6 mcg; maintain ribavirin dose at 1,200 or 1,000 mg; (d) If the

platelet count is $<25 \times 10^9$/L, discontinue interferon alfacon-1 and ribavirin.

11. The following are dose modifications for clients with anemia and who are taking interferon alfacon-1 and ribavirin: (a) If hemoglobin levels are <10 grams/dL and there is a history of cardiac or CV disease, reduce the dose of interferon alfacon-1 from 15 to 9 mcg or 9 to 6 mcg and the ribavirin dose by 200 mg/day if a decrease more than 2 grams/dL in hemoglobin is observed during any 4-week period. The second dose reduction of ribavirin, if needed, is by an additional 200 mg/day. Discontinue both drugs permanently if clients have hemoglobin levels less than 12 grams/dL after this ribavirin dose reduction; (b) If hemoglobin is <8.5 grams/dL and there is a history of cardiac or CV disease, permanently discontinue both drugs.
12. Store refrigerated but do not freeze. Avoid vigorous shaking and exposure to direct sunlight.

ASSESSMENT

1. Note reasons for therapy, clinical presentation, other therapies trialed/outcome, disease characteristics.
2. Note any cardiac disease, hypertension, severe psychiatric disorders; these preclude drug therapy.
3. Monitor VS, CBC, TSH, triglycerides, viral load, renal and LFTs closely.

CLIENT/FAMILY TEACHING

1. Review dose and method of administration (SC), care, disposal, and safe storage of drug and equipment; usually administered 3 times per week with 48 hr between doses unless retreatment.
2. Demonstrate proper technique for self-injection at visit. Store drug in refrigerator. Review medication guide to facilitate administration.
3. Use caution with activities that require mental alertness; may cause drowsiness or dizziness.
4. May experience flu-like symptoms, including headache, fatigue, fever, muscle/joint pain, rigors, increased sweating; may be minimized by taking at bedtime and analgesics.
5. Stop drug, report any S&S of depression, suicide thoughts/attempt, vision changes, hives, shortness of breath or difficult breathing, persistent fever, sore throat, unusual bleeding or bruising, or intolerable injection-site reaction.
6. Males and females must practice reliable contraception.
7. Do not change brands of interferon without provider approval.
8. Keep all F/U to assess response, labs, and for adverse SE.

OUTCOMES/EVALUATE

Improvement in LFTs; ↓ viral load

Interferon alfa-n3

(in-ter-**FEER**-on **AL**-fah)

Classification(s): Antineoplastic

Pregnancy Category: C

RX: Alferon N.

INDICATIONS/USES

Intralesional treatment of refractory or recurring external condylomata acuminata (genital or venereal warts) in clients 18 years of age or older. *Investigational:* Alpha interferons are being tested for use in a large number of neoplastic diseases and viral infections.

ACTION/KINETICS

Action

Is a sterile, aqueous formulation of purified, natural, human interferon alpha proteins. Binds to receptors on cell surfaces leading to a sequence of events including inhibition of virus replication and suppression of cell proliferation. Also, causes immunomodulation characterized by enhanced phagocytosis by macrophages, augmentation of the cytotoxicity of lymphocytes, and enhancement of human leukocyte antigen expression.

Pharmacokinetics

Intralesional use of interferon alfa-n3 does not result in detectable plasma levels of the drug.

CONTRAINDICATIONS

Hypersensitivity to human interferon alpha; clients who are allergic to mouse immunoglobulin (IgG), egg protein, or neomycin (the production process involves a nutrient medium containing neomycin although it has not been detected in the final product). Lactation. Use in clients less than 18 years of age.

SPECIAL CONCERNS

- Due to fever and flu-like symptoms, use caution in clients with debilitating diseases, including unstable angina, uncontrolled CHF, COPD, diabetes mellitus with ketoacidosis, thrombophlebitis, pulmonary embolism, hemophilia, severe myelosuppression, or seizure disorders.
- Use with caution in fertile men.
- Made from human blood; may carry risk of transmitting infections.
- Safety and effectiveness not determined in children less than 18 years of age.

SIDE EFFECTS

Most Common

Myalgias, fever, headache, fatigue, chills, malaise, dizziness, nausea, arthralgia, back pain.

Flu-like symptoms: Commonly, fever, headache, myalgias, which decrease with repeated doses. Also, chills, fatigue, malaise. **Hypersensitivity reaction:** Urticaria, angioedema, bronchoconstriction, ***anaphylaxis***. **CNS:** Dizziness, headache, lightheadedness, insomnia, depression, nervousness, decreased ability to concentrate. **GI:** N&V, heartburn, dyspepsia, diarrhea, tongue hyperesthesia, thirst, altered taste, increased salivation. **Musculoskeletal/Skin:** Arthralgia, myalgia, back pain, hot sensation at bottom of feet, tingling of legs/feet, muscle cramps. **Respiratory:** Nose or sinus drainage, nose bleed, throat tightness, pharyngitis. **Miscellaneous:** Pruritus, swollen lymph nodes, heat intolerance, visual disturbances, sensitivity to allergens, papular rash on neck, hot flashes, herpes labialis, dysuria, photosensitivity, sweating, vasovagal reaction.

NOTE: When used for treatment of cancer, the incidence of many of the preceding side effects was increased. Additional side effects were noted including: **GI:** Constipation, anorexia, stomatitis, dry mouth, mucositis, sore mouth. **Miscellaneous:** Insomnia, blurred vision, ocular rotation pain, sore injection site, chest pains, low BP.

LABORATORY TEST CONSIDERATIONS

↓ WBC. The following may be affected in cancer clients: Hemoglobin levels, WBC and platelet count, GGT, AST, alkaline phosphatase, and total bilirubin.

HOW SUPPLIED

Injection: 5 million international units/mL.

DOSAGE

INTRADERMAL

Condylomata acuminata.

0.05 mL (250,000 international units)/wart twice a week for up to 8 weeks. The maximum recommended dose per treatment session is 0.5 mL (2.5 million international units). The safety and effectiveness of a second course of treatment have not been determined.

NURSING IMPLICATIONS

IMPLEMENTATION/ADMINISTRATION/STORAGE

1. Inject drug into base of the wart using a 30-gauge needle.
2. For large warts, inject at several points around the wart periphery using a total of 0.05 mL/wart.
3. Do not give further drug or conventional therapy for 3 months after the initial 8-week course of treatment unless the warts enlarge or new warts appear.
4. Store drug at 2–8°C (36–46°F). Do not freeze or shake.

ASSESSMENT

1. Note reasons for therapy, onset, clinical presentation, other therapy trialed; assess for allergy to egg protein or neomycin (may have ↑ drug sensitivity).
2. List any pre-existing debilitating diseases; note functional level.
3. Do not change brands without approval; manufacturing process, strength, and type of interferon may vary.
4. For condylomata therapy, measure and document size, location, and number of lesions.
5. Assess for other STDs and treat as indicated.

CLIENT/FAMILY TEACHING

1. Intralesional treatment should be continued for 8 weeks.
2. Genital warts may disappear both during and after treatment has been completed. When this occurs, unless new warts appear or warts become enlarged, there should be a 3-month waiting period after the first 8-week course of therapy.
3. May use acetaminophen as needed if flu-like symptoms occur.

4. **Avoid activities that require mental alertness until drug effects realized; decreased mental status or dizziness may occur.**
5. **Practice reliable barrier contraception. May consider egg/sperm harvesting if pregnancy desired.**
6. **Report early signs of hypersensitivity reactions (e.g., hives, chest tightness, generalized urticaria, hypotension, wheezing, anaphylaxis).**
7. **Keep F/U to assess response, labs, and for adverse SE.**

OUTCOMES/EVALUATE

- ↓ Pain, number of genital warts
- Suppression of malignant cell proliferation

Interferon beta-1a
Interferon beta-1b (r1FN-B)

(in-ter-**FEER**-on **BAY**-tah)

Classification(s): Immunomodulator

Pregnancy Category: C

RX: Interferon beta-1a: Avonex, Rebif, **Interferon beta-1b:** Betaseron, Extavia.

INDICATIONS/USES

Interferon beta-1a: Treatment of relapsing forms of MS to slow the appearance of physical disability (and possibly mental decline) and decrease the frequency of clinical exacerbations. Safety and efficacy have not been established in those with chronic progressive MS.

Interferon beta-1b: Treatment of relapsing forms of MS to reduce the frequency of clinical exacerbations. Those in whom efficacy has been shown include clients who have experienced a first clinical episode and have magnetic resonance imaging features consistent with MS. Evidence of efficacy beyond 2 years is not known. Safety and efficacy in chronic progressive MS have not been studied.

Investigational: Treatment of AIDS, AIDS-related Kaposi's sarcoma, metastatic renal cell carcinoma, herpes of the lips or genitals, malignant melanoma, cutaneous T-cell lymphoma, and acute non-A/non-B hepatitis.

ACTION/KINETICS

Action

Interferon beta-1a is produced by mammalian cells into which the human interferon beta gene has been introduced. Interferon beta-1b is a genetically engineered plasmid containing the gene for human interferon beta$_{ser17}$. Interferon betas have antiviral, antiproliferative, and immunoregulatory effects. Mechanism for the beneficial effect in MS is unknown, although the effects are mediated through combination with specific cell receptors located on the cell membrane. The receptor-drug complex induces the expression of a number of interferon-induced gene products that are thought to be the mediators of the biologic effects of interferon beta-1a and beta-1b.

Pharmacokinetics

t½, interferon beta-1a: 10 hr. Kinetic information is not available for interferon beta-1a since serum levels are low or not detectable following SC administration to MS clients. **Peak serum levels of beta-1b:** Within 1–8 hr with a mean serum concentration of 40 international units/mL. Mean terminal half-lives ranged from 8 min to 4.3 hr.

CONTRAINDICATIONS

Hypersensitivity to natural or recombinant interferon beta or human albumin. Use of Avonex with other hepatotoxic drugs. Lactation.

SPECIAL CONCERNS

- **Use caution in clients with depression and other severe psychiatric symptoms as depression, attempted suicide, and suicide have occurred.**
- **Use caution with pre-existing seizure disorder.**
- **Potential abortifacient.**
- **Safety and efficacy for use in chronic progressive MS and in children less than 18 years of age not studied.**

SIDE EFFECTS

Most Common

Interferon beta-1a: Headache, flu-like symptoms, nausea, myalgia, arthralgia, URTI, fever, pain, asthenia, chills, infection, sleep difficulty, dizziness, diarrhea, sinusitis, bronchitis, skeletal/back pain, abnormal vision, xerophthalmia, chest pain, inflammatory ecchymosis, injection site reaction.

Interferon beta-1b: Injection site reaction, headache, fever, flu-like symptoms, pain, asthenia, chills, abdominal pain, mental symptoms, hypertonia, dizziness, diarrhea, constipation, vomiting, myalgia, arthralgia, myasthenia, dyspnea, chest pain, inflammatory ecchymosis, leg cramps, malaise, sinusitis.

- **Interferon beta-1a and beta-1b**

Body as a whole: Headache, fever, pain, asthenia, chills, reaction at injection site (including necrosis/inflammation/pain), malaise. **Flu-like symptoms:** Muscle aches, fever, chills, asthenia, headache, pain, nausea, diarrhea, infection, sleep difficulty, dizziness. **GI:** Abdominal pain, diarrhea, dry mouth, ***GI hemorrhage***, gingivitis, hepatomegaly, intestinal obstruction, periodontal abscess, proctitis. **CV:** Arrhythmia, hypotension, postural hypotension. **CNS:** Dizziness, depression, speech disorder, convulsion, ***suicide attempt***, abnormal gait, depersonalization, facial paralysis, hyperesthesia, neurosis, psychosis. **Respiratory:** Sinusitis, dyspnea, hemoptysis, hyperventilation. **Musculoskeletal:** Myalgia, arthritis, arthralgia, back pain, myasthenia, skeletal pain. **Dermatologic:** Contact dermatitis, furunculosis, seborrhea, skin ulcer, photosensitivity. **GU:** Epididymitis, gynecomastia, hematuria, kidney calculus, nocturia, ***vaginal hemorrhage***, ovarian cyst. **Miscellaneous:** Abscess, ascites, cellulitis, hernia, chest pain, hypothyroidism, ***sepsis***, hiccoughs, thirst, leukorrhea.

- **Interferon beta-1a**

Body as a whole: Infection, neutralizing antibodies (significance unknown). **GI:** Nausea, dyspepsia, anorexia, blood in stool, colitis, constipation, diverticulitis, gallbladder disorder, gastritis, gum hemorrhage, hepatoma, increased appetite, ***intestinal perforation***, periodontitis, tongue disorder. **Hepatic:** Autoimmune hepatitis. Avonex may cause hepatic injury (including hepatic failure), elevated serum LFTs (asymptomatic), and hepatitis. **CV:** Syncope, vasodilation, arteritis, ***heart arrest, hemorrhage, pulmonary embolus, CHF, cardiomyopathy, cardiomyopathy with CHF***, palpitation, pericarditis, peripheral ischemia, peripheral vascular disorder, spider angioma, telangiectasia. **CNS:** Sleep difficulty, muscle spasm, ataxia, amnesia, Bell's palsy, clumsiness, drug dependence, increased libido, new or worsening psychiatric disorders, ***seizures***. **Respiratory:** URTI, emphysema, laryngitis, pharyngeal edema, pneumonia. **Musculoskeletal:** Arthralgia, bone pain, myasthenia, osteonecrosis, synovitis. **Dermatologic:** Urticaria, alopecia, nevus, herpes zoster/simplex, basal cell carcinoma, blisters, cold clammy skin, erythema, genital pruritus, skin discoloration. **GU:** Vaginitis, fibroids, kidney pain, breast fibroadenosis/pain, dysuria, fibrocystic change of the breast, menopause, PID, penis disorder, Peyronie's disease, polyuria, postmenopausal hemorrhage, testis/prostatic disorder, pyelonephritis, urethral pain, urinary urgency/retention/incontinence, menorrhagia, metrorrhagia. **Hematologic:** Anemia, ecchymosis at injection site, eosinophils >10%, hematocrit <37%, increased coagulation time, ecchymosis, lymphadenopathy, petechia, rarely pancytopenia or thrombocytopenia, idiopathic thrombocytopenia, ***pancytopenia*** (rare). **Metabolic:** Dehydration, hypoglycemia/magnesemia/-kalemia, hypo-/hyperthyroidism. **Ophthalmic:** Abnormal vision, conjunctivitis, eye pain, vitreous floaters. **Miscellaneous:** Otitis media, decreased hearing, facial edema, fibrosis/hypersensitivity at injection site, rarely ***anaphylaxis, allergic reactions***, lipoma, neoplasm, photosensitivity, toothache, sinus headache, chest pain.

- **Interferon beta-1b**

Body as a whole: Generalized edema, hypothermia, ***anaphylaxis, shock***, adenoma, sarcoma. **GI:** Constipation, vomiting, GI disorder, aphthous stomatitis, cardiospasm, cheilitis, cholecystitis, cholelithiasis, duodenal ulcer, enteritis, esophagitis, fecal impaction or incontinence, flatulence, gastritis, glossitis, hematemesis, ileus, increased salivation, melena, nausea, oral leukoplakia/moniliasis, ***pancreatitis, rectal hemorrhage***, salivary gland enlargement, stomach ulcer, peritonitis, tenesmus. **Hepatic:** Autoimmune hepatitis, severe liver damage leading to hepatic failure and transplant, hepatic neoplasia, hepatitis. **CV:** Migraine, palpitation, hypertension, tachycardia, peripheral vascular disorder, ***hemorrhage***, angina pectoris, atrial fibrillation, cardiomegaly, ***cardiac arrest, cerebral hemorrhage, heart failure, MI, pulmonary embolus, ventricular fibrillation, cardiomyopathy, DVT***, cerebral ischemia, endocarditis, pericardial effusion, spider angioma, subarachnoid hemorrhage, syncope, thrombophlebitis, thrombosis, varicose veins, vasospasm, venous pressure increase, ventricular extrasystoles. **CNS:** Mental symptoms, hypertonia, somnolence, hyperkinesia, acute/chronic brain syndrome, agitation, apathy, aphasia, ataxia, confusion, depersonalization, emotional lability, paresthesia, ***seizures***, brain edema, ***coma***, delirium, delusions, dementia, dystonia, encephalopathy, euphoria, hallucinations, hemiplegia, hypalgesia, incoordination, intracranial hypertension, decreased libido, manic reaction, meningitis, neuralgia, neuropathy, paralysis, paranoid reaction, decreased reflexes, stupor, subdural hematoma, torticollis, tremor. **Respiratory:** Laryngitis, apnea, asthma, atelectasis, lung carcinoma, hypoventilation, interstitial pneumonia, ***bronchospasm***, lung edema, pleural effusion, pneumothorax. **Musculoskeletal:** Myasthenia, arthrosis, bursitis, leg cramps, muscle atrophy, myopathy, myositis, ptosis, tenosynovitis. **Dermatologic:** Sweating, alopecia, erythema nodosum, pruritus, skin discoloration, exfoliative dermatitis, hirsutism, leukoderma, lichenoid dermatitis, maculopapular rash, photosensitivity, psoriasis, benign skin neoplasm, urticaria, skin hypertrophy/necrosis/carcinoma, vesiculobullous rash. **GU:** Dysmenorrhea, menstrual disorder, metrorrhagia, cystitis, breast pain, menorrhagia, urinary urgency, fibrocystic breast, breast neoplasm, urinary retention, anuria, balanitis, breast engorgement, cervicitis, impotence, kidney failure, tubular disorder, nephritis, oliguria, polyuria, UTI, urosepsis, salpingitis, urethritis, urinary incontinence, enlarged uterine fibroids, uterine neoplasm. **Hematologic:** Lymphocytes <1,500/mm^3, active neutrophil count <1,500/mm^3, WBCs <3,000/mm^3, lymphadenopathy, CLL, petechia, hemoglobin <9.4 g/dL, platelets <75,000/mm^3, splenomegaly, anemia, thrombocytopenia. **Metabolic:** Weight gain/loss, goiter, glucose <55 mg/dL or >160 mg/dL, AST or ALT >5 times baseline, total bilirubin >2.5 times baseline, urine protein >1+, alkaline phosphatase >5 times baseline, BUN >40 mg/dL, calcium >11.5 mg/dL, increased GGT, hypocalcemia, hyperuricemia, increased triglycerides, cyanosis, edema, glycosuria, hypoglycemic reaction, hypoxia, ketosis. **Endocrine:** Hypo-/hyperthyroidism, thyroid dysfunction. **Ophthalmic:** Conjunctivitis, abnormal vision, diplopia, nystagmus, oculogyric crisis, papilledema, blepharitis, blindness, dry eyes, iritis, keratoconjunctivitis, mydriasis, photophobia, retinitis, visual field defect. **Hematologic**: Anemia, thrombocytopenia. **Miscellaneous:** Pelvic pain, hydrocephalus, alcohol intolerance, otitis/externa media, parosmia, taste loss/perversion, ***fatal capillary leak syndrome***.

LABORATORY TEST CONSIDERATIONS

↑ ALT, total bilirubin, AST, BUN, urine protein. Hypoglycemia or hyperglycemia. Ketosis.

Interferon beta-1b: ↑ GGT, triglycerides. Hypocalcemia, hyperuricemia.

HOW SUPPLIED

Interferon beta-1a. ***Injection (Rebif):*** 8.8 mcg/0.2 mL (2.4 million units), 22 mcg/0.5 mL (6 million units), 44 mcg/0.5 mL (12 million units); ***Powder for Injection, Lyophilized (Avonex):*** 33 mcg (6.6 million units [30 mcg/vial] when reconstituted); ***Prefilled Syringes (Avonex):*** 30 mcg/0.5 mL. **Interferon beta-1b.** ***Powder for Injection, Lyophilized (Betaseron or Extavia):*** 0.3 mg.

DOSAGE

Interferon beta-1a

IM; SC

Relapsing forms of MS.

Avonex: 30 mcg IM once a week. Sites include the thigh or upper arm. Do not substitute SC administration of Avonex for IM administration.

Rebif: Usually start with 20% of the final dose 3 times per week and increase over a 4-week period to the targeted dose, either 22 mcg or 44 mcg three times per week. For a prescribed dose of 44 mcg, give 8.8 mcg three times per week for weeks 1 and 2 and 22 mcg three times per week for weeks 3 and 4. For a prescribed dose of 22 mcg, give 4.4 mcg three times per week for weeks 1 and 2 and 11 mcg three times per week for weeks 3 and 4. Give the full prescribed dose beginning week 5. Give, if possible, at the same time (preferably late afternoon or evening) on the same days each week, at least 48 hr apart (e.g., Monday, Wednesday, Friday). Rotate injection sites.

Inteferon beta-1b

SC

Relapsing-remitting MS.

Goal: 0.25 mg SC every other day. Sites include arms, abdomen, hips, and thigh. Generally start clients at 0.0625 mg (0.25 mL) SC every other day for weeks 1 and 2; then, for weeks

3 and 4, give 0.125 mg (0.5 mL) every other day; for weeks 5 and 6, give 0.1875 mg (0.75 mL) every other day; and, beginning week 7, give 0.25 mg (1 mL) every other day.

NURSING IMPLICATIONS

IMPLEMENTATION/ADMINISTRATION/STORAGE

1. Avonex and Rebif are intended for use under the direction of a physician. Clients may self-inject only if the physician determines it is appropriate and with medical follow-up, as needed, after proper training in IM (for Avonex) or SC (for Rebif) injection technique.
2. To reconstitute and use Avonex (interferon beta-1a) use the following process:
   - Use a sterile syringe and *Micro Pin* to inject 1.1 mL of the supplied diluent, sterile water for injection, into the vial and swirl gently to dissolve. Do not shake.
   - The reconstituted solution should be clear to slightly yellow without particles. Discard if the product contains particulate matter or is discolored.
   - Each vial contains 30 mcg/mL of drug.
   - Withdraw 1 mL of reconstituted solution into a sterile syringe. Replace the cover on the *Micro Pin* and attach the sterile 23-gauge 1.25-inch needle and inject IM.
   - Vials must be stored in a refrigerator at 2–8°C (36–46°F).
   - Following reconstitution, use within 6 hr; store at same temperatures as unreconstituted drug. Do not freeze reconstituted Avonex.
3. If using Avonex prefilled syringes, allow to warm to room temperature (about 30 min) after removing from the refrigerator and use within 12 hr. Do not use external heat sources to warm prefilled Avonex syringes. To administer, hold the prefilled syringe upright (rubber cap facing up). Remove the protective cover by turning and gently pulling the rubber cap in a clockwise motion. Attach the 23-gauge, 1.25-inch needle, and inject IM. The prefilled syringe is for single use only.
4. When using Rebif, rotate injection sites. Leukopenia or elevated liver function tests may necessitate dose reduction or discontinuation of Rebif until toxicity is resolved.
5. Store Rebif from 2–8°C (36–46°F). Do not freeze. If refrigeration is not available, store Rebif at or below 25°C (77°F) for up to 30 days away from heat and light. Do not use beyond the expiration date. Discard unused portions.
6. Concurrent use of analgesics or antipyretics may help decrease flu-like symptoms on Rebif treatment days.
7. To reconstitute and use Betaseron (interferon beta-1b), use the following process:
   - Using the sterile single-use syringe and needle, slowly inject 1.2 mL of diluent provided (0.54% NaCl) into the vial. Swirl gently to dissolve the drug completely. Do not shake. Foaming may occur if the vial is swirled or shaken too vigorously.
   - Visually inspect reconstituted product; discard if it contains particulate matter or is discolored.
   - Withdraw the appropriate amount of the reconstituted solution from the vial into a sterile syringe fitted with a 27-gauge needle and inject SC. Injection sites include the arms, abdomen, hips, and thighs.
   - Since the reconstituted product contains no preservative, discard any unused portions after one use.
   - Before reconstitution, store from 2–8°C (36–46°F). After reconstitution, if not used immediately, refrigerate and use within 3 hr. Do not freeze. If refrigeration is not possible, keep vials and diluent as cool as possible below 30°C (86°F), away from heat and light; use within 7 days.

ASSESSMENT

1. List age at diagnosis, frequency of exacerbations, other therapies prescribed, outcome. Document brain MRI confirmation; degree of debilitation and frequency of relapse.
2. Note any hypersensitivity to human albumin or interferon beta. Assess psychological status noting depression or suicidal ideations; use with extreme caution.
3. Check for pregnancy; drug has abortifacient properties.
4. Determine any cardiac disease or seizure disorder; monitor closely.
5. Monitor hematologic profile and hepatic enzyme levels q 3 months.

6. Conduct LFTs 1, 3, and 6 months after beginning interferon beta-1b therapy and then periodically thereafter in the absence of clinical symptoms.

CLIENT/FAMILY TEACHING

1. Review guidelines for drug use, proper dose, administration, and care and disposal of equipment. Demonstrate proper technique for self-injection at visit. Do not change dose or administration schedule without approval.
2. If possible, give Rebif at the same time, preferably in the late afternoon or evening on the same 3 days (e.g., Monday, Wednesday, Friday) at least 48 hr apart each week.
3. For Rebif, a starter kit is available to titrate the dose during the first 4 weeks of therapy. Following the administration of each dose, discard any unused product in the syringe. Use Rebif only under the guidance and supervision of provider. Observe client technique to ensure correct self-administration SC using the prefilled syringes; rotate injection sites.
4. Flu-like symptoms are common; analgesics or antipyretics may help.
5. Report any mental status changes, depression, suicide thoughts.
6. Practice reliable birth control; drug may harm fetus.
7. May cause photosensitivity reactions; wear protective clothing, sunscreen, sunglasses, and a hat when sun exposed.
8. Avoid alcohol in any form.
9. With diabetes, monitor FS and report any overt changes.
10. Identify support groups that may assist to cope with chronic disease.
11. Keep all F/U visits to assess response, labs, and for adverse SE.

OUTCOMES/EVALUATE

↓ Frequency and severity of MS exacerbations

IV

Interferon gamma-1b

(in-ter-**FEER**-on **GAM**-uh)

Classification(s): Immunomodulator

Pregnancy Category: C

RX: Actimmune.

INDICATIONS/USES

(1) Decrease the frequency and severity of serious infections associated with chronic granulomatous disease. (2) Delay time to disease progression in severe, malignant osteoporosis.

ACTION/KINETICS

Action

Manifests potent phagocyte-activating effects including generation of toxic oxygen metabolites within phagocytes. Such metabolites result in the death of microorganisms such as *Staphylococcus aureus, Toxoplasma gondii, Leishmania donovani, Listeria monocytogenes,* and *Mycobacterium avium intracellulare.* Since interferon gamma regulates activity of immune cells, it is characterized as a lymphokine of the interleukin type. Interferon gamma interacts functionally with other interleukin molecules (e.g., interleukin-2) and all interleukins form part of a complex, lymphokine regulatory network. As an example, interferon gamma and interleukin-4 may interact reciprocally to regulate murine IgE levels; interferon gamma can suppress IgE levels and inhibit the production of collagen at the transcription level in humans.

Pharmacokinetics

Slowly absorbed after SC injection; more than 89% is absorbed. **t½, elimination: SC,** 5.9 hr. **Peak plasma levels:** 7 hr after SC.

CONTRAINDICATIONS

Hypersensitivity to interferon gamma, to *E. coli*-derived products, or any component of the product. Lactation.

SPECIAL CONCERNS

- Use caution in clients with pre-existing cardiac disease, including symptoms of ischemia, arrhythmia, or CHF, and in clients with myelosuppression or taking other potentially myelosuppressive drugs, seizure disorders, or compromised CNS function.
- Safety and efficacy not determined in children less than 1 year of age.

SIDE EFFECTS

Most Common

Fever, headache, rash, chills, injection site erythema/tenderness, fatigue, diarrhea, N&V, abdominal pain, myalgia.

The following side effects were noted in clients with chronic granulomatous disease or severe, malignant osteoporosis receiving the drug SC. **GI:** Diarrhea, N&V, abdominal pain, anorexia, **CNS:** Fever (over 50%), headache, fatigue, depression. Decreased mental status, gait disturbances, and dizziness in those with compromised CNS function or seizure disorders. **Musculoskeletal:** Arthralgia, myalgia, back pain. **Hematologic:** Myelosuppression, neutropenia, thrombocytopenia. **Miscellaneous:** Serious infections, rash, chills, injection site erythema or tenderness/pain, weight loss, hypersensitivity reactions (may be acute and serious).

When used in clients other than those with chronic granulomatous disease, in addition to the preceding, the following side effects were reported. **GI:** ***GI bleeding, pancreatitis***, hepatic insufficiency. **CNS:** Confusion, disorientation, symptoms of parkinsonism, gait disturbance, ***seizures***, hallucinations. **CV:** Hypotension, heart block, ***heart failure***, syncope, ***tachyarrhythmia, MI, DVT, pulmonary embolism***, TIAs. **Respiratory:** ***Bronchospasm***, tachypnea, interstitial pneumonitis. **Metabolic:** Hyperglycemia, hyponatremia, hypertriglyceridemia. **Miscellaneous:** Reversible renal insufficiency, worsening of dermatomyositis, chest discomfort, increased autoantibodies, lupus-like syndrome.

LABORATORY TEST CONSIDERATIONS

↑ AST, ALT, proteinuria.

OVERDOSE MANAGEMENT

Symptoms: CNS side effects, including decreased mental status, dizziness, and gait disturbances in cancer clients receiving more than 100 mcg/m^2/day IV or IM. Also, elevation of hepatic enzymes and triglycerides, reversible neutropenia, and thrombocytopenia. *Treatment:* CNS side effects are reversible within a few days upon reducing the dose or discontinuing therapy.

DRUG INTERACTIONS

CYP450 system / Potential ↓ microsomal CYP-450 levels → depression of hepatic metabolism of certain drugs that use this metabolic pathway

Myelosuppressive agents / Use with caution when combined with other potentially myelosuppressive agents

HOW SUPPLIED

Injection, Solution: 2 million international units (100 mcg)/0.5 mL.

DOSAGE

SC

Chronic granulomatous disease. Severe, malignant osteoporosis.

50 mcg/m^2 (1 million $units/m^2$) for clients whose body surface is greater than 0.5 m^2. If the body surface is less than 0.5 m^2, the dose of interferon gamma should be 1.5 mcg/kg/dose. The drug is given 3 times per week (e.g., Monday, Wednesday, Friday).

NURSING IMPLICATIONS

IMPLEMENTATION/ADMINISTRATION/STORAGE

1. Preferred injection sites: right and left deltoid; anterior thigh.
2. Does not contain a preservative. Use the vial only for a single dose and discard any unused portion.
3. Safety and efficacy not determined for doses greater or less than 50 mcg/m^2.
4. If severe side effects occur, dose can be reduced by 50% or therapy can be discontinued until these subside.
5. May be administered using either sterilized glass or plastic disposable syringes.
6. Do not shake the vial; avoid vigorous agitation.
7. May be given using either sterilized glass or plastic disposable syringes.
8. Discard vials stored at room temperature for more than 12 hr.
9. Do not store undiluted drug in syringes due to syringe adhesion.
10. Do not mix with other drugs in the same syringe.
11. Vials must be stored at 2–8°C (36–46°F) to ensure optimal retention of activity. Do not freeze vial.
12. IV Although not FDA approved, the drug has been given by continuous (10 days to 8 weeks) or intermittent (at 1, 6, or 24 hr) IV infusion as well as by IM injection.
13. COMPATIBILITY No information available.
14. INCOMPATIBILITY Administer separately.

ASSESSMENT

1. List age at onset, any treatments used in the past to reduce frequency/severity of infections; bone scan results.
2. Identify frequency and severity of serious infections associated with Chronic Granulomatous Disease.
3. Note history of CAD or CNS disorders; assess for S&S of seizure disorder or allergy to drug products made from *E. Coli* bacteria.
4. Obtain and monitor BNP, urinalysis, CBC, renal and LFTs q 3 months. If <1 y.o.; obtain monthly LFTs.

CLIENT/FAMILY TEACHING

1. Review reconstitution, preparation, method for administration (subcutaneously), storage (keep vial refrigerated), and disposal of drug/equipment. Observe client or significant other administer SC injection to ensure proper use.
2. Keep drug in the refrigerator; do *not* shake container.
3. Take at bedtime with acetaminophen to minimize flu-like symptoms (fever and headaches).
4. Avoid activities that require mental alertness until drug effects realized; may cause dizziness/drowsiness.
5. Sufferers of osteopetrosis have low osteoclasts, or too little bone being resorbed, resulting in too much bone being created which causes: marble bone disease and Albers-Schönberg disease.
6. Consume 2–3 L/day of fluids to ensure adequate hydration.
7. Avoid alcohol and any other CNS depressants.
8. Close medical supervision is imperative with this disease and genetically engineered drug therapy as dosage may require frequent adjustments.
9. Keep all F/U to assess response, labs, and adverse SE.

OUTCOMES/EVALUATE

- Suppression of infective organisms associated with chronic granulomatous disease
- Control of malignant osteopetrosis progression

IV

Ipilimumab

(ip-i-**LIM**-you-mab)

Classification(s): Antineoplastic agent, monoclonal antibody

Pregnancy Category: C

RX: Vervoy.

INDICATIONS/USES

Treatment of unresectable or metastatic melanoma.

ACTION/KINETICS

Action

Ipilimumab binds to the cytotoxic T-lymphocyte-associated antigen 4 (CTLA-4). CTLA-4 is a negative regulator of T-cell activation. Ipilimumab binds to CTLA-4 and blocks the interaction of CTLA-4 with its ligands. Blockade of CTLA-4 augments T-cell activation and proliferation. Ipilimumab's effect in those with melanoma is indirect, possibly through T-cell mediated antitumor immune responses.

Pharmacokinetics

Steady-state is reached by the third dose. There is minimal systemic accumulation. **t½, terminal:** 14.7 days. Clearance increases with increasing body weight; however, no dosage adjustment is needed for body weight after administration on a mg/kg basis.

CONTRAINDICATIONS

Lactation.

SPECIAL CONCERNS

(1) **Immune-mediated adverse reactions.** Ipilimumab can result in severe and fatal immune-mediated adverse reactions due to T-cell activation and proliferation. These immune-mediated reactions may involve any organ system; however, the most common severe immune-mediated adverse reactions are enterocolitis, hepatitis, dermatitis (including toxic epidermal necrolysis), neuropathy, and endocrinopathy. The majority of these immune-mediated reactions are initially manifested during treatment; however, a minority occurred weeks to months after discontinuation of ipilimumab. (2) Permanently discontinue ipilimumab and initiate systemic high-dose corticosteroid therapy for severe immune-mediated reactions. (3) Assess clients for signs and symptoms of enterocolitis, dermatitis, neuropathy, and endocrinopathy, and evaluate clinical chemistries, including liver

function tests and thyroid function tests, at baseline and before each dose. ■

- Safety and efficacy not determined in children.
- Approximately 10% of clients discontinue the drug due to adverse reactions.

ADDITIONAL SIDE EFFECTS

Most Common

Fatigue, pruritus, rash, diarrhea, immune-mediated reactions, colitis.

More common side effects are listed as well as those that are life-threatening. **Immune-mediated:** ***Enterocolitis***, hypopituitarism, endocrinopathy (e.g., hypopituitarism, adrenal insufficiency, hypogonadism, hypothyroidism), ***dermatitis*** (e.g., Stevens-Johnson syndrome, toxic epidermal necrolysis, or rash complicated by full-thickness dermal ulceration, or necrotic, bullous, or hemorrhagic manifestations), hepatitis, ***hepatotoxicity, neuropathy*** (e.g., myasthenia gravis, Guillain-Barré syndrome), ocular manifestations (e.g., iritis, uveitis). **CNS:** Meningitis. **Dermatologic:** Pruritus, rash, urticaria, erythema multiforme, psoriasis. **GI:** Diarrhea, colitis, large intestinal ulcer, esophagitis, pancreatitis. **CV:** ***Pericarditis,*** myocarditis, angiopathy, temporal arteritis, vasculitis, leukocytoclastic vasculitis. **Respiratory:** Pneumonitis, acute respiratory distress syndrome. **Musculoskeletal:** Polymyalgia rheumatica, arthritis. **GU:** Nephritis, renal failure. **Hematologic:** Eosinophilia, hemolytic anemia. **Ophthalmic:** Conjunctivitis, blepharitis, episcleritis, scleritis. **Body as a whole:** Fatigue, infusion reaction. **Miscellaneous:** Immunogenicity, autoimmune thyroiditis.

HOW SUPPLIED

Injection Solution, Concentrate: 5 mg/mL.

DOSAGE

IV

Melanoma.

Adults: 3 mg/kg over 90 min q 3 weeks for a total of 4 doses.

NURSING IMPLICATIONS

IMPLEMENTATION/ADMINISTRATION/STORAGE

1. IV Preparation for administration: Allow the vials to stand at room temperature for about 5 min prior to preparation of the infusion. Do not shake the vials. Withdraw the required volume of ipilimumab and transfer into an IV bag. Dilute with 0.9% NaCl injection or D5W injection to prepare a diluted solution with a final concentration from 1–2 mg/mL. Mix the diluted solution by gentle inversion.
2. Administer the diluted solution over 90 min through an IV line containing a sterile, non-pyrogenic, low-protein-binding in-line filter. Flush the IV line with 0.9% NaCl injection or D5W injection after each dose.
3. Withhold the scheduled dose for any moderate immune-mediated side effects or for symptomatic endocrinopathy. For those with complete or partial resolution of side effects (grade 0 to 1), and who are receiving less than 7.5 mg of prednisone or equivalent per day, resume ipilimumab at a dosage of 3 mg/kg q 3 weeks until administration of all 4 planned doses or 16 weeks from the first dose, whichever occurs earlier.
4. Permanently discontinue ipilimumab for any of the following:
   - Persistent moderate side effects or inability to reduce corticosteroid dose to 7.5 mg prednisone or equivalent per day;
   - Failure to complete a full treatment course within 16 weeks from administration of the first dose;
   - Severe or life-threatening side effects, including any of the following: (a) colitis with abdominal pain, fever, ileus, or peritoneal signs; (b) an increase in stool frequency (7 or more over baseline); (c) stool incontinence; (d) need for IV hydration for more than 24 hr; (e) GI hemorrhage or GI perforation; (f) AST or ALT more than 5 × ULN or total bilirubin more than 3 × ULN; (g) Stevens-Johnson syndrome or toxic epidermal necrolysis; (h) rash complicated by full-thickness dermal ulceration, or necrotic, bullous, or hemorrhagic manifestations; (i) severe immune-mediated reactions involving any organ system (e.g., nephritis, pneumonitis, pancreatitis, noninfectious myocarditis); or, (j) immune-mediated ocular disease that is unresponsive to topical immunosuppressive therapy.
5. Store under refrigeration from 2–8°C (36–46°F). Do not freeze; protect from light. Store the diluted solution for no more than 24

hr under refrigeration or at room temperature from 20–25°C (68–77°F). Discard partially used vials or empty vials.

6. COMPATIBILITY 0.9% NaCl, D5W.
7. INCOMPATIBILITY Do not mix with or administer as an infusion with other medicinal agents.

ASSESSMENT

1. Note melanoma onset, location, extent (metastasis), other agents trialed and outcome.
2. Assess for S&S of immune mediated reactions that may cause enterocolitis, dermatitis, neuropathy, and endocrinopathy (thyroid, adrenal). May occur during therapy or weeks to months following treatment. Initiate high dose systemic corticosteroid therapy and permanently discontinue therapy.
3. Monitor VS, chemistries, thyroid and LFTs.

CLIENT/FAMILY TEACHING

1. Drug is administered IV over 90 min every 3 weeks for a total of 4 doses; review patient medication guide regularly.
2. Use caution with activities that require mental alertness; may cause dizziness and drowsiness.
3. Review risks of immune mediated adverse reactions that may occur such as intestinal perforation, hepatitis leading to liver failure, dermatologic reactions, neuropathy, and inflammation of glands and eyes. If any of these reactions occur, do not continue therapy or receive retreatment–notify provider.
4. May experience rash, fatigue, itching and diarrhea; report if persistent or bothersome.
5. Practice reliable contraception, may cause fetal harm.
6. Keep all F/U to assess response, labs, and adverse SE.

OUTCOMES/EVALUATE

Treatment of unresectable or metastatic melanoma

Ipratropium bromide

(eye-prah-**TROH**-pee-um)

Classification(s): Cholinergic blocking drug

Pregnancy Category: B

RX: Atrovent, Atrovent HFA.

✱ **Rx:** Apo-Ipravent, Gen-Ipratropium, ratio-Ipratropium, ratio-Ipratropium UDV.

SEE ALSO ***CHOLINERGIC BLOCKING AGENTS***.

INDICATIONS/USES

Aerosol or solution for inhalation: Alone or with other bronchodilators, especially beta-adrenergics, as a bronchodilator for maintenance treatment of bronchospasm associated with COPD, including chronic bronchitis and emphysema.

Nasal spray: (1) Symptomatic relief (using 0.03%) of rhinorrhea associated with allergic and nonallergic perennial rhinitis in clients over 6 years of age. (2) Symptomatic relief (using 0.06%) of rhinorrhea associated with the common cold in those aged 5 and older. It does not relieve nasal congestion or sneezing associated with the common cold or seasonal allergic rhinitis.

ACTION/KINETICS

Action

Chemically related to atropine. Antagonizes the action of acetylcholine. Prevents the increase in intracellular levels of cyclic guanosine monophosphate, which is caused by the interaction of acetylcholine with muscarinic receptors in bronchial smooth muscle; this leads to bronchodilation which is primarily a local, site-specific effect.

Pharmacokinetics

Poorly absorbed into the systemic circulation (about 7%). About 50% of unchanged drug excreted through the urine. **t½, elimination:** 2 hr after use of the inhalation aerosol and 1.6 hr after use of the nasal spray.

CONTRAINDICATIONS

Hypersensitivity to atropine, ipratropium, or derivatives. Hypersensitivity to soy lecithin or related food products, including soybean or peanut (inhalation aerosol). Use for initial treatment of acute bronchospasms.

SPECIAL CONCERNS

- Use caution in clients with narrow-angle glaucoma, prostatic hypertrophy, or bladder neck obstruction and during lactation.
- Use as a single agent for the relief of bronchospasm in acute COPD has not been studied adequately.
- Safety and efficacy of the aerosol not determined in children; of the solution in children less than

12 years of age; of the nasal spray, 0.03%, in children less than 6 years of age; and of the nasal spray, 0.06%, in children less than 5 years of age.

SIDE EFFECTS

Most Common

Use of inhalation aerosol: Headache, dizziness, chest pain, URTI, nausea, bronchitis, coughing, dyspnea, pharyngitis, pain.

Use of nasal spray: Headache, pharyngitis, URTI, epistaxis, nasal dryness, nausea, nasal irritation. dry mouth/throat, taste perversion.

Inhalation aerosol. CNS: Cough, nervousness, dizziness, headache, fatigue, insomnia, drowsiness, difficulty in coordination, tremor. **GI:** Dryness of oropharynx, GI distress, dry mouth, nausea, constipation. **CV:** Palpitations, tachycardia, flushing. **Dermatologic:** Itching, hives, alopecia. **Miscellaneous:** Irritation from aerosol, worsening of symptoms, rash, hoarseness, blurred vision, difficulty in accommodation, drying of secretions, urinary difficulty, paresthesias, mucosal ulcers.

Inhalation solution. CNS: Dizziness, insomnia, nervousness, tremor, headache. **GI:** Dry mouth, nausea, constipation. **CV:** Hypertension, aggravation of hypertension, tachycardia, palpitations. **Respiratory:** Worsening of COPD symptoms, URTI, coughing, dyspnea, bronchitis, ***bronchospasm***, increased sputum, URI, pharyngitis, rhinitis, sinusitis. **Miscellaneous:** Urinary retention, UTIs, urticaria, pain, flu-like symptoms, back/chest pain, arthritis.

Nasal spray. CNS: Headache, dizziness. **GI:** Nausea, dry mouth, taste perversion. **CV:** Palpitation, tachycardia. **Respiratory:** URTI, epistaxis, pharyngitis, nasal dryness, miscellaneous nasal symptoms, nasal irritation, blood-tinged mucus, dry throat, cough, nasal congestion/burning, coughing. **Ophthalmic:** Ocular irritation, blurred vision, conjunctivitis. **Miscellaneous:** Hoarseness, thirst, tinnitis, urinary retention.

All products. Allergic: Skin rash, angioedema of the tongue, throat, lips, and face; urticaria, ***laryngospasm***, oropharyngeal edema, ***bronchospasm, anaphylaxis.*** **Anticholinergic reactions:** Precipitation or worsening of narrow-angle glaucoma, prostatic disorders, tachycardia, urinary retention, constipation, bowel obstruction, blurred vision, difficulty in accommodation. *NOTE:* Rarely, immediate hypersensitivity reactions may occur. Symptoms include urticaria, ***angioedema***, rash, ***bronchospasm, anaphylaxis, and oropharyngeal edema.***

DRUG INTERACTIONS

Potential additive interaction when used concomitantly with other anticholinergics

HOW SUPPLIED

Inhalation Aerosol: 17 mcg/inh (HFA aerosol); ***Nasal Spray:*** 0.03% (21 mcg/spray), 0.06% (42 mcg/spray); ***Solution for Inhalation:*** 0.02% (500 mcg/vial).

DOSAGE

INHALATION AEROSOL (HFA)

Treat bronchospasms.

Adults, initial: 2 inhalations (34 mcg) 4 times per day. Additional inhalations may be required but should not exceed 12 inhalations/day. Each actuation delivers 17 mcg of ipratropium.

SOLUTION FOR INHALATION

Treat bronchospasms.

Adults, usual: 500 mcg (1-unit-dose vial) given 3–4 times per day by oral nebulization with doses 6–8 hr apart. The unit-dose vials contain 500 mcg of ipratropium anhydrous in 2.5 mL of normal saline. Can be mixed in the nebulizer with albuterol or metaproterenol if used within 1 hr.

NASAL SPRAY, 0.03%

Perennial rhinitis.

Adults and children, 6 years and older: 2 sprays (42 mcg) per nostril 2–3 times per day for a total daily dose of 168–252 mcg/day. Optimum dose varies.

NASAL SPRAY, 0.06%

Rhinitis due to the common cold.

Adults and children, 12 years and older: 2 sprays (84 mcg) per nostril 3–4 times per day for a total daily dose of 504–672 mcg/day. **Children, 5–11 years:** 2 sprays (84 mcg) per nostril 3 times per day (total dose of 504 mcg/day). Safety and efficacy for use for the common cold for more than 4 days have not been determined.

Rhinorrhea associated with seasonal allergic rhinitis.

Adults and children, 5 years and older: 2 sprays (84 mcg) per nostril 4 times per day (total of 672 mcg/day). Safety and efficacy for use beyond 3 weeks have not been determined.

NURSING IMPLICATIONS

Do not confuse Atrovent with Alupent (a sympathomimetic).

IMPLEMENTATION/ADMINISTRATION/STORAGE

1. Use of a nebulizer with mouthpiece rather than a face mask may be preferable to reduce the chance of the nebulizer solution reaching the eyes.
2. Store the aerosol between 15–30°C (59–86°F); avoid excessive humidity.
3. Store solution between 15–30°C (59–86°F); protect from light. Store unused vials in the foil pouch.
4. Store nasal spray tightly closed between 15–30°C (59–86°F). Avoid freezing.

ASSESSMENT

1. List type, onset, characteristics of S&S, other agents used, outcome.
2. Note any glaucoma, prostate gland enlargement, difficulty urinating; may aggravate.
3. Perform full pulmonary/ENT assessment; monitor PFTs, O_2 sats, x-rays/subjective symptom reports.

CLIENT/FAMILY TEACHING

1. Take only as directed; shake well before using. Review administration technique. Rinse mouth and equipment after use. With inhalers do not exceed 12 inhalations in 24 hr; with nasal spray do not exceed 8 sprays in each nostril in 24 hr.
2. Prime or actuate the HFA inhalation aerosol before using for the first time by releasing 2 test sprays into the air away from the face. In cases where the inhaler has not been used for more than 3 days, prime the inhaler again by releasing 2 sprays into the air away from the face.
3. If using more than one inhalation per dose, wait 3 min before administering the second inhalation. If also prescribed steroid inhaler, use ipratropium and then wait 5 min before using the steroid inhaler.
4. With nasal inhaler: Initial pump priming: 7 actuations of the pump. No further priming is required with regular use but if not used for more than 24 hr, 2 pump actuations are needed. If not used for more than 7 days, 7 actuations are needed.
5. Transient dizziness, insomnia, blurred vision, or excessive weakness may occur, use caution.
6. Drug is not for use in terminating an acute attack; effects take up to 15 min. Have another prescribed agent readily available in this event.
7. Avoid contact with the eyes. A spacer may be useful with the inhaler and a mouthpiece with the nebulizer to help prevent solution (mist) contact with the eyes; also enhances lung dispersion.
8. May experience a bitter taste and dry mouth; use frequent mouth rinses and hard candy to relieve.
9. Stop smoking now to preserve current level of lung function and to prevent further damage; utilize smoking cessation program.
10. Keep all F/U to evaluate response, and for adverse SE.

OUTCOMES/EVALUATE

- Improved airway exchange and breathing patterns
- ↓ Wheezing, dyspnea
- Relief of rhinorrhea

Combination Drug

Ipratropium bromide and Albuterol sulfate

(eye-prah-**TROH**-pee-um, al-**BYOU**-ter-ohl)

Classification(s): Cholinergic blocking drug and sympathomimetic

Pregnancy Category: C

RX: Combivent, DuoNeb.

✱ **Rx:** ratio-Ipra Sal UDV.

SEE ALSO ***IPRATROPIUM BROMIDE*** AND ***ALBUTEROL SULFATE.***

INDICATIONS/USES

Treatment of COPD (including bronchospasms) in those who are on regular aerosol bronchodilator therapy and who require a second bronchodilator.

CONTENT

Combivent: Each actuation of the aerosol delivers: Ipratropium bromide (*cholinergic blocking drug*), 18 mcg; and Albuterol sulfate (*sympathomimetic*), 103 mcg. **DuoNeb:** Inhalation solution contains: Ipratropium bromide (*cholinergic blocking drug*), 0.5 mg, and Albuterol sulfate (*sympathomimetic*), 3 mg (equivalent to 2.5 mg albuterol base).

ACTION/KINETICS

Action

Ipratropium is an anticholinergic drug that acts to inhibit the effect of acetylcholine following vagal nerve stimulation. This results in bronchodilation that is primarily a local, site-specific effect. Albuterol is a beta-2-adrenergic agonist that also causes bronchodilation.

Pharmacokinetics

Ipratropium is poorly absorbed into the systemic circulation. About 50% of unchanged drug excreted in the urine. **t½, elimination:** 2 hr after inhalation. After inhalation, the onset for albuterol is within 5 min; peak effect occurs within 60–90 min and duration is 3–6 hr. Albuterol and metabolites are excreted in the urine and feces.

CONTRAINDICATIONS

History of hypersensitivity to soy lecithin or related food products, such as soybean and peanuts. Lactation.

SPECIAL CONCERNS

- **Use with caution in CV disorders, especially coronary insufficiency, cardiac arrhythmias, and hypertension.**
- **Use with caution in narrow-angle glaucoma, prostatic hypertrophy, bladder-neck obstruction, convulsive disorders, hyperthyroidism, diabetes mellitus, in those unusually responsive to sympathomimetic amines, and renal or hepatic disease.**
- **Safety and efficacy not determined in children.**

SIDE EFFECTS

Most Common

Bronchitis, URTI, headache, pain, dyspnea, coughing, nausea, pharyngitis, sinusitis.

Respiratory: ***Paradoxical bronchospasm***, bronchitis, dyspnea, coughing, respiratory disorders, pneumonia, URTI, pharyngitis, sinusitis, rhinitis. **CV:** ECG changes including flattening of T wave, prolongation of QTc interval, and ST segment depression. Also, arrhythmias, palpitation, tachycardia, angina, hypertension. **Hypersensitivity, immediate:** Urticaria, ***angioedema, bronchospasm, anaphylaxis, oropharyngeal edema***. **Body as a whole:** Headache, pain, flu, chest pain, edema, fatigue. **GI:** N&V, dry mouth, diarrhea, dyspepsia. **CNS:** Dizziness, nervousness, headache, paresthesia, tremor, dysphonia, insomnia. **Miscellaneous:** Arthralgia, increased sputum, taste perversion, UTI, dysuria, pain.

DRUG INTERACTIONS

See individual drugs.

HOW SUPPLIED

See *Content*.

DOSAGE

AEROSOL (COMBIVENT)

Chronic obstructive pulmonary disease (COPD).

2 inhalations q 6 hr not to exceed 12 inhalations/24 hr.

INHALATION SOLUTION (DUONEB)

COPD.

One 3 mL vial given 4 times per day via nebulization with up to 2 additional 3 mL doses daily, if needed.

NURSING IMPLICATIONS

Do not confuse Combivent with Combivir (combination antiviral drug to treat AIDS).

IMPLEMENTATION/ADMINISTRATION/STORAGE

1. **Aerosol canister provides sufficient medication for 200 inhalations.**
2. **Discard canister after labeled number of inhalations used.**
3. **Give DuoNeb via a jet nebulizer connected to an air compressor with an adequate air flow, equipped with mouthpiece or suitable face mask.**
4. **Store Combivent between 15–30°C (59–86°F). Avoid excessive humidity. Canister should be at room temperature before use.**

5. Store DuoNeb between 2–25°C (36–77°F). Protect from light.

ASSESSMENT

1. Note reasons for therapy, characteristics/frequency of symptoms/sputum production, other agents trialed, outcome.
2. Assess for soybean or peanut allergy.
3. Determine any cardiovascular disease, HTN, or arrhythmia.
4. Check BP and HR and assess for significant changes or hypersensitivity reaction.
5. Assess breath sounds, triggers; monitor CXR, symptoms, and PFTs. Stop therapy if bronchospasm worsens.

CLIENT/FAMILY TEACHING

1. Use as directed; do not increase dose or frequency of administration unless specifically directed.
2. To use inhaler: breathe out fully, hold inhaler 1 to 2 inches in front of mouth or attach a spacer to the inhaler, and place the spacer in your mouth (above tongue and past teeth to prevent drug from depositing tongue/throat). Take a deep, slow breath as you push down on the canister. Hold your breath for 10 seconds, then exhale slowly. If more than one puff ordered, wait for at least 1 full minute after each puff, then repeat the procedure. Avoid exhaling into mouthpiece to avoid moisture accumulation. Keep inhaler capped to avoid dirt getting inside. Rinse mouth and inhaler with water after use to prevent infections.
3. Avoid excessive humidity. For best results, have canister at room temperature before use. Shake inhaler well before using. Test canister spray 3 times before first use and again if the canister has not been used for 24 hr.
4. Report any loss of effectiveness, change in symptoms early to prevent exacerbation and resultant hospitalization. If steroid inhaler also prescribed, use Combivent first and wait 5 min before using the steroid to ensure better lung penetration.
5. Avoid eye contact; report any visual disturbances or eye irritation.
6. Drug is not for use in terminating an acute attack; effects take up to 15 min. Have another prescribed agent readily available.
7. Stop smoking to preserve current level of lung function and to prevent further damage; utilize smoking cessation program.
8. Record peak flows and identify critical zones.
9. Keep all F/U to assess response and for adverse SE.

OUTCOMES/EVALUATE

Improved airway exchange with ↓ cough/SOB/sputum production

Irbesartan

(ihr-beh-**SAR**-tan)

Classification(s): Antihypertensive, angiotensin II receptor blocker

Pregnancy Category: C (first trimester); **D** (second and third trimesters)

RX: Avapro.

SEE ALSO ***ANGIOTENSIN II RECEPTOR ANTAGONISTS*** AND ***ANTIHYPERTENSIVE DRUGS***.

INDICATIONS/USES

(1) Hypertension, alone or in combination with other antihypertensives. (2) Nephropathy in type 2 diabetics with an elevated serum creatinine and proteinuria (greater than 300 mg/day) with hypertension. Will reduce rate of progression of renal disease. *Investigational:* Heart failure.

ACTION/KINETICS

Action

Competitively blocks the angiotensin AT_1 receptor located in vascular smooth muscle and the adrenal glands, thus blocking the vasoconstrictor and aldosterone-secreting effects of angiotensin II (a potent vasoconstrictor). Thus, BP is reduced.

Pharmacokinetics

Rapid absorption after PO use. **Peak plasma levels:** 1.5–2 hr. Is 60–80% bioavailable; food does not affect bioavailability. Effect somewhat less in Blacks. t_{max}: 1.5–2 hr. **t½, terminal elimination:** 11–15 hr. Metabolized in liver by CYP2C9 and both unchanged drug and metabolites excreted through urine (20%) and feces (80%). **Plasma protein binding:** More than 90%.

SPECIAL CONCERNS

When used during the second and third trimesters of pregnancy, drugs that act directly on the renin-angiotensin system can cause injury and even death to the developing fetus. When pregnancy is detected, discontinue irbesartan as soon as possible.

Safety and efficacy not determined in children less than 6 years of age.

SIDE EFFECTS

Most Common

URTI, cough, fatigue, dyspepsia/heartburn, diarrhea.

GI: Diarrhea, dyspepsia, heartburn, abdominal distension/pain, N&V, constipation, oral lesion, gastroenteritis, flatulence. **CV:** Tachycardia, syncope, orthostatic hypotension, hypertension, hypotension (especially in volume- or salt-depletion), flushing, cardiac murmur, ***MI, cardiorespiratory arrest, heart failure, hypertensive crisis, CVA***, angina pectoris, arrhythmias, conduction disorder, TIA. **CNS:** Sleep disturbance, fatigue, anxiety, nervousness, dizziness, numbness, somnolence, emotional disturbance, depression, paresthesia, tremor. **Musculoskeletal:** Extremity swelling, muscle cramp/ache/weakness, arthritis, musculoskeletal pain, musculoskeletal chest pain, joint stiffness, bursitis. **Respiratory:** Cough, epistaxis, tracheobronchitis, congestion, pulmonary congestion, dyspnea, wheezing, URTI, rhinitis, pharyngitis, sinus abnormality. **GU:** Abnormal urination, prostate disorder, UTI, sexual dysfunction, libido change. **Dermatologic:** Pruritus, dermatitis, ecchymosis, facial erythema, urticaria. **Ophthalmic:** Vision disturbance, conjunctivitis, eyelid abnormality. **Otic:** Hearing abnormality, ear infection/pain/abnormality. **Miscellaneous:** Gout, fever, fatigue, chills, facial edema, upper extremity edema, headache, influenza, rash, chest pain.

LABORATORY TEST CONSIDERATIONS

↑ BUN (minor), serum creatinine. ↓ Hemoglobin. Neutropenia.

HOW SUPPLIED

Tablets: 75 mg, 150 mg, 300 mg.

DOSAGE

TABLETS

Hypertension.

Adults: 150 mg once daily with or without food, up to 300 mg once daily. Lower initial dose of 75 mg is recommended for clients with depleted intravascular volume or salt. If BP is not controlled by irbesartan alone, hydrochlorothiazide may have an additive effect. Clients not adequately treated by 300 mg irbesartan are unlikely to get benefit from higher dose or twice a day dosing. **Children, 6–12 years, initial:** 75 mg once daily. Titrate those requiring further reduction in BP to 150 mg once daily. **Children, 13–16 years, initial:** 150 mg once daily. Titrate those requiring further reduction in BP to 300 mg once daily.

Nephropathy in type 2 diabetics.

Adults: Target dose is 300 mg once daily. **Adolescents, 13–16 years of age, initial:** 150 mg once daily. Titrate those requiring further reduction in BP to 300 mg once daily. **Children, 6–12 years of age, initial:** 75 mg once daily. Titrate those requiring further reduction in BP to 150 mg once daily.

NURSING IMPLICATIONS

IMPLEMENTATION/ADMINISTRATION/STORAGE

1. Dose adjustment is not required in geriatric clients or in hepatic or renal impairment.
2. May be given with other antihypertensive drugs.
3. Correct volume depletion prior to administration of antihypertensive therapy; or, use a low starting dose (75 mg) of irbesartan. Monitor the client closely.
4. Store between 15–30°C (59–86°F).

ASSESSMENT

1. Note reasons for therapy, onset, duration, characteristics of symptoms, other agents trialed.
2. If pregnancy detected, stop drug as soon as possible.
3. Observe infants exposed to angiotensin II inhibitor in utero for hypotension, oliguria, and ↑ K.
4. Ensure adequately hydrated prior to starting therapy; reduce dose if volume/salt depleted.
5. Monitor VS, electrolytes, U/A, microalbumin, renal and LFTs; use cautiously with renal dysfunction.

CLIENT/FAMILY TEACHING

1. Take only as directed. May take with or without food.
2. Avoid tasks that require mental alertness until drug effects realized; may cause dizziness or drowsiness; change positions slowly to prevent sudden drop in BP.
3. Continue low-fat, low-cholesterol diet, regular exercise, tobacco cessation, salt restriction, limited alcohol use and lifestyle changes necessary to maintain lowered BP.
4. Practice reliable contraception. Stop drug and report if pregnancy suspected.
5. Report any fainting; swelling of the face, lips, eyelids, or tongue immediately. Also report persistent muscle/joint pains, anxiety, nervousness, cold symptoms, diarrhea, headaches, unusual tiredness, heartburn, stomach discomfort.
6. Ensure adequate hydration; report excessive perspiration, diarrhea, or vomiting as this can lead to drop in BP.
7. Keep all F/U (bring BP and HR log) to assess response, labs, and adverse SE.

OUTCOMES/EVALUATE

- ↓ BP
- Renal protection in DM

Combination Drug

Irbesartan and Hydrochlorothiazide

(ihr-beh-**SAR**-tan, **hy**-droh-klor-oh-**THIGH**-ah-zyd)

Classification(s): Antihypertensive (combination drug)

Pregnancy Category: C (first trimester); **D** (second and third trimesters)

RX: Avalide.

SEE ALSO ***IRBESARTAN*** AND ***HYDROCHLOROTHIAZIDE***.

INDICATIONS/USES

Treatment of hypertension. Not indicated for initial therapy.

CONTENT

Avalide 150/12.5: Irbesartan (*angiotensin II receptor blocker*), 150 mg, and hydrochlorothiazide (*thiazide diuretic*), 12.5 mg. *Avalide 300/12.5:* Irbesartan, 300 mg, and hydrochlorothiazide, 12.5 mg. *Avalide 300/25:* Irbesartan, 300 mg, and hydrochlorothiazide, 25 mg.

ACTION/KINETICS

Action

Irbesartan competitively blocks the angiotensin AT_1 receptor located in vascular smooth muscle and the adrenal glands, thus blocking the vasoconstrictor and aldosterone-secreting effects of angiotensin II (a potent vasoconstrictor). Thus, BP is reduced. The antihypertensive activity of hydrochlorothiazide is thought to be due to direct dilation of the areterioles, as well as to a reduction in the total fluid volume of the body and altered sodium balance.

Pharmacokinetics

Irbesartan is rapidly absorbed; absolute bioavailability is 60–80%. **Irbesartan, peak plasma levels:** 1.5–2 hr. **Maximum effect:** 4 hr; **duration:** 24 hr. Food does not affect bioavailability. **t½, terminal, irbesartan:** 11–15 hr. Irbesartan is mainly excreted unchanged (>80%) through the urine and feces.

Hydrochlorothiazide, onset: 2 hr; **peak effect:** 4–6 hr; **duration:** 6–12 hr. **t½:** 5.6–14.8 hr. Hydrochlorothiazide is not metabolized but is eliminated rapidly by the kidney; about 61% excreted unchanged within 24 hr. **Plasma protein binding:** Irbesartan is 90% bound to plasma proteins.

CONTRAINDICATIONS

Hypersensitivity to any component of the product. In clients with anuria or hypersensitivity to sulfonamide-derived drugs. Use of lithium with diuretics reduces renal clearance of lithium and adds a high risk of lithium toxicity. Lactation.

SPECIAL CONCERNS

When used in pregnancy during the second and third trimesters, drugs that act directly on the renin-angiotensin system can cause injury and even death to the developing fetus. When pregnancy is detected, discontinue Avalide as soon as possible.

- **Use with caution in impaired hepatic function or progressive liver disease since minor alterations of fluid and electrolyte imbalance can cause hepatic coma.**

- Safety and efficacy not determined in children less than 18 years of age.

SIDE EFFECTS

Most Common

Hypokalemia, lightheadedness, musculoskeletal pain, fatigue, dizziness, edema, N&V.

See *Irbesartan* and *Hydrochlorothiazide* for a list of possible side effects. Also, hypersensitivity reactions (with or without a history of allergy or bronchial asthma). Exacerbation or activation of systemic lupus erythematosus. Postmarketing side effects: Urticaria, ***angioedema*** (including swelling of the face, lips, pharynx, and/or tongue), hepatitis, jaundice (rare), ***rhabdomyolysis*** (rare).

LABORATORY TEST CONSIDERATIONS

Slight ↑ serum creatinine, BUN. Rarely, ↑ liver enzymes and/or serum bilirubin.

HOW SUPPLIED

See *Content*.

DOSAGE

TABLETS

Hypertension.

Adults, usual: One tablet daily (i.e., 150 or 300 mg irbesartan, and 12.5–25 mg hydrochlorothiazide). A lower initial dose of irbesartan (75 mg) is recommended in clients with depletion of intravascular volume.

NURSING IMPLICATIONS

Ⓢ Do not confuse Avalide with Avapro (irbesartan alone).

IMPLEMENTATION/ADMINISTRATION/STORAGE

1. No dosage adjustment is needed in mild to severe renal impairment (unless the client is also volume depleted) or in hepatic insufficiency.
2. Clients not responding adequately to 300 mg irbesartan once daily are not likely to derive additional benefit from a higher dose or twice-daily dosing.
3. It is usually appropriate to begin combination therapy only after monotherapy has failed.
4. Avalide may be given with other antihypertensive drugs.
5. Store from 25–30°C (59–86°F).

ASSESSMENT

1. Note reasons for therapy, disease onset, other therapies trialed, outcome. Ensure adequately hydrated.
2. List agents prescribed to ensure none interact. Assess for sulfonamide allergy.
3. Monitor BP, electrolytes, renal and LFTs; use caution with dysfunction. Determine if pregnant.

CLIENT/FAMILY TEACHING

1. May take with or without food with a full glass of water. Do not skip doses or double up if dose missed.
2. Take early in the day to prevent nighttime awakening to urinate.
3. May experience dizziness or drowsiness; avoid activities that require mental alertness until drug effects realized.
4. If lightheadedness or fainting occur, may be aggravated if diarrhea, vomiting, excessive sweating, poor fluid intake, or if on a low-salt diet; report if persistent.
5. Avoid alcohol or prolonged activities in hot weather; may cause dehydration and increased lightheadedness. Change positions slowly to prevent sudden drop in BP.
6. With diabetes may have elevated blood sugar; monitor finger sticks closely and adjust as directed.
7. Wear sunscreen and protective clothing if sun exposed; may cause photosensitivity reaction.
8. Practice reliable contraception; stop drug if pregnancy suspected.
9. Keep all F/U to assess response (bring BP and HR log), labs, and for adverse SE.

OUTCOMES/EVALUATE

Desired BP control

■ IV

Irinotecan hydrochloride

(**eye**-rih-noh-**TEE**-kan)

Classification(s): Antineoplastic, hormone

Pregnancy Category: D

RX: Camptosar.

SEE ALSO ***ANTINEOPLASTIC AGENTS***.

INDICATIONS/USES

(1) First-line therapy with 5-fluorouracil and leucovorin for metastatic colon or rectal carcinomas. (2) Metastatic carcinoma of the colon or rectum in those whose disease has recurred or progressed following 5-fluorouracil therapy.

ACTION/KINETICS

Action

The cytotoxic effect is due to double-strand DNA damage produced during DNA synthesis when replication enzymes interact with the ternary complex formed by topoisomerase I, DNA, and either irinotecan or SN-38 (its active metabolite). Conversion of irinotecan to SN-38 occurs in the liver.

Pharmacokinetics

t½, terminal, irinotecan: About 6 hr; **t½, terminal, SN-38:** About 10 hr. **Plasma protein binding:** SN-38: 95%.

CONTRAINDICATIONS

Use with the Mayo Clinic regimen of 5-FU/LV (i.e., administration for 4 to 5 days q 4 weeks) due to increased toxicity, including deaths. Lactation.

SPECIAL CONCERNS

(1) Give under the supervision of a physician experienced in the use of cancer chemotherapeutic drugs. Appropriate management of complications is possible only when adequate diagnostic and treatment facilities are readily available. (2) Irinotecan can cause both early and late forms of diarrhea that are mediated by different mechanisms. Both forms may be severe. Early diarrhea may be accompanied by cholinergic symptoms, including rhinitis, increased salivation, miosis, lacrimation, diaphoresis, flushing, and intestinal hyperperistalsis that may cause abdominal cramping. This type of diarrhea may be treated with atropine. Late diarrhea (occurring more than 24 hr after giving the drug) may be life-threatening because it may be prolonged and lead to dehydration, electrolyte imbalance, or sepsis. Treat late diarrhea promptly with loperamide. Monitor clients with diarrhea carefully and give fluid and electrolyte replacement if dehydration occurs, or give antibiotics if clients develop ileus, fever, or severe neutropenia. Stop irinotecan therapy and reduce subsequent dosage if severe diarrhea occurs. (3) Severe myelosuppression may occur.

- **Increased risk for severe myelosuppression in clients who have previously received pelvic or abdominal irradiation.**
- **Safety and efficacy not determined in children.**

SIDE EFFECTS

Most Common

Neutropenia, anemia, leukopenia, diarrhea, N&V, abdominal pain/cramping, constipation, rhinitis, dyspnea, cough, asthenia, pain, fever, headache, back pain, chills, flushing, edema, enlarged abdomen, infection, dehydration, weight loss.

NOTE: Side effects listed include symptoms of combination therapy with 5-FU and leucovorin. **GI:** Diarrhea (both early and late; may be life-threatening), cholinergic syndrome, N&V, anorexia, abdominal cramping or pain, constipation, flatulence, stomatitis, mucositis, dyspepsia, colitis (accompanied by ulceration, bleeding, ileus, infection), ileus. **Hematologic:** Severe myelosuppression, including leukopenia, anemia, neutropenia (including neutropenic fever/infection), serious thrombocytopenia (rare). **CNS:** Insomnia, dizziness, somnolence, confusion. **Respiratory:** Dyspnea, increased coughing, pneumonia, rhinitis, severe pulmonary events (rare). **CV:** Vasodilation, flushing, thromboembolism, orthostatic hypotension, ***hemorrhage***. **Dermatologic:** Alopecia, sweating, rashes, exfoliative dermatitis, hand and foot syndrome. **GU:** Acute renal failure. **Metabolic/nutritional:** Decreased body weight, dehydration. ***Body as a whole:*** Asthenia, fever, pain, headache, back pain, chills, minor infections (usually UTI), edema, abdominal enlargement, ascites, jaundice, cholinergic syndrome (flushing, bradycardia), hypersensitivity reactions (***anaphylaxis***, anaphylactoid reactions).

LABORATORY TEST CONSIDERATIONS

↑ AST, alkaline phosphatase, bilirubin.

OVERDOSE MANAGEMENT

Symptoms: Extension of side effects. *Treatment:* Maximum supportive care to prevent dehydration due to diarrhea. Treat any infections.

DRUG INTERACTIONS

Antineoplastic agents / ↑ Risk of myelosuppression and diarrhea

Dexamethasone / ↑ Risk of lymphocytopenia and hyperglycemia
Diuretics / ↑ Risk of dehydration secondary to diarrhea and vomiting
Phenytoin / ↓ AUC and ↑ irinotecan clearance
Prochlorperazine / ↑ Risk of akathisia

HOW SUPPLIED

Injection: 20 mg/mL.

DOSAGE

IV INFUSION

Metastatic carcinoma of the colon or rectum.

Combination agent dosage regimen 1: *Irinotecan:* 125 mg/m^2 given as an IV infusion over 90 min on days 1, 8, 15, and 22, followed by a 2-week rest period. *5-Fluorouracil:* 500 mg/m^2 by IV bolus on days 1, 8, 15, and 22 followed by a 2-week rest period. *Leucovorin:* 20 mg/m^2 by IV bolus on days 1, 8, 15, and 22, followed by a 2-week rest period. Next course begins on day 43.

Combination agent dosage regimen 2: *Irinotecan:* 180 mg/m^2 by IV infusion over 90 min on days 1, 15, and 29. *5-Fluorouracil:* 400 mg/m^2 by IV bolus on days 1, 2, 15, 16, 29, and 30. This is followed by an IV infusion over 22 hr of 600 mg/m^2 on days 1, 2, 15, 16, 29, and 30. *Leucovorin:* 200 mg/m^2 IV over 2 hr on days 1, 2, 15, 16, 29, and 30. Next course begins on day 43. *NOTE:* Modifications of the dosage are based on the degree of neutropenia, neutropenic fever, diarrhea, and other toxicities. Consult the package insert for specific dosage modifications.

Single-agent dosage schedule regimen 1, initial: Irinotecan 125 mg/m^2 IV over 90 min on days 1, 8, 15, and 22, followed by a 2-week rest period. Subsequent doses may be adjusted as high as 150 mg/m^2 or as low as 50 mg/m^2 in 25–50 mg/m^2 decrements depending on toxicity. If intolerable toxicity does not occur, courses of treatment may be continued indefinitely, as long as beneficial effects are noted.

Single-agent dosage schedule regimen 2: Irinotecan 350 mg/m^2 given IV over 90 min once every 3 weeks. Subsequent doses may be adjusted as low as 200 mg/m^2 in 50 mg/m^2 decrements, depending on toxicity.

NURSING IMPLICATIONS

IMPLEMENTATION/ADMINISTRATION/STORAGE

1. IV Avoid extravasation. If extravasation occurs, flush site with sterile water and apply ice.
2. Causes vomiting; give antiemetic therapy; this includes dexamethasone, 10 mg, and a 5-HT_3 blocker such as granisetron or ondansetron; give 30 min before giving irinotecan.
3. Prepare infusion solution by diluting in D5W (preferred) or 0.9% NaCl to a final concentration of 0.12–1.1 mg/mL; administer over 90 min.
4. Solutions diluted in D5W, stored in the refrigerator, and protected from light are stable for 48 hr. However, due to possible microbial contamination during dilution, use refrigerated admixtures within 24 hr or, if kept at room temperature, use within 6 hr. Do not refrigerate admixtures containing 0.9% NaCl. Freezing irinotecan or admixtures may cause drug precipitation.
5. COMPATIBILITY D5W, 0.9% NaCl.
6. INCOMPATIBILITY Do not mix with other solutions or medications.

ASSESSMENT

1. Note reasons for therapy; assess for any history of pelvic/abdominal irradiation and last 5-FU therapy.
2. List all drugs currently prescribed to ensure none exacerbate side effects.
3. Drug is emetogenic; administer antiemetics 30 min prior to therapy.
4. May need IV atropine for those who experience early-onset abdominal cramps, diarrhea, or diaphoresis (cholinergic symptoms). Late-onset diarrhea may be treated with loperamide and fluid and electrolyte replacement.
5. Assess infusion site carefully; flush site with sterile water and apply ice with extravasation.
6. Check VS, renal and LFTs, especially bilirubin elevations; adjust dose with dysfunction. Obtain CBC before each treatment. Hold if ANC

below 500/mm^3 or neutropenic fever occurs. Any significant reduction in WBC (<2,000/mm^3), neutrophil count (<1,000/mm^3), or platelet count (<100,000/mm^3) warrants dose reduction.

CLIENT/FAMILY TEACHING

1. Drug is administered IV usually weekly but depends on condition and reasons for treatment.
2. Diarrhea may occur within 24 hr of therapy; is cholinergic in nature and usually transient. Consume adequate fluids to prevent dehydration.
3. Report if temperature is over 38°C (101°F) or diarrhea, vomiting, or dehydration develop.
4. With late-onset diarrhea (usually 10 days after therapy) take 4 mg of loperamide, followed by 2 mg q 2 hr for 12 hr until diarrhea free (or other antidiarrheal prescribed). After the first treatment, delay weekly chemotherapy in clients with diarrhea until bowel function returns to pretreatment status. Consume extra fluids to prevent dehydration. Report if persistent or unresponsive to therapy; may be fatal. Avoid laxatives unless approved.
5. Practice birth control during and for several months following therapy.
6. Avoid crowds, those with active infections, and immunizations during drug therapy.
7. Report any unusual bruising/bleeding or S&S of infection. Avoid alcohol and OTC agents without approval.
8. Keep all F/U visits to assess response, labs, and for adverse SE.

OUTCOMES/EVALUATE

Inhibition of colon/rectal malignant cell proliferation

IV

Iron dextran parenteral

Classification(s): Antianemic, iron

Pregnancy Category: C

RX: DexFerrum, InFeD.

✤ **Rx:** Dexlron, Infufur.

INDICATIONS/USES

IV or IM treatment of documented iron deficiency where oral use is unsatisfactory or impossible. *Investigational:* Iron supplementation in clients receiving epoetin therapy.

ACTION/KINETICS

Action

A complex of ferric hydroxide and dextran that is removed from the plasma by the reticuloendothelial system which splits the complex into iron and dextran. The iron is bound to protein to form hemosiderin or ferritin, which replenishes hemoglobin and depleted iron stores.

Pharmacokinetics

After IM, absorbed into capillaries and the lymphatic system; most absorbed within 72 hr and the rest over 3–4 weeks. **t½:** From 5 hr (circulating iron dextran) to more than 20 hr (total iron, both circulating and bound). Dextran is either metabolized or excreted. Negligible amounts of iron in iron dextran are lost via the urine and feces.

CONTRAINDICATIONS

Hypersensitivity to the product. All anemias not associated with iron deficiency. Acute phase of infectious kidney disease. Use in infants less than 4 months of age.

SPECIAL CONCERNS

Parenteral complexes of iron and carbohydrates may cause anaphylactic reactions. Deaths have been reported; thus, use iron dextran injection only in those clients in whom the indications have been clearly established and laboratory tests confirm an iron-deficient acute state not amenable to oral iron therapy. Because fatal anaphylactic reactions have been reported after administration of iron dextran injection, give the drug only when resuscitation techniques and treatment of anaphylactic and anaphylactoid shock are readily available.

- Large IV or IM doses may cause arthralgia, backache, chills, dizziness, moderate to high fever, headache, malaise, myalgia, N&V (onset is 24–48 hr; symptoms usually subside within 3–4 days after IV and within 3–7 days after IM).
- Use with extreme caution in seriously impaired liver function.
- Use with caution during lactation and in clients with a history of significant allergies/asthma.

- Rheumatoid arthritis clients may have an acute exacerbation of joint pain and swelling after iron dextran.
- Side effects may exacerbate CV complications in clients with pre-existing CV disease.
- Unwarranted therapy will cause excess storage of iron with the possibility of exogenous hemosiderosis. Is most apt to occur in clients with hemoglobinopathies and other refractory anemias that might be erroneously diagnosed as iron deficiency anemia.

SIDE EFFECTS

Most Common

Flushing, headache, dizziness, tingling of hands/feet, N&V, diarrhea, shivering, injection site reaction, metallic taste.

Delayed reactions (1–2 days): Arthralgia, backache, chills, dizziness, moderate to high fever, headache, malaise, myalgia, N&V. **Hypersensitivity:** ***Anaphylaxis*** (often within the first several minutes of administration), including respiratory difficulty or ***CV collapse***. **GI:** Abdominal pain, N&V, diarrhea. **CNS:** Convulsions, syncope, headache, weakness, unresponsiveness, paresthesia, febrile episodes, dizziness, disorientation, numbness, unconsciousness, ***seizures***. **CV:** Chest pain, chest tightness, shock, ***cardiac arrest***, hyper-/hypotension, tachycardia, bradycardia, flushing, arrhythmias. Also, flushing and hypotension from too rapid IV injection. **Respiratory:** Dyspnea, bronchospasm, wheezing, ***respiratory arrest***. **Musculoskeletal:** Arthralgia, tingling of hands/feet, arthritis (including reactivation), myalgia, backache, sterile abscess, atrophy/fibrosis (at IM injection site), soreness or pain at or near IM injection site, cellulitis, swelling, inflammation, local phlebitis at or near IV injection site, brown skin or underlying tissue discoloration. **GU:** Hematuria. **Hematologic:** Leukocytosis, lymphadenopathy. **Dermatologic:** Urticaria, pruritus, purpura, rash, cyanosis. **Body as a whole:** Sweating, shivering, chills, fever, malaise. **Miscellaneous:** Altered taste (metallic), carcinogenesis after IM injection. *NOTE:* Unwarranted therapy with parenteral iron will cause excess storage of iron with possible exogenous hemosiderosis, especially in those with hemoglobinopathies and other refractory anemias that might be erroneously diagnosed as iron deficiency anemia.

LABORATORY TEST CONSIDERATIONS

Large doses of iron dextran (5 mL or more) give a brown color to serum from a blood sample drawn 4 hr after administration; may cause falsely ↑ values of serum bilirubin and falsely ↓ values of serum calcium.

OVERDOSE MANAGEMENT

Symptoms: Hemosiderosis. Probably no acute manifestations. Large IV doses (e.g., used with total dose infusions) may cause an increased frequency of side effects (usually delayed 1–2 days and subside within 3–4 days). Symptoms include arthralgia, backache, chills, dizziness, moderate to high fever, headache, malaise, myalgia, N&V. *Treatment:* Monitor serum ferritin levels periodically to determine a deleterious progressive accumulation of iron resulting from impaired uptake of iron from the reticuloendothelial system in concurrent medical conditions, such as chronic renal failure, Hodgkin's disease, and rheumatoid arthritis.

DRUG INTERACTIONS

If taken with chloramphenicol, may see ↑ serum iron levels R/T ↓ iron clearance and erythropoiesis R/T direct bone marrow toxicity.

HOW SUPPLIED

Injection: 50 mg iron/mL (as dextran).

DOSAGE

IM, IV

Iron deficiency.

Dosage is based on results of hematology data. The table in the package insert must be used to estimate the total iron required to restore hemoglobin to normal or near normal levels plus an additional allowance to replenish iron stores. The information in the table is to be used only in clients with iron deficiency anemia; it is not to be used to determine dosage in those needing iron replacement for blood loss.

IV injection. Prior to the first therapeutic dose, give an IV test dose of 0.5 mL slowly (over 30 seconds for InFeD or 5 minutes or more for Dex-Ferrum). To ensure the client does not experience an anaphylactic reaction, allow 1 hr or more to elapse before the remainder of the initial therapeutic dose is given. Individual doses of 2 mL or less may be given daily until the calculated total amount of iron required has been administered. Give undiluted and slowly 50 mg or less/min (1 mL or less/min).

IM injection. As with IV administration, give a 0.5 mL test dose as described previously. If no side effects occur, give injections as follows until the calculated total amount of iron has been administered. Do not exceed a daily dose of 25 mg iron (i.e., 0.5 mL) for infants less than 5 kg, 50 mg iron (i.e., 1 mL) for children less than 10 kg, and 100 mg iron (i.e., 2 mL) for all others.

NURSING IMPLICATIONS

IMPLEMENTATION/ADMINISTRATION/STORAGE

1. Perform IM test dose. For IM, inject into the upper outer quadrant of the buttock; never inject into the arm or other exposed areas. Inject deeply with a 2- or 3-inch 19- or 20-gauge needle.
2. No more than 2 mL (100 mg) should be given daily.
3. If client is standing, have client bear weight on the leg opposite the injection site. If in bed, have client lie in a lateral position with injection site uppermost.
4. To avoid leakage or injection into SC tissue, use a Z-track technique.
5. The correlation of body iron stores and serum ferritin may not be valid in those on chronic renal dialysis who are also receiving iron dextran complex.
6. **IV** Do not mix iron dextran with other drugs or add to parenteral nutrition solutions for IV infusion.
7. Perform IV test dose of 0.5 mL. Test dose should be administered at a gradual rate per product recommendations.
8. Give undiluted solution slowly; do not exceed rate of 1 mL/min (50 mg/min).
9. COMPATIBILITY D5W, 0.9% NaCl.
10. INCOMPATIBILITY Do not mix with other solutions.

ASSESSMENT

1. Note reasons for therapy (ensure iron deficiency anemia), onset, reason oral replacement not used, previous therapies trialed.
2. Assess for CAD, significant allergies, asthma, infectious kidney disease.
3. With rheumatoid arthritis may experience acute exacerbation of joint swelling and pain after dosing.
4. Ensure test dose performed as directed (0.5 mL given per product recommendations to assess response to drug; allow 1 hr to elapse before therapy). Delayed reactions may occur manifested by N&V, chills, fever, arthralgia, backache, malaise, myalgia.
5. May alter bone scans and discolor blood brown in samples drawn 4 hr after treatment.
6. Assess for sarcoma and sepsis with IM use.
7. May falsely elevate bilirubin and decrease calcium. Keep this in mind when monitoring lab values. Assess H&H and reticulocyte count. Serum iron levels not useful for 3 weeks; ferritin peaks in 7–9 days and reliable at 3 weeks.

CLIENT/FAMILY TEACHING

1. Iron is essential for red cell synthesis so is replaced when iron stores depleted.
2. May notice pain and brown staining at injection site. Stools usually appear black to dark green in color during therapy.
3. Do not consume oral iron or vitamins when receiving injections. Iron poisoning may occur if intake is excessive.
4. Report any bleeding sources, and unusual or adverse side effects. Therapy may end once anemia is corrected.
5. Fluids, fiber, and laxatives may help control constipation.
6. Keep all F/U to assess response, labs, adverse SE.

OUTCOMES/EVALUATE

Iron replacement with iron deficiency anemia

Isoniazid (INH, Isonicotinic acid hydrazide)

(eye-so-**NYE**-ah-zid)

Classification(s): Antitubercular drug

Pregnancy Category: C

RX: Nydrazid Injection.

Rx: Isotamine.

INDICATIONS/USES

(1) Tuberculosis caused by human, bovine, and BCG strains of *Mycobacterium tuberculosis.* Not to be used as the sole tuberculostatic agent. (2) Prophylaxis of tuberculosis in the following: HIV, close contacts with those newly diagnosed with infectious tuberculosis, recent converters, abnormal chest radiographs, IV drug users, those with increased risk of tuberculosis, those less than 35 years of age with tuberculin skin test reaction 10 mm or greater, and children less than 4 years of age if they have greater than 10 mm induration from a purified protein derivative Mantoux tuberculin skin test. *Investigational:* To improve severe tremor in clients with multiple sclerosis.

ACTION/KINETICS

Action

The most effective tuberculostatic agent. Probably interferes with lipid and nucleic acid metabolism of growing bacteria, resulting in alteration of the bacterial wall. Is tuberculostatic.

Pharmacokinetics

Readily absorbed after PO and parenteral (IM) administration and widely distributed in body tissues, including cerebrospinal, pleural, and ascitic fluids. **Peak plasma concentration: PO,** 1–2 hr. **t½, fast acetylators:** 0.5–6 hr; **t½, slow acetylators:** 2–5 hr. Liver and kidney impairment increase these values. Metabolized in liver and excreted primarily in urine. The metabolism of isoniazid is genetically determined. Clients fall into two groups, depending on the rapidity with which they metabolize isoniazid. As a rule, 50% of Caucasians and Blacks inactivate the drug slowly, whereas the majority of American Indians, Eskimos, Japanese, and Chinese are rapid acetylators (inactivators).

1. **Slow acetylators:** These clients show earlier, favorable response but have more toxic reactions (e.g., neuropathies because of higher blood levels of drug).
2. **Rapid acetylators:** These clients have possible poor clinical response due to rapid inactivation, which is 5–6 times faster than slow acetylators. This group requires an increased daily dose of the drug. They are more likely to develop hepatitis.

CONTRAINDICATIONS

Severe hypersensitivity to isoniazid or in clients with previous isoniazid-associated hepatic injury or side effects. Active liver disease.

SPECIAL CONCERNS

■ (1) Severe and sometimes fatal hepatitis may occur even after several months of therapy; incidence is age-related. Daily alcohol use increases the risk. (2) Carefully monitor and interview clients at monthly intervals. For people over 25 years, in addition to monthly interviews, measure AST and ALT prior to starting isoniazid therapy and periodically during therapy. Isoniazid-induced hepatitis usually occurs during the first 3 months of treatment. Enzyme levels generally return to normal even if continuing drug therapy; in some cases, however, progressive liver dysfunction occurs. (3) Other factors associated with an increased risk of hepatitis include daily use of alcohol, chronic liver disease, and injection drug use. There is an increased risk of fatal hepatitis in minority women, especially Blacks and Hispanics, as well as postpartum. Consider more careful monitoring in these groups. If abnormal liver function 3 to 5 times ULN occurs, consider discontinuing isoniazid. (4) Liver function tests are not a substitute for clinical evaluation at monthly intervals or for the prompt assessment of signs or symptoms of side effects occurring during regularly scheduled evaluations. Instruct clients to report immediately signs and symptoms consistent with liver damage or other side effects. These include: Unexplained anorexia, N&V, dark urine, icterus, rash, persistent paresthesias of the hands and feet, persistent fatigue, weakness or fever more than 3 days duration, or abdominal tenderness (especially right upper quadrant discomfort). If these symptoms appear or signs suggestive of hepatic damage are detected, discontinue isoniazid promptly as continued use may cause a more severe form of liver damage. (5) Treat clients with tuberculosis who have hepatitis due to isoniazid with appropriate alternative drugs. Reinstitute isoniazid after symptoms and lab abnormalities have become normal. Restart the drug in small doses; gradually increase doses and withdraw immediately if there is any indication of recurrent liver involvement. (6) Defer preventive treatment in those with acute hepatic diseases.

- **Use with extreme caution in clients with convulsive disorders, in whom the drug should be administered only when client is adequately controlled by anticonvulsant medication.**
- **Use with caution for the treatment of renal tuberculosis and, in the lowest dose possible, with impaired renal function and in alcoholics.**

SIDE EFFECTS

Most Common

Peripheral neuropathy, N&V, heartburn, dizziness, optic neuritis, hepatitis.

Neurologic: Peripheral neuropathy characterized by symmetrical numbness and tingling of extremities (dose-related). Rarely, toxic encephalopathy, optic neuritis, optic atrophy, ***seizures***, impaired memory, toxic psychosis. **GI:** N&V, epigastric distress, heartburn, xerostomia, hepatitis. **Hypersensitivity:** Fever, skin rashes and eruptions, vasculitis, lymphadenopathy. **Hepatic:** Liver dysfunction, jaundice, bilirubinemia, bilirubinuria, ***serious and sometimes fatal hepatitis (even many months after treatment)*** especially in clients over 50 years of age. Increases in serum AST and ALT. **Hematologic:** ***Agranulocytosis***, eosinophilia, thrombocytopenia; ***hemolytic, sideroblastic, or aplastic anemia***. **Metabolic/Endocrine:** Metabolic acidosis, pyridoxine deficiency, pellagra, hyperglycemia, gynecomastia. **Miscellaneous:** Tinnitus, dizziness, urinary retention, rheumatic syndrome, lupus-like syndrome, arthralgia. *NOTE:* Pyridoxine, 10–50 mg/day, may be given concomitantly with isoniazid to decrease CNS side effects. Ophthalmologic and liver function tests are recommended periodically.

OVERDOSE MANAGEMENT

Symptoms: N&V, dizziness, blurred vision, slurred speech, visual hallucinations within 30–180 min. Severe overdosage may cause respiratory distress, ***CNS depression (coma can occur), severe seizures***, metabolic acidosis, acetonuria, hyperglycemia. *Treatment:* Maintain respiration and undertake gastric lavage (within first 2–3 hr providing seizures are not present). To control seizures, give diazepam or a short-acting IV barbiturate followed by pyridoxine (1 mg IV/1 mg isoniazid ingested). Sodium bicarbonate IV to correct metabolic acidosis. Forced osmotic diuresis; monitor fluid I&O. For severe cases, consider hemodialysis or peritoneal dialysis.

DRUG INTERACTIONS

Al salts / ↓ Effect of isoniazid R/T ↓ GI tract absorption
Aminosalicylate / ↑ Effect of isoniazid by ↑ blood levels
Anticoagulants, oral / ↓ Anticoagulant effect
Atropine / ↑ Side effects of isoniazid
Benzodiazepines / ↑ Effect of benzodiazepines that undergo oxidative metabolism (e.g., diazepam, triazolam)
Carbamazepine / ↑ Risk of carbamazepine and isoniazid toxicity
Chlorzoxazone / ↑ Chlorzoxazone peak levels and plasma elimination t½ R/T ↓ liver metabolism
Cycloserine / ↑ Risk of cycloserine CNS side effects
Disulfiram / ↑ Risk of acute behavioral and coordination changes
Enflurane / May → high levels of hydrazine → ↑ defluorination of enflurane
Ethanol / ↑ Chance of isoniazid-induced hepatitis
Halothane / ↑ Risk of hepatotoxicity and hepatic encephalopathy
Hydantoins (phenytoin) / ↑ Hydantoins effect R/T ↓ liver breakdown
Ketoconazole / ↓ Serum ketoconazole levels → ↓ effect
Meperidine / ↑ Risk of hypotension or CNS depression
Niacin / Possible ↑ of niacin requirements
Pyridoxine / Possible ↑ of pyridoxine requirements
Rifampin / Additive liver toxicity

HOW SUPPLIED

Injection: 100 mg/mL; *Syrup:* 50 mg/5 mL; *Tablets:* 50 mg, 100 mg, 300 mg.

DOSAGE

SYRUP; TABLETS

Active tuberculosis.

Adults: 5 mg/kg/day (up to 300 mg/day) as a single dose; **children and infants:** 10–20 mg/kg/day (up to 300 mg total) in a single dose.

Prophylaxis of tuberculosis.
Adults: 300 mg/day in a single dose; **children and infants:** 10 mg/kg/day (up to 300 mg total) in a single dose.

IM

Active tuberculosis.
Adults: 5 mg/kg (up to 300 mg) once daily. **Pediatric:** 10–20 mg/kg (up to 300 mg) once daily.

Prophylaxis of tuberculosis.
Adults/adolescents: 300 mg/day. **Pediatric:** 10 mg/kg/day. *NOTE:* Pyridoxine, 10–50 mg/day, is recommended in the malnourished and those prone to neuropathy (e.g., alcoholics, diabetics).

NURSING IMPLICATIONS

IMPLEMENTATION/ADMINISTRATION/STORAGE

1. Store in dark, tightly closed containers.
2. Solutions for IM injection may crystallize at low temperature; warm to room temperature if precipitation evident.
3. Anticipate slight local irritation at injection site. Rotate and document injection sites.
4. Administer with pyridoxine, 10–50 mg/day, in malnourished, alcoholic, or diabetic clients to prevent symptoms of peripheral neuropathy.

ASSESSMENT

1. Note reasons for therapy, type/onset of symptoms; note birth origin, travel outside of country. List other therapies used, outcome.
2. New PPD converters without symptoms still require treatment and then periodic CXR. +AFB clients require treatment and isolation initially and tracking/treatment of contacts if +AFB or PPD converters.
3. Perform pulmonary assessment; note cough/sputum characteristics.
4. Severe and sometimes fatal hepatitis may occur during and many months after treatment. Risk is related to age and increased with daily alcohol consumption.
5. Obtain baseline labs, CXR, and AFB sputums; note date of PPD conversion if positive. Monitor renal and LFTs; reduce dose with dysfunction or alcohol overuse.

CLIENT/FAMILY TEACHING

1. Take on an empty stomach 1 hr before or 2 hr after meals; may take with food if GI upset.
2. Avoid activities that require mental alertness if dizziness or drowsiness occur.
3. Consume 2–3 L/day of fluids to ensure adequate hydration.
4. Treatment will be lengthy (6 months–2 years); must complete entire course of therapy. If therapy stopped prematurely, relapse of TB is higher.
5. Pyridoxine is given to prevent neurotoxic drug effects (peripheral neuritis). Report any numbness or tingling of hands or feet.
6. Avoid alcohol to prevent hepatic toxicity. May need to avoid certain foods (tyramine-containing) during therapy to prevent itching and redness of skin.
7. Withhold drug and report fatigue, weakness, malaise, yellow eyes/skin, dark urine, and loss of appetite (S&S of liver problems).
8. Report any visual disturbances; may precede optic neuritis.
9. With diabetes, monitor FS closely. Practice reliable contraception during therapy; may cause fetal defects.
10. Take drugs as ordered, missing doses may require retreatment; therapy may take 6 months to a year.
11. Keep all F/U to assess response, labs, eye exams and for adverse SE.

OUTCOMES/EVALUATE

- Negative sputum cultures for AFB
- ↓ Neurotoxic drug effects
- Symptomatic improvement (↓ fever, ↓ secretions, ↑ appetite)
- Prevention of TB in those exposed

Isophane insulin suspension (NPH)

(**EYE**-so-fayn **IN**-sue-lin)

Classification(s): Insulin product
Pregnancy Category: B
OTC: Human: Humulin N, Novolin N.
🍁 **Rx: Human:** Novolinge NPH.

SEE ALSO ***ANTIDIABETIC AGENTS: INSULINS.***

ACTION/KINETICS

Action

Contains zinc insulin crystals modified by protamine, appearing as a cloudy or milky suspension.

Not recommended for emergency use. Not suitable for IV administration or in the presence of ketosis.

Pharmacokinetics

Onset: 1–1.5 hr. **Peak:** 4–12 hr. **Duration: 24** hr. May be mixed with regular insulin.

SIDE EFFECTS

Most Common

Hypoglycemia, hypokalemia, injection site reaction, lipodystrophy, pruritus, rash, allergic reactions.

See *Antidiabetic Agents: Insulins* for a complete list of possible side effects.

HOW SUPPLIED

Injection: 100 units/mL.

DOSAGE

SC

Diabetes.

Adult, individualized, usual, initial: 7–26 units as a single dose 30–60 min before breakfast. A second smaller dose may be given, if needed, prior to the evening meal or at bedtime. If necessary, the daily dose may be increased in increments of 2–10 units at daily or weekly intervals until desired control is achieved. Clients on insulin zinc may be transferred directly to isophane insulin on a unit-for-unit basis. If client is being transferred from regular insulin, the initial dose of isophane should be from two-thirds to three-fourths the dose of regular insulin.

NURSING IMPLICATIONS

ASSESSMENT

1. Note reasons for therapy, age at onset, other therapies trialed, outcome.
2. Monitor BP, Wt, HbA1c, renal and LFTs, lipid panel, and microalbumin.

CLIENT/FAMILY TEACHING

1. Review technique for self-administration. Keep current with regular diabetes education class attendance.
2. Be alert for signs of hypoglycemia, loss of glucose control, and kidney, eye, or foot problems, and report promptly.
3. Record FS at different times during the day/night to assess response.
4. Continue BP and weight control, diet, smoking and alcohol cessation, and exercise to achieve glycemic and lipid control and to prevent complications.
5. Keep all F/U to assess response, labs, adverse SE.

OUTCOMES/EVALUATE

- Control of BS; HbA1c <8
- Prevention of target organ damage

Combination Drug

Isophane insulin suspension and Insulin injection

Classification(s): Insulin product

Pregnancy Category: B

OTC: Human Insulin: Humulin 50/50, Humulin 70/30, Novolin 70/30.

✦ **OTC:** Novolinge (10/90, 20/80, 30/70, 40/60, and 50/50).

SEE ALSO ***ANTIDIABETIC AGENTS: INSULINS.***

CONTENT

Humulin 50/50: Contains 50% isophane insulin and 50% regular insulin injection. **Humulin 70/30 and Novolin 70/30:** Contain 70% isophane insulin and 30% regular insulin injection. *NOTE:* Canadian products contain amounts of isophane and regular insulins that are different.

ACTION/KINETICS

Pharmacokinetics

Onset: 45 min. **Peak effect:** 7–12 hr. **Duration:** 16–24 hr. Insulin injection provides for a rapid onset while the long duration is due to isophane insulin.

SIDE EFFECTS

Most Common

Hypoglycemia, hypokalemia, injection site reaction, lipodystrophy, pruritus, rash.

See *Antidiabetic Agents: Insulins* for a complete list of possible side effects.

HOW SUPPLIED

See *Content*.

DOSAGE

SC

Diabetes.

Adults: Individualized and given once daily 15–30 min before breakfast, or as directed. **Children:** Individualized according to client size.

NURSING IMPLICATIONS

ASSESSMENT

1. Note reasons for therapy, age at onset, other agents trialed, outcome.
2. Education related to diet, medication, exercise, weight, lifestyle changes, disease should be initiated and reinforced.
3. Monitor BP, Wt, HbA1c, renal panel, LDL, and microalbumin.

CLIENT/FAMILY TEACHING

1. Review technique for self-administration. Keep current with regular diabetes education class attendance.
2. Be alert for signs of hypoglycemia, loss of glucose control, kidney, eye, or foot problems and report promptly.
3. Record FS at different times during the day/night to assess response.
4. Continue BP and weight control, diet, smoking and alcohol cessation, and exercise to achieve glycemic and lipid control and to prevent complications.
5. Keep all F/U to assess response, labs, and adverse SE.

OUTCOMES/EVALUATE

Control of BS; HbA1c <8

Isosorbide dinitrate

(eye-so-**SOR**-byd)

Classification(s): Coronary vasodilator

Pregnancy Category: C

RX: Capsules, Sustained-Release: Dilatrate-SR. **Tablets**: Isordil Titradose. **Tablets, Extended-Release**: Isochron. **Tablets, Sublingual**: Isosorbide dinitrate.

🍁 **Rx:** Apo-ISDN.

SEE ALSO ***ANTIANGINAL DRUGS—NITRATES/NITRITES***.

INDICATIONS/USES

(1) Treatment of angina pectoris (sublingual tablets only). (2) Prevention of angina pectoris caused by coronary artery disease. The onset is not sufficiently rapid for this product to be used to abort an acute anginal attack. *Investigational:* With hydralazine to increase survival among Black clients with advanced heart failure; treat acute angle-closure glaucoma in emergency situations (not for long-term management); achalasia.

ACTION/KINETICS

Action

Relaxes vascular smooth muscle by stimulating production of intracellular cyclic guanosine monophosphate. Dilation of postcapillary vessels decreases venous return to the heart due to pooling of blood; thus, LV end-diastolic pressure (preload) is reduced. Relaxation of areterioles results in a decreased systemic vascular resistance and arterial pressure (afterload).

Pharmacokinetics

Sublingual chewable. Onset: 2–5 min; **duration:** 1–3 hr. **Oral Capsules/Tablets. Onset:** 20–40 min; **duration:** 4–6 hr. **Extended-Release. Onset:** up to 4 hr; **duration:** 6–8 hr.

ADDITIONAL CONTRAINDICATIONS

Use to abort acute anginal attacks.

SPECIAL CONCERNS

- Use with caution during lactation.
- Safety and efficacy not established in children.

SIDE EFFECTS

Most Common

Headache, vascular headache, lightheadedness, hypotension.

See *Antianginal Drugs—Nitrates/Nitrites* for a complete list of possible side effects. Vascular headaches occur especially frequently.

ADDITIONAL DRUG INTERACTIONS

Acetylcholine / Acetylcholine effect antagonized
Norepinephrine / Norepinephrine effect antagonized
PDE5 inhibitors (e.g., sildenafil, tadalafil, vardenafil) / Possible fatal hypotension; absolute contraindication to use together

HOW SUPPLIED

Capsules, Sustained-Release: 40 mg; *Tablets:* 5 mg, 10 mg, 20 mg, 30 mg, 40 mg; *Tablets, Extended-Release:* 40 mg; *Tablets, Sublingual:* 2.5 mg, 5 mg.

DOSAGE

CAPSULES, SUSTAINED-RELEASE; TABLETS, EXTENDED-RELEASE

Antianginal.

Initial: 40 mg; **maintenance:** 40–80 mg q 8–12 hr. Tolerance may occur to these agents. Consider giving the short-acting products 2 or 3 times daily (last dose no later than 7 p.m.) and the sustained-release products once daily or twice daily at 8 a.m. and 2 p.m.

TABLETS

Antianginal.

Initial: 5–20 mg 2–3 times per day; **maintenance:** 10–40 mg 2–3 times per day. To minimize tolerance, a daily dose-free interval of at least 14 hr is recommended.

TABLETS, SUBLINGUAL

Antianginal, acute attack.

Initial: 2.5–5 mg. The dose can be titrated upward until angina is relieved or side effects occur. To minimize development of tolerance, a daily dose-free interval must be longer than 14 hr.

Prophylaxis of angina.

2.5–5 mg about 15 min before activity that is likely to cause angina. Sublingual tablets may be used to abort an acute anginal episode, but use is recommended only in those who fail to respond to sublingual nitroglycerin.

NURSING IMPLICATIONS

Do not confuse Isordil with Isuprel (a beta-adrenergic agonist) or Inderal (a beta-adrenergic blocker).

IMPLEMENTATION/ADMINISTRATION/STORAGE

1. Capsules, Sustained-Release: Store from 15–30°C (59–86°F) in a dry location.
2. Tablets: Store at room temperature protected from light. Keep bottles tightly closed. Dispense in a light-resistant, tight container.
3. Tablets, Extended-Release: Store from 15–30°C (59–86°F). Dispense in a well-closed container.
4. Tablets, Sublingual: Store from 15–30°C (59–86°F) protected from light and moisture. Dispense in a tight, light-resistant container.

ASSESSMENT

1. Note reasons for therapy; include onset, location, characteristics of chest pain; rate pain levels.
2. Assess VS and ECG; note stress thallium, catheterization, or IVUS findings as well as CAD history/interventions.

CLIENT/FAMILY TEACHING

1. Take tablets with meals or acetaminophen to eliminate/reduce headaches; otherwise, take on an empty stomach to facilitate absorption. Store product in original container.
2. Review method for administration. May take SL tablets at first symptom of chest pain. Do not chew or crush sublingual (SL) tablets or extended-release tablets or capsules. Do not stop abruptly; may cause heart spasms.
3. Swallow extended-release tablets/capsules whole; place SL tablet under the tongue and allow to dissolve.
4. Use caution; may cause dizziness, lightheadedness, or fainting, especially if used while standing or following consumption of alcohol. Avoid sudden position changes to prevent drop in BP.
5. Tolerance may develop (stay nitrate free for 14 hr for sublingual and oral tablets; at least 18 hr for extended-release tablets and capsules, usually at night, to prevent tolerance). Short-acting products can be given 2–3 times per day with the last dose no later than 6:00 p.m. The extended-release products can be given once or twice daily at 8:00 a.m. and 2:00 p.m. or as prescribed.
6. Take as directed before any stressful activity (sexual activity, exercise).
7. Acetaminophen (Tylenol) or aspirin may assist to relieve drug-induced headaches.
8. Avoid alcohol and any OTC agents without approval.
9. Do not take if also using erectile dysfunction drugs (phosphodiesterase type 5 inhibitors); severe hypotension may occur.
10. Keep all F/U to assess response and for adverse SE.

OUTCOMES/EVALUATE

- ↓ Frequency/severity of anginal attacks
- ↑ CO/Exercise tolerance

Isosorbide mononitrate

(eye-so-**SOR**-byd)

Classification(s): Coronary vasodilator

Pregnancy Category: C

RX: Tablets: ISMO, Monoket. **Tablets, Extended-Release**: Imdur.

Rx: Apo-ISMN.

SEE ALSO ***ANTIANGINAL DRUGS—NITRATES/NITRITES*** AND ***ISOSORBIDE DINITRATE***.

INDICATIONS/USES

(1) Treatment of angina pectoris (Monoket only). (2) Prophylaxis of angina pectoris caused by coronary artery disease. The onset of action of the mononitrate is not sufficiently rapid to be used in aborting an acute angina attach. *Investigational:* With nadolol to prevent recurrent variceal bleeding.

ACTION/KINETICS

Action

Isosorbide mononitrate is the major metabolite of isosorbide dinitrate. The mononitrate is not subject to first-pass metabolism. Relaxes vascular smooth muscle by stimulating production of intracellular cyclic guanosine monophosphate. Dilation of postcapillary vessels decreases venous return to the heart due to pooling of blood; thus, LV end-diastolic pressure (preload) is reduced. Relaxation of areterioles results in a decreased systemic vascular resistance and arterial pressure (afterload).

Pharmacokinetics

Bioavailability is nearly 100%. **Onset:** 30–60 min. **t_{max}, tablets:** 0.6–0.7 hr; **t_{max}, ER tablets:** 2.9–4.5 hr. **$t^{1/2}$, tablets:** About 5 hr; **$t^{1/2}$, ER tablets:** 6.2 hr.

CONTRAINDICATIONS

To abort acute anginal attacks. Use in acute MI or CHF.

SPECIAL CONCERNS

- Use with caution during lactation and in clients who may be volume depleted or are already hypotensive.
- Benefits not established in acute MI or CHF.
- Safety and efficacy not determined in children.

SIDE EFFECTS

Most Common

Dizziness, headache, hypotension, N&V, increased cough, allergic reaction.

CV: Hypotension (may be accompanied by paradoxical bradycardia and increased angina pectoris), CV disorder, chest pain. **CNS:** Headache, lightheadedness, dizziness, fatigue, emotional lability. **GI:** N&V, diarrhea, abdominal pain. **Dermatologic:** Pruritus, rash. **Respiratory:** Increased cough, URTI. **Miscellaneous:** Possibility of methemoglobinemia, allergic reactions, flushing, pain.

OVERDOSE MANAGEMENT

Symptoms: Increased intracranial pressure manifested by throbbing headache, confusion, moderate fever. Also, vertigo, palpitations, visual disturbances, N&V, syncope, air hunger, dyspnea (followed by reduced ventilatory effort), diaphoresis, skin either flushed or cold and clammy, heart block, bradycardia, paralysis, ***coma, seizures, death.*** *Treatment:* Direct therapy toward an increase in central fluid volume. Do *not* use vasoconstrictors.

DRUG INTERACTIONS

Ethanol / Additive vasodilation
Calcium channel blockers / Severe orthostatic hypotension
Organic nitrates / Severe orthostatic hypotension
Sildenafil / Severe hypotension → possible death; use together an absolute contraindication
Tadalafil / Severe hypotension → possible death; use together an absolute contraindication
Vardenafil / Severe hypotension → possible death; use together an absolute contraindication

HOW SUPPLIED

Tablets: 10 mg, 20 mg; ***Tablets, Extended-Release:*** 30 mg, 60 mg, 120 mg.

DOSAGE

TABLETS

Prophylaxis of angina.

20 mg twice a day with the two doses given 7 hr apart, with the first dose

upon awakening. A starting dose of 5 mg (one-half of the 10 mg tablet) may be appropriate for clients of particularly small stature; however, increase to at least 10 mg by the second or third day. This dosing regimen provides a daily nitrate-free interval to minimize tolerance development.

TABLETS, EXTENDED-RELEASE

Prophylaxis of angina.

Initial: 30 mg or 60 mg once daily; **then,** after several days dosage may be increased to 120 mg (given as a single 120 mg tablet or as 2 60 mg tablets). Rarely, 240 mg daily may be needed. The suggested regimen is to give the dose in the a.m. on arising.

NURSING IMPLICATIONS

Do not confuse Imdur with Imuran (an immunosuppressant) or Inderal (a beta-adrenergic blocker).

IMPLEMENTATION/ADMINISTRATION/STORAGE

1. The treatment regimen minimizes the development of refractory tolerance.
2. Tablets: Store from 15–30°C (59–86°F). Keep tightly closed.
3. Protect from excessive moisture.

ASSESSMENT

1. Note reasons for therapy, cardiac history, onset/frequency of angina, triggers, other agents trialed and outcome.
2. Monitor VS, ECG, cardiac status, family history, risk factors, and electrolytes.
3. List drugs prescribed to ensure none interact. Do not use if taking any drug for erectile dysfunction of phosphodiesterase type 5 inhibitors (e.g., sildenafil, tadalafil, vardenafil) because of the risk of severe low BP.

CLIENT/FAMILY TEACHING

1. Drug used to prevent chest pain in those with heart disease by decreasing workload of heart.
2. Take first dose in morning upon awakening with or without food.
3. Take the extended-release tablet in the morning upon arising as directed. Do not crush or chew; take with a half glass of water. Do not change brands.
4. Consume 1–2 L/day of fluids to ensure adequate hydration. Do not stop abruptly due to risk of angina attacks.
5. Ensure sublingual nitroglycerin available at all times for acute attacks.
6. May cause dizziness or lightheadedness. Alcohol, hot weather, exercise, and fever can increase these effects. Use caution performing activities that require mental alertness until drug effects realized. Change positions slowly to prevent dizziness.
7. Not to be used to stop an attack of angina; intended only for prevention of an attack.
8. Avoid alcohol. Report if chest pain persists/recurs.
9. Keep all F/U to assess response, labs, ECGs, and for adverse SE.

OUTCOMES/EVALUATE

Angina prophylaxis

Isotretinoin

(eye-so-**TRET**-ih-noyn)

Classification(s): Retinoid

Pregnancy Category: X

RX: Amnesteem, Claravis, Sotret.

✤ **Rx:** Accutane Roche.

INDICATIONS/USES

Severe recalcitrant nodular acne unresponsive to standard therapies. Severe refers to many nodules that are inflammatory with a diameter of 5 mm or more. Nodules may become suppurative or hemorrhagic. *NOTE:* To decrease further the chances of pregnancy during therapy, pharmacies, wholesalers, and clients must register with the iPLEDGE Program to obtain and distribute isotretinoin. *Investigational:* Pityriasis rubra pilaris, rosacea, psoriasis, prevention and treatment of basal cell carcinoma; adjunctive treatment of inoperable neoplasms such as squamous cell carcinoma of the lung; treatment of advanced squamous cell carcinoma of the skin; keratoacanthomas; cutaneous T-cell lymphomas.

ACTION/KINETICS

Action

Exact mechanism is unknown but the drug inhibits sebaceous gland function and keratinization.

Reduces sebaceous gland size and decreases sebum secretion.

Pharmacokinetics

Approximately 25% of the PO dosage form is bioavailable. Absorption is enhanced when given with a high-fat meal. **Peak plasma levels:** 3 hr in fasted clients and 5.3 hr in fed clients. **Steady-state blood levels following 80 mg/day:** 160 ng/mL. **t½, terminal:** 21 hr. Metabolized in the liver to 4-oxo-isotretinoin, which is also active, and other metabolites. **t½, terminal of 4-oxo-isotretinoin:** 17–50 hr. Approximately equal amounts are excreted through the urine and in the feces. **Plasma protein binding:** >99.9%.

CONTRAINDICATIONS

Due to the possibility of fetal abnormalities or spontaneous abortion at any dose, women who are pregnant or intend to become pregnant must not use the drug. Certain conditions for use should be met in women with childbearing potential (see package insert). Hypersensitivity to isotretinoin or any component of the product, including parabens (used as a preservative in the gelatin capsules of Accutane and Sotret). Lactation.

SPECIAL CONCERNS

(1) Isotretinoin must not be used by women and adolescents who are pregnant or who may become pregnant. There is an extremely high risk that severe birth defects can result if pregnancy occurs while taking isotretinoin in any amount, even for short periods of time. Potentially, any fetus exposed during pregnancy can be affected. There are no accurate means of determining whether an exposed fetus has been affected. (2) Birth defects that have been documented following isotretinoin exposure include abnormalities of the face, eyes, ears, skull, CNS, CV system, and thymus and parathyroid glands. Cases of intelligence quotient (IQ) scores less than 85 with or without other abnormalities have been reported. There is an increased risk of spontaneous abortion, and premature births have been reported. (3) Documented external abnormalities include skull abnormality; ear abnormalities (including anotia, micropinna, small or absent external auditory canals); eye abnormalities (including microphthalmia); facial dysmorphia; cleft palate. Documented internal abnormalities include CNS abnormalities (including cerebral abnormalities, cerebellar malformation, hydrocephalus, microcephaly, cranial nerve deficit); CV abnormalities; thymus gland abnormality; parathyroid hormone deficiency. In some cases death has occurred with some of the abnormalities previously noted. (4) If pregnancy does occur during treatment of a female client who is taking isotretinoin, isotretinoin must be discontinued immediately and she should be referred to an obstetrician-gynecologist experienced in reproductive toxicity for further evaluation and counseling. (5) Because of isotretinoin's teratogenicity and to minimize fetal exposure, isotretinoin is approved for marketing only under a special restricted distribution program approved by the FDA. This program is called iPLEDGE. Isotretinoin must only be prescribed by prescribers who are registered and activated with the iPLEDGE program. Isotretinoin must only be dispensed by a pharmacy registered and activated with iPLEDGE and must only be dispensed to clients who are registered and meet all the requirements of iPLEDGE. (6) Information for the pharmacist. Access the iPLEDGE system via the Internet (www.ipledgeprogram.com) or telephone (1-866-495-0654) to obtain an authorization and the "do not dispense to patient after" date. Isotretinoin must only be dispensed in no more than a 30-day supply. (7) Refills require a new prescription and a new authorization from the iPLEDGE system. (8) An isotretinoin Medication Guide must be given to the client each time isotretinoin is dispensed, as required by law. This isotretinoin Medication Guide is an important part of the risk management program for the client.

- **Intolerance to contact lenses may develop.**
- **Increased risks for birth defects, aggressive and/or violent behavior, psychiatric disorders (including suicidal tendencies). Give for no longer than the recommended duration.**
- **Avoid use during lactation.**
- **Check lipids before therapy, and then at intervals until response established (within 4 weeks).**
- **Monitor LFTs before therapy, weekly or biweekly until response established.**

- Avoid prolonged UV rays or sunlight, and donating blood up to 1 month after discontinuing therapy.
- Use with caution with genetic predisposition for age-related osteoporosis, history of childhood osteoporosis, osteomalacia, other bone metabolism disorders (i.e., anorexia nervosa).
- Use with caution with drugs that cause drug-induced osteoporosis/osteomalacia and affect vitamin D metabolism disorders (i.e., corticosteroids, phenytoin).
- The elderly may experience increased risk associated with isotretinoin therapy.
- Use in children less than 12 years of age has not been studied; carefully consider the use of isotretinoin to treat severe recalcitrant nodular acne in children 12 to 17 years of age, especially if a known metabolic or structural bone disease exists.

SIDE EFFECTS

Most Common

Dry skin, itching, dry nose, epistaxis, cheilitis, dry mouth, conjunctivitis, joint aches, depression, hallucinations, suicidal behavior, increased blood glucose and triglycerides.

Dermatologic: Cheilitis, itching, skin fragility, pruritus, dry skin/mouth/nose, alopecia, desquamation of facial skin, nail dystrophy, photoallergic/photosensitizing reactions, epistaxis, flushing, rash (including facial erythema, seborrhea, and eczema), hypo-/hyperpigmentation, urticaria, pruritus, erythema nodosum, hirsutism, excess granulation of tissues as a result of healing, petechiae, peeling of palms and soles, skin infections (including disseminated herpes simplex), paronychia, thinning of hair, nail dystrophy, pyogenic granuloma, bruising, acne fulminans, eruptive xanthomas, sweating, increased susceptibility to sunburn, abnormal wound healing (delayed healing or exuberant granulation tissue with crusting), vasculitis (including Wegener granulomatosis). **CNS:** Headache, fatigue, pseudotumor cerebri (i.e., headaches, papilledema, N&V, disturbances in vision, dizziness), depression, emotional instability, psychosis, hallucinations, suicidal ideation, ***suicide attempts, suicide***, drowsiness, insomnia, lethargy, malaise, nervousness, paresthesias, ***seizures, stroke***, syncope, weakness, emotional instability. Aggressive and/or violent behaviors. **GI:** Dry mouth, N&V, abdominal pain, nonspecific GI symptoms, hepatitis, hepatotoxicity, inflammatory bowel disease (including regional ileitis), anorexia, weight loss, ***acute pancreatitis***, inflammation and bleeding of gums, colitis, ileitis, esophageal ulceration, esophagitis. **CV:** Flushing, palpitation, ***stroke***, tachycardia, vascular thrombotic disease. **Neuromuscular:** Arthralgia, arthritis, myalgia, transient chest pain; muscle, bone and joint pain and stiffness; skeletal hyperostosis, calcification of tendons and ligaments, premature epiphyseal closure, arthritis, tendonitis, back pain, rhabdomyolysis (rare). Reports of osteoporosis, osteopenia, bone fractures, and delayed healing of bone fractures. Decrease in lumbar spine bone mineral density. **Hematologic:** Neutropenia, thrombocytopenia, anemia, ***agranulocytosis (rare)***. **GU:** White cells in urine, proteinuria, nonspecific urogenital findings, microscopic or gross hematuria, abnormal menses, glomerular nephritis. **Respiratory:** Bronchospasms with or without history of asthma, respiratory tract infections, voice alterations, epistaxis, dry nose. **Ocular/Ophthalmic:** Conjunctivitis, optic neuritis, corneal opacities, dry eyes, decrease in acuity of night vision (may persist), photophobia, eyelid inflammation, cataracts, visual disturbances, color vision disorder, keratitis. **Otic:** Impaired hearing, tinnitus. **Miscellaneous:** Disseminated herpes simplex, edema, fatigue, development of diabetes, lymphadenopathy, flushing, weight loss, severe allergic (hypersensitivity) reactions (including ***anaphylaxis***, cutaneous allergic reactions, allergic vasculitis, purpura).

LABORATORY TEST CONSIDERATIONS

↑ Plasma triglycerides, sedimentation rate, platelet counts, alkaline phosphatase, AST, ALT, GGTP, LDH, fasting blood glucose, uric acid in blood, serum cholesterol, CPK levels in clients who exercise vigorously. ↓ HDL, RBC parameters, WBC counts. Hypertriglyceridemia, hyperuricemia.

OVERDOSE MANAGEMENT

Symptoms: Abdominal pain, ataxia, cheilosis, dizziness, facial flushing, headache, vomiting. Symptoms are transient. *Treatment:* Symptoms are quickly resolved with drug cessation or decrease in dose.

DRUG INTERACTIONS

Alcohol / Potentiation of ↑ serum triglycerides
Corticosteroids, systemic / Possible interactive effect on bone loss; use together with caution

Minocycline / ↑ Risk of developing pseudotumor cerebri or papilledema
Oral contraceptives and injectable/implantable contraceptives, microdose progesterone products / Possible inadequate pregnancy protection
Phenytoin / Possible interactive effect on bone loss; use together with caution
H *St. John's wort* / May cause breakthrough bleeding with oral contraceptives
Tetracycline / ↑ Risk of developing pseudotumor cerebri or papilledema; avoid concomitant use
Vitamin A / ↑ Risk of additive toxicity

HOW SUPPLIED

Capsules: 10 mg, 20 mg, 30 mg, 40 mg; *Capsules, Softgel:* 10 mg, 20 mg, 30 mg, 40 mg.

DOSAGE

CAPSULES; CAPSULES SOFTGEL

Recalcitrant cystic acne.

Adults and children 12 years and older, individualized, initial:
0.5–1 mg/kg/day (range: 0.5–2 mg/kg/day) divided in two doses with food for 15–20 weeks. Adjust dose based on toxicity and clinical response; if cyst count decreases by 70% or more, drug may be discontinued. If necessary, a second course of therapy may be instituted after a rest period of 2 months. Long-term use, even in low doses, is not recommended. Doses of 0.05–0.5 mg/kg/day are effective but result in higher frequency of relapses.

Investigational: keratinization disorders.

Doses up to 4 mg/kg/day have been used.

Prevent second tumors in squamous-cell carcinoma of the head and neck.

50–100 mg/m^2.

NURSING IMPLICATIONS

Do not confuse Accutane with Accupril (ACE inhibitor).

IMPLEMENTATION/ADMINISTRATION/STORAGE

1. Monthly required iPLEDGE interactions include the following:
   - For females, the prescriber must register each client in the iPLEDGE program, confirm client counseling, record the two contraceptive methods chosen by the client, and record pregnancy test results.
   - For males, the prescriber must confirm client counseling.
   - Female clients must provide answer on educational questions before every prescription and record two forms of contraception.
   - For both female and male clients the pharmacist must be trained by the responsible site pharmacist concerning the program requirements, call the system to get authorization, and write the Risk Management Authorization number on the prescription.
2. Isotretinoin must be dispensed only:
   - In no more than a 30-day supply.
   - With an isotretinoin Medication Guide.
   - After authorization from the iPLEDGE program.
   - Prior to the "do not dispense to patient after" date provided by the iPLEDGE system (within 7 days of the office visit).
   - With a new prescription for refills and another authorization from the iPLEDGE program (no automatic refills allowed).
3. A rest period of 2 months is recommended if a second course of therapy is needed.
4. Store Amnesteem from 15–30°C (59–86°F); protect from light. Store Claravis and Sotret from 20–25°C (68–77°F); protect from light.

ASSESSMENT

1. Note clinical presentation, other agents/therapies trialed, outcome; use photos to document.
2. Document mental status and behavioral presentation; assess for changes, psychosis, depression, or suicide ideation.
3. Isotretinoin prescribed and dispensed by prescribers and pharmacies registered with and activated by the FDA-restricted distribution program, iPLEDGE.
4. May affect BS, hearing, vision, and bone mineral density; monitor closely.
5. Advise not to donate blood for transfusion during treatment and for 1 mo after discontinuing therapy.
6. Obtain 2 negative urine or serum pregnancy tests prior to receiving initial isotretinoin prescription and negative result for urine or serum pregnancy test each month; obtain pretreatment and follow-up lipids during fasting conditions; monitor liver function weekly or bi-

weekly until isotretinoin response has been established.

7. Monitor serum glucose levels, chemistry, CBC, urinalysis, LFTs, CPK, and lipid panels.

CLIENT/FAMILY TEACHING

1. Do not crush capsules. Should be given with food or milk; a high-fat meal will increase the absorption of isotretinoin.
2. Only prescribed through restricted access/distribution program called iPLEDGE.
3. Before receiving isotretinoin, clients must sign an informed consent form that details the risks associated with isotretinoin use. Clients will also receive a medication guide and information about contraceptive methods. Females must confirm they have a negative result for the second urine pregnancy request, conducted on the second day of the next menstrual period or 11 days or more after the last unprotected act of sexual intercourse, whichever is later. Drug is teratogenic; monthly pregnancy tests are required. Females of childbearing age should practice 2 reliable forms of birth control 1 month before, during, and 1 month following therapy; severe fetal damage may occur. Any pregnancy should be reported to iPLEDGE pregnancy registry at 1-866-495-0654 or visiting their website at www.ipledgeprogram.com.
4. A 30-day prescription will be dispensed with no refills to ensure compliance. It must be filled within 7 days of order date and prescription must have yellow qualification sticker.
5. Report if persistent headache, N&V, or visual disturbances occur. Avoid abrasive skin cleaners, medicated soaps, topical acne preparations/alcohol based products and peeling agents. Lubricants may help diminish symptoms of dry, chapped skin and lips.
6. Contact lens wearers may develop sensitivity to contacts during and after therapy. Excessively dry eyes may require an eye lubricant. Report vision changes.
7. Condition may become worse before healing starts. Report any muscle, joint, or bone pains. Avoid wax epilation and skin resurfacing procedures (e.g., dermabrasion, laser) during therapy and for at least 6 months after completion due to possible scarring.
8. Avoid OTC medications, especially vitamin A, without consent.
9. Eliminate or markedly reduce consumption of alcohol; may increase triglyceride levels.
10. Report any increased agitation/irritability, unusual behavioral changes, or suicide ideations.
11. Avoid prolonged sunlight exposure; may cause photosensitivity. Wear protective clothing, sunscreen, and sunglasses when exposed.
12. May aggravate intestinal problems and cause hearing loss; report if evident.
13. Avoid therapy with tetracycline (pseudotumor cerebri) and donating blood for 30 days after discontinuing drug therapy.
14. Keep all F/U to assess response, labs, for adverse SE, and monthly script.

OUTCOMES/EVALUATE

- ↓ Number/size and severity of cystic acne lesions
- Healing/clearing and restoration of skin integrity

Itraconazole

(**ih**-trah-**KON**-ah-zohl)

Classification(s): Antifungal

Pregnancy Category: C

RX: Sporanox.

INDICATIONS/USES

Capsules: (1) Onychomycosis of the toenail with or without fingernail involvement and onychomycosis of the fingernail because of dermatophytes (*Tinea unguium*) in nonimmunocompromised clients. (2) Pulmonary and extrapulmonary aspergillosis in nonimmunocompromised or immunocompromised clients who are intolerant of or refractory to amphotericin B therapy. (3) Pulmonary and extrapulmonary blastomycosis in nonimmunocompromised or immunocompromised clients. (4) Histoplasmosis, including chronic cavitary pulmonary disease and disseminated, nonmeningeal histoplasmosis in nonimmunocompromised or immunocompromised clients.

Capsules or Oral Solution: Oropharyngeal and esophageal candidiasis. *NOTE:* If clients with cystic fibrosis do not respond to the PO solution, consider switching to alternative therapy.

Oral Solution: For empiric therapy of febrile neutropenic clients with suspected fungal infections.

Investigational: (1) Solution (200 mg/day) as an alternative to fluconazole as secondary prevention of oropharyngeal, vaginal, or esophageal candidiasis in HIV-infected clients who have severe or frequent recurrences. (2) Capsules (200 mg/day) as an alternative to fluconazole for primary prevention of cryptococcosis in adults with advanced HIV disease (CD4 counts less than 50 cells/mcL). (3) Capsules as an alternative to fluconazole for lifelong secondary prevention of cryptococcal disease in HIV-infected adults. (4) Capsules (200 mg/day) as first-line therapy in the primary prevention of histoplasmosis in adults with advanced HIV disease (CD4 counts less than 100 cells/mcL) and live in endemic areas (rate greater than or equal to 10 cases/100 patient-years). Also as first-line drug (200 mg/day) for lifelong secondary prophylaxis. (5) Capsules (200 mg/day) as an alternate drug to fluconazole for lifelong secondary prevention of coccidioidomycosis in HIV-infected adults. (6) Oral products for secondary prevention of histoplasmosis (first line: 2–5 mg/kg q 12–48 hr), cryptococcal disease (alternative therapy: 2–5 mg/kg q 12–24 hr), and coccidioidomycosis (alternative therapy: 2–5 mg/kg q 12–48 hr) in children with HIV. (7) Oral products (2–5 mg/kg q 12–24 hr) for primary prevention of histoplasmosis (first-line drug) and cryptococcal disease (alternative drug) in children with HIV, severe immunosuppression, and live in endemic histoplasmosis areas.

ACTION/KINETICS

Action

Believed to inhibit cytochrome P-450-dependent synthesis of ergosterol, a necessary component of fungal cell membranes.

Pharmacokinetics

Oral bioavailability is maximum when capsules are taken with a full meal. Absorption was increased under fasting conditions in those with AIDS when taken with a cola beverage. Absorption is decreased in the presence of decreased gastric acidity. Concentrates in fatty tissues, omentum, liver, kidney, and skin. **T_{max}, capsules, steady-state:** 4.6 hr. **t½ for capsules at steady-state:** 64 hr. Extensively metabolized in the liver by CYP3A4; the major metabolite is hydroxyitraconazole, which also has antifungal activity. Metabolites are excreted in both the urine and feces.

Plasma protein binding: Itraconazole and hydroxyitraconazole: More than 99%.

CONTRAINDICATIONS

Concomitant use of dofetilide, pimozide, quinidine, triazolam, or oral midazolam due to possible serious CV events. Hypersensitivity to the drug or its excipients. Lactation. Use for the treatment of onychomycosis in pregnant women or in women wishing to become pregnant. Use with severe renal dysfunction (C_{CR} less than 30 mL/min). Use of capsules in clients with a history of cardiac dysfunction (e.g., CHF or a history of CHF) or other ventricular dysfunction. Use with HMG-CoA reductase inhibitors (e.g., lovastatin, simvastatin) or ergot alkaloids (e.g., dihydroergotamine, ergotamine, ergonovine, methylergonovine) metabolized by the CYP3A4 enzyme system. Initiation of therapy in clients with elevated or abnormal liver enzyme levels, active liver disease, or a previous incident of hepatotoxicity during therapy with any drug.

SPECIAL CONCERNS

(1) Do not give itraconazole to treat onychomycosis or dermatomycoses in clients with evidence of cardiac dysfunction, such as CHF or a history of CHF. Discontinue if S&S of CHF occur during treatment. If S&S of CHF occur during treatment for more serious fungal infections involving other parts of the body, continued use of itraconazole should be reassessed. Possible negative inotropic effects may occur. (2) Coadministration with dofetilide, pimozide, or quinidine is contraindicated. Itraconazole is a potent inhibitor of the CYP3A4 isoenzyme system and may raise plasma concentrations of drugs metabolized by this pathway. Serious CV events, including QT prolongation, torsades de pointes, ventricular tachycardia, cardiac arrest, or sudden death have occurred in those taking itraconazole with these drugs, which are inhibitors of the CYP3A4 system.

- Use with caution in clients with hypersensitivity to other azoles.
- Liver enzymes may be elevated more than twice that of normal.
- Safety and efficacy not determined in children 3–16 years of age although pediatric clients have been treated for systemic fungal infections.

SIDE EFFECTS

Most Common

N&V, rash, asthenia, headache, abdominal pain, diarrhea, dyspepsia, flatulence, rhinitis, sinusitis, URTI, coughing, fever.

GI: N&V, diarrhea, abdominal pain, anorexia, taste perversion, flatulence, general GI disorders, constipation, gingivitis, ulcerative stomatitis, gastritis, gastroenteritis, increased appetite, dyspepsia, dysphagia, hemorrhoids. **Hepatic:** Abnormal hepatic function, hepatitis, ***serious hepatotoxicity, liver failure***, jaundice. **CNS:** Headache, anxiety, depression, vertigo, dizziness, somnolence, decreased libido, abnormal dreaming, insomnia. **CV:** Hypertension, hypotension, orthostatic hypotension, vasculitis, ***CHF***, tachycardia, vein disorder. **Respiratory:** URTI, rhinitis, sinusitis, pharyngitis, coughing, dyspnea, pneumonia, increased sputum, pulmonary edema/infiltration. **Dermatologic:** Increased sweating, skin disorders, hot flushes, rash, pruritus, alopecia, erythematous rash, skin disorder, ***Stevens-Johnson syndrome.*** **Musculoskeletal:** Bursitis, chest/back pain, myalgia. **GU:** UTI, impotence, cystitis, menstrual disorders, abnormal renal function, gynecomastia, hematuria, male breast pain. **Allergic:** Rash, pruritus, urticaria, angioedema, ***anaphylaxis*** (rare). **Hematologic:** Neutropenia. **Ophthalmic:** Abnormal vision. **Otic:** Tinnitus. **Body as a whole:** Edema, fatigue, pain, fever, malaise, myalgia, rigors, asthenia, tremor, dehydration, infection, jaundice, fluid overload, unspecified infection. **Miscellaneous:** Injury, herpes zoster, *Pneumocystis carinii* infection, reaction at injection/application site, implantation complication, adrenal insufficiency, weight loss, peripheral edema, peripheral neuropathy.

LABORATORY TEST CONSIDERATIONS

↑ ALT, AST, alkaline phosphatase, BUN, serum creatinine, LDH, GGT. Hypertriglyceridemia, hypokalemia, hypocalcemia, hypomagnesemia, hypophosphatemia, albuminuria, bilirubinemia. Abnormal hepatic function.

OVERDOSE MANAGEMENT

Symptoms: Extension of side effects. *Treatment:* Use supportive measures, including gastric lavage and sodium bicarbonate. Dialysis will not remove itraconazole.

DRUG INTERACTIONS

Alfentanil / ↑ Alfentanil effect and toxicity R/T inhibition of metabolism
Almotriptan / ↑ Almotriptan levels → ↑ pharmacologic and side effects; do not take almotriptan within 7 days of itraconazole
Alprazolam / ↑ and prolonged alprazolam levels → ↑ CNS depression and psychomotor impairment
Amphotericin B / ↓ Activity of amphotericin B
Antacids / ↓ Itraconazole absorption R/T ↓ gastric acidity; give antacid at least 1 hr before or 2 hr after itraconazole capsules
Aripiprazole / ↑ Aripiprazole levels → ↑ pharmacologic and side effects; reduce aripiprazole dose by 50% if given with itraconazole
Buspirone / ↑ Buspirone levels → ↑ effects and toxicity
Busulfan / ↑ Busulfan levels → ↑ risk of toxicity (e.g., pancytopenia)
Calcium channel blockers / Inhibition of metabolism of felodipine, nifedipine, nisoldipine, and verapamil; also ↑ negative inotropic effects and possible edema
Carbamazepine / ↑ Carbamazepine levels → ↑ clinical and adverse effects; also, possible ↓ itraconazole levels
Cilostazol / ↑ Cilostazol levels → ↑ pharmacologic and side effects
Clarithromycin / ↑ Itraconazole levels R/T inhibition of metabolism by CYP3A4
Corticosteroids (budesonide, dexamethasone, methylprednisolone) / ↓ Corticosteroid metabolism → ↑ corticosteroid pharmacologic and toxic effects
Cyclosporine / ↑ Cyclosporine levels (dose of cyclosporine should be ↓ by 50% if itraconazole doses are much greater than 100 mg/day)
Diazepam / ↑ and prolonged diazepam levels → ↑ CNS depression and psychomotor impairment
Didanosine (buffered formulation) / ↓ Itraconazole effects; give itraconazole 2 hr or more before didanosine chewable tablets
Digoxin / ↑ Digoxin levels → ↑ pharmacologic and toxic effects
Disopyramide / ↑ Disopyramide levels; potential to ↑ QT interval
Docetaxel / Inhibition of docetaxel metabolism
Dofetilide / ↑ Dofetilide levels → possible serious CV events, including QT prolongation, torsades de pointes, ventricular tachycardia, cardiac arrest, or sudden death; do not use together

I

Eletriptan / ↑ Eletriptan levels → ↑ pharmacologic and side effects; do not take eletriptan within 72 hr of itraconazole
Eplerenone / ↑ Eplerenone levels → ↑ risk of hyperkalemia and associated serious arrhythmias; do not use together
Ergot alkaloids (dihydroergotamine, ergonovine, ergotamine, methylergonovine) / ↑ Risk of ergot toxicity (i.e., peripheral vasospasm, ischemia of the extremities, and/or cerebral ischemia)
Erythromycin / ↑ Itraconazole levels R/T inhibition of metabolism by CYP3A4
Felodipine / ↑ Felodipine levels (possible edema)
Grapefruit juice / ↓ Itraconazole bioavailability R/T inhibition of absorption
Haloperidol / ↑ Haloperidol levels → ↑ risk of side effects
H_2 antagonists / ↓ Itraconazole absorption R/T ↓ gastric acidity; give itraconazole with a cola beverage
HMG-CoA reductase inhibitors (atorvastatin, lovastatin, simvastatin) / ↑ Plasma levels and side effects of reductase inhibitors; possibility of rhabdomyolysis; do not use lovastatin or simvastatin with itraconazole
Indinavir / ↑ Indinavir levels R/T inhibition of metabolism by CYP3A4 → ↑ risk of toxicity; also, possible ↑ itraconazole levels
Isoniazid / ↓ Plasma itraconazole levels
Losartan / ↑ Losartan antihypertensive effect
Lovastatin / ↑ Lovastatin levels → possible rhabdomyolysis; do not use together
Methylprednisolone / Inhibition of methylprednisolone metabolism
Midazolam, oral / ↑ Prolonged levels of oral midazolam → ↑ CNS depression and psychomotor impairment
Neviripine / ↓ Itraconazole levels
Nisoldipine / ↑ Nisoldipine levels
Oral contraceptives / ↓ Oral contraceptive effect
Oral hypoglycemics / Possible severe hypoglycemia; monitor blood glucose
Phenobarbital / ↓ Itraconazole levels
Phenytoin / ↓ Effect of itraconazole and ↑ effect of phenytoin; do not use together
Pimozide / Possible serious CV events, including QT prolongation, torsades de pointes, ventricular tachycardia, cardiac arrest/sudden death; do not use together
Proton pump inhibitors / ↓ Itraconazole absorption R/T ↓ gastric acidity
Quinidine / Possible serious CV events, including QT prolongation, torsades de pointes, ventricular tachycardia, cardiac arrest and/or sudden death; do not use together
Rifampin, Rifabutin, Rifapentine / ↓ Itraconazole levels; possible ↑ rifabutin levels; do not use together
Ritonavir / ↑ Ritonavir levels R/T inhibition of metabolism by CYP3A4 → ↑ risk of toxicity; also, possible ↑ itraconazole levels
Sildenafil / ↑ Sildenafil levels → ↑ risk of side effects; give sildenafil with caution and at reduced doses
Simvastatin / ↑ Simvastatin levels → possible rhabdomyolysis; do not use together
Sirolimus / Possible ↑ sirolimus levels; monitor for sirolimus toxicity
Sulfonylureas / ↑ Hypoglycemia risk
Tacrolimus / ↑ Tacrolimus levels → ↑ toxicity
Tadalafil / ↑ Tadalafil levels → ↑ risk of side effects; give tadalafil with caution and at reduced doses
Tolterodine / ↑ Tolterodine levels; do not give more than 1 mg tolterodine twice a day
Triazolam / ↑ and prolonged triazolam levels → ↑ CNS depression and psychomotor impairment
Trimetrexate / Inhibition of trimetrexate metabolism
Vardenafil / ↑ Vardenafil levels → ↑ risk of side effects; give vardenafil with caution and at reduced doses
Vinca alkaloids / ↑ Risk of vinca alkaloid toxicity (e.g., constipation, myalgia, neutropenia) R/T inhibition of metabolism; do not use together
Warfarin / ↑ Anticoagulant effect; monitor PT and INR values q 2 days when adding or discontinuing an azole antifungal
Zolpidem / ↑ Zolpidem effects R/T inhibition of metabolism

HOW SUPPLIED

Capsules: 100 mg; ***Oral Solution:*** 10 mg/mL.

DOSAGE

CAPSULES

Blastomycosis or chronic pulmonary histoplasmosis.

Adults: 200 mg once daily. If there is no improvement or the disease is progressive, the dose may be increased in 100 mg increments to a maximum of

400 mg/day. Give doses greater than 200 mg/day in 2 divided doses. For life-threatening situations, a loading dose of 200 mg 3 times per day may be given for the first 3 days of treatment.

Aspergillosis.

200–400 mg daily.

Onychomycosis, fingernails only.

Two treatment pulses, each consisting of 200 mg twice a day for 1 week. Pulses are separated by a 3-week period without the drug.

Onychomycosis, toenails with or without fingernail involvement.

200 mg/day for 12 weeks.

Life-threatening situations.

Loading dose: 200 mg 3 times/day for the first 3 days of treatment; continue treatment for a minimum of 3 months and until clinical parameters and lab tests indicate the active fungal infection has subsided.

ORAL SOLUTION

Esophageal candidiasis.

100 mg/day (10 mL) for a minimum of 3 weeks. Continue treatment for 2 weeks following resolution of symptoms. Doses of 200 mg/day may be used based on medical judgment of response.

Empiric therapy of febrile neutropenia with suspected fungal infections.

After about 14 days of IV therapy, continue treatment with PO solution, 200 mg (20 mL) twice a day, until resolution of clinically significant neutropenia. Safety and efficacy for more than 28 days are not known.

Oropharyngeal candidiasis.

200 mg/day (20 mL) for 1–2 weeks. For those unresponsive or refractory to treatment with fluconazole tablets, the recommended dose of itraconazole is 100 mg twice a day. A response should occur within 2–4 weeks. Clients may relapse shortly after discontinuing therapy. Data on use for more than 6 months are lacking.

NURSING IMPLICATIONS

IMPLEMENTATION/ADMINISTRATION/STORAGE

1. Take capsules, but not oral solution, after a full meal to ensure maximal absorption. Swallow capsules whole. Swish solution in oral cavity and swallow; do not rinse after swallowing. Do not use capsules and oral solution interchangeably.
2. Give daily doses greater than 200 mg in two divided doses.
3. Continue treatment for a minimum of 3 months until symptoms and lab tests indicate the active fungal infection has subsided. Recurrence of active infection may occur with inadequate treatment period.
4. Absorption from capsules is impaired when gastric acidity is decreased (e.g., use of antacids, proton pump inhibitors, H_2-histamine blockers). Thus, give such drugs at least 2 hr after itraconazole.
5. Give with a cola beverage when coadministering with H_2-antagonists or other gastric acid suppressors.
6. Plasma levels using capsules are lower in neutropenic and AIDS clients than in healthy subjects due to hypochlorhydria. However, the bioavailability of the oral solution in AIDS clients is not different from healthy subjects.
7. Protect capsules from light and moisture. Do not freeze the oral solution; discard any unused oral solution 3 months after opening.

ASSESSMENT

1. Note reasons for therapy, location, onset, characteristics of S&S, clinical presentation, other agents prescribed, and compliance/outcome. Drug is extremely expensive and should not be used as first-line therapy with typical fungal infections.
2. Assess for ventricular dysfunction/CHF; precludes therapy. Obtain ECG and note QT prolongation.
3. Due to possibility of liver failure, confirm diagnosis of onychomycosis through scrapings/lab tests. If symptoms of CHF develop, stop drug.
4. List drugs currently prescribed to prevent any unfavorable effects. Note any previous liver dysfunction with any other therapy; precludes drug therapy.
5. Drug is not intended for pregnant or nursing mothers.

6. The response rate of histoplasmosis in HIV-infected clients is similar to non-HIV-infected clients, although the clinical course in HIV-infected clients is more severe and usually requires maintenance therapy to prevent relapse.
7. Absorption may be decreased in HIV-infected clients with hypochlorhydria.
8. Monitor CBC, electrolytes, fungal cultures/scrapings, renal and LFTs. Stop therapy if S&S of hepatotoxicity occur; do not reinstitute therapy.

CLIENT/FAMILY TEACHING

1. Take capsules with food to enhance absorption and only as directed (usually for 3 months). Do not take the oral solution with food; take on empty stomach to enhance absorption. Swish oral solution in mouth vigorously for 10 seconds and then swallow. Noncompliance or inadequate treatment period may lead to recurrence of active infection. Oral solution and capsules are not interchangeable.
2. Take capsules with 8 oz of a cola beverage in those HIV-infected or if taking gastric acid suppressive therapy (e.g., H_2-receptor antagonist, proton pump inhibitor) or with achlorhydria.
3. The Sporanox PulsePak comes with special instructions and contains 7 pouches—one for each day of treatment. Inside each pouch is a card containing 4 capsules. On the back of the card, fold along the dashed line and peel away the backing so that you can remove 2 capsules. Take 2 capsules in a.m. and 2 capsules in the p.m. for next 7 days. You rest for 3 weeks and then before end of week 4 obtain script for another PulsePak to take as the first to treat fungal infection.
4. Administer antacids at least 1 hr before or 2 hr after taking itraconazole capsules.
5. Practice reliable hygiene measures to prevent spread of infection and reinfection.
6. Avoid activities requiring mental alertness until drug effects realized; may cause drowsiness.
7. Stop drug and report S&S suggesting liver dysfunction; appetite loss, unusual fatigue, N&V, diarrhea, yellow skin/eyes, or dark urine. Avoid alcohol during therapy.
8. Report symptoms that may indicate reactivation of histoplasmosis, such as weight loss, chest pain, SOB, fever, crackles, and pain.
9. S&S of blastomycosis include SOB, rales, hemoptysis, chest pain, fever, cough, skin lesions, rashes, and weight loss; requires immediate attention.
10. Avoid alcohol and OTC agents without provider approval.
11. With fingernail fungus, treatment is usually twice a day for 1 week, rest for 3 weeks and then another course for 1 week. Toenails consists of 200 mg daily for 12 weeks. Usually takes about 6 months to grow a new fingernail and up to 12 months to grow a new toenail so immediate improvement may not be evident.
12. Women should use effective contraceptive measures during treatment and for 2 months following discontinuation of therapy.
13. Report hearing loss or numbness in hands or feet.
14. Keep all F/U to assess response, labs, and for adverse SE.

OUTCOMES/EVALUATE

- Treatment of blastomycosis/histoplasmosis/aspergillosis
- Eradication of infecting organisms with onychomycosis

IV

Ixabepilone

(ix-ab-**EP**-i-lone)

Classification(s): Antineoplastic agent, antimitotic (epothilone)

Pregnancy Category: D

RX: Ixempra.

SEE ALSO ***ANTINEOPLASTIC AGENTS.***

INDICATIONS/USES

(1) In combination with capecitabine to treat metastatic or locally advanced breast cancer resistant to treatment with an anthracycline or a taxane, or in those whose cancer is taxane-resistant and for whom further anthracycline therapy is contraindicated. (2) As monotherapy to treat metastatic or locally advanced breast cancer in clients whose tumors are resistant or refractory to anthracyclines, taxanes, and capecitabine.

ACTION/KINETICS

Action

Ixabepilone binds directly to β-tubulin subunits on microtubules, leading to suppression of microtubule dynamics. The drug blocks cells in the mitotic phase of the cell division cycle, leading to cell death.

Pharmacokinetics

Maximum plasma levels: 3 hr. Extensively metabolized in the liver by CYP3A4. Eliminated primarily as metabolites in the feces (65%) and urine (21%). **$t^{1/2}$, elimination:** 52 hr.

CONTRAINDICATIONS

In those with a history of severe (CTC grade 3/4) hypersensitivity reaction to drugs containing polyoxyethylated castor oil. Clients who have neutrophil counts less than 1,500 cells/mm^3 or a platelet count less than 100,000 cells/mm^3. In combination with capecitabine in those with AST or ALT greater than 2.5 times ULN or bilirubin greater than 1 times ULN. Lactation.

SPECIAL CONCERNS

■ Ixabepilone in combination with capecitabine is contraindicated in clients with AST or ALT greater than 2.5 times ULN or bilirubin greater than 1 times ULN because of an increased risk of toxicity and neutropenia-related death. ■

- Use caution in those with a history of cardiac disease.
- Incidence of toxicity higher in the elderly.
- Safety and efficacy not determined in children.

SIDE EFFECTS

Most Common

Alopecia, diarrhea, fatigue/asthenia, musculoskeletal pain, myalgia, arthralgia, peripheral neuropathy, stomatitis, mucositis, N&V, palmar-plantar erythrodysesthesia syndrome, nail disorder, hematologic abnormalities.

Side effects listed are for monotherapy as well as therapy combined with capecitabine. **GI:** Diarrhea, stomatitis, anorexia, mucositis, N&V, abdominal pain, constipation, GERD, taste disorder, colitis, dysphagia, enterocolitis, esophagitis, gastritis, ***GI hemorrhage***, ileus, impaired gastric emptying. **Hepatic:** ***Acute hepatic failure***, jaundice. **CNS:** Neuropathy (burning sensation, hyper-/hypoesthesia, paresthesia, discomfort, neuropathic pain), motor neuropathy, insomnia, dizziness, headache, abnormal coordination, ***cerebral hemorrhage***, cognitive disorder, lethargy, syncope. **Dermatologic:** Palmar-plantar erythrodysesthesia syndrome, alopecia, nail disorder, skin hyperpigmentation, skin exfoliation, pruritus, erythema multiforme. **Hematologic:** Anemia, leukopenia, thrombocytopenia, neutropenia, febrile neutropenia, coagulopathy, lymphopenia, neutropenic infection. **CV:** Hot flush, angina pectoris, atrial flutter, ***cardiomyopathy***, ***embolism***, ***hemorrhage***, hypotension, hypovolemic shock, left ventricular dysfunction, ***MI***, myocardial ischemia, supraventricular tachycardia, ***thrombosis***, vasculitis. **Musculoskeletal:** Myalgia, arthralgia, musculoskeletal pain, chest pain, muscle spasms, muscle weakness, trismus. **Respiratory:** Dyspnea, cough, URTI, acute pulmonary edema, dysphonia, hypoxia, laryngitis, lower RTI, pharyngolaryngeal pain, pneumonia, pneumonitis, ***respiratory failure***. **GU:** UTI, nephrolithiasis, renal failure. **Metabolic/Nutritional:** Decreased weight, dehydration. **Ophthalmic:** Increased lacrimation. **Body as a whole:** Fatigue, asthenia, edema, hypersensitivity reactions, pain, pyrexia, bacterial infection, chills, infection, ***sepsis***.

LABORATORY TEST CONSIDERATIONS

↑ Blood alkaline phosphatase, GGT, ALT, AST. Hypokalemia, hyponatremia, hypovolemia, metabolic acidosis.

DRUG INTERACTIONS

Azole antifungals (e.g., fluconazole, itraconazole, ketoconazole, voriconazole) / ↑ Ixabepilone levels R/T inhibition of CYP3A4; if alternative treatment not possible, consider dosage adjustment

Carbamazepine / ↓ Ixabepilone levels R/T induction of CYP3A4 → subtherapeutic levels

Delavirdine / ↑ Ixabepilone levels R/T inhibition of CYP3A4; avoid coadministration

Dexamethasone / ↓ Ixabepilone levels R/T induction of CYP3A4 → subtherapeutic levels

Grapefruit juice / ↑ Ixabepilone plasma levels; do not use together

Macrolide antibiotics (e.g., clarithromycin, erythromycin) / ↑ Ixabepilone levels R/T inhibition of CYP3A4; avoid coadministration

Nefazodone / ↑ Ixabepilone levels R/T inhibition of CYP3A4; avoid coadministration

Phenobarbital / ↓ Ixabepilone levels R/T induction of CYP3A4 → subtherapeutic levels

Phenytoin / ↓ Ixabepilone levels R/T induction of CYP3A4 → subtherapeutic levels
Protease inhibitors (e.g., amprenavir, atazanavir, indinavir, nelfinavir, ritonavir, saquinavir) / ↑ Ixabepilone levels R/T inhibition of CYP3A4; avoid coadministration
Rifamycins (e.g., rifabutin, rifamycin, rifampin) / ↓ Ixabepilone levels R/T induction of CYP3A4 → subtherapeutic levels
H ***St. John's wort*** / ↓ Ixabepilone levels unpredictably; avoid concomitant use
Telithromycin / ↑ Ixabepilone levels R/T inhibition of CYP3A4; avoid coadministration
Verapamil / ↑ Ixabepilone levels R/T inhibition of CYP3A4; use together with caution and monitor closely for toxicity

HOW SUPPLIED

Injection, Lyophilized Powder for Injection, Concentrate: 15 mg, 45 mg.

DOSAGE

IV ONLY

Breast cancer.

40 mg/m^2 given over 3 hr q 3 weeks. Doses for those with body surface area greater than 2.2 m^2 should be calculated based on 2.2 m^2.

NURSING IMPLICATIONS

IMPLEMENTATION/ADMINISTRATION/STORAGE

1. **IV** Premedicate clients with both an H_1- and H_2-antagonist about 1 hr before ixabepilone infusion and observe for hypersensitivity reactions. In cases of severe hypersensitivity reactions, stop the infusion and begin aggressive supportive treatment (e.g., epinephrine, corticosteroids).
2. The ixabepilone kit contains 2 vials—one labeled ixabepilone for injection that contains the drug and the other containing the diluent (use only this diluent to reconstitute). Before reconstituting, allow the kit to stand at room temperature for about 30 min. Each kit is for single use only.
3. To allow for withdrawal losses, the vial labeled 15 mg for injection contains 16 mg and the vial labeled 45 mg for injection contains 47 mg.
4. To reconstitute, aseptically withdraw the diluent with a suitable syringe and slowly inject it into the ixabepilone for injection vial. The 15 mg kit contains 8 mL of the diluent and the 45 mg kit contains 23.5 mL of the diluent. Gently swirl and invert the vial until the powder is completely dissolved. After reconstituting with the diluent, the concentration of ixabepilone is 2 mg/mL.
5. Before administration, the reconstituted solution must be further diluted only with Ringer's lactate injection, supplied in di-(2-ethylhexyl) phthalate-free bags. For most doses, a 250 mL bag of Ringer's lactate is sufficient. The final concentration of the diluted solution for infusion must be between 0.2 and 0.6 mg/mL. To calculate the final infusion concentration, use the following formulas:
   - Total infusion volume = mL of reconstituted solution + mL of Ringer's lactate injection
6. Administer the infusion solution through an appropriate inline filter with a microporous membrane of 0.2–1.3 microns. Discard any remaining solution. Administration of diluted ixabepilone must be completed within 6 hr.
7. To minimize the risk of dermal exposure, wear impervious gloves when handling vials containing ixabepilone.
8. Evaluate all clients receiving ixabepilone for toxicity and delay treatment to allow recovery. The following are dosage adjustments for monotherapy and combination therapy:
   - Decrease the dose by 20% in the event of grade 2 neuropathy (moderate) lasting 7 or more days.
   - Decrease the dose by 20% in the event of grade 2 neuropathy (severe) lasting less than 7 days.
   - Discontinue treatment in the event of grade 2 neuropathy (severe) lasting 7 or more days or disabling neuropathy.
   - Decrease dose by 20% for any grade 3 toxicity (severe) other than neuropathy.
   - No change in the dose of ixabepilone is needed in the event of transient grade 3 arthralgia/myalgia or fatigue or for grade 3 hand-foot syndrome (palmar-plantar erythrodysesthesia).
   - Discontinue treatment for any grade 4 toxicity (disabling).

- Decrease the dose by 20% if neutrophils are <500 cells/mm^3 for 7 or more days.
- Decrease the dose by 20% in the event of febrile neutropenia.
- Decrease the dose by 20% if platelets are <25,000/mm^3 or platelets are <50,000/mm^3 with bleeding.
- *NOTE:* If toxicities recur, reduce the dose by an additional 20%.

9. Dosage adjustment for capecitabine when used in combination with ixabepilone.
   - For nonhematologic toxicity, follow the guidelines on the capecitabine label.
   - If platelets are <25,000/mm^3 or <50,000/mm^3 with bleeding, hold for concurrent diarrhea or stomatitis until platelet count is >50,000/mm^3; then continue at the same dose.
   - If neutrophils are <500 cells/mm^3 for 7 days or longer or if febrile neutropenia, hold for concurrent diarrhea or stomatitis until neutrophil count is >1,000 cells/mm^3; then continue at the same dose.
10. Clients should not begin a new cycle of treatment unless the neutrophil count is at least 1,500 cells/mm^3, the platelet count is at least 100,000 cells/mm^3, and nonhematologic toxicities have improved to grade 1 (mild) or resolved.
11. All clients must be premedicated with a H_1-antagonist (e.g., diphenhydramine, 50 mg PO or equivalent) and a H_2-antagonist (e.g., ranitidine, 150–300 mg PO or equivalent) about 1 hr before the ixabepilone infusion begins. Those who experienced a hypersensitivity reaction required premedication with corticosteroids (e.g., dexamethasone, 20 mg IV 30 min before the infusion or PO 60 min before the infusion) in addition to pretreatment with H_1- and H_2-antagonists.
12. If a strong CYP3A4 inhibitor (see *Drug Interactions*) is required, reduce the dose of ixabepilone by 20 mg/m^2. If the strong inhibitor is discontinued, allow a washout period of about 1 week before the ixabepilone dose is adjusted upward to the indicated dose.
13. Store the ixabepilone kit from 2–8°C (36–46°F) in the original package to protect from light.
14. COMPATIBILITY LR, 0.9% NaCl (pH adjusted to between 6.0 and 9.0 by adding sodium bicarbonate), PLASMA-LYTE A Injection pH 7.4. Use in-line filter with a microporous membrane of 0.2–1.2 microns. DEHP-free infusion containers and administration sets must be used.
15. INCOMPATIBILITY Administer separately.

ASSESSMENT

1. Note reasons for therapy, clinical presentation, breast cancer staging and when therapy with anthracycline and taxane trialed and outcome. If resistance then usually administered in combination with capecitabine.
2. List all drugs prescribed to ensure none interact.
3. Perform clinical examination and identify findings. Identify any liver or heart disease; precludes therapy.
4. Assess for any allergy to taxol or castor oil and any evidence of neuropathy.
5. Obtain baseline CBC, renal and LFTs; monitor during therapy. If abnormal, adjust dosage as outlined in administration.

CLIENT/FAMILY TEACHING

1. Drug is generally given IV over 3 hrs every 3 weeks along with the medicine capecitabine. Will be premedicated 1 hr before infusion with Benadryl and Zantac to help prevent allergic reactions.
2. Infusion contains alcohol. Avoid activities that require mental alertness (i.e., driving or operating machinery) as dizziness or drowsiness may occur.
3. Do not drink grapefruit juice while receiving ixabepilone; may cause increased blood levels of ixabepilone and increase adverse side effects.
4. Report any numbness and tingling of extremities, fever over 38°C (100.5°F) or chills, cough, burning or pain on urination. If itching, rash, hives, flushing, swelling, difficulty breathing, chest tightness, palpitations, or other allergic reactions occur report immediately.
5. Use reliable contraception to prevent pregnancy and avoid nursing.
6. Any pain, difficulty breathing, palpitations or unusual weight gain should be evaluated.
7. Keep all F/U to assess response, labs, and for adverse SE.

OUTCOMES/EVALUATE

Tumor regression with metastatic breast cancer

K

Ketoconazole

(kee-toe-**KON**-ah-zohl)

Classification(s): Antifungal

Pregnancy Category: C

OTC: Nizoral, Nizoral A-D.

RX: Extina, Ketoconazole Cream, Shampoo, and Tablets, Kuric, Nizoral, Xolegel.

🍁 **Rx:** Apo-Ketoconazole, Ketoderm.

SEE ALSO ***ANTI-INFECTIVE DRUGS.***

INDICATIONS/USES

PO: (1) Candidiasis, chronic mucocutaneous candidiasis, candiduria, histoplasmosis, chromomycosis, oral thrush, blastomycosis, coccidioidomycosis, paracoccidioidomycosis. (2) Recalcitrant cutaneous dermatophyte infections not responding to other therapy. *Investigational:* Onychomycosis due to *Trichophyton* and *Candida.* CNS fungal infections (high doses). Cushing's syndrome.

Cream: (1) Tinea pedis (athlete's foot), tinea corporis (ringworm), and tinea cruris (jock itch) due to *Trichophyton rubrum, T. mentagrophytes,* and *Epidermophyton floccosum.* (2) Tinea versicolor (pityriasis) caused by *Pityrosporum orbiculare.* (3) Cutaneous candidiasis caused by *Candida* sp. (4) Seborrheic dermatitis.

Foam/Gel: Seborrheic dermatitis in immunocompetent adults and children 12 years and older. Safety and efficacy to treat fungal infections have not been established.

Shampoo, 1%: Reduce scaling, flaking, and itching due to dandruff.

Shampoo, 2%: Tinea versicolor due to or presumed to be due to *P. orbiculare.*

ACTION/KINETICS

Action

Inhibits synthesis of ergosterol (the main sterol of fungal cell membranes), damaging the cell membrane and resulting in loss of essential intracellular material. Also inhibits biosynthesis of triglycerides and phospholipids and inhibits oxidative and peroxidative enzyme activity. When used to treat *Candida albicans,* it inhibits transformation of blastospores into the invasive mycelial form. Inhibits growth of *Pityrosporum ovale* when used to treat dandruff. Use in Cushing's syndrome is due to its ability to inhibit adrenal steroidogenesis.

Pharmacokinetics

After PO use: Peak plasma levels: 3.5 mcg/mL 1–2 hr after a 200 mg dose. **t½, biphasic:** first, 2 hr; second, 8 hr. Requires acidity for dissolution. Metabolized in liver to inactive metabolites and most excreted through feces. Very little ketaconazole is absorbed after topical use of the cream, foam, gel, or shampoos.

CONTRAINDICATIONS

Hypersensitivity to ketaconazole or any component of the products. Fungal meningitis. Topical products are not for ophthalmic, PO, or intravaginal use. Lactation.

SPECIAL CONCERNS

■ PO ketoconazole has been associated with hepatic toxicity, including some fatalities. Closely monitor clients and inform them of the risk. ■

- **Use tablets with caution in children less than 2 years of age.**
- **Safety and efficacy of the cream not determined in children.**
- **Safety and efficacy of the foam, gel, and 2% shampoo not established in children younger than 12 years.**

SIDE EFFECTS

Most Common

Systemic use: N&V, abdominal pain, pruritus.
Topical use: Stinging, irritation, pruritus. Also, see the following for individual products.

Tablets. GI: N&V, abdominal pain, diarrhea, hepatotoxicity (including fatalities). **CNS:** Headache, dizziness, somnolence, fever, chills, suicidal tendencies, depression (rare). **Hematologic:** Thrombocytopenia, leukopenia, ***hemolytic anemia.*** **Miscellaneous:** Hepatotoxicity, photophobia, pruritus, gynecomastia, impotence, bulging fontanelles, urticaria, decreased serum testosterone levels, anaphylaxis (rare).

Topical cream. Stinging, irritation (may be severe), pruritus, contact dermatitis. Sulfites in the cream may cause allergic reactions, including anaphylactic symptoms and life-threatening or less severe asthmatic symptoms in susceptible individuals.

Topical foam. Application site burning or other reaction, contact sensitization.

Topical gel. Dermatologic: Application site burning, dermatitis, discharge, dryness, erythema, irritation, pain, pruritus, pustules, acne, facial swelling, impetigo, keratoconjunctivitis sicca, nail discoloration, pyogenic granuloma. **CNS:** Headache, dizziness, paresthesia. **Ophthalmic:** Eye irritation/swelling.

Shampoo, 1%. Increased or abnormal hair loss; mild irritation or stinging; itching; oiliness or dryness of the scalp and hair; scalp pustules; hair discoloration (rare); reddening, blistering, peeling, itching, or burning of the skin.

Shampoo, 2%. Application site reaction, dry skin, pruritus, increase in normal hair loss, irritation, abnormal hair texture, itching, mild dryness of the skin, oiliness or dryness of the hair and scalp, scalp pustules, hair discoloration (rare).

NOTE: Any of the topical products may cause hypersensitivity, including photoallergenicity.

LABORATORY TEST CONSIDERATIONS

Transient ↑ serum liver enzymes. ↓ Serum testosterone.

DRUG INTERACTIONS

Acyclovir / ↑ or synergistic antiviral effects
Almotriptan / ↑ AUC and plasma levels of almotriptan R/T ketoconazole inhibition of gut wall and hepatic first-pass metabolism of almotriptan
Antacids / ↓ Absorption of ketoconazole R/T ↑ pH
Anticoagulants / ↑ Anticoagulant effect
Benzodiazepines / Prolonged levels → ↑ CNS depression and psychomotor impairment
Buspirone / ↑ Buspirone levels
Carbamazepine / ↑ Carbamazepine levels
Corticosteroids / ↑ Risk of drug toxicity R/T ↑ bioavailability
Cyclosporine / ↑ Cyclosporine levels (ketaconazole may be used therapeutically to decrease cyclosporine dose) R/T inhibition of metabolism
Didanosinse / ↓ Ketoconazole effect R/T ↓ absorption
Docetaxel / ↓ Docetaxel clearance R/T ↓ metabolism by CYP3A4
Donepezil / ↑ Levels of donepezil R/T ↓ liver metabolism
Histamine H_2 antagonists / ↓ Ketoconazole absorption R/T ↑ gastric pH
Isoniazid / ↓ Bioavailability of ketoconazole
Nisoldipine / ↑ Nisoldipine levels R/T ↓ liver metabolism
Oral contraceptives / Possible ↓ effect of contraceptive
Protease inhibitors (Indinavir, Ritonavir, Saquinavir) / ↑ Levels of protease inhibitor
Proton pump inhibitors / ↓ Ketoconazole effect R/T ↓ bioavailability
Quinidine / ↑ Quinidine levels
Rifampin / ↓ Levels of either drug
Rosiglitazone / ↑ Rosiglitazone AUC and peak plasma levels and prolonged t½ R/T inhibition of CYP2C8 and CYP2C9
Sucralfate / ↓ Ketoconazole effect R/T ↓ bioavailability
Sulfonylureas / ↑ Hypoglycemic effect R/T ↑ serum levels
Theophyllines / ↓ Serum theophylline levels R/T ↓ absorption
Tolterodine / ↑ Tolterodine t½ and AUC in those deficient in CYP2D6 enzymes
Tricyclic antidepressants / ↑ TCA levels
Valacyclovir / ↑ or synergistic antiviral effects
Vinca alkaloids / ↑ Risk of vinca toxicity R/T inhibition of metabolism
Zolpidem / ↑ Half-life of zolpidem R/T ↓ liver metabolism

HOW SUPPLIED

Cream, Topical (Rx): 2%; ***Foam, Topical (Rx):*** 2%; ***Gel, Topical (Rx):*** 2%; ***Shampoo:*** 1% (OTC), 2% (Rx); ***Tablets (Rx):*** 200 mg.

DOSAGE

TABLETS

Fungal infections.

Adults: 200 mg once daily; in serious infections or if response is not sufficient, increase to 400 mg once daily.

Pediatric, over 2 years: 3.3–6.6 mg/kg once daily. Dosage has not been established for children less than 2 years of age.

K

CNS fungal infections.

Adults: 800–1,200 mg/day.

Cushing's syndrome.

800–1,200 mg/day.

CREAM, TOPICAL

Tinea corporis, tinea cruris, tinea versicolor, tinea pedis, cutaneous candidiasis.

Cover the affected and immediate surrounding areas once daily (twice daily for more resistant cases). Duration of treatment is usually 2 weeks for tinea versicolor and 6 weeks for tinea pedis.

Seborrheic dermatitis.

Apply to affected area twice a day for 4 weeks or until clinical clearing. If there is no improvement after the treatment period, re-evaluate the diagnosis.

FOAM

Seborrheic dermatitis.

Apply to the affected area twice daily for 4 weeks.

GEL, TOPICAL

Seborrheic dermatitis.

Apply once daily to affected area for 2 weeks.

SHAMPOO, 1%

Reduction of scaling due to dandruff.

Apply sufficient shampoo to produce enough lather to wash scalp and hair and gently massage it over the entire scalp area for about 1 minute. Rinse hair thoroughly with warm water and repeat leaving shampoo on the scalp for an additional 3 minutes. Repeat use q 3–4 days for up to 8 weeks or as directed by the provider. Then, use only as needed to control dandruff.

SHAMPOO, 2%

Tinea versicolor.

Apply shampoo to the damp skin of the affected area and a wide margin surrounding this area. Lather, leave in place for 5 minutes. Then, rinse off with water. One application of the shampoo should be sufficient to treat the condition.

NURSING IMPLICATIONS

IMPLEMENTATION/ADMINISTRATION/STORAGE

1. Give a minimum of 2 hr before administration of drugs that increase gastric pH (such as antacids, anticholinergics, or H_2 blockers).
2. The minimum treatment for candidiasis (using tablets) is 1–2 weeks; for other systemic mycoses 6 months. The minimum treatment for recalcitrant dermatophyte infections is 4 weeks in cases involving glabrous skin; palmar and plantar infections may respond more slowly.
3. Store cream from 20–25°C (66–77°F). Do not store above 25°C (77°F).
4. Store foam from 20–25°C (66–77°F). Do not refrigerate or expose containers to heat and/or storage above 49°C (120°F). Do not store in direct sunlight. Contents are flammable and under pressure. Do not puncture and/or incinerate the container.
5. Store gel from 15–30°C (59–86°F). Protect from light and freezing.
6. Store the 1% shampoo from 2–30°C (35–85°F); protect from light and freezing. Do not store the 2% shampoo above 25°C (77°F); protect from light.

ASSESSMENT

1. Note reasons for therapy, onset, characteristics of S&S, clinical presentation, other agents trialed, outcome.
2. List all drugs/agents prescribed to ensure none interact.
3. With lack of stomach acid, may dissolve each tablet in 4 mL aqueous solution of 0.2 N HCl; use a straw to avoid contact with teeth. Follow by drinking a full glass of water.
4. Monitor LFTs before/during therapy. Assess skin integrity and note any complications with therapy.

CLIENT/FAMILY TEACHING

1. Take tablets with food to decrease GI upset. Take 2 hr before drugs (antacids) that change gastric pH. Water, fruit juice, coffee, or tea provides an acid medium for dissolution and absorption.
2. Apply shampoo to wet hair in sufficient quantities to cover the entire scalp for 1 min. Rinse with warm water; repeat, leaving shampoo on the scalp for 3 min. After the second washing, rinse thoroughly and dry hair with towel or warm air flow. Use twice a week for 4 weeks with at least 3 days between treatments.
3. With topical product, avoid contact with eyes, nostrils, and mouth; wash hands after application and report if any severe itching, irritation, or stinging occurs after application.

4. To administer foam:
   - Hold container upright, dispense into cap of the can or other cool surface in an amount sufficient to cover affected area(s).
   - Do not dispense directly onto hands as foam will begin to melt immediately upon contact with warm skin.
   - Pick up small amounts of foam with fingertips; gently massage into affected area(s) until foam disappears.
   - For hair-bearing areas, part hair and apply foam directly to the skin.
   - Avoid contact with eyes and/or mucous membranes.
5. Report persistent fever, pain, rash, lack of clearing or worsening of condition, severe N&V, unusual bruising/bleeding, yellow skin or eyes, dark urine, pale stools, or diarrhea.
6. Use caution when driving or performing hazardous tasks; tablets may cause headaches, dizziness, and drowsiness. Avoid all forms of alcohol. Report adverse effects or lack of response.
7. Wear sunglasses, sunscreen, and protective clothing to prevent photosensitivity reactions.
8. Complete the full course of therapy. Long-term therapy is needed and beneficial effects may not be evident for several weeks. Interruption of therapy may cause recurrence of infection.
9. Keep all F/U to assess response, labs, and for adverse SE.

OUTCOMES/EVALUATE

- Eradication of fungal infections
- Clearing of skin lesions
- Control of dandruff with ↓ scaling

Ketoprofen

(kee-toe-**PROH**-fen)

Classification(s): Nonsteroidal anti-inflammatory drug

Pregnancy Category: B

🍁 **Rx:** Apo-Keto, Apo-Keto-E, Apo-Keto-SR.

SEE ALSO ***NONSTEROIDAL ANTI-INFLAMMATORY DRUGS.***

INDICATIONS/USES

(1) Management of the signs and symptoms of rheumatoid arthritis and osteoarthritis (both immediate-release and sustained-release capsules). (2) Primary dysmenorrhea (immediate-release capsules only). (3) Analgesic for mild to moderate pain (immediate-release capsule only). *Investigational:* Juvenile idiopathic arthritis.

ACTION/KINETICS

Action

Possesses anti-inflammatory, antipyretic, and analgesic properties. Known to inhibit both prostaglandin and leukotriene synthesis, to have antibradykinin activity, and to stabilize lysosomal membranes.

Pharmacokinetics

Onset: 15–30 min. **Peak plasma levels:** 0.5–2 hr. **Duration:** 4–6 hr. **t½:** 2–4 hr. **t½, geriatrics:** Approximately 5 hr. For Ketoprofen ER: **Peak:** 6–7 hr; **t½:** 5.4 hr. Food does not alter the bioavailability; however, the rate of absorption is reduced. **Plasma protein binding:** 99%.

CONTRAINDICATIONS

Use during late pregnancy, in children, and during lactation. Use of the extended-release product for acute pain in any client or for initial therapy in clients who are small, elderly, or who have renal or hepatic impairment.

SPECIAL CONCERNS

(1) **Cardiovascular risk.** NSAIDs may cause an increased risk of serious CV thrombotic events, MI, and stroke, which can be fatal. This risk may increase with duration of use. Clients with CV disease or risk factors for CV disease may be at greater risk. (2) NSAIDs are contraindicated for the treatment of perioperative pain in the setting of coronary artery bypass graft surgery. (3) **GI risk.** NSAIDs can cause an increased risk of serious GI adverse reactions, including bleeding, ulceration, and perforation of the stomach or intestines, which can be fatal. These reactions can occur at any time during use and without warning symptoms. Elderly clients are at great risk for serious GI reactions.

- Use caution in clients with a history of GI tract disorders, in fluid retention, hypertension, and heart failure.

- **Geriatric clients may manifest increased and prolonged serum levels due to decreased protein binding and clearance.**
- **Safety and effectiveness not established in children.**

SIDE EFFECTS

Most Common

Abdominal pain/cramps, diarrhea, N&V, constipation, flatulence, dyspepsia/indigestion, headache, CNS depression or excitation, impaired renal function, edema.

See *Nonsteroidal Anti-Inflammatory Drugs* for a complete list of possible side effects. Also, **GI:** Peptic ulcer, ***GI bleeding***, dyspepsia, nausea, diarrhea, constipation, abdominal pain, flatulence, anorexia, vomiting, stomatitis. **CNS:** Headache. **CV:** Peripheral edema, fluid retention.

ADDITIONAL DRUG INTERACTIONS

Acetylsalicylic acid / ↑ Plasma ketoprofen levels R/T ↓ plasma protein binding
Hydrochlorothiazide / ↓ Chloride and potassium excretion
Methotrexate / Concomitant use → toxic plasma levels of methotrexate
Probenecid / ↓ Plasma clearance of ketoprofen and ↓ plasma protein binding
Warfarin / Additive effect to cause bleeding

HOW SUPPLIED

Capsules, Extended-Release: 100 mg, 150 mg, 200 mg; ***Capsules, Immediate-Release:*** 50 mg, 75 mg.

DOSAGE

CAPSULES, EXTENDED-RELEASE; CAPSULES, IMMEDIATE-RELEASE

Rheumatoid arthritis, osteoarthritis.

Adults, initial: 75 mg 3 times per day or 50 mg 4 times per day for immediate release; for extended-release, 200 mg once a day. Doses above 300 mg/day for the immediate-release or 200 mg/day for the extended-release are not recommended.

CAPSULES, IMMEDIATE-RELEASE ONLY

Mild to moderate pain, dysmenorrhea.

Adults: 25–50 mg q 6–8 hr as required, not to exceed 300 mg/day. Reduce dose in smaller or geriatric clients and in those with liver or renal dysfunction. Doses greater than 75 mg do not provide any added therapeutic effect.

NURSING IMPLICATIONS

IMPLEMENTATION/ADMINISTRATION/STORAGE

1. **Use lower initial doses in smaller clients.**
2. **The maximum recommended daily dose in those with mild renal impairment is 150 mg. In those with a more severe renal impairment (C_{CR} <25 mL/min/1.73 m^2 or end-stage renal impairment) the maximum recommended daily dose is 100 mg.**
3. **Reduce initial dose of both immediate-release and extended-release capsules in elderly clients (>75 years old).**
4. **The maximum daily dose should be 100 mg in clients with impaired liver function and serum albumin levels <3.5 grams/L. If good tolerance is demonstrated, the dose may be increased to the recommended dosage for the general population.**
5. **Store from 15–30°C (59–86°F). Protect from direct light and excessive heat and humidity.**

ASSESSMENT

1. **List reasons for therapy, type, onset, location, ADL/pain level, ROM/physical limitations, symptom characteristics.**
2. **Note history of GI disorders/bleeding, cardiac failure, hypertension, or edema.**
3. **With cardiac disease determine risk factors; advise increased risk of thrombotic events, MI, and stroke, which can be fatal with prolonged use.**
4. **Determine if pregnant. Not for children under age 12.**
5. **Monitor CBC, renal and LFTs. In high doses, may prolong bleeding times by decreasing platelet aggregation. Reduce dose/stop with liver/renal dysfunction/GI bleeding; consider adding H_2 blocker.**

CLIENT/FAMILY TEACHING

1. **GI side effects may be minimized by taking with antacids, milk, or food. Swallow capsule whole, do not chew or crush.**
2. **Use caution; may cause dizziness and drowsiness. Review risks of prolonged therapy.**

3. Avoid alcohol; may increase risk for GI bleed. Report adverse effects or lack of response.
4. Do not take any OTC agents or aspirin products unless specifically prescribed/approved.
5. Report any new symptoms such as rash, headaches, black stools, disturbances in vision, unexplained bruising, or bleeding from the gums or nose.
6. Report any S&S of liver dysfunction such as fatigue, upper right quadrant pain, clay-colored stools, or yellowing of the skin and eyes.
7. Avoid prolonged sun exposure; use protection if exposed.
8. Keep all F/U to assess response, labs (CBC, renal and LFTS), and for adverse SE.

OUTCOMES/EVALUATE

- ↓ Joint pain/swelling; ↑ mobility
- ↓ Uterine cramping
- ↓ Pain ↓ fever

■ IV

Ketorolac tromethamine

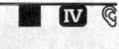

(kee-toh-**ROH**-lack)

Classification(s): Nonsteroidal anti-inflammatory drug

Pregnancy Category: C

RX: Acular, Acular LS, Acuvail, Sprix.

♣ **Rx:** Apo-Ketorolac, Apo-Ketorolac Ophthalmic Solution, ratio-Ketorolac, Toradol IM.

SEE ALSO ***NONSTEROIDAL ANTI-INFLAMMATORY DRUGS.***

INDICATIONS/USES

PO: Short-term (up to 5 days) management of severe, acute pain in adults who require analgesia at the opiate level, usually in a postoperative setting. Always initiate therapy with IV or IM followed by PO only as continuation treatment, if necessary. The combination of ketorolac tromethamine IV/IM and ketorolac tromethamine oral is not to exceed 5 days due to the potential of increased frequency and severity of side effects. Switch clients to alternative analgesics as soon as possible.

IM/IV: (1) In adults, as a single- or multiple-dose regimen on a regular or as needed schedule for the management of moderately severe acute pain that requires analgesia at the opioid level, usually in a postoperative setting. Switch to alternative analgesics as soon as possible, but no later than after 5 days. (2) In pediatric clients between 2 and 16 years of age as a single injection for the management of moderately severe acute pain that requires analgesia at the opioid level, usually postoperatively. *Investigational:* IV or IM to treat migraine headaches in adults.

Ophthalmic, Acular (0.5%): (1) Relieve itching caused by seasonal allergic conjunctivitis. (2) Postoperative inflammation following cataract surgery.

Ophthalmic, Acular LS (0.4%): Reduce ocular pain, burning, and stinging after corneal refractive surgery.

Ophthalmic, Acuvail (0.45%, preservative free): Treatment of pain and inflammation after cataract surgery.

Spray, Nasal: Short-term treatment (up to 5 days) of acute to moderate to moderately severe pain that requires analgesia at the opioid level.

K

ACTION/KINETICS

Action

Possesses anti-inflammatory, analgesic, and antipyretic effects.

Pharmacokinetics

Completely absorbed following IM use. **Onset:** Within 30 min after IM or IV. **Maximum effect:** 1–2 hr after IV or IM dosing. **Duration:** 4–6 hr after IM or IV. **Peak plasma levels:** 2.2–3.0 mcg/mL 50 min after a dose of 30 mg. **t½, terminal:** 3.8–6.3 hr in young adults and 4.7–8.6 hr in geriatric clients. Nasal spray is rapidly absorbed reaching peak blood levels as rapidly as IM administration. Metabolized in the liver with over 90% excreted in the urine and the remainder excreted in the feces. **Plasma protein binding:** More than 99%.

CONTRAINDICATIONS

Hypersensitivity to the drug or allergic symptoms (angioedema, bronchospasm) to aspirin or other NSAIDs. Active peptic ulcer disease, recent GI bleeding or perforation, history of peptic ulcer disease or GI bleeding. Advanced renal impairment and in those at risk for renal failure due to volume depletion. Suspected or confirmed cerebrovascular bleeding, hemorrhagic diathesis, or incomplete hemostasis and in those with a high risk of bleeding. As prophylactic analgesic before any major surgery or intraoperatively when hemostasis is critical (due to increased risk of bleeding). Intrathecal or epidural administration (due to alcohol content of product). Use of injection/tablets in labor, delivery, or during lactation. Use with aspirin or other NSAIDs. Use of the ophthalmic solution in clients wearing soft contact lenses.

SPECIAL CONCERNS

■ **PO, IM, or IV use.** (1) Indicated for the short-term (up to 5 days in adults) management of moderately severe acute pain that requires analgesia at the opioid level. It is not indicated for minor or chronic painful conditions. Ketorolac tromethamine is a potent NSAID analgesic; its administration carries many risks. The resulting NSAID-related adverse effects can be serious in certain clients for whom ketorolac is indicated, especially when the drug is used inappropriately. Increasing the dose beyond the label recommendations will not provide better efficacy but will result in increased risk of developing serious adverse effects. (2) **GI effects.** Ketorolac tromethamine is contraindicated in clients with active peptic ulcer disease, in clients with recent GI bleeding or perforation, and in those with a history of peptic ulcer disease or GI bleeding. (3) **Renal effects.** Ketorolac tromethamine is contraindicated in those with advanced renal impairment and in clients at risk for renal failure due to volume depletion. (4) **Risk of bleeding.** Ketorolac tromethamine inhibits platelet function and is, therefore, contraindicated in clients with suspected or confirmed cerebrovascular bleeding, hemorrhagic diathesis, incomplete hemostasis, and in those at high risk of bleeding. Ketorolac tromethamine is contraindicated as a prophylactic analgesic before any major surgery and is contraindicated intraoperatively when hemostasis is critical because of the increased risk of bleeding. (5) **Hypersensitivity.** Ketorolac is contraindicated in those with previously demonstrated hypersensitivity to ketorolac or allergic manifestations to aspirin or other NSAIDs. (6) **Labor, delivery, and nursing.** Ketorolac tromethamine is contraindicated in labor and delivery because, through its prostaglandin synthesis inhibitory effect, it may adversely affect fetal circulation and inhibit uterine contractions. The use of ketorolac tromethamine is contraindicated in nursing mothers because of the potential adverse effects of prostaglandin-inhibiting drugs on neonates. (7) **Concomitant use with NSAIDs.** Ketorolac tromethamine is contraindicated in clients currently receiving aspirin or NSAIDs because of the cumulative risks of inducing serious NSAID-related adverse effects. (8) **Dosage and administration**. Ketorolac tromethamine oral is indicated only as continuation therapy to ketorolac tromethamine IV/IM, and the combined duration of use of ketorolac tromethamine IV/IM and ketorolac tromethamine oral is not to exceed 5 days because of the increased risk of serious adverse effects. The recommended total daily dose of ketorolac tromethamine oral (maximum 40 mg) is significantly lower than that for ketorolac tromethamine IV/IM (maximum 120 mg). (9) **Special populations.** Dosage should be adjusted for clients 65 years of age and older, for clients less than 50 kg (110 lbs) of body weight, and for clients with moderately elevated serum creatine. Doses of ketorolac IV/IM are not to exceed 60 mg (total dose per day) in these clients. Ketorolac is indicated as a single-dose therapy in pediatric clients; not to exceed 30 mg for IM administration and 15 mg for IV administration. (10) **Intrathecal or epidural administration.** Ketorolac tromethamine is contraindicated for neuraxial (epidural or intrathecal) administration due to its alcohol content.

Intranasal use. (1) **Limitations of use.** Ketorolac nasal spray, an NSAID, is indicated for short-term (up to 5 days in adults) management of moderate to moderately severe pain that requires analgesia at the opioid level. Do not exceed a total combined duration of use of ketorolac nasal spray and other ketorolac formulations (IM, IV, PO) of 5 days. (2) Ketorolac spray is not intended for use in children, and it is not indicated for minor or chronic painful conditions. (3) **GI risk.** Ketorolac can cause peptic ulcers, GI bleeding, and/or perforation of the stomach or intestines, which can be fatal. These events can occur at any time during use and without warning symptoms. Therefore, ketorolac is contraindicated in clients with active peptic

K

ulcer disease, in clients wtih recent GI bleeding or perforation, and in clients with a history of peptic ulcer disease or GI bleeding. Elderly clients are at greater risk for serious GI events. (4) **Bleeding risk.** Ketorolac inhibits platelet function and is, therefore, contraindicated in clients with suspected or confirmed CV bleeding, hemorrhagic diathesis, or incomplete hemostasis, and those at high risk of bleeding. (5) **CV risk.** NSAIDs may cause an increased risk of serious CV thrombotic events, MI, and stroke, which can be fatal. This risk may increase with duration of use. Clients with CV disease or risk factors for CV disease may be at greater risk. (6) Ketorolac nasal spray is contraindicated for treatment of perioperative pain in the setting of coronary artery bypass graft surgery. (7) **Renal risk**. Ketorolac is contraindicated in clients with advanced renal impairment and in clients at risk for renal failure due to volume depletion. ■

- **Age of the client, dosage, and duration of therapy should receive special consideration when using this drug.**
- **Use of ophthalmic products in clients with complicated ocular surgeries, corneal denervation, corneal epithelial defects, diabetes mellitus, ocular surface diseases, rheumatoid arthritis, or repeat ocular surgeries within a short period of time may be at increased risk for corneal side effects that may be sight-threatening.**
- **Use ophthalmic products with caution during lactation.**
- **Safety and efficacy of the systemic products have not been determined in children less than 2 years of age and of the ophthalmic product in children less than 3 years of age.**

SIDE EFFECTS

Most Common

Systemic use: Headache, dizziness, drowsiness, diarrhea, nausea, dyspepsia/indigestion, epigastric/GI pain, edema.
Ophthalmic use: Transient burning/stinging upon administration, ocular irritation.
See *Nonsteroidal Anti-Inflammatory Drugs* for a complete set of possible side effects, as well as information under *Special Concerns.* Also, **CV:** Vasodilation, pallor. **GI:** GI pain, peptic ulcers, nausea, dyspepsia, flatulence, GI fullness, stomatitis, excessive thirst, GI bleeding (higher risk in geriatric clients), ***perforation.*** **CNS:** Headache, nervousness, abnormal thinking, depression, euphoria. **Hypersensitivity: *Bronchospasm, anaphylaxis.*** **Miscellaneous:** Purpura, asthma, abnormal vision, abnormal liver function. **Ophthalmic Solution.** Transient stinging and burning following instillation, ocular irritation, allergic reactions, superficial ocular infections, superficial keratitis.

DRUG INTERACTIONS

Ketorolac may ↑ plasma levels of salicylates due to ↓ plasma protein binding.

HOW SUPPLIED

Injection: 15 mg/mL, 30 mg/mL; *Ophthalmic Solution:* 0.4%, 0.5%; *Spray, Nasal:* 15.75 mg/spray; *Tablets:* 10 mg.

DOSAGE

IM, IV

Moderately severe acute pain, single dose.

Adults and children 17 years and older: One 60-mg dose IM or 1 30 mg dose IV. **Adults, elderly, in renal impairment, or weight less than 50 kg (110 lbs):** One 30 mg dose IM or one 15 mg dose IV. **Children, 2–16 years of age:** One dose of 1 mg/kg IM or 0.5 mg/kg IV, up to a maximum of 30 mg IM or 15 mg IV. *NOTE:* See dosing of tablets following conversion from a single IM or IV dose.

IM; IV

Moderately severe acute pain, multiple doses.

Adults: 30 mg IM or IV q 6 hr, not to exceed 120 mg daily. **Adults, elderly, in renal impairment, or weight less than 50 kg (110 lbs):** 15 mg IM or IV q 6 hr, not to exceed 60 mg daily. *NOTE:* See dosing of tablets following conversion from multiple IM or IV doses.

TABLETS

Moderate to severe pain: transition from IV/IM to PO.

Adults and children 16 years and older: 20 mg as a first PO dose following IM or IV therapy; **then,** 10 mg PO q 4–6 hr, up to a maximum of 40 mg in 24 hr. **Adults, elderly, in renal im-**

pairment, or weight less than 50 kg (110 lbs): 10 mg as a first PO dose following IM or IV therapy; **then,** 10 mg PO q 4–6 hr, up to a maximum of 40 mg in 24 hr.

ACULAR LS: OPHTHALMIC SOLUTION, 0.4%

Pain, burning, stinging following cataract extraction.

1 gtt 4 times per day in the operated eye, as needed for pain and burning/stinging for up to 4 days following corneal refractive surgery.

ACUVAIL: OPHTHALMIC SOLUTION, 0.45%, PRESERVATIVE FREE

Pain and inflammation following cataract surgery.

1 drop to the affected eye twice a day beginning 1 day prior to cataract surgery, continued on the day of surgery, and through the first 2 weeks after surgery. May be given with other topical ophthalmic medications. Give drops at least 5 min apart.

ACULAR: OPHTHALMIC SOLUTION, 0.5%

Ocular itching.

1 gtt (0.25 mg) 4 times per day.

Postoperative inflammation following cataract extraction.

1 gtt to the affected eye(s) 4 times per day beginning 24 hr after cataract surgery and continuing through the first 2 weeks of the postoperative period.

SPRAY, NASAL

Moderate to moderately severe pain.

Adults weighing more than 50 kg: One 15.75 mg spray in each nostril (total dose of 31.5 mg) q 6–8 hr, up to a maximum of 126 mg/day for no more than 5 days. **Adults weighing less than 50 kg, the elderly, and those with renal impairment:** One 15.75 mg spray in only 1 nostril q 6–8 hr, up to a maximum of 63 mg/day for no more than 5 days.

NURSING IMPLICATIONS

Do not confuse Toradol with tramadol.

IMPLEMENTATION/ADMINISTRATION/STORAGE

1. Use as part of a regular analgesic schedule rather than on an as-needed basis.
2. If given on PRN basis, base size of a repeat dose on the duration of pain relief from the previous dose. If pain returns within 3–5 hr, the next dose can be increased by up to 50% (as long as the total daily dose is not exceeded). If pain does not return for 8–12 hr, the next dose can be decreased by as much as 50% or the dosing interval can be increased to q 8–12 hr.
3. Give IM slowly and deeply into the muscle.
4. For breakthrough pain, supplement the lower end of the ketorolac IM or IV dosage range with low doses of narcotics as needed, unless otherwise contraindicated.
5. Shortening the dosing intervals recommended will lead to an increased frequency and duration of side effects.
6. Correct hypovolemia prior to administering.
7. Children should receive only a single doses of ketorolac injection.
8. Do not store any single bottle of the spray for more than 1 day as it will not deliver the intended dose after 24 hr. Thus, discard the bottle after 24 hr even if it still contains some liquid.
9. Store Acular and Acular LS from 15–30°C (59–86°F) protected from light. Store Acuvail from 15–25°C (59–77°F) protected from light.
10. Store tablets from 15–30°C (59–86°F).
11. Store unopened spray bottles from 2–8°C (36–46°F). Protect from light and freezing. During use keep from 15–30°C (59–86°F) and out of direct sunlight.
12. IV The IV bolus must be given over no less than 15 sec.
13. Store the injection from 15–30°C (59–86°F). Protect from light.
14. COMPATIBILITY D5W, NSS, D5/NSS, RL; administer undiluted.
15. INCOMPATIBILITY Do not mix IV/IM ketorolac in a small volume (i.e., a syringe) with morphine sulfate, meperidine HCl, promethazine HCl, or hydroxyzine HCl; will precipitate from solution.

ASSESSMENT

1. Identify reasons for therapy, onset, location, pain intensity/level, characteristics of S&S, clinical presentation.

K

2. Note any previous experience with NSAIDs and results.
3. Assess for any asthma, aspirin-induced allergy, PUD/recent GI bleed or nasal polyps.
4. Determine history of ulcers, heart disease, or cardiac failure. May cause an increased risk of serious CV thrombotic events, MI, and stroke; risk increased with longer use and with heart disease.
5. List drugs prescribed; note if any are ACE inhibitors, anticonvulsants, or antidepressants as they may cause adverse effects with prolonged therapy.
6. Check for liver or renal dysfunction, monitor and adjust dose; assess hydration status.

CLIENT/FAMILY TEACHING

1. Take only as directed; do not exceed prescribed dosage. May take with food/milk if GI upset occurs.
2. Drug may cause drowsiness and dizziness; avoid activities that require mental alertness until drug effects realized.
3. Avoid alcohol, aspirin, and all OTC agents without approval.
4. Report any unusual bruising/bleeding, weight gain, SOB, chest pain, swelling of feet/ankles, increased joint pain, change in urine patterns or lack of response.
5. With eyedrops, wash hands, do not allow dropper to touch eye. Tilt head back; looking up pull lower eyelid down and instill prescribed number of drops. Close eye for 1 to 2 min, apply gentle pressure to bridge of nose for 1 to 3 min. Do not rub eye or touch top of dropper bottle to eye, fingers, or other surface.
6. If more than 1 topical eye drug used, give at least 5 min apart administering the ointment last. May experience temporary stinging or burning; report if bothersome or if eye/eyelid inflammation noted.
7. If wearing contact lens, remove before instilling eye drops. Do not wear soft contact lens.
8. With nasal spray, clear nasal passage, place the tip of the spray container into the nose. Using a finger from other hand, press against the opposite nostril to close it off. Breathe gently through the open nostril and squeeze the spray container. Switch and do same to other nostril. Discard SPRIX bottle after 24 hours even if fluid remains as will not deliver intended dose. Do not exceed 5 days of this therapy as side effects increase significantly.
9. Keep all F/U to assess response, labs (CBC, renal and LFTs), and for adverse SE.

OUTCOMES/EVALUATE

- Effective pain control
- ↓ Ocular allergic manifestations
- ↓ Ocular pain/photophobia

L

IV

Labetalol hydrochloride

(lah-**BET**-ah-lohl)

Classification(s): Alpha-beta adrenergic blocking agent

Pregnancy Category: C

RX: Trandate.

✤ **Rx:** Apo-Labetalol.

SEE ALSO ***BETA-ADRENERGIC BLOCKING AGENTS*** AND ***ANTIHYPERTENSIVE AGENTS.***

INDICATIONS/USES

PO: Hypertension, alone or in combination with other drugs (especially thiazide and loop diuretics). **IV:** Control of BP in severe hypertension. *Investigational:* Pheochromocytoma (higher IV doses may be needed), clonidine withdrawal hypertension.

ACTION/KINETICS

Action

Decreases BP by blocking both alpha- and beta-adrenergic receptors. Standing BP is lowered more than supine. Significant reflex tachycardia and bradycardia do not occur, although AV conduction may be prolonged.

Pharmacokinetics

Completely absorbed after PO. Absolute bioavailability is 25%. Food increases bioavailability of the drug. **Steady state plasma levels:** About 3 days. **Onset, PO:** 2–4 hr; **IV:** 5 min. **Peak plasma levels, PO:** 1–2 hr. **Peak effects, PO, after single dose:** 2–4 hr. **Duration, PO:** 8–12 hr. **t½, elimination, PO:** 6–8 hr; **IV:** 5.5 hr. Significant first-pass effect; metabolized in liver. Excreted in the urine and feces. **Plasma protein binding:** About 50%.

CONTRAINDICATIONS

Cardiogenic shock, overt cardiac failure, bronchial asthma, severe bradycardia, greater than first-degree heart block.

SPECIAL CONCERNS

- **Use with caution during lactation, in impaired renal and hepatic function, in chronic bronchitis and emphysema, in those with a history of heart failure who are well compensated, and in diabetes (may prevent premonitory signs of acute hypoglycemia).**
- **Elderly clients may experience orthostatic hypotension, dizziness, and lightheadedness.**
- **Safety and efficacy in children not established.**

SIDE EFFECTS

Most Common

Headache, nausea, dizziness, impotence, tingling scalp, fatigue, dry itchy skin, insomnia, anxiety/nervousness.

See also *Beta-Adrenergic Blocking Agents*.

After PO Use. GI: Nausea, diarrhea, cholestasis with or without jaundice. **CNS:** Fatigue, dizziness, drowsiness, paresthesias, headache, anxiety/nervousness, insomnia, syncope (rare). **GU:** Impotence, priapism, ejaculation failure, difficulty in micturition, Peyronie's disease, acute urinary bladder retention. **Respiratory:** Dyspnea, nasal stuffiness, ***bronchospasm***. **Musculoskeletal:** Muscle cramps, asthenia, toxic myopathy. **Dermatologic:** Dry itchy skin, generalized maculopapular, lichenoid, or urticarial rashes; bullous lichen planus, psoriasis, facial erythema, reversible alopecia. **Ophthalmic:** Abnormal vision, dry eyes. **Miscellaneous:** SLE, positive antinuclear factor, antimitochondrial antibodies, fever, edema.

After parenteral use. CV: Ventricular arrhythmias. **CNS:** Numbness, somnolence, yawning, hypesthesia. **Renal:** Transient increases in BUN and serum creatinine associated with drops in BP usually in those with prior renal insufficiency. **Miscellaneous:** Pruritus, flushing, wheezing.

After PO or parenteral use. CV: Depression of myocardial contractility causing more heart failure, postural hypotension. **GI:** N&V, dyspepsia, taste distortion, jaundice or hepatic dysfunction (rare). **CNS:** Dizziness, tingling of skin or scalp, vertigo. **Miscellaneous:** Postural hypotension, increased sweating, hypersensitivity reactions.

LABORATORY TEST CONSIDERATIONS

False + increase in urinary catecholamines or for amphetamine when screening urine for drugs. Transient ↑ serum transaminases, BUN, serum creatinine.

OVERDOSE MANAGEMENT

Symptoms: Excessive hypotension and bradycardia. *Treatment:* Induce vomiting or perform gastric lavage. Place clients in a supine position with legs elevated. If required, the following treatment can be used:

- Epinephrine or a beta-2-agonist (aerosol) to treat bronchospasm.
- Atropine or epinephrine to treat bradycardia.
- Digitalis glycoside and a diuretic for cardiac failure; dopamine or dobutamine may also be used.
- Diazepam to treat seizures.
- Norepinephrine (or another vasopressor) to treat hypotension.
- Administration of glucagon (5–10 mg rapidly over 30 sec), followed by continuous infusion of 5 mg/hr, may be effective in treating severe hypotension and bradycardia.

DRUG INTERACTIONS

Beta-adrenergic bronchodilators / ↓ Bronchodilator drug effects; ↑ dose of bronchodilator may be required
Calcium channel blockers (e.g., verapamil) / Use together with caution
Cimetidine / ↑ Bioavailability of PO labetalol
Glutethimide / ↓ Labetalol effects R/T ↑ liver breakdown
Halothane / ↑ Risk of severe myocardial depression → hypotension; do not use together
Nitroglycerin / Additive hypotension; labetalol blunts reflex tachycardia due to nitroglycerin without preventing hypotension

Tricyclic antidepressants / ↑ Risk of tremors

HOW SUPPLIED

Injection: 5 mg/mL; *Tablets:* 100 mg, 200 mg, 300 mg.

DOSAGE

TABLETS

Hypertension.

Individualize. Initial: 100 mg twice a day alone or with a diuretic. After 2 or 3 days, using standing BP as a guide, titrate dosage in increments of 100 mg twice a day, q 2–3 days. **Maintenance:** 200–400 mg twice a day up to 1,200–2,400 mg/day for severe cases. Should side effects occur with twice a day dosing, the same total daily dose given 3 times/day may improve tolerance. Do not exceed titration increments of 200 mg/day. Geriatric clients will generally require lower maintenance doses.

IV, REPEATED INJECTIONS

Hypertension.

Individualize. Initial: 20 mg (0.25 mg/kg for an 80 kg client) slowly over 2 min; measure supine BP immediately before and at 5 and 10 min after injection. Additional injections of 40 or 80 mg q 10 min can be given until desired effect occurs or a total of 300 mg has been given. Maximum effect usually occurs within 5 min of each injection.

SLOW CONTINUOUS IV INFUSION

Hypertension.

Initial: 2 mg/min; **then,** adjust rate according to response. Continue until a satisfactory response is obtained, then discontinue infusion and start PO labetalol. **Effective cumulative IV dose range:** 50–200 mg, up to 300 mg.

Transfer from IV to PO therapy.

Begin PO dosing when supine diastolic BP begins to rise. **Initial:** 200 mg; **then,** 200 or 400 mg 6–12 hr later, depending on response. Thereafter, dosage based on response.

NURSING IMPLICATIONS

Do not confuse labetalol with lamotrigine or Lamictal (anticonvulsant), with Lomotil (an antidiarrheal), or with lamivudine (an antiviral drug).

IMPLEMENTATION/ADMINISTRATION/STORAGE

1. When transferring to PO labetalol from other antihypertensive therapy, slowly reduce dosage of current therapy.
2. Full antihypertensive effect is usually seen within the first 1–3 hr after the initial dose or dose increment.
3. IV For slow continuous infusion, use one of the following methods: (a) Add 200 mg to 160 mL of IV fluid to prepare a 1 mg/mL solution at a rate of 2 mL/min (2 mg/min), or (b) Add 200 mg to 250 mL of an IV fluid to prepare 2 mg/3 mL solution; give at a rate of 3 mL/min (2 mg/min).
4. Keep clients supine during IV injection. Before permitting ambulation, establish ability of client to tolerate the upright position.
5. To transfer from IV to PO therapy in hospitalized clients, begin when supine BP begins to increase.
6. May give IV undiluted (20 mg over 2 min) or reconstituted with dextrose or saline solutions (infuse at a rate of 2 mg/min). When given by IV infusion, use an infusion control device.
7. Store injection and tablets from 2–30°C (36–86°F). Protect the injection from light.
8. Store injection and tablets from 2–30°C (36–86°F); protect the injection from light.
9. COMPATIBILITY Labetalol, at a final concentration of 1.25–3.75 mg/mL is compatible with Ringer's, LR, D5/Ringer's, D5/LR, D5W, 0.9% NaCl, D5/0.2% NaCl, 2.5% Dextrose and 0.45% NaCl, D5/0.9% NaCl, and D5/0.33% NaCl.
10. INCOMPATIBILITY Not compatible with 5% sodium bicarbonate injection, furosemide, or other alkaline products.

ASSESSMENT

1. Note reasons for therapy, other agents trialed, outcome. List any conditions that may preclude therapy.
2. Assess effect of labetalol tablets on standing BP before hospital discharge. Obtain standing BP at different times (in left and right arm) during day to assess full effects.

3. To reduce chance of orthostatic hypotension, keep supine during IV administration and for 3 hr afterward.
4. Advise if positive urine test for amphetamine, confirmation should be made by using more specific methods, such as a gas chromatographic-mass spectrometer technique.
5. Assess for conditions that preclude therapy: severe bradycardia, second- and third-degree heart block, heart failure, cardiogenic shock, bronchial asthma, hepatic injury.
6. Monitor VS, ECG, BS, renal and LFTs.

CLIENT/FAMILY TEACHING

1. Take as directed with meals; tablets can be crushed.
2. If nausea and dizziness occur with twice-daily dosing of oral form, same total daily dose can be administered as divided doses 3 times per day.
3. Do not stop taking abruptly; may cause chest pain.
4. Use caution and change positions slowly; may precipitate sudden drop in BP and cause dizziness (support hose may help). Report any low heart rate, confusion, fever, swelling of extremities, difficulty breathing, night cough, or persistent dizziness. Record heart rate, weight, and BP for provider review.
5. May cause increased sensitivity to cold; dress appropriately. Transient scalp tingling may occur with initiation of therapy.
6. Avoid alcohol, OTC products (especially cold remedies), high sodium intake, and tobacco.
7. Continue lifestyle changes to ensure BP control: regular exercise, weight control, smoking cessation and moderate intake of alcohol and salt.
8. Keep all F/U to assess response and for adverse SE.

OUTCOMES/EVALUATE

↓ BP

IV

Lacosamide

(la-**KOE**-sa-mide)

Classification(s): Anticonvulsant

Pregnancy Category: C

RX: Vimpat, **C-V**

SEE ALSO ***ANTICONVULSANTS***.

INDICATIONS/USES

Adjunctive therapy in the treatment of partial-onset seizures in clients 17 years of age and older with epilepsy.

ACTION/KINETICS

Action

The mechanism is not fully known but is believed that the drug selectively enhances slow inactivation of voltage-gated sodium channels resulting in stabilization of hyperexcitable neuronal membranes and inhibition of repetitive neuronal firing.

Pharmacokinetics

Completely absorbed after PO administration with negligible first-pass effect. Absolute bioavailability is 100%. **Maximum plasma levels:** 1–4 hr. **t½, elimination:** 15–23 hr. Steady-state plasma levels are reached after 3 days of twice daily dosing. Metabolized in the liver by CYP2C19; unchanged drug and metabolites are excreted through the urine. **Plasma protein binding:** <15%.

CONTRAINDICATIONS

Lactation. Use in severely impaired hepatic function.

SPECIAL CONCERNS

- Increased risk of suicidal behavior and ideation.
- Use caution in dose titration in the elderly.
- Safety and efficacy not determined in children younger than 17 years of age.

SIDE EFFECTS

Most Common

Dizziness, ataxia, headache, N&V, fatigue, ataxia, somnolence, tremor, diplopia, blurred vision.

CNS: Dizziness, ataxia, headache, syncope, somnolence, euphoria, vertigo, tremor, balance disorder, depression, gait disturbance, memory impairment, cerebellar syndrome, cognitive disorder, confusional state, depressed mood, disturbance to attention, dysarthria, feeling drunk, hypoesthesia, irritability, altered mood, paresthesia, suicidal behavior and ideation. **GI:** N&V, diarrhea, constipation, dry mouth, dyspepsia, oral hypoesthesia. **CV:** Palpitations, prolongation of PR interval, atrial fibrillation/flutter, syncope, bradycardia. **Dermatologic:** Skin laceration, contusion, pruritus, rash. **Hematologic:** Anemia, neutropenia. **Ophthalmic:** Diplopia, blurred vision, nystagmus. **Body as a whole:** Fatigue, asthenia, pyrexia, contusion, muscle spasms. **Miscellaneous:** Fall, tinnitus, hypersensitivity reactions. *NOTE:* IV administration is associated with injection-site pain, discomfort, irritation, and erythema.

LABORATORY TEST CONSIDERATIONS

↑ ALT. LFT abnormalities.

OVERDOSE MANAGEMENT

Symptoms: Similar to side effects. *Treatment:* There is no specific antidote for lacosamide. Give general supportive care, including monitoring of vital signs and observation of the clinical status. Standard hemodialysis procedures remove up to 50% of the drug in 4 hours.

DRUG INTERACTIONS

Anti-epileptic drugs (e.g., carbamazepine, phenobarbital, phenytoin) / Small (15–20%) ↓ in lacosamide plasma levels

Contraceptives, hormonal / Ethinyl estradiol C_{max} ↑ 20%

Omeprazole / Plasma levels of the O-desmethyl metabolite of lacosamide ↓ 60% in presence of omeprazole

HOW SUPPLIED

Injection Solution: 10 mg/mL; ***Oral Solution:*** 10 mg/mL; ***Tablets:*** 50 mg, 100 mg, 150 mg, 200 mg.

DOSAGE

IV, ORAL SOLUTION, TABLETS

Partial-onset seizures.

Adults, 17 years and older, initial: 50 mg twice a day. Increase at weekly intervals by 100 mg/day, given as 2 divided doses, up to the recommended maintenance dose of 200–400 mg/day, based on client response and tolerability. **Maintenance:** 200–400 mg/day; doses of 600 mg/day were associated with a significantly higher incidence of side effects. *NOTE:* At the end of the IV treatment period, the client may be switched to PO administration of lacosamide at the equivalent daily dosage and frequency of the IV administration.

NURSING IMPLICATIONS

IMPLEMENTATION/ADMINISTRATION/STORAGE

1. No dosage adjustment is needed in those with mild to moderate renal impairment. However, a maximum dose of 300 mg/day is recommended for clients with severe renal impairment (C_{CR} of 30 mL/min or less), and in those with end-stage renal disease.
2. A maximum dose of 300 mg/day is recommended for those with mild or moderate impaired hepatic function. Do not administer to those with severely impaired hepatic function.
3. Gradually withdraw lacosamide over a minimum of 1 week to minimize the potential of increased seizure frequency.
4. Lacosamide is removed from plasma by hemodialysis. Following a 4-hr hemodialysis treatment, consider dosage supplementation of up to 50%.
5. At the end of IV administration, the client may be switched to PO lacosamide at the equivalent daily dose and frequency as IV use.
6. IV Injection can be given IV without further dilution, or may be mixed with diluents.
7. When switching from PO to IV dosing, the initial total daily dose and frequency of PO lacosamide should be infused IV over a 30- to 60-min period.
8. Store from 15–30°C (59–86°F). Do not freeze the oral solution. Discard any unused oral solution after 7 weeks of first opening the bottle.
9. COMPATIBILITY NSS, D5W or LR; stable for at least 24 hr and stored in glass or PVC bags at ambient room temperature.
10. INCOMPATIBILITY Use with other infusion solutions has not been evaluated.

ASSESSMENT

1. Note indications for therapy, characteristics of seizures, other agents trialed, outcome.
2. List drugs prescribed to ensure none interact.
3. With any heart disease or conduction problems, obtain ECG before starting treatment and after titrating dose; may cause ECG changes that cause irregular heartbeat and syncope.
4. Determine any history of depression or suicide ideations. Monitor for emergence or worsening of depression, suicidal thoughts or behavior.

5. The elderly may be more sensitive to drug's effects.
6. Ensure enrollment in UCB AED Pregnancy Registry at 1-888-537-7734 if client is pregnant to continue to study drug effects during pregnancy.
7. Obtain renal and LFTs; reduce dose with dysfunction.

CLIENT/FAMILY TEACHING

1. May be taken with or without food. When using the oral solution, use a calibrated measuring device. A household teaspoon or tablespoon is not an adequate measuring device.
2. Drug is used to help control seizures. Take as directed with other prescribed antiepileptic drugs (AEDs) and do not stop suddenly. Withdraw gradually to minimize potential for increased seizure frequency.
3. Avoid activities that require mental alertness until drug effects realized; may cause dizziness, loss of coordination/balance, blurred vision and drowsiness.
4. If partial loss of consciousness occurs lie down with legs raised to help recover; notify provider.
5. Practice reliable contraception. If pregnancy occurs enroll in UCB AED Pregnancy Registry at 1-888-537-7734 and also the North American Antiepileptic Drug Pregnancy Registry at 1-888-233-2334 so that drug effects on fetus can be followed.
6. Serious hypersensitivity reactions affecting multiple organs may occur. Report any S&S, including dark urine, fatigue, and jaundice, to provider.
7. Report any behavioral changes, including aggressiveness, anxiety, mood changes, irritability, trouble sleeping, rash, or thoughts of suicide immediately.
8. Keep all F/U to assess response, labs, ECG, and for adverse SE.

OUTCOMES/EVALUATE

Control of seizures

Lamivudine (3TC)

(lah-**MIH**-vyou-deen)

Classification(s): Antiviral, nucleoside reverse transcriptase inhibitor

Pregnancy Category: C

RX: Epivir, Epivir-HBV.

Rx: 3TC, Heptovir.

SEE ALSO ***ANTIVIRAL DRUGS***.

INDICATIONS/USES

Epivir. In combination with other antiretroviral drugs for the treatment of HIV infection. **Epivir-HBV.** (1) Chronic hepatitis B associated with evidence of hepatitis B replication and active liver inflammation. (2) Hepatitis B in children, 2–17 years of age. *Investigational:* Prevention of maternal-fetal HIV transmission.

ACTION/KINETICS

Action

Synthetic nucleoside analog effective against HIV. Converted to active 5'-triphosphate (L-TP) metabolite which inhibits HIV reverse transcription via viral DNA chain termination. L-TP also inhibits the RNA- and DNA-dependent DNA polymerase activities of reverse transcriptase. Lamivudine-resistant HIV-1 mutants are cross-resistant to didanosine and zalcitabine.

Pharmacokinetics

Rapidly absorbed after PO administration; absolute bioavailability is about 86%. Most eliminated unchanged through the urine.

CONTRAINDICATIONS

Hypersensitivity to any component of the product. Lactation. Use of Epivir-HBV tablets or oral solution to treat HIV infections (due to the lower amount of lamivudine compared with Epivir).

SPECIAL CONCERNS

(1) Lactic acidosis and severe hepatomegaly with steatosis, including fatal cases, have been reported with the use of nucleoside analogs alone or in combination, including lamivudine and other antiretroviral agents. Suspend treatment with lamivudine in any client who develops clinical or laboratory findings suggestive of lactic acidosis or pronounced hepatotoxicity. (2) Lamivudine tablets and oral solution (used to treat HIV) contain a higher dose of the active ingredient (lamivudine) than lamivudine-HBV tablets and oral solution (used to treat chronic hepatitis B). Clients with HIV infection should receive only dosing forms appropriate for treatment of HIV.

The formulation and dosage of lamivudine-HBV are not appropriate for those dually infected with HBV and HIV. (3) Offer HIV counseling and testing to all clients before beginning lamivudine-HBV and periodically during treatment because lamivudine-HBV tablets and oral solution contain a lower dose of the same active ingredient as lamivudine tablets and oral solution used to treat HIV. If treatment with lamivudine-HBV is prescribed for chronic hepatitis B for a client with unrecognized or untreated HIV infection, rapid emergence of HIV resistance is likely because of the subtherapeutic dose and inappropriate monotherapy. (4) Severe acute exacerbations of hepatitis B have been reported in clients who have discontinued anti-hepatitis B therapy (including lamivudine-HBV) or are coinfected with HBV and HIV and have discontinued lamivudine. Monitor hepatic function closely with both clinical and laboratory follow-up for at least several months in those who discontinue anti-hepatitis B therapy or who discontinue lamivudine and are coinfected with HIV and HBV. If appropriate, initiation of anti-hepatitis B therapy may be warranted.

- **Clients taking lamivudine and zidovudine may continue to develop opportunistic infections and other complications of HIV infection.**
- **Use with caution and at a reduced dose in those with impaired renal function.**
- **Use lamivudine with caution in pediatric clients with a history of prior antiretroviral nucleoside exposure, a history of pancreatitis, or other significant risk factors for the development of pancreatitis.**
- **Data on the use of lamivudine and zidovudine in pediatric clients are lacking; however, use the combination with extreme caution in children with pancreatitis.**
- **Safety and efficacy of Epivir-HBV not determined in those with decompensated liver disease or organ transplants, in children under age 2, or in clients dually infected with HBV and HIV, hepatitis delta, or HIV.**
- **Possible virologic failure and emergence of nucleoside reverse transcriptase-associated mutations with a regimen consisting of didanosine enteric-coated beadlets, lamivudine, and tenofovir disoproxil fumarate.**

SIDE EFFECTS

Most Common

When used for HIV treatment: Headache, dreams, fatigue and/or malaise, insomnia and other sleep disorders, nasal signs/symptoms, diarrhea, cough, nausea, skin rash.
When used for chronic hepatitis B: Ear/nose/throat infections, malaise, fatigue, headache, N&V, abdominal discomfort/pain.
Side effects include those when lamivudine is taken alone or with other antiretroviral drugs.

When used to treat HIV. Adults: CNS: Headache, neuropathy, insomnia and other sleep disorders, dizziness, depression, dreams. **GI:** N&V, diarrhea, anorexia/decreased appetite, abdominal pain/cramps, dyspepsia, ***severe hepatomegaly with steatosis***, ***pancreatitis***, posttreatment worsening of hepatitis B. **Dermatologic:** Skin rashes. **Musculoskeletal:** Myalgia, musculoskeletal pain, arthralgia. **Respiratory:** Nasal signs/symptoms, cough. **Hematologic:** Anemia, neutropenia. **GU:** UTI. **Body as a whole:** Malaise, fatigue, fever, chills. **Children: CNS:** Paresthesias, peripheral neuropathies. **GI:** Hepatomegaly, diarrhea, N&V, stomatitis, splenomegaly, jaundice, ***pancreatitis***. **Dermatologic:** Skin rashes. **Respiratory:** Cough, nasal discharge or congestion, abnormal breath sounds/wheezing, respiratory infections. **Otic:** Pain, discharge, erythema, or swelling of an ear. **Metabolic:** Electrolyte disturbances, hypoglycemia. **Body as a whole:** Fever, lymphadenopathy, ***sepsis***, immune reconstitution syndrome (infections such as *Mycobacterium avium,* cytomegalovirus, *Pneumocystis jirovecii* pneumonia or tuberculosis), fat redistribution (central obesity, dorsocervical fat enlargement, peripheral/facial wasting, breast enlargement, cushingoid appearance).

When used for chronic hepatitis B: Adults and children: CNS: Headache, paresthesia, peripheral neuropathy, dizziness, depressive disorders. **GI:** Abdominal discomfort/pain, N&V, diarrhea, stomatitis, ***severe hepatomegaly with steatosis, pancreatitis***. **Dermatologic:** Skin rashes, alopecia, pruritus, rash, urticaria. **Musculoskeletal:** Myalgia, arthralgia, rhabdomyolysis, muscle weakness. **Respiratory:** Sore throat, ear/nose/throat infections; cough, bronchitis, viral respiratory tract infections in children; abnormal breath sounds, wheezing. **Hematologic:** Anemia (including pure red cell aplasia and severe anemias), lymphadenopathy, splenomegaly, neutropenia.

Body as a whole: Fever, chills, fatigue, malaise, lactic acidosis, hyperglycemia, redistribution/accumulation of body fat, weakness, immune reconstitution syndrome (infections such as *Mycobacterium avium*, cytomegalovirus, *Pneumocystis jirovecii* pneumonia or tuberculosis), fat redistribution (central obesity, dorsocervical fat enlargement, peripheral/facial wasting, breast enlargement, cushingoid appearance). **Miscellaneous:** ***Anaphylaxis***, posttreatment worsening of hepatitis B. *NOTE:* Pediatric clients have an increased risk to develop ***pancreatitis.***

LABORATORY TEST CONSIDERATIONS

↑ ALT, AST, amylase, bilirubin, serum lipase, creatine kinase. ↓ Hemoglobin, ANC, platelets, neutrophils.

DRUG INTERACTIONS

Interferon alfa / May cause hepatic decompensation (some fatal) in HIV/HCV coinfected clients
Ribavirin / Possible ↓ phosphorylation of lamivudine
Trimethoprim-Sulfamethoxazole / Significant ↑ (44%) in lamivudine levels
Zalcitabine / Inhibition of the intracellular phosphorylation of one another; do not use together
Zidovudine / ↑ (about 39%) C_{max} of zidovudine

HOW SUPPLIED

Lamivudine (Epivir). *Oral Solution:* 10 mg/mL; *Tablets:* 150 mg, 300 mg.
Lamivudine-HBV (Epivir-HBV). *Oral Solution:* 5 mg/mL; *Tablets:* 100 mg.

DOSAGE

Lamivudine (Epivir)

ORAL SOLUTION; TABLETS

HIV infection.

Adults: 150 mg twice a day or 300 mg once daily in combination with other antiretroviral drugs. For adults with low body weight (<50 kg), recommended dose is 2 mg/kg twice a day in combination with other antiretroviral drugs. **Children, 3 months to 16 years old, usual:** 4 mg/kg twice a day (up to a maximum of 150 mg twice a day) in combination with other antiretroviral drugs. Use oral solution for children. Tablets can be used in children who weigh at least 14 kg and who can swallow tablets.

In clients over age 16, adjust dose as follows in impaired renal function: C_{CR} 50 mL/min or more: 150 mg twice a day or 300 mg once daily; C_{CR} 30–49 mL/min: 150 mg once daily; C_{CR} 15–29 mL/min: 150 mg for the first dose followed by 100 mg once daily; C_{CR} 5–14 mL/min: 150 mg for the first dose followed by 50 mg once daily; C_{CR} <5 mL/min: 50 mg for the first dose followed by 25 mg once daily.

Lamivudine-HBV (Epivir-HBV)

Chronic hepatitis B.

Adults: 100 mg once daily. **Children, 2–17 years:** 3 mg/kg once daily, not to exceed 100 mg daily. Safety and efficacy beyond 1 year in adults and children have not been determined.

Adjust dose in adults as follows in impaired renal function: C_{CR} 50 mL/min or more: 100 mg once daily; C_{CR} 30–49 mL/min: 100 mg for the first dose followed by 50 mg once daily; C_{CR} 15–29 mL/min: 100 mg for the first dose followed by 25 mg once daily; C_{CR} 5–14 mL/min: 35 mg for the first dose followed by 15 mg once daily; C_{CR} <5 mL/min: 35 mg for the first dose followed by 10 mg once daily.

Prevention of maternal-fetal HIV transmission.

Neonates 35 weeks of age and older: 2 mg/kg twice a day for 7 days in combination with zidovudine, 2 mg/kg PO q 6 hr starting within 12 hr after birth and continuing through 6 weeks of age. **Neonates between 30 and 35 weeks of age:** 2 mg/kg twice a day for 7 days in combination with zidovudine, 2 mg/kg PO q 12 hr, advanced to q 8 hr at 2 weeks of age and continued through 6 weeks of age. **Neonates, less than 30 weeks of age:** 2 mg/kg q 12 hr for 7 days in combination with zidovudine, 2 mg/kg PO q 12 hr advanced to q 8 hr at 4 weeks of age and continued through 6 weeks of age.

NURSING IMPLICATIONS

Do not confuse lamivudine with lamotrigine or Lamictal (anticonvulsant), with Lamisil (an antifungal), with labetalol (an alpha–beta adrenergic blocking drug), or with Lomotil (an antidiarrheal).

IMPLEMENTATION/ADMINISTRATION/STORAGE

1. Consult zidovudine or other antiviral drug prescribing information before using with lamivudine.
2. Use the following dosing recommendations for lamivudine, 150 mg tablets in children:
   - Weight: 14–21 kg: Give one half tablet (75 mg) in the a.m. and p.m. (total daily dose: 150 mg).
   - Weight: >21–<30 kg: Give one half tablet (75 mg) in the a.m. and 1 tablet (150 mg) in the p.m. (total daily dose: 225 mg).
   - Weight 30 kg or more: Give 1 tablet (150 mg) in the a.m. and p.m. (total daily dose: 300 mg).
3. If lamivudine is given to a client dually infected with HIV and HBV, the dosage indicated for HIV therapy should be used as part of the regimen. The formulation and dosage of lamivudine-HBV are not appropriate for those dually infected with HIV and HBV.
4. Safety and efficacy of twice-daily lamivudine in combination with other antiretroviral drugs have been established in children over 3 months of age.
5. There are insufficient data to recommend a specific dosage regimen for children with either HIV or HBV and who have impaired renal function. However, a dose reduction or an increase in the dosing interval should be considered.
6. Store Epivir Solution at 25°C (77°F). Store Epivir-HBV Solution from 20–25°C (68–77°F). Store Epivir and Epivir-HBV Tablets from 15–30°C (59–86°F).

ASSESSMENT

1. Note disease onset/confirmation, other agents trialed, outcome.
2. Monitor child for clinical symptoms of pancreatitis.
3. Assess for HIV, HCV, hepatitis delta when treating hepatitis B.
4. Monitor closely for lactic acidosis and severe hepatomegaly with steatosis, severe acute exacerbations of hepatitis B, hepatic decompensation in those co-infected with HIV-1 and hepatitis, and pancreatitis.
5. Monitor liver, renal, and hematologic parameters, including CD_4 and viral load. Adjust dose with impaired renal function.

CLIENT/FAMILY TEACHING

1. Take as prescribed with other antiretroviral drug(s) twice a day. Drug works by inhibiting replication of HIV and/or hepatitis B virus.
2. May take without regard to food. Drug is not a cure; may continue to experience illnesses and opportunistic infections associated with HIV/HBV.
3. Epivir-HBV tablets and oral solution contain a lower dose of the same active ingredient as Epivir oral solution and tablets, and lamivudine/zidovudine tablets. Do not take Epivir-HBV concurrently with Epivir or lamivudine/zidovudine.
4. Advise that each 15-mL dose of EPIVIR (lamivudine) Oral Solution contains 3 grams of sucrose.
5. Use caution with activities that require mental alertness. Report memory loss, confusion, or S&S of infection.
6. Use barrier protection with sexual partners to prevent HIV/hepatitis transmission. Practice reliable contraception, do not breast feed; drug may be transferred to the fetus through the placenta.
7. May experience fainting or dizziness; GI upset, and insomnia may resolve after 3–4 weeks of therapy.
8. Do not stop without provider approval; acute exacerbations of hepatitis B have occurred.
9. With children, report symptoms of pancreatitis (i.e., abdominal pain, N&V, fever, loss of appetite, yellow skin discoloration).
10. Redistribution or accumulation of body fat may occur during treatment with antiretroviral therapy.
11. Keep all F/U to assess response, for exams, labs, and adverse SE.

OUTCOMES/EVALUATE

- Control of HIV disease progression with other antiretroviral drugs
- ↓ Viral load ↑ CD4 levels
- Stabilization of hepatitis B disease

Combination Drug

Lamivudine/ Zidovudine

(lah-**MIH**-vyou-deen, zye-**DOH**-vyou-deen)

Classification(s): Antiviral, nucleoside reverse transcriptase inhibitors

Pregnancy Category: C

RX: Combivir.

SEE ALSO ***LAMIVUDINE AND ZIDOVUDINE*** AND ***ANTIVIRAL DRUGS***.

INDICATIONS/USES

Treatment of HIV-1 infection in combination with other antiretrovirals.

CONTENT

Each Combivir tablet contains: *Antiviral:* Lamivudine, 150 mg and *Antiviral:* Zidovudine, 300 mg.

ACTION/KINETICS

Action

Both drugs are reverse transcriptase inhibitors with activity against HIV. Combination results in synergistic antiretroviral effect.

Pharmacokinetics

Each drug is rapidly absorbed. **t½, lamivudine:** 5–7 hr; **t½, zidovudine:** 0.5–3 hr. Most lamivudine is excreted unchanged in the urine. Zidovudine is metabolized by the liver and unchanged drug and metabolites are excreted in the urine. **Plasma protein binding:** Less than 36% of lamivudine and less than 38% of zidovudine.

CONTRAINDICATIONS

Use in clients requiring dosage reduction of lamivudine/zidovudine (product is a fixed-dose combination), children <12 years old, C_{CR} <50 mL/min, body weight <50 kg, and in those experiencing dose-limiting side effects. Lactation.

SPECIAL CONCERNS

(1) Zidovudine has been associated with hematologic toxicity, including neutropenia and severe anemia, particularly in clients with advanced HIV disease. Prolonged use of zidovudine has been associated with symptomatic myopathy. (2) Lactic acidosis and severe hepatomegaly with steatosis, including deaths, have been reported with use of nucleoside analogs alone or in combination, including lamivudine, zidovudine, and other antiretrovirals. (3) Severe acute exacerbations of hepatitis B have been reported in clients who are coinfected with hepatitis B virus (HBV) and HIV and have discontinued lamivudine. Monitor hepatic function closely with both clinical and laboratory follow-up for at least several months in those who discontinue lamivudine/zidovudine and are coinfected with HIV and HBV. If appropriate, initiation of hepatitis B therapy may be warranted.

Use with caution in clients with bone marrow compromise as evidenced by granulocyte count <1,000 cells/mm³ or hemoglobin <9.5 grams/dL.

SIDE EFFECTS

Most Common

Headache, N&V, ear/nose/throat infections, malaise/fatigue, diarrhea, anorexia, dizziness, myalgia, musculoskeletal pain, neuropathy, cough, fever, chills.

See *Lamivudine* and *Zidovudine* for a complete list of possible side effects. Note especially, possibility of hematologic toxicity, lactic acidosis, myopathy and myositis, and severe hepatomegaly with steatosis. Hepatic decompensation (some fatal) has occurred in HIV/HCV coinfected clients receiving combination antiretroviral therapy for HIV and interferon alfa and ribavirin. Immune reconstitution syndrome is possible. Redistribution/accumulation of body fat, including central obesity, dorsocervical fat enlargement, peripheral wasting, facial wasting, breast enlargement, and cushingoid appearance are possible.

LABORATORY TEST CONSIDERATIONS

↑ ALT, AST, amylase, bilirubin. Anemia, neutropenia, thrombocytopenia.

ADDITIONAL DRUG INTERACTIONS

See ***Lamivudine*** and ***Zidovudine*** for a complete list of possible drug interactions.

Didanosine / The AUC of didanosine may be ↓ and the plasma level of zidovudine may be ↑

Trimethoprim, Trimethoprim/Sulfamethoxazole / ↑ Lamivudine plasma levels R/T inhibition of lamivudine renal secretion; also, ↑ serum levels of zidovudine and its metabolite especially in those with impaired hepatic glucuronidation

HOW SUPPLIED

See *Content.*

DOSAGE

TABLETS

HIV infection.

Adults and children over 12 years of age: One combination tablet—150 mg lamivudine/300 mg zidovudine—twice a day.

NURSING IMPLICATIONS

Do not confuse Combivir with Combivent (combination drug for COPD).

IMPLEMENTATION/ADMINISTRATION/STORAGE

1. May be taken without regard to food.
2. Since Combivir is a fixed-dose combination, do not use for those requiring dosage adjustment, such as with reduced renal function (C_{CR} <50 mL/min) or those experiencing dose-limiting side effects.
3. A decrease in dosage may be needed in those with mild to moderate impaired hepatic function or liver cirrhosis.
4. Store between 2–30°C (36–86°F).

ASSESSMENT

1. Note disease onset, clinical characteristics, other agents trialed, outcome.
2. Weigh client; not for use in those with low body weight (<30 kg) or C_{CR} <50 mL/min.
3. May experience severe anemia and neutropenia with zidovudine.
4. Assess for myopathy, cardiomyopathy, hepatomegaly and lactic acidosis (pH <7.35 or serum lactate >5–6 mEq/L).
5. Monitor liver, renal, and hematologic parameters, including CD_4 and viral load; reduce dose with dysfunction.

CLIENT/FAMILY TEACHING

1. Take as directed, with or without food, twice daily.
2. Report adverse effects including severe abdominal pain, fatigue, SOB, dizziness, or muscle pain/weakness or memory loss or confusion; drug may cause low white count and anemia.
3. Drug is not a cure; may experience opportunistic infections. May cause lactic acidosis and liver swelling/toxicity.
4. May experience fainting or dizziness; GI upset, and insomnia may resolve after 3–4 weeks of therapy. Do not stop without provider approval; acute exacerbations of hepatitis B have occurred.
5. Use caution with activities that require mental alertness. Report memory loss, confusion, or S&S of infection.
6. Report symptoms of pancreatitis (i.e., abdominal pain, N&V, fever, loss of appetite, yellow skin discoloration).
7. A redistribution of fat may occur including breast enlargement, central obesity, cushingoid appearance, dorsocervical fat enlargement (buffalo hump).
8. Practice barrier contraception; drug does not prevent disease transmission. Do not breastfeed.
9. Keep all F/U to assess response, labs, and for adverse SE.

OUTCOMES/EVALUATE

Control of HIV; ↓ HIV RNA (viral load)

Lamotrigine

(lah-**MOH**-trih-jeen)

Classification(s): Anticonvulsant, miscellaneous

Pregnancy Category: C

RX: Lamictal, Lamictal ODT, Lamictal ODT Patient Titration Kit, Lamictal Starter Kit, Lamictal XR, Lamictal XR Patient Titration Kit, Lamotrigine Starter Kit.

✱ **Rx:** Apo-Lamotrigine, Gen-Lamotrigine, PMS-Lamotrigine, ratio-Lamotrigine.

SEE ALSO ***ANTICONVULSANTS***.

INDICATIONS/USES

Immediate-Release: (1) Adjunct in treatment of partial seizures in adults and children 2 years and older. (2) Adjunct in treating seizures in adults and children 2 years and older with Lennox-Gastaut syndrome. (3) Adjunct to treat primary generalized tonic-clonic seizures in adults and children 2 years of age and older. Extended-release tablets are for use in clients aged 13 and older. (4) Conversion to monotherapy in adults with partial seizures who are receiving carbamazepine, phenytoin, phenobarbital, primidone, or valproate as the single antiepileptic drug. (5) Long-term maintenance of bipolar I disorder to delay occurrence of mood episodes in those treated for acute mood episodes (depression, mania, hypomania, mixed episodes) with standard therapy. The efficacy in the acute treatment of mood episodes has not been determined. *Investigational:* Children with absence seizures; juvenile myoclonic epilepsy; and temporal lobe seizures. Depression, obesity.

Extended-Release: (1) For primary generalized tonic-clonic seizures and partial-onset seizures with or without secondary generalization in clients 13 years of age and older. (2) Conversion to monotherapy in clients 13 years and older with partial seizures who are receiving treatment with a single antiepileptic drug.

ACTION/KINETICS

Action

Mechanism of anticonvulsant action not known. May act to inhibit voltage-sensitive sodium channels. This effect stabilizes neuronal membranes and modulates presynaptic transmitter release of excitatory amino acids such as glutamate and aspartate. The mechanism for efficacy in bipolar disorder has not been determined.

Pharmacokinetics

Rapidly and completely absorbed after PO use with negligible first-pass metabolism; absolute bioavailability is 98% and is not affected by food. **Peak plasma levels, immediate-release:** 1.4–4.8 hr. **T_{max}, immediate-release:** 1–1.5 hr. T_{max} for ER product depends on whether other antiepileptic drugs are taken concomitantly. The chewable/dispersible tablets are equivalent in terms of rate and extent of absorption whether they are given as dispersed in water, chewed and swallowed, or swallowed whole as compared with compressed tablets. Metabolized by the liver with metabolites and unchanged drug excreted mainly through the urine (94%). Lamotrigine induces its own metabolism following multiple doses. $t\frac{1}{2}$, elimination varies over a wide range depending on whether lamotrigine is taken with other antiepileptic drugs. Eliminated more rapidly in clients who have been taking antiepileptic drugs that induce liver enzymes. Also eliminated more rapidly, on a body weight basis, in children compared with adults. However, valproic acid decreases the clearance of lamotrigine. **Plasma protein binding:** About 55% (does not displace other antiepileptic drugs from protein-binding sites).

CONTRAINDICATIONS

Hypersensitivity to the drug or any component of the product. Lactation. Children less than 16 years of age, other than as adjunctive therapy for generalized seizures of Lennox-Gastaut syndrome or for generalized tonic-clonic seizures in children older than 2 years.

SPECIAL CONCERNS

■ (1) Skin reactions. Lamotrigine can cause serious rashes requiring hospitalization and discontinuation of treatment. The incidence of these rashes, which have included Stevens-Johnson syndrome, is approximately 0.8% (8/1,000) in children (2–16 years of age) receiving lamotrigine immediate release as adjunctive therapy for epilepsy and 0.3% (3/1,000) in adults receiving adjunctive therapy for epilepsy. In clinical trials of bipolar and other mood disorders, the rate of serious rash was 0.08% (0.8/1,000) in adult clients receiving lamotrigine as initial monotherapy and 0.13% (1.3/1,000) in adult clients receiving lamotrigine as adjunctive therapy. In a prospectively followed cohort of 1,983 children (2 to 16 years of age) with epilepsy taking adjunctive lamotrigine immediate release, there was one rash-related death. In worldwide postmarketing experience, rare cases of toxic epidermal necrolysis or rash-related death have been reported in adult and pediatric clients, but those numbers are too few to permit a precise estimate of the rate. (2) The risk of serious rash caused by treatment with lamotrigine ER is not expected to differ from that with the immediate-release formulation of lamotrigine. However, the relatively limited treatment experience with lamotrigine ER makes it difficult to characterize the frequency and risk of serious rashes caused by treatment with lamotrigine ER. Lamotrigine ER is not approved for clients younger than 13 years of age. (3) Other than age, there are no known factors identified to predict the risk of occurrence or the severity of rash associated with lamotrigine. There are suggestions, yet to be proven, that the risk of rash may also be increased by coadministration of lamotrigine with valproate (includes valproic acid and divalproex sodium), exceeding the recommended initial dose of lamotrigine, or exceeding the recommended dose escalation for lamotrigine. However, cases have been reported in the absence of these factors. (4) Nearly all cases of life-threatening rashes associated with lamotrigine have occurred within 2 to 8 weeks of treatment initiation. However, isolated cases have been reported after prolonged treatment (e.g., 6 months). Accordingly, duration of therapy cannot be relied upon as a means to predict the potential risk heralded by the first appearance of a rash. (5) Although benign rashes also occur with lamotrigine, it is not possible to predict reliably which rashes will prove to be serious or life-threatening. Accordingly, discontinue lamotrigine at the first sign of rash, unless the rash is clearly not drug related. Discontinuation of treatment may not prevent a rash from becoming life-threatening or permanently disabling or disfiguring.

- **Use with caution with diseases or conditions that could affect metabolism or elimination of the drug, such as in impaired renal, hepatic, or cardiac function, or in the elderly.**
- **Abrupt withdrawal may increase seizure frequency.**
- **Increased risk of suicidal behavior and ideation.**
- **Sudden unexplained death has occurred (rare).**
- **Use caution with dose selection in the elderly, starting at the low end of the dosing range.**
- **Safety and efficacy in children not determined for the following: Use of the immediate-release product in bipolar disorder in children less than 18 years; use of the extended-release product in children less than 13 years; use of the immediate-release product as adjunctive treatment for partial seizures in children 1–24 months.**

SIDE EFFECTS

Most Common

When used as adjunctive therapy in adults with epilepsy: Dizziness, ataxia, somnolence, headache, diplopia, blurred vision, N&V, rash.

When used as adjunctive therapy in children with epilepsy: Abdominal pain, accidental injury, asthenia, ataxia, bronchitis, diarrhea, diplopia, dizziness, fever, flu syndrome, infection, N&V, rash, somnolence, tremor.

When used as monotherapy in adults with epilepsy: N&V, abnormal coordination, anxiety, chest pain, dizziness, dysmenorrhea, dyspepsia, infection, insomnia, pain, rhinitis, weight decrease.

When used during conversion to monotherapy (add-on) period in adults with epilepsy: Dizziness, headache, N&V, asthenia, abnormal coordination, rash, somnolence, diplopia, ataxia, accidental injury, tremor, blurred vision, insomnia, nystagmus, diarrhea, lymphadenopathy, pruritus, sinusitis.

When used for bipolar disorder: Dizziness, rash, diarrhea, dream abnormality, headache, pruritus, insomnia, nausea, somnolence.

Side effects listed are for all uses and with an incidence of 0.1% or greater or a more serious side effect. **CNS:** Dizziness, headache, ataxia, anxiety, somnolence, incoordination, insomnia, depression, tremor, intention tremor, vertigo, mania, speech disorder, irritability, agitation, ***convulsions (including withdrawal seizures), status epilepticus***, disturbed concentration, seizure exacerbation, amnesia, migraine, decreased or increased reflexes, dream abnormality, increased/decreased libido, hypesthesia, emotional lability, dyspraxia, nervousness, abnormal thinking, confusion, paresthesia, akathisia, apathy, aphasia, depersonalization, dysarthria, dyskinesia, euphoria, hallucinations, hostility, hyperkinesia, hypoesthesia, hypertonia, decreased memory, mind racing, movement disorder, myoclonus, panic attack, paranoid reaction, personality disorder, psychosis, sleep disorder, tics, stupor, gait abnormality, mania/hypomania/mixed mood episodes (when used for bipolar I disorder), cerebellar coordination/balance disorder, aseptic meningitis, ***suicidal behavior/ideation and behavior***. **GI:** N&V, diarrhea, abdominal pain, dry mouth, dyspepsia, constipation, tooth disorder, anorexia, flatulence, peptic ulcer, dysphagia, eructation, gastritis, gingivitis, increased appetite, increased salivation, mouth ulceration, esophagitis, pancreatitis, ***rectal hemorrhage***. **CV:** Migraine, flushing, hot flashes, hypertension, palpitations, postural hypotension, syncope, tachycardia, vasodilation, vasculitis, ***hemorrhage*** (in children). **Dermatologic:** Rash (both serious and nonserious), pruritus, contact dermatitis, dry skin, sweating, eczema, acne, alopecia, hirsutism, maculopapular rash, skin discoloration, urticaria, ***Stevens-Johnson syndrome, toxic epidermal necrolysis***. **Musculoskeletal:** Arthralgia, myalgia, gait abnormality, arthritis, leg cramps, myasthenia, twitching, neck/back/chest pain, rhabdomyolysis (in those experiencing hypersensitivity reactions). **Respiratory:** Rhinitis, pharyngitis, sinusitis, increased cough/exacerbation of cough, respiratory disorder, bronchitis, ***bronchospasm***, dyspnea, epistaxis, yawn, apnea, pharyngolaryngeal pain. **Hematologic:** Lymphadenopathy (including that not associated with hypersensitivity disorder), ecchymosis, anemia, thrombocytopenia, leukopenia, agranulocytosis, ***aplastic anemia, disseminated intravascular coagulation***, hemolytic anemia, neutropenia, pancytopenia, red pure cell aplasia. **GU:** Amenorrhea, dysmenorrhea, vaginitis, menstrual disorder, UTI, penis disorder, urinary frequency, abnormal ejaculation, breast pain, hematuria, impotence, menorrhagia, polyuria, urinary abnormality, urinary incontinence. **Ophthalmic:** Diplopia, blurred vision, abnormal vision, nystagmus, amblyopia, abnormal accommodation, conjunctivitis, dry eye. **Otic:** Ear disorder, ear pain, tinnitus. **Metabolic:** Weight gain/loss, peripheral/facial edema. **Body as a whole:** Fever, flu syndrome, asthenia, fatigue, paresthesia, infection, accidental injury, pain, photosensitivity, allergic reaction, chills, malaise, hypersensitivity reaction. **Miscellaneous:** Halitosis, taste perversion, worsening of parkinsonism in those with pre-existing Parkinson's disease, lupus-like reaction, ***multiorgan failure***, progressive immunosuppression, ***sudden unexplained death***.

NOTE: Women are more likely to report side effects.

OVERDOSE MANAGEMENT

Symptoms: Ataxia, nystagmus, increased seizures, decreased level of consciousness, coma, intraventricular conduction delay, ***death***. *Treatment:* There is no specific antidote. Use the following general guidelines:

- Hospitalization with general supportive care.
- Frequent monitoring of vital signs and close observation.
- Perform gastric lavage.
- Protect the airway.
- Hemodialysis may or may not be effective.

DRUG INTERACTIONS

NOTE: Lamotrigine is metabolized predominantly by glucuronic acid conjugation; drugs that induce or inhibit glucuronidation may affect the apparent clearance of lamotrigine; lamotrigine doses may need adustment. Also, lamotrigine is a weak inhibitor of dihydrofolate reductase; be aware of this action when giving other drugs that inhibit folate metabolism.

Acetaminophen / ↓ Serum lamotrigine levels; lamotrigine dosage adjustment may be required
Carbamazepine / 40% ↓ in lamotrigine levels; possible ↑ in carbamazepine levels → ↑ carbamazepine toxicity; adjust lamotrigine and/or carbamazepine doses as needed
Clozapine / ↑ Clozapine plasma levels → ↑ risk of pharmacologic/toxic effects; monitor and adjust clozapine dose as needed
Contraceptives, hormone replacement therapy / ↓ Lamotrigene levels by 50% R/T ↑ lamotrigine clearance → ↓ seizure control; maintenance dose of lamotrigine may need to be ↑ by as much as 2-fold over the recommended target dose; during hormone-free weeks, plasma lamotrigine levels may ↑ leading to side effects (ataxia, diplopia, dizziness); also, ↓ level of oral contraceptive hormones
Folate inhibitors / Lamotrigine inhibits dihydrofolate reductase
Orlistat / ↓ Lamotrigine plasma levels → ↓ pharmacologic effect; monitor and adjust lamotrigine dose as needed
Oxcarbazepine / ↓ Lamotrigine levels by 29% R/T ↑ liver metabolism; adjust lamotrigine dose as needed
Phenobarbital / 40% ↓ in lamotrigine levels → ↓ therapeutic effect; observe clinical response and adjust dosage as needed
Phenytoin / 40% ↓ in lamotrigine levels → ↓ therapeutic effect; observe clinical response and adjust dosage as needed
Primidone / 40% ↓ in lamotrigine levels → ↓ therapeutic effect; observe clinical response and adjust dosage as needed
Protease inhibitors (e.g., ritonavir) / ↓ Lamotrigine levels → ↓ therapeutic response; monitor and adjust lamotrigine dose as needed
Rifamycins (e.g., Rifampin) / ↓ Lamotrigine levels R/T ↑ liver metabolism; adjust lamotrigine dose as needed
Sertraline / ↑ Lamotrigine levels → ↑ pharmacologic/toxic effects; monitor and adjust lamotrigine dosage as needed
Succinimides (e.g., ethosuximide) / ↓ Lamotrigine levels → ↓ therapeutic effects; adjust dosage as needed

Topiramate / 15% ↑ in topiramate levels; not likely to be clinically important but monitor clinical response
Valproic acid / Twofold ↑ in lamotrigine levels; 25% ↓ in valproic acid levels; ↓ lamotrigine dose to less than ½; monitor and adjust dose of one or both drugs as needed

HOW SUPPLIED

Tablets: 25 mg, 50 mg, 100 mg, 150 mg, 200 mg, 250 mg.
Starter Kits contains Tablets 25 mg; or, 25 mg and 100 mg; ***Tablets, Chewable Dispersible:*** 2 mg, 5 mg, 25 mg; ***Tablets, Extended-Release:*** 25 mg, 50 mg, 100 mg, 200 mg.

Patient Titration Kits contain Extended-Release Tablets 25 mg and 50 mg; 25 mg, 50 mg, and 100 mg; or, 50 mg, 100 mg, 200 mg; ***Tablets, Oral Disintegrating:*** 25 mg, 50 mg, 100 mg, 200 mg.

Patient Titration Kits contain Orally Disintegrating Tablets 25 mg and 40 mg; 50 mg and 100 mg; or, 25 mg, 50 mg, and 100 mg.

DOSAGE

TABLETS; TABLETS, CHEWABLE DISPERSIBLE; TABLETS, ORAL DISINTEGRATING

Partial seizures, ***lamotrigine immediate-release*** *added to valproic acid.*

Adults and children over 12 years of age: Weeks 1 and 2, 25 mg q other day. **Weeks 3 and 4,** 25 mg every day. **Week 5 onwards to maintenance:** Increase by 25–50 mg/day q 1 to 2 weeks. **Maintenance, usual:** 100–400 mg/day in 1 or 2 divided doses (100–200 mg/day with valproate alone). **Children, 2–12 years: Weeks 1 and 2,** 0.15 mg/kg/day in 1 or 2 divided doses, rounded down to the nearest whole tablet. **Weeks 3 and 4,** 0.3 mg/kg/day in 1 or 2 divided doses; round down to the nearest whole tablet. **Week 5 onwards to maintenance:** Increase dose q 1 to 2 weeks as follows: Calculate 0.3 mg/kg/day; round this amount down to the nearest whole tablet and add this amount to the previously administered daily dose. **Maintenance, usual:** 1–5 mg/kg/day in 1 or 2 divided doses, not to exceed 200 mg/day. Give 1–3 mg/kg/day with valproate alone. Maintenance doses in children weighing less than 30 kg may need to be increased by as much as 50%, based on clinical response.

If dosage is calculated on a weight basis in children 2–12 years of age, use the following guide:

- **6.7 to 14 kg: Weeks 1 and 2:** 2 mg every other day; **weeks 3 and 4**: 2 mg per day.
- **14.1 to 27 kg: Weeks 1 and 2:** 2 mg per day; **weeks 3 and 4:** 4 mg per day.
- **27.1 to 34 kg: Weeks 1 and 2:** 4 mg per day; **weeks 3 and 4:** 8 mg per day.
- **34.1 to 40 kg: Weeks 1 and 2:** 5 mg per day; **weeks 3 and 4:** 10 mg per day.

Give daily doses using the most appropriate combination of 2 mg and 5 mg tablets. **Maintenance:** 1–3 mg/kg/day (see above).

Partial seizures, ***lamotrigine immediate-release*** *in clients taking enzyme-inducing antiepileptic drugs (e.g., carbamazepine, phenobarbital, phenytoin, primidone) and not taking valproic acid.*

Adults and children over 12 years: Weeks 1 and 2, 50 mg/day. **Weeks 3 and 4,** 100 mg/day in 2 divided doses. **Week 5 onwards to maintenance:** Increase by 100 mg/day q 1–2 weeks. **Maintenance, usual:** 300–500 mg/day in 2 divided doses. **Children, 2–12 years: Weeks 1 and 2,** 0.6 mg/kg/day in 2 divided doses, rounded down to the nearest whole tablet. **Weeks 3 and 4,** 1.2 mg/kg/day in 2 divided doses, rounded down to the nearest whole tablet. **Week 5 onwards to maintenance:** Increase the dose as follows q 1–2 weeks: Calculate 1.2 mg/kg/day and round down to the nearest whole tablet; add this amount to the previously administered daily dose. **Maintenance, usual:** 5–15 mg/kg/day, to a maximum of 400 mg/day in 2 divided doses. Doses for those weighing less than 30 kg may need to be increased by as much as 50%, based on clinical response.

*Partial seizures, **lamotrigine immediate-release** in clients not taking carbamazepine, phenobarbital, phenytoin, primidone, or valproate.*

Adults and children older than 12 years of age: Weeks 1 and 2: 25 mg/day; **weeks 3 and 4:** 50 mg/day; **weeks 5 onwards to maintenance:** Increase by 50 mg/day q 1–2 weeks; **maintenance, usual:** 225–375 mg/day in 2 divided doses.

Children, 2–12 years of age: Weeks 1 and 2: 0.3 mg/kg/day in 1 or 2 divided doses, rounded down to the nearest whole tablet; **Weeks 3 and 4:** 0.6 mg/kg/day in 2 divided doses, rounded down to the nearest whole tablet; **Week 5 onward to maintenance:** Dose should be increased every 1–2 weeks as follows: Calculate 0.6 mg/kg/day and round this amount down to the nearest whole tablet, and add this amount to the previously administered daily dose; **maintenance, usual:** 4.5–7.5 mg/kg/day, up to a maximum of 300 mg/day in 2 divided doses. Maintenance doses in children weighing less than 30 kg may need to be increased by as much as 50%, based on clinical response.

*Conversion from adjunctive therapy with carbamazepine, phenytoin, phenobarbital, or primidone, as the single antiepileptic drug to monotherapy with **lamotrigene, immediate-release**, in clients 16 years and older with epilepsy.*

Clients 16 years and older: 500 mg/day (maintenance dose) in 2 divided doses. To convert, titrate lamotrigine to 500 mg/day in 2 divided doses (according to the escalation regimen) while maintaining the dose of the enzyme-inducing drug at a fixed level. Withdraw the enzyme-inducing drug by 20% decrements each week over a 4-week period.

*Conversion from adjunctive therapy with valproate to monotherapy with **lamotrigine, immediate-release**, in clients 16 years and older with epilepsy.*

Age, 16 years and older with epilepsy: The conversion requires four steps. **Step 1:** Achieve a dosage of 200 mg/day lamotrigine (if already not on 200 mg/day according to escalation regimen, see above). Maintain previous stable valproate dose. **Step 2:** Maintain lamotrigine at 200 mg/day. Decrease valproate dosage to 500 mg/day by decrements no greater than 500 mg/day per week and then maintain the dose of 500 mg/day for one week. **Step 3:** Increase the lamotrigine dose to 300 mg/day and maintain for one week. Simultaneously decrease the valproate dose to 250 mg/day and maintain for one week. **Step 4:** Increase the lamotrigine dose by 100 mg/day every week to achieve a maintenance dose of 500 mg/day. Discontinue valproate.

Bipolar disorder, escalation regimen for lamotrigine.

For clients not taking carbamazepine, phenytoin, phenobarbital, primidone, or valproate: Weeks 1 and 2: 25 mg/day; **weeks 3 and 4:** 50 mg/day; **week 5:** 100 mg/day; **weeks 6 and 7:** 200 mg/day.

For clients taking carbamazepine, phenytoin, phenobarbital, primidone, and not taking valproate: Weeks 1 and 2: 50 mg/day; **weeks 3 and 4:** 100 mg/day in divided doses; **week 5:** 200 mg/day in divided doses; **week 6:** 300 mg/day in divided doses; **week 7:** Up to 400 mg/day in divided doses.

For clients taking valproate: Weeks 1 and 2: 25 mg every other day; **weeks 3 and 4:** 25 mg/day; **week 5:** 50 mg/day; **weeks 6 and 7:** 100 mg/day.

NOTE: To avoid an increased risk of rash, do not exceed the recommended initial dose and subsequent dose escalations.

Bipolar disorder, adjustments to lamotrigine dosing following discontinuation of psychotropic medications.

Discontinuing of psychotropic drugs (excluding carbamazepine, phenobarbital phenytoin, primidone, and val-

proate). Weeks 1, 2, and 3 and beyond: Maintain current lamotrigine dosage.

After discontinuation of carbamazepine, phenobarbital, phenytoin, or primidone (current lamotrigine dose of 400 mg/day). Week 1: 400 mg/day; **week 2:** 300 mg/day; **week 3 and beyond:** 200 mg/day.

After discontinuation of valproate (current lamotrigine dose of 100 mg/day). Week 1: 150 mg/day; **week 2:** 200 mg/day; **week 3 and beyond:** 200 mg/day.

Depression in adults (investigational).

100–500 mg/day. Dose varies when used with other antiepileptic drugs.

Obesity in adults (investigational).

25 mg/day for 2 weeks, titrated to a maximum of 200 mg/day for up to 26 weeks.

TABLETS, EXTENDED-RELEASE

*Partial seizures, **lamotrigine extended-release**, added to valproate.*

Adults and children 13 years and older, weeks 1 and 2: 25 mg q other day; **weeks 3 and 4:** 25 mg/day; **week 5:** 50 mg/day; **week 6:** 100 mg/day; **week 7:** 150 mg/day; **maintenance range (week 8 and onward):** 200–250 mg/day. Dose increases at week 8 or later should not exceed 100 mg/day at weekly intervals.

*Partial seizures, **lamotrigine extended-release**, in clients taking enzyme-inducing drugs (carbamazepine, phenobarbital, phenytoin, or primidone) but not taking valproate.*

Adults and children, 13 years and older, weeks 1 and 2: 50 mg/day; **weeks 3 and 4:** 100 mg/day; **week 5:** 200 mg/day; **week 6:** 300 mg/day; **week 7:** 400 mg/day; **maintenance range (week 8 and onward):** 400–600 mg/day. Dose increases at week 8 or later should not exceed 100 mg/day at weekly intervals.

*Partial seizures, **lamotrigine extended-release** in clients not taking carbamazepine, phenobarbital, phenytoin, primidone, or valproate.*

Adults and children, 13 years and older, weeks 1 and 2: 25 mg/day; **weeks 3 and 4:** 50 mg/day; **week 5:** 100 mg/day; **week 6:** 150 mg/day; **week 7:** 200 mg/day; **maintenance range (week 8 and onward):** 300–400 mg/day. Dose increases at week 8 or later should not exceed 100 mg/day at weekly intervals.

Conversion to monotherapy in those with partial seizures receiving a single antiepileptic drug.

Clients 13 years and older: 250–300 mg given once daily.

NURSING IMPLICATIONS

Do not confuse lamotrigine or Lamictal with labetalol (an alpha-beta adrenergic blocking agent), Lamisil (an antifungal), lamivudine (an antiviral drug), or with Lomotil (an antidiarrheal).

IMPLEMENTATION/ADMINISTRATION/STORAGE

1. *Check dosing regimens carefully; they vary significantly depending on whether other antiepileptic medication is being taken concomitantly, as well as whether immediate- or extended-release products are being used.*
2. To avoid an increased risk of rash, do not exceed the recommended initial dose and subsequent dose escalations.
3. Lamotrigine starter kits, lamotrigine orally disintegrating tablet titration kits, and lamotrigine ER titration kits provide lamotrigine at doses consistent with the recommended titration schedule for the first 5 weeks of treatment. These are intended to help reduce the potential for rash.
4. It is recommended that lamotrigine not be restarted in those who discontinue due to rash associated with prior treatment unless potential benefits clearly outweigh risks. The greater the interval of time since the previous dose, the greater consideration that should be given to restarting with the initial dosing regimen.
5. Extended-release tablets are for adults and children 13 years and older with partial onset seizures; take once daily.
6. Clients may be converted directly from immediate-release to ER tablets. The initial dose of the ER tablets should match the total daily dose of the immediate-release. However some clients on concomitant enzyme-inducing drugs may have lower plasma levels of lamotrigine

on conversion and should be monitored. After conversion, monitor carefully for seizure control as the total daily dose may need to be adjusted.

7. Dose based on the therapeutic response since a therapeutic plasma level has not been determined.
8. Use caution in selecting doses for geriatric clients.
9. If the calculated dose cannot be achieved using whole tablets, round the dose down to the nearest whole tablet.
10. If a change in seizure control or worsening of side effects is noted in clients on lamotrigine in combination with other antiepileptics, reevaluate all drugs in the regimen.
11. Discontinuing an enzyme-inducing antiepileptic drug should prolong the drug half-life, whereas discontinuing valproic acid should shorten the half-life of lamotrigine.
12. If decided to discontinue lamotrigine therapy, a stepwise reduction of dose over 2 weeks (about 50% per week) is recommended unless safety concerns mandate a more rapid withdrawal.
13. For children, ages 2 to 12 years, smaller starting doses and lower dose escalation are recommended in order to reduce the risk of rash. Thus, maintenance doses will take longer to reach.
14. Initial, escalation, and maintenance doses should generally be reduced by 25% in clients with moderate and severe hepatic impairment (without ascites) and by 50% in clients with severe hepatic impairment.
15. In women starting on estrogen-containing oral contraceptives while taking a stable dose of lamotrigine, and not taking carbamazepine, phenobarbital, phenytoin, primidone, or other drugs (e.g., rifampin) that induce lamotrigine metabolism, the maintenance dose of lamotrigine may need to be increased by as much as 2-fold in order to maintain a consistent lamotrigine plasma level. Increase the dose at the same time that the oral contraceptive is introduced and continue, based on clinical response, no more rapidly than 50–100 mg/day every week. Do not exceed dose increases at the recommended rate unless lamotrigine plasma levels or clinical response support larger increases.
16. If discontinuing estrogen-containing contraceptive therapy in women not taking carbamazepine, phenobarbital, phenytoin, primidone, or other drugs (e.g., rifampin) that induce lamotrigine metabolism, the maintenance dose of lamotrigine will likely need to be decreased by as much as 50% in order to maintain a consistent lamotrigine plasma level. The decrease in lamotrigine dose should not exceed 25% of the total daily dose/week over a 2-week period unless clinical response or lamotrigine plasma levels indicate otherwise.
17. To produce information on the effects of lamotrigine in utero exposure, pregnant clients should enroll in the North American Antiepileptic Drug Pregnancy Registry by calling 1-888-233-2334. Registration must be done by clients themselves. Information on the registry may be found at http://www.aedpregnancyregistry.org.
18. Store all tablets from 15–30°C (59–86°F).

ASSESSMENT

1. Note type, onset, characteristics of seizures, previous agents used, outcome.
2. If also prescribed other antiepileptic drugs (AED) (i.e., valproate, carbamazepine), monitor closely for adverse effects. List drugs prescribed to ensure none interact.
3. With bipolar disorder assess clinical behavioral presentation including mood, mania, and ideation; monitor for suicide behaviors.
4. Discontinue drug at first sign of rash or hypersensitivity reaction.
5. During dosing adjustments with other agents, monitor drug levels closely.
6. Reduce dose with renal or liver dysfunction and in the elderly; monitor for hypersensitivity reaction (fever, enlarged lymph nodes), CBC, renal and LFTs. Assess for blood dyscrasias and multiorgan failure during therapy.

CLIENT/FAMILY TEACHING

1. Swallow chewable dispersible tablets whole, chewed, or dispersed in water or diluted fruit juice. If chewed, drink a small amount of water or diluted fruit juice to help in swallowing and to offset bitter taste. To disperse chewable tablets, add the tablets to 5 mL (or enough to cover the drug) of liquid. About 1 min later, when tablets are completely dispersed, swirl the solution and consume the

entire amount immediately. Do not take partial amounts of dispersed tablets.

2. Swallow extended-release tablets once daily with or without food. Swallow whole; do not chew, crush, or divide.
3. Drug will be started at a low dose and then gradually increased as tolerated until maximum benefits have been obtained. Take as directed.
4. Do not stop abruptly; may cause increased seizure frequency. Drug should be gradually decreased over at least 2 weeks unless safety concerns require rapid withdrawal. If stopped for any reason, do not restart drug without instruction from provider—a dosage adjustment may be indicated if medication is restarted.
5. Do not perform activities that require mental alertness and/or coordination until drug effects realized; may cause dizziness, drowsiness, walking problems, headache, and blurred vision.
6. Immediately report loss of or changes in seizure control, sudden changes in mood/behavior, suicide ideations, or occurrence of a rash.
7. Avoid alcohol and CNS depressants. Alert all providers to this therapy.
8. Report any fever, hives, painful mouth sores, skin rash, swelling of the lips or tongue, or swollen lymph glands.
9. May cause aseptic meningitis; report any S&S such as headache, fever, nausea, vomiting, stiff neck, rash, abnormal sensitivity to light, confusion, or drowsiness.
10. Do not start or stop using birth control pills or other female hormonal products during therapy; avoid pregnancy. Report unusual changes in menstrual cycle (i.e., break-through bleeding). Some estrogen-containing oral contraceptives have been shown to decrease serum concentrations of lamotrigine.
11. Avoid prolonged sun exposure, wear sunscreen and protective clothing if exposed to avoid photosensitivity reaction.
12. Keep all F/U to assess response, labs, counselling, and adverse SE.

OUTCOMES/EVALUATE

- Control of seizures
- Mood swing stabilization with bipolar disorder

IV

Lansoprazole

(lan-**SAHP**-rah-zohl)

Classification(s): Proton pump inhibitor

Pregnancy Category: B

OTC: Prevacid 24 Hour.

RX: Prevacid, Prevacid I.V.

INDICATIONS/USES

Rx, PO.

1. Short-term treatment (up to 4 weeks) for healing and symptomatic relief of active duodenal ulcer.
2. Maintain healing of duodenal ulcer.
3. With clarithromycin and amoxicillin (triple therapy) to eradicate *Helicobacter pylori* infection in duodenal ulcer disease (active or 1-year history of duodenal ulcer). Use lansoprazole and amoxicillin (dual therapy) in those who are either allergic to, intolerant of, or resistant to clarithromycin.
4. Short-term treatment (up to 8 weeks) for healing and symptomatic relief of active benign gastric ulcer.
5. Treatment of NSAID-associated gastric ulcer in those who continue NSAID use.
6. Reduce the risk of NSAID-associated gastric ulcer in those with a history of documented gastric ulcer who required an NSAID. Use for up to 12 weeks.
7. Short-term treatment (up to 8 weeks) for healing and symptomatic relief of all grades of erosive esophagitis. Maintain healing of erosive esophagitis for up to 12 weeks.
8. Long-term treatment of pathologic hypersecretory conditions, including Zollinger-Ellison syndrome (PO only).
9. Short-term treatment of symptomatic GERD and erosive esophagitis including in children, aged 1 to 17 years.
10. Heartburn and other symptoms of GERD.

Investigational: Prevention of GI bleeding in clients receiving antiplatelets.

IV: In those who cannot take PO lansoprazole formulations for short-term treatment of all grades of erosive esophagitis. Switch to a PO formulation as soon as possible and treat for a total of 6–8 weeks.

OTC, PO: Heartburn that occurs two or more days per week.

ACTION/KINETICS

Action

Drug is a gastric acid (proton) pump inhibitor in that it blocks the final step of acid production. Suppresses gastric acid secretion by inhibition of the (H^+, K^+)-ATPase system located at the secretory surface of the parietal cells in the stomach. Both basal and stimulated gastric acid secretion are inhibited, regardless of the stimulus. May have antimicrobial activity against *H. pylori.*

Pharmacokinetics

Absorption begins only after lansoprazole granules leave the stomach, but absorption is rapid. Bioavailability is greater than 80%. **Peak plasma levels:** 1.7 hr. **Mean plasma t½, PO:** 1.5 hr, **IV:** 1.3 hr. **Onset:** 1–3 hr. **Duration:** Over 24 hr. Food does not appear to affect the rate of absorption, if given before meals. If given after meals, both C_{max} and AUC are decreased. Metabolized in the liver with metabolites excreted through both the urine (33%) and feces (66%). Clearance is decreased in the elderly. **Plasma protein binding:** More than 97%.

CONTRAINDICATIONS

Hypersensitivity to lansoprazole or any component of the product. Lactation. Use with rabeprazole.

SPECIAL CONCERNS

- **Reduce dosage in impaired hepatic function.**
- **Symptomatic relief does not preclude the presence of gastric malignancy.**
- **Safety and efficacy not determined for IV use in initial treatment of erosive esophagitis.**
- **Safety and efficacy not determined in children less than 18 years.**

SIDE EFFECTS

Most Common

Diarrhea, headache, N&V, constipation, rash.

GI: Diarrhea, abdominal pain, abnormal stools, N&V, melena, anorexia, bezoar, cardiospasm, cholelithiasis, colitis, dry mouth, enlarged abdomen, dyspepsia, dysphagia, enteritis, eructation, esophageal stenosis/ulcer, esophagitis, fecal discoloration, flatulence, gastric nodules, fundic gland polyps, gastritis, gastroenteritis, GI anomaly/disorder, ***GI hemorrhage***, glossitis, gum hemorrhage, hematemesis, ***pancreatitis***, increased appetite/salivation, mouth ulceration, oral moniliasis, rectal disorder, ***rectal hemorrhage***, stomatitis, tenesmus, tongue disorder, ulcerative colitis/stomatitis, hepatotoxicity. **CV:** Angina, bradycardia, ***cerebral infarction***, hyper-/hypotension, ***CVA, MI, shock***, palpitations, syncope, tachycardia, vasodilation. **CNS:** Headache, agitation, amnesia, anxiety, apathy, confusion, ***convulsion,*** depersonalization, depression, dizziness, emotional lability, hallucinations, hemiplegia, aggravated hostility, hyperkinesia, hypertonia, hypesthesia, insomnia, decreased/increased libido, migraine, nervousness, neurosis, paresthesia, sleep disorder, somnolence, abnormal thinking, speech disorder, tremor, vertigo. **GU:** Abnormal menses, albuminuria, breast enlargement/tenderness/pain, dysmenorrhea, dysuria, glycosuria, gynecomastia, hematuria, impotence, kidney calculus/pain, leukorrhea, menorrhagia, menstrual disorder, polyuria, penis/testis disorder, urethral pain, urinary frequency/urgency/retention, urinary disorder, UTI, impaired urination, vaginitis. **Respiratory:** Asthma, bronchitis, increased cough, dyspnea, epistaxis, hemoptysis, hiccoughs, laryngeal neoplasia, pharyngitis, pleural/respiratory disorder, pneumonia, rhinitis, sinusitis, stridor, URTI/inflammation. **Endocrine:** Diabetes mellitus, goiter, hypo-/hyperglycemia, hypothyroidism. **Hematologic:** Anemia, eosinophilia, hemolysis, lymphadenopathy, leukopenia, neutropenia, ***pancytopenia***, agranulocytosis, ***aplastic anemia***, hemolytic anemia, thrombocytopenia. **Musculoskeletal:** Arthritis, arthralgia, bone/joint disorder, leg cramps, musculoskeletal pain, myalgia, myasthenia, synovitis. **Dermatologic:** Acne, alopecia, contact dermatitis, dry skin, fixed eruption, hair disorder, maculopapular rash, nail disorder, pruritus, rash, skin carcinoma/disorder, sweating, urticaria; severe dermatological reactions, including erythema multiforme, ***Stevens-Johnson syndrome, toxic epidermal necrolysis***, thrombocytopenia, thrombotic thrombocytopenic purpura. **Metabolic:** Dehydration, edema, gout, peripheral edema, thirst, weight loss/gain. **Ophthalmic:** Amblyopia, abnormal/blurred vision, diplopia, eye pain, visual field defect, conjunctivitis, dry eyes, photophobia, retinal degeneration. **Otic:** Deafness, otitis media, tinnitus, ear disorder. **Body as a whole:** Asthenia, candidiasis, chills, fever, flu syndrome, infection, malaise, ***carcinoma, allergic reaction, anaphylactoid-like re-***

action. **Miscellaneous:** Taste loss/perversion, chest/back/neck/pelvic pain, neck rigidity, fever, halitosis, parosmia, speech disorder.

LABORATORY TEST CONSIDERATIONS

Abnormal LFTs, RBCs. ↑ AST, ALT, creatinine, alkaline phosphatase, globulins, GGTP, glucocorticoids, LDH, gastrin. ↑, ↓, or abnormal WBC and platelets. Abnormal AG ratio, RBC. Abnormal bilirubinemia, hyperlipemia. ↑ or ↓ Electrolytes or cholesterol.

DRUG INTERACTIONS

Ampicillin / ↓ Ampicillin effect R/T ↓ absorption
Clarithromycin / ↑ Lansoprazole AUC and peak plasma levels R/T inhibition of metabolism by CYP2C19
Digoxin / ↓ Digoxin effect R/T ↓ absorption
Fluvoxamine / ↑ Lansoprazole AUC and prolonged elimination $t\frac{1}{2}$ R/T inhibition of metabolism by CYP2C19
Iron salts / ↓ Effect of iron salts R/T ↓ absorption
Ketoconazole / ↓ Ketoconazole effect R/T ↓ absorption
Sucralfate / Delayed absorption of lansoprazole
Tacrolimus / ↑ Tacrolimus whole blood levels → ↑ pharmacologic/toxic effects; monitor tacrolimus levels

HOW SUPPLIED

Capsules, Delayed-Release: 15 mg (OTC or Rx) 30 mg (Rx); *Rx: Granules for Oral Suspension, Delayed-Release:* 15 mg, 30 mg; *Rx: Tablets, Orally Disintegrating, Delayed-Release:* 15 mg, 30 mg; *Rx: Powder for Injection:* 30 mg single dose vial.

DOSAGE

RX: CAPSULES, DELAYED-RELEASE; ORAL SUSPENSION, DELAYED-RELEASE; TABLETS, ORALLY DISINTEGRATING, DELAYED-RELEASE

Treatment of duodenal ulcer.

Adults, initial: 15 mg once daily before breakfast for 4 weeks.

Maintenance of healed duodenal ulcer.

Adults: 15 mg once daily.

Duodenal ulcer associated with H. pylori *infections.*

The following regimens may be used: (1) *Triple therapy.* Lansoprazole, 30 mg, plus clarithromycin, 500 mg, plus amoxicillin, 1 gram, each taken twice a day (q 12 hr) for 10 or 14 days. (2) *Dual Therapy.* Lansoprazole, 30 mg plus amoxicillin, 1 gram each taken 3 times per day (q 8 hr) for 14 days (for clients intolerant or resistant to clarithromycin).

Treatment of gastric ulcer.

Adults: 30 mg once daily for up to 8 weeks.

Reduce risk of NSAID-associated gastric ulcer.

Adults: 15 mg once daily for up to 12 weeks.

Treatment of NSAID-associated gastric ulcer.

Adults: 30 mg once daily for 8 weeks.

Gastroesophageal reflux disease (GERD).

Adults and children, 12 years and older: 15 mg once daily for up to 8 weeks. An additional 8 weeks of therapy may be given to adults who do not heal within 8 weeks. **Children, 1–11 years of age, 30 kg or less, initial:** 15 mg/day for up to 12 weeks; if symptoms remain after 2 or more weeks, can increase the dose to 30 mg twice a day. **Children, 1–11 years of age, over 30 kg, initial:** 30 mg/day for up to 12 weeks; if symptoms remain after 2 or more weeks, can increase the dose to 30 mg twice a day.

Erosive esophagitis.

Adults, and children 12 years and older, initial: 30 mg once daily before meals for up to 8 weeks. For adults who do not heal in 8 weeks, an additional 8 weeks of therapy may be given. If there is a recurrence, an additional 8-week course may be considered. **Adults, maintenance:** 15 mg once daily. **Children, 1–11 years of age, initial, 30 kg or less:** 15 mg/day for up to 12 weeks; if symptoms remain after 2 or more weeks, can increase the dose to 30 mg twice a day. **Children, 1–11 years, initial, over 30 kg:** 30 mg/day for up to 12 weeks; if symptoms remain after 2 or more weeks, can increase the dose to 30 mg twice a day.

Pathologic hypersecretory conditions (including Zollinger-Ellison syndrome).

Adults, initial: 60 mg once daily. Adjust the dose to client need. Dosage may be continued as long as necessary. Doses up to 90 or 120 mg (in divided doses) daily have been given. Some clients have been treated for longer than 4 years.

IV

Erosive esophagitis for those unable to take PO lansoprazole.

Adults: 30 mg (1 vial)/day IV infused over 30 min for up to 7 days. Switch to PO lansoprazole as soon as possible and continue for a total of 6–8 weeks.

OTC: CAPSULES, DELAYED-RELEASE

Heartburn occurring 2 or more days per week.

Adults: 15 mg (1 capsule) once daily in the morning with a full glass of water before eating for 14 days. A 14-day course may be repeated q 4 months.

NURSING IMPLICATIONS

Do not confuse lansoprazole with aripiprazole (an antipsychotic). Also, do not confuse Prevacid with Pravachol (an antihyperlipidemic).

IMPLEMENTATION/ADMINISTRATION/STORAGE

1. Consider dosage reduction in those with severe liver disease.
2. Do not crush or chew any lansoprazole PO product. Take before meals.
3. The 15 mg delayed-release capsule contains phenylalanine. Do not administer to client with phenylketonuria without approval.
4. For those unable to swallow capsules, open delayed-release capsule and sprinkle contents on a tablespoon of applesauce, *Ensure,* pudding, cottage cheese, yogurt, or strained pears and swallow immediately. Alternatively, contents of the capsule can be mixed with about 2 oz of either apple, orange, or tomato juice, mixed briefly, and swallowed immediately. To ensure complete delivery of the medication, rinse the glass with 2 or more volumes of juice and swallow contents immediately. Do not chew or crush the granules.
5. To give capsules with an NG tube in place, open capsule and mix intact granules with 40 mL of apple juice; do not use other liquids. Instill through NG tube into the stomach, flushing with additional apple juice to clear the tube.
6. The delayed-release, orally disintegrating tablets may be given with an oral syringe or NG tube. To give via syringe or NG tube, dissolve a 15 mg tablet in 4 mL water or a 30 mg tablet in 10 mL water; shake gently and give within 15 min. Refill the syringe with approximately 5 mL of water, shake gently, and flush the NG tube.
7. For delayed-release oral suspension, open packet and empty contents into container containing 2 tablespoons of water. Stir well, and drink immediately without chewing granules. If any material remains after drinking, add more water, stir, and drink immediately. Do not mix oral suspension with any liquid other than water, or with food. Do not administer oral suspension via enteral administration tubes.
8. Store in a tight container protected from moisture. Store between 15–30°C (59–86°F).
9. IV To reconstitute the powder, inject 5 mL of sterile water for injection into the 30 mg vial; the resulting solution will contain 6 mg/mL lansoprazole. Failure to reconstitute with sterile water may cause formation of precipitation/particulates. The reconstituted solution is stable for 1 hr when stored at 25°C (77°F) prior to further dilution.
10. Dilute the reconstituted solution in either 50 mL of 0.9% NaCl injection, lactated Ringer's injection, or D5W injection. Administer within 24 hr if diluted with 0.9% NaCl injection or lactated Ringer's injection, and within 12 hr if diluted with D5W injection.
11. Store powder for injection from 15–30°C (59–86°F); protect from light.
12. COMPATIBILITY D5W, 0.9% NaCl, RL.
13. INCOMPATIBILITY Do not administer with other drugs or diluents; may cause incompatibilities.

ASSESSMENT

1. List reasons for therapy, onset, duration, characteristics of S&S, other agents trialed, triggers.
2. Note findings of abdominal assessment, US, UGI, barium swallow, endoscopy. Check *H. pylori* results.

3. Review increased risk for osteoporosis-related fractures of the hip, wrist, and spine with high-dose, (defined as multiple daily doses), and long-term PPI therapy (a year or longer).
4. Monitor CBC, electrolytes, triglycerides, renal and LFTs; reduce dose with severe liver disease.

CLIENT/FAMILY TEACHING

1. Acts by decreasing the amount of acid produced in the stomach. Take as prescribed (usually 30 min before meals); do not exceed dose or share medications. Place orally disintegrating tablets on the tongue and allow to dissolve and then swallow small particles.
2. Swallow capsules whole; do not open, chew, or crush. Those who have difficulty swallowing capsules may open capsule and sprinkle the contents onto applesauce, *Ensure,* yogurt, cottage cheese, strained pears, or juices.
3. To prepare the oral suspension, empty packet contents into 30 mL water (do not use other liquids or food). Stir well and drink immediately. Do not crush/chew the granules. If any material remains after drinking, add more water, stir, and drink immediately.
4. Avoid hazardous activities until drug effects realized; dizziness may occur.
5. Follow prescribed diet and activities to control S&S of GERD. Drug should be withdrawn once condition resolved; avoid triggers.
6. May have to stop drug if severe headaches, worsening of symptoms, fever, chills, persistent diarrhea occurs.
7. Avoid alcohol, aspirin, NSAIDs, and OTC agents unless prescribed; may increase GI irritation.
8. Keep all F/U to assess response. Drug is generally for short-term use and stopped once condition is healed. Long-term effects are not known; users should be assessed periodically for adverse SE and gastric malignancy.

OUTCOMES/EVALUATE

- Suppression of acid secretion
- Healing of ulcer/erosive esophagitis
- ↓ Pain; relief of heartburn

Leflunomide

(leh-**FLOON**-oh-myd)

Classification(s): Antiarthritic drug

Pregnancy Category: X

RX: Arava.

INDICATIONS/USES

Treatment of active rheumatoid arthritis in adults to reduce signs and symptoms, to inhibit structural damage as evidenced by x-ray erosions and joint-space narrowing, and to improve physical function. *Investigational:* Juvenile idiopathic arthritis.

ACTION/KINETICS

Action

Inhibits dihydroorotate dehydrogenase, an enzyme involved in de novo pyrimidine synthesis; has antiproliferative activity and anti-inflammatory and uricosuric effects.

Pharmacokinetics

After PO, is metabolized to an active metabolite (M1). **Peak levels, M1:** 6–12 hr. **t½, M1:** About 2 weeks. M1 is extensively bound to albumin. M1 is further metabolized and excreted through the kidney (more significant over the first 96 hr) and bile. *NOTE:* Due to the long t½ and 24-hr dosing interval, a loading dose is needed to provide steady-state levels more rapidly. **Plasma protein binding:** >99.3%.

CONTRAINDICATIONS

Hypersensitivity to the drug or any component of the product. Use in pregnancy or in women who may become pregnant, lactation, in children less than 18 years of age, in hepatic insufficiency, or positive hepatitis B or C. Also, use in those with severe immunodeficiency, bone marrow dysplasia, severe uncontrolled infections, or vaccination with live vaccines.

SPECIAL CONCERNS

(1) **Pregnancy.** Pregnancy must be excluded before the start of treatment with leflunomide. Leflunomide is contraindicated in pregnant women and women of childbearing potential who are not using reliable contraception. Pregnancy must be avoided during leflunomide treatment or prior to the completion of the drug elimination procedure after leflunomide treatment. (2) **Hepatotoxicity.** Severe liver injury, including fatal liver failure, has been reported in some clients treated with leflunomide. Clients with pre-existing acute or chronic

liver disease, or those with ALT more than twice the upper limit of normal (ULN) before initiating treatment, should not be treated with leflunomide. Use caution when leflunomide is given with other potentially hepatotoxic drugs. (3) Monitoring ALT levels is recommended at least monthly for 6 months after starting leflunomide, and every 6 to 8 weeks thereafter. If ALT elevation greater than 3 × the ULN occurs, interrupt leflunomide therapy while investigating the probable cause of the ALT elevation by close observation and additional tests. If the ALT elevation is likely leflunomide-induced, start cholestyramine washout and monitor liver tests weekly until normal. If leflunomide induced liver injury is unlikely because another probable cause has been found, resumption of leflunomide therapy may be considered.

- **Use with caution with renal insufficiency.**
- **Rare, serious hepatic injury (may be fatal) can occur within 6 months of therapy in clients with multiple risk factors for hepatotoxicity.**
- **Clients have died from interstitial lung disease that developed during therapy; onset or worsening of cough or dyspnea may require further evaluation; the drug elimination process may be required (See *Implementation/Administration/Storage*).**
- **Safety and efficacy not fully evaluated in children with polyarticular course juvenile rheumatoid arthritis.**

SIDE EFFECTS

Most Common

Diarrhea, respiratory infection, hypertension, alopecia, rash, headache, nausea, bronchitis, dyspepsia, GI/abdominal pain, back pain, UTI.

GI: Diarrhea, N&V, dyspepsia, abnormal liver enzymes, GI/abdominal pain, anorexia, constipation, dry mouth, esophagitis, flatulence, gastroenteritis, mouth ulcer, colitis, constipation, esophagitis, flatulence, gastritis, gingivitis, melena, oral moniliasis, ***pancreatitis***, pharyngitis, enlarged salivary gland, stomatitis or aphthous stomatitis, tooth disorder. **Hepatic:** Cholelithiasis, hepatitis, jaundice/cholestasis, acute hepatotoxicity with ***hepatic necrosis, hepatic failure, serious hepatic injury.*** **CNS:** Headache, dizziness, paresthesia, anxiety, depression, insomnia, neuralgia, neuritis, peripheral neuropathy, sleep disorder, vertigo. **CV:** Hypertension (as pre-existing condition was overrepresented in drug treatment groups), chest pain, angina pectoris, migraine, palpitation, tachycardia, vasculitis (including cutaneous necrotizing vasculitis), vasodilation, varicose vein. **Dermatologic:** Alopecia, rash, pruritus, eczema, dry skin, acne, contact/fungal dermatitis, hair discoloration, hematoma, herpes simplex/zoster, nail disorder, subcutaneous nodule, maculopapular rash, skin disorder/discoloration/ulcer/nodule, sweating, erythema multiforme, ***Stevens-Johnson syndrome, toxic epidermal necrolysis***. **Musculoskeletal:** Back pain, joint disorder, tenosynovitis, synovitis, arthralgia, leg/muscle cramps, arthrosis, bursitis, myalgia, bone pain/necrosis, tendon rupture. **Respiratory:** Respiratory tract infection, bronchitis, increased cough, URTI, pharyngitis, pneumonia, rhinitis, sinusitis, asthma, dyspnea, epistaxis, lung disorder, ***interstitial lung disease (including pneumonitis, pulmonary fibrosis)***. **GU:** Albuminuria, cystitis, dysuria, hematuria, menstrual disorder, vaginal moniliasis, prostate disorder, urinary frequency, UTI. **Hematologic:** Anemia, including iron deficiency anemia; ecchymosis, eosinophilia; rarely pancytopenia, agranulocytosis, leukopenia, thrombocytopenia (including transient). **Metabolic:** Weight loss, hypokalemia, peripheral edema, hyperglycemia, hyperlipidemia. **Ophthalmic:** Blurred vision, cataract, conjunctivitis, eye disorder. **Body as a whole:** Asthenia, allergic reaction, angioedema, flu syndrome, pain, abscess, cyst, fever, malaise, malignancies, ***sepsis.*** **Miscellaneous:** Diabetes mellitus, hyperthyroidism, taste perversion, injury accident, hernia, neck/pelvic pain. Increased susceptibility to infections, including opportunistic infections, especially *Pneumocystis jiroveci* pneumonia, tuberculosis (including extrapulmonary tuberculosis), and aspergillosis.

LABORATORY TEST CONSIDERATIONS

↑ ALT, AST, CPK. Uricosuric effect, hypophosphatemia.

OVERDOSE MANAGEMENT

Symptoms: See *Side Effects. Treatment:* Give cholestyramine or charcoal. Dose of cholestyramine is 8 grams 3 times per day PO for 24 hr. Dose of charcoal is 50 grams made into a suspension for PO or NGT given q 6 hr for 24 hr.

DRUG INTERACTIONS

Charcoal / Rapid and significant ↓ in leflunomide active M1 metabolite
Cholestyramine / Rapid and significant ↓ in leflunomide active M1 metabolite
Hepatotoxic drugs (e.g., methotrexate) / ↑ Side effects; undertake close clinical monitoring
NSAIDs (e.g., diclofenac, ibuprofen) / Possible ↑ in the free fraction of both diclofenac and ibuprofen; when used together, monitor clinical response and adjust the NSAID dose as needed
Rifampin / ↑ M1 peak levels; use together with caution
Tolbutamide / ↑ Tolbutamide free fraction; clinical significance not known
Warfarin / Rarely, ↑ INR; closely monitor coagulation parameters and adjust warfarin dose as needed

HOW SUPPLIED

Tablets: 10 mg, 20 mg.

DOSAGE

TABLETS

Rheumatoid arthritis.

Adults: loading dose: 100 mg once a day PO for 3 days. **Adults, maintenance:** 20 mg/day; if this dose is not well tolerated, decrease to 10 mg/day. Doses greater than 20 mg/day are not recommended due to increased risk of side effects.

NURSING IMPLICATIONS

IMPLEMENTATION/ADMINISTRATION/STORAGE

1. Aspirin, NSAIDs, or low-dose corticosteroids may be continued during leflunomide therapy.
2. Use the drug elimination procedure to achieve nondetectable plasma levels (<0.02 mcg/mL) after stopping treatment: Give cholestyramine, 8 grams 3 times per day for 11 days (no need to be consecutive unless need to lower plasma levels rapidly). Verify plasma levels by 2 separate tests at least 14 days apart. Without the drug elimination procedure, it may take 2 years or less to reach plasma M1 levels of 0.02 mcg/mL due to variations in drug clearance.
3. To monitor fetal outcomes, health care providers are encouraged to register pregnant women exposed to leflunomide by calling 1-877-311-8972.
4. To minimize any potential risk, males wishing to father a child should consider discontinuing use of leflunomide, and taking cholestyramine 8 grams 3 times per day for 11 days.
5. Store from 15–30°C (59–86°F); protect from light.

ASSESSMENT

1. Note reasons for therapy, pain level, functional limitations, ROM, quality of life, joint(s) characteristics, other agents trialed.
2. Assess for liver dysfunction, hepatitis B or C, severe immunodeficiency, bone marrow dysplasia, or severe, uncontrolled infections; precludes therapy.
3. Obtain negative pregnancy test. Review risk of malignancy related to drug therapy.
4. Drug metabolite M1 has an extremely long half-life (up to 2 years). Cholestyramine may accelerate drug elimination. Women of childbearing age desiring pregnancy should undergo the drug elimination procedure to prevent fetal death or damage. Advise men wishing to father a child to consider discontinuing leflunomide, and taking cholestyramine 8 g 3 times daily for 11 days.
5. Obtain platelets, WBC, H&H, and monitor monthly for 6 months following initiation of therapy, and every 6 to 8 weeks thereafter. If used with concomitant methotrexate and/or other potential immunosuppressive agents, monitor monthly. If evidence of bone marrow suppression occurs, stop treatment with leflunomide and initiate drug elimination procedure. Monitor SGPT (ALT) and SGOT (AST) monthly; adjust dosage with elevations. If elevations persist 2–3 times ULN and continued therapy is desired, consider liver biopsy.

CLIENT/FAMILY TEACHING

1. Therapy consists of a 3-day loading dose and then a daily maintenance dose. Drug used to reduce S&S of RA, for inhibition of structural damage and improvement in physical function in those with disease.
2. May take with or without food; takes up to 8 weeks for desired effects.
3. Drug will cause fetal damage. Practice reliable birth control. If pregnancy desired or suspected in females, or males wish to father a child,

start drug elimination procedure. Do not breast-feed during therapy.
4. Avoid live vaccines during therapy.
5. May experience dizziness, diarrhea, nausea, GI upset, URI, headache, and rash; report if evident or persistent. Report any S&S of lowered blood counts: easy bruising or bleeding, recurrent infections, fever, paleness or unusual tiredness or S&S of liver dysfunction: unusual tiredness, abdominal pain or jaundice.
6. Keep all F/U to assess response, labs (monthly CBC, LFTs) and for adverse SE.

OUTCOMES/EVALUATE
- ↓ Bone erosion/joint narrowing
- Slowed RA disease progression
- Improved functioning level/quality of life

Lenalidomide

(le-na-**LID**-oh-mide)

Classification(s): Immunomodulator

Pregnancy Category: X

RX: Revlimid.

SEE ALSO ***ANTINEOPLASTIC AGENTS***.

INDICATIONS/USES

(1) Treatment of transfusion-dependent anemia due to low- or intermediate-1 risk myelodysplastic syndrome associated with a deletion 5q cytogenetic abnormality with or without additional cytogenetic abnormalities. (2) In combination with dexamethasone to treat multiple myeloma in those who have received at least one prior therapy. *Investigational:* Behçet syndrome.

ACTION/KINETICS

Action

The mechanism of action is not fully understood; the drug possesses antineoplastic, immunomodulatory, and antiangiogenic properties. It is known to inhibit proinflammatory cytokines and increase the secretion of anti-inflammatory cytokines from peripheral blood mononuclear cells.

Pharmacokinetics

Rapidly absorbed. **Maximum plasma levels:** 0.63–1.5 hr. Food does not affect the AUC but does decrease C_{max}. About two-thirds excreted unchanged in the urine. **t½, elimination:** About 3 hr. Dosage adjustment is necessary in impaired renal function. **Plasma protein binding:** About 30%.

CONTRAINDICATIONS

Hypersensitivity to the drug or any component of the product. Pregnancy and women of childbearing potential since lenalidomide is structurally similar to thalidomide. Lactation.

SPECIAL CONCERNS

■ **Warnings.** (1) Potential for human birth defects. Lenalidomide is an analog of thalidomide. Thalidomide is a known human teratogen that causes severe, life-threatening human birth defects. If lenalidomide is taken during pregnancy, it may cause birth defects or death to a fetus. Advise women to avoid pregnancy while taking lenalidomide.
(2) **Special prescribing requirement.** Because of this potential toxicity and to avoid fetal exposure to lenalidomide, the drug is only available under a special restricted distribution program called RevAssist. Under this program, only health care providers and pharmacists registered with the program are able to prescribe and dispense the products. In addition, lenalidomide is only dispensed to clients who are registered and meet all the conditions of the RevAssist program. **Consult the package insert for a detailed description of Celgene's RevAssist Program for the requirements for prescribers, male clients, and especially use in women of childbearing age.** (3) **Hematologic toxicity (neutropenia and thrombocytopenia).** Lenalidomide is associated with significant neutropenia and thrombocytopenia. Eighty percent of clients with deletion 5q myelodysplastic syndromes had to have a dose delay/reduction during the major study. Thirty-four percent of clients had to have a second dose delay/reduction. Grade 3 or 4 hematologic toxicity was seen in 80% of clients enrolled in the study. Clients on therapy for deletion 5q myelodysplastic syndrome should have their complete blood count monitored weekly for the first 8 weeks of therapy and at least monthly thereafter. Clients may require dose interruption and/or reduction. Clients may require use of blood product support and/or growth factors.
(4) **Deep vein thrombosis (DVT) and pulmonary embolism (PE).** Lenalidomide is associ-

ated with significant DVT and PE in those with multiple myeloma who were treated with lenalidomide combination therapy. Clients and health care providers are advised to be observant for the signs and symptoms of thromboembolism. Instruct clients to seek medical care if they develop symptoms such as shortness of breath, chest pain, or arm or leg swelling. It is not known whether prophylactic anticoagulation or antiplatelet therapy prescribed in conjunction with lenalidomde may lessen the potential for venous thromboembolic events. The decision to take prophylactic measures should be done carefully after an assessment of an individual client's underlying risk factors. (5) Information about lenalidomide and the RevAssist program can be obtained at http://www.revlimid.com or by calling the manufacturer's toll-free number 1-888-423-5436.

- **Use with caution in impaired renal function and in the elderly (more likely to experience diarrhea, fatigue, pulmonary embolism, and syncope).**
- **Safety and efficacy not determined in children less than 18 years of age.**

SIDE EFFECTS

Most Common

Thrombocytopenia, neutropenia, diarrhea, pruritus, rash, fatigue, dizziness, headache, dry skin, constipation, N&V, arthralgia, back pain, muscle cramps, myalgia, cough, dyspnea, nasopharyngitis, URTI, asthenia, peripheral edema, pyrexia.

Side effects listed are for all uses. **GI:** Abdominal pain, upper abdominal pain, anorexia, constipation, diarrhea, dry mouth, dysgeusia, dyspepsia, loose stools, N&V, pseudomembranous colitis, ischemic colitis, colonic polyp, diverticulitis, dysphagia, gastritis, gastroenteritis, GERD, ***GI hemorrhage***, ***intestinal perforation***, IBS, melena, obstructive inguinal hernia, ***pancreatitis*** (including that due to biliary obstruction), perirectal abscess, ***rectal hemorrhage***, small intestinal obstruction, ***peptic ulcer hemorrhage***, ***UGI hemorrhage***. **Hepatic:** Cholecystitis (including acute), ***hepatic failure***, hyperbilirubinemia, toxic hepatitis. **CV:** Hyper-/hypotension, orthostatic hypotension, palpitations, pulmonary hypertension, ***pulmonary embolism***, angina pectoris, aortic disorder, atrial fibrillation (including aggravated), bradycardia, ***cardiac arrest/failure***, CHF, ***cardio-respiratory arrest***, ***cardiogenic shock***, ***cardiomyopathy***, ***DVT***, ischemia, ***MI***, myocardial/cerebral/peripheral ischemia, pulmonary edema, supraventricular arrhythmia, tachyarrhythmia, superficial thrombophlebitis, thrombosis, ventricular dysfunction, ***subarachnoid hemorrhage***, TIA, postprocedural hemorrhage, ***cerebellar/cerebral infarction***, ***CVA***, ***postprocedural hemorrhage***, ***intracranial venous sinus thrombosis*** (when used with dexamethasone), atrial flutter, circulatory collapse, phlebitis, subacute endocarditis, limb venous thrombosis, ***intracranial hemorrhage***. **CNS:** Depression, dizziness, fatigue, headache, hypesthesia, insomnia, peripheral neuropathy, rigors, syncope, aphasia, confusion, decreased level of consciousness, dysarthria, falls, abnormal gait, vertigo, migraine, spinal cord compression, paresthesia, tremor, delirium, delusion, encephalitis, leukoencephalopathy, impaired memory, changes in mental status, decreased performance status, psychotic disorder, somnolence, brain edema. **Dermatologic:** Dry skin, ecchymosis, erythema, pruritus, night sweats, rash, increased sweating, acute febrile neutrophilic dermatosis, skin desquamation, angioedema, ***Stevens-Johnson syndrome***, ***toxic epidermal necrolysis***. **GU:** Dysuria, UTI, azotemia, ureteric calculus, hematuria, kidney infection, renal failure (including acute), renal mass, pelvic pain, metastatic prostate cancer, acquired Fanconi syndrome, renal tubular necrosis, urinary retention. **Hematologic:** Anemia, febrile neutropenia, leukopenia, lymphopenia, neutropenia, thrombocytopenia, granulocytopenia, ***pancytopenia***, acute leukemia, acute myeloid leukemia, bone marrow depression, coagulopathy, hemolysis, hemolytic anemia, lymphoma, refractory anemia, splenic infarction, warm type hemolytic anemia, ***neutropenic sepsis***. **Musculoskeletal:** Arthralgia, back/limb pain, muscle cramps/weakness, myalgia, arthritis, aggravated arthritis, chondrocalcinosis pyrophosphate, gouty arthritis, neck pain, cervical vertebral fracture, femoral neck fracture, femur/pelvis/hip/rib fracture, pelvic pain, spinal compression fracture, cerebral vertebral fracture, myopathy (including that due to steroids). **Respiratory:** Bronchitis, cough, dyspnea, exertional dyspnea, epistaxis, hypoxia, nasopharyngitis, pharyngitis, pneumonia, rhinitis, sinusitis (including acute), URTI, respiratory tract infection, hypoxia, pleural effusion, pneumonia, pneumonitis, respiratory distress, exaggerated chronic

L

obstructive airway disease, exacerbated dyspnea, interstitial lung disease, lobar pneumonia, lung infiltration, pulmonary edema, ***respiratory failure***, wheezing, bronchopneumonia, bronchopneumopathy, bronchoaveolar carcinoma, metastatic lung cancer. **Infections:** Bacteremia, central line infection, clostridial infection, *Enterobacter* sepsis or bacteremia, fungal infection, herpes viral infection, influenza, kidney infection, *Klebsiella* sepsis, localized infection, oral infection, GI infection, *Pseudomonas* infection, *Staphylococcal* infection (including pneumonia), ***Streptococcal sepsis***, urosepsis, lung infection, *Escherichia* sepsis, *Pneumocystis carnii* pneumonia, bacterial pneumonia, cytomegaloviral pneumonia, pneumococcal pneumonia, primary atypical pneumonia, infective bursitis, herpes zoster, staphylococcal cellulitis, ***sepsis***, ***septic shock***. **Ophthalmic:** Blurred vision, blindness, ophthalmic herpes zoster. **Otic:** Ear infection. **Body as a whole:** Asthenia, cellulitis, edema, peripheral edema, pain, peripheral swelling, pyrexia (including intermittent), dehydration, rigors, hypersensitivity, increased/decreased weight, diabetes mellitus, diabetes with hyperosmolarity, diabetic ketoacidosis, tumor lysis syndrome. **Miscellaneous:** Acquired hypothyroidism, adrenal insufficiency, chest pain, ear infection, contusion, gout, ***multi-organ failure***, Basedow disease, nodule, cellulitis (including staphylococcal), transfusion reaction, ***sudden death***.

LABORATORY TEST CONSIDERATIONS

↑ AST, blood creatinine, troponin I, C-reactive protein, INR. ↓ Hemoglobin, WBC. Abnormal LFTs. Hypokalemia, hypomagnesemia, hypernatremia, hypo-/hyperglycemia, hypocalcemia.

DRUG INTERACTIONS

Digoxin / ↑ Digoxin C_{max} (AUC did not change)

HOW SUPPLIED

Capsules: 5 mg, 10 mg, 15 mg, 25 mg.

DOSAGE

CAPSULES

Myelodysplastic syndrome with transfusion-dependent anemia.

Initial: 10 mg daily with water. See *Implementation/Administration/Storage* for dosage information for clients who experience thrombocytopenia or neutropenia.

Multiple myeloma.

Lenalidomide, 25 mg/day with water given as a single 25 mg capsule on days 1 through 21 of repeated 28-day cycles. The dose of dexamethasone is 40 mg/day PO on days 1 through 4, 9 through 12, and 17 through 20 of each 28-day cycle for the first 4 cycles of therapy; then, 40 mg/day PO on days 1 through 4 every 28 days. Dosing is continued or modified based on clinical and lab findings.

NURSING IMPLICATIONS

IMPLEMENTATION/ADMINISTRATION/STORAGE

1. The following dosage schedule is used for those who are dosed initially at 10 mg/day lenalidomide for myelodysplastic syndrome and who experience thrombocytopenia *within* 4 weeks of starting treatment:
   - If baseline platelets are 100,000/mcL or more, interrupt lenalidomide treatment when platelets fall to fewer than 50,000/mcL. Resume lenalidomide at 5 mg/day when platelets return to 50,000/mcL or greater.
   - If baseline platelets are less than 100,000/mcL, interrupt lenalidomide treatment when platelets fall to 50% of baseline value. Resume lenalidomide at 5 mg/day if baseline is 60,000/mcL or greater and returns to 50,000/mcL or greater.
   - If baseline platelets are less than 100,000/mcL and return to 30,000/mcL or more, interrupt lenalidomide treatment when platelets fall to 50% of baseline value. Resume lenalidomide at 5 mg/day if baseline is <60,000/ mcL and returns to 30,000/mcL or more.
2. The following dosage schedule is used for those who are dosed initially at 10 mg/day lenalidomide for myelodysplastic syndrome and who experience thrombocytopenia *after* 4 weeks of starting treatment:
   - Interrupt lenalidomide treatment when platelets are <30,000/mcL or <50,000 mcL and platelet transfusions. Resume lenalidomide at 5 mg/day when platelets

return to 30,000/mcL or more (without hemostatic failure).

3. The following dosage schedule is used for those who experience thrombocytopenia at 5 mg/day when used for myelodysplastic syndrome:
   - Interrupt lenalidomide treatment when platelets are 30,000/mcL or less or 50,000/mcL or less and platelet transfusions. Resume lenalidomate at 5 mg every other day when platelets return to 30,000/mcL or more (without hemostatic failure).
4. The following dosage schedule is used for those who are dosed initially at 10 mg/day for myelodysplastic syndrome and experience neutropenia *within* 4 weeks of starting treatment:
   - If baseline ANC is 1,000/mcL or greater, interrupt lenalidomide treatment when neutrophils fall to <750/mcL. Resume lenalidomide at 5 mg/day when neutrophils return to 1,000/mcL or greater.
   - If baseline ANC is <1,000/mcL, interrupt lenalidomide treatment when neutrophils fall to <500/mcL. Resume lenalidomide at 5 mg/day when neutrophils return to 500/mcL or greater.
5. The following dosage schedule is used for those who are dosed initially at 10 mg/day for myelodysplastic syndrome and experience neutropenia *after* 4 weeks of starting treatment:
   - Interrupt lenalidomide treatment when neutrophils are <500/mcL for 7 days or more or neutrophils are <500/mcL associated with fever (38.5°C/101°F) or greater. Resume lenalidomide at 5 mg/day when neutrophils return to 500/mcL or more.
6. The following dosage schedule is used for those who experience neutropenia at 5 mg/day when used for myelodysplastic syndrome:
   - Interrupt lenalidomide treatment when neutrophils are <500/mcL for 7 days or more or neutrophils are <500/mcL associated with fever (38.5°C/101°F) or greater. Resume lenalidomide at 5 mg every other day when neutrophils return to 500 mcL or more.
7. When used to treat multipl[illegible]se the following dosage adjustme[illegible]rom-bocytopenia or neutropenia:
   - Interrupt lenalidomide trea[illegible]nd follow CBC weekly when plate[illegible]all to <30,000/mcL. Resume lenalidomde at 15 mg/day when platelets return to >30,000/mcL or more. For each subsequent platelet count drop to <30,000/mcL, interrupt lenalidomide therapy. When platelet counts return to 30,000/mcL or more after subsequent drops, resume treatment at 5 mg less than the previous dose; do not dose below 5 mg/day.
   - Interrupt lenalidomide treatment, add granulocyte colony-stimulating factor, and follow CBC weekly when neutrophils fall to <1,000/mcL. Resume lenalidomide at 25 mg/day when neutrophils return to 1,000/mcL or more and neutropenia is the only toxicity. When neutrophils return to >1,000/mcL and there is other toxicity, resume lenalidomide at 15 mg/day. Interrupt lenalidomide for each subsequent neutrophil count drop to <1,000/mcL. When neutrophils return to >1,000/mcL or more, resume lenalidomide at 5 mg less than the previous dose; do not dose below 5 mg/day.
8. For other grade 3/4 toxicities that are related to lenalidomide, hold treatment and restart at the next lower dose level when toxicity has resolved to grade 2 or less.
9. The lenalidomide starting dose is reduced in clients with C_{CR} <60 mL/min. The recommendations for initial starting doses for clients with myelodysplastic syndromes or multiple myeloma follow:
   - For moderate renal impairment (C_{CR} >30 to 59 mL/min), give 5 mg lenalidomide q 24 hr for myelodysplastic syndromes and 10 mg q 24 hr for multiple myeloma.
   - For severe renal impairment (C_{CR} <30 mL/min not requiring dialysis), give 5 mg lenalidomide q 48 hr for myelodysplastic syndromes and 15 mg q 48 hr for multiple myeloma.
   - For end-stage renal disease (C_{CR} <30 mL/min requiring dialysis), give 5 mg lenalidomide 3 times per week following each dialysis for myelodysplastic syn-

dromes and 5 mg once a day for multiple myeloma (on dialysis days, give the dose after dialysis).

10. Store from 15–30°C (59–86°F).

ASSESSMENT

1. Note reasons for therapy, myelodysplastic syndrome (MDS)/multiple myeloma (MM), other agents trialed, outcome.
2. List all drugs/agents consumed to ensure none interact. Identify all other medical conditions; assess renal function.
3. Ensure negative pregnancy test drug teratogenic and a derivative of thalidomide causing severe birth defects or death to fetus.
4. Review increased risk of DVT and PE with multiple myeloma therapy.
5. For uninsured or underinsured, drug company participates in Patient Support Solutions; provider may call for new case application forms at 1-888-423-5436.
6. Only available through restricted distribution system; only registered providers may prescribe and dispense lenalidomide to those clients registered and that meet program requirements.
7. Chromosomal abnormality involving 5q evident in 20–30% of all MDS clients.
8. Assess for liver and renal dysfunction and follow dosing guidelines. Obtain CBC weekly during first 8 weeks of therapy and then monthly thereafter with 5q MDS and q 2 weeks × 12 weeks then monthly with MM. Follow dosing guidelines carefully under *Implementation/Administration/Storage* based on blood count and platelet results. May require use of blood product support and/or growth factors.

CLIENT/FAMILY TEACHING

1. Myelodysplastic syndrome (5q MDS) has low red blood cell counts that require treatment with blood transfusions. This is caused by bone marrow that does not produce enough mature blood cells.
2. Take capsules whole with water daily. Do not break, chew or open capsules. Do not double up on dose. No more than a 28 day supply will be dispensed at one time.
3. All providers, dispensing pharmacies, and clients must enroll in the RevAssist program and follow all of the guidelines/requirements and sign the Patient-Physician Agreement form in order to get Revlimid. Information about lenalidomide and the RevAssist program can be obtained at http://www.revlimid.com or by calling the manufacturer's toll-free number 1-888-423-5436.
4. Use caution with tasks requiring mental alertness or coordination until tolerance is determined; may cause dizziness.
5. Do not donate blood during and for 4 weeks following drug therapy.
6. Females that can become pregnant will get regular pregnancy testing weekly for 4 weeks and must agree to use 2 separate forms of birth control at the same time: 4 weeks before, during and 4 weeks after stopping drug.
7. Males, even those who have had a vasectomy, must agree to use a latex condom during sexual contact with a female who can become or is pregnant. Do not donate sperm during and for 4 weeks following therapy.
8. May experience diarrhea, rash, fatigue, itching, hives, unexplained tiredness; report if evident. Other adverse effects include birth defects, low WBCs and platelets, blood clots in the veins and the lungs. Report immediately any SOB, chest pain or sudden swelling in hands and/or feet.
9. With MDS, blood counts are checked weekly for 8 weeks then monthly thereafter; with multiple myeloma, drug is administered with dexamethasone; blood counts should be checked every 2 weeks for the first 12 weeks and then at least monthly after that.
10. Keep all F/U to assess response, labs, and for adverse SE.

OUTCOMES/EVALUATE

- Restoration of blood cells (transfusion dependent anemia) without blood transfusion with MDS
- Treatment of MM with dexamethasone

IV

Lepirudin

(leh-**PEER**-you-din)

Classification(s): Anticoagulant, thrombin inhibitor

Pregnancy Category: B

RX: Refludan.

SEE ALSO *ANTICOAGULANTS*.

INDICATIONS/USES

Anticoagulation in heparin-induced thrombocytopenia (HIT) and associated thromboembolic disease to prevent further complications. *Investigational:* Adjunct to treat unstable angina, acute MI without ST elevation, prevent deep vein thrombosis, and in those undergoing percutaneous coronary intervention.

ACTION/KINETICS

Action

Lepirudin is a highly specific direct inhibitor of thrombin. One antithrombin unit (ATU) is the amount of lepirudin that neutralizes one unit of World Health Organization preparation 89/588 of thrombin. One molecule of lepirudin binds to one molecule of thrombin, blocking the thrombogenic activity of thrombin. Thus, all thrombin-dependent assays are affected (i.e., activated partial thromboplastin time [aPTT]), resulting in an increase in aPTT.

Pharmacokinetics

t½, distribution: About 10 min; **t½, elimination:** About 1.3 hr. Systemic clearance is dependent on glomerular filtration rate. About half is excreted in the urine as unchanged drug and other fragments. Thought to be metabolized by release of amino acids via catabolic hydrolysis of the parent drug. The systemic clearance in women is about 25% lower than in men and clearance in the elderly is 20% less than in younger clients. Dose must be adjusted based on C_{CR} as elimination half-lives in marked renal insufficiency and those on hemodialysis are prolonged up to 2 days.

CONTRAINDICATIONS

Hypersensitivity to hirudins or any components of the product. Lactation.

SPECIAL CONCERNS

- **Assess risk of therapy in those with an increased risk of bleeding, including recent puncture of large vessels or organ biopsy; anomaly of vessels or organs; recent CVA, stroke, intracerebral surgery or other neuraxial procedures; severe uncontrolled hypertension; bacterial endocarditis; advanced renal impairment; hemorrhagic diathesis; recent major surgery; recent intracranial, GI, intraocular, or pulmonary major bleeding; recent active peptic ulcer.**
- **Formation of antihirudin antibodies or serious hepatic injury may increase the anticoagulant effect.**
- **Increased risk of allergic reactions in those also receiving thrombolytic therapy (e.g., streptokinase) for acute MI or contrast media for coronary angiography.**
- **Intracranial bleeding following concomitant thrombolytic therapy with alteplase may be life-threatening.**
- **Renal impairment may cause a relative overdose.**
- **Safety and efficacy not determined in children.**

SIDE EFFECTS

Most Common

Bleeding from puncture sites/wounds, anemia, hematuria, GI/rectal bleeding, fever, abnormal liver function, pneumonia.

Hemorrhagic events: Bleeding from puncture sites and wounds, anemia or isolated drop in hemoglobin, hematoma, hematuria, GI/rectal bleeding, epistaxis, hemothorax, intracranial bleeding, hemoperitoneum, hemoptysis, liver/vaginal/lung/mouth/retroperitoneal bleeding. **CV:** ***Heart failure, pericardial effusion, ventricular fibrillation.*** **Allergic reactions:** Cough, ***bronchospasms***, stridor, dyspnea, pruritus, urticaria, rash, flushes, chills, ***anaphylaxis, angioedema, facial/tongue/larynx edema.*** **Miscellaneous:** Fever, pneumonia, anemia, ***sepsis***, allergic reactions (including the skin), abnormal kidney/liver function, unspecified infections, ***multiorgan failure.***

LABORATORY TEST CONSIDERATIONS

Thrombin-dependent coagulation assays may be changed.

OVERDOSE MANAGEMENT

Symptoms: Bleeding. *Treatment:* Immediately stop administration. Determine aPTT and other coagulation levels as appropriate. Determine hemoglobin and prepare for blood transfusion. Follow guidelines for treatment of shock. Hemofiltration or hemodialysis may be helpful.

DRUG INTERACTIONS

Coumarin derivatives (e.g., vitamin K antagonists) / ↑ Risk of bleeding

Thrombolytics (e.g., alteplase) / ↑ Risk of bleeding complications and ↑ effect on aPTT prolongation

HOW SUPPLIED

Powder for Injection: 50 mg.

DOSAGE

IV

Heparin-induced thrombocytopenia and associated thromboembolic disease.

Adults, initial: 0.4 mg/kg given slowly over 15–20 seconds as a bolus dose followed by 0.15 mg/kg/hr as a continuous IV infusion for 2–10 days or longer if needed. Normally the initial dose is based on body weight; this is valid for clients up to 110 kg; for those over 110 kg, do not increase the initial dosage beyond the 110 kg body weight dose (the maximum bolus dose is 44 mg and the maximal initial infusion dose is 16.5 mg/hr). Adjust dose according to the aPTT ratio (client aPTT at a given time over an aPTT reference value, usually median of the lab normal range for aPTT). The target range for aPTT is 1.5 to 2.5. To avoid initial overdosing, do not start therapy in clients with a baseline aPTT ratio of 2.5 or more. The bolus and infusion doses must be reduced in known or suspected renal insufficiency (C_{CR} <60 mL/min or serum creatinine >1.5 mg/dL).

Concomitant use with thrombolytics.

Initial IV bolus: 0.2 mg/kg; **continuous IV infusion:** 0.1 mg/kg/hr.

NURSING IMPLICATIONS

IMPLEMENTATION/ADMINISTRATION/STORAGE

1. **IV** If client is to receive coumarin derivatives for PO anticoagulation after lepirudin, gradually reduce lepirudin dose to reach an aPTT ratio just above 1.5 before initiating PO anticoagulation. As soon as an INR of 2 is reached, stop drug.
2. Reconstitution and further dilution are to be done under sterile conditions as follows:
   - Use D5W or water for injection for reconstitution.
   - For further dilution, 0.9% NaCl injection or D5W injection is suitable.
   - For rapid, complete reconstitution, inject 1 mL of diluent into the vial and shake gently. A clear, colorless solution is usually obtained in a few seconds, but <3 min.
   - Do not use solutions that are cloudy or contain particles.
   - Use reconstituted solution immediately; it is stable for 24 hr or less at room temperature (i.e., during infusion).
   - Warm product to room temperature before administration.
   - Discard any unused solution.
3. For the initial IV bolus, use a 5 mg/mL solution. Prepare as follows:
   - Reconstitute one vial (50 mg) with 1 mL of 0.9% NaCl or water for injection.
   - To obtain a final concentration of 5 mg/mL, transfer contents of the vial into a sterile, single-use syringe (10 mL or greater capacity); dilute solution to a total volume of 10 mL using water for injection, 0.9% NaCl, or D5W.
4. For continuous IV infusion, use a concentration of 0.2 or 0.4 mg/mL. Prepare as follows:
   - Reconstitute two vials (50 mg each) with 1 mL each using either 0.9% NaCl or water for injection.
   - To obtain a final concentration of 0.2 or 0.4 mg/mL, transfer contents of both vials into an infusion bag containing 500 or 250 mL of 0.9% NaCl or D5W.
   - The infusion rate (mL/hr) is determined according to body weight).
5. COMPATIBILITY Water for injection, D5W, or 0.9% NaCl.
6. INCOMPATIBILITY Do not mix with other drugs or solutions.

ASSESSMENT

1. Note reasons for therapy, clinical presentation of heparin-induced thrombocytopenia, and associated thromboembolic disease.
2. Assess for conditions that preclude therapy: recent surgery, bleed, ulcers, etc. Note allergic reactions with thrombolytic therapy.
3. If weight is more than 110 kg, do not increase dosage beyond that weight dose.
4. Monitor carefully at all sites for evidence of excessive bleeding. Have RBCs available for transfusion.
5. Get aPTT 4 hr after first dose and at least daily during therapy (more frequently with liver/renal impairment). If aPTT ratio >2.5, stop infusion (for at least 2 hr) report. Monitor LFTs, CBC, bleeding parameters, renal function studies; reduce dose with dysfunction.

CLIENT/FAMILY TEACHING

1. **Drug is used to thin the blood and prevent blood clots in those with low platelets caused by heparin.**
2. **Report any evidence of allergic reaction, bleeding, oozing from catheter sites, under skin or gums, in urine or stools, or adverse effects.**
3. **Use soft-bristled toothbrush, electric razor, night-light, and slippers to prevent injury; avoid contact sports or aggressive hugging, juggling, or wrestling.**
4. **May experience redness or pain at injection site.**
5. **Keep all F/U to assess response, labs, adverse SE.**

OUTCOMES/EVALUATE

- Inhibition of thromboembolic complications
- PTT ratio 1.5 to 2.5

Letrozole

(**LET**-roh-zohl)

Classification(s): Antineoplastic, hormone

Pregnancy Category: D

RX: Femara.

SEE ALSO ***ANTINEOPLASTIC AGENTS.***

INDICATIONS/USES

(1) First-line treatment of advanced or metastatic breast cancer in postmenopausal women who have hormone-receptor positive disease or hormone-receptor unknown disease and where there is progression following antiestrogen therapy. (2) Extended adjuvant treatment of early breast cancer in postmenopausal women who have received 5 years of adjuvant tamoxifen therapy. (3) First-line treatment of postmenopausal women with hormone receptor-positive or hormone receptor-unknown locally advanced or metastatic breast cancer with disease progression following antiestrogen therapy. *Investigational:* Stimulation of ovulation to improve chances of pregnancy.

ACTION/KINETICS

Action

A nonsteroidal competitive inhibitor of aromatase, resulting in inhibition of conversion of androgens to estrogens. It acts by competitively binding to heme of the cytochrome P450 subunit of aromatase, leading to decreased biosynthesis of estrogen in all tissues. Does not cause an increase in serum FSH and does not affect synthesis of adrenocorticosteroids, aldosterone, or thyroid hormones.

Pharmacokinetics

Rapidly and completely absorbed. **t½, terminal elimination:** About 2 days. Steady state plasma levels after daily doses of 2.5 mg reached in 2 to 6 weeks. Slowly broken down in the liver to inactive metabolites that are excreted in urine.

CONTRAINDICATIONS

Hypersensitivity to any component of the product.

SPECIAL CONCERNS

- **Use with caution during lactation and in those with severely impaired hepatic function.**
- **Safety and efficacy not determined in children.**

SIDE EFFECTS

Most Common

Bone pain, hot flashes, flushing, back pain, nausea, arthralgia/arthritis, dyspnea, fatigue/lethargy/asthenia, headache, weight increase, increased sweating, edema.

CNS: Headache, somnolence, insomnia, dizziness, vertigo, depression, anxiety, hemiparesis. **GI:** N&V, constipation, diarrhea, abdominal pain, anorexia, dyspepsia. **CV:** Hypertension, angina, coronary heart disease, thrombophlebitis, ***MI, pulmonary embolism, thrombotic or hemorrhagic strokes***, myocardial ischemia, portal vein thrombosis, TIAs, venous thrombosis. **GU:** Renal disorders, vaginal hemorrhage, vulvovaginal dryness, breast pain, UTIs. **Body as a whole:** Fatigue, lethargy, malaise, increased sweating, viral infections, infections and infestations, peripheral edema (including lower leg), asthenia, weakness, influenza, increased or decreased weight, nonspecific pain. **Dermatologic:** Hot flashes, flushing, rash (erythematous, maculopapular, psoriaform, vesicular), pruritus, alopecia, increased sweating. **Respiratory:** Dyspnea, coughing, pleural effusion. **Musculoskeletal:** Bone/back/limb pain, arthralgia, arthritis, myalgia, fracture. **Miscellaneous:** Chest wall pain, chest pain, peripheral edema, hypercholesterolemia, hypercalcemia, postmastectomy lymphedema.

LABORATORY TEST CONSIDERATIONS

↑ AST, ALT, GGT. ↓ Lymphocyte counts. Hypercholesterolemia, hypercalcemia.

DRUG INTERACTIONS

Tamoxifen may ↓ letrozole plasma levels by about 37%; clinical significance not known

HOW SUPPLIED

Tablets: 2.5 mg.

DOSAGE

TABLETS

All uses.

Adults and elderly: 2.5 mg once per day without regard to meals. Continue until tumor progression is evident; discontinue treatment at relapse. Dosage adjustment is not needed in renal impairment if C_{CR} is greater than or equal to 10 mL/min. **Severe hepatic impairment or cirrhosis:** 2.5 mg every other day (i.e., decrease dose by 50%).

NURSING IMPLICATIONS

Do not confuse Femara with Femhrt (an estrogen-progestin combination).

ASSESSMENT

1. **Note disease onset, clinical findings, previous antiestrogen therapy, and response.**
2. **Closely monitor for reduced letrozole antitumor effects (clinical and laboratory signs) in those taking letrozole immediately after tamoxifen.**
3. **Monitor bone mineral density via (DEXA) bone scan at baseline and annually during therapy; monitor BMD closely with osteopenia.**
4. **Obtain and monitor CBC, calcium, cholesterol, renal and LFTs; reduce dose with liver dysfunction. Stop drug if tumor progression evident.**

CLIENT/FAMILY TEACHING

1. **Take as directed; may take without regard to meals.**
2. **Report any severe rash, chills, fever, diarrhea, pain, severe depression, changes in color of urine/stool or skin/sclera, SOB, or chest pain. May experience hot flashes, headaches, lightheadedness, and nausea; report if persistent.**
3. **May experience drowsiness/dizziness; use caution with activities requiring mental alertness. Avoid alcohol and OTC agents without approval.**
4. **Practice reliable contraception; may cause serious fetal harm.**
5. **Keep all F/U to assess response, labs, and for adverse SE.**

OUTCOMES/EVALUATE

↓ Tumor mass; ↓ malignant cell proliferation

IV

Leucovorin calcium (Citrovorum factor, Folinic acid)

(loo-koh-**VOR**-in)

Classification(s): Folic acid derivative

Pregnancy Category: C

RX: Leucovorin calcium.

INDICATIONS/USES

PO and parenteral: (1) Prophylaxis and treatment of toxicity due to methotrexate and folic acid antagonists (e.g., pyrimethamine and trimethoprim). (2) Leucovorin rescue following high doses of methotrexate for osteosarcoma.

Parenteral: (1) Megaloblastic anemias due to nutritional deficiency, sprue, pregnancy, and infancy when oral folic acid is not appropriate. (2) Adjunct with 5-FU to prolong survival in the palliative treatment of metastatic colorectal carcinoma. *NOTE:* It is recommended for megaloblastic anemia caused by pregnancy even though the drug is pregnancy category C.

ACTION/KINETICS

Action

Is a mixture of the diastereoisomers of the 5-formyl derivative of tetrahydrofolic acid. Does not require reduction by dihydrofolate reductase to be active in intracellular metabolism; thus, it is not affected by dihydrofolate inhibitors. Quickly metabolized to 1,5-methyltetrahydrofolate, which is then metabolized by other pathways back to 5,10-methylene-tetrahydrofolate and then converted to 5-methyltetrahydrofolate using the cofactors $FADH_2$ and NADPH. Leucovorin can counteract the therapeutic and toxic effects of methotrexate (acts by inhibiting dihydrofolate reductase) but can enhance the effects of 5-fluorouracil (5-FU).

Pharmacokinetics

Rapidly absorbed following PO administration. Is rapidly absorbed. **Peak serum levels, PO:** Approximately 2.3 hr; **after IM:** 52 min; **after IV:** 10 min. **Onset, PO:** 20–30 min; **IM:** 10–20 min; **IV:** <5 min. **Terminal t½:** 5.7 hr (PO), 6.2 hr (IM and IV). **Duration:** 3–6 hr. Excreted by the kidney.

CONTRAINDICATIONS

Pernicious anemia or megaloblastic anemia due to vitamin B_{12} deficiency.

SPECIAL CONCERNS

- **Use with caution during lactation.**
- **May increase the frequency of seizures in susceptible children.**
- **When leucovorin is used with 5-FU for advanced colorectal cancer, use lower 5-FU doses as leucovorin enhances the toxicity of 5-FU.**
- **Benzyl alcohol in the parenteral form may cause a fatal gasping syndrome in premature infants.**

SIDE EFFECTS

Most Common

Urticaria, anaphylaxis (no other side effects attributed to leucovorin alone).

Leucovorin alone. Allergic reactions, including urticaria and ***anaphylaxis.*** **Leucovorin and 5-FU. GI:** N&V, diarrhea, stomatitis, constipation, anorexia. **Hematologic:** Leukopenia, thrombocytopenia. **CNS:** Fatigue, lethargy, malaise. **Miscellaneous:** Infection, alopecia, dermatitis.

DRUG INTERACTIONS

5-FU / ↑ 5-FU toxicity
Methotrexate / High doses ↓ effect of intrathecal methotrexate
PAS / ↓ Folate levels → folic acid deficiency
Phenobarbital / ↓ Phenobarbital effect → ↑ seizure frequency, especially in children
Phenytoin / ↓ Phenytoin effect R/T ↑ rate of liver breakdown; also, drug may ↓ folate levels
Primidone / ↓ Primidone effect → ↑ seizure frequency, especially in children
Sulfasalazine / ↓ Folate levels → folic acid deficiency

HOW SUPPLIED

Injection: 10 mg/mL; ***Injection, Lyophilized Powder for Solution:*** 200 mg, 500 mg; ***Powder for Injection:*** 50 mg, 100 mg, 350 mg; ***Tablets:*** 5 mg, 15 mg, 25 mg.

DOSAGE

IM; IV; TABLETS

Leucovorin rescue after high-dose methotrexate therapy.

The dose of leucovorin is based on a methotrexate dose of 12–15 mg/m² given by IV infusion over 4 hr. The dose of leucovorin is 15 mg (10 mg/m²) PO, IM, or IV q 6 hr for 10 doses starting 24 hr after the start of the methotrexate infusion. Give leucovorin parenterally if there is nausea, vomiting, or GI toxicity. If serum methotrexate levels are greater than 0.2 micromolar at 72 hr and greater than 0.05 micromolar at 96 hr after administration, leucovorin should be continued at a dose of 15 mg PO, IM, or IV q 6 hr until methotrexate levels are less than 0.05 μM. If serum methotrexate levels are equal to or greater than 50 μM at 24 hr, or equal to or greater than 5 μM at 48 hr after administration, or if there is a 100% or greater increase in serum creatinine levels at 24 hr after methotrexate administration, the dose of leucovorin should be 150 mg IV q 3 hr until methotrexate levels are less than 1 μM; **then,** give leucovorin, 15 mg IV q 3 hr until methotrexate levels are less than 0.05 μM. If significant clinical toxicity is seen following methotrexate, leucovorin rescue should total 14 doses over 84 hr in subsequent courses of methotrexate therapy.

Advanced colorectal cancer.

Either leucovorin, 200 mg/m² by slow IV over a minimum of 3 min followed by 5-FU, 370 mg/m² IV **or** leucovorin 20 mg/m² IV followed by 5-FU, 425 mg/m² IV. Treatment is repeated daily for 5 days with the 5-day treatment course repeated at 28-day intervals for two courses and then repeated at 4- to 5-week intervals as long as the client has recovered from the toxic effects.

Impaired methotrexate elimination or accidental overdose.

Start leucovorin rescue as soon as the overdose is discovered and within 24 hr of methotrexate administration when excretion is impaired. Give leucovorin, 10 mg/m^2 PO, IM, or IV q 6 hr until serum methotrexate levels are less than 10^{-8} M. If the 24-hr serum creatinine has increased 50% over baseline or if the 24- or 48-hr methotrexate level is more than 5×10^{-6} M or greater than 9×10^{-7} M, respectively, the dose of leucovorin should be increased to 100 mg/m^2 IV q 3 hr until the methotrexate level is less than 10^{-8} M. Urinary alkalinization with sodium bicarbonate solution (to maintain urine pH at 7 or greater) and hydration with 3 L/day should be undertaken at the same time.

Overdosage of folic acid antagonists.

5–15 mg/day.

Megaloblastic anemia due to folic acid deficiency.

Adults and children: Up to 1 mg/day.

NURSING IMPLICATIONS

Do not confuse folinic acid with folic acid (Vitamin B complex).

IMPLEMENTATION/ADMINISTRATION/STORAGE

1. Oral solution stable for 14 days refrigerated or 7 days stored at room temperature.
2. If used for methotrexate (MTX) rescue, hydrate well and alkalinize urine to reduce nephrotoxicity.
3. IV Dilute with 5 mL bacteriostatic water for injection and use within 1 week. If sterile water for injection is added, use the solution immediately.
4. Administer IV solution slowly, at rate of less than 160 mg/min, because of calcium content. Further dilution with 100 to 500 mL dextrose or saline solutions for intermittent infusion may be performed.
5. Give doses higher than 25 mg parenterally because PO absorption is saturated.
6. Do not use leucovorin calcium injection containing benzyl alcohol in doses greater than 10 mg/m^2.
7. Parenteral use is preferred if there is a possibility client may vomit or not absorb leucovorin.
8. In treating overdosage due to folic acid antagonists, give as soon as possible. As the time interval between the overdosage and administration of leucovorin increases, the effectiveness of leucovorin decreases.
9. Protect from light.
10. COMPATIBILITY D5W, D10W, 0.9% NaCl, Ringer's or LR.
11. INCOMPATIBILITY Administer separately.

ASSESSMENT

1. Note reasons for therapy: replacement or rescue. For overdose therapy, administer promptly (first dose within 1 hr) whereas for rescue, after high-dose methotrexate therapy, administer first dose 24 h after beginning methotrexate infusion.
2. Note history of B_{12} deficiency that has resulted in pernicious or megaloblastic anemia. Leucovorin may obscure the diagnosis of pernicious anemia if previously undiagnosed.
3. Determine any history of seizure disorders; assess for recurrence.
4. Urine pH should be >7.0; monitor q 6 hr during therapy. Urine alkalinization with $NaHCO_3$ or acetazolamide may be necessary to prevent nephrotoxic effects.
5. Monitor renal, B_{12}, folic acid, MTX, and hematologic values. Creatinine increases of 50% over pretreatment levels indicate severe renal toxicity. Obtain daily methotrexate levels when leucovorin is used for high-dose methotrexate rescue.

CLIENT/FAMILY TEACHING

1. This drug is used to save or "rescue" normal cells from the damaging effects of chemotherapy, allowing them to survive while the cancer cells die.
2. Report immediately any skin rash, itching, uneasiness, or difficulty breathing.
3. IV therapy is used following chemotherapy; N&V may prevent oral absorption.
4. Tablets can be crushed if necessary.
5. When high-dose therapy is used, be alert for mental confusion and impaired judgment.

Safety measures and supervision help ensure safety and protection.
6. Consume at least 3 L/day of fluids with rescue therapy.
7. Keep all F/U to assess response, labs, and for adverse SE.

OUTCOMES/EVALUATE

- Symptom improvement (↓ fatigue, ↑ weight, improved mentation)
- ↑ Normoblasts (with anemia)
- MTX level $<5 \times 10^{-8}$ M
- Prevention/reversal of GI, renal, and bone marrow toxicity in MTX therapy or during overdosage of folic acid antagonists

Leuprolide acetate

(loo-**PROH**-lyd)

Classification(s): Antineoplastic, hormone

Pregnancy Category: X

RX: Eligard, Lupron, Lupron Depot, Lupron Depot-3 Month, Lupron Depot-4 Month, Lupron Depot-6 Month, Lupron Depot-Ped, Lupron for Pediatric Use.

✤ **Rx:** Lupron Depot 3.75 mg/11.25 mg, Lupron Depot 3.75 mg/7.5 mg, Lupron Depot 7.5 mg, 22.5 mg, 30 mg, 45 mg.

SEE ALSO ***ANTINEOPLASTIC AGENTS.***

INDICATIONS/USES

(1) Palliative treatment in advanced prostatic cancer when orchiectomy or estrogen treatment are not appropriate (use injection or depot 7.5, 22.5, 30 mg, or 45 mg). (2) Endometriosis (use depot 3.75 or 11.25 mg). (3) Central precocious puberty (use pediatric injection or Lupron Depot-Ped). (4) In combination with iron supplements for the presurgical treatment of anemia caused by uterine leiomyomata (use depot form, 3.75 or 11.25 mg). *Investigational:* With flutamide for metastatic prostatic cancer.

ACTION/KINETICS

Action

Related to the naturally occurring GnRH. By desensitizing GnRH receptors, gonadotropin secretion is inhibited. Initially, however, LH and FSH levels increase, leading to increases of sex hormones; decreases in these hormones will be observed within 2–4 weeks. Levels of serum testosterone and prostate-specific antigen in men with advanced prostate cancer are decreased to castrate levels.

Pharmacokinetics

Peak plasma levels: 4 hr for various doses. **t½:** 3 hr. Chronic use results in a measurable increase in body length, return to prepubertal state of reproductive organs, and cessation of menses (if present). A miniature titanium implant is available which releases leuprolide over one year and provides an alternative to frequent injections. **Plasma protein binding:** From 43–49%.

CONTRAINDICATIONS

Pregnancy, in women who may become pregnant while receiving the drug, and during lactation. Sensitivity to benzyl alcohol (found in leuprolide injection). Undiagnosed abnormal vaginal bleeding. Hypersensitivity to GnRH or GnRH agonist analogs. Use of the 7.5 mg (monthly), 22.4 mg (3-month), and 30 mg (4-month) injections in women and children. Lactation.

SPECIAL CONCERNS

- Safety and efficacy not determined in children (except Lupron Depot-PED).
- With therapy for prostate cancer, may cause increased bone pain and difficulty in urination during the first few weeks of therapy.
- At beginning of therapy may see increased signs and symptoms of central precocious puberty, endometriosis/uterine leiomyomata, and advanced prostatic cancer.

SIDE EFFECTS

Most Common

Injection site reactions, peripheral edema, general pain, hot flashes/sweats, asthenia, malaise/fatigue, decreased bone density, GI disorders, edema, testicular atrophy, skin reactions, headache, depression/emotional lability, dizziness/vertigo, N&V, headache/migraine, vaginitis.

When used for central precocious puberty. Dermatologic: Acne, seborrhea, injection site reactions (including induration, abscess), rash (including erythema multiforme), alopecia, skin striae, rash, urticaria, photosensitivity reactions, hair growth. **GI:** Dysphagia, gingivitis, N&V, hepatic dysfunction. **CNS:** Emotional lability, nervousness, personality disorder, somnolence, peripheral neuropathy, spinal fracture/paralysis. **CV:**

Syncope, vasodilation, hypotension, ***pulmonary embolism***. **Respiratory:** Epistaxis, respiratory disorders. **Musculoskeletal:** Tenosynovitis-like symptoms, fibromyalgia, decreased bone density. **GU:** Vaginitis/bleeding/discharge, cervix disorder, gynecomastia, breast disorders, urinary incontinence, prostate pain. **Body as a whole:** Body odor, fever, headache, infection. **Miscellaneous:** General pain, accelerated sexual maturity, peripheral edema, weight gain, decreased WBCs, hearing disorder, hard nodule in throat, weight gain, increased uric acid.

When used for advanced prostate cancer (all dosage forms). CNS: Dizziness, lightheadedness, general pain, headache, insomnia/sleep disorders, anxiety, agitation, lethargy, memory disorder, mood swings, nervousness, numbness, paresthesia, peripheral neuropathy, syncope/blackouts, depression, spinal fracture/paralysis, disturbance of smell/taste, vertigo, delusions, hypesthesia, abnormal thinking, amnesia, confusion, ***convulsions***, dementia. **GI:** Anorexia, constipation, flatulence, N&V, diarrhea, dysphagia, GI bleeding, dyspepsia, GI disturbance, duodenal/peptic ulcer, rectal polyps, hepatic dysfunction, gastroenteritis, colitis, eructation, thirst/dry mouth, increased appetite, ***GI hemorrhage***, gingivitis, gum hemorrhage, hepatomegaly, intestinal obstruction, periodontal abscess. **CV:** CHF, EEG changes, ischemia, high BP, heart murmur, peripheral edema, phlebitis, thrombosis, hypo-/hypertension, TIA, angina, CHF, arrhythmia, bradycardia, varicose vein, atrial fibrillation, deep thrombophlebitis, ***heart failure***, ***stroke, pulmonary embolism***. **Dermatologic:** Dermatitis, carcinoma of skin/ear, dry skin, ecchymosis, hair loss/growth, alopecia, itching, local skin reactions, pigmentation, skin lesions, erythema, transient burning/stinging, pain, mild bruising, pruritus, induration/abscess at injection site, ulceration, hot flashes, sweating, night sweats, clamminess, herpes zoster, melanosis. **Musculoskeletal:** Bone/joint/neck pain, myalgia, ankylosing spondylosis, pelvic fibrosis, backache, tremor, changes in bone density, arthralgia, limb pain/cramps, muscle atrophy, fibromyalgia, tenosynovitis-like syndrome, pathological fracture. **Respiratory:** Dyspnea, sinus congestion, cough, pleural rub, pneumonia, pulmonary fibrosis, pulmonary infiltrate, respiratory disorders, emphysema, hemoptysis, increased sputum, lung edema, epistaxis, pharyngitis, pleural effusion, hypoxia, asthma, bronchitis, lung disorder, sinusitis, voice alteration, hiccough. **Endocrine:** Impotence, decreased/increased libido, thyroid enlargement. **GU:** Gynecomastia, breast enlargement, breast tenderness/pain/soreness, urinary frequency/urgency, urinary difficulty, hematuria, decreased testicular size/testicular atrophy, UTI, bladder spasms, dysuria, incontinence, testicular/prostate pain, urinary obstruction, scanty urination, penile swelling, nocturia, erectile dysfunction, reduced penis size, balanitis, prostate pain, impotence, bladder carcinoma, epididymitis. **Hematologic:** Anemia, decreased WBCs/RBCs, hemoptysis, decreased H&H, lymphedema, lymphadenopathy. **Ophthalmic:** Blurred vision, temporal bone swelling, abnormal vision, amblyopia, dry eyes, ptosis. **Otic:** Hearing disorder, tinnitus. **Hypersensitivity:** Rash, urticaria, photosensitivity, ***anaphylaxis***. **At site of injection:** Induration, abscess. **Body as a whole:** Asthenia, diabetes, fatigue, malaise, chills, fever, lethargy, weakness, rigors, generalized edema, dehydration, general pain, infection, cellulitis, flu syndrome. **Miscellaneous:** Taste disorder, infection, inflammation, hard nodule in throat, weight gain/loss, increased uric acid, enlarged abdomen, neoplasm, abnormal healing, abscess, accidental injury, allergic reaction, cyst, hernia.

When used for endometriosis (all dosage forms). GI: Appetite changes, dry mouth, GI disturbances, N&V, thirst, altered bowel function. **CV:** Hot flashes/sweats, palpitations, syncope, tachycardia. **CNS:** Anxiety, depression, headache/migraine, emotional lability, dizziness/vertigo, insomnia, sleep disorder, changes in libido, memory disorder, nervousness, delusions, personality disorder. **Musculoskeletal:** Neuromuscular disorders. **Dermatologic:** Alopecia, ecchymosis, hair disorder, skin/mucous membrane reaction. **GU:** Dysuria, lactation, breast pain/tenderness, menstrual disorders, vaginitis. **Body as a whole:** Asthenia, pain. **Miscellaneous:** Lymphadenopathy, ophthalmologic disorders, edema, weight changes, injection site reaction.

When used for uterine leiomyomata (all dosage forms). CV: Hot flashes, sweats, tachycardia. **GI:** Appetite changes, dry mouth, GI disturbances, N&V. **CNS:** Depression, emotional lability, headache/migraine, anxiety, decreased libido, dizziness, insomnia, nervousness, paresthesias. **Respiratory:** Rhinitis. **Dermatologic:** Androgen-like effects, nail disorder, skin reactions. **GU:** Vaginitis, breast changes, menstrual disorders. **Musculoskeletal:** Joint disorder, neuromuscular disorders, changes in bone density. **Body as a whole:** Asthenia, general pain, body odor, flu syndrome. **Miscellaneous:** Edema, weight changes, conjunctivitis, taste perversion, injection site reactions.

When used for endometriosis or uterine leiomyomata (all dosage forms). CNS: Mood swings including depression, peripheral neuropathy, spinal fracture/paralysis, decreased libido, dizziness/vertigo, nervousness, paresthesias, headache, anxiety, delusions, insomnia/sleep disorders, memory disorder, personality disorder, hypesthesia, agitation, ***suicidal ideation/attempt.*** **GI:** N&V, GI disturbances, appetite changes, dry mouth, thirst, glossitis, altered bowel function. **CV:** Hypotension, hot flashes, sweats, palpitations, syncope, tachycardia, ***pulmonary embolism.*** **Musculoskeletal:** Fibromyalgia, tenosynovitis-like symptoms, neuromuscular disorders, joint disorder, myalgia. **Dermatologic:** Skin reactions, acne, hirsutism, alopecia, hair/nail disorder. **Respiratory:** Rhinitis, laryngitis. **GU:** Prostate pain, breast changes/tenderness/pain, vaginitis, dysuria, lactation, menstrual disorders, pyelonephritis, urinary disorders, lactation. **Hematologic:** Decreased WBCs, ecchymosis, lymphadenopathy. **Ophthalmic:** Conjunctivitis, ophthalmologic disorders. **At injection site:** Induration, abscess. **Hypersensitivity:** Rash, urticaria, photosensitivity reactions, asthma-like symptoms, ***anaphylaxis.*** **Body as a whole:** Asthenia, general pain, body odor, flu syndrome. **Miscellaneous:** Edema, weight gain/loss, androgen-like effects, taste perversion, facial edema, ear pain.

LABORATORY TEST CONSIDERATIONS

Injection and Depot. ↑ Calcium. ↓ WBC. Hypoproteinemia. **Injection:** ↑ BUN, creatinine. **Depot:** ↑ LDH, alkaline phosphatase, AST, uric acid, cholesterol, LDL, triglycerides, PT, PTT, glucose, WBC. ↓ Platelets, potassium. Hyperphosphatemia, abnormal LFTs. Misleading results from tests of pituitary gonadotropic and gonadal function up to 4–8 weeks after discontinuing depot therapy.

HOW SUPPLIED

Injection: 5 mg/mL; ***Injection, Depot (Eligard):*** 22.5 mg (3-month), 30 mg (4-month), 45 mg (6-month); ***Microspheres for Injection, Lyophilized (Lupron Depot, Lupron Depot-Ped, Lupron Depot-3 Month, Lupron Depot-4 Month):*** 3.75 mg, 7.5 mg, 11.25 mg, 15 mg, 22.5 mg, 30 mg; ***Powder for Injection, Lyophilized (Eligard):*** 7.5 mg.

DOSAGE

INJECTION; DEPOT INJECTION

Advanced prostatic cancer.

Injection (SC): 1 mg/day using the syringes provided. **Depot (IM):** 7.5 mg monthly, 22.5 mg q 3 months, 30 mg q 4 months, or 45 mg q 6 months.

Central precocious puberty.

Individualize, based on a mg/kg ratio of drug to body weight. Younger children require higher doses on a mg/kg ratio. **Injection, initial:** 50 mcg/kg/day SC as a single dose. If down regulation is not achieved, titrate dose upward by 10 mcg/kg/day, which is the maintenance dose. **Lupron Depot-Ped, initial:** 0.3 mg/kg/4 weeks (minimum 7.5 mg) as a single IM dose. Determine the starting dose as follows: If weight is 25 kg or less, give 7.5 mg; if weight is 25–37.5 kg, give 11.25 mg; if weight is >37.5 kg, give 15 mg. If total down regulation is not reached, titrate upward in 3.75 mg increments q 4 weeks (which will be the maintenance dose). *NOTE:* The first dose to cause an adequate down regulation can probably be maintained for duration of therapy in most children.

Endometriosis.

Depot only: 3.75 mg IM once a month or 11.25 mg IM q 3 months for at least 6 months for endometriosis. If further treatment is contemplated, assess bone density prior to beginning therapy.

Uterine leiomyomata.

Use 3.75 mg of the depot only IM monthly or one 11.25 mg IM injection for 3 months with concomitant iron therapy. The 11.25 mg depot is for women for whom 3 months of hormonal suppression is needed. Duration of therapy is 3 months or less. If further treatment is contemplated, assess bone density prior to beginning therapy.

NURSING IMPLICATIONS

IMPLEMENTATION/ADMINISTRATION/STORAGE

1. Follow manufacturer's guidelines carefully to prepare the depot form. Reconstitute only with the diluent provided; after reconstitution, the preparation is stable for 24 hr. There is no preservative so discard if not used immediately.
2. Due to different release properties, a fractional dose of the 3-month and 4-month depot formulations is not equivalent to the same dose of the monthly product; thus, do not interchange.
3. When injecting depot form, do not use needles smaller than 22 gauge.
4. Give the injection using only the syringes provided. If alternate syringes are needed, use insulin syringes.
5. For a single IM injection, reconstitute the lyophilized microspheres with the diluent provided. Withdraw the appropriate amount of diluent from the ampule (1 or 1.5 mL) using a 22-gauge needle and inject into the vial. Shake well to obtain uniform suspension which will appear milky. Withdraw entire contents into the syringe and inject immediately.
6. If using the prefilled dual-chamber syringe, the suspension will be milky. If the microspheres adhere to the stopper, tap the syringe against a finger. Remove the needle guard and advance the plunger to expel air from the syringe. Inject the entire contents of the syringe IM (Lupron) or SC (Eligard). Mix and use immediately as the suspension settles quickly following reconstitution. Reshake suspension if settling occurs.
7. Injection: Store below room temperature at 25°C (77°F) or less. Avoid freezing and protect from light. Store vial in carton until use.
8. Depot: Store Lupron from 15–30°C (59–86°F). The product does not contain a preservative; thus, discard if not used immediately. Store Eligard from 2–8°C (35–46°F); once mixed, must be given within 30 min.

ASSESSMENT

1. Note reasons for therapy, onset/characteristics of S&S, other agents trialed, outcome.
2. After 1–2 months of initiating central precocious puberty (CPP) therapy or changing doses, monitor GnRH stimulation test, sex steroids, and Tanner staging to confirm down regulation.
3. Monitor measurements of bone age for advancement every 6–12 months.
4. Obtain and monitor CBC, lipid profile, uric acid, renal and LFTs. With prostate cancer therapy, monitor response by measuring testosterone levels, PSA, and prostatic acid phosphatase.

CLIENT/FAMILY TEACHING

1. With prostate cancer, drug is used as an alternative to orchiectomy but must be administered for lifetime. With central precocious puberty, drug is given continuously until before girl reaches age 11 and before boy reaches age 12. Undergo careful instruction before assuming responsibility to administer drug therapy.
2. Hot flashes may occur with drug therapy.
3. Record weight; report gains of more than 2 lb/day or 10 lbs per week.
4. Immediately report any weakness, numbness, respiratory difficulty, or impaired urination.
5. Altered sexual effects (impotence, decreased testes size) may occur; identify appropriate resources for counseling and support.
6. Women should expect menstrual irregularities; practice nonhormonal form of contraception.
7. Increased bone pain may be evident at the start of therapy; analgesics may be used for pain control. Decreased bone density may occur with depot therapy; may cause additional bone loss with long-term use.
8. Keep all F/U to assess response, labs, and for adverse SE.

OUTCOMES/EVALUATE

- ↓ Tumor size and spread
- Inhibition of early puberty
- Improved symptoms with endometriosis

IV ᴄ̧ 📷

Levetiracetam

(**lehv**-ah-ter-**ASS**-ah-tam)

Classification(s): Anticonvulsant, miscellaneous

Pregnancy Category: C

RX: Keppra, Keppra XR.

🍁 **Rx:** Apo-Levetiracetam, CO Levetiracetam.

SEE ALSO ***ANTICONVULSANTS.***

INDICATIONS/USES

Immediate-Release Tablets, Oral Solution. (1) Adjunctive treatment of partial onset seizures in adults and children 4 years and older with epilepsy. (2) Adjunctive treatment of myoclonic seizures in adults and adolescents, 12 years and older, with juvenile myoclonic epilepsy. (3) Adjunctive treatment of primary generalized tonic-clonic seizures in adults and children 6 years and older with idiopathic generalized seizures. **Extended-Release Tablets.** Adjunctive treatment of partial-onset seizures in adults and adolescents, 16 years of age and older with epilepsy. *Investigational:* Prevention of migraines in adults, adolescents, and children; bipolar disorder in adults and adolescents; neuroleptic-induced tardive dyskinesia.

IV. (1) Adjunctive treatment of partial-onset seizures in adults and children over 16 years of age with epilepsy. (2) Adjunctive treatment of myoclonic seizures in adults and children over 16 years of age with juvenile myoclonic epilepsy. (3) Adjunctive treatment of primary generalized tonic-clonic seizures in adults and children over 16 years of age with idiopathic generalized epilepsy.

ACTION/KINETICS

Action

Precise mechanism unknown. May act in synaptic plasma membranes in the CNS to prevent hypersynchronization of epileptiform burst firing and propagation of seizure activity without affecting normal neuronal excitability.

Pharmacokinetics

Absorption of immediate-release and PO solution is rapid and almost complete and are bioequivalent in rate and extent of absorption; oral bioavailability is 100%. Food does not affect the extent of absorption but it decreases C_{max} and delays time to T_{max}. **Peak plasma levels, immediate-release:** 1 hr during fasting; **extended-release**: 4 hr. **Steady state:** Within 2 days of twice a day dosing. Not extensively metabolized in the liver. **t½:** 7 hr. Excreted through the urine as metabolites and unchanged (66%) drug. Half-life is longer (by 2.5 hr) in elderly clients. Total body clearance is reduced in those with impaired renal function.

CONTRAINDICATIONS

Lactation.

SPECIAL CONCERNS

- **Reduce dosage in clients with impaired renal function.**
- **Clearance is increased in children.**
- **Use care in dose selection in the elderly due to possible decreased renal function.**
- **There is an increased risk of suicidal behavior and ideation.**
- **Safety and efficacy not determined in children less than 4 years of age for immediate-release tablets and in children younger than 16 years of age for IV use or extended-release tablets.**

SIDE EFFECTS

Most Common

Adults: Somnolence, behavioral disorders, asthenia, headache, infection, dizziness, pain, neck pain, pharyngitis, accidental injury.
Children: Somnolence, hostility, nervousness, asthenia, vomiting, anorexia, diarrhea, rhinitis, increased cough, pharyngitis, accidental injury, fatigue.

Adults: CNS: Somnolence, headache, irritability, depression, vertigo, dizziness, depression, nervousness, amnesia, anxiety, emotional lability, hostility, paresthesia, abnormal thinking, confusion, ***convulsion, generalized tonic-clonic seizure***, insomnia, tremor, coordination difficulties (abnormal gait, ataxia), psychotic symptoms, aggression, agitation, anger, anxiety, apathy, depersonalization, ***suicidal behavior (including completed suicide).*** **GI:** Abdominal pain, constipation, diarrhea, dyspepsia, gastroenteritis, gingivitis, N&V, mouth ulceration, weight gain, ***hepatic failure***, hepatitis, ***pancreatitis.*** **Respiratory:** Pharyngitis, influenza, rhinitis, increased cough, sinusitis, bronchitis, nasopharyngitis, ***respiratory failure.*** **Musculoskeletal:** Neck pain, arthralgia, back/chest pain. **Dermatologic:** Ecchymosis, rash, alopecia. **GU:** UTI. **Hematologic:** Leukopenia, neutropenia, ***pancytopenia*** (with bone marrow suppression), thrombocytopenia. **Ophthalmic:** Diplopia, amblyopia. **Body as a whole:** Asthenia, infection, pain, accidental injury, fever, fungal infection, weight loss. **Miscellaneous:** Anorexia, accidental injury.

Children: CNS: Somnolence, hostility, nervousness, personality disorder, dizziness, emotional lability, irritability, mood swings, agitation, depression, vertigo, confusion, increased reflexes, anxiety, depressed, hypersomnia, insomnia, agitation, apathy, depersonalization, hyperkinesia, neurosis. **GI:** Vomiting, diarrhea, gastroenteritis, constipation. **Respiratory:** Rhinitis, increased cough, pharyngitis, nasopharyngitis, asthma. **Musculoskeletal:** Neck pain. **Dermatologic:** Ecchymosis, pruritus, skin discoloration, vesiculobullous rash. **GU:** Urine abnormality. **Ophthalmic:** Conjunctivitis, amblyopia, diplopia. **Otic:** Ear pain. **Body as a whole:** Asthenia, fatigue, dehydration, flu syndrome, viral infection, pain. **Miscellaneous:** Accidental injury, anorexia, facial edema.

LABORATORY TEST CONSIDERATIONS

Infrequent abnormalities in hematologic parameters (significant ↓ in total mean RBC count, mean hemoglobin, and mean hematocrit) and LFTs. ↓ WBC and neutrophil counts in children. Albuminuria.

OVERDOSE MANAGEMENT

Symptoms: Drowsiness (most common), aggression, agitation, coma, depressed level of consciousness, respiratory depression, somnolence. *Treatment:* Emesis or gastric lavage; maintain airway. General supportive care. Monitor VS. Hemodialysis may be beneficial.

L

DRUG INTERACTIONS

Carbamazepine / ↑ Risk of carbamazepine toxicity
Probenecid / Doubling of the maximum steady-state plasma level of the levetiracetam metabolite

HOW SUPPLIED

Injection Solution, Concentrate: 100 mg/mL; ***Oral Solution:*** 100 mg/mL; ***Tablets, Immediate-Release:*** 250 mg, 500 mg, 750 mg, 1,000 mg; ***Tablets, Extended-Release:*** 500 mg, 750 mg.

DOSAGE

ORAL SOLUTION; IMMEDIATE-RELEASE TABLETS

Partial onset seizures in adults and children 4 to younger than 16 years.

Adults, 16 years and older, initial: 500 mg twice a day. Can increase dose by 1,000 mg/day q 2 weeks up to a maximum daily dose of 3,000 mg. There is no evidence that doses above 3,000 mg/day confer additional benefits. For impaired renal function, use the following doses: **C_{CR}, 50–80 mL/min:** 500–1,000 mg q 12 hr; **C_{CR}, 30–50 mL/min:** 250–750 mg q 12 hr; **C_{CR}, less than 30 mL/min:** 250–500 mg q 12 hr. **ESRD clients using dialysis:** 500–1,000 mg q 24 hr; following dialysis, a 250–500 mg supplemental dose is recommended.

Children, 4 to younger than 16 years of age, initial: 20 mg/kg in 2 divided dose (i.e.,10 mg/kg twice a day). Increase the daily dose q 2 weeks by increments of 20 mg/kg to a recommended daily maintenance dose of 60 mg/kg (30 mg/kg twice a day). If the client cannot tolerate a dose of 60 mg/kg, the daily dose can be reduced. Use the oral solution in those with a body weight of 20 kg or less.

Myoclonic seizures, 12 years and older.

Initial: 500 mg twice a day. Increase the daily dose by 1,000 mg/day q 2 weeks to the recommended daily dose of 3,000 mg. See above for dosing in those with impaired renal function.

Primary generalized tonic-clonic seizures.

Adults, 16 years and older, initial: 500 mg twice a day. Increase the daily dose by 1,000 mg/day q 2 weeks to the recommended daily dose of 3,000 mg. See above for dosing in those with impaired renal function. **Children, 6 years to younger than 16 years, initial:** 10 mg/kg twice a day. Increase the daily dose q 2 weeks by increments of 20 mg/kg to the recommended daily dose of 60 mg/kg (i.e., 30 mg/kg twice a day). Use the oral solution in those with a body weight less than 20 kg.

EXTENDED-RELEASE TABLETS

Partial onset seizures.

Adults and children over 16 years of age, initial: 1,000 mg once a day. Dose may be adjusted in increments of 1,000 mg q 2 weeks to a maximum daily dose of 3,000 mg. Adjust the dose as follows in those with impaired renal function: **C_{CR} 50–80 mL/min:** 1,000–2,000 mg q 24 hr; **C_{CR} 30–50 mL/min:** 500–1,500 mg q 24 hr; **C_{CR} <30 mL/min:** 500–1,000 mg q 24 hr.

IV ONLY

Adjunct to treat partial onset seizures.

Adults and children 16 years and older, initial: 500 mg twice a day. Dose may be increased by 1,000 mg/day every 2 weeks to a maximum of 3,000 mg/day. There is no evidence that doses greater than 3,000 mg/day provide additional benefit. *NOTE:* For doses to be used in the event of impaired renal function, see dosage for partial seizures above.

Myoclonic seizures.

Adults and children 16 years and older, initial: 500 mg twice a day. Increase dosage by 1,000/day every 2 weeks to the recommended daily dose of 3,000 mg. **Maintenance:** 3,000 mg/day. Doses above 3,000 mg/day have not been studied.

Primary generalized tonic-clonic seizures.

Adults and children 16 years and older, initial: 500 mg twice a day. Increase the dose by 1,000 mg/day every 2 weeks to the recommended daily dose of 3,000 mg/day. **Maintenance:** 3,000 mg/day. Doses higher than 3,000 mg/day have not been studied.

NURSING IMPLICATIONS

Do not confuse Keppra with Kaletra (combination antiretroviral drug containing ritonavir and lopinavir).

IMPLEMENTATION/ADMINISTRATION/STORAGE

1. Withdraw levetiracetam slowly to minimize the potential of increased seizure frequency.
2. The manufacturer has established the levetiracetam pregnancy registry. Either the client or health care provider can initiate enrollment by calling 1-888-537-7734. Clients may also enroll in the North American Antiepileptic Drug Pregnancy Registry by calling 1-888-233-2334.
3. **IV** For IV use, dilute in 100 mL of 0.9% NaCl injection, lactated Ringer's injection, or D5W injection prior to administration and infuse over 15-minutes.
4. When switching from PO levetiracetam, the initial total daily IV dose should be equivalent to the total daily dosage and frequency of PO levetiracetam. At the end of the IV treatment period, the client may be switched to PO levetiracetam at the equivalent daily dosage and frequency of the IV administration.
5. Do not use if the product shows particulate matter or discoloration.
6. The IV product is physically compatible and chemically stable for at least 24 hr if mixed with compatible diluents and antiepileptic drugs.
7. Store in polyvinyl bags from 15–30°C (59–86°F).
8. COMPATIBILITY D5W, LR, or 0.9% NaCl. Levetiracetam is compatible with lorazepam, diazepam, and valproate sodium.
9. INCOMPATIBILITY Administer separately.

ASSESSMENT

1. List age at onset, history and characteristics of seizures. Note other agents trialed and outcome.
2. Identify drugs currently prescribed.
3. Assess mental status and clinical presentation.
4. Monitor VS, CBC, renal and LFTs; with impaired renal function, drug dose based on C_{CR}.

CLIENT/FAMILY TEACHING

1. Take exactly as directed; swallow immediate- or extended-release tablets whole and do not crush, chew, or break. May take with food to ↓ GI upset. Continue to take with other prescribed seizure medications.
2. If using oral solution, measure dose using dosing syringe, dosing dropper, or medicine cup. Do not measure dose using a spoon.
3. Store from 15–30°C (59–86°F).
4. May cause incoordination, dizziness and sleepiness. Do not engage in activities that require mental alertness until drug effects realized. Rise slowly from a sitting or lying position.
5. Use reliable birth control. Notify provider if pregnant or planning to become pregnant.
6. Report any unusual side effects or loss of seizure control. Do not stop suddenly. Report coordination problems, extreme sleepiness, weakness, mood or behavior changes.
7. Drug may cause changes in behavior (e.g., aggression, agitation, anger, anxiety, hostility, hallucinations, irritability) and, in rare cases, psychotic symptoms and thoughts of suicide; report immediately if evident.

L

8. Keep all F/U to assess response, labs, and for adverse SE.

OUTCOMES/EVALUATE

Control of seizures

Levobunolol hydrochloride

(lee-voh-**BYOU**-no-lohl)

Classification(s): Beta-adrenergic blocking agent

Pregnancy Category: C

RX: AKBeta, Betagan Liquifilm.

Rx: PMS-Levobunolol, ratio-Levobunolol.

SEE ALSO ***BETA-ADRENERGIC BLOCKING AGENTS.***

INDICATIONS/USES

To decrease intraocular pressure in chronic open-angle glaucoma or ocular hypertension.

ACTION/KINETICS

Action

Both beta-1- and beta-2-adrenergic receptor agonist. May act by decreasing the formation of aqueous humor.

Pharmacokinetics

Onset: <60 min. **Peak effect:** 2–6 hr. **Duration:** 24 hr.

CONTRAINDICATIONS

Use of 2 or more topical ophthalmic beta-adrenergic blocking agents simultaneously.

SPECIAL CONCERNS

- Safety and efficacy not determined in children.
- Significant absorption in geriatric clients may result in myocardial depression.
- Use with caution in angle-closure glaucoma (use with a miotic), in clients with muscle weaknesses, and in those with decreased pulmonary function.

SIDE EFFECTS

Most Common

Transient burning/stinging, blepharoconjunctivitis.

Ophthalmic: Stinging and burning (transient), decreased corneal sensitivity, blepharoconjunctivitis, iridocyclitis. **CNS:** Ataxia, dizziness, headache, lethargy. **Dermatologic:** Urticaria, pruritus. **CV:** Bradycardia, arrhythmia, hypotension, syncope.

HOW SUPPLIED

Ophthalmic Solution: 0.25%, 0.5%.

DOSAGE

OPHTHALMIC SOLUTION

Decrease IOP.

Adults, usual: 1–2 gtt of 0.25% solution in affected eye(s) twice a day or 1–2 gtt of 0.5% solution in affected eye(s) once a day (use twice a day in more severe or uncontrolled glaucoma).

NURSING IMPLICATIONS

IMPLEMENTATION/ADMINISTRATION/STORAGE

1. If IOP is not decreased sufficiently, pilocarpine, epinephrine, or systemic carbonic anhydrase inhibitors may be used.
2. Due to diurnal IOP variations, a satisfactory response to twice-daily therapy is best determined by measuring IOP at different times during the day.
3. Do not give two or more ophthalmic beta-adrenergic blocking agents simultaneously.

ASSESSMENT

1. Note reasons for therapy, disease onset, other agents trialed, eye exam findings, and pressures recorded.
2. List other drops prescribed to ensure they are not beta blockers.
3. Assess for angle-closure glaucoma, clients with muscle weaknesses, cardiac failure, decreased pulmonary function, geriatric clients; use cautiously.

CLIENT/FAMILY TEACHING

1. Used to lower pressures in the eye and to prevent vision loss.
2. Wash hands. Apply gentle pressure to the inside corner of the eye for approximately 60 sec following instillation.
3. When instilling, do not touch dropper tip to any surface, as this may result in contamination.
4. Wait at least 5 min before instilling other eyedrops.

5. Do not close the eyes tightly or blink more frequently than usual after instillation of the drug.
6. May experience transient burning, stinging, itching; report if persistent.
7. Keep all F/U to assess response and for adverse SE.

OUTCOMES/EVALUATE

↓ IOP

Levocetirizine dihydrochloride

(lee-voe-se-**TIR**-i-zeen)

Classification(s): Antihistamine, second generation, piperazine

Pregnancy Category: B

RX: Xyzal.

SEE ALSO ***ANTIHISTAMINES (H_1 BLOCKERS)***.

INDICATIONS/USES

(1) Symptomatic relief of perennial allergic rhinitis in adults and children 6 months of age and older. (2) Symptomatic relief of seasonal allergic rhinitis in adults and children 2 years of age and older. (3) Uncomplicated skin manifestations of chronic idiopathic urticaria in adults and children 6 months of age and older.

ACTION/KINETICS

Action

Levocetirizine is metabolized to the active cetirizine which is an antagonist at the H_1-histamine receptor. Not expected to have QT/QTc effects.

Pharmacokinetics

Rapidly and extensively absorbed. **Peak plasma levels, adults:** 0.9 hr. **Steady state:** 2 days. A high fat meal delays T_{max} and decreases C_{max} but not significantly. Metabolized in part by CYP3A4. Excreted in the urine (about 85%) and feces (about 13%). **t½, plasma, adults:** 8 hr. **Plasma protein binding:** 91–92%.

CONTRAINDICATIONS

Hypersensitivity to levocetirizine or any component of the product. End-stage renal disease (C_{CR} <10 mL/min or those on hemodialysis). Children, 6–11 years of age with impaired renal function. Use during lactation is not recommended.

SPECIAL CONCERNS

- Use caution in dose selection in the elderly.
- Safety and efficacy not determined in children less than 6 years of age.

SIDE EFFECTS

Most Common

Adults: Somnolence, fatigue, asthenia, pharyngitis, nasopharyngitis, dry mouth.
Children, 6–12 years: Pyrexia, cough, somnolence, epistaxis.
See *Antihistamines (H_1-Blockers)* for a complete list of potential side effects. Also, **CNS:** Somnolence, ***convulsion***, aggression, agitation, hallucinations, ***suicidal ideation.*** **GI:** Dry mouth, nausea, hepatitis, cholestasis. **CV:** Syncope, palpitations, hypotension. **Dermatologic:** Pruritus, rash, urticaria. **Respiratory:** Pharyngitis, nasopharyngitis, epistaxis, cough, dyspnea. **Musculoskeletal:** Myalgia, orofacial dyskinesia. **Body as a whole:** Asthenia, fatigue, pyrexia, ***anaphylaxis***, hypersensitivity, ***angioneurotic edema***, fixed drug eruption, weight gain. **Miscellaneous:** Visual disturbances, glomerulonephritis, ***still birth.***

LABORATORY TEST CONSIDERATIONS

↑ Blood bilirubin, transaminases.

OVERDOSE MANAGEMENT

Symptoms: Drowsiness in adults and agitation and restlessness in children followed by drowsiness. *Treatment:* Symptomatic and supportive treatment. There is no specific antidote. The drug is not effectively removed by dialysis.

DRUG INTERACTIONS

Ritonavir / ↑ Cetirizine (active metabolite) AUC and t½; ↓ cetirizine clearance
Theophylline / Small (16%) ↓ clearance of cetirizine (active metabolite)

HOW SUPPLIED

Oral Solution: 2.5 mg/5 mL (0.5 mg/mL); ***Tablets:*** 5 mg.

DOSAGE

ORAL SOLUTION; TABLETS

Allergic rhinitis (perennial, seasonal), chronic idiopathic urticaria.

Adults and children, 12 years and older: 5 mg (1 tablet or 10 mL oral solution) once daily in the evening. Some may be controlled adequately by 2.5 mg (½ tablet or 5 mL oral solution) once daily in the evening. **Children, 6–11 years of age:** 2.5 mg (½ tablet or 5 mL oral solution) once daily in the evening; do not exceed this dose. **Children, 6 months to 5 years of age:** 1.25 mg (2.5 mL of oral solution) once daily in the evening. Do not exceed this dose.

NURSING IMPLICATIONS

IMPLEMENTATION/ADMINISTRATION/STORAGE

1. For mild impaired renal function (C_{CR} 50–80 mL/min), use a dose of 2.5 mg once daily. For moderate impaired renal function (C_{CR} 50–80 mL/min), use a dose of 2.5 mg every other day. For severe impaired renal function (C_{CR} 10–30 mL/min), use a dose of 2.5 mg given twice a week (once q 3–4 days). Do not use in clients with end-stage renal disease (C_{CR} <10 mL/min) or in hemodialysis clients.
2. No dosage adjustment is needed in those with only impaired hepatic function. Adjust the dose as recommended in clients with both hepatic and renal function impairment.
3. Store from 15–30°C (59–86°F).

ASSESSMENT

1. Note onset, characteristics of S&S, and clinical presentation; identify triggers/time of year.
2. List other agents trialed, length of use, outcome.
3. Assess renal and liver function; adjust dose with renal dysfunction.

CLIENT/FAMILY TEACHING

1. May take with or without food; take only prescribed dose as increased dose will increase risk of somnolence
2. Use caution when performing activities that require mental alertness; may cause drowsiness/sedation.
3. May cause dry mouth, fatigue; report adverse effects that prevent taking medications. Increase fluid intake to thin secretions.
4. Avoid alcohol/CNS depressants, and other OTC antihistamines; increases sedative effects.
5. Report any behavioral changes, aggressiveness, or evidence of seizures.
6. Practice reliable contraception; may cause still birth.
7. Review allergens that trigger symptoms, e.g., ragweed, dust mites, molds, animal dander, etc., and how to control/avoid contact.
8. Keep all F/U to assess response, labs, and for adverse SE.

OUTCOMES/EVALUATE

- Control of symptoms of seasonal allergic rhinitis (i.e., ↓ sneezing, pruritus, nasal congestion, watery/red eyes, itchy eyes/nose)
- ↓ Pruritus with idiopathic urticaria

Levodopa

(lee-voh-**DOH**-pah)

Classification(s): Antiparkinson drug

RX: L-Dopa.

INDICATIONS/USES

Idiopathic, arteriosclerotic, or postencephalitic parkinsonism due to carbon monoxide or manganese intoxication and in the elderly associated with cerebral arteriosclerosis. Not effective in drug-induced extrapyramidal symptoms. Levodopa only provides symptomatic relief and does not alter the course of the disease. When effective, it relieves rigidity, bradykinesia, tremors, dysphagia, seborrhea, sialorrhea, and postural instability. *NOTE:* Often used in combination with carbidopa. See *Carbidopa/Levodopa. Investigational:* Pain from herpes zoster; restless legs syndrome.

ACTION/KINETICS

Action

Depletion of dopamine in the striatum of the brain is thought to cause the symptoms of Parkinson's disease. Levodopa, a dopamine precursor, is able to cross the blood-brain barrier to enter the CNS. It is decarboxylated to dopamine in the basal ganglia, thus replenishing depleted dopamine stores.

Pharmacokinetics

Peak plasma levels: 0.5–2 hr (may be delayed if ingested with food). **t½, plasma:** 1–3 hr. **Onset:** 2–3 weeks, although some clients may require up to 6 months. Extensively metabolized (>95%)

both in the periphery and the liver; metabolites are excreted in the urine.

CONTRAINDICATIONS

Concomitant use with MAOIs, except MAO-B inhibitors (e.g., selegiline). History of melanoma or in clients with undiagnosed skin lesions. Lactation. Hypersensitivity to drug, narrow-angle glaucoma, blood dyscrasias, hypertension, coronary sclerosis.

SPECIAL CONCERNS

- **Use with extreme caution in clients with history of MIs, convulsions, arrhythmias, bronchial asthma, emphysema, active peptic ulcer, psychosis or neurosis, wide-angle glaucoma, and renal, hepatic, or endocrine diseases.**
- **Use during pregnancy only if benefits clearly outweigh risks.**
- **Elderly may require a lower dose due to a reduced tolerance for the drug and its side effects (including cardiac effects).**
- **Clients may experience an "on-off" phenomenon, i.e., an improved clinical status followed by loss of therapeutic effect.**
- **Safety not established in children less than 12 years of age.**

SIDE EFFECTS

Most Common

Choreiform and/or dystonic movements, anorexia, N&V, abdominal pain, dry mouth, dysphagia, dysgeusia, headache, dizziness, sialorrhea, malaise, fatigue, euphoria.

The side effects of levodopa are numerous and usually dose related. Some may abate with usage. **CNS:** Choreiform and/or dystonic movements, sudden sleep attacks, paranoid ideation, psychotic episodes, depression (with possibility of suicidal tendencies), dementia, ***seizures*** (rare), dizziness, headache, faintness, confusion, insomnia, nightmares, hallucinations, delusions, agitation, anxiety, malaise, fatigue, euphoria. **GI:** N&V, anorexia, abdominal pain, dry mouth, sialorrhea, dysphagia, dysgeusia, hiccoughs, diarrhea, constipation, burning sensation of tongue, bitter taste, flatulence, weight gain/loss, ***upper GI hemorrhage*** (in clients with a history of peptic ulcer), GI bleeding (rare), duodenal ulcer (rare). **CV:** Cardiac irregularities, palpitations, orthostatic hypo-/hypertension, phlebitis, hot flashes. **Ophthalmic:** Diplopia, dilated pupils, blurred vision, development of Horner's syndrome, oculogyric crisis. **Hematologic: *Hemolytic anemia, agranulocytosis***, leukopenia. **Musculoskeletal:** Muscle twitching (early sign of overdose), tonic contraction of the muscles of mastication, increased hand tremor, ataxia. **Miscellaneous:** Blepharospasm (early sign of overdose), urinary retention/incontinence, increased sweating, unusual breathing patterns, weakness, numbness, bruxism, alopecia, priapism, hoarseness, edema, dark sweat/urine, flushing, skin rash, sense of stimulation. Levodopa interacts with many other drugs (see *Drug Interactions*) and must be administered cautiously.

LABORATORY TEST CONSIDERATIONS

↑ BUN, AST, LDH, ALT, bilirubin, alkaline phosphatase, protein-bound iodine, uric acid (with colorimetric test). ↓ H&H, WBCs. False + Coombs' test. Interference with tests for urinary glucose and ketones.

OVERDOSE MANAGEMENT

Symptoms: Muscle twitching, blepharospasm. Also see *Side Effects. Treatment:* Immediate gastric lavage for acute overdose. Maintain airway and give IV fluids carefully. General supportive measures.

DRUG INTERACTIONS

Antacids / ↑ Effect of levodopa R/T ↑ absorption from GI tract
Anticholinergic drugs / Possible ↓ levodopa effect R/T ↑ levodopa breakdown in stomach (R/T delayed gastric emptying time)
Antidepressants, tricyclic / ↓ Levodopa effect R/T ↓ GI tract absorption; also, ↑ risk of hypertension
Benzodiazepines / ↓ Levodopa effect
Clonidine / ↓ Levodopa effect
Digoxin / ↓ Digoxin effect
Furazolidone / ↑ Levodopa effect R/T ↓ liver breakdown
Guanethidine / ↑ Hypotensive drug effect
Hypoglycemic drugs / Levodopa upsets diabetic control with hypoglycemic agents
H ***Indian snakeroot*** / ↓ Effect of levodopa but ↑ extrapyramidal symptoms
MAOIs / Concomitant administration may result in hypertension, light-headedness, and flushing R/T ↓ breakdown of dopamine and norepinephrine formed from levodopa
Methionine / ↓ Levodopa effect
Methyldopa / Additive effects including hypotension

Metoclopramide / ↑ Bioavailability of levodopa; ↓ metoclopramide effect
Papaverine / ↓ Levodopa effect
Phenothiazines / ↓ Levodopa effect R/T ↓ neuronal uptake of dopamine
Phenytoin / Antagonizes levodopa effect
Propranolol / May antagonize the hypotensive and positive inotropic effect of levodopa
Pyridoxine / Reverses levodopa-induced improvement in Parkinson's disease
Thioxanthines / ↓ Levodopa effect in Parkinson clients
Tricyclic antidepressants / ↓ Levodopa absorption and bioavailability → ↓ effect

HOW SUPPLIED

Capsules: 100 mg, 250 mg, 500 mg; *Tablets:* 100 mg, 250 mg.

DOSAGE

CAPSULES; TABLETS

Parkinsonism.

Adults, initial: 250 mg 2–4 times per day taken with food; **then,** increase total daily dose by no more than 750 mg/day q 3–7 days until optimum dosage reached (should not exceed 8 grams/day). Up to 6 months may be required to achieve a significant therapeutic effect.

NURSING IMPLICATIONS

IMPLEMENTATION/ADMINISTRATION/STORAGE

1. If unable to swallow tablets or capsules, crush tablets or empty the capsule into a small amount of fruit juice at the time of administration.
2. Often administered together with an anticholinergic agent.

ASSESSMENT

1. Assess condition, note onset, and document baseline rigidity, tremors, motor function, and involuntary movements R/T Parkinson's disease. Note mental status.
2. Review medical history for any contraindications to therapy. Stop drug 24 hr before surgery and note when drug is to be restarted.
3. Identify adverse effects that may require ↓ drug dose or "drug holiday." Very low dose therapy used with RLS.
4. Monitor VS, Wt, ECG, CBC, liver/renal function studies, and PBI tests.

CLIENT/FAMILY TEACHING

1. Take exactly as prescribed; may take with food to decrease GI upset. Dosage should not exceed 8 grams/day; do not stop abruptly.
2. May cause dizziness or drowsiness. Do not perform tasks that require mental alertness until drug effects realized. Change from a sitting or lying position slowly, and wear elastic hose to decrease dizziness.
3. Report headaches; may indicate drug-induced glaucoma. Twitching or eye spasms may indicate toxicity.
4. Avoid fortified cereals, taking multivitamin preparations containing 10–25 mg of B_6 as they may reverse the antiparkinson effect. *Larobec* is a form of multivitamin that does not contain pyridoxine.
5. Significant results may take up to 6 months to be realized.
6. Sweat and urine may appear dark; this is not harmful.
7. If sustained erection occurs; report immediately.
8. Report any evidence of depression or psychosis, other unusual mental or behavioral changes.
9. Keep all F/U to assess response, labs and for adverse SE.
10. Identify local support groups/services.

OUTCOMES/EVALUATE

- Improvement in motor function, reflexes, gait, strength of grip, amount of tremor, and quality of life
- Relief of S&S of RLS (restless leg syndrome)

■ IV

Levofloxacin

(**lee**-voh-**FLOX**-ah-sin)

Classification(s): Antibiotic, fluoroquinolone
Pregnancy Category: C
RX: Iquix, Levaquin, Quixin.

SEE ALSO *FLUOROQUINOLONES*.

INDICATIONS/USES

PO, Injection.

1. Acute bacterial sinusitis (5-day to 10–14-day treatment regimen) due to *Streptococcus*

pneumoniae, Haemophilus influenzae, or *Moraxella catarrhalis.*

2. Acute bacterial exacerbation of chronic bronchitis due to methicillin-susceptible *Staphylococcus aureus, S. pneumoniae, H. influenzae, Haemophilus parainfluenzae,* or *M. catarrhalis.*
3. Community acquired pneumonia (5-day treatment regimen) due to *S. pneumoniae* (excluding multidrug-resistant strains), *H. influenzae, H. parainfluenzae, M. pneumonia,* or *Chlamydophila pneumoniae.*
4. Community acquired pneumonia (7–14 day treatment regimen) due to *S. aureus, S. pneumoniae* (including multidrug resistant *S. pneumoniae*), *H. influenzae, H. parainfluenzae, Klebsiella pneumoniae, M. catarrhalis, C. pneumoniae, Legionella pneumophila, or Mycoplasma pneumoniae.*
5. Nosocomial (hospital acquired) pneumonia due to methicillin-susceptible *S. aureus, Pseudomonas aeruginosa, Serratia marcescens, Escherichia coli, Klebsiella pneumoniae, H. influenzae,* or *S. pneumoniae.* When *P. aeruginosa* is documented or presumed to be the pathogen, also use an antipseudomonal beta-lactam.
6. Uncomplicated mild to moderate infections of the skin and skin structures, including abscesses, cellulitis, furuncles, impetigo, pyoderma, and wound infections due to *S. aureus* or *Streptococcus pyogenes.*
7. Complicated skin and skin structure infections, including surgical incisions, infected bites and lacerations, major abscesses, and infected ulcers due to methicillin-sensitive *S. aureus, Enterococcus faecalis, S. pyogenes,* or *Proteus mirabilis.*
8. Complicated UTIs (5-day treatment regimen) due to *E. coli, K. pneumoniae,* or *P. mirabilis.*
9. Mild to moderate complicated UTIs (10-day treatment regimen) due to *E. faecalis, Enterobacter cloacae, E. coli, K. pneumoniae, P. mirabilis,* or *P. aeruginosa.*
10. Uncomplicated UTIs (mild to moderate) due to *E. coli, K. pneumoniae,* or *Staphylococcus saprophyticus.*
11. Acute mild to moderate pyelonephritis (5- or 10-day treatment regimen) due to *E. coli,* including cases with concurrent bacteremia.
12. Chronic bacterial prostatitis due to *E. coli, E. faecalis,* or *Staphylococcus epidermidis.*
13. Reduce the incidence or progression of inhalational anthrax following exposure to *Bacillus anthracis. Investigational:* An alternative regimen to treat disseminated gonococcal infections, traveler's diarrhea.

Ophthalmic.

1. Bacterial conjunctivitis caused by *S. aureus* (methicillin-susceptible strains only), *Corynebacterium* species, *S. epidermidis* (methicillin-susceptible strains only), *S. pneumoniae, Streptococcus* (Groups C/F and G), Viridans Group streptococci, *Acinetobacter lwoffii, H. influenzae, S. marcescens.*
2. Corneal ulcers caused by *S. aureus, S. epidermidis, S. pneumoniae, P. aeruginosa, S. marcescens.*

ACTION/KINETICS

Action

Interferes with DNA gyrase and topoisomerase IV. DNA gyrase is an enzyme needed for replication, transcription, and repair of bacterial DNA. Topoisomerase IV plays a key role in the partitioning of chromosomal DNA during bacterial cell division. Effective against both gram-positive and gram-negative organisms.

Pharmacokinetics

About 99% bioavailable. **t½, after multiple doses:** 7–8.8 hr. About 87% excreted unchanged in the urine after PO use.

CONTRAINDICATIONS

Lactation. IM, intrathecal, intraperitoneal, or SC administration. Rapid or bolus IV administration (hypotension may occur).

SPECIAL CONCERNS

Fluoroquinolones, including levofloxacin, are associated with an increased risk of tendinitis and tendon rupture in all ages. This risk is further increased in older clients (usually older than 60 years of age), in clients taking corticosteroid drugs, and in clients with kidney, heart, or lung transplants.

- **The dose must be reduced with impaired renal function. (See *Implementation/Administration/Storage.*)**
- **Safety and efficacy not determined in those less than 18 years of age.**

SIDE EFFECTS

Most Common

Headache, dizziness, insomnia, N&V, diarrhea, dyspepsia/heartburn, constipation.

See *Fluoroquinolones* for a complete list of possible side effects.

ADDITIONAL DRUG INTERACTIONS

↑ Risk of tendon rupture, especially in the elderly, if taken with corticosteroids

HOW SUPPLIED

Injection Solution, Concentrate: 5 mg/mL, 25 mg/mL; ***Ophthalmic Solution:*** 0.5%, 1.5%; ***Oral Solution:*** 25 mg/mL; ***Tablets:*** 250 mg, 500 mg, 750 mg.

DOSAGE

SLOW IV INFUSION; ORAL SOLUTION; TABLETS

Acute maxillary (bacterial) sinusitis.

750 mg once daily for 7 days or 500 mg once daily for 10–14 days.

Acute bacterial exacerbation of chronic bronchitis.

500 mg once daily for 7 days.

Community-acquired pneumonia due to methicillin-susceptible S. aureus, S. pneumoniae *(including multi-drug resistant strains),* H. influenzae, H. parainfluenzae, K. pneumoniae, M. catarrhalis, C. pneumoniae, L. pneumophila, *or* M. pneumoniae.

500 mg once daily for 7–14 days.

Community-acquired pneumonia due to S. pneumoniae *(excluding multidrug-resistant strains),* H. influenzae, H. parainfluenzae, M. pneumoniae, C. pneumoniae.

750 mg once daily for 5 days.

Nosocomial pneumonia.

750 mg once daily for 7–14 days.

Uncomplicated skin and skin structure infections.

500 mg once daily for 7–10 days.

Complicated skin and skin structure infections.

750 mg once daily for 7–14 days.

Complicated UTI or acute pyelonephritis (5-day treatment regimen).

750 mg once daily for 5 days.

Complicated UTI or acute pyelonephritis (10-day regimen).

250 mg once daily for 10 days.

Uncomplicated UTIs.

250 mg once daily for 3 days.

Chronic bacterial prostatitis.

500 mg once daily for 28 days.

Inhalation anthrax (postexposure).

Adults: 500 mg once daily for 60 days. **Children, >50 kg and 6 months of age or older:** 500 mg once daily for 60 days; **children, <50 kg and 6 months of age or older:** 8 mg/kg (not to exceed 250 mg per dose) q 12 hr for 60 days. For adults and children, begin therapy as soon as possible after suspected or confirmed exposure to aerosolized *B. anthracis.* Safety beyond use for 28 days for adults and 14 days for children has not been studied; only use prolonged therapy in adults or children when the benefit outweighs the risk.

Disseminated gonococcal infections.

IV: 250 mg once daily for 24–48 hr (after improvement begins); **then,** 500 mg/day PO for 7 days.

OPHTHALMIC SOLUTION

Bacterial conjunctivitis.

Days 1 and 2: 1–2 gtt in affected eye(s) q 2 hr while awake, up to 8 times per day; **Days 3 through 7:** 1–2 gtt in affected eye(s) q 4 hr while awake, up to 4 times per day.

Bacterial corneal ulcer.

Days 1 and 2: 1–2 gtt in the affected eye(s) q 30 min while awake. Awaken at about 4 and 6 hr after retiring and instill 1–2 gtt. **Days 3 through 7 to 9:** Instill 1–2 gtt hourly while awake. **Days 7 to 9 to treatment completion:** 1–2 gtt 4 times per day.

Corneal ulcer.

Days 1 through 3: 1–2 gtt in the affected eye(s) q 30 min to 2 hr while awake and about every 4–6 hr after retiring; **Days 4 through treatment completion:** 1–2 gtt in the affected eye(s) q 1 to 4 hr while awake.

NURSING IMPLICATIONS

Do not confuse levofloxacin with lomefloxacin (also a fluoroquinolone) or levofloxacin with levothyroxine (thyroid hormone).

IMPLEMENTATION/ADMINISTRATION/STORAGE

1. Sequential therapy (IV to PO) may be instituted at the discretion of the health care provider.
2. For PO or IV dosing, reduce dose with impaired renal function as follows: (a) **If the dosage is 750 mg q 24 hr in normal renal function:** If C_{CR} is 20–49 mL/min, give 750 mg q 48 hr; if C_{CR} is 10–19 mL/min, give 750 mg as the initial dose and then 500 mg q 48 hr; in hemodialysis or chronic ambulation peritoneal dialysis, give 750 mg as the initial dose and then 500 mg q 48 hr. (b) **If the dosage is 500 mg q 24 hr in normal renal function:** If C_{CR} is 20–49 mL/min, give 500 mg as the initial dose and then 250 mg q 24 hr; if C_{CR} is 10–19 mL/min, give 500 mg as the initial dose and then 250 mg q 48 hr; in hemodialysis or chronic ambulation peritoneal dialysis, give 500 mg as the initial dose and then 250 mg q 48 hr. (c) **If the dosage is 250 mg q 24 hr in normal renal function:** If C_{CR} is 20–49 mL/min, no dosage adjustment is required; if C_{CR} is 10–19 mL/min, give 250 mg q 48 hr (if treating uncomplicated UTI, no dosage adjustment is needed); in hemodialysis or chronic ambulation peritoneal dialysis: no information on dosing adjustment available.
3. Oral doses are given at least 2 hr before or 2 hr after antacids containing Mg or Al, as well as sucralfate, iron products, multivitamin preparations containing zinc, and didanosine (chewable/buffered tablets or pediatric powder for PO solution).
4. Store tablets in a tight container at 15–30°C (59–85°F).
5. IV Administer doses of 250 or 500 mg by slow infusion over 60 min q 24 hr or 750 mg given by slow infusion over 90 min q 24 hr. Avoid rapid or bolus IV infusion.
6. Diluted solutions for IV use are stable for 72 hr up to a concentration of 5 mg/mL when stored in IV containers at 25°C or less (77°F or less). Such solutions are stable for 14 days when stored under refrigeration at 5°C (41°F). Diluted solutions that are frozen in glass bottles or plastic IV containers are stable for 6 months when stored at -20°C (-4°F).
7. Thaw frozen solutions at room temperature or in refrigerator. Do not thaw in a microwave or by bath immersion. After initial thawing, do not refreeze.
8. COMPATIBILITY 0.9% NaCl, D5W, D5/0.9% NaCl, D5/RL, Plasma-Lyte 56 dextrose/5% injection, D5/0.45% NaCl, 0.15% KCl injection, or M/6 sodium lactate injection.
9. INCOMPATIBILITY Do not coadminister with any solution containing multivalent cations (e.g., magnesium) through the same IV tube; flush before and after drug infusion.

ASSESSMENT

1. Note reasons for therapy, onset, location, characteristics of S&S, clinical presentation and C&S. List drugs trialed/outcome.
2. Assess for seizure history or CNS disorders; may preclude therapy. If also prescribed corticosteroids, >60 yr of age, or with kidney, heart, or lung transplants may see increased risk of tendonitis and tendon rupture.
3. Obtain baseline cultures, CBC, BS, renal and LFTs, and monitor. Follow guidelines for reducing dosage with renal impairment based on C_{CR}.

CLIENT/FAMILY TEACHING

1. Tablets can be taken without regard to food. Consume plenty of fluids to prevent urinary crystal formation.
2. Take the oral solution 1 hr before or 2 hr after eating.
3. Take as directed for the time prescribed; different conditions require varying lengths of therapy.
4. Avoid activities that require mental alertness until effects realized, may cause dizziness or light-headedness.
5. With eye drops, wash hands and do not touch dropper to eye, fingers, or other surface. Tilt head back, pull lower lid out to make pocket, and instill medication into conjunctival sac. Close eyes and apply light finger pressure to bridge of nose for 1 to 2 min. Do not blink or rub eyes for at least 5 min after instillation. Do not wear contacts with S&S bacterial conjunctivitis.
6. If using other eye drops, separate each medication by at least 5 min.

7. Avoid multivitamins with zinc, iron products, sucralfate, and magnesium or aluminum-containing antacids 2 hr before and after dose.
8. Use caution until drug effects realized; may experience dizziness, drowsiness, or visual changes. May also experience N&V, abdominal pain, diarrhea/constipation, and photosensitivity.
9. Practice reliable birth control.
10. Avoid prolonged exposure to sunlight or UV light; use sunscreen and wear protective clothing.
11. Diabetics should monitor BS closely and report low/high blood sugars.
12. Report pain or inflammation in tendon of foot, rash, or if S&S do not improve or worsen after 72 hr of therapy.
13. Keep all F/U assess response, labs, and for adverse SE.

OUTCOMES/EVALUATE

- Symptomatic improvement
- Resolution of infection
- ↓ Disease progression after inhalational anthrax exposure

L

IV

Levoleucovorin calcium

(**LEE**-voe-**LOO**-koe-**VOE**-rin)

Classification(s): Folic acid derivative.

Pregnancy Category: C

RX: Fusilev, Levoleucovorin.

INDICATIONS/USES

(1) Rescue after high-dose methotrexate therapy in osteosarcoma. (2) Diminish the toxicity and counteract the effects of impaired methotrexate elimination and of inadvertant overdosage of folic acid antagonists. (3) Combination therapy with 5–fluorouracil in the palliative treatment of advanced metastatic colorectal cancer (Fusilev).

ACTION/KINETICS

Action

Levoleucovorin is the active isomer of 5-formyl tetrahydrofolic acid. It does not require reduction by the enzyme dihydrofolate reductase in order to participate in reactions utilizing folates as a source of one-carbon moieties. Levoleucovorin counteracts the therapeutic and toxic effects of folic acid antagonists, such as methotrexate.

Pharmacokinetics

Time to peak levels: 0.9 hr. **t½, terminal:** 5.1 hr for total tetrahydrofolate.

CONTRAINDICATIONS

Previous allergic reactions to folic acid or folinic acid.

SPECIAL CONCERNS

- Use with caution during lactation.
- Deaths from severe enterocolitis, diarrhea, and dehydration have been reported in elderly clients receiving weekly doses of d,l-leucovorin and 5-fluorouracil.

SIDE EFFECTS

Most Common

N&V, stomatitis, confusion, neuropathy, dyspepsia, diarrhea, asthenia, fatigue, malaise, anorexia, decreased appetite, dermatitis, alopecia.

CNS: Confusion, neuropathy. **GI:** Stomatitis, N&V, diarrhea, dyspepsia, abdominal pain, anorexia, decreased appetite, taste perversion, typhilitis. **Dermatologic:** Dermatitis, alopecia, pruritus, rash. **Respiratory:** Dyspnea. **GU:** Abnormal renal function. **Body as a whole:** Temperature change, asthenia, fatigue, malaise, rigors, allergic reactions.

DRUG INTERACTIONS

Anticonvulsants / Folic acid, in large amounts, may ↓ the antiepileptic effects of phenobarbital, phenytoin, and primidone → ↑ frequency of seizures in susceptible children; consider this possibility when using levoleucovorin

5-Fluorouracil / Enhanced toxicity of 5-fluorouracil

Trimethoprim and Sulfamethoxazole / Use of the combination for acute ***Pneumocystis carinii*** pneumonia in those with HIV infection → ↑ rates of treatment failure and morbidity

HOW SUPPLIED

Injection, Lyophilized Powder for Solution: 50 mg; *Injection Solution:* 10 mg/mL.

DOSAGE

IV

Rescue after high-dose methotrexate therapy.

The recommendations for levoleucovorin rescue are based on a methotrexate dose of 12 grams/m^2 given by IV infusion over 4 hours. Adjust or extend the levoleucovorin dose based on the following guidelines:

- **Normal methotrexate elimination:** Lab findings of serum methotrexate levels about 10 micromolar at 24 hr after administration, 1 micromolar at 48 hr, and <0.2 micromolar at 72 hr. The levoleucovorin dosage and duration would be 7.5 mg IV q 6 hr for 60 hr (10 doses starting at 24 hr after the start of the methotrexate infusion).
- **Delayed late methotrexate elimination:** Lab findings of serum methotrexate levels remaining above 0.2 micromolar at 72 hr, and >0.05 micromolar at 96 hr after administration. The levoleucovorin dosage and duration would be to continue 7.5 mg IV q 6 hr until the methotrexate level is <0.05 micromolar.
- **Delayed early methotrexate elimination and/or evidence of acute renal injury:** Lab findings of serum methotrexate levels of greater than or equal to 50 micromolar at 24 hr or greater than or equal to 5 micromolar at 48 hr after administration, or a 100% or greater increase in serum creatinine level at 24 hr after methotrexate administration (e.g., an increase from 0.5 mg/dL to a level of 1 mg/dL or more). The levoleucovorin dosage and duration would be 75 mg IV q 3 hr until the methotrexate level is <1 micromolar; then, 7.5 mg IV q 3 hr until the methotrexate level is <0.05 micromolar. *NOTE:* If significant clinical toxicity is observed, levoleucovorin rescue should be extended for an additional 24 hr (total of 14 doses over 84 hr) in subsequent courses of therapy. Consider that the client may be taking medications that interfere with methotrexate elimination or binding to serum albumin.

Impaired methotrexate elimination or inadvertant overdosage.

Administer levoleucovorin 7.5 mg (about 5 mg/m^2) IV q 6 hr until the serum methotrexate level is less than 10^{-8} molar. Begin levoleucovorin rescue as soon as possible after an inadvertant overdosage or within 24 hr of methotrexate administration when there is delayed excretion.

Determine serum creatinine and methotrexate levels at 24-hr intervals. If the 24-hr serum creatinine has increased 50% over baseline or if the 24-hr methotrexate level is more than 5×10^{-6} molar or the 48-hr level is more than 9×10^{-7} molar, increase the dose of levoleucovorin to 50 mg/m^2 q 3 hr until the methotrexate level is less than 10^{-8} molar. Hydration (3 liters/day) and urinary alkalinization with sodium bicarbonate should be employed concomitantly. Adjust the bicarbonate dose to maintain the urine at pH 7 or greater.

Fusilev administration with 5-fluorouracil to treat colorectal cancer.

Adults: (1) Regimen l: 100 mg/m^2 of Fusilev by slow IV injection over a minimum of 3 min followed by 5-fluorouracil at 370 mg/m^2 by IV injection each day for 5 days. (2) Regimen 2: 10 mg/m^2 of Fusilev IV followed by 5-fluorouracil at 425 mg/m^2 IV each day for 5 days. Administer separately to avoid formation of a precipitate. The five-day treatment course may be repeated at 4 week (28 day) intervals for 2 courses and then repeated at 4–5 week intervals (28–35 days) intervals provided that the client has completely recovered from the toxic effects of the prior treatment course.

NURSING IMPLICATIONS

IMPLEMENTATION/ADMINISTRATION/STORAGE

1. **IV** Clients who have delayed early methotrexate elimination are likely to develop reversible renal failure. In addition to levoleucovorin therapy, these individuals require continuing hydration and urinary alkalinization and close monitoring of fluid and electrolyte status until the serum methotrexate level has fallen to below 0.05 micromolar and the renal failure has resolved.

L

2. Delayed methotrexate excretion may be caused by accumulation in a third space fluid collection (i.e., ascites, pleural effusion), renal function impairment, or inadequate hydration. In such cases, higher doses of levoleucovorin or prolonged administration may be needed.
3. Levoleucovorin has no effect on other methotrexate toxicities, such as nephrotoxicity.
4. When combined with 5-fluorouracil (5-FU) to treat colorectal cancer, adjust the 5-FU dose based on client tolerance of the prior treatment course. Reduce the daily dose of 5-FU by 20% for clients who experienced moderate hematologic or GI toxicity in the prior treatment course, and by 30% for those who experienced severe toxicity. For clients who experienced no toxicity in the prior treatment course, the 5-FU dose may be increased by 10%. Fusilev dosages are not adjusted for toxicity.
5. Reconstitute the 50 mg vial with 5.3 mL of NaCl 0.9% injection to yield a levoleucovorin concentration of 10 mg/mL. The use of solutions other than NaCl 0.9% injection is not recommended.
6. The reconstituted levoleucovorin, 10 mg/mL, contains no preservative. Observe strict aseptic technique during reconstitution of the product.
7. Reconstituted levoleucovorin may be further diluted immediately to concentrations of 0.5 to 5 mg/mL in NaCl 0.9% injection or D5W injection. The initial reconstituted solution or diluted solution with NaCl 0.9% injection may be held at room temperature for not more than a total of 12 hr. Dilutions in D5W injection may be held at room temperature for no more than 4 hr.
8. Do not inject more than 16 mL of reconstituted solutions (i.e., levoleucovorin, 160 mg) per minute due to the calcium content of the product.
9. Store vials in the carton until used from 15–30°C (59–86°F); protect from light.
10. COMPATIBILITY 0.9% NaCl, D5W.
11. INCOMPATIBILITY Do not coadminister levoleucovorin with other agents in the same admixture.

ASSESSMENT

1. Note if for overdosage or rescue; include when antifolate given, dose of administration or overdose. Administer IV leucovorin as soon as possible following dosage guidelines.
2. List other drugs prescribed to ensure none interact; may counteract some AED drugs with resultant seizure activity.
3. If diarrhea occurs during combination therapy with 5-fluorouracil, monitor closely until diarrhea resolved.
4. Monitor serum methotrexate levels to determine dose and treatment duration required; usually treated until serum MTX level is $<10^{-8}$ molar.
5. To prevent reversible renal failure, ensure hydration and urinary alkalinization and close monitoring of fluid and electrolyte status until the serum methotrexate level falls below 0.05 micromolar and renal failure resolves.
6. Monitor CBC, electrolytes, renal and LFTs, during treatment; monitor B_{12} and folate levels.

CLIENT/FAMILY TEACHING

1. Drug is given IV to counteract the toxic effects of certain drugs (folic acid antagonists) or to assist in their elimination to prevent renal failure.
2. May be given daily for 5 days or more often and longer depending on toxic drug levels and elimination patterns.
3. Report N&V, diarrhea, fever, chills; consume plenty of fluids to prevent reversible renal failure.
4. Keep all F/U to assess response, labs, and for adverse SE.

OUTCOMES/EVALUATE

- Rescue after high dose MTX therapy in osteosarcoma
- Decreased toxicity with impaired MTX elimination

■ IV

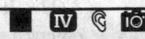

Levothyroxine sodium (T_4)

(lee-voh-thigh-**ROX**-een)

Classification(s): Thyroid product

Pregnancy Category: A

RX: Levothroid, Levoxyl, Synthroid, Thyro-Tabs, Tirosint.

Rx: Synthroid.

SEE ALSO ***THYROID DRUGS***.

INDICATIONS/USES

(1) Replacement or supplemental therapy for congenital or acquired hypothyroidism of any etiology, except transient hypothyroidism during the recovery phase of subacute thyroiditis. Specific uses include cretinism, myxedema, ordinary hypothyroidism, primary hypothyroidism due to functional deficiency; primary atrophy, partial or total absence of thyroid gland, or the effects of surgery, radiation, or drugs, with or without the presence of goiter; also secondary (pituitary) or tertiary (hypothalamus) hypothyroidism. (2) Treatment or prevention of various types of euthyroid goiters, including thyroid nodules, subacute or chronic lymphocytic thyroiditis, and multinodular goiter. (3) Adjunct to surgery and radioiodine therapy to manage thyrotropin-dependent well-differentiated thyroid cancer.

ACTION/KINETICS

Action

Levothyroxine is the synthetic sodium salt of the levo isomer of T_4 (tetraiodothyronine). Levothyroxine, 0.05–0.06 mg equals approximately 60 mg (1 grain) of thyroid. Is believed the effects of levothyroxine occur through control of DNA transcription and protein synthesis. Levothyroxine enhances oxygen consumption by most body tissues and increases the basal metabolic rate and metabolism of carbohydrates, lipids, and proteins in the body.

Pharmacokinetics

Absorption from the GI tract is incomplete and variable (from 40 to 80%), especially when taken with food. Has a slower onset but a longer duration than sodium liothyronine. More active on a weight basis than thyroid. Is usually the drug of choice. Effect is predictable as thyroid content is standard. **Time to peak therapeutic effect:** 3–4 weeks. **t½:** 6–7 days in a euthyroid person, 9–10 days in a hypothyroid client, and 3–4 days in a hyperthyroid client. **Duration:** 1–3 weeks after withdrawal of chronic therapy. 80% excreted in the feces. *NOTE:* All levothyroxine products are not bioequivalent; thus, changing brands is not recommended. **Plasma protein binding:** >99%.

SPECIAL CONCERNS

Drugs with thyroid hormone activity, alone or with other drugs, have been used to treat obesity. In euthyroid clients, doses within the range of daily hormonal requirements are ineffective for weight reduction. Larger doses may produce serious or even life-threatening manifestations of toxicity, especially when given with sympathomimetic amines such as those used for their anorectic effects.

- **Use with caution in those with underlying CV disease, in the elderly, and in those with concomitant adrenal insufficiency.**
- **Errors have occurred when prescribers have ordered 0.25 mg (250 mcg) instead of the correct dose of 0.025 mg (25 mcg). Be careful with decimal point placements and when converting a dose from micrograms to milligrams.**

SIDE EFFECTS

Most Common

Symptoms of hyperthyroidism

See *Thyroid Drugs* for a complete list of possible side effects.

DRUG INTERACTIONS

Al hydroxide / Adsorption of levothyroxine to the Al and increased fecal elimination of levothyroxine

Carbamazepine / ↑ Levothyroxine elimination R/T ↑ liver metabolism

Cholestyramine / ↓ Absorption of thyroxine R/T binding to cholestyramine in the GI tract

Digoxin / ↓ Digoxin levels and therapeutic effect

Imitinib / Hypothyroidism and ↑ TSH levels in those receiving levothyroxine after thyroidectomy

Iron salts / ↓ Absorption of levothyroxine R/T complex formation with iron in the GI tract

Raloxifene / ↓ Levothyroxine absorption

Sucralfate / ↓ Absorption of thyroxine R/T binding to sucralfate in the GI tract

Theophylline / ↓ Theophylline effect R/T ↑ elimination

Warfarin / ↑ Risk of bleeding; monitor INR and PT; may need to ↓ warfarin dose

HOW SUPPLIED

Capsules: 12.5 mcg, 25 mcg, 50 mcg, 75 mcg, 100 mcg, 125 mcg, 150 mcg; ***Powder for Injection, Lyophilized:*** 200 mcg, 500 mcg; ***Tablets:*** 25 mcg, 50 mcg, 75 mcg, 88 mcg, 100 mcg, 112 mcg, 125

mcg, 137 mcg, 150 mcg, 175 mcg, 200 mcg, 300 mcg.

DOSAGE

CAPSULES; TABLETS

Mild hypothyroidism.

Adults, initial: 50 mcg once daily; **then**, increase by 25–50 mcg q 2–3 weeks until desired clinical response is attained; **maintenance, usual:** 75–125 mcg/day (although doses up to 200 mcg/day may be required in some clients).

Severe hypothyroidism.

Adults, initial: 12.5–25 mcg once daily; **then** increase dose, as necessary, in increments of 25 mcg at 2- to 3-week intervals.

Congenital hypothyroidism.

Pediatric, 12 years and older: 2–3 mcg/kg once daily until the adult daily dose (usually 150 mcg) is reached. **6–12 years of age:** 4–5 mcg/kg/day or 100–150 mcg once daily. **1–5 years of age:** 5–6 mcg/kg/day or 75–100 mcg once daily. **6–12 months of age:** 6–8 mcg/kg/day or 50–75 mcg once daily. **Less than 6 months of age:** 8–10 mcg/kg/day or 25–50 mcg once daily.

IM; IV

Myxedematous coma.

Adults, initial: 400 mcg by rapid IV injection, even in geriatric clients; **then**, 100–200 mcg/day, IV. **Maintenance:** 100–200 mcg/day, IV. Smaller daily doses should be given until client can tolerate PO medication.

Hypothyroidism.

Adults: 50–100 mcg once daily; **pediatric, IV, IM:** A dose of 75% of the usual PO pediatric dose should be given.

TSH suppression in well-differentiated thyroid cancer or thyroid nodules.

Individualize dose. **Usual dose:** 2 mcg/kg/day.

NURSING IMPLICATIONS

(Sound Alike Drug) Do not confuse levothyroxine with levofloxacin (a fluoroquinolone antibiotic).

IMPLEMENTATION/ADMINISTRATION/STORAGE

1. Take with a full glass of water to prevent choking, gagging, dysphagia, or getting tablets stuck in the throat.
2. In infants with congenital or acquired hypothyroidism, institute therapy with full doses as soon as the diagnosis is made.
3. In infants and children who cannot swallow tablets, the correct dosage tablet may be crushed and suspended in a small amount of formula or water and given by dropper or spoon. The crushed tablet may also be sprinkled over cooked cereal or applesauce.
4. Transfer from liothyronine to levothyroxine: Administer replacement drug for several days before discontinuing liothyronine. Transfer from levothyroxine to liothyronine: Discontinue levothyroxine before starting low daily dose of liothyronine.
5. IV Prepare solution for injection immediately before administration.
6. Discard any unused portion of the IV medication.
7. COMPATIBILITY Reconstitute by adding 5 mL of 0.9% NaCl injection (shake to ensure complete mixing). Give immediately after reconstitution.
8. INCOMPATIBILITY Do not mix with other IV infusion solutions.

ASSESSMENT

1. List reasons for therapy, clinical presentation, laboratory confirmation, other agents/therapies trialed and outcome.
2. With thyroid disease, elderly clients are likely to have undetected cardiac problems.
3. If pregnant, must continue taking thyroid preparations throughout the pregnancy.
4. Note height, weight, and psychomotor development in child.
5. List drugs currently consumed to ensure none interact.
6. Errors have occurred when prescribers have ordered 0.25 mg (250 mcg) instead of the correct dose of 0.025 mg (25 mcg). Review orders carefully and question if unsure.
7. Obtain ECG prior to initiating therapy; monitor VS, ECG, TSH, Wt, and subjective symptoms. Adjust dose based on TSH.

CLIENT/FAMILY TEACHING

1. Used to replace a hormone that is low in the body, causing hypothyroidism. Drug is not a

cure for hypothyroidism; must be taken for life to control symptoms.

2. Take at the same time each day on an empty stomach 1 hr before or 2–3 hr after a meal. Take in the morning to prevent insomnia. However, it may be more effective if taken at night on an empty stomach instead of in the morning before breakfast. Do not take with food unless specifically instructed; may interfere with absorption. Avoid iodine-rich foods.
3. Do not switch brands; bioavailability may change.
4. Report severe headache, palpitations, chest pain, diarrhea, irritability, excitability, insomnia, intolerance to heat, significant weight loss, and/or excessive sweating.
5. Avoid OTC medications unless approved. Drug is NOT indicated for weight control.
6. Child may experience hair loss; hair should regrow. Return for evaluation of bone age, growth, labs, and psychomotor functioning.
7. If taking raloxifene, take levothyroxine at least 12 hr earlier in the day.
8. Keep all F/U to assess response, VS, labs, and adverse SE.

OUTCOMES/EVALUATE

- Promotion of normal metabolism
- ↑ Levels of T_3 and T_4, ↓ TSH

IV

Lidocaine hydrochloride

(**LYE**-doh-kayn)

Classification(s): Antiarrhythmic, Class IB

Pregnancy Category: B

RX: IM: LidoPen Auto-Injector. **Direct IV, IV Admixtures:** Lidocaine HCl for Cardiac Arrhythmias, Xylocaine HCl IV for Cardiac Arrhythmias. **IV Infusion:** Lidocaine HCl in 5% Dextrose.

✤ **Rx:** Xylocard.

SEE ALSO ***ANTIARRHYTHMIC AGENTS***.

INDICATIONS/USES

IM: Single doses in certain emergency situations (e.g., ECG equipment not available; by the client in the prehospital phase of suspected acute MI, directed by qualified medical personnel viewing the transmitted ECG).

IV: Acute ventricular arrhythmias (i.e., following MIs or occurring during surgery). Ineffective against atrial arrhythmias. *Investigational:* IV in children who develop ventricular couplets or frequent premature ventricular beats.

ACTION/KINETICS

Action

Shortens the refractory period and suppresses the automaticity of ectopic foci without affecting conduction of impulses through cardiac tissue. Increases the electrical stimulation threshold of the ventricle during diastole. It does not affect BP, CO, or myocardial contractility. Since lidocaine has little effect on conduction at normal antiarrhythmic doses, use in acute situations (instead of procainamide) in instances in which heart block might occur.

Pharmacokinetics

IV, Onset: 45–90 sec; **duration:** 10–20 min. **IM, Onset:** 5–15 min; **duration:** 60–90 min. **t½:** 1–2 hr. **Therapeutic serum levels:** 1.5–6 mcg/mL. **Time to steady-state plasma levels:** 3–4 hr (8–10 hr in clients with AMI). Ninety percent is rapidly metabolized in the liver to active metabolites. **Plasma protein binding:** 40–80%.

CONTRAINDICATIONS

Hypersensitivity to amide-type local anesthetics, Stokes-Adams syndrome, Wolff-Parkinson-White syndrome, severe SA, AV, or intraventricular block (when no pacemaker is present). Use of the IM autoinjector for children.

SPECIAL CONCERNS

- Use with caution during labor and delivery, during lactation, and in the presence of liver or severe kidney disease, CHF, marked hypoxia, digitalis toxicity with AV block, reduced cardiac output, severe respiratory depression, or shock.
- In the elderly, decrease the rate and dose for IV infusion by one-half; adjust slowly.
- Accelerated ventricular rate may occur when given to those with atrial flutter or fibrillation.
- Safety and efficacy not determined in children.

SIDE EFFECTS

Most Common

N&V, nervousness, anxiety, dizziness, drowsiness, sensation of heat or cold, numbness, injection site pain.

Body as a whole: Malignant hyperthermia characterized by tachycardia, tachypnea, labile BP, metabolic acidosis, temperature elevation. **GI:** N&V. **CV:** Precipitation or aggravation of arrhythmias (following IV use), hypotension, bradycardia ***(with possible cardiac arrest), CV collapse.*** **CNS:** Dizziness, apprehension, euphoria, light-headedness, nervousness, anxiety, drowsiness, confusion, changes in mood, hallucinations, twitching, "doom anxiety," ***convulsions***, unconsciousness. **Respiratory:** Difficulties in breathing or swallowing, ***respiratory depression or arrest.*** **Allergic:** Rash, cutaneous lesions, urticaria, edema, ***anaphylaxis.*** **Miscellaneous:** Tinnitus, blurred/double vision, vomiting, numbness, sensation of heat or cold, twitching, tremors, soreness at IM injection site, fever, ***venous thrombosis or phlebitis (extending from site of injection)***, extravasation. *NOTE:* During anesthesia, CV depression may be the first sign of lidocaine toxicity. During other usage, convulsions are the first sign of lidocaine toxicity.

LABORATORY TEST CONSIDERATIONS

↑ CPK following IM use.

OVERDOSE MANAGEMENT

Symptoms: Dependent on plasma levels. If plasma levels range from 4 to 6 mcg/mL, mild CNS effects are observed. Levels of 6 to 8 mcg/mL may result in significant CNS and CV depression while levels greater than 8 mcg/mL cause hypotension, decreased CO, respiratory depression, obtundation, ***seizures, and coma.*** *Treatment:* Discontinue the drug and begin emergency resuscitative procedures. Seizures can be treated with diazepam, thiopental, or thiamylal. Succinylcholine, IV, may be used if the client is anesthetized. IV fluids, vasopressors, and CPR are used to correct circulatory depression.

DRUG INTERACTIONS

Aminoglycosides / ↑ Neuromuscular blockade
Beta-adrenergic blockers / ↑ Lidocaine levels with possible toxicity
Cimetidine / ↓ Clearance of lidocaine → possible toxicity
Fluvoxamine / ↓ Lidocaine elimination; adding PO erythromycin further ↓ lidocaine elimination R/T inhibition of lidocaine metabolism by CYP3A4
Phenytoin / IV phenytoin → excessive cardiac depression
Procainamide / Additive cardiodepressant effects
Smoking / ↑ Hepatic metabolism of lidocaine
Succinylcholine / ↑ Succinylcholine action by ↓ plasma protein binding
Tocainide / ↑ Risk of side effects
Tubocurarine / ↑ Neuromuscular blockade

HOW SUPPLIED

IM Injection: 10% (300 mg/3 mL); ***IV Admixtures:*** 4% (40 mg/mL), 10% (100 mg/mL), 20% (200 mg/mL); ***IV Infusion:*** 0.2% (2 mg/mL), 0.4% (4 mg/mL), 0.8% (8 mg/mL); ***IV Injection, Direct:*** 1% (10 mg/mL), 2% (20 mg/mL).

DOSAGE

IM

Antiarrhythmic.

Adults: 4.5 mg/kg (approximately 300 mg for a 70-kg adult). Switch to IV lidocaine or oral antiarrhythmics as soon as possible although an additional IM dose may be given after 60–90 min.

IV BOLUS

Antiarrhythmic.

Adults: 50–100 mg at a rate of 25–50 mg/min. Bolus is used to establish rapid therapeutic plasma levels. Repeat if necessary after 5 min interval. Onset of action is 10 sec. **Maximum dose/hour:** 200–300 mg. Reduce the dose in those with CHF or reduced cardiac output and in the elderly; some recommended, however, that the usual loading dose be given and only the maintenance dose be reduced.

IV INFUSION

Antiarrhythmic.

20–50 mcg/kg at a rate of 1–4 mg/min. No more than 200–300 mg/hr should be given. Reduce maintenance doses in those with heart failure or liver disease or who are also receiving other drugs known to decrease lidocaine clearance or liver blood flow, and in clients over 70 years of age. **Pediatric, bolus dose:** 1 mg/kg IV or intrathecally q 5–10 min until desired effect reached (maximum total dose: 5 mg/kg); **maintenance:** 20–50 mcg/kg/min.

NURSING IMPLICATIONS

IMPLEMENTATION/ADMINISTRATION/STORAGE

1. For IM use, the deltoid muscle is preferred. Use only the 10% solution for IM injection.
2. IV *Do not add lidocaine to blood transfusion assembly.*
3. Do not use lidocaine solutions that contain epinephrine to treat arrhythmias. Make certain that vial states, "For Cardiac Arrhythmias." Check prefilled syringes closely to ensure appropriate dose has been obtained. (Lidocaine prefilled syringes come in both milligrams and grams.)
4. Use D5W to prepare solution; this is stable for 24 hr. Administer with an electronic infusion device.
5. Reduce IV bolus dosage in clients over 70 years old, with CHF or liver disease, and if taking cimetidine or propranolol (i.e., where metabolism of lidocaine is reduced).
6. For continuous infusion, use prediluted solution or add lidocaine 1 g to 500 mL of D5W to prepare 0.2% solution. Rate of administration should not exceed 1 to 4 mg/min. Adjust rate according to cardiac response.
7. COMPATIBILITY D5W.
8. INCOMPATIBILITY Administer separately.

ASSESSMENT

1. List reasons for therapy; any hypersensitivity to amide-type local anesthetics.
2. Those with hepatic or renal disease or who weigh less than 45.5 kg will need to be watched closely for adverse side effects; adjust dosage as directed.
3. Note CNS status. Report sudden changes in mental status, dizziness, visual disturbances, twitching, tremors; may precede convulsions.
4. Review pulmonary findings; assess for respiratory depression. Monitor VS, ECG; assess for hypotension, cardiac collapse.
5. View monitor strips for myocardial depression, variations of rhythm, aggravation of arrhythmia during infusion.
6. IM use may increase CPK levels. Monitor renal and LFTs, electrolytes.

CLIENT/FAMILY TEACHING

1. Drug is used to eradicate ventricular arrhythmias. It is generally administered IV in a continuously monitored environment.
2. Report any evidence of dizziness or altered mentation; may be S&S of toxicity and progress to seizures and coma.
3. Smoking is not permitted during drug therapy. Refer to smoking cessation for alternative therapy.
4. Reactions (i.e., confusion, convulsions, drowsiness, paresthesias, respiratory arrest) can occur and are a result of CNS toxicity.

OUTCOMES/EVALUATE

- Control of ventricular arrhythmias
- Therapeutic serum drug levels (1.5–6 mcg/mL)

Linagliptin

(lin-ah-**GLIP**-tin)

Classification(s): Antidiabetic agent, dipeptidyl peptidase-4 inhibitor

Pregnancy Category: B

RX: Tradjenta.

SEE ALSO ***ANTIDIABETIC AGENTS: HYPOGLYCEMIC AGENTS***

INDICATIONS/USES

Adjunct to diet and exercise to improve glycemic control in adults with type 2 diabetes mellitus as monotherapy or combination therapy.

ACTION/KINETICS

Action

Linagliptin increases the concentrations of active incretin hormones, thus stimulating the release of insulin in a glucose-dependent manner and decreasing the levels of circulating glucagon. Incretin hormones are secreted at a low basal level throughout the day but levels rise immediately after a meal. Incretins GLP-1 and GLP-2 increase insulin biosynthesis and secretion from pancreatic beta cells in the presence of normal and elevated blood glucose levels. Also, GLP-1 decreases glucagon secretion from pancreatic alpha cells resulting in a reduction of hepatic glucose output.

Pharmacokinetics

Absolute bioavailability: About 30%. **Peak plasma levels:** 1.5 hr. Steady-state plasma levels reached by the third dose. Plasma binding is not affected in those with renal or hepatic impairment. About 90% of the drug is excreted unchanged (85% via the enterohepatic system and

5% in the urine). **t½, terminal:** About 100 hr. No dosage adjustment is required in those with renal or hepatic impairment. **Plasma protein binding:** 89–99%.

CONTRAINDICATIONS

Hypersensitivity (e.g., angioedema, bronchial hyper reactivity) to linagliptin.

SPECIAL CONCERNS

- Use with caution during lactation.
- Elderly may show greater sensitivity to the drug; no dosage adjustment is recommended.
- Safety and efficacy not determined in children.

SIDE EFFECTS

Most Common

Hypoglycemia, arthralgia, back pain, headache, nasopharyngitis.

Side effects also include those when linagliptin is taken with other hypoglycemic drugs. **CNS:** Headache. **GI:** Pancreatitis. **Musculoskeletal:** Arthralgia, back pain. **Respiratory:** Nasopharyngitis, cough. **Metabolic:** Hypoglycemia, hyperlipidemia, hypertriglyceridemia, increased weight. **Hypersensitivity:** ***Angioedema***, bronchial hyperreactivity, localized skin exfoliation, urticaria.

LABORATORY TEST CONSIDERATIONS

↑ Uric acid, blood triglycerides.

OVERDOSE MANAGEMENT

Treatment: Initiate supportive measures, including removing unabsorbed drug from the GI tract. Monitor. The drug is not eliminated to a significant degree by hemodialysis or peritoneal dialysis.

DRUG INTERACTIONS

CYP3A4 strong inducers (e.g., rifampin) / ↓ Linagliptin levels → ↓ pharmacologic effect; alternative therapy recommended

P-glycoprotein strong inducers (e.g., rifampin) / ↓ Linagliptin levels → ↓ pharmacologic effect; alternative therapy recommended

Ritonavir / ↑ Linagliptin levels → ↑ pharmacologic/toxic effects; use together with caution and monitor

Sulfonylureas / ↑ Risk of hypoglycemia; monitor blood glucose and adjust dose as needed

HOW SUPPLIED

Tablets: 5 mg.

DOSAGE

TABLETS

Type 2 diabetes mellitus.

Adults, usual: 5 mg once a day. When linagliptin is used with an insulin secretagogue (e.g., a sulfonylurea), a lower dose of the secretagogue may be required to reduce the risk of hypoglycemia.

NURSING IMPLICATIONS

IMPLEMENTATION/ADMINISTRATION/STORAGE

Store from 15–30°C (59–86°F).

ASSESSMENT

1. Note reasons for therapy, onset, characteristics of S&S, other agents trialed, outcome.
2. List risk factors, weight, BP, eye and foot exam findings. Assess for organ damage, neuropathy or other diabetes related problems.
3. Observe carefully for S&S of pancreatitis.
4. Monitor lipids, renal and LFTs, HbA1c, microalbumin.

CLIENT/FAMILY TEACHING

1. Can be taken with or without food. Drug works to increase insulin secretion.
2. Drug is used alone or with other agents to control blood sugar in addition to diet, regular daily exercise and weight loss.
3. May experience upper respiratory tract infection, stuffy or runny nose, sore throat, and headache; report if persistent or bothersome.
4. Record finger sticks to share with provider.
5. Persistent, severe abdominal pain with/without vomiting may indicate acute pancreatitis and requires immediate reporting.
6. During periods of stress (e.g., fever, trauma, infection, surgery) may require different medication doses; report.
7. Hypoglycemia increased when drug added to a sulfonylurea or insulin; lower doses of the sulfonylurea or insulin may be required to reduce hypoglycemia.
8. Allergic reactions have been reported. If S&S of allergic reactions occur (rash, hives, and swelling of the face, tongue, and throat), stop drug and seek medical care.
9. Keep all F/U to assess response, labs, and for adverse SE.

OUTCOMES/EVALUATE

Control of diabetes; HbA1c <8

IV

Liothyronine sodium (T_3)

(lye-oh-**THIGH**-roh-neen)

Classification(s): Thyroid product

Pregnancy Category: A

RX: Cytomel, Sodium-L-Triiodothyronine, Triostat.

SEE ALSO ***THYROID DRUGS***.

INDICATIONS/USES

(1) Replacement or supplemental therapy for congenital or acquired hypothyroidism of any etiology, except transient hypothyroidism during the recovery phase of subacute thyroiditis. Specific indications include cretinism, myxedema, ordinary hypothyroidism, primary hypothyroidism resulting from functional deficiency; primary atrophy, partial, or total absence of thyroid gland; or, the effects of surgery, radiation, or drugs, with or without the presence of goiter; secondary or tertiary hypothyroidism. (2) Treatment or prevention of various types of euthyroid goiters, including thyroid nodules, subacute or chronic lymphocytic thyroiditis, and multinodular goiter. (3) Adjunct to surgery and radioiodine therapy to manage thyrotropin-dependent well-differentiated thyroid cancer. (4) Diagnostic agent in suppression tests to differentiate suspected mild hypothyroidism or thyroid gland autonomy.

ACTION/KINETICS

Action

Synthetic sodium salt of the levoisomer of T_3. Has more predictable effects due to standard hormone content. From 15 to 37.5 mcg is equivalent to about 60 mg of desiccated thyroid. May be preferred when a rapid effect or rapidly reversible effect is required. Has a rapid onset, which may result in difficulty in controlling the dosage as well as the possibility of cardiac side effects and changes in metabolic demands. However, its short duration allows quick adjustment of dosage and helps control overdosage.

Pharmacokinetics

t½: 24 hr for euthyroid clients, approximately 34 hr in hypothyroid clients, and approximately 14 hr in hyperthyroid clients. **Duration:** Up to 72 hr. Excreted mainly through the kidney. **Plasma protein binding:** 99%.

ADDITIONAL CONTRAINDICATIONS

Use in children with cretinism because there is some question about whether the hormone crosses the blood-brain barrier.

SPECIAL CONCERNS

Drugs with thyroid hormone activity, alone or with other drugs, have been used to treat obesity. In euthyroid clients, doses within the range of daily hormonal requirements are ineffective for weight reduction. Larger doses may produce serious or even life-threatening manifestations of toxicity, especially when given with sympathomimetic amines such as those used for their anorectic effects.

SIDE EFFECTS

Most Common

Symptoms of hyperthyroidism.

See *Thyroid Drugs* for a complete list of possible side effects.

HOW SUPPLIED

Injection: 10 mcg/mL; ***Tablets:*** 5 mcg, 25 mcg, 50 mcg.

DOSAGE

IV ONLY

Myxedema coma, precoma.

Adults, initial: 25–50 mcg. Base subsequent doses on continuous monitoring of client's clinical status and response. Doses should be given at least 4 hr, and no more than 12 hr, apart. Total daily doses of 65 mcg in initial days of therapy are associated with a lower incidence of mortality. In cases of known CV disease, give an initial dose of 10–20 mcg.

TABLETS

Mild hypothyroidism.

Adults, individualized, initial: 25 mcg/day. Increase by 12.5–25 mcg q 1–2 weeks until satisfactory response

L

has been obtained. **Usual maintenance:** 25–75 mcg/day (100 mcg may be required in some clients). Use lower initial dosage (5 mcg/day) for the elderly, children, and clients with CV disease. Increase only by 5 mcg increments.

Myxedema.

Adults, initial: 5 mcg/day increased by 5–10 mcg/day q 1–2 weeks until 25 mcg/day is reached; **then,** increase q 1–2 weeks by 12.5–50 mcg. **Usual maintenance:** 50–100 mcg/day.

Simple (nontoxic) goiter.

Adults, initial: 5 mcg/day; **then,** increase q 1–2 weeks by 5–10 mcg until 25 mcg/day is reached; **then,** dose can be increased by 12.5–25 mcg/week until the maintenance dose of 50–100 mcg/day is reached (usual is 75 mcg/day).

T_3 suppression test.

75–100 mcg/day for 7 days followed by a repeat of the I^{131} thyroid uptake test (a 50% or greater suppression of uptake indicates a normal thyroid-pituitary axis).

Congenital hypothyroidism.

Adults and children, initial: 5 mcg/day; **then,** increase by 5 mcg/day q 3–4 days until the desired effect is achieved. Approximately 20 mcg/day may be sufficient for infants a few months of age while children 1 year of age may require 50 mcg/day. Children above 3 years may require the full adult dose.

NURSING IMPLICATIONS

Do not confuse liothyronine with liotrix or levothyroxine (both thyroid products). Do not confuse Cytomel with Cytotec (a prostaglandin).

IMPLEMENTATION/ADMINISTRATION/STORAGE

1. *Transfer from other thyroid preparations to liothyronine:* Discontinue old preparation before starting on low daily dose of liothyronine. *Transfer from liothyronine to another thyroid preparation:* Start therapy with replacement drug several days prior to complete withdrawal of sodium liothyronine.
2. If symptoms of hyperthyroidism noted, the drug can be withdrawn for 2–3 days and can be reinstituted at a lower dose.
3. IV Available for emergency treatment of myxedema coma.
4. May administer undiluted at a rate of 10 mcg/mL as a bolus.
5. COMPATIBILITY Triostat injectable: Administer directly as prepared (comes 10 mcg/mL)
6. INCOMPATIBILITY Do not mix; give separately.

ASSESSMENT

1. Note reasons for therapy, other agents trialed, outcome. List drugs prescribed to ensure none interact or interfere with lab studies.
2. Stress importance of adherence to therapy and not to change brands once dosage stabilized.
3. Assess for any medicinal or dietary iodine intake.
4. Monitor VS, ECG, thyroid function tests and those with CAD for evidence of insufficiency and any diabetes or adrenal disorders.

CLIENT/FAMILY TEACHING

1. Take once a day at the same time, preferably before breakfast to prevent insomnia. Liothyronine's effects are more rapid than levothyroxine.
2. Used to control symptoms of hypothyroidism; requires replacement for life.
3. Report any chest pain, palpitations, fever, insomnia, irritability, unusual sweating, bruising/bleeding, heat intolerance, diarrhea, weight loss, and headaches.
4. Partial hair loss may be experienced by children in first few months of therapy, usually transient.
5. Record pulse; report signs of rapid heart rate or irregularity.
6. Do NOT take liothyronine for weight control; may cause life-threatening or serious consequences when used in large doses or in combination with other anorectics.
7. Keep all F/U to assess response, labs, physical exams, and adverse SE.

OUTCOMES/EVALUATE

Desired thyroid hormone replacement

Liotrix

(**LYE**-oh-trix)

Classification(s): Thyroid product

Pregnancy Category: A

RX: Thyrolar.

SEE ALSO ***THYROID DRUGS***.

INDICATIONS/USES

(1) Replacement or supplemental therapy for congenital or acquired hypothyroidism of any etiology, except transient hypothyroidism during the recovery phase of subacute thyroiditis. Specific indications include cretinism, myxedema, ordinary hypothyroidism, primary hypothyroidism resulting from functional deficiency; primary atrophy, partial, or total absence of thyroid gland; or, the effects of surgery, radiation, or drugs, with or without the presence of goiter; secondary or tertiary hypothyroidism. (2) Treatment or prevention of various types of euthyroid goiters, including thyroid nodules, subacute or chronic lymphocytic thyroiditis, and multinodular goiter. (3) Adjunct to surgery and radioiodine therapy to manage thyrotropin-dependent well-differentiated thyroid cancer. (4) Diagnostic agent in suppression tests to differentiate suspected mild hypothyroidism or thyroid gland autonomy.

ACTION/KINETICS

Action

Mixture of synthetic levothyroxine sodium (T_4) and liothyronine (T_3) in a 4:1 ratio by weight and in a 1:1 ratio by biologic activity. 50 mcg T_4/12.5 mcg T_3 is equivalent to 50–60 mcg of levothyroxine.

Pharmacokinetics

Primarily excreted through the kidneys. **Plasma protein binding:** >99%.

SPECIAL CONCERNS

Drugs with thyroid hormone activity, alone or with other drugs, have been used for the treatment of obesity. In euthyroid clients, doses within the range of daily hormonal requirements are ineffective for weight reduction. Larger doses may produce serious or even life-threatening manifestations of toxicity, especially when given in association with sympathomimetic amines such as those used for their anorectic effects.

SIDE EFFECTS

Most Common

Symptoms of hyperthyroidism.

See *Thyroid Drugs* for a complete list of possible side effects.

HOW SUPPLIED

Tablets: T_3/T_4: 3.1 mcg/12.5 mcg; 6.25 mcg/25 mcg; 12.5 mcg/50 mcg; 25 mcg/100 mcg; 37.5 mcg/150 mcg.

DOSAGE

TABLETS

Hypothyroidism.

Adults and children, initial: 50 mcg levothyroxine and 12.5 mcg liothyronine (Thyrolar); **then,** at monthly intervals, increments of like amounts can be made until the desired effect is achieved. **Usual maintenance:** 50–100 mcg of levothyroxine and 12.5–25 mcg liothyronine daily.

Congenital hypothyroidism.

Children, 0–6 months: 3.1 mcg/12.5 mcg (T_3/T_4) to 6.25 mcg/25 mcg (T_3/T_4); **6–12 months:** 6.25 mcg/25 mcg (T_3/T_4) to 9.35 mcg/37.5 mcg (T_3/T_4); **1–5 years:** 9.35 mcg/37.5 mcg (T_3/T_4) to 12.5 mcg/50 mcg (T_3/T_4); **6–12 years:** 12.5 mcg/50 mcg (T_3/T_4) to 18.75 mcg/75 mcg (T_3/T_4); **over 12 years:** more than 18.75 mcg/75 mcg (T_3/T_4).

NURSING IMPLICATIONS

IMPLEMENTATION/ADMINISTRATION/STORAGE

1. In infants with congenital hypothyroidism, begin therapy with full doses as soon as the diagnosis is made.
2. In children, make dosing increments q 2 weeks until desired response attained.
3. Protect tablets from light, heat, and moisture.

ASSESSMENT

1. Note reasons for therapy, disease onset, S&S, TFTs, dose at start of therapy.

2. **Monitor height, weight, and intellectual function in child to document normal development.**
3. **Assess VS, thyroid function tests before initiating dosage and with dosage changes, and check BS with diabetes.**

CLIENT/FAMILY TEACHING

1. **Take once a day as a single dose before breakfast. May split dose if nausea and diarrhea persist.**
2. **Used to control S&S of hypothyroidism; requires replacement for life. Do not stop suddenly.**
3. **Report any chest pain, palpitations, fever, insomnia, irritability, unusual sweating, heat intolerance, diarrhea, weight loss, and headaches. With diabetes, check FS often.**
4. **Partial hair loss may occur in child during first few months of therapy; usually reversible.**
5. **Keep all F/U to assess response, physical exam, labs, and for adverse SE.**

OUTCOMES/EVALUATE

Thyroid hormone replacement

Lisdexamfetamine dimesylate

(lis-**DEX**-am-**FET**-a-meen)

Classification(s): CNS stimulant

Pregnancy Category: C

RX: Vyvanse.

SEE ALSO ***AMPHETAMINES AND DERIVATIVES.***

INDICATIONS/USES

Treatment of attention-deficit/hyperactivity disorder (ADHD) in adults, adolescents 13 to 17 years of age, and children 6 to 12 years of age. Use of the drug is part of a total treatment program that may include psychological, educational, or social measures.

ACTION/KINETICS

Action

Lisdexamfetamine is a prodrug and is converted to dextroamphetamine, the active moiety. The mechanism of action for ADHD is not known. However, amphetamines are thought to block the reuptake of norepinephrine and dopamine into presynaptic neurons and increase the release of monoamines into the extraneuronal space leading to CNS effects.

Pharmacokinetics

Rapidly absorbed; T_{max}: 3.5 hr after a single dose. Food does not affect the AUC or C_{max} but prolongs the T_{max} by about 1 hr. Dextroamphetamine and metabolites (98%) are excreted in the urine. **t½, plasma elimination:** Less than 1 hr.

CONTRAINDICATIONS

Advanced arteriosclerosis, symptomatic CV disease (structural cardiac abnormalities, cardiomyopathy, serious heart rhythm abnormalities), recent MI, moderate to severe hypertension, hyperthyroidism, hypersensitivity or idiosyncrasy to sympathomimetics, glaucoma, agitated states, history of drug abuse, during or within 14 days following administration of MAOIs (hypertensive crisis may occur). Use not recommended during lactation and in children less than 3 years of age.

SPECIAL CONCERNS

(1) **Potential for abuse.** Amphetamines have a high potential for abuse. Administration of amphetamines for prolonged periods of time may lead to drug dependence. Pay particular attention to the possibility of subjects obtaining amphetamines for nontherapeutic use or distribution to others; prescribe or dispense the drugs sparingly. (2) Misuse of amphetamine may cause sudden death and serious cardiovascular adverse reactions.

- **Worsening behavior disturbance symptoms and thought disorder may occur with pre-existing psychotic disorder.**
- **Possible lowering of seizure threshold in those with prior history of seizures, without a history of seizures, and no prior EEG evidence of seizures.**
- **Use with caution with concomitant use of other sympathomimetic drugs.**
- **Tolerance, significant psychological dependence, and severe social disability may occur with amphetamine use/abuse.**
- **Safety and efficacy not determined in children less than 6 years or over 12 years of age.**

SIDE EFFECTS

Most Common

Decreased appetite, insomnia, upper abdominal pain, headache, irritability, decreased weight, N&V, dry mouth, dizziness.

CNS: Insomnia, headache, irritability, dizziness, somnolence, affect lability, tic, initial insomnia, psychomotor hyperactivity, treatment emergent psychotic or manic symptoms (e.g., hallucinations, delusional thinking, mania), overstimulation, restlessness, euphoria, dyskinesia, dysphoria, depression, tremor, aggressive behavior/hostility, worsening of motor and phonic tics and Tourette's syndrome, ***seizures***. **GI:** Decreased appetite, upper abdominal pain, N&V, dry mouth, diarrhea, constipation, unpleasant taste. **CV:** ↑ BP/HR, palpitations, tachycardia, ***cardiomyopathy*** with chronic use, ***CVA, MI***. **Dermatologic:** Rash. **Allergic:** Urticaria, ***angioedema***, ***anaphylaxis***, serious skin rashes including ***Stevens-Johnson syndrome*** and ***toxic epidermal necrolysis***. **Ophthalmic:** Accommodation difficulty, blurred vision. **Body as a whole:** Decreased weight, pyrexia, long-term suppression of growth. **Miscellaneous:** Impotence, changes in libido, ***sudden death***.

LABORATORY TEST CONSIDERATIONS

↑ Plasma corticosteroid levels. Interference with urinary steroid determinations.

OVERDOSE MANAGEMENT

SEE ALSO ***AMPHETAMINES AND DERIVATIVES***.

DRUG INTERACTIONS

Adrenergic blockers / ↓ Effect of adrenergic blockers
Antihistamines / Amphetamines may counteract the sedative effects of antihistamines
Antihypertensives / Amphetamines may antagonize the hypotensive effect of antihypertensives
Chlorpromazine / Inhibition of CNS stimulant effect of amphetamines R/T blockade of dopamine and norepinephrine receptors
Ethosuximide / Possible delayed absorption of ethosuximide
Haloperidol / ↓ Amphetamine effect R/T blockade of dopamine receptors
Lithium carbonate / ↓ Anorectic and stimulatory effect of amphetamine
MAOIs / ↓ Amphetamine metabolism → ↑ effect of amphetamine, including headaches and other signs of hypertensive crisis, malignant hyperpyrexia, death
Meperidine / Potentiation of meperidine's analgesic effect
Methenamine / ↓ Amphetamine effect R/T ↑ urinary excretion
Norepinephrine / ↑ Adrenergic effects of norepinephrine
Phenobarbital / Delayed phenobarbital absorption; also, synergistic anticonvulsant action
Phenytoin / Delayed phenytoin absorption; also, synergistic anticonvulsant action
Sympathomimetics / ↑ Effect of sympathomimetics
Tricyclic antidepressants / ↑ Effect of TCAs; also, significant ↑ amphetamine brain levels → potentiation of cardiac effects
Urinary acidifiers (e.g., ammonium chloride, sodium acid phosphate) / ↓ Amphetamine blood levels R/T ↑ urinary excretion → ↓ efficacy

HOW SUPPLIED

Capsules: 20 mg, 30 mg, 40 mg, 50 mg, 60 mg, 70 mg.

DOSAGE

CAPSULES

Attention deficit-hyperactivity disorder in adults, adolescents 13–17 years of age, and children 6–12 years of age.

Individualize. **Adults and children, 6–12 years of age, initial:** 30 mg once daily in the morning for those either starting treatment for the first time or switching from another drug. If a dosage increase is needed, adjust in increments of 10 mg or 20 mg at approximately weekly intervals. **Maximum daily dose:** 70 mg. A dose of 20 mg/day may be started in some children.

NURSING IMPLICATIONS

IMPLEMENTATION/ADMINISTRATION/STORAGE

1. The least amount of the drug should be prescribed or dispensed at one time in order to minimize possible overdosage.
2. When possible interrupt the drug occasionally to determine if there is a recurrence of behavioral symptoms to warrant continued use of the drug.
3. The efficacy for use longer than 4 weeks has not been determined.
4. Store from 15–30°C (59–86°F) in tight, light-resistant containers.

ASSESSMENT

1. Note reasons for therapy, onset/characteristics of S&S, other drugs trialed/outcome and those currently prescribed that may interact unfavorably.
2. Assess for conditions that may preclude therapy: advanced/symptomatic CV disease (structural cardiac abnormalities, cardiomyopathy, serious heart rhythm abnormalities), recent MI, moderate to severe hypertension, hyperthyroidism, hypersensitivity or idiosyncrasy to sympathomimetics, glaucoma, agitated states, history of drug abuse, during or within 14 days following administration of MAOIs.
3. Ensure psychologic evaluations show no evidence of psychotic disorder, excessive stimulation, or severe stress.
4. Assess growth (height and weight); provide periodic "drug holiday" to determine need for continued therapy.
5. Monitor scripts and evaluate for any drug overuse/abuse.
6. Obtain and monitor VS, Wt, CBC, CNS status (including behavioral presentation/changes and if indicated reports from school), ECG.

CLIENT/FAMILY TEACHING

1. May be taken whole with or without food. The capsule may be opened and the entire contents dissolved in a glass of water; do not divide the dose of a single capsule. Consume the solution immediately. Rinse to ensure that entire contents consumed.
2. Take in the morning to ensure ability to sleep at bedtime. Avoid afternoon doses to minimize insomnia.
3. Use caution when driving or operating hazardous machinery; drug may mask fatigue and/or cause physical incoordination, dizziness, blurred vision, drowsiness.
4. Record BP, HR, and weight 2 times per week; report any significant weight loss or changes.
5. Report changes in mood, attention span; seizure disorder. May cause treatment-emergent psychotic or manic symptoms.
6. Skin rashes, fever, or joint pains should be reported immediately.
7. Therapy may be interrupted every few months ("drug holiday") to determine if still needed in those responsive to therapy.
8. May require more rest as drug effects fade.
9. Chronic use may lead to psychic dependence and marked tolerance. Scripts will be carefully monitored to prevent overdose and abuse.
10. Review potential for serious CV risk (including stroke, hypertension, MI) with drug therapy.
11. Keep all F/U to assess response, therapy, VS, weight, ECG, adverse SE.

OUTCOMES/EVALUATE

↑ Ability to sit quietly/focus/concentrate in those with ADHD

Lisinopril

(lie-**SIN**-oh-prill)

Classification(s): Antihypertensive, ACE inhibitor

Pregnancy Category: C

RX: Prinivil, Zestril.

🍁 **Rx:** Apo-Lisinopril.

SEE ALSO ***ANGIOTENSIN-CONVERTING ENZYME INHIBITORS***.

INDICATIONS/USES

(1) Alone or in combination with a diuretic (usually a thiazide) to treat hypertension. (2) Hypertension in children, aged 6–16 years. (3) Adjunctive therapy to manage heart failure in those who are not responding adequately to diuretics and digitalis. (4) Use within 24 hr of acute MI to improve survival in hemodynamically stable clients (clients should receive the standard treatment, including thrombolytics, aspirin, and beta blockers). *Investigational:* Prophylaxis of migraine in adults.

ACTION/KINETICS

Action

Inhibits angiotensin-converting enzyme resulting in decreased plasma angiotensin II, which leads to decreased vasopressor activity and decreased aldosterone secretion. Both supine and standing BPs are reduced, although the drug is less effective in African Americans than in Caucasians.

Pharmacokinetics

Although food does not alter the bioavailability of lisinopril, only 25% of a PO dose is absorbed. **Onset:** 1 hr. **Peak serum levels:** 7 hr. **Peak effect:** 6 hr. **Duration:** 24 hr. **t½:** 12 hr. 100% of the drug is excreted unchanged in the urine. Impaired renal function (GFR <30 mL/min) decreases elimination, increases peak and trough levels, and increases T_{max}, and time to reach steady state is prolonged.

CONTRAINDICATIONS

Use in children less than 6 years of age or in children with a GFR less than 30 mL/min/1.73 m^2. Not recommended for use during lactation.

SPECIAL CONCERNS

When used during the second and third trimesters of pregnancy, ACE inhibitors can cause injury and even death to the developing fetus. When pregnancy is detected, discontinue lisinopril as soon as possible.

- **Geriatric clients may manifest higher blood levels.**
- **Reduce dosage in clients with impaired renal function.**
- **Safety and efficacy not established in children.**

SIDE EFFECTS

Most Common

Chest pain, dizziness, headache, hypotension, fatigue, diarrhea, URTI.

CV: Hypotension (especially following the first dose), orthostatic hypotension, palpitations, ***stroke***, chest pain, orthostatic effects, peripheral edema, ***MI, CVA***, worsening of heart failure, PVCs, TIAs, atrial fibrillation, bradycardia, ventricular/atrial tachycardia, arrhythmias, postinfarction angina, ***cardiac arrest***. **CNS:** Dizziness, headache, vertigo, insomnia, sleepiness, paresthesias, nervousness, confusion, ataxia, impaired memory, tremor, irritability, hypersomnia, peripheral neuropathy, spasm. **GI:** Diarrhea, N&V, dyspepsia, constipation, dry mouth, abdominal pain, flatulence, gastritis, heartburn, GI cramps, weight loss/gain, taste alterations, increased salivation. **Hepatic:** Hepatitis, hepatocellular/cholestatic jaundice, pancreatitis, hepatomegaly. **Respiratory:** URTI, cough (may be chronic), dyspnea, bronchitis, nasal congestion, sinusitis, pharyngeal pain, ***bronchospasm***, asthma, pulmonary edema infiltrates, ***pulmonary embolism/infarction***, PND, chest discomfort, common cold, pleural effusion, wheezing, painful respiration, epistaxis, laryngitis, pharyngitis, rhinitis, rhinorrhea, orthopnea, pneumonia, hemoptysis, ***malignant lung neoplasms***. **Musculoskeletal:** Muscle cramps, pain (neck, hip, leg, knee, arm, joint, shoulder, back, pelvic, flank), myalgia, arthralgia, arthritis, lumbago. **Dermatologic:** Rash, flushing, increased sweating, urticaria, alopecia, erythema, photosensitivity, pemphigus/pemphigoid, herpes zoster, skin lesions, skin infections; rarely, ***Stevens-Johnson syndrome or toxic epidermal necrolysis***. **GU:** Impotence, oliguria, progressive azotemia, decreased libido, acute renal failure, UTI, anuria, uremia, renal dysfunction, pyelonephritis, dysuria. **Hematologic:** Rarely, neutropenia, leukopenia, agranulocytosis, aplastic or hemolytic anemia, or bone marrow depression; eosinophilia. **Body as a whole:** Fatigue, fever, malaise, asthenia, influenza, gout, fluid overload, dehydration, chills, virus infection. **Ophthalmic:** Blurred vision, visual loss, diplopia, photophobia. **Otic:** Tinnitus. **Miscellaneous:** ***Angioedema (may be fatal if laryngeal edema occurs)***, hyperkalemia, syncope, vasculitis of the legs, diabetes mellitus, edema, facial edema, ***anaphylactoid reaction***, breast pain, gout.

LABORATORY TEST CONSIDERATIONS

↑ Serum potassium, BUN, serum creatinine. ↓ H&H.

OVERDOSE MANAGEMENT

Symptoms: Hypotension. *Treatment:* Supportive. To correct hypotension, IV normal saline is treatment of choice. Lisinopril may be removed by hemodialysis.

DRUG INTERACTIONS

See ***Angiotensin-Converting Enzyme (ACE) Inhibitors.***

Diuretics / Excess ↓ BP

Indomethacin / Possible ↓ lisinopril effect

Potassium-sparing diuretics / Significant ↑ serum potassium

HOW SUPPLIED

Tablets: 2.5 mg, 5 mg, 10 mg, 20 mg, 30 mg, 40 mg.

DOSAGE

TABLETS

Essential hypertension, used alone.

Adults, Initial: 10 mg once daily. Adjust dosage depending on response (range: 20–40 mg/day given as a single dose). Doses greater than 80 mg/day do not give a greater effect. **Children over**

6 years of age, initial: 0.07 mg/kg once daily up to 5 mg total. Adjust dose according to BP response; doses above 0.61 mg/kg (or in excess of 40 mg) have not been studied in children.

Essential hypertension in combination with a diuretic.

If BP is not controlled with lisinopril alone, a low dose of a diuretic may be added to the regimen. Hydrochlorothiazide, 12.5 mg, provides an additive effect. The dose of lisinopril may be reduced if a diuretic is used.

Congestive heart failure.

Initial: 5 mg once daily (2.5 mg/day in clients with hyponatremia) in combination with diuretics and digitalis. **Dosage range:** 5–20 mg/day (of Zestril) as a single dose, up to a maximum of 40 mg/day; do not use increments of more than 10 mg at intervals of no less than 2 weeks.

Acute myocardial infarction to improve survival.

First dose: 5 mg within 24 hr of the onset of symptoms; **then**, 5 mg after 24 hr, 10 mg after 48 hr, and then 10 mg daily. Continue dosing for 6 weeks. In clients with a systolic pressure less than 120 mm Hg when treatment is started or within 3 days after the infarct should be given 2.5 mg. If hypotension occurs (systolic BP less than 100 mm Hg), the dose may be temporarily reduced to 2.5 mg. If prolonged hypotension occurs, withdraw the drug.

NURSING IMPLICATIONS

Do not confuse lisinopril with Lioresal (a muscle relaxant). Also, do not confuse Prinivil with Prilosec (a proton pump inhibitor) or Proventil (a sympathomimetic). Do not confuse Zestril with Zetia (ezetimibe, an antihyperlipidemic).

IMPLEMENTATION/ADMINISTRATION/STORAGE

1. To prepare a suspension (200 mL) of a 1 mg/mL concentration, add 10 mL purified water to a polyethylene terephthalate bottle containing ten 20 mg tablets of lisinopril. Shake for at least 1 min. Add 30 mL Bicitra diluent and 160 mL of Ora-Sweet SF to the concentrate in the bottle; shake gently for several seconds to disperse the ingredients. Store the suspension at or below 25°C (77°F) for up to 4 weeks. Shake the suspension before each use.
2. When considering use of lisinopril in a client taking diuretics, discontinue the diuretic, if possible, 2–3 days before beginning lisinopril therapy. If diuretic cannot be discontinued, the initial dose of lisinopril should be 5 mg; observe closely for at least 2 hr.
3. Maximum antihypertensive effects may not be observed for 2–4 weeks.
4. When starting treatment for CHF, give under medical supervision, especially if SBP <100 mm Hg.
5. With clients whose BP is controlled with lisinopril, 20 mg, plus hydrochlorothiazide 25 mg, given separately, may trial Prinzide 12.5 mg or Zestoretic 10–12.5 mg before Prinzide 25 mg or Zestoretic 20–25 mg is used.
6. The maximum recommended daily dose of lisinopril is 80 mg in a single daily dose. Clients usually do not require hydrochlorothiazide in doses exceeding 50 mg/day, especially if combined with other antihypertensives.
7. Use of potassium supplements, potassium-sparing diuretics, or potassium salt substitutes with Prinzide or Zestoretic may lead to increases in serum potassium.
8. Prinzide or Zestoretic is recommended for those with a C_{CR} >30 mL/min.
9. Anticipate reduced dosage with renal insufficiency—initial dose of 10 mg/day if C_{CR} >30 mL/min, 5 mg/day if C_{CR} is between 10 and 30 mL/min, and 2.5 mg/day in dialysis clients (i.e., C_{CR} <10 mL/min).
10. Store tablets from 15–30°C (59–86°F); protect from moisture, freezing, and excessive heat. Store suspension below 25°C (77°F) for up to 4 weeks; protect from moisture.

ASSESSMENT

1. Note reasons for therapy, other agents trialed, and outcome.
2. Perform physical exam noting cardiopulmonary status, review history for any existing conditions, and labs for any organ dysfunction.
3. Identify risk factors and those that are modifiable to reduce CHD progression.

4. Start within 24 hr of AMI in addition to ASA, beta blockers, statins, and thrombolytics to reduce mortality.
5. Obtain ECG, VS, CXR, baseline labs (BUN, creatinine, BS, Na^+, and K^+) and monitor. Reduce dose with hyponatremia and renal dysfunction.

CLIENT/FAMILY TEACHING

1. Must be taken as directed at least once a day to control BP.
2. Avoid symptoms of low BP (i.e., rise slowly from sitting or lying position and wait until symptoms subside). May cause dizziness; use caution with activities requiring mental alertness until drug effects realized.
3. Avoid all potassium supplements and high potassium foods unless otherwise directed.
4. Record BP and weights; report any increase of more than 2 lb/day or 5 lb/week or loss of BP control. Ensure adequate hydration especially with excessive vomiting/diarrhea and sweating to prevent low BP effects.
5. Avoid prolonged sun/UV exposure; use protection if exposed, to prevent sensitivity reaction.
6. Report new or unusual side effects or aggravation of existing conditions, as well as sore throat, hoarseness, cough, chest pain, difficulty breathing, or swelling of hands, feet, tongue/throat, or face.
7. Avoid OTC agents without approval; may affect drug action.
8. Continue lifestyle changes to ensure BP/symptom control: weight loss/control; regular daily exercise; low-fat; low-salt diet; smoking cessation; alcohol moderation; and regular intake of prescribed medications. Record BP for provider review.
9. Use reliable contraception; harmful to fetus in second and third trimesters.
10. Keep all F/U to assess response, ECG, labs, and for adverse SE.

OUTCOMES/EVALUATE

- ↓ BP
- Control S&S CHF
- Improved survival with acute MI

Combination Drug

Lisinopril and Hydrochlorothiazide

(lie-**SIN**-oh-prill, **hy**-droh-klor-oh-**THIGH**-ah-zyd)

Classification(s): Antihypertensive (combination ACE inhibitor and thiazide diuretic)

Pregnancy Category: C (first trimester); **D** (second and third trimesters)

RX: Prinzide, Zestoretic.

SEE ALSO ***LISINOPRIL*** AND ***HYDROCHLOROTHIAZIDE.***

INDICATIONS/USES

Hypertension (not indicated for initial therapy).

CONTENT

Prinzide or Zestoretic: Lisinopril, an ACE inhibitor (amount listed first)/hydrochlorothiazide, a thiazide diuretic: 10/12.5; 20/12.5; 20/25.

ACTION/KINETICS

Action

Lisinopril inhibits angiotensin-converting enzyme, resulting in decreased plasma angiotensin II, which leads to decreased vasopressor activity and decreased aldosterone secretion. Hydrochlorothiazide promotes the excretion of sodium and chloride, and thus water, by the distal renal tubule. Also increases excretion of potassium and to a lesser extent bicarbonate. The antihypertensive activity is thought to be due to direct dilation of the areterioles, as well as to a reduction in the total fluid volume of the body and altered sodium balance.

Pharmacokinetics

Lisinopril, about 25% absorbed; peak serum levels: about 7 hr. Lisinopril absorption not affected by food. **Hydrochlorothiazide: Onset, 2 hr; peak effect:** 4 hr; **duration:** 6–12 hr. **t½, lisinopril:** 12 hr; **hydrochlorothiazide:** 5.6–14.8 hr. Lisinopril and hydrochlorothiazide are excreted unchanged in the urine.

CONTRAINDICATIONS

Use in clients hypersensitive to any components of the product, a history of angioedema related to

L

previous treatment with ACE inhibitors, hereditary or idiopathic angioedema, anuria, or hypersensitivity to other sulfonamide-derived drugs. Lactation.

SPECIAL CONCERNS

- **Angioedema and anaphylactoid reactions are possible with ACE inhibitors.**
- **Black clients receiving ACE inhibitors have a higher incidence of angioedema compared with non-Blacks.**
- **Use thiazides with caution in severe renal disease, impaired hepatic function, or progressive liver disease.**
- **Use lisinopril with caution in aortic stenosis or hypertrophic cardiomyopathy.**
- **Safety and efficacy not determined in children.**

SIDE EFFECTS

Most Common

Dizziness, headache, cough, fatigue, orthostatic hypotension, hypokalemia.

See *Angiotensin-Converting Enzyme Inhibitors* and *Diuretics, Thiazides* for a complete list of possible side effects.

DRUG INTERACTIONS

See ***Angiotensin-Converting Enzyme Inhibitors*** and ***Diuretics, Thiazides.***

HOW SUPPLIED

See *Content.*

DOSAGE

TABLETS

Hypertension.

Individualized, usual: 1 or 2 tablets daily of 1 of the strengths (depending on response; see strengths under *Content*). For geriatric clients, begin therapy at the low end of the dosage range.

NURSING IMPLICATIONS

Do not confuse Zestoretic with Zestril (lisinopril alone).

IMPLEMENTATION/ADMINISTRATION/STORAGE

1. **To minimize dose-independent side effects, in general, use combination therapy only after a client has failed to achieve the desired effect with monotherapy.**
2. **Clients whose BP is controlled adequately with 25 mg/day of hydrochlorothiazide, but who experience significant hypokalemia, may achieve similar or greater BP control with less potassium loss if they are switched to the 10/12.5 mg product.**
3. **Dosages higher than lisinopril, 80 mg, and hydrochlorothiazide, 50 mg, should not be used.**
4. **The usual dosage does not require adjustment if the client's C_{CR} is >30 mL/min/1.73 m^2. In those with more severe renal impairment, do not use thiazides.**
5. **Store from 15–30°C (59–86°F). Protect from excessive light and humidity.**

ASSESSMENT

1. **Note disease onset, other drugs trialed/outcome, age, other co-morbidities.**
2. **Assess for sulfa-based allergies; precludes therapy.**
3. **Use cautiously with aortic stenosis or hypertrophic cardiomyopathy.**
4. **Monitor VS, CBC, electrolytes, renal and LFTs; reduce dose with dysfunction.**

CLIENT/FAMILY TEACHING

1. **Take as directed with a full glass of water; do not skip or forget doses.**
2. **May cause dizziness/drowsiness use caution until drug effects realized; change positions slowly to ↓ dizziness.**
3. **Avoid activities that cause excessive overheating; may become dehydrated.**
4. **Do not use salt substitutes with potassium.**
5. **Use reliable contraception; harmful to fetus in second and third trimesters.**
6. **Record BP and weights; report any increase of more than 2 lb/day or 5 lb/week or loss of BP control. Ensure adequate hydration, especially with excessive vomiting/diarrhea and sweating, to prevent low BP effects.**
7. **Avoid prolonged sun/UV exposure; use protection if exposed, to prevent sensitivity reaction.**
8. **Report new or unusual side effects or aggravation of existing conditions, as well as sore throat, hoarseness, cough, chest pain, difficulty breathing, or swelling of hands, feet, tongue/throat, or face.**
9. **Avoid OTC agents without approval; may affect drug action.**
10. **Continue lifestyle changes to ensure BP/symptom control: weight loss/control; regular daily exercise; low-fat, low-salt diet; smoking**

Color Photo Quick Reference Guide

This color photo quick reference guide provides rapid identification of 98 most commonly prescribed drugs. Actual-sized tablets and capsules, with their strength, are organized alphabetically by generic name and include appropriate trade name and manufacturer. Page numbers to monograph within book are included for reference.

ALENDRONATE SODIUM

pg 51
Fosamax
MERCK

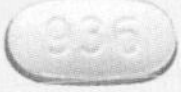

10 mg

Rx

AMPHETAMINE MIXTURES

pg 91
Adderall XR
SHIRE

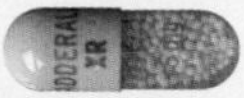

5 mg

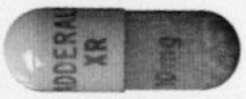

10 mg

20 mg

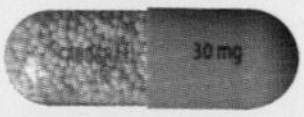

30 mg

Rx C-II

ATORVASTATIN CALCIUM

pg 146
Lipitor
PFIZER

10 mg

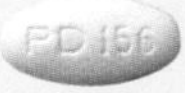

20 mg

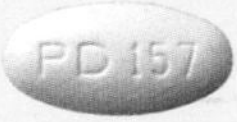

40 mg

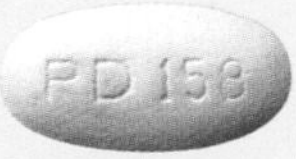

80 mg

Rx

CELECOXIB

pg 309
Celebrex
PFIZER

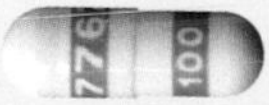

100 mg

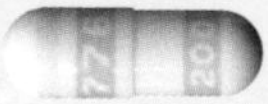

200 mg

Rx

CLOPIDOGREL BISULFATE

pg 381
Plavix
BRISTOL-MYERS SQUIBB

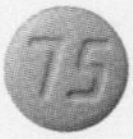

75 mg

Rx

DIGOXIN

pg 504

Lanoxin

GLAXO SMITH KLINE

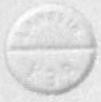

0.125 mg

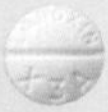

0.25 mg

Rx

ESCITALOPRAM OXALATE

pg 619

Lexapro

FOREST

5 mg

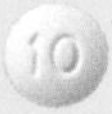

10 mg

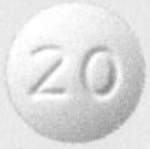

20 mg

Rx

ESOMEPRAZOLE MAGNESIUM

pg 624

Nexium

ASTRAZENECA

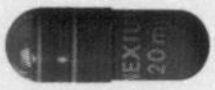

20 mg

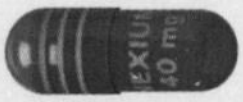

40 mg

Rx

ESTROGENS, CONJUGATED ORAL

pg 636

Premarin

PFIZER

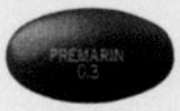

0.3 mg

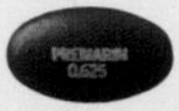

0.625 mg

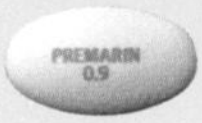

0.9 mg

Rx

ESZOPICLONE

pg 639

Lunesta

SUNOVION

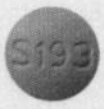

3 mg

Rx C-IV

EZETIMIBE AND SIMVASTATIN

pg 668

Vytorin

MERCK

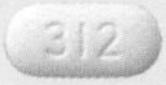

10/20 mg

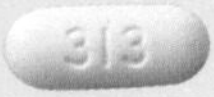

10/40 mg

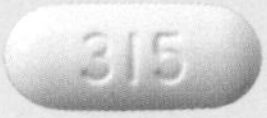

10/80 mg

Rx

FUROSEMIDE
pg 786
Lasix
SANOFI

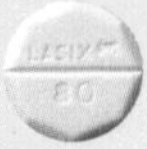

80 mg

Rx

IBANDRONATE SODIUM
pg 850
Boniva
ROCHE

150 mg

Rx

IRBESARTAN
pg 929
Avapro
BRISTOL-MYERS SQUIBB

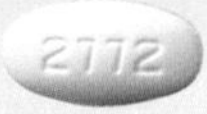

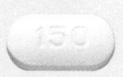

150 mg

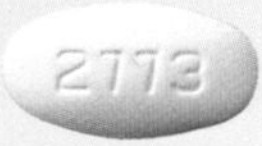

300 mg

Rx

LAMOTRIGINE
pg 977
Lamictal
GLAXO SMITH KLINE

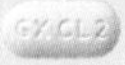

5 mg

25 mg

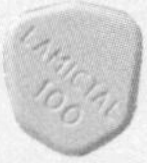

100 mg

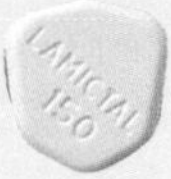

150 mg

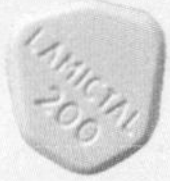

200 mg

Rx

LANSOPRAZOLE
pg 985
Prevacid
TAKEDA

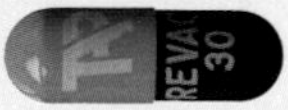

30 mg

Rx

LEVETIRACETAM
pg 1006
Keppra
UCB

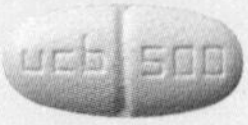

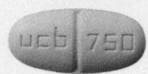

500 mg

750 mg

Rx

LEVOFLOXACIN
pg 1014
Levaquin
JANSSEN

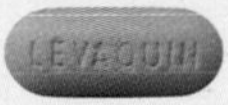

250 mg

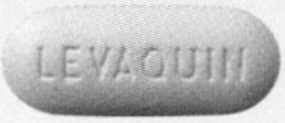

500 mg

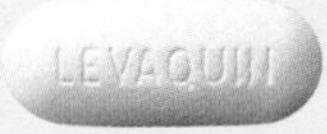

750 mg

Rx

LEVOTHYROXINE SODIUM

pg 1020

Synthroid
ABBOTT

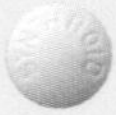

50 micrograms

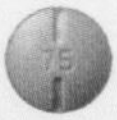

75 micrograms

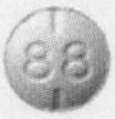

88 micrograms

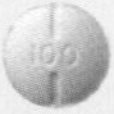

100 micrograms

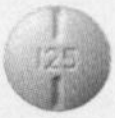

125 micrograms

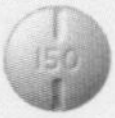

150 micrograms

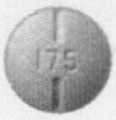

175 micrograms

Rx

LOSARTAN POTASSIUM

pg 1047

Cozaar
MERCK

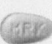

25 mg

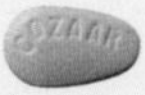

50 mg

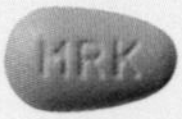

100 mg

Rx

MEMANTINE HYDROCHLORIDE

pg 1073

Namenda
FOREST

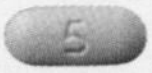

5 mg

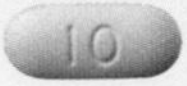

10 mg

Rx

METOPROLOL SUCCINATE

pg 1114

Toprol XL
ASTRAZENECA

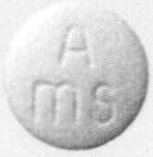

100 mg

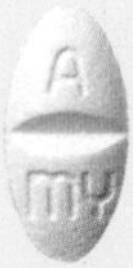

200 mg

Rx

MOXIFLOXACIN HYDROCHLORIDE

pg 1163

Avelox
BAYER SCHERING

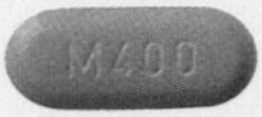

400 mg

Rx

OMEPRAZOLE

pg 1262
Prilosec
PROCTOR & GAMBLE

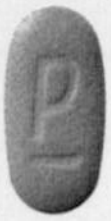

40 mg

Rx

PIOGLITAZONE HYDROCHLORIDE

pg 1372
Actos
TAKEDA

15 mg

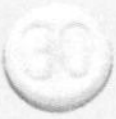

30 mg

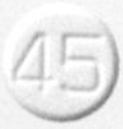

45 mg

Rx

QUETIAPINE FUMARATE

pg 1447
Seroquel
ASTRAZENECA

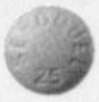

25 mg

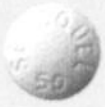

50 mg

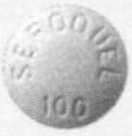

100 mg

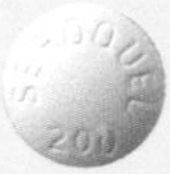

200 mg

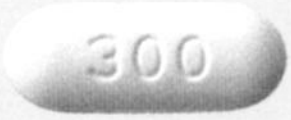

300 mg

Rx

RALOXIFENE HYDROCHLORIDE

pg 1465
Evista
ELI LILLY

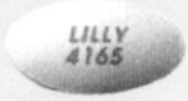

60 mg

Rx

ROSIGLITAZONE MALEATE

pg 1557
Avandia
GLAXO SMITH KLINE

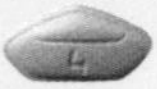

4 mg

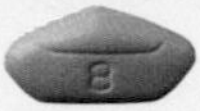

8 mg

Rx

ROSUVASTATIN CALCIUM

pg 1559

Crestor

ASTRA-ZENECA

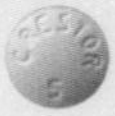

5 mg

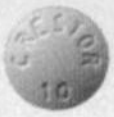

10 mg

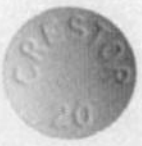

20 mg

Rx

SERTRALINE HYDROCHLORIDE

pg 1584

Zoloft

PFIZER

25 mg

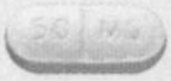

50 mg

Rx

SILDENAFIL CITRATE

pg 1588

Viagra

PFIZER

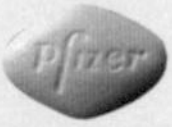

50 mg

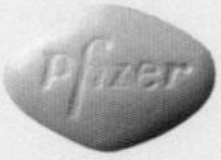

100 mg

Rx

TADALAFIL

pg 1657

Cialis

ELI LILLY

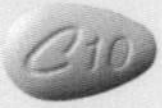

10 mg

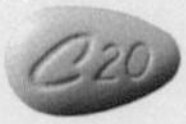

20 mg

Rx

TAMSULOSIN HYDROCHLORIDE

pg 1663

Flomax

BOEHRINGER INGELHEIM

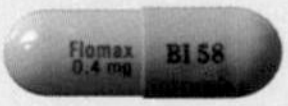

0.4 mg

Rx

TOLTERODINE TARTRATE

pg 1763
Detrol LA
PFIZER

1 mg

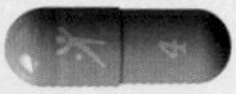

4 mg

Rx

TOPIRAMATE

pg 1764
Topomax
JANSSEN

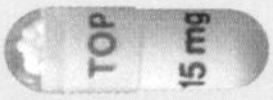

15 mg

25 mg

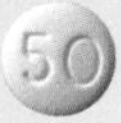

50 mg

Rx

VALSARTAN

pg 1829
Diovan
NOVARTIS

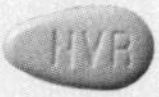

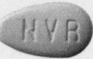

80 mg

160 mg

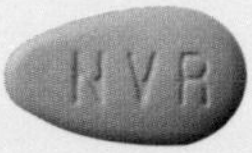

320 mg

Rx

VENLAFAXINE HYDROCHLORIDE

pg 1852
Effexor XR
PFIZER

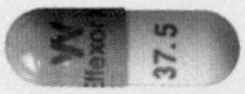

37.5 mg

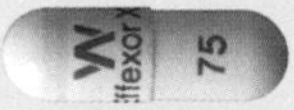

75 mg

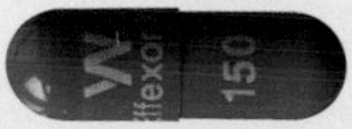

150 mg

Rx

WARFARIN SODIUM

pg 1876
Coumadin
BRISTOL-MYERS SQUIBB

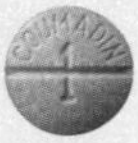

1 mg

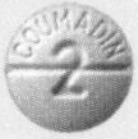

2 mg

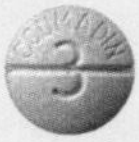

3 mg

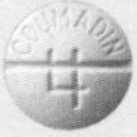

4 mg

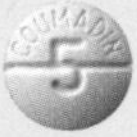

5 mg

Rx

ZOLPIDEM TARTRATE

pg 1909

Ambien
SANOFI

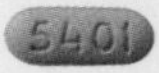

5 mg

10 mg

Rx C-IV

Ambien CR
SANOFI

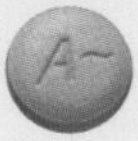

6.25 mg

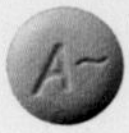

12.5 mg

Rx C-IV

A more comprehensive color photo quick reference guide can be found on the 2013 Delmar Nurse's Drug Handbook Website.

www.cengage.com/community/nursesdrughandbook

cessation; alcohol moderation; and regular intake of prescribed medications. Record BP for provider review.

11. Keep all F/U to assess response, ECG, labs and adverse SE.

OUTCOMES/EVALUATE

- Desired BP control
- BP <140/85 or <130/80 with diabetes, renal disease

Lithium carbonate

(**LITH**-ee-um)

Classification(s): Antimanic

Pregnancy Category: D

RX: Lithobid, Lithonate, Lithotabs.

✤ **Rx:** Apo-Lithium Carbonate, Apo-Lithium Carbonate SR, Carbolith, Duralith, PMS-Lithium Carbonate.

Lithium citrate

Pregnancy Category: D

✤ **Rx:** PMS-Lithium Citrate.

INDICATIONS/USES

Control of mania in manic-depressive clients. *Investigational:* To reverse neutropenia induced by cancer chemotherapy, in children with chronic neutropenia, and in AIDS clients receiving zidovudine. Prophylaxis of cluster headaches. Also for premenstrual tension, alcoholism accompanied by depression, tardive dyskinesia, bulimia, hyperthyroidism, excess ADH secretion, postpartum affective psychosis, corticosteroid-induced psychosis.

ACTION/KINETICS

Action

Mechanism for the antimanic effect of lithium is unknown. Various hypotheses include: (a) a decrease in catecholamine neurotransmitter levels caused by lithium's effect on Na^+-K^+ ATPase to improve transneuronal membrane transport of sodium ion; (b) a decrease in cyclic AMP levels caused by lithium which decreases sensitivity of hormonal-sensitive adenyl cyclase receptors; or (c) interference by lithium with lipid inositol metabolism ultimately leading to insensitivity of cells in the CNS to stimulation by inositol. Affects the distribution of Ca^{++}, Mg^{++}, and Na^+ ions and affects glucose metabolism.

Pharmacokinetics

Peak serum levels: regular release: 1–4 hr; **slow-release:** 4–6 hr. **Onset:** 5–14 days. **Therapeutic serum levels:** 0.4–1.0 mEq/L (must be carefully monitored because toxic effects may occur at these levels and significant toxic reactions occur at serum lithium levels of 2 mEq/L). **t½, plasma:** 24 hr (longer in presence of renal impairment and in the elderly). Lithium and sodium are excreted by the same mechanism in the proximal tubule. Thus, to reduce the danger of lithium intoxication, sodium intake must remain at normal levels.

CONTRAINDICATIONS

Cardiovascular or renal disease. Brain damage. Dehydration, sodium depletion, clients receiving diuretics. Lactation.

SPECIAL CONCERNS

Toxicity is closely related to serum lithium levels and can occur at therapeutic doses. Facilities to monitor serum lithium are required.

- Use with caution in the elderly as lithium is more toxic to the CNS in these clients. The elderly are more likely to develop lithium-induced goiter and clinical hypothyroidism and are more likely to manifest excessive thirst and larger volumes of urine.
- Safety and efficacy not established for children less than 12 years of age.

SIDE EFFECTS

Most Common

Due to initial therapy: Fine hand tremor, polyuria, thirst, transient and mild nausea, general discomfort.

The following side effects are dependent on the serum level of lithium. **CV:** Arrhythmia, hypotension, ***peripheral circulatory collapse***, bradycardia, sinus node dysfunction with ***severe bradycardia causing syncope***; reversible flattening, isoelectricity, or inversion of T waves. **CNS:** Blackout spells, epileptiform seizures, slurred speech, dizziness, vertigo, somnolence, psychomotor retardation, restlessness, sleepiness, confusion, stupor, ***coma***, acute dystonia, startled response, hypertonicity, slowed intellectual functioning, hallucinations, poor memory, tics, cog wheel rigidity, tongue movements. Pseudotumor cerebri leading to increased intracranial pressure and papilledema; if undetected may cause enlargement of the blind spot, constriction of visual fields, and eventual blindness. Diffuse slowing of EEG; widening of frequency spectrum of EEG; disorganization of background rhythm of EEG. **GI:** Anorexia, N&V, diarrhea, dry mouth, gastritis, salivary gland swelling, abdominal pain, excessive salivation, flatulence, indigestion, incontinence of urine or feces, dysgeusia/taste distortion, salty taste, swollen lips, dental caries. **Dermatologic:** Drying and thinning of hair, anesthesia of skin, chronic folliculitis, xerosis cutis, alopecia, exacerbation of psoriasis, acne, angioedema. **Neuromuscular:** Tremor, muscle hyperirritability (fasciculations, twitching, clonic movements), ataxia, choreoathetotic movements, hyperactive DTRs, polyarthralgia. **GU:** Albuminuria, oliguria, polyuria, glycosuria, decreased C_{CR}, symptoms of nephrogenic diabetes, impotence/sexual dysfunction. **Thyroid:** Euthyroid goiter or hypothyroidism, including myxedema, accompanied by lower T_3 and T_4. **Miscellaneous:** Fatigue, lethargy, dehydration, weight loss, transient scotomata, tightness in chest, hypercalcemia, hyperparathyroidism, thirst, swollen painful joints, fever.

The following symptoms are unrelated to lithium dosage. Transient EEG and ECG changes, leukocytosis, headache, diffuse nontoxic goiter with or without hypothyroidism, transient hyperglycemia, generalized pruritus with or without rash, cutaneous ulcers, albuminuria, worsening of organic brain syndrome, excessive weight gain, edematous swelling of ankles or wrists, thirst or polyuria (may resemble diabetes mellitus), metallic taste, symptoms similar to Raynaud's phenomenon.

LABORATORY TEST CONSIDERATIONS

False + urinary glucose test (Benedict's). ↑ Serum glucose, CK. False – or ↓ serum PBI, uric acid; ↑ TSH, I^{131} uptake; ↓ T_3, T_4.

OVERDOSE MANAGEMENT

Symptoms: Symptoms dependent on serum lithium levels. **Levels less than 2 mEq/L:** N&V, diarrhea, muscle weakness, drowsiness, loss of coordination. **Levels of 2–3 mEq/L:** Agitation, ataxia, blackouts, blurred vision, choreoathetoid movements, confusion, dysarthria, fasciculations, giddiness, hyperreflexia, hypertonia, agitation or manic-like behavior, myoclonic twitching or movement of entire limbs, slurred speech, tinnitus, urinary or fecal incontinence, vertigo. **Levels over 3 mEq/L:** Complex clinical picture involving multiple organs and organ systems. ***Arrhythmias, coma***, hypotension, ***peripheral vascular collapse, seizures (focal and generalized)***, spasticity, stupor, twitching of muscle groups. *Treatment:* Early symptoms are treated by decreasing the dose or stopping treatment for 24–48 hr. In severe cases, first eliminate lithium from the body:

- Use gastric lavage.
- Restore fluid and electrolyte balance (can use saline).
- Regulate and maintain kidney function.
- Increase lithium excretion by giving aminophylline, mannitol, or urea.
- Prevent infection. Maintain adequate respiration.
- Chest x-rays
- Monitor thyroid function.
- Institute hemodialysis, especially if lithium levels are >3.5 to 4 mEq/L.

DRUG INTERACTIONS

Acetazolamide / ↓ Lithium effect by ↑ renal excretion
Bumetanide / ↑ Lithium toxicity R/T ↓ renal clearance
Carbamazepine / ↑ Risk of lithium toxicity
Diazepam / ↑ Risk of hypothermia
Ethacrynic acid / ↑ Lithium toxicity R/T ↓ renal clearance
Fluoxetine / ↑ Serum lithium levels
Furosemide / ↑ Lithium toxicity R/T ↓ renal clearance
Haloperidol / ↑ Risk of neurologic toxicity
Iodide salts / Additive effect to cause hypothyroidism
Mannitol / ↓ Lithium effect by ↑ renal excretion
Mazindol / ↑ Chance of lithium toxicity R/T ↑ serum levels
Methyldopa / ↑ Chance of neurotoxic effects with or without ↑ lithium serum levels
Neuromuscular blocking agents / Lithium ↑ neuromuscular blockade → severe respiratory depression/apnea
NSAIDs / ↓ Lithium renal clearance, possibly R/T inhibition of renal prostaglandin synthesis
Phenothiazines / ↓ Phenothiazine levels or ↑ lithium levels
Phenytoin / ↑ Risk of lithium toxicity

Probenecid / ↑ Risk of lithium toxicity R/T ↑ serum levels
Sodium chloride / Excretion of lithium is proportional to amount of sodium chloride ingested; if client is on salt-free diet, may develop lithium toxicity since less lithium excreted
Sympathomimetics / ↓ Drug pressor effects
Theophyllines, including aminophylline / ↓ Lithium effect R/T ↑ renal excretion
Thiazide diuretics, triamterene / ↑ Risk of lithium toxicity R/T ↓ renal clearance
Tricyclic antidepressants / ↑ TCA effects
Urea / ↓ Lithium effect by ↑ renal excretion
Urinary alkalinizers / ↓ Lithium effect by ↑ renal excretion
Verapamil / ↓ Lithium levels and toxicity

HOW SUPPLIED

Lithium carbonate. ***Capsules:*** 150 mg, 300 mg, 600 mg; ***Oral Solution:*** 8 mEq lithium/5 mL (equivalent to 300 mg lithium carbonate/5 mL); ***Tablets:*** 300 mg; ***Tablets, Extended-Release:*** 300 mg, 400 mg.
Lithium citrate. ***Syrup:*** 300 mg/5 mL.

DOSAGE

Lithium carbonate, Lithium citrate

CAPSULES; ORAL SOLUTION; SYRUP; TABLETS; TABLETS, EXTENDED-RELEASE

Acute mania.

Adults: Individualized and according to lithium serum level (not to exceed 1.4 mEq/L) and clinical response. **Usual initial:** 300–600 mg 3 times per day or 600–900 mg twice per day of slow-release form; **elderly and debilitated clients:** 0.6–1.2 grams/day in three divided doses. **Maintenance:** 300 mg 3–4 times per day. Administration of drug is discontinued when lithium serum level exceeds 1.2 mEq/L and resumed 24 hr after it has fallen below that level.

To reverse neutropenia.

300–1,000 mg/day (to achieve serum levels of 0.5–1.0 mEq/L) for 7–10 days.

Prophylaxis of cluster headaches.

600–900 mg/day.

NURSING IMPLICATIONS

Do not confuse Lithonate, Lithobid, and Lithotabs (all trade names for lithium carbonate). Do not confuse lithium carbonate with lanthanum carbonate (a phosphate binder).

IMPLEMENTATION/ADMINISTRATION/STORAGE

1. To prevent toxic serum levels, determine blood levels 1–2 times per week during initiation of therapy, and monthly thereafter, on blood drawn 8–12 hr after dosage.
2. Full beneficial drug effects may not be noted for 6–10 days.

ASSESSMENT

1. Note reasons for therapy, other agents trialed, characteristics of S&S, behavioral presentation. Conduct a drug history; determine if taking other medications likely to interact, i.e., thiazide diuretics which may induce dehydration.
2. Use lower doses and more frequent monitoring in elderly. Toxicity closely related to serum concentrations and may occur at doses close to therapeutic levels.
3. Since drug decreases renal sodium absorption, ensure clients maintain adequate salt and fluid intake. Thyroid replacement may be required with chronic therapy. Chronic use may also lead to nephrogenic diabetes insipidus.
4. Assess mental and hydration status, CV function, VS, electrolytes, urinalysis, Wt, and ECG. Monitor lithium levels, kidney and thyroid function studies; assess for decreased function.

CLIENT/FAMILY TEACHING

1. Take with food or immediately after meals. Avoid any caffeinated beverages/foods; may aggravate mania.
2. Do not engage in physical activities that require alertness or physical coordination until drug effects realized; may cause drowsiness.
3. Maintain a constant level of salt intake to avoid fluctuations in lithium activity. Weight gain and swelling may be related to sodium retention; report if excessive.
4. Drink 10–12 glasses of water each day; avoid dehydration (e.g., vigorous exercise, sunbathing, sauna) to prevent increased concentrations of lithium in urine. Avoid excessive caf-

feine intake; may increase urinary excretion of drug.

5. **Report diarrhea (may need supplemental fluids or salt), vomiting, drowsiness, muscular weakness, or lack of coordination.**
6. **Will take several weeks to realize a behavioral benefit from therapy.**
7. **Do not change brands of drug. Avoid all OTC agents.**
8. **Lithium works well in the manic phase; concomitant antidepressant use may be necessary during depressive phases.**
9. **Transient acne eruptions, folliculitis, altered sexual function in men may occur.**
10. **Carry name and telephone number of persons to contact if needed or if family members note behavioral/physical changes contrary to expectations.**
11. **Keep all F/U to assess response, labs (drug levels), and for adverse SE.**

OUTCOMES/EVALUATE

- Stabilization of mood swings
- ↓ Symptoms of mania (↓ hyperactivity, ↓ sleeplessness; improved judgment)
- Therapeutic serum drug levels (0.4–1.0 mEq/L)

Lomustine

(loh-**MUS**-teen)

Classification(s): Antineoplastic, alkylating

Pregnancy Category: D

RX: CeeNu (Abbreviation: CCNU).

SEE ALSO ***ANTINEOPLASTIC AGENTS*** AND ***ALKYLATING AGENTS***.

INDICATIONS/USES

(1) Used alone or in combination to treat primary and metastatic brain tumors. (2) Secondary therapy in Hodgkin's disease (in combination with other antineoplastics).

ACTION/KINETICS

Action

Alkylating agent that inhibits DNA and RNA synthesis through DNA alkylation. It also affects other cellular processes, including RNA, protein synthesis and the processing of ribosomal and nucleoplasmic messenger RNA; DNA base component structure; the rate of DNA synthesis and DNA polymerase activity. Is cell cycle nonspecific.

Pharmacokinetics

Rapidly absorbed from the GI tract; crosses the blood-brain barrier resulting in concentrations higher than in plasma. **Peak plasma level:** 1–6 hr; **t½:** biphasic; **initial,** 6 hr; **postdistribution:** 1–2 days. From 15 to 20% of drug remains in body after 5 days. Fifty percent of drug excreted within 12 hr through the kidney, 75% within 4 days. Small amounts are excreted through the lungs and feces. Metabolites present in milk.

CONTRAINDICATIONS

Lactation.

SPECIAL CONCERNS

■ (1) Bone marrow suppression, especially thrombocytopenia and leukopenia, which may contribute to bleeding and overwhelming infections in an already compromised client, is the most common and severe toxic effect. (2) Because the major toxicity is delayed bone marrow suppression, monitor blood counts weekly for 6 or more weeks after a dose. Do not give courses of lomustine more frequently than every 6 weeks at the recommended dose. (3) Bone marrow toxicity is cumulative. Consider dosage adjustments on the basis of nadir blood counts from prior dosage. ■

SIDE EFFECTS

Most Common

N&V, sore mouth/lips/throat, alopecia, lethargy, ataxia, disorientation, bone marrow suppression.

See *Antineoplastic Agents* for a complete list of possible side effects. Also, high incidence of N&V 3–6 hr after administration and lasting for 24 hr. Renal and pulmonary toxicity. Dysarthria. Delayed bone marrow suppression may occur due to cumulative bone marrow toxicity. ***Thrombocytopenia and leukopenia may lead to bleeding and overwhelming infections.*** Secondary malignancies.

LABORATORY TEST CONSIDERATIONS

↑ LFTs (reversible).

HOW SUPPLIED

Capsules: 10 mg, 40 mg, 100 mg; ***Dose Pack:*** 2–100 mg capsules, 2–40 mg capsules, and 2–10 mg capsules.

DOSAGE

CAPSULES

Metastatic brain tumors; secondary therapy in Hodgkin's disease.

Adults and children, initial:
130 mg/m² as a single dose q 6 weeks. If bone marrow function is reduced, decrease dose to 100 mg/m² q 6 weeks. Subsequent dosage based on blood counts of clients (platelet count above 100,000/mm³ and leukocyte count above 4,000/mm³). Undertake weekly blood tests and do not repeat therapy before 6 weeks.

NURSING IMPLICATIONS

IMPLEMENTATION/ADMINISTRATION/STORAGE

1. Given alone or in combination with other drugs, surgery, or XRT.
2. Store below 40°C (104°F).

ASSESSMENT

1. Note reasons for therapy, onset, other agents/therapies trialed, outcome and mental status.
2. Obtain baseline PFTs during treatment. Those with baseline less than 70% of the predicted forced vital capacity (FVC) or carbon monoxide diffusing capacity (DLCO) are particularly at risk.
3. Antiemetics prior to dosing may diminish/prevent N&V. Nausea and vomiting may occur 3 to 6 hr after oral dose; usually lasts <24 hr. Also may reduce N&V if given while fasting.
4. Review CT/MRI and/or lab/bone marrow results.
5. Monitor CBC weekly for 6 weeks after a dose. Dose based on WBC and platelet counts. Monitor liver and renal function periodically; causes platelet and leukocyte suppression. Nadir: 3–7 weeks.

CLIENT/FAMILY TEACHING

1. Medication comes in capsules of three strengths and a combination of capsules will make up the correct dose in the dose pack; take all at one time preferably on an empty stomach to ↓ nausea. Wear gloves when handling capsules.
2. May have N&V up to 36 hr after treatment; may be followed by 2–3 days of anorexia. Take antiemetics as prescribed. GI distress may be reduced by taking antiemetics before drug therapy or by taking the drug after fasting.
3. Report feelings of depression caused by prolonged N&V so that various antiemetics can be tried and to ensure that psychological support is available as needed.
4. Report abnormal bruising or bleeding, sore throat, significant weight loss, swelling of feet or ankles, yellowing of skin or S&S of flu (fever, chills, fatigue).
5. Avoid all OTC agents and avoid alcohol for short periods after taking a dose of lomustine.
6. Practice reliable contraception during therapy.
7. Six-week intervals are needed between doses for optimum effect with minimal toxicity; hematologic profiles should be assessed frequently.
8. Keep all F/U to assess response, labs, and for adverse SE.

OUTCOMES/EVALUATE

Control/remission of metastatic processes

Loperamide hydrochloride

(loh-**PER**-ah-myd)

Classification(s): Antidiarrheal

Pregnancy Category: B

OTC: Diar-aid Caplets, Imodium, Imodium A-D Caplets and Liquid, K-Pek II, Neo-Diaral, Pepto Diarrhea Control.

RX: Imodium.

✱ **OTC:** Apo-Loperamide, Riva-Loperamide, Sandoz Loperamide.

INDICATIONS/USES

OTC: Control symptoms of diarrhea, including traveler's diarrhea. *Investigational:* With trimethoprim-sulfamethoxazole to treat traveler's diarrhea.

Rx: (1) Symptomatic relief of acute nonspecific diarrhea and of chronic diarrhea associated with inflammatory bowel disease. (2) Decrease the volume of discharge from ileostomies. *NOTE:* Not effective in improving symptoms of irritable bowel syndrome.

ACTION/KINETICS

Action

Slows intestinal motility by acting on the nerve endings and/or intramural ganglia embedded in the intestinal wall. The prolonged retention of the feces in the intestine results in reducing the volume of the stools, increasing viscosity, and decreasing fluid and electrolyte loss. Reportedly more effective than diphenoxylate.

Pharmacokinetics

Time to peak effect, capsules: 5 hr; **PO solution:** 2.5 hr. **t½:** 9.1–14.4 hr. Twenty-five percent excreted unchanged in the feces.

CONTRAINDICATIONS

In clients in whom constipation should be avoided. OTC if body temperature is over 38°C (101°F) and in presence of bloody diarrhea. Use in acute diarrhea associated with organisms that penetrate the intestinal mucosa, such as *E. coli, Salmonella,* and *Shigella.*

SPECIAL CONCERNS

- **Safe use in children under age 2 and during lactation not established.**
- **Fluid and electrolyte depletion may occur in clients with diarrhea.**
- **Children under age 3 are more sensitive to the narcotic effects of loperamide.**

SIDE EFFECTS

Most Common

Abdominal pain/distention/discomfort, constipation, dry mouth, N&V, epigastric distress, dizziness, drowsiness.

GI: Abdominal pain, distention, or discomfort. Constipation, dry mouth, N&V, epigastric distress. Toxic megacolon in clients with acute colitis. **CNS:** Drowsiness, dizziness, fatigue. **Miscellaneous:** Allergic skin rashes.

OVERDOSE MANAGEMENT

Symptoms: Constipation, CNS depression, GI irritation. *Treatment:* Give activated charcoal (it will reduce absorption up to ninefold). If vomiting has not occurred, perform gastric lavage followed by activated charcoal, 100 grams, through a gastric tube. Give naloxone for respiratory depression.

DRUG INTERACTIONS

Ritonavir / ↑ Loperamide AUC and peak plasma levels

Saquinavir / ↑ Loperamide levels and ↓ saquinavir levels perhaps R/T ↓ saquinavir absorption

HOW SUPPLIED

Capsules: 2 mg; *Liquid:* 1 mg/1 mL, 1 mg/5 mL, 1 mg/7.5 mL; *Tablets:* 2 mg.

DOSAGE

OTC: CAPSULES, LIQUID, TABLETS

Acute diarrhea.

Adults: 4 mg after the first loose bowel movement (LBM) followed by 2 mg after each subsequent bowel movement to a maximum of 8 mg/day for no more than 2 days. **Pediatric, 9–11 years:** 2 mg after the first LBM followed by 1 mg after each subsequent LBM, not to exceed 6 mg/day for no more than 2 days. **Pediatric, 6–8 years:** 1 mg after the first bowel movement followed by 1 mg after each subsequent LBM, not to exceed 4 mg/day for no more than 2 days.

RX: CAPSULES

Acute diarrhea.

Adults, initial: 4 mg, followed by 2 mg after each unformed stool, up to maximum of 16 mg/day. **Pediatric:** *Day 1 doses:* **8–12 years:** 2 mg 3 times per day; **6–8 years:** 2 mg twice a day; **2–5 years:** 1 mg 3 times per day using only the liquid. *After day 1:* 1 mg/10 kg after a loose stool (total daily dosage should not exceed day 1 recommended doses).

Chronic diarrhea.

Adults: 4–8 mg/day as a single or divided dose. Dosage not established for chronic diarrhea in children.

NURSING IMPLICATIONS

ASSESSMENT

1. **Note reasons for therapy, onset, frequency, characteristics of stools. Identify any contributing/causative factors, i.e., travel, drinking untreated water.**
2. **Note any experience with this drug or any allergy to piperidine derivatives.**
3. **Stop drug promptly and report if abdominal distention develops in clients with acute ulcerative colitis.**

4. Ensure colonoscopy completed with chronic diarrhea to note etiology.

CLIENT/FAMILY TEACHING

1. Take as directed; do not exceed 16 mg/24 hr.
2. May cause dry mouth; try ice, sugarless gum, and candy to alleviate. Ensure adequate fluid intake to prevent dehydration R/T diarrhea.
3. Use caution while driving or performing tasks requiring alertness; may cause dizziness/drowsiness.
4. OTC products are not intended for use in children less than 6 years of age unless provider prescribed. Avoid alcohol and CNS depressants during therapy with this drug.
5. Record number, frequency, and consistency of stools per day and the amount of drug consumed. Report if diarrhea lasts up to 5 days without relief.
6. In *acute diarrhea,* discontinue after 48 hr and report if ineffective.
7. If no improvement within 10 days after using up to 16 mg/day for *chronic diarrhea,* symptoms are not likely to improve with further use. Seek medical intervention.
8. Report if fever, nausea, abdominal pain/distention occurs; may require dosage adjustment.
9. In children, dietary treatment of diarrhea is preferred. Avoid apple juices, formulas, and high fat or spicy foods.
10. Keep all F/U to assess response, for adverse SE, and need for further workup.

OUTCOMES/EVALUATE

- Reduction/Control of diarrhea
- ↓ Volume of ileostomy output

Loratidine

(loh-**RAH**-tih-deen)

Classification(s): Antihistamine, second generation, piperidine

Pregnancy Category: B

OTC: Liqui-Gel: Claritin Non-Drowsy Liqui-Gels. **Syrup:** Alavert Children's, Children's Loratidine Syrup, Claritin, Claritin Allergy Children's, Clear-Atadine Children's, Dimetapp Children's ND Non-Drowsy Allergy, Loratidine Hive Relief, Non-Drowsy Allergy Relief for Kids. **Tablets:** Claritin 24-Hour Allergy, Claritin Hives Relief, Clear-Atadine. **Tablets, Chewable:** Claritin Children's Allergy. **Tablets, Orally Disintegrating:** Alavert, Claritin RediTabs, Dimetapp Children's ND Non-Drowsy Allergy, Non-Drowsy Allergy Relief, Triaminic Allerchews.

🍁 **Rx:** Apo-Loratidine, Claritin Kids.

SEE ALSO ***ANTIHISTAMINES.***

INDICATIONS/USES

Relief of nasal and nonnasal symptoms of seasonal allergic rhinitis, including runny nose, itchy and watery eyes, itchy palate, and sneezing. *Investigational:* Treatment of chronic idiopathic urticaria in clients 2 years of age and older.

ACTION/KINETICS

Action

Metabolized in the liver to active metabolite descarboethoxyloratidine. Low to no sedative and anticholinergic effects; no antiemetic effect. Does not alter cardiac repolarization and has not been linked to development of torsades de pointes as seen with astemizole and terfenadine.

Pharmacokinetics

Onset: 1–3 hr. **Maximum effect:** 8–12 hr. Food delays absorption. **t½, loratidine:** 8.4 hr; **t½, descarboethoxyloratidine:** 28 hr. **Duration:** 24 hr. Excreted through both the urine and feces.

CONTRAINDICATIONS

Use of antihistamines in children less than 2 years of age; studies are continuing for use in children, age 2–11 years.

SPECIAL CONCERNS

- **Use with caution, if at all, during lactation.**
- **Give a lower initial dose in liver impairment.**

SIDE EFFECTS

Most Common

Headache, somnolence, fatigue, dry mouth.

GI: Altered salivation, dry mouth, gastritis, dyspepsia, stomatitis, toothache, thirst, altered taste, flatulence. **CNS:** Headache, somnolence, hypoesthesia, hyperkinesia, migraine, anxiety, depression, agitation, paroniria, amnesia, impaired concentration. **Ophthalmic:** Altered lacrimation, conjunctivitis, blurred vision, eye pain, blepharospasm. **Respiratory:** URTI, epistaxis, pharyngitis, dyspnea, coughing, rhinitis, sinusitis, sneezing, bronchitis, ***bronchospasm***, hemoptysis, laryngitis.

Body as a whole: Fatigue, asthenia, increased sweating, flushing, malaise, rigors, fever, dry skin, aggravated allergy, pruritus, purpura. **Musculoskeletal:** Back/chest pain, leg cramps, arthralgia, myalgia. **GU:** Breast pain, menorrhagia, dysmenorrhea, vaginitis. **Miscellaneous:** Earache, dysphonia, dry hair, urinary discoloration.

HOW SUPPLIED

Liqui-Gels: 10 mg; *Syrup:* 5 mg/5 mL; *Tablets:* 10 mg; *Tablets, Chewable:* 5 mg; *Tablets, Orally Disintegrating:* 5 mg, 10 mg.

DOSAGE

LIQUI-GELS; SYRUP; TABLETS; TABLETS, CHEWABLE; TABLETS, ORALLY DISINTEGRATING

Allergic rhinitis, chronic idiopathic urticaria.

Adults and children, 6 and older: 10 mg once daily. **Children, 2–5 years of age:** 5 mg (chewable tablet or syrup) once daily. *In clients with impaired kidney function (GFR <30 mL/min):* **Adults and children years and older, initial:** 10 mg every other day; **children, 2–5 years of age, initial:** 5 mg every other day. Do not use in children less than 2 years of age.

NURSING IMPLICATIONS

IMPLEMENTATION/ADMINISTRATION/STORAGE

1. Use the liqui-gels, syrup, or chewable/orally disintegrating tablets for children ages 6 to 11.
2. Use caution. The concentration of the syrup is 5 mg/5 mL.
3. Protect unit dose packs, unit-of-use packs, and rapidly disintegrating tablets from excessive moisture.
4. Store tablets from 2–30°C (36–86°F). Store syrup and rapidly disintegrating tablets from 2–25°C (36–77°F).

ASSESSMENT

1. List reasons for therapy, type, onset, characteristics of S&S. clinical presentation. List other agents trialed; outcome.
2. Note pulmonary findings; assess lung sounds/secretions, throat, cervical nodes, turbinates, skin testing when necessary.
3. Identify triggers contributing to allergic S&S. Advise to remove carpet, enclose mattress and pillows in plastic, control dust, vacuum regularly, remove pets and plants from sleeping area.
4. Review drug profile. Cautiously coadminister with drugs that inhibit hepatic metabolism (i.e., macrolide antibiotics, cimetidine, ranitidine, ketoconazole, or theophylline).
5. Do not administer orally-disintegrating tablet to client with phenylketonuria without provider approval.
6. Monitor renal and LFTs; reduce dose or frequency of dosing with dysfunction. Assess elderly and clients with hepatic and renal impairment for increasing somnolence.

CLIENT/FAMILY TEACHING

1. Take with or without food. If stomach upset occurs, take with food.
2. If using rapidly disintegrating tablets, remove from blister pack just before using and place on the tongue. Disintegration occurs within seconds, after which the tablet contents may be swallowed with or without water. Use rapidly disintegrating tablets within 6 months of opening the foil pouch and immediately after opening the individual tablet blister.
3. With syrup, use dosing syringe/spoon, or dosing cup to measure and administer prescribed dose.
4. Do not perform activities that require mental alertness until drug effects realized; should not cause drowsiness.
5. Increase fluid intake to 1.5 to 2 qt/day to decrease viscosity of secretions.
6. Avoid intake of alcohol or other CNS depressants (e.g., sedatives, hypnotics, tranquilizers).
7. With allergy skin testing, avoid taking medication for 4 days before test.
8. Avoid prolonged or excessive exposure to direct or artificial sunlight.
9. Identify triggers, i.e., foods, detergents, or materials that may have induced allergic/itching response.
10. Keep all F/U to assess response and for adverse SE.

OUTCOMES/EVALUATE

- Relief of nasal congestion and seasonal allergic manifestations

- **Control of skin eruption R/T antigenic offender (unlabeled)**

IV

Lorazepam

(lor-**AYZ**-eh-pam)

Classification(s): Antianxiety drug, benzodiazepine

Pregnancy Category: D

RX: Ativan, Lorazepam Intensol, **C-IV**

Rx: Apo-Lorazepam, PMS-Lorazepam.

SEE ALSO ***TRANQUILIZERS/ANTIMANIC DRUGS/HYPNOTICS***.

INDICATIONS/USES

PO: Short-term relief of anxiety disorders or symptoms of anxiety with depression. *Investigational:* Short-term improvement of chronic insomnia.

Parenteral: (1) Preanesthetic medication to produce sedation, relief of anxiety, and a decreased ability to recall events related to surgery. (2) Status epilepticus.

ACTION/KINETICS

Action

Reduces anxiety by increasing or facilitating the inhibitory neurotransmitter activity of GABA.

Pharmacokinetics

Absorbed and eliminated faster than other benzodiazepines. **Peak plasma levels, PO:** 1–6 hr; **IM:** 1–1.5 hr. **t½:** 10–20 hr. Metabolized to inactive compounds, which are excreted through the kidneys.

ADDITIONAL CONTRAINDICATIONS

Narrow-angle glaucoma. Parenterally in children less than 18 years.

SPECIAL CONCERNS

- **PO dosage in children less than 12 years of age and IV dosage in children less than 18 years of age has not been established.**
- **Use cautiously in renal or hepatic disease.**

SIDE EFFECTS

Most Common

Drowsiness (transient), ataxia, confusion.

See *Tranquilizers/Antimanic Drugs/Hypnotics* for a complete list of possible side effects.

ADDITIONAL DRUG INTERACTIONS

Scopolamine / Sedation, hallucinations, and behavioral abnormalities when used with parenteral lorazepam

Valproic acid / ↑ Valproic acid levels

HOW SUPPLIED

Injection: 2 mg/mL, 4 mg/mL; ***Oral Solution, Concentrated:*** 2 mg/mL; ***Tablets:*** 0.5 mg, 1 mg, 2 mg.

DOSAGE

ORAL CONCENTRATE; TABLETS

Anxiety.

Adults, initial: 2–3 mg/day given 2 or 3 times per day. Dose range varies from 1 to 10 mg/day given in divided doses.

Insomnia due to anxiety or transient situational stress.

Single dose of 2–4 mg at bedtime.

IM

Preanesthetic.

0.05 mg/kg, up to a maximum of 4 mg. For optimum effect, give at least 2 hr before surgical procedure. Administer narcotic analgesics at their usual preoperative time.

IV

Status epilepticus.

Adults, 18 years and older, usual: 4 mg given slowly (2 mg/min). If seizures continue or recur after a 10–15 min period, an additional 4 mg IV may be given slowly.

Preanesthetic.

Initial: 2 mg total or 0.044 mg/kg (whichever is smaller). This will sedate most adults. Do not exceed dose in clients over 50 years of age. Doses as high as 0.05 mg/kg (up to a total of 4 mg) may be given if a greater lack of recall is desired. For optimum effect, give 15–20 min prior to procedure.

NURSING IMPLICATIONS

Do not confuse lorazepam (Ativan) with alprazolam (Xanax) or with hydroxyzine (Atarax), each of which is an anti-anxiety agent.

IMPLEMENTATION/ADMINISTRATION/STORAGE

1. Individualize dosage. If higher doses required, increase evening dose before the daytime doses. Increase gradually to minimize side effects.
2. For the elderly or debilitated, start with 1–2 mg/day of tablet or solution in divided doses. Adjust dose as needed and tolerated. When higher doses are needed, increase the evening dose before the daytime dose. The total daily dose should not exceed 3 mg in the elderly.
3. Intensol product is a concentrated PO solution. Mix with liquid or semi-solid foods such as water, juices, soda or soda-like beverages, applesauce, or puddings.
4. Use only the calibrated dropper provided with the Intensol solution. Draw prescribed amount into the dropper; squeeze contents onto the liquid or semi-solid food and stir gently for a few seconds. Consume entire amount of the mixture immediately. Do not store for future use.
5. For IM, inject deep into muscle mass.
6. IM administration is not recommended for status epilepticus as therapeutic levels may not be reached as quickly as with IV. IM can be used when an IV port is not available.
7. Reduce dose of lorazepam by 50% when given with probenecid or valproate.
8. It may be necessary to increase dose of lorazepam in females who are also taking oral contraceptives.
9. Refrigerate injection and oral solution from 2–8°C (36–46°F). Protect from light.
10. Store tablets at controlled room temperature from 15–30°C (59–86°F). Protect from moisture.
11. IV For IV use, dilute just before use with equal amounts of either sterile water, NaCl, or 5% dextrose injection. Do not shake vigorously; will result in air entrapment.
12. Inject directly into tubing of an existing IV infusion over 2–5 min.
13. Do not exceed 2 mg/min IV. Have available equipment to maintain a patent airway. Keep client supine after parenteral therapy and observe.
14. Do not use if solution is discolored or contains a precipitate.
15. COMPATIBILITY D5W, NSS.
16. INCOMPATIBILITY Give separately.

ASSESSMENT

1. Note reasons for therapy, onset, characteristics of S&S. Assess mental status; describe anxiety symptoms, any associated factors/triggers.
2. List other agents trialed, outcome.
3. Determine if psychological evaluation/counselling has been initiated.
4. Check for sleep apnea, severe respiratory conditions that may preclude therapy. Avoid with narrow angle glaucoma. Assess for fall risk and limit total daily dose to 3 mg in the elderly.
5. Prolonged therapy may lead to physical/psychological dependence.
6. Monitor CBC, renal and LFTs.

CLIENT/FAMILY TEACHING

1. Take as directed; may take with food if stomach upset occurs. Do not share meds.
2. If using concentrated oral solution, use calibrated dropper to measure prescribed dose and then add solution to a liquid (i.e., juice, water, soda) or semisolid food (i.e., applesauce, pudding); stir for a few seconds then immediately take (give) the entire mixture. Do not prepare mixtures ahead of time and store.
3. May cause dizziness, drowsiness, impaired judgment, loss of recall; avoid activities that require mental alertness until drug effects realized.
4. Report increased depression or suicidal ideations or any new onset rash immediately.
5. Avoid alcohol and CNS depressants.
6. With long-term therapy, do not stop suddenly; must be tapered to prevent severe withdrawal symptoms.
7. Report if symptoms (i.e., anxiety, panic attacks, seizures) do not appear to improve, get worse, or if bothersome side effects (i.e., drowsiness, memory impairment) persist.
8. Keep all F/U to assess response, counselling (need to continue therapy), and adverse SE.

OUTCOMES/EVALUATE

- ↓ Anxiety; ↓ Insomnia
- Termination of seizures
- Muscle relaxation/amnesia
- Control of alcohol withdrawal (unlabeled)
- Relief of chemotherapy-induced N&V (unlabeled)

Losartan potassium

(loh-**SAR**-tan)

Classification(s): Antihypertensive, angiotensin II receptor blocker

Pregnancy Category: C (first trimester); **D** (second and third trimesters)

RX: Cozaar.

SEE ALSO ***ANGIOTENSIN II RECEPTOR ANTAGONISTS*** AND ***ANTIHYPERTENSIVE AGENTS***.

INDICATIONS/USES

(1) Antihypertensive, alone or in combination with other antihypertensive drugs (including diuretics). (2) Reduce risk of stroke in clients with hypertension and left ventricular hypertrophy. Is evidence this use does not apply to African American clients. (3) Nephropathy in type 2 diabetics with an elevated serum creatinine and proteinuria.

ACTION/KINETICS

Action

Competitively blocks the angiotensin AT_1 receptor located in vascular smooth muscle and the adrenal glands, thus blocking the vasoconstrictor and aldosterone-secreting effects of angiotensin II (a potent vasoconstrictor). Thus, BP is reduced.

Pharmacokinetics

Undergoes significant first-pass metabolism (by CYP2C9 and CYP3A4) in the liver, where it is converted to an active carboxylic acid metabolite that is responsible for most of the angiotensin receptor blockade. About 33% is bioavailable. Rapidly absorbed after PO administration, although food slows absorption. **Peak plasma levels of losartan and metabolite:** 1 hr and 3–4 hr, respectively. When used alone, decrease in BP in African Americans was less than in non-African Americans. **t½, losartan:** 2 hr; **t½, metabolite:** 6–9 hr. **Maximum effects:** 1 week (3 to 6 weeks in some clients). Drug and metabolites are excreted through both the urine (35%) and feces (60%). **Plasma protein binding:** 98.7% of the drug and 99.8% of the metabolite.

CONTRAINDICATIONS

Use during second and third trimesters of pregnancy due to possible injury and death to developing fetus. Use in children less than 6 years of age or in children with a GFR <30 mL/min/1.73 m^2.

SPECIAL CONCERNS

When used in pregnancy during the second and third trimesters, drugs that act directly on the renin-angiotensin system can cause injury and even death to the developing fetus. When pregnancy is detected, discontinue losartan as soon as possible.

- **Risk, in severe CHF, of oliguria and/or progressive azotemia with acute renal failure and/or death (rare).**
- **Risk of increased serum creatinine or BUN in unilateral or bilateral renal artery stenosis**
- **Lower doses recommended in hepatic insufficiency.**

SIDE EFFECTS

Most Common

URTI, dizziness, cough, diarrhea, sinus disorder, nasal congestion, dyspepsia/heartburn, pain.

GI: Diarrhea, dyspepsia, anorexia, constipation, dental pain, dry mouth, flatulence, gastritis, vomiting, taste perversion. **CV:** Angina pectoris, second-degree AV block, vasculitis, ***CVA, MI, ventricular tachycardia, ventricular fibrillation***, hypotension, palpitation, sinus bradycardia, tachycardia, orthostatic effects. **CNS:** Dizziness, insomnia, anxiety, anxiety disorder, ataxia, confusion, depression, abnormal dreams, hypesthesia, decreased libido, impaired memory, migraine, nervousness, paresthesia, peripheral neuropathy, panic disorder, sleep disorder, somnolence, tremor, vertigo. **Respiratory:** URTI, cough, nasal congestion, sinus disorder, sinusitis, dyspnea, bronchitis, pharyngeal discomfort, epistaxis, rhinitis, respiratory congestion. **Musculoskeletal:** Muscle cramps, myalgia, joint swelling, musculoskeletal pain, stiffness, arthralgia, arthritis, fibromyalgia, muscle weakness; pain in the back, legs, arms, hips, knees, shoulders. **Dermatologic:** Alopecia, dermatitis, dry skin, ecchymosis, erythema, flushing, photosensitivity, pruritus, rash, sweating, urticaria. **GU:** Impotence, nocturia, urinary frequency, UTI. **Ophthalmic:** Blurred vision, burning/stinging in the eye, conjunctivitis, decrease in visual acuity. **Miscellaneous:** Gout, anemia, tinnitus, facial edema, fever, syncope, pain.

LABORATORY TEST CONSIDERATIONS

Minor ↑ BUN, serum creatinine. Occasional ↑ liver enzymes and/or serum bilirubin. Small ↓ H&H.

OVERDOSE MANAGEMENT

Symptoms: Hypotension, tachycardia, bradycardia (due to vagal stimulation). *Treatment:* Supportive treatment. Hemodialysis is not indicated.

DRUG INTERACTIONS

Grapefruit juice / ↓ Liver metabolism of losartan to its active form
Indomethacin / ↓ Antihypertensive effect of losartan
Phenobarbital / ↓ Plasma losartan levels (20%)

HOW SUPPLIED

Tablets: 25 mg, 50 mg, 100 mg.

DOSAGE

TABLETS

Hypertension.

Individualize dosage. **Adults, usual initial:** 50 mg once daily with or without food. Total daily doses range from 25 to 100 mg. In those with possible depletion of intravascular volume (e.g., clients treated with a diuretic) or in hepatic impairment, use 25 mg once daily. If the antihypertensive effect (measured at trough) is inadequate, a twice-a-day regimen, using the same dose, may be tried; or an increase in dose may give a more satisfactory result. If BP is not controlled by losartan alone, a diuretic (e.g., hydrochlorothiazide, 12.5 mg with losartan, 50 mg once daily) may be added.

Pediatric hypertension (age 6 years and older).

Initial: 0.7 mg/kg once daily (up to 50 mg total) given as a tablet or suspension. Adjust dose according to BP response. Doses above 1.4 mg/kg (or in excess of 100 mg) daily have not been evaluated in children.

Hypertension with left ventricular hypertrophy.

Initial: 50 mg once daily. Add hydrochlorothiazide, 12.5 mg/day, and/or increase the dose of losartan to 100 mg once daily followed by an increase in hydrochlorothiazide to 25 mg once daily based on BP response.

Nephropathy in type 2 diabetics.

Initial: 50 mg once daily. Increase to 100 mg once daily based on BP response. May be given with insulin and other hypoglycemic drugs.

NURSING IMPLICATIONS

Do not confuse Cozaar with Zocor (an antihyperlipidemic) or with Hyzaar (combination of losartan potassium and hydrochlorothiazide).

IMPLEMENTATION/ADMINISTRATION/STORAGE

1. No initial dosage adjustment is needed for the elderly or for those with renal impairment, including those on dialysis.
2. To prepare 200 mL of a 2.5 mg/mL suspension, add 10 mL of purified water to a 240 mL (8 oz) amber polyethylene terephthalate bottle containing ten 50 mg losartan tablets. Immediately shake for at least 2 min. Let the concentrate stand for 1 hr and then shake for 1 min to disperse the tablet contents. Separately prepare a 50/50 volumetric mixture of Ora-Plus and Ora-Sweet SF. Add 190 mL of the 50/50 Ora-Plus/Ora-Sweet SF mixture to the tablet and water slurry and shake for 1 min to disperse the ingredients. Refrigerate the suspension; can be stored for up to 4 weeks. Shake the suspension prior to each use and return promptly to the refrigerator.
3. Store tablets from 15–30°C (59–86°F) and protect from light. Keep container tightly closed.

ASSESSMENT

1. List reasons for therapy, onset, other agents used, other related conditions (diabetes, low EF), outcome.
2. Correct any volume depletion prior to using to prevent sympathomimetic hypotension. Reduce starting dose with volume depletion or renal/hepatic impairment. Observe for S&S of fluid or electrolyte imbalance.
3. When pregnancy is detected, discontinue as soon as possible.
4. Monitor CBC, microalbumin, renal and LFTs.

CLIENT/FAMILY TEACHING

1. Take as directed with or without food. Do not take with grapefruit juice. Avoid any OTC agents unless directed.
2. Do not change positions suddenly; dangle legs before rising, and rest until symptoms subside to prevent low BP and dizziness.
3. Avoid activities that require mental alertness until drug effects realized; may cause dizziness.
4. May cause photosensitivity reaction; avoid prolonged sun exposure and use precautions.
5. Use effective contraception; report immediately if pregnancy suspected. Drug associated with fetal injury.
6. Regular exercise, weight loss, low-salt diet, and lifestyle changes (i.e., no smoking, low alcohol, low-fat diet, low stress, adequate rest) may also contribute to enhanced BP control. Avoid salt substitutes containing potassium; may cause ↑ potassium levels.
7. Record BP and HR regularly for provider review.
8. Report any loss of response, swelling of the face/tongue, swallowing difficulty, or breathing problems immediately.
9. Keep all F/U to assess response, labs, and for adverse SE.

OUTCOMES/EVALUATE

- BP control
- Control of nephropathy in type 2 diabetics
- ↓ Stroke risk with HTN and LVH

Combination Drug

Losartan potassium and Hydrochlorothiazide

(loh-**SAR**-tan, **hy**-droh-klor-oh-**THIGH**-ah-zyd)

Classification(s): Antihypertensive (combination of angiotensin II receptor blocker and thiazide diuretic)

Pregnancy Category: C (first trimester); **D** (second and third trimesters)

RX: Hyzaar.

SEE ALSO ***LOSARTAN POTASSIUM AND HYDROCHLOROTHIAZIDE.***

INDICATIONS/USES

(1) Hypertension. Not indicated for initial therapy, except when hypertension is severe enough that the value of achieving prompt BP control exceeds the risk of initiating combination therapy. (2) Reduce risk of stroke in those with hypertension and left ventricular hypertrophy. Is evidence this benefit does not apply to Black clients.

CONTENT

Hyzaar: Losartan, an angiotensin II receptor blocker (listed first)/hydrochlorothiazide (thiazide diuretic): 50 mg/12.5 mg, 100 mg/12.5 mg, 100 mg/25 mg.

ACTION/KINETICS

Action

Losartan competitively blocks the angiotensin AT_1 receptor located in vascular smooth muscle and the adrenal glands, thus blocking the vasoconstrictor and aldosterone-secreting effects of angiotensin II (a potent vasoconstrictor). Thus, BP is reduced. Hydrochlorothiazide promotes the excretion of sodium and chloride, and thus water, by the distal renal tubule. Also increases excretion of potassium and to a lesser extent bicarbonate. The antihypertensive activity is thought to be due to direct dilation of the areterioles, as well as to a reduction in the total fluid volume of the body and altered sodium balance.

Pharmacokinetics

Losartan undergoes significant first-pass metabolism (by CYP2C9 and CYP3A4) in the liver, where it is converted to an active carboxylic acid metabolite that is responsible for most of the angiotensin receptor blockade. About 33% is bioavailable. Rapidly absorbed after PO administration, although food slows absorption. **Peak plasma levels of losartan and metabolite:** 1 hr and 3–4 hr, respectively. **t½, losartan:** 2 hr; **t½, metabolite:** 6–9 hr. **Maximum effects:** 1 week (3 to 6 weeks in some clients). Drug and metabolites are excreted through both the urine (35%) and feces (60%). Hydrochlorothiazide, **onset:** 2 hr; **peak effect:** 4–6 hr; **duration:** 6–12 hr. **t½:** 5.6–14.8 hr. Hydrochlorothiazide is not metabolized but is eliminated rapidly by the kidney.

CONTRAINDICATIONS

Hypersensitivity to any components of the product. In those with anuria or hypersensitivity to other sulfonamide-derived drugs. Not recommended for use during pregnancy or lactation. Not recommended for use in those with hepatic impairment who require titration with losartan (the lower starting dose of losartan recommended for use in such clients cannot be given using Hyzaar). Use with lithium.

SPECIAL CONCERNS

When used during the second and third trimesters of pregnancy, drugs that act directly on the renin-angiotensin system can cause injury and even death to the developing fetus. When pregnancy is detected, discontinue as soon as possible.

- **Use with caution in impaired hepatic function or progressive liver disease (minor alterations of fluid and electrolyte balance may precipitate hepatic coma).**
- **Hypersensitivity reactions to hydrochlorothiazide may occur in those with or without a history of allergy or bronchial asthma (more likely in clients with such a history).**
- **Thiazides may cause exacerbation/activation of systemic lupus erythematosus.**
- **Safety and efficacy not determined in children.**

SIDE EFFECTS

Most Common

Hypokalemia, dizziness, URTI, cough, back pain, rash, edema/swelling, palpitation.

See *Losartan potassium* and *Hydrochlorothiazide* for a complete list of possible side effects.

OVERDOSE MANAGEMENT

Symptoms: **Due to losartan:** Hypotension and tachycardia. Possible bradycardia due to parasympathetic stimulation. **Due to hydrochlorothiazide:** Hypokalemia, hypochloremia, hyponatremia, dehydration. *Treatment:* Supportive treatment. Hemodialysis does not remove losartan.

DRUG INTERACTIONS

See ***Losartan potassium*** and ***Hydrochlorothiazide*** for lists of possible drug interactions.

HOW SUPPLIED

See *Content.*

DOSAGE

TABLETS

Hypertension.

Individualize. Usual, initial: Losartan, 50 mg once daily (25 mg for those with intravascular volume depletion and in those with a history of hepatic impairment). **Losartan, range:** 25–100 mg once or twice a day. **Hydrochlorothiazide, usual:** 12.5–50 mg once daily and can be given at doses of 12.5–25 mg as Hyzaar. The usual dose of Hyzaar is one tablet of Hyzaar, 50–12.5 once daily. More than 2 tablets of Hyzaar, 50–12.5 once daily or more than 1 tablet of Hyzaar, 100–25 once daily is not recommended.

Severe hypertension.

Initial: 1 Hyzaar, 50–12.5 tablet once daily. For those who do not respond adequately to the 50–12.5 dose after 2–4 weeks of therapy, the dosage may be increased to Hyzaar, 100–25 once daily (maximum recommended dose).

Hypertension with left ventricular hypertrophy.

Initial: Losartan alone, 50 mg once daily. Add hydrochlorothiazide, 12.5 mg or Hyzaar 50–12.5 if further BP reduction is needed. If additional BP reduction is needed, Hyzaar 100–12.5 may be substituted followed by Hyzaar, 100–25. For further BP reduction, add other antihypertensives.

NURSING IMPLICATIONS

Do not confuse Hyzaar with Cozaar (contains only losartan potassium).

IMPLEMENTATION/ADMINISTRATION/STORAGE

1. **In clients who are intravascularly volume-depleted (e.g., those treated with diuretics), symptomatic hypotension may result after initiation of Hyzaar therapy. Correct this condition before administering Hyzaar.**
2. **To minimize dose-dependent side effects, begin combination therapy only after the client has failed to achieve the desired effect with monotherapy.**
3. **The maximal antihypertensive effect is reached about 3 weeks after beginning therapy.**
4. **The usual dosage regimen of Hyzaar may be followed as long as the client's C_{CR} is >30 mL/min. In clients with more severe renal impairment, loop diuretics are preferred to**

thiazides. Thus, Hyzaar is not recommended for these clients.

ASSESSMENT

1. Note disease onset, other agents trialed/outcome, all co-morbidities (diabetes, low EF).
2. When pregnancy is detected, discontinue as soon as possible.
3. Correct any volume depletion prior to using to prevent sympathomimetic hypotension. Reduce starting dose with volume depletion or renal/hepatic impairment. Observe for S&S of fluid or electrolyte imbalance.
4. Monitor VS, ECG, electrolyes, microalbumin, renal and LFTs.

CLIENT/FAMILY TEACHING

1. Take as directed with or without food with a full glass of water. Do not take with grapefruit juice. Avoid any OTC agents unless directed.
2. Do not change positions suddenly; dangle legs before rising, and rest until symptoms subside to prevent low BP and dizziness.
3. Avoid activities that require mental alertness until drug effects realized; may cause dizziness.
4. Ensure adequate hydration; avoid excessive overheating/perspiration.
5. Avoid prolonged sun exposure and use precautions.
6. Practice reliable contraception; do not use if pregnant. Drug associated with fetal injury/death.
7. Regular exercise, weight loss, low-salt diet, and lifestyle changes (i.e., no smoking, low alcohol, low-fat diet, low stress, adequate rest) may also contribute to enhanced BP control. Avoid salt substitutes containing potassium; may cause ↑ potassium levels.
8. Record BP and HR regularly for provider review.
9. Report any loss of response, swelling of the face/tongue, swallowing difficulty or breathing problems immediately.
10. Keep all F/U to assess response, labs, and for adverse SE.

OUTCOMES/EVALUATE

BP control

Lovastatin (Mevinolin)

(**LOW**-vah-**STAT**-in, me-**VIN**-oh-lin)

Classification(s): Antihyperlipidemic, HMG-CoA reductase inhibitor

Pregnancy Category: X

RX: Altoprev, Mevacor.

🍁 **Rx:** Apo-Lovastatin, CO Lovastatin, Gen-Lovastatin, Nu-Lovastatin, PMS-Lovastatin, RAN-Lovastatin, ratio-Lovastatin, Sandoz Lovastatin.

SEE ALSO ***ANTIHYPERLIPIDEMIC AGENTS-HMG-COA REDUCTASE INHIBITORS.***

INDICATIONS/USES

Immediate- and Extended Release: (1) Reduce the risk of MI, unstable angina, and in coronary revascularization procedures in clients without symptomatic CV disease, average to moderately elevated total-C and LDL-C, and below average HDL-C. (2) Slow the progression of coronary atherosclerosis in clients with coronary heart disease as part of a treatment regimen to decrease total-C and LDL-C to target levels. (3) Adjunct to diet to reduce elevated total-C and LDL-C levels in those with primary hypercholesterolemia (type IIa and IIb) when the response to diet restricted in fat and cholesterol and to other nonpharmacologic measures alone have been inadequate. (4) As an adjunct to diet to reduce total-C, LDL-C, and apo B levels in adolescent boys and girls (who are at least 1 year menarche) and 10–17 years old, with heterozygous familial hypercholesterolemia. Used in those after an adequate trial of diet, the LDL-C remains higher than 190 mg/dL or if LDL cholesterol remains higher than 160 mg/dL *and* there is a positive family history of premature CV disease or 2 or more CV disease risk factors present.

Extended-Release Only: Adjunct to diet to decrease elevated total and LDL cholesterol, apolipoprotein B, and triglycerides and to increase HDL cholesterol in those with primary hypercholesterolemia (heterozygous familial and nonfamilial and mixed dyslipidemia Fredrickson types IIa and IIb) when response to diet restricted in saturated fat and cholesterol and other nonpharmacological measures have been inadequate.

Investigational: Diabetic dyslipidemia, nephrotic hyperlipidemia, familial dysbetalipoproteinemia, and familial combined hyperlipidemia.

ACTION/KINETICS

Action

Competitively inhibits HMG-CoA reductase; this enzyme catalyzes the early rate-limiting step in the synthesis of cholesterol. Thus, cholesterol synthesis is inhibited/decreased. Decreases total cholesterol, triglycerides, LDL, and VLDL and increases HDL.

Pharmacokinetics

Approximately 35% of a dose is absorbed. Extensive first-pass metabolism (by CYP2C9); less than 5% reaches the general circulation. Food decreases the bioavailability of the extended-release product. Higher levels are seen in geriatric clients. **Onset:** Within 2 weeks using multiple doses. **Time to peak plasma levels:** 2–4 hr. **Time to peak effect:** 4–6 weeks using multiple doses. **t½:** 3–4 hr for immediate-release. **Duration:** 4–6 weeks after termination of therapy. Metabolized in the liver (its main site of action) to active metabolites by CYP3A4. Severe renal impairment increases plasma levels. 83% of a PO dose is excreted in the feces, via the bile, and 10% is excreted through the urine. **Plasma protein binding:** >95%.

L

ADDITIONAL CONTRAINDICATIONS

Use with mibefradil (Posicor).

SPECIAL CONCERNS

- **Carefully monitor clients with impaired renal function.**
- **Use with caution during lactation.**
- **Geriatric clients are at a higher risk of myopathy.**
- **Safety and efficacy of both immediate- and extended-release products not determined in children.**

SIDE EFFECTS

Most Common

Headache, diarrhea, flatulence, nausea, abdominal pain/cramps, sinusitis, accidental trauma, constipation, dyspepsia, myalgia, back pain, rash/pruritus, flu syndrome, infection, pain, asthenia, dizziness, UTI, arthralgia.

See *Antihyperlipidemic Agents-HMG-CoA Reductase Inhibitors* for a complete list of side effects. **CNS:** Headache, dizziness, paresthesia, insomnia. **GI:** Flatus, abdominal pain, cramps, diarrhea, constipation, dyspepsia, N&V, heartburn, dysgeusia, acid regurgitation, dry mouth. **Musculoskeletal:** Myalgia, muscle cramps/pain, arthralgia, back/leg/shoulder pain, localized pain, rhabdomyolysis with acute renal failure secondary to myoglobinemia. **Dermatologic:** Rash, pruritus, alopecia. **Ophthalmic:** Blurred vision, eye irritation, baseline lenticular opacities. **Miscellaneous:** Asthenia, chest pain.

LABORATORY TEST CONSIDERATIONS

↑ ALT, CPK. ↑ Risk of elevated serum transaminases in clients with homozygous familial hypercholesterolemia.

DRUG INTERACTIONS

Amiodarone / ↑ Risk of myopathy R/T ↓ lovastatin elimination R/T inhibition of CYP3A4; if concurrent use necessary, use the lowest possible lovastatin dose
Bosentan / ↓ Lovastatin effect R/T ↑ metabolism by CYP3A4; monitor closely and adjust lovastatin dose if necessary
Carbamazepine / ↓ Lovastatin effect R/T ↑ metabolism by CYP3A4; monitor closely and adjust lovastatin dose if necessary
Cilostazol / ↑ Risk of myopathy R/T ↓ lovastatin elimination R/T inhibition of CYP3A4; monitor closely and adjust lovastatin dose if necessary
Cyclosporine / ↑ Risk of myopathy or rhabdomyolysis R/T ↓ lovastatin elimination R/T inhibition of CYP3A4
Danazol / ↑ Risk of myopathy or rhabdomyolysis especially, if given with higher doses of lovastatin; if concurrent use necessary, decrease dose of lovastatin and monitor
Delavirdine / Possible ↑ risk of toxicity (e.g., myopathy) R/T ↓ lovastatin metabolism by CYP3A4
Efavirenz / Possible ↑ metabolism of lovastatin R/T induction of CYP3A4 → ↓ lovastatin therapeutic effect
Erythromycin / ↑ Risk of myopathy or rhabdomyolysis R/T ↓ lovastatin elimination R/T inhibition of CYP3A4
Grapefruit juice (>1 qt daily) / ↑ Risk of myopathy or rhabdomyolysis R/T ↓ lovastatin elimination R/T inhibition of CYP3A4
Imatinib / ↑ Risk of toxicity (e.g., myopathy) R/T ↓ lovastatin metabolism by CYP3A4
Isradipine / ↑ Clearance of lovastatin; monitor response and adjust lovastatin dose if necessary

Itraconazole / ↑ Risk of myopathy or rhabdomyolysis R/T ↓ lovastatin elimination R/T inhibition of CYP3A4
Ketoconaozle / ↑ Risk of myopathy or rhabdomyolysis R/T ↓ lovastatin elimination R/T inhibition of CYP3A4
Nefazodone / ↑ Risk of myopathy or rhabdomyolysis R/T ↓ lovastatin elimination R/T inhibition of CYP3A4
Nevirapine / Possible ↑ metabolism of lovastatin R/T induction of CYP3A4 → ↓ lovastatin therapeutic effect
Ritonavir / ↑ Risk of myopathy or rhabdomyolysis R/T ↓ lovastatin elimination R/T inhibition of CYP3A4
Saquinavir / ↑ Risk of myopathy or rhabdomyolysis R/T ↓ lovastatin elimination R/T inhibition of CYP3A4
H *St. John's wort* / Possible ↑ metabolism of lovastatin R/T induction of CYP3A4 → ↓ lovastatin therapeutic effect
Telithromycin / ↑ Risk of myopathy or rhabdomyolysis R/T ↓ lovastatin elimination R/T inhibition of CYP3A4
Verapamil / ↑ Risk of myopathy or rhabdomyolysis R/T ↓ lovastatin elimination R/T inhibition of CYP3A4
Warfarin / Possible ↑ warfarin anticoagulant effect; monitor anticoagulation parameters

HOW SUPPLIED

Tablets, Extended-Release: 10 mg, 20 mg, 40 mg, 60 mg; ***Tablets, Immediate-Release:*** 10 mg, 20 mg, 40 mg.

DOSAGE

TABLETS, EXTENDED-RELEASE

Primary hypercholesterolemia and mixed dyslipidemia.

Initial: 20, 40, or 60 mg once a day at bedtime; **range:** 10–60 mg/day in single doses. Start with 10 mg once a day for those requiring small reductions in lipid levels. Adjust dose at intervals of 4 weeks or more.

TABLETS, IMMEDIATE-RELEASE

Primary prevention of coronary heart disease, hypercholesterolemia, coronary heart disease.

Adults initial: 20 mg once daily with the evening meal. Initiate at 10 mg/day in clients who require smaller reductions. Initiate at 20 mg/day in those requiring reductions in LDL-C of 20% or more. **Dose range:** 10–80 mg (maximum)/day in single or two divided doses. Adjust dose at intervals of every 4 weeks, if necessary. If C_{CR} is less than 30 mL/min, use doses greater than 20 mg/day with caution.

Adolescents, age 10–17 years, with heterozygous familial hypercholesterolemia.

Dose range: 10–40 mg/day (maximum). Individualize dose depending on goal of therapy. Start clients with 20 mg/day who require decreases in LDL cholesterol of 20% or more to achieve their goal. For those requiring smaller reductions, start with 10 mg/day. Adjust dose at intervals of 4 weeks or more.

NURSING IMPLICATIONS

Do not confuse lovastatin with Lotensin (an ACE inhibitor).

IMPLEMENTATION/ADMINISTRATION/STORAGE

1. Immediate-release is effective alone or when used together with bile acid sequestrants. If lovastatin is used with gemfibrozil, other fibrates, or lipid-lowering doses of niacin (1 gram per day or more), do not exceed a dose of 20 mg/day of lovastatin R/T increased risk of myopathy.
2. If used with severe renal insufficiency (C_{CR} <30 mL/min), increase lovastatin doses above 20 mg/day carefully and only if deemed necessary.
3. Do not exceed dose of 40 mg/day of lovastatin if taking amiodarone or verapamil.
4. If lovastatin is used with cyclosporine, start with 10 mg lovastatin and do not exceed 20 mg/day lovastatin as there is an increased risk of myopathy.
5. Store immediate-release tablets between 5–30°C (41–86°F) protected from light in a well-closed, light-resistant container. Store extended-release tablets at controlled room temperature of 20–25°C (68–77°F); avoid excess heat and humidity.

ASSESSMENT

1. Note lipid profile, cardiac risk factors, family history, other therapies trialed, outcome.

2. Assess for hepatic disease, heavy alcohol consumption. List drugs prescribed to ensure none interact.
3. Determine if pregnant.
4. Request recent eye exam; slight changes have been noted in the lenses of some clients.
5. Assess lifestyle, including weight, diet (intake of fats, CHOs, and proteins), activity (regular exercise), alcohol consumption, smoking history. Identify areas that may contribute to increased cholesterol levels.
6. Assess LFTs q 4–6 weeks for the first 3 months of therapy, every 6 to 8 weeks during next 18 months, and every 6 months thereafter. A threefold increase in serum transaminase or new-onset abnormal LFTs is an indication to stop therapy as well as severe myalgia (check CPK). Note any renal dysfunction.

CLIENT/FAMILY TEACHING

1. Swallow extended-release tablets whole; do not crush, chew, or cut. Avoid coadministration with grapefruit juice due to increased serum levels of lovastatin. Continue cholesterol-lowering diet and exercise program. Cholesterol production by the liver is highest in the evening; usually taken with the evening meal.
2. Follow a standard cholesterol-lowering diet before starting lovastatin and continue during therapy. Adhere to dietary restrictions, daily exercise, and weight loss in the overall management and control of hypercholesterolemia/hyperlipidemia.
3. Practice reliable birth control; drug is pregnancy category X.
4. Report unexplained muscle pain, tenderness, or weakness, or fever. These may be mistaken for the flu, but could be serious side effects of drug therapy.
5. Any RUQ abdominal pain or yellowing of eyes, skin, stools should be reported.
6. Periodic LFTs and eye exams are mandatory; report early visual disturbances.
7. Keep all F/U to assess response, labs, and for adverse SE.

OUTCOMES/EVALUATE

- ↓ LDL and total cholesterol levels
- ↓ Progression of coronary atherosclerosis

■ IV

Lymphocyte immune globulin, anti-thymocyte globulin sterile solution (equine)

(**LIM**-foh-sight im-**MYOUN GLOH**-byou-lin, an-tih-**THIGH**-moh-sight **GLOH**-byou-lin **EE**-kwine)

Classification(s): Immunosuppressant

Pregnancy Category: C

RX: Atgam.

INDICATIONS/USES

(1) Management of allograft rejection in renal transplant clients, given either at the time of rejection or as an adjunct with other immunosuppressants to delay onset of the first rejection episode. (2) Treatment of moderate to severe aplastic anemia in those who are unsuitable for bone marrow transplantation. *Investigational:* As an immunosuppressant in liver, bone marrow, heart, or other organ transplants. Treatment of multiple sclerosis, pure red-cell aplasia, and scleroderma. *NOTE:* Only physicians with experience in immunosuppressive therapy in treating renal transplant or aplastic anemia should use this drug.

ACTION/KINETICS

Action

Obtained from hyperimmune serum of horses immunized with human thymus lymphocytes. Reduces the number of circulating, thymus-dependent lymphocytes that form rosettes from sheep erythrocytes. Antilymphocytic effect may be due to alteration of the function of T-lymphocytes, which are responsible, in part, for cell-mediated immunity.

Pharmacokinetics

t½, serum: 5.7 days when the drug is given with other immunosuppressants and measured as horse IgG.

CONTRAINDICATIONS

In those who have demonstrated a severe systemic reaction during prior administration of the drug or any other equine gamma globulin preparation.

SPECIAL CONCERNS

(1) Only physicians experienced in immunosuppressive therapy in the treatment of renal transplant or aplastic anemia clients should use this drug. (2) Treat clients receiving this drug in facilities equipped and staffed with adequate lab and supportive medical resources.

- Systemic reactions, such as a generalized rash, tachycardia, dyspnea, hypotension, or anaphylaxis, precludes any further administration of the drug.
- Potency may vary from lot to lot.
- Possible transmission of infectious agents.
- Use with caution during lactation.

SIDE EFFECTS

Most Common

When used for renal transplantation: Fever, chills, leukopenia, rash, pruritus, urticaria, wheal, flare, thrombocytopenia.

When used for aplastic anemia: Chills, arthralgia, headache, myalgia, nausea, chest pain, phlebitis.

General side effects. Body as a whole: Fever, chills, systemic or localized infection, malaise, serum sickness, edema, sweating. **GI:** N&V, diarrhea, ***GI bleeding or perforation***, sore mouth or throat, epigastric or stomach pain, abdominal pain. **CNS:** Headache, ***seizures***, confusion, disorientation, dizziness, faintness, paresthesias. **CV:** Hypertension or hypotension, tachycardia, DVT, thrombophlebitis, CHF, vasculitis, renal artery thrombosis. **Hematologic:** Thrombocytopenia, leukopenia, eosinophilia, neutropenia, granulocytopenia, anemia, lymphadenopathy, aplasia, pancytopenia, hemolysis, hemolytic anemia. **Dermatologic:** Rashes. **Respiratory:** Dyspnea, apnea, cough, ***pulmonary edema***, nosebleed. **Musculoskeletal:** Chest/back/flank pain; arthralgia, myalgias, abnormal involuntary movement or tremor, rigidity. **Miscellaneous:** Herpes simplex infection, swelling or redness at infusion site, ***anaphylaxis, laryngospasm/edema***, hyperglycemia, ***acute renal failure***, viral hepatitis, enlarged or ruptured kidney.

When used for renal transplantation with other immunosuppressants. Body as a whole: Fever, chills, weakness or faintness. **CNS:** Headache, dizziness, paresthesia, ***seizures***. **GI:** Diarrhea, nausea/vomiting, stomatitis, hiccoughs, epigastric pain, malaise. **Hematologic:** Leukopenia, thrombocytopenia. **Dermatologic:** Rash, pruritus, urticaria, wheal, flare. **CV:** Hypotension, peripheral thrombophlebitis, edema, hypertension, renal artery stenosis, tachycardia. **Musculoskeletal:** Arthralgia, chest or back pain (or both), myalgia. **Respiratory:** Dyspnea, laryngospasm, pulmonary edema. **Miscellaneous:** Clotted AV fistula, pain at infusion site, night sweats, ***anaphylaxis***, herpes simplex reactivation, hyperglycemia, iliac vein obstruction, localized infection, lymphadenopathy, serum sickness, systemic infection, ***toxic epidermal necrosis***, wound dehiscence.

When used for aplastic anemia with support therapy. Body as a whole: Fever, chills, diaphoresis, aches. **GI:** N&V, diarrhea. **CNS:** Headache, agitation, lethargy, listlessness, lightheadedness, ***seizures***, encephalitis or postviral encephalopathy. **CV:** Chest pain, phlebitis, bradycardia, myocarditis, cardiac irregularity, hypotension, CHF, hypertension. **Hematologic:** Lymphadenopathy, postcervical lymphadenopathy, tender lymph nodes. **Respiratory:** Bilateral pleural effusion, respiratory distress. **Musculoskeletal:** Arthralgia, myalgia, joint stiffness, muscle aches. **Miscellaneous:** Periorbital edema, edema, hepatosplenomegaly, burning soles/palms, foot sole pain, proteinuria, ***anaphylaxis.***

LABORATORY TEST CONSIDERATIONS

↑ ALT, AST, alkaline phosphatase, serum creatinine.

DRUG INTERACTIONS

Previously masked reactions to Atgam may appear when the drug is given concomitantly with corticosteroids or other immunosuppressants.

HOW SUPPLIED

Injection: 50 mg horse gamma globulin/mL.

DOSAGE

IV ONLY

Renal allograft recipients.

Adults: 10–30 mg/kg daily. **Children:** 5–25 mg/kg daily. Usually used concomitantly with azathioprine and corticosteroids. When used to delay the onset of allograft rejection, a fixed dose of 15 mg/kg for 14 days is used; then, the dose is given every other day for 14 days for a total of 21 doses in 28 days.

Give the first dose within 24 hr before or after the transplant. When used to treat allograft rejection, the first dose can be delayed until the first rejection episode is diagnosed. **Recommended dose:** 10–15 mg/kg daily for 14 days; additional alternate day therapy can be given for a total of 21 doses.

Aplastic anemia.

10–20 mg/kg daily for 8–14 days; additional alternate day therapy may be given for a total of 21 doses. Thrombocytopenia can be associated with Atgam use; thus, clients may need prophylactic platelet transfusions to maintain platelets at an acceptable level.

NURSING IMPLICATIONS

IMPLEMENTATION/ADMINISTRATION/STORAGE

1. IV Recommended that clients be skin tested with an intradermal injection of 0.1 mL of a 1:1,000 dilution (5 mcg horse IgG) of Atgam in NaCl and a contralateral NaCl injection. Observe every 15–20 min the first hour after intradermal injection. A local reaction of 10 mm or greater with a wheal or erythema (or both) with or without pseudopod formation and itching or a marked local swelling should be considered a positive test. A systemic reaction such as a generalized rash, tachycardia, dyspnea, hypotension, or anaphylaixs precludes any additional administration. *NOTE:* Allergic reactions and anaphylaxis have occurred following negative skin tests.
2. The product can be transparent to slightly opalescent, colorless to faintly pink or brown. A slight granular or flaky deposit may form during storage.
3. To avoid excessive foaming and/or denaturation of protein, do not shake either diluted or undiluted Atgam.
4. For IV infusion, dilute in an inverted bottle of sterile vehicle so the undiluted drug does not come in contact with the air inside. Do not exceed a 4 mg/mL concentration; gently rotate or swirl the diluted solution so it is thoroughly mixed. Allow diluted drug to come to room temperature before administration.
5. Administer drug into a vascular shunt, arterial venous fistula, or a high-flow central vein through an in-line filter with a pore size of 0.2–1.0 micron. The filter prevents administration of any insoluble material that may develop during product storage. Use of high-flow veins will minimize development of phlebitis and thrombosis.
6. Do not administer in less than 4 hr.
7. Diluted Atgam is stable for up to 24 hr at concentrations up to 4 mg/mL in 0.9% NaCl, D5/0.25% NaCl, and D5/0.45% NaCl. Store diluted solution in the refrigerator. Do not keep diluted form for more than 24 hr (including actual infusion time).
8. Store refrigerated from 2–8°C (36–46°F). Do not freeze; discard if frozen.
9. COMPATIBILITY 0.9% NaCl, D5/0.225% NaCl, and D5/0.45% NaCl.
10. INCOMPATIBILITY Dilution with dextrose not recommended (low sugar concentrations may cause precipitation). Avoid highly acidic infusion solutions due to the possibility of physical instability over time.

ASSESSMENT

1. List type of symptoms, date of transplant, hematologic profile and general physical condition.
2. Should only be administered by those trained in immunosuppressive therapy in the treatment of renal transplant or aplastic anemia.
3. Ensure intradermal skin test performed 1 hr before first dose and note results. Observe every 15 to 20 minutes over the first hour after intradermal injection. Observe for evidence of wheal >10 mm; indicates positive test and potential for severe systemic reactions. A systemic reaction (generalized rash, tachycardia, dyspnea, hypotension, or anaphylaxis) precludes any additional administration of Atgam. Some clients with negative skin test results have also experienced anaphylaxis.
4. Administer corticosteroids, antihistamines, and antipyretics to help control drug-induced side effects during therapy.
5. Observe for evidence of concurrent infection, pregnancy, thrombocytopenia, or leukopenia.
6. Continuously observe for possible allergic reactions. Respiratory distress and pain in the chest, back, or flank may indicate anaphylactoid reaction. Discontinue if any of the following occurs: (a) symptoms of anaphylaxis, (b)

severe and unremitting thrombocytopenia or leukopenia.

7. Clients with aplastic anemia may require platelet transfusions during therapy to maintain acceptable platelet levels. Monitor ECG, electrolytes, hematologic profile, renal, LFTs. Ensure lymphocyte count (total lymphocyte and/or T-cell subsets) is monitored during treatment to assess amount of T-cell depletion.

CLIENT/FAMILY TEACHING

1. Drug is used to prevent transplant rejection; medication will be prepared and administered in health care setting and may be used with other agents to attain desired results.
2. There are benefits and risks with this therapy including potential to transmit disease and unknown infectious agents.
3. Anticipate premedication with corticosteroids, acetaminophen, and/or antihistamine 1 hr before infusion of anti-thymocyte globulin which is given over 4 hr.
4. Report any fever, chills, fatigue, sore throat, chest/flank/back pain, night sweats or adverse side effects. Use reliable contraception during treatment.
5. Keep all F/U to assess response, labs, and for adverse SE.

OUTCOMES/EVALUATE

- Interruption of cell-mediated renal allograft rejection
- ↓ Rejection and graft loss
- Hematologic remission

M

IV

Mannitol

(**MAN**-nih-tol)

Classification(s): Diuretic, osmotic

Pregnancy Category: C

RX: Osmitrol.

INDICATIONS/USES

(1) Diuretic to prevent or treat the oliguric phase of acute renal failure before irreversible renal failure occurs. (2) Decrease ICP and cerebral edema by decreasing brain mass. (3) Decrease elevated intraocular pressure when the pressure cannot be lowered by other means. (4) To promote urinary excretion of toxic substances. *Investigational:* Prevent hemolysis during cardiopulmonary bypass surgery.

ACTION/KINETICS

Action

Increases the osmolarity of the glomerular filtrate, which decreases the reabsorption of water and increases excretion of sodium and chloride. It also increases the osmolarity of the plasma, which causes enhanced flow of water from tissues into the interstitial fluid and plasma. Thus, cerebral edema, increased ICP, and CSF volume and pressure are decreased.

Pharmacokinetics

Onset, IV: 30–60 min for diuresis and within 15 min for reduction of cerebrospinal and intraocular pressures. **Peak:** 30–60 min. **Duration:** 6–8 hr for diuresis and 4–8 hr for reduction of intraocular pressure. **t½:** 15–100 min. Over 90% excreted through the urine unchanged. A test dose is given in clients with impaired renal function or oliguria.

CONTRAINDICATIONS

Anuria, pulmonary edema, severe dehydration, active intracranial bleeding except during craniotomy, progressive heart failure or pulmonary congestion after mannitol therapy, progressive renal damage following mannitol therapy.

SPECIAL CONCERNS

- **Use with caution during lactation.**
- **If blood is given simultaneously with mannitol, add at least 20 mEq of sodium chloride to each liter of mannitol solution to avoid pseudoagglutination.**
- **Sudden expansion of the extracellular volume that occurs after rapid IV mannitol may lead to fulminating CHF.**

M

- **Mannitol may obscure and intensify inadequate hydration or hypovolemia.**

SIDE EFFECTS

Most Common

Headache, N&V, diarrhea, dry mouth, irritation/pain/swelling at injection site.

Electrolyte: Fluid and electrolyte imbalance, acidosis, loss of electrolytes, dehydration. **GI**: N&V, dry mouth, thirst, diarrhea. **CV**: Edema, hypo-/hypertension, increased heart rate, angina-like chest pain, CHF, thrombophlebitis. **At injection site:** Irritation, pain, swelling. **CNS**: Dizziness, headaches, blurred vision, ***seizures.*** **Miscellaneous**: Pulmonary congestion, marked diuresis, rhinitis, chills, fever, urticaria, pain in arms, skin necrosis.

LABORATORY TEST CONSIDERATIONS

↑ or ↓ Inorganic phosphorus. ↑ Ethylene glycol values because mannitol is oxidized to an aldehyde during test.

OVERDOSE MANAGEMENT

Symptoms: Increased electrolyte excretion, especially sodium, chloride, and potassium. Sodium depletion results in orthostatic tachycardia or hypotension and decreased CVP. Potassium loss can impair neuromuscular function and cause intestinal dilation and ileus. If urine flow is inadequate, pulmonary edema or water intoxication may occur. Other symptoms include hypotension, polyuria that rapidly becomes oliguria, stupor, ***seizures***, hyperosmolality, and hyponatremia. *Treatment:* Discontinue the infusion immediately and begin supportive measures to correct fluid and electrolyte imbalances. Hemodialysis is effective.

DRUG INTERACTIONS

May cause deafness when used in combination with kanamycin.

HOW SUPPLIED

Injection: 5%, 10%, 15%, 20%, 25%.

DOSAGE

IV INFUSION ONLY

Test dose (oliguria or reduced renal function).

Either 50 mL of a 25% solution, 75 mL of a 20% solution, or 100 mL of a 15% solution infused over 3–5 min. If urine flow is 30–50 mL/hr, therapeutic dose can be given. If urine flow does not increase, give a second test dose; if still no response, client must be reevaluated.

Prevention of acute renal failure (oliguria).

Adults: 50–100 grams, as a 5–25% solution, given at a rate to maintain urine flow of at least 30–50 mL/hr.

Treatment of oliguria.

Adults: 50–100 grams of a 15–25% solution.

Reduction of intracranial pressure and brain mass.

Adults: 1.5–2 grams/kg as a 15–25% solution, infused over 30–60 min.

Reduction of intraocular pressure.

Adults: 1.5–2 grams/kg as a 20% solution (7.5–10 mL/kg) or as a 15% solution (10–13 mL/kg) given over 30–60 min. When used preoperatively, the dose should be given 1–1.5 hr before surgery to maintain the maximum effect.

Antidote to remove toxic substances.

Adults: Dose depends on the fluid requirement and urinary output. IV fluids and electrolytes are given to replace losses. If a beneficial effect is not seen after 200 grams mannitol, the infusion should be discontinued.

NURSING IMPLICATIONS

IMPLEMENTATION/ADMINISTRATION/STORAGE

1. **IV Use a filter with concentrated mannitol (15%, 20%, and 25%).**
2. **Concentrations >15% may crystallize. To redissolve, warm bottle in a hot water bath or autoclave; cool to body temperature before administering.**
3. **If blood is administered concurrently, add 20 mEq of NaCl to each liter of mannitol to prevent pseudoagglutination.**
4. **COMPATIBILITY 0.9% NaCl.**
5. **INCOMPATIBILITY Do not add to other IV solutions, or mix with other medications.**

ASSESSMENT

1. **Note reasons for therapy, type/onset/characteristics of S&S and causes.**
2. **List other medications prescribed to ensure none alter drug effects.**

3. **Note mental status/neurologic findings. With severe renal impairment ensure test dose performed.**
4. **When used to reduce ICP and brain mass, evaluate circulatory and renal reserve, fluid/electrolyte balance, body weight, total I&O before/after infusion.**
5. **Monitor VS, I&O. Assess cardio-pulmonary status; report S&S of pulmonary edema manifested by dyspnea, cyanosis, rales, frothy sputum or any other adverse event.**
6. **Assess for S&S of electrolyte imbalances (Na^+, K^+), renal dysfunction, and dehydration; replace as needed. If renal failure or oliguria present, ensure test dose performed (under dosage).**

CLIENT/FAMILY TEACHING

1. **Drug is administered IV in a controlled setting to increase water excretion or to decrease intracranial or intraocular (eye) pressures.**
2. **May experience increased thirst or dry mouth; do not exceed amount of fluid provided.**
3. **Increased SOB or pain in chest, back, or legs should be reported immediately.**

OUTCOMES/EVALUATE

- **Desired diuresis with ↓ edema**
- **↓ ICP, intraocular pressures**

Maraviroc

(mare-ah-**VYE**-rock)

Classification(s): Cellular chemokine receptor antagonist

Pregnancy Category: B

RX: Selzentry.

INDICATIONS/USES

In combination with other antiretroviral agents to treat adult clients infected only with chemokine receptor 5-tropic HIV-1 detectable, who have evidence of viral replication and HIV-1 strains resistant to multiple antiretroviral agents.

ACTION/KINETICS

Action

Maraviroc selectively binds to the human chemokine receptor CCR5 present on the cell membrane, thus preventing the interaction of HIV-1 gp120 and CCR5 which is necessary for CCR5-tropic HIV-1 to enter cells.

Pharmacokinetics

Peak plasma levels: 0.5–4 hr, depending on the dose. Absolute bioavailability is 23–33%, depending on the dose. A high fat meal will decrease C_{max} and AUC, although it can be taken with or without food. Plasma levels may be higher in those with impaired hepatic function. Metabolized in the liver mainly by CYP3A. **t½, terminal:** 14–18 hr. Excreted in the feces (76%) and urine (20%). **Plasma protein binding:** About 76%.

CONTRAINDICATIONS

Use with severe renal impairment or ESRD (C_{CR} <30 mL/min) who are taking potent CYP3A inhibitors or inducers. Lactation.

SPECIAL CONCERNS

Hepatotoxicity has been reported with maraviroc use. Evidence of a systemic allergic reaction (e.g., eosinophilia or elevated immunoglobulin E, pruritic rash) prior to development of hepatotoxicity may occur. Immediately evaluate clients with signs or symptoms of hepatitis or allergic reactions following use of maraviroc.

- **Cross resistance is possible.**
- **Use with caution in the elderly, in those with preexisting impaired hepatic or renal function, in those who are coinfected with hepatitis B or C, and in those with a history of postural hypotension, a history of CV events, or on concomitant antihypertensive medications.**
- **Safety, efficacy, and pharmacokinetics not determined in children less than 16 years of age; do not use maraviroc in this population.**

SIDE EFFECTS

Most Common

Cough, dizziness, pyrexia, rash, URTI, diarrhea, edema, esophageal candidiasis, influenza, parasomnias, rhinitis, sleep disorders, urinary abnormalities, infections.

CNS: Dizziness, postural dizziness, syncope, disturbances in initiating and maintaining sleep, paresthesias, dysesthesias, disturbances in consciousness, depressive disorders, sensory abnormalities, anxiety, peripheral neuropathies, ***convulsions*** and epilepsy, facial palsy, loss of consciousness, tremor (excluding congenital). **GI:**

M

GI and abdominal pains, constipation, dyspeptic signs/symptoms, stomatitis (ulceration), abdominal neoplasm, anal cancer, colitis, esophageal carcinoma, tongue neoplasm. **Hepatic:** Hepatotoxicity with allergic features, cholestatic jaundice, jaundice, metastases to liver, portal vein thrombosis, hepatic cirrhosis, malignant bile duct neoplasms, ***hepatic failure***. **CV:** Vascular hypertensive disorders, ***CVA, acute cardiac failure***, coronary artery disease/occlusion, ***MI***, myocardial ischemia, unstable angina, postural hypotension, endocarditis. **Dermatologic:** Rash, apocrine/eccrine gland disorders, pruritus, erythema, folliculitis, dermatitis/eczema, lipodystrophies, benign skin neoplasms, basal cell carcinoma, squamous cell skin carcinoma, ***Stevens-Johnson syndrome.*** **GU:** Bladder/urethral symptoms, urinary tract S&S, *Condyloma acuminatum*. **Musculoskeletal:** Musculoskeletal and connective tissue S&S, joint-related S&S, muscle pains, myositis (including infective), osteonecrosis, rhabdomyolysis. **Respiratory:** URTI, URT S&S, coughing and associated symptoms, sinusitis, bronchitis, breathing abnormalities, ***bronchospasm and obstruction***, nasal congestion/inflammation, paranasal sinus disorders, pneumonia, respiratory tract disorders, nasopharyngeal carcinoma. **Hematologic:** Hypoplastic anemia, bone marrow depression. **Ophthalmic:** Conjunctivitis, ocular infections/inflammation, ocular associated manifestations, visual field defect. **Otic:** Otitis media. **Body as a whole:** Pyrexia, pain/discomfort, influenza, ***septic shock***. **Miscellaneous:** Immune reconstitution syndrome (including getting opportunistic infections), increased risk of infections (especially URTI and herpes virus), appetite disorders, herpes infection, *Clostridium difficile* colitis, meningitis, viral meningitis; benign/malignant/unspecified neoplasms (including cysts and polyps), anaplastic large cell lymphomas T- and null-cell type, Bowen disease, diffuse large B-cell lymphoma, malignant and unspecified endocrine neoplasms, lymphoma, squamous cell carcinoma, treponemal infections.

LABORATORY TEST CONSIDERATIONS

↑ ALT, AST, total bilirubin, amylase, lipase, blood creatine kinase. ↓ Absolute neutrophil count.

OVERDOSE MANAGEMENT

Symptoms: Postural hypotension. *Treatment:* Institute general supportive measures. Keep client in a supine position. Assess vital signs, BP, and ECG. Gastric lavage and activated charcoal can be used to aid in removal of the drug. Dialysis may also be beneficial.

DRUG INTERACTIONS

Carbamazepine / ↓ Maraviroc plasma levels R/T induction of CYP3A → ↑ metabolism; recommended dose is maraviroc, 600 mg twice/day
Clarithromycin / ↑ Maraviroc plasma levels R/T inhibition of CYP3A → ↓ metabolism
Delavirdine / ↑ Maraviroc plasma levels R/T inhibition of CYP3A → ↓ metabolism
Efavirenz /↓ Maraviroc plasma levels R/T induction of CYP3A → ↑ metabolism; recommended dose is maraviroc, 600 mg twice/day
Etravirine / ↓ Maraviroc plasma levels R/T induction of CYP3A → ↑ metabolism; recommended dose is maraviroc, 600 mg twice/day
Itraconazole / ↑ Maraviroc plasma levels R/T inhibition of CYP3A → ↓ metabolism
Ketoconazole / ↑ Maraviroc plasma levels R/T inhibition of CYP3A → ↓ metabolism
Nefazodone / ↑ Maraviroc plasma levels R/T inhibition of CYP3A → ↓ metabolism
Phenobarbital / ↓ Maraviroc plasma levels R/T induction of CYP3A → ↑ metabolism; recommended dose is maraviroc, 600 mg twice/day
Phenytoin / ↓ Maraviroc plasma levels R/T induction of CYP3A → ↑ metabolism; recommended dose is maraviroc, 600 mg twice/day
Protease inhibitors (except ritonavir/tipranavir) / ↑ Maraviroc plasma levels R/T inhibition of CYP3A → ↓ metabolism
Rifampin / ↓ Maraviroc plasma levels R/T induction of CYP3A → ↑ metabolism; recommended dose is maraviroc, 600 mg twice/day
H ***St. John's wort*** / ↓ Maraviroc levels → suboptimal maraviroc levels and loss of virologic response and possible resistance; do not use together
Telithromycin / ↑ Maraviroc plasma levels R/T inhibition of CYP3A → ↓ metabolism

HOW SUPPLIED

Tablets: 150 mg, 300 mg.

DOSAGE

TABLETS

HIV infection.

Adults and children, 16 years and older: As a result of drug interactions, the recommended dose of maraviroc differs based on use of concomitant drugs. The dose of maraviroc is 150 mg twice a day if given with protease inhibitors (except tipranavir/ritonavir), delavirdine, ketoconazole, itraconazole, clarithromycin, or other strong CYP3A inhibitors (e.g., nefazodone, telithromycin).

The dose of maraviroc is 300 mg twice a day if given with tipranavir/ritonavir, nevirapine, all nucleoside reverse transcriptase inhibitors, raltegravir, and enfuvirtide.

The dose of maraviroc is 600 mg twice a day if given with CYP3A inducers, including carbamazepine, phenobarbital, phenytoin, efavirenz, etravirine, or rifampin.

Dosage adjustment based on renal function. (1) If taken with potent CYP3A inhibitors, with or without a CYP3A inducer: 150 mg twice/day if the C_{CR} is anywhere from 30 mL/min to greater than 80 mL/min. Maraviroc is not recommended in this group if the C_{CR} is <30 mL/min or if the client is in ESRD on regular hemodialysis. (2) If taken with concomitant medications, including protease inhibitors (except tipranavir/ritonavir), clarithromycin, delavirdine, itraconazole, ketoconazole, nefazodone, telithromycin: 300 mg twice/day if the C_{CR} is anywhere from <30 mL/min to greater than 80 mL/min plus those with ESRD on regular hemodialysis. (3) If taken with CYP3A inducers, without a potent CYP3A inhibitor; drugs include carbamazepine, etravirine, phenobarbital, phenytoin, and rifampin: 600 mg twice/day if the C_{CR} is anywhere from 30 mL/min to greater than 80 mL/min. Maraviroc is not recommended in this group if the C_{CR} is <30 mL/min or if the client is in ESRD on regular hemodialysis.

NURSING IMPLICATIONS

IMPLEMENTATION/ADMINISTRATION/STORAGE

1. Maraviroc must be given in combination with other antiretroviral drugs.
2. May be taken with or without food.
3. Store from 15–30°C (59–86°F).

ASSESSMENT

1. Note reasons for therapy: CCR5-tropic HIV-1 detectable disease, other agents trialed/failed. It is used along with other HIV medicines to prevent virus from entering the cells.
2. List all drugs prescribed to ensure none interact.
3. Assess for history of liver problems, hepatitis B or C, heart or kidney problems.
4. Evaluate closely for S&S of hepatitis or allergic reaction and report immediately.
5. Monitor for fever/infection, BP, CBC, HIV RNA, renal and LFTs, at baseline and regularly.

CLIENT/FAMILY TEACHING

1. May take with or without food. Swallow whole; do not break, crush, or chew before swallowing. It is used together with other medications to treat CCR5-tropic human immunodeficiency virus (HIV) type 1.
2. Take even if feeling well; do not miss/skip any doses. Do not stop taking maraviroc, even for a short period of time. The virus may grow resistant to the medicine and become harder to treat.
3. Avoid activities that require mental alertness until drug effects realized; may cause dizziness.
4. Report any sore throat, weakness, cough, or evidence of infection. Avoid those with known infections; may still develop opportunistic infections.
5. Report any difficulty breathing, chest tightness/pain, swelling of the mouth, face, lips, or tongue, rash, bloody diarrhea, or confusion.
6. Drug does not prevent spread of HIV to others through blood or sexual contact; practice barrier protection. Do not share needles, injection supplies, toothbrushes or razors.
7. May cause liver dysfunction; report and yellow discoloration of skin, RUQ pain, fatigue or other adverse side effects.
8. To monitor maternal-fetal outcomes of pregnant women exposed to maraviroc and other antiretroviral drugs, an antiretrovial registry has been established. Health care providers are encouraged to register clients by calling 1-800-258-4263.
9. Keep all F/U to assess response, labs, and for adverse SE.

M

OUTCOMES/EVALUATE

- ↓ HIV RNA
- Inhibition of HIV viral replication

Mebendazole

(meh-**BEN**-dah-zohl)

Classification(s): Anthelmintic

Pregnancy Category: C

RX: Vermox.

INDICATIONS/USES

Single or mixed infections of whipworm, pinworm, roundworm, and common and American hookworm. Not effective for hydatid disease.

ACTION/KINETICS

Action

Anthelmintic effect occurs by blocking the glucose uptake of the organisms, thereby reducing their energy until death results. It also inhibits the formation of microtubules in the helminth.

Pharmacokinetics

Peak plasma levels: 2–4 hr. Poorly absorbed from the GI tract. Excreted in feces as unchanged drug or metabolites.

CONTRAINDICATIONS

Hypersensitivity to mebendazole.

SPECIAL CONCERNS

Use with caution in children under 2 years of age and during lactation.

SIDE EFFECTS

Most Common

Transient abdominal pain, diarrhea.

GI: Transient abdominal pain and diarrhea. **Hematologic:** Reversible neutropenia. **Miscellaneous:** Fever (possibly due to drug-induced tissue necrosis).

OVERDOSE MANAGEMENT

Symptoms: GI complaints (may last a few hours). *Treatment:* Induce vomiting and purging.

DRUG INTERACTIONS

Carbamazepine and hydantoin may ↓ effect due to ↓ plasma levels of mebendazole.

HOW SUPPLIED

Tablets, Chewable: 100 mg.

DOSAGE

TABLETS, CHEWABLE

Whipworm, roundworm, and hookworm.

Adults and children: 1 tablet morning and evening on 3 consecutive days.

Pinworms.

1 tablet, one time. All treatments can be repeated after 3 weeks if the client is not cured.

NURSING IMPLICATIONS

ASSESSMENT

1. Note reasons for therapy, clinical confirmation of organism, onset and characteristics of S&S, and any other contributing factors.
2. Identify source/all persons in contact and potentially infected.
3. Assess for any history of Crohn's, ulcerative colitis, or liver disease; precludes therapy.
4. Monitor CBC and LFT with prolonged therapy.

CLIENT/FAMILY TEACHING

1. Tablets may be chewed, swallowed, or crushed and mixed with food. Fasting or purging are not required.
2. Pinworms may be highly contagious. To prevent reinfection:
    - Carefully wash hands with soap and water frequently during the day and especially before and after eating and toileting; clean nails and keep out of mouth.
    - Advise school nurse of treatment.
    - Do not scratch the infected area or place your fingers in your mouth.
    - Do not share washcloths and towels. Wear tight underpants day and night; change daily. Sleep alone; wear shoes during waking hours.
    - Do not shake clothing/linens before washing. Change and wash underwear, bed linens, towels, clothes, and pajamas daily in hot water.
    - Clean toilet and seats with disinfectant daily; vacuum or wet-mop bedroom floors daily during treatment and for several days after treatment. Avoid dry sweeping; stirs up dust.

- All family members should be treated simultaneously to eradicate infestation.
- Second treatment may be necessary.

3. Hookworm, whipworm and roundworm also live in the bowel. Eggs from the worms are deposited in the soil if an infected person fails to use a toilet or bathroom. Eggs in the soil are usually carried to the mouth on food or by contact with dirty hands. With hookworms, a pre-adult form penetrates the skin (usually the foot) and burrows its way into the bloodstream. Once inside they grow and breed inside the bowel. New eggs are released in the feces. Poor sewage disposal or the use of human waste for fertilizer can contaminate the ground with new eggs, which can then reinfect people. Do not go barefoot.
4. Wash all fruits and vegetables. Thoroughly cook all meats and vegetables.
5. In hookworm and whipworm infections anemia may occur. May be advised to take iron supplements daily and for up to 6 months after completing therapy to help clear up the anemia.
6. Immobilization followed by death of parasites is slow. Complete clearance from the GI tract may take up to 3 days after initiation of treatment. Report if S&S do not improve or worsen after 3 weeks.
7. Keep all F/U to assess response, labs, need for retreatment, and for adverse SE.

OUTCOMES/EVALUATE

- Three consecutive negative stool and/or perianal swabs
- Organism expulsion/destruction
- Desired eradication

Meclizine hydrochloride

(**MEK**-lih-zeen)

Classification(s): Antiemetic

Pregnancy Category: B

OTC: Bonine, Dramamine Less Drowsy Formula, Zentrip.

RX: Antivert, Antivert/25 and /50, Antrizine.

✤ **OTC:** Bonamine.

SEE ALSO ***ANTIHISTAMINES*** AND ***ANTIEMETICS***.

INDICATIONS/USES

(1) Prevention and treatment of N&V. (2) Prevention of N&V or dizziness associated with motion sickness. (3) Vertigo associated with diseases of the vestibular system (possibly effective).

ACTION/KINETICS

Action

Meclizine has antiemetic, anticholinergic, and antihistaminic effects. Mechanism for the antiemetic effect may be due to a central anticholinergic effect to decrease vestibular stimulation and depress labyrinthine activity. May also act on the CTZ to decrease vomiting.

Pharmacokinetics

Onset: 30–60 min; **Duration:** 8–24 hr. **t½:** 6 hr.

SPECIAL CONCERNS

- Safety for use during lactation and in children less than 12 years of age not determined.
- Use with caution in glaucoma, obstructive disease of the GI or GU tract, and in prostatic hypertrophy.
- Pediatric and geriatric clients may be more sensitive to meclizine's anticholinergic effects.

SIDE EFFECTS

Most Common

Drowsiness, dry mouth, nervousness, insomnia, constipation.

CNS: Drowsiness, excitation, nervousness, restlessness, insomnia, euphoria, vertigo, auditory or visual hallucinations (especially when doses recommended are exceeded). **GI:** N&V, diarrhea, constipation, dry mouth, anorexia. **GU:** Urinary frequency or retention; difficulty in urination. **CV:** Hypotension, tachycardia, palpitations. **Dermatologic:** Rash, urticaria. **Miscellaneous:** Dry nose and throat, blurred or double vision, tinnitus.

OVERDOSE MANAGEMENT

Symptoms: Hyperexcitability alternating with drowsiness. Massive overdosage may cause ***convulsions***, hallucinations, and ***respiratory paryalysis***. *Treatment:* Appropriate supportive and symptomatic treatment. Do **not** use morphine or other respiratory depressants.

HOW SUPPLIED

Strips, Orally Dissolving: 25 mg; ***Tablets:*** 12.5 mg, 25 mg, 50 mg; ***Tablets, Chewable:*** 25 mg.

DOSAGE

TABLETS; TABLETS, CHEWABLE

Motion sickness, including N&V.

Adults: 25–50 mg 1 hr before travel; may be repeated q 24 hr during travel.

Vertigo.

Adults: 25–100 mg/day in divided doses.

STRIPS, ORALLY DISSOLVING

Prevention of N&V or dizziness associated with motion sickness.

Adults and children 12 years and older: 1–2 strips to dissolve on the tongue once a day (or as directed by provider).

NURSING IMPLICATIONS

ASSESSMENT

1. Note onset, duration, characteristics of symptoms and other agents trialed/outcome. Identify triggers if known, any recent cold or URI, fever.
2. Assess for adverse symptoms; drug may mask signs of drug overdose or pathology such as increased ICP or intestinal obstruction.
3. Determine any asthma, emphysema, enlarged prostate, glaucoma, intestinal or urinary tract blockage and report.

CLIENT/FAMILY TEACHING

1. Take as directed; report if condition does not improve or worsens.
2. With motion sickness, take 1 hr before departure to ensure best results.
3. Antiemetics tend to cause drowsiness and dizziness. Do not drive or perform other hazardous tasks until drug response evident.
4. For dryness of mouth, may try sugarless candy or gum, ice chips, or using a saliva substitute.
5. Consume plenty of fluids and bulk to prevent constipation.
6. Avoid CNS depressants and alcohol; markedly increases sedative effects.
7. Report if vomiting worsens, or persistent sedation, dizziness, palpitations, difficulty or inability to urinate occurs.
8. Keep all F/U to assess response and for adverse SE.

OUTCOMES/EVALUATE

- Prevention of motion sickness
- Control of vertigo

Medroxyprogesterone acetate

(meh-**drox**-see-proh-**JESS**-ter-ohn)

Classification(s): Progestin

Pregnancy Category: X

RX: Depo-Provera, depo-subQ provera 104, Provera.

Rx: Apo-Medroxy, Gen-Medroxy, ratio-MPA.

SEE ALSO ***PROGESTERONE AND PROGESTINS*** AND ***ANTINEOPLASTIC AGENTS.***

INDICATIONS/USES

104 mg SC and 150 mg/mL IM: Prevention of pregnancy.

400 mg/mL IM: Adjunctive therapy and palliative treatment of inoperable, recurrent, and metastatic endometrial or renal carcinoma.

PO Tablets: (1) Secondary amenorrhea. (2) Abnormal uterine bleeding due to hormonal imbalance in the absence of organic pathology, such as fibroids or uterine cancer. (3) Reduce the incidence of endometrial hyperplasia in nonhysterectomized postmenopausal women receiving conjugated estrogen, 0.625 mg. *Investigational:* Treatment of advanced breast cancer.

ACTION/KINETICS

Action

Synthetic progestin devoid of estrogenic and androgenic activity. Prevents stimulation of endometrium by pituitary gonadotropins. Priming with estrogen is necessary before response is noted. **150 mg/mL product:** Inhibits secretion of gonadotropins which prevent follicular maturation and ovulation and thus results in endometrial thinning and thus the contraceptive effect. **400 mg/mL product:** When given to women with adequate endogenous estrogen, it transforms proliferative endometrium into secretory endometrial. As with the 150 mg/mL product, follicular maturation and ovulation are prevented.

Pharmacokinetics

Rapidly absorbed from GI tract. **Maximum levels:** 1–2 hr. **t½, after PO:** 2–3 hr for first 6 hr; then, 8–9 hr. **t½, long-acting forms IM:** About 50 days with maximum levels within 24 hr.

CONTRAINDICATIONS

Known hypersensitivity to medroxyprogesterone acetate or any component of the product. Clients with CV disease or current or past history of thromboembolic disease, active thrombophlebitis, cerebral apoplexy. Liver dysfunction or disease. Known or suspected malignancy of the breasts or genital organs. Missed abortion; as a diagnostic for pregnancy. Undiagnosed vaginal bleeding. Use during the first 4 months of pregnancy. Parenteral forms to treat secondary amenorrhea or dysfunctional uterine bleeding (PO therapy is recommended).

SPECIAL CONCERNS

(1) The use of progestins during the first 4 months of pregnancy is not recommended. There is the possibility that intrauterine exposure to progestational drugs in the first trimester of pregnancy may cause genital abnormalities in female and male fetuses. If the client is exposed to progestational drugs during the first 4 months of pregnancy or if the woman becomes pregnant while taking a progestational drug, apprise her of the potential risks to the fetus. (2) Significant bone mineral density loss has been associated with the use of the drug; loss may be greater with increased duration of use. Bone loss may not be completely reversible. (3) Use is not recommended for long-term birth control (longer than 2 years) unless other methods are inadequate. (4) Counsel clients that the contraceptive injection does not protect against HIV infection (AIDS) or other sexually transmitted diseases.

- **The overall risk of breast, liver, ovarian, endometrial, and cervical cancer is not thought to increase with use of the injectable long-acting contraceptive preparation.**
- **Possibility of ectopic pregnancy.**
- **Use with caution with a history of depression.**
- **Due to the possibility of fluid retention, use with caution in clients with epilepsy, migraine, asthma, or cardiac or renal dysfunction.**
- **Safety and efficacy not established in children.**

SIDE EFFECTS

Most Common

Breast tenderness, breakthrough bleeding, spotting, change in menstrual flow, urticaria/pruritus, acne, generalized rash.

GU: Amenorrhea or infertility for up to 18 months, breast tenderness/pain, galactorrhea, breakthrough bleeding, change in menstrual flow (irregular or unpredictable bleeding or spotting; rarely heavy or continuous bleeding), changes in cervical erosion and cervical secretions, decreased libido, anorgasmia, pelvic pain, vaginitis. **CV:** Thrombophlebitis, CV disorder, ***pulmonary embolism***. **GI:** Nausea, abdominal pain/discomfort, cholestatic jaundice (including neonatal jaundice). **CNS:** Nervousness, drowsiness, somnolence, insomnia, fatigue, dizziness, depression (in those with a history of such), headache, ***seizures*** (with use of the injection). **Dermatologic:** Pruritus, urticaria, generalized rash (including allergic rash with and without pruritus), acne, hirsutism, alopecia, angioneurotic edema. **Musculoskeletal:** Bone mineral density changes (risk factor for developing osteoporosis), arthralgia, backache, leg cramps. **Metabolic:** Decrease in glucose tolerance. **Ophthalmic:** Sudden or partial or complete loss of vision, sudden onset of proptosis, diplopia, or migraine, retinal thrombosis. **Body as a whole:** Hyperpyrexia, fluid retention, fatigue, asthenia, bloating, weight gain or loss, ***anaphylaxis. and anaphylactoid reaction.*** **Miscellaneous:** Leukorrhea, hot flashes.

LABORATORY TEST CONSIDERATIONS

↓ Plasma and urinary steroid levels (e.g., cortisol, estradiol, pregnanediol, progesterone, testosterone). ↓ Levels of gonadotropin, sex-hormone binding globulin, T_3 uptake values. ↑ Protein bound iodine and butanol extractable protein bound iodine. ↑ Prothrombin, Factors VII, VIII, IX, and X. ↑ BSP and other LFTs. ↑ or ↓ Total cholesterol, triglycerides, LDL cholesterol, and HDL cholesterol.

DRUG INTERACTIONS

Aminoglutethimide may ↑ metabolism of medroxyprogesterone → ↓ effect

HOW SUPPLIED

Injection: 104 mg/0.65 mL, 150 mg/mL, 400 mg/mL; ***Tablets:*** 2.5 mg, 5 mg, 10 mg.

DOSAGE

IM

Endometrial or renal carcinoma using the 400 mg/mL product.

Initial: 400–1,000 mg/week; **then,** if improvement noted within a few weeks or months and the disease appears stabilized it may be possible to maintain improvement using 400 mg/month. Medroxyprogesterone is not intended to be the primary therapy.

Long-acting contraceptive using the 150 mg/mL product.

150 mg of depot form q 3 months (13 weeks) by deep IM injection into the gluteal or deltoid muscle. Given only during the first 5 days after the onset of a normal menstrual period, within 5 days postpartum if not breast-feeding, or 6 weeks postpartum if breast-feeding.

SC

Long-acting contraceptive using the 104 mg product.

Recommended dose: 104 mg q 3 months (12–14 weeks) given SC into the anterior thigh or abdomen.

TABLETS

Secondary amenorrhea.

Adults: 5–10 mg/day for 5–10 days, with therapy beginning at any time during the menstrual cycle. If endometrium has been estrogen primed: 10 mg medroxyprogesterone/day for 10 days beginning any time. Withdrawal bleeding usually begins within 3–7 days after therapy ends.

Abnormal uterine bleeding caused by hormonal imbalance in the absence of organic pathology.

Adults: 5 or 10 mg/day for 5–10 days, with therapy beginning on day 16 or 21 of the menstrual cycle. If endometrium has been estrogen primed: 10 mg/day for 10 days, beginning on day 16 of the menstrual cycle. Withdrawal bleeding usually begins within 3–7 days after discontinuing therapy.

Endometrial hyperplasia.

Adults: 5 or 10 mg/day for 12–14 consecutive days per month, beginning either day 1 or 16 of the cycle.

NURSING IMPLICATIONS

℘ Do not confuse Amen with Ambien (sedative-hypnotic). Also, do not confuse Provera with Premarin (an estrogen).

IMPLEMENTATION/ADMINISTRATION/STORAGE

1. When switching from other contraceptive methods, give medroxyprogesterone in a way that ensures continuous contraceptive protection. For example, clients switching from an estrogen/progestin product should have their first injection within 7 days after the last day of taking the last active tablet, removing the patch or ring. Similarly contraceptive protection will be maintained in switching from 150 mg IM to 104 mg SC provided the next injection is given within the prescribed dosing period for the IM (150 mg) product.
2. Use special care to avoid contamination when using multi-dose vials.
3. Consider a lower PO dose or less frequent administration for those with mild to moderate hepatic impairment.
4. Store tablets from 20–25°C (68–77°F).

ASSESSMENT

1. Note reasons for therapy, type, onset, and characteristics of S&S.
2. List any thromboembolic disease, liver dysfunction, malignancy of the breasts or genital organs; precludes therapy.
3. Monitor BMD, calcium, BS, thyroid, renal and LFTs. With severe hypercalcemia, have IV fluids, diuretics, corticosteroids, and phosphate supplements available; monitor closely once corrected.

CLIENT/FAMILY TEACHING

1. With oral administration may take with food to ↓ GI upset; mark calendar to ensure dosing. IM injection may be painful. After repeated injections, infertility and amenorrhea may last as long as 18 months.
2. With cancer therapy, the combined effect of the drug and osteolytic metastases may result in hypercalcemia. Report insomnia, lethargy, anorexia, and N&V. Increase fluids to minimize hypercalcemia.
3. Keep scheduled appointments for contraceptive evaluation and regular GYN exams. Additional barrier protection is necessary to prevent STDs and HIV transmission. Practice regular breast exams. May induce mild masculinization of the external genitalia of the female fetus, as well as hypospadias in the male fetus; avoid use during the first 4 months of pregnancy.

4. Report pain/swelling in calves, sudden chest pain, shortness of breath as well as any other unusual side effects.
5. Keep all F/U to assess response, labs, and for adverse SE.

OUTCOMES/EVALUATE

- Prevention of pregnancy
- Control of tumor size and spread
- Regular menses; normal hormone levels
- ↓ Endometrial hyperplasia in postmenopausal women receiving estrogen

Mefloquine hydrochloride

(meh-**FLOH**-kwin)

Classification(s): Antimalarial
Pregnancy Category: C

INDICATIONS/USES

(1) Mild to moderate acute malaria caused by mefloquine-susceptible strains of *Plasmodium falciparum* (both chloroquine susceptible and resistant strains) or *P. vivax.* Data are not available regarding effectiveness in treating *P. ovale* or *P. malariae.* (2) Prophylaxis of *P. falciparum* and *P. vivax* infections, including prophylaxis of chloroquine-resistant strains of *P. falciparum.* (3) In case of life-threatening, serious, or overwhelming malaria infections due to *P. falciparum,* treat with an IV antimalarial drug. Following completion of the IV therapy, mefloquine may be given to complete the course of therapy. *NOTE:* Clients with acute *P. vivax* malaria are at a high risk for relapse as mefloquine does not eliminate the exoerythrocytic (hepatic) parasites. Thus, these clients should also be treated with primaquine. Strains of *P. falciparum* are reported to be resistant to mefloquine.

ACTION/KINETICS

Action

Related chemically to quinine and acts as a blood schizonticide although the exact mechanism is unknown. It may increase intravesicular pH in acid vesicles of parasite. It shows myocardial depressant activity with about 20% of the antifibrillatory activity of quinidine and 50% of the increase in the PR interval noted with quinine.

Pharmacokinetics

Food significantly increases the rate and extent of absorption leading to about a 40% increase in bioavailability. **Peak plasma levels:** 6–24 hr in healthy volunteers. A dose of 250 mg once weekly produces maximum steady-state plasma levels of 1,000 to 2,000 mcg/L which are reached in 7–10 weeks. The erythrocyte-to-plasma concentration ratio is about 2:1. Thus, the drug is concentrated in blood erythrocytes (i.e., the target cells in treatment of malaria). Metabolized in the liver and excreted mainly in the bile and feces. **t½:** 13–24 days (average 3 weeks) **Plasma protein binding:** 98%.

CONTRAINDICATIONS

Hypersensitivity to mefloquine or related compounds (e.g., quinine, quinidine). Use as prophylaxis with active or recent history of depression, anxiety, generalized anxiety disorder, psychosis or schizophrenia, or other major psychiatric disorder, or with a history of convulsions. Lactation.

SPECIAL CONCERNS

- Monitor LFTs and perform ophthalmic exams if therapy >1 year.
- Use with extreme caution with cardiovascular disease.
- Use with caution with hepatic dysfunction, psychiatric disturbances (may cause emotional disturbances), and epilepsy (may increase risk of seizures).
- If used in clients with *P. vivax,* there is high risk of relapse as mefloquine does not eliminate the exoerythrocytic phase of the parasite.
- Safety and efficacy not established to treat malaria in children less than 6 months of age.

SIDE EFFECTS

Most Common

N&V, diarrhea/loose stools, abdominal pain, dizziness, vertigo, myalgia, chills, skin rash, fever, loss of balance, headache, somnolence, insomnia, abnormal dreams, fatigue, loss of appetite, tinnitus. *NOTE:* At the doses used, it is difficult to distinguish side effects due to the drug from symptoms attributable to the disease itself.

Side effects listed are for either prophylaxis and/or treatment of malaria. **GI**: N&V, diarrhea, abdominal pain, dyspepsia, loss of appetite. **CNS:**

M

Dizziness, syncope, paranoia, hallucinations, psychotic behavior, vertigo, confusion, anxiety, depression, headache, emotional problems, agitation, restlessness, aggression psychotic or paranoid reactions, mood changes, panic attacks, insomnia, somnolence, abnormal dreams, forgetfulness, motor and sensory neuropathy (e.g., paresthesia, tremor, ataxia), encephalopathy of unknown origin, ***seizures***. *CV*: Hypertension, hypotension, tachycardia, bradycardia, palpitations, chest pain, bradycardia, irregular pulse, extrasystoles, AV block, ECG alterations, other transient cardiac conduction alterations (rare). **Dermatologic**: Flushing, urticaria, sweating, erythema multiforme, ***Stevens-Johnson syndrome***, skin rash, exanthema, erythema, pruritus, edema, hair loss. **Musculoskeletal**: Muscle weakness, muscle cramps, myalgia, arthralgia (rare). **Miscellaneous**: Loss of balance, chills, asthenia, visual disturbances, vestibular disorders (including tinnitus, hearing impairment), dyspnea, malaise, fatigue, fever, chills, hypersensitivity reactions (including mild cutaneous events to ***anaphylaxis***).

LABORATORY TEST CONSIDERATIONS

When used for prophylaxis: Transient ↑ transaminases, leukocytosis, thrombocytopenia. **When used for treatment of acute malaria:** ↓ Hematocrit, transient ↑ transaminases, leukopenia, thrombocytopenia.

OVERDOSE MANAGEMENT

Symptoms: Cardiotoxic effects, vomiting, diarrhea. *Treatment:* Induce vomiting and administer fluid therapy to treat vomiting and diarrhea.

DRUG INTERACTIONS

Anticonvulsants (e.g., carbamazepine, phenobarbital, phenytoin, valproic acid) / Loss of seizure control R/T ↓ anticonvulsant blood levels

Bacterial vaccines, live attenuated (e.g., oral live typhoid vaccines) / Possible attenuation of immunization; complete vaccinations with attenuated live bacteria 3 days before the first dose of mefloquine

Drugs known to alter cardiac conduction (i.e., antiarrhythmic or beta-adrenergic blocking agents, calcium channel blockers, H_1-antihistamines, tricyclic antidepressants and phenothiazines) / May contribute to a prolongation of the QTc interval

Chloroquine / ↑ Risk of seizures

Halofantrine / Potentially fatal prolongation of the QTc interval; do not use together

Quinidine / ↑ Risk of ECG abnormalities or cardiac arrest; delay mefloquine dose for at least 12 hr after the last dose of quinidine

Quinine / ↑ Risk of seizures, ECG abnormalities, or cardiac arrest; delay mefloquine dose for at least 12 hr after the last dose of quinine

HOW SUPPLIED

Tablets: 250 mg.

DOSAGE

TABLETS

Mild to moderate malaria caused by P. vivax *or mefloquine-susceptible strains of* P. falciparum.

Adults: 1,250 mg (5 tablets) as a single dose with at least 8 oz of water (not to be taken on an empty stomach). Take with food. **Children, 6 months and older:** 20–25 mg/kg, split in 2 doses. Take 6–8 hrs apart (may decrease the occurrence or severity of side effects). Do not take on an empty stomach and should be taken with ample water. If vomiting occurs <30 minutes after dose, give a second full dose. If vomiting occurs 30–60 minutes after dose, give additional half-dose.

Prophylaxis of malaria.

Adults: 250 mg once a week. Start 1 week before departure to endemic area and continue weekly while in area. Continue for 4 weeks after leaving the area. Take with food and 8 oz of water. **Children:** 5 mg/kg once a week. One 250 mg tablet should be taken in clients weighing >45 kg. In children weighing <45 kg, the weekly doses decrease in proportion to body weight: **31–45 kg**: $\frac{3}{4}$ tab/week; **21–30 kg**: $\frac{1}{2}$ tab/week; **11–20 kg**: $\frac{1}{4}$ tab/week; **5–10 kg**: $\frac{1}{8}$ tab/week. Take with food and water. May crush and mix with water.

NURSING IMPLICATIONS

IMPLEMENTATION/ADMINISTRATION/STORAGE

1. **If a full treatment course does not lead to improvement within 48–72 hr, mefloquine should not be used for retreatment. Use an alternative treatment. Also, if previous prophy-**

laxis with mefloquine has failed, do not use mefloquine for curative treatment.

2. When a traveler is taking other medications, it may be desirable to start prophylaxis 2–3 weeks prior to departure to ensure that the drug combination is well tolerated.
3. Vaccinations with attenuated live bacteria (e.g., typhoid vaccine) should be completed at least 3 days before the first dose of mefloquine.
4. Store tablets at 15–30°C (59–86°F).

ASSESSMENT

1. Note if for prophylaxis or treatment; dosages differ. List travel location and time of visit.
2. Country-specific information on malaria can be obtained from the CDC.
3. Note any psychiatric disturbances or severe emotional lability, assess for anxiety, depression, restlessness, or confusion. With seizure disorder, monitor anticonvulsant blood levels.
4. With life-threatening *P. falciparum* infection, treat with an IV antimalarial and follow with mefloquine to complete therapy.
5. Assess for CAD and get baseline ECG. To reduce cardiotoxic effects, induce vomiting with overdose. Obtain eye exam with prolonged therapy.
6. Obtain laboratory confirmation of causative organism; monitor CBC/LFTs.

CLIENT/FAMILY TEACHING

1. Do not take on an empty stomach; take with at least 8 oz of water and at same time each day. May be crushed and put in water, milk, or juice if necessary.
2. Avoid activities that require mental alertness until drug effects realized.
3. Report any unusual side effects, S&S of infection, mental status changes, visual disturbances; obtain periodic eye exams.
4. For prophylaxis, the CDC recommends a single dose taken weekly starting 1 week before travel, continued weekly during travel, and for 4 weeks after leaving malarious areas on the same day of the week.
5. If also prescribed other meds, start prophylaxis 2–3 weeks prior to departure to ensure that the drug combination is well tolerated. Report if acute anxiety, depression, restlessness, confusion, paranoia, hallucinations, or change in behavior occur. Alternative therapy will be necessary if mefloquine is discontinued.
6. Protective clothing, insect repellant, and bed nets are important components of malaria prophylaxis.
7. Practice reliable contraception during therapy.
8. Report if fever or "flu-like" S&S occur during your travels or within 2 to 3 months after you leave the area.
9. Keep all F/U to assess response and for adverse SE.

OUTCOMES/EVALUATE

Treatment/prophylaxis of malaria (with drug-sensitive malarial parasites)

Megestrol acetate

(meh-**JESS**-trohl)

Classification(s): Progestin

Pregnancy Category: D

RX: Megace, Megace ES.

✤ **Rx:** Apo-Megestrol, Megace OS.

SEE ALSO ***PROGESTERONE AND PROGESTINS*** AND ***ANTINEOPLASTIC AGENTS***.

INDICATIONS/USES

Oral suspension: Treatment of anorexia, cachexia, or an unexplained, significant weight loss in clients with a diagnosis of AIDS.

Tablets: Palliative treatment of advanced endometrial or breast cancer–recurrent, inoperable, or metastatic disease. Do not use in place of chemotherapy, radiation, or surgery.

Investigational: Appetite stimulant for cachexia in advanced cancer. Treatment of hot flashes.

ACTION/KINETICS

Action

Antineoplastic activity is due to suppression of gonadotropins (antiluteinizing effect). Has appetite-enhancing properties (mechanism unknown). Contains tartrazine, which can cause allergic-type reactions, including asthma, often occurring in aspirin sensitivity.

CONTRAINDICATIONS

Use as a diagnostic aid test for pregnancy, in known or suspected pregnancy, or for prophylaxis to avoid weight loss. Use during the first 4 months of pregnancy. Use for other types of neoplasms.

SPECIAL CONCERNS

■ The use of progestins during the first 4 months of pregnancy is not recommended. There is the possibility that intrauterine exposure to progestational drugs in the first trimester of pregnancy may cause genital abnormalities in female and male fetuses. If the client is exposed to progestational drugs during the first 4 months of pregnancy or if the woman becomes pregnant while taking a progestational drug, apprise her of the potential risks to the fetus. ■

- Use with caution in clients with a history of thromboembolic disease.
- Use in HIV-infected women with endometrial or breast cancer not widely studied.
- Long-term use may increase the risk of respiratory infections and may cause secondary adrenal suppression.
- Safety and efficacy in children not determined.

SIDE EFFECTS

Most Common

Diarrhea, impotence, rash, flatulence, hypertension, asthenia, insomnia, nausea, anemia, fever, headache.

GI: Diarrhea, flatulence, nausea, dyspepsia, vomiting, constipation, dry mouth, hepatomegaly, increased salivation, abdominal pain, oral moniliasis. **CV:** Hypertension, ***cardiomyopathy***, palpitation. **CNS:** Insomnia, headache, paresthesia, confusion, ***seizures***, depression, neuropathy, hypesthesia, abnormal thought process. **Respiratory:** Pneumonia, dyspnea, cough, pharyngitis, chest pain, lung disorder, increased risk of respiratory infection with chronic use. **Dermatologic:** Rash, alopecia, herpes, pruritus, vesiculobullous rash, sweating, skin disorder. **GU:** Impotence, decreased libido, urinary frequency, albuminuria, urinary incontinence, UTI, gynecomastia. **Body as a whole:** Asthenia, anemia, fever, pain, moniliasis, infection, sarcoma. **Miscellaneous:** Leukopenia, edema, peripheral edema, amblyopia.

LABORATORY TEST CONSIDERATIONS

Hyperglycemia, ↑ LDH.

HOW SUPPLIED

Oral Suspension: 40 mg/mL, 125 mg/mL; ***Tablets:*** 20 mg, 40 mg.

DOSAGE

ORAL SUSPENSION

Appetite stimulant in AIDS clients.

Adults, initial: 800 mg/day (20 mL/day of the 40 mg/mL oral suspension) or 625 mg/day (5 mL/day of the 125 mg/mL extra strength oral suspension). *NOTE:* Daily doses of 400 and 800 mg/day of the 40 mg/mL oral suspension are clinically effective.

TABLETS

Breast cancer.

Adults: 40 mg 4 times per day for palliation. At least 2 months of continuous treatment is considered an adequate period to determine efficacy.

Endometrial cancer.

Adults: 40–320 mg/day in divided doses. To determine efficacy, treatment should be continued for at least 2 months.

Hot flashes (investigational).

Adults: 20 mg twice a day. Alternatively, 20 mg/day or less may also be beneficial. Use the lowest effective dose.

NURSING IMPLICATIONS

IMPLEMENTATION/ADMINISTRATION/STORAGE

1. Megestrol is also a teratogen. Follow safe handling procedures when preparing, administering, or dispensing the drug.
2. The oral suspension is available in a lemon-lime flavor that contains 40 mg of micronized megestrol acetate/mL; shake well before using.
3. Store suspension from 15–25°C (59–77°F); dispense in a tight container. Protect from heat.
4. Store tablets from 15–30°C (59–86°F). Protect from temperatures above 40°C (104°F).

ASSESSMENT

1. Note reasons for therapy, other agents trialed, symptom onset and characteristics, weight history.

2. List any sensitivity to tartrazines or thromboembolic disease.
3. Determine if pregnant; avoid if pregnant.
4. Monitor VS, also Wt, appetite, and intake in those with HIV.
5. Note any pain, swelling or tenderness in legs; assess for DVT.
6. With long-term therapy, assess for respiratory infections and adrenal suppression.

CLIENT/FAMILY TEACHING

1. Shake the suspension well before using.
2. Take exactly as prescribed; do not skip or double up doses. May take with meals if GI upset occurs. Consume plenty of fluids to prevent dehydration.
3. Report vaginal bleeding, headaches, breast tenderness, back/abdominal pain or pain/weakness in hands (CTS).
4. Practice reliable birth control during and for several months following therapy. Do not breastfeed during therapy.
5. Report any pain, swelling or warmth in calves (S&S of DVT); as well as any other unusual side effects.
6. Monitor weights when used to stimulate appetite.
7. Keep all F/U to assess response, labs, adverse SE; with cancer therapy may take up to 2 months to determine effectiveness.

OUTCOMES/EVALUATE

- ↓ Tumor size and spread
- ↑ Appetite and weight gain especially in HIV-related cachexia

Meloxicam

(meh-**LOX**-ih-kam)

Classification(s): Nonsteroidal anti-inflammatory drug

Pregnancy Category: C

RX: Mobic.

🍁 **Rx:** Apo-Meloxicam, CO Meloxicam, Gen-Meloxicam, Mobicox, Novo-Meloxicam, PMS-Meloxicam, ratio-Meloxicam.

SEE ALSO ***NONSTEROIDAL ANTI-INFLAMMATORY DRUGS.***

INDICATIONS/USES

(1) Relief of signs and symptoms of osteoarthritis. (2) Relief of signs and symptoms of rheumatoid arthritis in adults. (3) Relief of signs and symptoms of pauciarticular or polyarticular course juvenile rheumatoid arthritis in clients 2 years of age and older. *Investigational:* Treatment of ankylosing spondylitis and acute shoulder pain.

ACTION/KINETICS

Action

Anti-inflammatory effect is likely due to inhibition of cyclo-oxygenase. Inhibition of cyclo-oxygenase results in decreased prostaglandin synthesis. Effective in reducing joint swelling, pain, and morning stiffness, as well as to increase mobility in those with inflammatory disease. Does not alter the course of the disease, however.

Pharmacokinetics

Prolonged drug absorption. 89% is bioavailable. Steady state reached in 5 days. Metabolized in the liver by P450-mediated metabolism. **Peak:** 4–5 hr. **t½, elimination:** 15–20 hr. Excreted in about equal amounts in the urine and feces. **Plasma protein binding:** More than 99%.

CONTRAINDICATIONS

Use in those who have exhibited asthma, urticaria, or allergic-type reactions after taking aspirin or other NSAIDs (anaphylaxis is possible). Use for treatment of perioperative pain in the setting of coronary artery bypass graft surgery. Use in advanced renal disease or late pregnancy (may cause premature closure of the ductus arteriosus). Lactation.

SPECIAL CONCERNS

(1) **Cardiovascular risk.** NSAIDs may cause an increased risk of serious CV thrombotic events, MI, and stroke, which can be fatal. The risk may increase with duration of use. Clients with CV disease or risk factors for CV disease may be at higher risk. (2) Meloxicam is contraindicated for the treatment of perioperative pain in the setting of coronary artery bypass graft surgery. (3) **GI risk.** NSAIDs cause an increased risk of serious GI adverse reactions, including bleeding, ulceration, and perforation of the stomach or intestines, which can be fatal. These reactions can occur at any time during use and without warning

symptoms. Elderly clients are at higher risk for serious GI reactions. ■

- Use with caution in pre-existing kidney disease.
- Use with caution in those 65 years and older.
- Safety and efficacy not determined in children less than 18 years.

SIDE EFFECTS

Most Common

Headache, dizziness, insomnia, rash, abdominal pain/cramps, diarrhea, N&V, constipation, flatulence, dyspepsia/indigestion, UTI, edema, URTI, pharyngitis.

See also *Nonsteroidal Anti-Inflammatory Drugs* for a complete list of possible side effects. Side effects listed are those with an incidence of 2% or greater. **GI:** Abdominal pain, cramps, diarrhea, dyspepsia, indigestion, constipation, flatulence, N&V. **CNS:** Dizziness, headache, insomnia. **Respiratory:** Pharyngitis, URTI, coughing. **GU:** Renal papillary necrosis, micturition frequency, UTI. **Hematologic:** Anemia. **Musculoskeletal:** Arthralgia, back pain. **Dermatologic:** Pruritus, rash. **Body as a whole:** Fluid retention, edema, pain, flu-like symptoms, accidents.

LABORATORY TEST CONSIDERATIONS

Elevation of LFTs.

DRUG INTERACTIONS

ACE Inhibitors / ↓ Antihypertensive effect of ACE inhibitors
Aspirin / ↑ Risk of GI side effects, including GI ulceration or other complications
Cholestyramine / ↑ Meloxicam clearance
Lithium / ↑ Plasma lithium levels
Warfarin / ↑ Risk of bleeding

HOW SUPPLIED

Oral Suspension: 7.5 mg/5 mL; *Tablets:* 7.5 mg, 15 mg.

DOSAGE

ORAL SUSPENSION; TABLETS

Osteoarthritis, rheumatoid arthritis in adults.

Adults, initial and maintenance: 7.5 mg once daily. Some may gain additional benefit from 15 mg once daily. Maximum recommended daily dose: 15 mg.

Pauciarticular/polyarticular course juvenile rheumatoid arthritis.

Recommended PO dose: 0.125 mg/kg once daily, up to a maximum of 7.5 mg daily. The following dosage recommendations are based on weight using the oral suspension (1.5 mg/mL): **12 kg (26 lbs):** 1 mL (1.5 mg); **24 kg (54 lbs):** 2 mL (3 mg); **36 kg (80 lbs):** 3 mL (4.5 mg); **48 kg (106 lbs):** 4 mL (6 mg); **greater or equal to 60 kg (132 lbs):** 5 mL (7.5 mg).

NURSING IMPLICATIONS

IMPLEMENTATION/ADMINISTRATION/STORAGE

1. Consider the potential benefits and risks before deciding to use meloxicam.
2. Use the lowest dose for the shortest duration consistent with individual client treatment goals. Adjust dose to suit the individual client's needs.
3. Use of the PO suspension is recommended to improve dosing accuracy in lower weight children.
4. The oral suspension, 7.5 mg/5 mL or 15 mg/10 mL, may be substituted for meloxicam tablets, 7.5 or 15 mg, respectively.
5. The maximum recommended daily dose is 15 mg, regardless of the formulation.
6. May be taken without regard to meals.
7. Store at 15–30°C (59–86°F). Keep in a dry place in a tight container.

ASSESSMENT

1. Identify reasons for therapy, onset, characteristics of disease, ROM, deformity/loss of function, level of pain, other agents trialed, outcome. List drugs prescribed to ensure none interact.
2. Check for any GI bleed or ulcer history, CAD, aspirin or other NSAID-induced asthma, urticaria, or allergic-type reactions.
3. May cause an increased risk of serious CV thrombotic events, MI, and stroke that can be fatal.
4. Monitor CBC, electrolytes, renal and LFTs, within 3 months of starting therapy and then q 6 months. Avoid with severe liver/renal dysfunction, perioperative CABG pain, pregnancy.

CLIENT/FAMILY TEACHING

1. Take as directed at the same time each day. May take with or without food. Shake the oral suspension gently before using and use dosing spoon, syringe, or cup to measure and administer dose.
2. The lowest dose for symptom control will be used. Class of drugs may cause serious CV side effects, such as MI or stroke.
3. Avoid activities that require mental alertness until drug effects realized; may cause dizziness or drowsiness.
4. Report unusual or persistent side effects including dyspepsia, abdominal pain, dizziness, weight gain, skin rash, swelling of ankles, chest pain, SOB, or lack of effect. and changes in stool or skin color. Alcohol and tobacco may aggravate GI S&S, so avoid smoking, alcohol, and self-administration of aspirin-containing medications while taking meloxicam.
5. Avoid therapy during pregnancy; may cause premature closure of baby's heart duct.
6. Keep all F/U to assess response, labs, and for adverse SE.

OUTCOMES/EVALUATE

- Relief of joint pain and inflammation with improved mobility

Memantine hydrochloride

(meh-**MAN**-teen)

Classification(s): Drug for Alzheimer's disease

Pregnancy Category: B

RX: Namenda, Namenda XR.

INDICATIONS/USES

Moderate-to-severe dementia of the Alzheimer's type. When combined with donepezil (Aricept), the decline of mental and physical function may be less. *Investigational:* Treatment of vascular dementia.

ACTION/KINETICS

Action

It is believed that activation of N-methyl-D-aspartate (NMDA) receptors in the brain by glutamate, an excitatory amino acid, contributes to the symptomatology of Alzheimer's disease. Memantine is believed to have low to moderate affinity as an antagonist for open-channel NMDA receptors thus preventing activation by glutamate. The drug does not prevent or slow neurodegeneration in Alzheimer's disease. The drug also shows antagonistic effects at the $5HT_3$ receptor and for nicotinic acetylcholine receptors.

Pharmacokinetics

Well absorbed after PO administration; **peak levels:** 3–7 hr for immediate–release tablets and 9–12 hr for extended–release capsules. Food has no effect on the absorption. About 50% excreted unchanged in the urine. **t½, terminal:** 60–80 hr. **Plasma protein binding:** 45%.

CONTRAINDICATIONS

Known hypersensitivity to memantine or any excipients in the formulation, including lactose monohydrate. Conditions that raise urine pH may decrease the urinary elimination of memantine resulting in increased plasma levels.

SPECIAL CONCERNS

- Higher levels possible in clients with moderate to severe renal impairment; consider dose reduction.
- Use with caution in renal tubular acidosis, severe UTIs, and during lactation.
- Safety and efficacy not determined in children.

SIDE EFFECTS

Most Common

Fatigue, pain, increased BP, dizziness, headache, constipation, vomiting, back pain, confusion, somnolence, hallucinations, coughing, dyspnea.

Immediate-Release and/or Extended-Release. CNS: Dizziness, confusion, headache, hallucinations (both auditory and visual), somnolence, agitation, anxiety, depression, dementia of the Alzheimer's type, disorientation, dyskinesia, abnormal gait, insomnia, aggressive reaction, ataxia, hypokinesia, irritability, vertigo, abnormal coordination, abnormal crying, abnormal thinking, amnesia, apathy, aphasia, ***cerebral hemorrhage, intracranial hemorrhage, convulsions (including tonic/clonic)***, delirium, delusions, depersonalization, depressed levels of consciousness, LOC, emotional lability, extrapyramidal disorder, hemiplegia, hyperkinesia, hypertonia, hypesthesia, nervousness, neuralgia, neuropathy, neurosis, paranoid reaction, paresthesia, parkinsonism, paroniria, personality disorder, psychosis, restlessness, sleep disorder, stupor, ***suicide attempt/ideation***, tremor, tardive dyskinesia, ***neuroleptic malignant syndrome***. **GI:** Constipation, vomiting, abdominal pain, colitis, diarrhea, fecal incontinence, N&V, diverticulitis, dysphagia, esophageal ulceration, gastritis, gastroenteritis, gastroesophageal reflux, ***GI hemorrhage***, ileus, melena, pancreatitis. **Hepatic:** Cholelithiasis, hepatic failure, hepatitis, cytolytic and cholestatic hepatitis. **CV:** Hyper-/hypotension, ***cardiac failure/infarction, CVA***, syncope, TIA, angina pectoris, atrial fibrillation, bradycardia, ***cardiac arrest,*** hypotension, ***MI,*** postural hypotension, thrombophlebitis, atrial fibrillation, AV block (including 2nd and ***3rd degree block***), claudication, DVT, EEG QT prolongation, increased INR ratio, supraventricular tachycardia, tachycardia, ***torsades de pointes***. **Respiratory:** Coughing, dyspnea, bronchitis, URTI, pulmonary edema/***embolism,*** pneumonia, ***apnea***, asthma, hemoptysis, nasopharyngitis, aspiration pneumonia. **Musculoskeletal:** Arthralgia, involuntary muscle contractions, pain in extremity, bone fracture, carpal tunnel syndrome, myoclonus. **Dermatologic:** Rash, alopecia, cellulitis, dermatitis, eczema, erythematous rash, pruritus, skin ulceration, urticaria, ***Stevens-Johnson syndrome***. **GU:** Urinary incontinence, UTI, increased libido, frequent micturition, dysuria, hematuria, urinary retention, acute renal failure, impotence. **Hematologic:** Anemia, leukopenia, agranulocytosis, neutropenia, pancytopenia, thrombocytopenia, thrombotic thrombocytopenic purpura. **Metabolic:** Decreased weight, anorexia, increased/decreased appetite, aggravated diabetes mellitus, dehydration. **Ophthalmic:** Ptosis, cataract, conjunctivitis, abnormal lacrimation, blepharitis, blurred vision, conjunctival hemorrhage, corneal opacity, decreased visual acuity, diplopia, eye pain, glaucoma, macula lutea degeneration, myopia retinal detachment, retinal hemorrhage, xerophthalmia. **Otic:** Decreased hearing, tinnitus. **Body as a whole:** Fatigue, asthenia, lethargy, malaise, pain, pyrexia, fall, inflicted injury, influenza-like symptoms, hypothermia, ***sepsis, sudden death***. **Miscellaneous:** Back/chest pain, peripheral edema, allergic reaction, inappropriate antidiuretic hormone secretion.

LABORATORY TEST CONSIDERATIONS

↑ Alkaline phosphatase. Hyper-/hypoglycemia, hyperlipidemia, hyponatremia.

OVERDOSE MANAGEMENT

Symptoms: See *Side Effects*. *Treatment:* Use general supportive measures; treat symptoms. Can enhance elimination by acidification of the urine.

DRUG INTERACTIONS

Amantadine / Use with memantine with caution as amantadine is also an NMDA antagonist
Carbonic anhydrase inhibitors / Accumulation of memantine → ↑ side effects; use together with caution
Cimetidine / Possible altered plasma levels of both drugs
Dextromethorphan / Use with memantine with caution as dextromethorphan is also an NMDA antagonist
Hydrochlorothiazide / Bioavailability of hydrochlorothiazide is decreases 20%; monitor and adjust thiazide dose if needed
Ketamine / Use with caution as ketamine is also an NMDA antagonist
Nicotine / Possible altered plasma levels of both drugs
Quinidine / Possible altered plasma levels of both drugs
Ranitidine / Possible altered plasma levels of both drugs
Sodium bicarbonate / Accumulation of memantine → ↑ side effects; use together with caution
Triamterene / Possible altered plasma levels of both drugs

HOW SUPPLIED

Capsules, Extended-Release (Namenda XR): 7 mg, 14 mg, 21 mg, 28 mg; ***Oral Solution (Namenda):*** 2 mg/mL; ***Tablets (Namenda):*** 5 mg, 10 mg.

DOSAGE

ORAL SOLUTION; TABLETS, IMMEDIATE-RELEASE

Alzheimer's disease, moderate to severe.

Adults, initial: 5 mg/day. Dose should be increased in 5 mg increments to 10 mg/day (5 mg twice a day), then 15 mg/day (5 mg and 10 mg as separate doses), and finally 20 mg/day (10 mg twice a day). The minimum recommended interval between dose increases is 1 week. Reduce the dose in clients with moderate renal impairment.

CAPSULES, EXTENDED-RELEASE

Alzheimer's disease, moderate to severe.

Adults, initial: 7 mg once a day; increase in 7 mg increments up to a maximum of 28 mg once a day. The minimum recommended interval between dose increases is 1 week and only if the previous dose has been well tolerated. Those taking the 10 mg immediate-release tablets twice a day may switch to the 28 mg extended-release capsules once a day the day following the last dose of an intermediate-release 10 mg tablet.

NURSING IMPLICATIONS

Do not confuse memantine with amantadine (antiviral and antiparkinson drug).

IMPLEMENTATION/ADMINISTRATION/STORAGE

1. The usual dose in severe renal impairment (C_{CR} 5–29 mL/min) is 5 mg twice a day. Clients taking the 5 mg tablet twice a day may switch to the 14 mg extended-release capsule once a day the day following the last dose of an immediate-release 5 mg tablet.
2. Store from 15–30°C (59–86°F).

ASSESSMENT

1. Note reasons for therapy, when diagnosed with Alzheimer's disease and when treatment began.
2. Assess for other medical conditions that require careful monitoring, i.e., seizure disorder, liver or renal dysfunction.
3. List all drugs prescribed to ensure none interact. Review MMSE score before therapy and then several months after to assess cognitive function and drug effectiveness.
4. Monitor Wt, VS, CBC, renal and LFTs; reduce dose with dysfunction.

CLIENT/FAMILY TEACHING

1. May take with or without food; with food if GI upset.
2. Drug started at a low dose and gradually increased at 1 week intervals.
3. Used in Alzheimer's disease to improve level of cognitive functioning; does not cure or alter disease but assists with symptoms. Improvement in cognitive functioning may take months before evident.
4. The ER capsules should be swallowed whole. If unable to swallow, the capsules may be opened and sprinkled on applesauce and the entire contents consumed. Do not divide, chew, or crush capsules.
5. If oral solution prescribed, client or caregiver should be instructed on how to attach the green cap and plastic tube to new bottles of oral solution and how to withdraw prescribed dose using the dosing syringe, and how to administer the dose.
6. Avoid alcohol and any OTC products or herbals without provider approval to prevent interactions.
7. May cause dizziness/drowsiness; avoid activities that require mental alertness until effects realized.
8. Keep all F/U to assess response, labs, and adverse SE.

OUTCOMES/EVALUATE

- ↑ Cognitive functioning, ↓ confusion with severe Alzheimer dementia
- Treatment of vascular dementia (unlabeled)

IV

Meperidine hydrochloride (Pethidine hydrochloride)

(meh-**PER**-ih-deen)

Classification(s): Narcotic analgesic

Pregnancy Category: C

RX: Demerol Hydrochloride, **C-II**

SEE ALSO ***NARCOTIC ANALGESICS***.

INDICATIONS/USES

PO, Parenteral: Analgesic for moderate-to-severe pain. **Parenteral:** (1) Preoperative medication. (2) Adjunct to support anesthesia. (3) Obstetrical analgesia (except 10 mg/mL).

ACTION/KINETICS

Action

One-tenth as potent an analgesic as morphine. Its analgesic effect is only one-half when given PO

M

rather than parenterally. Has no antitussive effects and does not produce miosis. Less smooth muscle spasm, constipation, and antitussive effect than equianalgesic doses of morphine. Produces both psychologic and physical dependence; overdosage causes severe respiratory depression (see *Narcotic Overdose).*

Pharmacokinetics

Onset: 10–45 min. **Peak effect:** 30–60 min. **Duration:** 2–4 hr (duration is less than that of most opiates; keep in mind when establishing a dosing schedule). **t½:** 3–6 hr for meperidine and <20 hr for normeperidine (active metabolite).

ADDITIONAL CONTRAINDICATIONS

Hypersensitivity to drug, convulsive states as in epilepsy, tetanus, and strychnine poisoning, children under 6 months, diabetic acidosis, head injuries, shock, liver disease, respiratory depression, increased intracranial pressure, and before labor during pregnancy. Use with sibutramine.

SPECIAL CONCERNS

- **Use with caution during lactation, in older, or debilitated clients.**
- **Due to decreased renal function may accumulate in the elderly leading to an increased risk of seizures. Also causes confusion in the elderly.**
- **Use with extreme caution in clients with asthma.**
- **Atropine-like effects may aggravate glaucoma, especially when given with other drugs used with caution in glaucoma.**

SIDE EFFECTS

Most Common

Constipation, dry mouth, N&V, anorexia, dizziness, fatigue, lightheadedness, muscle twitches, sweating, itching, decreased urination, decreased libido.

See *Narcotic Analgesics* for a complete list of possible side effects. Also, transient hallucinations, transient hypotension (high doses), visual disturbances, shock. Active metabolite may accumulate in renal dysfunction, leading to an increased risk of CNS toxicity.

OVERDOSE MANAGEMENT

Symptoms: Severe respiratory depression. See *Narcotic Analgesics. Treatment:* Naloxone 0.4 mg IV is effective in the treatment of acute overdosage. In PO overdose, gastric lavage and induced emesis are indicated. Treatment, however, is aimed at combating the progressive respiratory depression usually through artificial ventilation.

ADDITIONAL DRUG INTERACTIONS

Antidepressants, tricyclic / Additive anticholinergic side effects
Cimetidine / ↑ Respiratory and CNS depression
Hydantoins / ↓ Meperidine effect R/T ↑ liver breakdown
MAOIs / ↑ Risk of severe symptoms including hyperpyrexia, restlessness, hyper- or hypotension, convulsions, or coma; do not use together
Protease inhibitors / Avoid combination
Sibutramine / Possibility of life-threatening serotonin syndrome
Smoking / ↓ Analgesia R/T ↑ hepatic metabolism; takes several weeks to occur

HOW SUPPLIED

Injection: 25 mg/mL, 50 mg/mL, 75 mg/mL, 100 mg/mL; ***Oral Solution:*** 50 mg/5 mL; ***Syrup:*** 50 mg/5 mL; ***Tablets:*** 50 mg, 100 mg.

DOSAGE

ORAL SOLUTION; SYRUP; TABLETS

Analgesic.

Adults: 50–100 mg q 3–4 hr as needed; **pediatric:** 1.1–1.75 mg/kg, up to adult dosage, q 3–4 hr as needed.

IM, SC

Analgesic.

Adults: 50–150 mg q 3–4 hr, as needed. For elderly clients, use the lower end of the dosage range and observe closely. **Children:** 1.1–1.75 mg/kg, up to the adult dose, q 3–4 hr, as needed.

Preoperatively.

Adults: 50–100 mg 30–90 min before beginning anesthesia. Use the lower end of the dosage range for elderly clients and observe closely. **Children:** 1.1–2.2 mg/kg, up to the adult dose, 30–90 min before beginning anesthesia.

Obstetrical analgesia.

Adults: 50–100 mg when the pain becomes regular; may repeat at 1 to 3 hr intervals.

IV

Analgesia.

Adults: 15–35 mg/hr by continuous infusion.

Analgesic using a compatible Hospira infusion device.

Adults, initial: 10 mg using the 10 mg/mL strength; **range:** 1–5 mg/incremental dose. The recommended lockout interval is 6–10 min with the minimum recommended lockout interval of 5 min. Dose may be adjusted upward or downward or the lockout interval may be increased or decreased, depending on client response.

Support of anesthesia.

Continuous IV infusion: 1 mg/mL or **slow IV injection:** 10 mg/mL until client needs met.

NURSING IMPLICATIONS

IMPLEMENTATION/ADMINISTRATION/STORAGE

1. Adjust the dose depending on the severity of the pain and the client response.
2. For repeated doses, IM administration is preferred over SC use.
3. More effective when given parenterally than when given PO.
4. Take the syrup with half a glass of water to minimize anesthetic effect on mucous membranes.
5. If used concomitantly with phenothiazines or antianxiety agents, reduce the PO or parenteral dose by 25–50%.
6. Adjust parenteral doses according to the severity of pain and client response. Reduce the dose in poor-risk clients, in the very young or very old, in those with impaired renal or hepatic function, and in clients receiving other CNS depressants.
7. For surgical clients, adjust parenteral doses based on response of the client, other premedications and concomitant medications, the anesthetic being used, and the nature and duration of the surgery.
8. IV IV doses should be decreased and the injection given very slowly, preferably using a diluted solution (e.g., 10 mg/mL). Rapid injection increases the incidence of side effects.
9. When given parenterally, especially IV, the client should be lying down.
10. Store PO forms from 15–30°C (59–86°F). Store parenteral forms (except the 10 mg/mL) at room temperature (up to 25°C, 77°F). Store the 10 mg/mL injection from 20–25°C (68–77°F).
11. COMPATIBILITY D5/RL, dextrose-saline combinations, dextrose (2.5%, 5%, 10%) in water; Ringer's, LR, 0.45% or 0.9% NaCl; or 1/6 M sodium lactate.
12. INCOMPATIBILITY Aminophylline, barbiturates, heparin, iodide, methicillin, morphine sulfate, phenytoin, sodium bicarbonate, sulfadiazine, and sulfisoxazole.

ASSESSMENT

1. Note reasons for therapy, with pain location, onset, characteristics of pain; rate pain level. List drugs prescribed to ensure none interact unfavorably.
2. List any head injury, seizure disorder, glaucoma, asthma, or conditions that may compromise respirations.
3. Assess bowel function and increase fluids and bulk in addition to laxatives to reduce constipating drug effects.
4. Monitor cognitive functioning, VS, renal and LFTs; note dysfunction.

CLIENT/FAMILY TEACHING

1. Take drug within ordered intervals to prevent pain recurring; report pain levels and lack of effectiveness.
2. With oral solution, each dose should be carefully measured and taken in one-half glass of water. If taken undiluted may exert a slight topical anesthetic effect to oral cavity.
3. Drug causes dizziness and drowsiness; do not engage in activities that require mental alertness.
4. Due to low BP effects, rise slowly and do not change positions abruptly.
5. Increase fluid intake and bulk and take laxatives as directed; report constipation if evident.
6. Avoid alcohol and other CNS depressants.
7. Store safely away from bedside; record dose and time of administration. Drug causes dependence and may be targeted for abuse/diversion. May cause delirium in the elderly assess for fall risk.
8. Keep all F/U to assess response, labs, adverse SE.

OUTCOMES/EVALUATE

Desired level of analgesia/pain control

M

Mercaptopurine (6-Mercaptopurine, 6-MP)

(mer-kap-toe-**PYOUR**-een)

Classification(s): Antineoplastic, antimetabolite

Pregnancy Category: D

RX: Purinethol.

SEE ALSO ***ANTINEOPLASTIC AGENTS.***

INDICATIONS/USES

(1) Remission, induction, and maintenance therapy of acute lymphocytic leukemia. Use combination therapy (e.g., L-asparaginase, prednisone, vincristine). (2) Acute myelogenous and myelomonocytic leukemia. Use combination therapy. Effectiveness varies depending on use. *NOTE:* Not effective for leukemia of the CNS, solid tumors, lymphomas, or chronic lymphocytic leukemia.

ACTION/KINETICS

Action

Mercaptopurine competes with hypoxanthine and guanine for the enzyme hypoxanthine-guanine phosphoribosyltransferase and is itself converted to thioinosinic acid (TIMP). Thioinosinic acid inhibits several reactions involving inosinic acid, including the conversion of inosinic acid to xanthylic acid and the conversion of inosinic acid to adenylic acid. In addition, 6-methylthioinosinate (MTIMP) is formed. Both TIMP and MTIMP allegedly inhibit glutamine-5-phosphoribosylpyrophosphate amidotransferase, the first enzyme unique to the de novo pathway for purine ribonucleotide synthesis.

Pharmacokinetics

Absorption is incomplete and variable, averaging about 50%. **Plasma t½:** 47 min in adults and 21 min in children. Metabolites are excreted in urine with up to 39% excreted unchanged. Cross-resistance with thioguanine has been observed. **Plasma protein binding:** About 19%.

CONTRAINDICATIONS

Use in resistance to mercaptopurine or thioguanine. Prophylaxis or treatment of CNS leukemia, CLL, lymphomas (including Hodgkin's disease), solid tumors. Not to be used unless a diagnosis of acute lymphatic leukemia has been adequately established. Concomitant use with azathioprine due to risk of severe myelosuppression. Lactation.

SPECIAL CONCERNS

■ Mercaptopurine is a potent drug. It should not be used unless a diagnosis of acute lymphatic leukemia has been adequately established, and the responsible physician is knowledgeable in assessing response to chemotherapy. ■

- **Use with caution in clients with impaired renal function; start with lower doses**
- **Use during lactation only if benefits clearly outweigh risks.**
- **Severe bone marrow depression (anemia, leukopenia, thrombocytopenia) may occur.**
- **Increased risk of pancreatitis when used for inflammatory bowel disease.**
- **Usually complete cross resistance between mercaptopurine and thioguanine.**

SIDE EFFECTS

Most Common

Myelosuppression (anemia, leukopenia, thrombocytopenia), alopecia, skin rash, hyperpigmentation, fatigue, weakness, yellow eyes/skin, N&V, anorexia, abdominal pain.

See *Antineoplastic Agents* for a complete list of possible side effects. **GI:** Oral lesions, intestinal ulceration, ***hepatotoxicity***. Pancreatitis (when used for inflammatory bowel disease). Produces less GI toxicity than folic acid antagonists. **Dermatologic:** Skin rashes, hyperpigmentation, alopecia. **Hematologic:** Myelosuppression, including anemia, leukopenia, and/or thrombocytopenia. **Miscellaneous:** Immunosuppression, drug fever, hyperuricemia, oligospermia. Side effects are less frequent in children than in adults.

OVERDOSE MANAGEMENT

Symptoms: Immediate symptoms include N&V, diarrhea, and anorexia while delayed symptoms include myelosuppression, gastroenteritis, and liver dysfunction. *Treatment:* Induction of emesis if detected soon after ingestion. Supportive measures.

DRUG INTERACTIONS

Allopurinol / ↑ Methotrexate effect R/T ↓ liver breakdown (reduce methotrexate dose from 25–33%)

Azathioprine / Mercaptopurine is a metabolite of azathioprine; do not use together due to ↑ risk of severe myelosuppression
Balsalazide / Possible leukopenia and ↑ in whole blood 6-thioguanine nucleotide levels in clients with Crohn's disease
Mesalamine / Possible leukopenia and ↑ in whole blood 6-thioguanine in clients with Crohn's disease
Sulfasalazine / Possible leukopenia and ↑ in whole blood 6-thioguanine nucleotide levels in clients with Crohn's disease
Thioguanine / Complete cross-resistance with mercaptopurine
Trimethoprim-Sulfamethoxazole / ↑ Risk of bone marrow suppression

HOW SUPPLIED

Tablets: 50 mg.

DOSAGE

TABLETS

Leukemias, induction therapy.

Highly individualized. **Adults and children, initial:** 2.5 mg/kg/day; the usual adult daily dose is 100–200 mg and the usual pediatric dose is 50 mg in an average 5-year-old child. If after 4 weeks at the preceding dose, there is no improvement and no definite evidence of leukocyte or platelet depression, the dose may be increased to 5 mg/kg/day. Calculate the dose to the nearest multiple of 25 mg. Dose may be given all at once. Dosage is increased until symptoms of toxicity appear.

Leukemias, maintenance therapy.

Maintenance therapy is essential once a complete hematologic remission is obtained. Maintenance doses vary from client to client. **Maintenance, usual:** 1.5–2.5 mg/kg/day as a single dose. *NOTE:* Children with acute lymphatic leukemia in remission obtain superior results when mercaptopurine is combined with other drugs (usually methotrexate) for remission maintenance.

NURSING IMPLICATIONS

Do not confuse Purinethol (mercaptopurine) with propylthiouracil (antithyroid drug).

IMPLEMENTATION/ADMINISTRATION/STORAGE

1. Start with lower doses in clients with impaired renal function.
2. When used for acute lymphocytic leukemia, combine with vincristine, prednisone, and L-asparaginase which induces complete remission more frequently than mercaptopurine alone. Remission is brief without use of maintenance therapy; although mercaptopurine alone can prolong complete remission, combination therapy has proven more effective.
3. In children with acute lymphoblastic leukemia, there is lowered risk of relapse if drug is given in the evening rather than morning.
4. Since maximum effect on blood count may be delayed and the count may drop for several days after drug has been discontinued, stop therapy at first sign of abnormally large drop in leukocyte count. Nadir: 14 days.
5. Reduce the dose of mercaptopurine one third to one quarter of the usual dose if allopurinol is given concurrently.
6. Because the drug may have a delayed action, discontinue at the first sign of an abnormally large or rapid fall in the leukocyte or platelet count. If subsequently, the leukocyte count or platelet count remains constant for 2 or 3 days, or rises, resume treatment.
7. Store tablets from 15–25°C (59–77°F) in a dry place.

ASSESSMENT

1. Note reasons for therapy, characteristics of S&S, other agents trialed, outcome. Note subclassification of ALL and age of client.
2. Once desired hematologic response obtained, maintenance therapy is required to maintain remission.
3. Obtain CBC, uric acid, renal and LFTs; reduce dose with dysfunction. Bone marrow examination for the evaluation of marrow status. Drug causes granulocyte and platelet suppression. Nadir: 10–14 days; recovery: 21–28 days.

CLIENT/FAMILY TEACHING

1. Take as directed with or without food.
2. Drink 8–10 glasses of water/fluids each day. Avoid alcoholic beverages.
3. Report any S&S of infection, dizziness, SOB, mouth sores, fever, chills, unusual bruising/bleeding, rash, hives, pain, N&V, diarrhea, or appetite loss.

M

4. **Avoid persons with infections; avoid activities that may cause bruising or injury.**
5. **Practice reliable contraception.**
6. **Keep all F/U to assess response, labs, adverse SE.**

OUTCOMES/EVALUATE

- Improved hematologic profile
- ↓ Malignant cell proliferation
- Disease remission

Mesalamine (5-Aminosalicylic acid)

(mes-**AL**-ah-meen)

Classification(s): Anti-inflammatory drug

Pregnancy Category: B

RX: Apriso, Asacol, Asacol HD, Canasa, Lialda, Pentasa, Rowasa, sfRowasa.

✤ **Rx:** Mesasal, Novo-5 ASA, Salofalk.

INDICATIONS/USES

PO. *Apriso:* Maintenance of remission of ulcerative colitis in clients 18 years and older. *Asacol:* Treat mild to moderate active ulcerative colitis and to maintain remission of ulcerative colitis. *Asacol HD:* Treatment of moderately active ulcerative colitis. *Lialda:* Induction of remission in clients with active, mild to moderate ulcerative colitis and for maintenance of remission of ulcerative colitis. *Pentasa:* Induction of remission and to treat mild to moderate active ulcerative colitis.

Rectal, Enema. *Rowasa:* Treatment of active mild to moderate distal ulcerative colitis, proctosigmoiditis, or proctitis. **Rectal, Suppository.** *Canasa:* Treatment of active ulcerative colitis.

ACTION/KINETICS

Action

Chemically related to acetylsalicylic acid. Thought to act locally in the colon to inhibit cyclo-oxygenase and therefore prostaglandin synthesis, resulting in a reduction of inflammation of colitis. Mesalamine may also inhibit a nuclear transcription factor that regulates the transcription of many genes for proinflammatory proteins.

Pharmacokinetics

Following PR administration, between 10% and 30% is absorbed and is excreted in the urine as the N-acetyl-5-aminosalicylic acid metabolite; the remainder is excreted in the feces. PO tablets are coated with an acrylic-based resin that prevents release of mesalamine until it reaches the terminal ileum and beyond. Approximately 28% of the drug found in tablets is absorbed with the remaining drug available for action in the colon. Capsules are methylcellulose coated, controlled-release designed to release the drug throughout the GI tract; from 20–30% is absorbed. **t½, mesalamine:** 0.5–1.5 hr; **t½, N-acetyl mesalamine:** 5–10 hr. **Time to reach maximum plasma levels:** 4–12 hr for both mesalamine and metabolite. Excreted mainly through the kidneys.

CONTRAINDICATIONS

Hypersensitivity to mesalamine, salicylates, or any component of the product.

SPECIAL CONCERNS

- **Use with caution in clients with sulfasalazine sensitivity, in those with impaired renal function or history of renal disease, in those with conditions predisposing to development of myocarditis/pericarditis, and during lactation.**
- **Pyloric stenosis may delay the drug in reaching the colon.**
- **Determine doses in the elderly with caution.**
- **Safety and efficacy not determined in children less than 18 years of age.**

SIDE EFFECTS

Most Common

After use of capsules: Headache, rash/spots, abdominal pain/cramps, diarrhea, N&V.
After use of rectal enema/suppositories: Dizziness, fever, headache, malaise/fatigue, itching, rash/spots, abdominal pain/cramps, diarrhea, flatulence, nausea, cold/sore throat, flu syndrome.
After use of tablets: Asthenia, chills, dizziness, fever, headache, rash/spots, abdominal pain/cramps, diarrhea, constipation, dyspepsia, eructation, nausea, arthralgia, back pain, hypertonia, pharyngitis, pain.

NOTE: The various products may have different side effects. The following is a compilation of all possible side effects. **Sulfite sensitivity:** Hives, wheezing, itching, ***anaphylaxis***. **Acute intolerance syndrome:** Cramping, acute abdominal pain, bloody diarrhea, fever, headache, malaise, pruritus, conjunctivitis, and rash. **GI:** N&V, abdominal pain/cramps or discomfort, flatulence, cramps, dyspepsia, nausea, diarrhea, hemorrhoids, rectal pain/burning/urgency, constipation, bloating, worsening of colitis, eructation, pain following insertion of enema, anorexia, gastritis, gastroenteritis, dry mouth, increased appetite, oral ulcers, tenesmus, ***perforated peptic ulcer***, bloody diarrhea, duodenal ulcer, dysphagia, esophageal ulcer, fecal incontinence, GI bleeding, oral moniliasis, rectal bleeding, abnormal stool color and texture, rectal polyp, hemorrhoids, rectal pain/soreness/burning after use of rectal product, pancolitis, ***pancreatitis***. **Hepatic:** Cholecystitis, hepatitis, jaundice, cholestatic jaundice, cirrhosis, hepatocellular damage (including ***liver necrosis, liver failure***). **CNS:** Headache, dizziness, insomnia, asthenia, anxiety, depression, hyperesthesia, nervousness, confusion, peripheral neuropathy, somnolence, emotional lability, vertigo, paresthesia, migraine, tremor, transverse myelitis, Guillain-Barré syndrome. **CV:** Pericarditis, myocarditis, vasodilation, palpitations, hyper-/hypotension, tachycardia, ***fatal myocarditis***, chest pain, T-wave abnormalities. **Respiratory:** Cold, sore throat, increased cough, pharyngitis, rhinitis, worsening of asthma, sinusitis, interstitial pneumonitis, pulmonary infiltrates, fibrosing alveolitis, pharyngolaryngeal pain, eosinophilic pneumonia, pleuritis. **Dermatologic:** Acne, pruritus, urticaria, prurigo, itching, alopecia, rash, sweating, dry skin, psoriasis, pyoderma gangrenosum, urticaria, erythema nodosum, eczema, photosensitivity, lichen planus, nail disorder, ecchymosis. **Musculoskeletal:** Back pain, hypertonia, arthralgia, myalgia, leg/joint pain, leg cramps, arthritis. **GU:** Nephropathy, acute and chronic interstitial nephritis, urinary urgency/burning/frequency, dysuria, hematuria, menorrhagia, epididymitis, amenorrhea, hypomenorrhea, metrorrhagia, dysmenorrhea, nephrotic syndrome, albuminuria, acute and chronic renal failure, UTI. Infertility in men, nephrotoxicity, oligospermia after use of rectal products. **Hematologic:** ***Agranulocytosis***, anemia, eosinophilia, leukopenia, granulocytopenia, thrombocytopenia, lymphadenopathy, thrombocythemia, ecchymosis, pancytopenia, leukocytosis, ***aplastic anemia***. **Ophthalmic:** Eye pain, blurred vision, conjunctivitis. **Otic:** Ear pain, tinnitus. **Body as a whole:** Chills, fatigue, malaise, fever, tiredness, drug fever, asthenia, angioedema, flu-like symptoms, pain, lupus-like syndrome, hypersensitivity reactions. **Miscellaneous:** Anorexia, peripheral edema, taste perversion, neck/breast/chest pain, enlargement of abdomen, facial edema, gout, thirst, hypersensitivity pneumonitis, Kawasaki-like syndrome, increased appetite. *NOTE:* An acute intolerance syndrome may occur; symptoms include cramping, acute abdominal pain, blood diarrhea, fever, headache, malaise, pruritus, conjunctivitis, and rash.

LABORATORY TEST CONSIDERATIONS

↑ AST, ALT, BUN, LDH, alkaline phosphatase, serum creatinine, amylase, lipase, gamma-glutamyl transpeptidase, total bilirubin. ↓ Platelet count. Albuminuria.

OVERDOSE MANAGEMENT

Symptoms: Salicylate toxicity manifested by tinnitus, vertigo, headache, confusion, drowsiness, sweating, hyperventilation, vomiting, and diarrhea. Severe toxicity results in disruption of electrolyte balance and blood pH, ***hyperthermia***, and ***dehydration***. *Treatment:* Therapy to treat salicylate toxicity, including emesis, gastric lavage, fluid and electrolyte replacement (if necessary), maintenance of adequate renal function.

DRUG INTERACTIONS

Azathioprine / ↑ Risk of blood disorders; monitor blood cell counts; adjust dosage as necessary
Mercaptopurine / ↑ Risk of blood disorders; monitor blood cell counts; adjust dosage as necessary
Nephrotoxic drugs (e.g., NSAIDs) / ↑ Risk of renal reactions
Warfarin / ↓ Anticoagulant effect of warfarin; monitor

HOW SUPPLIED

Capsules, Controlled-Release (Pentasa): 250 mg, 500 mg; ***Capsules, Extended-Release (Apriso):*** 375 mg; ***Enema, Rectal (Rowasa):*** 4 grams/60 mL; ***Suppositories, Rectal (Canasa):*** 1,000 mg; ***Suspension, Rectal (sfRowasa):*** 4 grams/60 mL; ***Tablets, Delayed-Release (Asacol, Asacol HD, Lialda):*** 400 mg, 800 mg, 1.2 grams.

M

DOSAGE

CAPSULES, CONTROLLED-RELEASE; CAPSULES, EXTENDED-RELEASE; TABLETS, DELAYED-RELEASE

Induction of remission in active, mild to moderate ulcerative colitis in adults.

Lialda, usual: Two to four 1.2-gram tablets taken once daily with food for a total daily dose of 2.4 or 4.8 grams. **Duration:** Up to 8 weeks.

Pentasa, usual: One gram (four 250 mg capsules or two 500 mg capsules) 4 times a day for a total of 4 grams. **Duration:** Up to 8 weeks.

Maintenance of remission of ulcerative colitis in adults.

Apriso, usual: 1.5 grams (four capsules) once daily in the morning. May be taken without regard to meals. **Duration:** Up to 6 months. Not to be taken with antacids.

Asacol, usual: 1.6 grams a day in divided doses. **Duration:** Up to 6 months.

Lialda, usual: Two 1.2 gram tablets once a day with a meal for a total daily dose of 2.4 grams.

Treatment of mildly to moderately active ulcerative colitis in adults.

Asacol, usual: Two 400 mg tablets 3 times a day for a total daily dose of 2.4 grams. **Duration:** 6 weeks.

Pentasa, usual: 1 gram (four 250 mg capsules or two 500 mg capsules) 4 times a day for a total dose of 4 grams. **Duration:** Up to 8 weeks.

Treatment of moderately active ulcerative colitis in adults.

Asacol HD, usual: Two 800 mg tablets 2 times a day with or without food, for a total daily dose of 4.8 grams. **Duration:** 6 weeks. *NOTE:* One Asacol HD 800 mg tablet not shown to be bioequivalent to two Asacol 400 mg tablets.

ENEMA, RECTAL

Mild to moderate distal ulcerative colitis, proctosigmoiditis, proctitis.

Rowasa: 4 grams in 60 mL once daily, usually given at bedtime for 3–6 weeks; retain for 8 hr.

SUPPOSITORIES, RECTAL

Active ulcerative proctitis.

Canasa: One 1-gram (1,000 mg) suppository a day at bedtime for 3–6 weeks, depending on symptoms and sigmoidoscopic results. Retain in the rectum for 1–3 hr or more.

NURSING IMPLICATIONS

Do not confuse Asacol with Avelox (fluoroquinolone antibiotic).

IMPLEMENTATION/ADMINISTRATION/STORAGE

1. Shake bottle well to ensure suspension is homogeneous.
2. Use caution in dose selection for the elderly; start at the low end of the dosage range.
3. Beneficial effects using the suppository or enema may occur within 3–21 days, with a full course of therapy lasting up to 6 weeks.
4. Store Asacol and Asacol HD from 20–25°C (68–77°F), Apriso, Lialda and Pentasa from 15–30°C (59–86°F), and Canasa below 25°C (77°F). Keep suppositories away from direct heat, light, or humidity and do not freeze.

ASSESSMENT

1. Note onset, character/frequency of stools. Assess abdomen for bowel sounds, distension, pain/tenderness.
2. Check for sulfite sensitivity. Use with caution in the elderly and in those with any renal or liver impairment.
3. Monitor I&O, electrolytes, renal and LFTs, U/A; abdominal films.

CLIENT/FAMILY TEACHING

1. Do not chew; take tablets whole, being careful not to break the outer coating. It must remain intact to pass through stomach and travel to sigmoid colon. Report to HCP if any remnant of capsule or tablet is seen in stool.
2. Apriso may be taken without regard to meals but do not take with antacids. Take Lialda with food.
3. Review technique for enema/suppository administration.
   - Prior to use, shake Rowasa bottle until all contents are thoroughly mixed.
   - Contents may darken with time; does not affect potency.

- Lie on the left side with the lower leg extended and the upper right leg flexed forward. The knee-chest position may also be used for suppository administration.
- Remove cap, insert tip into rectum, and squeeze steadily to completely discharge contents.
- Retain the enema for 8 hr to ensure proper absorption; may best be accomplished by administering at bedtime, after BM; retain throughout the sleep cycle.
- May cause staining of direct contact surfaces, including fabrics, floor covering, painted surfaces, marble, granite, vinyl, and enamel; use care.
- Remove foil wrapper from suppository; avoid excess handling as the suppository will melt at body temperature.
- Insert the pointed end first into the rectum.
- For maximal effect, retain suppository for 1–3 hr or more.
- Protect bed linens with towels or rubber pads.

4. Hold drug and report severe abdominal pain, cramping, bloody diarrhea, rash, fever, itching, hives, or wheezing.
5. Avoid smoking and cold foods; increases bowel motility.
6. The therapy may last 3–6 weeks; follow as prescribed.
7. Keep all F/U to assess response, labs, and adverse SE.

OUTCOMES/EVALUATE

- Relief of pain and diarrhea
- Normalization of bowel patterns

IV

Mesna

(**MEZ**-nah)

Classification(s): Antidote for ifosfamide toxicity

Pregnancy Category: B

RX: Mesnex.

✤ Rx: Uromitexan.

INDICATIONS/USES

Prophylactically to reduce the incidence of hemorrhagic cystitis caused by ifosfamide. *Investigational:* Reduce incidence of hemorrhagic cystitis in bone marrow transplantation in those receiving high-dose cyclophosphamide. As a uroprotective drug in those receiving antimetabolite regimens containing high-dose cyclophosphamide and in a limited number of clients receiving cyclophosphamide for immunologically mediated disorders (e.g., systemic lupus erythematosus, polyarteritis, Wegener's granulomatosis, dermatomyositis).

ACTION/KINETICS

Action

Ifosfamide is metabolized to products that cause hemorrhagic cystitis. In the kidney, mesna disulfide is reduced to the free thiol compound, mesna, which reacts chemically with the urotoxic ifosfamide metabolites resulting in their detoxification.

Pharmacokinetics

Following IV use, mesna is rapidly oxidized to mesna disulfide (dimesna), which is eliminated by the kidneys. **t½ in blood, mesna:** 0.36 hr; **dimesna:** 1.17 hr. **t½, terminal:** 7 hr.

CONTRAINDICATIONS

Hypersensitivity to thiol compounds. Lactation.

SPECIAL CONCERNS

- Contains benzyl alcohol, which may cause a fatal "gasping syndrome" in infants.
- Does not prevent hemorrhagic cystitis in all clients.
- Use caution with selection in the elderly.
- Safety and efficacy not determined in children.

SIDE EFFECTS

Most Common

N&V, headache, injection site reactions, flushing, dizziness, somnolence, diarrhea, anorexia, fever, pharyngitis, hyperesthesia, flu-like symptoms, cough.

Since mesna is used with ifosfamide and other antineoplastic agents, it is difficult to identify those side effects that are due to mesna. The following symptoms are believed possible. **GI:** N&V, constipation, anorexia, abdominal pain, diarrhea, dyspepsia, flatulence. **CNS:** Dizziness, headache, somnolence, anxiety, confusion, insomnia, hyperesthesia. **CV:** Chest pain, hypotension, hypertension, tachycardia, tachypnea, increased HR, ST-segment elevation. **Hematologic**: Leukopenia, thrombocytopenia, anemia, granulocytopenia, decreased platelet counts (associated with allergic reactions). **Dermatologic**: Alopecia, injection site reaction (including pain and erythema), pallor, flushing, increased sweating. **Respiratory:** Dyspnea, pharyngitis, pneumonia, coughing, tachypnea, rhinitis. **Musculoskeletal:** Back/limb pain, myalgia, arthralgia. **Metabolic:** Peripheral edema, edema, dehydration. **Ophthalmic:** Conjunctivitis. **Body as a whole:** Fatigue, fever, asthenia, malaise, rigors, pain, flu-like symptoms, allergic/hypersensitivity reactions (including ***anaphylax-is***). **Miscellaneous**: Facial edema.

LABORATORY TEST CONSIDERATIONS

False + test for urinary ketones. ↑ Liver enzymes. Hematuria, hypokalemia.

HOW SUPPLIED

Injection: 100 mg/mL; *Tablets:* 400 mg.

DOSAGE

IV BOLUS

Prophylaxis of ifosfamide-induced hemorrhagic cystitis.

Dosage of mesna equal to 20% of the ifosfamide dose given at the same time as ifosfamide and at 4 and 8 hr after each dose of ifosfamide. Thus, the total daily dose of mesna is 60% of the ifosfamide dose (e.g., an ifosfamide dose of 1.2 grams/m^2 would mean doses of mesna would be 240 mg/m^2 at the time the ifosfamide dose was given, 240 mg/m^2 after 4 hr, and 240 mg/m^2 after 8 hr). This dosage should be given on each day that ifosfamide is administered.

IV AND TABLETS

Prophylaxis of ifosfamide-induced hemorrhagic cystitis.

Initial: IV mesna equal to 20% of the ifosfamide dose, given at the time of ifosfamide, followed 2 and 6 hr later by PO doses of mesna equal to 40% of the ifosfamide dose. The total daily dose of mesna is 100% of the ifosfamide dose. For example, if the ifosfamide dose is 1.2 grams/m^2, give mesna IV, 240 mg/m^2, followed by mesna tablets, 480 mg/m^2, 2 and 6 hr after the ifosfamide dose. Give a repeat PO mesna dose if client vomits within 2 hr of ingesting mesna. Or, a replacement IV dose may be given. PO mesna therapy has not been thoroughly evaluated for ifosfamide doses greater than 2 grams/m^2.

NURSING IMPLICATIONS

IMPLEMENTATION/ADMINISTRATION/STORAGE

1. IV If the dosage of ifosfamide is increased or decreased, adjust mesna dosage accordingly.
2. Reconstitute to a final concentration of 20 mg mesna/mL fluid by adding compatible solution.
3. Diluted solutions are stable for 24 hr at 25°C (77°F) but refrigeration is recommended. When mesna is exposed to oxygen, dimesna is formed; use a new ampule for each administration.
4. Mesna multidose vials may be stored and used for up to 8 days.
5. Store tablets from 20–25°C (68–77°F).
6. COMPATIBILITY D5W, D5/0.2% NaCl, D5/0.33% NaCl, D5/0.45% NaCl, 0.9% NaCl, RL and ifosfamide.
7. INCOMPATIBILITY Cisplatin or carboplatin.

ASSESSMENT

1. Note reasons for ifosfamide therapy, onset, other agents trialed. Drug must be administered with each dose of ifosfamide and at 4 and 8 hr intervals following the initial dose to be effective against drug-induced hemorrhagic cystitis.
2. Note age and any sensitivity to benzyl alcohol.
3. Analyze morning urine specimen each day before ifosfamide therapy for hematuria. May alter tests for ketones in urine.

CLIENT/FAMILY TEACHING

1. Drug is used to prevent ifosofamide-induced hemorrhagic cystitis; will not prevent any other drug-associated adverse reactions or toxicities.
2. May experience a bad taste in the mouth during drug therapy; use hard candy to mask taste.
3. N&V and diarrhea are frequent side effects of drug therapy; report those and headaches if persistent or bothersome. If vomiting occurs

M

within 2 hrs of oral administration report as dose may need to be repeated or given IV.

4. Consume at least 1 quart of fluids/day during mesna therapy.
5. Immediately report any of the following: red or pink-colored urine, rash, itching, hives.
6. Keep all F/U to assess response, labs, and for adverse SE.

OUTCOMES/EVALUATE

Prevention of ifosfamide-induced hemorrhagic cystitis

Metformin hydrochloride

(met-**FOR**-min)

Classification(s): Antidiabetic, oral; biguanide

Pregnancy Category: B

RX: Fortamet, Glucophage, Glucophage XR, Glumetza, Riomet.

✦ **Rx:** Apo-Metformin, CO Metformin, Gen-Metformin, Novo-Metformin, Nu-Metformin, PMS-Metformin, RAN-Metformin, ratio-Metformin, Sandoz Metformin FC.

INDICATIONS/USES

(1) As monotherapy, as an adjunct to diet and exercise, to improve glycemic control in clients with type 2 diabetes. The immediate-release tablets and PO solution can be used in clients 10 years of age and older. (2) Extended-release form used to treat type 2 diabetes as initial therapy or in combination with a sulfonylurea or insulin in clients aged 17 years and older. *Investigational:* Polycystic ovary syndrome to improve rate of ovulation, cervical scores, and pregnancy rates. Treat antipsychotic-induced weight gain.

ACTION/KINETICS

Action

Decreases hepatic glucose production, decreases intestinal absorption of glucose, and increases peripheral uptake and utilization of glucose. Does not cause hypoglycemia in either diabetic or nondiabetic clients, and it does not cause hyperinsulinemia. Insulin secretion remains unchanged, while fasting insulin levels and day-long plasma insulin response may decrease. In contrast to sulfonylureas, the body weight of clients treated with metformin remains stable or may decrease somewhat.

Pharmacokinetics

Bioavailability of immediate-release tablets is 50–60%. Food decreases and slightly delays the absorption of metformin. Steady-state plasma levels (less than 1 mcg/mL) are reached within 24–48 hr. Excreted unchanged in the urine; no biliary excretion. **t½, plasma elimination:** 6.2 hr. The plasma and blood half-lives are prolonged with decreased renal function and in the elderly. **Plasma protein binding:** Negligible.

CONTRAINDICATIONS

Renal disease or dysfunction (serum creatinine levels greater than 1.5 mg/dL in males and greater than 1.4 mg/dL in females) or abnormal C_{CR} due to cardiovascular collapse, acute MI, or septicemia. In CHF requiring pharmacologic intervention. In clients undergoing radiologic studies using iodinated contrast media, because use of such products may cause alteration of renal function, leading to acute renal failure and lactic acidosis. Acute or chronic metabolic acidosis, including diabetic ketoacidosis, with or without coma. Abnormal hepatic function. Acute hemodynamic compromise of hypoxic states. Dehydration. Lactation.

SPECIAL CONCERNS

(1) Lactic acidosis is a rare, but serious, metabolic complication that can occur due to metformin accumulation during treatment with metformin. When it occurs, it is fatal in approximately 50% of cases. Lactic acidosis may also occur in association with a number of pathophysiologic conditions, including diabetes mellitus, and whenever there is significant tissue hypoperfusion and hypoxemia. (2) Lactic acidosis is characterized by elevated blood lactate levels (>5 mmol/L), decreased blood pH, electrolyte disturbances with an increased anion gap, and an increased lactate/pyruvate ratio. When metformin is implicated as the cause of lactic acidosis, metformin plasma levels >5 mcg/mL are generally found. (3) The incidence of lactic acidosis in those receiving metformin is approximately 0.03 cases/1,000 client years, with approximately 0.015 fatal cases/1,000 client years. Reported cases have occurred

M

primarily in diabetic clients with significant renal insufficiency, including both intrinsic renal disease and renal hypoperfusion, often in the setting of multiple concomitant medical/surgical problems and multiple concomitant medications. (4) Clients with CHF requiring pharmacologic management, in particular those with unstable or acute CHF who are at risk of hypoperfusion and hypoxemia, are at increased risk of lactic acidosis. The risk of lactic acidosis increases with the degree of renal dysfunction and the client's age. The risk of lactic acidosis, therefore, may be significantly decreased by regular monitoring of renal function in clients taking metformin and by use of the minimum effective dose of metformin. (5) In particular, treatment of the elderly should be accompanied by careful monitoring of renal function. Metformin treatment should not be initiated in clients >80 years of age unless measurement of creatinine clearance demonstrates that renal function is not reduced, as these clients are more susceptible to developing lactic acidosis. (6) Metformin should be promptly withheld in the presence of any condition associated with hypoxemia, dehydration, or sepsis. (7) Because impaired hepatic function may significantly limit the ability to clear lactate, metformin should generally be avoided in clients with clinical or laboratory evidence of hepatic disease. (8) Clients should be cautioned against excessive alcohol intake, either acute or chronic, when taking metformin, since alcohol potentiates the effects of metformin on lactate metabolism. (9) In addition, metformin should be temporarily discontinued prior to any intravascular radiocontrast study and for any surgical procedure. (10) The onset of lactic acidosis often is subtle, and accompanied only by nonspecific symptoms such as malaise, myalgias, respiratory distress, increasing somnolence, and nonspecific abdominal distress. There may be associated hypothermia, hypotension, and resistant bradyarrhythmias with more marked acidosis. The client and the client's provider must be aware of the possible importance of such symptoms, and the client should be instructed to notify the provider immediately if they occur. Metformin should be withdrawn until the situation is clarified. (11) Serum electrolytes, ketones, blood glucose, and if indicated, blood pH, lactate levels, and even blood metformin, are unlikely to be drug related. (12) Later occurrence of GI symptoms could be due to lactic acidosis or other serious disease. (13) Levels of fasting venous plasma lactate above the upper limit of normal but less than 5 mmol/L in clients taking metformin do not necessarily indicate impending lactic acidosis and may be explained by other mechanisms, such as poorly controlled diabetes or obesity, vigorous physical activity, or technical problems in sample handling. (14) Lactic acidosis should be suspected in any diabetic client with metabolic acidosis lacking evidence of ketoacidosis (ketonuria and ketonemia). (15) Lactic acidosis is a medical emergency that must be treated in a hospital setting. In a client with lactic acidosis taking metformin, the drug should be discontinued immediately and general supportive measures promptly instituted. Because metformin is dialyzable (with a clearance of up to 170 mL/min under good hemodynamic conditions), prompt hemodialysis is recommended to correct the acidosis and remove the accumulated metformin. Such management often results in prompt reversal of symptoms and recovery. ■

- **Use of oral hypoglycemic agents may increase the risk of *cardiovascular mortality.***
- **Hypoglycemia does not usually occur with metformin; it may result with deficient caloric intake, with strenuous exercise not supplemented by increased intake of calories, or when metformin is taken with sulfonylureas or alcohol.**
- **Use with caution as age increases due to age-related decreased renal function.**
- **Safety and efficacy of extended-release tablets not determined in children.**

SIDE EFFECTS

Most Common

Hypoglycemia, diarrhea, N&V, asthenia, flatulence, headache, abdominal pain/discomfort.

Metabolic: ***Lactic acidosis*** (fatal in approximately 50% of cases). **GI:** Diarrhea, N&V, abdominal bloating/pain/discomfort, flatulence, anorexia, unpleasant or metallic taste, abnormal stools, taste disorder. **CNS:** Light-headedness, headache. **Hematologic:** Asymptomatic subnormal serum vitamin B_{12} levels. **Body as a whole:** Asthenia, rash, chills, flu syndrome, flushing, increased sweating. **Miscellaneous:** Hypoglycemia, myalgia, dyspnea, nail disorder, chest discomfort, palpitation. *NOTE:* Common side effects for metformin, extended-release, include N&V, diarrhea, constipation, abdominal distention/pain, dyspepsia, heartburn, flatulence, dizziness, headache, URTI, taste disturbance.

OVERDOSE MANAGEMENT

Symptoms: Lactic acidosis, hypoglycemia. *Treatment:* Hemodialysis since metformin is dialyzable with a clearance up to 170 mL/min.

DRUG INTERACTIONS

Alcohol / ↑ Metformin effect on lactate metabolism
Cimetidine / ↑ (by 60%) Peak metformin plasma and whole blood levels and a 40% ↑ in AUC
Furosemide / ↑ Metformin plasma and blood levels; also, metformin ↓ the half-life of furosemide
Iodinated contrast media / ↑ Risk of acute renal failure and lactic acidosis
Nifedipine / ↑ Absorption of metformin, leading to ↑ plasma metformin levels
Propantheline / ↑ Absorption of metformin R/T slowed GI motility

HOW SUPPLIED

Oral Solution: 500 mg/5 mL; *Tablets:* 500 mg, 850 mg, 1,000 mg; *Tablets, Extended-Release:* 500 mg, 750 mg, 1,000 mg.

DOSAGE

ORAL SOLUTION

Type 2 diabetes.

Individualize dosage. **Adults and adolescents over 16 years of age:** Up to 2,550 mg/day; **Children, 10–16 years of age:** up to 2,000 mg/day.

TABLETS; TABLETS, EXTENDED-RELEASE

Type 2 diabetes.

Individualize dosage regimen. Adults, using 500 mg immediate-release tablet: Starting dose is one 500 mg tablet twice a day given with the morning and evening meals. Dosage increases may be made in increments of 500 mg every week, given in divided doses, up to a maximum of 2,500 mg/day. If a 2,500 mg daily dose is required, it may be better tolerated when given in divided doses 3 times per day with meals. The extended-release tablet is given once daily. **Adults, using 850 mg immediate-release tablet:** Starting dose is 850 mg once daily given with the morning meal. Dosage increases may be made in increments of 850 mg every other week, given in divided doses, up to a maximum of 2,550 mg/day. **Usual maintenance dose:** 850 mg twice a day with the morning and evening meals. However, some may require 850 mg 3 times per day with meals. **Adults, using 500 mg extended-release tablet: Initial:** 500 mg once daily with the evening meal. Adjust dose, if needed, in increments of 500 mg/week, up to a maximum of 2,000 mg once daily with the evening meal. If glycemic control is not achieved on 2,000 mg once daily, consider 1,000 mg twice a day. If higher doses are needed, use total daily dose up to 2,550 mg given in divided doses. **Adults using 1,000 mg extended-release tablet: Initial:** 1,000 mg once daily with the evening meal. Dosage may be increased weekly in 500 mg increments, based on efficacy and tolerance, but must not exceed 2,500 mg/day. *NOTE:* Initial dose of metformin immediate release in children is 500 mg twice a day given with meals. Increase dose, if necessary, in increments of 500 mg/week, up to a maximum of 2,000 mg daily given in divided doses. Safety and efficacy of metformin extended-release have not been determined in children.

NURSING IMPLICATIONS

Do not confuse Glucophage with Glucovance (combination antidiabetic product containing metformin and glyburide). Also, do not confuse metformin with metronidazole (a trichomonacide/amebicide).

IMPLEMENTATION/ADMINISTRATION/STORAGE

1. Individualize dosage based on tolerance and effectiveness.
2. Give with meals starting at a low dose with gradual escalation. This will reduce GI side effects and allow determination of the minimal dose necessary for adequate BS control.
3. May safely switch from metformin to metformin extended-release (ER) once daily at the same total daily dose, up to 2,000 mg once daily. Once switched, closely monitor glycemic control and make dosage adjustments as needed.
4. No transition period required when transferring from standard oral hypoglycemic drugs (other than chlorpropamide) to metformin. When transferring from chlorpropamide, exercise caution during first 2 weeks R/T chlorpropamide's long duration of action.
5. Glumetza, 500 mg, is an extended-release tablet with a novel drug-delivery system that provides controlled and prolonged release of metformin. Can be used alone or as combination therapy (e.g., sulfonylurea or insulin).
6. If maximum dose of metformin for 4 weeks does not provide adequate control of blood glucose, gradual addition of an oral sulfonylurea (data are available for glyburide, chlorpropamide, tolbutamide, and glipizide) may be considered, while maintaining maximum dose of metformin. Desired control of blood glucose may be attained by adjusting the dose of each drug.
7. If initiating metformin or metformin ER, continue current insulin dose. Start metformin or metformin ER at 500 mg once daily. For those not responding, increase metformin or metformin ER dose by 500 mg after about 1 week and by 500 mg every week thereafter until adequate control reached. Maximum recommended daily dose is 2,500 mg for metformin and 2,000 mg for metformin ER. Decrease insulin dose by 10–25% when fasting glucose levels decrease to less than 120 mg/dL in those receiving both metformin/metformin extended-release and insulin.
8. Be conservative with initial and maintenance doses in the elderly, because of possible decreased renal function. Generally, do not titrate geriatric clients to the maximum dose. Do not start metformin or metformin ER in clients 80 years and older unless tests show renal function is not decreased.
9. If no response to 1–3 months of concomitant metformin and oral sulfonylurea therapy, consider initiating insulin therapy and discontinuing oral agents.
10. If exposed to stress (e.g., fever, trauma, infection, surgery), may experience loss of glycemic control. May be necessary to withhold metformin and administer insulin temporarily.
11. Temporarily suspend metformin for dye and surgical procedures (unless minor and not associated with restricted intake of food and fluids). Do not restart until oral intake has resumed and renal function is normal.
12. Store tablets and oral solution from 15–30°C (59–86°F).

ASSESSMENT

1. Note age at diabetes onset, BMI, family Hx, previous therapies utilized, outcome.
2. Withhold for surgery and iodinated procedures (usually 48 hr before and 48 hr after). May administer when normal diet and fluids resumed or the day after the procedure.
3. If anemia develops, exclude vitamin B_{12} deficiency; may interfere with B_{12} absorption—monitor levels every 1–2 yr.
4. A small dose with insulin therapy may enhance glucose control.
5. Avoid with CHF; may alter furosemide effects. During acute stress, monitor carefully; may require insulin therapy.
6. Monitor BP, Wt, CBC, BS, electrolytes, HbA1c, urinalysis, microalbumin, renal and LFTs. Assess for liver/renal failure; may precipitate lactic acidosis (i.e., serum lactate levels greater than 5 mmol/L, decreased blood pH, increased anion gap).

CLIENT/FAMILY TEACHING

1. Take with food to ↓ GI upset. Do not crush or chew extended-release tablets.
2. May cause a metallic taste; should subside.
3. The inactive components in the extended-release tablets may pass into the feces and appear as a soft, hydrated mass.
4. Regular exercise, decreased caloric intake, and weight loss are required to reduce blood glucose levels; medication neither replaces nor excuses compliance with these modalities.

5. Inadequate caloric intake or strenuous exercise without caloric replacement may precipitate hypoglycemia.
6. Do regular blood sugar monitoring (fingersticks), especially 1–2 hr after meals, if symptomatic, and maintain record for provider review.
7. Avoid alcohol and situations that may precipitate dehydration.
8. Consume plenty of fluids; report when illnesses with fever, vomiting, and diarrhea are persistent/severe.
9. Practice reliable contraception; report if pregnancy suspected.
10. Stop drug and immediately report any symptoms of difficulty breathing, severe weakness, muscle pain, increased sleepiness, dizziness, palpitation, or sudden increased abdominal distress.
11. Keep all F/U visits to assess response, labs, and for adverse SE.

OUTCOMES/EVALUATE

- Control of BS; prevention of microvascular complications
- HbA1c <8%
- Treatment of anovulation with polycystic ovary syndrome (unlabeled)
- Treatment of antipsychotic-induced weight gain (unlabeled)

Methadone hydrochloride

(**METH**-ah-dohn)

Classification(s): Narcotic analgesic

Pregnancy Category: C

RX: Dolophine Hydrochloride, Methadone HCl Diskets, Methadose, **C-II**

✤ **Rx:** Metadol.

SEE ALSO ***NARCOTIC ANALGESICS***.

INDICATIONS/USES

(1) Moderate to severe pain not responsive to nonnarcotic analgesics. Oral concentrate and tablets for suspension not used for this purpose. (2) Detoxification treatment of opioid addiction (heroin or other morphine-type drugs). (3) For maintenance treatment of opioid addiction (heroin and other morphine-type drugs) in conjunction with appropriate social and medical services. *NOTE:* Outpatient maintenance and detoxification treatment may be provided only by Opioid Treatment Programs certified by the Federal Substance Abuse and Mental Health Services Administration and registered by the Drug Enforcement Administration. This does not preclude the maintenance treatment of a client with concurrent opioid addiction who is hospitalized for conditions other than opioid addiction and who requires temporary maintenance during the critical period of stay, or of a client whose enrollment has been verified in a program that has been certified for maintenance treatment with methadone.

ACTION/KINETICS

Action

Produces only mild euphoria, which is the reason it is used as a heroin withdrawal substitute and for maintenance programs. Peak respiratory depressant effects occur later and persist longer than its peak analgesic effects. Produces physical dependence; withdrawal symptoms develop more slowly and are less intense but more prolonged than those associated with morphine. Does not produce sedation or narcosis. Not effective for preoperative or obstetric anesthesia. Only one-half as potent PO as when given parenterally.

Pharmacokinetics

PO administration results in a delay of onset, lower peak, and an increased duration of analgesic effect. **Onset, PO:** 30–60 min; **parenteral**: 10–20 min. **Peak effects:** 30–60 min. **Duration:** 4–8 hr. **t½, elimination:** 8–59 hr. Full analgesic effects may not occur for 3–5 days. Both the duration and half-life increase with repeated use due to cumulative effects as it is retained in the liver. Metabolized in the liver primarily by CYP3A4 and to a lesser extent by CYP2D6. Excreted in the urine and feces.

ADDITIONAL CONTRAINDICATIONS

IV use, liver disease, during pregnancy, in children, or in obstetrics (due to long duration of action and chance of respiratory depression in the neonate). Use to relieve general anxiety.

SPECIAL CONCERNS

(1) Deaths have been reported during initiation of methadone treatment for opioid dependence. In some cases, drug interactions

with other drugs, both licit and illicit, have been suspected. However, in other cases, deaths appear to have occurred because of the respiratory or cardiac effects of methadone and too-rapid titration without appreciation for the accumulation of methadone over time. It is critical to understand the pharmacokinetics of methadone and to exercise vigilance during treatment initiation and dose titration. Clients must also be strongly cautioned against self-medicating with CNS depressants during initiation of methadone treatment. (2) Respiratory depression is the chief hazard associated with methadone administration. Methadone's peak respiratory depressant effects typically occur later and persist longer than its peak analgesic effects, particularly in the early dosing period. These characteristics can contribute to the cases of iatrogenic overdose, particularly during treatment initiation and dose titration. (3) Cases of QT interval prolongation and serious arrhythmia (torsades de pointes) have been observed during treatment with methadone. Most cases involve clients being treated for pain with large, multiple daily doses of methadone, although cases have been reported in clients receiving doses commonly used for maintenance treatment of opioid addiction. (4) Conditions for distribution and use of methadone products for the treatment of opioid addiction: Methadone products, when used for the treatment of opioid addiction in detoxification or maintenance programs, shall be dispensed only by opioid treatment programs (and agencies, practitioners, or institutions by formal agreement with the program sponsor) certified by the Substance Abuse and Mental Health Services Administration and approved by the designated state authority. Certified treatment programs shall dispense and use methadone in oral form only and according to the treatment requirements stipulated in the Federal Opioid Treatment Standards (42 CFR 8.12). See the following information for important regulatory exceptions to the general requirement for certification to provided opioid agonist treatment. (5) Failure to abide by the requirements in these regulations may result in criminal prosecution, seizure of the drug supply, revocation of the program approval, and injunction precluding operation of the program. (6) Regulatory exceptions to the general requirement for certification to provide opioid agonist treatment include the following: (a) During inpatient care, when the client was admitted for any condition other than concurrent opioid addiction (pursuant to 21 CFR 1306.07[c]), to facilitate the treatment of the primary admitting diagnosis. (b) During an emergency period of no longer than 3 days while definitive care for the addiction is being sought in an appropriately licensed facility (pursuant to 21 CFR 1306.07[b]). ■

- **Use with caution during lactation.**
- **Methadone can build up in the body to toxic levels if taken too often, if the amount taken is too high, or if taken with other drugs or supplements.**

SIDE EFFECTS

Most Common

Insomnia, dizziness, anxiety, nervousness, weakness, drowsiness, N&V, diarrhea, anorexia, constipation, dry mouth, impotence, decreased libido. See *Narcotic Analgesics* for a complete list of possible side effects. Also, marked constipation, excessive sweating, visual disturbances, edema, shock, pulmonary edema, choreic movements. Possible ***Q-T prolongation*** and ***torsades de pointes***, especially in those with predisposing factors.

LABORATORY TEST CONSIDERATIONS

↑ Immunoglobulin G.

ADDITIONAL DRUG INTERACTIONS

Cimetidine / ↑ Respiratory and CNS depression
Desipramine / ↑ Desipramine blood levels
Nelfinavir / ↓ Methadone plasma levels
Phenytoin / ↓ Methadone effect R/T ↑ liver metabolism
Protease inhibitors / ↑ Respiratory and CNS depression
Rifampin / ↓ Methadone effect R/T ↑ liver metabolism; may precipitate withdrawal
Ritonavir / ↓ Methadone plasma levels

HOW SUPPLIED

Injection: 10 mg/mL; ***Oral Concentrate:*** 10 mg/mL; ***Oral Solution:*** 5 mg/5 mL, 10 mg/5 mL; ***Tablets:*** 5 mg, 10 mg; ***Tablets, Dispersible for Suspension:*** 40 mg (distribution restricted to hospitals and facilities authorized to treat opiate addiction).

DOSAGE

INJECTION; ORAL CONCENTRATE; ORAL SOLUTION; TABLETS; TABLETS FOR SUSPENSION

Analgesia.

Adults, individualized (when PO methadone is used as the first analgesic in those not already being treated with, and tolerant to opioids): 2.5–10 mg q 8–12 hr. Slowly titrate to effect. More frequent administration may be needed during methadone imitation in order to maintain adequate analgesia. Use extreme caution to avoid overdose (i.e., take into account methadone's long half-life). *NOTE:* Do not use dispersible tablets or oral concentrate for analgesia.

Narcotic withdrawal (detoxification).

Initial: A single dose of 20–30 mg often suppresses withdrawal symptoms. Do not exceed an initial dose of 30 mg. Administer the initial dose under supervision when there are no signs of sedation or intoxication and the individual shows signs of withdrawal. Do not determine initial doses by previous treatment episodes or dollars spent per day on illict drug use. Consider loss of tolerance in a client who has not taken opioids for more than 5 days.

If same day adjustments in dose are to be made, wait 2–4 hr for further evaluation, when peak levels have been reached. An additional 5–10 mg may be given if withdrawal symptoms have not been suppressed or if symptoms reappear. The total dose of methadone on the first day of treatment should not ordinarily exceed 40 mg. Make dosage adjustments over the first week of treatment based on control of withdrawal symptoms at the time of expected peak activity (i.e., 2–4 hr after dosing). Make dosage adjustments cautiously as deaths have occurred in early treatment due to the cumulative effects of the first several days of dosing.

Maintenance following narcotic withdrawal.

Titrate to a dose where opioid symptoms are prevented for 24 hr, drug hunger or craving is reduced, the euphoric effects of self-administered opioid are blocked or attenuated, and the client is tolerant to the sedative effects of methadone. **Adults, individualized, initial, usual:** 20–40 mg PO 4–8 hr after heroin is stopped; **then,** adjust dosage as required up to 80–120 mg/day.

NURSING IMPLICATIONS

IMPLEMENTATION/ADMINISTRATION/STORAGE

1. There is high interpatient variability in methadone's absorption, metabolism, and relative analgesic potency. This necessitates a cautious and highly individualized approach to prescribing. Special attention is needed during initiation of treatment, conversion from one opioid to another, and dose titration.
2. Dilute solution in at least 90 mL of water prior to administration.
3. Dispersible tablets are formulated with insoluble excipients to deter use by injection. Dissolve each tablet in 1 oz of liquid (other than grapefruit juice); allow at least 1 min for complete drug dispersion before swallowing. Do not swallow tablets whole or chew tablets.
4. For repeated analgesic doses, IM administration is preferred over SC administration due to local irritation. Inspect sites for signs of irritation.
5. A methadone dose will hold for a longer period of time as tissue stores of methadone accumulate.
6. A high degree of opioid tolerance does not eliminate the possibility of methadone overdosage.
7. There is significant variability in the appropriate rate of tapering of methadone in clients choosing medically supervised withdrawal from methadone treatment. Usually dose reductions should be less than 10% of the established tolerance or maintenance doses, and that 10- to 14-day intervals should elapse between dose reductions. Appraise

M

clients of the high risk of relapse to illicit drug use associated with discontinuing methadone treatment.

8. Methadone clearance may be increased during pregnancy (i.e., lower trough levels and shorter half-lives). During pregnancy the methadone dose may need to be increased or their dosing interval decreased. However, use in pregnancy only if the potential benefit outweighs the potential risk to the fetus.
9. Switching from another chronically administered opioid to methadone requires caution due to the uncertainty of dose conversion ratios and incomplete cross-tolerance. Deaths have occurred in opioid-tolerant clients during conversion to methadone. Always individualize dosage of methadone taking into account the client's achievement of adequate pain relief, balanced against tolerability of opioid side effects.
10. Store from 15–30°C (59–86°F).

ASSESSMENT

1. Note reasons for therapy: opioid withdrawal or chronic pain control, other therapies/agents trialed, outcome. List characteristics of pain, location, onset and pain level.
2. Strict federal guidelines must be followed with any detoxification/maintenance program (see *Special Concerns).*
3. Assess for CAD, arrhythmia, interactions with drugs, respiratory/cardiac effects of methadone, and too-rapid titration of methadone during therapy. Avoid with acute bronchial asthma or hypercarbia and in those who have or are suspected of having a paralytic ileus.
4. With long-term therapy, assess ECG, VS, and monitor for QT prolongation. With chronic therapy the usual dose generally will not control acute pain.
5. Monitor renal and LFTs.

CLIENT/FAMILY TEACHING

1. Take as prescribed for pain control.
2. Methadone Diskets and tablets for oral suspension should not be chewed or swallowed before dispersing in liquid.
3. Prior to administration, the desired dose of the Diskets or tablet for oral suspension should be dispersed in approximately 120 mL of water, orange juice, Tang, citrus flavors of Kool-Aid, or other acidic fruit beverage. If residue remains in the cup after initial administration, a small amount of liquid should be added and the resulting mixture should be ingested by client.
4. If ambulatory and not suffering acute pain, side effects may be more pronounced.
5. Avoid activities that require mental alertness until drug effects realized; causes sedation, drowsiness, impaired vision. Change positions slowly to prevent sudden drop in BP.
6. With dosing adjustments use caution; deaths have occurred in early treatment because of the cumulative effects of the first several days dosing. When dose is being titrated avoid overdosage as methadone has long elimination half-life.
7. Avoid alcohol. Report N&V; a lower drug dose may relieve symptoms. Practice reliable contraception.
8. To minimize constipation, exercise regularly, increase intake of fluids, fruit, and bulk, and use stool softener/laxative regularly.
9. May adversely affect employment R/T type of drug consumed and drug association. Drug causes tolerance and dependence with long-term use. Do not stop drug suddenly; it must be weaned slowly.
10. For clients on narcotic withdrawal therapy, store drug out of the reach of children. Continue to attend group therapy such as Narcotics Anonymous. Identify social service groups for assistance in child care, food and living arrangements, and expenses.
11. Keep all F/U to assess response, labs, adverse SE, and scripts as needed.

OUTCOMES/EVALUATE

- Control of severe/chronic pain
- Detoxification and maintenance in narcotic-dependent individual

IV

Methocarbamol

(meth-oh-**KAR**-bah-mohl)

Classification(s): Skeletal muscle relaxant, centrally-acting

Pregnancy Category: C

RX: Robaxin, Robaxin-750.

SEE ALSO ***SKELETAL MUSCLE RELAXANTS, CENTRALLY ACTING.***

INDICATIONS/USES

(1) Adjunct to rest, physical therapy, and other measures for the relief of acute, painful musculoskeletal conditions (e.g., sprains, strains). (2) Adjunct to treat neuromuscular symptoms of tetanus. Methocarbamol does not replace the usual treatment of debridement, tetanus antitoxin, penicillin, tracheotomy, appropriate fluid balance, and supportive care.

ACTION/KINETICS

Action

Beneficial effect may be related to the sedative properties of the drug. Has no direct effect on the contractile mechanism of striated muscle, the motor endplate, or the nerve fiber, and it does not directly relax tense skeletal muscles.

Pharmacokinetics

Onset: 30 min. **Peak plasma levels:** 2 hr after 2 grams. **t½:** 1–2 hr. Inactive metabolites are excreted in the urine with small amounts in the feces.

CONTRAINDICATIONS

Hypersensitivity, when muscle spasticity is required to maintain upright position, seizure disorders, pregnancy. Renal disease (parenteral dosage form only since it contains polyethylene glycol 300). SC use.

SPECIAL CONCERNS

- **Use with caution in suspected or known epileptics and during lactation.**
- **Except for tetanus, safety and efficacy not determined in children less than 12 years of age.**

SIDE EFFECTS

Most Common

Drowsiness, dizziness, GI upset/nausea, blurred vision, fever.

After PO/IV Use. CNS: Lightheadedness, dizziness, drowsiness, headache, vertigo, fainting, seizures after IV use. **GI:** Nausea, GI upset, metallic taste. **CV:** Syncope, hypotension, bradycardia, thrombophlebitis. **Dermatologic:** Urticaria, pruritus, rash, flushing. **Ophthalmic:** Conjunctivitis with nasal congestion, blurred vision, nystaymus, diplopia. **Miscellaneous:** Fever, sloughing or pain at injection site, ***anaphylactic reaction.***

LABORATORY TEST CONSIDERATIONS

Color interference in certain screening tests for 5-HIAA and VMA.

OVERDOSE MANAGEMENT

Symptoms: CNS depression, including coma, is often seen when methocarbamol is used with alcohol or other CNS depressants. *Treatment:* Supportive, depending on the symptoms.

DRUG INTERACTIONS

CNS depressants (including alcohol) may ↑ the effect of methocarbamol.

HOW SUPPLIED

Injection: 100 mg/mL; ***Tablets:*** 500 mg, 750 mg.

DOSAGE

TABLETS

Skeletal muscle disorders.

Adults, initial: 1.5 grams 4 times/day, for the first 2–3 days (for severe conditions, 8 grams/day may be given); **maintenance:** 1 gram 4 times/day, 0.75 gram q 4 hr, or 1.5 grams 3 times/day.

IM OR IV ONLY

Musculoskeletal conditions.

Do not exceed a total adult dosage of 3 grams for more than 3 consecutive days, except to treat tetanus (see the following). Repeat dose after 48 hr if condition persists. Base dosage and frequency of dosage on the response and severity of the condition. For some, 1 gram may be adequate. For severe cases or in postoperative conditions where PO use is not feasible, 2–3 grams may be needed.

Tetanus.

Adults: Inject 1 or 2 grams directly into the IV tubing. An additional 1 or 2 grams may be added to the infusion bottle so that a total of 3 grams or less is given as the initial dose. Repeat q 6 hr until conditions allow for insertion of a nasogastric tube. Crushed methocarbamol tablets may be suspended in water or saline and given through the nasogastric tube. Total daily PO doses of 24 grams or less may be required. **Children:** A minimum initial dose of 15 mg/kg. Give into IV tubing or by IV infusion with an appropriate amount of fluid. Dose may be repeated q 6 hr as needed.

M

NURSING IMPLICATIONS

IMPLEMENTATION/ADMINISTRATION/STORAGE

1. IV Give undiluted directly IV at a maximum rate of 3 mL/min. Avoid vascular extravasation (solution is hypertonic); may cause thrombophlebitis.
2. May also be added to an IV drip of NaCl injection or D5W injection. Do not dilute one vial given as a single dose to more than 250 mL for IV infusion.
3. Client should be recumbent during and for at least 10–15 min following injection.
4. COMPATIBILITY D5W, 0.9% NaCl.
5. INCOMPATIBILITY Administer separately.

ASSESSMENT

1. Note reasons for therapy, location, onset, characteristics of S&S, associated factors, other agents trialed, outcome.
2. Rate pain level, assess range of motion, tenderness, impaired mobility/gait/movement, muscle stiffness, x-ray if indicated, note neuromuscular findings, clinical presentation, and renal function.
3. During IV administration monitor VS. Observe seizure precautions.
4. Assess IV site may cause thrombophlebitis; avoid extravasation. Assess for fall risk; supervise activity. Keep side rails up or bed in low-level position, supervise ambulation of elderly or those who have been immobilized prior to drug therapy.
5. Monitor renal function with prolonged parenteral therapy.

CLIENT/FAMILY TEACHING

1. Take as directed with meals or milk for muscle spasms or limited mobility. Do not exceed dosage parameters; usually tapered off over 1–2 weeks with extended use.
2. Causes drowsiness; do not operate dangerous machinery or drive a car.
3. Rise slowly from a recumbent position and dangle legs before standing up to minimize low BP effects.
4. Double/blurred vision, and involuntary eye movement may occur; report if persistent.
5. Report skin eruptions/rash or itching (allergic responses which may require drug withdrawal), persistent dizziness or excessive sedation.
6. Nausea, anorexia, metallic taste may occur; report if severe or interferes with nutrition.
7. Avoid alcohol/CNS depressants during therapy.
8. Urine may turn black, brown, or green (upon standing); will resolve once drug stopped.
9. Drug for short-term use during acute sprain/strain. Use as needed and perform exercises/stretching, rest, and PT/exercises as directed.
10. Keep all F/U to assess response, ROM, labs, and for adverse SE.

OUTCOMES/EVALUATE

- ↓ Muscle spasticity, pain; ↑ ROM, mobility
- Control of tetanus-induced neuromuscular manifestations

■ IV

Methotrexate, Methotrexate sodium (Amethopterin, MTX)

(meth-oh-**TREKS**-ayt)

Classification(s): Antineoplastic, antimetabolite; Antipsoriasis drug

Pregnancy Category: X

RX: Methotrexate LPF Sodium, Rheumatrex, Rheumatrex Dose Pack, Trexall.

Rx: Apo-Methotrexate, ratio-Methotrexate Sodium.

SEE ALSO *ANTINEOPLASTIC AGENTS*.

INDICATIONS/USES

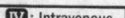

(1) Certain carcinomas including uterine choriocarcinoma (curative), chorioadenoma destruens, hydatidiform mole, acute lymphocytic and lymphoblastic leukemia, lymphosarcoma, and other disseminated neoplasms in children. (2) Meningeal leukemia. (3) Some beneficial effect in regional chemotherapy of head and neck tumors, breast tumors, and lung cancer. (4) In combination for advanced stage non-Hodgkin's lymphoma. (5) Advanced mycosis fungoides. (6) High doses followed by leucovorin rescue in combination with other drugs for prolonging relapse-free survival in nonmetastatic osteosarcoma in individuals who have had surgical resection or amputation for the primary tumor. (7) Severe, recalcitrant, disabling psoriasis not responsive to other therapy. Use only when diagnosis has been

established by biopsy or after dermatologic consultation. (8) Rheumatoid arthritis (severe, active, classical, or definite) in clients who have had inadequate response to NSAIDs and at least one or more antirheumatic drugs (disease modifying). *Investigational:* Severe corticosteroid-dependent asthma to reduce corticosteroid dosage; adjunct to treat osteosarcoma. Psoriatic arthritis and Reiter's disease. SC to treat rheumatoid arthritis.

ACTION/KINETICS

Action

Cell-cycle specific for the S phase of cell division. Acts by inhibiting dihydrofolate reductase, which prevents reduction of dihydrofolate to tetrahydrofolate; this results in decreased synthesis of purines and consequently DNA. The most sensitive cells are bone marrow, fetal cells, dermal epithelium, urinary bladder, buccal mucosa, intestinal mucosa, and malignant cells. When used for rheumatoid arthritis it may affect immune function. In psoriasis, the rate of production of epithelial cells in the skin is greater than normal skin; methotrexate interferes with DNA synthesis, repair, and cellular replication, especially in actively proliferating tissues.

Pharmacokinetics

Variable absorption from GI tract. Food may delay the absorption and reduce peak levels. **Peak serum levels, IM:** 30–60 min; **PO:** 1–2 hr. **t½:** initial, 1 hr; intermediate, 2–3 hr; final, 8–12 hr. May accumulate in the body. Excreted by kidney (55–92% in 24 hr).

CONTRAINDICATIONS

Clients with psoriasis or rheumatoid arthritis (1) with alcoholism, alcoholic liver disease, or other chronic liver disease; (2) who have overt or lab evidence of immunodeficiency syndromes; or (3) who have pre-existing blood dyscrasias (e.g., bone marrow hypoplasia, leukopenia, thrombocytopenia, significant anemia). Pregnancy and lactation.

SPECIAL CONCERNS

(1) The high doses required for treating osteosarcoma require meticulous care. (2) Use only in life-threatening, neoplastic diseases, or in those with psoriasis, *Pneumocystis carinii*, pneumonia, or rheumatoid arthritis (RA) with severe, recalcitrant, disabling disease that is not adequately responsive to other types of therapy. Deaths have occurred with the use of methotrexate in malignancy, psoriasis, and RA. Closely monitor clients for bone marrow, liver, lung, and kidney toxicities. (3) Marked bone marrow depression may occur with resultant anemia, leukopenia, or thrombocytopenia. (4) Unexpected severe (sometimes fatal) bone marrow suppression, aplastic anemia, and GI toxicity have occurred with coadministration of methotrexate (usually high doses) with some NSAIDs. (5) Monitor periodically for toxicity, including CBC with differential and platelet counts; liver and renal function testing is mandatory. Periodic liver biopsies may be necessary in some situations. Monitor those at increased risk for impaired methotrexate elimination (e.g., renal dysfunction, pleural effusion, ascites) more frequently. (6) Causes hepatotoxicity, fibrosis, and cirrhosis, usually only after prolonged use. Acutely, liver enzyme elevations are frequent but are usually transient and asymptomatic; they do not seem predictive of subsequent liver disease. Liver biopsy after sustained use often shows histologic changes, and fibrosis and cirrhosis have occurred; these latter lesions are not preceded by symptoms of abnormal LFTs. Thus, periodic liver biopsies are usually recommended for those who are treated long-term. Persistent abnormalities in LFTs may precede appearance of fibrosis or cirrhosis in those with RA. (7) Methotrexate-induced lung disease is a potentially dangerous lesion that may occur acutely at any time during therapy; has occurred at doses as low as 7.5 mg/week. It is not always fully reversible. Pulmonary symptoms (especially a dry, nonproductive cough) may require interruption of treatment and careful investigation. (8) Fetal death and/or congenital anomalies have occurred; do not use in women of childbearing age unless benefits outweigh possible risks. Pregnant women with psoriasis or RA should not receive methotrexate. (9) Use with extreme caution in clients with impaired renal function and at reduced dosage because renal dysfunction will prolong elimination. (10) Diarrhea and ulcerative stomatitis require interruption of therapy. Hemorrhagic enteritis and death from intestinal perforation may occur. (11) Do not

use methotrexate formulations and diluents containing preservatives for intrathecal or experimental high dose methotrexate therapy. (12) Malignant lymphomas, which may regress following withdrawal of methotrexate, may occur in those receiving low-dose methotrexate; they may not require cytotoxic treatment. Discontinue methotrexate first and, if the lymphoma does not regress, start appropriate treatment. (13) Methotrexate may induce tumor lysis syndrome in clients with rapidly growing tumors. (14) Severe, occasionally fatal skin reactions have been reported following single or multiple doses of methotrexate. Reactions have occurred within days of PO, IM, IV, or intrathecal administration. Recovery occurs with discontinuation of therapy. (15) Potentially fatal opportunistic infections, especially *Pneumocystis carinii* pneumonia, may occur with methotrexate therapy. (16) May increase the risk of soft tissue necrosis and osteonecrosis when given concomitantly with radiotherapy. (17) Because of the possibility of severe toxic reactions (that may be fatal), inform clients fully of the risks involved and ensure constant supervision. ■

- **Use with caution in impaired renal function and the elderly.**
- **Use with extreme caution in the presence of active infection and in debilitated clients.**
- **Safety and efficacy not established for children other than in cancer chemotherapy and in polyarticular-course juvenile rheumatoid arthritis.**
- **Read prescription order carefully; do not give daily when the order reads weekly dosing.**

SIDE EFFECTS

Most Common

Ulcerative stomatitis, leukopenia, nausea, abdominal distress, malaise, fatigue, chills, fever, dizziness, decreased resistance to infection.

GI: Gingivitis, stomatitis, anorexia, N&V, diarrhea, hematemesis, melena, GI ulceration/perforation, GI bleeding, ***enteritis (including hemorrhagic), pancreatitis***. **CNS:** Headache, drowsiness, aphasia, dizziness, hemiparesis, paresis, ***convulsions***, speech impairment (including dysarthria). Following low doses: Transient subtle cognitive dysfunction, mood alteration, unusual cranial sensations, leukoencephalopathy, encephalopathy. **CV:** Pericarditis, ***pericardial effusion***, hypotension, thromboembolic events (including, arterial thrombosis, ***cerebral thrombosis***, DVT, retinal vein thrombosis, thrombophlebitis, vasculitis, ***pulmonary embolism)***. **Pulmonary:** Chronic interstitial pulmonary disease, ***respiratory fibrosis***, ***respiratory failure***, interstitial pneumonitis, URTI, cough, epistaxis. **Dermatologic:** Erythematous rashes, pruritus, urticaria, photosensitivity, pigmentary changes, sweating, alopecia, ecchymosis, telangiectasia, acne, furunculosis, erythema multiforme, ***toxic epidermal necrolysis, Stevens-Johnson syndrome***, skin necrosis, skin ulceration, exfoliative dermatitis, "burning skin" lesions, plaque erosions (rare). **Hematologic:** Bone marrow depression, leukopenia, thrombocytopenia, suppressed hematopoiesis causing anemia, ***aplastic anemia***, pancytopenia, neutropenia, decreased hematocrit, lymphadenopathy, lymphoproliferative disorders, hypogammaglobulinemia (rare). **GU:** Renal failure (acute), cystitis, hematuria, severe nephropathy, defective oogenesis or spermatogenesis, transient oligospermia, menstrual dysfunction, vaginal discharge, infertility, ***abortion***, fetal defects, gynecomastia, dysuria. **Hepatic:** Hepatotoxicity, acute hepatitis, chronic fibrosis, cirrhosis. **Musculoskeletal:** Stress fractures, arthralgia, myalgia, chest pain, osteoporosis (rare). **Ophthalmic:** Blurred vision, transient blindness, conjunctivitis, serious visual changes of unknown etiology, eye discomfort. **Body as a whole:** Malaise, fatigue, chills, fever, decreased resistance to infection, soft tissue necrosis, osteonecrosis. **Miscellaneous:** Diabetes, ***sudden death, anaphy-laxis***, nodulosis, loss of libido/impotence, reversible lymphomas, ***tumor lysis syndrome***, opportunistic infections, including *Pneumocystis carinii* (some may be fatal). **Following intrathecal use.** Acute chemical arachnoiditis (headache, back pain, nuchal rigidity, fever). Subacute myelopathy (paraparesis/paraplegia with involvement of spinal nerve roots). Chronic leukoencephalopathy (confusion, irritability, somnolence, ataxia, dementia, ***seizures, coma***).

LABORATORY TEST CONSIDERATIONS

Azotemia. ↑ Liver enzymes. ↓ Serum albumin.

OVERDOSE MANAGEMENT

Symptoms: See *Antineoplastic Agents*. *Treatment:* Leucovorin, given as soon as possible, may decrease toxic effects. The dose used is 10 mg/m^2

PO or parenterally followed by 10 mg/m^2 PO q 6 hr for 72 hr. In massive overdosage, routine hemodialysis and hemoperfusion are ineffective. Hydration and urinary alkalinization are needed to prevent precipitation of methotrexate and metabolites in the renal tubules.

DRUG INTERACTIONS

Alcohol, ethyl / Additive hepatotoxicity; combination can → coma
Aminoglycosides, oral / ↓ Absorption of PO methotrexate
Anticoagulants, oral / Additive hypoprothrombinemia
Azathioprine / ↑ Risk of hepatotoxicity; monitor closely
Caffeine / Ingestion of more than 180 mg/day of caffeine may ↓ effect of methotrexate compared with ingestion of less than 120 mg/day
Cephalosporins / ↓ Methotrexate elimination R/T ↓ urinary pH → precipitation in renal tubules → acute nephrotoxicity
Charcoal / ↓ Methotrexate absorption and ↑ removal from systemic circulation
Chloramphenicol, oral / ↓ Methotrexate intestinal absorption or interference with enterohepatic circulation by inhibiting bowel flora and suppressing metabolism of the drug by bacteria
Cyclosporine / ↑ Methotrexate peak plasma levels and AUC and ↓ AUC and urinary excretion of the 7-hydroxy-methotrexate metabolite
Digoxin / ↓ Serum digoxin levels
Doxycycline / GI and hematologic toxicity after high-dose methotrexate
Etretinate / Possible hepatotoxicity if used together for psoriasis; monitor closely
Folic-acid-containing vitamin preparations / ↓ Methotrexate systemic response
Glutamine ↓ Urinary pH → ↑ plasma methotrexate levels and nephrotoxicity due to precipitation of methotrexate in renal tubules
Ibuprofen / ↑ Methotrexate effect by ↓ renal secretion
NSAIDs / ↓ Methotrexate elimination R/T ↓ urinary pH → precipitation in renal tubules → acute nephrotoxicity
PABA / ↑ Methotrexate effect by ↓ plasma protein binding
Penicillins / ↓ Methotrexate elimination R/T ↓ urinary pH → precipitation in renal tubules → acute nephrotoxicity
Phenytoin / ↓ Serum phenytoin levels → ↓ therapeutic effect
Probenecid / ↓ Methotrexate elimination R/T ↓ urinary pH → precipitation in renal tubules → acute nephrotoxicity
Procarbazine / Possible ↑ nephrotoxicity
Pyrimethamine / ↑ Methotrexate toxicity
Salicylates (aspirin) / ↓ Methotrexate elimination R/T ↓ urinary pH → precipitation in renal tubules → acute nephrotoxicity
Smallpox vaccination / Methotrexate impairs immunologic response to smallpox vaccine
Sulfasalazine / ↑ Risk of hepatotoxicity; monitor closely
Sulfonamides / ↑ Risk of methotrexate-induced bone marrow suppression
Tetracyclines / ↑ Methotrexate effect by ↓ plasma protein binding
Theophylline / ↓ Theophylline clearance
Thiopurines (e.g., azathioprine) / ↑ Plasma drug levels
Trimethoprim / ↑ Risk of methotrexate-induced bone marrow suppression and megaloblastic anemia; do not use together
Vancomycin / ↑ Methotrexate serum levels and markedly delayed methotrexate excretion

HOW SUPPLIED

Methotrexate. ***Tablets:*** 2.5 mg, 5 mg, 7.5 mg, 10 mg, 15 mg.
Methotrexate Sodium. ***Injection:*** 25 mg/mL (as base); ***Powder for Injection, Lyophilized:*** 20 mg/vial (as base-preservative free), 1 gram/vial (as base-preservative free).

DOSAGE

IA; IM; INTRATHECAL; IV; TABLETS

Choriocarcinoma and similar trophoblastic diseases.

Dose individualized. PO, IM: 15–30 mg/day for 5 days. May be repeated 3–5 times with 1-week rest period between courses.

Acute lymphatic (lymphoblastic) leukemia.

Initial: 3.3 mg/m^2 (with 60 mg/m^2 prednisone daily); **maintenance: PO, IM,** 30 mg/m^2 2 times per week or **IV,** 2.5 mg/kg q 14 days.

Meningeal leukemia.

Intrathecal: 12 mg/m^2 q 2–5 days until cell count returns to normal.

M

Lymphomas.

PO: 10–25 mg/day for 4–8 days for several courses of treatment with 7- to 10-day rest periods between courses.

Mycosis fungoides.

PO: 2.5–10 mg/day for several weeks or months; **alternatively, IM:** 50 mg once weekly or 25 mg twice weekly.

Lymphosarcoma.

0.625–2.5 mg/kg/day in combination with other drugs.

Osteosarcoma.

Used in combination with other drugs, including doxorubicin, cisplatin, bleomycin, cyclophosphamide, and dactinomycin. **Usual IV starting dose for methotrexate:** 12 grams/m^2; dose may be increased to 15 grams/m^2 to achieve a peak serum level of 10^{-3} mol/L at the end of the methotrexate infusion.

Psoriasis.

Adults, usual: PO, IM, IV: 10–25 mg/week, continued until beneficial response observed. Weekly dose should not exceed 30 mg. **Alternate regimens:** PO, 2.5 mg q 12 hr for three doses or q 8 hr for four doses each week (not to exceed 30 mg/week). Once beneficial effects are noted, reduce dose to lowest possible level with longest rest periods between doses.

Rheumatoid arthritis.

Initial: Single PO doses of 7.5 mg/week or divided PO doses of 2.5 mg at 12-hr intervals for three doses given once a week; **then,** adjust dosage to achieve optimum response, not to exceed a total weekly dose of 20 mg. Once response has been reached, reduce the dose to the lowest possible effective dose.

NURSING IMPLICATIONS

Do not confuse methotrexate with metolazone (a thiazide diuretic).

IMPLEMENTATION/ADMINISTRATION/STORAGE

1. Use only sterile, preservative-free NaCl injection to reconstitute powder for intrathecal administration.
2. Prevent inhalation of drug particles and skin exposure.
3. When used for rheumatoid arthritis, improvement is thought to be maintained for up to 2 years with continuous therapy. When discontinued, arthritis usually worsens within 3–6 weeks.
4. IV Six hours prior to initiation of a methotrexate infusion, hydrate with 1 L/m^2 of IV fluid. Continue hydration at 125 mL/m^2/hr during methotrexate infusion and for 2 days after infusion completed.
5. Alkalinize urine (see *Sodium Bicarbonate*) to a pH >7 during infusion.
6. Follow guidelines provided for leucovorin rescue schedule following high doses of methotrexate.
7. COMPATIBILITY 0.9% NaCl, D5W, or D5/0.9% NaCl.
8. INCOMPATIBILITY Administer separately.

ASSESSMENT

1. Note reasons for therapy, onset, characteristics of S&S. With arthritis, note joint findings, ROM, pain level, other agents trialed, outcome.
2. List drugs prescribed. Identify if receiving other organic acids, such as aspirin, phenylbutazone, probenecid, and/or sulfa drugs; these affect renal clearance of methotrexate and increase thrombocytopenia and GI side effects. Note any acute infections.
3. Monitor I&O, weight, and VS. Administer antiemetic as needed.
4. Have calcium leucovorin—a potent antidote for folic acid antagonists—readily available in case of overdosage. Antidotes are ineffective if not administered within 4 hr of overdosage; may give corticosteroids concomitantly with initial dose of methotrexate. Allow maximum rest between doses.
5. Renal function tests are recommended before initiation of therapy; perform daily leukocyte counts during therapy. Monitor CBC, uric acid, renal and LFTs; report oliguria. Drug causes granulocyte and platelet suppression. Nadir: 10 days; recovery: 14 days.

CLIENT/FAMILY TEACHING

1. Take at bedtime with an antacid to minimize GI upset. Prepare calendar to ensure correct dosage days. Do not consume OTC vitamins.

2. If taking for rheumatoid arthritis or psoriasis, prescribed dose is taken once weekly, on the same day each week. More frequent use may result in serious toxicity.
3. Use caution with activities that require mental alertness until tolerance determined; may cause dizziness or drowsiness.
4. Avoid aspirin (salicylates) and alcohol as liver toxicity/bleeding may result. Avoid contact sports.
5. Report oral ulcerations, 1 of the first signs of toxicity. May experience hair loss; should regrow once therapy completed.
6. Avoid crowds, those with infections, vaccinations (esp. smallpox); impaired immunologic response may result in vaccinia.
7. Consume 2–3 L/day of fluids to prevent renal damage and facilitate drug excretion.
8. Test urine pH, report if less than 6.5; bicarbonate tablets may be prescribed to assist in alkalinizing urine.
9. Drug may precipitate gouty arthritis; allopurinol may be added to reduce uric acid levels.
10. Avoid sun exposure, use sunscreens, sunglasses, and appropriate clothing when necessary. Report if psoriasis lesions worsen.
11. Practice reliable contraception during and for at least 8 weeks following therapy. A female partner of male receiving therapy should use effective contraception during and for at least 3 mo after therapy has been completed by her partner.
12. Keep all F/U to assess response, labs, and for adverse SE.

OUTCOMES/EVALUATE

- Suppression of malignant cell proliferation, ↓ tumor size/spread
- Improvement in skin lesions
- ↓ Joint swelling/pain; ↑ mobility
- Improved hematologic parameters

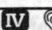

IV

Methyldopa

(meth-ill-**DOH**-pah)

Classification(s): Antihypertensive, centrally-acting

Pregnancy Category: B (PO); **C** (IV)

✤ **Rx:** Apo-Methyldopa.

Methyldopate hydrochloride

Pregnancy Category: B (PO); **C** (IV)

RX: Aldomet Hydrochloride.

SEE ALSO ***ANTIHYPERTENSIVE AGENTS.***

INDICATIONS/USES

PO (Methyldopa): Moderate to severe hypertension. Particularly useful for clients with impaired renal function, renal hypertension, resistant cases of hypertension complicated by stroke, CAD, or nitrogen retention. **IV (Methyldopate HCl):** Hypertensive crisis. *Investigational:* Hypertension in pregnancy.

ACTION/KINETICS

Action

The active metabolite, alpha-methylnorepinephrine, lowers BP by stimulating central inhibitory alpha-adrenergic receptors, false neurotransmission, and/or reduction of plasma renin. Little change in CO.

Pharmacokinetics

PO, Onset: 7–12 hr. **Duration:** 12–24 hr. All effects terminated within 48 hr. Absorption is variable. **IV, Onset:** 4–6 hr. **Duration:** 10–16 hr. Seventy percent of drug excreted in urine. **Full therapeutic effect:** 1–4 days. **t½:** 1.7 hr. Metabolites excreted in the urine.

CONTRAINDICATIONS

Sensitivity to drug (including sulfites), labile and mild hypertension, pregnancy, active hepatic disease (e.g., acute hepatitis, active cirrhosis), use with MAOIs, or pheochromocytoma. Use if previous methyldopa therapy has been associated with liver disorders.

SPECIAL CONCERNS

- Use with caution in clients with a history of liver or kidney disease.
- A decrease in dose in the elderly may prevent syncope.

SIDE EFFECTS

Most Common

Dizziness, drowsiness, headache, flatulence, dry mouth, N&V, fatigue, stomach upset, menstrual irregularities, rash, impotence.

CNS: Sedation (transient), drowsiness, weakness, headache, asthenia, dizziness, paresthesias, Parkinson-like symptoms, psychic disturbances, symptoms of CV impairment, choreoathetotic movements, Bell's palsy, decreased mental acuity, verbal memory impairment. **CV:** Bradycardia, orthostatic hypotension, hypersensitivity of carotid sinus, worsening of angina, paradoxical hypertensive response (after IV), myocarditis, CHF, pericarditis, vasculitis. **GI:** N&V, stomach upset, abdominal distention, diarrhea or constipation, flatus, colitis, dry mouth, sore or "black tongue," pancreatitis, sialoadenitis, hepatotoxicity, jaundice. **Hematologic:** ***Hemolytic anemia***, leukopenia, granulocytopenia, thrombocytopenia, ***bone marrow depression***. **Endocrine:** Gynecomastia, amenorrhea, galactorrhea, lactation, hyperprolactinemia. **GU:** Impotence, menstrual irregularities, failure to ejaculate, decreased libido. **Dermatologic:** Rash, ***toxic epidermal necrolysis***. **Hepatic:** Jaundice, hepatitis, liver disorders, abnormal LFTs. **Miscellaneous:** Edema, weight gain, fever, lupus-like symptoms, nasal stuffiness, arthralgia, myalgia, ***septic shock-like syndrome***.

LABORATORY TEST CONSIDERATIONS

Positive Coombs' test. Hepatotoxicity may cause ↑ alkaline phosphatase, AST, ALT, bilirubin, and prothrombin time; also, eosinophilia. Interference with urinary uric acid by phosphotungstate method; serum creatinine by the alkaline picrate method; AST by colorimetric methods.

OVERDOSE MANAGEMENT

Symptoms: CNS, GI, and CV effects, including sedation, weakness, light-headedness, dizziness, coma, bradycardia, acute hypotension, impairment of AV conduction, constipation, diarrhea, distention, flatus, N&V. *Treatment:* Induction of vomiting or gastric lavage if detected early. General supportive treatment with special attention to HR, CO, blood volume, urinary function, electrolyte imbalance, paralytic ileus, and CNS activity. In severe cases, hemodialysis is effective.

DRUG INTERACTIONS

Anesthetics, general / Additive hypotension
Antidepressants, tricyclic / May block methyldopa hypotensive effects
Ferrous gluconate or sulfate / ↓ Bioavailability of methyldopa
Haloperidol / ↑ Haloperidol toxic effects
Levodopa / ↑ Effect of both drugs
Lithium / ↑ Possibility of lithium toxicity
MAOIs / Accumulation of methyldopa metabolites may → excessive sympathetic stimulation
Methotrimeprazine / Additive hypotensive effect
Phenothiazines / Possible ↑ BP
Propranolol / Paradoxical hypertensive crisis
Sympathomimetics / Potentiation of pressor effects → hypertension
Thiazide diuretics / Additive hypotensive effect
Thioxanthenes / Additive hypotensive effect
Tolbutamide / ↑ Hypoglycemia R/T ↓ liver breakdown
Tricyclic antidepressants / ↓ Methyldopa effect
Vasodilator drugs / Additive hypotensive effect
Verapamil / ↑ Methyldopa effect

HOW SUPPLIED

Methyldopa. *Tablets:* 250 mg, 500 mg.
Methyldopate hydrochloride. *Injection:* 50 mg/mL.

DOSAGE

Methyldopa

TABLETS

Hypertension.

Initial: 250 mg 2–3 times per day for 2 days. Adjust dose q 2 days. If dose increased, start with evening dose. **Usual maintenance:** 0.5–2.0 grams/day in two to four divided doses; **maximum:** 3 grams/day. Gradually transfer to and from other antihypertensive agents, with initial dose of methyldopa not exceeding 500 mg. *NOTE:* Do not use combination medication to initiate therapy. **Pediatric, initial:** 10 mg/kg/day in 2–4 divided doses, adjusting maintenance to a maximum of 65 mg/kg/day (or 3 grams/day, whichever is less).

Methyldopate HCl

IV INFUSION

Hypertensive crisis.

Adults: 250–500 mg q 6 hr; **maximum:** 1 gram q 6 hr for hypertensive crisis. Switch to PO methyldopa, at same dosage level, when BP is brought under control. **Pediatric:** 20–40 mg/kg/day in divided doses q 6 hr;

maximum: 65 mg/kg/day (or 3 grams/day, whichever is less).

NURSING IMPLICATIONS

Do not confuse Aldomet with Aldoril (also an antihypertensive). Do not confuse methyldopa with levodopa.

IMPLEMENTATION/ADMINISTRATION/STORAGE

1. Tolerance may occur following 2–3 months of therapy. Increasing the dose or adding a diuretic often restores effect on BP.
2. IV For IV, mix with 100 mL of D5W or administer in D5W at a concentration of 10 mg/mL. Infuse over 30–60 min.
3. COMPATIBILITY D5W.
4. INCOMPATIBILITY Administer separately.

ASSESSMENT

1. Note reasons for therapy, onset/characteristics of S&S, other agents trialed, outcome.
2. Avoid during pregnancy. Note if jaundiced; avoid with active hepatic disease.
3. Assess for depression, drug tolerance; may occur during the second or third month of therapy.
4. If blood transfusion required, check direct and indirect Coombs' tests; if positive, consult hematologist.
5. Obtain CBC to detect for anemia before therapy. Monitor BP, I&O, CBC, renal and LFTs.

CLIENT/FAMILY TEACHING

1. Drug is used to lower BP; take as directed throughout the day.
2. To prevent dizziness and fainting, rise slowly to a sitting position and dangle legs over the bed edge; hot baths or showers may aggravate dizziness. Use caution, sedation may occur initially; should disappear once maintenance dose established.
3. Nausea, vomiting, or diarrhea may cause increase in hypotensive effect because of dehydration. Keep record of BP and HR.
4. Withhold and report any of the following symptoms: tiredness, fever, depression, or yellowing of eyes/skin. May darken or turn urine blue; not harmful.
5. Continue regular exercise, weight reduction, sodium and alcohol restriction, cessation of smoking, stress reduction, in the overall goal of BP control. Keep log of BP recordings and weight for provider review.
6. Avoid alcohol. Do not take any other medications or remedies unless approved.
7. Report any S&S of infection such as fever, or sore throat. May use ice chips or sugarless gums/candy to relieve dry mouth.
8. Avoid prolonged sun exposure, use sunscreen/wear protective clothing to avoid photosensitivity reaction.
9. Keep all F/U to assess response, labs, and for adverse SE.

OUTCOMES/EVALUATE

BP control

IV

Methylergonovine maleate

(meth-ill-er-**GON**-oh-veen)

Classification(s): Oxytocic drug

Pregnancy Category: C

RX: Methergine.

INDICATIONS/USES

(1) Management and prevention of postpartum and postabortal hemorrhage by producing firm uterine contractions and decreasing uterine bleeding. (2) During the second stage of labor following delivery of the anterior shoulder, but only under full obstetric supervision. *Investigational:* Ergonovine has been used to diagnose Prinzmetal's angina (variant angina).

ACTION/KINETICS

Action

Synthetic drug related to ergonovine. Acts directly on the uterine smooth muscle to stimulate the rate, tone, and amplitude of uterine contractions. It induces a rapid, sustained tetanic uterotonic effect that shortens the third stage of labor and reduces blood loss. The uterus becomes more sensitive to the drug toward the end of pregnancy.

Pharmacokinetics

Decrease in bioavailability after PO use probably due to first-pass metabolism in the liver. **Onset** (uterine contractions), **PO:** 5–10 min; **IM:** 2–5 min; **IV:** immediate. **t½, IV:** 2–3 min (initial) and 20–30 min (final). **Duration, PO, IM:** 3 hr; **IV:** 45 min. **t½, elimination:** 3.4 hr.

CONTRAINDICATIONS

Pregnancy, toxemia, hypertension. Ergot hypersensitivity. To induce labor or threatened spontaneous abortions. Administration before delivery of the placenta. Use with CYP3A4 inhibitors (e.g., protease inhibitors, macrolide antibiotics, azole antifungal drugs).

SPECIAL CONCERNS

- **Use with caution in sepsis, obliterative vascular disease, impaired renal or hepatic function, during the second stage of labor, and during lactation.**
- **Do not routinely use IV due to possible induction of sudden hypertension and CVA.**

SIDE EFFECTS

Most Common

Hypertension associated with seizure or headache.

CV: Hypertension that may be associated with seizure or headache; hypotension, ***acute MI***, thrombophlebitis, palpitation, transient chest pains. **GI:** N&V, diarrhea, foul taste. **CNS:** Dizziness, headache, tinnitus, hallucinations, seizures. **Miscellaneous:** Sweating, dyspnea, hematuria, water intoxication, leg cramps, nasal congestion. *NOTE:* ***Use of methylergonovine during labor may result in uterine tetany with rupture, cervical and perineal lacerations, embolism of amniotic fluid as well as hypoxia and intracranial hemorrhage in the infant.***

OVERDOSE MANAGEMENT

Symptoms: Initially, N&V, abdominal pain, increase in BP, tingling of extremities, numbness. Symptoms of severe overdose include hypotension, hypothermia, ***respiratory depression, seizures, coma.*** *Treatment:* Induce vomiting or perform gastric lavage. Administer a cathartic; institute diuresis. Maintain respiration, especially if seizures or coma occur. Treat seizures with anticonvulsant drugs. Warm extremities to control peripheral vasospasm.

DRUG INTERACTIONS

Azole antifungals (itraconazole, ketoconazole, voriconazole) / ↑ Risk of vasospasm leading to cerebral ischemia and/or ischemia of the extremities; do not use together

Clarithromycin / ↑ Risk of vasospasm leading to cerebral ischemia and/or ischemia of the extremities; do not use together

Erythromycin / ↑ Risk of vasospasm leading to cerebral ischemia and/or ischemia of the extremities; do not use together

Protease inhibitors / ↑ Risk of vasospasm leading to cerebral ischemia and/or ischemia of the extremities; do not use together

Reverse transcriptase inhibitors / ↑ Risk of vasospasm leading to cerebral ischemia and/or ischemia of the extremities; do not use together

Sympathomimetics / Hypertension R/T additive vasoconstriction

Troleoandomycin / ↑ Risk of vasospasm leading to cerebral ischemia and/or ischemia of the extremities; do not use together

HOW SUPPLIED

Injection: 0.2 mg/mL; ***Tablets:*** 0.2 mg.

DOSAGE

IM; IV (EMERGENCIES ONLY)

Prevention and treatment of postpartum and postabortal hemorrhage; during second stage of labor following delivery of anterior shoulder.

0.2 mg q 2–4 hr following delivery of placenta, of the anterior shoulder, or during the puerperium.

TABLETS

Prevention and treatment of postpartum and postabortal hemorrhage.

0.2 mg 3–4 times per day in the puerperium for a maximum of 1 week.

NURSING IMPLICATIONS

IMPLEMENTATION/ADMINISTRATION/STORAGE

1. **Store tablets below 25°C (77°F) in tight, light-resistant containers.**
2. **IV Administer slowly over 1 min (may give undiluted or diluted in 5 mL of 0.9% NaCl over 5 min); check VS for evidence of shock or hypertension after IV administration. Have emergency drugs available. Not for routine use.**
3. **Give only if solution is clear and colorless; discard ampules if discolored.**
4. **Store ampules from 2–8°C (36–46°F). Protect from light.**
5. **COMPATIBILITY 0.9% NaCl.**
6. **INCOMPATIBILITY Administer separately.**

ASSESSMENT

1. Note reasons for therapy, onset, characteristics of S&S. Avoid with liver or renal dysfunction. List drugs prescribed to ensure none interact.
2. Assess fundal tone and nonphasic contractures; massage to check for relaxation or severe cramping.
3. With postpartum bleeding, report frequency, amount, color, and any associated S&S. Ensure placenta completely passed/removed.
4. Monitor VS, CBC, and calcium; correct if low to improve drug effectiveness. Monitor prolactin levels; assess for decreased milk production.

CLIENT/FAMILY TEACHING

1. Take only as directed; do not exceed dosage.
2. Avoid smoking; nicotine constricts blood vessels.
3. Report any S&S of ergotism (cold/numb fingers/toes, N&V, headache, muscle or chest pain, weakness) or infection.
4. Abdominal cramps may be experienced; report any severe cramping, headaches, or increased bleeding.
5. Stop drug and report if numbness, tingling, coldness, or paleness in the fingers or toes, muscle pain in arms or legs, weakness in the legs, chest pain, tightness, or pressure, or changes in heart rate.
6. Keep all F/U to assess response and for adverse SE.

OUTCOMES/EVALUATE

Improved uterine tone; control of postpartum hemorrhage

Methylphenidate hydrochloride

(meth-ill-**FEN**-ih-dayt)

Classification(s): CNS stimulant

Pregnancy Category: C

RX: Capsules, Extended-Release: Metadate CD, Ritalin LA. **Oral Solution**: Methylin. **Tablets, Chewable**: Methylin. **Tablets, Extended-Release**: Concerta, Metadate ER, Methylin ER, Ritalin-SR. **Tablets, Immediate-Release**: Methylin, Ritalin. **Transdermal Patch**: Daytrana, **C-II**

✤ **Rx:** Apo-Methylphenidate, Apo-Methylphenidate SR, PMS-Methylphenidate.

INDICATIONS/USES

(1) Attention-deficit disorders (ADD) and attention-deficit hyperactivity disorders (ADHD) in children as part of overall treatment regimen. Syndrome characterized by moderate to severe distractibility, short attention span, hyperactivity, emotional lability, and impulsivity. Transdermal patch used only for ADHD. (2) Narcolepsy (Concerta, Metadate CD, Ritalin LA only). *Investigational:* Depression in medically ill (including stroke) elderly clients. Alleviation of neurobehavioral symptoms after traumatic brain injury. Improvement in pain control, sedation, or both in those receiving opiates.

ACTION/KINETICS

Action

Mechanism unknown; may activate the brain stem arousal system and cortex to produce stimulation. In children with attention-deficit disorders, methylphenidate causes decreases in motor restlessness with an increased attention span. In narcolepsy the drug acts on the cerebral cortex and subcortical structures (e.g., thalamus) to increase motor activity and mental alertness and decrease fatigue.

Pharmacokinetics

Rapidly and well absorbed from the GI tract. Food delays peak levels of the chewable tablets by about 1 hr. **Peak blood levels, children:** 1.9 hr for tablets; 1–2 hr for chewable tablets; and, 4.7 hr for extended-release tablets. **Duration:** 4–6 hr. **t½ tablets, chewable tablets, Concerta tablets:** 1–3.5 hr; **t½, Metatate CD:** 6.8 hr. Metabolized by the liver and excreted by the kidney. *NOTE:* The various methylphenidate products have different pharmacokinetic properties. For example, the extended-release capsules (Ritalin LA) are taken once daily to eliminate the need for dosing during school hours. Drug is released in 2 parts—the second dose 4 hr after the first dose. Ritalin-SR is also for once daily dosing but provides continuous release over 8 hr.

CONTRAINDICATIONS

Marked anxiety, tension and agitation, glaucoma. Severe depression (either endogenous or exogenous), to prevent or treat normal fatigue, diagnosis or family history of Tourette's syndrome, motor tics. In children who manifest symptoms of primary psychiatric disorders (psychoses) or acute stress. Concurrent treatment of Concerta, Metadate CD, Ritalin, Ritalin LA, and Ritalin-SR with monoamine oxidase inhibitors and within a minimum of 14 days after stopping MAOI therapy (hypertensive crisis may occur). Use in children less than 6 years of age.

SPECIAL CONCERNS

■ (1) Give cautiously to emotionally unstable clients, such as those with a history of drug dependence or alcoholism, because such clients may increase dosage on their own initiative. (2) Chronic abuse can lead to marked tolerance and psychic dependence with varying degrees of abnormal behavior. Frank psychotic episodes can occur, especially after parenteral abuse. (3) Careful supervision is required during drug withdrawal because severe depression, as well as the effects of chronic overactivity, can be unmasked. (4) Long-term follow-up may be required due to the client's basic personality disturbances. (5) There is an increased risk of serious CV events and sudden death with CNS stimulants of this class. ■

- **Use with caution during lactation.**
- **Use with great caution in clients with history of hypertension or convulsive disease or to emotionally unstable clients (e.g., those with history of drug dependence or alcoholism).**
- **Lowers seizure threshold in those with a history of seizures or with prior EEG abnormalities in the absence of seizures.**
- **May worsen symptoms of behavior disturbances and thought disorder.**
- **Safety and efficacy not established in children less than 6 years of age.**

SIDE EFFECTS

Most Common

Headache, URTI, abdominal pain, anorexia, insomnia, vomiting, accidental injury, nervousness, anxiety/irritability.

CNS: Nervousness, insomnia, headaches, dizziness, drowsiness, chorea, depressed mood (transient). Toxic psychosis, dyskinesia, Tourette's syndrome, neuroleptic malignant syndrome (rare). Psychologic dependence. **CV:** Palpitations, tachycardia, angina, arrhythmias, hyper-/hypotension, cerebral arteritis and/or occlusion. **GI:** N&V, anorexia, abdominal pain, weight loss (chronic use). GI obstruction (Concerta only as it is nondeformable and does not change shape appreciably in the GI tract.) **Respiratory:** URTI, increased cough, pharyngitis, sinusitis. **Allergic:** Skin rashes, fever, urticaria, arthralgia, exfoliative dermatitis, erythema multiforme with necrotizing vasculitis, erythema. **Hematologic:** Thrombocytopenic purpura, leukopenia, anemia. **Ophthalmic:** Accommodation difficulty, blurred vision. **Miscellaneous:** Scalp hair loss, accidental injury, rash at application site (for transdermal product), abnormal liver function (including transaminase elevation to ***hepatic coma***). **In children, in addition to the preceding side effects, the following side effects are common:** Loss of appetite, abdominal pain, weight loss during chronic use, insomnia, tachycardia, dysmenorrhea, rhinitis, fever.

OVERDOSE MANAGEMENT

Symptoms: Characterized by CNS overstimulation and excessive sympathomimetic effects including: Vomiting, agitation, tremors, hyperreflexia, muscle twitching, ***convulsions (may be followed by coma), hyperpyrexia***, euphoria, confusion, hallucinations, delirium, sweating, flushing, headache, tachycardia, palpitations, cardiac arrhythmias, hypertension, mydriasis, dry mucous membranes. *Treatment:* Symptomatic. Treat excess CNS stimulation by keeping the client in quiet, dim surroundings to reduce external stimuli. Protect the client from self-injury. A short-acting barbiturate may be used. Undertake emesis or gastric lavage if the client is conscious. Adequate circulatory and respiratory function must be maintained. Hyperpyrexia may be treated by cooling the client (e.g., cool bath, hypothermia blanket).

DRUG INTERACTIONS

Anticoagulants, oral (coumarin) / ↑ Anticoagulant effect R/T ↓ liver breakdown
Anticonvulsants (phenobarbital, phenytoin, primidone) / ↑ Anticonvulsant effect and ↑ toxic effects R/T ↓ liver breakdown
Carbamazepine / ↓ Methylphenidate levels

Clonidine / Possible serious side effects
Guanethidine / ↓ Guanethidine effect by displacement from its action site
MAOIs / Possibility of hypertensive crisis, hyperthermia, convulsions, coma; do not use with Concerta, Metadate CD, Ritalin, Ritalin LA, Ritalin SR
Selective serotonin reuptake inhibitors / ↑ Serum levels of SSRIs
Tricyclic antidepressants / ↑ Plasma levels and TCA effect R/T ↓ liver breakdown

HOW SUPPLIED

Capsules, Extended-Release: 10 mg, 20 mg, 30 mg, 40 mg, 50 mg, 60 mg; ***Oral Solution:*** 5 mg/5 mL, 10 mg/5 mL; ***Tablets, Chewable:*** 2.5 mg, 5 mg, 10 mg; ***Tablets, Extended-Release:*** 10 mg, 18 mg, 20 mg, 27 mg, 36 mg, 54 mg; ***Tablets, Immediate-Release:*** 5 mg, 10 mg, 20 mg; ***Tablets, Sustained-Release:*** 20 mg; ***Transdermal Patch:*** 10 mg, 15 mg, 20 mg, 30 mg (each strength is the amount delivered over 9 hr).

DOSAGE

CAPSULES, EXTENDED-RELEASE; ORAL SOLUTION; TABLETS, CHEWABLE; TABLETS, EXTENDED-RELEASE; TABLETS, IMMEDIATE-RELEASE

Narcolepsy.

Adults, average dose: 20–30 mg/day in 2 to 3 divided doses (range: 10–15 to 40–60 mg/day), preferably 30–45 min before meals. For those unable to sleep if the medication is given late in the day, take the last dose before 6 p.m.

Attention-deficit/hyperactivity disorder.

Individualize dose. Children, 6 years and older, initial: 5 mg twice a day before breakfast and lunch; **then,** increase gradually by 5–10 mg/week to a maximum of 60 mg/day. If no improvement is noted after a 1-month period, discontinue the drug. *NOTE:* See *Implementation/Administration/Storage* for additional dosing information.

TRANSDERMAL PATCH

Attention-deficit/hyperactivity disorder.

Children, 6–17 years of age, initial: 10 mg over 9 hr for the first week with the patch is applied to the client's hip 2 hr before an effect is needed; remove after 9 hr. **Week 2:** 15 mg over 9 hr; **week 3:** 20 mg over 9 hr; **week 4 and thereafter:** 30 mg over 9 hr.

NURSING IMPLICATIONS

Do not confuse Metadate CD and Metadate ER (both are extended-release forms of methylphenidate).

IMPLEMENTATION/ADMINISTRATION/STORAGE

1. Discontinue periodically to assess condition as drug therapy is not indefinite; discontinue at puberty.
2. Sustained-release (SR) and Methylin ER tablets are effective for 8 hr and may be substituted for regular-release tablets if the 8-hr dosage of the sustained-release tablets is the same as the titrated 8-hr dosage of regular tablets. ER tablets must be swallowed whole, never crushed or chewed.
3. If paradoxical aggravation of symptoms or other side effects occur, reduce dose or discontinue drug.
4. Give Concerta once daily in the a.m. with or without food. Swallow tablets whole with liquids; do not chew, divide, or crush.
5. The recommended starting dose for Concerta is 18 mg/day for those not currently taking methylphenidate or if on stimulants other than methylphenidate. Dose may be adjusted in 18 mg increments at weekly intervals up to a maximum of 54 mg/day taken once in the a.m. For adolescents, aged 13–17 years, maximum dose may be 72 mg/day, but not more than 2 mg/kg/day, taken once in the morning.
6. The recommended dose for Concerta for clients currently taking methylphenidate 2 or 3 times per day, or SR at doses from 10–60 mg/day:
   - 18 mg every a.m. if previously taking methylphenidate 5 mg 2 or 3 times per day or methylphenidate-SR, 20 mg/day.
   - 36 mg every a.m. if previously taking methylphenidate 10 mg 2 or 3 times per day or methylphenidate-SR, 40 mg/day.
   - 54 mg every a.m. if previously taking methylphenidate 15 mg 2 or 3 times per day or methylphenidate-SR, 60 mg/day.

M

7. For Metadate CD form, give once daily in the a.m. before breakfast. Swallow capsules whole with liquids; do not chew, divide, or crush. May also be given by sprinkle administration (e.g., on applesauce).
8. If Metadate CD is to be sprinkled onto soft food, the entire capsule contents must be used as a single 20 mg dose. Dose cannot be split because the immediate-release and continuous-release beads cannot be physically distinguished from one another. Give dose immediately after sprinkling; do not store for future use. The beads must not be crushed or chewed.
9. For Metadate CD, the dosage form is extended-release capsules. The 40 mg dose contains 12 mg immediate-release and 28 mg extended-release; the 50 mg dose contains 15 mg immediate-release and 35 mg extended-release; and, the 60 mg dose contains 18 mg immediate-release and 42 mg extended-release.
10. For Ritalin LA, start with 20 mg q day. Adjust dose, if needed, in 10 mg increments weekly up to a maximum of 60 mg/day taken once daily in the a.m. If a lower initial dose is appropriate, begin with an immediate-release methylphenidate. After titration to 10 mg twice a day, switch to Ritalin LA according to the following guidelines:
    - If previous methylphenidate dose was 10 mg twice a day or 20 mg methylphenidate SR, give 20 mg Ritalin LA once daily.
    - If previous methylphenidate dose was 15 mg twice a day, give 30 mg Ritalin LA once daily.
    - If previous methylphenidate dose was 20 mg twice a day or 40 mg methylphenidate SR, give 40 mg Ritalin LA once daily.
    - If previous methylphenidate dose was 30 mg twice a day or 60 mg methylphenidate SR, give 60 mg Ritalin LA once daily.
11. Each methylphenidate chewable tablet, 2.5 mg, contains phenylalanine, 0.42 mg; each 5 mg chewable tablet contains phenylalanine, 0.84 mg; and, each 10 mg chewable tablet contains phenylalanine, 1.68 mg.
12. Do not store Ritalin above 30°C (86°F). Protect from light, dispense in tight, light-resistant container.
13. Store Concerta, Metadate CD, and Ritalin LA from 25–30°C (59–86°F). Protect from humidity; store in a tight container.
14. Store Metadate ER, Methylin, and Methylin ER from 15–30°C (59–86°F). Protect from moisture and light. Dispense in a tight, light-resistant container.

ASSESSMENT

1. Note reasons for therapy, onset/characteristics of S&S, clinical presentation, other drugs prescribed, outcome. Note any drugs prescribed that may interact unfavorably.
2. Ensure psychologic evaluations show no evidence of psychotic disorder, excessive stimulation, or severe stress. Assess growth (height and weight) in child; provide periodic *drug holiday* to determine need for continued therapy.
3. Monitor for appearance of hostility or aggressive behavior at the beginning of therapy.
4. May cause Tourette's syndrome in child; monitor effects carefully.
5. Obtain/monitor BP, CBC, CNS status, and ECG.

CLIENT/FAMILY TEACHING

1. With ADD, take IR tablets before breakfast and lunch to avoid interference with sleep. Take ER e.g., Ritalin SR and Concerta tablets whole once daily; do not chew or crush. May notice the tablet shell in the stool (passes through intestine and is not absorbed). The capsules may be swallowed whole or sprinkled onto a small amount of applesauce and taken immediately.
2. Review the form prescribed and dosing and application guidelines. With patch, avoid exposing application site to direct external heat sources (e.g., heating pads, electric blankets, hair dryers) while wearing; may increase absorption rate. Clean patch area after patch removal to remove any remaining adhesive.
3. Avoid touching adhesive during application, and immediately wash hands if adhesive is touched. Use only intact patches and do not cut the patches. Fold patch over onto itself upon removal and dispose of as directed (closed container).
4. With solution, take 30 to 45 min before a meal. Use the accompanying dosing cup/spoon provided to ensure accurate dosing.

5. If using chewable tablets, take 30 to 45 min before meal with a full glass of water; prevents choking.
6. Notify school and nurse of use in school age child.
7. Immediately seek medical attention if experiencing any of the following after taking the chewable tablet: chest pain, vomiting, or difficulty swallowing or breathing.
8. Chewable tablet contains phenylalanine; caution those with phenylketonuria.
9. Use caution when driving or operating hazardous machinery; drug may mask fatigue and/or cause physical incoordination, dizziness, blurred vision, drowsiness.
10. Record weight 2 times per week; report any significant loss.
11. Report changes in mood/behavior, attention span; seizure disorder.
12. Skin rashes, fever, or joint pains should be reported immediately.
13. Therapy may be interrupted periodically (*drug holiday*) to determine need in those responsive to therapy.
14. Avoid caffeine in any form. May require more rest as drug effects fade.
15. Chronic use may lead to psychic dependence and marked tolerance. Scripts will be carefully monitored.
16. With ADD and ADHD, ensure psychological, educational, and social interventions are incorporated into care plan.
17. Report any visual changes, appetite loss, nervousness, or difficulty sleeping.
18. Keep all F/U to assess response, labs, ECG, weight, diversion, and for adverse SE.

OUTCOMES/EVALUATE

- ↑ Ability to sit quietly/concentrate
- ↓ Daytime sleeping
- Alleviation of neurobehavioral S&S after TBI (unlabeled)
- Improved pain control/sedation in those receiving opiates (unlabeled)

IV

Methylprednisolone

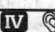

(meth-ill-pred-**NISS**-oh-lohn)

Classification(s): Glucocorticoid
Pregnancy Category: C
RX: Tablets: Medrol.

Methylprednisolone acetate

Pregnancy Category: C

RX: Parenteral: Depo-Medrol.

Methylprednisolone sodium succinate

Pregnancy Category: C

RX: A-Methapred, Solu-Medrol.

SEE ALSO ***CORTICOSTEROIDS***.

ADDITIONAL USES

(1) Severe hepatitis due to alcoholism. (2) Within 8 hr of severe spinal cord injury (to improve neurologic function). (3) Septic shock (controversial).

ACTION/KINETICS

Action

The anti-inflammatory effect is due to inhibition of prostaglandin synthesis. The drug also inhibits accumulation of macrophages and leukocytes at sites of inflammation and inhibits phagocytosis and lysosomal enzyme release. Low incidence of increased appetite, peptic ulcer, psychic stimulation, and sodium and water retention. May mask negative nitrogen balance.

Pharmacokinetics

Onset: Slow, 12–24 hr. **t½, plasma:** 78–188 min. **Duration:** Long, up to 1 week. Rapid onset of sodium succinate by both IV and IM routes. Long duration of action of the acetate due to low solubility.

SPECIAL CONCERNS

Use during pregnancy only if benefits outweigh risks.

SIDE EFFECTS

Most Common

After PO use: GI upset, headache, dizziness, changes in menstrual cycle, insomnia, weight gain.
After parenteral use: Nausea, increased appetite, indigestion, dizziness, weight gain, weakness, sleep disturbances.
See *Corticosteroids* for a complete list of possible side effects.

M

LABORATORY TEST CONSIDERATIONS

↓ Immunoglobulins A, G, M.

ADDITIONAL DRUG INTERACTIONS

Aprepitant / ↑ Methylprednisolone AUC, peak levels, and t½ R/T ↓ metabolism by CYP3A4
Erythromycin / ↑ Methylprednisolone effect R/T ↓ liver metabolism
Grapefruit juice / ↑ AUC, peak levels, and t½ of methylprednisolone R/T ↓ liver metabolism
Nefazodone / ↑ Methylprednisolone AUC and prolonged t½ R/T ↓ metabolism
Troleandomycin / ↑ Methylprednisolone effect R/T ↓ liver metabolism

HOW SUPPLIED

Methylprednisolone. *Tablets:* 2 mg, 4 mg, 8 mg, 16 mg, 24 mg, 32 mg.
Methylprednisolone acetate. *Injection, Suspension:* 20 mg/mL, 40 mg/mL, 80 mg/mL.
Methylprednisolone sodium succinate. *Injection, Powder for Solution:* 40 mg, 125 mg, 500 mg, 1 gram, 2 grams (all per vial).

DOSAGE

NOTE: Initial dosage of methylprednisolone tablets varies from 4 to 96 mg/day, depending on the specific disease. Maintain or adjust the initial dose until a satisfactory response is noted. If there is lack of a response, discontinue and transfer the client to other therapy.

Methylprednisolone

TABLETS

Rheumatoid arthritis.

Adults: 6–16 mg/day. Decrease gradually when condition is under control. **Pediatric:** 6–10 mg/day.

SLE.

Adults, acute: 20–96 mg/day; **maintenance:** 8–20 mg/day.

Acute rheumatic fever.

1 mg/kg body weight daily. Drug is always given in four equally divided doses after meals and at bedtime.

Methylprednisolone acetate

IM ONLY

Adrenogenital syndrome.

40 mg q 2 weeks.

Rheumatoid arthritis.

40–120 mg/week.

Dermatologic lesions, dermatitis.

40–120 mg/week for 1–4 weeks; for severe cases, a single dose of 80–120 mg should provide relief. In chronic contact dermatitis, repeated injections q 5–10 days may be needed.

Seborrheic dermatitis.

80 mg/week.

Asthma, allergic rhinitis.

80–120 mg.

Intra-articular and soft tissue.

Large joints: 20–80 mg; **medium joints:** 10–40 mg; **small joints:** 4–10 mg. **Ganglion, tendinitis, epicondylitis, bursitis:** 4–30 mg.

Intralesional.

20–60 mg.

Methylprednisolone sodium succinate

IM; IV

Most conditions.

Adults, initial: 10–40 mg, depending on the disease; **then,** adjust dose depending on response, with subsequent doses given either **IM, IV.**

Severe conditions.

Adults: 30 mg/kg infused IV over 10–20 min; may be repeated q 4–6 hr for 2–3 days only. **Pediatric:** Not less than 0.5 mg/kg/day.

NURSING IMPLICATIONS

Do not confuse Medrol with Haldol (an antipsychotic). Do not confuse Solu-Medrol with Solu-Cortef (a hydrocortisone product). Do not confuse methylprednisolone with medroxyprogesterone (a progestin).

IMPLEMENTATION/ADMINISTRATION/STORAGE

1. Dosage must be individualized.
2. Methylprednisolone acetate is not for IV use. Should be used as a temporary substitute for PO therapy; give the total daily dose as a single IM injection. For a prolonged effect, give a single weekly dose.
3. For alternate day therapy, twice the usual PO dose is given every other morning (client re-

ceives beneficial effect while minimizing side effects).

4. Store methylprednisolone tablets and methylprednisolone sodium succinate injection from 20–25°C (68–77°F).
5. IV Use only the accompanying diluent or bacteriostatic water for injection with benzyl alcohol when reconstituting methylprednisolone sodium succinate. Use within 48 hr after preparation.
6. COMPATIBILITY D5W, 0.9% NaCl, D5/0.9% NaCl.
7. INCOMPATIBILITY Administer separately.

ASSESSMENT

1. List location, reasons for treatment, onset, characteristics of S&S, other agents trialed; describe clinical presentation.
2. Note any aspirin allergy; the 24 mg tablets distributed as Medrol contain tartrazine which may cause allergic reaction.
3. Document any scans, MRIs, or radiographic findings.
4. Assess for hypothalamic-pituitary-adrenal (HPA) axis suppression, Cushing syndrome, and hyperglycemia in those on long-term therapy. Monitor IOP if therapy continued for more than 6 weeks. Monitor/record linear growth in children.
5. Monitor VS, Wt, CBC, HbA1c, glucose, renal/LFTs, thyroid function tests (TFTs), cholesterol, and electrolytes with prolonged therapy.

CLIENT/FAMILY TEACHING

1. Take as directed; take with food or milk to diminish GI upset. Do not ↑, ↓, or stop taking suddenly after prolonged use (must be tapered off) without provider consent; may cause rebound symptoms/adrenal crisis. Usually if administered before 9 a.m. may mimic normal peak body corticosteroid levels and prevent insomnia.
2. Report unusual weight gain, mood swings, extremity swelling (cushingoid symptoms), fatigue, nausea, anorexia, joint pain, muscle weakness, dizziness, fever (adrenal insufficiency), black or tarry stools, acne and skin flushing, prolonged sore throat/colds, infections, or worsening of problem.
3. With joint (intra-articular) injections do not overuse joint with relief of symptoms, may re-injure or aggravate condition.
4. Avoid live vaccines and persons with infections or diseases.
5. Severe stress or trauma may require increased dosage.
6. Prolonged use may cause bone weakening; and glucose intolerance requiring treatment with insulin or oral agents.
7. Keep all F/U to assess response, labs, and for adverse SE.

OUTCOMES/EVALUATE

- Relief of allergic manifestations
- ↓ Pain/inflammation; ↑ mobility
- ↓ Nerve fiber destruction in spinal cord injury (SCI)

IV

Metoclopramide

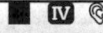

(meh-toe-kloh-**PRAH**-myd)

Classification(s): Gastrointestinal stimulant

Pregnancy Category: B

RX: Metozolv ODT, Reglan.

♣ Rx: Apo-Metoclop, Nu-Metoclopramide.

INDICATIONS/USES

PO: (1) Short-term (4 to 12 weeks) therapy for adults with symptomatic documented gastroesophageal reflux who fail to respond to conventional treatment. (2) Symptomatic relief of acute and recurrent diabetic gastroparesis in adults. Relief of vomiting and anorexia may precede the relief of abdominal fullness by 1 week or more. *Investigational:* Gastroparesis in adults, hiccoughs, improve lactation.

Parenteral: (1) Prevention of N&V associated with emetogenic cancer chemotherapy. (2) Prevention of postoperative N&V when nasogastric suction is undesirable. (3) Facilitate small bowel intubation in adults and children when the tube does not pass the pylorus with conventional methods (use single doses). (4) Stimulate gastric emptying and intestinal transit of barium in clients where delayed emptying interferes with radiological examination of the stomach and/or small intestine. (5) Symptomatic relief of acute and recurrent diabetic gastroparesis. *Investigational:* Hiccoughs, treatment of migraine in adults.

ACTION/KINETICS

Action

Dopamine antagonist that acts by increasing sensitivity to acetylcholine; results in increased motility of the upper GI tract and relaxation of the pyloric sphincter and duodenal bulb. Gastric emptying time and GI transit time are shortened. No effect on gastric, biliary, or pancreatic secretions. Facilitates intubation of the small bowel and speeds transit of a barium meal. Produces sedation, induces release of prolactin, increases circulating aldosterone levels (is transient), may produce extrapyramidal symptoms, and is an antiemetic. The antiemetic effect may be due to antagonism of central and peripheral dopamine receptors which produce N&V by stimulating the chemoreceptor trigger zone.

Pharmacokinetics

Rapidly and well absorbed after PO administration; relative bioavailability about 8%. **Onset, IV:** 1–3 min; **IM:** 10–15 min; **PO:** 30–60 min. **Peak plasma levels, after PO:** 1–2 hr. **Duration:** 1–2 hr. **t½, elimination:** 5–6 hr. Significant first-pass effect following PO use; unchanged drug and metabolites excreted in urine. Renal impairment decreases clearance of the drug. In children, the pharmacodynamics of both PO and IV use are highly variable. **Plasma protein binding:** About 30%.

M

CONTRAINDICATIONS

Known sensitivity to the drug or components of the product. Gastrointestinal hemorrhage, obstruction, or perforation; epilepsy; clients taking drugs likely to cause extrapyramidal symptoms, such as phenothiazines (severity of seizures or extrapyramidal reactions may be increased). Pheochromocytoma (drug may cause hypertensive crisis).

SPECIAL CONCERNS

■ (1) Treatment with metoclopramide can cause tardive dyskinesia, a serious movement disorder that is often irreversible. The risk of developing tardive dyskinesia increases with duration of treatment and cumulative dose. (2) Discontinue metoclopramide therapy in clients who develop signs or symptoms of tardive dyskinesia. There is no known treatment for tardive dyskinesia. In some clients, symptoms may lessen or resolve after metoclopramide treatment is stopped. (3) Avoid treatment with metoclopramide for longer than 12 weeks in all but rare cases in which therapeutic benefit is thought to outweigh the risk of developing tardive dyskinesia. ■

- **Use with caution during lactation and in hypertension.**
- **Extrapyramidal effects more likely to occur in children and geriatric clients.**
- **Safety and efficacy not established in children except to facilitate small bowel intubation. Use with care in neonates due to possibility of increased serum levels.**

SIDE EFFECTS

Most Common

Extrapyramidal symptoms, restlessness, drowsiness, fatigue, lassitude, akathisia, dizziness, nausea, diarrhea.

CNS: Restlessness, drowsiness, fatigue, lassitude, akathisia (including feelings of anxiety, agitation, jitteriness, insomnia, inability to sit still, pacing, foot-tapping), confusion, headaches, dizziness, extrapyramidal symptoms (especially acute dystonic reactions including facial grimacing, torticollis, oculogyric crisis, rhythmic protrusion of the tongue, bulbar type of speech, trismus, opisthotonos, stridor, dyspnea), Parkinson-like symptoms (including cogwheel rigidity, mask-like facies, bradykinesia, tremor), dystonia, myoclonus, ***depression (with suicidal ideation and suicide)***, tardive dyskinesia (including involuntary movements of the tongue, face, mouth, or jaw), ***seizures***, hallucinations (rare). **GI:** Nausea, bowel disturbances (usually diarrhea), **Hepatic:** Hepatotoxicity (including jaundice, altered LFTs), porphyria. **CV:** Hypertension (may lead to hypertensive crisis), hypotension, SVT, bradycardia, acute CHF, AV block. **Hematologic: *Agranulocytosis***, leukopenia, neutropenia, sulfhemoglobinemia (in adults). Methemoglobinemia in premature and full-term infants at doses of 1–4 mg/kg/day IM, IV, or PO for 1–3 or more days. **Endocrine:** Galactorrhea, amenorrhea, gynecomastia, impotence (due to hyperprolactinemia), fluid retention (due to transient elevation of aldosterone). **Neuroleptic malignant syndrome: *Hyperthermia***, altered consciousness, autonomic dysfunction, muscle rigidity, ***death***. **Allergic:** Rash, urticaria, bronchospasm (especially with a history of asthma), angioneurotic edema (including glossal or laryngeal edema—

rare). **GU:** Urinary frequency, incontinence. **Ophthalmic:** Visual disturbances. **Miscellaneous:** Flushing of the face and upper body.

OVERDOSE MANAGEMENT

Symptoms: Agitation, irritability, hypertonia of muscles, drowsiness, disorientation, EPS. *Treatment:* Treat extrapyramidal effects by giving anticholinergic drugs, antiparkinson drugs, or antihistamines with anticholinergic effects. General supportive treatment. Reverse methemoglobinemia by giving methylene blue.

DRUG INTERACTIONS

Acetaminophen / ↑ Acetaminophen absorption from the small intestine
Alcohol / ↑ Absorption of alcohol R/T ↓ time for alcohol to reach the small intestine where it is rapidly absorbed; also, additive CNS depression
Anticholinergics / ↓ Metoclopramide effect
Cimetidine / Bioavailability of cimetidine may be ↓ R/T ↓ absorption as a result of faster gastric transit time
CNS depressants (e.g., hypnotics, sedatives, tranquilizers) / Additive sedative effects
Cyclosporine / ↑ Cyclosporine absorption R/T faster gastric emptying time → ↑ immunosuppressive and toxic effects
Digoxin / ↓ Digoxin effect R/T ↓ GI tract absorption; capsules, elixir, and tablets with a high dissolution rate are least affected
Insulin / Possible action of insulin before food leaves the stomach → hypoglycemia
Levodopa / ↑ Levodopa GI absorption and ↓ metoclopramide effects on gastric emptying and lower esophageal pressure; metoclopramide is relatively contraindicated in Parkinson's clients
MAOIs / ↑ Release of catecholamines → toxicity; use metoclopramide with caution, if at all, with MAOI use
Narcotic analgesics / ↓ Metoclopramide effect; also, additive CNS depressant effects
Sertraline / Possible serotonin syndrome with EPS
Succinylcholine / ↑ Succinylcholine effect R/T plasma cholinesterase inhibition
Tetracyclines / ↑ Tetracycline GI absorption from the small intestine
Venlafaxine / Possible serotonin syndrome with EPS

HOW SUPPLIED

Injection: 5 mg/mL; ***Syrup:*** 5 mg/5 mL; ***Tablets:*** 5 mg, 10 mg; ***Tablets, Oral Disintegrating (Metozolv ODT):*** 5 mg, 10 mg.

DOSAGE

SYRUP; TABLETS; TABLETS, ORALLY DISINTEGRATING

Symptomatic gastroesophageal reflux.

Adults, usual: 10–15 mg 4 times per day, 30 min before meals and at bedtime. If symptoms occur only intermittently, single doses up to 20 mg prior to the provoking situation may be used. Avoid treatment longer than 12 weeks except in rare cases where the benefit is believed to counterbalance the risks to the client of developing tardive dyskinesia. *NOTE:* Elderly clients and those who are more sensitive to the therapeutic or side effects of metoclopramide should receive 5 mg/dose.

Diabetic gastroparesis.

Adults: 10 mg 30 min before meals and at bedtime up to 4 times/day for 2–8 weeks, depending on response and the likelihood of continued well-being after the drug is discontinued. Do not exceed 12 weeks of therapy.

Gastroparesis in adults (investigational).

Adults: 10–20 mg PO 4 times/day 30 min before meals and bedtime for 2–8 weeks as adjunctive therapy.

Prophylaxis and treatment of hiccoughs (investigational).

Prophylaxis. Adults: 10 mg PO q 6–8 hr starting the day of or 1 day before the anticipated hiccough-precipitating event. **Treatment. Adults:** 10 mg PO q 6–8 hr. Therapy may begin with parenteral dosing (5–10 mg IV or IM q 8 hr) and then transition to PO dosing when hiccoughs are controlled.

Enhance lactation (investigational).

Adults: 10–15 mg 3 times/day for 2 weeks.

IM; IV

Prophylaxis of vomiting due to emetogenic cancer chemotherapy.

Adults, initial: 2 mg/kg IV if highly emetogenic drugs such as cisplatin or dacarbazine are used alone or in combination. For less emetogenic regiments, 1 mg/kg may be adequate. Give 30 min before beginning cancer chemotherapy

M

and repeat q 2 hr for 2 dose; **then,** q 3 hr for 3 doses. Inject slowly IV over 15 min.

Prophylaxis of postoperative N&V.

Adults: 10–20 mg IM near the end of surgery.

Facilitate small bowel intubation.

Adults: If the tube has not passed the pylorus with conventional maneuvers in 10 min, give a single dose (undiluted) of 10 mg slowly by IV over 1–2 min. **Pediatric, age 14 years and older:** Use adult dose; **pediatric, 6–14 years:** If the tube has not passed the pylorus with conventional maneuvers in 10 min, give a single dose (undiluted) of 2.5–5 mg slowly IV over 1–2 min; **pediatric, less than 6 years:** If the tube has not passed the pylorus with conventional maneuvers in 10 min, give a single dose (undiluted) of 0.1 mg/kg slowly IV over 1–2 min.

Radiologic examinations to increase intestinal transit time.

Adults: 10 mg as a single dose given IV over 1–2 min.

Diabetic gastroparesis.

Adults, usual: 10 mg given by slow IV over 1–2 min. Up to 10 days may be required before symptoms subside; then, PO therapy may be instituted.

Treatment of migraine in adults (investigational).

Adults: 10 mg infused over 15 min IV. A 20 mg dose given IV has also been investigated.

NURSING IMPLICATIONS

Ⓢ Do not confuse metoclopramide with metoprolol (a beta-adrenergic blocker) or with metolazone (a thiazide diuretic).

IMPLEMENTATION/ADMINISTRATION/STORAGE

1. Determine route of administration to treat diabetic gastroparesis by the severity of symptoms. With only the earliest symptoms, begin PO therapy. If symptoms are severe, begin with parenteral therapy. Administer 10 mg over 1–2 min.
2. If C_{CR} is <40 mL/min, begin therapy at approximately one-half the recommended dosage. Depending on efficacy and safety, the dose may be increased or decreased as needed.
3. After PO use, absorption of certain drugs from the GI tract may be affected (see *Drug Interactions*).
4. For outpatient treatment when PO dosing is not possible, suppositories containing 25 mg metoclopramide have been made extemporaneously. Give 1 suppository 30–60 min before each meal and at bedtime.
5. IV Inject undiluted solutions of 10 mg slowly IV over 1–2 min to prevent transient feelings of anxiety/restlessness followed by drowsiness.
6. For doses in excess of 10 mg, dilute in 50 mL of sodium chloride injection. Inject slowly over a period of not less than 15 min.
7. If extrapyramidal symptoms occur after parenteral use, inject diphenhydramine, 50 mg IM.
8. Store PO and IV from from 20–25°C (68–77°F). Store vials in their carton until use. Do not store open single-dose vials for later use, as they contain no preservative. Dilutions may be stored unprotected from light up to 24 hr after preparation.
9. COMPATIBILITY Give undiluted or with sodium chloride injections.
10. INCOMPATIBILITY Cephalothin, chloramphenicol, sodium bicarbonate. Metoclopramide is physically/chemically incompatible with a number of drugs; check package insert if drug is to be admixed.

ASSESSMENT

1. Note reasons for therapy, type, onset, characteristics of S&S. List drugs prescribed, ensuring none interact.
2. Assess for any tardive dyskinesia (repetitive, involuntary, purposeless movements of face and extremities). Stop drug as this may be irreversible.
3. During IV therapy if dystonic movements noted, give diphenhydramine IV/IM and report.
4. Assess abdomen for bowel sounds, distention, N&V. Monitor BP, HR, and LFTs.

CLIENT/FAMILY TEACHING

1. Take as directed 30 min before meals; may dilute syrup in water, juice or carbonated beverage just before taking.

2. Take the orally disintegrating tablets on an empty stomach at least 30 min before eating because food can decrease peak levels of the drug in the bloodstream and/or the time it takes to reach maximum drug levels in the bloodstream. Do not repeat the dose if taken inadvertantly with food.
3. Because the orally disintegrating tablets absorb moisture rapidly, remove each dose from the package just prior to taking. Handle the tablet with dry hands and place on the tongue. If the tablet should break or crumble while handling, discard and remove a new tablet. Do not take with any liquid; tablets are designed to disintegrate on the tongue in about 1 minute (range of 10 seconds to 14 min).
4. Drug increases movements/contractions of the stomach and intestines.
5. Do not operate a car or hazardous machinery until drug effects realized; drug has a sedative effect up to 2 hr after dosing.
6. Avoid alcohol and CNS depressants.
7. Extrapyramidal effects (trembling hands, facial grimacing) should be reported; may be treated with parenteral diphenhydramine.
8. Keep all F/U to assess response and for adverse SE.

OUTCOMES/EVALUATE

- Prevention of N&V
- Enhanced gastric motility
- Promotion of gastric emptying
- Prophylaxis of gastric bezoars

Metolazone

(meh-**TOH**-lah-zohn)

Classification(s): Diuretic, thiazide

Pregnancy Category: B

RX: Zaroxolyn.

SEE ALSO ***DIURETICS, THIAZIDE.***

INDICATIONS/USES

(1) Treatment of mild to moderate hypertension alone or in combination with other drugs of a different class. (2) Treatment of salt and water retention, including edema accompanying CHF, edema accompanying renal diseases, including the nephrotic syndrome and states of diminished renal function. *Investigational:* Diuretic in children, osteoporosis, diabetes insipidus.

ACTION/KINETICS

Pharmacokinetics

Onset: 1 hr. **Peak blood levels:** 2–4 hr; **t½, elimination:** About 14 hr. **Duration:** 24 hr or more. Most excreted unchanged through the urine.

CONTRAINDICATIONS

Anuria, prehepatic and hepatic coma, allergy or hypersensitivity to metolazone. Routine use during pregnancy. Lactation.

SPECIAL CONCERNS

- Use with caution in severely impaired renal function and in the elderly.
- Safety and efficacy not determined in children.

SIDE EFFECTS

Most Common

Dizziness, headache, muscle cramps, malaise, lethargy, lassitude, joint pain/swelling, chest pain.

See *Diuretics, Thiazide* for a complete list of possible side effects. Also, ***toxic epidermal necrolysis*** and ***Stevens-Johnson syndrome.***

ADDITIONAL DRUG INTERACTIONS

Alcohol / ↑ Hypotensive effect
Barbiturates / ↑ Hypotensive effect
Narcotics / ↑ Hypotensive effect
NSAIDs / ↓ Hypotensive effect of metolazone
Salicylates / ↓ Hypotensive effect of metolazone

HOW SUPPLIED

Tablets: 2.5 mg, 5 mg, 10 mg.

DOSAGE

TABLETS

Hypertension.

Adults: 2.5–5 mg once daily.

Salt and water retention.

Adults: 5–20 mg once daily. For those who experience paroxysmal nocturnal dyspnea, a larger dose may be required to ensure prolonged diuresis and saluresis for a 24-hr period. **Children (investigational):** 0.2–0.4 mg/kg/day given once a day or in 2 divided doses.

NURSING IMPLICATIONS

Do not confuse metolazone with methotrexate (an antineoplastic) or with metoclopramide (a GI stimulant).

IMPLEMENTATION/ADMINISTRATION/STORAGE

1. The antihypertensive effect may be observed from 3–4 days to 3–6 weeks.
2. If other antihypertensive drugs or diuretics are given together with metolazone, more careful dosage adjustment may be necessary.
3. Reduce the dose or discontinue if side effects are moderate or severe.
4. Store tablets from 15–30°C (59–86°F); protect from light.

ASSESSMENT

1. Note reasons for therapy, onset, duration, clinical characteristics; has synergistic effect with furosemide.
2. List drugs prescribed to ensure none interact. Assess for sulfonamide allergy.
3. Monitor Wt, BP, ECG, CBC, electrolytes, BS, Ca^{++}, uric acid, renal and LFTs; assess for S&S of electrolyte imbalance (i.e., ↓ Na^+/K^+/Mg^{++}/P and hypochloremic alkalosis).

M

CLIENT/FAMILY TEACHING

1. Take with/without food exactly as directed; early in the day to prevent nighttime awakening for urination.
2. May cause sudden drop in BP and syncope; use caution and change positions slowly. Avoid alcohol during therapy.
3. Record BP and check weight regularly; report increases of more than 3 lb/day or 5 lb/week or lack of response to extremity swelling.
4. Avoid exposure to sun or bright lights; may cause photosensitivity.
5. May cause potassium depletion; eat a K^+-rich diet (whole grain cereals, legumes, meat, bananas, apricots, orange juice, potatoes, raisins); report S&S of hypokalemia (muscle weakness, cramping).
6. Keep all F/U to assess response, labs, and for adverse SE.

OUTCOMES/EVALUATE

- ↓ Edema
- ↓ BP

Metoprolol succinate

(me-toe-**PROH**-lohl)

Classification(s): Beta-adrenergic blocking agent

Pregnancy Category: C

RX: Toprol XL.

Metoprolol tartrate

Pregnancy Category: B

RX: Lopressor.

Rx: Apo-Metoprolol, Apo-Metoprolol SR, Betaloc, Betaloc Durules, Gen-Metoprolol (Type L), Novo-Metoprol, Nu-Metop, PMS-Metoprolol-L, Sandoz Metoprolol (Type L).

SEE ALSO ***BETA-ADRENERGIC BLOCKING AGENTS***.

INDICATIONS/USES

Metoprolol Succinate: (1) Alone or with other drugs to treat hypertension. (2) Chronic management of angina pectoris. (3) Treatment of stable, symptomatic (NYHA Class II or III) heart failure of ischemic, hypertensive, or cardiomyopathic origin. *Investigational:* Prophylaxis of migraine in adults (both succinate and tartrate).

Metoprolol Tartrate, PO: (1) Hypertension (either alone or with other antihypertensive agents, such as thiazide diuretics). (2) To reduce CV mortality in hemodynamically stable clients with definite or suspected acute MI. (3) Long-term treatment of angina pectoris. **IV:** To reduce CV mortality in hemodynamically stable clients with definite or suspected acute MI. Begin treatment as soon as the clinical condition allows.

ACTION/KINETICS

Action

Combines reversibly mainly with $beta_1$-adrenergic receptors to block the response to sympathetic nerve impulses, circulating catecholamines, or adrenergic drugs. Blockade of beta-1 receptors decreases HR, myocardial contractility, and CO and slows AV conduction, all of which lead to a decrease in BP. Beta-1 activity is diminished as the dose is increased. Beta-2 receptors are blocked at high doses. Has no membrane-stabilizing or intrinsic sympathomimetic effects.

Pharmacokinetics

Moderate lipid solubility. **Onset:** 15 min. **Peak plasma levels:** 90 min. **t½:** 3–7 hr. Effect of drug is cumulative. Food increases bioavailability. Exhibits significant first-pass effect. Metabolized in liver and excreted in urine.

ADDITIONAL CONTRAINDICATIONS

Myocardial infarction in clients with an HR of less than 45 bpm, in second- or third-degree heart block, or if SBP is less than 100 mm Hg. Moderate to severe cardiac failure.

SPECIAL CONCERNS

Ischemic heart disease. Following abrupt cessation of therapy with certain beta-blocking agents, exacerbations of angina pectoris and, in some cases, myocardial infarction have occurred. When discontinuing chronically administered metoprolol, particularly in clients with ischemic heart disease, gradually reduce the dosage over a period of 1 to 2 weeks and carefully monitor the client. If angina markedly worsens or acute coronary insufficiency develops, reinstate metoprolol administration promptly, at least temporarily, and take other measures appropriate for the management of unstable angina. Warn clients against interruption or discontinuation of therapy without the physician's advice. Because coronary artery disease is common and may be unrecognized, it may be prudent not to discontinue metoprolol therapy abruptly, even in clients treated only for hypertension.

- **Safety and efficacy not established in children.**
- **Use with caution in impaired hepatic function and during lactation.**

SIDE EFFECTS

Most Common

Fatigue, dizziness, depression, shortness of breath, bradycardia, diarrhea.

See *Beta-Adrenergic Blocking Agents* for a complete list of possible side effects.

LABORATORY TEST CONSIDERATIONS

↑ Serum transaminase, LDH, alkaline phosphatase.

ADDITIONAL DRUG INTERACTIONS

Cimetidine / May ↑ plasma metoprolol levels
Contraceptives, oral / May ↑ metoprolol effects
Diphenhydramine / ↓ Metoprolol clearance → prolonged negative chronotropic and inotropic effects in extensive metabolizers
Hydroxychloroquine / ↑ Bioavailability of metoprolol in homozygous extensive metabolizers
Methimazole / May ↓ metoprolol effects
Phenobarbital / ↓ Metoprolol effect R/T ↑ liver metabolism
Propylthiouracil / May ↓ metoprolol effects
Quinidine / May ↑ metoprolol effects
Rifampin / ↓ Metoprolol effect R/T ↑ liver metabolism

HOW SUPPLIED

Metoprolol succinate. *Tablets, Extended-Release:* 25 mg, 50 mg, 100 mg, 200 mg (all are equivalent to metoprolol tartrate).

Metoprolol tartrate. *Injection:* 1 mg/mL; *Tablets:* 25 mg, 50 mg, 100 mg.

DOSAGE

Metoprolol Succinate

TABLETS, EXTENDED-RELEASE

Hypertension.

Initial: 50–100 mg/day in a single dose with or without a diuretic. Dosage may be increased in weekly intervals until maximum effect is reached. Doses above 400 mg/day have not been studied.

Angina pectoris.

Individualized, Initial: 100 mg/day in a single dose. Dose may be increased slowly, at weekly intervals, until optimum effect is reached or there is a pronounced slowing of HR. Doses above 400 mg/day have not been studied. If the drug is to be discontinued, reduce dosage gradually over a period of 1 to 2 weeks.

Congestive heart failure.

Individualize dose. **Initial:** 25 mg once daily for 2 weeks in clients with NYHA Class II heart failure and 12.5 mg once daily in those with more severe heart failure. Double the dose q 2 weeks to the highest dose level tolerated or up to 200 mg.

Metoprolol Tartrate

TABLETS

Hypertension.

Adults, initial: 100 mg/day in single or divided doses; **then,** dose may be increased weekly to maintenance level of 100–450 mg/day. A diuretic may also be used. The dose may be increased at weekly (or longer) intervals until optimum BP reduction occurs. The maximum effect of any change in dose will be apparent within 1 week.

Long-term treatment of angina pectoris.

Adults, initial: 100 mg/day in 2 divided doses. Dose may be increased gradually at weekly intervals until optimum response is obtained or a pronounced slowing of HR occurs. Effective dose range: 100–400 mg/day. If treatment is to be discontinued, reduce dose gradually over 1–2 weeks.

Prophylaxis of migraine (Investigational).

100–200 mg daily.

INJECTION (IV); TABLETS

Early and maintenance treatment of Myocardial Infarction (MI).

Three IV bolus injections of 5 mg each at approximately 2 min intervals. If clients tolerate the full IV dose, give 50 mg tablets q 6 hr PO beginning 15 min after the last IV dose (or as soon as client's condition allows). This dose is continued for 48 hr followed by 100 mg tablets twice a day as soon as feasible (see *Late Treatment of MI*). In clients who do not tolerate the full IV dose, begin with 25–50 mg tablets q 6 hr PO beginning 15 min after the last IV dose or as soon as client's condition allows.

Late treatment of MI.

Clients with contraindications to treatment during the early phase of suspected or definite MI, those who appear not to tolerate the full early treatment, and those in whom the health care provider wishes to delay therapy for any other reason, should be started on metoprolol tablets, 100 mg twice a day, as soon as their clinical condition allows. Continue therapy for at least 3 months. However, therapy may be continued for 1 to 3 years.

NURSING IMPLICATIONS

Do not confuse metoprolol with metoclopramide (GI stimulant), metaproterenol (bronchodilator), or with misoprostol (prostaglandin derivative). Also, do not confuse Toprol-XL with Topamax (an antiepileptic, antimigraine drug) or Tegretol and Tegretol-XR (an antiepileptic).

IMPLEMENTATION/ADMINISTRATION/STORAGE

1. Individualize the dosage.
2. Once-daily dosing is effective and can maintain a reduction in BP throughout the day. However, lower doses (e.g., 100 mg) may not maintain a full effect at the end of a 24 hr period; larger or more frequent daily doses may be needed.
3. If transient worsening of heart failure occurs, treat with increased doses of diuretics. May need to lower dose of metoprolol or temporarily discontinue.
4. For CHF, do not increase dose until symptoms of worsening CHF have been stabilized. Initial difficulty with titration should not preclude attempts later to use metoprolol. Prior to beginning metoprolol extended-release tablets, stabilize the dosage of ACE inhibitors, diuretics, and digitalis, if any are used.
5. During the early phase of definite or suspected acute MI, metoprolol treatment can be initiated as soon as possible after arrival at the hospital. Initiate treatment in a coronary care or similar unit immediately after the hemodynamic condition has been stabilized. If CHF clients experience symptomatic bradycardia, reduce dose.
6. When switching from immediate-release tablets to extended-release tablets, the same total daily dose of metoprolol should be used.
7. Store tablets from 15–30°C (59–86°F); protect from moisture. Store the injection below 30°C (86°F); protect from light.
8. IV IV bolus injection undiluted of 5 mg given slowly (over 1 min) during acute MI; may be repeated slowly every 2 min up to 15 mg. During the IV use of metoprolol, carefully monitor BP, HR, and ECG.
9. COMPATIBILITY Give undiluted.

10. INCOMPATIBILITY Administer separately.

ASSESSMENT

1. Note reasons for therapy: ↑ BP, headache, angina/CAD, recent MI (NYHA class) and clinical response.
2. Assess for asthma, emphysema, depression, myasthenia gravis, circulation problems, CHF, or greater than 1° AVB, thyroid, liver or kidney disorders; may preclude drug therapy.
3. Monitor VS, EF, CXR, CBC, liver/renal function studies, ECG, echocardiogram. Hold if HR <50, and assess rhythm.

CLIENT/FAMILY TEACHING

1. Take at same time each day; do not stop suddenly: reduce dose gradually over 1–2 weeks.
2. Take with food. Do not crush or chew the extended-release products; swallow tablets whole.
3. Avoid activities that require mental alertness until drug effects realized; may cause drowsiness. Alcohol may intensify these effects.
4. Before taking any OTC agents, obtain medical advice; some may affect action of metoprolol.
5. Continue with low fat/cholesterol/salt diet, regular exercise, and weight loss in the overall goal of BP control. Record BP and HR for review.
6. Report any symptoms of fluid overload such as sudden weight gain, SOB, or swelling of extremities. Avoid salt.
7. Dress appropriately; may cause an increased sensitivity to cold. Do not smoke.
8. Keep all F/U to assess response, Wt, BP, and HR readings (report heart rate <50 or irregular) and adverse SE.

OUTCOMES/EVALUATE

- ↓ BP; ↓ anginal attacks
- Prevention of myocardial reinfarction and associated mortality

Metronidazole

IV

(meh-troh-**NYE**-dah-zohl)

Classification(s): Trichomonacide, amebicide
Pregnancy Category: B

RX: Injection: Metronidazole, Metronidazole in Sodium Chloride. **PO**: Flagyl, Flagyl 375, Flagyl ER, Metric 21, Protostat. **Topical**: MetroCream, MetroGel, MetroLotion, Noritate, Vitazol. **Vaginal Gel/Jelly**: MetroGel Vaginal, Vandazole.

✤ **Rx:** Apo-Metronidazole, NidaGel.

SEE ALSO ***ANTI-INFECTIVE DRUGS.***

INDICATIONS/USES

Systemic:

1. Serious infections due to susceptible anaerobic bacteria, including *Bacteroides fragilis* resistant to clindamycin, chloramphenicol, and penicillin.
2. Peritonitis, intra-abdominal abscess and liver abscess due to *B. fragilis, B. distasonis, B. ovatus, B. thetaiotaomicron, B. vulgatus, Clostridium* species, *Eubacterium* species, *Peptostreptococcus* species, and *Peptococcus niger.*
3. Skin and skin structure infections due to *Bacteroides* species including *B. fragilis* group, *Clostridium* species, *Peptostreptococcus* species, *Fusobacterium* species, and *Peptococcus niger.*
4. Endometritis, endomyometritis, tubo-ovarian abscess, and postsurgical vaginal cuff infection due to *Bacteroides* species including the *B. fragilis* group, *Clostridium* species, *Peptococcus* species, and *Peptostreptococcus* species.
5. Bacterial vaginosis (use Flagyl ER only). Symptomatic trichomoniasis in males and females (endocervicitis, cervicitis, cervical erosion).
6. Bacterial septicemia due to *Bacteroides* species including the *B. fragilis* group and *Clostridium* species.
7. Adjunct therapy to treat bone and joint infections due to *Bacteroides* species including the *B. fragilis* group.
8. Meningitis and brain abscess due to *Bacteroides* species including the *B. fragilis* group.
9. Pneumonia, empyema, and lung abscess due to *Bacteroides* species including the *B. fragilis* group.
10. Endocarditis due to *Bacteroides* species including the *B. fragilis* group.
11. Amebiasis. Symptomatic and asymptomatic trichomoniasis; to treat asymptomatic partner.
12. To reduce postoperative anaerobic infection following colorectal surgery, elective hysterectomy, and emergency appendectomy.

M

13. As part of combination therapy to eradicate *Helicobacter pylori* infections.
14. Hepatic encephalopathy.
15. Crohn's disease.
16. Diarrhea associated with *Clostridium difficile.*
17. Recurrent and persistent urethritis.
18. Pelvic inflammatory disease as an alternative parenteral regimen.
19. Prophylaxis after sexual assault.
20. Bacterial vaginosis.

Investigational: Giardiasis, *Gardnerella vaginalis.*

Topical: Inflammatory papules, pustules, and erythema of rosacea. *Investigational:* Infected decubitus ulcers (use gel or 1% solution or suspension). Perioral dermatitis using the topical cream or gel.

Vaginal: Bacterial vaginosis.

ACTION/KINETICS

Action

Effective against anaerobic bacteria and protozoa. Specifically inhibits growth of trichomonae and amoebae by binding to DNA, resulting in loss of helical structure, strand breakage, inhibition of nucleic acid synthesis, and cell death. The mechanism for its effectiveness in reducing the inflammatory lesions of acne rosacea is not known but may include an antibacterial or anti-inflammatory effect.

Pharmacokinetics

Well absorbed from GI tract and widely distributed in body tissues. Rate of absorption of extended-release tablet is increased in the fed state resulting in alteration of the extended-release characteristics. **Peak serum concentration, PO:** 6–40 mcg/mL, depending on the dose, after 1–2 hr. **$t_{1/2}$, PO:** 6–12 hr; average: 8 hr. $t_{1/2}$ is inversely related to gestational age in newborns. Eliminated primarily in urine (20% unchanged), which may be red-brown in color following either PO or IV use. Is minimally absorbed after topical use.

CONTRAINDICATIONS

Blood dyscrasias, active organic disease of the CNS, trichomoniasis during the first trimester of pregnancy, lactation. Is carcinogenic in rodents; avoid unnecessary use. Topical use if hypersensitive to parabens or other ingredients of the formulation. Consumption of alcohol during use. For the vaginal gel, hypersensitivity to the drug, parabens, or other.

SPECIAL CONCERNS

Metronidazole is carcinogenic in rats; avoid unnecessary use.

- **Use with caution in those with evidence or history of blood dyscrasias or in those with impaired hepatic function.**
- **Safety and efficacy have not been established in children except for treating amebiasis.**
- **Those with candidiasis may show more pronounced symptoms during metronidazole therapy; treat with a candicidal drug.**

SIDE EFFECTS

Most Common

Following topical use: Erythema, contact dermatitis, local allergic reaction.

Systemic Use. GI: Nausea, metallic taste, abdominal pain, diarrhea, dry mouth, anorexia, vomiting, epigastric distress, abdominal cramping, constipation, proctitis, modification of the taste of alcoholic beverages, furry tongue, glossitis, stomatitis, ***pancreatitis*** (rare). **CNS:** Headache, dizziness, vertigo, incoordination, ataxia, confusion, irritability, depression, weakness, insomnia, syncope, ***seizures***, peripheral neuropathy, including paresthesia. **CV:** Flattening of the T-wave in ECG tracings, thrombophlebitis after IV infusion. **GU:** Vaginitis, genital pruritus, abnormal urine, dysmenorrhea, UTI, dysuria, cystitis, polyuria, incontinence, sense of pelvic pressure, proliferation of *Candida* in the vagina, dyspareunia, decreased libido, dark brown color to urine. **Hematologic:** Leukopenia (reversible), reversible thrombocytopenia (rare). **Respiratory:** URTI, rhinitis, sinusitis, pharyngitis. **Hypersensitivity:** Urticaria, erythematous rash, flushing, nasal congestion, dry mouth/vagina/vulva, fever. **Body as a whole:** Bacterial infection, flu-like symptoms, moniliasis. **Miscellaneous:** Fleeting joint pain sometimes resembling serum sickness.

Topical Use. Dermatologic: Acne, burning/stinging, contact dermatitis, dryness, erythema, local allergic reaction, metallic taste, pruritus, rash, skin irritation, tingling/numbness of extremities, severe flare of comedonal acne, transient redness, worsening of rosacea. **GI:** Nausea, constipation, metallic taste. **CNS:** Headache, paresthesia. **Ophthalmic:** Conjunctivitis, watery eyes if gel applied too closely to this area.

Vaginal Use. GI: Nausea, metallic taste, abdominal pain, diarrhea, dry mouth. **CNS:** Headache, dizziness. **GU:** Vaginitis, genital pruritus, abnormal urine, dysmenorrhea, UTI. **Respiratory:** URTI, rhinitis, sinusitis, pharyngitis **Body as a whole:** Bacterial infection, flu-like symptoms, moniliasis.

LABORATORY TEST CONSIDERATIONS

May interfere with chemical analyses for AST, ALT, LDH, triglycerides, and glucose hexokinase; zero values may result.

OVERDOSE MANAGEMENT

Symptoms: Ataxia, N&V, peripheral neuropathy, ***seizures*** up to 5–7 days. *Treatment:* Supportive treatment.

DRUG INTERACTIONS

Barbiturates / Possible therapeutic failure of metronidazole R/T ↑ elimination
Busulfan / ↑ Busulfan trough plasma levels; ↑ risk of toxicity
Cimetidine / ↑ Serum metronidazole levels R/T ↓ clearance
Coumarin / ↑ Anticoagulant effect → prolonged prothrombin time
Disulfiram / Concurrent use may cause confusion or acute psychosis; do not give metronidazole to clients who have taken disulfiram within the past 2 weeks
Ethanol / Possible disulfiram-like reaction, including flushing, palpitations, tachycardia, and N&V
Hydantoins / ↑ Hydantoins effect R/T ↓ clearance
Lithium / ↑ Lithium levels and toxicity
Phenytoin / Possible therapeutic failure of metronidazole R/T ↑ elimination
Warfarin / ↑ Anticoagulant effect → prolonged prothrombin time

HOW SUPPLIED

Capsules: 375 mg; ***Cream, Topical:*** 0.75%, 1%; ***Gel, Topical:*** 0.75%, 1%; ***Injection:*** 5 mg/mL; ***Lotion:*** 0.75%; ***Tablets:*** 250 mg, 500 mg; ***Tablets, Extended-Release:*** 750 mg; ***Vaginal Gel/Jelly:*** 0.75%.

DOSAGE

CAPSULES; TABLETS

Amebiasis: Acute amebic dysentery or amebic liver abscess.

Adult: 500–750 mg 3 times per day for 5–10 days; **pediatric:** 35–50 mg/kg/day in three divided doses for 10 days.

Trichomoniasis, female.

Female: 250 mg if using tablets 3 times per day for 7 days, 2 grams given on 1 day in single or divided doses, or 375 mg if using capsules twice a day for 7 days. **Pediatric:** 5 mg/kg 3 times per day for 7 days. An interval of 4–6 weeks should elapse between courses of therapy. *NOTE:* Do not treat pregnant women during the first trimester. **Male:** Individualize dosage; usual, 250 mg 3 times per day for 7 days.

Treat Helicobacter pylori *infections.*

One of the following regimens may be used: (1) Metronidazole, 500 mg twice a day; clarithromycin, 500 mg twice a day; and, either lansoprazole, 30 mg twice a day or omeprazole, 20 mg twice a day. All drugs given with meals for 2 weeks. (2) Metronidazole, 500 mg twice a day for 2 weeks, or amoxicillin, 1 gram twice a day for 2 weeks, or tetracycline, 500 mg twice a day for 2 weeks; plus, clarithromycin, 500 mg twice a day for 2 weeks and ranitidine bismuth citrate, 400 mg twice a day for 2 weeks. (3) Tetracycline, 500 mg 4 times per day; metronidazole, 500 mg 3 times per day for 2 weeks with meals and at bedtime; bismuth subsalicylate, 525 mg 4 times per day with meals and at bedtime for 2 weeks; and, either lansoprazole, 30 mg once daily for 2 weeks or omeprazole, 20 mg once daily for 2 weeks. (4) Tetracycline, 500 mg 4 times per day for 2 weeks; metronidazole, 250 mg 4 times per day with meals and at bedtime for 1 week; bismuth subsalicylate, 525 mg 4 times per day with meals and at bedtime for 2 weeks; and, a H_2-receptor antagonist as directed for 2 or more weeks. (5) Amoxicillin, 1 gram twice a day with meals; metronidazole, 500 mg twice a day with meals; and, omeprazole, 20 mg twice a day before meals. Each drug is given for 2 weeks.

Giardiasis.

250 mg 3 times per day for 7 days.

G. vaginalis.

500 mg twice a day for 7 days.

TABLETS, EXTENDED-RELEASE

Bacterial vaginosis.

One 750-mg tablet per day for 7 days.

IV

Anaerobic bacterial infections.

Adults, initially: 15 mg/kg infused over 1 hr; **then,** after 6 hr, 7.5 mg/kg q 6 hr for 7–10 days (daily dose should not exceed 4 grams). Treatment may be necessary for 2–3 weeks, although PO therapy should be initiated as soon as possible.

Prophylaxis of anaerobic infection during surgery.

Adults: 15 mg/kg given over a 30- to 60-min period, with completion 1 hr prior to surgery and 7.5 mg/kg infused over 30–60 min 6 and 12 hr after the initial dose.

TOPICAL CREAM; TOPICAL GEL; TOPICAL LOTION

Rosacea.

After washing, apply a thin film and rub in well either once (1% cream or gel) daily or twice a day in the morning and evening for 4–9 weeks.

VAGINAL GEL (0.75%)

Bacterial vaginosis.

One applicatorful (5 grams which contains 37.5 mg metronidazole) once or twice daily for 5 days. Metro-Gel Vaginal allows for once-daily dosing at bedtime.

NURSING IMPLICATIONS

(Sound Alike Drug) Do not confuse metronidazole with metformin (an oral hypoglycemic).

IMPLEMENTATION/ADMINISTRATION/STORAGE

1. Reduce dose in those with hepatic disease. Dosage reduction may be necessary in geriatric clients.
2. For topical use, therapeutic results should be seen within 3 weeks with continuing improvement through 9 weeks of therapy.
3. Metronidazole used vaginally may be absorbed in sufficient quantities to produce systemic effects.
4. Cosmetics may be used after application of topical metronidazole.
5. Store the 0.75% cream and gel from 15–30°C (59–86°F) and the 1% cream and 1% gel from 20–25°C (68–77°F).
6. **IV** Do not give by IV bolus. Administer each single dose over 1 hr.
7. Do not use syringes with Al needles or hubs.
8. Discontinue primary IV infusion during infusion of metronidazole.
9. The order of mixing to prepare powder for injection is important:
   - Reconstitute.
   - Dilute in IV solutions in glass or plastic containers.
   - Neutralize pH with $NaHCO_3$ solution. Do not refrigerate neutralized solutions.
10. Premixed, ready-to-use Flagyl comes as 5 mg/mL (500 mg metronidazole in 100 mL of solution) in plastic bags; administer over 1 hr.
11. Drug has a high sodium content.
12. COMPATIBILITY Give infusion undiluted.
13. INCOMPATIBILITY Administer separately.

ASSESSMENT

1. Note reasons for therapy, onset, location, symptom characteristics and culture results.
2. With amebiasis, monitor stool number/characteristics and 3 consecutive samples several days apart several weeks after therapy to assess results. With IV therapy assess for sodium retention and neurologic problems. With pregnancy use the 7-day regimen for trichomoniasis. Use only after *T. vaginalis* or *E. histolytica* has been confirmed by wet smear/culture/identification process.
3. Review associated risks and evidence of carcinogenic activity in mice and rats with this therapy.
4. Monitor VS, I&O, CBC, LFTs, and cultures. Reduce dose with liver dysfunction.

CLIENT/FAMILY TEACHING

1. Take tablets with food or milk to reduce GI upset; may cause a metallic taste. Take ER tablets at least 1 hr before or 2 hr after meals; do not crush, chew or split.
2. Report lack of response, any symptoms of CNS toxicity, i.e., uncoordinated movements/tremors, numbness, seizures, any unusual bruising/bleeding.
3. Do not perform tasks that require mental alertness until drug effects are realized; dizziness may occur.

4. Drug may turn urine brown; do not be alarmed.
5. No alcohol until at least 48 hr after therapy completed; a disulfiram-like reaction may occur (abdominal cramps, vomiting, flushing, and headache).
6. During treatment for trichomoniasis, treat partner also since organisms may be in the male urogenital tract and reinfect partner. Use condom to prevent reinfections.
7. With gel, review how to fill and care for applicator and how to administer. If gel accidentally comes in contact with the eye(s): rinse eye(s) with copious amounts of cool tap water and report if eye irritation persists after rinsing. Avoid vaginal intercourse during treatment.
8. With topical therapy: clean areas to be treated before applying. Then apply and rub in a thin film twice daily to entire affected areas. May apply cosmetics after application of medication. If using lotion, allow it to dry first. Avoid contact of topical products with the eyes.
9. Keep all F/U to assess response, labs/cultures, and adverse SE.

OUTCOMES/EVALUATE

- Symptomatic improvement
- Negative culture reports

Mexiletine hydrochloride

(mex-**ILL**-eh-teen)

Classification(s): Antiarrhythmic, Class IB

Pregnancy Category: C

RX: Mexitil.

✦ **Rx:** Novo-Mexiletine.

SEE ALSO ***ANTIARRHYTHMIC DRUGS***.

INDICATIONS/USES

Documented life-threatening ventricular arrhythmias (such as ventricular tachycardia). *Investigational:* Prophylactically to decrease the incidence of ventricular tachycardia and other ventricular arrhythmias in the acute phase of MI. To reduce pain, dysesthesia, and paresthesia associated with diabetic neuropathy.

ACTION/KINETICS

Action

Similar to lidocaine but is effective PO. Inhibits the flow of sodium into the cell, thereby reducing the rate of rise of the action potential. The drug decreases the effective refractory period in Purkinje fibers. BP and pulse rate are not affected following use, but there may be a small decrease in CO and an increase in peripheral vascular resistance. Also has both local anesthetic and anticonvulsant effects.

Pharmacokinetics

Bioavailability: About 90%. **Onset:** 30–120 min. **Peak blood levels:** 2–3 hr. **Therapeutic plasma levels:** 0.5–2 mcg/mL. **Plasma t½:** 10–12 hr. Metabolized in the liver mainly by CYP2D6. Approximately 10% excreted unchanged in the urine; acidification of the urine enhances excretion, whereas alkalinization decreases excretion.

CONTRAINDICATIONS

Cardiogenic shock, pre-existing second- or third-degree AV block (if no pacemaker is present). Use with lesser arrhythmias. Lactation.

SPECIAL CONCERNS

Clients with asymptomatic, non-life-threatening ventricular arrhythmias who had an MI more than 6 days but less than 2 years previously may show an excessive mortality or nonfatal cardiac arrest. Use of mexiletine should be reserved for those with life-threatening ventricular arrhythmias.

- Use with caution in hypotension, severe CHF, or known seizure disorders.
- Safety and efficacy not determined in children.

SIDE EFFECTS

Most Common

Upper GI distress, tremor, lightheadedness, dizziness, coordination difficulties, nervousness, headache, blurred vision, paresthesias, N&V, heartburn, fatigue, constipation.

CV: ***Worsening of arrhythmias***, palpitations, chest pain, increased ventricular arrhythmias (PVCs), CHF, angina or angina-like pain, hypotension, bradycardia, syncope, ***AV block or conduction disturbances***, atrial arrhythmias, hypertension, ***cardiogenic shock***, hot flashes, edema, worsening of CHF in those with pre-existing compromised ventricular function. **GI:** High incidence of UGI distress, N&V, heartburn. Also, diarrhea/constipation, changes in appetite, dry mouth, abdominal cramps/pain/discomfort, salivary changes, dysphagia, altered taste, pharyngitis, changes in oral mucous membranes, UGI bleeding, peptic ulcer, esophageal ulceration, dyspepsia, pancreatitis (rare). **CNS:** High incidence of lightheadedness, dizziness, tremor, coordination difficulties, and nervousness. Also, changes in sleep habits, headache, fatigue, weakness, tinnitus, paresthesias, numbness, depression, confusion, difficulty with speech, short-term memory loss, hallucinations, malaise, psychosis, drowsiness, ataxia, ***seizures***, loss of consciousness. **Hematologic:** Leukopenia, neutropenia, agranulocytosis, thrombocytopenia. **GU:** Decreased libido, impotence, urinary hesitancy/retention. **Dermatologic:** Rash, dry skin. Rarely, exfoliative dermatitis, and ***Stevens-Johnson syndrome***. **Pulmonary:** Dyspnea, laryngeal or pharyngeal changes, pulmonary fibrosis, pulmonary infiltration. **Ophthalmic:** Blurred vision, visual disturbances, nystamus. **Miscellaneous:** Arthralgia, fever, diaphoresis, loss of hair, hiccoughs, syndrome of SLE, myelofibrosis, hypersensitivity reaction.

LABORATORY TEST CONSIDERATIONS

↑ AST. Positive ANA. Abnormal LFTs.

OVERDOSE MANAGEMENT

Symptoms: Nausea. CNS symptoms (dizziness, drowsiness, confusion, paresthesias, seizures) usually precede CV symptoms (hypotension, sinus bradycardia, intermittent LBBB, ***temporary asystole, AV heart block, ventricular tachyarrhythmias, CV collapse). Massive overdoses cause coma and respiratory arrest.*** *Treatment:* General supportive treatment. Give atropine to treat hypotension or bradycardia. Give anticonvulsants for seizures. Transvenous cardiac pacing may be helpful. Acidification of the urine may increase rate of excretion.

DRUG INTERACTIONS

Al hydroxide / ↓ Mexiletine absorption
Atropine / ↓ Mexiletine absorption
Caffeine / ↓ Drug clearance (50%)
Cimetidine / ↑ or ↓ Plasma mexiletine levels
Fluvoxamine / ↓ Oral clearance and ↑ in AUC and peak serum levels of mexiletine R/T ↓ liver metabolism by CYP1A2
Mg hydroxide / ↓ Mexiletine absorption
Metoclopramide / ↑ Mexiletine absorption
Narcotics / ↓ Mexiletine absorption
Phenobarbital / ↓ Plasma mexiletine levels
Phenytoin / ↑ Mexiletine clearance → ↓ plasma mexiletine levels
Propafenone / ↓ Metabolic clearance of mexiletine in extensive metabolizers → no differences between extensive and poor metabolizers
Rifampin / ↑ Clearance → ↓ plasma mexiletine levels
Smoking / ↑ Mexiletine clearance → ↓ $t^{1/2}$
Theophylline / ↑ Drug effect R/T ↑ serum levels
Urinary acidifiers / ↑ Rate of mexiletine excretion
Urinary alkalinizers / ↓ Rate of mexiletine excretion

HOW SUPPLIED

Capsules: 150 mg, 200 mg, 250 mg.

DOSAGE

CAPSULES

Antiarrhythmic.

Adults, individualized, initial: 200 mg q 8 hr if rapid control of arrhythmia not required; dosage adjustment may be made in 50- or 100-mg increments q 2–3 days, if required. **Maintenance:** 200–300 mg q 8 hr, depending on response and tolerance of client. If adequate response is not achieved with 300 mg or less q 8 hr, 400 mg q 8 hr may be tried although the incidence of CNS side effects increases. If the drug is effective at doses of 300 mg or less q 8 hr, the same total daily dose may be given in divided doses q 12 hr (e.g., 450 mg q 12 hr). Maximum total daily dose: 1,200 mg.

Rapid control of arrhythmias.

Initial loading dose: 400 mg followed by a 200-mg dose in 8 hr.

Diabetic neuropathy.

Initial: 150 mg/day for 3 days; **then,** 300 mg/day for 3 days. **Maintenance:** 10 mg/kg/day.

NURSING IMPLICATIONS

IMPLEMENTATION/ADMINISTRATION/STORAGE

1. If transferring to mexiletine from other class I antiarrhythmics, initiate mexiletine at a dose

of 200 mg and then titrate according to the response at the following times: 6–12 hr after the last dose of quinidine sulfate, 3–6 hr after the last dose of procainamide, 6–12 hr after the last dose of disopyramide, or 8–12 hr after the last dose of tocainide.

2. Hospitalize client when transferring to mexiletine if there is a chance that withdrawal of the previous antiarrhythmic may produce life-threatening arrhythmias.
3. When transferring from lidocaine to mexiletine, stop the lidocaine infusion when the first PO dose of mexiletine is given. Maintain the IV line until suppression of the arrhythmia appears satisfactory.
4. Avoid concurrent drugs or diets that may markedly affect urinary pH.

ASSESSMENT

1. Identify life-threatening ventricular arrhythmia, other agents trialed, outcome.
2. Note evidence of CHF; assess ECG for AV block.
3. Assess pulmonary status; note SaO_2/PO_2, respiratory rate.
4. Check urinary pH; alkalinity decreases/acidity increases renal drug excretion.
5. Monitor ECG, CXR, CBC, electrolytes, renal and LFTs. Reduce dose with severe liver disease, marked right-sided CHF.

CLIENT/FAMILY TEACHING

1. Take with food or an antacid to ↓ GI upset. Drug controls, but does not cure, abnormal heart rhythm.
2. Do not perform tasks that require mental alertness until drug effects realized; may cause dizziness. Change positions slowly to prevent any sudden drop in BP.
3. Report any bruising, bleeding, fevers, or sore throat or adverse CNS effects such as dizziness, tremor, impaired coordination, N&V. Immediately report any increase in heart palpitations, irregularity, low BP or HR <50 bpm.
4. Record BP and HR and bring to each visit.
5. Keep all F/U to assess response, labs, and for adverse SE.
6. Ensure family/significant other know CPR.

OUTCOMES/EVALUATE

- Control of ventricular arrhythmias
- Therapeutic drug levels (0.5–2 mcg/mL)

IV

Micafungin sodium

(me-ka-**FUN**-jin)

Classification(s): Antifungal

Pregnancy Category: C

RX: Mycamine.

INDICATIONS/USES

(1) Treatment of esophageal candidiasis. (2) Prophylaxis of *Candida* infections in clients undergoing hematopoietic stem cell transplantation. (3) Treatment of candidemia, acute disseminated candidiasis, *Candida* peritonitis, and abscesses.

ACTION/KINETICS

Action

Micafungin, a semisynthetic lipopeptide, inhibits the synthesis of 1,3-β-D-glucan, an essential component of fungal cell walls; it is not present in mammalian cells.

Pharmacokinetics

t½: 14–17.2 hr, depending on the use and dose. Metabolized to M-1 (catechol form) and subsequently to M-2 (methoxy form) by CYP450 isoenzymes. Excreted mainly through the feces. **Plasma protein binding:** >99% mainly to albumin.

CONTRAINDICATIONS

Hypersensitivity to micafungin, other components of the product, or to other echinocandins.

SPECIAL CONCERNS

- Use with caution during lactation.
- Safety and efficacy not determined in children.

SIDE EFFECTS

Most Common

Headache, N&V, phlebitis, rash, diarrhea, leukopenia, neutropenia, pyrexia, rigors, hypokalemia. Side effects listed are for all uses. **Histamine-mediated symptoms:** Rash, pruritus, facial swelling, vasodilation. **Injection site reactions:** Phlebitis, thrombophlebitis, thrombosis. **GI:** N&V, diarrhea, dysgeusia, dyspepsia, constipation, hiccoughs, abdominal pain, upper abdominal pain. **Hepatic:** Significant hepatic dysfunction, hepatitis, hepatomegaly, jaundice, hepatocellular damage, ***hepatic failure***. **CNS:** Headache, delirium, anxiety, dizziness, somnolence, insomnia, ***convulsions***, encephalopathy, nervous system disorders.

M

intracranial hemorrhage*.** **CV:** Hyper-/hypotension, flushing, arrhythmias, atrial fibrillation, bradycardia, ***cardiac arrest, cyanosis, ***DVT***, ***MI***, tachycardia, phlebitis, cardiac and/or vascular disorders. **Dermatologic:** Rash, pruritus, erythema multiforme, skin necrosis, urticaria, decubitus ulcer. **GU:** Significant renal dysfunction, acute renal failure, anuria, renal tubular necrosis, oliguria. **Respiratory:** Apnea, dyspnea, cough, epistaxis, hypoxia, pneumonia, ***pulmonary embolism***. **Hematologic:** Leukopenia, anemia, aggravated anemia, neutropenia, thrombocytopenia, lymphopenia, febrile neutropenia, coagulopathy, hemolysis, pancytopenia, thrombotic thrombocytopenic purpura; ***acute intravascular hemolysis*** and hemoglobinuria when used with PO prednisolone. Also hemolysis and ***hemolytic anemia*** when used alone. **Hypersensitivity reactions:** Rash, pruritus, facial swelling, vasodilation, ***anaphylaxis*** and anaphylactoid reactions, including ***shock***. **Body as a whole**: Rigors, pyrexia, fatigue, decreased appetite, acidosis, arthralgia, infections, fluid overload/retention, ***septic shock***, ***sepsis***. **Miscellaneous:** Mucosal inflammation, bacteremia, peripheral edema, anorexia/decreased appetite, back pain.

LABORATORY TEST CONSIDERATIONS

↑ ALT, AST, BUN, creatinine, blood alkaline phosphatase, aspartate aminotransferase, LDH. ↓ WBCs. Hypomagnesemia, hyperbilirubinemia, hypocalcemia, hypo-/hyperkalemia, hypo-/hypernatremia, hypoglycemia, hemoglobinuria. Abnormal LFTs.

DRUG INTERACTIONS

Cyclosporine / ↑ Cyclosporine PO clearance and ↑ single-dose cyclosporine whole blood levels R/T inhibition of CYP3A metabolism

Itraconazole / ↑ Itraconazole AUC and C_{max}; monitor for itraconazole toxicity and adjust dose if necessary

Nifedipine / ↑ Nifedipine AUC and C_{max}; monitor for nifedipine toxicity and adjust dose if necessary

Sirolimus / ↑ Sirolimus AUC; monitor for sirolimus toxicity and adjust dose if necessary

HOW SUPPLIED

Injection, Lyophilized Powder for Solution: 50 mg, 100 mg.

DOSAGE

IV INFUSION

Esophageal candidiasis.

150 mg/day. Mean duration of treatment is 15 days.

Prophylaxis of Candida infections in hematopoietic stem cell transplantation.

50 mg/day. Mean duration of treatment is 19 days.

Candidemia, acute disseminated candidiasis, Candida *peritonitis, and abscesses.*

100 mg/day. Mean duration of treatment is 15 days.

NURSING IMPLICATIONS

IMPLEMENTATION/ADMINISTRATION/STORAGE

1. **IV** Give over a period of 1 hr. More rapid infusion may cause more frequent histamine-mediated reactions.
2. For administration, an existing IV line should be flushed with 0.9% NaCl injection prior to infusion of micafungin.
3. Solutions for infusion are prepared as follows:
   - Aseptically add 5 mL of 0.9% NaCl injection (without a bacteriostatic agent) to each 50 mg vial to yield a preparation containing about 10 mg/mL micafungin and add 10 mL of 0.9% NaCl injection (without a bacteriostatic agent) to each 100 mg vial to yield a preparation containing about 10 mg/mL micafungin.
   - To minimize excess foaming, gently dissolve the micafungin powder by swirling the vial. Do not shake vigorously. Visually inspect the vial for particulate matter.
   - Protect the diluted solution from light, although it is not necessary to cover the infusion drip chamber or the tubing.
4. For prophylaxis of *Candida* infections, add 50 mg of reconstituted micafungin in 5 mL NaCl injection into 100 mL of 0.9% NaCl; infuse over 1 hr.
5. For treatment of candidemia, acute disseminated candidiasis, *Candida* peritonitis, and abscesses, add 100 mg reconstituted micafungin into 100 mL of 0.9% NaCl or 100 mL of D5W injection and infuse over 1 hr.
6. For treatment of esophageal candidiasis, add micafungin, 150 mg (i.e., from 3–50 mg vials) reconstituted in 15 mL NaCl injection into 100 mL of 0.9% NaCl injection; infuse over 1 hr.
7. Since micafungin is preservative free, discard partially used vials.

8. Store unopened vials of lyophilized drug at room temperature. The reconstituted drug may be stored in the original vial for up to 24 hr at room temperature. Protect the diluted infusion solution from light; it may be stored for up to 24 hr at room temperature.
9. COMPATIBILITY 0.9% NaCl, D5W.
10. INCOMPATIBILITY Do not mix or coinfuse micafungin with other drugs. Micafungin will precipitate when mixed directly with a number of other commonly used drugs.

ASSESSMENT

1. Note reasons for therapy and characteristics of S&S: treatment or prophylaxis, schedule for hematopoietic stem cell transplantation (HSCT), or cause of infection, other agents trialed and those currently prescribed.
2. Monitor during infusion for S&S of hypersensitivity reaction or IV site reactions.
3. Assess cultures, K^+, Ca^{++}, Mg^{++}, CBC, renal and LFTs. If any dysfunction occurs, stop drug and report. Drug is highly protein bound and not dialyzable.

CLIENT/FAMILY TEACHING

1. Drug is administered intravenously to treat or prevent a type of fungal infection. Therapy usually is anywhere from 7-21 days.
2. Report any headaches, skin rashes, N&V, diarrhea, pain at injection site, swelling of extremities, unusual bruising/bleedings, itching, cough, fever or chills.
3. Keep all F/U to assess response, labs, and for adverse SE.

OUTCOMES/EVALUATE

- Resolution of esophageal and/or other types of *Candida* infections
- Prophylaxis of *Candida* infections in HSCT recipients

Miconazole nitrate

(my-**KON**-ah-zohl)

Classification(s): Antifungal

Pregnancy Category: C

OTC: Topical: Desenex, Desenex Liquid Spray, Fungoid Tincture, Lotrimin AF, Micatin, Neosporin AF, Tetterine, Ting, Triple Paste AF, Zeasorb-AF. **Vaginal:** Monistat 7, Monistat 7 Combination Pack, Vagistat-3 Combination Pack.

RX: Tablet, Buccal: Oravig. **Vaginal:** Monistat 1 Combination Pack, Monistat 3, Monistat 3 Combination Pack, Monistat Dual-Pak.

✦ **Rx:** Micozole, Monazole 7.

SEE ALSO ***ANTI-INFECTIVE DRUGS***.

INDICATIONS/USES

Tablet, Buccal: Oropharyngeal candidiasis in adults and children, 16 years and older.

Topical, OTC: Tinea pedis (athlete's foot), tinea cruris (jock itch), tinea corporis (ringworm) caused by *Trichophyton rubrum*, *T. mentagrophytes*, and *Epidermophyton floccosum*. Relieves itching, burning, cracking, and scaling.

Vaginal, OTC and Rx: Vulvovaginal candidiasis (suppositories). Relief of external vulvar itching and irritation associated with a yeast infection (cream).

ACTION/KINETICS

Action

Broad-spectrum fungicide that inhibits the enzyme CYP450 alpha–demethylase; this leads to inhibition of ergosterol synthesis, an essential component of the fungal cell membrane. The drug also inhibits biosynthesis of triglycerides and phospholipids and also inhibits oxidative and peroxidative enzyme activity increasing the amount of reactive oxygen species in the cell. May be fungistatic or fungicidal, depending on the concentration.

Pharmacokinetics

The duration of buccal adhesion averages 15 hr following a single dose application. Most of the drug that is absorbed is metabolized by the liver. **t½, terminal:** 24 hr following systemic use.

CONTRAINDICATIONS

Hypersensitivity to miconazole, milk protein concentrate (buccal tablets), or any component of the product. Use of topical products in or around the eyes or mucous membranes. Use of topical products in children less than 2 years of age unless directed by a physician. Use of buccal tablets in young children due to risk of choking.

SPECIAL CONCERNS

- **Use buccal tablets with caution in impaired hepatic function.**

- Use with caution during lactation.
- Safe use of topical products not established in children less than 1 year of age and use of buccal tablets in children less than 16 years of age.

SIDE EFFECTS

Most Common

Following use of buccal tablets: Headache, N&V, infections/infestations, diarrhea, dysgeusia.
Following topical use: Irritation, burning, maceration, allergic contact dermatitis.
Following vaginal use: Irritation, sensitization, vulvovaginal burning.
Use of vaginal products. At vaginal administration site: Burning, irritation, sensitization, vulvovaginal burning, pruritus, discharge, edema, pain. **GI:** GI cramping, nausea, dry mouth, flatulence. **GU:** Genital erythema, vaginal tenderness, dysuria, perianal burning, pelvic cramping. **CNS:** Headache. **Dermatologic:** Rash, urticaria, skin irritation. **Ophthalmic:** Periorbital edema, conjunctival pruritus. **Miscellaneous:** Allergic reaction, hypersensitivity reactions (e.g., ***anaphylaxis***).

Use of buccal tablets. At oral administration site: Altered taste, application site pain/discomfort, dry mouth, gingival pain/pruritus/swelling, glossodynia, loss of taste, mouth ulceration, toothache. **CNS:** Headache, ageusia, dysgeusia. **GI:** N&V, dry mouth, diarrhea, glossodynia, oral discomfort, upper abdominal pain, gastroenteritis. **Dermatologic:** Pruritus. **Hematologic:** Anemia, ***lymphopenia, neutropenia***. **Respiratory:** Cough, pharyngeal pain, URTI. **Body as a whole:** Fatigue, infections/infestations, pain.

DRUG INTERACTIONS

NOTE: Drug interactions listed are for use of miconazole buccal tablets.

CYP2C9 and CYP3A4 substrates (e.g., ergot derivatives, hydantoins, oral hypoglycemic drugs) / Potential for an interaction of miconazole with these drugs cannot be ruled out

Warfarin / Possible enhanced anticoagulant effect of warfarin; monitor PT and INR closely if used together

HOW SUPPLIED

Oral, Rx. *Tablet, Buccal:* 50 mg.
Topical, OTC. *Cream:* 2%; *Gel:* 2%; *Ointment:* 2%; *Powder:* 2%; *Solution:* 2%; *Spray Liquid:* 2%; *Spray Powder:* 2%.
Vaginal, OTC and Rx. *Cream:* 2%; ***Suppositories and Topical Cream (Combination Pack or Dual-Pack):*** Suppositories, 100 mg and Topical Cream, 2%; Suppositories, 200 mg and Topical Cream, 2%; Suppositories, 1,200 mg, and Topical Cream, 2%; ***Suppositories:*** 100 mg, 200 mg.

DOSAGE

TABLET, BUCCAL

Oropharyngeal candidiasis.

Adults and children, 16 years and older: 50 mg once daily place for 14 consecutive days in the upper gum region (canine fossa) in the morning after brushing the teeth.

TOPICAL: CREAM; GEL; OINTMENT; POWDER; SOLUTION; SPRAY LIQUID/POWDER

Athlete's foot, jock itch, ringworm.

Clean the affected area and dry thoroughly. Apply or spray a thin layer of the product to cover affected areas in morning and evening for 2 weeks for tinea cruris and for 4 weeks for tinea pedis and tinea corporis. Topical products are not effective on the scalp or nails.

VAGINAL CREAM; VAGINAL SUPPOSITORIES

Suppositories: One suppository daily at bedtime for 7 days (100-mg suppositories), 3 consecutive days (200-mg suppositories), or 1 day (1,200 mg).
Cream: 1 applicator-full intravaginally once daily at bedtime for 3–7 days. For topical use, apply cream to affected areas twice a day (morning and evening) for up to 7 days or as needed. Repeat course, if needed, after ruling out other pathogens.

NURSING IMPLICATIONS

IMPLEMENTATION/ADMINISTRATION/STORAGE

1. The lotion is preferred for intertriginous areas.
2. Store topical and vaginal products and buccal tablets from 15–30°C (59–86°F). Protect tablets from moisture.

ASSESSMENT

1. Note indications for therapy, location, clinical presentation, size/number/extent of lesions. List any previous experience/sensitivity with this drug; response obtained.
2. Monitor cultures/skin scraping, CBC, electrolytes, LFTs and healing/clearing progress.

CLIENT/FAMILY TEACHING

1. Review administration technique; use only as directed. Complete full course of therapy despite symptom improvement. To ensure success, tinea cruris, tinea corporis, and candida should be treated for 2 weeks; tinea pedis should be treated for 1 month.
2. Sprays are under pressure; do not puncture or incinerate. The mixture is flammable; do not use near fire or flame. Do not expose to temperatures above 49°C (120°F).
3. When used for vaginal infections, use at bedtime, refrain from intercourse or use a condom to prevent reinfection. Use sanitary pads to protect clothing and linens when using cream or suppositories. When used vaginally, continue treatment during menses.
4. With buccal tablet, use immediately after removal from the bottle. Do not crush, chew, or swallow tablet.
   - Place rounded side of tablet to upper gum in the a.m. after brushing teeth. Hold tablet in place for 30 sec to make it stick to the gum. Leave in place—will dissolve as tablet gains moisture from mouth. Alternate sides of gum with each dose.
   - If tablet does not stick or falls off within the first 6 hr, may reposition tablet. If it still does not adhere, replace with a new tablet. If tablet is accidently swallowed within the first 6 hr, then drink a glass of water and apply a new tablet only once. If a tablet falls off or is swallowed after in place for 6 hr or more, do not apply a new tablet until the next regularly scheduled dose.
   - When tablet is in place may eat and drink normally.
   - Avoid situations that could interfere with sticking of the tablet, such as chewing gum, wearing an upper denture, or hitting tablet when brushing teeth.
   - May experience diarrhea, headache, nausea, and change in taste; report if persistent or bothersome.
5. If pregnant or breast-feeding, avoid use without approval.
6. Report if exposed to HIV and recurrent vaginal infections occur.
7. Report lack of response, persistent N&V, diarrhea, dizziness, itching, or other adverse SE.
8. Keep all F/U to assess response and for adverse SE.

OUTCOMES/EVALUATE

- Negative culture reports
- Clearing of fungal infection
- Resolution of vaginitis evidenced by ↓ itching/burning; ↓ discharge
- ↓ Size and number of lesions

IV

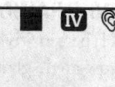

Midazolam hydrochloride

(my-**DAYZ**-oh-lam)

Classification(s): Benzodiazepine, adjunct to general anesthesia

Pregnancy Category: D, C-IV

SEE ALSO ***TRANQUILIZERS/ANTIMANIC DRUGS/HYPNOTICS***.

INDICATIONS/USES

IV, IM: Preoperative sedation, anxiolysis, and amnesia. **IV:** (1) Sedation, anxiolysis, and amnesia prior to or during short diagnostic, therapeutic, or endoscopic procedures (either alone or with other CNS depressants). (2) Induction of general anesthesia before administration of other anesthetics. (3) Supplement to nitrous oxide and oxygen in balanced anesthesia. (4) Sedation of intubated and mechanically ventilated clients as a component of anesthesia or during treatment in a critical care setting. **Syrup:** Preprocedural sedation and anxiolysis in children. *Investigational:* Treat epileptic seizures. Alternative to terminate refractory status epilepticus.

ACTION/KINETICS

Action

Short-acting benzodiazepine with sedative-general anesthetic properties. Depresses the response of the respiratory system to carbon dioxide stimula-

M

tion, which is more pronounced in clients with COPD. Possible mild to moderate decreases in CO, mean arterial BP, SV, and systemic vascular resistance. HR may rise somewhat in those with slow HRs (<65 bpm) and decrease in others (especially those with HRs >85 bpm).

Pharmacokinetics

Onset, IM: 15 min; **IV:** 2–2.5 min for induction (if combined with a preanesthetic narcotic, induction is about 1.5 min). If preanesthetic medication (morphine) is given, the **peak plasma levels, IM:** 45 min. **Maximum effect:** 30–60 min. **Time to recovery:** Usually within 2 hr, although up to 6 hr may be required. **t½, elimination:** 1.2–12.3 hr. Rapidly metabolized in the liver to inactive compounds; excreted through the urine. **Plasma protein binding:** About 97%.

CONTRAINDICATIONS

Hypersensitivity to benzodiazepines. Acute narrow-angle glaucoma. Use in obstetrics, coma, shock, or acute alcohol intoxication where VS are depressed. IA injection.

SPECIAL CONCERNS

■ (1) IV midazolam has been associated with respiratory depression and respiratory arrest. In some cases, when not recognized and treated effectively, death or hypoxic encephalopathy resulted. (2) Use IV midazolam in a hospital or ambulatory care setting, including physicians' offices, that provide for continuous monitoring of respiratory and cardiac function. Ensure immediate availability of resuscitative drugs and equipment and personnel trained in their use. (3) The initial IV dose for conscious sedation may be as little as 1 mg, and should not exceed 2.5 mg in a normal healthy adult. Lower doses are necessary for older (over 60 years) or debilitated clients and in clients receiving concomitant narcotics or other CNS depressants. (4) Never give the initial dose and all subsequent doses as a bolus; rather, give over at least 2 min and allow an additional 2 or more min to evaluate fully the sedative effect. Use of a 1 mg/mL formulation or dilution of 1 mg/mL or 5 mg/mL formulation is recommended to facilitate slower injection. ■

- Use with caution during lactation.
- Children may require higher doses than adults.
- Severe hypotension and seizures are possible in neonates after rapid IV injection, especially with concurrent fentanyl; do not give by rapid IV injection in this group.
- Hypotension may be more common in conscious sedated clients who have received a preanesthetic narcotic.
- Geriatric and debilitated clients require lower doses to induce anesthesia; they are more prone to side effects.
- Use IV with extreme caution in severe fluid or electrolyte disturbances.

SIDE EFFECTS

Most Common

Following IM or IV use: Fluctuations in VS, including decreased respiratory rate and tidal volume; apnea.
Following IM use: Headache, pain at injection site, muscle stiffness, induration, redness.
Following IV use: Coughing, oversedation, headache, drowsiness, bronchospasm.

Fluctuations in VS, including decreased respiratory rate and tidal volume, apnea, variations in BP and pulse rate are common. The following are general side effects regardless of the route of administration. **CV**: Hypotension, ***cardiac arrest***. **CNS**: Oversedation, headache, drowsiness, grogginess, confusion, retrograde amnesia, euphoria, nervousness, agitation, anxiety, argumentativeness, restlessness, emergence delirium, increased time for emergence, dreaming during emergence, nightmares, insomnia, tonic-clonic movements, ataxia, muscle tremor, involuntary or athetoid movements, dizziness, dysphoria, dysphonia, slurred speech, paresthesia. **GI**: Hiccoughs, N&V, acid taste, retching, excessive salivation. **Ophthalmic:** Double/blurred vision, nystagmus, pinpoint pupils, visual disturbances, cyclic eyelid movements, difficulty in focusing. **Dermatologic**: Hives, swelling or feeling of burning, warmth or cold feeling at injection site, hive-like wheal at injection site, pruritus, rash. **Miscellaneous**: Blocked ears, loss of balance, chills, weakness, faint feeling, lethargy, yawning, toothache, hematoma. **More common following IM use:** Pain at injection site, headache, induration and redness, muscle stiffness.

More common following IV use: Respiratory: ***Bronchospasm***, coughing, dyspnea, ***laryngospasm***, hyperventilation, shallow respirations, tachypnea, ***airway obstruction***, wheezing, respiratory depression and ***respiratory arrest*** when used for conscious sedation. **CV:** PVCs, bigeminy, bradycardia, tachycardia, vasovagal episode, nodal rhythm. **At injection site:** Tenderness, pain, redness, induration, phlebitis.

DRUG INTERACTIONS

Alcohol / ↑ Risk of apnea, airway obstruction, desaturation, or hypoventilation
Anesthetics, inhalation / ↓ Dose if midazolam used as an induction agent
Antifungals, azole / ↑ Effect of midazolam R/T ↓ liver metabolism
Aprepitant / ↑ Midazolam AUC, peak, plasma levels, and t½ R/T inhibition of metabolism by CYP3A4
Cimetidine / ↑ Sedation
Clarithromycin / ↑ Effect of midazolam R/T ↓ liver metabolism
CNS depressants / ↑ Risk of apnea, airway obstruction, desaturation, or hypoventilation
Contraceptives, oral / Prolongation of midazolam half-life
Droperidol / ↑ Hypnotic effect of midazolam when used as a premedication
Erythromycin / ↑ Effect of midazolam R/T ↓ liver metabolism
Fentanyl / ↑ Hypnotic effect of midazolam when used as a premedication
Fluvoxamine / ↑ Serum midazolam levels, reduced clearance, and prolonged half-life
Indinavir / Possible prolonged sedation and respiratory depression
Meperidine / See **Narcotics**; also, ↑ risk of hypotension
Narcotics / ↑ Hypnotic effect of midazolam when used as premedication
Propofol / ↑ Effect of propofol
Protease inhibitors / ↑ Effect of midazolam R/T ↓ liver metabolism
Rifamycins / Possible pharmacokinetic changes of midazolam
Ritonavir / Possible prolonged sedation and respiratory depression
Selective serotonin reuptake inhibitors / ↑ Effect of midazolam R/T ↓ liver metabolism
Theophyllines / Antagonism of midazolam's sedative effects
Thiopental / ↓ Dose if midazolam used as an induction agent
Valproic acid / Possible ↓ liver metabolism of midazolam
Verapamil / Possible ↑ CNS depression and prolonged midazolam effects

HOW SUPPLIED

Injection: 1 mg/mL, 5 mg/mL; ***Syrup:*** 2 mg/mL.

DOSAGE

IM

Preoperative sedation, anxiolysis, amnesia.

Adults: 0.07–0.08 mg/kg IM (average: 5 mg) 1 hr before surgery. **Children:** 0.1–0.15 mg/kg (up to 0.5 mg/kg may be needed for more anxious clients).

IV

Conscious sedation, anxiolysis, amnesia for endoscopic or cardiovascular procedures in healthy adults under age 60.

Using the 1 mg/mL (can be diluted with 0.9% sodium chloride or D5W) product, titrate slowly to the desired effect (usually slurred speech); initial dose should be no higher than 2.5 mg IV (may be as low as 1 mg IV) within a 2-min period; wait an additional 2 min to evaluate the sedative effect. If additional sedation is necessary, give small increments waiting an additional 2 min or more after each increment to evaluate the effect. Total doses greater than 5 mg are usually not required. **Children:** Dosage must be individualized by the physician.

Conscious sedation for endoscopic or CV procedures in debilitated or chronically ill clients or clients aged 60 or over.

Slowly titrate to the desired effect using no more than 1.5 mg initially IV (may be as little as 1 mg IV) given over a 2-min period; wait an additional 2 min or more to evaluate the effect. If additional sedation is needed, no more than 1 mg should be given over 2 min; wait an additional 2 min or more after each increment in dose. Total doses greater than 3.5 mg are usually not needed.

Induction of general anesthesia, before use of other general anesthetics, in unmedicated clients.

Adults, unmedicated clients up to 55 years of age, IV, initial:
0.3–0.35 mg/kg given over 20–30 sec, waiting 2 min for effects to occur. If

needed, increments of about 25% of the initial dose can be used to complete induction; or, induction can be completed using a volatile liquid anesthetic. Up to 0.6 mg/kg may be used but recovery will be prolonged. **Adults, unmedicated clients over 55 years of age who are good risk surgical clients, initial IV:** 0.15–0.3 mg/kg given over 20–30 sec. **Adults, unmedicated clients over 55 years of age with severe systemic disease or debilitation, initial IV:** 0.15–0.25 mg/kg given over 20–30 sec. **Pediatric:** 0.05–0.2 mg/kg IV.

Induction of general anesthesia, before use of other general anesthetics, in medicated clients.

Adults, premedicated clients up to 55 years of age, IV, initial: 0.15–0.35 mg/kg. If less than 55 years of age, 0.25 mg/kg may be given over 20–30 sec, allowing 2 min for effect. **Adults, premedicated clients over 55 years of age who are good risk surgical clients, initial, IV:** 0.2 mg/kg. **Adults, premedicated clients over 55 years of age with severe systemic disease or debilitation, initial, IV:** 0.15 mg/kg may be sufficient.

Maintenance of balanced anesthesia for short surgical procedures.

IV: Incremental injections about 25% of the dose used for induction when signs indicate anesthesia is lightening. *NOTE:* Narcotic preanesthetic medication may include fentanyl, 1.5–2 mcg/kg IV 5 min before induction; morphine, up to 0.15 mg/kg IM; meperidine, up to 1 mg/kg IM; or, Innovar, 0.02 mL/kg IM. Sedative preanesthetic medication may include secobarbital sodium, 200 mg PO or hydroxyzine pamoate, 100 mg PO. Except for fentanyl, give all preanesthetic medications 1 hr prior to midazolam. Always individualize doses.

SYRUP

Preprocedural sedation and anxiolysis in children.

Children: 0.25–1 mg/kg, not to exceed 20 mg.

NURSING IMPLICATIONS

Do not confuse Versed with Vistaril (an antianxiety drug) or with VePesid (an antineoplastic).

IMPLEMENTATION/ADMINISTRATION/STORAGE

1. When used for procedures via the mouth, use a topical anesthetic.
2. Give IM doses in a large muscle mass.
3. IV When used for conscious sedation, do not give by rapid or single bolus IV; may cause respiratory depression.
4. When used for induction of general anesthesia, give the initial dose over 20–30 sec.
5. If preanesthetic medications with a depressant component are given (e.g., narcotic analgesics or CNS depressants), reduce the midazolam dosage by 50% compared with healthy, young unmedicated clients.
6. Give maintenance doses to all clients in increments of 25% of the dose first required to achieve the sedative endpoint.
7. Give a narcotic preanesthetic for bronchoscopic procedures.
8. Carefully monitor all IV doses with the immediate availability of oxygen, resuscitative equipment, and personnel who are skilled in maintaining a patent airway and ventilation support; continue monitoring during recovery period.
9. At a concentration of 0.5 mg/mL midazolam is compatible with D5W and 0.9% NaCl for up to 24 hr and with RL solution for up to 4 hr.
10. COMPATIBILITY D5W, 0.9% NaCl.
11. INCOMPATIBILITY Administer separately with compatible drugs. May be mixed in the same syringe with atropine, meperidine, morphine, or scopolamine.

ASSESSMENT

1. Note reasons for therapy, general client condition, level of sedation/consciousness, VS, airway integrity, oxygen saturation during procedure.
2. Determine method for administration and verify dosage.
3. Use caution and monitor closely with renal dysfunction, and in the elderly and debilitated.
4. Have oxygen and resuscitative equipment readily available in the event of respiratory depression. Effects may be reversed with flumazenil (Romazicon).

CLIENT/FAMILY TEACHING

1. Drug may cause dizziness and drowsiness. Avoid alcohol, CNS depressants, and activities that require mental alertness for 24–48 hr following drug administration.
2. Repeat post-procedure instructions and provide in writing, as may not fully recall instructions; transient amnesia is normal and memory of procedure may be minimal.
3. With continuous infusions in ICU over extended periods of time, client may experience symptoms of withdrawal following abrupt discontinuation.
4. Assess for fall risk and incorporate safety precautions.

OUTCOMES/EVALUATE

Desired level of sedation and amnesia; ↓ anxiety

Mifepristone

(mih-feh-**PRIS**-tohn)

Classification(s): Abortifacient

Pregnancy Category: X

RX: Mifeprex

INDICATIONS/USES

Medical termination of intrauterine pregnancy through day 49 of pregnancy. Pregnancy is dated from the first day of the last menstrual period in a presumed 28-day cycle with ovulation occurring at mid-cycle. When mifepristone and misoprostol fail to cause termination of intrauterine pregnancy, pregnancy termination by surgery is recommended. Not effective to treat ectopic pregnancy. *Investigational:* Emergency contraception, uterine leiomyomata.

ACTION/KINETICS

Action

Competes with progesterone at progesterone-receptor sites, thus inhibiting the activity of endogenous or exogenous progesterone. During pregnancy, the drug sensitizes the myometrium to the contraction-inducing activity of prostaglandins. Termination of pregnancy results. Also exhibits antiglucocorticoid and weak antiandrogenic activity.

Pharmacokinetics

Rapidly absorbed. **Peak plasma levels:** 1.98 mg/L after 90 min. Absolute bioavailability is 69%. **t½, elimination:** 50% eliminated between 12 and 72 hr followed by a more rapid phase with a terminal t½ of 18 hr. Metabolized in the liver by CYP3A4 with most eliminated in the feces. **Plasma protein binding:** 98%.

CONTRAINDICATIONS

Use for termination of pregnancy in any one of the following conditions: Confirmed or suspected ectopic pregnancy or undiagnosed adnexal mass; IUD in place; chronic adrenal failure; concurrent long-term corticosteroid therapy; history of allergy to mifepristone, misoprostol, or other prostaglandins; hemorrhagic disorders or concurrent anticoagulant therapy; pregnancy termination >49 days; inherited porphyrias. Use if client does not have adequate access to medical facilities equipped to provide emergency treatment of incomplete abortion, blood transfusions, and emergency resuscitation during the period from the first visit until discharged by the administering physician. Use in those who cannot understand the effects of the treatment procedure or comply with its regimen.

SPECIAL CONCERNS

(1) Serious and sometimes fatal infections and bleeding occur very rarely following spontaneous, surgical, and medical abortions, including following mifepristone use. Before prescribing mifepristone, inform the client about the risk of these serious events and discuss the Medication Guide and the Patient Agreement. Ensure that the client knows whom to call and what to do, including going to an emergency room, if none of the provided contacts are reachable, or if she experiences sustained fever, severe abdominal pain, prolonged heavy bleeding, or syncope. (2) Clients with serious bacterial infections and sepsis can present without fever, bacteremia, or significant findings on pelvic examination following an abortion. No causal relationship between the use of mifepristone and misoprostol and these events has been established. A high index of suspicion is needed to rule out sepsis. (3) Prolonged heavy bleeding may be a sign of incomplete abortion or other complications, and prompt medical or surgical intervention may be needed. Advise

clients to seek immediate medical attention if they experience prolonged heavy vaginal bleeding. (4) Advise clients to take their Medication Guide with them if they visit an emergency room or another health care provider who did not prescribe mifepristone, so that provider will be aware that the client is undergoing a medical abortion. ■

- **Clients should expect vaginal bleeding or spotting for an average of 9–16 days.**
- **Safety and efficacy not determined for use in cardiovascular, hypertensive, hepatic, respiratory, or renal disease; IDDM; severe anemia; heavy smoking; or pediatric clients.**
- **Use with caution during lactation; consider discarding breast milk for a few days following use.**

SIDE EFFECTS

Most Common

Bleeding, uterine cramping, abdominal pain/cramping, N&V, diarrhea, headache, back pain, fatigue, dizziness.

NOTE: Bleeding and cramping are expected results of therapy. **GI**: N&V, diarrhea, abdominal pain, dyspepsia. **GU**: Uterine cramping/bleeding/hemorrhage, vaginitis, leukorrhea, pelvic pain, endometritis, salpingitis, pelvic inflammatory disease, postabortal infection, ***ruptured ectopic pregnancy***. **CV:** Hypotension (including orthostatic), shortness of breath, tachycardia (including racing pulse, heart palpitations, heart pounding). **CNS**: Headache, dizziness, insomnia, anxiety, syncope, lightheadedness, loss of consciousness. **Hematologic:** Anemia, decreased hemoglobin. **Body as a whole:** Asthenia, fatigue, fever, viral infection, chills/shaking, allergic reaction (including rash, hives, itching). **Miscellaneous**: Fainting, pelvic/back/leg pain, sinusitis, serious infection (including ***septic shock***), ***MI***.

LABORATORY TEST CONSIDERATIONS

Rarely, ↑ AST, ALT, alkaline phosphatase, GGT. ↓ H&H, RBCs in women who bleed heavily.

DRUG INTERACTIONS

Carbamazepine / Possible ↓ mifepristone levels R/T ↑ liver metabolism
Dexamethasone / Possible ↓ mifepristone levels R/T ↑ liver metabolism
Erythromycin / Possible ↑ mifepristone levels R/T ↓ liver metabolism
Grapefruit juice / Possible ↑ mifepristone levels R/T ↓ liver metabolism
Itraconazole / Possible ↑ mifepristone serum levels R/T ↓ liver metabolism
Ketoconazole / Possible ↑ mifepristone levels R/T ↓ liver metabolism
Misoprostol / ↑ Risk of bacterial infection and sepsis with possible death
Phenobarbital / Possible ↓ mifepristone levels R/T ↑ liver metabolism
Phenytoin / Possible ↓ mifepristone serum levels R/T ↑ liver metabolism
Rifampin / Possible ↓ mifepristone serum levels R/T ↑ liver metabolism
H ***St. John's wort*** / Possible ↓ mifepristone levels R/T ↑ liver metabolism

NOTE: When used with mifepristone, possible increase in serum levels of drugs that are CYP3A4 substrates. Use with caution with such drugs that have a narrow therapeutic range (e.g., some agents used during general anesthesia).

HOW SUPPLIED

Tablets: 200 mg.

DOSAGE

TABLETS

Termination of intrauterine pregnancy.

Treatment includes both mifepristone and misoprostol and requires three office visits. **Day 1:** Three 200-mg tablets (600 mg) of mifepristone taken as a single dose. **Day 3:** Unless abortion has occurred and has been confirmed by clinical examination or ultrasonographic scan, clients must take misoprostol, 400 mcg (two 200-mcg tablets) PO. **Day 14:** Client returns for follow-up visit to confirm by clinical examination or ultrasonographic scan that complete termination of pregnancy has occurred.

NURSING IMPLICATIONS

Do not confuse mifepristone with misoprostol (prostaglandin used with mifepristone to terminate pregnancy).

IMPLEMENTATION/ADMINISTRATION/STORAGE

1. **The drug is supplied only to licensed physicians who sign and return a Prescriber's**

Agreement. It is not available to the public through licensed pharmacies.

2. Remove any IUD before beginning mifepristone treatment.
3. Available only in single-dose packaging.
4. Administration must be under the supervision of a qualified provider.
5. Clients must read the Medication Guide and read and sign the Patient Agreement before mifepristone is given. Review risk of serious and sometimes fatal infections and bleeding that could occur following mifepristone use.
6. Mifepristone may be less effective if misoprostol is given more than 2 days after mifepristone use.

ASSESSMENT

1. The duration of pregnancy can be determined from menstrual history and clinical examination. Use an ultrasonographic scan if the duration of pregnancy is uncertain or if ectopic pregnancy is suspected.
2. Ensure client fully understands the results of treatment and is in concurrence. Provide a copy of the Medication Guide and the Patient Agreement. May obtain by contacting Danco Laboratories.
3. List drugs prescribed to ensure none interact unfavorably (CYP3A4 metabolism).
4. Obtain history to assess for CAD, HTN, IDDM, smoking, hepatic/respiratory/renal disease, or severe anemia as drug has not been studied in these groups.
5. Assess for any heavy or prolonged bleeding. Monitor CBC, LFTs.

CLIENT/FAMILY TEACHING

1. Review Medication Guide and Patient Agreement to understand the treatment procedure and its effects. Request clarification or pose questions as needed and sign agreement.
2. The treatment consists of three visits to the provider. On day 1 a dose of mifepristone (600 mg) PO is administered. Return on day 3 to determine if abortion has occurred by clinical exam or by ultrasound. If not, misoprostol 400 mcg will be administered orally. Finally, must return on day 14–16 to confirm termination of pregnancy.
3. Carry instructions on whom to call, including phone number and what to do in the event of an emergency following administration of both mifepristone and misoprostol.
4. Take Medication Guide with you if you visit an emergency room or another health care provider who did not prescribe mifepristone.
5. Onset of action usually occurs between 2 and 24 hr of initial treatment. Menses should begin within 5 days of treatments and will last 1–2 weeks.
6. Bleeding and spotting usually last for 9 to 16 days but could last longer. Immediately notify provider using supplied phone number if severe abdominal pain, fever of 100.4°F or higher that lasts for more than 4 hr, or excessive vaginal bleeding (i.e., soak through 2 thick full-size sanitary pads per hour for 2 consecutive hr) experienced.
7. Prolonged, heavy bleeding does not confirm a complete expulsion. With treatment failure, there is an increased risk of fetal malformation.
8. If medical treatment fails, these cases are managed by surgical termination (D&C).
9. Any sustained fever, severe abdominal pain, prolonged heavy bleeding, or syncope require medical care.
10. Contraception must be initiated as soon as the termination of pregnancy has been confirmed or before sexual intercourse is resumed as pregnancy can occur before resumption of normal menses.
11. In addition to uterine bleeding and cramping, may experience N&V, pelvic pain, diarrhea, fainting, headaches, and dizziness. Bleeding and spotting may occur for over 2 weeks after treatment. Report immediately if persistent or significant side effects.
12. Keep all F/U to assess response and for adverse SE.

OUTCOMES/EVALUATE

Termination of pregnancy

Miglitol

(**MIG**-lih-tohl)

Classification(s): Antidiabetic, oral; alpha-glucosidase inhibitor

Pregnancy Category: B

RX: Glyset.

SEE ALSO ***ANTIDIABETIC AGENTS: HYPOGLYCEMIC AGENTS***.

M

INDICATIONS/USES

(1) Alone as adjunct to diet to treat non-insulin-dependent diabetes when hyperglycemia cannot be managed with diet alone. (2) With a sulfonylurea when diet plus either miglitol or a sulfonylurea alone do not result in adequate control (effects of sulfonylurea and miglitol are additive).

ACTION/KINETICS

Action

Acts by delaying digestion of ingested carbohydrates resulting in smaller rise in blood glucose levels after meals. Effect is due to reversible inhibition of membrane-bound intestinal glucoside hydrolase enzymes which hydrolyze oligosaccharides and disaccharides to glucose and other monosaccharides. Reduces levels of glycosylated hemoglobin in type 2 diabetes. Does not enhance insulin secretion or increase insulin sensitivity. Does not cause hypoglycemia when given in fasted state.

Pharmacokinetics

Absorption is saturable at high doses (i.e., only 50 to 70% of 100 mg dose is absorbed while 25 mg dose is 100% absorbed). **Peak levels:** 2–3 hr. Drug is not metabolized and is eliminated unchanged in urine. Reduce dose in impaired renal function.

M

CONTRAINDICATIONS

Lactation, diabetic ketoacidosis, IBD, colonic ulceration, partial intestinal obstruction, those predisposed to intestinal obstruction, chronic intestinal diseases associated with marked disorders of digestion or absorption, conditions that may deteriorate due to increased gas formation in the intestine, hypersensitivity to drug.

SPECIAL CONCERNS

- When given with sulfonylurea or insulin, miglitol causes further decrease in blood sugar and increased risk of hypoglycemia.
- Safety and efficacy not determined in children.

SIDE EFFECTS

Most Common

Flatulence, diarrhea, abdominal pain.

GI: Flatulence, diarrhea, abdominal pain/discomfort, soft stools. **Dermatologic:** Skin rash (transient). **Miscellaneous:** Low serum iron.

DRUG INTERACTIONS

Amylase / ↓ Miglitol effect
Charcoal / ↓ Miglitol effect; do not take together
Digestive enzymes / ↓ Miglitol absorption
Digoxin / May ↓ digoxin levels
Pancreatin / ↓ Miglitol effect
Propranolol / Significant ↓ in propranolol bioavailability
Ranitidine / Significant ↓ in ranitidine bioavailability

HOW SUPPLIED

Tablets: 25 mg, 50 mg, 100 mg.

DOSAGE

TABLETS

Type 2 diabetes.

Individualize dosage. **Initial:** 25 mg 3 times per day with first bite of each main meal (some may benefit from starting with 25 mg once daily to minimize GI side effects). After 4 to 8 weeks of 25 mg 3 times per day dose, increase dosage to 50 mg 3 times per day for about 3 months. Measure glycosylated hemoglobin; if not satisfactory, increase dose to 100 mg 3 times per day. **Maintenance:** 50 mg 3 times per day, up to 100 mg 3 times per day (maximum).

NURSING IMPLICATIONS

ASSESSMENT

1. Note age, onset, characteristics of disease, other agents trialed, outcome.
2. List any IBD, colonic ulceration, intestinal obstruction, severe digestion/absorption problems from colonoscopy.
3. Note drugs prescribed to ensure none interact.
4. Use glucose (dextrose) and not cane sugar (table sugar) or fruits/fruit juices to treat hypoglycemia.
5. Monitor BP, BS, HbA1c, lipids, urine for albumin, renal function; reduce dose with impaired function; avoid if creatinine >2 mg/dL.

CLIENT/FAMILY TEACHING

1. Take with first bite of each meal, 3 times per day as directed.
2. Attend diabetic education program to enhance understanding of disease, dietary control, weight loss, foot/eye care, BP, and exercise as it relates to overall health. Continue prescribed diet and regular exercise.

3. **May experience abdominal pain and diarrhea which should diminish with continued treatment.**
4. **Any stress, fever, trauma, infection, or surgery may alter glucose control; monitor/record FS regularly.**
5. **Drug inhibits breakdown of table sugar; have glucose available for episodes of marked hypoglycemia.**
6. **Do not use if pregnant; report as insulin is the agent preferred to control BS during pregnancy.**
7. **Keep all F/U to assess response, labs, and for adverse SE.**

OUTCOMES/EVALUATE

↓ BS; HbA1c <8

Milnacipran hydrochloride

(mil-**NAY**-si-pran **HYE**-droe-**KLOR**-ide)

Classification(s): Antidepressant, serotonin and norepinephrine reuptake inhibitor

Pregnancy Category: C

RX: Savella.

INDICATIONS/USES

Management of fibromyalgia.

ACTION/KINETICS

Action

The exact mechanism of milnacipran to improve the symptoms of fibromyalgia is not known. The drug is a potent inhibitor of neuronal reuptake of norepinephrine and serotonin.

Pharmacokinetics

Absolute bioavailability is 85–90%. **Maximum concentration:** 2–4 hr. **Steady state levels:** 36–48 hr. Unchanged drug (55%) and metabolites excreted in the urine. **t½, terminal:** 6–8 hr. AUC and terminal elimination t½ increased in mild, moderate, or severe impaired renal function. **Plasma protein binding:** 13%.

CONTRAINDICATIONS

Concomitant use with MAOIs or within 14 days of discontinuing treatment with an MAOI. Uncontrolled narrow-angle glaucoma, end-stage renal disease, substantial alcohol use or chronic liver disease, lactation, use in children.

SPECIAL CONCERNS

Suicidality and antidepressant drugs. Milnacipran is a selective serotonin and norepinephrine reuptake inhibitor, similar to some drugs used for the treatment of depression and other psychiatric disorders. Antidepressants increased the risk, compared with placebo, of suicidal thinking and behavior (suicidality) in children, adolescents, and young adults in short-term studies of major depressive disorder and other psychiatric disorders. Anyone considering the use of such drugs in a child, adolescent, or young adult must balance this risk with the clinical need. Short-term studies did not show an increase in the risk of suicidality with antidepressants compared with placebo in adults older than 24 years of age; there was a reduction in risk with antidepressants compared with placebo in adults 65 years of age and older. Depression and certain other psychiatric disorders are themselves associated with increases in the risk of suicide. Appropriately monitor clients of all ages who are started on milnacipran and observe closely for clinical worsening, suicidality, or unusual changes in behavior. Advise families and caregivers of the need for close observation and communication with the prescriber. Milnacipran is not approved for use in the treatment of major depressive disorder. Milnacipran is not approved for use in children.

- **Contains tartrazine which may cause allergic reactions (including bronchial asthma) in susceptible individuals.**
- **Use with caution in severe hepatic impairment, in controlled narrow-angle glaucoma, with a history of seizure disorders or mania, with a history of dysuria (e.g., men with prostatic hypertrophy), and when taken in combination with other CNS drugs.**
- **May produce physical dependence as evidenced by development of withdrawal symptoms.**
- **Possible significant hyponatremia in the elderly who are prone to this side effect.**
- **Safety and efficacy not determined in children younger than 17 years of age with fibromyalgia.**

M

SIDE EFFECTS

Most Common

N&V, constipation, hot flush, headache, dizziness, insomnia, hyperhidrosis, palpitations, ↑ HR, hypertension, dry mouth, URTI.

CNS: Headache, insomnia, dizziness, migraine, aggressiveness, akathisia, anxiety, hostility, hypomania, impulsivity, insomnia, irritability, mania, panic attacks, paresthesia, tension headache, tremor, hypesthesia, depression, fall, irritability, pyrexia, somnolence, stress, ***convulsions (including tonic–clonic)***, delirium, hallucination, loss of consciousness, ***neuroleptic malignant syndrome***, Parkinsonism, worsening of depression and/or emergence of ***suicidal ideation and suicidality***, unusual changes in behavior, withdrawal symptoms. **Serotonin syndrome:** Agitation, coma, hallucinations, hyperthermia, labile BP, tachycardia, hyperreflexia, incoordination, diarrhea, N&V. **GI:** N&V, constipation, dry mouth, abdominal pain, decreased appetite, abdominal distension, diarrhea, dysgeusia, dyspepsia, flatulence, GERD. **Hepatic:** Hepatitis, hepatotoxicity, ***fulminant hepatitis***. **CV:** Palpitations, increased HR, hypertension, tachycardia, flushing, increased BP, ***hypertensive crisis***, SVT, increased risk of bleeding events. **Respiratory:** URTI, dyspnea, chest discomfort/pain. **Dermatologic:** Hyperhidrosis, pruritus, rash, erythema multiforme, ***Stevens-Johnson syndrome***. **GU:** Cystitis, UTI, acute renal failure, galactorrhea.

In men: Dysuria, ejaculation disorder/failure, erectile dysfunction, decreased libido, prostatitis, scrotal pain, testicular pain/swelling, urethral pain, urinary hesitation/retention, decreased urine flow. **Metabolic/Nutritional:** Hypercholesterolemia, peripheral edema, decreased/increased weight, anorexia, hyponatremia. **Hematologic:** Leukopenia, neutropenia, thrombocytopenia. **Ophthalmic:** Blurred vision, accommodation disorder, mydriasis. **Body as a whole:** Hot flush, fatigue, chills, night sweats. **Miscellaneous:** Contusion, rhabdomyolysis, withdrawal symptoms upon drug discontinuation.

LABORATORY TEST CONSIDERATIONS

↑ ALT, AST. Hyperprolactinemia, hyponatremia.

OVERDOSE MANAGEMENT

Symptoms: Increased BP, ***cardiorespiratory arrest***, changes in the level of consciousness (from somnolence to coma), confusion, dizziness, and increased hepatic enzymes. *Treatment:* There is no specific antidote. Ensure an adequate airway, oxygenation, and ventilation. Monitor cardiac rhythm and vital signs. Gastric lavage with a large-bore orogastric tube with appropriate airway protection may be used if performed soon after ingestion or in symptomatic clients. Activated charcoal may also be used. Induction of emesis is not recommended. Forced diuresis, dialysis, hemoperfusion, and exchange transfusion are not likely to be beneficial.

DRUG INTERACTIONS

Alcohol / May aggravate pre-existing liver disease; do not give to those with substantial alcohol use or chronic liver disease

Amphetamine / Use with caution if given with amphetamine; closely monitor

Antipsychotic drugs (e.g., risperidone) / ↑ Risk of serotonin syndrome; closely monitor if coadministration is necessary

Aspirin / ↑ Bleeding effects of aspirin; use together with caution

Clomipramine / ↑ Euphoria and postural hypotension in those who switched from clomipramine to milnacipran

Clonidine / May ↓ antihypertensive effect of clonidine

Cyclobenzaprine / Possible additive serotonergic effects and serotonin syndrome; monitor closely if coadministration necessary

Digoxin / Possible postural hypotension and tachycardia in combination with IV digoxin; avoid coadministration

Epinephrine / Possible paroxysmal hypertension and arrhythmia; use together with caution

Lithium / Possible serotonin syndrome; closely monitor if coadministration is necessary

MAOIs (e.g., phenelzine, rasagiline) / Possible serotonin syndrome; see ***Implementation/Administration/Storage***

Methylene blue / ↑ Risk of CNS toxicity including serotonin syndrome; avoid coadministration

Metoclopramide / Possible serotonin syndrome; closely monitor if coadministration is necessary

Norepinephrine / Possible paroxysmal hypertension and arrhythmia; use together with caution

NSAIDs / ↑ Bleeding effects of NSAIDs; use together with caution

Serotonergic drugs (e.g., SNRIs, SSRIs, tramadol, triptans) / Possible hypertension and coronary artery vasoconstriction R/T additive serotonergic effects

l-Tryptophan / Possible symptoms of serotonin syndrome (e.g., headache, sweating, dizziness, N&V); do not give together

Warfarin / ↑ Bleeding effects of warfarin; use together with caution

HOW SUPPLIED

Tablets: 12.5 mg, 25 mg, 50 mg, 100 mg.

DOSAGE

TABLETS

Fibromyalgia.

Adults, usual: 50 mg twice a day. **Dose titration:** Give 12.5 mg once on day 1, 12.5 mg twice a day on days 2 and 3, 25 mg twice a day on days 4–7, and 50 mg twice a day after day 7. May increase dose to 100 mg twice a day based on individual response. **Maximum dose:** 200 mg/day (i.e., 100 mg twice a day).

NURSING IMPLICATIONS

IMPLEMENTATION/ADMINISTRATION/STORAGE

1. Give with or without food, although may improve tolerability if taken with food.
2. After extended use, taper the dose; do not abruptly discontinue.
3. For those with severe renal impairment (i.e., C_{CR} from 5–29 mL/min), reduce the maintenance dose by 50% to 25 mg twice a day.
4. At least 14 days should elapse between discontinuation of an MAOI and initiation of milnacipran therapy. In addition, at least 5 days should elapse after stopping milnacipran before starting an MAOI.
5. To provide information regarding exposure to milnacipran during pregnancy, health care providers are voluntary asked to register clients by calling 1-877-643-3010 or by email at www.registrieskendle.com. Data forms may also be downloaded from the registry website at http://www.savellapregnancyregistry.com
6. Store from 15–30°C (59–86°F).

ASSESSMENT

1. Note reasons for therapy, onset, characteristics of S&S, ROM/mobility, other agents trialed, outcome.
2. Document clinical presentation and assess for any behavioral changes or depression; rate pain levels.
3. List drugs prescribed to ensure none interact.
4. Note medical history, especially seizures, CAD. Assess ECG for arrhythmia.
5. Drug contains FD&C yellow No. 5 (tartrazine); use caution.
6. Assess for withdrawal symptoms when discontinuing treatment with milnacipran.
7. Monitor BP, HR, Wt, CBC, electrolytes, renal and LFTs; adjust dose with dysfunction.

CLIENT/FAMILY TEACHING

1. Take twice a day as directed with or without food to control symptoms of fibromyalgia. Taking the drug with food may improve tolerability.
2. Avoid activities that require mental alertness until effects realized; may experience diminished mental and physical capacities.
3. Do not stop taking abruptly, should be tapered if stopping therapy to prevent withdrawal symptoms.
4. Avoid alcohol, NSAIDS, and aspirin during therapy; may affect clotting.
5. Report increased anxiety, agitation, panic attacks, aggressiveness, or other unusual behavioral changes, worsening of depression, and suicidal ideation.
6. Monitor BP and heart rate and report if persistently elevated.
7. Practice reliable contraception and avoid pregnancy.
8. Keep all F/U to assess response, labs, and for adverse SE.

OUTCOMES/EVALUATE

↓ Pain and ↑ mobility with fibromyalgia

IV

Milrinone lactate

(**MILL**-rih-nohn)

Classification(s): Inotropic drug

Pregnancy Category: C

M

INDICATIONS/USES

Short-term IV treatment of acute decompensated heart failure.

ACTION/KINETICS

Action

Selective inhibitor of peak III cyclic AMP phosphodiesterase isozyme in cardiac and vascular muscle, resulting in a direct inotropic effect and a direct arterial vasodilator activity. Also improves diastolic function as manifested by improvements in LV diastolic relaxation. In clients with depressed myocardial function, produces a prompt increase in CO and a decrease in pulmonary wedge pressure and vascular resistance, without a significant increase in HR or myocardial oxygen consumption. Causes an inotropic effect in clients who are fully digitalized without causing signs of glycoside toxicity. Also, LV function has improved in clients with ischemic heart disease.

Pharmacokinetics

Steady state plasma levels after about 6–12 hr of infusion of 0.5 mcg/kg/min are about 200 ng/mL. **Therapeutic plasma levels:** 150–250 ng/mL. **t½:** 2.3 hr following doses of 12.5–125 mcg/kg to clients with CHF. Metabolized in the liver and excreted primarily through the urine. **Plasma protein binding:** 70%.

M

CONTRAINDICATIONS

Hypersensitivity to the drug. Use in severe obstructive aortic or pulmonary valvular disease in lieu of surgical relief of the obstruction.

SPECIAL CONCERNS

- Use with caution during lactation.
- Safety and efficacy not determined in children.

SIDE EFFECTS

Most Common

Ventricular arrhythmias (see below), hypotension, angina/chest pain, headaches.

CV: ***Ventricular and supraventricular arrhythmias, including ventricular ectopic activity, nonsustained ventricular tachycardia, sustained ventricular tachycardia, and ventricular fibrillation.*** Infrequently, ***life-threatening arrhythmias associated with pre-existing arrhythmias***, metabolic abnormalities, abnormal digoxin levels, and catheter insertion. Also, hypotension, angina, chest pain. **Miscellaneous:** Mild to moderately severe headaches, tremor, thrombocytopenia, bronchospasm (rare).

LABORATORY TEST CONSIDERATIONS

Abnormal LFTs. Hypokalemia.

OVERDOSE MANAGEMENT

Symptoms: Hypotension. *Treatment:* If hypotension occurs, reduce or temporarily discontinue administration of milrinone until the condition of the client stabilizes. Use general measures to support circulation.

HOW SUPPLIED

Injection: 1 mg/mL.

DOSAGE

IV INFUSION

CHF in clients receiving digoxin and diuretics.

Adults, loading dose: 50 mcg/kg administered slowly over 10 min. **Maintenance, minimum:** 0.59 mg/kg/24 hr (infused at a rate of 0.375 mcg/kg/min); **maintenance, standard:** 0.77 mg/kg/24 hr (infused at a rate of 0.5 mcg/kg/min); **maintenance, maximum:** 1.13 mg/kg/24 hr (infused at a rate of 0.75 mcg/kg/min). *NOTE:* The doses per 24 hr are presented in **milligrams** while the infusion rate per minute is presented in **micrograms**.

NURSING IMPLICATIONS

Ⓢ Do not confuse milrinone with inamrinone (an inotropic drug).

IMPLEMENTATION/ADMINISTRATION/STORAGE

1. IV Should be given with a loading dose followed by a continuous infusion (maintenance dose).
2. Give IV infusions at rates described in the package insert.
3. Reduce infusion rate in renal impairment (see package insert for chart).
4. Adjust rate depending on the hemodynamic and clinical response.
5. Prepare dilutions using compatible fluids.
6. Discard unused portion after initial use.
7. Store at room temperatures of 15–30°C (59–86°F). Avoid freezing and avoid excessive heat.
8. COMPATIBILITY NSS, D5W.

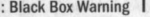

9. INCOMPATIBILITY Furosemide—a precipitate will form; administer separately.

ASSESSMENT

1. Note onset, characteristics of S&S. Identify NYHA class, other therapies used, outcome.
2. List heart and lung assessments and monitor for evidence of CHF. Observe ECG on monitor (for increased supraventricular and ventricular arrhythmias), HR and BP during infusion.
3. Monitor VS; review parameters for interruption of infusion (e.g., SBP <80; HR <50).
4. Document ECG, CO, CVP, and pulmonary artery wedge pressure (PAWP); rule out acute MI.
5. Monitor I&O, Wt, CBC, electrolytes, renal and LFTs. Potassium loss due to excessive diuresis may cause arrhythmias in digitalized clients; correct hypokalemia.

CLIENT/FAMILY TEACHING

1. Given IV to treat heart failure; treatment usually does not exceed 5 days.
2. May experience headaches; report as mild analgesics may alleviate, i.e., acetaminophen. Also report if tremors occur. Report any increased chest pain, SOB, or worsening of symptoms.

OUTCOMES/EVALUATE

- ↑ CO and ↓ pulmonary artery wedge pressure (PAWP)
- Resolution of S&S of CHF
- Therapeutic drug levels (150–250 ng/mL)

IV

Minocycline hydrochloride

(mih-no-**SYE**-kleen)

Classification(s): Antibiotic, tetracycline

Pregnancy Category: D

RX: Arestin, Cleervue-M, Dynacin, Minocin, Myrac, Solodyn.

✤ **Rx:** Apo-Minocycline, Gen-Minocycline, ratio-Minocycline, Sandoz Minocycline.

SEE ALSO ***ANTI-INFECTIVE DRUGS*** AND ***TETRACYCLINES.***

INDICATIONS/USES

PO, Systemic.

1. Gram-negative infections due to *Haemophilis ducreyi* (chancroid); *Francisella tularensis* (tularemia); *Yersinia pestis* (plague); *Bartonella bacilliformis* (bartonellosis); *Campylobacter fetus; Vibrio cholerae* (cholera); *Brucella* species (used with streptomycin); *Neisseria gonorrhoeae* (uncomplicated urethritis in men). Do not use extended-release products for these infections.
2. Infections caused by the following miscellaneous organisms: *Rickettsiae* (Rocky Mountain spotted fever, typhus fever and the typhus group); Q fever; rickettsiapox; tick fevers); *Mycoplasma pneumoniae* (respiratory tract infections); *Chlamydia trachomatis* (lymphogranuloma venereum; trachoma, inclusive conjunctivitis), *Chlamydia psittaci* (psittacosis); *Borellia recurrentis* (relapsing fever); *Ureaplasma urealyticum* (nongonococcal urethritis). Do not use extended-release products for these infections.
3. Following susceptibility testing (resistance has been shown): *Escherichia coli; Enterobacter aerogenes; Acinetobacter* and *Shigella* species; *Haemophilus influenzae* (respiratory tract infections); *Klebsiella* species (respiratory and urinary tract infections); *Streptococcus pneumoniae* (upper respiratory infections); *Staphylococcus aureus* (skin and skin structure infections).
4. Alternative therapy for the following infections when penicillin is contraindicated: *Neisseria gonorrhoeae* infections; syphilis due to *Treponema pallidum;* yaws due to *Treponema pertenue;* listeriosis due to *Listeria monocytogenes;* anthrax due to *Bacillus anthracis;* Vincent's infections due to *Fusobacterium fusiforme;* actinomycosis due to *Actinomyces israelii;* infections due to *Clostridium* species. Do not use extended-release products for these infections.
5. As an adjunct to amebicides to treat acute intestinal amebiasis. Do not use extended-release products for these infections.
6. As an adjunct to treat severe acne.
7. Treat asymptomatic meningococcal carriers due to *N. meningitidis*. Do not use extended-release products for this infection.
8. Inflammatory lesions of moderate to severe acne vulgaris without nodules in clients ages 12 years and older.

Investigational: Early rheumatoid arthritis; gallbladder infections due to *E. coli;* alternative drug for nocardiosis in those who cannot take sulfa drugs; chronic malignant pleural effusion; *Mycobacterium marinum* infections.

Dental: Adjunctive treatment to scaling and root planing procedures to reduce pocket depth adult periodontitis (Arestin). May be used as part of a periodontal maintenance program that includes good oral hygiene and scaling and root planning.

Injection.

1. Infections due to the following susceptible strains: Rocky Mountain spotted fever; typhus fever and the typhus group; Q fever; rickettsial pox and tick fevers caused by rickettsia; respiratory tract infections due to *Mycoplasma pneumoniae;* lymphogranuloma venereum due to *Chlamydia trachomatis;* psittacosis (ornithosis) due to *Chlamydia psittaci;* trachoma due to *C. trachomatis* (infection not always eliminated); inclusion conjunctivitis due to *C. trachomatis;* nongonococcal urethritis, endocervical, or rectal infections in adults due to *Ureaplasma urealyticum* or *C. trachomatis;* relapsing fever due to *Borrelia recurrentis;* chancroid due to *Haemophilus ducreyi;* plague due to *Yersinia pestis;* tularemia due to *Francisella tularensis;* cholera due to *Vibrio cholerae; Campylobacter fetus* infections due to *C. fetus;* brucellosis due to *Brucella* species (in conjunction with streptomycin); bartonellosis due to *Bartonella bacilliformis;* granuloma inguinale due to *Calymmatobacterium granulomatis.*
2. Infections due to the following gram-negative microorganisms susceptible to the drug: *E. coli; Enterobacter aerogenes; Shigella species; Acinetobacter species;* respiratory tract infections due to *Haemophilus influenzae;* respiratory tract and urinary tract infections due to *Klebsiella* species.
3. Infections due to the following gram-positive microorganisms susceptible to the drug: Upper respiratory tract infections due to *Streptococcus pneumoniae;* skin and skin structure infections due to *Staphylococcus aureus* (minocycline is not the drug of choice).
4. As an alternative drug for the following infections when penicillin is contraindicated: Uncomplicated urethritis in men due to *Neisseria gonorrhoeae* and to treat other gonococcal infections; infections in women due to *N. gonorrhoeae;* meningitis due to *Neisseria meningitidis;* syphilis due to *Treponema pallidum* subspecies *pallidum;* yaws due to *T. pallidum* subspecies *pertenue;* listeriosis due to *Listeria monocytogenes;* anthrax due to *Bacillus anthracis;* Vincent infection due to *Fusobacterium fusiforme;* actinomycosis due to *Actinomyces israelii;* infections due to *Clostridium* species.
5. Adjunct to amebicides to treat acute intestinal amebiasis.
6. Adjunct therapy to treat severe acne.

NOTE: Do not use tetracyclines for streptococci infections unless the organism has been shown to be susceptible. Tetracyclines are not the drugs of choice to treat any type of staphylococcal infection.

ACTION/KINETICS

Action

Inhibits protein synthesis by binding to the ribosomal 30S subunit, thereby interfering with protein synthesis. Blocks the binding of aminoacyl transfer RNA to the messenger RNA complex. Cell wall synthesis is not inhibited.

Pharmacokinetics

In fasting adults, 90–100% of an oral dose is absorbed. **Peak plasma levels:** 1–4 hr. Absorption is less affected by milk or food than for other tetracyclines. **t½, elimination:** 11–26 hr after PO use and 15–23 hr after IV use. Metabolized in the liver. 5–10% excreted in the urine. **Plasma protein binding:** 75%.

SPECIAL CONCERNS

Use the dental product (Arestin) with caution in clients with a history of predisposition to oral candidiasis.

SIDE EFFECTS

Most Common

Diarrhea, dizziness, unsteadiness, drowsiness, headache, vomiting.

See *Tetracyclines* for a complete list of possible side effects. Also, blue-gray pigmentation areas of cutaneous inflammation, vertigo, ataxia, drowsiness, ***Stevens-Johnson syndrome*** (rare). **When used for adult periodontitis:** Tooth discoloration, periodontitis, tooth disorder, tooth caries, dental pain, stomatitis, infection, headache, gingivitis, flu syndrome, pharyngitis, dental infection, pain, mucous membrane disorder, dyspepsia, mouth ulceration. Also, overgrowth of nonsusceptible microorganisms, including fungi.

HOW SUPPLIED

Capsules: 50 mg, 75 mg, 100 mg; ***Capsules, Pellet-Filled:*** 50 mg, 100 mg; ***Oral Suspension:*** 50 mg/5 mL; ***Powder for Injection, Lyophilized:*** 100 mg/vial; ***Powder, Extended-Release, Dental:*** 1 mg; ***Tablets:*** 50 mg, 75 mg, 100 mg; ***Tablets, Extended-Release:*** 45 mg, 65 mg, 90 mg, 115 mg, 135 mg.

DOSAGE

CAPSULES, IMMEDIATE-RELEASE; CAPSULES, PELLET-FILLED; ORAL SUSPENSION; TABLETS

Infections against which effective.

Adults, initial: 200 mg; **then,** 100 mg q 12 hr. An alternative regimen is 100–200 mg initially followed by 50 mg q 6 hr. **Children over 8 years of age, initial:** 4 mg/kg; **then,** 2 mg/kg q 12 hr. When used parenterally do not exceed 400 mg per day in adults; for children, do not exceed the adult dose.

Uncomplicated urethral infections in adults due to C. trachomatis *or* Ureaplasma urealyticum.

Adults: 100 mg q 12 hr for at least 7 days.

Uncomplicated gonococcal urethritis in men.

100 mg q 12 hr for 5 days.

Uncomplicated gonococcal infections except urethritis and anorectal infections in men.

Initial: 200 mg; **then,** 100 mg q 12 hr for at least 4 days, with posttherapy cultures within 2–3 days.

Meningococcal carrier state.

100 mg q 12 hr for 5 days.

Mycobacterium marinum *infections.*

Usual: 100 mg q 12 hr for 6–8 weeks.

DENTAL: MICROSPHERES, EXTENDED-RELEASE

Adult periodontitis.

Amount given depends on the size, shape, and number of pockets being treated. The unit-dose cartridge is inserted into a cartridge handle in order to administer. Up to 121 unit-dose cartridges have been used in a single visit; also, up to 3 treatments, at 3-month intervals were administered in pockets with a depth of 5 mm or more.

TABLETS, EXTENDED-RELEASE

Moderate-to-severe acne vulgaris without nodules.

Adults and children, 12 years and older: 91–136 kg (200–300 lbs): 0.99–1.48 mg/kg (use 135 mg strength); **60–90 kg (132–100 lbs):** 1–1.5 mg/kg (use 90 mg strength); **45–59 kg (99–131 lbs):** 0.76–1 mg/kg (use 45 mg strength).

IV

Infections against which effective.

Adults, initial: 200 mg; **then,** 100 mg q 12 hr, not to exceed 400 mg in 24 hr. **Children, age 8 years and older, initial:** 4 mg/kg; **then,** 2 mg/kg q 12 hr, not to exceed the usual adult dose.

NOTE: Exceeding the recommended dose may cause an increased incidence of side effects.

NURSING IMPLICATIONS

Do not confuse Minocin with Indocin (NSAID).

IMPLEMENTATION/ADMINISTRATION/STORAGE

1. Minocycline microspheres (Arestin) are delivered directly into the infected periodontal pocket after scaling and root planing. No refrigeration or mixing is needed and the product does not require removal.
2. Decrease the recommended dose and/or increase the dosing intervals in clients with renal impairment. Do not exceed a dose of 200 mg/day of Minocin (whether using PO or injection) in these clients.
3. When used for syphilis, give usual dose over a period of 10–15 days. Close follow-up, including lab tests, is recommended.
4. Store capsules, suspension, tablets, and microspheres from 15–30°C (59–86°F). Do not freeze. Protect from light, moisture and excessive heat.
5. IV Avoid rapid administration. Use parenteral therapy only when PO therapy is inadequate

or not tolerated. Institute PO therapy as soon as possible. Thrombophlebitis may occur if IV therapy is given over a prolonged period.

6. Do not dissolve in solutions containing calcium; forms a precipitate. Also, check the package insert for the large number of drugs that should not be mixed before or during administration of minocycline.
7. Reconstitute the cryodesiccated powder with 5 mL sterile water for injection; immediately dilute further to 500–1,000 mL with NaCl injection, dextrose injection, dextrose and NaCl injection, Ringer's injection, or RL injection. When diluted in 500 to 1,000 mL the pH usually ranges from 2.5 to 4, except when using RL where the pH ranges from 4.5 to 6.
8. Administer immediately although reconstituted solutions may be stored at room temperature up to 24 hr. Discard any unused portions after 24 hr at room temperature.
9. Store the Powder for Injection from 20–25°C (68–77°F). Protect from light, moisture, and excessive heat.
10. COMPATIBILITY NaCl, D5W, dextrose and NaCl solutions, RL, Ringer's solution.
11. INCOMPATIBILITY Solutions containing calcium.

ASSESSMENT

1. List reasons for therapy, onset, location, clinical presentation, characteristics of S&S, cultures, other agents trialed/outcome.
2. Identify contacts when treating contagious diseases; get infectious disease referral.
3. Assess infusion site due to increased risk of thrombophlebitis; convert to oral therapy as soon as possible.
4. Monitor C&S, renal and LFTs, CBC; reduce dose/dosing intervals with renal dysfunction.

CLIENT/FAMILY TEACHING

1. Take with or without food, with a full glass of water and at least 1 hr prior to bedtime to prevent esophageal irritation. Check expiration date; discard any outdated products to prevent adverse effects.
2. Take 1 hr before or 2 hr after antacids containing aluminum, calcium, or magnesium, or preparations containing iron or zinc.
3. With oral suspension, measure and administer prescribed dose using dosing spoon/syringe, or medicine cup.
4. Use caution, avoid activities that require mental alertness until drug effects realized; may cause dizziness or blurred vision.
5. With STDs, use condoms during therapy to prevent reinfections and obtain periodic cultures.
6. Avoid in children under 8 years old during tooth development; may stain teeth.
7. Practice reliable non-hormonal birth control may make birth control pills less effective; drug may cause fetal harm.
8. Avoid prolonged sunlight exposure; may cause photosensitivity reaction.
9. Report any dizziness, unusual bruising/bleeding, severe skin rash/hives, or diarrhea, difficulty breathing, blurred vision, dark urine or light stools, severe cramps, and lack of improvement after 72 hr.
10. With Microspheres SR: avoid touching treated areas and avoid brushing for 12 hr following treatment. Do not eat hard, crunchy, or sticky foods for 1 wk following treatment; avoid interproximal cleaning devices (floss) for 10 days.
11. Mild to moderate sensitivity is expected after treatment; report to dental provider immediately if pain, swelling, or other problems occur.
12. Keep all F/U to assess response, labs, and for adverse SE.

OUTCOMES/EVALUATE

Symptomatic improvement; resolution of infection

Minoxidil, topical solution

(mih-**NOX**-ih-dil)

Classification(s): Hair growth stimulant

Pregnancy Category: C

OTC: Minoxidil Extra Strength for Men, Rogaine, Rogaine Extra Strength for Men, Rogaine Men's Extra Strength.

OTC: Apo-Gain.

INDICATIONS/USES

To treat androgenetic alopecia as expressed in males as baldness of the vertex of the scalp and in females as diffuse hair loss or thinning of the frontoparietal areas. At least 4 months of twice daily application is necessary before evidence of hair growth can be expected. *Investigational:* Alopecia areata.

ACTION/KINETICS

Action

The topical solution stimulates vertex hair growth in clients with male pattern baldness or in women with androgenetic alopecia. Mechanism may be related to dilation of areterioles and stimulation of resting hair follicles into active growth.

Pharmacokinetics

Following topical administration, approximately 1.4% is absorbed into the systemic circulation. **Onset:** 4 months but is variable. **Duration:** New hair growth may be lost 3–4 months after withdrawal of therapy. Minoxidil and its inactive metabolites are excreted in the urine. Also, see *Minoxidil, oral.*

CONTRAINDICATIONS

Hypersensitivity to minoxidil or any components of the product. Lactation.

SPECIAL CONCERNS

- **Use with caution in clients with hypertension, coronary heart disease, or predisposition to heart failure.**
- **Contains alcohol that will cause burning and irritation of the eyes.**
- **Possible increased systemic absorption if the scalp is irritated or there are abrasions.**
- **Safety and efficacy not determined in clients under 18 years of age.**

SIDE EFFECTS

Most Common

Allergic contact dermatitis, irritant dermatitis, diarrhea, N&V, headache, dizziness, lightheadedness, faintness.

Dermatologic: Allergic contact dermatitis, irritant dermatitis, pruritus, dry skin, flaking of scalp, alopecia, hypertrichosis, local erythema, eczema, worsening of hair loss. **Allergic:** Hives, facial swelling, allergic rhinitis, nonspecific allergic reactions. **GI:** N&V, diarrhea. **CNS:** Dizziness, lightheadedness, headache, faintness, anxiety, depression, fatigue. **CV:** Edema, chest pain, BP increase or decrease, palpitations, increase/decrease in pulse rate. **Respiratory:** Sinusitis, bronchitis, URTI. **Endocrine:** Menstrual changes, breast symptoms. **GU:** UTI, renal calculi, urethritis, prostatitis, epididymitis, vaginitis, vulvitis, vaginal discharge, itching, sexual dysfunction, menstrual changes, breast symptoms. **Hematologic:** Lymphadenopathy, thrombocytopenia, anemia. **Musculoskeletal:** Fractures, back pain, tendonitis, aches and pains. **Ophthalmic:** Conjunctivitis, visual disturbances, decreased visual acuity. **Miscellaneous:** Vertigo, ear infections, edema, weight gain. *NOTE:* The incidence of side effects due to placebos is often similar to the incidence of side effects R/T the drug itself.

DRUG INTERACTIONS

Corticosteroids, topical / Enhances absorption of topical minoxidil

Guanethidine / Possible ↑ risk of orthostatic hypotension

Petrolatum / Enhances absorption of topical minoxidil

Retinoids / Enhances absorption of topical minoxidil

HOW SUPPLIED

Aerosol Foam, Topical: 5%; ***Solution, Topical:*** 2%, 5%.

DOSAGE

AEROSOL FOAM 5%, TOPICAL

Stimulate hair growth.

Apply ½ capful 2 times per day to the scalp in the hair loss area. Continued use is necessary to increase and retain hair regrowth, or hair loss will begin again.

TOPICAL SOLUTION: 2%

Stimulate hair growth.

Adults: Apply 1 mL twice a day to the affected areas of the scalp. Do not exceed a total daily dosage of 2 mL. Twice daily application for 4 or more months may be needed before evidence of hair growth is observed. If hair regrowth is realized, twice daily applications are needed for additional and continued hair regrowth.

TOPICAL SOLUTION: 5%

Stimulate hair growth.

Apply 1 mL twice a day directly onto the scalp in the area of hair thinning or loss. Spread the liquid evenly over the hair loss area. Using more often will not improve results. Continued use is need-

M

ed to increase and maintain hair regrowth or hair loss will begin again.

NURSING IMPLICATIONS

IMPLEMENTATION/ADMINISTRATION/STORAGE

1. Use only in clients with normal, healthy scalps. Dermatitis, scalp abrasions, scalp psoriasis, or severe sunburn may increase the absorption of topical minoxidil and lead to systemic side effects (See *Minoxidil, oral*).
2. Do not use in conjunction with other topical agents, including topical corticosteroids, retinoids, or petroleum or agents that are known to enhance cutaneous drug absorption.
3. Hair may be shampooed before treatment, but dry the hair and scalp prior to topical application.
4. The product comes with a metered spray attachment (for application to large areas of the scalp), extender spray attachment (for application to small scalp areas or under the hair), and a rub-on applicator tip (to spread the solution on the scalp). Follow directions on the package insert carefully for each of these methods of application. Warn not to inhale the spray mist.
5. If the fingertips are used to apply the drug, wash hands thoroughly after application.
6. At least 4 months of continuous therapy is necessary before evidence of hair growth can be expected. Further hair growth continues through 1 year of treatment.
7. Avoid inhaling the spray mist.

ASSESSMENT

1. Note reasons for therapy, onset, location, extent, age at onset, clinical presentation, and family history.
2. List any drugs or treatments to ensure no relationship to condition. Assess psychological presentation.
3. Assess scalp to ensure skin intact and infection/lesion free.

CLIENT/FAMILY TEACHING

1. Review method and frequency for application. Solution may dry and leave a residue on the hair; this is harmless. Dry head and scalp before application; wash hands after application.
2. May permanently discolor linens, hats and pillows with prolonged use/contact.
3. More frequent than prescribed applications will not enhance hair growth but will increase systemic side effects. Review drug info booklet.
4. Product contains alcohol as base; avoid contact with eyes, mucous membranes, or sensitive/irritated areas. If accidental contact occurs, rinse area with large amounts of cool tap water and report if symptomatic.
5. New hair growth will be soft and hard to see and is not permanent. Drug is a treatment, not a cure; stopping therapy will lead to hair loss within a few months. Topical minoxidil must be used indefinitely to sustain the effect.
6. Treatment has positive benefits for only approximately one-half the population. May take up to 4 months of continuous therapy before any response is noted.
7. Do not use in conjunction with other topical scalp medications. Apply drug only to healthy areas of scalp and do not use if scalp becomes irritated or sunburned, and do not use it on other parts of body.
8. Report any evidence of irritation or rash. Do not apply any other topical products to the scalp without approval. In case of accidental contact with sensitive surfaces, such as eyes, abraded skin, or mucous membranes, wash the area with large quantities of cool water.
9. Consult provider before using if no family history of gradual hair loss, if hair loss is sudden or patchy, if hair loss is accompanied by other symptoms, or if the reasons for hair loss are not clear.
10. Keep all F/U to assess response and for adverse SE.

OUTCOMES/EVALUATE

Stimulation of hair growth

Mirtazapine

(mir-**TAZ**-ah-peen)

Classification(s): Antidepressant, tetracyclic

Pregnancy Category: C

RX: Remeron, Remeron SolTab.

Rx: Apo-Mirtazapine, CO Mirtazapine, Gen-Mirtazapine, Novo-Mirtazapine OD, PMS-

Mirtazapine, ratio-Mirtazapine, Sandoz Mirtazapine, Sandoz Mirtazapine FC.

INDICATIONS/USES

Treatment of major depressive disorder. *Investigational:* Chronic urticaria, pruritus associated with cancer.

ACTION/KINETICS

Action

Enhances central noradrenergic and serotonergic activity, perhaps by antagonism at central presynaptic alpha$_2$-adrenergic inhibitory autoreceptors and heteroreceptors. Also a potent antagonist of 5-HT$_2$, 5-HT$_3$, and histamine H$_1$ receptors. Moderate antagonist of peripheral alpha$_1$-adrenergic receptors and muscarinic receptors. Causes high degree of sedation and moderate degree of orthostatic hypotension and anticholinergic effects.

Pharmacokinetics

Rapidly and completely absorbed from the GI tract; about 50% bioavailable. **Peak plasma levels:** Within 2 hr. **t½, elimination:** 20–40 hr. Time to reach steady state: 5 days. Extensively metabolized in the liver by CYP2D6, CYP1A2, and CYP3A; excreted in both the urine (75%) and feces (15%). Females exhibit significantly longer elimination half-lives than males. Geriatric clients, especially men, have a slower clearance compared with younger men. **Plasma protein binding:** About 85%.

CONTRAINDICATIONS

Use in combination with an MAOI or within 14 days of initiating or discontinuing therapy with a MAOI. Known or suspected seizure disorders. During acute phase of MI.

SPECIAL CONCERNS

Suicidality and antidepressant drugs. Antidepressants increased the risk, compared with placebo, of suicidal thinking and behavior (suicidality) in children, adolescents, and young adults in short-term studies of major depressive disorder and other psychiatric disorders. Anyone considering the use of mirtazapine or any other antidepressant in a child, adolescent, or young adult must balance this risk with the clinical need. Short-term studies did not show an increase in the risk of suicidality with antidepressants compared with placebo in adults older than 24 years of age; there was a reduction in risk with antidepressants compared with placebo in adults 65 years of age and older. Depression and certain other psychiatric disorders are associated with increases in suicide risk. Appropriately monitor and closely observe clients of all ages who are started on antidepressant therapy for clinical worsening, suicidality, or unusual changes in behavior. Advise families and caregivers of the need for close observation and communication with the prescriber. Mirtazapine is not approved for use in children.

- **Use with caution in impaired renal or hepatic disease, in geriatric clients, during lactation, in CV or cerebrovascular disease that can be exacerbated by hypotension (e.g., history of MI, angina, ischemic stroke), and in conditions that would predispose to hypotension (e.g., dehydration, hypovolemia, treatment with antihypertensive medications).**
- **The effect of mirtazapine for longer than 6 weeks has not been evaluated, although treatment is indicated for 6 months or longer.**
- **Safety and efficacy have not been determined in children.**
- **Suicide attempts and suicidal thinking have occurred in pediatric clients taking antidepressant drugs for major depressive disorder.**

SIDE EFFECTS

Most Common

Somnolence, dry mouth, constipation, increased appetite, dizziness, weight gain, asthenia, abnormal dreams.

Side effects with an incidence of 0.1% or greater are listed. **CNS**: Somnolence, dizziness, activation of mania or hypomania, ***suicidal ideation***, sedation, drowsiness, abnormal dreams, abnormal thinking, confusion, tremor, agitation, anxiety, ataxia, amnesia, apathy, depression, hyperkinesia, hypesthesia, hypokinesia, paresthesia, vertigo, extrapyramidal symptoms, hallucinations, abnormal coordination, delirium, delusions, depersonalization, dysarthria, dyskinesia, dystonia, emotional lability, euphoria, hostility, increased libido, increased reflexes, neurosis, paranoid reaction. **GI:** Dry mouth, increased appetite, constipation, N&V, abdominal pain, acute abdominal syndrome, anorexia, cholecystitis, colitis, enlarged abdomen, eructation, glossitis, gum hemorrhage, stomatitis, ulcer. **CV**: Hypertension, hypotension, orthostatic hypotension, vasodilation, angina pectoris, bradycardia, ***MI***, syncope, migraine, ventricular extrasystoles. **Hematologic**: Agranulocytosis. **Respiratory:** Increased cough, dyspnea, sinusitis, asthma, bronchitis, epistaxis, pneumonia. **Dermatologic:** Pruritus, rash, alopecia, acne, dry skin, exfoliative dermatitis, herpes simplex. **GU:** UTI, amenorrhea, breast pain, urinary frequency, cystitis, dysmenorrhea, dysuria, hematuria, impotence, kidney calculus, leukorrhea, urinary incontinence, urinary retention, vaginitis. **Musculoskeletal:** Myasthenia, arthralgia, myalgia, arthritis, tenosynovitis, neck pain/rigidity. **Metabolic/nutritional:** Weight gain/loss, peripheral edema, edema, thirst, dehydration. **Ophthalmic:** Abnormality of accommodation, conjunctivitis, eye pain, glaucoma, keratoconjunctivitis, lacrimation disorder. **Otic:** Ear pain, deafness, hyperacusis. **Body as a whole:** Asthenia, weakness, fatigue, flu syndrome, malaise, chills, fever, photosensitivity reaction. **Miscellaneous:** Back pain, facial edema.

LABORATORY TEST CONSIDERATIONS

↑ ALT and nonfasting cholesterol and triglycerides. Altered liver function.

OVERDOSE MANAGEMENT

Symptoms: Disorientation, drowsiness, impaired memory, tachycardia. *Treatment:* General supportive measures. If the client is unconscious, establish and maintain an airway. Consider gastric lavage and administration of activated charcoal. Monitor cardiac and vital signs. Induction of emesis is not recommended.

DRUG INTERACTIONS

Alcohol / Possible enhanced impairment of cognitive and motor skills; do not use together
Benzodiazepines (e.g., diazepam) / Possible enhanced impairment of cognitive and motor skills; do not use together
Clonidine / Possible ↓ clonidine's hypertensive effect
CNS depressants / Enhanced CNS depressant effect
Fluvoxamine / Possible ↑ mirtazapine serum levels
MAOIs / Do not use mirtazapine with MAOIs or within 14 days of initiating or discontinuing therapy with an MAOI
Phenytoin / ↓ Plasma mirtazapine levels R/T ↑ liver metabolism

HOW SUPPLIED

Tablets: 7.5 mg, 15 mg, 30 mg, 45 mg; ***Tablets, Oral Disintegrating:*** 15, 30, 45 mg.

DOSAGE

TABLETS; TABLETS, ORAL DISINTEGRATING

Treatment of depression.

Adults, initial: 15 mg/day given as a single dose, preferably in the evening before sleep. **Dose range:** 15–45 mg/day. Those not responding to the 15-mg dose may respond to doses up to a maximum of 45 mg/day. Do not make dose changes at intervals of less than 1 to 2 weeks. **Maintenance:** Acute episodes of depression require several months or longer of sustained therapy. Mirtazapine has been given for up to 40 weeks, following the initial 8 to 12 weeks of therapy. Periodically assess clients to determine the need for continued therapy.

Chronic urticaria (investigational).

Adults, initial: 15–30 mg/day.

Pruritus associated with cancer (investigational).

Adults, initial: 15–30 mg/day. Most are controlled at a dose of 15 mg/day.

NURSING IMPLICATIONS

IMPLEMENTATION/ADMINISTRATION/STORAGE

1. The oral disintegrating tablet (SolTab) can be swallowed with or without water, chewed, or allowed to disintegrate.
2. Clearance is decreased in the elderly and in clients with moderate to severe renal or hepatic impairment.
3. If discontinuing therapy, a gradual reduction in dosage over several weeks is recommended, rather than abrupt cessation.
4. If intolerable symptoms occur following a decrease in dose or discontinuation of therapy, manage dose titration based on clinical response.
5. At least 2 weeks should elapse between discontinuing an MAOI and starting mirtazapine

therapy. Also, 14 or more days should elapse after stopping mirtazapine and starting an MAOI.

6. Store from 15–30°C (59–86°F). Protect from light and moisture.

ASSESSMENT

1. Note reasons for therapy, onset, triggers, behavioral manifestations and clinical presentation. Identify events that may be R/T to depression, i.e., death, divorce, illness, or job loss.
2. List drugs prescribed; ensure no MAOI use within past 2 weeks.
3. Assess for history of MI, angina, seizures, alcohol abuse, ischemic stroke; and any evidence of dehydration or hypovolemia. Monitor closely if treated with antihypertensives.
4. Monitor mental status, VS, Wt, ECG, CBC, renal and LFTs, cholesterol, and triglyceride levels. Use caution with renal and liver dysfunction and in the elderly.

CLIENT/FAMILY TEACHING

1. Take as directed; do not exceed prescribed dosing schedule. Bedtime dosing may minimize problems with drowsiness.
2. For the orally disintegrating tablet, open tablet blister pack with dry hands and place tablet on tongue; it will disintegrate within 30 seconds and can be swallowed with saliva or chewed. Do not split the tablet and do not open the blister pack until just before use.
3. Do not engage in activities that require mental alertness until drug effects realized; dizziness and drowsiness may occur.
4. Report any S&S of infection or flu (fever, sore throat, stomatitis, etc.); drug may cause (↓ WBCs) agranulocytosis.
5. Avoid alcohol and OTC agents; may potentiate drug's cognitive and motor skill impairment.
6. Monitor weight and dietary intake; may note increased appetite and weight gain.
7. Parents should consult medication guide and keep weekly visits during first 4 weeks of therapy then every other week for the next 4 weeks until child stabilized. Report any clinical worsening, suicidality, and unusual changes in behavior to provider.
8. Report any evidence of aggressiveness, agitation, anxiety, hostility, hypomania, impulsivity, insomnia, irritability, mania, panic attacks, suicide ideation, or psychomotor restlessness.
9. Report for F/U to assess response, labs, counselling, and adverse SE.

OUTCOMES/EVALUATE

Improved sleeping and eating patterns; improved mood, ↑ interest in social activities, ↓ depression

Misoprostol

(my-soh-**PROST**-ohl)

Classification(s): Prostaglandin

Pregnancy Category: X

RX: Cytotec.

✱ **Rx:** Apo-Misoprostol.

INDICATIONS/USES

(1) Prevention of aspirin and other nonsteroidal anti-inflammatory-induced gastric ulcers in clients with a high risk of gastric ulcer complications (e.g., geriatric clients with debilitating disease) or in those with a history of ulcer. (2) In combination with mifepristone to terminate pregnancy. *Investigational:* Vaginally to produce cervical ripening and induction of labor and to treat serious postpartum hemorrhage in the presence of uterine atony. Chronic, idiopathic constipation.

ACTION/KINETICS

Action

Synthetic prostaglandin E_1 analog that inhibits gastric acid secretion, protects the gastric mucosa by increasing bicarbonate and mucus production, and decreases pepsin levels during basal conditions. May also stimulate uterine contractions that may endanger pregnancy.

Pharmacokinetics

Extensively absorbed and rapidly converted to the active misoprostol acid. **Time for peak levels of misoprostol acid:** 12 min. **t½, misoprostol acid:** 20–40 min. Excreted in the urine. **Plasma protein binding:** Less than 90%.

NOTE: Misoprostol does not prevent development of duodenal ulcers in clients on NSAIDs.

CONTRAINDICATIONS

Allergy to prostaglandins, during lactation (may cause diarrhea in nursing infants). Use in pregnancy to reduce risk of ulcers induced by NSAIDs.

SPECIAL CONCERNS

■ (1) If given to pregnant women, can cause abortion, premature birth, or birth defects. Uterine rupture has been reported if given to pregnant women to induce labor or to induce abortion beyond week 8 of pregnancy.
(2) Not to be taken by pregnant women to reduce risk of ulcers induced by NSAIDs.
(3) Advise clients of the abortifacient property and warn them not to give the drug to others.
(4) Should not be used to reduce risk of NSAID-induced ulcers in women of childbearing age unless the client is at high risk of developing complications from gastric ulcers associated with NSAID use, or is at high risk of developing gastric ulceration. In such clients, misoprostol may be prescribed if the client:

- Has had a negative serum pregnancy test within 2 weeks prior to beginning therapy.
- Is capable of complying with effective contraceptive measures.
- Has received both oral and written warnings of the hazards of misoprostol, the risk of possible contraception failure, and the danger to other women of childbearing age should the drug be taken by mistake.
- Will begin misoprostol only on the second or third day of the next normal menstrual period. ■

SIDE EFFECTS

Most Common

Diarrhea, abdominal pain, N&V, flatulence, dyspepsia, headache, uterine cramping.

GI: Diarrhea (may be severe, but is usually self-limiting), abdominal pain, nausea, dyspepsia, flatulence, vomiting, constipation. **GU**: Spotting, cramps, dysmenorrhea, hypermenorrhea, menstrual disorders, postmenopausal vaginal bleeding. **Miscellaneous:** Headache.

OVERDOSE MANAGEMENT

Symptoms: Abdominal pain, diarrhea, dyspnea, sedation, tremor, fever, palpitations, bradycardia, hypotension, ***seizures.*** *Treatment:* Use supportive therapy.

HOW SUPPLIED

Tablets: 100 mcg, 200 mcg.

DOSAGE

TABLETS

Reduce risk of NSAID-induced gastric ulcers.

Adults: 200 mcg 4 times per day with food for the duration of NSAID therapy. Dose can be reduced to 100 mcg if the larger dose cannot be tolerated. In renal impairment, the 200 mcg dose can be reduced if necessary.

With mifepristone to terminate pregnancy.

Treatment includes both mifepristone and misoprostol and requires three office visits. **Day 1:** Three 200-mg tablets (600 mg) of mifepristone taken as a single dose. **Day 3:** Unless abortion has occurred and has been confirmed by clinical examination or ultrasonographic scan, clients must take misoprostol, 400 mcg (two 200-mcg tablets) PO. **Day 14:** Client returns for follow-up visit to confirm by clinical examination or ultrasonographic scan that complete termination of pregnancy has occurred.

NURSING IMPLICATIONS

Do not confuse misoprostol with mifepristone (an abortifacient) or with metoprolol (a beta-adrenergic blocker). Also, do not confuse Cytotec with Cytoxan (an antineoplastic) or with Cytosar (an antineoplastic).

IMPLEMENTATION/ADMINISTRATION/STORAGE

1. Reduce diarrhea by giving after meals and at bedtime; avoid Mg-containing antacids. Diarrhea is usually self-limiting.
2. Maximum plasma levels are decreased if drug is taken with food.
3. Take for the duration of NSAID therapy.
4. Drug may increase gastric bicarbonate and mucus production.

ASSESSMENT

1. List reasons for therapy, note any ulcer disease (for gastric ulcer prevention); assess GI S&S, clinical presentation, other agents trialed. Identify any tests or studies used to confirm diagnosis.
2. Obtain a negative pregnancy test unless being used with mifepristone to induce abortion. Usually started on 2nd or 3rd day of menstrual

M

cycle following negative test. Advise of abortifacient properties and effect on fertility.

3. If for termination of pregnancy monitor cramps and bleeding during therapy.
4. Monitor CBC and renal function; may reduce dose in elderly and those with renal dysfunction if dosage not tolerated.

CLIENT/FAMILY TEACHING

1. Drug reduces stomach acid and protects stomach. Not used to treat stomach ulcers but is being used to prevent the NSAID from causing stomach ulcers so medication must be taken regularly, as prescribed, for this beneficial effect to occur.
2. Take with or after a meal to reduce risk of diarrhea. Diarrhea is the most common adverse reaction of misoprostol; taking each dose with or after meals and avoiding magnesium-containing antacids may minimize this problem.
3. Advise client to take the last dose of the day just before bedtime.
4. Avoid foods/spices that may aggravate condition: caffeine, alcohol, and black pepper.
5. Take exactly as prescribed for the duration of aspirin or NSAID therapy to prevent ulcer formation.
6. Report persistent diarrhea, postmenopausal bleeding, or increased menstrual bleeding. Also report any S&S of stomach ulcer (i.e., ↑ indigestion, stomach pain), or intolerable adverse reactions (i.e., diarrhea, cramping) develop.
7. All women of childbearing age must practice effective contraceptive measures during therapy, and for 1 mo or for 1 menstrual cycle after misoprostol has been discontinued; drug has abortifacient properties. Never share medications.
8. With abortion, report any increased bleeding, pain, or fever; administered 2 days after mifepristone if no activity.
9. Keep all F/U to assess response, labs, and for adverse SE.

OUTCOMES/EVALUATE

- Prevention of NSAID-induced gastric ulcers
- Termination of pregnancy

IV

Mitomycin (MTC)

(my-toe-**MY**-sin)

Classification(s): Antineoplastic, antibiotic

Pregnancy Category: X

RX: MitoExtra.

SEE ALSO ***ANTINEOPLASTIC AGENTS***.

INDICATIONS/USES

Palliative treatment and adjunct to surgical or radiologic treatment of disseminated adenocarcinoma of the stomach and pancreas when other treatment fails. Used in combination with other agents (not recommended as a single agent for primary treatment or in place of surgery and/or radiotherapy). *Investigational:* Superficial bladder cancer (by the intravesical route). As an ophthalmic solution as an adjunct to surgical excision in primary or recurrent pterygia.

ACTION/KINETICS

Action

Antibiotic produced by *Streptomyces caespitosus* that inhibits DNA synthesis. The guanine and cytosine content correlates with the degree of mitomycin-induced cross-linking. At high doses both RNA and protein synthesis are inhibited. Most active during late G_1 and early S stages.

Pharmacokinetics

Rapidly cleared from the serum. **t½, initial:** 17 min after a 30 mg bolus injection; **final:** 50 min. Metabolized in liver; 10% excreted unchanged in urine, more when dose is increased.

CONTRAINDICATIONS

Primary therapy as a single agent. Use to replace surgery or radiotherapy. Hypersensitivity or idiosyncratic reaction to mitomycin. Pregnancy and lactation. Thrombocytopenia, coagulation disorders, increase in bleeding tendency due to other causes. In clients with a serum creatinine level greater than 1.7 mg/dL.

SPECIAL CONCERNS

(1) Bone marrow suppression, especially thrombocytopenia and leukopenia, which may contribute to overwhelming infection in an already compromised client, is the most common and severe toxic effect. (2) Hemolytic uremic syndrome, a serious syndrome of microangiopathic hemolytic anemia, thrombocytopenia, and irreversible renal failure has occurred.

Use with extreme caution in presence of impaired renal function.

M

SIDE EFFECTS

Most Common

Thrombocytopenia, leukopenia, cellulitis at injection site, stomatitis, alopecia, fever, anorexia, N&V.

See *Antineoplastic Agents* for a complete list of possible side effects. Also, severe bone marrow depression, especially leukopenia and thrombocytopenia. Pulmonary toxicity including dyspnea with nonproductive cough. ***Microangiopathic hemolytic anemia with renal failure and hypertension (hemolytic uremic syndrome)***, especially when used long-term in combination with fluorouracil. Cellulitis. Extravasation causes severe necrosis of surrounding tissue. ***Acute respiratory distress syndrome in adults***, especially when used with other chemotherapy.

DRUG INTERACTIONS

Severe bronchospasm and SOB when used with vinca alkaloids

HOW SUPPLIED

Powder for Injection: 5 mg, 20 mg, 40 mg.

DOSAGE

IV ONLY

Adenocarcinoma of the stomatch and pancreas.

After hematological recovery from previous chemotherapy, give 20 mg/m^2 as a single dose via infusion q 6–8 wk. Subsequent courses of treatment are based on hematologic response; do not repeat until leukocyte count is at least 4,000/mm^3 and platelet count is at least 100,000/mm^3. Adjust the dose as follows depending on the nadir after prior dose/mm^3: If leukocytes are between 3,000 and 3,999 and platelets are between 75,000 and 99,999, give 100% of the prior dose; if leukocytes are between 2,000 and 2,999 and platelets are between 25,000 and 74,999, give 70% of the prior dose; if leukocytes are less than 2,000 and platelets are less than 25,000, give 50% of the prior dose.

NURSING IMPLICATIONS

IMPLEMENTATION/ADMINISTRATION/STORAGE

1. **IV** Drug is toxic; avoid extravasation. Observe infusion site closely for evidence of erythema or complaints of discomfort. Apply ice and use thiosulfate for infiltrate.
2. Reconstitute 5-, 20-, or 40-mg vial with 10, 40, or 80 mL sterile water for injection, respectively, as indicated and administer IVP over 5–10 min; will dissolve if allowed to remain at room temperature.
3. Drug concentration of 0.5 mg/mL is stable for 14 days under refrigeration or 7 days at room temperature.
4. Diluted concentrations of 20–40 mcg/mL, are stable for 3 hr in D5W, for 12 hr in isotonic saline, and for 24 hr in sodium lactate injection.
5. Mitomycin (5–15 mg) and heparin (1,000–10,000 units) in 30 mL of isotonic saline are stable for 48 hr at room temperature.
6. COMPATIBILITY 0.9% NaCl, D5W or sodium lactate injection.
7. INCOMPATIBILITY Administer separately.

ASSESSMENT

1. Note reasons for therapy, other agents trialed/failed, anticipated length of therapy. Monitor VS and I&O and ensure adequate hydration and antiemetics.
2. List pulmonary function. Obtain CXR; pulmonary infiltrates and fibrosis can occur with cumulative doses. Observe closely for early evidence of pulmonary complications, such as dyspnea, nonproductive cough, and abnormal ABGs/lung sounds.
3. Obtain baseline CBC, PT, PTT, LFT, and renal function; do not initiate if serum creatinine level is >1.7 mg/dL. Drug may cause platelet and granulocyte suppression. Nadir: 28 days; recovery: 40–55 days. Follow dosing schedule based on platelets and leukocytes.

CLIENT/FAMILY TEACHING

1. Drug is used with other agents to treat disseminated adenocarcinoma of stomach and pancreas.
2. Report any adverse side effects, S&S of cold/flu or respiratory distress. May lose hair; should regrow.
3. Avoid vaccinations during active therapy. Mitomycin may lower your body's resistance and there is a chance you might get the infection the immunization is meant to prevent. In addition, other persons living in your household should not take oral polio vaccine since there

is a chance they could pass the polio virus on to you. Also, avoid persons who have taken oral polio vaccine. Do not get close to them, and do not stay in the same room with them for very long. If you cannot take these precautions, you should consider wearing a protective face mask that covers the nose and mouth.

4. Mitomycin can temporarily lower the number of WBCs increasing chances of getting an infection. It can also lower the number of platelets, which are necessary for proper blood clotting. If this occurs, report and take the following precautions, especially when your blood count is low, to reduce the risk of infection or bleeding:
   - Avoid people with infections. Report immediately: fever or chills, cough or hoarseness, lower back or side pain, or painful or difficult urination.
   - Report any unusual bleeding or bruising; black, tarry stools; blood in urine or stools; or pinpoint red spots on your skin.
   - Be careful with regular toothbrush, dental floss, or toothpick. Use a soft bristled toothbrush and waxed dental floss. Check before having any dental work done.
   - Do not touch your eyes or the inside of your nose unless you have just washed your hands and have not touched anything else in the meantime.
   - Be careful not to cut yourself when using sharp objects such as a safety razor or fingernail or toenail cutters.
   - Avoid contact sports or other situations where bruising or injury could occur.
5. If mitomycin accidentally seeps out of the vein into which it is injected, it may damage the skin and cause scarring. In some, this may occur weeks or even months after this medicine is given. Report if you notice redness, pain, or swelling at the place of injection or anywhere else on your skin.
6. Avoid alcohol and agents that may cause increased bleeding i.e., aspirin, NSAIDS.
7. Practice reliable contraception throughout therapy; may negatively affect fetus.
8. Keep all F/U to assess response, labs, and for adverse SE.

OUTCOMES/EVALUATE

↓ Tumor size/spread

Mometasone furoate

(moh-**MET**-ah-sohn)

Classification(s): Glucocorticoid

Pregnancy Category: C

RX: Cream, Lotion, Ointment, Topical Solution: Elocon, Momexin. **Powder for Inhalation**: Asmanex Twisthaler.

✤ **Rx:** PMS-Mometasone, ratio-Mometasone, Taro-Mometasone.

Mometasone furoate monohydrate

RX: Nasonex.

SEE ALSO ***CORTICOSTEROIDS***.

INDICATIONS/USES

Mometasone furoate. Cream, Lotion, Ointment, Topical Solution: Dermatoses. **Powder for Oral Inhalation:** Maintenance treatment of chronic asthma in clients 4 years and older. For asthma clients who require PO corticosteroid therapy, where adding mometasone may reduce or eliminate the need for PO corticosteroids.

Mometasone furoate monohydrate. Nasal Spray: (1) Treatment of the nasal symptoms of seasonal allergic rhinitis and perennial allergic rhinitis in adults and children 2 years and older. (2) Prophylaxis of nasal symptoms of seasonal allergic rhinitis in adults and adolescents 12 years and older. (3) Treatment of nasal polyps in clients 18 years and older.

ACTION/KINETICS

Action

Anti-inflammatory due to ability to inhibit prostaglandin synthesis. Also inhibits accumulation of macrophages and leukocytes at sites of inflammation as well as to inhibit phagocytosis and lysosomal enzyme release.

Pharmacokinetics

Undetected in plasma although some may be swallowed after use. No effect on adrenal function. Metabolized in the liver by CYP3A4 enzymes. **t½:** 5.8 hr. Excreted in the feces and urine. **Plasma protein binding:** 98–99%.

CONTRAINDICATIONS

Use in those with recent nasal septum ulcers, nasal surgery, or nasal trauma until healing has occurred. Not indicated to relieve acute bronchospasms. Mometasone furoate for the relief of acute bronchospasms or for children younger than 4 years of age.

SPECIAL CONCERNS

- **Use with caution, if at all, in active or quiescent tuberculosis infection of the respiratory tract, in untreated fungal, bacterial, systemic viral infections, or ocular herpes simplex.**
- **Safety and efficacy of Nasonex not determined in children less than 2 years for use in allergic rhinitis and in children less than 18 years to treat nasal polyps.**
- **Use with caution during lactation.**

SIDE EFFECTS

Most Common

For Asmanex: Dry/irritated throat, hoarseness, cough, dry mouth, taste alteration.
For Nasonex: Headache, pharyngitis, epistaxis, nasal burning/irritation, diarrhea, dyspepsia, N&V.

Respiratory: Pharyngitis, epistaxis, nasal burning/irritation/ulceration, dry/irritated throat, hoarseness, blood-tinged mucus, cough, URTI, sinusitis, rhinitis, asthma symptoms, bronchitis, wheezing. Rarely, nasal ulcers/perforation and nasal/oral candidiasis. **GI:** Diarrhea, dyspepsia, N&V, dry mouth, taste alteration. **Respiratory:** Musculoskeletal pain, arthralgia, chest pain, myalgia. **Ophthalmic:** Conjunctivitis, increased IOP. **Otic:** Earache, otitis media. **Body as a whole:** Flu-like symptoms, infection, viral infection, angioedema, ***anaphylaxis***. **Miscellaneous:** Headache, dysmenorrhea, loss of taste/smell (rare).

HOW SUPPLIED

Mometasone furoate. ***Cream, Lotion, Ointment, Topical Solution:*** Each is 0.1%; ***Powder for Oral Inhalation (Asmanex Twisthaler):*** 110 mcg (delivers 100 mcg/actuation), 220 mcg (delivers 200 mcg/actuation).
Mometasone furoate monohydrate. ***Nasal Spray Suspension (Nasonex):*** 0.05% (50 mcg/actuation).

DOSAGE

Mometasone furoate

CREAM, LOTION, OINTMENT

Dermatoses.

Apply sparingly to affected area(s) 2–4 times per day.

TOPICAL SOLUTION

Dermatoses.

Adults and children 12 years and older: Apply a few drops to the affected skin once a day; massage lightly until solution disappears.

POWDER FOR ORAL INHALATION (ASMANEX TWISTHALER)

Chronic asthma for prophylactic therapy.

Recommended starting doses.
(1) Previous therapy in clients 12 years and older who received bronchodilators alone or inhaled corticosteroids: 220 mcg once daily in the evening; **highest recommended daily dose:** 440 mcg given in divided doses of 220 mcg twice daily or as 440 mcg once daily. (2) **Previous therapy in clients 12 years and older who received oral corticosteroids:** 440 mcg twice daily; **highest recommended daily dose:** 880 mcg. Reduce prednisone no faster than 2.5 mg/day on a weekly basis beginning after at least 1 week of mometasone therapy. Monitor carefully. (3) **Children, 4–11 years of age:** 110 mcg once daily in the evening, not to exceed 110 mcg/day.

Mometasone furoate monohydrate

NASAL SPRAY (NASONEX)

Prophylaxis and treatment of seasonal/perennial allergic rhinitis.

Adults and children over 12 years: 2 sprays (50 mcg in each spray) in each nostril once daily (i.e., total daily dose: 200 mcg). In those with a known seasonal allergen that precipitates seasonal allergic rhinitis, give prophylactically, 200 mcg/day, 2 to 4 weeks prior to the anticipated start of the pollen season.
Children 2–11 years of age: One spray (50 mcg) in each nostril once daily (total daily dose: 100 mcg).

Treatment of nasal polyps.

Adults 18 years and older: 2 sprays (100 mcg) into each nostril twice a day (i.e., total daily dose of 400 mcg). In some, a dose of 2 sprays once daily in each nostril (i.e., total daily dose of 200 mcg) may be effective.

NURSING IMPLICATIONS

IMPLEMENTATION/ADMINISTRATION/STORAGE

1. For asthma, titrate to the lowest effect dose once asthma stability has been reached.
2. Improvement is usually seen within 11 hours to 2 days after the first dose. Maximum benefit: Within 1 to 2 weeks. For those 12 years of age or older who do not respond adequately to the starting dose after 2 weeks, higher doses may be tried.
3. Giving mometasone by the orally inhaled route will result in a variable time to onset and degree of symptom relief.
4. Store nasal spray from 15–30°C (59–86°F) protected from light. Avoid prolonged exposure to direct light when removed from cardboard container.
5. Store oral inhaler in a dry place from 15–30°C (59–86°F). Avoid prolonged exposure to light.

ASSESSMENT

1. Note onset, duration, and characteristics of S&S. List other agents trialed.
2. Assess EENT/lungs and describe clinical presentation. Check nasal mucosa with nasal therapy.
3. Check for changes in vision or a history of glaucoma, increased IOP, and/or cataracts.
4. Monitor growth of children on prolonged therapy.
5. With skin condition describe presentation.
6. Attempt to identify triggers with seasonal allergy and asthma.

CLIENT/FAMILY TEACHING

1. Used to control allergic symptoms.
2. Shake nasal spray well before using. Review enclosed instructions for proper use and cleaning.
3. Prior to initial use, prime the pump by actuating 10 times or until a fine spray appears.
4. The pump may be stored, unused, for up to 1 week without repriming. If more than one week has elapsed between use, reprime by actuating 2 times, or until a fine spray appears.
5. Do not spray into the eyes or directly onto the nasal septum. If on immunosuppressant doses of corticosteroids, avoid exposure to chickenpox or measles, and report if exposed.
6. Protect nasal spray from sunlight.
7. Discard oral inhaler 45 days after opening the foil pouch or when the dose counter reads "00," whichever comes first.
8. When using oral inhaler, inhale deeply and rapidly and hold breath for about 10 seconds, or as long as possible. Do not breathe out through the inhaler. Rinse mouth/equipment after inhalation use.
9. Use regularly as directed. Do not increase dose/frequency; does not increase effectiveness. Use in the evening with once daily dosing. A spacer facilitates oral inhaler administration. Rinse with water after use.
10. With topical products and skin problems, wash hands after using finger to apply medicine. Avoid contact with eyes, but if it accidentally gets in eyes, flush carefully with water. Do not bandage or cover skin area being treated or use on face, groin, or under arms unless directed.
11. Identify triggers and practice avoidance. Report if condition does not improve or worsens after 3–5 days of therapy.
12. Keep all F/U to assess response, condition status, and for adverse SE.

OUTCOMES/EVALUATE

- Prophylaxis/relief of allergic rhinitis/nasal polyps
- Control of asthma S&S
- Clearing of skin lesions

Montelukast sodium

(mon-teh-**LOO**-kast)

Classification(s): Antiasthmatic, leukotriene receptor antagonist

Pregnancy Category: B

RX: Singulair.

INDICATIONS/USES

(1) Prophylaxis and chronic treatment of asthma in adults and children 12 months of age and old-

er. (2) Relief of symptoms of seasonal allergic rhinitis in adults and children 2 years of age and older. (3) Relief of symptoms of perennial allergic rhinitis in adults and children 6 months of age and older. (4) Prevention of exercise-induced bronchoconstriction in clients 15 years of age and older. *Investigational:* Chronic urticaria. Atopic dermatitis. Nonsteroidal anti-inflammatory drug-induced urticaria.

ACTION/KINETICS

Action

Cysteinyl leukotrienes and leukotriene receptor occupation are associated with symptoms of asthma, including airway edema, smooth muscle contraction, and inflammation. Montelukast binds with cysteinyl leukotriene receptors, thus preventing the action of cysteinyl leukotrienes.

Pharmacokinetics

Rapidly absorbed after PO use; bioavailability of film-coated tablets is 64%. **Time to peak levels:** 3–4 hr for 10 mg tablet, 2–2.5 hr for 5 mg tablet, and 2 hr for the 4 mg chewable tablet in children, 2–5 years of age in the fasted state. The 4 mg oral granule formulation is bioequivalent to the 4 mg chewable tablet in adults in the fasted state. Metabolized extensively in the liver by cytochromes CYP3A4 and CYP2C9; mainly excreted in feces. **t½:** 2.7–5.5 hr for healthy, young adults. 86% excreted in the feces. **Plasma protein binding:** More than 99%.

CONTRAINDICATIONS

Hypersensitivity to any component of the product. Use to reverse bronchospasm in acute asthma attacks, including status asthmaticus. Use to abruptly substitute for inhaled or oral corticosteroids. Use as monotherapy to treat and manage exercise-induced bronchospasm. Use with known aspirin or NSAID sensitivity.

SPECIAL CONCERNS

- **Safety and efficacy not determined in children less than 12 months of age with asthma and younger than 6 months of age with perennial allergic rhinitis.**
- **Those with known sensitivity to aspirin should continue to avoid aspirin and NSAIDs if taking montelukast.**
- **Use with caution during lactation.**

SIDE EFFECTS

Most Common

URTI, fever, headache, pharyngitis, cough, abdominal pain, diarrhea, otitis media, influenza, rhinorrhea, sinusitis, otitis.

Adolescents and adults aged 15 and older: GI: Abdominal pain, dyspepsia, infectious gastroenteritis, dental pain. **CNS:** Headache, dizziness, somnolence. **Body as a whole:** Asthenia, fatigue, fever, trauma. **Respiratory:** Cough, nasal congestion, URTI, epistaxis, sinus headache, sinusitis. **Dermatologic:** Rash. **Miscellaneous:** Influenza, pyuria, fever, trauma.

Children, aged 6 to 14 years: GI: Nausea, diarrhea, dyspepsia, gastroenteritis, tooth infection. **CNS:** Headache. **Otic:** Otitis media. **Respiratory:** Pharyngitis, laryngitis, sinusitus, infective rhinitis, acute bronchitis, URTI. **Dermatologic:** Atopic dermatitis, skin infection, varicella. **Miscellaneous:** Viral infection, influenza, fever, myopia, eosinophilic conditions consistent with Churg-Strauss syndrome.

Children, aged 2 to 5 years: Respiratory: Rhinorrhea, cough, sinusitis, pneumonia, pharyngitis, URTI. **GI:** Abdominal pain, diarrhea, gastroenteritis. **CNS:** Headache. **Dermatologic:** Rash, urticaria, eczema, varicella, dermatitis. **Otic:** Otitis media, ear pain. **Ophthalmic:** Conjunctivitis. **Miscellaneous:** Fever, influenza.

Children, aged 6 to 23 months: Respiratory: URTI, wheezing, pharyngitis, tonsillitis, rhinitis, cough. **Otic:** Otitis media.

Postmarketing side effects: CNS: Dream abnormalities, hallucinations, drowsiness, psychomotor hyperactivity, irritability, agitation, aggressive behavior or hostility, restlessness, insomnia, anxiousness, disorientation, somnambulism, ***seizures (very rare)***, paresthesia, hypesthesia, tremor, depression, suicidal thinking/behavior, ***suicide***. **GI:** N&V, dyspepsia, diarrhea, ***pancreatitis (very rare)***. **Hepatic:** Cholestatic hepatitis, hepatocellular liver injury, mixed-pattern liver injury. **Hypersensitivity:** Urticaria, pruritus, angioedema, ***anaphylaxis***, hepatic eosinophilic infiltration (very rare). **Musculoskeletal:** Arthralgia; myalgia, including muscle cramps. **Dermatologic:** Bruising, erythema nodosum. **Miscellaneous:** Increased bleeding tendency, systemic eosinophilia, vasculitis (consistent with Churg-Strauss syndrome), palpitations, edema, epistaxis, palpitations.

LABORATORY TEST CONSIDERATIONS

↑ ALT, AST in adults/adolescents 15 years and older.

OVERDOSE MANAGEMENT

Symptoms: Headache, vomiting, psychomotor hyperactivity, thirst, somnolence, mydriasis, hyperkinesia, abdominal pain. *Treatment:* Usual supportive measures, including removing unabsorbed drug from GI tract and clinical monitoring.

DRUG INTERACTIONS

Gemfibrozil / ↑ Montelukast plasma levels → ↑ pharmacologic/toxic effects; monitor and adjust dose if needed
Phenobarbital / ↓ Montelukast plasma levels → ↓ effect; monitor and adjust montelukast dose if needed
Prednisone / ↑ Prednisone adverse effects (e.g., edema); monitor and consider reducing one or both drugs
Rifampin / ↓ Montelukast plasma levels → ↓ effect; monitor and adjust montelukast dose if needed

HOW SUPPLIED

Granules, Oral: 4 mg/packet; ***Tablets:*** 10 mg; ***Tablets, Chewable:*** 4 mg, 5 mg.

DOSAGE

GRANULES

Asthma.

Children 12–23 months of age: One packet of 4 mg granules once daily in the evening.

Perennial allergic rhinits.

Children, 6–23 months of age: 1 packet of 4 mg once daily in the evening.

GRANULES; TABLETS, CHEWABLE

Asthma, Seasonal/perennial allergic rhinitis.

Pediatric clients aged 6 to 14 years: One 5 mg chewable tablet once daily in the evening. **Pediatric clients aged 2 to 5 years:** One 4 mg chewable tablet or one 4 mg oral granule packet taken once daily in the evening.

TABLETS

Asthma, Seasonal/perennial allergic rhinitis, Prophylaxis of exercise-induced bronchoconstriction.

Adults and adolescents, 15 years and older: One 10 mg tablet once daily (in the evening for asthma; anytime for allergic rhinits). To prevent exercise-induced bronchoconstriction, take at least 2 hr before exercise. An additional dose is not to be taken within 24 hr of a previous dose.

NURSING IMPLICATIONS

Do not confuse Singulair with Sinequan (doxepin, a tricyclic antidepressant).

IMPLEMENTATION/ADMINISTRATION/STORAGE

1. Take daily as prescribed, even when symptom free. Contact provider if asthma is not well controlled.
2. The 4 and 5 mg chewable tablets contain phenylalanine (a component of aspartame).
3. Do not abruptly substitute montelukast for inhaled or oral corticosteroids.
4. The manufacturer maintains a registry to monitor the pregnancy outcomes of women being treated with montelukast during pregnancy. Clients and health care providers are asked to report any prenatal exposure by calling the pregnancy registry at 1-800-986-8999.
5. Store from 15–30°C (59–86°F); protect from moisture and light.

ASSESSMENT

1. List reasons for therapy, onset, triggers, characteristics of disease, assess EENT/lungs and note findings. List other agents trialed, outcome.
2. Review other agents prescribed for asthma; identify which should be continued.
3. Do not use with aspirin or NSAID allergy.
4. Chewable 5 mg tablet contains 0.842 mg of phenylalanine and 4 mg tablet contains 0.674 mg phenylalanine; not to be used with phenylketonurics.
5. Note behavioral presentation, and assess for any changes in behavior or depression.
6. Assist to identify and eliminate/minimize triggers.
7. Monitor LFTs, lung assessments, PFTs, and x-rays.

CLIENT/FAMILY TEACHING

1. Take once daily in the evening for asthma; for seasonal allergic rhinitis, the time of administration can be individualized. For those with combined asthma and seasonal allergic rhinitis, give one tablet daily in the evening.
2. Granules can be given directly in the mouth or mixed with a spoonful of cold or room-temperature food such as applesauce, carrots, rice, or ice cream. Do not open packet until ready to use. The full dose must be given within 15 min. Do not store drug mixed with food. Oral granules are not intended to be dissolved in liquid. Granules can be given without regard to meals; may take with food to decrease stomach upset.
3. The 4 and 5 mg chewable tablets contain phenylalanine; make parents aware.
4. Those taking montelukast, 1 tablet daily, for another indication (including chronic asthma) should not take an additional dose to prevent exercise-induced bronchoconstriction. Use short-acting prescribed beta-agonist inhalers to treat acute asthma attacks. Report if increased use/frequency of inhalers needed for symptom control.
5. Continue drug during acute attacks as well as during symptom-free periods, and continue other prescribed antiasthma medications during this therapy.
6. With exercise-induced asthma, continue to use prescribed inhaler for prophylaxis.
7. Report unusual side effects, changes in disease, or significant drop in peak flow readings.
8. Notify provider if pregnancy suspected or planned. Monitor pregnancy outcomes of women exposed to montelukast during pregnancy; providers should report prenatal exposure to the pregnancy registry by calling 1-800-986-8999.
9. Report any changes in thinking, behavior, or suicide ideations.
10. Assess environment for triggers, and take steps to minimize or avoid exposures.
11. Keep all F/U to assess respiratory status, response, and for adverse SE.

OUTCOMES/EVALUATE

- Asthma control/prophylaxis
- Control of seasonal/perennial allergic rhinitis
- Prevention of exercise-induced bronchoconstriction
- Chronic urticaria, atopic dermatitis (unlabeled use)

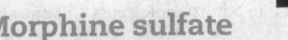

■ IV ©

Morphine sulfate

(**MOR**-feen **SUL**-fayt)

Classification(s): Narcotic analgesic

Pregnancy Category: C

RX: Capsules, Extended-Release Pellets: Avinza, Kadian. **Injection**: Astramorph PF, Duramorph, Infumorph 200 and 500, Morphine Sulfate in 5% Dextrose. **Injection, Extended-Release Liposomal**: DepoDur. **Oral Solution**: MSIR, Roxanol, Roxanol 100, Roxanol T. **Rectal Suppository**: RMS. **Tablets, Controlled-Release**: MS Contin, Oramorph SR, **C-II.**

🍁 **Rx:** M.O.S.-Sulfate, M-Eslon, Morphine HP Injection, Morphine LP Epidural, PMS-Morphine Sulfate, ratio-Morphine SR.

SEE ALSO ***NARCOTIC ANALGESICS.***

INDICATIONS/USES

Oral: (1) Immediate-Release Tablets/Solution: Relief of moderate to severe pain. (2) Controlled-/Extended-Release Capsules/Tablets: Relief of moderate to severe pain in those requiring continuous, around-the-clock opioid therapy for an extended period of time. Not indicated for use as an as-needed analgesic.

IV: (1) Relief of severe pain (MI, severe injuries, severe chronic pain associated with terminal cancer after all nonnarcotic analgesics have failed). (2) Preoperatively for sedation and to reduce apprehension. (3) Facilitate induction of anesthesia and reduce anesthetic dose. (4) Control postoperative pain. (5) Relieve anxiety and reduce left ventricular work by reducing preload pressure. (6) Treat dyspnea associated with acute left ventricular failure and pulmonary edema. (7) Anesthesia for open-heart surgery.

SC, IM: (1) Relief of moderate to severe pain. (2) Reduce preoperative apprehension and produce sedation. (3) Control postoperative pain. (4) Supplement to anesthesia. (5) Analgesia during labor. (6) Acute pulmonary edema. (7) Allay anxiety.

Epidural, Intrathecal: (1) Management of pain not responsive to nonnarcotic analgesics. (2) Treat intractable chronic pain (Infumorph only).

ER Epidural: Treatment of pain following major surgery. Is a liposomal preparation for single-dose administration by the epidural route, at the lumbar level. Is given prior to surgery or after clamping the umbilical cord during cesarean section.

Rectal: Severe acute and chronic pain.

Investigational: Combined with gabapentin to treat diabetic neuropathy or postherpetic neuralgia.

ACTION/KINETICS

Action

Morphine is the prototype for opiate analgesics. Morphine combines with specific receptors located in the CNS to produce various effects. The mechanism is believed to involve decreased permeability of the cell membrane to sodium, which results in diminished transmission of pain impulses and therefore analgesia.

Pharmacokinetics

Onset, IM/SC: 10–30 min. **Peak effect, PO:** 60 min; **epidural:** 10–15 min. **Duration, SC:** 4–5 hr. **t½, elimination:** 1.5–2 hr. Oral morphine is only one-third to one-sixth as effective as parenteral products. Metabolized in the liver by glucuronidation. Excreted in the urine.

ADDITIONAL CONTRAINDICATIONS

Epidural or intrathecal morphine: If infection is present at injection site; with anticoagulant therapy; bleeding diathesis; if client has received parenteral corticosteroids within the past 2 weeks. **Morphine injection:** Heart failure secondary to chronic lung disease, cardiac arrhythmias, brain tumor, acute alcoholism, delirium tremens, convulsive states. **Immediate-release oral solution of morphine:** Respiratory insufficiency, severe CNS depression, heart failure secondary to chronic lung disease, cardiac arrhythmias, increased intracranial or CSF pressure, head injuries, brain tumor, acute alcoholism, delirium tremens, after biliary tract surgery, suspected surgical abdomen, convulsive disorders, surgical anastomosis, with MAOIs or within 14 days of these drugs.

SPECIAL CONCERNS

(1) **Avinza.** These capsules are a modified-release formulation of morphine indicated for once daily administration for relief of moderate to severe pain requiring continuous, around-the-clock opioid therapy for an extended period of time. Avinza capsules are to be swallowed whole or the contents of the capsules sprinkled on applesauce. The capsule beads are not to be chewed, crushed, or dissolved because of the risk of rapid release and absorption of a potentially fatal dose of morphine. (2) Morphine release is increased when Avinza capsules are exposed to ethanol. Clients must not use prescription or nonprescription medications containing alcohol while on Avinza therapy. Consumption of alcohol while taking Avinza may result in the rapid release and absorption of a potentially fatal dose of morphine. (3) **Kadian.** Morphine has an abuse liability similar to other opioid analgesics. Morphine can be abused in a manner similar to other opioid agonists, legal or illicit. Consider this when prescribing or dispensing Kadian in situations in which the health care provider or pharmacist is concerned about an increased risk of misuse, abuse, or diversion. (4) Kadian capsules are an extended-release oral formulation of morphine indicated for the management of moderate to severe pain requiring a continuous, around-the-clock opioid analgesic for an extended period of time. (5) Kadian capsules are NOT for use as an as-needed analgesic. Kadian 100 and 200 mg capsules are for use in opioid-tolerant clients only. Ingestion of these capsules or of the pellets within the capsules may cause fatal respiratory depression when administered to clients not already tolerant to high doses of opioids. Kadian capsules are to be swallowed whole or the contents of the capsules sprinkled on applesauce. The pellets in the capsules are not to be chewed, crushed, or dissolved because of the risk of rapid release and absorption of a potentially fatal dose of morphine. (6) **Astromorph PF, Duramorph, Infumorph.** Because of the risk of severe adverse effects when the epidural or intrathecal route of administration is employed, clients must be observed in a fully equipped and staffed environment for at

M

least 24 hr after the initial dose. (7) **Infumorph.** Is not recommended for single-dose IV, IM, or SC administration because of the very large amount of morphine in the ampule and the associated risk of overdosage. ■

- **May increase the length of labor.**
- **Clients with known seizure disorders may be at greater risk for morphine-induced seizure activity.**
- **Respiratory depression may be delayed up to 24 hr after epidural or intrathecal use.**
- **Use with extreme caution in aged or debilitated clients; lower doses are usually satisfactory.**

SIDE EFFECTS

Most Common

N&V, constipation, somnolence, headache.

See *Narcotic Analgesics* for a complete list of possible side effects. Also, diplopia, nystagmus, taste perversion, visual disturbances, chills, edema, dehydration, fever, flu syndrome, infection, malaise, ***sepsis, shock***.

ADDITIONAL DRUG INTERACTIONS

Amitriptyline / ↑ CNS and respiratory depression
Cimetidine / ↑ CNS and respiratory depression
Clomipramine / ↑ CNS and respiratory depression
Nortriptyline / ↑ CNS and respiratory depression
Smoking / ↓ Analgesia R/T ↑ hepatic metabolism; takes several weeks to occur
Warfarin / ↑ Warfarin anticoagulant effect

HOW SUPPLIED

Capsules, Extended-Release Pellets: 10 mg, 20 mg, 30 mg, 45 mg, 50 mg, 60 mg, 75 mg, 80 mg, 90 mg, 100 mg, 120 mg, 200 mg; ***Injection:*** 0.5 mg/mL, 1 mg/mL, 2 mg/mL, 4 mg/mL, 5 mg/mL, 8 mg/mL, 10 mg/mL, 15 mg/mL, 25 mg/mL, 50 mg/mL; 1 mg/mL in 5% Dextrose; ***Injection, Extended-Release Liposomal:*** 10 mg/mL; ***Oral Solution:*** 10 mg/5 mL, 20 mg/mL (concentrate), 20 mg/5 mL, 100 mg/5 mL (concentrate); ***Suppository, Rectal:*** 5 mg, 10 mg, 20 mg, 30 mg; ***Tablets:*** 15 mg, 30 mg; ***Tablets for Injection, Soluble:*** 10 mg, 15 mg, 30 mg; ***Tablets, Controlled-Release:*** 15 mg, 30 mg, 60 mg, 100 mg, 200 mg; ***Tablets, Extended-Release:*** 15 mg, 30 mg, 60 mg, 100 mg, 200 mg.

DOSAGE

ORAL SOLUTION; TABLETS; TABLETS, SOLUBLE

Analgesia.

5–30 mg (solution or tablets) on a regularly scheduled basis q 4 hr at the lowest dosage level that will achieve adequate analgesia.

CAPSULES, EXTENDED-RELEASE PELLETS

Analgesia.

Avinza. Initial, no proven opioid tolerance: 30 mg once daily (at 24-hour intervals). Increase the dose conservatively in these clients; adjust the dose in increments not greater than 30 mg q 4 days. Some degree of tolerance may develop requiring a dosage adjustment until a balance is reached between analgesia and opioid side effects. If necessary, increase the total daily dose until pain relief is reached or clinically significant opioid-related side effects occur. If breakthrough pain occurs, Avinza may be supplemented with a small dose (5–15% of the total daily dose of morphine) of a short-acting analgesic.

Limit the daily dose of Avinza to a maximum of 1,600 mg; doses over 1,600 mg/day contain an amount of fumaric acid that has not been shown to be safe and may cause serious renal toxicity. The 60, 90, and 120 mg capsules are for use only in opioid-tolerant clients. All doses are intended to be given once daily.

Kadian. Initial: 20 mg daily in clients who do not have a proven tolerance to opioids. The first dose may be taken with the last dose of any immediate-release morphine product because of the long delay until the peak effect occurs with Kadian. Increase the dose at a rate of up to 20 mg every other day. Individualize dosage. The 100 mg and 200 mg capsules are for use only in opioid-tolerant clients.

Give one-half of the estimated daily PO morphine dose q 12 hr (twice a day) or give the total daily PO morphine dose q 24 hr (once a day). To avoid accumulation, do not reduce the dosing interval below 12 hr. Titrate the dose no more frequently than every other day to allow clients to stabilize before escalating the dose. If breakthrough pain occurs, the dose of Kadian may be supplemented with a small dose (less than 20% of the total daily dose) of a short-acting analgesic.

Clients who are excessively sedated after a once-daily dose of Kadian or who regularly experience inadequate analgesia before the next dose should be switched to a twice-daily dose. Most clients will rapidly develop some degree of tolerance, requiring adjustment of dosage until a balance between baseline analgesia and opioid side effects have occurred. Increase the total daily dose of Kadian until the desired therapeutic end point is reached or clinically significant opioid-related side effects occur.

TABLETS, CONTROLLED-RELEASE; TABLETS, EXTENDED-RELEASE

Analgesia.

Titrate first to analgesia using an immediate-release product dosing q 4–6 hr. Transfer to a long-acting controlled- or extended-release product in either of 2 ways. (1) Give one-half the total 24-hr PO morphine dose as MS Contin or Oramorph SR q 12 hr or (2) give one-third of the client's 24-hr requirement using MS Contin on an every 8-hr schedule. Use the 15 mg extended-release MS Contin tablet for initial conversion if the client's total daily requirement is expected to be less than 60 mg. The 30 mg extended-release product of Oramorph SR is recommended for those with a daily morphine requirement of 60 to 120 mg. When the total daily dose is expected to be greater than 120 mg, the appropriate tablet strength should be used. The MS Contin 200 mg tablet is only for narcotic-tolerant clients requiring daily morphine equivalent doses of 400 mg or more.

IM; SC

Analgesia.

Adults: 10 mg (range: 5–20 mg)/70 kg q 4 hr as needed. **Pediatric:** 0.1–0.2 mg/kg q 4 hr, up to a maximum of 15 mg/dose. For analgesia during labor, 10 mg is the usual dose. If using soluble tablets, prepare in sterile water and filter through a 0.22 micron membrane filter. For preanesthetic medication: **Adults:** 10 mg (range: 5–20 mg)/70 mg kg body weight; **children, 1 year of age and older:** 0.1 mg/kg, up to a maximum dose of 10 mg.

IV

Analgesia.

Adults: 2–10 mg/70 kg. A strength of 2.5–15 mg can be used in 4–5 mL of water for injection (administer slowly over 4–5 min).

Relief of pain and as a preanesthetic.

Adult, usual: 10 mg q 4 hr, depending on the severity of the condition and the client response. Individual dose range: 5–15 mg; usual daily dose range: 12–120 mg. **Children (as an analgesic):** 50–100 micrograms/kg (0.05–0.1 mg/kg) given very slowly, not to exceed 10 mg/dose.

Chronic severe pain associated with terminal cancer.

Initial: Loading dose of 15 mg or more of morphine by IV push followed by the infusion of 0.2–1 mg/mL. Infusion amount may range from 0.8–80 mg/hr, up to 144 mg/hr. Thus, for the 1 mg/mL solution, the infusion may be run from 0.8–80 mL/hr and for the 0.5 mg/mL solution, the infusion may be run from 1.6–160 mL/hr. A constant infusion rate must be maintained with an infusion pump in order to ensure proper control of dosage. Avoid overdosage (respiratory depression) or abrupt cessation of therapy, which may cause withdrawal symptoms.

Open-heart surgery.

0.5–3 mg/kg (large doses) as the sole anesthetic or with a suitable anesthetic. Give oxygen and adequate ventilation to maintain CV function.

M

MI pain.

8–15 mg. For very severe pain, additional smaller doses may be given q 3–4 hr, as needed.

INTRATHECAL

Pain not responsive to nonnarcotic analgesics.

Adults: 0.2–1 mg as a single daily injection; may provide relief for up to 24 hr. NOTE: The dose is only 0.4–2 mL of the 0.5 mg/mL potency or 0.2–1 mL of the 1 mg/mL product. Do not inject intrathecally more than 2 mL of the 0.5 mg/mL potency or 1 mL of the 1 mg/mL potency product. Use in lumbar area only. Repeated intrathecal injections are not recommended. A constant IV infusion of naloxone, 0.6 mg/hr, for 24 hr after intrathecal injection may reduce the incidence of potential side effects. Continue client monitoring for at least 24 hr after each dose due to the possibility of delayed respiratory depression. *NOTE:* The intrathecal dose is usually one tenth the epidural dose.

EPIDURAL

Pain not responsive to nonnarcotic analgesics.

Initial: 5 mg/day in the lumbar region may provide pain relief for up to 24 hr; if analgesia is not manifested in 1 hr, increasing doses of 1–2 mg can be given, not to exceed 10 mg/day. Thoracic use has been shown to dramatically increase the incidence of early and late respiratory depression even at doses of 1 to 2 mg. Administer with extreme caution to aged or debilitated clients; doses less than 5 mg may provide satisfactory analgesia for up to 24 hr. For continuous infusion, 2–4 mg/day with additional doses of 1–2 mg if analgesia is not satisfactory. Usual starting dose of Infumorph for those not tolerant to opiates ranges from 2.5–7.5 mg/day whereas the usual starting dose for continuous epidural infusion in those who have some degree of opiate tolerance is 4.5–10 mg/day. Dose requirements may increase significantly (i.e., up to 20–30 mg/day) during treatment.

INJECTION, EXTENDED-RELEASE LIPOSOMAL (DEPO-DUR)

Pain resulting from major surgery.

One-time dose of DepoDur: 15 mg for major orthopedic surgery of the lower extremity, 10–15 mg for lower abdominal or pelvic surgery, and 10 mg for cesarean section. DepoDur is not intended for intrathecal, IV, or IM use. Give via needle or catheter at the lumbar level. May be given undiluted or diluted up to 5 mL total volume with preservative-free 0.9% NaCl. Do not use an in-line filter during administration of DepoDur. *NOTE:* Use in clients 65 years and older only after careful evaluation of their underlying medication condition and the risks associated with use. The dose for such clients should be at the low end of the dose range.

RECTAL SUPPOSITORY

Severe chronic and acute pain.

Adults, usual: 10–20 mg q 4 hr or as directed by prescriber. Give on a regular schedule and at the lowest dose that will achieve adequate analgesia. During the first 2 to 3 days of effective pain relief, the client may sleep for many hours. This may be misinterpreted as an excessive analgesic dose rather than the first sign of relief of a pain-exhausted client. Therefore, maintain dosage for at least 3 days before reduction. Following successful relief of severe pain, periodic attempts to reduce dose of narcotic should be made as lower doses may be feasible due to a physiologic change or improved mental status of the client.

NURSING IMPLICATIONS

(1) Do not confuse morphine with hydromorphone (also a narcotic analgesic). (2) Do not confuse Avinza (extended-release morphine sulfate) with Evista (raloxifene—used to treat and prevent osteoporosis in postmenopausal women). (3) Do not confuse Roxanol with Uroxatral (drug for benign prostatic hypertrophy) or Oxytrol (drug for overactive bladder).

IMPLEMENTATION/ADMINISTRATION/STORAGE

1. Begin therapy using an immediate-release morphine product as it may be more difficult to titrate a client to adequate analgesia using a controlled- or extended-release product.
2. During the first 2 to 3 days of immediate-release morphine therapy, the client may sleep for many hours. This may be the first sign of relief in a pain-exhausted client rather than the effect of excessive dosing. Thus, if respiratory activity and other vital signs are adequate, maintain the dose for at least 3 days before reduction. Following successful relief of severe pain, reduce the narcotic dose periodically. Smaller doses or complete discontinuation of the narcotic may be feasible due to a physiologic change or the improved mental state of the client.
3. If signs of excessive opioid effects are seen early in the dosing interval when using controlled-/extended-release products, the next dose should be decreased. If this dosage reduction leads to breakthrough pain late in the dosing interval, the dosing interval may be shortened. If breakthrough pain occurs when Kadian is given on an every 24-hr dosing regimen, consider dosing q 12 hr. Alternatively, a supplemental dose of a short-acting analgesic may be given.
4. The MS Contin 200 mg tablet is for use only in opioid-tolerant clients requiring daily morphine-equivalent doses of 400 mg or more. Reserve this strength for those who have already been titrated to a stable analgesic regimen using lower strengths of MS Contin or other opioids.
5. The contents of the immediate-release capsule may be delivered through an NG or a gastric tube.
6. Conversion from parenteral morphine or parenteral or PO other opioids to controlled-/extended-release PO morphine: Initial dosing regimens should be conservative since there is intersubject variation in relative estimates of opioid potency and cross-tolerance (i.e., an underestimation of the 24-hr PO morphine requirement is preferred to an overestimate). In clients whose daily PO requirements are expected to be no more than 120 mg, the 30 mg tablet is recommended for the initial titration period. Once a stable dose regimen is reached the client can be converted to the 60 or 100 mg tablet or appropriate combination of tablet strengths.
7. From 2 to 6 mg of PO morphine may be required to provide analgesia equivalent to 1 mg of parenteral morphine. A dose of PO morphine 3 times the daily parenteral morphine requirement may be sufficient for chronic use. A reasonable initial dose of Avinza would be about 3 times the previous daily parenteral morphine requirement.
8. Conversion from controlled-/extended-release PO morphine to parenteral opioids: Assume that the parenteral-to-PO potency is high. To estimate the required 24-hr dose of morphine for IM use, a conversion of 1 mg morphine IM for every 6 mg morphine as a controlled-release tablet can be used. The IM 24-hr dose is divided by six (6) and given on an every 4-hr regimen. This approach is least likely to cause an overdose.
9. When converting from Avinza or Kadian to parenteral opioids, calculate an equivalent parenteral dose and then begin treatment at one-half of this calculated value. For example, an estimated 24-hr parenteral morphine requirement of a client receiving Avinza or Kadian is one-third of the dose of Avinza or Kadian. This estimated dose should then be divided in half and this last calculated dose is the total daily dose. This value should be further divided by six (6) if the desire is to dose with parenteral morphine every 4 hr. This approach may require a dosage increase in the first 24 hr for many clients. However, this method is less likely to result in overdose. *Example:* A client takes 360 mg of Avinza or Kadian per day. The estimated total 24-hr parenteral morphine requirement would be one-third of 360 mg (i.e., 120 mg). Dividing by two (2) gives the total daily dose of 60 mg. If parenteral morphine is to be given at 4-hr intervals, 10 mg (60 mg divided by 6) would be given q 4 hr.
10. Conversion of extended-release morphine (Avinza or Kadian) to other controlled-/extended-release PO morphine products: Kadian is *not* equivalent to other extended-release morphine products. For a given dose, the same total amount of morphine is available from Avinza or Kadian as from PO morphine solution

M

or controlled-/extended-release morphine tablets. However, the slower release of Kadian results in reduced maximum and increased minimum plasma levels than with shorter-acting morphine products. Conversion from Kadian or Avinza to the same total daily dose of another controlled-/extended-release morphine formulation may lead to either excessive sedation at peak or inadequate analgesia at trough. Close observation and appropriate dosing adjustments are recommended. *NOTE:* Persistence of Avinza-derived plasma morphine levels may be in excess of 36 hr when making a conversion to other pain control therapies.

11. For intrathecal use, do not give more than 2 mL of the 0.5-mg/mL preparation or 1 mL of the 1-mg/mL product.
12. Give intrathecally only in the lumbar region; repeated injections are not recommended.
13. To reduce chance of side effects with intrathecal administration, a constant IV infusion of naloxone (0.6 mg/hr for 24 hr after intrathecal injection) is recommended.
14. For Infumorph, Duramorph, and Astromorph PF use epidural doses of 20 mg or more with caution R/T the increased possibility of serious side effects.
15. In certain circumstances (e.g., tolerance, severe pain), provider may prescribe doses higher than those listed under *Dosage*.
16. Dose may be lower in geriatric clients or those with respiratory disease.
17. Intraventricular administration may be effective in select clients with a short life expectancy and recalcitrant pain due to head and neck malignancies and tumors and breast cancer that affect the brachial plexus. Only 1–2 doses/day are usually needed.
18. Use caution interpreting dosage, especially for concentrated morphine sulfate oral solutions. **Do not interchange milligrams for milliliters.** Prescription should contain concentration of morphine oral solution to be dispensed and intended dose of morphine in milligrams with the corresponding volume in milliliters written out in the directions. As an example, a prescription should look as follows: "Roxanol Concentrated Oral Solution, 20 mg/mL" at a dose of "15 mg (0.75 mL) q 4 hr as needed."
19. Store PO solution, soluble tablets for injection, and capsules at controlled room temperature of 15–30°C (59–86°F) protected from light and moisture. Solutions made from soluble tablets for injection may darken with age; do not use if solution is darker than pale yellow, discolored in any way, or contains a precipitate.
20. IV For IV use, dilute 2–10 mg with at least 5 mL sterile water or NSS and administer over 4–5 min. For continous infusions, reconstitute to concentration of 0.1–1 mg/mL and administer as prescribed to control symptoms.
21. Rapid IV administration increases risk of adverse effects; do not give IV unless a narcotic antagonist (e.g., naloxone) is immediately available.
22. When therapy is no longer required, taper doses gradually to prevent S&S of withdrawal in the physically-dependent client.
23. Store injections at controlled room temperature; do not use if injection is darker than pale yellow, discolored in any way, or contains a precipitate.
24. Store Infumorph, Duramorph, or Astromorph PF injections from 15–30°C (59–86°F) protected from light; do not freeze. Discard any unused portion as products contain no preservative or antioxidant. Do not heat sterilize.
25. Store DepoDur in the refrigerator at 2–8°C (36–46°F). May be held at 15–30°C (59–86°F) for up to 7 days in sealed, intact (unopened) vials. Product is sterile but does not contain bacteriostatic agents; thus, give within 4 hr after withdrawal from vial. Do not heat or gas sterilize. Protect from freezing; do not give if suspected that the vial has been frozen.
26. COMPATIBILITY D5W, D10W, 0.9% NaCl, 0.45% NaCl, Ringer's, RL, and combinations of these solutions.
27. INCOMPATIBILITY Administer separately.

ASSESSMENT

1. Identify reasons for and type of therapy, onset, location and characteristics of pain. Rate pain level using a pain-rating scale.
2. List other agents prescribed, outcome. Giving with other nonopioid analgesics may have additive analgesic effects.
3. Note any seizure disorder or head trauma. With continuous IV drips follow established

protocols for infusion (i.e. Resp Rate >10). With patient controlled analgesia (PCA) ensure facility procedure is followed and client/family instructed in use. Record on sedation-monitoring tool for those using PCA.

4. Discontinue gradually to ensure no S&S of withdrawal with long term therapy.
5. Monitor VS and respiratory status. Have naloxone readily availably to treat overdose.
6. Assess for falls and fall risk; ensure call bell is close and instruct to call before attempting ambulation.
7. Consider dosage reduction in the elderly and with renal or liver dysfunction.

CLIENT/FAMILY TEACHING

1. May take with food to diminish GI upset. Do not crush or chew controlled- or extended-release capsules or tablets as this will lead to the rapid release and absorption of a potentially fatal dose of morphine.
2. Avinza or Kadian beads sprinkled over applesauce are bioequivalent to Avinza or Kadian capsules swallowed whole under fasting conditions. Capsules may be opened and the entire bead contents sprinkled on a small amount of applesauce immediately prior to ingestion. The applesauce should be at room temperature or cooler. Clients should ingest the mixture immediately without chewing or crushing the beads; clients should then rinse their mouths and swallow to ensure all beads have been ingested. Do not divide the applesauce into separate doses.
3. The entire capsule contents of Kadian may also be administered through a 16-French gastrostomy tube. Flush the tube with water to ensure that it is wet. Sprinkle the Kadian pellets into 10 mL of water. Using a swirling motion pour the pellets and water into the gastrostomy tube through a funnel. Rinse the beaker with a further 10 mL of water and pour this into the funnel. Repeat rinsing until no pellets remain in the beaker. Do not administer Kadian pellets through a nasogastric tube.
4. Immediate-release capsules may be swallowed intact or the contents of the capsule may be sprinkled on food or stirred in juice to avoid the bitter taste.
5. Drug may cause dizziness and drowsiness; avoid activities that require mental alertness.
6. Practice cough and deep-breathing exercises and incentive spirometry to decrease risk of atelectasis. Ensure that bedside and path to bathroom are unrestricted to prevent falls; have those at risk call for help with ambulation.
7. May experience constipation; use softener/laxative, high fiber diet, increased fluids and exercise.
8. Record drug use for breakthrough pain when SR therapy prescribed, to ensure adequate dosage.
9. Avoid alcohol/CNS depressants and OTC agents. Keep out of reach of children and away from bedside.
10. PCA pumps should be free-flow-protected and allow for easy programming. The client and family should be educated on how to use the PCA pump and provided with written instructions as well.
11. Secure drug to prevent inadvertent diversion or misuse.
12. Keep all F/U to assess response and for adverse SE.

OUTCOMES/EVALUATE

- ↓ Pain rating/ ↑ pain control
- Control of respirations during mechanical ventilation

IV

Moxifloxacin hydrochloride

(**mox**-ee-**FLOX**-ah-sin)

Classification(s): Antibiotic, fluoroquinolone

Pregnancy Category: C

RX: Avelox, Avelox I.V., Moxeza, Vigamox.

SEE ALSO ***FLUOROQUINOLONES.***

INDICATIONS/USES

Systemic. All uses are for adults at least 18 years of age.

1. Acute bacterial sinusitis due to *Streptococcus pneumoniae, Haemophilus influenzae,* or *Moraxella catarrhalis.*
2. Acute bacterial exacerbation of chronic bronchitis due to *S. pneumoniae, H. influenzae, Haemophilus parainfluenzae, Klebsiella pneumoniae, Staphylococcus aureus* (methicillin-susceptible), or *M. catarrhalis.*

3. Community-acquired pneumonia due to *S. pneumoniae* (including multidrug-resistant strains), *H. influenzae, Mycoplasma pneumoniae, Chlamydia pneumoniae, M. catarrhalis, K. pneumoniae* (including multi-drug–resistant strains), or *S. aureus* (methicillin-susceptible).
4. Uncomplicated skin and skin structure infections due to *S. aureus* (methicillin-susceptible) or *Streptococcus pyogenes.*
5. Complicated skin and skin structure infections due to *S. aureus* (methicillin-susceptible), *E. coli, K. pneumoniae, Enterobacter cloacae,* or methicillin–susceptible *S. aureus.*
6. Complicated intra-abdominal infections, including polymicrobial infection such as abscess due to *E. coli, Bacteroides fragilis, Streptococcus anginosus, Streptococcus constellatus, Proteus mirabilis, Clostridium perfringens, Bacteroides thetaiotaomicron, Enterococcus faecalis,* or *Peptostreptococcus* species.

Investigational: Hospital–acquired pneumonia, infective endocarditis in adults, tuberculosis.

Ophthalmic. Bacterial conjunctivitis due to (a) gram positive organisms, including *Corynebacterium* species, *Micrococcus luteus, S. aureus, S. epidermidis, S. haemolyticus, S. hominis, S. warneri, S. pneumoniae, Streptococcus viridans* group, *Aerococcus viridans, Corynebacterium macginleyi, Enterococcus faecalis, Staphylococcus arlettae, Staphylococcus saprophyticus, Streptococcus mitis, Streptococcus parasanguinis, Propionibacterium acnes, Staphylococcus capitis*; (b) gram negative organisms, including *Acinetobacter lwoffi, E. coli, H. influenzae, Klebsiella pneumoniae, H. influenzae;* and (c) *Chlamydia trachomatis.*

M

ACTION/KINETICS

Action

Interferes with DNA gyrase and topoisomerase IV. DNA gyrase is an enzyme needed for replication, transcription, and repair of bacterial DNA. Topoisomerase IV plays a key role in the partitioning of chromosomal DNA during bacterial cell division. Effective against both gram-positive and gram-negative organisms.

Pharmacokinetics

Well absorbed from the GI tract (about 90% bioavailable). A high-fat meal does not affect absorption. **t½, elimination:** About 12 hr. Steady state is reached in 3 days (400 mg/day). Widely distributed in the body. Metabolized in the liver; metabolites and unchanged drug are excreted in the feces and urine.

CONTRAINDICATIONS

Hypersensitivity to moxifloxacin or any quinolone antibiotic. Use with moderate to severe hepatic insufficiency. Use in clients with known prolongation of the QT interval (the drug prolongs the QT interval in some), with uncorrected hypokalemia, and in those receiving class IA (e.g., quinidine, procainamide) or Class III (e.g., amiodarone, sotalol) antiarrhythmic drugs. IM, intrathecal, IP, or SC use. Lactation.

SPECIAL CONCERNS

■ (1) Fluoroquinolones, including moxifloxacin, are associated with an increased risk of tendinitis and tendon rupture in clients of all ages. This risk is further increased in older clients (usually older than 60 years), in clients taking corticosteroid drugs, and in clients with kidney, heart, or lung transplants. (2) Fluoroquinolones, including moxifloxacin, may exacerbate muscle weakness in persons with myasthenia gravis. Avoid moxifloxacin in clients with known history of myasthenia gravis. ■

- **Use with caution in clinically significant bradycardia or acute myocardial ischemia, with known or suspected CNS disorders (e.g., severe cerebral arteriosclerosis, epilepsy), or with risk factors that predispose to seizures or lower the seizure threshold.**
- **Use with caution with drugs that may affect the QTc interval (e.g., cisapride, erythromycin, antipsychotics, tricyclic antidepressants).**
- **Safety and efficacy of PO and IV use not determined in children, adolescents less than 18 years of age, in pregnancy, and during lactation. Safety of the ophthalmic product not determined in children less than 1 year.**

SIDE EFFECTS

Most Common

N&V, diarrhea, dizziness, headache, dyspepsia/heartburn.

Hypersensitivity: ***Anaphylaxis after the first dose, CV collapse***, loss of consciousness, tingling, pharyngeal or facial edema, dyspnea, urticaria, itching. **CNS**: Dizziness, headache, convulsions, confusion, tremors, hallucinations, depression, insomnia, nervousness, anxiety, depersonalization, hypertonia, incoordination, somnolence, vertigo, paresthesia, psychotic reaction, syncope, suicidal thoughts/acts (rare). **GI**: N&V, diarrhea, abdominal pain, taste perversion, dyspepsia, heartburn, dry mouth, constipation, oral moniliasis, anorexia, stomatitis, gastritis, glossitis, GI disorder, pseudomembranous colitis, cholestatic jaundice, hepatitis. **CV**: Palpitation, vasodilation, tachycardia, hypertension, peripheral edema, hypotension, QTc prolongation. **Body as a whole:** Asthenia, moniliasis, pain, malaise, allergic reaction, leg/pelvic/back/chest/hand pain, chills, infection. **Hematologic**: Thrombocytopenia, thrombocythemia, eosinophilia, leukopenia. **Respiratory:** Asthma, dyspnea, increased cough, pneumonia, pharyngitis, rhinitis, sinusitis. **Musculoskeletal**: Arthralgia, myalgia, tendon ruptures. **Dermatologic**: Rash, pruritus, sweating, urticaria, dry skin, ***Stevens-Johnson syndrome***. **GU**: Vaginal moniliasis, vaginitis, cystitis. **Miscellaneous**: Tinnitus, amblyopia.

LABORATORY TEST CONSIDERATIONS

↑ GGTP, LDH, MCH, WBCs, PT ratio, ionized calcium, chloride, albumin, globulin, bilirubin. ↓ Hemoglobin, RBCs, eosinophils, basophils, glucose, pO_2. Either ↑ or ↓ Amylase, PT, bilirubin, neutrophils. Hyperglycemia, hyperlipidemia. Abnormal LFTs and kidney function.

OVERDOSE MANAGEMENT

Symptoms: Possible prolongation of the QT interval. *Treatment:* Empty the stomach and monitor ECG. Carefully observe and provide supportive treatment. Maintain adequate hydration. Not known if moxifloxacin is dialyzable.

DRUG INTERACTIONS

Antacids / Significant ↓ bioavailability of moxifloxacin
Antidepressants, tricyclic / Potential to add to the QTc prolonging effect of moxifloxacin
Antipsychotics / Potential to add to the QTc prolonging effect of moxifloxacin
Didanosine / ↓ Absorption of moxifloxacin
Erythromycin / Potential to add to the QTc prolonging effect of moxifloxacin
Iron products / Significant ↓ bioavailability of moxifloxacin
NSAIDs / ↑ Risk of CNS stimulation and convulsions
Sucralfate / ↓ Absorption of moxifloxacin
Warfarin / ↑ Anticoagulant effect of warfarin

HOW SUPPLIED

Injection Solution (Premix): 400 mg/250 mL; ***Ophthalmic Solution:*** 0.5% (5 mg/mL); ***Tablets:*** 400 mg.

DOSAGE

IV; TABLETS

Acute bacterial sinusitis.

Adults 18 years and older: 400 mg q 24 hr for 10 days.

Acute bacterial exacerbation of chronic bronchitis.

Adults 18 years and older: 400 mg q 24 hr for 5 days.

Community-acquired pneumonia.

Adults 18 years and older: 400 mg q 24 hr for 7–14 days.

Uncomplicated skin and skin structure infections.

Adults 18 years and older: 400 mg q 24 hr for 7 days.

Complicated skin and skin structure infections.

Adults 18 years and older: 400 mg q 24 hr for 7–21 days.

Complicated intra-abdominal infections.

Adults 18 years and older: 400 mg q 24 hr for 5–14 days. Begin therapy with the IV formulation.

Hospital-acquired pneumonia (investigational).

Adults 18 years and older: 400 mg IV once daily given over 60 min; switch to 400 mg PO once daily. The switch from IV to PO is made at the discretion of the health care provider. **Duration of treatment:** 7–8 days.

Infective endocarditis in adults (investigational).

Adults: Specific dosing not available but the usual dose is 400 mg daily. *NOTE:* Moxifloxacin can be substituted for ciprofloxacin for 4 weeks in native valve infections and for 6 weeks in prosthetic valve infections.

Tuberculosis (investigational).

Adults: 400 mg PO once daily.

M

OPHTHALMIC SOLUTION

Bacterial conjunctivitis.

Moxeza. Adults and children 4 months and older: 1 gtt in the affected eye(s) 2 times a day for 7 days.

Vigamox. Adults and children at least 1 year of age: 1 gtt in affected eye(s) 3 times a day for 7 days.

NURSING IMPLICATIONS

Do not confuse Avelox with Asacol (mesalamine, an anti-inflammatory drug).

IMPLEMENTATION/ADMINISTRATION/STORAGE

1. Avoid high humidity when storing tablets. Not for IM, SC, intrathecal, or intraperitoneal use.
2. The ophthalmic product is not to be used as an injection.
3. Store tablets from 15–30°C (59–86°F) avoiding high humidity and the ophthalmic solution from 2–25°C (36–77°F).
4. IV No dosage adjustment needed when switching from IV to PO dosing.
5. Give only by IV infusion over 60 min through a Y-type IV infusion set. Avoid rapid or bolus IV infusion. If Y-type or piggyback method used, temporarily discontinue administration of other solutions during moxifloxacin IV administration.
6. Do **not** give by the following routes: Intra--arterial, IM, intrathecal, IP, or SC.
7. The premix containers are for single use only; discard any unused portion.
8. Store IV solution from 15–30°C (59–86°F); do not refrigerate as the product precipitates upon refrigeration.
9. COMPATIBILITY With the following at ratios from 1:10 to 10:1: 0.9% NaCl, 1 molar NaCl injection, D5W, D10W, LR, sterile water for injection.
10. INCOMPATIBILITY Administer separately; flush line before and after moxifloxacin infusion with a compatible solution.

ASSESSMENT

1. Note onset, location, characteristics of S&S, clinical presentation, and culture results. List drugs prescribed to ensure none interact.
2. Avoid with uncorrected hypokalemia, prolonged QT intervals, if receiving class 1A or III antiarrhythmic agents, or seizure disorder.
3. Monitor cultures, electrolytes, CBC, renal and LFTs; avoid with moderate to severe liver dysfunction.

CLIENT/FAMILY TEACHING

1. Take tablets once daily at the same time, as directed. May take with/without meals. Drink fluids liberally.
2. Take at least 4 hr before or 8 hr after multivitamins containing iron or zinc, antacids containing Mg^{++}/calcium/aluminum, sucralfate, or didanosine (chewable/buffered tablets or the pediatric powder for PO solution).
3. Do not perform activities that require mental alertness until drug effects realized.
4. May cause GI upset, dizziness, and headaches. Report pain or inflammation in a tendon, muscle weakness, paralysis, pain, numbness, or a burning sensation.
5. Avoid excess sunlight and tanning beds to prevent photosensitivity reactions.
6. With eye drops: wash hands, tilt head back looking up, pull lower eyelid down and instill drops as prescribed. Avoid any contact with dropper. Close eye for 1–2 min; press gently on bridge of nose for 3–5 min. Do not rub eyes. Do not wear contact lenses during therapy. If more than 1 eye drop is being used, give at least 5 min apart.
7. May experience blurred vision, eye itching/pain/discomfort; report if persistent or bothersome, if eye or eyelid inflammation occurs or if eye S&S do not improve or worsen.
8. Complete the entire course of therapy to ensure max benefit even if S&S have resolved.
9. Stop drug and report skin rash immediately. Report adverse SE, lack of effectiveness, or worsening of condition.
10. Keep all F/U to assess response, labs, and adverse SE.

OUTCOMES/EVALUATE

- Resolution of infection
- Symptomatic improvement
- Clearing of eye infection
- Negative culture results

Mupirocin

(myou-**PEER**-oh-sin)

Classification(s): Antibiotic, topical

Pregnancy Category: B

RX: Bactroban Nasal, Bactroban Ointment, Centany Ointment.

✤ **Rx:** Taro-Mupirocin.

Mupirocin calcium

Pregnancy Category: B

RX: Bactroban Cream, Bactroban Nasal, Centany.

SEE ALSO ***ANTI-INFECTIVE DRUGS.***

INDICATIONS/USES

Nasal Ointment: Eradication of nasal colonization with methicillin-resistant *S. aureus* in adult clients and health care workers as part of a comprehensive infection control program to reduce risk of infection among clients at high risk of methicillin-resistant *S. aureus* infection during institutional outbreaks of infections.

Topical Cream: Secondarily infected traumatic skin lesions (up to 10 cm in length or 100 cm^2) due to susceptible strains of *S. aureus* and *Streptococcus pyogenes.* **Topical Ointment:** Impetigo due to *S. aureus, Streptococcus pyogenes,* and beta-hemolytic streptococcus. *Investigational:* Topical products to treat diaper dermatitis due to *Candida.*

ACTION/KINETICS

Action

Binds to bacterial isoleucyl transfer RNA synthetase, which results in inhibition of protein synthesis by the organism. Not absorbed into the systemic circulation. Serum present in exudative wounds decreases the antibacterial activity. No cross resistance with other antibiotics such as chloramphenicol, erythromycin, gentamicin, lincomycin, methicillin, neomycin, novobiocin, penicillin, streptomycin, or tetracyclines.

Pharmacokinetics

Any drug reaching the systemic circulation is rapidly metabolized to inactive monic acid which is excreted by the kidneys.

CONTRAINDICATIONS

Hypersensitivity to any component of the product. Ophthalmic use. Use if absorption of large quantities of polyethylene glycol is possible (i.e., large, open wounds). Use with other nasal products. Should not be used for general prophylaxis of any infection.

SPECIAL CONCERNS

- **Superinfection may result from chronic use.**
- **Safety and efficacy not established in children less than 12 years for mupirocin nasal or for the cream and ointment in children 2 months to 16 years.**
- **Use with caution during lactation.**

SIDE EFFECTS

Most Common

Use of nasal ointment: Headache, rhinitis, upper respiratory tract congestion, pharyngitis, taste perversion, burning/stinging, cough.

Use of topical cream: Headache, rash, nausea.

Use of topical ointment: Burning, stinging, pain, itching.

- **NASAL USE**

Headache, rhinitis, respiratory disorder (including upper respiratory tract congestion), pharyngitis, taste perversion, burning, stinging, cough, pruritus, blepharitis, diarrhea, dry mouth, ear pain, epistaxis, nausea, rash.

- **TOPICAL CREAM**

Headache, rash, nausea, abdominal pain, burning at application site, cellulitis, dermatitis, dizziness, pruritus, secondary wound infection, ulcerative stomatitis.

- **TOPICAL OINTMENT**

Burning, stinging or pain, itching, rash, nausea, erythema, dry skin, tenderness, swelling contact dermatitis, increased exudate.

HOW SUPPLIED

Nasal Ointment: 2%; ***Topical Cream:*** 2%; ***Topical Ointment:*** 2%.

DOSAGE

NASAL OINTMENT

Eradication of nasal colonization with methicillin-resistant S. aureus.

Adults and adolescents 12 years and older: Divide about one-half of the ointment from the single-use tube between the nostrils and apply in the morning and evening for 5 days. The single-use tube will deliver about 0.25 gram/nostril.

M

TOPICAL CREAM

Traumatic skin lesions due to S. aureus *or* S. pyogenes.

Apply to affected area 3 times per day for 10 days. May be covered with a gauze dressing. If no response in 3–5 days, re-evaluate.

TOPICAL OINTMENT

Impetigo due to S. aureus, S. pyogenes, *or beta-hemolytic streptococcus.*

A small amount of ointment is applied to the affected area 3 times per day. Area may be covered with a gauze dressing. If no response in 3–5 days, re-evaluate.

NURSING IMPLICATIONS

Do not confuse Bactroban with bacitracin (also a topical antibacterial agent).

IMPLEMENTATION/ADMINISTRATION/STORAGE

1. After application of the nasal product, close the nostrils by pressing them together for about 1 min.
2. Store the topical ointment between 15–30°C (59–86°F); store the topical cream or nasal ointment below 25°C (77°F). Do not freeze the cream.

ASSESSMENT

1. Note reasons for therapy, onset, duration, characteristics of S&S, clinical presentation, and skin integrity. Note other agents/therapies trialed and outcome.
2. Assess labs, swab/culture results.

CLIENT/FAMILY TEACHING

1. Review technique for administering topical and/or nasal medications; use aseptic measures and hand washing before and after therapy to prevent contamination. For external use only; avoid contact with eyes and mucous membranes.
2. Report any symptoms of chemical irritation or hypersensitivity such as increased rash, itching, pain at site, or lack of healing.
3. Clear nasal passages and do not use other nasal products during nasal therapy.
4. Notify school nurse to ensure appropriate screening is performed when treating school-aged children with impetigo.
5. Review hygiene measures to help prevent spread of impetigo. Keep fingernails well trimmed to prevent scratching.
6. Keep all F/U to assess response, cultures, healing, and for adverse SE.

OUTCOMES/EVALUATE

- Healing of lesions; symptomatic improvement
- Eradication of MRSA nasal colonization

IV

Mycophenolate mofetil

(**my**-koh-**FEN**-oh-layt)

Classification(s): Immunosuppressant

Pregnancy Category: D

RX: CellCept.

Mycophenolate mofetil hydrochloride

Pregnancy Category: D

RX: CellCept.

Mycophenolate sodium

Classification(s): Immunosuppressant

Pregnancy Category: D

RX: Myfortic.

INDICATIONS/USES

Mycophenolate mofetil (PO). With cyclosporine and corticosteroids to prevent organ rejection in those receiving allogeneic renal, heart, or liver transplants. May be used in children with renal transplants. *Investigational:* In combination with previous corticosteroid, cyclosporine, or tacrolimus therapy to treat refractory uveitis. In combination with prednisolone to treat diffuse proliferative lupus nephritis. Secondary therapy for Churg-Strauss syndrome.

Mycophenolate mofetil hydrochloride (IV). With cyclosporine and corticosteroids to prevent organ rejection in those receiving allogeneic renal, heart, or liver transplants. Is alternative dosage form for those unable to take PO medication.

Mycophenolate sodium (PO). With cyclosporine and corticosteroids for prophylaxis of organ rejection in clients receiving allogeneic renal transplants.

ACTION/KINETICS

Action

Is hydrolyzed to the active mycophenolic acid (MPA). MPA is a potent, selective, uncompetitive, and reversible inhibitor of inosine monophosphate dehydrogenase and thus inhibits the de novo pathway of guanosine nucleotide synthesis without incorporation into DNA. MPA has potent cytostatic effects on lymphocytes. Inhibits proliferative responses of T- and B-lymphocytes to both mitogenic and allospecific stimulation. MPA also suppresses antibody formation of B-lymphocytes. MPA also inhibits recruitment of leukocytes into sites of inflammation and graft rejection.

Pharmacokinetics

Rapidly absorbed after PO administration. The enteric-coated delayed-release tablets do not release mycophenolic acid under a pH of 5 (e.g., in the stomach) but is highly soluble in neutral pH of the intestine. Food has no effect on absorption of the mofetil salt but decreases C_{max} of the sodium salt. Metabolized in the liver by glucuronyl transferase. **t½, MPA:** 8–16 hr after PO administration and 16.6 hr after IV administration. MPA and additional metabolites excreted mainly in the urine (93%). Levels of MPA and the glucuronide increase significantly in impaired renal function. **Plasma protein binding:** Mycophenolate acid (MPA) at clinical doses: 97%.

CONTRAINDICATIONS

Hypersensitivity to mycophenolate, mycophenolic acid, or polysorbate 80 (Tween; IV only). Use in those with rare hereditary deficiency of hypoxanthine-guanine phosphoribosyl transferase, such as Lesch-Nyhan and Kelley-Seegmiller syndrome. Lactation.

SPECIAL CONCERNS

(1) Increased susceptibility to infection and possible development of lymphoma and other neoplasms may result from immunosuppression. Only health care providers experienced in immunosuppressive therapy and management of organ transplant clients should use mycophenolate. Manage those receiving mycophenolate in facilities equipped and staffed with adequate lab and supportive medical resources. The health care provider responsible for maintenance therapy should have complete information requisite for the follow-up of the client. (2) Women of childbearing potential must use contraception. Use of mycophenolate mofetil during pregnancy is associated with increased risk of miscarriage and congenital malformations.

- **Higher blood levels are seen in those with severe impaired renal function.**
- **Use with caution in active serious digestive system disease.**
- **Elderly are particularly prone to certain infections, including CMV tissue invasive disease and possibly GI hemorrhage and pulmonary edema; use care in dose selection in the elderly.**
- **Use the oral suspension with caution in those with phenylketonuria (product contains aspartame, a source of phenylalanine).**
- **Avoid the use of live, attenuated vaccines during treatment; vaccinations may be less effective.**
- **Clients receiving immunosuppressants involving combinations of drugs, including mycophenolate, are at an increased risk of developing lymphomas and other malignancies, especially of the skin.**
- **Safety and efficacy not determined in children receiving allogeneic cardiac or hepatic transplants. Limited data available for stable pediatric renal transplant clients from ages 5–16 years.**

SIDE EFFECTS

Most Common

Hypertension, constipation, diarrhea, N&V, UTI, anemia, leukopenia, peripheral edema, infection, abdominal pain, fever, headache, infections (viral, fungal), pain, asthenia, back/chest pain, sepsis.

Hematologic: Severe neutropenia, anemia, leukopenia, thrombocytopenia, hypochromic anemia, leukocytosis, ecchymosis, ***hemorrhage***, polycythemia, pancytopenia, coagulation disorder, petechiae, lymphocele, ***thrombosis (after IV)***. **GI:** ***GI tract bleeding/hemorrhage/perforations***, diarrhea, abdominal pain, constipation, N&V, dyspepsia, flatulence, enlarged abdomen, anorexia, cholangitis, hepatitis, cholestatic jaundice, oral/GI moniliasis, esophagitis, gastritis, gastroenteritis, ***GI hemorrhage***, gingivitis, gum hyperplasia, ileus, infection, mouth ulceration, rectal disorder, GI disorder, liver damage, dysphagia, jaundice, stomatitis, thirst, melena, stomach ulcer, peritonitis, colitis, intestinal villous atrophy, abdominal distention, upper/lower abdominal pain, loose stool, sore throat, GERD, duodenal/gastric ulcers, ***pancreatitis***. **CNS:** Headache, tremor, insomnia, anxiety, paresthesia, hypertonia, depression, agitation, somnolence, confusion, nervousness, dizziness, emotional lability, neuropathy, convulsions, hallucinations, abnormal thinking, vertigo, delirium, dry mouth, hypesthesia, psychosis. Also, possible ***progressive multifocal leukoencephalopathy*** (vision changes, loss of coordination, clumsiness, memory loss, difficulty speaking, weakness in the legs). **GU:** UTI, hematuria, abnormal kidney function, oliguria, kidney tubular necrosis, dysuria, albuminuria, hydronephrosis, impotence, pain, pyelonephritis, urinary frequency, nocturia, kidney failure, urine abnormality, urinary incontinence, prostate disorder, urinary retention, urinary tract disorder, dysuria, acute kidney failure, scrotal edema, hernia, bladder spasm, impaired renal function, renal tubular necrosis. **CV:** Hypertension, hypotension, CV disorder, tachycardia, arrhythmia, bradycardia, pericardial effusion, ***cardiac failure, angina pectoris***, atrial fibrillation, palpitation, peripheral vascular disorder, postural hypotension, thrombosis, vasodilation, ventricular extrasystole, CHF, supraventricular tachycardia, ventricular tachycardia, atrial flutter, pulmonary hypertension, ***cardiac arrest, arterial thrombosis***, increased venous pressure, syncope, supraventricular extrasystoles, extrasystoles, pallor, vasospasm, phlebitis. IV use may cause phlebitis and thrombosis. **Respiratory:** Infection, dyspnea (including exertional), increased cough, pharyngitis, lung disorder, sinusitis, rhinitis, pleural effusion, asthma, atelectasis, pneumonia, lung edema, hiccough, pneumothorax, increased sputum, epistaxis, apnea, voice alteration, pain, hemoptysis, ***neoplasm***, respiratory acidosis, bronchitis, respiratory disorder, hyperventilation, respiratory moniliasis, nasopharyngitis, pharyngolaryngeal pain, sinus congestion, URTI, ***fatal pulmonary fibrosis, respiratory failure***. **Dermatologic:** Alopecia, rash, fungal dermatitis, hirsutism, acne, pruritus, benign skin neoplasm, skin hypertrophy, skin ulcer, hemorrhage, skin carcinoma, vesiculobullous rash, contusion. **Metabolic/Endocrine:** Peripheral edema, edema, dehydration, fluid overload, weight gain, diabetes mellitus, parathyroid disorder, Cushing's syndrome, hypothyroidism. **Musculoskeletal:** Leg/muscle cramps, myasthenia, myalgia, arthralgia, joint disorder, osteoporosis, pain in limb, peripheral swelling. **Ophthalmic:** Cataract, conjunctivitis, abnormal/blurred vision, lacrimation disorder, eye hemorrhage, amblyopia. **Otic:** Ear pain, deafness, ear disorder, tinnitus. **Body as a whole:** Pain, fever, ***sepsis, infection (may be fatal)***, asthenia, accidental injury, chills, ascites, edema, flu syndrome, fatigue, malaise, cellulitis (with IV), abnormal healing, abscess, gout. **Miscellaneous:** Increased incidence of lymphoma/lymphoproliferative disease, nonmelanoma skin carcinoma, and other malignancies. Increased incidence of opportunistic infections, including herpes simplex, CMV disease/infection, herpes zoster, tissue invasive disease, fungemia/disseminated disease, cryptococcosis, *Candida, Aspergillus/Mucor* invasive disease, and *Pneumocystis carinii*. ***Life-threatening infections, including meningitis and infectious endocarditis***. Tuberculosis, atypical mycobacterial infection, enlarged abdomen, cyst, facial edema, chest/back/pelvic/neck pain, postoperative pain, weight gain, congenital malformations (including ear malformations), delayed graft function, complications of transplant surgery (including infection).

LABORATORY TEST CONSIDERATIONS

↑ Creatinine, BUN, LDH, AST, ALT, alkaline phosphatase, GGT, prothrombin, thromboplastin. Hypophosphatemia, hypo-/hyperkalemia, hypo-/hyperglycemia, bilirubinemia, hypervolemia, hyperuricemia, hypomagnesemia, acidosis, hyponatremia, hyperlipemia, hypo-/hypercalcemia, hypochloremia, hypoproteinemia, hypercholesterolemia. Abnormal LFTs.

OVERDOSE MANAGEMENT

Symptoms: Nausea, vomiting, diarrhea, hematologic abnormalities, especially neutropenia. *Treatment:* Reduce dose of the drug. Removal of MPA by bile acid sequestrants (e.g., cholestyramine).

DRUG INTERACTIONS

NOTE: Drugs that alter the GI flora may interact with mycophenolate by disrupting enterohepatic recirculation. Interference with mycophenolic acid glucuronide hydrolysis may lead to less mycophenolic acid available for absorption.

Acyclovir / ↑ Plasma levels of both drugs R/T competition for renal tubular excretion
Antacids containing Al or Mg^{++} / ↓ Absorption of mycophenolate; avoid simultaneous administration

Azathioprine / Avoid concomitant use R/T ↑ risk of bone marrow suppression
Charcoal, activated / ↓ Mycophenolic acid exposure R/T interruption of enterohepatic recirculation; do not give together
Cholestyramine / ↓ Mycophenolic acid exposure R/T interruption of enterohepatic recirculation; do not give together
Cyclosporine / ↓ Mycophenolic acid levels; monitor
H ***Echinacea*** / Do not give with mycophenolate
Ganciclovir / ↑ Plasma levels of both drugs in those with renal impairment R/T competition for renal tubular excretion
Iron / ↓ Mycophenolate absorption; do not use together
Levonorgestrel (including oral contraceptives containing levonorgestrel) / Significant ↓ in levonorgestrel AUC; consider additional birth control measures
Metronidazole & Norfloxacin / ↓ Mycophenolic acid and mycophenolic acid glucuronide AUC
Phenytoin / ↓ Plasma protein binding of phenytoin → ↑ free phenytoin levels
Probenecid / Significant ↑ plasma levels of MPA
Rifamycins (e.g., rifabutin, rifampin / Possible ↓ mycophenolic acid levels; monitor and adjust dose as needed
Salicylates / ↑ Free fraction of MPA
Sirolimus / Mycophenolic acid trough levels may be increased → ↑ risk of side effects; monitor plasma mycophenolic acid levels
Tacrolimus / Mycophenolic acid trough levels may be increased → ↑ risk of side effects; monitor plasma mycophenolic acid levels
Theophylline / ↓ Plasma protein binding of theophylline → ↑ free theophylline levels
Vaccines, life attenuated / Vaccinations may be less effective
Valacyclovir / ↑ Plasma levels of both drugs in those with renal impairment R/T competition for renal tubular excretion

HOW SUPPLIED

Mycophenolate mofetil. *Capsules:* 250 mg; *Powder for Oral Suspension:* 200 mg/mL (reconstituted); *Tablets:* 250 mg, 500 mg.
Mycophenolate mofetil hydrochloride. *Injection, Lyophilized Powder for Solution Concentrate:* 500 mg.
Mycophenolate sodium. *Tablets, Delayed-Release:* 180 mg, 360 mg.

DOSAGE

Mycophenolate mofetil (PO), Mycophenolate mofetil hydrochloride (IV)

CAPSULES; IV; ORAL SUSPENSION; TABLETS

Renal transplantation.

Adults: 1 gram twice a day (a dose of 1.5 grams twice a day is also safe and effective). Give IV dose over 2 hr. **Children, 3 months to 18 years of age:** 600 mg/m^2 twice a day, up to a maximum daily dose of 2 grams/10 mL oral suspension. Those with a body surface area of 1.25–1.5 m^2 may be dosed with mycophenolate capsules, 750 mg twice a day (i.e., 1.5 grams daily dosage). Clients with a body surface area greater than 1.5 m^2 may be dosed with capsules or tablets, 1 gram twice a day (i.e., 2 grams daily dosage).

In clients with severe chronic impaired renal function (GFR <25 mL/min) outside the immediate posttransplant period, avoid doses greater than 1 gram twice a day. No dosage adjustments are needed in renal transplant clients experiencing delayed graft function postoperatively.

Cardiac transplantation.

Adults: 1.5 grams twice a day. Give IV dose over 2 hr or more.

Hepatic transplantation.

1 gram twice a day IV given over 2 hr or 1.5 grams twice a day PO.

Mycophenolate sodium

TABLETS, DELAYED-RELEASE

Renal transplantation.

Adults: 720 mg twice a day (1,440 maximum total daily dose) on an empty stomach, 1 hr before or 2 hr after food. For the elderly, give no more than 720 mg twice daily. **Children:** 400 mg/m^2 twice a day in stable pediatric clients, up to a maximum of 720 mg twice a day. Clients with a body surface area (BSA) of 1.19 to 1.58 m^2 may be dosed with either three 180 mg extended-release tablets or one 180 mg ex-

M

tended-release tablet plus one 360 mg extended-release tablet twice a day. Clients with a BSA of more than 1.58 m^2 may be dosed with either four 180 mg extended-release tablets or two 360 mg extended-release tablets. Pediatric doses for clients with a BSA less than 1.19 m^2 cannot be accurately given the drug using currently available extended-release formulations.

NURSING IMPLICATIONS

IMPLEMENTATION/ADMINISTRATION/STORAGE

1. For PO dosage forms, start therapy as soon as possible following transplantation.
2. Give on an empty stomach as food decreases mycophenolic acid maximum plasma levels. In stable renal transplant clients, may be given with food if necessary.
3. The oral suspension may be given via a nasogastric tube with a minimum size of 8 French catheter.
4. Two 500 mg tablets are bioequivalent to four 250 mg capsules. Five mL of the 200 mg/mL PO suspension are bioequivalent to four 250 mg capsules. Mycophenolate sodium delayed-release tablets and mycophenolate mofetil capsules and tablets are not interchangeable; do not interchange without health care supervision since the rate of absorption following administration of the mofetil and sodium products is not equivalent.
5. Mycophenolate is teratogenic; do not open or crush capsules. Avoid inhalation or direct contact with the skin or mucous membranes; wash area thoroughly with soap and water if contact occurs. Rinse eyes with plain water.
6. Dispense tablets in light-resistant containers, i.e., manufacturer's original container.
7. To prepare oral suspension tap the closed bottle several times to loosen the powder. Measure 94 mL water and add one half the total amount of water to the bottle and shake well for about 1 min. Add the remainder of the water and shake the closed bottle well for about 1 min. Remove child-resistant cap and push the bottle adapter into the neck of bottle. Close bottle with child-resistant cap tightly to ensure proper seating of the bottle adapter and the child-resistant status of the cap.
8. Do not mix the PO suspension with any other medication.
9. If neutropenia develops (ANC $<1.3 \times 10^3$/mcL), interrupt or reduce dose; perform appropriate diagnostic tests and manage appropriately.
10. Store capsules, dry powder for oral suspension, tablets, or delayed-release tablets from 15–30°C (59–86°F). Store constituted suspension from 15–30°C (59–86°F) for up to 60 days; may also be stored from 2–8°C (36–46°F). Do not freeze. Discard any unused portion of the oral suspension 60 days after reconstitution.
11. IV Give IV over 2 or more hours by a peripheral or central vein. Do not give by rapid or IV bolus. IV recommended for those unable to take capsules, oral suspension, or tablets.
12. Begin 24 or fewer hours after transplantation and give for 14 days or fewer; switch to PO mycophenolate as soon as PO medication can be tolerated.
13. Reconstitute for IV administration as follows:
    - Step 1: Two vials of mycophenolate are used for preparing each 1 gram dose, whereas 3 vials are needed for each 1.5 gram dose. Reconstitute the contents of each vial by injecting 14 mL of D5W injection. Gently shake the vial to dissolve the drug. Inspect the resulting slightly yellow solution for particulate matter and discoloration prior to further dilution. Discard if particulate matter or discoloration is observed.
    - Step 2: To prepare a gram dose, further dilute the contents of the 2 reconstituted vials (about 2 × 15 mL) into 140 mL of D5W injection. To prepare a 1.5 gram dose, further dilute the contents of the 3 vials (about 3 × 15 mL) into 210 mL of D5W. The final concentration of both solutions is 6 mg/mL mycophenolate. As with Step 1, inspect for particulate matter or discoloration and discard if any is observed. Use within 4 hr of reconstitution and dilution.
14. Because the drug is teratogenic in animals, use caution in handling and preparing IV solu-

tions. If contact occurs, wash thoroughly with soap and water; rinse eyes with plain water.

15. Store lyophilized powder and infusion solutions from 15–30°C (59–86°F).
16. COMPATIBILITY D5W.
17. INCOMPATIBILITY Do not mix or give with any other IV drugs or infusion admixtures.

ASSESSMENT

1. Note date/type of transplant, other procedures trialed/agents used and outcome. Usually given within 24 hr of transplant.
2. Document negative pregnancy test 1 week prior to initiating therapy in all women of childbearing age.
3. Assess carefully for S&S of infections and organ rejection.
4. Review risk of malignancies/lymphoma and infections R/T ↑ immunosuppression.
5. CellCept Oral Suspension contains aspartame; use caution with phenylketonuria.
6. Obtain CBC weekly during the first month, twice monthly during the second and third months of treatment, then monthly through the first year of therapy.
7. Monitor VS, ECG, renal and LFTs, and hematologic profiles; observe closely for severe neutropenia (day 31 to day 180) posttransplant. If ANC is less than 1.3×10^3/mcL, then drug therapy must be interrupted or decreased. With chronic renal failure monitor those with GFR <25 mL/min for adverse SE.

CLIENT/FAMILY TEACHING

1. Take exactly as directed on an empty stomach twice a day; taken with cyclosporine and steroids. Must take for life to prevent transplant rejection.
2. Do not remove from manufacturer's original container. Do not break/crush, chew, or open capsules as powder may be teratogenic if inhaled or contact with skin/mucous membranes. Wash immediately with soap and water and rinse with plain water if contact occurs.
3. Use caution with activities that require mental alertness until effects realized; may cause drowsiness or dizziness.
4. With increased immunosuppression the susceptibility to infection and the risk of lymphoproliferative disease and other malignancies may be increased. Report any new/unusual side effects or fever/infections. Avoid live vaccines, crowds, and contact with persons with contagious disease or infection. Vaccinations may be less effective.
5. With ↑ risk of skin cancer, limit sun and UV exposure; wear protective clothing and sunscreen.
6. Practice two reliable forms of contraception simultaneously before, during, and for 6 weeks following therapy.
7. Keep all F/U to assess response, labs, and for adverse SE. Need CBC weekly during first month, twice monthly for the second and third months, and then monthly thereafter for the first year.

OUTCOMES/EVALUATE

- Prevention of allogeneic transplant rejection
- Treatment of refractory uveitis; diffuse proliferative lupus nephritis (unlabeled)

N

Nadolol

(**NAY**-doh-lohl)

Classification(s): Beta-adrenergic blocking agent

Pregnancy Category: C

RX: Corgard.

✤ **Rx:** Apo-Nadol.

SEE ALSO ***BETA-ADRENERGIC BLOCKING AGENTS.***

INDICATIONS/USES

(1) Hypertension, either alone or with other drugs (e.g., especially thiazide diuretic). (2) Long-term management of angina pectoris. *Investigational:* Prophylaxis of migraine.

N

ACTION/KINETICS

Action

Manifests both beta-1-/beta-2-adrenergic blocking activity. Has no membrane stabilizing or intrinsic sympathomimetic activity. Low lipid solubility.

Pharmacokinetics

Peak serum concentration: 3–4 hr. **t½:** 20–24 hr (permits once-daily dosage). **Duration:** 17–24 hr. Absorption variable, averaging 30%; steady plasma level achieved after 6–9 days of administration. Excreted unchanged by the kidney.

CONTRAINDICATIONS

Use in bronchial asthma or bronchospasm, including severe COPD.

SPECIAL CONCERNS

■ Exacerbation of ischemic heart disease following abrupt withdrawal. Hypersensitivity to catecholamines has been observed in clients withdrawn from beta-blocker therapy; exacerbation of angina and, in some cases, myocardial infarction, have occurred after abrupt discontinuation of such therapy. When discontinuing chronically administered nadolol, particularly in clients with ischemic heart disease, gradually reduce the dosage over a period of 1 to 2 weeks and carefully monitor the client. If angina markedly worsens or acute coronary insufficiency develops, reinstitute nadolol administration promptly, at least temporarily, and take other measures appropriate for the management of unstable angina. Warn clients against interruption or discontinuation of therapy without the physician's advice. Because coronary artery disease is common and may be unrecognized, it may be prudent not to discontinue nadolol therapy abruptly, even in clients treated only for hypertension. ■

Dosage not established in children.

SIDE EFFECTS

Most Common

Nausea, decreased libido, impotence, insomnia, malaise, anxiety, nervousness.

See *Beta-Adrenergic Blocking Agents* for a complete list of possible side effects.

HOW SUPPLIED

Tablets: 20 mg, 40 mg, 80 mg, 120 mg, 160 mg.

DOSAGE

TABLETS

Hypertension.

Adults, initial: 40 mg once daily whether used alone or with a diuretic; **then,** dose may be increased in 40 to 80 mg increments until optimum response obtained. **Maintenance, usual:** 40–80 mg once daily, although up to 240–320 mg/day may be needed.

Angina.

Adults, initial: 40 mg once daily; **then,** increase dose in 40 to 80 mg increments every 3–7 days until optimum response obtained or there is a pronounced slowing of HR. **Maintenance, usual:** 40–80 mg once daily, although up to 160–240 mg/day may be needed.

Prophylaxis of migraine (investigational).

Adults: 80–240 mg/day for 2–18 months.

NURSING IMPLICATIONS

© Do not confuse Corgard with Coreg (an alpha/beta adrenergic blocking agent).

IMPLEMENTATION/ADMINISTRATION/STORAGE

1. Dosage must be individualized.
2. Adjust dose as follows in clients with renal impairment: If C_{CR} is >50 mL/min/1.73 m^2, use a dosing interval of 24 hr. If C_{CR} is 31-50 mL/min/1.73 m^2, use a dosing interval of 24-36 hr. If C_{CR} is 10-30 mL/min/1.73 m^2, use a dosing interval of 24-48 hr. If C_{CR} is <10 mL/min/1.73 m^2, use a dosing interval of 40-60 hr.
3. If treatment is to be discontinued, reduce the dose gradually over 1-2 weeks.
4. Store tablets from 15-30°C (59-86°F) protected from light and excessive heat. Keep bottle tightly closed.

ASSESSMENT

1. Note reasons for therapy (angina, BP), medical history, characteristics of S&S, other agents trialed.
2. Assess for asthma, CAD, severe COPD. Monitor VS, I&O, weight and for drop in BP with changes in position.

N

3. List baseline VS, electrolytes, uric acid, renal function, and ECG; reduce dose with renal dysfunction.

CLIENT/FAMILY TEACHING

1. May be given without regard to meals; may crush and add to food if swallowing problems.
2. Take only as directed; do not stop abruptly.
3. Report any rapid weight gain, increased SOB, or extremity swelling.
4. Do not perform tasks that require mental alertness until drug effects realized; may cause dizziness/drowsiness. Change positions slowly to prevent sudden drop in BP.
5. May cause increased sensitivity to cold; dress appropriately.
6. Keep log of BP and HR for provider review. Hold dose and report if HR <50 or BP <80, or as directed.
7. To help control BP: maintain healthy diet and limit intake of caffeine, avoid alcohol, salt substitutes, or high Na^+ and high K^+ foods, perform regular exercise, maintain weight, and stop smoking.
8. Report if any major surgery planned; may be withdrawn before procedure to help reduce anesthesia risks.
9. With diabetes may mask S&S of hypoglycemia; monitor BS regularly. Avoid OTC meds without provider approval.
10. Keep all F/U to assess response, VS, labs, and for adverse SE.

OUTCOMES/EVALUATE

- ↓ BP, ↓ HR
- ↓ Frequency/intensity of angina

Nafarelin acetate

(**NAF**-ah-rel-in)

Classification(s): Gonadotropin-releasing hormone

Pregnancy Category: X

RX: Synarel.

INDICATIONS/USES

(1) Endometriosis (including reduction of endometriotic lesions) in clients aged 18 or older (400 mcg/day is clinically comparable to 3.75 mg/month of Lupon Depot). (2) Central precocious puberty in children of both sexes.

ACTION/KINETICS

Action

Produced through biotechnology; differs by only one amino acid from naturally occurring GnRH. Stimulates the release of LH and FSH from the adenohypophysis. Causes estrogen and progesterone synthesis in the ovary, resulting in the maturation and subsequent release of an ovum. With repeated use of the drug, however, the pituitary becomes desensitized and no longer produces endogenous LH and FSH; thus endogenous estrogen is not produced, leading to a regression of endometrial tissue, cessation of menstruation, and a menopausal-like state.

Pharmacokinetics

Broken down by the enzyme peptidase. **Peak serum levels:** 10–40 min. **t½:** 3 hr. **Plasma protein binding:** 80%.

CONTRAINDICATIONS

Hypersensitivity to GnRH or analogs. Abnormal vaginal bleeding of unknown origin. Pregnancy or possibility of becoming pregnant. Lactation.

SPECIAL CONCERNS

- Rule out pregnancy before initiating therapy.
- Safety and efficacy not established in children.

SIDE EFFECTS

Most Common

Hot flashes, decreased libido, vaginal dryness, headaches, emotional lability, acne, myalgia, reduced breast size, nasal irritation.

Due to hypoestrogenic effects: Hot flashes, decreased libido, vaginal dryness, headaches, emotional lability, insomnia. **Due to androgenic effects:** Acne, myalgia, reduced breast size, edema, seborrhea, weight gain, increased libido, hirsutism. **Musculoskeletal:** Decrease in vertebral trabecular bone density and total vertebral bone mass. **Miscellaneous:** Nasal irritation, depression, weight loss.

LABORATORY TEST CONSIDERATIONS

↑ Cholesterol and triglyceride levels, plasma phosphorus, eosinophils. ↓ Serum calcium, WBCs.

HOW SUPPLIED

Nasal Spray: 2 mg/mL (200 mcg/inh).

DOSAGE

NASAL SPRAY

Endometriosis.

200 mcg into one nostril in the morning and 200 mcg into the other nostril at night (400 mcg twice a day may be required for some women).

Central precocious puberty.

400 mcg (2 sprays) into each nostril in the morning (i.e., 4 sprays total) and in the evening (total of 8 sprays/day). If adequate suppression is not achieved, 3 sprays (600 mcg) into alternating nostrils 3 times per day (i.e., a total of 9 sprays/day).

NURSING IMPLICATIONS

IMPLEMENTATION/ADMINISTRATION/STORAGE

1. Initiate therapy between days 2 and 4 of the menstrual cycle.
2. Use longer than 6 months not recommended R/T the lack of safety data.
3. Store at room temperature in an upright position protected from light.

ASSESSMENT

1. Note reasons for therapy. Perform history, noting any osteoporosis, alcohol, tobacco, or corticosteroid use; major risk factors for bone mineral loss that would preclude any repeated courses.
2. With central precocious puberty (CPP) review history and physical exam and ensure complete endocrinologic exam. Obtain labs, pelvic/testicular/adrenal ultrasound and CT/MRI of the head; monitor after 6 weeks and then every 3–6 months during therapy. Monitor bone growth/age velocity during therapy (hand, wrist x-rays, ht and Wt). Stop drug at onset of normal puberty. Assess menstrual cycle, reproductive functioning and final adult height.
3. Note description of menstrual cycles and start between days 2 and 4 of cycle with endometriosis and continue for up to 5 months. Document abdominal/vaginal assessments and ultrasound findings.
4. Assess for sudden headache, vomiting, visual changes, altered mental status, and cardiovascular collapse; S&S of pituitary apoplexy.
5. Determine if pregnant; drug is teratogenic.
6. Obtain testosterone or estradiol levels, adrenal steroid level, GnRH stimulation test, beta human chorionic gonadotropin level.

CLIENT/FAMILY TEACHING

1. With endometriosis, begin treatment between the second and fourth day of the menstrual cycle. Keep accurate records of menstrual patterns and cycles.
2. To use nasal spray, gently blow nose then wash hands. While sitting, tilt head back and place the tip of the spray container into the nose. Using a finger from your other hand, press against the opposite nostril to close it off. Breathe gently through the open nostril and squeeze the spray container. If using more than 1 spray, wait for at least 30 seconds between sprays.
3. After using the medicine, rinse the tip of the spray unit in hot water and dry with a clean tissue to prevent contamination.
4. If a topical nasal decongestant is required during treatment, use 2 hr after nafarelin to prevent interference with drug absorption
5. Menses should cease while on therapy; report if regular menses continues. Breakthrough bleeding may occur if successive doses are missed.
6. Use nonhormonal contraception; drug may cause fetal harm.
7. May cause hypoestrogenic and androgenic side effects; report, as a change in dosage or therapy may be indicated. May experience hot flashes.
8. Signs of puberty may occur during the first month of therapy (vaginal bleeding, breast enlargement); should resolve after the first month. Drug is discontinued when puberty onset is desired.
9. Keep all F/U to assess response, labs, and for adverse SE.

OUTCOMES/EVALUATE

- Restoration of pituitary-gonadal function in 4–8 weeks
- ↓ Number/size of endometriotic lesions
- Inhibition of early puberty

Naloxone hydrochloride

(nal-**OX**-ohn)

IV

Classification(s): Narcotic antagonist

Pregnancy Category: B

RX: Narcan.

SEE ALSO ***NARCOTIC ANTAGONISTS.***

INDICATIONS/USES

(1) Complete or partial reversal of narcotic depression, including respiratory depression induced by natural and synthetic narcotics, methadone, nalbuphine, butorphanol, and pentazocine. Drug of choice when nature of depressant drug is not known. (2) Diagnosis of acute opiate overdosage. Not effective when respiratory depression is induced by hypnotics, sedatives, or anesthetics and other nonnarcotic CNS depressants. *Investigational:* Treatment of Alzheimer's dementia, alcoholic coma, and schizophrenia. Improve circulation in refractory shock.

ACTION/KINETICS

Action

Combines competitively with opiate receptors and blocks or reverses the action of narcotic analgesics. The drug reverses respiratory depression, sedation, and hypotension. Also, naloxone will reverse psychotomimetic and dysphoric effects of agonist-antagonists (e.g., pentazocine). Since the duration of action of naloxone is shorter than that of the narcotic analgesics, the respiratory depression may return when the narcotic antagonist has worn off. In usual doses, has virtually no pharmacologic effects in the absence of opioids. When given to a client with opioid dependence, withdrawal symptoms will appear in minutes and subside in about 2 hr.

Pharmacokinetics

Onset, IV: 2 min; **SC, IM:** <5 min. **Time to peak effect:** 5–15 min. **Duration:** Dependent on dose and route of administration but may be as short as 45 min. **t½, serum:** Average of 64 min in adults and 3.1 hr in neonates. Metabolized in the liver to inactive products; eliminated through the kidneys.

CONTRAINDICATIONS

Sensitivity to drug. Narcotic addicts (drug may cause severe withdrawal symptoms). Use in neonates.

SPECIAL CONCERNS

- If given during labor, may cause severe hypertension in the mother with mild to moderate hypertension.
- Hypotension, hypertension, pulmonary edema, ventricular tachycardia and fibrillation may occur in clients, most often in those who had pre-existing CV disorders or had received other drugs that may have similar adverse CV effects.
- Absorption after IM or SC use in neonates and children may be erratic.
- Administer cautiously to individuals dependent on opiates.
- Use with caution during lactation.

SIDE EFFECTS

Most Common

Virtually no pharmacologic effects in the absence of opioids.

N&V, sweating, hypertension, tremors, sweating due to reversal of narcotic depression. If used postoperatively, excessive doses may cause ***VT and fibrillation***, hypo-/hypertension, pulmonary edema, and ***seizures*** (infrequent).

HOW SUPPLIED

Injection: 0.4 mg/mL, 1 mg/mL.

DOSAGE

IM; IV; SC

Narcotic overdose.

Initial: 0.4–2 mg IV; if necessary, additional IV doses may be repeated at 2- to 3-min intervals. If no response after 10 mg, reevaluate diagnosis. Higher doses may be needed to reverse buprenorphine-induced respiratory depression. **Children, initial:** 0.01 mg/kg IV; **then,** 0.1 mg/kg IV, if needed. The SC or IM route may be used if an IV route is not available.

To reverse postoperative narcotic depression.

Adults, initial, 0.1 to 0.2 mg increments at 2- to 3-min intervals; **then,** repeat at 1- to 2-hr intervals if necessary. Supplemental IM dosage increases the

N

duration of reversal. **Children, initial:** 0.005–0.01 mg IV at 2- to 3-min intervals until desired response is obtained.

Reverse narcotic-induced depression in neonates.

Initial: 0.01 mg/kg IV, IM, or SC. May be repeated using adult administration guidelines.

NURSING IMPLICATIONS

Do not confuse naloxone with naltrexone (also a narcotic antagonist).

IMPLEMENTATION/ADMINISTRATION/STORAGE

1. IV The duration of action of some narcotics may exceed that of naloxone necessitating additional naloxone doses.
2. May administer undiluted at a rate of 0.4 mg over 15 sec with narcotic overdosage. May reconstitute 2 mg in 500 mL of NSS or D5W to provide a 4 mcg/mL (0.004 mg/mL) concentration. Administration rate varies with client response.
3. When mixed with other solutions, use within 24 hr.
4. Not effective against respiratory depression due to nonopioid drugs.
5. Employ other supportive therapy to counteract acute narcotic overdosage (e.g., maintain a free airway, provide artificial respiration, cardiac massage, and vasopressor drugs).
6. COMPATIBILITY D5W, NSS.
7. INCOMPATIBILITY Do not mix with preparations containing bisulfite, metabisulfite, long-chain or high molecular weight anions, or alkaline pH solutions.

ASSESSMENT

1. List type and amount of agent used, duration, half-life, when administered/ingested. Identify opioid addiction.
2. List cardiopulmonary and neurologic assessments.
3. Duration of narcotic may exceed naloxone (the antagonist). Therefore, more than one dose may be necessary to counteract the effects of the narcotic.
4. Monitor VS at 5-min intervals, then every 30 min once stabilized.
5. Titrate to avoid interfering with pain control or readminister narcotic at a lower dosage to maintain pain control.
6. Make appropriate referrals for those requiring substance-abuse counseling.

CLIENT/FAMILY TEACHING

1. Drug works by blocking opiate receptor sites, which reverses or prevents toxic effects of narcotic (opioid) analgesics. Administered by injection in hospital setting.
2. Do not perform activities that require mental alertness until drug effects realized; may cause dizziness, drowsiness.
3. May experience N&V, fever, headaches, chills, pain, dizziness, tachycardia and withdrawal symptoms if narcotic dependent.
4. If return of symptoms (i.e., drowsiness or difficulty breathing) experienced, report immediately.

OUTCOMES/EVALUATE

Reversal of narcotic-induced respiratory depression

Naltrexone

(nal-**TREX**-ohn)

Classification(s): Narcotic antagonist

Pregnancy Category: C

RX: ReVia, Vivitrol.

SEE ALSO ***NARCOTIC ANTAGONISTS***.

INDICATIONS/USES

PO. (1) Blockade of the effects of exogenously given opioids. Has not been shown to produce any therapeutic benefit except as part of an appropriate plan of management for opioid dependence. *NOTE:* Use of naltrexone does not eliminate or diminish the alcohol withdrawal syndrome. (2) Treatment of alcohol dependence. *Investigational:* Treat eating disorders; postconcussional syndrome not responding to other approaches; posttraumatic stress disorder; pruritus; pathological gambling; smoking cessation.

IM. (1) Treatment of alcohol dependence in those who are able to abstain from alcohol in an outpatient setting prior to initiation of naltrexone treatment. Clients should not be actively drinking at the time of beginning naltrexone. Treatment with naltrexone should be part of a comprehensive management program that includes psychosocial support. (2) Prevention of relapse to opioid dependence following opioid detoxification.

ACTION/KINETICS

Action

A pure opioid antagonist that competitively binds to opiate receptors, thereby reversing or preventing the effects of narcotics. Has few, if any, intrinsic effects besides its ability to block opioid receptors. The drug will precipitate withdrawal if given to an individual physically dependent on a narcotic. The blockade to naltrexone is surmountable; attempts by clients to overcome blockade by taking opioids is dangerous and may lead to a fatal overdose. The mechanism in alcoholism is not understood but may involve the endogenous opioid system.

Pharmacokinetics

Following PO administration, absorption is rapid and nearly complete (96% absorbed). **Peak plasma levels:** 1 hr after PO; 2 hr after IM for first peak and 2–3 days for second peak. Significant first-pass metabolism; thus, PO bioavailability ranges from 5–40%. **Duration:** 24–72 hr after PO. Metabolized in the liver; a major metabolite-6-beta-naltrexol-is active. **Peak serum levels, after 50 mg PO: naltrexone,** 8.6 ng/mL; **6-beta-naltrexol,** 99.3 ng/mL. **t½, after PO: naltrexone,** approximately 4 hr; **6-beta-naltrexol,** 13 hr. **t½, terminal, after IM, naltrexone:** 5–10 days; **6-beta-naltrexol:** 5–10 days. Naltrexone and its metabolites are excreted mainly in the urine. Liver disease increases naltrexone AUC. **Plasma protein binding:** About 21%.

CONTRAINDICATIONS

Those taking narcotic analgesics, dependent on narcotics (including those maintained on methadone), in acute withdrawal from narcotics, failed naloxone challenge test, positive urine screen for opioids, or history of hypersensitivity to naltrexone or any component of the product. Liver failure, acute hepatitis. Parenteral product not recommended during lactation.

SPECIAL CONCERNS

(1) **Hepatotoxicity.** Naltrexone has the capacity to cause hepatocellular injury when given in excessive doses. Naltrexone is contraindicated in acute hepatitis or liver failure and its use in clients with active liver disease must be carefully considered in light of its hepatotoxic effects. (2) The margin of separation between the apparently safe dose of naltrexone and the dose causing hepatic injury appears to be only 5-fold or less. Naltrexone does not appear to be a hepatotoxin at the recommended doses. (3) Warn clients of the risk of hepatic injury and advise them to stop the use of naltrexone and seek medical attention if they experience symptoms of acute hepatitis.

- **Use with caution during lactation if used PO.**
- **If using IM, administer with caution to those with thrombocytopenia or any coagulation disorder (e.g., hemophilia, severe hepatic failure).**
- **Use with caution with impaired renal or hepatic function.**
- **Possible unintended precipitation of abstinence syndrome; ensure client is opioid-free for 7–10 days before starting naltrexone.**
- **The risk of suicide is not decreased by treatment with naltrexone.**
- **Safety not established in children under 18 years of age.**

SIDE EFFECTS

Most Common

Naltrexone, in opioid-free individuals, produces almost no side effects. Effects seen are due to narcotic withdrawal.

Side effects listed are for both PO and parenteral use. High doses of naltrexone may produce hepatotoxicity. **Effects due to narcotic withdrawal or alcohol dependence.** A severe narcotic withdrawal syndrome may be precipitated if naltrexone is administered to a dependent individual. The syndrome may begin within 5 min and may last for up to 2 days. **Injection-site reactions:** Pain, tenderness, induration, swelling, erythema, bruising, nodules, pruritus, cellulitis, ecchymosis, hematoma, abscess, sterile abscess, necrosis. **CNS:** Insomnia, difficulty sleeping, anxiety, delirium, disturbance in attention, somnolence, nervousness, "feeling down," irritability, agitation, dizziness, depression, paranoia, fatigue, headache, mental impairment, migraine, paresthesia, restlessness, confusion, euphoria, disorientation, abnormal thinking, hallucinations, nightmares, abnormal/bad dreams, ***convulsions, suicidality (suicidal ideation, suicide attempts, completed suicides)***. **GI:** N&V, abdominal pain/cramps/discomfort, anorexia, diarrhea, colitis, constipation, dry mouth, dysgeusia, increased thirst, excessive gas, flatulence, gastroenteritis, GERD, ***GI hemor-***

rhage, hemorrhoids, ***acute pancreatitis***, ulcer, paralytic ileus, perirectal abscess, toothache. **Hepatic:** Hepatitis, hepatotoxicity, acute cholecystitis, cholelithiasis. **Musculoskeletal:** Joint/muscle pain, painful shoulders/legs/knees, tremors, twitching, chest pain/tightness, hyperkinesia, myalgia, arthralgia, arthritis, joint stiffness, back pain/stiffness, muscle cramps/spasms, pain in limb. **CV:** Nosebleeds, phlebitis, edema, hypertension, BP changes, nonspecific ECG changes, palpitations, tachycardia, angina pectoris, atrial fibrillation, CHF, coronary artery atherosclerosis, ***cerebral artery aneurysm***, ***DVT***, ischemic stroke, ***MI***, ***pulmonary embolism***, unstable angina. **Respiratory:** Nasal congestion, itching, rhinorrhea, sneezing, sore throat, excess mucus/phlegm, sinus trouble, heavy breathing, hoarseness, cough, shortness of breath, dyspnea, eosinophilic pneumonia, pharyngitis, nasopharyngitis, bronchitis, COPD, laryngitis, pharyngolaryngeal pain, pneumonia, sinusitis, sinus congestion, URTI. **GU:** Delayed ejaculation, increased frequency of or discomfort during urination, increased/decreased libido, inguinal pain, missed abortion, UTI. **Dermatologic:** Skin rash, oily skin, pruritus, acne, athlete's foot, cold sores, alopecias, hot flashes, increased sweating, night sweats. **Hematologic:** Lymphadenopathy (including cervical adenitis). **Hypersensitivity:** Urticaria, angioedema, angioneurotic edema, ***anaphylaxis***. **Ophthalmic:** Blurred vision, burning, light sensitivity, swollen/aching/strained eyes, conjunctivitis, retinal artery occlusion. **Otic:** Aching/clogged ears, tinnitus. **Body as a whole:** Low or high energy, chills, fever, rigors, swollen glands, asthenia, lethargy, malaise, tremor, increased sweating, influenza, dehydration, heat exhaustion. **Miscellaneous:** Increased/decreased appetite, anorexia, weight loss/gain, yawning, head "pounding," cold feet, "hot spells," side pains, facial edema, advanced HIV disease in HIV-infected clients. *NOTE:* Death has resulted from ultra rapid opiate detoxification.

LABORATORY TEST CONSIDERATIONS

↑ Eosinophil counts (returned to normal over several months), WBCs. ↑ AST, ALT, CPK, GGT, bilitrubin. ↓ Platelet count. Abnormal hepatic function. Hypercholesterolemia.

DRUG INTERACTIONS

Opioid analgesics / ↓ Or attenuated analgesic effect → a severe opioid withdrawal syndrome; do not coadminister naltrexone with opioid analgesics

Opioid-containing products (e.g., cough/cold, antidiarrheals, opioid analgesics) / No beneficial effect may be obtained due to blockade of opioid effect by naltrexone; amount of opioid required may be greater than usual; the resulting respiratory depression may be deeper and more prolonged.

Thioridazine / Possible lethargy and somnolence

HOW SUPPLIED

Suspension for Injection, Extended-Release: 380 mg/vial; *Tablets:* 50 mg.

DOSAGE

TABLETS

Opiate dependence: Blockade of opiate actions.

Adults, initial: 25 mg; if no withdrawal signs occur after initiation of therapy, the client may be started on 50 mg/day thereafter. **Alternate dosing schedule:** The weekly dose of 350 mg may be given as: (a) 50 mg/day on weekdays and 100 mg on Saturday; (b) 100 mg q other day; or (c) 150 mg q third day. *NOTE:* The degree of blockade may be reduced by using extended dosing intervals. Also, there may be a higher risk of hepatocellular injury with single doses above 50 mg.

Alcohol dependence.

Adults: 50 mg once daily for up to 12 weeks. Treatment for longer than 12 weeks has not been studied. **Alternative dosage:** See information under *Opioid dependence.*

IM

Alcohol dependence, Opioid dependence.

Adults: 380 mg IM q 4 weeks or once a month.

NURSING IMPLICATIONS

Do not confuse naltrexone and naloxone (another narcotic antagonist).

IMPLEMENTATION/ADMINISTRATION/STORAGE

1. ***Never*** **initiate therapy until determined that client is not dependent on narcotics (i.e., naloxone challenge test should be negative).**

2. A candidate for treatment for alcohol dependence should meet the following:
   - Be willing to take the drug to help with alcohol dependence;
   - Is opioid free for 7–10 days;
   - Does not have severe or active liver or kidney problems (i.e., LFTs no greater than 3 times ULN and bilirubin normal);
   - Is not allergic to naltrexone; and,
   - No other contraindications are present.
3. A candidate for treatment for opiate dependence should meet the following:
   - Must be opiate free for at least 7–10 days before beginning therapy;
   - Verify self-reporting of abstinence by analysis of the client's urine for absence of opioids;
   - No manifestations of withdrawal signs or reporting of withdrawal symptoms;
   - Perform a naloxone challenge test if there is any question of occult opioid dependence. If signs of opioid withdrawal are observed following naloxone challenge, do not attempt treatment with naltrexone. The naloxone challenge can be repeated in 24 hr.
4. Use the following procedure for the naloxone challenge test:
   - Do not undertake in a client showing signs or symptoms of opioid withdrawal or in someone whose urine contains opioids.
   - Administer the test either by IV or SC routes.
   - Individual clients, especially those who are opioid dependent, may respond to lower naloxone doses.
   - If using the IV route, give 0.2 mg naloxone; observe for 30 seconds for signs and symptoms of withdrawal. If no evidence of withdrawal is observed, inject 0.6 mg naloxone and observe for an additional 20 min. In some cases, 0.1 mg naloxone has produced a response.
   - If using the SC route, inject 0.8 mg naloxone; observe for 20 min for signs and symptoms of withdrawal.
   - If signs or symptoms of withdrawal appear, the test is positive; no additional naloxone should be given and do not initiate naltrexone therapy. Repeat the challenge in 24 hr.
   - If the test is negative, naltrexone therapy may be started if no other contraindications are present. If there is any doubt about the naloxone challenge test, hold naltrexone and repeat the challenge in 24 hr.
5. Due to its hepatotoxic effects, carefully consider use of naltrexone in clients with active liver disease.
6. The blockade produced by naltrexone may be overcome by taking large doses of narcotics; such doses may be fatal.
7. Clients taking naltrexone may not respond to preparations containing narcotics for use in coughs, diarrhea, or pain.
8. When used parenterally, give as a deep IM gluteal injection, alternating buttocks, using the components provided. Do not give IV.
9. If an IM dose is missed, give as soon as possible. Pretreatment with PO naltrexone is not required before using parenteral naltrexone.
10. To prepare the IM injection, allow the drug to reach room temperature (about 45 min). Suspend only in the diluent provided in the carton; give only with the needle supplied. All components (i.e., microspheres, diluent, preparation needle, and administration needle) are required for administration. Do not substitute any other components.
11. Inspect the product for particulate matter and discoloration prior to administration. A properly mixed suspension will be milky white, will not contain clumps, and will move freely down the wall of the vial.
12. Store the entire IM dose pack from 2–8°C (36–46°F). Unrefrigerated, can be stored for no more than 7 days at temperatures not exceeding 25°C (77°F). Do not freeze. Store tablets from 20–25°C (68–77°F).

ASSESSMENT

1. Note if opiate addicted and when last dose was ingested; must be opiate free for 7–10 days before initiating therapy. Check urine to confirm absence of opiates; note naloxone challenge test results.
2. Report if respirations severely lowered or client has difficulty breathing.
3. A nonopioid analgesic should be used when analgesia is necessary. Consider alternative maintenance plan for those with compliance problems.

4. Follow administration guidelines carefully. Vivitrol should be mixed with diluent just prior to administration and will appear milky white. Use only provided diluent and needles. If the needle clogs during injection, remove from site. Apply the supplied needle and readminister in an adjacent site.
5. Monitor for the development of depression or suicidal thinking and report if evident.
6. Review risks of therapy and caution against any client attempts to overcome opioid block as dose required may be lethal.
7. Assess for hepatitis; monitor ECG and VS. Obtain renal and LFTs; monitor monthly during the first 6 months of therapy and use cautiously with any dysfunction.

CLIENT/FAMILY TEACHING

1. This drug blocks the effects of narcotics and opiates. It also may help to prevent alcohol consumption. Taking an opiate with this therapy may prove fatal as the amount needed to overcome the blockade is quite high.
2. May take with food or milk to diminish GI upset. Request list of nonopiod drugs that may be used for pain, cough, or diarrhea.
3. Headaches, restlessness, and irritability may be caused by naltrexone.
4. Report loss of appetite, unusual fatigue, yellowing of skin or sclera, or itching. Abdominal pain or difficulty with bowel function may warrant a dosage reduction.
5. Injectable Vivitrol appears milky white when mixed. Will be administered in clinic once monthly into buttocks. Report any injection site reactions or changes.
6. May cause allergic pneumonia; report any S&S of shortness of breath, coughing, wheezing.
7. Get medical attention for worsening skin reactions, especially if reaction does not improve 1 month after injection.
8. Remain drug/alcohol free; identify individuals, agencies, and support groups that may assist you in remaining drug free. Attend support groups and behavioral therapy sessions.
9. Report any increased depression or suicide thoughts immediately.
10. Always carry/wear medical ID to alert medical personnel that you take naltrexone.
11. Keep all F/U to assess response, labs, and for adverse SE.

OUTCOMES/EVALUATE

- Maintenance of narcotic-free state in detoxified addicts
- Successful alcohol abstinence in outpatients

Naproxen

(nah-**PROX**-en)

Classification(s): Nonsteroidal anti-inflammatory drug

Pregnancy Category: B

RX: EC-Naprosyn, Naprosyn.

Rx: Apo-Naproxen, Apo-Naproxen EC, Apo-Naproxen SR, Gen-Naproxen EC, Novo-Naprox, Novo-Naprox EC, Nu-Naprox.

Naproxen sodium

Pregnancy Category: B

OTC: Aleve, Midol Extended Relief.

RX: Anaprox, Anaprox DS, Naprelan.

Rx: Apo-Napro-Na, Apo-Napro-Na DS, Novo-Naprox Sodium, Novo-Naprox Sodium DS, Novo-Naprox SR.

SEE ALSO ***NONSTEROIDAL ANTI-INFLAMMATORY DRUGS***.

INDICATIONS/USES

Rx. (1) Mild to moderate pain. (2) Treatment of rheumatoid arthritis, osteoarthritis, ankylosing spondylitis. (3) Juvenile rheumatoid arthritis. Use of the suspension is recommended in order to obtain the maximum dosage flexibility based on client weight. (4) Treatment of bursitis, tendonitis. (5) Primary dysmenorrhea. (6) Acute gout. *NOTE:* The delayed-release or enteric-coated products are not recommended for initial treatment of pain because, compared to other naproxen products, absorption is delayed. *Investigational:* Analgesia in children.

OTC. (1) Relief of minor aches and pains due to the common cold, headache, toothache, muscular aches, backache, minor arthritis pain, pain due to menstrual cramps. (2) Antipyretic.

ACTION/KINETICS

Action

Anti-inflammatory effect is likely due to inhibition of cyclo-oxygenase. Inhibition of cyclo-oxygenase results in decreased prostaglandin synthesis. Effective in reducing joint swelling, pain, and morning stiffness, as well as to increase mobility in those with inflammatory disease. Does not alter the course of the disease, however. The antipyretic action occurs by decreasing prostaglandin synthesis in the hypothalamus resulting in an increase in peripheral blood flow and heat loss, as well as promoting sweating.

Pharmacokinetics

The various dosage forms have different pharmacokinetic properties that may affect onset of action. 95% is bioavailable. **Peak serum levels of naproxen:** 2–4 hr; **for sodium salt:** 1–2 hr. **t½ for naproxen:** 12–15 hr; **for sodium salt:** 12–13 hr. **Onset, immediate release for analgesia:** 1–2 hr. **Duration, analgesia:** Approximately 7 hr. **Onset (both immediate and delayed release):** 30 min; **duration:** 24 hr. **Onset, anti-inflammatory effects:** Up to 2 weeks; **duration:** 2–4 weeks. Food delays the rate but not the amount of drug absorbed. 95% excreted in the urine. **Plasma protein binding:** More than 99%.

CONTRAINDICATIONS

Simultaneous use of naproxen and naproxen sodium. Lactation. Use of delayed-release product for initial treatment of acute pain.

SPECIAL CONCERNS

(1) **Cardiovascular risk.** NSAIDs may cause an increased risk of serious CV thrombotic events, MI, and stroke, which can be fatal. This risk may increase with duration of use. Clients with CV disease or risk factors for CV disease may be at a greater risk. (2) Naproxen (except for controlled-released tablets) is contraindicated for treatment of perioperative pain in the setting of coronary artery bypass graft surgery. (3) **Gastrointestinal risk.** NSAIDs cause an increased risk of serious GI adverse events including bleeding, ulceration, and perforation of the stomach or intestines, which can be fatal. These events can occur at any time during use and without warning symptoms. Elderly clients are at greater risk for serious GI events.

- Safety and efficacy of naproxen not determined in children less than 2 years of age; the safety and efficacy of naproxen sodium not established in children.
- Geriatric clients may manifest increased total plasma levels of naproxen.
- Higher doses and use in those at risk of developing Alzheimer's disease may increase the risk of strokes and heart attacks.

SIDE EFFECTS

Most Common

Headache, dizziness, drowsiness, pruritus, skin eruptions, constipation, dyspepsia/indigestion, ecchymoses, edema, dyspnea, tinnitus.

See *Nonsteroidal Anti-Inflammatory Drugs* for a complete list of possible side effects.

LABORATORY TEST CONSIDERATIONS

Naproxen may increase urinary 17-ketosteroid values. Both forms may interfere with urinary assays for 5-HIAA.

DRUG INTERACTIONS

Alendronate / ↑ Risk of gastric ulcers
Methotrexate / Possibility of a fatal interaction
Probenecid / ↓ Plasma clearance of naproxen

HOW SUPPLIED

Naproxen (all Rx). *Oral Suspension:* 125 mg/mL; *Tablets:* 250 mg, 375 mg, 500 mg; *Tablets, Delayed-Release:* 375 mg, 500 mg.
Naproxen Sodium. *Capsules, Gelcaps:* **OTC:** 220 mg; *Tablets:* **OTC:** 220 mg; **Rx:** 275 mg, 550 mg; *Tablets, Controlled-Release:* **Rx:** 412.5 mg, 550 mg, 825 mg.

DOSAGE

Naproxen, Naproxen Sodium

RX: NAPROXEN ORAL SUSPENSION; NAPROXEN TABLETS; NAPROXEN SODIUM TABLETS; NAPROXEN DELAYED-RELEASE TABLETS; NAPROXEN SODIUM CONTROLLED-RELEASE TABLETS

Management of pain.

Naproxen Sodium Tablets, initial: 550 mg, not to exceed 1,275 mg; thereafter do not exceed a daily dose of 1,100 mg. **Usual:** 550 mg q 12 hr or 275 mg q 6–8 hr as required.

Rheumatoid arthritis, osteoarthritis, anklyosing spondylitis.

Naproxen Suspension/Tablets.
Adults: 250–500 mg twice a day. **Na-**

proxen Sodium Tablets. Adults: 275–550 mg twice a day. **Naproxen Controlled-Release/Delayed-Release Tablets. Adults:** 375 mg or 500 mg twice a day. For long-term use, the dose may be adjusted up or down depending on the clinical response. In those who tolerate lower doses well, the dose may be increased to 1,500 mg/day when a higher anti-inflammatory effect/analgesic is needed. The morning and evening doses do not have to be the same size. Giving the drug more frequently than twice a day does not generally make a difference in the response.

Juvenile rheumatoid arthritis.

Naproxen Suspension. Usual: 10 mg/kg/day in two divided doses. The following dosage of the suspension can be used: **13 kg (29 lb):** 62.5 mg twice a day given as 2.5 mL twice a day; **25 kg (55 lb):** 125 mg twice a day given as 5 mL twice a day; **38 kg (84 lb):** 187.5 mg twice a day given as 7.5 mL twice a day. **Maximum dose:** 15 mg/kg/day.

Bursitis, acute tendonitis, primary dysmenorrhea.

Naproxen Sodium Tablets. Adults, initial: 550 mg; **then,** 550 mg q 12 hr or 275 mg q 6–8 hr as needed. Do not exceed an initial daily dose of 1,375 mg of naproxen sodium; thereafter, do not exceed a total daily dose of 1,100 of naproxen sodium.

Acute gout.

Naproxen Tablets. Adults, initial: 750 mg; **then,** 250 mg q 8 hr until symptoms subside. **Naproxen Sodium Tablets. Adults, initial:** 825 mg; **then,** 275 mg q 8 hr until symptoms subside.

Analgesia in children (investigational).

Children, 2 years and older: 5–7 mg/kg per dose q 8–12 hr.

OTC: CAPSULES, GELCAPS; TABLETS

Analgesic, antipyretic.

Adults: 220 mg q 8–12 hr with a full glass of liquid. For some clients, 440 mg initially followed by 220 mg 12 hr later will provide better relief. Do not exceed 660 mg in a 24-hr period. Do not exceed 220 mg q 12 hr for geriatric clients. Not for use in children less than 12 years of age unless directed by provider.

NURSING IMPLICATIONS

IMPLEMENTATION/ADMINISTRATION/STORAGE

1. Do not use naproxen delayed-release tablets for initial treatment of acute pain because absorption is delayed compared with other naproxen-containing products.
2. Use lower doses in the elderly and in those with hepatic or renal impairment.
3. To be taken in the morning and in the evening. The doses do not have to be equal.
4. Do not give to children under age 2.
5. Do not use the OTC product for more than 10 days for pain or 3 days for fever unless prescribed.
6. Store all products from 15–30°C (59–86°F) in well-closed containers. Avoid excessive heat.

ASSESSMENT

1. List reasons for therapy, onset, characteristics of S&S. Rate pain level using a pain-rating scale. Note any joint swelling, pain, trauma, inflammation, or decreased ROM.
2. Assess for allergy history, GI bleeding, or ulcer history; use GI protectant if needed. Enteric-coated product (EC-Naprosyn) reduces GI side effects.
3. Determine history of heart disease or cardiac failure.
4. This class of drugs has been associated with increased risk of heart attacks/stroke (those with CV disease or risk factors for CV disease may be at higher risk); monitor for S&S and advise client as risk may increase with length of therapy.
5. Monitor for GI bleeding, ulceration, and perforation of the stomach or intestines, which can be fatal. Elderly clients are at higher risk for serious GI events.
6. Monitor CBC, renal and LFTs, with chronic therapy.

CLIENT/FAMILY TEACHING

1. Take with food and a full glass of water to ↓ GI upset; take in the morning and evening for

N

optimal effects. Do not break, chew, or crush delayed-release tablets.
2. May cause dizziness or drowsiness; avoid activities that require mental alertness until effects realized.
3. Report lack of response, worsening of symptoms, unusual bruising/bleeding, persistent abdominal pain, fatigue, lethargy, itching, jaundice, right upper quadrant tenderness, sore throat, fever, rash, altered vision, joint pain/swelling, or dark-colored stools. May need periodic eye exams with prolonged therapy.
4. Desired response may take 2 to 4 weeks with naproxen and 1 to 2 days with naproxen sodium (Aleve) for anti-inflammatory effects.
5. Avoid alcohol, aspirin, corticosteroids and all other OTC agents without approval.
6. NSAIDs have been associated with serious, possibly fatal, heart and blood vessel risks such as heart attack and stroke.
7. Keep all F/U to assess response, labs, and for adverse SE.

OUTCOMES/EVALUATE

- Improved joint pain and mobility
- Relief of headaches/pain
- ↓ Uterine cramping
- Relief of sunburn, migraine, PMS (unlabeled use)

Naratriptan hydrochloride

(**NAR**-ah-trip-tan)

Classification(s): Antimigraine drug
Pregnancy Category: C
RX: Amerge.

INDICATIONS/USES

Acute treatment of migraine attacks in adults with or without aura.

ACTION/KINETICS

Action

Binds to serotonin 5-HT_{1D} receptors. Activation of these receptors located on intracranial blood vessels, including those on arteriovenous anastomoses, leads to vasoconstriction and thus relief of migraine. Also possible that activation of these receptors on sensory nerve endings in trigeminal system causes inhibition of pro-inflammatory neuropeptide release.

Pharmacokinetics

Well absorbed from GI tract. Bioavailability is 74%. **Time to onset:** 1 hr. **Time to peak effect:** 2–3 hr. Unchanged drug and metabolites are primarily eliminated in urine. **t½:** 5.5 hr. Excretion is decreased in moderate liver or renal impairment. **Plasma protein binding:** About 28%.

CONTRAINDICATIONS

Use for prophylaxis of migraine, for management of hemiplegic or basilar migraine, in those with ischemic bowel disease. Use in clients with ischemic cardiac, cerebrovascular, or peripheral vascular syndromes; coronary artery vasospasm, uncontrolled hypertension. Use in severe renal impairment (C_{CR} less than 15 mL/min); severe hepatic impairment (Child-Pugh grade C); within 24 hr of treatment with another 5-HT_1 agonist, dihydroergotamine, or methysergide. Concurrent use with a MAOI or within 2 weeks of discontinuing a MAOI.

SPECIAL CONCERNS

- Safety and efficacy not determined for use in cluster headaches (usually in older males) or for use in children.
- Use with caution during lactation and with diseases that may alter the absorption, metabolism, or excretion of drugs, such as impaired renal or hepatic function.

SIDE EFFECTS

Most Common

Paresthesia, dizziness, drowsiness, malaise, fatigue, nausea, throat and neck symptoms, pain and pressure sensation.

Side effects that occurred in 0.1% to 1% of clients. GI: Hyposalivation, vomiting, dyspeptic symptoms, diarrhea, GI discomfort and pain, gastroenteritis, constipation. **CNS:** Vertigo, tremors, cognitive function disorders, sleep disorders, disorders of equilibrium, anxiety, depression, detachment. **CV:** Palpitations, increased BP, tachyarrhythmias, syncope, abnormal ECG (PR prolongation, QTc prolongation, ST/T wave abnormalities, premature ventricular contractions, atrial flutter, or atrial fibrillation). **Musculoskeletal:** Muscle pain, arthralgia, articular rheumatism, muscle cramps and spasms, joint and muscle stiffness, tightness, and rigidity. **Dermatologic:**

N

Sweating, skin rashes, pruritus, urticaria. **GU:** Bladder inflammation, polyuria, diuresis. **Body as a whole:** Chills, fever, descriptions of odor or taste, edema and swelling, allergies, allergic reactions, warm/cold temperature sensations, feeling strange, burning/stinging sensation. **Respiratory:** Bronchitis, cough, pneumonia. **Ophthalmic:** Photophobia, blurred vision. **ENT:** Ear, nose, and throat infections; phonophobia, sinusitis, upper respiratory inflammation, tinnitus. **Endocrine/Metabolic:** Thirst, polydipsia, dehydration, fluid retention. **Hematologic:** Increased WBCs.

OVERDOSE MANAGEMENT

Symptoms: Increased BP, chest pain. *Treatment:* Standard supportive treatment. Possible use of antihypertensive therapy. Monitor ECG if chest pain presents.

DRUG INTERACTIONS

Dihydroergotamine / Prolonged vasospastic reaction; effects additive
Methysergide / Prolonged vasospastic reaction; effects additive
Oral contraceptives / ↑ Mean plasma levels of naratriptan
SSRIs / Possible weakness, hyperreflexia, and incoordination
Serotonin 5-HT_1 agonists / Additive effects
Sibutramine / Possible serotonin syndrome, including CNS irritability, motor weakness, shivering, myoclonus, and altered consciousness

HOW SUPPLIED

Tablets: 1 mg, 2.5 mg.

DOSAGE

TABLETS

Acute treatment of migraine headaches with/without aura.

Adults: Single doses of 1 mg or 2.5 mg taken with fluid. If headache returns or client has had only partial response, dose may be repeated once after 4 hr, for maximum of 5 mg in a 24-hr period. Doses of 5 mg/24 hr do not provide greater relief than 2.5 mg/24 hr.

NURSING IMPLICATIONS

IMPLEMENTATION/ADMINISTRATION/STORAGE

1. A dose of 2.5 mg is usually more effective than 1 mg but causes more side effects. Choice of dose made on individual basis, weighing possible benefit of 2.5-mg dose with greater risk for side effects.
2. Safety of treating, on average, more than four headaches in 30-day period has not been established.
3. In clients with mild-to-moderate renal or hepatic impairment, do not exceed a dose of 2.5 mg over a 24-hr period. Consider lower starting dose.
4. Store medication at controlled room temperature away from light.

ASSESSMENT

1. *Note onset, frequency, duration, characteristics of migraines and any symptoms associated with migraines. If not clear, assess for neuro documentation of migraine: drug is not intended for preventing migraines or treating basilar migraines, cluster or hemiplegic headaches.*
2. List all drugs consumed to ensure none interact.
3. Assess baseline cardiac function. Drug may cause coronary vasospasm, elevated BP; avoid with CAD, risk factors for CAD, HTN, arrhythmias.
4. Monitor BP, ECG, renal and LFTs; assess for dysfunction/dosage adjustment. In mild to moderate renal or hepatic impairment, do not exceed a dose of 2.5 mg over a 24-hr period. Consider lower initial dose.

CLIENT/FAMILY TEACHING

1. Take as soon as symptoms of migraine appear. Will not reduce or prevent number of attacks experienced.
2. Use caution while driving or performing activities requiring mental alertness; may cause fatigue/dizziness.
3. Review package insert; do not use with other similar headache medications. May repeat once after 4 hr if headache returns or if only partial response attained. Do not exceed 5 mg/24 hr.
4. Report any unusual side effects including chest pain, SOB, palpitations, lack of response. Practice reliable contraception.
5. Avoid prolonged sun exposure or tanning lamps; use sunscreen/protective clothing to avoid photosensitivity reactions.
6. Report if pregnancy suspected; use reliable contraceptive.

N

7. **Avoid alcohol (causes vasodilation)—may aggravate migraine.**
8. **Attempt to identify migraine triggers. Keep a headache diary (identifying factors surrounding each headache) for provider review. Continue other remedies (i.e., noise reduction, reduced lighting, bed rest) that assist to control S&S.**
9. **Keep all F/U to assess response and for adverse SE.**

OUTCOMES/EVALUATE
Relief of migraine headache

IV

Natalizumab

(na-ta-**LIZ**-u-mab)

Classification(s): Immunomodulator

Pregnancy Category: C

RX: Tysabri.

INDICATIONS/USES

(1) As monotherapy in adults to treat relapsing forms of multiple sclerosis to delay the accumulation of physical disability and reduce the frequency of clinical exacerbations. (2) Treatment of adults with moderate to severe active Crohn's disease with evidence of inflammation who have had an inadequate response to, or are unable to tolerate, conventional Crohn's disease therapies and inhibitors of tumor necrosis factor alpha.

NOTE: Natalizumab is on a special restricted distribution program due to possible progressive multifocal leukoencephalopathy.

ACTION/KINETICS

Action

Natalizumab is a recombinant, humanized $IgG4_{k}$ monoclonal antibody. The specific mechanism for its effects in multiple sclerosis are not known. However, the effect may be secondary to blockade of the molecular interaction of $\alpha 4\beta 1$-integrin expressed by inflammatory cells on vascular endothelial cells and with CS-1 and/or osteopontin expressed by parenchymal cells in the brain. The drug increases the number of circulating leukocytes due to inhibition of transmigration out of the vascular space; it does not affect the number of circulating neutrophils.

Pharmacokinetics

Maximum serum level, after repeated IV administration of 300 mg: 110 mcg/mL in those with multiple sclerosis and 101 mcg/mL in those with Crohn's disease. **Time to steady state:** 16 to 24 weeks. **t½:** About 10–11 days.

CONTRAINDICATIONS

Hypersensitivity to the drug or any of its components. History of or currently has progressive multifocal leukoencephalopathy. Use with other MS medications or in combination with immunosuppressants (e.g., azathioprine, cyclosporine, methotrexate, 6-mercaptopurine) or inhibitors of tumor necrosis factor alpha. Lactation. Use in children.

SPECIAL CONCERNS

(1) **Progressive multifocal leukoencephalopathy (PML).** Natalizumab increases the risk of progressive multifocal leukoencephalopathy, an opportunistic viral infection of the brain that usually leads to death or severe disability. Cases of PML have been reported in clients taking natalizumab who were recently or concomitantly treated with immunomodulators or immunosuppressants, as well as in clients receiving natalizumab as monotherapy. (2) Because of the risk of PML, natalizumab is available only through a special restricted distribution program called the TOUCH prescribing program. Under the TOUCH prescribing program, only prescribers, infusion centers, and pharmacies associated with infusion centers registered with the program are able to prescribe, distribute, or infuse the product. In addition, natalizumab must be administered only to clients who are enrolled in and meet all the conditions of the TOUCH prescribing program. (3) Monitor clients on natalizumab for any new sign or symptom that may be suggestive of PML. Withhold natalizumab dosing immediately at the first sign or symptom suggestive of PML. For diagnosis, and evaluation that includes a gadolinium-enhanced magnetic resonance imaging scan of the brain and, when indicated, cerebrospinal fluid analysis for John Cunningham viral DNA are recommended.

- **Safety and efficacy not established in those with chronic, progressive multiple sclerosis; in combi-**

N

nation with other immunosuppressive agents; or in children less than 18 years of age.

- **Use of live vaccines during natalizumab administration may reduce vaccine effectiveness. Defer live vaccines until immune function has improved. Immune globulin or inactivated vaccine may be effective immunization alternatives.**

SIDE EFFECTS

Most Common

Headache, fatigue, UTI, depression, upper/lower respiratory tract infection, joint pain, abdominal discomfort, diarrhea, gastroenteritis, arthralgia, vaginitis, pain in extremities, nausea, vaginitis.

Hypersensitivity reactions: Urticaria, dizziness, fever, rash, rigors, pruritus, nausea, flushing, hypotension, dyspnea, chest pain, ***anaphylaxis/anaphylactoid reaction.*** **Infusion-related reactions:** Headache, dizziness, fatigue, hypersensitivity, urticaria, pruritus, rigors. **GI:** Cholelithiasis, abdominal discomfort, diarrhea, constipation, dyspepsia, flatulence, nausea, gastroenteritis, liver injury, abnormal LFTs, jaundice, tooth infections, intestinal obstruction/stenosis, abdominal adhesions, aphthous stomatitis, lower abdominal pain. **CNS:** Depression, including ***suicidal ideation/attempt;*** headache, somnolence, vertigo, tremor, ***progressive multifocal leukoencephalopathy***. **Respiratory:** Lower/upper respiratory tract infection, pneumonia, tonsillitis, cough, pharyngolaryngeal pain, sinusitis, nasopharyngitis. **Musculoskeletal:** Pain in extremities, arthralgia, joint swelling, limb injury, muscle cramps, back pain. **GU:** UTI, vaginitis, vaginal infections, urinary urgency/frequency, urinary incontinence, irregular menstruation, amenorrhea, dysmenorrhea, ovarian cyst. **Dermatologic:** Rash, dermatitis, pruritus, night sweats, skin laceration, thermal burn, dry skin. **Body as a whole:** Pneumonia, fatigue, rigors, syncope, weight increased/decreased, presence of anti-natalizumab antibodies, increased risk of infections, immunosuppression, immunogenicity, seasonal allergy, flu-like illness, peripheral edema. **Miscellaneous:** Chest discomfort, local bleeding, herpes infection, viral infection, opportunistic infections.

LABORATORY TEST CONSIDERATIONS

↑ ALT, AST, total bilirubin. ↑ Circulating lymphocytes, monocytes, eosinophils, basophils, and nucleated RBCs; increases are reversible and return to baseline levels within 16 weeks after the last dose. Mild ↓ hemoglobin (often transient).

DRUG INTERACTIONS

Antineoplastic agents / ↑ Risk of infection
Corticosteroids / ↑ Risk of infection in clients with Crohn's disease
Immunomodulating agents (e.g., peginterferon alfa–2a) / Potential for increased risk of progressive multifocal leukoencephalopathy; do not use immunosuppressants in clients with Crohn's disease receiving natalizumab
Immunosuppressants (e.g., azathioprine, cyclosporine, 6-mercaptopurine, methotrexate) / ↑ Risk of progressive multifocal leukoencephalopathy; do not use together
Interferon beta-1a / ↓ Natalizumab clearance by about 30%
Tissue necrosis factor alpha inhibitors (e.g., adalimumab, etanercept, golimumab, infliximab) / ↑ Risk of progressive multifocal leukoencephalopathy; do not use together

HOW SUPPLIED

Injection Solution, Concentrate: 300 mg/15 mL (20 mg/mL).

DOSAGE

IV INFUSION

Relapsing multiple sclerosis.

Adults: 300 mg infused over 1 hr q 4 weeks. **Maximum dose:** 300 mg q 4 weeks.

Crohn's disease in adults.

Adults: 300 mg over 1 hr q 4 weeks. If no therapeutic benefit occurs by 12 weeks of induction therapy, discontinue natalizumab. For those with Crohn's disease who start natalizumab while on chronic PO corticosteroids, begin steroid tapering as soon as a therapeutic benefit of natalizumab occurs. If the Crohn's disease client cannot be tapered off PO corticosteroids within 6 months of starting natalizumab, discontinue natalizumab. Other than the initial 6-month taper, consider discontinuing natalizumab for those who require additional steroid use that exceeds 3 months in a calendar year to control their Crohn's disease. *NOTE:* Do not use natalizumab with concomitant immunosuppressants (e.g., azathioprine, cyclosporine, methotrexate, 6-mercaptopu-

N

rine) or concomitant TNF-alpha inhibitors. Aminosalicylates may be continued during natalizumab treatment.

NURSING IMPLICATIONS

IMPLEMENTATION/ADMINISTRATION/STORAGE

1. IV Only prescribers registered in the TOUCH prescribing program may prescribe natalizumab for multiple sclerosis or Crohn's disease. To enroll in the TOUCH program, call 1-800-456-2255.
2. To prepare the infusion, withdraw 15 mL of natalizumab concentrate from the vial using a sterile needle and syringe. Inject the concentrate into 100 mL of 0.9% NaCl injection. The final dosage solution has a concentration of 2.6 mg/mL. No other IV diluents may be used to prepare the infusion. Invert solution gently to mix, do not shake.
3. Natalizumab is a colorless, clear to slightly opalescent concentrate. Inspect the vial for particulate matter and discoloration; if visible particles are observed and/or the liquid is discolored, do not use the vial.
4. Infuse 300 mg over about 1 hr in 100 mL of NaCl 0.9% injection (infusion rate of about 5 mg/min). After the infusion is complete, flush with 0.9% NaCl injection. Do not administer as an IV push or bolus injection.
5. Inspect the solution for particular matter prior to administration
6. Discontinue the infusion promptly upon the first observation of any signs or symptoms consistent with a hypersensitivity-type reaction.
7. Store undiluted vials from 2–8°C (36–46°F). Infuse the prepared diluted infusion solution immediately or refrigerate from 2–8°C (36–46°F) and use within 8 hr of preparation. If refrigerated, allow the solution to warm to room temperature prior to infusion. Do not shake or freeze. Protect from light.
8. COMPATIBILITY 0.9% NaCl.
9. INCOMPATIBILITY Do not inject or mix other drugs with natalizumab.

ASSESSMENT

1. Note disease onset, other therapies trialed, outcome. Drug is reserved for those with inadequate response or intolerance to alternative therapies for MS or Crohn's disease.
2. Observe during infusion and for 1–2 hr after infusion complete. Promptly discontinue infusion with any S&S associated with a hypersensitivity reaction. Do not attempt to retreat those who have experienced an allergic reaction as they may have antibodies to natalizumab.
3. Obtain MRI scan prior to starting therapy. Drug increases the risk of progressive multifocal leukoencephalopathy (PML) a viral infection of the brain that causes severe disability or death. Any suggestive symptoms warrants a repeat MRI with gadolinium and/or if indicated CSF for John Cunningham viral DNA.
4. Only providers, infusion centers, pharmacies associated with infusion centers will be permitted to prescribe, distribute or infuse this product through a restricted distribution program: TOUCH Prescribing Program. Signed permission by client is required. They must be enrolled in the program and meet all the requirements to be eligible for this therapy. TOUCH Prescribing Program through Biogen Idec at 1-800-456-2255 (EST M–F 8:00 a.m.–4:30 p.m.).
5. Will evaluate at 3 months and 6 months after first infusion, and every 6 months thereafter. Will be checked every 6 months to determine if treatment should be reauthorized. Questionnaire and reauthorization forms are required for treatment.
6. Monitor LFTs and for toxicity.

CLIENT/FAMILY TEACHING

1. Drug is administered intravenously to reduce the frequency of exacerbations of relapsing MS and/or Crohn's disease. It is used after other therapies have been proven ineffective or client intolerant.
2. Report any dizziness, itching, fever, rash, chills, nausea, flushing, SOB or chest pain (S&S allergic reaction) immediately.
3. May experience depression, infections (lowers immune system ability to fight these so report any S&S), and gallstones; report especially if suicidal ideations occur.
4. With Crohn's disease, if prescribed steroid therapy, this will be tapered off. If unable to come off oral corticosteroids within 6 months

N

of starting natalizumab, therapy will be discontinued.

5. Drug requires authorization and acceptance into the TOUCH Prescribing Program. There have been reports of increased risk of a viral brain infection. This requires that client understands all the benefits and risks of therapy.
6. A scan of the brain is required as well as careful review of the medication guide before beginning therapy. A signed permit will be required if therapy is to be administered. Review risks of therapy before considering infusion.
7. Report any RUQ pain, yellow skin discoloration, fevers, or S&S of liver dysfunction; may cause damage.
8. Must F/U with provider at 3 months, and 6 months after first infusion and every 6 months thereafter.
9. Call with any questions, problems or adverse side effects immediately.
10. Keep all F/U to assess response, labs, scans, and for adverse SE.

OUTCOMES/EVALUATE

- ↓ Frequency of relapsing MS exacerbations
- Control of symptoms of Crohn's disease

Nateglinide

(nah-**TEG**-lin-eyed)

Classification(s): Antidiabetic agent, oral

Pregnancy Category: C

RX: Starlix.

SEE ALSO ***ANTIDIABETIC AGENTS: HYPOGLYCEMIC AGENTS.***

INDICATIONS/USES

Type 2 diabetes: (1) **Monotherapy:** To lower BG in clients whose hyperglycemia cannot be controlled adequately by diet and physical exercise and who have not been treated chronically with other antidiabetic drugs and (2) **Combination Therapy:** In clients whose hyperglycemia is inadequately controlled with metformin or after a therapeutic response to a thiazolidinedione, nateglinide may be added to, but not substituted for, metformin. Do not switch clients to nateglinide when hyperglycemia is not adequately controlled with glyburide or other insulin secretagogues; do not add nateglinide to their treatment.

ACTION/KINETICS

Action

Lowers blood glucose and reduces post-mealtime glucose spikes by stimulating insulin secretion from the pancreas. Action depends on functioning beta-cells in pancreatic islets. Interacts with the ATP-sensitive potassium (K^+_{ATP}) channel on pancreatic beta cells causing depolarization of the beta cells. This opens the calcium channel producing calcium influx and insulin secretion. Drug is highly tissue selective with a low affinity for heart and skeletal muscle.

Pharmacokinetics

Peak plasma levels: 1 hr with a fall to baseline by 4 hr after dosing. Extent of absorption unaffected by food but there is a delay in the rate of absorption. Peak plasma levels are significantly reduced if administered 10 min prior to a liquid meal. Metabolized in the liver by CYP2C9 and CYP3A4 with most excreted through the urine. **t½, elimination:** About 1.5 hr.

CONTRAINDICATIONS

Use in type 1 diabetes or diabetic ketoacidosis. Lactation.

SPECIAL CONCERNS

- Use with caution in chronic liver disease or moderate to severe liver disease.
- Transient loss of glycemic control with fever, infection, trauma, surgery; insulin therapy may be required.
- Safety and efficacy not determined in children.

SIDE EFFECTS

Most Common

URTI, back pain, bronchitis, flu symptoms, diarrhea.

Metabolic: Hypoglycemia. **Respiratory:** URTI, bronchitis, coughing. **Hypersensitivity (rare):** Rash, itching, urticaria. **Miscellaneous:** Diarrhea, arthropathy, dizziness, flu symptoms, back pain, accidental trauma.

LABORATORY TEST CONSIDERATIONS

↑ Mean uric acid levels.

OVERDOSE MANAGEMENT

Symptoms: Hypoglycemia, including coma, seizure, neurological symptoms. *Treatment:* Treat severe symptoms with IV glucose.

DRUG INTERACTIONS

NOTE: Nateglinide is a potential inhibitor of CYP2C9.

Beta-adrenergic blocking agents, nonselective / Possible potentiation of hypoglycemic effect
Corticosteroids / Possible reduction of hypoglycemic effect
Fluconazole / ↑ Nateglinide AUC and t½ R/T inhibition of CYP2C9 metabolism
NSAIDs / Possible potentiation of hypoglycemic effect
MAOIs / Possible potentiation of hypoglycemic effect
Rifamycins (rifampin) / ↓ Nateglinide plasma levels and pharmacologic effects
Salicylates / Possible potentiation of hypoglycemic effect
Sulfinpyrazone / ↑ Nateglinide AUC R/T ↓ metabolism by CYP2C9
Sympathomimetics / Possible reduction of hypoglycemic effect
Thiazides / Possible reduction of hypoglycemic effect
Thyroid products / Possible reduction of hypoglycemic effect

HOW SUPPLIED

Tablets: 60 mg, 120 mg.

DOSAGE

TABLETS

Type 2 diabetes mellitus, monotherapy or combination with metformin or a thiazolidinedione.

Initial: 120 mg 3 times per day before meals, with or without metformin. Use the 60 mg dose, alone or with metformin, in those who are near their HbA1c goal when treatment is initiated.

NURSING IMPLICATIONS

IMPLEMENTATION/ADMINISTRATION/STORAGE

1. For type 2 diabetes, diet and exercise are the primary form of treatment. Use of nateglinide is in addition to diet and exercise.
2. Store at 15–30°C (59–86°F). Dispense in a tight container.

ASSESSMENT

1. Note disease onset/type of symptoms, HbA1c range, BMI, and all therapies trialed.
2. List drugs prescribed to ensure none interact.
3. Assess understanding of disease and refer for diabetes, nutrition, and exercise education.
4. Obtain VS, Wt, lipids, BS, HbA1c, urine for protein, renal and LFTS, noting any liver dysfunction and uric acid level; monitor throughout therapy.

CLIENT/FAMILY TEACHING

1. Food delays absorption. Take 1–30 min before meals. Do not take while eating, as drug will cause hypoglycemia. May take extra dose with extra meal; may skip dose if meal missed, thus reducing the risk of hypoglycemia.
2. Avoid activities that require mental alertness until drug effects realized.
3. Drug helps to control blood sugar by stimulating the pancreas to release insulin. Must continue diet, exercise, BP control, eye exams, and lifestyle changes conducive to diabetes control.
4. Report unusual side effects, GI upset, or lack of glucose control. Check finger sticks regularly; bring glucometer to visits.
5. Drug is generally used initially when diet and exercise fail. May be added to metformin therapy but not in those whose DM is not adequately controlled with glyburide or other related agents.
6. Do not take aspirin or use alcohol while taking this drug, unless provider approved.
7. Use reliable form of contraception other than oral contraceptives. If pregnant, use insulin during pregnancy.
8. Keep all F/U to assess response, labs, and for adverse SE.

OUTCOMES/EVALUATE

Control of blood sugar; HbA1c <8

Nebivolol

(ne-**BIV**-oh-lol)

Classification(s): Beta-adrenergic blocking agent

Pregnancy Category: C

RX: Bystolic.

SEE ALSO ***BETA-ADRENERGIC BLOCKING AGENTS.***

N

INDICATIONS/USES

Hypertension, alone or in combination with other antihypertensive drugs.

ACTION/KINETICS

Action

At doses of 10 mg in extensive metabolizers (most of the population), nebivolol is β-1 selective. In poor metabolizers and at higher doses, the drug inhibits both β-1 and β-2 adrenergic receptors. The mechanism for the antihypertensive effect is not known but may include (1) decreased HR; (2) decreased cardiac contractility; (3) decreased tonic sympathetic outflow to the periphery from cerebral vasomotor centers; (4) suppression of renin activity; and (5) vasodilation and decreased peripheral resistance.

Pharmacokinetics

Mean peak plasma levels: 1.5–4 hr. Metabolized to the active d-nebivolol and other metabolites by CYP2D6 and by N-dealkylation. Food does not affect the pharmacokinetics. **t½, active metabolite:** 12 hr in extensive metabolizers and 19 hr in poor metabolizers. Excreted in both the feces and urine. **Plasma protein binding:** Approximately 98%.

CONTRAINDICATIONS

Severe bradycardia, greater than first degree heart block, cardiogenic shock, decompensated cardiac failure, sick sinus syndrome (unless a permanent pacemaker is in place), severe hepatic impairment (Child-Pugh >8), bronchospastic disease, in clients hypersensitive to any component of the product. Use not recommended during lactation.

SPECIAL CONCERNS

- Use with caution in severe renal impairment, moderate hepatic impairment, in those with compensated CHF (beta blockade may result in further depression of myocardial contractility and cause more severe failure), and in peripheral vascular disease (possible precipitation or aggravation of symptoms of arterial insufficiency).
- May mask some manifestations of hypoglycemia or thyrotoxicosis, especially tachycardia.
- Safety and efficacy not determined in children 18 years of age and younger.

SIDE EFFECTS

Most Common

Headache, nausea, diarrhea, bradycardia, fatigue, dizziness.

See also *Beta-Adrenergic Blocking Agents* for a complete list of possible side effects. **CNS:** Headache, dizziness, insomnia, paresthesia. **GI:** Nausea, diarrhea, abdominal pain. **CV:** Bradycardia. **Body as a whole:** Fatigue, asthenia. **Miscellaneous:** Chest pain, dyspnea, rash, peripheral edema, anaphylaxis in those with a history of such.

LABORATORY TEST CONSIDERATIONS

↑ BUN, uric acid, triglycerides. ↓ HDL, cholesterol, platelets. Hypercholesterolemia, hyperuricemia.

OVERDOSE MANAGEMENT

SEE ALSO *BETA-ADRENERGIC BLOCKING AGENTS.*

DRUG INTERACTIONS

NOTE: Drugs that inhibit (e.g., fluoxetine, paroxetine, propafenone, quinidine) or induce CYP2D6 can be expected to alter plasma levels of nebivolol. Monitor clients closely; adjust the nebivolol dose according to the BP response.

Cimetidine / ↑ Nebivolol plasma levels by 23%
Clonidine / Discontinue nebivolol several days before gradually tapering the dose of clonidine
Cyclopropane / ↑ Risks of general anesthesia R/T additive depression of myocardial function
Digitalis glycosides / Both slow AV conduction → ↑ risk of bradycardia
Diltiazem / Significant negative inotropic and chronotropic effects; monitor ECG and BP
Disopyramide / Significant negative inotropic and chronotropic effects; monitor ECG and BP
Fluoxetine / ↑ Nebivolol AUC by 8-fold and C_{max} by 3-fold
Guanethidine / Possible reduction of sympathetic activity
Insulin / Potential to ↑ insulin-induced hypoglycemia and delay recovery of serum glucose levels
Sildenafil / ↓ Sildenafil AUC by 21% and C_{max} by 23%
Trichloroethylene / ↑ Risks of general anesthesia R/T additive depression of myocardial function
Verapamil / Significant negative inotropic and chronotropic effects; monitor ECG and BP

HOW SUPPLIED

Tablets: 2.5 mg, 5 mg, 10 mg, 20 mg.

N

DOSAGE

TABLETS

Hypertension.

Individualize dose. **Adults, initial:** 5 mg once daily, with or without food, as monotherapy or in combination with other drugs. Dose can be increased at 2-week intervals up to 40 mg in those requiring further reduction in BP. In those with C_{CR} <30 mL/min or moderate hepatic impairment, the initial dose is 2.5 mg once daily; undertake upward titration cautiously.

NURSING IMPLICATIONS

IMPLEMENTATION/ADMINISTRATION/STORAGE

1. In those with known or suspected pheochromocytoma, an alpha-blocker should be given prior to use of any beta-blocker.
2. When discontinuing therapy, taper dosage over 1–2 weeks when possible. If angina worsens or acute coronary insufficiency develops, promptly reinstitute nebivolol, at least temporarily.
3. If nebivolol is to be continued postoperatively, monitor clients closely when anesthetic agents were used that depress the myocardium (e.g., cyclopropane, ether, trichloroethylene). If the beta-blocker is withdrawn prior to major surgery, the impaired ability of the heart to respond to reflex adrenergic stimuli may increase the risks of general anesthesia and surgical procedures.
4. Store from 20–25°C (68–77°F). Dispense in a tight, light-resistant container.

ASSESSMENT

1. Note onset, other agents trialed and outcome. List drugs prescribed to ensure none interact.
2. Identify any conditions that may preclude therapy (i.e., >1° AVB, severe liver failure, marked bradycardia, decompensated cardiac failure, or SSS without permanent pacemaker).
3. Assess for pulmonary or CAD, diabetes, thyroid disease, CHF, or peripheral vascular disease.
4. Monitor BP, ECG, HR, lipids, renal and LFTS; reduce dose with dysfunction.

CLIENT/FAMILY TEACHING

1. May be taken with or without food. If dose is missed, take only the next scheduled dose (i.e., do not double the dose).
2. Those with coronary artery disease should not stop nebivolol therapy abruptly.
3. When medications are discontinued, decrease slowly and avoid physical overexertion.
4. Avoid activities that require mental alertness until drug effects realized, may cause dizziness. Change positions slowly to prevent sudden drop in BP.
5. Report any breathing difficulty, weight gain >2 lb day or >5 lb/week, SOB, or excessive slow heart rate.
6. Those on insulin or oral hypoglycemic agents, should be aware that β-blockers may mask S&S of hypoglycemia, especially tachycardia. Monitor FS closely.
7. Record BP and HR for provider review.
8. Keep all F/U to assess response, labs, and for adverse SE.

OUTCOMES/EVALUATE

- Desired BP reduction
- BP <130/80

Nedocromil sodium

(neh-**DAH**-kroh-mill)

Classification(s): Antiasthmatic drug

Pregnancy Category: B

RX: Alocril.

INDICATIONS/USES

Ophthalmic. Itching associated with allergic conjunctivitis in adults and children over 3 years old.

ACTION/KINETICS

Action

Is a mast cell stabilizer. Thus, inhibits the release of various mediators, such as histamine, leukotriene C_4, and prostaglandin D_2, from a variety of cell types associated with asthma. Has no intrinsic bronchodilator, antihistamine, or glucocorticoid activity; also, systemic bioavailability is low.

Pharmacokinetics

Only about 4% of the ophthalmic product is absorbed systemically. Not metabolized; eliminated primarily unchanged in urine (70%) and feces (30%).

CONTRAINDICATIONS
Hypersensitivity to nedocromil sodium or any component of the product.

SPECIAL CONCERNS
- Use with caution during lactation.
- Safety and efficacy not determined in children less than 3 years of age.

SIDE EFFECTS
Most Common
After ophthalmic use: Headache, nasal congestion, ocular burning/irritation/stinging, unpleasant taste.

Headache, ocular burning, irritation, stinging, unpleasant taste, nasal congestion, asthma, conjunctivitis, eye redness, photophobia, rhinitis.

LABORATORY TEST CONSIDERATIONS
↑ ALT.

HOW SUPPLIED
Ophthalmic Solution: 2% (20 mg/mL).

DOSAGE
OPHTHALMIC SOLUTION
Allergic conjunctivitis.

Adults and children, 3 years of age and older: 1 or 2 gtt in each eye twice a day. Continue treatment until pollen season is over or until exposure to allergen is terminated. Use even when symptoms are absent.

NURSING IMPLICATIONS
IMPLEMENTATION/ADMINISTRATION/STORAGE
1. Must be used regularly, even during symptom-free period, in order to achieve beneficial effects.
2. Store ophthalmic solution between 2–25°C (36–77°F). Keep tightly closed; out of the reach of children.

ASSESSMENT
1. Note reasons for therapy, type, onset, characteristics of S&S, triggers. List other agents trialed; outcome.
2. Review drug usage/time between prescriptions to ensure proper use.

CLIENT/FAMILY TEACHING
1. Review procedure for administration; use the step-by-step instructions provided with the drug.
2. Use eye solution as directed throughout pollen season. With eye drops, wash hands; tilt head back; looking up, pull lower eyelid down and instill prescribed number of drops. Close eye for 1 to 2 min, apply gentle pressure to bridge of nose for 1 to 3 min. Do not rub eye or touch top of dropper bottle to eye, fingers, or other surface. If more than 1 topical eye drug used, give at least 5 min apart administering the ointment last. May experience temporary stinging or burning; report if bothersome or if eye/eyelid inflammation noted. If wearing contact lens, remove before instilling eye drops.
3. Keep all F/U to assess response and for adverse SE.

OUTCOMES/EVALUATE
↓ Eye itching/irritation

Nefazodone hydrochloride

(nih-**FAY**-zoh-dohn)

Classification(s): Antidepressant, miscellaneous

Pregnancy Category: C

INDICATIONS/USES
Treatment of depression.

ACTION/KINETICS
Action
Exact antidepressant mechanism not known. Inhibits neuronal uptake of serotonin and norepinephrine (to a lesser extent) and antagonizes central 5-HT_2 receptors and alpha-1-adrenergic receptors (which may cause postural hypotension). Produces none to slight anticholinergic effects, moderate sedation, and slight orthostatic hypotension.

Pharmacokinetics
Rapidly and completely absorbed. **Peak plasma levels:** 1 hr. **t½:** 2–4 hr. **Time to reach steady**

state: 4–5 days. Extensively metabolized by the liver with less than 1% excreted unchanged in the urine. Food delays the absorption of nefazodone and decreases the bioavailability by approximately 20%.

CONTRAINDICATIONS

Use with pimozide, carbamazepine, or triazolam. In combination with an MAOI or within 14 days of discontinuing MAOI therapy. Use in active liver disease, elevated baseline serum transaminases, or those who were withdrawn from nefazodone due to evidence of liver injury. Clients hypersensitive to nefazodone or other phenylpiperazine antidepressants.

SPECIAL CONCERNS

(1) Life-threatening hepatic failure has occurred. The reported rate in the U.S. is about 1 case of liver failure resulting in death or transplant per 250,000 to 300,000 client-years of nefazodone treatment. (2) Ordinarily, do not initiate treatment in those with active liver disease or with elevated baseline serum transaminases. There is no evidence that preexisting liver disease increases the likelihood of developing liver failure; however, baseline abnormalities can complicate client monitoring. (3) Advise clients to be alert for signs and symptoms of liver dysfunction (e.g., jaundice, anorexia, GI complaints, malaise) and to report them to their provider immediately if they occur. (4) Discontinue if clinical signs or symptoms suggest liver failure. Those who develop evidence of hepatocellular injury, such as increased serum AST or serum ALT levels greater than 2 times ULN should be withdrawn from the drug. These clients should be presumed to be at increased risk for liver injury if nefazodone is reintroduced. Do not consider such clients for retreatment. (5) Antidepressants, including nefazodone, have the ability to increase the risk of suicidal thinking and behavior in children and adolescents with major depressive disorder and other psychiatric disorders. Anyone considering the use of nefazodone or any other antidepressant in a child or adolescent must balance this risk with the clinical need. Clients who are started on therapy should be observed closely for clinical worsening, suicidality, or unusual changes in behavior. Families and caregivers should be advised of the need for close observation and communication with the prescriber. Nefazodone is not approved for use in pediatric clients. (6) Placebo-controlled trials in children and adolescents with major depressive disorder, obsessive-compulsive disorder, or other psychiatric disorders revealed a greater risk of adverse reactions representing suicidal thinking or behavior (suicidality) during the first few months of treatment in those receiving antidepressants. The average risk of such reactions in those receiving antidepressants was 4%, twice the placebo risk of 2%. No suicides occurred in these trials.

- **Use with caution in clients with known CV or cerebrovascular disease (e.g., history of MI, angina, ischemic stroke), conditions that predispose to hypotension (e.g., dehydration, hypovolemia, antihypertensive medications), or a history of mania.**
- **Use with caution during lactation.**
- **Possible suicide attempts that may persist until significant remission occurs. Both adult and pediatric clients may experience worsening of their depression.**
- **Suicide attempts and suicidal thinking have occurred in children, adolescents, and young adults taking antidepressant drugs for major depressive disorder.**
- **From 2 weeks to 6 months may elapse between the time from liver injury to liver failure, resulting in death or transplant.**
- **Safety and efficacy not determined in individuals below 18 years of age.**

SIDE EFFECTS

Most Common

Somnolence, dizziness, insomnia, dry mouth, nausea, constipation, headache, asthenia, dyspepsia, diarrhea, abnormal/blurred vision, infection.

CNS: Dizziness, insomnia, agitation, somnolence, light-headedness, activation of mania/hypomania, confusion, memory impairment, paresthesia, abnormal dreams, decreased concentration, ataxia, incoordination, psychomotor retardation, tremor, hypertonia, decreased/increased libido, vertigo, twitching, depersonalization, hallucinations, ***suicide thoughts/attempt***, apathy, euphoria, hostility, abnormal gait/thinking, decreased attention, derealization, neuralgia, paranoid reaction, dys-

N

arthria, myoclonus, hyperkinesia, hyperesthesia, hypotonia, increased libido, ***suicide, neuroleptic malignant syndrome (rare)***. **CV:** Postural hypotension, hypo-/hypertension, sinus bradycardia, tachycardia, syncope, ventricular extrasystoles, angina pectoris, AV block, CHF, hemorrhage, varicose vein, pallor, ***CVA*** (rare). **GI:** Nausea, dry mouth, constipation, dyspepsia, diarrhea, increased appetite, vomiting, eructation, periodontal abscess, gingivitis, colitis, gastritis, mouth ulceration, stomatitis, esophagitis, glossitis, hepatitis, hepatotoxicity, dysphagia, ***GI hemorrhage***, oral moniliasis, ulcerative colitis, peptic ulcer, rectal hemorrhage, gastroenteritis, ***hepatic failure***. **Dermatologic:** Pruritus, dry skin, acne, alopecia, urticaria, maculopapular/vesiculobullous rash, eczema. **Musculoskeletal:** Arthralgia, arthritis, tenosynovitis, muscle stiffness, bursitis, tendinous contracture. **Respiratory:** Pharyngitis, increased cough, dyspnea, bronchitis, asthma, pneumonia, laryngitis, voice alteration, epistaxis, hiccoughs, hyperventilation, yawn. **Hematologic:** Ecchymosis, anemia, leukopenia, lymphadenopathy. **Ophthalmic:** Blurred vision, scotoma, visual trails, abnormal vision/accommodation, visual field defect, dry eye, eye pain, diplopia, conjunctivitis, mydriasis, keratoconjunctivitis, photophobia, night blindness, glaucoma, ptosis. **Otic:** Ear pain, hyperacusis, deafness, tinnitus. **GU:** Urinary frequency/retention/urgency/incontinence, UTI, vaginitis, breast pain, cystitis, metrorrhagia, amenorrhea, polyuria, vaginal/uterine hemorrhage, breast enlargement, menorrhagia, abnormal ejaculation, hematuria, nocturia, kidney calculus, enlarged uterine fibroids, anorgasmia, oliguria, impotence, priaprism (rare). **Body as a whole:** Headache, asthenia, infection, flu syndrome, chills, fever, neck rigidity, allergic reaction, malaise, photosensitivity, facial edema, hangover effect, enlarged abdomen, hernia, pelvic pain, halitosis, cellulitis, weight loss, gout, dehydration. **Miscellaneous:** Peripheral edema, thirst, taste loss.

N

LABORATORY TEST CONSIDERATIONS

↑ AST, ALT, LDH. ↓ Hematocrit. Hypercholesterolemia, hypoglycemia. Abnormal LFTs.

OVERDOSE MANAGEMENT

Symptoms: N&V, somnolence, increased incidence of severity of any of the reported side effects.

Treatment: Symptomatic and supportive in the cases of hypotension or excessive sedation. Gastric lavage with a large-bore orogastric tube with appropriate airway protection may be used; induction of emesis is not recommended. Ensure an adequate airway, oxygenation, and ventilation. Monitor cardiac rhythm and vital signs. Administer activated charcoal.

DRUG INTERACTIONS

Alprazolam / ↑ Alprazolam levels R/T inhibition of metabolism by CYP3A4
Anesthetics, general / Discontinue nefazodone for as long as clinically feasible before using general anesthetics since little is known about potential interactions
Atorvastatin / ↑ Atorvastatin levels R/T inhibition of metabolism by CYP3A4; ↑ risk of rhabdomyolysis
Benzodiazepines / Possible ↑ CNS depression
Buspirone / ↑ Levels of both drugs R/T inhibition of metabolism by CYP3A4; ↑ risk of light-headedness, somnolence, dizziness, asthenia
Carbamazepine / ↑ Carbamazepine plasma levels → ↑ side effects
Cyclosporine / ↑ Cyclosporine levels → ↑ toxicity
Digoxin / ↑ Digoxin plasma levels; monitor digoxin plasma levels
Ethanol / Do not use together in depressed clients
HMG-CoA reductase inhibitors / ↑ Risk of rhabdomyolysis and myositis
MAOIs / Serious and possibly fatal reactions including symptoms of hyperthermia, rigidity, myoclonus, autonomic instability with possible rigid fluctuations of VS, and mental status changes that may include extreme agitation progressing to delirium and coma
Methylprednisolone / ↑ Methylprednisolone AUC and t½ R/T inhibition of metabolism
Pimozide / ↑ Plasma levels of pimozide resulting in QT prolongation and possible serious CV events, including death due to ventricular tachycardia of the torsades de pointes type
Propranolol / ↓ Propranolol plasma levels
H ***St. John's wort*** / ↑ Sedative-hypnotic effects
Sibutramine / Serotonin syndrome, including CNS irritability, motor weakness, shivering, myoclonus, and altered consciousness
Simvastatin / ↑ Simvastatin levels R/T inhibition of metabolism by CYP3A4; ↑ risk of rhabdomyolysis

Sumatriptan / Possible serotonin syndrome, including CNS irritability, increased muscle tone, shivering, myoclonus, and altered consciousness
Trazodone / Serotonin syndrome, including CNS irritability, motor weakness, shivering, myoclonus, and altered consciousness
Triazolam / ↑ Triazolam plasma levels; reduce initial triazolam dosage by 75% if used together; avoid coadministration for most clients, including the elderly

HOW SUPPLIED

Tablets: 50 mg, 100 mg, 150 mg, 200 mg, 250 mg.

DOSAGE

TABLETS

Depression.

Adults, initial: 200 mg/day given in two divided doses. Increase dose in increments of 100–200 mg/day at intervals of no less than 1 week. Continue treatment for 6 or more months. The effective dose range is 300–600 mg/day. The initial dose for elderly or debilitated clients is 100 mg/day given in two divided doses.

NURSING IMPLICATIONS

IMPLEMENTATION/ADMINISTRATION/STORAGE

1. May take several weeks for full beneficial effect to be observed.
2. Although long-term use has not been studied, it is usually recommended that the drug be given for a period of 6 months or longer.
3. At least 14 days should elapse between discontinuation of an MAOI and initiation of therapy with nefazodone; also, at least 7 days should elapse after stopping nefazodone and before starting an MAOI.
4. Store at room temperature below 40°C (104°F); dispense in a tight container.

ASSESSMENT

1. Note reasons for therapy, characteristics of S&S, any precipitating factors/triggers, clinical presentation, behavioral manifestations. Assess depression regularly, record mood changes; note any evidence of suicidal ideations.
2. Before initiating treatment, adequately screen those with depressive symptoms to determine if at risk for bipolar disorder.
3. Evaluate for history of drug abuse and follow clients closely, observing for signs of misuse or abuse.
4. List any seizure history, drugs currently prescribed to ensure none interact unfavorably. Assess for CAD, recent MI, or conditions requiring digoxin administration.
5. Monitor VS, CBC, ECG, renal and LFTs. If AST or ALT increase to levels >3 × ULN, stop drug and do not restart.

CLIENT/FAMILY TEACHING

1. Take before meals; food may inhibit absorption.
2. Do not perform activities that require mental alertness or coordination until drug effects realized; may cause dizziness, drowsiness, confusion, incoordination, decreased concentration/response time. Change positions slowly to prevent drop in BP.
3. Avoid all OTC agents, alcohol and any other CNS depressants. Use reliable birth control.
4. Avoid prolonged or excessive exposure to direct or artificial sunlight.
5. May take several weeks (2–4) before any effects are realized; do not become discouraged. Continue counselling sessions.
6. Report any unusual sensations or side effects, rash, memory problems, S&S of liver dysfunction (stomach pain, yellowing of skin, loss of appetite or fatigue), increased depression, sexual dysfunction, or suicidal thoughts/behavior.
7. Keep all F/U to assess response, labs, and for adverse SE review.

OUTCOMES/EVALUATE

- Symptomatic improvement
- ↓ Depression, improved sleeping and eating patterns
- ↑ Social interaction, ↓ fatigue

Nelfinavir mesylate

(nel-**FIN**-ah-veer)

Classification(s): Antiviral, protease inhibitor
Pregnancy Category: B
RX: Viracept.

SEE ALSO ***ANTIVIRAL DRUGS***.

INDICATIONS/USES

HIV infections in combination with other antiretroviral drugs. *Investigational:* Part of a three-drug regimen for occupational HIV postexposure prophylaxis where there is an increased risk of transmission. For HIV infection in neonates. Twice-daily dosing in children over age 6 with HIV infection.

ACTION/KINETICS

Action

HIV-1 protease inhibitor, resulting in prevention of cleavage of gagpol polyprotein resulting in production of immature, noninfectious viruses. Activity is increased when used with didanosine, lamivudine, stavudine, zalcitabine, or zidovudine.

Pharmacokinetics

Peak plasma levels: 2–4 hr. **Steady-state plasma levels:** 3–4 mcg/mL. Food increases plasma levels 2–3 fold. **t½, terminal:** 3.5–5 hr. Metabolites (one of which is as active as parent compound) and unchanged drug excreted mainly in feces.

CONTRAINDICATIONS

Use with drugs that are highly dependent on CYP3A4 for metabolism and for which elevated plasma levels are associated with serious and/or life-threatening events. Drugs include amiodarone, ergot derivatives, lovastatin, midazolam, pimozide, quinidine, simvastatin, and triazolam. Lactation.

SPECIAL CONCERNS

- Use with caution with hepatic impairment.
- Increased bleeding in those with hemophilia type A and B in clients treated with protease inhibitors.
- Safety and efficacy not determined in children less than 2 years of age.

SIDE EFFECTS

Most Common

Diarrhea, nausea, flatulence, rash, anemia, leukopenia.

NOTE: Side effects were determined when used in combination with other antiviral drugs. **GI:** N&V, diarrhea, flatulence, abdominal pain, anorexia, dyspepsia, epigastric pain, GI bleeding, hepatitis, mouth ulcers, pancreatitis. **CNS:** Anxiety, depression, dizziness, emotional lability, hyperkinesia, insomnia, migraine, paresthesia, ***seizures***, sleep disorder, somnolence, ***suicide ideation***. **CV:** Prolongation of QTc; ***torsades de pointes***. **Hematologic:** Anemia, leukopenia, thrombocytopenia. **Respiratory:** Dyspnea, rhinitis, sinusitis, pharyngitis. **GU:** Kidney calculus, sexual dysfunction, urine abnormality. **Ophthalmic:** Eye disorder, acute iritis. **Musculoskeletal:** Arthralgia, arthritis, cramps, myalgia, myasthenia, myopathy. **Dermatologic:** Dermatitis, folliculitis, fungal dermatitis, maculopapular rash, pruritus, urticaria, sweating. **Hypersensitivity:** ***Bronchospasm***, moderate to severe rash, fever, edema, jaundice. **Miscellaneous:** Asthenia, dehydration, allergic reaction, back pain, fever, headache, malaise, pain, accidental injury, new-onset diabetes mellitus or exacerbation of pre-existing diabetes mellitus, hyperglycemia.

LABORATORY TEST CONSIDERATIONS

↑ ALT, AST, creatine CPK, alkaline phosphatase, amylase, LDH, GGT. Hyperlipidemia, hyperuricemia, hypoglycemia, bilirubinemia, metabolic acidosis. Abnormal LFTs.

OVERDOSE MANAGEMENT

Symptoms: See *Side Effects*. *Treatment:* Emesis or gastric lavage, followed by activated charcoal.

DRUG INTERACTIONS

Amiodarone / Possible inhibition of metabolism via CYP3A4 isoenzyme; do not give together
Anticonvulsants / Possible ↓ nelfinavir plasma levels
Azithromycin / ↓ AUC and C_{max} of nelfinavir and ↑ AUC and C_{max} of azithromycin
Azole antifungal drugs / Possible inhibition of metabolism of nelfinavir
Benzodiazepines / Possible severe sedation and respiratory depression R/T ↓ metabolism
Didanosine / ↓ Absorption of nelfinavir; give on an empty stomach
Delavirdine / ↑ AUC and C_{max} of nelfinavir and a ↓ AUC and C_{max} of delavirdine
Efavirenz / ↑ AUC and C_{max} of nelfinavir and a ↓ AUC and C_{max} of efavirenz
Ergot alkaloids / Possible inhibition of metabolism of ergot alkaloids via CYP3A4 isoenzyme; do not give together due to possible severe side effects, including peripheral vasospasm and ischemia of the extremities and other tissues

Felodipine / Possible leg edema and orthostatic hypotension R/T ↓ nelfinavir metabolism by CYP3A4
Fentanyl / Possible ↓ fentanyl metabolism; monitor and adjust dose if needed
HMG-CoA reductase inhibitors / ↑ in C_{max}; potential for serious reactions, such as ↑ risk of myopathy including rhabdomyolysis
Indinavir / Significant ↑ AUC of nelfinavir and indinavir
Interleukins / Possible inhibition of nelfinavir metabolism; dosage adjustment may be needed
Lamivudine / ↑ Lamivudine AUC and C_{max}
Methadone / ↓ Methadone plasma levels → possible withdrawal S&S
Nevirapine / ↑ Hepatic metabolism of nelfinavir; monitor levels and adjust dose if needed
Oral contraceptives / ↓ Drug effects; use other contraceptive measures
Phenytoin / ↓ Phenytoin AUC and C_{max}; dosage adjustment may be needed
Pimozide / Do not give together due to potential for serious or life-threatening reactions, including cardiac arrhythmias
Quinidine / Possible inhibition of metabolism via CYP3A4 isoenzyme; do not give together
Rifabutin / ↑ Rifabutin levels; reduce rifabutin dose one-half; also, ↓ nelfinavir AUC
Rifampin / Significant ↓ in nelfinavir levels; do not coadminister
Ritonavir / Significant ↑ nelfinavir AUC
Saquinavir / ↑ In both nelfinavir and saquinavir AUCs
Sildenafil / ↓ Sildenafil metabolism; coadminister carefully; do not exceed a maximum single dose of sildenafil of 25 mg/48 hr
Sirolimus / ↑ Sirolimus plasma levels; monitor carefully with possible dosage adjustment
H ***St. John's wort*** / ↑ Nelfinavir metabolism by CYP3A4 → loss of virologic response
Tacrolimus / ↑ Tacrolimus plasma levels; monitor carefully with possible dosage adjustment
Zidovudine / ↓ Zidovudine AUC

HOW SUPPLIED

Oral Powder: 50 mg/1 gram; ***Tablets, Film-Coated:*** 250 mg, 625 mg.

DOSAGE

ORAL POWDER; TABLETS, FILM-COATED

HIV infections.

Adults: 1,250 mg (five 250 mg tablets or two 625 mg tablets) twice a day or 750 mg (three 250 mg tablets) 3 times per day in combination with nucleoside analogs. **Children, 2 to 13 years:** 20–30 mg/kg/dose 3 times per day. Doses as high as 45 mg/kg q 8 hr have been used.

NURSING IMPLICATIONS

Do not confuse nelfinavir with nevirapine (also an antiviral drug).

IMPLEMENTATION/ADMINISTRATION/STORAGE

1. Nelfinavir powder contains 11.2 mg phenylalanine/gram of powder.
2. Store tablets and powder at controlled room temperature 59°–86°F (15°–30°C).

ASSESSMENT

1. Note disease onset, characteristics of S&S of disease, other agents trialed.
2. List drugs prescribed/consumed to ensure none interact unfavorably.
3. Monitor CBC, for any evidence/history of increased bleeding tendencies, CD_4 counts, viral load, renal and LFTs.

CLIENT/FAMILY TEACHING

1. Drug is not a cure but helps to manage disease symptoms; unless postexposure prophylaxis.
2. Take as prescribed with snack or light meal to enhance absorption. Must take drug with other nucleoside analogs as prescribed.
3. Do not reconstitute powder with water in its original container. Mix powder with small amount of water, milk, formula, soy formula/milk or dietary supplement. Once mixed, consume entire amount for full dose or may be refrigerated for up to 6 hr. Do not mix with acidic foods or juice (e.g., orange or apple juice, applesauce) due to their bitter taste. Powder contains 11.2 mg phenylalanine/gram of powder.
4. Report any evidence of increased bruising/bleeding, severe headache/fatigue/lethargy, N&V, rash, breathing problems, redistribution of body fat, or changes in stool/urine color. Diarrhea may be controlled with loperamide.
5. Oral contraceptives may be ineffective; additionally use barrier contraception. Men may experience adverse effects with Viagra, use cautiously and do not exceed 25 mg of Viagra

in a 48 hr period. Drug does not prevent disease transmission; practice safe sex. Avoid OTC agents without approval.

6. Keep all F/U to assess response, labs, and for adverse SE.

OUTCOMES/EVALUATE

- Control of HIV symptoms
- ↓ Viral load
- Improved CD_4 count

Neomycin sulfate

(nee-oh-**MY**-sin)

Classification(s): Antibiotic, aminoglycoside

Pregnancy Category: D

RX: Mycifradin Sulfate, Neo-fradin, Neo-Tabs.

SEE ALSO ***ANTI-INFECTIVE DRUGS*** AND ***AMINOGLYCOSIDES.***

INDICATIONS/USES

PO: (1) Hepatic coma. (2) Sterilization of gut prior to surgery. (3) Inhibition of ammonia-forming bacteria in GI tract in hepatic encephalopathy. (4) Therapy of intestinal infections due to pathogenic strains of *Escherichia coli*, primarily in children. *Investigational:* Hypercholesterolemia.

ACTION/KINETICS

Pharmacokinetics

Peak plasma levels: PO, 1–4 hr; **therapeutic serum level:** 5–10 mcg/mL. **t½:** 2–3 hr.

ADDITIONAL CONTRAINDICATIONS

Intestinal obstruction (PO). Use of topical products in or around the eyes.

SPECIAL CONCERNS

- Safe use during pregnancy not determined.
- Use with caution in clients with extensive burns, trophic ulceration, or other conditions where significant systemic absorption is possible.

SIDE EFFECTS

Most Common

N&V, diarrhea, skin rashes.

See *Anti-Infective Drugs* and *Aminoglycosides* for a complete list of possible side effects. Also, N&V, ototoxicity, skin rashes, nephrotoxicity. Sprue-like syndrome with steatorrhea, malabsorption, and electrolyte imbalance.

ADDITIONAL DRUG INTERACTIONS

Digoxin / ↓ Digoxin effect R/T ↓ GI tract absorption

Penicillin V / ↓ PCN effect R/T ↓ GI tract absorption

Procainamide / ↑ Muscle relaxation produced by neomycin

HOW SUPPLIED

Oral Solution: 125 mg/5 mL; ***Tablets:*** 500 mg.

DOSAGE

ORAL SOLUTION; TABLETS

Hepatic coma, adjunct.

Adults, 4–12 grams/day in divided doses for 5–6 days; **children:** 50–100 mg/kg/day in divided doses for 5–6 days.

Preoperatively in colorectal surgery.

1 gram each of neomycin and erythromycin base for a total of three doses: the first two doses 1 hr apart the afternoon before surgery and the third dose at bedtime the night before surgery.

NURSING IMPLICATIONS

ASSESSMENT

1. List reasons for therapy; note any experience with this drug. Include clinical presentation, abdominal assessments, and symptom characteristics.
2. Check all drugs prescribed to ensure none interact.
3. Assess hearing before and after therapy. Review risk of renal, neuro and ototoxicity; may be increased by dehydration or advanced age.
4. Note fluid and electrolyte status, CBC, renal function, C&S.

CLIENT/FAMILY TEACHING

1. Take as directed. Consume 2-3 L/day of fluids to prevent dehydration.
2. Carefully follow procedure to prepare the GI tract for surgery (suppression of intestinal bacteria).

3. Expect slight laxative effect produced by PO neomycin. Withhold and report with S&S of intestinal obstruction.
4. With hepatic coma (portal-systemic encephalopathy) drug used to reduce ammonia-forming bacteria in the intestinal tract with neurologic improvement.
5. Report any hearing changes such as loss, ringing, roaring, or dizziness or numbness, vestibular symptoms (e.g., dizziness, incoordination), skin tingling, muscle twitching and convulsions (S&S neurotoxicity).
6. Anticipate low-residue diet for preoperative disinfection and a laxative immediately preceding PO administration of neomycin sulfate.
7. Keep all F/U to assess response, labs, adverse SE.

OUTCOMES/EVALUATE

- Improved level of consciousness
- Bowel sterilization before surgery

IV

Nesiritide

(nih-**SIR**-ih-tide)

Classification(s): Vasodilator, peripheral

Pregnancy Category: C

RX: Natrecor.

INDICATIONS/USES

IV treatment of acutely decompensated CHF in those who have dyspnea at rest or with minimal activity.

ACTION/KINETICS

Action

Nesiritide is a human B-type natriuretic peptide (hBNP) that binds to the particulate guanylate cyclase receptor in vascular smooth muscle and endothelial cells, leading to increased intracellular levels of guanosine 3'5'-cyclic monophosphate (cGMP) and smooth muscle cell relaxation. Cyclic GMP serves as a second messenger to dilate veins and arteries. In acutely decompensated CHF, the drug reduces pulmonary capillary wedge pressure and improves dyspnea.

Pharmacokinetics

t½, initial elimination: About 2 min; **t½, mean terminal, elimination:** About 18 min. Human BNP is cleared from the circulation by three mechanisms: (1) Binding to cell surface clearance receptors with subsequent cellular internalization and lysosomal proteolysis; (2) Proteolytic cleavage of the peptide by endopeptidases, such as neutral endopeptidase (present on the vascular lumenal surface); and (3) renal filtration.

CONTRAINDICATIONS

Use as primary therapy for those with cardiogenic shock or in those with a systolic BP <90 mm Hg. Hypersensitivity to any of the product components. Use in those suspected of having, or known to have, low cardiac filling pressures. Use in those for whom vasodilating agents are not appropriate, including valvular stenosis, restrictive or obstructive cardiomyopathy, constrictive pericarditis, pericardial tamponade, or other conditions in which cardiac output is dependent on venous return.

SPECIAL CONCERNS

- Use with caution during lactation.
- Increased risk of death.
- Safety and efficacy not determined in children.

SIDE EFFECTS

Most Common

Hypotension (both symptomatic and asymptomatic), ventricular tachycardia, nonsustained ventricular tachycardia, ventricular extrasystole, headache, insomnia, dizziness, anxiety, N&V, angina pectoris, abdominal pain, back pain.

CV: Hypotension (symptomatic, asymptomatic), ***ventricular tachycardia***, nonsustained ventricular tachycardia, ventricular extrasystoles, angina pectoris, bradycardia, tachycardia, atrial fibrillation, AV node conduction abnormalities. **CNS:** Headache, insomnia, dizziness, anxiety, confusion, paresthesia, somnolence, tremor. **GI:** N&V, abdominal pain. **Dermatologic:** Sweating, pruritus, rash. **Respiratory:** Increased cough, hemoptysis, apnea. **Miscellaneous:** Back pain, abdominal pain, hypersensitivity reactions, catheter pain, fever, injection site reaction, leg cramps, amblyopia, anemia, ***worsened renal function (may be fatal), increased risk of death.***

LABORATORY TEST CONSIDERATIONS

↑ Creatinine.

N

DRUG INTERACTIONS

↑ Symptomatic hypotension when used with ACE inhibitors.

HOW SUPPLIED

Powder for Injection, Lyophilized: 1.58 mg.

DOSAGE

IV ONLY

Acutely decompensated CHF.

IV bolus of 2 mcg/kg, followed by a continuous IV infusion of 0.01 mcg/kg/min.

NURSING IMPLICATIONS

Do not confuse Natrecor with Norcuron (a neuromuscular blocker).

IMPLEMENTATION/ADMINISTRATION/STORAGE

1. IV Do not start nesiritide higher than the recommended dose.
2. Prime IV tubing with an infusion of 5 mL before connecting to the client's vascular access port and prior to giving the bolus or starting the infusion.
3. After preparing the infusion bag, withdraw bolus volume and give over about 60 seconds through an IV port in the tubing. Immediately following the bolus, infuse nesiritide at a flow rate of 0.1 mL/kg/hr (this will deliver an infusion dose of 0.01 mcg/kg/min).
4. To calculate the appropriate bolus volume and infusion flow rate to deliver 0.01 mcg/kg/min dose, use the following formulas: Bolus volume (mL) = 0.33 × client weight (kg). Infusion flow rate (mL/hr) = 0.1 × client weight (kg).
5. To prepare infusion, use the following procedure:
   - Reconstitute one 1.5 mg vial by adding 5 mL of diluent removed from a prefilled 250 mL plastic IV bag containing the compatible diluent.
   - Do not shake vial but rock gently so that all surfaces, including the stopper, are in contact with diluent to ensure complete reconstitution. Use only a clear, essentially colorless solution.
   - Withdraw entire contents of the reconstituted vial and add to the 250 mL plastic IV bag. This will yield a solution with a nesiritide concentration of about 6 mcg/mL. Invert the IV bag several times to ensure complete mixing of the solution.
   - Use the reconstituted solution within 24 hr, as there are no preservatives in the product. Inspect visually for particulate matter and discoloration prior to use.
6. If hypotension occurs during administration, reduce or discontinue the dose and begin other measures to support BP (e.g., IV fluids, changes in body position). The drug may be restarted at a dose that is reduced by 30% (with no bolus given). Hypotension may be prolonged; thus, before restarting the drug, a period of observation may be needed.
7. Store at controlled room temperature between 20–25°C (68–77°F) or refrigerated at 2–8°C (36–46°F). Reconstituted vials may be left at controlled room temperature or refrigerated for 24 hr or less. Keep in carton until time of use.
8. Nesiritide binds to heparin. Thus, **do not** give through a central line heparin-coated catheter.
9. COMPATIBILITY D5W, 0.9% NaCl, D5/0.45% NaCl, or D5/0.2% NaCl.
10. INCOMPATIBILITY Heparin, insulin, ethacrynate sodium, bumetanide, enalaprilat, hydralazine, and furosemide. Do not give injectable drugs that contain sodium metabisulfate in the same infusion line. Flush catheter between administration of nesiritide and incompatible drugs.

ASSESSMENT

1. Note reasons for therapy, clinical presentation, other agents trialed, ejection fraction, and NYHA class.
2. For IV use only; avoid infusing through central line heparin-coated catheters.
3. Review list of drugs not compatible for co-administration.
4. Administer in a closely monitored environment by trained individuals; monitor heart pressures and assess closely for arrhythmias. Review risks of therapy.
5. Monitor cardiac status, ECG, I&O, renal function, VS; if SBP <90 mm Hg, reduce dose or stop infusion and report.

CLIENT/FAMILY TEACHING

1. Given IV in ICU for decompensated CHF in those with dyspnea at rest or with minimal activity.

2. May experience dizziness, blurred vision, lightheadedness or sweating; report if evident.

OUTCOMES/EVALUATE

Improved exercise tolerance; ↓ PACWP; ↓ SOB with mild exertion and at rest

Nevirapine

(neh-**VYE**-rah-peen)

Classification(s): Antiviral, non-nucleoside reverse transcriptase inhibitor

Pregnancy Category: B

RX: Viramune, Viramune XR.

SEE ALSO ***ANTIVIRAL DRUGS***.

INDICATIONS/USES

In combination with nucleoside analogues (e.g., zidovudine, lamivudine, didanosine, zalcitabine) or protease inhibitors (e.g., saquinavir, indinavir, nelfinavir, aritonavir) for HIV-1 infections in adults who have experienced clinical and immunologic deterioration. Always use in combination with at least one other antiretroviral agent, as resistant viruses emerge rapidly when nevirapine is used alone. *NOTE:* Use of antiretroviral drugs (nonoccupational, postexposure) for prophylaxis of HIV should be restricted to treatment no more than 72 hr after high-risk exposure with a person known to be HIV-infected.

ACTION/KINETICS

Action

A nonnucleoside reverse transcriptase inhibitor. By binding tightly to reverse transcriptase, nevirapine prevents viral RNA from being converted into DNA. In combination with a nucleoside analogue, it reduces the amount of virus circulating in the body and increases CD4+ cell counts.

Pharmacokinetics

Immediate-Release: Readily absorbed (more than 90%); absolute bioavailability is 93% in adults. **Peak plasma levels:** 4 hr after a 200-mg dose. **Extended-Release:** Bioavailability is 75%. T_{max}: About 24 hr. Extensively metabolized in the liver by CYP3A4 and CYP2B6. Excreted through both the urine (about 90%) and the feces (about 10%). Induces hepatic CYP3A4 and CYP2B6; also, induces its own metabolism. Following chronic use the half-life decreases from about 45 hr following a single dose to 25 to 30 hr following multiple dosing with 200 or 400 mg daily. **Plasma protein binding:** 63%.

CONTRAINDICATIONS

Hypersensitivity to nevirapine or any component of the products. Moderate or severe (Child–Pugh B or C, respectively) hepatic impairment. Beginning therapy in women with CD4+ counts greater than 250 cells/mm^3 or men with counts greater than 400 cells/mm^3 unless benefits outweigh risks. Use as a single agent to treat HIV or add on as a sole agent to a failing regimen (due to emergence of resistant strains). Use as part of occupational and nonoccupational postexposure prophylaxis regimens. Lactation.

SPECIAL CONCERNS

(1) **Hepatotoxicity.** Severe, life-threatening and, in some cases, fatal hepatotoxicity, particularly in the first 18 weeks, has been reported in clients treated with nevirapine. In some cases, clients presented with nonspecific prodromal signs or symptoms of hepatitis and progressed to hepatic failure. These events are often associated with rash. Women and clients with higher CD4+ counts at initiation of therapy are at increased risk. Women with CD4+ counts higher than 250 cells/mm^3, including pregnant women receiving nevirapine in combination with other antiretrovirals for treatment of HIV infection, are at greatest risk. However, hepatotoxicity associated with nevirapine use can occur in both genders, all CD4+ counts, and at any time during treatment. Hepatic failure has also been reported in clients without HIV taking nevirapine for postexposure prophylaxis. Use of nevirapine for occupational and nonoccupational postexposure prophylaxis is contraindicated. Clients with signs or symptoms of hepatitis or with increased transaminases combined with rash or other systemic symptoms must discontinue nevirapine and seek medical evaluation immediately. (2) **Skin reactions.** Severe, life-threatening skin reactions, including fatal cases, have occurred in clients treated with nevirapine. These have included cases of Stevens–Johnson syndrome, toxic epidermal necrolysis, and hypersensitivity reactions characterized by rash, constitutional findings, and organ dysfunction. Clients

developing signs or symptoms of severe skin reactions or hypersensitivity reactions must discontinue nevirapine and seek medical evaluation immediately. Check transaminase levels immediately for all clients who develop a rash in the first 18 weeks of treatment. The 14-day lead-in period with immediate-release nevirapine 200 mg daily dosing has been observed to decrease the incidence of rash and must be followed. (3) **Monitoring.** It is essential that clients be monitored intensively during the first 18 weeks of therapy with nevirapine to detect potentially life-threatening hepatotoxicity or skin reactions. Extra vigilance is warranted during the first 6 weeks of therapy, which is the period of greatest risk of these reactions. Do not restart nevirapine following clinical hepatitis, or transaminase elevations combined with rash or other systemic symptoms, or following severe skin rash or hypersensitivity reactions. In some cases, hepatic injury has progressed despite discontinuation of treatment. ■

- **Is not a cure for HIV infections; clients may continue to experience illnesses associated with HIV infections, including opportunistic infections.**
- **Not been shown to reduce the risk of transmitting HIV to others through sexual contact or blood contamination.**
- **Use with caution in moderately impaired renal or hepatic function. Use caution in dose selection in the elderly.**
- **Women who received single-dose nevirapine during labor and delivery to prevent prenatal potential transmission of HIV-1 are more likely to manifest virologic failure if nevirapine is prescribed within 6 months of labor; delaying the use of nevirapine for 6 months may improve control.**
- **Although used in children, safety and efficacy have not been established.**

SIDE EFFECTS

Most Common

Rash, fever, nausea, headache, abnormal LFTs, diarrhea.

Side effects listed are for both immediate-release and extended-release tablets and the suspension. **GI:** N&V, diarrhea, abdominal pain, ulcerative stomatitis. **Hepatic:** Hepatitis; ***severe, life-threatening (sometimes fatal) hepatotoxicity, including fulminant and cholestatic hepatitis, necrosis, and failure*** (especially during the first 12 weeks of therapy), jaundice, abnormal LFTs. **CNS:** Headache, fatigue, paresthesia, somnolence. **Hematologic:** Granulocytopenia (occurs more in children), anemia (more common in children), esosinophilia, neutropenia, thrombocytopenia. **Dermatologic:** Angioedema, bullous eruptions, ulcerative stomatitis, urticaria, rash (may be severe and life-threatening), maculopapular erythematous cutaneous eruptions, pruritus. Possible ***severe, life-threatening skin reactions, including Stevens-Johnson syndrome, toxic epidermal necrolysis, and hypersensitivity reactions.*** **Musculoskeletal:** Myalgia, arthralgia, rhabdomyolysis associated with skin and/or liver reactions. **Hypersensitivity**: Severe rash or rash accompanied by fever, angioedema, general malaise, fatigue, muscle or joint aches, blisters, oral lesions, conjunctivitis, facial edema, hepatitis, eosinophilia, granulocytopenia, lymphadenopathy, renal dysfunction, ***anaphylaxis***, angioedema, bullous eruptions, ulcerative stomatitis, urticaria. **Miscellaneous:** Fever, peripheral neuropathy, opportunistic infections, immune reconstitution syndrome, drug withdrawal. Redistribution/accumulation of body fat, including central obesity, dorsocervical fat enlargement, peripheral wasting, breast enlargement, and "cushingoid appearance."

LABORATORY TEST CONSIDERATIONS

↑ ALT, AST, GGT, alkaline phosphatase, amylase, total bilirubin, LDL, cholesterol, triglycerides. ↓ Hemoglobin, neutrophils, platelets. Abnormal LFTs.

OVERDOSE MANAGEMENT

Symptoms: Edema, erythema nodosum, fatigue, fever, headache, insomnia, nausea, pulmonary infiltrates, rash, vertigo, vomiting, weight loss. *Treatment:* There is no known antidote. Symptoms of overdosage subsided following discontinuation of nevirapine.

DRUG INTERACTIONS

Antiarrhythmics (e.g., amiodarone, disopyramide, systemic lidocaine) / ↓ Plasma levels of antiarrhythmic

Anticonvulsants (e.g., carbamazepine, clonazepam, ethosuximide) / ↓ Plasma levels of anticonvulsant

Cabazitaxel / ↓ Cabazitaxel plasma levels → ↓ pharmacologic effect

Calcium channel blockers (e.g., diltiazem, nifedipine, verapamil) / ↓ Plasma levels of calcium channel blocker
Cisapride / ↓ Plasma levels of cisapride
Clarithromycin / ↓ Clarithromycin levels and ↑ levels of active metabolite (14–OH clarithromycin; consider using azithromycin
Cyclophosphamide / ↓ Plasma levels of cyclophosphamide
Efavirenz / ↓ Efavirenz plasma levels; also, ↑ side effects and no improvement efficacy; do not use together
Ergot alkaloids / ↓ Plasma levels of ergot alkaloids
Exemestane / ↓ Plasma exemestane levels → ↓ pharmacologic effect
Fluconazole / ↑ Nevirapine levels; use together with caution and monitor for side effect
Immunosuppressants (e.g., cyclosporine, sirolimus, tacrolimus) / ↓ Plasma levels of immunosuppressant
Itraconazole / ↓ Plasma levels of itraconazole; do not use together
Ketoconazole / Significant ↓ ketoconazole levels; do not use together
Lurasidone / ↓ Lurasidone plasma levels → ↓ pharmacologic effect; do not use together
Maraviroc / ↑ Maraviroc plasma levels
Narcotic analgesics (e.g., fentanyl, methadone) / ↓ Fentanyl and methadone levels R/T ↑ metabolism; narcotic withdrawal syndrome reported; ↑ dose of the analgesic
Oral contraceptives / ↓ Estrogen and progestin levels → ↓ effect; use a nonhormonal contraceptive or an additional method of contraception
Protease inhibitors (e.g., atazanavir, darunavir, fosamprenavir, indinavir, lopinavir, nelfinavir, ritonavir, saquinavir) / ↓ Plasma levels and clinical efficacy of protease inhibitors; dosage ↑ may be necessary
Rifabutin / ↑ Rifabutin and metabolites
Rifampin / ↓ Nevirapine plasma levels; possible slight ↑ rifampin AUC; coadministration not recommended
H ***St. John's wort*** / ↓ Nelfinavir levels R/T ↑ hepatic metabolism → loss of virologic response; coadministration not recommended
Tyrosine kinase receptor inhibitors (e.g., lapatinib, nilotinib, pazopanib) / ↓ Tyrosine kinase receptor plasma levels → ↓ pharmacologic effect
Warfarin / Possible ↑ anticoagulant activity; monitor coagulation parameters and adjust dose if necessary
Zidovudine / ↓ Zidovudine AUC and C_{max}; monitor clinical response and adjust zidovudine dose if needed

HOW SUPPLIED

Suspension: 50 mg/5 mL; *Tablets:* 200 mg; *Tablets, Extended-Release:* 400 mg.

DOSAGE

SUSPENSION; TABLETS

HIV-1 infections.

Adults, initial: 200 mg/day of the immediate-release tablet for the first 14 days; use this lead-in period to lessen the frequency of rash. **Maintenance:** 200 mg twice a day of the immediate-release tablets (e.g., 7:00 a.m. and 7:00 p.m.) or 400 mg/day of the extended-release tablet in combination with a nucleoside analogue antiretroviral agent. **Children, 15 days and older, initial:** 150 mg/m² once a day for 14 days; **maintenance:** 150 mg/m² twice a day, up to a maximum dose of 400 mg/day.

NURSING IMPLICATIONS

Do not confuse nevirapine with nelfinavir (also an antiviral drug).

IMPLEMENTATION/ADMINISTRATION/STORAGE

1. **If nevirapine dosing interrupted for more than 7 days, should restart therapy using one 200-mg tablet daily (150 mg/m² for children) for the first 14 days, followed by 200 mg twice a day or 400 mg of the extended-release tablet once a day (150 mg/m² twice a day for children).**
2. **Discontinue if severe rash or rash accompanied by constitutional findings noted. Clients experiencing rash during the 14-day lead-in period should have their nevirapine dose decreased until the rash has resolved. The total duration of the once-daily lead-in dosing period should not exceed 28 days, at which time an alternative regimen should be considered.**
3. **If symptomatic hepatitis occurs, permanently discontinue nevirapine; do not restart after recovery.**
4. **Shake suspension gently prior to administration. Give entire measured dose of suspension by using an oral dosing syringe or dosing cup.**

If dosing cup used, thoroughly rinse with water and give rinse to client.

5. An additional dose of nevirapine, 200 mg, is given following each dialysis treatment. Clients with a C_{CR} of 20 mL/min or greater do not require any adjustment in nevirapine dosage.
6. Use caution in selecting doses for the elderly due to greater frequency of decreased hepatic, renal, or cardiac function and of concomitant disease or other drug therapy.
7. Store tablets and suspension in a tightly closed bottle at 15–30°C (59–86°F).

ASSESSMENT

1. Note disease onset, symptom characteristics, other agents trialed, outcome. List drugs currently prescribed to ensure none interact unfavorably.
2. Assess closely for any skin rash or liver reactions, hepatitis B or C; monitor for the first 18 weeks of therapy. Do not increase dose if rash evident and stop therapy if not resolved within 28 days.
3. To monitor maternal-fetal outcomes, pregnant women exposed to nevirapine, an antiretroviral pregnancy registry has been established. Register clients by calling 1-800-258-4263.
4. Monitor CBC, CD4 counts, viral load, renal and LFTs. Most serious hepatic side effects occur during the first 12 weeks of therapy. Perform LFTs at least monthly during the first 12 weeks, especially at baseline, before, and 2 weeks after a dose increase. Monitor liver function frequently thereafter. Stop drug and do not resume at the first sign of liver toxicity.

CLIENT/FAMILY TEACHING

1. Drug is not a cure but helps control disease symptoms. Take exactly as directed. Should be taken with other HIV drugs and antiretroviral agent to prevent emergence of resistant viruses.
2. Can be taken with or without food. Swallow ER tablets whole; do not crush, chew, or divide. Shake the suspension gently before administering. If dose skipped, take the next dose as soon as possible; do not double dose.
3. A rash may occur in the first few weeks of therapy; do not increase dosage until rash subsides. Generally a 14-day lead-in period (lower dose) is used to reduce frequency of rash; do not exceed prescribed dose during this period.
4. May notice fat redistribution; report significant appetite loss, blisters, dark or decreased urination, facial swelling, fatigue, general body discomfort or muscle/joint aches, mouth sores, nausea, pale stools, red or inflamed eyelids, severe skin rash or rash accompanied by fever, swollen lymph nodes, tenderness on right side below ribs, or yellowing of skin or eyes.
5. Drug does not prevent transmission through sexual contact or blood contamination. Practice barrier contraception and nonhormonal form of birth control.
6. Avoid OTC agents without provider approval.
7. Keep all F/U to assess response, labs, and for adverse SE.

OUTCOMES/EVALUATE

Improved CD4 cell counts; ↓ viral load

Niacin (Nicotinic acid)

(**NYE**-ah-sin, nih-koh-**TIN**-ick **AH**-sid)

Classification(s): Vitamin B complex

Pregnancy Category: C (if used in doses above the RDA)

OTC: Niacin Flush-Free, Niacin No Flush, Slo-Niacin.

RX: Advicor, Niacor, Niaspan.

Niacinamide (Nicotinamide)

(nye-ah-**SIN**-ah-myd)

Pregnancy Category: C (Pregnancy category A. However, Category C if used in doses higher than the RDA.)

INDICATIONS/USES

Niacin. OTC: (1) Treatment of niacin deficiency. (2) Prevention and treatment of pellagra.

OTC/Rx: (1) Adjunct therapy in adults with very high serum triglycerides (Types IV and V hyperlipidemia) who are at risk of pancreatitis and who do not respond adequately to diet. (2) Adjunct to diet to reduce elevated total and LDL levels in primary hypercholesterolemia when the response to diet and other nonpharmacologic measures alone have been inadequate. (3) Prevention of recurring MI in those with a history of MI and hypercholesterolemia. (4) In combination with a bile acid binding resin to slow progression or promote regression of atherosclerotic disease in those with a history of CAD and hypercholesterolemia.

Niacinamide. (1) Dietary supplement when niacin intake may be inadequate. (2) Prophylaxis and treatment of pellagra. *Investigational:* Treatment of various dermatologic disorders. There is no evidence to support the use of niacin to treat schizophrenia.

ACTION/KINETICS

Action

Niacin (nicotinic acid) and niacinamide are water-soluble, heat-resistant vitamins prepared synthetically. Niacin (after conversion to the active niacinamide) is a component of the coenzymes nicotinamide-adenine dinucleotide and nicotinamide-adenine dinucleotide phosphate, which are essential for oxidation-reduction reactions involved in lipid metabolism, glycogenolysis, and tissue respiration. Deficiency of niacin results in pellagra, the most common symptoms of which are dermatitis, diarrhea, and dementia. In high doses niacin also produces vasodilation.

Niacin, but not nicotinamide, reduces total and LDL cholesterol, triglycerides, and VLDL, and increases HDL cholesterol. Mechanism is unknown but may involve partial inhibition of release of free fatty acids from adipose tissue and increased lipoprotein lipase activity, which may increase the rate of chylomicron triglyceride removal from plasma.

Pharmacokinetics

Niacin is rapidly and extensively absorbed from the GI tract. **Peak serum levels:** 30–60 min, after 1 gram; **t½, elimination:** 20–45 min. About 88% of a PO dose of niacin is eliminated by the kidneys unchanged or as nicotinuric acid.

CONTRAINDICATIONS

Hypersensitivity to niacin or any component of products. Gallbladder disease, gout, arterial bleeding, glaucoma, diabetes, significant or unexplained impaired liver function, active peptic ulcer disease, pregnancy, or lactation, Use of the extended-release tablets and capsules in children.

SPECIAL CONCERNS

- Extended-release niacin may be hepatotoxic.
- Use with caution in those who consume a large amount of alcohol.
- Niacin should be taken only under the supervision of a health care provider in those with heart disease (especially with recurrent chest pain or angina) or who recently suffered a MI (especially if taking nitrates, calcium channel blockers, or adrenergic blocking agents).
- Safety and efficacy not determined in children in doses that exceed the RDA.

SIDE EFFECTS

Most Common

Niacin: Flushing, pruritus, GI distress, redness, itching, tingling.

Niacin. GI: N&V, diarrhea, peptic ulcer activation, abdominal pain, GI distress, dyspepsia, severe hepatic toxicity (including ***fulminating hepatic necrosis*** with high doses). **Dermatologic:** Flushing (begins 20 min after ingestion and lasts 30–60 min), warm feeling, skin rash, pruritus, dry skin, itching and tingling feeling, sweating, keratosis nigricans. **CNS:** Headache, dizziness. **CV:** Hypotension, orthostasis, atrial fibrillation, tachycardia, palpitations. **Respiratory:** Shortness of breath, rhinitis. **Body as a whole:** Chills, edema, pain. **Miscellaneous:** Cystoid macular edema, toxic amblyopia, decreased glucose tolerance, rhabdomyolysis using lipid-altering doses (rare). *NOTE:* Megadoses are accompanied by serious toxicity including the symptoms listed in the preceding as well as liver damage, hyperglycemia, hyperuricemia, arrhythmias, tachycardia, and dermatoses.

Side effects due to Niaspan Extended-Release Tablets. *NOTE:* Use of Niaspan extended-release tablets may also cause the preceding side effects. **GI:** Activation of peptic ulcers and peptic ulceration, jaundice. **CNS:** Dizziness, insomnia. **CV:** Atrial fibrillation, other cardiac arrhythmias, tachycardia, palpitations, orthostasis, syncope, hypotension. **Dermatologic:** Hyperpigmentation, acanthosis nigricans, maculopapular rash, urticaria, dry skin, sweating. **Hematologic:** Slight ↓ platelet count and ↑ PT. **Musculoskeletal:** Myalgia. **Ophthalmic:** Toxic amblyopia, cystoid macular edema. **Body as a whole:** Edema, asthenia, chills, migraine. **Miscellaneous:** Decreased glucose tolerance, gout; increases in serum transaminases,

LDH, fasting glucose, uric acid, total bilirubin, and amylase; reductions in phosphorus.

Side effects due to Niacor Tablets. *NOTE:* Use of Niacor tablets may also cause the preceding side effects. **GI:** Dyspepsia, vomiting, diarrhea, peptic ulceration, jaundice, abnormal LFTs. **CNS:** Headache. **CV:** Atrial fibrillation, other cardiac arrhythmias, orthostasis, hypotension. **Dermatologic:** Mild to severe cutaneous flushing, pruritus, hyperpigmentation, acanthosis nigricans, dry skin. **Ophthalmic:** Toxic amblyopia, cystoid macular edema. **Miscellaneous:** Decreased glucose tolerance, hyperuricemia, gout.

Niacinamide. GI: N&V, diarrhea, abdominal pain, dyspepsia, liver dysfunction at high doses.

LABORATORY TEST CONSIDERATIONS

↑ Uric acid. ↓ Phosphorus levels using doses of 2,000 mg/day. Abnormal LFTs (↑ ALT, AST).

DRUG INTERACTIONS

Alcohol / ↑ Flushing and pruritus; avoid alcohol at the time of nicotinic acid ingestion
Anticoagulants / Small but significant ↓ in platelet counts
Aspirin / ↓ Clearance of nicotinic acid
Chenodiol / ↓ Effect of chenodiol
Cholestyramine/Colestipol / Binds nicotinic acid; 4–6 hr should elapse between ingestion of bile acid-binding resins and ingestion of nicotinic acid
Ganglionic blocking agents / Potentiation of effects of ganglionic blocking agents
HMG-CoA reductase inhibitors / ↑ Risk of myopathy and rhabdomyolysis
Probenecid / Niacin may ↓ uricosuric effect of probenecid
Sulfinpyrazone / Niacin ↓ uricosuric effect of sulfinpyrazone
Sympathetic blocking agents / Additive vasodilating effects → postural hypotension

HOW SUPPLIED

NOTE: Some products designated as OTC may also be available Rx; it is up to distributor discretion. Most products are marketed as nutritional supplements.
OTC: Niacin (Nicotinic acid). ***Capsules:*** 250 mg; ***Capsules, Extended-Release:*** 250 mg, 400 mg; ***Capsules, Sustained-Release:*** 125 mg, 500 mg; ***Capsules, Timed-Release:*** 250 mg, 500 mg; ***Tablets:*** 50 mg, 100 mg, 250 mg, 400 mg, 500 mg; ***Tablets, Controlled-Release:*** 250 mg, 500 mg, 750 mg; ***Tablets, Extended-Release:*** 50 mg, 750 mg, 1,000 mg; ***Tablets, Sustained-Release:*** 500 mg; ***Tablets, Timed-Release:*** 250 mg, 500 mg.
Niacinamide (Nicotinamide). ***Tablets:*** 100 mg, 500 mg.
Rx: Niacin (Nicotinic acid). ***Tablets, Immediate-Release (Niacor):*** 500 mg; ***Tablets, Extended-Release (Niaspan):*** 500 mg, 750 mg, 1000 mg.

DOSAGE

Niacin (Nicotinic acid)

OTC: CAPSULES; CAPSULES, EXTENDED-RELEASE; CAPSULES, SUSTAINED-RELEASE; CAPSULES, TIMED-RELEASE; TABLETS; TABLETS, SUSTAINED-RELEASE; TABLETS, TIMED-RELEASE

RDA for niacin.

Adult males: 15–20 mg; **adult females:** 13–15 mg.

Pellagra.

Up to 500 mg/day.

Hyperlipidemia.

One to two grams 2 or 3 times per day, not to exceed 6 grams/day.

OTC: TABLETS, CONTROLLED-RELEASE (SLO-NIACIN)

Adults: One 250- or 500-mg tablet morning or evening, or as directed by provider. Or, one-half a 750 mg tablet morning or evening or as directed by provider. Consult provider before using more than 500 mg daily.

RX: TABLETS, IMMEDIATE-RELEASE (NIACOR)

Hyperlipidemia.

Adults: 1–2 grams 2–3 times per day. Individualize the dose depending on client response. Initiate at 250 mg as a single dose following the evening meal. The frequency of dosing and total daily dose may be increased q 4–7 days until the desired LDL or triglyceride level is reached or the first-level therapeutic dose of 1.5–2 grams/day is reached. If hyperlipidemia is not controlled adequately after 2 months at this level, increase dosage at 2- to 4-week intervals to 1 gram 3 times per day. Do not exceed 6 grams/day.

RX: TABLETS, EXTENDED-RELEASE (NIASPAN)

Hyperlipidemia.

Initial: 500 mg at bedtime (to reduce incidence and severity of side effects). Escalate dose as follows: **Weeks 1–4:** 500 mg (one Niaspan 500 mg tablet) at bedtime; **weeks 5–8:** 1,000 mg (two Niaspan 500 mg tablets at bedtime). **After 8 weeks:** Titrate to client response and tolerance. If response to 1,000 mg/day is inadequate, increase the dose to 1,500 mg/day (two Niaspan 750 mg tablets or three Niaspan 500 mg tablets at bedtime). The dose may subsequently be increased to 2,000 mg/day (two Niaspan 1,000 mg tablets or four Niaspan 500 mg tablets at bedtime). Doses above 2,000 mg/day are not recommended. Women may respond to lower doses. Do not increase the daily dose of Niaspan by more than 500 mg in any 4-week period.

Niacinamide

OTC: TABLETS

RDA for niacinamide.

Individualize dosage. **RDA, males, 14 years and older:** 16 mg/day; **RDA, females, 14 years and older:** 14 mg/day. **RDA, children 1–3 years of age:** 6 mg/day; **children, 4–8 years of age:** 8 mg/day; **children, 9–13 years of age:** 12 mg/day. **RDA, during pregnancy:** 18 mg/day; **during lactation:** 17 mg/day. **Supplemental dosage:** 20–100 mg/day.

Niacinamide deficiency.

Dose determined by provider determined by severity of the deficiency.

NURSING IMPLICATIONS

IMPLEMENTATION/ADMINISTRATION/STORAGE

1. Before starting therapy with niacin, attempt to control hyperlipidemia with appropriate diet, exercise, and weight reduction in obese clients. Also, treat other underlying medical conditions.
2. Do not substitute sustained-release niacin products for equivalent doses of immediate-release niacin.
3. To reduce flushing associated with niacin therapy, start by slowly increasing the dose by 100 mg 3 times a day each week. Flushing can be reduced with aspirin or NSAIDs. Tolerance to flushing occurs rapidly over the course of several weeks.
4. Niacin, 100 mg/day, plus a statin may increase HDL levels.
5. Store nicotinic acid from 20–25°C (68–77°F). Store Niacor and Slo-Niacin from 15–30°C (59–86°F).

ASSESSMENT

1. Note reasons for therapy, other agents trialed, outcome. Note any history of CAD, PUD, liver or gallbladder dysfunction.
2. Assess diet, exercise, and lifestyle changes necessary to decrease coronary risk factors and if trialed.
3. If and when used with statins, monitor LFTs closely; both utilize same metabolic pathway.
4. With the extended-release tablets, titrate up and advise to take at bedtime with an ASA or small snack to diminish side effects (flushing/hot flashes).
5. If also taking a bile acid sequestrant (e.g., cholestyramine) instruct to take niacin at least 2 hr before or 4 hr or more after the sequestrant.
6. Monitor glucose, HbA1c, LFTs, CPK, uric acid, and cholesterol panel.

CLIENT/FAMILY TEACHING

1. Take tablet with cold water (no hot beverages) at bedtime after a low-fat snack. Swallow tablet whole; may be broken if scored; do not crush or chew.
2. May experience a warm flushing in the face and ears within 2 hr after taking. To prevent/reduce, take one aspirin (325 mg) or a small low-fat snack 30–60 min prior to dosing. Hot showers, exercise, hot/spicy foods, and alcohol may increase these effects.
3. If awakened during the night with flushing, rise slowly to reduce the risk of dizziness or fainting.
4. Lie down if feeling weak and dizzy after taking niacin (until this feeling passes), avoid activi-

N

ties that require mental alertness and report if feeling persists.

5. Identify food sources high in niacin (dairy products, meats, tuna, and eggs); assess consumption. No unsupervised excessive vitamin ingestion; high doses may impair liver function.
6. With diabetes, avoid niacin unless specifically ordered; monitor BS levels closely for hyperglycemia; monitor urine for ketonuria and glucosuria. Antidiabetic agents may require adjustment.
7. With elevated triglycerides, continue dietary restrictions (fat, cholesterol, alcohol, and CHO), regular exercise, smoking cessation to accomplish desired goal.
8. Report any skin color changes, abdominal pain, or yellowing of the sclera. Avoid alcohol.
9. Clients predisposed to gout may experience flank, joint, or stomach pains; report immediately.
10. Report if blurred vision or skin lesions occur, remain out of direct sunlight.
11. Keep all F/U visits to assess response, labs, and for adverse SE.

OUTCOMES/EVALUATE

- ↓ Triglyceride, apolipoprotein B (Apo B), LDL, and total cholesterol levels
- ↑ HDL cholesterol
- Relief of symptoms of pellagra and niacin deficiency

IV

Nicardipine hydrochloride

(nye-**KAR**-dih-peen)

Classification(s): Calcium channel blocker

Pregnancy Category: C

RX: Cardene I.V., Cardene SR.

SEE ALSO ***CALCIUM CHANNEL BLOCKING AGENTS***.

INDICATIONS/USES

Immediate-release: Chronic stable angina (effort-associated angina) alone or in combination with beta-adrenergic blocking agents.

Immediate- and sustained-release: Hypertension alone or in combination with other antihypertensive drugs.

IV: Short-term treatment of hypertension when PO therapy is not desired or possible. For prolonged BP control, transfer clients to PO therapy as soon as possible.

ACTION/KINETICS

Action

Moderately increases CO and HR and significantly decreases peripheral vascular resistance. Slight increase in QT interval and slight to no decrease in myocardial contractility. No effect on QRS complex or PR interval.

Pharmacokinetics

Nearly 100% absorbed. **Onset of action:** 20 min. **Maximum plasma levels:** 30–120 min. Significant first-pass metabolism. Food (especially fats) will decrease the amount of drug absorbed from the GI tract. Steady-state plasma levels are reached after 2–3 days of therapy. **Therapeutic serum levels:** 0.028–0.050 mcg/mL. **t½, at steady state:** 8.6 hr. **Maximum BP-lowering effects, immediate-release:** 1–2 hr; **maximum BP-lowering effects, sustained-release:** 2–6 hr. **Duration:** 8 hr. Metabolized by the liver with excretion through both the urine and feces. **Plasma protein binding:** More than 95%.

CONTRAINDICATIONS

Use in advanced aortic stenosis due to the effect on reducing afterload. Lactation.

SPECIAL CONCERNS

- Use with caution in clients with CHF, especially in combination with a beta blocker (possible negative inotropic effect).
- Use with caution in clients with severely impaired liver function, reduced hepatic blood flow, or impaired renal function.
- Initial increase in frequency, duration, or severity of angina.
- Use caution in dose selection in the elderly.
- Safety and efficacy not established in children less than 18 years of age.

SIDE EFFECTS

Most Common

Flushing, increased angina, hypotension, palpitations, tachycardia, vasodilation, anxiety, dizziness, lightheadedness, headache, N&V.

CV: Pedal edema, flushing, increased angina, palpitations, vasodilation, tachycardia, other edema, abnormal ECG, hypotension, postural hypotension, syncope, ***MI, AV block***, ventricular extrasystoles, PVD. **CNS:** Dizziness, lightheadedness, headache, somnolence, malaise, nervousness, insomnia, abnormal dreams, vertigo, depression, confusion, amnesia, anxiety, weakness, psychoses, hallucinations, paranoia. **GI:** N&V, dyspepsia, dry mouth, constipation, sore throat. **Neuromuscular:** Asthenia, myalgia, paresthesia, hyperkinesia, arthralgia. **Miscellaneous:** Rash, dyspnea, SOB, nocturia, polyuria, allergic reactions, abnormal LFTs, hot flashes, impotence, rhinitis, sinusitis, nasal congestion, chest congestion, tinnitus, equilibrium disturbances, abnormal or blurred vision, infection, atypical chest pain.

OVERDOSE MANAGEMENT

Symptoms: Marked hypotension, bradycardia, palpitations, flushing, drowsiness, confusion, and slurred speech following PO overdose. Lethal overdose may cause systemic hypotension, bradycardia (following initial tachycardia) and progressive AV block. *Treatment:*

- Treatment is supportive. Monitor cardiac and respiratory function.
- If client is seen soon after ingestion, emetics or gastric lavage should be considered, followed by cathartics.
- *Hypotension*: IV calcium, dopamine, isoproterenol, metaraminol, or norepinephrine. Also, provide IV fluids. Place client in Trendelenburg position.
- *Ventricular tachycardia*: IV procainamide or lidocaine; cardioversion may be necessary. Also, provide slow-drip IV fluids.
- *Bradycardia, asystole, AV block*: IV atropine sulfate (0.6–1 mg), calcium gluconate (10% solution), isoproterenol, norepinephrine; also, cardiac pacing may be indicated. Provide slow-drip IV fluids.

DRUG INTERACTIONS

Beta-blockers / Additive or synergistic effects; possible ↓ metabolism of certain beta-blockers
Cimetidine / ↑ Bioavailability of nicardipine → ↑ plasma levels
Cyclosporine / ↑ Plasma levels of cyclosporine possibly leading to renal toxicity
Grapefruit juice / ↑ Bioavailability of nicardipine R/T ↓ liver metabolism of nicardipine in the gut wall
Ranitidine / ↑ Bioavailability of nicardipine
Rifampin / ↓ Nicardipine effects

HOW SUPPLIED

Capsules, Immediate-Release: 20 mg, 30 mg; ***Capsules, Sustained-Release:*** 30 mg, 45 mg, 60 mg; ***Injection Solution:*** 2.5 mg/mL.

DOSAGE

CAPSULES, IMMEDIATE-RELEASE

Angina, hypertension.

Individualize. Adults, initial, usual: 20 mg 3 times per day (range: 20–40 mg 3 times per day). Wait 3 days before increasing dose to ensure steady-state plasma levels. The maximum BP-lowering effect occurs about 1–2 hr after dosing.

CAPSULES, SUSTAINED-RELEASE

Hypertension.

Individualize. Adults, initial: 30 mg twice a day (range: 30–60 mg twice a day). The maximum BP-lowering effect at steady state is sustained 2–6 hr after dosing.

IV

Hypertension.

Individualize dose. Initial: 5 mg/hr; if using the premixed injection, 0.1 mg/mL, give 50 mL/hr; if using the premixed injection, 0.2 mg/mL, give 25 mL/hr; if using vials (each vial containing 25 mg in 10 mL must be diluted with 240 mL of a compatible IV diluent, resulting in 250 mL of a solution containing 0.1 mg/mL), give 50 mL/hr. **Maximum dose:** 15 mg/hr (150 mL/hr) of the 0.1 mg/mL premixed injection; 15 mg/hr (75 mL/hr) of the 0.2 mg/mL premixed injection; and, 15 mg/hr (150 mL/hr of the diluted vial–see above).

NURSING IMPLICATIONS

Do not confuse nicardipine with nimodipine or nifedipine (also calcium channel blockers). Also, do not confuse Cardene with Cardura or Cardizem (also calcium channel blockers).

IMPLEMENTATION/ADMINISTRATION/STORAGE

1. Initial dose in renal impairment: 20 mg 3 times per day of immediate-release or 30 mg twice a day for sustained-release. Initial dose

of immediate-release capsules in hepatic impairment: 20 mg twice a day. The sustained-release capsules have not been studied in severe liver impairment.
2. The total daily dose of immediate-release capsules may not be a useful guide in judging the effective dose of the sustained-release product. Clients currently taking the immediate-release form may be titrated with the extended-release form starting at their current total daily dose of nicardipine immediate-release and then reexamined to assess adequacy of BP control.
3. When used for treating angina, may be given safely along with SL nitroglycerin, long-acting nitrates, or beta blockers.
4. When used to treat hypertension, may be given safely along with diuretics or beta blockers.
5. During initial therapy and when dosage is increased, may experience an increase in frequency, duration, or severity of angina.
6. If transfer to PO antihypertensives other than nicardipine is planned, initiate therapy after discontinuing infusion. If PO nicardipine is used at a dosage regimen of three times daily, give the first dose 1 hr prior to discontinuing infusion.
7. Store capsules from 15–30°C (59–86°F).
8. IV Administer by slow continuous IV infusion. Change the infusion site q 12 hr if given via a peripheral vein.
9. If using the premixed injection, do not use plastic containers in series connection as this could result in air embolism due to residual air being drawn from the primary container before administration of the fluid from the secondary container is complete.
10. If transferring from PO nicardipine to IV infusion therapy of nicardipine, use the following equivalents: 20 mg q 8 hr is equivalent to 0.5 mg/hr IV; 30 mg q 8 hr is equivalent to 1.2 mg/hr; and, 40 mg q 8 hr is equivalent to 2.2 mg/hr.
11. When treating acute hypertensive episodes in clients with chronic hypertension, discontinuation of the infusion is followed by a 50% offset of action in about 30 min; however, plasma levels of the drug and gradually decreasing antihypertensive effects exist for about 50 hr.
12. If there is concern of impending hypotension or tachycardia, discontinue the infusion. When BP has stabilized, the infusion may be restarted at low doses as follows: (a) 30–50 mL/hr (3–5 mg/hr) using the premixed solution, 0.1 mg/mL; (b) 15–25 mL/hr (3–5 mg/hr) using the premixed solution, 0.2 mg/mL/mL; (c) 30–50 mL/hr (3–5 mg/hr) using the diluted solution (0.1 mg/mL) from vials. Adjust to maintain BP.
13. Continue IV use as long as BP control is needed. Change the infusion site q 12 hr if given via a peripheral vein.
14. **Dose titration with the premixed injection, 0.1 mg/mL:** If the desired BP decrease is not achieved at the initial dose, the infusion rate may be increased by 25 mL/hr (2.5 mg/hr) q 15 min until the desired BP is reached. For more rapid BP reduction, initiate therapy at 50 mL/hr (5 mg/hr). If the desired BP decrease is not reached at this dose, the infusion rate may be increased by 25 mL/hr (2.5 mg/hr) q 5 min until the desired BP is achieved. Following achievement of the BP goal, decrease the infusion rate to 30 mL/hr (3 mg/hr).
15. **Dose titration with the premixed injection, 0.2 mg/mL:** If the desired BP decrease is not achieved at the initial dose, the infusion rate may be increased by 12.5 mL/hr (2.5 mg/hr) q 15 min until the desired BP is reached. For a more rapid BP reduction, initiate therapy at 25 mL/hr (5 mg/hr). If the desired BP decrease is not reached at this dose, the infusion rate may be increased by 12.5 mL/hr (2.5 mg/hr) q 5 min until the desired BP is achieved. Following achievement of the BP goal, decrease the infusion rate to 15 mL/hr (3 mg/hr).
16. **Dose titration using vials (i.e., diluted to 0.1 mg/mL):** If the desired BP decrease is not achieved at the initial dose, the infusion rate may be increased by 25 mL/hr (2.5 mg/hr) q 15 min until the desired BP response is achieved. For more rapid BP reduction, titrate q 5 min.
17. The diluted product is stable at room temperature for 24 hr.
18. The premixed container is for single-use only; discard any unused portion.

19. Store ampules at room temperature. Protect from freezing although freezing does not affect the product in vials. Protect ampules from light and excessive heat. Store ampules in their carton until used.
20. COMPATIBILITY Stable in polyvinyl chloride containers for 24 hr at controlled room temperature with D5W, D5/0.9% NaCl, D5W + 40 mEq KCL, 0.9% NaCl, and 0.45% NaCl solutions.
21. INCOMPATIBILITY Do not combine with any product in the same IV line or premixed container. Sodium bicarbonate 5% injection or lactated Ringer's injection.

ASSESSMENT

1. Note reasons for therapy, other agents prescribed, outcome.
2. Assess for CAD, and angina; use with caution. With angina note onset, location, duration, and precipitating factors. Avoid with CHF.
3. List drugs prescribed to ensure none interact.
4. Monitor VS. When the immediate-release product is used for hypertension, maximum lowering of BP occurs 1–2 hr after dosing. Evaluate BP at trough (8 hr after dosing). When the sustained-release product is used, maximum lowering of BP occurs 2–6 hr after dosing. Monitor BP frequently during and following IV infusion. Avoid too rapid or excessive decrease in BP and discontinue infusion if significant hypotension or tachycardia.
5. Monitor BP, ECG, I&O, Wt, K^+, renal and LFTs; note any dysfunction and follow reduced dosing guidelines.

CLIENT/FAMILY TEACHING

1. Take at the same time each day. Swallow sustained-release capsules whole; do not crush or chew.
2. Avoid activities that require mental alertness until drug effects realized.
3. Report any persistent/bothersome side effects such as dizziness, flushing, increased chest pain, SOB, weight gain, or swelling of extremities. Maintain proper intake of fluids to avoid constipation. Avoid alcohol; limit caffeine.
4. Record BP and HR.
5. Anginal attacks may persist up to 30 min following drug ingestion due to reflex tachycardia; use nitrates as prescribed. Do not stop taking drug abruptly.
6. Report any change in psychologic state (i.e., depression, anxiety, sleep problems, or decreased mental acuity). Particularly important when working with elderly clients since there is a tendency to misdiagnose as senility.
7. With BP control, maintain healthy diet and limit intake of caffeine; avoid alcohol, salt substitutes, or high Na^+ and high K^+ foods; perform regular exercise; maintain weight; and stop smoking.
8. Keep all F/U to assess response, labs, and for adverse SE.

OUTCOMES/EVALUATE

- Control of hypertension
- ↓ Frequency/intensity of anginal attacks

Nicotine inhalation system

(**NIK**-oh-teen)

Classification(s): Smoking deterrent

Pregnancy Category: D

RX: Nicotrol Inhaler.

Nicotine nasal spray

Pregnancy Category: D

RX: Nicotrol NS.

SEE ALSO ***NICOTINE POLACRILEX***.

INDICATIONS/USES

As an aid in smoking cessation for the relief of nicotine withdrawal symptoms. Both products are to be used as part of a comprehensive behavioral smoking cessation program.

ACTION/KINETICS

Action

The nicotine from the inhalation system or spray provides blood levels of nicotine approximating those produced by smoking cigarettes.

Pharmacokinetics

Time to peak levels, inhalation system or nasal spray: 15 min. **Peak plasma levels, inhalation system:** 6 ng/mL; **nasal spray:** 12 ng/mL. **t½, inhalation system:** Not determined; **nasal spray:** 1–2 hr. Nicotine is rapidly and extensively metabolized by the liver; excreted in the urine.

N

CONTRAINDICATIONS

Not recommended for use during lactation even though nicotine levels in breast milk are lower with inhaler or spray therapy, when used as directed, compared with cigarette smoking. Use of the nasal spray in severe reactive airway disease (e.g., asthma, bronchospasm).

SPECIAL CONCERNS

- **Use the inhaler with caution in those with bronchospastic disease.**
- **Safety and efficacy not evaluated in children/adolescents less than 18 years of age who smoke.**

SIDE EFFECTS

Most Common

Use of the inhaler: Irritation of mouth/throat, coughing, rhinitis, dyspepsia, headache.

Use of the nasal spray: Irritation of mouth/throat, headache, back pain, dyspnea, nausea, arthralgia, menstrual disorder, palpitations, flatulence, tooth/gum disorder.

INHALER. Respiratory: Irritation of mouth/throat, coughing, rhinitis, sinusitis. **GI:** Dyspepsia, taste/tooth disorders, flatulence, nausea, diarrhea, hiccough. **CNS:** Headache, paresthesia. **Miscellaneous:** Pain in jaw/neck/back, flu-like symptoms, fever, allergy. **Withdrawal from nicotine:** Dizziness, anxiety, sleep disorder, depression, drug dependence, fatigue, myalgia. **Smoking-related symptoms:** Chest discomfort, bronchitis, hypertension.

NASAL SPRAY. Respiratory: Irritation of mouth/throat, dyspnea, bronchitis, bronchospasm, increased sputum. **GI:** Nausea, flatulence, tooth/gum disorder, abdominal pain, dry mouth, hiccough, diarrhea. **CNS:** Headache, confusion, aphasia, amnesia, migraine, numbness, calming. **CV:** Palpitations, peripheral edema. **Musculoskeletal:** Arthralgia, myalgia, back pain. **Miscellaneous:** Menstrual disorder, pain, allergy, purpura, rash, abnormal vision, feelings of dependence. **Withdrawal from nicotine:** Anxiety, irritability, restlessness, cravings, dizziness, impaired concentration, emotional lability, somnolence, fatigue, increased weight/appetite/dreaming/sweating, insomnia, confusion, depression, apathy, tremor, incoordination. **Smoking-related symptoms:** Chest tightness, dyspepsia, paresthesia in limbs, constipation, stomatitis.

HOW SUPPLIED

Nicotine inhalation system (Nicotrol Inhaler). *Inhaler:* 4 mg delivered (10 mg/cartridge). **Nicotine nasal spray (Nicotrol NS).** *Spray Pump:* 0.5 mg/actuation (10 mg/mL).

DOSAGE

Nicotine inhalation system (Nicotrol Inhaler)

INHALER

Smoking deterrent.

Individualize initial dose; clients may self-titrate to the level of nicotine they require. **Usual:** Between 6 and 16 cartridges/day. The best effect occurs by frequent continuous puffing (20 minutes). **Recommended duration:** 3 months, after which clients may be weaned from the inhaler by gradual reduction of the daily dose over 6–12 weeks. *NOTE:* The goal of inhaler therapy is complete abstinence. If a client is unable to stop smoking by the fourth week of therapy, discontinue use of the inhaler.

Nicotine nasal spray (Nicotrol NS)

SPRAY PUMP

Smoking deterrent.

Each actuation delivers a metered 50 mcL spray containing 0.5 mg nicotine; one dose is 1 mg of nicotine (2 sprays, 1 in each nostril). **Initial dose:** 1 or 2 doses/hr, which may be increased up to a maximum recommended dose of 40 mg (80 sprays) per day. Clients should use at least the recommended minimum of 8 doses/day, as less is likely to be ineffective. **Maximum duration of treatment:** 3 months with a maximum of 5 doses/hr and 40 doses/day. *NOTE:* Clients should stop smoking completely when they begin using the spray. If the client is unable to stop smoking by the fourth week of therapy, discontinue use of the nasal spray.

NURSING IMPLICATIONS

IMPLEMENTATION/ADMINISTRATION/STORAGE

INHALER:

1. Encourage clients to use at least 6 cartridges/day for the first 3–6 weeks of treatment. Regular use of the inhaler during the first week of treatment may help clients adapt to the irritant effects of the product.
2. With the inhaler, some clients may exhibit S&S of nicotine withdrawal or excess that will require dosage adjustment.
3. After using the inhaler, carefully separate the mouthpiece, remove the used cartridge, and throw it away, out of the reach of children and pets. Store the mouthpiece in the plastic storage case for further use. Clean mouthpiece regularly with soap and water.
4. Store the inhaler at room temperature not to exceed 25°C (77°F). Protect from light.

NASAL SPRAY:

1. No tapering strategy has been developed for the nasal spray. Recommended procedure for discontinuation of use include: Use only half a dose (1 spray at a time); use the spray less frequently; keep a tally of daily usage; try to meet a steadily reducing usage target; skip a dose by not medicating every hour; and, set a planned "quit date" for stopping use of the spray.
2. Regular use of the spray during the first week of treatment may help clients adapt to the irritant effects.
3. Those who are successfully abstinent on the nasal spray should be treated at the selected dosage for up to 8 weeks; then, discontinue the spray over the next 4–6 weeks. Safety of the spray has not been established for more than 6 months of use.
4. If the spray pump is dropped and breaks, clean up the spill immediately with an absorbent cloth/paper towel. Avoid contact of the solution with the skin; wash the area several times. Should even a small amount of the solution come in contact with the skin, lips, mouth, eyes, or ears, immediately rinse the affected area with water.
5. Dispose of used bottles in a way so as to prevent access by children or pets.
6. Store the nasal spray at room temperature not to exceed 30°C (86°F).

ASSESSMENT

1. Note onset/duration of addiction, readiness to quit, amount consumed, other agents trialed, outcome.
2. Assess for any conditions that may preclude therapy: severe COPD/CAD, recent MI, severe chest pain/arrhythmia.
3. Have formal smoking cessation program available to provide support and encouragement to ensure success.

CLIENT/FAMILY TEACHING

1. For spray: Do not sniff, swallow, or inhale through the nose as the spray is being administered. Administer spray with the head tilted back slightly. Dose is 8–40 doses/day for 3–6 months.
2. Use Nicotine Spray whenever you feel the urge to smoke.
3. With inhaler, therapy consists of a mouthpiece and a plastic cartridge delivering 4 mg of nicotine from a porous plug containing 10 mg nicotine. The cartridge is inserted into the mouthpiece prior to use. Continuously puff on mouthpiece (approximately 20 minutes). Discard used container in safe place.
4. Clean mouthpiece regularly with soap and water; store mouthpiece in plastic case between uses.
5. Stop smoking completely when initiating Nicotrol Inhaler or spray therapy; if smoking continues, may experience adverse effects due to peak nicotine levels higher than those experienced from smoking alone. If clinically significant increase in cardiovascular or other effects attributable to nicotine, stop treatment. Other medications may also need dosage adjustment
6. May experience mild irritation of the mouth or throat and cough when you first use the Nicotrol Inhaler; should subside with use. Stomach upset may occur.
7. Do not use more than 16 cartridges each day or longer than 6 months.
8. Store cartridges at room temperature, not to exceed 77°F (25°C). If you keep cartridges in car, use care as interiors heat up quickly. Protect from light.
9. Store spray and cartridges away from children or pets; dispose of properly.
10. Attempt to stop smoking completely when beginning to use products; attend smoking cessation therapy program and keep all F/U to assess response and for adverse SE.

OUTCOMES/EVALUATE

Smoking cessation aid; control of S&S nicotine withdrawal symptoms

Nicotine polacrilex (Nicotine resin complex)

(**NIK**-oh-teen)

Classification(s): Smoking deterrent

Pregnancy Category: C

OTC: Commit, Nicorette, Nicotine Gum, Thrive.

INDICATIONS/USES

Adjunct with behavioral modification in smokers wishing to give up the smoking habit in those 18 years and older. Is considered only as an initial aid, with the ultimate goal being abstention from all forms of nicotine. Most likely to benefit are individuals with the following characteristics: (a) smoke brands of cigarettes containing more than 0.9 mg nicotine; (b) smoke more than 15 cigarettes daily; (c) inhale cigarette smoke deeply and frequently; (d) smoke most frequently during the morning; (e) smoke the first cigarette of the day within 30 min of arising; (f) indicate cigarettes smoked in the morning are the most difficult to give up; (g) smoke even if the individual is ill and confined to bed; (h) find it necessary to smoke in places where smoking is not allowed. *NOTE:* Nicotine may be effective in improving the course of difficult-to-treat ulcerative colitis.

ACTION/KINETICS

Action

Following chewing, nicotine is released from an ion exchange resin in the gum product, providing blood nicotine levels approximating those produced by smoking cigarettes.

Pharmacokinetics

The amount of nicotine released depends on the rate and duration of chewing. **Time to peak levels:** 15–30 min. **Peak plasma levels:** 5–10 ng/mL. If the gum is swallowed, only a minimum amount of nicotine is released. **t½:** 3–4 hr. Metabolized mainly by the liver, with about 10–20% excreted unchanged in the urine.

CONTRAINDICATIONS

Pregnancy, lactation, nonsmokers, serious arrhythmias, angina, vasospastic disease, MI, active temporomandibular joint disease. Use in individuals less than 18 years of age.

SPECIAL CONCERNS

- **Safety and efficacy not determined in children and adolescents who smoke.**
- **Use with caution in hypertension, PUD, oral or pharyngeal inflammation, gastritis, stomatitis, hyperthyroidism, IDDM, and pheochromocytoma.**

SIDE EFFECTS

Most Common

Sore mouth/throat, nausea, salivation, dizziness.

CNS: Dizziness, irritability, headache. **GI:** N&V, indigestion, GI upset, salivation, eructation. **Miscellaneous:** Sore mouth or throat, hiccoughs, sore jaw muscles.

OVERDOSE MANAGEMENT

Symptoms: **GI:** N&V, diarrhea, salivation, abdominal pain. **CNS:** Headache, dizziness, confusion, weakness, fainting, ***seizures***. **Respiratory:** Labored breathing, ***respiratory paralysis (cause of death)***. **Other:** Cold sweat, disturbed hearing and vision, hypotension, and rapid, weak pulse. *Treatment:* Institute gastric lavage and/or activated charcoal. Maintenance of respiration, maintenance of CV function.

DRUG INTERACTIONS

Caffeine / Possibly ↓ caffeine blood levels R/T ↑ rate of liver breakdown
Catecholamines / ↑ Catecholamine levels
Cortisol / ↑ Cortisol levels
Furosemide / Possible ↓ diuretic effect of furosemide
Imipramine / Possibly ↓ imipramine blood levels R/T ↑ rate of liver breakdown
Pentazocine / Possibly ↓ pentazocine blood levels R/T ↑ rate of liver breakdown
Theophylline / Possibly ↓ theophylline blood levels R/T ↑ rate of liver breakdown

HOW SUPPLIED

Gum: 2 mg/square, 4 mg/square; ***Lozenges:*** 2 mg/lozenge, 4 mg/lozenge. *NOTE:* Some are mint flavored.

DOSAGE

GUM

Smoking deterrent.

If the client smokes less than 25 cigarettes/day, start with the 2 mg nicotine gum. If the client smokes more than 25 cigarettes/day, start with the 4 mg nicotine gum. **Weeks 1–6:** 1 piece of gum q 2 hr; **Weeks 7–9:** 1 piece of gum q 2–4 hr; **Weeks 10–12:** 1 piece of gum q 4–8 hr.

LOZENGES

Smoking deterrent.

If first cigarette is smoked more than 30 min after waking, start with the 2 mg lozenge. If the first cigarette is smoked within 30 min of waking, start with the 4 mg lozenge. **Weeks 1–6:** 1 lozenge q 2 hr; **Weeks 7–9:** 1 lozenge q 2–4 hr; **Weeks 10–12:** 1 lozenge q 4–8 hr.

NURSING IMPLICATIONS

IMPLEMENTATION/ADMINISTRATION/STORAGE

1. All products are over-the-counter.
2. Client must stop smoking completely when beginning to use the gum.
3. Those who smoke more than 25 cigarettes/day should be started on the 4-mg dose.
4. Have client chew gum slowly until it tingles; then, park it between the cheek and gum. When the tingle is gone, have client begin chewing again until the tingle returns. Repeat the process until most of the tingle is gone (about 30 min).
5. Advise client to place the lozenge in the mouth and allow it to dissolve slowly (20–30 min). Minimize swallowing. Client should not chew or swallow the lozenge. A warm or tingling sensation may be felt. Advise to occasionally move the lozenge from one side of the mouth to the other.
6. Advise client not to eat or drink for 15 min before chewing the nicotine gum or while using the lozenge.
7. To improve chances of quitting, have client chew at least 9 pieces/day for the first 6 weeks. If there are strong and frequent cravings, use a second piece within the hour. Do not have client use continuously 1 piece after the other as hiccoughs, heartburn, nausea, and other side effects may occur.
8. Do not use more than 24 pieces/day. Stop using nicotine gum at the end of 12 weeks.
9. After gum has been chewed, place used chewing pieces in a wrapper and dispose so that children or pets cannot obtain them.
10. If the lozenge must be removed, wrap in paper and dispose in the trash. Lozenges have enough nicotine to make pets and children ill.

ASSESSMENT

1. Note nicotine profile: type and brand (cigarettes, chewing tobacco, or cigars), amount used per day, readiness to quit, when used, and what triggers/increases usage.
2. List any temporomandibular joint syndrome or cardiac arrhythmia; precludes gum therapy.

CLIENT/FAMILY TEACHING

1. Must want to stop smoking and be willing to do so immediately.
2. Avoid activities, persons, and locations that stimulate the desire to smoke (i.e., drinking, bars, smokers).
3. With lozenge, place in mouth and allow to dissolve slowly. Do not chew or swallow. Move from side to side in mouth until dissolved; may feel a warm tingly sensation.
4. Use gum only as directed. When the urge to smoke occurs, chew one piece at a time, slowly and chew intermittently for about 30 min. If a slight tingling becomes evident, stop chewing until sensation subsides. Has a tobacco pepper like taste.
5. Acidic beverages, such as coffee, juices, soft drinks, and wine, interfere with buccal absorption of nicotine; thus, avoid eating and drinking 15 min before and during chewing.
6. Gum will not stick to dentures or appliances. Gradually decrease the number of pieces chewed per day; may take up to 3 months to be completely free of nicotine.
7. Dispose of unit carefully (wrap in paper) and keep out of the reach of children. May be harmful to pregnant woman and/or fetus.
8. Identify individuals and local support groups that can help with smoking cessation and provide emotional and psychologic support throughout the endeavor. Participate in formal smoking program.
9. Keep all F/U to assess response, need for additional counselling, and for adverse SE.

N

OUTCOMES/EVALUATE
Control of nicotine withdrawal symptoms with smoking cessation

Nicotine transdermal system

(**NIK**-oh-teen)

Classification(s): Smoking deterrent

Pregnancy Category: D

OTC: Nicoderm CQ Step 1, Step 2, and Step 3, Nicotine Transdermal System Step 1, Step 2, and Step 3, Nicotrol Step 1, Step 2, and Step 3.

INDICATIONS/USES
As an aid to stopping smoking for the relief of nicotine withdrawal symptoms in those 18 years and older. Should be used in conjunction with a comprehensive behavioral smoking cessation program.

ACTION/KINETICS
Action
Nicotine transdermal system is a multilayered film that provides systemic delivery of varying amounts of nicotine over a 24-hr period after applying to the skin. Nicotine's reinforcing activity is due to stimulation of the cortex (via the locus ceruleus), producing increased alertness and cognitive performance and a "reward" effect due to an action in the limbic system. At low doses the stimulatory effects predominate, whereas at high doses the reward effects predominate. The nicotine transdermal system produces an initial (first day of use) increase in BP, an increase in HR (3–7%), and a decrease in SV after 10 days.

Pharmacokinetics
Time to peak levels: 2–12 hr. **Peak plasma levels:** 5–17 ng/mL. **t½:** 3–4 hr. Metabolized in the liver to a large number of metabolites, all of which are less active than nicotine.

CONTRAINDICATIONS
Hypersensitivity or allergy to nicotine or any components of the therapeutic system. Use in children and during pregnancy, labor, delivery, and lactation. Use in those with heart disease, hypertension, a recent MI, severe or worsening angina pectoris, those taking certain antidepressants or antiasthmatic drugs, or in severe renal impairment.

SPECIAL CONCERNS
- **Encourage pregnant smokers to try to stop smoking using educational and behavioral interventions before using the nicotine transdermal system.**
- **Use during pregnancy only if the potential benefit outweighs the potential risk of nicotine to the fetus.**
- **Use for longer than 3 months has not been studied.**
- **Before use, screen clients with coronary heart disease (history of MI and/or angina pectoris), serious cardiac arrhythmias, or vasospastic diseases (e.g., Buerger's disease, Prinzmetal's variant angina) carefully.**
- **Use with caution with hyperthyroidism, pheochromocytoma, IDDM (nicotine causes the release of catecholamines), in active peptic ulcers, in accelerated hypertension, and during lactation.**

SIDE EFFECTS
Most Common
Erythema, pruritus, or burning at site of application; headache.

NOTE: The incidence of side effects is complicated by the fact that clients manifest effects of nicotine withdrawal or by concurrent smoking. **Dermatologic:** Erythema, pruritus, or burning at the site of application; cutaneous hypersensitivity, sweating, rash at application site. **Body as a whole:** Allergy, back pain. **GI:** Diarrhea, dyspepsia, dry mouth, abdominal pain, constipation, N&V. **Musculoskeletal:** Arthralgia, myalgia. **CNS:** Abnormal dreams, somnolence, dizziness, impaired concentration, headache, insomnia. **CV:** Tachycardia, hypertension. **Respiratory:** Increased cough, pharyngitis, sinusitis. **GU:** Dysmenorrhea.

OVERDOSE MANAGEMENT
Symptoms: Pallor, cold sweat, N&V, abdominal pain, salivation, diarrhea, headache, dizziness, disturbed hearing and vision, mental confusion, weakness, tremor. Large overdoses may cause prostration, hypotension, ***respiratory failure, seizures, and death.*** *Treatment:* Remove the transdermal system immediately. The surface of the skin may be flushed with water and dried; soap

should not be used, as it may increase the absorption of nicotine. Diazepam or barbiturates may be used to treat seizures, and atropine can be given for excessive bronchial secretions or diarrhea. Respiratory support for respiratory failure and fluid support for hypotension and CV collapse. If transdermal systems are ingested PO, activated charcoal should be given to prevent seizures. If the client is unconscious, the charcoal should be administered by an NGT. A saline cathartic or sorbitol added to the first dose of activated charcoal may hasten GI passage of the system. Doses of activated charcoal should be repeated as long as the system remains in the GI tract as nicotine will continue to be released for many hours.

HOW SUPPLIED

Nicoderm CQ Step 1, Step 2, Step 3, and Nicotine Transdermal System Step 1, Step 2, Step 3. *Film, Extended-Release:* Amount absorbed/24 hr: 21 mg/24 hr (Step 1), 14 mg/24 hr (Step 2), 7 mg/24 hr (Step 3).
Nicotrol Step 1, Step 2, Step 3. *Patch, Extended-Release:* Amount absorbed/16 hr: 15 mg/16 hr (Step 1), 10 mg/16 hr (Step 2), 5 mg/16 hr (Step 3).

DOSAGE

Nicoderm CQ, Nicotine Transdermal System

TRANSDERMAL SYSTEM

Smoking deterrent.

21 mg/day for the first 6 weeks, 14 mg/day for the next 2 weeks, and 7 mg/day for the last 2 weeks. Total course of therapy: 8–10 weeks. Start with 14 mg/day for 6 weeks for those who smoke less than 10 cigarettes/day. Decrease dose to 7 mg/day for the final 2 weeks.

Nicotrol

TRANSDERMAL SYSTEM

Smoking deterrent.

15 mg/16 hr for the first 6 weeks, 10 mg/16 hr for the next 2 weeks, and 5 mg/16 hr for the last 2 weeks. Total course of therapy: 10 weeks.

NURSING IMPLICATIONS

IMPLEMENTATION/ADMINISTRATION/STORAGE

1. All products are over-the-counter.
2. There will be differences in the duration and length of therapy, depending on the product selected.
3. The goal of therapy with nicotine transdermal systems is complete abstinence. If still smoking by the fourth week of therapy, discontinue treatment.
4. Do not store Nicotrol above 30°C (86°F). Store Nicoderm CQ at 20–25°C (68–77°F).

ASSESSMENT

1. Detail nicotine profile: type and brand (cigarettes, chewing tobacco, or cigars), readiness to quit, amount used per day, when used, and what increases usage. Determine any CAD, liver or renal dysfunction.
2. List medications currently prescribed. Cessation of smoking, with or without nicotine replacement, may alter the response to certain drugs.
3. Note any skin disorders; nicotine transdermal systems may be irritating with skin disorders such as atopic or eczematous dermatitis.

CLIENT/FAMILY TEACHING

1. Follow manufacturer's guidelines for proper system application. Review information sheet that comes with the product for instructions on how to use and dispose of the transdermal systems.
2. May cause dizziness or drowsiness; assess drug effects before engaging in activities that require mental alertness.
3. Use extreme caution during application; remove old patch first then immediately apply the new one to a clean, nonhairy, dry skin site on upper arm or torso. Avoid eye contact. These systems can be a skin irritant and cause contact dermatitis. Report any persistent skin irritations such as redness, swelling, or itching at the application site as well as any generalized skin reactions such as large red skin elevations, or a generalized rash; remove system.
4. Stop smoking completely. If smoking continues, may experience adverse side effects due to higher nicotine levels in the body. Nicotine in any form can be toxic and addictive; transdermal systems may lead to depen-

N

dence. To minimize this risk, withdraw system gradually after 4–8 weeks of use.

5. Participate in a formal smoking program. The success or failure of smoking cessation depends on the quality, intensity, and frequency of supportive care.
6. Symptoms of nicotine withdrawal include craving, nervousness, restlessness, irritability, mood lability, anxiety, drowsiness, sleep disturbances, impaired concentration, increased appetite, headache, myalgia, constipation, fatigue, and weight gain; report as dosage may require adjustment.
7. Change site of application daily; do not reuse same site for 1 week. With Nicotrol, remove patch at bedtime and apply upon arising.
8. Keep all products (used and unused) away from children and pets; sufficient nicotine is still present in used systems to cause toxicity.
9. Apply the transdermal system promptly after its removal from the protective pouch to prevent loss of nicotine due to evaporation. Only use systems where the pouch is intact.
10. Apply system once daily to a nonhairy, clean, and dry site on the trunk or upper, outer arm. Hold for 10 seconds. Wash hands thoroughly after application. Do not wear more than 1 patch at a time. Do not cut the patch in half or in smaller pieces.
11. For Nicoderm CQ, remove the used system after 16–24 hr and apply a new system to alternate skin site. Do not leave the patch on for more than 24 hr as skin irritation may occur and potency is lost. Apply at the same time each day. If vivid dreams or other sleep disturbances, patch may be removed at bedtime and a new patch applied in the morning.
12. For Nicotrol, apply a new system each day upon waking and remove at bedtime. If you forget to remove patch at bedtime, vivid dreams or other sleep disturbances may result. Do not wear patch more than 16 hr.
13. When a used system is removed, fold over and place in the protective pouch from the new system. Dispose of the used system to prevent access by children or pets.
14. If therapy is unsuccessful after 4–6 weeks, discontinue and identify reasons for failure so that a later attempt may be more successful.
15. Keep all F/U to assess response, need for additional counselling, and for adverse SE.

OUTCOMES/EVALUATE

Smoking cessation; control of nicotine withdrawal symptoms

N

Nifedipine

(nye-**FED**-ih-peen)

Classification(s): Calcium channel blocker

Pregnancy Category: C

RX: Adalat CC, Afeditab CR, Nifediac CC, Nifedical XL, Procardia, Procardia XL.

Rx: Adalat XL, Apo-Nifed, Apo-Nifed PA, Novo-Nifedin.

SEE ALSO ***CALCIUM CHANNEL BLOCKING AGENTS***.

INDICATIONS/USES

(1) Vasospastic (Prinzmetal's or variant) angina (**except** Adalat CC, Afeditab CR, or Nifediac CC). (2) Classic effort-associated angina without vasospasm in those who remain symptomatic despite adequate doses of beta blockers or organic nitrates and who cannot tolerate these drugs (**except** Adalat CC, Afeditab CR, or Nifediac CC). (3) Essential hypertension (extended-release only) alone or in combination with other antihypertensive drugs. *Investigational:* Anal fissures, Raynaud phenomenon.

ACTION/KINETICS

Action

Inhibits the influx of calcium through the cell membrane, resulting in a depression of automaticity and conduction velocity leading to a depression of contraction. Also dilates coronary vessels in both normal and ischemic tissues and inhibits spasms of coronary arteries. Decreases total peripheral resistance thus reducing energy and oxygen requirements of the heart. Variable effects on AV node effective and functional refractory periods. CO is slightly increased while peripheral vascular resistance is significantly decreased. Slight to no increase in HR and slight to no decrease in myocardial contractility.

Pharmacokinetics

Onset: 20 min. **Peak plasma levels:** 30 min (up to 4 hr for extended-release). **t½:** 2–5 hr. **Therapeutic serum levels:** 0.025–0.1 mcg/mL. **Duration:** 4–8 hr (12 hr for extended-release). Low-fat meals may slow the rate but not the extent of absorption. Metabolized in the liver to inactive metabolites with 60–80% excreted in the urine and 15% excreted in the feces. **Plasma protein binding:** 92–95%.

CONTRAINDICATIONS

Hypersensitivity. Lactation.

SPECIAL CONCERNS

- **Use with caution in impaired hepatic or renal function and in elderly clients.**
- **Initial increase in frequency, duration, or severity of angina (may also be seen in clients being withdrawn from beta blockers and who begin taking nifedipine).**

SIDE EFFECTS

Most Common

Flushing, headache, fatigue/lethargy, edema, peripheral edema, weakness, muscle cramps, dizziness/lightheadedness, disturbed equilibrium.

CV: Peripheral and pulmonary edema, ***MI***, hypotension, palpitations, syncope, CHF (especially if used with a beta blocker), decreased platelet aggregation, arrhythmias, tachycardia. Increased frequency, length, and duration of angina when beginning nifedipine therapy. **GI:** Nausea, diarrhea, constipation, flatulence, abdominal cramps, dysgeusia, vomiting, dry mouth, eructation, gastroesophageal reflux, melena. **CNS:** Dizziness, lightheadedness, giddiness, nervousness, sleep disturbances, headache, weakness, depression, migraine, psychoses, hallucinations, disturbances in equilibrium, somnolence, insomnia, abnormal dreams, malaise, anxiety. **Dermatologic:** Rash, dermatitis, urticaria, pruritus, photosensitivity, erythema multiforme, ***Stevens-Johnson syndrome***. **Respiratory:** Dyspnea, cough, wheezing, SOB, respiratory infection; throat, nasal, or chest congestion. **Musculoskeletal:** Muscle cramps or inflammation, joint pain or stiffness, arthritis, ataxia, myoclonic dystonia, hypertonia, asthenia. **Hematologic:** Thrombocytopenia, leukopenia, purpura, anemia. **Miscellaneous:** Fever, chills, sweating, weakness, fatigue/lethargy, blurred vision, sexual difficulties, flushing, transient blindness, hyperglycemia, hypokalemia, gingival hyperplasia, allergic hepatitis, hepatitis, tinnitus, gynecomastia, polyuria, nocturia, erythromelalgia, weight gain, epistaxis, facial and periorbital edema, hypoesthesia, gout, abnormal lacrimation, breast pain, dysuria, hematuria.

LABORATORY TEST CONSIDERATIONS

↑ Alkaline phosphatase, CPK, LDH, AST, ALT. Positive Coombs' test.

ADDITIONAL DRUG INTERACTIONS

Anticoagulants, oral / Possibility of ↑ PT
Barbiturates / ↓ Nifedipine effects
Cimetidine / ↑ Bioavailability of nifedipine
Cyclosporine / ↑ Cyclosporine levels and toxicity
Digoxin / ↑ Effect of digoxin by ↓ excretion by kidney
Diltiazem / ↑ Plasma levels of both nifedipine and diltiazem
H ***Ginkgo biloba*** / ↑ Nifedipine plasma levels R/T inhibition of nifedipine CYP3A4 metabolism
Grapefruit juice / ↑ Nifedipine plasma levels R/T ↓ metabolism; do not use together
Itraconazole / ↑ Nifedipine serum levels
Mg sulfate / ↑ Neuromuscular blockade and hypotension
Melatonin / Melatonin may ↓ antihypertensive effect
Nafcillin / Significant ↓ nifedipine plasma levels
Quinidine / Possible ↓ quinidine effect R/T ↓ plasma levels; ↑ risk of hypotension, bradycardia, AV block, pulmonary edema, and VT
Quinupristin/Dalfopristin / ↑ Nifedipine plasma levels
Ranitidine / ↑ Nifedipine bioavailability
Rifampin ↑ Nifedipine effects
H ***St. John's wort*** / ↓ Nifedipine plasma levels R/T ↑ metabolism
Tacrolimus / ↑ Tacrolimus levels → ↑ toxicity
Theophylline / Possible ↑ effect of theophylline
Vincristine / ↑ Vincristine levels → ↑ toxicity

HOW SUPPLIED

Capsules: 10 mg, 20 mg; ***Tablets, Extended-Release:*** 30 mg, 60 mg, 90 mg.

DOSAGE

CAPSULES

Angina.

Individualized. Initial: 10 mg 3 times per day (range: 10–20 mg 3 times per day); **maintenance:** 10–30 mg 3–4 times per day. Those with coronary artery spasm may respond better to 20–30 mg 3–4 times per day. Doses greater than 120 mg/day are rarely needed while doses greater than

N

180 mg/day (maximum dose) are not recommended. *NOTE:* Titrate throughout 7–14 days to assess response to each dose level; monitor BP before proceeding to a higher dose. If symptoms warrant, titrate more rapidly but assess frequently. Increase dose from 10–20 mg 3 times per day and then 30 mg 3 times per day throughout 3 days.

Angina, hospitalized clients.

In hospitalized clients under close supervision, the dose may be increased in 10 mg increments throughout 4- to 6-hr period, as needed, to control pain and arrhythmias due to ischemia. Do not exceed a single dose of 30 mg.

Raynaud phenomenon (investigational).

Adults: 5–20 mg 3 times per day of the immediate-release formulation or 20 mg 2 times per day of a slow-release formulation.

TABLETS, EXTENDED-RELEASE

Angina.

Nifedical XL or Procardia XL, initial: 30 or 60 mg once daily. Titrate over a 7–14 day period, although titration may occur more rapidly if the client is assessed frequently. Titration to doses above 120 mg is not recommended. Angina clients maintained on immediate-release capsules may be switched to the extended-release tablet at the nearest equivalent total daily dose. Experience with doses greater than 90 mg daily in angina are limited.

Hypertension.

Adalat CC, Afeditab CR, or Nifediac CC, initial: 30 mg once daily. Titrate over a 7–14 day period. Base upward titration on efficacy and safety. **Maintenance, usual:** 30–60 mg once daily. Titration to doses above 90 mg/day is not recommended for Nifedical XL or Procardia XL and 30 mg once daily for Adalat CC. Titrate over a 7- to 14-day period. Dosage can be increased as required and as tolerated to a maximum of 90 mg/day.

NURSING IMPLICATIONS

Do not confuse nifedipine with nicardipine (also a calcium channel blocker).

IMPLEMENTATION/ADMINISTRATION/STORAGE

1. Do not exceed a single dose (other than sustained-release) of 30 mg.
2. Before increasing dose, carefully monitor BP.
3. Use only the sustained-release tablets to treat hypertension.
4. Sublingual nitroglycerin and long-acting nitrates may be used concomitantly with nifedipine.
5. Concomitant therapy with beta-adrenergic blocking agents may be used. In these cases, note any potential drug interactions.
6. Clients withdrawn from beta blockers may manifest symptoms of increased angina which cannot be prevented by nifedipine; in fact, nifedipine may increase the severity of angina in this situation.
7. Clients with angina may be switched to the sustained-release product at the nearest equivalent total daily dose. Use doses greater than 90 mg/day with caution.
8. No rebound effect noted when nifedipine discontinued. If drug to be discontinued, decrease dosage gradually with supervision.
9. Protect capsules from light and moisture; store at room temperature in original container.
10. During initial therapy and when dosage increased, may experience increase in frequency, duration, or severity of angina.
11. Food may decrease rate but not extent of absorption; can be taken without regard to meals.
12. Store capsules from 15–25°C (59–77°F). Protect from light, moisture, and humidity. Prevent freezing of capsules, as they may be liquid-filled. Store tablets below 30°C (86°F); protect from moisture and humidity.

ASSESSMENT

1. List reasons for therapy, other agents trialed/outcome, any sensitivity to calcium channel blockers.
2. Note pulmonary edema, ECG abnormalities, or palpitations.
3. Document cardiopulmonary assessment findings.

4. During titration period, note any hypotensive response, increased HR that result from peripheral vasodilation; may precipitate angina.
5. Although beta-blocking drugs may be used concomitantly with chronic stable angina, the combined drug effects cannot be predicted (especially with compromised LV function or cardiac conduction abnormalities). Pronounced hypotension, heart block, and CHF may occur.
6. If therapy with a beta blocker is to be discontinued, gradually decrease dosage to prevent withdrawal syndrome.
7. Monitor ECG, BP, K^+, platelets, renal and LFTs.

CLIENT/FAMILY TEACHING

1. May take with or without food. Sustained-release tablets should not be chewed, crushed, or divided. Grapefruit juice may cause increased serum drug levels.
2. Avoid activities that require mental alertness until drug effects realized; may cause dizziness or lightheadedness.
3. Maintain fluid intake of 2–3 L/day to avoid constipation. No cause for concern if a tablet coating appears in the stool.
4. Do not switch brands; Adalat CC and Procardia XL are not interchangeable; not equivalent.
5. Do not use OTC agents unless approved; avoid alcohol and caffeine.
6. Report persistent headache, flushing, nausea, palpitations, weight gain, dizziness, rash, palpitations, or lack of response.
7. Brush teeth and floss regularly to reduce swelling and tenderness of your gums.
8. Keep log of BP. Perform weekly weights, note any extremity swelling. This may result from arterial vasodilation precipitated by nifedipine, or the swelling may indicate increasing ventricular dysfunction and should be reported.
9. If also receiving beta-adrenergic blocking agents, report any evidence of hypotension, exacerbation of angina, or evidence of heart failure. Once beta-blocking agents have been discontinued, report increased anginal pain.
10. Keep all F/U to assess response, labs, and for adverse SE.

OUTCOMES/EVALUATE

- ↓ Frequency and intensity of anginal episodes ↓ BP
- Improved peripheral circulation
- Prevention of strokes and ↓ risk of CHF in geriatric hypertensives

Nilutamide

(nye-**LOO**-tah-myd)

Classification(s): Antineoplastic, hormone

Pregnancy Category: C

RX: Nilandron.

🍁 **Rx:** Anadron.

SEE ALSO *ANTINEOPLASTIC AGENTS*.

INDICATIONS/USES

In combination with surgical castration to treat metastatic prostate cancer (Stage D_2). *Investigational:* Treat prostate cancer alone or in combination with luteinizing hormone-releasing hormone agonists.

ACTION/KINETICS

Action

Antiandrogen with no estrogen, progesterone, mineralocorticoid, or glucocorticoid effects. Binds to the androgen receptor, thus blocking effects of testosterone and preventing the normal androgenic response.

Pharmacokinetics

Rapidly and completely absorbed from the GI tract. **Steady-state:** 2–4 weeks. Extensively metabolized by the liver; one of the five metabolites is active. Excreted mainly in the urine. **t½, elimination:** Approximately, 41–49 hr. **Plasma protein binding:** Moderately bound.

CONTRAINDICATIONS

Severe hepatic impairment, severe respiratory deficiency, hypersensitivity to nilutamide or any product components. Use in women.

SPECIAL CONCERNS

(1) Interstitial pneumonitis has been reported in 2% of clients in controlled clinical trials in clients exposed to nilutamide. A small study in Japanese clients showed that 17% of clients developed interstitial pneumonitis. Re-

ports of interstitial changes, including pulmonary fibrosis that led to hospitalization and death, have been reported rarely in postmarketing. Symptoms included exertional dyspnea, cough, chest pain, and fever. X-rays showed interstitial or alveolo-interstitial changes, and pulmonary function tests revealed a restrictive pattern with decreased diffusing capacity of lungs for carbon monoxide. Most cases occurred within the first 3 months of treatment with nilutamide, and most reversed with discontinuation of therapy. (2) Perform a routine chest x-ray prior to initiating treatment with nilutamide. Consider baseline pulmonary function tests. Instruct clients to report any new or worsening shortness of breath that they experience while taking nilutamide. If symptoms occur, immediately discontinue nilutamide until it can be determined if the symptoms are drug-related. ■

Safety and efficacy not determined in children.

SIDE EFFECTS

Most Common

When used with leuprolide: Hot flashes, impaired adaptation to dark, pain, insomnia, headache, dizziness, nausea, constipation, testicular atrophy, gynecomastia, dyspnea, asthenia, back pain.

CV: Hypertension, angina, ***heart failure***, syncope. **GI:** N&V, abdominal pain, anorexia, constipation, diarrhea, dry mouth, dyspepsia, GI disorder, ***GI hemorrhage***, melena, hepatotoxicity, ***hepatitis*** (rare). **CNS:** Dizziness, depression, headache, hypesthesia, insomnia, nervousness, paresthesia, decreased libido. **Respiratory:** Increased cough, interstitial pneumonitis, lung disorder, rhinitis, dyspnea, pneumonia, URTI. **Hematologic:** Leukopenia, anemia, aplastic anemia (rare). **GU:** UTI, impotence, gynecomastia, hematuria, nocturia, testicular atrophy, urinary tract disorder. **Musculoskeletal:** Arthritis, back/bone/chest pain. **Dermatologic:** Pruritus, body hair loss, dry skin, rash, sweating. **Metabolic/Nutritional:** Edema, peripheral edema, weight loss, intolerance to alcohol. **Ophthalmic:** Cataract, photophobia, impaired adaptation to dark/light, abnormal vision, colored vision, chromatopsia. **Body as a whole:** Malaise, asthenia, fever, flu syndrome, pain. **Miscellaneous:** Hot flashes.

NOTE: Certain side effects may be due to the effect of surgical castration.

LABORATORY TEST CONSIDERATIONS

↑ Haptoglobin, alkaline phosphatase, BUN, creatinine, AST, ALT. Hyperglycemia.

DRUG INTERACTIONS

NOTE: Nilutamide, in vitro, inhibits the activity of CYP450 isoenzymes; thus, the metabolism of compounds requiring these enzymes may be reduced.

Phenytoin / Possible phenytoin delayed elimination and ↑ serum t½ → toxic levels

Theophylline / Possible theophylline delayed elimination and ↑ serum t½ → toxic levels

Vitamin K antagonists / Possible vitamin K antagonist delayed elimination and ↑ serum t½ → toxic levels

HOW SUPPLIED

Tablets: 150 mg.

DOSAGE

TABLETS

Metastatic prostate cancer.

Adults: 300 mg once daily for 30 days followed by 150 mg once daily.

NURSING IMPLICATIONS

IMPLEMENTATION/ADMINISTRATION/STORAGE

1. **To ensure maximum beneficial effects, initiate treatment on the same day as or the day after surgical castration.**
2. **Nilutamide is a hormonal drug and is considered a potential teratogen; follow safe handling procedures when preparing, administering, or dispensing the drug.**
3. **Protect from light and store at room temperature at 15–30°C (59–86°F).**

ASSESSMENT

1. **Note prostate cancer onset, other agents/therapies trialed, outcome. Anticipate first dosing on or the day after surgical castration.**
2. **Obtain CBC, LFTs, and CXR. Assess cardiopulmonary status closely; may cause interstitial pneumonitis.**
3. **Monitor VS, PSA, LFTs, PFTs, ECG; assess for dysfunction.**

CLIENT/FAMILY TEACHING

1. **Take daily as directed, with or without food. Start nilutamide tablets on the day of, or the day after, surgical castration. Do not stop or interrupt dose without provider approval.**
2. **May experience difficulty driving at night or through tunnels (delayed dark adaptation); tinted glasses may alleviate this effect.**
3. **Immediately report any symptoms of chest pain, SOB, cough with fever, jaundice, dark urine, fatigue, or unusual side effects.**
4. **Avoid alcohol if facial flushing, malaise, or hypotension occurs after consuming alcoholic beverages (drug-induced alcohol intolerance).**
5. **Keep all F/U to assess response, labs, and for adverse SE.**

OUTCOMES/EVALUATE

Control of malignant cell proliferation

Nitrofurantoin

(**nye**-troh-fyour-**AN**-toyn)

Classification(s): Urinary anti-infective

Pregnancy Category: B

RX: Capsules (as macrocrystals): Macrodantin. **Capsules (as monohydrate/macrocrystals):** Macrobid. **Oral Suspension:** Furadantin.

✤ **Rx:** Apo-Nitrofurantoin, Novo-Furantoin.

SEE ALSO ***ANTI-INFECTIVE DRUGS.***

INDICATIONS/USES

UTIs due to susceptible strains of *Escherichia coli, Staphylococcus aureus,* Enterococci, and certain strains of *Enterobacter* and *Klebsiella.* Not indicated to treat pyelonephritis or perinephric abscesses. *NOTE:* Nitrofurantoin monohydrate/macrocrystals is indicated only for treatment of uncomplicated UTIs (e.g., acute cystitis) caused by susceptible strains of *E. coli* or *Staphylococcus saprophyticus* in clients 12 years of age and older.

ACTION/KINETICS

Action

Nitrofurantoin is reduced by bacterial flavoproteins to reactive intermediates that inactivate or alter bacterial ribosomal proteins and other macromolecules. As a result, vital biochemical processes of protein synthesis, aerobic energy metabolism, DNA and RNA synthesis, and cell wall synthesis are inhibited. Is bactericidal in urine at therapeutic doses. Development of resistance has not been a significant problem.

Pharmacokinetics

Absorption of macrocrystals is slower when compared with the oral suspension (which is readily absorbed from the GI tract). Each monohydrate/macrocrystal capsule contains two forms of nitrofurantoin: 25% is macrocrystalline, which has slower dissolution and absorption than the monohydrate, and 75% is the monohydrate. Upon exposure to gastric and intestinal fluids the monohydrate forms a gel matrix that releases nitrofurantoin over time. Bioavailability is increased by food. **t½:** 20 min (60 min in anephric clients). **Urine levels:** 50–250 mcg/mL. The oral suspension is rapidly excreted in urine while excretion of macrocrystals and the monohydrate/macrocrystals is somewhat less.

CONTRAINDICATIONS

Anuria, oliguria, and clients with impaired renal function (C_{CR} below 40 mL/min), and clinically significant elevated serum creatinine. Also, during pregnancy, especially near term; during labor; infants less than 1 month of age; and lactation.

SPECIAL CONCERNS

- **Use with extreme caution in anemia, diabetes, electrolyte imbalance, avitaminosis B, or a debilitating disease.**
- **There may be a higher proportion of pulmonary reactions, including fatalities, in the elderly (See *Side Effects*).**
- **Safety and efficacy of the monohydrate/macrocrystals not determined in children less than 12 years.**

SIDE EFFECTS

Most Common

Headache, dizziness, N&V, anorexia, diarrhea, drowsiness, rust-colored or brownish urine.

Nitrofurantoin is a potentially toxic drug with many side effects. **GI:** Abdominal pain, anorexia, diarrhea, emesis, N&V, ***pancreatitis***, sialadenitis, pseudomembranous colitis. **Hepatic:** Hepatitis, cholestatic jaundice, chronic active hepatitis, ***hepatic necrosis***. **CNS:** Asthenia, confusion, depression, dizziness, drowsiness, headache, nystagmus, psychotic reactions, vertigo. **CV:** Benign intracranial hypertension (pseudotumor cerebri), nonspecific ST/T wave changes, bundle branch block (in association with pulmonary reactions). **Pulmonary, acute (usually within first week of treatment):** Fever, chills, cough, chest pain, dyspnea, pulmonary infiltration with consolidation or pleural effusion on x-ray, eosinophilia. **Pulmonary, subacute use:** Fever and eosinophilia occur less often. **Pulmonary, chronic use (6 months or longer):** Malaise, dyspnea on exertion, cough, altered pulmonary function, diffuse interstitial pneumonitis or fibrosis (or both). **Dermatologic:** Erythema multiforme (including ***Stevens-Johnson syndrome***), exfoliative dermatitis (rare), alopecia. **Hypersensitivity:** ***Angioedema***, arthralgia, chills, drug fever, anaphylaxis, lupus-like syndrome (associated with pulmonary reactions), myalgia, pruritus, urticaria; eczematous, erythematous, or maculopapular eruptions. **Hematologic:** Hemolytic anemia (similar to the primaquine-sensitivity type), agranulocyosis, eosinophilia, glucose-6-phosphate dehydrogenase deficiency anemia, granulocytopenia, hemolytic anemia, leukopenia, megaloblastic anemia, thrombocytopenia, ***aplastic anemia*** (rare). **Ophthalmic:** Optic neuritis (rare). **Miscellaneous:** Peripheral neuropathy, super infections caused by resistant organisms, rust-colored or brownish urine.

Monohydrate/macrocrystals. GI: Nausea, flatulence, abdominal pain, constipation, diarrhea, dyspepsia, emesis. **CNS:** Headache, amblyopia, drowsiness, dizziness. **Dermatologic:** Alopecia. **Respiratory:** Acute pulmonary hypersensitivity reactions (see above). **Miscellaneous:** Chills, fever, malaise.

N

LABORATORY TEST CONSIDERATIONS

↑ ALT, AST, serum phosphorus. ↓ Hemoglobin. False + glucose using Benedict and Fehling solutions.

OVERDOSE MANAGEMENT

Symptoms: Vomiting (most common). *Treatment:* Induce emesis. High fluid intake to promote urinary excretion. The drug is dialyzable.

DRUG INTERACTIONS

Anticholinergics / ↑ Nitrofurantoin bioavailability R/T delaying gastric emptying and increasing absorption
Magnesium salts / Delay or ↓ nitrofurantoin absorption
Uricosurics / High doses of probenecid ↓ nitrofurantoin renal clearance and ↑ serum levels → possible toxicity

HOW SUPPLIED

Nitrofurantoin. *Oral Suspension:* 25 mg/5 mL.
Nitrofurantoin Macrocrystals. *Capsules:* 25 mg, 50 mg, 100 mg.
Nitrofurantoin Monohydrate/Macrocrystals. *Capsules:* 100 mg.

DOSAGE

CAPSULES (MACROCRYSTALS), ORAL SUSPENSION

UTIs.

Adults: 50–100 mg 4 times per day, not to exceed 600 mg/day. The lower dose is for uncomplicated UTIs. **Children, 1 month of age and older:** 5–7 mg/kg/day given in 4 divided doses. The following dosages in children, using the oral suspension, are based on average weight in each range receiving 5–6 mg/kg/day given in 4 divided doses: **7–11 kg (15–26 lb):** 2.5 mL 4 times per day; **12–21 kg (27–46 lb):** 5 mL 4 times per day; **22–30 kg (47–68 lb):** 7.5 mL 4 times per day; **31–41 kg (69–91 lb):** 10 mL 4 times per day.

Long-term suppressive therapy.

Adults: 50–100 mg at bedtime may be sufficient. **Children:** 1 mg/kg per day, given in a single dose or in 2 divided doses, may be adequate.

CAPSULES (MONOHYDRATE/MACROCRYSTALS)

Uncomplicated UTIs (cystitis).

Adults: 100 mg q 12 hr for 7 days. **Pediatric, 1 month of age and over:** 5–7 mg/kg/day in four equal doses.

NURSING IMPLICATIONS

IMPLEMENTATION/ADMINISTRATION/STORAGE

1. Continue therapy for UTIs for 1 week or for at least 3 days after urine sterility obtained.
2. Avoid exposure of oral suspension to strong light (may darken drug). Is stable when stored

from 20–25°C (68–77°F). Protect from freezing. Dispense in glass amber bottles.

3. Store capsules from 15–30°C (59–86°F). Dispense in a tight container using child-resistant closures.

ASSESSMENT

1. Note reasons for therapy, onset, and characteristics of S&S.
2. Observe for acute or delayed-onset anaphylactic reaction. Assess for pulmonary reactions or symptoms.
3. Monitor bowel function and for recurrent UTI symptoms; superinfections may occur.
4. Blacks and ethnic groups of Mediterranean and Near Eastern origin should be assessed for symptoms of anemia (G6PD).
5. Monitor CBC, urine C&S, renal and LFTs, also CXR and PFTs with chronic therapy.

CLIENT/FAMILY TEACHING

1. Do not crush or chew tablets; swallow whole.
2. Take with food or milk to minimize gastric irritation and enhance absorption; complete full course of therapy to prevent bacterial resistance.
3. Increase fluid intake; drink at least 2 qt/day of water. Avoid alcohol. Acidic foods (prunes, cranberry juice, plums) enhance drug action whereas alkaline foods (milk products) minimize drug action. May turn urine a dark yellow or brown color.
4. Any numbness and tingling of extremities or flu-like symptoms must be reported; indications for drug withdrawal as condition may worsen and become irreversible. Breathing problems require immediate help. RUQ pain, yellow skin discoloration, fatigue may indicate liver dysfunction. Persistent N&V, diarrhea; may be symptoms of a GI superinfection.
5. Avoid prolonged sun exposure, use sunscreen/wear protective clothing to prevent photosensitivity reaction.
6. Keep all F/U to assess response, labs, and adverse SE.

OUTCOMES/EVALUATE

- Negative urine culture results
- Resolution of infection
- Symptomatic improvement (↓ dysuria, frequency)

IV

Nitroglycerin IV

(nye-troh-**GLIH**-sir-in)

Classification(s): Vasodilator, coronary

Pregnancy Category: C

RX: Nitroglycerin in 5% Dextrose.

SEE ALSO ***ANTIANGINAL DRUGS-NITRATES/NITRITES.***

INDICATIONS/USES

(1) Perioperative hypertension. (2) CHF associated in the setting of acute MI. (3) Angina unresponsive to sublingual nitroglycerin and beta-adrenergic blocking agents. (4) Induction of intraoperative hypotension. *Investigational:* Management of an acute MI; treatment of hypertensive emergencies; with vasopressin to treat variceal bleeding; treat cocaine-induced acute coronary syndrome; management of Prinzmetal's angina that occurs in those without coronary heart disease.

ACTION/KINETICS

Pharmacokinetics

Onset: 1–2 min; **duration:** 3–5 min (dose-dependent).

SPECIAL CONCERNS

Dosage not established in children.

SIDE EFFECTS

Most Common

Headache (may be severe and persistent), lightheadedness, hypotension.

See *Antianginal Drugs-Nitrates/Nitrites* for a complete list of possible side effects.

HOW SUPPLIED

Injection: 100 mcg/mL, 200 mcg/mL, 400 mcg/mL; ***Solution for Injection:*** 5 mg/mL (requires dilution).

DOSAGE

IV INFUSION ONLY

All uses.

Initial: When using a nonabsorbing infusion set, start with 5 mcg/min delivered through an infusion pump capable of exact and constant delivery of the drug. May be increased by 5 mcg/min q 3–5 min until response is seen. If no re-

N

sponse seen at 20 mcg/min, dose can be increased by 10 or even 20 mcg/min until response noted. Monitor titration continuously until client reaches desired level of response. Then, reduce the dose and lengthen the interval between increments.

NURSING IMPLICATIONS

Do not confuse nitroglycerin with nitroprusside (drug for hypertensive emergencies).

IMPLEMENTATION/ADMINISTRATION/STORAGE

1. IV There is no fixed optimum dose due to variations in responsiveness. Thus, titrate to the desired level of hemodynamic function. Continuously monitor BP, HR, and other measurements to achieve the correct dosage. Maintain adequate systemic blood and coronary perfusion pressures.
2. The solution for injection is not for direct IV use; must first be diluted. Transfer contents of 1 nitroglycerin vial (containing nitroglycerin 25 or 50 mg, i.e., 5 mg/mL) into a 500 mL glass bottle of either D5W or 0.9% NaCl. This yields a final concentration of 50 mcg/mL or 100 mcg/mL.
3. After the initial dosage titration, the concentration of the solution may be increased to limit the volume of fluids given. Do not exceed a nitroglycerin concentration of 400 mcg/mL.
4. Use glass IV bottle only, and administration set provided by the manufacturer; is readily absorbed onto many plastics. Avoid adding unnecessary plastic to IV system.
5. Aspirate medication into a syringe, and then inject immediately into a glass bottle (or polyolefin bottle) to minimize contact with plastic. Greater absorption occurs with low flow rates, high concentrations, and long tubing.
6. If the concentration is adjusted, the infusion set must be flushed or replaced before a new concentration is used. If the set is not flushed or replaced, it may take minutes to hours (depending on flow rate and the dead space of the set) for new concentration to reach the client.
7. Administer solution with infusion device (volumetric) in a closely monitored environment.
8. Store from 15–30°C (59–86°F). Discard unused portion. Do not freeze. Protect from light.
9. The premixed nitroglycerin with dextrose can be stored at room temperature (25°C). Brief exposure up to 40°C does not affect potency. Avoid excessive heat and protect from freezing.
10. COMPATIBILITY D5W, 0.9% NaCl.
11. INCOMPATIBILITY Do not admix with any other medications. Do not interrupt IV nitroglycerin for administration of a bolus of any other medication.

ASSESSMENT

1. Note reasons/goals of therapy. Assess and rate pain, noting location, onset, duration, and any precipitating factors.
2. Assess VS, ECG, history, cardiopulmonary assessments.
3. Pericardial tamponade, restrictive cardiomyopathy, or constrictive pericarditis preclude therapy.
4. Monitor BP and HR continuously during IV therapy. Obtain written parameters for BP and pulse; monitor during therapy. Note any evidence of hypotension, N&V, or sweating. Monitor CVP/PA pressure as ordered; document presence of tachycardia or bradycardia:
   - Elevate the legs to restore BP.
   - Reduce the rate of flow or administer additional IV fluids.
5. Assess for thrombophlebitis at the IV site; remove if reddened.
6. After the initial positive response to therapy, dosage increments will be smaller and made at longer intervals.
7. Sinus tachycardia may occur in client with angina receiving a maintenance dose of nitroglycerin (HR of 80 beats/min or less reduces myocardial demand).
8. Check that topical, PO, or SL doses are adjusted/held if on concomitant IV nitroglycerin.
9. Wean from IV nitroglycerin by gradually decreasing doses to avoid posttherapy CV distress. Usually initiated when the client is receiving the peak effect from PO or topical vasodilators; monitor for hypertension and angina.
10. Administer nonnarcotic analgesic (usually acetaminophen) because headache is a common side effect of drug therapy.

CLIENT/FAMILY TEACHING

1. Drug is used IV to lower BP during surgery, control chest pain, and/or reduce cardiac

workload. Report pain and level so dose may be adjusted to control.
2. Administered in a monitored setting. Change to upright position slowly and if dizzy, lie down.
3. Report any headaches so medications to relieve them can be administered/ordered.

OUTCOMES/EVALUATE

- Resolution/control of angina
- ↓ BP; ↑ activity tolerance
- ↓ LVEDP (preload) and ↓ systemic vascular resistance (afterload)
- Improvement in S&S of CHF (↑ output, ↓ rales, ↓ CVP)

Nitroglycerin sublingual

(nye-troh-**GLIH**-sir-in)

Classification(s): Vasodilator, coronary

Pregnancy Category: C

RX: Nitrostat.

✱ **Rx:** Gen-Nitro.

SEE ALSO ***ANTIANGINAL DRUGS-NITRATES/NITRITES***.

INDICATIONS/USES

Acute relief or prophylaxis of angina pectoris caused by coronary artery disease.

ACTION/KINETICS

Action

Relax vascular smooth muscle by stimulating production of intracellular cyclic guanosine monophosphate. Dilation of postcapillary vessels decreases venous return to the heart due to pooling of blood; thus, LV end-diastolic pressure (preload) is reduced. Relaxation of areterioles results in a decreased systemic vascular resistance and arterial pressure (afterload).

Pharmacokinetics

Rapidly absorbed. Absolute bioavailability is 40% (but is variable). **Onset:** 1–3 min; **mean peak plasma levels:** 6–7 min. **duration:** 30–60 min. **t½, elimination:** About 2–3 min. Rapidly metabolized to dinitrates and mononitrates by a liver reductase enzyme. Also metabolized by red blood cells and vascular walls.

SPECIAL CONCERNS

Dosage not established in children.

SIDE EFFECTS

Most Common

Headache (may be severe and persistent), dizziness, palpitations, vertigo, weakness, postural hypotension, syncope.

See *Antianginal Drugs-Nitrates/Nitrites* for a complete list of possible side effects.

ADDITIONAL DRUG INTERACTIONS

Do not use nitroglycerin with PDE5 inhibitors (e.g., sildenafil, tadalafil, vardenafil) R/T significant hypotension and possible death.

HOW SUPPLIED

Tablets, Sublingual: 0.3 mg, 0.4 mg, 0.6 mg.

DOSAGE

TABLETS, SUBLINGUAL

Dissolve 1 tablet under the tongue or in the buccal pouch at first sign of attack; may be repeated in 5 min if necessary (no more than 3 tablets should be taken within 15 min). For prophylaxis, tablets may be taken 5–10 min prior to activities that may precipitate an attack.

NURSING IMPLICATIONS

IMPLEMENTATION/ADMINISTRATION/STORAGE

Store sublingual tablets from 15–30°C (59–86°F).

ASSESSMENT

1. Note reasons for therapy, assess and rate pain, noting location, onset, duration, and any precipitating factors. Document cardiac history/assessments.
2. Assess for anemia, heart failure, overactive thyroid, recent head trauma, recent heart attack or stroke.
3. List drugs prescribed to ensure none interact.
4. Monitor VS, ECG, and response.

CLIENT/FAMILY TEACHING

1. Sit down and place sublingual tablet under the tongue and allow to dissolve; do not swallow until entirely dissolved. Do not crush, chew, or swallow sublingual tablets. May sting when it comes in contact with the mucosa. Avoid eating or drinking until tablet dissolved.

N

2. Remain sitting or lie down if dizziness or lightheadedness occurs.
3. Take 5–10 min *before* stressful activity, i.e., exercise, sex. Check with provider, may consider additional dose before anticipated stressful activity or if chest pain at night.
4. Report immediately if pain is not controlled with prescribed dosage (usually 1 tab q 5 min × 3). Call 911 or for an ambulance as directed by provider if relief not attained. Stop drug and report if vision blurring or dry mouth occurs.
5. Date sublingual container upon opening. Keep medicine tightly closed in original glass bottle; discard cotton once bottle is opened. Protect from moisture. Discard unused tablets if 6 months has elapsed since the original container opened.
6. Do not smoke and enroll in smoking cessation program if not able to quit.
7. Encourage family members to learn CPR. Keep all F/U to assess response and adverse SE.

OUTCOMES/EVALUATE
- Angina prophylaxis
- Termination of anginal attack

Nitroglycerin sustained-release capsules

(nye-troh-**GLIH**-sir-in)

Classification(s): Vasodilator, coronary

Pregnancy Category: C

RX: Nitro-Time.

SEE ALSO ***ANTIANGINAL DRUGS-NITRATES/NITRITES***.

INDICATIONS/USES
Prophylaxis and long-term treatment of recurrent angina. Onset of effect of capsules is not sufficiently rapid to be useful in aborting an acute anginal attack.

ACTION/KINETICS
Pharmacokinetics

Sustained-release. Onset: 20–45 min; **duration:** 3–8 hr.

SPECIAL CONCERNS
Dosage not established in children.

SIDE EFFECTS
Most Common

Headache (may be severe and persistent), lightheadedness, hypotension.

See *Antianginal Drugs-Nitrates/Nitrites* for a complete list of possible side effects.

HOW SUPPLIED
Capsules, Sustained-Release: 2.5 mg, 6.5 mg, 9 mg.

DOSAGE

CAPSULES, SUSTAINED-RELEASE
Angina pectoris, prophylaxis.

Initial: 2.5–6.5 mg 3–4 times per day. Titrate upward to an effective dose until side effects limit dose. Upward dose titration in 2.5–6.5 mg increments 2–4 times per day over a period of days or weeks can be attempted. Doses as high as 26 mg given 4 times per day have been effective. However, give the smallest effective dose 2–4 times per day.

NURSING IMPLICATIONS

ASSESSMENT
1. Note reasons for therapy, cardiac history/assessments.
2. Assess and rate pain, noting location, onset, duration, and any precipitating factors.

CLIENT/FAMILY TEACHING
1. Drug is used to control/prevent chest pain. Take as directed and have SL NTG available for acute use.
2. Do not break, chew, or crush sustained-release capsules–swallow whole; not intended for sublingual use.
3. Take smallest effective dose 2–4 times per day with a glass of water. Report if tolerance/lack of response evident.
4. Avoid alcohol; may cause dizziness, lightheadedness, or fainting, especially while standing or following consumption of alcohol.
5. Acetaminophen can be used to relieve headache without reducing the medications antianginal effectiveness.

6. Keep all F/U to assess response and for adverse SE.

OUTCOMES/EVALUATE

Angina prophylaxis

Nitroglycerin topical ointment

(nye-troh-**GLIH**-sir-in)

Classification(s): Vasodilator, coronary

Pregnancy Category: C

RX: Nitro-Bid, Rectiv.

SEE ALSO ***ANTIANGINAL DRUGS-NITRATES/NITRITES***.

INDICATIONS/USES

(1) Prophylaxis and treatment of angina pectoris due to CAD. *NOTE:* Onset of action of the ointment is not rapid enough to be used to abort an acute anginal attack. (2) Chronic to severe pain associated with chronic anal fissures. *Investigational:* Management of acute MI; erectile dysfunction; Raynaud disease; management of Prinzmetal's angina that occurs in clients without CAD.

ACTION/KINETICS

Pharmacokinetics

Onset: 30–60 min; **duration:** 2–12 hr (depending on amount used per unit of surface area).

SPECIAL CONCERNS

Dosage not established in children.

SIDE EFFECTS

Most Common

Headache (may be severe and persistent), flushing, dizziness, weakness, hypotension, paresthesia.

See *Antianginal Drugs-Nitrates/Nitrites* for a complete list of possible side effects.

HOW SUPPLIED

Ointment: 0.4%, 2%.

DOSAGE

OINTMENT

Two daily ½ inch (7.5 mg) doses; apply one on rising in morning and apply one 6 hr later. The dose can be doubled and even doubled again in those tolerating this dose but failing to respond to it.

NURSING IMPLICATIONS

Do not confuse Nitro-Bid with Nitro-Tab (also a nitroglycerin product).

IMPLEMENTATION/ADMINISTRATION/STORAGE

Store from 15–30°F (59–86°F).

ASSESSMENT

1. Note reasons for therapy, cardiac history/assessments, VS and ECG.
2. Assess and rate pain, noting location, onset, duration, and any precipitating factors.

CLIENT/FAMILY TEACHING

1. Squeeze ointment carefully onto dose-measuring application papers (packaged with the medicine). Use applicator to spread ointment or fold paper in half and rub back and forth. Clean around tube opening and tightly cap tube after use.
2. Place the paper with the ointment onto a nonhairy area of skin and tape into place. Avoid rubbing ointment into skin. Application to the chest may be psychologically helpful, but may be applied to other nonhairy areas. Avoid distal extremities or any cut, callused, or irritated skin area.
3. Rotate sites to prevent irritation. Keep a record of areas used to avoid unnecessary repetitive use of sites. Carry SL NTG for acute chest pain relief.
4. Apply ointment in a thin, even layer covering an area of skin 3–6 inches in diameter; remove last dose. Date and tape the application paper over the area, or cover the area with a piece of clear plastic cover (plastic kitchen wrap) to prevent staining of clothing by ointment, reduce leakage of ointment, decrease skin irritation and increase absorption.
5. Once the dose is established, use the same type of covering to ensure that the same amount of drug is absorbed during each application.
6. To prevent systemic absorption, protect skin from contact with ointment, prevent contact with hands and wash hands thoroughly after application to avoid headache.

7. Remove at bedtime or as directed to prevent tolerance or loss of drug effect. Remember to reapply upon awakening the next morning.
8. Change positions slowly and avoid alcohol to prevent to prevent lightheadedness.
9. Do not take Viagra during therapy.
10. Use caution (wrap or secure) as discarded patches are potential hazard to children and pets.
11. Keep all F/U to assess response and for adverse SE.

OUTCOMES/EVALUATE

Prevention of anginal episodes

Nitroglycerin transdermal system

(nye-troh-**GLIH**-sir-in)

Classification(s): Vasodilator, coronary

Pregnancy Category: C

RX: Minitran 0.1 mg/hr, 0.2 mg/hr, 0.4 mg/hr, and 0.6 mg/hr, Nitrek 0.2 mg/hr, 0.4 mg/hr, and 0.6 mg/hr, Nitro-Dur 0.1 mg/hr, 0.2 mg/hr, 0.3 mg/hr, 0.4 mg/hr, 0.6 mg/hr, and 0.8 mg/hr.

SEE ALSO *ANTIANGINAL DRUGS-NITRATES/NITRITES.*

INDICATIONS/USES

Prophylaxis of angina pectoris due to CAD. The onset of action is not sufficiently rapid to be used in aborting an acute anginal attack. *Investigational:* Management of acute MI; erectile dysfunction; Raynaud's disease; management of Prinzmetal's angina that occurs in those without coronary heart disease.

ACTION/KINETICS

Pharmacokinetics

Onset: 30–60 min; **duration:** 8–24 hr. The amount released each hour is indicated in the name.

SPECIAL CONCERNS

Dosage not established in children.

SIDE EFFECTS

Most Common

Headache (may be severe and persistent), lightheadedness, hypotension.

See *Antianginal Drugs-Nitrates/Nitrites* for a complete list of possible side effects.

HOW SUPPLIED

Transdermal Patch (Extended-Release): To release: 0.1 mg/hr, 0.2 mg/hr, 0.3 mg/hr, 0.4 mg/hr, 0.6 mg/hr, 0.8 mg/hr.

DOSAGE

TRANSDERMAL PATCH (EXTENDED-RELEASE)

Angina pectoris, prophylaxis.

Initial: 0.2–0.4 mg/hr (initially the smallest available dose in the dosage series) applied each day to skin site free of hair and free of excessive movement (e.g., chest, upper arm). Doses between 0.4 and 0.8 mg/hr are effective for 10–12 hr/day for at least 1 month of intermittent administration. A nitrate-free interval of 10–12 hr is sufficient. Thus, an appropriate dosing schedule would include a daily "patch-on" period of 10–12 hr and a "patch-off" period of 10–12 hr. **Maintenance:** Additional systems or strengths may be added depending on the clinical response.

NOTE: Tolerance is a major limiting factor to efficacy when the system is used constantly for more than 12 hr/day.

NURSING IMPLICATIONS

IMPLEMENTATION/ADMINISTRATION/STORAGE

1. Follow instructions for specific products on package insert.
2. Remove patch before defibrillating, as patch may explode.
3. The various products differ in the mechanism for the delivery system; the most important factor is the amount of drug released per hour. A wide range of client variability will be noted. Variables in the absorption rate include skin, physical exercise, and elevated ambient temperature.

4. Store from 15–30°C (59–86°F). Avoid extremes of temperature/humidity. Do not refrigerate or store outside of protective package.

ASSESSMENT

1. Note reasons for therapy, cardiac history/assessments, VS and ECG.
2. Assess and rate pain, noting location, onset, duration, and any precipitating factors.
3. Do not cardiovert/defibrillate through paddle that overlies a transdermal patch. May damage the paddles and burn the client. Remove patch before performing this activity.

CLIENT/FAMILY TEACHING

1. Apply as directed at the same time each day. Remove patch from foil pouch immediately prior to application and remove protective liner from patch and apply to any area of the body except the extremities below the knee or elbow (chest is preferred site).
2. Press patch onto skin and smooth down. Dry skin completely before applying to a hair-free site. *Do not change brands or attempt to trim or cut system.*
3. Rotate application sites each day to avoid skin irritation. Do not apply to irritated, abraded, or scarred skin or immediately after showering or bathing.
4. If patch becomes dislodged, discard it and put a new one on at a different skin site. Date patch as a reminder that drug has been administered. Once applied, do not disturb or open patch. Do not stop abruptly.
5. Remove at bedtime or as directed (12–14 hr) to prevent a diminished response (tolerance) to the drug. Remember to reapply a new system upon awakening the next morning.
6. Acetaminophen can be used to relieve headache without reducing the medications antianginal effectiveness.
7. Report adverse effects or breakthrough pain. Bathing or swimming should not interfere with therapy. Carry SL NTG for acute pain relief.
8. When terminating therapy, gradually reduce the dose and frequency of application over 4–6 weeks.
9. Avoid taking Viagra during therapy; may cause severe drop in BP.
10. Remove patch before defibrillating, as patch may explode. Have family/significant other learn CPR.
11. Keep all F/U to assess response and for adverse SE.

OUTCOMES/EVALUATE

Control/prevention of anginal episodes

Nitroglycerin translingual spray

(nye-troh-**GLIH**-sir-in)

Classification(s): Vasodilator, coronary
Pregnancy Category: C
RX: Nitrolingual, NitroMist.

SEE ALSO ***ANTIANGINAL DRUGS-NITRATES/NITRITES.***

INDICATIONS/USES

(1) Terminate an acute anginal attack due to coronary artery disease. (2) Prophylactically 10–15 min before beginning activities that can cause an acute anginal attack due to coronary artery disease.

ACTION/KINETICS

Pharmacokinetics

Onset: 2 min; **duration:** 30–60 min.

SPECIAL CONCERNS

Dosage not established in children.

SIDE EFFECTS

Most Common

Headache (may be severe and persistent), flushing, dizziness, weakness, hypotension, paresthesia.

See *Antianginal Drugs-Nitrates/Nitrites* for a complete list of possible side effects. Also, **hypersensitivity:** N&V, pallor, perspiration, restlessness, weakness, collapse. **Dermatologic:** Rash, exfoliative dermatitis. **Miscellaneous:** Abdominal pain, asthenia, dyspnea, peripheral edema, pharyngitis, rhinitis, vasodilation.

HOW SUPPLIED

Aerosol Spray, Lingual: 0.4 mg (400 mcg)/metered dose (spray).

DOSAGE

AEROSOL SPRAY, LINGUAL

Termination of acute attack.

One to two metered doses (400–800 mcg) on or under the tongue q 5 min as

N

needed; no more than three metered doses should be administered within a 15-min period.

Prophylaxis of angina.

One to two metered doses (400–800 mcg) 5–10 min before beginning activities that might precipitate an acute attack.

NURSING IMPLICATIONS

IMPLEMENTATION/ADMINISTRATION/STORAGE

1. Each metered spray delivers 48 mg of solution containing 400 mcg nitroglycerin, after an initial priming of 1 spray. The container will remain adequately primed for 6 weeks.
2. If the product is not used within 6 weeks, reprime with 1 spray.
3. There are 60–200 doses/bottle. The total number of available sprays depends on the number of sprays per use (1 or 2 sprays) and the frequency of repriming.
4. Store from 15–30°C (59–86°F).

ASSESSMENT

1. Note reasons for therapy, cardiac history/assessments, VS and ECG.
2. Assess and rate pain, noting location, onset, duration, and any precipitating factors.

CLIENT/FAMILY TEACHING

1. Do not shake container before administering dose. Prime aerosol unit initially with 1 spray. (Reprime with 1 spray if unit has not been used for 6 or more weeks). Hold container upright as close to open mouth as possible, press button firmly to release spray onto or under the tongue.
2. Do not inhale spray; avoid: swallowing immediately after administering spray or expectorating or rinsing the mouth for 5–10 min following administration.
3. Sit upright during application. Spray under or on the tongue 5–10 min before anticipated activity or when pain is experienced. Wait 10 sec and then swallow.
4. If pain remains, may repeat dose every 5 min until 3 sprays are taken. Seek immediate medical attention (911) if pain becomes more intense or persists after a total of 3 sprays.
5. Aerosol spray contains alcohol; do not spray toward flames or forcefully open or burn container after use. Discard aerosol and replace with new unit when end of pump is no longer covered by fluid.
6. Avoid sudden changes in position to prevent dizziness.
7. Acetaminophen can be used to relieve headache without reducing the medication's antianginal effectiveness.
8. Avoid drugs for erection during therapy (phosphodiesterase inhibitors), may cause severe drop in BP.
9. Have family/significant other learn CPR.
10. Keep all F/U to assess response and for adverse SE.

OUTCOMES/EVALUATE

Control/prevention of acute anginal episodes

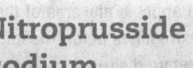

■ IV ℗

Nitroprusside sodium

(nye-troh-**PRUS**-eyed)

Classification(s): Antihypertensive, peripheral vasodilator

Pregnancy Category: C

RX: Nitropress.

INDICATIONS/USES

(1) Hypertensive crisis to reduce BP immediately. (2) To produce controlled hypotension during anesthesia to reduce bleeding. (3) Acute CHF. *Investigational:* In combination with dopamine for acute MI. Left ventricular failure with coadministration of oxygen, morphine, and a loop diuretic.

ACTION/KINETICS

Action

Direct action on vascular smooth muscle, leading to peripheral vasodilation of arteries and veins. Acts on excitation-contraction coupling of vascular smooth muscle by interfering with both influx and intracellular activation of calcium. No effect on smooth muscle of the duodenum or uterus and is more active on veins than on arteries. May also improve CHF by decreasing systemic resistance, preload and afterload reduction, and improved CO. Caution must be exercised as nitroprusside injection can result in toxic levels of cyanide. However, when used briefly or at low infusion rates, the cyanide produced reacts with thiosulfate to produce thiocyanate, which is excreted in the urine.

Pharmacokinetics

Onset (drug must be given by IV infusion): 0.5–1 min; **peak effect:** 1–2 min; **t½:** 2 min; **duration:** Up to 10 min after infusion stopped. Reacts with hemoglobin to produce cyanmethemoglobin and cyanide ion.

CONTRAINDICATIONS

Compensatory hypertension where the primary hemodynamic lesion is aortic coarctation or AV shunting. Use to produce controlled hypotension during surgery in clients with known inadequate cerebral circulation or in moribund clients. Clients with congenital optic atrophy or tobacco amblyopia (both of which are rare). Acute CHF associated with decreased peripheral vascular resistance (e.g., high-output heart failure that may be seen in endotoxic sepsis). Lactation.

SPECIAL CONCERNS

(1) After reconstitution, nitroprusside is not suitable for direct injection. The reconstituted solution must be further diluted in D5W before infusion. (2) Can cause a precipitous drop in BP. In clients not properly monitored, these decreases can lead to irreversible ischemic injuries or death. Use only when available equipment and personnel allow BP to be monitored continuously. (3) Nitroprusside injection gives rise to important quantities of cyanide except when used briefly or at low (less than 2 mcg/kg/min) infusion rates. This can lead to toxic and potentially lethal levels. The usual dose rate is 0.5-10 mcg/kg/min, but infusion at the maximum rates should never last beyond 10 minutes. If BP has not been adequately controlled after 10 min of infusion at the maximum rate, terminate administration immediately. (4) Monitor acid-base balance and venous oxygen levels; they may indicate cyanide toxicity but these tests provide imperfect guidance.

- **Use with caution in hypothyroidism, liver or kidney impairment, during lactation, and in the presence of increased ICP.**
- **Elderly may be more sensitive to the hypotensive effects of nitroprusside; also, a decrease in dose may be necessary in the elderly due to age-related decreases in renal function.**

SIDE EFFECTS

Most Common

Excessive hypotension, dizziness, nausea, restlessness, headache, sweating, palpitations, abdominal pain, muscle twitching, retrosternal discomfort.

Large doses may lead to cyanide toxicity. **Following rapid BP reduction:** Dizziness, nausea, restlessness, headache, sweating, muscle twitching, palpitations, abdominal pain, apprehension, retching, retrosternal discomfort. **Other side effects:** Bradycardia, tachycardia, ECG changes, venous streaking, rash, vomiting, methemoglobinemia, decreased platelet aggregation, flushing, ileus, irritation at injection site, hypothyroidism. **Symptoms of thiocyanate toxicity:** Blurred vision, tinnitus, confusion, hyperreflexia, seizures. **CNS symptoms (transitory):** Restlessness, agitation, increased ICP, and muscle twitching.

OVERDOSE MANAGEMENT

Symptoms: Excessive hypotension, cyanide toxicity, thiocyanate toxicity. *Treatment:*

- Measure cyanide levels and blood gases to determine venous hyperoxemia or acidosis.
- To treat cyanide toxicity, discontinue nitroprusside and give sodium nitrite, 4–6 mg/kg (about 0.2 mL/kg) over 2–4 min (to convert hemoglobin into methemoglobin); follow by sodium thiosulfate, 150–200 mg/kg (about 50 mL of the 25% solution). This regimen can be given again, at half the original doses, after 2 hr.

DRUG INTERACTIONS

Concomitant use of other antihypertensives, volatile liquid anesthetics, or certain depressants ↑ nitroprusside response.

HOW SUPPLIED

Powder for Injection: 50 mg/vial.

DOSAGE

IV INFUSION ONLY

Hypertensive crisis.

Adults: Average, 3 mcg/kg/min. **Range:** 0.3–10 mcg/kg/min. Smaller dose is required for clients receiving other antihypertensives. **Pediatric:** 1.4 mcg/kg/min adjusted slowly depending on the response.

Monitor BP and use as guide to regulate rate of administration to maintain desired antihypertensive effect. Do not exceed a rate of administration of 10 mcg/kg/min.

NURSING IMPLICATIONS

Do not confuse nitroprusside with nitroglycerin (a coronary vasodilator).

IMPLEMENTATION/ADMINISTRATION/STORAGE

1. IV Dissolve contents of the vial (50 mg) in 2–3 mL of D5W. Must be further diluted in 250–1,000 mL D5W.
2. If protected from light, reconstituted solution is stable for 24 hr. Discard solutions that are any color but light brown.
3. Protect dilute solutions during administration by wrapping bag and tubing with opaque material such as aluminum foil or foil-lined bags; change setup every 24 hr. Explain that covering the IV bag protects the medication from light and maintains drug stability. Administer IV solution with an electronic infusion device in a monitored environment.
4. Cyanide toxicity is possible if more than 500 mcg/kg nitroprusside is given faster than 2 mcg/kg/min. To reduce this possibility, sodium thiosulfate can be co-infused with nitroprusside at rates of 5–10 times that of nitroprusside.
5. Protect drug from heat, light, and moisture. Store at 15–30°C (59–86°F).
6. COMPATIBILITY D5W.
7. INCOMPATIBILITY Do not add any other drug or preservative to solution.

ASSESSMENT

1. Note onset and etiology of hypertensive crisis, S&S, other therapies trialed, outcome.
2. Note any hypothyroidism or B_{12} deficiency. Assess for any increased ICP, electrolyte disturbance, liver or renal dysfunction or conditions that would preclude drug therapy (i.e., AV shunt, coarctation of aorta, etc.).
3. Monitor BP closely and titrate infusion. Administer only in a continuously monitored environment by trained personnel.
4. Observe for symptoms of thiocyanate toxicity. Evaluate thiocyanate levels daily with prolonged infusions of >3 mcg/kg/min or in anuric clients and q 48–72 hr otherwise. Levels should be <100 mcg thiocyanate/mL or 3 μmol cyanide/mL. Metabolic acidosis may precede cyanide toxicity.
5. With cyanide toxicity, administer sodium nitrite 4–6 mg/kg over 2–4 min (as a 3% solution). Then use sodium thiosulfate 150–200 mcg/kg as a 25% or 50% solution to convert cyanide to thiocyanate so the body can eliminate it.
6. Monitor VS, I&O, ECG, CBC, electrolytes, ABGs, PAWP, renal and LFTs. With prolonged infusions monitor plasma thiocyanate levels daily. Serum lactate levels usually higher than 10 mmol/L may provide a quicker determination.

CLIENT/FAMILY TEACHING

1. Drug is given in a monitored environment to rapidly lower BP and to reduce the workload of the heart.
2. To maintain drug stability, it will be protected from light, using supplied opaque sleeve, aluminum foil, or other opaque material. Not necessary to cover the infusion chamber or the tubing.
3. Avoid sudden changes in position to prevent significant drop in BP.
4. Report any ringing in the ears, headache, dizziness or blurred vision as well as any other adverse side effects or pain at injection site immediately.

OUTCOMES/EVALUATE

- ↓ BP; ↓ Preload/afterload
- Improved S&S of refractory CHF

Nizatidine

(nye-**ZAY**-tih-deen)

Classification(s): Histamine H_2 receptor blocking drug

Pregnancy Category: B

OTC: Axid AR.

RX: Axid, Axid Pulvules.

Rx: Apo-Nizatidine, Gen-Nizatidine, PMS-Nizatidine.

SEE ALSO ***HISTAMINE H_2 ANTAGONISTS***.

INDICATIONS/USES

Rx: (1) Treatment of acute duodenal ulcer (up to 8 weeks) and maintenance following healing of a duodenal ulcer. (2) GERD, including erosive and ulcerative esophagitis and associated heartburn. Has been used for up to 12 weeks in adults and 8 weeks in children 12 years and older. (3) Short-term (up to 8 weeks) treatment of benign gastric ulcer.

OTC: Prevention and relief of heartburn, acid indigestion, and sour stomach due to certain foods and beverages.

Investigational: Prevention of olanzapine-induced weight gain. Prevention of NSAID-induced gastroduodenal ulcer. In combination with amoxicillin and clarithromycin for *Helicobacter pylori* infection.

ACTION/KINETICS

Action

Decreases gastric acid secretion by blocking the effect of histamine on histamine H_2 receptors. Does not affect the P-450 and P-448 drug metabolizing enzymes.

Pharmacokinetics

Greater than 70% bioavailable. **Onset:** 30 min. **Peak plasma levels:** 0.5–3 hr after a PO dose. **Time to peak effect:** 0.5–3 hr. **Duration, nocturnal:** Up to 12 hr; **basal:** Up to 8 hr. **$t^{1/2}$:** 1–2 hr. Approximately 60% of a PO dose is excreted unchanged in the urine. Clients with moderate to severe renal impairment manifest a significant prolongation of $t^{1/2}$ with decreased clearance. **Plasma protein binding:** About 35%.

CONTRAINDICATIONS

Hypersensitivity to H_2 receptor antagonists. Cirrhosis of the liver, impaired renal or hepatic function. Lactation.

SPECIAL CONCERNS

Use oral solution and OTC tablets only for those 12 years of age and older.

SIDE EFFECTS

Most Common

Headache, dizziness, insomnia, agitation/anxiety, somnolence, fatigue, rash, nausea, diarrhea.

CNS: Headache, fatigue, somnolence, insomnia, dizziness, abnormal dreams, agitation/anxiety, nervousness, confusion (rare). **GI:** N&V, diarrhea, pancreatitis, constipation, abdominal discomfort, flatulence, dyspepsia, anorexia, dry mouth. **Dermatologic:** Rash, exfoliative dermatitis, erythroderma, pruritus, urticaria, erythema multiforme. **CV:** Asymptomatic VT; ***rarely, cardiac arrhythmias or arrest following rapid IV use.*** **Respiratory:** Rhinitis, pharyngitis, sinusitis, cough. **Body as a whole:** Asthenia, back/chest pain, infection, fever, myalgia. **Miscellaneous:** Impotence, loss of libido, thrombocytopenia, sweating, gynecomastia, hyperuricemia, eosinophilia, gout, and cholestatic or hepatocellular effects (resulting in increased AST, ALT, or alkaline phosphatase).

LABORATORY TEST CONSIDERATIONS

False + test for urobilinogen.

DRUG INTERACTIONS

Antacids containing Al and Mg⁺⁺ hydroxides / ↓ Nizatidine absorption by about 10%
Aspirin, high doses / ↑ Salicylate levels
Simethicone / ↓ Nizatidine absorption by about 10%

HOW SUPPLIED

Capsules (Rx): 150 mg, 300 mg; *Oral Solution (Rx):* 15 mg/mL; *Tablets (OTC):* 75 mg.

DOSAGE

Axid, Axid Pulvules

RX: CAPSULES, ORAL SOLUTION

Acute therapy for duodenal ulcer.

Adults: Either 300 mg once daily at bedtime or 150 mg 2 times per day. Most heal within 4 weeks. **Maintenance therapy:** 150 mg once daily at bedtime.

GERD, including erosive and ulcerative esophagitis.

Adults and children 12 years and older: 150 mg twice a day.

Treatment of benign gastric ulcer.

Adults: Either 150 mg twice a day or 300 mg once daily at bedtime

Axid AR

OTC: TABLETS

Heartburn, acid indigestion, sour stomach.

For relief of symptoms: 1 tablet with a full glass of water. To prevent symptoms: 1 tablet with a full glass of water before eating or up to 60 minutes before consuming foods and beverages that cause heartburn. *NOTE:* Can be used up to two times per day (i.e., 2 tablets in 24 hr).

NURSING IMPLICATIONS

IMPLEMENTATION/ADMINISTRATION/STORAGE

1. Use the following doses for moderate to severe renal insufficiency for treating active duodenal ulcer, GERD, or benign gastric ulcer: If the C_{CR} is 20–50 mL/min: 150 mg/day and 150 mg every other day for maintenance; if C_{CR} <20 mL/min: 150 mg every other day and 150 mg every 3 days for maintenance.
2. Maintain treatment for active duodenal ulcer for up to 8 weeks.
3. Gastric malignancy may be present even though a clinical response to nizatidine has occurred.
4. Doses of 150 and 300 mg can be mixed with commercial juices (apple juice, Gatorade, Ocean Spray, and others); such preparations are stable for 48 hr when refrigerated. However, a 10% loss in potency is seen if mixed with V8 or Cran-Grape juices.
5. Store capsules from 20–25°C (68–77°F) in tightly closed container. Store solution from 15–30°C (59–86°F).

N

ASSESSMENT

1. List type, onset, characteristics of S&S, other agents trialed, outcome.
2. Note any experience/intolerance to H_2 receptor antagonists; assess abdomen, mouth/throat, teeth, and symptoms.
3. List drugs prescribed to ensure none interact.
4. Note *H. pylori* results and diagnostic findings, i.e., radiographic/endoscopic.
5. Monitor hepatic and renal function studies; reduce dosage/frequency with renal dysfunction.

CLIENT/FAMILY TEACHING

1. Take at bedtime if sedative effects noted. Continue to take as ordered even if symptoms subside to ensure adequate healing. With erosive esophagitis expect prolonged therapy.
2. Use caution when performing tasks that require mental alertness until drug effects realized.
3. Report any rashes, flaking of skin, extreme sleepiness, blood in stool/vomit, or lack of response. Stay active and increase fluid and roughage in diet to prevent constipation.
4. Avoid alcohol, caffeine, spicy foods, and aspirin-containing products. Do not smoke, as this aggravates condition by increasing gastric acid secretion.
5. OTC use: To relieve heartburn, take 1 tablet (75 mg) with a full glass of water. To prevent heartburn, take 1 tablet with a full glass of water just before eating or up to 60 min before consuming food/beverages that cause heartburn.
6. Keep all F/U to assess response and for adverse SE.

OUTCOMES/EVALUATE

Improvement in ulcer pain/irritation with healing; ↓ GERD S&S

■ IV

Norepinephrine bitartrate (Levarterenol)

(nor-ep-ih-**NEF**-rin)

Classification(s): Sympathomimetic

Pregnancy Category: C

RX: Levophed.

SEE ALSO ***SYMPATHOMIMETIC DRUGS***.

INDICATIONS/USES

(1) Hypotensive states caused by septicemia, blood transfusions, drug reactions, spinal anesthesia, poliomyelitis, sympathectomy, MI, and pheochromocytomectomy. (2) Adjunct to treatment of cardiac arrest and profound hypotension. Used during cardiac resuscitation after cardiac arrest to restore and maintain an adequate BP after an effective heartbeat and ventilation have been established.

ACTION/KINETICS

Action

Norepinephrine is a powerful peripheral vasoconstrictor due to stimulation of alpha-adrenergic receptors; it is also a potent inotropic agent due to its action on B_1 receptors in the heart. Coronary vasodilation occurs secondary to enhanced myocardial contractility. The result is an increase in systemic BP and coronary artery blood flow. Cardiac output changes vary but is usually increased in hypotension when BP is raised to optimal levels. Venous return is increased and the heart tends to have a more normal rate and rhythm compared with the hypotensive state. Minimal hyperglycemic effect.

Pharmacokinetics

Onset: immediate; **duration:** 1–2 min after discontinuation of the infusion. Metabolized in liver and other tissues by the enzymes MAO and catechol-O-methyltransferase; however, the pharmacologic activity is terminated by uptake and metabolism in sympathetic nerve endings. Metabolites excreted in urine.

CONTRAINDICATIONS

Use in hypotension due to blood volume deficits, except as an emergency measure to maintain coronary and cerebral artery perfusion until blood volume replacement therapy can be completed. Use in clients with mesenteric or peripheral vascular thrombosis (due to increased risk of ischemia and extending the area of infarction) unless use is necessary as a life-saving procedure. Use during cyclopropane and halothane anesthesia or in those with profound hypoxia or hypercarbia (due to risk of producing ventricular tachycardia or fibrillation).

SPECIAL CONCERNS

Antidote for extravasation ischemia. To prevent sloughing and necrosis in areas in which extravasation has taken place, the area should be infiltrated as soon as possible with 10–15 mL of saline solution containing from 5–10 mg of phentolamine, an adrenergic blocking agent. A syringe with a fine hypodermic needle should be used, with the solution being infiltrated liberally throughout the area, which is easily identified by its cold, hard, and pallid appearance. Sympathetic blockade with phentolamine causes immediate and conspicuous local hyperemic changes if the area is infiltrated within 12 hours. Therefore, phentolamine should be given as soon as possible after the extravasation is noted.

- **Use is not a substitute for replacement of blood, plasma, fluids, and electrolytes.**
- **Some products contain sulfites that may cause allergic effects, including anaphylaxis or life-threatening or less severe asthmatic episodes.**
- **Use with caution during lactation.**
- **Select doses carefully in the elderly.**
- **Safety and efficacy not demonstrated in children.**

SIDE EFFECTS

Most Common

Bradycardia, headache, anxiety.

CV: Bradycardia (probably as a reflex due to a rise in BP), arrhythmias. **CNS:** Headache (may be a symptom of overdosage and severe hypertension), transient headache, anxiety. **Miscellaneous:** Ischemic injury due to potent vasoconstriction and tissue hypoxia, respiratory difficulty, extravasation necrosis at injection site, gangrene (when infused into an ankle vein). *NOTE:* Prolonged administration may result in plasma volume depletion which should be continuously corrected by appropriate fluid and electrolyte replacement. If plasma volume is not corrected, hypotension may recur when norepinephrine injection is discontinued.

OVERDOSE MANAGEMENT

Symptoms: Dangerously high BP, headache, reflex bradycardia, marked increase in peripheral resistance, decreased cardiac output. Prolonged administration may result in plasma volume depletion. *Treatment:* Appropriate fluid and electrolyte replacement. If plasma volumes are not corrected, hypotension may result when norepinephrine is discontinued or BP may be maintained at the risk of severe peripheral vasoconstriction with diminution of blood flow and tissue perfusion.

DRUG INTERACTIONS

Anesthetics, halogenated hydrocarbon (e.g., halothane) / Sensitization of heart to the effects of norepinephrine → possible ventricular tachycardia and fibrillation; do not use together

Bretylium / Potentiation of action of vasopressors on adrenergic receptors → possible arrhythmias

Guanethidine / ↑ Pressor response of norepinephrine → possible severe hypertension

MAOIs / Possible severe, prolonged hypertension; use together with extreme caution

Oxytocic drugs / In obstetrics, if norepinephrine is used either to correct hypotension or added to the local anesthetic solution → possible severe persistent hypertension

Tricyclic antidepressants / Potentiation of pressor response; use together with caution

HOW SUPPLIED

Injection: 1 mg (as base)/mL.

DOSAGE

IV INFUSION ONLY

Restoration of BP in acute hypotensive states.

Correct blood volume as much as possible before giving any vasopressor. In emergency situations when intra-aortic pressures must be maintained to prevent cerebral or coronary artery ischemia, give norepinephrine before and concurrently with blood volume replacement.

Effect on BP determines dosage, initial: 8–12 mcg base/min or 2–3 mL of a 4-mcg/mL solution. Adjust the rate of flow to establish and maintain a low normal BP (usually 80–100 mm Hg systolic). In previously hypertensive clients, raise the BP no more than 40 mm Hg below the pre-existing systolic pressure. **Average maintenance**: 2–4 mcg base/min with the dose determined by client response.

N

NURSING IMPLICATIONS

IMPLEMENTATION/ADMINISTRATION/STORAGE

1. **IV** Norepinephrine is a potent, concentrated drug that must be diluted in dextrose solution before infusion.
2. Monitor BP q 2 min from the time administration is started until desired BP is obtained; then, monitor q 5 min if administration is continued. Constantly watch flow rate. Never leave client unmonitored during infusion.
3. Whenever possible, infuse into a large vein, particularly an antecubital or femoral vein to minimize necrosis from overlying skin and prolonged vasoconstriction.
4. If extravasation occurs, infiltrate as soon as possible with 10–15 mL of saline solution containing 5–10 mg phentolamine to prevent sloughing and necrosis. Infiltrate liberally, using a syringe with a fine needle, throughout the ischemic area.
5. Avoid a catheter tie-in technique because obstruction to blood flow around the tubing may cause stasis and increased local concentration of the drug.
6. Avoid leg veins in elderly clients or in those suffering from such disorders due to an increased risk of atherosclerosis, arteriosclerosis, diabetic endarteritis, or Buerger's disease.
7. If large fluid volumes are needed at a flow rate involving an excessive dose of the drug per unit of time, use a solution more diluted than 4 mcg/mL. When large fluid volumes are undesirable, a higher concentration may be given.
8. Continue the norepinephrine infusion until adequate BP and tissue perfusion are maintained without therapy. Reduce infusion gradually, avoiding abrupt withdrawal.
9. When used to restore BP in hypotensive states, add 4 mL of the solution to 1,000 mL D5W in water or saline solution for a concentration of 4 mcg base/mL.
10. Do not administer through the same tube as blood products. However, a Y-tube and individual flasks may be used.
11. Store at room temperature protected from light. Discard solutions that are brown or that have a precipitate.
12. COMPATIBILITY D5W, or D5 and saline solutions.
13. INCOMPATIBILITY Do not use saline solution alone (dextrose protects against oxidation and loss of potency). Administer separately.

ASSESSMENT

1. Note reasons for therapy; ensure adequately hydrated.
2. Administer in a monitored environment. Monitor BP by arterial line or electronically continuously until stable then q 5 min during drug therapy. Assess I&O, ECG, VS, CVP, and PA wedge pressures.
3. Observe infusion site frequently for extravasation; ischemia and sloughing may occur. Blanching along the course of the vein may indicate permeability of the vein wall, which could allow leakage to occur. If evident, change IV site and give phentolamine at extravasation site.
4. Withdraw drug gradually; may experience an initial rebound drop in BP. Extra fluids paren-

terally may diminish rebound hypotension and help stabilize BP during withdrawal. Keep atropine on hand for reflex bradycardia, and propranol for arrhythmias.

CLIENT/FAMILY TEACHING

1. Drug is given by infusion in a closely monitored environment to restore BP.
2. Avoid sudden position changes to prevent sudden drop in BP (orthostatic hypotension).
3. Report any pain or discomfort at IV site, difficulty breathing, dizziness, nausea, abdominal pain, chest pain or confusion.

OUTCOMES/EVALUATE

- ↑ BP/CO
- Improved tissue perfusion

Norfloxacin

(nor-**FLOX**-ah-sin)

Classification(s): Antibiotic, fluoroquinolone

Pregnancy Category: C

RX: Noroxin.

✤ **Rx:** Apo-Norflox.

SEE ALSO ***ANTI-INFECTIVE DRUGS*** AND ***FLUOROQUINOLONES***.

INDICATIONS/USES

(1) Uncomplicated UTIs (including cystitis) caused by *Escherichia coli, Klebsiella pneumoniae, Enterobacter cloacae, Proteus mirabilis, P. vulgaris, Pseudomonas aeruginosa, Citrobacter freundii, Staphylococcus aureus, S. epidermidis, Enterococcus faecalis, Enterobacter aerogenes, S. saprophyticus,* and *S. agalactiae.* (2) Complicated UTIs caused by *Enterococcus faecalis, E. coli, K. pneumoniae, P. mirabilis, P. aeruginosa,* or *Serratia marcescens.*
(3) Urethral gonorrhea and endocervical gonococcal infections due to penicillinase- or non-penicillinase-producing *Neisseria gonorrhoeae.*
(4) Prostatitis due to *E. coli. Investigational:* Traveler's diarrhea.

ACTION/KINETICS

Action

Active against gram-positive and gram-negative organisms by inhibiting bacterial DNA synthesis. Not effective against obligate anaerobes.

Pharmacokinetics

Peak plasma levels: 1.4–1.6 mcg/mL after 1–2 hr following a dose of 400 mg and 2.5 mcg/mL 1–2 hr after a dose of 800 mg. **t½:** 3–4.5 hr. Food decreases the absorption of norfloxacin. Approximately 30% excreted unchanged in the urine and 30% through the feces.

CONTRAINDICATIONS

Hypersensitivity to nalidixic acid, cinoxacin, or norfloxacin. Lactation, infants, and children.

SPECIAL CONCERNS

(1) **Tendonitis and tendon rupture.** Fluoroquinolones, including norfloxacin, are associated with an increased risk of tendonitis and tendon rupture in all ages. This risk is further increased in older clients, usually older than 60 years of age, in clients taking corticosteroid drugs, and in clients with kidney, heart, or lung transplants. (2) **Myasthenia gravis.** Fluoroquinolones, including norfloxacin, may exacerbate muscle weakness in persons with myasthenia gravis. Avoid norfloxacin in clients with known history of myasthenia gravis.

- Use with caution with a history of seizures and in impaired renal function.
- Elderly eliminate norfloxacin more slowly.

SIDE EFFECTS

Most Common

Headache, dizziness, N&V, diarrhea, dyspepsia/heartburn, eosinophilia, neutropenia.

See *Fluoroquinolones* for a complete list of possible side effects. **GI:** N&V, diarrhea, abdominal pain/discomfort, dry/painful mouth, dyspepsia/heartburn, flatulence, constipation, pseudomembranous colitis, stomatitis. **CNS:** Headache, dizziness, fatigue, malaise, drowsiness, depression, insomnia, confusion, psychoses. **Hematologic:** Decreased hematocrit, eosinophilia, leukopenia, neutropenia, increased/decreased platelets. **Dermatologic:** Photosensitivity, rash, pruritus, exfoliative dermatitis, ***toxic epidermal necrolysis***, erythema, erythema multiforme, ***Stevens-Johnson syndrome***. **Miscellaneous:** Paresthesia, hypersensitivity, fever, visual disturbances, hearing loss, crystalluria, cylindruria, candiduria, myoclonus (rare), hepatitis, pancreatitis, arthralgia.

LABORATORY TEST CONSIDERATIONS

↑ AST, ALT, alkaline phosphatase, BUN, serum creatinine, and LDH.

ADDITIONAL DRUG INTERACTIONS

Metronidazole and Mycophenolate / ↓ Mycophenolic and mycophenolic acid glucuronide when all three taken together

Nitrofurantoin / ↓ Norfloxacin antibacterial effect

HOW SUPPLIED

Tablets: 400 mg.

DOSAGE

TABLETS

Uncomplicated UTIs due to E. coli, K. pneumoniae, *or* P. mirabilis.

Adults: 400 mg q 12 hr for 3 days.

Uncomplicated UTIs due to other indicated organisms.

Adults: 400 mg q 12 hr for 7–10 days.

Complicated UTIs.

Adults: 400 mg q 12 hr for 10–21 days.

NOTE: Maximum dose for UTIs should not exceed 800 mg/day.

Uncomplicated gonorrhea.

Adults: 800 mg as a single dose.

Acute or chronic prostatitis due to E. coli.

Adults: 400 mg q 12 hr for 28 days.

Impaired renal function, with C_{CR} equal to or less than 30 mL/min/1.73 m^2.

400 mg/day for appropriate duration for infection present; includes elderly clients.

Traveler's diarrhea.

Adults: 400 mg twice a day for 3 days.

NURSING IMPLICATIONS

Ⓢ Do not confuse Noroxin with Floxin (also a fluoroquinolone) or Neurontin (an anticonvulsant).

IMPLEMENTATION/ADMINISTRATION/STORAGE

Store from 15–30°C (59–86°F); keep container tightly closed.

ASSESSMENT

1. Note reasons for therapy, characteristics of S&S, C&S results, other agents trialed, outcome. List drugs prescribed to ensure none interact unfavorably.
2. List any seizure disorder or impaired renal/liver function. Determine if pregnant. Assess CBC, cultures, renal and LFTs; reduce dose with impaired renal function.

CLIENT/FAMILY TEACHING

1. Take 1 hr before or 2 hr after meals, with a glass of water; food decreases drug absorption. Take drug at evenly spaced intervals, generally every 12 hr.
2. Multivitamins, products containing iron or zinc, antacids containing magnesium and aluminum, sucralfate, or didanosine pediatric powder for oral solution should not be taken within 2 hr of administration of norfloxacin.
3. Use caution if operating equipment or driving a motor vehicle; may cause dizziness.
4. To prevent dehydration and crystalluria, consume 2–3 L/day of fluids.
5. Report pain, inflammation, or rupture of tendon; rest or refrain from exercise until diagnosis of tendonitis or tendon rupture is excluded.
6. Avoid prolonged sun exposure, wear sunscreen and protective clothing if exposed to avoid photosensitivity reaction.
7. Females of childbearing age should practice reliable contraception.
8. Keep all F/U to assess response, labs, and for adverse SE.

OUTCOMES/EVALUATE

- Negative culture reports
- Symptomatic improvement

N

■ Ⓢ

Nortriptyline hydrochloride

(nor-**TRIP**-tih-leen)

Classification(s): Antidepressant, tricyclic

Pregnancy Category: C

RX: Aventyl, Pamelor.

🍁 **Rx:** Apo-Nortriptyline, Gen-Nortriptyline, ratio-Nortriptyline.

SEE ALSO *ANTIDEPRESSANTS, TRICYCLIC*.

INDICATIONS/USES

Treatment of symptoms of depression. Endogenous depressions are more likely to be helped than other depressive illnesses. *Investigational:* Adjunct to analgesia, panic disorder, premenstrual symptoms, dermatologic disorders.

ACTION/KINETICS

Action

Inhibits reuptake of norepinephrine or serotonin at the presynaptic neuron. Also blocks the amine pump. Manifests moderate anticholinergic and sedative effects but slight orthostatic hypotensive effects.

Pharmacokinetics

Well absorbed; significant first-pass effect. Long serum **t½** (thus once daily dosing may suffice). **Effective plasma levels:** 50–150 ng/mL. **t½:** 18–44 hr. **Time to reach steady state:** 4–19 days. Partially metabolized in the liver; primarily excreted in the urine.

SPECIAL CONCERNS

(1) Antidepressants increased the risk of suicidal thinking and behavior (suicidality) in short-term studies in children, adolescents, and young adults with major depressive disorder and other psychiatric disorders. Anyone considering the use of nortriptyline or any other antidepressant in a child, adolescent, or young adult must balance this risk with the clinical need. Clients who are started on therapy should be observed closely for clinical worsening, suicidality, or unusual changes in behavior. Families and caregivers should be advised of the need for close observation and communication with the prescriber. Nortriptyline is not approved for use in pediatric clients. (2) Short-term placebo-controlled trials of 9 antidepressant drugs in children and adolescents with major depressive disorder, obsessive-compulsive disorder, or other psychiatric disorders revealed a greater risk of adverse reactions during the first few months of treatment. The average risk of such reactions in clients receiving antidepressants was 4%, twice the placebo risk of 2%. No suicides occurred in these trials.

- Safety and efficacy not determined in children.
- Cross sensitivity may occur between tricyclic antidepressants.
- Use with caution during lactation.

SIDE EFFECTS

Most Common

Tachycardia, blurred vision, urinary retention, dry mouth, weight gain/loss, orthostatic hypotension. See *Antidepressants, Tricyclic* for a complete list of possible side effects.

LABORATORY TEST CONSIDERATIONS

↓ Urinary 5-HIAA.

ADDITIONAL DRUG INTERACTIONS

↑ Nortriptyline levels if used together with valproic acid

HOW SUPPLIED

Capsules: 10 mg, 25 mg, 50 mg, 75 mg; ***Oral Solution:*** 10 mg base/5 mL.

DOSAGE

CAPSULES; ORAL SOLUTION

Depression.

Adults: 25 mg 3–4 times per day. Dose individualized; begin at a low dosage and increase as needed. **Doses above 150 mg/day are not recommended.**

Adolescent and elderly clients: 30–50 mg/day in divided doses or total daily dose may be given once a day.

NURSING IMPLICATIONS

Do not confuse nortriptyline (Aventyl, Pamelor) with amitriptyline or norpramin, each of which is a tricyclic antidepressant. Do not confuse Pamelor with Tambocor (an antiarrhythmic).

IMPLEMENTATION/ADMINISTRATION/STORAGE

1. The total daily dose may be given at bedtime.
2. Monitor plasma levels if doses greater than 100 mg/day are given. Maintain plasma levels in the range of 50–150 nanograms/mL.
3. Store at controlled room temperatures.

ASSESSMENT

1. List reasons for therapy, clinical presentation, onset, age, characteristics of S&S, mental status, other agents trialed. Identify causative factors; rate pain if indicated.
2. Avoid after acute MI; monitor ECG before and during therapy.
3. Stop several days before surgery to prevent hypertensive episodes; reduce dose if psychosis occurs/increases.

N

4. Monitor VS, Wt, BS, CBC, renal and LFTs. Reduce dose with dysfunction and in elderly, debilitated clients.

CLIENT/FAMILY TEACHING

1. Take after meals and at bedtime to minimize GI upset. May take several weeks before beneficial effects noted. Do not stop suddenly after long term use.
2. Take entire dose at bedtime with drowsiness and chronic pain conditions to minimize daytime sedation. Avoid activities that require mental alertness until drug effects realized. Move slowly; may experience drop in BP with sudden changes in position.
3. Report unusual/intolerable side effects. May require dosage adjustment or change in therapy. Report visual changes; ensure regular eye exams.
4. May experience sun sensitivity; use sunscreen and protective clothing.
5. Avoid alcohol, and CNS depressants; may potentiate effects. May experience dry mouth; use sugar free candy/gum, frequent sips of water/ice chips to offset.
6. Report worsened depression, suicidal thoughts, or changes in behavior ASAP.
7. Keep all F/U to assess response, labs, and for adverse SE.

OUTCOMES/EVALUATE

- Control of symptoms of depression (↓ fatigue, improved sleeping/eating patterns, effective coping)
- ↓ Nocturnal pruritus (UL)
- Control of chronic neurogenic pain (UL)

O

IV

Ofatumumab

(**OH**-fah-**TYOO**-myoo-mab)

Classification(s): Antineoplastic drug, monoclonal antibody

Pregnancy Category: C

RX: Arzerra.

INDICATIONS/USES

Treatment of chronic lymphocytic leukemia refractory to fludarabine and alemtuzumab.

ACTION/KINETICS

Action

Ofatumumab binds specifically to the small and large extracellular loops of the CD20 molecule. The CD20 molecule is expressed on normal B lymphocytes and on B-cell chronic lymphocytic leukemia. The Fab domain of ofatumumab binds to the CD20 molecule and the Fe domain mediates immune effector functions resulting in B-cell lysis. Possible mechanisms for cell lysis include complement-dependent cytotoxicity and antibody-dependent, cell-mediated toxicity.

Pharmacokinetics

Maximum plasma levels are higher after the 8th infusion compared with after the 4th infusion. There is dose-dependent clearance of the drug with clearance being slower after subsequent infusions compared with the first infusion. **t½, mean:** 2.3 hr for the 4th infusion and 61.5 days for the 12th infusion.

CONTRAINDICATIONS

Administration of live viral vaccines in those who have recently received ofatumumab.

SPECIAL CONCERNS

- The safety of immunization with live viral vaccines during or after ofatumumab administration not studied.
- Infusion reactions are more common with the first 2 infusions.
- Use with caution during lactation.
- Safety and efficacy not determined in children.

SIDE EFFECTS

Most Common

Anemia, bronchitis, cough, diarrhea, dyspnea, fatigue, nausea, neutropenia, pneumonia, pyrexia, rash, URTI.

CNS: Insomnia, headache. **GI:** Diarrhea, nausea, intestinal obstruction. **Hepatic:** Reactivation of hepatitis B, including fulminant hepatitis and ***death***. **CV:** Peripheral edema, hyper-/hypotension, tachycardia. **Respiratory:** Pneumonia, cough, dyspnea, bronchitis, URTI, nasopharyngitis, sinusitis. **Dermatologic:** Rash (including macular, vesicular), urticaria, hyperhidrosis, herpes zoster. **Musculoskeletal:** Back pain, muscle spasms. **Hematologic:** Anemia, neutropenia, thrombocytopenia. **Infusion reactions:** ***Bronchospasm***, dyspnea, ***laryngeal edema***, pulmonary edema, flushing, hypertension, hypotension, syncope, cardiac ischemia/***infarction***, back pain, abdominal pain, pyrexia, rash, urticaria, angioedema. **Body as a whole:** Fatigue, chills, pyrexia, infections (bacterial, viral, fungal), ***sepsis (including neutropenic sepsis, bacteremia, septic shock)***. **Miscellaneous:** Immunogenicity, ***progressive multifocal leukoencephalopathy***.

HOW SUPPLIED

Injection Solution, Concentrate: 20 mg/mL.

DOSAGE

IV

Chronic lymphocytic leukemia.

Adults, usual: 12 doses given IV according to the following: 300 mg initial dose (dose 1), followed 1 week later by 2,000 mg weekly for 7 doses (doses 2 to 8), followed 4 weeks later by 2,000 mg q 4 weeks for 4 doses (doses 9 to 12).

NURSING IMPLICATIONS

IMPLEMENTATION/ADMINISTRATION/STORAGE

1. IV Do not give as an IV push or bolus.
2. Premedicate 30–120 min before each dose with PO acetaminophen, 1,000 mg (or equivalent), PO or IV antihistamine (cetirizine, 10 mg or equivalent), and IV corticosteroid (prednisolone, 100 mg or equivalent).
3. Do not reduce the corticosteroid dose for doses 1, 2, and 9. Corticosteroid dose may be reduced as follows for doses 3–8 and 10–12: For doses 3 through 8, gradually reduce corticosteroid dose with successive infusions if grade 3 or greater infusion reaction did not occur with the preceding dose. For doses 10 through 12, give prednisolone, 50–100 mg (or equivalent), if a grade 3 or greater infusion reaction did not occur with dose 9.
4. Interrupt infusion for infusion reactions of any severity. For grade 4 infusion reactions, do not resume the infusion. For grade 1, 2, or 3 infusion reaction, if the infusion reaction resolves or remains grade 2 or less, resume infusion with the following modifications according to the initial grade of the infusion reaction. For grade 1 or 2, infuse at one-half the previous infusion rate. For grade 3, infuse at a rate of 12 mL/hr. After resuming the infusion, the infusion rate may be increased based on client tolerance.
5. Prepare all doses in 1,000 mL of NaCl, 0.9% injection.
6. Prepare the solution as follows: For the *300 mg dose*, withdraw and discard 15 mL from a 1,000 mL polyolefin bag of NaCl, 0.9% injection. Withdraw 5 mL from each of 3 vials of ofatumumab and add to the bag. Mix diluted solution by gentle inversion. Do not shake. For the *2,000 mg dose*, withdraw and discard 100 mL from a 1,000 mL bag of NaCl, 0.9% injection. Withdraw 5 mL from each of the 20 vials of ofatumumab and add to the bag. Mix diluted solution by gentle inversion. Do not shake.
7. Administer using an infusion pump, the in-line filter provided with the product, and PVC administration sets. Flush the IV line with NaCl, 0.9% injection before and after each dose.
8. Start the infusion within 12 hr of preparation of the solution.
9. Use the following infusion rates: **Dose 1:** Initiate infusion at a rate of 3.6 mg/hr (12 mL/hr). **Dose 2:** Initiate infusion at a rate of 24 mg/hr (12 mL/hr). **Doses 3 through 12:** Initiate infusion at a rate of 50 mg/hr (25 mL/hr). In the absence of infusion toxicity, the rate of infusion may be increased q 30 min. Do not exceed the infusion rates.
10. Discontinue in those who develop viral hepatitis or reactivation of viral hepatitis; institute appropriate treatment.
11. Do not mix with, or administer as an infusion with, other drug products.
12. Store from 2–8°C (36–46°F). Do not freeze; protect vials from light. Discard prepared solution after 24 hr.
13. COMPATIBILITY 0.9% NaCl.
14. INCOMPATIBILITY Do not mix or administer with any other medicinal products.

ASSESSMENT

1. Note reasons for therapy, disease onset (CLL), characteristics of S&S, when failed fludarabine and alemtuzumab therapy.
2. Premedicate with acetaminophen, an antihistamine, and a corticosteroid. Interrupt infusion for any infusion reaction.
3. Consider progressive multifocal leukoencephalopathy (PML) with new onset or changes in baseline neurological presentation or S&S. Stop arzerra if suspected, and initiate PML workup with neurologist, brain MRI, and lumbar puncture (LP).
4. Assess for HBV; therapy may reactivate disease. Monitor carriers of hepatitis B for clinical and laboratory signs of active hepatitis B virus infection during and for 6 to 12 mo following the last infusion.
5. Monitor pulmonary status and assess for any evidence of pneumonia or infections.
6. Monitor VS, ECG, CBC, renal and LFTs.

CLIENT/FAMILY TEACHING

1. Drug is administered by IV infusion in those whose cancer does not respond to other chemotherapy.
2. Will receive pre-medications to reduce risk of infusion reaction which is manifested by SOB, fever, chills or rash within 24 hr of infusion; report.
3. Avoid vaccinations with live vaccines during therapy as more prone to infections.
4. Report any confusion, dizziness, loss of balance, difficulty talking or walking, or vision problems.
5. May reactivate other infections, report any yellow discoloration of skin or eyes, ↑ fatigue (S&S hepatitis).
6. Practice reliable contraception during therapy.
7. Keep all F/U to assess response, labs, and for adverse SE.

OUTCOMES/EVALUATE

Treatment of refractory CLL; inhibition of malignant cell proliferation

Ofloxacin

(oh-**FLOX**-ah-sin)

Classification(s): Antibiotic, fluoroquinolone

Pregnancy Category: C

RX: Floxin, Floxin Otic, Ocuflox.

🍁 **Rx:** Apo-Oflox, Apo-Ofloxacin.

SEE ALSO ***ANTI-INFECTIVE DRUGS*** AND ***FLUOROQUINOLONES***.

INDICATIONS/USES

Systemic (PO):

1. Community-acquired pneumonia or acute bacterial exacerbations of chronic bronchitis due to *Haemophilus influenzae* or *Streptococcus pneumoniae.*
2. Acute, uncomplicated urethral and cervical gonorrhea due to *Neisseria gonorrhoeae;* nongonococcal urethritis, and cervicitis due to *Chlamydia trachomatis.* Mixed infections of the urethra and cervix due to *N. gonorrhoeae* and *C. trachomatis.*
3. Uncomplicated mild to moderate skin and skin structure infections due to *Staphylococcus aureus* methicillin–susceptible), *Streptococcus pyogenes,* or *Proteus mirabilis.*
4. Uncomplicated cystitis due to *Citrobacter diversus, Enterobacter aerogenes, Escherichia coli, Klebsiella pneumoniae, Proteus mirabilis,* or *Pseudomonas aeruginosa.*
5. Complicated UTIs due to *E. coli, K. pneumoniae, P. mirabilis, C. diversus,* or *P. aeruginosa.*
6. Prostatitis due to *E. coli.*
7. Acute PID (including severe infection) due to *C. trachomatis* or *N. gonorrhoeae.*

Investigational: Epididymitis, traveler's diarrhea.

Ophthalmic: (1) Treatment of conjunctivitis caused by *S. aureus, Staphylococcus epidermidis, S. pneumoniae, Enterobacter cloacae, H. influenzae, P. mirabilis,* and *P. aeruginosa.* (2) Corneal ulcers caused by *S. aureus, S. epidermidis, S. pneumoniae, P. aeruginosa,* and *Serratia marcescens.*

Otic: (1) Otitis externa due to *S. aureus, E. coli,* and *P. aeruginosa* in adults and children, 6 months of age and older. (2) Acute otitis media due to *S. aureus, S. pneumoniae, H. influenzae, Moraxella catarrhalis,* and *P. aeruginosa* in children 1 year and older with tympanostomy tubes. (3) Chronic suppurative otitis media due to *S. aureus, P. mirabilis,* and *P. aeruginosa* in clients 12 years and older who have perforated tympanic membranes.

ACTION/KINETICS

Action

Effective against a wide range of gram-positive and gram-negative aerobic and anaerobic bacteria.

Penicillinase has no effect on the activity of ofloxacin.

Pharmacokinetics

Widely distributed to body fluids. **Maximum serum levels:** 1–2 hr. **t½, first phase:** 5–7 hr; **second phase:** 20–25 hr. **Peak serum levels at steady state, after PO doses:** 1.5 mcg/mL after 200-mg doses, 2.4 mcg/mL after 300-mg doses, and 2.9 mcg/mL after 400-mg doses. Between 70% and 80% is excreted unchanged in the urine.

CONTRAINDICATIONS

Hypersensitivity to quinolone antibacterial agents. Use for syphilis (ineffective). Ophthalmic use in dendritic keratitis, vaccinia, varicella, mycobacterial infections of the eye, fungal diseases of the eye, and with steroid combinations after uncomplicated removal of a corneal foreign body. Lactation. Interchangeable use of the otic and ophthalmic solutions.

SPECIAL CONCERNS

(1) **Tendonitis and tendon rupture.** Fluoroquinolones, including ofloxacin, are associated with an increased risk of tendonitis and tendon rupture in all ages. This risk is further increased in older clients (usually older than 60 years), clients taking glucocorticoid drugs, and clients with kidney, heart, or lung transplants. (2) **Myasthenia gravis.** Fluoroquinolones, including ofloxacin, may exacerbate muscle weakness in persons with myasthenia gravis. Avoid ofloxacin in clients with a known history of myasthenia gravis.

- Safety and efficacy of the systemic forms not established in children, adolescents under the age of 18 years, pregnant women, and during lactation.
- Safety and efficacy of the ophthalmic form not established in children less than 1 year of age.
- Use with caution in known or suspected CNS disorders (e.g., severe cerebral atherosclerosis, epilepsy, or factors that predispose to seizures).

SIDE EFFECTS

Most Common

After systemic use: N&V, abdominal pain/discomfort, diarrhea, dry/painful mouth, constipation, flatulence, headache, dizziness, fatigue/malaise, depression, insomnia, rash, pruritus, fever, vaginitis, visual disturbances.

After ophthalmic use: Transient irritation/burning/stinging, itching, inflammation.

After otic use: Pruritus, application site reaction, dizziness, earache, vertigo.

See *Fluoroquinolones* for a complete list of possible side effects. **GI:** N&V, diarrhea, abdominal pain/discomfort, dry/ painful mouth, dyspepsia, flatulence, constipation, flatulence, pseudomembranous colitis, dysgeusia, decreased appetite. **CNS:** Headache, dizziness, fatigue, malaise, somnolence, depression, insomnia, seizures, sleep disorders, nervousness, anxiety, cognitive change, dream abnormality, euphoria, hallucinations, vertigo. **CV:** Chest pain, edema, hypertension, palpitations, vasodilation. **Hypersensitivity reactions:** Dyspnea, ***CV collapse***, loss of consciousness, angioedema (including laryngeal, pharyngeal, or facial edema), airway obstruction, urticaria, itching, ***anaphylaxis***. **GU:** External genital pruritus in women, vaginitis, vaginal discharge; burning, irritation, pain, and rash of the female genitalia; glucosuria, proteinuria, hematuria, pyuria, dysmenorrhea, menorrhagia, metrorrhagia, urinary frequency or pain. **Respiratory:** Cough, rhinorrhea. **Dermatologic:** Diaphoresis, vasculitis, photosensitivity, rash, pruritus. **Hematologic:** Leukocytosis, lymphocytopenia, eosinophilia. **Musculoskeletal:** Asthenia, extremity pain, arthropathy, arthralgia, myalgia, possibility of osteochondrosis. **Miscellaneous:** Fever, chills, malaise, syncope, hyperglycemia or hypoglycemia, whole body pain, thirst, weight loss, photophobia, trunk pain, paresthesia, visual disturbances, hypersensitivity, hearing loss, superinfection.

After ophthalmic use: Visual disturbances, transient ocular burning or discomfort, stinging, redness, itching, photophobia, tearing, and dryness.

After otic use: Pruritus, application site reaction, dizziness, earache, vertigo, taste perversion, paresthesia, rash, diarrhea, otorrhagia, dry mouth, headache, tinnitus, fever, N&V.

HOW SUPPLIED

Ophthalmic Solution: 0.3% (3 mg/mL); ***Otic Solution:*** 0.3% (3 mg/mL); ***Tablets:*** 200 mg, 300 mg, 400 mg.

DOSAGE

TABLETS

Community-acquired pneumonia, exacerbation of chronic bronchitis.

Adults: 400 mg q 12 hr for 10 days.

O

Acute uncomplicated urethral or cervical gonorrhea.

Adults: One 400-mg dose. The CDC also recommend adding doxycycline or azithromycin.

Nongonococcal cervicitis/urethritis due to C. trachomatis *or mixed infection of the urethra/cervix due to* C. trachomatis *and* N. gonorrhoeae.

Adults: 300 mg q 12 hr for 7 days.

Mild to moderate skin and skin structure infections.

Adults: 400 mg q 12 hr for 10 days.

Uncomplicated cystitis due E. coli *or* K. pneumoniae.

Adults: 200 mg q 12 hr for 3 days.

Uncomplicated cystitis due to other organisms.

Adults: 200 mg q 12 hr for 7 days.

Complicated UTIs.

Adults: 200 mg q 12 hr for 10 days.

Prostatitis due to E. coli.

Adults: 300 mg q 12 hr for 6 weeks.

Acute PID.

Adults: 400 mg PO q 12 hr for 10–14 days plus metronidazole.

Traveler's diarrhea (investigational).

Adults: 200 mg twice a day for 3 days.

Epididymitis (investigational).

Adults: 300 mg q 12 hr for 10 days.

OPHTHALMIC SOLUTION, (0.3%)

Conjunctivitis.

Initial: 1–2 gtt in the affected eye(s) q 2–4 hr for the first 2 days; **then,** 1–2 gtt 4 times per day for 7 additional days.

Bacterial corneal ulcer.

1–2 gtt q 30 min while awake. Awaken at about 4 and 6 hr after retiring and instill 1–2 gtt. **Then,** instill 1–2 gtt hourly while awake for days 3 through 7–9; for days 7–9 through treatment completion, instill 1–2 gtt 4 times per day.

OTIC SOLUTION (0.3%)

Otitis externa.

Adults and children over 13 years: 0.5 mL (10 drops) of the 0.3% solution instilled into the affected ear once daily for 7 days. **Children, 6 months to 13 years:** 0.25 mL (5 drops) of the 0.3% solution instilled into the affected ear once daily for 7 days.

Acute otitis media in children with tympanostomy tubes.

Children 1–12 years: 0.25 mL (5 drops) in the affected ear twice a day for 10 days.

Chronic suppurative otitis media with perforated tympanic membranes.

Adults and children, 12 years and older: 0.5 mL (10 drops) instilled into the affected ear twice a day for 14 days.

NURSING IMPLICATIONS

Do not confuse Ocuflox with Ocufen (an ophthalmic NSAID).

IMPLEMENTATION/ADMINISTRATION/STORAGE

1. Do not take with food.
2. Do not exceed a daily PO dose of 400 mg in those with a Child-Pugh score of 10–15.
3. Adjust the dose as follows for clients with impaired renal function. If the C_{CR} is 20–50 mL/min, give the usual recommended unit dose once a day. If the C_{CR} is <20 mL/min, give half the usual recommended unit dose once a day.
4. Do not inject the ophthalmic solution subconjunctivally and do not introduce directly into the anterior chamber of the eye.
5. Do not confuse the ophthalmic and otic dosage forms; they are not interchangeable.
6. Store tablets in tightly closed containers at a temperature <30°C (86°F). Store otic solution from 15–30°C (59–86°F); protect from light.

ASSESSMENT

1. Note reasons for therapy, characteristics of S&S, any sensitivity to quinolone derivatives.
2. Review other prescribed agents; probenecid may block renal tubular excretion.
3. Assess for any CNS disorders. Report tremors, restlessness, confusion, hallucinations; may need to stop therapy. Avoid with myasthenia gravis.
4. Consult provider if diabetic and a hypoglycemic reaction occurs when treated with ofloxacin and insulin or an oral hypoglycemic.

5. Review risk of tendon rupture with fluoroquinolones.
6. Monitor CBC, BS, cultures, renal and LFTs; reduce dose with renal dysfunction.

CLIENT/FAMILY TEACHING

1. Can be taken without regard to meals. Drink 2–3 L/day of fluids to assist in drug elimination.
2. Avoid vitamins, iron, or mineral combinations, aluminum- or magnesium-based antacids 2 hr before and 2 hr after ingestion of ofloxacin.
3. Do not perform activities that require mental alertness until drug effects realized; may cause drowsiness and lightheadedness.
4. Wash hands before and after use. Avoid contamination of the eye or ear applicator tip with material from the eye, ear, or fingers. Do not confuse eye and ear dosage forms; not interchangeable.
5. Before using, warm ear drops by rolling the bottle in hands; instillation of cold drops may cause dizziness. When used in the ear, lie with the affected ear upward. Instill drops and maintain this position for 5 min to ensure penetration of the drops into the ear canal. When used for acute otitis media or chronic suppurative otitis media, pump the earlobe 4 times after instillation by pushing inward to facilitate penetration into the middle ear. If ordered, repeat for the opposite ear.
6. With eye drops, tilt head back looking up and pull lower eyelid down and instill prescribed number of drops. Close eye for 1 to 2 min, apply gentle pressure to bridge of nose for 1 to 3 min. May experience temporary stinging or burning; report if bothersome or if eye/eyelid inflammation noted. If wearing contact lens, remove before instilling eye drops.
7. May experience N&V and diarrhea, stinging/burning; report any pain, inflammation, or rupture of tendon; rest or refrain from exercise until diagnosis of tendonitis or tendon rupture is excluded.
8. Avoid direct sun exposure as photosensitivity reaction may occur. If exposed, wear sunglasses, protective clothing, and sunscreen.
9. Practice reliable contraception and do not nurse during therapy.
10. Keep all F/U to assess response, labs, and for adverse SE.

OUTCOMES/EVALUATE

Negative culture reports; symptomatic improvement

Olanzapine

(oh-**LAN**-zah-peen)

Classification(s): Antipsychotic

Pregnancy Category: C

RX: Zyprexa, Zyprexa IntraMuscular, Zyprexa Zydis.

✱ **Rx:** Novo-Olanzapine.

Olanzapine pamoate

Classification(s): Antipsychotic.

Pregnancy Category: C

RX: Zyprexa Relprevv.

INDICATIONS/USES

PO: (1) Short- and long-term management (including maintenance of treatment response) of schizophrenia. (2) As monotherapy to treat acute mixed, or manic episodes associated with bipolar I disorder and for maintenance monotherapy of bipolar disorder. (3) In combination with lithium or valproate for the short-term treatment of acute mixed or manic episodes associated with bipolar I disorder. (4) In combination with fluoxetine to treat depressive episodes associated with bipolar I disorder in adults. (5) In combination with fluoxetine to treat treatment-resistant depression (major depressive disorder) in those who do not respond to 2 separate trials of different antidepressants of adequate dose and duration in the current episode. (6) Pediatric schizophrenia and bipolar I disorder only after a thorough diagnostic evaluation along with careful consideration of the risks associated with drug treatment.

IM (10 mg/mL product): Agitation associated with schizophrenia and bipolar I mania.

IM (Olanzapine pamoate): Treatment of schizophrenia.

Investigational: (1) Tourette's disorder in adults, adolescents, and children. (2) OCD refractory to selective serotonin reuptake inhibitors. (3) Delusional parasitosis. (4) Psychosis/agitation in dementia or Alzheimer's disease. (5) Stuttering.

ACTION/KINETICS

Action

A thienobenzodiazepine antipsychotic believed to act by antagonizing dopamine D_{1-4} and serotonin ($5HT_{2A}$ and $5HT_{2C}$) receptors. Also has high affinity for muscarinic M_{1-4} receptors, histamine H_1, and alpha$_1$-adrenergic receptors, which can explain many of the side effects. Has weak affinity for $GABA_A$, benzodiazepine, and beta–adrenergic receptors. Some effect on the QTc interval may result in sudden cardiac death and torsades de pointes. High incidence of weight gain; moderate incidence of sedation, anticholinergic effects, and orthostatic hypotension; and, low incidence of extrapyramidal symptoms.

Pharmacokinetics

Well absorbed from the GI tract; about 60% bioavailable. **Peak plasma levels:** 6 hr after PO dosing. Undergoes significant first-pass metabolism with about 40% metabolized before it reaches the systemic circulation; about 60% bioavailable. Food does not affect the rate or extent of absorption. Metabolized in the liver through glucuronidation and oxidation by CYP1A2 and CYP2D6. **t½:** 21–54 hr after PO and 30 days for the ER injection. Elimination t½ 1.5 times greater in clients 65 years and older and 30% greater in women. Also, clearance is 2 times greater in Japanese clients and 40% higher in smokers. Unchanged drug and metabolites are excreted through both the urine (57%) and feces (30%). **Plasma protein binding:** About 93%.

CONTRAINDICATIONS

Lactation. IV or SC use of the parenteral product. Treatment of bipolar disorder or schizophrenia in children less than 13 years of age.

SPECIAL CONCERNS

■ **Increased mortality in elderly clients with dementia-related psychosis.** Elderly clients with dementia-related psychosis treated with atypical antipsychotic drugs are at an increased risk of death. Analyses of 17 placebo-controlled trials (modal duration of 10 weeks), largely in clients taking atypical antipsychotic drugs, revealed a risk of death in the drug-treated clients between 1.6–1.7 times that seen in placebo-treated clients. Over the course of a typical 10-week controlled trial, the rate of death in drug-treated clients was about 4.5%, compared with a rate of about 2.6% in the placebo group. Although the causes of death were varied, most of the deaths appeared to be either cardiovascular (e.g., heart failure, sudden death) or infectious (e.g., pneumonia) in nature. Observational studies suggest that, similar to atypical antipsychotic drugs, treatment with conventional antipsychotic drugs may increase mortality. The extent to which the findings of increased mortality in observational studies may be attributed to antipsychotic drug as opposed to some characteristic(s) of the client is not clear. Olanzapine is not approved for the treatment of clients with dementia-related psychosis.

Olanzapine pamoate: In addition to the preceding concerns: Adverse events with signs and symptoms consistent with olanzapine overdose, in particular, sedation (including coma) and/or delirium, have been reported following injections of olanzapine extended–release (ER) injection. Olanzapine ER injection must be administered in a registered health care facility with ready access to emergency response services. After each injection, clients must be observed at the health care facility by a health care provider for at least 3 hours. Because of this risk, olanzapine ER is available only through a restricted distribution program called *Zyprexa Relprevv* Patient Care Program, and requires health care provider, health care facility, client, and pharmacy enrollment. ■

- **Use with caution in geriatric clients (drug may be excreted more slowly); consider lower starting doses.**
- **Use with caution in impaired hepatic function and where there is a chance of increased core body temperature (e.g., strenuous exercise, exposure to extreme heat, concomitant anticholinergic drug administration, dehydration).**
- **Due to anticholinergic side effects, use with caution in clients with significant prostatic hypertrophy, narrow-angle glaucoma, or a history of paralytic ileus.**
- **Use with caution in those at risk of aspiration pneumonia.**
- **Those with Parkinson's disease or dementia have an increased sensitivity to antipsychotic medications.**

- Maximal dose of IM (short-acting) olanzapine (e.g., 3 doses of 10 mg given 2 to 4 hr apart) may be associated with significant orthostatic hypotension.
- There is an increased risk of hyperglycemia and diabetes.
- Safety and efficacy not determined for use in combination with fluoxetine or for the injection formulations in children less than 18 years of age.

SIDE EFFECTS

Most Common

Asthenia, dizziness, drowsiness/sedation/somnolence, constipation, dry mouth, dyspepsia, weight gain, increased cough, hypotension, personality disorder, accidental injury.

Listed are side effects with an incidence of 0.1% or more. **Neuroleptic malignant syndrome:** Hyperpyrexia, muscle rigidity, altered mental status, irregular pulse/BP, tachycardia, diaphoresis, cardiac dysrhythmia, rhabdomyolysis, ***acute renal failure, death***. **CNS:** Drowsiness/sedation/somnolence, dizziness, insomnia, personality disorder, abnormal gait, impaired articulation, tremor, dystonia, akathisia, akinesia, dyskinesia, abnormal/bizarre/increased dreams, euphoria, paresthesia, suicide attempt/thought, amnesia, ataxia, delirium, dysarthria, hypesthesia, hypokinesia, incoordination, increased libido, migraine, neuropathy, pseudoparkinsonism, tardive dyskinesia, vertigo, antisocial reaction, CNS stimulation, obsessive compulsive symptoms, phobias, ***suicide***. **CV:** Hypotension (including orthostatic), tachycardia, hypertension, bradycardia, ***cardiac arrest, CVA, hemorrhage***, CHF, palpitation, ***pulmonary embolism***, vasodilation, cerebrovascular adverse events (e.g., ***stroke***, TIA, ***death***), atrial contractions (premature/atrial fibrillation/flutter), arteritis. **GI:** Dry mouth, constipation, dyspepsia, increased appetite, weight gain, N&V, polydipsia, salivation, abdominal distention/enlargement, dysphagia, eructation, fecal impaction, flatulence, gastritis, gastroenteritis, gingivitis, fecal incontinence, melena, mouth ulceration, rectal hemorrhage, stomatitis, tooth caries, dental pain, tongue edema. **Hepatic:** Hepatitis. **Dermatologic:** Ecchymosis, acne, alopecia, dermatitis, eczema, maculopapular skin reactions, pallor, photosensitivity, pruritus, vesiculobullous rash, seborrhea, urticaria. **GU:** Mastalgia, amenorrhea, hematuria, metrorrhagia, urinary incontinence, ejaculation disorders, galactorrhea, glycosuria, impotence, menorrhagia, polyuria, priapism, urinary frequency, increased urgency, urinary retention, vaginal hemorrhage, UTI. **Musculoskeletal:** Arthralgia, joint/back/chest pain, arthritis, bursitis, cogwheel rigidity, neck pain/rigidity, pelvic pain, arthrosis. **Respiratory:** Rhinitis, increased cough, pharyngitis, dyspnea, apnea, asthma, epistaxis, hemoptysis, pneumonia, laryngitis. **Hematologic:** Leukopenia, anemia, leukocytosis, lymphadenopathy, thrombocythemia, thrombocytopenia. **Metabolic:** Hyperglycemia, diabetes mellitus, dehydration. **Ophthalmic:** Abnormal accommodation, amblyopia, conjunctivitis, blepharitis, cataracts, diplopia, dry eyes, eye hemorrhage. **Otic:** Tinnitus. **Body as a whole:** Asthenia, malaise, fever, chills, flu syndrome, diaphoresis, peripheral edema, allergic reaction, cyanosis, angioedema, weight gain (especially in young clients), ***anaphylaxis***. **Miscellaneous:** Accidental injury, hyper–/hypotonia, withdrawal syndrome, extremity pain (not joint), intentional injury, hyper-/hypotonia, facial edema, moniliasis, thyroiditis, voice alteration, tobacco misuse.

NOTE: After injection of olanzapine pamoate (olanzapine ER), the following symptoms may occur necessitating observation of the client at a health care facility for 3 hr: Sedation (ranging from mild in severity to coma) and/or delirium (including confusion, disorientation, agitation, anxiety, and other cognitive impairment). Other symptoms may include extrapyramidal symptoms, dysarthria, ataxia, aggression, dizziness, weakness, hypertension, or convulsions. The risk of a reaction is greatest during the first hour after the injection.

LABORATORY TEST CONSIDERATIONS

↑ ALT, AST, GGT, alkaline phosphatase, serum prolactin, eosinophils, CPK. Hyperprolactinemia. Greater risk of ↑ lipid levels, prolactin, AST, ALT in adolescents. Hypercholesterolemia, hyper–/hypoglycemia, hyper–/hypokalemia, hyperlipemia, hyponatremia, hypoproteinemia.

OVERDOSE MANAGEMENT

Symptoms: Drowsiness, slurred speech. Possible obtundation, seizures, dystonic reaction of the head and neck. CV symptoms, arrhythmias. *Treatment:* Establish and maintain an airway and ensure adequate oxygenation and ventilation. Gastric lavage followed by activated charcoal and a

O

laxative can be considered, although dystonic reaction may cause aspiration with induced emesis. Begin CV monitoring immediately with continuous ECG monitoring to detect possible arrhythmias. Hypotension and circulatory collapse are treated with IV fluids or sympathomimetic agents. Do not use epinephrine, dopamine, or other sympathomimetics with beta-agonist activity, as beta stimulation may worsen hypotension.

DRUG INTERACTIONS

Antihypertensive agents / ↑ Antihypertensive effect R/T blockade of alpha-adrenergic receptors
Carbamazepine / ↑ Olanzapine clearance R/T ↑ metabolism; adjust olanzapine dose as needed
Charcoal / ↓ Olanzapine absorption
CNS depressants, including alcohol / ↑ CNS depressant effect; possible dystonic reactions precipitated by alcohol; use together with caution or not at all
Divalproex / ↑ Hepatic enzyme levels to a greater degree than either drug used alone
Fluoxetine / ↑ Olanzapine peak levels and ↓ clearance
Fluvoxamine / ↑ Olanzapine plasma levels R/T inhibition of CYP1A2
Levodopa and Dopamine agonists / May antagonize the effects of levodopa and dopamine agonists
Omeprazole / Possible ↓ olanzapine serum levels R/T induction of CYP1A2
Probenecid / ↑ Olanzapine rate of absorption, AUC, and peak plasma level
Rifampin / Possible ↓ olanzapine serum levels R/T induction of CYP1A2
Ritonavir / ↑ Olanzapine oral clearance and ↓ systemic exposure R/T ↑ metabolism
H ***St. John's wort*** / Possible ↓ olanzapine plasma levels R/T ↑ metabolism
Smoking / ↓ Olanzapine effect R/T ↑ liver metabolism by CYP1A2

HOW SUPPLIED

Olanzapine. ***Injection, Powder for Solution:*** 10 mg/mL; ***Tablets:*** 2.5 mg, 5 mg, 7.5 mg, 10 mg, 15 mg, 20 mg; ***Tablets, Oral Disintegrating:*** 5 mg, 10 mg, 15 mg, 20 mg.
Olanzapine pamoate. ***Injection, Powder for Suspension, Extended-Release:*** 210 mg, 300 mg, 405 mg.

DOSAGE

TABLETS; TABLETS, ORAL DISINTEGRATING

Schizophrenia.

Adults, initial: 5–10 mg once daily without regard to meals. Goal is 10 mg daily within several days of initiation. Adjust dosage, if needed, at 5 mg/day increments or decrements in intervals of not less than 1 week. Doses higher than 10 mg daily are recommended only after clinical assessment and should not be greater than 20 mg/day. The recommended initial dose is 5 mg in those who are debilitated, who have a predisposition to hypotensive reactions, who may have factors that cause a slower metabolism of olanzapine (e.g., nonsmoking female clients over 65 years of age), or who may be more sensitive to the drug. It is recommended that clients who respond to the drug be continued on it at the lowest possible dose to maintain remission with periodic evaluation to determine continued need for the drug. Periodically reassess to determine the need for maintenance treatment.

Bipolar mania, monotherapy.

Initial: 10–15 mg/day without regard to meals. Adjust dose, if needed, at 5 mg increments in intervals not less than 24 hr, if needed. **Dose range:** 5–20 mg/day for short-term (3 to 4 weeks) use. The safety of doses above 20 mg/day has not been determined. **Maintenance:** 5–20 mg/day, after reaching an effective dose for an average duration of 2 weeks. Periodically reevaluate in those taking the drug for extended periods.

Bipolar mania when combined with lithium or valproate.

Initial: 10 mg once daily without regard to meals; **then** 5–20 mg/day.

With fluoxetine to treat depressive episodes associated with bipolar I disorder or with fluoxetine for treatment-resistant depression.

Initial: Olanzapine 5 mg and fluoxetine 20 mg once/day in the evening, without regard to meals. Dosage adjustments, if needed, can be made according to efficacy and tolerance within the dose ranges of PO olanzapine 5–12.5 mg and fluoxetine 20–50 mg. The disorder is a chronic illness requiring long-term treatment. Periodically assess to determine continued need for treatment. *NOTE:* The starting dose of PO olanzapine 2.5–5 mg with fluoxetine 20 mg should be used for those with a predisposition to hypotensive reactions or those who exhibit a combination of factors that may slow the metabolism of olanzapine or fluoxetine in combination (e.g., women, elderly, nonsmokers), or those clients who may be sensitive to olanzapine. When indicated undertake dose escalation with caution in these clients.

Pediatric schizophrenia or bipolar I disorder.

Children, 13 years and older, initial: 2.5 or 5 mg once/day without regard to meals. When dosage adjustments are needed, dose increments/decrements of 2.5 or 5 mg are recommended. **Maintenance:** 10 mg/day. Continue responding clients beyond the acute response but at the lowest dose needed to maintain remission. Periodically assess to determine continued need for treatment.

IM ONLY, 10 mg/mL PRODUCT

Agitation associated with schizophrenia and bipolar I mania.

Usual recommended: 10 mg; a lower dose of 5 or 7.5 mg may be given when clinical factors warrant. If agitation warrants, additional IM doses up to 10 mg may be given (efficacy of repeated doses has not been evaluated systematically). **Maximum dose:** 30 mg/day. Consider a dose of 5 mg/injection for geriatric clients or when other clinical factors indicate. Consider a dose of 2.5 mg/injection for those who otherwise might be debilitated, predisposed to hypotensive reactions, or more sensitive to olanzapine. Maximal dosing (e.g., three 10 mg doses given 2 to 4 hr apart) may cause significant orthostatic hypotension.

Olanzapine pamoate

IM ONLY

Treatment of schizophrenia.

Adults, usual: 150–300 mg q 2 weeks or 405 mg q 4 weeks. Efficacy demonstrated over 24 weeks. Periodically assess to determine need for continued treatment.

The following is the recommended dosing for extended-release olanzapine based on correspondence to oral olanzapine doses: (a) **Target PO dose: 10 mg/day.** For dosing of olanzapine ER during the first 8 weeks, give 210 mg per 2 weeks or 405 mg per 4 week; then, for maintenance, give 150 mg per 2 weeks or 300 mg per 4 weeks. (b) **Target PO dose: 15 mg/day.** For dosing of olanzapine ER during the first 8 weeks, give 300 mg per 2 weeks; then, for maintenance, give 210 mg per 2 weeks or 405 mg per 4 weeks. (c) **Target PO dose: 20 mg/day.** For dosing of olanzapine ER during the first 8 weeks, give 300 mg per 2 weeks; then, for maintenance, give 300 mg per 2 weeks.

NOTE: The recommended initial dose is 150 mg per 4 weeks in those who are debilitated, who have a predisposition to hypotensive reactions, who otherwise show a combination of factors that may result in slower metabolism of olanzapine (e.g., nonsmoking women over 65 years of age and older), or who may be more sensitive to olanzapine. When needed, undertake dose escalation with caution.

NURSING IMPLICATIONS

Do not confuse Zyprexa with Zyrtec (an antihistamine) or Celexa (an antidepressant). Do not confuse olanzapine with olsalazine (an anti-inflammatory).

IMPLEMENTATION/ADMINISTRATION/STORAGE

1. **There are two olanzapine IM formulations with different dosing schedules. Do not con-**

fuse the short-acting formulation (10 mg/mL) with olanzapine ER (i.e., Zyprexa Relprevv).

2. The safety of parenteral total daily doses greater than 30 mg, or 10 mg given more frequently than every 2 hr after the initial dose and 4 hr after the second dose, have not been evaluated.
3. If ongoing olanzapine is indicated after IM therapy, PO olanzapine may be initiated at doses from 5–20 mg/day.
4. To prepare for IM use, dissolve the contents of the vial with 2.1 mL of sterile water for injection (results in a solution containing about 5 mg/mL olanzapine). The solution should be clear and yellow. Use within 1 hr after reconstitution and discard any unused portion. Do **not** give by IV or SC routes.
5. IM injection volumes: If the olanzapine dose is 10 mg, withdraw the total contents of the reconstituted drug; if the dose is 7.5 mg, withdraw 1.5 mL; if the dose is 5 mg, withdraw 1 mL; and, if the dose is 2.5 mg, withdraw 0.5 mL.
6. Follow the package instructions carefully for preparation of olanzapine pamoate (olanzapine ER) for injection.
7. Olanzapine ER must be suspended using only the diluent provided in the convenience kit.
8. Administer olanzapine ER IM deep into gluteal muscle; do not inject IV or SC.
9. For administration of olanzapine ER select the 19-gauge, 1.5 inch *Hypodermic Needle-Pro* needle with needle protection device. For obese clients, a 2-inch, 19-gauge or larger needle (not included in the convenience kit) may be used.
10. Before giving olanzapine ER confirm there will be someone to accompany the client after the 3-hr observation period. If this cannot be confirmed, do not give the injection.
11. Protect tablets from light and moisture and store at a controlled room temperature of 20–25°C (68–77°F). Orally disintegrating tablets contain phenylalanine.
12. Protect the 10 mg/mL injection from light; do not freeze. Before reconstitution and up to 1 hr after reconstitution, store from 20–25°C (68–77°F). Discard any unused portion of reconstituted olanzapine.
13. Store olanzapine ER vials at room temperature, not to exceed 30°C (86°F). When the drug is suspended in the solution, it may be held at room temperature for 24 hr. Agitate the vial immediately before withdrawing the drug. Once the suspension is withdrawn into the syringe, inject immediately.
14. Do not combine the 10 mg/mL product in a syringe with diazepam injection as precipitation will occur. Also, do not use lorazepam injection to reconstitute olanzapine injection as this combination results in a delayed reconstitution time. Do not combine olanzapine injection with haloperidol injection as the resulting low pH will degrade olanzapine over time.

ASSESSMENT

1. Note onset, duration, characteristics of S&S, presenting behaviors, reasons for therapy; list agents trialed and outcome.
2. Assess mental status and monitor for any significant changes in behavior or depression.
3. Temperature regulation may be impaired especially with strenuous exercise or if exposed to extreme heat. Assess carefully for dehydration especially in the elderly. If neuroleptic malignant syndrome (altered mental status, diaphoresis, hyperpyrexia, irregular BP/pulse, muscle rigidity, and tachycardia) occurs, stop drug therapy immediately.
4. Assess for BPH, glaucoma (narrow-angle) or history of paralytic ileus as these conditions may cause ↑ adverse SE. Voiding before drug administration may decrease anticholinergic effects of urinary retention.
5. With injection (ensure correct form is ordered/selected) of the ER formula, client must be observed for at least 3 hr after each injection. The provider, health care facility, client, and dispensing pharmacy must be enrolled in the Zyprexa Relprevv Patient Care Program. Olanzapine ER injection is only available through this restricted distribution program.
6. Assess for S&S of diabetes mellitus. Monitor weights closely to ensure no overt increases. After prolonged use, monitor for tardive dyskinesia (irreversible, involuntary dyskinetic movements) which may occur months or years after therapy and may persist for lifetime or disappear suddenly, despite stopping therapy.

7. Do not use with dementia-related psychosis or in the elderly due to increased risk of death from heart failure and pneumonia.
8. Monitor VS, Wt, ECG, CBC, BS, lipids, renal and LFTs.

CLIENT/FAMILY TEACHING

1. Take only as directed; do not share medications or exceed prescribed dosage.
2. To take disintegrating tablets, peel back foil on blister; do not push tablet through foil. Using dry hands, remove from foil and place entire tablet in the mouth; will disintegrate with or without liquid in about 2 min. Disintegrating tablets contain phenylalanine (aspartame).
3. Avoid activities or situations where overheating may occur, e.g., strenuous exercise, hot baths. Heat exposure may impair ability to reduce core body temperatures.
4. Do not drive or perform activities that require mental alertness until drug effects realized; may experience drowsiness, trouble thinking, trouble controlling movements, or trouble seeing clearly.
5. Avoid changing positions suddenly, especially from lying to standing position R/T low BP effects.
6. Avoid prolonged/excessive exposure to direct or artificial light.
7. Report any suicidal ideations, abnormal bleeding, sudden muscle pain/weakness, irregular heartbeat.
8. Avoid alcohol, CNS depressants or OTC agents.
9. Practice reliable birth control. Record BP and weight for provider review.
10. Keep all F/U to assess response, for medication renewals, therapy, VS, Wt, and for adverse SE.

OUTCOMES/EVALUATE

Improved patterns of behavior with ↓ agitation, ↓ hostility, and fewer delusions with schizophrenia and bipolar disorder.

Olmesartan medoxomil

(**ohl**-meh-**SAR**-tan)

Classification(s): Antihypertensive agent-angiotension II receptor antagonist

Pregnancy Category: C

RX: Benicar.

SEE ALSO ***ANGIOTENSIN II RECEPTOR ANTAGONISTS.***

INDICATIONS/USES

Hypertension in adults and children, age 6 years and older. Can be used alone or in combination with other antihypertensives.

ACTION/KINETICS

Action

Selectively blocks the binding of angiotensin II to the AT_1 receptor in vascular smooth muscle, resulting in a decrease in BP. Angiotensin II is a pressor agent causing vasoconstriction, stimulation of the synthesis of and release of aldosterone, cardiac stimulation, and renal reabsorption of sodium.

Pharmacokinetics

Rapid and complete conversion of olmesartan medoxomil to olmesartan occurs during absorption from the GI tract. Olmesartan itself is not further metabolized. Is about 26% bioavailable. **Peak plasma levels:** 1–2 hr. Food does not affect bioavailability. **Steady-state levels:** Within 3 to 5 days, with no drug accumulation following once-daily dosing. **t½, terminal:** 13 hr. Excreted through the urine (35–50%) and feces (50–65%). **Plasma protein binding:** More than 99%.

CONTRAINDICATIONS

Hypersensitivity to the drug or any component of the product. Lactation.

SPECIAL CONCERNS

When pregnancy is detected, discontinue olmesartan as soon as possible. Drugs that act directly on the renin-angiotensin system can cause injury and even death to the developing fetus.

Safety and efficacy have not been determined in children.

SIDE EFFECTS

Most Common

Dizziness, diarrhea, GI upset, insomnia, headache.

CV: Hypotension, especially in volume- and/or salt-depleted clients, tachycardia. **GI:** Diarrhea, abdominal pain, dyspepsia, gastroenteritis, GI upset, nausea. **CNS:** Dizziness, headache, vertigo, in-

O

somnia. **GU:** Oliguria, progressive azotemia, hematuria, ***acute renal failure (rare)***. **Musculoskeletal:** Arthralgia, arthritis, myalgia, skeletal pain. **Respiratory:** Bronchitis, pharyngitis, rhinitis, sinusitis, URTI. **Body as a whole:** Inflicted injury, flu-like symptoms, fatigue, pain, peripheral edema, rash. **Miscellaneous:** Back/chest pain, facial edema, ***angioedema***.

LABORATORY TEST CONSIDERATIONS

↑ CPK. Slight ↓ H&H. Hyperglycemia, hypertriglyceridemia, hypercholesterolemia, hyperlipemia, hyperuricemia.

OVERDOSE MANAGEMENT

Symptoms: Hypotension, tachycardia. *Treatment:* If needed, supportive treatment for symptomatic hypotension.

HOW SUPPLIED

Tablets: 5 mg, 20 mg, 40 mg.

DOSAGE

TABLETS

Hypertension.

Individualize dosage. **Adults, initial:** 20 mg once daily when used as monotherapy in those not volume-depleted. After 2 weeks of therapy, if further reduction in BP is required, dose may be increased to 40 mg. Doses above 40 mg appear not to have a greater effect. **Children, 6–16 years of age, 20– <35 kg, initial:** 10 mg once/day. After 2 weeks of therapy, the dose may be increased to a maximum of 20 mg/day. **Children, 6–16 years of age, 35 kg or more, initial:** 20 mg once/day. After 2 weeks of therapy, the dose may be increased to a maximum of 40 mg/day. Consider a lower starting dose, with close monitoring, in those who are volume- and salt-depleted (e.g., those treated with diuretics, especially clients with impaired renal function).

NURSING IMPLICATIONS

Ⓢ **Do not confuse Benicar (olmesartan alone) with Benicar HCT (olmesartan combined with hydrochlorothiazide).**

IMPLEMENTATION/ADMINISTRATION/STORAGE

1. Twice-daily dosing has no advantage over once-daily dosing.
2. No initial dosage adjustment is recommended for the elderly or those with moderate to severe renal or hepatic dysfunction.
3. May be given with or without food.
4. If BP is not controlled with olmesartan alone, a diuretic or other antihypertensive drugs may be added.
5. For children who cannot swallow tablets, an extemporaneous suspension may be prepared as follows: Add 50 mL of purified water to an amber polyethylene terephthalate bottle containing 20 olmesartan 20 mg tablets. Allow to stand for a minimum of 5 min. Shake the container for at least 1 min and allow the suspension to stand for at least 1 min. Repeat 1 min shaking and 1 min standing 4 additional times. Add 100 mL Ora-Sweet and 50 mL Ora-Plus to the suspension and shake well for 1 min. Shake the suspension well before each use.
6. Store tablets from 20–25°C (68–77°F). Store the prepared suspension in the refrigerator from 2–8°C (36–46°F) for up to 4 weeks.

ASSESSMENT

1. Note disease onset, reasons for therapy, characteristics of S&S, risk factors, all medical conditions, other agents trialed, outcome. List drugs prescribed to ensure none interact.
2. Ensure client is well hydrated.
3. Assess renal function in heart failure or post-MI clients regularly.
4. Monitor BP, CBC, electrolytes, renal and LFTs; reduce dose with dysfunction/dehydration.

CLIENT/FAMILY TEACHING

1. May take with food to ↓ GI upset; continue all other prescribed BP medications.
2. Change positions slowly and avoid dehydration to prevent sudden drop in BP and dizziness. Consume plenty of fluids to ensure adequate hydration.
3. Practice reliable contraception; report if pregnancy suspected, as drug may cause fetal death.
4. Continue low-fat, low-sodium diet, regular exercise, weight loss, smoking and alcohol cessation, and stress weight reduction to regain BP control.

5. **May experience headaches, altered glucose readings with diabetes, coughing, diarrhea, nausea, and joint aches; report if persistent. Report any swelling of face, lips, or tongue.**
6. **Keep all F/U to assess response, labs, review log of BP and HR readings, and for adverse SE.**

OUTCOMES/EVALUATE

Control of hypertension

Combination Drug

Olmesartan medoxomil and Hydrochlorothiazide

(**ohl**-meh-**SAR**-tan, **hy**-droh-klor-oh-**THIGH**-ah-zyd)

Classification(s): Antihypertensive combination drug

Pregnancy Category: C (first trimester); **D** (second and third trimesters)

RX: Benicar HCT.

SEE ALSO ***OLMESARATN MEDOXOMIL*** AND ***HYDROCHLOROTHIAZIDE***.

INDICATIONS/USES

Treatment of hypertension. Not indicated for initial therapy; begin combination therapy only after a client has failed to achieve the desired effect with monotherapy.

CONTENT

Benicar HCT contains olmesartan medoxomil *(angiotensin II receptor antagonist)*, amount listed first, and hydrochlorothiazide *(thiazide diuretic)*, amount listed second: 20 mg/12.5 mg tablets, 40 mg/12.5 mg tablets, and 40 mg/25 mg tablets.

ACTION/KINETICS

Action

Olmesartan selectively blocks the binding of angiotensin II to the AT_1 receptor in vascular smooth muscle, resulting in a decrease in BP. Angiotensin II is a pressor agent causing vasoconstriction, stimulation of the synthesis of and release of aldosterone, cardiac stimulation, and renal reabsorption of sodium. Hydrochlorothiazide promotes the excretion of sodium and chloride, and thus water, by the distal renal tubule. Also increases excretion of potassium and to a lesser extent bicarbonate. The antihypertensive activity is thought to be due to direct dilation of the areterioles, as well as to a reduction in the total fluid volume of the body and altered sodium balance.

Pharmacokinetics

Olmesartan. Absolute bioavailability is about 26%; food does not affect bioavailability. Olmesartan medoxomil is rapidly and completely bioactivated by ester hydrolysis to olmesartan during absorption from the GI tract. **Peak plasma levels:** 1–2 hr. **t½, elimination, terminal:** 13 hr. Steady state levels reached within 3–5 days; no accumulation in plasma occurs with once-daily dosing. Olmesartan is excreted in both the urine (35–50%) and feces (50–65%).

Hydrochlorothiazide. t½, plasma: 5.6–14.8 hr. **Onset of diuresis:** 2 hr; **peak:** About 4 hr; **duration:** 6–12 hr. Not metabolized; eliminated rapidly by the kidney (61% within 24 hr). **Plasma protein binding:** Olmesartan: 99% bound to plasma proteins.

CONTRAINDICATIONS

Hypersensitivity to any component of the product. Clients with anuria or hypersensitivity to other sulfonamide-derived drugs. Use during lactation is not recommended.

SPECIAL CONCERNS

Use of drugs during the second and third trimesters of pregnancy that act directly on the renin-angiotensin system can cause injury and even death to the fetus. When pregnancy is detected, discontinue as soon as possible.

- **Symptomatic hypotension may occur after beginning treatment in those who are volume- or salt-depleted.**
- **Use with caution in those with impaired hepatic function, progressive liver disease (minor alterations of fluid and electrolyte balance may precipitate hepatic coma), or severe renal disease.**
- **Hypersensitivity reactions to hydrochlorothiazide may occur in those with or without a history of allergy or bronchial asthma (but are more likely in those with such a history).**
- **Safety and efficacy not established in children.**

O

SIDE EFFECTS

Most Common

Dizziness, URTI, nausea, hyperuricemia, headache, UTI.

See *Olmesartan medoxomil* and *Diuretics, Thiazides* for a complete list of possible side effects. **GU:** Oliguria and/or progressive azotemia with acute renal failure and/or ***death*** (rare). **Miscellaneous:** Thiazides may cause exacerbation or activation of systemic lupus erythematosus.

LABORATORY TEST CONSIDERATIONS

↑ Cholesterol, triglycerides, creatinine, BUN. ↓ H&H. ↓ Urinary calcium and ↑ serum calcium. Possible hypokalemia, hyponatremia, hypochloremic alkalosis, hyperuricemia, hypomagnesemia.

OVERDOSE MANAGEMENT

Symptoms: Olmesartan: Hypotension, tachycardia, bradycardia (if vagal stimulation occurs). Hydrochlorothiazide: Electrolyte depletion and dehydration. *Treatment:* Institute supportive treatment.

DRUG INTERACTIONS

See ***Drug Interactions*** for Olmesartan medoxomil and Diuretics, Thiazides. ***NOTE:*** Olmesartan is not metabolized by the cytochrome P450 system and has no effects on P450 enzymes; thus, interactions with drugs that inhibit, induce, or are metabolized by those enzymes are not expected.

HOW SUPPLIED

See *Content.*

DOSAGE

TABLETS

Hypertension.

Once daily dosing with either 20 mg/12.5 mg, 40 mg/12.5 mg, or 40 mg/25 mg. Individualize dosage based on BP response. Titrate in 2–4 week intervals.

NURSING IMPLICATIONS

Do not confuse Benicar (olmesartan alone) with Benicar HCT (olmesartan and hydrochlorothiazide).

IMPLEMENTATION/ADMINISTRATION/STORAGE

1. In diabetics, the dosage of insulin or oral hypoglycemics may need to be increased due to hyperglycemia.
2. For those with possible depletion of intravascular volume, initiate Benicar HCT under close medical supervision. Consider use of a lower starting dose.
3. No initial dosage adjustment is recommended for elderly clients, for those with marked renal impairment (C_{CR} <40 mL/min), or with moderate to marked hepatic dysfunction.

ASSESSMENT

1. Note reasons for therapy, disease onset, characteristics of S&S, risk factors, other agents trialed, outcome. List drugs prescribed to ensure none interact.
2. Assess for any drug allergies; list all medical conditions.
3. Ensure client is well hydrated.
4. Assess renal function in heart failure or post-MI clients regularly.
5. Monitor BP, hydration status, CBC, electrolytes, renal and LFTs; reduce dose with dysfunction/dehydration.

CLIENT/FAMILY TEACHING

1. May take on an empty stomach or with food.
2. Can cause dizziness or drowsiness, avoid activities that require mental alertness until drugs effects realized.
3. Change positions slowly to prevent sudden drop in BP and dizziness.
4. Continue low-fat, low-sodium diet, regular exercise, weight loss, smoking and alcohol cessation, and stress weight reduction to regain BP control.
5. May experience headaches, altered glucose readings with diabetes, coughing, diarrhea, nausea, and joint aches; report if persistent. Report any swelling of face, lips, or tongue.
6. Avoid alcohol and OTC drugs without provider approval.
7. Consume plenty of fluids to ensure well hydrated. Avoid strenuous exercise in hot weather or situations that may cause ↑ sweating.
8. May experience abdominal/stomach pain, cough, diarrhea, dizziness, headache, unusual tiredness; report if persistent or bothersome. Report any swelling of face, lips or tongue.
9. Practice reliable contraception. Report if pregnancy suspected or desired.
10. Keep all F/U to assess response, labs, BP and HR log, and for adverse SE.

OUTCOMES/EVALUATE

Desired BP control

Olsalazine sodium

(ohl-**SAL**-ah-zeen)

Classification(s): Anti-inflammatory drug

Pregnancy Category: C

RX: Dipentum.

INDICATIONS/USES

Maintain remission of ulcerative colitis in clients intolerant of sulfasalazine.

ACTION/KINETICS

Action

A salicylate that is converted by bacteria in the colon to 5-ASA (5-para-aminosalicylic acid), which exerts an anti-inflammatory effect for the treatment of ulcerative colitis. 5-ASA is slowly absorbed resulting in a high concentration of drug in the colon. The anti-inflammatory activity is likely due to blockade of cyclooxygenase and inhibition of synthesis of prostaglandins in the bowel mucosa.

Pharmacokinetics

After PO use the drug is only slightly absorbed (2.4%) into systemic circulation (98–99% reaches the colon). **t½, serum:** 0.9 hr. **Plasma protein binding:** More than 99%.

CONTRAINDICATIONS

Hypersensitivity to salicylates.

SPECIAL CONCERNS

- Use with caution during lactation.
- May cause worsening of symptoms of colitis.
- Safety and efficacy not established in children.

SIDE EFFECTS

Most Common

Diarrhea, pain/cramps, headache, nausea, dyspepsia, rash.

GI: Diarrhea, pain or cramps, N&V, dyspepsia, bloating, anorexia, stomatitis, blood in stool, pancreatitis, rectal bleeding, rectal discomfort, epigastric discomfort, flatulence, granulomatous hepatitis, nonspecific reactive hepatitis. **CNS:** Headache, drowsiness, lethargy, fatigue, depression, dizziness, vertigo, insomnia, paresthesia, tremors, mood swings, irritability. **CV:** Pericarditis, second degree heart block, hypertension, orthostatic hypotension, peripheral edema, chest pains, tachycardia, palpitations. **Dermatologic:** Rash, itching, erythema nodosum, photosensitivity, erythema, hot flashes, alopecia. **Respiratory:** URTI, bronchospasm, shortness of breath. **Musculoskeletal:** Arthralgia, muscle cramps. **GU:** Renal tubular damage, urinary frequency, dysuria, impotence, menorrhagia. **Hematologic:** Leukopenia, neutropenia, lymphopenia, eosinophilia, thrombocytopenia, anemia, reticulocytosis. **Ophthalmic:** Dry eyes, watery eyes, blurred vision. **Miscellaneous:** Worsening of symptoms of ulcerative colitis, fever, chills. *NOTE:* The following symptoms have been reported on withdrawal of therapy: Diarrhea, nausea, abdominal pain, rash, itching, headache, heartburn, insomnia, anorexia, dizziness, lightheadedness, rectal bleeding, depression.

LABORATORY TEST CONSIDERATIONS

↑ ALT, AST.

OVERDOSE MANAGEMENT

Symptoms: Diarrhea, decreased motor activity. *Treatment:* Treat symptoms.

HOW SUPPLIED

Capsules: 250 mg.

DOSAGE

CAPSULES

Maintain remission of ulcerative colitis.

Adults: Total of 1 gram/day in two divided doses.

NURSING IMPLICATIONS

Do not confuse olsalazine with olanzapine (an antipsychotic).

ASSESSMENT

1. Note reasons for therapy, type, onset, characteristics of S&S (stools). List sensitivity to salicylates/intolerance to sulfasalazine, other agents trialed, outcome.
2. Review radiographic/endoscopic findings; assess abdomen.
3. Monitor I&O; ensure adequate fluid intake to prevent dehydration.
4. Assess stool frequency, quantity and consistency; note abdominal pain and findings.

5. With renal disease, monitor urinalysis, BUN, creatinine. With chronic therapy, monitor CBC (every 3 to 6 mo), renal and LFTs.

CLIENT/FAMILY TEACHING

1. Drug works by reducing inflammation of the colon by possibly preventing the production of substances that cause inflammation.
2. Take with food and in evenly divided doses. Consume adequate fluids to prevent dehydration.
3. Report any persistent diarrhea, lethargy, pain, fatigue, fever, blood in the stools, or lack of desired response.
4. Practice reliable contraception; report if pregnancy suspected.
5. Keep all F/U to assess response, labs, adverse SE.

OUTCOMES/EVALUATE

Symptom remission with ulcerative colitis; ↓ mucus in stools ↓ abdominal pain

Omalizumab

(oh-mah-lye-**ZOO**-mab)

Classification(s): Monoclonal antibody-antiasthmatic

Pregnancy Category: B

RX: Xolair.

INDICATIONS/USES

Moderate to severe persistent asthma in adults and adolescents 12 years and older who have a positive skin test or in vitro reactivity to a perennial aeroallergen with symptoms not adequately controlled with inhaled corticosteroids. Safety and efficacy have not been determined for other allergic conditions. *Investigational:* Seasonal allergic rhinitis; use to treat asthma in children less than 12 years of age.

ACTION/KINETICS

Action

Omalizumab is a recombinant monoclonal antibody that binds selectively to human IgE. Omalizumab inhibits binding of IgE to the high affinity IgE receptor on the surface of mast cells and basophils. Reduction in the surface-bound IgE on IgE receptor-bearing cells limits the degree of release of mediators of the allergic response. The drug also reduces the number of IgE receptors on basophils in atopic clients. After the drug was discontinued, the increase in total IgE and decrease in free IgE receptor levels were reversible but did not return to pretreatment levels for up to 1 year after discontinuing omalizumab.

Pharmacokinetics

About 62% of the drug is bioavailable but it is slowly absorbed; **peak serum levels:** 7–8 days. Drug is metabolized in the liver and excreted in the bile. **t½, elimination:** 26 days.

CONTRAINDICATIONS

Severe hypersensitivity to omalizumab. Use to treat acute bronchospasm or status asthmaticus.

SPECIAL CONCERNS

■ Anaphylaxis, presenting as bronchospasm, hypotension, syncope, urticaria, and/or angioedema of the throat or tongue, has been reported to occur after administration of omalizumab. Anaphylaxis has occurred as early as after the first dose of omalizumab but also has occurred beyond 1 year after beginning regularly administered treatment. Because of the risk of anaphylaxis, closely observe clients for an appropriate period of time after omalizumab administration, and be prepared to manage anaphylaxis that can be life-threatening. Also inform clients of the signs and symptoms of anaphylaxis and instruct them to seek immediate medical care if symptoms occur. ■

- Use with caution during lactation.
- Safety and efficacy not determined in children less than 12 years of age.

SIDE EFFECTS

Most Common

Injection site reactions, viral infections, URTI, headache, sore throat, pharyngitis, sinusitis.

Respiratory: URTI, sinusitis, pharyngitis, sore throat, cold symptoms. **CNS:** Dizziness, fatigue. **Dermatologic:** Pruritus, dermatitis, hair loss. **Musculoskeletal:** Arthralgia, leg/arm pain, fracture. **Injection Site:** Bruising, redness, warmth, burning, stinging, itching, hive formation, pain, indurations, mass, and inflammation. **Hematologic:** Severe thrombocytopenia. **Hypersensitivity:** Urticaria, dermatitis, pruritus, ***anaphylaxis***. **Miscellaneous:** Leg/arm/ear pain, earache, viral infections, headache, cold symptoms, possible parasitic (helminth) infections. Most serious side effects include malignancies and ***anaphylaxis***.

HOW SUPPLIED

Injection, Lyophilized Powder for Solution: 202.5 mg (delivers 150 mg/1.2 mL after reconstitution).

DOSAGE

SC

Moderate to severe persistent asthma.

Adults and adolescents 12 years and older: 150–375 mg q 2–4 weeks. Doses and dosing frequency are determined by serum total immunoglobulin E (IgE) level (units/mL), measured before starting treatment and body weight (kg). See package insert for appropriate dose assignment.

NURSING IMPLICATIONS

IMPLEMENTATION/ADMINISTRATION/STORAGE

1. The injection may take 5–10 seconds to administer because solution is slightly viscous.
2. Doses of more than 150 mg are divided among more than 1 injection site; no more than 150 mg should be given in any one site.
3. Total IgE levels are elevated during treatment and remain elevated for up to 1 year after termination of therapy. Thus, retesting of IgE levels during treatment cannot be used as a guide for dose determinations. Base dose determinations after treatment interruptions lasting <1 year on serum IgE levels obtained at the initial dose determination.
4. Total serum IgE levels may be retested for dose determination if treatment with omalizumab has been interrupted for 1 year or more.
5. Adjust doses for significant changes in body weight.
6. Prepare omalizumab for SC use as follows:
   - Use only sterile water for injection.
   - The lyophilized product takes 15–20 min to dissolve. The fully reconstituted product appears clear or slightly opalescent and may have a few small bubbles or foam around the edge of the vial.
   - Draw 1.4 mL sterile water for injection into a 3 mL syringe equipped with a 1-inch 18-gauge needle.
   - Place the vial upright on a flat surface and, using a standard aseptic technique, insert the needle and inject sterile water directly into product.
   - Keeping vial upright, gently swirl vial for about 1 min to evenly wet powder. Do not shake.
   - Gently swirl vial for 5–10 sec about every 5 min to dissolve any remaining solids. There should be no visible gel-like particles in the solution. Some vials may take longer than 20 min to dissolve completely. Do not use if contents do not dissolve completely by 40 min.
   - Invert vial for 15 sec to allow the solution to drain toward the stopper. Using a new 3 mL syringe equipped with a 1-inch 18-gauge needle, insert needle into the inverted vial. Before removing needle from vial, pull plunger all the way back to the end of the syringe barrel in order to remove all of the solution from the inverted vial.
   - Replace 18-gauge needle with a 25-gauge needle for SC injection.
   - To obtain the full 1.2 mL dose, all of the product must be withdrawn from the vial before expelling any air or excess solution from the syringe.
   - Expel air, large bubbles, and any excess solution to obtain the required 1.2 mL dose
7. A vial delivers 1.2 mL (150 mg) of omalizumab. For a 75 mg dose, draw up 0.6 mL into the syringe and discard the remaining product. For doses higher than 150 mg, use the following: Dose of 225 mg: Inject 1.8 mL (2 injections); dose of 300 mg: Inject 2.4 mL (2 injections); dose of 375 mg: Inject 3 mL (3 injections).
8. Do not abruptly discontinue systemic or inhaled corticosteroids when starting omalizumab therapy. Perform decreases (may need to be done gradually) in corticosteroids under direct provider supervision.
9. Omalizumab is for single use only as it contains no preservatives. Solution may be used SC within 8 hr following reconstitution when stored in the vial from 2–8°C (36–46°F) or

O

within 4 hr of reconstitution when stored at room temperature. Protect reconstituted vials from direct sunlight.

10. Store omalizumab under refrigeration from 2–8°C (36–46°F).

ASSESSMENT

1. Note reasons for therapy, onset, clinical presentation, characteristics of S&S, other inhaled corticosteroid agents trialed, outcome.
2. Assess lungs sounds and respiratory function; document PFTs, CXR.
3. Note any allergic symptom presentation or evidence of anaphylaxis. Anaphylaxis, presenting as bronchospasm, hypotension, syncope, urticaria, and/or angioedema of the throat or tongue, has been reported. This has occurred with first dose as well as after a year of regularly administered treatment.
4. Increased risk for parasitic infection (e.g., hookworm, roundworm, threadworm, whipworm) in those at high risk for geohelminth infection; monitor during therapy.
5. Monitor injection site for evidence of any reactions.
6. Dose is determined by total IgE level (international units/mL) which is measured before therapy and by body weight (kg). Doses >150 mg should be divided and administered into different injection sites.

CLIENT/FAMILY TEACHING

1. Drug administered once every 2 to 4 weeks SC after dosage determined by weight and IgE level.
2. Self-administer following written guidelines after injection demonstration and practice. Solution is thick so it may take 5 to 10 sec to administer. May experience bruising, burning/stinging, itching, redness, warmth, and induration at injection site. Usually occurs within 1 hr of injection, and lasts less than 8 days; should decrease with repeated use.
3. Do not decrease dose or stop other systemic or inhaled antiasthmatics unless directed by provider.
4. Use peak flow meter to evaluate breathing patterns, and to identify volumes to call for medication adjustment and for hospitalization. Identify triggers; practice avoidance.
5. Report S&S of anaphylaxis: swelling of throat/tongue, bronchospasm, chest tightness, cough. Also report skin changes/wheals/hives, increased SOB, low BP, or syncope.
6. Practice reliable contraception; report if pregnant to pregnancy registry established by Genetech to monitor outcomes.
7. Not for use with acute bronchospasms or acute asthma attack.
8. Stool may be monitored in those at high risk for geohelminth infection.
9. Keep all F/U visits to assess response, VS, weight, and for adverse SE.

OUTCOMES/EVALUATE

Improved breathing patterns; control of asthma

Omeprazole

(oh-**MEH**-prah-zohl)

Classification(s): Proton pump inhibitor

Pregnancy Category: C

OTC: Prilosec OTC.

RX: Prilosec.

Rx: Apo-Omeprazole, Losec, Losec MUPS.

INDICATIONS/USES

Rx:

1. Short-term treatment of active duodenal ulcer. Most clients heal in 4 weeks; others require an additional 4 weeks of therapy.
2. With clarithromycin to treat duodenal ulcer associated with *Helicobacter pylori*. With clarithromycin and amoxicillin in those with a 1-year history of duodenal ulcers or active duodenal ulcers to eradicate *H. pylori*.
3. Short-term (4–8 weeks) treatment of erosive esophagitis diagnosed by endoscopy. Maintain healing of erosive esophagitis.
4. Short-term (4–8 weeks) treatment of active benign gastric ulcer in adults.
5. Long-term treatment of hypersecretory conditions (e.g., Zollinger-Ellison syndrome, multiple endocrine adenomas, systemic mastocytosis) in adults.
6. Treatment of heartburn and other symptoms associated with GERD in adults and children.

Investigational: GERD-related laryngitis. GERD in infants and children. In combination with amoxicillin/clarithromycin to eradicate *H. pylori* in children with *H. pylori*-induced gastritis. Improve pancreatic enzyme absorption in cystic fibrosis clients with intestinal malabsorption. Alternate-day dosing to maintain remission of ulcers or GERD during long-term treatment after clients have healed via a short course (4 to 8 weeks) of daily therapy. Reduce the risk of GI bleeding in those who are at high risk for GI bleeding and are receiving antiplatelet therapy (e.g., clopidogrel).

OTC. Frequent heartburn occurring 2 or more days/week. Not intended for immediate relief. *NOTE:* There is an OTC product (Zegerid OTC) that contains omeprazole, 20 mg, and sodium bicarbonate, 1,000 mg, to be used to treat frequent heartburn (i.e., 2 or more days per week).

ACTION/KINETICS

Action

Thought to be a gastric pump inhibitor in that it blocks the final step of acid production by inhibiting the H^+/K^+ ATPase system at the secretory surface of the gastric parietal cell. Both basal and stimulated acid secretions are inhibited. Serum gastrin levels are increased during the first 1 or 2 weeks of therapy and are maintained at such levels during the course of therapy.

Pharmacokinetics

Because omeprazole is acid-labile, the product contains an enteric-coated granule formulation; however, absorption is rapid once the granules leave the stomach. Bioavailability is 30–40%. **Peak plasma levels:** 0.5–3.5 hr. **Onset:** Within 1 hr. **t½:** 0.5–1 hr. **Duration:** Up to 72 hr (due to prolonged binding of the drug to the parietal H^+/K^+ ATPase enzyme). Extensively metabolized in the liver and inactive metabolites are excreted through the urine (77%). Consider dosage adjustment in Asians. **Plasma protein binding:** About 95%.

CONTRAINDICATIONS

Lactation. Use as maintenance therapy for duodenal ulcer disease. Use with clopidogrel. OTC use in those who have trouble or pain swallowing food, are vomiting blood, or are excreting bloody or black stools.

SPECIAL CONCERNS

- Bioavailability may be increased in geriatric clients.
- Use with caution during lactation.
- Symptomatic effects with omeprazole do not preclude gastric malignancy.
- Safety and efficacy have not been determined in children.

SIDE EFFECTS

Most Common

Headache, abdominal pain, diarrhea, N&V, URTI, dizziness, rash.

CNS: Headache, dizziness. Possibly anxiety disorders, abnormal dreams, agitation, vertigo, insomnia, nervousness, apathy, paresthesia, somnolence, depression, aggression, hallucinations, hemifacial dysesthesia, tremors, confusion. **GI:** Diarrhea, N&V, abdominal pain/swelling, constipation, flatulence, anorexia, fecal discoloration, esophageal candidiasis, mucosal atrophy of the tongue, dry mouth, irritable colon, gastric fundic gland polyps, gastroduodenal carcinoids, atrophic gastritis, taste alteration, stomatitis. **Hepatic**: ***Pancreatitis.*** Overt liver disease, including hepatocellular, cholestatic, or mixed hepatitis; ***liver necrosis, hepatic failure***, hepatic encephalopathy, jaundice. **CV:** Angina, chest pain, tachycardia, bradycardia, palpitation, peripheral edema, elevated BP. **Respiratory:** URTI, pharyngeal pain, bronchospasms, cough, epistaxis. **Dermatologic:** Rash, severe generalized skin reaction including ***toxic epidermal necrolysis, Stevens-Johnson syndrome***; erythema multiforme, skin inflammation, urticaria, pruritus, alopecia, dry skin, hyperhidrosis, purpura and/or petechiae. **GU:** UTI, acute interstitial nephritis, urinary frequency, hematuria, proteinuria, glycosuria, testicular pain, microscopic pyuria, gynecomastia. **Hematologic:** Pancytopenia, thrombocytopenia, anemia, leukocytosis, neutropenia, hemolytic anemia, ***agranulocytosis***. **Musculoskeletal:** Asthenia, back pain, myalgia, joint/leg pain, muscle cramps/weakness, increased risk for osteoporosis-related fractures of the hip, wrist, or spine. **Hypersensitivity:** Angioedema, allergic reactions, ***anaphylactic shock***, ***anaphylaxis*** (rare). **Otic:** Tinnitus, anterior ischemic optic neuropathy, optic atrophy/neuritis. **Ophthalmic:** Blurred vision, double vision, dry eye syndrome, ocular irritation, optic atrophy, optic neuritis, photosensitivity. **Body as a whole:** Rash, fever,

O

gout, fatigue, malaise, pain, weight gain. When used with clarithromycin, the following *additional* side effects were noted: Tongue discoloration, rhinitis, pharyngitis, and flu syndrome. *NOTE:* Data are lacking on the effect of long-term hypochlorhydria and hypergastrinemia on the risk of developing tumors.

LABORATORY TEST CONSIDERATIONS

↑ ALT, AST, alkaline phosphatase, bilirubin, serum creatinine, GGTP. Hyponatremia, hypoglycemia.

OVERDOSE MANAGEMENT

Symptoms: Confusion, drowsiness, blurred vision, tachycardia, nausea, diaphoresis, flushing, headache, dry mouth. *Treatment:* Symptomatic and supportive. Omeprazole is not readily dialyzable.

DRUG INTERACTIONS

Ampicillin (esters) / Possible ↓ absorption of ampicillin esters R/T ↑ stomach pH
Calcium / Possible ↓ fractional calcium absorption from calcium carbonate
Carbamazepine / ↑ Carbamazepine plasma levels → ↑ toxicity; monitor and adjust carbamazepine dose if needed
Cilostazol / ↑ Cilostazol plasma levels → ↑ pharmacologic/toxic effects; consider cilostazol dose adjustment
Clarithromycin / Possible ↑ plasma levels of both drugs
Clopidogrel / ↓ Effect of clopidogrel R/T ↑ metabolism by CYP2C19; do not give together
Clozapine / ↑ Clozapine plasma levels → ↑ pharmacologic/toxic effects; monitor and adjust clozapine dose if needed
Cyanocobalamin / ↓ Cyanocobalamin absorption R/T ↑ gastric pH
Diazepam / ↑ Diazepam plasma levels R/T ↓ rate of liver metabolism
Digoxin / ↓ Digoxin absorption R/T ↑ gastric pH
Disulfiram / Possible ↑ neurotoxicity; if an interaction is suspected, discontinue both drugs
Escitalopram / ↑ Escitalopram AUC and t½ R/T inhibition of metabolism
H ***Ginkgo biloba*** / ↑ Omeprazole metabolism by CYP2C19
Iron salts / Possible ↓ absorption of iron salts R/T ↑ stomach pH
Ketoconazole / Possible ↓ ketoconazole absorption R/T ↑ stomach pH
Phenytoin / ↑ Plasma phenytoin levels R/T ↓ rate of liver metabolism
Sucralfate / ↓ Omeprazole absorption; take 30 min before sucralfate
Sulfonylureas / Possible ↑ serum sulfonylurea levels → ↑ hypoglycemic effects
Tacrolimus / ↓ Tacrolimus dose/weight normalized trough levels in renal transplant clients
Theophylline / ↑ Rate of absorption from slow-release theophylline forms; monitor and adjust theophylline dose if needed
Tolterodine / ↑ Peak concentration of tolterodine R/T ↑ gastric pH due to omeprazole administration
Triazolam / ↑ Triazolam plasma levels R/T ↓ rate of liver metabolism
Warfarin / Prolonged rate of warfarin elimination R/T ↓ rate of liver metabolism

HOW SUPPLIED

RX. ***Capsules, Delayed-Release:*** 10 mg, 20 mg, 40 mg (each contains enteric-coated granules); ***Granules for Suspension, Delayed-Release:*** 2.5 mg, 10 mg.
OTC. ***Tablets, Delayed-Release (as omeprazole magnesium):*** 20 mg.

DOSAGE

RX: CAPSULES, DELAYED-RELEASE; SUSPENSION, DELAYED-RELEASE

Active duodenal ulcer.

Adults: 20 mg/day for 4–8 weeks. Some may require an additional 4 weeks of therapy.

Duodenal ulcer associated with H. pylori.

The following regimens may be used in adults: **Triple Therapy:** Omeprazole, 20 mg, plus clarithromycin, 500 mg, plus amoxicillin, 1,000 mg, each given twice daily for 10 days. If an ulcer is present at the beginning of therapy, continue omeprazole, 20 mg once daily, for an additional 18 days. **Dual Therapy:** Omeprazole, 40 mg once daily plus clarithromycin, 500 mg, 3 times per day for 14 days. If an ulcer is present at the beginning of therapy, continue omeprazole, 20 mg daily, for an additional 14 days. Omeprazole with clarithromycin is more likely to be associated with clarithromycin resistance compared with triple therapy.

GERD with erosive esophagitis.

Adults, initial: 20 mg/day for 4–8 weeks; **maintenance of healing:** 20 mg/day. Controlled studies do not exceed 1 year. **Children, 1 year and older, 5–<10 kg:** 5 mg once a day; **10–20 kg:** 10 mg once a day; **20 kg or more:** 20 mg once a day. *NOTE:* On a per kg basis, the doses of omeprazole needed to heal erosive esophagitis are greater for children than for adults.

GERD without esophageal lesions.

Adults: 20 mg/day for up to 4 weeks.

GERD in children.

Children, 1 year and older, 5–<10 kg: 5 mg once a day; **10–20 kg:** 10 mg once a day; **20 kg or more:** 20 mg once a day.

Gastric ulcers.

Adults, usual: 40 mg once daily for 4–8 weeks.

Pathologic hypersecretory conditions.

Adults, initial: 60 mg/day; then dose individualized, although doses up to 120 mg 3 times/day have been used. Daily doses greater than 80 mg should be divided. Continue treatment for as long as needed; some have been treated for more than 5 years.

OTC: TABLETS, DELAYED-RELEASE

Frequent heartburn, greater than 2 or more days/week.

20 mg (1 tablet) taken with a full glass of water once daily before the first meal of the day, every day, for 14 days. **Maximum daily dose:** 20 mg. Takes 1 to 4 days for the full effect; some may get complete relief within 24 hr. The 14-day course may be repeated q 4 months.

NURSING IMPLICATIONS

Do not confuse Prilosec with Prozac (an antidepressant) or Prinivil (ACE inhibitor).

IMPLEMENTATION/ADMINISTRATION/STORAGE

1. Give daily doses more than 80 mg in divided doses.
2. Efficacy for more than 8 weeks has not been determined. However, if a client does not respond to 8 weeks of therapy, an additional 4 weeks may help. If there is a recurrence of erosive or symptomatic GERD poorly responsive to usual treatment, an additional 4 to 8 weeks of therapy may be tried.
3. Consider dosage adjustment in Asian clients or in those with impaired hepatic function especially when used for maintaining clients with erosive esophagitis.
4. For clients with a nasogastric or gastric tube, add 5 mL water to a catheter tipped syringe and then add the contents of a 2.5 mg packet (or 15 mL of water for the 10 mg packet). Use only catheter tipped syringes. Immediately shake the syringe and leave 2 to 3 min to thicken. Shake the syringe and inject through the nasogastric or gastric tube, French size 6 or larger, into the stomach within 30 min. Refill the syringe with an equal amount of water. Shake and flush any remaining contents from the tube into the stomach.
5. Store capsules from 15–30°C (59–86°F) in a tight container protected from light and moisture. Store oral suspension from 15–30°C (59–86°F). Store tablets from 20–25°C (68–77°F) protected from high heat, humidity, and moisture.

ASSESSMENT

1. List reasons for therapy, triggers, frequency, characteristics of S&S, other agents trialed.
2. Identify other conditions that may be basis for treatment, i.e. CF with malabsorption, chronic laryngitis, reduce drug-induced bleeding risk, or long-term alternative day dosing with ulcers or GERD.
3. Record abdominal assessments, radiographic/endoscopic findings, and *H. pylori* results.
4. Note age and associated conditions; if receiving high-dose/long-term therapy >1-yr increased risk for osteoporosis-related fractures reported of hip, wrist, or spine. Obtain BMD testing with high risk group.
5. Determine if pregnant.
6. Monitor U/A, CBC, and LFTs; adjust dosage with hepatic dysfunction.

O

CLIENT/FAMILY TEACHING

1. Take at least 1 hr before eating and swallow whole; do not open, chew, or crush. Antacids can be administered with omeprazole.
2. For those who have difficulty swallowing capsules, add 1 tablespoon of applesauce to an empty bowl. Open omeprazole capsule, and empty pellets onto applesauce. Mix pellets with the applesauce, and swallow immediately. Do not heat or chew the applesauce, and do not chew or crush the pellets. Do not store mixture for future use.
3. Take oral suspension on an empty stomach at least 1 hr before a meal. To prepare the oral suspension, empty the contents of the 2.5 mg packet into a small cup containing 5 mL of water or empty the contents of the 10 mg packet into 10 mL of water. Do not use other liquids or foods. Leave for 2–3 min to thicken. Stir well and drink within 30 min. Refill cup with water and drink.
4. Report any changes in urinary elimination, pain, discomfort, or persistent diarrhea.
5. Avoid alcohol and OTC agents as well as foods known to cause GI upset/irritation.
6. Avoid activities that require mental alertness, until drug effects realized; may cause dizziness.
7. Do not use OTC product for more than 14 days unless directed by provider.
8. Use reliable contraception; potential risk to the fetus.
9. For short-term use only, drug inhibits total gastric acid secretion. Side effects of prolonged therapy and suppression of acid secretion alter bacterial colonization and lead to hypochlorhydria and hypergastrinemia, which may cause an increased risk for gastric tumors.
10. Keep all F/U to assess response, labs, and for adverse SE.

OUTCOMES/EVALUATE

- Control of GERD S&S
- Promotion of ulcer healing; relief of pain
- ↓ Gastric acid production
- Control of GERD-related laryngitis, improved pancreatic enzyme absorption with CF, ↓ bleeding with antiplatelet therapy, remission of ulcers/GERD with alternate day therapy (UL)

OnabotulinumtoxinA (Botulinum toxin A)

(on-a-**BOT**-you-**LYE**-num-**TOX**-in-ay)

Classification(s): Botulinum Toxin Type A

Pregnancy Category: C

RX: Botox, Botox Cosmetic.

INDICATIONS/USES

Botox. (1) Severe primary axillary hyperhidrosis that is inadequately managed with topical agents. (2) Cervical dystonia in adults to reduce the severity of abnormal head position and neck pain associated with cervical dystonia. (3) Prophylaxis of headaches in adults with chronic migraine (at least 15 days/month with headache lasting 4 hr/day or longer). (4) Strabismus and blepharospasm associated with dystonia, including benign essential blepharospasm or VII nerve disorders in those 12 years and older. (5) Upper limb spasticity in adults to decrease the severity of increased muscle tone in elbow flexors (biceps), wrist flexors (flexor carpi radialis and flexor carpi ulnaris), and finger flexors (flexor digitorum profundus and flexor digitorum sublimis). (6) Urinary incontinence due to detrusor overactivity associated with a neurologic condition (e.g., spinal cord injury) or multiple sclerosis in adults who have an inadequate response to or who are intolerant of an anticholinergic medication.

Botox Cosmetic. Temporary improvement in the appearance of moderate to severe glabellar lines associated with corrugator and/or procerus muscle activity in adults 65 years and younger.

Investigational: (1) Achalasia. (2) Facial lines and wrinkles. (3) Gustatory sweating (Frey syndrome). (4) Hand dystonia. (5) Tension headaches. (6) Palmar hyperhidrosis. (7) Tourette syndrome. (8) Drooling in adults and children. (9) Spasticity of cerebral palsy in children and adolescents. (10) Tardive dyskinesia.

ACTION/KINETICS

Action

OnabotulinumtoxinA blocks neuromuscular transmission by binding to receptor sites on motor nerve or sympathetic nerve terminals. The drug then enters nerve terminals and inhibits the release of acetylcholine. When injected intradermally, onabotulinumtoxinA products a temporary chemical denervation of the sweat gland resulting in local reduction of sweating. Following intradetrusor injection, the drug affects efferent pathways of detrusor activity by inhibiting acetylcholine release. The drug is also believed to inhibit afferent neurotransmitters and sensory pathways.

Pharmacokinetics

Using current technology it is not possible to detect onabotulinumtoxinA in the peripheral blood following IM injection at recommended doses.

CONTRAINDICATIONS

Infection at the proposed site(s). Hypersensitivity to any botulinum toxin preparation or any component of the product. Those with detrusor overactivity associated with neurologic conditions who have acute urinary tract infection, and in those with acute urinary retention who are not routinely performing clean intermittent self catheterization.

SPECIAL CONCERNS

Spread of toxin effect. Postmarketing reports indicate that the effects of all botulinum toxin products may spread from the area of injection to produce symptoms consistent with botulinum toxin effects. These may include asthenia, generalized muscle weakness, diplopia, ptosis, dysphagia, dysphonia, dysarthria, urinary incontinence, and breathing difficulties. These symptoms have been reported hours to weeks after injection. Swallowing and breathing difficulties can be life-threatening, and there have been reports of death. The risk of symptoms is probably greatest in children treated for spasticity, but symptoms can also occur in adults treated for spasticity and other conditions, particularly in those clients who have underlying conditions that would predispose them to these symptoms. In unapproved uses, including spasticity in children and adults, and in approved indications, cases of spread of effect have been reported at doses comparable with those used to treat cervical dystonia and at lower doses.

- **Use with caution in those who have excessive weakness or atrophy in the target muscle(s), marked facial asymmetry, inflammation of the injection site(s), ptosis, excessive dermatochalasis, deep dermal scarring, thick sebaceous skin, or the inability to substantially lessen glabellar lines by physically spreading them apart.**
- **Use with caution during lactation.**
- **In general use caution with dose selection in the elderly starting at the low end of the dosage range.**
- **The products contain albumin, a derivative of human blood. Based on effective screening and product manufacturing processes, the products carry an extremely remote risk for transmission of viral diseases as well as for Creutzfeldt-Jakob disease. No cases of transmission have been reported.**
- **Safety and efficacy not established in children younger than 12 years for blepharospasm or strabismus; younger than16 years for cervical dystonia; or younger than 18 years for axillary hyperhidrosis, spasticity, urinary incontinence due to detrusor overactivity associated with a neurologic condition, or chronic migraine.**

SIDE EFFECTS

Most Common

When used for blepharospasm: Ptosis, eye dryness, and superficial punctate keratitis.
When used for cervical dystonia: Dysphagia, dyspnea, URTI, headache, neck pain.
When used for chronic migraine: Neck pain, headache, worsening of migraine, muscle weakness, ptosis.

Botox, all uses. At local site: Bleeding/bruising, erythema, infection, inflammation, pain, swelling, tenderness. Needle–related anxiety and/or pain may cause hypotension or syncope. **GI:** Constipation, abdominal pain, anorexia, diarrhea, vomiting. **CNS:** Insomnia, new onset or recurrent ***seizures***, facial palsy/paresis, hypoesthesia, localized numbness, paresthesia, radiculopathy, vertigo. **CV:** Arrhythmia, ***MI***. **Respiratory:** Dyspnea, dysphagia, breathing difficulties. **GU:** Dysuria. **Dermatologic:** Hyperhidrosis, skin rash including erythema multiform and psoriasiform eruption. **Musculoskeletal:** Gait disturbance, fall, muscle spasm/weakness, myalgia, local weakness of injected muscle(s) (expected) and adjacent muscles, brachial plexopathy. **Hypersensitivity:** Serum sickness, urticaria, soft tissue edema, dyspnea, ***anaphylaxis***. **Ophthalmic:** Visual disturbances; reduced blinking from injection into the orbicularis muscle can lead to corneal exposure, persistent epithelial defect, and corneal ulceration especially in those with VII nerve disorders. **Otic:** Hyperacusis, tinnitus. **Body as a whole:** Malaise, pyrexia, death (associated with dysphagia, pneumonia, other debility, anaphylaxis). **Miscellaneous:** Immunogenicity.

When used for blepharospasm. Ophthalmic: Ptosis, eye dryness, superficial punctate keratitis, irritation, tearing, lagophthalmos, photophobia, electropion, keratitis, diplopia, entropion, local swelling of the eyelid skin lasting for several days. **Miscellaneous:** Diffuse skin rash, focal facial paralysis, exacerbation of myasthenia gravis, syncope.

When used for cervical dystonia. GI: Dysphagia, oral dryness, nausea. **CNS:** Headache, dizziness, speech disorder, drowsiness. **Respiratory:** URTI, cough, rhinitis, dyspnea. **Musculoskeletal:** Neck/back pain, hypertonia, stiffness, numbness. **Ophthalmic:** Diplopia, ptosis. **Body as a whole:** Flu syndrome, asthenia, fever. **Miscellaneous:** Soreness at injection site, dysphonia.

When used for chronic migraine. Musculoskeletal: Neck pain, muscle weakness/spasms, musculoskeletal pain/stiffness, myalgia, jaw pain. **CNS:** Headache, worsening of migraine, facial paresis, vertigo. **GI:** Dysphagia, **CV:** Hypertension. **Respiratory:** Bronchitis. **Ophthalmic:** Eyelid ptosis, dry eye, eyelid edema, eye infection. **Miscellaneous:** Injection site pain.

When used for hyperhidrosis. CNS: Anxiety, headache. **Musculoskeletal:** Neck/back pain. **Respiratory:** Pharyngitis. **Dermatologic:** Nonaxillary sweating, pruritus. **Body as a whole:** Fever, flu syndrome, infection. **Miscellaneous:** Injection site pain and hemorrhage.

When used for strabismus. Ophthalmic: Extraocular muscles adjacent to the injection site can be affected causing vertical deviation, especially with higher doses. Ptosis, retrobulbar hemorrhage.

When used for upper limb spasticity. Musculoskeletal: Muscle weakness, pain in extremity. **GI:** Nausea. **Respiratory:** Bronchitis, URTI. **Body as a whole:** Fatigue.

When used for urinary incontinence. CNS: Insomnia. **GU:** Hematuria, urinary retention, UTI, autonomic dysreflexia. **Body as a whole:** Fatigue.

Botox Cosmetic. At local site: Bleeding, bruising, erythema, infection, inflammation, pain, swelling, tenderness, weakness of adjacent muscles to those being treated. **CNS:** Focal facial paralysis, localized numbness, vertigo with nystagmus. **GI:** Abdominal pain, diarrhea, loss of appetite, vomiting. **Musculoskeletal:** Myalgia, myasthenia gravis, brachial plexopathy. **Dermatologic:** Erythema multiforme, pruritus, psoriasiform eruption, sweating. **Ophthalmic:** Blurred vision, transient ptosis, glaucoma, retinal vein occlusion. **Otic:** Decrease hearing, ear noise. **Body as a whole:** Malaise, fever, syncope.

When used for glabellar lines. GI: Nausea, dyspepsia, tooth disorder. **CNS:** Headache, syncope. **CV:** Hypertension. **Musculoskeletal:** Muscle weakness, facial pain, focal facial paralysis, weakness of adjacent muscles to those being treated, exacerbation of myasthenia gravis. **Dermatologic:** Skin tightness. **Respiratory:** Respiratory injection. **Ophthalmic:** Acute angle closure glaucoma when used for blepharospasm. **Body as a whole:** Paresthesia, flu syndrome, pain. **Miscellaneous:** Blepharoptosis.

DRUG INTERACTIONS

Aminoglycosides (e.g., gentamicin) / Enhanced neuromuscular action → protracted respiratory depression; use together with caution
Anticholinergic drugs (e.g., atropine) / Potentiation of systemic anticholinergic effects (e.g., blurred vision); use together with caution
Cholinesterase inhibitors / Enhanced neuromuscular action → protracted respiratory depression; use together with caution
Magnesium sulfate / Enhanced neuromuscular action → protracted respiratory depression; use together with caution
Muscle relaxants (e.g., metaxalone) / Exaggeration of excessive weakness; use together with caution
Nondepolarizing muscle relaxants (e.g., tubocurarine) / Enhanced neuromuscular activity → protracted respiratory depression; use together with caution
Other botulinum neurotoxins (e.g., botulinum toxin B) / Administration at the same time or within several months of each other → exacerbation of excessive neuromuscular weakness
Quinidine / Enhanced neuromuscular action → protracted respiratory depression; use together with caution

HOW SUPPLIED

Botox. ***Injection, Lyophilized Powder for Solution:*** 100 units, 200 units.

Botox Cosmetic. ***Injection, Lyophilized Powder for Injection:*** 50 units, 100 units.

DOSAGE

Botox

Blepharospasm.

Adults and children over 12 years, initial: 1.25–2.5 units (0.05–0.1 mL volume at each site) injected into the medial and lateral pretarsal orbicularis oculi of the upper lid and into the lateral pretarsal orbicularis oculi of the lower lid. **Maximum:** 300 units in a 30–day period. The initial effect is seen within 3 days and reaches a peak at 1–2 weeks posttreatment. Each treatment lasts about 3 months following which the procedure can be repeated. The dose may be increased up to 2-fold if the response from the initial dose is insufficient (i.e., the effect does not last longer than 2 months). Some tolerance may be noted if treatments are given more frequently than q 3 months.

Cervical dystonia.

Adults, botulinum toxin-experienced: Individualize initial and sequential dosing for each client based on the client's head and neck position, localization of pain, muscle hypertrophy, client response, and history of side effects. The mean dose administered to clients in one study was 236 units (25th to 75th percentile range was 198 to 300 units). **Adults and children 16 years and older, botulinum toxin-naive:** Initial dose should be lower with subsequent dosing based on individual response. Limiting the total dose injected into the sternocleidomastoid muscles to 100 units or less may decrease the incidence of dysphagia. For all clients, improvement usually begins within the first 2 weeks with maximum benefit at approximately 6 weeks postinjection. **Maximum dose, all clients:** No more than 50 units per site.

Chronic migraine.

Adults, usual: 155 units IM as 0.1 mL (5 units) injections per each site. Divide injections across 7 specific head/neck muscle areas. The following are recommended dose by muscle for chronic migraine (doses for each muscle -except for procerus-are distributed bilaterally): **Frontalis:** 20 units divided in 4 sites; **Corrugator:** 10 units divided in 2 sites; **Procerus:** 5 units in 1 site; **Occipitalis:** 30 units divided in 6 sites; **Temporalis:** 40 units divided in 8 sites; **Trapezius:** 30 units divided in 6 sites; **Cervical paraspinal muscle group:** 20 units divided in 4 sites. **Total dose:** 155 units divided in 31 sites. The recommended retreatment schedule is q 12 weeks.

Primary axillary hyperhidrosis.

Adults, usual: 50 units per axilla. Determine the hyperhidrotic area to be injected using standard staining techniques. Inject 50 units intradermally in 0.1–0.2 mL aliquots to each axilla, evenly distributed in multiple sites (10–15) about 1–2 cm apart. Administer repeat injections when the clinical effect of the previous injection diminishes.

Strabismus.

Adults and children 12 years and older. *Vertical muscles and for horizontal strabismus of less than 20 prism diopters:* 1.25–2.5 units in any 1 muscle. *Horizontal strabismus of 20–50 prism diopters:* 2.5–5 units in any 1 muscle. *Persistent VI nerve palsy of 1 month or longer duration:* 1.25–2.5 units in the medial rectus muscle. **Initial dose:** Use the lower listed doses for the treatment of small deviations and the larger doses only for large deviations. **Maximum dose:** 25 units for any 1 muscle as a single injection. The initial doses create paralysis of injected muscles 1–2 days after injection that increases in intensity during the first week. Paralysis lasts for 2–6 weeks. About 50% of clients will require subsequent doses because of inadequate paralytic response of the muscle to the initial dose or because mechanical factors such as large deviations or restrictions, or lack of binocular motor fusion to stabilize the alignment.

O

Examine clients 7–14 days after each injection to assess the effect. Subsequent doses for those experiencing incomplete paralysis of the target muscle may be increased up to 2-fold compared with the previously administered dose. Do not give subsequent injections until the effects of the previous injection have dissipated as evidenced by substantial function in the injected and adjacent muscles.

Upper limb spasticity.

Adults, usual: Ranges from 75–360 units divided among selected muscles at a given treatment session. The recommended dose ranges per muscle for upper limb spasticity are as follows: *Biceps brachii:* 100–200 units divided in 4 sites; *flexor carpi radialis:* 12.5–50 units in 1 site; *flexor carpi ulnaris:* 12.5–50 units in 1 site; *flexor digitorum profundus:* 30–50 units in 1 site; *flexor digitorum sublimis:* 30–50 units in 1 site. Generally, no more than 50 units per site should be administered. The lowest recommended starting dose should be used. Tailor sequential treatment to the individual based on the size, number, and location of muscles involved; also, severity of spasticity; presence of local muscle weakness; and, client's response to previous treatment or side event history. When the effect of a previous injection has diminished (but generally no sooner than 12 weeks after the previous injection), repeat treatment may be given. The degree and pattern of muscle spasticity at the time of reinjection may necessitate alterations in the dose and muscles to be injected.

Urinary incontinence.

Adults, usual: 30 injections of 1 mL (about 6.7 units) each (i.e., total dose of 200 units—30 mL—) into the detrusor. **Maximum dose:** 200 units/treatment. Clients should not have an acute UTI prior to treatment. Prophylactic antibiotics (except aminoglycosides) should be given 1–3 days pretreatment, on the treatment day, and 1–3 days posttreatment. Consider clients for reinjection when the clinical effect of the previous injection diminishes but no sooner than 12 weeks from the prior bladder injection.

Botox Cosmetic

Glabellar lines.

Adults, usual: 0.1 mL into each of the 5 sites, 2 in each corrugator muscle and 1 in the procerus muscle for a total dose of 20 units. An effective dose for facial lines is determined by gross observation of the client's ability to activate the superficial muscles injected. Usually the initial doses induce a chemical denervation of the injected muscles 1–2 days after injection, increasing in intensity during the first week. Duration of activity is about 3–4 months; more frequent dosing is not recommended. Injection intervals should be no more frequent than q 3 months and should be undertaken using the lowest effective dose.

NURSING IMPLICATIONS

IMPLEMENTATION/ADMINISTRATION/STORAGE

1. See package insert for depictions for preparation for various uses.
2. Potency units are specific to the preparation and assay method used. They are not interchangeable with other products of botulinum toxin. Thus, units of biological activity of onabotulinumtoxinA cannot be compared with or converted into units of any other botulinum toxin products assessed with any other specific assay method.
3. In treating adults for 1 or more indications, do not exceed the maximum cumulative Botox dose of 300 units in a 3-month period.
4. If used for urinary incontinence, discontinue antiplatelet therapy at least 3 days before injection of onabotulinumtoxinA. Those on anticoagulant therapy must be managed appropriately to decrease the risk of bleeding.
5. **Administration for blepharospasm.** IM use only. Inject reconstituted toxin using a sterile 27- to 30-gauge needle without EMG guidance. Avoiding injection near the levator palpebrae superioris may reduce the complication of ptosis. Avoiding medial lower lid injections and thereby reduction of diffusion

O

into the inferior oblique may reduce complications of diplopia. Ecchymosis occurs easily in the soft eyelid tissues; prevent by applying pressure to the injection site immediately after injection.

6. **Administration for cervical dystonia.** IM use only. Use a 25- to 30-gauge needle for superficial muscles and a longer 22-gauge needle for deeper musculature. Localization of the involved muscles with EMG guidance may be useful.
7. **Administration for chronic migraine.** IM using a sterile 30-gauge, 0.5-inch needle as 0.1 mL (5 units) injections per each site. Divide injections across 7 specific head/neck muscle areas. A 1-inch needle may be needed in the neck region for those with thick neck muscles. With the exception of the procerus muscle, which should be injected at 1 site (midline), inject all muscles bilaterally with half the number of injections given to the left and half to the right side of the head and neck.
8. **Administration for axillary hyperhidrosis.** Give intradermally using a 30-gauge needle. Each dose is injected to a depth of about 2 mm and at a 45-degree angle to the skin surface, with the bevel side up to minimize leakage and to ensure the injections remain intradermal. If injection sites are marked in ink, do not inject directly through the ink mark to avoid a permanent tattoo effect. Each injection site has a ring effect up to about 2 cm in diameter. To minimize the area of no effect, evenly space the injection sites. Clients should shave underarms and abstain from the use of over-the-counter deodorants or antiperspirants for 24 hr prior to the test. Clients should rest comfortably without exercise or hot drinks for about 30 min prior to the test.
9. **Administration for strabismus.** IM use only. Use is intended for injection into extraocular muscles using the electrical activity recorded from the tip of the injection needle as a guide to placement within the target muscle. Do not attempt injecting without surgical exposure or EMG guidance. To prepare the eye for injection, it is recommended that several drops of a local anesthetic and an ocular decongestant be given several minutes prior to injection. The volume injected for treatment of strabismus should be between 0.05 to 0.15 mL per muscle.
10. **Administration for upper limb spasticity.** IM use only. Use a 25- to 30-gauge needle for superficial muscles and a longer 22-gauge needle for deeper musculature. Localization of the involved muscles with EMG guidance or nerve stimulation techniques is recommended.
11. **Administration for urinary incontinence.** Prior to the injection, an intravesical instillation of diluted local anesthetic with or without sedation or general anesthesia may be used. If a local anesthetic instillation is performed, the bladder should be drained and irrigated with sterile saline before the injection. Reconstituted onabotulinumtoxinA (200 units/30 mL) is injected into the detrusor muscle via a flexible or rigid cystoscope, avoiding the trigone. The bladder should be instilled with enough saline to achieve adequate visualization for the injections, but over-distension should be avoided. Insert the needle about 2 mm into the detrusor and 30 injections of 1 mL (about 6.7 units) each (total volume of 30 mL) should be spaced about 1 cm apart. For the final injection, about 1 mL of sterile sodium chloride 0.9% should be injected so the full dose is delivered. After the injections are given, the saline used for bladder wall visualization should be drained. Observe the client for at least 30 min postinjection.
12. **Administration of Botox Cosmetic.** IM use only. Use a 30- to 33-gauge needle. To reduce the complication of ptosis, use the following steps: Avoid injection near the levator palpebrae superioris, particularly in those with larger brow depressor complexes; place lateral corrugator injections at least 1 cm above the boy supraorbital ridge; ensure the injected volume/dose is accurate and, where feasible, kept to a minimum; do not inject toxin closer than 1 cm above the central eyebrow.
13. Store unopened vials in a refrigerator (2–8°C; 36–46°F) for up to 24 months (Botox 200 unit vial and Botox Cosmetic 50 unit vial) or for up to 36 months (Botox 100 unit vial or Botox Cosmetic 100 unit vial). The product and diluent do not contain a preservative; thus, once opened and reconstituted, administer within 24 hr. During this time period,

O

store reconstituted toxin in a refrigerator. Discard any remaining solution; do not freeze.

ASSESSMENT

1. Note reasons for therapy, (i.e., cervical dystonia, hyperhidrosis, glabellar lines, migraine prophylaxis, upper limb spasticity, strabismus, blepharospasm, urinary incontinence/frequency) associated characteristics, appropriate dose for use, other agents/therapies trialed. Document clinical presentation as indicated.
2. Assess carefully for evidence/history of neuropathic, neurologic, or neuromuscular disorders.
3. For use/administration only by those individuals trained to administer.
4. Monitor carefully for post injection effects (hours to weeks later) which may spread from the area of injection to other body areas to produce symptoms consistent with botulinum toxin effects.
5. Review associated risk factors to ensure client understanding. Drug contains albumin which may present the remote risk of viral disease transmission.

CLIENT/FAMILY TEACHING

1. Drug has many uses: may be used to relieve abnormal muscle spasms/contractures of the head and neck, or spasticity of extremities permitting more controlled movement, improved posture, and increased activity, to decrease frown lines and skin wrinkles, to inhibit migraine headaches, to control urination, for eye twitching and severe sweating (underarm). Review FDA-Approved Medication Guide which trained provider will go over with you.
2. Do not perform activities that require mental alertness until drug effects realized; may cause drowsiness. Resume activity slowly and carefully following administration.
3. The clostridium bacteria (A) that makes the toxin is not being injected directly; a sterilized by-product of the bacteria is utilized. May experience slight sting with injections.
4. Report any swallowing problems, SOB, respiratory disorders/infections, injection site abnormalities, facial/eye drooping, or weakness immediately.
5. For cervical dystonia, improvement should occur within the first 2 wk following treatment, and maximum improvement should occur within about 6 wk. Beneficial effects may last 3 months before retreatment is needed.
6. For blepharospasm, improvement should occur within the first 3 days following treatment, and maximum improvement should occur within about 1 to 2 wk. Beneficial effects may last 3 months before retreatment is needed.
7. For strabismus, improvement should occur within the first 2 days following treatment, and maximum improvement should occur within the first week. Beneficial effects may last 2 to 6 wk before the effects begin to wear off.
8. May cause reduced blinking or effectiveness of blinking; seek immediate medical attention if eye pain or irritation occurs following treatment.
9. For glabellar lines, improvement should occur within the first 2 days following treatment, and maximum improvement should occur within the first week. Beneficial effects may last 3 to 4 months.
10. Report any difficulties in voiding after bladder injection for urinary incontinence.
11. Upper arm spasticity may require multiple injections and dosing based on size, number, and location of muscles involved, severity of spasticity and presence of local muscle weakness.
12. Provider will review additional information related to conditions being treated and the associated time frames for improvement.
13. Practice reliable contraception.
14. An antitoxin is available in the event of significant overdose or misinjection. Contact Allergan Inc. (Pharmacovigilance Department) at 1-800-433-8871 or the CDC directly at 1-770-488-7100. The antitoxin will not reverse any botulinum toxin induced effects already apparent by the time of antitoxin administration. The antitoxin needs to be administered within 20 hr of overdosage. More information may be found at http://www.cdc.gov/mmwr/preview/mmwrhtml/mm5232a8.htm.
15. Keep all F/U to assess response and for adverse SE.

OUTCOMES/EVALUATE

Improvement in underlying symptoms or conditions requiring treatment

IV

Ondansetron hydrochloride

(on-**DAN**-sih-tron)

Classification(s): Antiemetic

Pregnancy Category: B

RX: Zofran, Zofran ODT, Zuplenz.

✦ **Rx:** Apo-Ondansetron, PMS-Ondansetron, ratio-Ondansetron, Sandoz Ondansetron.

INDICATIONS/USES

Oral Film/Solution/Tablets: (1) Prevent N&V associated with highly emetogenic cancer chemotherapy, including cisplatin, greater than 50 mg/m^2. (2) Prevent N&V associated with initial and repeat courses of moderately emetogenic cancer chemotherapy. (3) Prevent N&V associated with radiotherapy in clients receiving either total body irradiation, single high-dose fraction to the abdomen, or daily fractions to the abdomen. (4) Prevent postoperative N&V. Routine prophylaxis is not recommended if there is little chance N&V will occur postoperatively. (5) Postoperatively in clients in whom N&V must be avoided, even when the incidence of postoperative N&V is low. Use oral solution, oral disintegrating tablets, or tablets. *Investigational:* Reduce alcohol consumption/effects; cholestatic pruritus.

Parenteral: (1) Prevent N&V associated with initial and repeat courses of emetogenic cancer chemotherapy, including high-dose cisplatin. Efficacy of the 32 mg single dose beyond 24 hr has not been determined. (2) Prevention of N&V postoperatively for those in whom nausea and/or vomiting must be avoided, even when the incidence of postoperative N&V is low. For those who do not receive prophylactic ondansetron injection and experience nausea and/or vomiting postoperatively, the injection may be given to prevent further episodes. *Investigational:* Treat radiation-induced N&V, postanesthetic shivering, cholestasis-related pruritus, opioid-related pruritus.

ACTION/KINETICS

Action

Cytotoxic chemotherapy is thought to release serotonin from enterochromaffin cells of the small intestine. The released serotonin may stimulate the vagal afferent nerves through the 5-HT_3 receptors, thus stimulating the vomiting reflex. Ondansetron, a 5-HT_3 antagonist, blocks this effect of serotonin. Whether the drug acts centrally and/or peripherally to antagonize the effect of serotonin is not known.

Pharmacokinetics

Time to peak plasma levels, after PO: 1.7–2.1 hr. **t½, after IV use:** 3.5–4.7 hr; **after PO use:** 3.1–6.2 hr, depending on the age. A decrease in clearance and increase in half-life are observed in clients over 75 years of age, although no dosage adjustment is recommended. Clients less than 15 years of age show a shortened plasma half-life after IV use (2.4 hr). Significantly metabolized with 5% of a dose excreted unchanged in the urine.

SPECIAL CONCERNS

- **Use with caution during lactation.**
- **Safety and efficacy in children 3 years of age and younger not known.**

SIDE EFFECTS

Most Common

Diarrhea, headache, dizziness, malaise/fatigue, constipation, bradycardia, hypotension, drowsiness/sedation, anxiety/agitation, gynecological disorder, urinary retention, hypoxia, pruritus, pyrexia, shivers.

GI: Diarrhea, constipation, xerostomia, abdominal pain. **CNS:** Headache, dizziness, drowsiness, sedation, malaise, fatigue, anxiety, agitation, extrapyramidal syndrome, ***clonic-tonic seizures***. **CV:** Tachycardia, chest pain, hypotension, ECG alterations, angina, bradycardia, syncope, vascular occlusive events. **Dermatologic:** Pain, redness, and burning at injection site; cold sensation, pruritus, paresthesia. **Hypersensitivity (rare):** ***Anaphylaxis, bronchospasm, shock***, SOB, hypotension, angioedema, urticaria. **Miscellaneous:** Rash, ***bronchospasm***, transient blurred vision, hypokalemia, weakness, fever, musculoskeletal pain, shivers, dysuria, postoperative carbon-dioxide-related pain, akathisia, acute dystonic reactions, gynecologic disorder, urinary retention, wound problem.

LABORATORY TEST CONSIDERATIONS

↑ AST, ALT.

DRUG INTERACTIONS

Rifampin / ↓ ondansetron plasma levels R/T ↑ liver metabolism.

O

HOW SUPPLIED

Ondansetron (as hydrochloride). ***Film, Oral:*** 4 mg, 8 mg; ***Injection:*** 2 mg/mL, 32 mg/50 mL (premixed); ***Oral Solution:*** 4 mg/5 mL; ***Tablets:*** 4 mg, 8 mg, 16 mg, 24 mg.
Ondansetron (as base). ***Tablets, Orally Disintegrating:*** 4 mg, 8 mg.

DOSAGE

IM; IV

Prevention of N&V due to chemotherapy.

Adults: A single 32 mg dose or three 0.15 mg/kg doses. A single 32 mg dose is infused over 15 min beginning 20 min prior to the start of emetogenic chemotherapy. For the 3-dose regimen, the first dose is infused over 15 min starting 30 min before the start of chemotherapy; the second and third doses are given 4 hr and 8 hr, respectively, after the first dose. **Children, 6 months to 18 years:** Three 0.15 mg/kg doses. The first dose is infused over 15 min starting 30 min before the start of chemotherapy; the second and third doses are given 4 hr and 8 hr, respectively, after the first dose.

Prevent postoperative N&V.

Adults: 4 mg undiluted given IV over 2–5 min (but not less than 30 seconds) immediately before induction of anesthesia or postoperatively as needed. Alternatively, 4 mg undiluted may be given IM as a single injection. Alternatively, 4 mg undiluted given IM as a single injection. **Children, 1 month to 12 years, less than 40 kg:** Single dose of 0.1 mg/kg IV given over 2–5 min, but not less than 30 seconds. **Children, 2–12 years weighing over 40 kg:** Single dose of 4 mg IV given over 2–5 min, but not less than 30 seconds. For children, give immediately prior to or following anesthesia induction, or postoperatively as needed.

Postanesthetic shivering.

Single IV dose of 4 or 8 mg given during induction of anesthesia.

ORAL FILM; ORAL SOLUTION; TABLETS; TABLETS, ORAL DISINTEGRATING

Prevent N&V associated with highly emetogenic cancer chemotherapy.

Adults: Single 24 mg tablet or three 8 mg films once a day given 30 min before the start of single-day highly emetogenic chemotherapy, including cisplatin greater than or equal to 50 mg/m^2. *NOTE:* There is no experience using the 24 mg tablet in children.

Prevent N&V associated with moderately emetogenic cancer chemotherapy.

Adults and children over 12 years of age: One 8-mg tablet, orally disintegrating tablet, or oral film; or 10 mL (equivalent to 8 mg ondansetron) oral solution twice a day. Give the first dose 30 min before treatment followed by a second 8-mg dose 8 hr after the first dose; **then,** 8 mg twice a day for 1–2 days after chemotherapy. **Children, 4–11 years:** One 4-mg tablet, orally disintegrating tablet, or oral film; or 5 mL (equivalent to 4 mg ondansetron) oral solution 3 times per day. The first dose is given 30 min before chemotherapy with subsequent doses 4 and 8 hr after the first dose. **Then,** 4 mg q 8 hr for 1–2 days after completion of chemotherapy.

Prevention of N&V associated with radiotherapy.

Adults: One 8-mg tablet, orally disintegrating tablet, or oral film; or 10 mL (equivalent to 8 mg ondansetron) oral solution 3 times per day. For total body irradiation give the preceding dose 1–2 hr before each fraction of radiotherapy administered each day.

Prevention of N&V in single high-dose fraction radiotherapy to the abdomen or for daily fractions to the abdomen.

Adults: One 8-mg tablet, orally disintegrating tablet, or oral film; or 10 mL (equivalent to 8 mg ondansetron) oral solution 1–2 hr before radiotherapy, with subsequent doses 8 hr after the first dose for each day radiotherapy is given. *NOTE:* There is no experience in children to prevent radiation-induced N&V.

Prevention of postoperative N&V.

Adults: 16 mg given as a single dose of two 8-mg tablets, 2 orally disintegrating tablets, or 2 oral films; or 20 mL (equivalent to 16 mg ondansetron) 1 hr before induction of anesthesia. *NOTE:* There is no experience giving ondansetron to children to prevent postoperative N&V.

Cholestasis-related pruritus.

4 mg twice a day or 8 mg 2 or 3 times a day for up to 5 months.

NURSING IMPLICATIONS

Do not confuse Zofran with Zoloft (an antidepressant), Zosyn (an antibiotic), or Zantac (an H_2 receptor blocker).

IMPLEMENTATION/ADMINISTRATION/STORAGE

1. With impaired hepatic function, do not exceed 8 mg PO or 8 mg IV daily infused over 15 min, 30 min prior to starting chemotherapy.
2. Tablets may be used to prepare a liquid product with cherry syrup, Syrpalta, Ora Sweet, or Ora Sweet Sugar Free. The concentration is 4 mg/5 mL and is stable for 42 days at 4°C (39°F).
3. Suppositories can be made by adding pulverized tablets to a melted fatty acid base, mixing thoroughly, and pouring into suppository molds. They are stable for 30 or more days if stored in light-resistant containers under refrigeration.
4. If more than one oral film is to be given, allow each oral film to dissolve completely before administering the next film.
5. Store tablets and orally disintegrating tablets from 2–30°C (36–86°F). Protect the 4 mg tablets from light. Store blisters in cartons. Store oral solution from 15–30°C (59–86°F) protected from light. Store upright in cartons. Store oral films from 20–25°C (68–77°F); store pouches in cartons. Keep product in pouch until ready to use.
6. IV When used to prevent chemotherapy-induced N&V, dilute the 2 mg/mL injection in 50 mL of D5W or 0.9% NaCl injection and infuse over 15 min. The 32 mg premixed injection in 50 mL D5W requires no dilution.
7. Ondansetron injection, 2 mg/mL, requires no dilution for administration for postoperative N&V.
8. In clients with severe hepatic function impairment (Child-Pugh score of 10 or more), a single maximum daily dose of 8 mg is recommended to be infused over 15 min beginning 30 min before the start of emetogenic chemotherapy.
9. Do not use flexible plastic containers in series connections. Ondansetron injection premixed in flexible plastic containers is to be given by IV drip infusion only.
10. Inspect visually for particulate matter and discoloration before administration. Do not administer unless solution is clear and the container is undamaged.
11. Occasionally ondansetron precipitates at the stopper/vial interface in vials stored upright. This does not affect safety or potency. Resolubilize by shaking the vial vigorously.
12. Do not mix the premixed solutions or the injection for which physical and chemical compatibility have not been established.
13. The diluted drug is stable at room temperature, with normal lighting, for 48 hr after dilution with compatible solution.
14. Store the premixed injection and injection between 2–30°C (36–86°F). Protect from light. Avoid excessive heat; do not freeze.
15. COMPATIBILITY D5W, 0.9% NaCl, D5/0.9% NaCl, D5/0.45% NaCl, 3% NaCl.
16. INCOMPATIBILITY Alkaline solutions (precipitate may form).

ASSESSMENT

1. Note reasons for therapy (agent, conditions, procedure, or therapy involved), characteristics of S&S, agents trialed, outcome.
2. Determine any QT abnormality; obtain ECG and monitor for QT prolongation and any conditions that may predispose to this condition.
3. Assess for dehydration, electrolyte imbalance with diarrhea/N&V, monitor I&O, adjust dose as needed.
4. If used after abdominal surgery or with chemotherapy-induced N&V, be alert as may mask gastric distension and/or progressive ileus. Check BS, for distension or N&V. Note any abnormal or uncontrolled movements.

O

5. Monitor ECG, electrolytes, renal and LFTs; adjust dosage with dysfunction.

CLIENT/FAMILY TEACHING

1. Drug is used to prevent N&V; take exactly as prescribed in order to ensure desired results.
2. The orally disintegrating tablets (ODT) contain phenylalanine (component of aspartame). Each 4-mg and 8-mg orally disintegrating tablet contains <0.03 mg phenylalanine (information for phenylketonurics).
3. With the ODT therapy do not remove tablets from the blister until just before dosing. With dry hands, remove blister backing completely off the package. Gently remove the tablet and immediately place it on the tongue to dissolve and be swallowed with the saliva. Never push the tablet through the foil.
4. Keep the oral film in the pouch until ready to use; do not chew or swallow the film. With dry hands, fold the pouch along the dotted line to expose the tear notch. While still folded, tear the pouch carefully along the edge and remove the soluble film from the pouch. Immediately place the film on top of the tongue where it dissolves in 4–20 seconds; then, swallow with saliva. Once the film dissolves, you can swallow liquid but it is not required. After taking Zuplenz, wash hands.
5. May cause drowsiness or dizziness. Do not perform activities that require mental alertness until drug effects realized. Using ondansetron solution alone, with certain other medicines, or with alcohol may lessen your ability to drive or perform other potentially dangerous tasks.
6. Report any rash, diarrhea, constipation, altered respirations (bronchospasms), or loss of response.
7. Keep all F/U to assess response, labs, adverse SE.

OUTCOMES/EVALUATE

- Prevention/control of chemo/radiotherapy-induced N&V
- Prophylaxis/relief of postoperative N&V

Oprelvekin (Interleukin 11, IL-11)

(oh-**PREL**-veh-kin)

Classification(s): Interleukin, human recombinant

Pregnancy Category: C

RX: Neumega.

INDICATIONS/USES

Prevention of severe thrombocytopenia and reduction of the need for platelet transfusions following myelosuppressive chemotherapy in adults with nonmyeloid malignancies who are at high risk of severe thrombocytopenia.

ACTION/KINETICS

Action

Produced by DNA recombinant technology. Interleukin 11 is a thrombopoietic growth factor that directly stimulates proliferation of hematopoietic stem cells and megakaryocyte progenitor cells and induces megakaryocyte maturation. This results in increased platelet production.

Pharmacokinetics

Absolute bioavailability is greater than 80%. **Peak serum levels:** 3.2 hr. **t½, terminal:** 6.9 hr. Metabolized and excreted through urine.

CONTRAINDICATIONS

Hypersensitivity to the drug or any component of the product. Use following myeloablative chemotherapy. Lactation.

SPECIAL CONCERNS

Oprelvekin has caused allergic or hypersensitivity reactions, including anaphylaxis. Permanently discontinue administration of oprelvekin in any client who develops an allergic or hypersensitivity reaction.

- Use with caution in CHF or in those who may be susceptible to developing CHF, and in those with history of heart failure who are well compensated and receiving appropriate medical therapy.
- Use with caution in those with history of atrial arrhythmia, in pre-existing papilledema or with tumors involving CNS.
- Safety and efficacy not determined for use in children.

SIDE EFFECTS

Most Common

N&V, edema, neutropenic fever, mucositis, diarrhea, headache, dizziness, insomnia, dyspnea, rhinitis, tachycardia, increased cough, pharyngitis, rash, conjunctival injection, palpitations, atrial arrhythmias, pleural effusions.

O

Body as a whole: Edema, neutropenic fever, headache, fever, conjunctival infection, asthenia, chills, pain, infection, flu-like symptoms, fluid retention (may be serious and cause peripheral edema, dyspnea on exertion, pulmonary edema, capillary leak syndrome, atrial arrhythmias, and worsening of pre-existing pleural effusions), hypersensitivity reactions (including ***anaphylaxis***). **GI:** N&V, mucositis, diarrhea, oral moniliasis, abdominal pain, constipation, dyspepsia. **CV:** Tachycardia, vasodilation, palpitations, syncope, atrial fibrillation or flutter, ***CHF, ventricular arrhythmias***, thrombocytosis, thrombotic events. **CNS:** Dizziness, headache, insomnia, nervousness. **Respiratory:** Dyspnea, rhinitis, increased cough, pharyngitis, pleural effusion, pneumonia, pulmonary edema, rhinitis. **Dermatologic:** Rash, alopecia. **Injection site reactions:** Dermatitis, pain, discoloration. **Ophthalmic:** Conjunctival injection, mild visual blurring (transient), blindness, optic neuropathy. **Miscellaneous:** Anorexia, ecchymosis, myalgia, bone pain, papilledema (more common in children 12 years and younger), renal failure.

In children: The following side effects occurred more commonly in children than in adults: Tachycardia, conjunctival injections, radiographic and echocardiographic evidence of cardiomegaly, and periosteal changes.

In cancer clients: The following side effects occurred more commonly in cancer clients: Amblyopia, dehydration, exfoliative dermatitis, eye hemorrhage, paresthesia, skin discoloration.

LABORATORY TEST CONSIDERATIONS

↑ Fibrinogen. ↓ H&H, RBCs, serum albumin, transferrin, gamma globulins (all due to expansion of plasma volume), calcium.

OVERDOSE MANAGEMENT

Symptoms: Increased incidence of cardiovascular events if doses greater than 50 mcg/kg are given. *Treatment:* Discontinue drug and observe for signs of toxicity.

HOW SUPPLIED

Powder for Injection, Lyophilized: 5 mg.

DOSAGE

SC INJECTION

Prevent thrombocytopenia.

Adults: 50 mcg/kg once daily SC either in the abdomen, thigh, or hip. Initiate dosing 6–24 hr after completion of chemotherapy. Doses generally given in courses of 10 to 21 days; dosing beyond 21 days is not recommended. The dose in adults with severe impaired renal function (C_{CR} <30 mL/min) is 25 mcg/kg.

NURSING IMPLICATIONS

IMPLEMENTATION/ADMINISTRATION/STORAGE

1. Initiate dosing 6 to 24 hr after completion of chemotherapy. Continue until post-nadir platelet count is 50,000 cells/mcL or more. Duration of dosing is usually 10 to 21 days; beyond 21 days is not recommended.
2. Discontinue treatment 2 or more days before starting next planned cycle of chemotherapy.
3. Reconstitute with 1 mL of sterile water for injection without preservative. Direct water at side of vial and swirl gently. Avoid excessive or vigorous shaking.
4. Reconstituted solution contains 5 mg/mL and is clear, colorless, and isotonic with a pH of 7. Use within 3 hr as there is no preservative. Store vial either in refrigerator or at room temperature. Do not shake or freeze reconstituted solution.
5. Do not re-enter or reuse single-use vial. Discard unused portion.
6. Store lyophilized drug and diluent at 2–8°C (36–46°F). Protect from light; do not freeze.

ASSESSMENT

1. Note reasons for therapy, onset, duration, clinical manifestations.
2. Monitor I&O and VS; assess for fluid retention (DOE, edema). Advise most develop anemia.
3. List chemotherapy agent and platelet nadir; initiate therapy 6–24 hr after chemotherapy completed. Continue until post-nadir platelet count is 50,000 cells/mcL. Stop oprelvekin at least 2 days before next round of chemotherapy.
4. Monitor electrolytes, CBC, platelet counts and renal function; reduce dose if C_{CR}<30 mL/min (↓ dose to 25 mcg/kg).

CLIENT/FAMILY TEACHING

1. Drug is used to prevent chemotherapy-induced low platelets by stimulating bone mar-

O

row to increase platelet production. Low platelets may cause increased bleeding.

2. Review administration and dosage guidelines that come with product. Keep product refrigerated. Dispose of syringes in sealed container to prevent tampering.
3. After instruction and demonstration, wash hands and administer SC, into abdomen, thigh, or hip; rotate sites. Follow administration step by step guidelines carefully. Pinch skin with thumb and forefinger, insert needle at a 45 degree angle, release skin, aspirate and inject drug if no blood return. Use a new bottle of Neumega powder and a new prefilled syringe every time you give yourself a dose.
4. Use caution may cause dizziness or blurred vision; assess response before engaging in activities that require mental alertness.
5. Report any unusual side effects, SOB, swelling of extremities, fatigue/weakness, irregular heartbeat, chest pain, swelling of face, feet or ankles, rapid weight gain, vision changes, or increased bruising/bleeding. May develop anemia.
6. Practice reliable contraception; may harm fetus.
7. Keep all F/U to assess response, labs, and for adverse SE.

OUTCOMES/EVALUATE

- Thrombocytopenia prophylaxis
- ↑ Platelet production 50,000 cells/mcL

O

Orlistat

(**OR**-lih-stat)

Classification(s): Antiobesity drug

Pregnancy Category: B

OTC: Alli.

RX: Xenical.

INDICATIONS/USES

OTC. Weight loss in overweight adults 18 years of age and older along with a reduced calorie, low-fat diet.

Rx. (1) Management of obesity, including weight loss and weight maintenance when used with a reduced-calorie diet. (2) To reduce risk for weight regain after prior weight loss. Orlistat is indicated for obese clients with an initial body mass index of 30 kg/m^2 or more, or 27 kg/m^2 or more in the presence of risk factors such as hypertension, diabetes, dyslipidemia.

ACTION/KINETICS

Action

Reversible inhibitor of lipases resulting in inhibition of absorption of dietary fats. Acts in the lumen of the stomach and small intestine to form a covalent bond with the active serine residue site of gastric and pancreatic lipases. Inactivated enzymes are not available to hydrolyze dietary fat, in the form of triglycerides, into absorbable free fatty acids and monoglycerides. At therapeutic doses, it inhibits dietary fat absorption by about 30%. Effect on absorption of lipids seen as soon as 24–48 hr after dosing. Weight loss was seen within 2 weeks of starting therapy and continued for 6–12 months.

Pharmacokinetics

Systemic absorption is not needed for activity, although a small amount is absorbed. Metabolism occurs mainly in the GI wall. Unabsorbed drug is excreted through the feces. Weight loss caused by orlistat delayed the onset of type 2 diabetes in obese clients with impaired glucose tolerance.

CONTRAINDICATIONS

Use in chronic malabsorption syndrome or cholestasis; known hypersensitivity to the drug. Lactation.

SPECIAL CONCERNS

- Exclude organic causes of obesity (e.g., hypothyroidism) before prescribing.
- GI side effects may increase when taken with a high-fat diet.
- Potential exists for misuse (e.g., in those with anorexia nervosa or bulimia).
- Use with caution with a history of hyperoxaluria or calcium oxalate nephrolithiasis.
- Safety and efficacy determined in children aged 12 to 16 but has not been studied in children less than 12 years of age.

SIDE EFFECTS

Most Common

Headache, oily spotting, flatus with discharge, fecal urgency, fatty/oily stool, oily evacuation, increased defecation, abdominal pain/discomfort, influenza, URTI.

GI: Oily spotting, flatus with discharge, fecal urgency, fatty/oily stool, oily evacuation, increased defecation, fecal incontinence, abdominal pain or discomfort, N&V, infectious diarrhea, rectal pain or discomfort, tooth disorder, gingival disorder. **CNS:** Headache, dizziness, psychiatric anxiety, depression. **Respiratory:** Influenza, URTI, lower respiratory infection, ENT symptoms. **Musculoskeletal:** Back pain, arthritis, myalgia, joint disorder, lower extremity pain, tendonitis. **Dermatologic:** Rash, dry skin. **GU:** Menstrual irregularity, vaginitis, UTI. **Hypersensitivity (rare):** Pruritus, rash, urticaria, angioedema, ***anaphylaxis***. **Miscellaneous:** Fatigue, sleep disorder, otitis, pedal edema.

DRUG INTERACTIONS

Beta-carotene / 30% ↓ absorption of beta-carotene supplement
Cyclosporine / ↓ Cyclosporine levels R/T ↓ absorption
Pravastatin / Additive lipid-lowering effects
Vitamin A / Possible malabsorption of Vitamin A
Vitamin D / Possible malabsorption of Vitamin D
Vitamin E / 60% ↓ absorption of vitamin E acetate supplement
Vitamin K / Possible ↓ vitamin K absorption
Warfarin / Possible ↑ INR following chronic orlistat dosing

HOW SUPPLIED

Capsules: 60 mg (OTC), 120 mg (Rx).

DOSAGE

OTC: CAPSULES

Management of obesity.

Adults, 18 years and older: 60 mg 3 times per day with each meal containing fat, not to exceed 3 capsules/day.

RX: CAPSULES

Management of obesity.

120 mg (1 capsule) 3 times per day with each main meal containing fat; give during or up to 1 hr after the meal. Doses greater than 120 mg 3 times per day have not been shown to produce additional benefit. Safety and effectiveness beyond 2 yr have not been determined.

NURSING IMPLICATIONS

Do not confuse Zenical with Xeloda (an antineoplastic drug).

IMPLEMENTATION/ADMINISTRATION/STORAGE

1. When the Rx form is used, the client should be on a nutritionally balanced, reduced-calorie diet that contains about 30% of calories from fat. Distribute over 3 main meals the daily intake of fat, carbohydrate, and protein.
2. To ensure adequate nutrition, clients on either the OTC or Rx product should take a multivitamin containing fat-soluble vitamins and beta-carotene. The supplement should be taken at least 2 hr before or after the administration of orlistat (i.e., at bedtime).
3. Weight lost due to orlistat may be accompanied by improved metabolic control in diabetics; this might require a reduction in dose of oral hypoglycemic drugs or insulin.

ASSESSMENT

1. Note reasons for therapy, length of weight problem, other agents/therapies trialed, and outcome.
2. Assess for history of cholestasis, eating disorders, or malabsorption syndrome. Note any thyroid dysfunction or kidney stones (drug may increase urinary oxalate). Instruct patients not to take orlistat if they are organ transplant patients or are taking cyclosporine, have been diagnosed with problems absorbing food, or are not overweight.
3. Instruct not to take orlistat if organ transplant or taking cyclosporine, have been diagnosed with problems absorbing food, or not overweight.
4. List medical conditions/risk factors necessitating treatment (i.e, DM, HTN, hyperlipidemia). Obtain baseline BMI, Wt, VS, waist and hip circumference.
5. Assess electrolytes, cholesterol profile, BS, urinalysis, renal and LFTs.

CLIENT/FAMILY TEACHING

1. Drug acts by inhibiting absorption of some of the dietary fat intake. Take with or within 1 hr following each main meal. If a meal is occasionally missed or contains no fat, the dose of orlistat can be omitted.
2. In order to be successful in losing weight, follow a nutritionally balanced, reduced-calorie diet containing 30% of calories from fat and

perform 20 min of daily exercise. Distribute the daily intake of CHO, protein, and fat over three main meals.
3. Drug may reduce absorption of fat-soluble vitamins (A, D, E) and beta-carotene. Take supplements at least 2 hr after therapy or at bedtime daily.
4. Diabetics should monitor FS; improved metabolic control may require a reduction of the dose of hypoglycemic agents.
5. May cause GI S&S, gas with discharge, fecal urgency/incontinence, oily or spotty discharge, abdominal pain/discomfort, diarrhea. Should subside with continued use; report any persistent side effects.
6. Keep all F/U to assess response, BP, labs, and for adverse SE.

OUTCOMES/EVALUATE

- ↓ Risk of weight gain after prior loss
- ↓ BMI
- Desired weight loss

Oseltamivir phosphate

(oh-sell-**TAM**-ih-vir)

Classification(s): Antiviral

Pregnancy Category: C

RX: Tamiflu.

INDICATIONS/USES

(1) Prophylaxis of influenza A and B in adults and children, 1 year of age and older. (2) Treatment of uncomplicated acute influenza in adults and children over 1 year of age who have been symptomatic for 2 days or less. *NOTE:* Oseltamivir is not a substitute for early vaccination on an annual basis as recommended by the CDC. *Investigational:* Chemoprophylaxis and treatment of H1N1 influenza A (swine flu) virus infection, including clients with confirmed, probable, or suspected H1N1 infection and their close contacts.

ACTION/KINETICS

Action

Hydrolyzed by hepatic esterases to the active oseltamivir carboxylate. May act by inhibiting the flu virus neuraminidase with possible alteration of virus particle aggregation and release. Drug resistance to influenza A virus is possible.

Pharmacokinetics

Readily absorbed from the GI tract and extensively converted to oseltamivir carboxylate by liver esterases. About 75% of an oral dose reaches the systemic circulation as the carboxylate. **t½, oseltamivir:** 1–3 hr; **t½, oseltamivir carboxylate:** 6–10 hr. Over 99% is eliminated in the urine as oseltamivir carboxylate. Children up to 12 years of age clear the prodrug and the active metabolite (carboxylate) faster than adults. **Plasma protein binding:** 42% of oseltamivir but only 3% of oseltamivir carboxylate are bound to plasma proteins.

CONTRAINDICATIONS

Hypersensitivity to any component of the product. Administration of live attenuated influenza vaccine within 2 weeks before or 48 hr after administration of oseltamivir (unless medically indicated).

SPECIAL CONCERNS

- Use during lactation only if potential benefits outweigh the potential risk to the infant.
- Efficacy has not been determined in clients who begin treatment after 40 hr of symptoms, for prophylactic use to prevent influenza, for repeated treatment courses, or for use in those with chronic cardiac or respiratory disease.
- Not been shown to prevent bacterial infections.
- Not been shown to prevent complications from serious bacterial infections.
- Efficacy not determined for prophylaxis or treatment in immunocompromised clients.
- Safety and efficacy to prevent or treat influenza not determined in children less than 1 year of age or of repeated prophylaxis or treatment.

SIDE EFFECTS

Most Common

When used in adults: N&V, headache, diarrhea, dizziness, abdominal pain, bronchitis.

When used in children: Diarrhea, N&V, abdominal pain, asthma, epistaxis, otitis media.

Adults and children 13 years and older. CNS: Headache, dizziness, insomnia, vertigo, abnormal behavior. **GI:** Nausea (with or without vomiting), diarrhea, abdominal pain, pseudomembranous colitis. **CV:** Unstable angina. **Respiratory:** Cough, bronchitis, peritonsillar abscess, pneumonia. **Body as a whole:** Fatigue, pyrexia. **Miscellaneous:** Anemia, humerus fracture.

Children, 1–12 years of age. CNS: Delirium, abnormal behavior (leading to injury), ***death***. **GI:** Diarrhea, N&V, abdominal pain. **Respiratory:** Asthma (including aggravated), epistaxis, bronchitis, pneumonia, sinusitis. **Dermatologic:** Dermatitis. **Ophthalmic:** Conjunctivitis. **Otic:** Otitis media, ear disorder, tympanic membrane disorder. **Miscellaneous:** Lymphadenopathy.

Postmarketing. CNS: Abnormal behavior, agitation, anxiety, confusion, delirium (including altered level of consciousness), delusions, hallucinations, nightmares, ***seizures***. **GI:** GI bleeding, hemorrhagic colitis. **Hepatic:** Abnormal liver function, hepatitis. **CV:** Arrhythmia. **Dermatologic:** Dermatitis, eczema, erythema multiforme, rash, urticaria. **Hypersensitivity:** Allergy, anaphylactic/anaphylactoid reactions, swelling of the face/tongue, erythema multiforme, ***Stevens-Johnson syndrome, toxic epidermal necrolysis***. **Miscellaneous:** Aggravation of diabetes.

LABORATORY TEST CONSIDERATIONS

Abnormal LFTs.

DRUG INTERACTIONS

Live attenuated influenza vaccine / Possible inhibition of replication of live vaccine virus; do not give the vaccine within 2 weeks before or 48 hr after oseltamivir administration (unless medically indicated)

Probenecid / About a 2-fold ↑ in exposure to oseltamivir carboxylate R/T ↓ in kidney tubular secretion

HOW SUPPLIED

Capsules: 30 mg, 45 mg, 75 mg; *Powder for Oral Suspension:* 6 mg/mL (after reconstitution).

DOSAGE

CAPSULES; ORAL SUSPENSION

Prophylaxis of influenza.

Adults and children 13 years and older following close contact with an infected individual: 75 mg once daily for at least 10 days. Begin treatment within 2 days of exposure to flu. The recommended daily dose for prophylaxis during a community outbreak of influenza is 75 mg once daily; safety and efficacy have been demonstrated for up to 6 weeks. For clients with a C_{CR} between 10 and 30 mL/min, reduce dose to 75 mg every other day or 30 mg of the oral suspension every day.

Children, 1–12 years of age following close contact with an infected individual: 15 kg or less (33 lbs or less): 30 mg once a day; **>15–23 kg (>33–51 lbs):** 45 mg once daily; **>23–40 kg (>31–55 lbs):** 60 mg once a day; **>40 kg (>88 lbs):** 75 mg once a day. Prophylaxis in children has not been evaluated for longer than 10 days duration. Begin therapy within 2 days of exposure.

NOTE: The commercially available suspension is 6 mg/mL and the pharmacy-compounded suspension is 15 mg/mL.

Treatment of influenza.

Adults and children 13 years and older: 75 mg twice a day for 5 days. For clients with a C_{CR} between 10 and 30 mL/min, reduce dose to 75 mg once daily for 5 days. **Children 1 year and older: 15 kg or less (33 lbs or less):** 30 mg twice a day; **>15–23 kg (>33–51 lbs):** 45 mg twice a day; **>23–40 kg (>51–88 lbs):** 60 mg twice a day; **>40 kg (>88 lbs):** 75 mg twice a day. Duration: 5 days. Begin treatment in all clients within 2 days of onset of flu symptoms.

NOTE: The commercially available suspension is 6 mg/mL and the pharmacy-compounded suspension is 15 mg/mL.

Investigational: Prophylaxis of H1N1 influenza A (swine flu).

Adults: 75 mg once a day for at least 10 days following close contact with an infected person. For prophylaxis during a community outbreak of influenza the dose is 75 mg once a day; safety and efficacy have been demonstrated for up to 6 weeks. **Children, 12 months and older: >40 kg (>88 lbs, 10 years of age and older):** 75 mg once a day for 10 days; **>23–40 kg (>51–88 lbs, 6–9 years of age):** 60 mg once a day for 10 days; **>15–23 kg (>33–51 lbs, 3–5 years of age):** 45 mg once a day for 10

O

days; **15 kg or less (33 lbs or less, 1–2 years of age):** 30 mg once a day for 10 days. **Children, younger than 12 months of age: 6–11 months of age:** 25 mg once a day for 10 days; **3–5 months:** 20 mg once a day for 10 days; **younger than 3 months:** Due to limited data on use in this age group, use not recommended unless situation judged critical. For all ages, begin treatment within 2 days of exposure.

Investigational: Treatment of H1N1 influenza A (swine flu).

Adults: 75 mg twice a day for 5 days. Begin treatment within 2 days of onset of influenza symptoms. **Children, 12 months and older: >40 kg (>88 lbs, 10 years of age and older):** 75 mg twice a day for 5 days; **>23–40 kg (>51–88 lbs, 6–9 years of age):** 60 mg twice a day for 5 days; **>15–23 kg (>33–51 lbs, 3–5 years of age):** 45 mg twice a day for 5 days; **15 kg or less (33 lbs or less, 1–2 years of age):** 30 mg twice a day for 5 days. **Children, younger than 12 months of age: 6–11 months of age:** 25 mg twice a day for 5 days; **3–5 months:** 20 mg twice a day for 5 days; **younger than 3 months:** 12 mg twice a day for 5 days. For all ages, begin treatment within 2 days of onset of flu symptoms.

O

NURSING IMPLICATIONS

IMPLEMENTATION/ADMINISTRATION/STORAGE

1. *NOTE:* **The commercially available suspension is 12 mg/mL while the pharmacy-compounded product results in a 15 mg/mL suspension. Calculate the volume to be given carefully.**
2. Prepare the commercially available oral suspension (will be 12 mg/mL) as follows:
   - Tap the closed bottle several times to loosen powder.
   - Measure 23 mL of water into a graduated cylinder.
   - Add the total amount of water for reconstitution to the bottle and shake the closed bottle well for 15 seconds.
   - Remove child-resistant cap and push bottle adapter into the neck of the bottle.
   - Close bottle with child-resistant cap tightly to ensure proper seating of the bottle adapter in the bottle and child-resistant status of the cap.
3. An oral dosing dispenser with 30, 45, and 60 mg graduations is provided with the oral suspension available commercially; the 75 mg dose can be measured using a combination of 30 and 45 mg. In the event the dispenser provided is lost or damaged, another dosing syringe or other device may be used to deliver the following volumes: 2.5 mL (½ teaspoon) for children weighing 15 kg or less; 3.8 mL (¾ teaspoon) for children weighing 15–23 kg; 5 mL (1 teaspoon) for children weighing 23–40 kg; and, 6.2 mL (1¼ teaspoon) for children weighing more than 40 kg.
4. When dispensing the oral suspension for infants less than 1 year of age, remove the oral dosing dispenser included in the product package and replace with an appropriate measuring device.
5. If the oral suspension is not available, oseltamivir capsules may be opened and mixed with sweetened liquids, such as regular or sugar-free chocolate syrup.
6. The directions for emergency compounding of an oral suspension from oseltamivir capsules (final concentration of 15 mg/mL) are found in the package insert.
7. Adjust dosage in clients with a C_{CR} <30 mL/min.
8. A bottle of 13 grams Tamiflu for oral suspension contains approximately 11 grams sorbitol. One dose of 75 mg Tamiflu for oral suspension delivers 2 grams sorbitol.
9. Use the reconstituted solution within 10 days of preparation.
10. For information on use of oseltamivir in preventing or treating H1N1 influenza, refer to the CDC guidelines at http://www.cdc.gov/h1n1flu/recommendations.htm.
11. Store capsules and the dry powder for suspension from 15–30°C (59–86°F). Store the reconstituted suspension under refrigeration from 2–8°C (36–46°F). Do not freeze.

ASSESSMENT

1. Note onset, characteristics of S&S, C&S results, and if for prevention or treatment of influenza as dosing is different.

2. Assess medical conditions, VS, clinical presentation, and history.
3. Avoid live attenuated influenza vaccine administration within 2 weeks before or 48 hr after oseltamivir dosing.
4. Ensure proper dosing apparatus for pediatrics; serious skin reactions, and neuropsychiatric events (self-injury and delirium), primarily in children have been reported. Monitor for signs of abnormal behavior throughout the treatment period.
5. Assess CBC, renal function; reduce dose with dysfunction.

CLIENT/FAMILY TEACHING

1. Initiate treatment at the onset of S&S and within 40 hr of onset of influenza S&S or exposure to influenza-infected individual in order to be effective. Drug is used to diminish side effects and duration of illness. An annual flu shot is still required. Avoid administration of live attenuated influenza vaccine within 2 weeks before or 48 hr after dosing.
2. Do not double up on doses. Take any missed dose as soon as remembered. If the missed dose is remembered within 2 hr of the next scheduled dose, take at the usual time and resume usual schedule.
3. Shake suspension well before use; refrigerate and complete within 10 days of preparation. May aggravate diabetes control (oral suspension contains sorbitol); monitor FS. Any child dosing requires special measurement device to ensure accuracy of dose.
4. If unable to swallow capsules, and if the oral suspension is not available, the capsules may be opened and mixed with sweetened liquids (e.g., regular or sugar-free chocolate syrup).
5. May be taken with or without food. Tolerability may be enhanced if taken with food. Continue hydration, OTC antipyretics/analgesics, and rest to help alleviate flu S&S.
6. May cause dizziness or lightheadedness; alcohol, hot weather, exercise, or fever may increase effects. To prevent, sit up or stand slowly. Sit or lie down at the first sign of these effects.
7. An increased risk of confusion and unusual behavioral changes has been noted including self-injury, hallucinations, and delirium, primarily in children. Report symptoms of confusion or any other unusual behavioral changes.
8. May cause more adverse effects than benefits in children.
9. Report if S&S do not improve or worsen, or if new symptoms develop during or after treatment.
10. Keep all F/U to assess response and for adverse SE.

OUTCOMES/EVALUATE

- ↓ Intensity/duration of S&S of influenza A and B or prophylaxis
- Prevention/treatment of confirmed, probable, or suspected H1N1 influenza A (swine flu) virus infection (unlabeled)

Oxaprozin
Oxaprozin potassium

(**ox**-ah-**PROH**-zin)

Classification(s): Nonsteroidal anti-inflammatory drug

Pregnancy Category: C

RX: Daypro, Daypro ALTA.

✤ **Rx:** Apo-Oxaprozin.

SEE ALSO ***NONSTEROIDAL ANTI-INFLAMMATORY DRUGS***.

INDICATIONS/USES

(1) Relief of signs and symptoms of rheumatoid arthritis and osteoarthritis. (2) Relief of signs and symptoms of juvenile rheumatoid arthritis. *NOTE:* Before deciding to use oxaprozin, carefully consider the potential benefits and risks as well as other treatment options.

ACTION/KINETICS

Pharmacokinetics

Is 95% bioavailable. **Peak effect:** 3–5 hr. **t½:** 42–50 hr. Excreted in the urine (65%) and feces (35%). **Plasma protein binding:** More than 99%.

CONTRAINDICATIONS

Use in clients who have had asthma, urticaria, or an allergic-type reaction after taking aspirin or other NSAIDs. Treatment of perioperative pain in coronary artery bypass graft. Use of oxaprozin potassium in those with advanced renal disease.

SPECIAL CONCERNS

■ (1) **Cardiovascular risk.** NSAIDs may cause an increased risk of serious cardiovascular thrombotic events, MI, and stroke, which can be fatal. This risk may increase with duration of use. Clients with cardiovascular disease or risk factors for cardiovascular disease may be at greater risk. (2) Oxaprozin is contraindicated for treatment of perioperative pain in the setting of coronary artery bypass graft surgery. (3) **GI risk.** NSAIDs cause an increased risk of serious GI adverse events including bleeding, ulceration, and perforation of the stomach or intestines, which can be fatal. These events can occur at any time during use and without warning symptoms. Elderly clients are at greater risk for serious GI events. ■

Use oxaprozin potassium with caution in those with severe hepatic dysfunction.

SIDE EFFECTS

Most Common

Rash, diarrhea, N&V, constipation, dyspepsia/indigestion, anorexia, dysuria, urinary frequency, tinnitus.

See *Nonsteroidal Anti-Inflammatory Drugs* for a complete list of possible side effects. Also, weight changes and nephrotic syndrome.

HOW SUPPLIED

Tablets: 600 mg (oxaprozin); 678 mg (oxaprozin potassium - equivalent to 600 mg oxaprozin).

DOSAGE

TABLETS

Rheumatoid arthritis, osteoarthritis.

Adults, usual: 1,200 mg once daily. For clients of low body weight or those with severe renal impairment/dialysis, an initial dose of 600 mg once daily may be appropriate. **Maximum dose:** 1,800 mg/day or 26 mg/kg, whichever is lower given in divided doses. A one-time loading dose may be considered by administering 1,200 to 1,800 mg, not to exceed 26 mg/kg; may be important where a quick onset of action is important.

Juvenile rheumatoid arthritis.

Children, 6–16 years of age. Body weight 22–31 kg: 600 mg once daily; **32–54 kg:** 900 mg once daily; **55 kg or more:** 1,200 mg once daily. *NOTE:* Safety and efficacy of oxaprozin not established in children less than 6 years of age. Safety and efficacy of oxaprozin potassium not established in children.

NURSING IMPLICATIONS

IMPLEMENTATION/ADMINISTRATION/STORAGE

1. Regardless of the use, individualize and use the lowest effective dose to minimize side effects.
2. Reserve doses greater than 1,200 mg/day for those who weigh more than 50 kg, have normal renal and hepatic function, are at low risk of peptic ulcer, and whose disease severity justifies maximal therapy.
3. Daily divided doses may be tried in those who cannot tolerate once daily dosing.
4. Store from 15–30°C (59–86°F) in tightly closed bottles. Protect from light.

ASSESSMENT

1. Note reasons for therapy, characteristics of S&S, pain level, quality of life. List other agents used, outcome.
2. Assess involved joint(s), baseline ROM, extent of inflammation and functionality.
3. List any history of diabetes, stomach or bowel problems (e.g., bleeding, perforation, ulcers), peripheral edema, asthma, nasal polyps, mouth inflammation; may preclude drug therapy.
4. Determine history of ulcers, heart disease, or cardiac failure. May cause an increased risk of serious CV thrombotic events, MI, and stroke.
5. Monitor BP, CBC, renal and LFTs; adjust dose with dysfunction.

CLIENT/FAMILY TEACHING

1. Take exactly as directed with a full glass of water to enhance absorption; do not share medications. May take with food or milk if GI upset occurs.
2. May cause dizziness or drowsiness; assess effects before driving or performing activities that require alertness.

3. Report S&S of kidney problems: Wt gain, edema, increased joint pain, fever, blood in the urine.
4. Avoid prolonged sun exposure; use protection when exposed to prevent reaction.
5. Report any evidence of unusual bruising/bleeding, blurred vision, ringing or roaring in ears (may indicate toxicity).
6. If surgery scheduled should stop 2 weeks before surgery.
7. May cause an increased risk of serious CV thrombotic events, MI, and stroke.
8. Avoid aspirin, alcohol, or other OTC meds without approval.
9. Keep all F/U to assess response, labs, adverse SE. May take up to 1 month to note positive effects.

OUTCOMES/EVALUATE

Relief of joint pain/inflammation with improved mobility

Oxcarbazepine

(ox-kar-**BAY**-zeh-peen)

Classification(s): Anticonvulsant, miscellaneous

Pregnancy Category: C

RX: Trileptal.

SEE ALSO ***ANTICONVULSANTS.***

INDICATIONS/USES

(1) Adjunctive therapy or monotherapy to treat partial seizures in adults. (2) Monotherapy to treat partial seizures in children 4 years of age and older. (3) Adjunctive therapy to treat partial seizures in children 2 years of age and older. *Investigational:* Alternative treatment for bipolar disorder. Diabetic neuropathy.

ACTION/KINETICS

Action

Anticonvulsant mechanism not known with certainty but effect is primarily through the active 10-monohydroxy metabolite. May block voltage-sensitive sodium channels, resulting in stabilization of hyperexcited neural membranes, inhibition of repetitive neuronal firing, and decreased propagation of synaptic impulses. These effects are thought to be important in preventing seizure spread. Also, increased potassium conductance and modulation of high-voltage activated calcium channels may contribute to the anticonvulsant effects.

Pharmacokinetics

Oxcarbazepine (active) is completely absorbed and extensively metabolized to the active 10-monohydroxy metabolite (MHD). Maximum plasma levels are higher in geriatric clients. **Peak levels:** 4.5 hr for oxcarbazepine and 6 hr for MHD. Steady-state plasma levels reached in 2–3 days. MHD is further metabolized to inactive compounds. **t½, oxcarbazepine:** About 2 hr; **t½, MHD:** About 9 hr. MHD and inactive metabolites are excreted mainly in the urine.

CONTRAINDICATIONS

Hypersensitivity to the drug or any of its components. Lactation.

SPECIAL CONCERNS

- About 25–30% of clients who experience hypersensitivity reactions to carbamazepine will experience hypersensitivity to oxcarbazepine.
- Clinically significant hyponatremia may occur usually during the first 3 months of treatment.
- Use with caution in severe hepatic impairment.
- Increased risk of suicidal behavior and ideation.

SIDE EFFECTS

Most Common

Adults: Headache, dizziness, somnolence, ataxia, N&V, abdominal pain, dyspepsia, diplopia, abnormal vision, fatigue, abnormal gait, tremor.
Children: Headache, somnolence, dizziness, ataxia, nystagmus, N&V, rhinitis, diplopia, abnormal vision, fatigue.

Side effects listed include those clients on adjunctive therapy treated with oxcarbazepine, monotherapy previously treated with other antiepileptic drugs, and those on monotherapy not previously treated with other antiepileptic drugs. **CNS:** Psychomotor slowing, concentration difficulty, somnolence, fatigue, speech/language problems, abnormal coordination (ataxia, gait disturbances), headache, dizziness, anxiety, ataxia, vertigo, abnormal gait, nystagmus, insomnia, tremor, amnesia, ***aggravated convulsions, status epilepticus***, emotional lability, hypoesthesia, nervousness, agitation, abnormal coordination, abnormal EEG, speech disorder, confusion, dysmetria, abnormal thinking, vertigo, aggressive reaction, anguish, apathy, aphasia, aura, delirium, delusion, dysphonia, dystonia, depressed level of consciousness, euphoria, extrapyramidal disorder, feeling "drunk," hemiplegia, hyperkinesia, hyperreflexia, hypesthesia, hypokinesia, hyporeflexia, hypotonia, hysteria, decreased or increased libido, mania, migraine, nervousness, neuralgia, panic disorder, paralysis, paroniria, personality disorder, psychosis, stupor, suicidal behavior/ideation. **GI:** N&V, abdominal pain, anorexia, dry mouth, ***rectal hemorrhage***, toothache, diarrhea, dyspepsia, constipation, gastritis, increased appetite, blood in stool, cholelithiasis, colitis, duodenal ulcer, dysphagia, enteritis, eructation, esophagitis, flatulence, gastric ulcer, gingival bleeding, gum hyperplasia, hematemesis, hemorrhoids, hiccough, biliary pain, retching, right hypochondrium pain, sialoadenitis, stomatitis, ulcerative stomatitis. **CV:** Bradycardia, ***cardiac failure, cerebral hemorrhage***, hypertension, postural hypotension, palpitations, syncope, tachycardia. **Respiratory:** Rhinitis, URTI, coughing, bronchitis, pharyngitis, epistaxis, chest infection, sinusitis, rhinitis, pneumonia, asthma, dyspnea, laryngismus, pleurisy. **GU:** UTI, frequent urination, vaginitis, dysuria, hematuria, intermenstrual bleeding, leukorrhea, menorrhagia, micturition frequency, renal pain, urinary tract pain, polyuria, priapism, renal calculus. **Hematologic:** Leukopenia, thrombocytopenia. **Dermatologic:** Acne, hot flushes, purpura, rash, alopecia, angioedema, bruising, increased sweating, contact dermatitis, eczema, facial rash, flushing, folliculitis, heat rash, hot flushes, photosensitivity, genital pruritus, psoriasis, purpura, erythematous rash, maculopapular rash, vitiligo, erythema multiforme, urticaria, ***Stevens-Johnson syndrome, toxic epidermal necrolysis***. **Musculoskeletal:** Muscle weakness, back pain, sprains, strains, involuntary muscle contractions, tetany, muscle hypertonia. **Metabolic:** Generalized edema, leg edema, weight increase/decrease. **Ophthalmic:** Diplopia, nystagmus, abnormal vision, abnormal accommodation, oculogyric crisis, ptosis, cataract, conjunctival hemorrhage, eye edema, hemianopia, mydriasis, xerophthalmia, photophobia, scotoma. **Otic:** Earache, ear infection, otitis externa, tinnitus. **Body as a whole:** Fatigue, fever, malaise, allergy, rigors, asthenia, abnormal feeling, falling down, viral infection, infection. **Miscellaneous:** Thirst, precordial chest pain, lymphadenopathy, taste perversion, systemic lupus erythematosus. Multiorgan hypersensitivity reaction with symptoms of rash, fever, lymphadenopathy, abnormal LFTs, eosinophilia and arthralgia.

LABORATORY TEST CONSIDERATIONS

↑ GGT, liver enzymes, serum transaminase. ↓ Serum sodium, T_4. Hyponatremia, hypocalcemia, hyper-/hypoglycemia, hypokalemia.

DRUG INTERACTIONS

Carbamazepine / ↓ Plasma MHD (oxcarbazepine) levels R/T ↑ liver metabolism
Felodipine / ↓ Felodipine levels
Lamotrigine / ↓ Lamotrigine levels
Oral contraceptives / ↓ Plasma levels of both estrogen and progestin
Phenobarbital / ↓ MHD (oxcarbazepine) levels R/T ↑ liver metabolism; ↑ levels of phenobarbital
Phenytoin / ↓ MHD (oxcarbazepine) levels R/T ↑ liver metabolism; ↑ levels of phenytoin
Valproic acid / ↓ MHD (oxcarbazepine) levels
Verapamil / ↓ MHD (oxcarbazepine) levels

HOW SUPPLIED

Oral Suspension: 60 mg/mL; ***Tablets:*** 150 mg, 300 mg, 600 mg.

DOSAGE

ORAL SUSPENSION; TABLETS

Adjunctive therapy for partial seizures in adults.

Adults, initial: 600 mg per day given as a twice daily regimen. If indicated, may increase by a maximum of 600 mg/day at approximately weekly intervals; recommended daily dose is 1,200 mg. Doses greater than 2,400 mg/day are not well tolerated due to CNS effects.

Conversion to monotherapy for partial seizures in adults.

Adults, initial: 300 mg twice a day while simultaneously reducing other anticonvulsant drug(s) over 3–6 weeks. Achieve maximum oxcarbazepine dose in 2–4 weeks. Dose may be increased by a maximum of 600 mg/day at approximately weekly intervals to a maximum daily dose of 2,400 mg.

Initiation of monotherapy for partial seizures in adults.

Adults: 600 mg/day given as a twice daily regimen. May increase by 300 mg/day every third day to a dose of 1,200 mg/day.

Adjunctive therapy for partial seizures in children, 2–16 years of age.

Children, aged 4–12 years, initial: 8–10 mg/kg, not to exceed 300 mg twice a day. Achieve target maintenance dose over 2 weeks according to client weight as follows:
20–29 kg: 900 mg/day;
29.1–39 kg: 1,200 mg/day;
over 39 kg: 1,800 mg/day.
Children, 2–4 years of age, initial: 8–10 mg/kg, not to exceed 300 mg twice a day. For those weighing less than 20 kg, consider a starting dose of 16–20 mg/kg. Achieve a target maintenance dose over 2 weeks, not to exceed 60 mg/kg/day as a twice daily regimen. *NOTE:* Children 2 to younger than 4 years may require twice the dose of oxcarbazepine per body weight compared with adults; children 4 to 12 years of age may require a 50% higher oxcarbazepine dose per body weight compared with adults.

Conversion to monotherapy in children 4-16 years of age.

Initial: 8–10 mg/kg/day in 2 divided doses while simultaneously reducing the dose of the concomitant antiepileptic drug. The concomitant drug can be completely withdrawn over 3–6 weeks, while oxcarbazepine may be increased, up to a maximum increment of 10 mg/kg/day at approximately weekly intervals to reach the recommended daily dose.

Initiation of monotherapy in children 4-16 years of age.

Initial: 8–10 mg/kg/day in 2 divided doses. Increase the dose by 5 mg/kg/day every third day to the recommended daily maintenance dose as follows:
20 kg: 600–900 mg/day;
25 kg and 30 kg: 900–1,200 mg/day;
35 kg and 40 kg: 900–1,500 mg/day;
45 kg: 1,200–1,500 mg/day;
50 kg and 55 kg: 1,200–1,800 mg/day;
60 kg and 65 kg: 1,200–2,100 mg/day;
70 kg: 1,500–2,100 mg/day.
NOTE: Initiate therapy at 300 mg/day in those with a C_{CR} less than 30 mL/min. May then increase slowly to achieve the desired response.

NURSING IMPLICATIONS

IMPLEMENTATION/ADMINISTRATION/STORAGE

1. Dosage adjustment is recommended for clients with impaired renal function. Initiate therapy at one-half the usual starting dose and increase, if needed, at a slower than usual rate until the desired response is obtained.
2. If withdrawal is needed, do so gradually to prevent increased seizure frequency.

ASSESSMENT

1. Note behaviors, with seizures identify type, onset/frequency, characteristics. Note other agents trialed, outcome.
2. If hypersensitivity reaction to carbamazepine may also have one to oxcarbazepine.
3. Assess neuro status. Monitor electrolytes, renal and LFTs. Assess for hyponatremia; adjust dose with renal dysfunction.

CLIENT/FAMILY TEACHING

1. Take exactly as directed with or without food. Do not double or skip doses.
2. Shake oral suspension well. May mix with water or swallow directly from syringe.
3. May cause dizziness/drowsiness. Do not perform activities that require mental alertness until drug effects realized. Get up slowly to prevent low BP effects.
4. Avoid alcohol; may increase sedative effect.
5. Report adverse effects or seizure recurrence or worsening. Do not stop therapy without approval. Report any S&S of low sodium, i.e., headache, confusion, nausea, malaise, or lethargy as well as fever, persistent nausea, skin reactions, speech language problems, or difficulty with concentration.
6. Avoid prolonged sun exposure and wear protective clothing to prevent photosensitivity reaction.
7. Practice reliable contraception; hormonal forms may be ineffective.
8. Keep all F/U visits to assess response, labs (sodium), and for adverse SE.

OUTCOMES/EVALUATE

- Absence or ↓ seizure activity

O

- Alternative treatment: bipolar disorder, diabetic neuropathy (unlabeled use)

Combination Drug

Oxycodone and Acetaminophen

(ox-ee-**KOH**-dohn, ah-**SEAT**-ah-**MIN**-oh-fen)

Classification(s): Analgesic

Pregnancy Category: C

RX: Endocet, Magnacet, Percocet, Perloxx, Primlev, Roxicet, Roxicet 5/500 Capsules, Roxilox, Tylox, **C-II**

Rx: Percocet-Demi, PMS-Oxycodone-Acetaminophen, ratio-Oxycocet.

SEE ALSO ***ACETAMINOPHEN*** AND ***NARCOTIC ANALGESICS***.

INDICATIONS/USES

Relief of moderate to moderately severe pain.

CONTENT

Oxocodone hydrochloride (*Narcotic analgesic*) and Acetaminophen (*Nonnarcotic analgesic*). *NOTE:* The amount of oxycodone hydrochloride is listed first followed by the amount of acetaminophen. **Endocet Tablets:** 5 mg/325 mg, 7.5 mg/325 mg, 10 mg/325 mg, 10 mg/650 mg. **Generic Tablets:** 7.5 mg/325 mg, 7.5 mg/500 mg, 10 mg/325 mg, 10 mg/650 mg. **Magnacet Tablets:** 5 mg/400 mg, 7.5 mg/400 mg, 10 mg/400 mg. **Percocet Tablets:** 2.5 mg/325 mg, 7.5 mg/325 mg, 7.5 mg/500 mg, 10 mg/325 mg, 10 mg/650 mg. **Perloxx Tablets:** 2.5 mg/300 mg, 5 mg/300 mg, 7.5 mg/300 mg, 10 mg/300 mg. **Primlev Tablets:** 5 mg/300 mg, 7.5 mg/300 mg, 10 mg/300 mg. **Roxicet Oral Solution:** 5 mg/325 mg per 5 mL. **Roxicet Tablets:** 2.5 mg/325 mg. **Roxicet 5/500 Caplets, Roxilox Capsules, Tylox Capsules:** 5 mg/500 mg.

ACTION/KINETICS

Action

Oxycodone is a semisynthetic opiate that combines with specific receptors located in the CNS to produce various effects. The mechanism is believed to involve decreased permeability of the cell membrane to sodium, which results in diminished transmission of pain impulses and therefore analgesia. Causes mild sedation and little or no antitussive effect. Most effective in relieving acute pain. Acetaminophen may cause analgesia by inhibiting CNS prostaglandin synthesis. Does not cause any anticoagulant effect or ulceration of the GI tract. Antipyretic and analgesic effects are comparable to those of aspirin.

Pharmacokinetics

Oxycodone. Onset: 15–30 min. **Peak effect:** 60 min. **Duration, immediate-release:** 3–4 hr; **controlled-release:** 12 hr. **t½, elimination:** 3.2 hr. Metabolized in the liver (somewhat involves CYP2D6 enzymes); excreted in the urine. **Acetaminophen. Peak plasma levels:** 30–120 min. **t ½:** 45 min-3 hr. **Therapeutic serum levels** (analgesia): 5–20 mcg/mL. Metabolized in the liver and excreted in the urine as glucuronide and sulfate conjugates. However, an intermediate hydroxylated metabolite is hepatotoxic following large doses of acetaminophen.

CONTRAINDICATIONS

Hypersensitivity to either oxycodone or acetaminophen.

SPECIAL CONCERNS

See *Oxycodone hydrochloride*.

- Can produce drug dependence and has abuse potential.
- The respiratory depressant effects of oxycodone can be exaggerated in clients with head injury, other intracranial lesions, or a pre-existing increase in intracranial pressure.
- Use with caution in clients who are elderly, debilitated, have severely impaired hepatic or renal function, are hyperthyroid, have Addison's disease, have prostatic hypertrophy, or have urethral stricture.
- Use for acute abdominal conditions may obscure the diagnosis or clinical course.
- Use with caution during lactation.
- Safety and efficacy not established in children.

SIDE EFFECTS

Most Common

Dizziness, light-headedness, N&V, sedation, sweating, itching, dry mouth, constipation.

See *Acetaminophen* and *Narcotic Analgesics* for a complete list of possible side effects. Preceding side effects are more common in ambulatory clients than nonambulatory clients. Other side effects include euphoria, dysphoria, skin rash, and pruritus.

DRUG INTERACTIONS

Anticholinergic drugs / Production of paralytic ileus
Antidepressants, tricyclic / ↑ Effect of either the TCAs or oxycodone
CNS depressants (including other narcotic analgesics, phenothiazines, antianxiety drugs, sedative-hypnotics, anesthetics, alcohol) / Additive CNS depression
MAOIs / ↑ Effect of either the MAOI or oxycodone

HOW SUPPLIED

See *Content.*

DOSAGE

CAPLETS; CAPSULES; ORAL SOLUTION; TABLETS

Analgesic.

Adults: 5 mL of the oral solution q 6 hr or 1 caplet, capsule, or tablet q 6 hr as needed for pain. From 6 to 12 caplets, capsules, or tablets may be taken per day, depending on the strength. *NOTE:* Check strength and maximum daily dose carefully for each dosages form.

NURSING IMPLICATIONS

Do not confuse Percocet (oxycodone/acetaminophen combination) with Percodan (oxycodone/aspirin combination). Do not confuse Roxicet (oxycodone/acetaminophen combination) with Roxicodone (oxycodone alone). Do not confuse oxycodone (generic name) with OxyContin (trade name for oxycodone).

ASSESSMENT

1. List reasons for therapy, type, onset, characteristics of S&S. Use a pain-rating scale to rate pain level. List other agents prescribed, outcome.
2. Monitor if prescribed anticholinergics; use with opioids may produce paralytic ileus.
3. Assess for head injury, increased ICP, hypothyroidism, acute asthma, Addison's disease, BPH, urethral strictures, or drug-seeking behaviors; may preclude drug therapy.
4. Note VS, x-rays, CNS assessment findings, ROM, level of consciousness, TSH, renal and LFTs; reduce dose with dysfunction.

CLIENT/FAMILY TEACHING

1. Take only as directed; may take with food to decrease GI upset. Do not share drugs; store in a safe place.
2. Drug may cause dizziness and drowsiness; do not perform activities that require mental or physical alertness and do not change positions abruptly.
3. May cause constipation (↑ fluid intake, stool softeners to prevent), N&V, dry mouth, rash/itching, and physical dependence (withdrawal S&S include N&V, cramps, fever, fainting, and anorexia); report.
4. Avoid alcohol and any other CNS depressants without provider approval. (*NOTE:* Oral solution contains small amounts of alcohol.)
5. Tolerance may occur; report loss of effectiveness. Do not stop suddenly with long-term therapy, to prevent withdrawal effects.
6. Keep all F/U to assess response and for adverse SE.

OUTCOMES/EVALUATE

Desired pain control

Oxycodone hydrochloride

(ox-ee-**KOH**-dohn)

Classification(s): Narcotic analgesic

Pregnancy Category: C

RX: Capsules, Immediate-Release: OxyIR. **Solution, Concentrate**: OxyFAST, Roxicodone Intensol. **Solution, Oral**: Roxicodone. **Tablets, Controlled-Release**: Oxy-Contin. **Tablets, Immediate-Release**: M-oxy, Oxecta, Roxicodone, **C-II**

Rx: Supeudol.

SEE ALSO ***NARCOTIC ANALGESICS***.

INDICATIONS/USES

Immediate-release: Management of moderate to severe pain. *Investigational:* Acute pain due to herpes zoster (shingles).

Controlled-release: Management of moderate to severe pain when a continuous, around-the-clock analgesic is required for an extended period of time. To be used postoperatively if the client has received the drug prior to surgery or if the postoperative pain is expected to be moderate to severe and last for an extended period of time. Not intended for use as an "as needed" analgesic. Not for pain in the immediate postoperative period (i.e., first 12–24 hr following surgery) or if the pain is mild or not expected to persist for a long period of time. Individualize treatment moving from parenteral to PO analgesics as appropriate.

ACTION/KINETICS

Action

Semisynthetic opiate that combines with specific receptors located in the CNS to produce various effects. The mechanism is believed to involve decreased permeability of the cell membrane to sodium, which results in diminished transmission of pain impulses and therefore analgesia. Causes mild sedation and little or no antitussive effect. Most effective in relieving acute pain.

Pharmacokinetics

Onset: 15–30 min. **Peak effect:** 60 min. **Duration, immediate-release:** 3–4 hr; **controlled-release:** 12 hr. **t½, elimination:** 3.2 hr for immediate-release product and 4.5 hr for extended-release. Metabolized in the liver (somewhat involves CYP2D6 enzymes); excreted in the urine. Oxycodone terephthalate is available but only in combination with aspirin (e.g., Percodan) or acetaminophen. **Plasma protein binding:** 45%.

O

ADDITIONAL CONTRAINDICATIONS

Use in hypercarbia, paralytic ileus, children, or during labor.

SPECIAL CONCERNS

(1) Controlled-release oxycodone is an opiate and a Schedule II drug with an abuse liability similar to morphine. (2) Oxycodone can be abused in a manner similar to other opiates, legal or illicit. Consider this when prescribing or dispensing oxycodone controlled-release tablets in situations where there is concern about an increased risk of misuse, abuse, or diversion. (3) Controlled-release tablets are for the management of moderate-to-severe pain when a continuous, around-the-clock analgesic is needed for an extended period of time. (4) Controlled-release tablets are not intended for use as an as-needed analgesic. (5) Oxycodone 80 mg controlled-release tablets are for use in opiate-tolerant clients only. This tablet strength may cause fatal respiratory depression when given to clients not previously exposed to opiates. (6) Controlled-release tablets are to be swallowed whole and are not to be broken, chewed, or crushed. Taking broken, chewed, or crushed oxycodone controlled-release tablets leads to rapid release and absorption of a potentially fatal dose of oxycodone.

Chewing, snorting, or injecting oxycodone can lead to death. Is a widely abused drug.

SIDE EFFECTS

Most Common

Constipation, dry mouth, N&V, mild itching, drowsiness, lightheadedness, anorexia, weakness.

See *Narcotic Analgesics* for a complete list of possible side effects.

ADDITIONAL DRUG INTERACTIONS

Use with protease inhibitors → ↑ CNS and respiratory depression.

HOW SUPPLIED

Capsules, Immediate-Release: 5 mg; ***Oral Solution:*** 5 mg/5 mL; ***Solution, Concentrate:*** 20 mg/mL; ***Tablets, Controlled-Release:*** 10 mg, 15 mg, 20 mg, 30 mg, 40 mg, 60 mg, 80 mg; ***Tablets, Immediate-Release:*** 5 mg, 7.5 mg, 10 mg, 15 mg, 20 mg, 30 mg.

DOSAGE

CAPSULES, IMMEDIATE-RELEASE; ORAL SOLUTION; SOLUTION, CONCENTRATE; TABLETS, CONTROLLED-RELEASE; TABLETS, IMMEDIATE-RELEASE

Analgesia.

Individualize dose depending on severity of pain, client response, and client size. **Adults:** 10–30 mg q 4 hr (5 mg q 6 hr for OxyIR, oxycodone IR capsules, ETH-Oxydose, and OxyFAST) as needed. More severe pain may require 30 mg or more q 4 hr. If pain increases in severity, analgesia is not adequate, or tolerance occurs, a gradual increase in dosage may be required. **Not recommended for use in children.**

Analgesia in opioid-naive clients.

Adults, initial: 5–15 mg q 4–6 hr, as needed for pain. Titrate dose based on client response to the initial dose of IR product. To prevent recurrence of pain, use an around-the-clock regimen for those with chronic pain.

NURSING IMPLICATIONS

Do not confuse OxyContin (oxycodone hydrochloride controlled-release tablets) with oxycodone hydrochloride immediate-release tablets. Do not confuse Roxicodone (oxycodone alone) with Roxicet (oxycodone/acetaminophen combination).

IMPLEMENTATION/ADMINISTRATION/STORAGE

1. Give around-the-clock dosing with chronic pain. For control of severe chronic pain, give immediate-release products on a regularly scheduled basis, q 4–6 hr at the lowest dose level that will provide adequate analgesia.
2. It is critical to individualize the dosing regimen taking into account the client's prior analgesic treatment. Attention must be given to: the general condition of the client; the daily dose, potency, and characteristics of a pure agonist or mixed agonist/antagonist the client has taken previously; the reliability of the relative potency estimate to calculate the dose of oxycodone required; the degree of opioid tolerance; special safety issues associated with conversion to CR tablet doses at or exceeding 160 mg q 12 hr; and, the balance between pain control and side effects.
3. When converting from a fixed-ratio opioid/nonopioid regimen, determine whether or not to continue the nonopioid drug. If the nonopioid drug is to be discontinued, it may be necessary to titrate the dose of immediate-release tablets in response to the level of analgesia and side effects experienced. If the nonopioid drug is to be continued, base the oxycodone starting dose on the most recent dose of opioid as a baseline.
4. If taking opiates prior to taking immediate-release oxycodone, factor the potency of the prior opiate into the selection of the total daily dose of oxycodone.
5. Continuous evaluation of those receiving immediate-release or controlled-release oxycodone is required. Supplemental doses for breakthrough or incident pain and titration of the total daily dose may be required, especially in those with rapidly changing disease states.
6. When client no longer requires therapy with immediate-release or controlled-release tablets, gradually discontinue over time to prevent development of withdrawal symptoms. Generally decrease therapy by 25–50% per day and monitor carefully for signs of withdrawal. If withdrawal symptoms develop, raise the dose to the previous level and titrate down more slowly.
7. For controlled-release tablets, swallow whole; do not break, chew, or crush. Controlled-release tablets are intended for moderate to severe pain when a continuous, around-the-clock analgesic is needed for an extended period of time.
8. For controlled-release tablets, the dosing regimen must be individualized based on prior opioid and nonopioid drug treatment, as well as the general condition and medical status of the client. For clients not already taking opiates, a reasonable starting dose is 10 mg q 12 hr; nonopiate analgesics (e.g., aspirin, acetaminophen, NSAIDs) may be continued.
9. Follow manufacturer's guidelines carefully for conversion from other opiates.
10. Controlled-release tablets, 80 mg, are for use only in opioid-tolerant clients requiring daily oxycodone equivalent dosages of 160 mg or more for the 80 mg tablets.
11. Oral concentrate solutions (ETH-Oxydose, OxyFAST, and Roxicodone) are highly concentrated solutions. Care must be taken in prescribing and dispensing this solution strength. Fill dropper to the level of the prescribed dose (1 mL = 20 mg; 0.75 mL = 15 mg; 0.5 mL = 10 mg; and, 0.25 mL = 5 mg). Add the dose to approximately 30 mL (1 fl. oz) or more of juice or other liquid. May also be added to applesauce, pudding, or other semi-solid foods. Use the drug-food mixture immediately; do not store for future use.
12. Oxecta is formulated using commonly used pharmaceutical agents to stop potential abus-

O

ers from crushing, chewing, snorting, or injecting the opioid.

13. Store from 15–30°C (59–86°F). Discard open bottles of oral solution after 90 days.

ASSESSMENT

1. List reasons for therapy; onset, location, duration of pain, ROM, characteristics of S&S.
2. Use a pain-rating scale to rate pain levels. Note other agents trialed and the outcome.
3. Note ability to function and perform daily activities. Review x-rays, CT/MRIs, and Hx.
4. Assess carefully for drug seeking behaviors: visits near end of office hours, not making appointments for full exam, emergency calls, severe pain, repeated loss or accidental destruction of drugs. They often doctor shop for multiple prescriptions.
5. Those with severe chronic pain deserve to be medicated and pain controlled appropriately; use opioids accordingly and in doses strong enough to control their pain. Have client keep record of *break thru pain* so that dosage can be adjusted accordingly; and/or break thru medication provided.

CLIENT/FAMILY TEACHING

1. Take medication with food to minimize GI upset.
2. Swallow controlled-release tablets whole. Ingesting broken, crushed, or chewed extended-release tablets may lead to rapid release/absorption and possibility of toxic effects.
3. Use caution; do not perform activities that require mental alertness as drowsiness may occur.
4. May cause constipation, N&V, dry mouth, and physical dependence (withdrawal S&S include N&V, cramps, fever, fainting and anorexia); increase bulk in diet, increase water intake and use stool softeners regularly.
5. Do not share medications; store in a safe, protected location. Drug has a high abuse potential. Tolerance may develop; report loss of effectiveness and do not stop suddenly with long term therapy.
6. Avoid alcohol in any form during therapy.
7. The extended-release 80 mg tablets should not be used in anyone not currently prescribed opioids. This tablet strength may cause fatal respiratory depression/death.
8. Keep all F/U to assess response, labs, and for adverse SE.

O

OUTCOMES/EVALUATE

Relief/control of pain

■ IV ©

Oxytocin, parenteral

(ox-eh-**TOE**-sin)

Classification(s): Oxytocic drug

Pregnancy Category: X

RX: Pitocin, Syntocinon.

INDICATIONS/USES

(1) *Antepartum:* Induction or stimulation of labor at term. To overcome true primary or secondary uterine inertia. Induction of labor with oxytocin is indicated only under certain *specific* conditions and is not usual because serious toxic effects can occur. Oxytocin is indicated:

- For uterine inertia.
- For induction of labor in cases of erythroblastosis fetalis, maternal diabetes mellitus, preeclampsia, and eclampsia.
- For induction of labor after premature rupture of membranes in last month of pregnancy when labor fails to develop spontaneously within 12 hr.
- To hasten uterine involution.
- To complete inevitable abortions after the 20th week of pregnancy.

(2) *Postpartum:* Produce uterine contractions during the third stage of labor and to control postpartum bleeding or hemorrhage.

ACTION/KINETICS

Action

Acts on smooth muscle of the uterus to stimulate contractions; response depends on the uterine threshold of excitability. Is selective for the uterus, especially toward the end of pregnancy, during labor, and immediately following delivery. Oxytocin stimulates rhythmic contractions of the uterus, increases the frequency of existing contractions, and raises the tone of uterine musculature.

Pharmacokinetics

Onset, IV: Immediate; **Duration:** Within 1 hr after infusion stopped. **IM:** 3–5 min; **Duration:** 2–3 hr. **t½:** 1–6 min. Plasma clearance occurs mainly by the kidney and liver; only small amounts excreted unchanged in the urine.

CONTRAINDICATIONS

Hypersensitivity to drug. Significant cephalopelvic disproportion; unfavorable fetal positions or presentations that are undeliverable without conversion prior to delivery. In obstetric emergencies where the benefit-to-risk ratio for either the mother or fetus favors surgical intervention. Fetal distress where delivery is not imminent, prolonged use in uterine inertia or severe toxemia, hypertonic or hyperactive uterine patterns, when adequate uterine activity does not achieve satisfactory progress. Induction of augmentation of labor where vaginal delivery is contraindicated, including invasive cervical cancer, cord presentation or prolapse, total placenta previa and vasa previa, active herpes genitalis. Also, predisposition to thromboplastin and amniotic fluid embolism (dead fetus, abruptio placentae), history of previous traumatic deliveries, or women with four or more deliveries. Never give oxytocin IV undiluted or in high concentrations.

SPECIAL CONCERNS

■ Oxytocin is indicated for the medical rather than elective induction of labor. Data and information are not available to define the benefit-to-risk consideration for using oxytocin for elective induction. ■

SIDE EFFECTS

Most Common

When used in the mother: N&V, cramping, stomach pain, headache, dizziness.

Mother. CV: Cardiac arrhythmia, hypertensive episodes, PVCs. **GI:** N&V, stomach pain, cramping. **CNS:** Headache, dizziness. **GU:** Pelvic hematoma, postpartum hemorrhage. Rupture of the uterus, spasm, tetanic contraction, uterine hypertonicity may occur due to excessive dosage or hypersensitivity to the drug. **Miscellaneous:** ***Anaphylaxis, fatal afibrinogenemia, subarachnoid hemorrhage, severe water intoxication with seizures, coma, death.***

Fetus. CV: Bradycardia, PVCs, other arrhythmias. **CNS:** Permanent CNS or brain damage, ***neonatal seizures*.** **Miscellaneous**: ***Fetal death***, low Apgar scores at 5 min, neonatal jaundice, neonatal retinal hemorrhage.

OVERDOSE MANAGEMENT

Symptoms: Hyperstimulation of the uterus resulting in hypertonic or tetanic contractions. Or, a resting tone of 15–20 cm water between contractions can result in uterine rupture, cervical and vaginal lacerations, tumultuous labor, uteroplacental hypoperfusion, ***postpartum hemorrhage***, and a variable deceleration of fetal heart rate, fetal hypoxia, hypercapnia, or ***death.*** Water intoxication with seizures can occur if large doses (40–50 mL/min) of the drug are infused for long periods of time. *Treatment:* Discontinue the drug and restrict fluid intake. Start diuresis and give a hypertonic saline solution IV. Correct electrolyte imbalance and control seizures with a barbiturate. If the client is comatose, provide special nursing care.

DRUG INTERACTIONS

Sympathomimetic amines / Severe hypertension and possible stroke

Vasoconstrictors/Caudal block anesthesia / Severe hypertension possible

HOW SUPPLIED

Injection: 10 units/mL.

DOSAGE

IV INFUSION (DRIP METHOD)

Induction or stimulation of labor.

Initial: 0.5–2 milliunits/min. Increase dose gradually in increments of no more than 1–2 milliunits/min at 30–60 min intervals until a contraction pattern has been established that is similar to normal labor. Rates exceeding 9–10 milliunits/min are rarely required.

Control of postpartum bleeding.

Add 10–40 units (maximum of 40 units) to 1,000 mL of a nonhydrating diluent and run at a rate needed to control uterine atony.

Treatment of incomplete or inevitable abortion.

Infuse 10 units of oxytocin with 500 mL physiological saline solution or D5W in physiological saline infused at a rate of 10–20 milliunits (20–40 drops/min). Do not exceed 30 units in a 12-hr period due to the risk of water intoxication.

O

IM

Control of postpartum bleeding.

Give 10 units after delivery of the placenta.

NURSING IMPLICATIONS

Do not confuse Pitocin (oxytocin) with Pitressin (vasopressin). Do not confuse oxytocin with oxyContin (a narcotic analgesic).

IMPLEMENTATION/ADMINISTRATION/STORAGE

1. IV To reconstitute add 1 mL (10 units) to 1,000 mL of 0.9% NaCl or Ringer's lactate. Solution contains 10 milliunits/mL (0.01 units/mL).
2. Use Y-tubing system, with one bottle containing IV solution and oxytocin, and the other containing only the IV solution. This allows for the discontinuation of the drug while maintaining the patency of the vein when it is decided to change to the drug-free infusion bottle. Use a constant infusion pump to control the rate of infusion accurately.
3. Oxytocin is rapidly broken down by sodium bisulfite. Have Mg^{++} sulfate immediately available to relax the uterus in case of tetanic uterine contractions.
4. Have the provider immediately available during drug administration.
5. COMPATIBILITY 0.9% NaCl, RL.
6. INCOMPATIBILITY Administer separately.

ASSESSMENT

1. Note reasons for therapy (i.e., induction for medical reasons, stimulation/reinforcement of labor, control bleeding), onset, characteristics of S&S. Note any sensitivity to drug.
2. Carefully review history and document all medical conditions; some may preclude oxytocin therapy.
3. Determine fetal maturity (size), pelvic adequacy, fetal presentation/position and lack of complications prior to initiating drug therapy.
4. Provide continuous observation of client checking for dilation, resting uterine tone, characteristics of uterine contractions, e.g., tonus, time, duration, amplitude and frequency. Record maternal/fetal HRs; intrauterine pressures. Assess for any distress.
5. Obtain guidelines for and parameters to stop infusion (i.e., contractions <2 min apart and >50–65 mm Hg; duration of 60–90 sec or longer or sudden drop in fetal HR). Stop infusion and report while positioning client on left side to protect fetus.
6. Assess closely for water intoxication, monitor electrolytes and record BP and HR; monitor fetal HR continuously during infusion.

INTERVENTIONS

For induction and stimulation of labor and/or oxytocin challenge test:

1. Before initiating therapy, inform client of rationale for using oxytocic agents and reassure that this procedure is not unusual. Explain drug will induce contractions that may feel like menstrual cramps initially but can be very painful; analgesics may be given as needed.
2. Apply oxygen and remain with client during induction period and throughout the stimulation of labor. Titrate oxytocin to establish uterine contractions that are similar to normal labor; continuously monitor rate and strength of contractions. Monitor VS, check I&O q 15 min.
3. Note resting uterine tone and assess contractions for frequency, duration, and strength. Monitor fetal HR and rhythm at least every 10 min. Document and immediately report any alterations.
4. Prevent uterine rupture and fetal damage by clamping off IV oxytocin, starting medication-free IV fluids, turning client on left side to prevent fetal anoxia, providing oxygen, and reporting when the following events occur:
   - If contractions occur more frequently than every 2 min and last longer than 60–90 sec with no period of uterine relaxation in between.
   - If the contractions are excessively strong and/or exceed 50–65 mm Hg or if they stop.
   - If resting uterine tone is 15–20 mm Hg or more.
   - If the fetal HR indicates bradycardia, tachycardia, or irregularities of rhythm.
5. The fetal heart rate (via fetal scalp electrode), resting uterine tone, and the frequency, duration, and amplitude/force of contractions should be monitored.
6. The oxytocin infusion should be discontinued immediately in the event of uterine hyperactivity or fetal distress. Give oxygen to the mother.
7. Assess for water intoxication following prolonged administration; drug has intrinsic anti-

diuretic effect, acting to increase water reabsorption from the glomerular filtrate. Monitor I&O and serum electrolytes closely. Observe for lethargy, confusion, and stupor.

8. Note any neuromuscular hyperexcitability with increased reflexes and muscular twitching. Report symptoms immediately; convulsions and coma may occur if left untreated. Mg^{++} sulfate should be readily available for IV administration. Stop infusion and report any uterine hyperactivity or fetal distress.

During the fourth stage of labor when oxytocin is administered for prevention or control of hemorrhage:

1. Describe location, size, and firmness of the uterus. Report if uterus is displaced or boggy; follow designated facility protocol.
2. In clients with spinal anesthesia, visually inspect for any evidence of bleeding. Sensation is diminished and hemorrhage may occur insidiously.
3. Note amount and color of lochia. Report bright red lochia, excessive bleeding, or the passage of clots.
4. Monitor VS until stable. Closely monitor I&O. Observe for S&S of water intoxication; document and report immediately.

CLIENT/FAMILY TEACHING

1. Drug is a uterine stimulant. It works by causing uterine contractions by changing calcium concentrations in the uterine muscle cells.
2. Cramps will feel like strong menstrual cramps but will continue to increase in intensity. Report increased blood/fluid loss, severe headaches, fever, foul-smelling drainage, or severe abdominal cramps.
3. Review potential adverse effects associated with this therapy.

OUTCOMES/EVALUATE

- Induction of labor with effective uterine contractions
- ↑ Uterine tone with ↓ postpartum bleeding

P

IV

Paclitaxel

(**PACK**-lih-**tax**-el)

Classification(s): Antineoplastic, miscellaneous

Pregnancy Category: D

RX: Abraxane, Onxol.

SEE ALSO ***ANTINEOPLASTIC AGENTS***.

INDICATIONS/USES

Abraxane. Breast cancer after failure of combination chemotherapy (that should have included an anthracycline, unless contraindicated) for metastatic disease or relapse within 6 months of adjuvant chemotherapy. **Onxol.** (1) Advanced carcinoma of the ovary as subsequent therapy. (2) Breast cancer after failure of combination chemotherapy for metastases (including use of an anthracycline unless contraindicated) or relapse within 6 months of adjuvant chemotherapy. **Paclitaxel generic.** (1) Advanced carcinoma of the ovary as first-line or subsequent therapy. When used as first-line therapy, combine with cisplatin. (2) Adjuvant treatment of node-positive breast cancer given sequentially to doxorubicin-containing combination therapy. (3) Treatment of breast cancer after failure of combination chemotherapy (including use of an anthracycline unless contraindicated) for metastases or relapse within 6 months of adjuvant chemotherapy. (4) Combined with cisplatin for first-line treatment of non-small-cell lung cancer in those not candidates for potentially curative surgery or radiation therapy. (5) Second-line therapy for AIDS-related Kaposi's sarcoma. *Investigational:* Alone or in combination with other chemotherapeutic drugs for advanced head and neck cancer, small-cell lung cancer, adenocarcinoma of the upper GI tract, hormone-refractory prostate cancer, non-Hodgkin's lymphoma, transitional cell carcinoma of the urothelium, pancreatic cancer, polycystic kidney disease.

ACTION/KINETICS

Action

Naturally occurring antineoplastic agent that promotes the assembly of microtubules from tubulin

P

dimers and stabilizes microtubules by preventing depolymerization. The stabilization results in the inhibition of the normal dynamic reorganization of the microtubule network that is required for vital interphase and mitotic cellular functions. Also induces abnormal "bundles" of microtubules throughout the cell cycle and multiple esters of microtubules during mitosis.

Pharmacokinetics

Following IV administration, there is a biphasic decline in plasma levels. The initial rapid decline is due to distribution to the peripheral compartment and significant elimination, whereas the second phase is due, in part, to a slow efflux of the drug from the peripheral compartment. Both forms (injection and albumin-bound) are metabolized in the liver by CYP2C8 (major) and CYP3A4 (minor). About 70% is excreted through the feces and 14% (including a small amount of unchanged drug) excreted in the urine. The clearance of protein-bound paclitaxel particles is larger (43%) than the clearance of paclitaxel injection.

CONTRAINDICATIONS

Onxol/Taxol: Hypersensitivity to paclitaxel, in those with a hypersensitivity to products containing polyoxymethylated castor oil (Cremophor EL), clients with solid tumors when baseline neutrophil counts are below 1,500 cells/mm^3, and those with AIDS-related Kaposi's sarcoma with baseline neutrophil counts below 1,000 cells/mm^3. **Abraxane:** Use in clients who have baseline neutrophil counts of less than 1,500 cells/mm^3. Lactation (all products).

P

SPECIAL CONCERNS

(1) Give under the supervision of a physician experienced in the use of cancer chemotherapeutic drugs. Appropriate management of complications is possible only when adequate diagnostic and treatment facilities are readily available. (2) Onxol/Taxol. Do not give paclitaxel therapy to those with solid tumors who have baseline neutrophil counts of less than 1,500 cells/mm^3, and do not give to clients with AIDS-related Kaposi's sarcoma if the baseline neutrophil count is less than 1,000 cells/mm^3. In order to monitor the occurrence of bone marrow suppression, primarily neutropenia, which may be severe and result in infection, perform frequent peripheral blood cell counts on all clients receiving paclitaxel. (3) Anaphylaxis and severe hypersensitivity reactions characterized by dyspnea and hypotension requiring treatment, angioedema, and generalized urticaria have occurred in 2–4% of clients receiving paclitaxel in clinical trials. Fatal reactions have occurred in clients despite premedication. Pretreat all clients with corticosteroids, diphenhydramine, and H_2 antagonists to prevent such reactions. Do not readminister to those who experience severe hypersensitivity reactions. (4) **Abraxane**. Do not give paclitaxel to those with metastatic breast cancer who have baseline neutrophil counts of less than 1,500 cells/mm^3. In order to monitor the occurrence of bone marrow suppression (primarily neutropenia) which may be severe and result in infection, perform frequent peripheral blood cell counts on all who receive the drug. (5) An albumin form of paclitaxel may substantially affect a drug's functional properties relative to those of drug in solution. Do not substitute for or use with other paclitaxel formulations.

- **Use with caution in clients with moderate to severe impaired hepatic function.**
- **Safety and efficacy not determined in children.**

SIDE EFFECTS

Most Common

Alopecia, peripheral neuropathy, N&V, mucositis, diarrhea, anemia, leukopenia, neutropenia, hypersensitivity, abnormal ECG, myalgia/arthralgia, infections.

Abraxane. GI: N&V, diarrhea, mucositis. Rarely, intestinal obstruction, ***intestinal perforation, pancreatitis***, neutropenic enterocolitis, ischemic colitis, ***hepatic necrosis, hepatic encephalopathy leading to death***. **CNS:** Sensory neuropathy. **CV:** Abnormal ECG (including nonspecific repolarization abnormalities, sinus tachycardia, premature beats), hypotension, severe CV events (***cardiac arrest***, chest pain, edema, hypertension, ***pulmonary emboli, pulmonary thromboembolism***, SVT, ***thrombosis***), bradycardia. Rarely, ***cardiac ischemia/infarction***. **Hematologic:** Neutropenia, anemia hemoglobin, thrombocytopenia, febrile neutropenia, bleeding. **Dermatologic:** Alopecia, changes in nail pigmentation or discoloration of nail bed, skin abnormalities related to radiation recall, ***toxic epidermal necrolysis***. **Musculoskeletal:** Arthralgia, myalgia. **Respiratory:** Dyspnea, cough. Rarely, pneumothorax. **Ophthalmic:** Conjunctivitis, increased lacrimation, ocular and visual disturbances (e.g., keratitis, blurred vision). **Infections:** Oral candidiasis, respiratory tract infections, pneumonia. **Body as a whole:** Asthenia, fluid retention/edema, infections, injection site reaction. **Miscellaneous:** Ototoxicity (hearing loss, tinnitus).

Onxol/Taxol. GI: N&V, diarrhea, mucositis. Rarely, paralytic ileus, intestinal obstruction, ***intestinal perforation, pancreatitis***, ischemic colitis, neutropenic enterocolitis, and dehydration. **CNS:** Peripheral neuropathy, neurotoxicity, neuromotor/sensory toxicity, ataxia, ***tonic-clonic seizures*** (rare), neuroencephalopathy, syncope. **Hematologic:** Leukopenia, neutropenia, febrile neutropenia, anemia hemoglobin, thrombocytopenia, bleeding, packed cell transfusions, platelet transfusions. **CV:** Abnormal ECG (including nonspecific repolarization abnormalities, sinus tachycardia, premature beats), bradycardia, hypotension, significant CV events (e.g., syncope, rhythm abnormalities, hypertension, venous thrombosis), bradycardia, atrial fibrillation, SVT, ***CHF, MI*** (rare). **Dermatologic:** Alopecia, transient skin changes, changes in nail pigmentation or discoloration of nail bed. **Musculoskeletal:** Myalgia, arthralgia. **Respiratory:** Rarely, interstitial pneumonia, ***lung fibrosis, pulmonary embolism***. **GU:** Renal insufficiency. **Ophthalmic:** Optic nerve or visual disturbances (e.g., scintillating scotomata), conjunctivitis, increased lacrimation. **Hypersensitivity:** Severe symptoms, including ***anaphylaxis***, usually occur during the first hour of therapy and occur during both the first or second course of therapy despite premedication. Severe symptoms include dyspnea, ***angioedema***, hypotension, or generalized urticaria all of which require immediate cessation of the drug and aggressive treatment therapy. Symptoms not requiring treatment include milder dyspnea, flushing, skin reactions, hypotension, or tachycardia. **Infections:** Cytomegalovirus, herpes simplex, *Mycobacterium avium intracellulare* infection, *Pneumocystis carinii* infection, esophageal candidiasis, cryptosporidiosis, cryptococcal meningitis. Also, infections of the urinary tract, GI tract (e.g., peritonitis) and upper respiratory tract (e.g., pneumonia), as well as ***sepsis due to neutropenia***. **Body as a whole:** Asthenia, malaise, edema, fever without infection. **Injection site reaction:** Erythema, extravasation, tenderness, skin discoloration, swelling. Rarely, phlebitis, cellulitis, induration, skin exfoliation, necrosis, fibrosis. **Accidental inhalation of injection:** Burning eyes, chest pain, dyspnea, nausea, sore throat; tingling, burning, and redness following topical exposure.

LABORATORY TEST CONSIDERATIONS

↑ Bilirubin, alkaline phosphatase, ALT, AST, creatinine.

OVERDOSE MANAGEMENT

Symptoms: ***Bone marrow suppression***, peripheral neurotoxicity, mucositis. Accidental inhalation may cause dyspnea, chest pain, burning eyes, sore throat, and nausea. *Treatment:* Treat symptomatically.

DRUG INTERACTIONS

Carbamazepine / ↑ Paclitaxel metabolism by CYP3A4

Cisplatin / More profound myelosuppression when paclitaxel was given after cisplatin than when paclitaxel was given before cisplatin R/T a ⅓ decrease in paclitaxel clearance

Cyclosporine / ↓ Paclitaxel metabolism R/T inhibition of CYP3A4

Diazepam / ↓ Paclitaxel metabolism R/T inhibition of CYP2C8

Doxorubicin / ↑ Levels of doxorubicin and doxorubicinol; also, ↓ paclitaxel metabolism R/T inhibition of CYP2C8 and CYP3A4

Ethinyl estradiol / ↓ Paclitaxel metabolism R/T inhibition of CYP2C8

Felodipine / ↓ Paclitaxel metabolism R/T inhibition of CYP2C8

Gemcitabine / ↓ Gemcitabine clearance and volume distribution → ↑ gemcitabine levels

Ketoconazole / ↓ Paclitaxel metabolism R/T inhibition of CYP2C8 and CYP3A4

Midazolam / ↓ Paclitaxel metabolism R/T inhibition of CYP2C8

Phenobarbital / ↑ Paclitaxel metabolism by CYP3A4

Retinoic acid / ↓ Paclitaxel metabolism R/T inhibition of CYP2C8

Troleandomycin / ↓ Paclitaxel metabolizing enzymes R/T inhibition of drug metabolism

P

HOW SUPPLIED

Abraxane. *Powder for Injection, Lyophilized:* 100 mg (albumin-bound).
Onxol, Paclitaxel generic. *Injection:* 6 mg/mL.

DOSAGE

Abraxane

IV INFUSION

Metastatic breast cancer or relapse.

After failure of combination chemotherapy for metastatic breast cancer or relapse within 6 months of adjuvant chemotherapy: 260 mg/m^2 of paclitaxel protein-bound particles given over 30 min q 3 weeks.

Onxol

IV INFUSION

Ovarian cancer.

In clients previously treated with chemotherapy for ovarian cancer, use the following regimen: 135 mg/m^2 or 175 mg/m^2 over 3 hr q 3 weeks.

Breast cancer.

After failure of initial chemotherapy for metastatic disease or relapse within 6 months of adjuvant chemotherapy: 175 mg/m^2 over 3 hr q 3 weeks. Repeat courses; do not give paclitaxel until the neutrophil count is at least 1,500 cells/mm^3 and the platelet count is at least 100,000 cells/mm^3.

Paclitaxel generic.

IV INFUSION

Ovarian cancer.

In clients untreated previously for ovarian cancer, use one of the following regimens given every three weeks: (1) **Adults:** Paclitaxel, 175 mg/m^2 given IV over 3 hr followed by cisplatin, 75 mg/m^2. (2) **Adults:** Paclitaxel, 135 mg/m^2 IV over 24 hr followed by cisplatin, 75 mg/m^2. In clients previously treated with chemotherapy for ovarian cancer, the recommended regimen is paclitaxel, either 135 mg/m^2 or 175 mg/m^2, IV over 3 hr every 3 weeks.

Adjuvant treatment of node-positive breast cancer.

Adults: 175 mg/m^2 given IV over 3 hr q 3 weeks for 4 courses given sequentially to doxorubicin-containing combination therapy. After failure of initial chemotherapy for metastatic disease or relapse within 6 months of adjuvant chemotherapy, paclitaxel, 175 mg/m^2, given IV over 3 hr q 3 weeks has been effective.

Non-small-cell lung carcinoma.

135 mg/m^2 over 24 hr followed by cisplatin, 75 mg/m^2, q 3 weeks. Do not repeat courses of Taxol until the neutrophil count is at least 1,500 cells/mm^3 and the platelet count is at least 100,000 cells/mm^3.

AIDS-related Kaposi's sarcoma.

135 mg/m^2 given IV over 3 hr q 3 weeks or 100 mg/m^2 given IV over 3 hr q 2 weeks. The former regimen is more toxic than the latter.

NURSING IMPLICATIONS

Do not confuse paclitaxel with paroxetine (an antidepressant) or Paxil (trade name for paroxetine). Also, do not confuse Taxol with Taxotere (an antineoplastic) or Paxil.

IMPLEMENTATION/ADMINISTRATION/STORAGE

1. **IV Do not allow the undiluted concentrate to come in contact with plasticized PVC equipment or devices used to prepare solutions for infusion.**
2. **Premedicate before use to prevent severe hypersensitivity reactions. Premedication may consist of oral dexamethasone, 20 mg, given 12 and 6 hr before paclitaxel; diphenhydramine (or equivalent), 50 mg IV, 30–60 min before; and cimetidine, 300 mg IV, or ranitidine, 50 mg IV, 30–60 min before paclitaxel.**
3. **In those with advanced HIV disease, reduce dose of dexamethasone to 10 mg PO; initiate or repeat treatment only if neutrophil count is 1,000 cells/mm^3 or greater; reduce the dose of subsequent courses of paclitaxel 20% for clients who experience severe neutropenia (neutrophil <500 cells/mm^3 for a week or longer); begin concomitant hematopoietic growth factor as needed.**
4. **Dilute paclitaxel concentrate prior to infusion in 0.9% NSS, D5W, D5/0.9% NaCl, or D5/RL to a final concentration of 0.3–1.2 mg/mL.**

Diluted solutions are stable for up to 24 hr at room temperature.

5. Paclitaxel protein-bound particles (Abraxane) is suppled as a sterile lyophilized powder. To reconstitute:
   - Aseptically reconstitute each vial by injecting 20 mL of 0.9% NaCl injection.
   - Slowly inject the 20 mL of 0.9% NaCl injection over a minimum of 1 min, using sterile syringe to direct solution flow onto inside wall of the vial.
   - Do not inject NaCl injection directly onto lyophilized cake; will result in foaming.
   - Once injection complete, allow the vial to sit for a minimum of 5 min to ensure proper wetting of lyophilized cake/powder.
   - Gently swirl/invert the vial slowly for at least 2 min until complete dissolution of any cake/powder occurs. Avoid generation of foam.
   - If foaming or clumping occurs, stand solution for at least 15 min until foam subsides.
   - Each mL of the reconstituted formulation will contain paclitaxel, 5 mg/mL.
   - The reconstituted product should be milky and homogenous without visible particulates. If particulates or settling are visible, gently invert vial again to ensure complete resuspension prior to use.
6. Administer Onxol through an in-line filter with a microporous membrane not greater than 0.22 μm. Use of filter devices, such as IVEX-2 filters that incorporate short inlet and outlet PVC-coated tubing, has not resulted in significant leaching of DEHP.
7. Do not use the Chemo Dispensing Pin device or similar devices with spikes with vials of paclitaxel because they can cause the stopper to collapse, resulting in loss of sterile integrity of the paclitaxel solution.
8. The dilutions may show haziness, which is due to the formulation vehicle. No significant loss of potency has been noted following simulated delivery of the solution through IV tubing containing an in-line (0.22-μm) filter.
9. To minimize client exposure to the plasticizer DHEP which may be leached from PVC infusion bags or sets, store diluted paclitaxel solutions in bottles (glass, polypropylene) or plastic bags (polypropylene, polyolefin) and administer through polyethylene-lined administration sets.
10. Unopened vials of the concentrate are stable when stored under refrigeration, protected from light, in the original package.
11. Do not undertake repeat courses until the neutrophil count is at least 1,500 cells/mm^3 and the platelet count is at least 100,000 cells/mm^3. When using Taxol or Onxol, reduce dose by 20% for subsequent courses in those who experience a neutrophil count <500 cells/mm^3 for 1 week or more or if there is severe peripheral neuropathy during therapy.
12. When using Abraxane, reduce the dose to 220 mg/m^2 for subsequent doses if the neutrophil count is <500 cells/mm^3 for 1 week or longer or severe sensory neuropathy has occurred. For recurrence of severe neutropenia or severe sensory neuropathy, make an additional dose reduction to 180 mg/m^2. For grade 3 sensory neuropathy, hold treatment until resolution to grade 1 or 2, followed by a dose reduction for all subsequent courses of paclitaxel protein-bound particles.
13. Use gloves when handling drug. If solution comes in contact with the skin, wash immediately and thoroughly with soap and water. If the drug comes in contact with mucous membranes, thoroughly flush the membranes with water. Due to possible extravasation, monitor infusion site closely for possible infiltration.
14. *Treatment of Hypersensitivity Reactions:* Stop infusion and treat with bronchodilators (such as albuterol or theophylline), epinephrine, antihistamines, and corticosteroids.
15. Store Onxol at 20–25°C (68–77°F) in the original package. Upon refrigeration, components in the vial may precipitate but will redissolve upon reaching room temperature with little or no agitation. If the solution remains cloudy or if an insoluble precipitate is noted, discard the vial. Solutions for infusion prepared as recommended are stable at ambient temperature (25°C, 77°F) and lighting conditions for up to 27 hr.
16. Unopened vials of Abraxane are stable when stored at 20–25°C (68–77°F) in the original package. Use reconstituted Abraxane immediately, although it may be refrigerated at 2–8°C (36–46°F) for a maximum of 8 hr. Ensure complete resuspension by mild agitation

P

before use. Discard reconstituted suspension if precipitates are observed.

17. COMPATIBILITY 0.9% NaCl.
18. INCOMPATIBILITY Administer separately.

ASSESSMENT

1. Note indications for therapy, tumor type, location, previous therapy (include agents, dosage, duration, radiation); may enhance myelosuppressive drug effects. Check if client has received this drug and response.
2. Give pretreatment meds (corticosteroids, diphenhydramine, and H_2 antagonists). If S&S of severe hypersensitivity reaction (dyspnea, hypotension, angioedema, generalized urticaria) appear, interrupt infusion and report. These reactions usually occur during first hour and despite premedication. Document any severe reaction so that client is *NOT* rechallenged with paclitaxel.
3. Reduce dose if severe peripheral neuropathy symptoms occur.
4. Monitor cardio-pulmonary and neurologic status, ECG, VS, I&O, CBC, renal, LFTs regularly; ensure neutrophil count is 1,500 cells/mm^3 before giving drug (with AIDS-related Kaposi's sarcoma with baseline neutrophil counts >1,000 cells/mm^3) and platelet count at least 100,000 cells/mm^3. Neutrophil nadir: 11 days; platelet nadir 8–9 days.

CLIENT/FAMILY TEACHING

1. Drug is administered every 2–3 weeks IV to inhibit/control rapid cell division of abnormal cells. Anticipate premedication with other agents to prevent hypersensitivity reactions.
2. Anticipate hair loss; should regrow. Avoid crowds and those with infections during therapy.
3. Joint pain and discomfort may be experienced 2–3 days after therapy but should resolve in several days. Report persistent nausea, vomiting, diarrhea, or appetite loss and persistent muscle or joint pain.
4. Report any severe N&V, fever, chills, sore throat, infection, abnormal bruising/bleeding, mouth sores, yellow discoloration of skin, or numbness and tingling in fingers/toes.
5. Avoid alcohol, aspirin, and NSAIDs. Ensure adequate hydration.
6. Use reliable contraception during and for 4 months following therapy.
7. Keep all F/U visits to assess BP, HR, labs, response to therapy, and for adverse SE.

OUTCOMES/EVALUATE

↓ Tumor size and spread

Paliperidone

(pal-ee-**PER**-i-done)

Classification(s): Antipsychotic

Pregnancy Category: C

RX: Invega, Invega Sustenna.

INDICATIONS/USES

Tablets, Extended-Release: (1) Acute and maintenance treatment of schizophrenia in adults and adolescents, age 12–17 years. (2) Acute treatment of schizoaffective disorder as monotherapy or as an adjunct to mood stabilizers and/or antidepressants. **Injection Suspension, Extended-Release:** Acute and maintenance treatment of schizophrenia in adults.

ACTION/KINETICS

Action

Paliperidone is the major active metabolite of risperidone. The mechanism of action is unknown but the drug may act through a combination of central dopamine type 2 (D_2) and serotonin type 2 ($5HT_{2A}$) receptor antagonism. It is also an antagonist at alpha-1, alpha-2, and histamine H_1 receptors. The drug also has antiemetic effects and a low incidence of sedation.

Pharmacokinetics

Absolute bioavailability: 28%. **Peak plasma levels:** 24 hr after PO and 13 days after IM. A high fat/high caloric meal increases both C_{max} and AUC. Steady state levels reached in 4–5 days. Metabolized to a limited extent by CYP2D6 and CYP3A4. **t½, terminal:** About 23 hr after PO and 25–49 days after IM. Unchanged drug and metabolites are excreted in the urine (70%) and feces (14%).

CONTRAINDICATIONS

Hypersensitivity to paliperidone or risperidone (paliperidone is a metabolite of risperidone). Use with drugs that prolong QTc (see *Drug Interactions*), in those with congenital long QT syn-

P

drome, in those with a history of cardiac arrhythmias. Use of alcohol. IV or SC administration.

SPECIAL CONCERNS

Increased mortality in elderly clients with dementia-related psychosis. Elderly clients with dementia-related psychosis treated with antipsychotic drugs are at an increased risk of death. Analysis of 17 placebo-controlled trials (modal duration of 10 weeks), largely in clients taking atypical antipsychotic drugs, revealed a risk of death in the drug-treated subjects between 1.6 to 1.7 times that seen in placebo-treated subjects. Over the course of a typical 10-week controlled trial, the rate of death in drug-treated subjects was about 4.5%, compared to a rate of about 2.6% in the placebo group. Although the causes of death were varied, most of the deaths appeared to be either cardiovascular (e.g., heart failure, sudden death) or infectious (e.g., pneumonia) in nature. Observational studies suggest that, similar to atypical drugs, treatment with conventional antipsychotic drugs may increase mortality. The extent to which the findings of increased mortality in observational studies may be attributed to the antipsychotic drug as opposed to some characteristic(s) of the clients is not clear. Paliperidone is not approved for the treatment of clients with dementia-related psychosis.

- **Dosage adjustment may be needed in elderly clients.**
- **Use with caution in those with history of MI or ischemic heart disease, heart failure, conduction abnormalities, CV disease, conditions that would predispose to hypotension (e.g., dehydration, hypovolemia, antihypertensive drugs), or mitral insufficiency.**
- **Use with caution in those at risk of aspiration pneumonia.**
- **Usually not given to those with pre-existing severe pathologic or iatrogenic GI narrowing because paliperidone tablets are nondeformable and thus may cause GI obstruction.**
- **Clients with Parkinson's disease or dementia have an increased sensitivity to antipsychotic drugs.**
- **Use during pregnancy only if the potential benefit outweighs the potential risk to the fetus.**
- **Use with caution during lactation or when used with other CNS drugs and alcohol.**
- **Safety and efficacy not determined in children less than 18 years of age.**

SIDE EFFECTS

Most Common

Headache, tachycardia, extrapyramidal disorder, dizziness, somnolence, akathisia, tremor, hypertonia, dry mouth, upper abdominal pain, orthostatic hypotension, bundle branch block, asthenia, fatigue.

GI: Upper abdominal pain, dry mouth, dyspepsia, nausea, salivary hypersecretion, abdominal discomfort/pain, swollen tongue, GI obstruction, dysphagia. **CNS:** Headache, dizziness, drowsiness, sedation, somnolence, akathisia, anxiety, confusion, extrapyramidal disorder/symptoms (dyskinesia, hyperkinesia), incoordination, insomnia, tremor, dystonia, hypertonia, parkinsonism, pseudoparkinsonism, tardive dyskinesia, cognitive and motor impairment, tremor, ***seizures, suicide***. **Neuroleptic malignant syndrome:** Hyperpyrexia, muscle rigidity, altered mental status, irregular pulse or BP, tachycardia, diaphoresis, cardiac dysrhythmia, acute renal failure. **CV:** Tachycardia, BBB, sinus arrhythmia, first degree AV block, hypertension, orthostatic hypotension, syncope, bradycardia, palpitations, ***pulmonary embolus***, ischemia, QTc interval prolongation, abnormal ECG T–wave, venous thrombosis, ***CVA/TIA in elderly clients with dementia-related psychosis***. **GU:** Priapism. **Respiratory:** Bronchopneumonia, increased cough, dyspnea. **Hematologic:** Thrombotic thrombocytopenic purpura, thrombocytopenia. **Metabolic:** Hyperglycemia, diabetes mellitus, increased blood insulin. **Ophthalmic:** Blurred vision. **Body as a whole:** Asthenia, fatigue, edema, fever, weight gain (with higher doses), back pain, hypotonia, pain in extremity. **Miscellaneous:** ***Anaphylaxis, increased mortality in elderly clients with dementia-related psychosis***, angioneurotic edema, impaired regulation of body temperature, injection site reactions.

LABORATORY TEST CONSIDERATIONS

Hyperprolactinemia. ↑ Prolactin, sensitivity with Lewy bodies.

OVERDOSE MANAGEMENT

Symptoms: Extrapyramidal symptoms, gait unsteadiness, drowsiness, sedation, tachycardia, hypotension, QT prolongation. *Treatment:* There is no specific antidote to paliperidone. Use the following approaches:

- Institute supportive measures.
- Provide close medical supervision and monitoring until the client recovers.
- In cases of acute overdosage, establish and maintain an airway; ensure adequate oxygenation and ventilation.
- Begin CV monitoring immediately. If antiarrhythmic therapy is instituted, note that disopyramide, procainamide, and quinidine may add to QT prolongation.
- Treat hypotension and circulatory collapse with IV fluids and/or sympathomimetic agents (do not use epinephrine or dopamine since beta stimulation may worsen hypotension)
- Gastric lavage (after intubation if client is unconscious).
- Consider giving activated charcoal with a laxative.
- In cases of severe extrapyramidal symptoms, give an anticholinergic.

DRUG INTERACTIONS

Amiodarone / Prolongs QTc → possible torsades de pointes; do not use together
Chlorpromazine / Prolongs QTc → possible torsades de pointes; do not use together
Dopamine agonists / Possible antagonism of dopamine agonist effects
Gatifloxacin / Prolongs QTc → possible torsades de pointes; do not use together
Levodopa / Possible antagonism of levodopa effects
Moxifloxacin / Prolongs QTc → possible torsades de pointes; do not use together
Procainamide / Prolongs QTc → possible torsades de pointes; do not use together
Quinidine / Prolongs QTc → possible torsades de pointes; do not use together
Risperidone / Additive effects R/T paliperidone is the major active metabolite of risperidone
Sotalol / Prolongs QTc → possible torsades de pointes; do not use together
Thioridazine / Prolongs QTc → possible torsades de pointes; do not use together

HOW SUPPLIED

Paliperidone. *Tablets, Extended-Release (Invega):* 1.5 mg, 3 mg, 6 mg, 9 mg.

Paliperidone palmitate. *Injection Suspension, Extended-Release (Invega Sustenna):* 39 mg, 78 mg, 117 mg, 156 mg, 234 mg.

DOSAGE

Paliperidone

TABLETS, EXTENDED-RELEASE

Schizophrenia.

Adults: 6 mg once daily given in the morning. Initial dose titration is not necessary. Some clients may benefit from doses up to 12 mg/day (side effects are increased) and others from a lower dose of 3 mg/day. Increase the dose above 6 mg/day only after clinical assessment and should occur at intervals of more than 5 days. When dose increases are indicated, small increments of 3 mg/day are recommended. **Maximum dose:** 12 mg/day. Prescribe at the lowest effective dose for maintaining clinical stability. Evaluate periodically to determine the need for continued therapy. **Adolescents, 12–17 years of age, usual:** 3 mg once daily; initial dose titration not required. If necessary, dose increases should be made only after clinical reassessment and should occur at increments of 3 mg/day at intervals of more than 5 days.

Schizoaffective disorder.

Adults: 6 mg once daily, given in the morning. Initial dose titration is not required. Some may benefit from lower or higher doses within the recommended dosage range of 3 to 12 mg once daily. Adjust dosage, if needed, only after clinical reassessment. Increase dosage, if needed, only at intervals of more than 4 days; increments of 3 mg/day are recommended, up to a maximum of 12 mg/day.

Paliperidone palmitate

INJECTION SUSPENSION, EXTENDED-RELEASE

Schizophrenia.

IM only. Adults, initial: 234 mg on treatment day 1 and 156 mg 1 week later, both given in the deltoid muscle. **Maintenance, monthly:** 117 mg; some may benefit from lower or higher doses with the range of 39 to 234 mg based on individual client tolerability and/or efficacy. Following the second dose, monthly maintenance doses can be given in either the deltoid or gluteal muscle. Continue responding clients at the lowest dose needed; periodically reassess to determine need for continued treatment. *NOTE:* Full beneficial effect may not be noted for several months.

NURSING IMPLICATIONS

IMPLEMENTATION/ADMINISTRATION/STORAGE

1. Paliperidone is the major active metabolite of risperidone. Thus, additive effects may occur if risperidone is coadministered with paliperidone.
2. Incidence of side effects is dose-related.
3. **Extended-Release Tablets and Renal Impairment.** For clients with C_{CR} from 50-<80 mL/min, the recommended initial dose is 3 mg once daily; the dose may then be increased to a maximum of 6 mg once daily, based on tolerability. For those with C_{CR} from 10 to <50 mL/min, the recommended initial dose is 1.5 mg/day with a maximum recommended dose of 3 mg once daily. Use is not recommended in those with C_{CR} <10 mL/min. **Extended-Release Suspension.** For those with mild renal impairment (C_{CR} at least 50 to <80 mL/min, the recommended initial dose is 156 mg on treatment day 1 and 117 mg 1 week later, both given in the deltoid muscle. Thereafter, follow with monthly injections of 78 mg in either the deltoid or gluteal muscle. Not recommended in those with moderate or severe renal impairment (C_{CR} <50 mL/min).
4. No dosage adjustment is necessary in clients with mild-moderate hepatic impairment (Child-Pugh score of A or B). Paliperidone has not been studied in those with severe hepatic impairment.
5. Establish tolerability with oral risperidone or paliperidone prior to beginning paliperidone injection for those who have never taken PO paliperidone injection or oral or injectable risperidone.
6. When switching from previous long-acting injectable antipsychotics, begin paliperidone injection in place of the next scheduled injection.
7. If paliperidone injection is discontinued, consider its prolonged release characteristics.
8. Inject IM slowly, deep into the muscle. Alternate deltoid injections between the 2 deltoid muscles. Avoid inadvertent injection into a blood vessel. Give as a single injection; do not administer in divided injections.
9. Needle size is important. For those weighing 90 kg or more (200 lb or more), the recommendation for the deltoid muscle is a 1½-inch, 22-gauge needle. For those weighing less than 90 kg, the 1-inch, 23-gauge needle is recommended for the deltoid muscle. The recommended needle size for the gluteal muscle is a 1½-inch, 22-gauge needle. Give into the upper outer quadrant of the gluteal area. Alternate gluteal injections between the 2 gluteal muscles.
10. Use the following guidelines for missed injectable doses of paliperidone:
    - To avoid a missed dose, the client may be given the second dose 2 days before or after the 1-week time point.
    - To avoid a missed monthly dose, give the injection up to 7 days before or after the monthly time point.
    - Missed dose (1 month to 6 weeks): After initiation, the recommended injection cycle of paliperidone is monthly. If less than 6 weeks have elapsed since the last injection, then the previously stabilized dose should be given as soon as possible, followed by injections at monthly intervals.
    - Missed dose (more than 6 weeks to 6 months): If more than 6 weeks has elapsed since the last injection, resume the same dose the client was previously stabilized on unless the client was stabilized on a dose of 234 mg, then the first 2 injections should each be 156 mg given as follows: Deltoid injection as soon as practical, followed by another deltoid injection (same dose) a week later and then resumption of either deltoid or gluteal dosing at monthly intervals.
    - Missed dose (more than 6 months): Initiate dosing as described under initial dosing.

P

11. Store the injection and tablets from 15–30°C (59–86°F); protect tablets from moisture. The injection is for single use only.

ASSESSMENT

1. List reasons for therapy, onset, duration, characteristics of S&S, presenting behavioral manifestations, mental status. Note all drugs prescribed to ensure none interact.
2. Perform appropriate baseline assessments. Monitor weight, BP, electrolyte imbalance, bradycardia, and concomitant administration with drugs that prolong the QT interval may increase risk of torsades de pointes. Monitor ECG and any cardiac conditions closely.
3. Observe for altered mental status, muscle rigidity, dyskinetic movements, or overt changes in VS. Monitor metabolic function and for S&S of diabetes. **Not** for use with dementia-related psychosis in the elderly; may increase mortality.
4. Review risk of NMS, irreversible tardive dyskinesia, and other associated adverse effects.
5. The antiemetic effect of risperidone may mask S&S of overdose with certain drugs or conditions such as intestinal obstruction, Reye's syndrome, brain tumor.
6. Reduce dose with renal dysfunction; monitor BP, CBC, cholesterol levels, serum prolactin, renal and LFTs.

CLIENT/FAMILY TEACHING

1. Take with or without food; do not chew, divide, or crush the extended-release tablets.
2. Since drug is contained with a nonabsorbable shell, the tablet shell is eliminated from the body. Do not be concerned if something that looks like a tablet is noted in the stool.
3. Use caution while driving, riding a bike, or performing other tasks requiring mental alertness until tolerance determined; may cause drowsiness, impaired judgment/thinking skills. Avoid alcohol.
4. Avoid sudden position changes to prevent sudden drop in BP. Rise slowly from a sitting or lying position.
5. During periods of high temperature or humidity avoid strenuous activity to prevent overheating and dehydration.
6. Report any mental status changes, suicide ideations, muscle rigidity, ↑HR/BP, or fever.
7. Practice reliable contraception; report if pregnancy suspected.
8. Keep all F/U to assess response, labs/ECG, and for adverse SE.

OUTCOMES/EVALUATE

- Improved behavior patterns with ↓ agitation, ↓ hyperactivity, and reality orientation
- Improved concentration and self-control

Palivizumab

(**pal**-ih-**VIZ**-you-mab)

Classification(s): Monoclonal antibody

Pregnancy Category: C

RX: Synagis.

INDICATIONS/USES

Prevention of serious lower respiratory tract disease due to RSV in pediatric clients at high risk of RSV disease. May be used (1) in children with hemodynamically significant congenital heart disease to prevent hospitalization due to RSV, (2) in infants with bronchopulmonary dysplasia, and (3) infants 35 weeks or less gestational age.

ACTION/KINETICS

Action

Humanized monoclonal antibody that exhibits neutralizing and fusion-inhibitory activity against respiratory syncytial virus (RSV), leading to a reduction in the quantity of RSV in the lower respiratory tract.

Pharmacokinetics

t½, children: 20 days.

CONTRAINDICATIONS

Use in adults. Pediatric clients with a history of severe reaction to palivizumab or other components of the product.

SPECIAL CONCERNS

- Safety and efficacy have not been determined for treatment of established RSV disease.
- Rare cases of anaphylaxis have been noted following initial or re-exposure to the drug.
- Side effects after a sixth or greater dose are similar in character and frequency than those after the initial five doses.

SIDE EFFECTS

Most Common

N&V, fever, URTI, otitis media, rhinitis, rash, pain, hernia, pharyngitis.

Respiratory: URTI, rhinitis, pharyngitis, cough, wheezing, bronchiolitis, pneumonia, bronchitis, asthma, croup, dyspnea, sinusitis, apnea. **GI:** Diarrhea, N&V, gastroenteritis, abnormal liver function, oral monilia. **CNS:** Nervousness. **Dermatologic:** Rash, fungal dermatitis, eczema, seborrhea, injection site reaction. **Hematologic:** Anemia. **Hypersensitivity:** Dyspnea, cyanosis, ***respiratory failure***, urticaria, pruritus, angioedema, hypotonia, unresponsiveness, ***anaphylaxis*** (following reexposure). **Ophthalmic:** Conjunctivitis. **Otic:** Otitis media. **Body as a whole:** Fever, pain, failure to thrive, viral infection, flu syndrome, allergic reactions. **Miscellaneous:** Hernia.

LABORATORY TEST CONSIDERATIONS

↑ AST, ALT.

HOW SUPPLIED

Injection: 100 mg/mL.

DOSAGE

IM

Prevention of RSV disease.

Children: 15 mg/kg per month IM (preferably in the anterolateral part of the thigh) throughout the RSV season. To calculate the monthly dose: [client weight (kg) × 15 mg/kg divided by 100 mg/mL of palivizumab]

NURSING IMPLICATIONS

IMPLEMENTATION/ADMINISTRATION/STORAGE

1. Give injection volumes >1 mL in divided doses.
2. The injection does not have to be reconstituted and is available for injection immediately.
3. Palivizumab is supplied in single-use vials. Do not reenter vial. Give immediately after withdrawal from the vial. Discard any unused portion.
4. Serum levels are decreased after cardiopulmonary bypass. Administer a dose of palivizumab to clients undergoing cardiopulmonary bypass as soon as possible after procedure (even if sooner than 1 month from previous dose). Thereafter give doses monthly.
5. Store between 2–8°C (36–46°F) in its original container. Do not freeze.

ASSESSMENT

1. Note candidates for therapy, i.e., premature infants at 35 weeks or less gestation without BPD and infants with BPD requiring intervention for RSV in the past 6 months.
2. Assess for congenital defects, coagulation disorders or liver dysfunction; may preclude therapy.
3. Give monthly doses throughout the RSV season. In the northern hemisphere, the RSV season usually begins in November and lasts through April (may be different in some communities). Give the first dose prior to the beginning of the RSV season to ensure protection.
4. Due to possibility of sciatic nerve damage, do not use the gluteal site routinely as the injection site. Administer IM into the anterolateral aspect of thigh. Give volumes greater than 1 mL in divided doses and in different sites. Follow dosing guidelines for correct dosage.

CLIENT/FAMILY TEACHING

1. Therapy consists of monthly injections based on body weight, during the RSV season. In the northern hemisphere, the RSV season typically starts in November and lasts through April, but it may begin earlier or last later in certain communities. Drug is used to prevent RSV, not to treat the disease.
2. Protect child from exposure to infection while on therapy, i.e., limit visitors, and avoid infected persons. Providers may need to wear masks and gloves.
3. May experience URI, runny nose, sore throat, ear infections, rash, or pain at injection site; report fever, other infections, difficulty breathing, swelling of the face, lips, or tongue, hives, or wheezing.
4. Keep all F/U visits to assess response, for monthly injection, and adverse SE.

OUTCOMES/EVALUATE

RSV prophylaxis in high risk infants

IV

Palonosetron hydrochloride

(pal-oh-**NOE**-see-tron)

Classification(s): Antiemetic, 5-HT_3 receptor antagonist

Pregnancy Category: B

RX: Aloxi.

INDICATIONS/USES

IV. (1) Prevention of acute and delayed N&V associated with initial and repeat courses of moderately and highly emetogenic cancer chemotherapy. (2) Prevention of postoperative N&V for up to 24 hr following surgery. Efficacy beyond 24 hr not demonstrated. Useful for clients in whom N&V must be avoided during the postoperative period, even where the incidence of postoperative nausea and/or vomiting is low.

ACTION/KINETICS

Action

It is believed cancer chemotherapeutic drugs cause N&V by releasing serotonin from the enterochromaffin cells of the small intestine and that released serotonin activates 5-HT_3 receptors on vagal afferent nerves to initiate the vomiting reflex. Palonosetron is a selective 5-HT_3 receptor antagonist with a strong binding affinity for this receptor. Thus, by blocking serotonin on these receptors, N&V are reduced.

Pharmacokinetics

About 50% of a dose is metabolized in the liver to inactive metabolites. Unchanged drug and metabolites are excreted mainly in the urine. **t½, elimination:** 40 hr. **Plasma protein binding:** About 62%.

CONTRAINDICATIONS

Hypersensitivity to palonosetron or any component of the product. Lactation.

SPECIAL CONCERNS

- Use with caution in those who have or may develop prolongation of cardiac conduction intervals (i.e., QTc) (i.e., those with hypokalemia or hypomagnesia, those taking diuretics with potential for inducing electrolyte abnormalities, those with congenital QT syndrome, those taking anti-arrhythmic drugs or other drugs which lead to QT prolongation, and cumulative high dose anthracycline therapy).
- Effects unknown in women undergoing labor or delivery.
- Safety and efficacy not determined in children less than 18 years of age.

SIDE EFFECTS

Most Common

Headache, constipation, dizziness, diarrhea, bradycardia, hypotension, hyperkalemia, weakness.

CNS: Headache, dizziness, insomnia, somnolence, hypersomnia, paresthesia, anxiety, euphoria. **CV:** Non-sustained tachycardia, bradycardia, hypotension, hypertension, myocardial ischemia, extrasystoles, sinus tachycardia, sinus arrhythmia, supraventricular extrasystoles, QT prolongation, vein discoloration, vein distention. **GI:** Constipation, diarrhea, abdominal pain, dyspepsia, dry mouth, hiccoughs, flatulence. **Body as a whole:** Fatigue, weakness, fever, hot flashes, flu-like syndrome, arthralgia. **Metabolic:** Hyperkalemia, electrolyte fluctuations, hyperglycemia, metabolic acidosis, glycosuria, decreased appetite, anorexia. **Ophthalmic:** Eye irritation, amblyopia. **Otic:** Motion sickness, tinnitus. **Dermatologic:** Allergic dermatitis, rash. **GU:** Urinary retention.

LABORATORY TEST CONSIDERATIONS

↑ ALT, AST, bilirubin.

HOW SUPPLIED

Injection (IV): 0.05 mg/mL.

DOSAGE

IV

Chemotherapy-induced N&V.

Adults: A single 0.25 mg dose about 30 min before the start of chemotherapy.

Postoperative N&V.

Adults: A single 0.075 mg IV dose given over 10 seconds immediately before the induction of anesthesia.

NURSING IMPLICATIONS

IMPLEMENTATION/ADMINISTRATION/STORAGE

1. IV Routine prophylaxis is not recommended in those where there is little expectation that

nausea and/or vomiting will occur postoperatively.

2. Repeated dosing within a 7 day period is now recommended as safety and efficacy of frequent dosing has been evaluated.
3. Supplied ready for IV injection. Flush infusion line with isotonic sodium chloride solution before and after palonosetron administration.
4. Inspect visually for particulate matter and discoloration before administration.
5. Store injection from 20–25°C (68–77°F); protect from freezing and light. Store capsules from 15–30°C (59–86°F); protect from light.
6. COMPATIBILITY NSS.
7. INCOMPATIBILITY Do not mix with other drugs.

ASSESSMENT

1. Note reasons for therapy, chemotherapy prescribed, other agents trialed, outcome.
2. Administer 30 min before chemo on day one of each cycle. Also may need other agents (corticosteroids) to help control N&V especially with highly emetogenic agents. May also require additional antiemetic agents for breakthrough N&V.
3. Monitor abdominal assessments, bowel sounds, N&V.
4. Assess hydration status, LFTs, electrolytes, and ECG findings.

CLIENT/FAMILY TEACHING

1. IV therapy is administered 30 min before chemotherapy. If ordered, take tablets 1 hour before anti-cancer medicine (chemotherapy) with or without food. Consume adequate fluids to prevent dehydration.
2. Drug may prolong the QT interval with other agents, so report any new drugs prescribed or any cardiac conduction problems.
3. Report if intolerable headache, or persistent/intolerable constipation or diarrhea or lack of desired response.
4. May be prescribed additional antiemetic for N&V that is not controlled with this therapy.
5. Keep all F/U visits to assess response and for adverse SE.

OUTCOMES/EVALUATE

Prevention of chemotherapy-induced N&V

IV

Pamidronate disodium

(pah-**MIH**-droh-nayt)

Classification(s): Bone growth regulator, bisphosphonate

Pregnancy Category: D

RX: Aredia.

INDICATIONS/USES

(1) In conjunction with hydration to treat moderate to severe hypercalcemia of malignancy associated with breast and lung cancers and multiple myeloma (with or without bone metastases). (2) Moderate to severe Paget's disease. (3) With standard therapy to treat osteolytic bone metastases of breast cancer or osteolytic lesions of multiple myeloma. *Investigational:* Postmenopausal osteoporosis; hyperparathyroidism; prophylaxis of glucocorticoid-induced osteoporosis; reduce bone pain in clients with prostatic carcinoma; treat immobilization-induced hypercalcemia; osteoporosis with spinal cord injury.

ACTION/KINETICS

Action

Inhibits both normal and abnormal bone resorption without inhibiting bone formation and mineralization. Precise mechanism is not known, but the drug may inhibit dissolution of hydroxyapatite crystal or have an effect on bone reabsorbing cells. Causes decreased serum phosphate levels probably due to a decreased release of phosphate from bone and increased renal excretion as parathyroid levels return to normal. Urinary calcium/creatinine and urinary hydroxyproline/creatinine ratios decrease and usually return to normal or below normal after treatment.

Pharmacokinetics

t½, elimination: 28 hr (beta). Approximately 50% of an IV infused dose is excreted unchanged in the urine within 72 hr. Rate of elimination from bone not determined.

CONTRAINDICATIONS

Hypersensitivity to bisphosphonates.

SPECIAL CONCERNS

- Use with caution during lactation.

P

- **Safety and efficacy not determined in children or to treat hypercalcemia associated with hyperparathyroidism or non-tumor-related conditions.**
- **Pamidronate not tested in clients who have creatinine levels greater than 5 mg/dL.**

SIDE EFFECTS

Most Common

N&V, anemia, bone/skeletal pain, dyspnea, fatigue, fever, headache, anorexia, diarrhea, dyspepsia, abdominal pain, headache, insomnia.

GI: N&V, diarrhea, constipation, abdominal pain, dyspepsia, anorexia, irritation of upper GI mucosa, ***GI hemorrhage***, ulcerative stomatitis. **CNS:** Somnolence, anxiety, insomnia, dizziness, headache, hypesthesia, paresthesia, psychosis, slight possibility of ***seizures***. **CV:** Hypertension, atrial fibrillation, syncope, tachycardia, ***cardiac failure***. **Respiratory:** Dyspnea, coughing, pleural effusion, rales, rhinitis, sinusitis, URTI. **GU:** UTI, decreased renal function (after IV), renal failure, uremia. **Musculoskeletal:** Bone/back/skeletal pain, osteonecrosis of the jaw, arthralgia, arthrosis, myalgia. **At site of administration:** Redness, swelling or induration, pain on palpation. **Hematologic:** Anemia, granulocytopenia, leukopenia, neutropenia, thrombocytopenia. **Metabolic/Electrolytes:** Hypocalcemia, hypokalemia, hypomagnesemia, hypophosphatemia. **Ophthalmic:** Abnormal vision. **Allergic:** Hypotension, dyspnea, ***angioedema***, ***anaphylaxis***. **Body as a whole:** Fatigue, asthenia, fever, malaise, metastases, slight increase in body temperature, fluid overload, edema, peripheral edema, generalized pain, moniliasis. **Miscellaneous:** Hypothyroidism, sweating.

P

HOW SUPPLIED

Injection: 3 mg/mL, 6 mg/mL, 9 mg/mL; *Powder for Injection, Lyophilized:* 30 mg, 90 mg.

DOSAGE

IV INFUSION

Moderate hypercalcemia (corrected serum calcium of about 12–13.5 mg/dL) of malignancy.

Initial therapy: 60–90 mg given as a single dose over 2–24 hr. Infusions more than 2 hr may reduce the risk for renal toxicity, especially in those with pre-existing renal insufficiency.

Severe hypercalcemia (corrected serum calcium greater than 13.5 mg/dL) of malignancy.

Initial therapy: 90 mg as a single initial infusion given over 2–24 hr. Infusions longer than 2 hr may reduce the risk for renal toxicity, especially in those with pre-existing renal insufficiency. If retreatment is necessary, use the same dose as for initial therapy; at least 7 days should elapse before retreatment.

Moderate to severe Paget's disease.

30 mg/day given as a 4-hr infusion on 3 consecutive days (total dose: 90 mg). If retreatment is necessary, the same dosage schedule is used.

Osteolytic bone lesions of breast cancer.

90 mg given as a 2-hr infusion every 3–4 weeks. Pamidronate has been frequently used with doxorubicin, fluorouracil, cyclophosphamide, methotrexate, mitoxantrone, vinblastine, dexamethasone, prednisone, melphalan, vincristine, megestrol, and tamoxifen.

Osteolytic bone lesions of multiple myeloma.

90 mg given as a 4-hr infusion every month. Those with marked Bence Jones proteinuria and dehydration should receive adequate hydration before infusion of pamidronate.

NOTE: Single doses should not exceed 90 mg due to renal toxicity and potential renal failure.

NURSING IMPLICATIONS

Do not confuse Aredia with Meridia (antiobesity drug) or Adriamycin (antineoplastic).

IMPLEMENTATION/ADMINISTRATION/STORAGE

1. **IV Hydrate clients adequately throughout treatment; overhydration, however, must be avoided, especially in those clients who have cardiac failure. Do not use diuretic therapy before correcting hypovolemia.**
2. **If hypercalcemia recurs, may retreat provided a minimum of 7 days has elapsed to allow full response to initial dose.**
3. **Reconstitute drug by adding 10 mL sterile water, which results in a concentration of 30 mg/10 mL or 90 mg/10 mL with a pH of 6–7.4.**

4. For hypercalcemia of malignancy, dilute recommended dose in 1,000 mL of sterile 0.45% or 0.9% NaCl or D5W. This solution stable for 24 hr at room temperature.
5. For treating Paget's disease, dilute the daily dose of 30 mg in 500 mL of 0.45% or 0.9% NaCl or D5W; give over a 4-hr period for 3 consecutive days.
6. For treating osteolytic bone lesions of breast cancer, dilute the dose of 90 mg dose in 250 mL of 0.45% or 0.9% NaCl or D5W; give over a 2-hr period every 3–4 weeks.
7. For treating osteolytic bone lesions of multiple myeloma, dilute the dose of 90 mg in 500 mL of sterile 0.45% or 0.9% NaCl or D5W; give over a 4-hr period on a monthly basis.
8. Visually inspect parenteral drug products for particulate matter or discoloration prior to administration.
9. Infusing over 2 or more hr reduces risk of renal toxicity.
10. Do not store above 30°C (86°F). May be stored from 2–8°C (36–46°F) for up to 24 hr when reconstituted with sterile water for injection.
11. COMPATIBILITY 0.45% or 0.9% NaCl, D5W.
12. INCOMPATIBILITY Give as single IV solution in a separate line. Do not mix with calcium-containing infusion solutions such as Ringer's solution.

ASSESSMENT

1. Note reasons for therapy, (i.e., hypercalcemia of malignancy, symptomatic Paget's disease, osteolytic bone lesions/pain), onset, presenting symptoms, any bisphosphonate hypersensitivity.
2. Due to possible osteonecrosis of the jaw (primarily in cancer clients who have received bisphosphonates as part of their therapy), consider dental exam before treating with bisphosphonates, and in those with concomitant risk factors such as cancer, chemotherapy, corticosteroids, or poor oral hygiene. Steroids may increase the risk of jaw bone problems.
3. List any cardiac disease. Monitor VS and I&O. Ensure adequate fluids to correct hypovolemia/volume deficits before giving diuretics.
4. During drug therapy, vigorous saline hydration should be undertaken for moderate to severe hypercalcemia to restore urine output to about 2 L/day. Avoid doses of over 90 mg to reduce risk of renal impairment. For less severe hypercalcemia, more conservative approaches can be taken, including saline hydration with or without loop diuretics. Overhydration should be avoided, especially with CHF. Weigh daily; observe for edema.
5. Assess for seizure activity; incorporate seizure precautions.
6. Monitor x-rays, BMD, ECG, serum Ca^{++}, Mg^{++}, K^+, PO_4, CBC, and renal function studies. Those with renal dysfunction are at greater risk for adverse side effects; obtain creatinine prior to each treatment. With bone metastases, withhold dose if renal function deteriorated. Replace calcium if needed and ensure aggressive hydration with NSS.

CLIENT/FAMILY TEACHING

1. Drug works to decrease calcium levels with cancer. Review dietary sources of calcium (dark green vegetables, yogurt, cheese, milk, etc.) that should be avoided with hypercalcemia.
2. Avoid activities that require mental alertness; may cause dizziness or drowsiness.
3. May experience transient mild temperature elevations for up to 48 hr following therapy. Maintain adequate hydration; keep log of I&O.
4. Report any increase in N&V, bone/jaw pain, thirst, or lethargy R/T hypercalcemia.
5. Practice reliable contraception; may cause fetal harm.
6. Keep all F/U to assess response, labs, and for adverse SE.

OUTCOMES/EVALUATE

- Desired calcium levels
- ↓ Bone pain/instability

Pancrelipase (Lipancreatin)

(pan-kree-**LY**-payz)

Classification(s): Digestive enzyme

Pregnancy Category: C

RX: Creon Delayed-Release Capsules, Lipram UL12, UL 18, or UL 20 Delayed-Release Capsules, PAN-2400 Capsules, Pancrease MT 4, MT 10, MT 16, or MT 20 Capsules,

Pancreaze, Pancrecarb MS-4, MS-8, or MS-16 Delayed-Release Capsules, Pangestyme MT 16 Delayed-Release Capsules, Panocaps MT 16 or MT 20 Delayed-Release Capsules, Panokase Tablets, Tri-Pase 8 and 16 Tablets, Ultrase Capsules, Ultrase MT 12, MT 18, or MT 20 Capsules, Viokase 8 or 16 Tablets, Zenpep Delayed-Release Capsules.

Rx: Creon 5, 10, 20, 25 Minimicrospheres, Pancrease MT, Ultrase, Ultrase MT.

INDICATIONS/USES

(1) Pancreatic deficiency diseases such as chronic pancreatitis, cystic fibrosis of the pancreas, pancreatectomy, ductal obstructions caused by cancer of the pancreas or common bile duct, steatorrhea of malabsorption syndrome, postgastrectomy, or postgastrointestinal surgery. (2) Presumptive test for pancreatic function, especially in insufficiency due to chronic pancreatitis.

ACTION/KINETICS

Action

Enzyme concentrate from hog pancreas, which contains lipase, amylase, and protease, enzymes that replace or supplement naturally occurring enzymes. More active at neutral or slightly alkaline pH. Has 12 times the lipolytic activity and 4 times both the proteolytic and amylolytic activity of pancreatin.

Pharmacokinetics

Certain products have an enteric coating that protects the enzymes from deactivation in the stomach.

CONTRAINDICATIONS

Hog protein sensitivity. Acute pancreatitis, acute exacerbation of chronic pancreatic disease.

SPECIAL CONCERNS

- **Safety for use during lactation and in children less than 6 months of age not established.**
- **Methacrylic acid copolymer, which is found in the enteric coating of certain products, may cause fibrosing colonopathy.**

SIDE EFFECTS

Most Common

N&V, diarrhea, abdominal cramps (after high doses), flatulence, bloating.

GI: N&V, diarrhea, abdominal cramps (after high doses), colonic strictures, intestinal obstruction, intestinal stenosis, constipation, flatulence, melena, bloating, cramping, perianal irritation. **Miscellaneous:** Dermatitis, weight decrease, pain. Inhalation of the powder is irritating to the skin and mucous membranes and may result in an asthma attack. High doses cause hyperuricemia and hyperuricosuria.

OVERDOSE MANAGEMENT

Symptoms: Diarrhea, intestinal upset.

DRUG INTERACTIONS

Calcium carbonate / ↓ Effect of pancreatic enzymes
Folic acid / ↓ Folic acid absorption may → folic acid deficiency
Iron / Response to oral iron may ↓ if given with pancreatic enzymes
Mg hydroxide / ↓ Effect of pancreatic enzymes

HOW SUPPLIED

Capsules, Powder, Tablets: with varying amounts of lipase, protease, and amylase (check label carefully).

DOSAGE

CREON 5

Pancreatic deficiency diseases.

Adults and children over 6 years of age: Usual starting dose is 2–4 capsules per meal or snack. **Children, under 6 years:** Select exact dose based on clinical experience with this age group. Start with 1 to 2 capsules per meal or snack. **Cystic fibrosis clients:** Usual doses are 1,500–3,000 lipase units/kg/meal. Doses in excess of 6,000 lipase units/kg/meal are not recommended.

CREON 10

Pancreatic deficiency diseases.

Adults and children over 6 years: Usual starting dose is 1–2 capsules per meal or snack. **Children, under 6 years:** Usual starting dose is up to 1 capsule per meal or snack. **Cystic fibrosis clients:** Usual doses are 1,500–3,000 lipase units/kg/meal. Doses in excess of 6,000 lipase units/kg/meal are not recommended.

CREON 20

Pancreatic deficiency diseases.

Adults and children over 6 years: Usual starting dose is 1 capsule per meal or snack. **Children under 6 years:** Select the exact dose based on clinical experience with this age group. **Cystic fibrosis clients:** Usual doses are 1,500–3,000 lipase units/kg/meal. Doses in excess of 6,000 units are not recommended.

PANCRECARB, ULTRASE, ULTRASE MT

Pancreatic deficiency diseases.

Initiate with 1 or 2 capsules with each meal or snack.

LIPRAM, PANCRELIPASE

Pancreatic deficiency diseases.

Children, 6 months to less than 1 year of age: 2,000 lipase units/meal. **Children, 1–6 years:** 4,000–8,000 lipase units with each meal and 4,000 units with snacks. **Children, 7–12 years:** 4,000–12,000 lipase units with each meal and with snacks. **Adults:** 4,000–20,000 lipase units with each meal and with snacks.

PANCREASE, PANCREASE MT4

Pancreatic deficiency diseases.

Infants, up to 12 months: 2,000–4,000 lipase units/120 mL of formula or breast milk. **Children under 4 years of age:** Initiate with 1,000 lipase units/kg/meal, up to a maximum of 2,500 lipase units/kg/meal. **Children over 4 years of age:** Initiate with 400 lipase units/kg/meal, up to a maximum of 2,500 lipase units/kg/meal. Doses greater than 2,500 lipase units/kg/meal should be used with caution and only if they are documented to be effective by 3-day fecal measures.

PANOKASE, VIOKASE TABLETS

Pancreatic deficiency diseases.

Cystic fibrosis and chronic pancreatitis clients: Dose ranges from 8,000–32,000 lipase units (1–4 tablets of Panokase or Viokase 8 or 1–2 tablets of Viokase 16). Take with meals. **Pancreatectomy or obstruction of pancreatic ducts:** 1–2 tablets (Panokase or Viokase 8) or 1 tablet (Viokase 16) q 2 hr.

VIOKASE POWDER

Pancreatic deficiency diseases.

0.7 gram (¼ teaspoon) with meals.

NURSING IMPLICATIONS

Do not confuse Ultrase with Ultram (an analgesic).

IMPLEMENTATION/ADMINISTRATION/STORAGE

1. When administering to young children, may sprinkle capsule contents on food.
2. After several weeks of use, adjust dosage according to therapeutic response.
3. Store unopened preparations in tight containers at a temperature not to exceed 25°C (77°F).
4. Do not crush or chew enteric-coated products (i.e., microspheres, microtablets). If unable to swallow, the capsule may be opened and shaken on a small amount of soft, cold food (e.g., applesauce, gelatin) that does not require chewing. Swallow immediately without chewing (enzymes may irritate the mucosa). Follow with a glass of juice or water to ensure complete swallowing of the product. Enteric-coated products that come in contact with foods with a pH greater than 5.5 will dissolve.
5. Generally, 300 mg of pancrelipase is required to digest every 17 grams of dietary fat. Products are not bioequivalent; do not interchange without approval.
6. Store Creon, Ultrase, and Ultrase MT from 15–25°C (59–86°F) in a dry place. Protect from high humidity; do not refrigerate.
7. Store Lipram, Pancrease, Pancrease MT, Pancrecarb, Pancrelipase, Panokase, and Viokase at room temperature not exceeding 25°C (77°F) in a dry place. Protect from high humidity; store in tight containers. Do not refrigerate.

ASSESSMENT

1. Note condition requiring enzyme replacement therapy; obtain thorough medical/surgical history.
2. Assess for any sensitivity or allergy to pork, since hog protein is the main constituent of pancrelipase.

3. Perform nutritional assessment noting ht, wt, BMI, muscle tone.
4. Assess abdomen noting tenderness, BS, quality/frequency of stooling (foul-smelling, frothy, fatty, frequency) and pancreatic function tests (amylase, lipase).

CLIENT/FAMILY TEACHING

1. Drug is used to help absorb and digest fat, proteins, and CHO. Review appropriate dietary recommendations (usually low fat, high calorie, high protein); utilize dietitian for dietary counseling/help in meal planning. Do not take with antacid containing calcium carbonate or magnesium hydroxide.
2. Take just before or with meals and snacks and with plenty of liquids to prevent oral mucosal irritation and enhance drug effectiveness. Do not crush or chew enteric-coated capsules; drug will deactivate in acid stomach environment; swallow whole. Avoid inhaling powder forms; may cause severe side effects.
3. Report any joint pain/swelling/soreness, significant weight loss, or breathing difficulty. With nausea, cramping, or diarrhea, dosage may need adjustment to control steatorrhea (fat in stool). May experience diarrhea and abdominal discomfort; report if persistent.
4. Keep all F/U to assess response, labs, adverse SE.

OUTCOMES/EVALUATE

- Improved digestion/nutritional status with deficiency states
- Control of diarrhea, ↓ steatorrhea

P

■ IV

Pancuronium bromide

(pan-kyou-**ROH**-nee-um)

Classification(s): Neuromuscular blocking drug

Pregnancy Category: C

RX: Pavulon.

SEE ALSO ***NEUROMUSCULAR BLOCKING AGENTS***.

INDICATIONS/USES

(1) Adjunct to anesthesia to facilitate tracheal intubation. (2) To provide skeletal muscle relaxation during surgery or mechanical ventilation.

ACTION/KINETICS

Action

Five times as potent as d-tubocurarine. Anticholinesterase agents will reverse effects. Possesses vagolytic activity although it is not likely to cause histamine release.

Pharmacokinetics

Onset: Within 45 sec. **Time to peak effect:** 3–4.5 min (depending on the dose). **Duration:** 35–45 min (increased with multiple doses). **t½, elimination:** 89–161 min. Forty percent is excreted through the urine either unchanged or as metabolites; 10% is excreted through the bile. In clients with renal failure, the t½ is doubled. **Plasma protein binding:** About 87%.

SPECIAL CONCERNS

■ Give in carefully adjusted doses only by, or under the supervision of, experienced clinicians. Do not give unless reversal agents and facilities for intubation, artificial respiration, and oxygen therapy are immediately available. Be prepared to assist or control respiration. ■

- Children up to 1 month of age may be more sensitive to the effects of pancuronium.
- Clients with myasthenia gravis or Eaton-Lambert syndrome may have profound effects from small doses.

SIDE EFFECTS

Most Common

Skeletal muscle weakness, prolonged skeletal muscle relaxation, respiratory insufficiency/apnea.

See *Neuromuscular Blocking Agents* for a complete list of possible side effects. Also, **Respiratory:** ***Apnea, respiratory insufficiency***. **CV:** Increased HR and MAP. **Miscellaneous:** Salivation, skin rashes, ***hypersensitivity reactions*** (e.g., ***bronchospasm***, flushing, hypotension, redness, tachycardia).

ADDITIONAL DRUG INTERACTIONS

Azathioprine / Reverses effects of pancuronium
Bacitracin / Additive muscle relaxation
Enflurane / ↑ Muscle relaxation
Isoflurane / ↑ Muscle relaxation
Metocurine / ↑ Muscle relaxation but duration is not prolonged
Phenytoin / Possible pancuronium shorter duration of action or less effective
Quinidine, Quinine / ↑ Effect of pancuronium

Sodium colistimethate / ↑ Muscle relaxation
Succinylcholine / ↑ Intensity and duration of action of pancuronium
Tetracyclines / Additive muscle relaxation
Theophyllines / ↓ Effects of pancuronium; also, possible cardiac arrhythmias
Tricyclic antidepressants with halothane / Administration of pancuronium may cause severe arrhythmias
Tubocurarine / ↑ Muscle relaxation but duration is not prolonged

HOW SUPPLIED

Injection: 1 mg/mL, 2 mg/mL.

DOSAGE

IV

Muscle relaxation during balanced anesthesia.

Adults and children over 1 month of age, initial: 0.04–0.1 mg/kg. Additional doses of 0.01 mg/kg may be administered as required (usually q 20–60 min). **Neonates:** Administer a test dose of 0.02 mg/kg first to determine responsiveness.

ET intubation.

0.06–0.1 mg/kg as a bolus dose. Can undertake intubation in 2 to 3 min.

NURSING IMPLICATIONS

IMPLEMENTATION/ADMINISTRATION/STORAGE

1. IV Administer IV in a monitored environment.
2. COMPATIBILITY D5W, NSS, D5/NSS, RL.
3. INCOMPATIBILITY Administer separately.

ASSESSMENT

1. Note reasons for therapy, expected duration, other agents/therapies trialed. Review conditions/drugs that antagonize and enhance neuromuscular blockade; assess for presence.
2. Drug should only be used on a short-term basis and in a continuously monitored environment. Drug blocks the effect of acetylcholine at the myoneural junction, thus preventing neuromuscular transmission.
3. Provide ventilatory support.
4. Monitor and record VS, ECG, and I&O. Drug can cause vagal stimulation resulting in bradycardia, hypotension, and cardiac arrhythmias.
5. Use peripheral nerve stimulator to evaluate neuromuscular response and recovery. Before reversing with neostigmine, ensure evidence of spontaneous recovery present.
6. Consciousness and pain threshold are not affected by pancuronium. Explain all procedures and provide emotional support and pain and anxiety medications. Do not conduct any discussions that should not be overheard.
7. With short-term therapy, reassure that client will be able to talk and move once the drug effects are reversed.
8. Muscle fasciculations may cause soreness or injury after recovery. Administer prescribed nondepolarizing agent and reassure that soreness is likely caused by the unsynchronized contractions of adjacent muscle fibers just before the onset of paralysis.
9. Position for comfort and so that the body is in proper alignment. Turn and perform mouth care and eye care frequently (protect eyes and instill liquid tears q 2 hr as blink reflex is suppressed).
10. Assess airway at frequent intervals. Have a suction machine at the bedside.
11. Check to be certain that the ventilator alarms are set and on at all times.
12. *Never* leave client unmonitored. Determine client need and administer medications for anxiety, pain, and/or sedation regularly (Valium, morphine). Store this medication away from any other drugs to prevent confusion.

CLIENT/FAMILY TEACHING

1. Drug used to control movement and permit procedures/treatments and will make you feel like you are paralyzed; sensation will return once drug is discontinued and wears off.
2. Will be unable to move or talk and a machine will do breathing. This will be in a setting that permits continous monitoring; response assessed with a peripheral nerve stimulator.
3. During therapy will be able to see and hear; medication will be given for pain and anxiety. All functions will return once the medication is discontinued.
4. May experience some burning at IV site. Site will be assessed and changed regularly.

OUTCOMES/EVALUATE

- Desired level of paralysis; suppression of twitch response

P

- Facilitation of ET intubation; tolerance of mechanical ventilation

IV

Panitumumab

(pan-ih-tuh-**MYOO**-mab)

Classification(s): Monoclonal antibody-antineoplastic drug

Pregnancy Category: C

RX: Vectibix.

SEE ALSO *ANTINEOPLASTIC AGENTS*.

INDICATIONS/USES

Treatment of epidermal growth factor receptor (EGFR)-expressing, metastatic colorectal carcinoma with disease progression or following fluoropyrimidine-, oxaliplatin-, and irinotecan-containing chemotherapy regimens. *NOTE:* Efficacy is based on progression-free survival.

ACTION/KINETICS

Action

A recombinant, human immunoglobulin G2 kappa monoclonal antibody that binds to the human epidermal growth factor receptor (EGFR). EGFR is a member of a subfamily of type 1 receptor tyrosine kinases. Overexpression of EGFR is detected in many human cancers, including the colon and rectum. Panitumumab binds specifically to EGFR and competitively inhibits the binding of ligands for EGFR. This results in inhibition of cell growth, induction of apoptosis, decreased proinflammatory cytokine and vascular growth factor production, and internalization of EGFR. It is believed panitumumab inhibits growth and survival of selected human tumor cell lines expressing EGFR.

Pharmacokinetics

Drug levels reach steady-state levels by the third infusion. **t½, elimination:** About 7.5 days (3.6–10.9 days).

CONTRAINDICATIONS

During lactation and for 2 months following the last dose of panitumumab.

SPECIAL CONCERNS

(1) **Dermatologic toxicity.** Dermatologic toxicities, related to panitumumab blockade of epidermal growth factor-binding and subsequent inhibition of epidermal growth factor receptor (EGFR)-mediated signaling pathways were reported in 89% of clients and were severe (NCI Common Toxicity Criteria, grade 3 and higher) in 12% of clients receiving panitumumab monotherapy. The clinical manifestations included, but were not limited to, dermatitis acneiform, pruritus, erythema, rash, skin exfoliation, paronychia, dry skin, and skin fissures. Severe dermatologic toxicities were complicated by infections including sepsis, septic death, and abscesses requiring incisions and drainage. Withhold or discontinue panitumumab and monitor for inflammatory or infectious sequelae in those with severe dermatologic toxicities. (2) **Infusion reactions.** Severe infusion reactions occurred with the administration of panitumumab in approximately 1% of clients. Severe infusion reactions were identified by reports of anaphylactic reaction, bronchospasm, fever, chills, and hypotension. Although fatal infusion reactions have not been reported with panitumumab, fatalities have occurred with other monoclonal antibody products. Stop the infusion if a severe infusion reaction occurs. Depending on the severity and/or persistence of the reaction, permanently discontinue panitumumab.

Safety and efficacy not determined in children.

SIDE EFFECTS

Most Common

Skin rashes/toxicity, hypomagnesemia, paronychia, fatigue, abdominal pain, nausea, constipation, diarrhea (may result in dehydration), infusion reactions, eye toxicities.

Dermatologic: Skin rashes, erythema, pruritus, acneiform dermatitis, skin exfoliation/fissures, paronychia, other nail disorders, photosensitivity, acne, dry skin, growth of eyelashes, abscesses requiring incisions and drainage, ***sepsis, septic death***. **Infusion reactions:** Fever, chills, dyspnea, hypotension, ***anaphylactoid reaction***. **GI:** N&V, abdominal pain, constipation, diarrhea (may result in dehydration), stomatitis, oral mucositis, mucosal inflammation. **Metabolic:** Hypomagnesemia, hypocalcemia, peripheral edema. **Respiratory:** Cough, pulmonary fibrosis. **Ophthalmic:** Conjunctivitis, ocular hyperemia, increased lacrimation, eye/eyelid irritation. **Body as a whole:**

P

Fatigue, general deterioration, ***sepsis, septic death***, abscesses requiring incisions and drainage, immunogenicity.

DRUG INTERACTIONS

Frequency and severity of diarrhea may ↑ when given with irinotecan.

HOW SUPPLIED

Injection, Solution: 20 mg/mL.

DOSAGE

IV INFUSION

EGFR-expressing, metastatic colorectal carcinoma.

Adults: 6 mg/kg given over 60 min every 14 days. Give doses higher than 1,000 mg over 90 min. For the duration of the infusion, reduce the infusion rate 50% in clients experiencing a mild or moderate (grade 1 or 2) reaction.

NURSING IMPLICATIONS

IMPLEMENTATION/ADMINISTRATION/STORAGE

1. **IV** Discontinue immediately and permanently in those experiencing severe (grade 3 or 4) infusion reactions.
2. Withhold for dermatologic toxicities that are grade 3 or higher or are considered intolerable. If toxicity does not improve to grade 2 or lower within 1 month, stop permanently. If dermatologic toxicity improves to grade 2 or lower, and the client is symptomatically improved after withholding up to 2 doses of panitumumab, resume treatment at 50% of the original dose. If toxicities recur, stop permanently. If toxicities do not recur, subsequent doses may be increased by increments of 25% of the original dose until the recommended dose of 6 mg/kg is reached.
3. To prepare the solution for infusion, withdraw the necessary amount of panitumumab for a dose of 6 mg/kg. Dilute to a total volume of 100 mL with NaCl 0.9% injection. Doses higher than 1,000 mg should be diluted to 150 mL with NaCl 0.9% injection. Final concentration should not exceed 10 mg/mL. Mix diluted solution by gentle inversion. Do not shake.
4. Do not administer panitumumab as an IV push or bolus. Must be given by an IV infusion pump using a low-protein binding 0.2 or 0.22 μm in-line filter. Infuse through peripheral line or indwelling catheter.
5. Store in the original carton from 2–8°C (36–46°F) until time of use. Protect from direct sunlight; do not freeze. Discard any unused portion as the product contains no preservatives.
6. Use the diluted infusion solution within 6 hr of preparation if stored at room temperature or within 24 hr if refrigerated. Do not freeze the solution.
7. COMPATIBILITY 0.9% NaCl.
8. INCOMPATIBILITY Do not mix with or administer as an infusion with other drugs; flush the line before and after panitumumab administration with NaCl 0.9% to avoid mixing with other drug products or IV solutions.

ASSESSMENT

1. List reasons for therapy, onset, other therapies trialed/failed.
2. Assess skin turgor and condition; monitor for any reaction (skin, pulmonary toxicity).
3. Monitor VS, lung sounds, I&O, infusion site, Mg^{++}, Ca^{++}, electrolytes, renal and LFTs.

CLIENT/FAMILY TEACHING

1. Drug is used to treat cancer that has metastasized following standard chemotherapy. Panitumumab is a monoclonal antibody. Monoclonal antibodies are made in the laboratory and can locate and bind to cancer cells. Panitumumab binds to the epidermal growth factor receptor (EGFR) and may block tumor cell growth.
2. May experience skin rash, fatigue, abdominal pain, nausea, and diarrhea. Report any skin or eye changes, new onset SOB, or breathing problems (pulmonary fibrosis), severe skin rash especially if complicated by infections, infusion reactions, and vomiting.
3. Skin may be more sensitive to sunlight and may easily burn. Use sunscreen (minimum SPF 15), wear protective clothing if must be out in the sun (for 2 mo following therapy).
4. Males and females should practice reliable contraception for 6 mo after therapy completed. May affect female's fertility; consider egg/sperm harvesting prior to therapy. May also cause irregular menstrual periods.

P

5. **Keep all F/U to assess response, labs, and for adverse SE.**

OUTCOMES/EVALUATE

Inhibition of malignant cell proliferation

IV

Pantoprazole sodium

(pan-**TOH**-prah-zohl)

Classification(s): Proton pump inhibitor

Pregnancy Category: B

RX: Protonix, Protonix I.V.

♣ **Rx:** Panto IV, Pantoloc, PMS Pantoprazole IV.

INDICATIONS/USES

PO: (1) Short-term treatment (up to 8 weeks) in the healing and symptomatic relief of erosive esophagitis. (2) Maintenance of healing of erosive esophagitis and reduction in relapse rates of day- and night-time heartburn symptoms in those with GERD. (3) Long-term treatment of pathological hypersecretory conditions, including Zollinger-Ellison syndrome. *Investigational:* Chronic laryngitis, prevention of GI bleeding in those receiving antiplatelets.

IV: (1) Short-term (7–10 days) treatment of GERD associated with a history of erosive esophagitis, as an alternative to PO therapy in those who are unable to continue taking the delayed-release tablets. (2) Pathological hypersecretory conditions associated with Zollinger-Ellison syndrome or other neoplastic conditions.

P

ACTION/KINETICS

Action

Proton pump inhibitor that suppresses the final step in gastric acid production by forming a covalent bond to two sites of the H^+/K^+-ATPase enzyme system at the secretory surface of the gastric parietal cell. Results in inhibition of both basal and stimulated gastric acid secretion regardless of the stimulus. Duration greater than 24 hr due to binding to ATPase. Gastrin levels increase.

Pharmacokinetics

About 77% is bioavailable. Absorption begins only after the tablet leaves the stomach although it occurs rapidly. Absorption is not affected by antacids, although food may delay absorption up to 2 hr or longer. **T_{max}:** 2.5 hr after PO. **Duration:** Over 24 hr. Extensively metabolized in the liver by the CYP system. **$t^{1/2}$:** About 1 hr. Excreted in both the urine (71%) and feces (18%). AUC and C_{max} are increased in the elderly. **Plasma protein binding:** About 98%.

CONTRAINDICATIONS

Hypersensitivity to any component of the formulation. Lactation.

SPECIAL CONCERNS

- **Safety and efficacy of IV use as initial treatment for GERD not established.**
- **Symptomatic response to therapy does not preclude the presence of gastric malignancy.**
- **Use with caution in severe hepatic impairment; modest drug accumulation may occur if dosed once/day.**
- **Safety and efficacy for children or for maintenance therapy (i.e., beyond 16 weeks) not established.**

SIDE EFFECTS

Most Common

Headache, diarrhea, flatulence, abdominal pain.

Side effects listed are those with an incidence of 1% or more or that may be life–threatening. **GI:** Diarrhea, flatulence, abdominal pain, eructation, constipation, dyspepsia, gastroenteritis, GI disorder, N&V, rectal disorder, ***esophageal/GI/rectal hemorrhage, hepatic failure*. CNS**: Headache, insomnia, anxiety, dizziness, migraine, ***convulsion*. CV: *Hemorrhage, MI*. Respiratory**: Bronchitis, increased cough, dyspnea, pharyngitis, rhinitis, sinusitis, URTI. **Musculoskeletal:** Arthralgia, back/chest/neck pain. **Dermatologic:** Rash, ***Stevens-Johnson syndrome, toxic epidermal necrolysis*. GU**: Urinary frequency, UTI. **Hypersensitivity: *Angioedema, anaphylaxis*. Body as a whole:** Asthenia, flu syndrome, infection, pain, hypertonia, ***allergic reaction, heat stroke*. Miscellaneous**: Injection–site reaction after IV (abscess, thrombophlebitis).

LABORATORY TEST CONSIDERATIONS

↑ ALT, AST, creatinine, alkaline phosphatase, creatine phosphokinase, GGTP. Hyperlipemia, hyperglycemia, hypercholesterolemia, hyperuricemia. Abnormal LFTs.

DRUG INTERACTIONS

NOTE: Pantoprazole may interfere with the absorption of drugs where gastric pH is an important determinant of bioavailabity.

Ampicillin esters / ↓ Ampicillin absorption R/T ↓ bioavailability R/T inhibition of gastric acid secretion → ↑ gastric pH
Cyanocobalamin / ↓ Cyanocobalamin absorption R/T ↓ bioavailability R/T inhibition of gastric acid secretion → ↑ gastric pH
Digoxin / ↓ Digoxin absorption R/T ↓ bioavailability R/T inhibition of gastric acid secretion → ↑ gastric pH
Iron salts / ↓ Iron absorption R/T ↓ bioavailability R/T inhibition of gastric acid secretion → ↑ gastric pH
Itraconazole / ↓ Itraconazole absorption R/T ↓ bioavailability R/T inhibition of gastric acid secretion → ↑ gastric pH
Ketoconazole / ↓ Ketoconazole absorption R/T ↓ bioavailability R/T inhibition of gastric acid secretion → ↑ gastric pH
Warfarin / Possible ↑ INR and PT; monitor carefully

HOW SUPPLIED

Granules for Oral Suspension, Delayed-Release: 40 mg; *Injection, Lyophilized Powder for Solution:* 40 mg (as base)/vial; *Tablets, Delayed-Release:* 20 mg (as base), 40 mg (as base).

DOSAGE

SUSPENSION, DELAYED-RELEASE, ORAL; TABLETS, DELAYED-RELEASE

Short-term treatment of erosive esophagitis associated with GERD.

Adults: 40 mg once daily for up to 8 weeks; an additional 8 weeks of therapy may be considered for those who have not healed after 8 weeks of treatment.

Maintenance of healing of erosive esophagitis.

Adults: 40 mg once daily.

Pathological hypersecretory conditions, including Zollinger-Ellison syndrome.

Individualize. **Adults, initial:** 40 mg twice a day. Adjust dose as needed as dosage varies with each individual; up to 240 mg/day may be given, if needed. Treatment in some has continued for more than 2 years.

IV ONLY

GERD associated with a history of erosive esophagitis.

Adults: 40 mg once daily for 7–10 days. Safety and efficacy for more than 10 days have not been shown. **Children, 2–16 years of age** (investigational): 0.32–1.88 mg/kg/dose IV given up to two times a day. **Maximum dose:** 80 mg per IV dose.

Pathological secretory conditions.

Individualize dose. **Adults, usual:** 80 mg q 12 hr. In those needing a higher dosage, 80 mg q 8 hr is expected to maintain acid output below 10 mEq/hr. Doses higher than 240 mg or given for more than 6 days have not been evaluated.

NURSING IMPLICATIONS

IMPLEMENTATION/ADMINISTRATION/STORAGE

1. Store delayed-release suspension and tablets from 15–30°C (59–86°F).
2. The delayed-release oral suspension may be given PO or via a nasogastric tube after being mixed with apple juice or applesauce.
3. Store PO products from 15–30°C (59–86°F).
4. IV IV pantoprazole may be given as follows:
   - *Two minute infusion.* Reconstitute IV pantoprazole with 10 mL of 0.9% NaCl injection for a final concentration of 4 mg/mL. For both uses, give over at least 2 min using the filter provided. Reconstituted solution may be stored for up to 24 hr at room temperature before administration. The solution does not need to be protected from light.
   - *Fifteen minute infusion used for GERD associated with a history of erosive esophagitis.* Reconstitute IV pantoprazole with 10 mL of 0.9% NaCl injection, and further dilute (admix) with 100 mL of D5W injection, 0.9% NaCl injection, or LR injection to a final concentration of about 0.4 mg/mL. The admixed solution may be stored at room temperature and must be used within 24 hr. Neither the reconstituted solution nor the admixed solution has to be protected from light.

P

- *Fifteen minute infusion used for hypersecretory conditions.* Reconstitute each vial with 10 mL of 0.9% NaCl injection. Combine the contents of the 2 vials and further dilute (admix) with 80 mL of D5W, 0.9% NaCl, or lactated Ringer's injection to a total volume of 100 mL, with a final concentration of about 0.8 mg/mL. Give the admixture over about 15 min at a rate of approximately 7 mg/min using the filter provided. The reconstituted solution may be stored for up to 6 hr at room temperature prior to further dilution; the admixed solution may be stored for up to 24 hr at room temperature prior to IV infusion. Give the admixture IV over approximately 15 min at a rate of about 7 mL/min using the filter provided. Do not freeze reconstituted drug. It is not necessary to protect the reconstituted or admixed solutions from light.

5. Give by IV infusion through a dedicated line using the filter provided. The filter must be used to remove precipitate that may form when the drug is reconstituted or mixed with IV solution.
6. If administration is through a Y-site, the in-line filter must be positioned below the Y-site that is closest to the client. Immediately stop use if precipitation or discoloration occurs.
7. Discontinue IV therapy as soon as able to resume PO therapy with the delayed-release tablets. Transition from IV to PO and PO to IV should be undertaken to ensure continuity of suppression of gastric acid secretion.
8. Store IV product at 2–8°C (36–46°F). Protect from light.
9. COMPATIBILITY D5W, 0.9% NaCl, LR.
10. INCOMPATIBILITY Flush line before and after administration of pantoprazole with either D5W or RL. Do not give with other IV solutions. Midazolam is incompatible with Y-site administration of pantoprazole IV. May not be compatible with zinc-containing products.

ASSESSMENT

1. Note reasons for therapy (short or long term), onset, duration, triggers, characteristics of S&S. Record abdominal assessment, skin lesions, urea breath, *H. Pylori* AB, UGI/endoscopic and biopsy results.
2. List drugs prescribed to ensure none require acidity for metabolism.
3. There have been reports of false + screening tests for tetrahydrocannabinol (THC) in those receiving most proton pump inhibitors. May require more selective testing to confirm results.
4. Review risk of osteoporosis related fractures with IV therapy as well as zinc deficiency with prolonged therapy.
5. Monitor CBC, B12, renal and LFTs; may reduce dose to every other day with dysfunction to prevent drug accumulations.

CLIENT/FAMILY TEACHING

1. Take as directed at the same time each day. Do not split, crush, or chew the delayed release tablets; swallow whole. If unable to swallow a 40-mg tablet, two 20 mg tablets may be taken.
2. Give the delayed-release oral suspension only in apple juice or applesauce, not in water or other liquids or food. Give 30 min before a meal.
3. May take with or without food in the stomach. Antacid consumption will not affect.
4. Avoid alcohol, aspirin or NSAIDs, and foods that may cause GI irritation.
5. Report abdominal pains, evidence of bleeding (bright blood or black tarry stools) and any unusual side effects, worsening of S&S, or lack of response; keep F/U appointments.
6. Avoid long term consumption unless indicated; may mask GI malignancies.
7. May cause false + THC drug test; ask for confirmatory testing.
8. Keep all F/U to assess response and for adverse SE.

OUTCOMES/EVALUATE

- Reduced gastric acidity with relief of S&S of erosive esophagitis/GERD
- Treatment of hypersecretory conditions (e.g., Zollinger-Ellison syndrome)
- Relief of laryngitis (unlabeled use)

Paroxetine hydrochloride, Paroxetine mesylate

(pah-**ROX**-eh-teen)

Classification(s): Antidepressant, selective serotonin reuptake inhibitor

P

Pregnancy Category: D

RX: Paroxetine hydrochloride: Paxil, Paxil CR. **Paroxetine mesylate:** Pexeva.

✤ **Rx:** Apo-Paroxetine, CO Paroxetine, Gen-Paroxetine, Novo-Paroxetine, PMS-Paroxetine, ratio-Paroxetine, Sandoz Paroxetine.

SEE ALSO ***SELECTIVE SEROTONIN REUPTAKE INHIBITORS***.

INDICATIONS/USES

Hydrochloride (Paxil CR). Immediate- and Controlled-Release: (1) Treatment of major depressive episodes as defined in the DSM-III (immediate-release) or DSM-IV (controlled-release). (2) Panic disorder with or without agoraphobia (as defined in DSM-IV). (3) Treatment of social anxiety disorder (social phobia) as defined in the DSM-IV. **Immediate-Release:** (1) Obsessive-compulsive disorders in clients with OCD (as defined in DSM-IV). (2) Generalized anxiety disorder (as defined in DSM-IV); up to 24 weeks for maintenance therapy. (3) Posttraumatic stress disorder as defined in DSM-IV. **Controlled-Release:** Premenstrual dysphoric disorder as defined in DSM-IV. *Investigational:* Hot flashes in men and women, premenstrual disorder, pruritus, stuttering.

Mesylate (Pexeva), Immediate-Release. (1) Treatment of major depressive disorder. Periodically evaluate the long-term usefulness. (2) Treatment of obsessive-compulsive disorder as defined in DSM-III-R. (3) Panic disorder as defined in DSM-IV.

ACTION/KINETICS

Action

Antidepressant effect likely due to inhibition of CNS neuronal uptake of serotonin and to a lesser extent norepinephrine and dopamine. Results in increased levels of serotonin in synapses. No anticholinergic or orthostatic hypotensive effects; none to slight sedative effect.

Pharmacokinetics

Completely absorbed from the GI tract; bioavailability is 100%. **Time to peak plasma levels:** 5.2 hr for immediate-release and 6–10 hr for controlled-release. **Peak plasma levels:** 61.7 ng/mL for immediate-release and 30 ng/mL for controlled-release. **$t^{1/2}$:** 21 hr for immediate-release and 15–20 hr for controlled-release. **Time to reach steady state:** About 10 days for immediate-release and 14 days for controlled-release. Plasma levels are increased in impaired renal and hepatic function as well as in geriatric clients. Extensively metabolized in the liver to inactive metabolites. Approximately two-thirds of the drug is excreted through the urine and one-third is excreted in the feces. *NOTE:* A generic form of paroxetine (Pexeva) is available as paroxetine mesylate, not paroxetine HCl (Paxil). **Plasma protein binding:** About 93–95%.

ADDITIONAL CONTRAINDICATIONS

Use during the first trimester of pregnancy. Use of alcohol. Concomitant use of thioridazine. Use in children and adolescents less than 18 years of age with major depressive disorder due to increased risk of suicidal thoughts and attempts.

SPECIAL CONCERNS

(1) Antidepressants increased the risk of suicidal thinking and behavior (suicidality) in short-term studies in children, adolescents, and young adults with major depressive disorder and other psychiatric disorders. Anyone considering the use of paroxetine or any other antidepressant in a child, adolescent, or young adult must balance this risk with the clinical need. Clients who are started on therapy should be observed closely for clinical worsening, suicidality, or unusual changes in behavior. Families and caregivers should be advised of the need for close observation and communication with the health care provider. Paroxetine is not approved for use in children. (2) Short-term placebo-controlled trials of nine antidepressant drugs in children and adolescents with major depressive disorder, obsessive-compulsive disorder, or other psychiatric disorders revealed a greater risk of adverse reactions representing suicidal thinking or behavior (suicidality) during the first few months of treatment. The average risk of such reactions in clients receiving antidepressants was 4%, twice the placebo risk of 2%. No suicides occurred in these trials.

- **Use with caution and initially at reduced dosage in elderly clients, as well as in impaired hepatic or renal function, with a history of mania, with a history of seizures, with diseases or conditions that could affect metabolism or hemodynamic responses.**

- **Undertake with caution concurrent administration of paroxetine with lithium or digoxin.**
- **Allow at least 14 days between discontinuing an MAOI and starting paroxetine or stopping paroxetine and starting an MAOI.**
- **Infants exposed to paroxetine during the third trimester of pregnancy may develop complications requiring prolonged hospitalization, respiratory support, and tube feeding.**
- **Carefully consider the potential risks and benefits of treating women during their third trimester; consider tapering paroxetine during the third trimester.**

SIDE EFFECTS

Most Common

Insomnia, somnolence, nausea, dry mouth, asthenia, headache, dizziness, tremor, excessive sweating, diarrhea/loose stools, constipation, abnormal ejaculation.

The side effects listed were observed with a frequency up to 1 in 1,000 clients. **CNS:** Headache, somnolence, insomnia, agitation, ***seizures***, tremor, anxiety, activation of mania/hypomania, dizziness, nervousness, paresthesia, drugged feeling, myoclonus, CNS stimulation, confusion, amnesia, impaired concentration, depression, emotional lability, vertigo, abnormal thinking, akinesia, alcohol abuse, ataxia, ***convulsions, possibility of suicide attempt***, depersonalization, hallucinations, hyperkinesia, hypertonia, incoordination, lack of emotion, manic reaction, paranoid reaction. **GI:** Nausea, abdominal pain, diarrhea/loose stools, dry mouth, vomiting, constipation, decreased appetite, flatulence, oropharynx disorder ('lump' in throat, tightness in throat), dyspepsia, increased appetite, bruxism, dysphagia, eructation, gastritis, glossitis, increased salivation, mouth ulceration, ***rectal hemorrhage***, abnormal LFTs. **Hematologic:** Anemia, leukopenia, lymphadenopathy, purpura. **CV:** Palpitation, vasodilation, postural hypotension, hypertension, syncope, tachy-/bradycardia, conduction abnormalities, abnormal ECG, migraine, peripheral vascular disorder. **Dermatologic:** Sweating, rash, pruritus, acne, alopecia, dry skin, ecchymosis, eczema, furunculosis, urticaria. **Metabolic/Nutritional:** Edema, weight gain/loss, hyperglycemia, peripheral edema, thirst. **Respiratory:** Respiratory disorder (cold symptoms or URI), pharyngitis, yawn, increased cough, rhinitis, asthma, bronchitis, dyspnea, epistaxis, hyperventilation, pneumonia, respiratory flu, sinusitis. **GU:** Abnormal ejaculation (usually delay), erectile difficulties, sexual dysfunction, impotence, decreased libido, urinary frequency/difficulty/hesitancy, anorgasmia in women, difficulty in reaching climax/orgasm in women, abortion, amenorrhea, breast pain, cystitis, dysmenorrhea, dysuria, menorrhagia, nocturia, polyuria, urethritis, urinary incontinence/retention, vaginitis. **Musculoskeletal:** Asthenia, back/neck pain, myopathy, myalgia, myasthenia, arthralgia, arthritis. **Ophthalmic:** Blurred vision, abnormality of accommodation, eye pain, mydriasis. **Otic:** Ear pain, otitis media, tinnitus. **Miscellaneous:** Asthenia, fever, chest pain, trauma, taste perversion/loss, chills, malaise, allergic reaction, ***carcinoma***, face edema, moniliasis, anorexia. *NOTE:* Over a 4- to 6-week period, there was evidence of adaptation to side effects such as nausea and dizziness but less adaptation to dry mouth, somnolence, and asthenia.

OVERDOSE MANAGEMENT

Symptoms: N&V, drowsiness, sinus tachycardia, dilated pupils. *Treatment:*

- Establish and maintain an airway.
- Ensure adequate oxygenation and ventilation.
- Induction of emesis, lavage, or both; following evacuation, 20–30 grams activated charcoal may be given q 4–6 hr during the first 24–48 hr after ingestion.
- Take an ECG and monitor cardiac function if evidence of abnormality.
- Provide supportive care with monitoring of VS.

ADDITIONAL DRUG INTERACTIONS

Antiarrhythmics, Type IC / Possible ↑ effect R/T ↓ liver breakdown
Cimetidine / ↑ Paroxetine effect R/T ↓ liver breakdown
Digoxin / Possible ↓ plasma levels
Phenobarbital / Possible ↓ paroxetine effect R/T ↑ liver breakdown
Phenytoin / Possible ↓ paroxetine effect R/T ↑ liver breakdown; also, ↓ phenytoin levels
Procyclidine / ↓ Procyclidine dose R/T significant anticholinergic effects
Risperidone / ↑ Risperidone levels R/T ↓ metabolism
H ***St. John's wort*** / Possible CNS depression
Tamoxifen / ↓ Plasma levels of the active metabolite (endoxifen) → ↓ therapeutic effect

P

Theophylline / ↑ Theophylline levels
Thioridazine / ↑ Thioridazine levels → possible prolongation of QTc interval
Valproic acid / ↑ Paroxetine levels

HOW SUPPLIED

Hydrochloride. ***Oral Suspension:*** 10 mg/5 mL; ***Tablets, Controlled-Release:*** 12.5 mg, 25 mg, 37.5 mg; ***Tablets, Immediate-Release:*** 10 mg, 20 mg, 30 mg, 40 mg.
Mesylate. ***Tablets, Immediate-Release:*** 10 mg, 20 mg, 30 mg, 40 mg.

DOSAGE

Paroxetine hydrochloride.

ORAL SUSPENSION; TABLETS, CONTROLLED-RELEASE; TABLETS, IMMEDIATE-RELEASE

Major depressive disorder.

Adults, initial, immediate-release: 20 mg/day, usually given as a single dose in the morning. Some clients not responding to the 20 mg dose may benefit from increasing the dose in 10 mg/day increments, up to a maximum of 50 mg/day. Make dose changes at intervals of at least 1 week. **Adults, initial, controlled-release:** 25 mg/day. Some clients not responding to the 25 mg dose may benefit from dose increases in 12.5 mg day increments, up to a maximum of 62.5 mg/day. Make dose changes at intervals of at least 1 week. **Maintenance:** Several months of therapy, possibly up to 1 year. Doses average about 30 mg/day.

Panic disorders with or without agoraphobia.

Adults, initial, immediate-release: 10 mg/day usually given in the morning; may be increased by 10 mg increments each week until a dose of 40 mg/day (dose range: 10–60 mg/day) is reached. **Maximum daily dose:** 60 mg. **Adults, initial, controlled-release:** 12.5 mg/day; may be increased in 12.5 mg/day increments at intervals of at least 1 week. **Dose range:** 12.5–75 mg/day (maximum daily dose). **Maintenance:** Since panic disorder is a chronic condition; long-term therapy is appropriate for responding clients.

Social anxiety disorder.

Adults, initial, immediate-release: 20 mg/day, given as a single dose with or without food, usually in the morning. **Dose range:** 20–60 mg/day. **Adults, initial, controlled-release:** 12.5 mg/day. **Dose range:** 12.5–37.5 mg/day. Make dosage increments at intervals of at least 1 week in increments of 12.5 mg/day. **Maintenance:** Social anxiety disorder is a chronic condition; long-term therapy is appropriate for responding clients.

Obsessive-compulsive disorders.

Adults, initial, immediate-release: 20 mg/day; **then** increase by 10 mg increments a day in intervals of at least 1 week until a dose of 40 mg/kg (range is 20–60 mg/day) is reached. Maximum daily dose: 60 mg. **Maintenance:** OCD is a chronic condition; consider long-term therapy for responding clients.

Generalized anxiety disorder.

Adults, initial, immediate-release: 20 mg/day, given as a single dose with or without food, usually in the morning. Dose range is 20–50 mg/day. Change doses in 10 mg/day increments at intervals of 1 week or more. Doses greater than 20 mg/day do not provide additional benefit. **Maintenance:** Adjust dose to maintain the client on the lowest effective dosage; periodically reassess to determine need for continued treatment. Found to be effective for up to 24 weeks.

Posttraumatic stress disorder.

Adults, initial, immediate-release: 20 mg/day given as a single daily dose with or without food. **Dose range:** 20–50 mg/day. If needed, can increase dose by 10 mg/day at intervals of 1 week. **Maintenance:** Adjust dose to maintain the client on the lowest effective dosage; periodically reassess to determine need for continued treatment.

P

Premenstrual dysphoric disorder.

Adults, initial, controlled-release: 12.5 mg/day. Give either daily throughout the menstrual cycle, or limit to the luteal phase of the menstrual cycle, depending on provider assessment. Both 12.5 mg/day and 25 mg/day have been shown to be effective. Make dosage changes at intervals of at least 1 week. **Maintenance:** Continue regimen for those clients responding.

Hot flashes.

Menopausal clients: 12.5 mg or 25 mg/day using the controlled-release product or 10 mg or 20 mg/day using the immediate-release product. **Breast cancer clients:** 20 mg daily or nightly.

Paroxetine mesylate.

TABLETS, IMMEDIATE-RELEASE

Major depressive disorder.

Adults, initial: 20 mg/day as a single dose, usually in the morning, with or without food. Some clients not responding to the 20 mg/day dose may benefit from dose increases, in 10 mg/day increments, up to a maximum of 50 mg/day. Make dosage changes in intervals of at least 1 week. **Dose range:** 20–50 mg/day. **Maintenance:** Acute episodes usually require several months or longer of therapy. Efficacy has been shown for up to 1 year with average daily doses of 30 mg.

Obsessive-compulsive disorder.

Adults, initial: 20 mg/day given as a single daily dose usually in the morning. Dosage can be increased to 40 mg/day (recommended dosage) in increments of 10 mg/day made no more often than weekly. **Maintenance:** OCD is a chronic condition; long-term therapy is warranted in responding clients.

Panic disorder.

Adults, initial: 10 mg/day, up to the target dosage of 40 mg/day. Make dosage changes in 10 mg/day increments no more often than weekly. **Dose range:** 10–60 mg/day. **Maintenance:** Panic disorder is a chronic condition; long-term therapy is warranted in responding clients. Adjust dosage to maintain the client on the lowest effective dose.

NURSING IMPLICATIONS

Do not confuse paroxetine with paclitaxel (an antineoplastic). Also, do not confuse Paxil with either paclitaxel (an antineoplastic) or Taxol (an antineoplastic).

IMPLEMENTATION/ADMINISTRATION/STORAGE

1. Geriatric or debilitated clients, those with severe hepatic or renal impairment, **initial:** 10 mg/day of immediate-release or 12.5 mg/day of controlled-release, up to a maximum of 40 mg/day of immediate-release or 50 mg/day of controlled-release for all uses.
2. Even though beneficial effects may be seen in 1–4 weeks, continue therapy as prescribed. Effectiveness is maintained for up to 1 year with daily doses averaging 30 mg of immediate-release or 37.5 mg of controlled-release.
3. Periodically assess clients to determine the need for continued therapy. Adjust dose to maintain the client on the lowest effective dose.
4. If discontinuing therapy, decrease dose incrementally. Abrupt cessation may cause dizziness, sensory disturbances, agitation, anxiety, nausea, and sweating.
5. At least 14 days should elapse between discontinuation of an MAOI and initiation of paroxetine. Also, allow at least 14 days after stopping paroxetine and beginning an MAOI.
6. Store immediate-release tablets between 15–30°C (59–86°F) and controlled-release tablets and suspension at or below 25°C (77°F).

ASSESSMENT

1. Note reasons for therapy, type, onset, characteristics of S&S, other therapy trialed, outcome. Assess clinical presentation and behavioral manifestations.
2. Document mania, altered metabolic or hemodynamic states, seizures.
3. List drugs currently prescribed to ensure none interact. Avoid use with an MAOI or within 14 days of discontinuing treatment with an MAOI.

4. Closely monitor infants born to mothers who took paroxetine during pregnancy due to the possibility of a withdrawal syndrome and baby heart defects.
5. During management of overdose, always entertain the possibility of multiple drug involvement.
6. Women who are or who may become pregnant and who are currently taking paroxetine should discuss the risks and benefits of continuing the drug with their provider; alternative therapies should be considered.
7. Monitor weight, BP, ECG, electrolytes, CBC, renal and LFTs; reduce dose with dysfunction.

CLIENT/FAMILY TEACHING

1. Administer as a single daily dose. Shake suspension well before using. May be given with or without food. Swallow controlled-release tablet whole; do not crush or chew.
2. Take only as directed. Prescriptions may be for small quantities to ensure compliance and to discourage overdose. Allow up to 4 weeks for therapeutic effects.
3. Do not engage in tasks that require mental alertness until drug effects realized; may cause dizziness or drowsiness. Avoid alcohol; OTC products without provider approval.
4. Report excessive weight loss/gain, and adjust diet and exercise to compensate.
5. Notify provider if pregnancy is suspected or planned. Practice reliable birth control, and avoid breastfeeding during therapy.
6. Report any thoughts of suicide or increased suicide ideations. Advise family not to leave severely depressed individuals alone; possibility of a suicide attempt is inherent in depression and may persist until significant remission is observed. Also report increased agitation, anxiety, hostility, aggression, impulsivity, irritability, or panic attacks.
7. Participate in counselling/therapy sessions to assist with underlying problems.
8. Do not stop suddenly; with prolonged use, titrate dose down to prevent withdrawal S&S.
9. Keep all F/U to assess response and for adverse SE.

OUTCOMES/EVALUATE

- ↓ Anxiety/depression, PTSD symptoms
- ↓ Panic attacks; ↓ palpitations; ↓ obsessive repetitive behaviors
- Resolution/control of postmenopausal hot flashes (unlabeled)

Pazopanib hydrochloride

(paz-**OH**-pah-nib)

Classification(s): Antineoplastic drug (tyrosine kinase inhibitor)

Pregnancy Category: D

RX: Votrient.

INDICATIONS/USES

Treatment of advanced renal cell carcinoma.

ACTION/KINETICS

Action

Pazopanib is an inhibitor of a number of tyrosine kinases, including vascular endothelial growth factor receptors 1, 2, and 3. The drug inhibits vascular endothelial growth factor-induced phosphorylation. Is thought to inhibit tumor growth.

Pharmacokinetics

Peak levels: 2–4 hr. High- or low-fat meals increase systemic exposure; thus, administer 1 hr before or 2 hr after a meal. Metabolized in the liver mainly by CYP3A4 (with a minor role of CYP1A2 and CYP2C8). Excreted mainly through the feces. **t½, mean:** 30.9 hr. Clearance is decreased by 50% in those with moderate hepatic impairment; dosage adjustment is necessary. **Plasma protein binding:** >99%.

CONTRAINDICATIONS

Severe hepatic impairment. Use in those who cannot avoid long-term use of strong CYP3A4 inducers. Use in those who have a history of hemoptysis, cerebral, or clinically significant GI hemorrhage in the past 6 months. Lactation.

SPECIAL CONCERNS

Hepatotoxicity. Severe and fatal hepatotoxicity has been observed in clinical studies. Monitor hepatic function and interrupt, reduce, or discontinue dosing as recommended.

- Clients older than 60 years may be at greater risk for an ALT >3 times ULN.

P

- **Possible additive effect with other drugs that prolong the QT interval. Use with caution in clients with a history of QT interval prolongation, in those taking antiarrhythmics or other drugs that may prolong the QT interval, and in those with pre-existing cardiac disease.**
- **Safety and efficacy not determined in children.**

SIDE EFFECTS

Most Common

Diarrhea, N&V, ↑ ALT/AST, anorexia, fatigue, hypertension, hair color changes, leukopenia, neutropenia, thrombocytopenia, lymphocytopenia.

CNS: Headache, ***cerebral/intracranial hemorrhage***. **GI:** Diarrhea, N&V, anorexia, abdominal pain, ***hepatic toxicity***, dysgeusia, dyspepsia, GI fistula, ***rectal hemorrhage, GI perforation***. **CV:** Hypertension, QT prolongation, ***torsades de pointes, MI***, myocardial ischemia, ***ischemic stroke***, ***CVA***, TIA, angina, ***hemorrhage, arterial thrombotic events***. **Dermatologic:** Alopecia, palmar-plantar erythrodysesthesia, rash, skin depigmentation. **Respiratory:** Epistaxis. **GU:** Hematuria. **Hematologic:** Leukopenia, neutropenia, thrombocytopenia, lymphocytopenia. **Body as a whole:** Fatigue, asthenia, weight decreased. **Miscellaneous:** Hair color changes, chest pain, facial edema, hypothyroidism, hemoptysis, hemorrhagic events (pulmonary, GI, GU).

LABORATORY TEST CONSIDERATIONS

↑ ALT, AST, total bilirubin, lipase. ↓ Magnesium, phosphorus, sodium. ↑ or ↓ Glucose. Proteinuria.

OVERDOSE MANAGEMENT

Symptoms: Possible fatigue, hypertension. *Treatment:* There is no specific antidote. Implement general supportive measures. Hemodialysis is not expected to increase elimination.

DRUG INTERACTIONS

NOTE: There is the possibility of an additive effect of pazopanib with other drugs that prolong the QT interval. Coadminister with caution and monitor for QT prolongation. The following drugs may prolong the QT interval and ↑ the risk of life-threatening cardiac arrhythmias, including torsades de pointes: Amiodarone, arsenic trioxide, bretylium, chlorpromazine, cisapride, disopyramide, dofetilide, dolasetron, droperidol, gatifloxacin, halofantrine, levomethadyl, mefloquine, mesoridazine, moxifloxacin, pentamidine, pimozide, probucol, procainamide, quinidine, sotalol, sparfloxacin, thioridazine, and ziprasidone.

Pazopanib inhibits OATP1B1 and UGT1A1 and thus may increase plasma levels of drugs eliminated by these means.

Drugs with a narrow therapeutic index metabolized by CYP3A4 (e.g., cyclosporine), CYP2C8, or CYP2D6 / ↑ Plasma levels of these drugs → ↑ pharmacologic effects and ↑ risk of side effects; do not use together
Grapefruit juice / ↑ Pazopanib plasma levels → ↑ pharmacologic effects and ↑ risk of side effects; do not use together
Lapatinib / ↑ Pazopanib AUC and C_{max} after 800 mg 50 to 60% when taken with 1,500 mg lapatinib; reduce pazopanib dose if needed
Midazolam / ↑ AUC and C_{max} of midazolam by about 30%; monitor and adjust midazolam dose as needed
Paclitaxel / ↑ AUC and C_{max} of paclitaxel by 26% and 31% respectively when given with 80 mg/m^2 paclitaxel once/week; monitor and adjust paclitaxel dose as needed
Rifampin / ↓ Pazopanib plasma levels → ↓ efficacy; do not use together
Strong CYP3A4 inhibitors (e.g., clarithromycin, ketoconazole, ritonavir) / ↑ Plasma pazopanib levels → ↑ pharmacologic effects and ↑ risk of side effects; do not use together. If coadministration is necessary, ↓ pazopanib dose to 400 mg once a day

HOW SUPPLIED

Tablets: 200 mg, 400 mg.

DOSAGE

TABLETS

Advanced renal cell carcinoma.

Adults, usual: 800 mg once a day without food (1 hr before or 2 hr after a meal). **Maximum dose:** 800 mg once a day. Initial dose reduction should be 400 mg; additional dose decrease or increase should be in 200 mg steps based on client tolerability.

NURSING IMPLICATIONS

- **Do not confuse pazopanib hydrochloride with pegaptanib sodium (to treat macular degeneration)**

IMPLEMENTATION/ADMINISTRATION/STORAGE

1. Do not crush tablets due to the potential for increased rate of absorption which may increase systemic levels.
2. If coadministration of a strong CYP3A4 inhibitor (see *Drug Interactions*) is warranted, reduce the pazopanib dose to 400 mg a day. Further dose reduction may be needed if side effects occur during therapy.
3. The use of strong CYP3A4 inducers may decrease pazopanib levels and should be avoided.
4. For moderate hepatic impairment, use a dose of 200 mg/day. Do not use in those with severe hepatic impairment.
5. Discontinue in those with wound dehiscence.
6. Store from 15–30°C (59–86°F).

ASSESSMENT

1. Note reasons for therapy, other agents trialed/failed and disease staging.
2. List drugs prescribed to ensure none interact.
3. Assess for evidence of GI fistula or perforation or any evidence of GI bleed in past 6 months; precludes therapy.
4. Temporarily interrupt therapy at least 7 days before surgical procedures; stop therapy with any wound dehiscence.
5. Obtain ECG to assess QT interval. Monitor BP, TSH, CBC, electrolytes, U/A, renal and LFTs; reduce dose or avoid with liver dysfunction. Monitor LFTs at least once every 4 wk for the first 4 months of therapy and periodically thereafter.

CLIENT/FAMILY TEACHING

1. Take once daily without food 1 hr before or 2 hr after meal. Do not chew, crush, or break tablets. Crushing tablets may increase the rate of absorption affecting systemic exposure.
2. If dose is missed, do not take if less than 12 hr until the next dose.
3. Report any S&S of liver problems immediately: yellowing of the skin or eyes, dark urine, unusual tiredness, right upper abdominal pain.
4. Diarrhea, nausea, and vomiting may occur. Report if moderate to severe diarrhea occurs.
5. Depigmentation of skin or hair may occur during therapy.
6. Use reliable contraception and avoid pregnancy; potential hazard to fetus.
7. Report any evidence of unusual bleeding.
8. Keep all F/U to assess response, labs and for adverse SE.

OUTCOMES/EVALUATE

Inhibition of malignant cell proliferation with advanced renal cell cancer

Pegaptanib sodium

(peh-**GAP**-tih-nib)

Classification(s): Selective vascular endothelial growth factor antagonist

Pregnancy Category: B

RX: Macugen.

INDICATIONS/USES

Treatment of neovascular (wet) age-related macular degeneration. *Investigational:* Diabetic macular edema.

ACTION/KINETICS

Action

Pegaptanib is a selective vascular endothelial growth factor antagonist. Vascular endothelial growth factor selectively binds and activates its receptors located mainly on the surface of vascular endothelial cells. It induces angiogenesis and increases vascular permeability and inflammation, which are believed to contribute to the progression of the wet form of age-related macular degeneration. Pegaptanib binds to vascular endothelial growth factor, thereby inhibiting its binding to receptors, thus decreasing the effect of vascular endothelial growth factor.

Pharmacokinetics

Slowly absorbed into the systemic circulation from the eye. The drug is metabolized by endo- and exonucleases.

CONTRAINDICATIONS

Ocular or periocular infections. Hypersensitivity to the drug or any component of the product.

SPECIAL CONCERNS

- Safety and efficacy of pegaptanib administered to both eyes, concurrently, not determined.
- Use with caution during lactation.
- Safety and efficacy not determined in children.

P

SIDE EFFECTS

Most Common

Anterior chamber inflammation, blurred vision, cataract, conjunctival hemorrhage, corneal edema, eye discharge/irritation/pain, hypertension, increased intraocular pressure, ocular discomfort, punctuate keratitis, reduced visual acuity, visual disturbance, vitreous floaters/opacities.

Ophthalmic: Endophthalmitis, increased intraocular pressure (within 30 min of administration), anterior chamber inflammation, blurred vision, cataract, conjunctival hemorrhage, corneal edema, eye discharge/irritation/pain, ocular discomfort, punctuate keratitis, reduced visual acuity, visual disturbance, vitreous floaters/opacities, blepharitis, conjunctivitis, photopsia, vitreous disorder, allergic conjunctivitis, conjunctival edema, corneal abrasion/deposits, corneal epithelium disorder, endophthalmitis, eye inflammation/swelling, eyelid irritation, mydriasis, periorbital hematoma, retinal edema, vitreous hemorrhage. **CNS:** Dizziness, headache, vertigo. **GI:** Diarrhea, nausea, dyspepsia, vomiting. **CV:** Hypertension, carotid artery occlusion, ***CVA***, TIA. **Musculoskeletal:** Arthritis, bone spur. **GU:** UTI, urinary retention. **Miscellaneous:** Bronchitis, chest pain, contact dermatitis, contusion, diabetes mellitus, pleural effusion, hearing loss, meibomianitis, ***anaphylaxis/anaphylactoid reactions***, including ***angioedema.***

HOW SUPPLIED

Injection: 0.3 mg.

DOSAGE

INTRAVITREOUS INJECTION

Age-related macular degeneration.

0.3 mg once every 6 weeks by intravitreous injection into the eye to be treated.

NURSING IMPLICATIONS

Do not confuse pegaptanib sodium with pazopanib hydrochloride (to treat advanced renal cell carcinoma).

IMPLEMENTATION/ADMINISTRATION/STORAGE

1. Inspect visually for particulate matter and discoloration prior to administration.
2. Carry out the injection under controlled aseptic conditions. Adequate anesthesia and a broad-spectrum antibiotic should be given prior to the injection.
3. Administration of the contents of the syringe involves attaching the threaded plastic plunger rod to the rubber stopper inside the syringe barrel. Do not pull back on the plunger. Then remove the syringe needle cap to allow administration of the drug.
4. Store from 2–8°C (36–46°F). Do not freeze or shake vigorously.

ASSESSMENT

1. List reasons for therapy, age at onset, other therapies trialed, outcome.
2. Note clinical presentation, any erythema, drainage, IOP, and level of vision.
3. Ensure that adequate anesthesia and a broad-spectrum microbicide have been administered prior to injection.
4. Drug is only administered by those trained to manage wet AMD. After proper aseptic injection, monitor IOP and for endophthalmitis. May check perfusion of the optic nerve head immediately after injection, tonometry within 30 min of administration and biomicroscopy between 2 and 7 days following injection.

CLIENT/FAMILY TEACHING

1. Drug is administered into the affected eye with a needle once every 6 weeks to prevent blindness from macular degeneration.
2. Seek immediate care from provider if a change in vision, redness of the eye, pain, or light sensitivity develops.
3. Therapy will require checkups to ensure that no infection develops, and if there is an increase in ocular pressure after the injection, the client may require more frequent monitoring procedures.

OUTCOMES/EVALUATE

Suppression of age-related neovascular macular degeneration (AMD) progression

IV

Pegaspargase (PEG-L-asparaginase)

(peg-**ASS**-pair-gays)

Classification(s): Antineoplastic, miscellaneous

Pregnancy Category: C

RX: Oncaspar.

SEE ALSO ***ANTINEOPLASTIC AGENTS.***

INDICATIONS/USES

(1) As a component of a multiagent chemotherapeutic regimen for clients with acute lymphoblastic leukemia who have developed hypersensitivity to the native forms of L-asparaginase. (2) As a component of a multiagent chemotherapeutic regimen for the first-line treatment of acute lymphoblastic leukemia.

ACTION/KINETICS

Action

Pegaspargase is a modification of the enzyme L-asparaginase. Some leukemic cells are not able to synthesize asparagine due to a lack of the enzyme asparaginase synthetase and are thus dependent on exogenous asparaginase for survival. Rapid depletion of asparagine, due to administration of asparaginase, kills leukemic cells. Normal cells, which can synthesize their own asparagine, are less affected.

Pharmacokinetics

t½, elimination: About 5.8 days during the induction.

CONTRAINDICATIONS

History of serious allergic reactions to pegaspargase (e.g., generalized urticaria, bronchospasm, laryngeal edema, hypotension, or other side effects); serious thrombosis, pancreatitis, and/or serious hemorrhagic events with prior L-asparaginase therapy. Lactation.

SPECIAL CONCERNS

- **Clients taking pegaspargase are at a higher risk for bleeding problems, especially with simultaneous use of other drugs that have anticoagulant properties (e.g., aspirin, NSAIDs).**
- **Safety and efficacy not determined in clients, 1 to 21 years of age with known previous hypersensitivity to L-asparaginase.**

SIDE EFFECTS

Most Common

Chemical hepatotoxicity, coagulopathies, hypersensitivity reactions, clinical pancreatitis, hyperglycemia requiring insulin therapy, thrombosis.
Most commonly hypersensitivity reactions, chemical hepatotoxicity, and coagulopathies. **Allergic reactions:** ***Hypersensitivity reactions*** (acute or delayed), including ***life-threatening anaphylaxis***, may occur during therapy, especially in clients with known hypersensitivity to other forms of L-asparaginase. Also, skin rashes, erythema, edema, pain, fever, chills, urticaria, dyspnea, ***bronchospasm***, increased ALT, N&V, malaise, arthralgia, induration, hives, tenderness, swelling, lip edema. **GI:** ***Pancreatitis*** (may be severe), GI/abdominal pain, anorexia, diarrhea, constipation, flatulence, indigestion, mucositis, mouth tenderness, severe colitis. **Coagulation disorders:** Decreased anticoagulant effect, ***DIC***, decreased fibrinogen, increased thromboplastin, increased coagulation time, prolonged PT/PTTs, ***clinical hemorrhage (may be fatal)***, decreased antithrombin III, superficial and deep venous thrombosis, sagittal sinus thrombosis, venous catheter thrombosis, atrial thrombosis, decreased platelet count, purpura, ecchymosis, easy bruisability. **Hepatic:** Jaundice, abnormal LFTs, fatty liver deposits, hepatomegaly, ascites, ***liver failure***. **CV:** Hypotension (may be severe), tachycardia, thrombosis (including sagittal sinus thrombosis), chest pain, hypertension, subacute bacterial endocarditis, edema. **Hematologic**: ***Hemolytic anemia***, leukopenia, pancytopenia, thrombocytopenia, ***agranulocytosis***, anemia. **CNS**: ***Convulsions, status epilepticus***, temporal lobe seizures, headache, paresthesia, mild to severe confusion, thrombosis/***hemorrhage***, disorientation, dizziness, emotional lability, somnolence, ***coma***, mental status changes, Parkinson-like syndrome. **Respiratory**: Dyspnea, ***bronchospasm***, increased cough, epistaxis, URI. **Dermatologic**: Injection site hypersensitivity, rash, petechial rash, erythema simplex, pruritus, itching, alopecia, fever blister, hand whiteness, fungal changes, nail whiteness and ridging. **GU**: Hematuria, increased urinary frequency, abnormal kidney function, severe hemorrhagic cystitis, ***renal failure***, uric acid nephropathy. **Musculoskeletal**: Arthralgia, myalgia, bone pain, joint disorder, local/diffuse musculoskeletal pain, joint stiffness, cramps. **Miscellaneous**: Pain in the extremities, injection site reaction (including pain, swelling, or redness), night sweats, peripheral edema, increased/decreased appetite, excessive thirst, weight loss, face/lesional edema, ***septic shock, sepsis***, infection, malaise, fatigue, metabolic acidosis, glucose intolerance, immunogenicity.

P

LABORATORY TEST CONSIDERATIONS

↑ AST, ALT, amylase, lipase, gamma-glutamyltranspeptidase, BUN, creatinine. Hyperbilirubinemia, hyperglycemia, hyperuricemia, hypoglycemia, hypoproteinemia, hyperammonemia, hyponatremia, hypoalbuminemia, proteinuria.

DRUG INTERACTIONS

Depletion of serum proteins by pegaspargase may ↑ the toxicity of other drugs which are protein bound. ↑ Predisposition to bleeding when used with warfarin, heparin, dipyridamole, aspirin, or NSAIDs. May ↓ the effect of methotrexate.

HOW SUPPLIED

Injection: 750 units/mL.

DOSAGE

IM (PREFERRED); IV

Acute lymphoblastic leukemia.

Adults: 2,500 international units/m^2 no more frequently than q 14 days. This dose is also used if the drug is given as a sole agent. **Children with a BSA greater than 0.6 m^2:** 2,500 international units/m^2 no more frequently than q 14 days. **Children with a BSA less than 0.6 m^2:** 82.5 international units/kg no more frequently than q 14 days.

NURSING IMPLICATIONS

Do not confuse pegaspargase (Oncaspar) with asparaginase (Elspar), each of which is an antineoplastic drugs.

IMPLEMENTATION/ADMINISTRATION/STORAGE

1. The preferred route of administration is IM due to a lower risk of hepatotoxicity, coagulopathy, and GI and renal disorders.
2. Do not give if there is any indication drug has been frozen; freezing destroys pegaspargase activity.
3. When given IM, do not exceed 2 mL to a single injection site; if more than 2 mL is necessary, use multiple injection sites.
4. When remission is obtained, appropriate maintenance therapy may be instituted.
5. Do not shake; avoid excessive agitation. Do not use if cloudy, if a precipitate is present, or if drug has been stored at room temperature for more than 48 hr.
6. Store at 2–8°C (36–46°F).
7. Use only one dose per vial; do not reenter the vial. Discard any unused portions.
8. IV When used IV, administer over a 1- to 2-hr period in 100 mL of NSS or D5W, through an infusion tube of a solution that is already running.
9. COMPATIBILITY D5W, NSS.
10. INCOMPATIBILITY Do not admix with other medications or solutions.

ASSESSMENT

1. List disease onset, characteristics of S&S, other agents trialed/failed.
2. Note previous therapy and outcome. Use the National Cancer Institute Common Toxic Criteria to grade the severity of any hypersensitivity reaction.
3. Anticipate giving with other antineoplastic agents. Monitor continuously for anaphylaxis during the first hour of therapy.
4. Drug may be a contact irritant. Wear gloves and avoid inhalation of vapors and contact with skin or mucous membrane. In case of contact, wash with copious amounts of water for at least 15 min.
5. Assess for early S&S of infection due to immunosuppressive effects; or pancreatitis (↑ amylase). Ensure adequate hydration to prevent hyperuricemia.
6. IM administration may decrease many of the drug-associated adverse systemic effects.
7. Assess for evidence of pancreatitis or bone marrow depression.
8. Monitor CBC, glucose, amylase, uric acid level, renal and LFTs.

CLIENT/FAMILY TEACHING

1. Given IM or IV as chemotherapy with or without other agents depending on condition being treated.
2. Avoid agents that may increase bleeding (e.g., aspirin/NSAIDs, alcohol). Report bruising or bleeding, and any early S&S of infection.
3. Report any persistent N&V, yellow skin discoloration, difficulty breathing, swelling, severe headaches, chest pain, rash, or severe abdominal pain immediately. Report any altered mental status or evidence of seizure activity.

4. **Increase fluid intake to 2–3 L/day to prevent urate deposits/calculi formation. Consume diet low in purines to maintain alkaline urine.**
5. **Drug lowers resistance to infections; avoid situations that may put one at risk (i.e., crowds, persons with infectious diseases, vaccinia).**
6. **Keep all F/U to assess response, labs, adverse SE.**

OUTCOMES/EVALUATE

Improved hematologic parameters; remission of acute lymphoblastic leukemia

Pegfilgrastim

(peg-fill-**GRAH**-stim)

Classification(s): Hematopoietic agent

Pregnancy Category: C

RX: Neulasta.

INDICATIONS/USES

Decrease incidence of infection, as demonstrated by febrile neutropenia, in clients with nonmyeloid malignancies who are receiving myelosuppressive anticancer drugs associated with a significant incidence of febrile neutropenia.

ACTION/KINETICS

Action

A colony stimulating factor that binds to specific cell surface receptors of hematopoietic cells resulting in proliferation, differentiation, commitment, and end cell function activation. Has same mechanism of action as filgrastim but has decreased renal clearance and prolonged activity compared with filgrastim.

Pharmacokinetics

A single SC dose will stimulate hematopoiesis for up to 14 days. Clients with higher body weights experienced higher systemic exposure after receiving a dose normalized for body weight. **t½:** 15–80 hr after SC.

CONTRAINDICATIONS

Known hypersensitivity to *Escherichia coli*-derived proteins, pegfilgrastim, filgrastim, or any component of the product. Use of the 6 mg fixed-dose single-use syringe formulation in infants, children, and smaller adolescents weighing less than 45 kg. Use between 14 days before and 24 hr after cytotoxic chemotherapy due to the potential for an increase in sensitivity of rapidly dividing myeloid cells to cytotoxic chemotherapy.

SPECIAL CONCERNS

- **Pegfilgrastim may act as a growth factor for any tumor type.**
- **Safety and efficacy not determined for peripheral blood progenitor cell mobilization; do not use for this purpose.**
- **Potential for immunogenicity.**
- **Use with caution during lactation.**
- **Safety and efficacy not established in children.**

SIDE EFFECTS

Most Common

Most side effects appear to be due to the underlying malignancy or cytotoxic chemotherapy. Medullary bone pain.

GI: Nausea, diarrhea, vomiting, constipation, anorexia, taste perversion, dyspepsia, abdominal pain, stomatitis, mucositis, ***splenic rupture***. **CNS**: Headache, insomnia, dizziness. **Allergic**: ***Anaphylaxis***, skin rash, urticaria. **Musculoskeletal:** Arthralgia, bone pain, myalgia, medullary bone pain. **Respiratory:** Hypoxia, ***ARDS***. **Dermatologic:** Alopecia, generalized erythema and flushing, acute febrile neutrophilic dermatosis. **Hematologic:** Granulocytopenia, leukocytosis, neutropenic fever. **Body as a whole**: Fatigue, fever, generalized weakness/asthenia, peripheral edema. **Miscellaneous**: Sickle cell crisis with sickle cell disease, injection site reactions (pain, induration, local erythema).

LABORATORY TEST CONSIDERATIONS

↑ LDH, alkaline phosphatase, uric acid (all are reversible).

OVERDOSE MANAGEMENT

Symptoms: Leukocytosis. *Treatment:* Consider leukapheresis in symptomatic clients.

DRUG INTERACTIONS

Lithium may potentiate the release of neutrophils; if used together with pegfilgrastim, monitor neutrophil counts more frequently.

HOW SUPPLIED

Injection Solution: 10 mg/mL (preservative-free).

P

DOSAGE

SC

Myelosuppressive chemotherapy.

Adults: Single 6 mg dose given once per chemotherapy cycle. Do not give the 6 mg fixed-dose formulation in infants, children, or smaller adolescents weighing less than 45 kg. For children weighing more than 45 kg, give 6 mg SC once per chemotherapy cycle.

NURSING IMPLICATIONS

IMPLEMENTATION/ADMINISTRATION/STORAGE

1. Not to be given during the 14 days preceding a dose of cytotoxic drugs through the first 24 hr afterward.
2. Visually inspect for discoloration and particulate matter before administration. Do not give if discoloration/particulate matter are noted.
3. Refrigerate at 2–8°C (36–46°F) and keep syringes in their carton to protect from light until use.
4. Avoid shaking. May be allowed to reach room temperature for a maximum of 48 hr before use, but protect from light. Discard any drug left at room temperature for more than 48 hr.
5. Avoid freezing. If accidentally frozen, allow to thaw in the refrigerator before administration. Discard if frozen a second time.

ASSESSMENT

1. Note reasons for therapy and chemotherapeutic agents being used.
2. Assess for any conditions that may preclude therapy, e.g. , sickle cell anemia, fever, respiratory distress, enlarged spleen. Document any S&S of splenic enlargement (e.g., LUQ pain, or shoulder tip pain).
3. Monitor bone pain, and assess pulmonary status noting any S&S of ARDS (e.g., fever, respiratory distress).
4. Obtain CBC with platelet count before giving chemotherapy; monitor regularly with alkaline phosphatase, LDH, uric acid.

CLIENT/FAMILY TEACHING

1. Review S&S of allergic drug reactions and appropriate actions to take. Report abdominal pain, shoulder pain, fever, or breathing problems immediately.
2. Ensure product is refrigerated as directed. Do not freeze. Must be compliant with therapy; have regular monitoring of blood counts.
3. May be given at home if instruction on the proper use of the drug is completed. Do not reuse syringes, needles, or drug products and follow proper disposal techniques. Use puncture-resistant container and guidelines for proper disposal of used needles and syringes.
4. Usually given SC during chemotherapy cycle; do not give 14 days before and 24 hr after cytotoxic chemotherapy. Do not shake syringe or use if particulate matter, cloudiness, or discoloration noted in solution.
5. Immediately report any adverse side effects or high fevers. Potential exists for tumor cell growth with this product.
6. Keep all F/U visits to assess response, labs, and for adverse SE.

OUTCOMES/EVALUATE

- Reduced incidence of infection during myelosuppressive chemotherapy
- ↑ Neutrophil production within bone marrow

Peginterferon alfa-2a

(**peg**-in-ter-**FEAR**-on)

Classification(s): Immunomodulator

Pregnancy Category: C

RX: Pegasys.

INDICATIONS/USES

(1) Chronic hepatitis B. Adults with HbeAg-positive and HbeAg-negative chronic hepatitis B virus infection who have compensated liver disease and evidence of viral replication and liver inflammation. (2) Chronic hepatitis C virus infection in adults who have compensated liver disease and have not been previously treated with interferon alpha. Efficacy demonstrated in those with compensated liver disease and histological evidence of cirrhosis (Child-Pugh class A) and those with HIV disease that is clinically stable (i.e., antiretroviral therapy not required, receiving stable antiretroviral therapy). *Investigational:* Renal cell carcinoma, chronic myelogenous leukemia.

ACTION/KINETICS

Action

Interferons bind to specific receptors on the cell surface initiating intracellular signaling via a complex cascade of protein-protein interactions; this leads to rapid activation of gene transcription. Interferon-stimulated genes modulate many biological effects, including inhibition of viral replication in infected cells, inhibition of cell proliferation, and immunomodulation. Peginterferon alfa-2a stimulates production of effector proteins (e.g., serum neopterin and 2',5"-oligoadenylate synthetase), raises body temperature, and causes reversible decreases in leukocyte and platelet counts.

Pharmacokinetics

Maximum serum levels: 72–96 hr (sustained for up to 168 hr). **Steady-state:** Serum levels reached in 5–8 weeks. **t½, terminal:** 80 hr (range: 50–140 hr). AUC is increased in clients over 62 years of age. Is a 25–45% reduction in clearance in those with end-stage renal disease. Clearance in children is nearly 4-fold lower compared with that in adults.

CONTRAINDICATIONS

Peginterferon alfa-2a alone: Hypersensitivity to peginterferon alfa-2a or any of its components; autoimmune hepatitis; hepatic decompensation (Child-Pugh score greater than 6–class B and C) in cirrhotic hepatitis C clients coinfected with HIV before or during treatment with peginterferon alfa-2a. Use in neonates and infants (contains benzyl alcohol). **Peginterferon alfa-2a with ribavirin:** Hypersensitivity to ribavirin tablets or to any component; pregnancy; men whose female partners are pregnant; those with hemoglobinopathies (e.g., thalessemia major, sickle-cell anemia). Lactation (alone or with ribavirin).

SPECIAL CONCERNS

(1) Alpha interferons, including peginterferon alfa-2a may cause or aggravate fatal or life-threatening neuropsychiatric, autoimmune, ischemic, or infectious disorders. Monitor clients closely with periodic clinical and lab evaluations. Withdraw therapy in clients with persistently severe or worsening signs or symptoms of these conditions. In many, but not all cases, these disorders resolve after stopping peginterferon alfa-2a therapy. (2) Combination therapy with ribavirin. Ribavirin may cause birth defects and/or death of the fetus. Extreme care must be taken to avoid pregnancy in women taking peginterferon alfa-2a and in female partners of men taking peginterferon alfa-2a. (3) Ribavirin causes hemolytic anemia. The anemia associated with ribavirin therapy may result in a worsening of cardiac disease. (4) Because ribavirin is genotoxic and mutagenic, consider it a potential carcinogen.

- **Use with caution in pre-existing cardiac disease, in those with a history of depression, in those with a creatinine clearance less than 50 mL/min, and in those with baseline neutrophil counts under 1,500 cells/mm^3, baseline platelet counts less than 90,000/mm^3, or baseline hemoglobin less than 10 grams/dL.**
- **Contains benzyl alcohol which is associated with an increased incidence of neurological and other complications in neonates and infants (may be fatal).**
- **Side effects may be more severe in the elderly.**
- **Safety and efficacy not determined in children under age 18.**

SIDE EFFECTS

Most Common

Peginterferon alfa-2a used alone: Depression, dizziness, fatigue/asthenia, headache, insomnia, irritability/anxiety, alopecia, pruritus, abdominal pain, diarrhea, N&V, neutropenia, anorexia, arthralgia, myalgia, injection site reaction, pyrexia, rigors.

NOTE: If used with ribavirin, consult information on that drug as well. **CNS:** Depression, irritability, anxiety, nervousness, headache, insomnia, dizziness, impaired concentration/memory, depressed mood. Neuropsychiatric reactions, including aggressive behavior, psychoses, hallucinations, bipolar disorders, mania, suicidal ideation, ***suicide***, homicidal ideation, depression, relapse of drug addiction, drug overdose. **GI:** N&V, anorexia, diarrhea, abdominal pain, dry mouth, dyspepsia, hepatic dysfunction, fatty liver, cholangitis, peptic ulcer, GI bleeding, ***pancreatitis, colitis (hemorrhagic/ischemic)***, exacerbations of hepatitis during hepatitis B therapy. **Hematologic:** Neutropenia, thrombocytopenia, lymphopenia, aplastic anemia (rare). **CV:** Arrhythmia, endocarditis, hypertension, supraventricular arrhythmias, chest pain, ***MI, pulmonary embolism, cerebral***

P

hemorrhage. **Dermatologic:** Alopecia, pruritus, increased sweating, dermatitis, rash, dry skin, eczema. **Musculoskeletal:** Myalgia, arthralgia, back pain, myositis. **Respiratory:** Pneumonia, cough, interstitial pneumonitis, dyspnea, pulmonary infiltrates, bronchiolitis obliterans, sarcoidosis. **Ophthalmic:** Corneal ulcer, decrease/loss of vision, macular edema, retinal artery or vein thrombosis, retinal hemorrhage, cotton wool spots, optic neuritis, papilledema. **Hypersensitivity:** Urticaria, angioedema, bronchoconstriction, ***anaphylaxis***. **Body as a whole:** Flu-like symptoms (fatigue, pyrexia, myalgia, headache, rigors), pain, asthenia, autoimmune phenomena, decreased weight, infections, hypo-/hyperglycemia, bacterial infections (sepsis, osteomyelitis, endocarditis, pyelonephritis). **Miscellaneous:** Injection site reaction, diabetes mellitus, peripheral neuropathy, impaired renal function, coma, aggravation of hypo-/hyperthyroidism. Development of or exacerbation of autoimmune disorders, including hepatitis, idiopathic thrombocytopenia purpura, interstitial nephritis, myositis, psoriasis, rheumatoid arthritis, systemic lupus erythematosus, thrombotic thrombocytopenic purpura, thyroiditis.

LABORATORY TEST CONSIDERATIONS

↑ ALT (transient), triglycerides. ↓ WBC, ANC, platelet counts. Abnormal thyroid lab values.

OVERDOSE MANAGEMENT

Symptoms: Fatigue, elevated liver enzymes, neutropenia, thrombocytopenia. *Treatment:* There is no specific antidote. Hemodialysis and peritoneal dialysis are ineffective.

P

DRUG INTERACTIONS

Methadone / ↑ (10–15%) Methadone levels after 4 weeks of treatment with peginterferon alfa-2a

Nucleoside reverse transcriptase inhibitors (didanosine, stabudine, zidobudine) / ↑ Hematologic toxicity; possible fatal hepatic decomposition

Theophylline / ↑ Theophylline AUC R/T inhibition of CYP1A2; monitor theophylline levels

HOW SUPPLIED

Injection: 180 mcg/mL.

DOSAGE

SC

Chronic hepatitis B.

Peginterferon alfa-2a monotherapy: 180 mcg once weekly for 48 weeks by SC injection in the abdomen or thigh.

Chronic hepatitis C in adults.

Peginterferon alfa-2a monotherapy: 180 mcg once a week for 48 weeks by SC injection in the abdomen or thigh. If dosage reduction is needed due to moderate to severe side effects, reduce dose to 135 mcg; in some cases drug reduction to 90 mcg may be necessary. Following improvement of side effects, re-escalation of dose may be considered. **When combined with ribavirin:** Dose depends on viral genotype. **Genotype 1, 4:** Peginterferon alfa-2a, 180 mcg as above. If weight is less than 75 kg, give ribavirin 1,000 mg/day. If weight is 75 kg or more, give ribavirin 1,200 mg/day. Duration of therapy is 48 weeks. **Genotype 2, 3:** Peginterferon alfa-2a, 180 mcg once a week with ribavirin 800 mg/day for 24 weeks.

Chronic hepatitis C with HIV.

Peginterferon alfa-2a monotherapy: 180 mcg once weekly for 48 weeks by SC injection into the abdomen or thigh. **Combination therapy with ribavirin:** 180 mcg peginterferon alfa-2a weekly and 800 mg ribavirin PO every day for 48 weeks, regardless of genotype.

NURSING IMPLICATIONS

IMPLEMENTATION/ADMINISTRATION/STORAGE

1. For the 180 mcg dose, can use either the 1 mL vial or the 0.5 mL prefilled syringe, each of which contains 180 mcg of the drug.
2. There are no safety and efficacy data for treating chronic HCV or HBV for longer than 48 weeks. For those with HCV, consider discontinuing after 12–24 weeks if there is no demonstrable response.
3. Consider dose reduction to 135 mcg if the neutrophil count is <750 cells/mm^3. If ANC falls below 500 cells/mm^3, suspend treatment until ANC values return to >1,000 cells/mm^3. Initially reinstitute therapy at 90 mcg and monitor neutrophil count.
4. Reduce dose to 135 mcg in clients with end-stage renal disease requiring hemodialysis.
5. If platelets decrease to <50,000/mm^3, reduce dose to 90 mcg. Discontinue peginter-

feron alfa-2a if the platelet count decreases to <25,000/mm^3.

6. In end-stage renal disease requiring hemodialysis, reduce the dose to 135 mcg. Monitor S&S of interferon toxicity closely. Do not use ribavirin in clients with a C_{CR} <50 mL/min.
7. In chronic hepatitis C clients with progressive ALT increases above baseline values, reduce dose to 135 mcg. Perform more frequent monitoring of liver function. Therapy can be resumed after ALT flares subside.
8. In chronic hepatitis B clients with elevations of ALT >5 times ULN, perform more frequent monitoring of liver function and consider either reducing the dose to 135 mcg or temporarily discontinuing treatment. Therapy can be resumed after ALT flares subside.
9. In hepatitis B clients with persistent, severe ALT values >10 times ULN, consider discontinuing treatment.
10. Check manufacturer's guidelines for modification or discontinuation of peginterferon alfa-2a for clients with depression.
11. Vials are for single use only; discard any unused portion. Prefilled syringes are available for ease of administration.
12. Store in the refrigerator but do not freeze. Do not shake. Protect from light.

ASSESSMENT

1. Note reasons for therapy, disease onset, genotype with hepatitis C, hepatitis Be antibody (HBeAg) positive and HBeAg negative with HBV, liver biopsy results, clinical presentation, other agents trialed, outcome.
2. Assess for CAD, depression, renal failure. Monitor BP, CBC, viral load, uric acid, renal, thyroid, LFTs and clinical presentation. Reduce dose as directed for specific deficits under *Implementation/Administration/Storage* and for adverse effects. May increase/reestablish dose once these subside.
3. List drugs prescribed to ensure none interact; with hepatitis C, ensure have not been treated previously with interferon alfa.
4. Review treatment criteria, i.e., platelets >90,000 cells/mm^3; ANC >1,500 cells/mm^3; creatinine <1.5 × ULN and TSH/T_4 WNL or controlled function.
5. Obtain baseline labs (hematologic, liver, and biochemical) and monitor: CBC q 2 weeks, chemistries/LFTs q 4 weeks, and TSH every 12 weeks. Progressive increases in ALT and bilirubin require interruption of therapy, as well as do severe depression/suicide ideations.

CLIENT/FAMILY TEACHING

1. Drug is used to prevent progressive liver destruction from the hepatitis C or hepatitis B virus (HBV). It is not known for sure if treatment will cure hepatitis C or prevent cirrhosis, liver failure, or liver cancer from infection with HCV/HBV. It is also not known if the drug will prevent transmission of HCV/HBV or HIV infection to others. Use protection and reliable birth control.
2. To minimize flu-like symptoms, administer drug at bedtime once a week (or as prescribed). Use antipyretics as needed.
3. Review procedure for storage (refrigeration), preparation, injection, and disposal of drug/equipment. Proper disposal of needles is imperative; do not reuse needles or syringes. A puncture-resistant container will be supplied for proper disposal of used needles and syringes at home.
4. Do not perform activities that require mental alertness until drug effects realized.
5. May experience depression, flu-like symptoms, bleeding abnormalities, visual problems, dizziness, disorientation, sleepiness, joint/muscle pains, fever, abdominal pain, bloody diarrhea, breathing problems, chills, and fatigue; report if persistent.
6. Must commit to a monitoring program for standard blood testing. Labs are required before beginning therapy and at periodic set intervals in order to continue drug therapy.
7. Practice reliable contraception during and for 6 months following combination therapy; may cause fetal death or birth defects.
8. Schedule activities/work to provide rest periods as fatigue accompanies therapy.
9. Report any severe depression, mood or behavioral changes or suicide thoughts immediately.
10. Keep all F/U to assess response, labs, adverse SE.

OUTCOMES/EVALUATE

- Inhibition of viral replication/proliferation with hepatitis C and hepatitis B
- ↓ HCV/HBV/HIV RNA; ↓ liver inflammation/fibrosis

P

Peginterferon alfa-2b

(peg-**in**-ter-**FEER**-on)

Classification(s): Immunomodulator

Pregnancy Category: C; X (when used with ribavirin)

RX: PegIntron, Sylatron.

INDICATIONS/USES

PegIntron. (1) Monotherapy (for those intolerant to ribavirin) to treat chronic hepatitis C in those with compensated liver disease who have not been previously treated with interferon alpha and who are 18 years of age and older. (2) In combination with ribavirin capsules to treat chronic hepatitis C in adults who have compensated liver disease and have not been treated previously with interferon alfa and are 3 years of age and older. *NOTE:* When used with ribavirin, consult ribavirin information as well.

Sylatron. For adjuvant treatment of melanoma with microscopic or gross nodal involvement within 84 days of definitive surgical resection, including complete lymphadenectomy.

Investigational: Renal cell carcinoma, chronic myelogenous leukemia, metastatic melanoma.

ACTION/KINETICS

Action

The drug induces innate antiviral immune response. Peginterferon alfa-2b binds to and activates the human type 1 interferon receptor. Upon binding, the receptor subunits dimerize and activate multiple intracellular signal transduction pathways. This initiates a complex series of intracellular effects, including suppression of cell cycle progression/cell proliferation, induction of apoptosis, anti-angiogenic activities, enhancement of phagocytic activity of macrophages, activation of natural killer cells, stimulation of cytotoxic T-lymphocytes, upregulation of the Th1 T-helper cell subset, and inhibition of virus replication in virus-infected cells. The mechanism for its effect in clients with melanoma is unknown.

Pharmacokinetics

PegIntron. Mean absorption t½ after SC: 4.6 hr. **Maximum serum levels:** 15–44 hr; serum levels sustained for 48 hr (or less) to 72 hr. Both AUC and C_{max} increased by 70% when drug is given with ribavirin capsules and a high-fat meal. **t½, elimination:** About 40 hr. About 30% excreted in the urine. Clearance is decreased by about one-half in those with impaired renal function. **Sylatron. t½, mean terminal:** After a dose of 3 and 6 mcg/kg once a weak, the mean terminal t½ was about 43 hr and 51 hr respectively.

CONTRAINDICATIONS

Hypersensitivity to peginterferon alfa, interferon alfa, or any component of the product. Autoimmune hepatitis. Lactation. **Peginterferon alfa-2b:** Decompensated liver disease (Child-Pugh class B and C) in cirrhotic chronic hepatitis C clients before or during treatment. Lactation. **Peginterferon alfa-2b and ribavirin:** In addition to above, hypersensitivity to ribavirin capsules or any other component of the product; pregnancy; men whose female partners are pregnant; those with hemoglobinopathies (e.g., thalessemia major, sickle-cell anemia), C_{CR} <50 mL/min; use with a history of significant or unstable cardiac disease. Neonates and infants (product contains benzyl alcohol). **Sylatron:** Hepatic decompensation (Child–Pugh score >6, i.e., Class B and C).

SPECIAL CONCERNS

■ (1) **PegIntron**. Alpha interferons, including PegIntron, may cause or aggravate fatal or life-threatening neuropsychiatric, autoimmune, ischemic, and infectious disorders. Closely monitor clients with periodic clinical and lab evaluations. Withdraw clients with persistently severe or worsening signs or symptoms of these conditions from therapy. In many, but not all cases, these disorders resolve after stopping PegIntron. (2) **Ribavirin use.** Ribavirin may cause birth defects and/or death of the fetus. Take extreme care to avoid pregnancy in women and in female partners of men. Ribavirin causes hemolytic anemia. The anemia associated with ribavirin therapy may result in worsening of cardiac disease. Ribavirin is genotoxic and mutagenic; consider it a potential carcinogen. (3) **Sylatron. Depression and other neuropsychiatric disorders.** The risk of serious depression with suicidal ideation, completed suicides, and other serious neuropsychiatric disorders are increased with alpha interferons, including Sylatron. Permanently discontinue Sylatron in clients with persistently severe or worsening signs or symptoms of depression, psychosis,

P

or encephalopathy. These disorders may not resolve after stopping Sylatron.

- **Serious, acute hypersensitivity reactions, although rare, may occur.**
- **When combined with ribavirin, side effects are common and severe.**
- **Use with extreme caution in those with a history of psychiatric disorders; use with caution in those with debilitating medical conditions, such as history of pulmonary disease (e.g., COPD).**
- **Use with caution in those with a C_{CR} less than 50 mL/min, in the elderly, and in CV disease.**
- **May be development or worsening of autoimmune disorders (e.g., thyroiditis, thrombocytopenia, rheumatoid arthritis, interstitial nephritis, SLE, psoriasis).**
- **Chronic hepatitis C clients with cirrhosis may be at risk of hepatic decompensation and death.**
- **Weight and height gain of children treated with peginterferon alfa-2b plus ribavirin lags behind that predicted by normative population data for the entire time of treatment.**
- **Safety and efficacy not determined for the treatment of clients with HCV coinfected with HIV or HBV or to treat hepatitis C in clients who have received liver or other organ transplants.**
- **Safety and efficacy not determined when used alone or in combination with ribavirin capsules to treat hepatitis C in those who have received liver or other organ transplants.**
- **Use with caution in the elderly; side effects may be greater in those with impaired renal function.**
- **Safety and efficacy not determined using peginterferon alfa-2b alone or in combination with ribavirin in those who have failed other alpha interferon therapy.**
- **Safety and efficacy not determined in children less than 3 years of age.**

SIDE EFFECTS

Most Common

PegIntron, Adults: Headache, fatigue/asthenia, myalgia, injection site inflammation/reaction, anxiety/irritability, depression, insomnia, alopecia, anorexia, nausea, arthralgia, musculoskeletal pain, fever, rigors, dizziness, impaired concentration, dry skin, pruritus, abdominal pain, pharyngitis, weight loss.

PegIntron, Children, 3 years and older: Pyrexia, headache, vomiting, neutropenia, fatigue, anorexia, injection-site erythema, abdominal pain

Sylatron: Fatigue, ↑ ALT/AST, depression, pyrexia, headache, anorexia, myalgia, nausea, chills, injection–site reaction.

Side effects also include use with ribavirin. **PegIntron. CNS:** Headache, depression, dizziness, emotional lability, irritability, insomnia, agitation, anxiety, aggressive reaction, anger, loss of consciousness, nerve palsy (e.g., facial, oculomotor), impaired concentration, nervousness, psychosis, relapse of drug addiction/overdose, memory loss, migraine, paresthesia, peripheral neuropathy, ***seizures***, vertigo, ***suicide, suicidal ideation, suicide attempts, homicidal ideation***. **GI:** N&V, abdominal pain, upper abdominal pain, anorexia, diarrhea, dry mouth, dyspepsia, constipation, gastroenteritis, ***pancreatitis***, aphthous stomatitis, dental/periodontal disorders, ***ulcerative or hemorrhagic/ischemic colitis***. **CV:** Angina, ***cardiomyopathy, MI***, pericardial effusion, supraventricular arrhythmias, TIA, vasculitis, palpitations, hyper-/hypotension, ischemic/hemorrhagic CV events, ***stroke, cardiac arrest***. **Hepatic:** Hepatomegaly, ***hepatic decompensation and death*** in those with cirrhosis. **Musculoskeletal:** Myalgia, musculoskeletal pain, arthralgia, rigors, rheumatoid arthritis, myositis, rhabdomyolysis. **Dermatologic:** Alopecia, dry skin, flushing, pruritus, rash, increased sweating, aggravated psoriasis, phototoxicity, urticaria, erythema multiforme, ***Stevens-Johnson syndrome, toxic epidermal necrolysis***. **Respiratory:** Pharyngitis, coughing, dyspnea, rhinitis, sinusitis, bronchiolitis obliterans, emphysema, pleural effusion, pulmonary hypertension, interstitial pneumonitis, pneumonia, pulmonary infiltrates, sarcoidosis. **GU:** Menstrual disorder, interstitial nephritis, renal failure/insufficiency. **Hematologic:** Neutropenia, anemia, hemolytic anemia, leukopenia, thrombocytopenia, autoimmune thrombocytopenia with/without purpura, idiopathic thrombocytopenic purpura, pure red cell aplasia, thrombotic thrombocytopenic purpura. **Metabolic/Endocrine:** Hyper-/hypothyroidism, thyroiditis, gout, hyperglycemia, diabetes, diabetic ketoacidosis, dehydration. **Hypersensitivity:** ***Angioedema***, bronchoconstriction, urticaria, ***anaphylaxis***. **Injection site:** Inflammation, bruising, erythema, itchiness, irritation, necrosis, pain. **Ophthalmic:** Conjunctivitis, blurred vision, blindness, decreased visual acuity, decreased/loss of vision, optic neuritis, retinal artery or vein thrombosis, retinal ischemia/hemorrhages, serious retinal detachment, retinopathy (including macular edema), cotton wool spots, neuritis, papilledema. **Otic:** Hearing loss/ impairment. **Body as a whole:** Fatigue, asthenia, chills, malaise, fever/pyrexia, weight loss, flu–like illness, bacterial/fungal/viral infections, infection (abscess, cellulitis, pneumonia, ***sepsis***), ***death***. **Miscellaneous:** Taste perversion, chest pain, right upper quadrant pain, unspecified pain, systemic lupus erythematosus, lupus-like syndrome, pain in extremity, Vogt-Koyanagi-Harada syndrome, immunogenicity.

Sylatron. CNS: Headache, depression, dizziness, paresthesia, olfactory nerve disorder. **GI:** N&V, diarrhea, dysgeusia. **Hepatic:** Hepatic decompensation and death in those with cirrhosis. **CV:** BBB, ***MI,*** ventricular tachycardia, supraventricular arrhythmia, hypotension, ***cardiomyopathy***, angina pectoris. **Metabolic/Endocrine:** Anorexia, decreased weight. New onset or worsening of hypothyroidism, hyperthyroidism, and diabetes mellitus. **Ophthalmic:** Decreased/loss of vision, blurred vision, decreased visual acuity, retinopathy (including macular edema), retinal artery/vein thrombosis, retinal hemorrhages, cotton wool spots, optic neuritis, papilledema, serious retinal detachment. **Body as a whole:** Fatigue, pyrexia, chills. **Miscellaneous:** Injection site reaction, immunogenicity.

LABORATORY TEST CONSIDERATIONS

PegIntron: ↑ ALT, triglycerides, total bilirubin, serum creatinine (especially in those with renal impairment). ↓ Neutrophils, hemoglobin, platelets. TSH abnormalities. Appearance of serum neutralizing antibodies. When used with ribavirin: Hyperbilirubinemia, hyperuricemia (with hemolysis). **Sylatron:** ↑ ALT, AST, GGT, blood alkaline phosphatase.

DRUG INTERACTIONS

CYP2C8/9 substrates (e.g., phenytoin, warfarin) / ↓ Therapeutic effect of these substrates → ↓ pharmacologic effect; evaluate the response and adjust dose if needed

CYP2D6 substrates (e.g., flecainide) / ↓ Therapeutic effect of these substrates → ↓ pharmacologic effect; evaluate the response and adjust dose if needed

Didanosine / Possible fatal hepatic failure, peripheral neuropathy, pancreatitis, and symptomatic hyperlactatemia/lactic acidosis; do not use together

Methadone / ↑ Methadone plasma levels → ↑ pharmacologic/toxic effects; monitor S&S and adjust dose as needed

Nucleoside reverse transcriptase inhibitors (NRTI) used with peginterferon alfa-2b with/without ribavirin / Treatment toxicities, including hepatic decompensation, anemia, especially in cirrhotic HIV/HCV coinfected clients; closely monitor and discontinue the NRTI; discontinue ribavirin/interferon if toxicity develops

Pyrimidine nucleoside analogs (e.g., lamivudine, stavudine, zidovudine) with peginterferon alfa-2b with ribavirin / Possible severe neutropenia and anemia may develop in HIV/HCV coinfected clients; closely monitor

Telbivudine / Peripheral neuropathy possible; safety and efficacy of the combination not shown

HOW SUPPLIED

Injection, Powder for Solution, Lyophilized (PegIntron): 50 mcg/0.5 mL, 80 mcg/0.5 mL, 120 mcg/ 0.5 mL, 150 mcg/0.5 mL (all strengths are after reconstitution); ***Injection, Powder for Solution, Lyophilized (Sylatron):*** 40 mcg/0.1 mL, 60 mcg/ 0.1 mL, 120 mcg/0.1 mL (all strengths are after reconstitution).

DOSAGE

PegIntron.

SC

Chronic hepatitis C in adults (PegIntron with/ without ribavirin).

Adults, monotherapy, initial: Based on weight. Dose of 1 mcg/kg is given once weekly (on the same day of each week) for 1 year. Doses, based on body weight, are: **45 kg or less:** 40 mcg (0.4 mL of the 50 mcg/0.5 mL strength); **46–56 kg:** 50 mcg (0.5 mL of the 50 mcg/0.5 mL strength); **57–72 kg:** 64 mcg (0.4 mL of the 80 mcg/ 0.5 mL strength); **73–88 kg:** 80 mcg (0.5 mL of the 80 mcg/0.5 mL strength); **89–106 kg:** 96 mcg (0.4 mL of the 120 mcg/0.5 mL strength); **107–136 kg:** 120 mcg (0.5 mL of the 120 mcg/0.5 mL strength); **137–160 kg:** 150 mcg (0.5 mL of the 150 mcg/ 0.5 mL strength).

Adults, when used with ribavirin: 1.5 mcg/kg/week of peginterferon alfa-

2b when given with ribavirin 800–1,400 mg capsules. Doses of peginterferon alfa-2b, based on body weight, are: **<40 kg:** 50 mcg (0.5 mL of the 40 mcg/0.5 mL strength) plus ribavirin, 800 mg/day (400 mg in the a.m. and 400 mg in the p.m.); **40–50 kg:** 64 mcg (0. 4 mL of the 80 mcg/0.5 mL strength) plus ribavirin, 800 mg/day (400 mg in the a.m. and 400 mg in the p.m.); **51–60 kg:** 80 mcg (0.5 mL of the 80 mcg/0.5 mL strength) plus ribavirin, 800 mg/day (400 mg in the a.m. and 400 mg in the p.m.): **61–65 kg:** 96 mcg (0.4 mL of the 120 mcg/0.5 mL strength) plus ribavirin, 800 mg/day (400 mg in the a.m. and 400 mg in the p.m.); **66–75 kg:** 96 mcg (0.4 mL of the 120 mcg/0.5 mL strength) plus ribavirin, 1,000 mg/day (400 mg in the a.m. and 600 mg in the p.m.); **76–80 kg:** 120 mcg (0.5 mL of the 120 mcg/ 0.5 mL strength) plus ribavirin, 1,000 mg/day (400 mg in the a.m. and 600 mg in the p.m.; **81–85 kg:** 120 mcg (0.5 mL of the 120 mcg/0.5 ml strength) plus ribavirin, 1,200 mg (600 mg in the a.m. and 600 mg in the p.m.); **86–105 kg:** 150 mcg (0.5 mL of the 150 mcg/0.5 mL strength) plus ribavirin, 1,200 mg/day (600 mg in the a.m. and 600 mg in the a.m.); **>105 kg:** 1.5 mcg/kg/week based on client weight plus ribavirin, 1,400 mg/day (600 mg in the a.m. and 800 mg in the p.m.). *NOTE:* Do not use ribavirin in clients with C_{CR} less than 50 mL/min. The duration of treatment for those with genotype 1 is 48 weeks. Clients with genotype 2 and 3 should be treated for 24 weeks. The duration of treatment for those who previously failed therapy is 48 weeks, regardless of HCV genotype.

Chronic hepatitis C in children (PegIntron only with ribavirin).

Determine children's dosage by body surface area for peginterferon alfa-2b and by body weight for ribavirin. Children, 3–17 years of age, usual: Peginterferon alfa-2b, 60 mcg/m²/week SC in combination with ribavirin, 15 mg/kg/day PO or in 2 divided doses. **Recommended ribavirin dosing in combination therapy (to be used with peginterferon alfa-2b, 60 mcg/ m²/week. <47 kg:** Ribavirin, 15 mg/kg/day (use oral solution); **47–59 kg:** Ribavirin, 800 mg/kg/day (2 × 200 mg capsules in the a.m. and 2 × 200 mg capsules in the p.m.); **60–73 kg:** Ribavirin, 1,000 mg/kg/day (2 × 200 mg capsules in the a.m. and 3 × 200 mg capsules in the p.m.); **>73 kg:** Ribavirin, 1,200 mg/kg/day (3 × 200 mg capsules in the a.m. and 3 × 200 mg capsules in the p.m.). The treatment duration for clients with genotype 1 is 48 weeks and those with genotypes 2 and 3 should be treated for 24 weeks. Clients receiving peginterferon alfa-2b with ribavirin (excluding those with HCV genotype 2 and 3) should be discontinued from therapy at 12 weeks if their treatment week 12 HCV RNA dropped less than 2 $\log_{10}$ compared with pretreatment, or at 24 weeks if they have detectable HCV RNA at treatment week 24. *NOTE:* Children who reach 18 years of age while receiving combination therapy should remain on the pediatric dosing regimen.

Sylatron

SC

Melanoma.

Adults, usual: 6 mcg/kg/week SC for 8 doses, followed by 3 mcg/kg/week SC for up to 5 years. Premedicate with acetaminophen 500–1,000 mg PO 30 min prior to the first dose of peginterferon alfa-2b and as needed for subsequent doses. Permanently discontinue the drug for persistent or worsening severe neuropsychiatric disorders; grade 4 nonhematologic toxicity; inability to tolerate a dosage of 1 mcg/kg/week; or, new or worsening retinopathy.

NURSING IMPLICATIONS

IMPLEMENTATION/ADMINISTRATION/STORAGE

1. **PegIntron is available only through the PegIntron Access Assurance Program. Pharmacists**

or clients may call 1-888-437-2608 to register and obtain an authorization number and order information.

2. Reconstitute with 0.7 mL of supplied diluent (sterile water for injection). Swirl gently to hasten complete dissolution. Diluent vial is for single use only; discard any remaining diluent. Do not reconstitute with any other diluent.
3. Administer SC; rotate injection sites. When PegIntron is taken as part of combination therapy, take ribavirin with food.
4. Use immediately after reconstitution as the product contains no preservative; do not freeze.
5. Reconstituted solution should be clear and colorless. Do not use the solution if it is discolored, cloudy, or contains particulate matter.
6. Peginterferon alfa-2b is also available in an easier to use product called Redipen. To reconstitute, hold the Redipen upright (dose button down) and press the two halves of the pen together until there is an audible click. Gently invert the pen to mix the solution; do not shake. Keeping the pen upright, attach the supplied needle and select the appropriate peginterferon alfa-2b dose by pulling back on the dosing button until the dark bands are visible and turning the button until the dark band is aligned with the correct dose. Redipen is for single use only.
7. Do not add other medications to peginterferon alfa-2b solutions.
8. Consider discontinuing therapy in those who do not achieve at least a 2 $\log_{10}$ drop or loss of hepatitis C virus RNA at 12 weeks of therapy or whose HCV RNA levels remain detectable after 24 weeks of therapy.
9. In children receiving PegIntron, 60 mcg/m^2/week SC, exposure may be about 50% higher than that seen in adults receiving PegIntron, 1.5 mcg/kg/week SC.
10. Dose reduction in children of peginterferon alfa-2b is accomplished by modifying the recommended dose in a 2-step process from the original starting dose of 60 mcg/m^2/week to 40 mcg/m^2/week, then to 20 mcg/m^2/week, if needed.
11. If renal function decreases during therapy, discontinue peginterferon alfa-2b therapy. When peginterferon alfa-2b is given with ribavirin, those with impaired renal function or those older than 50 years should be monitored more carefully with respect to development of anemia.
12. Reduce the dose of peginterferon alfa-2b by 25% in those with a C_{CR} 30–50 mL/min and by 50% in those with a C_{CR} 10–29 mL/min.
13. Consult package insert for dose reduction instructions if adverse reactions (e.g., depression, hematologic toxicity) develop.
14. Store PegIntron and Sylatron vials of unreconstituted drug between 15–30°C (59–86°F). After reconstitution use immediately, but may be stored for 24 hr or less between 2–8°C (36–46°F). Do not freeze. Keep PegIntron vials away from heat.
15. Store PegIntron Redipen at 2–8°C (36–46°F). After reconstitution, use immediately; or, it may be stored up to 24 hr from 2–8°C (36–46°F).
16. The reconstituted solution contains no preservative; it is clear and colorless. Do not freeze.

ASSESSMENT

1. Note reasons for therapy, onset/characteristics of disease, other agents trialed. Assess mental status, history of depression. Note results of liver biopsy.
2. Ensure adequate hydration, especially during initial stages of treatment.
3. List any other medical conditions that may require monitoring during therapy; drug may aggravate hypo-/hyperthyroidism or diabetes control.
4. If Ribavirin also prescribed, may cause birth defects and fetal death. Use caution to avoid pregnancy in women and in female partners of men. Ribavirin causes hemolytic anemia, which may result in worsening of cardiac disease. It is also genotoxic and mutagenic and should be considered a potential carcinogen.
5. Ensure an eye exam prior to the start of therapy and periodically thereafter in those with diabetic or hypertensive retinopathy.
6. Monitor bilirubin, ALT, AST, alkaline phosphatase, and LDH at 2- and 8-week intervals, and 2 and 3 months following initiation of therapy, then every 6 months while receiving treatment.

7. With renal impairment assess for peginterferon toxicity, including increases in serum creatinine.
8. Evaluate CBC and blood chemistry before treatment, at weeks 2 and 4 of therapy, and periodically thereafter.
9. Obtain ECG in those with pre-existing cardiac abnormalities before treatment.
10. Determine any worsening depression, suicidal thoughts or ideation, aggressive behavior, or other psychiatric symptoms every 3 weeks during first 8 weeks of treatment, and every 6 months thereafter (monitor for these S&S for at least 6 months after the last dose.)
11. Check TSH levels within 4 wk prior to initiation of treatment, at 3 and 6 months following initiation, then every 6 months.
12. Obtain HCV levels before starting therapy and after 12 and 24 weeks of therapy. Be prepared to stop therapy in those who do not achieve a 2 log_{10} drop or loss of HCV-RNA at 12 weeks, or if HCV-RNA remains detectable after 24 weeks of therapy.
13. Persistent, severe, or worsening signs or symptoms may necessitate discontinuation of therapy.
14. Permanently discontinue peginterferon alfa-2b with persistently severe or worsening signs or symptoms of depression, psychosis, or encephalopathy. Understand that these disorders may not resolve after stopping peginterferon alfa-2b.
15. Monitor CBC, eye exams, TSH, renal, LFTs, viral load. Assess clients with impaired renal function for S&S of interferon toxicity; adjust dose or stop therapy accordingly.

CLIENT/FAMILY TEACHING

1. To minimize flu-like symptoms, administer the drug at bedtime once a week. Use antipyretics as needed to minimize these symptoms (take 500 to 1,000 mg of acetaminophen 30 min prior to first Sylatron dose and as needed for subsequent doses). After instruction may self administer SC; rotate sites. Follow "Instructions for use and administration guidelines" carefully.
2. Hepatitis C therapy (peginterferon) may last from 24 to 48 weeks whereas melanoma therapy may last up to 5 years depending on response (Sylatron).
3. It is not known if PegIntron treatment will cure hepatitis C or prevent cirrhosis, liver failure, or liver cancer that may result from infection with the hepatitis C virus. It is also not known if the drug will prevent transmission of HCV infection to others.
4. Sylatron is used as an adjuvant treatment of melanoma with microscopic or gross nodal involvement within 84 days of definitive surgical resection.
5. Once reconstituted, may only store in the refrigerator up to 24 hr. Pens can be stored refrigerated until use. Sylatron is for single use only; discard any unused portion.
6. Proper disposal of needles is imperative; do not reuse needles or syringes. A puncture-resistant container will be supplied for disposal of used needles and syringes at home.
7. Drug may cause depression, flu-like symptoms, bleeding abnormalities, sleep problems, fatigue, and autoimmune dysfunction. Report any unusual/adverse side effects.
8. Any worsening depression, or thoughts of hurting yourself, aggressive behavior towards others, or thoughts of hurting others, memory changes and confusion require immediate reporting.
9. Practice reliable contraception; may cause fetal harm/death.
10. Keep all F/U to assess response, labs and for adverse SE.

OUTCOMES/EVALUATE

- Inhibition of progression of hepatitis C; improved LFTs ↓ HCV RNA
- Prevention of recurrence of melanoma (Sylatron)

P

IV

Pemetrexed

(pem-e-**TREKS**-ed)

Classification(s): Antineoplastic, folic acid antagonist

Pregnancy Category: D

RX: Alimta.

INDICATIONS/USES

(1) In combination with cisplatin to treat malignant pleural mesothelioma that is unresectable or for clients who are not candidates for curative surgery. (2) Alone for locally advanced or metastatic

non-small-cell lung cancer after prior chemotherapy. (3) With cisplatin for the initial treatment of locally advanced or metastatic non-small-cell lung cancer. (4) Maintenance treatment of locally advanced or metastatic nonsquamous non-small-cell lung cancer where the disease has not progressed after 4 cycles of platinum-based first-line chemotherapy.

ACTION/KINETICS

Action

Pemetrexed acts by disrupting folate-dependent metabolic processes needed for cell replication. The drug is transported into cells by the reduced folate carrier and membrane folate binding protein transport systems. Once inside the cell, the drug is converted to polyglutamate forms by the enzyme folylpolyglutamate synthase. The polyglutamate forms are retained in cells and are inhibitors of thymidylate synthase and glycinamide ribonucleotide formyltransferase. Polyglutamation is a time- and concentration-dependent process that occurs in tumor cells (and to a lesser extent in normal cells). Polyglutamated metabolites have an increased intracellular half life, resulting in prolonged drug activity in malignant cells. Synergistic effects occur when combined with cisplatin.

Pharmacokinetics

Pemetrexed is not metabolized significantly; from 70–90% of a dose is eliminated in the urine within 24 hr. **t½, elimination:** 3.5 hr in clients with normal renal function. Plasma clearance in the presence of cisplatin decreases as renal function decreases. **Plasma protein binding:** About 81%.

P

CONTRAINDICATIONS

History of severe hypersensitivity to pemetrexed or any ingredient of the formulation. Use in clients whose C_{CR} is less than 45 mL/min. Lactation.

SPECIAL CONCERNS

- **Use with caution when given concurrently with NSAIDs to clients whose C_{CR} is less than 80 mL/min.**
- **Use care in dose selection in the elderly due to possible decreased renal function.**
- **Safety and efficacy not determined in children.**

SIDE EFFECTS

Most Common

N&V, anorexia, fatigue, dyspnea, sensory neuropathy, constipation, diarrhea, stomatitis, pharyngitis, anemia, myalgia, chest pain, edema, fever, infection without neutropenia.

NOTE: Side effects include those manifested when combined with cisplatin. **GI:** N&V, constipation, dyspepsia/heartburn, abdominal pain, anorexia, stomatitis, pharyngitis, diarrhea (without colostomy), colitis, dehydration, dysphagia, esophagitis, odynophagia, taste disturbance. **CNS:** Sensory/motor neuropathy, depression, mood alteration. **Hematologic:** Neutropenia, leukopenia, anemia, thrombocytopenia, febrile neutropenia. **CV:** Hypertension, thrombosis, embolism, arrhythmia, supraventricular arrhythmias, ***cardiac ischemia***. **Respiratory:** Dyspnea, chest pain, interstitial pneumonitis. **Dermatologic:** Alopecia, rash (higher incidence in men), desquamation, urticaria, pruritus/itching, erythema multiforme. **GU:** Renal failure, decreased glomerular filtration rate. **Musculoskeletal:** Arthralgia, myalgia. **Metabolic:** Dehydration, edema. **Ophthalmic:** Conjunctivitis, increased lacrimation, ocular surface disease. **Body as a whole:** Fatigue, fever, infection without neutropenia, infection with grade 3 or 4 neutropenia, febrile neutropenia, other infection, allergic reaction, hypersensitivity, radiation recall (in those who previously received radiotherapy).

LABORATORY TEST CONSIDERATIONS

↑ ALT, AST, GGT, creatinine. ↓ Creatinine clearance.

OVERDOSE MANAGEMENT

Symptoms: Neutropenia, anemia, thrombocytopenia, mucositis, rash, bone marrow suppression, infection with or without fever, diarrhea. *Treatment:* Institute general supportive measures. Possibly leucovorin for CTC grade 4 leukopenia lasting at least 3 days, CTC grade 4 neutropenia lasting at least 3 days, and immediately for CTC grade 4 thrombocytopenia, bleeding associated with grade 3 thrombocytopenia, or grade 3 or 4 mucositis. IV dose of leucovorin is 100 mg/m^2 once, followed by 50 mg/m^2 q 6 hr for 8 days.

DRUG INTERACTIONS

NSAIDs (e.g., ibuprofen) / Closely monitor for toxicity, especially myelosuppression, renal, and GI toxicity; interrupt dosing in those taking NSAIDs with long elimination t½s for at least 5 days before, the day of, and 2 days after pemetrexed administration

Nephrotoxic drugs / Possible delayed clearance of pemetrexed
Probenecid / Possible delayed clearance of pemetrexed

HOW SUPPLIED

Injection, Lyophilized Powder for Solution: 100 mg, 500 mg.

DOSAGE

IV INFUSION ONLY

Malignant pleural mesothelioma.

Adults: Pemetrexed, 500 mg/m^2, infused over 10 min on day 1 of each 21-day cycle plus cisplatin, 75 mg/m^2, infused over 2 hr beginning about 30 min after the end of the pemetrexed administration. Dose adjustments at the start of a subsequent cycle should be based on nadir hematologic counts or maximum nonhematologic toxicity from the preceding cycle of therapy. Treatment may be delayed to allow sufficient time for recovery. See *Implementation/Administration/Storage* for information on premedication therapy.

Clients should not begin a new cycle of treatment unless the ANC is 1,500 cells/mm^3 or more, the platelet count is 100,000 cells/mm^3 or more, and C_{CR} is 45 mL/min or more. If clients develop nonhematologic toxicities (excluding neurotoxicity) of grade 3 or higher, withhold treatment until resolution is less than or equal to the clients pretherapy value.

Non-small-cell lung cancer.

Adults: 500 mg/m^2 over 10 min on day 1 of each 21-day cycle when used as a single agent or in combination with cisplatin. For use with cisplatin, see "*Malignant pleural mesothelioma*". See *Implementation/Administration/Storage* for information on premedication therapy.

NURSING IMPLICATIONS

IMPLEMENTATION/ADMINISTRATION/STORAGE

1. IV The following protocol for premedication therapy is followed for administration of pemetrexed:

- **Folic acid, 350–1,000 mcg PO. At least 5 daily doses must be taken during the 7-day period preceding the first dose of pemetrexed; continue dosing during the full course of therapy and for 21 days after the last dose. The most common dose of folic acid is 400 mcg.**
- **Vitamin B_{12}, 1,000 mcg IM. Begin 1 week prior to treatment, continue through treatment, and for every 3 cycles thereafter. Give subsequent vitamin B_{12} injections on the same day as pemetrexed.**
- **Dexamethasone, 4 mg 2 times per day PO. Give the day before, the day of, and the day after treatment to help prevent skin rash.**

2. In clients with third space fluid (e.g., pleural effusion, ascites), consider draining the effusion prior to pemetrexed administration.

3. Reconstitute 100 mg vials with 4.2 mL 0.9% NaCl injection (preservative-free) to give a solution containing 25 mg/mL pemetrexed. Reconstitute 500 mg vials with 20 mL 0.9% NaCl injection (preservative-free) to give a solution containing 25 mg/mL pemetrexed. Gently swirl each vial until powder is completely dissolved. The resulting solution is clear and ranges in color from colorless to yellow or green-yellow. The pH of the reconstituted solution ranges from 6.8 to 7.8. Further dilute the appropriate volume of reconstituted solution to 100 mL with 0.9% NaCl injection (preservative-free) and give as an IV infusion over 10 min.

4. Pemetrexed is compatible with standard PVC administration sets and IV solution bags.

5. If a pemetrexed solution contacts the skin, wash skin immediately and thoroughly with soap and water. If contact with mucous membranes occurs, flush thoroughly with water.

6. Be sure clients receive consistent hydration prior to and after receiving cisplatin. Consult cisplatin monograph.

7. Base dosage adjustments at the start of a subsequent cycle on nadir hematologic counts or maximum nonhematologic toxicity from the preceding cycle of therapy. Treatment may be delayed to allow sufficient time for recovery. Do not begin a new cycle of treatment unless the ANC is 1,500 cells/mm^3 or more, the platelet count is 100,000 cells/mm^3, and C_{CR} is 45 mL/min or more.

P

8. Hematologic toxicities: Use the following dose reduction schedule for pemetrexed (single agent or in combination with cisplatin):
   - Give 75% of the previous doses of both drugs if the nadir ANC is <500/mm^3 and nadir platelets are 50,000/mm^3 or more.
   - Give 75% of the previous dose of both drugs if the nadir platelets are <50,000/mm^3 without bleeding regardless of nadir ANC.
   - Give 50% of the previous dose of both drugs if the nadir platelets are <50,000/mm^3 with bleeding regardless of the nadir ANC.
9. Nonhematologic toxicity (excluding neurotoxicity) except grade 3 transaminase elevations). Use the following dose reduction schedule for pemetrexed (single agent or in combination) and cisplatin:
   - Give 75% (as mg/m^2) of the previous doses of both pemetrexed and cisplatin for any grade 3 (except grade 3 transaminase elevations) or 4 toxicities except mucositis.
   - Give 75% (as mg/m^2) of the previous doses of both pemetrexed and cisplatin for any diarrhea requiring hospitalization (irrespective of grade) or grade 3 or 4 diarrhea.
   - Give 50% (as mg/m^2) of the previous dose of pemetrexed and 100% (as mg/m^2) of the previous dose of cisplatin for any grade 3 or 4 mucositis.
10. Neurotoxicity. Use the following dose reduction schedule for pemetrexed (single agent or in combination with cisplatin):
    - If the CTC grade for neurotoxicity is 0 to 1, give 100% (as mg/m^2) of the previous doses of both pemetrexed and cisplatin.
    - If the CTC grade for neurotoxicity is 2, give 100% of the previous dose of pemetrexed and 50% of the previous dose of cisplatin.
    - If the CTC grade for neurotoxicity is 3 or 4, discontinue both drugs.
11. Discontinue pemetrexed therapy if the client shows any hematologic or nonhematologic grade 3 or 4 toxicity after 2 dose reductions (except grade 3 transaminase elevations). Discontinue immediately if grade 3 or 4 neurotoxicity occurs.
12. Avoid giving NSAIDs with short elimination half-lives 2 days before, the day of, and 2 days after pemetrexed. Stop dosing in all clients taking NSAIDs with long elimination half lives for at least 5 days before, the day of, and 2 days after pemetexed administration.
13. Consider draining the effusion prior to pemetrexed administration in those with clinically significant third space fluid.
14. Store vials from 15–30°C (59–86°F). Reconstituted and infusion solutions may be stored for up to 24 hr from 2–8°C (36–46°F). Discard unused portion as reconstituted as infusion solutions contain no preservatives.
15. COMPATIBILITY 0.9% NaCl injection (preservative-free).
16. INCOMPATIBILITY Diluents containing calcium, LR injection and Ringer's injection. Avoid coadministration with other drugs and diluents.

ASSESSMENT

1. Note reasons for therapy, other agents used, when disease determined unresectable, physical status of client.
2. List all drugs prescribed to ensure none interact. Avoid/monitor use carefully with NSAIDs during therapy; may cause myelosuppression, renal and GI toxicity.
3. Determine if present and if draining third-space fluid (e.g., pleural effusion and ascites) prior to administering pemetrexed considered.
4. Ensure corticosteroid is prescribed and taken for 3 days during treatment to reduce skin reactions from pemetrexed. To reduce toxicity, a low-dose folic acid preparation or multivitamin containing folic acid should be taken. At least 5 daily doses of folic acid must be taken during the 7-day period preceding the first pemetrexed dose, and daily dosing for 21 days after the last dose. IM vitamin B_{12} shot must be given the week before the first pemetrexed dose and every 3 cycles thereafter. Subsequent vitamin B_{12} injections may be given the same day as pemetrexed.
5. Monitor chemistry, renal, LFTs, CBC during therapy (before each dose and on days 8 and 15 of each cycle). Dosage adjustments at the start of a subsequent cycle are based on nadir hematologic counts or maximum nonhematologic toxicity from the preceding cycle of therapy. Treatment may be delayed to allow sufficient time for recovery. Do not begin a new cycle of treatment unless the ANC is 1,500

cells/mm^3 or more, the platelet count is 100,000 cells/mm^3, and C_{CR} is 45 mL/min or more. Upon recovery from hematologic toxicity, follow dose reduction schedule for pemetrexed and cisplatin as directed.

CLIENT/FAMILY TEACHING

1. Drug is administered IV and used to treat malignant pleural mesothelioma and lung cancer, usually in combination with cisplatin.
2. Take steroid pill for 3 days during therapy to help reduce risk of rash occurrence.
3. To minimize chances of side effects, take folic acid tablets in doses of 350–1,000 mcg for at least 5 of the 7 days prior to starting pemetrexed, daily during treatment, and for 21 days following treatment. Also vitamin B_{12} injections will be administered the week before starting therapy and then about every 9 weeks or every 3 cycles during therapy. Corticosteroid will also be used to reduce toxic effects of chemotherapy.
4. Practice reliable contraception. Drug is fetal toxic; do not nurse during therapy. Identify egg/sperm donor candidates.
5. Avoid OTC meds and NSAIDS without provider approval; especially with mild renal insufficiency.
6. May experience GI upset, diarrhea, fatigue, mouth/throat/lip sores, appetite loss, low blood cell counts and rash. Report any fever, chills, or S&S of infection, unusual bruising/bleeding or injection site reactions.
7. Keep all F/U to assess response, labs (to determine dose or delay in therapy), and adverse SE.

OUTCOMES/EVALUATE

Inhibition of malignant cell proliferation with pleural mesothelioma/lung cancer

Penciclovir

(pen-**SIGH**-kloh-veer)

Classification(s): Antiviral

Pregnancy Category: B

RX: Denavir.

SEE ALSO ***ANTIVIRAL DRUGS***.

INDICATIONS/USES

Treatment of recurrent herpes labialis (cold sores) in adults and children, 12 years and older.

ACTION/KINETICS

Action

Active against herpes simplex viruses (HSVs), including HSV-1 and HSV-2. In infected cells, viral thymidine kinase phosphorylates penciclovir to a monophosphate form which then is converted to penciclovir triphosphate by cellular kinases. Penciclovir triphosphate inhibits HSV polymerase competitively with deoxyguanosine triphosphate which inhibits herpes viral DNA synthesis and replication.

Pharmacokinetics

Not absorbed through the skin.

CONTRAINDICATIONS

Lactation. Application of the drug to mucous membranes.

SPECIAL CONCERNS

- Use with caution if applied around the eyes due to the possibility of irritation.
- The effect in immunocompromised clients not determined.
- Safety and efficacy not determined in children.

SIDE EFFECTS

Most Common

Application site reaction, hypesthesia, local anesthesia.

Dermatologic: Application site reaction, hypesthesia, local anesthesia, erythematous rash, mild erythema, pruritus, pain, allergic reaction. **Miscellaneous:** Headache, taste perversion.

HOW SUPPLIED

Cream: 1%.

DOSAGE

CREAM

Cold sores.

Apply q 2 hr while awake for 4 days.

NURSING IMPLICATIONS

IMPLEMENTATION/ADMINISTRATION/STORAGE

1. Start treatment as soon as possible during prodrome or when lesions appear.

P

2. Use only on the lips and face.

ASSESSMENT

1. Note onset, location, description, extent of lesions.
2. List frequency of occurrence, any triggers or prodrome.

CLIENT/FAMILY TEACHING

1. Wash hands before and after application. Apply q 2 hr while awake for 4 days at first cold sore symptoms.
2. Avoid contact with mucous membranes and eyes; apply to lips and face only.
3. Use sunscreens and lip balms with a sunscreen when sun exposed to prevent recurrence and to diminish intensity of outbreaks.
4. Avoid additional OTC creams or ointments; may delay healing process or cause disease spread.
5. Report if lesions do not improve or if a foul odor or purulent drainage appears.
6. Keep all F/U to assess response and for adverse SE.

OUTCOMES/EVALUATE

↓ Intensity/pain; clearing of herpes lesions

Penicillamine

(pen-ih-**SILL**-ah-meen)

Classification(s): Antirheumatic

Pregnancy Category: D

RX: Cuprimine, Depen.

INDICATIONS/USES

(1) Wilson's disease. (2) Cystinuria. (3) Rheumatoid arthritis (severe active disease unresponsive to conventional therapy). (4) Heavy metal antagonist. *Investigational:* Primary biliary cirrhosis. Scleroderma.

ACTION/KINETICS

Action

A chelating agent for mercury, lead, iron, and copper; forms soluble complexes, thus decreasing toxic levels of the metal (e.g., copper in Wilson's disease). Anti-inflammatory activity may be due to its ability to inhibit T-lymphocyte function and therefore decrease cell-mediated immune response. May also protect lymphocytes from hydrogen peroxide generated at the site of inflammation by inhibiting release of lysosomal enzymes and oxygen radicals. Beneficial effects may not be seen for 2 to 3 months when used for rheumatoid arthritis. In cystinuria, reduces excess cystine excretion, probably by disulfide interchange between penicillamine and cystine. This results in penicillamine-cysteine disulfide, which is a complex that is more soluble than cystine and is thus readily excreted.

Pharmacokinetics

Well-absorbed from the GI tract and excreted in urine. Food decreases the absorption of penicillamine over 50%. **Peak plasma levels:** 1–3 hr. **t½:** Approximately 2 hr. Metabolites excreted through the urine. **Plasma protein binding:** About 80%.

CONTRAINDICATIONS

Pregnancy, lactation, penicillinase-related aplastic anemia or agranulocytosis, hypersensitivity to drug. Clients allergic to penicillin may cross-react with penicillamine. Renal insufficiency or history thereof.

SPECIAL CONCERNS

- Use for juvenile rheumatoid arthritis not established.
- Clients older than 65 years may be at greater risk of developing hematologic side effects.

SIDE EFFECTS

Most Common

Anorexia, altered taste perception, epigastric pain, N&V, diarrhea, thrombocytopenia, leukopenia, generalized pruritus, early/late rashes, lupus erythematous-like syndrome, proteinura.

NOTE: This drug manifests a large number of potentially serious side effects. Clients should be carefully monitored. **GI:** Altered taste perception, N&V, diarrhea, anorexia, epigastric pain, stomatitis, oral ulcerations, reactivation of peptic ulcer, glossitis, cheilosis, colitis, gingivostomatitis (rare). **CNS:** Tinnitus, myasthenia gravis, peripheral sensory and motor neuropathies (with or without muscle weakness), reversible optic neuritis, polyradiculopathy (rare). **Hematologic:** Thrombocytopenia, leukopenia, ***agranulocytosis, aplastic anemia***, eosinophilia, monocytosis, red cell aplasia, ***hemolytic anemia***, leukocytosis, thrombocytosis. **Renal:** Proteinuria, hematuria, nephrotic syndrome, ***Goodpasture's syndrome*** (a severe and ultimately fatal glomerulonephritis). **Allergic:**

Rashes (common), lupus-like syndrome, drug fever, pruritus, pemphigoid-type symptoms (e.g., bullous lesions), arthralgia, lymphadenopathy, dermatoses, urticaria, thyroiditis, hypoglycemia, migratory polyarthralgia, polymyositis, allergic alveolitis. **Respiratory:** Obliterative bronchiolitis, pulmonary fibrosis, pneumonitis, bronchial asthma, interstitial pneumonitis. **Dermatologic:** Increased skin friability, early/late rashes, excessive skin wrinkling, development of small white papules at venipuncture and surgical sites, alopecia or falling hair, lichen planus, dermatomyositis, nail disorders, ***toxic epidermal necrolysis***, cutaneous macular atrophy. **Hepatic:** Pancreatitis, hepatic dysfunction, intrahepatic cholestasis, ***toxic hepatitis (rare)***. **Miscellaneous:** Thrombophlebitis, hyperpyrexia, polymyositis, mammary hyperplasia, renal vasculitis (may be fatal), hot flashes, lupus erythematosus-like syndrome.

LABORATORY TEST CONSIDERATIONS

↑ Serum alkaline phosphatase, LDH. Proteinuria. Positive thymol turbidity test and cephalin flocculation test.

DRUG INTERACTIONS

Antacids / ↓ Effect of penicillamine R/T ↓ absorption from GI tract
Antimalarial drugs / ↑ Risk of blood dyscrasias and adverse renal effects
Cytotoxic drugs / ↑ Risk of blood dyscrasias and adverse renal effects
Digoxin / ↓ Effect of digoxin
Gold therapy / ↑ Risk of blood dyscrasias and adverse renal effects
Iron salts / ↓ Effect of penicillamine R/T ↓ absorption from GI tract
Pyridoxine / ↑ Pyridoxine requirements

HOW SUPPLIED

Capsules: 250 mg; *Tablets, Titratable:* 250 mg.

DOSAGE

CAPSULES; TABLETS, TITRATABLE

Wilson's disease.

Dosage is usually calculated on the basis of the urinary excretion of copper. One gram of penicillamine promotes excretion of 2 mg of copper. **Adults and adolescents, usual, initial:** 250 mg 4 times per day. Dosage may have to be increased to 2 grams/day. A further increase does not produce additional excretion. **Pediatric, 6 months to young children:** 250 mg as a single dose given in fruit juice.

Cystinuria.

Individualized and based on excretion rate of cystine (100–200 mg/day in clients with no history of stones, below 100 mg with clients with history of stones or pain). Initiate at low dosage (250 mg/day) and increase gradually to minimum effective dosage. **Adult, usual:** 2 grams/day (range: 1–4 grams/day); **pediatric:** 7.5 mg/kg 4 times per day. If divided in fewer than four doses, give larger dose at night.

Rheumatoid arthritis.

Adults, individualized, initial: 125–250 mg/day. Dosage may be increased at 1- to 3-month intervals by 125- to 250-mg increments until adequate response is attained. **Maximum:** 500–750 mg/day. Up to 500 mg/day can be given as a single dose; higher dosages should be divided. **Maintenance, individualized. Range:** 500–750 mg/day. If the client is in remission for 6 or more months, a gradual stepwise decrease in dose of 125 or 250 mg/day at about 3-month intervals can be attempted.

Antidote for heavy metals.

Adults: 0.5–1.5 grams/day for 1–2 months; **pediatric:** 30–40 mg/kg/day (600–750 mg/m^2/day) for 1–6 months.

Primary biliary cirrhosis.

Adults: 600–900 mg/day.

NURSING IMPLICATIONS

Do not confuse penicillamine with penicillin (an antibiotic).

IMPLEMENTATION/ADMINISTRATION/STORAGE

1. If unable to tolerate dosage for cystinuria, the bedtime dosage should be larger and should be continued.
2. Administer contents of the capsule in 15–30 mL of chilled juice or pureed fruit if unable to swallow capsules or tablets.

P

3. When treating rheumatoid arthritis, discontinue if doses up to 1.5 grams/day for 2–3 months do not produce improvement.
4. Alternative dosage forms may be prepared if needed. An elixir containing 50 mg/mL may be prepared by dissolving the contents of 48 capsules in 100 mL of water. This is then filtered, and 100 mL of cherry syrup and 30 mL of alcohol stirred in. The volume is then brought up to 240 mL with water. The preparation is shaken well and stored in the refrigerator. Suppositories (750 mg) may be prepared by melting 51 grams of cocoa butter and dissolving the contents of 150 capsules in the cocoa butter; the mixture is poured into a prelubricated suppository mold and then frozen and stored in a refrigerator.

ASSESSMENT

1. Note indications, presenting symptoms, other therapies prescribed, outcome.
2. List any meds consumed with which penicillamine will interact unfavorably; impedes absorption of many drugs. White papules appearing at the site of venipuncture or at surgical sites may indicate sensitivity to penicillamine or presence of infection.
3. Assess CNS/neurologic status. Test hearing to detect any evidence of hearing loss.
4. With arthritis, assess joints for pain, stiffness, erythema, soreness, swelling, and ↓ ROM.
5. Test for pregnancy; drug can cause fetal damage.
6. If to undergo surgery, anticipate dosage reduction to 250 mg/day until wound healing complete.
7. A positive ANA test indicates client may develop a lupus-like syndrome in the future. The drug need not be discontinued.
8. Monitor CBC, LFTs, urinalysis. If WBC falls below 3,500/mm^3 or platelet count falls below 100,000/mm^3, withhold drug and report. If counts are low for three successive lab tests, a temporary interruption of therapy is indicated.

CLIENT/FAMILY TEACHING

1. Give on an empty stomach 1 hr before or 2 hr after meals; wait 1 hr after ingestion of any other food, milk, or drug. With Wilson's disease take 30–60 min before meals and at bedtime.
2. Take temperature nightly during the first few months of therapy. A fever may indicate a hypersensitivity reaction. Report any evidence of fever, sore throat, chills, skin rash, bruising/bleeding; early S&S of granulocytopenia.
3. If mouth inflammation occurs, report immediately and stop drug. Practice regular oral hygiene i.e., brushing teeth with a soft toothbrush, flossing daily, using alcohol free mouth rinses.
4. Inspect skin surfaces at regular intervals. Skin tends to become friable and susceptible to injury; avoid activities that could injure skin. Elderly should avoid excessive pressure on the shoulders, elbows, knees, toes, and buttocks. Report if ulcers appear and are severe or persistent; may need to reduce drug dose as may interfere with wound healing.
5. Penicillamine increases the body's need for pyridoxine; add pyridoxine (vitamin B_6 25 mg/day PO).
6. A loss of taste perception or a metallic taste may develop; relates to zinc chelation and may last for 2 months or more. With N&V or diarrhea, monitor weight and I&O. Report jaundice or other signs of hepatic dysfunction.
7. If to receive an oral iron preparation, at least 2 hr should elapse between ingestion of penicillamine and dose of therapeutic iron. Iron decreases the copper lowering effects of penicillamine.
8. Report cloudy urine or urine that is smoky brown (signs of proteinuria and hematuria). Practice reliable birth control; report missed menstrual period or other symptoms of pregnancy.
9. With Wilson's disease:
   - Eat a diet low in copper. Exclude foods such as chocolate, nuts, shellfish, mushrooms, liver, molasses, broccoli, and copper-enriched cereals.
   - Use distilled or demineralized water if drinking water contains more than 0.1 mg/L copper.
   - Unless taking iron supplements, take sulfurated potash or Carbo-Resin with meals to minimize the absorption of copper.
   - It may take 1–3 months for neurologic improvements to occur. Therefore, continue the therapy even if no improvements seem evident.

- Check any vitamin preparations being used to ensure that they do not contain copper.

10. If excess cystine in urine, do the following:
    - Drink large amounts of fluid to prevent the formation of renal calculi. Drink 500 mL of fluid at bedtime and another pint during the night, when the urine tends to be the most concentrated and most acidic. The greater the fluid intake, the lower the required dose of penicillamine.
    - Measure urine specific gravity (SG) and determine pH. The urine SG should be maintained at <1.010 and the pH maintained at 7.5–8.0.
    - Obtain yearly x-ray of the kidneys to detect presence of renal calculi.
    - Eat a diet low in methionine, a major precursor of cystine. Exclude foods high in cystine such as rich meat, soups and broths, milk, eggs, cheeses, and peas.
    - If client is pregnant or a child, diets low in methionine are also low in calcium; consider calcium supplementation.
11. With rheumatoid arthritis, continue using other therapies and medications to achieve relief from symptoms; penicillamine may take 4–6 months to have therapeutic effect. As improvement begins, analgesic drugs and NSAIDs may be slowly tapered.
12. Keep all F/U to assess response, labs, and for adverse SE.

OUTCOMES/EVALUATE

- ↑ Urinary excretion of copper
- ↓ Cystine excretion and prevention of renal calculi in cystinuria
- ↓ Joint pain, swelling, inflammation, and stiffness with ↑ mobility

IV

Penicillin G Aqueous

(pen-ih-**SILL**-in)

Classification(s): Antibiotic, penicillin

Pregnancy Category: B

RX: Pfizerpen.

SEE ALSO ***ANTI-INFECTIVE DRUGS*** AND ***PENICILLINS***.

INDICATIONS/USES

Streptococci of groups A, C, G, H, L, and M are sensitive to penicillin G. High serum levels are effective against streptococci of the D group.

ACTION/KINETICS

Pharmacokinetics

The first choice for treatment of many infections due to low cost. Rapid onset makes it especially suitable for fulminating infections. Is neither penicillinase resistant nor acid stable. **Peak plasma levels: IM or SC,** 6–20 units/mL after 15–30 min. **t½:** 30 min.

SIDE EFFECTS

Most Common

Hypersensitivity reactions, N&V, diarrhea, abdominal cramps, thrush/yeast infection, sore mouth/tongue.

See *Penicillins* for a complete list of possible side effects. Also, rapid IV administration may cause hyperkalemia and cardiac arrhythmias. Renal damage occurs rarely.

ADDITIONAL DRUG INTERACTIONS

Aspirin, ethacrynic acid, furosemide, indomethacin, sulfonamides, or thiazide diuretics may compete with penicillin G for renal tubular secretion → prolongation of serum t½ of penicillin

HOW SUPPLIED

Injection (Premix): 1 million units/vial, 2 million units/vial, 3 million units/vial; ***Powder for Injection:*** 5 million units, 20 million units.

DOSAGE

IM; IV, INFUSION (CONTINUOUS)

Serious streptococcal infections (empyema, endocarditis, meningitis, pericarditis, pneumonia).

Adults: 5–24 million units/day in divided doses q 4 to 6 hr. **Pediatric:** 150,000 units/kg/day given in equal doses q 4 to 6 hr. **Infants over 7 days of age:** 75,000 units/kg/day in divided doses q 8 hr. **Infants less than 7 days of age:** 50,000 units/kg/day given in divided doses q 12 hr. For group B streptococcus, give 100,000 units/kg/day.

P

Meningococcal meningitis/septicemia.

Adults: 1–2 million units IM q 2 hr or 20–30 million units/day continuous IV drip for 14 days or until afebrile for 7 days. Or, 200,000–300,000 units/kg/day q 2–4 hr in divided doses for a total of 24 doses.

Meningitis due to susceptible strains of Pneumococcus *or* Meningococcus.

Children: 250,000 units/kg/day divided in equal doses q 4 to 6 hr for 7 to 14 days (maximum total daily dose: 12–20 million units). **Infants over 7 days of age:** 200,000–300,0000 units/kg/day divided into equal doses given q 6 hr. **Infants less than 7 days of age:** 100,000–150,000 units/kg/day.

Anthrax.

Adults: A minimum of 5 million units/day (up to 12–20 million units have been used).

Clostridial infections.

Adults: 20 million units/day in divided doses q 4–6 hr used with an antitoxin.

Actinomycosis.

Adults: *Cervicofacial:* 1–6 million units/day. *Thoracic and abdominal disease:* **Initial,**10–20 million units/day divided into equal doses given q 4–6 hr IV for 6 weeks followed by penicillin V, PO, 500 mg 4 times/day for 2–3 months.

Rat-bite fever, Haverhill fever.

Adults: 12–20 million units/day q 4 to 6 hr for 3–4 weeks. **Children:** 150,000–250,000 units/kg/day in equal doses q 4 hr for 4 weeks.

Endocarditis due to Listeria.

Adults: 15–20 million units/day q 4 to 6 hr for 4 weeks.

Endocarditis due to Erysipelothrix rhusiopathiae.

Adults: 12–20 million units/day q 4 to 6 hr for 4–6 weeks.

Meningitis due to Listeria.

Adults: 15–20 million units/day q 4 to 6 hr for 2 weeks.

Pasteurella *infections causing bacteremia and meningitis.*

Adults: 4–6 million units/day q 4 to 6 hr for 2 weeks.

Severe fusospirochetal infections of the oropharynx, lower respiratory tract, and genital area.

Adults: 5–10 million units/day q 4 to 6 hr.

Pneumococcal infections causing empyema.

Adults: 5–24 million units/day in divided doses q 4–6 hr.

Pneumococcal infections causing meningitis.

Adults: 20–24 million units/day for 14 days.

Pneumococcal infections causing endocarditis, pericarditis, peritonitis, suppurative arthritis, osteomyelitis, mastoiditis.

Adults: 12–20 million units/day for 2–4 weeks.

Adjunct with antitoxin to prevent diphtheria.

Adults: 2–3 million units/day in divided doses q 4 to 6 hr for 10–12 days. **Children:** 150,000–250,000 units/kg/day in equal doses q 6 hr for 7–10 days.

Neurosyphilis.

Adults: 18–24 million units/day (3–4 million units q 4 hr) for 10–14 days (can be followed by benzathine penicillin G, 2.4 million units IM weekly for 3 weeks).

Disseminated gonococcal infections.

Adults: 10 million units/day q 4 to 6 hr (for meningococcal meningitis/septicemia, give q 2 hr). **Children, less than 45 kg:** *Arthritis*: 100,000 units/kg/day in 4 equally divided doses for 7 to 10 days. *Endocarditis:* 250,000 units/kg/day in equal doses q 4 hr for 4 weeks. *Meningitis:* 250,000 units/kg/day in equal doses q 4 hr for 10 to 14 days. **Children, over 45 kg:** *Arthritis, endocarditis, meningitis:* 10 million units/day in 4 equally divided doses (duration depends on type of infection).

Syphilis (congenital, neurosyphilis) after the newborn period.

200,000–300,000 units/kg/day (given as 50,000 units/kg q 4–6 hr) for 10–14 days.

P

Symptomatic or asymptomatic congenital syphilis in infants.

Infants: 50,000 units/kg/dose IV q 12 hr the first 7 days; then, q 8 hr for a total of 10 days. **Children:** 50,000 units/kg q 4–6 hr for 10 days.

NURSING IMPLICATIONS

Do not confuse penicillin G with penicillin V (another penicillin type) or with penicillamine (a heavy metal antagonist).

IMPLEMENTATION/ADMINISTRATION/STORAGE

1. Depending on the route of administration, prepare injections with sterile water, isotonic sodium chloride, or dextrose injection. Penicillin is rapidly inactivated in carbohydrate solutions at alkaline pH.
2. IM administration is preferred; discomfort is minimized by using solutions of up to 100,000 units/mL. Keep the total volume of the IM injection small.
3. Use 1–2% lidocaine solution as diluent for IM (if ordered) to lessen pain at injection site. Do not use procaine as diluent for aqueous penicillin.
4. Electrolyte contents: Pfizerpen contains 0.3 mEq sodium and 1.68 mEq potassium/million units.
5. If penicillin G is to be given by intrapleural or other local infusion and fluid is aspirated, give infusion in a volume equal to one fourth or one half the amount of fluid aspirated. Otherwise, prepare as for the IM injection.
6. Intrathecal use must be highly individualized and used only with full consideration of possible irritating effects of penicillin when given intrathecally. The preferred route in bacterial meningitis is IV supplemented by IM.
7. IV Use sterile water, isotonic saline, or D5W and mix with recommended volume for desired strength. When larger doses are needed, give by continuous IV infusion.
8. For intermittent IV administration (q 6 hr) reconstitute with 100 mL of dextrose or saline solution; infuse over 1 hr.
9. Loosen powder by shaking bottle before adding diluent. Hold vial horizontally and rotate slowly while directing the stream of diluent against the vial wall, then shake vigorously.
10. Solutions may be stored at room temperature for 24 hr or in refrigerator for 1 week. Discard remaining solution.
11. The dry powder does not require refrigeration. Sterile solutions may be kept in the refrigerator for 1 week. Solutions prepared for IV infusion are stable at room temperature for 24 or more hr.
12. For the premixed, frozen solution, thaw at room temperature or in a refrigerator. Do not force thaw by immersion in water baths or by microwave irradiation. The thawed solution is stable for 24 hr at room temperature or for 14 days under refrigeration. Do not refreeze thawed solutions.
13. COMPATIBILITY Dextrose or saline solutions.
14. INCOMPATIBILITY The following drugs should NOT be mixed with penicillin during IV administration: Aminophylline, amphotericin B, ascorbic acid, chlorpheniramine, chlorpromazine, gentamicin, heparin, hydroxyzine, lincomycin, metaraminol, novobiocin, oxytetracycline, phenylephrine, phenytoin, polymyxin B, prochlorperazine, promazine, promethazine, sodium bicarbonate, sodium salts of barbiturates, sulfadiazine, tetracycline, tromethamine, vancomycin, vitamin B complex.

ASSESSMENT

1. Identify condition requiring therapy, onset, characteristics of S&S; check culture results.
2. Assess drug allergies. Order drug by specifying sodium or potassium salt.
3. Monitor I&O. Dehydration decreases drug excretion and may raise blood level of penicillin G to dangerously high levels causing kidney damage. GI disturbances may lead to dehydration.
4. Very high doses (>20 million units) may cause seizures or platelet dysfunction, especially with impaired renal function.
5. Assess electrolytes, CBC, renal, LFTs. Monitor cardiac and vascular status during prolonged therapy with high doses of IV penicillin G.

CLIENT/FAMILY TEACHING

1. With IM dosing, drug must be given by injection into the muscle to clear up infection. May experience pain at injection site; apply ice to relieve pain.
2. Report any unusual bruising, bleeding, N&V, sore mouth, diarrhea, rash, fever, difficulty

P

breathing, adverse side effects, or lack of improvement.

3. Use nonhormonal form of contraception during therapy.
4. Keep all F/U to assess response, labs, and for adverse SE.

OUTCOMES/EVALUATE

- Symptomatic improvement; negative culture reports
- Resolution of infective process

Penicillin G benzathine, intramuscular

(pen-ih-**SILL**-in, **BEN**-zah-theen)

Classification(s): Antibiotic, penicillin

Pregnancy Category: B

RX: Bicillin L-A, Permapen.

SEE ALSO ***ANTI-INFECTIVE DRUGS*** AND ***PENICILLINS***.

INDICATIONS/USES

(1) URTI (mild to moderate) due to susceptible streptococci. (2) Sexually transmitted diseases, such as syphilis, yaws, bejel, and pinta. (3) Prophylaxis of rheumatic fever or chorea. (4) Follow-up prophylactic therapy for rheumatic heart disease and acute glomerulonephritis.

ACTION/KINETICS

Action

Penicillin G is neither penicillinase resistant nor acid stable. The product is a long-acting (repository) form of penicillin in an aqueous vehicle; it is administered as a sterile suspension.

Pharmacokinetics

Peak plasma levels, IM: 0.03–0.05 unit/mL.

CONTRAINDICATIONS

IV use. Injection into or near an artery or nerve.

SPECIAL CONCERNS

This product is not intended for IV administration.

SIDE EFFECTS

Most Common

Hypersensitivity reactions, N&V, diarrhea, abdominal cramps, thrush/yeast infection, sore mouth/tongue.

See *Penicillins* for a complete list of possible side effects.

ADDITIONAL DRUG INTERACTIONS

Aspirin, ethacrynic acid, furosemide, indomethacin, sulfonamides, or thiazide diuretics may compete with penicillin G for renal tubular secretion → prolongation of serum $t^{1/2}$ of penicillin

HOW SUPPLIED

Injection (Suspension): 600,000 units/dose; 1,200,000 units/dose; 2,400,000 units/dose.

DOSAGE

IM ONLY (SUSPENSION)

URTI due to Group A streptococcus.

Adults: 1,200,000 units as a single dose; **older children:** 900,000 units as a single dose; **children under 27 kg:** 300,000–600,000 units as a single dose.

Early syphilis (primary, secondary, or latent).

Adults: 2,400,000 units as a single dose. **Children:** 50,000 units/kg, up to the adult dose.

Gummas and cardiovascular syphilis (latent).

Adults: 2,400,000 units q 7 days for 3 weeks. **Children:** 50,000 units/kg, up to adult dose.

Neurosyphilis.

Adults: Aqueous penicillin G, 18,000,000–24,000,000 units IV/day (3–4 million units q 4 hr) for 10–14 days followed by penicillin G benzathine, 2,400,000 units IM q week for 3 weeks. An alternative regimen is procaine penicillin G, 2,400,000 units/day plus probenecid, 500 mg PO, 4 times per day, both for 10–14 days. Some recommend benzathine G penicillin, 2.4 million units following completion of this regimen.

Congenital syphilis.

Children less than 2 years of age: 50,000 units/kg. **Children, 2–12 years:** Adjust dose based on adult dosage schedule.

Yaws, bejel, pinta.
1,200,000 units in a single dose.

Prophylaxis of rheumatic fever and glomerulonephritis.
Following an acute attack, 1,200,000 units once a month or 600,000 units q 2 weeks.

NURSING IMPLICATIONS

Do not confuse Bicillin L-A with Bicillin C-R (combination of benzathine and procaine penicillin).

IMPLEMENTATION/ADMINISTRATION/STORAGE

1. Shake multiple-dose vial vigorously before withdrawing desired dose as drug tends to clump on standing. Check that all medication is dissolved and no residue present at bottom of bottle.
2. Use a 20-gauge needle and do not allow medication to remain in the syringe and needle for long periods of time before administration; needle may become plugged and the syringe "frozen."
3. Inject slowly and steadily into muscle; *do not massage* injection site. For adults, use upper outer quadrant of the buttock; for infants and small children, the midlateral aspect of the thigh should be used. Do not administer in the gluteal region in children less than 2 years of age. Rotate and chart site of injections. Divide between two injection sites if dose is large or available muscle mass is small.
4. *Do not administer IV.* Before injection of medication, aspirate to ensure that needle is not in a vein.
5. Bicillin C-R should not be given in place of Bicillin L-A.
6. Refrigerate, but do not freeze.

ASSESSMENT

1. Note reasons for therapy, onset, characteristics of S&S, other agents trialed, outcome.
2. Use caution, quadriceps femoris fibrosis and atrophy can occur following repeated IM injections of penicillin into the anterolateral thigh.
3. List client history, allergies; review lab and culture results.

CLIENT/FAMILY TEACHING

1. Must return as scheduled for repository penicillin injections.
2. With STDs obtain sexual counseling. Sexual partner(s) should also undergo treatment.
3. Report any unusual side effects, lack of response or worsening of condition.
4. Keep all F/U to assess response, labs, and adverse SE.

OUTCOMES/EVALUATE

- Prophylaxis of poststreptococcal rheumatic fever
- Resolution of infection/STD

Combination Drug

Penicillin G benzathine/ Penicillin G procaine

(pen-ih-**SILL**-in, **BEN**-zah-theen, **PROH**-kain)

Classification(s): Antibiotic, penicillin

Pregnancy Category: B

RX: Bicillin C-R, Bicillin C-R 900/300.

SEE ALSO ***ANTI-INFECTIVE DRUGS*** AND ***PENICILLINS***.

INDICATIONS/USES

(1) Moderately severe to severe infections of the upper respiratory tract, skin, soft tissues, and scarlet fever due to susceptible streptococci in groups A, C, G, H, L, and M. (2) Moderately severe pneumonia and otitis media due to susceptible pneumococci. *NOTE:* For severe pneumonia, empyema, bacteremia, pericarditis, meningitis, peritonitis, arthritis of pneumococcal etiology, and streptococcal infections with bacteremia, use penicillin G sodium or potassium. Not to be used to treat venereal diseases, including syphilis, gonorrhea, yaws, bejel, and pinta.

CONTENT

Bicillin C-R: *600,000 units/dose:* 300,000 units each of penicillin G benzathine and penicillin G procaine. *1,200,000 units/dose:* 600,000 units each of penicillin G benzathine and penicillin G procaine. **Bicillin C-R 900/300:** 900,000 units of penicillin G benzathine and 300,000 units of penicillin G procaine.

P

CONTRAINDICATIONS

Use to treat syphilis, gonorrhea, yaws, bejel, and pinta. IV use. Injection into or near an artery or nerve. Use with IV solutions.

SPECIAL CONCERNS

■ This product is not for IV administration. Do not inject IV or admix with other IV solutions. There have been reports of inadvertent IV administration of penicillin G benzathine, which has been associated with cardiorespiratory arrest and death. Prior to administration of this drug, carefully read the labeling. ■

SIDE EFFECTS

Most Common

Hypersensitivity reactions, N&V, diarrhea, abdominal cramps, thrush/yeast infection, sore mouth/tongue.

See *Penicillins* for a complete list of possible side effects.

ADDITIONAL DRUG INTERACTIONS

Aspirin, ethacrynic acid, furosemide, indomethacin, sulfonamides, or thiazide diuretics may compete with penicillin G for renal tubular secretion → prolongation of serum t½ of penicillin

HOW SUPPLIED

See *Content.*

DOSAGE

IM ONLY

Streptococcal infections (upper respiratory tract, skin, soft tissue, scarlet fever).

Bicillin C-R. Adults and children over 27 kg: 2,400,000 units, given at a single session using multiple injection sites or, alternatively, in divided doses on days 1 and 3 (as long as client cooperation is assured); **children 13.5–27 kg:** 900,000–1,200,000 units; **infants and children under 13.5 kg:** 600,000 units. *NOTE:* A single injection of Bicillin C-R 900/300 is usually sufficient to treat group A streptococcal infections in children.

Pneumococcal infections (pneumonia, otitis media), except pneumococcal meningitis.

Bicillin C-R. Adults: 1,200,000 units; **pediatric:** 600,000 units. Give q 2–3 days until temperature is normal for 48 hr. **Bicillin C-R 900/300:** One Tubex cartridge repeated at 2- or 3-day intervals until the temperature is normal for 48 hr. For severe cases, other forms of penicillin may be needed.

NURSING IMPLICATIONS

Do not confuse Bicillin C-R with Bicillin L-A (benzathine penicillin).

IMPLEMENTATION/ADMINISTRATION/STORAGE

1. For adults, administer by deep IM injection in the upper outer quadrant of the buttock. For infants and children, use the midlateral aspect of the thigh. Rotate injection sites for repeated doses.
2. Refrigerate. Protect from freezing.

ASSESSMENT

1. Note reasons for therapy, symptom type/onset/location, disease confirmation.
2. Assess for drug allergies, culture results.

CLIENT/FAMILY TEACHING

1. Drug must be given by injection into the muscle to clear up infection. May experience pain at injection site; apply ice to relieve pain.
2. Report any unusual bruising, bleeding, N&V, sore mouth, diarrhea, rash, fever, difficulty breathing, adverse side effects, or lack of improvement.
3. Keep all F/U to assess response, labs, adverse SE.

OUTCOMES/EVALUATE

Resolution of infection

Penicillin G procaine, intramuscular

(pen-ih-**SILL**-in, **PROH**-caine)

Classification(s): Antibiotic, penicillin

Pregnancy Category: B

RX: Wycillin.

SEE ALSO ***ANTI-INFECTIVE DRUGS*** AND ***PENICILLINS***.

INDICATIONS/USES

(1) Penicillin-sensitive staphylococci, pneumococci, streptococci, and bacterial endocarditis (for

Streptococcus viridans and *S. bovis* infections). (2) Gonorrhea and all stages of syphilis. (3) *Prophylaxis:* Rheumatic fever, pre- and postsurgery. (4) Diphtheria, anthrax, fusospirochetosis (Vincent's infection), erysipeloid, rat-bite fever. *NOTE:* Severe pneumonia, empyema, bacteremia, pericarditis, meningitis, peritonitis, and purulent or septic arthritis due to pneumococcus are better treated with aqueous penicillin G during the acute stage.

ACTION/KINETICS

Action

Long-acting (repository) form in aqueous or oily vehicle. Destroyed by penicillinase. Because of slow onset, a soluble penicillin is often administered concomitantly for fulminating infections.

CONTRAINDICATIONS

Use in newborns due to possible sterile abscesses and procaine toxicity. Injection into or near an artery or nerve. IV use.

SIDE EFFECTS

Most Common

Hypersensitivity reactions, N&V, diarrhea, abdominal cramps, thrush/yeast infection, sore mouth/tongue.

See *Penicillins* for a complete list of possible side effects.

ADDITIONAL DRUG INTERACTIONS

Aspirin / May compete with penicillin G for renal tubular secretion → prolongation of serum t½ of penicillin

Ethacrynic acid / May compete with penicillin G for renal tubular secretion → prolongation of serum t½ of penicillin

Furosemide / May compete with penicillin G for renal tubular secretion → prolongation of serum t½ of penicillin

Indomethacin / May compete with penicillin G for renal tubular secretion → prolongation of serum t½ of penicillin

Oral contraceptives / ↓ Effectiveness of oral contraceptives

Sulfonamides / May compete with penicillin G for renal tubular secretion → prolongation of serum t½ of penicillin

Thiazide diuretics / May compete with penicillin G for renal tubular secretion → prolongation of serum t½ of penicillin

HOW SUPPLIED

Injection: 600,000 units/vial, 1,200,000 units/vial.

DOSAGE

DEEP IM ONLY

Pneumococcal, streptococcal (Group A, including tonsillitis, erysipelas, scarlet fever, URTI, and skin and skin structure infections), staphylococcal infections (moderate to severe of the skin and soft tissues).

Adults, usual: 600,000–1 million units/day for 10–14 days. **Children, less than 27.2 kg:** 300,000 units/day.

Bacterial endocarditis (only very sensitive S. viridans *or* S. bovis *infections).*

Adults: 600,000–1 million units/day.

Diphtheria carrier state.

300,000 units/day for 10 days.

Diphtheria, adjunct with antitoxin.

300,000–600,000 units/day for 14 days.

Anthrax (cutaneous), erysipeloid, rat-bite fever.

600,000 to 1 million units/day.

Fusospirochetosis: Vincent's gingivitis, pharyngitis.

600,000 to 1 million units/day. Obtain necessary dental care in infections involving gum tissue.

Gonococcal infections.

4.8 million units divided into at least two doses at one visit and given with 1 gram PO probenecid (given 30 min before the injections).

Neurosyphilis.

2.4 million units/day for 10 to 14 days (given at two sites) with probenecid 500 mg PO 4 times per day; **then,** benzathine penicillin G, 2.4 million units/week for 3 weeks. *NOTE:* For yaws, bejel, and pinta, treat the same as syphilis in corresponding stage of disease.

Congenital syphilis in children (less than 32 kg), symptomatic and asymptomatic.

50,000 units/kg/day given as a single dose for 10–14 days.

Syphilis: Primary, secondary, latent with negative spinal fluid.

Adults and children over 12 years: 600,000 units/day for 8 days (total of 4.8 million units).

P

Syphilis: Tertiary, neurosyphilis, latent with positive spinal fluid examination or no spinal fluid examination.

Adults: 600,000 units/day for 10 to 15 days (total of 6 to 9 million units).

Anthrax, cutaneous.

600,000–1,000,000 units/day. Continue prophylaxis until exposure to *Bacillus anthracis* has been excluded. If exposure is confirmed and vaccine is available, continue prophylaxis for 4 weeks and until 3 doses of vaccine have been given, or for 30–60 days if vaccine is not available.

NURSING IMPLICATIONS

IMPLEMENTATION/ADMINISTRATION/STORAGE

1. Shake multiple-dose vial thoroughly to ensure uniform suspension before injection. If it is clumped at the bottom of the vial, shake until clump dissolves.
2. Use a 20-gauge needle and aspirate immediately after withdrawing medication from the vial; otherwise needle may become clogged and syringe may "freeze." Aspirate to check that the needle is not in a vein.
3. Administer into two sites if dose is large or available muscle mass is small. Inject slowly, deep into the muscle. For IM use only. Rotate and chart injection sites. Do not massage site.
4. Inspect visually for particulate matter and discoloration prior to administration.
5. Store from 2–8°C (36–46°F). Do not freeze.

P

ASSESSMENT

Note reasons for therapy, onset, characteristics of S&S, any drug allergies, other therapies trialed, lab and culture results.

CLIENT/FAMILY TEACHING

1. Drug can only be given IM. Report a wheal or other skin reactions at injection site, or mental disturbances; may indicate reaction to procaine as well as to penicillin.
2. Report N&V, diarrhea, mouth sores, severe pain at injection site, unusual bruising/bleeding, or difficulty breathing.
3. With STDs obtain sexual counseling; have sexual partner also undergo treatment. Use an additional non-hormonal form of birth control due to decreased effectiveness.
4. Keep all F/U to assess response, labs, adverse SE.

OUTCOMES/EVALUATE

- Resolution of infection
- Infection prophylaxis

Penicillin V potassium (Phenoxymethyl-penicillin potassium)

(pen-ih-**SILL**-in)

Classification(s): Antibiotic, penicillin

Pregnancy Category: B

RX: Penicillin VK, Veetids.

🍁 **Rx:** Apo-Pen-VK.

SEE ALSO ***ANTI-INFECTIVE DRUGS*** AND ***PENICILLINS***.

INDICATIONS/USES

1. Mild to moderate upper respiratory tract streptococcal infections, including scarlet fever and erysipelas.
2. Mild to moderate upper respiratory tract pneumococcal infections, including otitis media.
3. Mild staphylococcal infections of the skin and soft tissue.
4. Mild to moderate fusospirochetosis (Vincent's infection) of the oropharynx, pharyngitis.
5. Prophylaxis of recurrence following rheumatic fever or chorea.

Investigational: Prophylactic treatment of children with sickle cell anemia or splenectomy to reduce the incidence of *S. pneumoniae* septicemia; actinomycosis; early Lyme disease; postexposure prophylaxis to anthrax (confirmed or suspected).

NOTE: Streptococci in groups A, C, G, H, L, and M are very sensitive to penicillin. Other groups, including group D (enterococci), are resistant. An increasing number of staphylococcal strains are resistant to penicillin; culture and susceptibility studies are important.

ACTION/KINETICS

Action

Binds to penicillin-binding proteins (PBP-1 and PBP-3) in the cytoplasmic membranes of bacteria, thus inhibiting cell wall synthesis. Cell division and growth are inhibited and often lysis and elongation of susceptible bacteria occur. Related closely to penicillin G. Products are not penicillinase resistant but are acid stable and resist inactivation by gastric secretions.

Pharmacokinetics

Well absorbed from the GI tract and not affected by foods. **Peak plasma levels: PO:** 1–9 mcg/mL after 30–60 min. **t½:** 30 min. Periodic blood counts and renal function tests are indicated during long-term usage.

CONTRAINDICATIONS

PO penicillin V to treat severe pneumonia, empyema, bacteremia, pericarditis, meningitis, and arthritis during the acute stage. Prophylactic uses for GU instrumentation or surgery, sigmoidoscopy, or childbirth.

SPECIAL CONCERNS

More and more strains of staphylococci are resistant to penicillin V, necessitating culture and sensitivity studies.

SIDE EFFECTS

Most Common

Hypersensitivity reactions, N&V, diarrhea, abdominal cramps, thrush/yeast infection, sore mouth/tongue.

See *Penicillins* for a complete list of possible side effects.

ADDITIONAL DRUG INTERACTIONS

Contraceptives, oral / ↓ Effectiveness of oral contraceptives

Neomycin, oral / ↓ Absorption of penicillin V

HOW SUPPLIED

Powder for Oral Solution: 125 mg/5 mL (when reconstituted), 250 mg/5 mL (when reconstituted); *Tablets:* 250 mg, 500 mg.

DOSAGE

ORAL SOLUTION; TABLETS

Streptococcal infections of the upper respiratory tract, including scarlet fever and mild erysipelas.

Adults and children over 12 years: 125–250 mg q 6–8 hr for 10 days.

Pharyngitis in children, usual: 25–50 mg/kg/day divided q 6 hr for 10 days.

Staphylococcal infections (mild infections of the skin and soft tissue); fusospirochetosis of oropharynx (mild to moderate infections).

Adults and children over 12 years: 250 mg q 6–8 hr.

Pneumococcal infections, mild to moderate respiratory tract infections, including otitis media.

Adults and children over 12 years: 250 mg q 6 hr until afebrile for at least 2 days.

Prophylaxis of recurrence of rheumatic fever/chorea.

Adults and children over 12 years: 125–250 mg twice a day, on a continuing basis.

Prophylactic treatment of children with sickle cell anemia or splenectomy to reduce incidence of S. pneumoniae septicemia.

Children, 3 months to 5 years: 125 mg twice a day. **Children, over 5 years of age:** 250 mg twice a day.

Actinomycosis.

Penicillin G, 10–20 mg/kg/day IV for 4–6 weeks; then, Penicillin V, 2–4 grams/day for 6–12 months.

Anthrax, postexposure prophylaxis (confirmed or suspected exposure to B. anthracis*).*

Adults: 7.5 mg/kg 4 times per day. **Children, less than 9 years of age:** 50 mg/kg/day divided 4 times per day. Continue prophylaxis until exposure to *B. anthracis* has been excluded. If exposure is confirmed and vaccine is available, continue prophylaxis for 4 weeks and until 3 doses of vaccine have been given or for 30–60 days if vaccine is not available.

Early Lyme disease (Borrelia burgdorferi)*.*

Adults and children over 12 years of age: 500 mg 4 times per day for 10–20 days.

NURSING IMPLICATIONS

Do not confuse penicillin V with penicillin G or with penicillamine (a heavy metal antagonist).

P

IMPLEMENTATION/ADMINISTRATION/STORAGE

1. To reconstitute the solution, tap bottle until all powder flows freely. Add about one-half of the total amount of water for reconstitution and shake well to wet powder. Add the remainder of the water and shake well again.
2. Store reconstituted solution in the refrigerator; discard unused portion after 14 days.

ASSESSMENT

1. Note reasons for therapy, onset, exposures, characteristics of S&S, any drug allergies, other therapies trialed, and culture results.
2. List drugs prescribed to ensure none interact.
3. Monitor VS, CBC, clinical presentation, and culture results.

CLIENT/FAMILY TEACHING

1. Blood levels may be slightly higher when administered on an empty stomach. Take 1 hr before or 2 hr after meal with full glass of water (avoid fruit juice or carbonated beverages). Complete entire prescription to prevent bacterial resistance.
2. With suspension, refrigerate and shake well before administering.
3. Clients with history of rheumatic fever or congenital heart disease need to use and understand the importance of antibiotic prophylaxis prior to any invasive medical or dental procedure.
4. Report lack of response, adverse SE, bloody stools, severe diarrhea, or stomach cramps/pain or if throat/ear S&S do not improve after 48 hr of therapy; may need to reevaluate and alter therapy.
5. With oral administration, if reaction is going to occur, you usually see it after the second dose. Seek care immediately if respiratory distress or skin wheals appear.
6. Use an additional nonhormonal form of birth control if taking oral contraceptives because their effectiveness may be diminished.
7. Keep all F/U to assess response, VS, labs, cultures, and for adverse SE.

OUTCOMES/EVALUATE

- Resolution of symptoms
- Negative C&S reports
- Infection prophylaxis (bacterial endocarditis) with valvular or congenital heart disease with dental procedures or surgical procedures of upper respiratory tract
- Recurrence prevention of rheumatic fever/chorea

P

IV

Pentamidine isethionate

(pen-**TAM**-ih-deen)

Classification(s): Antibiotic, miscellaneous

Pregnancy Category: C

RX: NebuPent, Pentacarinate, Pentam 300.

INDICATIONS/USES

Parenteral: Pneumonia caused by *Pneumocystis carinii.* **Inhalation:** Prophylaxis of *P. carinii* in high-risk HIV-infected clients defined by one or both of the following: (a) a history of one or more cases of pneumonia caused by *P. carinii* and/or (b) a peripheral CD4+ lymphocyte count <200/mm^3. *Investigational:* Trypanosomiasis, visceral leishmaniasis.

ACTION/KINETICS

Action

Inhibits synthesis of DNA, RNA, phospholipids, and proteins, thereby interfering with cell metabolism. May also interfere with folate transformation.

Pharmacokinetics

Plasma levels following inhalation are significantly lower than after a comparable IV dose. About one-third of the dose excreted unchanged in the urine.

CONTRAINDICATIONS

Anaphylaxis to inhaled or parenteral pentamidine.

SPECIAL CONCERNS

Use with caution in clients with hepatic or kidney disease, hyper-/hypotension, hyper-/hypoglycemia, hypocalcemia, leukopenia, thrombocytopenia, anemia, ventricular tachycardia, pancreatitis, Stevens-Johnson syndrome.

SIDE EFFECTS

Most Common

When used parenterally: Sterile abscess/pain/induration at IM injection site, leukopenia, nausea, anorexia, hypotension, fever, hypoglycemia, rash, bad taste in mouth, confusion, hallucinations.

When used as aerosol: Fatigue, metallic taste, shortness of breath, decreased appetite, dizziness, rash, cough, N&V, pharyngitis, chest pain/congestion, night sweats, chills, bronchospasm.
Parenteral. CV: Hypotension, ***ventricular tachycardia***, phlebitis. **GI:** Nausea, anorexia, bad taste in mouth. **Hematologic:** Leukopenia, thrombocytopenia, anemia. **Electrolytes/glucose:** Hypoglycemia, hypocalcemia, hyperkalemia. **CNS:** Dizziness without hypotension, confusion, hallucinations. **Miscellaneous:** Acute renal failure, ***Stevens-Johnson syndrome***, elevated serum creatinine, elevated LFTs, fever, sterile abscess/pain/induration at IM injection site, rash, neuralgia.

Inhalation. Most frequent include the following: **GI:** Decreased appetite, N&V, metallic taste, diarrhea, abdominal pain. **CNS**: Fatigue, dizziness, headache. **Respiratory**: SOB, cough, pharyngitis, chest pain/congestion, ***bronchospasm***, pneumothorax. **Miscellaneous**: Rash, night sweats, chills, myalgia, headache, anemia, edema.

DRUG INTERACTIONS

Cidofovir / ↑ Risk of nephrotoxicity
Foscarnet / Hypocalcemia possible

HOW SUPPLIED

Aerosol (for Inhalation): 300 mg; *Injection:* 300 mg; *Powder for Injection, Lyophilized:* 300 mg.

DOSAGE

IM, (DEEP); IV

Pneumonia due to Pneumocystis carinii.

Adults and children: 4 mg/kg/day for 14 days. Dosage should be reduced in renal disease.

INHALATION AEROSOL

Prevention of P. carinii *pneumonia.*

300 mg q 4 weeks given via the Respirgard II nebulizer.

NURSING IMPLICATIONS

IMPLEMENTATION/ADMINISTRATION/STORAGE

1. For use in the nebulizer, reconstitute by dissolving vial contents in 6 mL sterile water for injection. Avoid saline solution as it causes the drug to precipitate. Do not mix with other medications in the nebulizer chamber.
2. Deliver the dose using the nebulizer until the chamber is empty (30–45 min). The suggested flow rate is 5–7 L/min from a 40- to 50-psi (pounds per square inch) air or oxygen source.
3. When used for nebulization, do not mix with any other drug. The solution for nebulization is stable at room temperature for 48 hr if protected from light.
4. To prepare IM solution, dissolve one vial in 3 mL of sterile water for injection.
5. For IM administration, inject deeply and rotate sites.
6. IV To prepare IV solution, dissolve one vial in 3–5 mL of sterile water for injection or D5W. The drug is then further diluted in 50–250 mL of D5W.
7. Infuse pentamidine slowly IV over 1 hr with client supine to minimize severe hypotension and arrhythmias.
8. IV solutions in concentrations of 1 and 2.5 mg/mL in D5W are stable for 48 hr at room temperature.
9. COMPATIBILITY D5W.
10. INCOMPATIBILITY Administer separately.

ASSESSMENT

1. Note reasons for therapy, onset, S&S; assess extent of infection.
2. Check for history of kidney disease, hypertension, past blood disorders.
3. List results of TB skin test. Auscultate lungs; document VS, CXR, respiratory assessment findings.
4. Observe for S&S of hypoglycemia, hypocalcemia, hyperkalemia.
5. During IV therapy monitor BP (q 15 min during therapy and q 2 hr after therapy until stable), VS and I&O. Obtain apical pulse; auscultate for evidence of arrhythmia.
6. During administration of aerosolized pentamidine, follow precautions to protect health care worker. Do not administer if pregnant; remove contact lenses. Administer with the Respirgard II nebulizer. Document worker exposure(s) and report any persistent or unusual symptoms, especially chronic URIs. Wear:
   - Eye protection with side shields
   - Disposable gowns
   - Respiratory protective equipment such as an organic dust-mist respirator unless

P

client is under hood stalls or in a ventilated booth
- Gloves

7. Follow appropriate institutional guidelines and Occupational Safety and Health Administration (OSHA) standards for administration of drug/exposure. Incorporate Standard Precautions.
8. Monitor ECG, VS, cultures, CBC, electrolytes, glucose, calcium, CD_4 counts, renal and LFTs.

CLIENT/FAMILY TEACHING

1. Parenteral drug therapy must be given every day (IV/IM). Use warm soaks for IM site pain. Inhalation therapy must be used once every 4 weeks. Use aerosol device until chamber is empty. Follow appropriate guidelines for administration.
2. Use caution, avoids activities that require mental alertness until drug effects realized. Rise from a prone position slowly and dangle legs before standing as drug may cause dizziness and low BP.
3. Report any blood in urine/stools, or unusual bruising/bleeding. Expect frequent blood tests and BP checks. Consume 2–3 L/day of fluids.
4. Avoid aspirin-containing compounds, alcohol, IM injections, or rectal thermometers. Use a soft toothbrush, electric razor, and night light to prevent injury and falls.
5. Be alert for S&S of low sugar level (which may be severe). Report early signs of Stevens-Johnson syndrome (characterized by high fever, severe headaches, mouth, eye, nose or penis inflammation or swelling).
6. During inhalation, a metallic taste and GI upset may be experienced. Eat small, frequent meals and perform regular mouth care to offset. Report any breathing difficulty or adverse side effects immediately. Stop smoking; if continued during therapy, then may trigger bronchospasms and increased coughing.
7. Administer inhalation therapy in a well ventilated area and if bronchodilator ordered, then give 5–10 min before pentamidine therapy.
8. Avoid crowds and persons with known infections.
9. Keep all F/U to assess response, labs, adverse SE.

OUTCOMES/EVALUATE

- (Parenteral) Improvement in symptoms of PCP
- (Inhalation) *Pneumocystis jiroveci* pneumonia prophylaxis

Phenazopyridine hydrochloride (Phenylazodiaminopyridine HCl)

(fen-**AY**-zoh-**PEER**-ih-deen)

Classification(s): Urinary tract drug

Pregnancy Category: B

OTC: AZO Standard Maximum Strength, Azo-Standard, Baridium, Prodium.

RX: Geridium, Pyridin, Pyridium, Pyridium Plus, Urodine, Urogesic, UTI Relief.

Rx: Phenazo.

INDICATIONS/USES

Relief of pain, urgency, frequency, burning, and other discomforts due to irritation of the lower urinary tract mucosa caused by infection, trauma, surgery, endoscopic procedures, or passage of sounds or catheters. Use may eliminate the need for systemic analgesics or narcotics. The drug treats painful symptoms but does not treat the source or cause of the disorder causing the pain.

ACTION/KINETICS

Action

An azo dye with local analgesic effect on the urinary tract mucosa. Mechanism of action is unknown.

Pharmacokinetics

Rapidly excreted by the urine; 65% excreted unchanged within 24 hr.

CONTRAINDICATIONS

Renal insufficiency. Use in children less than 12 years of age. Chronic use to treat undiagnosed pain of the urinary tract.

SPECIAL CONCERNS

No information available on the effect of phenazopyridine on lactation.

SIDE EFFECTS

Most Common

Headache, itching, rash, GI upset.

GI: Nausea, GI upset, indigestion, stomach cramps/pain. **CNS:** Headache, dizziness, confusion. **Hematologic:** Methemoglobinemia, hemolytic anemia (especially in clients with G6PD deficiency). **Respiratory:** SOB, chest tightness, wheezing, troubled breathing. **Dermatologic:** Yellowish tinge of the skin or sclerae may indicate accumulation of drug due to renal insufficiency, blue or blue-purple skin color, pruritus, rash, itching. **Body as a whole:** Fever, unusual tiredness or weakness, weight gain. **Miscellaneous:** Renal and hepatic toxicity, anaphylactoid reaction, staining of contact lenses, sudden decrease in amount of urine; swelling of face, fingers, feet, and/or lower legs.

OVERDOSE MANAGEMENT

Symptoms: Methemoglobinemia following massive overdoses. Hemolysis due to G6PD deficiency. *Treatment:* Methylene blue, 1–2 mg/kg IV or 100–200 mg PO of ascorbic acid to treat methemoglobinemia.

HOW SUPPLIED

OTC. Tablet: 95 mg, 97.5 mg, 100 mg; *Rx. Tablet:* 97.2 mg, 100 mg, 150 mg, 200 mg.

DOSAGE

OTC OR RX: TABLETS

Symptomatic relief of pain, burning, urgency, frequency, discomfort.

Adults: 200 mg 3 times per day after meals for not more than 2 days when used together with an antibacterial agent for UTI. **Pediatric, 6–12 years:** 4 mg/kg 3 times per day with food for 2 days.

NURSING IMPLICATIONS

IMPLEMENTATION/ADMINISTRATION/STORAGE

Do not use for more than 2 days; there is no evidence that combined administration of phenazopyridine and an antibacterial provides greater benefit than administration of the antibacterial alone after 2 days.

ASSESSMENT

1. Note reasons for therapy, type, onset, characteristics of S&S, other agents used.
2. Assess frequency, urgency, and pain with urination. May stop therapy after pain relieved (or 2 days) but continue antibiotic as prescribed.
3. Review culture results and renal function; assess for G-6-PD, liver/renal dysfunction.

CLIENT/FAMILY TEACHING

1. Take with or after meals to prevent GI upset. Consume 2–3 L/day of fluids. Do not crush or chew tablets. Permanent teeth discoloration may occur.
2. Generally used for only 2 days when taken together with an antibacterial agent for UTIs; complete entire antibiotic prescription.
3. With diabetes, check finger sticks regularly.
4. May cause staining of contact lenses; do not wear during therapy, wear glasses instead.
5. Drug turns urine orange-red; may stain fabrics. Wear a sanitary napkin to avoid staining garments. A 0.25% sodium dithionate or sodium hydrosulfite solution, available from a pharmacy, will remove these stains.
6. Report itching/yellowing of skin/eyes, bluish skin hue, lack of response, headache, rash, pruritus, or upset stomach.
7. Keep all F/U to assess response, labs, adverse SE.

OUTCOMES/EVALUATE

Relief of pain and discomfort with UTI

IV

Phenobarbital

(fee-no-**BAR**-bih-tal)

Classification(s): Sedative-hypnotic, barbiturate

Pregnancy Category: D

RX: Bellatal, Solfoton, **C-IV**

✤ **Rx:** PMS-Phenobarbital.

Phenobarbital sodium

Pregnancy Category: D

RX: Luminal Sodium, **C-IV**

INDICATIONS/USES

PO: (1) Sedative or hypnotic (short-term). (2) Anticonvulsant (partial and generalized tonic-clonic or cortical focal seizures). (3) Emergency control of acute seizure disorders due to status epilepticus, meningitis, tetanus, eclampsia, toxicity of local anesthetics.

Parenteral: (1) Sedative or hypnotic (short-term). (2) Preanesthetic. (3) Anticonvulsant (generalized tonic-clonic and cortical focal seizures). (4) Emergency control of acute seizure disorders (e.g., tetanus, eclampsia, status epilepticus).

ACTION/KINETICS

Action

Depressant and anticonvulsant effects may be related to its ability to increase and/or mimic the inhibitory activity of GABA on nerve synapses. Is not an analgesic; not to be given to relieve pain.

Pharmacokinetics

Onset: 30 to more than 60 min. **Duration:** 10–16 hr. **Anticonvulsant therapeutic serum levels:** 15–40 mcg/mL. **Time for peak effect, after IV:** Up to 15 min. Distributed more slowly than other barbiturates due to lower lipid solubility. Long-acting. **t½:** 53–140 hr. Twenty-five percent eliminated unchanged in the urine. **Plasma protein binding:** 50–60%.

CONTRAINDICATIONS

Hypersensitivity to barbiturates, severe trauma, pulmonary disease when dyspnea or obstruction is present, edema, uncontrolled diabetes, history of porphyria, and impaired liver function and for clients in whom they produce an excitatory response. Also, clients who have been addicted previously to sedative-hypnotics.

SPECIAL CONCERNS

- Use with caution during lactation and in clients with CNS depression, hypotension, marked asthenia (characteristic of Addison's disease, hypoadrenalism, and severe myxedema), porphyria, fever, anemia, hemorrhagic shock, cardiac, hepatic or renal damage, and a history of alcoholism in suicidal clients.
- Geriatric clients usually manifest increased sensitivity to barbiturates, as evidenced by confusion, excitement, mental depression, and hypothermia.
- Reduce the dose in geriatric and debilitated clients, as well as with impaired hepatic or renal function.
- When given in the presence of pain, restlessness, excitement, and delirium may result.

SIDE EFFECTS

Most Common

Somnolence, headache, agitation, confusion, ataxia, dizziness.

CNS: Sleepiness, drowsiness, agitation, confusion, hyperkinesia, ataxia, CNS depression, nightmares, nervousness, psychiatric disturbances, hallucinations, insomnia, anxiety, dizziness, headache, abnormal thinking, vertigo, lethargy, hangover, excitement, appearance of being inebriated. Irritability and hyperactivity in children. **Musculoskeletal:** Localized or diffuse myalgic, neuralgic, or arthritic pain, especially in psychoneurotic clients. Pain is often most intense in the morning and is frequently located in the neck, shoulder girdle, and arms. **Respiratory:** Hypoventilation, ***apnea, respiratory depression***. **CV:** Bradycardia, hypotension, syncope, ***circulatory collapse***. **GI:** N&V, constipation, liver damage (especially with chronic use of phenobarbital). **Allergic:** Skin rashes, ***angioedema***, exfoliative dermatitis (including ***Stevens-Johnson syndrome and toxic epidermal necrolysis***). Allergic reactions are most common in clients who have asthma, urticaria, angioedema, and similar conditions. Symptoms include localized swelling (especially of the lips, cheeks, or eyelids) and erythematous dermatitis.

- **AFTER IV USE**

CV: Circulatory depression, thrombophlebitis, ***peripheral vascular collapse, seizures with cardiorespiratory arrest, myocardial depression, cardiac arrhythmias***. **Respiratory: *Apnea, laryngospasm, bronchospasm***, dyspnea, rhinitis, sneezing, coughing. **CNS:** Emergence delirium, headache, anxiety, prolonged somnolence and recovery, restlessness, ***seizures***. **GI:** N&V, abdominal pain, diarrhea, cramping. **Hypersensitivity: *Acute allergic reactions***, including erythema, pruritus, ***anaphylaxis***. **Miscellaneous:** Pain or nerve injury at injection site, salivation, hiccoughs, skin rashes, shivering, skeletal muscle hyperactivity, ***immune hemolytic anemia with renal failure***, and radial nerve palsy.

- **AFTER IM USE**

Pain at injection site.

NOTE: Although barbiturates can induce physical and psychologic dependence if high doses are used regularly for long periods of time, the incidence of dependence on phenobarbital is low. Withdrawal symptoms usually begin after 12–16 hr of abstinence. Manifestations of withdrawal include anxiety, weakness, N&V, muscle cramps, delirium, and even tonic-clonic seizures. Chronic use may result in headache, fever, and megaloblastic anemia.

LABORATORY TEST CONSIDERATIONS

Interference with test method: ↑ 17-Hydroxycorticosteroids. ↑ CPK, alkaline phosphatase, serum transaminase, serum testosterone (in certain women), urinary estriol, porphobilinogen, coproporphyrin, uroporphyrin. ↓ PT in clients on coumarin. ↑ or ↓ Bilirubin. False + lupus erythematosus test.

OVERDOSE MANAGEMENT

Symptoms: Acute Toxicity: Characterized by cortical and ***respiratory depression; anoxia; peripheral vascular collapse;*** feeble, rapid pulse; pulmonary edema; decreased body temperature; clammy, cyanotic skin; depressed reflexes; stupor; and ***coma.*** After initial constriction the pupils become dilated. ***Death results from respiratory failure or arrest followed by cardiac arrest.*** *Chronic Toxicity:* Prolonged use of barbiturates at high doses may lead to physical and psychologic dependence, as well as tolerance. Symptoms of dependence are similar to those associated with chronic alcoholism, and withdrawal symptoms are equally severe. Withdrawal symptoms usually last for 5–10 days and are terminated by a long sleep. *Treatment: Acute Toxicity:*

- Maintenance of an adequate airway, oxygen intake, and carbon dioxide removal are essential.
- After PO ingestion, gastric lavage or gastric aspiration may delay absorption. Emesis should not be induced once the symptoms of overdosage are manifested, as the client may aspirate the vomitus into the lungs. Also, if the dose of barbiturate is high enough, the vomiting center in the brain may be depressed.
- Absorption following SC or IM administration of the drug may be delayed by the use of ice packs or tourniquets.
- Maintain renal function.
- Removal of the drug by peritoneal dialysis or an artificial kidney should be carried out.
- Supportive physiologic methods have proven superior to use of analeptics.

Chronic Toxicity: Cautious withdrawal of the hospitalized addict over a 2–4-week period. A stabilizing dose of 200–300 mg of a short-acting barbiturate is administered q 6 hr. The dose is then reduced by 100 mg/day until the stabilizing dose is reduced by one-half. The client is then maintained on this dose for 2–3 days before further reduction. The same procedure is repeated when the initial stabilizing dose has been reduced by three-quarters. If a mixed spike and slow activity appear on the EEG, or if insomnia, anxiety, tremor, or weakness is observed, the dosage is maintained at a constant level or increased slightly until symptoms disappear.

DRUG INTERACTIONS

General Considerations: Phenobarbital stimulates the activity of enzymes responsible for the metabolism of a large number of other drugs by a process known as enzyme induction. As a result, when phenobarbital is given to clients receiving such drugs, their therapeutic effectiveness may be markedly reduced or even abolished.

The CNS depressant effect of the barbiturates is potentiated by many drugs. Concomitant administration may result in coma or fatal CNS depression. Barbiturate dosage should either be reduced or eliminated when other CNS drugs are given. Barbiturates also potentiate the toxic effects of many other agents.

Acetaminophen / ↑ Risk of hepatotoxicity when used with large or chronic doses of barbiturates
Alcohol / Potentiation or addition of CNS depressant effects. Concomitant use may lead to drowsiness, lethargy, stupor, respiratory collapse, coma, or death
Anesthetics, general / See ***Alcohol***
Anorexiants / ↓ Effect of anorexiants R/T opposite effects
Antianxiety drugs / See ***Alcohol***
Anticoagulants, oral (including warfarin) / ↓ Effect of anticoagulants R/T ↓ GI tract absorption and ↑ liver breakdown; monitor PT and INR
Antidepressants, tricyclic / ↓ Antidepressant effects R/T ↑ liver breakdown
Antidiabetic agents / Prolong the effects of barbiturates
Antihistamines / See ***Alcohol***
Beta-adrenergic agents / ↓ Beta blockade R/T ↑ liver breakdown
Carbamazepine / ↓ Carbamazepine levels may occur

P

Charcoal / ↓ Absorption of barbiturates from the GI tract
Chloramphenicol / ↑ Effect of barbiturates R/T ↓ liver breakdown and ↓ effect of chloramphenicol by ↑ liver breakdown
Clonazepam / Barbiturates may ↑ excretion of clonazepam → loss of efficacy
Clozapine / ↓ Clozapine levels R/T ↑ liver metabolism
CNS depressants / See ***Alcohol***
Corticosteroids / ↓ Effect of corticosteroids R/T ↑ liver breakdown
Doxorubicin / ↓ Effect of doxorubicin R/T ↑ excretion
Doxycycline / ↓ Effect of doxycycline R/T ↑ liver breakdown (effect may last up to 2 weeks after barbiturates are discontinued)
Estrogens / ↓ Effect of estrogen R/T ↑ liver breakdown
Felodipine / ↓ Felodipine levels → ↓ effect
Fenoprofen / ↓ Bioavailability of fenoprofen
Furosemide / ↑ Risk or intensity of orthostatic hypotension
Griseofulvin / ↓ Effect of griseofulvin R/T ↓ absorption from GI tract
Haloperidol / ↓ Effect of haloperidol R/T ↑ liver breakdown
H ***Indian snakeroot*** / Additive CNS depression
H ***Kava kava*** / Potentiation of CNS depression
MAOIs / ↑ Effect of barbiturates R/T ↓ liver breakdown
Meperidine / CNS depressant effects may be prolonged
Methadone / ↓ Effect of methadone
Methoxyflurane / ↑ Kidney toxicity R/T ↑ liver breakdown of methoxyflurane to toxic metabolites
Metronidazole / ↓ Effect of metronidazole
Narcotic analgesics / See ***Alcohol***
Oral contraceptives / ↓ Effect of contraceptives R/T ↑ liver breakdown
Phenothiazines / ↓ Effect of phenothiazines R/T ↑ liver breakdown; also see ***Alcohol***
Phenytoin / Effect variable and unpredictable; monitor carefully
Procarbazine / ↑ Effect of barbiturates
Quinidine / ↓ Effect of quinidine R/T ↑ liver breakdown
Rifampin / ↓ Effect of barbiturates R/T ↑ liver breakdown
Sedative-hypnotics, nonbarbiturate / See ***Alcohol***
Theophyllines / ↓ Effect of theophyllines R/T ↑ liver breakdown
Valproic acid / ↑ Effect of barbiturates R/T ↓ liver breakdown
Verapamil / ↑ Excretion of verapamil → ↓ effect
Vitamin D / Barbiturates may ↑ requirements for vitamin D R/T ↑ liver breakdown

HOW SUPPLIED

Phenobarbital. *Capsules:* 16 mg; ***Elixir:*** 15 mg/5 mL, 20 mg/5 mL; ***Tablets:*** 15 mg, 16 mg, 16.2 mg, 30 mg, 60 mg, 90 mg, 100 mg.
Phenobarbital sodium. *Injection:* 30 mg/mL, 60 mg/mL, 65 mg/mL, 130 mg/mL.

DOSAGE

Phenobarbital, Phenobarbital Sodium

CAPSULES; ELIXIR; TABLETS

Sedation.
Adults: 30–120 mg/day in two to three divided doses. Or, a single dose of 30–120 mg may be given at intervals; frequency is determined by response, but no more than 400 mg per day. **Pediatric:** 8–32 mg.

Hypnotic.
Adults: 100–200 mg at bedtime. **Pediatric:** Dose should be determined by provider, based on age and weight.

Anticonvulsant.
Adults: 60–200 mg/day in single or divided doses. **Pediatric:** 3–6 mg/kg/day in single or divided doses. In infants and children, a loading dose of 15–20 mg/kg achieves blood levels of about 20 mcg/mL shortly after administration. To reach therapeutic blood levels of 10–25 mcg/mL, higher doses per kilogram are generally necessary compared with adults.

IM; IV

Sedation.
Adults: 30–120 mg/day IM or IV in two to three divided doses.

Preoperative sedation.
Adults: 100–200 mg IM only, 60–90 min before surgery. **Pediatric:** 1–3 mg/kg IM or IV 60–90 min prior to surgery.

Hypnotic.
Adults: 100–320 mg IM or IV.
Acute convulsions.
Adults: 200–320 mg IM or IV; may be repeated in 6 hr if needed. **Pediatric:** 4–6 mg/kg/day for 7–10 days to achieve a blood level of 10–15 mcg/mL (or 10–15 mg/kg/day, IV or IM).
Status epilepticus.
Adults: 15–20 mg/kg IV (given over 10–15 min); may be repeated if needed. **Pediatric:** 15–20 mg/kg given over a 10 to 15 min period. *NOTE:* Use the minimal amount required and wait for the anticonvulsant effect to occur before giving a second dose.

NURSING IMPLICATIONS

Do not confuse phenobarbital with pentobarbital (a shorter-acting barbiturate) or with phenytoin (an anticonvulsant).

IMPLEMENTATION/ADMINISTRATION/STORAGE

1. Use parenterally only when PO use is impossible or impractical.
2. Reduce dose in the elderly, debilitated, or those with impaired hepatic or renal function.
3. When used for seizures, give major part of the dose according to when seizures are likely to occur (i.e., on arising for daytime seizures; at bedtime when seizures occur at night).
4. When used IM, inject into large muscle (e.g., gluteus maximus, vastus lateralis). Injection into/near peripheral nerves may cause permanent neurologic deficit.
5. In most cases, when used for epilepsy, drug must be taken regularly to avoid seizures, even when no seizures are imminent. Give lowest dose possible to avoid adding to the depression that may follow seizures.
6. IV Reserve IV use for conditions when other routes are not feasible. There is the possibility of overdose, including respiratory depression, even with slow injection of fractional doses.
7. In convulsive states, minimize dosage to avoid compounding the depression that may follow seizures. Make the injection slowly.
8. Administer preferably into a larger vein to minimize the possibility of thrombosis. Do not give into varicose veins due to slowed circulation.
9. Inadvertant injection into or adjacent to an artery may cause gangrene requiring amputation of the extremity or portion thereof. Aspirate to avoid inadvertent intra-arterial injection.
10. Freshly prepare aqueous solution for injection and inject slowly at a rate of 50 mg/min.
11. Some ready-dissolved solutions for injection are available; the vehicle is propylene glycol, water, and alcohol.
12. Avoid any extravasation as tissue damage and necrosis may result.
13. COMPATIBILITY Reconstitute with sterile water and administer slowly.
14. INCOMPATIBILITY Administer separately.

ASSESSMENT

1. List reasons for therapy, type, onset, characteristics of S&S/seizures, other agents trialed. Note clinical presentation; list drugs prescribed to ensure none interact.
2. Assess mental status, pulmonary status, any fall potential, and behavioral presentation.
3. Monitor VS, CBC, folate levels, renal and LFTs. Reduce dose with dysfunction and in debilitated/elderly clients.

CLIENT/FAMILY TEACHING

1. Take as directed. Store away from bedside and out of child's reach.
2. May initially cause drowsiness; assess effects before performing tasks that require mental alertness.
3. Phenobarbital may require an increase in vitamin D consumption; consume foods high in vitamin D. May also contribute to folate deficiency requiring supplemental folic acid and vitamin D.
4. Drug decreases effects of oral contraceptives; practice other nonhormonal forms of birth control. Avoid alcohol, CNS depressants, and OTC agents without approval.
5. Do not stop abruptly following long term use; may precipitate seizures. Tolerance may develop and require dosage adjustment.
6. Report any loss of effects, adverse effects or fever, sore throat, rash or bruising/bleeding. Brush teeth frequently and carefully to prevent gingivitis and have regular dental exams.
7. Keep all F/U to assess response, labs, adverse SE.

OUTCOMES/EVALUATE

- Sedation; control of seizures

P

- Therapeutic anticonvulsant drug levels (15–40 mcg/mL)

■ IV Sound Alike

Phenytoin

(**FEN**-ih-toyn)

Classification(s): Antiarrhythmic, Class IB; anticonvulsant, hydantoin

Pregnancy Category: D

RX: Dilantin Infatab, Dilantin-125.

🍁 **Rx:** Dilantin-30 Suspension, Taro-Phenytoin.

Phenytoin sodium, extended

Pregnancy Category: D

RX: Dilantin, Phenytek.

Phenytoin sodium, parenteral

Pregnancy Category: D

RX: Phenytoin Sodium Injection Solution.

SEE ALSO ***ANTICONVULSANTS*** AND ***ANTIARRHYTHMIC DRUGS***.

INDICATIONS/USES

PO: (1) Control of generalized tonic-clonic seizures. (2) Control of complex partial (psychomotor, temporal lobe) seizures. (3) Prevent or treat seizures during or following neurosurgery (tablets only). **Parenteral:** (1) Prevent or treat seizures during or following neurosurgery. (2) IV to treat status epilepticus.

P

ACTION/KINETICS

Action

Acts in the motor cortex of the brain to reduce the spread of electrical discharges from the rapidly firing epileptic foci in this area. This is accomplished by stabilizing hyperexcitable cells possibly by promoting sodium efflux. Also, phenytoin decreases activity of centers in the brain stem responsible for the tonic phase of grand mal seizures. Has few sedative effects. As an antiarrhythmic, phenytoin increases the electrical stimulation threshold of heart muscle, although it is less effective than quinidine, procainamide, or lidocaine. It also decreases the QT interval.

Pharmacokinetics

Phenytoin is available as chewable tablets, extended-release (ER) capsules, oral suspension, and injection. There is about an 8% increase in drug content with the free acid form over that of the sodium salt. **Peak serum levels:** 1.5–3 hr for chewable tablets and PO suspension, 4–12 hr for ER capsules, and 24 hr for IM injection. Since the rate and extent of absorption depend on the particular preparation, the same product should be used for a particular client. **Therapeutic serum levels:** 10–20 mcg/mL following any of the dosage forms. **t½, plasma:** Average of 14 hr for chewable tablets, 22 hr for ER capsules and PO suspension, and 10–15 hr following IV use. **Steady state:** 7–10 days after initiation of therapy with doses of 300 mg/day. Biotransformed in the liver. Both inactive metabolites and unchanged (less than 5%) drug are excreted in the urine and feces. A small number of clients metabolize phenytoin slowly; may be genetic. As an antiarrhythmic: **Onset:** 30–60 min. **Duration:** 24 hr or more. **t½:** 22–36 hr. **Plasma protein binding:** About 90% (range: 69–96%).

CONTRAINDICATIONS

Hypersensitivity to hydantoins, exfoliative dermatitis. Use of parenteral phenyton in sinus bradycardia, second- and third-degree AV block, clients with Adams-Stokes syndrome, SA block. IM use for status epilepticus. Lactation.

SPECIAL CONCERNS

■ **Parenteral.** Phenytoin sodium injection must be administered slowly. In adults, do not exceed 50 mg per minute IV. In neonates, administer the drug at a rate not exceeding 1 to 3 mg/kg/min. ■

- **Use with caution in acute, intermittent porphyria.**
- **Administer with extreme caution with history of asthma or other allergies, impaired renal or hepatic function, and heart disease (hypotension, severe myocardial insufficiency).**
- **Abrupt withdrawal may cause status epilepticus.**
- **Combined drug therapy required if petit mal seizures also present.**

SIDE EFFECTS

Most Common

Ataxia, drowsiness, slurred speech, confusion, N&V, rash, constipation/diarrhea, gum/gingival hyperplasia.

After PO use. CNS: Ataxia, decreased coordination, dizziness, headache, insomnia, mental confusion, motor twitchings, nervousness, peripheral polyneuropathy, slurred speech, dyskinesias (rare). **CV:** Periarteritis nodosa. **GI:** Constipation, gum/gingival hypertrophy, N&V. **Hepatic:** Toxic hepatitis, acute hepatotoxicity, hepatic failure, hepatomegaly, jaundice. **Dermatologic:** Dermatitis (bullous, exfoliative, or purpuric), dermatitis, hypertrichosis, morbilliform rash, scarlatiniform rash, skin rash, ***toxic epidermal necrolysis***. **Hematologic:** Agranulocytosis, benign lymph node hyperplasia, granulocytopenia, Hodgkin's disease, leukopenia, lymphadenopathy, lymphoma, macrocytosis, megaloblastic anemia, pancytopenia (with or without bone marrow suppression), pseudolymphoma, thrombocytopenia, leukocytosis. **Hypersensitivity:** Hypersensitivity syndrome (arthralgia, eosinophilia, fever, liver dysfunction, lymphadenopathy, rash), ***Stevens-Johnson syndrome***. **Ophthalmic:** Nystagmus. **Body as a whole:** Immunoglobulin abnormalities, lupus erythematosus (including systemic), Peyronie's disease. **Miscellaneous:** Coarsening of facial features, enlargement of lips.

After parenteral use. CNS: Ataxia, CNS depression, decreased coordination, dizziness, headache, insomnia, mental confusion, motor twitchings, nervousness, peripheral polyneuropathy, slurred speech, dyskinesias (rare). **CV:** Hypotension, periarteritis nodosa, ***ventricular fibrillation***. Rapid parenteral administration may cause serious CV effects, including hypotension, arrhythmias, atrial/ventricular conduction depression, ***CV collapse***, and heart block, as well as CNS depression. **GI:** Constipation, gum/gingival hypertrophy, N&V. **Hepatic:** Toxic hepatitis, acute hepatotoxicity, hepatic failure, hepatomegaly, jaundice. **Dermatologic:** Dermatitis (bullous, exfoliative, or purpuric), dermatitis, hypertrichosis, morbilliform rash, scarlatiniform rash, skin rash, ***toxic epidermal necrolysis***. **Hematologic:** Agranulocytosis, benign lymph node hyperplasia, granulocytopenia, Hodgkin's disease, leukopenia, lymphadenopathy, lymphoma, macrocytosis, megaloblastic anemia, pancytopenia (with or without bone marrow suppression), pseudolymphoma, thrombocytopenia, eosinophilia, leukocytosis. **At site of injection:** Inflammation, local irritation, necrosis, sloughing, tenderness, pain. **Hypersensitivity:** ***Stevens-Johnson syndrome***. **Ophthalmic:** Nystagmus. **Body as a whole:** Immunoglobulin abnormalities, lupus erythematosus (including systemic), Peyronie's disease. **Miscellaneous:** Coarsening of facial features, enlargement of lips.

LABORATORY TEST CONSIDERATIONS

↑ Serum alkaline phosphatase, GGT, glucose.

OVERDOSE MANAGEMENT

Symptoms: Initially, ataxia, dysarthria, and nystagmus followed by unresponsive pupils, hypotension, and coma. Delirium, psychosis, or encephalopathy. Plasma levels greater than 40 mcg/mL result in significant decreases in mental capacity. *Treatment:* Treat symptoms. Hemodialysis may be effective. In children, total-exchange transfusion has been used.

DRUG INTERACTIONS

Acetaminophen / ↓ Acetaminophen effect R/T ↑ liver breakdown; possible ↑ hepatotoxicity
Alcohol, ethyl / ↑ Phenytoin serum levels with acute alcohol use; ↓ Phenytoin serum levels with chronic alcohol use
Alprazolam / Possible ↑ phenytoin serum levels → toxicity; monitor phenytoin levels
Amiodarone / ↑ Phenytoin levels with possible toxicity; ↓ amiodarone serum levels with loss of effect
Antacids / ↓ Phenytoin effect R/T ↓ GI absorption; stagger ingestion times
Anticoagulants, oral / ↑ Phenytoin effect R/T ↓ liver breakdown. Also, possible ↑ anticoagulant effect
Bleomycin / ↓ Phenytoin levels → loss of therapeutic effect; monitor phenytoin levels
Carbamazepine / ↓ Phenytoin or carbamazepine effect R/T ↑ liver breakdown
Carboplatin / ↓ Phenytoin levels → loss of therapeutic effect; monitor phenytoin levels
Carmustine / ↓ Phenytoin levels → loss of therapeutic effect; monitor phenytoin levels
Chloral hydrate / ↑ Phenytoin clearance → ↓ therapeutic effects
Chloramphenicol / ↑ Phenytoin effect R/T ↓ liver breakdown; possible phenytoin toxicity
Chlordiazepoxide / Possible ↑ phenytoin serum levels → toxicity; monitor phenytoin levels
Cimetidine / ↑ Phenytoin effect R/T ↓ liver breakdown

P

Cisplatin / ↓ Phenytoin levels → loss of therapeutic effect; monitor phenytoin levels
Contraceptives, hormonal / ↑ Phenytoin levels; ↓ effect of hormonal contraceptives
Corticosteroids / ↓ Corticosteroid effect R/T ↑ liver breakdown; also, corticosteroids may mask hypersensitivity reactions due to phenytoin
Cyclosporine / ↓ Cyclosporine levels → ↓ effect R/T ↑ liver breakdown
Diazepam / Possible ↑ phenytoin serum levels → toxicity; monitor phenytoin levels
Diazoxide / ↓ Phenytoin effect R/T ↑ liver breakdown
Digoxin / ↓ Digoxin effect R/T ↑ liver breakdown; possibly ↑ digoxin dose
Disopyramide / ↓ Disopyramide effect R/T ↑ liver breakdown
Disulfiram / ↑ Phenytoin effect R/T ↓ liver breakdown → ↑ pharmacologic/toxic effects
Dopamine / IV phenytoin → profound hypotension and possible cardiac arrest; use together with extreme caution
Doxycycline / ↓ Doxycycline effect R/T ↑ liver breakdown; doxycycline dose may need to be doubled
Estrogens (conjugated estrogens, estradiol, ethinyl estradiol) / Possible ↑ metabolism of estrogens → breakthrough bleeding, spotting, and loss of efficacy; protein binding of phenytoin may be affected with loss of seizure control
Felbamate / ↑ Phenytoin serum levels → ↑ pharmacologic/toxic effects; also, possible ↓ felbamate levels with changes in seizure control
Felodipine / ↓ Felodipine effects; higher doses may be required
Fluconazole / ↑ Phenytoin effect R/T ↓ liver breakdown → possible toxicity
Folic acid / Possible ↓ phenytoin levels with loss of seizure control; monitor phenytoin levels; also, ↓ serum folate levels → possible megaloblastic anemia
Furosemide / ↓ Furosemide effect R/T ↓ absorption
Haloperidol / ↓ Haloperidol effect R/T ↑ liver breakdown
Halothane / ↑ Serum phenytoin levels
Ibuprofen / ↑ Serum phenytoin levels → ↑ pharmacologic/toxic effects
Itraconazole / ↑ Phenytoin effect R/T ↓ liver breakdown → possible toxicity; possible ↓ itraconazole plasma levels → ↓ efficacy
Isoniazid / ↑ Phenytoin effect R/T ↓ liver breakdown → ↑ pharmacologic/toxic effects
Levodopa / ↓ Levodopa effect
Methadone / ↓ Methadone effect R/T ↑ liver breakdown
Methotrexate / ↓ Phenytoin levels → loss of therapeutic effect; monitor phenytoin levels
Methylphenidate / ↑ Serum phenytoin levels
Metronidazole / ↑ Phenytoin effect R/T ↓ liver breakdown
Metyrapone / ↓ Metyrapone effect R/T ↑ liver breakdown
Mexiletine / ↓ Mexiletine effect R/T ↑ liver breakdown
Midazolam / ↑ Midazolam clearance
Mirtazapine / ↓ Plasma mirtazapine levels R/T ↑ metabolism → ↓ effects
Molindone / ↓ Serum phenytoin levels R/T calcium ions in the product ↓ PO phenytoin absorption
Muscle relaxants, nondepolarizing (e.g., cisatracurium, pancuronium, vecuronium) / ↓ Duration of action of muscle relaxants; dose may need to be increased
Nisoldipine / ↓ Nisoldipine effects; monitor CV status
Omeprazole / ↑ Phenytoin effect R/T ↓ liver breakdown → ↑ pharmacologic/toxic effects
Oxazepam / ↑ Oxazepam clearance
Phenobarbital / Effect on phenytoin unpredictable; possible ↑ phenobarbital levels; monitor serum levels of both drugs
Phenothiazines (e.g., fluphenazine, prochlorperazine, thioridazine) / ↑ Phenytoin effect R/T ↓ liver breakdown; possible ↓ thioridazine effects
Praziquantel / ↓ Praziquantel serum levels → treatment failures
Primidone / ↑ Serum primidone levels
Progestins (e.g., levonorgestrel, norgestrel) / ↓ Efficacy of progestins → ↑ risk of contraceptive failure
Protease inhibitors (e.g., fosamprenavir, lopinavir, ritonavir) / ↓ Plasma levels of phenytoin and certain protease inhibitors → ↓ therapeutic effect of both drugs
Quetiapine / ↓ Peak and trough quetiapine levels R/T ↑ liver metabolism
Quinidine / ↓ Quinidine efficacy; monitor serum quinidine levels

P

Rifabutin, Rifampin / ↓ Phenytoin effect R/T ↑ liver breakdown; phenytoin may ↓ rifampin efficacy
Salicylates (e.g., aspirin, bismuth subsalicylate) / ↑ Phenytoin effect R/T ↓ plasma protein binding
Selective serotonin reuptake inhibitors (e.g., fluoxetine, fluvoxamine, sertraline) / ↑ Phenytoin serum levels → ↑ pharmacologic/toxic effects; possible ↓ paroxetine efficacy
Succinimides (e.g., ethosuximide, methsuximide) / ↑ Serum phenytoin levels → ↑ pharmacologic/toxic effects
Sucralfate / ↓ Phenytoin effect R/T ↓ absorption from GI tract
Sulfonamides / ↑ Phenytoin effect R/T ↓ liver breakdown → ↑ pharmacologic/toxic effects
Tacrolimus / ↑ Serum phenytoin levels and ↓ serum tacrolimus levels; monitor serum levels of both drugs
Theophylline / ↓ Effect of both drugs R/T ↑ liver breakdown
Ticlopidine / ↑ Serum phenytoin levels → possible toxic effects
Tolbutamide / ↑ Serum phenytoin levels; ↑ blood glucose levels → need for higher dose of tolbutamide
Topiramate / ↑ Phenytoin effects and ↓ topiramate effects
Trazodone / ↑ Phenytoin plasma levels → toxicity
Trimethoprim / ↑ Phenytoin serum levels → ↑ pharmacologic/toxic effects
Valproic acid, sodium valproate, divalproex sodium / ↑ Phenytoin effect R/T ↓ liver breakdown and ↓ plasma protein binding → ↑ toxicity; phenytoin may also ↓ effect of valproic acid R/T ↑ liver breakdown
Vinblastine / ↓ Phenytoin levels → loss of therapeutic effect; monitor phenytoin levels
Vitamin D / ↓ Vitamin D efficacy → possible osteomalacia
Voriconazole / ↑ Phenytoin effect R/T ↓ liver breakdown → possible toxicity; possible ↓ itraconazole plasma levels → ↓ efficacy
Warfarin / ↑ or ↓ Effect of warfarin

HOW SUPPLIED

Phenytoin. *Oral Suspension:* 125 mg/5 mL; *Tablets, Chewable:* 50 mg.
Phenytoin sodium, extended. *Capsules, Extended-Release:* 30 mg, 100 mg, 200 mg, 300 mg.
Phenytoin sodium, injection solution. *Injection Solution:* 50 mg/mL.

DOSAGE

Phenytoin
ORAL SUSPENSION; TABLETS, CHEWABLE

Seizures.

Individualize dosage. **Adults, initial:** 100 mg (2 tablets) or 125 mg (5 mL of the suspension) 3 times per day in those who have not received previous treatment; adjust dosage at 7- to 10-day intervals until seizures are controlled; **usual, maintenance:** 300–400 mg/day, although 600 mg/day (625 mg of the suspension) may be required in some. **Children, initial:** 5 mg/kg/day in two to three divided doses; **maintenance,** 4–8 mg/kg (up to maximum of 300 mg/day). Children over 6 years may require up to 300 mg/day. **Geriatric:** 3 mg/kg initially in divided doses; **then**, adjust dosage according to serum levels and response. Once dosage level has been established, the extended capsules may be used for once-a-day dosage.

Phenytoin sodium
CAPSULES, EXTENDED-RELEASE

Seizures.

Adults, initial, no previous treatment: 100 mg 3 times per day; adjust dose at 7- to 10-day intervals until control is achieved. For most adults, satisfactory maintenance dosage will be 100 mg (1 capsule) 3–4 times per day. An increase up to 2–100 mg capsules or one 200 mg capsule 3 times per day may be necessary. If seizure control is established with divided doses of three 100 mg extended-release capsules/day, once daily dosage with phenytoin, 300 mg extended-release may be considered.
NOTE: Some advocate use of an oral loading dose in adults who require rapid steady-state serum levels and in whom IV use is not desirable. Reserve this regimen for those in a clinic or hospital setting where phenytoin serum levels can be monitored closely. **Loading dose:** 1 gram of phenytoin capsules divided into 3 doses (400, 300, and

P

300 mg) given at 2-hr intervals. Normal maintenance dosage is begun 24 hr after the loading dose. **Pediatric:** See dose for Oral Suspension and Chewable Tablets.

IV

Status epilepticus.

Adults, loading dose: 10–15 mg/kg at a rate not to exceed 50 mg/min; **then,** 100 mg PO or IV q 6–8 hr. **Pediatric, loading dose:** 15–20 mg/kg in divided doses of 5–10 mg/kg given at a rate of 1–3 mg/kg/min. *NOTE:* Coadministration of an IV benzodiazepine (e.g., diazepam) or an IV short–acting barbiturate will usually be necessary for rapid control of seizures because of the required slow rate of administration of phenytoin.

IM

Prevention of seizures during neurosurgery.

Adults, usual: 100–200 mg (2–4 mL) IM at approximately 4–hr intervals during surgery and continued during the postoperative period. When IM administration is required for a client previously stabilized on PO medication, compensating dosage adjustments are needed to maintain therapeutic plasma levels. An IM dose of 50% more than the PO dose is necessary to maintain these levels. When returned to PO administration, reduce the dose by 50% of the original PO dose for 1 week to prevent excessive plasma levels due to sustained release from IM tissue sites. *NOTE:* Although the manufacturer recommends IM administration for prevention of seizures during neurosurgery, most providers avoid IM use because of severe pain and the potential for tissue necrosis and crystallization at the injection site.

NURSING IMPLICATIONS

Do not confuse phenytoin with fosphenytoin or mephyton (also anticonvulsants); also, do not confuse phenytoin with phenobarbital (barbiturate). Do not confuse Dilantin with Dilaudid (a narcotic analgesic).

IMPLEMENTATION/ADMINISTRATION/STORAGE

1. Individualize dosage. Serum blood levels may be necessary for optimal adjustments of dosage. Clinically effective serum level is usually from 10 to 20 mcg/mL.
2. Tablets are not for once-daily dosing. Only phenytoin sodium extended-release capsules are recommended for once-daily dosing.
3. When given in equal doses, phenytoin yields higher plasma levels than phenytoin sodium. Thus, dosage adjustments and serum level monitoring may be necessary when switching from phenytoin to phenytoin sodium and vice versa.
4. Full effectiveness of PO administered hydantoins is delayed and may take 7–10 days to be fully established. A similar period of time will elapse before effects disappear completely.
5. When hydantoins are substituted for or added to another anticonvulsant medication, their dosage is gradually increased, while dosage of the other drug is decreased proportionally.
6. Avoid IM, SC, or perivascular injections. Pain, inflammation, and necrosis may be caused by the highly alkaline solutions.
7. If receiving tube feedings of Isocal or Osmolite, the PO absorption of phenytoin may be decreased. Do not administer together.
8. Due to potential differences in bioavailability between PO products, do not interchange brands. Also, when switching from extended to prompt products, dosage adjustments may be required.
9. Abrupt withdrawal may precipitate status epilepticus. Discontinue or substitute alternative antiepileptic medication gradually.
10. Store chewable tablets from 15–30°C (59–86°F); protect from moisture. Store the suspension and extended–release capsules from 20–25°C (68–77°F); protect from freezing and light.
11. IV Use of IV infusion is not recommended, as the drug is poorly soluble and may form a precipitate. Inject slowly and directly into a large vein through a large-gauge needle or IV catheter.
12. For parenteral preparations:
    - Use only a clear solution.
    - Dilute with special diluent supplied by manufacturer.

- Shake the vial until the solution is clear. It may take about 10 min for the drug to dissolve.
- To hasten the process, warm the vial in warm water after adding the diluent.

13. The loading dose for obese clients may be calculated using an adjusted body weight of the following formula: Dosing weight (kg) = ideal body weight (IBW) + 1.33 × (measured weight – IBW).
14. If IV infusion is used, a rate of 50 mg/min should not be exceeded in adults or 1–3 mg/kg/min in neonates.
15. Give into a large vein through a large-gauge needle or IV catheter. Following IV administration, administer NSS through the same needle or IV catheter to avoid local irritation of the vein due to alkalinity of the solution.
16. For treatment of status epilepticus, inject IV slowly at a rate not to exceed 50 mg/min. May repeat the dose 30 min after the initial administration if needed. Usually coadministration of an IV benzodiazepine (e.g., diazepam) or IV short-acting barbiturate will be necessary for rapid control of seizures due to the slow rate of administration of phenytoin.
17. Store the injection from 15–30°C (59–86°F); do not freeze.
18. COMPATIBILITY NSS.
19. INCOMPATIBILITY Dextrose and acid solutions; do *not* admix with other meds or solutions.

ASSESSMENT

1. List reasons for therapy, onset, characteristics of S&S, clinical presentation, blood levels, other agents trialed, outcome.
2. Note history and nature of seizures, addressing location, frequency, duration, causes/characteristics, triggers and EEG findings.
3. Check ECG; avoid with sinus bradycardia, sino-atrial block, second- and third-degree A-V block.
4. Consider monitoring free phenytoin levels for those with low albumin levels, renal or hepatic impairment, or a critical illness. Alternatively, equations may be used that take into account the serum albumin level of clients and renal function may be used to estimate the serum phenytoin level that would have been observed if serum albumin and renal function were normal. The therapeutic range of free phenytoin is 1–2 mcg/mL.
5. During IV administration, assess for hypotension.
6. Monitor serum drug levels; serum concentrations of phenytoin increase disproportionately as dosage is increased:
   - Seven to 10 days may be required to achieve recommended serum levels. Drug is highly protein bound; may order free and bound drug levels to better assess response. Drug is metabolized much slower by the elderly; may be managed with once a day dosing.
   - If receiving drugs that interact with hydantoins or have impaired liver function, obtain level more frequently. Dilantin induces hepatic microsomal enzymes for drug metabolism.
7. Oral form has variable absorption; do not administer with tube feedings. Administer separately, flush, and clamp tube for 20 min to ensure absorption.
8. Determine if hypersensitive to hydantoins or has exfoliative dermatitis. Consider fosphenytoin in those unable to tolerate phenytoin. Avoid breast-feeding following delivery.
9. Monitor ECG, VS, CBC, phenytoin drug levels, TSH, CPK, U/A, renal and LFTs; reduce dose with dysfunction. May lower serum Mg^{++}, folate, calcium and vitamin D; consider replacement.

CLIENT/FAMILY TEACHING

1. May take with food to minimize GI upset. Do not take antacids within 1 hr of ingestion. Tablets can be chewed thoroughly before swallowing or swallowed whole. Do not use discolored capsules.
2. Use care when performing tasks that require mental alertness. Drug may cause drowsiness, dizziness, and blurred vision.
3. Do not substitute products or exchange brands; bioavailability of phenytoin may vary. Seizure control may be lost or toxic blood levels may develop with substitutions.
4. Prompt-release forms cannot be substituted for another unless the dosage is also adjusted.
   - If taking phenytoin extended, do not substitute chewable tablets for capsules. Medication strengths are not equal.

P

- If taking phenytoin extended, check bottle carefully. Chewable tablets are never extended form.
- With extended release, take only a single dose daily; take only as directed and only in the brand prescribed.

5. If dose is missed, take as soon as remembered; then resume the usual schedule. Do not double up to make up for the missed dose. If the doses of drug are scheduled throughout the day, and one of the doses is missed, take the drug as soon as it is realized unless it's within 4 hr of the next dose. In that case, omit unless otherwise instructed.
6. Do not take any other agents. Hydantoins interact with many other medications; may require adjustment of the anticonvulsant dose. Avoid alcohol in any form and CNS depressants.
7. With diabetes, monitor FS and report changes; may have to adjust insulin dosage and/or diet.
8. May cause urine to appear pink, red, or brown; do not be alarmed.
9. To minimize bleeding from the gums and prevent gingival hyperplasia, practice good oral hygiene. Brush teeth with a soft toothbrush, massage the gums, and floss every day. Advise dentist of therapy.
10. Hydantoin has an androgenic effect on the hair follicle. Acne may develop; practice good skin care. Report any excessive hair growth on the face and trunk and any discolorations or skin rash; may require dermatologist referral.
11. Complaints of weakness, ease of fatigue, headaches, or feeling faint may be signs of folic acid deficiency or megaloblastic anemia. Dietitian evaluation as well as hematologic evaluations may be indicated.
12. Report for labs as ordered, including CBC, drug levels, and renal and liver function studies. May alter thyroid function results; if thyroid studies are conducted, for ensured accuracy, they should be repeated 10 days after therapy has been discontinued.
13. Do not stop abruptly; report all side effects as may be dose-related.
14. Report worsening S&S of depression, any unusual changes in mood or behavior, or the emergence of suicidal thoughts, behavior, or thoughts about self-harm.
15. Practice reliable birth control; may decrease effectiveness of oral contraceptives.
16. Keep all F/U to assess response, labs, and for adverse SE.

OUTCOMES/EVALUATE

- Control of seizures
- Therapeutic drug levels (10–20 mcg/mL)

■ IV

Phytonadione (Vitamin K_1)

(fye-toe-nah-**DYE**-ohn)

Classification(s): Vitamin K derivative

Pregnancy Category: C

RX: Mephyton.

INDICATIONS/USES

Coagulation disorders due to faulty formation of factors II, VII, IX, and X when caused by vitamin K deficiency or interference with vitamin K activity.

PO. (1) Anticoagulant-induced PT deficiency due to coumarin or indandione derivatives. (2) Hypoprothrombinemia secondary to antibacterial therapy or salicylates. (3) Secondary to obstructive jaundice and biliary fistulas (use only if bile salts are given together with phytonadione so phytonadione will be absorbed).

Parenteral. (1) Anticoagulant-induced prothrombin deficiency caused by coumarin or indandione derivatives. (2) Hypoprothrombinemia secondary to conditions limiting absorption or synthesis of vitamin K (e.g., obstructive jaundice, biliary fistula, sprue, ulcerative colitis, celiac disease, intestinal resection, cystic fibrosis of the pancreas, regional enteritis). (3) Drug-induced hypoprothrombinemia due to interference with vitamin K metabolism (e.g., salicylates, antibacterial therapy). (4) Prophylaxis and therapy of hemorrhagic disease in newborns.

ACTION/KINETICS

Action

Vitamin K is essential for the hepatic synthesis of factors II, VII, IX, and X, all of which are essential for blood clotting. Vitamin K deficiency causes an increase in bleeding tendency, demonstrated by ecchymoses, epistaxis, hematuria, GI bleeding, and postoperative and intracranial hemorrhage.

Phytonadione is similar to natural vitamin K. GI absorption occurs only via intestinal lymphatics and requires the presence of bile salts. Vitamin K is not effective in reversing the anticoagulant effect of heparin. Frequent determinations of PT are indicated during therapy.

Pharmacokinetics
IM, Onset: 1–2 hr. **Control of bleeding:** Parenteral, 3–6 hr. **Normal PT:** 12–14 hr. **PO, Onset:** 6–10 hr.

CONTRAINDICATIONS

Severe liver disease.

SPECIAL CONCERNS

IV or IM use. Severe reactions, including death, have occurred during and immediately after IV injection, even with precautions to dilute the injection and to avoid rapid infusion. Severe reactions, including fatalities, have also been reported following IM administration. These severe reactions have resembled hypersensitivity or anaphylaxis, including shock and cardiac or respiratory arrest. Some clients exhibit these severe reactions on receiving vitamin K for the first time. Thus, restrict the IV route to those situations where other routes are not feasible and the serious risk involved is considered justified.

- **Use with caution in clients with sulfite sensitivity and during lactation.**
- **Benzyl alcohol, contained in some preparations, may cause toxicity in newborns.**
- **Safety and efficacy not determined in children.**

SIDE EFFECTS

Most Common

After PO use: N&V, stomach upset, headache, transient flushing of face, sweating, chills, fever.
After parenteral use: Flushing, sweating, hypotension, dizziness, pain/swelling/tenderness at injection site.

May be transient flushing of the face, sweating, a sense of constriction of the chest, and weakness. Cramp-like pain, weak and rapid pulse, convulsive movements, chills and fever, hypotension, cyanosis, or hemoglobinuria has been reported occasionally. ***Shock and cardiac and respiratory failure may be observed.*** **Allergic:** Rash, urticaria, anaphylaxis.

After PO use: N&V, stomach upset, headache.

After parenteral use: Flushing, alteration of taste, sweating, hypotension, dizziness, rapid and weak pulse, dyspnea, cyanosis, delayed skin reactions. Pain, swelling, and tenderness at injection site. ***IV administration may cause severe reactions (e.g., shock, cardiac or respiratory arrest, anaphylaxis) leading to death.*** These effects may occur when receiving vitamin K for the first time. **Newborns:** ***Fatal kernicterus***, hemolysis, jaundice, hyperbilirubinemia (especially in premature infants).

DRUG INTERACTIONS

Antibiotics / May inhibit vitamin K production → bleeding; give vitamin K supplements
Anticoagulants, oral / Antagonizes anticoagulant effect
Cholestyramine / ↓ Phytonadione effect R/T ↓ GI tract absorption
Colestipol / ↓ Phytonadione effect R/T ↓ GI tract absorption
Hemolytics / ↑ Potential for toxicity
Mineral oil / ↓ Phytonadione effect R/T ↓ GI tract absorption
Quinidine, Quinine / ↑ Requirement for vitamin K
Salicylates / High doses → ↑ vitamin K requirements
Sulfonamides / ↑ Requirements for vitamin K
Sucralfate / ↓ Phytonadione effect R/T ↓ GI tract absorption

HOW SUPPLIED

Injection, Aqueous Colloidal Solution: 2 mg/mL, 10 mg/mL; ***Tablets:*** 5 mg.

DOSAGE

IM, IV, SC; TABLETS

Hypoprothrombinemia, anticoagulant-induced (coumarin or indandione derivatives).

Adults: 2.5–10 mg (up to 25 mg). Dose may be repeated after 6–8 hr (parenteral use) or 12–48 hr (PO use) if PT has not been shortened sufficiently.

Hypoprothrombinemia due to other causes (antibiotics, salicylates or other drugs, factors limiting absorption or synthesis).

Adults, PO: 2.5–25 mg (rarely up to 50 mg). If possible, discontinue or reduce the dose of drugs interfering with coagulation mechanisms that is an alternative to administering concurrent phytonadione. Amount and route of administration depend on severity of condition and client response. Avoid PO route when condition would prevent proper absorption.

Hemorrhagic disease of the newborn.

Prophylaxis: Single IM dose of 0.5–1 mg within 1 hr of birth. **Treatment:** 1 mg SC or IM (higher doses may be necessary) if the mother has been receiving PO anticoagulants.

NURSING IMPLICATIONS

IMPLEMENTATION/ADMINISTRATION/STORAGE

1. Whenever possible, give by SC injection.
2. Store tablets from 15–30°C (59–86°F). Protect from light.
3. Heparin may be used to reverse effects from overdosage.
4. IV If IV use is unavoidable, inject very slowly, not exceeding 1 mg/min.
5. When dilutions are indicated, begin administration immediately after mixing with the diluent and discard any unused portion of the dilution, as well as unused contents of the ampule.
6. The product contains aluminum that may be toxic with prolonged parenteral administration if kidney function is impaired. Premature neonates are particularly at risk as their kidneys are immature and they require large amounts of calcium and phosphate solutions, which contain aluminum.
7. Protect vitamin K from light. Store injectable emulsion or colloidal solutions in cool, 5–15°C (41–59°F), dark place. Do not freeze.
8. COMPATIBILITY 0.9% NaCl, D5W, or D5W/0.9% NaCl. All the diluents should be preservative-free.
9. INCOMPATIBILITY Administer separately.

ASSESSMENT

1. Note reasons for therapy, other agents trialed, outcome; assess for any sensitivity to sulfites.
2. List drugs prescribed to ensure none interact.
3. It takes a minimum of 1–2 hr for measurable improvement in the PT after IV phytonadione is given.
4. Note any frank bleeding. Test stools, urine, and GI drainage for occult blood.
5. Observe hospitalized clients with poor nutrition (receiving TPN), uremia, recent surgery, and multiple antibiotic therapy for vitamin K deficiency. Administer slowly. Rapid parenteral administration can produce dyspnea, chest and back pain, and even death.
6. With decreased bile secretion, administer bile salts to ensure absorption of PO phytonadione. If receiving bile acid-binding resins such as colestipol or cholestyramine, monitor PT and assess carefully for malabsorption of vitamin K.
7. Monitor PT/PTT, liver, B_{12}, hematologic values; determine history or lab evidence of advanced liver disease. This results in loss of protein synthesis and is not responsive to vitamin K.

CLIENT/FAMILY TEACHING

1. Take only as directed. Dietary sources high in vitamin K include dairy products, meats, and green leafy vegetables. The dietary requirement is low since it is also synthesized by colonized bacteria in the intestine.
2. Report any evidence of unusual bruising or bleeding. Use a soft toothbrush, electric razor, and a night light at night. Wear shoes and avoid IM shots and flossing to prevent injury with bleeding.
3. If possible, discontinue or reduce the dose of drugs interfering with coagulation mechanism (e.g., salicylates, antibiotics).
4. Avoid alcohol, aspirin, and ibuprofen compounds (NSAIDs) as well as any other OTC preparations. May experience flushing sensation and alteration in taste; should subside.
5. Keep all F/U to assess response, labs, and for adverse SE.

OUTCOMES/EVALUATE

- Prevention/control of bleeding
- Prophylaxis of hypoprothrombinemia during prolonged TPN
- Prevention of hemorrhagic disease in the newborn

Pioglitazone hydrochloride

(**pie**-oh-**GLIT**-ah-zohn)

Classification(s): Antidiabetic, oral; thiazolidinedione

Pregnancy Category: C

RX: Actos.

SEE ALSO ***ANTIDIABETIC AGENTS: HYPOGLYCEMIC AGENTS***.

INDICATIONS/USES

(1) Type 2 diabetes as monotherapy as an adjunct to diet and exercise. (2) Type 2 diabetes in combination with a sulfonylurea, metformin, or insulin as an adjunct to diet and exercise. Used when diet and exercise plus the single drug does not adequately control blood glucose. *Investigational:* Polycystic ovary syndrome.

ACTION/KINETICS

Action

Depends on the presence of insulin to act. Decreases insulin resistance in the periphery and liver resulting in increased insulin-dependent glucose disposal and decreased hepatic glucose output. It is not an insulin secretagogue. Is an agonist for peroxisome proliferator-activated receptor (PPAR) gamma, which is found in adipose tissue, skeletal muscle, and liver. Activation of these receptors modulates the transcription of a number of insulin responsive genes that control glucose and lipid metabolism. Reduces fasting plasma glucose 39–65 mg/dL from placebo and HbA1c 1–1.6% from placebo.

Pharmacokinetics

After PO, steady state serum levels are reached within 7 days. **Peak levels:** 2 hr; food slightly delays the time to peak serum levels to 3–4 hr, but does not change the extent of absorption. Metabolized by CYP2C8, CYP3A4, and CYP1A1 to both active and inactive metabolites. Unchanged drug and metabolites are excreted in the urine (15–30%) and feces. **t½, elimination:** 3–7 hr (pioglitazone); 16–24 hr (total pioglitazone). Those with Child-Pugh class B/C have about 45% reduction in mean peak levels. Mean C_{max} and AUC values are increased 20–60% in women. **Plasma protein binding:** Over 99%.

CONTRAINDICATIONS

In type 1 diabetes, diabetic ketoacidosis, active liver disease, with ALT levels that exceed 2.5 times ULN, in clients with NYHA Class III or IV heart failure, lactation, or in pediatric clients less than 18 years of age. Use in those with active bladder cancer.

SPECIAL CONCERNS

(1) Thiazolidinediones, including pioglitazone, cause or exacerbate CHF in some clients. After initiation of pioglitazone, and after dose increases, observe clients carefully for signs and symptoms of heart failure (including excessive, rapid weight gain, dyspnea, and/or edema). If these signs and symptoms develop, the heart failure should be managed according to the current standards of care. Furthermore, discontinuation or dose reduction of pioglitazone must be considered. (2) Pioglitazone is not recommended in clients with symptomatic heart failure. Initiation of pioglitazone in clients with established NYHA Class III or IV heart failure is contraindicated.

- **Treatment may result in resumption of ovulation in premenopausal anovulatory clients with insulin resistance.**
- **Increased risk for hypoglycemia when combined with insulin or other oral hypoglycemics.**
- **Use with caution with edema (drug causes fluid retention that can worsen or lead to CHF).**
- **May cause osteoporosis.**
- **There is an increased risk of heart disease.**
- **Use for over 1 year may be associated with an increased risk of bladder cancer. Use with caution in those with a prior history of bladder cancer.**
- **Safety and efficacy not determined in children.**

SIDE EFFECTS

Most Common

URTI, headache, sinusitis, hypoglycemia, aggravated diabetes mellitus, tooth disorder, pharyngitis, myalgia, edema.

CNS: Headache. **Musculoskeletal:** Increased risk of bone fracture (more common in women), osteoporosis, myalgia, arthralgia. **Metabolic:** Hypoglycemia, aggravation of diabetes mellitus, weight gain (dose-related). **Respiratory:** URTI, sinusitis, pharyngitis. **Hepatic:** ↑ Hepatic enzymes to 3 or more times ULN, ***hepatic failure*** with and without fatal outcome, hepatitis. **CV:** Hypertension; fluid retention leading to heart failure (especially when used as monotherapy or with insulin), usually in those with underlying cardiac disease or a history of CV conditions; CHF, ***pleural effusions and pulmonary edema*** with or without a fatal outcome. **Dermatologic:** Angioedema, pruritus, rash, urticaria, ***Steven-Johnson syndrome***. **Ophthalmic:** Macular edema, blurred vision, de-

P

creased visual acuity. **Miscellaneous:** Tooth disorder, anemia, edema, ***anaphylactic reaction.***

LABORATORY TEST CONSIDERATIONS

↑ ALT, creatine phosphokinase, HDL. ↓ Alkaline phosphatase, AST, GGT, H&H, triglycerides.

DRUG INTERACTIONS

Atorvastatin / ↓ Serum levels of both drugs when used for 7 days
Contraceptives, hormonal (e.g., ethinyl estradiol) / ↓ Ethinyl estradiol AUC and C_{max}
CYP2C8 inducers (e.g., rifampin) / ↓ Pioglitazone levels → ↓ glycemic control
Gatifloxacin / Severe and persistent hypoglycemia; do not use together
Gemfibrozil / ↑ Pioglitazone AUC R/T inhibition of CYP2C8 isoenzyme metabolism
Insulin / ↑ Incidence of edema; possible additive or synergistic pharmacologic effects
Ketoconazole / ↑ Pioglitazone AUC and C_{max} R/T inhibition of CYP2C8 isoenzyme metabolism
Midazolam / Possible ↓ midazolam C_{max} and AUC
Nifedipine (extended release) / ↓ Nifedipine levels
Oral contraceptives (containing ethinyl estradiol/norethindrone) / ↓ Plasma levels of both hormones; possible loss of contraception
Trimethoprim / ↑ Pioglitazone AUC R/T inhibition of CYP2C8 isoenzyme metabolism

HOW SUPPLIED

Tablets: 15 mg, 30 mg, 45 mg.

DOSAGE

TABLETS

Type 2 diabetes as monotherapy.

Adults, initial: 15 mg or 30 mg once daily in clients not adequately controlled with diet and exercise. Initial dose can be increased in increments up to 45 mg once daily for those who respond inadequately. Consider combination therapy for those not responding adequately to monotherapy.

Type 2 diabetes as combination therapy.

If combined with a sulfonylurea: Initiate pioglitazone at 15 or 30 mg once daily. The current sulfonylurea dose can be continued unless hypoglycemia occurs; then, reduce the sulfonylurea dose.

If combined with metformin: Initiate pioglitazone at 15 or 30 mg once daily. The current metformin dose can be continued; it is unlikely the metformin dose will have to be adjusted due to hypoglycemia.

If combined with insulin: Initiate pioglitazone at 15 or 30 mg once daily. The current insulin dose can be continued unless hypoglycemia occurs or plasma glucose levels decrease to less than 100 mg/dL; then, decrease the insulin dose by 10–25%. Individualize further dosage adjustments based on glucose-lowering response.

NOTE: Daily dose of pioglitazone should not exceed 45 mg either as monotherapy or if combined with a sulfonylurea, metformin, or insulin.

Polycystic ovary syndrome (Investigational). Used as monotherapy or combination therapy at a single dose of 15–30 mg/day without regard to meals.

NURSING IMPLICATIONS

Do not confuse Actos with Actonel (bone growth regulator).

IMPLEMENTATION/ADMINISTRATION/STORAGE

1. It is recommended that clients be treated with pioglitazone for a period of time (3 months) adequate to evaluate changes in HbA1c unless glycemic control deteriorates or evidence of CHF.
2. Do not initiate if there is clinical evidence of active liver disease or increased ALT levels more than 2.5 ULN at the start of therapy.
3. Discontinue if signs of heart failure emerge.
4. Initiate at the lowest approved dose if prescribed for those with systolic heart failure (NYHA class II). If subsequent dose escalation is necessary, increase dose gradually only after several months of treatment with careful monitoring for weight gain, edema, or signs and symptoms of CHF exacerbation.
5. Store at 15–30°C (59–86°F) in a tightly closed container protected from moisture and humidity.

ASSESSMENT

1. List reasons for therapy, onset, characteristics of disease, other agents trialed, outcome. List drugs prescribed to ensure none interact.

2. Review diet, exercise, and other lifestyle changes to ensure good glucose control.
3. Ensure no evidence of heart failure or NYHA III or IV disease. May cause fluid accumulation and worsening of failure.
4. Counsel anovulatory premenopausal women that ovulation may result with this therapy (use reliable contraception); may see increased lower and distal limb fracture risk in females.
5. Obtain BP, Wt, CBC, HbA1c, microalbumin, renal and LFTs. Ensure clients undergo periodic monitoring of liver enzymes. Evaluate ALT prior to initiation of therapy, every 2 months for the first year of therapy, and periodically thereafter. Obtain LFTs if symptoms suggest hepatic dysfunction. Discontinue if jaundice noted or elevated LFTs.

CLIENT/FAMILY TEACHING

1. Take once daily without regard to meals. Follow dietary guidelines, perform regular exercise, weight loss, dietary restrictions, and other lifestyle changes consistent with controlling diabetes.
2. May cause swelling of extremities, resumption of ovulation (in premenopausal, anovulatory women), and hypoglycemia. Report if dark urine, lack of BS control, abdominal pain, fatigue or unexplained N&V occur.
3. Immediately report onset of an unusually rapid increase in weight or extremity swelling, SOB, or other symptoms of heart failure.
4. Practice reliable nonhormonal contraception to prevent pregnancy.
5. Monitor FS at different times during the day, and maintain log for provider review.
6. Keep all F/U to assess response, labs (HbA1c, LFTs), and for adverse SE.

OUTCOMES/EVALUATE

- Control of NIDDM by ↓ insulin resistance
- Normalization of glucose and HbA1c <8

Combination Drug

IV

Piperacillin sodium and Tazobactam sodium

(pie-**PER**-ah-**sill**-in, tay-zoh-**BAC**-tam)

Classification(s): Antibiotic, penicillin

Pregnancy Category: B

RX: Zosyn.

✤ **Rx:** Tazocin.

SEE ALSO ***PENICILLINS*** AND ***PIPERACILLIN SODIUM***.

INDICATIONS/USES

1. Appendicitis complicated by rupture or abscess and peritonitis caused by piperacillin-resistant, beta-lactamase-producing strains of *Escherichia coli, Bacteroides fragilis, B. ovatus, B. thetaiotaomicron,* or *B. vulgatus.*
2. Uncomplicated and complicated skin and skin structure infections (including cellulitis, cutaneous abscesses, and ischemic/diabetic foot infections) caused by piperacillin-resistant, beta-lactamase-producing strains of *Staphylococcus aureus.*
3. Postpartum endometritis or PID caused by piperacillin-resistant, beta-lactamase-producing strains of *E. coli.*
4. Community-acquired pneumonia of moderate severity caused by piperacillin-resistant, beta-lactamase-producing strains of *Haemophilus influenzae.*
5. Moderate to severe nosocomial pneumonia caused by piperacillin-resistant, beta-lactamase-producing strains of *S. aureus* and by susceptible strains of *Acinetobacter baumanii, H. influenzae, K. pneumoniae,* and *Pseudomonas aeruginosa* (*P. aeruginosa* should be treated in combination with an aminoglycoside).
6. Infections caused by piperacillin-susceptible organisms for which piperacillin is effective may also be treated with this combination.

NOTE: The treatment of mixed infections caused by piperacillin-susceptible organisms and piperacillin-resistant, beta-lactamase-producing organisms susceptible to this combination does not require addition of another antibiotic. The exception is treatment of *P. aeruginosa* in nosocomial pneumonia which should be treated in combination with an aminoglycoside.

ACTION/KINETICS

Action

A combination of piperacillin sodium and tazobactam sodium, a beta-lactamase inhibitor. Tazobactam inhibits beta-lactamases, thus ensuring activity of piperacillin against beta-lactamase-pro-

P

ducing microorganisms. Thus, tazobactam broadens the antibiotic spectrum of piperacillin to those bacteria normally resistant to it.

Pharmacokinetics

Peak plasma levels: Attained immediately after completion of an IV infusion. **t½, piperacillin and tazobactam:** 0.7–1.2 hr. Both drugs are eliminated through the kidney with piperacillin and tazobactam both excreted unchanged and as inactive metabolites. The t½ of both drugs is increased in clients with renal impairment and in hepatic cirrhosis (dose adjustment not required).

CONTRAINDICATIONS

Hypersensitivity to penicillins, cephalosporins, or beta-lactamase inhibitors.

SPECIAL CONCERNS

- **Use with caution during lactation.**
- **Safety and efficacy not determined in children less than 12 years of age.**

SIDE EFFECTS

Most Common

Diarrhea, constipation, N&V, dyspepsia, headache, rash, rhinitis, dyspnea, abdominal pain.

See *Penicillins* for a complete list of possible side effects. The highest incidence of side effects include the following: **GI:** Diarrhea, constipation, N&V, dyspepsia, stool changes, abdominal pain. **CNS:** Headache, insomnia, fever, agitation, dizziness, anxiety. **Dermatologic:** Rash, including maculopapular, bullous, urticarial, and eczematoid; pruritus. **Hematologic:** Thrombocytopenia, eosinophilia, leukopenia, neutropenia, hemolytic anemia. **Miscellaneous:** Pain, moniliasis, hypertension, chest pain, edema, rhinitis, dyspnea.

LABORATORY TEST CONSIDERATIONS

↓ H&H. Transient ↑ AST, ALT, alkaline phosphatase, and bilirubin. ↑ Serum creatinine, BUN. Prolonged PT and PTT. Positive direct Coombs' test. Proteinuria, hematuria, pyuria, abnormalities in electrolytes (↑ and ↓ sodium, potassium, calcium), hyperglycemia. ↓ Total protein or albumin.

DRUG INTERACTIONS

Heparin / Possible ↑ heparin effect

Oral anticoagulants / Possible ↑ anticoagulant effect

Tobramycin / ↓ AUC, renal clearance, and urinary recovery of tobramycin

Vecuronium / Prolongation of neuromuscular blockade

HOW SUPPLIED

Injection, Solution (first number refers to amount of piperacillin sodium): 2 grams-0.25 gram, 3 grams-0.375 gram, 4 grams-0.5 gram; ***Injection, Powder for Solution (first number refers to amount of piperacillin sodium):*** 2 grams-0.25 gram; 3 grams-0.375 gram; 4 grams-0.5 gram; 36 grams-4.5 grams.

DOSAGE

IV INFUSION

Susceptible infections.

Adults: 12 grams/day piperacillin and 1.5 grams/day tazobactam, given as 3.375 grams (i.e., 3 grams piperacillin and 0.375 gram tazobactam) q 6 hr for 7–10 days. In clients with renal insufficiency, the IV dose is adjusted depending on the extent of impaired function. If C_{CR} is 20–40 mL/min, the dose is 8 grams/day piperacillin and 1 gram/day tazobactam in divided doses of 2.25 grams q 6 hr. If the C_{CR} <20 mL/min, the dose is 6 grams/day piperacillin and 0.75 gram/day tazobactam in divided doses of 2.25 grams q 8 hr. In hemodialysis clients or continuous ambulatory peritoneal dialysis, give 2.25 grams q 12 hr; give 0.75 gram following each hemodialysis session on hemodialysis days.

Moderate to severe nosocomial pneumonia due to piperacillin-resistant, beta-lactamase-producing S. aureus.

Adults: 4.5 grams piperacillin q 6 hr with an aminoglycoside for 7 to 14 days. Adjust the piperacillin dose as follows in clients with impaired renal function: If C_{CR} is 20–40 mL/min, give 3.375 grams q 6 hr; if C_{CR} <20 mL/min, give 2.25 grams q 6 hr. If the client is on hemodialysis or continuous ambulatory peritoneal dialysis, give 2.25 grams q 8 hr; give 0.75 gram following each hemodialysis session on hemodialysis days.

Children, 2 months and older, with appendicitis and/or peritonitis, weighing up to 40 kg, and with healthy renal function.

Children, 9 months and older: 100 mg piperacillin/12.5 mg of tazobactam/kg q 8 hr. **Children, 2–9 months:** 80 mg piperacillin/10 mg tazobactam/kg q 8 hr. Children weighing more than 40 kg with healthy renal function should receive the adult dose.

NURSING IMPLICATIONS

Do not confuse Zosyn with Zofran (an antiemetic).

IMPLEMENTATION/ADMINISTRATION/STORAGE

1. IV For IV administration or by infusion, reconstitute conventional vials with 5 mL suitable diluent per gram piperacillin. Thus, piperacillin/tazobactam 2.25, 3.375, and 4.5 grams should be reconstituted with 10, 15, and 20 mL respectively. IV diluents listed under compatibility. After the diluent is added, shake vial well until the powder is dissolved. May further dilute to the desired final volume with the diluent.
2. If intermittent IV infusion is used, the 5 mL diluent per gram piperacillin is further diluted to a volume of at least 50 mL. Give the infusion over a period of 30 min. During the infusion, discontinue the primary infusion solution.
3. To prevent unintentional overdose, do not use piperacillin/tazobactam in Galaxy containers for children who require less than the full adult dose.
4. Use single-dose vials immediately after reconstitution. Discard any unused drug after 24 hr if stored at room temperature or after 48 hr if stored in the refrigerator at 2–8°C (36–46°F). Do not refreeze thawed antibiotics.
5. After reconstitution, is stable in glass and plastic syringes, IV bags, and tubing. Is stable in IV bags for up to 24 hr at room temperature and up to 1 week in the refrigerator. Is stable in an ambulatory IV infusion pump for 24 hr at room temperature.
6. COMPATIBILITY 0.9% NaCl, sterile water for injection, dextran 6% in saline, D5W, KCl 40 mEq, bacteriostatic saline/parabens, bacteriostatic water/parabens, bacteriostatic saline/benzyl alcohol, bacteriostatic water/benzyl alcohol. A formulation contains edetate disodium dihydrate and the buffer sodium citrate; it is compatible with lactated Ringer's injection and, under certain conditions, with amikacin or gentamicin.
7. INCOMPATIBILITY RL. If concomitant therapy with aminoglycosides is indicated, give piperacillin/tazobactam and the aminoglycoside separately, as penicillin can inactivate the aminoglycoside if they are mixed.

ASSESSMENT

1. Note reasons for therapy, type, location, characteristics of S&S and culture results.
2. List any sensitivity to penicillins, cephalosporins, beta-lactamase inhibitors, or other allergens.
3. List drugs prescribed to ensure none interact unfavorably. Use of heparin and oral anticoagulants may require dosage adjustments.
4. Monitor C&S, lytes, urinalysis, hematologic, coagulation profile, renal and LFTs; reduce dosage with renal impairment.

CLIENT/FAMILY TEACHING

1. Drug is given IV every 8–12 hrs as directed. Follow dilution, dosage guidelines.
2. Report any pain at injection site, fever/chills, rash/hives, SOB, diarrhea, GI upset, lack of response or worsening of condition.
3. Keep all F/U visits to assess response, labs, and for adverse SE.

OUTCOMES/EVALUATE

Resolution of infection

Pirbuterol acetate

(peer-**BYOU**-ter-ohl)

Classification(s): Sympathomimetic

Pregnancy Category: C

RX: Maxair Autohaler.

SEE ALSO ***SYMPATHOMIMETIC DRUGS***.

INDICATIONS/USES

Alone or with theophylline or corticosteroids in clients 12 years and older for prophylaxis and treatment of bronchospasm in asthma and other conditions with reversible bronchospasms, including exercise-induced bronchospasm, bronchitis, emphysema, bronchiectasis, obstructive pulmonary disease.

P

ACTION/KINETICS

Action

Causes bronchodilation by stimulating $beta_2$-adrenergic receptors. Has minimal effects on $beta_1$ receptors. Also inhibits histamine release from mast cells, causes vasodilation, and increases ciliary motility.

Pharmacokinetics

Onset, inhalation: Approximately 5 min. **Time to peak effect:** 30–60 min. **Duration:** 5 hr.

CONTRAINDICATIONS

Cardiac arrhythmias due to tachycardia; tachycardia caused by digitalis toxicity.

SPECIAL CONCERNS

■ (1) Long-acting beta-2 agonists may increase the risk of asthma-related death. Data from a large placebo-controlled U.S. study that compared the safety of salmeterol or placebo added to usual asthma therapy showed an increase in asthma-related deaths in clients receiving salmeterol. This finding is considered a class effect of long-acting beta-2 agonists. All long-acting beta-2 agonists are contraindicated in clients with asthma without the use of a long-term asthma control medication. Currently available data are inadequate to determine whether current use of inhaled corticosteroids or other long-term asthma control drugs mitigates the increased risk of asthma related-death from long-acting beta-2 adrenergic agonists. (2) Once asthma control is achieved and maintained, assess the client at regular intervals and step down therapy (e.g., discontinue long-acting beta-2 agonist) if possible without loss of asthma control and maintain the client on a long-term asthma control medication, such as an inhaled corticosteroid. Do not use long-acting beta-2 agonists for clients whose asthma is adequately controlled on low- or medium-dose inhaled corticosteroids. (3) **Children and adolescents.** Available data from controlled clinical trials suggest that long-acting beta-2 agonists increase the risk of asthma-related hospitalization in children and adolescents. For children and adolescents with asthma, who require addition of a long-acting beta-2 agonist to an inhaled corticosteroid, a fixed-dose combination product containing both an inhaled corticosteroid and a long-acting beta-2 agonist should ordinarily be used to ensure adherence with both drugs. In cases where use of a separate long-term asthma control medication (e.g., inhaled corticosteroid) and a long-acting beta-2 agonist is clinically indicated, appropriate steps must be taken to ensure adherence with both treatment components. If adherence combination product containing both an inhaled corticosteroid and a long-acting beta-2 agonist is recommended. ■

- **Lower doses may be required in the elderly.**
- **Use with caution in CV disorders, including coronary insufficiency, ischemic heart disease, coronary artery disease, cardiac arrhythmias, CHF, and hypertension.**
- **Safety and efficacy not determined in children less than 12 years of age.**

SIDE EFFECTS

Most Common

Palpitations, tachycardia, tremor, dizziness/vertigo, nervousness/shakiness, headache, N&V, diarrhea, dry mouth, cough.

CV: Palpitations, chest tightness/pain/discomfort, angina, tachycardia, PVCs, arrhythmias, missed beats, tachycardia, hypotension. **CNS**: Dizziness/vertigo, nervousness, shakiness, tension, hyperactivity, headache, hyperkinesia, excitement, insomnia, anxiety, confusion, depression, fatigue, tremor, syncope, weakness. **GI**: N&V, diarrhea, dry mouth, anorexia, loss of appetite, bad taste or taste change, abdominal pain/cramps, stomatitis, glossitis. **Respiratory:** Cough, dry throat, throat irritation, pharyngitis, paradoxical bronchospasm. **Dermatologic**: Rash, flushing, edema, pruritus, alopecia, bruising. **Metabolic:** Edema, weight gain. **Miscellaneous**: Numbness in extremities, unusual/bad taste, smell change.

LABORATORY TEST CONSIDERATIONS

Hypokalemia.

HOW SUPPLIED

Inhalation Aerosol (Autoinhaler): 200 mcg/actuation.

DOSAGE

AUTOINHALER

Asthma/bronchospasm.

Adults and children over 12 years, usual: 2 inhalations (400 mcg) q 4–6 hr,

P

not to exceed 12 inhalations (2,400 mcg) daily. Some may benefit from one inhalation (200 mcg) q 4–6 hr.

NURSING IMPLICATIONS

IMPLEMENTATION/ADMINISTRATION/STORAGE

1. For optimal results, the canister should be at room temperature (15–30°C; 59–86°F) before use. Failure to use the product at room temperature may result in improper dosing. Shake well before using.
2. Test spray inhaler into the air before using for the first time and in case where the aerosol has not been used for a prolonged period of time.
3. The light blue plastic actuator supplied with the aerosol should not be used with any other product canisters. Also, actuators from other products should not be used with pirbuterol acetate inhalation canisters.
4. Store from 15–30°C (59–86°F). Exposure to a temperature above 120°F (50°C) may cause bursting.

ASSESSMENT

1. Note reasons for therapy, onset, duration, characteristics of S&S.
2. List other agents and asthma therapy prescribed; observe for adverse SE.
3. Assess lungs; note ECG, CXR, oxygen saturation, PFTs/spirometry readings.

CLIENT/FAMILY TEACHING

1. Review methods, frequency, and reasons for therapy. Taking therapy in the morning and after meals may reduce fatigue and improve lung ventilation.
2. Increase fluid intake to help liquefy secretions.
3. Shake well and prime the unit by releasing three test sprays into the air before using for the first time or resuming use after 2 or more weeks of nonuse. Use a spacer (chamber) to enhance dispersion. Wash in warm water and dry equipment after use and rinse mouth to prevent fungal infections. Do not exceed prescribed dosage.
4. If a previously effective dose does not provide relief, seek medical advice immediately as this is often a sign of seriously worsening asthma.
5. Report if condition or peak flows deteriorate, bronchospasm increases after treatment, or if inhaler is ineffective in relieving symptoms at prescribed dosage. Avoid triggers.
6. If using more than one corticosteroid inhaler, use the pirbuterol first, wait 5 min and then use the other inhaler. If more than one inhalation prescribed, wait at least 2 min before the next inhalation.
7. Report if dizziness, chest pain, SOB, palpitations, muscle spasms, difficulty urinating, or nervous tremors occur.
8. Avoid smoking, smoke-filled rooms, and persons with respiratory infections.
9. Keep all F/U appointments to evaluate response and adverse SE.

OUTCOMES/EVALUATE

Improved airway exchange; ↓ airway resistance; ↓ bronchospasm

Piroxicam

(peer-**OX**-ih-kam)

Classification(s): Nonsteroidal anti-inflammatory drug

Pregnancy Category: C

RX: Feldene.

🍁 **Rx:** Apo-Piroxicam, Gen-Piroxicam.

SEE ALSO ***NONSTEROIDAL ANTI-INFLAMMATORY DRUGS***.

INDICATIONS/USES

Acute and chronic treatment of rheumatoid arthritis and osteoarthritis. *Investigational:* Juvenile rheumatoid arthritis, primary dysmenorrhea.

ACTION/KINETICS

Action

May inhibit prostaglandin synthesis. Effect is comparable to that of aspirin, but with fewer GI side effects and less tinnitus. May be used with gold, corticosteroids, and antacids.

Pharmacokinetics

Peak plasma levels: 1.5–2 mcg/mL after 3–5 hr (single dose). **Steady-state plasma levels** (after 7–12 days): 3–8 mcg/mL. **t½:** 50 hr. **Analgesia, onset:** 1 hr; **duration:** 2–3 days. **Anti-inflammatory activity, onset:** 7–12 days; **duration:** 2–3 weeks. Metabolites and unchanged drug excreted

P

in urine and feces. **Plasma protein binding:** 98.5%.

CONTRAINDICATIONS

Safe use during pregnancy has not been determined. Use not recommended in those with advanced impaired renal function. Use in children less than 14 years old. Lactation.

SPECIAL CONCERNS

(1) **CV risk.** NSAIDs may cause an increased risk of serious cardiovascular thrombotic events, MI, and stroke, which can be fatal. This risk may increase with duration of use. Clients with cardiovascular disease or risk factors for cardiovascular disease may be at greater risk. (2) Piroxicam is contraindicated for treatment of perioperative pain in the setting of coronary artery bypass graft surgery. (3) **GI risk.** NSAIDs cause an increased risk of serious GI adverse events including bleeding, ulceration, and perforation of the stomach or intestines, which can be fatal. These reactions can occur at any time during use and without warning symptoms. Elderly clients are at greater risk for serious GI events.

- Increased plasma levels and elimination t½ possible in the elderly (especially women).
- Safety and efficacy not established in children.

SIDE EFFECTS

Most Common

Headache, dizziness, rash, pruritus, abdominal pain/cramps, diarrhea, N&V, constipation, flatulence, dyspepsia/indigestion, heartburn, gross bleeding/perforation, peptic ulcer, impaired renal function, anemia, abnormal LFTs, increased bleeding time, edema, tinnitus.

See *Nonsteroidal Anti-Inflammatory Drugs* for a complete list of possible side effects.

LABORATORY TEST CONSIDERATIONS

Reversible ↑ BUN.

ADDITIONAL DRUG INTERACTIONS

Ritonavir may ↑ piroxicam levels and possibly toxicity R/T inhibition of metabolism

HOW SUPPLIED

Capsules: 10 mg, 20 mg.

P

DOSAGE

CAPSULES

Rheumatoid arthritis, osteoarthritis.

Adults: 20 mg/day in one or more divided doses. Do not assess the effect of therapy for 2 weeks.

NURSING IMPLICATIONS

IMPLEMENTATION/ADMINISTRATION/STORAGE

1. Use the lowest effective dose for the shortest duration based on individual client treatment goals, especially in the elderly.
2. Steady-state plasma levels may not be reached for 2 weeks.
3. Clients over 70 years of age generally require one-half the usual adult dose of medication.
4. Store from 20–25°C (68–77°F).

ASSESSMENT

1. Note reasons for therapy, symptom characteristics, other agents prescribed, outcome. Rate pain level and quality of life.
2. Assess involved joints, note ROM, erythema, swelling/warmth, pain, spasm. Include any radiographic reports.
3. Determine history of ulcers, heart disease, or cardiac failure. May cause an increased risk of serious CV thrombotic events, MI, stroke and GI bleed.
4. Monitor CBC, renal, LFTs, as well as auditory function with prolonged therapy; reduce dose with dysfunction.

CLIENT/FAMILY TEACHING

1. Take as directed with food or milk to decrease GI upset. A stomach protectant (i.e., Cytotec, or H_2 blocker) may be prescribed for those with a history of ulcer disease.
2. Take an anti-inflammatory dose to prevent further joint destruction during acute exacerbations. Therapeutic effects of the medication cannot be evaluated fully for at least 2–4 weeks after treatment onset. Drug side effects may not be evident for 7–10 days.
3. Avoid activities that require mental alertness until drug effects realized; may experience dizziness/drowsiness.
4. Aspirin decreases the effectiveness of piroxicam and may increase the occurrence of side effects. Avoid concomitant aspirin, ethanol, other NSAIDs, and OTC products. Report any

increased abdominal pain, abnormal bruising or bleeding, malaise, or changes in the color of the stool immediately.

5. Avoid prolonged exposure to sunlight; use sunscreen or protective clothing to prevent photosensitivity reaction.
6. Keep all F/U to assess response, labs, and adverse SE.

OUTCOMES/EVALUATE

↓ Joint pain and inflammation with improved mobility

Pitavastatin

(**pit**-ah-vah-**STAT**-in)

Classification(s): Antihyperlipidemic, HMG-CoA reductase inhibitor

Pregnancy Category: X

RX: Livalo.

SEE ALSO ***ANTIHYPERLIPIDEMIC AGENTS—HMG-COA REDUCTASE INHIBITORS***

INDICATIONS/USES

Adjunctive therapy to diet to reduce elevated total cholesterol, LDL-C, Apo B, triglycerides, and to increase HDL-C in adults with primary hyperlipidemia or mixed dyslipidemia.

ACTION/KINETICS

Action

Competitively inhibits HMG-CoA reductase, which is the rate determining enzyme involved with biosynthesis of cholesterol. Cholesterol synthesis is inhibited in the liver. The sustained inhibition of cholesterol synthesis in the liver decreases levels of VLDL.

Pharmacokinetics

Peak plasma levels: 1 hr. Absolute bioavailability is 51%. C_{max} and AUC are higher in women. Marginally metabolized by CYP2C9 and to a lesser extent by CYP2C8. 79% excreted in the liver and 15% in the urine. **t½, elimination from plasma:** 12 hr. **Plasma protein binding:** >99%.

CONTRAINDICATIONS

Known hypersensitivity to pitavastatin or any component of the product. Active liver disease, which may include unexplained persistent increases in hepatic transaminase levels. Women who are pregnant or may become pregnant. Coadministration with cyclosporine. Use in clients with glomerular filtration rate <30 mL/min/1.73 m^2 or in those on hemodialysis. Use with lopinavir/ritonavir combination therapy. Lactation.

SPECIAL CONCERNS

- **Use with caution in clients with predisposing factors to myopathy (e.g., >65 years of age, renal impairment, inadequately treated hypothyroidism) and in clients with impaired renal function, the elderly, or when used together with fibrates or lipid-modifying doses of niacin.**
- **Elderly clients may manifest greater sensitivity to pitavastatin.**
- **Safety and efficacy not determined in children.**

SIDE EFFECTS

Most Common

Myalgia, back pain, diarrhea, constipation, pain in extremities.

See *Antihyperlipidemic Agents-HMG CoA Reductase Inhibitors* for a complete list of possible side effects. **Musculoskeletal:** Myopathy and rhabdomyolysis with acute renal failure secondary to myoglobinuria. Myalgia, arthralgia, back pain, pain in extremity. **GI:** Constipation, diarrhea. **CNS:** Headache. **Respiratory:** Nasopharyngitis. **Hypersensitivity:** Rash, pruritus, urticaria. **Body as a whole:** Influenza.

LABORATORY TEST CONSIDERATIONS

↑ ALT, AST, creatine kinase, alkaline phosphatase, bilirubin, glucose.

DRUG INTERACTIONS

Cyclosporine / Significant ↑ pitavastatin levels; do not use together
Erythromycin / Significant ↑ pitavastatin levels; reduce pitavastatin dose to 1 mg once/day
Fibrate / Concomitant use ↑ risk of adverse skeletal muscle effects
Lopinavir/Ritonavir / Possible significant ↑ pitavastatin levels; do not use together
Niacin (lipid-lowering doses) / ↑ Risk of skeletal muscle effects; decrease pitavastatin dose
Rifampin / Significant ↑ pitavastatin levels; reduce pitavastatin dose to 2 mg once/day
Warfarin / Possible ↑ anticoagulant effect; monitor

HOW SUPPLIED

Tablets: 1 mg, 2 mg, 4 mg.

DOSAGE

TABLETS

Primary hyperlipidemia and mixed dyslipidemia.

Adults, initial: 2 mg once daily; **maintenance:** 1–4 mg (maximum) once daily at any time of the day with or without food. After initiation or upon titration of dosage, analyze lipid levels after 4 weeks and adjust the dose accordingly.

NURSING IMPLICATIONS

IMPLEMENTATION/ADMINISTRATION/STORAGE

1. Doses greater than 4 mg/day are associated with an increased risk of severe myopathy.
2. Clients with moderate renal impairment (GFR 30–<60 mL/min/1.73 m^2) and end stage renal disease receiving hemodialysis should receive a starting dose of 1 mg once daily and a maximum dose of 2 mg once daily.
3. In clients taking erythromycin, do not exceed a pitavastatin dose of 1 mg once daily.
4. In clients taking rifampin, do not exceed a pitavastatin dose of 2 mg once daily.
5. Store from 15–30°C (59–86°F); protect from light.

ASSESSMENT

1. Note reasons for therapy: prophylaxis, plaque stability or elevated TG/LDL cholesterol in CAD.
2. List all medications prescribed; ensure none interact. Reduce dose with certain drugs. Identify/list risk factors for CHD.
3. Assess level of adherence to weight reduction, regular exercise, cholesterol-lowering diet, BP, BS control. Note any alcohol abuse.
4. Assess for any secondary causes for hypercholesterolemia (e.g., hypothyroidism, nephrotic syndrome, dysproteinemias, obstructive liver disease, other drug therapy, alcoholism).
5. Monitor CBC, lipid profile, renal and LFTs; reduce dose with dysfunction. Schedule LFTs after 4 weeks of therapy, with dosage changes and adjust dosage accordingly.

CLIENT/FAMILY TEACHING

1. Take once daily without regard to meals. More preferable to take in the evening.
2. A low-cholesterol diet must be followed during drug therapy. Consult dietitian for assistance in meal planning and food preparation.
3. Report any S&S of infections, unexplained muscle pain, tenderness/weakness (especially if accompanied by fever or malaise), surgery, trauma, yellowing of skin or eyes.
4. Review importance of regular exercise, weight loss/control, low alcohol consumption, smoking abstinence, and following a low-cholesterol diet in the overall plan to reduce serum cholesterol levels and inhibit progression of CAD.
5. Not for use during pregnancy or while nursing; use barrier contraception.
6. Keep all F/U to assess response, labs, eye exams, and for adverse SE.

OUTCOMES/EVALUATE

- ↓ Elevated total-C, LDL-C, Apo B, and TG
- ↑ HDL; cardiovascular risk reduction

Polidocanol

(pol-ee-**DOE**-ka-nole)

Classification(s): Sclerosing agent

Pregnancy Category: C

RX: Asclera.

INDICATIONS/USES

Treat uncomplicated spider veins (varicose veins 1 mm or less in diameter) and uncomplicated reticular veins (varicose veins 1–3 mm in diameter) in the lower extremity.

ACTION/KINETICS

Action

Polidocanol locally damages the endothelium of blood vessels. When injected IV, the drug induces endothelial damage. Platelet then aggregate at the site of damage and attach to the venous wall. Eventually a dense network of platelets, cellular debris, and fibrin occludes the vessel. Then, the occluded vein is replaced with connective fibrous tissue.

Pharmacokinetics

There are low systemic blood levels of polidocanol.

CONTRAINDICATIONS

Hypersensitivity to polidocanol or any component of the product. Acute thromboembolic diseases. Lactation.

SPECIAL CONCERNS

Safety and efficacy not established in children.

SIDE EFFECTS

Most Common

Local discoloration, irritation, pain, pruritus, warmth, hematoma.

At local site of injection: Hematoma, irritation, discoloration, pain, pruritus, warmth, neovascularization, thrombosis, necrosis, nerve injury. **Dermatologic:** Allergic dermatitis, hypertrichosis (in the area of sclerotherapy), skin hyperpigmentation. **CV:** ***Cardiac arrest, CVA, circulatory collapse***, DVT, hot flush, palpitations, ***pulmonary embolism***, vasovagal syncope, vasculitis. **CNS:** Confusion, dizziness, LOC, migraine, paresthesia (local). Hypersensitivity: Anaphylactic shock, ***angioedema***, asthma, generalized urticaria. **Respiratory:** Dyspnea. **Body as a whole:** Pyrexia.

HOW SUPPLIED

Injection Solution: 0.5%, 1%.

DOSAGE

IV ONLY

Varicose veins.

Adults, usual, reticular veins (1 to 3 mm in diameter): 0.1–0.3 mL of the 1% solution per injection; **spider veins (1 mm or less in diameter):** 0.1–0.3 mL of the 0.5% solution. **Maximum dose:** 10 mL per session. Repeat treatments may be necessary if the extent of the varicose vein requires more than 10 mL. Separate treatments by 1–2 weeks.

NURSING IMPLICATIONS

IMPLEMENTATION/ADMINISTRATION/STORAGE

1. Small IV blood clots that develop may be removed by stab incision and thrombus expression (microthrombectomy).
2. Keep the client under observation to detect any anaphylactic or allergic reaction.
3. Use a glass or plastic syringe with a fine needle (usually 26- or 30-gauge). Insert the needle tangentially into the vein and inject the solution slowly while the needle is still in the vein. Apply only gentle pressure during the injection to prevent vein rupture. After the needle has been removed and the injection site covered, apply compression in the form of a stocking or bandage. After the treatment session, encourage the client to walk for 15–20 min.
4. Maintain compression for 2–3 days after treatment of spider veins and for 5–7 days for reticular veins. For extensive varicosities, longer compression treatment with compression bandages or a gradient compression stocking of a higher compression class is recommended. Posttreatment compression is necessary to reduce the risk of deep vein thrombosis.
5. Intra-arterial injection can cause severe necrosis, ischemia, or gangrene. If this occurs, consult a vascular surgeon immediately.
6. Inadvertant perivascular injection can cause pain. If pain is severe, a local anesthetic (without epinephrine) may be injected.
7. Severe local side effects, including tissue necrosis, may result following extravasation. Take care in IV needle placement and use the smallest effective volume at each injection site.
8. Store from 15–30°C (59–86°F). Each ampule is intended for immediate use; each unopened ampule is stable for up to 3 years.

ASSESSMENT

1. Note size and extent of spider/varicose veins requiring treatment.
2. After the treatment session, apply compression with a stocking or bandage. Have client walk for 15–20 minutes. Keep under observation to detect any anaphylactic or allergic reaction.
3. Maintain compression for 2 to 3 days after treatment of spider veins and for 5 to 7 days for reticular veins. For extensive varicosities, longer compression treatment with compression bandages or a gradient compression stocking of a higher compression class is recommended. Posttreatment compression is necessary to reduce the risk of DVT.

P

4. **Repeat treatments may be necessary if the extent of the varicose veins requires more than 10 ml. These treatments should be separated by 1 to 2 weeks.**

CLIENT/FAMILY TEACHING

1. **Drug is injected into veins to minimize size by sclerosing vessel.**
2. **Will need to wear compression stockings or support hose on the treated legs continuously for 2 to 3 days and for 2 to 3 weeks during the daytime. Compression stockings or support hose should be thigh or knee high depending upon the area treated in order to provide adequate coverage.**
3. **Walk for 15–20 minutes immediately after the procedure and daily for the next few days.**
4. **Avoid heavy exercise, sunbathing, long plane flights, and hot baths or sauna for 2 to 3 days following treatment.**
5. **Report any chest pain, SOB, severe leg pain or evidence of infection.**
6. **Keep all F/U to assess response and for adverse SE.**

OUTCOMES/EVALUATE

Minimized/resolution of spider/varicose veins

IV

Polymyxin B sulfate, parenteral

(pol-ee-**MIX**-in)

Classification(s): Antibiotic, polymyxin
Pregnancy Category: C

SEE ALSO ***ANTI-INFECTIVE DRUGS***.

INDICATIONS/USES

Systemic: (1) Acute infections of the urinary tract and meninges; septicemia caused by *Pseudomonas aeruginosa.* (2) Meningeal infections caused by *Haemophilus influenzae,* UTIs caused by *Escherichia coli,* bacteremia caused by *Enterobacter aerogenes* or *Klebsiella pneumoniae.* (3) Combined with neomycin for irrigation of the urinary bladder to prevent bacteriuria and bacteremia from indwelling catheters.

ACTION/KINETICS

Action

Bactericidal against most gram-negative organisms; rapidly inactivated by alkali, strong acid, and certain metal ions. Increases the permeability of the plasma cell membrane of the bacterium (i.e., similar to detergents), causing leakage of essential metabolites and ultimately inactivation.

Pharmacokinetics

Peak serum levels: IM, 2 hr. **t½:** 4.3–6 hr. Longer in presence of renal impairment. Sixty percent of drug excreted in urine. Virtually unabsorbed from the GI tract except in newborn infants. Remains in plasma after parenteral administration.

CONTRAINDICATIONS

Hypersensitivity. A potentially toxic drug to be reserved for the treatment of severe, resistant infections in hospitalized clients. Not indicated for clients with severely impaired renal function or nitrogen retention. Use with nephro- or neurotoxic drugs.

SPECIAL CONCERNS

(1) When given IM or intrathecally, give only to hospitalized clients to provide constant physician supervision. (2) Carefully determine renal function; reduce dosage in those with renal damage and nitrogen retention. Clients with nephrotoxicity due to polymyxin B sulfate usually show albuminuria, cellular casts, and azotemia. Diminishing urine output and a rising BUN are indications to discontinue therapy. (3) Neurotoxic reactions may be manifested by irritability, weakness, drowsiness, ataxia, perioral paresthesia, numbness of the extremities, and blurring of vision. These are usually associated with high serum levels found in those with impaired renal function or nephrotoxicity. Avoid concurrent use of other nephrotoxic and neurotoxic drugs, especially colistin, gentamicin, kanomycin, neomycin, paromomycin, streptomycin, and tobramycin. (4) Neurotoxicity can result in respiratory paralysis from neuromuscular blockade, especially when the drug is given soon after anesthesia or muscle relaxants.

Safe use during pregnancy not established.

SIDE EFFECTS

Most Common

When used parenterally: N&V, diarrhea, nephrotoxicity, facial flushing, dizziness, paresthesias, drowsiness, abdominal cramps.

Nephrotoxic: Albuminuria, cylindruria, azotemia, hematuria, proteinuria, leukocyturia, electrolyte loss. **Neurologic:** Dizziness, flushing of face, mental confusion, irritability, nystagmus, muscle weakness, drowsiness, paresthesias, blurred vision, slurred speech, ataxia, ***coma, seizures. Neuromuscular blockade may lead to respiratory paralysis.*** **GI:** N&V, diarrhea, abdominal cramps. **Miscellaneous:** Fever, urticaria, skin exanthemata, eosinophilia, ***anaphylaxis.***

Intrathecal use: Meningeal irritation with fever, stiff neck, headache, increase in leukocytes and protein in the CSF. Nerve-root irritation may result in neuritic pain and urine retention.

IM use: Irritation, severe pain.

IV use: Thrombophlebitis.

LABORATORY TEST CONSIDERATIONS

False + or ↑ levels of urea nitrogen and creatinine. Casts and RBCs in urine.

DRUG INTERACTIONS

Aminoglycoside antibiotics / Additive nephrotoxic effects

Anesthetics / Additive muscle relaxation → respiratory paralysis

Cephalosporins / ↑ Risk of renal toxicity

Phenothiazines / ↑ Risk of respiratory depression

Skeletal muscle relaxants (surgical) / Additive muscle relaxation → respiratory paralysis

HOW SUPPLIED

Powder for Injection: 500,000 units.

DOSAGE

IV

Infections.

Adults and children: 15,000–25,000 units/kg/day (maximum) in divided doses q 12 hr. **Infants,** up to 40,000 units/kg/day.

IM (NOT USUALLY RECOMMENDED DUE TO PAIN AT INJECTION SITE)

Infections.

Adults and children: 25,000–30,000 units/kg/day in divided doses q 4–6 hr. **Infants,** up to 40,000 units/kg/day.

Both IV and IM doses should be reduced in renal impairment.

INTRATHECAL

Meningitis.

Adults and children over 2 years: 50,000 units/day for 3–4 days; **then,** 50,000 units every other day until 2 weeks after cultures are negative; **children under 2 years,** 20,000 units/day for 3–4 days or 25,000 units once every other day; dosage of 25,000 units should be continued every other day for 2 weeks after cultures are negative.

NURSING IMPLICATIONS

IMPLEMENTATION/ADMINISTRATION/STORAGE

1. Store and dilute as directed on package insert.
2. Lessen pain on IM injection by reducing drug concentration as much as possible. It is preferable to give drug more frequently in more dilute doses. If ordered, procaine hydrochloride (2 mL of a 0.5–1.0% solution per 5 units of dry powder) may be used for mixing the drug for IM injection.
3. Only give intrathecally for meningeal infections.
4. IV For IV administration, reconstitute 500,000 units with 300–500 mL of D5W and infuse over 60–90 min.
5. COMPATIBILITY D5W.
6. INCOMPATIBILITY Administer separately.

ASSESSMENT

1. Note reasons for therapy, onset, characteristics of S&S, C&S results.
2. Assess respiratory function; note any prior problems/conditions.
3. Observe for any muscle weakness and early signs of muscle paralysis R/T neuromuscular blockade; withhold drug and report. Ambulatory or bedridden clients with neurologic disturbances require supervision.
4. Evaluate for nephrotoxicity, characterized by albuminuria, urinary casts, nitrogen retention, and hematuria.
5. Monitor I&O, CBC, cultures and renal function; reduce dose with impaired function.

CLIENT/FAMILY TEACHING

1. Drug is used to treat infections. Administered parenterally and intrathecally under medical supervision to hospitalized clients.

2. Avoid hazardous tasks until drug effects realized; may cause dizziness, vertigo, and gait problems.
3. Consume at least 2 L/day of fluids.
4. Report any neurologic disturbances, i.e., dizziness, blurred vision, irritability, circumoral and peripheral numbness and tingling, weakness, and ataxia; usually gone 24–48 hr after drug discontinued; associated with high drug levels.
5. Keep all F/U to assess response, labs, and adverse SE.

OUTCOMES/EVALUATE

Negative cultures; resolution of infection; symptomatic improvement

Posaconazole

(**POE**-sah-**KON**-ah-zole)

Classification(s): Antifungal, triazole
Pregnancy Category: C
RX: Noxafil.

INDICATIONS/USES

(1) Prophylaxis of invasive *Aspergillus* and *Candida* infections in clients 13 years and older who are at high risk of developing these infections because of being severely immunocompromised, such as hematopoietic stem cell transplant recipients with graft-versus-host disease or those with hematologic malignancies with prolonged neutropenia from chemotherapy. (2) Oropharyngeal candidiasis, including oropharyngeal candidiasis refractory to itraconazole and/or fluconazole.

ACTION/KINETICS

Action

Posaconazole blocks the synthesis of ergosterol, a key component of the fungal cell membrane, inhibiting the enzyme lanosterol 14α-demethylase and accumulation of methylated sterol precursors.

Pharmacokinetics

T_{max}: 3–5 hr. AUC and C_{max} are about 4 times higher when the drug is given with a high-fat meal (about 50 grams of fat) and about 3 times higher when given with a liquid nutritional supplement (14 grams of fat). Metabolized by glucuronidation. Metabolites and parent drug excreted through the feces (71%) and urine (13%). **t½, elimination:** 35 hr. **Plasma protein binding:** Greater than 98% bound to plasma proteins (mainly albumin).

CONTRAINDICATIONS

Use with drugs that prolong the QTc interval. Lactation.

SPECIAL CONCERNS

- Closely monitor clients with severe impaired renal function for breakthrough fungal infections.
- Use with caution in impaired hepatic function, in those with potential proarrhythmic conditions, or in those hypersensitive to other azoles.
- Safety and efficacy not determined in children less than 13 years of age.

SIDE EFFECTS

Most Common

Fever, N&V, diarrhea, hypokalemia, headache, abdominal pain, constipation, anemia, febrile neutropenia, thrombocytopenia, rigors, coughing, dyspnea, hypertension, fatigue, insomnia, rash, mucositis, bilirubinemia, hepatocellular damage.

CV: Hyper-/hypotension, tachycardia, QT/QTc prolongation. **CNS:** Headache, fatigue, insomnia, dizziness, anxiety, weakness, tremor. **GI:** Diarrhea, N&V, abdominal pain, dry mouth, constipation, mucositis, dyspepsia, anorexia, hepatocellular damage, clinical hepatitis, abnormal hepatic function, hepatomegaly, jaundice. **Dermatologic:** Rash, pruritus, increased sweating. **GU:** Vaginal hemorrhage, acute renal failure. **Hematologic:** Febrile neutropenia, thrombocytopenia, anemia, neutropenia, petechiae, thrombotic thrombocytopenia (rare), hemolytic uremic syndrome (rare). **Musculoskeletal:** Rigors, musculoskeletal pain, arthralgia, myalgia, back pain, rigors. **Respiratory:** Coughing, dyspnea, epistaxis, pharyngitis, URTI, pneumonia, ***pulmonary embolus (rare)***. **Body as a whole:** Fever, bacteremia, asthenia, cytomegalovirus infection, edema, dehydration, weight decrease, allergic/***hypersensitivity reactions***. **Miscellaneous:** Herpes simplex, edema in legs, taste perversion, blurred vision, adrenal insufficiency, oral candidiasis.

LABORATORY TEST CONSIDERATIONS

↑ ALT, AST, GGT, hepatic enzymes, alkaline phosphatase, bilirubin, blood creatine, total bilirubin. Bilirubinemia, hypokalemia, hypomagnesemia, hyperglycemia, hypocalcemia.

DRUG INTERACTIONS

Benzodiazepines, selected (alprazolam, midazolam, triazolam) / Prolonged levels of certain benzodiazepine → ↑ CNS depression and psychomotor impairment
Calcium channel blockers metabolized by CYP3A4 (e.g., felodipine) / Monitor frequently for side effects and toxicity; dose reduction of CCB may be needed
Cimetidine / ↓ (39%) Posaconazole C_{max} and AUC; avoid use together unless benefit outweighs risk
Cyclosporine / ↑ Cyclosporine levels → possible nephrotoxicity, leukoencephalopathy, and death; reduce cyclosporine dose by three fourths; monitor plasma levels
Ergot alkaloids (ergotamine, dihydroergotamine) / ↑ Ergot alkaloid plasma levels → possible ergotism; do not use together
Glipizide / ↓ Glucose levels; monitor glucose concentrations
HMG-CoA reductase inhibitors metabolized by CYP3A4 (e.g., atorvastatin) / ↑ Statin levels → possible rhabdomyolysis; consider statin dose reduction
Midazolam / ↑ Midazolam AUC (83%); monitor and consider midazolam dose reduction
Phenytoin / ↓ Posaconazole C_{max} (41%) and AUC (50%) and ↑ (16%) phenytoin C_{max} and AUC; avoid use together unless benefit outweighs risk and monitor frequently
Quinidine / ↑ Quinidine levels → QT prolongation and rarely torsades de pointes; do not use together
Rifabutin / ↓ Posaconazole C_{max} (43%) and AUC (49%) and ↑ rifabutin C_{max} (31%) and AUC (72%); avoid use together unless benefit outweighs risk and monitor frequently
Sirolimus / ↑ Sirolimus plasma levels → possible serious side effects; monitor sirolimus blood levels frequently
Tacrolimus / ↑ Tacrolimus plasma levels → possible serious side effects; reduce tacrolimus dose by one-third and monitor frequently
Vinca alkaloids (vinblastine, vincristine) / ↑ Vinca alkaloids plasma levels → neurotoxicity; consider alkaloid dosage adjustment

HOW SUPPLIED

Oral Suspension: 40 mg/mL.

DOSAGE

ORAL SUSPENSION

Prophylaxis of invasive Aspergillus *or* Candida *fungal infection.*

Adults and children, 13 years and older: 200 mg (5 mL) three times per day. Duration is based on recovery from neutropenia or immunosuppression.

Oropharyngeal candidiasis.

Loading dose: 100 mg (2.5 mL) twice the first day; **then,** 100 mg (2.5 mL) once daily for 13 days.

Oropharyngeal candidiasis refractory to itraconazole and/or fluconazole.

400 mg (10 mL) twice a day. Base duration of therapy on the severity of the client's underlying disease and clinical response.

NURSING IMPLICATIONS

IMPLEMENTATION/ADMINISTRATION/STORAGE

1. Use the following guidelines to enhance oral absorption and optimize plasma levels:
   - Give each dose with a full meal or liquid nutritional supplement. For those who cannot eat a full meal or tolerate an oral nutritional supplement, consider alternative antifungal therapy or monitor closely for breakthrough fungal infections.
   - Those who have severe diarrhea or vomiting should be monitored closely for breakthrough fungal infections.
   - Coadministration of drugs that can decrease the plasma levels of posaconazole should be avoided unless the benefit outweighs the risk. If such drugs are required, monitor closely for breakthrough fungal infections.
2. Store from 15–30°C (59–86°F). Do not freeze.

ASSESSMENT

1. Note reasons for therapy, onset, duration, characteristics of S&S, clinical presentation, other agents trialed, cultures, outcome.
2. With oropharyngeal candidiasis refractory to itraconazole and/or fluconazole, note when treated.

3. List drugs, herbals consumed to ensure none interact.
4. Monitor those with severe renal dysfunction, severe diarrhea, or vomiting for breakthrough fungal infections.
5. Assess VS, CBC, electrolytes, renal and LFTs; note any liver dysfunction to prevent further damage.

CLIENT/FAMILY TEACHING

1. Take each dose with a full meal or liquid nutritional supplement, or an acidic carbonated beverage (e.g., ginger ale).
2. Shake well before each use and measure dose with enclosed measuring spoon. Rinse spoon with water after each use and before storage.
3. Take on regular schedule to get the most benefit (at the same times each day). Continue to take even if you feel well. Do not miss any doses; do not take 2 doses at once.
4. May cause dizziness or blurred vision. May be worse if taken with alcohol or certain medicines. Do not drive or perform other possibly unsafe tasks until drug effects realized.
5. Drug only works against fungi; it does not treat viral infections; complete full course of treatment. The fungus could become less sensitive to this or other medicines making the infection harder to treat in the future. May experience secondary infections; report if evident.
6. Report severe diarrhea or vomiting (may change serum drug levels).
7. Birth control pills may not work as well while using posaconazole suspension. To prevent pregnancy, use additional non-hormonal form of BC (e.g., condoms). Harm to the fetus unknown; report if pregnant, planning to become pregnant, or breast-feeding.
8. With diabetes, check blood sugar levels closely.
9. Use with extreme caution in children younger than 13 years old; safety and effectiveness have not been confirmed.
10. Keep all F/U to assess response, labs, and adverse SE.

OUTCOMES/EVALUATE

Resolution of fungal infection

IV ©

Potassium salts

Classification(s): Electrolyte

Pregnancy Category: C

Potassium acetate, parenteral

Potassium acetate, Potassium bicarbonate, and Potassium citrate (Trikates)

RX: Oral Solution: Tri-K.

Potassium bicarbonate

RX: Effervescent Tablets: Potassium Bicarbonate Effervescent Tablets.

Potassium bicarbonate and Potassium chloride

RX: Tablets, Effervescent: Effervescent Potassium/Chloride, Klor-Con/EF, Klorvess, K-Lyte/Cl 50.

Potassium bicarbonate and Potassium citrate

RX: Tablets, Effervescent: Effer-K, K-Lyte.

Potassium chloride

RX: Capsules, Extended-Release: Micro-K 10 Extencaps, Micro-K Extencaps. **Tablets, Extended-Release**: Kaon-Cl, Kaon-Cl-10, K-Dur 10 and 20, Klor-Con 8 and 10, Klor-Con M10, M15, and M20, Klotrix, K-Tab, Ten-K. **Injection**: Potassium Chloride for Injection Concentrate. **Oral Solution**: Cena-K 10% and 20%, Kaon-Cl 20% Liquid, Klorvess 10% Liquid, Potasalan. **Powder for Oral Solution**: Gen-K, K-Lor, Klor-Con Powder, Klor-Con/25 Powder, K-Lyte/Cl Powder, Mirco-K LS.

🍁 **Rx: Tablets, Extended-Release**: Apo-K, K-Lyte/Cl. **Oral Solution**: K-10.

Potassium chloride, Potassium bicarbonate, and Potassium citrate

RX: Granules, Effervescent: Klorvess Effervescent Granules.

Potassium gluconate

RX: Elixir: Kaon, Kaylixir, K-G Elixir.

INDICATIONS/USES

PO: (1) Treat hypokalemia due to digitalis intoxication, diabetic acidosis, diarrhea and vomiting, attacks of familial periodic paralysis, certain cases of uremia, hyperadrenalism, starvation and debilitation, and corticosteroid or diuretic therapy. (2) Hypokalemia with or without metabolic acidosis and following surgical conditions accompanied by nitrogen loss, vomiting and diarrhea, suction drainage, and increased urinary excretion of potassium. (3) Prophylaxis of potassium depletion when dietary intake is not adequate in the following conditions: Clients on digitalis and diuretics for CHF, hepatic cirrhosis with ascites, excess aldosterone with normal renal function, significant cardiac arrhythmias, potassium-losing nephropathy, and certain states accompanied by diarrhea. *Investigational:* Mild hypertension. *NOTE:* Use potassium chloride when hypokalemia is associated with alkalosis; potassium bicarbonate, citrate, acetate, or gluconate should be used when hypokalemia is associated with acidosis.

IV: (1) Prophylaxis and treatment of moderate to severe potassium loss when PO therapy is not feasible. (2) Potassium acetate is used as an additive for preparing specific IV formulas when client needs cannot be met by usual nutrient or electrolyte preparations. (3) Potassium acetate is also used in the following conditions: Marked loss of GI secretions due to vomiting, diarrhea, GI intubation, or fistulas; prolonged parenteral use of potassium-free fluids (e.g., dextrose or NSS); diabetic acidosis, especially during treatment with insulin and dextrose infusions; prolonged diuresis; metabolic alkalosis; hyperadrenocorticism; primary aldosteronism; overdose of adrenocortical steroids, testosterone, or corticotropin; attacks of hereditary or familial periodic paralysis; during the healing phase of burns or scalds; and cardiac arrhythmias, especially due to digitalis glycosides.

ACTION/KINETICS

Action

Potassium is required to maintain intracellular tonicity; for transmission of nerve impulses; contraction of cardiac, skeletal, and smooth muscle; and, maintenance of normal renal function. Potassium participates in carbohydrate utilization and protein synthesis. It is critical in regulating nerve conduction and muscle contraction, especially the heart.

Potassium is readily and rapidly absorbed from the GI tract. Though a number of salts can be used to supply the potassium cation, potassium chloride is the agent of choice since hypochloremia frequently accompanies potassium deficiency. Dietary measures can often prevent and even correct potassium deficiencies. Potassium-rich foods include most meats (beef, chicken, ham, turkey, veal), fish, beans, broccoli, brussels sprouts, lentils, spinach, potatoes, milk, bananas, dates, prunes, raisins, avocados, watermelon, cantaloupe, apricots, and molasses.

Pharmacokinetics

From 80 to 90% of potassium intake is excreted by the kidney and is partially reabsorbed from the glomerular filtrate. A deficit of either potassium or chloride will lead to the deficit of the other.

CONTRAINDICATIONS

Severe renal function impairment with azotemia or oliguria, postoperatively before urine flow has been reestablished, early postoperative oliguria except during GI drainage. Crush syndrome, Addison's disease, hyperkalemia from any cause, anuria, heat cramps, acute dehydration, severe hemolytic reactions, adynamia episodica hereditaria, clients receiving potassium-sparing diuretics or aldosterone-inhibiting drugs, renal failure and conditions in which potassium retention is present. Solid dosage forms in clients in whom there is a reason for delay or arrest in passage of tablets through the GI tract.

SPECIAL CONCERNS

- **Safety during lactation, pregnancy (give during pregnancy only if clearly needed), and in children not established.**
- **Geriatric clients are at greater risk of developing hyperkalemia due to age-related changes in renal function.**
- **Use with caution with cardiac disease, especially in digitalized clients, or in the presence of renal disease; metabolic acidosis; Addison's disease, acute dehydration, prolonged or severe diarrhea, familial periodic paralysis, hypoadrenalism, hyperkalemia, hyponatremia, and, myotonia congenita.**

P

- **Potassium loss is often accompanied by an obligatory loss of chloride resulting in hypochloremic metabolic alkalosis; thus, treat the underlying cause of potassium loss.**

SIDE EFFECTS

Most Common

N&V, diarrhea, flatulence, abdominal discomfort.

GI: N&V, diarrhea, flatulence, abdominal discomfort, GI obstruction, GI bleeding, GI ulceration or perforation. **Nutritional:** Hyperkalemia. **Dermatologic:** Skin rash.

Symptoms of hyperkalemia. CNS: Mental confusion, listlessness, weakness. **Musculoskeletal:** Paresthesias of extremities, flaccid paralysis, muscle or respiratory paralysis, areflexia, weakness and heaviness of legs. **CV:** Hypotension, cardiac arrhythmias, heart block, ECG abnormalities (e.g., disappearance of P waves, spreading and slurring of QRS complex with development of a biphasic curve), ***cardiac arrest***.

Effects due to solution or IV technique used: Fever, infection at injection site, venous thrombosis, phlebitis extending from injection site, extravasation, venospasm, hypervolemia, hyperkalemia.

OVERDOSE MANAGEMENT

Symptoms: Mild (5.5–6.5 mEq/L) to moderate (6.5–8 mEq/L) hyperkalemia (may be asymptomatic except for ECG changes). ECG changes include progression in height and peak of T waves, lowering of the R wave, decreased amplitude and eventually disappearance of P waves, prolonged PR interval and QRS complex, shortening of the QT interval, ***ventricular fibrillation, death. Muscle weakness that may progress to flaccid quadriplegia and respiratory failure***, although dangerous cardiac arrhythmias usually occur before onset of complete paralysis. *Treatment: (plasma potassium levels greater than 6.5 mEq/L):* All measures must be monitored by ECG. Measures consist of actions taken to shift potassium ions from plasma into cells by:

- **Sodium bicarbonate:** IV infusion of 50–100 mEq over period of 5 min. May be repeated after 10–15 minutes if ECG abnormalities persist.
- **Glucose and insulin:** IV infusion of 3 grams glucose to 1 unit regular insulin to shift potassium into cells.
- **Calcium gluconate or other calcium salt** (only for clients not on digitalis or other cardiotonic glycosides): IV infusion of 0.5–1 grams (5–10 mL of a 10% solution) over a period of 2 min. Dosage may be repeated after 1–2 min if ECG remains abnormal. When ECG is approximately normal, the excess potassium should be removed from the body by administration of polystyrene sulfonate, hemodialysis, or peritoneal dialysis (clients with renal insufficiency) or other means.
- **Sodium polystyrene sulfonate, hemodialysis, peritoneal dialysis:** To remove potassium from the body.

DRUG INTERACTIONS

ACE inhibitors / May cause potassium retention → hyperkalemia in certain clients
Digitalis glycosides / Possible cardiac arrhythmias
Potassium-sparing diuretics / Severe hyperkalemia with possibility of cardiac arrhythmias or arrest

GENERAL STATEMENT

Potassium is the major cation of the body's intracellular fluid. It is essential for the maintenance of important physiologic processes, including cardiac, smooth, and skeletal muscle function, acid-base balance, gastric secretions, renal function, protein and carbohydrate metabolism. Symptoms of hypokalemia include weakness, cardiac arrhythmias, fatigue, ileus, hyporeflexia or areflexia, tetany, polydipsia, and, in severe cases, flaccid paralysis and inability to concentrate urine. Loss of potassium is usually accompanied by a loss of chloride resulting in hypochloremic metabolic alkalosis. The usual adult daily requirement of potassium is 40–80 mg. In adults, the normal extracellular concentration of potassium ranges from 3.5 to 5 mEq/L with the intracellular levels being 150–160 mEq/L. Extracellular concentrations of up to 5.6 mEq/L are normal in children. Both hypokalemia and hyperkalemia, if uncorrected, can be fatal; thus, potassium must always be administered cautiously.

HOW SUPPLIED

Potassium acetate, parenteral. ***Injection:*** 2 mEq/mL, 4 mEq/mL.
Potassium acetate, potassium bicarbonate, and potassium citrate. ***Liquid:*** 45 mEq/15 mL.
Potassium bicarbonate. ***Tablets, Effervescent:*** 25 mEq, 650 mg.

P

Potassium bicarbonate and potassium chloride. ***Granules for Reconstitution:*** 20 mEq; ***Tablets, Effervescent:*** 25 mEq, 50 mEq.
Potassium bicarbonate and potassium citrate. ***Tablets, Effervescent:*** 10 mEq, 20 mEq, 25 mEq.
Potassium chloride. ***Capsules, Extended-Release:*** 8 mEq, 10 mEq; ***Injection:*** 1.5 mEq/mL, 2 mEq/mL, 10 mEq/50 mL, 10 mEq/100 mL, 20 mEq/50 mL, 20 mEq/100 mL, 30 mEq/100 mL, 40 mEq/100 mL, 100 mEq/L, 200 mEq/L; ***Liquid:*** 20 mEq/15 mL, 30 mEq/15 mL, 40 mEq/15 mL; ***Powder for Reconstitution:*** 20 mEq, 25 mEq, 200 mEq; ***Tablets:*** 180 mg; ***Tablets, Extended-Release:*** 8 mEq, 10 mEq, 15 mEq, 20 mEq.
Potassium gluconate. ***Elixir:*** 20 mEq/15 mL; ***Tablets:*** 486 mg, 500 mg, 550 mg, 595 mg, 610 mg, 620 mg; ***Tablets, Extended-Release:*** 595 mg.

DOSAGE

Highly individualized. Oral administration is preferred because the slow absorption from the GI tract prevents sudden, large increases in plasma potassium levels. Dosage is usually expressed as mEq/L of potassium. The bicarbonate, chloride, citrate, and gluconate salts are usually administered PO. The chloride, acetate, and phosphate may be administered by **slow IV** infusion.

IV INFUSION

Serum K less than 2.0 mEq/L.

400 mEq/day at a rate not to exceed 40 mEq/hr. Use a maximum concentration of 80 mEq/L.

Serum K more than 2.5 mEq/L.

200 mEq/day at a rate not to exceed 20 mEq/hr. Use a maximum concentration of 40 mEq/L. **Pediatric:** Up to 3 mEq potassium/kg (or 40 mEq/m^2) daily. Adjust the volume administered depending on the body size.

CAPSULES, EXTENDED-RELEASE; ELIXIR; GRANULES, EFFERVESCENT; GRANULES, EXTENDED-RELEASE; ORAL SOLUTION; POWDER FOR ORAL SOLUTION; TABLETS; TABLETS, EFFERVESCENT; TABLETS, EXTENDED-RELEASE

Prophylaxis of hypokalemia.

16–24 mEq/day.

Potassium depletion.

Usual additive dilution of potassium chloride is 40–80 mEq/L of IV fluid. If serum K^+ is >2.5 mEq/L, the maximum infusion rate is 10 mEq/hr, the maximum concentration is 40 mEq/L and the maximum 24 hour dose is 200 mEq. If serum K^+ is <2 mEq/L, the maximum infusion rate is 40 mEq/hr, the maximum concentration is 80 mEq/L, and the maximum 24 hr dose is 400 mEq.

Children: 3 mEq/kg or 40 mEq/m^2/day; adjust volume of administered fluids to body size.

NOTE: Usual dietary intake of potassium is 40–250 mEq/day. For clients with accompanying metabolic acidosis, use an alkalizing potassium salt (potassium bicarbonate, potassium citrate, potassium acetate, or potassium gluconate).

NURSING IMPLICATIONS

Do not confuse K-Phos Neutral with Neutra-Phos-K or K-dur with Imdur.

IMPLEMENTATION/ADMINISTRATION/STORAGE

1. Give PO doses 2–4 times per day. Correct hypokalemia slowly over a period of 3–7 days to minimize risk of hyperkalemia.
2. With esophageal compression, administer dilute liquid solutions of potassium rather than tablets.
3. IV Do not administer potassium IV undiluted. Usual method is to administer by slow IV infusion in dextrose solution at a concentration of 40–80 mEq/L and at a rate not to exceed 10–20 mEq/hr.
4. Do not infuse rapidly; high plasma levels of potassium may result in death due to cardiac depression, arrhythmias, or arrest.
5. IV administration can cause fluid or solute overloading resulting in dilution of serum electrolyte levels, overhydration, congested states, or pulmonary edema.
6. Avoid 'layering' by inverting container during addition of potassium solution and properly agitating the prepared IV solution. Squeezing the plastic container will not prevent KCl from

settling to the bottom. Never add potassium to an IV bottle that is hanging.

7. Check site of administration frequently for pain and redness because drug is extremely irritating.
8. Discontinue administration if signs of renal insufficiency develop during infusions.
9. In critical clients, KCl may be given by slow IV in a solution of saline (unless contraindicated) since dextrose may lower serum potassium levels by producing an intracellular shift.
10. Administer all concentrated potassium infusions and riders with an infusion control device.
11. Have sodium polystyrene sulfonate (Kayexalate) available for oral or rectal administration in the event of hyperkalemia.
12. COMPATIBILITY Dextrose, saline, Ringer's solution, RL, dextrose/saline and dextrose/RL solutions.
13. INCOMPATIBILITY Administer separately.

ASSESSMENT

1. Identify reasons for therapy; document electrolytes and ECG. List all drugs prescribed and OTC agents consumed.
2. Note any impaired renal function or conditions that may preclude therapy.
3. Assess for adequate urinary flow before administering; dysfunction can lead to hyperkalemia.
4. Withhold and report: abdominal pain, distention, or GI bleeding.
5. Complaints of weakness, fatigue, or the presence of cardiac arrhythmias may be S&S of hypokalemia indicating a low *intracellular* potassium level, although serum level may appear WNL.
6. Withhold drug and report oliguria, anuria, or azoturia.
7. Observe for S&S of adrenal insufficiency or extensive tissue breakdown.
8. Report complaints of weakness or heaviness of the legs, the presence of a gray pallor, cold skin, listlessness, mental confusion, flaccid paralysis, hypotension, or cardiac arrhythmias (S&S of hyperkalemia).
9. Monitor I&O, renal function, serum potassium levels during parenteral therapy; normal level is 3.5–5.0 mEq/L.

CLIENT/FAMILY TEACHING

1. Dilute or dissolve PO liquids, effervescent tablets, or soluble powders in 3–8 oz of cold water, fruit or vegetable juice, or other suitable liquid and drink slowly. Chill to improve taste. Take all products with plenty of water.
2. If GI upset occurs, products can be taken after meals or with food—with a full glass of water.
3. Swallow enteric-coated tablets and extended-release capsules and tablets; do not chew or dissolve in the mouth.
4. Do not use salt substitutes concomitantly with potassium preparations.
5. If receiving potassium-sparing diuretics, such as spironolactone or triamterene, do not take potassium supplements or eat foods high in potassium.
6. Identify high-potassium sources in the diet: Spinach, potatoes, collards, brussels sprouts, beet greens, tomato juice, celery. Once parenteral potassium is discontinued, ingest potassium-rich foods such as citrus juices, bananas, apricots, raisins, and nuts. The daily adult requirement is usually 40–80 mg. A dietitian may assist with meal planning.
7. Avoid self-prescribed enemas, and large amounts of licorice.
8. Keep all F/U to assess response, labs, and for adverse SE.

OUTCOMES/EVALUATE

Correction of potassium deficiency; potassium levels within desired range

Pramipexole

(prah-mih-**PEX**-ohl)

Classification(s): Antiparkinson drug

Pregnancy Category: C

RX: Mirapex, Mirapex XR.

INDICATIONS/USES

(1) Signs and symptoms of idiopathic Parkinson's disease. (2) Moderate to severe restless legs syndrome (immediate-release tablets only).

ACTION/KINETICS

Action

Thought to act by stimulating dopamine (especially D_3) receptors in striatum.

Pharmacokinetics

Rapidly absorbed. **Peak levels:** 2 hr. Food increases time for maximum levels to occur. **t½, terminal:** About 8 hr (12 hr in geriatric clients). Excreted mainly unchanged in urine. Clearance decreases with age.

CONTRAINDICATIONS

Use of extended-release tablets in severe renal impairment (C_{CR} <30 mL/min) or in those on hemodialysis. Lactation.

SPECIAL CONCERNS

- **Possible sudden, overwhelming urge to sleep; driving and operating machinery may prove dangerous.**
- **Use with caution in renal impairment; dosage adjustment required.**
- **Safety and efficacy not determined in children.**

SIDE EFFECTS

Most Common

Postural hypotension, dyskinesia, extrapyramidal syndrome, insomnia, dizziness, hallucinations, abnormal dreams, confusion, constipation, dry mouth, accidental injury, asthenia.

Side effects listed also include those when pramipexole is given with levodopa. **CNS:** Hallucinations (especially in elderly), dyskinesia, extrapyramidal syndrome, aggravated parkinsonism, dizziness, somnolence, insomnia, abnormal dreams, hallucinations, confusion, amnesia, hypesthesia, dystonia, akathisia, abnormal thinking, decreased libido, myoclonus, abnormal gait/hypokinesia, hypertonia, amnesia, tremor/twitching, akathisia, paranoid reaction, delusions, sleep disorders, sudden uncontrolled sedation. **GI:** Nausea, constipation, anorexia, dysphagia, dry mouth. **CV:** Postural hypotension. **GU:** Urinary frequency/infection/incontinence, impotence. **Musculoskeletal:** Arthritis, twitching, bursitis, myasthenia, chest pain. **Respiratory:** Dyspnea, rhinitis, pneumonia. **Ophthalmic:** Abnormal accommodation, vision abnormalities, diplopia. **Metabolic:** Peripheral edema, general edema, decreased weight. **Body as a whole:** Asthenia, malaise, fever. **Miscellaneous:** Accidental injury, disorders.

DRUG INTERACTIONS

Butyrophenones / Possible ↓ effect of pramipexole
Cimetidine / ↑ Levodopa levels and half-life
CNS depressants / Additive CNS depression
Levodopa / ↑ Levodopa levels; also, may cause or worsen pre-existing dyskinesia
Metoclopramide / Possible ↓ effect of pramipexole
Phenothiazines / Possible ↓ effect of pramipexole
Thioxanthines / Possible ↓ effect of pramipexole

HOW SUPPLIED

Tablets: 0.125 mg, 0.25 mg, 0.5 mg, 0.75 mg, 1 mg, 1.5 mg; *Tablets, Extended-Release:* 0.375 mg, 0.75 mg, 1.5 mg, 2.25 mg, 3 mg, 3.75 mg, 4.5 mg.

DOSAGE

TABLETS, IMMEDIATE-RELEASE

Parkinsonism.

Adults. Week 1: 0.125 mg 3 times per day. **Week 2:** 0.25 mg 3 times per day. **Week 3:** 0.5 mg 3 times per day. **Week 4:** 0.75 mg 3 times per day. **Week 5:** 1 mg 3 times per day. **Week 6:** 1.25 mg 3 times per day. **Week 7:** 1.5 mg 3 times per day. **Maintenance:** 1.5–4.5 mg/day in equally divided doses 3 times per day with or without concomitant levodopa (about 800 mg/day).

Impaired renal function: C_{CR} >60 mL/min: Start with 0.125 mg 3 times per day, up to maximum of 1.5 mg 3 times per day. **C_{CR} 35–59 mL/min:** Start with 0.125 mg twice/day, up to maximum of 1.5 mg twice/day. **C_{CR} 15–34 mL/min:** Start with 0.125 mg once daily, up to maximum of 1.5 mg once daily. **C_{CR} <15 mL/min and hemodialysis clients:** Pramipexole not adequately studied in this group.

Restless legs syndrome.

Adults, initial: 0.125 mg once daily 2–3 hr before bedtime. For those requiring additional relief, the dose may be increased as follows after the initial dose is given for 4–7 days: 0.25 mg for 4–7 days followed by 0.5 mg for 4–7 days. Increase the duration between titration steps to 14 days in those with severe and moderate impaired renal function (C_{CR} from 20–60 mL/min).

TABLETS, EXTENDED-RELEASE

Parkinson's disease.

Adults, initial: 0.375 mg once a day. Based on efficacy and tolerability, may increase the dose gradually not more frequently than q 5–7 days, first to 0.75 mg/day and then by 0.75 mg increments, up to a maximum of 4.5 mg/day. If therapy is to be discontinued, taper gradually over 1 week.

In clients with moderate renal impairment (i.e., C_{CR} between 30 and 50 mL/min), initially take pramipexole every other day. Carefully assess efficacy and tolerability before increasing daily dosing after 1 week and before any additional titration in 0.375 mg increments, up to 2.25 mg/day.

NURSING IMPLICATIONS

IMPLEMENTATION/ADMINISTRATION/STORAGE

1. Gradually titrate dosage; increase the dose to reach a maximum therapeutic effect, balanced against the main side effects of dyskinesia, hallucinations, somnolence, and dry mouth.
2. If there is significant interruption of therapy, retitration may be warranted.
3. Consider a decrease in levodopa dose if taken with pramipexole.
4. Do not increase dosage more frequently than every 5–7 days.
5. Clients may be switched overnight from immediate-release to extended-release pramipexole at the same daily dose. When switching, monitor to determine if dosage adjustment is needed.
6. Discontinue pramipexole over a 1 week period. However, clients taking doses up to 0.75 mg once daily for restless legs syndrome were discontinued without taper.
7. Store from 15–30°C (59–86°F). Protect from light. Protect ER tablets from exposure to high humidity.

ASSESSMENT

1. Note disease onset, extent of motor function, reflexes, gait, strength of grip, rigidity, amount of tremor.
2. With tremor, assess for muscle weakness, muscle rigidity, difficulty walking, or changing directions with Parkinson's disease.
3. Use very low dose for control of RLS symptoms (immediate release tabs).
4. Assess sleep habits and patterns and frequency of disturbances.
5. Obtain dermatological screening periodically.
6. Check for S&S of orthostatic hypotension especially during dose escalation; note any drowsiness or sleepiness.
7. Monitor mental status (note any confusion or hallucinations), neurologic evaluations, VS, ECG, renal and LFTs; reduce dose with dysfunction.

CLIENT/FAMILY TEACHING

1. Take only as prescribed; may take with food to decrease nausea.
2. Do not chew, crush, or divide ER tablets.
3. Rise slowly from sitting or lying position to prevent drop in BP.
4. Do not drive or perform activities that require mental/motor alertness until stabilized on drug. May cause dizziness, fainting, blackouts, hypotension, sudden urge to sleep, and sedation.
5. Practice reliable contraception.
6. Report lack of response, worsening of condition, or any vision problems; obtain regular eye exams.
7. May cause hallucinations especially in the elderly.
8. Impulse control disorders such as pathological gambling, compulsive eating, or hypersexuality can occur.
9. Report headaches, mood/mental changes, persistent nausea, or uncontrolled movements.
10. Do not stop abruptly; must taper over 1 week period.
11. Avoid alcohol and any other CNS depressants, may exaggerate drowsiness and dizziness.
12. Keep all F/U visits to evaluate response, labs, and for adverse SE.

OUTCOMES/EVALUATE

- Control of parkinsonian symptoms (e.g., improvement in motor function, reflexes, gait, strength of grip, and amount of tremor)
- Relief of RLS S&S

P

Pramlintide acetate

(**PRAM**-lin-tide)

Classification(s): Antidiabetic, amylin analog

Pregnancy Category: C

RX: Symlin.

INDICATIONS/USES

(1) Adjunct treatment in type 1 diabetes mellitus in clients who use mealtime insulin therapy and who have failed to achieve desired glucose control despite optimal insulin therapy. (2) Adjunct treatment in type 2 diabetes mellitus in clients who use mealtime insulin therapy and who have failed to achieve desired glucose control despite optimal insulin therapy, with or without a concurrent sulfonylurea agent and/or metformin. *NOTE:* Proper client selection is critical to safe and effective use of pramlintide.

ACTION/KINETICS

Action

Pramlintide is a synthetic analog of human amylin, a naturally occurring neuroendrocrine hormone synthesized by pancreatic beta cells; it contributes to glucose control during the postprandial period. Amylin is stored with insulin in secretory granules and cosecreted with insulin by pancreatic beta cells in response to food intake. Amylin affects the rate of postprandial glucose appearance through a variety of mechanisms. It slows gastric emptying without altering the overall absorption of nutrients. Also, amylin suppresses glucagon secretion which leads to suppression of endogenous glucose output from the liver. It also regulates food intake caused by centrally-mediated modulation of appetite. Thus, pramlintide, by acting as an amylinomimetic agent, has the following effects: (1) modulation of gastric emptying; (2) prevention of the postprandial rise in plasma glucagon; and, (3) satiety leading to decreased caloric intake and potential weight loss.

Pharmacokinetics

The bioavailability of a SC dose is about 30–40%. Not extensively bound to plasma proteins. Metabolized primarily by the kidneys; the primary metabolite is biologically active. **t½, parent drug and active metabolite:** 48 min.

CONTRAINDICATIONS

Hypersensitivity to pramlintide acetate or any of its components, including metacresol. Diagnosis of gastroparesis. Hypoglycemia. Use when taking drugs that alter GI motility (e.g., atropine) or agents that slow GI absorption of nutrients (e.g., alpha-glucosidase inhibitors).

SPECIAL CONCERNS

■ Pramlintide is used with insulin and has been associated with an increased risk of insulin-induced severe hypoglycemia, particularly in clients with type 1 diabetes. When severe hypoglycemia associated with pramlintide use occurs, it is seen within 3 hr following a pramlintide injection. If severe hypoglycemia occurs while operating a motor vehicle, heavy machinery, or while engaging in other high-risk activities, serious injuries may occur. Appropriate client selection, careful client instruction, and insulin dose adjustments are critical elements for reducing this risk. ■

- **Potential to delay the absorption of coadministered PO drugs; when rapid onset of a PO coadministered drug is a critical determinant of efficacy (e.g., analgesics), administer the drug at least 1 hr prior to or 2 hr after pramlintide injection.**
- **May delay the absorption of coadministered PO medications.**
- **Increased risk of severe hypoglycemia in the elderly.**
- **Use during lactation only if potential benefit outweighs the potential risk to the infant.**
- **Safety and efficacy not determined in children.**

SIDE EFFECTS

Most Common

Hypoglycemia, headache, N&V, abdominal pain, anorexia, inflicted injury, fatigue, coughing.

Side effects listed are associated with administration of pramlintide with insulin. **GI:** N&V, abdominal pain, anorexia. **CNS:** Headache, dizziness. **Respiratory:** Coughing, pharyngitis. **At injection site:** Redness, swelling, itching. **Body as a whole:** Fatigue, ***systemic allergic reaction***. **Miscellaneous:** ***Hypoglycemia (may be severe)***, inflicted injury, arthralgia. *NOTE:* Pramlintide alone does not cause hypoglycemia but when mixed with insulin, the risk of hypoglycemia is increased.

P

OVERDOSE MANAGEMENT

Symptoms: Hypoglycemia, severe nausea, vomiting, diarrhea, vasodilation, dizziness. *Treatment:* Severe hypoglycemia treatment may include glucagon injection, IV glucose, hospitalization, paramedic assistance, or ER visit. Supportive measures.

DRUG INTERACTIONS

Alpha-glucosidase inhibitors / Do not use together with pramlintide due to effects on gastric emptying
Anticholinergic drugs, including atropine / Do not use together with pramlintide due to effects on gastric emptying
Drugs that increase susceptibility to hypoglycemia / ↑ Risk of hypoglycemia
Insulins / ↑ Risk of hypoglycemia
Sulfonylureas / ↑ Risk of hypoglycemia

HOW SUPPLIED

Solution for Injection: 0.6 mg/mL.

DOSAGE

SC

Type 1 diabetes mellitus.

Initial: 15 mcg; **then,** titrate at 15 mcg increments to a maintenance dose of 30 or 60 mcg, as tolerated. Increase the pramlintide dose to the next increment (30, 45, or 60 mcg) when no clinically significant nausea has occurred for at least 3 days.

Type 2 diabetes mellitus.

Initial: 60 mcg; **then,** increase the dose, as tolerated, to 120 mcg. Increase the pramlintide dose to 120 mcg when no clinically significant nausea has occurred for 3–7 days. If significant nausea persists at the 120 mcg dose, decrease the dose to 60 mcg.

NURSING IMPLICATIONS

IMPLEMENTATION/ADMINISTRATION/STORAGE

1. Proper client selection is critical to the safe and effective use of pramlintide.
2. When used for type 1 or type 2 diabetes, reduce preprandial, rapid-acting, or short-acting insulin dosages, including fixed-mix insulins (e.g. 70/30) by 50%.
3. If significant nausea persists at the 45 or 60 mcg dose when used for type 1 diabetics, decrease the dose to 30 mcg. If the 30 mcg dose is not tolerated, consider discontinuing pramlintide.
4. Both type 1 and type 2 diabetics should only make pramlintide dose adjustments as directed by their provider.
5. Both type 1 and type 2 diabetics should adjust insulin doses to optimize glycemic control once the target dose of pramlintide is achieved and nausea has subsided. Only make insulin dose changes as directed by the provider.
6. Administer pramlintide SC immediately prior to each major meal (250 or more kcal or containing 30 grams or more of carbohydrate). If a pramlintide dose is missed, the client should not be given an additional injection. Wait until the next scheduled dose and give the usual amount.
7. To give SC from a vial, use a U-100 insulin syringe (preferably a 0.3 mL) size for optimal accuracy. Check package insert for conversion of pramlintide dose to insulin unit equivalents.
8. The *Pen-injector* is available as a 60 pen-injector for doses of 15, 30, 45, and 60 mcg and a 120 pen-injector for doses of 60 and 120 mcg. Advise clients of the following:
   - Confirm they are using the correct pen-injector that will deliver the prescribed dose.
   - Proper use of the pen-injector, emphasizing how and when to set up a new pen-injector.
   - Not to transfer pramlintide from the pen-injector to a syringe as this could result in a higher dose than intended because pramlintide in the pen-injector is a higher concentration than pramlintide in the vial.
   - Not to share the pen-injector and needles with others.
   - Needles are not included with the pen-injector and must be purchased separately.
   - Which needle length and gauge should be used.
   - Use a new needle for each injection.
9. SC administration should be into the abdomen or thigh. The arm is not recommended because of variable absorption. Rotate injection sites. The injection site should be distinct from the site chosen for any concomitant insulin injection.

10. Clients should always use a new syringe and needle to give pramlintide and insulin injections.
11. Pramlintide and insulin should always be given as separate injections. Mixing may alter the pharmacokinetic parameters.
12. Discontinue pramlintide if any of the following occur:
    - Recurrent unexplained hypoglycemia that requires medical assistance.
    - Persistent clinically significant nausea.
    - Noncompliance with self-monitoring of blood glucose concentrations.
    - Noncompliance with insulin dose adjustments.
    - Noncompliance with scheduled health care professional contacts or recommended clinic visits.
13. Store unopened (not in-use) vials or pen-injectors in the refrigerator at 2–8°C (36–46°F) protected from light. Do not freeze; if a vial has been frozen or overheated, discard it. Keep opened (in-use) vials or pen-injectors refrigerated or at room temperature for up to 30 days as long as the temperature is not more than 30°C (86°F). Discard after 28 days.
14. To reduce the potential for injection-site reactions, pramlintide should be at room temperature before injection.

ASSESSMENT

1. Note reasons for therapy, onset and characteristics of disease, other agents trialed, outcome.
2. Monitor weight, VS, HbA1c, glucose monitoring results, insulin or antihypoglycemic regimen followed and client compliance.
3. Assess for conditions that would preclude drug therapy: gastroparesis, poor compliance or HbA1c >9%, hypoglycemia unawareness, hospitalized with hypoglycemia in past 6 months, requires drug to stimulate gastric motility, poor compliance with insulin administration or blood sugar monitoring, or a child.
4. Monitor HbA1c, CBC, lipids, renal and LFTs, microalbuminuria, eye and foot exams.

CLIENT/FAMILY TEACHING

1. Drug administered by injection under the skin to help better control blood sugar. It cannot be administered or mixed with insulin and cannot be injected within 2 inches of the insulin administration site.
2. Rotate pramlintide and insulin injection sites (abdomen and thigh). Do not inject pramlintide into arm because of variable absorption and effectiveness.
3. Injections are given at mealtimes and do not replace the daily or more frequent insulin injections, but may lower the amount of insulin or antihypoglycemic agent required.
4. Pramlintide and insulin must be administered as separate injections at separate injection sites; pramlintide cannot be mixed with any insulin product.
5. Avoid activities that require mental alertness until drug effects realized. May significantly lower blood glucose levels especially if adequate food and carbohydrates not consumed.
6. Most frequent side effect is nausea and can be managed with reduction in dosage.
7. Follow dietary guidelines, perform regular exercise, weight loss, dietary restrictions and other lifestyle changes consistent with controlling diabetes.
8. May experience profound hypoglycemia. Early S&S include: hunger, headaches, sweating, tremor, irritability, difficulty concentrating. These S&S may vary or be less noticeable with long history of diabetes, diabetic nerve disease, or when on certain drugs such as clonidine, or beta blockers.
9. Follow and refer to pramlintide Medication Guide for additional information and guidelines for things such as omitted dose, inadequate food intake, missed meals, or accidental excess dose of insulin.
10. Must monitor finger sticks regularly and follow schedule for mealtimes, injections, caloric consumption, and exercise.
11. Avoid alcohol, may cause increase in low blood sugar and associated symptoms.
12. Keep all F/U to assess response, labs, and for adverse SE.

OUTCOMES/EVALUATE

Control of blood glucose; HbA1c <8

P

Prasugrel hydrochloride

(prah-soo-**GREL HYE**-droh-**KLOR**-ide)

Classification(s): Antiplatelet agent (aggregation inhibitor)

Pregnancy Category: B

RX: Effient.

INDICATIONS/USES

Reduce the rate of thrombotic CV events (including stent thrombosis) in those with acute coronary syndrome who are to be managed with percutaneous coronary intervention as follows: (1) Clients with unstable angina or non-ST elevation MI or (2) those with ST elevation MI when managed with primary or delayed percutaneous coronary intervention.

ACTION/KINETICS

Action

Inhibits platelet activation and aggregation through irreversible binding of the active metabolite to the $P2Y_{12}$ class of ADP receptors on platelets. Platelet inhibition is rapid and irreversible (lasts for the life of the platelet).

Pharmacokinetics

At least 79% of a dose is absorbed. Prasugrel is a prodrug and is rapidly metabolized by CYP3A4 and CYP2B6 (and to a lesser extent by CYP2C9 and CYP2C19) to an active metabolite. **Peak plasma levels, active metabolite:** About 30 min. Mean steady-state inhibition of platelet aggregation is about 70% following 3–5 days of dosing at 10 mg/day after a 60 mg loading dose. **t½, elimination:** About 7 hr for the active metabolite. Inactive metabolites excreted in the urine (68%) and feces (27%). **Plasma protein binding:** 98% (of the active metabolite).

CONTRAINDICATIONS

Hypersensitivity (e.g., anaphylaxis) to the drug or any component of the product. Active pathological bleeding (e.g., peptic ulcer, intracranial hemorrhage). Prior TIA or stroke. Generally not recommended in those 75 years of age and older except in high risk situations (See *Black Box Warning*).

SPECIAL CONCERNS

■ **Bleeding risk.** (1) Prasugrel can cause significant, sometimes fatal, bleeding. (2) Do not use prasugrel in clients with active pathological bleeding or a history of TIA or stroke. (3) In clients 75 years of age and older, prasugrel is generally not recommended because of the increased risk of fatal and intracranial bleeding and uncertain benefit, except in high-risk situations (those with diabetes or a history of prior MI) in which its effect appears to be greater and its use may be considered. (4) Do not start prasugrel in clients likely to undergo urgent coronary artery bypass graft surgery. When possible, discontinue prasugrel at least 7 days prior to any surgery. (5) Additional risk factors for bleeding include body weight less than 60 kg, propensity to bleed, and concomitant use of medications that increase the risk of bleeding (e.g., warfarin, heparin, fibrinolytic therapy, long-term use of NSAIDs). (6) Suspect bleeding in any client who is hypotensive and has recently undergone coronary angiography, percutaneous coronary intervention, coronary artery bypass graft surgery, or other surgical procedures in the setting of prasugrel. (7) If possible, manage bleeding without discontinuing prasugrel. Discontinuing prasugrel, particularly in the first few weeks after acute coronary syndrome, increases the risk of subsequent CV events. ■

- **Use during lactation only if the potential benefit to the mother justifies the potential risk to the fetus.**
- **Clients with severe hepatic impairment and those with body weight less than 60 kg are generally at a higher risk of bleeding.**
- **Use generally not recommended in those 75 years and older due to an increased risk of fatal bleeding events. Exceptions include high-risk situations (e.g., diabetes, history of MI) where effect appears to be greater and use of prasugrel may be considered.**
- **Safety and efficacy not determined in children.**

SIDE EFFECTS

Most Common

Bleeding (minor or major), hypertension, headache, dyspnea, nausea, hypercholesterolemia, hyperlipidemia.

CV: Bleeding (minor, major, ***life-threatening***), ***symptomatic intracranial hemorrhage, thrombosis in MI, GI hemorrhage***, hemoptysis, SC hematoma, ***postprocedural hemorrhage, retroperitoneal hemorrhage, pericardial effusion/hemorrhage/tamponade***, retinal hemorrhage, epistaxis. Hyper-/hypotension, atrial fibrillation, bradycardia. **CNS:** Headache, dizziness. **GI:** Nausea, diarrhea. **Respiratory:** Dyspnea, cough. **Dermatologic:** Rash. **Hematologic:** Leukopenia, severe thrombocytopenia, anemia, thrombotic thrombocytopenic purpura (including thrombocytopenia, microangiopathic hemolytic anemia). **Hypersensitivity:** Allergic reactions, ***angioedema, anaphylaxis***. **Body as a whole:** Fatigue, peripheral edema, pyrexia, pain in extremity. **Miscellaneous:** Back pain, noncardiac chest pain, malignancies (e.g., colon, lung).

NOTE: Factors that increase the risk of bleeding if using prasugrel include: Clients 75 years of age and older; coronary artery bypass graft or other surgical procedures; body weight less than 60 kg (use lower dose); propensity to bleed (e.g., recent trauma, recent surgery, recent or recurrent GI bleeding, active peptic ulcer disease, severe hepatic impairment); drugs that increase the risk of bleeding (e.g., PO anticoagulants, chronic use of NSAIDs, fibrinolytic drugs).

LABORATORY TEST CONSIDERATIONS

Hypercholesterolemia, hyperlipidemia. Abnormal liver function.

OVERDOSE MANAGEMENT

Symptoms: Platelet inhibition is rapid and irreversible and lasts for the life of the platelet; inhibition is unlikely to be increased in an overdose. *Treatment:* Platelet transfusions may restore clotting ability. Dialysis is not likely to remove the active metabolite.

DRUG INTERACTIONS

Heparin / ↑ Risk of bleeding although coadministration can be undertaken
NSAIDs (chronic use) / ↑ Risk of bleeding
Tenecteplase / ↑ Risk of bleeding
Warfarin / ↑ Risk of bleeding; use together with caution

HOW SUPPLIED

Tablets: 5 mg, 10 mg.

DOSAGE

TABLETS

Acute coronary syndrome.

Adults weighing 60 kg or more, usual: 10 mg once a day; **adults weighing less than 60 kg, usual:** 5 mg once a day should be considered. **Loading dose:** 60 mg single dose. *NOTE:* Prasugrel should be taken with aspirin, 75–325 mg a day.

NURSING IMPLICATIONS

IMPLEMENTATION/ADMINISTRATION/STORAGE

1. May be given with or without food. Do not break the tablet.
2. The optimal duration of therapy is unknown.
3. Discontinue prasugrel for active bleeding, elective surgery, stroke, or TIA.
4. In clients managed with percutaneous coronary intervention and stent placement, premature discontinuation of prasugrel results in an increased risk of stent thrombosis, MI, and death. If prasugrel must be temporarily discontinued due to a side effect, restart therapy as soon as possible.
5. Store from 15–30°C (59–86°F). Keep the product in its original container.

ASSESSMENT

1. Note reasons for therapy: MI or unstable angina managed by percutaneous coronary intervention (PCI). Administered with aspirin to reduce risk of MI/damage related to clots.
2. Avoid with any history of stroke or TIA, active bleeding, severe hepatic impairment, or potential for high risk of bleeding that could outweigh benefits. Also if >75 y.o., weight <60 kg, significant renal impairment, or if undergoing CABG, avoid therapy.
3. Drug inhibits platelet aggregation for the lifetime of the platelet (7–10 days).
4. Drug is similar to Plavix and seems to work better but has a much higher bleeding risk.
5. Monitor BP, HR, ECG, CBC, renal and LFTs.

CLIENT/FAMILY TEACHING

1. Take once daily with aspirin; do not break tabs. May take with food if GI upset. Drug helps prevent platelets from sticking together and forming a clot that can block an artery or a stent.

P

2. It takes longer than usual to stop bleeding and may bruise much easier.
3. Stop drug 7 days before any planned surgery or dental procedures.
4. Report any fever, weakness, extreme paleness or purple skin patches, yellowing of the skin or eyes, or neurologic changes.
5. Avoid alcohol and OTC agents, including NSAIDs without approval.
6. Keep all F/U to assess response, labs, and adverse SE.

OUTCOMES/EVALUATE

↓ Thrombotic events with acute coronary syndrome (ACS)

Pravastatin sodium

(prah-vah-**STAH**-tin)

Classification(s): Antihyperlipidemic, HMG-CoA reductase inhibitor

Pregnancy Category: X

RX: Pravachol.

Rx: Apo-Pravastatin, CO Pravastatin, Gen-Pravastatin, Novo-Pravastatin, Nu-Pravastatin, PMS-Pravastatin, ratio-Pravastatin, Sandoz Pravastatin.

SEE ALSO ***ANTIHYPERLIPIDEMIC—HMG-COA REDUCTASE INHIBITORS.***

INDICATIONS/USES

1. Adjunct to diet for reducing elevated total and LDL cholesterol and triglyceride levels in clients with primary hypercholesterolemia (type IIa and IIb) and mixed dyslipidemia when the response to a diet with restricted saturated fat and cholesterol has not been effective. Treat elevated serum triglyceride levels (Fredrickson Type IV) and primary dysbetalipoproteinemia (Fredrickson Type III). Reduction of apolipoprotein B serum levels.
2. Reduce the risk of recurrent MI in those with previous MI and normal cholesterol levels; reduce risk of undergoing myocardial revascularization procedures; reduce risk of stroke or TIA.
3. Reduce risk of MI in hypercholesterolemia without evidence of coronary heart disease; reduce risk of CV mortality with no increase in death from noncardiovascular causes.
4. Slow the progression of coronary atherosclerosis, and reduce risk of acute coronary events in hypercholesterolemia with clinically evident CAD, including prior MI.
5. Adjunct to diet and lifestyle modification to treat heterozygous familial hypercholesterolemia in children and adolescents 8 years of age and older if after an adequate trial of diet the following are present: LDL-C remains 190 mg/dL or greater, or LDL-C remains 160 mg/dL and there is a positive family history of premature CV disease or two or more other cardiovascular disease factors are present.
6. *Investigational:* To lower cholesterol levels in those with heterozygous familial hypercholesterolemia, familial combined hyperlipidemia, diabetic dyslipidemia in non-insulin-dependent diabetics, hypercholesterolemia secondary to nephrotic syndrome, homozygous familial hypercholesterolemia in those not completely devoid of LDL receptors but who have a decreased level of LDL receptor activity.

ACTION/KINETICS

Action

Competitively inhibits HMG-CoA reductase; this enzyme catalyzes the early rate-limiting step in the synthesis of cholesterol. Thus, cholesterol synthesis is inhibited/decreased. Decreases total cholesterol, triglycerides, LDL, and VLDL, and increases HDL. Drug increases survival in heart transplant recipients. Drug effect greater in geriatric clients.

Pharmacokinetics

Rapidly absorbed from the GI tract; absolute bioavailability is 17%. **Peak plasma levels:** 1–1.5 hr. Significant first-pass extraction and metabolism in the liver, which is the site of action of the drug; thus, plasma levels may not correlate well with lipid-lowering effectiveness. **t½, elimination:** 77 hr (including metabolites). Metabolized in the liver; excreted in the urine (about 20%) and feces (70%). Potential accumulation of drug with renal or hepatic insufficiency. **Plasma protein binding:** About 50%.

ADDITIONAL CONTRAINDICATIONS

To treat hypercholesterolemia due to hyperalphaproteinemia.

SPECIAL CONCERNS

- **Use with caution in clients with a history of liver disease or renal insufficiency.**
- **Possible effect on basal steroid hormone levels.**
- **Safety and efficacy not determined in children less than 8 years of age.**

SIDE EFFECTS

Most Common

Muscle cramps/pain, localized pain, N&V, diarrhea, abdominal cramps/pain, constipation, flatulence, heartburn, fatigue, rhinitis, rash/pruritus, cardiac chest pain, dizziness, headache, fatigue, angina pectoris.

Musculoskeletal: Muscle cramps/pain, localized pain, myalgia, myopathy, rhabdomyolysis (including with renal dysfunction secondary to myoglobinuria), arthralgia, arthritis, muscle weakness, polymyalgia, rheumatica. **CNS:** Dizziness, headache, depression, insomnia, paresthesia, vertigo, memory impairment, neuropathy (including peripheral neuropathy), tremor. **Neurologic:** Dysfunction of certain cranial nerves, including alteration of taste, facial paresis, and impairment of extraocular movement; peripheral nerve palsy. **GI:** Dyspepsia, N&V, flatulence, abdominal pain/cramps, constipation, diarrhea, heartburn, decreased appetite, ***pancreatitis***. **Hepatic:** Cholestatic jaundice, cirrhosis, fatty change in liver, ***fulminant hepatic necrosis***, hepatitis (including chronic active hepatitis), hepatoma. **CV:** Angina pectoris, cardiac chest pain, vasculitis. **GU:** Urinary abnormality, libido change, sexual dysfunction, gynecomastia. **Dermatologic:** Rash, alopecia, pruritus, flushing, dermatomyositis, erythema multiforme (including ***Stevens-Johnson syndrome***), ***toxic epidermal necrolysis***, skin changes (changes to hair/nails, discoloration, dryness of mucous membranes, nodules). **Respiratory:** Dyspnea, URTI, cough, rhinitis. **Hematologic:** Hemolytic anemia. **Ophthalmic:** Visual disturbance, lens opacity. **Hypersensitivity: *Anaphylaxis***, angioedema. **Body as a whole:** Fatigue, allergy/hypersensitivity, pain, asthenia, fever, chills, malaise, lupus erythematosus-like syndrome, photosensitivity. **Miscellaneous:** Edema of the head/neck, taste disturbance.

LABORATORY TEST CONSIDERATIONS

↑ CPK, AST, ALT, alkaline phosphatase, bilirubin, erythrocyte sedimentation rate. Positive ANA. Transient asymptomatic eosinophilia. Abnormalities in thyroid and liver function tests.

ADDITIONAL DRUG INTERACTIONS

Bile acid sequestrants (cholestyramine, colestipol) / ↓ Bioavailability of pravastatin R/T ↓ GI absorption
Nonnucleoside reverse transcriptase inhibitors (e.g., delavirdine, efavirenz, nevirapine) / ↑ Risk of pravastatin toxicity (e.g., myopathy) R/T inhibition of metabolism by CYP3A4
Rifamycins (e.g., rifampin) / Possible ↑ or ↓ pravastatin levels

HOW SUPPLIED

Tablets: 10 mg, 20 mg, 40 mg, 80 mg.

DOSAGE

TABLETS

Antihyperlipidemic.

Adults, initial: 40 mg once daily. A dose of 80 mg/day can be used if the 40 mg dose does not achieve desired results. Use a starting dose of 10 mg/day at bedtime in renal/hepatic dysfunction, in those taking concomitant immunosuppressants, and in the elderly (maximum maintenance dose for these clients is 20 mg/day). **Children, 8–13 years of age (inclusive):** 20 mg once daily. Doses greater than 20 mg have not been studied in this population. **Adolescents, 14–18 years of age, initial:** 40 mg once daily. Doses greater than 40 mg have not been studied in this population. *NOTE:* Reevaluate children and adolescents treated with pravastatin in adulthood, and make appropriate changes to their regimen for lowering cholesterol to achieve adult goals for LDL-C.

P

NURSING IMPLICATIONS

Do not confuse Pravachol with Prevacid (proton pump inhibitor) or propranolol (a beta-adrenergic blocking agent).

IMPLEMENTATION/ADMINISTRATION/STORAGE

1. **Place on a standard cholesterol-lowering diet for 3–6 months before (unless documented CAD) beginning pravastatin, and continue during therapy.**

2. In clients taking immunosuppressants (e.g., cyclosporine), begin pravastatin therapy at 10 mg/day at bedtime and titrate to higher doses with caution. Usual maximum dose is 20 mg/day.
3. Drug may be taken as a single dose anytime of the day without regard to meals.
4. The lipid-lowering effects are enhanced when combined with a bile-acid binding resin. When given with a bile-acid binding resin (e.g., cholestyramine, colestipol), give pravastatin either 1 hr or more before or 4 or more hr after the resin. Only use this combination if further changes in lipid levels are likely to outweigh the increased risk of the drug combination.
5. The maximum effect is seen within 4 weeks, during which time periodic lipid determinations should be undertaken.
6. Pravastatin is not indicated when hypercholesterolemia is due to hyperalphalipoproteinemia (elevated HDL-C).
7. Store from 15–30°C (59–86°F); protect from light and moisture.

ASSESSMENT

1. Note reasons for therapy, other agents trialed/outcome. Rule out secondary causes for hypercholesterolemia; these include hypothyroidism, poorly controlled diabetes mellitus, dysproteinemias, obstructive liver disease, nephrotic syndrome, alcoholism, other drug therapy.
2. Determine if pregnant or planning pregnancy. Note mental status and cognitive functioning level.
3. Assess for liver disease, if alcohol has been abused, before initiating therapy, before increasing the dose, and as clinically indicated.
4. Document all CAD risk factors. Initiate therapy during hospitalization for MI/angioplasty procedure to improve clinical outcomes.
5. Stop pravastatin temporarily in clients experiencing an acute or serious condition (e.g., sepsis, hypotension, major surgery, trauma, uncontrolled epilepsy, or severe metabolic, endocrine, or electrolyte disorders) predisposing to the development of renal failure R/T rhabdomyolysis.
6. Pravastatin should be discontinued if markedly elevated CPK levels occur or myopathy is diagnosed.
7. Monitor lipid profile, CBC, renal and LFTs. Obtain LFTs prior to therapy, 6 weeks after starting therapy, with any dose increases, and periodically thereafter as condition indicates; if WNL may monitor at 6-month intervals.

CLIENT/FAMILY TEACHING

1. Take at the same time each day with or without food.
2. Continue regular exercise program; strive to attain recommended weight loss. Stop smoking, follow dietary restrictions (reduced saturated fat intake, increase soluble fiber intake), and control stress in overall goal of cholesterol control.
3. Report unexplained muscle pain, tenderness, or weakness, especially if accompanied by malaise or fever.
4. Practice reliable barrier contraception; report if pregnancy is suspected, as drug therapy is hazardous to a developing fetus.
5. Report severe GI upset, unusual bruising/bleeding, vision changes, dark urine, or light-colored stools.
6. Stop drug and report if mental status changes or cognitive impairment noted.
7. Keep all F/U to assess response, labs, and for adverse SE.

OUTCOMES/EVALUATE

↓ Serum cholesterol and LDL levels; MI prophylaxis in those with atherosclerosis and hypercholesterolemia

Prazosin hydrochloride

(**PRAY**-zoh-sin)

Classification(s): Antihypertensive, alpha-1-adrenergic blocking drug

Pregnancy Category: C

RX: Minipress.

🍁 **Rx:** Apo-Prazo.

SEE ALSO ***ALPHA-1-ADRENERGIC BLOCKING AGENTS*** AND ***ANTIHYPERTENSIVE AGENTS***.

INDICATIONS/USES

Mild to moderate hypertension alone or in combination with other antihypertensive drugs (e.g., diuretics, beta-adrenergic blocking agents). *Investigational:* Raynaud phenomenon.

ACTION/KINETICS

Action

Produces selective blockade of postsynaptic alpha-1-adrenergic receptors. Dilates areterioles and veins, thereby decreasing total peripheral resistance and decreasing DBP more than SBP. CO, HR, and renal blood flow are not affected. Can be used to initiate antihypertensive therapy; most effective when used with other agents (e.g., diuretics, beta-adrenergic blocking agents).

Pharmacokinetics

Onset: 2 hr. Absorption not affected by food. **Maximum effect:** 2–3 hr; **duration:** 6–12 hr. **t½:** 2–3 hr. Full therapeutic effect: 4–6 weeks. Metabolized extensively; excreted primarily in feces.

SPECIAL CONCERNS

- **Use with caution during lactation.**
- **Elderly may be more sensitive to the hypotensive and hypothermic effects; may need to decrease the dose due to age-related decreases in renal function.**
- **Syncopal episodes may occur 30–90 min after the initial dose, including rapid dosage increases or adding another antihypertensive drug to the regimen.**
- **Safe use in children not established.**

SIDE EFFECTS

Most Common

Dizziness, drowsiness, headache, lack of energy, weakness, palpitations, nausea.

First-dose effect: ***Marked hypotension*** and syncope 30–90 min after administration of initial dose (usually 2 or more mg), increase of dosage, or addition of other antihypertensive agent. **CNS:** Dizziness, drowsiness, headache, fatigue, paresthesias, depression, vertigo, nervousness, hallucinations, insomnia. **CV:** Palpitations, syncope, tachycardia, orthostatic hypotension/hypotension, aggravation of angina, angina pectoris, bradycardia, vasculitis. **GI:** N&V, diarrhea or constipation, dry mouth, abdominal pain, abnormal liver function, ***pancreatitis***. **GU:** Urinary frequency/incontinence, impotence, priapism, gynecomastia. **Respiratory:** Dyspnea, nasal congestion, epistaxis. **Musculoskeletal:** Arthralgia, myalgia. **Dermatologic:** Pruritus, rash, alopecia, lichen planus, diaphoresis, flushing, urticaria. **Ophthalmic:** Blurred vision, reddening of sclera, eye pain, conjunctivitis. **Body as a whole:** Lack of energy, weakness, asthenia, malaise, pain, edema, fever. **Miscellaneous:** Symptoms of lupus erythematosus, tinnitus, allergic reaction.

LABORATORY TEST CONSIDERATIONS

↑ Urinary metabolites of norepinephrine, VMA.

OVERDOSE MANAGEMENT

Symptoms: Hypotension, shock. *Treatment:* Keep client supine to restore BP and HR. If shock is manifested, use volume expanders and vasopressors; maintain renal function.

DRUG INTERACTIONS

Antihypertensives (other) / ↑ Antihypertensive effect
Beta-adrenergic blocking agents / Enhanced acute postural hypotension after first dose of prazosin
Clonidine / ↓ Antihypertensive effect of clonidine
Diuretics / ↑ Antihypertensive effect
Indomethacin / ↓ Effect of prazosin
Nifedipine / ↑ Hypotensive effect
Propranolol / Especially pronounced additive hypotensive effect
Verapamil / ↑ Hypotensive effect of prazosin; ↑ sensitivity to prazosin-induced postural hypotension

HOW SUPPLIED

Capsules: 1 mg, 2 mg, 5 mg.

DOSAGE

CAPSULES

Hypertension.

Individualize depending on BP response. Adults, initial, 1 mg 2–3 times per day; **maintenance:** if necessary, increase gradually to 6–15 mg/day in two to three divided doses. Do not exceed 20 mg/day, although some clients have benefitted from doses of 40 mg daily. If used with diuretics or other antihypertensives, reduce dose to 1–2 mg 3 times per day.

Raynaud phenomenon.

Adults: 1 mg 3 times a day.

NURSING IMPLICATIONS

IMPLEMENTATION/ADMINISTRATION/STORAGE

Store from 15–30°C (59–86°F). Protect from moisture and light.

P

ASSESSMENT

1. Note reasons for therapy, characteristics of S&S, other agents trialed, outcome.
2. Assess for fall risk, cardiopulmonary status, VS, and renal function.

CLIENT/FAMILY TEACHING

1. Take the first dose at bedtime. Also, take the first dose of each dosage increment at bedtime to reduce the incidence of syncope.
2. Do not drive or operate machinery for 24 hr after the first or incremental dose change; may cause dizziness and drowsiness.
3. Food may delay absorption and minimize side effects of the drug.
4. Avoid rapid changes in body position that may precipitate weakness, dizziness, and syncope. Lie down or sit down and put head below knees to avoid fainting if a rapid heartbeat is felt. Avoid dangerous situations that may lead to fainting.
5. Report any bothersome side effects because reduction in dosage may be indicated. Use sips of water and sugarless gum or candies for dry mouth effects.
6. Do not stop medication unless directed.
7. Avoid cold, cough, and allergy medications. The sympathomimetic component of such medications will interfere with the action of prazosin.
8. To help control BP: maintain healthy diet and limit intake of caffeine, avoid alcohol, salt substitutes, or high Na^+ and high K^+ foods, perform regular exercise, maintain weight, and stop smoking.
9. Comply with prescribed drug regimen; full drug effect may not be evident for 4–6 weeks.
10. Keep all F/U to assess response and for adverse SE.

OUTCOMES/EVALUATE

- ↓ BP
- Control Raynaud phenomenon

IV

Prednisolone

(pred-**NISS**-oh-lohn)

Classification(s): Glucocorticoid

Pregnancy Category: C

RX: Oral Solution: AsmalPred Plus. **Syrup:** Prelone. **Tablets:** Delta-Cortef, Millipred.

Prednisolone acetate

Pregnancy Category: C

RX: Ophthalmic Suspension: Omnipred Ophthalmic, Pred Forte Ophthalmic, Pred Mild Ophthalmic, Prednisolone Acetate Ophthalmic. **Oral Suspension:** Flo-Pred. **Parenteral:** Predcor-50.

🍁 **Rx:** ratio-Prednisolone Ophthalmic Suspension, Sandoz Prednisolone Ophthalmic/Otic.

Prednisolone sodium phosphate

Pregnancy Category: C

RX: Ophthalmic Solution: Prednisone Sodium Phosphate Ophthalmic. **Oral Liquid/Solution:** Orapred, Pediapred, Veripred 20. **Tablets, Orally Disintegrating:** Orapred ODT.

Prednisolone tebutate

Pregnancy Category: C

RX: Prednisol TPA.

SEE ALSO ***CORTICOSTEROIDS***.

INDICATIONS/USES

Prednisolone acetate: (1) See *Corticosteroids* for systemic uses. (2) Corneal injury from chemical, radiation, or thermal burns or penetration of foreign bodies. (3) Steroid-responsive inflammatory conditions of the palpebral and bulbar conjunctiva, cornea, and anterior segment of the globe (e.g., acne rosacea, allergic conjunctivitis, eyelitis, herpes zoster keratitis, iritis, superficial punctate keratitis, and selective infective conjunctivitis, noninfectious uveitis affecting the posterior segment of the eye, postoperative inflammation/pain following ocular surgery). Corneal injury from chemical, radiation, or thermal burns, or penetration of foreign bodies.

Prednisolone sodium phosphate: (1) See *Corticosteroids* for systemic uses. (2) Moderate to severe inflammations, especially when unusually rapid control is desired as in anterior segment eye disease. (3) Steroid-responsive inflammatory conditions of the palpebral and bulbar conjunctiva, cornea, and anterior segment of the globe (e.g., acne rosacea, allergic conjunctivitis, eyelitis, herpes zoster keratitis, iritis, superficial punctate keratitis, and selective infective conjunctivitis. (4)

The 1% ophthalmic solution is recommended for moderate to severe inflammations, especially when rapid control is desired.

ACTION/KINETICS

Action

Intermediate-acting. Is five times more potent than hydrocortisone and cortisone. Minimal side effects except for GI distress. Moderate mineralocorticoid activity.

Pharmacokinetics

Plasma t½: Over 200 min.

CONTRAINDICATIONS

Lactation.

SPECIAL CONCERNS

- **Use with particular caution in diabetes.**
- **The acetate contains sodium bisulfate that may cause allergic reactions in susceptible people.**

SIDE EFFECTS

Most Common

Insomnia, N&V, GI upset, fatigue, dizziness, muscle weakness, increased hunger/thirst, joint pain, decreased diabetic control.

See *Corticosteroids* for a complete list of possible side effects. Prolonged ophthalmic use may result in glaucoma with damage to the optic nerve, defects in visual acuity and fields of vision, corneal and scleral thinning, and posterior subcapsular cataract formation. Formation of cataracts.

HOW SUPPLIED

Prednisolone. *Oral Solution:* 10 mg/5 mL. 15 mg/5 mL; *Syrup:* 15 mg/5 mL; *Tablets:* 5 mg.
Prednisolone acetate. *Injection:* 25 mg/mL, 50 mg/mL; *Ophthalmic Suspension:* 0.12%, 1%; *Oral Suspension:* 5.6 mg/5 mL (equivalent to 5 mg prednisolone), 16.7 mg/5 mL (equivalent to 15 mg prednisolone).
Prednisolone sodium phosphate. *Ophthalmic Solution:* 1%; *Oral Liquid/Solution:* 5 mg/5 mL, 15 mg/5 mL, 20 mg/5 mL; *Tablets, Orally Disintegrating:* 10 mg, 15 mg, 30 mg.
Prednisolone tebutate. *Injection:* 20 mg/mL.

DOSAGE

Prednisolone

ORAL SOLUTION; SYRUP; TABLETS

Most uses.

5–60 mg/day, depending on disease being treated.

Multiple sclerosis (exacerbation).

200 mg/day for 1 week; **then,** 80 mg on alternate days for 1 month.

Pleurisy of tuberculosis.

0.75 mg/kg/day (then taper) given concurrently with antituberculosis therapy.

Prednisolone acetate

IM

4–60 mg/day. **Not for IV use.**

Multiple sclerosis (exacerbation).

See *Prednisolone.*

INJECTION, SOFT TISSUE; INTRA-ARTICULAR; INTRALESIONAL

4–100 mg (larger doses for large joints).

OPHTHALMIC SUSPENSION (0.12%, 1%)

Corneal injury, inflammatory conditions.

Adults: Instill 2 gtt into the eye(s) 4 times per day. Reevaluate if symptoms fail to improve after 2 days. For Pred Mild or Pred Forte, instill 1–2 gtt in the conjunctival sac 2–4 times a day. During the first 24 to 48 hr, the frequency of dosing may be increased if necessary. **Children (investigational): Initial:** 1–2 gtt q hr during the day and q 2 hr at night. After a favorable response is obtained, reduce the dose to1 gtt q 4 hr; dose may be further reduced to 1 gtt 3–4 times per day.

ORAL SUSPENSION

Most uses.

Initial: 5–60 mg/day, depending on the specific disease being treated.

Multiple sclerosis.

Adults: 200 mg followed by 80 mg every other day for 1 month. **Children, initial:** 0.14–2 mg/kg per day in 3 or 4 divided doses (i.e., 4–60 mg/m^2 per day).

Nephrotic syndrome.

Children: 60 mg/m^3/day in 3 divided doses for 4 weeks; then, 4 weeks of single dose alternate day therapy at 40 mg/m^2/day.

Asthma.

Children: 1–2 mg/kg/day in single or divided doses. Short course or "burst" therapy must be continued until a child

P

achieves a peak expiratory flow rate of 80% of his or her personal best or symptoms resolve. This usually is achieved in 3 to 10 days of treatment, although it can take longer.

Prednisolone sodium phosphate

ORAL LIQUID/SOLUTION; TABLETS, ORALLY DISINTEGRATING

Most uses.

5–60 mg/day in single or divided doses (10–60 mg/day of orally disintegrating tablets).

Multiple sclerosis.

Adults: 200 mg/day for 1 week followed by 80 mg every other day (or dexamethasone 4 to 8 mg every other day) for 1 month. **Children:** 0.14–2 mg/kg/day in 3 or 4 divided doses (i.e., 4–60 mg/m^2/day). *NOTE:* This pediatric dose is also used in children for other diseases.

Nephrotic syndrome.

Children: 60 mg/m^2/day in 3 divided doses for 4 weeks, followed by 4 weeks of single-dose alternate-day therapy at 40 mg/m^2/day.

Asthma, uncontrolled.

Children: 1–2 mg/kg/day in single or divided doses. Continue short-course, or "burst" therapy until the child achieves a peak expiratory flow of 80% of his or her personal best or until symptoms resolve. This usually takes 3 to 10 days, although it can take longer.

OPHTHALMIC SOLUTION (1%)

Corneal injury, inflammatory conditions.

Adults: Depending on the severity of inflammation, instill 1–2 gtt into the conjunctival sac q hr during the day and q 2 hr during the night; **then,** after response obtained, decrease dose to 1 gtt q 4 hr and then later 1 gtt 3–4 times per day. The duration of therapy varies with the type of lesion and may extend from a few days to several weeks, depending on the therapeutic response. **Children, investigational, initial:** 1–2 gtt q hr during the day and q 2 hr during the night. After a favorable response is obtained, reduce the dose to 1 gtt q 4 hr; dose may be further reduced to 1 gtt 3–4 times per day.

Prednisolone tebutate

INJECTION, SOFT TISSUE; INTRA-ARTICULAR; INTRALESIONAL

4–30 mg, depending on site and severity of disease. Doses higher than 40 mg are not recommended.

NURSING IMPLICATIONS

Ⓢ Do not confuse prednisolone with prednisone (also a corticosteroid).

IMPLEMENTATION/ADMINISTRATION/STORAGE

1. For systemic use in adults and children, individualize dosage according to the severity of the disease and client response.
2. Before administering, check spelling and dose carefully; frequently confused with prednisone.
3. Check if provider wants PO form administered with an antacid.
4. Prednisolone sodium phosphate oral solution produces a 20% higher peak plasma level than tablets.
5. Shake suspension well before using.
6. In cases of bacterial infections of the eye, concomitant use of anti-infective agents is mandatory. Re-evaluate if signs and symptoms fail to improve after 2 days.
7. If a period of spontaneous remission occurs in a chronic condition, discontinue treatment. If, after long-term therapy, the drug is to be discontinued, it is recommended that it be withdrawn gradually rather than abruptly.
8. Store prednisolone acetate ophthalmic suspensions from 8–24°C (46–75°F) in an upright position. Store Pred Mild from 15–30°C (59–86°F); protect from freezing. Store Pred Forte up to 25°C (77°F).
9. Store prednisolone acetate oral suspension from 20–25°C (68–77°F). Do not transfer the bottle contents to other containers to prevent loss of the viscous formulation. Do not refrigerate.
10. Store prednisolone sodium phosphate ophthalmic suspension from 15–30°C (59–86°F); protect from light.
11. Store prednisolone sodium phosphate orally disintegrating tablets from 20–25°C (68–77°F); do not break or use a partial tab-

let. Store the 5 mg/5 mL oral solution from 4–25°C (39–77°F); may be refrigerated. Store the 15 mg/5 mL oral solution from 2–8°C (36–48°F).

12. **IV** The IV form (sodium phosphate) may be administered at a rate not to exceed 10 mg/min.
13. COMPATIBILITY D5W, 0.9% NaCl.
14. INCOMPATIBILITY Administer separately.

ASSESSMENT

1. Note reasons for therapy, onset, characteristics of S&S, any previous experiences with this drug, outcome.
2. Obtain CXR at regular intervals during prolonged therapy.
3. Check linear growth of infants and children on prolonged therapy; UGI in those with PUD.
4. If ophthalmic product used for more than 10 days or oral product more than 6 weeks, routinely monitor IOP. Review risk of visual changes and cataract formation with prolonged use.
5. Monitor mental status, weight, BP, CBC, electrolytes, and blood sugar.

CLIENT/FAMILY TEACHING

1. Take as directed and do not stop suddenly without provider approval; adrenal crisis may occur.
2. May take with food to decrease GI upset. Report any loss of effect; dose may need adjustment.
3. Avoid exposure to infected persons and crowds.
4. Report nausea, anorexia, fatigue, joint pain, weakness, dizziness, or SOB; S&S of adrenal insufficiency.
5. With joint injections, do not overuse joint after therapy despite improvement in ROM and pain.
6. Assess for weight gain, swelling of extremities, and adjust diet/salt intake and exercise to control.
7. Do not break or use partial prednisolone sodium phosphate orally disintegrating tablets. Remove the tablet from the blister just prior to use. Place the tablet on the tongue where tablets may be swallowed whole (as any conventional tablet) or allowed to dissolve in the mouth with or without water.
8. With eye drops, wash hands, and do not allow dropper to touch eye. Tilt head back looking up pull lower eyelid down and instill prescribed number of drops. Close eye for 1 to 2 min, apply gentle pressure to bridge of nose for 1 to 3 min. Do not rub eye or touch top of dropper bottle to eye, fingers, or other surface. If more than 1 topical eye drug used, give at least 5 min apart administering the ointment last. May experience temporary stinging or burning; report if bothersome or if eye/eyelid inflammation noted.
9. Do not drive right after using eye drops; vision may be blurred initially. May also cause sensitivity to bright light; use sunglasses to minimize effect.
10. Keep all F/U to assess response, labs, for adverse SE.

OUTCOMES/EVALUATE

- Replacement therapy during adrenocortical hypofunction
- Symptomatic relief of allergic, immune, and inflammatory manifestations
- ↓ Ocular inflammation

Prednisone

(**PRED**-nih-sohn)

Classification(s): Glucocorticoid

Pregnancy Category: C

RX: Prednisone Intensol Concentrate.

✦ **Rx: Tablets**: Apo-Prednisone, Winpred.

SEE ALSO ***CORTICOSTEROIDS***.

INDICATIONS/USES

See *Corticosteroids*. Also, (1) COPD. (2) Ophthalmopathy due to Graves' disease. (3) Duchenne's muscular dystrophy.

ACTION/KINETICS

Action

The anti-inflammatory effect is due to inhibition of prostaglandin synthesis. The drug also inhibits accumulation of macrophages and leukocytes at sites of inflammation and inhibits phagocytosis and lysosomal enzyme release.

Pharmacokinetics

Three to five times as potent as cortisone or hydrocortisone. May cause moderate fluid retention. Metabolized in the liver to prednisolone, the active form.

SPECIAL CONCERNS

- Dose must be highly individualized.
- Carefully monitor growth and development of infants and children on prolonged corticosteroid therapy.

SIDE EFFECTS

Most Common

Insomnia, N&V, GI upset, fatigue, dizziness, muscle weakness, increased hunger/thirst, joint pain, decreased diabetic control.
See *Corticosteroids* for a complete list of possible side effects.

HOW SUPPLIED

Oral Solution: 5 mg/mL, 5 mg/5 mL; ***Tablets:*** 1 mg, 2.5 mg, 5 mg, 10 mg, 20 mg, 50 mg.

DOSAGE

ORAL SOLUTION; TABLETS

Replacement.

Pediatric: 0.1–0.15 mg/kg/day.

Acute, severe conditions.

Initial: 5–60 mg/day in four equally divided doses after meals and at bedtime. After an adequate response is reached, determine the proper maintenance dose by decreasing the initial dose in small decrements (e.g., 5–10 mg q 4–5 days) to establish the lowest dose that will maintain an adequate clinical response. Constant monitoring is required.

COPD.

30–60 mg/day for 1–2 weeks; then taper.

Multiple sclerosis.

Initial: 200 mg per day for 1 week; **then,** 2× 80 mg every other day for 1 month.

Ophthalmopathy due to Graves' disease.

60 mg/day; **then,** taper to 20 mg/day.

Duchenne's muscular dystrophy.

0.75–1.5 mg/kg/day (used to improve strength).

NURSING IMPLICATIONS

Ⓢ Do not confuse prednisone with prednisolone (also a corticosteroid) or prednisone with primidone (an anticonvulsant).

IMPLEMENTATION/ADMINISTRATION/STORAGE

1. For all age groups, individualize dosage depending on severity, prognosis, expected duration of the disease, and client reaction to the medication.
2. Decrease or discontinue dosage gradually when the drug has been given for more than a few days.
3. If after a reasonable period of time there is an unsatisfactory response, discontinue and initiate other therapy.
4. After a favorable response is obtained, determine the maintenance dosage by decreasing the initial dosage in small decrements until the lowest dose that will maintain an adequate response is reached.
5. Alternate day therapy can be considered to minimize undesirable side effects, including pituitary-adrenal suppression.
6. Store from 15–30°C (59–86°F).

ASSESSMENT

1. Note reasons for therapy, type, onset, characteristics of S&S, clinical presentation. List other agents trialed/prescribed, outcome.
2. With chronic back pain, titrate dose to assess for relief; if relief attained may send for trigger point injections. Generally, if pain is diffuse/severe or involves joints other than spine, trigger point injections are usually not effective. Titrate to lowest dose possible to control symptoms and to ensure adequate physical functioning level. Address benefits versus risks with client/family.
3. With asthma/COPD, provide rescue doses and instruct client how and when to use, i.e., during acute exacerbation when sputum is clear to white and no fever, short-term high-dose therapy may be used. If no relief, advise to call for instructions or seek hospitalization depending on severity of symptoms/peak flow readings. Generally more than 2 weeks of higher dose corticosteroid therapy needs to be taken before developing drug-induced adrenal suppression.
4. Monitor CBC, ESR, electrolytes, BP, blood sugar, weights, and mental status.

CLIENT/FAMILY TEACHING

1. Take in the morning to prevent insomnia and with food to decrease GI upset.
2. Do not stop abruptly with long-term therapy. Take as directed, and wean as directed. Once

stabilized, every other day dosing may assist to reduce adverse effects.

3. Report any S&S of adrenal insufficiency (N&V, confusion, appetite loss, low BP, fever, muscle pain, dizziness, faintness) or loss of effectiveness.
4. Avoid alcohol and OTC agents.
5. With weight gain, adjust caloric intake and exercise to control.
6. Avoid live vaccines, skin tests, crowds, and infected individuals when on suppressive therapy; more susceptible to illnesses.
7. With long-term therapy, may experience cataracts, glaucoma, eye infections, bone weakening that may lead to osteoporosis, elevation in BP, diabetes, salt and water retention, and increased potassium loss. Consume adequate calcium and vitamin D supplements.
8. Keep all F/U to assess response, labs, and for adverse SE.

OUTCOMES/EVALUATE

- Relief of allergic, immune, and inflammatory manifestations
- Control of pain
- Treatment of Duchenne's muscular dystrophy, Graves' ophthalmopathy, COPD

Pregabalin

(pre-**GAB**-a-lin)

Classification(s): Anticonvulsant, miscellaneous

Pregnancy Category: C

RX: Lyrica, **C-V**

INDICATIONS/USES

(1) Management of neuropathic pain associated with diabetic peripheral neuropathy. (2) Adjunctive therapy for adults with partial-onset seizures. (3) Management of postherpetic neuralgia. (4) Management of fibromyalgia. *Investigational:* Generalized anxiety disorder.

ACTION/KINETICS

Action

Binds with high affinity to the alpha$_2$-delta site (subunit of voltage-gated calcium channels) in CNS tissues. Precise mechanism unknown; the drug may reduce the calcium-dependent release of several neurotransmitters, possibly by modulation of calcium channel function.

Pharmacokinetics

Well absorbed after PO use; rate of absorption is decreased when given with food. **Peak plasma levels:** 1.5 hr. Is more than 90% bioavailable; does not bind to plasma proteins. **Steady state:** 24–48 hr. More than 90% excreted in the urine unchanged. **t½, elimination:** About 6.3 hr. Dose reduction is necessary in those with impaired renal function.

CONTRAINDICATIONS

Hypersensitivity to any component of the product, including lactose. Lactation.

SPECIAL CONCERNS

- Dosage reduction may be needed in geriatric clients with age-related decreased renal function. The following neurological side effects occur more frequently in the elderly: Abnormal coordination, balance disorder, blurred vision, confusional state, dizziness, lethargy, and tremor.
- Withdraw the drug gradually in seizure disorders to minimize the potential of increased seizure frequency or symptoms such as insomnia, nausea, headache, and diarrhea.
- Use with caution with CHF.
- Discontinue if myopathy is diagnosed or suspected or if markedly elevated creatine kinase levels occur.
- There is an increased risk of suicidal behavior and ideation.
- Safety and efficacy not determined in children.

P

SIDE EFFECTS

Most Common

Dizziness, somnolence, dry mouth, peripheral edema, asthenia, ataxia, abnormal gait, confusion, headache, blurred vision, diplopia, flu syndrome, infection, pain, amnesia, incoordination, speech disorder, abnormal thinking, tremor, twitching, constipation, weight gain.

Side effects most commonly resulting in discontinuation: Dizziness, somnolence, asthenia, ataxia, blurred vision, diplopia, headache, nausea, tremor, vertigo, confusion, incoordination, peripheral edema, abnormal thinking, balance disorder, fatigue, increased weight. **The following side effects have a frequency of more than 0.1% or may be life-threatening. CNS:** Dizziness, somnolence, neuropathy, vertigo, headache, ataxia, abnormal gait, confusion, abnormal thinking, impaired memory, amnesia, myoclonus, euphoria, speech disorder, attention disturbance, balance disorder, depression, disorientation, feeling abnormal/drunk, incoordination, tremor, twitching, nervousness, anxiety, depersonalization, hypertonia, hypesthesia, decreased/increased libido, paresthesia, stupor, twitching, abnormal dreams, agitation, apathy, aphasia, euphoria, circumoral paresthesia, dysarthria, hallucinations, hostility, hyperalgesia, hyperesthesia, hyperkinesis, hypoesthesia, hypokinesia, hypotonia, myoclonus, neuralgia, ***suicidal behavior and ideation, suicide attempt***. **GI:** Dry mouth, constipation, flatulence, N&V, diarrhea, increased appetite, abdominal pain/distention, gastroenteritis, cholecystitis, cholelithiasis, colitis, dysphagia, esophagitis, gastritis, ***GI hemorrhage***, melena, mouth ulceration, ***pancreatitis, rectal hemorrhage***, tongue edema. **CV:** Deep thrombophlebitis, ***heart failure***, hypotension, postural hypotension, retinal vascular disorder, syncope, prolonged PR interval. **Respiratory:** Dyspnea, bronchitis, pharyngolaryngeal pain, sinusitis. **Dermatologic:** Pruritus, alopecia, dry skin, eczema, hirsutism, skin ulcer, urticaria, vesiculobullous rash. **GU:** Anorgasmia, impotence, urinary frequency/incontinence/retention, abnormal ejaculation, amenorrhea, dysmenorrhea, dysuria, hematuria, kidney calculus, leukorrhea, menorrhagia, metrorrhagia, nephritis, oliguria, urine abnormality. **Musculoskeletal:** Myasthenia, arthralgia, arthrosis, leg cramps, myalgia, back/chest/pelvic pain, muscle spasms, neck rigidity. **Hematologic/Lymphatic:** Ecchymosis, anemia, eosinophilia, hypochromic anemia, leukocytosis, leukopenia, lymphadenopathy, thrombocytopenia. **Metabolic/Nutritional:** Peripheral edema, facial edema, weight gain, increased appetite, edema, hypoglycemia. **Ophthalmic:** Blurred/abnormal vision, diplopia, conjunctivitis, abnormal accommodation, blepharitis, dry eyes, eye hemorrhage/disorder, photophobia, retinal edema, nystagmus. **Otic:** Otitis media, tinnitus. **Hypersensitivity:** Blisters, dyspnea, hives, rash, red skin, wheezing, angioedema. **Body as a whole:** Asthenia, fatigue, accidental injury, flu syndrome, infection, pain, fever, ***allergic reaction***, abscess, cellulitis, chills, malaise, lethargy, photosensitivity reaction. **Miscellaneous:** Hyperacusis, taste loss/perversion.

LABORATORY TEST CONSIDERATIONS

↑ Creatine kinase. ↓ Platelet count. Albuminuria.

OVERDOSE MANAGEMENT

Symptoms: Similar to usual side effects. *Treatment:* There is no specific antidote. Elimination of unabsorbed drug may be attempted by emesis or gastric lavage. Use general supportive care, including monitoring of vital signs and observation of the clinical status.

DRUG INTERACTIONS

ACE inhibitors (e.g., captopril) / ↑ Risk of swelling and hives; contact provider immediately if this occurs

Antidiabetic drugs, thiazolidinedione class / Weight gain and/or fluid retention can exacerbate or lead to heart failure; use together with caution

CNS depressants (including lorazepam, oxycodone) / Additive effects on cognitive and gross motor functioning

Ethanol / Additive effects on cognition and gross motor function; avoid alcohol

HOW SUPPLIED

Capsules: 25 mg, 50 mg, 75 mg, 100 mg, 150 mg, 200 mg, 225 mg, 300 mg; ***Oral Solution:*** 20 mg/mL.

DOSAGE

CAPSULES; ORAL SOLUTION

Neuropathic pain associated with diabetic peripheral neuropathy.

Adults, initial: 50 mg 3 times per day; may be increased to 100 mg 3 times/day within 1 week based on efficacy and tolerability. **Maximum dose:** 100 mg 3 times per day provided clients have a C_{CR} of at least 60 mL/min.

Partial-onset seizures.

Adults, initial: 75 mg twice a day or 50 mg 3 times per day. Based on individual client response and tolerability, may be increased to a maximum dose of 600 mg/day in 2 or 3 divided doses.

Maintenance, usual: 150–600 mg/day divided and given 2 or 3 times/day.

Postherpetic neuralgia.

Adults, initial: 75 mg twice a day or 50 mg 3 times per day in those with a

C_{CR} of at least 60 mL/min. Based on efficacy and tolerability, dose may be increased in 1 week to 75–150 mg twice a day or 50–100 mg 3 times per day.
Maximum daily dose: 300 mg/day. Clients whose pain is not relieved following 2–4 weeks of treatment with 300 mg/day and who are able to tolerate pregabalin, may be given up to 300 mg twice a day or 200 mg 3 times per day (i.e., total of 600 mg/day).

Fibromyalgia.

Adults, initial: 75 mg two times a day; may increase to 150 mg two times a day (300 mg/day) within 1 week. **Maximum dose:** 225 mg two times a day (450 mg/day). Doses greater than 450 mg/day offered no additional benefit and side effects were increased.

NURSING IMPLICATIONS

IMPLEMENTATION/ADMINISTRATION/STORAGE

1. Adjust dosage, as follows, in clients with impaired renal function:
   - For a C_{CR} at 30–60 mL/min, give 75 to 300 mg/day in 2 or 3 divided doses.
   - For a C_{CR} at 15–30 mL/min, give 25–150 mg/day in a single daily dose or 2 divided doses.
   - For a C_{CR} less than 15 mL/min, give 25–75 mg/day in a single daily dose.
2. For clients undergoing hemodialysis, the daily dose should be adjusted based on renal function. In addition to the daily dose adjustment, a supplemental dose should be given immediately following every 4-hr hemodialysis treatment. For clients on the 25 mg single daily dose regimen, give 1 supplemental dose of 25 or 50 mg. For clients on the 25–50 mg single daily dose regimen, give 1 supplemental dose of 50 or 75 mg. For clients on the 50–75 mg single daily dose regimen, give 1 supplemental dose of 75 or 100 mg. For clients on the 75 mg single daily dose regimen, give 1 supplemental dose of 100 or 150 mg.
3. A dosage decrease may be needed in those who have age-related compromised renal function.
4. When discontinuing, taper gradually over a minimum of 1 week to minimize the potential of increased seizures.
5. Health care providers should recommend to pregnant clients that they enroll in the North American Antiepileptic Drug Pregnancy Registry by calling 1-888-233-2334. This must be done by clients themselves. Information on the registry can also be obtained at the website: http://www.aedpregnancyregistry.org.
6. Store from 15–30°C (59–86°F). For the oral solution, use within 45 days of opening the bottle.

ASSESSMENT

1. Note reasons for therapy, onset, characteristics of S&S, other agents trialed, outcome. Document clinical presentation, seizure frequency or rate pain level.
2. Assess mental status and behavioral presentation; note any depression or suicide thoughts.
3. Note medical history, especially seizures, CAD. Assess ECG, note NYHA class; avoid or use cautiously with NYHA class III and IV.
4. Assess for history of drug abuse. Drug is Schedule V. Observe for evidence or S&S of pregabalin misuse or abuse (i.e., tolerance development, drug-seeking behavior, dose escalation).
5. Monitor VS, weight, HbA1c, liver, CK, CBC, and renal function studies; adjust dose with dysfunction. May note decrease in platelet counts.

CLIENT/FAMILY TEACHING

1. May take with or without food as directed. Do not stop drug abruptly; may experience insomnia, nausea, headache, or diarrhea.
2. Drug is used to help manage nerve pain with diabetes or for pain after shingles outbreak. It is also used with other seizure medicine to help control partial seizures. Do not stop suddenly, may precipitate seizure activity.
3. Review patient information pamphlet prior to taking drug.
4. Do not perform activities that require mental alertness until drug effects realized; may cause dizziness, blurred vision, and sleepiness.
5. May experience weight gain and swelling of extremities. If already taking another antidiabetic thiaglitazone agent may increase effects

P

of swelling and weight gain and with heart conditions, may increase risk of heart failure.

6. Report any unexplained muscle pain, weakness, or tenderness especially if accompanied by fever or increased tiredness. Report any changes in vision, significant weight gain, trouble concentrating, worsening of depression or suicide thoughts.
7. Avoid alcohol and CNS depressants as these may potentiate sedation and impairment of motor skills. If CNS depressants prescribed, expect additive side effects such as sleepiness.
8. Practice reliable contraception; report if pregnancy suspected. If pregnant enroll in the North American Antiepileptic Drug Pregnancy Registry by calling 1-888-233-2334. Males intending to father a child should be advised of risk of male mediated teratogenicity.
9. With diabetes, special attention to skin integrity should be maintained. Report any ulcerations or rashes.
10. Keep all F/U to assess response, labs, and adverse SE.

OUTCOMES/EVALUATE

- Management of partial seizures/fibromyalgia
- Relief of post herpetic neuralgia
- Control of neuropathic pain in diabetics
- Anxiety disorder (unlabeled use)

Primaquine phosphate

(**PRIM**-ah-kwin)

Classification(s): Antimalarial, 8-aminoquinolone

Pregnancy Category: C

INDICATIONS/USES

(1) Radical cure of *Plasmodium vivax* malaria. (2) Prophylaxis of relapse in *P. vivax* malaria. (3) Following the termination of chloroquine phosphate suppressive therapy in areas where *P. vivax* is endemic.

ACTION/KINETICS

Action

Mechanism of action not known, but the drug binds to and may alter the properties of DNA leading to decreased protein synthesis. Both the gametocyte and exoerythrocyte forms are inhibited. Some gametocytes are destroyed while others cannot undergo maturation division in the gut of the mosquito.

Pharmacokinetics

Well absorbed from GI tract. **Peak plasma levels:** 1–3 hr. Poorly distributed in body tissues. **t½, elimination:** 4 hr. Rapidly metabolized.

CONTRAINDICATIONS

Concomitant use with quinacrine. In clients with rheumatoid arthritis or lupus erythematosus who are acutely ill or who have a tendency to develop granulocytopenia. Concomitant use with other bone marrow depressants or hemolytic drugs.

SPECIAL CONCERNS

Use during pregnancy only when benefits outweigh risks.

SIDE EFFECTS

Most Common

N&V, abdominal cramps, epigastric distress, leukopenia.

GI: Abdominal cramps, epigastric distress, N&V. **Hematologic:** Leukopenia. Methemoglobinemia in NADH-methemoglobin reductase deficient individuals. Blacks and members of certain Mediterranean ethnic groups (Sardinians, Sephardic Jews, Greeks, Iranians) manifest a high incidence of G6PD deficiency and as a result have a low tolerance for primaquine. These individuals manifest ***marked hemolytic anemia*** following primaquine administration. **Miscellaneous:** Headache, pruritus, interference with visual accommodation, ***cardiac arrhythmias***, hypertension.

OVERDOSE MANAGEMENT

Symptoms: Abdominal cramps, vomiting, burning and epigastric distress, cyanosis, methemoglobinemia, anemia, moderate leukocytosis or leukopenia, CNS and CV disturbances. Granulocytopenia and ***acute hemolytic anemia*** in sensitive clients. *Treatment:* Treat symptoms.

DRUG INTERACTIONS

Bone marrow depressants, hemolytic drugs / Additive side effects

Quinacrine / ↓ Metabolic degradation of primaquine → ↑ effects. **Do not give primaquine** to clients who are receiving or have received quinacrine within the past 3 months

HOW SUPPLIED
Tablets: 26.3 mg.

DOSAGE

TABLETS
Acute attack of vivax malaria, clients with parasitized RBCs.

26.3 mg (15 mg base) daily for 14 days together with chloroquine phosphate (to destroy erythrocytic parasites).

Suppression of malaria.

Adults: 26.3 mg (15 mg base) daily for 14 days or 78.9 mg once a week for 8 weeks; **children:** 0.5 mg/kg/day (0.3 mg/kg base) for 14 days.

NURSING IMPLICATIONS

IMPLEMENTATION/ADMINISTRATION/STORAGE
1. Store in tightly closed containers.
2. For suppression therapy, initiate during the last 2 weeks of or after suppressive therapy with chloroquine or a similar drug.

ASSESSMENT
1. Note reasons for therapy, other agents trialed, history of rheumatoid arthritis or lupus. Documents dates of exposure and locations.
2. List other drugs prescribed to ensure no unfavorable interactions.
3. Determine if pregnant. Do not give during first trimester and preferably not until after delivery.
4. Assess dark-skinned clients closely. Because of a possible inborn deficiency of G6PD, these clients are particularly susceptible to hemolytic anemia while on primaquine.
5. Obtain hematologic profile and cultures. Monitor for indications to withdraw drug: dark urine may indicate hemolysis.

CLIENT/FAMILY TEACHING
1. Take immediately before or after meals or with antacids to minimize gastric irritation.
2. Drug works by preventing the development of the blood forms of the organism, which cause relapses of vivax malaria.
3. For suppressive therapy, take drug on same day each week.
4. Monitor color of urine; report darkening or brown discoloration.
5. Must complete a full course of therapy for effective results.
6. If visual disturbances experienced, avoid driving or hazardous activities.
7. Report any GI, neurologic, and cardiovascular disturbances; symptoms of overdose.
8. Keep all F/U to assess response, labs, for adverse SE.

OUTCOMES/EVALUATE
Termination of acute malarial attacks; suppression of malarial symptoms.

Primidone

(**PRIH**-mih-dohn)

Classification(s): Anticonvulsant, miscellaneous

Pregnancy Category: D

RX: Mysoline.

✱ **Rx:** Apo-Primidone.

INDICATIONS/USES
Alone or with other anticonvulsants to treat psychomotor, focal, or tonic-clonic seizures (including those refractory to anticonvulsant regimens). *Investigational:* Benign familial tremor (essential tremor).

ACTION/KINETICS

Action
Closely related to the barbiturates; however, the anticonvulsant mechanism is unknown. Produces a greater sedative effect than barbiturates when used for seizure treatment. Side effects usually subside with use.

Pharmacokinetics
Rapidly and almost completely absorbed after PO. **Peak plasma levels:** 3 hr. Primidone is converted in the liver to two active metabolites, phenobarbital and phenylethylmalonamide (PEMA). **Peak plasma levels (PEMA):** 7–8 hr. **t½ (primidone):** 5–15 hr; **t½ (PEMA):** 10–18 hr; **t½ (phenobarbital):** 53–140 hr. The appearance of phenobarbital in the plasma may be delayed several days after initiation of therapy. **Therapeutic plasma levels, primadone:** 5–12 mcg/mL; **phenobarbital,** 15–40 mcg/mL. Primidone and metabolites are excreted through the kidneys, although 40% of

primidone is excreted unchanged. **Plasma protein binding:** 20–25%.

CONTRAINDICATIONS

Porphyria. Hypersensitivity to phenobarbital. Lactation.

SPECIAL CONCERNS

- **Safe use during pregnancy not determined.**
- **Use during lactation may result in drowsiness in the neonate.**
- **Children and the elderly may manifest restlessness and excitement.**
- **Abrupt withdrawal may precipitate status epilepticus.**
- **Neonatal hemorrhage, with coagulation defect resembling vitamin K deficiency, may occur in newborns whose mothers were taking primidone.**

SIDE EFFECTS

Most Common

Ataxia, vertigo, fatigue, N&V, anorexia, hyperirritability.

CNS: Drowsiness, ataxia, vertigo, fatigue, hyperirritability, emotional disturbances, personality disturbances with mood changes and paranoia. **GI:** N&V, anorexia, painful gums. **Hematologic:** Megaloblastic anemia, thrombocytopenia; rarely granulocytopenia, agranulocytosis, and red-cell hyperplasia. **Ophthalmic:** Diplopia, nystagmus. **Miscellaneous:** Impotence, morbilliform and maculopapular skin rashes. Occasionally has caused hyperexcitability, especially in children. ***Postpartum hemorrhage and hemorrhagic disease of the newborn***. Symptoms of SLE.

P

DRUG INTERACTIONS

SEE ALSO ***BARBITURATES***.

Acetazolamide / ↓ Effect of primidone R/T ↓ levels
Carbamazepine / ↓ Levels of primidone and phenobarbital and ↑ levels of carbamazepine
Doxycycline / ↓ Doxycycline t½ and serum levels with possible ↓ effect; may persist for weeks following primidone discontinuation; consider an alternate tetracycline
Ethanol / Impaired hand-eye coordination, additive CNS effects, and possible death upon acute ingestion; avoid concomitant use
Felodipine / ↓ Effects of felodipine; may need ↑ felodipine doses if used chronically
Hydantoins / ↑ Levels of primidone, phenobarbital, and PEMA
Isoniazid / ↑ Effect of primidone R/T ↓ liver breakdown
Methadone / ↓ Methadone effects; those on chronic methadone therapy may experience withdrawal symptoms
Metronidazole / Possible metronidazole therapeutic failure; higher metronidazole doses may be needed
Nicotinamide / ↑ Effect of primidone R/T ↓ rate of clearance from body
Nifedipine / Possible ↓ nifedipine serum levels → ↓ efficacy; titrate dose according to response
Oral contraceptives / ↓ Levels of estrogens → contraceptive failure; consider use of alternative contraceptive
Prednisone / ↓ Effect of prednisone; avoid concomitant use
Propranolol / ↓ Effect of propranolol; may need to ↑ propranolol dose
Quinidine / ↓ Quinidine levels and elimination t½
Succinimides / ↓ Levels of primidone and phenobarbital
Theophylline / ↓ Theophylline levels → ↓ therapeutic effect; may need to ↑ theophylline dose
Valproic acid / ↑ Primidone levels → ↑ pharmacologic and side effects; in some, decreased primidone dose may be needed
Warfarin / ↓ Effect of warfarin; monitor warfarin dose and adjust dose as needed

HOW SUPPLIED

Tablets: 50 mg, 250 mg.

DOSAGE

TABLETS

Seizures, in clients on no previous anticonvulsant medication.

Adults and children over 8 years, initial, no previous treatment: Days 1–3, 100–125 mg at bedtime; days 4–6, 100–125 mg twice a day (morning and evening); days 7–9, 100–125 mg 3 times per day (morning, noon, and evening); day 10 to maintenance: 250 mg 3–4 times per day (morning, noon, evening). **Usual maintenance:** 250 mg 3–4 times daily. Dose may be increased to 250 mg 5–6 times per day, not to exceed 500 mg 4 times per day. **Children**

under 8 years, initial: Days 1–3, 50 mg at bedtime; days 4–6, 50 mg twice a day; days 7–9, 100 mg twice a day; day 10 to maintenance: 125 mg twice a day to 250 mg 3 times per day. **Usual maintenance:** 125–250 mg 3 times daily or 10–25 mg/kg in divided doses.

Clients already receiving other anticonvulsants, initial: 100–125 mg at bedtime; gradually increase to maintenance level as the other drug is gradually decreased. Continue this regimen until a satisfactory dosage level is reached for the combination or the other drug is completely withdrawn. The transition from concomitant therapy should not be completed in less than 2 weeks.

Seizures, in clients receiving other anticonvulsants.

Initial: 100–125 mg at bedtime; **then,** increase to maintenance levels as other drug is slowly withdrawn (transition should take at least 2 weeks).

Benign familial tremor.

750 mg/day.

NURSING IMPLICATIONS

Do not confuse primidone with prednisone (a corticosteroid).

IMPLEMENTATION/ADMINISTRATION/STORAGE

1. Pregnant women should receive prophylactic vitamin K therapy for 1 month prior to and during delivery.
2. Due to bioequivalence problems, brand interchange is not recommended unless bioavailability data are available.
3. May take several weeks for therapeutic effect.

ASSESSMENT

1. Note age at seizure onset, frequency/characteristics of seizures, and cause if known. Note other agents trialed, outcome.
2. List other agents prescribed to ensure none interact unfavorably.
3. Monitor CBC, renal and LFTs; assess for dysfunction.

CLIENT/FAMILY TEACHING

1. May be taken with food if GI upset occurs.
2. Do not stop abruptly as withdrawal symptoms/seizures may occur.
3. Avoid alcohol, OTC agents, and CNS depressants. Do not perform activities that require mental alertness until drug effects realized; may cause dizziness and drowsiness.
4. Report any of the following: hyperexcitability in children; visual disturbances; swelling of eyes or face; mental status changes; mood/behavioral changes or depression; impotence; or increased seizure activity.
5. Practice reliable contraception. Vitamin K may be prescribed during the last month of pregnancy to prevent postpartum hemorrhage in the mother and hemorrhagic disease of the newborn. Enroll in the North American Antiepileptic Drug (NAAED) Pregnancy Registry. Must be done by client that is taking drug and can be done by calling toll-free number 1-888-233-2334.
6. Report immediately if rash or fever occur.
7. Keep all F/U to assess response, labs, and adverse SE.

OUTCOMES/EVALUATE

- Control of refractory seizures
- Therapeutic drug levels (5–12 mcg/mL)

Probenecid

(proh-**BEN**-ih-sid)

Classification(s): Antigout drug, uricosuric

Pregnancy Category: B

RX: Benemid.

♣ **Rx:** Benuryl.

INDICATIONS/USES

(1) Hyperuricemia in chronic gout and gouty arthritis. (2) Adjunct in therapy with penicillins or cephalosporins to elevate and prolong plasma antibiotic levels.

ACTION/KINETICS

Action

A uricosuric agent that increases the excretion of uric acid by inhibiting the tubular reabsorption of uric acid; this results in a decreased serum level of uric acid. Also inhibits the renal secretion of penicillins and cephalosporins; this effect is often taken advantage of in the treatment of infections be-

P

cause concomitant administration of probenecid will increase plasma levels of antibiotics.

Pharmacokinetics

Peak plasma levels: 2–4 hr. **Time to peak effect, uricosuric:** 0.5 hr; **for suppression of penicillin excretion:** 2 hr. **Therapeutic plasma levels for inhibition of antibiotic secretion:** 40–60 mcg/mL; **therapeutic plasma levels for uricosuric effect:** 100–200 mcg/mL. **t½:** Approximately 5–8 hr. **Duration for inhibition of penicillin excretion:** 8 hr. Metabolized in the liver to active metabolites; excreted in urine (5–10% unchanged). Excretion is increased in alkaline urine.

CONTRAINDICATIONS

Hypersensitivity to drug, blood dyscrasias, uric acid, and kidney stones. Use for hyperuricemia in neoplastic disease or its treatment. Use in children less than 2 years of age. Concomitant use of salicylates or use with penicillin in renal impairment.

SPECIAL CONCERNS

Use with caution in renal disease, porphyria, G6PD deficiency, history of allergy to sulfa drugs, and peptic ulcer.

SIDE EFFECTS

Most Common

Headache, dizziness, anorexia, N&V, diarrhea, constipation, skin rash, abdominal discomfort, urinary frequency.

CNS: Headaches, dizziness. **GI:** Anorexia, N&V, diarrhea, constipation, and abdominal discomfort. **Allergic:** Skin rash, dermatitis, pruritus, drug fever, and rarely ***anaphylaxis***. **GU:** Nephrotic syndrome, uric acid stones with or without hematuria, urinary frequency, renal colic, or costovertebral pain. **Miscellaneous:** Flushing, ***hemolytic anemia (possibly related to G6PD deficiency)***, anemia, sore gums, ***hepatic necrosis***, ***aplastic anemia***. Initially, the drug may increase frequency of acute gout attacks due to mobilization of uric acid.

DRUG INTERACTIONS

Acyclovir / ↓ Renal excretion of acyclovir
Allopurinol / Additive effects to ↓ uric acid serum levels
Benzodiazepines / More rapid onset and longer duration of benzodiazepine effects
Carbamazepine / ↑ Carbamazepine metabolism R/T induction of CYP2C8 and CYP3A4
Cephalosporins / ↑ Cephalosporin effect R/T ↓ kidney excretion
Ciprofloxacin / 50% ↑ in systemic levels of ciprofloxacin
Clofibrate / ↑ Clofibric acid (active) levels → ↑ effects
Dapsone / ↑ Dapsone effects
Dyphylline / ↑ Dyphylline effect R/T ↓ kidney excretion
Fexofenadine / ↑ Fexofenadine AUC and ↓ renal clearance R/T inhibition of P-glycoprotein transport
Ganciclovir / ↑ Ganciclovir plasma levels and ↓ renal clearance
Methotrexate / ↑ Methotrexate effect and toxicity R/T ↓ kidney excretion
Niacin / ↓ Uric acid-lowering effects of probenecid
NSAIDs / ↑ NSAID effects R/T ↓ kidney excretion
Olanzapine / ↑ AUC, peak plasma levels, and rate of olanzapine absorption R/T inhibition of olanzapine metabolism
Pantothenic acid / ↑ Pantothenic acid effects
Penicillamine / ↓ Penicillamine effects
Penicillins / ↑ Penicillin effects R/T ↓ kidney excretion
Pyrazinamide / Inhibits hyperuricemia produced by pyrazinamide
Rifampin / ↑ Rifampin effects R/T ↓ kidney excretion
Salicylates / Inhibits uricosuric activity of probenecid
Sulfinpyrazone / ↑ Sulfinpyrazone effects R/T ↓ kidney excretion
Sulfonamides / ↑ Sulfonamide effects R/T ↓ plasma protein binding
Sulfonylureas, oral / ↑ Sulfonylurea effect → ↑ hypoglycemia
Thiopental / ↑ Thiopental effects
Zidovudine (AZT) / ↑ Bioavailability of AZT; possible malaise, myalgia, fever

HOW SUPPLIED

Tablets: 500 mg.

DOSAGE

TABLETS

Gout.

Adults, initial: 250 mg twice a day for 1 week. **Maintenance:** 500 mg twice a day. Dosage may have to be increased further (by 500 mg/day q 4 weeks to maximum of 2 grams) until urate excretion <700 mg in 24 hr. Colbenemid, a combination tablet containing colchicine (0.5 mg) and probenecid (500 mg), is also available.

Adjunct to penicillin or cephalosporin therapy.

Adults: 500 mg 4 times per day. Dosage is decreased for elderly clients with renal damage. **Pediatric, 2–14 years, initial:** 25 mg/kg (or 700 mg/m^2); **maintenance,** 10 mg/kg 4 times per day (or 300 mg/m^2 4 times per day). **For children 50 kg or more:** Give adult dosage.

Gonorrhea, uncomplicated.

Adults: 1 gram (as a single dose) 30 min before 4.8 million units of penicillin G procaine aqueous; **pediatric, less than 45 kg:** 25 mg/kg (up to a maximum of 1 gram) with appropriate antibiotic therapy.

Neurosyphilis.

Adults: 0.5 gram 4 times per day with penicillin G procaine aqueous, 2.4 million units/day IM, both for 10–14 days.

Pelvic inflammatory disease.

Adults: 1 gram (as a single dose) plus cefoxitin, 2 grams IM given concurrently.

NURSING IMPLICATIONS

IMPLEMENTATION/ADMINISTRATION/STORAGE

1. Do not start therapy until acute gouty attack has subsided. If an acute attack is precipitated during therapy, continue drug.
2. To prevent kidney stones, take at least 6 to 8 (8-oz) glasses of water.
3. Maintain an alkaline urine by taking sodium bicarbonate, 3–7.5 grams/day, or potassium citrate, 7.5 grams/day.

ASSESSMENT

1. Note reasons for therapy, onset, characteristics of S&S, other agents trialed, triggers if evident.
2. List any PUD, G6PD deficiency, uricemia R/T neoplastic disease, kidney stones, sulfa allergy, blood dyscrasia.
3. Assess involved joints, noting pain, inflammation, heat, swelling, deformity, tophaceous deposits, ROM.
4. Hypersensitivity reactions may occur more frequently with intermittent therapy.
5. Assess for toxic plasma antibiotic levels if excretion inhibited by probenecid; adjust dosage.
6. Monitor CBC, uric acid, renal and LFTs. Note urate excretion levels, urine alkalinity; urates crystalize in acid urine.

CLIENT/FAMILY TEACHING

1. Take with food or milk to minimize gastric irritation. Report gastric intolerance so dosage may be corrected without loss of therapeutic effect. Drug works by increasing the excretion of uric acid from the body.
2. Take a liberal amount of fluid (2.5–3 L/day) to prevent the formation of sodium urate stones. Avoid cranberry juice or vitamin C preparations, which acidify urine. Sodium bicarbonate may be used to maintain an alkaline urine to prevent urates from crystallizing and forming kidney stones.
3. Acute gout attacks may initially be more frequent due to mobilization of uric acid. Report increase in the number of acute attacks at initiation of therapy since colchicine may need to be added. Continue to take during acute attacks with colchicine unless otherwise specified.
4. Report any unexplained fever, fatigue, skin rash, persistent GI upset, painful urination, bloody urine, severe lower back pain, difficulty breathing, flushing, increased sweating, headaches, or dizziness.
5. Do not take OTC meds, salicylates or use caffeine or alcohol during uricosuric therapy. Acetaminophen preparations may be used for analgesia.
6. Monitor FS closely; drug may increase hypoglycemic effects of PO antidiabetic agents.
7. Keep all F/U to assess response, labs, and for adverse SE.

OUTCOMES/EVALUATE

- ↓ Uric acid levels; ↓ gout attacks
- ↓ Joint pain/swelling
- Elevated/prolonged antibiotic (penicillin or cephalosporin) levels

P

IV

Procainamide hydrochloride

(proh-**KAYN**-ah-myd)

Classification(s): Antiarrhythmic, Class IA

Pregnancy Category: C

SEE ALSO ***ANTIARRHYTHMIC DRUGS***.

INDICATIONS/USES

Documented ventricular arrhythmias (e.g., sustained ventricular tachycardia) that may be life threatening in clients where benefits of treatment clearly outweigh risks. *NOTE:* Antiarrhythmic drugs have not been shown to improve survival in clients with ventricular arrhythmias. *Investigational:* Atrial fibrillation/flutter.

ACTION/KINETICS

Action

Produces a direct cardiac effect to prolong the refractory period of the atria and to a lesser extent the bundle of His-Purkinje system and ventricles. Large doses may cause AV block. Some anticholinergic and local anesthetic effects.

Pharmacokinetics

Onset, PO: 30 min; **IV:** 1–5 min. **Time to peak effect, PO:** 90–120 min; **IM:** 15–60 min; **IV:** Immediate. **Duration:** 3 hr. **$t^{1/2}$:** 2.5–4.7 hr. **Therapeutic serum level:** 4–8 mcg/mL. **Toxic serum levels:** Over 16 mcg/mL. From 40–70% excreted unchanged. Metabolized in the liver (16–21% by slow acetylators and 24–33% by fast acetylators) to the active N-acetylprocainamide (NAPA); has antiarrhythmic properties with a longer half-life than procainamide. **Plasma protein binding:** 14–23%.

CONTRAINDICATIONS

Hypersensitivity to drug, complete AV heart block, lupus erythematosus, torsades de pointes, asymptomatic ventricular premature depolarizations. Lactation.

SPECIAL CONCERNS

(1) Prolonged use of procainamide often leads to development of a positive antinuclear antibody (ANA) test, with or without symptoms of lupus erythematosus-like syndrome. If a positive ANA titer develops, assess the benefit/risk ratio related to continued procainamide therapy. (2) Use should be reserved for those with life-threatening ventricular arrhythmias. (3) Agranulocytosis, bone marrow depression, neutropenia, hypoplastic anemia, and thrombocytopenia have been reported. Most cases occurred after recommended dosage. Fatalities have occurred (usually with agranulocytosis). Because most of these events occur during the first 12 weeks of therapy, it is recommended that CBC, including WBC, differential, and platelet counts be performed weekly for the first 3 months of therapy and periodically thereafter. Perform CBC promptly if the client develops any signs of infection (e.g., fever, chills, sore throat, stomatitis), bruising, or bleeding. If any of these hematologic disorders occur, discontinue therapy. Blood counts usually return to normal within 1 month after discontinuation. Use caution in those with pre-existing bone marrow failure or cytopenia of any type.

- **Increased risk of death in those with non-life-threatening arrhythmias.**
- **Although used in children, safety and efficacy not established.**
- **Use with extreme caution in clients for whom a sudden drop in BP could be detrimental, in CHF, acute ischemic heart disease, or cardiomyopathy.**
- **Use with caution in clients with liver or kidney dysfunction, pre-existing bone marrow failure or cytopenia of any type, development of first-degree heart block while on procainamide, myasthenia gravis, and those with bronchial asthma or other respiratory disorders.**
- **May cause more hypotension in geriatric clients; dose may have to be decreased due to age-related decreases in renal function.**

SIDE EFFECTS

Most Common

Dizziness, fatigue, bitter taste, GI upset, nausea, anorexia, diarrhea, headache, blurred vision, giddiness, depression.

CV: Following IV use: Hypotension, ***ventricular asystole or fibrillation, partial or complete heart block***. Rarely, second-degree heart block after PO use. **GI**: N&V, diarrhea, anorexia, bitter taste, GI upset, abdominal pain. **Hematologic**: Thrombocytopenia, ***agranulocytosis***, neutropenia, hypoplastic anemia. Rarely, hemolytic anemia. **Dermatologic**: Urticaria, pruritus, angioneurotic edema, flushing, maculopapular rash. **CNS** Depression, headache, dizziness, weakness, giddiness, psychoses with hallucinations. **Body as a whole:** Lupus erythematosus-like syndrome especially in those on maintenance therapy and who are slow acetylators. Symptoms include arthralgia, pleural or abdominal pain, arthritis, pleural effusion, pericarditis, fever, chills, myalgia, skin lesions, hematologic changes. **Miscellaneous:** Granulomatous hepatitis, weakness, fever, chills, blurred vision.

LABORATORY TEST CONSIDERATIONS

May affect LFTs. False + ↑ in serum alkaline phosphatase. Positive ANA test. High levels of lidocaine and meprobamate may inhibit fluorescence of procainamide and NAPA.

OVERDOSE MANAGEMENT

Symptoms: Plasma levels of 10–15 mcg/mL are associated with toxic symptoms. Progressive widening of the QRS complex, prolonged QT or PR intervals, lowering of R and T waves, increased AV block, increased ventricular extrasystoles, ***ventricular tachycardia or fibrillation.*** IV overdose may result in hypotension, CNS depression, tremor, respiratory depression. *Treatment:*

- Induce emesis or perform gastric lavage followed by administration of activated charcoal.
- To treat hypotension, give IV fluids and/or a vasopressor (dopamine, phenylephrine, or norepinephrine).
- Infusion of ⅙ molar sodium lactate IV reduces the cardiotoxic effects.
- Hemodialysis (but not peritoneal dialysis) is effective in reducing serum levels.
- Renal clearance can be enhanced by acidification of the urine and with high flow rates.
- A ventricular pacing electrode can be inserted as a precaution in the event AV block develops.

DRUG INTERACTIONS

Acetazolamide / ↑ Procainamide effect R/T ↓ kidney excretion
Amiodarone / ↑ Procainamide levels
Antiarrhythmics (e.g., lidocaine, disopyramide, quinidine) / Additive effects on the heart; quinidine may also ↑ procainamide and metabolite levels
Anticholinergic agents, atropine / Additive antivagal effects on AV conduction
Antihypertensive agents / Additive hypotensive effect
Cholinergic agents / Anticholinergic activity of procainamide antagonizes effect of cholinergic drugs
Cimetidine / ↑ Procainamide effect R/T ↓ renal clearance
Disopyramide / ↑ Risk of enhanced prolongation of conduction or depression of contractility and hypotension
Ethanol / Effect of procainamide may be altered, but because the main metabolite is active as an antiarrhythmic, specific outcome not clear
H ***Henbane leaf*** / ↑ Anticholinergic effects
Kanamycin / ↑ Kanamycin-induced muscle relaxation
Lidocaine / Additive cardiodepressant effects
Magnesium salts / ↑ Mg-induced muscle relaxation
Neomycin / ↑ Neomycin-induced muscle relaxation
Ofloxacin / See ***Quinolones;*** also, possible ↑ procainamide levels
Propranolol / ↑ Serum procainamide levels
Quinidine / ↑ Risk of enhanced prolongation of conduction or depression of contractility and hypotension
Quinolones / ↑ Risk of life-threatening cardiac arrhythmias, including torsades de pointes
Ranitidine / ↑ Procainamide effect R/T ↓ renal clearance
Sodium bicarbonate / ↑ Procainamide effect R/T ↓ kidney excretion
Succinylcholine / ↑ Succinylcholine-induced muscle relaxation
Thioridazine / Possible synergistic or additive prolongation of the QTc interval and ↑ risk for life-threatening cardiac arrhythmias, including torsades de pointes
Trimethoprim / ↑ Procainamide effect R/T ↑ serum levels
Ziprasidone / Possible synergistic or additive prolongation of the QTc interval and ↑ risk for life-threatening cardiac arrhythmias, including torsades de pointes

HOW SUPPLIED

Injection: 100 mg/mL, 500 mg/mL; ***Tablets, Immediate-Release:*** 250 mg, 375 mg, 500 mg.

P

DOSAGE

IM

Ventricular arrhythmias.

Adults, initial: 50 mg/kg/day divided into fractional doses of 1/8–1/4 given q 3–6 hr until PO therapy is possible. If more than 3 injections are given, assess client factors such as age, renal function, clinical response, and blood procainamide and N-acetylprocainamide levels in adjusting further doses.

Arrhythmias associated with surgery or anesthesia.

Adults: 100–500 mg.

IV

Ventricular arrhythmias.

Initial loading infusion: Slowly inject into a vein or tubing at a rate not to exceed 50 mg/min; doses of 100 mg may be given q 5 min until arrhythmia is suppressed or until 500 mg has been given. Wait at least 10 min to allow for more distribution into tissues before resuming. Alternatively, a loading infusion containing 20 mg/mL (1 gram diluted to 50 mL with D5W) may be given at a constant rate of 1 mL/min for 25–30 min to deliver 500–600 mg. Maximum dosage either by repeated bolus injections or loading infusion is 1 gram. **Maintenance infusion:** 2–6 mg/min.

TABLETS, IMMEDIATE-RELEASE

Adults, initial: Up to 50 mg/kg/day in divided doses q 3 hr. **Usual, 40–50 kg:** 250 mg q 3 hr or 500 mg q 6 hr; **60–70 kg:** 375 mg q 3 hr or 750 mg q 6 hr; **80–90 kg:** 500 mg q 3 hr or 1 gram q 6 hr; **over 100 kg:** 625 mg q 3 hr or 1.25 grams q 6 hr.

NURSING IMPLICATIONS

IMPLEMENTATION/ADMINISTRATION/STORAGE

1. IM therapy may be used as an alternative to PO in clients with less threatening arrhythmias but who are nauseated or vomiting, who cannot take anything PO (e.g., preoperatively), or who have malabsorptive problems.
2. If more than three IM injections are required, assess the age, renal function, and blood levels of procainamide and NAPA; adjust dosage accordingly.
3. IV Reserve IV use for emergency situations.
4. For IV initial therapy, dilute the drug with D5W; give a maximum of 1 gram slowly to minimize side effects by one of the following methods:
   - Direct injection into a vein or into tubing of an established infusion line at a rate not to exceed 50 mg/min. Dilute either the 100- or 500-mg/mL vials prior to injection to facilitate control of the dosage rate. Doses of 100 mg may be given q 5 min until arrhythmia is suppressed or until 500 mg has been given (then wait 10 or more min before resuming administration).
   - Loading infusion containing 20 mg/mL (1 gram diluted with 50 mL of D5W) given at a constant rate of 1 mL/min for 25–30 min to deliver 500–600 mg.
5. For IV maintenance infusion, dose is usually 2–6 mg/min. Administer with electronic infusion device.
6. Discard solutions that are darker than light amber or otherwise colored. Solutions that have turned slightly yellow on standing may be used. Consult pharmacist if unsure.
7. COMPATIBILITY D5W.
8. INCOMPATIBILITY Administer separately.

ASSESSMENT

1. Note reasons for therapy, type, onset, characteristics of S&S. List other agents prescribed, outcome. Use reserved for life-threatening ventricular arrhythmias.
2. Assess cardiopulmonary status and note findings. List any sensitivity to tartrazine, pregnancy, CHF, or heart block. May cause or aggravate CHF or produce severe hypotension, especially with CHF, acute ischemic heart disease, or cardiomyopathy.
3. Place supine during IV infusion and monitor BP. Discontinue if SBP falls 15 mm Hg or more during administration or if increased SA or AV block noted.
4. Reduce dose with liver or renal dysfunction, or if client <120 lb.
5. Assess for symptoms of SLE, manifested by polyarthralgia, arthritis, pleuritic pain, fever, myalgia, and skin lesions. ANA titer may be-

come positive in 60% of those taking this drug without lupus-like S&S; may progress to SLE if drug is not discontinued.

6. Monitor VS, ECG, CBC, electrolytes, ANA titers, renal, LFTs. Approximately 50% of clients will develop positive ANA titer within 2 to 18 mo of starting therapy.

CLIENT/FAMILY TEACHING

1. Take with a full glass of water to lessen GI symptoms. Take either 1 hr before or 2 hr after meals.
2. Use caution when driving or performing activities requiring mental alertness; may cause dizziness.
3. If GI symptoms are severe and persistent, may take with meals or with a snack to ensure adherence.
4. Report any sore throat, fever, rash, chills, bruising, diarrhea, or increased palpitations. With long term use may note loss of effectiveness.
5. Do not take any OTC drugs, do not stop suddenly.
6. Keep all F/U to assess response, labs, and for adverse SE.

OUTCOMES/EVALUATE

- Termination of arrhythmias with restoration of stable cardiac rhythm
- Therapeutic drug levels (4–8 mcg/mL)

Procarbazine hydrochloride (PCB, MIH, N-Methylhydrazine)

(pro-**KAR**-bah-zeen)

Classification(s): Antineoplastic, miscellaneous

Pregnancy Category: D

RX: Matulane.

SEE ALSO ***ANTINEOPLASTIC AGENTS***.

INDICATIONS/USES

Adjunct in the treatment of Hodgkin's disease (stage III and stage IV) as part of MOPP (nitrogen mustard, vincristine, procarbazine, prednisone) or ChIVPP (chlorambucil, vinblastine, procarbazine, prednisone) therapies. *Investigational:* Non-Hodgkin's lymphomas, malignant melanoma, primary brain tumors, lung cancer.

ACTION/KINETICS

Action

May inhibit synthesis of protein, RNA, and DNA and inhibit transmethylation of methyl groups of methionine into t-RNA. Absence of t-RNA could result in cessation of protein synthesis and subsequently DNA and RNA synthesis. Also, hydrogen peroxide formed during auto-oxidation of the drug may attack protein sulfhydryl groups found in residual protein that is tightly bound to DNA.

Pharmacokinetics

Rapidly and completely absorbed from GI tract. Drug quickly equilibrates between plasma and CSF (peak CSF levels occur within 30–90 min and peak plasma levels occur within 60 min). **t½, after IV:** 10 min. Metabolized in the liver and kidneys to cytotoxic products. About 70% eliminated in urine, mostly as metabolites, after 24 hr.

CONTRAINDICATIONS

Inadequate bone marrow reserve as shown by bone marrow aspiration (i.e., in clients with leukopenia, thrombocytopenia, or anemia). Lactation. Hypersensitivity to drug.

SPECIAL CONCERNS

- Use with caution in impaired kidney or liver function.
- Monitor closely in children due to possible tremors, convulsions, and coma.

SIDE EFFECTS

Most Common

N&V, constipation, dry mouth, difficulty swallowing, fatigue, weakness, drowsiness, dizziness, darkening of skin, muscle twitching, insomnia, temporary alopecia.

GI: N&V, anorexia, stomatitis, dry mouth, dysphagia, difficulty swallowing, abdominal pain, hematemesis, melena, diarrhea, constipation. **CNS:** Paresthesias, neuropathies, headache, dizziness, depression, apprehension, nervousness, insomnia, nightmares, hallucinations, falling, weakness, fatigue, lethargy, drowsiness, unsteadiness, ataxia, foot drop, decreased reflexes, tremors, confusion, ***coma, convulsions***. **CV:** Hypotension, tachycardia, syncope. **Respiratory:** Pleural effusion, pneumonitis, cough. **Hematologic:** Leukopenia, ane-

P

mia, thrombocytopenia, pancytopenia, eosinophilia, ***hemolytic anemia***, petechiae, purpura, epistaxis, hemoptysis. **GU:** Hematuria, urinary frequency, nocturia. **Dermatologic:** Dermatitis, pruritus, rash, urticaria, herpes, hyperpigmentation, flushing, alopecia (temporary). **Ophthalmic:** Retinal hemorrhage, nystagmus, photophobia, diplopia, inability to focus, papilledema. **Hepatic:** Jaundice, hepatic dysfunction. **Miscellaneous:** Gynecomastia in prepubertal and early pubertal boys, muscle twitching, pain, myalgia and arthralgia, pyrexia, diaphoresis, chills, intercurrent infections, edema, hoarseness, generalized allergic reactions, hearing loss, slurred speech, second nonlymphoid malignancies (including AML, malignant myelosclerosis) and azoospermia in those treated with procarbazine combined with other chemotherapy or radiation.

OVERDOSE MANAGEMENT

Symptoms: N&V, diarrhea, enteritis, hypotension, tremors, seizures, coma, hematologic and hepatic toxicity. *Treatment:* Induce vomiting or undertake gastric lavage. IV fluids. Perform frequent blood counts and LFTs.

DRUG INTERACTIONS

Alcohol / Antabuse-like reaction
Antihistamines / Additive CNS depression
Antihypertensive drugs / Additive CNS depression
Barbiturates / Additive CNS depression
Chemotherapy / Depressed bone marrow activity
Digoxin / ↓ Digoxin levels
Guanethidine / Excitation and hypertension
Hypoglycemic agents, oral / ↑ Hypoglycemic effect
Insulin / ↑ Hypoglycemic effect
Levodopa / Flushing and hypertension within 1 hr of administration
MAO inhibitors / Possibility of hypertensive crisis
Methotrexate / ↑ Methotrexate nephrotoxicity; wait 72 hr after the last dose of procarbazine before first dose of methotrexate infusion
Methyldopa / Excitation and hypertension
Narcotics / Significant CNS depression → possible deep coma/death
Phenothiazines / Additive CNS depression; possible hypertensive crisis
Sympathomimetics, indirectly acting / Possibility of hypertensive crisis
Tricyclic antidepressants / Possible toxic and fatal reactions, including excitability, fluctuations in BP, seizures, and coma
Tyramine-containing foods / Possibility of hypertensive crisis

HOW SUPPLIED

Capsules: 50 mg.

DOSAGE

CAPSULES

When used alone for Hodgkin's disease.

Adults: 2–4 mg/kg/day for first week; **then,** 4–6 mg/kg/day until leukocyte count falls below 4,000/mm^3 or platelet count falls below 100,000/mm^3. If toxic symptoms appear, discontinue drug until satisfactory recovery, and resume treatment at rate of 1–2 mg/kg/day; **maintenance:** 1–2 mg/kg/day. **Children, highly individualized:** 50 mg/m^2/day for first week; then 100 mg/m^2 (to nearest 50 mg) until maximum response obtained or until leukopenia or thrombocytopenia occurs. When maximum response is reached, maintain the dose at 50 mg/m^2/day.

When used in combination with other antineoplastic drugs (e.g., MOPP or ChlVPP therapies) for Hodgkin's disease.

100 mg/m^2 for 14 days.

NURSING IMPLICATIONS

ASSESSMENT

1. Note reasons for therapy, disease stage, other agents/treatments prescribed.
2. Assess cardiopulmonary and neurologic status.
3. Discontinue if any CNS S&S (paresthesias, neuropathies, seizures) occur, if stomatitis or diarrhea with frequent bowel movements or watery stools occur, or if there is hemorrhage or bleeding tendencies.
4. Monitor VS, urinalysis, BS, BUN, creatinine, uric acid, transaminases, and alkaline phosphatase before starting and every week during treatment. Assess reticulocyte count and CBC with differential and platelet count before starting and every 3 to 4 days during treat-

ment. May cause granulocyte and platelet suppression. Nadir: 14 days; recovery: 21–28 days.

CLIENT/FAMILY TEACHING

1. Consult provider before taking any other medication because procarbazine has MAO inhibitory activity. Avoid sympathomimetic drugs and foods with a high tyramine content (yeasts, yogurt, caffeine, chocolate, aged cheese, liver, smoked or pickled fish, fermented sausage, etc.) during and for 2 weeks after completing therapy; may precipitate a hypertensive crisis.
2. Do not drive or perform tasks that require mental alertness until drug effects realized; may cause drowsiness and dizziness.
3. Consume adequate fluids (2–3 L/day) to prevent dehydration.
4. Drug increases effect of insulin and oral hypoglycemic agents; report symptoms as medication adjustment may be necessary.
5. Avoid exposure to sun or to ultraviolet rays because a photosensitive skin reaction may occur. Wear sunscreen, sunglasses, and protective clothing if exposure is necessary.
6. Avoid CNS depressants, decongestants, and alcohol; a disulfiram-type reaction may occur.
7. Practice reliable contraception. Determine those that may benefit from sperm/egg harvesting.
8. Avoid crowds and persons with known infections. Report fever, rash, chills, SOB, abnormal bruising/bleeding, persistent constipation (especially if diet, increased fluids, and bulk are ineffective); laxatives may be needed.
9. Advise those who smoke that a second malignancy, including lung cancer, can develop following treatment and that tobacco use increases the risk. Offer help to quit.
10. Keep all F/U to assess response, labs, and for adverse SE.

OUTCOMES/EVALUATE

Suppression of malignant cell proliferation

IV

Prochlorperazine

(proh-klor-**PAIR**-ah-zeen)

Classification(s): Antipsychotic, phenothiazine

Pregnancy Category: C

RX: Compro Suppositories, Prochlorperazine.

Prochlorperazine edisylate

Pregnancy Category: C

RX: Prochlorperazine Edisylate.

Prochlorperazine maleate

Pregnancy Category: C

RX: Prochlorperazine maleate.

✱ **Rx:** Apo-Prochlorazine.

SEE ALSO ***ANTIPSYCHOTIC AGENTS, PHENOTHIAZINES.***

INDICATIONS/USES

(1) Schizophrenia. (2) Short-term treatment of generalized nonpsychotic anxiety (not drug of choice). (3) N&V. *Investigational:* IM for abortive treatment of migraine attacks in adults.

ACTION/KINETICS

Action

Has affinity for the following receptors: Dopamine D_2, histamine H_1, alpha–adrenergic, and serotonin 5-HT_2. Causes a high incidence of extrapyramidal and antiemetic effects, moderate sedative effects, and a low incidence of anticholinergic effects and orthostatic hypotension.

Pharmacokinetics

t½: 3.5 hr after PO and 6.9 hr after IV.

CONTRAINDICATIONS

Use in clients who weigh less than 44 kg. Use for severe N&V in children weighing less than 9 kg (20 lbs) or who are under 2 years of age. Use in pediatric surgery. Lactation.

SPECIAL CONCERNS

- Use with caution in those with CV disease.
- Geriatric, emaciated, and debilitated clients usually require a lower initial dose.
- Safe use during pregnancy not established.

SIDE EFFECTS

Most Common

Drowsiness, dizziness, amenorrhea, blurred vision, skin reactions, hypotension, extrapyramidal reactions.

CNS: Agitation, akathisia, catatonic-like states, cerebral edema, ***convulsions***, dizziness, abnormal/bizarre/increased dreams, dystonia, drowsiness, sedation, somnolence, extrapyramidal symptoms,

P

staggering/shuffling gait, headache, hyperactivity, hyperreflexia, insomnia, jitteriness, motor restlessness, neuroleptic malignant syndrome, pseudoparkinsonism, psychosis, dyskinesia, tardive dyskinesia, ***suicide***, tardive dystonia, tremor, trismus. **GI:** Adynamic ileus, increased appetite, atonic colon, constipation, drooling, dry mouth, dysphagia, nausea, obstipation, salivation, tongue protrusion, increased weight. **Hepatic:** Biliary stasis, jaundice, impaired liver function. **CV:** ECG changes, hypotension, Q- and T-wave distortions, ***cardiac arrest***. **Dermatologic:** Dermatitis (including exfoliative dermatitis), eczema, erythema, photosensitivity, pruritus, thrombocytopenic purpura, skin pigmentation changes, urticaria. **GU:** Amenorrhea, ejaculation disorders, galactorrhea, glycosuria, gynecomastia, impotence, menstrual irregularities, priapism, urinary retention. **Musculoskeletal:** Muscle rigidity, opisthotonos, carpopedal spasms, spasm of neck muscles, torticollis. **Respiratory:** Asphyxia, asthma, failure of cough reflex, bronchopneumonia, ***laryngeal edema***, nasal congestion, **Hematologic:** Agranulocytosis, ***aplastic anemia***, hemolytic anemia, blood dyscrasias, eosinophilia, leukopenia, pancytopenia. **Hypersensitivity:** Allergic reactions, angioneurotic edema, ***anaphylactoid reactions***. **Ophthalmic:** Lenticular/corneal opacities, miosis, mydriasis, oculogyric crisis, pigmentary retinopathy, blurred vision. **Body as a whole:** Cogwheel rigidity, fever, hyperpyrexia, hyperthermia, peripheral edema, systemic lupus erythematosus-like syndrome. **Miscellaneous:** Epithelial keratopathy, mask-like face, pill rolling motion, ***sudden death***.

P

LABORATORY TEST CONSIDERATIONS

Glycosuria, hyper/hypoglycemia, hyperprolactinemia. Abnormal CSF proteins.

ADDITIONAL DRUG INTERACTIONS

↑ Dofetilide levels with ↑ risk of ventricular arrhythmias, including torsades de pointes; do not use together

HOW SUPPLIED

Prochlorperazine. *Suppositories:* 2.5 mg, 5 mg, 25 mg.
Prochlorperazine edisylate. *Injection:* 5 mg/mL; *Syrup:* 5 mg/5 mL.
Prochlorperazine maleate. *Capsules, Sustained-Release:* 30 mg; *Tablets:* 5 mg, 10 mg, 25 mg.

DOSAGE

EDISYLATE SYRUP; MALEATE SUSTAINED-RELEASE CAPSULES; MALEATE TABLETS

Schizophrenia.

Adults and adolescents: 5 or 10 mg 3 or 4 times per day for mild conditions. For moderate to severe conditions, for hospitalized, or adequately supervised clients: 10 mg 3 or 4 times per day. Dose can be increased gradually q 2–3 days as needed and tolerated. For extended-release capsules, up to 100–150 mg/day can be given for severe conditions. **Pediatric, 2–12 years:** 2.5 mg 2–3 times per day. Do not give more than 10 mg on the first day. For children, aged 2–5 years, the usual daily dose does not exceed 20 mg; for children, aged 6–12 years, the usual daily dose does not exceed 25 mg.

Anxiety, nonpsychotic.

Adults and adolescents: 5 mg 3–4 times per day on arising. Or, 15 mg sustained release on arising or 10 mg sustained release q 12 hr. Do not give more than 20 mg/day for more than 12 weeks. Do not use in pediatric clients under 20 lb or under 2 years old.

N&V.

Adults and adolescents: 5–10 mg 3–4 times per day (up to 40 mg/day). For extended-release capsules, the dose is 15–30 mg once daily in the morning (or 10 mg q 12 hr, up to 40 mg/day). **Pediatric, 18–39 kg:** 2.5 mg (base) 3 times per day (or 5 mg twice a day), not to exceed 15 mg/day; **14–17 kg:** 2.5 mg (base) 2–3 times per day, not to exceed 10 mg/day; **9–13 kg:** 2.5 mg (base) 1–2 times per day, not to exceed 7.5 mg/day. The total daily dose for children should not exceed 10 mg the first day; on subsequent days, the total daily dose should not exceed 20 mg for children 2–5 years of age or 25 mg for children 6–12 years of age.

IM, EDISYLATE INJECTION

Psychotic disorders, for immediate control of severely disturbed clients.

Adults and adolescents, initial: 10–20 mg; dose can be repeated q 2–4

hr as needed (usually up to three or four doses). If prolonged therapy is needed: 10–20 mg q 4–6 hr. **Children, less than 12 years of age:** 0.03 mg/kg by deep IM injection. After control is achieved (usually after 1 injection), switch to PO at same dosage level or higher.

N&V.

Adults and adolescents: 5–10 mg; repeat the dose q 3–4 hr as needed, not to exceed 40 mg/day. **Pediatric, 2–12 years:** 0.132 mg/kg by deep IM.

N&V during surgery.

Adults and adolescents: 5–10 mg (base) given 1–2 hr before induction of anesthesia; may be repeated once in 30 min. Also, to control acute symptoms during and after surgery (may repeat once).

RECTAL SUPPOSITORY

Adults: 25 mg twice a day. **Pediatric, 2–12 years:** 2.5 mg 2–3 times per day with no more than 10 mg given on the first day. Then no more than 20 mg/day for children 2–5 years of age and 25 mg/day for children 6–12 years of age.

IV

Severe N&V.

Injection: 5–10 mg, 15–30 min before induction of anesthesia, or to control symptoms during or after surgery. Repeat once if needed. Do not exceed 5 mg/mL/min. Do not use bolus injection. **Infusion:** 20 mg/L of isotonic solution.

NURSING IMPLICATIONS

Do not confuse prochlorperazine with chlorpromazine or promethazine, both of which are also antipsychotics.

IMPLEMENTATION/ADMINISTRATION/STORAGE

1. Use doses in the lower range for the elderly, as they are more susceptible to hypotension and neuromuscular reactions.
2. Store all forms of the drug in tight-closing amber-colored bottles; store suppositories below 37°C (98.6°F).
3. Due to local irritation, do not give SC.
4. Do not mix with other agents in a syringe.
5. Do not dilute with any material containing the preservative parabens.
6. When given IM to children for N&V, the duration of action may be 12 hr.
7. Parenteral prescribing limits are 20 mg/day for children 2–5 years of age and 25 mg/day for children 6–12 years of age.
8. IV Administer IV dose by slow injection or infusion at rate not exceeding 5 mg/mL. May administer undiluted or diluted in isotonic solution (e.g., NSS, D5W). Do not administer as bolus.
9. COMPATIBILITY D5W, NSS.
10. INCOMPATIBILITY Administer separately.

ASSESSMENT

1. Note reasons for therapy, onset/characteristics of S&S, clinical presentation, any triggers evident.
2. Assess mental status; note behavioral presentation/manifestations or evidence of severe depression.
3. Monitor I&O and VS. Auscultate bowel sounds; assess function.
4. Use caution with CV disease or mitral insufficiency, history of glaucoma, EEG abnormalities or seizure disorders, prior brain damage, hepatic or renal function impairment, or those who will be exposed to extreme heat.
5. Incorporate safety precautions during treatment of overdose. If taking spansules, continue treatment until all signs of overdosage are no longer evident. Saline laxatives may hasten the evacuation of pellets that have not yet released their medication.
6. Some parenteral products may contain sulfites. If injection is spilled on skin or clothing, rinse area immediately with water to prevent contact dermatitis.
7. Assess for involuntary body and facial movements, especially with elderly and females.
8. Position to prevent aspiration; cough reflex suppressed.
9. Monitor CBC, renal, LFTs, ECG.

CLIENT/FAMILY TEACHING

1. Do not exceed prescribed dose. Avoid skin contact with solution. Take sustained-release capsules whole 1 hr before or 2 hr after meals; do not crush bite or chew capsule. May take with food if GI upset occurs.

P

2. Check child suppository dose: (2.5 mg) to avoid confusion with adult dose (25 mg).
3. Withhold drug and report if child shows signs of restlessness and excitement. Report symptoms of extrapyramidal effects and tardive dyskinesia (tremor, involuntary twitching).
4. Report fainting or loss of consciousness, palpitations, dizziness, high fever, muscle rigidity, altered mental status, irregular pulse, sore throat, unusual bruising, yellowing of the skin or eyes.
5. Do not drive or operate machinery until drug effects are realized; drowsiness or dizziness may occur. Rise and change positions slowly to prevent low BP effects.
6. Avoid alcohol and CNS depressants.
7. Consume adequate fluids to prevent dehydration; avoid strenuous activity during periods of high temperature or humidity and use precautions in hot weather. When in the sun, use protection to prevent photosensitivity reaction. Avoid high temperature exposures; may precipitate heat stroke.
8. Urine may be discolored pink to reddish-brown. False + urine pregnancy tests may occur.
9. Report fever, sore throat, rashes, tremors, dark urine, pale stools, impaired vision, excessive drowsiness, or lack of response.
10. Keep all F/U to assess response, labs, and for adverse SE.

OUTCOMES/EVALUATE

- Control of N&V
- Reduction in agitation, excitability, withdrawn behaviors

P

Progesterone gel

(pro-**JES**-ter-ohn)

Classification(s): Progesterone

RX: Prochieve.

SEE ALSO ***PROGESTERONE AND PROGESTINS.***

INDICATIONS/USES

(1) Progesterone supplementation or replacement as part of assisted reproductive technology treatment for infertile women with progesterone deficiency. (2) Secondary amenorrhea. The 4% gel is to treat secondary amenorrhea and the 8% gel is for women who have failed to respond to treatment with the 4% gel.

ACTION/KINETICS

Action

Pharmacokinetics

t½, absorption: 25–50 hr. **t½, elimination:** 5–20 min. Metabolized in liver; excreted through urine and feces. **Plasma protein binding:** Extensively bound.

CONTRAINDICATIONS

Undiagnosed vaginal bleeding, liver disease or dysfunction, known or suspected malignancy of breast or genital organs, missed abortion, active thrombophlebitis or thromboembolic disease (or history of such). Concurrent use with other local intravaginal therapy.

SPECIAL CONCERNS

- See *Progesterone and Progestins.*
- Safety and efficacy not determined in children.

SIDE EFFECTS

Most Common

Breast enlargement, somnolence, constipation, nausea, headache, perineal pain, nervousness, depression, abdominal pain, decreased libido.

See *Progesterone and Progestins* for a complete list of possible side effects.

HOW SUPPLIED

Vaginal Gel/Jelly: 45 mg/1.125 grams (Prochieve 4%), 90 mg/1.125 grams (Prochieve 8%).

DOSAGE

Prochieve 4%

VAGINAL GEL/JELLY

Secondary amenorrhea.

45 mg (1 applicator of the 4% gel) every other day up to total of 6 doses. For women who fail to respond, the 8% gel (90 mg) may be given every other day up to total of 6 doses.

Prochieve 8%

VAGINAL GEL/JELLY

Assisted reproductive technology.

90 mg (1 applicator of the 8% gel) once daily for women who require progesterone supplementation. Administer 90 mg twice a day in women with par-

tial or complete ovarian failure who require progesterone replacement. If pregnancy occurs, treatment may be continued until placental autonomy has been achieved (up to 10–12 weeks).

NURSING IMPLICATIONS

IMPLEMENTATION/ADMINISTRATION/STORAGE

1. Dosage increase from 4% gel can only be accomplished by using 8% gel. Increasing volume of gel does not increase amount absorbed.
2. If other local intravaginal therapy is to be used, wait at least 6 hr before or after Prochieve administration.
3. Store from 15–30°C (59–86°F).

ASSESSMENT

1. Note reasons for therapy, physical and gynecologic findings including PAP smear. Alert pathologist when progesterone therapy used.
2. Assess for liver disease, breast or genital malignancy, undiagnosed vaginal bleeding, missed abortion, liver dysfunction, or history of thromboembolic disease; precludes drug therapy. Note menstrual history and review risk of thrombotic disorders associated with therapy.
3. Check for history of psychic depression; if present, observe carefully and stop drug if the depression recurs to a serious degree.
4. Determine any history of epilepsy, migraines, severe depression, asthma, and heart or kidney dysfunction; may preclude drug therapy.
5. Monitor CBC, TSH, lipid panel, and LFTs.

CLIENT/FAMILY TEACHING

1. Review product information sheet on how to use product; use only as directed.
2. Used to treat progesterone deficiency in women undergoing infertility treatment and/or to restore menstruation in women whose menstrual periods have stopped.
3. Administer gel using prefilled disposable applicator. Discard applicator after delivering dose. Do not save for future use.
4. Small, white globules may appear as a discharge, even several days after using gel; this is normal and of no concern.
5. Do not use with other intravaginal products; if concurrent therapy prescribed, wait for 6 hr.
6. If being used at altitudes above 762 meters, review special instructions for preparing the applicator to prevent partial release of gel before vaginal insertion.
7. May experience breast enlargement, constipation, headaches, sleepiness, and perineal pain. Report any depression, chest pain, SOB, pain in groin or calves, dizziness or fainting or abnormal vaginal bleeding.
8. Keep all F/U to assess response and for adverse SE.

OUTCOMES/EVALUATE

- Progesterone replacement/supplementation with ART (assistive reproductive technology)
- Restoration of menses with amenorrhea

IV

Promethazine hydrochloride

(proh-**METH**-ah-zeen)

Classification(s): Antihistamine, first generation, phenothiazine

Pregnancy Category: C

RX: Phenadoz, Phenergen, Promethegan.

SEE ALSO ***ANTIHISTAMINES*** AND ***ANTIEMETICS***.

INDICATIONS/USES

PO, Rectal. (1) Perennial and seasonal allergic rhinitis; vasomotor rhinitis. (2) Allergic conjunctivitis due to inhalant allergens and foods. (3) Mild, uncomplicated allergic skin manifestations of urticaria and angioedema. (4) Relief of allergic reactions to blood or plasma. (5) Dermatographism. (6) Adjunct to epinephrine and other measures to treat anaphylactic reactions after acute symptoms have been controlled. (7) Preoperative, postoperative, or obstetric sedation. (8) Prevention and control of N&V associated with certain types of anesthesia and surgery. (9) Adjunct to meperidine or other analgesics to control postoperative pain. (10) Sedation in both children and adults. (11) Relief of apprehension and production of light sleep from which the client can be easily aroused. (12) Active and prophylactic treatment of motion sickness. (13) Antiemetic in postoperative clients. *Investigational:* N&V of pregnancy.

Parenteral. (1) Adjunct to control postoperative pain. (2) Prevention and control of N&V associated with certain types of anesthesia and sur-

P

gery and in postoperative clients. (3) Relief of allergic reactions to blood or plasma; in anaphylaxis as an adjunct to epinephrine and other standard measures after the acute symptoms have been controlled; for other uncomplicated allergic conditions of the immediate type when PO therapy is impossible or contraindicated. (4) Preoperative, postoperative, or obstetric sedation. (5) Relief of apprehension and production of light sleep from which the client can be easily aroused. (6) IV with reduced amounts of meperidine or other narcotic analgesic as an adjunct to anesthesia and analgesia in special surgical situations (e.g., repeated bronchoscopy, ophthalmic surgery, and poor risk clients). (7) Active treatment of motion sickness. *Investigational:* N&V of pregnancy; opioid-induced N&V.

ACTION/KINETICS

Action

Antiemetic effects are likely due to inhibition of the CTZ. Effective in vertigo by its central anticholinergic effect, which inhibits the vestibular apparatus and the integrative vomiting center as well as the CTZ. May cause severe drowsiness. Significant anticholinergic and antiemetic effects.

Pharmacokinetics

Onset, PO, IM, PR: 20 min; **IV:** 3–5 min. **Duration, antihistaminic:** 6–12 hr; **sedative:** 2–8 hr. Slowly eliminated through urine and feces.

CONTRAINDICATIONS

Lactation. Comatose clients, CNS depression due to drugs (including barbituates, general anesthetics, tranquilizers, alcohol, narcotics), previous phenothiazine idiosyncrasy or hypersensitivity, acutely ill or dehydrated children (due to greater susceptibility to dystonias). Children up to 2 years of age. Treatment of uncomplicated vomiting in children. Use in children whose signs and symptoms may suggest Reye's syndrome or other hepatic diseases. SC or intra-arterial use due to tissue necrosis and gangrene. Use in the treatment of lower respiratory tract symptoms, including asthma.

SPECIAL CONCERNS

PO and Rectal Use. (1) Do not use promethazine in pediatric clients younger than 2 years of age, because of the potential for fatal respiratory depression. (2) Postmarketing cases of respiratory depression, including fatalities, have been reported with use of promethazine in pediatric clients younger than 2 years of age. A wide range of weight-based doses of promethazine have resulted in respiratory depression in these clients. (3) Exercise caution when administering promethazine to pediatric clients 2 years of age and older. It is recommended that the lowest effective dose of promethazine be used in pediatric clients 2 years of age and older and that coadministration of other drugs with respiratory depressant effects be avoided. **Injection.** (1) Do not use promethazine in pediatric clients younger than 2 years of age because of the potential for fatal respiratory depression. (2) Postmarketing cases of respiratory depression, including fatalities, have been reported with use of promethazine in pediatric clients younger than 2 years of age. Exercise caution when administering promethazine to pediatric clients 2 years of age and older. (3) Promethazine can cause severe chemical irritation and damage to tissues regardless of the route of administration. Irritation and damage can result from perivascular extravasation, unintentional intra-arterial injection, and intraneuronal or perineuronal infiltration. Adverse reactions include burning, pain, thrombophlebitis, tissue necrosis, and gangrene. In some cases, surgical intervention, including fasciotomy, skin graft, and/or amputation have been required. (4) Due to the risks of IV injection, the preferred route of administration is deep IM injection. Subcutaneous injection is contraindicated.

- **Geriatric clients are more likely to experience confusion, dizziness, hypotension, and sedation.**
- **The extrapyramidal symptoms that can occur following promethazine use may be confused with the CNS signs of undiagnosed primary diseases, such as encephalopathy or Reye's syndrome.**
- **Safe use during pregnancy not established.**
- **Use in children may cause paradoxical hyperexcitability and nightmares.**

SIDE EFFECTS

Most Common

Drowsiness, dizziness, confusion, blurred vision, dry mouth, tinnitus, N&V, photosensitivity.

CNS: Drowsiness, sedation, somnolence, dizziness, confusion, disorientation, extrapyramidal symptoms, lassitude, incoordination, fatigue, euphoria, nervousness, insomnia, tremors, ***seizures***, excitation, catatonic-like states, hysteria, hallucinations. **CV:** Increased or decreased BP, tachycardia, bradycardia, faintness. **GI:** Dry mouth, N&V, jaundice. **Dermatologic:** Dermatitis, photosensitivity, urticaria. **Hematologic:** Leukopenia, thrombocytopenia, thrombocytopenic purpura, ***agranulocytosis***. **Respiratory:** Asthma, nasal stuffiness, ***respiratory depression***, ***apnea***. **Ophthalmic:** Blurred vision, diplopia. **Miscellaneous:** Tinnitus, angioneurotic edema, ***neuroleptic malignant syndrome***, hyperexcitability, abnormal movements.

HOW SUPPLIED

Injection: 25 mg/mL, 50 mg/mL (IM only); ***Oral Solution:*** 6.25 mg/5 mL; ***Suppositories:*** 12.5 mg, 25 mg, 50 mg; ***Tablets:*** 12.5 mg, 25 mg, 50 mg.

DOSAGE

ORAL SOLUTION; SUPPOSITORIES; TABLETS

Allergic conditions.

Adults and children over 2 years of age, usual: 25 mg at bedtime or 12.5 mg before meals and at bedtime. Alternate dosage: 6.25–12.5 mg 3 times per day. *NOTE:* 25 mg doses will usually control minor transfusion reactions of an allergic nature. Adjust dose to the smallest amount needed to relieve symptoms. If given rectally, resume PO administration as soon as possible if continued therapy is needed.

Sedation.

Adults: 25–50 mg at bedtime for nighttime, presurgical, or obstetrical sedation. **Children, over 2 years of age:** 12.5–25 mg at bedtime or pre- or postoperatively for sedation. *NOTE:* If used for preoperative sedation, give the night before surgery to relieve apprehension and to produce quiet sleep.

Antiemetic.

Adults, usual: 12.5–25 mg q 4–6 hr as needed. **Children, over 2 years of age, initial:** 1 mg/kg q 4–6 hr; **then,** adjust the dose to the age and weight of the client and the severity of the condition being treated. The prophylactic dosage for adults and children is 25 mg q 4–6 hr as needed during surgery and the postoperative period.

Motion sickness.

Adults, initial: 25 mg 30–60 min before anticipated travel repeated 8–12 hr later if needed; **maintenance:** 25 mg twice a day, on arising and before the evening meal, on succeeding days of travel. **Children, over 2 years of age, initial:** 12.5–25 mg 30–60 min before anticipated travel repeated 8–12 hr if needed; **maintenance:** 12.5–25 mg twice a day, on arising and before the evening meal, on succeeding days of travel.

Analgesia.

Adults, preoperatively: 50 mg with an appropriately reduced dose of narcotic or barbiturate and the required amount of an atropine-like drug; **postoperatively:** 25–50 mg with analgesics. **Children, over 2 years of age, preoperatively:** 1 mg/kg in combination with an appropriately reduced dose of narcotic or barbiturate and the appropriate dose of an atropine-like drug; **postoperatively**: 12.5–25 mg with analgesics. To produce quiet sleep and to relieve apprehension, give 12.5–25 mg the night before surgery.

N&V of pregnancy (investigational).

12.5–25 mg q 4 hr PO or rectally.

IM (PREFERRED); IV

Allergic conditions.

Adults: 25 mg by deep IM (preferred) or IV; may repeat dose within 2 hr, if needed. The average adult dose for amelioration of allergic reactions to blood or plasma is 25 mg. After initiation of treatment, adjust the dose to the smallest amount needed to relieve symptoms. Resume PO therapy as soon as possible. **Children, 2 years and older, initial:** Up to 12.5 mg by deep IM (preferred) or IV; may repeat dose within 2 hr, if needed. After initiation of treatment, adjust the dose to the smallest amount needed to relieve symptoms. Resume PO therapy as soon as possible as circumstances permit.

P

Sedation.

Adults: 25–50 mg, preferably IM, at bedtime for nighttime sedation. Doses of 50 mg IM provide sedation and relieve apprehension during early stages of labor. When labor is definitely established, may give 25–75 mg (usual is 50 mg) IM; if used IV, do not exceed a concentration of 25 mg/mL at a rate no greater than 25 mg/min. Appropriately reduce the dose of any desired narcotic. If needed, promethazine with a reduced dose of analgesic may be repeated once or twice at 4-hr intervals, not to exceed 100 mg/24 hr for clients in labor. **Children, 2–12 years of age, initial:** Up to 12.5–25 mg deep IM (preferred) or IV at bedtime; **maximum:** 25 mg/dose.

Antiemetic.

Adults, usual: 12.5–25 mg deep IM (preferred) or IV; may repeat q 4 hr as needed. **Children, 2–12 years of age, usual:** Up to 6.25–12.5 mg by deep IM (preferred) or IV; may repeat q 4 hr as needed. Maximum dose for children: 12.5 mg/dose. For adults and children, reduce dose of concomitant analgesics or barbiturates accordingly if used postoperatively. Do not use when etiology of vomiting is unknown.

Pre- and postoperative use.

Adults, usual: 25–50 mg by deep IM (preferred) or IV in combination with an appropriately reduced dose of analgesics, hypnotics, and atropine-like drugs; if given IV, do not exceed a concentration of 25 mg/mL at a rate no greater than 25 mg/min. For elderly clients, consider limiting the dose to 6.25–12.5 mg as the starting IV dose. **Children, 2–12 years of age, usual:** 1 mg/kg by deep IM (preferred) or IV in combination with an appropriately reduced dose of narcotic or barbiturates and atropine-like drugs. Maximum dose in children: 25 mg/dose.

N&V of pregnancy (investigational).

12.5–25 mg q 4 hr IV.

P

NURSING IMPLICATIONS

Do not confuse promethazine with chlorpromazine or with prochlorperazine, both of which are antipsychotics.

IMPLEMENTATION/ADMINISTRATION/STORAGE

1. The extrapyramidal symptoms that can occur secondary to promethazine administration may be confused with the CNS signs of undiagnosed primary disease (e.g., encephalopathy, Reyes syndrome). Avoid promethazine in such situations.
2. Decrease dosage in dehydrated or oliguric clients.
3. Store PO formulations from 20–25°C (68–77°F). Protect from light.
4. Refrigerate suppositories between 2–8°C (36–46°F). Dispense in well-closed container.
5. Store injection at controlled room temperature from 20–25°C (68–77°F). Protect from light. Keep covered in carton until used. Do not use if solution has developed color or contains a precipitate.
6. Ampules may contain sulfite. Inject IM deep into large muscle mass, rotating sites. Not for SC or intra-arterial administration; may cause tissue necrosis.
7. IV If given correctly, IV doses are well tolerated; however, IV use is associated with increased risks. Do not exceed a concentration of 25 mg/mL at a rate of greater than 25 mg/min.
8. It is recommended to inject through the tubing of an IV infusion set that is known to be functioning satisfactorily. If the client complains of pain during IV injection, stop the injection immediately and evaluate for possible arterial injection or perivascular extravasation.
9. COMPATIBILITY 0.9% NaCl, D5W.
10. INCOMPATIBILITY Alkaline substances (causes precipitation of promethazine base). Administer separately.

ASSESSMENT

1. List reasons for therapy, onset/characteristics of S&S, triggers, other agents trialed. Assess for sedation and fall risk.
2. Note age; avoid in those under 2 years of age; older clients may manifest more adverse side effects. Assess for respiratory depression and level of sedation following dosing.

3. If tremors, drooling, shuffling gait, dysphagia (parkinsonism-like effects); restlessness (akathisia) or muscle spasms and twisting like motions (dystonia) occur, hold drug and report.
4. With chronic therapy, may experience blood dyscrasias.
5. Stop drug 48 hr prior to scheduled myelogram, and do not resume for 24 hr following procedure; ↑ risk seizure activity.
6. When used as adjunct to analgesics, be aware drug has no analgesic ability (only sedative effects); may be pronounced.
7. Monitor VS, BS, and CBC.

CLIENT/FAMILY TEACHING

1. Take only as directed and do not exceed dose; cardiac arrhythmias may occur. May take with food or milk to decrease GI upset.
2. When used to prevent motion sickness, take 30–60 min before travel. On successive travel days, take on rising and again before the evening meal.
3. Avoid activities requiring mental alertness until drug effects realized; may cause sedation. Change positions slowly to prevent sudden drop in BP.
4. Do not consume alcohol, CNS depressants, or OTC agents unless provider approved.
5. Drug may alter skin testing; stop 72 hr before testing.
6. Consume adequate fluids to prevent dehydration; use caution in hot weather to prevent heat stroke.
7. Avoid prolonged sun exposure; may cause photosensitivity reaction. Wear sunscreen and protection if exposed.
8. Report any involuntary muscle movements, palpitations, high fever, muscle rigidity, altered mental status (e.g., confusion, disorientation), excessive dizziness/drowsiness, sore throat, unusual bruising/bleeding, or yellowing of the skin or eyes.
9. Keep all F/U to assess response, labs, and for adverse SE.

OUTCOMES/EVALUATE

- Prevention of vertigo/motion sickness
- Relief of N&V
- Sedation
- Control of allergic manifestations

Propafenone hydrochloride

(proh-pah-**FEN**-ohn)

Classification(s): Antiarrhythmic, Class IC

Pregnancy Category: C

RX: Rythmol, Rythmol SR.

♣ **Rx:** Apo-Propafenone, Gen-Propafenone.

INDICATIONS/USES

Immediate-Release. (1) Prolong the time to recurrence of paroxysmal atrial fibrillation/flutter associated with disabling symptoms in clients without structural heart disease. (2) To prolong the time to recurrence of paroxysmal supraventricular tachycardia associated with disabling symptoms in clients without structural heart disease. (3) Treatment of ventricular arrhythmias, such as sustained ventricular tachycardia, that are life-threatening.

Extended-Release. Prolong the time to recurrence of symptomatic atrial fibrillation in clients without structural heart disease. *NOTE:* Antiarrhythmic drugs have not been shown to improve survival in clients with ventricular arrhythmias.

Investigational: Arrhythmias associated with Wolff-Parkinson-White syndrome.

ACTION/KINETICS

Action

Manifests local anesthetic effects and a direct stabilizing action on the myocardium. Reduces upstroke velocity (Phase O) of the monophasic action potential, reduces the fast inward current carried by sodium ions in the Purkinje fibers, increases diastolic excitability threshold, and prolongs the effective refractory period. Also, spontaneous activity is decreased. Slows AV conduction and causes first-degree heart block. Has slight beta-adrenergic blocking activity.

Pharmacokinetics

Almost completely absorbed after PO administration. **Peak plasma levels:** 3.5 hr. **Therapeutic serum levels:** 0.06–1 mcg/mL. Significant first-pass effect. Most metabolize rapidly (**t½:** 2–10 hr) to two active metabolites: 5-hydroxypropafenone and N-depropylpropafenone. However, approximately 10% (as well as those taking quinidine) metabolize the drug more slowly (**t½:** 10–32 hr).

P

Less than 1% excreted unchanged. Because the 5-hydroxy metabolite is not formed in slow metabolizers and because steady-state levels are reached after 4–5 days in all clients, the recommended dosing regimen is the same for all clients. **Plasma protein binding:** 97%.

CONTRAINDICATIONS

Uncontrolled CHF, cardiogenic shock, sick sinus node syndrome or AV block in the absence of an artificial pacemaker, bradycardia, marked hypotension, bronchospastic disorders, electrolyte disorders, hypersensitivity to the drug. MI more than 6 days but less than 2 years previously. Use to control ventricular rate during atrial fibrillation. Use with lesser ventricular arrhythmias, even if clients are symptomatic. Lactation.

SPECIAL CONCERNS

The National Heart, Lung, and Blood Institute's Cardiac Arrhythmia Suppression Trial (CAST) reported that in clients with asymptomatic non-life-threatening ventricular arrhythmias who had an MI more than 6 days but less than 2 years previously, an increased rate of death or reversed cardiac arrest rate was seen in clients treated with encainide or flecainide (Class 1C antiarrhythmics) compared with that seen in those receiving a placebo. The applicability of the CAST results to other populations (e.g., those without recent MI) or other antiarrhythmic drugs is uncertain, but at present, it is prudent to consider any 1C antiarrhythmic to have a significant risk in clients with structural heart disease. Given the lack of any evidence that these drugs improve survival, antiarrhythmic drugs should generally be avoided in those with non-life-threatening ventricular arrhythmias, even if the clients are experiencing unpleasant, but not life-threatening symptoms or signs.

- May cause new or worsened arrhythmias or CHF.
- Use with caution during labor and delivery.
- Use with caution in clients with impaired hepatic or renal function.
- Geriatric clients may require lower dosage.
- Monitor clients taking propafenone and an inhibitor of CYP1A2, CYP2D6, or CYP3A4 metabolizing enzymes; dosage adjustment may be necessary.
- Safety and effectiveness not determined in children.

SIDE EFFECTS

Most Common

Dizziness, N&V, unusual taste, constipation, blurred vision, angina, CHF, palpitations, proarrhythmia, fatigue, headache, dyspnea, rash, weakness.

CV: ***New or worsened arrhythmias.*** First-degree AV block, intraventricular conduction delay, palpitations, PVCs, proarrhythmia, bradycardia, atrial fibrillation, angina, syncope, CHF, ***ventricular tachycardia, second-degree AV block***, increased QRS duration, chest pain, hypotension, bundle branch block. Less commonly, atrial flutter, AV dissociation, flushing, hot flashes, sick sinus syndrome, sinus pause or arrest, SVT, prolongation of the PR and QRS interval, ***cardiac arrest.*** **CNS:** Dizziness, headache, anxiety, drowsiness, fatigue, loss of balance, ataxia, insomnia. Less commonly, abnormal speech/dreams/vision, confusion, depression, memory loss, ***apnea***, psychosis/mania, vertigo, ***seizures, coma***, numbness, paresthesias. **GI:** Unusual taste, constipation, nausea and/or vomiting, dry mouth, anorexia, flatulence, abdominal pain, cramps, diarrhea, dyspepsia. Less commonly, gastroenteritis and liver abnormalities (cholestasis, hepatitis, elevated enzymes). **Hematologic**: ***Agranulocytosis***, increased bleeding time, anemia, granulocytopenia, bruising, leukopenia, purpura, thrombocytopenia. **Miscellaneous:** Blurred vision, dyspnea, weakness, rash, edema, tremors, diaphoresis, joint pain, possible decrease in spermatogenesis. Less commonly, tinnitus, unusual smell sensation, alopecia, eye irritation, hyponatremia, inappropriate ADH secretion, impotence, increased glucose, kidney failure, lupus erythematosus, muscle cramps or weakness, nephrotic syndrome, pain, pruritus, exacerbation of myasthenia gravis.

LABORATORY TEST CONSIDERATIONS

↑ ANA titers, alkaline phosphatase, AST, ALT.

OVERDOSE MANAGEMENT

Symptoms: Bradycardia, hypotension, IA and intraventricular conduction disturbances, somnolence. ***Rarely, high-grade ventricular arrhythmias and seizures.*** *Treatment:* To control BP and cardiac rhythm, defibrillation and infusion of dopamine or isoproterenol. If seizures occur, diazepam, IV, can be given. External cardiac massage and mechanical respiratory assistance may be required.

P

DRUG INTERACTIONS

Drugs that inhibit CYP2D6, CYP1A2, and CYP3A4 may lead to increased plasma levels of propafenone; monitor such situations carefully.

Beta-adrenergic blockers / ↑ Levels of beta blockers metabolized by the liver
Cimetidine / ↑ Propafenone levels → ↑ effects
Cyclosporine / ↑ Cyclosporine trough levels; ↓ renal function
Desipramine / ↑ Desipramine levels
Digoxin / ↑ Digoxin levels → ↓ digoxin dose
Local anesthetics / May ↑ risk of CNS side effects
Mexiletine / ↓ Metabolic clearance of mexiletine in extensive metabolizers → no differences between extensive and poor metabolizers
Quinidine / ↑ Propafenone levels in rapid metabolizers → possible ↑ effect
Rifamycins / ↓ Propafenone effect R/T ↑ clearance
Ritonavir / Large ↑ in propafenone levels; do not use together
SSRIs / Certain SSRIs may inhibit the metabolism (by CYP2D6) of propafenone
Theophylline / ↑ Theophylline levels → possible toxicity
Warfarin / May ↑ warfarin levels; ↓ warfarin dose

HOW SUPPLIED

Capsules, Extended-Release: 225 mg, 325 mg, 425 mg; ***Tablets, Immediate-Release:*** 150 mg, 225 mg.

DOSAGE

CAPSULES, EXTENDED-RELEASE

Symptomatic atrial fibrillation without structural heart disease.

Individualize dosage based on response and tolerance. **Initial:** 225 mg q 12 hr; increase in 5 day or more intervals to 325 mg q 12 hr. Increase to 425 mg q 12 hr if needed.

TABLETS, IMMEDIATE-RELEASE

Titrate on basis of response and tolerance. **Adults, initial:** 150 mg q 8 hr; dose may be increased at a minimum of q 3–4 days to 225 mg q 8 hr and, if necessary, to 300 mg q 8 hr. The safety and efficacy of doses exceeding 900 mg/day have not been established.

NURSING IMPLICATIONS

IMPLEMENTATION/ADMINISTRATION/STORAGE

1. Always initiate therapy in a hospital setting.
2. Consider dose reduction in those in whom significant widening of the QRS complex or second- or third-degree AV block occurs. Consider dose reduction in those with hepatic impairment.
3. Increase the dose of the immediate-release tablets more gradually during the initial treatment phase in the elderly or in those with marked previous myocardial damage.
4. There is no evidence that the use of propafenone affects the survival or incidence of sudden death with recent MI or SVT.

ASSESSMENT

1. List reasons for therapy noting ECG and baseline arrhythmias; note any cardiac problems, list drugs prescribed to ensure none interact.
2. Report any significant QT prolongation, any evidence of second- or third-degree AV block and assess for CHF. May induce new or more severe arrhythmias; titrate dose based on client response and tolerance. Avoid in those with non-life-threatening ventricular arrhythmias despite S&S.
3. May alter both pacing and sensing thresholds of artificial pacemakers; monitor and program pacemakers accordingly during therapy.
4. Increase dose more gradually in elderly clients as well as those with previous myocardial damage.
5. Evaluate hematologic studies for anemia, agranulocytosis, leukopenia, thrombocytopenia, altered prothrombin and coagulation times.
6. Will be initiated in hospital in monitored setting. Avoid with bronchospastic disease.
7. Monitor VS, I&O, CBC, electrolytes, renal, and LFTS. Assess for renal or hepatic disease.

CLIENT/FAMILY TEACHING

1. The sustained-release capsules can be taken with or without food. Do not crush or further divide the contents of the capsule. Drug is used to prevent serious heart rhythm disorders.
2. Avoid activities that require mental alertness until drug effects realized, may experience dizziness and drowsiness.

P

3. May experience dizziness or unusual taste in the mouth; report if interferes with walking, eating, or nutritional status.
4. Drink adequate quantities of fluid (2–3 L/day) and add bulk to the diet to avoid constipation.
5. Report increased chest pain, SOB, blurred vision, palpitations, unusual bruising/bleeding, or S&S of liver failure such as yellow eyes, dark-yellow urine, or yellow skin. Also report any urinary tract problems or decreased urinary output. Record BP and pulse readings for provider review. Ensure family know CPR.
6. Keep all F/U to assess response, labs, and for adverse SE.

OUTCOMES/EVALUATE

- Termination of life-threatening VT; restoration of stable rhythm
- Therapeutic drug levels (0.06–1 mcg/mL)

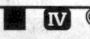

■ IV

Propranolol hydrochloride

(proh-**PRAN**-oh-lohl)

Classification(s): Beta-adrenergic blocking agent

Pregnancy Category: C

RX: Inderal LA, InnoPran XL.

✦ **Rx:** Apo-Propranolol.

SEE ALSO ***BETA-ADRENERGIC BLOCKING AGENTS***.

P

INDICATIONS/USES

PO. Propranolol is approved for use in adults for the following: (1) To decrease angina frequency and increase exercise tolerance in angina pectoris due to coronary atherosclerosis (*excluding InnoPran XL*). (2) Control ventricular rate in atrial fibrillation and a rapid ventricular response (*excluding extended-release products*). (3) Management of familial and hereditary essential tremor (*excluding extended-release products*). (4) Management of hypertension alone or in combination with other antihypertensive drugs, especially thiazide diuretics. Not to be used for hypertensive emergencies. (5) Improvement of New York Heart Association functional class in symptomatic clients with hypertrophic subaortic stenosis (*excluding InnoPran XL*). (6) Prophylaxis of common migraine headache (*excluding InnoPran XL*). Not to be used for an established migraine attack. (7) Reduce CV mortality in those who have survived the acute phase of MI and are clinically stable (*excluding extended-release products*). (8) Adjunct to alpha-adrenergic blockade to control BP and reduce symptoms of catecholamine-secreting tumors. *Investigational:* Traumatic brain injury.

IV. (1) Short-term treatment of supraventricular tachycardia, including Wolff-Parkinson-White syndrome and thyrotoxicosis (to decrease ventricular rate). (2) Ventricular tachycardias. (3) Control ventricular rate in life-threatening digitalis-induced arrhythmias (severe bradycardia may occur). (4) Treatment of persistent premature ventricular extrasystoles that impair the well-being of the client and do not respond to conventional measures. (5) Resistant tachyarrhythmias due to excessive catecholamine action during anesthesia.

ACTION/KINETICS

Action

Combines reversibly with beta-adrenergic receptors to block the response to sympathetic nerve impulses, circulating catecholamines, or adrenergic drugs. Manifests both beta-1- and beta-2-adrenergic blocking activity. Is also an antiarrhythmic, type II. Antiarrhythmic action is due to both beta-adrenergic receptor blockade and a direct membrane-stabilizing action on the cardiac cell; decreases HR. Has no intrinsic sympathomimetic activity and has high lipid solubility.

Pharmacokinetics

Bioavailability is 30% for immediate-release and 9–18% for the long-acting product. **Onset, PO:** 30 min; **IV:** immediate. **Maximum effect:** 1–1.5 hr. **Duration:** 3–5 hr. **t½:** 2–3 hr (8–11 hr for long-acting). **Therapeutic serum level, antiarrhythmic:** 0.05–0.1 mcg/mL. Completely metabolized by liver and excreted in urine. Although food increases bioavailability, absorption may be decreased. **Plasma protein binding:** 90–95%.

CONTRAINDICATIONS

Bronchial asthma, bronchospasms including severe COPD. Treatment of hypertensive emergencies.

SPECIAL CONCERNS

■ **Angina pectoris.** There have been reports of exacerbation of angina and, in some cases, myocardial infarction, following abrupt discontinuance of propranolol therapy. Therefore, when discontinuance of propranolol is planned, the dosage should be gradually reduced over at least a few weeks, and the client should be cautioned against interruption or cessation of therapy without a health care provider's advice. If propranolol therapy is interrupted and exacerbation of angina pectoris occurs, it is usually advisable to reinstitute propranolol therapy and take other measures appropriate for the management of angina pectoris. Because coronary artery disease may be unrecognized, it may be prudent to follow the preceding advice in clients considered at risk of having occult atherosclerotic heart disease who are given propranolol for other indications. ■

It is dangerous to use propranolol for pheochromocytoma unless an alpha-adrenergic blocking agent is already in use.

SIDE EFFECTS

Most Common

Insomnia, anxiety, impotence, nervousness, fatigue, dizziness, drowsiness, lightheadedness, diarrhea, vision problems.

See *Beta-Adrenergic Blocking Agents* for a complete list of possible side effects. Also, psoriasis-like eruptions, skin necrosis, SLE (rare).

LABORATORY TEST CONSIDERATIONS

↑ Blood urea, serum transaminase, alkaline phosphatase, LDH. Interference with glaucoma screening test.

ADDITIONAL DRUG INTERACTIONS

Gabapentin / Possible paroxysmal dystonic movements in the hands
Haloperidol / Severe hypotension
Hydralazine / ↑ Effect of both agents
Methimazole / May ↑ propranolol effects
Phenobarbital / ↓ Propranolol effect R/T ↑ liver breakdown
Propylthiouracil / May ↑ propranolol effects
Rifampin / ↓ Propranolol effect R/T ↑ liver breakdown
Rizatriptan / ↑ AUC and peak rizatriptan levels R/T ↓ rizatriptan metabolism
Smoking / ↓ Serum levels and ↑ clearance of propranolol R/T ↑ hepatic metabolism

HOW SUPPLIED

Capsules, Extended-Release: 60 mg, 80 mg, 120 mg, 160 mg; ***Injection:*** 1 mg/mL; ***Oral Solution:*** 4 mg/mL, 8 mg/mL; ***Tablets:*** 10 mg, 20 mg, 40 mg, 60 mg, 80 mg.

DOSAGE

ORAL SOLUTION; TABLETS, IMMEDIATE-RELEASE

Angina pectoris due to coronary atherosclerosis.

Adults, initial: 80–320 mg 2–4 times per day; **dose range:** 80–320 mg 2-, 3-, or 4 times per day. Gradually increase initial dose at 3–7 day intervals until optimum response is obtained). Do not exceed 320 mg/day. If therapy is to be discontinued, reduce dose gradually over several weeks.

Atrial fibrillation

Adults: 10–30 mg 3–4 times per day given before meals and at bedtime.

Essential tremor.

Adults, initial: 40 mg twice a day; **then,** 120 mg/day up to 240–320 mg/day.

Hypertension.

Adults, initial: 40 mg twice a day whether used alone or with a diuretic. **Maintenance:** Increase initial dose to maintenance level of 120–240 mg/day given in two to three divided doses; some may require 640 mg/day. Do not exceed 640 mg/day. Some clients may experience a rise in BP after 12 hr; thus, daily dosage may be given 3 times/day to achieve better control. Dosage may be increased gradually until adequate BP control is reached; this may take a few days to several weeks.

Hypertrophic subaortic stenosis.

Adults: 20–40 mg 3–4 times per day before meals and at bedtime.

Migraine prophylaxis.

Adults, initial: 80 mg/day in divided doses; **usual dosage:** 160–240 mg/day. Dosage may be increased gradually to achieve optimal migraine prophylaxis. If a satisfactory response has not been

P

observed after 4–6 weeks, discontinue the drug and withdraw gradually over several weeks.

Pheochromocytoma, preoperatively.

Adults: 60 mg/day for 3 days before surgery, given concomitantly with an alpha-adrenergic blocking agent.

Myocardial infarction.

Adults, initial: 40 mg 3 times per day; after 1 month, titrate to 60–80 mg 3 times/day as tolerated. **Maintenance:** 180–240 mg/day. Efficacy and safety of doses greater than 240 mg/day have not been established.

Pheochromocytoma, preoperatively.

Adults: 60 mg/day in divided doses for 3 days prior to surgery, together with an alpha-adrenergic blocking agent.

Pheochromocytoma, inoperable tumors.

Adults: 30 mg/day in divided doses together with an alpha-adrenergic blocking agent.

CAPSULES, EXTENDED-RELEASE *(excluding InnoPran XL)*

Angina pectoris.

Adults, initial: 80 mg once daily; increase dosage gradually at 3- to 7-day intervals until optimal response is reached. **Average dose:** 160 mg once daily; doses exceeding 320 mg daily have not been evaluated. If treatment is to be discontinued, reduce dosage gradually over a few weeks.

Hypertension.

Adults, initial: 80 mg once daily whether used alone or with a diuretic; dosage may be increased to 120 mg once daily or higher over a period of a few days to several weeks until adequate BP control is reached. **Usual maintenance dose:** 120–160 mg once a day; up to 640 mg may be required in some clients.

Hypertrophic subaortic stenosis.

Adults: 80–160 mg once daily.

Migraine, prophylaxis.

Adults, initial: 80 mg once daily; dosage may be increased gradually to achieve optimal migraine prophylaxis. **Usual dose range:** 160–240 mg once daily. If a satisfactory response is not reached within 4 to 6 weeks after reaching the maximum dose, discontinue therapy. Withdraw the drug gradually over several weeks.

CAPSULES, EXTENDED-RELEASE *(InnoPran XL only)*

Hypertension.

Adults: 80 mg once a day at bedtime (approximately 10 p.m.). Titration may be needed to a dose of 120 mg. The time for a full antihypertensive effect is variable but is usually reached in 2–3 weeks.

IV

Life-threatening arrhythmias or those occurring under anesthesia.

Adults: 1–3 mg under careful monitoring, not to exceed 1 mg/min; a second dose may be given after 2 min, with subsequent doses q 4 hr. Begin PO therapy as soon as possible. **Children:** Although use in pediatrics is not recommended, investigational doses of 0.01–0.25 mg/kg given over 10 min, up to a maximum of 1 mg/dose in infants and 3 mg/dose in children; give at a rate not to exceed 1 mg/min. Repeat q 6–8 hr as needed.

NURSING IMPLICATIONS

Do not confuse propranolol with Pravachol (antihyperlipidemic). Also, do not confuse Inderal with Inderide (an antihypertensive) or with Isordil (a coronary vasodilator).

IMPLEMENTATION/ADMINISTRATION/STORAGE

1. Regardless of the route of administration, when discontinuance is planned, gradually reduce the dose over at least a few weeks.
2. Do not administer for a minimum of 2 weeks after MAO drug use.
3. Protect products from light, moisture, freezing, and excessive heat. Store in tight, light-resistant containers.
4. For the elderly, start at the low end of the dosing range.
5. The pharmacokinetics of the extended-release product have not been studied in impaired renal or hepatic function.

6. The extended-release capsules are not a simple mg-for-mg substitute for propranolol immediate-release tablets. Retitration may be necessary if switching from tablets to capsules, especially to maintain effectiveness at the end of the 24-hr dosing regimen for extended-release capsules.
7. Store PO products 15–30°C (59–86°F). Protect the ER capsules from light, moisture, freezing, and excessive heat.
8. IV Reserve IV use for life-threatening arrhythmias or those occurring during anesthesia.
9. If signs of serious myocardial depression occur, slowly infuse isoproterenol (Isuprel) IV.
10. Consider reducing the IV dose in those with hepatic insufficiency.
11. Dilute 1 mg in 10 mL of D5W and administer IV over at least 1 min. May be further reconstituted in 50 mL of dextrose or saline solution and infused IVPB over 10–15 min. The rate of administration should not exceed 1 mg/min.
12. After IV administration, have emergency drugs and equipment available to combat hypotension or circulatory collapse.
13. Store the injection at about 25°C (77°F); protect from light, freezing, and excessive heat. Store in carton until time of use. Discard any unused portion.
14. COMPATIBILITY Dextrose or saline solutions.
15. INCOMPATIBILITY Administer separately.

ASSESSMENT

1. List reasons for therapy, onset, duration, characteristics of S&S, other agents trialed, outcome. Assess mental status and note any depression.
2. Note ECG, and cardiopulmonary findings. Assess for pulmonary disease, bronchospasms, CAD, bradycardia, heart block, depression; may preclude therapy.
3. Continuously monitor ECG and BP with IV infusion. Do not exceed 1 mg (1 mL)/minute to diminish possibility of lowering BP and causing cardiac standstill.
4. Report rash, fever, and/or purpura; S&S of hypersensitivity reaction.
5. List all drugs prescribed to ensure none interact.
6. Observe for S&S of CHF (e.g., SOB, rales, edema, and weight gain).
7. Monitor glucose, uric acid, TSH, K^+, renal/LFTs, (monitor closely with dysfunction), VS, I&O.

CLIENT/FAMILY TEACHING

1. Sustained-release products are usually taken at bedtime. It is recommended that InnoPran XL be taken about 10 p.m. on an empty stomach or with food.
2. Mix the concentrated oral solution with liquid or semi-solid food (e.g., water, juices, soda or soda-like beverages, applesauce, and puddings). Draw into dropper the amount prescribed for a single dose; squeeze the dropper contents into the liquid or semi-solid food. Stir for a few seconds. Consume the entire amount of the mixture immediately. Do not store for future use.
3. May cause drowsiness; assess drug response before performing activities that require mental alertness.
4. Do not smoke; smoking decreases serum levels and interferes with drug clearance.
5. May mask signs of low blood sugar, such as a rapid heartbeat; monitor FS carefully. Report any skin rashes, abnormal bleeding, unusual crying, or feelings of depression.
6. Keep log of BP and pulse for provider review; report significant changes. To help control BP: maintain healthy diet and limit intake of caffeine, avoid alcohol, salt substitutes, or high Na^+ and high K^+ foods, perform regular exercise, maintain weight, and stop smoking.
7. Do not stop abruptly or without provider approval; may precipitate hypertension, angina, heart attack, or cardiac arrhythmias. Must taper off dose over several weeks.
8. Dress appropriately; may cause increased sensitivity to cold.
9. Avoid alcohol and any OTC agents containing alpha-adrenergic stimulants or sympathomimetics.
10. Keep all F/U to assess response, labs, and for adverse SE.

OUTCOMES/EVALUATE

- ↓ BP, ↓ HR
- ↓ Angina; prophylaxis of myocardial reinfarction
- Prophylaxis of vascular headaches
- Management of thyrotoxicosis
- Control of tachyarrhythmias
- ↓ Tremors; ↓ S&S PTSD

P

Propylthiouracil

(proh-pill-thigh-oh-**YOUR**-ah-sill)

Classification(s): Antithyroid drug

Pregnancy Category: D

Rx: Propyl-Thyracil.

INDICATIONS/USES

(1) Long-term therapy for hyperthyroidism. (2) Hyperthyroidism prior to surgery for subtotal thyroidectomy or radiotherapy. *NOTE:* Reserve propylthiouracil for those who are intolerant of methimazole and for whom surgery (including thyroidectomy) or radioactive iodine is not an appropriate treatment regimen. *Investigational:* Reduce mortality due to alcoholic liver disease.

ACTION/KINETICS

Action

Inhibits (partially or completely) the production of thyroid hormones by the thyroid gland by preventing the incorporation of iodide into tyrosine and coupling of iodotyrosines. Does not affect release or activity of preformed hormone; thus, it may take several weeks for the therapeutic effect to become established. May be preferred for treatment of thyroid storm, as it inhibits peripheral conversion of thyroxine to triiodothyronine.

Pharmacokinetics

Rapidly absorbed from the GI tract and concentrated in the thyroid gland. Is 80–95% bioavailable. **Duration:** 2–3 hr. **t½:** 1–2 hr. **Onset:** 10–20 days. **Time to peak effect:** 2–10 weeks. Metabolized by the liver and excreted through the kidneys. **Plasma protein binding:** 75–80%.

CONTRAINDICATIONS

Hypersensitivity to antithyroid drugs. Lactation (may cause hypothyroidism in infant). Use in children unless methimazole is not well tolerated and surgery or radioactive iodine therapy are not appropriate.

SPECIAL CONCERNS

■ (1) **Hepatotoxicity.** Severe liver injury and acute liver failure, in some cases fatal, have been reported in clients treated with propylthiouracil. These reports of hepatic reactions include cases requiring liver transplantation in adults and children. Reserve propylthiouracil for clients who cannot tolerate methimazole and in whom radioactive iodine therapy or surgery are not appropriate treatment for management of hyperthyroidism. (2) **Pregnancy.** Because of the risk of fetal abnormalities associated with methimazole, propylthiouracil may be the treatment of choice when an antithyroid drug is indicated during or just prior to the first trimester of pregnancy. ■

- **Incidence of vasculitis is increased.**
- **Use with caution in the presence of CV disease.**
- **Monitor PT due to possible hypoprothrombinemia and bleeding.**

SIDE EFFECTS

Most Common

Rash, itching, urticaria, N&V, heartburn, loss of taste, swelling, joint/muscle aches, headache, numbness.

Hematologic: ***Agranulocytosis***, thrombocytopenia, granulocytopenia, hypoprothrombinemia and bleeding, ***aplastic anemia***, leukopenia. **GI:** N&V, taste loss, epigastric pain, sialadenopathy. **Hepatic:** Jaundice, hepatitis, hepatic injury leading to ***liver failure***, liver transplantation, or ***death***. **CNS:** Headache, paresthesias, drowsiness, vertigo, depression, CNS stimulation, neuritis, neuropathies, vertigo. **CV:** Periarteritis, leukocytoplastic vasculitis. **Dermatologic:** Skin rash/ulcers, urticaria, alopecia, lupus-like syndrome (including splenomegaly and vasculitis), skin pigmentation, pruritus, exfoliative dermatitis, erythema nodosum. **Musculoskeletal:** Arthralgia, myalgia, myopathy. **Respiratory:** Interstitial pneumonitis, ***alveolar hemorrhage***, pulmonary infiltrates. **GU:** Glomerulonephritis, nephritis. **Metabolic:** Hypothyroidism, edema. **Body as a whole:** Drug fever, abnormal hair loss. **Miscellaneous:** Lymphadenopathy, antineutrophil cytoplasmic antibody-positive vasculitis (may include rapidly progressive glomerulonephritis sometimes leading to acute renal failure, arthralgia, drug fever, edema, and insulin autoimmune syndrome resulting in hypoglycemic coma).

OVERDOSE MANAGEMENT

Symptoms: N&V, headache, fever, pruritus, epigastric distress, arthralgia, pancytopenia, ***agranulocytosis*** (most serious). Rarely, exfoliative dermatitis, hepatitis, neuropathies, CNS stimulation or depression. *Treatment:* Maintain a patent airway and support ventilation and perfusion. Very carefully monitor and maintain VS, blood gases, and serum electrolytes. Monitor bone marrow function.

DRUG INTERACTIONS

Propylthiouracil may produce hypoprothrombinemia, adding to the effect of anticoagulants

HOW SUPPLIED

Tablets: 50 mg.

DOSAGE

TABLETS

Hyperthyroidism.

Adults, initial: 300 mg/day, usually given in 3 equally divided doses about 8 hr apart. In those with severe hyperthyroidism, very large goiters or both, the initial dose is usually 400 mg/day; occasionally a client will require 600–900 mg/day. **Maintenance, usual:** 100–150 mg/day. *NOTE:* Propylthiouracil is generally not recommended for use in children, except in rare instances where other alternative therapies are not appropriate options. **Pediatric, 6 years and older, initial:** 50 mg/day in three equal doses about 8 hr apart; carefully titrate upward based on clinical response and evaluation of TSH and free T4 levels. Maintenance for all pediatric use is based on response.

Investigational: **Alternative dose for children, older than 10 years, initial:** 150–300 mg/day in divided doses q 8 hr or 5–7 mg/kg/day divided q 8 hr; **maintenance:** ⅓-⅔ the initial dose divided q 8–12 hr when client is euthyroid (usually after 2 months). **Alternative dose for children, 6–10 years, initial:** 50–150 mg/day divided q 8 hr or 5–7 mg/kg/day divided q 8 hr; **maintenance:** ⅓–⅔ the initial dose divided q 8–12 hr when client is euthyroid (usually after 2 months). **Alternative dose for children, less than 6 years and infants, initial:** 5–7 mg/kg/day divided q 8 hr; **maintenance:** ⅓–⅔ the initial dose divided q 8–12 hr when client is euthyroid (usually after 2 months). **Alternative dose for neonates:** 5–10 mg/kg/day divided q 8 hr.

Reduce mortality due to alcoholic liver disease (investigational).

Adults: 300 mg/day.

NURSING IMPLICATIONS

IMPLEMENTATION/ADMINISTRATION/STORAGE

1. Cases of severe liver injury have been reported in adults and children. In children, doses as low as 50 mg/day have caused liver injury, although most cases were associated with doses of 300 mg/day or higher.
2. Store tablets from 15–30°C (59–86°F). Protect from light and moisture.

ASSESSMENT

1. Note onset, symptoms experienced, physical presentation, any underlying cause. Identify if for long term management of hyperthyroidism or prep for other therapy (i.e., subtotal thyroidectomy or radioactive iodine therapy).
2. Check if pregnant; may require reduced dosage as pregnancy progresses (may cause fetal harm).
3. Assess thyroid gland noting any enlargement, pain, asymmetry, nodules, or bruits and scan results.
4. Check children every 6 months for appropriate growth and development; plot on a graph.
5. Monitor VS, I&O, and weights; PT, CBC, LFT, ECG, and thyroid function studies. Assess carefully for agranulocytosis.

CLIENT/FAMILY TEACHING

1. Take with meals to minimize GI irritation.
2. It takes 6–12 weeks for the drug to produce full effect. Take regularly and exactly as directed q 8 hr around the clock. Hyperthyroidism may recur if not taken properly. Regularly record heart rate and weight.
3. May cause drowsiness, avoid activities that require mental alertness until effects realized.
4. Report symptoms of hyperthyroidism or thyrotoxicosis (palpitations, increased HR, nervousness, sleeplessness, sweating, diarrhea, weight loss, fever). Report symptoms of hypothyroidism (weak, listless, tired, headache, dry

P

skin, cold intolerance, constipation) as dosage may require adjustment.

5. Any sore throat, skin eruptions, enlargement of the cervical lymph nodes, GI disturbances, fever, skin rashes, itching, or jaundice should be reported; may require either a dosage reduction or withdrawal of the drug. Hepatic dysfunction, such as unexplained nausea, vomiting, abdominal pain, fatigue, anorexia, or jaundice and/or dark urine require immediate reporting.
6. Report symptoms of iodism (cold symptoms, skin lesions, stomatitis, GI upset, metallic taste)
7. Identify dietary sources of iodine (iodized salt, shellfish, turnips, cabbage, kale) that may need to be omitted from the diet.
8. Report unusual bleeding, alopecia, nausea, loss of taste, or epigastric pain.
9. When drug is taken for 1 year, more than half the clients achieve a permanent remission. Those who relapse are usually treated with radioiodine.
10. Carry ID listing medical problems and currently prescribed medications.
11. Read labels carefully for sources of iodine. Avoid all OTC agents without approval.
12. Keep all F/U to assess response, labs, and for adverse SE.

OUTCOMES/EVALUATE

- Normal metabolism; control of S&S hyperthyroidism (↑ weight, ↓ sweating, ↓ HR)
- Suppression of thyroid hormones (↓ T_3, T_4); thyroid function studies within desired range (euthyroid)

P

IV

Protamine sulfate

(**PROH**-tah-meen)

Classification(s): Heparin antagonist

Pregnancy Category: C

INDICATIONS/USES

Only for treatment of heparin overdose.

ACTION/KINETICS

Action

A strong basic polypeptide that complexes with strongly acidic heparin to form an inactive stable salt. The complex has no anticoagulant activity. Heparin is neutralized within 5 min after IV protamine.

Pharmacokinetics

Onset: Rapid. **Duration:** 2 hr (but depends on body temperature). The t½ of protamine is shorter than heparin; thus, repeated doses may be required. Upon metabolism, the complex may liberate heparin (heparin rebound).

CONTRAINDICATIONS

Previous intolerance to protamine. Use to treat spontaneous hemorrhage, postpartum hemorrhage, menorrhagia, or uterine bleeding. Administration of over 50 mg over a short period.

SPECIAL CONCERNS

- Use with caution during lactation.
- Hyperheparinemia or bleeding may occur up to 18 hr after cardiac surgery (under cardiopulmonary bypass) in spite of complete neutralization of heparin by adequate protamine sulfate doses.
- Rapid administration may cause severe hypotension and anaphylaxis.
- Safety and efficacy not determined in children.

SIDE EFFECTS

Most Common

Sudden fall in BP, bradycardia, transitory flushing, warm feeling, dyspnea, N&V, lassitude.

CV: Sudden fall in BP, bradycardia, transitory flushing, warm feeling, ***acute pulmonary hypertension, circulatory collapse (possibly irreversible) with myocardial failure*** and decreased CO. Pulmonary edema in clients on cardiopulmonary bypass undergoing CV surgery. **Anaphylaxis:** Severe respiratory distress, ***circulatory collapse***, capillary leak, and noncardiogenic pulmonary edema. **GI:** N&V. **CNS:** Lassitude. **Miscellaneous:** Dyspnea, back pain in conscious clients undergoing cardiac catheterization, hypersensitivity reactions.

OVERDOSE MANAGEMENT

Symptoms: Bleeding. Rapid administration may cause dyspnea, bradycardia, flushing, warm feeling, severe hypotension, hypertension. In assessing overdose, there may be the possibility of multiple drug overdoses leading to drug interactions and unusual pharmacokinetics. *Treatment:* Replace blood loss with blood transfusions or fresh frozen plasma. Fluids, epinephrine, dobutamine, or dopamine to treat hypotension

DRUG INTERACTIONS

Protamine sulfate is incompatible with certain antibiotics, including certain cephalosporins and penicillins.

HOW SUPPLIED

Injection: 10 mg/mL.

DOSAGE

SLOW IV

Heparin overdose.

Give no more than 50 mg of protamine sulfate over 10-min by very slow IV infusion. One mg of protamine sulfate, calculated on a dried basis, can neutralize not less than 100 units of heparin. *NOTE:* The dose of protamine sulfate depends on the amount of time that has elapsed since IV heparin administration. For example, if 30 min has elapsed, one-half the usual dose of protamine sulfate may be sufficient because heparin is cleared rapidly from the circulation.

NURSING IMPLICATIONS

IMPLEMENTATION/ADMINISTRATION/STORAGE

1. IV Incompatible with several penicillins and with cephalosporins. Do not mix with other drugs.
2. To minimize side effects, give slowly over 10 min. Rapid administration can cause severe hypotensive and anaphylactoid reactions.
3. Is intended to be injected without further dilution. However, it may be diluted in 50 mL of D5W or saline solution and administered at a rate of 50 mg over 10–15 min. Do not store diluted solutions as they do not contain a preservative.
4. Previous exposure to protamine through use of protamine-containing insulins or during heparin neutralization may cause development of side effects from subsequent use of protamine.
5. Store at 15–30°C (59–86°F); do not freeze.
6. COMPATIBILITY D5W, 0.9% NaCl.
7. INCOMPATIBILITY Administer separately.

ASSESSMENT

1. Note amount, time of overdose, source to ensure appropriate antidote dosing.
2. Request type and crossmatch; assess need for fresh frozen plasma or whole blood.
3. Coagulation studies should be performed 5–15 min after protamine has been administered; repeat in 2–8 hr to assess for heparin rebound (increased bleeding, lowered BP, and/or shock).
4. Bleeding may occur up to 18 hr after cardiac surgery (under cardiopulmonary bypass) in spite of complete neutralization of heparin by adequate protamine sulfate doses; assess closely for any evidence for bleeding or hemorrhage.
5. Monitor VS, I&O, CBC, PT/PTT; assess for sudden fall in BP, bradycardia, dyspnea, transitory flushing, or sensations of warmth.

CLIENT/FAMILY TEACHING

1. Drug is administered IV to offset the effects of too much heparin which can lead to hemorrhage and shock due to fluid volume loss.
2. Report immediately any bleeding, SOB, dizziness, or swelling.
3. Avoid activities that could damage blood vessels or precipitate bleeding (e.g., shaving, vigorous toothbrushing, ambulation) until hemorrhage risk has passed.

OUTCOMES/EVALUATE

Stable H&H; control of heparin-induced hemorrhage

Pseudoephedrine hydrochloride

(soo-doh-eh-**FED**-rin)

Classification(s): Sympathomimetic
Pregnancy Category: B
OTC: Capsules: Sinustop. **Drops:** Kid Kare, Nasal Decongestant Oral. **Liquid/Syrup:** ElixSure Children's Congestion, Unifed. **Tablets:** Congestaid, Genaphed, Simply Stuffy, Sudafed Non-Drowsy Maximum Strength, SudoGest Non-Drowsy. **Tablets, Controlled Release or Extended-Release:** Dimetapp Maximum Strength 12-Hour Non-Drowsy Extentabs, Sudafed Non-Drowsy 12 Hour Long-Acting, Sudafed Non-Drowsy 24 Hour Long-Acting.
✤ **OTC:** Eltor 120.

SEE ALSO ***SYMPATHOMIMETIC DRUGS***.

P

INDICATIONS/USES

Temporary relief of nasal congestion due to hay fever, common cold, or other upper respiratory allergies associated with sinusitis.

ACTION/KINETICS

Action

Produces direct stimulation of both alpha- (pronounced) and beta-adrenergic receptors, as well as indirect stimulation through release of norepinephrine from storage sites. Results in decongestant effect on the nasal mucosa. Systemic administration eliminates possible damage to the nasal mucosa.

Pharmacokinetics

Onset: 15–30 min. **Time to peak effect:** 30–60 min. **Duration:** 3–4 hr. **Extended-release, duration:** 8–12 hr. Urinary excretion slowed by alkalinization, causing reabsorption of drug.

ADDITIONAL CONTRAINDICATIONS

Lactation. Not recommended for use in children less than 6 years of age. Use of sustained-release products in children less than 12 years of age.

SPECIAL CONCERNS

- **Geriatric clients may be more prone to age-related prostatic hypertrophy.**
- ***NOTE:* Pseudoephedrine products must be kept behind the counter in pharmacies, thus requiring clients to ask for the product.**

SIDE EFFECTS

Most Common

Somnolence, insomnia, nervousness, excitability, dizziness, anxiety, skin rashes, nausea, gastric irritation.

See *Sympathomimetic Drugs* for a complete list of possible side effects.

HOW SUPPLIED

Pseudoephedrine hydrochloride. ***Capsules:*** 60 mg; ***Drops:*** 7.5 mg/0.8 mL; ***Liquid/Syrup:*** 15 mg/5 mL, 30 mg/5 mL; ***Tablets:*** 30 mg, 60 mg; ***Tablets, Chewable:*** 15 mg; ***Tablets, Controlled-Release:*** 240 mg (60 mg immediate-release and 180 mg controlled-release); ***Tablets, Extended-Release:*** 120 mg.

DOSAGE

Pseudoephedrine Hydrochloride

CAPSULES; DROPS; LIQUID/SYRUP; TABLETS; TABLETS, CHEWABLE

Decongestant.

Adults, and children over 12 years: 60 mg q 4–6 hr, not to exceed 240 mg in 24 hr. **Pediatric, 6–12 years:** 30 mg using the drops, liquid, syrup or chewable tablets q 4–6 hr, not to exceed 120 mg in 24 hr; **2–6 years:** Use not recommended.

TABLETS, CONTROLLED-RELEASE (24 HR); TABLETS, EXTENDED-RELEASE (12 HR)

Decongestant.

Adults and children over 12 years: 120 mg of the sustained-release q 12 hr or 240 mg of the controlled-release q 24 hr. Do not exceed 240 mg/24 hr.

NURSING IMPLICATIONS

Do not confuse Sudafed (containing pseudoephedrine) with Sudafed PE (containing phenylephrine). Also, do not confuse Sudafed with Sotalol (an antiarrhythmic drug).

ASSESSMENT

1. **Note reasons for therapy, onset, characteristics of S&S, clinical presentation, other agents trialed, outcome.**
2. **Assess ENT, lung/heart sounds, palpate sinuses, check BP, HR; note allergy history and any triggers.**

CLIENT/FAMILY TEACHING

1. **Drug acts by constricting (shrinking) blood vessels (veins and arteries) in the nose, lungs, and other mucous membranes.**
2. **Avoid taking near bedtime; stimulation may produce insomnia.**
3. **With hypertension, report headaches, dizziness, or increased BP. Any extreme restlessness or sensitivity reactions should be reported.**

4. Take exactly as directed. Do not crush or chew extended-release products. Continuous use or excessive dosing may cause rebound congestion.
5. Use enclosed calibrated measuring device to administer liquid and calibrated dropper to administer drops to prevent excess dosing.
6. Avoid OTC medications; may also contain ephedrine or other sympathomimetic amines and intensify drug action.
7. Report if symptoms do not improve after 3–5 days or worsen. Identify triggers and practice avoidance especially with seasonal allergies.
8. Keep all F/U to assess response and for adverse SE.

OUTCOMES/EVALUATE

Relief of nasal, sinus, or eustachian tube congestion

Psyllium hydrophilic muciloid

(**SILL**-ee-um hi-droh-**FILL**-ik)

Classification(s): Laxative, bulk-forming

OTC: Fiberall Natural Flavor, Fiberall Orange Flavor, Fiberall Tropical Fruit Flavor, Fiberall Wafers, Genfiber, Genfiber Orange Flavor, Hydrocil Instant, Konsyl, Konsyl Easy Mix Formula, Konsyl Orange, Konsyl Orange Sugar Free, Konsyl-D, Metamucil, Metamucil Lemon-Lime Flavor, Metamucil Orange Flavor, Metamucil Orange Flavor-Original Texture, Metamucil Orange Flavor-Smooth Texture, Metamucil Original Texture, Metamucil Sugar Free, Metamucil Sugar Free Orange Flavor, Metamucil Sugar Free-Smooth Texture, Metamucil Sugar-Free Orange Flavor-Smooth Texture, Modane, Natural Fiber Laxative, Natural Psyllium Fiber, Natural Psyllium Fiber-Orange, Perdiem Fiber Therapy, Reguloid, Reguloid Orange, Reguloid Sugar Free Orange, Reguloid Sugar Free Regular, Serutan, Syllact.

SEE ALSO ***LAXATIVES***.

INDICATIONS/USES

(1) Prophylaxis of constipation in clients who should not strain during defecation. (2) Short-term treatment of constipation; useful in geriatric clients with diminished colonic motor response and during pregnancy and postpartum to reestablish normal bowel function. (3) To soften feces during fecal impaction.

ACTION/KINETICS

Action

The powder forms a gelatinous mass with water, which adds bulk to the stools and stimulates peristalsis. Also has a demulcent effect on an inflamed intestinal mucosa. Products may also contain dextrose, sodium bicarbonate, monobasic potassium phosphate, citric acid, and benzyl benzoate.

Pharmacokinetics

Laxative effects usually occur in 12–24 hr. The full effect may take 2–3 days. Dependence may occur.

CONTRAINDICATIONS

Severe abdominal pain or intestinal obstruction.

SIDE EFFECTS

Most Common

Diarrhea, N&V, perianal irritation, bloating, flatulence, cramps.

GI: Diarrhea, N&V, perianal irritation, bloating, flatulence, cramps. Obstruction of the esophagus, stomach, small intestine, and rectum. **CNS:** Fainting.

DRUG INTERACTIONS

Do not use concomitantly with salicylates, nitrofurantoin, or cardiac glycosides (e.g., digitalis)

HOW SUPPLIED

Caplets, Capsules: 0.5 gram, 0.52 gram; ***Effervescent Powder; Granules; Powder; Wafers:***

DOSAGE

Dose depends on the product. General information on adult dosage follows.

GRANULES; POWDER

Laxative.

Adults: 1–2 teaspoons 1–3 times per day; spread on food or take with a 8 oz of water or other liquid.

EFFERVESCENT POWDER

Laxative.

Adults: 1 packet in water 1–3 times per day.

WAFERS

Adults: 2 wafers followed by a glass of water 1–3 times per day.

P

NURSING IMPLICATIONS

ASSESSMENT

1. Note reasons for therapy, characteristics of S&S, abdominal/rectal assessment, other agents trialed, outcome.
2. Monitor consistency of bowel movement, color, consistency, amount and frequency.
3. Assess diet, prescribed medications, fluid intake, and activity levels.

CLIENT/FAMILY TEACHING

1. Bulk-forming laxatives are not digested but absorb liquid in the intestines and swell to form a soft, bulky stool. The stimulates the bowel normally by the presence of the bulky mass.
2. Mix powder with 8 oz of liquid just prior to administering; otherwise, the mixture may become thick and difficult to drink. Wash down with another glass of water/juice.
3. The powder may be noxious and irritating when removing from the packets or canister. Open in a well-ventilated area and avoid inhaling particulate matter.
4. Take exactly as directed. Report lack of response, severe stomach pain, N&V, or intolerable side effects.
5. Do not take other oral medicines within 2 hours before or 2 hours after taking psyllium.
6. May take 12–24 hrs for desired response or up to 3 days. If taken before meals may reduce appetite. Check contents—some contain sugar.
7. Ensure adequate fluid intake and consume other dietary sources of fiber such as bran, cereals with this listed, fresh fruits and vegetables as well as regular exercise.
8. Keep all F/U to assess response and for adverse SE.

OUTCOMES/EVALUATE

Prophylaxis/relief of constipation

P

Pyrantel pamoate

(pie-**RAN**-tell **PAM**- oh-ate)

Classification(s): Anthelmintic

Pregnancy Category: C

OTC: Pin-Rid, Pin-X, Reese's Pinworm.

🍁 **Rx:** Combantrin.

INDICATIONS/USES

Pinworm (enterobiasis) and roundworm (ascariasis) infestations. *Investigational:* Treatment of hairworm.

ACTION/KINETICS

Action

Has neuromuscular blocking effect which paralyzes the helminth, allowing it to be expelled through the feces. Also inhibits cholinesterases.

Pharmacokinetics

Poorly absorbed from GI tract. **Peak plasma levels:** 0.05–0.13 mcg/mL after 1–3 hr. Partially metabolized in liver. Fifty percent is excreted unchanged in feces and less than 7% excreted unchanged or as metabolites in urine.

CONTRAINDICATIONS

Pregnancy. Hepatic disease (unless directed by health care provider).

SPECIAL CONCERNS

Safe use not established in children less than 2 years of age.

SIDE EFFECTS

Most Common

Anorexia, N&V, diarrhea, headache, dizziness.

GI: Anorexia, N&V, abdominal cramps, diarrhea. **Hepatic:** Transient elevation of AST. **CNS:** Headache, dizziness, drowsiness, insomnia. **Miscellaneous:** Skin rashes.

DRUG INTERACTIONS

Piperazine / Use with piperazine for ascariasis → antagonism of the effect of both drugs

Theophylline / ↑ Theophylline serum levels in children

HOW SUPPLIED

Capsules, Soft Gel: 180 mg (equivalent to 62.5 mg pamoate base); ***Oral Suspension:*** 50 mg (as pamoate)/mL, 144 mg/mL (equivalent to 50 mg/mL); ***Tablets:*** 180 mg (equivalent to 62.5 mg pyrantel base); ***Tablets, Chewable:*** 720.5 mg (equivalent to 250 mg pyrantel base).

DOSAGE

CAPSULES, SOFT GEL; ORAL SUSPENSION; TABLETS; TABLETS, CHEWABLE

Helminth infections.

Individualize dose by weight. **Adults and children:** One dose of 11 mg/kg (5 mg/lb) given as a single dose. **Maximum total dose:** 1.0 gram (16 tablets/capsules or 20 mL suspension for adults and 16 tablets/capsules or 20 mL suspension for children).

NURSING IMPLICATIONS

IMPLEMENTATION/ADMINISTRATION/STORAGE

Store from 15–30°C (59–86°F).

ASSESSMENT

1. Note reasons for therapy, symptom characteristics, causative organism(s), and/or stool culture results.
2. Identify close contacts/travel, note type of organism and assess for hepatic dysfunction–avoid use if evident.
3. Assess for malnutrition, anemia or liver dysfunction.

CLIENT/FAMILY TEACHING

1. Drug works by paralyzing the nervous system of intestinal parasites (worms); the parasite is then passed in the stool.
2. May be taken without regard to food intake at any time of the day. Can take with milk or fruit juices. Shake the suspension well before taking.
3. Use of a laxative is not necessary prior to, during, or after the medication.
4. Depending on organism being treated may require one to three consecutive daily doses of drug. Depending on stool cultures may require retreatment.
5. Dizziness or drowsiness may occur; do not engage in activities that require mental alertness.
6. Report rash, severe headaches/GI upset, joint pain, or prolonged dizziness.
7. When treating pinworms, review client/family precautions R/T transmission:
   - Strict handwashing and hygiene measures with daily cleansing of perianal area and cleaning of fingernails.
   - Wash hands before meals and after each bowel movement carefully.
   - Do not prepare food for others when infested.
   - Change underwear and pajamas daily.
   - Launder undergarments, bed linens, sleep clothes in hot water daily.
   - Disinfect toilet facilities and bathroom floors daily.
   - Wet mop bedroom floors to prevent egg spread.
   - Do not share towels or wash clothes.
   - Treat all family members.
8. Keep all F/U to assess response, labs, and for adverse SE.

OUTCOMES/EVALUATE

Resolution of infection/infestation; negative stool and perianal swabs

IV

Pyridoxine hydrochloride (Vitamin B_6)

(peer-ih-**DOX**-een)

Classification(s): Vitamin B complex

Pregnancy Category: A (C for doses that exceed the RDA)

OTC: Aminoxin.

RX: Pyridoxine HCl Injection.

INDICATIONS/USES

Pyridoxine deficiency including poor diet, drug-induced (e.g., oral contraceptives, hydralazine, isoniazid), and inborn errors of metabolism. *Investigational:* Hydrazine poisoning, PMS, hyperoxaluria type I, N&V due to pregnancy, carpal tunnel syndrome, tardive dyskinesia due to antipsychotic drugs.

ACTION/KINETICS

Action

A water-soluble, heat-resistant vitamin that is destroyed by light. Acts as a coenzyme in the metabolism of protein, carbohydrates, and fat. As the amount of protein increases in the diet, the pyri-

P

doxine requirement increases. Vitamin B_6 is essential to make hemoglobin and helps increase the amount of oxygen carried by hemoglobin. Vitamin B_6 is also involved in maintaining the health of the thymus, spleen, and lymph nodes that make WBCs. The vitamin maintains normal levels of blood glucose by helping convert stored carbohydrates or other nutrients to glucose. However, pyridoxine deficiency alone is rare.

Pharmacokinetics

t½: 2–3 weeks. Metabolized in the liver and excreted through the urine.

SPECIAL CONCERNS

Safety and efficacy not established in children for doses that exceed the RDA.

SIDE EFFECTS

Most Common

Paresthesia, numbess of feet, perioral numbness, unstable gait.

CNS: Unstable gait; decreased sensation to touch, temperature, and vibration; paresthesia, sleepiness; numbness of feet; awkwardness of hands; perioral numbness, photoallergic reaction, ataxia. *NOTE:* Abuse and dependence have been noted in adults administered 200 mg/day.

OVERDOSE MANAGEMENT

Symptoms: Ataxia, severe sensory neuropathy, numbness of the hands and feet. *Treatment:* Discontinue pyridoxine; allow up to 6 months for CNS sensation to return.

DRUG INTERACTIONS

Chloramphenicol / ↑ Pyridoxine requirements
Contraceptives, oral / ↑ Pyridoxine requirements
Cycloserine / ↑ Pyridoxine requirements
Ethionamide / ↑ Pyridoxine requirements
Hydralazine / ↑ Pyridoxine requirements
Immunosuppressants / ↑ Pyridoxine requirements
Isoniazid / ↑ Pyridoxine requirements
Levodopa / Doses exceeding 5 mg/day ↓ levodopa effectiveness R/T ↑ peripheral metabolism → ↓ levels available for CNS penetration
Penicillamine / ↑ Pyridoxine requirements
Phenobarbital / ↓ Serum phenobarbital levels
Phenytoin / ↓ Serum phenytoin levels

HOW SUPPLIED

Injection: 100 mg/mL; ***Tablets:*** 25 mg, 50 mg, 100 mg, 250 mg, 500 mg.

P

DOSAGE

TABLETS

Recommended daily allowance.

Males and females, 14–50 years of age: 1.2–1.3 mg/day; **males and females >50 years of age:** 1.5–1.7 mg/day. **Children, 1–3 years of age:** 0.5 mg/day; **4–8 years of age:** 0.6 mg/day; **9–13 years of age:** 1 mg/day. **Pregnancy:** 1.9 mg/day; **lactation:** 2 mg/day. Avoid excess pyridoxine use during pregnancy and lactation.

Nutritional supplementation.

Usual: 100–200 mg/day.

Isoniazid-induced deficiency.

Adults, prophylaxis: 6–100 mg/day for isoniazid. **Adults, treatment:** 50–200 mg/day for 3 weeks followed by 25–100 mg/day to prevent relapse. **Adults, alcoholism:** 50 mg/day for 2–4 weeks; if anemia responds, continue pyridoxine indefinitely.

PMS.

40–500 mg/day.

Hyperoxaluria type I.

25–300 mg/day.

Carpal tunnel syndrome.

100–200 mg/day for 12 or more weeks.

Tardive dyskinesia due to antipsychotic drugs.

100 mg/day for 4 weeks.

IM; IV

Isoniazid-induced deficiency.

Adults: 50–200 mg/day for 3 weeks followed by 25–100 mg/day as needed.

Cycloserine poisoning.

Adults: 300 mg/day.

Isoniazid poisoning.

Adults: 1 gram for each gram of isoniazid taken.

NURSING IMPLICATIONS

IMPLEMENTATION/ADMINISTRATION/STORAGE

1. **If receiving levodopa, avoid preparations of vitamins containing B_6 as this decreases the availability of levodopa to the brain.**
2. **IV May be administered by direct IV or placed in infusion solutions.**
3. **COMPATIBILITY Standard IV solutions.**

4. INCOMPATIBILITY Alkaline solutions.

ASSESSMENT

1. Note reasons for therapy, e.g., to prevent toxicity (peripheral neuropathy) with long term isoniazid or contraceptive therapy, to replace vitamin B_6 with inborn errors of metabolism or with poor nutrition, or other conditions, characteristics of S&Ss, nutritional status.
2. Take a complete dietary/drug history. Report cycloserine, isoniazid, or oral contraceptive use as these increase pyridoxine requirements.
3. Monitor uric acid levels, renal, LFTs; assess for dysfunction.

CLIENT/FAMILY TEACHING

1. Take enteric-coated tabs whole; do not break, crush or chew. Do not take excessive doses; overdosing may cause unsteady gait, impaired hand coordination and numbness of feet.
2. Foods high in vitamin B_6 include potatoes, lima beans, broccoli, bananas, chicken breast, liver, yeast, wheat germ, whole-grain cereals. Well-balanced diets are the best source of vitamins. Those on high protein diets increase pyridoxine requirements.
3. Avoid activities that require mental alertness until drug effects realized; may cause drowsiness.
4. If prescribed levodopa, avoid vitamin supplements containing vitamin B_6. More than 5 mg of the vitamin antagonizes levodopa effect. At the same time, concomitant carbidopa administration will prevent effects of vitamin B_6 on levodopa.
5. If taking phenobarbital and/or phenytoin, obtain serum drug levels routinely, as pyridoxine alters serum concentrations.
6. Pyridoxine may inhibit lactation. Protein rich diet increases pyridoxine needs. Usual RDA for adults is 2.2 mg; in pregnancy/lactation, 2.6 mg.
7. Do not take OTC vitamin preparations without provider approval.
8. Keep all F/U to assess response, labs, and for adverse SE.

OUTCOMES/EVALUATE

- Relief of symptoms of pyridoxine deficiency
- Prophylaxis of drug-induced deficiency; ↓ toxic drug side effects

Q

Quetiapine fumarate

(kweh-**TYE**-ah-peen)

Classification(s): Antipsychotic

Pregnancy Category: C

RX: Seroquel, Seroquel XR.

INDICATIONS/USES

Immediate- and Extended-Release: (1) Treatment of schizophrenia. (2) Acute treatment of manic episodes associated with bipolar I disorder either as monotherapy or adjunct therapy with divalproex or lithium. (3) Maintenance of bipolar I disorder as adjunct therapy to lithium or divalproex. (4) Treatment of depressive episodes associated with bipolar disorder. **Extended-Release:** (1) Treatment of mixed episodes associated with bipolar I disorder as an adjunct to lithium or divalproex. (2) Treatment of adults with major depressive disorder as an adjunct to other antidepressants. *Investigational:* Alcohol dependence. Obsessive-compulsive disorder.

ACTION/KINETICS

Action

Mechanism unknown but may act as an antagonist at dopamine D_2 and serotonin $5HT_2$ receptors. Side effects may be due to antagonism of other receptors (e.g., histamine H_1, dopamine D_1, adrenergic $alpha_1$ and $alpha_2$, serotonin $5HT_{1A}$). Produces high incidence of weight gain, moderate sedation and orthostatic hypotension, few to no anticholinergic effects, and no extrapyramidal symptoms.

Pharmacokinetics

Rapidly absorbed. Bioavailability is 73% or more. **Peak plasma levels:** 1.5 hr. Metabolized by liver by CYP3A4 and sulfoxidation and oxidation to inactive metabolites that are excreted through urine (about 73%) and feces (about 20%). **$t^{1/2}$, terminal:** About 6 hr. Oral clearance is less in clients 65 years of age and older. **Plasma protein binding:** About 83%.

CONTRAINDICATIONS

Lactation.

SPECIAL CONCERNS

■ **Increased mortality in elderly clients and dementia-related psychosis.** (1) Elderly clients with psychosis treated with atypical antipsychotic drugs are at an increased risk of death. Analyses of 17 placebo-controlled trials (modal duration of 10 weeks), largely in clients taking atypical antipsychotic drugs, revealed a risk of death in the drug-treated clients between 1.6 and 1.7 times that seen in placebo-treated clients. Over the course of a typical 10-week controlled trial, the rate of death in drug-treated clients was about 4.5%, compared with a rate of about 2.6% in the placebo group. Although the causes of death were varied, most of the deaths appeared to be either cardiovascular (e.g., heart failure, sudden death) or infectious (e.g., pneumonia) in nature. Observational studies suggest that, similar to atypical antipsychotic drugs, treatment with conventional antipsychotic drugs may increase mortality. The extent to which the findings of increased mortality in observational studies may be attributed to the antipsychotic drug as opposed to some characteristic(s) of the clients is not clear. Quetiapine is not approved for the treatment of clients with dementia-related psychosis. (2) **Suicidality and antidepressant drugs.** Antidepressants increased the risk compared with placebo of suicidal thinking and behavior (suicidality) in short-term studies in children, adolescents, and young adults with major depressive disorder and other psychiatric disorders. Anyone considering the use of quetiapine or any other antidepressant in a child, adolescent, or young adult must balance this risk with the clinical need. Short-term studies did not show an increase in the risk of suicidality with antidepressants compared with placebo in adults older than 24 years of age; there was a reduction in risk with antidepressants compared with placebo in adults 65 years of age and older. Depression and certain other psychiatric disorders are themselves associated with increases in the risk of suicide. Monitor clients of all ages who are started on antidepressant therapy appropriately, and observe these clients closely for clinical worsening, suicidality, or unusual changes in behavior. Advise families and caregivers of the need for close observation and communication with the prescriber. (3) Quetiapine is not approved for use in children younger than 10 years of age (immediate-release) or younger than 18 years of age (extended-release [ER]). ■

- **Use with caution in liver disease, in those at risk for aspiration pneumonia, and in those with history of seizures or conditions that lower seizure threshold (e.g., Alzheimer's).**
- **Increased risk of hyperglycemia and diabetes associated with quetiapine.**
- **Use with caution in geriatric clients; drug may be excreted more slowly in this population; rate of death due to CV events or infections is higher in clients with dementia.**

SIDE EFFECTS

Most Common

Headache, drowsiness/sedation/somnolence, dizziness, akathisia, hypotension, tachycardia, constipation, dry mouth, dyspepsia.

Side effects with an incidence of 0.1% or more are listed. **CNS:** Headache, drowsiness, sedation, somnolence, dizziness, akathisia, dystonia, syncope, amnesia, apathy, ataxia, catatonic-like states, confusion, dysarthria, dyskinesia, abnormal gait, hallucinations, hemiplegia, hostility, hyperkinesia, incoordination, insomnia, libido increased, manic reaction, migraine, nervousness, paranoid reaction, delusions, depersonalization, paresthesia, psychosis, suicide attempt/thought, involuntary movements, stupor, tremor, abnormal thinking, twitch. **CV:** Hypotension, tachycardia, bradycardia, bundle branch block, ***CVA,*** cerebral ischemia, hypertension, irregular pulse, increased QRS duration, palpitations, QTc interval prolongation, T-wave flattening, T-wave inversion, thrombophlebitis (including deep), vasodilation. **GI:** Dry mouth, constipation, dyspepsia, dysphagia, abdominal discomfort/pain, anorexia, appetite increased, diarrhea, flatulence, gastritis, gastroenteritis, gastroesophageal reflux, gingivitis, gum hemorrhage, hemorrhoids, fecal incontinence, melena, mouth ulceration, N&V, polydipsia, rectal hemorrhage, salivation, stomatitis, taste altered, tooth caries, bruxism. **Dermatologic:** Rash, acne, dermatitis, diaphoresis, dry skin, ecchymosis, eczema, maculopapular skin reactions, photosensitivity, pruritus, seborrhea, skin ulcer. **GU:** Amenorrhea, cystitis, dysmenorrhea, ejaculation disorders, galactorrhea, impotence, urinary incontinence, metrorrhagia, orchitis, urinary frequency, increased urgency, urinary retention, vaginal hemorrhage, UTI, vaginitis, vulvovaginitis dysuria. **Hematologic:** Leukopenia, hypochromic anemia, eosinophilia, leg cramps, leukorrhea, leukocytosis, lymphadenopathy. **Musculoskeletal:** Myalgia, arthralgia/joint pain, arthritis, back/chest pain, bone pain, muscle weakness, myoclonus, neck pain/rigidity, pelvic pain, pathological fracture. **Respiratory:** Rhinitis, increased cough, dyspnea, pharyngitis, asthma, epistaxis, pneumonia. **Metabolic:** Peripheral edema, facial/tongue edema, cyanosis, diabetes mellitus. **Ophthalmic:** Blurred vision, blepharitis, conjunctivitis, dry eyes, abnormal vision, eye pain. **Otic:** Tinnitus, ear pain. **Body as a whole:** Asthenia, chills, dehydration, fever, flu syndrome, malaise, pain, weight gain/loss. **Miscellaneous:** Accidental injury, hypertonia, hypothyroidism, moniliasis, alcohol intolerance.

LABORATORY TEST CONSIDERATIONS

↑ ALT during initial therapy, AST, alkaline phosphatase, creatinine, GGT, cholesterol, triglycerides. ↓ Total and free thyroxine. Hyperglycemia, hyperlipemia, hypoglycemia,

OVERDOSE MANAGEMENT

Symptoms: Drowsiness, sedation, deep sleep from which the client cannot be aroused, tachycardia, hypotension, dystonic reaction of the head and neck, seizures, obtundation, agitation, autonomic reactions, cardiac arrest, cardiac arrhythmias, coma, confusion, death, delirum, dilated or constricted pupils, dry mouth, ECG changes, fever, hyperpyrexia, hyperthermia, hypothermia, ileus, respiratory depression/failure, neuroleptic malignant syndrome, restlessness, salivation, slurred speech, tachycardia, vomiting. *Treatment:* Cardiovascular monitoring for arrhythmias. If antiarrhythmic therapy is used, disopyramide, procainamide, and quinidine increase risk of prolongation of QT. Treat hypotension and circulatory shock with IV fluids or sympathomimetic drugs (do not use epinephrine or dopamine as they may worsen hypotension). Use anticholinergic drugs to treat severe extrapyramidal symptoms.

DRUG INTERACTIONS

Alcohol / ↑ CNS depression, especially impaired motor skills; also, possible dystonic reaction; avoid concurrent use
Barbiturates / ↓ Quetiapine effect R/T ↑ liver breakdown; higher maintenance doses may be needed
Carbamazepine / ↓ Quetiapine effect R/T ↑ liver breakdown; higher maintenance doses may be needed
Charcoal / ↓ GI absorption
Cimetidine / ↓ Quetiapine oral clearance
CNS depressants / ↑ CNS depression, especially impaired motor skills
Dopamine agonists / Quetiapine antagonizes effect
Erythromycin / ↑ Quetiapine peak plasma levels, AUC, and t½ R/T inhibition of metabolism by CYP3A4
Glucocorticoids / ↓ Quetiapine effect R/T ↑ liver breakdown
Ketoconazole / ↑ Quetiapine plasma levels R/T inhibition of CYP3A4
Levodopa / Quetiapine antagonizes effect
Lorazepam / ↓ Lorazepam oral clearance
Phenobarbital / ↓ Quetiapine effect R/T ↑ liver breakdown; higher maintenance doses may be needed
Phenytoin / ↓ Quetiapine effect R/T ↑ liver breakdown; higher maintenance doses may be needed
Rifampin / ↓ Quetiapine effect R/T ↑ liver breakdown
Thioridazine / ↑ Quetiapine clearance significantly

HOW SUPPLIED

Tablets, Extended-Release: 50 mg, 150 mg, 200 mg, 300 mg, 400 mg; ***Tablets, Immediate-Release:*** 25 mg, 50 mg, 100 mg, 200 mg, 300 mg, 400 mg.

DOSAGE

TABLETS, EXTENDED-RELEASE; TABLETS, IMMEDIATE-RELEASE

Schizophrenia.

Adults, Immediate-Release. Initial: 25 mg 2 times per day, with increases of 25 to 50 mg 2–3 times per day on the second and third day, as tolerated. Target dose range, by fourth day, is 300 to 400 mg divided into 2 or 3 doses. Further dosage adjustments can occur at intervals of two or more days. The antipsychotic dose range is 150 to 750 mg/day. If dosage adjustments are needed, increments/decrements of 25–50 mg twice daily are recommended. **Adults, Extended-Release. Initial:** 300 mg/day given once a day, preferably in the evening. Titrate within a dose range of 400–800 mg/day, depending on client response and tolerance. Dose increases can be made at intervals of 1 day and in increments of 300 mg/day. **Maximum dose:** 800 mg/day. Periodically assess to determine the need for continued treatment.

Children, 13–17 years of age, Immediate-Release: The total daily dose (given twice/day but can be given 3 times/day if needed) for the initial 5 days of therapy using immediate-release tablets, is: **Day 1:** 50 mg; **Day 2:** 100 mg; **Day 3:** 200 mg; **Day 4:** 300 mg; and **Day 5:** 400 mg. After day 5, adjust the dose within the recommended dose range of 400–800 mg/day based on response and tolerability. Make dosage adjustments in increments no greater than 100 mg/day. The efficacy for longer than 6 weeks has not been evaluated; however, it is generally recommended that responding clients be continued beyond the acute response but at the lowest dose needed to maintain remission. Periodically assess the need for maintenance treatment.

Bipolar disorder, acute manic episodes.

Immediate-Release, Adults: When used as either monotherapy or adjunct therapy (with lithium or divalproex), begin quetiapine with a total of 100 mg/day on day 1 (given in 2 doses); increase to 400 mg/day on day 4 in increments of up to 100 mg/day in twice daily divided doses. Further dosage adjustments, up to 800 mg/day by day 6, should be in increments of no more than 200 mg/day. The majority of clients respond at doses between 400 and 800 mg/day. The safety of doses above 800 mg/day has not been evaluated. **Extended-Release, Adults:** When used as monotherapy or adjunct therapy (with lithium or divalproex), give quetiapine once daily in the evening starting with 300 mg on day 1 and 600 mg on day 2. Quetiapine can be adjusted between 400 and 800 mg beginning on day 3, depending on the response and tolerance of the client. Clients can be maintained on the same dose on which they were stabilized during the stabilization phase.

Immediate-Release, Children, 10–17 years of age: The total daily dose (given twice/day but can be given 3 times/day if needed) for the initial 5 days of therapy using immediate-release tablets is: **Day 1:** 50 mg; **Day 2:** 100 mg; **Day 3:** 200 mg; **Day 4:** 300 mg; and **Day 5:** 400 mg. After day 5, adjust the dose within the recommended dose range of 400–600 mg/day based on response and tolerability. Make dosage adjustments in increments no greater than 100 mg/day. The efficacy for longer than 3 weeks has not been evaluated; however, it is generally recommended that responding clients be continued beyond the acute response but at the lowest dose needed to maintain remission. Periodically assess the need for maintenance treatment.

Bipolar disorder, depressive episodes.

Adults, Immediate-Release, initial: Day 1: 50 mg; **Day 2:** 100 mg; **Day 3:** 200 mg; **Day 4:** 300 mg given once dailiy at bedtime. The usual dosage is 300 or 600 mg/day; no additional benefit was seen at doses above 600 mg/day. **Adults, Extended-Release: Day 1,** 50 mg; **Day 2:** 100 mg; **Day 3:** 200 mg; **Day 4:** 300 mg given once daily in the evening.

Maintenance treatment of bipolar I disorder.

Immediate-Release, Adults: Total of 400–800 mg/day given twice daily as

Q

adjunct therapy to lithium or divalproex. The dose for maintenance therapy is generally the same on which the client was stabilized during stabilization therapy. **Extended-Release, Adults:** The dose for maintenance therapy is generally the same on which the client was stabilized during stabilization therapy.

Major depressive disorder, adjunctive therapy with antidepressants.

Extended-Release. Adults, initial: 50 mg once/day in the evening. On day 3, the dose can be increased to 150 mg once daily in the evening. **Dose range:** 150–300 mg/day. Doses above 300 mg not studied.

Alcohol dependence (investigational).

Adults, initial: 25–50 mg nightly. Can be titrated to a maximum of 300 mg nightly based on tolerance and efficacy.

Obsessive-compulsive disorder (investigational).

Adults, initial: 50 mg/day. Increase dose based on therapeutic effect and tolerance. **Dose range:** 25–400 mg/day. Once successful management is reached, continue therapy for 1–2 years before attempting to taper the dose. During tapering, doses may be reduced by 10–25% q 1–2 months while monitoring for symptom worsening or return.

NURSING IMPLICATIONS

Do not confuse Seroquel with Serzone (an antidepressant).

IMPLEMENTATION/ADMINISTRATION/STORAGE

1. Once daily therapy may be possible if using the extended-release tablets.
2. Continue clients who respond to quetiapine using the lowest dose needed to maintain remission. Periodically reassess.
3. Start clients with impaired hepatic function on 25 mg/day of immediate-release. Increase the dose daily by 25–50 mg/day immediate-release to an effective dosage, depending on the clinical response and client tolerability. Start those with impaired hepatic function on 50 mg/day quetiapine ER; dose can be increased in increments of 50 mg/day, depending on tolerance and clinical response.
4. Start elderly clients on quetiapine ER 50 mg/day. Dose can be increased in increments of 50 mg/day, depending on tolerance and response.
5. Consider a slower rate of titration and a lower target dose in elderly, debilitated clients, or in those who have a predisposition to hypotensive reactions.
6. Titration is not required when restarting clients who have had an interval of less than 1 week off immediate-release quetiapine. Initial titration schedule is followed if clients have been off drug for more than 1 week.
7. When restarting clients who have been off quetiapine ER for less than 1 week, gradual dose escalation may not be required and the maintenance dose may be reinitiated. If the client has been off ER for more than 1 week, follow the initial dosing schedule.
8. Schizophrenic clients being treated with divided daily doses of immediate-release tablets may be switched to the extended-release drug at equivalent daily doses taken once a day.
9. The period of overlapping antipsychotic drugs should be minimized. When switching clients from depot antipsychotics, if medically appropriate, start quetiapine therapy in place of the next scheduled injection. In other instances, more gradual discontinuation may be more appropriate. Periodically reevaluate clients.
10. Gradual withdrawal of quetiapine is advisable. Rarely, acute withdrawal symptoms have been observed, including insomnia, N&V.
11. Store from 15–30°C (59–86°F). Protect from moisture.

ASSESSMENT

1. List reasons for therapy, clinical presentation, cognitive functioning, and behavioral manifestations. Note age and other agents trialed. List other agents prescribed.
2. Note any predisposition to hypotensive reactions if debilitated; if hepatic impairment present.
3. Document ophthalmic exam initially, and at 6-month intervals, to assess for cataract formation.
4. Assess mental status and for S&S of Alzheimer's disease, history of seizures, cardiovascular disease. Use cautiously in the elderly; do

not clear drug normally and have increased mortality with dementia-related psychosis.

5. Monitor weight, VS, ECG, BS, CBC, renal and LFTs; reduce dose with dysfunction.

CLIENT/FAMILY TEACHING

1. May take immediate-release tabs with or without food. Total daily dose is divided and given two or three times a day unless using the extended-release tablets.
2. Extended-release tablets should be swallowed whole and not split, chewed, or crushed. May be taken without food or with a light meal (approx. 300 calories).
3. Do not perform activities that require mental alertness until after titration period and until drug effects realized; may impair judgment and motor skills, and cause sleepiness. Change positions slowly to prevent low BP effects.
4. Avoid alcohol and any OTC agents without approval. May induce/aggravate diabetes control.
5. Use reliable contraception; report if pregnancy suspected. Do not breastfeed.
6. Report any evidence of tardive dyskinesia (involuntary movements) and extrapyramidal symptoms (tremors, jerking movements).
7. Report any altered mental status, increased depression or suicide thoughts, high fever, irregular or fast pulse, muscle rigidity, rash, seizures, or ↑ sweating. Avoid situations where overheating or dehydration may occur.
8. Long-term usefulness must be evaluated periodically while on lowest dose to maintain remission.
9. Determine any unusual weight gain or need for nutritional management.
10. Keep all F/U to assess response, labs (CBC, renal and LFTs), VS, weight, and for adverse SE.

OUTCOMES/EVALUATE

- Control of S&S of psychotic disorders i.e., ↓ Paranoia/delusions/hallucinations/emotional lability
- Control of bipolar mania/depression
- Alcohol dependence (unlabeled use)

■ ℗

Quinapril hydrochloride

(**KWIN**-ah-prill)

Classification(s): Antihypertensive, ACE inhibitor

Pregnancy Category: D (Category C: First trimester; Category D: Second and third trimesters)

RX: Accupril.

SEE ALSO ***ANGIOTENSIN-CONVERTING ENZYME INHIBITORS.***

INDICATIONS/USES

(1) Alone or in combination with a thiazide diuretic for the treatment of hypertension. (2) Adjunct with a diuretic or digitalis to treat CHF in those not responding adequately to diuretics or digitalis. *Investigational:* Pediatric hypertension.

ACTION/KINETICS

Action

Inhibits angiotensin-converting enzyme resulting in decreased plasma angiotensin II, which leads to decreased vasopressor activity and decreased aldosterone secretion. Also appears to improve endothelial function, an early marker of coronary atherosclerosis.

Pharmacokinetics

Onset: 1 hr. **Time to peak serum levels:** About 1 hr for quinaprilat. **Peak effect:** 2–4 hr. Bioavailability is about 60%. Metabolized to quinaprilat, the active metabolite. **t½, elimination, quinaprilat:** About 2 hr. **Duration:** 24 hr. Food reduces absorption. Metabolized with approximately 60% excreted through the urine and 40% excreted in the feces. Levels are decreased in those with alcoholic cirrhosis due to impaired esterification of quinapril. Elimination t½ may be decreased in those 65 years and older and increased as C_{CR} decreases. **Plasma protein binding:** About 97%.

CONTRAINDICATIONS

Lactation.

SPECIAL CONCERNS

■ When used in pregnancy during the second and third trimesters, ACE inhibitors can cause injury and even death to the developing fetus.

Q

When pregnancy is detected, discontinue the ACE inhibitor as soon as possible.

- **May cause a profound fall in BP following the first dose.**
- **Use with caution during lactation.**
- **Safety and efficacy not determined in children.**
- **Geriatric clients may be more sensitive to the effects of quinapril and manifest higher peak quinaprilat blood levels.**

SIDE EFFECTS

Most Common

Dizziness, headache, fatigue, chest pain, hypotension, dyspnea, N&V.

CV: Vasodilation, tachycardia, ***heart failure***, palpitations, chest pain, hypotension (may be profound following the first dose), ***MI, CVA, hypertensive crisis***, angina pectoris, orthostatic hypotension, cardiac rhythm disturbances, ***cardiogenic shock***. **GI:** Dry mouth or throat, constipation, diarrhea, dyspepsia, flatulence, N&V, abdominal pain, hepatitis, pancreatitis, ***GI hemorrhage***. **Hepatic:** Hepatitis; rarely, cholestatic jaundice progressing to ***fulminant hepatic necrosis*** and sometimes ***death***. **CNS:** Dizziness, somnolence, drowsiness, vertigo, insomnia, sleep disturbances, paresthesias, nervousness, depression, headache. **Hematologic**: ***Agranulocytosis***, anemia, bone marrow depression, hemolytic anemia, thrombocytopenia. **Dermatologic**: ***Angioedema of the lips, tongue, glottis, and larynx;*** alopecia, sweating, pruritus, exfoliative dermatitis, pemphigus/pemphigoid, photosensitivity, dermatopolymyositis, flushing, rash, urticaria. **GU:** Oliguria and/or progressive azotemia and rarely ***acute renal failure and/or death in severe heart failure***. Impotence, UTI. Worsening renal failure. **Respiratory:** Pharyngitis, cough (may be chronic), asthma, bronchospasm, dyspnea. **Musculoskeletal:** Myalgia, arthralgia. **Hypersensitivity:** ***Anaphylactoid*** reactions, angioedema. **Body as a whole:** Malaise, fatigue, edema, back pain. **Miscellaneous:** Oligohydramnios in fetuses exposed to the drug in utero. Syncope, amblyopia, viral infection.

LABORATORY TEST CONSIDERATIONS

Hyperkalemia.

OVERDOSE MANAGEMENT

Symptoms: Commonly, hypotension. *Treatment:* IV infusion of normal saline to restore blood pressure.

DRUG INTERACTIONS

Potassium-containing salt substitutes / ↑ Risk of hyperkalemia
Potassium-sparing diuretics / ↑ Risk of hyperkalemia
Potassium supplements / ↑ Risk of hyperkalemia
Tetracyclines / ↓ Absorption R/T high Mg^{++} content of quinapril tablets

HOW SUPPLIED

Tablets: 5 mg, 10 mg, 20 mg, 40 mg.

DOSAGE

TABLETS

Hypertension, client not on diuretics.

Initial: 10 or 20 mg once daily; **then,** adjust dosage based on BP response at peak (2–6 hr) and trough (predose) blood levels. The dose should be adjusted at 2-week intervals. **Maintenance:** 20, 40, or 80 mg daily as a single dose or in two equally divided doses; usual dose is 10–40 mg/day. With impaired renal function, the maximal initial dose should be 10 mg if the C_{CR} is greater than 60 mL/min, 5 mg if the C_{CR} is between 30 and 60 mL/min, and 2.5 mg if the C_{CR} is between 10 and 30 mL/min. If the initial dose is well tolerated, the drug may be given the following day as a twice a day regimen.

Hypertension, client on diuretics.

Initial: 5 mg with careful supervision for several hr until BP stabilizes.

CHF.

Initial: 5 mg twice a day. If this dose is well tolerated, titrate clients at weekly intervals until an effective dose, usually 20–40 mg daily in two equally divided doses, is attained. Undesirable hypotension, orthostasis, or azotemia may prevent this dosage level from being reached. For dosage adjustment in those with heart failure and impaired renal function or hyponatremia, see dosage for hypertension. *NOTE:* Quinapril is indicated as an adjunctive drug when added to conventional therapy including diuretics and digitalis.

Q

NURSING IMPLICATIONS

Do not confuse Accupril with Accutane (antiacne drug) or with Aciphex (proton pump inhibitor).

IMPLEMENTATION/ADMINISTRATION/STORAGE

1. If taking a diuretic, discontinue diuretic 2–3 days prior to beginning quinapril. If BP is not controlled, reinstitute the diuretic. If the diuretic cannot be discontinued, the initial dose of quinapril should be 5 mg.
2. If the antihypertensive effect decreases at the end of the dosing interval with once-daily therapy, consider either twice-daily administration or increasing the dose.
3. In the elderly, the recommended initial dose to treat hypertension is 10 mg once daily followed by titration.
4. If the initial dose is well tolerated for treating CHF, quinapril may be given as a twice a day regimen. In the absence of excessive hypotension or significant renal function deterioration, the dose may be increased at weekly intervals, based on clinical and hemodynamic responses.
5. The antihypertensive effect may not be observed for 1–2 weeks.
6. Store from 15–30°C (59–86°F).

ASSESSMENT

1. Note reasons for therapy, disease onset, all medical conditions, other agents trialed.
2. Observe infants exposed to quinapril in utero for the development of hypotension, oliguria, and hyperkalemia.
3. If angioedema occurs, stop drug, assess airway, and observe until swelling resolved. Antihistamines may help relieve symptoms.
4. Agranulocytosis and bone marrow depression seen more often with renal impairment, especially if collagen vascular disease (e.g., SLE, scleroderma) present. Check BP before and 2–6 hr after therapy to assess BP control.
5. Clients with unilateral or bilateral renal artery stenosis may manifest increased BUN and creatinine if given quinapril. Assess renal function closely especially during first few weeks of therapy; reduce dose with dysfunction. Monitor BP, renal function and serum K^+ during therapy. Ensure adequately hydrated.
6. Monitor VS, I&O, weights, electrolytes, CBC, microalbumin, renal and LFTs; may need to reduce dose with dysfunction.

CLIENT/FAMILY TEACHING

1. Take as directed; 1–2 hr before food or antacids as they will reduce absorption. Avoid foods high in potassium/potassium supplements. Consume adequate fluids to prevent dehydration; hot weather and exercise may increase loss.
2. Avoid activities that require mental alertness until drug effects realized; may cause dizziness or drowsiness. Change positions slowly to prevent sudden low BP.
3. Report unusual bruising/bleeding, fever, sore throat, cough, or persistent side effects. Consume adequate fluids to prevent dehydration.
4. Any increased SOB, palpitations, swelling, or persistent nonproductive cough should be evaluated as well as rash and altered taste perception. Immediately report any sudden breathing difficulty, swelling of eyes, tongue, lips or face.
5. Keep a log of BP and HR readings at different times during the day for provider review.
6. Practice reliable contraception; report if pregnancy suspected.
7. Some OTC drugs may affect the action of quinapril; consult provider before taking OTC drugs.
8. Avoid prolonged sun exposure, wear sunscreen and protective clothing to avoid photosensitivity reaction.
9. Continue activities to help control BP: maintain healthy diet, limit intake of caffeine, avoid alcohol, salt and high sodium or potassium foods, perform regular exercise, maintain weight and stop smoking.
10. Keep all F/U to assess response, labs, and for adverse SE.

OUTCOMES/EVALUATE

↓ BP

IV

Quinidine gluconate

(**KWIN**-ih-deen)

Classification(s): Antiarrhythmic, Class IA
Pregnancy Category: C
RX: Quinidine Gluconate Injection.

Quinidine sulfate

Pregnancy Category: C

SEE ALSO ***ANTIARRHYTHMIC AGENTS***.

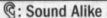

INDICATIONS/USES

(1) Premature atrial, AV junctional, and ventricular contractions. (2) Treatment and control of atrial flutter, established atrial fibrillation, paroxysmal atrial tachycardia, paroxysmal AV junctional rhythm, paroxysmal and chronic atrial fibrillation, paroxysmal ventricular tachycardia not associated with complete heart block. (3) Maintenance therapy after electrical conversion of atrial flutter or fibrillation. The parenteral route is indicated when PO therapy is not feasible or immediate effects are required. *Investigational:* Gluconate salt for life-threatening *Plasmodium falciparum* malaria.

ACTION/KINETICS

Action

Reduces the excitability of the heart and depresses conduction velocity and contractility. Prolongs the refractory period and increases conduction time. It also decreases CO and possesses anticholinergic, antimalarial, antipyretic, and oxytocic properties.

Pharmacokinetics

PO: Onset: 0.5–3 hr. **Maximum effects, after IM:** 30–90 min. **t½:** 6–7 hr. **Time to peak levels, PO:** 3–5 hr for gluconate salt and 1–1.5 hr for sulfate salt. **IM:** 1 hr. **Therapeutic serum levels:** 2–6 mcg/mL. **Duration:** 6–8 hr for tablets/capsules and 12 hr for extended-release tablets. Metabolized by liver. Urine pH affects rate of urinary excretion (10–50% excreted unchanged). **Plasma protein binding:** 60–80%.

CONTRAINDICATIONS

Hypersensitivity to drug or other cinchona drugs. Myasthenia gravis, history of thrombocytopenic purpura associated with quinidine use, digitalis intoxication evidenced by arrhythmias or AV conduction disorders. Also, complete heart block, left bundle branch block, or other intraventricular conduction defects manifested by marked QRS widening or bizarre complexes. Complete AV block with an AV nodal or idioventricular pacemaker, aberrant ectopic impulses and abnormal rhythms due to escape mechanisms. History of drug-induced torsades de pointes or long QT syndrome.

SPECIAL CONCERNS

- **Safety in children and during lactation not established.**
- **Use with extreme caution in clients in whom a sudden change in BP might be detrimental or in those suffering from extensive myocardial damage, subacute endocarditis, bradycardia, coronary occlusion, disturbances in impulse conduction, chronic valvular disease, considerable cardiac enlargement, frank CHF, and renal or hepatic disease.**
- **Use with caution in acute infections, hyperthyroidism, muscular weakness, respiratory distress, and bronchial asthma.**
- **Elderly dosage may have to be reduced due to age-related changes in renal function.**

SIDE EFFECTS

Most Common

Diarrhea, anorexia, bitter taste in mouth, dizziness, headache, tinnitus, blurred vision, GI upset, fever, rash, arrhythmias, N&V, asthenia, cerebral ischemia.

CV: Widening of QRS complex, hypotension, ***cardiac asystole***, ectopic ventricular beats, ***ventricular tachycardia/flutter or fibrillation, torsades de pointes***, paradoxical tachycardia, ***arterial embolism***, ventricular extrasystoles (one or more every 6 beats), prolonged QT interval, cerebral ischemia, ***complete AV block***. **GI:** N&V, GI upset, abdominal pain, anorexia, diarrhea, urge to defecate as well as urinate, bitter taste in mouth, esophagitis (rare). **CNS:** Syncope, headache, dizziness, confusion, excitement, vertigo, apprehension, delirium, dementia, ataxia, depression. **Dermatologic:** Rash, urticaria, exfoliative dermatitis, photosensitivity, flushing with intense pruritus, eczema, psoriasis, pigmentation abnormalities. **Musculoskeletal:** Arthritis, myalgia, increase in serum skeletal muscle CPK. **Allergic:** Acute asthma, angioneurotic edema, ***respiratory arrest***, dyspnea, fever, ***vascular collapse***, purpura, vasculitis, hepatic dysfunction (including granulomatous hepatitis), ***hepatic toxicity***. **Hematologic:** Hypoprothrombinemia, ***acute hemolytic anemia***, thrombocytopenic purpura, ***agranulocytosis***, thrombocytopenia, leukocytosis, neutropenia, shift to left in WBC differential. **Ophthalmic:** Blurred vision, mydriasis, alterations in color perception, decreased field of vision, double vision, photophobia, optic neuritis, night blindness, sco-

Q

tomata. **Miscellaneous:** Fever, asthenia, liver toxicity including hepatitis, lupus nephritis, tinnitus, decreased hearing acuity, lupus erythematosus.

LABORATORY TEST CONSIDERATIONS

False + or ↑ PSP, 17-ketosteroids, PT.

OVERDOSE MANAGEMENT

Symptoms: **CNS:** Lethargy, confusion, ***coma, seizures, respiratory depression or arrest***, headache, paresthesia, vertigo. CNS symptoms may be seen after onset of CV toxicity. **GI:** Vomiting, diarrhea, abdominal pain, hypokalemia, nausea. **CV:** Sinus tachycardia, ***ventricular tachycardia or fibrillation, torsades de pointes, depressed automaticity and conduction*** (including bundle branch block, sinus bradycardia, SA block, prolongation of QRS and QTc, sinus arrest, AV block, ST depression, T inversion), syncope, ***heart failure***. Hypotension due to decreased conduction and CO and vasodilation. **Miscellaneous:** Cinchonism, visual and auditory disturbances, hypokalemia, tinnitus, acidosis. *Treatment:*

- Perform gastric lavage, induce vomiting, and administer activated charcoal if ingestion is recent.
- Monitor ECG, blood gases, serum electrolytes, and BP.
- Institute cardiac pacing, if necessary.
- Acidify the urine.
- Use artificial respiration and other supportive measures.
- Infusions of 1/6 molar sodium lactate IV may decrease the cardiotoxic effects.
- Treat hypotension with metaraminol or norepinephrine after fluid volume replacement.
- Use phenytoin or lidocaine to treat tachydysrhythmias.
- Hemodialysis is effective but not often required.

DRUG INTERACTIONS

Acetazolamide, Antacids / ↑ Quinidine effect R/T ↓ renal excretion
Amiodarone / ↑ Quinidine levels with possible fatal cardiac dysrhythmias
Anticholinergic agents, Atropine / Additive effect on blockade of vagus nerve action
Anticoagulants, oral / Additive hypoprothrombinemia with possible hemorrhage
Barbiturates / ↓ Quinidine effect R/T ↑ liver breakdown
H ***Belladonna leaf/root*** / Increased anticholinergic effect
Cholinergic agents / Quinidine antagonizes effect of cholinergic drugs
Cimetidine / ↑ Quinidine effect R/T ↓ liver breakdown
Digoxin / ↑ Symptoms of digoxin toxicity
Disopyramide / Either ↑ disopyramide levels or ↓ quinidine levels
Guanethidine / Additive hypotensive effect
Grapefruit juice / ↓ Quinidine absorption and inhibition of quinidine metabolism; effects on the QTc interval delayed and reduced
H ***Henbane leaf*** / ↑ Anticholinergic effects
Itraconazole / ↑ Risk of tinnitus and ↓ hearing
H ***Lily-of-the-valley*** / ↑ Effect and side effects of quinidine
Methyldopa / Additive hypotensive effect
Metoprolol / ↑ Metoprolol effect in fast metabolizers
Neuromuscular blocking agents / ↑ Respiratory depression
Nifedipine / ↓ Quinidine effect
H ***Pheasant's eye herb*** / ↑ Effect and side effects of quinidine
Phenobarbital, Phenytoin / ↓ Quinidine effect R/T ↑ rate of liver metabolism
Potassium / ↑ Quinidine effect
Procainamide / ↑ Procainamide effects with possible toxicity
Propafenone / ↑ Serum propafenone levels in rapid metabolizers
Propranolol / ↑ Propranolol effect in fast metabolizers
Rifampin / ↓ Quinidine effect R/T ↑ liver breakdown
H ***Scopolia root*** / ↑ Quinidine effect
Skeletal muscle relaxants / ↑ Skeletal muscle relaxation
Sodium bicarbonate / ↑ Quinidine effect R/T ↓ renal excretion
H ***Squill*** / ↑ Effect and side effects of quinidine
Sucralfate / ↓ Serum quinidine levels → ↓ effect
Thiazide diuretics / ↑ Quinidine effect R/T ↓ renal excretion
Tricyclic antidepressants / ↑ TCA effect R/T ↓ clearance

Verapamil / ↓ Verapamil clearance → ↑ hypotension, bradycardia, AV block, VT, and pulmonary edema

HOW SUPPLIED

Quinidine gluconate. *Injection:* 80 mg/mL; *Tablets, Extended-Release:* 324 mg.
Quinidine sulfate. *Tablets:* 100 mg, 200 mg, 300 mg; *Tablets, Extended-Release:* 300 mg.

DOSAGE

Quinidine Gluconate Injection

IM; IV

Acute tachycardia.

Adults, initial: 600 mg IM; **then,** 400 mg IM repeated as often as q 2 hr.

Arrhythmias.

Adults: 330 mg IM or less IV (as much as 500–750 mg may be required).

P. falciparum *malaria.*

Two regimens may be used. (1) *Loading dose:* 15 mg/kg in 250 mL NSS given over 4 hr; **then,** 24 hr after beginning the loading dose, institute 7.5 mg/kg infused over 4 hr and given q 8 hr for 7 days or until PO therapy can be started. (2) **Loading dose:** 10 mg/kg in 250 mL NSS infused over 1–2 hr followed immediately by 0.02 mg/kg/min for up to 72 hr or until parasitemia decreases to less than 1% or PO therapy can be started.

Quinidine Gluconate or Quinidine Sulfate

TABLETS, EXTENDED-RELEASE

All uses.

Adults: 300–600 mg q 8–12 hr.

Quinidine Sulfate

TABLETS

Premature atrial and ventricular contractions.

Adults: 200–300 mg 3–4 times per day.

Paroxysmal SVTs.

Adults: 400–600 mg q 2–3 hr until the paroxysm is terminated.

Conversion of atrial flutter.

Adults: 200 mg q 2–3 hr for five to eight doses; daily doses can be increased until rhythm is restored or toxic effects occur.

Conversion of atrial flutter, maintenance therapy.

Adults: 200–300 mg 3–4 times per day. Large doses or more frequent administration may be required in some clients.

NURSING IMPLICATIONS

Do not confuse quinidine with quinine (an antimalarial) or with clonidine (an antihypertensive).

IMPLEMENTATION/ADMINISTRATION/STORAGE

1. A preliminary test dose may be given. **Adults:** 200 mg quinidine sulfate or quinidine gluconate administered PO or IM. **Children:** Test dose of 2 mg/kg of quinidine sulfate.
2. The extended-release forms are not interchangeable.
3. **IV** Prepare IV solution by diluting 10 mL of quinidine gluconate injection (800 mg) with 50 mL of D5W; give at a rate of 1 mL/min.
4. Use only colorless, clear solution for injection. Light may cause quinidine to crystallize, which turns solution brownish.
5. COMPATIBILITY D5W.
6. INCOMPATIBILITY Administer separately.

ASSESSMENT

1. Note any allergic reactions to antiarrhythmic drugs or tartrazine, which is found in some formulations. Perform a test dose; observe for hypersensitivity reactions and check for intolerance.
2. List reasons for therapy, onset, characteristics S&S, other agents/therapies trialed, outcome.
3. Assess VS, ECG, CXR, cardiopulmonary findings and monitor.
4. Report any increased AV block, prolonged PR or QT intervals, cardiac irritability, or rhythm suppression during IV administration and stop drug therapy.
5. Monitor I&O, VS; observe for ↓ BP. Drug induces urinary alkalization. Report any persistent diarrhea.
6. Report any neurologic deficits/sensory impairment (i.e., numbness, confusion, psychosis, depression, or involuntary movements).
7. Among the elderly, there is a higher risk of toxicity, reduced CO, and unpredictable drug effects.

Q

8. Clients with long-standing atrial fibrillation or CHF with atrial fibrillation run a risk of embolization from mural thrombi when converting to sinus rhythm. Assess echocardiogram and ensure antiocoagulated to prevent thromboembolism.
9. Ensure client aware of studies R/T increased mortality rates when used to treat non-life-threatening arrhythmias.
10. Monitor VS, lytes, CBC, PT/INR, renal and LFTs.

CLIENT/FAMILY TEACHING

1. Drug works by stabilizing the heart rhythm when the heart is beating too fast or with an irregular rhythm.
2. Take with food to minimize GI effects. Do not crush or chew sustained-release tablets.
3. Avoid activities that require mental alertness until drug effects realized; may cause dizziness or blurred vision.
4. Add fruit and grain to diet. A high intake of fruits and vegetables (alkaline-ash foods) may prolong drug half-life. However, avoid grapefruit juice if taking quinidine sulfate extended-release tablets. Intake of salt may increase the plasma levels of quinidine.
5. Report any skin rash, hives, itching. severe headache, unexplained fever, ringing in the ears, buzzing, or hearing loss, unusual bruising or bleeding, blurred vision, irregular heartbeat, palpitations, or faintness or continued diarrhea.
6. Wear dark glasses both indoors and outside if light sensitive. Avoid exposure to sunlight and use sunscreen, and protective clothing to avoid photosensitivity reaction.
7. Avoid OTC drugs or other agents without provider approval.
8. Ensure family/significant other know CPR.
9. Keep all F/U to assess response, labs, ECG, PFTs, eye exams, and for adverse SE.

OUTCOMES/EVALUATE

- Restoration of stable rhythm
- Therapeutic drug levels (2–6 mcg/mL)
- Malaria treatment (UL)

Quinine sulfate

(**KWYE**-nine)

Classification(s): Antimalarial

Pregnancy Category: D (Category C per manufacturer's prescribing guidelines)

RX: Qualaquin.

Rx: Quinine-Odan.

INDICATIONS/USES

Only for treatment of uncomplicated *Plasmodium falciparum* malaria. Shown to be effective in geographical regions where chloroquine resistance has been documented. *Investigational:* Prevention and treatment of nocturnal recumbency leg cramps; malaria caused by *P. falciparum.*

ACTION/KINETICS

Action

Natural alkaloid having antimalarial, antipyretic, analgesic, and oxytocic properties. Antimalarial mechanism not known precisely; is known to inhibit nucleic acid synthesis, protein synthesis, and glycolysis in *P. falciparum.* Eradicates the erythrocytic stages of plasmodia. Increases the refractory period of skeletal muscle, decreases the excitability of the motor end-plate region, and affects the distribution of calcium within the muscle fiber, thus making it useful for nocturnal leg cramps. Is oxytocic and may cause congenital malformations.

Pharmacokinetics

Rapidly and completely absorbed from the upper small intestine; widely distributed in body tissues. Oral bioavailability is 76–88% in healthy adults. **Peak plasma levels:** 1–3 hr; **plasma levels following chronic use:** 7 mcg/mL. **t½:** 4–5 hr. Metabolized in the liver by CYP450 enzymes with about 20% excreted unchanged in urine. Small amounts found in saliva, bile, feces, and gastric juice. Acidifying the urine increases the rate of excretion. Pharmacokinetics of quinine are affected by malaria, with a decrease in volume of distribution and systemic clearance. **Plasma protein binding:** 69–92%.

CONTRAINDICATIONS

Use with a prolonged QT interval; G6PD deficiency; myasthenia gravis; optic neuritis; known hypersensitivity to quinine, mefloquine, or quinidine; history of potential hypersensitivity reactions associated with previous quinine use (i.e., thrombotic thrombocytopenic purpura or hemolytic uremic syndrome); thrombocytopenia; blackwater fever (acute intravascular hemolysis, hemoglobinuria, hemoglobinemia). Pregnancy.

SPECIAL CONCERNS

- **Use with caution in clients with cardiac arrhythmias (e.g., atrial flutter/fibrillation) and during lactation.**
- **Hemolysis, with a potential for hemolytic anemia, may occur in clients with G6PD deficiency; use in these clients only if essential and under close supervision.**
- **Tinnitus and impaired hearing may occur at plasma quinine levels >10 mcg/mL (a level not normally reached with daily doses of quinine) but in a hypersensitive client, as little as 300 mg may produce tinnitus.**
- **Safety and efficacy not established in children less than 16 years of age.**

SIDE EFFECTS

Most Common

Headache, vasodilation, sweating, nausea, tinnitus, impaired hearing, vertigo/dizziness, blurred vision, disturbed color perception.

Use of quinine may result in a syndrome referred to as cinchonism. Mild cinchonism is characterized by tinnitus, hearing impairment, headache, vasodilation, sweating, nausea, vertigo/dizziness, blurred vision, disturbance of color perception. Larger doses, however, may cause severe CNS, CV, GI, or dermatologic effects.

Hypersensitivity reactions: Flushing, cutaneous rashes (papular, scarlatinal, urticarial), fever, angioedema, facial edema, ***bronchospasm***, pruritus, dyspnea, tinnitus, sweating, asthmatic symptoms, visual impairment, gastric upset, ***anaphylactoid reactions, anaphylaxis, Stevens-Johnson syndrome, toxic epidermal necrolysis***. **GI:** N&V, epigastric pain, GI disturbance, abdominal pain, diarrhea, esophagitis, gastric irritation. **Hepatic:** Hepatitis, granulomatous hepatitis, jaundice. **CNS:** Headache, confusion, restlessness, vertigo, syncope, fever, apprehension, excitement, delirium, hypothermia, dizziness, acute dystonic reactions, altered mental status, aphasia, ataxia, coma, confusion, disorientation, tremors, ***suicide, convulsions***. **CV:** Atrial fibrillation, AV block, bradycardia, ***cardiac arrest***, chest pain, hypotension, irregular rhythm, palpitations, postural hypotension, nodal escape beats, ***QT prolongation***, syncope, tachycardia, ***torsades de pointes***, unifocal premature ventricular contractions, U waves, vasodilation, ***ventricular fibrillation***, ventricular tachycardia. **Respiratory:** Symptoms of asthma, dyspnea, pulmonary edema. **Dermatologic:** Cutaneous rashes (including urticarial, papular, or scarlatinal rashes), acral necrosis, allergic contact dermatitis, bullous dermatitis, cutaneous vasculitis, erythema multiforme, exfoliative dermatitis, fixed drug eruption, photosensitivity reactions, pruritus, sweating, ***Stevens-Johnson syndrome, toxic epidermal necrolysis***. **Musculoskeletal:** Muscle weakness, myalgias. **GU:** Acute interstitial nephritis, renal failure, renal impairment. **Hematologic:** Acute hemolysis, hemolytic anemia, agranulocytosis, hypoprothrombinemia, hemolysis in clients with G-6–PD deficiency, ***aplastic anemia, blackwater fever***, coagulopathy, ***DIC***, ecchymosis, hemolytic uremic syndrome, ***hemorrhage***, idiopathic thrombocytopenic purpura, leukopenia, lupus anticoagulant, neutropenia, pancytopenia, petechiae, thrombocytopenia, thrombotic thrombocytopenic purpura. **Ophthalmic:** Diplopia, blurred vision with scotomata, photophobia, blindness/night blindness, decreased visual fields, impaired color vision and perception, amblyopia, mydriasis, optic atrophy, fixed pupillary dilatation, optic neuritis, photophobia, sudden loss of vision. **Otic:** Tinnitus and impaired hearing at plasma levels >10 mcg/mL; deafness, vertigo. **Body as a whole:** Asthenia, chills, fever, flushing, lupus-like syndrome. **Miscellaneous:** Hypoglycemia, lichenoid photosensitivity, anorexia.

LABORATORY TEST CONSIDERATIONS

↑ Urinary 17-ketogenic steroid values when the Zimmerman method is used. Hypoglycemia.

OVERDOSE MANAGEMENT

Symptoms: Dizziness, intestinal cramping, skin rash, tinnitus. With higher doses, symptoms include apprehension, confusion, fever, headache, vomiting, and seizures. *Treatment:*

- Induce vomiting or undertake gastric lavage.
- Maintain BP and renal function.
- If necessary, provide artificial respiration.
- Sedatives, oxygen, and other supportive measures may be required.
- Give IV fluids to maintain fluid and electrolyte balance.
- Treat angioedema or asthma with epinephrine, corticosteroids, and antihistamines.
- Urinary acidification will hasten excretion; however, in the presence of hemoglobinuria, acidification of the urine will increase renal blockade.

Q

DRUG INTERACTIONS

NOTE: An additive effect of quinine with other drugs that prolong the QT interval cannot be excluded. The following drugs may prolong the QT interval and increase the risk of life-threatening cardiac arrhythmias, included torsades de pointes: Amiodarone, arsenic trioxide, bretylium, chlorpromazine, cisapride, disopyramide, dofetilide, dolasetron, droperidol, halofantrine, mefloquine, mesoridazine, moxifloxacin, pentamidine, pimozide, procainamide, quinidine, sotalol, tacrolimus, thioridazine, ziprasidone.

Acetazolamide / ↑ Blood levels with potential for quinine toxicity R/T ↓ rate of elimination
Al-containing antacids / ↓ Or delayed quinine absorption; do not use together
Anticoagulants, oral / ↑ Warfarin action → additive hypoprothrombinemia R/T ↓ synthesis of vitamin K-dependent clotting factors
Carbamazepine / ↓ Plasma quinine levels; also, ↑ carbamazepine C_{max} and AUC
Cimetidine / ↑ Quinine effect R/T ↓ rate of excretion (↑ elimination $t^{1/2}$)
Desipramine / Inhibition of desipramine metabolism by CYP2D6; monitor
Dextromethorphan / Inhibition of dextromethorphan metabolism by CYP2D6; monitor
Digoxin / ↑ Digoxin serum levels; periodically monitor digoxin levels
Erythromycin / ↑ Quinine plasma levels; do not use together
Flecainide / Inhibition of flecainide metabolism by CYP2D6; monitor
Heparin / ↑ Heparin effect R/T depression of hepatic enzyme synthesis of vitamin K-dependent coagulation pathway proteins; monitor PT, PTT, and INR
HMG-CoA reductase inhibitors (e.g., atorvastatin, lovastatin, simvastatin) / ↑ Plasma HMG-CoA reductase inhibitor → possible myopathy and rhabdomyolysis
Ketoconazole / ↑ Quinine plasma levels
Mefloquine / ↑ Risk of ECG abnormalities or cardiac arrest; also, ↑ risk of convulsions. **Do not** use together; delay mefloquine administration at least 12 hr after the last dose of quinine.
Metoprolol / Inhibition of metoprolol metabolism by CYP2D6; monitor
Neuromuscular blocking agents (depolarizing and nondepolarizing) / ↑ Neuromuscular blockade → Respiratory depression and apnea
Phenobarbital / ↓ Plasma quinine levels
Phenytoin / ↓ Plasma quinine levels
Rifabutin, Rifampin / ↑ Hepatic clearance of quinine R/T induction of hepatic microsomal enzymes; can persist for several days after discontinuing rifampin
Smoking / Significantly greater quinine clearance R/T ↑ hepatic metabolism
Succinylcholine / ↓ Succinylcholine metabolism rate due to ↓ plasma cholinesterase activity
Tetracycline / ↑ Plasma quinine levels by 2-fold; monitor for quinine side effects
Troleandomycin / ↑ Quinine plasma levels; do not use together
Urinary alkalinizers (e.g., acetazolamide, sodium bicarbonate) / ↑ Quinine blood levels with potential for quinine toxicity R/T ↓ elimination rate
Warfarin / ↑ Warfarin effect R/T depression of hepatic enzyme synthesis of vitamin K-dependent coagulation pathway proteins; monitor PT, PTT, and INR
Xanthine derivatives (e.g., aminophylline, theophylline) / ↓ Plasma theophylline levels; monitor plasma theophylline levels

HOW SUPPLIED

Capsules: 324 mg.

DOSAGE

CAPSULES

Uncomplicated P. falciparum *malaria in adults.*
Adults and children, 16 years and older: 648 mg (2 capsules) q 8 hr for 7 days.

Malaria caused by Plasmodium falciparum *or species unknown.*
8.3 mg base/kg (=10 mg salt/kg) 3 times a day for 3–7 days plus one of the following: clindamycin 20 mg base/kg/day 3 times daily for 7 days *or* doxycycline 2.2 mg/kg q 12 hr for 7 days *or* tetracycline 25 mg/kg/day 4 times a day for 7 days.

Prevention and treatment of nocturnal recumbency leg cramps.
260–300 mg at bedtime.

Malaria caused by Plasmodium vivax.
8.3 mg base/kg (= 10 mg salt/kg) 3 times a day for 3–7 days and primaquine 0.5 mg base/kg/day for 14 days plus one of the following: doxycycline

Q

2.2 mg/kg q 12 hr for 7 days or tetracycline 25 mg/kg/day 4 times a day for 7 days.

NURSING IMPLICATIONS

Do not confuse quinine with quinidine (an antiarrhythmic).

IMPLEMENTATION/ADMINISTRATION/STORAGE

1. For severe, chronic renal failure, give a loading dose of 648 mg followed 12 hr later by maintenance doses of 324 mg q 12 hr.
2. Rule out clients at risk for G-6PD deficiency before breastfeeding.
3. The parenteral form is available from the Centers for Disease Control if client unable to take PO.
4. Dispense in a light-resistant and child-resistant container; store at controlled room temperatures of 25–30°C (77–86°F).

ASSESSMENT

1. List reasons for therapy, onset, duration, symptoms, travel dates, lab results, other agents trialed.
2. Note any history or evidence of liver dysfunction, cardiac arrhythmias or CAD.
3. Monitor ECG, LFTs, CBC, labs, and eye exams.

CLIENT/FAMILY TEACHING

1. Drug is an antimalarial; works by killing the malaria parasite.
2. Do not take with antacids. Take with food or after meals with a full glass of water to minimize GI irritation. Stop smoking.
3. Do not drive a car or operate machinery until drug effects realized; may cause dizziness or blurred vision.
4. Use sunglasses to protect from photophobia.
5. Avoid tonic water and OTC agents, especially cold remedies. If also taking cimetidine or digoxin, may require dosage adjustment; report side effects.
6. Females should use non-hormonal contraception; drug may harm fetus.
7. Report adverse effects, lack of response, ringing in the ears, blurring of vision, and headache, which may be followed by digestive disturbances, confusion, and delirium. May indicate intolerance or overdosage and requires immediate medical intervention.
8. Keep all F/U to assess response, labs, and for adverse SE.

OUTCOMES/EVALUATE

Termination of acute malarial attack/control of malaria symptoms

Combination Drug

IV

Quinupristin/ Dalfopristin

(**kwin**-oo-**PRIS**-tin, **DAL**-foh-**pris**-tin)

Classification(s): Antibiotic, streptogramin

Pregnancy Category: B

RX: Synercid.

INDICATIONS/USES

(1) Serious or life-threatening infections associated with vancomycin-resistant *Enterococcus faecium* bacteremia. (2) Complicated skin and skin structure infections caused by *Staphylococcus aureus* (methicillin-sensitive) or *Streptococcus pyogenes.*

ACTION/KINETICS

Action

A sterile, lyophilized product of two semisynthetic pristinamycin derivatives-quinupristin (30 parts) and dalfopristin (70 parts). The two act synergistically so the microbiologic activity is greater than each individually. Metabolites of the two are also active. The drugs act at the bacterial ribosome: Dalfopristin inhibits the early phase of protein synthesis while quinupristin inhibits the late phase of protein synthesis. Vancomycin-resistant infections may also be resistant to this product.

Pharmacokinetics

t½, quinupristin and metabolites: 3.07 hr; **t½, dalfopristin and metabolites:** 1.04 hr. Both can interfere with the metabolism of other drugs that are associated with QTc prolongation; however, they do not themselves induce QTc prolongation. Excreted through the feces (about 75% for both drugs) and urine (about 17% for both drugs).

CONTRAINDICATIONS

Hypersensitivity to quinupristin/dalfopristin or prior hypersensitivity to other streptogramins. Use

Q

with drugs metabolized by the CYP3A4 enzyme system that may prolong the QTc interval.

SPECIAL CONCERNS

■ This drug was approved through FDA's accelerated approval regulations for serious or life-threatening infections associated with vancomycin-resistant *Enterococcus faecium* bacteremia. Approval is based on a demonstrated effect on a surrogate endpoint that is likely to predict clinical benefit. Clearance of vancomycin-resistant *E. faecium* from the bloodstream with clearance of bacteremia is considered to be a surrogate endpoint. No results from well-controlled clinical studies confirm the validity of this surrogate marker, although such studies are underway. ■

- Use with caution during lactation.
- Although sometimes used for emergencies in children, safety and efficacy not determined in clients less than 16 years of age.

SIDE EFFECTS

Most Common

Inflammation/pain/edema at infusion site, N&V, diarrhea, rash, thrombophlebitis, pain, arthralgia, myalgia, pruritus.

At infusion site: Inflammation, pain, edema, infusion site reaction. **GI:** Pseudomembranous colitis (mild to life-threatening), N&V, diarrhea, constipation, dyspepsia, oral moniliasis, pancreatitis, stomatitis. **CNS:** Headache, anxiety, confusion, dizziness, hypertonia, insomnia, leg cramps, paresthesia. **CV:** Thrombophlebitis, palpitation, phlebitis, vasodilation. **Dermatologic:** Rash, pruritus, maculopapular rash, sweating, urticaria. **Musculoskeletal:** Arthralgia, myalgia, myasthenia. **GU:** Hematuria, vaginitis. **Respiratory:** Dyspnea, pleural effusion. **Miscellaneous:** Pain, abdominal pain, worsening of underlying illness, allergic reaction, chest pain, fever, infection, superinfection.

LABORATORY TEST CONSIDERATIONS

↑ AST, ALT, bilirubin, conjugated bilirubin, LDH, alkaline phosphatase, GGT, CPK, creatinine, BUN, hematocrit. ↓ Hemoglobin. ↑ or ↓ Blood glucose, bicarbonates, CO_2, sodium, potassium, platelets. Hyperbilrubinemia.

DRUG INTERACTIONS

Quinupristin/dalfopristin may cause increased plasma levels of drugs primarily metabolized by the CYP3A4 enzyme system. These drugs include: Carbamazepine, cisapride, cyclosporine, delavirdine, diazepam, diltiazem, disopyramide, docetaxel, HMG-CoA reductase inhibitors, indinavir, lidocaine, methylprednisolone, midazolam, nevirapine, nifedipine, paclitaxel, quinidine, ritonavir, tacrolimus, verapamil, vinca alkaloids.

HOW SUPPLIED

Injection, Lyophilized: 500 mg (150 mg quinupristin and 350 mg dalfopristin)/10 mL.

DOSAGE

IV INFUSION

Vancomycin-resistant Enterococcus faecium *infections.*

7.5 mg/kg q 8 hr. Base treatment duration on the site and severity of the infection.

Complicated skin and skin structure infections.

7.5 mg/kg q 12 hr for 7 days.

NURSING IMPLICATIONS

IMPLEMENTATION/ADMINISTRATION/STORAGE

1. IV Give by IV infusion in D5W over a 60-min period.
2. Central venous access may be used to decrease venous irritation.
3. Use infusion pump/device to control infusion rate.
4. Prepare and give as follows:
   - Reconstitute the single dose vial by slowly adding 5 mL D5W or sterile water for injection under strict aseptic conditions (e.g., laminar flow hood).
   - To ensure dissolution, gently swirl the vial by manual rotation without shaking (limits foam formation).
   - Allow solution to sit for a few minutes until all the foam has disappeared. Solution should be clear. Concentration is 100 mg/mL. Further dilution is required before administration; dilute within 30 min of reconstitution.
   - According to the client's weight, add the reconstituted solution to 250 mL of D5W (about 2 mg/mL). An infusion volume of 100 mL may be used for central line infusions.

- If moderate-to-severe venous irritation occurs following peripheral administration, consider increasing the infusion volume to 500 or 750 mL, changing the infusion site, or inserting a central venous catheter.

5. With intermittent infusion of these drugs and other drugs through a common IV line, flush the line before and after administration with D5W.
6. Before reconstitution, refrigerate vials at 2–8°C (36–46°F).
7. Prior to infusion, diluted solution stable for 5 hr at room temperature or 54 hr if refrigerated. Do not freeze the solution.
8. COMPATIBILITY D5W.
9. INCOMPATIBILITY Saline solutions. Do not mix with or physically add these drugs to other drugs except for the following: Aztreonam (20 mg/mL), ciprofloxacin (1 mg/mL), fluconazole (2 mg/mL), haloperidol (0.2 mg/mL), metoclopramide (5 mg/mL), and potassium chloride (40 mEq/L).

ASSESSMENT

1. Note reasons for therapy, characteristics of infection, culture and sensitivity results. Obtain blood cultures to verify *E. faecium* and not *E. faecalis. [vancomycin-resistant Enterococcus faecium (VREF)].*
2. If these drugs are used with drugs that are CYP3A4 substrates (see *Drug Interactions*) and possess a narrow therapeutic index, monitor liver function and client carefully.
3. If client develops diarrhea, test for *C. difficile* colitis.
4. Isolate client, and take special precautions to identify source and to prevent spread of organism.

CLIENT/FAMILY TEACHING

1. Drug is given parenterally to clear up infection that is resistant to vancomycin (VRE). May require isolation and care to prevent transmission throughout facility.
2. Report any pain redness or irritation at injection site, diarrhea, pain in joints/muscles. With persistent muscle and joint pains, may reduce severity by reducing the dosing interval to every 12 hrs. If S&S worsen, report.
3. Keep all F/U to assess response, labs, and adverse SE.

OUTCOMES/EVALUATE

- Resolution of VRE infection
- Treatment of infections R/T VREF bacteremia

R

Rabeprazole sodium

(rah-**BEP**-rah-zohl)

Classification(s): Proton pump inhibitor

Pregnancy Category: B

RX: Aciphex.

✤ **Rx:** Pariet.

INDICATIONS/USES

(1) Short-term (4–8 weeks) treatment in the healing and symptomatic relief of erosive or ulcerative gastroesophageal reflux disease (GERD). (2) Maintenance of healing and reduction in relapse rates of heartburn symptoms in clients with erosive or ulcerative GERD. (3) Short-term (up to 4 weeks) treatment in healing and symptomatic relief of duodenal ulcers. (4) Long-term treatment of pathological hypersecretory symptoms, including Zollinger-Ellison syndrome. (5) Daytime and nighttime heartburn and other symptoms of GERD in adults and adolescents 12 years of age and older. (6) In combination with amoxicillin and clarithromycin (triple therapy) to treat *H. pylori* infection and duodenal ulcer disease (active or history of within the past 5 years) to eradicate *H. pylori*. *Investigational:* Prevention of GI bleeding in those receiving antiplatelets.

ACTION/KINETICS

Action

Suppresses gastric secretion by inhibiting gastric H^+/K^+ ATPase at the secretory surface of parietal cells; it is a gastric proton-pump inhibitor. Blocks the final step of gastric acid secretion.

Pharmacokinetics

Is about 52% bioavailable. When taken with a high fat meal, T_{max} is variable and may delay absorption up 4 hr or longer; C_{max} and AUC not affected significantly. **Peak plasma levels:** 2–5 hr. **t½, plasma:** 1–2 hr. **Onset:** Less than 1 hr. **Duration:** Over 24 hr. Extensively metabolized in the liver by CYP3A4 and CYP2C19. Excreted mainly (90%) in the urine. In those with mild to severe hepatic impairment, AUC and t½ elimination are increased while total body clearance decreased. Also, AUC and C_{max} are increased in the elderly compared with younger clients. **Plasma protein binding:** 96.3%.

CONTRAINDICATIONS

Known sensitivity to rabeprazole or substituted benzimidazoles. Lactation.

SPECIAL CONCERNS

- **Greater sensitivity in some geriatric clients is possible.**
- **Symptomatic response to therapy does not preclude presence of gastric malignancy.**
- **Use with caution in severe hepatic impairment.**
- **Safety and efficacy not determined in children.**

SIDE EFFECTS

Most Common

Headache, GI upset, diarrhea, insomnia, nervousness, rash, itching.

GI: Diarrhea, N&V, abdominal pain, enlarged abdomen, GI upset, dyspepsia, flatulence, constipation, dry mouth, eructation, gastroenteritis, ***GI hemorrhage***, ***rectal hemorrhage***, melena, anorexia, cholelithiasis, cholangitis, duodenitis, mouth ulceration, stomatitis, dysphagia, gingivitis, cholecystitis, increased appetite, abnormal stools, bloody diarrhea, colitis, esophagitis, glossitis, pancreatitis, proctitis, enlarged salivary gland. **Hepatic:** Hepatic encephalopathy, hepatitis, hepatoma, liver fatty deposit. **CNS:** Insomnia, headache, anxiety, dizziness, depression, nervousness, somnolence, hypertonia, neuralgia, vertigo, ***convulsions***, abnormal dreams, decreased libido, neuropathy, paresthesia, tremor, coma, disorientation, delirium, agitation, amnesia, confusion, extrapyramidal syndrome, hyperkinesia. **CV:** Hypertension, ***MI***, abnormal EEG, migraine, syncope, angina pectoris, bradycardia, bundle branch block, palpitation, sinus bradycardia, QTc prolongation, SVT, tachycardia, thrombophlebitis, vasodilation, ventricular tachycardia. **Musculoskeletal:** Myalgia, arthritis, leg cramps, bone pain, arthrosis, twitching, bursitis, neck rigidity, ***rhabdomyolysis***. **Respiratory:** Dyspnea, asthma, epistaxis, laryngitis, apnea, hiccough, hyper-/hypoventilation, interstitial pneumonia, pulmonary embolus. **Dermatologic:** Rash, pruritus, sweating, urticaria, alopecia, dry skin, jaundice, bullous and other skin eruptions, erythema multiforme, herpes zoster, psoriasis, skin discoloration, ***toxic epidermal necrolysis, Stevens-Johnson syndrome***. **GU:** Cystitis, urinary frequency, dysmenorrhea, dysuria, kidney calculus, metorrhagia, polyuria, breast enlargement, hematuria, impotence, menorrhagia, orchitis, urinary incontinence, urine abnormality, interstitial nephritis. **Endocrine:** Hyper-/hypothyroidism. **Hematologic:** Anemia, ecchymosis, lymphadenopathy, hypochromic anemia, agranulocytosis, hemolytic anemia, leukopenia, pancytopenia, thrombocytopenia. **Metabolic:** Peripheral/facial edema, edema, weight gain/loss, gout, dehydration, hyper–/hypothyroidism. **Hypersensitivity:** Allergic reaction, angioedema, ***anaphylaxis***. **Ophthalmic:** Cataract, amblyopia, glaucoma, dry eyes, abnormal/blurred vision, corneal opacity, diplopia, eye pain, retinal degeneration, strabismus. **Otic:** Tinnitus, otitis media, deafness. **Body as a whole:** Asthenia, fever, chills, malaise, thirst, substernal chest pain, photosensitivity reaction, hangover effect, jaundice, ***sudden death***.

LABORATORY TEST CONSIDERATIONS

↑ CPK, AST, ALT, TSH, PSA. ↑ PT and INR in those also receiving warfarin. Abnormal platelets, erythrocytes, LFTs, urine, WBCs. Albuminuria, hypercholesterolemia, hyperglycemia, hyperlipemia, hypokalemia, hyponatremia, leukocytosis, leukorrhea, hyperammonemia.

DRUG INTERACTIONS

Ampicillin / ↓ Plasma levels of ampicillin R/T changes in gastric pH
Clarithromycin / Possible ↑ clarithromycin and rabeprazole serum levels
Cyanocobalamin / ↓ Plasma levels of cyanocobalamin R/T changes in gastric pH
Digoxin / ↑ Plasma levels of digoxin R/T changes in gastric pH
Itraconazole / ↓ Plasma levels of itraconazole R/T changes in gastric pH
Ketoconazole / ↓ Plasma levels of ketoconazole R/T changes in gastric pH
Iron salts / ↓ Plasma levels of iron salts R/T changes in gastric pH
Warfarin / ↑ PT and INR

HOW SUPPLIED

Tablets, Delayed-Release: 20 mg.

DOSAGE

TABLETS, DELAYED-RELEASE

Healing of erosive or ulcerative GERD.

Adults: 20 mg once daily for 4–8 weeks. An additional 8 weeks of therapy may be considered for those who have not healed.

Maintenance of healing of erosive or ulcerative GERD.

Adults: 20 mg once daily.

Healing of duodenal ulcers.

Adults: 20 mg once daily after the morning meal for up to 4 weeks. A few clients may require additional time to heal.

Treatment of pathological hypersecretory conditions.

Individualized. Adults, initial: 60 mg once a day. Adjust dosage to individual client needs (doses up to 100 mg/day and 60 mg 2 times per day have been used). Continue as long as clinically needed; some have been treated for up to 1 year.

Heartburn and other symptoms related to GERD.

Adults: 20 mg once daily for 4 weeks. If symptoms do not resolve after 4 weeks, an additional course of treatment may be considered. **Adolescents, 12 years and older:** 20 mg once daily for up to 8 weeks.

H. pylori *eradication to reduce risk of duodenal ulcer recurrence.*

Triple therapy. Rabeprazole, 20 mg two times a day for 7 days; amoxicillin, 1,000 mg two times a day for 7 days; clarithromycin, 500 mg two times a day for 7 days. All three medications should be taken with the morning and evening meals.

NURSING IMPLICATIONS

Do not confuse Aciphex with Accupril (ACE inhibitor) or with Aricept (drug for Alzheimer's disease).

IMPLEMENTATION/ADMINISTRATION/STORAGE

1. No dosage adjustment is needed in elderly clients, those with renal disease, or in mild to moderate hepatic impairment.
2. Protect tablets from moisture.
3. Store from 15–30°C (59–86°F).

ASSESSMENT

1. List reasons for therapy (short or long term), onset, duration, triggers, characteristics of S&S, other agents tried, outcome. List drugs prescribed to ensure none interact.
2. Note ECG, UGI/endoscopy findings/biopsies, abdominal assessment and any evidence of bleeding.
3. Monitor CBC, B12, TSH, *H. pylori,* renal and LFTs; note dysfunction.

CLIENT/FAMILY TEACHING

1. Take as directed. Swallow tablets whole with or without food; do not crush, chew, or split tablets.
2. Report unusual bruising/bleeding, acid reflux, abdominal pain, severe light-headedness, diarrhea, rash, or lack of effectiveness. Prolonged therapy may mask GI malignancies.
3. Avoid alcohol, NSAIDs, and salicylates; may increase GI upset.
4. Do not perform activities that require mental alertness until drug effects realized.
5. Keep all F/U to assess response, labs, and for adverse SE.

OUTCOMES/EVALUATE

- Reduced gastric acidity with relief of S&S of erosive esophagitis/GERD
- Healing of duodenal ulcers
- Treatment of hypersecretory conditions (e.g., Zollinger-Ellison syndrome)

Raloxifene hydrochloride

(ral-**OX**-ih-feen)

Classification(s): Estrogen receptor modulator

Pregnancy Category: X

RX: Evista.

INDICATIONS/USES

(1) Prevention and treatment of osteoporosis in postmenopausal women. (2) Reduce the risk of

invasive breast cancer in postmenopausal women with osteoporosis. (3) Reduce the risk of invasive breast cancer in postmenopausal women at high risk of invasive breast cancer. *Investigational:* Treatment of uterine leiomyomas (with gonadotropin-releasing hormone agonist therapy). Treatment of pubertal gynecomastia. Prevent bone loss in men with prostate cancer (with gonadotropin-releasing hormone agonist therapy).

ACTION/KINETICS

Action

Selective estrogen receptor modulator that is considered both an agonist and antagonist that combines with estrogen receptors. Acts as an agonist in bone in that it reduces bone resorption and decreases overall bone turnover, increases bone mineral density, and decreases fracture incidence. Has not been associated with endometrial proliferation, breast enlargement, breast pain, increased risk of breast cancer, or increased risk of heart attack and other heart problems. Also decreases total and LDL cholesterol levels.

Pharmacokinetics

Absorbed rapidly after PO (60% is absorbed); significant first-pass effect. Not metabolized by the CYP450 pathways. **t½:** 27.7 hr (multiple doses). Excreted primarily in feces with small amounts excreted in urine.

CONTRAINDICATIONS

In women who are or who might become pregnant, active or history of venous thromboembolic events (e.g., DVT, pulmonary embolism, retinal vein thrombosis). Use in premenopausal women, during lactation, in pediatric clients or in men (some investigational work is ongoing). Concurrent use with systemic estrogen or hormone replacement therapy. Use for the primary or secondary prevention of CV disease.

SPECIAL CONCERNS

■ (1) Increased risk of deep vein thrombosis (DVT) and pulmonary embolism have been reported with raloxifene. Women with active venous thromboembolism or a history of venous thromboembolism should not take raloxifene. (2) Increased risk of death caused by stroke occurred in a trial in postmenopausal women with documented coronary heart disease or increased risk for major coronary reactions. Consider the risk-benefit balance in women at risk for stroke. ■

- **Use with caution with highly protein-bound drugs, including clofibrate, diazepam, diazoxide, ibuprofen, indomethacin, and naproxen.**
- **Use with caution in moderate or severe impaired renal function and in those with impaired hepatic function.**
- **Effect on bone mass density beyond 2 years of treatment not known.**
- **Safety and efficacy not determined in children.**

SIDE EFFECTS

Most Common

Hot flashes, leg cramps, weight gain, nausea, dyspepsia, arthralgia, myalgia, sinusitis, pharyngitis, infection, flu syndrome.

CV: Hot flashes, migraine, venous thromboembolic events (e.g., ***pulmonary embolism, DVT***, retinal vein thrombosis/occlusion), ***stroke/death associated with venous thromboembolism***, syncope, varicose vein. **CNS:** Depression, headache, insomnia, vertigo, neuralgia, hypesthesia. **GI:** N&V, dyspepsia, diarrhea, flatulence, GI disorder, gastroenteritis, abdominal pain, cholelithiasis. **GU:** Vaginitis, UTI, cystitis, leukorrhea, endometrial disorder, uterine disorder, vaginal hemorrhage, urinary tract disorder, breast pain. **Respiratory:** Sinusitis, rhinitis, pharyngitis, bronchitis, increased cough, pneumonia, laryngitis. **Musculoskeletal:** Arthralgia, myalgia, leg cramps/muscle spasms, arthritis, tendon disorder. **Dermatologic:** Rash, sweating. **Body as a whole:** Infection, flu syndrome, headache, chest pain, fever, weight gain, peripheral edema, infection. **Miscellaneous:** Conjunctivitis.

LABORATORY TEST CONSIDERATIONS

↑ Apolipoprotein A1, steroid-binding globulin, thyroxine-binding globulin, corticosteroid-binding globulin. ↓ Total cholesterol, LDL cholesterol, fibrinogen, apolipoprotein B, lipoprotein.

DRUG INTERACTIONS

Cholestyramine / ↓ Raloxifene absorption by 60%; do not use together
Diazepam / Use with caution R/T both drugs highly protein bound
Diazoxide / Use with caution R/T both drugs highly protein bound
Estrogens, systemic / Safety has not been studied; do not use together

Levothyroxine / ↓ Levothyroxine absorption
Lidocaine / Use with caution R/T both drugs highly protein bound
Warfarin / ↓ PT; monitor PT closely

HOW SUPPLIED

Tablets: 60 mg.

DOSAGE

TABLETS

Prevention and treatment of osteoporosis in postmenopausal women; reduce risk of invasive breast cancer in postmenopausal women with osteoporosis or those at high risk of invasive breast cancer.

Adults: 60 mg once daily.

NURSING IMPLICATIONS

Do not confuse Evista with Avinza (an extended-release morphine sulfate).

IMPLEMENTATION/ADMINISTRATION/STORAGE

1. May be taken without regard for meals.
2. Take supplemental calcium (1,500 mg/day) and vitamin D (400–800 units/day) if daily dietary intake is inadequate in postmenopausal women.

ASSESSMENT

1. Note reasons for therapy; bone mineral density, onset of menopause, family history, any history of chronic steroid therapy.
2. Assess for history/evidence of CHF, CAD, active cancer; ↑ risk of breast cancer in high risk postmenopausal women, blood clots in legs, lungs, or eyes. Review risk of death due to stroke, (may be ↑ in postmenopausal women with documented coronary heart disease or at increased risk of major coronary events).
3. Monitor VS, bone density, lipids (triglycerides), renal and LFTs; assess for any dysfunction.

CLIENT/FAMILY TEACHING

1. Take as directed once daily with calcium (1,500 mg) and vitamin D supplements (400 international units). May take without regard to food, avoid all forms of estrogen therapy during treatment.
2. Drug is used by women after menopause to prevent bones from becoming weak and thin when bone mineral density is very low or to reduce risk or to inhibit invasive breast cancer in those at high risk with osteoporosis.
3. Avoid prolonged immobilization and movement restrictions as with travel, due to increased risk of blood clots. Stop 3 days prior to and during prolonged immobilization as with surgery or prolonged bed rest and only restart once client fully mobile.
4. Drug is not effective in reducing hot flashes or flushes associated with low estrogen; does not stimulate breast or uterus.
5. Regular weight-bearing exercises as well as tobacco cessation and alcohol modification should be practiced.
6. Have breast exams and mammograms performed before starting therapy and regularly thereafter.
7. Report pain in calves or swelling in legs, fever, insomnia, acute migraines, emotional distress, unexplained uterine bleeding, breast abnormalities, sudden chest pain, SOB, or coughing up blood, as well as any vision changes.
8. Keep all F/U to assess response, labs, BMD, and for adverse SE.

OUTCOMES/EVALUATE

- Treatment of postmenopausal osteoporosis with reduction in bone turnover/resorption
- Reduce risk of breast cancer in high risk postmenopausal women (unlabeled use)

Raltegravir potassium

(ral-**TEG**-ra-vir poe-**TAS**-ee-um)

Classification(s): Antiretroviral agent, integrase inhibitor.

Pregnancy Category: C

RX: Isentress.

R

INDICATIONS/USES

In combination with other antiretroviral agents for the treatment of HIV-1 infection in treatment-experienced or treatment-naive adults who have evidence of viral replication and HIV-1 strains resistant to multiple antiretroviral drugs.

ACTION/KINETICS

Action

Inhibits the catalytic activity of HIV-1 integrase, and HIV-1 encoded enzyme that is required for viral replication. Inhibition of integrase prevents the covalent insertion or integration of unintegrated linear HIV-1 DNA into the host cell genome, preventing the formation of HIV-1 provirus. Inhibiting the integration prevents propagation of the viral infection.

Pharmacokinetics

Maximum concentration: About 3 hr in fasting clients. With twice-daily dosing, pharmacokinetic steady-state is reached in about 2 days. **t½, terminal:** 9 hr. UGT1A1 is the main enzyme responsible for formation of the glucuronide metabolite. Parent drug is excreted in the feces (51%) and parent drug and metabolites are excreted in the urine (32%). **Plasma protein binding:** 83%.

CONTRAINDICATIONS

Lactation.

SPECIAL CONCERNS

- **Immune reconstitution syndrome: Clients responding to antiretroviral therapy may develop an inflammatory response to indolent or residual opportunistic infections, including *Mycobacterium avium* complex, cytomegalovirus, *Pneumocystis jiroveci* pneumonia, *Mycobacterium* tuberculosis, or reactivation of varicella zoster virus.**
- **Use with caution in clients at increased risk of myopathy or rhabdomyolysis.**
- **Dose selection in the elderly should be cautious.**
- **Safety and efficacy not determined in children.**

SIDE EFFECTS

Most Common

Headache, diarrhea, nausea, pyrexia.

GI: Diarrhea, nausea, abdominal pain, vomiting, gastritis, hepatitis. **CNS:** Headache, dizziness, depression, anxiety, insomnia, suicidal ideation/behaviors. **CV:** ***MI***. **GU:** Toxic nephropathy, renal failure, chronic renal failure, renal tubular necrosis, genital herpes. **Dermatologic:** Acquired lipodystrophy, rash, ***Stevens-Johnson syndrome***. **Musculoskeletal:** Myopathy, rhabdomyolysis. **Hematologic:** Anemia, neutropenia. **Body as a whole:** Pyrexia, asthenia, fatigue, hypersensitivity. **Miscellaneous:** Herpes simplex/zoster; development of cancers, including Kaposi's sarcoma, lymphoma, squamous cell carcinoma, hepatocellular carcinoma, anal cancer (although most clients had other risk factors for cancer); immune reconstitution syndrome.

R

LABORATORY TEST CONSIDERATIONS

↑ ALT, AST, total serum bilirubin, serum alkaline phosphatase, serum pancreatic amylase, serum lipase, serum creatine kinase. ↓ Absolute neutrophil count, hemoglobin, platelet count. Hyperglycemia.

DRUG INTERACTIONS

Raltegravir is eliminated mainly via UGT1A1-mediated glucuronidation; coadministration of raltegravir with drugs that inhibit UGT1A1 may ↑ raltegravir plasma levels.

Atazanavir / ↑ Raltegravir plasma levels R/T inhibition of UGT1A1; monitor client response
Atazanavir/Ritonavir / ↑ Raltegravir plasma levels R/T inhibition of UGT1A1; monitor client response
Efavirenz / ↓ Plasma raltegravir levels; monitor client response
Etravirine / ↓ Plasma raltegravir levels; monitor client response
Omeprazole / ↑ Raltegravir plasma levels R/T ↑ raltegravir solubility at higher pH
Rifampin / ↓ Raltegravir plasma levels R/T induction of UGT1A1; coadminister with caution; adjust raltegravir dose to 800 mg twice/day; coadminister with caution
Tipranavir/Ritonavir / The combination ↓ raltegravir plasma levels; monitor client response

HOW SUPPLIED

Tablets: 400 mg.

DOSAGE

TABLETS

HIV infection.

Adults: 400 mg twice a day, with or without food. *NOTE:* If used with rifampin, the recommended dose of raltegravir is 800 mg twice a day.

NURSING IMPLICATIONS

IMPLEMENTATION/ADMINISTRATION/STORAGE

1. **To monitor maternal-fetal outcomes of pregnant individuals exposed to raltegravir, an antiretroviral registry has been established. Health care providers are encouraged to register clients by calling 1-800-258-4263.**
2. **Store from 15–30°C (59–86°F).**

ASSESSMENT

1. Note disease onset, characteristics of S&S, other agents trialed/failed.
2. List drugs prescribed; ensure none interact.
3. Note mental status, and presence of depression or anxiety.
4. Assess for S&S of lactic acidosis, muscle pain, opportunistic infections.
5. Check CBC, lipids, CPK, renal and LFTs; may reduce dose with dysfunction. Monitor CD4+ cell count and HIV RNA load.

CLIENT/FAMILY TEACHING

1. Drug works by blocking HIV-1 integrase, an enzyme needed for the HIV virus to replicate.
2. Take with or without food as directed; do not skip or double doses.
3. Avoid activities that require mental alertness until drug effects realized; may cause dizziness.
4. Report symptoms of unexplained muscle pain, tenderness, or weakness.
5. Practice reliable contraception; stop drug and report if pregnancy suspected. An Antiretroviral Pregnancy Registry has been established to monitor maternal-fetal outcomes (1-800-258-4263). Does not prevent disease transmission or STDs; use protection.
6. Keep all F/U to evaluate response to therapy and adverse SE.

OUTCOMES/EVALUATE

- Management of HIV infection
- ↓ HIV RNA

Ramelteon

(ram-**EL**-tee-on)

Classification(s): Sedative-hypnotic, nonbarbiturate

Pregnancy Category: C

RX: Rozerem.

INDICATIONS/USES

Insomnia due to difficulty with sleep onset. *NOTE:* Has been shown to be effective in elderly clients with a low incidence of side effects.

ACTION/KINETICS

Action

Ramelteon is a melatonin receptor agonist with high affinity for melatonin MT_1 and MT_2 receptors. The activity at melatonin receptors is thought to contribute to its sleep-promoting properties, as these receptors are thought to be involved in the maintenance of the circadian rhythm underlying the normal sleep-wake cycle.

Pharmacokinetics

Rapidly absorbed. **Median peak levels:** 0.75 hr (0.5–1.5 hr) after fasting and PO administration. Significant first-pass metabolism is primarily oxidation to hydroxyl and carbonyl derivatives by CYP1A2. Excreted mainly in the urine. Repeated once-daily administration does not result in significant accumulation because of the short elimination **t½** (about 1–2.6 hr).

CONTRAINDICATIONS

Hypersensitivity to the drug or any component of the product. Use with severely impaired hepatic function. Use in clients with severe sleep apnea or chronic COPD as the drug has not been evaluated in these populations. Lactation.

SPECIAL CONCERNS

- Use with caution in moderate impaired hepatic function.
- Use with caution in those taking less strong CYP1A2 inhibitors.

SIDE EFFECTS

Most Common

Somnolence, dizziness, nausea, diarrhea, fatigue, headache, insomnia.

CNS: Somnolence, dizziness, headache, insomnia, depression. **GI:** Diarrhea, nausea, dysgeusia. **Respiratory:** URTI. **Body as a whole:** Fatigue, influenza, myalgia, arthralgia.

DRUG INTERACTIONS

Alcohol / Additive CNS depressant effects
Azole antifungals (e.g., fluconazole, ketoconazole) / Significant ↑ ramelteon AUC and C_{max}
Fluvoxamine / Significant (190-fold) ↑ ramelteon AUC; do not use together
Rifampin / ↓ Ramelteon AUC and C_{max}

HOW SUPPLIED

Tablets: 8 mg.

DOSAGE

TABLETS

Insomnia due to difficulty with sleep onset.

Adults: 8 mg taken within 30 min of going to bed.

R

NURSING IMPLICATIONS

IMPLEMENTATION/ADMINISTRATION/STORAGE

1. Should not be taken with or immediately after a high-fat meal.
2. Store from 15–30°C (59–86°F). Protect from moisture and humidity; keep container tightly closed.

ASSESSMENT

1. Note reasons for therapy, onset, characteristics of S&S, contributing factors, other agents trialed, outcome.
2. Assess for any history of breathing problems (bronchitis, emphysema, sleep apnea), psychiatric illness, or liver disease; may preclude drug therapy.
3. List drugs prescribed to ensure none interact unfavorably.
4. If GU dysfunction or problems with fertility surface, consider reviewing prolactin/testosterone levels.

CLIENT/FAMILY TEACHING

1. Take drug as prescribed within 30 min of going to bed; confine activities to those for sleep preparation. Never attempt to engage in hazardous activities (i.e., operate machinery or drive a car) after dose.
2. Ramelteon acts like a natural substance called melatonin that is produced by your body. It helps regulate your sleep-wake cycle (circadian rhythm).
3. Avoid alcohol and do not consume ramelteon with or immediately after consuming a high fat meal; fat may interfere with drug action. Do not break tablet, swallow it whole.
4. May experience sedation; avoid activities that require mental alertness upon awakening.
5. Report any problems with menses or breast drainage, decreased libido, or fertility problems. Also advise provider of any adverse side effects, behavioral changes, or worsening of insomnia.
6. Advise of reports of people getting out of bed after taking a sleep medication and driving their cars while not fully awake, often with no memory of the event. Other complex behaviors (e.g., preparing and eating food, making phone calls, having sex) have also been reported in those who were not fully awake after taking a sleep medicine.
7. Reinforce activities/changes that may facilitate sleep: quiet and dark environment, avoidance of caffeine and nicotine, warm water bath, relaxation techniques.
8. Keep all F/U to assess response and for adverse SE.

OUTCOMES/EVALUATE

- Ability to get to sleep
- Relief of insomnia

Ramipril

(**RAM**-ih-prill)

Classification(s): Antihypertensive, ACE inhibitor

Pregnancy Category: D (Category C during first trimester and Category D during second and third trimesters)

RX: Altace.

✤ **Rx:** Apo-Ramipril, Novo-Ramipril, ratio-Ramipril.

SEE ALSO ***ANGIOTENSIN-CONVERTING ENZYME INHIBITORS***.

INDICATIONS/USES

(1) Alone or in combination with other antihypertensive agents (especially thiazide diuretics) for the treatment of hypertension. (2) Treatment of CHF following MI to decrease risk of CV death and decrease the risk of failure-related hospitalization and progression to severe or resistant heart failure. (3) Reduce risk of stroke, MI, and death from CV causes in clients over 55 years with a history of CAD, stroke, peripheral vascular disease, or with diabetes and one other risk factor (e.g., elevated total cholesterol, cigarette smoking, hypertension, low HDL levels, documented microalbuminuria). Can be used in addition to other therapy, including antihypertensive, antiplatelet, or lipid-lowering therapy. *Investigational:* Reduce progression of nondiabetic nephropathy.

ACTION/KINETICS

Action

Inhibits angiotensin-converting enzyme resulting in decreased plasma angiotensin II, which leads to decreased vasopressor activity and decreased aldosterone secretion.

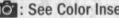

Pharmacokinetics

Onset: 1–2 hr. From 50–60% bioavailable. **Time to peak serum levels:** 1 hr (1–2 hr for ramiprilat, the active metabolite). **Peak effect:** 3–6 hr. Ramiprilat has approximately six times the ACE inhibitory activity than ramipril. **t½:** 1–2 hr (9–18 hr for ramiprilat); prolonged in impaired renal function. **Duration:** 24 hr. Metabolized in the liver with 60% excreted through the urine and 40% in the feces. Food decreases the rate, but not the extent, of absorption of ramipril. Peak levels are approximately doubled and trough levels may be as much as five times higher in those with a C_{CR} <40 mL/min. Metabolism is slowed in those with hepatic impairment. Peak levels and AUC are higher in the elderly. **Plasma protein binding:** Ramipril: about 73%; ramiprilat: 56%.

CONTRAINDICATIONS

Lactation.

SPECIAL CONCERNS

> When used in pregnancy during the second and third trimesters, ACE inhibitors can cause injury and even death to the developing fetus. When pregnancy is detected, discontinue as soon as possible.

- **Geriatric clients may manifest higher peak blood levels of ramiprilat.**
- **May cause hyperkalemia, especially when used with salt substitutes.**

SIDE EFFECTS

Most Common

Hypotension, headache, dizziness, N&V, cough.

CV: Hypotension (may be profound especially after the first dose), bradycardia, ***cardiac arrest,*** chest pain, palpitations, angina pectoris, orthostatic hypotension, CHF, TIA, ***MI, CVA, arrhythmias,*** tachycardia. **GI:** N&V, abdominal pain, diarrhea, dysgeusia, anorexia, constipation, dry mouth, dyspepsia, enzyme changes suggesting pancreatitis, dysphagia, gastroenteritis, increased salivation, jaundice, taste disturbance. **Hepatic:** Hepatitis, hepatic failure, ***fatal fulminant hepatic necrosis.*** **CNS:** Headache, dizziness, fatigue, insomnia, sleep disturbances, somnolence, drowsiness, depression, nervousness, malaise, vertigo, anxiety, amnesia, ***convulsions,*** tremor. **Respiratory:** Cough (may be chronic), dyspnea, URI, asthma, ***bronchospasm.*** **Hematologic:** Leukopenia, anemia, eosinophilia, pancytopenia, hemolytic anemia, thrombocytopenia. Rarely, decreases in hemoglobin or hematocrit. **Dermatologic:** Diaphoresis, photosensitivity, pruritus, rash, dermatitis, purpura, onycholysis, alopecia, erythema multiforme, urticaria, ***Stevens–Johnson syndrome, toxic epidermal necrolysis.*** **Musculoskeletal:** Muscle cramps, myalgia, arthralgia, arthritis. **GU:** Impotence, abnormal renal function. **Body as a whole:** Paresthesias, angioedema, asthenia, syncope, fever, neuralgia, neuropathy, influenza, edema, vasculitis. **Miscellaneous:** Impotence, tinnitus, hearing loss, vision disturbances, epistaxis, weight gain, proteinuria, angioneurotic edema, edema, flu syndrome.

LABORATORY TEST CONSIDERATIONS

↑ Blood glucose (rare), uric acid. ↓ H&H. Hyperkalemia, proteinuria, hypoglycemia.

ADDITIONAL DRUG INTERACTIONS

Hypoglycemic drugs, oral / Possible hypoglycemia
Insulin / Possible hypoglycemia

HOW SUPPLIED

Capsules: 1.25 mg, 2.5 mg, 5 mg, 10 mg; *Tablets:* 1.25 mg, 2.5 mg, 5 mg, 10 mg.

DOSAGE

CAPSULES; TABLETS

Hypertension.

Initial: 2.5 mg once daily in clients not taking a diuretic; **maintenance:** 2.5–20 mg/day as a single dose or two equally divided doses.

Congestive heart failure (CHF) following myocardial infarction (MI).

Initial: 2.5 mg twice a day. Clients intolerant of this dose may be started on 1.25 mg twice a day. The target maintenance dose is 5 mg twice a day.

Reduce risk of MI, stroke, death in clients 55 and over with risk factors.

Initial: 2.5 mg/day for 1 week followed by 5 mg/day for the next 3 weeks.
Maintenance: 10 mg/day. If the client is hypertensive or post-MI, the dose can be divided.

NOTE: In clients with a C_{CR} of 40 $mL/min/m^2$ or less, doses of 25% of those normally used should cause full

R

therapeutic levels of ramiprilat. For use in hypertension, start with 1.25 mg once daily; dose may be titrated upward until BP is controlled or to a maximum of 5 mg/day. For use in heart-failure post-MI, start with 1.25 mg once daily. Dose may be increased to 1.25 mg twice a day, up to a maximum of 2.5 mg twice a day, depending on response and tolerability.

NURSING IMPLICATIONS

Do not confuse Altace with Artane (cholinergic blocking agent).

IMPLEMENTATION/ADMINISTRATION/STORAGE

1. If antihypertensive effect decreases at the end of the dosing interval with once-daily dosing, consider either twice-daily administration or an increase in dose.
2. If taking diuretic, discontinue 2–3 days prior to beginning ramipril. If BP is not controlled, reinstitute diuretic. If the diuretic cannot be discontinued, consider an initial dose of ramipril of 1.25 mg.
3. Dosage adjustment may be needed in those with impaired renal function.

ASSESSMENT

1. Note reasons for therapy, other agents trialed, other medical conditions, and outcome.
2. List drugs prescribed to ensure none interact.
3. Assess for other medical conditions that may preclude therapy; renal artery stenosis, severe autoimmune disease, lupus, scleroderma, or bone marrow depression.
4. Monitor BP, K^+, microalbumin, CBC, renal and LFTs to ensure no abnormality; adjust dose with dysfunction.

CLIENT/FAMILY TEACHING

1. For ease of swallowing, may mix contents of the capsule with water, apple juice, or applesauce.
2. Use caution; drug may cause drowsiness or dizziness and low BP effects with sudden changes in position.
3. Report persistent, dry, nonproductive cough, increased SOB, sore throat, fever, swelling of hands or feet, irregular heartbeat, chest pains, significant weight gain, unusual bruising/bleeding or swelling of the face, lips, or tongue.
4. Avoid prolonged sun/UV exposure; wear protection if exposed, may cause sensitivity reaction.
5. Practice reliable birth control; report if pregnancy suspected or desired as drug will need to be stopped.
6. For BP control, continue additional modalities (e.g., weight control, regular exercise, smoking cessation, and moderate intake of alcohol and salt) to ensure success.
7. Do not take OTC agents, including potassium/potassium-based salt supplements without approval.
8. Keep all F/U to assess response, review BP and HR record, labs, and for adverse SE.

OUTCOMES/EVALUATE

- ↓ BP
- ↓ Mortality with AMI/DM
- ↓ Risk of MI, stroke, or death from CV causes in high risk clients

Ranibizumab

(ran-ih-**BIZ**-oo-mab)

Classification(s): Selective vascular endothelial growth factor antagonist.

Pregnancy Category: C

RX: Lucentis.

INDICATIONS/USES

(1) Neovascular (wet) age-related macular degeneration. (2) Macular edema following retinal vein occlusion.

ACTION/KINETICS

Action

Binds to the receptor-binding site of active forms of vascular endothelial growth factor A (VEGF-A). VEGF-A causes neovascularization and leakage and is thought to contribute to the progression of the neovascular form of age-related macular degeneration. The binding of ranibizumab to VEGF-A prevents the interaction of VEGF-A with its receptors on the surface of endothelial cells, reducing endothelial cell proliferation, vascular leakage, and new blood vessel formation.

Pharmacokinetics

Small amounts are absorbed systemically. **t½, vitreous elimination:** 9 days.

CONTRAINDICATIONS

Ocular or periocular infections. Hypersensitivity to any component of the product.

SPECIAL CONCERNS

- **Use with caution during lactation.**
- **Safety and efficacy not determined in children.**

SIDE EFFECTS

Most Common

Conjunctival hemorrhage, eye irritation/pain, foreign body sensation in eyes, intraocular inflammation, increased intraocular pressure, retinal hemorrhage, blurred/decreased visual acuity, vitreous detachment/floaters, headache, arthralgia, nasopharyngitis, URTI, hypertension.

Ophthalmic: Blepharitis, cataract, conjunctival hemorrhage, conjunctival hyperemia, dry eye, eye irritation, eye pain, eye pruritus, foreign body sensation in eyes, injection–site hemorrhage, intraocular inflammation, increased intraocular pressure, increased lacrimation, maculopathy, ocular discomfort, ocular hyperemia, posterior capsule opacification, retinal degeneration, retinal disorder, retinal exudates, retinal hemorrhage, subretinal fibrosis, blurred/decreased visual acuity, visual disturbance, vitreous detachment, vitreous floaters, increased intraocular pressure, endophthalmitis, retinal detachments. **CNS:** Headache, dizziness, insomnia. **GI:** Nausea, constipation, viral gastroenteritis. **CV:** Hypertension/elevated BP, arterial thromboembolic reactions, atrial fibrillation, possible increased risk of stroke. **Musculoskeletal:** Arthralgia, arthritis, back pain, pain in extremity. **Respiratory:** Bronchitis, COPD, cough, dyspnea, nasopharyngitis, sinusitis, URTI. **Miscellaneous:** Anemia, influenza, hypersensitivity, immunogenicity, UTI.

LABORATORY TEST CONSIDERATIONS

Hypercholesterolemia.

DRUG INTERACTIONS

When used adjunctively with verteporfin photodynamic therapy, possible serious intraocular inflammation

HOW SUPPLIED

Injection Solution, Intravitreal (Ophthalmic): 10 mg/mL.

DOSAGE

INTRAVITREAL INJECTION ONLY

Neovascular (wet) age-related macular degeneration, macular edema following retinal vein occlusion.

Administer 0.5 mg (0.05 mL) by intravitreal injection once a month (about 28 days). To treat macular degeneration, although less effective, treatment may be reduced to 1 injection every 3 months after the first 4 injections, if monthly injections are not feasible.

NURSING IMPLICATIONS

IMPLEMENTATION/ADMINISTRATION/STORAGE

1. **For ophthalmic intravitreal injection only.**
2. **Using aseptic technique, all (0.2 mL) of the ranibizumab vial contents are withdrawn through a 5-micron, 19-gauge filter needle attached to a 1 mL tuberculin syringe. Discard filter needle after withdrawal from the vial; do not use for intravitreal injection. Replace filter needle with a sterile 30-gauge × ½-inch needle for the intravitreal injection. Expel the contents until plunger tip is aligned with the line that marks 0.05 mL on the syringe.**
3. **Carry out intravitreal injection under controlled aseptic conditions, including use of sterile gloves, sterile drape, and a sterile eyelid speculum. Give adequate anesthesia and a broad-spectrum microbicide prior to the injection.**
4. **Use each vial only to treat a single eye. If the contralateral eye requires treatment, use a new vial. Change the sterile field, syringe, gloves, drapes, eyelid speculum, filter, and injection needles.**
5. **Refrigerate from 2–8°C (36–46°F). Do not freeze; protect from light. Store in original container until use.**

ASSESSMENT

1. **Note onset, symptoms, history, baseline IOP and vision level.**
2. **List drugs prescribed to ensure none interact.**

R

3. Assess eye area to ensure infection free and post injection IOP. (Monitor IOP, and for endophthalmitis.)
4. Monitoring may consist of a check for perfusion of the optic nerve head immediately after the injection and tonometry within 30 min following the injection. Monitor during the week following the injection to permit early treatment in case an infection occurs. Monitor IOP as well as the perfusion of the optic nerve head.
5. Add daily supplement of vitamins A, C, and E, along with beta-carotene, zinc, and copper.
6. Identify agencies and support groups that can assist with low vision.

CLIENT/FAMILY TEACHING

1. Drug is injected into eye by retinal specialist to maintain/improve vision with macular degeneration (wet). A post-injection exam will be done before leaving office. Have friend/family member accompany so they can drive you home after injection. Bring sunglasses/hat to wear after injection; may be light sensitive (eyes were dilated).
2. May experience red eye, eye pain, small specks in vision, sensation of something in eye, and increased tears. Other side effects may include high blood pressure, nose and throat infection, and headache.
3. Can track progress in-between visits (using an Amsler grid). By using an Amsler grid once a week, you may be able to see changes to your vision. Ask retinal specialist for one or download one from http://www.lucentis.com/lucentis/about_and_monitor.html.
4. Macular degeneration is usually seen in white females over 55 years old who have a family history, are obese, smoke, consume a diet low in minerals such as zinc, and vitamins A, C, and E and have cardiovascular disease.
5. Report if eyes become red, sensitive to light, painful, or vision changes.
6. Generally the injections are given once a month. Keep all F/U visits to evaluate progress, maintain/improve vision, and to assess for any adverse SE.

OUTCOMES/EVALUATE

Maintenance/improvement in vision with macular degeneration

IV

Ranitidine hydrochloride

(rah-**NIH**-tih-deen)

Classification(s): Histamine H_2 receptor blocking drug

Pregnancy Category: B

OTC: Zantac 150 Maximum Strength Acid Reducer, Zantac 75 Acid Reducer.

RX: Zantac, Zantac EFFERdose.

Rx: Apo-Ranitidine, CO Ranitidine, Gen-Ranitidine, Novo-Ranitidine, Nu-Ranit, PMS-Ranitidine, ratio-Ranitidine, Sandoz Ranitidine.

SEE ALSO ***HISTAMINE H_2 ANTAGONISTS***.

INDICATIONS/USES

Rx: (1) Short-term (4–8 weeks) and maintenance treatment of duodenal ulcer. (2) Pathologic hypersecretory conditions such as Zollinger-Ellison syndrome and systemic mastocytosis. (3) Short-term treatment of active, benign gastric ulcers and maintenance treatment after healing of the acute ulcer. (4) Treatment of GERD. (5) Treatment of endoscopically diagnosed erosive esophagitis and for maintenance of healing of erosive esophagitis. (6) IV in some hospitalized clients with pathological hypersecretory conditions or intractable duodenal ulcers, or as an alternative to PO doses for short-term use in those who are unable to take PO medication.

Investigational: **PO or IM/IV:** As part of a multidrug regimen to eradicate *Helicobacter pylori* in the treatment of peptic ulcer; perioperatively to suppress gastric acid secretion, prevent stress ulcers, and prevent aspiration pneumonitis; in combination with H_1 histamine antagonists to treat certain types of urticaria; and, as prophylaxis to reduce the incidence of NSAID-induced duodenal ulcers.

IV: Prevent paclitaxel hypersensitivity; reduce the incidence of GI hemorrhage associated with stress-related ulcers.

OTC: (1) Relief of heartburn associated with acid indigestion and sour stomach. (2) Prophylaxis of heartburn associated with acid indigestion and sour stomach due to certain foods and beverages.

ACTION/KINETICS

Action

Competitively inhibits gastric acid secretion by blocking the effect of histamine on histamine H_2 receptors. Both daytime and nocturnal basal gastric acid secretion, as well as food- and pentagastrin-stimulated gastric acid are inhibited. Weak inhibitor of cytochrome P-450 (drug-metabolizing enzymes); thus, drug interactions involving inhibition of hepatic metabolism are not expected to occur.

Pharmacokinetics

Bioavailability is 50% after PO administration and 90–100% after IM. Food increases the bioavailability. **Peak effect, PO:** 2–3 hr; **IM; IV:** 15 min. **t½:** 2.5–3 hr. **Duration, nocturnal:** 13 hr; **basal:** 4 hr. **Serum level to inhibit 50% stimulated gastric acid secretion:** 36–94 ng/mL. From 30% to 35% of a PO dose and from 68% to 79% of an IV dose excreted unchanged in urine. **Plasma protein binding:** 15%.

CONTRAINDICATIONS

Cirrhosis of the liver, impaired renal or hepatic function.

SPECIAL CONCERNS

- **Use with caution during lactation, in the elderly, and with decreased hepatic or renal function.**
- **Safety and efficacy not established in children.**

SIDE EFFECTS

Most Common

Headache, abdominal pain, constipation, diarrhea, N&V.

GI: Constipation, N&V, diarrhea, abdominal pain, pancreatitis (rare). **CNS:** Headache, dizziness, malaise, insomnia, vertigo, confusion, anxiety, agitation, depression, fatigue, somnolence, hallucinations. **CV:** Bradycardia or tachycardia, premature ventricular beats following rapid IV use (especially in clients predisposed to cardiac rhythm disturbances), vasculitis, ***cardiac arrest***. **Hematologic:** Thrombocytopenia, granulocytopenia, leukopenia, pancytopenia (sometimes with marrow hypoplasia), ***agranulocytosis, autoimmune hemolytic or aplastic anemia***. **Hepatic:** Hepatotoxicity, jaundice, hepatitis, increase in ALT. **Dermatologic:** Erythema multiforme, rash, alopecia. **Allergic:** ***Bronchospasm, anaphylaxis***, angioneurotic edema (rare), rashes, fever, eosinophilia. **Miscellaneous:** Arthralgia, gynecomastia, impotence, loss of libido, blurred vision, pain at injection site, local burning or itching following IV use.

DRUG INTERACTIONS

Antacids / May ↓ ranitidine absorption
Cyanocobalamin / ↓ Cyanocobalamin absorption R/T ↑ gastric pH
Diazepam / ↓ Diazepam effects R/T ↓ GI tract absorption
Glipizide / ↑ Glipizide effects
Procainamide / ↓ Procainamide excretion → possible ↑ effect
Smoking / ↓ Rate of ulcer healing
Theophylline / Possible ↑ theophylline pharmacologic and toxicologic effects
Warfarin / May ↑ warfarin hypoprothrombinemic effects

HOW SUPPLIED

Rx. ***Capsules:*** 150 mg, 300 mg; ***Injection:*** 1 mg/mL (premixed), 25 mg/mL; ***Oral Solution:*** 15 mg/mL; ***Syrup:*** 15 mg/mL; ***Tablets:*** 150 mg, 300 mg; ***Tablets, Effervescent:*** 25 mg.
OTC. ***Tablets:*** 75 mg, 150 mg.

DOSAGE

RX: CAPSULES; ORAL SOLUTION; SYRUP; TABLETS; TABLETS, EFFERVESCENT

Duodenal ulcer, short-term.

Adults: 150 mg twice a day or 300 mg after the evening meal or at bedtime. A dose of 100 mg twice daily is as effective as the 150 mg dose in inhibiting gastric acid secretion. **Maintenance:** 150 mg at bedtime. **Children:** 2–4 mg/kg/day given twice a day, up to a maximum of 300 mg/day. For maintenance in children, 2–4 mg/kg once daily, up to a maximum of 150 mg/day.

Pathologic hypersecretory conditions.

Adults: 150 mg twice a day (up to 6 grams/day has been used in severe cases). **Children:** 5–10 mg/kg/day, usually in 2 divided doses.

Benign gastric ulcer.

Adults: 150 mg twice a day for active ulcer. **Maintenance:** 150 mg at bedtime. **Children:** 2–4 mg/kg/day given

R

twice a day, up to a maximum of 300 mg/day. For maintenance in children, 2–4 mg/kg once daily, up to a maximum of 150 mg/day.

Gastroesophageal reflux disease.

Adults: 150 mg twice a day. **Children:** 5–10 mg/kg/day, usually given as 2 divided doses.

Erosive esophagitis.

Adults: 150 mg 4 times per day.

Maintenance of healing of erosive esophagitis.

Adults: 150 mg twice a day. **Maintenance:** 150 mg twice a day. **Children:** 5–10 mg/kg/day, usually in 2 divided doses.

IM; IV

Treatment and maintenance for duodenal ulcer, hypersecretory conditions, gastroesophageal reflux.

Adults, IM: 50 mg q 6–8 hr. **Intermittent bolus:** 50 mg q 6–8 hr (dilute 50 mg in 0.9% NaCl or other compatible IV solution to a concentration no greater than 2.5 mg/mL [20 mL]). Inject at a rate no greater than 4 mL/min (5 minutes). **Intermittent IV infusion:** 50 mg q 6–8 hr. Dilute 50 mg in 5% dextrose injection or other compatible IV solution to a concentration no greater than 0.5 mg/mL (100 mL) and infuse at a rate no greater than 5–7 mL/min (15–20 min) or use 50 mL of 1 mg/mL premixed solution and infuse over 15–20 min. Do not exceed 400 mg/day. **Continuous IV infusion:** Add the injection to 5% dextrose injection or other compatible IV solution. Give at a rate of 6.25 mg/hr (e.g., 150 mg ranitidine injection in 250 mL of 5% dextrose injection at 10.7 mL/hr).

Children, IV: 2–4 mg/kg/day in divided doses q 6–8 hr, up to a maximum of 50 mg q 6–8 hr.

Zollinger-Ellison clients.

Continuous IV infusion: Dilute ranitidine in 5% dextrose injection or other compatible IV solution to a concentration no greater than 2.5 mg/mL with an initial infusion rate of 1 mg/kg/hr. If after 4 hr the client shows a gastric acid output of greater than 10 mEq/hr or if symptoms appear, increase the dose by 0.5 mg/kg/hr increments and measure the acid output. Doses up to 2.5 mg/kg/hr may be necessary.

OTC: TABLETS

Treat heartburn.

Treatment: 75 mg or 150 mg with a glass of water. **Maintenance:** Use up to 2 times per day (up to 2 tablets in 24 hr).

Prevent heartburn.

75 mg or 150 mg with a glass of water 30–60 min before eating food or drinking beverages that cause heartburn.

NURSING IMPLICATIONS

(Sound Alike Drug) Do not confuse Zantac with Xanax (an antianxiety drug) or with Zyrtec (an H_1 receptor blocker). Do not confuse ranitidine with rimantadine (an antiviral).

IMPLEMENTATION/ADMINISTRATION/STORAGE

1. If the C_{CR} is less than 50 mL/min, give 50 mg PO q 24 hr or 50 mg parenterally q 18–24 hr. Parenteral dosing may be increased to q 12 hr or further with caution.
2. Give antacids concomitantly for gastric pain although they may interfere with ranitidine absorption.
3. Dissolve EFFERdose tablets and granules in 6–8 oz of water before taking. The 25 mg EFFERdose tablets (for use in infants) are dissolved in at least 5 mL of water; solution may be given with dosing cup, medicine dropper, or oral syringe.
4. About one-half of clients may heal completely within 2 weeks; thus, endoscopy may show no need for further treatment.
5. No dilution is required for IM use.
6. Store tablets from 15–30°C (59–86°F) in a dry place protected from light. Store effervescent tablets and granules from 2–30°C (36–86°F). Store the syrup from 4–25°C (39–77°F). Dispense in a light-resistant container.
7. IV The premixed injection does not require dilution; give by slow IV drip over 15–20 min. Do not introduce additives into the solution. If

R

used with a primary IV fluid system, discontinue primary solution during drug infusion.

8. Drug is stable for 48 hr at room temperature when mixed with 0.9% NaCl, 5% or 10% dextrose injection, RL, or 5% $NaHCO_3$ injection.
9. Undiluted ranitidine injection tends to manifest a yellow color that may intensify over time without adversely affecting potency.
10. Visually inspect parenteral drug product for particulate matter and discoloration before administration.
11. Premixed ranitidine injection (50 mg/50 mL), in 0.45% NaCl, is available as a sterile, premixed solution for IV use in single-dose, flexible plastic containers. The product does not contain preservatives.
12. Store the premixed injection from 2–25°C (36–77°F) and the injection from 4–25°C (39–77°F) protected from light.
13. COMPATIBILITY 0.45% NaCl, 0.9% NaCl, D5W or D10W, RL, or 5% $NaHCO_3$ injection.
14. INCOMPATIBILITY Administer separately.

ASSESSMENT

1. List reasons for therapy, onset, duration, triggers, characteristics of S&S.
2. Record abdominal assessment, skin lesions, urea breath, labs, UGI/endoscopic and biopsy results.
3. Assess for infections. Determine if pregnant.
4. Skin tests using allergens may elicit false negative results; stop drug 24–72 hr prior to testing.
5. Monitor CBC, B12, renal and LFTs.

CLIENT/FAMILY TEACHING

1. Take as directed with or immediately following meals. May take with antacid for stomach pain but interferes with drug absorption.
2. For EFFERdose tablets and granules, dissolve each dose in 6–8 oz of water before drinking. Do not chew, swallow whole or dissolve effervescent tablets on the tongue. A liquid (syrup) is available if unable to swallow pills; may use this preparation with feeding tubes.
3. Do not drive or operate machinery until drug effects are realized; dizziness or drowsiness may occur.
4. Avoid alcohol, aspirin-containing products, and beverages that contain caffeine (tea, cola, coffee); these increase stomach acid. Avoid things that may aggravate symptoms, i.e., alcohol, aspirin, NSAIDs, caffeine, chocolate, and black pepper. Avoid herbals such as garlic, ginseng, ginkgo, or vitamin E with ulcer.
5. Do not smoke; interferes with healing and drug's effectiveness.
6. Report any evidence of yellow discoloration of skin or eyes, or diarrhea. Maintain adequate hydration. Report any confusion/disorientation, unusual bruising or bleeding, black tarry stools, diarrhea or rash immediately.
7. Symptoms of breast tenderness will usually disappear after several weeks; report if persistent may need to stop drug.
8. Keep all F/U to assess extent of healing, expected length of therapy, labs, and for adverse SE.

OUTCOMES/EVALUATE

- ↓ Gastric acid production
- ↓ Abdominal pain/discomfort
- Endoscopic/radiographic evidence of duodenal ulcer healing

Ranolazine

(rah-**NOH**-la-zeen)

Classification(s): Antianginal drug

Pregnancy Category: C

RX: Ranexa.

INDICATIONS/USES

Treat chronic angina. May be used with beta-blockers, nitrates, calcium channel blockers, antiplatelet therapy, lipid-lowering therapy, angiotensin-converting enzyme inhibitors, and angiotensin-receptor blockers. *NOTE:* Ranolazine prolongs the QT interval; thus, reserve use for those who have not achieved an adequate response with other antianginal drugs.

R

ACTION/KINETICS

Action

Mechanism is not known. The drug has antianginal and anti-ischemic effects that do not depend on decreases in HR or BP. The drug does not increase the rate-pressure product, a measure of myocardial work at maximal exercise. QTc prolongation effect on the surface ECG is the result of inhibition of I_{Kr}, which prolongs the ventricular action potential.

Pharmacokinetics

Absorption is highly variable. **Peak plasma levels:** Between 2–5 hr. Bioavailability is 76%. Steady state is usually reached in 3 days with twice daily dosing. Food has no significant effect on C_{max} or AUC. **t½, terminal:** 7 hr. Metabolized rapidly and extensively in the liver (mainly by CYP3A and CYP2D6) and intestine. Excreted in the urine (75%) and feces (25%). **Plasma protein binding:** About 62%.

CONTRAINDICATIONS

Use in pre-existing QT prolongation, in impaired hepatic function (Child-Pugh classes A, B, or C), in severe impaired renal function, if on QT-prolonging drugs, and if on potent and moderately potent CYP3A inhibitors (e.g., diltiazem, HIV protease inhibitors, ketoconazole, macrolide antibiotics, verapamil), or CYP3A inducers. Lactation.

SPECIAL CONCERNS

Safety and efficacy not determined in children.

SIDE EFFECTS

Most Common

Dizziness, headache, constipation, nausea, lightheadedness.

CV: Palpitations, bradycardia, hypotension, orthostatic hypotension, palpitations, prolongation of QTc interval (may cause ***torsades de pointes-type arrhythmias, and sudden death***). **GI:** N&V, constipation, abdominal pain, dry mouth. **CNS:** Dizziness, headache, lightheadedness, vertigo, hypesthesia, paresthesia, tremor, syncope, confusion. **Respiratory:** Dyspnea, pulmonary fibrosis. **GU:** Hematuria, renal failure. **Hematologic:** Eosinophilia, leukopenia, pancytopenia, thrombocytopenia. **Ophthalmic:** Blurred vision. **Otic:** Tinnitus. **Body as a whole:** Asthenia, angioedema. **Miscellaneous:** Peripheral edema.

LABORATORY TEST CONSIDERATIONS

Small, reversible ↑ BUN and serum creatinine. Small, mean ↓ hematocrit. Transient esosinophilia.

OVERDOSE MANAGEMENT

Symptoms: Expected symptoms include confusion, diplopia, dizziness, N&V, paresthesia, syncope with prolonged loss of consciousness. *Treatment:* Continuous ECG monitoring (due to increase in QTc interval). Initiate general supportive measures. Complete clearance by hemodialysis is not likely.

DRUG INTERACTIONS

Amiodarone / Prolongation of QT interval → ↑ risk of life-threatening cardiac arrhythmias, including torsades de pointes
Aprepitant / ↑ Ranolazine plasma levels and QTc prolongation; adjust ranolazine dosage
Arsenic trioxide / Prolongation of QT interval → ↑ risk of life-threatening cardiac arrhythmias, including torsades de pointes
Azole antifungals / ↑ Ranolazine levels and QTc prolongation R/T inhibition of metabolism by CYP3A; do not use together
Bretylium / Prolongation of QT interval → ↑ risk of life-threatening cardiac arrhythmias, including torsades de pointes
Carbamazepine / ↑ Ranolazine clearance → ↓ plasma levels
Chlorpromazine / Prolongation of QT interval → ↑ risk of life-threatening cardiac arrhythmias, including torsades de pointes
Clarithromycin / ↑ Ranolazine plasma levels and QTc prolongation; do not use together
Cyclosporine ↑ / Ranolazine absorption; down titrate ranolazine dosage as needed
Digoxin / ↑ Digoxin levels 1.5 fold; may need to ↓ digoxin dose
Diltiazem / ↑ Ranolazine steady-state levels by about 1.8–2.3 fold R/T inhibition of metabolism by CYP3A; do not use together
Disopyramide / Prolongation of QT interval → ↑ risk of life-threatening cardiac arrhythmias, including torsades de pointes
Dofetilide / Prolongation of QT interval → ↑ risk of life-threatening cardiac arrhythmias, including torsades de pointes
Dolasetron / Prolongation of QT interval → ↑ risk of life-threatening cardiac arrhythmias, including torsades de pointes
Droperidol / Prolongation of QT interval → ↑ risk of life-threatening cardiac arrhythmias, including torsades de pointes
Grapefruit juice / ↑ Ranolazine levels and QTc prolongation R/T inhibition of metabolism by CYP3A; do not use together
Ketoconazole / ↑ Ranolazine steady-state levels 3.2 fold R/T inhibition of metabolism by CYP3A; do not use together

R

Macrolide antibiotics (e.g., erythromycin) / ↑ Ranolazine levels and QTc prolongation R/T inhibition of metabolism by CYP3A; do not use together
Mefloquine / Prolongation of QT interval → ↑ risk of life-threatening cardiac arrhythmias, including torsades de pointes
Mesoridazine / Prolongation of QT interval → ↑ risk of life-threatening cardiac arrhythmias, including torsades de pointes
Moxifloxacin / Prolongation of QT interval → ↑ risk of life-threatening cardiac arrhythmias, including torsades de pointes
Nefazodone / ↑ Ranolazine plasma levels and QTc prolongation; do not use together
Paroxetine / ↑ Ranolazine steady-state plasma levels 1.2 fold
Pentamidine / Prolongation of QT interval → ↑ risk of life-threatening cardiac arrhythmias, including torsades de pointes
Phenobarbital / ↑ Ranolazine clearance → ↓ plasma levels
Phenytoin / ↑ Ranolazine clearance → ↓ plasma levels
Pimozide / Prolongation of QT interval → ↑ risk of life-threatening cardiac arrhythmias, including torsades de pointes
Procainamide / Prolongation of QT interval → ↑ risk of life-threatening cardiac arrhythmias, including torsades de pointes
Protease inhibitors (e.g., indinavir, nelfinavir, ritonavir, saquinavir) / ↑ Ranolazine levels and QTc prolongation R/T inhibition of metabolism by CYP3A; do not use together
Quinidine / Prolongation of QT interval → ↑ risk of life-threatening cardiac arrhythmias, including torsades de pointes
Rifamycins (e.g., rifampin) / ↓ Ranolazine plasma levels by 95%
Simvastatin / ↑ Levels of simvastatin and its active metabolites; may need to ↓ simvastatin dose
Sotalol / Prolongation of QT interval → ↑ risk of life-threatening cardiac arrhythmias, including torsades de pointes
H ***St. John's wort*** / ↑ Ranolazine clearance → ↓ plasma levels
Tacrolimus / Prolongation of QT interval → ↑ risk of life-threatening cardiac arrhythmias, including torsades de pointes
Thioridazine / Prolongation of QT interval → ↑ risk of life-threatening cardiac arrhythmias, including torsades de pointes
Verapamil / ↑ Ranolazine steady-state levels by about 2 fold R/T inhibition of metabolism by CYP3A; do not use together
Ziprasidone / Prolongation of QT interval → ↑ risk of life-threatening cardiac arrhythmias, including torsades de pointes

HOW SUPPLIED

Tablets, Extended-Release: 500 mg, 1,000 mg.

DOSAGE

TABLETS, EXTENDED-RELEASE

Chronic angina.

Adults, initial: 500 mg two times a day; increase to a maximum of 1,000 mg two times a day, as needed based on clinical symptoms. Dosage adjustments are usually not needed on the basis of age, gender, in those with CHF (NYHA, class I-IV), or diabetes mellitus.

NURSING IMPLICATIONS

IMPLEMENTATION/ADMINISTRATION/STORAGE

1. For the elderly, use caution when selecting the dose; start at the low end of the dosage range.
2. If a dose is missed, the prescribed dose should be taken at the next scheduled time; do not double the dose.
3. Avoid using ranolazine with potent or moderately potent inhibitors of CYP3A because coadministration will increase ranolazine plasma levels and QTc prolongation. Inhibitors include azole antifungals (e.g., ketoconazole), diltiazem, grapefruit juice (or grapefruit-containing products), HIV protease inhibitors, macrolide antibiotics, and verapamil. Limit the dose of ranolazine in such instances to 500 mg twice a day.
4. Store from 15–30°C (59–86°F).

ASSESSMENT

1. Note reasons for therapy, generally used for those not responding adequately to other antianginal drugs; list all other therapies, procedures, and outcome.

R

2. Check baseline ECG and monitor; may cause QTc interval prolongation. Assess for any personal or family history of QTc prolongation, congenital long QT syndrome, or proarrhythmic conditions such as hypokalemia.
3. List drugs prescribed; note if receiving drugs that prolong the QTc interval such as Class Ia (e.g., quinidine) or Class III (e.g., dofetilide, sotalol) antiarrhythmic agents, erythromycin, and certain antipsychotics (e.g., thioridazine, ziprasidone).
4. If receiving drugs that are potent or moderately potent inhibitors of CYP3A, i.e., ketoconazole, HIV protease inhibitors, macrolide antibiotics, diltiazem, and verapamil do not use this drug.
5. Avoid using doses of Ranexa higher than 1,000 mg twice a day and in the elderly.
6. Generally used in combination with another medicine (i.e., amlodipine, beta-blockers, nitrates).
7. Monitor ECG, electrolytes, renal/LFTs; avoid use with dysfunction, or QT prolongation.

CLIENT/FAMILY TEACHING

1. May take with or without meals. Grapefruit juice or grapefruit products should be avoided.
2. Swallow tablets whole; do not crush, break, or chew tablets. Drug is used with others such as amlodipine, beta-blockers, nitrates to control angina symptoms.
3. Avoid activities that require mental alertness, may cause dizziness, lightheadedness, or fainting. Alcohol, hot weather, exercise, and fever can increase these effects. To prevent, sit up or stand slowly, especially in the morning. Report any palpitations or fainting spells.
4. If dose of drug is missed, take the next dose at the next scheduled time. The next dose should not be doubled.
5. Ranexa will not stop an acute angina episode (have SL NTG readily available); use other therapy for acute angina and notify provider.
6. Keep all F/U to assess response, labs, ECG, and for adverse SE.

OUTCOMES/EVALUATE

Control of resistant angina

Rasagiline

(rah-**SA**-jih-leen)

Classification(s): Antiparkinson drug.

Pregnancy Category: C

RX: Azilect.

INDICATIONS/USES

Treat signs and symptoms of idiopathic Parkinson's disease as initial monotherapy and as adjunct therapy to levodopa. The drug may slow progression of Parkinson's disease.

ACTION/KINETICS

Action

Rasagiline is a potent, irreversible monoamine oxidase (MAOI) of MAO type B. The precise mechanism in treating parkinsonism is not known but may include an increase in extracellular levels of dopamine in the striatum. Elevated dopamine levels and subsequent increased dopaminergic activity likely mediate rasagiline's beneficial effects.

Pharmacokinetics

Rapidly absorbed. **Peak plasma levels:** 1 hr. Absolute bioavailability is about 36%. Food does not affect the time to reach T_{max}, although T_{max} and AUC are decreased by about 60% and 20%, respectively when the drug is taken with a high-fat meal. Undergoes almost complete metabolism in the liver mainly by CYP1A2. Excreted in the urine (62%) and feces (7%).

CONTRAINDICATIONS

Hypersensitivity to any component of the product. Tyramine-rich foods, beverages, or dietary supplements and amines (from OTC cough/cold medications) to prevent a possible hypertensive crisis. Pheochromocytoma. Coadministration with meperidine, methadone, propoxyphene, tramadol, dextromethorphan, St. John's wort, mirtazapine, cyclobenzaprine, sympathomimetic amines (including amphetamines, nasal and oral decongestants, cold products, and weight-reducing products), other MAOIs, cocaine, and local or general anesthetics. Moderate or severe impaired hepatic function.

SPECIAL CONCERNS

- Use with caution during lactation.
- Safety and efficacy not determined in children.

SIDE EFFECTS

Most Common

When used as monotherapy: Headache, dyspepsia, flu syndrome, depression, fall, dyspepsia, arthralgia, gastroenteritis, rhinitis, fever.

R

When used as an adjunct to levodopa therapy: Dyskinesia, accidental injury, weight loss, postural hypotension, N&V, anorexia, arthralgia, abdominal pain, constipation, dry mouth, rash, ecchymosis, somnolence, paresthesia.

Monotherapy. CNS: Hallucinations, depression, headache, malaise, paresthesia, vertigo, dizziness, hallucinations, syncope. **GI:** Dyspepsia, gastroenteritis, diarrhea, anorexia, vomiting. **CV:** Angina pectoris. **Musculoskeletal:** Arthralgia, arthritis. **Respiratory:** Rhinitis, asthma. **Dermatologic:** Ecchymosis, alopecia, skin carcinoma, vesiculobullous rash. **GU:** Impotence, decreased libido. **Hematologic:** Leukopenia. **Miscellaneous:** Fall, flu syndrome, conjunctivitis, fever, neck/chest pain, allergic reaction.

Adjunct to levodopa therapy. CNS: Hallucinations, dyskinesia, somnolence, paresthesia, headache, ataxia, dystonia, amnesia, confusion, abnormal gait, anxiety, hyperkinesia, neuropathy, tremor, agitation, aphasia, circumoral paresthesia, convulsions, delusions, dementia, dysarthria, dysautonomia, dysesthesia, emotional lability, facial paralysis, foot drop, hemiplegia, hypesthesia, incoordination, manic reaction, migraine, myoclonus, neuritis, neurosis, paranoid reaction, personality disorder, psychosis, wrist drop, apathy, delirium, hostility, manic depressive reaction, myelitis, neuralgia, psychotic depression, stupor. **GI:** Diarrhea, N&V, anorexia, abdominal pain, constipation, dry mouth, dyspepsia, gingivitis, dysphagia, ***GI hemorrhage***, colitis, esophageal ulcer, esophagitis, fecal incontinence, intestinal obstruction, mouth ulceration, stomach ulcer, stomatitis, tongue edema, hematemesis, ***hemorrhagic gastritis***, ***intestinal perforation***, intestinal stenosis, jaundice, ***large intestine perforation***, megacolon, melena. **CV:** Postural hypotension, hemorrhage, ***CVA***, bundle branch block, deep thrombophlebitis, ***heart failure***, ***MI***, phlebitis, ventricular tachycardia, ***arterial thrombosis***, atrial arrhythmia, complete AV block, second degree AV block, bigeminy, ***cerebral hemorrhage***, cerebral ischemia, ***ventricular fibrillation***. **Hematologic:** Anemia, macrocytic anemia, purpura, thrombocythemia. **Respiratory:** Dyspnea, epistaxis, increased cough, apnea, emphysema, laryngismus, pleural effusion, pneumothorax, interstitial pneumonia, ***larynx edema***, lung fibrosis. **Musculoskeletal:** Arthralgia, tenosynovitis, myasthenia, arthritis, bursitis, leg cramps, bone necrosis, muscle atrophy, arthrosis. **Dermatologic:** Rash, ecchymosis, sweating, skin carcinoma/ulcer, pruritus, eczema, urticaria, exfoliative dermatitis, leukoderma, increased risk of melanoma. **GU:** Hernia, hematuria, urinary incontinence, abnormal sexual function, acute kidney failure, dysmenorrhea, dysuria, kidney calculus, nocturia, polyuria, scrotal edema, urinary retention, impaired urination, ***vaginal hemorrhage***, vaginal moniliasis, vaginitis, abnormal ejaculation, amenorrhea, anuria, epididymitis, gynecomastia, hydroureter, leukorrhea, priapism. **Ophthalmic:** Blepharitis, diplopia, eye hemorrhage, eye pain, glaucoma, keratitis, ptosis, retinal degeneration, visual field defect, blindness, retinal detachment, retinal hemorrhage, strabismus. **Otic:** Deafness, vestibular disorder. **Body as a whole:** Weight loss, infection, asthenia, chills, photosensitivity. **Miscellaneous:** Accidental injury/falls, hernia, neck pain, taste perversion, parosmia, photophobia, taste loss.

LABORATORY TEST CONSIDERATIONS

Monotherapy: Albuminuria, leukopenia. **Adjunct to levodopa therapy:** Albuminuria. hypocalcemia.

OVERDOSE MANAGEMENT

Symptoms: Possible symptoms include drowsiness, dizziness, faintness, irritability, hyperactivity, agitation, severe headache, hallucinations, trismus, opisthotonos, ***convulsions***, ***coma***, rapid and irregular pulse, hypertension, hypotension, ***vascular collapse***, precordial pain, respiratory depression/failure, hyperpyrexia, diaphoresis, cool/clammy skin. *Treatment:* Treatment is symptomatic and supportive. Support respiration, including management of the airway, supplemental oxygen, and mechanical ventilatory assistance, if needed. Monitor body temperature closely. Intensive management of hyperpyrexia may be required. Maintain fluid and electrolyte balance.

DRUG INTERACTIONS

Anesthetics / Do not use together; discontinue rasagiline at least 14 days prior to elective surgery

Antidepressants (e.g., tricyclic antidepressants, mirtazapine, SNRIs, SSRIs) / Severe CNS toxicity with hyperpyrexia and death; at least 14 days should elapse between discontinuing rasagiline and beginning an antidepressant

Ciprofloxacin / ↑ Rasagiline AUC by 83%

R

CNS stimulants / Possible hypertensive crisis; do not use together
Cocaine / Possible hypertensive crisis; do not use together
Cyclobenzaprine / Do not use together as cyclobenzaprine is structurally related to tricyclic antidepressants
CYP1A2 inhibitors (e.g., atazanavir, mexiletine, tacrine) / Possible 2-fold ↑ in rasagiline plasma levels → ↑ side effects
Dextromethorphan / Possible brief episodes of psychosis and bizarre behavior; do not use together; ↑ risk of serotonin syndrome
Fluoxetine / Possible CNS toxicity with hyperpyrexia and death; at least 5 weeks should elapse between discontinuing fluoxetine and beginning rasagiline
Levodopa / Possible potentiation of dopaminergic side effects and exacerbation of dyskinesia; possibly reduce levodopa dose
MAOIs / Possible hypertensive crisis; at least 14 days should elapse between discontinuing rasagiline and starting MAOIs
Meperidine / Possible coma, severe hypertension or hypotension, severe respiratory depression, convulsions, death; at least 14 days should elapse between discontinuing rasagiline and beginning meperidine
Methadone / Possible coma, severe hypertension or hypotension, severe respiratory depression, convulsions, death
H ***St. John's wort*** / Do not use together
Sympathomimetic (e.g., amphetamines, cold products, anorexiants) / Possible severe hypertensive reactions
Tramadol / Possible coma, severe hypertension or hypotension, severe respiratory depression, convulsions, death
Tricyclic antidepressants / ↑ Risk of serotonin syndrome
Tryptophan / ↑ Risk of serotonin syndrome
Tyramine-containing foods/beverages / Possible severe hypertensive crisis

HOW SUPPLIED

Tablets: 0.5 mg (as base), 1 mg (as base).

DOSAGE

TABLETS

Idiopathic Parkinson's disease.

Monotherapy: 1 mg once daily. **Adjunctive therapy, initial:** 0.5 mg once daily; if satisfactory response is not obtained, may increase the dose to 1 mg once daily.

NURSING IMPLICATIONS

IMPLEMENTATION/ADMINISTRATION/STORAGE

1. When used wtih levodopa, consider a decrease in the levodopa dosage, depending on individual client response.
2. Use a dose of 0.5 mg in clients with mild impaired hepatic function. Do not give rasagiline to those with moderate or severe impaired hepatic function.
3. Plasma levels of rasagiline may double in those taking concomitant ciprofloxacin or other CYP1A2 inhibitors. Thus, in such clients, use rasagiline, 0.5 mg/day.
4. Store form 15–30°C (59–86°F).

ASSESSMENT

1. Note onset, duration and reasons for therapy, other agents trialed, outcome.
2. List drugs prescribed to ensure none interact especially, SSRI antidepressants, sympathomimetic amine drugs, Ciprofloxacin inhibits the enzymes in the liver that eliminate rasagiline, thereby increasing blood levels and possibly adverse SE of rasagiline.
3. With Parkinson's, note range of motion, rigidity, tremor, gait, and facial expressions. Decrease dose of levodopa if used together.
4. Perform periodic skin examinations for melanoma.
5. Belongs to a class of drugs called monoamine oxidase inhibitors (MAOI) that also includes selegiline and tranylcypromine. Use cautiously especially with other drugs.
6. Monitor VS, CBC, and LFTs.

CLIENT/FAMILY TEACHING

1. Used alone or in combination with levodopa to treat S&S of Parkinson's disease. Avoid foods high in tyramine; hypertensive crisis may occur.
2. Use caution, do not drive or perform other tasks that require mental alertness until drug effects realized. May cause dizziness, drowsiness, lightheadedness, or fainting; alcohol, hot weather, exercise, or fever may increase these effects. To minimize, sit up or stand slowly, especially in the a.m.

R

3. Eating foods high in tyramine (e.g., aged cheeses, red wines, beer, certain meats and sausages, liver, sour cream, soy sauce, raisins, bananas, avocados) while you use an MAOI may cause severe high blood pressure. This could occur for up to 2 weeks after you stop taking an MAOI. Do not eat foods high in tyramine while you take rasagiline.
4. Report if severe headache, fast or irregular heartbeat, sore or stiff neck, nausea, vomiting, sweating, enlarged pupils, or sensitivity to light occur.
5. Avoid CNS stimulants e.g., pseudoephedrine, phenylephrine, or ephedrine while using rasagiline.
6. Rasagiline should be discontinued at least 14 days before elective surgery.
7. If advised to stop taking rasagiline, you will need to wait at least 14 days before beginning to take certain other medicines (e.g., medicines for depression, anxiety, pain, cough, congestion, weight loss, Parkinson disease; muscle relaxants).
8. Review S&S of marked BP elevation; severe headache or other atypical or unusual symptoms that could be caused by hypertensive crisis and report.
9. Rasagiline may increase your risk of developing skin cancer (melanoma). Report any skin changes (e.g., change in color or thickness).
10. Keep all F/U to assess response, BP, labs, skin exams, and for adverse SE.

OUTCOMES/EVALUATE

Improved S&S of Parkinson's disease with improved function

IV

Rasburicase

(ras-**BYOUR**-ih-kase)

Classification(s): Antimetabolite, purine analog

Pregnancy Category: C

RX: Elitek.

SEE ALSO ***ANTINEOPLASTIC AGENTS***.

INDICATIONS/USES

Initial treatment to reduce plasma uric acid levels in adults and children with leukemia, lymphoma, and solid tumor malignancies who are receiving anticancer therapy expected to cause tumor lysis and thus increases in plasma uric acid.

ACTION/KINETICS

Action

A recombinant urate-oxidase enzyme that catalyzes enzymatic oxidation of uric acid into an inactive and soluble metabolite (allantoin), thus decreasing plasma levels.

Pharmacokinetics

t½, terminal, adults and children: 15.7–22.5 hr. No accumulation of drug has been noted.

CONTRAINDICATIONS

Use in G6PD deficient clients, known history of anaphylaxis or hypersensitivity reactions, hemolytic reactions, methemoglobinemia reactions to rasburicase or any components of the product. Lactation.

SPECIAL CONCERNS

(1) **Anaphylaxis.** Rasburicase may cause hypersensitivity reactions, including anaphylaxis. Immediately and permanently discontinue rasburicase in any client developing clinical evidence of a serious hypersensitivity reaction. (2) **Hemolysis.** Do not administer rasburicase to clients with glucose-6-phosphate dehydrogenase (G6PD) deficiency. Immediately and permanently discontinue rasburicase in clients developing hemolysis. It is recommended that clients at higher risk for G6PD deficiency (e.g., those of African or Mediterranean ancestry) be screened prior to starting rasburicase. (3) **Methemoglobinemia.** Rasburicase can result in methemoglobinemia in some clients. Immediately and permanently discontinue rasburicase in clients developing methemoglobinemia. (4) **Interference with uric acid measurements.** Rasburicase enzymatically degrades uric acid in blood samples left at room temperature. Collect blood samples into prechilled tubes containing heparin and immediately immerse and maintain in an ice water bath. Assay plasma samples within 4 hr of collection.

- Safety and efficacy established only for a single course of treatment once daily for 5 days.
- Children less than 2 years of age had a lower rate of success by 48 hr after treatment and also experienced more toxicity.

SIDE EFFECTS

Most Common

N&V, fever, headache, abdominal pain, constipation, diarrhea, mucositis, rash.

Allergic reaction: Chest pain/tightness, dyspnea, hypoxia, hypotension, urticaria, shock, ***bronchospasm, anaphylaxis*.** **Hematologic:** Hemolysis, methemoglobinemia, neutropenia with fever, neutropenia, pancytopenia. **GI:** N&V, diarrhea, ileus, intestinal obstruction, abdominal pain, constipation. **CNS:** ***Convulsions***, headache. **CV:** Arrhythmia, ***cardiac failure/arrest, MI***, cerebrovascular disorder, hot flushes, ***hemorrhage***, thrombosis, thrombophlebitis. **Respiratory:** Respiratory distress, pneumonia, pulmonary edema, ***pulmonary hypertension*.** **Ophthalmic:** Retinal hemorrhage. **Body as a whole:** Rash, fever, cyanosis, dehydration, infection, paresthesia, rigors. **Miscellaneous:** Mucositis, acute renal failure, cellulitis, immunogenicity.

LABORATORY TEST CONSIDERATIONS

At room temperature, rasburicase causes enzymatic degradation of uric acid in blood, plasma, or serum samples that may cause low plasma uric acid assay readings.

HOW SUPPLIED

Powder for Injection, Lyophilized: 1.5 mg/vial, 7.5 mg/vial.

DOSAGE

IV

Decrease plasma uric acid in adults and children treated for cancer.

Adults and children: 0.2 mg/kg/day as a 30-min IV infusion for up to 5 days. Dosing beyond 5 days or administration of more than 1 course is not recommended.

R

NURSING IMPLICATIONS

IMPLEMENTATION/ADMINISTRATION/STORAGE

1. IV Begin chemotherapy 4–24 hr after the first rasburicase dose.
2. Give as an IV infusion over 30 min; **do not give as bolus infusion.** Do not use filters for infusion.
3. Infuse through a different line than that used for other drugs. If use of a separate line not possible, flush line with at least 15 mL of saline solution before and after infusion with rasburicase.
4. Determine number of vials of drug required based on weight and dose/kg. Must reconstitute with the diluent provided. Reconstitute the 1.5 mg vial with 1 mL of the diluent and reconstitute the 7.5 mg vial with 5 mL of the diluent. Mix by swirling gently. Do not shake or vortex.
5. After reconstitution, remove dose to be given and inject into an infusion bag containing an amount of 0.9% NaCl to achieve a final volume of 50 mL.
6. Visually inspect for particulate matter and discoloration before administering. Discard if particulate matter visible or if there is discoloration.
7. IV hydration of clients is needed to manage plasma uric acid in those at risk for tumor lysis syndrome.
8. There are no preservatives in the product; thus, give within 24 hr of reconstitution. The reconstituted or diluted solution can be stored at 2–8°C (36–46°F) up to 24 hr. Do not freeze; protect from light. Discard any unused product.
9. COMPATIBILITY 0.9% NaCl-flush before and after dosing.
10. INCOMPATIBILITY Administer separately.

ASSESSMENT

1. Note age, onset, type of cancer/chemotherapy regimen. Monitor VS.
2. Alert lab to collect blood in prechilled tubes containing heparin. Immediately immerse in ice water bath; specimen must be analyzed within 4 hr of draw (otherwise results not reliable). Rasburicase enzymatically degrades uric acid in blood samples left at room temperature.
3. Assess for G6PD; screen those of African or Mediterranean ancestry prior to therapy as prone to hemolysis. Assess all recipients carefully for allergic reaction, hemolysis and methoglobinemia. If evident stop drug and never reuse in this client.
4. Assess GI symptoms; N&V, severe diarrhea may signal toxicity. Ensure well hydrated and administer antiemetic 1 hr before therapy and as needed.

5. Monitor oral/auxilliary temperature, CBC, serum uric acid level, lytes, renal and LFTs.

CLIENT/FAMILY TEACHING

1. Drug is given to lower the uric acid levels from tumor breakdown during chemotherapy.
2. Generally given once daily IV × 5 days.
3. Report temperature elevations, unusual bruising/bleeding, N&V, diarrhea or adverse side effects immediately.
4. Keep all F/U to assess response, labs, adverse SE.

OUTCOMES/EVALUATE

↓ Uric acid levels R/T chemotherapy

IV

Remifentanil hydrochloride

(rem-ih-**FEN**-tah-nil)

Classification(s): Narcotic analgesic

Pregnancy Category: C

RX: Ultiva, **C-II**

SEE ALSO ***NARCOTIC ANALGESICS***.

INDICATIONS/USES

(1) As an analgesic during the induction and maintenance of general anesthesia for inpatient and outpatient procedures and for continuation as an analgesic in the immediate postoperative period. (2) Analgesic component of monitored anesthesia care. *NOTE:* Not indicated as the sole agent for general anesthesia because loss of consciousness cannot be guaranteed and also due to a high incidence of apnea, muscle rigidity, and tachycardia.

ACTION/KINETICS

Action

Narcotic analgesic that binds with mu-opioid receptors. Depresses respiration in a dose-dependent manner and causes muscle rigidity.

Pharmacokinetics

Rapidly metabolized by nonspecific blood and tissue esterases; not metabolized appreciably by the liver or lung. **Onset:** 1 min. **Peak effect:** 1 min. **t½, elimination:** 10–20 min. **Recovery:** Within 5–10 min. Metabolized in the liver by hydrolysis by esterases. Excreted in the urine.

CONTRAINDICATIONS

Epidural or intrathecal use due to the presence of glycine in the formulation. Hypersensitivity to fentanyl analogues. Use as the sole agent in general anesthesia because LOC cannot be ensured and due to a high incidence of apnea, muscle rigidity, and tachycardia.

SPECIAL CONCERNS

- Use with caution in obese clients and during lactation.
- Respiratory depression and other narcotic effects may be seen in newborns whose mothers are given remifentanil shortly before delivery.
- Elderly are twice as sensitive as younger clients to drug effects.
- Not studied in children less than one year of age, in children for use in the immediate postoperative period, or for use as a component of monitored anesthesia care.
- Possible intraoperative awareness in clients less than 55 years old when given with propofol infusion rates of 75 mcg/kg/min or less.

SIDE EFFECTS

Most Common

Hypotension, apnea, headache, itching/pruritus, dizziness, shivering, sweating, N&V, muscle rigidity, flank pain.

GI: N&V, constipation, abdominal discomfort, xerostomia, gastroesophageal reflux, dysphagia, diarrhea, heartburn, ileus. **CNS:** Shivering, fever, dizziness, headache, agitation, chills, warm sensation, anxiety, involuntary movement, prolonged emergence from anesthesia, tremors, disorientation, dysphoria, nightmares, hallucinations, paresthesia, nystagmus, twitch, sleep disorder, seizures, amnesia. **CV:** Hypo-/hypertension, brady-/tachycardia, atrial and ventricular arrhythmias, ***heart block***, ECG change consistent with myocardial ischemia, syncope. **Musculoskeletal:** Muscle rigidity/stiffness, flank pain, musculoskeletal chest pain, delayed recovery from neuromuscular block. **Respiratory:** Respiratory depression, ***apnea***, hypoxia, cough, dyspnea, ***bronchospasm***, ***laryngospasm***, rhonchi, stridor, nasal congestion, pharyngitis, pleural effusion, hiccoughs, pulmonary edema, rales, bronchitis, rhinorrhea. **Dermatologic:** Pruritus, itching, rash, urticaria, erythema, sweating, flushing, pain at IV site. **GU:** Urine retention/incontinence, oliguria, dysuria. **Hematologic:** Ane-

R

mia, lymphopenia, leukocytosis, thrombocytopenia. **Metabolic:** Abnormal liver function, hyperglycemia, electrolyte disorders. **Miscellaneous:** Decreased body temperature, ***anaphylactic reaction***, visual disturbances, postoperative pain, injection site pain/reaction.

LABORATORY TEST CONSIDERATIONS

↑ CPK-MB levels.

OVERDOSE MANAGEMENT

Symptoms: Apnea, chest-wall rigidity, seizures, hypoxemia, hypotension, bradycardia. *Treatment:* Discontinue administration, maintain a patent airway, initiate assisted or controlled ventilation with oxygen, and maintain adequate CV function. A neuromuscular blocking agent or a mu-opiate receptor antagonist may be used to treat muscle rigidity. IV fluids, vasopressors, and other supportive measures are indicated to treat hypotension. Bradycardia or hypotension may also be treated with atropine or glycopyrrolate. IV naloxone is used to treat respiratory depression or muscle rigidity. Reversal of the opioid effects may lead to acute pain and sympathetic hyperactivity.

DRUG INTERACTIONS

Remifentanil is synergistic with other anesthetics. Doses of thiopental, propofol, isoflurane, and midazolam have been reduced by up to 75% with the coadministration of remifentanil.

HOW SUPPLIED

Powder for Injection: 1 mg (as base), 2 mg (as base), 5 mg (as base).

DOSAGE

CONTINUOUS IV INFUSION

Induction of anesthesia through intubation.

0.5–1 mcg/kg/min given with a hypnotic or volatile agent. If endotracheal intubation is to occur less than 8 min after the start of the infusion of remifentanil, the initial dose of 1 mcg/kg may be given over 30 to 60 sec.

Maintenance of nitrous oxide (66%) anesthesia.

The dose of remifentanil is 0.4 mcg/kg/min by continuous IV infusion (dose range for IV infusion is 0.1–2 mcg/kg/min). A supplemental IV bolus dose of 1 mcg/kg may be given q 2–5 min in response to light anesthesia or transient episodes of intense surgical stress.

Maintenance of isoflurane (0.4 to 1.5 MAC) or propofol (100–200 mcg/kg/min) anesthesia.

The dose of remifentanil is 0.25 mcg/kg/min by continuous IV infusion (dose range is 0.05–2 mcg/kg/min). A supplemental IV bolus dose of 1 mcg/kg may be given.

Continuation as an analgesic into the immediate postoperative period.

0.1 mcg/kg/min (range of 0.025–0.2 mcg/kg/min). The infusion rate may be adjusted every 5 min in 0.025-mcg/kg/min increments to balance the client's level of analgesia and respiratory rate. Infusion rates more than 0.2 mcg/kg/min are associated with respiratory depression (less than 8 breaths/min). The use of bolus injections to treat pain during the postoperative period is not recommended.

Analgesic component of monitored anesthesia care.

Adults only. Single IV dose: 1 mcg/kg administered over 30 to 60 sec and given 90 sec before the local anesthetic. If remifentanil is given with midazolam (2 mg), the dose is 0.5 mcg/kg given over 30–60 sec. **Continuous IV infusion:** 0.1 mcg/kg beginning 5 min before the local anesthetic. After the local anesthetic, the dose of remifentanil is 0.05 mcg/kg/min (range 0.025–0.2 mcg/kg/min) at 5-min intervals in order to balance the level of analgesia and respiratory rate. If remifentanil is given with midazolam (2 mg), the dose is 0.025 mcg/kg/min (range 0.025–0.2 mcg/kg/min).

Coronary artery bypass surgery.

Induction of anesthesia through intubation: 1 mcg/kg/min by continuous IV infusion. **Maintenance of anesthesia:** 1 mcg/kg/min (range: 0.125–4 mcg/kg/min) by continuous IV infusion. A supplemental bolus dose of 0.5–1 mcg/kg may be given. **Continuation as an analgesic into ICU:** 1

R

mcg/kg/min (range: 0.05–1 mcg/kg/min) by continuous IV infusion.

Pediatric clients, 1 year of age and older, with physical status of I, II, or III.

Maintenance of anesthesia (given with halothane, 0.3–1.5 MAC; sevoflurane, 0.3–1.5 MAC; or, isoflurane, 0.4–1.5 MAC): 0.25 mcg/kg/min (range: 0.05–3 mcg/kg/min) by continuous IV infusion. A supplemental IV bolus dose of 1 mcg/kg may be given. *NOTE:* Remifentanil was given with nitrous oxide or nitrous oxide in combination with halothane, sevoflurane, or isoflurane.

NURSING IMPLICATIONS

IMPLEMENTATION/ADMINISTRATION/STORAGE

1. IV Individualize choice of anesthetic and need for preanesthetic drugs.
2. Use under the direct supervision of an anesthesia practitioner in a postoperative anesthesia care unit or intensive care setting.
3. Decrease starting dose by 50% in clients over age 65. Cautiously titrate to desired effect.
4. In obese clients (i.e., greater than 30% over ideal body weight [IBW]) base the starting dose on IBW.
5. The need for premedication and the choice of anesthetic agents must be individualized.
6. Give continuous infusions only by an infusion device. Have the injection site close to the venous cannula.
7. Give IV bolus injections only during the maintenance of general anesthesia.
8. Do not give remifentanil into the same IV tubing with blood.
9. Due to the rapid onset and short duration, administration during anesthesia can be titrated upward in 25% to 100% increments or downward in 25% to 50% decrements every 2 to 5 min to attain the desired opiate effect. With light anesthesia or transient periods of intense surgical stress, supplemental bolus doses of 1 mcg/kg may be given q 2–5 min.
10. Administer under close anesthesia supervision into the immediate postoperative period. Infusion rates greater than 0.2 mcg/kg/min are associated with respiratory depression. Manage respiratory depression by decreasing the rate of infusion by 50% or discontinue the infusion temporarily.
11. When infusion is discontinued, clear the IV tubing to prevent inadvertant administration at a later time.
12. Due to its short duration, no opioid activity will be present within 5–10 min of discontinuation.
13. Stable for 24 hr at room temperature after reconstitution and further dilution to concentrations of 20–250 mcg/mL with compatible solutions. Is stable for 4 hr at room temperature after reconstitution and further dilution to concentrations of 20–250 mcg/mL with lactated Ringer's injection.
14. Store at 2–25°C (36–77°F).
15. COMPATIBILITY D5W, D5/0.9% NaCl, 0.9% and 0.45% NaCl, or LR/D5W. Propofol when coadministered into a running IV administration set.
16. INCOMPATIBILITY Blood; administer separately.

ASSESSMENT

1. Used during anesthesia to control pain; note any previous experience with this therapy. Not recommended as the sole agent in general anesthesia.
2. Have resuscitative and intubation equipment readily available. Monitor oxygen sats continuously during therapy.
3. Manage respiratory depression in spontaneously breathing clients by decreasing rate of Ultiva infusion by 50% or by temporarily discontinuing the infusion.
4. Monitor renal and LFTs. Observe closely for progressive respiratory depression. Assess level of consciousness, VS, I&O and for any evidence of allergic reaction.

CLIENT/FAMILY TEACHING

1. Drug is administered in a monitored environment to ensure no adverse side effects.
2. Call caregiver for assistance. Do not perform activities that require mental alertness for 24 hr; drug causes dizziness, drowsiness, and impaired physical and mental performance.
3. Breathing will be monitored closely and supported during administration; breathing and function will quickly return to normal after medication has been discontinued.

R

4. Avoid alcohol and any other CNS depressants for 24 hr after procedure.
5. May experience N&V, itching, or headaches during recovery period.
6. Change positions slowly to prevent postural effects (low BP).

OUTCOMES/EVALUATE

Pain control; maintenance of anesthesia

Repaglinide

(re-**PAY**-glin-eyed)

Classification(s): Antidiabetic, oral; meglitinide

Pregnancy Category: C

RX: Prandin.

Rx: GlucoNorm.

SEE ALSO ***ANTIDIABETIC AGENTS: HYPOGLYCEMIC AGENTS.***

INDICATIONS/USES

(1) Adjunct to diet and exercise in type 2 diabetes mellitus where hyperglycemia cannot be controlled by diet and exercise alone. (2) In combination with metformin, pioglitazone or rosiglitazone to lower blood glucose where hyperglycemia cannot be controlled by exercise, diet, or metformin, sulfonylureas, repaglinide, or thiazolidinediones used alone.

ACTION/KINETICS

Action

Lowers blood glucose by stimulating release of insulin from the pancreas. Action depends on functioning beta cells in pancreatic islets. Drug closes ATP-dependent potassium channels in beta-cell membrane due to binding at sites. Blockade of potassium channel depolarizes beta cells, which leads to opening of calcium channels. This causes calcium influx which induces insulin secretion. Is highly tissue selective with low affinity for heart and skeletal muscle.

Pharmacokinetics

Rapidly and completely absorbed from GI tract, although food decreases mean C_{max} and AUC. Mean absolute bioavailability is 56%. **Peak plasma levels:** 1 hr. **t½:** 1 hr. Completely metabolized in liver with 90% excreted in feces and 8% excreted in the urine.

CONTRAINDICATIONS

Lactation. Diabetic ketoacidosis, with or without coma. Type 1 diabetes. Known hypersensitivity to any component of the product. Use in combination with NPH insulin.

SPECIAL CONCERNS

- Use with caution in impaired hepatic function.
- Oral hypoglycemics are associated with increased CV mortality compared with diet alone or diet plus insulin.
- May need to discontinue repaglinide and give insulin if the client is exposed to stress (e.g., fever, trauma, infection, surgery); known as secondary failure.
- Safety and efficacy not determined in children.

SIDE EFFECTS

Most Common

Hypoglycemia, headache, paresthesia, N&V, diarrhea, constipation, dyspepsia, back pain, arthralgia, bronchitis, rhinitis, sinusitus, URTI, chest pain, tooth disorder, UTI, allergy.

CNS: Headache, paresthesia. **CV:** Chest pain, angina, ischemia, hypertension, abnormal ECG, arrhythmias, palpitations, ***MI***. **GI:** N&V, diarrhea, constipation, dyspepsia, ***pancreatitis***, severe hepatic dysfunction. **Hematologic:** Thrombocytopenia, leukopenia, hemolytic anemia. **Respiratory:** URTI, sinusitis, rhinitis, bronchitis. **Musculoskeletal:** Arthralgia, back pain. **Miscellaneous:** Hypoglycemia, chest pain, UTI, tooth disorder, allergy, alopecia, ***Stevens-Johnson syndrome, anaphylaxis***.

OVERDOSE MANAGEMENT

Symptoms: Hypoglycemia. Symptoms of severe hypoglycemia include coma, seizure, or other neurologic impairment; this is a medical emergency. *Treatment:* Oral glucose. Also adjust drug dosage or meal patterns. For severe hypoglycemia, give a rapid IV injection of 50% glucose solution followed by a continuous infusion of more dilute (10%) glucose solution at a rate that will maintain BG at a level above 100 mg/dL.

DRUG INTERACTIONS

See ***Antidiabetic Agents: Hypoglycemic Agents.***

Beta blockers / Potentiation of repaglinide action, including by drugs highly protein bound

R

Calcium channel blockers / Calcium channel blockers cause hyperglycemia → loss of glycemic control
Chloramphenicol / Potentiation of repaglinide action, including by drugs highly protein bound
Clarithromycin / Possible ↑ peak plasma levels and t½ of repaglinide
Corticosteroids / Corticosteroids cause hyperglycemia → loss of glycemic control
Coumarins / Potentiation of repaglinide action, including by drugs highly protein bound
Cyclosporine / ↑ Repaglinide plasma levels R/T inhibition of metabolism by CYP3A4
CYP3A4 inducers (e.g., barbiturates, carbamazepine, rifampin) / ↓ Repaglinide AUC and plasma levels R/T induction of its metabolism
CYP3A4 inhibitors (e.g., ketoconazole, macrolide antibiotics, miconazole) / ↑ Repaglinide AUC and plasma levels R/T inhibition of its metabolism
Estrogens / Estrogens cause hyperglycemia → loss of glycemic control
Gemfibrozil / Enhanced and prolonged BG lowering effects of repaglinide R/T inhibition of metabolism → ↑ repaglinide blood levels; repaglinide dosage adjustment may be needed
Gemfibrozil/Itraconazole / Combination has a synergistic metabolic inhibitory effect on repaglinide; do not take itraconazole with repaglinide and gemfibrozil
Isoniazid / Isoniazid cause hyperglycemia → loss of glycemic control
Levonorgestrel/ethinyl estradiol / 20% ↑ in repaglinide, levonorgestrel, and ethinyl estradiol C_{max}; also 20% ↑ in ethinyl estradiol AUC
Nicotinic acid / Nicotinic acid causes hyperglycemia → loss of glycemic control
MAOIs / Potentiation of repaglinide action, including by drugs highly protein bound
NSAIDs / Potentiation of repaglinide action, including by drugs highly protein bound
Oral contraceptives / Oral contraceptives cause hyperglycemia → loss of glycemic control
Phenothiazines / Phenothiazines cause hyperglycemia → loss of glycemic control
Phenytoin / Phenytoin causes hyperglycemia → loss of glycemic control
Probenecid / Potentiation of repaglinide action, including by drugs highly protein bound
Rifampin / ↓ Plasma levels and effects of repaglinide R/T ↑ liver metabolism
Salicylates / Potentiation of repaglinide action, including by drugs highly protein bound
Simvastatin / ↑ Repaglinide C_{max} by 26%
Sulfonamides / Potentiation of repaglinide action, including by drugs highly protein bound
Sympathomimetics / Sympathomimetics cause hyperglycemia → loss of glycemic control
Thiazides (and other diuretics) / Thiazides and other diuretics cause hyperglycemia → loss of glycemic control
Thyroid drugs / Thyroid drugs cause hyperglycemia → loss of glycemic control

HOW SUPPLIED

Tablets: 0.5 mg, 1 mg, 2 mg.

DOSAGE

TABLETS

Diabetes mellitus, type 2.

Individualize dosage as there is no fixed dosage. **Initial:** In those not previously treated or whose HbA1c is less than 8%, give 0.5 mg with each meal. For those previously treated or whose HbA1c is 8% or more, give 1 or 2 mg before each meal. **Dose range:** 0.5–4 mg taken with meals. May also be dosed preprandially 2, 3, or 4 times a day in response to changes in the client's meal pattern. **Maximum daily dose:** 16 mg. Start those with severe renal impairment at 0.5 mg taken with meals.

NURSING IMPLICATIONS

Do not confuse Prandin with Avandia (also an oral hypoglycemic).

IMPLEMENTATION/ADMINISTRATION/STORAGE

1. Usually taken within 15 min of meal but time may vary from immediately preceding meal to as long as 30 min before meal.
2. In renal impairment, initial dose adjustments not required. Make subsequent increases in dose carefully in impaired renal function or in renal failure requiring hemodialysis.
3. When used to replace another oral hypoglycemic, may be started the day after the last dose of other drug. Observe carefully for hypoglycemia as drug effects may overlap. When transferring from a longer-acting sulfonylurea

R

(e.g., chlorpropamide), monitor for up to 1 week or longer.
4. If combined with metformin, starting dose and dose adjustments are the same as if repaglinide was used alone.
5. If glucose control has not been achieved after a suitable trial of combination therapy, consider discontinuing these drugs and starting insulin.
6. Fever, trauma, infection, or surgery may result in loss of glycemic control (known as secondary failure). At these times, it may be necessary to discontinue repaglinide and administer insulin.
7. Do not store above 25°C (77°F). Protect from moisture.

ASSESSMENT

1. Note onset, duration, characteristics of disease, age at onset, other agents/methods trialed, outcome.
2. Monitor Wt, VS, CBC, HbA1c, BS, lipids, electrolytes, U/A, microalbumin, Ca^{++}, renal and LFTs.

CLIENT/FAMILY TEACHING

1. Take as prescribed within 15 min of the meal up to as long as 30 min before the meal for glucose control. Do not take if meal is skipped.
2. Continue regular exercise, diabetic diet, and lifestyle modifications (smoking cessation, moderate alcohol use and stress reduction) to control BS and prevent organ damage.
3. Record FS for provider review; report any unusual side effects or lack of response. Have regular foot and eye exams. Strive for BP and weight control.
4. Report fever, sore throat, unusual bruising/bleeding, severe abdominal pain, or lack of effectiveness. Attend diabetic education classes and dietary instruction.
5. Keep all F/U to assess response, labs, and for adverse SE.

OUTCOMES/EVALUATE

HBA1c <8, control of DM

IV

Reteplase recombinant

(**REE**-teh-place)

Classification(s): Thrombolytic, tissue plasminogen activator

Pregnancy Category: C

RX: Retavase.

INDICATIONS/USES

Acute MI in adults for improvement of ventricular function, reduction of the incidence of CHF, and reduction of mortality. *Investigational:* Clearance of occluded venous catheters, thrombolytic treatment of acute and chronic DVT, treatment of massive pulmonary embolism with a double bolus, with heparin and percutaneous transluminal angioplasty to treat thrombosed polytetrafluoroethylene hemodialysis arteriovenous grafts.

ACTION/KINETICS

Action

Plasminogen activator that catalyzes the cleavage of endogenous plasminogen to generate plasmin. Plasmin, in turn, degrades the matrix of the thrombus, causing a thrombolytic effect.

Pharmacokinetics

t½: 13 to 16 min. Cleared primarily by the liver and kidney.

CONTRAINDICATIONS

Active internal bleeding; history of CVA; recent intracranial or intraspinal surgery or trauma; intracranial neoplasm, arteriovenous malformation, or aneurysm; known bleeding diathesis; severe uncontrolled hypertension.

SPECIAL CONCERNS

- Use with caution during lactation.
- Safety and efficacy not determined in children.

SIDE EFFECTS

Most Common

Bleeding disorders.

See *NOTE* below. **Bleeding disorders:** From internal bleeding sites, including intracranial, retroperitoneal, GI, GU, or respiratory. ***Hemorrhage may occur*** from superficial bleeding sites, including venous cutdowns, arterial punctures, sites of recent surgery. **CV:** ***Cholesterol embolism***, coronary thrombolysis resulting in arrhythmias associated with perfusion (no different from those seen in the ordinary course of acute MI), ***cardiogenic shock***, sinus bradycardia, accelerated idioventricular rhythm, ventricular premature depolarizations, SVT, ventricular ***tachycardia/fibrillation***, AV block, pulmonary edema, ***heart failure, cardiac arrest, recurrent ischemia, myocardial rupture, cardiac tamponade, venous thrombosis or embolism, electromechanical dissociation, mitral regurgitation, pericardial effusion, pericarditis.*** **Hypersensitivity:** Serious allergic reactions. *NOTE:* Many of the CV side effects listed are frequent sequelae of MI and may or may not be attributable to reteplase recombinant.

LABORATORY TEST CONSIDERATIONS

↓ Plasminogen, fibrinogen. Degradation of fibrinogen in blood samples removed for analysis.

DRUG INTERACTIONS

Use with abciximab, aspirin, dipyridamole, heparin, or vitamin K antagonists may increase the risk of bleeding.

HOW SUPPLIED

Powder for Injection, Lyophilized: 10.4 international units (18.1 mg).

DOSAGE

IV ONLY

Acute MI.

Adults: 10 + 10 unit double-bolus injection. Each bolus is given over 2 min, with the second bolus given 30 min after initiation of the first bolus injection.

NURSING IMPLICATIONS

IMPLEMENTATION/ADMINISTRATION/STORAGE

1. IV Initiate treatment as soon as possible after symptom onset.
2. Have available antiarrhythmic therapy for bradycardia and/or ventricular irritability.
3. Reconstitution is performed using the diluent, syringe, needle, and dispensing pin provided with the drug as follows:
   - Remove the flip-cap from one vial of sterile water (preservative free), and, with the syringe provided, withdraw 10 mL of the sterile water.
   - Open the package containing the dispensing pin. Remove the needle from the syringe and discard. Remove the protective cap from the spike end of the dispensing pin and connect the syringe to the dispensing pin. Remove the protective flip-cap from one vial of reteplase.
   - Remove the protective cap from the spike end of the dispensing pin, and insert the spike into the vial of reteplase. Transfer the 10 mL of sterile water through the dispensing pin into the vial.
   - With the dispensing pin and syringe still attached to the vial, gently swirl the vial to dissolve the reteplase. *Do not shake.*
   - Withdraw the 10 mL of reconstituted reteplase back into the syringe (a small amount will remain due to overfill).
   - Detach the syringe from the dispensing pin, and attach the sterile 20-gauge needle provided. The solution is ready to administer.
4. Since reteplase contains no antibacterial preservatives, reconstitute just prior to use. When reconstituted as directed, the solution may be used within 4 hr when stored at 2–30°C (36–86°F).
5. Keep the kit sealed until use and store at 2–25°C (36–77°F).
6. COMPATIBILITY If given through IV line containing heparin, flush normal saline or D5W through line prior to and following reteplase injection.
7. INCOMPATIBILITY Administer separately; avoid other meds or infusions.

ASSESSMENT

1. Note reasons for therapy (location of MI), onset, pain level, characteristics of chest pain.
2. List drugs currently prescribed to ensure none interact unfavorably.
3. Assess for evidence of CVA, internal bleeding, trauma, neurosurgery, or bleeding disorders.
4. During administration, continuously monitor cardiac rhythm. Have medications available for management of arrhythmias. Record VS every 15 min during infusion and for 2 hr following.
5. Administer first bolus dose (10 + 10 unit double-bolus injection) over 2 min, the second dose 30 min later if no serious bleeding is observed. In the event of any uncontrolled bleeding, terminate heparin infusion and withhold second dose.
6. Avoid: unnecessary client handling, IM injections, and invasive procedures. Observe all puncture sites and areas for evidence of bleeding. Arterial sticks require 30 min of

R

manual pressure followed by application of a pressure dressing.

7. Assess for reperfusion reactions such as:
   - Arrhythmias usually of short duration, which may include bradycardia or ventricular tachycardia
   - Reduction of chest pain
   - Return of elevated ST segment and smaller Q waves
8. Maintain bed rest and observe for S&S of abnormal bleeding (hematuria, hematemesis, melena, CVA, cardiac tamponade).
9. Obtain CBC, type/cross, coagulation times, cardiac enzyme panel, renal and LFTs. Monitor VS, cardiopulmonary assessments, ECG.

CLIENT/FAMILY TEACHING

1. Review goals of therapy and inherent risks of drug therapy during acute coronary artery occlusion. Administered IV in a monitored setting.
2. Drug used to dissolve blood clots that have formed in certain blood vessels.
3. To be effective, must initiate therapy as soon as possible after symptom onset.
4. Call for assistance before getting out of bed during treatment.
5. Encourage family members to learn CPR.

OUTCOMES/EVALUATE

Improved ventricular function; ↓ incidence of CHF, and ↓ mortality with AMI

■ IV

Rh_o(D) Immune Globulin IM (Rh_o(D) IGIM)

(roh (dee) im-**MYOUN GLOH**-byou-lin)

Classification(s): Immunosuppressant

Pregnancy Category: C

RX: HyperRHO S/D Full Dose, RhoGAM Ultra Filtered Plus.

Rh_o(D) Immune Globulin IV (Rh_o(D) IGIV)

Pregnancy Category: C

RX: Rhophylac, WinRho SDF.

Rh_o(D) Immune Globulin Microdose Injection

RX: HyperRHO S/D Mini-Dose, MICRhoGAM Ultra-Filtered Plus.

INDICATIONS/USES

Rh_o(D) IGIM: (1) HyperRHO S/D Full Dose. Prevention of Rh hemolytic disease of the newborn by its administration to the Rh_o(D)-negative mother within 72 hr of the birth of an Rh_o(D)-positive infant, provided the following criteria are met:

- The mother is Rh_o(D) negative and not already sensitized to the Rh_o(D) factor and
- Her child is Rh_o(D) positive and has a negative direct antiglobulin test.If given antepartum, the mother must receive another dose after delivery of an Rh_o(D)-positive infant. If the father can be determined to be Rh_o(D) negative, Rh_o(D) immune globulin does not need to be given.

Administer Rh_o(D) immune globulin within 72 hr to all nonimmunized Rh_o(D)-negative women who have undergone spontaneous or induced abortion following ruptured tubal pregnancy, amniocentesis, or abdominal trauma, unless the blood group of the fetus or the father is known to be Rh_o(D) negative. If the fetal blood group cannot be determined, assume that it is Rh_o(D) positive and administer Rh_o(D) immune globulin to the mother.

(2) RhoGAM Ultra Filtered Plus. For administration to Rh-negative women not previously sensitized to the Rh_o(D) factor, unless the father or baby are conclusively Rh negative, in the following situations:

- Delivery of an Rh-positive baby irrespective of the ABO groups of the mother and baby.
- Antepartum prophylaxis at 26 to 28 weeks of gestation;
- Antepartum fetomaternal hemorrhage (suspected or proven) as a result of placenta previa, amniocentesis, chorionic villus sampling, percutaneous umbilical blood sampling.
- Other obstetrical manipulative procedure (e.g, version) or abdominal trauma.
- Actual or threatened pregnancy loss at any stage of gestation.
- Ectopic pregnancy. Also, used to prevent Rh immunization in any Rh_o(D)-negative individid-

ual after incompatible transfusion of Rh-positive blood or blood products (e.g., RBCs, platelet or granulocyte concentrates).

Investigational (controversial): Prior to external version attempts for breech presentation (due to induced fetomaternal hemorrhage) and following tubal ligation after delivery of a Rh_oD positive infant (to prevent problems should sterilization fail or subsequent tubal reanastomoses occur).

Rh_o(D) IGIV: Rhophylac. (1) Immune thrombocytopenic purpura: Treatment of Rh_o(D)-positive, nonsplenectomized adults with chronic ITP to raise platelet counts. (2) Suppression of Rh isoimmunization. Pregnancy and obstetric conditions: Suppression of Rh isoimmunization in nonsensitized Rh_o(D)-negative women with an Rh-incompatible pregnancy, including routine antepartum and postpartum Rh prophylaxis, and Rh prophylaxis in cases of obstetric complications (e.g., miscarriage, abortion, threatened abortion, ectopic pregnancy or hydatidiform mole, transplacental hemorrhage resulting from antepartum hemorrhage), invasive procedures during pregnancy (e.g., amniocentesis, chorionic biopsy), or obstetric manipulative procedures (e.g., external version, abdominal trauma). (3) Transfusion: Suppression of Rh isoimmunization in Rh_o(D)-negative individuals transfused with Rh_o(D)-positive red blood cells or blood components containing Rh_o(D)-positive red blood cells.

Rh_o(D) IGIV: WinRho SDF. (1) Immune thrombocytopenic purpura: Treatment of nonsplenectomized, Rh_o(D)-positive children with long-term or acute ITP, adults with long-term ITP, or children and adults with TIP secondary to HIV infection. (2) Suppression of Rh isoimmunization. Pregnancy and obstetric conditions: Suppression of Rh isoimmunization in nonsensitized Rh_o(D)-negative women within 72 hr after spontaneous or induced abortions, amniocentesis, chorionic villus sampling, ruptured tubal pregnancy, abdominal trauma or transplacental hemorrhage, or in the normal course of pregnancy, unless the blood type of the fetus or father is known to be Rh_o(D)-negative. (3) Transfusion: Suppression of Rh isoimmunization in Rh_o(D)-female children and women in their childbearing years transfused with RH_o(D)-positive red blood cells or blood components containing RH_o(D)-positive red blood cells.

Rh_o(D) Immune Globulin Microdose: (1) Prevention of isoimmunization of Rh_o(D)-negative women at the time of spontaneous or induced abortion up to 12 weeks of gestation, provided the following criteria are met: (a) the mother is Rh_o(D) negative and not already sensitized to the Rh_o(D) antigen, (b) the father is not known to be Rh_o(D) negative, and/or (c) gestation is not more than 12 weeks at termination. Prophylaxis is not indicated if the fetus or father can be determined to be Rh negative. If the Rh status of the fetus is not known, the fetus must be assumed to be Rh_o(D) positive, and the dose should be administered to the mother. *NOTE:* If abortions or miscarriages occur after 12 weeks of gestation, a standard dose of Rh_o(D) immune globulin is indicated. (2) To prevent Rh immunization in any Rh_o(D)-negative individual after incompatible transfusion of Rh-positive blood or blood products (e.g., red blood cells, platelet or granulocyte concentrates).

ACTION/KINETICS

Action

Sterile, freeze-dried gamma globulin (IgG) fraction containing antibodies to Rh_o(D) derived from human plasma. The manufacturing process is effective in inactivating lipid-enveloped viruses, including hepatitis B and C and HIV. Contains approximately 2 mcg IgA/1,500 international units (300 mcg). It suppresses the immune response of nonsensitized Rh_o(D) antigen-negative individuals following Rh_o(D) antigen-positive red blood cell exposure. Mechanism for ITP may be due to formation of anti-Rh_o(D) (anti-D) coated RBC complexes resulting in Fc receptor blockade; this spares antibody-coated platelets. Suppression of Rh isoimmunization decreases the possibility of hemolytic disease in an Rh_o(D) antigen-positive fetus in present and future pregnancies.

Pharmacokinetics

For Rh_o(D) IGIV, **Peak levels, after IV:** 2 hr; **after IM:** 5–10 days. **t½, after IV:** 24 days; **after IM:** 30 days.

CONTRAINDICATIONS

History of anaphylactic or severe systemic reaction to human globulin (i.e., due to the presence of trace amounts of IgA). Administration to Rh_o(D) antigen-negative or splenectomized individuals, as efficacy has not been shown. Use in Rh_o(D) antigen-negative clients who are Rh immunized (Rh

R

antibody-positive), as evidenced by standard manual Rh antibody screening tests. IV use of Rh$_o$(D) IGIM. Use of IGIM in those who have severe thrombocytopenia or any coagulation disorder that would contraindicate IM use. Injection of Rh$_o$(D) IGIV, Rh$_o$(D) IGIM, or Rh$_o$(D) IG micro-dose in infants.

SPECIAL CONCERNS

■ These products have been associated with renal dysfunction, acute renal failure, osmotic nephrosis, and death. Clients predisposed to acute renal failure include those with any degree of preexisting renal insufficiency, diabetes mellitus, those over 65 years of age, volume depletion, sepsis, paraproteinemia, or those receiving known nephrotoxic drugs. IGIV should be given in such clients at the minimum concentration available and the minimum rate of infusion practical. While reports of renal dysfunction and acute renal failure have been associated with many of the IGIV products, those containing sucrose as a stabilizer account for a disproportionate share of the total number.

For Rh$_o$(D) Immune Globulin: Intravenous (IGIV): (1) Intravascular hemolysis. Intravascular hemolysis leading to death has been reported in clients treated for immune thrombocytopenic purpura (ITP) with Rh$_o$(D) immune globulin. (2) Intravascular hemolysis can lead to clinically compromising anemia and multisystem organ failure, including acute respiratory distress syndrome. (3) Serious complications, including severe anemia, acute renal insufficiency, renal failure, and disseminated intravascular coagulation, have been reported. (4) Closely monitor clients with ITP in a health care setting for at least 8 hours after administration. Perform a dipstick urinalysis at baseline, 2 and 4 hours after administration, and prior to the end of the monitoring period. Alert clients and monitor for signs and symptoms of intravascular hemolysis, including back pain, shaking chills, fever, and discolored urine or hematuria. Absence of these signs and/or symptoms of intravascular hemolysis within 8 hours do not indicate intravascular hemolysis cannot occur subsequently. If signs and/or symptoms of intravascular hemolysis are present or suspected after administration, perform posttreatment laboratory tests, including plasma hemoglobin, haptoglobin, lactate dehydrogenase, and plasma bilirubin (direct and indirect). ■

- **Use with extreme caution with a hemoglobin level <8 grams/dL due to the possibility of increasing the severity of anemia.**
- **Risk of transmitting infectious agents as products are made from human plasma.**
- **Safety for use during lactation not established.**
- **Safety and efficacy not established in children.**

SIDE EFFECTS

Most Common

Rho(D) IGIM: Headache, muscle aches/pains, pain/tenderness at injection site.
Rho(D) IGIV: Fever, chills, wheezing, muscle aches/pains, back pain, pain/tenderness at injection site.

Side effects are infrequent. At injection site: Pain/tenderness at injection site, discomfort and slight swelling at the injection site. **CNS:** Headache. **Musculoskeletal:** Muscle aches/pains, back pain. **GU:** Symptoms following IGIV include anuria, acute renal failure, acute tubular necrosis, proximal tubular nephropathy, osmotic nephrosis. **Hematologic:** Decreased hemoglobin. **Body as a whole:** Fever, chills, wheezing, ***anaphylaxis***. *NOTE:* Immune thrombocytopenic clients positive for Rho antigen D-(positive) may show symptoms of intravascular hemolysis, clinically compromising anemia, and renal insufficiency.

DRUG INTERACTIONS

Antibodies present in immune globulin products may interfere with the immune response to live virus vaccines, such as mumps, rubella, and especially measles. As a general rule, give live virus vaccines 14 to 30 days before or 6 to 12 weeks after immune globulin administration.

HOW SUPPLIED

HyperRHO S/D Full Dose (IGIM). ***Solution for Injection:*** 15–18% protein (greater than or equal to 1,500 units).
RhoGAM Ultra Filtered Plus (IGIM). ***Solution for Injection:*** 300 mcg (1,500 units).
Rhophylac (IGIV). ***Injection Solution:*** 1,500 units (300 mcg).

WinRho SDF (IGIV). ***Liquid Injection:*** 1,500 units (300 mcg); 2,500 units (500 mcg); 5,000 units (1,000 mcg); 15,000 units (3,000 mcg).
HyperRHO S/D Mini-Dose (Rh_0(D) Globulin Microdose). ***Injection Solution:*** 15–18% protein (250 or more units).
MICRhoGAM Ultra-Filtered Plus (Rh_0(D) Globulin Microdose). ***Injection Solution:*** 50 mcg (250 units/dose).

DOSAGE

HyperRHO S/D Full Dose, RhoGAM Ultra Filtered Plus.

IM ONLY

Postpartum prophylaxis.

Give 1 syringe (1,500 units) preferably within 72 hr of delivery. Although a lesser degree of protection is afforded if Rh antibody is given beyond the 72-hr period, Rh_0(D) immune globulin may still be given. Full-term deliveries can vary in their dosage requirements, depending on the magnitude of fetomaternal bleeding. One full-dose syringe provides sufficient antibody to prevent Rh sensitization if the volume of RBCs that has entered the circulation is 15 mL or less. If a large fetomaternal hemorrhage is suspected (more than 30 mL of whole blood or 15 mL of RBCs), a fetal RBC count by an approved laboratory technique should be undertaken to determine the dosage of immune globulin requirement.

The RBC volume of the calculated fetomaternal hemorrhage is divided by 15 mL to obtain the number of syringes needed. If more than 15 mL of RBCs is suspected or if the dose calculation results in a fraction, administer the next higher whole number of syringes.

Antenatal prophylaxis.

One syringe (1,500 units) is given at about 26 to 28 weeks gestation. Must be followed by another full dose (1,500 units), preferably within 72 hr after delivery if infant is Rh positive.

Threatened abortion/miscarriage; termination of ectopic pregnancy.

Give 1 syringe (1,500 units). If more than 15 mL RBCs is suspected due to fetomaternal hemorrhage, give a dose as described under postpartum prophylaxis. Following miscarriage, abortion, or termination of ectopic pregnancy at or beyond 13 weeks gestation, one syringe (1,500 units) should be given. If more than 15 mL of RBCs is suspected because of fetomaternal hemorrhage, the same dose modification as in postpartum prophylaxis applies. If pregnancy is terminated prior to 13 weeks of gestation, where licensed, a single dose of Rh_0(D) immune globulin micro-dose may be used instead of Rh_0(D) IGIM.

Following amniocentesis at either 13–18 weeks gestation or during the third trimester; following abdominal trauma in the second or third trimester; obstetrical manipulation; chorionic villus sampling or percutaneous umbilical blood sampling.

Give 1 syringe (1,500 units) within 72 hr of suspected or proven exposure to Rh-positive RBCs. If more than 15 mL of RBCs is suspected because of fetomaternal hemorrhage, the same dose modification as in postpartum prophylaxis applies. If abdominal trauma, amniocentesis, or other side effects require the administration of Rh_0(D) immune globulin at 13 to 18 weeks of gestation, another dose should be given at 26 to 28 weeks of gestation.

To maintain protection throughout pregnancy, the level of passively acquired anti-Rh_0(D) should not be allowed to fall below the level required to prevent an immune response to Rh-positive RBCs. A dose of Rh_0(D) immune globulin should be given within 72 hr of delivery if the baby is Rh positive. If delivery occurs within 3 weeks of the last dose, the postpartum dose may be withheld unless there is fetomaternal hemorrhage in excess of 15 mL of RBCs.

Transfusion in adults.

The volume or Rh-positive whole blood administered is multiplied by the hematocrit of the donor unit giving the volume of RBCs transfused. The volume of RBCs is divided by 15 mL,

R

which provides the number of syringes of Rh_o(D) globulin to be given. If the dose calculated results in a fraction, the next higher whole number of syringes should be given (e.g., if 1.4, give 2 syringes). Administer Rh_o(D) immune globulin within 72 hr of an incompatible transfusion, but preferably as soon as possible.

Rhophylac

IV

ITP.

Adults: 50 mcg (250 units)/kg given as a single IV injection given at a rate of 2 mL/15–60 seconds. Use the following formula to calculate the amount of Rhophylac to administer:

dose (units) × body weight (kg) = total units/1,500 units per syringe = number of syringes.

IM, IV

Suppression of Rh isoimmunization (Rh-incompatible pregnancy; incompatible transfusions).

NOTE: A 1,500 unit (300 mcg) dose of Rhophylac will suppress the immunizing potential of 15 or more mL of Rh_o(D)-positive RBCs. The dose must be increased if the client is exposed to >15 mL of Rh_o(D)-positive RBCs; follow the dosing guidelines for excessive fetomaternal hemorrhage.

Adults (all uses). (1) Routine antepartum prophylaxis: 1,500 units (300 mcg) IM or IV at weeks 28 to 30 of gestation.

(2) Postpartum prophylaxis (only if the newborn is Rh_o(D)-positive): 1,500 units (300 mcg) IM or IV within 72 hr of birth.

(3) Obstetric complications (See ***Uses*****):** 1,500 units (300 mcg) IM or IV within 72 hr of the complication.

(4) Invasive procedures during pregnancy e.g., amniocentesis, chorionic biopsy) or obstetric manipulation procedures (e.g., external version, abdominal trauma): 1,500 units (300 mcg) IM or IV within 72 hr of procedure.

(5) Excessive fetomaternal hemorrhage (>15 mL): 1,500 units (300 mcg) IM or IV within 72 hr of complication plus 100 units (20 mcg)/mL fetal RBCs in excess of 15 mL if excess transplacental bleeding is quantified OR an additional 1,500 units (300 mcg) if excess transplacental bleeding cannot be quantified.

(6) Incompatible transfusions: 100 units (20 mcg)/2 mL of transfused blood OR per 1 mL of erythrocyte concentrate within 72 hr of exposure. Give IM or IV.

WinRho SDF

IV ONLY

ITP.

Adults and children. Initial after confirming the client is Rh_o(D) positive: 250 units (50 mcg)/kg body weight, given as a single IV injection. The initial dose may be given in 2 divided doses given on separate days, if desired. If the client has a hemoglobin level that is less than 10 grams/dL, a reduced dose of 125–200 units/kg (25–40 mcg/kg) should be given to minimize the risk of increasing the severity of anemia. If subsequent dosing is required to elevate platelet counts, give an IV dose of 125–300 units/kg body weight (25–60 mcg/kg). **Maintenance:** Determine the frequency and dose used in maintenance therapy by the clinical response by assessing platelet counts, RBC counts, hemoglobin, and reticulocyte levels. If the client responded to the initial dose with a satisfactory response in platelets, a maintenance dose of 125–300 units/kg (25–60 mcg/kg) is individualized based on platelet and hemoglobin levels. If the client did not respond to the initial dose, give a subsequent dose based on hemoglobin levels. If hemoglobin is between 8–10 grams/dL, redose from 125–200 units/kg (25–40 mcg/kg). If hemoglobin is greater than 10 grams/dL, redose from 250–300 mcg/kg (50–60 mcg/kg). If hemoglobin is less than 8 grams/dL, use

R

with caution. *NOTE:* Safety and efficacy of doses exceeding 300 units/kg (60 mcg/kg) have not been established.

IM OR IV

Suppression of Rh isoimmunization, pregnancy and obstetric conditions.

Routine antepartum prophylaxis: 1,500 units (300 mcg) given IM or IV at 28 weeks gestation. If WinRho SDF is given early in the pregnancy, give at 12-week intervals to maintain an adequate level of passively acquired anti-Rh.

Postpartum (if newborn Rh_o(D)-positive): 600 units (120 mcg) given IM or IV within 72 hr of birth. If the Rh status of the baby is unknown at 72 hr, give WinRho SDF to the mother at 72 hr after delivery. If more than 72 hr have passed, do not withhold WinRho SDF but give as soon as possible up to 28 days after delivery.

Threatened abortion at any time: 1,500 units (300 mcg) given IM or IV immediately.

Amniocentesis and chorionic villus sampling before 34 weeks' gestation: 1,500 units (300 mcg) given immediately after the procedure. Repeat q 12 weeks during pregnancy.

Abortion, amniocentesis, or any other manipulation after 34 weeks' gestation: 600 units (120 mcg) given within m72 hr of the event.

Transfusion.

NOTE: Give WinRho SDF within 72 hr after exposure for treatment of incompatible blood transfusions or massive fetal hemorrhage.

Adults and children. IM: 60 units (12 mcg)/mL blood if exposed to Rh_o(D)-positive whole blood. Or, 120 units (24 mcg)/mL cells if exposed to Rh_o(D)-positive RBCs. Administer 6,000 units (1,200 mcg) q 12 hr IM until the total calculated dose is given.

Adults and children. IV: 45 units (9 mcg)/mL blood if exposed to Rh_o(D)-positive whole blood. Or, 90 units (18 mcg)/mL cells if exposed to Rh_o(D)-positive RBCs. Administer 3,000 units (600 mcg) q 8 hr IV until the total calculated dose is given.

Rh_o(D) Immune Globulin Microdose

IM ONLY (NEVER INJECT IV)

Actual or threatened termination of pregnancy (spontaneous or induced) at 12 weeks or less gestation.

50 mcg (250 units) within 72 hr. This dose will suppress the immune response of up to 2.5 mL of Rh-positive red blood cells or the equivalent of 5 mL of whole blood. *NOTE:* Full dose Rh_o(D) immune globulin may be given if the microdose product is not available.

Transfusion of Rh-incompatible blood or blood products (<2.5 mL of Rh-positive red blood cells).

MICRhoGam Ultra-Filtered Plus only: 50 mcg (250 units) within 72 hours.

NURSING IMPLICATIONS

IMPLEMENTATION/ADMINISTRATION/STORAGE

1. Never inject Rh_o(D) IGIM Full Dose or Microdose IV.
2. Do not give Rh_o(D) IGIM or IGIV to a neonate.
3. IV To maintain an adequate level of anti-D, Rh_o(D) immune globulin IM, should be given q 12 weeks. The timing for the injection is based on 12-week intervals starting from the administration of the first injection. If delivery of the baby does not occur 12 weeks after the administration of the standard antepartum dose (at 26–28 weeks), a second dose is recommended for maximum protection antepartum. If delivery occurs within 3 weeks of the last antepartum dose, the postpartum dose may be withheld, but a test for fetomaternal hemorrhage should be performed to determine if exposure to more than 15 mL of RBCs has occurred.
4. In the case of postpartum use, the product is intended for maternal administration. Inject the entire contents of the syringe IM, preferably in the anterolateral aspects of the upper thigh and the deltoid muscle of the upper arm. Do not use the gluteal area routinely due

R

to possible injury to the sciatic nerve. If used, only the upper, outer quadrant should be used.

5. If using multiple syringes, calculate total number of syringes needed. The total volume can be given in divided doses at different sites at 1 time or the total dose may be divided and given at intervals, provided the total dose is given within 72 hr of the fetomaternal hemorrhage or transfusion.
6. Use the following administration procedure for a syringe containing Rh_0(D) IGIM:
   - Remove the prefilled syringe from the package. Lift by the barrel, not the plunger.
   - Twist the plunger rod clockwise until the threads are seated.
   - With the rubber needle shield secured on the syringe tip, push the plunger rod forward a few millimeters to break any friction seal between the rubber stopper and the glass syringe barrel.
   - Remove needle shield and expel air bubbles.
   - Proceed with puncture with the needle.
   - Aspirate prior to injection to ensure needle is not in an artery or vein.
   - Inject the drug. Withdraw the needle and destroy it.
7. For IM use of Rh_0(D) IGIV: Reconstitute the 600 international units and the 1,500 international units product aseptically with 1.25 mL of 0.9% NaCl injection and the 5,000 international units product with 8.5 mL 0.9% NaCl, using the same method as for IV use. Administer into the deltoid muscle of the upper arm or the anterolateral aspects of the upper thigh. Do not use the gluteal region routinely, due to the risk of sciatic nerve injury; if used, give only in the upper, outer quadrant.
8. Reduce dose (125–200 international units/kg) of Rh_0(D) IGIV if hemoglobin level is less than 10 grams/dL, to reduce the risk of increasing the severity of anemia.
9. For Rh_0(D) IGIV: Must be given IV for treating ITP, as the SC or IM routes are not effective.
10. The following formulas are to be used to calculate the dose and number of vials of WinRho SDF needed to treat immune thrombocytopenic purpura:
    - weight in lbs/2.2083 = weight in kg
    - weight in kg × selected mcg (units) dosing level = dose
    - dosage/vial size = number of vials needed
11. Rhophylac preparation for administration: Bring to room temperature before use. If more than 5 mL is required and IM injection is chosen, give in divided doses at different sites. Give IV at a rate of 2 mL/15 to 60 seconds for ITP clients.
12. WinRho SDF preparation for administration: No reconstitution is required. Remove the entire contents of the vial to obtain the labeled dosage. If partial vials are required for dosage calculation, the entire contents of the vial should be withdrawn to ensure accurate calculation of the required dose. For IV administration, the entire dose may be injected into a suitable vein as rapidly as over 3 to 5 min. For IM administration, give into the deltoid muscle of the upper arm or the anterolateral aspects of the upper thigh. Due to the possibility of sciatic nerve injury, do not use the gluteal region as a routine injection site. If the gluteal region is used, use only the upper outer quadrant. If using the liquid for IV or IM injection, reconstitution is not required.
13. If using Rh_0(D) Immune Globulin Microdose, give IM only preferably in the anterolateral aspects of the upper thigh and the deltoid muscle of the upper arm. Do not use the gluteal region because of the risk of injury to the sciatic nerve. If the gluteal region is used, only the upper, outer quadrant should be used. Administer only to women post abortion or post miscarriage of up to 12 weeks gestation.
14. The maximum dose of Rh_0(D) Immune Globulin Microdose is 50 mcg (250 units).
15. Store IGIM and IGIV products from 2–8°C (36–46°F); do not freeze. Discard any unused portion. Keep Rhophylac in original carton to protect from light.
16. COMPATIBILITY 0.9% NaCl.
17. INCOMPATIBILITY Administer WinRho SDF separately from other drugs.

ASSESSMENT

1. Note reasons and condition requiring therapy. Review history of Rh-positive exposure in Rh-negative client, any reactions to immunizations and allergies.
2. Determine Rh factor to ensure client is not antibody positive. Obtain blood sample for

type and cross from mother and the neonate's cord. The neonate should be $Rh_0(D)$ positive and the mother must be $Rh_0(D)$ negative and (D^u) negative. A large fetomaternal hemorrhage late in pregnancy or following delivery may cause a weak mixed field positive (D^u) test result. Assess for a large fetomaternal hemorrhage and adjust the dose of $Rh_0(D)$ immune globulin accordingly. Give drug if there is any doubt about the blood type of the mother.

3. Monitor Rh_0 clients for S&S of intravascular hemolysis, clinically compromising anemia, and renal insufficiency. Observe for at least 20 minutes after administration.
4. Reduce dose if hemoglobin is <10 or there is evidence of a large fetomaternal hemorrhage.
5. When used to treat ITP, monitor clinical response by assessing platelet counts, red cell counts, hemoglobin, and reticulocyte levels.

CLIENT/FAMILY TEACHING

1. When an Rh-negative mother carries an Rh-positive fetus, the fetal RBCs cross the placenta and enter the mother's circulation, evoking maternal antibody production against the Rh factor. When these antibodies cross to the fetal circulation, they destroy fetal RBCs, hence the need for monitoring and administration with all subsequent pregnancies. The medication prevents sensitization of an Rh-negative mother by an Rh-positive fetus, ultimately preventing hemolytic disease of the newborn.
2. Avoid immunizations with live-virus vaccines for at least 3 months after receiving drug.
3. Report new onset abdominal/back/muscle pains, chills, decreased urine output, discolored urine, fever, fluid retention, lethargy, shaking, SOB, and sudden weight loss during therapy.
4. Keep all F/U to assess response, labs, and for adverse SE.

OUTCOMES/EVALUATE

- Suppression of Rh isoimmunization
- Prevention of hemolytic disease of the newborn
- ↑ Platelets

Ribavirin

(rye-bah-**VYE**-rin)

Classification(s): Antiviral

Pregnancy Category: X

RX: Copegus, Rebetol, Ribaspheres, Virazole.

SEE ALSO ***ANTIVIRAL DRUGS***.

INDICATIONS/USES

Aerosol (Virazole): Hospitalized pediatric clients (including infants) with severe lower respiratory tract infections (viral pneumonia including bronchiolitis) due to RSV. Underlying conditions, such as prematurity or cardiopulmonary disease, may increase the severity of the RSV infection. Ribavirin is intended to be used along with standard treatment (including fluid management) for such clients with severe lower respiratory tract infections. *Investigational:* Treatment of influenza A and B viruses and herpes simplex virus.

Capsules and Oral Solution (Rebetol): In combination with interferon alfa-2b (pegylated and nonpegylated) for the treatment of chronic hepatitis C virus in clients 3 years and older with compensated liver disease. *NOTE:* Consider evidence of disease progression (such as hepatic inflammation and fibrosis), as well as prognostic factors for response, HCV genotype, and viral load, when deciding to treat a child. Weigh the benefits of treatment against the safety for children.

Capsules (Ribasphere): (1) In combination with interferon alfa-2b for the treatment of chronic hepatitis C virus in those 18 years of age and older with compensated liver disease previously untreated with alpha interferon and in those 18 years of age and older who have relapsed following alpha interferon therapy. (2) In combination with peginterferon alfa-2b for the treatment of chronic HCV in those with compensated liver disease who have not previously been treated with interferon alpha and are at least 18 years of age.

Tablets (Copegus, Ribasphere): In combination with peginterferon alfa-2a to treat adults with chronic hepatitis C virus infections who have compensated liver disease and have not been treated previously with interferon alpha. Is effective in those with compensated liver disease and histological evidence of cirrhosis (Child-Pugh Class A). Efficacy of Copegus was also shown in clients with HIV disease that is clinically stable (e.g., antiretroviral therapy not required or receiving stable antiretroviral therapy).

Investigational: Treatment of viral hemorrhagic fevers such as Crimean-Congo hemorrhagic fever.

NOTE: Ribavirin capsules, oral solution, or tablets as monotherapy are not effective to treat chronic HCV infection.

ACTION/KINETICS

Action

Has antiviral activity against respiratory syncytial virus (RSV), influenza virus, and HSV. Precise mechanism not known; may act as a competitive inhibitor of cellular enzymes that act on guanosine and xanthosine. Ribavirin increases the mutation frequency in the genomes of several viruses and ribavirin triphosphate inhibits HCV polymerase in a biochemical reaction. Ribavirin alone is not effective to treat chronic HCV infections.

Pharmacokinetics

Ribavirin is distributed to the plasma, respiratory tract, and RBCs and is rapidly taken up by cells. The capsules are rapidly and extensively absorbed but due to first-pass metabolism the bioavailability averages 64%. Ribavirin tablets reach T_{max} in 1 (single dose of 600 mg solution) to 3 (multiple dose 600 mg twice daily capsules) hr. Drug accumulation occurs with multiple doses. Steady state is reached in about 4 weeks using capsules. A high-fat meal increases the AUC and C_{max} following ingestion of capsules or tablets. **t½ of tablets:** 120–170 hr; **of capsules:** 298 hr; **t½, plasma, after inhalation:** 9.5 hr. There is little or no CYP450-mediated metabolism of ribavirin. Eliminated through both the urine and feces.

CONTRAINDICATIONS

Aerosol: Pregnancy or the potential for pregnancy during drug exposure. Lactation.

Capsules/Oral Solution/Tablets: Women who are pregnant or in men whose female partners are pregnant. Clients with hemoglobinopathies (e.g., thalessemia major or sickle-cell anemia). As monotherapy to treat chronic hepatitis C. Use to treat HIV infection, adenovirus, respiratory syncytial virus, parainfluenza, or influenza infections. Use in clients with C_{CR} <50 mL/min. Lactation.

Aerosol, Capsules, and Tablets: Lactation. In those with hemoglobinopathies (e.g., thalessemia major, sickle-cell anemia) or pancreatitis. Use in those with a history of significant or unstable cardiac disease.

Capsules/Oral Solution and peginterferon alfa-2b: Autoimmune hepatitis as this combination makes the hepatitis worse. Lactation.

Tablets and peginterferon alfa-2a: Clients with autoimmune hepatitis, in cirrhotic chronic HCV noninfected clients with hepatic decompensation (Child-Pugh score >6; class B and C) before or during treatment, and in cirrhotic chronic HCV clients coinfected with HIV who have hepatic decompensation with a Child-Pugh score of 6 or more before or during treatment. Lactation.

SPECIAL CONCERNS

■ **Capsules/Tablets.** (1) Ribavirin monotherapy is not effective for the treatment of chronic hepatitis C virus (HCV) infection and should not be used alone for this indication. (2) The primary clinical toxicity of ribavirin is hemolytic anemia, which may result in worsening of cardiac disease and lead to fatal and nonfatal myocardial infarctions. Do not treat clients with a history of significant or unstable cardiac disease with ribavirin. (3) Significant teratogenic and/or embryocidal effects have been demonstrated in all animal species exposed to ribavirin. In addition, ribavirin has a multiple-dose half-life of 12 days, and it may persist in nonplasma compartments for as long as 6 months. Therefore, ribavirin therapy is contraindicated in women who are pregnant and in the male partners of women who are pregnant. Extreme care must be taken to avoid pregnancy during therapy and for 6 months after completion of treatment in women receiving ribavirin therapy and female partners of men who are taking ribavirin therapy. At least 2 reliable forms of effective contraception must be used during treatment and during the 6-month posttreatment follow-up period.

Inhalation. (1) Use of ribavirin in clients requiring mechanical ventilator assistance should be undertaken only by health care providers and support staff familiar with this mode of administration and the specific ventilator being used. Strict attention must be paid to procedures that have been shown to minimize the accumulation of drug precipitate, which can result in mechanical ventilator dysfunction and associated increases in pulmonary pressures. (2) Sudden deterioration of respiratory function has been associated with the initiation of aerosolized ribavirin use in infants. Carefully monitor respiratory function during treatment. If the initiation of aerosolized ribavirin treatment appears to produce sudden deterioration of respiratory function, stop treatment and reinstitute it only with extreme caution, continuous monitoring, and consideration of coadministration of bronchodilators. (3) Aerosolized ribavirin is not indicated for use in adults. Be aware that ribavirin has been shown to produce testicular lesions in rodents and to be teratogenic in all animal species in which adequate studies have been conducted (rodents and rabbits).

- **Use with caution in the elderly as the capsules or oral solution cause a higher frequency of anemia. Do not use ribavirin in elderly clients with C_{CR} <50 mL/min.**
- **Use the tablets with caution in those with preexisting cardiac disease.**
- **Safety and efficacy of ribavirin and interferon alfa-2b or peginterferon alfa-2a combination therapy for hepatitis C not determined in clients coinfected with HIV or HBV or in those who have received liver or other organ transplants.**
- **Safety and efficacy of ribavirin and peginterferon alfa-2a, interferon alfa-2b, and peginterferon alfa-2b combination therapy not established to treat HIV infection, adenovirus RSV, parainfluenza, or influenza infections.**
- **Safety and efficacy of ribavirin and interferon alfa-2b or peginterferon alfa-2b not determined for treatment of HCV in liver or other organ transplant clients.**
- **Safety and efficacy of the tablets not determined in children less than 18 years of age.**
- **Safety and efficacy of Rebetol/peginterferon alfa-2b not established in children less than 3 years of age. Safety and efficacy of Ribasphere/peginteferon alfa-2b not established in children.**

SIDE EFFECTS

Most Common

Capsules/Oral Solution used with interferon alfa-2b or peginterferon alfa-2b: Fatigue, asthenia, headache, myalgia, depression, rigors, nausea, arthralgia, insomnia, irritability, anorexia, alopecia, injection site reactions, fever.
Tablets used with peginterferon alfa-2b: Anxiety, depression, insomnia, irritability, fatigue, headache, myalgia, pyrexia, rigors, alopecia, anorexia, arthralgia, diarrhea, N&V, injection site reactions, pruritus.

Aerosol. Respiratory: Worsening of respiratory status, pneumothorax, apnea, bacterial pneumonia, dependence on ventilator, ***bronchospasm***, pulmonary edema/hypertension, hypoventilation, cyanosis, dyspnea, atelectasis, increased positive and expiratory pressure and increased positive inspiratory pressure (due to precipitation of the drug within the ventilatory apparatus). **CV:** Hypotension, ***cardiac arrest***, manifestations of digitalis toxicity, bradycardia, bigeminy, tachycardia. **Hematologic:** Anemia (with IV or PO ribavirin), hemolytic anemia that may worsen cardiac disease leading to nonfatal and ***fatal MI***, reticulocytosis. **Miscellaneous:** Conjunctivitis, rash, ***seizures***, asthenia, ***death***. *NOTE:* The following symptoms were noted in health care workers exposed to the aerosol: Headache, conjunctivitis, rhinitis, nausea, rash, dizziness, pharyngitis, lacrimation, bronchospasm and/or chest pain, damage to contact lenses after prolonged close exposure.

Capsules or Oral Solution in combination with interferon alfa-2b, or peginterferon alfa-2b. CNS: Headache, dizziness, agitation, aggression, anger, anxiety, emotional lability, irritability, impaired concentration, depression (may be severe), insomnia, nervousness, vertigo, ***suicidal ideation/suicide attempts*** (especially in adolescents). **GI:** N&V, anorexia, decreased appetite, dyspepsia, constipation, abdominal pain, upper abdominal pain, diarrhea, dry mouth, hepatomegaly, pancreatitis. **CV:** Nonfatal and ***fatal MI, cardiac arrest***. **Musculoskeletal:** Myalgia, arthralgia, musculoskeletal pain, pain in extremity. **Hematologic:** Hemolytic anemia, anemia, ***aplastic anemia***, pure red cell aplasia, leukopenia, neutropenia, thrombocytopenia, suppression of bone marrow function. **Respiratory:** Dyspnea, sinusitis, coughing, pharyngitis, rhinitis, pulmonary infiltrates, pneumonitis, pneumonia, pulmonary dysfunction, ***pulmonary hypertension***, sarcoidosis (including exacerbation). **Dermatologic:** Alopecia, injection site inflammation/erythema/reaction, pruritus, rash, flushing, dry skin, increased sweating. **Hypersensitivity reactions:** ***Angioedema***, ***anaphylaxis***, urticaria, rashes, bronchoconstriction, vesiculobullous eruptions, ***Stevens-Johnson syndrome***, exfoliative dermatitis. **Ophthalmic:** Conjunctivitis, blurred vision, decrease/loss of vision, retinopathy (including macular edema), retinal artery/vein thrombosis, retinal hemorrhages, cotton wool spots, optic neuritis, papilledema, serious retinal detachment. **Otic:** Hearing disorder/loss. **Body as a whole:** Fungal or viral infection, asthenia, chills, fatigue, fever, pyrexia, flu-like symptoms, rigors, malaise, decreased weight, dehydration, diabetes. **Miscellaneous:** Chest pain, taste perversion, menstrual disorder, hypothyroidism, right upper quadrant pain, autoimmune and infectious disorders, fungal/viral infection, dental/periodontal disorders.

Tablets in combination with peginterferon alfa-2a. CNS: Depression (may be severe), ***suicide, suicidal ideation***, relapse of drug abuse/overdose, irritability, anxiety, impaired concentration, dizziness (excluding vertigo), headache, insomnia, irritability, nervousness, insomnia, impaired memory, altered mood, aggression, hallucination, peripheral neuropathy, psychosis, psychotic disorder. **Hematologic:** Neutropenia, leukopenia, thrombocytopenia, anemia, lymphopenia, hemolytic anemia, suppression of bone marrow function, thrombotic thrombocytopenic purpura, pure red cell aplasia, ***aplastic anemia***. **GI:** N&V, anorexia, diarrhea, decreased weight, abdominal pain, dyspepsia, dry mouth, colitis, peptic ulcer, ***GI bleeding***. **Hepatic:** Pancreatitis, hepatitis decompensation, cholangitis, fatty liver, hepatic dysfunction. **CV:** Nonfatal and ***fatal MI,*** angina, arrhythmia, ***cerebral hemorrhage***. **Dermatologic:** Alopecia, injection site reaction, pruritus, dermatitis, dry skin, rash, increased sweating, eczema. **Musculoskeletal:** Myalgia, arthralgia, back pain, rheumatoid arthritis, myositis. **Respiratory:** Dyspnea, cough, exertional dyspnea, pneumonitis, pneumonia, pulmonary dysfunction, ***pulmonary embolism***, sarcoidosis (including exacerbation). **Hypersensitivity reactions:** Angioedema, ***anaphylaxis***, urticaria, rashes, bronchoconstriction, vesiculobullous eruptions, ***Stevens-Johnson syndrome***, exfoliative dermatitis. **Metabolic:** Diabetes mellitus. **Ophthalmic:** Blurred vision, decrease/loss of vision, retinopathy (including macular edema), retinal artery/vein thrombosis, retinal hemorrhages, cotton wool spots, optic neuritis, papilledema, serious retinal detachment, corneal ulcer. **Otic:** Hearing disorder/loss. **Body as a whole:** Fatigue, asthenia, lethargy, pyrexia, chills, dehydration, rigors, fever, overall resistance mechanism disorder, pain, flu-like symptoms (e.g., fatigue, pyrexia, lethargy, myalgia, headache, rigors), bacterial infection (e.g., sepsis, osteomyelitis, endocarditis, pyelonephritis, pneumonia), autoimmune disorders (e.g., systemic lupus erythematosus), diabetes. **Miscellaneous:** Hyper-/hypothyroidism, dental/periodontal disorders, coma.

LABORATORY TEST CONSIDERATIONS

When combined with interferon alfa-2a: ↓ Hemoglobin (<10 grams/dL).

When combined with interferon alfa-2b: ↑ Bilirubin, uric acid. ↓ Hemoglobin, leukocytes, neutrophils, platelets.

When combined with peginterferon alfa-2a: ↓ Hemoglobin.

When combined with peginterferon alfa-2b: ↑ ALT, total bilirubin. ↓ Hemoglobin, leukocytes. Severe ↓ neutrophils and platelets.

OVERDOSE MANAGEMENT

Symptoms: Following overdose of the capsules: Hepatic enzyme abnormalities, renal failure, hemorrhage, MI. *Treatment:* No specific antidote; hemodialysis and peritoneal dialysis are not effective.

DRUG INTERACTIONS

Al- or Mg⁺⁺-containing products / ↓ Mean ribavirin AUC using ribavirin capsules or oral solution

Azathioprine / ↑ Risk of azathioprine-related myelosuppression (e.g., pancytopenia); do not use together

Didanosine / Possible fatal hepatic failure or peripheral neuropathy, pancreatitis, and symptomatic hyperlactatemia/lactic acidosis when used with ribavirin/peginterferon alfa-2b; do not use together

Lamivudine / Possible antagonism of antiviral activity of lamivudine when used with ribavirin/peginterferon-alfa 2b

Mercaptopurine / ↑ Risk of mercaptopurine-related myelosuppression (e.g., pancytopenia); do not use together

Simethicone / ↓ Mean ribavirin AUC

Stavudine / Ribavirin/peginterferon alfa-2b antagonizes the antiviral activity of stavudine against HIV

Warfarin / ↓ Anticoagulant effect of warfarin; monitor INR during first 4 weeks of combination therapy and upon discontinuation

Zidovudine / Combination of ribavirin, zidovudine, and peginterferon alfa-2a → severe neutropenia and severe anemia

R

HOW SUPPLIED

Capsules (Rebetol, Ribasphere): 200 mg; ***Inhalation, Lyophilized Powder for Solution (Virazole):*** 6 grams/100 mL vial; ***Oral Solution (Rebetol):*** 40 mg/mL; ***Tablets (Copegus, Ribasphere):*** 200 mg, 400 mg, 600 mg.

DOSAGE

Ribavirin

NOTE: Carefully examine the dosages to follow as ribavirin may be combined with interferon alfa-2b, peginterferon alfa-2a, or peginterferon alfa-2b.

AEROSOL ONLY, TO AN INFANT OXYGEN HOOD USING THE SMALL PARTICLE AEROSOL GENERATOR-2 (SPAG-2)

Severe lower respiratory tract infections due to RSV in infants.

The concentration administered is 20 mg/mL and the average aerosol concentration for a 12-hr period is 190 mcg/L of air. Treatment is continued for 12–18 hr a day for 3 (minimum)-7 days (maximum). See *Implementation/Administration/Storage.*

COPEGUS OR RIBASPHERE TABLETS PLUS PEGINTERFERON ALFA-2A

Chronic hepatitis C virus infection.

Individualize dosage based on disease characteristics (e.g., genotype), response to therapy, and tolerability to the drug regimen. **Adults, usual:** 800–1,200 mg ribavirin PO in 2 divided doses. The following are dosing recommendations based on genotype: **Genotype 1, 4:** Ribavirin, 1,000 mg/day in 2 divided doses in those <75 kg plus peginterferon alfa-2a, 180 mcg, each for 48 weeks. The dose of ribavirin is 1,200 mg/day in 2 divided doses in those weighing 75 kg or more plus peginterferon alfa-2a, 180 mcg, each for 48 weeks. **Genotype 2, 3:** 800 mg ribavirin/day plus peginterferon alfa-2a, 180 mcg, each given for 24 weeks. Duration of treatment listed is for those previously untreated with ribavirin and interferon.

Chronic hepatitis C virus with HIV coinfection.

Adults, usual: Copegus, 800 mg/day plus peginterferon alfa–2a, 180 mcg once a week given SC. **Duration:** 48 weeks regardless of genotype.

REBETOL OR RIBASPHERE CAPSULES PLUS INTERFERON ALFA-2B

Chronic hepatitis C viral infection.

Adults, using Rebetol or Ribasphere Capsules plus Interferon alfa-2b. Adults, usual, 76 kg or more: Ribavirin, 600 mg in the morning and 600 mg in the evening with interferon alfa-2b, 3 million units 3 times a week given SC; **75 kg or less:** Ribavirin, 400 mg in the morning and 600 mg in the evening with interferon alfa-2b, 3 million units 3 times a week given SC. **Duration:** 24–48 weeks for those previously untreated with interferon; 24 weeks for those who relapsed following nonpegylated interferon monotherapy.

Children, using Rebetol plus Interferon alfa-2b. Usual dose is provided. **Children, 76 kg or more:** Ribavirin, 600 mg in the morning and 600 mg in the evening plus interferon alfa-2b, 3 million units 3 times a week given SC; **62–75 kg:** Ribavirin, 400 mg in the morning and 600 mg in the evening plus interferon alfa-2b, 3 million units 3 times a week given SC; **25–61 kg:** Ribavirin, 15 mg/kg/day (divided dose in the morning and in the evening) plus interferon alfa-2b, 3 million units 3 times a week given SC. **Duration:** 48 weeks for children with genotype 1 and 24 weeks for children with genotype 2 and 3.

REBETOL PLUS PEGINTERFERON ALFA-2B

Chronic hepatitis C viral infection.

Dosage is based on body weight; the usual adult dose is provided. **Body weight <40 kg:** Rebetol, 800 mg/day (given as 2 × 200 mg capsules in the morning and 2 × 200 mg capsules in the evening) plus peginterferon alfa-2b, 50 mcg/week (0.5 mL of the 50 mcg/

0.5 mL injection); **40–50 kg:** Rebetol, 800 mg/day (given as 2 × 200 mg capsules in the morning and 2 × 200 mg capsules in the evening) plus peginterferon alfa-2b, 64 mcg/week (0.4 mL of the 80 mcg/0.5 mL injection); **51–60 kg:** Rebetol, 800 mg/day (given as 2 × 200 mg capsules in the morning and 2 × 200 mg capsules in the evening) plus peginterferon alfa-2b, 80 mcg/week (0.5 mL of the 80 mcg/0.5 mL injection); **61–65 kg:** Rebetol, 800 mg/day (given as 2 × 200 mg capsules in the morning and 2 × 200 mg capsules in the evening) plus peginterferon alfa-2b, 96 mcg/week (0.4 mL of the 120 mcg/0.5 mL injection); **66–75 kg:** Rebetol, 1,000 mg/day (given as 2 × 200 mg capsules in the morning and 3 × 200 mg capsules in the evening) plus peginterferon alfa-2 b, 96 mcg/week (0.4 mL of the 120 mcg/0.5 mL injection); **76–80 kg:** Rebetol, 1,000 mg/day (given as 2 × 200 mg capsules in the morning and 3 × 200 mg capsules in the evening) plus peginterferon alfa-2b, 120 mcg/week (0.5 mL of the 120 mcg/0.5 mL injection); **81–85 kg:** Rebetol, 1,200 mg/day (given as 3 × 200 mg capsules in the morning and 3 × 200 mg capsules in the evening) plus peginterferon alfa-2b, 120 mcg/week (0.5 mL of the 120 mcg/0.5 mL injection); **86–105 kg:** Rebetol, 1,200 mg/day (given as 3 × 200 mg capsules in the morning and 3 × 200 mg capsules in the evening) plus peginterferon alfa-2b, 150 mcg/week (0.5 mL of the 150 mcg/0.5 mL injection); **105 kg or more:** Rebetol, 1,400 mg/day (given as 3 × 200 mg capsules in the morning and 4 × capsules in the evening) plus peginterferon alfa-2b, 1.5 mcg/kg/week. **Duration:** 48 weeks in interferon alpha-naive clients with genotype 1; 24 weeks for those with genotypes 2 and 3. Duration of 48 weeks for retreatment with peginterferon alfa-2b of prior treatment failures, regardless of HCV genotype.

Chronic hepatitis C viral infection in children, 3-17 years of age.

Dosage is based on body weight. **Body weight <47 kg:** Ribavirin, 15 mg/kg/day using the oral solution plus peginterferon alfa-2b, 60 mcg/m^2/week; **47–59 kg:** Ribavirin, 800 mg/day (2 × 200 mg capsules in the morning and 2 × 200 mg capsules in the evening) plus peginterferon alfa-2b, 60 mcg/m^2/week; **60–73 kg:** Ribavirin, 1,000 mg/day (2 × 200 mg capsules in the morning and 3 × 200 mg capsules in the evening) plus peginterferon alfa-2b, 60 mcg/m^2/week; **>73 kg:** Ribavirin, 1,200 mg/day (3 × 200 mg capsules in the morning and 3 × 200 mg capsules in the evening) plus peginterferon alfa-2b, 60 mcg/m^2/week. **Duration:** 48 weeks for those with genotype 1 and 24 weeks for those with genotypes 2 and 3. *NOTE:* (1) The oral solution may be used for any client regardless of body weight. (2) Clients who reach their 18th birthday while receiving these drugs should remain on the pediatric dosing regimen.

NURSING IMPLICATIONS

Do not confuse ribavirin with riboflavin (vitamin B_2).

IMPLEMENTATION/ADMINISTRATION/STORAGE

1. **Ribavirin is considered a teratogen. Follow safe procedures when preparing, administering, or dispensing the drug.**
2. **Treatment is most effective if initiated within the first 3 days of the RSV that causes lower respiratory tract infections.**
3. **Administer ribavirin aerosol using only the SPAG-2 aerosol generator. Administration should be undertaken only by providers and support staff familiar with the mode of administration.**
4. **Do *not* institute therapy in clients requiring artificial respiration.**
5. **Do not give any other aerosolized medications if using ribavirin aerosol.**
6. **Reconstitute the aerosol with a minimum of 75 mL sterile water (USP) for injection or inhalation in the original 100-mL vial. Shake**

well, and transfer the solution to the 500 mL SPAG-2 reservoir utilizing a sterilized 500-mL wide-mouth Erlenmeyer flask, and further dilute to a final volume of 300 mL with sterile water. Use water that has no antimicrobial agent, or other substance added. The final concentration should be 20 mg/mL.

7. Replace solutions in the SPAG-2 reservoir daily. Also, if the liquid level is low, discard before new drug solution is added.
8. The dose and administration schedule for infants who require mechanical ventilation are the same as for those who do not.
9. For nonmechanically ventilated infants, the aerosol is delivered to an infant oxygen hood from the SPAG-2 aerosol generator. If a hood cannot be used, the aerosol is given by face mask or oxygen tent. However, due to the larger size of a tent, the delivery dynamics may be altered.
10. Do not administer ribavirin aerosol in a mixture for combined aerosolization, or simultaneously with other aerosolized medications.
11. Store reconstituted solutions at room temperature up to 24 hr.
12. Women of childbearing age are not to administer the drug. *Post* this advisement so they do not come in contact with the drug.
13. Once ribavirin tablets have been withheld because of a lab abnormality or clinical manifestation, the drug may be restarted at 600 mg/day with a further increase to 800 mg/day, depending on the provider's judgment. It is not recommended that ribavirin tablets be increased to the original assigned dose of 1,000–1,200 mg/day.
14. Dosage modification guidelines for ribavirin tablets are:
    - If hemoglobin with no cardiac disease is <10 grams/dL, reduce only the ribavirin tablet dose to 600 mg/day (1 × 200 mg tablet in the morning and 2 × 200 mg tablets in the evening). If hemoglobin is <8.5 grams/dL, discontinue ribavirin tablets.
    - If there is a 2 or more grams/dL decrease in hemoglobin during any 4-week treatment period in clients with a history of stable cardiac disease, reduce only the ribavirin tablet dose to 600 mg/day (1 × 200 mg tablet in the morning and 2 × 200 mg tablets in the evening). If hemoglobin <12 grams/dL despite 4 weeks at a reduced ribavirin dose, discontinue ribavirin tablets.
    - Once ribavirin has been withheld due to a laboratory abnormality or clinical manifestation, attempt to restart ribavirin at 600 mg/day and further increase to 800 mg/day, depending on the judgment of the health care provider. However, it is not recommended that ribavirin be increased to the original assigned dose of 1,000 to 1,200 mg per day.
    - Discontinue ribavirin tablets in those who develop hepatic decompensation during treatment.
15. The following are guidelines for use of ribavirin capsules, or oral solution with interferon alfa-2b.
    - In adults and children, assess the virologic response after 24 weeks.
    - Discontinuation of treatment should be considered in any client who has not achieved an HCV RNA below the limit of detection of the assay by 24 weeks.
    - In adults who relapse following nonpegylated interferon monotherapy, the recommended duration of treatment is 24 weeks.
    - For children weighing 25 kg or less, consider using the oral solution (40 mg/mL). For children weighing 25 kg or more, either the oral solution or 200 mg capsule may be used.
    - The recommended duration of treatment for children with genotype 2/3 is 24 weeks. There are no safety and efficacy data for treatment longer than 48 weeks in children.
16. When using ribavirin/peginterferon alfa-2b combination, consider discontinuation in those who do not achieve at least a 2 $\log_{10}$ drop from baseline in HCV-RNA at 12 weeks, or undetectable HCV-RNA after 24 weeks of therapy. Retreated clients who do not achieve undetectable HCV-RNA at week 12 therapy, or whose HCV-RNA remains detectable after 24 weeks of therapy are unlikely to reach a sustained virologic response; consider discontinuation of therapy.
17. Check the package insert for Rebetol to determine dose modification and discontinuation of combination therapy with peginterferon

R

alfa-2b or interferon alfa-2b in adults and children.

18. A ribavirin pregnancy registry has been established to monitor maternal-fetal outcomes of pregnancies of female clients, and female partners of male clients exposed to ribavirin during treatment, and for 6 months following discontinuation of treatment. Health care providers and clients should call 1-800-593-2214.
19. Store capsules and tablets between 15–30°C (59–86°F), and store lyophilized drug powder for the aerosol from 15–30°C (59–86°F). Store oral solution from 2–8°C (36–46°F), or from 15–30°C (59–86°F). Store reconstituted solutions under sterile conditions at room temperature for 24 hr or less.

ASSESSMENT

1. Note reasons for therapy, form of therapy prescribed, onset, characteristics of S&S, any experience with this drug, outcome. Document laboratory confirmation of disease/need; screen for cardiac disease and obtain ECG.
2. When using the aerosol, carefully monitor respiratory function. If sudden deterioration occurs, stop drug and restart only with extreme caution. When restarted, consider concurrent therapy with bronchodilators.
3. If aerosol used ensure client aware of potential for testicular changes/tumors.
4. Health care workers administering aerosolized drug should use goggles and respirator to protect mucous membranes; remove contact lens, and monitor exposure times. Review drug-related side effects.
5. It is essential that constant monitoring be undertaken for both the fluid and respiratory status of the client. For ventilator-assisted clients be sure to drain tubing and suction ET often (q 1-2 hr) to prevent obstruction and impaired ventilation.
6. For pressure and volume ventilators, heated wire connective tubing and bacteria filters in series in the expiratory limb of the system (which must be changed q 4 hr) must be used to minimize the risk of ribavirin precipitation in the system and the subsequent risk of ventilator dysfunction. Water column pressure release valves should be used in the ventilator circuit for pressure-cycled ventilators and may be utilized with volume-cycled ventilators.
7. Assess frequently for evidence of respiratory distress; stop therapy and report if distress occurs. Do not leave child unattended and unstimulated in the tent for long periods. Administration by face mask or oxygen tent may be necessary if a hood cannot be employed.
8. Monitor and record VS and I&O and H&H, especially in the elderly.
9. Assess for co-infection with HIV.
10. Anticipate limited use in infants and adults with COPD or asthma.
11. With prolonged therapy assess for anemia; monitor VS, ECG, and CBC.
12. With hepatitis C document genotype, other meds prescribed, viral load, CBC, renal and LFTs. Document weight, clinical presentation; assess carefully for anemia with therapy—may require transfusion.

CLIENT/FAMILY TEACHING

1. Drug is an antiviral that has been used to successfully treat a variety of conditions. The aerosol form is used for infections caused by the RSV.
2. Oral agents have been used in combination with other drugs to treat chronic hepatitis C infections.
3. Take with food; do not open, crush, or break the capsules. Ensure well hydrated, especially during the initial stages of treatment.
4. Use caution with activities requiring mental alertness until tolerance determined, may cause confusion, dizziness and/or drowsiness.
5. For children weighing 25 kg or less or who cannot swallow capsules, use ribavirin oral solution. For children weighing more than 25 kg, give either the 200 mg capsule or the oral solution.
6. Avoid activities that require mental alertness until drug effects realized; may cause confusion, dizziness, or drowsiness.
7. Practice two reliable forms of contraception; report immediately if pregnancy suspected. Pregnancy tests will be performed before starting therapy, monthly during therapy, and then monthly for 6 months following completion of therapy. Males under treatment need to have female partners take extreme care to avoid pregnancy during his therapy and for 6 months after completion of therapy because of significant risk of birth defects and/or death of fetus.

8. Keep all meds stored safely out of reach. Do not share with anyone.
9. Report any unusual bruising/bleeding, change in vision, chest pain, depression or suicidal thoughts, high fever, hives or swelling, severe stomach or low back pain, trouble breathing, weight loss, skin rash, or unusual illness.
10. Do not consume alcohol—worsens liver disease; avoid OTC agents unless approved.
11. Keep all F/U to assess response, labs, and for adverse SE.

OUTCOMES/EVALUATE

- Improved airway exchange; resolution of RSV pneumonia
- Improved liver condition with Hepatitis C; ↓ HCV-RNA

Rifabutin

(**rif**-ah-**BYOU**-tin)

Classification(s): Antitubercular drug

Pregnancy Category: B

RX: Mycobutin.

INDICATIONS/USES

Prevention of disseminated *Mycobacterium avium* complex (MAC) disease in clients with advanced HIV infection. *Investigational:* Eradicate *H. pylori* as part of a triple-therapy (amoxicillin, pantoprazole, rifabutin), 10-day regimen.

ACTION/KINETICS

Action

Inhibits DNA-dependent RNA polymerase in susceptible strains of *Escherichia coli* and *Bacillus subtilis.*

Pharmacokinetics

Rapidly absorbed from the GI tract. **Peak plasma levels after a single dose:** 3.3 hr. **Mean terminal t½:** 45 hr. High-fat meals slow the rate, but not the extent, of absorption. About 30% of a dose is excreted in the feces and 53% in the urine, primarily as metabolites. The 25-O-desacetyl metabolite is equal in activity to rifabutin. **Plasma protein binding:** About 85%.

CONTRAINDICATIONS

Hypersensitivity to rifabutin or other rifamycins (e.g., rifampin). Use in active tuberculosis. Lactation.

SPECIAL CONCERNS

Safety and efficacy not determined in children, although it has been used in HIV-positive children.

SIDE EFFECTS

Most Common

Discolored urine, rash, abdominal pain, diarrhea, N&V, dyspepsia, eructation, headache, taste perversion.

GI: Anorexia, abdominal pain, diarrhea, dyspepsia, eructation, flatulence, N&V, taste perversion. **Respiratory:** Chest pain, chest pressure or pain with dyspnea. **CNS:** Insomnia, ***seizures***, paresthesia, aphasia, confusion. **Musculoskeletal:** Asthenia, myalgia, arthralgia, myositis. **Body as a whole:** Fever, headache, generalized pain, flu-like syndrome. **Dermatologic:** Rash, skin discoloration. **Hematologic:** Neutropenia, leukopenia, anemia, eosinophilia, thrombocytopenia. **Miscellaneous:** Discolored urine, nonspecific T wave changes on ECG, hepatitis, hemolysis, uveitis.

LABORATORY TEST CONSIDERATIONS

↑ AST, ALT, alkaline phosphatase.

OVERDOSE MANAGEMENT

Symptoms: Worsening of side effects. *Treatment:* Gastric lavage followed by instillation into the stomach of an activated charcoal slurry.

DRUG INTERACTIONS

Although less potent than rifampin, rifabutin induces liver enzymes and may be expected to have similar interactions as does rifampin.

Amprenavir / ↓ Rifabutin clearance; ↓ rifabutin dose by 50%

Cyclosporine / ↓ Cyclosporine plasma levels R/T ↑ liver breakdown

Oral contraceptives / May ↓ OC effectiveness

Saquinavir / ↓ AUC and peak levels of saquinavir (after giving soft-gelatin capsules) and ↑ AUC and peak levels of rifabutin

Zidovudine (AZT) / ↓ AZT steady-state plasma levels after repeated rifabutin dosing

HOW SUPPLIED

Capsules: 150 mg.

DOSAGE

CAPSULES

Prophylaxis of MAC disease in clients with advanced HIV infection.

Adults: 300 mg/day.

R

NURSING IMPLICATIONS

ASSESSMENT

1. Note reasons for therapy, type, onset, characteristics of S&S.
2. List drugs prescribed to ensure none interact.
3. Ensure CXR, PPD, and sputum AFB cultures have been performed to rule out active tuberculosis. Clients who develop active TB during therapy must be covered with appropriate antituberculosis medications.
4. Monitor CBC for neutropenia/thrombocytopenia. Monitor renal and LFTs; reduce dose with dysfunction.

CLIENT/FAMILY TEACHING

1. Take as directed and do not interrupt therapy. If N&V or other GI upset occurs, may take doses of 150 mg twice a day with food.
2. Urine, feces, saliva, sputum, perspiration, tears, skin, and mucous membranes may be colored brown-orange. Soft contact lenses may be permanently stained.
3. Report any S&S of muscle or eye pain, irritation, light sensitivity, or inflammation as well as any persistent vomiting or abnormal bruising/bleeding.
4. Avoid crowds and those with infections.
5. Practice nonhormonal form of birth control.
6. Keep all F/U to assess response, labs, and for adverse SE.

OUTCOMES/EVALUATE

Prevention of disseminated *Mycobacterium avium* complex (MAC) with advanced HIV

IV

Rifampin

(rih-**FAM**-pin)

Classification(s): Antitubercular drug

Pregnancy Category: C

RX: Rifadin, Rimactane.

✤ **Rx:** Rofact.

INDICATIONS/USES

(1) All types of tuberculosis. Must be used in conjunction with at least one other tuberculostatic drug (such as isoniazid, ethambutol, pyrazinamide) but is the drug of choice for retreatment. (2) Treatment of asymptomatic meningococcal carriers to eliminate *Neisseria meningitis*.
Investigational: Used in combination for infections due to *Staphylococcus aureus* and *S. epidermidis* (endocarditis, osteomyelitis, prostatitis); Legionnaire's disease; in combination with dapsone for leprosy; prophylaxis of meningitis due to *Haemophilus influenzae* and gram-negative bacteremia in infants.

ACTION/KINETICS

Action

Suppresses RNA synthesis by binding to the beta subunit of DNA-dependent RNA polymerase. This prevents attachment of the enzyme to DNA and blockade of RNA transcription. Both bacteriostatic and bactericidal; most active against rapidly replicating organisms.

Pharmacokinetics

Well absorbed from the GI tract; widely distributed in body tissues. **Peak plasma concentration:** 4–32 mcg/mL after 2–4 hr. **t½:** 1.5–5 hr (higher in clients with hepatic impairment). In normal clients t½ decreases with usage. Metabolized in liver; 60% is excreted in feces.

CONTRAINDICATIONS

Hypersensitivity; not recommended for intermittent therapy.

SPECIAL CONCERNS

- Safe use during lactation not established.
- Use with extreme caution with hepatic dysfunction.
- Use with caution, if at all, with pyrazinamide in a 2 month regimen to treat latent tuberculosis in those not infected with human immunodeficiency virus.
- Safety and efficacy not determined in children less than 5 years of age.

SIDE EFFECTS

Most Common

Diarrhea, N&V, dizziness, headache, drowsiness, anorexia, sore mouth/tongue, flushing.

GI: N&V, diarrhea, anorexia, pseudomembranous colitis, pancreatitis, sore mouth and tongue, cramps, heartburn, flatulence. **CNS:** Headache, drowsiness, fatigue, ataxia, dizziness, confusion, generalized numbness, fever, difficulty in concentrating. **Hepatic:** Jaundice, hepatitis, ***severe/fatal liver injury when used with pyrazinamide.*** Increases in AST, ALT, bilirubin, alkaline phosphatase. **Hematologic:** Thrombocytopenia, eosinophilia, hemolysis, leukopenia, ***hemolytic anemia.***

Allergic: Flu-like symptoms, dyspnea, wheezing, SOB, purpura, pruritus, urticaria, skin rashes, sore mouth and tongue, conjunctivitis. **Renal:** Hematuria, hemoglobinuria, renal insufficiency, acute renal failure. **Miscellaneous:** Visual disturbances, flushing, muscle weakness or pain, arthralgia, decreased BP, osteomalacia, menstrual disturbances, edema of face and extremities, adrenocortical insufficiency, increases in BUN and serum uric acid. *NOTE:* Urine, saliva, tears, sweat, and feces may be red-orange to red-brown in color.

OVERDOSE MANAGEMENT

Symptoms: Shortly after ingestion, N&V, and lethargy will occur. Followed by severe hepatic involvement (liver enlargement with tenderness, increased direct and total bilirubin, change in hepatic enzymes) with unconsciousness. Also, brownish red or orange discoloration of urine, saliva, tears, sweat, skin, and feces. *Treatment:* Gastric lavage followed by activated charcoal slurry introduced into the stomach. Antiemetics to control N&V. Forced diuresis to enhance excretion. If hepatic function is seriously impaired, bile drainage may be required. Extracorporeal hemodialysis may be necessary.

DRUG INTERACTIONS

Acetaminophen / ↓ Acetaminophen effects R/T ↑ liver breakdown
Aminophylline / ↓ Aminophylline effects R/T ↑ liver breakdown
Amiodarone / ↓ Amiodarone serum levels R/T ↑ liver breakdown
Aminosalicylic acid / ↓ Rifampin effect; give 2 agents 8–12 hr apart
Amprenavir / Significant ↑ amprenavir clearance; do not use together
Anticoagulants, oral / ↓ Anticoagulant effects R/T ↑ liver breakdown
Antidiabetics, oral / ↓ Antidiabetic effects R/T ↑ liver breakdown
Barbiturates / ↓ Barbiturate effects R/T ↑ liver breakdown
Benzodiazepines / ↓ Benzodiazepine effects R/T ↑ liver breakdown
Beta-adrenergic blocking agents / ↓ Beta-blocking effects R/T ↑ liver breakdown
Buspirone / ↓ Buspiron effect R/T ↑ liver metabolism
Chloramphenicol / ↓ Chloramphenicol effects R/T ↑ liver breakdown
Clofibrate / ↓ Clofibrate effects R/T ↑ liver breakdown
Contraceptives, oral / ↓ OC effects R/T ↑ liver breakdown
Corticosteroids / ↓ Corticosteroid effects R/T ↑ liver breakdown
Cyclosporine / ↓ Cyclosporine effects R/T ↑ liver breakdown
Delaviridine / ↓ Delaviridine effect R/T ↑ liver metabolism
Digoxin / ↓ Digoxin serum levels
Disopyramide / ↓ Disopyramide effects R/T ↑ liver breakdown
Doxycycline / ↓ Doxycycline serum level and t½ possible; ↓ effect
Enalapril / ↓ Enalapril effect
Estrogens / ↓ Estrogen effects R/T ↑ liver breakdown
Fluconazole / Rifampin ↑ fluconazole metabolism
Fluoroquinolones / Possible ↑ fluoroquinolone liver metabolism
Haloperidol / ↓ Haloperidol plasma levels and effect
Halothane / ↑ Risk of hepatotoxicity and hepatic encephalopathy
Hydantoins / ↓ Hydantoin effects R/T ↑ liver breakdown
Imatinib / ↓ Imatinib peak plasma levels and AUC R/T ↑ metabolism by CYP3A4
Isoniazid / ↑ Risk of hepatotoxicity
Ketoconazole / Rifampin ↑ ketoconazole metabolism; ketoconazole ↓ rifampin absorption → ↓ effect of both drugs
Lamotrigine / ↓ Lamotrigine AUC and t½ due to ↑ liver metabolism
Linezolid / ↓ Linezolid serum levels after IV use R/T induction of P-glycoprotein which may increase linezolid secretion into the intestine
Losartan / Rifampin may ↑ losartan liver metabolism
Macrolide antibiotics (e.g., clarithromycin) / Possible ↑ clarithromycin liver metabolism and ↓ rifamycin liver metabolism
Methadone / ↓ Methadone effects R/T ↑ liver breakdown
Mexiletine / ↓ Mexiletine effects R/T ↑ liver breakdown
Morphine / ↓ Morphine analgesia

R

Nevirapine / ↓ AUC and peak plasma nevirapine levels in HIV-infected clients
Nifedipine / ↓ Nifedipine effects
Ondansetron / ↓ Ondansetron plasma levels R/T ↑ liver breakdown
Propafenone / ↓ Propafenone serum levels R/T ↑ liver breakdown
Protease inhibitors (e.g., indinavir, nelfinavir, ritonavir) / Possible ↓ liver metabolism of both drugs
Pyrazinamide / Possible severe hepatitis
Quinine / ↑ Quinine liver metabolism
Quinidine / ↓ Quinidine effects R/T ↑ liver breakdown
Repaglinide / ↓ Repaglinide plasma levels and effects R/T ↑ liver metabolism
Rosiglitazone / ↓ Rosiglitazone AUC, peak plasma levels, and elimination $t^{1/2}$ R/T ↑ rosiglitazone metabolism by CYP2C8
Sertraline / ↓ Sertraline effect R/T ↑ liver metabolism
Sulfapyridine / ↓ Sulfapyridine plasma levels
Sulfones / ↓ Sulfone effects R/T ↑ liver breakdown
Tacrolimus / ↓ Tacrolimus immunosuppressant effects
Theophylline / ↓ Theophylline effects R/T ↑ liver breakdown
Thyroid hormones / TSH levels may ↑ → hypothyroidism
Tocainide / ↓ Tocainide effects R/T ↑ liver breakdown
Tricyclic antidepressants / ↓ TCA levels R/T ↑ liver metabolism
Trimethoprim/Sulfamethoxazole / ↓ AUC and serum levels of trimethoprim and sulfamethoxazole
Verapamil / ↓ Verapamil effects R/T ↑ liver breakdown
Zidovudine / ↓ Zidovudine effect R/T ↑ liver metabolism
Zolpidem / ↓ Zolpidem plasma levels and effect

HOW SUPPLIED

Capsules: 150 mg, 300 mg; ***Injection, Lyophilized Powder for Solution:*** 600 mg.

DOSAGE

CAPSULES; IV

Pulmonary tuberculosis.

Adults: 10 mg/kg in a single daily dose, not to exceed 600 mg/day; **children over 5 years:** 10–20 mg/kg/day, not to exceed 600 mg/day.

Meningococcal carriers.

Adults: 600 mg q 12 hr for 2 days; **children, over 1 month:** 10–20 mg/kg q 12 hr for four doses, not to exceed 600 mg/day.

NURSING IMPLICATIONS

IMPLEMENTATION/ADMINISTRATION/STORAGE

1. Give capsules once daily 1 hr before or 2 hr after meals to ensure maximum absorption.
2. A PO suspension (10 mg/mL) may be prepared as follows: The contents of either four 300-mg rifampin capsules or eight 150-mg capsules are emptied into a 4-oz amber glass bottle. Add 20 mL of simple syrup; shake vigorously; then add 100 mL of simple syrup and shake again. The suspension is stable for 4 weeks when stored at room temperature or in the refrigerator.
3. Check to ensure there's a desiccant in the bottle containing capsules of rifampin because these are relatively moisture sensitive.
4. If administered concomitantly with PAS, give drugs 8–12 hr apart; the acid interferes with the absorption of rifampin.
5. When used for tuberculosis, continue therapy for 6–9 months.
6. IV IV use is restricted for initial treatment and retreatment of tuberculosis when the drug cannot be taken PO.
7. Reconstitute the 600-mg vial using 10 mL of sterile water for injection; swirl gently to dissolve. The resultant solution contains 60 mg/mL rifampin; stable at room temperature for 24 hr.
8. Add the volume of reconstituted solution needed to 500 mL of D5W and infuse over 3 hr, or may be added to 100 mL D5W and infused over 30 min. Sterile saline may be used when dextrose is contraindicated; however, the stability of rifampin is slightly less.
9. Use diluted solution within 4 hr or drug may precipitate from solution.
10. Injectable solution appears dark reddish brown.
11. COMPATIBILITY D5W, NSS.
12. INCOMPATIBILITY Administer separately.

ASSESSMENT

1. Note reasons for therapy, type, onset, characteristics of S&S. List drugs prescribed to en-

sure none interact; note any previous therapy, outcome.

2. Assess for GI disturbances or auditory nerve impairment.
3. Obtain baseline CXR; auscultate and describe lung sounds/characteristics of sputum. Note PPD skin test results.
4. Monitor CBC, cultures, renal and LFTs; note any dysfunction.

CLIENT/FAMILY TEACHING

1. Take drug on an empty stomach 1 hr before or 2 hr after meals; report if GI upset occurs.
2. Must take daily for months to effectively treat tuberculosis. Do not stop or skip doses of medication or relapse may occur.
3. Use caution with activities that require mental alertness; may cause drowsiness.
4. Avoid alcohol; increases risk of liver toxicity.
5. Use caution: headache, drowsiness, confusion, fever, muscle/joint aches may occur during the first few weeks of therapy; report if symptoms persist or increase in intensity.
6. Rifampin may impart a red-orange color to urine, feces, saliva, sputum, and tears; may *permanently* discolor contact lenses.
7. Practice alternative birth control since oral contraceptives are not effective; drug has teratogenic properties.
8. Keep all F/U to assess response, labs, and for adverse SE.

OUTCOMES/EVALUATE

- Adjunct in treating tuberculosis
- Elimination of meningococci from nasopharynx in *Neisseria meningitidis* carriers.

Rifapentine

(rih-fah-**PEN**-teen)

Classification(s): Antitubercular drug
Pregnancy Category: C
RX: Priftin.

INDICATIONS/USES

Pulmonary tuberculosis. Must be used with at least one other antituberculosis drug.

ACTION/KINETICS

Action

Similar activity to rifampin. Inhibits DNA-dependent RNA polymerase in susceptible strains of *Mycobacterium tuberculosis,* but not in mammalian cells. Is bactericidal against both intracellular and extracellular organisms.

Pharmacokinetics

Food increases amount absorbed. **Maximum levels:** 5–6 hr. **Steady state conditions:** 10 days after 600 mg/day. Metabolized to the active 25-desacetyl rifapentine. **t½:** 13.2 hr for parent drug, 13.4 hr for active metabolite. Excreted in the feces (70%) and the urine (17%). **Plasma protein binding:** Both the parent drug and active metabolite are significantly bound to plasma proteins.

CONTRAINDICATIONS

Hypersensitivity to other rifamycins (e.g., rifampin or rifabutin). Porphyria, lactation.

SPECIAL CONCERNS

- Experience is limited in HIV-infected clients.
- Organisms resistant to other rifamycins are likely to be resistant to rifapentine.
- Use only if necessary and with caution with abnormal liver tests or liver disease.
- Use caution in dose selection for the elderly.
- Use during pregnancy only if the potential benefit justifies the potential risk to the fetus.
- Safety and efficacy not determined in children less than 12 years of age.

SIDE EFFECTS

Most Common

When combined with other antituberculosis drugs: Hyperuricemia, lymphopenia, proteinuria, hematuria, pyuria, urinary casts, pruritus, rash, anorexia, N&V, anemia, neutropenia, arthralgia, pain.

Side effects listed occurred in 1% or more of clients and were seen when rifapentine was used in combination with other antituberculosis drugs (e.g., isoniazid, pyrazinamide, ethambutol). **GI:** N&V, anorexia, dyspepsia, diarrhea, hemoptysis, pseudomembranous colitis, constipation, esophagitis, gastritis, hepatitis, ***pancreatitis.*** **CNS:** Headache, dizziness, aggressive reaction, fatigue. **GU:** Pyuria, proteinuria, hematuria, urinary casts. **Dermatologic:** Rash, acne, maculopapular rash, pruritus, skin discoloration, urticaria. **Hematologic:** Neutropenia, lymphopenia, anemia, leukopenia, thrombocytosis, hematoma, leukocytosis, neutrophilia, purpura, thrombocytopenia. **Musculoskeletal:** Arthrosis, gout, arthralgia. **Miscellaneous:** Hyperuricemia (probably due to pyrazi-

R

namide), hyperbilirubinemia, hypertension, pain, red coloration of body tissues and fluids, peripheral edema.

LABORATORY TEST CONSIDERATIONS

↑ ALT, AST, alkaline phosphatase, LDH. Hyperkalemia, hypovolemia. Inhibition of standard microbiological assays for serum folate and vitamin B_{12}.

DRUG INTERACTIONS

Cytochrome P450 / Rifapentine is an inducer of certain cytochromes P450 → reduced activity of a number of drugs (See *Rifampin*). Dosage adjustment may be required
Indinavir / Three fold ↑ in clearance of indinavir

HOW SUPPLIED

Tablets: 150 mg.

DOSAGE

TABLETS

Tuberculosis, intensive phase.

600 mg (four 150 mg tablets) twice weekly with an interval of 72 hr or more between doses; continue for 2 months.

Tuberculosis, continuation phase.

Continue rifapentine therapy once weekly for 4 months in combination with isoniazid or another antituberculosis drug. If the client is still sputum-, smear-, or culture-positive, if resistant organisms are present, or if the client is HIV-positive, follow ATS/CDC treatment guidelines.

R

NURSING IMPLICATIONS

IMPLEMENTATION/ADMINISTRATION/STORAGE

1. Give rifapentine in combination as part of a regimen that includes other antituberculosis drugs, especially on days when rifapentine is not given.
2. For the elderly, start at the low end of the dosage range.
3. Store from 15–30°C (59–87°F) protected from heat and humidity.

ASSESSMENT

1. Note onset, duration, S&S of disease. List medical history, other attempts at treatment, outcome.
2. List other drugs prescribed to ensure none interact.
3. Give concomitant pyridoxine in the malnourished, those predisposed to neuropathy (e.g., alcoholics, diabetics), and in adolescents.
4. Obtain chemistries, CBC, and LFTs; assess sputum culture. Monitor LFTs every two to four weeks during therapy and assess regularly for adverse SE.

CLIENT/FAMILY TEACHING

1. Take exactly as directed. May take with food if stomach upset, nausea, or vomiting occurs.
2. Vitamin B_6 is prescribed for those malnourished or predisposed to neuropathy, and in adolescents.
3. May stain body fluids/tissues (tears, urine, saliva, sweat, skin, feces, tongue) a red-orange color.
4. Drug is administered less frequently and in conjunction with other antitubercular agents. During the two-month intensive phase, drug is taken every three days. Following this phase, rifapentine is given once a week for four months in combination with isoniazid or other agent for susceptible organisms called the continuation phase for TB. A more frequent dosing pattern is used in HIV infected clients. Adherence to prescribed regimen is of utmost importance.
5. Report any unusual tiredness/fatigue, SOB, N&V, fever, darkened urine, pain or swelling of the joints, or yellow discolorations of the skin and eyes. Avoid crowds and persons with infections.
6. Practice nonhormonal method of contraception.
7. Keep all F/U to assess response, labs, and for adverse SE.

OUTCOMES/EVALUATE

- Treatment of pulmonary TB
- Negative sputum cultures

Rifaximin

(rif-AX-i-min)

Classification(s): Drug for traveler's diarrhea

Pregnancy Category: C

RX: Xifaxan.

INDICATIONS/USES

(1) **200 mg:** Treatment of traveler's diarrhea due to noninvasive strains of *Escherichia coli* in clients 12 years of age and older. Not useful for traveler's diarrhea caused by *Campylobacter jejuni, Shigella* species, or *Salmonella* species. (2) **550 mg:** Reduction in risk of overt hepatic encephalopathy recurrence in clients 18 years and older. *Investigational:* Relieve symptoms of irritable bowel syndrome.

ACTION/KINETICS

Action

Rifaximin binds to the beta subunit of bacterial DNA-dependent RNA polymerase causing inhibition of bacterial RNA synthesis. For hepatic encephalopathy, rifaximin is thought to have an effect on the GI flora.

Pharmacokinetics

Less than 0.4% is absorbed; thus, it is not useful for treating systemic bacterial infections. **Peak plasma levels:** 1 hr. When used for hepatic encephalopathy, there is a high variability in pharmacokinetic parameters. Excreted mainly in the feces predominantly as unchanged drug. **Plasma protein binding:** 62% after a dose of 550 mg.

CONTRAINDICATIONS

Use in those with diarrhea complicated by fever, blood in the stool, or diarrhea caused by pathogens other than *E. coli.* Hypersensitivity to rifaximin, any of the rifamycin antimicrobial drugs, or any components of the product. Lactation.

SPECIAL CONCERNS

- Use may promote development of superinfection.
- Use with caution in severe hepatic impairment.
- Safety and efficacy of the 200 mg dose not determined in children less than 12 years of age and of the 550 mg dose in clients younger than 18 years of age.

SIDE EFFECTS

Most Common

When used for traveler's diarrhea: Dizziness, headache, N&V, abdominal pain, flatulence, constipation, defecation urgency, rectal tenesmus, fever, rash.

When used for hepatic encephalopathy: Nausea, peripheral edema, fatigue, ascites, anemia, abdominal pain/distention, pruritus.

When used for traveler's diarrhea. GI: Flatulence, rectal tenesmus, abdominal pain, defecation urgency, N&V, constipation, abdominal distension, anorexia, blood in stool, diarrhea, dry lips, dry throat, dysentery, fecal abnormality, gingival disorder, inguinal hernia, stomach discomfort, loss of taste, *Clostridium difficile*-associated diarrhea (may range in severity from mild diarrhea to ***fatal colitis***). **CNS:** Abnormal dreams, dizziness, insomnia, migraine, syncope. **Respiratory:** Dyspnea, irritated nasal passages, nasopharyngitis, pharyngitis, pharyngolaryngeal pain, RTI, rhinitis, rhinorrhea, URTI. **Dermatologic:** Clamminess, rash, sunburn, increased sweating. **Hematologic:** Lymphocytosis, monocytosis, neutropenia. **GU:** Blood in urine, choluria, dysuria, hematuria, polyuria, proteinuria, urinary frequency. **Musculoskeletal:** Arthralgia, muscle spasms, myalgia, chest/neck pain. **Otic:** Ear pain, tinnitus. **Hypersensitivity:** Allergic dermatitis, angioneurotic edema, flushing, pruritus, rash, urticaria, exfoliative dermatitis, ***anaphylaxis***. **Metabolic:** Dehydration, weight loss. **Body as a whole:** Fever, motion sickness, fatigue, hot flashes, malaise, pain, weakness.

When used for hepatic encephalopathy. GI: Nausea, abdominal pain/distention, upper/lower abdominal pain, constipation, abdominal tenderness, anorexia, dry mouth, esophageal variceal bleed, stomach discomfort. **CNS:** Dizziness, depression, insomnia, amnesia, confusional state, disturbance in attention, hypoesthesia, impaired memory, tremor. **CV:** Hypotension, **Respiratory:** Cough, nasopharyngitis, dyspnea, epistaxis, pneumonia, rhinitis, URTI. **Dermatologic:** Pruritus, rash. **Hematologic:** Anemia. **Musculoskeletal:** Muscle spasms, back/chest pain, arthralgia, myalgia, pain in extremity. **Metabolic:** Dehydration, peripheral edema, generalized edema, weight increased. **Body as a whole:** Ascites, cellulitis, flu-like illness, pyrexia, pain, procedural pain. **Miscellaneous:** Contusion, fall.

LABORATORY TEST CONSIDERATIONS

↑ Aspartate aminotransferase.

OVERDOSE MANAGEMENT

Symptoms: Similar to side effects. *Treatment:* Discontinue the drug. Treat symptomatically and institute supportive care as needed.

R

HOW SUPPLIED

Tablets: 200 mg, 550 mg.

DOSAGE

TABLETS, 200 MG

Traveler's diarrhea.

Adults and children over 12 years: 200 mg 3 times per day for 3 days given with or without food.

Irritable bowel syndrome (investigational).

Adults: 400 mg 2 or 3 times per day for 10 days.

TABLETS, 550 MG

Hepatic encephalopathy.

Adults and clients 18 years and older: 550 mg twice a day.

NURSING IMPLICATIONS

Ⓢ Do not confuse rifaximin with rifampin (an anti-tuberculosis drug).

IMPLEMENTATION/ADMINISTRATION/STORAGE

Store from 15–30°C (59–86°F).

ASSESSMENT

1. Note reasons for therapy, onset/characteristics of S&S, culture results.
2. Attempt to identify source of infection; note all travel areas.

CLIENT/FAMILY TEACHING

1. Drug may be taken with or without food.
2. Although it is common to feel better early in the course of therapy, must continue to take medication as directed.
3. To prevent traveler's diarrhea, eat only thoroughly cooked foods, drink bottled water, boiled water, or other beverages made with boiled water; drink carbonated beverages in bottles or cans; avoid tap water, fountain drinks, and beverages containing ice.
4. Take medication only if you get diarrhea while traveling; do not take it in an effort to prevent diarrhea.
5. Stop drug and report if blood noted in stools, fever develops, or if diarrhea worsens or persists for more than 24 to 48 hr.
6. Keep all F/U to assess response and for adverse SE.

OUTCOMES/EVALUATE

Relief of *E. coli* traveler's diarrhea

Rilpivirine hydrochloride

(ril-pi-**VIR**-een)

Classification(s): Antiviral drug, non-nucleoside reverse transcriptase inhibitor

Pregnancy Category: B

RX: Edurant.

INDICATIONS/USES

Treatment of HIV-1 infection in antiretroviral treatment-naive adults in combination with other antiretroviral drugs.

ACTION/KINETICS

Action

Inhibits HIV-1 replication by noncompetitive inhibition of HIV-1 reverse transcriptase. Rilpivirine does not inhibit human cellular DNA polymerases alpha, beta, and gamma.

Pharmacokinetics

Maximum plasma levels: 4–5 hr. Food increases the percent absorbed. Is metabolized primarily by CYP3A. Unchanged drug and metabolites excreted in both the feces (85%) and urine (about 6%). **t½, elimination:** 50 hr. No dosage adjustment is necessary in those with mild or moderate renal or hepatic impairment. **Plasma protein binding:** 99.7%.

CONTRAINDICATIONS

Lactation. Coadministration with anticonvulsants (e.g., carbamazepine, oxcarbazepine, phenobarbital, phenytoin), antimycobacterials (e.g., rifabutin, rifampin, rifapentine), proton pump inhibitors (e.g., esomeprazole, lansoprazole, omeprazole, pantoprazole, rabeprazole), systemic glucocorticoid (more than a single dose of dexamethasone), and St. John's wort.

SPECIAL CONCERNS

- Use with caution in severe renal impairment or end-stage renal disease.
- Cross resistance is possible to efavirenz, etravirine, and/or nevirapine.
- Use with caution in the elderly due to decreased renal and hepatic function and of concomitant disease or other drug therapy.
- Safety and efficacy not established in children.

SIDE EFFECTS

Most Common

Depressive disorders, headache, insomnia, rash.

CNS: Headache, insomnia, depressed mood, depression, dysphoria, major depression, altered mood, negative thoughts, ***suicide attempt/ideation***, abnormal dreams, dizziness, anxiety, sleep disorders, somnolence. **GI:** Abdominal pain/discomfort, N&V, decreased appetite, diarrhea. **Hepatic:** Cholecystitis, cholelithiasis. **Dermatologic:** Rash. **GU:** Membranous glomerulonephritis, mesangioprolilferative glomerulonephritis. **Body as a whole:** Fatigue, immune reconstitution syndrome (inflammatory response to indolent or residual opportunistic infections, such as *Mycobacterium avium* complex, cytomegalovirus, *Pneumocystis jiroveci* pneumonia, and tuberculosis). **Miscellaneous:** Adrenal insufficiency, redistribution/accumulation of body fat, including central obesity, dorsocervical fat enlargement (buffalo hump), peripheral wasting, facial wasting, breast enlargement, and 'cushingoid appearance.'

LABORATORY TEST CONSIDERATIONS

↑ Creatinine, AST, ALT, total bilirubin, total cholesterol (fasted), LDL cholesterol (fasted), triglycerides (fasted), triglycerides (fasted).

OVERDOSE MANAGEMENT

Treatment: No specific antidote. Treatment consists of general supportive measures, including monitoring of vital signs and ECG (QT interval), as well as the clinical status. Gastric lavage or activated charcoal may be used to eliminate unabsorbed drug. Dialysis is unlikely to result in significant removal of the drug since it is highly bound to plasma protein.

DRUG INTERACTIONS

(1) Rilpivirine is metabolized mainly by the CYP3A enzyme systems; thus, substances known to inhibit these enzymes may decreases metabolism or increase bioavailability of rilpivirine. Also, drugs known to induce these enzyme systems may result in an increased metabolism of rilpivirine or decreased bioavailability.

(2) An additive effect of rilpivirine with other drugs that prolong the QT interval cannot be excluded. The following drugs may prolong the QT interval and increase the risk of life-threatening cardiac arrhythmias, including torsades de pointes: Amiodarone, arsenic trioxide, bretylium, chlorpromazine, cisapride, disopyramide, dofetilide, dolasetron, droperidol, gatifloxacin, halofantrine, levomethadyl, mefloquine, mesoridazine, moxifloxacin, pentamidine, pimozide, probucol, procainamide, quinidine, sotalol, sparfloxacin, thioridazine, and ziprasidone.

Antacids (e.g., aluminum or magnesium hydroxide, calcium carbonate) / ↓ Rilpivirine plasma levels; give antacids at least 2 hr before or at least 4 hr after rilpivirine

Carbamazepine / ↓ Rilpivirine plasma levels → loss of virologic response and possible resistance to rilpivirine or to the class of non–nucleoside reverse transcriptase inhibitors; coadministration contraindicated

Delavirdine / ↑ Rilpivirine plasma levels; coadministration not recommended

Didanosine, buffered / ↓ Rilpivirine plasma levels; give didanosine at least 2 hr before or 4 hr after rilpivirine

Efavirenz / ↓ Rilpivirine plasma levels; coadministration not recommended

Etravirine / ↓ Rilpivirine plasma levels; coadministration not recommended

Fluconazole / ↑ Rilpivirine plasma levels; dosage adjustment not needed; monitor for breakthrough fungal infection

Glucocorticoids (e.g., dexamethasone) / More than a single dexamethasone dose may ↓ rilpivirine plasma levels → loss of virologic response and possible resistance to rilpivirine or the class of non–nucleoside reverse transcriptase inhibitors; coadministration contraindicated

H_2-receptor antagonists (e.g., cimetidine, famotidine, nizatidine, ranitidine) / ↑ Gastric pH → ↓ rilpivirine plasma levels; give H_2-receptor antagonist at least 12 hr before or at least 4 hr after rilpivirine

Itraconazole / ↑ Rilpivirine plasma levels; dosage adjustment not needed; monitor for breakthrough fungal infection

Ketoconazole / ↑ Rilpivirine plasma levels; dosage adjustment not needed; monitor for breakthrough fungal infection

Macrolide antibiotics (e.g., clarithromycin, erythromycin) / ↑ Rilpivirine plasma levels; when possible consider using azithromycin

Methadone / ↓ Plasma levels of both methadone and rilpivirine; no dosage adjustments needed but monitor

R

Nevirapine / ↓ Rilpivirine plasma levels; coadministration not recommended
Oxcarbazepine / ↓ Rilpivirine plasma levels → loss of virologic response and possible resistance to rilpivirine or to the class of non–nucleoside reverse transcriptase inhibitors; coadministration contraindicated
Phenobarbital / ↓ Rilpivirine plasma levels → loss of virologic response and possible resistance to rilpivirine or to the class of non–nucleoside reverse transcriptase inhibitors; coadministration contraindicated
Phenytoin / ↓ Rilpivirine plasma levels → loss of virologic response and possible resistance to rilpivirine or to the class of non–nucleoside reverse transcriptase inhibitors; coadministration contraindicated
Posaconazole / ↑ Rilpivirine plasma levels; dosage adjustment not needed; monitor for breakthrough fungal infection
Protease inhibitors (e.g., atazanavir, atazanavir/ritonavir, darunavir/ritonavir, fosamprenavir, fosamprenavir/ritonavir, indinavir, lopinavir/ritonavir, nelfinavir, saquinavir/ritonavir, tipranavir/ritonavir) / Possible ↑ rilpivirine plasma levels; monitor clinical response; no rilpivirine dosage adjustment needed when rilpivirine coadministered with darunavir/ritonavir or lopinavir/ritonavir
Proton pump inhibitors (e.g., esomeprazole, lansoprazole, omeprazole, pantoprazole, rabeprazole) / Possible ↓ rilpivirine plasma levels → loss of virologic response and possible resistance to rilpivirine or the class of non–nucleoside reverse transcriptase inhibitors; coadministration contraindicated
QT prolonging drugs (for list see beginning of this section) / Use rilpivirine with caution when given with a drug with a known risk of torsades de pointes
Rifamycins (e.g., rifabutin, rifampin, rifapentine) / Possible ↓ rilpivirine plasma levels → loss of virologic response and possible resistance to rilpivirine or the class of non–nucleoside reverse transcriptase inhibitors; coadministration contraindicated
H ***St. John's wort*** / Possible ↓ rilpivirine plasma levels → loss of virologic response and possible resistance to rilpivirine or the class of non–nucleoside reverse transcriptase inhibitors; coadministration contraindicated
Voriconazole / ↑ Rilpivirine plasma levels; dosage adjustment not needed; monitor for breakthrough fungal infection

HOW SUPPLIED

Tablets: 25 mg.

DOSAGE

TABLETS

HIV-1 infections.

Adults: 25 mg once a day given in combination with other antiretroviral drugs.

NURSING IMPLICATIONS

IMPLEMENTATION/ADMINISTRATION/STORAGE

Store in the original bottle (to protect from light) from 15–30°C (59–86°F).

ASSESSMENT

1. Note reasons for therapy, date confirmed, other agents trialed, outcome.
2. List drugs prescribed to ensure none interact. Assess for development of any rash.
3. Determine any history of psychiatric disorders or depression; may aggravate these conditions.
4. Obtain ECG; assess for Q-T prolongation; avoid drugs that may contribute to this condition.
5. Monitor lipid profile, renal, and LFTs with history of hepatitis B and/or C. Record viral load, CD4 counts during therapy.

CLIENT/FAMILY TEACHING

1. Take as directed and with other antiretroviral agents. Should be taken with a meal once a day.
2. Drug does not cure disease but works to reduce viral load.
3. Practice reliable contraception (use latex or polyurethane condoms) as drug does not prevent transmission of disease. Do not breast feed. Advise if pregnancy occurs so provider can report to the Antiretroviral Pregnancy Registry by calling 1-800-258-4263.
4. Immediately report if S&S of serious psychiatric adverse reactions occur; i.e., increased depression, or suicide thoughts.
5. Redistribution of fat may occur. May notice an increased amount of fat in the upper back and neck, breast, and around the middle of body. Loss of fat from the legs, arms, and face may also occur.

6. Avoid alcohol, prescribed and OTC meds without provider approval.
7. Keep all F/U to assess response and for adverse SE. Long-term effects and adverse reactions are not known.

OUTCOMES/EVALUATE

- Treatment of HIV-1 infection in combination with other antiretroviral agents
- ↓ HIV-RNA levels; ↑ CD_4 cell counts

Riluzole

(**RIL**-you-zohl)

Classification(s): Drug for amyotropic lateral sclerosis

Pregnancy Category: C

RX: Rilutek.

INDICATIONS/USES

Amyotropic lateral sclerosis (ALS) to extend both survival and time to tracheostomy.

ACTION/KINETICS

Action

Mechanism not known. Possible effects include (a) inhibition of glutamate release, (b) inactivation of voltage-dependent sodium channels, and (c) interference with intracellular events that follow transmitter binding at excitatory amino acid receptors.

Pharmacokinetics

Well absorbed (90%) following PO use; high-fat meals decrease absorption. **t½, elimination, after repeated doses:** 12 hr. Extensively metabolized by CYP450 enzymes in the liver; excreted in the urine. Women may have a lower metabolic capacity to eliminate riluzole than men. **Plasma protein binding:** About 96%.

CONTRAINDICATIONS

History of severe hypersensitivity reactions to riluzole or any of the product components. Lactation.

SPECIAL CONCERNS

- Use with caution in hepatic and renal impairment due to decreased excretion and higher plasma levels.
- Use with caution in the elderly, as age-related changes in renal and hepatic function may cause a decreased clearance.
- Clearance is 50% lower in Japanese clients compared with Caucasians; clearance may also be lower in women.
- Safety and efficacy not determined in children.

SIDE EFFECTS

Most Common

Abdominal pain, anorexia, asthenia, circumoral paresthesia, decreased lung function, diarrhea, dizziness, N&V, pneumonia, somnolence, vertigo.

Side effects listed occurred at a frequency of 0.1% or more or are life-threatening. **GI:** N&V, diarrhea, anorexia, abdominal pain, enlarged abdomen, dyspepsia, flatulence, dry mouth, stomatitis, tooth disorder, oral moniliasis, dysphagia, constipation, increased appetite, intestinal obstruction, increased sputum, fecal impaction, ***GI hemorrhage***, GI ulceration, gastritis, fecal incontinence, jaundice, hepatitis, glossitis, ***gum hemorrhage, pancreatitis***, tenesmus, esophageal stenosis. **CNS:** Dizziness (more common in women), vertigo, somnolence, circumoral paresthesia, headache, aggravation reaction, hypertonia, depression, insomnia, agitation, tremor, hallucination, personality disorders, abnormal thinking, coma, paranoid reaction, manic reaction, ataxia, extrapyramidal syndrome, hypokinesis, emotional lability, delusions, apathy, hypesthesia, incoordination, confusion, ***convulsion***, amnesia, attempted suicide, decreased/increased libido, stupor, subdural hematoma, abnormal gait, delirium, depersonalization, facial paralysis, hemiplegia, decreased libido, hostility. **CV:** Hypertension, tachycardia, phlebitis, palpitation, postural hypotension, ***heart arrest, heart failure***, syncope, hypotension, migraine, PVD, angina pectoris, ***MI***, ventricular extrasystoles, ***cerebral hemorrhage***, atrial fibrillation, BBB, CHF, pericarditis, lower extremity embolus, peripheral vascular disease, ***myocardial ischemia, shock***. **Hematologic:** Neutropenia, anemia, leukocytosis, leukopenia, ecchymosis. **Respiratory:** Decreased lung function, pneumonia, hypersensitivity pneumonitis, rhinitis, increased cough, sinusitis, apnea, bronchitis, dyspnea, respiratory disorder, increased sputum, hiccup, pleural disorder, asthma, epistaxis, hemoptysis, yawn, hyper-/hypoventilation, lung edema, interstitial lung disease, ***lung carcinoma***, hypoxia, laryngitis, pleural effusion, pneumothorax, respiratory moniliasis, stridor. **Musculoskeletal:** Arthralgia, back pain, leg cramps, dysarthria, myoclonus, arthrosis, myasthenia, ***bone neoplasm***. **GU:** Urinary retention/urgency/incontinence, dysuria, UTI, urine abnormality, kidney calculus, hematuria, impotence, ***prostate carcinoma***, kidney pain, menorrhagia, metrorrhagia, priapism. **Dermatologic:** Pruritus, eczema, alopecia, exfoliative dermatitis, skin ulceration, urticaria, psoriasis, seborrhea, skin disorder, fungal dermatitis. **Metabolic:** Gout, respiratory acidosis, edema, thirst, hypokalemia, hyponatremia, peripheral edema, facial edema, weight loss/gain. **Ophthalmic:** Amblyopia, ophthalmitis. **Body as a whole:** Asthenia, malaise, flu syndrome, abscess, ***sepsis***, photosensitivity reaction, cellulitis, hernia, peritonitis, reaction at injection site, chills, ***attempted suicide***, enlarged abdomen, neoplasm, anaphylactic reaction, ***anaphylaxis***. **Miscellaneous:** Accidental or intentional injury, ***death***, diabetes mellitus, thyroid neoplasia, neoplasm.

LABORATORY TEST CONSIDERATIONS

↑ ALT, GGT, alkaline phosphatase, gamma globulins. ↓ H&H, erythrocyte counts, Abnormal LFTs, positive direct Coombs' test.

DRUG INTERACTIONS

NOTE: Potential interactions may occur when riluzole is given together with other agents that are also metabolized primarily by CYP1A2.

Alcohol / Not known if risk of serious hepatotoxicity occurs; discourage drinking excessive amounts of alcohol

Amitriptyline / ↓ Elimination of riluzole → higher plasma levels; monitor and ↓ riluzole dose if necessary

Caffeine / ↓ Elimination of riluzole → higher plasma levels; monitor and ↓ riluzole dose if necessary

Carbamazepine / Marked, rapid ↑ liver enzymes with jaundice and bilirubin 4 months after starting riluzole; use together with caution and monitor

Charcoal-broiled foods / ↑ Elimination of riluzole → lower plasma levels

Omeprazole / ↑ Elimination of riluzole → lower plasma levels; monitor and ↑ riluzole dose if necessary

Quinolones / ↓ Elimination of riluzole → higher plasma levels; monitor and ↓ riluzole dose if necessary

Phenobarbital / Marked, rapid ↑ liver enzymes with jaundice and bilirubin 4 months after starting riluzole; use together with caution and monitor

Rifampin / ↑ Elimination of riluzole → lower plasma levels; monitor and ↑ riluzole dose if necessary

Smoking (cigarettes) / ↑ Elimination of riluzole → lower plasma levels by 20%; dosage adjustment not necessary

Theophyllines / ↓ Elimination of riluzole → higher plasma levels; monitor and ↓ riluzole dose if necessary

HOW SUPPLIED

Tablets: 50 mg.

DOSAGE

TABLETS

Treatment of ALS.

Adults: 50 mg q 12 hr. Higher daily doses will not increase the beneficial effect but will increase the incidence of side effects.

NURSING IMPLICATIONS

IMPLEMENTATION/ADMINISTRATION/STORAGE

1. Protect from bright light.
2. Store from 20–25°C (68–77°F).

ASSESSMENT

1. List symptom onset, characteristics, ethnic background, familial associations. Note clinical presentation and respiratory assessment.
2. List drugs prescribed to ensure none interact.
3. Review potential side effects R/T therapy with client. Women may have a lower metabolic capacity to eliminate riluzole than men.
4. Assess renal, LFTs. Elevations of several liver functions, especially bilirubin, should preclude drug use.
5. Monitor LFTs. Measure ALT every month for first 3 months of therapy, every 3 months for the remainder of the first year, and then periodically.

CLIENT/FAMILY TEACHING

1. Take 1 hr before or 2 hr after meals with a full glass of water to maintain drug bioavailability. Take at the same time each day. Do not double up if dose is missed or forgotten, take the next tablet as originally planned.

R

2. **Avoid activities that require mental alertness until drug effects realized; may cause dizziness, drowsiness, or vertigo.**
3. **Report any nausea, diarrhea, respiratory problems, febrile illnesses. Severe dry mouth symptoms may require oral replacement i.e., Salagen.**
4. **Do not smoke. Avoid alcohol; may potentiate liver toxicity.**
5. **Avoid drinking alcohol in excess during therapy.**
6. **Keep all F/U to assess response, labs, and for adverse SE.**

OUTCOMES/EVALUATE

↑ Survival/time to tracheostomy with ALS

Rimantadine hydrochloride

(rih-**MAN**-tih-deen)

Classification(s): Antiviral

Pregnancy Category: C

RX: Flumadine.

SEE ALSO ***ANTIVIRAL DRUGS*** AND ***AMANTADINE HYDROCHLORIDE.***

INDICATIONS/USES

Adults: Prophylaxis and treatment against strains of influenza A virus. **Children:** Prophylaxis against influenza A virus. *NOTE:* Rimantadine is not a substitute for early vaccination on an annual basis. *Investigational:* H1N1 influenza A (swine flu). Treatment of influenza A in children.

NOTE: Recommendations for prophylaxis:

- High risk clients vaccinated after flu outbreak has begun. Consider prophylaxis until immunity from the flu vaccine has developed (up to 2 weeks).
- Caretakers of those at high risk: Consider prophylaxis for unvaccinated caretakers of high-risk clients during peak flu activity.
- Clients with immune deficiency: Consider prophylaxis for high-risk clients who are expected to have inadequate antibody response to flu vaccine (e.g., HIV).
- Consider prophylaxis in high-risk clients who should not be vaccinated. Prophylaxis may be offered to those who desire to avoid the flu.

NOTE: The H1N1 virus is resistant to rimantadine.

ACTION/KINETICS

Action

May act early in the viral replication cycle, possibly by inhibiting the uncoating of the virus. A virus protein specified by the virion M_2 gene may play an important role in the inhibition of the influenza A virus by rimantadine. Has little or no activity against influenza B virus.

Pharmacokinetics

Suspension and tablet equally absorbed after PO use. Plasma trough levels following 100 mg twice a day for 10 days range from 118 to 468 ng/mL; however, levels are higher in clients over the age of 70 years. **Time to peak levels:** About 6 hr. Metabolized in the liver, and both unchanged drug (25%) and metabolites excreted through the urine. **Single dose t½:** 25.4 hr for young adults and 32 hr for elderly clients. **Plasma protein binding:** About 40% bound to plasma proteins.

CONTRAINDICATIONS

Hypersensitivity to amantadine, rimantadine, or other drugs in the adamantane class. Use of live attenuated intranasal flu vaccine before 48 hr after cessation of rimantadine. Lactation.

SPECIAL CONCERNS

- **Use with caution with renal or hepatic insufficiency.**
- **Possible increased incidence of seizures in those with a history of epilepsy who have received amantadine.**
- **Influenza A virus strains resistant to rimantadine can emerge during treatment and be transmitted, causing symptoms of influenza.**
- **Serious bacterial infections may begin with flu-like symptoms or may coexist with or occur as complications during a course of the flu.**
- **The incidence of side effects is higher in the elderly.**
- **Safety and efficacy not established in children for the treatment of symptomatic influenza infections.**
- **Safety and efficacy not determined for prophylaxis of infections in children less than 1 year of age.**

R

SIDE EFFECTS

Most Common

Insomnia, nervousness, impaired concentration, dizziness, asthenia, nervousness, N&V, anorexia, dry mouth, abdominal pain.

GI: N&V, anorexia, dry mouth, abdominal pain, diarrhea, dyspepsia, constipation, dysphagia, stomatitis. **CNS:** Insomnia, dizziness, headache, nervousness, fatigue, impaired concentration, ataxia, somnolence, agitation, depression, gait abnormality, euphoria, hyperkinesia, tremor, hallucinations, confusion, ***convulsions***, agitation, diaphoresis, hypesthesia. **Respiratory:** Dyspnea, ***bronchospasm***, cough. **CV:** Pallor, palpitation, hypertension, ***cerebrovascular disorder, cardiac failure***, pedal edema, heart block, tachycardia, syncope. **GU:** Nonpuerperal lactation, increased micturition frequency. **Ophthalmic:** Eye pain, increased lacrimation. **Body as a whole:** Rash, fever, rigors, asthenia, diaphoresis. **Miscellaneous:** Tinnitus, taste loss or change, parosmia. *NOTE:* Geriatric clients experience more GI and CNS side effects, including dizziness, anxiety, headache, asthenia, fatigue, N&V, and abdominal pain.

OVERDOSE MANAGEMENT

Symptoms: Extensions of side effects including the possibility of agitation, hallucinations, ***cardiac arrhythmias, and death.*** *Treatment:* Supportive therapy. IV physostigmine at doses of 1–2 mg IV in adults and 0.5 mg in children, not to exceed 2 mg/hr, has been reported to be beneficial in treating overdose for amantadine (a related drug).

DRUG INTERACTIONS

Acetaminophen / ↓ Rimantadine peak concentration and AUC; a clinically important interaction unlikely
Aspirin / ↓ Rimantadine peak plasma levels and AUC; a clinically important interaction unlikely
Cimetidine / ↑ Rimantadine AUC and ↓ clearance; a clinically important interaction unlikely

HOW SUPPLIED

Tablets: 100 mg.

DOSAGE

TABLETS

Prophylaxis of influenza A virus.

Adults and children over 10 years of age: 100 mg twice a day. **Children, 1–9 years of age:** 5 mg/kg once a day, up to a maximum of 150 mg/day. In clients with severe hepatic dysfunction, renal failure (C_{CR} <10 mL/min), and in elderly nursing home clients, reduce the dose to 100 mg/day.

Treatment of influenza A virus.

Adults: 100 mg twice a day. In clients with severe hepatic dysfunction, renal failure (C_{cr} less than or equal to 10 mL/min), and in elderly nursing home clients, reduce the dose to 100 mg/day. Initiate therapy as soon as possible, preferably within 48 hr after the onset of S&S of influenza A infection. Continue therapy for about 7 days from the initial onset of symptoms.

Treatment of influenza A virus in children (investigational).

Children, 10 years of age and older, 40 kg or more: 100 mg twice a day. Initiate within 48 hr of onset of illness; treat for 5–7 days. **Children, 10 years and older, less than 40 kg:** 5 mg/kg/day in 1 or 2 divided doses, up to a maximum of 150 mg/day. Initiate within 48 hr of onset of illness; treat for 5–7 days. **Children, 1–9 years of age:** 5 mg/kg once a day, up to a maximum of 150 mg/day. Initiate within 48 hr of onset of illness; treat for 5–7 days.

NURSING IMPLICATIONS

IMPLEMENTATION/ADMINISTRATION/STORAGE

1. For treatment of influenza A virus infections, initiate therapy as soon as possible, preferably within 48 hr after onset of S&S. Continue treatment for approximately 7 days from the initial onset of symptoms.
2. In those who have trouble swallowing tablets or if a dose lower than 100 mg is required, an oral suspension (10 mg/mL) may be compounded from the oral tablets using Ora-Sweet (see manufacturer's prescribing information for further directions).
3. Store tablets between 15–30°C (59–86°F). The compounded suspension is stable for 14 days when stored at ambient room temperature.

R

ASSESSMENT

1. Note reasons for therapy, onset, duration of symptoms/exposure. Determine when immunized/exposed. H1N1 virus is resistant to rimantadine.
2. List other drugs prescribed to ensure none interact unfavorably. With epilepsy; assess for loss of seizure control.
3. Assess renal and LFTs to note any dysfunction; reduce dosage with severe renal/hepatic dysfunction and with elderly nursing home clients.

CLIENT/FAMILY TEACHING

1. Take only as directed; do not share medications. Taking several hours before bedtime may help minimize insomnia.
2. If using the compounded oral suspension, shake gently prior to use.
3. Initiate within 48 hr of when symptoms appear and continue for 7 days after S&S noted. Still able to spread disease so use care.
4. Drug may cause dizziness; avoid activities that require mental alertness until drug effects realized. Report any adverse side effects or psychosis.
5. Early annual vaccination is the method of choice for influenza prophylaxis. The 2- to 4-week time frame required to develop an antibody response can be managed with rimantadine.
6. Do not take until 2 weeks after live intranasal flu vaccine, and do not receive a live nasal flu vaccine within 48 hr of taking medication.
7. Keep all F/U to assess response, labs, and for adverse SE.

OUTCOMES/EVALUATE

Prevention/ ↓ severity of influenza A virus

Risedronate sodium

(rih-**SEH**-droh-nayt)

Classification(s): Bone growth regulator, bisphosphonate

Pregnancy Category: D

RX: Actonel, Atelvia.

INDICATIONS/USES

Immediate-Release. (1) Treatment of Paget's disease in men and women who (a) have a serum alkaline phosphatase level at least two times the ULN, (b) are symptomatic, or (c) are at risk for future complications from the disease. (2) Prophylaxis and treatment of postmenopausal osteoporosis. The drug increases bone mineral density and reduces the incidence of vertebral fractures and a composite end point of nonvertebral osteoporosis-related fractures. (3) Prophylaxis and treatment of glucocorticoid-induced osteoporosis in men and women taking the daily dosage equivalent of 7.5 mg or more of prednisone for chronic diseases. Adequate amounts of calcium and vitamin D must be given as well. (4) To increase bone mass in men with osteoporosis.

Delayed-Release. Treatment of osteoporosis in postmenopausal women.

ACTION/KINETICS

Action

Binds to bone hydroxyapatite and inhibits osteoclast activity, thereby preventing bone resorption. Bone turnover returns to normal in a majority of clients as evidenced by reductions in serum alkaline phosphatase and in urinary hydroxyproline/creatinine and deoxypyridinoline/creatinine. Appears to reduce fracture risk and reverse the progression of osteoporosis. Does not inhibit bone mineralization.

Pharmacokinetics

Rapidly absorbed; food decreases absorption. $\mathbf{T_{max}}$**:** 1 hr for immediate-release and 3 hr for delayed-release. **t½, initial:** 1.5 hr; **terminal:** 220 hr. Excreted unchanged in the urine.

CONTRAINDICATIONS

Hypersensitivity to risedronate or any component of the product. Use in those with C_{CR} less than 30 mL/min. Abnormalities of the esophagus (e.g., stricture, achalasia) that delay emptying. Inability to stand or sit upright for at least 30 min. Hypocalcemia. Lactation.

SPECIAL CONCERNS

- **May cause upper GI disorders, including dysphagia, esophagitis, esophageal ulcer, or gastric ulcer.**
- **Use with caution in those with a history of upper GI disorders.**
- **Safety and efficacy not determined in children less than 18 years of age.**

R

SIDE EFFECTS

Most Common

Infection, hypertension, chest pain, dizziness, headache, rash, abdominal pain, constipation, diarrhea, nausea, arthralgia, pharyngitis, edema, pain

GI: Diarrhea, abdominal pain, dyspepsia, flatulence, N&V, constipation, belching, colitis, GI irritation/disorders, duodenitis, esophagitis, esophageal/gastric ulcers, glossitis. **CNS:** Headache, depression, dizziness, insomnia. **CV:** Angina pectoris, CV disorder, chest pain, hypertension. **Body as a whole:** Flu syndrome, chest pain, pain, asthenia, infection, neoplasm. **Musculoskeletal:** Arthralgia, arthritis, back/neck pain, bone/joint/muscle/skeletal pain, joint disorder, leg/muscle cramps, myasthenia, osteonecrosis, jaw osteonecrosis, musculoskeletal pain. **Respiratory:** Sinusitis, bronchitis, pharyngitis. **Dermatologic:** Skin rash. **Hypersensitivity:** Angioedema, generalized rash, bullous skin reactions. **Ophthalmic:** Amblyopia, conjunctivitis, dry eye, iritis, uveitis. **Otic:** Tinnitus. **Body as a whole:** Asthenia, edema, infection, influenza, influenza–like symptoms, pain, peripheral edema. **Miscellaneous:** Accidental injury.

LABORATORY TEST CONSIDERATIONS

↓ Serum Ca and P. Abnormal LFTs.

OVERDOSE MANAGEMENT

Symptoms: Hypocalcemia. *Treatment:* Gastric lavage to remove unabsorbed drug. Milk or antacids to bind risedronate. IV calcium.

DRUG INTERACTIONS

Aluminum-containing products / ↓ Absorption of risedronate; take at a different time of day than risedronate
Antacids, calcium-containing / ↓ Absorption of risedronate; take at a different time of day than risedronate
Bone imaging agents / Risedronate interferes with these agent
Calcium / ↓ Absorption of risedronate; take at a different time of day than risedronate
Iron products / ↓ Absorption of risedronate; take at a different time of day than risedronate
Laxatives / ↓ Absorption of risedronate; take at a different time of day than risedronate
Magnesium-containing products / ↓ Absorption of risedronate; take at a different time of day than risedronate
NSAIDs / Possible additive GI side effects

HOW SUPPLIED

Tablets: 5 mg, 30 mg, 35 mg, 150 mg; ***Tablets, Delayed-Release:*** 35 mg.

DOSAGE

TABLETS, IMMEDIATE-RELEASE

Paget's disease in men and women.

Adults: 30 mg once daily for 2 months. Retreatment may be considered following posttreatment observation for at least 2 months if relapse occurs or if treatment fails to normalize serum alkaline phosphatase. For retreatment, the dose and duration of therapy are the same as for initial treatment.

Prevention and treatment of postmenopausal osteoporosis.

Adults: 5 mg once daily or one 35 mg tablet taken once weekly or 75 mg taken on 2 consecutive days for a total of 2 tablets (150 mg) per month, or 150 mg taken once a month.

Prevention and treatment of glucocorticoid-induced osteoporosis in men and women.

Adults: 5 mg once daily.

Osteoporosis in men.

Adults: 35 mg once per week.

TABLETS, DELAYED-RELEASE

Treatment of osteoporosis in postmenopausal women.

Adults: 35 mg once a week.

NURSING IMPLICATIONS

Do not confuse Actonel with Actos (oral hypoglycemic).

IMPLEMENTATION/ADMINISTRATION/STORAGE

1. **Before starting therapy, treat hypocalcemia, other disturbances of bone, and mineral metabolism. Use supplemental calcium and vitamin D.**
2. **Dosage adjustment is not necessary in clients with a C_{CR} 30 mL/min or greater.**
3. **If clients miss a dose of risedronate, 35 mg once weekly, they should take 1 tablet on the**

morning after they remember and return to taking 1 tablet once weekly, as originally prescribed, on their chosen day. Clients should not take 2 tablets on the same day.

4. If the dose of risedronate, 150 mg once a month, is missed and the next month's scheduled dose is more than 7 days away, instruct the client to take the missed tablet on the morning after the day it is remembered. Instruct the client to return to taking their risedronate, 150 mg once a month, as originally prescribed. Instruct the client not to take more than one 150 mg tablet within 7 days. If the dose of risedronate, 150 mg once a month, is missed and the next month's scheduled dose is within 7 days, instruct the client to wait until their next month's scheduled dose and then continue taking risedronate, 150 mg once a month, as originally prescribed.
5. Store from 20–25°C (68–77°F).

ASSESSMENT

1. Note reasons for therapy, onset, characteristics of disease; list other agents trialed. Assess for GI disease/dysfunction.
2. Assess nutritional status, vitamin D, calcium intake. Assess bone density (BMD), for low bone mass, evidence of fracture on x-ray, history of osteoporotic fracture, height loss or kyphosis indicative of vertebral fracture.
3. Obtain chemistries, alkaline phosphatase, parathyroid hormone, phosphorus, Ca^{++}, lipids, renal and LFTs; assess for dysfunction, avoid if C_{CR} <30 mL/min.

CLIENT/FAMILY TEACHING

1. Take immediate-release tablets while sitting or standing with a full glass of water at least 30 min before the first food or drink of the day. To facilitate delivery to the stomach and minimize esophageal irritation, take in an upright position with 8 oz of water. Avoid lying down for 30 min after taking drug. Mark calendar to ensure weekly or monthly dosing not missed.
2. Take delayed-release tablets immediately following breakfast, i.e. not under fasting conditions. Swallow whole while in an upright position and with at least 4 oz of water. Do not cut, chew, or crush delayed-release tablets. Do not lie down for 30 min after taking the drug.
3. Consume daily supplemental calcium and vitamin D. Antacids and calcium may interfere with drug so take them at different times during the day with food.
4. May experience nausea, diarrhea, bone pain, headache, and rash. Report so appropriate analgesics and skin care may be prescribed.
5. Regular weight bearing exercise and cessation of alcohol and tobacco is advised.
6. Report any swallowing difficulty, GI bleeding, throat/abdominal pain, muscle spasms, fractures, or dark-colored urine.
7. Osteonecrosis of the jaw has been reported rarely; severe bone, joint, or muscle pain may occur report if persistent.
8. Keep all F/U visits to assess response, BMD, and for adverse SE.

OUTCOMES/EVALUATE

- ↓ Bone resorption, ↓ pain, ↓ alkaline phosphatase levels, ↑ bone mass
- Inhibition of bone resorption/progression of osteoporosis

Risperidone

(ris-**PAIR**-ih-dohn)

Classification(s): Antipsychotic

Pregnancy Category: C

RX: Risperdal, Risperdal Consta, Risperdal M-Tab.

✤ **Rx:** Apo-Risperidone, CO Risperidone, Gen-Risperidone, Novo-Risperidone, PMS-Risperidone, ratio-Risperidone, Sandoz Risperidone.

INDICATIONS/USES

PO. (1) Acute and maintenance treatment of schizophrenia in adults. (2) Treatment of schizophrenia in adolescents, 13–17 years of age. (3) Monotherapy in adults and children (10–17 years of age) for short-term treatment of acute manic or mixed episodes associated with bipolar I disorder. (4) In combination with lithium or valproate for the short-term treatment of adults with acute manic or mixed episodes associated with bipolar I disorder. (5) Irritability associated with autistic disorder in children and adolescents (5–16 years of age), including symptoms of aggression toward others, deliberate self-injuriousness, temper tantrums, and quickly changing moods. *Investigational:* OCD refractory to selective serotonin reuptake inhibitors, stuttering, Tourette's syndrome, psychosis/agitation in dementia or Alzheimer disease.

IM. (1) Treatment of schizophrenia. (2) Monotherapy or adjunctive therapy to lithium or valproate for maintenance treatment of bipolar I disorder.

NOTE: Has not been shown to be safe or effective to treat dementia-related psychosis.

ACTION/KINETICS

Action

Mechanism may be due to a combination of antagonism of dopamine (D_2) and serotonin ($5\text{-}HT_2$) receptors. Also has low to moderate affinity for $5\text{-}HT_{1c}$, $5\text{-}HT_{1D}$, $5\text{-}HT_{1A}$, $alpha_1$-, $alpha_2$-, and $histamine_1$ receptors. Low incidence of sedation and anticholinergic effects, moderate incidence of extrapyramidal effects and orthostatic hypotension, and a high incidence of weight gain.

Pharmacokinetics

Metabolized significantly in the liver to the active metabolite 9-hydroxyrisperidone, which has equal receptor-binding activity as risperidone. Thus, the effect is likely due to both the parent compound and the metabolite. Food does not affect either the rate or extent of absorption. Bioavailability is 70%. The ability to convert risperidone to 9-hydroxyrisperidone is subject to genetic variation. A low percentage of Asians have the ability to metabolize the drug. **Peak plasma levels, risperidone:** 1 hr; **peak plasma levels, 9-hydroxyrisperidone:** 3 hr for extensive metabolizers and 17 hr for poor metabolizers. **t½, risperidone and 9-methylrisperidone:** 3 and 20 hr, respectively, for extensive metabolizers and 20 and 30 hr, respectively, for poor metabolizers. Metabolized by CYP2D6 and by N-dealkylation. Excreted in the feces (about 70%) and urine (about 14%). Clearance is decreased in geriatric clients and in clients with hepatic and renal impairment. The orally disintegrating tablets are bioequivalent to the original-formulation tablets. **Plasma protein binding:** 90%.

CONTRAINDICATIONS

Lactation.

SPECIAL CONCERNS

Increased mortality in elderly clients with dementia-related psychoses. Elderly clients with dementia-related psychosis treated with atypical antipsychotic drugs are at an increased risk of death. Analyses of placebo-controlled trials (modal duration of 10 weeks), largely in clients taking atypical antipsychotic drugs, revealed a risk of death in the drug-treated clients between 1.6–1.7 times that seen in placebo-treated clients. Over the course of a typical 10-week controlled trial, the rate of death in drug-treated clients was about 4.5%, compared with a rate of about 2.6% in the placebo group. Although the causes of death were varied, most of the deaths appeared to be either cardiovascular (e.g., heart failure, sudden death) or infectious (e.g., pneumonia) in nature. Observational studies suggest that, similar to atypical antipsychotic drugs, treatment with conventional antipsychotic may increase mortality. The extent to which the findings of increased mortality in observational studies may be attributed to the antipsychotic drug as opposed to some characteristic(s) of the clients is not clear. Risperidone is not approved for the treatment of clients with dementia-related psychosis.

- **Use with caution with known CV disease (including history of MI or ischemia, heart failure, conduction abnormalities), cerebrovascular disease, in conditions that predispose client to hypotension (e.g., dehydration, hypovolemia, use of antihypertensive drugs), and in the elderly predisposed to aspiration pneumonia.**
- **Use with caution in clients exposed to extreme heat or when taken with other CNS drugs or alcohol.**
- **Greater risk of orthostatic hypotension, aspiration pneumonia, and toxic effects in geriatric clients with impaired renal function.**
- **Effectiveness of risperidone for more than 6–8 weeks not studied.**
- **Children appear to be at greater risk than adults for extrapyramidal and metabolic side effects.**
- **Safety and efficacy not determined in children younger than 5 years of age with autistic disorder.**

SIDE EFFECTS

Most Common

Agitation, anxiety, extrapyramidal symptoms, headache, insomnia, constipation, dyspepsia, diar-

rhea, dry mouth, N&V, weight gain, impotence, menorrhagia, ejaculation disorders, rhinitis, lymphedema.
Except for life-threatening side effects, those with an incidence of 0.1% or greater are listed. **Neuroleptic malignant syndrome.** Hyperpyrexia, muscle rigidity, altered mental status, autonomic instability (i.e., irregular pulse or BP, tachycardia, diaphoresis, cardiac dysrhythmia), elevated CPK, rhabdomyolysis, ***acute respiratory failure, death***. **CNS:** Agitation, anxiety, extrapyramidal symptoms, headache, decreased/loss of libido, insomnia, drowsiness, sedation, somnolence, dizziness, amnesia, apathy, catatonic-like states, confusion, depression, aggressive reaction, abnormal/bizarre/increased dreams, dysarthria, euphoria, increased/decreased/loss of libido, nervousness, paresthesia, pseudoparkinsonism, stupor, vertigo, impaired concentration. **CV:** Tachycardia, bradycardia, AV block, ***CVA***, hyper-/hypotension, ***MI***, palpitations, ***pulmonary embolus***, cerebrovascular disorder, prolongation of the QT interval that might lead to ***torsades de pointes and sudden cardiac death, stroke or ischemic attacks in elderly clients with dementia***. **GI:** Constipation, dyspepsia, abdominal discomfort/pain, anorexia, diarrhea, increased appetite, dry mouth, N&V, dysphagia, flatulence, gastritis, hemorrhoids, intestinal obstruction, melena, polydipsia, salivation, stomatitis, weight gain/loss, toothache, jaundice. **Dermatologic:** Rash, eczema, acne, alopecia, dermatitis, photosensitivity, pruritus, seborrhea, hyperkeratosis, skin exfoliation. **GU:** Impotence, menorrhagia, ejaculation disorders, dysmenorrhea, amenorrhea, galactorrhea, hematuria, urinary incontinence, mastalgia, polyuria, priapism, urinary retention, vaginal hemorrhage. **Respiratory:** Rhinitis, increased cough, URTI, pharyngitis, sinusitis, epistaxis, hyperventilation, apnea, pneumonia, bronchospasm. **Hematologic:** Anemia, hypochromic anemia, nonthrombocytopenic purpura. **Musculoskeletal:** Arthralgia, joint pain, back/chest pain, myalgia, rigidity. **Hypersensitivity:** Angioedema, allergic reaction, ***anaphylaxis***. **Ophthalmic:** Accommodation abnormality, abnormal vision, xerothalmia. **Body as a whole:** Lymphedema, fatigue, malaise, fever, edema, diaphoresis, flu syndrome, stridor, ***sudden death***. **Miscellaneous:** Increased risk of diabetes mellitus, hyperpigmentation.

LABORATORY TEST CONSIDERATIONS

↑ CPK, serum prolactin, AST, ALT, creatinine. Hypokalemia, hyponatremia, hyper-/hypoglycemia, hypoproteinemia.

OVERDOSE MANAGEMENT

Symptoms: Exaggeration of known effects, especially drowsiness, sedation, tachycardia, hypotension, and extrapyramidal symptoms. *Treatment:* Establish and secure airway, and ensure adequate oxygenation and ventilation. Follow gastric lavage with activated charcoal and a laxative. Monitor CV system, including continuous ECG readings. Provide general supportive measures. Treat hypotension and circulatory collapse with IV fluids or sympathomimetic drugs; however, do not use epinephrine and dopamine, as beta stimulation may worsen hypotension due to risperidone-induced alpha blockade. Anticholinergic drugs can be given for severe extrapyramidal symptoms.

DRUG INTERACTIONS

Alcohol / ↑ Risk of dystonic reactions
Carbamazepine / ↑ Risperidone clearance → ↓ therapeutic effect R/T ↑ metabolism; titrate dosage accordingly
Clozapine / ↑ Clozapine pharmacologic/toxic effects; adjust dose as needed
CNS depressants / Enhanced CNS depression, especially impaired motor skills
Dopamine agonists / Risperidone antagonizes the effect of dopamine agonists
Fluoxetine / ↑ Risperidone levels → ↑ risk of side effects; titrate dose of risperidone accordingly
Levodopa / Risperidone antagonizes the effects of levodopa
Maprotiline / ↑ Maprotiline levels R/T ↓ metabolism
Paroxetine / Significant ↑ in risperidone levels → ↑ risk of side effects R/T ↓ liver metabolism; titrate dose of risperidone accordingly
Phenobarbital / ↑ Risperidone clearance R/T ↑ metabolism; titrate dosage accordingly
Phenytoin / ↑ Risperidone clearance R/T ↑ metabolism; titrate dosage accordingly
Rifampin / ↑ Risperidone clearance R/T ↑ metabolism; titrate dosage accordingly
Ritonavir / ↑ Risperidone levels → ↑ risk of toxicity
Thioridazine / ↑ Risperidone levels and ↓ 9-hydroxyrisperidone levels R/T inhibition of CYP2D6

R

Valproate / ↑ Valproate C_{max} by 20%; adjust therapy as needed

HOW SUPPLIED

Oral Solution: 1 mg/mL; *Powder for Suspension (Injection), Extended-Release:* 12.5 mg, 25 mg, 37.5 mg, 50 mg; *Tablets:* 0.25 mg, 0.5 mg, 1 mg, 2 mg, 3 mg, 4 mg; *Tablets, Oral Disintegrating:* 0.5 mg, 1 mg, 2 mg, 3 mg, 4 mg.

DOSAGE

ORAL SOLUTION; TABLETS; TABLETS, ORAL DISINTEGRATING

Schizophrenia in adults.

Adults, initial: 2 mg/day given once daily or half the total daily dose given twice a day. Make dosage increases at intervals of no less than 24 hr in increments of 1–2 mg/day to a recommended dosage of 4–8 mg/day. In some, slower titration may be appropriate. Efficacy has been shown in a dose range of 4–16 mg/day. However, doses greater than 6 mg/day for twice-daily dosing were not shown to be more effective than lower doses and were associated with more extrapyramidal symptoms and other side effects. **Maintenance:** Use lowest dose that will maintain remission; doses from 2–8 mg/day have been shown to be effective for longer-term therapy. Periodically assess for the need for continued treatment.

Schizophrenia in adolescents, 13–17 years of age.

Adolescents, 13 to 17 years, initial: 0.5 mg once daily, given as a single daily dose either in the morning or evening. Make dosage adjustments, if needed, at intervals of no less than 24 hr in increments of 0.5 or 1 mg/day, as tolerated to the recommended dose of 3 mg/day. Although doses up to 6 mg/day have been used, they have not been shown to be more effective than 3 mg/day and were associated with more side effects. **Maintenance:** There are no studies supporting use beyond 8 weeks. If longer term therapy is used, periodically evaluate.

Bipolar mania in adults and children.

Adults, initial: 2–3 mg/day. If needed, adjust dose at intervals of not less than 24 hr in increments/decrements of 1 mg/day. There are no data to support use for more than 3 weeks with a dose range from 1–6 mg/day. **Children, 10–17 years of age, initial:** 0.5 mg once daily, as a single dose either in the morning or evening. If needed, adjust dose at intervals of not less than 24 hr in increments of 0.5 or 1 mg/day, as tolerated, to the recommended dose of 2.5 mg/day. Doses up to 6 mg/day may be used but no additional benefit was seen with doses higher than 2.5 mg/day. There are no data to support use for more than 3 weeks. Whether used long-term in adults or children, periodically evaluate the long-term risks and benefits.

Irritability associated with autistic disorder in children 5–16 years of age.

Individualize dose according to response and client tolerability. **Children and adolescents, 5–16 years of age, initial:** 0.25 mg/day for those weighing less than 20 kg and 0.5 mg/day for those at least 20 kg. After a minimum of 4 days, the dose may be increased to the recommended dose of 0.5 mg/day for those weighing less than 20 kg and 1 mg/day for those at least 20 kg. Maintain these doses for a minimum of 14 days. In those not achieving a sufficient response, the dose may be increased at intervals of at least 2 weeks in increments of 0.25 mg/day for those weighing less than 20 kg or 0.5 mg/day for those at least 20 kg. Use caution for smaller children who weigh less than 15 kg. The total daily dose can be given once daily or half the total daily dose can be given twice daily. For those experiencing somnolence, the dose can be given once daily at bedtime. **Maintenance:** Once a satisfactory response has been obtained, consider lowering the dose gradually to achieve the optimal balance of safety and efficacy. *NOTE:*

R

The safety and efficacy in children younger than 5 years of age with autistic disorder have not been determined.

IM

Schizophrenia.

Adults: 25 mg q 2 weeks by deep IM injection. Some not responding to 25 mg may benefit from doses of 37.5 mg or 50 mg. Do not exceed a dose of 50 mg q 2 weeks. PO risperidone (or another antipsychotic drug) should be given with the first risperidone injection and continued for 3 weeks and then discontinued (this is to ensure adequate therapeutic plasma levels are maintained prior to the main release phase from the injection site). Do not make upward dosage adjustments more frequently than q 4 weeks. Periodically reassess to determine need for continued therapy. For the elderly, the recommended dosage is 25 mg IM q 2 weeks. Treat clients with hepatic or renal impairment with titrated doses of PO risperidone prior to beginning risperidone injections. **Maintenance:** Responding clients can be continued at the lowest dose needed. Periodically assess the need for continued treatment. *NOTE:* For those with a history of poor tolerability to psychotropic drugs, a lower initial dose of 12.5 mg IM may be more appropriate.

Maintenance treatment of bipolar I disorder, either monotherapy or adjunctive therapy to lithium or valproate.

Adults: 25 mg IM q 2 weeks; some may benefit from a higher dose of 37.5 mg or 50 mg (maximum) q 2 weeks. Doses above 50 mg q 2 weeks have not been studied in this group. Periodically evaluate the benefits and risks for each client.

NURSING IMPLICATIONS

Do not confuse Risperdal with Restoril (a hypnotic).

IMPLEMENTATION/ADMINISTRATION/STORAGE

1. For clients with severe renal impairment, the initial PO dose is 0.5 mg twice a day. Make increments of no more than 0.5 mg twice a day. Increases to dosages greater than 1.5 mg twice a day should usually occur at intervals of at least 1 week. In some clients, slower titration may be appropriate.
2. The initial PO dose is 0.5 mg twice a day for clients who are elderly or debilitated, and in those predisposed to hypotension or in whom hypotension would pose a risk. Dosage increases in these clients should be in increments of 0.5 mg twice a day. Dosage increases above 1.5 mg twice a day should occur at intervals of about 1 week. If a once-daily dosing regimen is being considered, the client should be titrated on a twice-a-day regimen for 2–3 days at the target dose. Subsequent switch to a once daily dosing can be done thereafter.
3. The PO solution may ease administration to geriatric clients and those in an acute-care setting.
4. If discontinuation is needed, some clients may be withdrawn immediately while others require a more gradual withdrawal.
5. When restarting clients who have had an interval of risperidone, follow the initial titration schedule.
6. If switching from other antipsychotic drugs to risperidone, stop other antipsychotic drug when starting risperidone therapy. When switching from a depot antipsychotic injection, initiate risperidone in place of the next scheduled injection.
7. For those who have never taken PO risperidone, establish tolerability with PO risperidone before beginning treatment with the injectable form.
8. Coadministration of carbamazepine and other CYP3A4 enzyme inducers (e.g., phenobarbital, phenytoin, rifampin) with risperidone will likely cause decreases in plasma levels of both risperidone and its active metabolite; this could result in decreased efficacy of risperidone treatment. Monitor clients closely during the first 4–8 weeks, because the risperidone dose may need to be adjusted. Titrate the dose of risperidone accordingly in this situation. If the CYP3A4 inducer is discontinued, the dose of risperidone may need to be decreased.

R

9. If risperidone is given with CYP2D6 inhibitors (e.g., fluoxetine, paroxetine), risperidone plasma levels may increase from 3- to 9-fold. Thus, the dose of risperidone needs to be titrated accordingly. If the CYP2D6 inhibitor drug is discontinued, the dose of risperidone may need to be increased.
10. Give PO risperidone or another antipsychotic drug with the first risperidone injection and continue for 3 weeks (then discontinue) to ensure adequate therapeutic plasma levels are maintained prior to the main release phase of risperidone from the injection site.
11. When using the drug IM in clients with impaired renal or hepatic function, clients should be treated with titrated doses of PO risperidone prior to beginning treatment with risperidone injection. The recommended starting dose of PO risperidone is 0.5 mg twice a day during the first week. The dose can be increased to 1 mg twice a day or 1 mg once a day during the second week. If a total daily dose of at least 2 mg of PO risperidone is well tolerated, an IM injection of risperidone, 25 mg, can be given q 2 weeks. PO supplementation should be continued for 2 weeks after the first injection until the main release of risperidone from the injection site has begin. In some clients, a slower titration may be more appropriate. Alternatively, a starting dose of 12.5 mg risperidone IM may be appropriate.
12. For IM use, suspend only in the diluent provided in the dose pack; doses must be given using the needle supplied in each dose pack. Do not substitute any components of the dose pack. Remove the dose pack from the refrigerator and allow to come to room temperature prior to reconstitution.
13. After reconstitution, it is recommended to use immediately. However, the suspension must be used within 6 hr. Resuspension will be necessary prior to administration if the drug is not given within 2 min of reconstitution, as settling will occur over time. Keeping the vial upright, shake vigorously back and forth for as long as it takes to resuspend the microspheres.
14. IM injections should be given by a health care provider using the safety needle provided. Give injections by deep IM q 2 weeks in the deltoid or gluteal region. For deltoid administration, use the 1-inch needle, alternating injections between the 2 arms. For gluteal administration, use the 2-inch needle, alternating between the 2 buttocks. Do not give IV. Do not combine 2 different dosage strengths of risperidone in a single administration.
15. Store tablets, orally disintegrating tablets, and solution between 15–25°C (59–77°F) away from children. Protect from light and moisture. Protect PO solution from freezing.
16. Refrigerate entire injection dose pack from 2–8°C (36–46°F) and protect from light. If refrigeration is not available, store at temperatures not exceeding 25°C (77°F) for no more than 7 days prior to use. Once in suspension, do not expose to temperatures above 25°C (77°F); use within 6 hr.

ASSESSMENT

1. List reasons for therapy, onset, duration, characteristics of S&S, presenting behavioral manifestations, mental status. Note history of drug dependency.
2. Perform appropriate baseline assessments. Electrolyte imbalance, bradycardia, and concomitant administration with drugs that prolong the QT interval may increase risk of torsades de pointes.
3. Reduce dose with the elderly, severe liver, cardiac, or renal dysfunction; monitor closely.
4. Observe for altered mental status, muscle rigidity, dyskinetic movements, or overt changes in VS. Monitor for S&S of diabetes.
5. Avoid in the treatment of dementia-related psychosis due to high risk of mortality.
6. The antiemetic effect of risperidone may mask S&S of overdose with certain drugs or conditions such as intestinal obstruction, Reye's syndrome, brain tumor.
7. Risperidone Orally Disintegrating Tablets contain phenylalanine.
8. Monitor CBC, BS, renal and LFTs.

CLIENT/FAMILY TEACHING

1. May mix oral solution with water, coffee, orange juice, or lowfat milk; do not mix with cola or tea as drug is incompatible. Take only as directed; do not share medications or stop abruptly.
2. Do not open blister containing orally disintegrating tablets until ready to administer. For single tablet removal, separate 1 of the 4 blis-

R

ter units by tearing apart at the perforation. Bend the corner where indicated and peel back foil to expose the tablet. Do not push tablet through the foil as this could damage the tablet. Using dry hands, remove tablet from blister unit and immediately place entire tablet on the tongue. Consume tablet immediately; cannot be stored once removed from the blister unit. Tablets disintegrate in the mouth within seconds and can be subsequently swallowed with or without liquid. Do not split or chew tablet. Orally disintegrating tablet contains phenylalanine.

3. Drug may cause drowsiness and impair judgment, motor skills, thinking, and cause blurred vision; determine drug effects before engaging in activities that require mental alertness. Rise slowly from a lying to a sitting position, dangle legs before standing; may cause drop in BP. Hot tubs and hot showers or baths may aggravate dizziness.
4. Wear protective clothing, sunscreen, hat, and sunglasses when sun exposure is necessary; may cause a photosensitivity reaction. Avoid prolonged or excessive exposure to direct or artificial sunlight. May alter temperature regulation. Avoid exposure to extreme heat or overheating in hot weather; heatstroke may occur
5. Report abnormal bruising/bleeding, yellow skin discoloration, or adverse effects. Avoid alcohol, CNS depressants or OTC agents.
6. Report if any muscle problems with your arms, legs, tongue, face, mouth, or jaw occur (e.g., tongue sticking out, puffing of cheeks, mouth puckering, chewing movements); may become irreversible.
7. Practice reliable birth control; report if pregnancy suspected/desired.
8. Risperidone elevates serum prolactin levels evidenced by unusual breast milk production, missed menstrual period, decreased sexual ability, decreased ability to produce sperm, or enlarged breasts. The potential relationships of prolactin and human breast cancer development are being explored; report evidence/history of breast cancer.
9. Fever, stiff muscles, confusion, abnormal thinking, fast or irregular heartbeat, and sweating may be S&S of neuroleptic malignant syndrome; seek help immediately.
10. Report any suicide ideations or bizarre behavior immediately. Due to the possibility of suicide attempts with schizophrenia, close supervision is necessary and prescriptions may be written for the smallest quantity of tablets.
11. With diabetes, monitor blood glucose closely. Report loss of BS control and any unusual weight gain.
12. Keep all F/U to assess response, BP, weight, and for adverse SE. Participate in counselling/therapy sessions designed to assist with underlying problems.

OUTCOMES/EVALUATE

- Improved behavior patterns with ↓ agitation, ↓ hyperactivity, and reality orientation
- Improved concentration and self-control
- ↓ Irritability, mood swings, aggressiveness, temper tantrums associated with autistic disorder

Ritonavir

(rih-**TOH**-nah-veer)

Classification(s): Antiviral, protease inhibitor

Pregnancy Category: B

RX: Norvir.

🍁 **Rx:** Norvir Sec.

SEE ALSO ***ANTIVIRAL DRUGS.***

INDICATIONS/USES

In combination with other antiretroviral drugs to treat HIV infection. Use of ritonavir may result in a reduction in both mortality and AIDS-defining clinical events.

ACTION/KINETICS

Action

A peptidomimetic inhibitor of both the HIV-1 and HIV-2 proteases. Inhibition of HIV protease results in the enzyme incapable of processing the "gag-pool" polyprotein precursor that leads to production of noninfectious immature HIV particles. The drug prolongs the PR interval.

Pharmacokinetics

Peak concentrations after 600 mg of the solution: 2 hr after fasting and 4 hr after nonfasting. Absorption from the capsule is increased when taken with food but absorption from tablets decreased when taken with food. **t½:** 3–5 hr. Metabolized by both CYP3A and CYP2D6. Metabolites and unchanged drug are excreted through both the feces and urine. The pharmacokinetic profile has not been determined in children less than 2 years of age. Some cross resistance has been noted among protease inhibitors. **Plasma protein binding:** 98–99%.

CONTRAINDICATIONS

Hypersensitivity to ritonavir or any component of the product. Use of ritonavir concurrently with any of the following drugs because competition for the drug-metabolizing system CYP3A by ritonavir may result in inhibition of metabolism, creating the potential for serious or life-threatening side effects (e.g., cardiac arrhythmias, prolonged or increased sedation, respiratory depression): Alfuzosin hydrochloride, amiodarone, bepridil, dihydroergotamine, ergonovine, ergotamine, flecainide, lovastatin, methylergonovine, midazolam (oral), pimozide, propafenone, quinidine, St. John's wort, sildenafil (only Revatio when used to treat pulmonary arterial hypertension), simvastatin, triazolam, and voriconazole. Use in severe hepatic impairment. Lactation.

SPECIAL CONCERNS

■ Coadministration of ritonavir with sedative hypnotics, antiarrhythmics, or ergot alkaloid products may result in potentially serious or life-threatening adverse effects due to possible effects of ritonovir on the hepatic metabolism of certain drugs. The following drugs are contraindicated with ritonavir: Alfuzosin, amiodarone, astemizole, bepridil, cisapride, dihydroergotamine, ergonovine, ergotamine, flecainide, methylergonovine, midazolam, pimozide, propafenone, quinidine, terfenadine, triazolam, voriconazole. ■

- **Not considered a cure for HIV infection; clients may continue to manifest illnesses associated with advanced HIV infection, including opportunistic infections.**
- **Has not been shown to decrease the risk of transmitting HIV to others through sexual contact or blood contamination.**
- **Use with caution in those with pre-existing liver diseases, liver enzyme abnormalities, hepatitis, and impaired hepatic function.**
- **Hemophiliacs treated with protease inhibitors may manifest spontaneous bleeding episodes.**
- **Varying degrees of cross resistance have been noted among protease inhibitors.**
- **For the elderly, start at the low end of the dosing range.**
- **Safety and efficacy have been established in children from 1 to 17 years of age.**

SIDE EFFECTS

Most Common

N&V, diarrhea, anorexia, abdominal pain, taste perversion, circumoral/peripheral paresthesias, dizziness, headache, insomnia, somnolence, sweating, malaise, asthenia.

Side effects listed are those with a frequency of 2% or greater or which are serious and must be monitored. **GI:** N&V, diarrhea, taste perversion, anorexia, flatulence, constipation, abdominal pain, dyspepsia, local throat irritation, fecal incontinence, ***pancreatitis***, impaired hepatic function. **CNS:** Anxiety, circumoral paresthesia, confusion, depression, dizziness, headache, insomnia, paresthesia, peripheral paresthesia, somnolence, abnormal thinking. **CV:** Syncope, vasodilation, prolonged PR interval. Increased bleeding, including spontaneous skin hematomas and hemarthrosis in those with hemophilia type A and B. **Hypersensitivity:** Urticaria, mild skin eruptions, ***bronchospasms***, angioedema. Rarely, ***anaphylaxis, Stevens-Johnson syndrome***. **Musculoskeletal:** Arthralgia, myalgia. **Dermatologic:** Sweating, rash. **Respiratory:** Pharyngitis. **Metabolic:** New onset or exacerbation of existing diabetes mellitus, hyperglycemia. **Body as a whole:** Asthenia, headache, malaise, fever, weight loss, redistribution/accumulation of body fat (e.g., central obesity, dorsocervical fat enlargement, peripheral wasting, breast enlargement, 'cushingoid' appearance). **Miscellaneous:** Hyperlipidemia, nocturia, unspecified pain, immune reconstitution syndrome (inflammatory response to indolent or residual opportunistic infections such as *Mycobacterium avium*, cytomegalovirus, *Pneumocystis jiroveci* pneumonia, or tuberculosis), resistance/cross resistance among protease inhibitors.

The following abnormalities occurred in 3% or more of children treated with ritonavir alone or with other antiviral drugs: Neutropenia, hyperamylasemia, thrombocytopenia, anemia, and ↑ AST. Also, in children, 2% or more experienced vomiting, diarrhea, and skin rash/allergy.

LABORATORY TEST CONSIDERATIONS

↑ Triglycerides, total cholesterol, AST, ALT, GGT, CPK, uric acid. ↓ Hematocrit, hemoglobin, neutrophils, RBCs, WBCs.

OVERDOSE MANAGEMENT

Symptoms: Extension of side effects. Accidental ingestion of the solution by a child could result in significant alcohol related toxicity and could approach the lethal dose of alcohol. *Treatment:* General supportive measures, including monitoring of VS and observing the clinical status. Elimination of unabsorbed drug may be assisted by emesis or gastric lavage, with attention given to maintaining a patent airway. Activated charcoal may also help in removing any unabsorbed drug. Dialysis is not likely to be of benefit in removing the drug from the body.

DRUG INTERACTIONS

(1) Ritonavir is expected to produce large ***increases*** in the plasma levels of a number of drugs, including amiodarone, amlodipine, bupropion, carbamazepine, clozapine, cyclosporine, dexamethasone, diltiazem, dronabinol, ethosuximide, methamphetamine, metoprolol, nefazodone, nifedipine, perphenazine, pimozide, piroxicam, prednisone, quinine, risperidone, sirolimus, tacrolimus, thioridazine, timolol, tricyclic antidepressants, trimethoprim, verapamil, and zolpidem. This may lead to an increased risk of arrhythmias, hematologic complications, seizures, or other serious adverse effects.

(2) Ritonavir may produce a ***decrease*** in the plasma levels of the following drugs: Atovaquone, clofibrate, daunorubicin, diphenoxylate, divalproex, lamotrigine, metoclopramide, olanzapine, phenytoin, sedative/hypnotics, sulfamethoxazole, and zidovudine.

(3) Coadministration of ritonavir with the following drugs may cause extreme sedation and respiratory depression and thus should **not** be combined: Alprazolam, clonazepam, clorazepate, diazepam, estazolam, flurazepam, midazolam, triazolam, and zolpidem. Thus, it is important to monitor plasma levels and make appropriate dosage adjustments when such drugs are used concomitantly with ritonavir.

Aldesleukin / ↑ Ritonavir levels → ↑ risk of toxicity; adjust ritonavir dose as needed

Alfentanil / ↑ Alfentanil plasma levels → possible toxicity; alfentanil dose decrease may be needed

Alfuzosin / ↑ Alfuzosin blood levels → ↑ pharmacologic & side effects (e.g., hypotension); do not use together

Antiarrhythmics (e.g., amiodarone, bepridil, disopyramide, flecainide, lidocaine, mexiletine, propafenone, quinidine) / ↑ Plasma level of antiarrhythmic → serious and/or life-threatening cardiac arrhythmias; do not use together with amiodarone, bepridil, flecainide, propafenone, or quinidine; use together with caution with disopyramide, lidocaine, and mexiletine

Antipsychotics (e.g., aripiprazole, perphenazine, quetiapine, risperidone, thioridazine) / ↑ Plasma levels of antipsychotics listed; adjust dose as needed

Atovaquone / ↓ Atovaquone levels; dosage ↑ may be needed

Azole antifungals (fluconazole, itraconazole, ketoconazole, voraconazole) / ↑ Ritonavir plasma levels → ↑ risk of toxicity; also, itraconazole and ketoconazole levels may be ↑ while voraconazole levels may be ↓ → possible loss of antifungal activity

Bosentan / ↑ Bosentan levels → ↑ risk of side effects; concomitant use contraindicated

Bupropion / Possible ↓ bupropion dose needed; monitor levels

Buspirone / ↑ Buspirone levels; ↓ buspirone dose may be needed

Calcium channel blockers (e.g, amlodipine, diltiazem, nifedipine, verapamil) / Possible ↑ level of calcium channel blocker; use with caution/monitor; possible ↓ blocker dose may be needed

Carbamazepine / ↓ Ritonavir levels → treatment failure; also, possible ↑ carbamazepine levels; closely monitor carbamazepine plasma levels

Cisapride / ↑ Risk of cardiac arrhythmias; do not use together

Clarithromycin / ↑ Clarithromycin and ritonavir levels; reduce clarithromycin dose by 50% in those with C_{CR} 30–60 mL/min and by 75% in those with C_{CR} <30 mL/min

Clonazepam / ↑ Clonazepam levels; ↓ dose may be needed

Clorazepate / ↑ Clorazepate levels; ↓ dose may be needed

Clozapine / Large ↑ clozapine serum levels possible → ↑ toxicity; use together with caution

Colchicine / ↑ Colchicine plasma levels → ↑ risk of toxicity; coadministration contraindicated in those with hepatic/renal impairment; in normal

R

renal function, use together with caution at a maximum dose of 0.3 mg/day twice a day
Conivaptan / Use contraindicated R/T ↑ risk of side effects
Corticosteroids (e.g., dexamethasone, fluticasone, prednisone) / ↑ Steroid levels; dose ↓ may be needed; use of fluticasone and ritonavir together is not recommended
Cyclosporine / ↑ Cyclosporine and ritonavir levels → ↑ pharmacologic effects; monitor clinical response and adjust dose if needed
Darunavir / ↑ Darunavir AUC and C_{max}; use with caution in those with hepatitis B or C coinfection; adjust dose of either drug or both as needed
Deferasirox / ↓ Deferasirox plasma levels and pharmacologic effects; use together contraindicated
Delavirdine / ↑ Ritonavir AUC and C_{max}; appropriate doses of the combination not established
Desipramine / Significant ↑ desipramine AUC (145%) and C_{max} (32%); reduce desipramine dose and monitor levels
Diazepam / ↑ Diazepam levels; ↓ dose may be needed
Didanosine / ↓ Didanosine AUC and C_{max}; separate dosing by 2.5 hr
Digoxin / ↑ Digoxin levels → ↑ risk of toxicity; monitor digoxin levels closely and adjust dose as needed
Disulfiram / Ritonavir products contain alcohol → disulfiram-like serious reactions
Divalproex / ↓ Divalproex levels; dose ↑ may be needed
Dronabinol / ↑ Dronabinol levels; ↓ dose may be needed
Dronedarone / ↑ Dronedarone plasma levels → ↑ risk of pharmacologic/toxic effects; concomitant use contraindicated
Efavirenz / ↓ Ritonavir plasma levels; appropriate doses of the combination not established
Eplerenone / ↑ Eplerenone levels → ↑ risk for hyperkalemia and associated arrhythmias; use together contraindicated
Ergot derivatives (dihydroergotamine, ergonovine, ergotamine, methylergonovine) / ↑ Plasma levels of ergot derivatives → ↑ risk of ergot toxicity (e.g., vasospasm, ischemia of extremities and other tissues including the CNS); use together contraindicated
Estazolam / ↑ Estazolam levels; ↓ dose may be needed
Ethinyl estradiol / ↓ Ethinyl estradiol levels; consider alternative nonhormonal contraceptive
Ethosuximide / ↑ Ethosuximide levels; ↓ dose may be needed
Eszopiclone / ↑ Eszopiclone plasma levels → ↑ pharmacologic and toxic effects; monitor and consider dose ↓ of eszopiclone
Fentanyl / ↑ Plasma levels of fentanyl → ↑ risk of fentanyl-induced respiratory depression due to ↓ liver metabolism; dose ↓ may be needed
Fluoxetine / Possible ↓ fluoxetine dose needed; monitor levels; also, ↑ ritonavir levels
Flurazepam / ↑ Flurazepam levels; ↓ dose may be needed
Fluticasone / ↑ Fluticasone (using nasal spray) AUC by 350-fold and C_{max} by 25-fold and a significant ↓ of 86% in plasma cortisol AUC; do not use together
Fosamprenavir / ↑ Fosamprenavir AUC and C_{max}; adjust dose of either drug or both as needed
Foscarnet / ↑ Risk of nephrotoxicity
Grapefruit juice / ↑ Plasma ritonavir levels → ↑ pharmacologic effects; if grapefruit juice cannot be avoided, monitor carefully and adjust ritonavir dose as needed
HMG-CoA reductase inhibitors (e.g., atorvastatin, lovastatin, pravastatin, rosuvastatin, simvastatin) / ↑ Plasma levels of HMG-CoA reductase inhibitor → ↑ risk of myopathy, including rhabdomyolysis; do not use ritonavir with lovastatin or simvastatin; if using atorvastatin, start with lowest dose and monitor
HMG-CoA reductase inhibitors + Saquinavir / Coadministered with ritonavir → ↑ AUC of atorvastatin and simvastatin and ↓ AUC of pravastatin
Iloperidone / ↑ Iloperidone plasma levels and pharmacologic effects; ↓ iloperidone dose by ½ when given with ritonavir
Indinavir / ↑ Indinavir plasma levels → ↑ toxicity; adjust dose of one or both drugs as needed
Ixabepilone / ↑ Ixabepilone plasma levels → ↑ pharmacologic effects; concomitant use contraindicated
Lamotrigine / ↓ Lamotrigine levels; dose ↑ may be needed; closely monitor
Levothyroxine / ↑ or ↓ Serum thyroxine levels → hyperthyroidism or hypothyroidism; monitor when starting or stopping ritonavir; adjust levothyroxine dose as needed

R

Lidocaine / Possible ↑ lidocaine plasma levels → cardiac arrhythmias
Maraviroc / ↑ Maraviroc plasma levels; dose adjustment may be needed
Mefloquine / ↓ Ritonavir plasma levels → ↓ efficacy; monitor and adjust dose as needed
Meperidine / ↓ Plasma meperidine levels but ↑ plasma levels of normeperidine → ↑ risk of neurologic toxicity (e.g., seizures); do not use together
Methadone / ↓ Plasma levels of methadone; consider ↑ dose
Methamphetamine / ↑ Methamphetamine levels; dose ↓ may be needed
Methadone / Possible ↓ Methadone levels; consider dosage ↑ of methadone
Metoprolol / ↑ Metoprolol levels; ↓ metoprolol dose may be needed; use together with caution and monitor
Metronidazole / Ritonavir products contain alcohol → serious disulfiram-like reactions
Midazolam / ↑ Risk of prolonged or increased sedation or respiratory depression; use together contraindicated
Muscarinic receptor antagonists (e.g., darifenacin, fesoterodine, solifenacin, tolterodine) / ↑ Plasma levels of the muscarinic receptor antagonist; if used together, do not exceed a dose of darifenacin, 7.5 mg/day; fesoterodine, 4 mg/day; solifenacin, 5 mg/day; tolterodine, 2 mg/day.
Nefazodone / Possible ↓ nefazodone dose needed; monitor levels
Nevirapine / ↓ Ritonavir plasma levels; appropriate doses of the combination not established
Nilotinib / ↑ Nilotinib plasma levels → ↑ pharmacologic/toxic effects; concomitant use contraindicated
Oral contraceptives or patch (ethinyl estradiol) / ↓ Ethinyl estradiol AUC by 40% and C_{max} by 32%; consider alternate nonhormonral contraceptives
Phenothiazines (e.g., perphenazine, thioridazine) / ↑ Phenothiazine levels; dose ↓ may be needed
Phenytoin / ↓ Phenytoin levels; dose ↑ may be needed; closely monitor
Pimozide / ↑ Potential for cardiac arrhythmias; use together contraindicated
Prednisone / ↑ Prednisone plasma levels; ↓ dose may be needed
Quinine / ↑ Quinine levels; quinine dose ↓ may be needed
Ranolazine / ↑ Ranolazine levels may → ↑ risk of QT prolongation, torsades de pointes, and sudden death; do not use together
Rapamycin / ↑ Plasma levels of both drugs within 3 days; monitor and adjust dosage as needed
Rifabutin / ↑ Levels of rifabutin and its metabolite; reduce rifabutin dose by at least 75%; further dosage reduction may be needed
Rifampin / ↓ Ritonavir serum levels → loss of virologic response; consider use of rifabutin
Risperidone / ↑ Risperidone levels; dose ↓ may be needed
Salmeterol / ↑ Salmeterol pharmacologic effects → ↑ risk of CV toxicity (e.g., QT prolongation, palpitations, sinus tachycardia); coadministration contraindicated
H ***St. John's wort*** / ↓ Ritonavir plasma levels R/T ↑ hepatic metabolism by CYP3A4 → loss of virologic response and possible resistance to ritonavir; do not use together
Saquinavir / Significant ↑ in saquinavir blood levels; do not coadminister saquinavir/ritonavir with rifampin due to ↑ risk of severe hepatotoxicity
Selective 5-HT$_1$ receptor agonists (e.g., eletriptan) / ↑ Plasma levels of the selective 5-HT$_1$ receptor agonist → ↑ pharmacologic effects; do not give eletriptan within 72 hr of ritonavir
Selective serotonin reuptake inhibitors (e.g., fluoxitine) / Possible ↓ SSRI dose; monitor levels
Sildenafil / ↑ Sildenafil levels → severe and potentially fatal hypotension when used for pulmonary arterial hypertension; do not exceed a dose of 25 mg of sildenafil within 48 hr when used for erectile dysfunction
Sirolimus / ↑ Plasma levels of both drugs within 3 days; monitor and adjust dose as needed
Sufentanil / ↑ Sufentanil plasma levels → possible toxicity; sufentanil dose decrease may be needed
Sulfamethoxazole / Coadministration of ritonavir with sulfamethoxazole/trimethoprim ↓ sulfamethoxazole AUC; not likely clinically important
Tacrolimus / ↑ Plasma levels of both drugs within 3 days; monitor and adjust dosage as needed
Tadalafil / Possible hypotension; do not exceed a dose of 10 mg of tadalafil every 72 hr
Theophylline / ↓ Theophylline AUC 43% and C_{max} 32%; monitor theophylline levels as an ↑ dose may be needed
Timolol / ↑ Timolol levels; ↓ timolol dose may be needed; use together with caution and monitor

R

Tipranavir / ↑ Tipranavir AUC and C_{max}; adjust dose of either drug or both as needed
Tramadol / ↑ Tramadol plasma levels → ↑ risk of toxicity; dose ↓ may be needed
Trazodone / ↓ Clearance, prolonged t½, and ↑ peak plasma levels of trazodone R/T ↓ metabolism; consider ↓ trazodone dosage
Triazolam / ↑ Risk of prolonged or increased sedation or respiratory depression; use together contraindicated
Tricyclic antidepressants (TCAs) / Possible ↓ TCA dose needed; monitor levels
Trimethoprim / Coadministration with sulfamethoxazole/trimethoprim → ↑ trimethoprim AUC by 20%
Tyrosine kinase receptor inhibitors (e.g., dasatinib) / ↑ Plasma levels of tyrosine kinase receptor inhibitor → ↑ risk of pharmacologic/toxic effects; closely monitor and adjust dose as needed
Vardenafil / Possible hypotension; do not exceed a dose of 2.5 mg vardenafil every 72 hr
Vinblastine/Vincristine / ↑ Vinblastine/vincristine levels; consider withholding ritonavir-containing regimens or use alternative treatment
Warfarin / ↓ or ↑ Warfarin anticoagulant effect; monitor INR frequently
Zidovudine / ↓ Zidovudine AUC 25% and C_{max} 27%; monitor and adjust dose as needed
Zolpidem / ↑ Zolpidem levels → possible severe sedation and respiratory depression; closely monitor and adjust zolpidem dose as needed

HOW SUPPLIED

Capsules, Soft Gelatin: 100 mg; ***Oral Solution:*** 80 mg/mL; ***Tablets:*** 100 mg.

DOSAGE

CAPSULES; ORAL SOLUTION; TABLETS

HIV infection.

Adults, initial: 300 mg twice a day. Use of a dose titration schedule may help reduce treatment-emergent side effects while maintaining appropriate ritonavir plasma levels. Increase at 2- to 3-day intervals by 100 mg twice daily. If nausea is experienced upon initiation of therapy, dose escalation may be tried as follows: 300 mg twice a day for 1 day, 400 mg twice a day for 2 days, 500 mg twice a day for 1 day, and then 600 mg twice a day thereafter. **Maintenance:** 600 mg twice a day.

Children: Should be used in combination with other antiretroviral drugs. **Children, 1 month and older, initial:** 250 mg/m²; increase at 2- to 3-day intervals by 50 mg/m² twice a day. **Maintenance:** 350–400 mg/m² twice a day, PO, not to exceed 600 mg/day. If 400 mg/m² is not tolerated, give the highest tolerated dose for maintenance in combination with other antiretroviral drugs; alternate therapy may also be considered. Check the package insert for pediatric dosage guidelines. **Children, less than 1 month of age (investigational):** 450 mg/m² BSA twice a day.

NURSING IMPLICATIONS

(Sound Alike) Do not confuse ritonavir with Retrovir (zidovudine, also an antiviral drug). Also do not confuse Norvir (the trade name for ritonavir) with Retrovir or Norvasc (a calcium channel blocker).

IMPLEMENTATION/ADMINISTRATION/STORAGE

1. Mild to moderate GI disturbances and paresthesias may decrease as therapy continues. Clients prescribed combination regimens with reverse transcriptase inhibitors may improve GI tolerance by starting therapy with ritonavir alone and then adding the reverse transcriptase inhibitors before completing 2 weeks of ritonavir monotherapy.
2. Those who take ritonavir capsules may experience more GI side effects (e.g., N&V, abdominal pain, diarrhea) when switching from the capsule to the tablet due to greater maximum plasma levels achieved with the tablet formulation. These side effects (GI or paresthesias) may decrease as therapy continues.
3. No dosage adjustment is needed in mild or moderate impaired hepatic function; however, there is the potential for lower ritonovir levels in those with moderate impaired hepatic function.
4. Dose reduction of ritonavir is needed when used with other protease inhibitors (e.g., amprenavir, atazanavir, darunavir, fosamprenavir, saquinavir, and tipranavir).

5. If saquinavir and ritonavir are used together, reduce the dose of saquinavir to 400 mg twice a day. The optimum dosage level of ritonavir (400 or 600 mg twice a day), in combination with saquinavir has not been determined. However, this combination is better tolerated in those who received ritonavir, 400 mg twice a day.
6. To monitor maternal-fetal outcomes, an antiretroviral pregnancy registry has been established. Health care providers are encouraged to register clients by calling 1-800-258-4263.
7. Until dispensed, store soft gelatin capsules in refrigerator at 2–8°C (36–46°F) and protect from light and excessive heat. Capsule refrigeration is recommended after dispensing; however, this is not necessary if used within 30 days, and kept below 25°C (77°F).
8. Store the solution at room temperature between 20–25°C (68–77°F). Do not refrigerate. Shake well before each use. Store and dispense in the original container and keep cap tightly closed. Avoid exposure to excessive heat.
9. Store tablets from 15–30°C (59–86°F). Dispense in original container or equivalent tight container. Do not expose to high humidity outside the original or equivalent tight container for longer than 2 weeks.

ASSESSMENT

1. Note onset, characteristics of S&S, serum confirmation of diagnosis, other agents trialed, outcome.
2. List other agents prescribed to ensure none interact unfavorably; especially note if using Viagra because side effects may be enhanced and may cause severe drop in BP; advise against or not to exceed 25 mg every 2 days.
3. Monitor CBC, T-lymphocytes (CD_4), viral load, cholesterol panel, and LFTs. Note impaired liver function; drug hepatically metabolized via cytochrome P450 system.

CLIENT/FAMILY TEACHING

1. Take with meals. Taste may be improved by mixing with chocolate milk, Ensure, or Advera within 1 hr of dosing. Give the pediatric dose using a calibrated dosage syringe.
2. Swallow tablets whole; do not chew, break, or crush.
3. Take each day as prescribed. Do not alter dosage or discontinue without approval. If dose is missed, take the next dose as soon as possible; if dose is skipped, do not double the next dose.
4. Use reliable birth control and barrier protection; drug does not reduce the risk of transmitting disease through sexual contact or blood contamination. If using estrogen-based hormonal contraceptive use additional form.
5. Drug is not a cure for HIV; illnesses associated with advanced HIV infection may still occur, including opportunistic infections.
6. Report any sensations of burning, prickling, or numbness; dose may require reduction. Any persistent abdominal pain, nausea, vomiting should be evaluated.
7. May produce ECG changes (eg, PR prolongation); report symptoms such as dizziness, light-headedness, abnormal heart rhythm, and loss of consciousness to provider.
8. Do not take any OTC meds without provider approval.
9. Keep all F/U visits to assess response, labs, disease progression and for adverse SE.

OUTCOMES/EVALUATE

Inhibition of disease progression and early death with HIV infection

IV

Rituximab

(rih-**TUK**-sih-mab)

Classification(s): Antineoplastic, monoclonal antibody

Pregnancy Category: C

RX: Rituxan.

SEE ALSO ***ANTINEOPLASTIC AGENTS.***

INDICATIONS/USES

1. As a single drug to treat relapsed or refractory low-grade or follicular, CD20 positive, B-cell non-Hodgkin's lymphoma.
2. For previously untreated follicular, CD20 positive, B-cell non-Hodgkin's lymphoma in combination with first–line chemotherapy and, in those achieving a complete or partial response to rituximab in combination with chemotherapy, as single–agent maintenance chemotherapy.

R

3. For non progressing (including stable disease) low-grade CD20-positive, B-cell non-Hodgkin's lymphoma as a single agent following first-line treatment with cyclophosphamide, vincristine, and prednisone chemotherapy.
4. For previously untreated diffuse large B-cell, CD20-positive non-Hodgkin's lymphoma in combination with cyclophosphamide, doxorubin, vincristine, and prednisone or other anthracycline-based chemotherapy regimens.
5. With methotrexate to reduce signs and symptoms of moderate-to-severe rheumatoid arthritis in adult clients who have had an inadequate response to one or more tissue necrosis factor antagonist therapies.
6. In combination with fludarabine and cyclophosphamide to treat previously untreated and previously treated CD20-positive chronic lymphocytic leukemia.
7. In combination with glucocorticoids to treat adults with microscopic polyangiitis.
8. In combination with glucocorticoids to treat adults with Wegener granulomatosis.

Investigational: Waldenström macroglobulinemia. Peripheral ulcerative keratitis. Idiopathic thrombocytopenic purpura. Juvenile idiopathic arthritis.

ACTION/KINETICS

Action

A chimeric murine/human monoclonal antibody that binds specifically to the CD20 antigen found on the surface of normal and malignant B lymphocytes causing cell lysis. Cell lysis may result due to complement-dependent cytotoxicity and antibody-dependent cellular cytotoxicity. Circulating B cells are almost completely depleted for up to 9 months. CD20 regulates early steps in the activation process for cell cycle initiation and differentiation and possibly functions as a calcium ion channel.

Pharmacokinetics

Following a dose of 375 mg/m^2 by IV infusion at weekly intervals for 4 doses, rituximab was detected in the serum 3–6 months after completion of treatment. **Mean terminal t½, elimination:** 22 days for lymphoma clients, 32 days for leukemia clients, and 18 days for rheumatoid arthritis clients.

CONTRAINDICATIONS

Use in known IgE-mediated hypersensitivity or anaphylactic reactions to murine proteins or any component of product. Use not recommended in those with rheumatoid arthritis who have **no** prior inadequate response to one or more tissue necrosis factor antagonists. Use in those with severe active infections. Lactation.

SPECIAL CONCERNS

■ (1) **Fatal infusion reactions.** Rituximab administration can result in serious, including fatal, infusion reactions. Deaths within 24 hr of rituximab infusion have been reported. Approximately 80% of fatal infusion reactions occurred in association with the first infusion. Carefully monitor clients during infusions. Discontinue rituximab infusion and administer medical treatment in clients who develop severe (grade 3 or 4) infusion reactions. (2) **Tumor lysis syndrome.** Acute renal failure requiring dialysis, with instances of fatal outcome, has been reported in the setting of tumor-lysis syndrome following rituximab treatment in clients with non-Hodgkin lymphoma. (3) **Severe mucocutaneous reactions.** Severe, including fatal, mucocutaneous reactions can occur in clients receiving rituximab treatment. (4) **Progressive multifocal leukoencephalopathy.** John Cunningham virus infection, resulting in progressive multifocal leukoencephalopathy and death, can occur in clients treated with rituximab. ■

- **Use with caution in preexisting cardiac conditions, including arrhythmias and angina.**
- **Infusion-related symptoms may occur from 30 to 120 min at beginning of first infusion and with less frequency with subsequent infusions.**
- **Use is associated with severe infusion and hypersensitivity reactions.**
- **Possible reactivation of hepatitis B virus with fulminant hepatitis, hepatic failure, and death.**
- **Safety of immunization with any vaccine, especially live viral vaccines, not studied, and therefore not recommended.**
- **Elderly are more likely to experience cardiac side effects (especially supraventricular arrhythmias) and serious pulmonary side effects (e.g., pneumonia, pneumonitis).**
- **Safety and efficacy not determined in children.**

SIDE EFFECTS

Most Common

Infusion reactions, fever, chills, infection, asthenia, headache, hypo-/hypertension, night sweats, rash, pruritus, N&V, diarrhea, lymphopenia, leukopenia, neutropenia, thrombocytopenia, angioedema, myalgia, arthralgia, increased cough, rhinitis, abdominal/back pain, pain.

This list also includes side effects when rituximab is used in combination with other drugs, including cyclophosphamide, doxorubicin, prednisone, and vincristine. **Infusion reactions:** Fever, chills, and rigors are most common. Also, N&V, urticaria, fatigue, dizziness, headache, pruritus, rash, myalgia, ***bronchospasm***, hypotension, ***angioedema***, dyspnea, rhinitis, flushing, pain at disease sites, hyper-/hypotension, hypoxia, pulmonary infiltrates, ***acute respiratory distress syndrome, MI, ventricular fibrillation, cardiogenic shock, anaphylactic/anaphylactoid events***. **Retreatment events:** Asthenia, throat irritation, flushing, tachycardia, anorexia, leukopenia, thrombocytopenia, anemia, peripheral edema, dizziness, depression, respiratory symptoms, night sweats, pruritus. **Tumor lysis syndrome:** From 12–24 hr after the first dose for non Hodgkin's lymphoma: Acute renal failure, hyperkalemia, hypocalcemia, hyperphosphatemia, ***death***. **CV**: Arrhythmias, including VT and SVTs; trigeminy, angina, hypo-/hypertension, tachycardia, postural hypotension, bradycardia, cardiac disorder, systemic vasculitis, ***cardiac failure***. **Hematologic:** Thrombocytopenia (up to 30 days following last dose), severe anemia, neutropenia (including febrile and late onset), leukopenia, lymphopenia, anemia, coagulation disorder, marrow hypoplasia, prolonged pancytopenia, hyperviscosity syndrome in Waldenström macroglobulinemia. **GI:** Abdominal pain (including upper abdominal pain), enlarged abdomen, N&V, diarrhea, dyspepsia, throat irritation, taste perversion, ***bowel obstruction/perforation***. **Hepatic:** Reactivation of hepatitis B with related fulminant hepatitis, hepatobiliary toxicity. **CNS:** Headache, dizziness, paresthesia, anxiety, agitation, insomnia, hypesthesia, nervousness, migraine, paresthesia. Reactivation of hepatitis B virus with fulminant hepatitis, ***hepatic failure, and death***. **Respiratory**: ***Bronchospasm***, increased cough, rhinitis, dyspnea, epistaxis, ***bronchiolitis obliterans***, hypoxia, asthma, sinusitis, respiratory disorder, bronchitis, lung disorder, pneumonitis (including interstitial), ***interstitial lung disease***, URTI, pleuritis. **Musculoskeletal:** Myalgia, arthralgia, chest/back pain, chest tightness, muscle spasms, polyarticular arthritis and vasculitis with rash. **Dermatologic:** Pruritus, rash, urticaria, flushing, night sweats, ***mucocutaneous skin reactions***, including lichenoid dermatitis, paraneoplastic pemphigus, ***Stevens–Johnson syndrome, toxic epidermal necrolysis***, and vesiculobullous dermatitis. **GU:** ***Acute renal failure*** (may require dialysis). **Ophthalmic:** Optic neuritis, conjunctivitis, lacrimation disorder, uveitis. **Hypersensitivity:** Hypotension, ***bronchospasm***, ***angioedema***. **Body as a whole:** Asthenia, pain, fatigue, fever, pain, serious infections (bacterial, viral, fungal), chills, malaise, peripheral sensory neuropathy, viral infections, weight gain, ***severe mucocutaneous reactions***, serum sickness, disease progression of Kaposi's sarcoma. **Miscellaneous:** Tumor pain, peripheral edema, anorexia, pain at injection site, hypertonia, immunogenicity, lupus-like syndrome, increase in ***fatal infections*** in HIV-associated lymphoma, disease progression of Kaposi's sarcoma, progressive multifocal leukoencephalopathy, posterior reversible encephalopathy syndrome/reversible posterior leukoencephalopathy syndrome.

LABORATORY TEST CONSIDERATIONS

↑ LDH. Hyperglycemia, hypocalcemia, hypophosphatemia, hyperuricemia.

DRUG INTERACTIONS

Biologic agents / Closely observe for signs of infection

Cisplatin / Renal toxicity; concomitant use not approved

Disease modifying antirheumatic drugs / Closely observe for signs of infection

Tocilizumab / ↑ Risk of serious infection; avoid concomitant use

Vaccines, live virus / Vaccination with live viruses is not recommended

HOW SUPPLIED

Injection Solution, Concentrate: 10 mg/mL.

DOSAGE

IV INFUSION

Relapsed or refractory, low-grade or follicular, CD20-positive B cell non-Hodgkin's lymphoma.

Adults, usual: 375 mg/m^2 as an IV infusion once a week for 4 or 8 doses.

R

Progressive disease may be retreated at the same dose, once weekly for 4 doses.
Retreatment: 375 mg/m^2 by IV infusion once weekly for 4 doses in responding clients who developed progressive disease after previous rituximab therapy.

Previously untreated follicular, CD20-positive, B-cell non-Hodgkin's lymphoma.

Adults, usual: 375 mg/m^2 by IV infusion given on day 1 of each cycle of cyclophosphamide, vincristine, and prednisone chemotherapy for up to 8 doses.
Maintenance: In those with complete or partial response, initiate rituximab maintenance 8 weeks following completion of rituximab in combination with chemotherapy as a single–agent at a dose of 375 mg/m^2 by IV infusion once q 8 weeks for 12 doses.

Non progressing low-grade, CD20-positive, B-cell non-Hodgkin lymphoma.

Adults: 375 mg/m^2 rituximab by IV infusion once weekly for 4 doses every 6 months to a maximum of 16 doses following completion of 6 to 8 cycles of cyclophosphamide, vincristine, and prednisone chemotherapy.

Diffuse, large B cell non-Hodgkin's lymphoma.

Adults: 375 mg/m^2 by IV infusion on day 1 of each cycle of chemotherapy, for up to 8 infusions.

With methotrexate to treat moderate to severe rheumatoid arthritis.

Adults: A single treatment course of two infusions of rituximab, 1,000 mg each, on days 1 and 15 combined with stable doses of methotrexate. To reduce the incidence of infusion reactions, also give methylprednisolone, 100 mg IV (or its equivalent) 30 min prior to each infusion. Subsequent courses should be given q 24 weeks or based on clinical evaluation, but not sooner than q 16 weeks.

Chronic lymphocytic leukemia.

Adults: 375 mg/m^2 by IV infusion the day prior to the initiation of fludarabine and cyclophosphamide chemotherapy; **then,** 500 mg/m^2 on day 1 of cycles 2–6 (q 28 days). *NOTE: Pneumocystis jiroveci* pneumonia and antiherpetic viral prophylaxis is recommended for those with chronic lymphocytic leukemia during treatment and for up to 12 months following treatment as appropriate.

Microscopic polyangiitis, Wegener granulomatosis.

Adults, usual: 375 mg/m^2 once a week for 4 weeks. To treat severe vasculitis symptoms, give methylprednisolone 1,000 mg/day IV for 1–3 days followed by PO prednisone 1 mg/kg/day, not to exceed 80 mg/day and tapered per clinical need. Begin this regimen within 14 days prior to or with initiation of rituximab and may continue during and after the 4–week course of rituximab treatment. *P. jiroveci* pneumonia prophylaxis is recommended for at least 6 months following the last rituximab infusion.

Rituximab as part of the ibritumomab tiuxetan therapeutic regimen.

Rituximab, 250 mg/m^2, infused within 4 hr prior to the administration of indium IN 11 ibritumomab tiuxetan and within 4 hr prior to the administration of yttrium Y-90-ibritumomab tiuxetan. Administration of rituximab and indium IN 111 ibritumomab tiuxetan should precede rituximab and Y-90-ibritumomab tiuxetan by 7–9 days. *NOTE:* Refer to the Ibritumomab tiuxetan monograph for complete information.

Peripheral ulcerative keratitis (investigational).

Adults: Infusions of 1,000 mg/week for 2 doses although there are safety concerns.

Waldenström macroglobulinemia (investigational).

Adults: 375 mg/m^2 once weekly for 4 doses. An extended dose regimen of 375 mg/m^2 twice weekly for 4 weeks (weeks 1 through 4), repeated at week 12 (weeks 12 through 15) has also been used. Has also been studied for maintenance treatment.

R

Idiopathic thrombocytopenic purpura (investigational).

Adults: 375 mg/m^2 IV once a week for 4 doses. Lower weekly doses (100 mg) have been documented as effective but with a longer time of response. Some trials have also administered antihistamines, acetaminophen, and/or hydrocortisone prior to the rituximab infusion.

Juvenile idiopathic arthritis (investigational).

Has been given as a 2–dose regimen with 1 gram on days 1 and 15. In some, treatment was repeated 6–12 months later.

NURSING IMPLICATIONS

IMPLEMENTATION/ADMINISTRATION/STORAGE

1. IV The maximum dose of rituximab for treatment of non-Hodgkin lymphoma is 375 mg/m^2 per dose while the maximum dose to treat rheumatoid arthritis is 1,000 mg per dose.
2. To prepare for administration, withdraw necessary amount of rituximab and dilute to final concentration of 1 to 4 mg/mL into infusion bag containing either 0.9% NaCl or D5W. Gently invert the bag to mix the solution. Discard any unused portion left in vial.
3. Premedicate with acetaminophen and an antihistamine (e.g., diphenhydramine) to attenuate infusion reactions. For rheumatoid arthritis clients, methylprednisolone, 100 mg IV or its equivalent, is recommended 30 min prior to each infusion to reduce the incidence and severity of infusion reactions. IV saline and vasopressors may also be used to slow or interrupt an infusion reaction. Consider withdrawing antihypertensive medication 12 hr prior to rituximab infusion due to rituximab-induced transient hypotension.
4. Administer aggressive IV hydration and antihyperuricemic therapy to those at high risk for tumor lysis syndrome.
5. For first infusion, give at initial rate of 50 mg/hr. If hypersensitivity or infusion-related events do not occur, escalate infusion rate in 50 mg/hr increments every 30 min to maximum of 400 mg/hr. If hypersensitivity or infusion-related events occur, temporarily slow or interrupt infusion; infusion can continue at one-half previous rate until symptoms improve. Subsequent infusions can be given at initial rate of 100 mg/hr, and increased by 100 mg/hr increments at 30 min intervals to maximum of 400 mg/hr (as long as tolerated).
6. **Do not administer as an IV push or bolus; administer only as an IV infusion.** Do not mix or dilute with other drugs.
7. Protect vials from direct sunlight. Do not freeze.
8. Solutions for infusion are stable at 2–8°C (36–46°F) for 24 hr (preferred since there is no preservative in the preparation). Because there is no preservative, refrigerate diluted solutions at 2–8°C (36–46°F).
9. COMPATIBILITY D5W, 0.9% NaCl.
10. INCOMPATIBILITY Do not mix or dilute with other drugs.

ASSESSMENT

1. Note any cardiac disease and assess for arrhythmias.
2. Screen persons at high risk for hepatitis B viral infections before initiation of therapy. Monitor for S&S of hepatitis B virus in carriers during therapy and for several months following therapy.
3. Therapy usually consists of once-weekly infusions for four doses. Due to the possibility of transient hypotension during infusion, consider withholding antihypertensive medication 12 hr prior to rituximab. Infusion-related reaction consisting of fever and chills/rigors may occur with first infusion.
4. Due to the potential of hypersensitivity reactions, consider premedication with acetaminophen and diphenhydramine. Interrupt infusion if severe reaction occurs; may resume infusion at 50% initial rate once symptoms resolved. Also, institute supportive care (IV fluids, vasopressors, oxygen, bronchodilators, diphenhydramine, acetaminophen).
5. Monitor CBC, renal, LFTs, CD20 positive B lymphocytes, BP, and ECG.

CLIENT/FAMILY TEACHING

1. Drug is administered IV once a week for about 4–8 weeks to eradicate malignant cells or with methotrexate every 2 weeks for resistant rheumatoid arthritis control.

R

2. Practice reliable contraception during and for up to 12 months following therapy.
3. Report any chest pain, SOB, unusual bruising/bleeding, S&S of infection, hives, rash, mouth sores, N&V, diarrhea, loss of appetite, persistent or worsening general body weakness.
4. Counsel clients with NHL about the possible risk of tumor lysis syndrome while receiving rituximab.
5. Keep all F/U visits to assess response, labs, for adverse SE.

OUTCOMES/EVALUATE

- Control of malignant cell proliferation
- Depletion of B lymphocytes
- Treatment of resistant rheumatoid arthritis

Rivaroxaban

(riv-a-**ROX**-a-ban)

Classification(s): Anticoagulant, selective factor Xa inhibitor

Pregnancy Category: C

RX: Xarelto.

INDICATIONS/USES

Prophylaxis of deep vein thrombosis (DVT) which may lead to pulmonary embolism in clients undergoing knee or hip replacement.

ACTION/KINETICS

Action

Rivaroxaban selectively blocks the active site of factor Xa and does not require a cofactor (e.g., anti-thrombin) for activity. Activation of factor X to factor Xa via the intrinsic and extrinsic pathways plays a central role in the cascade of blood coagulation.

Pharmacokinetics

Absolute bioavailability of 80–100% for the 10 mg dose. C_{max}: 2–4 hr. Metabolized by CYP3A4/5 and CYP2J2 and hydrolysis. Rivaroxaban is also a substrate for P-gp and ABCG2. Both unchanged drug and inactive metabolites are excreted in the feces and urine. **t½, terminal:** 5–9 hr in healthy individuals age 20–45 years and 11–13 hr in elderly clients. Healthy Japanese subjects have a 50% higher exposure compared with other ethnicities, including Chinese subjects. **Plasma protein binding:** 92–95%.

CONTRAINDICATIONS

Hypersensitivity to rivaroxaban or any component of the product. Active major bleeding. Lactation. Avoid use in severe renal impairment (C_{CR} <30 mL/min) and in those with moderate to severe (Child-Pugh class B or C) hepatic impairment or with any hepatic disease associated with coagulopathy.

SPECIAL CONCERNS

Spinal/Epidural hematoma. (1) Epidural or spinal hematomas may occur in clients who are anticoagulated and are receiving neuraxial anesthesia or undergoing spinal puncture. These hematomas may result in long-term or permanent paralysis. Consider these risks when scheduling clients for spinal procedures. Factors that can increase the risk of developing epidural or spinal hematomas in these clients include: use of indwelling epidural catheters; concomitant use of other drugs that affect hemostasis, such as NSAIDs, platelet inhibitors, other anticoagulants; a history of traumatic or repeated epidural or spinal punctures; a history of spinal deformity or spinal surgery. (2) Monitor clients frequently for signs and symptoms of neurological impairment. If neurological compromise is noted, urgent treatment is necessary. (3) Consider the benefits and risks before neuraxial intervention in clients who are anticoagulated or are to be anticoagulated for thromboprophylaxis.

- Bleeding can occur at any site during rivaroxaban therapy.
- Geriatric clients exhibit an increase in exposure that may be caused by age-related changes in renal function.
- Safety and efficacy not established in children.

SIDE EFFECTS

Most Common

Bleeding complications.

Bleeding complications: Major bleeding event (intracranial, GI, retinal, adrenal bleeding), ***fatal bleeding***, bleeding that requires re-operation, bleeding into a critical organ, extra surgical site bleeding requiring transfusion of >2 units of whole blood or packed cells, ***retroperitoneal hemorrhage***, epidural/spinal hematoma. **CNS:** ***Cerebral hemorrhage***, subdural hematoma, epidural hematoma, hemiparesis. **Hepatic:** Jaundiced cholestasis, cytolytic hepatitis. **Dermatologic:** Pruritus, blister. **Musculoskeletal:** Pain in extremity, muscle spasm. **GU:** Dysuria. **Hypersensitivity:** Anaphylactic reaction, ***anaphylactic shock, Steven-Johnson syndrome***. **Miscellaneous:** Syncope, wound secretion, agranulocytosis.

OVERDOSE MANAGEMENT

Symptoms: Overdosage may result in ***hemorrhage***. *Treatment:* A specific antidote is not available. Discontinue rivaroxaban and begin appropriate therapy if bleeding complications associated with overdose occur. Consider use of activated charcoal to reduce absorption. Due to high plasma protein binding, dialysis is not effective.

DRUG INTERACTIONS

(1) Because rivaroxaban is metabolized by CYP3A4/5 enzyme systems, substances known to inhibit these enzymes may decrease metabolism or increase bioavailability of rivaroxaban and cause changes in rivaroxaban exposure.
(2) Clients with impaired renal function who receive rivaroxaban with drugs that are combined CYP3A4 and P-gp inhibitors (e.g., amiodarone, azithromycin, diltiazem, dronedarone, erythromycin, felodipine, quinidine, ranolazine, verapamil) may cause increases in rivaroxaban exposure compared with those with normal renal function. The risk of bleeding may be increased; avoid coadministration of rivaroxaban unless the benefit justifies the potential risk.

Aspirin / Bleeding risk may be ↑; if coadministration can not be avoided, monitor closely
Carbamazepine / ↓ Rivaroxaban AUC and C_{max} R/T ↑ metabolism due to induction of CYP3A4 and P-gp inhibitor
Clopidogrel / ↑ Bleeding time; coadministration contraindicated
Conivaptan / Possible ↑ rivaroxaban exposure → ↑ risk of bleeding R/T CYP3A4 inhibition and P-gp inhibitor
Desirudin / ↑ Risk of bleeding; coadministration contraindicated
Heparins (e.g., enoxaparin) / Possible additive effect on anti-factor Xa → ↑ risk of bleeding; avoid concurrent use
Indinavir/Ritonavir / Possible ↑ rivaroxaban exposure → ↑ risk of bleeding R/T CYP3A4 inhibition and P-gp inhibitor
Itraconazole / Possible ↑ rivaroxaban exposure → ↑ risk of bleeding R/T CYP3A4 inhibition and P-gp inhibitor
Ketoconazole / Possible ↑ rivaroxaban exposure → ↑ risk of bleeding R/T CYP3A4 inhibition and P-gp inhibitor
Lopinavir/Ritonavir / Possible ↑ rivaroxaban exposure → ↑ risk of bleeding R/T CYP3A4 inhibition and P-gp inhibitor
NSAIDs (e.g., naproxen) / Possible ↑ risk of bleeding; if coadministration cannot be avoided monitor closely
Phenytoin / ↓ Rivaroxaban AUC and C_{max} R/T ↑ metabolism due to induction of CYP3A4 and P-gp inhibition
Rifampin / ↓ Rivaroxaban AUC and C_{max} R/T ↑ metabolism due to induction of CYP3A4 and P-gp inhibition
Ritonavir / Possible ↑ rivaroxaban exposure → ↑ risk of bleeding R/T CYP3A4 inhibition and P-gp inhibitor
St. John's wort / ↓ Rivaroxaban AUC and C_{max} R/T ↑ metabolism due to induction of CYP3A4 and P-gp inhibition
Warfarin / Concomitant use not studied; avoid concurrent use due to ↑ risk of bleeding

HOW SUPPLIED

Tablets: 10 mg.

DOSAGE

TABLETS

Prophylaxis of deep vein thrombosis.

Adults, usual: 10 mg once a day. Take initial dose 6–10 hr after surgery once hemostasis has been established. **Duration of therapy:** 35 days for hip replacement and 12 days for knee replacement.

NURSING IMPLICATIONS

IMPLEMENTATION/ADMINISTRATION/STORAGE

1. **If a dose is not taken at the scheduled time, the dose should be taken as soon as possible on the same day and continued on the following day with the once daily intake as recommended.**

R

2. Avoid concomitant use with drugs that are combined P-glycoprotein (P-gp) and strong CYP3A4 inducers (e.g., carbamazepine, phenytoin, rifampin, St. John's wort). Consider a rivaroxaban dose of 20 mg if these drugs must be coadministered.
3. Absorption of rivaroxaban is dependent on the site of drug release in the GI tract (i.e., gastric versus small intestine). When giving rivaroxaban as a crushed tablet via a feeding tube, confirm gastric placement of the tube; avoid administration via a method that could deposit the drug directly into the proximal small intestine.
4. Store from 15–30°C (59–86°F).

ASSESSMENT

1. Note condition(s) requiring therapy, onset, estimated duration of therapy. Give initial dose (po) at least 6 to 10 hr after surgery once hemostasis has been established. Usual duration of therapy is 35 days following hip replacement or 12 days following knee replacement surgery.
2. List drugs prescribed to ensure none interact.
3. Monitor all sites, incisions, orifices for bleeding. Assess mobility and adherence to exercise program.
4. Assess carefully for S&S of neurologic impairment (e.g., midline back pain, numbness or weakness in lower extremities, bowel and/or bladder dysfunction); anticoagulated clients undergoing epidural/spinal anesthesia may sustain a spinal/epidural hematoma that could result in paralysis. Risk increased with postoperative use of indwelling epidural catheters, or concomitant use of other drugs affecting hemostasis such as NSAIDs.
5. Monitor CBC, renal and LFTs; avoid with moderate liver failure.

R

CLIENT/FAMILY TEACHING

1. Drug is used to prevent the formation of blood clots in those extremities that have compromised functioning due to a surgical procedure or in those that have atrial fibrillation, where clots may form in the heart. Clots may enter the circulation, and be transported to the lung causing a pulmonary embolus that can be lethal.
2. Take the 10 mg oral dose with or without food; the 20 mg oral dose (with atrial fibrillation) should be taken with the evening meal.
3. May bruise easier and bleeding from scratches may take longer to stop. Report if excessive bruising or prolonged bleeding occurs.
4. Report S&S of spinal or epidural hematoma, such as tingling, numbness (especially in the lower limbs), and muscular weakness.
5. Do not stop therapy suddenly as this increases risk of stroke occurrence. If need to stop rivaroxaban, provider may prescribe another blood thinner to prevent clot formation.
6. Report adverse effects, as well as extremity pain, chest pain, SOB, S&S bleeding (e.g., black, tarry stools, blood in the urine, dizziness when standing, excessive bruising, nosebleed, paleness).
7. Avoid OTC agents including aspirin, NSAIDs, and other agents without provider approval.
8. Practice reliable contraception; report immediately if pregnancy suspected or any unusual blood loss.
9. Keep all F/U to assess response, labs, adverse SE.

OUTCOMES/EVALUATE

- DVT prophylaxis with hip/knee replacement
- ↓ Risk of stroke/clots with atrial fibrillation

Rivastigmine tartrate

(rih-vah-**STIG**-meen)

Classification(s): Treatment of Alzheimer's disease

Pregnancy Category: B

RX: Exelon.

INDICATIONS/USES

PO, Transdermal: (1) Mild to moderate dementia of the Alzheimer's type. (2) Mild to moderate dementia associated with Parkinson's disease. *Investigational:* Treat behavioral effects in Lewy-body dementia.

ACTION/KINETICS

Action

Probably acts by enhancing cholinergic function by increasing levels of acetylcholine through reversible inhibition of its hydrolysis by acetylcholinesterase. There is no evidence that the drug alters the course of the underlying disease.

Pharmacokinetics

After PO, is rapidly and completely absorbed. Absolute bioavailability is 40% (after 3 mg). Absorption from the patch is greatest from the back, chest, or upper arm. Administration with food delays absorption by 90 min, lowers C_{max} by about 30%, and increases AUC by about 30%. **Peak plasma levels, after PO:** 1 hr; **from the patch:** 8 hr. Is rapidly and extensively metabolized by cholinesterase-mediated hydrolysis. **t½, elimination:** About 1.5 hr. Excreted mainly in the urine. **Plasma protein binding:** 40%.

CONTRAINDICATIONS

Hypersensitivity to rivastigmine or other carbamate derivatives, or other components of the product.

SPECIAL CONCERNS

- **Use with caution during lactation; not known if rivastigmine is excreted in breast milk.**
- **Use with caution with a history of asthma or obstructive pulmonary disease.**
- **Drugs that increase cholinergic activity may have vagotonic effects on the heart, cause urinary obstruction, and may cause seizures.**
- **Safety and efficacy not determined in children.**

SIDE EFFECTS

Most Common

N&V, dizziness, headache, diarrhea, anorexia, weight loss, abdominal pain, insomnia, confusion, asthenia, dyspepsia, accidental trauma, fatigue, UTI, tremor.

Side effects listed are those with a frequency of 1% or greater and those that may be life-threatening. Significant GI side effects may occur. **GI:** N&V, diarrhea, anorexia, weight loss, abdominal pain (including upper), peptic ulcers, GI bleeding (active or occult), dyspepsia, constipation, flatulence, eructation, fecal incontinence, gastritis. **CNS:** Dizziness, headache, insomnia, confusion, depression, anxiety, somnolence, hallucination, tremor, aggressive reaction, syncope, abnormal gait, ataxia, paresthesia, agitation, nervousness, delusion, ***convulsions***, paranoid reaction, confusion, vertigo, worsening of Parkinson's disease, bradykinesia, dyskinesia, restlessness. **CV:** Hypotension, postural hypotension, hypertension, ***cardiac failure, MI***, atrial fibrillation, bradycardia, palpitation, angina pectoris, TIA. **Body as a whole:** Accidental trauma, fatigue, asthenia, malaise, increased sweating, flu-like symptoms, syncope, dehydration, fever, edema, allergy, hot flushes, general infection, pain. **Dermatologic:** Rashes, including maculopapular, eczema, bullous, exfoliative, psoriaform, erythematous; pruritus. **GU:** UTI, urinary obstruction, hematuria, urinary incontinence. **Musculoskeletal:** Arthritis, leg cramps, myalgia, back pain, arthralgia, bone fracture. **Respiratory:** Rhinitis, epistaxis, URTI, coughing, pharyngitis, nasopharyngitis, bronchitis, dyspnea, pneumonia. **Miscellaneous:** Anemia, hypokalemia, tinnitus, cataract, rigors, chest pain, peripheral edema.

LABORATORY TEST CONSIDERATIONS

Hematuria, hypokalemia.

OVERDOSE MANAGEMENT

Symptoms: Cholinergic crisis, including symptoms of severe nausea, vomiting, salivation, sweating, bradycardia, hypotension, respiratory depression, collapse, seizures. Increasing muscle weakness with possible death if respiratory muscles are involved. *Treatment:* General supportive measures. Treat severe nausea and vomiting with antiemetics.

DRUG INTERACTIONS

Anticholinergics / Rivastigmine interferes with anticholinergic activity
Bethanechol / Synergistic effect
Neuromuscular blocking agents / Synergistic effect
Nicotine / ↑ PO clearance of rivastigmine by 23%
NSAIDs / Rivastigmine ↑ gastric acid secretion; monitor for active or occult GI bleeding
Succinylcholine / Exaggeration of succinylcholine-induced muscle relaxation during anesthesia

HOW SUPPLIED

Capsules: 1.5 mg, 3 mg, 4.5 mg, 6 mg; *Oral Solution:* 2 mg/mL (all concentrations as the base); *Transdermal Patch:* 4.6 mg/24 hr, 9.5 mg/24 hr.

DOSAGE

CAPSULES; ORAL SOLUTION

Mild-to-moderate dementia due to Alzheimer's disease.

Initial: 1.5 mg twice a day to minimize GI side effects. If the dose is well tolerated after a minimum of 2 weeks, may increase dose to 3 mg twice a day. Attempt subsequent increases to 4.5 mg

R

and 6 mg twice a day only after a minimum of 2 weeks at the previous dose. If side effects are intolerable, discontinue treatment for several doses and then restart at the same or next lower dose level. If treatment is interrupted for longer than several days, reinitiate treatment with the lowest daily dose and titrate as described above. **Maximum dose:** 6 mg twice a day.

Dementia associated with Parkinson's disease.

Initial: 1.5 mg twice a day; **then,** the dose may be increased to 3 mg twice a day and further to 4.5 mg twice a day and 6 mg twice a day, based on tolerability. There should be a minimum of 4 weeks at each dose. **Dose range:** 1.5–6 mg twice a day.

TRANSDERMAL PATCH

Dementia due to Alzheimer's disease or Parkinsons' disease.

Initial: 4.6 mg/24 hr. After a minimum of 4 weeks and if well tolerated, the dose should be increased to 9.5 mg/24 hr (the recommended effective dose).

Maintenance: Increase doses only after a minimum of 4 weeks at the previous dose and only if the previous dose has been well tolerated. The maximum recommended dose is 9.5 mg/24 hr; higher doses offer no significant additional benefit but there is a significant increase in side effects.

NURSING IMPLICATIONS

IMPLEMENTATION/ADMINISTRATION/STORAGE

1. If side effects develop during treatment, discontinue treatment for several doses; restart at the lowest daily dose (to prevent severe vomiting) and titrate back to the maintenance dose.
2. The capsules and oral solution may be interchanged at equal doses.
3. Clients with a body weight less than 50 kg may experience more side effects using the transdermal patch. Use particular caution in titrating these clients above the recommended maintenance dose of 9.5 mg/24 hr.
4. Clients on capsules or oral solution may be switched to the transdermal patch as follows: (a) a client who is on a total daily dose of less than 6 mg PO can be switched to the 4.6 mg/24 hr patch; (b) A client who is on a total daily dose of 6–12 mg PO may be directly switched to the 9.5 mg/24 hr transdermal patch. Apply the first transdermal patch on the day following the last PO dose.
5. Store the oral solution, tablets, and transdermal patches from 15–30°C (59–86°F). Store solution in an upright position; protect from freezing. When combined with cold fruit juice or soda, the mixture is stable at room temperature for up to 4 hr. Keep patches in the individually sealed pouches until use.

ASSESSMENT

1. Note onset, characteristics of S&S, performance of ADLs, other agents trialed, outcome. Identify caregiver and start therapy as soon as diagnosed.
2. Describe clinical presentation, cognitive functioning, mini mental exam score or similar test of cognitive ability.
3. Note history of asthma, seizures, BPH, or COPD.
4. Assess for S&S occult GI bleeding especially in those at increased risk for developing ulcers e.g., taking NSAIDS.
5. Obtain baseline weight, VS, ECG, lytes and metabolic panel, B12, CBC, rapid plasma reagin (RPR), U/A, and BS; monitor.

CLIENT/FAMILY TEACHING

1. Take with food in divided doses in the morning and evening. Establish reasonable expectations.
2. If using the oral solution, remove the oral dosing syringe provided and withdraw the correct amount of drug from the container. Each dose of rivastigmine may be swallowed directly from the syringe or first mixed with a small glass of water, cold fruit juice, or soda. When mixed with fruit juice or soda, the mixture is stable for 4 hr or less.
3. Use caution, patch may cause drowsiness or dizziness, at start of treatment and when increasing dose. Avoid activities that require mental alertness until drug effects realized and/or assessed by provider.
4. Apply the transdermal patch once a day to clean, dry, hairless, intact healthy skin in a location that will not be rubbed by tight clothing. Press down on the patch firmly until the

edges stick well. The patch can be used in situations that include bathing and hot weather. Do not apply to a skin area where cream, lotion, or powder has been applied recently.

5. The upper or lower back is recommended for patch placement since less likely to remove patch. When sites on the back are not accessible, patch can be applied to the upper arm or chest. Do not apply to skin that is red, irritated, or cut. Change site of patch application daily to avoid potential irritation, although consecutive patches can be applied to the same anatomic site (i.e., another site on the upper back). Do not use the same site within 14 days.
6. Used patches should be folded, with the adhesive surfaces pressed together; discard safely.
7. Drug may cause a high incidence of GI effects (N&V); monitor weight and report if loss significant or appetite affected so therapy can be reassessed. Stop drug and report any evidence of seizures, urinary obstruction, dizziness, and low heart rate.
8. Dosage may be gradually increased by provider if drug is tolerated and desired effects not evident. Report evidence of behavioral disturbances or psychosis and agitation.
9. Keep all F/U to assess response, labs, and for adverse SE.

OUTCOMES/EVALUATE

- Improved daily and cognitive functioning with Alzheimer's disease
- Reduced caregiver time and reduced institutionalization

Rizatriptan benzoate

(rise-ah-**TRIP**-tan)

Classification(s): Antimigraine drug

Pregnancy Category: C

RX: Maxalt, Maxalt-MLT.

✤ **Rx:** Maxalt RPD.

INDICATIONS/USES

Acute treatment of migraine attacks in adults with or without aura.

ACTION/KINETICS

Action

Binds to 5-$HT_{IB/ID}$ receptors, resulting in cranial vessel vasoconstriction, inhibition of neuropeptide release, and reduced transmission in trigeminal pain pathways.

Pharmacokinetics

Completely absorbed after PO use; rate of absorption of Maxalt-MLT is somewhat slower. 40% is bioavailable. **Time to onset of action:** 45 min. **Peak plasma levels, Maxalt:** 1–1.5 hr; **Maxalt-MLT:** 1.6–2.5 hr. Food has no effect on bioavailability, but will delay time to reach peak levels by one hr. **t½:** 2–3 hr. Metabolized by MAO-A; most is excreted through the urine. Is a significant first-pass effect. **Plasma protein binding:** About 14%.

CONTRAINDICATIONS

Use in children less than 18 years of age, as prophylactic therapy of migraine, or use in the management of hemiplegic or basilar migraine. Use in those with ischemic heart disease or vasospastic coronary artery disease, uncontrolled hypertension, within 24 hr of treatment with another 5-HT_1 agonist or an ergotamine-containing or ergot-type medication (e.g., dihydroergotamine, methysergide). Use concurrently with MAOIs or use of rizatriptan within 2 weeks of discontinuing an MAOI. Strongly recommended the drug not be given in unrecognized coronary artery disease (CAD) predicted by the presence of risk factors, including hypertension, hypercholesterolemia, smoking, obesity, diabetes, strong family history of CAD, female with surgical or physiological menopause, or males over 40, unless a CV evaluation reveals the client is free from CAD or ischemic myocardial disease.

SPECIAL CONCERNS

- Safety and efficacy not determined for use in cluster headache or in children.
- Use with caution during lactation, with diseases that may alter the absorption, metabolism, or excretion of drugs; in dialysis clients, and in moderate hepatic insufficiency.
- Maxalt-MLT tablets contain phenylalanine; may be of concern to phenylketonurics.
- Serious cardiac events may occur within a few hours after giving Maxalt.
- The safety of treating more than 4 headaches in a 30-day period not established.

R

SIDE EFFECTS

Most Common

Palpitations, dizziness, fatigue, headache, somnolence, chest tightness/pressure/heaviness, neck/throat/jaw heaviness, dry mouth, N&V, hypesthesia, decreased mental acuity, euphoria, tremor, flushing, diarrhea, hot flashes, dsypnea, warm/cold sensations.

CV: ***Acute MI, coronary artery vasospasm, life-threatening disturbances in cardiac rhythm (VT, ventricular fibrillation), death, cerebral hemorrhage, subarachnoid hemorrhage, stroke, hypertensive crisis.*** Also, transient myocardial ischemia, peripheral vascular ischemia, colonic ischemia with abdominal pain and bloody diarrhea, palpitations, tachycardia, cold extremities, hypertension, arrhythmia, bradycardia. **GI:** N&V, diarrhea, dry mouth, abdominal distention, dyspepsia, thirst, acid regurgitation, dysphagia, constipation, flatulence, tongue edema. **CNS:** Somnolence, headache, dizziness, paresthesias, hypesthesia, decreased mental acuity, euphoria, tremor, nervousness, vertigo, insomnia, anxiety, depression, disorientation, ataxia, dysarthria, confusion, dream abnormality, abnormal gait, irritability, impaired memory, agitation, hypesthesia. **Pain and pressure sensations:** Chest tightness/pressure/heaviness; pain, tightness, or pressure in the precordium, neck, throat, jaw; regional pain, tightness, pressure, or heaviness; or unspecified pain. **Musculoskeletal:** Muscle weakness, stiffness, myalgia, muscle cramps, musculoskeletal pain, arthralgia, muscle spasm. **Respiratory:** Dyspnea, pharyngitis, nasal irritation, nasal congestion, dry throat, URI, yawning, dry nose, epistaxis, sinus disorder. **GU:** Urinary frequency, polyuria, menstrual disorder. **Dermatologic:** Flushing, sweating, pruritus, rash, urticaria. **Body as a whole:** Asthenia, fatigue, chills, heat sensitivity, hangover effect, warm/cold sensations, dehydration, hot flashes. **Ophthalmic:** Blurred vision, dry eyes, burning eye pain, eye irritation, tearing. **Miscellaneous:** Facial edema, tinnitus, ear pain.

DRUG INTERACTIONS

Dihydroergotamine / Additive vasospastic reactions; do not use within 24 hr of each other
MAOIs / ↑ Rizatriptan plasma levels; do not use together
Methysergide / Additive vasospastic reactions; do not use within 24 hr of each other
Propranolol / ↑ Rizatriptan levels
Selective serotonin reuptake inhibitors / Possible weakness, hyperreflexia, and incoordination
Sibutramine / Possible serotonin syndrome, including CNS irritability, motor weakness, shivering, myoclonus, and altered consciousness

HOW SUPPLIED

Tablets: 5 mg, 10 mg; *Tablets, Oral Disintegrating:* 5 mg, 10 mg.

DOSAGE

TABLETS; TABLETS, ORAL DISINTEGRATING

Acute treatment of migraine.

Adults: Single dose of 5 mg or 10 mg of Maxalt or Maxalt-MLT. Doses should be separated by at least 2 hr, with no more than 30 mg taken in any 24-hr period.

NURSING IMPLICATIONS

IMPLEMENTATION/ADMINISTRATION/STORAGE

1. In clients receiving propranolol, use the 5 mg dose of Maxalt, up to a maximum of 3 doses in any 24-hr period.
2. There is little evidence that the 10 mg dose provides a greater effect than the 5 mg dose. Individualize dose, weighing the potential benefits of the 10 mg dose with the potential risks.
3. Store Maxalt and Maxalt-MLT tablets at room temperature (15–20°C or 59–86°F).

ASSESSMENT

1. Note characteristics of migraines, when diagnosed, neurologist findings, other agents trialed, outcome.
2. List any evidence of CAD, uncontrolled HTN, DM, or allergies. Assess risk factors for CAD. Clients over age 40 should be carefully screened for CAD.
3. List all medications consumed to ensure none interact. Reduce dose if prescribed propranolol.
4. Advise that the MLT formulation contains phenylalanine. Monitor BP.

CLIENT/FAMILY TEACHING

1. Take as soon as symptoms of migraine appear. If headache returns or only a partial re-

R

sponse is attained, may repeat dose after waiting at least 2 hr. Taking with food may delay drug onset. Do not exceed 30 mg in a 24-hr period.

2. For Maxalt-MLT, do not remove the blister from the outer pouch until just before dosing. Peel open the blister (do not push through the blister) with dry hands, and place the orally disintegrating tablet on the tongue. It will dissolve in the saliva and be swallowed; fluids are not needed, which eases administration.
3. May cause dizziness, drowsiness, or pressure sensation in the upper chest; do not operate equipment or drive until effects realized.
4. Do not take within 24 hr of any other prescription drug used to treat headaches or depression.
5. Review "patient information sheet" provided for side effects; report if persistent or intolerable. May experience rebound headaches if taken >2–3 times per week.
6. Use alternative birth control if oral contraceptives prescribed. Report if pregnancy suspected.
7. Prevent photosensitivity by using sunscreen and protective clothing.
8. Keep a headache diary and attempt to identify triggers.
9. Report any chest pain that does not go away, sudden and/or severe stomach pain, SOB, wheezing, or swelling of eyelids, face, or lips.
10. Ensure phenylketonuric clients aware that each 5 mg of the oral disintegrating tablets contain 1.05 mg phenylalanine.
11. Keep all F/U to assess response, labs, and for adverse SE.

OUTCOMES/EVALUATE
Relief of migraine headache

IV

Rocuronium bromide

(**roh**-kyou-**ROH**-nee-um)

Classification(s): Neuromuscular blocking drug

Pregnancy Category: C

RX: Zemuron.

SEE ALSO ***NEUROMUSCULAR BLOCKING AGENTS***.

INDICATIONS/USES
(1) As an adjunct to general anesthesia to facilitate rapid sequence and routine tracheal intubation. (2) To cause relaxation of skeletal muscle during surgery or mechanical ventilation.

ACTION/KINETICS
Action
A nondepolarizing neuromuscular blocking agent that acts by competing with acetylcholine for receptors at the motor end-plate. Causes histamine release in a small number of clients. Use must be accompanied by adequate anesthesia or sedation, as the drug has no effect on consciousness, pain threshold, or cerebration. Drug action is antagonized by acetylcholinesterase inhibitors (e.g., neostigmine, edrophonium).

Pharmacokinetics
Depending on the dose, it has a rapid to intermediate onset and an intermediate duration of action. **t½, rapid distribution phase:** 1–2 min; **t½, slower distribution phase:** 14–18 min. Metabolized by the liver. **Plasma protein binding:** About 30%.

CONTRAINDICATIONS
Hypersensitivity to rocuronium or other neuromuscular blocking drugs.

SPECIAL CONCERNS
The drug should be given by adequately trained individuals familiar with its actions, characteristics, and hazards.

- Use with caution in clients with pulmonary hypertension, valvular heart disease, or significant hepatic disease.
- Clients with renal failure may have a greater variation in duration of effect.
- Burns, disuse atrophy, denervation, or direct muscle trauma are associated with resistance to nondepolarizing neuromuscular blocking agents.
- Elderly clients may exhibit a slightly prolonged medical clinical duration of action.
- Small doses of nondepolarizing neuromuscular blocking drugs have profound effects in clients with either myasthenia gravis or Eaton-Lambert syndrome.
- Severe acid-base and/or electrolyte abnormalities may potentiate or cause resistance to the neuromuscular blocking effects of rocuronium.

- **Although not studied, apparent tolerance may develop during chronic administration in the ICU.**
- **The effects of the amount of rocuronium excreted into breast milk are probably not clinically significant.**
- **Use in children less than 3 months of age has not been studied.**

SIDE EFFECTS

Most Common

Transient hypotension and hypertension.

CV: Arrhythmias, abnormal ECG, transient hypotension and hypertension, tachycardia, increase in pulmonary vascular resistance, prolongation of QTc interval in children. **GI:** N&V. **Respiratory:** Symptoms of asthma, including ***bronchospasm***, wheezing, rhonchi, hiccup. **Dermatologic:** Rash, edema at injection site, pruritus. **Miscellaneous:** Malignant hyperthermia; severe allergic reactions, including ***anaphylaxis, anaphylactoid reactions, and shock***.

OVERDOSE MANAGEMENT

Symptoms: Neuromuscular blockade longer than needed for anesthesia and surgery. *Treatment:* Careful monitoring of client. Artificial respiration may be required. Once evidence of recovery from neuromuscular blockade has been observed, recovery may be facilitated by giving an anticholinesterase drug. The use of a nerve stimulator to document recovery is recommended.

DRUG INTERACTIONS

Anesthetics, inhalation (enflurane, halothane, isoflurane) / ↑ Neuromuscular blockade; may need to ↓ rate of infusion by 30–50% at 45–60 min after the intubating dose
Anesthetics, local / ↑ Duration of neuromuscular block and ↓ infusion requirements of neuromuscular blocking drugs
Antibiotics (aminoglycosides, bacitracin, colistin, polymyxin, sodium colistimethate, tetracycles, vancomycin) / ↑ Neuromuscular blocking action of rocuronium
Azathioprine / Reversal of neuromuscular blocking effects
Carbamazepine / Shorter duration of action or ↓ efficacy of rocuronium
Diuretics / Diuretics may cause electrolyte imbalance which may modify neuromuscular blockade
Ketamine / ↑ Neuromusclar blockade → profound and severe respiratory depression
Lithium / ↑ Duration of neuromuscular blockade and ↓ infusion requirements of neuromuscular blocking drugs
Mg^{++} sulfate / Potentiation of the effects of rocuronium
Phenytoin / Shorter duration or less effectiveness of rocuronium
Procainamide / ↑ Duration of neuromuscular blockade and ↓ infusion requirements of neuromuscular blocking drugs
Quinidine / Possibility of recurrent paralysis
Succinylcholine / ↑ Rocuronium blockade and duration of action; if used together, delay rocuronium administration until recovery from succinylcholine observed
Theophyllines / Dose-dependent reversal of neuromuscular blockade
Verapamil / Possible enhanced effects of rocuronium → prolonged respiratory depression

HOW SUPPLIED

Injection Solution: 10 mg/mL.

DOSAGE

IV ONLY

Rapid sequence intubation.

Adults: 0.6–1.2 mg/kg in appropriately premedicated and adequately anesthetized clients will result in good intubating conditions in less than 2 min. Rapid sequence intubation using rocuronium is not recommended for children.

Tracheal intubation.

Adults, initial, regardless of anesthetic technique: 0.6 mg/kg. Maximum blockade is noted in less than 3 min with a mean duration of 31 min. However, a dose of 0.45 mg/kg may also be used with maximum blockade in less than 4 min with a mean duration of 22 min. A large bolus dose of 0.9 or 1.2 mg/kg can be given under opioid/nitrous oxide/oxygen anesthesia without side effects to the CV system.

Children, initial: 0.6 mg/kg; a dose of 0.45 mg/kg may be used, depending on the anesthetic and the client age. For sevoflurane induction, doses of 0.45 mg/kg and 0.6 mg/kg generally produce excellent to good intubating conditions within 75 sec. Also, initial doses of 0.6 mg/kg in children under halothane anesthesia produce excellent to good intubating conditions within 1 min. When sevoflurane is used for induction and isoflurane/nitrous oxide for maintenance of general anesthesia, rocuronium can be given as a bolus dose of 0.15 mg/kg at reappearance of T_3 in all pediatric ages. Maintenance dosing can also be given at the reappearance of T_2 at a rate of 7–10 mcg/kg/min, with the lowest dose requirement for neonates (birth to younger than 28 days) and the highest dose for children (older than 2 years of age to 11 years of age).

When halothane is used for general anesthesia, clients from 3 months through adolescence can be given rocuronium maintenance doses of 0.075–0.125 mg/kg, given on return of T_1 to 25% of control, providing clinical relaxation for 7–10 min.

Alternatively, a continuous infusion of rocuronium, initiated at a rate of 12 mcg/kg/min on return of T_1 to 10% of control (1 twitch present in the train-of-four) may also be used to maintain neuromuscular blockade in children.

Maintenance doses.

Adults: 0.1, 0.15, and 0.2 mg/kg, given at 25% recovery of control T_1 (defined as three twitches of train-of-four), provide a median of 12 (2 to 31), 17 (6 to 50), and 24 (7 to 69) min of duration under opioid/nitrous oxide/oxygen anesthesia. Do not administer the dose until recovery of neuromuscular function is evident.

Continuous infusion.

Initial: 0.01–0.02 mg/kg/min only after early evidence of spontaneous recovery from an intubating dose. Upon reaching the desired level of neuromuscular blockade, the infusion must be individualized for each client; adjust the rate based on the twitch response (monitored with the use of a peripheral nerve stimulator) of the client. **Maintenance, usual:** 0.004–0.016 mg/kg/min.

NURSING IMPLICATIONS

Do not confuse rocuronium with vecuronium (another neuromuscular blocking drug).

IMPLEMENTATION/ADMINISTRATION/STORAGE

1. **IV Initiate infusion at a rate of 10–12 mcg/kg/min only after early evidence of recovery from an intubating dose. Because of rapid redistribution and the associated rapid spontaneous recovery, initiation of the infusion after substantial return of neuromuscular function (more than 10% of control T_1) may necessitate additional bolus doses to maintain adequate block for surgery.**
2. **Upon reaching the desired level of neuromuscular block, individualize infusion of rocuronium for each client. Adjust the rate of administration according to the client's twitch response, as monitored with the use of a peripheral nerve stimulator. Infusion rates, in clinical trials, have ranged from 4 to 16 mcg/kg/min. Consult the manufacturer's information for rocuronium infusion rates based on client's weight, and the rate of drug delivery desired.**
3. **In obese clients, base the initial dose of 0.6 mg/kg on the client's actual body weight.**
4. **Inhalation anesthetics (especially enflurane or isoflurane) may enhance the effects of rocuronium. When inhalation anesthetics are used, it may be necessary to reduce the rate of infusion by 30–50% 45–60 min after the intubating dose.**
5. **Do not increase the initial dose in those with prolonged circulation time to reduce onset time; rather, when feasible, allow more time for the drug to achieve onset of effects.**
6. **In myasthenia gravis or Lambert-Eaton syndrome clients, a peripheral nerve stimulator and use of a small test dose may be of value in monitoring the response to muscle relaxants, as these clients are very sensitive to nondepolarizing neuromuscular blockers.**
7. **To prevent complications from residual paralysis, extubate only after the client has recovered sufficiently from neuromuscular block. Also, consider other factors that could cause residual paralysis after intubation in the postoperative phase (e.g., drug interactions, client condition).**
8. **Prepare solutions for infusion by mixing with compatible solutions.**

R

9. If given via the same infusion line that is also used for other drugs, adequately flush the infusion line between administration of rocuronium and drugs for which incompatibility with rocuronium has been shown, or for which compatibility has not been established.
10. Is compatible in solution at concentrations up to 5 mg/mL for 24 hr at room temperature in plastic bags, glass bottles, and plastic syringe pumps when mixed with the appropriate solution.
11. Spontaneous recovery occurs at about the same rate in children 3–12 months as in adults, but is more rapid in children 1–12 years old.
12. If extravasation occurs, terminate the injection immediately, and restart in another vein.
13. Store at 2–8°C (36–46°F); do not freeze. When removed from refrigeration to room temperature, use within 60 days. Use opened vials within 30 days. Use infusion solutions within 24 hr of mixing. Discard any unused portions of infusion solutions.
14. COMPATIBILITY D5W, RL, 0.9% NaCl, D5/NSS.
15. INCOMPATIBILITY Is physically incompatible when mixed with amphotericin, amoxicillin azathioprine, cefazolin, cloxacillin, dexamethasone, diazepam, erythyromycin, famotidine, furosemide, hydrocortisone, sodium succinate, insulin, intralipid, ketorolac, lorazepam, methohexital, methylprednisolone, thiopental, trimethoprim, and vancomycin. Do not mix rocuronium, which has an acid pH, with alkaline solutions (e.g., barbiturates) in the same syringe, or give at the same time during IV infusion through the same needle.

ASSESSMENT

1. Note reasons for therapy, other agents trialed and anticipated duration of therapy. Clients with burns, hemiparesis/paraparesis, or liver disease may require a higher dosage for desired response, and may have prolonged drug effects.
2. In the critically ill, intubate prior to rocuronium administration. Use a peripheral nerve stimulator/train of four to assess neuromuscular function, and to confirm recovery from neuromuscular blockade. Reversal/recovery R/T dosage amounts and repetitive number of doses.
3. Medicate for pain and anxiety as drug does not affect these conditions, and client may be unable to convey. Reassure that once drug is stopped, client may resume breathing, moving, and talking again.
4. Monitor VS, ECG, renal and LFTs.

INTERVENTIONS

1. Provide ventilatory support. Monitor and record VS, ECG, and I&O. Drug can cause vagal stimulation resulting in bradycardia, hypotension, and cardiac arrhythmias. A peripheral nerve stimulator/train of four monitoring may be used to evaluate neuromuscular response and recovery.
2. Perform frequent neurovascular assessments. Prolonged use of neuromuscular blocking agents may cause profound weakness and paralysis; may precipitate an acute myopathy.
3. Monitor VS frequently and pulmonary status continuously. Cardiac monitor and ventilator alarms should be set and checked frequently. Observe for excessive bronchial secretions or respiratory wheezing; suction to maintain patent airway.
4. Consciousness and pain thresholds are not affected by neuromuscular blocking agents; clients can still hear, feel, and see while receiving these agents. Avoid discussions that should not be overheard. Explain all contacts, injections, therapies, and procedures. Adequate anxiolytic therapy and analgesics should be administered for pain and/or fear with procedures and situations requiring this therapy. Anxiety levels may be very high, but client cannot communicate this.
5. Observe for drug interactions which may potentiate muscular relaxation and prove fatal.
6. Administer eye drops and patches to protect corneas during prolonged therapy; explain why this is done (i.e., blink reflex suppressed).
7. Muscle fasciculations may cause soreness or injury after recovery. Administer prescribed nondepolarizing agent and reassure that soreness likely caused by the unsynchronized contractions of adjacent muscle fibers just before the onset of paralysis.
8. Position for comfort and so that the body is in proper alignment. Turn and perform mouth care and eye care frequently (protect eyes and instill liquid tears q 2 hr).

R

CLIENT/FAMILY TEACHING

1. Causes body to be paralyzed. Reassure that once the drug is discontinued, will regain use of body, and be able to walk, talk, and breathe on own again.
2. Reassure that they will be continuously monitored during therapy.
3. Explain all procedures and exams as consciousness is not affected by rocuronium. Reassure will be medicated for pain and anxiety.

OUTCOMES/EVALUATE

- Desired level of skeletal muscle relaxation/paralysis
- Control of breathing during mechanical ventilation

Roflumilast

(roe-**FLUE**-mi-last)

Classification(s): Selective phosphodiesterase 4 inhibitor.

Pregnancy Category: C

RX: Daliresp.

INDICATIONS/USES

To reduce the risk of chronic obstructive pulmonary disease (COPD) exacerbations in clients with severe COPD associated with chronic bronchitis and a history of exacerbations.

ACTION/KINETICS

Action

Roflumilast and its active metabolite (roflumilast N-oxide) are selective inhibitors of phosphodiesterase 4 (PDE4). Inhibition of PDE4 leads to accumulation of intracellular cyclic AMP. Although the mechanism of action of roflumilast and its active metabolite are not known with certainty, it is believed the action is related to the effects of increased intracellular cyclic AMP in lung cells.

Pharmacokinetics

Absolute bioavailability is 80% after a 500 mcg dose. **C_{max}, roflumilast:** About 1 hr in the fasted state; **C_{max}, active metabolite:** About 8 hr. Steady state plasma levels of roflumilast and the active metabolite reached in about 4 days and 6 days, respectively. Food has no effect on total drug absorption but delays T_{max} by 1 hr and reduces C_{max} by 40%; however T_{max} and C_{max} of the active metabolite are not affected. Metabolized to the active metabolite by CYP1A2 and CYP3A4. **t½, median plasma:** 17 and 30 hr, respectively for roflumilast and its active metabolite. About 70% excreted in the urine. **Plasma protein binding:** Roflumilast: 99%; active metabolite: 97%.

CONTRAINDICATIONS

Moderate to severe liver impairment (Child-Pugh class B or C). Use during labor and delivery. Lactation.

SPECIAL CONCERNS

- Elderly may be more sensitive to the drug.
- Safety and efficacy not determined in children although COPD does not normally occur in children.

SIDE EFFECTS

Most Common

Diarrhea, nausea, back pain, dizziness, headache, insomnia, decreased weight, influenza.

CNS: Headache, insomnia, dizziness, anxiety, depression, tremor, ***suicidal ideation/behavior***, ***completed suicide***. **GI:** Diarrhea, decreased weight, N&V, decreased appetite, ***acute pancreatitis***, abdominal pain, dyspepsia, gastritis. **CV:** Atrial fibrillation. **Musculoskeletal:** Back pain, muscle spasms. **Respiratory:** Rhinitis, sinusitis, lung cancer. **GU:** URI, acute renal failure, prostate cancer. **Body as a whole:** Influenza.

OVERDOSE MANAGEMENT

Symptoms: Headache, GI disorders, dizziness, palpitations, lightheadedness, clamminess, arterial hypotension. *Treatment:* Appropriate supportive care. Hemodialysis is not likely to be effective due to high percentage of protein binding.

DRUG INTERACTIONS

Carbamazepine / ↓ Roflumilast plasma levels R/T induction of CYP3A4 → ↓ drug exposure and ↓ efficacy; avoid coadministration

Cimetidine / ↑ Roflumilast plasma level R/T inhibition of CYP3A4 and CYP1A2 → ↑ drug exposure and ↑ risk of side effects; assess risk vs benefit of concomitant use

Erythromycin / ↑ Roflumilast plasma level R/T inhibition of CYP3A4 and CYP1A2 → ↑ drug exposure and ↑ risk of side effects; assess risk vs benefit of concomitant use

Fluvoxamine / ↑ Roflumilast plasma level R/T inhibition of CYP3A4 and CYP1A2 → ↑ drug exposure and ↑ risk of side effects; assess risk vs benefit of concomitant use
Ketoconazole / ↑ Roflumilast plasma level R/T inhibition of CYP3A4 and CYP1A2 → ↑ drug exposure and ↑ risk of side effects; assess risk vs benefit of concomitant use
Oral contraceptives containing ethinyl estradiol and gestodene / ↑ Roflumilast exposure → ↑ risk of side effects; assess risk vs benefit of concomitant use
Phenobarbital / ↓ Roflumilast plasma levels R/T induction of CYP3A4 → ↓ drug exposure and ↓ efficacy; avoid coadministration
Phenytoin / ↓ Roflumilast plasma levels R/T induction of CYP3A4 → ↓ drug exposure and ↓ efficacy; avoid coadministration
Rifampin / ↓ Roflumilast plasma levels R/T induction of CYP3A4 → ↓ drug exposure and ↓ efficacy; avoid coadministration

HOW SUPPLIED

Tablets: 500 mcg.

DOSAGE

TABLETS

Chronic obstructive pulmonary disease.

Adults: 500 mcg (micrograms) per day.

NURSING IMPLICATIONS

IMPLEMENTATION/ADMINISTRATION/STORAGE

1. No dosage adjustment is needed for renal impairment, the elderly, gender, race, or smokers versus nonsmokers.
2. Store from 15–30°C (59–86°F).

ASSESSMENT

1. Note disease onset, characteristics, frequency of exacerbations, other agents trialed and outcome.
2. Assess clinical presentation, pulmonary function and determine any evidence of psychiatric problems, including depression or history of suicide ideations as drug may aggravate.
3. Monitor PFTs/spirometry, VS, weight, renal and LFTs; avoid with severe liver dysfunction.

CLIENT/FAMILY TEACHING

1. Drug is administered once a day with or without food.
2. It is used to reduce the flare-ups associated with COPD; use other drugs prescribed (bronchodilator) for sudden breathing problems.
3. Report any mood changes, lack of impulse control, insomnia, or new onset or increased depression and any thoughts of suicide immediately.
4. Continue all other prescribed therapy to control chronic bronchitis/COPD. Use incentive spirometer to assess for changes in lung function.
5. Weight loss is a common adverse effect; monitor weight regularly and report any significant changes.
6. Keep all F/U to assess response, lung function, weight, and for adverse SE.

OUTCOMES/EVALUATE

↓ Risk COPD exacerbations

IV

Romidepsin

(**ROE**-mih-**DEP**-sin)

Classification(s): Antineoplastic agent, histone deacetylase inhibitor

Pregnancy Category: D

RX: Istodax.

INDICATIONS/USES

Treatment of cutaneous or peripheral T-cell lymphoma in those who have received at least 1 prior systemic therapy.

ACTION/KINETICS

Action

Mechanism of action not fully characterized. The drug causes the accumulation of acetylated histones and induces cell cycle arrest and apoptosis of some cancer cell lines.

Pharmacokinetics

C_{max}, after recommended dose: 377 ng/mL; **AUC, after recommended dose:** 1,549 ng/mL. Extensively metabolized in the liver, mainly by CYP3A4 with minor contributions by CYP3A5, CYP1A1, CYP2B6, and CYP2C19. **t½, terminal:** About 3 hr. **Plasma protein binding:** 92–94%.

CONTRAINDICATIONS

Lactation.

SPECIAL CONCERNS

- **Use with caution in end-stage renal disease or in those with moderate or severe impaired hepatic function.**
- **Safety and efficacy not determined in children.**

SIDE EFFECTS

Most Common

Hypotension, ECG ST-T wave changes, pruritus, dermatitis/exfoliative dermatitis, anorexia, constipation, dysgeusia, N&V, anemia, neutropenia, leukopenia, lymphopenia, thrombocytopenia, asthenia, fatigue, hyperglycemia, infections, pyrexia, electrolyte changes.

CV: ECG ST-T wave changes, hypotension, supraventricular arrhythmia, QT prolongation, ***ventricular arrhythmia, cardiopulmonary failure, myocardial ischemia*.** **GI:** N&V, anorexia, constipation, diarrhea, dysgeusia. **Dermatologic:** Pruritus, dermatitis/exfoliative dermatitis. **Respiratory:** Acute respiratory distress syndrome, dyspnea. **GU:** Acute renal failure. **Hematologic:** Anemia, thrombocytopenia, neutropenia, lymphopenia, leukopenia. **Body as a whole:** Asthenia, fatigue, infections, pyrexia, edema, ***sepsis***.

LABORATORY TEST CONSIDERATIONS

↑ ALT, AST. Hypermagnesemia, hyperuricemia, hyperglycemia. Hypoalbuminemia, hypocalcemia, hypokalemia, hypomagnesemia, hyponatremia, hypophosphatemia.

OVERDOSE MANAGEMENT

Symptoms: See side effects. *Treatment:* No known antidote. Employ usual supportive measures. Not known if dialyzable.

DRUG INTERACTIONS

(1) Because romidepsin is metabolized mainly by CYP3A enzymes, substances known to inhibit these enzymes may ↓ metabolism or ↑ bioavailability of romidepsin (i.e., ↑ whole blood or plasma levels). Drugs known to induce these enzymes may cause an ↑ metabolism of romidepsin or ↓ bioavailability (i.e., ↓ whole blood or plasma levels). Monitor blood levels; dosage adjustment is essential when such drugs are used concomitantly. (2) It is possible for an additive effect of romidepsin with other drugs that prolong the QT interval → ↑ risk of life-threatening cardiac arrhythmias, including torsades de pointes. Drugs include the following: Amiodarone, arsenic trioxide, bretylium, chlorpromazine, cisapride, disopyramide, dofetilide, dolasetron, droperidol, mefloquine, mesoridazine, moxifloxacin, pentamidine, pimozide, procainamide, quinidine, sotalol, tacrolimus, thioridazine, and ziprasidone.

Aprepitant / ↑ Romidepsin plasma levels R/T inhibition of metabolism by CYP3A4; use together with caution

Atazanavir / ↑ Romidepsin plasma levels R/T inhibition of metabolism by CYP3A4 → ↑ pharmacologic and toxic effects; avoid coadministration if possible

Carbamazepine / ↓ Romidepsin plasma levels R/T ↑ metabolism by CYP3A4; avoid coadministration if possible

Clarithromycin / ↑ Romidepsin plasma levels R/T inhibition of metabolism by CYP3A4 → ↑ pharmacologic and toxic effects; avoid coadministration if possible

Cyclosporine / ↑ Romidepsin plasma levels R/T inhibition of P-glycoprotein efflux transport; possible ↑ pharmacologic and toxic effects; use together with caution

Dexamethasone / ↓ Romidepsin plasma levels R/T ↑ metabolism by CYP3A4; avoid coadministration if possible

Diltiazem / ↑ Romidepsin plasma levels R/T inhibition of metabolism by CYP3A4; use together with caution

Fluconazole / ↑ Romidepsin plasma levels R/T inhibition of metabolism by CYP3A4; use together with caution

Grapefruit juice / ↑ Romidepsin plasma levels R/T inhibition of metabolism by CYP3A4; use together with caution

Indinavir / ↑ Romidepsin plasma levels R/T inhibition of metabolism by CYP3A4 → ↑ pharmacologic and toxic effects; avoid coadministration if possible

Itraconazole / ↑ Romidepsin plasma levels R/T inhibition of metabolism by CYP3A4 → ↑ pharmacologic and toxic effects; avoid coadministration if possible

Ketoconazole / ↑ Romidepsin plasma levels R/T inhibition of metabolism by CYP3A4 → ↑ pharmacologic and toxic effects; avoid coadministration if possible

Nefazodone / ↑ Romidepsin plasma levels R/T inhibition of metabolism by CYP3A4 → ↑ pharmacologic and toxic effects; avoid coadministration if possible

Nelfinavir / ↑ Romidepsin plasma levels R/T inhibition of metabolism by CYP3A4 → ↑ pharmacologic and toxic effects; avoid coadministration if possible
Phenobarbital / ↓ Romidepsin plasma levels R/T ↑ metabolism by CYP3A4; avoid coadministration if possible
Phenytoin / ↓ Romidepsin plasma levels R/T ↑ metabolism by CYP3A4; avoid coadministration if possible
QT interval prolonging drugs (see #2 above for list) / ↑ Risk of QT prolongation → cardiac arrhythmias, including torsades de pointes; consider CV monitoring
Ranolazine / ↑ Romidepsin plasma levels R/T inhibition of P-glycoprotein efflux transport; possible ↑ pharmacologic and toxic effects; use together with caution
Rifabutin, Rifampin, Rifapentine / ↓ Romidepsin plasma levels R/T ↑ metabolism by CYP3A4; avoid coadministration if possible
Ritonavir / ↑ Romidepsin plasma levels R/T inhibition of metabolism by CYP3A4 → ↑ pharmacologic and toxic effects; avoid coadministration if possible
Saquinavir / ↑ Romidepsin plasma levels R/T inhibition of metabolism by CYP3A4 → ↑ pharmacologic and toxic effects; avoid coadministration if possible
H ***St. John's wort*** / ↓ Romidepsin plasma levels → ↓ pharmacologic effect; if possible do not use together
Telithromycin / ↑ Romidepsin plasma levels R/T inhibition of metabolism by CYP3A4 → ↑ pharmacologic and toxic effects; avoid coadministration if possible
Voriconazole / ↑ Romidepsin plasma levels R/T inhibition of metabolism by CYP3A4 → ↑ pharmacologic and toxic effects; avoid coadministration if possible
Warfarin / Possible PT prolongation and ↑ INR; monitor PT and INR and adjust dose if needed

HOW SUPPLIED

Injection, Lyophilized Powder for Solution: 10 mg.

DOSAGE

IV

Cutaneous T-cell lymphoma.

Adults: 14 mg/m^2 IV over a 4-hr period on days 1, 8, and 15 of a 28-day cycle. Repeat cycles every 28 days provided the client continues to benefit from and tolerates the therapy.

NURSING IMPLICATIONS

Do not confuse romidepsin with romiplostim (drug for thrombocytopenia).

IMPLEMENTATION/ADMINISTRATION/STORAGE

1. **IV Reconstitute with the 2 mL of the supplied diluent. Aseptically, using a suitable syringe, withdraw 2 mL from the supplied diluent vial and inject slowly into the romidepsin vial. Swirl the contents of the vial until there are no visible particles in the solution. The reconstituted solution contains 5 mg/mL of romidepsin.**
2. **Extract the appropriate amount of romidepsin from the reconstituted vial(s) to deliver the desired dose, using aseptic technique. Further dilute in 500 mL of NaCl 0.9% injection before IV infusion.**
3. **Adjust dose as follows for nonhematologic toxicities, except alopecia: (a) *Grade 2 or 3 toxicity:* Delay treatment until toxicity returns to grade 1 or less or baseline. Then restart therapy at 14 mg/m^2. If grade 3 toxicity recurs, delay treatment until toxicity returns to grade 1 or less or baseline; the dose should be permanently reduced to 10 mg/m^2. (b) *Grade 4 toxicity:* Delay treatment until toxicity returns to grade 1 or less or baseline; then, permanently reduce the dose to 10 mg/m^2.**
4. **Adjust the dose as follows for hematologic toxicities: (a) *Grade 3 or 4 neutropenia or thrombocytopenia:* Delay treatment until the specific cytopenia returns to ANC of 1.5 × 10^9/L or higher and/or platelet count of 75 × 10^9/L or higher or baseline; then, restart therapy at 14 mg/m^2. (b) *Grade 4 febrile (38.5°C or higher) neutropenia or thrombocytopenia that requires platelet transfusion:* Delay treatment until the specific cytopenia returns to grade 1 or less or baseline; then, permanently reduce the dose to 10 mg/m^2.**
5. **Store from 15–30°C (59–86°F). Reconstituted solution is stable for 8 hr at room temperature. Diluted reconstituted solution is stable for at least 24 hr at room temperature. Administer as soon after dilution as possible.**

R

6. COMPATIBILITY 0.9% NaCl. The diluted solution is compatible with polyvinyl chloride, ethylene vinyl acetate, polyethylene infusion bags, and glass bottles.
7. INCOMPATIBILITY Administer separately.

ASSESSMENT

1. Note type, onset, clinical presentation, and staging; other therapy failed and outcome. Identify date of prior systemic therapy.
2. List drugs prescribed to ensure none interact.
3. Closely monitor those with advanced stage disease and/or high tumor burden and take appropriate precautions.
4. Monitor ECG assess for QT prolongation, CBC, K^+ and Mg^{++}, renal and LFTs.

CLIENT/FAMILY TEACHING

1. Drug is administered by IV infusion over 4 hours on days 1, 8, and 15 of a 28-day cycle. Cycles are repeated every 28 days as long as tolerated and beneficial.
2. Report vomiting, chest pain, SOB, palpitations, or bleeding to provider.
3. Practice reliable contraception; avoid pregnancy during therapy. May reduce effectiveness of estrogen related contraceptives.
4. Infections may occur during therapy; report fever, cough, shortness of breath, (with or without chest pain), flu-like symptoms, muscle aches, or worsening of skin problems.
5. Keep all F/U to assess response, labs, and for adverse SE.

OUTCOMES/EVALUATE

Inhibition of malignant cell proliferation

Ropinirole hydrochloride

(roh-**PIN**-ih-roll)

Classification(s): Antiparkinson drug

Pregnancy Category: C

RX: Requip, Requip XL.

SEE ALSO ***ANTIPARKINSON AGENTS.***

INDICATIONS/USES

(1) Signs and symptoms of idiopathic Parkinson's disease (PD), both as initial therapy and adjunctive therapy with levodopa. (2) Moderate to severe restless legs syndrome (immediate-release only).

ACTION/KINETICS

Action

Mechanism is not known but believed to involve stimulation of postsynaptic D_2 dopamine receptors in caudate-putamen in brain. Causes decreases in both systolic and diastolic BP at doses above 0.25 mg.

Pharmacokinetics

Rapidly absorbed. **Peak plasma levels:** 1–2 hr. Food reduces maximum concentration. **t½, elimination:** 6 hr. First pass effect; extensively metabolized in liver.

CONTRAINDICATIONS

Lactation.

SPECIAL CONCERNS

Safety and efficacy not determined in children.

SIDE EFFECTS

Most Common

Dyskinesia, dizziness, somnolence, headache, hallucinations, falls, N&V, abdominal pain, pneumonia, fatigue, viral infection, increased sweating, edema, confusion.

CNS: Hallucinations, cause and/or exacerbate preexisting dyskinesia, dizziness, anxiety, somnolence, headache, abnormal dreams, confusion, falls, abnormal gait/hypokinesia, amnesia, tremor/twitching, nervousness, paresthesia, paresis, sudden uncontrolled sedation. **GI:** N&V, constipation, abdominal pain, diarrhea, dysphagia, increased salivation, dry mouth, anorexia, flatulence. **CV:** Syncope (sometimes with bradycardia), postural hypotension. **GU:** UTI, urinary incontinence, pyuria, impotence. **Musculoskeletal:** Arthritis, twitching. **Respiratory:** Pharyngitis, rhinitis, sinusitis, bronchitis, dyspnea, pneumonia. **Ophthalmic:** Abnormal vision, eye abnormality, xerophthalmia. **Metabolic:** Peripheral edema, edema, decreased weight. **Body as a whole:** Asthenia, fatigue, viral infection, pain, malaise, fever. **Miscellaneous:** Increased sweating, anemia, chest pain, peripheral ischemia.

LABORATORY TEST CONSIDERATIONS

↑ Alkaline phosphatase.

OVERDOSE MANAGEMENT

Symptoms: Agitation, increased dyskinesia, grogginess, sedation, orthostatic hypotension, chest pain, confusion, N&V. *Treatment:* General supportive measures. Maintain vital signs. Gastric lavage.

DRUG INTERACTIONS

Ciprofloxacin / Significant ↑ ropinirole levels
Estrogens / ↓ Oral clearance of ropinirole

HOW SUPPLIED

Tablets, Immediate-Release: 0.25 mg, 0.5 mg, 1 mg, 2 mg, 3 mg, 4 mg, 5 mg; *Tablets, Extended-Release:* 2 mg, 4 mg, 6 mg, 8 mg, 12 mg.

DOSAGE

TABLETS, IMMEDIATE-RELEASE

Parkinson's disease.

Adults. Titrate dosage in weekly increments. **Week 1:** 0.25 mg 3 times per day. **Week 2:** 0.5 mg 3 times per day. **Week 3:** 0.75 mg 3 times per day. **Week 4:** 1 mg 3 times per day. After week 4, daily dose, if necessary, may be increased by 1.5 mg/day on weekly basis up to dose of 9 mg/day. This may be followed by increases of up to 3 mg/day weekly to total dose of 24 mg/day.

Restless legs syndrome.

Adults. Days 1 and 2: 0.25 mg. **Days 3–7:** 0.5 mg. **Week 2:** 1 mg. **Week 3:** 1.5 mg. **Week 4:** 2 mg. **Week 5:** 2.5 mg. **Week 6:** 3 mg. **Week 7:** 4 mg. *NOTE:* Dose is to be taken once daily 1–3 hr before bedtime. The safety and efficacy of doses greater than 4 mg have not been established for treating restless legs syndrome. Discontinue gradually over 7 days.

TABLETS, EXTENDED-RELEASE

Parkinson's disease.

Adults, initial: 2 mg once a day for 1 to 2 weeks, followed by increases of 2 mg/day at 1-week or longer intervals (depends on response and tolerability), up to a maximum daily dose of 24 mg. Assess for efficacy and tolerability at a minimal interval of 1 week or longer after each dose increase. *NOTE:* Use caution during dose titration; a too rapid rate of titration may increase the risk of side effects.

NURSING IMPLICATIONS

IMPLEMENTATION/ADMINISTRATION/STORAGE

1. If taken with L-dopa, decrease dose of L-dopa gradually, as tolerated.
2. Clients may be switched directly from the immediate-release to the extended-release formulation. The initial dose of the extended-release tablets should most closely match the total daily dose of the immediate-release formulation. For example, if the total daily dose of the immediate-release tablets is 0.75 to 2.25, use the 2 mg extended-release tablet and if the total daily dose of the immediate-release tablets is 3 to 4.5 mg, use the 4 mg extended-release tablet.
3. When discontinuing the immediate-release tablet, do so gradually over 7-day period. Reduce frequency of administration to twice daily for 4 days. For remaining 3 days, reduce frequency to once daily prior to complete withdrawal. For the extended-release tablet, discontinue gradually over a 7-day period.
4. Titrate dose with caution in clients with impaired hepatic function.
5. If there is a significant interruption in therapy, retitration may be warranted.
6. Store immediate-release tablets from 20–25°C (68–77°F) and extended-release tablets from 15–30°C (59–86°F). Protect from light and moisture.

ASSESSMENT

1. Note reasons for therapy (PD, restless legs syndrome, periodic limb movements of sleep), disease onset, symptom occurrence, extent of motor function, stiffness, reflexes, gait, strength of grip, amount of tremor. Assess clinical presentation.
2. Note neurological assessment and mental status. With tremor, note extent, muscle weakness/rigidity, difficulty walking or changing direction.
3. Monitor VS, weight, ECG, renal and LFTs. With long-term therapy obtain CXR, eye exams.

CLIENT/FAMILY TEACHING

1. May be taken with or without food. Drug will be gradually increased at weekly intervals to control symptoms.
2. Take extended-release tablets whole; do not chew, crush, or divide.

R

3. Change positions slowly to prevent sudden drop in BP.
4. Avoid tasks that require mental alertness until drug effects realized. May cause dizziness and drowsiness so use caution; report if persists.
5. Report any loss of effectiveness or worsening of condition. Avoid alcohol during therapy.
6. Do not smoke: increases drug clearance. Report if start/stop smoking while taking ropinirole.
7. Practice reliable birth control and do not nurse. Report if pregnancy suspected.
8. Do not stop abruptly. Drug must be gradually withdrawn over 7-day period.
9. Report if hallucinations (unreal visions, sounds, or sensations) occur as well as involuntary body or facial movements, mood or mental status changes or persistent or frequent nausea or vomiting.
10. May affect impulse control including compulsive behaviors; pathological gambling and hypersexuality, have been reported.
11. Keep all F/U to assess response, labs, CXR, eye exams and for adverse SE.

OUTCOMES/EVALUATE

- Control of tremor, bradykinesia, and rigidity in PD
- Improvement in periodic limb movements of sleep (PLMD) and restless leg syndrome (RLS) resulting in improved sleep efficiency

Rosiglitazone maleate

(**roh**-sih-**GLIH**-tah-zohn)

Classification(s): Antidiabetic, oral; thiazolidinedione

Pregnancy Category: C

RX: Avandia.

SEE ALSO ***ANTIDIABETIC AGENTS: HYPOGLYCEMIC AGENTS.***

INDICATIONS/USES

(1) Monotherapy as an adjunct to diet and exercise to improve glycemic control in type 2 diabetes. (2) In combination with a sulfonylurea, insulin, or metformin in clients with type 2 diabetes when diet and exercise and either single agent does not achieve adequate control. In clients inadequately controlled with a maximum dose of a sulfonylurea or metformin, add rosiglitazone to the regimen, rather than substitute for the sulfonylurea or metformin. (3) In combination with a sulfonylurea plus metformin when diet, exercise, and both agents do not result in adequate glycemic control. *Investigational:* Increased ovulation frequency in women with polycystic ovary syndrome; reduced in-stent restenosis in clients with diabetes.

ACTION/KINETICS

Action

Improves blood glucose levels by improving insulin sensitivity in type 2 diabetes insulin resistant. Active only in the presence of insulin. A highly selective and potent agonist for the peroxisome proliferator-activated receptor (PPAR)-gamma which is found in adipose tissue, skeletal muscle, and liver. Activation of these receptors regulates the transcription of insulin-responsive genes involved in the control of glucose production, transport, and use. The genes also participate in regulation of fatty acid metabolism. Fasting blood glucose decreases from 31–64 mg/dL from placebo and HbA1c decreases from 0.8–1.5% from placebo.

Pharmacokinetics

Peak plasma levels: 1 hr (over 99% bioavailable). Food decreases the rate of absorption but not the total amount absorbed. **t½, elimination:** 3–4 hr. Extensively metabolized in the liver by CYP2C8 and CYP2C9; excreted in the urine (64%) and feces (23%). Clearance is lower in moderate to severe liver disease. The drug does not inhibit any of the major P450 enzymes at clinical doses. *NOTE:* A product called Avandamet is available that contains 1 gram metformin with either 2 or 4 mg rosiglitazone. **Plasma protein binding:** Approximately 99.8%.

CONTRAINDICATIONS

Type 1 diabetes, diabetic ketoacidosis, coadministration of insulin and rosiglitazone, use with nitrates, use with metformin in renal impairment, active liver disease, if serum ALT levels are 2.5 times ULN, in clients with NYHA Class III and IV heart failure, during lactation, and in children less than 18 years of age.

R

SPECIAL CONCERNS

(1) Thiazolidinediones, including rosiglitazone, cause or exacerbate CHF in some clients. After initiation of rosiglitazone, and after dose increases, observe clients carefully for signs and symptoms of heart failure (including excessive, rapid weight gain, dyspnea, and/or edema). If these signs and symptoms develop, the heart failure should be managed according to current standards of care. Furthermore, consider discontinuation or dose reduction of rosiglitazone. (2) Rosiglitazone is not recommended in clients with symptomatic heart failure. Initiation of rosiglitazone in such clients with established NYHA Class III or IV heart failure is contraindicated.

- **Treatment may result in resumption of ovulation in premenopausal anovulatory clients with insulin resistance.**
- **Use with caution in clients with edema, at risk for heart failure, or hepatic impairment.**
- **Increased risk of MI and CV events, especially in long-term users of insulin and those taking nitrates.**
- **May cause osteoporosis.**
- **Safety and efficacy not determined in clients under 18 years of age.**

SIDE EFFECTS

Most Common

Headache, edema, back pain, injury, URTI, hyperglycemia, fatigue, sinusitis, diarrhea, anemia.

CV: ***Cardiac failure***, cardiac effects, fluid retention that may worsen or cause CHF, pleural effusions, ***pulmonary edema*** with or without fatal outcome, hypertension, increased risk of ***MI, death from CV causes***. **GI:** Diarrhea, hepatitis, elevated hepatic enzymes to 3 or more times the ULN, ***hepatic failure*** with or without fatal outcome. **Respiratory:** URTI, sinusitis, nasopharyngitis. **Musculoskeletal:** Back pain, osteoporosis, increase incidence of bone fractures in women, arthralgia. **Dermatologic:** Angioedema, pruritus, rash, urticaria, ***Steven-Johnson syndrome***. **Metabolic:** Hypoglycemia/hyperglycemia, dose-related weight gain. **Miscellaneous:** Injury, headache, fatigue, anemia, edema, macular edema, new or worsening diabetic macular edema with decreased visual acuity, ***anaphylaxis***.

R

LABORATORY TEST CONSIDERATIONS

↑ ALT, total cholesterol, LDL, HDL, bilirubin. ↓ H&H, free fatty acids, white blood cells. Hyperbilirubinemia.

DRUG INTERACTIONS

Gemfibrozil / ↑ Rosiglitazone AUC R/T inhibition of CYP2C8 isoenzyme
Ketoconazole / ↑ Rosiglitazone AUC, peak plasma levels, prolongation in $t_{1/2}$, and ↓ PO clearance R/T inhibition of metabolism by CYP2C8 and CYP2C9
Trimethoprim / ↑ Rosiglitazone plasma levels R/T inhibition of metabolism by CYP2C8

HOW SUPPLIED

Tablets: 2 mg, 4 mg, 8 mg.

DOSAGE

TABLETS

Type 2 diabetes, monotherapy.

Individualize dosage. **Adults, initial:** 4 mg once daily or in divided doses twice a day. If the response is inadequate after 8–12 weeks, the dose can be increased to 8 mg (maximum daily dose) as a single dose once daily or in divided doses twice a day. A dose of 4 mg twice a day resulted in the greatest decrease in fasting blood glucose and HbA1c.

Type 2 diabetes, combination therapy with sulfonylurea, insulin, or metformin.

Adults, initial: 4 mg once daily or in divided doses twice a day. The current dose(s) of existing therapy can be continued upon initiation of rosiglitazone. If the response is inadequate after 8–12 weeks, the dose can be increased to 8 mg (maximum daily dose) as a single dose once daily or in divided doses twice a day.

NURSING IMPLICATIONS

Do not confuse Avandia with Coumadin (an anticoagulant) or with Prandin (also an oral hypoglycemic drug).

IMPLEMENTATION/ADMINISTRATION/STORAGE

1. **Metformin is contraindicated in clients with renal impairment, as is coadministration with**

rosiglitazone. However, no dosage adjustment is required when rosiglitazone is used as monotherapy in those with renal impairment.

2. Do not begin rosiglitazone therapy in clients with active liver disease or increased serum transaminase levels (ALT more than 2.5 times ULN at start of therapy).
3. Doses of rosiglitazone higher than 4 mg daily in combination with insulin are not recommended. It is recommended that the insulin dose be decreased 10–25% if the client reports hypoglycemia or if the FBS concentrations decrease to less than 100 mg/dL. Make further adjustments based on glucose-lowering response.
4. Store between 15–30°C (59–86°F) in a tight, light-resistant container.

ASSESSMENT

1. Note disease onset, degree of control, other agents trialed, dietary/exercise adherence.
2. List any history of macular edema, CAD, CHF; NYHA class as drug may aggravate. List agents prescribed to ensure none interact.
3. Assess for S&S of heart failure (SOB, swelling of lower extremities). Stop drug if symptoms appear.
4. Monitor LFTs following initiation of therapy, every 2 months during first year of use, and periodically thereafter. If ALT increase to 3× ULN at any time, recheck LFTs as soon as possible. If ALT levels remain >3× ULN, stop therapy. Check BS, microalbumin, HbA1c levels regularly.

CLIENT/FAMILY TEACHING

1. Take once or twice daily as prescribed with meals (may also be taken without regard to meals). If dose missed may be taken at next meal.
2. May cause swelling of extremities, resumption of ovulation in premenopausal women with insulin resistance, and hypoglycemia.
3. Report if dark urine, abdominal pain, fatigue, or unexplained N&V occur. Also report any fever, sore throat, unusual bleeding/bruising, rash, or hypoglycemic reactions.
4. Practice reliable barrier contraception if using hormonal contraception and pregnancy is not desired.
5. Follow dietary guidelines, perform regular daily exercise, weight loss, and other lifestyle changes consistent with controlling diabetes. Ensure annual foot exam and eye exam and keep SBP below 130 and DBP below 80; LDL below 100 and TG below 150. Record BP and monitor FS at different times during the day for provider review.
6. Report any new onset visual changes, SOB, chest pain, significant weight gain or swelling of extremities.
7. There is an increased risk of MI and CV events, especially in long-term users of insulin and those taking nitrates.
8. Must report as scheduled for regular monitoring of renal and LFTs q 2 months and A1C, BP, foot, and eye exams.
9. Keep all F/U to assess response, labs, and for adverse SE.

OUTCOMES/EVALUATE

- Control of NIDDM by ↓ insulin resistance
- HbA1c <8
- ↑ Ovulation frequency with polycystic ovary syndrome (unlabeled use)
- ↓ In-stent restenosis in those with diabetes (UL)

Rosuvastatin calcium

(roe-**SUE**-vuh-stah-tin)

Classification(s): Antihyperlipidemic, HMG-CoA reductase inhibitor

Pregnancy Category: X

RX: Crestor.

SEE ALSO ***ANTIHYPERLIPIDEMIC AGENTS, HMG-COA REDUCTASE INHIBITORS.***

INDICATIONS/USES

1. As an adjunct to diet to reduce elevated total cholesterol, LDL-C, Apo B, non-high-density HDL-C, and triglyceride levels, and to increase HDL-C in primary hyperlipidemia and mixed dyslipidemia.
2. Reduce LDL-C, total cholesterol, and Apo B in homozygous familial hypercholesterolemia in adults as an adjunct to other lipid-lowering treatments (e.g., LDL apheresis) or if such treatments are not available.
3. Adjunct to diet in adults with hypertriglyceridemia.
4. Adjunctive therapy to diet to slow the progression of atherosclerosis in adults as part

of the regimen to lower total cholesterol and LDL-C to target levels.

5. Adjunct to diet to treat primary dysbetalipoproteinemia (type III hyperlipoproteinemia).
6. Adjunct to diet to reduce total cholesterol, LDL-C, and APO-B levels in adolescent boys and girls, who are at least 1 year postmenarche, 10–17 years of age with heterozygous familial hypercholesterolemia if after an adequate trial of diet therapy the following are present: LDL-C more than 190 mg/dL or more than 160 mg/dL if there is a positive family history of premature CV disease *or* two or more other CV disease risk factors.
7. Reduce the risk of stroke, MI, and arterial revascularization procedures in those without clinically evident coronary heart disease, but with an increased risk of CV disease based on age of 50 years and older in men and 60 years and older in women, high-sensitivity C-reactive protein of at least 2 mg/mL, and the presence of at least 1 additional CV disease risk factor, such as hypertension, low HDL-C, smoking, or a family history of premature coronary heart disease.

ACTION/KINETICS

Action

Competitively inhibits HMG-CoA reductase; this enzyme catalyzes the early rate-limiting step in the synthesis of cholesterol. Thus, cholesterol synthesis is inhibited/decreased. Reduces total cholesterol, LDL-C, Apo B, and non-HDL-C in clients with homozygous and heterozygous familial hypercholesterolemia, nonfamilial forms of hypercholesterolemia, and mixed dyslipidemia. Also, reduces triglycerides and increases HDL-C.

Pharmacokinetics

Peak plasma levels: 3–5 hr. Absolute bioavailability is about 20%. Food decreases the rate (20%) but not the extent of absorption. About 10% metabolized by CYP2C9 to N-desmethyl rosuvastatin. Excreted primarily (90%) in the feces. **t½, elimination:** About 19 hr. Severe renal or hepatic insufficiency significantly increases plasma levels. **Plasma protein binding:** About 95%.

CONTRAINDICATIONS

Pregnancy and lactation. Use in clients with active liver disease or with unexplained persistent elevations of serum transaminases.

SPECIAL CONCERNS

- **Use with caution in clients who consume substantial amounts of alcohol and/or have a history of liver disease.**
- **Use with caution in those 65 years and older, in hypothyroidism, and renal insufficiency (all predispose clients to myopathy).**
- **Cases (rare) of rhabdomyolysis with acute renal failure secondary to myoglobinuria have been reported.**

SIDE EFFECTS

Most Common

Muscle cramps/pain, arthralgia, myalgia, constipation, asthenia, dizziness, abdominal pain/cramps, gastroenteritis/gastritis, nausea, headache, pain, peripheral edema.

Musculoskeletal: Muscle cramps/pain, arthralgia, myalgia, myopathy, rhabdomyolysis, arthritis. **CNS:** Headache, dizziness, memory loss. **GI:** Nausea, abdominal pain/cramps, constipation, gastroenteritis/gastritis, ***pancreatitis***. **Dermatologic:** Pruritus, rash. **Hepatic:** ***Hepatic failure***, hepatitis, jaundice. **GU:** Hematuria. **Body as a whole:** Asthenia, allergy, hypersensitivity (rare), pain, peripheral edema.

LABORATORY TEST CONSIDERATIONS

↑ Serum transaminases (up to 3 or more times ULN), creatine kinase, bilirubin, glutamyl transpeptidase, glucose, alkaline phosphatase. Proteinuria. Thyroid function abnormalities.

DRUG INTERACTIONS

Antacids, Al/Mg combination / ↓ Rosuvastatin levels; give antacid 2 hr after rosuvastatin
Cyclosporine / Significant ↑ of rosuvastatin C_{max} and AUC → ↑ risk of myopathy
Digoxin / Possible ↑ plasma digoxin levels; monitor digoxin levels and adjust dose if necessary
Gemfibrozil / Significant ↑ of rosuvastatin C_{max} and AUC → ↑ risk of myopathy
Oral contraceptives / ↑ Levels of ethinyl estradiol and norgestrel
Warfarin / Significant ↑ INR

HOW SUPPLIED

Tablets: 5 mg, 10 mg, 20 mg, 40 mg.

DOSAGE

TABLETS

Hyperlipidemia, mixed dyslipidemia, hypertriglyceridemia, atherosclerosis, primary dysbetalipoproteinemia.

Individualize therapy. **Initial:** 10 mg once daily (use 5 mg once daily for those requiring less aggressive LDL-C reductions or who have predisposing factors for myopathy). For clients with marked hypercholesterolemia (LDL-C >190 mg/dL) and aggressive lipid targets, consider a 20 mg starting dose. After initiation and/or upon titration, analyze lipid levels within 2 to 4 weeks; adjust dosage accordingly. Reserve the 40 mg dose for those who have not achieved goal LDL-C at 20 mg.

Homozygous familial hypercholesterolemia.

Initial: 20 mg once daily. **Dose range:** 5–40 mg; **maximum recommended dose:** 40 mg daily. Use rosuvastatin as an adjunct to other lipid-lowering treatments (e.g., LDL apheresis) or if other treatments are not available. Estimate response to therapy from preapheresis LDL-C levels.

Primary prevention of cardiovascular disease.

Initial dose: 10–20 mg once a day. **Usual dosage range:** 5–40 mg once a day.

Heterozygous familial hypercholesterolemia in children 10–17 years of age after failing an adequate trial of diet therapy.

Children, 10–17 years of age: 5–20 mg once a day.

NURSING IMPLICATIONS

IMPLEMENTATION/ADMINISTRATION/STORAGE

1. Before beginning rosuvastatin therapy, try to control hypercholesterolemia with appropriate diet and exercise, weight reduction in obese clients, and treatment of underlying medical problems. Continue cholesterol-lowering diet during drug treatment.
2. Temporarily withhold rosuvastatin in clients with an acute, serious condition suggestive of myopathy or predisposing to the development of renal failure secondary to rhabdomyolysis (e.g., sepsis, hypotension, major surgery, trauma, uncontrolled seizures, severe metabolic, endocrine, and electrolyte disorders).
3. For clients with severe renal impairment (C_{CR} less than 30 mL/min/1.73 m^2 not on hemodialysis), use an initial dose of 5 mg once daily; dosage should not exceed 10 mg once daily.
4. Due to the possibility of myopathy and rhabdomyolysis, reserve 40 mg dose for clients who have not achieved their LDL-C goal with the 20 mg regimen.
5. In clients taking cyclosporine, limit rosuvastatin dose to 5 mg once daily.
6. In clients taking a combination of lopinavir/ritonavir or atazanavir/ritonavir, limit the dose of rosuvastatin to 10 mg once daily.
7. The effect of rosuvastatin on LDL-C and total cholesterol may be enhanced if used with niacin or fenofibrate; consider a reduction in rosuvastatin dosage. Avoid combination therapy with gemfibrozil due to an increase in rosuvastatin exposure if used together. If gemfibrozil is used with rosuvastatin, limit the dose of rosuvastatin to 10 mg once daily.
8. In Asian clients, initiate therapy with 5 mg once daily.
9. Consider dose reduction in clients on 40 mg rosuvastatin therapy with unexplained persistent proteinuria during routine urinalysis.
10. Store at controlled room temperature (20–25°C; 68–77°F) protected from moisture.

ASSESSMENT

1. Note reasons for therapy: CHD prophylaxis, plaque stability or elevated TG/LDL cholesterol in CAD. Review other therapy/meds trialed, risk factors, ancestry, and family history.
2. List all medications prescribed to ensure none interact unfavorably.
3. Assess adherence to weight reduction, exercise, cholesterol-lowering diet, and BP/BS control. Note any alcohol abuse and liver or renal dysfunction.
4. Monitor BS, CBC, lipid profile, TSH, CPK, renal and LFTs. Schedule LFTs at the beginning of therapy, in 3 months, and semiannually for the first year of therapy. Special attention

R

should be paid to elevated ALT/AST and CPK levels.

CLIENT/FAMILY TEACHING

1. Take once daily with or without food as directed. Do not use antacid for 2 hr after consuming drug.
2. Report any S&S of infections, unexplained muscle pain, tenderness/weakness (especially if accompanied by fever or malaise), surgery, trauma, or metabolic disorders; stop therapy.
3. Review importance of following a low-cholesterol diet, regular exercise, weight control, and smoking cessation, in the overall goal to inhibit progression of CAD.
4. Not for use during pregnancy; use barrier contraception.
5. Report for F/U to assess response, labs, and for adverse SE.

OUTCOMES/EVALUATE

- ↓ Total and LDL cholesterol, non-HDL cholesterol, apolipoprotein B (Apo B), and triglyceride levels
- ↑ HDL cholesterol

Rufinamide

(roo-**FIN**-ah-mide)

Classification(s): Anticonvulsant.
Pregnancy Category: C
RX: Banzel.

INDICATIONS/USES

Adjunctive treatment of seizures associated with Lennox-Gastaut syndrome in adults and children, 4 years of age and older.

ACTION/KINETICS

Action

The precise mechanism is unknown. The drug may modulate activity of sodium channels and, in particular, prolongation of the inactive state of the channel, thus limiting sustained repetitive firing of sodium-dependent action potentials.

Pharmacokinetics

Well absorbed (85%) after PO administration but rate of absorption is slow. Food increases the extent of absorption. **Peak plasma levels:** 4–6 hr, under both fed and fasting conditions. **t½:** 6–10 hr. Metabolized in the liver by CYP450 enzymes. Rufinamide is a weak inducer of CYP3A4 and can decrease exposure to drugs that are substrates of CYP3A4. **t½, plasma:** 6–10 hr. Excreted mainly (85%) by the kidney. **Plasma protein binding:** 34%.

CONTRAINDICATIONS

Familial short QT syndrome. Severe hepatic impairment. Lactation.

SPECIAL CONCERNS

- Use with caution with mild to moderate hepatic impairment.
- Increased risk of suicidal behavior and ideation.
- Use caution in dose selection in the elderly.
- Safety and efficacy not determined in children less than 4 years of age.

SIDE EFFECTS

Most Common

Adults: Ataxia, diplopia, dizziness, fatigue, nausea, blurred vision, somnolence.
Children: Headache, somnolence, vomiting.
CNS: Somnolence, headache, fatigue, coordination abnormalities, dizziness, gait disturbances, ataxia, anxiety, aggression (children), disturbance in attention (children), psychomotor hyperactivity (children), tremor, vertigo, ***seizures, status epilepticus***. **GI:** N&V, upper abdominal pain, constipation, dyspepsia. **CV:** Shortening of the QT interval, first-degree AV block, right bundle branch block. **Hematologic:** Anemia, iron deficiency anemia, leukopenia, lymphadenopathy, neutropenia, thrombocytopenia. **Dermatologic:** Rash, pruritus. **Respiratory:** Bronchitis, sinusitis, nasopharyngitis. **GU:** Pollakiuria, dysuria, enuresis, hematuria, incontinence, nephrolithiasis, nocturia, polyuria, urinary incontinence. **Hypersensitivity:** Rash, fever, hematuria, lymphadenopathy, elevated LFTs. **Ophthalmic:** Diplopia, nystagmus, blurred vision. **Otic:** Ear infection. **Miscellaneous:** Influenza, back pain, decreased/increased appetite.

DRUG INTERACTIONS

Carbamazepine / ↓ Rufinamide plasma levels; also, ↓ carbamazepine plasma levels
Contraceptives, hormonal / ↓ Ethinyl estradiol/norethindrone AUC and C_{max}; additional nonhormonal contraceptives are recommended

Lamotrigine / ↓ Lamotrigine levels (especially in children)
Phenobarbital / ↓ Rufinamide plasma levels (especially in children); also, ↑ phenobarbital plasma levels (especially in children)
Phenytoin / ↓ Rufinamide plasma levels (especially in children); also, ↑ phenytoin plasma levels (especially in children)
Primidone / ↓ Rufinamide plasma levels (especially in children)
Triazolam / ↓Triazolam AUC and C_{max}
Valproate / ↑ Rufinamide plasma levels (especially in children)

HOW SUPPLIED

Suspension, Oral: 40 mg/mL; ***Tablets:*** 200 mg, 400 mg.

DOSAGE

TABLETS

Seizures associated with Lennox-Gastaut syndrome.

Adults, initial: 400–800 mg/day, given in 2 equally divided doses. Increase the dose by 400 to 800 mg/day q 2 days until a maximum daily dose of 3,200 mg/day is reached; give in 2 equally divided doses. It is not known if doses less than 3,200 are effective. **Maintenance:** 3,200 mg/day. **Children, 4 years and older, initial:** About 10 mg/kg/day, given in 2 equally divided doses. Increase the dose by approximately 10 mg/kg increments every other day to a target dose of 45 mg/kg/day or 3,200 mg/day, whichever is less. Give in 2 equally divided doses. Maintenance: 45 mg/kg/day or 3,200 mg/day, whichever is less, given in 2 equally divided doses. It is not known if lesser doses are effective.

NURSING IMPLICATIONS

IMPLEMENTATION/ADMINISTRATION/STORAGE

1. To minimize the risk of precipitating seizures, seizure exacerbation, or status epilepticus, withdraw gradually. If abrupt discontinuation is medically necessary, transfer to another antiepileptic drug under close medical supervision.
2. Consider adjusting the dose during hemodialysis.
3. Clients on valproate should begin rufinamide at a lower dose than 400 mg/day for adults and 10 mg/kg/day for children.
4. To provide information regarding the effects of in utero exposure to rufinamide, pregnant women should enroll in the North American Antiepileptic Drug Pregnancy Registry. Clients should call 1-888-233-2334. This must be done by the women themselves. Registry information can also be found at the web site: www.aedpregnancyregistry.org.
5. Store from 15–30°C (59–86°F); protect tablets from moisture.

ASSESSMENT

1. Note reasons for therapy, onset, characteristics of seizure S&S, other agents trialed, outcome.
2. List all meds prescribed to ensure none interact.
3. Assess mental status, note any evidence or history of depression, psychiatric problems, or familial shortened QT syndrome.
4. Observe those who develop a rash while receiving treatment closely.
5. Monitor VS, Wt, ECG, CBC, renal and LFTs; adjust dose with dysfunction.

CLIENT/FAMILY TEACHING

1. Rufinamide tablets are scored on both sides and can be cut in half for dosing flexibility. May be given whole, in half, or crushed and should be taken with food.
2. Shake the oral suspension well before use. Administer using the provided adapter and calibrated PO dosing syringe. Insert the adapter firmly into the neck of the bottle before use; it should remain in place for the duration of usage of the bottle. Insert the dosing syringe into the adapter and withdraw the dose from the inverted bottle. Replace the cap after each use; the cap fits properly when the adapter is in place.
3. Avoid activities that require mental alertness until drug effects realized; may cause dizziness and drowsiness.
4. Report any fever, rash, elevated liver function studies, hematuria, and/or lymph node enlargement; multi-organ hypersensitivity syndrome has occurred and requires discontinuation of therapy.

R

5. **Avoid alcohol and CNS depressants.**
6. **Notify provider if a rash associated with fever experienced.**
7. **Report loss of seizure control and any unusual changes in mood or behavior, or the emergence of suicidal thoughts/self-harm feelings immediately.**
8. **Women should practice reliable contraception; with hormonal therapy advise to use additional non-hormonal forms of contraception. Pregnant women should enroll in the North American Antiepileptic Drug Pregnancy Registry. Clients should call 1-888-233-2334. This must be done by the women themselves. Registry information can also be found at the web site: www.aedpregnancyregistry.org.**
9. **Keep all F/U to assess response, labs, and for adverse SE.**

OUTCOMES/EVALUATE

Control of seizures

Ruxolitinib phosphate

(rux-oh-**LI**-ti-nib)

Classification(s): Tyrosine kinase inhibitor.

Pregnancy Category: C

RX: Jakafi.

INDICATIONS/USES

Treatment of intermediate or high-risk myelofibrosis, including primary myelofibrosis, post-polycythemia vera myelofibrosis, and post-essential thrombocythemia myelofibrosis.

ACTION/KINETICS

Action

Ruxolitinib, a kinase inhibitor, inhibits Janus-associated kinases (Jak1 and Jak2) which mediate the signaling of a number of cytokines and growth factors that are important for hematopoiesis and immune function. Myelofibrosis is a myeloproliferative neoplasm known to be associated with dysregulated Jak1 and Jak2 signaling. Thus, inhibition of Jak1 and Jak2 kinases should relieve myelofibrosis.

Pharmacokinetics

Rapidly absorbed; at least 95% absorbed. C_{max}: 1–2 hr postdose. A high fat meal does not affect the pharmacokinetics. CYP3A4 is the major enzyme responsible for ruxolitinib metabolism; two metabolites are active but less so than the parent drug. Excreted in both the urine (74%) and feces (22%). **t½, mean elimination:** About 3 hr for ruxolitinib alone and 5.8 hr for ruxolitinib plus its metabolites. **Plasma protein binding:** 97%.

CONTRAINDICATIONS

Coadministration with strong CYP3A4 inhibitors in those with platelet counts <100 × 10^9/L. Moderate to severe renal impairment with platelet counts <100 × 10^9/L. Hepatic impairment with platelet counts <100 × 10^9/L. Lactation.

SPECIAL CONCERNS

- **Herpes zoster is a possible adverse effect; inform clients of early signs and symptoms of herpes zoster and advise them to seek treatment as early as possible.**
- **Safety and efficacy not determined in children.**

SIDE EFFECTS

Most Common

Thrombocytopenia, anemia, neutropenia, bruising, dizziness, headache.

CNS: Dizziness, headache, vertigo, balance disorder, Ménière's disease labyrinthitis, postural dizziness. **GI:** Flatulence, weight gain, abnormal weight gain, hepatic abnormalities. **Dermatologic:** Bruising, contusion, ecchymosis, hematoma, petechiae, purpura. **Hematologic:** Thrombocytopenia, anemia, neutropenia. **GU:** UTI, cystitis, urosepsis, bacterial UTI, kidney infection, pyuria, bacteria in urine, nitrite urine present. **Ophthalmic:** Periorbital hematoma. **At injection site:** Hematoma, puncture–site hematoma. **Body as a whole:** Herpes zoster, postherpetic neuralgia; serious bacterial, mycobacterial, fungal, and viral infections.

LABORATORY TEST CONSIDERATIONS

↑ Cholesterol, ALT, AST.

OVERDOSE MANAGEMENT

Symptoms: Increased myelosuppression, including thrombocytopenia, leukopenia, and anemia. *Treatment:* There is no known antidote. Provide appropriate supportive treatment. Hemodialysis is not expected to enhance ruxolitinib elimination.

DRUG INTERACTIONS

The starting dose of ruxolitinib is decreased in clients coadministered the following CYP3A4 inhibitors: Boceprevir, clarithromycin, conivaptan, grapefruit juice, indinavir, itraconazole, ketoconazole, lopinavir/ritonavir, mibefradil, nefazodone, nelfinavir, posaconazole, ritonavir, saquinavir, telaprevir, telithromycin, and voriconazole.

CYP3A4 inducers (e.g., rifampin) / ↓ Ruxolitinib C_{max} and AUC R/T ↑ metabolism; no dosage adjustment is required; monitor and adjust ruxolitinib dose based on safety and efficacy

CYP3A4 mild or moderate inhibitors (e.g., erythromycin) / ↑ Ruxolitinib plasma levels; no dosage adjustment is needed

CYP3A4 strong inhibitors (see list above) / ↑ Ruxolitinib plasma levels R/T inhibition of metabolism → ↑ pharmacologic/toxic effects; avoid coadministration

Grapefruit juice / ↑ Ruxolitinib plasma levels R/T inhibition of metabolism → ↑ pharmacologic/toxic effects; avoid coadministration

HOW SUPPLIED

Tablets: 5 mg, 10 mg, 15 mg, 20 mg, 25 mg.

DOSAGE

TABLETS

Myelofibrosis.

Adults, initial dose, platelet count >200 × 10⁹/L: 20 mg twice a day; **platelet count 100 × 10⁹ L to 200 × 10⁹ L:** 15 mg twice a day. **Maximum dose:** 50 mg/day. Dosage may be increased in 5 mg twice daily increments to a maximum of 25 mg twice a day. Do not increase doses during the first 4 weeks of therapy and not more frequently than q 2 weeks. Long-term maintenance at a 5 mg twice daily dosage has not shown response; limit continued use at this dose to clients in whom the benefits outweigh the potential risks.

NURSING IMPLICATIONS

IMPLEMENTATION/ADMINISTRATION/STORAGE

1. Dose increases should be considered in clients who meet all of the following conditions:
   - Failure to achieve a reduction from pretreatment baseline in either palpable spleen length of 50% or a 35% reduction in spleen volume as measured by computed tomography or MRI;
   - Platelet count greater than 125×10^9/L at 4 weeks and platelet count never below 100×10^9/L;
   - Absolute neutrophil count (ANC) levels greater than 0.75×10^9/L.
2. **Dose interruption for thrombocytopenia.** Interrupt treatment for platelet counts less than 50×10^9/L. After recovery of platelet counts above this level, dosing may be restarted or increased following recovery of platelet counts to acceptable levels. The following are ruxolitinib maximum restarting doses after interruption for thrombocytopenia. Maximum doses are indicated. When restarting, begin with a dose at least 5 mg twice a day below the dose at interruption.
   - Current platelet count: Greater than or equal to 125×10^9/L, the maximum restarting dose is 20 mg twice a day.
   - Current platelet count: 100 to <125×10^9/L, the maximum restarting dose is 15 mg twice a day.
   - Current platelet count: 75 to <100×10^9/L, the maximum restarting dose is 10 mg twice a day for at least 2 weeks; if stable, may increase to 15 mg twice a day.
   - Current platelet count: 50 to <75×10^9/L, the maximum restarting dose is 5 mg twice a day for at least 2 weeks; if stable, may increase to 10 mg twice a day.
   - Current platelet count: <50×10^9/L, continue to hold the drug.
3. **Dose reduction for thrombocytopenia.** To avoid dose interruptions for thrombocytopenia, consider dose reductions if the platelet counts decrease as follows:
   - Platelet count: 100 to <125×10^9/L: If dose at the time of platelet decline is 25 mg twice a day, the new dose should be 20 mg twice a day. If dose at the time of platelet decline is 20 mg twice a day, the new dose should be 15 mg twice a day. If the dose at the time of platelet decline is 15 mg, 10 mg, or 5 mg twice a day at the time of platelet decline, do not change the dose.
   - Platelet count: 75 to <100×10^9/L: If dose at the time of platelet decline is 25 mg twice a day, the new dose should be 10 mg twice a day. If dose at the time of platelet decline is 20 mg twice a day, the new dose should be 10 mg twice a

R

day. If dose at the time of platelet decline is 15 mg twice a day, the new dose should be 10 mg twice a day. If dose at the time of platelet decline is either 10 mg or 5 mg twice a day, do not change the dose.

- Platelet count 50 to <75×10^9/L: If dose at the time of platelet decline is 25 mg, 20 mg, 15 mg, or 10 mg twice a day, the new dose should be 5 mg twice a day. If dose at the time of platelet decline is 5 mg twice a day, do not change the dose.
- Platelet count <50×10^9/L: Hold the ruxolitinib dose regardless of the twice daily dose.

4. When giving ruxoliltinib with strong CYP3A4 inhibitors (see *Drug Interactions* for the list), the recommended starting dose is 10 mg twice a day for clients with a platelet count greater than or equal to 100×10^9/L. Additional dose modifications can be made with careful monitoring of safety and efficacy.
5. When discontinuing ruxolitinib for reasons other than thrombocytopenia, gradual tapering of the dose may be considered (e.g., 5 mg twice a day each week).
6. If a dose is missed, the client should not take an additional dose but take the next usual prescribed dose.
7. In clients with moderate to severe renal impairment, the recommended starting dose is 10 mg twice a day for those with a platelet count between 100×10^9/L and 150×10^9/L and moderate creatinine clearance (C_{CR} from 30–59 mL/min) or severe renal impairment (C_{CR} 15–29 mL/min). Additional dose modifications can be made with careful monitoring of safety and efficacy.
8. In clients with end-stage renal disease who are on dialysis, the recommended starting dose is 15 mg for those with a platelet count between 100×10^9/L and 200×10^9/L or 20 mg for clients with a platelet count >200 $\times 10^9$/L. Subsequent doses should be given on dialysis days following each dialysis session. Additional dose modifications can be made with careful monitoring of safety and efficacy.
9. In clients with impaired hepatic function, the recommended starting dose is 10 mg twice a day for clients with a platelet count between 100×10^9/L and 150×10^9/L. Additional dose modifications can be made with careful monitoring of safety and efficacy.
10. For those unable to ingest tablets, ruxolitinib can be given through a nasogastric tube (8 French or greater) as follows: Suspend 1 tablet in approximately 40 mL of water and stir for about 10 min; within 6 hr after the tablet has dispersed, the suspension can be given through a nasogastric tube using an appropriate syringe. Rinse the tube with approximately 75 mL of water.
11. Store from 15–30°C (59–86°F).

ASSESSMENT

1. Note disease onset, clinical presentation, and associated symptoms. Dosage based on platelet counts,(those with platelet counts of less than 200×10^9/L at the start of therapy are more likely to develop thrombocytopenia during treatment).
2. Ensure infection-free prior to initiating therapy. Observe for S&S of infection and initiate therapy promptly if evident. Review risk of developing serious bacterial, mycobacterial, fungal and viral infections.
3. Assess for symptoms of herpes zoster and stress importance of early treatment.
4. Obtain CBC/platelets before therapy and monitor every two to four weeks until doses stabilized; monitor renal and LFTs and reduce dose or avoid with dysfunction.

CLIENT/FAMILY TEACHING

1. Take twice a day with or without food as directed. Avoid grapefruit juice. Dose based on hematologic parameters and may require adjustment.
2. Report any signs of infection: fever, chills, sore throat, painful urination, etc.
3. Practice reliable contraception; report if pregnancy occurs.
4. Drug associated with thrombocytopenia, anemia, and neutropenia so labs will occur often.
5. Report any unusual bruising or bleeding, yellow skin or eyes, RUQ pain, or LLQ pain.
6. Avoid contact sports with enlarged spleen.
7. Report S&S of herpes zoster infections and seek medical care/treatment.
8. Keep all F/U to assess response, regularly scheduled labs, and adverse SE.

OUTCOMES/EVALUATE

- Treatment of myelofibrosis symptoms
- ↓ Spleen size ↑ RBCs/platelets

R

S

Salmeterol xinafoate

(sal-**MET**-er-ole)

Classification(s): Sympathomimetic

Pregnancy Category: C

RX: Serevent Diskus.

SEE ALSO ***SYMPATHOMIMETIC DRUGS***.

INDICATIONS/USES

(1) Treatment of asthma and the prevention of bronchospasm only as concomitant therapy with a long-term asthma control medication, such as an inhaled corticosteroid, in clients age 4 years and older with reversible obstructive airway disease, including those with symptoms of nocturnal asthma. (2) Chronic maintenance (twice daily) treatment of bronchospasms associated with COPD, including emphysema and chronic bronchitis. (3) Prevention of exercise-induced bronchospasm in clients 4 years of age and older. Use of salmeterol as a single agent for prevention of exercise-induced bronchospasm in those who do not have persistent asthma.

ACTION/KINETICS

Action

Selective for $beta_2$-adrenergic receptors located in the bronchi and heart. Only minimal activity for beta-1-receptors. Acts by stimulating intracellular adenyl cyclase, the enzyme that converts ATP to cyclic AMP. Increased AMP levels cause relaxation of bronchial smooth muscle and inhibition of release of mediators of immediate hypersensitivity, especially from mast cells.

Pharmacokinetics

Onset, inhalation: Within 5–45 min. **Duration:** 12 hr. Cleared by hepatic metabolism. **Plasma protein binding:** Significantly bound.

CONTRAINDICATIONS

Use in clients who can be controlled by short-acting, inhaled $beta_2$-agonists or in those whose asthma can be successfully managed by inhaled corticosteroids or other controller medications, along with occasional use of inhaled, short-acting $beta_2$-agonists. Use to treat acute symptoms of asthma or in those who have worsening or deteriorating asthma. Lactation.

SPECIAL CONCERNS

(1) Long-acting $beta_2$-adrenergic agonists, such as salmeterol, may increase the risk of asthma-related death. Data from a large placebo-controlled U.S. study that compared the safety of salmeterol or placebo added, to usual asthma therapy showed an increase in asthma-related deaths in clients receiving salmeterol. This finding is considered a class effect of long-acting $beta_2$ agonists. All long-acting $beta_2$ agonists are contraindicated in clients with asthma without the use of a long-term asthma control medication. Currently available data are inadequate to determine whether concurrent use of inhaled corticosteroids or other long-term asthma control drugs mitigates the increased risk of asthma-related death from long-acting $beta_2$-adrenergic agonists. (2) Once asthma control is achieved and maintained, assess the client at regular intervals and step down therapy (e.g., discontinue salmeterol) if possible without loss of asthma control and maintain the client on a long-term asthma control medication, such as an inhaled corticosteroid. Do not use salmeterol for clients whose asthma is adequately controlled on low- or medium-dose inhaled corticosteroids. (3) **Children and adolescents.** Available data from controlled clinical trials suggest that long-acting $beta_2$-adrenergic agonists increase the risk of asthma-related hospitalization in pediatric and adolescent clients. For children and adolescents with asthma who require addition of a long-acting $beta_2$ agonist to an inhaled corticosteroid, a fixed-dose combination product containing both an inhaled corticosteroid and a long-acting $beta_2$-adrenergic agonist should ordinarily be used to ensure adherence with both drugs. In cases where use of a separate long-term asthma control medication (e.g., inhaled corticosteroid) and a long-acting $beta_2$-adrenergic agonist is clinically indicated, appropriate steps must be taken to en-

S

sure adherence with both treatment components. If adherence cannot be ensured, a fixed-dose combination product containing both an inhaled corticosteroid and a long-acting $beta_2$-adrenergic agonist is recommended. ■

- **Not a substitute for PO or inhaled corticosteroids.**
- **The safety and efficacy of using salmeterol with a spacer or other devices not studied adequately.**
- **Use with caution in impaired hepatic function; with cardiovascular disorders, including coronary insufficiency, cardiac arrhythmias, ischemic heart disease, coronary artery disease, CHF, and hypertension; with convulsive disorders or thyrotoxicosis; and in clients who respond unusually to sympathomimetic amines.**
- **Due to potential of the drug interfering with uterine contractility, use of salmeterol during labor should be restricted to those in whom benefits clearly outweigh risks.**
- **Safety and efficacy not determined in children less than 4 years of age.**

SIDE EFFECTS

Most Common

Palpitations, tachycardia, tremor, dizziness/vertigo, nervousness, headache, N&V, heartburn, diarrhea, cough, dry/irritated throat, pharyngitis, URTI, nasopharyngitis.

Respiratory: ***Paradoxical bronchospasms***, upper or lower respiratory tract infection, asthma, nasopharyngitis, nasal cavity/sinus disease, dry/irritated throat, nasal/sinus congestion, sinus headache, cough, pharyngitis, allergic rhinitis, rhinitis, laryngitis, sinusitis, tracheitis, bronchitis; ***increased risk of severe, fatal asthma episodes***. **Allergic:** ***Immediate hypersensitivity reactions***, including urticaria, rash, and ***bronchospasm***. **CV:** Palpitations, chest pain, increased BP, hypertension, tachycardia, arrhythmias (atrial fibrillation, SVT, extrasystoles). **CNS:** Headache, sinus headache, tremors, nervousness, shakiness, tension, dizziness/vertigo, giddiness, anxiety, giddiness, migraine, paresthesia, sleep disturbance. **GI:** N&V, diarrhea, heartburn, GI distress, stomachache, viral gastroenteritis, candidiasis of the mouth/throat, dyspeptic symptoms, hyposalivation, dental discomfort/pain, GI infections, oral mucosal abnormality. **Dermatologic:** Skin eruption, urticaria, rash, contact dermatitis, eczema, photodermatitis. **Musculoskeletal:** Joint/back pain, muscle cramps/contractions/soreness, myalgia, myositis, arthralgia, articular rheumatism, muscle pain, bone and skeletal pain, musculoskeletal inflammation, muscle stiffness, tightness, rigidity. **Respiratory:** Tracheitis, bronchitis, lower respiratory signs/symptoms, viral respiratory infection; upper airway symptoms of laryngeal spasm, irritation, or swelling such as stridor or choking; oropharyngeal irritation. **GU:** Dysmenorrhea, possible inhibition of uterine contractions during labor/delivery. **Ophthalmic:** Conjunctivitis, keratitis. **Otic:** Ear signs/symptoms. **Body as a whole:** Malaise, fatigue, influenza syndrome, edema, pain, pyrexia of unknown origin. **Miscellaneous:** Swelling, ***anaphylaxis,*** rarely anaphylactic reaction in those with severe milk protein allergy.

LABORATORY TEST CONSIDERATIONS

Hypokalemia.

OVERDOSE MANAGEMENT

Symptoms: Tachycardia, arrhythmia, tremors, headache, muscle cramps, hypokalemia, hyperglycemia. *Treatment:* Supportive therapy. Consider judicious use of a beta-adrenergic blocking agent, although these drugs can cause bronchospasms. Cardiac monitoring is necessary. Dialysis is not an appropriate treatment of overdosage.

DRUG INTERACTIONS

NOTE: An additive effect of salmeterol with other drugs that prolong the QT interval cannot be excluded.

Atazanavir / ↑ Salmeterol plasma levels; coadministration not recommended

Clarithromycin / ↑ Salmeterol plasma levels; coadministration not recommended

Diuretics / Worsening of diuretic-induced ECG changes and hypokalemia

Erythromycin / ↑ Salmeterol C_{max}, HR, and QTc interval; use together with caution

Indinavir / ↑ Salmeterol plasma levels → prolongation of QT interval; coadministration not recommended

Itraconazole / ↑ Salmeterol plasma levels → prolongation of QT interval; coadministration not recommended

Ketoconazole / ↑ Salmeterol plasma levels → prolongation of QT interval; coadministration not recommended

MAOIs / ↑ Salmeterol effect
Nefazodone / ↑ Salmeterol plasma levels → prolongation of QT interval; coadministration not recommended
Nelfinavir / ↑ Salmeterol plasma levels → prolongation of QT interval; coadministration not recommended
Ritonavir / ↑ Salmeterol plasma levels → prolongation of QT interval; coadministration not recommended
Saquinavir / ↑ Salmeterol plasma levels → prolongation of QT interval; coadministration not recommended
Telithromycin / ↑ Salmeterol plasma levels → prolongation of QT interval; coadministration not recommended
Tricyclic antidepressants / ↑ Salmeterol effect

HOW SUPPLIED

Powder for Inhalation: 50 mcg (base)/inhalation.

DOSAGE

POWDER FOR INHALATION

Bronchospasm; asthma, including nocturnal asthma.

Adults and children 4 years and over: 1 inhalation (50 mcg) twice a day (morning and evening, approximately 12 hr apart). If a previously effective dose fails to provide the usual response, seek medical advice immediately as this is often a sign of destabilization of asthma. If symptoms arise in the period between doses, use a short-acting, inhaled $beta_2$-agonist for immediate relief.

Bronchospasm associated with chronic obstructive pulmonary disease (COPD).

Adults: 1 inhalation (50 mcg) of the powder twice a day in the morning and evening (about 12 hr apart).

Prevention of exercise-induced bronchospasms.

Adults and children over 4 years of age: 1 inhalation (50 mcg) at least 30 min before exercise. Protection may last up to 9 hr in adolescents and adults and up to 12 hr in those 4–11 years of age. Additional doses should not be used for 12 hr. In those who are receiving salmeterol twice daily, do not use additional salmeterol for prevention of exercise-induced bronchospasm.

NURSING IMPLICATIONS

Do not confuse Serevent with Seroquel (an antipsychotic).

IMPLEMENTATION/ADMINISTRATION/STORAGE

1. Ensure doses are spaced 12 hr apart. Side effects are more likely to occur with higher doses or more frequent administration.
2. The safety of more than 8 inhalations per day of short-acting $beta_2$-agonists with salmeterol has not been established. If a previously effective dose fails to provide the usual response, contact provider immediately.
3. Do not exhale into the inhalation device; only activate and use the inhalation device in a level, horizontal position. Do not use a spacer.
4. When beginning salmeterol in those receiving PO or inhaled corticosteroids to treat asthma, clients should be continued on a suitable corticosteroid dose to maintain clinical stability even if they feel better as a result of initiating salmeterol.
5. The client should also be prescribed an inhaled, short-acting $beta_2$-agonist (e.g., albuterol) to treat symptoms that occur acutely despite regular twice-daily (morning and evening) use of salmeterol.
6. When beginning treatment with salmeterol, instruct clients who have been taking inhaled, short-acting $beta_2$-agonists on a regular basis (e.g., 4 times per day) to discontinue the regular use of such drugs and to use them only for symptomatic relief of acute asthma or COPD symptoms.
7. Store the inhalation powder from 20–25°C (68–77°F) in a dry place away from direct heat or sunlight. Keep the mouthpiece dry and never wash the mouthpiece or any part of the device.
8. For the inhalation of powder (Diskus), a built-in dose counter shows the number of doses remaining. The inhalation device is not reusable; discard after every blister has been used or 6 weeks after removal from the moisture-protective foil overwrap, whichever comes first.

S

ASSESSMENT

1. Note indications for therapy, onset, characteristics of S&S, triggers, clinical presentation; list agents trialed without desired control.
2. Assess for cardiac/liver dysfunction, thyrotoxicosis, hypertension, seizure disorders; may preclude therapy. Check ECG and use with caution in those with cardiac disease.
3. Advise of risk of asthma-related death. Salmeterol is contraindicated when used without a concomitant long-term asthma control medication (e.g., inhaled corticosteroid) for the treatment of asthma.
4. Review CXR and cardiopulmonary findings. Monitor VS, lung sounds, liver enzymes, electrolytes, PFTs (ABGs, FEV).

CLIENT/FAMILY TEACHING

1. Review proper use (with actuator) and obtain instruction. Shake well. Use the inhalation device in a level, horizontal position. Do not use a spacer. Record peak flows and identify critical zones.
2. Use only as directed; do not exceed prescribed dosage and administration frequency (drug effects last 12 hr).
3. Do not use drug during an acute asthma attack.
4. Review procedure for use of the short-acting $beta_2$-agonist (i.e., albuterol) prescribed to treat symptoms of asthma that occur between the salmeterol dosing schedule. Increased utilization warrants medical evaluation.
5. May experience palpitations, chest pain, headaches, tremors, nervousness, dizziness, drowsiness as side effects. Report immediately if chest pain, fast pounding irregular heartbeat, hives, increased wheezing, or difficulty breathing occurs.
6. Acetaminophen or other analgesic may relieve drug related headaches.
7. Take 30–60 min before activity to prevent acute bronchospasms. If already prescribed twice daily, do not take additional dose before exercise.
8. Salmeterol does not replace inhaled or systemic steroids; do not stop prescribed steroid therapy abruptly without approval.
9. Identify appropriate support groups that may assist to cope and live a normal life with asthma.
10. Stop smoking; avoid smoky environments and any other triggers that may aggravate breathing condition.
11. Be aware that when added to usual asthma therapy there may be an increase in asthma-related deaths.
12. Keep all F/U to assess response, labs, and for adverse SE.

OUTCOMES/EVALUATE

- Prevention/control of bronchospasm with COPD and asthma (e.g., decreased wheezing, dyspnea, orthopnea, and cough)
- Prevention of exercise-induced bronchospasms

Saquinavir mesylate ■

(sah-**KWIN**-ah-veer)

Classification(s): Antiviral, protease inhibitor

Pregnancy Category: B

RX: Invirase.

SEE ALSO ***ANTIVIRAL DRUGS.***

INDICATIONS/USES

In combination with ritonavir and other antiretroviral drugs to treat HIV-1 infection in adults older than 16 years of age. *NOTE:* Must be combined with ritonavir because ritonavir significantly inhibits metabolism of saquinavir to achieve increased plasma saquinavir levels.

ACTION/KINETICS

Action

HIV protease cleaves viral polyprotein precursors to form functional proteins in HIV-infected cells. Cleavage of viral polyprotein precursors is required for maturation of the infectious virus. Saquinavir inhibits the activity of HIV protease and prevents the cleavage of viral polyproteins, resulting in the formation of immature noninfectious viral particles.

Pharmacokinetics

Has a low bioavailability (4%) after PO use, probably due to incomplete absorption and first-pass metabolism. A high-fat meal or high-calorie meal increases the amount of drug absorbed. Women have a higher AUC than men. More than 90% of the hepatic metabolism is by CYP3A4. Saquinavir is also a substrate for P-glycoprotein; thus drugs that affect CYP3A4 or P-glycoprotein may change

S

the pharmacokinetics of saquinavir. Both metabolites and unchanged drug are excreted mainly through the feces. Higher levels seen in those with severe renal impairment or end-stage renal disease; there is a decrease in exposure in those with moderate hepatic impairment. **Plasma protein binding:** More than 98%.

CONTRAINDICATIONS

Hypersensitivity (e.g., anaphylactic reaction or Stevens–Johnson syndrome) to saquinavir, ritonavir, or any component of the product. Use in severe hepatic impairment when given with ritonavir. Congenital long QT syndrome; refractory hypokalemia or hypomagnesemia; complete AV block without implanted pacemakers, or those who are at high risk of complete AV block. Coadministration with drugs that both increase saquinavir plasma levels and prolong the QT interval. Coadministration with CYP3A substrates (e.g., alfuzosin, amiodarone, bepridil, cisapride, dihydroergotamine, dofetilide, ergonovine, ergotamine, flecainide, systemic lidocaine, lovastatin, methylergonovine, PO midazolam, pimozide, propafenone, quinidine, rifampin, sildenafil when used for pulmonary arterial hypertension, simvastatin, trazodone, and triazolam due to possible life–threatening reactions, such as cardiac arrhythmias or prolonged sedation (See *Drug Interactions*). Lactation.

SPECIAL CONCERNS

Saquinavir mesylate capsules and tablets and saquinavir soft gelatin capsules are not bioequivalent and cannot be used interchangeably. Use saquinavir mesylate only if it is combined with ritonavir, which significantly inhibits saquinavir's metabolism to provide plasma saquinavir levels at least equal to those achieved with saquinavir soft gelatin capsules. When using saquinavir as the sole protease inhibitor in an antiviral regimen, saquinavir soft gelatin capsules are the recommended formulation.

- **Photoallergy or phototoxicity may occur; take protective measures against exposure to ultraviolet or sunlight until tolerance is assessed.**
- **Use with caution in those with hepatic or renal insufficiency and in the elderly.**
- **Hemophiliacs treated with protease inhibitors for HIV infections may manifest spontaneous bleeding episodes.**
- **Cross resistance is possible among protease inhibitors.**
- **Safety and efficacy not determined in HIV-infected children or adolescents less than 16 years of age.**

SIDE EFFECTS

Most Common

N&V, fatigue, diarrhea, abdominal pain, pneumonia, pruritus, rash, fever, hyperglycemia, bronchitis, influenza, sinusitis.

GI: N&V, constipation, diarrhea, abdominal pain/discomfort, ascites, dry mouth, dysgeusia, dyspepsia, dysphagia, esophagitis, eructation, flatulence, gastralgia, gastritis, ***GI hemorrhage***, GI inflammation, gingivitis, glossitis, rectal hemorrhage, hemorrhoids, infectious diarrhea, melena, mucosa ulceration, intestinal obstruction, blood stained feces, frequent bowel movements, cheilitis, abdominal colic, pelvic pain, painful defecation, pancreatitis, parotid disorder, salivary glands disorder, stomach upset, stomatitis, toothache, tooth disorder. **Hepatic:** Hepatitis, chronic active hepatitis, hepatomegaly, hepatosplenomegaly, jaundice, portal hypertension, liver enzyme disorder. **CNS:** Agitation, amnesia, anxiety, coordination abnormal, depression, dizziness, excessive dreaming, euphoria, hallucinations, headache, insomnia, decreased intellectual ability, irritability, lethargy, libido disorder, loss of consciousness, paresthesia, peripheral neuropathy, psychosis, sleep disorder, somnolence, speech disorder, ***suicide attempt***, ataxia, confusion, ***convulsions***, dysarthria, dysesthesia, facial numbness, hyperesthesia, hypoesthesia, hyper-/hyporeflexia, lightheadedness, myelopolyradiculoneuritis, paresis, poliomyelitis, prickly sensation, progressive multifocal leukoencephalopathy, spasms, tremor, unconsciousness. **CV:** Cyanosis, heart murmur, heart rate/heart valve disorder, hyper-/hypotension, ***intracranial hemorrhage***, peripheral vasoconstriction, thrombophlebitis, PR interval prolongation ***(second– or third–degree heart block)***, QT interval prolongation (rarely, ***torsades de pointes***), syncope, spontaneous bleeding in those with hemophilia, vein distended. **Dermatologic:** Acne, dry lips/skin, pruritus, rash, alopecia, chalazion, dermatitis, drug eruption, eczema, erythema, folliculitis, furunculosis, hair changes, hot flushes, maculopapu-

S

lar rash, nail disorder, papillomatosis, photosensitivity reaction, bullous/seborrheic dermatitis, skin disorder/nodule/pigment changes, severe cutaneous reaction associated with increased LFTs, skin ulceration, increased sweating, ***Stevens–Johnson syndrome***, urticaria, verruca, xeroderma. **GU:** Impotence, enlarged prostate, nephrolithiasis, vaginal discharge. **Musculoskeletal:** Arthralgia, arthritis, back pain, leg cramps, facial pain, generalized weakness, muscle cramps/spasms, myalgia, musculoskeletal disorders, polyarthritis, stiffness, tissue changes, trauma. **Respiratory:** Bronchitis, cough, dyspnea, epistaxis, hemoptysis, laryngitis, pharyngitis, pneumonia, pulmonary disease, respiratory disorder, rhinitis, sinusitis, URTI. **Hematologic:** Thrombocytopenia, anemia, acute myeloid leukemia, hemolytic anemia, leukopenia, neutropenia, dermal bleeding, microhemorrhages, pancytopenia, splenomegaly. **Metabolic:** Dehydration, diabetes mellitus (new onset or exacerbation of existing), hyperglycemia, weight decrease/increase, lipodystrophy. **Ophthalmic:** Blepharitis, dry eye syndrome, eye irritation, visual disturbance, xerophthalmia. **Otic:** Decreased hearing, earache, ear pressure, otitis, tinnitus. **Body as a whole**: ***Allergic reaction***, increased/decreased appetite, asthenia, edema, fatigue, influenza, fever, intoxication, lethargy, shivering, wasting syndrome. **Resistance mechanism:** Abscess, angina tonsillaris, candidiasis, cellulitis, herpes simplex/zoster, bacterial/mycotic/staphylococcal infection, influenza, lymphadenopathy, moniliasis, tumor. **Miscellaneous:** Taste alteration, anorexia, chest pain, external parasites, night sweats, immune reconstitution syndrome, redistribution/accumulation of body fat (including breast enlargement, central obesity, "cushingoid appearance," dorsocervial fat enlargement, facial/peripheral wasting), retrosternal pain.

LABORATORY TEST CONSIDERATIONS

↑ ALT, AST, GGT, TSH, alkaline phosphatase, amylase, lactic dehydrogenase, creatinine phosphokinase, cholesterol, triglycerides. Hyper-/hypoglycemia, hypertriglyceridemia, hypocalcemia, hypophosphatemia, hyper-/hypokalemia, hyper-/hyponatemia, hyperbilirubinemia.

DRUG INTERACTIONS

NOTE: An additive effect of saquinavir with other drugs that prolong the QT interval cannot be excluded. The following drugs may prolong the QT interval and increase the risk of life-threatening cardiac arrhythmias, including torsades de pointes: Amiodarone, arsenic trioxide, bretylium, chlorpromazine, cisapride, clozapine, disopyramide, dofetilide, dolasetron, gatifloxacin, halofantrine, haloperidol, ibutilide, levomethadyl, mefloquine, mesoridazine, moxifloxacin, pentamidine, phenothiazines, pimozide, probucol, procainamide, quinidine, sotalol, sparfloxacin, tacrolimus, thioridazine, and ziprasidone.

Aldesleukin / ↑ Saquinavir levels; ↑ risk of toxicity; adjust aldesleukin dose as needed
Alfuzosin / ↑ Alfuzosin plasma levels; coadministration contraindicated
Amiodarone / Use together contraindicated due to potential for serious and/or life-threatening side effects
Amitriptyline / ↑ Amitriptyline levels; monitor amitriptyline plasma levels and adjust dose as needed
Aripiprazole / ↑ Aripiprazole levels and pharmacologic effects; avoid coadministration; consider ↓ aripiprazole dose by 50%
Atazanavir / Possible ↑ saquinavir plasma levels
Atorvastatin / ↑ Atorvastatin plasma levels → ↑ risk of myopathy, including rhabdomyolysis; use the lowest dose of atorvastatin with careful monitoring; consider using fluvastatin
Benzodiazepines (alprazolam, clorazepate, diazepam, flurazepam) / ↑ Benzodiazepine levels R/T inhibition of CYP3A4; ↓ dose may be needed
Bepridil / Use together contraindicated due to potential for serious and/or life-threatening side effects
Bosentan / ↑ Bosentan plasma levels (See ***Implementation/Administration/Storage***)
Buprenorphine / ↑ Buprenorphine plasma levels → ↑ risk of side effects, including respiratory depression; closely monitor
Buspirone / ↑ Buspirone plasma levels → ↑ pharmacologic/toxic effects; monitor closely
Calcium channel blockers (all) / ↑ Calcium channel blocker levels; use with caution and monitor; adjust calcium channel blocker dose as needed
Cabazitaxel / ↑ Cabazitaxel plasma levels → ↑ pharmacologic/toxic effects; avoid concurrent use
Carbamazepine / ↓ Saquinavir blood levels R/T ↑ metabolism; also, ↑ carbamazepine levels → ↑ risk of toxicity
Cimetidine / ↑ Saquinavir AUC and peak plasma levels R/T inhibition of CYP3A4 metabolism

S

Clarithromycin / ↑ Blood levels of both drugs and ↓ levels of 14-OH clarithromycin (active); reduce clarithromycin dose for those with impaired renal function
Colchicine / Do not coadminister to those with hepatic or renal impairment (See Implementation/Administration/Storage)
Cyclosporine / ↑ Cyclosporine and saquinavir blood levels; monitor levels and adjust cyclosporine dose
Darifenacin / ↑ Darifenacin plasma levels; do not exceed a dose of 7.5 mg darifenacin/day
Delavirdine / Significant ↑ in saquinavir plasma levels and ↓ delavirdine plasma levels; possibly ↓ saquinavir dose and ↑ delavirdine dose
Dexamethasone / ↓ Saquinavir blood levels → ↓ efficacy; use with caution
Digoxin / ↑ Digoxin plasma levels → ↑ risk of toxicity; use together with caution; monitor digoxin levels
Docetaxel / ↑ Docetaxel plasma levels → ↑ pharmacologic/toxic effects; avoid concurrent use; if concurrent use necessary, consider ↓ docetaxel dose by 50% with close monitoring
Dofetilide / Use together contraindicated due to potential for serious and/or life-threatening side effects
Dronedarone / Use together contraindicated due to potential for serious and/or life-threatening side effects
Efavirenz / ↓ Saquinavir and/or efavirenz blood levels; do not use saquinavir as the sole protease inhibitor
Eplerenone/ ↑ Eplerenone plasma levels → ↑ pharmacologic/toxic effect; monitor closely
Ergot derivatives (dihydroergotamine, ergonovine, ergotamine, methylergonovine) / Possibility of serious and life-threatening reactions, including acute ergot toxicity (peripheral vasospasm and ischemia of the extremities and other tissues)
Erlotinib / ↑ Erlotinib plasma levels → ↑ toxic effects; reduce erlotinib dose if necessary
Erythromycin / ↑ Erythromycin plasma levels; additive effects on prolongation of QT and/or PR interval; avoid coadministration
Eszopiclone / ↑ Eszopiclone plasma levels → ↑ pharmacologic/toxic effects; reduce eszopiclone dose
Everolimus / ↑ Everolimus plasma levels → ↑ pharmacologic/toxic effects; avoid coadministration
Fentanyl / ↑ Fentanyl plasma levels → ↑ risk of side effects, including respiratory depression; closely monitor
Fesoterodine / ↑ Fesoterodine plasma levels; do not exceed a dose of 4 mg fesoterodine a day
Flecainide / Use together contraindicated due to potential for serious and/or life-threatening side effects
Fluoxetine / ↑ Fluoxetine and saquinavir plasma levels → ↑ risk of toxicity (e.g., serotonin syndrome)
Fluticasone (inhaled/nasal) / ↑ Plasma fluticasone levels → significant reduced serum cortisol levels; do not use together unless benefits outweighs risk
Foscarnet / ↑ Risk of nephrotoxicity
H ***Garlic (capsules)*** / ↓ Saquinavir plasma levels; do not use if taking saquinavir as the sole protease inhibitor
Grapefruit juice / ↑ Bioavailability and blood levels of saquinavir R/T inhibition of metabolism by CYP3A4; avoid coadministration
5-HT$_1$ receptor agonists (selected ones, including eletriptan) / ↑ Triptan plasma levels and pharmacologic effects; do not give triptans within 72 hr of ritonavir
Iloperidone / ↑ Iloperidone plasma levels and pharmacologic effects; ↓ iloperidone dose by 50%
Imipramine / ↑ Imipramine levels; monitor imipramine plasma levels and adjust dose as needed
Indinavir / ↑ Saquinavir blood levels
Itraconazole / ↑ Saquinavir blood levels R/T ↓ metabolism; also ↑ itraconazole blood levels; monitor and adjust saquinavir dose if necessary; do not give more than 200 mg/day itraconazole
Ixabepilone / ↑ Ixabepilone plasma levels → ↑ risk of toxicity; avoid coadministration
Ketoconazole / ↑ Saquinavir blood levels R/T ↓ metabolism; also ↑ ketoconazole blood levels; monitor and adjust saquinavir dose if necessary; do not give more than 200 mg/day ketoconazole
Levothyroxine / ↑ or ↓ Thyroxine levels → hyperthyroidism or hypothyroidism; monitor carefully and adjust levothyroxine dose as needed
Lidocaine, systemic / Use together contraindicated due to potential for serious and/or life-threatening side effects
Loperamide / ↑ Loperamide plasma levels → ↑ pharmacologic/toxic effect; ↓ saquinavir plasma levels R/T ↓ saquinavir absorption; closely monitor for ↓ antiretroviral activity

S

Lopinavir/Ritonavir / See ***Implementation/Administration/Storage***
Lovastatin / ↑ Lovastatin plasma levels → ↑ risk of myopathy, including rhabdomyolysis; do not use together
Maraviroc / ↑ Maraviroc plasma levels; maraviroc dose should be 150 mg twice a day if given together
Methadone / ↓ Methadone levels; may need to ↑ methadone dosage when given with saquinavir/ritonavir; additive effects on QT and/or PR interval prolongation with saquinavir/ritonavir
Midazolam / Possible serious and/or life-threatening side effects, such as prolonged or increased sedation or respiratory depression; do not use together
Nelfinavir / ↑ Saquinavir and nelfinavir blood levels
Nevirapine / ↓ Saquinavir blood levels → ↓ efficacy
Nilotinib / ↑ Nilotinib plasma levels; avoid coadministration; if concurrent use necessary, monitor for side effects, including QT prolongation; nilotinib dosage adjustment may be needed
Oral contraceptives containing ethinyl estradiol / ↓ Ethinyl estradiol levels; use alternative or additional contraception
Oxycodone / ↑ Oxycodone plasma levels → ↑ risk of side effects, including respiratory depression; closely monitor
Phenobarbital / ↓ Saquinavir blood levels R/T ↑ metabolism
Phenytoin / ↓ Saquinavir blood levels R/T ↑ metabolism
Pimozide / Possible serious and/or life-threatening reactions; do not use together
Propafenone / Use together contraindicated due to potential for serious and/or life-threatening side effects
Proton pump inhibitors (e.g., omeprazole) / ↑ Saquinavir plasma levels and ↓ proton pump inhibitor levels; use together with caution and monitor for saquinavir toxicity
Quetiapine / ↑ Quetiapine plasma levels and pharmacologic effects
Quinidine / Use together contraindicated due to potential for serious and/or life-threatening side effects
Ranitidine / ↑ Saquinavir AUC and peak plasma levels R/T inhibition of CYP3A4 metabolism
Ranolazine / ↑ Plasma ranolazine levels → ↑ risk of dose-related prolongation of the QTc interval, torsades de pointes-type arrhythmias, and sudden death; coadministration contraindicated
Rapamycin / ↑ Rapamycin levels; monitor rapamycin levels and adjust dose as needed
Rifampin / ↓ Saquinavir blood levels and ↑ rifampin levels. Also, ↑ risk of severe hepatocellular toxicity; rifampin is contraindicated in those taking ritonavir, 100 mg/saquinavir, 1,000 mg twice daily
Risperidone / ↑ Risperidone plasma levels; ↑ risk of toxicity
Ritonavir / ↑ Saquinavir blood levels R/T inhibition of metabolism; must be used together
Ritonavir/Tipranavir / ↓ Saquinavir plasma levels; do not use together
Romidepsin / ↑ Romidepsin plasma levels → ↑ pharmacologic/toxic effects, including QT prolongation; avoid coadministration
Rosuvastatin / ↑ Rosuvastatin plasma level → ↑ risk of myopathy, including rhabdomyolysis; use the lowest dose of rosuvastatin
Salmeterol / ↑ Salmeterol plasma levels → ↑ risk of CV side effects, including QT prolongation, palpitations, and sinus tachycardia; coadministration not recommended
Sildenafil / ↑ Sildenafil plasma levels → severe and potentially fatal hypotension; use sildenafil with caution and do not exceed a dose of 25 mg q 48 hr; monitor
Silodosin / ↑ Silodosin plasma levels; coadministration contraindicated
Simvastatin / ↑ Simvastatin plasma levels → ↑ risk of myopathy, including rhabdomyolysis; do not use together
Solifenacin / ↑ Solifenacin plasma levels; do not exceed a dose of 5 mg solifenacin a day
H ***St. John's wort*** / ↓ Saquinavir plasma levels R/T ↑ CYP3A4 metabolism; do not use together
Tacrolimus / ↑ Tacrolimus levels; monitor tacrolimus levels and adjust dose as needed
Tadalafil / ↑ Tadalafil plasma levels; → severe and potentially fatal hypotension; use tadalafil with caution and do not exceed a dose of 10 mg q 72 hr; monitor
Tamsulosin / ↑ Tamsulosin plasma levels; coadministration contraindicated
Temsirolimus / ↑ Temsirolimus plasma levels → ↑ pharmacologic/toxic effects; avoid coadministration

S

Tolterodine / ↑ Tolterodine plasma levels; do not exceed a dose of 2 mg tolterodine a day
Trazodone / ↑ Trazodone levels → side effects R/T inhibition of CYP3A4; coadministration contraindicated
Triazolam / Possible serious and/or life-threatening side effects, such as prolonged or increased sedation or respiratory depression; do not use together
Tyrosine kinase inhibitors (e.g., dasatinib, lapatinib) / ↑ Tyrosine kinase inhibitor plasma levels → ↑ pharmacologic/toxic effects; closely monitor and adjust tyrosine kinase inhibitor dose as needed
Vardenafil / ↑ Vardenafil plasma levels → severe and potentially fatal hypotension; use vardenafil with caution and do not exceed a dose of 2.5 mg q 72 hr; monitor
Vasopressin receptor antagonists (e.g., conivaptan, tolvaptan) / ↑ Vasopressin receptor antagonist plasma levels and pharmacologic effect; coadministration contraindicated
Warfarin / Warfarin levels may be ↑ or ↓; monitor INR; adjust warfarin dose as needed

HOW SUPPLIED

Capsules: 200 mg (as mesylate); ***Tablets:*** 500 mg (as mesylate).

DOSAGE

CAPSULES; TABLETS

HIV infection, saquinavir given with ritonavir.

Adults, age 16 years and older: Saquinavir 1,000 mg twice a day (5 × 200 mg capsules or 2 × 500 mg tablets) in combination with ritonavir 100 mg twice a day. Take ritonavir at the same time as saquinavir and within 2 hr of a meal.

NURSING IMPLICATIONS

IMPLEMENTATION/ADMINISTRATION/STORAGE

1. If severe toxicity occurs, interrupt saquinavir until the cause of the event is identified or toxicity resolves. At that time, resumption of treatment may be considered.
2. Take within 2 hr of a full meal. If taken without food, blood levels may not be sufficiently high to exert an antiviral effect.
3. Doses less than 200 mg 3 times per day are not recommended; lower doses have not shown antiviral activity.
4. Interrupt therapy for serious toxicities associated with saquinavir mesylate. Base dosage adjustments on the known toxicity profile of the individual agent and the pharmacokinetic interaction between saquinavir and the coadministered drug. Doses of saquinavir mesylate less than 1,000 mg with ritonavir 100 mg twice a day are not recommended since lower doses do not have antiviral activity.
5. In clients receiving saquinavir/ritonavir for at least 10 days when bosentan is started, start bosentan at 62.5 mg once a day or every other day, based on tolerability. In clients receiving bosentan, discontinue bosentan at least 36 hr before starting saquinavir/ritonavir. At last 10 days after starting saquinavir/ritonavir, resume bosentan at a dose of 62.5 mg once a day or every other day, based on tolerability.
6. For treatment of gout flares, coadminister colchicine 0.6 mg followed by 0.3 mg 1 hr later. Do not repeat the dose earlier than 3 days. For prophylaxis of gout flares, if the original colchicine regimen was 0.6 mg twice a day, adjust the dose to 0.3 mg once a day. If the original colchicine dosage was 0.6 mg once a day, adjust the regimen to colchicine 0.3 mg every other day. For treating Mediterranean fever, coadminister colchicine at a maximum of 0.3 mg twice a day.
7. When given with lopinavir 400 mg/ritonavir 100 mg twice a day, the appropriate dosage of saquinavir mesylate is 1,000 mg twice a day (with no additional ritonavir).
8. To monitor maternal-fetal outcomes of pregnant women exposed to antiretroviral medication, an antiretroviral pregnancy registry has been established. Register clients by calling 1-800-258-4263.
9. Store Invirase from 15–30°C (59–86°F) in tightly closed bottles.

ASSESSMENT

1. Note onset, duration, characteristics of S&S, lab confirmation, other therapies trialed.
2. List drugs currently prescribed; drug is metabolized hepatically via cytochrome P450 system.

3. If serious or severe toxicity occurs, stop therapy until cause is determined or toxicity resolves. Monitor for opportunistic infections; treat appropriately.
4. Monitor CBC, chemistry, T-lymphocytes/viral load, triglycerides, renal and LFTs.

CLIENT/FAMILY TEACHING

1. Take only as prescribed and with or within 2 hr of a full meal with ritonavir; blood levels markedly reduced when taken without food. Invirase and Fortavase are not interchangeable; dosage differs.
2. Drug is not a cure for HIV infections. It does not prevent the occurrence or decrease the frequency of opportunistic infections associated with HIV but may prolong life.
3. May affect heart rhythm and electrical activity (in the heart). Report any S&S such as dizziness, fainting, light-headedness, or sensation of abnormal heartbeats, immediately.
4. Avoid sun exposure; take protective measures against UV or sunlight until tolerance assessed to avoid photosensitivity reaction.
5. Continue to use barrier contraception and practice safe sex; drug does not inhibit disease transmission. If pregnancy occurs, register on antiretroviral pregnancy registry by calling 1-800-258-4263.
6. May cause redistribution or accumulation of body fat.
7. Long-term drug effects still unknown; report side effects. May use analgesics, antidiarrheal, or antiemetics as prescribed/needed. Avoid any unprescribed or OTC agents; Viagra may cause adverse side effects, visual changes, and low BP. If needed, use once every 2 days and in doses not exceeding 25 mg.
8. Keep all F/U to assess response, labs, and for adverse SE.

OUTCOMES/EVALUATE

Control of HIV infections with ↓ viral load and ↑ CD4 count

S

IV

Sargramostim

(sar-**GRAM**-oh-stim)

Classification(s): Granulocyte colony-stimulating factor, human

Pregnancy Category: C

RX: Leukine.

INDICATIONS/USES

(1) Increase myeloid recovery in clients with non-Hodgkin's lymphoma, ALL, and Hodgkin's disease undergoing autologous bone marrow transplantation. (2) Bone marrow transplantation failure or engraftment delay. (3) Shorten recovery time to neutrophil recovery and to decrease the incidence of severe and life-threatening infections in older adult clients with AML. Safety and efficacy have not been determined in those less than 55 years of age. (4) Mobilize hematopoietic progenitor cells into peripheral blood collection by leukapheresis. (5) Acceleration of myeloid recovery in allogeneic bone marrow transplantation from human lymphocyte antigen-matched related donors. *Investigational:* Increase WBC counts in clients with myelodysplastic syndrome and in AIDS clients taking AZT; correct neutropenia in clients with aplastic anemia; decrease the nadir of leukopenia secondary to myelosuppressive chemotherapy and decrease myelosuppression in preleukemic clients; and, decrease organ system damage following transplantation, especially in the liver and kidney.

ACTION/KINETICS

Action

A granulocyte-macrophage colony-stimulating factor (rhu GM-CSF) that stimulates the proliferation and differentiation of hematopoietic progenitor cells. It stimulates partially committed progenitor cells to divide and differentiate in the granulocyte-macrophage pathways. Division, maturation, and activation are induced through GM-CSF binding to specific receptors located on the surface of target cells. Also activates mature granulocytes and macrophages. Increases the cytotoxicity of monocytes toward certain neoplastic cell lines as well as activates polymorphonuclear neutrophils, thus inhibiting the growth of tumor cells. Sargramostim differs from the naturally occurring GM-CSF by one amino acid and by a different carbohydrate moiety.

Pharmacokinetics

Peak levels: 2–3 hr, depending on the dose. **t½, initial:** 12–17 min; **t½, terminal:** 1.6–2.6 hr, depending on the dose. Neutralizing antibodies have been detected in a small number of clients.

CONTRAINDICATIONS

Use in more than 10% leukemic myeloid blasts in the bone marrow or peripheral blood. Known hypersensitivity to GM-CSF, yeast-derived products, or any component of the product. Simultaneous use with cytotoxic chemotherapy or radiotherapy or use within 24 hr preceding or following chemotherapy or radiotherapy.

SPECIAL CONCERNS

- **Use with caution in clients with pre-existing cardiac disease and hypoxia and during lactation.**
- **May aggravate fluid retention in clients with pre-existing peripheral edema, or pleural or pericardial effusion.**
- **Insufficient data on efficacy of sargramostim in increasing myeloid recovery after peripheral blood stem cell transplantation.**
- **Is possible that sargramostim can act as a growth factor for any tumor type, especially myeloid malignancies; thus, use with caution in any malignancy with myeloid characteristics.**
- **Safety and efficacy not determined in children although it appears the drug is no more toxic in children than in adults.**

SIDE EFFECTS

Most Common

Hypertension, hemorrhage, headache, rash, alopecia, N&V, diarrhea, abdominal pain, bone pain, GI disorder, stomatitis, anorexia, GI hemorrhage, blood dyscrasias, dyspnea, fever, mucous membrane disorder, malaise, weight loss, chills, asthenia, edema, myalgia, increased glucose.

First-dose effects (rare): Respiratory distress, hypoxia, flushing, hypotension, syncope, tachycardia. **CV:** Hyper-/hypotension, ***hemorrhage***, edema, peripheral edema, cardiac event, tachycardia, pericardial effusion, pleural effusion, ***capillary leak syndrome***, transient supraventricular arrhythmia, thrombosis. **GI:** N&V, diarrhea, abdominal pain, GI disorder, stomatitis, dyspepsia, anorexia, hematemesis, dysphagia, ***GI hemorrhage***, constipation, abdominal distension, liver damage, transient liver function abnormalities. **CNS:** Neuroclinical, neuromotor, neuropsychiatric, and neurosensory side effects. Paresthesia, headache, CNS disorder, insomnia, anxiety, fainting, dizziness. **Respiratory:** Pulmonary event, pharyngitis, lung disorder, epistaxis, dyspnea, rhinitis. **Hematologic:** Blood dyscrasias, thrombocytopenia, leukopenia, petechia, ***agranulocytosis***, coagulation disorders, eosinophilia. **Musculoskeletal:** Bone pain, arthralgia. **Dermatologic:** Rash, alopecia, pruritus, sweating. **GU:** Urinary tract disorder, hematuria, abnormal kidney function. **Body as a whole:** Asthenia, fever, infection, malaise, weight loss/gain, chills, pain, allergy, edema, mucous membrane disorder, metabolic disorder, ***sepsis, hypersensitivity reactions including anaphylaxis***. **Miscellaneous:** Chest/back/joint pain, eye hemorrhage, peripheral edema, injection site reactions.

LABORATORY TEST CONSIDERATIONS

↑ Glucose, BUN, cholesterol, bilirubin, serum creatinine, ALT, alkaline phosphatase. ↓ Albumin, calcium. Hypomagnesemia.

OVERDOSE MANAGEMENT

Symptoms: Dyspnea, malaise, nausea, fever, rash, sinus tachycardia, chills, headache. Increases in WBC less than or equal to 200,000 cells/mm^3. *Treatment:* Discontinue therapy. Monitor for increases in WBCs and for respiratory symptoms.

DRUG INTERACTIONS

Drugs such as corticosteroids and lithium may ↑ the myeloproliferative effects of sargramostim. The effect of sargramostim may be limited in those who have received alkylating agents, anthracycline antibiotics, or antimetabolites.

HOW SUPPLIED

Injection: 500 mcg/mL; ***Powder for Injection, Lyophilized:*** 250 mcg.

DOSAGE

IV INFUSION; SC

Myeloid reconstitution after autologous or allogenic bone marrow transplantation.

250 mcg/m^2/day as a 2-hr infusion beginning 2–4 hr after the autologous bone marrow infusion and greater than 24 hr after the last dose of chemotherapy and 12 hr after the last dose of radiotherapy. Do not give drug until the postmarrow infusion absolute neutrophil count (ANC) is less than 500 cells/mm^3. Continue until ANC is >1,500 cells/mm^3 for 3 consecutive days. To avoid complications of excessive leukocytosis, a CBC with differential is rec-

S

ommended twice weekly during therapy; interrupt or reduce the dose by 50% if the ANC >20,000 cells/m^3.

Bone marrow transplantation failure or engraftment delay.

250 mcg/m^2/day for 14 days as a 2-hr IV infusion. If engraftment has not occurred, therapy may be repeated after 7 days off therapy. A third course of 250 mcg/m^2/day may be undertaken after another 7 days off therapy. However, if no response occurs after three courses, it is unlikely the drug will be beneficial. To avoid complications of excessive leukocytosis, a CBC with differential is recommended twice weekly during therapy; interrupt or reduce the dose by 50% if the ANC >20,000 cells/m^3.

Neutrophil recovery following chemotherapy in acute myelogenous leukemia.

250 mcg/m^2/day given over a 4-hr period starting at about day 11 or 4 days following completion of induction chemotherapy. Use if the day 10 bone marrow is hypoplastic with less than 5% blasts. If a second cycle of therapy is needed, give about 4 days after the completion of chemotherapy if the bone marrow is hypoplastic with less than 5% blasts. Continue therapy until an absolute neutrophil count >1,500/mm^3 is noted for 3 consecutive days or a maximum of 42 days. If a severe adverse reaction occurs, decrease the dose by 50% or discontinue temporarily until the drug reaction is reduced. To avoid complications of excessive leukocytosis, a CBC with differential is recommended twice weekly during therapy; interrupt or reduce the dose by 50% if the ANC >20,000 cells/m^3.

Mobilization of peripheral blood progenitor cells (PBPCs).

250 mcg/m^2/day IV over 24 hr or SC once daily. Use this dose throughout the PBPC collection period. If the WBC count is >50,000 cells/mm^3, reduce the dose by 50%. If sufficient numbers of progenitor cells are not collected, use other mobilization therapy.

Postperipheral blood progenitor cell transplantation.

250 mcg/m^2/day IV over 24 hr or SC once daily beginning immediately after infusion of progenitor cells and continuing until an absolute neutrophil count >1,500 is reached for 3 consecutive days.

NURSING IMPLICATIONS

IMPLEMENTATION/ADMINISTRATION/STORAGE

1. Use for SC injection with no further dilution.
2. IV Give daily dosage as a 2-hr IV infusion beginning 2–4 hr after the autologous bone marrow infusion. Ensure at least 24 hr have elapsed after last dose of chemotherapy and 12 hr elapsed since the last dose of XRT.
3. Reduce dose or discontinue if severe adverse reactions occur; may resume once reactions abate.
4. Reconstitute lyophilized powder with 1 mL of sterile water for injection without preservatives. Direct sterile water at the side of the vial, followed by a gentle swirling of the contents to avoid foaming. Avoid excessive or vigorous agitation. Reconstituted solutions are clear, colorless, and isotonic with a pH of 7.4.
5. Dilute for IV infusion in 0.9% NaCl injection. If the final concentration is less than 10 mcg/mL, add human albumin at a final concentration of 0.1% to the saline prior to the addition of sargramostim (prevents adsorption of the drug delivery system). For a final concentration of 0.1% human albumin, add 1 mg human albumin/1 mL of 0.9% NaCl (use 1 mL of 5% human albumin) in 50 mL 0.9% NaCl injection.
6. Do not use an in-line membrane filter for IV infusion. Do not reenter or reuse the vial; discard unused portion.
7. Contains no preservatives; thus, give as soon as possible, but within 6 hr, following reconstitution or dilution for IV infusion. Store the sterile powder, reconstituted solution, and dilution solution in the refrigerator at 2–8°C (36–46°F). Do not freeze or shake solutions or use beyond the expiration date on the vial.
8. Sargramostim liquid may be stored for up to 20 days at 2–8°C (36–46°F). Do not freeze or shake.

S

9. COMPATIBILITY 0.9% NaCl.
10. INCOMPATIBILITY Do not add other drugs to infusion.

ASSESSMENT

1. Note sensitivity to yeast-derived products. List any cardiac disease, hypoxia, peripheral edema, pleural or pericardial effusion, or myeloid-type malignancy. Drug can act as tumor growth factor with myeloid cancers.
2. Assess cardiopulmonary status, lung sounds, and for any breathing difficulty.
3. List any therapy with drugs or radiation. Drug should *not* be administered 24 hr before or after cytotoxic chemotherapy or radiation therapy. Give within 2–4 hr of bone marrow infusion.
4. Monitor I&O, VS, and weight; assess for fluid retention or edema.
5. Assess for respiratory symptoms during or immediately following infusion, especially with pre-existing lung disease. Reduce rate of infusion by one-half if dyspnea occurs.
6. Monitor hematologic response with a CBC twice weekly. If the ANC exceeds 20,000/mm^3 or the platelet count exceeds 500,000/mm^3 or a severe reaction occurs, stop therapy and reduce dose by one-half. Excessive blood counts have returned to normal levels within 3–7 days following termination of therapy.
7. Renal and hepatic function should be monitored every 2 weeks with hepatic/renal dysfunction.
8. Drug effectiveness may be limited in clients who, before autologous bone marrow transplantation, received extensive radiotherapy in the chest or abdomen to treat the primary disease; effectiveness is also limited in those who have received multiple myelotoxic agents such as antimetabolites, alkylating agents, or anthracycline antibiotics.
9. Monitor CBC (ANC and platelets twice weekly during therapy- examine for blast cells), renal and LFTs as indicated.

CLIENT/FAMILY TEACHING

1. Drug is administered by injection to improve recovery time with transplant or chemotherapy. It helps to increase the number and function of your white blood cells.
2. Report any dyspnea, wheezing, chest pain, congestion, fever, fainting, rash or hives, rapid heart rate, chills, fluid in hands or feet, or other adverse side effects immediately.
3. Practice reliable contraception, report if pregnancy suspected.

OUTCOMES/EVALUATE

- Improved hematologic parameters; neutrophil recovery
- Mobilization of peripheral blood progenitor cells

Saxagliptin

(**SAX**-ah-**GLIP**-tin)

Classification(s): Antidiabetic drug, dipeptidyl peptidase-4 inhibitor

Pregnancy Category: B

RX: Onglyza.

INDICATIONS/USES

Adjunct to diet and exercise to improve glycemic control in adults with type 2 diabetes mellitus.

ACTION/KINETICS

Action

Increased levels of the incretin hormones (e.g., glucagon like peptide-1 and glucose-dependent insulinotropic polypeptide) are released into the bloodstream from the small intestine in response to meals. These hormones cause insulin release from the pancreatic beta cells in a glucose-dependent manner; however, they are inactivated by the dipeptidyl peptidase-4 (DPP4) enzyme within minutes. In clients with type 2 diabetes, concentrations of glucagon-like peptide-1 are reduced but the insulin response to this hormone is preserved. Saxagliptin is a competitive DPP4 inhibitor that slows the inactivation of the incretin hormones, thus increasing their bloodstream levels and reducing fasting and postprandial concentrations of glucose.

Pharmacokinetics

T_{max}, after 5 mg: 2 hr for saxagliptin and 4 hr for its active metabolite. A high-fat meal will increase T_{max} for about 20 min compared with fasting; however, no dosage adjustment is needed. Metabolized primarily by CYP3A4/5. The major metabolite of saxagliptin is also a DPP4 inhibitor, which is one-half as potent as saxagliptin. Excreted in both the urine and feces. **t½, terminal plasma:**

S

2.5 hr for saxagliptin and 3.1 hr for the active metabolite. **Plasma protein binding:** Negligible.

SPECIAL CONCERNS

- **Use caution in dose selection in the elderly.**
- **Use with caution during lactation.**
- **Safety and efficacy not determined in children.**

SIDE EFFECTS

Most Common

Hypoglycemia, headache, URTI, UTI, nasopharyngitis (when coadministered with metformin).

CNS: Headache. **GI:** Abdominal pain, vomiting. **Respiratory:** URTI, sinusitis. **Dermatologic:** Rash. **GU:** UTI. **Hematologic:** Lymphopenia, thrombocytopenia. **Metabolic:** Hypoglycemia. **Hypersensitivity:** Urticaria, facial edema. **Miscellaneous:** Peripheral edema, fractures.

LABORATORY TEST CONSIDERATIONS

↑ Blood creatinine, blood creatine phosphokinase. ↓ Absolute lymphocyte counts.

OVERDOSE MANAGEMENT

Symptoms: See side effects. *Treatment:* Supportive treatment determined by client's clinical status. Saxagliptin and its active metabolite are removed by hemodialysis.

DRUG INTERACTIONS

NOTE: Saxagliptin is metabolized by CYP3A4/5; thus, strong CYP3A4/5 inhibitors and inducers will alter the pharmacokinetics of saxagliptin and its active metabolite. Monitor the clinical response and adjust saxagliptin dosage if needed.

Aluminum hydroxide/magnesium hydroxide/simethicone / Coadministration of this mixture with saxagliptin ↓ C_{max} of saxagliptin but not AUC
Amprenavir / ↑ Saxagliptin exposure R/T inhibition of CYP3A4/5 metabolism; dosage adjustment not recommended but adjust dosage if interaction suspected
Antidiabetic agents (e.g., sulfonylureas) / ↑ Risk of hypoglycemia; lower dose may be needed
Aprepitant / ↑ Saxagliptin exposure R/T inhibition of CYP3A4/5 metabolism; dosage adjustment not recommended but adjust dosage if interaction suspected
Atazanavir / ↑ Saxagliptin C_{max} and AUC and ↓ C_{max} and AUC of the active metabolite R/T inhibition of metabolism by CYP3A4/5; reduce dose of saxagliptin to 2.5 mg a day; monitor client response
Clarithromycin / ↑ Saxagliptin C_{max} and AUC and ↓ C_{max} and AUC of the active metabolite R/T inhibition of metabolism by CYP3A4/5; reduce dose of saxagliptin to 2.5 mg a day; monitor client response
CYP3A4/5 inducers (e.g., rifampin) / ↓ C_{max} but not AUC; dosage adjustment not necessary unless an interaction is suspected
Diltiazem / ↑ Saxagliptin exposure R/T inhibition of CYP3A4/5 metabolism; dosage adjustment not recommended but adjust dosage if interaction suspected; also, ↑ diltiazem C_{max} but did not alter AUC
Erythromycin / ↑ Saxagliptin exposure R/T inhibition of CYP3A4/5 metabolism; dosage adjustment not recommended but adjust dosage if interaction suspected
Famotidine / ↑ Saxagliptin C_{max} but did not alter AUC
Fluconazole / ↑ Saxagliptin exposure R/T inhibition of CYP3A4/5 metabolism; dosage adjustment not recommended but adjust dosage if interaction suspected
Fosamprenavir / ↑ Saxagliptin exposure R/T inhibition of CYP3A4/5 metabolism; dosage adjustment not recommended but adjust dosage if interaction suspected
Glyburide / ↑ Saxagliptin and glyburide C_{max} but not the AUC of either drug
Grapefruit juice / ↑ Saxagliptin exposure; dosage adjustment not recommended
Indinavir / ↑ Saxagliptin C_{max} and AUC and ↓ C_{max} and AUC of the active metabolite R/T inhibition of metabolism by CYP3A4/5; reduce dose of saxagliptin to 2.5 mg a day; monitor client response
Itraconazole / ↑ Saxagliptin C_{max} and AUC and ↓ C_{max} and AUC of the active metabolite R/T inhibition of metabolism by CYP3A4/5; reduce dose of saxagliptin to 2.5 mg a day; monitor client response
Ketoconazole / ↑ Saxagliptin C_{max} and AUC and ↓ C_{max} and AUC of the active metabolite R/T inhibition of metabolism by CYP3A4/5; reduce dose of saxagliptin to 2.5 mg a day; monitor client response; also, ↓ ketoconazole C_{max} and AUC
Metformin / ↓ Saxagliptin C_{max} but did not alter AUC

S

Nefazodone / ↑ Saxagliptin C_{max} and AUC and ↓ C_{max} and AUC of the active metabolite R/T inhibition of metabolism by CYP3A4/5; reduce dose of saxagliptin to 2.5 mg a day; monitor client response
Nelfinavir / ↑ Saxagliptin C_{max} and AUC and ↓ C_{max} and AUC of the active metabolite R/T inhibition of metabolism by CYP3A4/5; reduce dose of saxagliptin to 2.5 mg a day; monitor client response
Pioglitazone / ↑ C_{max} of pioglitazone but did not alter AUC
Ritonavir / ↑ Saxagliptin C_{max} and AUC and ↓ C_{max} and AUC of the active metabolite R/T inhibition of metabolism by CYP3A4/5; reduce dose of saxagliptin to 2.5 mg a day; monitor client response
Saquinavir / ↑ Saxagliptin C_{max} and AUC and ↓ C_{max} and AUC of the active metabolite R/T inhibition of metabolism by CYP3A4/5; reduce dose of saxagliptin to 2.5 mg a day; monitor client response
Simvastatin / ↑ Saxagliptin C_{max} but did not alter AUC
Telithromycin / ↑ Saxagliptin C_{max} and AUC and ↓ C_{max} and AUC of the active metabolite R/T inhibition of metabolism by CYP3A4/5; reduce dose of saxagliptin to 2.5 mg a day; monitor client response
Verapamil / ↑ Saxagliptin exposure R/T inhibition of CYP3A4/5 metabolism; dosage adjustment not recommended but adjust dosage if interaction suspected

HOW SUPPLIED

Tablets: 2.5 mg, 5 mg.

DOSAGE

TABLETS

Type 2 diabetes mellitus.

Adults: 2.5 or 5 mg once a day.

NURSING IMPLICATIONS

Do not confuse saxagliptin with sitagliptin (also an antidiabetic drug).

IMPLEMENTATION/ADMINISTRATION/STORAGE

1. Take without regard to meals.
2. Reduce the dose to 2.5 mg once a day in those with moderate to severe renal impairment (C_{CR} 50 mL/min or less) or if coadministered with strong CYP3A4/5 inhibitors (see *Drug Interactions).*
3. Administer a dose of 2.5 mg once daily after hemodialysis in those with end-stage renal disease requiring hemodialysis.
4. Store from 15–30°C (59–86°F).

ASSESSMENT

1. Note age at diabetes onset, BMI, family Hx, previous therapies utilized, outcome.
2. List drugs prescribed to ensure none interact.
3. Monitor BP, Wt, CBC, BS, HbA1c, microalbumin, renal and LFTs.

CLIENT/FAMILY TEACHING

1. Drug acts to lower blood sugar by helping the body release insulin after meals.
2. Regular exercise, decreased caloric intake, and weight loss are required to reduce blood glucose levels; medication neither replaces nor excuses compliance with these modalities.
3. May experience headache, URI or UTI; report if bothersome or persistent.
4. Practice reliable contraception, report if pregnancy suspected.
5. Review reports of pancreatitis with saxagliptin and symptoms, such as persistent severe abdominal pain (may radiate to the back and may be accompanied by vomiting, which can indicate pancreatitis). Stop taking saxagliptin and contact provider immediately if these occur
6. Keep all F/U to assess response, labs, and adverse SE.

OUTCOMES/EVALUATE

Control of BS; HbA1c <8%

IV

Scopolamine hydrobromide (Hyoscine hydrobromide)

(scoh-**POLL**-ah-meen)

Classification(s): Cholinergic blocking drug; antiemetic

Pregnancy Category: C

RX: Isopto Hyoscine Ophthalmic, Scopace.

S

Scopolamine transdermal therapeutic system

Pregnancy Category: C

RX: Transderm-Scop.

🍁 **Rx:** Transderm-V.

SEE ALSO ***CHOLINERGIC BLOCKING AGENTS***.

INDICATIONS/USES

Ophthalmic: (1) For cycloplegia and mydriasis in diagnostic procedures. (2) For some preoperative and postoperative states in the treatment of iridocyclitis.

Oral: (1) Prevention of motion sickness. (2) Inhibits excessive motility and hypertonus of the GI tract, including conditions such as irritable bowel syndrome, mild dysentery, diverticulitis, pylorospasm, and cardiospasm. (3) Symptomatic treatment of postencephalitic parkinsonism and paralysis agitans. (4) Spastic states.

Parenteral: (1) Preanesthetic sedation for sedative, tranquilizing, and antisecretory effects. (2) Antiemetic. (3) Treat maniacal states. (4) Delirium tremens. (5) Obstetrics. (6) Mydriasis/cycloplegia.

Transdermal: In adults for prevention of N&V associated with motion sickness or recovery from anesthesia and surgery.

ACTION/KINETICS

Action

Anticholinergic with CNS depressant effects; produces amnesia when given with morphine or meperidine. Inhibits excessive motility and hypertonus of the GI tract. In the presence of pain, delirium may be produced. Causes pupillary dilation and paralyzes the muscle required to accommodate for close vision (cycloplegia). This enables the physician to examine the inner structure of the eye, including the retina, as well as to examine refractive errors of the lens without automatic accommodation by the client. Tolerance may develop if scopolamine is used alone.

Pharmacokinetics

When used for refraction: **Peak for mydriasis:** 20–30 min; **peak for cycloplegia:** 30–60 min; **recovery:** 24 hr (residual cycloplegia and mydriasis may last for 3–7 days). Recovery time can be reduced by using 1–2 gtt pilocarpine (1% or 2%). To reduce absorption, apply pressure over the nasolacrimal sac for 2–3 min. The transdermal therapeutic system contains 1.5 mg scopolamine, which is slowly released from a mineral oil-polyisobutylene matrix. Approximately 0.5 mg is released from the system per day. **Parenteral use effect:** 1–2 hr; **duration:** About 4 hr.

ADDITIONAL CONTRAINDICATIONS

Hypersensitivity to any component of the products. Use of the transdermal system in children or lactating women. Ophthalmic use in glaucoma (e.g., narrow anterior chamber angle). Adhesions between the iris and the lens. PO use in those with impaired hepatic or renal function.

SPECIAL CONCERNS

- **Use with caution in children, infants, geriatric clients, diabetes, hypo- or hyperthyroidism, narrow anterior chamber angle.**
- **Increased sensitivity possible in those with Down syndrome, children with brain damage, and in the elderly.**
- **Use with caution during lactation.**
- **Safety and efficacy of ophthalmic use not determined in children.**

SIDE EFFECTS

Most Common

When used systemically: Dizziness, drowsiness, dry mouth, flushing, blurred vision, headache, nausea.

When used ophthalmically: Transient stinging/burning, increased intraocular pressure, blurred vision, light sensitivity, dry mouth, dizziness, drowsiness.

See *Cholinergic Blocking Agents* for a complete list of possible side effects. Disorientation, delirium, increased HR, decreased respiratory rate. **Ophthalmic:** Increased intraocular pressure, transient stinging/burning, blurred vision, photophobia with or without corneal staining, irritation with long–term use (e.g., allergic lid reactions, hyperemia, follicular conjunctivitis, blepharoconjunctivitis, vascular congestion, edema, exudate, eczematoid dermatitis). Systemic side effects after ophthalmic use are possible and include dry mouth and skin, tachycardia, headache, parasympathetic stimulation, somnolence, visual hallucinations. **Transdermal:** Frequently, dry mouth, drowsiness, blurred vision, dilation of pupils. Infrequently, disorientation, memory disturbances, dizziness, restlessness, hallucinations, confusion, difficulty

S

urinating, rashes or erythema, narrow-angle glaucoma; dry, itchy, or red eyes.

NOTE: Elderly and debilitated clients may respond to the usual doses with agitation, confusion, drowsiness, or excitement.

OVERDOSE MANAGEMENT

Symptoms: See side effects. *Treatment:* For ocular overdose, flush the eye(s) with water or normal saline. Use of a topical miotic may be required.

ADDITIONAL DRUG INTERACTIONS

Grapefruit juice / ↑ Scopolamine bioavailability and time to reach peak plasma levels

HOW SUPPLIED

Scopolamine hydrobromide: *Injection:* 0.3 mg/mL, 0.4 mg/mL, 0.86 mg/mL, 1 mg/mL; *Ophthalmic Solution:* 0.25%; *Tablets, Soluble:* 0.4 mg.

Scopolamine transdermal therapeutic system: *Film, Extended-Release, Transdermal:* 1.5 mg (delivers about 1 mg over 3 days).

DOSAGE

OPHTHALMIC SOLUTION

Cycloplegia/mydriasis.

Adults: 1–2 gtt of the 0.25% solution in the conjunctiva 1 hr prior to refraction.

Iridocyclitis.

Adults: 1 gtt of the 0.25% solution 1–4 times per day as required.

IM; IV; SC

Antiemetic.

Adults: 0.6–1 mg SC. **Pediatric:** 0.006 mg/kg (0.2 mg/m^2) SC. Maximum dose: 0.3 mg.

Preoperative sedation.

Adults: 0.32–0.65 mg. **Children, 3–6 years:** 0.2–0.3 mg; **6 months–3 years:** 0.1–0.15 mg.

Obstetric amnesia.

0.32–0.65 mg.

Sedation/Tranquilization.

Adults: 0.6 mg 3 or 4 times/day. **Children, 3–6 years:** 0.2–0.3 mg; **6 months–3 years:** 0.1–0.15 mg

TABLETS, SOLUBLE

Prevent motion sickness. GI tract disorders. Postencephalitic parkinsonism.

Adults, usual: 0.4–0.8 mg.

TRANSDERMAL SYSTEM

Antiemetic, antivertigo.

Adults: 1 transdermal system placed on the postauricular skin to deliver 1 mg over 3 days (apply at least 4 hr before antiemetic effect is required). The Canadian product should be applied about 12 hr before the antiemetic effect is desired.

NURSING IMPLICATIONS

IMPLEMENTATION/ADMINISTRATION/STORAGE

1. Give drops into the conjunctival sac followed by digital pressure for 2–3 min after instillation.
2. Do not give alone for pain because it may cause delirium; use an analgesic or sedative as needed.
3. Lower doses may be required in the elderly and debilitated
4. Store ophthalmic solution from 8–27°C (46–80°F). Store tablets and injection from 15–30°C (59–86°F). Protect the ophthalmic solution and injection from light.
5. IV Protect solution from light.
6. Dilute dose with equal volume of diluent and inject slowly over 2–3 min.
7. COMPATIBILITY Dilute with sterile water for injection prior to administration.
8. INCOMPATIBILITY Administer separately. Incompatible with alkaline solutions.

ASSESSMENT

1. Note reasons for therapy, onset, characteristics of S&S. List any conditions that may preclude therapy (acute hemorrhage, BPH, pyloric obstruction etc.).
2. With eye drops, check for angle-closure glaucoma; may precipitate glaucoma crisis.
3. Determine presence of pain before using as drug may act as stimulant and precipitate delirium if used without opioid analgesics in this condition. Assess for urinary retention during therapy.
4. Some clients may experience toxic delirium with therapeutic doses. Observe closely and

S

have physostigmine available to reverse effects.

5. Monitor HR during parenteral therapy; assess for N&V when using as antiemetic. Assess for thyroid abnormalities and use with caution.

CLIENT/FAMILY TEACHING

1. Use exactly as directed. Take oral agents 30 min before meals. Do not share; store safely out of reach of children.
2. Do not drive or operate dangerous machinery until drug effects realized; may cause drowsiness, confusion, disorientation, and, with eye drops, blurred vision and dilated pupils.
3. Wash hands before and after use. Do not permit dropper to come in contact with eye.
4. Tilt head back, looking up, pull lower eyelid down to form pocket and place prescribed number of drops in the pocket. Look downward before closing eye and compress lacrimal sac for 2 to 3 min after instillation; do not rub eye(s).
5. If other eye drops prescribed, wait 5 min before instilling.
6. Wear dark glasses if photosensitivity occurs; report if eye pain occurs. May temporarily impair vision.
7. With the transdermal system:
   - Wash hands before and after application.
   - Apply at least 4 hr before desired effect.
   - Apply to a clean, nonhairy site, behind the ear.
   - To minimize exposure to the newborn baby, apply 1 hr prior to cesarean section.
   - Use pressure to apply the patch to ensure contact with the skin.
   - Replace with a new system on another site if patch becomes dislodged.
   - System is waterproof so bathing and swimming are permitted.
   - System effects last for 3 days; change patch every 72 hr if continuation of therapy is required and rotate application sites.
   - NOT for use in children.
   - Wear only one patch at the time; do not cut the patch.
   - After applying on dry skin behind the ear, wash hands thoroughly with soap and water and dry. Discard the removed patch and wash hands and old application site thoroughly with soap and water. May cause pupillary dilation if eye is touched and hand contaminated with drug.
8. Report any unusual movements, urinary retention, constipation and lack of response. Increase fluids and bulk to prevent constipation and ensure adequate hydration. Avoid hot temperatures; may become heat intolerant.
9. Avoid alcohol and any other CNS depressants. Use gum, sugarless candies, and frequent mouth rinses to alleviate symptoms of dry mouth.
10. Keep all F/U to assess response, labs, and for adverse SE.

OUTCOMES/EVALUATE

- Control of vomiting
- Preoperative sedation; postoperative amnesia
- Desired mydriasis
- Prevention of motion sickness

Sertraline hydrochloride

(**SIR**-trah-leen)

Classification(s): Antidepressant, selective serotonin reuptake inhibitor

Pregnancy Category: C

RX: Zoloft.

Rx: Apo-Sertraline, Novo-Sertraline, ratio-Sertraline.

SEE ALSO ***SELECTIVE SEROTONIN REUPTAKE INHIBITORS.***

INDICATIONS/USES

1. Major depressive disorder as defined in the DSM-III.
2. Obsessive-compulsive disorders in adults and children as defined in the DSM-III-R.
3. Panic disorder, with or without agoraphobia, as defined in the DSM-IV.
4. Posttraumatic stress disorder in men and women as defined in the DSM-III-R.
5. Premenstrual dysphoric disorder as defined in the DSM-III-R/IV.
6. Social anxiety disorder (social phobia) as defined by DSM-IV.

Investigational: Nocturnal enuresis, hot flashes in men and women, cholestatic pruritus.

ACTION/KINETICS

Action

Antidepressant effect likely due to inhibition of CNS neuronal uptake of serotonin and to a less extent norepinephrine and dopamine. Results in increased levels of serotonin in synapses. No anticholinergic or orthostatic hypotensive effects; slight sedative effect.

Pharmacokinetics

Steady-state plasma levels are usually reached after 1 week of once-daily dosing, but is increased to 2–3 weeks in older clients. May cause slight sedation. **Time to peak plasma levels:** 4.5–8.4 hr. **Peak plasma levels:** 20–55 ng/mL. **Time to reach steady state:** 7 days. **Terminal elimination t½:** 1–4 days (including active metabolite). Washout period is 7 days. Food decreases the time to reach peak plasma levels. Undergoes significant first-pass metabolism. Excreted through the urine (40–45%) and feces (40–45%). Metabolized to N-desmethylsertraline, which has minimal antidepressant activity. **Plasma protein binding:** 98%.

CONTRAINDICATIONS

Use with pimozide or MAOIs due to increased risk of QT prolongation.

SPECIAL CONCERNS

Suicidality in children and adolescents. (1) Antidepressants increased the risk of suicidal thinking and behavior (suicidality) in short-term studies in children, adolescents, and young adults with major depressive disorder and other psychiatric disorders. Anyone considering the use of sertraline or any other antidepressant in a child, adolescent, or young adults must balance this risk with the clinical need. Clients who are started on therapy should be observed closely for clinical worsening, suicidality, or unusual changes in behavior. Families and caregivers should be advised of the need for close observation and communication with the prescriber. Sertraline is not approved for use in pediatric clients except for clients with obsessive-compulsive disorder (OCD). (2) Pooled analyses of short-term placebo-controlled trials of 9 antidepressant drugs (SSRIs and others) in children and adolescents with major depressive disorder, obsessive-compulsive disorder, or other psychiatric disorders have revealed a greater risk of adverse reactions representing suicidal thinking or behavior (suicidality) during the first few months of treatment in those receiving antidepressants. The average risk of such reactions in clients receiving antidepressants was 4%, twice the placebo risk of 2%. No suicides occurred in these trials.

- **Use with caution in hepatic or renal dysfunction, and with seizure disorders.**
- **Plasma clearance may be lower in elderly clients.**
- **Neonates exposed to sertraline late in the third trimester have developed serious complications requiring prolonged hospitalization, respiratory support, and tube feeding; when treating pregnant women with sertraline during the third trimester, carefully consider the potential risks and benefits.**
- **Discontinuation of sertraline may cause the following symptoms: Dysphoric mood, irritability, agitation, dizziness, sensory disturbances, anxiety, confusion, headache, lethargy, emotional lability, insomnia, and hypomania.**
- **Risk of a suicide attempt is possible in depression and may persist until significant remission occurs.**

SIDE EFFECTS

Most Common

Nausea, diarrhea/loose stools, headache, insomnia, somnolence, rash, dry mouth, dizziness, anorexia, abnormal ejaculation.

A large number of side effects is possible; listed are those side effects with a frequency of 0.1% or greater. **GI:** Nausea, diarrhea/loose stools, dry mouth, constipation, dyspepsia, vomiting, flatulence, anorexia, abdominal pain, thirst, increased salivation/appetite, gastroenteritis, dysphagia, eructation, taste perversion/change, teeth-grinding. **CV:** Palpitations, hot flushes, edema, hyper-/hypotension, peripheral ischemia, postural hypotension or dizziness, syncope, tachycardia. **CNS:** Headache, insomnia, somnolence, agitation, nervousness, activation of mania/hypomania, ***seizures***, anxiety, dizziness, tremor, fatigue, impaired concentration, yawning, paresthesia, hyper-/hypoesthesia, twitching, hypertonia, confusion, ataxia or abnormal coordination/gait, hyper-/hypokinesia, abnormal dreams, aggressive reaction, amnesia, apathy, delusion, depersonalization, depression, aggravated depression, emotional lability, euphoria, hallucinations, neurosis, paranoid

S

reaction, ***suicidal ideation or attempt***, abnormal thinking, migraine, nystagmus, vertigo. **Dermatologic:** Rash, acne, excessive sweating, alopecia, pruritus, cold/clammy skin, facial edema, erythematous rash, maculopapular rash, dry skin. **Musculoskeletal:** Myalgia, arthralgia, arthrosis, dystonia, muscle cramps/weakness. **GU:** Urinary frequency/incontinence, UTI, abnormal ejaculation, micturition/menstrual disorders, dysmenorrhea, dysuria, painful menstruation, intermenstrual bleeding, sexual dysfunction and decreased libido, nocturia, polyuria, dysuria. **Respiratory:** Rhinitis, pharyngitis, bronchospasm, coughing, dyspnea, epistaxis. **Ophthalmic:** Blurred/abnormal vision, abnormal accommodation, conjunctivitis, diplopia, eye pain, xerophthalmia. **Otic:** Tinnitus, earache. **Body as a whole:** Asthenia, fever, chest/back pain, chills, weight loss/gain, generalized edema, malaise, flushing, hot flashes, rigors, lymphadenopathy, purpura.

LABORATORY TEST CONSIDERATIONS

↑ AST or ALT, total cholesterol, triglycerides. ↓ Serum uric acid. Altered platelet function. Hyponatremia.

OVERDOSE MANAGEMENT

Symptoms: Intensification of side effects. *Treatment:*

- Establish and maintain an airway, ensuring adequate oxygenation and ventilation.
- Activated charcoal, with or without sorbitol, may be as or more effective than emesis or lavage.
- Monitor cardiac and vital signs.
- Provide general supportive measures and symptomatic treatment.
- Since sertraline has a large volume of distribution, it is unlikely that dialysis, forced diuresis, hemoperfusion, or exchange transfusion will benefit.

ADDITIONAL DRUG INTERACTIONS

Because sertraline is highly bound to plasma proteins, its use with other drugs that are also highly protein bound may lead to displacement, resulting in higher plasma levels of the drug and possibly increased side effects.

Alcohol / Concurrent use is not recommended in depressed clients

Benzodiazepines / ↓ Clearance of benzodiazepines metabolized by hepatic oxidation

Carbamazepine / Possible ↓ sertraline effect R/T ↑ liver metabolism

Cimetidine / ↑ Half-life and blood levels of sertraline

Clozapine / ↑ Serum clozapine levels

Diazepam / ↑ Levels of desmethyldiazepam (significance not known)

Erythromycin / Possibility of "Serotonin Syndrome"

Hydantoins / Possible ↑ hydantoin levels

MAOIs / ↑ Risk of QT prolongation; do not use together

Pimozide / ↑ Pimozide levels → QT prolongation; do not use together

Rifampin / Possible ↓ sertraline levels

HOW SUPPLIED

Solution, Oral Concentrate: 20 mg/mL (as base); ***Tablets:*** 25 mg, 50 mg, 100 mg (all as base).

DOSAGE

SOLUTION, ORAL CONCENTRATE; TABLETS

Major depressive disorder.

Adults, initial: 50 mg once daily either in the morning or evening. Clients not responding to a 50 mg dose may benefit from doses ranging from 50–200 mg/day (average: 70 mg/day). Generally several months or longer of sustained therapy is required.

Obsessive-compulsive disorder.

Adults, initial: 50 mg once daily either in the morning or evening; a dose range 50–200 mg/day may be required. **Children, 6 to 12 years, initial:** 25 mg once a day; **adolescents, 13 to 17 years, initial:** 50 mg once a day. **Dose range, children 6 to 17 years:** 25–200 mg/day. Those not responding may require doses up to a maximum of 200 mg/day. OCD requires several months or longer of sustained drug therapy. Periodically assess to determine the need for continued therapy.

Panic disorder.

Adults, initial: 25 mg/day for the first week; **then** increase the dose to 50 mg once daily. Dose ranges from 50–200 mg/day have been used. Panic disorder requires several months or

S

longer of sustained drug therapy. Periodically assess to determine the need for continued therapy.

Post-traumatic stress disorder.

Adults, initial: 25 mg once daily. After 1 week, increase dose to 50 mg once daily. **Dose range:** 50–200 mg/day. Posttraumatic stress disorder requires several months or longer of sustained drug therapy. Periodically assess to determine the need for continued therapy.

Premenstrual dysphoric disorder.

Adults, initial: 50 mg/day either daily throughout the menstrual cycle or limited to the luteal phase, depending on provider assessment. Those not responding at the 50 mg/day dose may benefit from dose increases, at 50 mg increments per menstrual cycle, up to 150 mg/day when dosing daily throughout the menstrual cycle or 100 mg/day when dosing during the luteal phase. If a 100 mg/day dose has been established with luteal phase dosing, use a 50 mg/day titration step for 3 days at the beginning of each luteal phase dosing period. **Dose range:** 50–150 mg/day. Efficacy has not been determined for more than 3 menstrual cycles. However, longer periods of treatment are reasonable.

Social anxiety disorder.

Adults, initial: 25 mg once daily. After 1 week, increase to 50 mg once daily. **Dose range:** 50–200 mg/day. Social anxiety disorder requires several months or longer of sustained drug therapy. Periodically assess to determine the need for continued therapy.

NURSING IMPLICATIONS

Do not confuse Zoloft with Zocor (an antihyperlipidemic) or sertraline with selegiline.

IMPLEMENTATION/ADMINISTRATION/STORAGE

1. Give once daily in the morning or evening. Due to the 24-hr elimination t½, dose changes should not occur at intervals of less than 1 week.
2. It is generally recognized that acute periods of depression and other disorders require several months or longer of sustained drug therapy. Periodically reassess clients to determine the need for maintenance therapy.
3. Beneficial effects may not be observed for 2–4 weeks after starting.
4. The use of this drug for more than 12 weeks for panic attacks has not been studied.
5. Lower the dose or change dosing intervals in those with hepatic or renal impairment.
6. Neonates exposed to SSRIs late in the third trimester of pregnancy have developed complications requiring prolonged hospitalization, respiratory support, and tube feeding. Carefully consider the risks and benefits of treating women during their third trimester. Consider tapering the dose in the third trimester.
7. At least 14 days should elapse between discontinuing an MAOI and starting sertraline therapy. Also, allow at least 14 days after discontinuing sertraline and starting an MAOI.
8. When discontinuing sertraline, a gradual reduction in dose rather than abrupt cessation is recommended whenever possible.
9. The oral concentrate is contraindicated with disulfiram due to the alcohol content of the concentrate.
10. Store tablets and oral concentrate at controlled room temperature from 15–30°C (59–86°F).

ASSESSMENT

1. Note reasons for therapy, onset, triggers, symptom/behavioral characteristics/presentation, other agents/therapies trialed. List drugs prescribed to ensure none interact/compete.
2. Assess lifestyle, i.e., recent loss (death of loved one), stress, job change/loss, alcohol/drug use, traumatic events, or other factors that may contribute to symptoms.
3. List any other concomitant illness or disease that may affect metabolism or response.
4. Determine if at risk for bipolar disorder; assess detailed psychiatric history, including a family history of suicide, bipolar disorder, and depression and monitor closely.
5. Assess for hepatitis, alcohol overuse, seizure disorder. Monitor clinical response, ECG, weight, renal and LFTs; reduce dose with dysfunction/elderly.

CLIENT/FAMILY TEACHING

1. Take only as directed; do not share medications, store safely, and remain under close medical supervision. Take once daily in the morning or evening. May take with/without food and in the evening if sedation is noted.
2. Prior to use of the oral concentrate, dilute with 4 oz of water, ginger ale, lemon/lime soda, lemonade, or orange juice only. Take immediately after mixing; do not mix in advance. Dropper may contain latex; avoid using if allergic.
3. Do not perform activities that require mental and physical alertness until drug effects are realized.
4. Review side effects, noting those that require immediate medical attention, especially yellow eyes/skin, abdominal pain, N&V, or light stool color. Loss of appetite, persistent nausea, and diarrhea with excessive weight loss should be reported.
5. Report any suicidal thoughts/behavior, aggression, anxiety, agitation, panic attacks, insomnia, hostility, impulsivity. Risk of suicide is tantamount in a depressive phase; may take 2–4 weeks to work. Do not stop suddenly; drug should be titrated down with prolonged use.
6. Ensure regular attendance at counselling/therapy sessions.
7. Report any persistent or unusual sweating, headache, drowsiness, nausea, diarrhea, or changes in sexual function.
8. Avoid OTC agents, alcohol, and any other CNS depressants. If alcohol consumed, wait and take dose in the a.m.
9. Use reliable contraception; report if pregnancy suspected.
10. Keep all F/U to assess response, labs, and for adverse SE.

OUTCOMES/EVALUATE

- Improved symptoms of depression, OCD, PTSD, panic disorder
- ↓ Levels of agitation and anxiety

IV 📷

Sildenafil citrate

(sill-**DEN**-ah-fill)

Classification(s): Drug for erectile dysfunction or pulmonary arterial hypertension

Pregnancy Category: B

RX: Revatio, Viagra.

INDICATIONS/USES

(1) **Viagra:** Erectile dysfunction. Has no effect in the absence of sexual stimulation. (2) **Revatio:** Pulmonary arterial hypertension (World Health Organization Group 1) to improve ability to exercise. Injection also used to delay clinical worsening. Efficacy not adequately evaluated in those taking bosentan concurrently. *Investigational:* Antipsychotic-induced sexual dysfunction; female sexual dysfunction.

ACTION/KINETICS

Action

Nitric oxide activates the enzyme guanylate cyclase, which causes increased levels of guanosine monophosphate (cGMP) and subsequently smooth muscle relaxation in the corpus cavernosum allowing inflow of blood. Sildenafil enhances effect of nitric oxide by inhibiting phosphodiesterase type 5 which is responsible for degradation of cGMP in the corpus cavernosum. When sexual stimulation causes local release of nitric oxide, inhibition of phosphodiesterase type 5 by sildenafil causes increased levels of cGMP in the corpus cavernosum and thus smooth muscle relaxation and inflow of blood resulting in an erection. Drug has no effect in absence of sexual stimulation.

Pharmacokinetics

Rapidly absorbed after PO use; about 40% is bioavailable. Absorption is decreased when taken with high-fat meal. Increased plasma levels will occur in clients older than 65 years (40% increase in AUC), hepatic impairment (e.g., cirrhosis, 80% increase), severe renal impairment (C_{CR} under 30 mL/min, 100% increase), and concomitant use of potent cytochrome CYP 3A4 inhibitors (see *Drug Interactions*); in these clients, start with a 25 mg dose. T_{max}: 0.5–2 hr. **Onset:** About 30 min. **Duration:** 4 or more hr. Metabolized in liver by CYP3A4 (major) and CYP2C9 (minor). Is converted to active metabolite (N-desmethyl sildenafil). **t½, sildenafil and metabolite:** 4 hr. Excreted mainly in feces (80%) with about 13% excreted in urine. Reduced clearance is seen in geriatric clients. **Plasma protein binding:** About 96%.

CONTRAINDICATIONS

Concomitant use with organic nitrates (potentiate hypotensive effects) in any form or with other treatments for erectile dysfunction. Use in men for whom sexual activity is not advisable due to underlying cardiovascular status. Use in newborns, children, or women. Severe hepatic impairment (Child-Pugh score from 10–15).

SPECIAL CONCERNS

- **Use with caution with anatomical deformation of penis, with predisposition to priapism (e.g., sickle cell anemia, multiple myeloma, leukemia), in bleeding disorders or active peptic ulceration, and with genetic disorders of retinal phosphodiesterases.**
- **Drug is potentially hazardous in those with acute coronary ischemia but not on nitrates; have CHF, borderline low BP, or borderline low volume status; are on complicated antihypertensive therapy with several drugs; are taking erythromycin or cimetidine; or have impaired hepatic or renal function.**
- **Is said to be safe in those with stable coronary artery disease managed without nitrites.**

SIDE EFFECTS

Most Common

Headache, flushing, dyspepsia, nasal congestion, UTI, abnormal vision, diarrhea, dizziness, rash.

CNS: Headache, dizziness, ataxia, hypertonia, neuralgia, neuropathy, paresthesia, tremor, vertigo, depression, insomnia, somnolence, abnormal dreams, decreased reflexes, hypesthesia, migraine, seizures, anxiety. **GI:** Dyspepsia, diarrhea, vomiting, glossitis, colitis, dysphagia, gastritis, gastroenteritis, esophagitis, stomatitis, dry mouth, rectal hemorrhage, gingivitis. **CV:** Hypertension, TIA, ***MI, sudden cardiac death, ventricular arrhythmia, CVA, subarachnoid and intracerebral hemorrhage, pulmonary hemorrhage***, especially with pre-existing CV risk factors. Also, angina pectoris, AV block, syncope, tachycardia, palpitation, hypotension, postural hypotension, myocardial ischemia, cerebral thrombosis, ***cardiac arrest, heart failure, cardiomyopathy***, abnormal ECG. **Dermatologic:** Flushing, rash, urticaria, herpes simplex, pruritus, sweating, skin ulcer, contact dermatitis, exfoliative dermatitis. **GU:** UTI, cystitis, nocturia, urinary frequency/incontinence, abnormal ejaculation, genital edema and anorgasmia, prolonged erection, priaprism, hematuria, breast enlargement. **Ophthalmic:** Mild and transient predominantly color tinge to vision, increased sensitivity to light, blurred vision, mydriasis, conjunctivitis, photophobia, eye pain, eye hemorrhage, cataract, dry eyes, diplopia, sudden vision loss (related to nonarteritic anterior ischemic optic neuropathy especially in those with underlying anatomic or vascular risk factors), temporary vision loss, ocular redness/burning/swelling/pressure or bloodshot appearance, increased intraocular pressure, retinal vascular disease or bleeding, vitreous detachment/traction, paramacular edema. **Otic:** Tinnitus, deafness, ear pain. **Respiratory:** Nasal congestion, respiratory tract infection, asthma, dyspnea, laryngitis, pharyngitis, sinusitis, bronchitis, increased sputum, increased cough. **Musculoskeletal:** Arthritis, arthrosis, arthralgia, myalgia, tendon rupture, tenosynovitis, bone pain, myasthenia, synovitis. **Metabolic:** Thirst, edema, gout, unstable diabetes, hyperglycemia, peripheral edema, hyperuricemia, hypoglycemic reaction, hypernatremia. **Miscellaneous:** Flu syndrome, facial edema, shock, asthenia, pain, chills, accidental fall/injury, back/abdominal pain, allergic reaction, chest pain, anemia, leukopenia. *NOTE:* Death has occurred in some clients following use of the drug.

LABORATORY TEST CONSIDERATIONS

Abnormal LFTs.

OVERDOSE MANAGEMENT

Symptoms: Extension of side effects. *Treatment:* Standard supportive measures.

DRUG INTERACTIONS

Alcohol (substantial amount) / ↓ BP, postural dizziness, and orthostatic hypotension
Alpha-adrenergic blockers / Symptomatic hypotension
Amlodipine / Additional ↓ in BP in clients with pulmonary arterial hypertension R/T induction of CYP3A4 metabolism
Barbiturates / Possible alteration of plasma levels of either or both drugs; dosage adjustments may be necessary
Bosentan / Possible alteration of plasma levels of either or both drugs; dosage adjustments may be necessary

S

Carbamazepine / Possible alteration of plasma levels of either or both drugs; dosage adjustments may be necessary
Cimetidine / ↑ Sildenafil levels by 56%
Diuretics, loop or potassium-sparing / ↑ Sildenafil AUC by 62%
Efavirenz / Possible alteration of plasma levels of either or both drugs; dosage adjustments may be necessary
Erythromycin / Significant ↑ sildenafil levels R/T inhibition of sildenafil first-pass metabolism
Fluvoxamine / ↑ Sildenafil levels and $t_{1/2}$ R/T inhibition of CYP3A4 first-pass metabolism
Grapefruit juice / ↑ Sildenafil levels R/T ↓ metabolism
Indinavir / ↑ Sildenafil levels → severe and possibly fatal hypotension
Itraconazole / ↑ Sildenafil levels R/T ↓ CYP3A4 metabolism; concomitant use not recommended with Revatio
Ketoconazole / ↑ Sildenafil levels R/T ↓ CYP3A4 metabolism; concomitant use not recommended with Revatio
Mibefradil / ↑ Sildenafil levels
Nevirapine / Possible alteration of plasma levels of either or both drugs; dosage adjustments may be necessary
Nitrites / Potentiation of vasodilatory effects → significant and potential fatal ↓ BP; do not use together
Phenytoin / Possible alteration of plasma levels of either or both drugs; dosage adjustments may be necessary
Rifabutin/Rifampin / Possible alteration of plasma levels of either or both drugs; dosage adjustments may be necessary
Ritonavir / ↑ Sildenafil levels → severe and possibly fatal hypotension; concomitant use not recommended with Revatio
Saquinavir / ↑ Sildenafil levels → severe and possibly fatal hypotension
Tacrolimus / ↑ Tacrolimus AUC, peak levels, and prolonged $t_{1/2}$ R/T inhibition of metabolism
Thiazide diuretics / ↓ BP

HOW SUPPLIED

Revatio. ***Tablets:*** 20 mg; ***Injection:*** 10 mg/12.5 mL.
Viagra. ***Tablets:*** 25 mg, 50 mg, 100 mg.

DOSAGE

TABLETS

Treat erectile dysfunction.

Viagra. Adults: For most clients, 50 mg no more than once daily, as needed, about 1 hr before sexual activity. Take anywhere from 0.5 hr to 4 hr before sexual activity. Depending on tolerance and effectiveness, dose may be increased to maximum of 100 mg or decreased to 25 mg. The maximum recommended dosing frequency is once daily.

Pulmonary arterial hypertension.

Revatio. Adults: 20 mg 3 times per day. Take doses about 4–6 hr apart with or without food. Doses higher than 20 mg 3 times per day are not recommended.

IV BOLUS

Pulmonary arterial hypertension.

Revatio. Adults: 10 mg (i.e., in 12.5 mL) given as an IV bolus injection 3 times per day. Dose does not need to be adjusted for body weight. The 10 mg dose is equivalent to that of a 20 mg PO dose.

NURSING IMPLICATIONS

IMPLEMENTATION/ADMINISTRATION/STORAGE

1. Consider starting dose of 25 mg in the following situations associated with higher plasma levels of sildenafil: Over 65 years of age, mild hepatic impairment (Child-Pugh score of 5 or 6), severe renal impairment (C_{CR} <30 mL/min), and concomitant use of cytochrome CYP3A4 inhibitors (including erythromycin, itraconazole, ketoconazole, ritonavir, and saquinavir).
2. Do not exceed a maximum single dose of 25 mg sildenafil in a 48 hr period with concomitant use of protease inhibitors (e.g., ritonavir) for HIV disease.
3. Do not take 50 or 100 mg of sildenafil within 4 hr of alpha-blocker administration. A 25 mg dose may be taken at any time.
4. Store tablets and injection from 15–30°C (59–86°F).

S

5. IV The injection is used for the continued treatment of those with pulmonary arterial hypertension who are currently prescribed PO sildenafil but who are temporarily unable to take PO medication.
6. The recommended dose is 10 mg (corresponding to 12.5 mL) administered as an intravenous bolus injection three times a day.
7. The 10 mg injection provides the pharmacological effect equivalent to a 20 mg PO dose.
8. Store the injection from 15–30C (59–86°F).
9. COMPATIBILITY Administer undiluted.
10. INCOMPATIBILITY Administer separately.

ASSESSMENT

1. List reasons for therapy, onset/cause of erectile dysfunction, i.e., organic, psychogenic, or combined; pulmonary artery pressure, distance able to walk.
2. Assess cardiovascular status; get ECG. Clients using nitrates/nitrites should not use this drug; should be nitrate free for 24 hr prior to use.
3. List drugs prescribed; some may potentiate drug effects.
4. Assess for any retinal, bleeding disorders, active ulcers.
5. Ensure client aware of potential for sudden visual loss.
6. Check for conditions that may predispose to priapism, i.e., multiple myelomas, sickle cell anemia, or leukemia.
7. Assess for any anatomical deformation of penis (Peyronie's disease, angulation, or cavernosal fibrosis).
8. Drug for pulmonary hypertension will be a different color.

CLIENT/FAMILY TEACHING

1. Take Viagra only as directed on an empty stomach 1–3 hr prior to intercourse; high-fat meal may slow drug absorption. May split drug if dose is adequate. May take with food if GI upset. Revatio may be taken with or without food.
2. Plan some form of sexual stimulation after ingestion to ensure desired erection obtained.
3. May experience headache, flushing, upset stomach, stuffy nose, dizziness (from drop in BP), drowsiness, or abnormal vision (especially blue/green color discrimination); report any unusual, persistent, or bothersome effects including chest pain, dizziness, prolonged/painful erections (>4 hr), or sudden loss of vision in 1 or both eyes.
4. Do not use any other agent for erections with this therapy. Effects may be evident the day after therapy; assess before taking additional drug. Do not use more than once a day.
5. Report all medications currently prescribed to ensure none alter effects. Stop smoking; may inhibit drug effect. If taking medications for BP or prostate be aware-may cause lowered BP; also alpha blockers (e.g., Hytrin) should be taken 4 hr apart from Viagra.
6. Practice safe sex; drug does not prevent disease transmission.
7. Do not share medications or prescriptions due to potential for adverse interactions and effects. *Never* use this drug if taking nitrates/nitrites in any form; avoid using poppers (e.g., amyl nitrate, butyl nitrate) while taking Viagra.
8. When used for pulmonary hypertension drug is called Revatio and is produced in a different shape, color and dosage. It is usually prescribed 3 times daily (separate doses by at least 4 to 6 hr). This vascular disease is characterized by fatigue, shortness of breath on exertion, chest pain, and dizziness. If untreated, median survival time after diagnosis may be as short as three years. May be administered IV if temporarily unable to take oral medication.
9. Keep all F/U to assess response, labs, and for adverse SE.

OUTCOMES/EVALUATE

- Improvement in S&S of ED (Viagra)
- ↓ Pulmonary arterial hypertension; improved exercise tolerance (Revatio)

Silodosin

(sil-**OH**-doe-sin)

Classification(s): Alpha-1 adrenergic receptor antagonist

Pregnancy Category: B

RX: Rapaflo.

INDICATIONS/USES

Treat signs and symptoms of benign prostatic hyperplasia.

S

ACTION/KINETICS

Action

Silodosin is a selective antagonist of post-synaptic alpha-1 adrenergic receptors. Blockade of these receptors causes smooth muscle in the prostate, bladder base and neck, prostatic capsule and prostatic urethra to relax, thus resulting in an improvement in urine flow and a reduction in BPH symptoms.

Pharmacokinetics

Absolute bioavailability is about 32%. **t_{max}:** 2.6 hr. **t½:** 13.3 hr. Is extensively metabolized, including by CYP3A4. The drug is a P-glycoprotein (P-gp) substrate. Excreted in both the feces (about 55%) and urine (about 33.5%). The AUC and elimination t½ are greater in geriatric clients than in younger individuals. **Plasma protein binding:** 97%.

CONTRAINDICATIONS

Treatment of hypertension. Use in women. Use in clients with severe renal impairment (C_{CR} <30 mL/min) or severe hepatic impairment (Child-Pugh score of 10 or more). Concomitant use with strong CYP3A4 inhibitors (e.g., clarithromycin, itraconazole, ketoconazole, ritonavir).

SPECIAL CONCERNS

- **Use caution during concomitant use with antihypertensive drugs due to possible dizziness and orthostatic hypotension.**
- **Safety and efficacy not determined in children.**

SIDE EFFECTS

Most Common

Retrograde ejaculation, dizziness, diarrhea, orthostatic hypotension, headache, nasopharyngitis, nasal congestion.

CNS: Dizziness, headache, insomnia. **GI:** Diarrhea, abdominal pain, jaundice, impaired hepatic function (with increased transaminase levels). **CV:** Orthostatic hypotension (with or without symptoms as dizziness), syncope. **GU:** Retrograde ejaculation. **Respiratory:** Nasopharyngitis, nasal congestion, sinusitis, rhinitis, rhinorrhea. **Dermatologic:** Toxic skin eruption, purpura. **Body as a whole:** Asthenia.

LABORATORY TEST CONSIDERATIONS

↑ ALT, AST, PSA.

OVERDOSE MANAGEMENT

Symptoms: Orthostatic hypotension. *Treatment:* Restore BP and normalization of HR by maintaining the client in a supine position. If this is not adequate, consider IV fluids. Vasopressors can be used. Monitor renal function and support as needed. Dialysis is unlikely to be of benefit since silodosin is highly protein bound.

DRUG INTERACTIONS

Alpha adrenergic blockers / Interactions expected; do not use together
Clarithromycin / ↑ Silodosin plasma levels R/T inhibition of metabolism by CYP3A4
Cyclosporine / Possible ↑ silodosin levels R/T inhibition of P-gp by cyclosporine
Diltiazem / Possible ↑ silodosin plasma levels R/T inhibition of metabolism by CYP3A4
Erythromycin / Possible ↑ silodosin plasma levels R/T inhibition of metabolism by CYP3A4 and P-gp
Itraconazole / ↑ Silodosin plasma levels R/T inhibition of metabolism by CYP3A4
Ketoconazole / ↑ Silodosin plasma levels by 3.2 fold R/T inhibition of metabolism by CYP3A4
Ritonavir / ↑ Silodosin plasma levels R/T inhibition of metabolism by CYP3A4
Sildenafil / ↑ Incidence of orthostatic side effects
Tadalafil / ↑ Incidence of orthostatic side effects
Verapamil / Possible ↑ silodosin plasma levels R/T inhibition of metabolism by CYP3A4 and P-gp

HOW SUPPLIED

Capsules: 4 mg, 8 mg.

DOSAGE

CAPSULES

Benign prostatic hyperplasia.

Men: 8 mg once daily with a meal.

NURSING IMPLICATIONS

IMPLEMENTATION/ADMINISTRATION/STORAGE

1. **Reduce the dose to 4 mg once daily in those with moderate renal impairment (C_{CR} 30–50 mL/min). No dosage adjustment is needed in those with mild renal impairment (C_{CR} 50–80 mL/min).**
2. **No dosage adjustment is needed in clients with mild or moderate hepatic impairment.**

3. Store from 15–30°C (59–86°F). Protect from light and moisture.

ASSESSMENT

1. Note reasons for therapy, onset, characteristics of S&S (BPH), other agents trialed.
2. Carcinoma of the prostate and BPH have similar symptoms; rule out the presence of carcinoma of the prostate before beginning treatment with silodosin. Document DRE findings.
3. List all drugs prescribed to ensure none interact.
4. Obtain BP (lying and standing to R/O orthostasis), PSA, U/A, renal and LFTs; reduce dose with dysfunction.

CLIENT/FAMILY TEACHING

1. Take with a meal to decrease the risk of side effects.
2. Use caution, may cause dizziness. Change positions slowly to prevent sudden drop in BP and avoid activities that require mental alertness until drug effects realized.
3. May cause retrograde ejaculation (orgasm with reduced semen); subsides once drug stopped.
4. Notify eye doctor of drug use before cataract surgery or other procedures involving the eye, even if the drug has been discontinued.
5. Keep all F/U to assess response, labs, BP, and for adverse SE.

OUTCOMES/EVALUATE

- Improved urine flow
- ↓ BPH symptoms

Simvastatin

(**sim**-vah-**STAH**-tin)

Classification(s): Antihyperlipidemic, HMG-CoA reductase inhibitor

Pregnancy Category: X

RX: Zocor.

✱ **Rx:** Apo-Simvastatin, CO Simvastatin, Gen-Simvastatin, Novo-Simvastatin, PMS-Simvastatin, ratio-Simvastatin, Sandoz Simvastatin, Taro-Simvastatin.

SEE ALSO ***ANTIHYPERLIPIDEMIC AGENTS, HMG-COA REDUCTASE INHIBITORS.***

INDICATIONS/USES

1. Reduce elevated total cholesterol, LDL-C, Apo B, and triglyceride levels and increase HDL-C in primary hypercholesterolemia (heterozygous familial and nonfamilial) and mixed dyslipidemia (Fredrickson types IIa and IIb).
2. Treat hypertriglyceridemia (Fredrickson type IV hyperlipidemia).
3. Treat primary dysbetalipoproteinemia (Fredrickson type III hyperlipidemia).
4. As an adjunct to other lipid-lowering treatments (e.g., LDL apheresis) to reduce total cholesterol and LDL-C in homozygous familial hypercholesterolemia.
5. As an adjunct to diet to reduce total and LDL-C and Apo B levels in adolescent boys and girls who are at least 1 year postmenarche, 10–17 years of age, with heterozygous familial hypercholesterolemia. Given if after an adequate trial of diet therapy, LDL-C remains 190 mg/dL or greater or LDL-C remains 160 mg/dL or greater and there is a positive family history of premature CV disease or 2 or more other CV disease risk factors are present in the adolescent client. The minimum goal is to achieve a mean LDL-C less than 130 mg/dL.
6. In those with a high risk of coronary events due to existing coronary heart disease, diabetes, peripheral vessel disease, or a history of stroke or other cerebrovascular disease, simvastatin is given to reduce the risk of total mortality by reducing coronary heart disease deaths; reduce the risk of nonfatal MI and stroke; and reduce the need for coronary and noncoronary revascularization procedures. *NOTE:* Simvastatin reduces risks of fatal and nonfatal heart attacks and strokes, as well as reduces the need for bypass surgery and angioplasty.

ACTION/KINETICS

Action

Competitively inhibits HMG-CoA reductase; this enzyme catalyzes the early rate-limiting step in the synthesis of cholesterol. Thus, cholesterol synthesis is inhibited/decreased. Decreases cholesterol, triglycerides, VLDL, LDL, and increases HDL. Does not reduce basal plasma cortisol or testosterone levels or impair renal reserve.

S

Pharmacokinetics

Time to peak levels: 1.3–2.4 hr. **Peak therapeutic response:** 4–6 weeks. Approximately 85% absorbed; significant first-pass effect (CYP3A4) with less than 5% of a PO dose reaching the general circulation. **t½:** 3 hr. Metabolites (some active) excreted in the feces (60%) and urine (13%). Increased levels seen in those with hepatic and severe renal insufficiency. **Plasma protein binding:** About 95%.

CONTRAINDICATIONS

Use if pregnant, planning to become pregnant, or while breastfeeding.

SPECIAL CONCERNS

- **Use with caution in clients who have a history of liver disease/consume large quantities of alcohol or with drugs that affect steroid levels or activity.**
- **Greater risk of muscle injury, including rhabdomyolysis, when using the 80 mg dose.**
- **Higher plasma levels may be observed in clients with hepatic and severe renal insufficiency.**
- **Elderly clients are at a greater risk to develop myopathy (due to higher blood levels); use with caution in these clients.**
- **Safety and efficacy not determined in children less than 10 years of age.**

SIDE EFFECTS

Most Common

Adults: Headache, abdominal pain/cramps, constipation, URTI, N&V, gastroenteritis/gastritis, myalgia, bronchitis, sinusitis, vertigo, atrial fibrillation, insomnia, eczema, UTI, diabetes mellitus, edema/swelling.

Children: URTI, headache, abdominal pain, nausea.

Musculoskeletal: Myalgia, arthralgia, muscle cramps/pain, myopathy, rhabdomyolysis (with renal dysfunction secondary to myoglobinuria). **GI:** Abdominal cramps/pain, constipation, N&V, gastroenteritis/gastritis, dyspepsia, flatulence, ***pancreatitis***. **Hepatic:** ***Hepatic failure***, hepatitis, jaundice. **CNS:** Headache, vertigo, insomnia, depression, dizziness, paresthesia, impaired memory. **Respiratory:** URTI, bronchitis, sinusitis. **Dermatologic:** Eczema, alopecia, pruritus, rash, pruritus, skin changes (e.g., changes to hair/nails, discoloration, dryness of skin/mucous membranes, nodule). **GU:** UTI. **Hematologic:** Anemia. **Hypersensitivity:** Although rare, the following symptoms have been noted: ***Angioedema, anaphylaxis***, lupus erythematous-like syndrome, vasculitis, purpura, thrombocytopenia, leukopenia, ***hemolytic anemia***, polymyalgia rheumatica, positive ANA, ESR increase, arthritis, arthralgia, asthenia, urticaria, photosensitivity, chills, fever, flushing, malaise, dyspnea, ***toxic epidermal necrolysis, erythema multiforme (including Stevens-Johnson syndrome)***. **Body as a whole:** Asthenia, edema, swelling. **Miscellaneous:** Diabetes mellitus, peripheral neuropathy.

LABORATORY TEST CONSIDERATIONS

↑ CPK, AST, ALT.

ADDITIONAL DRUG INTERACTIONS

Amiodarone / Possibility of myopathy, muscle weakness, and rhabdomyolysis R/T ↓ metabolism by CYP3A4; if used together, do not give client more than 20 mg/day of simvastatin

Bosentan / ↓ Simvastatin levels R/T ↑ metabolism

Carbamazepine / ↓ Simvastatin AUC, peak levels, and shortened t½ R/T ↑ metabolism by CYP3A4; monitor closely and adjust dose as needed

Cilostazole / ↑ Risk of toxicity (e.g., myopathy) R/T ↓ metabolism by CYP3A4; monitor closely and adjust dose as needed

Cyclosporine / ↑ Risk of myopathy or rhabdomyolysis R/T ↓ simvastatin elimination

Danazol / ↑ Risk of myopathy or rhabdomyolysis; if concurrent use cannot be avoided, consider ↓ simvastatin dose

Digoxin / Possible ↑ digoxin plasma levels; monitor digoxin levels and adjust dose if needed

Diltiazem ↑ Risk of myopathy R/T ↓ metabolism by CYP3A4

Erythromycin / ↑ Risk of myopathy or rhabdomyolysis R/T ↓ simvastatin elimination

Grapefruit juice (>1 qt/day) / Chronic use of grapefruit juice ↑ simvastatin levels R/T ↓ liver metabolism

Hydantoins (e.g., phenytoin) / ↓ Simvastatin plasma levels R/T ↑ metabolism → ↓ therapeutic effect

Imatinib / ↑ Risk of toxicity (e.g., myopathy) R/T ↓ metabolism by CYP3A4

Itraconazole / ↑ Risk of myopathy or rhabdomyolysis R/T ↓ simvastatin elimination

Nefazodone / ↑ Risk of myopathy or rhabdomyolysis R/T ↓ simvastatin elimination

S

Nonnucleoside reverse transcriptase inhibitors (e.g., delavirdine, efavirenz, nevirapine) / Possible ↓ (e.g., delavirdine) → ↑ toxicity (e.g., myopathy) or ↑ (e.g., efavirenz, nevirapine) metabolism
Protease inhibitors (e.g., nelfinavir, ritonavir) / ↑ Risk of myopathy or rhabdomyolysis R/T ↓ simvastatin elimination
H ***St. John's wort*** / ↓ Simvastatin levels R/T ↑ metabolism → ↓ therapeutic effect
Telithromycin / ↑ Risk of toxicity (e.g., myopathy) R/T ↓ metabolism by CYP3A4
Verapamil / ↑ Risk of toxicity (e.g., myopathy) R/T ↓ metabolism by CYP3A4
Warfarin / ↑ INR; monitor anticoagulation parameters

HOW SUPPLIED

Tablets: 5 mg, 10 mg, 20 mg, 40 mg, 80 mg; *Tablets, Orally Disintegrating:* 10 mg, 20 mg, 40 mg, 80 mg.

DOSAGE

TABLETS

Hyperlipidemia, coronary heart disease.

Adults, initially: 20–40 mg once daily in the evening; **maintenance:** 5–80 mg/day as a single dose in the evening. Consider a starting dose of 10 mg/day for clients with LDL greater than 190 mg/dL. Consider a starting dose of 40 mg as an alternative for those who require a reduction of more than 45% in their LDL cholesterol (most often those with CAD).

Homozygous familial hypercholesterolemia.

Adults: 40 mg/day in the evening or 80 mg/day in 3 divided doses of 20 mg, 20 mg, and an evening dose of 40 mg. Use as an adjunct to other lipid-lowering treatments (e.g., LDL apheresis) or if such treatments are unavailable.

Adolescents 10–17 years of age with heterozygous familial hypercholesterolemia.

Initial: 10 mg once a day in the evening. **Dose range:** 10–40 mg/day (maximum). Individualize dose. Adjust at intervals of 4 weeks or more.

Prevention of coronary events.

Initial: 20–40 mg once a day in the evening. The recommended initial dose is 40 mg/day for those at high risk for a coronary heart disease event caused by existing coronary heart disease, diabetes, peripheral vessel disease, history of stroke, or other CV disease.

NURSING IMPLICATIONS

Do not confuse Zocor with Cozaar (an antihypertensive) or with Zoloft (an antidepressant).

IMPLEMENTATION/ADMINISTRATION/STORAGE

1. If no more than two risk factors, place on a standard cholesterol-lowering diet for 3–6 months before starting simvastatin (unless CAD); continue diet during drug therapy.
2. Consider a starting dose of 5 mg/day in those with LDL less than 190 mg/dL.
3. For geriatric clients, the starting dose should be 5 mg/day with maximum LDL reductions seen with 20 mg or less daily.
4. May give without regard to meals.
5. Dosage may be adjusted at intervals of at least 4 weeks.
6. In clients taking cyclosporine or danazol together with simvastatin, begin therapy with 5 mg/day of simvastatin; do not exceed 10 mg/day simvastatin.
7. In clients taking amiodarone or verapamil together with simvastatin, the dose of simvastatin should not exceed 20 mg/day.
8. In clients with severely impaired renal function, start at 5 mg/day simvastatin; monitor closely.
9. Simvastatin is effective alone or together with bile acid sequestrants. Avoid use of simvastatin with gemfibrozil, other fibrates, or lipid-lowering doses (1 gram/day or more) of niacin unless the benefit of further alteration in lipid levels is likely to outweigh the increased risk of the drug combination. However, if simvastatin is used together with fibrates or niacin, monitor carefully; do not exceed 10 mg/day of simvastatin.
10. In clients with coronary heart disease or at high risk of coronary heart disease, simvastatin orally disintegrating tablets may be started simultaneously with diet.
11. Store from 5–30°C (41–86°F).

ASSESSMENT

1. Note reasons for therapy: prophylaxis, plaque stability or elevated TG/LDL cholesterol in CAD.

S

2. List all medications prescribed; ensure none interact. Reduce dose with certain drug combinations. Identify/list risk factors for CHD.
3. Assess level of adherence to weight reduction, regular exercise, cholesterol-lowering diet, BP, BS control. Note any alcohol abuse.
4. Assess for any secondary causes for hypercholesterolemia (e.g., hypothyroidism, nephrotic syndrome, dysproteinemias, obstructive liver disease, other drug therapy, alcoholism).
5. Monitor CBC, lipid profile, CPK, renal and LFTs; reduce dose with dysfunction. Schedule LFTs, CPK after 4–6 weeks of therapy (with any dose increases) and semiannually for the first year of therapy. Special attention should be paid to elevated serum transaminase levels.

CLIENT/FAMILY TEACHING

1. Take once or twice daily as directed without regard to meals. More preferable in evening.
2. Place orally disintegrating tablets on the tongue where it will dissolve and then be swallowed with saliva. Follow with water, if necessary.
3. A low-cholesterol diet must be followed during drug therapy. Consult dietitian for assistance in meal planning and food preparation. Do not take with large quantities of grapefruit juice.
4. Report any S&S of infections, unexplained muscle pain, tenderness/weakness (especially if accompanied by fever or malaise), surgery, trauma, yellowing of skin or eyes.
5. Review importance of regular exercise, weight loss/control, low alcohol consumption, smoking abstinence, and following a low-cholesterol diet in the overall plan to reduce serum cholesterol levels and inhibit progression of CAD.
6. Not for use during pregnancy; use barrier contraception.
7. Keep all F/U to assess response, labs, eye exams, and for adverse SE.

OUTCOMES/EVALUATE

- ↓ Elevated total-C, LDL-C, Apo B, and TG
- ↑ HDL; cardiovascular risk reduction

Sirolimus

(sir-oh-**LIH**-mus)

Classification(s): Immunosuppressant

Pregnancy Category: C

RX: Rapamune.

INDICATIONS/USES

Use with corticosteroids and cyclosporine to prevent organ rejection in renal transplants, including for cyclosporine-sparing immunosuppression in those with kidney transplants who are at low or moderate risk of organ rejection. Use only in clients 13 years of age and older. *Investigational:* Treat psoriasis.

ACTION/KINETICS

Action

Inhibits both T-lymphocyte activation and proliferation that occurs in response to antigenic and interleukin IL-2, IL-4, and IL-15 stimulation. Also inhibits antibody production. Thus, there is a significant reduction in the incidence of organ rejection.

Pharmacokinetics

Rapidly absorbed after PO use. **Peak levels:** About 1 hr in healthy clients and about 2 hr in renal transplant clients. Bioavailability is low (15% for the oral solution and 27% for tablets). High-fat meals increase AUC and alter the bioavailability of sirolimus. The majority of the drug is sequestered in formed blood elements resulting in much higher blood levels compared with plasma levels. Extensively metabolized by CYP3A4 and P-glycoprotein in the liver and gut wall. Over 90% is excreted in the feces with a small amount excreted in the urine. Adjust dosage for mild-to-severe hepatic impairment. **t½, terminal, after multiple dosing in renal transplant clients:** About 62 hr. **Plasma protein binding:** Approximately 92%.

CONTRAINDICATIONS

Hypersensitivity to sirolimus, its derivatives, or any component of the drug product. Use as an immunosuppressant in liver or lung transplants. Lactation.

SPECIAL CONCERNS

■ (1) **Immunosuppression.** Increased susceptibility to infection and possible development of lymphoma may result from immunosuppression. Only health care providers experienced in immunosuppressive therapy and management of renal transplant clients

S

should use sirolimus. Manage clients receiving the drug in facilities equipped and staffed with adequate lab and supportive medical resources. The physician responsible for maintenance therapy should have complete information needed for the follow-up of the client. (2) **Liver transplantation.** The use of sirolimus in combination with tacrolimus was associated with excess mortality and graft loss in a study in de novo liver transplant recipients. Many had evidence of infection at or near the time of death. (3) In this and another study in de novo liver transplant recipients, the use of sirolimus in combination with cyclosporine or tacrolimus was associated with an increase in hepatic artery thrombosis; most cases of hepatic artery thrombosis occurred within 30 days post transplantation, and most led to graft loss or death. The safety and efficacy of sirolimus as immunosuppressive therapy have not been established in liver transplant clients; therefore, use is not recommended in these clients. (4) **Lung transplantation.** Cases of bronchial anastomotic dehiscence, most fatal, have been reported in de novo lung transplant clients when sirolimus has been used as part of an immunosuppressive regimen. The safety and efficacy of sirolimus as immunosuppressive therapy have not been established in lung transplant clients; therefore, use in these clients is not recommended.

- **Use with caution in those with impaired renal function or when used with drugs that impair renal function (e.g., aminoglycosides, amphotericin B).**
- **Increased susceptibility to infection and possible development of lymphoma due to immunosuppression.**
- **De novo use of sirolimus without cyclosporine not established in renal transplant clients.**
- **Use caution with dose selection in the elderly.**
- **Safety and efficacy not determined in combination with other immunosuppressant drugs or in children less than 13 years of age.**

SIDE EFFECTS

Most Common

Abdominal pain, anemia, arthralgia, constipation, creatinine increased, diarrhea, fever, headache, hypercholesterolemia, hypertension, hypertriglyceridemia, nausea, pain, peripheral edema, thrombocytopenia, UTI.

GI: Diarrhea, N&V, constipation, abdominal pain, dyspepsia, anorexia, dysphagia, eructation, esophagitis, flatulence, gastritis, gastroenteritis, gingivitis, gum hyperplasia, ileus, mouth ulceration, oral moniliasis, stomatitis, rectal disorder, ***pancreatitis, fatal hepatic necrosis***. **CNS:** Tremor, headache, insomnia, anxiety, confusion, depression, dizziness, emotional lability, hyper-/hypotonia, hypesthesia, insomnia, neuropathy, paresthesia, somnolence. **CV:** Hyper-/hypotension, atrial fibrillation, CHF, ***hemorrhage***, hypervolemia, palpitation, peripheral vascular disorder, postural hypotension, syncope, tachycardia, thrombophlebitis, thrombosis, vasodilation, venous thromboembolism (including DVT), pericardial effusion (including hemodynamically significant effusions and tamponade requiring intervention in adults and children), ***hepatic artery thrombosis*** (in liver transplants). **Dermatologic:** Acne, rash, fungal dermatitis, hirsutism, pruritus, skin hypertrophy, skin ulcer, sweating, photosensitivity, skin cancer (including basal cell carcinoma, melanoma, squamous cell carcinoma), exfoliative dermatitis. **Respiratory:** Dyspnea, URTI, pharyngitis, asthma, atelectasis, bronchitis, bronchiolitis obliterans organizing pneumonia, pneumonitis, increased cough, epistaxis, hypoxia, lung edema, pleural effusion, pneumonia, rhinitis, sinusitis, interstitial lung disease, bronchial anastomotic dehiscence (in lung transplants), interstitial lung disease, alveolar proteinosis, ***pulmonary fibrosis***, ***pulmonary embolism, pulmonary hemorrhage***. **Hematologic:** Anemia, thrombocytopenia, ecchymosis, leukopenia, leukocytosis, lymphadenopathy, polycythemia, lymphoma, lymphoproliferative disease, thrombotic thrombocytopenic purpura (***hemolytic uremic syndrome***), pancytopenia (rare), lymphedema (rare). **GU:** UTI, bladder pain, dysuria, hematuria, hydronephrosis, impotence, kidney pain, kidney tubular necrosis, nocturia, oliguria, pyuria, scrotal edema, testis disorder, pyelonephritis, ***toxic nephrotoxicity***, nephrotic syndrome, azoospermia, impaired renal function, urinary frequency/incontinence/retention, menorrhagia, metrorrhagia, polyuria, focal segmental glomerulosclerosis, azoospermia. **Musculoskeletal:** Arthralgia, arthrosis, bone necrosis, leg cramps, myalgia, osteoporosis, tetany. **Endocrine:** Cushing's syndrome, diabetes mellitus, glycosuria. **Ophthalmic:** Abnormal vision, cataract, conjunctivitis. **Otic:** Deafness, ear pain, otitis media, tinnitus. **Hypersensitivity:** Angioedema, ***anaphylactic/anaphylactoid reactions***, hypersensitivity vasculitis. **Metabolic:** Peripheral edema, generalized edema, facial edema, acidosis, ascites, dehydration, weight gain/loss. **Body as a whole:** Asthenia, fever, abnormal healing, abscess, cellulitis, chills, flu syndrome, infection, malaise, mycobacterial infections (including *Mycobacterium tuberculosis),* Epstein-Barré viral infections, angioedema, ***sepsis***. **Miscellaneous:** Pain (abdominal, pelvic, back, chest), enlarged abdomen, ascites, hernia, lymphocele, herpes simplex/zoster, ***peritonitis***, increased susceptibility to infection (including *Pneumocystis carinii*) and possible development of lymphoma and other malignancies, activation of latent viral infections, CMV infections, posttransplant lymphoproliferative disorder, graft loss, fluid accumulation, impaired or delayed wound healing, calcineurin inhibitor-induced reactions (e.g., hemolytic uremic syndrome, thrombotic thrombocytopenic purpura, thrombotic microangiopathy), ***BK virus-associated nephropathy.***

LABORATORY TEST CONSIDERATIONS

↑ Alkaline phosphatase, BUN, CPK, LDH, ALT, AST, serum cholesterol, triglycerides, serum creatinine. ↓ Mean GFR, platelets, hemoglobin. Abnormal LFTs. Acidosis, albuminuria, proteinuria, hyper-/hypophosphatemia, hyper-/hypocalcemia, hyper-/hypoglycemia, hyper-/hypokalemia, hyperlipemia, hypomagnesemia, hyponatremia.

OVERDOSE MANAGEMENT

Symptoms: Symptoms due to overdosage are consistent with those listed under *Side Effects. Treatment:* Institute general supportive measures. Sirolimus is not dialyzable to any extent.

DRUG INTERACTIONS

Sirolimus is metabolized by the CYP3A4 and P-gp enzyme systems; thus, substances known to inhibit these enzymes may decrease metabolism or increase bioavailability of sirolimus. Drugs known to induce these enzyme systems may increase metabolism or decrease bioavailability of sirolimus.

Amiodarone / ↑ Sirolimus levels → ↑ risk of toxicity; consider lowering sirolimus dose and monitor blood levels frequently

Angiotensin-converting enzyme (ACE) inhibitors / Possible angioneurotic edema-type reactions; monitor and provide treatment as needed

Azole antifungal drugs (e.g., fluconazole, itraconazole, ketoconazole, voriconazole) / ↑ Sirolimus levels R/T inhibition of CYP3A4 or P-gp → ↑ toxicity; do not use together

Bromocriptine / ↑ Sirolimus levels → ↑ risk of side effects R/T inhibition of CYP3A4 metabolism; monitor sirolimus levels and adjust dose if necessary

Carbamazepine / ↓ Sirolimus levels R/T induction of CYP3A4 metabolism; use together with caution; monitor sirolimus levels and adjust dose if needed

Cimetidine / ↑ Sirolimus levels → ↑ risk of side effects R/T inhibition of CYP3A4 metabolism; monitor sirolimus levels and adjust dose if necessary

Clarithromycin / ↑ Sirolimus levels →↑ risk of toxicity R/T ↓ metabolism; do not use together

Clotrimazole / ↑ Sirolimus levels → ↑ risk of side effects R/T inhibition of CYP3A4 metabolism; monitor sirolimus levels and adjust dose if necessary

Cyclosporine / ↑ Risk of hepatic artery thrombosis → graft loss or death; also, ↑ sirolimus levels → ↑ toxicity, including hemolytic uremic syndrome, thrombotic thrombocytopenia purpura, thrombotic microangiopathy (give sirolimus 4 hr after cyclosporine); monitor sirolimus levels and adjust dosage if needed

Dalfopristin / ↑Sirolimus levels → ↑ pharmacologic/toxic effects; monitor sirolimus levels and adjust dose if necessary

Danazol / ↑ Sirolimus levels → ↑ risk of side effects R/T inhibition of CYP3A4 metabolism; monitor sirolimus levels and adjust dose if necessary

Diltiazem / ↑ Sirolimus levels; monitor sirolimus levels and adjust dose if necessary

Disulfiram / Sirolimus PO solution contains alcohol; may produce acute and severe alcohol intolerance; do not use together

Erythromycin / ↑ Sirolimus levels → ↑ risk of toxicity; also, ↑ erythromycin levels; do not use together

Furazolidone / Sirolimus PO solution contains alcohol; may produce acute and severe alcohol intolerance; do not use together

Grapefruit juice / ↑ Sirolimus levels R/T ↓ CYP3A4-mediated metabolism of sirolimus; do not give together
Metoclopramide / ↑ Sirolimus levels → ↑ risk of side effects R/T inhibition of CYP3A4 metabolism; monitor sirolimus levels and adjust dose if necessary
Metronidazole / Sirolimus PO solution contains alcohol; may produce acute and severe alcohol intolerance; do not use together
Mycophenolate mofetil / ↑ Mycophenolic acid exposure → ↑ risk of side effects; monitor mycophenolic acid levels and adjust dose if necessary
Nicardipine / ↑ Sirolimus levels →↑ risk of side effects R/T inhibition of CYP3A4 metabolism; monitor sirolimus levels and adjust dose if necessary
Phenobarbital / ↓ Sirolimus levels R/T induction of CYP3A4 metabolism; use together with caution; monitor sirolimus levels and adjust dose as necessary
Phenytoin / ↓ Sirolimus levels R/T induction of CYP3A4 metabolism; use together with caution; monitor sirolimus levels and adjust dose as necessary
Pimecrolimus / ↑ Sirolimus levels → ↑ pharmacologic/toxic effects; monitor sirolimus levels and adjust dose if necessary
Protease inhibitors (e.g., indinavir, ritonavir) / ↑ Sirolimus levels →↑ risk of side effects R/T inhibition of CYP3A4 metabolism; monitor sirolimus levels and adjust dose if necessary
Quinupristin / ↑ Sirolimus levels → ↑ pharmacologic/toxic effects; monitor sirolimus levels and adjust dose if necessary
Rifamycins (rifabutin, rifampin, rifapentine) / ↓ Sirolimus levels R/T ↑ metabolism by CYP3A4 or P-gp; do not use together
H ***St. John's wort*** / ↓ Sirolimus levels R/T ↑ metabolism; possible transplant rejection; monitor sirolimus levels and adjust dose as necessary
Tacrolimus / ↑ Sirolimus levels → ↑ pharmacologic/toxic effects; monitor sirolimus levels and adjust dose if necessary; also, ↓ trough tacrolimus levels → ↑ risk of organ transplant rejection
Telithromycin / ↑ Sirolimus levels →↑ risk of side effects R/T ↓ metabolism; do not use together
Tacrolimus / ↑ Risk of hepatic artery thrombosis → graft loss or death; ↓ tacrolimus AUC and peak plasma levels in pediatric renal transplant clients; also, ↑ risk of hemolytic uremic syndrome, thrombotic thrombocytopenia purpura, thrombotic microangiopathy
Troleandomycin / ↑ Sirolimus levels → ↑ risk of side effects R/T inhibition of CYP3A4 metabolism; monitor sirolimus levels and adjust dose if necessary
Vaccines / Vaccines may be less effective
Verapamil / ↑ Sirolimus levels R/T ↓ metabolism; also, ↑ S (-) verapamil levels; monitor sirolimus levels and adjust dose if necessary

HOW SUPPLIED

Oral Solution: 1 mg/mL; ***Tablets:*** 0.5 mg, 1 mg, 2 mg.

DOSAGE

ORAL SOLUTION; TABLETS

Prophylaxis of rejection following kidney transplantation in adults.

Adults. High immunologic risk. Loading dose, initial: Up to 15 mg on day 1 post transplantation; **maintenance dose:** 5 mg/day beginning on day 2. **Maximum dose:** 40 mg/day. A trough level should be obtained between days 5 and 7, and the daily dose adjusted thereafter. Once the maintenance dose is adjusted, continue clients on the new maintenance dose for 7–14 days before making further adjustments. In most clients, dosage adjustments can be based on a simple proportion:

new dose = current dose × (target concentration/current concentration).

Consider a loading dose in addition to a new maintenance dose when it is necessary to increase sirolimus trough levels:

sirolimus loading dose = 3 × (new maintenance dose − current maintenance dose).

If an estimated daily dose exceeds 40 mg because of the addition of a loading dose, administer the loading dose over 2 days.

NOTE: Use in combination with cyclosporine and corticosteroids for the first 12 months following transplantation. The starting dose of cyclosporine should be up to 7 mg/kg/day in

S

divided doses; adjust dosage subsequently to achieve target whole blood trough levels. Administer prednisone at a minimum of 5 mg/day. Antibody induction therapy may be used.

Adults. Low to moderate immunologic risk. Loading dose: 6 mg; **maintenance dose:** 2 mg/day. **Maximum dose:** 40 mg/day. For dosage adjustment, see earlier information for "high immunologic risk."

NOTE: It is recommended that sirolimus be used initially in a regimen with cyclosporine and corticosteroids. At 2 to 4 months following transplantation, discontinue cyclosporine progressively over 4–8 weeks; adjust the sirolimus dose to obtain whole blood trough levels within the target range. Because cyclosporine inhibits the metabolism and transport of sirolimus, sirolimus levels may decrease when cyclosporine is discontinued unless the sirolimus dose is increased.

Prophylaxis of rejection following kidney transplantation in children.

Low to moderate immunologic risk. Children, 13 years and older, initial loading dose: 6 mg for those weighing 40 kg or more and 3 mg/m^2 for those weighing less than 40 kg; **maintenance:** 2 mg for those weighing 40 kg or more and 1 mg/m^2 for those weighing less than 40 kg. For dosage adjustments and concomitant therapy, see preceding "Adults Low to Moderate Immunologic Risk".

Psoriasis (investigational).

Adults: 3 mg/m^2/day in combination with subtherapeutic doses of cyclosporine.

S

NURSING IMPLICATIONS

IMPLEMENTATION/ADMINISTRATION/STORAGE

1. Use sirolimus with cyclosporine and corticosteroids. Give sirolimus 4 hr after cyclosporine. Give initial dose of sirolimus as soon as possible after transplantation.
2. Reduce the dose of sirolimus by about one-third in those with mild to moderate hepatic impairment and by about one-half in those with severe hepatic impairment. Dose reduction is not required in those with impaired renal function.
3. Note that 2 mg of oral solution is equivalent to 2 mg oral tablets, making them interchangeable on a mg-to-mg basis. It is not known if higher doses of oral solutions are clinically equivalent to higher doses of tablets on a mg-to-mg basis.
4. Take once daily consistently with or without food. Give sirolimus 4 hr after administration of cyclosporine. Grapefruit juice reduces CYP3A4-mediated metabolism; do not give sirolimus with grapefruit juice.
5. Sirolimus is an immunosuppressant. Follow safe handling procedures when preparing, administering, or dispensing sirolimus.
6. After dilution, use the product immediately. Discard syringe after one use.
7. Dilute and administer oral solution in *bottles* as follows:
   - Use the amber oral dose syringe to withdraw the prescribed amount of solution from the bottle.
   - Empty the correct amount from the syringe into a glass or plastic (only) container holding at least 2 ounces of water or orange juice. No other liquids (including grapefruit juice) should be used for the dilution.
   - Stir vigorously and drink at once.
   - Refill the container with an additional volume (minimum of 4 ounces) of water or orange juice, stir vigorously, and drink at once.
8. Protect the oral solution bottles from light. Refrigerate at 2–8°C (36–46°F). The oral solution is stable for 24 months under these storage conditions. Use the contents within 1 month once the bottle has been opened. If necessary, the bottles may be stored at room temperature (25°C; 77°F) for no more than 24 hr. If the oral solution in bottles develops a slight haze when refrigerated, allow to stand at room temperature and shake gently until haze disappears. Haze does not affect the quality of the product.
9. Store tablets from 20–25°C (68–77°F). Use cartons to protect blister cards and strips from light.

ASSESSMENT

1. Note date of transplant and for what reasons required (not recommended for use with lung and liver transplants at this time due to bronchial anastomotic dehiscence/hepatic artery thrombosis). Ensure F/U provided by transplant center as drugs require careful monitoring for adverse effects.
2. Monitor sirolimus levels closely in pediatric clients, in those with impaired hepatic function, during concurrent administration of strong CYP3A4 inhibitors and inducers, and if cyclosporine is markedly reduced or discontinued.
3. Determine need for antibiotic prophylaxis for *Pneumocystis* pneumonia and CMV after transplant.
4. Assess VS, ensure BP well controlled. Due to immunosuppressant effect, assess for infections and development of lymphoma.
5. Monitor CBC, lipids, renal, and LFTs as well as cyclosporine and sirolimus drug levels, clinical signs/symptoms, urinary protein excretion, and tissue biopsy. Reduce dose with liver dysfunction.

CLIENT/FAMILY TEACHING

1. Take sirolimus as prescribed. If taking with cyclosporine, take sirolimus 4 hr after cyclosporine to prevent variations in sirolimus levels. Follow directions carefully for storage, dilution, and dosing of drug.
2. Do not crush, chew, or split the tablets. Take consistently with or without food to minimize variability in blood levels and efficacy. Grapefruit juice reduces metabolism; do not give sirolimus with grapefruit juice. Use water or orange juice and rinse glass to ensure entire dose consumed.
3. Initial dose of sirolimus will be given as soon as possible after transplantation. Review drug insert carefully.
4. If the oral solution in bottles develops a slight haze when refrigerated, allow to stand at room temperature and shake gently until haze disappears. Haze does not affect the quality of the product.
5. Report any unusual side effects including rash, fever, chills, sore throat, diarrhea, or infections. Do not permit solution to touch skin or eyes; if contact occurs rinse eyes with plain water and wash skin with soap and water.
6. May also be prescribed antibiotics for 1 year to prevent *P. carinii* and CMV prophylaxis for 3 months post transplant.
7. Females must use reliable contraception before, during and for 12 weeks after therapy has been discontinued.
8. Avoid prolonged sun exposure; use protective sun screen, clothing and glasses if exposed.
9. While receiving immunosuppressive drugs, one may be more susceptible to infections and possibly lymphoma. Avoid crowds, infected persons and report any symptoms of illness.
10. Report any S&S of transplant rejection (fever, pain over transplant site, rapid weight gain), fever or other signs of infection.
11. Vaccinations may be less effective during treatment with immunosuppressants; avoid live vaccines.
12. Keep all F/U to assess response, labs, and for adverse SE.

OUTCOMES/EVALUATE

- Prophylaxis of renal transplant rejection
- Therapeutic serum drug levels

Sitagliptin phosphate

(**SI**-tah-glip-tin)

Classification(s): Antidiabetic agent, dipeptidyl peptidase-4 inhibitor

Pregnancy Category: B

RX: Januvia.

INDICATIONS/USES

Adjunct to diet and exercise to improve glycemic control in type 2 diabetes mellitus either as monotherapy or in combination with metformin or a thiazolidinedione when the single agent alone, with diet and exercise, does not provide adequate glycemic control.

ACTION/KINETICS

Action

Incretin hormones are released by the intestine throughout the day; levels increase in response to a meal. The incretins are involved in the physiologic regulation of glucose homeostasis. When blood glucose levels are normal or elevated, incretins increase insulin synthesis and release from

S

pancreatic beta cells. One of the incretins also lowers glucagon secretion from pancreatic alpha cells, leading to reduced hepatic glucose production. The incretins are normally rapidly inactivated by the enzyme, dipeptidyl peptidase-4. Sitagliptin is a specific inhibitor of dipeptidyl peptidase-4 and acts by slowing inactivation of incretin hormones. By increasing and prolonging active incretin levels, sitagliptin increases insulin release and decreases glucagon levels in the circulation in a glucose-dependent manner.

Pharmacokinetics

Rapidly absorbed; **peak plasma levels:** 1–4 hr. Absolute bioavailability is about 87%. About 79% excreted unchanged in the urine with metabolites excreted in the urine and feces. The primary enzyme responsible for the limited metabolism is CYP3A4 with some contribution from CYP2C8. **t½, terminal:** 12.4 hr. **Plasma protein binding:** 38%.

CONTRAINDICATIONS

Use in type 1 diabetes mellitus or to treat diabetic ketoacidosis as the drug is not effective for these conditions.

SPECIAL CONCERNS

- Use with caution during lactation.
- Use with sulfonylureas or insulin not adequately studied.
- Take care with dose selection in the elderly.
- Safety and efficacy not established in children less than 18 years of age.

SIDE EFFECTS

Most Common

Headache, nasopharyngitis, URTI.

GI: Abdominal pain, nausea, diarrhea. **CNS:** Headache. **Respiratory:** Nasopharyngitis, URTI. **Metabolic:** Hypoglycemia. **Miscellaneous:** ***Anaphylaxis***, ***angioedema***, exfoliative skin reactions (including ***Stevens-Johnson syndrome***).

LABORATORY TEST CONSIDERATIONS

Small ↑ WBCs and serum creatinine.

HOW SUPPLIED

Tablets: 25 mg, 50 mg, 100 mg.

DOSAGE

TABLETS

Type 2 diabetes mellitus.

Adults: 100 mg once daily either as monotherapy or in combination with metformin or a thiazolidinedione.

NURSING IMPLICATIONS

IMPLEMENTATION/ADMINISTRATION/STORAGE

1. Give a dose of 50 mg once daily for those with moderately impaired renal function: C_{CR} greater than or equal to 30 mL/min to <50 mL/min, approximately corresponding to serum creatinine levels less than or equal to 1.7 mg/dL in men and less than or equal to 1.5 mg/dL in women.
2. Give a dose of 25 mg once daily for severely impaired renal function: C_{CR} <30 mL/min, corresponding to serum creatinine levels of >3 mg/dL in men and >2.5 mg/dL in women or with end stage renal disease requiring hemodialysis or peritoneal dialysis. Sitagliptin can be given without regard to the timing of hemodialysis.
3. Dosage adjustment not needed in clients with mild or moderate impaired hepatic function. There is no clinical experience for use in those with a Child-Pugh score >9.
4. Store from 15–30°C (59–86°F).

ASSESSMENT

1. Note reasons for therapy, onset, characteristics of S&S, other agents trialed, outcome.
2. Assess renal function in the elderly before initiating sitagliptin therapy; reduce dose with renal dysfunction.
3. List risk factors, weight, BP, eye and foot exam findings. Assess for organ damage, neuropathy or other diabetes related problems.
4. Observe carefully for S&S of pancreatitis.
5. Monitor lipids, renal and LFTs, HbA1c, microalbumin; reduce dose with liver/renal dysfunction.

CLIENT/FAMILY TEACHING

1. Can be taken with or without food. Acts by slowing the inactivation of incretin hormones.
2. Drug is used alone or with other agents to control blood sugar in addition to diet, regular daily exercise and weight loss.

S

3. May experience upper respiratory tract infection, stuffy or runny nose, sore throat, and headache; report if persistent or bothersome.
4. Record finger sticks to share with provider.
5. Persistent severe abdominal pain with/without vomiting may indicate acute pancreatitis and requires immediate reporting.
6. During periods of stress (e.g., fever, trauma, infection, surgery) may require different medication doses; report.
7. Hypoglycemia increased when drug added to a sulfonylurea or insulin; lower doses of the sulfonylurea or insulin may be required to reduce hypoglycemia.
8. Reports of allergic reactions have been reported. If S&S of allergic reactions occur (rash, hives, and swelling of the face, tongue, and throat), stop drug and seek medical care.
9. Keep all F/U to assess response, labs, and for adverse SE.

OUTCOMES/EVALUATE

Control of diabetes; HbA1c <8

IV

Sodium bicarbonate

(**SO**-dee-um bye-**KAR**-bon-ayt)

Classification(s): Alkalinizing agent, Antacid, Electrolyte

Pregnancy Category: C

OTC: Arm and Hammer Pure Baking Soda, Bell/ans, Citrocarbonate, Soda Mint.

RX: Neut.

INDICATIONS/USES

(1) Treatment of hyperacidity. (2) Severe diarrhea (where there is loss of bicarbonate). (3) Alkalization of the urine to treat drug toxicity (e.g., due to barbiturates, salicylates, methanol). (4) Treatment of acute mild to moderate metabolic acidosis due to shock, severe dehydration, anoxia, uncontrolled diabetes, renal disease, cardiac arrest, extracorporeal circulation of blood, severe primary lactic acidosis. (5) Prophylaxis of renal calculi in gout. (6) During sulfonamide therapy to prevent renal calculi and nephrotoxicity. (7) Neutralizing additive solution to decrease chemical phlebitis and client discomfort due to vein irritation at or near the site of infusion of IV acid solutions. *Investigational:* Sickle cell anemia.

ACTION/KINETICS

Action

The antacid action is due to neutralization of hydrochloric acid by forming sodium chloride and carbon dioxide (1 gram of sodium bicarbonate neutralizes 12 mEq of acid). Provides temporary relief of peptic ulcer pain and of discomfort associated with indigestion. Although widely used by the public, sodium bicarbonate is rarely prescribed as an antacid because of its high sodium content, short duration of action, and ability to cause alkalosis (sometimes desired). Is also a systemic and urinary alkalinizer by increasing plasma and urinary bicarbonate, respectively.

CONTRAINDICATIONS

Chloride loss due to vomiting or from continuous GI suction. With diuretics known to produce a hypochloremic alkalosis. Metabolic and respiratory alkalosis. Hypocalcemia in which alkalosis may cause tetany. Hypertension, convulsions, CHF, and other situations where administration of sodium can be dangerous. As a systemic alkalinizer when used as a neutralizing additive solution. As an antidote for strong mineral acids because carbon dioxide is formed, which may cause discomfort and even perforation.

SPECIAL CONCERNS

Use with caution in impaired renal function; toxemia of pregnancy; with oliguria or anuria; during lactation; in edema; CHF; liver cirrhosis; with low-salt diets; and, in geriatric or postoperative clients with renal or CV insufficiency with or without CHF.

SIDE EFFECTS

Most Common

Rebound hyperacidity, milk-alkali syndrome.

GI: Rebound hyperacidity, gastric distention. **Milk-alkali syndrome:** Hypercalcemia, metabolic alkalosis (dizziness, cramps, thirst, anorexia, N&V, hyperexcitability, tetany, diminished breathing, ***seizures***), renal dysfunction. **Miscellaneous:** Systemic alkalosis after prolonged use. **Following rapid infusion:** Hypernatremia, alkalosis, hyperirritability, tetany, fluid or solute overload. Extravasation following IV use may manifest ulceration, sloughing, cellulitis, or tissue necrosis at the site of injection.

S

OVERDOSE MANAGEMENT

Symptoms: Severe alkalosis that may be accompanied by tetany or hyperirritability. *Treatment:* Discontinue sodium bicarbonate. Reverse symptoms of alkalosis by rebreathing expired air from a paper bag or using a rebreathing mask. Use an IV infusion of ammonium chloride solution, 2.14%, to control severe cases. Treat hypokalemia by IV sodium chloride or potassium chloride. Calcium gluconate will control tetany.

DRUG INTERACTIONS

Amphetamines / ↑ Amphetamine effect by ↑ renal tubular reabsorption
Antidepressants, tricyclic / ↑ TCA effect by ↑ renal tubular reabsorption
Benzodiazepines / ↓ Benzodiazepine effect R/T ↑ urine alkalinity
Chlorpropamide / ↑ Chlorpropamide excretion rate R/T urine alkalinization
Ephedrine / ↑ Ephedrine effect by ↑ renal tubular reabsorption
Erythromycin / ↑ Erythromycin effect in urine R/T ↑ urine alkalinity
Flecainide / ↑ Flecainide effect R/T ↑ urine alkalinity
Iron products / ↓ Iron effects R/T ↑ urine alkalinity
Ketoconazole / ↓ Ketoconazole effect R/T ↑ urine alkalinity
Lithium carbonate / Excretion of lithium proportional to amount of sodium ingested. If client on sodium-free diet, may develop lithium toxicity R/T ↓ lithium excreted
Mecamylamine / ↓ Mecamylamine excretion R/T alkalinization of the urine
Methenamine compounds / ↓ Methenamine effect R/T ↑ urine alkalinity
Methotrexate / ↑ Renal methotrexate excretion R/T alkalinization of the urine
Nitrofurantoin / ↓ Nitrofurantoin effect R/T ↑ urine alkalinity
Procainamide / ↑ Procainamide effect R/T ↓ kidney excretion
Pseudoephedrine / ↑ Pseudoephedrine effect R/T ↑ tubular reabsorption
Quinidine / ↑ Quinidine effect by ↑ renal tubular reabsorption
Salicylates / ↑ Rate of salicylate excretion R/T alkalinization of the urine
Sulfonylureas / ↓ Sulfonylurea effect R/T ↑ urine alkalinity
Sympathomimetics / ↓ Sympathomimetic renal excretion R/T alkalinization of the urine
Tetracyclines / ↓ Tetracycline effect R/T ↑ kidney excretion

HOW SUPPLIED

Injection: 4%, 4.2%, 5%, 7.5%, 8.4%; ***Powder; Tablets:*** 325 mg, 520 mg, 650 mg.

DOSAGE

EFFERVESCENT POWDER

Antacid.

Adults: 3.9–10 grams in a glass of cold water after meals. **Geriatric and pediatric, 6–12 years:** 1.9–3.9 grams after meals.

ORAL POWDER

Antacid.

Adults: ½ teaspoon in a glass of water q 2 hr; adjust dosage as required.

Urinary alkalinizer.

Adults: 1 teaspoon in a glass of water q 4 hr; adjust dosage as required. Dosage not established for this form for children.

TABLETS

Antacid.

Adults: 0.325–2 grams 1–4 times per day; **pediatric, 6–12 years:** 520 mg; may be repeated once after 30 min.

Urinary alkalinizer.

Adults, initial: 0.325–2 grams up to 4 times per day; **then**, maximum of 15 grams in those under age 60 and 8 grams in those over age 60.

IV

Cardiac arrest.

Adults: 200–300 mEq given rapidly as a 7.5% or 8.4% solution. In emergencies, 300–500 mL of a 5% solution given as rapidly as possible without overalkalinizing the client. **Infants, less than 2 years of age, initial:** 1–2 mEq/kg/min given over 1–2 min; **then,** 1 mEq/kg q 10 min of arrest. Do not exceed 8 mEq/kg/day.

Severe metabolic acidosis.

90–180 mEq/L (about 7.5–15 grams) at a rate of 1–1.5 L during the first hour. Adjust to needs of client.

Less severe metabolic acidosis.
Add to other IV fluids. **Adults and older children:** 2–5 mEq/kg given over a 4 to 8 hr period.
Neutralizing additive solution.
One vial of neutralizing additive solution added to 1 L of commonly used parenteral solutions, including dextrose, NaCl, and Ringer's.

NURSING IMPLICATIONS

IMPLEMENTATION/ADMINISTRATION/STORAGE

1. IV Hypertonic solutions must be administered by trained personnel. Avoid extravasation as tissue irritation or cellulitis may result.
2. Determine IV dose by arterial blood pH, pCO_2, and base deficit; may be given by IV push in arrest situation or diluted in dextrose or saline solution and given over 4–8 hr.
3. Administer isotonic solutions slowly; too rapid administration may result in death due to cellular acidity. Check rate of flow frequently.
4. If only the 7.5% or 8.4% solution is available, dilute 1:1 with D5W when used in infants for cardiac arrest.
5. Do not exceed a rate of administration of 8 mEq/kg/day in infants with cardiac arrest to guard against hypernatremia, induction of intracranial hemorrhage, and decreasing CSF pressure.
6. In the event of severe alkalosis or tetany, have available a parenteral solution of calcium gluconate and 2.14% ammonium chloride.
7. Do not add to calcium-containing solutions, except where compatibility has been established.
8. Norepinephrine and dobutamine are incompatible with $NaHCO_3$.
9. COMPATIBILITY D5W, saline and dextrose/saline solutions.
10. INCOMPATIBILITY Ringer's solution, RL; administer separately.

ASSESSMENT

1. Note reasons for therapy, any history of renal impairment or CHF.
2. Assess for edema, which may indicate inability to utilize $NaHCO_3$. May try potassium bicarbonate (sodium content is 27%).
3. If on low continuous or intermittent NG suctioning or vomiting, assess for evidence of excessive chloride loss.
4. Record I&O. Observe for dry skin/mucous membranes, polydipsia, polyuria, and air hunger; may indicate a reversal of metabolic acidosis. With acidosis, assess relief of dyspnea and hyperpnea.
5. If prescribed to counteract metabolic acidosis, monitor electrolytes and ABGs (pH, pCO_2, and HCO_3). For urine, test q 4–8 hr with nitrazine paper to determine if becoming alkaline (pH >7).

CLIENT/FAMILY TEACHING

1. Chew tablets thoroughly and take only as prescribed. Follow with a full glass of water. Do not take with milk or yogurt—will fizz up and may cause renal calculi. Consuming sodium bicarbonate with milk or calcium may result in a milk-alkali syndrome.
2. If routinely taking excessive PO preparations of sodium bicarbonate to relieve gastric distress, a rebound reaction may occur, resulting either in an increased acid secretion or systemic alkalosis. Persistent symptoms of gastric distress especially with chest pain, SOB, diarrhea or dark tarry BMs require medical care.
3. Continuous, routine ingestion of sodium bicarbonate may cause formation of phosphate crystals in the kidney, kidney stones, and fluid retention.
4. Report immediately if anorexia, N&V, or mental confusion occurs.
5. Avoid OTC preparations that contain sodium bicarbonate, such as Alka/Bromo-Seltzer, Gaviscon, or Fizrin.
6. Keep all F/U to assess response, labs, and for adverse SE.

OUTCOMES/EVALUATE

- Reversal of metabolic acidosis
- ↑ Urinary and serum pH
- ↓ Gastric discomfort

IV

Sodium chloride

(**SO**-dee-um **KLOR**-eyed)

Classification(s): Electrolyte

Pregnancy Category: C

S

OTC: Nasal Gel: Ayr Saline, Nasal Moist, Rhinaris. **Nasal Drops/Nasal Solution/Nasal Spray:** Ayr Saline, Breathe Free, Entsol, HuMIST Moisturizing Mist, Mycinaire Saline Mist, NaSal, Nasal Moist, Ocean Mist, Pretz Irrigation, Pretz Moisturizing, Salinex Nasal Mist, Simply Saline. **Ophthalmic:** Adsorbonac Ophthalmic, AK-NaCl, Hypersal 5%, Muro-128 Ophthalmic, Muroptic-5. **Tablets:** Slo-Salt.

RX: Parenteral: Concentrated Sodium Chloride Injection (14.6%, 23.4%), Sodium Chloride Diluent (0.9%), Sodium Chloride Injection for Admixtures (50, 100, 625 mEq/vial), Sodium Chloride IV Infusions (0.45%, 0.9%, 3%, 5%).

🍁 **OTC:** Rhinaris Saline Pediatric Drops/Saline Spray.

INDICATIONS/USES

PO: (1) Prophylaxis of heat prostration or muscle cramps. (2) Chloride deficiency due to diuresis or salt restriction. (3) Prevention or treatment of extracellular volume depletion.

Parenteral: 0.9% (Isotonic) NaCl. (1) Restore sodium and chloride losses. (2) Dilute or dissolve drugs for IV, IM, or SC use or for inhalation. (3) Flushing of IV catheters, including the indwelling venipuncture device where the drug is to be given is incompatible with heparin. (4) Extracellular fluid replacement. (5) Priming solution for hemodialysis. (6) Initiate and terminate blood transfusions so RBCs will not hemolyze. (7) Metabolic alkalosis when there is fluid loss and mild sodium depletion.

0.45% (Hypotonic) NaCl. (1) Fluid replacement when fluid loss exceeds depletion of electrolytes. (2) Hyperosmolar diabetes when dextrose should not be used (need for large volume of fluid but without excess sodium ions). (3) Dissolve drugs for IM, IV, or SC injection or for inhalation.

0.45% and 0.9% flexible plastic containers. Parenteral replenishment of fluid and NaCl as required by the clinical condition of the client.

0.45% and 0.9% vial: (1) Diluting or dissolving drugs for IM, IV, or SC injection or for inhalation according to instructions of the manufacturer of the drug to be given. (2) Flushing of IV catheters and for tracheal lavage.

3% or 5% (Hypertonic) NaCl. (1) Hyponatremia and hypochloremia due to electrolyte and fluid loss replaced with sodium-free fluids. (2) Drastic dilution of extracellular body fluid following excessive water intake sometimes resulting from multiple enemas or perfusion of irrigating fluids into open venous sinuses during transurethral prostatic resections. (3) Emergency treatment of severe salt depletion due to excessive sweating, vomiting, diarrhea, or other conditions.

Concentrated NaCl (14.6%). Electrolyte replenisher in parenteral fluid therapy. Serves as a sodium supplement in hyponatremia or low salt syndrome, as an additive for TPN, and as an additive for carbohydrate-containing IV fluids. Conditions include extensive burns, failure of gastric secretion, and postoperative intestinal paralysis.

Concentrated NaCl (23.4%). Additive in parenteral fluid therapy for those who have special problems of sodium electrolyte intake or excretion.

Bacteriostatic NaCl. Used only to dilute or dissolve drugs for IM, IV, or SC injection.

Nasal Topical Gel/Drops/Mist/Spray: (1) Relief of inflamed, dry, or crusted nasal membranes. (2) Nasal wash for sinuses and to restore moisture.

Ophthalmic: (1) Hypertonic solutions to decrease corneal edema due to bullous keratitis. (2) An aid to facilitate ophthalmoscopic examination in gonioscopy, biomicroscopy, and funduscopy.

ACTION/KINETICS

Action

Sodium is the major cation of the body's extracellular fluid. It plays a crucial role in maintaining the fluid and electrolyte balance. Excess retention of sodium results in overhydration (edema, hypervolemia), which is often treated with diuretics. Abnormally low levels of sodium result in dehydration. Normally, the plasma contains 136–145 mEq sodium/L and 98–106 mEq chloride/L. The average daily requirement of salt is approximately 5 grams.

CONTRAINDICATIONS

Congestive heart failure, severely impaired renal function, hypernatremia, fluid retention. Use of the 3% or 5% solutions in elevated, normal, or only slightly depressed levels of plasma sodium and chloride. Use of bacteriostatic NaCl injection in newborns.

SPECIAL CONCERNS

- **Use with caution in CV, cirrhotic, or renal disease; in presence of hyperproteinemia, hyper-**

volemia, urinary tract obstruction, and CHF; in those with concurrent edema and sodium retention; in clients receiving corticosteroids or corticotropin; and, during lactation.

- **Use with caution in geriatric or postoperative clients with renal or CV insufficiency with or without CHF.**
- **Safety and efficacy of NaCl injection have not been determined in children, although 0.45% and 0.9% flexible plastic containers are used in children.**
- **In neonates or very small infants, the volume of fluid may affect fluid and electrolyte balance.**
- **Only preservative-free NaCl solution should be used in newborns.**

SIDE EFFECTS

Most Common

When used IV: Reactions at site of IV administration, hypernatremia, local pain/irritation from too rapid infusion.

Hypernatremia: Excessive NaCl may lead to hypopotassemia and acidosis. Hypokalemia due to excessive administration of potassium-free solutions. Fluid and solute overload leading to dilution of serum electrolyte levels, CHF, overhydration, ***acute pulmonary edema*** (especially in clients with CV disease or in those receiving corticosteroids or other drugs that cause sodium retention). Too rapid administration may cause local pain and venous irritation. Ion excess or deficit due to ions present/not present in the solution. Sodium overload can result from administration of concentrated NaCl solutions.

Postoperative intolerance of NaCl: Cellular dehydration, weakness, asthenia, disorientation, anorexia, nausea, oliguria, increased BUN levels, distention, deep respiration.

Symptoms due to solution or administration technique: Fever, abscess, tissue necrosis, infection at injection site, venous thrombosis or phlebitis extending from injection site, local tenderness, extravasation, hypervolemia. ***Inadvertent administration of concentrated NaCl (i.e., without dilution) will cause sudden hypernatremia with the possibility of CV shock, extensive hemolysis, CNS problems, necrosis of the cortex of the kidneys, local tissue necrosis (if given extravascularly).***

OVERDOSE MANAGEMENT

Symptoms: Irritation of GI mucosa, N&V, abdominal cramps, diarrhea, edema. Hypernatremia symptoms include: irritability, restlessness, ***weakness, seizures***, coma, tachycardia, hypertension, fluid accumulation, ***pulmonary edema, respiratory arrest.*** *Treatment:* Supportive measures, including gastric lavage, induction of vomiting, provide adequate airway and ventilation, maintain vascular volume and tissue perfusion. Mg sulfate given as a cathartic.

DRUG INTERACTIONS

Use solutions containing sodium with caution in clients receiving corticosteroids or corticotropin.

HOW SUPPLIED

Injection: 0.45%, 0.9%, 2.5%, 3%, 5%, 14.6%, 23.4%; ***Inhalation Solution:*** 0.45%, 0.9%, 3%, 10%; ***Irrigation Solution:*** 0.45%, 0.9%; ***Nasal Drops:*** 0.4%, 0.65%; ***Nasal Gel:*** 0.2%, 0.65%; ***Nasal Drops/Mist/Spray:*** 0.4%, 0.65%; ***Ophthalmic Ointment:*** 5%; ***Ophthalmic Solution:*** 0.44%, 2%, 5%; ***Tablets:*** 600 mg, 1 gram, 2.25 grams; ***Tablets, Slow Release:*** 600 mg; ***Powder for Reconstitution.***

DOSAGE

TABLETS; TABLETS, SLOW RELEASE

Heat cramps/dehydration.

0.5–1 gram with 8 oz water up to 10 times/day; total daily dose should not exceed 4.8 grams.

IV

Individualized. Daily requirements of sodium and chloride can be met by administering 1 L of 0.9% NaCl.

To calculate sodium deficit. Amount of sodium to be given to raise serum sodium to the desired level:

Total body water (TBW): sodium deficit (mEq) = TBW × (desired plasma Na − observed plasma Na)

NASAL DROPS, SOLUTION, SPRAY

Nasal wash, restore moisture, thin nasal secretions.

2 to 6 drops/sprays in each nostril q 2 hr, as often as needed, or as directed by provider.

OPHTHALMIC SOLUTION 2% OR 5%

1–2 gtt in eye q 3–4 hr.

S

OPHTHALMIC OINTMENT

A small amount (approximately ¼ in.) to the inside of the affected eye(s) (i.e., by pulling down the lower eyelid) q 3–4 hr.

NURSING IMPLICATIONS

IMPLEMENTATION/ADMINISTRATION/STORAGE

1. IV Give hypertonic injections of NaCl slowly through a small-bore needle placed well within the lumen of a large vein (to minimize irritation). Avoid infiltration.
2. Flush IV catheters before and after the medications are given using 0.9% NaCl for injection.
3. Incompatibilities may occur when mixing NaCl injection with other additives; inspect the final product for cloudiness or a precipitate immediately after mixing, before administration, and periodically during administration. Do not store these mixtures.
4. When using the 3% and 5% concentrates, do not use plastic container in series connection.
5. If administration is controlled by a pumping device, take care to discontinue pumping action before the container runs dry or air embolism may result.
6. When a hypertonic solution is to be given peripherally, infuse slowly through a small bore needle, placed well within the lumen of a large vein to minimize venous irritation. Carefully avoid infiltration.
7. The maximum IV dosage of the 3% or 5% concentrate should be 100 mL given over a period of 1 hr. Before an additional amount is given, determine the serum electrolyte concentrations, including chloride and bicarbonate in order to evaluate the need for more sodium chloride. Do not exceed 400 mL given in 24 hr.
8. The 14.6% concentrate is given IV, but only after dilution in a larger volume of fluid. The actual dose of sodium chloride given depends on specific client needs, which are usually determined by review of serial blood samples and clinical evaluations. In solutions for total parenteral nutrition, adults typically receive 120 mEq of sodium/day (range: 75–180 mEq/day), whereas preterm infants receive 3–4 mEq/kg/day.
9. The 23.4% concentrate is strongly hypertonic and must be diluted prior to administration. The dosage is determined by the particular need of the client after clinical and laboratory information is considered. The appropriate volume is then withdrawn for proper dilution. Having determined the mEq of sodium chloride to be added, divide by 4 to calculate the number of mL of concentrated solution to be used. Withdraw this volume aseptically and transfer this additive solution into appropriate IV solutions (e.g., D5W injection). The properly diluted solution may be given IV or SC.
10. INCOMPATIBILITY Dextrose and saline solutions, Ringer's and RL solutions and combinations.
11. INCOMPATIBILITY Concentrated NaCl injection must be diluted before use.

ASSESSMENT

1. Note reasons for therapy, onset, characteristics of S&S; Note level of consciousness; assess heart and lung sounds.
2. Monitor VS and I&O. Assess urine specific gravity and serum sodium levels. Report if urine specific gravity is above 1.020 and serum sodium level is above 146 mEq/L.
3. When administering IV the 0.45% NaCl is hypotonic, the 0.9% NaCl is isotonic, and the 3% and 5% NaCl solutions are hypertonic.
4. Observe for S&S of hypernatremia: flushed skin, elevated temperature, rough dry tongue, and edema. S&S of hyponatremia include N&V, muscle cramps, dry mucous membranes, increased HR, and headaches.
5. Monitor electrolytes, ECG, renal and LFTs.

CLIENT/FAMILY TEACHING

1. Infusions usually given in monitored facility. Review form of drug prescribed and when and how to use.
2. May take tablet with a full glass of water. Undigested tablets may pass in stool. Liquid electrolyte solutions for replacement preferred.
3. Review situations that may predispose one to dehydration; exercise in high temperatures and when to take tablets.
4. Report swelling of extremities, dizziness, headaches, or confusion.
5. Keep all F/U to assess response, labs, and for adverse SE

S

OUTCOMES/EVALUATE

- Prophylaxis of heat prostration during exposure to high temperatures or during increased activity
- Prevention of chloride deficiency R/T excessive diuresis or salt restriction or excessive sweating

Solifenacin succinate

(sol-i-**FEN**-a-cin)

Classification(s): Cholinergic blocking drug

Pregnancy Category: C

RX: Vesicare.

SEE ALSO ***CHOLINERGIC BLOCKING AGENTS.***

INDICATIONS/USES

Treatment of overactive bladder with symptoms of urge urinary incontinence, urgency, and urinary frequency.

ACTION/KINETICS

Action

Solifenacin is a competitive muscarinic receptor antagonist. Muscarinic receptors play an important role in contraction of urinary bladder smooth muscle. Thus, blockade of such receptors will decrease an overactive bladder.

Pharmacokinetics

Peak plasma levels: 3–8 hr. Absolute bioavailability is about 90%. C_{max}, AUC, and t½ values are 20 to 25% higher in clients 65 to 80 years of age compared with younger clients. Is extensively metabolized by CYP3A4 isoenzymes. About 70% is excreted in the urine and 22.5% in the feces. **t ½, elimination:** 45–68 hr. **Plasma protein binding:** About 98%.

CONTRAINDICATIONS

Use in those with urinary retention, gastric retention, uncontrolled narrow-angle glaucoma, severe hepatic impairment (Child-Pugh score 10–15), and in those with hypersensitivity to the drug or any components of the product. Lactation.

SPECIAL CONCERNS

- Use with caution in those with reduced renal and hepatic function and in those with clinically significant bladder outflow obstruction, GI obstructive disorders or decreased GI motility, or in clients being treated for narrow-angle glaucoma.
- Use with caution in those with a known history of QT prolongation or in those who are taking medications known to prolong the QT interval.
- Safety and efficacy not determined in children.

SIDE EFFECTS

Most Common

Dry mouth, dry eyes, constipation, blurred vision, influenza, urinary retention, UTI, upper abdominal pain, dizziness.

GI: Dry mouth, constipation, N&V, upper abdominal pain, dyspepsia. **CNS:** Dizziness, depression, confusion, hallucinations, headache. **CV:** Hypertension, QT prolongation, torsades de pointes. **GU:** UTI, urinary retention. **Respiratory:** Pharyngitis, cough. **Hypersensitivity:** ***Angioedema*** of the face, lips, tongue, and/or larynx (even after the first dose); airway obstruction, pruritus, rash, urticaria. **Ophthalmic:** Blurred vision (accommodation abnormalities), dry eyes. **Body as a whole:** Fatigue, influenza. **Miscellaneous:** Lower limb edema, peripheral edema.

OVERDOSE MANAGEMENT

Symptoms: **Acute:** Severe anticholinergic effects. **Chronic:** Intolerable anticholinergic side effects, including fixed and dilated pupils, blurred vision, failure of heel-to-toe exam, tremors, dry skin. *Treatment:* Gastric lavage. Appropriate supportive measures.

DRUG INTERACTIONS

Atazanavir / ↑ Solifenacin plasma levels → ↑ pharmacologic/toxic effects; do not exceed a 5 mg/day dose of solifenacin
Clarithromycin / ↑ Solifenacin plasma levels → ↑ pharmacologic/toxic effects; do not exceed a 5 mg/day dose of solifenacin
CYP3A4 inducers (e.g., rifampin) / ↓ Solifenacin plasma levels → ↓ pharmacologic effect
Indinavir / ↑ Solifenacin plasma levels → ↑ pharmacologic/toxic effects; do not exceed a 5 mg/day dose of solifenacin
Itraconazole / ↑ Solifenacin plasma levels → ↑ pharmacologic/toxic effects; do not exceed a 5 mg/day dose of solifenacin
Ketoconazole / ↑ Solifenacin plasma levels → ↑ pharmacologic/toxic effects; do not exceed a 5 mg/day dose of solifenacin
Nefazodone / ↑ Solifenacin plasma levels → ↑ pharmacologic/toxic effects; do not exceed a 5 mg/day dose of solifenacin

S

Nelfinavir / ↑ Solifenacin plasma levels → ↑ pharmacologic/toxic effects; do not exceed a 5 mg/day dose of solifenacin
Potassium preparations (e.g., potassium chloride) / Passage of solid KCl dose forms through the GI trace may be delayed or arrested R/T slowing of GI motility by solifenacin; coadministration is contraindicated; use KCl liquid products
Ritonavir / ↑ Solifenacin plasma levels → ↑ pharmacologic/toxic effects; do not exceed a 5 mg/day dose of solifenacin
Saquinavir / ↑ Solifenacin plasma levels → ↑ pharmacologic/toxic effects; do not exceed a 5 mg/day dose of solifenacin
Telithromycin / ↑ Solifenacin plasma levels → ↑ pharmacologic/toxic effects; do not exceed a 5 mg/day dose of solifenacin
Voriconazole / ↑ Solifenacin plasma levels → ↑ pharmacologic/toxic effects; do not exceed a 5 mg/day dose of solifenacin

HOW SUPPLIED

Tablets: 5 mg, 10 mg.

DOSAGE

TABLETS

Overactive bladder.

Adults: 5 mg once daily. If the 5 mg dose is well tolerated, the dose may be increased to 10 mg once daily.

NURSING IMPLICATIONS

IMPLEMENTATION/ADMINISTRATION/STORAGE

1. Do not exceed a dose of 5 mg daily in clients with severe renal impairment (C_{CR} <30 mL/min), with moderate hepatic impairment (Child-Pugh score 7 to 9), or when administered with therapeutic doses of ketoconazole or other CYP3A4 inhibitors.
2. Store from 15–30°C (59–86°F).

ASSESSMENT

1. Note reasons for therapy, characteristics of S&S, other agents trialed, urologic findings.
2. List drugs prescribed to ensure none interact. Review urinary patterns, S&S of overactive bladder (frequency, urgency, incontinence) and triggers.
3. Note history of CAD, urinary/gastric retention, ulcerative colitis, BPH, narrow angle glaucoma, myasthenia gravis or severe liver/renal disease; may preclude drug therapy.
4. Monitor renal and LFTs; reduce dose with dysfunction.

CLIENT/FAMILY TEACHING

1. Read the "Patient Information Leaflet" before using solifenacin, and each time you get a refill. Take at the same time each day. If dose is missed, skip that dose, and take the next dose at regularly scheduled time. Never take 2 doses to catch up, or 2 doses in the same day.
2. Take by mouth, with or without food, usually once a day, as directed. Swallow tablet whole with a full glass of liquid; do not break, crush, or chew.
3. Avoid activities that require mental alertness until drug effects realized; may experience dizziness and blurred vision.
4. Stop drug and report inability to urinate, severe abdominal pain, or sudden eye pain.
5. Wear dark glasses to make bright lights or sunlight tolerable; may cause pupils to dilate, resulting in intolerance to bright lights or sunlight.
6. Dry mouth, constipation, blurred vision, stomach upset/pain, dry eyes, or unusual tiredness/weakness may occur. Report if side effects persistent or bothersome.
7. To relieve dry mouth, suck on (sugarless) hard candy or ice chips, chew (sugarless) gum, drink water, or use a saliva substitute.
8. May cause angioedema, which could result in life-threatening airway obstruction. If evident, stop drug and seek medical attention immediately if edema of the tongue or throat, or difficulty breathing is experienced.
9. Avoid strenuous activities in hot weather; avoid overheating.
10. Maintain a diet adequate in fiber, drink plenty of water, and exercise to prevent constipation. If constipated, may need stimulant-type laxative with stool softener.
11. Practice reliable contraception; report if pregnancy suspected or desired.
12. Keep all F/U to assess response, labs, and for adverse SE.

OUTCOMES/EVALUATE

Control of urination with ↓ frequency and ↓ urgency

Somatropin

(so-mah-**TROH**-pin)

Pregnancy Category: B (**B:** Genotropin, Omnitrope, Saizen, Serostim, Zorbtive. **C:** Accretropin, Humatrope, Norditropin, Nutropin, Nutropin AQ, Tev-Tropin)

RX: Accretropin, Genotropin, Genotropin Miniquick, Humatrope, HumatroPen, Norditropin, Norditropin FlexPro, Nutropin, Nutropin AQ, Nutropin AQ NuSpin 5, NuSpin 10, and NuSpin 20, Omnitrope, Saizen, Serostim, Tev-Tropin, Zorbtive.

INDICATIONS/USES

1. Growth failure associated with chronic renal insufficiency up to the time of renal transplantation (Nutropin or Nutropin AQ in combination with optimal management of chronic renal insufficiency).
2. Growth failure (i.e., children with short stature) associated with Noonan syndrome (Norditropin).
3. Growth failure associated with Prader-Willi syndrome (Genotropin). Confirm diagnosis by appropriate genetic testing.
4. Growth failure associated with Turner syndrome in those who have open epiphyses (Accretropin, Genotropin, Humatrope, HumatroPen, Norditropin, Nutropin, Nutropin AQ).
5. Growth failure in children caused by an inadequate secretion of endogenous growth hormone (Accretropin, Genotropin, Humatrope, HumatroPen, Norditropin, Nutropin, Nutropin AQ, Omnitrope, Saizen, Tev-Tropin). Genotropin is also used for children born small for gestational age who fail to manifest catch-up growth by 2 years of age. Norditropin is used to treat children with short stature born small for gestational age with no catch-up growth by 2 to 4 years of age.
6. Growth hormone deficiency in adults who either (a) have growth hormone deficiency, either alone or associated with multiple hormone deficiencies, as a result of pituitary disease, hypothalamic disease, surgery, radiation, or trauma or (b) those who were growth hormone deficient during childhood as a result of congenital, genetic, acquired, or idiopathic causes (Genotropin, Humatrope, HumatroPen, Norditropin, Nutropin, Nutropin AQ, Omnitrope, Saizen). Usually, confirmation of the diagnosis of adult growth hormone deficiency in both groups requires an appropriate growth hormone stimulation test.
7. Long-term treatment of idiopathic short stature (Humatrope, HumatroPen, Nutropin, Nutropin AQ).
8. Short bowel syndrome in clients receiving specialized nutritional support (Zorbtive: used in conjunction with optimal management of short bowel syndrome).
9. Short stature homeobox-containing gene deficiency where epiphyses are not closed (Humatrope, HumatroPen).
10. Wasting or cachexia associated with HIV to increase lean body mass and body weight, and improve physical endurance (Serostim). Must be used concomitantly with antiretroviral therapy (Serostim).

ACTION/KINETICS

Action

Derived from recombinant DNA technology. Somatropin has the identical sequence of amino acids as does human growth hormone of pituitary origin. The drug stimulates linear growth by increasing somatomedin-C serum levels, which, in turn, increases the incorporation of sulfate into proteoglycans, thereby stimulating skeletal growth. It also increases the number and size of muscle cells, increases synthesis of collagen, increases protein synthesis, and increases internal organ size. Serum insulin levels increase (indicative of insulin resistance), and there is acute mobilization of lipid. A small percentage of clients may develop antibodies to the protein. *NOTE:* The response in children tends to decrease with time.

Pharmacokinetics

The various products have different pharmacokinetic properties. Check the package insert carefully.

CONTRAINDICATIONS

- Known hypersensitivity to somatropin, growth hormone, or any component of the products.
- Use for growth promotion in children with closed epiphyses; in those with active proliferative, preproliferative, or severe nonproliferative

diabetic retinopathy; hypersensitivity to growth hormone; evidence of active malignancy.

- Use in those with any evidence of progression or recurrence of an underlying intracranial tumor.
- Initiation of growth hormone to treat clients with acute critical illness due to complications following open-heart surgery or abdominal surgery or multiple accidental trauma, or to treat those having acute respiratory failure.
- When reconstituted with bacteriostatic water for injection in clients with a known sensitivity to benzyl alcohol.
- Humatrope: Those with a known sensitivity to metacresol or glycerin should not be given Humatrope reconstituted with the supplied diluent.
- Genotropin, Humatrope, Norditropin, Nutropin, Nutropin AQ, Omnitrope, Saizen, and Tev-Tropin: Use in clients with Prader-Willi syndrome who are severely obese or have severe respiratory impairment.
- Use of Humatrope, Norditropin, Nutropin, Nutropin AQ, Omnitrope, Saizen, or Tev-Tropin in clients with Prader-Willi syndrome unless they also have a diagnosis of growth hormone deficiency.

SPECIAL CONCERNS

- **Antimalignancy treatment must be complete with evidence of remission before instituting therapy. Discontinue somatropin if there is evidence of recurrent activity.**
- **Use with caution during lactation.**
- **Concomitant use of glucocorticoids may decrease response to growth hormone.**
- **Safety and efficacy not determined for use in individuals 65 years and older.**
- **Obese clients are more likely to manifest side effects when treated with a weight-based regimen.**
- **Women may need higher doses than men. Oral estrogen uses may increase dose requirements in women.**
- **After somatropin therapy, fatalities have occurred in children with Prader-Willi syndrome who also had one or more of the following risk factors: Severe obesity, history of upper airway obstructions or sleep apnea, or unidentified respiratory infection. Males are at greater risk than females.**
- **Benzyl alcohol, a preservative in bacteriostatic water for injection, has been associated with toxicity in newborns. When giving somatropin to newborns, use sterile water for injection.**

SIDE EFFECTS

NOTE: Due to the large number of somatropin products with varying side effects, each product will be listed separately. However, there are side effects that are common to most somatropin products. These include: Glucose intolerance; new onset type 2 diabetes mellitus or exacerbation of pre-existing diabetes mellitus; intracranial hypertension (including symptoms of papilledema, visual changes, headache, N &/or V); fluid retention in adults; slipped capital femoral epiphyses in clients with endocrine disorders; progression of renal osteodystrophy; progression of pre-existing scoliosis; tissue atrophy if somatropin is given at the same site over a long period of time; hypersensitivity reactions.

Accretropin. Injection site reactions: Bruising, edema, erythema, hemorrhage, pain, pruritus, rash, swelling. **CNS:** Headache, fatigue. **GI:** Nausea. **Miscellaneous:** Scoliosis.

Genotropin. Injection site reactions: Pain/burning on injection, fibrosis, nodules, rash, inflammation, pigmentation, bleeding. **CNS:** Headache, aggressiveness, paresthesia, hypoesthesia, central precocious puberty. **Musculoskeletal:** Arthralgia, myalgia, joint pain, jaw prominence, aggravation of pre-existing scoliosis, pain and stiffness of the extremities, back pain, carpal tunnel syndrome. **Respiratory:** URTI, sinusitis, tonsillitis. **GU:** Hematuria, UTI. **Metabolic:** Hypothyroidism, mild hyperglycemia, diabetes mellitus. **Body as a whole:** Development of antibodies to the protein, edema, fluid retention, peripheral edema, peripheral swelling, fatigue, flu syndrome. **Miscellaneous:** Lipoatrophy, hair loss in children, benign intracranial hypertension, leukemia in children.

Humatrope. Injection site reactions: Pain. **GI:** Gastritis, pancreatitis (rare). **CNS:** Headache, paresthesia, hypesthesia. **CV:** Hypertension. **Musculoskeletal:** Bone disorder, scoliosis, aching joints, hip/muscle/joint/back pain, joint disorder, arthralgia, arthrosis, myalgia, localized muscle pain, carpal tunnel syndrome. **Respiratory:** Increased cough, rhinitis, respiratory tract disorder, pharyngitis. **GU:** Gynecomastia. **Otic:** Otitis media, ear disorders. **Ophthalmic:** Conjunctival edema. **Dermatologic:** Increased nevi or increased growth of pre-existing nevi, acne. **Metabolic:**

Glucosuria, hyper-/hypothyroidism, hyperlipidemia, changes in mean fasting insulin levels, hyperglycemia. **Body as a whole:** Development of antibodies to the protein, edema (conjunctival, nonspecific, facial, peripheral), lymphedema, weakness, pain, flu syndrome, asthenia. **Miscellaneous:** Leukemia, increases in serum insulin-like growth factor-1, increased ALT and AST.

Norditropin. Body as a whole: Development of antibodies to the protein, weakness, fluid retention, peripheral edema. **Injection site reactions:** Rashes, lipoatrophy, hypersensitivity reactions (rare). **CNS:** Headache, paresthesia, ***intracranial tumors***. **GI:** Gastroenteritis, ***pancreatitis*** in children. **CV:** Hypertension, intracranial hypertension. **Musculoskeletal:** Localized muscle pain, arthralgia, myalgia, skeletal pain, leg edema, slipped capital femoral epiphysis in children. **Respiratory:** Bronchitis, laryngitis. **Ophthalmic:** Diabetic retinopathy. **Metabolic:** Fluid retention/edema, peripheral edema, unmasking of latent central hypothyroidism, glucose intolerance. **Body as a whole:** Flu-like symptoms, increased sweating, nonviral infection. **Miscellaneous:** Mild hyperglycemia, glucosuria, leukemia in children, gynecomastia in children, ***sudden death in children with Prader-Willi syndrome***.

Nutropin, Nutropin AQ. Body as a whole: Development of antibodies to the protein, peripheral edema (mild, transient), edema. **CNS:** CNS tumor, **CV:** Intracranial hypertension. **At injection site:** Discomfort, pain. **GI:** Pancreatitis (rare). **Musculoskeletal:** Arthralgia, arthritis, carpal tunnel syndrome, joint disorders, abnormal bone or other growth, fracture, new onset or progression of scoliosis, new or recurrent slipped capital femoral epiphyses, avascular necrosis. **Dermatologic:** Increased growth of pre-existing nevi (rare but possible malignant transformation). **Metabolic:** Diabetes mellitus, edema, peripheral edema. **GU:** Renal osteodystrophy, gynecomastia. **Miscellaneous:** Increased median fasting insulin, leukemia, new onset or recurring benign tumor, new onset or recurrence cancer.

Omnitrope. Injection site reaction: Rashes, lipoatrophy, hypersensitivity reactions (rare). **CNS:** Headache, paresthesia, hypesthesia, ***intracranial tumors***, especially meningiomas in teenagers/adults. **GI:** Pancreatitis in children. **CV:** Intracranial hypertension. **Musculoskeletal:** Leg pain, arthralgia, myalgia, pain and stiffness of the extremities, slipped capital femoral epiphyses in children, progression of pre-existing scoliosis in children. **GU:** Gynecomastia in children. **Hematologic:** Eosinophilia, hematoma. **Metabolic:** Glucose intolerance, fluid retention, peripheral edema, unmasking of latent central hypothyroidism, elevated glycosylated hemoglobin, hypertriglyceridemia, hypothyroidism. **Ophthalmic:** Significant diabetic retinopathy. **Miscellaneous:** ***Sudden death in children with Prader-Willi syndrome***.

Saizen. Body as a whole: Development of antibodies to the protein, disturbances in fluid balance, flu-like symptoms. **Injection site reactions:** Pain, numbness, redness, swelling. **CNS:** Paresthesia, hypesthesia, depression, dizziness, headache, insomnia, ***seizures***. **GI:** Nausea. **Musculoskeletal:** Myalgia, arthralgia, carpal tunnel syndrome, skeletal pain, back/chest pain. **Respiratory:** Rhinitis, URTI. **Metabolic:** Edema, peripheral edema, hypothyroidism. **Miscellaneous:** Hypothyroidism, hypoglycemia, leukemia, exacerbation of pre-existing psoriasis.

Serostim. GI: Diarrhea, nausea, abdominal pain, anorexia, constipation, dyspepsia, gastroenteritis, vomiting, ***pancreatitis***. **CNS:** Insomnia, paresthesia, hypesthesia, headache, peripheral neuropathy, dizziness, hypertonia, depression, anxiety, somnolence. **CV:** Hypertension, tachycardia. **Musculoskeletal:** Increased tissue turgor (swelling, especially of the hands and feet), musculoskeletal discomfort (pain, swelling, stiffness), carpal tunnel syndrome, arthralgia, myalgia, arthrosis, back/leg/chest pain, arthropathy. **Respiratory:** Rhinitis, URTI, bronchitis, cough, sinusitis, pharyngitis, pneumonia. **Dermatologic:** Folliculitis, rash, verruca, maculopapular rash, night sweats. **GU:** Gynecomastia, renal calculus, UTI, male breast neoplasm. **Hematologic:** Lymphadenopathy. **Ophthalmic:** Conjunctivitis. **Metabolic:** Elevated glucose/triglyceride levels, glucose intolerance, new onset or exacerbation of existing diabetes mellitus, diabetic ketoacidosis, ***diabetic coma***. **Body as a whole:** Edema (generalized, peripheral, dependent, periorbital), fatigue, rigors, fever, night sweats, pain, flu-like syndrome, asthenia. **Miscellaneous:** Herpes simplex, moniliasis, viral infection.

Tev-Tropin. CNS: Headaches. **Injection site reactions:** Bruising, pain.

S

Zorbtive. GI: Abdominal pain, flatulence, N&V, constipation, ***pancreatitis***, tenesmus, hemorrhoids, dry mouth, enlarged abdomen, aggravated Crohn's disease, gastric ulcer, GI fistula, melena, ***rectal hemorrhage***, mouth disorder, steatorrhea, abnormal hepatic function. **Injection site reactions:** Pain, injection site disorders, inflammation, reaction pain. **CNS:** Dizziness, headache, hypesthesia, depression, insomnia, paresthesia, phantom pain, psychiatric disorders. **CV:** Vascular disorder, vasodilation, tachycardia. **Dermatologic:** Rash, pruritus, nail disorder, skin disorder, increased sweating, alopecia, bullous eruption. **Respiratory:** Rhinitis, laryngitis, pharyngitis, bronchospasm, dsypnea, respiratory tract disorder/infection. **Musculoskeletal:** Increased tissue turgor (swelling, especially of the hands and feet), musculoskeletal discomfort (pain, swelling, stiffness), carpal tunnel syndrome, arthralgia, myalgia, chest/back pain, arthritis, arthropathy, bursitis, cramps. **GU:** Pyelonephritis, breast pain/enlargement (females), vaginal fungal infection, renal calculus, dysuria, UTI, abnormal urine, vaginal fungal infection. **Hematologic:** Purpura, decreased prothrombin. **Ophthalmic:** Visual field defect. **Otic:** Hearing/ear problems. **Body as a whole:** Dehydration, thirst, edema (peripheral, facial, generalized, periorbital), pain, fever, flu-like disorder, malaise, fatigue, rigors, allergic reaction. **Miscellaneous:** Infection (bacterial, viral, fungal), moniliasis, hypomagnesemia, enlarged abdomen, ***sepsis.***

LABORATORY TEST CONSIDERATIONS

↑ Inorganic phosphorus, alkaline phosphatase, parathyroid hormone, IGF-1.

OVERDOSE MANAGEMENT

Symptoms: In acute overdose, hypoglycemia followed by hyperglycemia. Long-term overdose can result in S&S of acromegaly or gigantism.

DRUG INTERACTIONS

Estrogens / Larger dose may be needed in women on PO estrogen replacement

Drugs metabolized by P450 liver enzymes (e.g., anticonvulsants, corticosteroids, cyclosporine, sex steroids) / ↑ P450-mediated clearance of these drugs; monitor carefully

Glucocorticoids (e.g., cortisol, cortisone, prednisone) / Inhibition of the effect of somatrem on growth; somatropin may also impact the metabolism of cortisol and cortisone

Insulin / ↓ Sensitivity to insulin especially at high doses in susceptible clients; adjustment of dosage may be required

Oral hypoglycemic drugs / Adjustment of dosage may be required

HOW SUPPLIED

Accretropin. *Injection Solution:* 5 mg (15 units)/mL.

Genotropin. *Injection, Lyophilized Powder for Solution:* 5.8 mg (about 17.4 units)/cartridge, 13.8 mg (about 41.4 units)/cartridge.

Genotropin Miniquick. *Injection, Lyophilized Powder for Solution:* 0.2 mg (about 0.6 units)/cartridge, 0.4 mg (about 1.2 units)/cartridge, 0.6 mg (about 1.8 units)/cartridge, 0.8 mg (about 2.4 units)/cartridge, 1 mg (about 3 units)/cartridge, 1.2 mg (about 3.6 units)/cartridge, 1.4 mg (about 4.2 units)/cartridge, 1.6 mg (about 4.8 units)/cartridge, 1.8 mg (about 5.4 units)/cartridge, 2 mg (about 6 units)/cartridge.

Humatrope. *Injection Lyophilized Powder for Solution:* 5 mg (about 15 units)/vial.

HumatroPen. *Injection, Lyophilized Powder for Solution:* 6 mg (18 units)/cartridge, 12 mg (36 units)/cartridge, 24 mg (72 units)/cartridge.

Norditropin. *Injection Solution:* 5 mg/1.5 mL, 10 mg/1.5 mL, 15 mg/1.5 mL, 30 mg/3 mL.

Norditropin FlexPro. *Injection Solution:* 5 mg/1.5 mL, 10 mg/1.5 mL, 15 mg/1.5 mL.

Nutropin. *Injection, Lyophilized Powder for Solution:* 5 mg (about 15 units)/vial, 10 mg (about 30 units)/vial.

Nutropin AQ. *Injection Solution:* 10 mg (about 30 units)/vial or cartridge, 20 mg (about 60 units)/cartridge.

Nutropin AQ NuSpin 5, 10, and 20. *Injection Solution:* 5 mg (about 15 units)/mL, 10 mg (about 30 units)/vial or cartridge, 20 mg (about 60 units)/cartridge.

Omnitrope. *Injection Solution:* 5 mg/1.5 mL, 10 mg/1.5 mL; *Injection, Lyophilized Powder for Solution:* 1.5 mg (about 4.5 units)/vial, 5.8 mg (about 17.4 units)/vial.

Saizen. *Injection, Lyophilized Powder for Solution:* 5 mg (about 15 units)/vial, 8.8 mg (about 26.4 units)/vial.

Serostim. *Injection, Lyophilized Powder for Solution:* 4 mg (about 12 units)/vial, 5 mg (about 15

S

units)/vial, 6 mg (about 18 units)/vial, 8.8 mg (about 26.4 units)/vial.
Tev-Tropin. *Injection, Lyophilized Powder for Solution:* 5 mg (about 15 units)/vial.
Zorbtive. *Injection, Powder for Solution:* 8.8 mg (about 26.4 units)/vial.

DOSAGE

Accretropin

SC

Growth failure in children.

Weekly dose: 0.18–0.3 mg/kg (0.9 unit/kg). Divide the dose into equal daily doses given 6 or 7 times per week. Do not continue therapy if epiphyseal fusion has occurred.

Growth failure associated with Turner syndrome.

Weekly dose: 0.36 mg/kg divided into equal daily doses given 6 or 7 times per week.

Genotropin; Genotropin Miniquick

SC

Growth failure in children.

Weekly dose: 0.16–0.24 mg/kg divided into 6 or 7 daily injections for children with growth hormone deficiency. For children born small for gestational age, the dosage is 0.48 mg/kg/week divided into 6 or 7 injections. Do not continue therapy if epiphyseal fusion has occurred.

Growth failure due to Prader-Willi syndrome in children.

Weekly dose, usual: 0.24 mg/kg divided into 6–7 SC injections.

Growth failure associated with Turner syndrome.

Weekly dose, usual: 0.33 mg/kg divided into 6–7 SC injections.

Growth hormone deficiency in adults.

Individualize. Weekly dose, initial: No more than 0.04 mg/kg given in 7 divided daily injections. May increase dose at 4- to 8-week intervals according to client response, up to a maximum of 0.08 mg/kg/week. *NOTE:* IGF-1 levels may be used as a guide in dose titration. **Alternative dose, initial:** 0.2 mg/day (range: 0.15–0.3 mg/day) without consideration of body weight. Can increase the dose q 1–2 months by increments of about 0.1–0.2 mg/day, depending on clinical response on serum IGF-1 levels. Decrease the dose if side effects and/or serum IGF-1 levels are above the age- and gender-specific normal range.

Idiopathic short stature.

Weekly dose: Up to 0.47 mg/kg divided into 6 or 7 SC injections.

Humatrope and HumatroPen

IM; SC

Growth hormone deficiency in children.

Individualize. Weekly dose usual: 0.18 mg/kg (0.54 units/kg), up to a maximum of 0.3 mg/kg/week (0.90 units/kg/week). Divide weekly dose into 6 or 7 equal daily doses. SC is preferred. Do not continue therapy if epiphyseal fusion has occurred.

Children small for gestational age.

Individualize. Weekly dose, usual: 0.47 mg/kg divided into 6 or 7 daily SC injections. Daily dose is 0.067 mg/kg/day.

Growth failure associated with Turner syndrome.

Weekly dose, usual: 0.375 mg/kg (1.125 units/kg) divided into 6 or 7 daily SC injections. Daily dose is 0.054 mg/kg/day.

Growth hormone deficiency in adults.

Adults, initial: No more than 0.006 mg/kg/day (0.0198 units/kg/day) SC. Dose may be increased, depending on individual requirements, to a maximum of 0.0125 mg/kg/day (0.0375 units/kg/day). **Alternative dose, initial:** 0.2 mg/day (range: 0.15–0.3 mg/day). Dose can be increased gradually q 1–2 months by increments of about 0.1–0.2 mg/day, based on individual client needs, clinical response, and IGF-1 levels. *NOTE:* IGF-1 levels may be used as a guide in dose titration. Titrate dose based on side effects or to maintain the insulin-like growth factor response below the ULN levels matched

S

for age and gender. Dose reductions may be needed in clients with advancing age or excessive body weight.

Idiopathic short stature.

Weekly dose, usual: Up to 0.37 mg/kg SC. Divide into equal doses given 6–7 times per week. Daily dose is 0.053 mg/kg/day.

Short stature homeobox-containing gene deficiency.

Weekly dose: 0.35 mg/kg divided into 6 or 7 daily SC injections. Daily dose is 0.05 mg/kg/day.

Norditropin, Norditropin FlexPro

SC

Growth hormone deficiency in children or children with short stature born small for gestational age.

Individualize. Daily dose, usual: 0.024–0.034 mg/kg 6 to 7 times per week in children with growth hormone deficiency. For children with short stature born small for gestational age with no catch-up growth by 2 to 4 years of age, a dose up to 0.067 mg/kg/day is recommended. Give injections in the thighs; vary injection site in the thigh on a rotating basis. Do not continue therapy if epiphyseal fusion has occurred.

Growth failure associated with Noonan syndrome.

Up to 0.066 mg/kg/day by SC injection. Not all clients with Noonan syndrome have short stature. Thus, prior to treatment establish that the client has short stature.

Growth failure associated with Turner syndrome.

Up to 0.067 mg/kg/day by SC injection.

Growth hormone deficiency in adults.

Adults, initial: Not more than 0.004 mg/kg/day. The dose may be increased to not more than 0.016 mg/kg/day after about 6 weeks depending on client requirements. **Alternative dose, initial:** 0.2 mg/day (range: 0.15–0.3 mg/day) used without consideration of body weight. Dose may be increased gradually q 1–2 months by increments of about 0.1–0.2 mg/day, according to client requirements, clinical response, and serum IGF-1 levels above the age- and gender-specific normal range. *NOTE:* IGF-1 levels may be used as a guide in dose titration.

Nutropin, Nutropin AQ

SC

Growth hormone deficiency in adults or children.

Adults, initial: Not more than 0.006 mg/kg/day SC, up to a maximum of 0.025 mg/kg/day in those less than 35 years of age and to a maximum of 0.0125 mg/kg/day in those over 35 years of age. Lower doses may be needed in older or overweight clients. Decrease dose if needed due to side effects or excessive IGF-I levels. **Alternative dose, initial:** 0.2 mg/day (range: 0.15–0.3 mg/day). Dose can be increased gradually q 1–2 months by increments of about 0.1–0.2 mg/day, based on individual client needs, clinical response, and IGF-1 levels. IGF-1 levels may be used as a guide in dose titration. *NOTE:* The Nutropin AQ pen allows for administration of a minimum dose of 0.1 mg to a maximum dose of 4 mg, in 0.1 increments. **Children:** Up to 0.3 mg/kg/week divided into daily SC injections. In pubertal children, a dose of 0.7 mg/kg/week divided daily may be used. Do not continue therapy if epiphyseal fusion has occurred.

Growth failure associated with chronic renal insufficiency.

Weekly dose: Up to 0.35 mg/kg divided into daily SC injections. May continue therapy up to renal transplantation. The following guidelines are recommended for clients who require dialysis: Hemodialysis clients should receive their injection at night just prior to going to sleep or at least 3–4 hr after their hemodialysis to prevent hematoma formation due to the heparin. Chronic cyclic peritoneal dialysis clients should receive their injection in the morning after they have completed dialysis. Chronic ambulatory peritoneal dialysis clients should receive their injection in the evening at the time of the overnight exchange.

Growth failure associated with Turner syndrome.

Weekly dose: Up to 0.375 mg/kg divided into equal doses given 3–7 times per week SC.

Idiopathic short stature.

Weekly dose: Up to 0.3 mg/kg divided into daily SC injections.

Omnitrope

SC

Growth failure in children.

Weekly dose, usual: 0.16–0.24 mg/kg divided into 6 or 7 daily doses. Do not continue therapy if epiphyseal fusion has occurred.

Growth hormone deficiency in adults.

Individualize. Weekly dose, initial: No more than 0.04 mg/kg given in 7 divided daily injections. May increase dose at 4- to 8-week intervals according to client response, up to a maximum of 0.08 mg/kg/week. *NOTE:* IGF-1 levels may be used as a guide in dose titration. **Alternative dose, initial:** 0.2 mg/day (range: 0.15–0.3 mg/day) without consideration of body weight. Can increase the dose q 1–2 months by increments of about 0.1–0.2 mg/day, depending on clinical response on serum IGF-1 levels. Decrease the dose if side effects and/or serum IGF-1 levels are above the age- and gender-specific normal range.

Saizen

IM; SC

Growth failure in children.

Individualize. Usual: 0.06 mg/kg (about 0.18 units/kg) 3 times weekly by SC or IM injection. Do not continue therapy if epiphyseal fusion has occurred.

Growth hormone deficiency in adults.

Adults, initial: Not more than 0.005 mg/kg/day by SC. The dose may be increased to not more than 0.01 mg/kg/day after 4 weeks, depending on individual client needs. **Alternative dose, initial:** 0.2 mg/day (range: 0.15–0.3 mg/day). Dose can be increased gradually q 1–2 months by increments of about 0.1–0.2 mg/day, based on individual client needs, clinical response, and IGF-1 levels. *NOTE:* IGF-1 levels may be used as a guide in dose titration.

Serostim

SC

HIV clients with wasting or cachexia.

Initial, usual: 0.1 mg/kg daily, up to 6 mg, given at bedtime. Use the following dosage recommendations: **Weight >55 kg (>121 lbs):** 6 mg daily SC; **45–55 kg (99–121 lbs):** 5 mg daily SC; **35–45 kg (75–99 lbs):** 4 mg daily SC; **less than 35 kg (<75 lbs):** 0.1 mg/kg. Giving Serostim every other day (0.1 mg/kg) produced fewer side effects with similar improvement in work output compared with 0.1 mg/kg daily; consider this dosage regimen in those at increased risk for side effects. **Maintenance:** Effects on work output and lean body mass usually apparent after 12 weeks of therapy. Dosage can be maintained for an additional 12 weeks. Rotate injection sites. Safety and efficacy not determined in children.

Tev-Tropin

SC

Growth failure in children.

Up to 0.1 mg/kg (0.3 units/kg) given 3 times per week. SC injection of more than 1 mL of reconstituted solution is not recommended. Do not continue therapy if epiphyseal fusion has occurred.

Zorbtive

SC

Short-bowel syndrome.

Adults, usual: About 0.1 mg/kg/day, up to a maximum of 8 mg/day, for 4 weeks. Rotate injection sites. Monitor for side effects. Treat moderate fluid retention and arthralgias symptomatically or reduce dose by 50%. Discontinue

Zorbtive for up to 5 days for severe toxicity. Upon resolution of symptoms, resume at 50% of the original dose. Permanently discontinue treatment if severe toxicity recurs and does not disappear within 5 days. Safety and efficacy have not been determined in children with short bowel syndrome.

NURSING IMPLICATIONS

Do not confuse Somatrem with Somatropin (human growth hormone) or Sumatriptan (an antimigraine agent).

IMPLEMENTATION/ADMINISTRATION/STORAGE

1. **Pay close attention to the dose. Depending on the product, the dose may be in milligrams or units and may be expressed as a weekly or daily dose.**
2. Somatrem should be prescribed only by a physician experienced in the diagnosis and treatment of pituitary disorders. Dosage must be adjusted for each client.
3. Due to the development of insulin resistance, evaluate for possible glucose intolerance.
4. Clinical response, side effects, and determination of age- and gender-adjusted serum insulin-like growth factor 1 (IGF-1) levels may be used as guidelines in titration of dose.
5. Maintenance doses vary significantly from client to client.
6. Response to growth hormone in children tends to decrease with time. However, failure to increase growth rate in children, especially during the first year of therapy, suggests the need for assessment of compliance and other reasons for growth failure (e.g., hypothyroidism, under nutrition, advanced bone age).
7. When used for growth hormone deficiency in geriatric clients, use a lower starting dose as these individuals are more prone to side effects than younger clients. Obese clients are more likely to manifest side effects when treated with a weight-based (i.e., per kg) regimen. In order to reach treatment goals, estrogen-replete women may need higher doses than men. Oral estrogen administration may increase the dose requirements in women.
8. If used in newborns, reconstitute somatrem with water for injection because benzyl alcohol can be toxic to newborns.
9. The following guidelines are for preparation for administration of all products. To reconstitute vials, inject the diluent into the vial by aiming the stream of liquid against the glass wall. Swirl the vial with a gentle rotary motion until contents are dissolved completely. Do not shake (shaking may cause denaturation of the protein resulting in a cloudy solution).
10. Inject only reconstituted somatrem solution that is clear and without particulate matter. If the solution is cloudy or contains particulate matter, do not inject. However, some products will become cloudy if refrigerated; this is not unusual. Allow the product to warm to room temperature before use. If cloudiness persists or particulate matter is noted, do not use the contents.
11. For multi use vials, about 10% mechanical loss can be associated with reconstitution and administration.
12. Be sure needle used for injection is at least 1 inch so that the injection reaches muscle layer.
13. Use reconstituted somatrem within 7 days; do not freeze.
14. The following information is applicable to *Accretropin:*
    - Store vials from 2–8°C (36–46°F). Avoid freezing and shaking. Once opened, vials may be stored from 2–8°C (36–46°F) for up to 14 days. Discard 14 days after first use. Protect from light.
    - Do not inject IV.
    - If the solution is cloudy or contains particles, do not inject the contents.
15. The following information is applicable to *Genotropin*:
    - Store the lyophilized powder under refrigeration from 2–8°C (36–46°F). Do not freeze. Protect from light.
    - *Genotropin* is supplied in a two-chamber cartridge with the drug in the front chamber and the diluent in the rear chamber. Use a reconstitution device to co-mix the drug and diluent following the directions on the package. Gently tip the cartridge upside down a few times until complete dissolution occurs. Do not shake.
    - The 1.5-mg cartridge may be refrigerated for 24 hr or less because it contains no preservative. Use once and discard any re-

S

maining solution. The 5.8- and 13.8-mg cartridges contain a preservative and may be stored under refrigeration for up to 28 days.

- Refrigerate the *Genotropin Miniquick* delivery device before dispensing; may be stored below 25°C (77°F) for up to 3 months after dispensing. The product contains no preservative. After reconstitution, may be stored refrigerated for 24 hr before use. Use only once and then discard.
- May be given in the thigh, buttocks, or abdomen; rotate site of injection daily to help prevent lipoatrophy.
- Do not inject IV.

16. The following information is applicable to *Humatrope and/or HumatroPen:*

- Reconstitute by adding 1.5–5 mL of the diluent for *Humatrope* supplied for each 5-mg vial. Use a small enough syringe to ensure accuracy when the solution is withdrawn from the vial.
- Before reconstitution, vials and diluent of *Humatrope* are stable when refrigerated from 2–8°C (36–46°F).
- After reconstitution, vials are stable for 14 days or less when reconsituted with diluent for *Humatrope* or bacteriostatic water for injection and refrigerated at 2–8°C (36–46°F).
- After reconstitution of vials with sterile water, use only one dose per *Humatrope* vial and discard the unused portion. If the solution is not used immediately, refrigerate at 2–8°C (36–46°F) and use within 24 hr.
- Before reconstitution, cartridges and diluent for *Humatrope* are stable when refrigerated at 2–8°C (36–46°F).
- After reconstitution, cartridges of *Humatrope* are stable for up to 28 days when reconstituted with diluent for *Humatrope* and refrigerated at 2–8°C (36–46°F). Avoid freezing.
- Store the *Humatrope* injection device without the needle attached.
- Reconstitute each cartridge with the diluent syringe that accompanies the cartridge; do not reconstitute with the diluent for *Humatrope* provided with the vials.
- Administer using sterile, disposable syringes and needles. The syringes should be of small enough volume that the prescribed dose can be drawn from the vial with reasonable accuracy.
- Avoid freezing the diluent and reconstituted vials and cartridges.

17. The following information is applicable to *Norditropin:*

- Give in the thighs and vary injection site on the thigh on a rotating basis to prevent lipoatrophy.
- Refrigerate unused *Norditropin* cartridges at 2–8°C (36–46°F). Do not freeze; avoid direct light.
- *Norditropin* cartridges must be administered using the *NordiPen* delivery systems. Each cartridge has a corresponding color-coded pen that is graduated to deliver the appropriate dose based on the concentration of *Norditropin* in the cartridge.
- After a *Norditropin* cartridge (5 mg/1.5 mL) has been inserted into the *NordiPen* delivery system, it may be stored in the pen in the refrigerator (2–8°C; 36–46°F) and used within 4 weeks or stored for up to 3 weeks at no more than 25°C (77°F). Discard unused portion.
- After a *Norditropin* cartridge (15 mg/1.5 mL) has been inserted into the *NordiPen* delivery system, it may be stored in the pen in the refrigerator (2–8°C; 36–46°F) and used within 4 weeks. Discard unused portion after 4 weeks.
- Unused *Norditropin NordiFlex* prefilled pens must be refrigerated at 2–8°C (36–46°F). Do not freeze; avoid direct light.
- After the initial injection, a *Norditropin NordiFlex* (5 mg/1.5 mL or 10 mg/1.5 mL) prefilled pen may be refrigerated (2–8°C; 36–46°F) and used within 4 weeks or stored for up to 3 weeks at not more than 25°C (77°F). Discard unused portion.
- After the initial injection, a *Norditropin NordiFlex* (15 mg/1.5 mL) prefilled pen may be refrigerated (2–8°C; 36–46°F) and used within 4 weeks. Discard unused portion after 4 weeks.
- Rotate injection site lipoatrophy.

18. The following information is applicable to *Nutropin, Nutropin AQ:*

S

- To reconstitute *Nutropin,* after the dose has been determined, add 1–5 mL bacteriostatic water for injection (benzyl alcohol preserved) per each 5 mg vial and 1–10 mL bacteriostatic water per each 10 mg vial.
- Before reconstitution, refrigerate. *Nutropin* and diluent must be stored at 2–8°C; (36–46°F) under refrigeration. Avoid freezing.
- For *Nutropin,* vial contents are stable for 14 days when reconstituted with bacteriostatic water for injection (benzyl alcohol preserved) and stored at 2–8°C (36–46°F) under refrigeration. Avoid freezing.
- For *Nutropin AQ,* vial, cartridge and *NuSpin* contents are stable for 28 days after initial use when stored in the refrigerator at 2–8°C (36–46°F). Avoid freezing the vial or cartridge. The vials and cartridge are light sensitive; protect from light. Store the vial and the cartridge refrigerated in a dark place when they are not in use.
- Administer using a sterile, disposable syringe and needle; syringes should be of small volume so the dose can be drawn accurately.
- Follow guidelines in the package insert carefully for reconstitution and administration.

19. The following information is applicable to *Omnitrope:*

- Each Omnitrope cartridge must be inserted into its corresponding Omnitrope Pen 5 or Omnitrope Pen 10 deliver system.
- Refrigerate from 2–8°C (36–46°F); do not freeze. Product is light sensitive; store in carton.
- Omnitrope cartridges: After the first use, keep the cartridge in the pen and refrigerate at 2–8°C (36–46°F) for a maximum of 21 days (5 mg/1.5 mL) or 28 days (10 mg/1.5 mL).
- Omnitrope 1.5 mg vials are supplied with diluent without preservative. After reconstitution, the vial may be refrigerated for up to 24 hr. Use once and discard any remaining solution.
- Omnitrope 5.8 mg vials are supplied with a diluent containing benzyl alcohol as a preservative. After reconstitution, use the product within 3 weeks. After the first injection, the vial should be stored in the carton in a refrigerator.
- May be injected in the thigh, buttocks, or abdomen; rotate injection sites daily to help prevent lipoatrophy.
- Do not inject IV.
- Do not use if the solution is cloudy or contains particulate matter; use only if it is clear and colorless.

20. The following information is applicable to *Saizen:*

- Before reconstitution store at room temperature (15–30°C; 59–86°F).
- Reconstitute the 5 mg vial with 1–3 mL bacteriostatic water for injection (benzyl alcohol preserved). Reconstitute the 8.8 mg vial with 2–3 mL of bacteriostatic water for injection. About 10% mechanical loss can be expected with reconstitution and multi-dose administration.
- The 5 mg and 8.8 mg vials reconstituted with bacteriostatic water for injection should be refrigerated for up to 14 days.
- The 8.8 mg click-easy cartridge reconstituted with bacteriostatic water for injection (metacresol 0.3%) should be refrigerated at 2–8°C (36–46°F) for up to 21 days. Avoid freezing reconstituted vials or cartridges.
- Administer using sterile, disposable syringes and needles. The syringes should be of small enough volume that the prescribed dose can be drawn from the vial with reasonable accuracy.

21. The following information is applicable to *Serostim:*

- Before reconstitution, store vials of Serostim and diluent at room temperature (15–30°C; 59–86°F).
- After reconstitution with sterile water for injection, use immediately and discard any unused portion.
- After reconstitution with bacteriostatic water for injection, refrigerate for up to 14 days. Avoid freezing reconstituted product.
- Each vial of 4, 5, or 6 mg is reconstituted with 0.5–1 mL of sterile water for injection. Each 8.8 mg vial is reconstituted with

1–2 mL of bacteriostatic water for injection (benzyl alcohol 0.9% preserved).
- Serostim 4, 5, or 6 mg single-use vials should be given to those requiring 4, 5, or 6 mg daily, respectively, as per the weight-based dosing table.
- Do not inject if the reconstituted solution is cloudy immediately after reconstitution or after refrigeration for up to 14 days.
- Rotate injection sites to prevent lipoatrophy.

22. The following information is applicable to *Tev-Tropin:*
- Before reconstitution refrigerate vials at 2–8°C (36–46°F).
- Reconstitute with 1–5 mL of bacteriostatic sodium chloride, 0.9% for injection (benzyl alcohol preserved).
- When administering to newborns, reconstitute with sterile isotonic sodium chloride solution for injection. Do not use bacteriostatic isotonic sodium chloride solution because it contains benzyl alcohol which has been associated with toxicity in newborns.
- After reconstitution, vials are stable for up to 14 days when reconstituted with bacteriostatic sodium chloride 0.9% and refrigerated. Do not freeze the reconstituted product.
- After refrigeration, some cloudiness may occur; this is not unusual. Allow product to warm to room temperature. If cloudiness persists or particulate matter is noted, do not use.
- Administer using a sterile, disposable syringe and needle; syringes should be of small volume so the dose can be drawn accurately.

23. The following information is applicable to *Zorbtive:*
- Before reconstitution, store at room temperature at 15–30°C (59–86°F).
- After reconstitution with bacteriostatic water for injection, refrigerate for up to 14 days. Avoid freezing reconstituted solutions.
- Reconstitute the 8.8 mg vial with 1–2 mL bacteriostatic water for injection (benzyl alcohol preserved). About 10% mechanical loss can be expected with reconstitution and administration from multidose vials.
- Allow refrigerated solution to come to room temperature prior to administration. If cloudiness persists or particulate matter is noted, do not use.
- Use a standard insulin-type syringe for administration.

ASSESSMENT

1. Note reasons for therapy, age of client, conditions requiring treatment, other therapy trialed.
2. Determine that x-ray evidence of bone growth (wrists, hands) has been conducted. Record height and weight monthly. Generally a growth increase of 2 cm/year should be attained in order for treatment to be continued. Observe for acromegaly.
3. If growth is slow in absence of rising antibody titers, hypopituitarism should be ruled out; untreated hypothyroidism or excessive glucocorticoid replacement can impair growth.
4. With pre-existing tumors or GHD secondary to an intracranial lesion monitor for progression or recurrence of the underlying disease process. In those with a history of scoliosis monitor for progression of condition. Monitor standard hormonal replacement therapy closely when administering somatropin to those with hypopituitarism. Carefully assess for any malignant transformation of skin lesions. Monitor clients with Turner syndrome for CV disorders (e.g., stroke).
5. Note any limps or knee/hip pain because a slipped capital epiphysis may occur.
6. Monitor VS, height, weight, renal and LFTs. Check blood sugar and thyroid function studies and assess for S&S of respiratory infection, diabetes or hypothyroidism. With diabetes, assess for hyperglycemia and acidosis.

CLIENT/FAMILY TEACHING

1. Keep and review drug literature with guidelines for administration, drug preparation, name, and storage, after instructed by provider. Somatrem is usually given once a week whereas somatropin is given more often parenterally.
2. Store before/after administration in refrigerator. Individual agents may differ. Use reconstituted drug within 14 days; refrigerate until used or otherwise directed; avoid freezing.

3. **Report any adverse effects or any limping or knee or hip pain. May experience sudden growth spurts with increased appetite.**
4. **Report if headache, weakness, localized muscle pain, or mild, transient edema occur.**
5. **Keep all F/U visits to assess response, to review growth record and for adverse SE.**

OUTCOMES/EVALUATE

- **Desired skeletal growth; (growth hormone replacement with deficiency)**
- **↑ Stature associated with Turner syndrome**

Sorafenib tosylate

(sor-ah-**FEE**-nib)

Classification(s): Antineoplastic, multikinase inhibitor

Pregnancy Category: D

RX: Nexavar.

INDICATIONS/USES

(1) Treatment of advanced renal cell carcinoma. (2) Treatment of unresectable hepatocellular carcinoma.

ACTION/KINETICS

Action

A multikinase inhibitor that decreases tumor cell proliferation. Sorafenib interacts with multiple intracellular and cell surface kinases, several of which are thought to be involved in angiogenesis. The drug inhibits tumor growth and angiogenesis of human hepatocellular carcinoma and renal cell carcinoma.

Pharmacokinetics

Mean relative bioavailability is 38–49%. Bioavailability is reduced by 29% following a high-fat meal. Asian clients (limited study) show a 45% lower systemic exposure compared with white clients. **Steady-state plasma levels:** 7 days. **Peak plasma levels:** 3 hr. Metabolized primarily in the liver by CYP3A4, as well as glucuronidation mediated by UGT1A9. One of the metabolites is as active as sorafenib. About 77% is excreted in the feces and 19% in the urine. Unchanged sorafenib (51%) is excreted in the feces but none in the urine. **t½, elimination:** 25–48 hr. In hepatocellular clients with mild or moderate impaired hepatic function, 400 mg sorafenib doses appear to be associated with AUC values 23–65% lower than clients without hepatic impairment. **Plasma protein binding:** About 99.5%.

CONTRAINDICATIONS

Severe hypersensitivity to sorafenib or any component of the product. Lactation.

SPECIAL CONCERNS

- **Use with caution with drugs that are metabolized/eliminated predominantly by glucuronidation mediated by UGT1A9.**
- **Possible greater sensitivity in the elderly.**
- **Safety and efficacy not demonstrated in children.**

SIDE EFFECTS

Most Common

Rash, hand-foot skin reaction, hypertension, alopecia, diarrhea, N&V, fatigue, sensory neuropathy, anorexia, asthenia, pain, constipation, hemorrhage (all sites), dyspnea, cough, weight loss, abdominal pain.

GI: Diarrhea, N&V, anorexia, constipation, abdominal pain, dyspepsia, dysphagia, mucositis, stomatitis, glossodynia, dry mouth, gastritis, GI reflux, pancreatitis, liver dysfunction, ***GI perforation*** (rare). **CNS:** Sensory neuropathy, headache, depression, tinnitus, reversible posterior leukoencephalopathy. **CV:** Hypertension, increased risk of bleeding/hemorrhage, ***myocardial ischemia/infarction***, ***hypertensive crisis***, arrhythmia, ***cardiac failure, cerebral hemorrhage***, TIA, thromboembolism, CHF. **Dermatologic:** Rash/desquamation, hand-foot skin reaction, alopecia, pruritus, dry skin, erythema, acne, exfoliative dermatitis, flushing, eczema, erythema multiforme, folliculitis, keratocanthomas/squamous cell carcinoma. **Respiratory:** Dyspnea, cough, hoarseness, rhinorrhea. **GU:** Erectile dysfunction, gynecomastia, acute renal failure. **Musculoskeletal:** Arthralgia, myalgia. **Hematologic:** Hemorrhage (all sites, including GI, respiratory tract, cerebral), leukopenia, lymphopenia, anemia, neutropenia, thrombocytopenia, abnormal INR. **Body as a whole:** Fatigue, joint pain, weight loss, hypersensitivity reaction including skin reactions and urticaria, dehydration, asthenia, pyrexia, infection. **Miscellaneous:** Pain (including mouth/bone/muscle/tumor pain), decreased appetite, flu-like illness, hypothyroidism.

S

LABORATORY TEST CONSIDERATIONS

↑ Lipase, amylase, transaminases (transient), bilirubin, alkaline phosphatase (transient). Hypophosphatemia, hyponatremia, hypothyroidism.

OVERDOSE MANAGEMENT

Symptoms: Diarrhea, dermatologic events. *Treatment:* Withhold sorafenib and institute supportive treatment.

DRUG INTERACTIONS

Carbamazepine / ↓ Sorafenib levels R/T ↑ metabolism by CYP3A4; a sorafenib dose increase may be considered but monitor carefully for toxicity
Dexamethasone / ↓ Sorafenib levels R/T ↑ metabolism by CYP3A4; a sorafenib dose increase may be considered but monitor carefully for toxicity
Docetaxel / ↑ Docetaxel plasma levels; use together with caution
Doxorubicin / ↑ Doxorubin plasma levels; use together with caution
Drugs metabolized by CYP2B6 (e.g., bupropion, paclitaxel, rosiglitazone) / Possible ↑ in levels of drugs metabolized by CYP2B6 R/T inhibition by sorafenib
Drugs metabolized by CYP2C8 (e.g., bupropion, paclitaxel, rosiglitazone) / Possible ↑ in levels of drugs metabolized by CYP2C8 R/T inhibition by sorafenib
Fluorouracil / Both ↑ and ↓ fluorouracil AUC seen; use together with caution
Irinotecan / Use together with caution as both drugs are metabolized by a similar pathway (e.g., UGT1A1)
Phenobarbital / ↓ Sorafenib levels R/T ↑ metabolism by CYP3A4; a sorafenib dose increase may be considered but monitor carefully for toxicity
Phenytoin / ↓ Sorafenib levels R/T ↑ metabolism by CYP3A4; a sorafenib dose increase may be considered but monitor carefully for toxicity
Rifabutin/Rifampin / ↓ Sorafenib levels R/T ↑ metabolism by CYP3A4; a sorafenib dose increase may be considered but monitor carefully for toxicity
H ***St. John's wort*** / ↓ Sorafenib levels R/T ↑ metabolism by CYP3A4; a sorafenib dose increase may be considered but monitor carefully for toxicity
Warfarin / Infrequent bleeding events or ↑ INR; monitor regularly for changes in PT, INR, or clinical bleeding episodes

HOW SUPPLIED

Tablets: 200 mg.

DOSAGE

TABLETS

Advanced renal cell carcinoma; unresectable hepatocellular carcinoma.

400 mg (2–200 mg tablets) twice a day, at least 1 hr before or 2 hr after eating. Continue treatment until the client is no longer benefiting from the drug or until unacceptable side effects occur. When dose reduction is necessary, due to side effects, reduce dose to 400 mg once daily. If additional dose reduction is needed, reduce to a single 400 mg dose every other day.

NURSING IMPLICATIONS

IMPLEMENTATION/ADMINISTRATION/STORAGE

1. Temporary interruption of therapy and/or dose reduction may be necessary for side effects. For skin toxicity, the following dose modifications are recommended:
   - **Grade 1:** Any occurrence of numbness, paresthesia, dysesthesia, tingling, painless swelling, erythema, discomfort of the hands or feet that do not disrupt normal living. Continue treatment and consider topical therapy for symptomatic relief.
   - **Grade 2:** First occurrence of painful erythema and swelling of the hands or feet and/or discomfort affecting normal activities. Continue treatment and consider topical therapy for symptomatic relief. If no improvement in 7 days (or if there is a second or third occurrence), interrupt treatment until toxicity resolves to grade 0 or 1. When resuming treatment, decrease dose by one dose level (400 mg per day or 400 mg every other day). If a fourth occurrence occurs, discontinue sorafenib.
   - **Grade 3:** First or second occurrence of moist desquamation, ulceration, blistering, or severe pain of the hands or feet, or severe discomfort that causes inability to work or perform activities of daily living. Interrupt treatment until toxicity resolves to 0 or 1. When resuming treatment, decrease dose by one dose level (400 mg per day or

S

400 mg every other day). For a third occurrence, discontinue sorafenib.

2. Consider temporary or permanent discontinuation of sorafenib in those who develop cardiac ischemia or infarction.
3. Temporary interruption of therapy is recommended in those undergoing major surgical procedures. Base the decision on when to resume sorafenib therapy on a judgment of adequate wound healing.
4. Store from 15–30°C (59–86°F); store in a dry place.

ASSESSMENT

1. Note reasons for therapy, disease onset, stage, other agents/therapies trialed, outcome.
2. List any bleeding disorders, HTN, kidney, liver or heart disease; may preclude drug therapy. Assess for any skin lesions/disorders or rashes.
3. May increase risk of bleeding, temporarily interrupt therapy during major surgery.
4. Stop drug if client develops cardiac ischemia and/or infarction.
5. Monitor BP weekly during first 6 weeks of therapy; ECG, CBC, renal and LFTs; reduce dose with dysfunction.

CLIENT/FAMILY TEACHING

1. Drug used to treat advanced renal and unresectable liver cancer. Take as directed 1 hr before or 2 hr after meals with a full glass of water.
2. Do not chew, crush, or break tablets.
3. Use reliable contraception in both male and females during and for a least 2 weeks after completing therapy. May cause birth defects or fetal loss.
4. May develop hand-foot skin reaction and rash during treatment. Follow guidelines for skin toxicity under *Implementation/Administration/Storage*.
5. Elevated BP may develop during treatment, especially during the first 6 weeks; monitor regularly during treatment.
6. Report any episodes of bleeding; drug increases risk and may even cause GI perforation.
7. May experience ischemia to the heart or heart attack during treatment; immediately report any chest pain or SOB.
8. If diarrhea, flushing, impaired wound healing, skin rash, increased sweating, suppressed skin test reaction or thin fragile skin evident—report.
9. Keep all F/U to assess response, labs, and for adverse SE.

OUTCOMES/EVALUATE

Inhibition of malignant cell proliferation

■ IV ©

Sotalol hydrochloride

(**SOH**-tah-lol)

Classification(s): Antiarrhythmic, class III; beta-adrenergic blocking agent

Pregnancy Category: B

RX: Betapace, Betapace AF, Sotalol HCl AF.

🍁 **Rx:** Apo-Sotalol, CO Sotalol, Gen-Sotalol, PMS-Sotalol, ratio-Sotalol, Sandoz Sotalol.

SEE ALSO ***BETA-ADRENERGIC BLOCKING AGENTS.***

INDICATIONS/USES

Sotalol hydrochloride tablets (Betapace): Treatment of documented ventricular arrhythmias such as life-threatening sustained ventricular tachycardia. Survival has shown to be enhanced with this drug. **Sotalol hydrochloride AF tablets (Betapace AF):** Maintenance of normal sinus rhythm in those with symptomatic atrial fibrillation/atrial flutter who are in sinus rhythm; since Betapace AF can cause life-threatening ventricular arrhythmias, reserve use for those who are highly symptomatic. *Do not substitute Betapace for Betapace AF.* **Sotalol hydrochloride injection:** (1) As a substitute for PO sotalol in clients who are unable to take sotalol orally. (2) Maintenance of normal sinus rhythm in clients with symptomatic atrial fibrillation/atrial flutter who are currently in sinus rhythm. Reserve for those in whom atrial fibrillation/atrial flutter is highly symptomatic (due to possible life-threatening ventricular arrhythmias). Those with atrial fibrillation should be anticoagulated according to usual medical practice. (3) Treatment of documented life-threatening ventricular arrhythmias. Due to possible torsades de pointes or new ventricular tachycardia, do not use in clients with less severe arrhythmias, even if the individual is symptomatic.

ACTION/KINETICS

Action

Blocks both $beta_1$- and $beta_2$-adrenergic receptors; has no membrane-stabilizing activity or intrinsic sympathomimetic activity. Has both Group II and Group III antiarrhythmic properties (dose dependent). Significantly increases the refractory period of the atria, His-Purkinje fibers, and ventricles. Also prolongs the QTc and JT intervals and decreases heart rate.

Pharmacokinetics

t½: 12 hr. Not metabolized; excreted unchanged in the urine.

CONTRAINDICATIONS

Use in asymptomatic PVCs or supraventricular arrhythmias due to the proarrhythmic effects of sotalol. Congenital or acquired long QT syndromes. Use in clients with hypokalemia or hypomagnesemia until the imbalance is corrected, as these conditions aggravate the degree of QT prolongation and increase the risk for torsades de pointes.

SPECIAL CONCERNS

Sotalol hydrochloride tablets (Betapace or Betapace AF): (1) To minimize the risk of induced arrhythmia, those initiated or reinitiated on Betapace or Betapace AF should be placed for a minimum of 3 days (on their maintenance dose) in a facility that can provide cardiac resuscitation, continuous electrocardiographic monitoring, and calculations of creatinine clearance. Consult the package insert for detailed instructions regarding dose selection and special cautions for those with renal impairment. (2) Do not substitute Betapace for Betapace AF because of significant differences in labeling (e.g., patient package insert, dosing administration, and safety information). **Sotalol hydrochloride injection:** (1) To minimize the risk of induced arrhythmia, clients initiated or reinitiated on IV sotalol, and clients who are converted from IV to PO administration should be hospitalized in a facility that can provide cardiac resuscitation, continuous ECG monitoring, and calculations of creatinine clearance. (2) Sotalol can cause life-threatening ventricular tachycardia associated with QT-interval prolongation. Do not initiate sotalol therapy if the baseline QTc is longer than 450 msec. If the QT interval prolongs to 500 msec or greater, the dose must be reduced, the duration of the infusion prolonged, or the drug discontinued. Adjust the dosing interval based on creatinine clearance.

- **Possible higher risk for serious proarrhythmias in clients with sustained ventricular tachycardia and a history of CHF.**
- **Dose, presence of sustained ventricular tachycardia, females, excessive prolongation of the QTc interval, and history of cardiomegaly or CHF are risk factors for torsades de pointes.**
- **Use with caution in clients with chronic bronchitis or emphysema and in asthma if an IV agent is required.**
- **Use with extreme caution in clients with SSS associated with symptomatic arrhythmias due to the increased risk of sinus bradycardia, sinus pauses, or sinus arrest.**
- **Reduce dosage in impaired renal function.**
- **Safety and efficacy in children not established.**
- **Do *not* interchange Betapace and Betapace AF due to significant differences in dosage and safety, although clients can be transferred to Betapace AF from Betapace.**

SIDE EFFECTS

Most Common

Angina, abnormal ECG, diarrhea, N&V, fatigue, hyperhidrosis, weakness, musculoskeletal pain, dizziness, headache, dyspnea, fever, insomnia, URTI, tracheobronchitis.

See *Beta-Adrenergic Blocking Agents* for a complete list of possible side effects. ***CV: New or worsened ventricular arrhythmias, including sustained VT or ventricular fibrillation that might be fatal. Torsades de pointes.***

HOW SUPPLIED

Sotalol HCl (Betapace). *Tablets:* 80 mg, 120 mg, 160 mg, 240 mg.
Sotalol HCl AF (Betapace AF). *Tablets:* 80 mg, 120 mg, 160 mg.
Sotalol HCl Injection. *Injection Solution, Concentrate:* 15 mg/mL.

DOSAGE

Sotalol hydrochloride: Betapace

TABLETS

Ventricular arrhythmias.

Adults, initial: 80 mg twice a day. The dose may be increased to 240 or

S

320 mg/day (120 to 160 mg twice a day) after appropriate evaluation. **Usual:** 160–320 mg/day given in two or three divided doses. Clients with life-threatening refractory ventricular arrhythmias may require doses ranging from 480 to 640 mg/day (due to potential proarrhythmias; use these doses only if the potential benefit outweighs the increased risk of side effects). Use the following doses in clients with impaired renal function: 80 mg twice a day if C_{CR} is greater than 60 mL/min, 80 mg once daily if the C_{CR} is between 30 and 59 mL/min, and 80 mg every 36–48 hr if the CCR is between 10 and 29 mL/min. Individualize dose if the C_{CR} is less than 10 mL/min. *NOTE:* Dosage increments in renal impairment should be made after administration of at least 5–6 doses at appropriate intervals.

Betapace AF

TABLETS

Maintenance of normal sinus rhythm in those with symptomatic atrial fibrillation/flutter who are in sinus rhythm.

Dose individualized according to calculated creatinine clearance. Initial: 80 mg. **Maintenance:** 80 mg twice a day if C_{CR} is greater than 60 mL/min and 80 mg once daily if the C_{CR} is between 40 and 60 mL/min. Do not use in clients with a C_{CR} less than 40 mL/min. Can be titrated upward to 120 mg during initial hospitalization or after discharge on 80 mg in the event of recurrence, by rehospitalization and repeating the same steps used during initiation of therapy. An increase in dose to 160 mg twice a day or daily can be considered if the 120 mg dose does not reduce the frequency of early relapse of AFIB/AF and is tolerated without excessive QT interval prolongation. Doses higher than 160 mg twice a day are associated with an increased incidence of torsade de pointes. *NOTE:* Follow dosing guidelines provided by the manufacturer carefully.

Sotalol hydrochloride injection

IV

Ventricular arrhythmias.

Initial dose: 75 mg infused over 5 hr once or twice a day based on creatinine clearance. The dose may be increased in increments of 75 mg/day q 3 days. The usual therapeutic effect is seen at doses of 75 to 150 mg IV. Doses as high as 225–300 mg IV have been used in clients with refractory life-threatening arrhythmias.

Symptomatic atrial fibrillation/atrial flutter.

IV dose of 112.5 mg was found to be the most effective in prolonging the time to ECG-documented symptomatic recurrence of atrial fibrillation/atrial flutter. If this dose, at steady state, does not reduce the frequency of relapse of arrhythmia and is tolerated without excessive QTc prolongation (greater than 520 msec), increase the dose to 150 mg IV.

NURSING IMPLICATIONS

Do not confuse Sotalol with Sorbitol (GU irrigant), Stadol (opioid analgesic), or Sudafed (pseudoephedrine).

IMPLEMENTATION/ADMINISTRATION/STORAGE

1. Adjust dosage gradually, allowing 2–3 days between increments in dosage. This allows steady-state plasma levels to be reached, and QT intervals to be monitored.
2. Undertake dosage initiation and increases in a hospital with facilities for cardiac rhythm monitoring. Dosage must be individualized only after appropriate clinical assessment.
3. Proarrhythmias can occur during initiation of therapy, and with each dosage increment.
4. Before initiating sotalol, withdraw previous antiarrhythmic therapy with careful monitoring, for a minimum of 2–3 plasma half-lives if condition permits.
5. Do not initiate sotalol after amiodarone is discontinued until the QT interval is normalized.
6. For children about 2 years of age and older, with healthy renal function, doses normalized for body surface area are appropriate for both initial and incremental dosing. For initiation of treatment, 30 mg/m^2 three times a day (i.e.,

90 mg/m^2 total daily dose) is approximately equivalent to the initial 160 mg total PO daily dose for adults. Subsequent titration to a maximum of 60 mg/m^2 (approximately equal to the 360 mg total daily dose for adults) can then occur. Guide dosage by clinical response, HR, and QTc, with increased dosing carried out in a hospital. Allow at least 36 hr between dose increments to allow steady-state plasma levels in those with age-adjusted healthy renal function. For children less than 2 years of age, carefully follow the guidelines provided by the manufacturer.

Initiation and Maintenance of Betapace AF Therapy

1. Determine the QT interval prior to initiation of therapy using an average of 5 beats. If the baseline QT is greater than 450 msec (QT equal to or greater than 330 msec if QRS over 100 msec), do not use Betapace AF.
2. Calculate the creatinine clearance.
3. Initiate correct dose of Betapace AF, depending on the creatinine clearance (see *Dosage*).
4. Begin continuous ECG monitoring with QT interval measurements 2–4 hr after each dose.
5. If the 80 mg dose is tolerated, and QT interval remains <500 msec after at least 3 days (after 5 or 6 doses if client receiving once daily dosing), client can be discharged. Alternatively, during hospitalization, the dose can be increased to 120 mg twice a day if the 80 mg dose does not reduce the frequency and relapses of atrial fibrillation/atrial flutter (AFIB/AFL). Once again, client is followed for 3 days on this dose (or 5 or 6 doses if receiving once daily dosing).
6. If the 120 mg dose twice a day or daily does not reduce the frequency of early relapses of AFIB/AFL, and is tolerated without excessive QT interval prolongation (520 msec or longer), Betapace AF can be increased to 160 mg twice a day or daily, provided appropriate monitoring is undertaken.
7. Re-evaluate renal function and QT regularly, if medically warranted. If QT is 520 msec or greater (JT 430 msec or greater if QRS >100 msec), reduce dose of Betapace AF, and monitor carefully until QT returns to <520 msec.
8. If the QT interval is 520 msec or greater while on the lowest maintenance dose (80 mg), discontinue drug.
9. If renal function decreases, reduce daily dose in half, and administer drug once daily.
10. If a dose is missed, the next dose should not be doubled. The next dose should be taken at the usual time.
11. Before starting Betapace AF, withdraw previous antiarrhythmic therapy, with careful monitoring, for a minimum of 2 or 3 plasma half-lives if the clinical condition permits.
12. Do not initiate Betapace AF after amiodarone until the QT interval is normalized.

General Dosing Considerations for IV Administration

1. IV Use the same safety measures for IV administration as described earlier for PO use.
2. Perform a baseline ECG to determine the QT interval, and measure and normalize serum potassium and magnesium levels before beginning sotalol therapy.
3. Measure serum creatinine, and calculate an estimated creatinine clearance in order to determine the appropriate dosing interval.
4. Begin sotalol therapy only if the baseline QT interval is less than 450 msec. During initiation and titration, monitor the QT interval after the completion of each infusion. If the QT interval prolongs to 500 msec or greater, reduce the dose, decrease the infusion rate, or discontinue sotalol.
5. Sotalol IV is not recommended in clients with a creatinine clearance less than 40 mL/min.
6. The bioavailability of PO sotalol is 90 to 100%. Thus, the corresponding IV dose is slightly less than the PO dose. Monitor the effects of the initial IV dose and the dose titrated upward or downward, if needed, based on clinical effects, QT interval, or side effects.
7. IV sotalol must be diluted prior to administration with compatible solutions.
8. IV sotalol has not been studied in children.
9. The adult starting dose of intravenous sotalol is 75 mg infused over 5 hours, once or twice daily based on the creatinine clearance. Monitor ECG for excessive increase in QT interval.
10. If tolerated, may increase the dose to 112.5 mg infused over 5 hours, once or twice daily depending upon the creatinine clearance and QT interval.
11. COMPATIBILITY D5W, 0.9% NaCl, Ringer's lactate.
12. INCOMPATIBILITY Administer separately.

S

ASSESSMENT

1. Note reasons for therapy, onset and characteristics of S&S. List other agents trialed and outcome.
2. Perform nursing history; note any cardiomegaly or CHF.
3. The following conditions preclude therapy: sinus bradycardia (HR <50) SSS, 2nd or 3rd degree AV block if no pacemaker in place, congenital or acquired long QT syndromes, QT interval >450 ms; cardiogenic shock, uncontrolled heart failure, C_{CR} <40 mL/min, K^+ <4 meq/L (determine CrCl to establish the appropriate dosing interval for sotalol), or bronchial asthma or related bronchospastic conditions.
4. Obtain ECG, document QT interval (must be ≤450 msec). Monitor q 2–4 hr and report if QTc interval >500 msec; reduce/stop therapy. Monitor QT interval after each infusion.
5. Administer infusion in a continuously monitored environment with VS and ECG monitored during initiation and dosage adjustment of sotalol.
6. Monitor VS, weight., I&O, electrolytes, uric acid, lipids, Mg^{++}, renal and LFTs.

CLIENT/FAMILY TEACHING

1. Take on an empty stomach; food decreases absorption. Betapace is used to treat rhythm disorders of ventricles and Betapace AF controls heart rhythm disorders of the upper part of the heart (atria); they are not interchangeable.
2. Take exactly as directed, do not stop abruptly; drug controls symptoms but does not cure condition.
3. Avoid activities that require mental alertness until drug effects realized; may cause dizziness/drowsiness. Report syncopal events or new pre-syncopal symptoms, may be signs of either hypotension or torsades de pointes.
4. Report increased chest pain/SOB, night cough, swelling of feet and ankles, increased fatigue, low heart rate (<60), or unsteady gait.
5. Continue dietary and exercise guidelines as prescribed and healthy lifestyle changes. Avoid alcohol and OTC agents. Drug may mask S&S of hypoglycemia.
6. Do not stop drug suddenly; dosage will be decreased over 1 to 2 wk.
7. Keep all F/U to assess response, labs, and for adverse SE.

OUTCOMES/EVALUATE

- Control/conversion of life-threatening arrhythmias to stable cardiac rhythm
- Maintenance of sinus rhythm with symptomatic AF

Spironolactone

(speer-oh-no-**LAK**-tohn)

Classification(s): Diuretic, potassium-sparing

Pregnancy Category: C (**D** if used in gestational hypertension)

RX: Aldactone.

Rx: Novo-Spiroton.

SEE ALSO ***DIURETICS, THIAZIDES***.

INDICATIONS/USES

1. Primary hyperaldosteronism, including diagnosis, short-term preoperative treatment, long-term maintenance therapy for those who are poor surgical risks and those with bilateral micronodular or macronodular adrenal hyperplasia.
2. Congestive heart failure to manage edema and sodium retention when the client is only partially responsive to, or is intolerant of other therapeutic measures. Also for those with CHF taking digitalis when other therapies are considered inappropriate.
3. Essential hypertension (usually in combination with other drugs) when treatment with other drugs is inadequate or inappropriate.
4. Cirrhosis of the liver accompanied by edema and/or ascites. Used together with bed rest and restriction of fluid and sodium.
5. Nephrotic syndrome when treatment of the underlying disease, restriction of fluid and sodium intake and the use of other diuretics do not provide an adequate response.
6. Treatment of hypokalemia when other measures are inappropriate or inadequate.
7. Prophylaxis of hypokalemia in clients taking digitalis when other measures are inadequate or inappropriate.
8. Severe heart failure (NYHA class III to IV) to increase survival and reduce the need for

S

hospitalization. Used in addition to standard therapy.

Investigational: Hirsutism in women.

ACTION/KINETICS

Action

Antagonist of aldosterone; acts mainly through competitive binding of receptors at the aldosterone-dependent sodium-potassium exchange site in the distal convoluted renal tubule. Causes increased amounts of sodium and water to be excreted while potassium is retained. Also has antihypertensive effects; lowers systolic and diastolic BP in those with primary hyperaldosteronism. May be given alone or with other diuretic drugs that act more proximally in the renal tubule.

Pharmacokinetics

Food increases bioavailability of unmetabolized spironolactone by almost 100%. **Onset:** 24–48 hr. **Peak:** 2–3 days. **Duration:** 2–3 days, and declines thereafter. Metabolized to an active metabolite (canrenone). **t½:** 13–24 hr for canrenone. Canrenone is excreted through the urine (primary) and the bile. **Plasma protein binding:** 98% or more.

CONTRAINDICATIONS

Acute renal insufficiency, progressive renal failure, hyperkalemia, and anuria. Clients receiving potassium supplements, amiloride, or triamterene; may cause hyperkalemia which can be fatal.

SPECIAL CONCERNS

> Spironolactone has been shown to be tumorigenic in chronic toxicity studies in rats. Use only in those conditions described under *Indications/Uses*. Avoid unnecessary use of the drug.

- **Use during pregnancy only if benefits clearly outweigh risks. Diuretics do not prevent toxemia of pregnancy.**
- **Use with caution in impaired renal function and in impaired hepatic function (minor alterations in fluid and electrolyte balance may cause hepatic coma).**
- **Geriatric clients may be more sensitive to the usual adult dose.**
- **Safety and efficacy not determined in children.**

SIDE EFFECTS

Most Common

Dizziness, blurred vision, N&V, fatigue, anorexia, insomnia, nasal congestion, gynecomastia.

Electrolyte: Hyperkalemia, hyponatremia (characterized by lethargy, dry mouth, thirst, drowsiness), hyperchloremic metabolic acidosis (usually in association with hyperkalemia in those with decompensated hepatic cirrhosis). **GI:** Diarrhea, cramps, ulcers, gastritis, gastric bleeding, N&V, anorexia, mixed cholestatic/hepatocellular toxicity (rare). **CNS:** Drowsiness, dizziness, ataxia, lethargy, mental confusion, headache, fatigue, insomnia. **GU:** Gynecomastia, inability to achieve or maintain an erection, renal dysfunction (including renal failure), menstrual irregularities, amenorrhea, bleeding in postmenopausal women, breast carcinoma (cause and effect not determined). **Hypersensitivity:** ***Anaphylactic reactions***, fever, maculopapular or erythematous cutaneous eruptions, urticaria, vasculitis. **Miscellaneous:** Blurred vision, nasal congestion, hirsutism, drug fever, deepening of voice, ***agranulocytosis***. *NOTE*: Spironolactone has been shown to be tumorigenic in chronic rodent studies.

LABORATORY TEST CONSIDERATIONS

↑ BUN (transient). Mild acidosis. Spironolactone and metabolites may interfere with digoxin radioimmunoassays.

OVERDOSE MANAGEMENT

Symptoms: Drowsiness, mental confusion, maculopapular or erythematous rash, N&V, dizziness, diarrhea. Rarely, hyponatremia, hyperkalemia, hepatic coma (in those with severe liver disease). *Treatment:* Undertake gastric lavage. Further treatment is supportive to maintain hydration, electrolyte balance, and vital functions. Hyperkalemia may be treated by IV calcium chloride solution, sodium bicarbonate solution, and/or the PO or parenteral administration of glucose with a rapid-acting insulin preparation. These are temporary measures and are to be repeated as needed. Cationic exchange resins (e.g., sodium polystyrene sulfonate) may be given PO or rectally. Persistent hyperkalemia may require dialysis.

DRUG INTERACTIONS

ACE inhibitors (e.g., losartan) / Significant hyperkalemia; use together with caution

Alcohol / Potentiation of orthostatic hypotension

S

Anesthetics, general / Additive hypotension; use caution in those subjected to regional or general anesthesia
Anticoagulants, oral (e.g., warfarin) / ↓ Anticoagulant hypoprothrombinemic effect
Antihypertensives / ↑ Hypotensive effect of both agents; ↓ dosage, especially of ganglionic blockers, by one-half
Barbiturates / Potentiation of orthostatic hypotension
Captopril / ↑ Risk of significant hyperkalemia
Corticosteroids, Corticotropin / Intensified electrolyte depletion, especially potassium
Digoxin / ↑ Half-life of digoxin → possible toxicity; monitor carefully
Diuretics, others / Often given together R/T potassium-sparing effect of spironolactone. Possible severe hyponatremia; monitor closely
Eplerenone / Significant hyperkalemia; use together contraindicated
Lithium / ↑ Risk of lithium toxicity R/T ↓ renal clearance
Mitotane / Adrenolytic effects of mitotane blocked by spironolactone
Narcotics / Potentiation of orthostatic hypotension
Norepinephrine / ↓ Vascular response to NE
NSAIDs (e.g., diclofenac, indomethacin) / ↓ Spironolactone effect; also possible severe hyperkalemia
Potassium salts / Hyperkalemia R/T spironolactone conserving potassium excessively → cardiac arrhythmias and possible death
Salicylates / ↓ Spironolactone effects
Skeletal muscle relaxants, nondepolarizing (e.g., tubocurarine) / Possible ↑ responsiveness to the muscle relaxant
Triamterene / Possible hazardous hyperkalemia

HOW SUPPLIED

Tablets: 25 mg, 50 mg, 100 mg.

S

DOSAGE

TABLETS

Diagnosis of primary hyperaldosteronism.

Adults: 400 mg/day for either 4 days (short-test) or 3–4 weeks (long-test). With the short test, if serum potassium increases during spironolactone administration but drops when the drug is discontinued, a presumptive diagnosis of primary hyperaldosteronism should be considered. With the long test, correction of hypokalemia and of hypertension provides presumptive evidence for the diagnosis of primary hyperaldosteronism. **Pediatric:** 125–375 mg/m^2/day divided 2–4 times/day. *NOTE:* Use to diagnose primary hyperaldosteronism in children is considered investigational.

Hyperaldosteronism.

Adults: 100–400 mg/day in 2 to 4 doses in preparation for surgery. For those unsuitable for surgery, give long-term maintenance therapy at the lowest effective dose individualized for each client.

Edema conditions.

Adults, initial: 100 mg/day (range: 25–200 mg/day) in 2 to 4 divided doses for at least 5 days at the initial dosage level; dose may then be adjusted to the optimal therapeutic or maintenance level given as either single or divided daily doses. If, after 5 days an adequate diuretic response has not occurred, a second diuretic may be added to the regimen. The dose of spironolactone should remain unchanged when another diuretic is added. **Pediatric, older than 29 days:** 1–3.3 mg/kg/day divided 1–4 times daily; **pediatric, less than 29 days:** 1–3 mg/kg/day divided once or twice daily. *NOTE:* Use as a diuretic in children is considered investigational.

Essential hypertension.

Adults, initial: 50–100 mg/day as a single dose or as 2 to 4 divided doses-give for at least 2 weeks; **maintenance:** adjust to individual response. May be given with diuretics that act more proximally in the renal tubule or with other antihypertensive drugs.

Hypokalemia.

Adults: 25–100 mg/day as a single dose or 2 to 4 divided doses.

Severe heart failure (NYHA Class III to IV).

Adults, initial: 25 mg once a day if serum potassium is 5 mEq/L or less and the serum creatinine is 2.5 mg/dl or less. Clients who tolerate 25 mg once a day may have their dosage increased to 50 mg once a day if needed. Those who do not tolerate the 25 mg once-daily dose may have their dose decreased to 25 mg every other day.

Hirsutism in women.

50–200 mg/day in 1–2 divided dose; used as either monotherapy or in combination therapy.

NURSING IMPLICATIONS

Do not confuse Aldactone with Aldactazide (combination antihypertensive/diuretic).

IMPLEMENTATION/ADMINISTRATION/STORAGE

1. When used as sole drug to treat edema, maintain initial dose for at least 5 days. After that, adjustments may be made. If dosage not effective, a second diuretic may be added, especially one that acts in the proximal tubules.
2. When administered to small children, tablets may be crushed and given as a suspension in cherry syrup.
3. Food may increase absorption of spironolactone.
4. Protect drug from light.

ASSESSMENT

1. Note reasons for therapy, other agents prescribed, outcome.
2. With cardiac disease, be alert for hypokalemia. Monitor VS, I&O, weights.
3. Assess for drug tolerance characterized by edema/reduced urine output. Ensure client informed that studies show drug tumorigenic in rats.
4. If client develops dysuria, urinary frequency, or renal spasm, obtain a urinalysis and urine culture.
5. Monitor ABGs, ECG, CBC, blood sugar, uric acid, serum electrolytes, renal and LFTs.

CLIENT/FAMILY TEACHING

1. Take as directed with a snack/meal to minimize GI upset. Report if nausea, bloating, anorexia, vomiting, or diarrhea persist. Take early in day to prevent frequent nighttime urination.
2. Avoid foods or salt substitutes high in potassium; drug is potassium-sparing. Record BP and weight twice a week for provider review. Report any increased swelling of extremities or weight gain of more than 5 lb (2.2 kg) weekly.
3. The full diuretic effect may not be achieved for 1 to 2 wk. May feel tired for several weeks because body needs to adjust to lowered BP.
4. Do not drive/operate dangerous machinery until drug effects realized; may cause drowsiness or unsteady gait.
5. Drug may cause breast swelling and diminished sex drive by reducing testosterone levels.
6. Report if deep, rapid respirations, headaches, or mental slowing occurs; may indicate hyperchloremic metabolic acidosis.
7. Drug is metabolized in the liver. Report jaundice, tremors, or mental confusion; may develop hepatic encephalopathy with liver disease. Avoid alcohol.
8. Keep all F/U to assess response, labs, and for adverse SE.

OUTCOMES/EVALUATE

- Enhanced diuresis with ↓ edema
- ↓ BP
- Antagonism of high levels of aldosterone
- Prevention of hypokalemia
- Reduced mortality in CAD with CHF

Stavudine

(**STAH**-vyou-deen)

Classification(s): Antiviral, nucleoside reverse transcriptase inhibitor

Pregnancy Category: C

RX: Zerit.

SEE ALSO ***ANTIVIRAL AGENTS***.

INDICATIONS/USES

Treatment of HIV-1 infection in combination with other antiretroviral drugs.

ACTION/KINETICS

Action

The drug causes antiviral activity and inhibition of HIV replication by two known mechanisms: (1) Inhibition of HIV reverse transcriptase by competing with the natural substrate deoxythymidine triphospate and (2) Inhibition of viral DNA synthesis by its incorporation into viral DNA,

S

causing DNA chain elongation termination (because stavudine lacks the 3'-hydroxyl group necessary for DNA elongation). Stavudine triphosphate also inhibits cellular DNA polymerase beta and gamma, and markedly decreases mitochondrial DNA synthesis.

Pharmacokinetics

Rapidly absorbed; about 86% bioavailable. **Peak plasma levels:** Within 1 hr. No significant accumulation with repeated administration. **t½, elimination:** Approximately 2.3 hr after a single PO dose in adults. Excreted mainly unchanged in the urine (95%) and feces (3%).

CONTRAINDICATIONS

Clinically significant hypersensitivity to stavudine or any component of the product. Avoid use of stavudine and hydroxyurea, with or without didanosine. Lactation.

SPECIAL CONCERNS

(1) **Lactic acidosis and hepatomegaly with steatosis.** Lactic acidosis and severe hepatomegaly with steatosis, including fatal cases, have been reported for nucleoside analogs used alone or in combination, including stavudine and other antiretrovirals. (2) Fatal lactic acidosis has been reported in pregnant women who received stavudine and didanosine with other antiretroviral drugs. Use the combination of stavudine and didanosine with caution during pregnancy; use is recommended only if the potential benefit clearly outweighs the potential risk. (3) **Pancreatitis.** Fatal and nonfatal pancreatitis have occurred during therapy when stavudine was part of a combination regimen that included didanosine in both treatment-naive and treatment-experienced clients, regardless of the degree of immunosuppression.

- **The effect of stavudine on the clinical progression of HIV infection, such as incidence of opportunistic infections or survival, has not been determined.**
- **Early signs of lactic acidosis include fatigue, nausea, respiratory symptoms, and neurologic symptoms (including motor weakness).**
- **HIV clients have a significantly increased risk for developing symptomatic sensory neuropathies.**

SIDE EFFECTS

Most Common

When used in combination therapy: Dizziness, peripheral neurologic symptoms/neuropathy, abnormal dreams, diarrhea, nausea, headache, rash, somnolence, insomnia.

Neurologic: Peripheral neuropathy, including numbness, tingling, or pain in feet or hands; severe motor weakness. **CNS:** Insomnia, abnormal dreams, headache, anxiety, depression, nervousness, dizziness, confusion, migraine, somnolence, tremor, neuralgia, dementia. **GI:** Diarrhea, N&V, abdominal pain, anorexia, dyspepsia, constipation, ulcerative stomatitis, aphthous stomatitis. **Hepatic:** Hepatitis, ***pancreatitis and severe hepatomegaly with steatosis, hepatic failure/death in HIV clients.*** **CV:** Chest pain, vasodilation, hypertension, peripheral vascular disorder, syncope. **Hematologic:** Anemia, leukopenia, macrocytosis, neutropenia, thrombocytopenia. **GU:** Dysuria, genital pain, dysmenorrhea, vaginitis, urinary frequency, hematuria, impotence, urogenital neoplasm. **Respiratory:** Dyspnea, pneumonia, asthma. **Dermatologic:** Rash, sweating, pruritus, maculopapular rash, benign skin neoplasm, urticaria, exfoliative dermatitis. **Metabolic:** Diabetes mellitus, hyperglycemia, lipoatrophy, lipodystrophy. **Ophthalmic:** Conjunctivitis, abnormal vision. **Body as a whole:** Lactic acidosis (especially in pregnancy when combined with didanosine with other antiretroviral drugs), headache, chills, fever, asthenia, abdominal/back pain, malaise, weight loss, ***allergic reactions***, flu syndrome, lymphadenopathy, pelvic pain, myalgia, ascending neuromuscular weakness, ***neoplasms, death.*** **Miscellaneous:** Redistribution/accumulation of body fat, including central obesity, dorsocervical fat enlargement, peripheral wasting, facial wasting, breast enlargement, and 'cushinoid appearance.' Immune reconstitution syndrome, including development of an inflammatory response to indolent or residual opportunistic infections (e.g., *Mycobacterium avium* infection, cytomegalovirus, *Pneumocystis jiroveci* pneumonia, tuberculosis). *NOTE:* Clients treated with stavudine and didanosine with or without hydroxyurea may be at increased risk for pancreatitis and hepatoxicity, which may be fatal; also severe peripheral neuropathy is possible.

LABORATORY TEST CONSIDERATIONS

↑ AST, ALT, amylase, bilirubin, GGT, lipase.

DRUG INTERACTIONS

Didanosine / ↑ Risk for lactic acidosis, hepatotoxicity, pancreatitis, or peripheral neuropathy; use this combination with caution during pregnancy
Doxorubicin / Inhibition of phosphorylation of stavudine → toxicities (especially hepatic decompensation); coadminister with caution
Hydroxyurea / ↑ Risk for lactic acidosis, hepatotoxicity, pancreatitis, or peripheral neuropathy; avoid coadministration of stavudine and hydroxyurea with or without didanosine
Methadone / ↓ AUC and peak drug levels of stavudine; adjust stavudine dose as needed
Ribavirin / Inhibition of phosphorylation of stavudine → toxicities (especially hepatic decompensation); coadminister with caution
Zidovudine / Competitive inhibition of intracellular phosphorylation of stavudine; do not use together

HOW SUPPLIED

Capsules: 15 mg, 20 mg, 30 mg, 40 mg; ***Powder for Oral Solution:*** 1 mg/mL (after reconstitution).

DOSAGE

CAPSULES, ORAL SOLUTION

HIV infections.

Adults, 60 kg or more: 40 mg q 12 hr; **less than 60 kg:** 30 mg q 12 hr. **Children, 14 days and older, less than 30 kg:** 1 mg/kg q 12 hr; **30 to <60 kg:** 30 mg q 12 hr; **60 kg or more:** 40 mg q 12 hr. **Birth to 13 days of age:** 0.5 mg/kg q 12 hr.

The dosage adjustment for renal impairment follows: **C_{CR}, >50 mL/min, weight 60 kg or more:** 40 mg q 12 hr; **<60 kg:** 30 mg q 12 hr; **C_{CR} 26–50 mL/min, weight 60 kg or more:** 20 mg q 12 hr; **<60 kg:** 15 mg q 12 hr. **C_{CR} 10–25 mL/min, weight 60 kg or more:** 20 mg q 24 hr; **<60 kg:** 15 mg q 24 hr. **Hemodialysis clients, weight 60 kg or more:** 20 mg q 24; **<60 kg:** 15 mg q 24 hr given after completion of hemodialysis on dialysis days and at the same time of day on nondialysis days.

NURSING IMPLICATIONS

IMPLEMENTATION/ADMINISTRATION/STORAGE

1. If peripheral neuropathy recurs after resumption of stavudine, consider permanent discontinuation.
2. The interval between doses should be 12 hr.
3. To monitor maternal/fetal outcomes of pregnant women exposed to stavudine and other antiretroviral agents, an antiretroviral registry has been established. Register clients by calling 1-800-258-4263.
4. Store capsules and powder for solution in tightly closed containers from 15–30°C (59–86°F). After reconstitution, store oral solution in tightly closed containers from 2–8°C (36–46°F). Discard any unused portion after 30 days.

ASSESSMENT

1. List reasons for therapy, onset, other agents trialed/prescribed, date confirmed; note intolerance. List drugs prescribed to ensure none interact.
2. Note clinical presentation, other medical problems, any history of neuropathy while prescribed other drugs for this condition or if undergoing chemotherapy with cytotoxic drugs.
3. Assess closely for S&S of lactic acidosis, pancreatitis, infections, or peripheral neuropathy during therapy.
4. Obtain baseline CBC, CD_4 counts/viral load, PT/PTT, renal, LFTs. Reduce dose with impaired function and peripheral neuropathy.

CLIENT/FAMILY TEACHING

1. May be taken without regard to meals. Take exactly as prescribed q 12 hr RTC, do not exceed prescribed dose, do not share medications. Contact a poison control center or emergency room right away if dosage exceeded.
2. Advise those with diabetes that oral solution contains sucrose 50 mg/mL.
3. Drug is not a cure, but alleviates/manages the symptoms of HIV infections and may help prolong life. May continue to acquire illnesses associated with AIDS or ARC, including opportunistic infections; must remain under close medical supervision.
4. The risk of transmission of HIV to others through blood or sexual contact is not reduced with drug therapy. Review the criteria

S

and precautions for safe sex and do not share needles.

5. Report any S&S of infection (i.e., sore throat, swollen glands, fever). Abdominal pain, N&V, weight loss and fatty material in stool may indicate pancreatitis; fatigue, SOB or faster breathing may signal lactic acidosis, pain, burning, feeling of pins and needles in hands/feet may indicate peripheral neuropathy and should all be reported immediately as drug will need to be stopped. Symptoms may temporarily worsen following cessation of drug therapy but, once resolved, drug may be reintroduced at a lower dose.
6. Insomnia and GI upset usually resolve after 3–4 weeks of therapy. Identify local support groups that may assist client/family to understand and cope with this disease.
7. Notify provider immediately if symptoms of symptomatic hyperlactemia or lactic acidosis, including unexplained weight loss, abdominal discomfort, nausea, vomiting, fatigue, dyspnea, and motor weakness occur.
8. Avoid alcohol during therapy; may increase risk of pancreatitis or liver failure.
9. Redistribution of body fat may occur; report if evident.
10. The CDC recommends that HIV infected mothers *not* nurse newborns to reduce postnatal transmission of disease.
11. Keep all F/U to assess response, labs, and for adverse SE.

OUTCOMES/EVALUATE

Clinical/immunologic improvement with HIV infection

IV

Succinylcholine chloride

(suck-sin-ill-**KOH**-leen)

Classification(s): Neuromuscular blocking drug, depolarizing

Pregnancy Category: C

RX: Anectine, Anectine Flo-Pack, Quelicin, Quelicin-1000.

SEE ALSO ***NEUROMUSCULAR BLOCKING AGENTS***.

INDICATIONS/USES

Adjunct to general anesthesia to facilitate ET intubation and to induce relaxation of skeletal muscle during surgery or mechanical ventilation. *Investigational:* Reduce intensity of electrically induced seizures or seizures due to drugs.

ACTION/KINETICS

Action

Initially excites skeletal muscle by combining with cholinergic receptors preferentially to acetylcholine. Subsequently, it prevents the muscle from contracting by prolonging the time during which the receptors at the neuromuscular junction cannot respond to acetylcholine. The order of paralysis is levator muscles of the eyelid, mastication muscles, limb muscles, abdominal muscles, glottis muscles, the intercostals, the diaphragm, and all other skeletal muscles. Prolonged use may change from a depolarizing neuromuscular block (phase I block) to a block that resembles a nondepolarizing block (phase II block). This may be associated with prolonged respiratory depression and apnea. No effect on pain threshold, cerebration, or consciousness; use with sufficient anesthesia. Effects are not blocked by anticholinesterase drugs and may even be enhanced by them. May cause a change in myocardial rhythm due to vagal stimulation due to surgical procedures (especially in children) and from potassium-mediated alterations in electrical conductivity (enhanced by halogenated anesthetics).

Pharmacokinetics

Onset, IV: 30–60 sec; **duration:** 4–6 min; **recovery:** 8–10 min. **Onset, IM:** 2–3 min; **duration:** 10–30 min. Metabolized by plasma pseudocholinesterase to succinylmonocholine, which is a nondepolarizing muscle relaxant, and then to succinic acid and choline. About 10% excreted unchanged in the urine.

CONTRAINDICATIONS

Use in genetically determined disorders of plasma pseudocholinesterase. Personal or family history of malignant hyperthermia. Myopathies associated with elevated CPK values. Acute narrow-angle glaucoma or penetrating eye injuries. Use of IV infusion in children due to the risk of malignant hyperpyrexia.

SPECIAL CONCERNS

■ Use only if skilled in the management of artificial respiration and when facilities are instantly available for tracheal intubation and for providing adequate ventilation of the client, including the administration of oxygen under positive pressure and the elimination of carbon dioxide. The clinician must be prepared to assist or control ventilation. ■

- **Use with caution during lactation.**
- **Pediatric clients may be especially prone to myoglobinemia, myoglobinuria, and cardiac effects.**
- **Use with caution in clients with severe liver disease, severe anemia, malnutrition, impaired cholinesterase activity, fractures.**
- **Use with caution in CV, pulmonary, renal, or metabolic diseases.**
- **Use with great caution in those with severe burns, electrolyte imbalance, hyperkalemia, those receiving quinidine, and those who are digitalized or recovering from severe trauma, as serious cardiac arrhythmias or cardiac arrest may result.**
- **Clients with myasthenia gravis may show resistance to succinylcholine.**
- **Those with fractures or muscle spasms may manifest additional trauma due to succinylcholine-induced muscle fasciculations.**

SIDE EFFECTS

Most Common

Respiratory depression, bradycardia, hypo-/hypertension, salivation, postoperative muscle pain.

Skeletal muscle: May cause ***severe, persistent respiratory depression or apnea***. Muscle fasciculations, postoperative muscle pain. **CV:** Hyper-/hypotension, brady-/tachycardia, ***arrhythmias, cardiac arrest***. **Respiratory:** ***Apnea, respiratory depression***. **Miscellaneous:** Fever, salivation, hyperkalemia, ***anaphylaxis***, myoglobinemia, myoglobinuria, skin rashes, increased intraocular pressure, myalgia, jaw rigidity, perioperative dreams in children, ***rhabdomyolysis*** with possible myoglobinuric acute renal failure. Repeated doses may cause ***tachyphylaxis***. **Malignant hyperthermia:** Muscle rigidity (especially of the jaw), tachycardia, tachypnea unresponsive to increased depth of anesthesia, increased oxygen requirement and carbon dioxide production, increased body temperature, metabolic acidosis.

OVERDOSE MANAGEMENT

Symptoms: Skeletal muscle weakness, decreased respiratory reserve, low tidal volume, apnea.
Treatment: Maintain a patent airway and respiratory support until normal respiration is ensured.

DRUG INTERACTIONS

Aminoglycoside antibiotics / Additive skeletal muscle blockade
Amphotericin B / ↑ Succinylcholine effect R/T induced electrolyte imbalance
Antibiotics, nonpenicillin / Additive skeletal muscle blockade
Beta-adrenergic blocking agents / Additive skeletal muscle blockade
Chloroquine / Additive skeletal muscle blockade
Cimetidine / Inhibits pseudocholinesterase
Clindamycin / Additive skeletal muscle blockade
Cyclophosphamide / ↑ Succinylcholine effect by ↓ breakdown by plasma pseudocholinesterase
Diazepam / ↓ Succinycholine effect
Digitalis glycosides / ↑ Risk of cardiac arrhythmias, including VF; possible ↑ in toxic effects of both drugs
Echothiophate iodide / ↑ Succinylcholine effect by ↓ breakdown by plasma pseudocholinesterase
Furosemide / ↑ Skeletal muscle blockade
Halothane / ↑ Risk of bradycardia, arrhythmias, sinus arrest, apnea, and malignant hyperthermia
Isoflurane / Additive skeletal muscle blockade
Lidocaine / Additive skeletal muscle blockade
Lincomycin / Additive skeletal muscle blockade
Lithium carbonate / ↑ Skeletal muscle blockade
Mg salts / Additive skeletal muscle blockade
Muscle relaxants, nondepolarizing / Possible synergistic or antagonistic effect of succinylcholine
Narcotics / ↑ Risk of bradycardia and sinus arrest
Nitrous oxide / ↑ Risk of bradycardia, arrhythmias, sinus arrest, apnea, and malignant hyperthermia
Oxytocin / ↑ Succinylcholine effect
Phenelzine / ↑ Succinylcholine effect
Phenothiazines / ↑ Succinylcholine effect
Polymyxin / Additive skeletal muscle blockade
Procainamide / ↑ Succinylcholine effect
Procaine / ↑ Succinylcholine effect by inhibiting plasma pseudocholinesterase
Promazine / ↑ Succinylcholine effect
Quinidine / Additive skeletal muscle blockade
Quinine / Additive skeletal muscle blockade
Tacrine / ↑ Succinylcholine effect

S

Thiazide diuretics / ↑ Succinylcholine effect due to induced electrolyte imbalance
Thiotepa / ↑ Succinylcholine effect by ↓ breakdown by plasma pseudocholinesterase
Trimethaphan / ↑ Succinylcholine effect by inhibiting plasma pseudocholinesterase

HOW SUPPLIED

Injection: 20 mg/mL, 100 mg/mL; *Powder for Infusion:* 500 mg, 1 gram.

DOSAGE

IM; IV

Short or prolonged surgical procedures.

Adults, IV, initial: 0.3–1.1 mg/kg (average: 0.6 mg/kg); **then,** repeated doses can be given based on client response. **Adults, IM:** 3–4 mg/kg, not to exceed a total dose of 150 mg.

Electroshock therapy.

Adults, IV: 10–30 mg given 1 min prior to the shock (individualize dosage). **IM:** Up to 2.5 mg/kg, not to exceed a total dose of 150 mg.

ET intubation.

Pediatric, IV: 1–2 mg/kg; if necessary, dose can be repeated. **IM:** 3–4 mg/kg, not to exceed a total dose of 150 mg.

IV INFUSION (PREFERRED)

Prolonged surgical procedures.

Adults: Average rate ranges from 2.5 to 4.3 mg/min. Most commonly used are 0.1–0.2% solutions in D5W, sodium chloride injection, or other diluent given at a rate of 0.5–10 mg/min depending on client response and degree of relaxation desired, for up to 1 hr.

IV, INTERMITTENT

Prolonged muscle relaxation.

Initial: 0.3–1.1 mg/kg; **then,** 0.04–0.07 mg/kg at appropriate intervals to maintain required level of relaxation.

NURSING IMPLICATIONS

IMPLEMENTATION/ADMINISTRATION/STORAGE

1. IV Give an initial test dose of 0.1 mg/kg to assess sensitivity and recovery time; if no or transient respiratory depression lasting less than 5 min, may give drug.
2. Do not mix with anesthetic. To reduce salivation, premedicate with atropine or scopolamine.
3. For IV infusion, use 1 or 2 mg/mL in compatible solution.
4. Refrigerate drug at 2–8°C (36–46°F). Multidose vials stable for 14 days or less at room temperature without significant loss of potency.
5. COMPATIBILITY D5W, 0.9% NaCl.
6. INCOMPATIBILITY Alkaline solutions (pH greater than 8.5); administer separately.

ASSESSMENT

1. List reasons for therapy, agents currently prescribed to ensure that none interact unfavorably. Note if taking digitalis products or quinidine; these clients sensitive to the release of intracellular potassium.
2. Note any evidence/history of MS, malignant hyperthermia, CPK myopathy, acute glaucoma, or eye injury; drug generally contraindicated.
3. Medicate for pain and anxiety as drug does not affect these symptoms; client unable to speak. Reassure they will regain function once therapy completed.
4. A peripheral nerve stimulator/train of four should be used to assess neuromuscular response and recovery (twitch response). The order of paralysis is levator muscles of the eyelid, mastication muscles, limb muscles, abdominal muscles, glottis muscles, the intercostals, the diaphragm, and all other skeletal muscles. This is reversed with recovery. Tests of muscle strength indicate recovery, such as return of hand grip, head lift, and ability to cough.
5. Monitor VS and ECG; can cause vagal stimulation resulting in bradycardia, hypotension, and cardiac arrhythmias, especially in children.
6. Muscle fasciculations may cause soreness and feelings of injury after recovery. Administer prescribed nondepolarizing agent (i.e., tubocurarine) and reassure that the soreness is likely caused by unsynchronized contractions of adjacent muscle fibers just before onset of paralysis.
7. Observe for excessive, transient increase in intraocular pressure. Monitor for evidence of

S

malignant hyperthermia, unresponsive tachycardia, jaw spasm, or lack of laryngeal relaxation.

8. Drug should be used only on a short-term basis in a continuously monitored environment by those trained in its use. Prolonged use may change from a depolarizing neuromuscular block (phase I block) to a block that resembles a nondepolarizing block (phase II block) which may be associated with prolonged respiratory depression and apnea.
9. Client is fully conscious and aware of surroundings/conversations. Drug does not affect pain or anxiety. Explain all procedures and provide emotional support. Do not conduct any discussions that should not be overheard. Reassure that client will be able to talk and move once drug effects reversed. Determine client need and administer medications for anxiety, pain, and/or sedation regularly (Valium, morphine).
10. When used for seizures, ensure that serum level of anticonvulsant agent is therapeutic. Succinylcholine does not cross the blood-brain barrier and will only suppress peripheral manifestations of seizures, not the central process.
11. Obtain baseline ECG, electrolytes, renal and LFTs. Those with low plasma pseudocholinesterase levels are sensitive to the effects of succinylcholine and require lower doses.

CLIENT/FAMILY TEACHING

1. Reassure will be continuously monitored and protected, a machine will breathe for them, and procedures/tests explained.
2. Once drug withdrawn will regain ability to move and talk again. May feel stiff and sore but should soon subside.
3. Medication for anxiety and pain will also be given, as this drug does not affect consciousness or alter pain threshold.

OUTCOMES/EVALUATE

- Muscle relaxation/paralysis
- Suppression of the twitch response
- Facilitation of ET intubation; control of breathing during mechanical ventilation
- ↓ Muscle contractions with drug/electroshock induced seizures

Sulfacetamide sodium

(sul-fah-**SEAT**-ah-myd)

Classification(s): Sulfonamide, topical

Pregnancy Category: C

RX: AK-Sulf, Bleph-10, Carmol Scalp Treatment, Isopto-Cetamide, Klaron 10%, Ocusulf-10, Ovace, Ovace Plus, Sebizon, Seb-Prev, Sodium Sulamyd, Storz Sulf, Sulf-10, Sulster.

SEE ALSO ***SULFONAMIDES***.

INDICATIONS/USES

(1) Topically for conjunctivitis, corneal ulcer, and other superficial ocular infections. (2) Adjunct to systemic sulfonamides to treat trachoma. (3) Secondary bacterial infections of the skin due to organisms susceptible to sulfonamides. (4) Topical application for seborrheic dermatitis and seborrhea sicca (dandruff).

ACTION/KINETICS

Pharmacokinetics

Significant absorption through the skin is possible, especially if applied to large, infected, abraded, denuded, or severely burned areas.

CONTRAINDICATIONS

Known or suspected sensitivity to sulfonamides or any component of the products. Use in infants less than 2 months of age. Use in the presence of epithelial herpes simplex keratitis, vaccinia, varicella, and other viral diseases of the cornea and conjunctiva. Mycobacterial or fungal infections of the ocular structures. After uncomplicated removal of a corneal foreign body.

SPECIAL CONCERNS

- Use with caution in clients with dry eye syndrome.
- Ophthalmic ointments may retard corneal wound healing.
- Cross-sensitivity with other sulfonamides is possible.
- Safe use not established during pregnancy, lactation, or in children less than 12 years of age.

SIDE EFFECTS

Most Common

Itching, local irritation, headache, burning, transient stinging, redness, swelling

S

Ophthalmic: Itching, local irritation, redness, swelling, periorbital edema, burning and transient stinging, headache, bacterial or fungal corneal ulcers. **CNS:** Headache.

Systemic side effects. Severe hypersensitivity reactions: Fever, skin rash, GI disturbances, bone marrow depression, ***Stevens-Johnson syndrome, toxic epidermal necrolysis***, exfoliative dermatitis, photosensitivity. Fatalities have occurred. **Miscellaneous:** Systemic lupus erythematosus, superinfection, irritation.

DRUG INTERACTIONS

Preparations containing silver are incompatible.

HOW SUPPLIED

Ophthalmic Ointment: 10%; ***Ophthalmic Solution:*** 1%, 10%, 15%, 30%; ***Topical Cream:*** 10%; ***Topical Foam:*** 10%; ***Topical Lotion:*** 10%; ***Topical Pads:*** 10%; ***Topical Shampoo:*** 10%; ***Topical Soap:*** 10%; ***Topical Suspension:*** 10%.

DOSAGE

OPHTHALMIC SOLUTION

Conjunctivitis or other superficial ocular infections.

For all strengths, 1–2 gtt in the conjunctival sac q 1–4 hr. Doses may be tapered by increasing the time interval between doses as the condition improves.

Trachoma.

2 gtt q 2 hr with concomitant systemic sulfonamide therapy.

OPHTHALMIC OINTMENT

Conjunctivitis, corneal ulcer, and other superficial ocular infections.

Apply approximately ¼ inch into the lower conjunctival sac 3–4 times per day and at bedtime. Alternatively, ½–1 inch is placed in the conjunctival sac at bedtime along with use of drops during the day.

LOTION

For cutaneous infections.

Apply locally (10%) to affected area 2–4 times per day

Seborrheic dermatitis.

Apply 1–2 times per day (for mild cases, apply overnight).

Cutaneous bacterial infections.

Apply 2–4 times per day until infection clears.

NURSING IMPLICATIONS

IMPLEMENTATION/ADMINISTRATION/STORAGE

Solutions will darken in color if left standing for long periods; discard these products.

ASSESSMENT

1. Note reasons for therapy, onset, duration, characteristics of S&S, clinical presentation.
2. List other agents prescribed, outcome.
3. Assess sites for irritation or sensitization during long-term therapy.
4. Note any allergy to sulfa drugs.

CLIENT/FAMILY TEACHING

1. Use only as directed. Wash hands before and after instillation.
2. Shake suspension well before using. For external use only.
3. Apply lotion at bedtime and allow to remain overnight. May shampoo if the hair or scalp is oily or greasy or if there is considerable debris before applying lotion.
4. Gently massage foam into affected areas of the scalp until foam disappears. Allow treated area to air dry. Do not wash the treated area immediately after applying foam.
5. With pads, wash affected areas twice daily (morning and evening). Massage into skin, work into a full lather, rinse thoroughly, and pat dry.
6. Medicated pads or wash may darken after prolonged exposure. Slight discoloration does not affect efficacy or safety.
7. Stop use and report if condition being treated becomes worse, if a rash develops, or if arthritis, fever, or mouth sores develop.
8. Ophthalmic products may cause sensitivity to bright light; wear sunglasses to minimize.
9. Report lack of response and any purulent eye drainage as this inactivates sulfacetamide.
10. If prescribed additional eye drops, wait 5 min after sulfacetamide instillation.
11. Do not wear contact lenses until infection is resolved.
12. Discard any cloudy or dark solutions. Do not let dropper/tip touch any part of eye so as to

S

prevent contamination of bottle/tube contents.

13. A slight yellowish discoloration may occur when excessive amounts of the product is used and comes in contact with white fabrics. Discoloration is readily removed by ordinary laundering without bleach.
14. Keep all F/U to assess response, labs, and for adverse SE.

OUTCOMES/EVALUATE

- Resolution of inflammation/infection
- Control of skin condition

Sulfadiazine

(sul-fah-**DYE**-ah-zeen)

Classification(s): Antibiotic, sulfonamide

Pregnancy Category: C

RX: Microsulfon.

SEE ALSO ***SULFONAMIDES***.

INDICATIONS/USES

(1) UTIs (primarily pyelonephritis, pyelitis, and cystitis) in the absence of obstructive uropathy or foreign bodies caused by *Escherichia coli, Klebsiella* species, *Enterobacter* species, *Staphylococcus aureus, Proteus mirabilis,* and *Proteus vulgaris. NOTE:* Use for UTIs only when the use of more soluble sulfonamides has been unsuccessful. (2) Chancroid. (3) Inclusion conjunctivitis. (4) Adjunct to treat chloroquine-resistant strains of *Plasmodium falciparum* when used as adjunctive therapy. (5) Meningitis caused by *Haemophilus influenzae,* meningococcal meningitis for sulfonamide-sensitive group A strains. (6) Nocardiosis. (7) With penicillin to treat acute otitis media caused by *H. influenzae.* (8) Prophylaxis of recurrences of rheumatic fever. (9) Adjunct with pyrimethamine for toxoplasmosis encephalitis in clients with or without AIDS. (10) Trachoma.

ACTION/KINETICS

Pharmacokinetics

Short-acting; often combined with other anti-infectives.

CONTRAINDICATIONS

Use in infants less than 2 months of age, except to treat congenital toxoplasmosis as adjunctive therapy with pyrimethamine. Treatment of group A beta-hemolytic streptococcal infections. Lactation.

SPECIAL CONCERNS

- Safe use during pregnancy not established.
- Possible cross-sensitivity with other sulfonamides.
- Use with caution with allergies and in those with renal or hepatic impairment.

SIDE EFFECTS

Most Common

Diarrhea, dizziness, headache, insomnia, rash, anorexia, stomach pain, tinnitus, myalgia.

See *Sulfonamides* for a complete list of possible side effects. Fatalities, although rare, due to severe reactions, including ***Stevens-Johnson syndrome, toxic epidermal necrolysis, fulminant hepatic necrosis, agranulocytosis, aplastic anemia***, and other blood dyscrasias. Pseudomembranous colitis can occur with any sulfonamide.

HOW SUPPLIED

Tablets: 500 mg.

DOSAGE

TABLETS

General use.

Adults, initial dose: 2–4 grams; **maintenance:** 2–4 grams/day in 3 to 6 divided doses; **infants over 2 months, initial dose:** 75 mg/kg/day (2 grams/m^2); **maintenance:** 150 mg/kg/day (4 grams/m^2/day) in 4 to 6 divided doses, not to exceed 6 grams/day.

Rheumatic fever prophylaxis.

Under 30 kg (66 lbs): 0.5 gram/day; **over 30 kg (66 lbs):** 1 gram/day.

NURSING IMPLICATIONS

Do not confuse sulfadiazine with sulfasalazine (also a sulfonamide).

IMPLEMENTATION/ADMINISTRATION/STORAGE

Store from 20–25°C (68–77°F).

ASSESSMENT

1. Note reasons for therapy, onset, duration, characteristics of S&S, and clinical presentation.
2. Assess for severe allergy or bronchial asthma, and use with caution if present.

S

3. Obtain appropriate labs: cultures, CBC, renal and LFTs; note dysfunction.

CLIENT/FAMILY TEACHING

1. Take as directed with a full glass of water (8 oz). Consume at least 2 L fluids/day to prevent dehydration and crystalluria. Do not share medications; complete entire prescription.
2. Avoid prolonged sun exposure, and use protection; may cause photosensitivity reaction.
3. No OTC medications, especially aspirin or vitamin C without provider approval.
4. Report any unusual bruising/bleeding, rash/hives, fever, sore throat, purple spots on skin, blood in urine, yellowing of the skin or eyes, or lack of effectiveness.
5. Practice reliable contraception to prevent pregnancy.
6. Discontinue at the first appearance of skin rash, or any signs of an adverse reaction.
7. Keep all F/U to assess response, labs, and for adverse SE.

OUTCOMES/EVALUATE

- Negative culture reports
- Infection prophylaxis

Sulfasalazine

(sul-fah-**SAL**-ah-zeen)

Classification(s): Antibiotic, sulfonamide

Pregnancy Category: B

RX: Azulfidine, Azulfidine EN-Tabs.

✤ **Rx:** PMS-Sulfasalazine, PMS-Sulfasalazine EC, Salazopyrin, Salazopyrin En-Tabs.

SEE ALSO ***SULFONAMIDES***.

INDICATIONS/USES

Tablets and Delayed-Release Tablets. (1) Mild-to-moderate ulcerative colitis. (2) Adjunctive in severe ulcerative colitis. (3) Prolongation of the remission period between acute attacks of ulcerative colitis. **Delayed-Release Tablets.** (1) Treat rheumatoid arthritis in adults who have responded inadequately to salicylates or other NSAIDs. (2) Pediatric clients with polyarticular-course juvenile rheumatoid arthritis who have responded inadequately to salicylates or other NSAIDs. *Investigational:* Ankylosing spondylitis, granulomatous colitis, Crohn's disease, regional enteritis.

ACTION/KINETICS

Pharmacokinetics

Bioavailability is less than 15% for the parent drug. The drug passes to the colon, where it is split to 5-aminosalicylic acid (5-ASA) and sulfapyridine. The drug does not affect the microflora. Peak plasma levels of both sulfasalazine and 5-aminosalicylic acid occur after about 10 hr. Sulfapyridine is metabolized by acetylation. **Mean plasma t½, fast acetylators:** 10.4 hr; **mean plasma t½, slow acetylators:** 14.8 hr. 5-ASA is metabolized by the liver and intestine. Absorbed sulfapyridine and 5-ASA and their metabolites are excreted primarily in the urine. However, the majority of 5-ASA remains in the colon and is excreted with the feces.

ADDITIONAL CONTRAINDICATIONS

In persons with marked sulfonamide, salicylate, or related drug hypersensitivity. Intestinal or urinary obstruction. Children less than 2 years of age.

SPECIAL CONCERNS

- Use with caution during lactation and in those with severe allergy or bronchial asthma.
- Observe those with G6PD deficiency closely for signs of hemolytic anemia (reaction is frequently dose-related).
- Possible cross-sensitivity with other sulfonamides.
- Safety and efficiency not determined in children less than 2 years of age with ulcerative colitis.

SIDE EFFECTS

Most Common

Anorexia, headache, N&V, dyspepsia, gastric distress, rash, reversible oligospermia.

GI: Anorexia, N&V, dyspepsia, gastric distress, stomatitis, diarrhea, hepatitis, pancreatitis, bloody diarrhea, impaired folic acid absorption, impaired digoxin absorption, abdominal pain, neutropenic enterocolitis, hepatotoxicity, jaundice, cholestatic jaundice, cirrhosis, ***liver necrosis, liver failure***. **CNS:** Headache, dizziness, transverse myelitis, ***convulsions, meningitis***, transient lesions of the posterior spinal column, cauda equina syndrome, Guillain-Barré syndrome, peripheral neuropathy, mental depression, vertigo, hearing loss, insomnia, ataxia, hallucinations, tinnitus, drowsiness. **Der-**

matologic: Pruritus, urticaria, skin rash/discoloration. **GU:** Oligospermia (reversible), infertility in men, toxic nephrosis with oliguria and anuria, nephritis, nephrotic syndrome, hematuria, crystalluria, proteinuria, hemolytic-uremic syndrome, urine discoloration. **Hematologic:** ***Agranulocytosis, aplastic anemia***, leukopenia, thrombocytopenia, suppression of immunoglobulin, megaloblastic anemia, purpura, hypoprothrombinemia, methemoglobinemia, congenital neutropenia, myelodysplastic syndrome. **Hypersensitivity:** ***Stevens-Johnson syndrome***, exfoliative dermatitis, epidermal necrolysis with corneal damage, ***anaphylaxis***, serum sickness syndrome, pneumonitis with or without eosinophilia, vasculitis, fibrosing alveolitis, pleuritis, ***pericarditis with or without tamponade***, allergic myocarditis, polyarteritis nodosa, lupus erythematosus-like syndrome, hepatitis, ***hepatic necrosis with or without immune complexes***, ***fulminant hepatitis*** (possible liver transplant necessary), parapsoriasis, varioliformis acute, rhabdomyolysis, photosensitivity, arthralgia, periorbital edema, conjunctival and scleral injection, alopecia. **Miscellaneous:** Fever, Heinz body anemia, ***hemolytic anemia***, cyanosis.
NOTE: Symptoms of sore throat, fever, pallor, purpura or jaundice may be signs of serious blood disorders.

LABORATORY TEST CONSIDERATIONS

↑ AST, ALT, GGT, lactic dehydrogenase, alkaline phosphatase, bilirubin. Abnormal LFTs.

OVERDOSE MANAGEMENT

Symptoms: N&V, gastric distress, abdominal pain, drowsiness, convulsions. *Treatment:*

- Gastric lavage or emesis plus catharsis.
- Alkalinize the urine to hasten excretion.
- Force fluids if kidney function is normal.
- If anuria is present, restrict fluids and salt and treat appropriately.
- Catherization of the ureters may be indicated for complete renal blockage by crystals.
- The low molecular weight of sulfasalazine and its metabolites may help their removal by dialysis.

DRUG INTERACTIONS

Azathioprine / High rate of leukopenia and ↑ whole blood 6-thioguanine in Crohn's disease clients
Cyclosporine / ↓ Cyclosporine levels; ↑ risk of nephrotoxicity
Digoxin / ↓ Digoxin absorption
Folic acid / ↓ Folic acid absorption; folic acid dosage adjustment may be needed
Mercaptopurine / High rate of leukopenia and ↑ whole blood 6-thioguanine in Crohn's disease clients
Methotrexate / ↑ Risk of methotrexate-induced bone marrow suppression R/T displacement of methotrexate from plasma protein binding sites; also, ↑ GI side effects, especially nausea
Sulfonylureas (e.g., glipizide) / ↑ Sulfonylurea levels R/T impaired hepatic metabolism or altered plasma protein binding; monitor and possibly decrease sulfonylurea dose
Warfarin / ↑ Warfarin anticoagulant effect; monitor carefully

HOW SUPPLIED

Tablets: 500 mg; ***Tablets, Delayed-Release:*** 500 mg.

DOSAGE

TABLETS; TABLETS, DELAYED-RELEASE

Ulcerative colitis.

Adults, initial: 3–4 grams/day in evenly divided doses with dosage intervals not exceeding 8 hr. A lower initial dosage (1–2 grams/day) may decrease side effects; **maintenance:** 500 mg 4 times per day. Doses greater than 4 grams/day increase the risk of toxicity. **Pediatric, over 6 years of age, initial:** 40–60 mg/kg/day in 3 to 6 equally divided doses; **maintenance:** 30 mg/kg/day in 4 divided doses.

Adult rheumatoid arthritis.

Delayed-Release Tablets: To reduce GI intolerance, **initial:** 0.5 gram in the evening for the first week, increased to 0.5 gram in the morning and evening the second week, 0.5 gram in the morning and 1 gram in the evening the third week; then, beginning week 4, 1 gram in the morning and evening. Consider increasing the daily dose to 3 grams if the clinical response after 12 weeks is inadequate. Monitor closely for doses over 2 grams/day.

S

Juvenile rheumatoid arthritis, polyarticular course.

Children, 6 years and older:
30–50 mg/kg daily in 2 evenly divided doses (maximum 2 grams/day). To reduce GI intolerance, begin with a quarter to a third of the planned maintenance dose and increase weekly until reaching the maintenance dose at 1 month.

Collagenous colitis.
2–3 grams/day.

Psoriasis.
3–4 grams/day.

Psoriatic arthritis.
2 grams/day.

NURSING IMPLICATIONS

Do not confuse sulfasalazine with salsalate (salicylate), sulfisoxazole or sulfadiazine (both sulfonamides).

IMPLEMENTATION/ADMINISTRATION/STORAGE

1. Adjust dose individually to each client's response and tolerance.
2. The enteric-coated delayed-release tablets are indicated particularly for those clients with ulcerative colitis who cannot take uncoated sulfasalazine tablets due to GI intolerance (e.g., N&V with the first few doses, clients in whom a reduction in dosage does not alleviate the adverse GI effects).
3. Rest and physiotherapy should be continued in adults and children with rheumatoid arthritis.
4. The delayed-release tablets do not produce an immediate response. Concurrent treatment with analgesics or NSAIDs is recommended, at least until the effect of sulfasalazine delayed-release tablets is apparent.
5. When used for rheumatoid arthritis, a therapeutic response has been seen as early as 4 weeks after initiating treatment with delayed-release tablets; however, treatment for 12 weeks may be needed in some before a clinical benefit is noted. Give consideration to increasing the daily dose of the delayed-release tablets to 3 grams if the clinical response after 12 weeks is inadequate; monitor carefully.
6. It is possible, in isolated instances, for delayed-release tablets to be excreted undisintegrated. If this occurs, discontinue the delayed-release tablets immediately.
7. Store from 15–30°C (59–86°F).

ASSESSMENT

1. Note reasons for therapy, onset, characteristics of S&S. List other agents trialed; outcome.
2. List frequency, quantity, and consistency of stool production; assess abdomen and pain with ulcerative colitis. Review colonoscopy, biopsy results.
3. Note joint deformity, pain, ROM, inflammation, and swelling with rheumatoid arthritis.
4. Monitor CBC, U/A, folate, renal and LFTs, (every 2 weeks during first 3 months of therapy, then every month during the next 3 months, then every 3 months thereafter). With colitis, send stool for regular analysis.

CLIENT/FAMILY TEACHING

1. Take exactly as ordered at the same time each day; even if using intermittent therapy (2 weeks on, 2 weeks off). Take with or after meals with a full glass of water, at evenly spaced intervals to reduce GI upset.
2. Swallow delayed-release tablets whole and not to crush, chew, or break.
3. Avoid activities that require mental alertness until drug effects realized; may cause dizziness.
4. Take at least 2–3 L/day of water to decrease incidence of dehydration and crystalluria/stone formation. Drug may discolor urine or skin a yellow-orange color. May permanently discolor soft contact lenses.
5. Avoid prolonged exposure to sunlight; may increase sensitivity. Wear protective clothing, sunglasses, and sunscreen.
6. Report any unusual bruising/bleeding, rash, fever, sore throat, intact tablet in stool, or worsening of symptoms.
7. Keep all F/U to assess response, labs, and for adverse SE.

OUTCOMES/EVALUATE

- ↓ Frequency of loose stools; ↓ abdominal pain; ↓ colon inflammation
- Relief of pain from joint deformity, swelling, and inflammation

S

Sulindac

(sul-**IN**-dak)

Classification(s): Nonsteroidal anti-inflammatory drug

RX: Clinoril.

🍁 **Rx:** Apo-Sulin.

SEE ALSO ***NONSTEROIDAL ANTI-INFLAMMATORY DRUGS.***

INDICATIONS/USES

Acute or chronic use for the relief of signs and symptoms of the following: (1) Rheumatoid arthritis (acute and long-term use). *NOTE:* Safety and efficacy have not been determined for those designated by the American Rheumatism Association classification as Functional Class IV. (2) Osteoarthritis (acute and long-term use). (3) Anklyosing spondylitis (acute and long–term use). (4) Acute or long–term use for painful shoulder (acute subacromial bursitis/supraspinatus tendinitis). (5) Acute gouty arthritis (acute and long-term use). *Investigational:* Juvenile rheumatoid arthritis.

ACTION/KINETICS

Pharmacokinetics

Bioavailability is 90%. Biotransformed in the liver to a sulfide, the active metabolite. **Peak plasma levels of sulfide:** After fasting, 2 hr; after food, 3–4 hr. **Onset, anti-inflammatory effect:** Within 1 week; **duration, anti-inflammatory effect:** 1–2 weeks. **t½,** of sulindac: 7.8 hr; of metabolite: 16.4 hr. Excreted in both urine (50%) and feces (25%). **Plasma protein binding:** More than 93%.

CONTRAINDICATIONS

Use with active GI lesions or a history of recurrent GI lesions.

SPECIAL CONCERNS

(1) **Cardiovascular risk.** NSAIDs may cause an increased risk of serious cardiovascular thrombotic events, MI, and stroke, which can be fatal. This risk may increase with duration of use. Clients with cardiovascular disease or risk factors for cardiovascular disease may be at greater risk. (2) Sulindac is contraindicated for treatment of perioperative pain in the setting of coronary artery bypass graft surgery. (3) **GI risk.** NSAIDs cause an increased risk of serious GI adverse events including bleeding, ulceration, and perforation of the stomach or intestines, which can be fatal. These reactions can occur at any time during use and without warning symptoms. Elderly clients are at greater risk for serious GI events.

- Safe use during pregnancy not established.
- Use with caution during lactation.
- Safety and efficacy not established for children.

SIDE EFFECTS

Most Common

Headache, dizziness, rash, abdominal pain, diarrhea, nausea, constipation.

See *Nonsteroidal Anti-Inflammatory Drugs* for a complete list of possible side effects. Also, hypersensitivity, pancreatitis, GI pain (common), maculopapular rash. Stupor, ***coma***, hypotension, and diminished urine output.

ADDITIONAL DRUG INTERACTIONS

Sulindac / ↑ Warfarin effect R/T ↓ plasma protein binding

HOW SUPPLIED

Tablets: 150 mg, 200 mg.

DOSAGE

TABLETS

Osteoarthritis, rheumatoid arthritis, ankylosing spondylitis.

Adults, initial: 150 mg twice a day wtih food. Individualize dosage based on response, but not to exceed 400 mg/day.

Acute painful shoulder, acute gouty arthritis.

Adults, usual: 200 mg twice a day with food. In acute painful shoulder, usual therapy is for 7–14 days; for acute gouty arthritis, therapy for 7 days is usually adequate.

NURSING IMPLICATIONS

- Do not confuse Clinoril with Clozaril (an antipsychotic).

IMPLEMENTATION/ADMINISTRATION/STORAGE

1. Use the lowest effective dose for the shortest duration consistent with individual client treatment goals.
2. A response within 1 week can be expected in about one-half of clients with osteoarthritis, rheumatoid arthritis, or ankylosing spondylitis.
3. For acute conditions, reduce dosage when satisfactory response is attained.
4. A lower dose may be needed in those with impaired hepatic or renal function.
5. Store from 15–30°C (59–86°F) in a tightly closed container.

ASSESSMENT

1. Note reasons for therapy, location, onset, and characteristics of S&S. List other agents/therapies trialed.
2. List baseline ROM; describe location, inflammation, swelling; rate pain level, note functional class of arthritis.
3. Assess all clients receiving therapy for GI bleeding. Review x-rays/MRI/CT.
4. Determine history of ulcers, heart disease, or cardiac failure. May cause an increased risk of serious CV thrombotic events, MI, and stroke; risk increased with longer use, in the elderly, and with heart disease.
5. Monitor BP, vision, CBC, uric acid, chemistry, renal and LFTs; reduce dose with dysfunction.

CLIENT/FAMILY TEACHING

1. Take with food to decrease GI upset; consume plenty of water. A stomach protectant (i.e., misoprostol) may be prescribed with history of ulcer disease.
2. Drug may cause dizziness/drowsiness; assess response prior to any activity requiring mental alertness or driving.
3. Do not take aspirin because plasma levels of sulindac will be reduced. Avoid alcohol.
4. Record BP for provider review; BP may increase due to drug induced sodium retention.
5. Report changes in urine pattern, weight gain, swelling of extremities, fever or any incidence of unexplained bleeding (oozing of blood from the gums, nosebleeds, or excessive bruising), blurred vision, or ringing/noise in ears.
6. When used for arthritis, a favorable response usually occurs within 1 week.
7. NSAIDs have been associated with serious, possibly fatal, heart and blood vessel risks such as heart attack and stroke.
8. Avoid use in late pregnancy because of possible premature closure of the ductus arteriosus (fetus).
9. Keep all F/U to assess response, labs, and for adverse SE.

OUTCOMES/EVALUATE

↓ Pain and inflammation with ↑ mobility

Sumatriptan succinate

(**soo**-mah-**TRIP**-tan)

Classification(s): Antimigraine drug

Pregnancy Category: C

RX: Imitrex, Sumavel DosePro.

✤ **Rx:** Apo-Sumatriptan, CO Sumatriptan, Gen-Sumatriptan, Novo-Sumatriptan, PMS-Sumatriptan, ratio-Sumatriptan, Sandoz Sumatriptan.

INDICATIONS/USES

PO, Nasal Spray: Acute treatment of migraine attacks in adults, with or without aura. Not intended for prophylaxis therapy of migraine or for use in the management of hemiplegic or basilar migraine. Safety and efficacy have not been established to treat cluster headache. *Investigational:* Migraines in children and adolescents.

Injection: (1) Acute treatment of migraine attacks with or without aura. Not for use to manage hemiplegic or basilar migraine. (2) Acute treatment of cluster headache episodes. *Investigational:* Migraines in children and adolescents; postdural puncture headache.

ACTION/KINETICS

Action

Selective agonist for a vascular 5-HT_1 receptor subtype (probably 5-HT_{1D}) located on cranial arteries, on the basilar artery, and the vasculature of the dura mater. Activates the 5-HT_1 receptor, causing vasoconstriction and therefore relief of migraine. Transient increases in BP may be observed. Weak activity against 5-HT_{1A}, 5-HT_{5A}, and 5-HT_7 receptors. No significant activity at 5-HT_2 or 5-HT_3 receptor subtypes.

Pharmacokinetics

Bioavailablity ranges from 14–19% after PO, nasal, or rectal use and 96% after SC administration. **Time to onset after SC:** 10 min after a 6 mg SC dose; **time to onset after PO:** 30 min; **time to onset after intranasal:** 15 min. **Time to peak effect after SC:** 12 min; **time to peak effect after PO:** 2.5 hr; **time to peak effect after intranasal:** 1–1.5 hr. **t½ distribution, after SC:** 15 min; **terminal t½:** 2.5 hr. Approximately 22% of a SC dose is excreted in the urine as unchanged drug and 38% as metabolites. Rapidly absorbed after PO administration, although bioavailability is low due to incomplete absorption and a first-pass effect (bioavailability may be significantly increased in those with impaired liver function). **PO, elimination t½:** About 2.5 hr. About 60% of a PO dose is excreted through the urine and 40% in the feces. **Plasma protein binding:** 14–21%.

CONTRAINDICATIONS

Hypersensitivity to sumatriptan. Tablets and spray for prophylactic therapy of migraine or for cluster headache. IV use due to the possibility of coronary vasospasm. SC use in clients with ischemic heart disease, history of MI, documented silent ischemia, Prinzmetal's angina, or uncontrolled hypertension. Concomitant use with ergotamine-containing products or MAOI therapy (or within 2 weeks of discontinuing an MAOI). Use in clients with hemiplegic or basilar migraine. Use in women who are pregnant, think they may be pregnant, or are trying to get pregnant. Not recommended for the elderly due to increased risk for coronary artery disease and increases in BP.

SPECIAL CONCERNS

- Use with caution during lactation, in clients with impaired hepatic or renal function, and in clients with heart conditions.
- Screen clients with risk factors for CAD (e.g., men over 40, smokers, postmenopausal women, hypertension, obesity, diabetes, hypercholesterolemia, family history of heart disease) before initiating treatment.
- Safety and efficacy not determined for use in children.

SIDE EFFECTS

Most Common

Paresthesia, warm/cold sensation, chest pain/tightness, vertigo, malaise/fatigue, neck/throat/jaw pain or pressure, N&V, headache, dizziness.

Side effects listed are for either SC or PO use of the drug. CV: Coronary vasospasm in clients with a history of CAD. ***Serious and/or life-threatening arrhythmias, including atrial fibrillation, ventricular fibrillation, ventricular tachycardia, MI, marked ischemic ST elevations***, chest and arm discomfort representing angina pectoris. Flushing, pallor, hyper-/hypotension, brady-/tachycardia, palpitations, pulsating sensations, ECG changes (including nonspecific ST- or T-wave changes, prolongation of PR or QTc intervals, sinus arrhythmia, nonsustained ventricular premature beats, isolated junctional ectopic beats, atrial ectopic beats, and delayed activation of the right ventricle), syncope, abnormal pulse, atherosclerosis, cerebral ischemia, CV lesion, ***heart block***, peripheral cyanosis, thrombosis, transient myocardial ischemia, vasodilation, Raynaud syndrome. **Injection site:** Pain, redness. **Atypical sensations:** Sensation of warmth, cold, tingling, or paresthesia. Localized or generalized feeling of pressure, burning, numbness, and tightness. Feeling of heaviness, feeling strange, tight feeling in head. **CNS:** Fatigue, dizziness, drowsiness, vertigo, sedation, headache, anxiety, malaise, confusion, euphoria, agitation, relaxation, chills, tremor, shivering, prickling or stinging sensations, phonophobia, depression, euphoria, facial pain, heat sensitivity, incoordination, monoplegia, sleep disturbances, shivering. **EENT:** Throat discomfort, discomfort in nasal cavity or sinuses. Vision alterations, eye irritation, photophobia, lacrimation, otalgia, feeling of fullness in ear, disorders of sclera, mydriasis. **GI:** Abdominal discomfort, N&V, dysphagia, discomfort of mouth and tongue, gastroesophageal reflux, diarrhea, peptic ulcer, retching, flatulence, eructation, gallstones, taste disturbances, GI bleeding, hematemesis, melena. **Respiratory:** Dyspnea, diseases of the lower respiratory tract, hiccoughs, influenza, asthma. **Dermatologic:** Erythema, pruritus, skin rashes/eruptions/tenderness, dry/scaly skin, tightness/wrinkling of skin. **GU:** Dysuria, dysmenorrhea, urinary frequency, renal calculus, breast tenderness, increased urination, intermenstrual bleeding, nipple discharge, abortion, hematuria. **Musculoskeletal:** Weakness, neck pain/stiffness, myalgia, muscle cramps, joint disturbances (pain, stiffness, swelling, ache), muscle stiffness, need to flex calf muscles, backache, muscle tiredness, swelling of the extremities, tetany. **Endocrine:** Elevated TSH levels, galactorrhea, hyper-/hypoglycemia, hypothyroidism, weight gain/loss. **Miscellaneous:** Chest,

S

jaw, or neck tightness. Sweating, thirst, polydipsia, chills, fever, dehydration.

LABORATORY TEST CONSIDERATIONS

Disturbance of LFTs.

OVERDOSE MANAGEMENT

Symptoms: Tremor, ***convulsions***, inactivity erythema of extremities, reduced respiratory rate, cyanosis, ataxia, mydriasis, injection site reactions (desquamation, hair loss, scab formation), paralysis. *Treatment:* Continuous monitoring of client for at least 10 hr and especially when signs and symptoms persist.

DRUG INTERACTIONS

Ergot drugs / Prolonged vasospastic reactions
MAOIs / ↑ Bioavailability of sumatriptan
Selective serotonin reuptake inhibitors (SSRIs) / Rarely, weakness, hyperreflexia, and incoordination
Sibutramine / Possible serotonin syndrome, including CNS irritability, motor weakness, shivering, myoclonus, and altered consciousness

HOW SUPPLIED

Injection: 4 mg/0.5 mL (as part of STATdose System), 6 mg/0.5 mL (as part of STAT dose System or as Sumavel DosePro); ***Nasal Solution Spray:*** 5 mg, 20 mg; ***Tablets:*** 25 mg, 50 mg, 100 mg.

DOSAGE

Imitrex

TABLETS

Migraine headaches.

Adults: A single dose of 25 mg, 50 mg, or 100 mg with fluids as soon as symptoms of migraine appear. Doses of 50 mg or 100 mg may provide a greater effect than 25 mg. A second dose may be taken if symptoms return but no sooner than 2 hr following the first dose. **Maximum recommended dose:** 100 mg, with no more than 200 mg taken in a 24-hr period. The safety of treating an average of more than 4 headaches in a 30-day period has not been determined. **Children and adolescents (investigational):** 50 mg for those 12 years and younger and 100 mg for those 12 years and older.

NASAL SPRAY

Migraine headaches.

Adults: A single dose of 5, 10, or 20 mg given in one nostril. The 20 mg dose increases the risk of side effects, although it is more effective. The 10 mg dose may be given as a single 5 mg dose in each nostril. If the headache returns, repeat the dose once after 2 hr, not to exceed a total daily dose of 40 mg. The safety of treating an average of more than 4 headaches in a 30 day period has not been studied. **Children and adolescents (investigational):** Doses of 5, 10, or 20 mg have been given.

SC

Migraine headaches, Cluster headaches.

Adults: 6 mg. A second injection may be given if symptoms of migraine come back but no more than two injections (6 mg each) should be taken in a 24-hr period and at least 1 hr should elapse between doses. **Children and adolescents (investigational):** 3 mg for those weighing less than 30 kg, and 6 mg for those weighing over 30 kg. Or, determine amount to be given using a dose of 0.06 mg/kg.

Sumavel DosePro

SC

Migraine headaches.

Adults: 1 Sumavel DosePro (6 mg) to the abdomen or thigh, up to 2 doses/day, separated by at least 1 hr.

NURSING IMPLICATIONS

IMPLEMENTATION/ADMINISTRATION/STORAGE

1. No increased beneficial effect found with administration of a second 6-mg dose SC in clients not responding to the first injection.
2. If side effects are dose limiting, a dose lower than 6 mg SC dose may be given; in such cases, use the single-dose 6 mg vial. An autoinjection device can be used to deliver the drug.
3. Consideration should be given to administering the first dose of sumatriptan in the provider's office due to the possibility (although

rare) of coronary events R/T undiagnosed CAD.
4. Is equally effective at whatever stage of the attack given; advisable to take as soon as possible after the onset of migraine attack.
5. Do not give more than 50 mg as a single dose in those with hepatic disease/impairment.
6. The SC dose should be decreased in those also taking an MAOI.
7. Store all dosage forms from 2–30°C (36–86°F). Protect the injection and nasal spray from light.

ASSESSMENT

1. Note headache characteristics, onset/duration, frequency. Rate pain levels, other agents used/outcome.
2. Assess neurologic exam/findings; review headache diary, triggers, and MRI/CT scans.
3. Parenteral form for SC use only—may see erythema at injection site. IV use may cause coronary vasospasm, MI.
4. Check for cardiac problems/disease, ischemic CV disease, history of stroke or TIAs, PVD, Raynaud syndrome, or if BP not controlled; precludes therapy.
5. Use caution, may cause coronary artery vasospasm. If angina occurs following dosing report so the presence of CAD or a predisposition to Prinzmetal variant angina may be assessed before additional therapy. Other S&S suggestive of decreased arterial flow, such as ischemic bowel syndrome or Raynaud syndrome following therapy should also be evaluated for atherosclerosis by provider.
6. Monitor ECG, renal and LFTs, VS; expect transient increases in BP.

CLIENT/FAMILY TEACHING

1. Review appropriate method for administration. Drug is used to terminate headaches not to prevent them. Take with plenty of water. With SC form, observe client; administer first dose in office to assess response and administration technique.
2. Printed instructions concerning how to load the autoinjector, administer the medication, and remove the syringe, are provided by the manufacturer. The injection is given just below the skin as soon as migraine symptoms appear or any time during the attack. A second injection may be administered 1 hr later if migraine symptoms return; do NOT exceed two injections in 24 hr. Report lack of response or loss of effectiveness. Practice safe handling, storage, and disposal of syringes. Pain and tenderness may be evident at injection site for up to an hour after administration.
3. The nasal spray contains only 1 spray/container; do not test before use. While sitting down, blow the nose to clear nasal passages. Keep head in an upright position and gently close one nostril with the index finger. Breathe out gently through the mouth. With the other hand, hold the container with the thumb supporting it at the bottom and the index and middle fingers on either side of the nozzle. Insert the nozzle into the open nostril about a half inch. Keep the head upright and close the mouth. While gently taking a breath through the nose, release the spray dosage by firmly pressing the blue plunger. Remove the nozzle from the nostril. At the same time, keep the head level for 10–20 seconds while gently breathing through the nose and breathing out through the mouth. Do not breathe in deeply.
4. May cause fatigue/dizziness; avoid activities that require mental alertness until effects realized.
5. For tablets, take a single dose with fluids as soon as symptoms appear; a second dose may be taken if symptoms return, but no sooner than 2 hr after the first dose. If there is no response to the first tablet, do not take a second tablet without consulting provider.
6. With nasal spray, use one spray in one nostril at onset of symptoms; may repeat in 2 hr if headache returns but not if pain persists after initial dose.
7. Check expiration date before use and discard all outdated drugs.
8. Report if chest, jaw, throat, and neck pain occur after injection; this should be medically evaluated before using more drug. Severe chest pain, SOB, wheezing, palpitations, facial swelling, or rashes/hives should be immediately reported.
9. Symptoms of flushing, tingling, heat, and heaviness; dizziness or drowsiness may occur and should be reported before taking more sumatriptan.
10. Practice barrier contraception and do not use drug if pregnancy is suspected.

S

11. Avoid prolonged or excessive exposure to direct or artificial sunlight.
12. Keep all F/U to assess response, review headache diary, identify triggers, and for adverse SE.

OUTCOMES/EVALUATE

Termination of acute migraine/cluster headaches with relief of symptoms

Sunitinib maleate

(soo-**NI**-tih-nib)

Classification(s): Antineoplastic, protein-tyrosine kinase inhibitor
Pregnancy Category: D
RX: Sutent.

INDICATIONS/USES

(1) Treatment of GI stromal tumor after disease progression on or intolerance to imatinib. (2) Treatment of advanced renal cell carcinoma. (3) Treatment of progressive, well–differentiated pancreatic neuroendocrine tumors in clients with unresectable locally advanced or metastatic disease.

ACTION/KINETICS

Action

Inhibits multiple receptor tyrosine kinases, some of which are implicated in tumor growth, pathologic angiogenesis, and metastatic progression of cancer. The primary metabolite exhibits similar potency to the parent compound. Sunitinib inhibits tumor growth or tumor regression and/or inhibited metastases.

Pharmacokinetics

Maximum plasma levels: 6–12 hr. Food has no effect on the bioavailability; thus the drug may be taken with or without food. Metabolized primarily by CYP3A4 to a primary active metabolite, which is further metabolized by CYP3A4. **Steady state:** 10–14 days. Excreted primarily by the feces (61%) with a smaller amount in the urine (16%). **t½, terminal:** 40–60 hr for sunitinib and 80–110 hr for the primary active metabolite. **Plasma protein binding:** 95% (sunitinib) and 90% (primary metabolite).

CONTRAINDICATIONS

Hypersensitivity to sunitinib or any component of the product. Lactation.

SPECIAL CONCERNS

■ **Hepatotoxicity.** Hepatotoxicity has been observed in clinical trials and postmarketing experience. Hepatotoxicity may be severe, and deaths have been reported. ■

Safety and efficacy not determined in children.

SIDE EFFECTS

Most Common

Abdominal pain, altered taste, anorexia, arthralgia, asthenia, back pain, bleeding, constipation, cough, diarrhea, dry skin, dyspepsia, dyspnea, extremity pain, fatigue, fever, hair color changes, hand–foot syndrome, headache, hypertension, mucositis/stomatitis, N&V, peripheral edema, rash, skin discoloration.

GI: Altered taste, abdominal pain, anorexia, diarrhea, dysgeusia, dyspepsia, flatulence, GERD/reflux esophagitis, glossodynia, N&V, mucositis, stomatitis, oral pain, constipation, abdominal pain, glossodynia, hemorrhoids, ***GI perforation***. **Hepatic:** Hepatoxicity (jaundice, encephalopathy, coagulopathy), ***pancreatitis, liver failure, death***. **CNS:** Fatigue, headache, depression, dizziness, insomnia. **CV:** Hypertension, peripheral edema, left ventricular dysfunction, decline in left ventricular ejection fraction, DVT, ***heart failure, cardiomyopathy***, myocardial disorders, bleeding events (including epistaxis; rectal, gingival, upper GI, genital, respiratory, urinary tract, ***brain hemorrhage***, and wound bleeding), QT interval prolongation, ***torsades de pointes, tumor-related hemorrhage***, arterial thrombotic events (e.g., ***CVA***, TIA, ***cerebral infarction***), thrombotic microangiopathy, ***pulmonary embolism***. **Hematologic:** Neutropenia, thrombocytopenia, lymphopenia, anemia. **Dermatologic:** Skin discoloration/yellow skin, rash, hand-foot syndrome, hair color changes, alopecia, dry skin, erythema, pruritus. **Musculoskeletal:** Arthralgia, back/chest pain, myalgia, limb pain, extremity pain, myopathy, rhabdomyolysis. **Respiratory:** Dyspnea, cough, nasopharyngitis, oropharyngeal pain, URTI. **GU:** Renal impairment and/or ***renal failure***, proteinuria, nephrotic syndrome (rare). **Endocrine:** Hypothyroidism, adrenal toxicity. **Hypersensitivity:** ***Angioedema***, hypersensitivity reactions. **Body as a whole:** Asthenia, chills, fever, bleeding (all sites), dehydration, decreased weight, flu–like illness. **Miscellaneous:** Impaired wound healing, reversible posterior leukoencephalopathy syndrome, serious infection with or without neutropenia, fistula formation, tumor necrosis and/or regression.

LABORATORY TEST CONSIDERATIONS

↑ ALT, AST, alkaline phosphatase, total bilirubin, indirect bilirubin, amylase, lipase, creatinine, creatine kinase, uric acid, pancreatic enzymes, uric acid. ↓ Hemoglobin, albumin, potassium, phosphorus, lymphocytes, magnesium, neutrophils, platelets. ↑ or ↓ Glucose, calcium, potassium, sodium. ↑ LFTs.

DRUG INTERACTIONS

NOTE: An additive effect of sunitinib with other drugs that prolong the QT interval cannot be excluded. The following drugs may prolong the QT interval and increase the risk of life–threatening cardiac arrhythmias, including torsades de pointes: Amiodarone, arsenic trioxide, bretylium, chlorpromazine, cisapride, disopyramide, dofetilide, dolasetron, droperidol, gatifloxacin, halofantrine, levomethadyl, mefloquine, mesoridazine, moxifloxacin, pentamidine, pimozide, probucol, procainamide, quinidine, sotalol, sparfloxacin, thioridazine, ziprasidone.

Atazanavir / Possible ↑ sunitinib levels R/T inhibition of metabolism by CYP3A4 → ↑ risk of side effects, including ventricular arrhythmias (e.g., torsades de pointes)

Bevacizumab / Possible unexpected severe toxicity; coadministration contraindicated

Carbamazepine / Possible ↓ sunitinib levels R/T ↑ metabolism by CYP3A4

Chloroquine / Prolongation of the QT interval with possible cardiac arrhythmias, including torsades de pointes; coadministration not advised

Clarithromycin / Possible ↑ sunitinib levels R/T inhibition of metabolism by CYP3A4 → ↑ risk of side effects, including ventricular arrhythmias (e.g., torsades de pointes)

Dasatinib / Prolongation of the QT interval with possible cardiac arrhythmias, including torsades de pointes; coadministration not advised

Dexamethasone / Possible ↓ sunitinib levels R/T ↑ metabolism by CYP3A4

Doxepin / Prolongation of the QT interval with possible cardiac arrhythmias, including torsades de pointes; coadministration not advised

Grapefruit / Possible ↑ sunitinib plasma levels

Haloperidol / Prolongation of the QT interval with possible cardiac arrhythmias, including torsades de pointes; coadministration not advised

Iloperidone / Prolongation of the QT interval with possible cardiac arrhythmias, including torsades de pointes; coadministration not advised

Indinavir / Possible ↑ sunitinib levels R/T inhibition of metabolism by CYP3A4 → ↑ risk of side effects, including ventricular arrhythmias (e.g., torsades de pointes)

Itraconazole / Possible ↑ sunitinib levels R/T inhibition of metabolism by CYP3A4 → ↑ risk of side effects, including ventricular arrhythmias (e.g., torsades de pointes)

Ketoconazole / Possible ↑ sunitinib levels R/T inhibition of metabolism by CYP3A4 → ↑ risk of side effects, including ventricular arrhythmias (e.g., torsades de pointes)

Lapatinib / Prolongation of the QT interval with possible cardiac arrhythmias, including torsades de pointes; coadministration not advised

Lithium / Prolongation of the QT interval with possible cardiac arrhythmias, including torsades de pointes; coadministration not advised

Maprotiline / Prolongation of the QT interval with possible cardiac arrhythmias, including torsades de pointes; coadministration not advised

Methadone / Prolongation of the QT interval with possible cardiac arrhythmias, including torsades de pointes; coadministration not advised

Modafinil / Possible ↓ sunitinib levels R/T ↑ metabolism by CYP3A4

Nefazodone / Possible ↑ sunitinib levels R/T inhibition of metabolism by CYP3A4→ ↑ risk of side effects, including ventricular arrhythmias (e.g., torsades de pointes)

Nelfinavir / Possible ↑ sunitinib levels R/T inhibition of metabolism by CYP3A4→ ↑ risk of side effects, including ventricular arrhythmias (e.g., torsades de pointes)

Nevirapine / Possible ↓ sunitinib levels R/T ↑ metabolism by CYP3A4

Paliperidone / Prolongation of the QT interval with possible cardiac arrhythmias, including torsades de pointes; coadministration not advised

Pazopanib / Prolongation of the QT interval with possible cardiac arrhythmias, including torsades de pointes; coadministration not advised

Phenobarbital / Possible ↓ sunitinib levels R/T ↑ metabolism by CYP3A4

Phenytoin / Possible ↓ sunitinib levels R/T ↑ metabolism by CYP3A4

Rifabutin, Rifampin, Rifapentine / Possible ↓ sunitinib levels R/T ↑ metabolism by CYP3A4

Ritonavir / Possible ↑ sunitinib levels R/T inhibition of metabolism by CYP3A4→ ↑ risk of side

T

effects, including ventricular arrhythmias (e.g., torsades de pointes)
Romidepsin / Prolongation of the QT interval with possible cardiac arrhythmias, including torsades de pointes; coadministration not advised
Saquinavir / Possible ↑ sunitinib levels R/T inhibition of metabolism by CYP3A4→ ↑ risk of side effects, including ventricular arrhythmias (e.g., torsades de pointes)
H ***St. John's wort*** / Possible ↓ sunitinib levels R/T ↑ metabolism by CYP3A4
Tacrolimus / Prolongation of the QT interval with possible cardiac arrhythmias, including torsades de pointes; coadministration not advised
Telithromycin / Possible ↑ sunitinib levels R/T inhibition of metabolism by CYP3A4 → ↑ risk of side effects, including ventricular arrhythmias (e.g., torsades de pointes)
Temsirolimus / Possible unexpected toxicity; use together with caution and monitor
Toremifine / Prolongation of the QT interval with possible cardiac arrhythmias, including torsades de pointes; coadministration not advised
Vandetanib / Prolongation of the QT interval with possible cardiac arrhythmias, including torsades de pointes; coadministration not advised
Voriconazole / Possible ↑ sunitinib levels R/T inhibition of metabolism by CYP3A4 → ↑ risk of side effects, including ventricular arrhythmias (e.g., torsades de pointes)

HOW SUPPLIED

Capsules: 12.5 mg (as base), 25 mg (as base), 50 mg (as base).

DOSAGE

CAPSULES

GI stromal tumor, advanced renal cell carcinoma.

Adults: One-50 mg capsule once daily on a schedule of 4 weeks on treatment followed by 2 weeks off. Dose increases or reductions of 12.5 mg increments are recommended based on individual safety and tolerability.

Advanced pancreatic neuroendocrine tumors.

Adults, usual: 37.5 mg once a day continuously without a scheduled off–treatment period; **maximum dose:** 50 mg/day. Dose interruption and/or dose modification in 12.5 mg increments or decrements is based on individual safety and tolerability.

NURSING IMPLICATIONS

IMPLEMENTATION/ADMINISTRATION/STORAGE

1. Sunitinib is a cytotoxic agent. Follow safe handling procedures when preparing, administering, or dispensing the drug.
2. Consider a dosage increase to a maximum of 87.5 mg/day (if treating GI stromal tumor or advanced renal cell carcinoma), or 62.5 mg/day (if treating advanced pancreatic neuroendocrine tumors) if the drug must be coadministered with a CYP3A4 inducer (see *Drug Interactions*). If dose increased, monitor carefully for toxicity.
3. Consider a dosage reduction of sunitinib to a minimum of 37.5 mg/day (if treating GI stromal tumor or advanced renal cell carcinoma), or 25 mg/day (if treating advanced pancreatic neuroendocrine tumors) if the drug must be coadministered with a strong CYP3A4 inhibitor (see *Drug Interactions*).
4. No adjustment in starting dose is required when given to clients with mild, moderate, or severe renal impairment, or in those with end-stage renal disease on hemodialysis.
5. Use the following guidelines for dosage adjustment for toxicity:
   - **CV:** If the ejection fraction decreases to 20 to 50% from baseline, without signs of heart failure, or if there is severe hypertension (SBP >200 mm Hg, DBP >110 mm Hg): Reduce dose or temporarily interrupt therapy; when symptoms resolve, resume therapy at reduced doses. If CHF occurs, discontinue therapy.
   - **GI:** If pancreatitis occurs, discontinue therapy.
   - **Hepatic:** If grade 3 or 4 hepatic toxicity occurs, interrupt dosage; discontinue therapy if there is no resolution. Do not restart sunitinib if clients subsequently experience changes in LFTs, or have other S&S of liver failure. If hepatic failure occurs, discontinue therapy.
   - **Hematologic:** If thrombotic microangiopathy occurs, suspend therapy; following resolution, treatment may be resumed.
   - **Neurologic:** If reversible posterior leukoencephalopathy occurs, temporarily suspend therapy. Following resolution, therapy may be resumed.
   - **Renal:** If a nephrotic syndrome occurs, discontinue therapy.

6. Store from 15-30°C (59-86°F).

ASSESSMENT

1. Note reasons for therapy, characteristics of S&S, other agents trialed/failed. Identify disease progression, or intolerance to imatinib with GI stromal tumor.
2. List drugs prescribed to ensure none interact.
3. Assess for active bleeding, history of heart problems (e.g., congestive heart failure, angina), blood vessel disease, bleeding problems, high blood pressure, adrenal gland problems, blood clot in the lung, or hypothyroidism, heart attack or stroke, or at risk for heart problems (ejection fraction <50%, prolonged QT interval), and avoid.
4. Identify if any severe infection, recently injured, or will be having surgery. With severe stress, monitor for adrenal insufficiency.
5. Check for elevated BP; treat with standard anti-hypertensive therapy. If severe hypertension occurs, stop therapy until BP controlled.
6. Monitor baseline: VS, ECG, BMP, TSH, CBC, phosphate, urine protein, renal and LFTs. Obtain LFTs (AST, ALT, and bilirubin) before starting therapy, during each cycle of treatment, and as clinically indicated. Hepatotoxicity has occurred and may be severe or fatal.

CLIENT/FAMILY TEACHING

1. May be taken with or without food. Eating grapefruit or drinking grapefruit juice may affect the amount of sunitinib in your blood.
2. Dizziness may occur; avoid activities that require mental alertness until drug effects realized.
3. Avoid OTC drugs (St. John's wort), and alcohol; may lessen cognitive functioning, and affect liver function. RUQ abdominal pain, abnormal yellow discoloration of skin/eyes should be reported; may result in fatal liver failure.
4. Drug may reduce number of clot-forming cells (platelets) in your blood. To prevent bleeding, avoid situations in which bruising or injury may occur. Report any unusual bleeding, bruising, blood in stools, or dark, tarry stools.
5. Avoid contact with people with colds or other infections. Report any signs of infection, including fever, sore throat, rash, or chills.
6. Skin or hair discoloration (yellow) may occur during therapy.
7. Practice reliable contraception; may cause fetal harm.
8. May experience diarrhea, N&V; report so meds can be ordered to offset. Fatigue, high blood pressure, mouth pain/irritation, and taste disturbance may also occur. Report blistering, pain, redness, or swelling of palms of hands or soles of feet. Rapid Wt gain, swelling of hands or feet, or unusual SOB should also be reported.
9. Keep all F/U to assess response, labs, heart/liver function tests, and for adverse SE.

OUTCOMES/EVALUATE

- Inhibition of malignant cell proliferation with GI stromal tumor
- Treatment of advanced renal cell carcinoma.

T

IV

Tacrolimus

(tah-**KROH**-lih-mus)

Classification(s): Immunosuppressant

Pregnancy Category: C

RX: Prograf, Protopic.

INDICATIONS/USES

Systemic (PO and Injection): Prophylaxis of organ rejection in allogeneic liver, heart, and kidney transplants; usually used with corticosteroids. In heart and kidney transplants, use in conjunction with azathioprine or mycophenolate mofetil. *Investigational:* Prevention and treatment of acute graft vs. host disease following hematopoietic stem cell transplantation. Also, rheumatoid arthritis, Crohn's disease, pyoderma gangrenosum.

Topical: Second-line therapy for short-term and intermittent long-term therapy to treat moderate to severe atopic dermatitis in nonimmunocompromised adults and children unable to take traditional agents or who do not respond to conventional therapy. *Investigational:* Vitiligo in children; facial, flexural, and intertriginous psoriasis.

T

ACTION/KINETICS

Action

Mechanism of action for either systemic or topical use is not known, but it inhibits T-lymphocyte activation by first binding to FKBP-12 (an intracellular protein). A complex of tacrolimus-FKBP-12, calcium, calmodulin, and calcineurin is formed, leading to inhibition of phosphatase activity of calcineurin. This effect prevents dephosphorylation and translocation of nuclear factor of activated T-cells (NF-AT), which is a nuclear component thought to initiate gene transcription to form lymphokines. Tacrolimus also inhibits transcription for genes that encode factors involved in the early states of T-cell activation. The net result is inhibition of T-lymphocyte activation (i.e., immunosuppression).

Pharmacokinetics

Absorption from the GI tract is variable; absorption is greatest under fasting conditions. Minimally absorbed after topical use. Absolute bioavailability ranges from 17–23%, depending on the organ transplant. **T_{max}** varies depending on whether used for heart (1.5–2.1 hr), kidney (1.5–3 hr), or liver (2.3 hr) transplants. **t½, terminal elimination:** 11.7 hr in liver transplant clients, 18.8 hr in kidney transplant clients, 23.6 hr in heart transplant clients, and 34 hr in healthy volunteers. The t½ is increased significantly in those with hepatic impairment. Food decreases both the absorption and bioavailability of tacrolimus. Extensively metabolized by the liver by CYP3A enzymes and excreted mainly through the feces (about 93%). **Plasma protein binding:** Approximately 99%.

CONTRAINDICATIONS

Hypersensitivity to tacrolimus or HCO-60 polyoxyl 60 hydrogenated castor oil (vehicle used for the injection). Concomitant use with cyclosporine. Use of the ointment in Netherton syndrome or other skin diseases where there is an increased potential for systemic absorption of tacrolimus. Use in children younger than 2 years of age. Use in children or adults with weakened or compromised immune systems. Lactation.

T

SPECIAL CONCERNS

■ (1) Increased susceptibility to infection and possible development of lymphoma may result from immunosuppression. Only health care providers experienced in immunosuppressive therapy and management of organ transplant clients should prescribe tacrolimus. Manage those receiving the drug in facilities equipped and staffed with adequate lab and supportive medical resources. The physician responsible for maintenance therapy should have complete information necessary for follow-up of the client. (2) Long-term safety of topical calcineurin inhibitors has not been determined. Although a causal relationship has not been established, rare cases of malignancy (i.e., skin cancer and lymphoma) have been reported in those treated with topical calcineurin inhibitors, including tacrolimus. Therefore, (a) avoid continuous long-term use of topical calcineurin inhibitors, including tacrolimus ointment, in any age group, and limit application to areas of involvement with atopic dermatitis; (b) tacrolimus ointment is not indicated for use in children younger than 2 years of age. Only tacrolimus 0.03% ointment is indicated for use in children 2–15 years of age. ■

- **Safety and efficacy of the ointment to treat infected atopic dermatitis not studied.**
- **With ointment, clients are predisposed to superficial skin infections, including eczema herpeticum, chickenpox or shingles, and herpes simplex virus infection.**
- **There is a potential cancer risk; thus, use tacrolimus only as indicated in clients who have failed treatment with other therapies.**
- **Should only be used for short periods of time, not continuously, as the long-term safety is not known.**
- **Safety and efficacy not established for concomitant use with sirolimus.**

SIDE EFFECTS

Most Common

After systemic use, liver transplants: Tremor, headache, diarrhea, hypertension, nausea, abnormal renal function, hyperglycemia, posttransplant diabetes mellitus.

After systemic use, kidney transplants: Infection, tremor, hypertension, abnormal renal function, constipation, diarrhea, headache, abdominal pain, insomnia, posttransplant diabetes mellitus.

After systemic use, heart transplants: Abnormal renal function, hypertension, CMV infection, tremor, hyperglycemia, leukopenia, infection, hyperlipemia, posttransplant diabetes mellitus. **After topical use:** Skin burning/erythema, flu-like symptoms, allergic reaction, headache, acne, folliculitis, rash, dysmenorrhea, peripheral edema, asthma, sinusitis, fever.

After Systemic Use. Listed are the more common and/or more serious side effects including when tacrolimus is used with steroids, cyclosporine, azathioprine, and others. **CNS**: Headache, tremor, insomnia, paresthesia, ***seizures***, ***coma***, delirium, abnormal dreams, anxiety, agitation, confusion, depression, dizziness, emotional lability, hallucinations, hypertonia, incoordination, myoclonus, nervousness, psychosis, somnolence, abnormal thinking, cerebral infection, hemiparesis, leukoencephalopathy, mental disorder, mutism, quadriplegia, speech disorder, syncope. **Neurotoxicity:** Changes in motor/sensory function, and mental status; tremor, headache. **GI:** Diarrhea, N&V, abdominal pain, constipation, anorexia, dyspepsia, dysphasia, flatulence, ***GI hemorrhage/perforation***, ileus, increased appetite, oral moniliasis, colitis, enterocolitis, gastroenteritis, GERD, impaired gastric emptying, mouth/stomach ulceration. **Hepatic:** Hepatitis, cholangitis, cholestatic jaundice, jaundice, liver damage, bile duct stenosis, abnormal LFTs, hepatic cytolysis, hepatotoxicity, fatty liver, venoocclusive liver disease, ***hemorrhagic pancreatitis, necrotizing pancreatitis, hepatic necrosis***. **CV:** Chest pain, abnormal ECG, ***hemorrhage, QT-interval prolongation, torsades de pointes***, hyper-/hypotension, tachycardia, myocardial hypertrophy, pericardial effusion, atrial fibrillation/flutter, cardiac arrhythmia, ***cardiac arrest***, ECG T-wave abnormality, MI, myocardial ischemia, pericardial effusion, deep limb venous thrombosis, ventricular extrasystoles, ***ventricular fibrillation***. **Hematologic:** Anemia, thrombocytopenia, leukocytosis, coagulation disorder, ecchymosis, hypochromic anemia, leukopenia, decreased prothrombin, disseminated intravascular coagulation, neutropenia, pancytopenia, thrombocytopenic purpura, thrombotic thrombocytopenic purpura. **GU:** Abnormal kidney function, nephrotoxicity, UTI, oliguria, hematuria, hemorrhagic cystitis, hemolytic uremic syndrome, micturition disorder, ***kidney failure (acute)***. **Metabolic:** Acidosis, alkalosis, posttransplant diabetes mellitus (insulin-dependent), glycosuria. **Respiratory:** Pleural effusion, atelectasis, dyspnea, asthma, bronchitis, increased cough, pulmonary edema, pharyngitis, pneumonia, lung/respiratory disorder, rhinitis, sinusitis, alteration in voice, acute respiratory distress syndrome, lung infiltration, ***respiratory distress/failure***. **Musculoskeletal:** Arthralgia, leg cramps, myalgia, myasthenia, osteoporosis, generalized spasm, carpal tunnel syndrome. **Dermatologic:** Pruritus, rash, alopecia, herpes simplex, sweating, skin disorder, hot flashes, ***Stevens-Johnson syndrome, toxic epidermal necrolysis***. **Ophthalmic:** Abnormal vision, amblyopia, blindness, cortical blindness. **Otic:** Hearing loss including deafness, tinnitus. **Body as a whole:** Hypersensitivity reactions (including anaphylaxis), increased incidence of malignancies, lymphoma, pain, fever, asthenia, ascites, abscess, chills, edema, photosensitivity, abnormal healing, decreased weight, photophobia, feeling hot and cold, feeling jittery, serious bacterial infections, opportunistic infections, *Candida* infection. **Miscellaneous:** Peripheral edema, back/abdominal pain, enlarged abdomen, hernia, peritonitis, lymphoproliferative disorder related to Epstein-Barr virus infection, latent viral infections, CMV infection, primary graft dysfunction, incision site complication, postprocedural pain, cushingoid features, ***multiorgan failure***.

After Topical Use. Dermatologic: Phototoxicity, herpes simplex, skin erythema/burning/infection, pruritus, eczema herpeticum, pustular/maculopapular/vesiculobullous rash, folliculitis, urticaria, fungal dermatitis, acne, alopecia, cellulitis, sunburn, skin disorder/tingling, dry skin, benign skin neoplasm, contact dermatitis, eczema, exfoliative dermatitis, varicella zoster/herpes zoster. **GI:** N&V, diarrhea, abdominal pain, gastroenteritis, dyspepsia. **Respiratory:** Increased cough, asthma, pharyngitis, rhinitis, sinusitis, bronchitis, pneumonia. **CNS:** Headache, insomnia, asthenia, depression, paresthesia. **GU:** Dysmenorreha, UTI, acute renal failure (rare). **Musculoskeletal:** Arthralgia, back pain, myalgia. **Miscellaneous:** Flu-like symptoms, allergic reaction, headache, fever, infection, accidental injury, otitis media, ear pain, alcohol intolerance, conjunctivitis, pain, herpes simplex, lymphadenopathy, facial/peripheral edema, hyperesthesia, asthenia, periodontal abscess, tooth disorder, cyst.

T

LABORATORY TEST CONSIDERATIONS

↑ Alkaline phosphatase, AST, ALT, serum urea nitrogen, creatinine, GGT. ↓ WBCs, platelets.

Hyper-/hypokalemia, hyperglycemia, hyperlipemia, hypomagnesemia, hypophosphatemia, hyperuricemia, hypocalcemia, hyper-/hypoproteinemia, hyponatremia, bilirubinemia, hypertriglyceridemia, hypercholesterolemia, hyperlipidemia. Abnormal LFTs.

DRUG INTERACTIONS

NOTE: (1) Tacrolimus is metabolized mainly by the CYP3A enzyme system; thus, substances known to inhibit these enzymes may decrease metabolism or increase bioavailability of tacrolimus as indicated by whole blood or plasma levels. Drugs known to induce these enzyme systems may cause an increased metabolism of tacrolimus or decreased bioavailability as indicated by whole blood or plasma levels. (2) It is possible for an additive effect of tacrolimus with other drugs that prolong the QT interval. The following drugs may prolong the QT interval and increase the risk of life-threatening cardiac arrhythmias, including torsades de pointes: Amiodarone, arsenic trioxide, bretylium, chlorpromazine, cisapride, disopyramide, dofetilide, dolasetron, droperidol, flecainide, lapatinib, mefloquine, mesoridazine, methadone, moxifloxacin, nilotinib, paliperidone, pentamidine, perflutren, pimozide, procainamide, propafenone, quinidine, quinupristin/dalfopristin, sotalol, tetrabenazine, thioridazine, ziprasidone.

Al-Mg hydroxide combinations / ↑ Tacrolimus AUC and ↓ C_{max}

Amiodarone / ↑ Tacrolimus plasma levels → ↑ risk of toxicity; consider lower tacrolimus doses and monitor plasma levels

Aminoglycosides / Additive or synergistic impairment of renal function

Amphotericin B / Additive or synergistic impairment of renal function

Antifungal drugs (clotrimazole, fluconazole, itraconazole, ketoconazole, voriconazole) / ↑ Tacrolimus levels → ↑ risk of toxicity

Atazanavir / Possible ↑ Tacrolimus levels → toxicity; reduce dose of tacrolimus

Bromocriptine / ↑ Tacrolimus levels → ↑ risk of toxicity

Calcium channel blockers (e.g., diltiazem, nicardipine, nifedipine, verapamil) / ↑ Tacrolimus levels → ↑ risk of toxicity

Carbamazepine / ↓ Tacrolimus levels → ↑ risk of organ transplant rejection

Caspofungin / ↓ Tacrolimus levels → ↑ risk of organ transplant rejection

Chloramphenicol / ↑ Tacrolimus levels → ↑ risk of toxicity

Cimetidine / ↑ Tacrolimus levels → ↑ risk of toxicity

Cisapride / ↑ Tacrolimus levels → ↑ risk of toxicity

Cisplatin / Additive or synergistic impairment of renal function

Clarithromycin / ↑ Tacrolimus levels → ↑ risk of toxicity

Cyclosporine / Additive or synergistic nephrotoxicity; also, ↑ tacrolimus blood levels; give the first tacrolimus dose no sooner than 24 hr after the last cyclosporine dose

Danazol / ↑ Tacrolimus levels → ↑ risk of toxicity

Diuretics, potassium-sparing / Tacrolimus causes hyperkalemia; avoid using potassium-sparing diuretics

H ***Echinacea*** / Do not give with tacrolimus

Erythromycin / ↑ Tacrolimus levels → ↑ risk of toxicity

Ethinyl estradiol / ↑ Tacrolimus levels → ↑ risk of toxicity

Fosphenytoin / ↓ Tacrolimus levels → ↑ risk of organ transplant rejection

Ganciclovir / Additive myelosuppression

Grapefruit juice / ↑ Tacrolimus trough levels in liver transplant clients; do not use together

HMG-CoA reductase inhibitors (e.g., lovastatin, simvastatin) / ↑ Plasma levels of tacrolimus and certain statins; fluvastatin and pravastatin may be less likely to interact and may be safer alternatives

Lansoprazole / ↑ Tacrolimus levels → ↑ risk of toxicity

Methylprednisolone / ↑ Tacrolimus levels → ↑ risk of toxicity

Metoclopramide / ↑ Tacrolimus levels → ↑ risk of toxicity

Metronidazole / ↑ Tacrolimus levels → ↑ risk of toxicity

Mycophenolate mofetil / ↑ Mycophenolate trough levels → ↑ risk of side effects

Nefazodone / ↑ Tacrolimus levels → ↑ risk of toxicity

Nelfinavir / ↑ Tacrolimus levels → ↑ risk of toxicity (probably due to ↓ liver metabolism); monitor in liver-transplant clients

Omeprazole / ↑ Tacrolimus levels → ↑ risk of toxicity

Phenobarbital / ↓ Tacrolimus levels → ↑ risk of organ transplant rejection

T

Phenytoin / ↓ Tacrolimus levels → ↑ risk of organ transplant rejection; also, ↑ phenytoin levels
Prednisone/Prednisolone / ↓ Tacrolimus levels → ↑ risk of organ transplant rejection
Protease inhibitors (e.g., ritonavir) / ↑ Tacrolimus levels → ↑ risk of toxicity
Rifamycins (rifabutin, rifampin) / ↓ Tacrolimus levels → ↑ risk of organ transplant rejection
H ***St. John's wort*** / ↓ Tacrolimus levels R/T induction of CYP3A4 and P-glycoprotein
Sildenafil / ↑ Sildenafil AUC, peak levels, and half-life
Sirolimus / ↓ Tacrolimus levels; do not use together; also, ↑ risk of wound healing complications, renal impairment, and insulin-dependent posttransplant diabetes mellitus in heart transplant clients
Sirolimus/Corticosteroids / Use of tacrolimus and sirolimus with corticosteroids → possible fatal cases of bronchial anastomotic dehiscence in lung transplant clients
Troleandomycin / ↑ Tacrolimus levels → ↑ risk of toxicity
Vaccines / ↓ Effectiveness of vaccines; avoid use of live vaccines
Valganciclovir / Additive myelosuppression
Ziprasidone / ↑ Risk of life-threatening cardiac arrhythmias, including torsades de pointes; do not use together

HOW SUPPLIED

Capsules: 0.5 mg, 1 mg, 5 mg; ***Injection Solution, Concentrate:*** 5 mg/mL; ***Ointment:*** 0.03%, 0.1%.

DOSAGE

CAPSULES

Heart transplantation.

Adults, initial: 0.075 mg/kg/day given q 12 hr in 2 divided doses. **Typical whole blood trough levels, month 1–3:** 10–20 ng/mL; **month 4 and beyond:** 5–15 ng/mL. If possible initiate therapy with tacrolimus capsules. If IV therapy is necessary, convert from IV to PO tacrolimus as soon as PO therapy can be tolerated (usually 2–3 days). Give the initial dose no sooner than 6 hr after transplantation. If using an IV infusion, the first PO dose should be given 8–12 hr after discontinuing the IV infusion. Base dosing on clinical assessment of rejection and tolerance. Lower doses may be sufficient as maintenance therapy. Adjunct therapy with corticosteroids is recommended early after transplantation. It is recommended that tacrolimus be used in conjunction with azathioprine or mycophenolate mofetil.

Kidney transplantation.

Adults, initial: 0.2 mg/kg/day (when used with azathioprine) given q 12 hr in 2 divided doses. When used with mycophenolate mofetil and an interleukin-2 receptor antagonist, use a dose of 0.1 mg/kg/day of tacrolimus. **Whole blood trough levels, if used with azathioprine, month 1–3:** 7–20 ng/mL; **month 4–12:** 5–15 ng/mL. **Whole blood trough levels, if used with mycophenolate mofetil and interleukin-2 receptor antagonist, months 1–12:** 4–11 ng/mL. The initial dose may be given within 24 hr of transplantation but should be delayed until renal function has recovered (i.e., serum creatinine less than or equal to 4 mg/dL). Black clients may require higher doses to achieve comparable blood levels. It is recommended that tacrolimus be used in conjunction with azathioprine or mycophenolate mofetil and interleukin-2 receptor antagonist.

Liver transplantation.

Adults, initial: 0.1–0.15 mg/kg/day given in 2 divided doses q 12 hr. **Children, initial:** 0.15–0.2 mg/kg/day given in 2 divided doses q 12 hr. **Whole blood trough levels, adults/children, months 1–12:** 5–20 ng/mL. If possible initiate therapy with tacrolimus capsules. If IV therapy is necessary, convert from IV to PO tacrolimus as soon as PO therapy can be tolerated (usually 2–3 days). Give the initial dose no sooner than 6 hr after transplantation. If using an IV infusion, the first PO dose should be given 8–12 hr after discontinuing the IV infusion. Lower doses may be sufficient for maintenance therapy. Adjunct therapy with corticosteroids is recommended early posttransplant.

Crohn disease (investigational).

Adults: 0.1 mg/kg twice a day; adjust dose to maintain serum levels of 10–20 ng/mL.

CONTINUOUS IV INFUSION

Heart, liver, kidney transplantation.

In those unable to take capsules, therapy may be initiated with the injection. Give the initial dose no sooner than 6 hr after transplantation; continue only until the client can tolerate PO administration. **Initial, adults, heart transplants:** 0.01 mg/kg/day; **initial, adults, kidney/liver transplants:** 0.03–0.05 mg/kg/day. For children, start at 0.03–0.05 mg/kg/day for liver transplants; dosage adjustments may be needed. Concomitant corticosteroid therapy is recommended early posttransplantation.

OINTMENT (0.03%, 0.1%)

Atopic dermatitis.

Adults: Apply a thin layer of either the 0.03% or 0.1% ointment to the affected skin areas twice a day. **Children, 2–15 years of age:** Apply a thin layer of only the 0.03% ointment to the affected skin areas twice a day. Stop when signs and symptoms of atopic dermatitis resolve. If signs and symptoms (e.g., itch, rash, redness) do not improve within 6 weeks, reassess to confirm the diagnosis of atopic dermatitis.

NURSING IMPLICATIONS

IMPLEMENTATION/ADMINISTRATION/STORAGE

1. An oral suspension may be compounded. For a 0.5 mg/mL PO suspension of tacrolimus, open six of the 5 mg capsules and pour out capsule contents. Combine into a paste with equal amounts of *Ora-Plus* and simple syrup. Then, further dilute with equal amounts of *Ora-Plus* and simple syrup for a final total volume of 60 mL. The PO suspension is stable for 56 days at room temperature in amber glass or plastic bottles.
2. The safety of using tacrolimus ointment with occlusive dressings has not been evaluated; thus, do not use with occlusive dressings.
3. Store capsules and ointment from 15–30°C (59–86°F).
4. IV IV therapy may be started if unable to take capsules. Continue IV therapy only until client can be switched to PO therapy (usually within 2–3 days). Give the first PO dose 8–12 hr after stopping the IV infusion.
5. Use the minimum amount of tacrolimus to control client symptoms; the risk of cancer increases with increased exposure to the drug.
6. For both IV and PO administration, give doses for adult clients at the lower end of the dosage range. Initiate doses for pediatric clients at the higher end of the dosage range (i.e., 0.03–0.05 mg/kg/day for IV use and 0.15–0.2 mg/kg/day for PO use).
7. Give the initial dose no sooner than 6 hr after implantation.
8. Children receiving liver transplants generally require higher doses of tacrolimus to maintain blood trough levels similar to those of adults.
9. Prior to use, dilute with either 0.9% NaCl or D5W to a concentration between 0.004 and 0.02 mg/mL. Where more dilute solutions are needed (e.g., children), polyvinyl chloride-free tubing should be used to minimize significant drug adsorption onto the tubing.
10. With renal or hepatic impairment administer at the lowest level of the dosage range.
11. Do not use tacrolimus and cyclosporine simultaneously unless specifically ordered; discontinue either agent at least 24 hr before initiating the other.
12. Store from 5–25°C (41–77°F). Store the diluted solution for infusion in glass or polyethylene containers and discard after 24 hr. Do not use PVC containers for storage due to decreased stability and the possibility of extraction of phthalates.
13. COMPATIBILITY 0.9% NaCl or D5W.
14. INCOMPATIBILITY Do not mix with solutions of pH 9 or greater (e.g., acyclovir, ganciclovir).

ASSESSMENT

1. Note reasons for use and form prescribed; assess clinical condition.

2. Identify time of transplantation; monitor in facilities equipped and staffed with adequate lab and supportive medical resources.
3. Injection contains castor oil derivatives; note any sensitivity.
4. Assess skin lesions with atopic dermatitis during therapy.
5. Monitor VS, I&O, tremors, or changes in mental and CV status. Anticipate higher dosages in children to maintain trough levels and reduced dosage with impaired renal function.
6. During IV therapy, observe continuously for the first 30 min and at frequent intervals until infusion completed; interrupt infusion if S&S of anaphylaxis occur.
7. Advise of risk of lymphoma and increased susceptibility to infection.
8. Note any combinations of headache, seizures, vision changes, HTN and altered mental status, S&S of PRES (posterior reversible encephalopathy syndrome). Maintain BP and confirm by CT/MRI.
9. Monitor serum electrolytes, CBC, uric acid, blood sugar, renal and LFTs. Obtain tacrolimus levels; helpful in clinical evaluation of rejection and toxicity.

CLIENT/FAMILY TEACHING

1. Review risk of therapy associated with neoplasia (lymphomas and other malignancies). Practice reliable contraception due to potential fetal risks.
2. Take capsules 30 min before or 2 hr after meals. May take with a full glass of water if GI upset; food diminishes effectiveness. Avoid grapefruit juice.
3. Must follow written guidelines for medication therapy explicitly. Call with questions or if problems arise. Drug must be taken throughout one's lifetime to prevent transplant rejection.
4. Because this drug is so important in preventing rejection, a written list of all possible side effects and how to identify which side effects need to be reported will be provided.
5. Perform daily weights and I&O. Take BP and keep a log of these values for provider review. Report any persistent diarrhea, N&V, and other adverse effects. May cause diabetes; monitor carefully.
6. Report as scheduled to specialist/transplant center for assessment and labs to evaluate drug effectiveness, since dosage is based on clinical assessments of rejection and tolerability.
7. Avoid crowds, infections, and those with infections. Report any S&S of infection or if injury occurs.
8. With skin disorders and topical application: wash hands, apply a thin film to cover involved areas only, rub ointment in gently and completely; report adverse effects. Do not use with occlusive dressings.
9. Avoid contact with eyes. Wash eyes with large amounts of cool water if contact occurs.
10. May experience burning sensations, stinging, soreness, or itching at the application site; report if persistent.
11. Stop therapy once S&S of dermatitis resolved. Avoid topical agents (e.g., medicated soaps, astringents, cosmetics) on treated skin.
12. Topical therapy may increase risk of shingles/chickenpox occurrence.
13. Limit exposure to sunlight and UV light due to the potential to increase risk of malignant skin changes.
14. Practice reliable contraception; report if pregnancy suspected.
15. Keep all F/U to assess response, dose, labs, and for adverse SE.

OUTCOMES/EVALUATE

- Prophylaxis of organ transplant rejection
- Improvement in atopic dermatitis presentation (topically)
- Median trough blood concentrations of 5–20 ng/mL

Tadalafil

(tah-**DA**-la-fil)

Classification(s): Drug for erectile dysfunction or pulmonary arterial hypertension

Pregnancy Category: B

RX: Adcirca, Cialis.

INDICATIONS/USES

Adcirca: Pulmonary arterial hypertension (WHO Group 1) to improve exercise ability. **Cialis:** Treat erectile dysfunction. *Investigational:* Raynaud's phenomenon.

ACTION/KINETICS

Action

During sexual stimulation, nitric oxide is released from nerve endings and endothelial cells in the corpus cavernosum of the penis. Nitric oxide activates the enzyme guanylate cylase, causing an increased synthesis of cyclic guanosine monophosphate (cGMP) in the smooth muscle cells of the corpus cavernosum. The cGMP in turn causes smooth muscle relaxation, allowing increased blood flow to the penis, resulting in erection. Tissue levels of cGMP are regulated by both the rate of synthesis and degradation via phosphodiesterases (PDEs). The most abundant PDE in the human corpus cavernosum is the cGMP-specific phosphodiesterase type 5 (PDE5). Thus, tadalafil, which is a selective inhibitor of PDE5, enhances erectile function by increasing the amount of cGMP.

Pharmacokinetics

Onset: About 30 min. **Maximum plasma levels:** 0.5–6 hr. **Duration:** 36 hr. Rate and extent of absorption are not affected by food. Predominantly metabolized by CYP3A4. **t½, terminal:** 17.5 hr. Excreted mainly as metabolites in the feces (61%) and urine (36%). **Plasma protein binding:** About 94%.

CONTRAINDICATIONS

Use in those with severe hepatic impairment. Use, either regularly or intermittently, in those taking any form of nitrates (due to potential for severe hypotension) or in those taking alpha-adrenergic blockers (except 0.4 mg daily of tamsulosin). Use in men for whom sexual activity is inadvisable due to their underlying CV status. Use in those with MI within the last 90 days, unstable angina or angina occurring during sexual intercourse, those with NYHA Class II or greater heart failure in the last 6 months, uncontrolled arrhythmias, hypotension, uncontrolled hypertension, those with a stroke within the last 6 months, and hereditary degenerative retinal disorders (including retinitis pigmentosa). Use in women or children. Lactation.

SPECIAL CONCERNS

Older clients or those with significant left ventricular outflow obstruction or severely impaired autonomic control of BP may be more sensitive to the drug. Use with caution in conditions that might predispose clients to priapism (e.g., such as sickle cell anemia, multiple myeloma, or leukemia) or anatomical deformation of the penis (e.g., angulation, cavernosal fibrosis, Peyronie's disease). Use in clients with bleeding disorders or significant active peptic ulcerations should be based on a careful risk to benefit assessment and caution. Safety and efficacy have not been determined in clients less than 18 years of age.

SIDE EFFECTS

Most Common

Headache, dyspepsia, nasal congestion, back pain, flushing, limb pain, myalgia, hypotension.

CV: Chest pain, hypotension, hypertension, ***angina pectoris***, ***MI***, palpitations, syncope, tachycardia. **GI:** Dyspepsia, diarrhea, dry mouth, dysphagia, esophagitis, gastroesophageal reflux, gastritis, loose stools, N&V, upper abdominal pain. **CNS:** Headache, dizziness, hypesthesia, insomnia, paresthesia, somnolence, vertigo. **Musculoskeletal:** Back pain, myalgia, arthralgia, neck pain, pain in limb. **Respiratory:** Nasal congestion, dyspnea, epistaxis, pharyngitis. **Dermatologic:** Flushing, pruritus, rash, sweating. **Ophthalmic:** Impaired blue/green color discrimination, blurred vision, conjunctivitis (including conjunctival hyperemia), eye pain, increased lacrimation, swelling of eyelids, sudden loss of vision, visual field defect, retinal vein occlusion, vision loss related to nonarteritic anterior ischemic optic neuropathy (especially in those with underlying anatomic or vascular risk factors). **GU:** Prolonged erections (more than 4 hr), priapism (greater than 6 hr), spontaneous penile erection. **Hypersensitivity:** Exfoliative dermatitis, ***Stevens-Johnson syndrome***, urticaria. **Body as a whole:** Asthenia, facial edema, fatigue, pain.

LABORATORY TEST CONSIDERATIONS

↑ GGTP. Abnormal LFTs.

DRUG INTERACTIONS

Alcohol / Possible ↓ BP with postural dizziness and orthostatic hypotension

Alpha-adrenergic blockers / Possible significant hypotension; do not use together

Amlodipine / ↑ Hypotensive effect

Angiotensin II receptor blockers / ↑ Hypotensive effect

Antacids, Mg- or calcium-containing / Possible ↓ rate of tadalafil absorption

T

Doxazosin / Significant ↓ BP
Enalapril / Mean ↓ of supine BP
Erythromycin / Possible ↑ tadalafil levels R/T ↓ hepatic metabolism
Grapefruit juice / Possible ↑ tadalafil levels R/T ↓ hepatic metabolism
Indinavir / ↑ Tadalafil levels R/T ↓ hepatic metabolism; possible severe (or even fatal) hypotension
Itraconazole / Possible ↑ tadalafil levels R/T ↓ hepatic metabolism
Ketoconazole / ↑ Tadalafil plasma levels R/T ↓ hepatic metabolism
Nitrates / Possible severe hypotension; **do not use together**
Rifampin / ↓ Tadalafil levels R/T ↑ hepatic metabolism
Ritonavir / ↑ Tadalafil levels R/T ↓ hepatic metabolism; possible severe (or even fatal) hypotension
Saquinavir / ↑ Tadalafil levels R/T ↓ hepatic metabolism; possible severe (or even fatal) hypotension

HOW SUPPLIED

Adcirca: *Tablets:* 20 mg.
Cialis: *Tablets:* 2.5 mg, 5 mg, 10 mg, 20 mg.

DOSAGE

Adcirca

TABLETS

Pulmonary arterial hypertension.

Adults: 40 mg (two 20-mg tablets) once a day. Dividing the dose over the course of the day is not recommended. For those with mild (C_{CR} 51–80 mL/min) or moderate (C_{CR} 31–50 mL/min) renal insufficiency, start with 20 mg once a day. Increase to 40 mg once a day based on tolerability. Avoid tadalafil in those with severe renal insufficiency (C_{CR} <30 mL/min) or those on hemodialysis due to increased exposure to the drug. Consider a starting dose of 20 mg once a day in those with mild or moderate (Child-Pugh class A or B) impaired hepatic function; avoid use in those with severe hepatic cirrhosis (Child-Pugh class C).

Cialis

TABLETS

Erectile dysfunction.

Adults, initial, as-needed use: 10 mg taken prior to anticipated sexual activity. Dose may be increased to 20 mg or decreased to 5 mg based on individual efficacy and tolerability. The maximum recommended dosing frequency is once per day for most clients. **Adults, once-daily use:** 2.5 mg taken at about the same time each day, without regard to timing of sexual activity; the dose may be increased to 5 mg once daily based on efficacy and tolerability. **Maximum dose:** 20 mg for as-needed use and 2.5 mg for once-daily use.

Renal/hepatic function impairment. Erectile dysfunction, as-needed use: No dosage adjustment is needed for those with mild (C_{CR} 51–80 mL/min) renal insufficiency; for those with moderate (C_{CR} 31–50 mL/min) renal insufficiency, use a starting dose of 5 mg, not more than once daily; limit the maximum dose to 10 mg not more than once q 48 hr. For those with severe renal insufficiency (C_{CR} <30 mL/min) and those on hemodialysis, the maximum recommended dose is 5 mg once q 72 hr. Do not exceed 10 mg once a day in those with mild or moderate (Child-Pugh class A or B) impaired hepatic function; use is not recommended in those with severe hepatic impairment (Child-Pugh class C).

Renal/hepatic function impairment. Erectile dysfunction, once-daily use: No dose adjustment is needed in those with mild or moderate renal insufficiency. For those with severe renal insufficiency and on hemodialysis, once-daily use is not recommended. Use with caution in those with mild or moderate impaired hepatic function; use is not recommended in those with severe hepatic impairment.

NURSING IMPLICATIONS

IMPLEMENTATION/ADMINISTRATION/STORAGE

1. Tadalafil improves erectile function up to 36 hr following dosing.
2. May be taken without regard to food.

T

3. Although clients 65 years and older may be more sensitive to the drug, no dosage adjustment is necessary.
4. Concomitant use of nitrates in any form is contraindicated. At least 48 hr should elapse between the last dose of tadalafil and beginning nitrate therapy.
5. **Adcirca:** In those receiving ritonavir for at least 1 week, start Adcirca at 20 mg once a day. Increase to 40 mg once a day based on tolerability. Avoid use of Adcirca during initiation of ritonavir. Stop Adcirca 24 hr before starting ritonavir. After at least 1 week following the initiation of ritonavir, resume Adcirca 20 mg once a day. Increase to 40 mg once a day based on tolerability.
6. **Cialis:** For as-needed use of Cialis, the dose should be limited to 10 mg no more than once every 72 hr in those taking potent inhibitors of CYP3A4 (i.e., itraconazole, ketoconazole, ritonavir). For once-daily use of Cialis, do not exceed 2.5 mg if taking potent CYP3A4 inhibitors.
7. **Cialis:** The client should be stable on an alpha-blocker prior to beginning Cialis; initiate Cialis at the lowest recommended dose whether taking Cialis for as-needed or once-daily use.
8. **Cialis:** Concomitant use of nitrates is contraindicated. In a life-threatening situation, at least 48 hr should elapse after the last dose of tadalafil (whether taking for as-needed or once-daily use) before nitrate use is considered.
9. Store from 15–30°C (59–86°F) and away from children.

ASSESSMENT

1. Note onset and characteristics of S&S; with erectile dysfunction, determine cause, i.e., organic, psychogenic, or combined, any contributing factors. With pulmonary arterial hypertension (PAH), note hemodynamic parameters, activity tolerance and list other agents trialed and outcome.
2. Assess cardiovascular status; obtain ECG. List drugs prescribed; some may potentiate drug effects.
3. Note conditions that may predispose client to priapism, i.e., multiple myelomas, sickle cell anemia, leukemia.
4. Assess for anatomical deformation of penis (Peyronie's disease, angulation, or cavernosal fibrosis).
5. Evaluate response to therapy, noting any changes in BP or heart rate, and hearing or vision loss.
6. Monitor testosterone initially with ED, exercise tolerance and pressures with PAH, renal and LFTs; reduce dose with dysfunction and if prescribed potent CYP3A4 inhibitors.

CLIENT/FAMILY TEACHING

1. Take as directed 30–60 min before anticipated act with ED and plan some form of sexual stimulation to ensure desired erection obtained. With pulmonary hypertension, take once daily with or without food.
2. May experience headache, flushing, stuffy nose, GI upset, back/limb pain or muscle pains, dizziness (from drop in BP) drowsiness, or abnormal vision; report any unusual (vision changes, hearing loss dizziness), persistent or bothersome effects. If chest pain experienced, seek medical care.
3. Report all medications currently prescribed to ensure none alter effects. Avoid OTC agents, alcohol in large amounts, and stop smoking; may inhibit drug effect. Allow at least 4 hr between alpha blocker (e.g., terazosin) use and avoid use of nitrates. Avoid using poppers (e.g., amyl nitrate, butyl nitrate) while taking this medication.
4. Practice safe sex; drug does not prevent disease transmission.
5. Effects may be evident the day after therapy; assess before taking additional drug dose. Do not use more than once a day. Erections lasting more than 4 hr or painful erections lasting more than 6 hr require immediate medical care; penile damage may result.
6. Do not share medications or prescriptions due to potential for adverse interactions and effects. *Never* use this drug if currently taking nitrates in any form; may cause significant drop in BP and increase the risk of heart attack or stroke.
7. Keep all F/U to assess response and for adverse SE.

OUTCOMES/EVALUATE

- Desired erection
- Improved activity tolerance with pulmonary hypertension

Tamoxifen citrate

(tah-**MOX**-ih-fen)

Classification(s): Antiestrogen

Pregnancy Category: D

RX: Soltamox.

✦ **Rx:** Apo-Tamox, Gen-Tamoxifen, Nolvadex-D, Tamofen.

SEE ALSO ***ANTINEOPLASTIC AGENTS***.

INDICATIONS/USES

(1) Adjuvant treatment of axillary node-negative or node-positive breast cancer in women following total or segmental mastectomy, axillary dissection, and breast irradiation. *NOTE:* The estrogen receptor and progesterone receptor values may help to predict whether adjuvant tamoxifen therapy is likely to be beneficial. (2) Metastatic breast cancer in premenopausal women as an alternative to oophorectomy or ovarian irradiation (especially in women with estrogen-positive tumors). (3) Reduce risk of invasive breast cancer following breast surgery and radiation in women with ductal carcinoma in situ. (4) Advanced metastatic breast cancer in men. (5) To reduce the incidence of breast cancer in high-risk women, taking into account age, previous breast biopsies, age at first live birth, number of first-degree relatives with breast cancer, age at first menstrual period, and a history of lobular carcinoma in situ. *NOTE:* See the package insert for examples of combinations of factors in various age groups predicting a 5-year risk greater than or equal to 1.67%. *Investigational:* Mastalgia, sympatomatic gynecomastia (to treat pain and size), malignant carcinoid tumor, and carcinoid syndrome. Migraine associated with menstruation, metastatic malignant melanoma, oligozoospermia, McCune-Albright syndrome in pediatric females (in combination with other drugs), metastatic melanoma, desmoid tumors. Stimulate ovulation in certain anovulatory women desiring pregnancy, especially those with amenorrhea or oligomenorrhea who previously took oral contraceptives.

ACTION/KINETICS

Action

Antiestrogen believed to compete with estrogen for estrogen-binding sites in target tissue (breast); also blocks uptake of estradiol.

Pharmacokinetics

The rate and extent of absorption of the oral solution is bioequivalent to that of the tablets under fasting conditions. **Steady-state plasma levels (after 10 mg twice a day for 3 months):** 120 ng/mL for tamoxifen and 336 ng/mL for N-desmethyltamoxifen (active metabolite). **Steady-state levels, tamoxifen:** About 4 weeks; **for N-desmethyltamoxifen:** About 8 weeks. **t½ for metabolite:** about 14 days. Tamoxifen is metabolized by CYP3A4, CYP2C9, and CYP2D6; tamoxifen and metabolites are excreted mainly through the feces. Objective response may be delayed 4–10 weeks with bone metastases.

CONTRAINDICATIONS

Lactation. Concomitant coumarin anticoagulant therapy or women with a history of deep vein thrombosis or pulmonary embolus.

SPECIAL CONCERNS

(1) Serious and life-threatening events associated with tamoxifen in the risk-reduction setting (women at high risk for cancer and women with ductal carcinoma in situ) include uterine malignancies, stroke, and pulmonary embolism. Incidence rates for these events were estimated from the National Surgical Adjuvant Breast and Bowel Project P-1 trial. Uterine malignancies consist of both endometrial adenocarcinoma (incidence rate per 1,000 women years of 2.2 for tamoxifen versus 0.71 for placebo) and uterine sarcoma (incidence rate per 1,000 women years of 0.17 for tamoxifen versus 0.4 for placebo). (2) For stroke, the incidence rate per 1,000 women years was 1.43 for tamoxifen versus 1 for placebo. For pulmonary embolism, the incidence rate per 1,000 women years was 0.75 for tamoxifen versus 0.25 for placebo. Some of the strokes, pulmonary embolisms, and uterine malignancies were fatal. (3) Discuss the potential benefits versus the potential risks of these serious events with women at high risk of breast cancer and with women with ductal carcinoma in situ considering tamoxifen to reduce their risks of developing breast cancer. (4) The benefits of tamoxifen outweigh its risks in women already diagnosed with breast cancer.

T

- **Use with caution in clients with leukopenia or thrombocytopenia.**
- **Women should not become pregnant while taking tamoxifen.**
- **Safety and efficacy not studied beyond 1 year of treatment in girls 2–10 years of age with McCune-Albright syndrome and precocious puberty.**

SIDE EFFECTS

Most Common

Flushing/hot flashes, altered/irregular menses, amenorrhea, vaginal discharge/bleeding, skin changes, fluid retention, mood changes.

GI: N&V, distaste for food, anorexia, diarrhea, abdominal cramps, constipation, pancreatitis. **CV:** Peripheral edema, flushing, superficial phlebitis, DVT, ***pulmonary embolism***, ***thromboembolic disorders*** (especially when tamoxifen is combined with other cytotoxic agents). **CNS:** Depression, dizziness, lightheadedness, headache, fatigue, mood changes. **Hepatic:** Rarely, fatty liver, cholestasis, hepatitis, liver cancer, ***hepatic necrosis***. **GU:** Hot flashes, vaginal bleeding/discharge, menstrual irregularities, amenorrhea, altered menses, oligomenorrhea, vaginal dryness, pruritus vulvae, ovarian cysts, hyperplasia of the uterus, polyps, endometrial cancer and uterine sarcoma. **Dermatologic:** Flushing/hot flashes, skin rash, skin changes, hair thinning or partial loss, alopecia. Rarely, erythema multiforme, ***Stevens-Johnson syndrome***, bullous pemphigoid. **Respiratory:** Coughing, throat irritation, interstitial pneumonitis (rare). **Musculoskeletal:** Bone pain, musculoskeletal pain. **Ophthalmic:** Corneal changes, cataracts, decrease in color vision perception, retinal vein thrombosis, retinopathy. **Hematologic:** Leukopenia, thrombocytopenia, neutropenia, pancytopenia, anemia. **Miscellaneous:** Hypercalcemia, edema, pain, hyperlipidemias, weight gain/loss, increased bone/tumor pain, fluid retention, allergy, hypersensitivity (including angioedema), infection/***sepsis***. In men, may be loss of libido and impotence after discontinuing therapy.

T

LABORATORY TEST CONSIDERATIONS

↑ Serum calcium (transient), thyroid-binding globulin and thyroxine in postmenopausal women, BUN, AST, alkaline phosphatase, bilirubin, creatinine, serum triglycerides. ↓ Platelet count in breast cancer clients. Hyperlipidemias (rare). In oligospermic men: ↑ LH, FSH, testosterone, estrogen.

DRUG INTERACTIONS

Aminoglutethimide / ↓ Tamoxifen and N-desmethyltamoxifen levels R/T ↑ metabolism by CYP3A4
Anticoagulants / ↑ Hypoprothrombinemic effect; carefully monitor PT
Bromocriptine / ↑ Serum tamoxifen and N-desmethyltamoxifen levels
Bupropion / ↓ Conversion of tamoxifen to the active endoxifen R/T inhibition of CYP2D6; use together contraindicated
Cytotoxic drugs / ↑ Risk of thromboembolic event
Fluoxetine / ↓ Conversion of tamoxifen to the active endoxifen R/T inhibition of CYP2D6; use together contraindicated
Letrozole / ↓ Plasma letrozole levels by 37%
Medroxyprogesterone / ↓ Plasma N-desmethyltamoxifen levels but not tamoxifen levels
Paroxetine / ↓ Conversion of tamoxifen to the active endoxifen R/T inhibition of CYP2D6; use together contraindicated
Rifamycins / ↓ Plasma tamoxifen levels R/T ↑ metabolism by CYP3A4; may need to ↑ dose

HOW SUPPLIED

Oral Solution: 10 mg/5 mL; ***Tablets:*** 10 mg, 20 mg.

DOSAGE

ORAL SOLUTION; TABLETS

Breast cancer.

10–20 mg twice a day (morning and evening) or 20 mg daily. If using the oral solution, give 10 mL for a 20 mg dose. Doses of 10 mg 2–3 times per day for 2 years and 10 mg twice a day for 5 or more years have been used. There is no evidence that doses greater than 20 mg daily are more effective.

Reduction in incidence of breast cancer in high-risk women.

20 mg/day for 5 years. There are no data to support use beyond 5 years.

Ductal carcinoma in situ.

20 mg/day for 5 years.

Mastalgia.

10 mg/day for 10 months.

NURSING IMPLICATIONS

IMPLEMENTATION/ADMINISTRATION/STORAGE

1. Initiate tamoxifen during menses in sexually active women of child-bearing age. In those with menstrual irregularities, a negative B-hCG just before starting therapy is sufficient.
2. If hypercalcemia occurs (may occur in breast cancer with bone metastases), take appropriate measures; if severe, discontinue tamoxifen.
3. Store tablets from 20–25°C (68–77°F) in a well-closed, light-resistant container. Do not store the oral solution above 25°C (77°F); store in the original container protected from light. Use within 3 months of opening; do not freeze or refrigerate the oral solution.

ASSESSMENT

1. Note onset, type, location, characteristics of S&S, surgery, biopsy results. List other therapies received. With increased pain, administer adequate analgesics and ensure adequate hydration.
2. Assess for history of thromboembolic events, may potentiate.
3. Document annual GYN exam. Review potential risks associated with therapy, including potential liver and other malignancy and eye changes.
4. The effect of the steroid and osteolytic metastases may result in hypercalcemia, which may require interruption of therapy. Monitor calcium level and report symptoms of hypercalcemia (insomnia, lethargy, anorexia, N&V, coma, and vascular collapse).
5. Monitor Ca^{++}, CBC, TFTs, and periodic LFTs, triglycerides and cholesterol levels. Drug may cause granulocyte suppression. Nadir: 14 days; recovery: 21 days.

CLIENT/FAMILY TEACHING

1. Review side effects that should be reported; a reduction in dosage or discontinuation may be indicated. Drug reduces incidence of breast cancer but may not eliminate risk.
2. Increased bone and lumbar pain or local disease flares should subside; take analgesics as needed and report if not responsive. Continue to have regular gynecologic exam to assess for any evidence of uterine cancer and regular mammograms.
3. Consume 2–3 L/day of fluids to minimize hypercalcemia. Exercise to reduce calcium levels, improve circulation, and prevent thrombophlebitis. (Perform ROM exercises if bedridden.) Record weights weekly; report excessive weight gain or evidence of extremity swelling.
4. May experience hot flashes; stay in cool environment. Wear protective clothing, sunscreens, and sunglasses to prevent photosensitivity reactions.
5. Obtain regular gynecologic exams; report menstrual irregularities, abnormal vaginal bleeding, change in discharge, or pelvic pain/pressure.
6. Practice safe, barrier or nonhormonal methods of contraception during and for 1 month following therapy; tamoxifen can induce ovulation.
7. Report headaches or decreased visual acuity; may be irreversible. Have regular eye exams, especially if higher than usual dosage.
8. Although the risk of breast cancer is significantly lowered, there is also an increased risk of endometrial cancer, pulmonary embolism, and DVT. Report any pain/swelling/tenderness of legs or calves, increased SOB, chest pain, mental confusion, or sleepiness to ensure no stroke or blood clot. Do NOT smoke.
9. Keep all F/U visits to assess response, labs and adverse SE.

OUTCOMES/EVALUATE

- Suppression of tumor growth and malignant cell proliferation
- Relief of breast pain
- Prophylaxis of breast cancer in high-risk women
- Ovulation, mastalgia, symptomatic gynecomastia, malignant carcinoid tumor (unlabeled use)

Tamsulosin hydrochloride

(tam-**SOO**-loh-sin)

Classification(s): Alpha-adrenergic blocking drug

Pregnancy Category: B

RX: Flomax.

✤ **Rx:** Novo-Tamsulosin, Sandoz Tamsulosin.

INDICATIONS/USES

Signs and symptoms of BPH. Rule out prostatic carcinoma before using tamsulosin. *Investigational:* Adjunctive therapy to manage ureteral stones.

ACTION/KINETICS

Action

Blockade of alpha-1-receptors (probably alpha-1a) in the prostate results in relaxation of smooth muscles in the bladder neck and prostate; thus, urine flow rate is improved and there is a decrease in symptoms of BPH.

Pharmacokinetics

Bioavailability is >90% when fasting; food interferes with the rate of absorption. **Peak levels:** 4–5 hr when fasting; 6–7 hr in fed state. Higher levels seen in the elderly. **t½, elimination:** 9–15 hr. Extensively metabolized in liver by CYP450 enzymes; excreted through urine (76%) and feces (21%). **Plasma protein binding:** 94–99%.

CONTRAINDICATIONS

Use to treat hypertension, with other alpha-adrenergic blocking agents, or in women or children.

SPECIAL CONCERNS

- **Use with caution with concurrent use of warfarin.**
- **Possible development of intraoperative floppy iris syndrome during phacoemulsification cataract surgery.**
- **Safety and efficacy not determined in children.**

SIDE EFFECTS

Most Common

Headache, dizziness, pharyngitis/rhinitis, infection, abnormal ejaculation, shoulder/neck/back/extremity pain, asthenia, diarrhea, chest pain.

CV: Marked hypotension (especially postural hypotension and syncope) with sudden loss of consciousness with the first few doses. Postural hypotension/hypotension, syncope, palpitations. **GI:** Diarrhea, nausea, tooth disorder, constipation, vomiting (rare). **CNS:** Dizziness, headache, vertigo, somnolence, insomnia. **Respiratory:** Rhinitis, pharyngitis, increased cough, sinusitis. **Musculoskeletal:** Chest pain, shoulder/neck/back/extremity pain. **GU:** Abnormal ejaculation, decreased libido, sexual dysfunction, priapism (rare). **Allergic reactions:** Skin rash, pruritus; angioedema of the tongue, lips, and face; urticaria. **Body as a whole:** Infection, asthenia. **Miscellaneous:** Amblyopia.

OVERDOSE MANAGEMENT

Symptoms: Hypotension. *Treatment:* Keep client in supine position to restore BP and normalize HR. If this is inadequate, consider IV fluids. Vasopressors may also be used; monitor renal function.

DRUG INTERACTIONS

Alcohol / ↑ Risk of hypotension; avoid alcohol use
Cimetidine / Significant ↓ in clearance of tamsulosin.

HOW SUPPLIED

Capsules: 0.4 mg.

DOSAGE

CAPSULES

Benign prostatic hypertrophy.

Adult males: 0.4 mg once daily given about 30 min after same meal each day. If, after 2 to 4 weeks, clients have not responded, dose can be increased to 0.8 mg daily.

NURSING IMPLICATIONS

Do not confuse Flomax with Fosamax (a bisphosphonate), Flonase (a corticosteroid), or Volmax (a sympathomimetic).

IMPLEMENTATION/ADMINISTRATION/STORAGE

1. **If dose is discontinued or interrupted for several days after either the 0.4 mg or 0.8 mg dose, start therapy again with 0.4 mg dose.**
2. **Store at 20–25°C (68–77°F).**

ASSESSMENT

1. **List reasons for therapy, onset, characteristics/frequency of symptoms. Note BPH score, prostate size, voiding diary.**
2. **Identify drugs prescribed to ensure none interact; especially cimetidine and coumadin.**
3. **Note PSA levels, family history of prostate cancer, results of digital rectal exam (DRE) to ensure no prostate cancer.**
4. **Obtain BP and monitor R/T syncope and orthostatic effects with first dose.**
5. **Monitor DRE, CBC, I&O, VS, weight, urodynamic studies.**

CLIENT/FAMILY TEACHING

1. **Take as directed, do not chew, crush, or open capsule. May take with a full glass of water,**

30 minutes after the same meal each day (to decrease GI upset). Report any loss of effectiveness or increased nighttime voiding.

2. Do not perform activities that require mental/physical alertness until drug effects realized; may cause dizziness, drowsiness, and syncope. Change positions slowly to prevent sudden drop in BP.
3. Stop fluid intake at least 4 hr before bedtime. Report if urinary S&S do not improve, or worsen.
4. Report any painful persistent erection lasting >4 hr.
5. Keep all F/U visits to evaluate response and adverse SE.

OUTCOMES/EVALUATE
Improvement in BPH symptoms; decreased nocturia

Tapentadol hydrochloride

(tah-**PEN**-tah-dol)

Classification(s): Narcotic analgesic.

Pregnancy Category: C

RX: Nucynta, Nucynta ER, **C-II**

SEE ALSO ***NARCOTIC ANALGESICS.***

INDICATIONS/USES
Relief of moderate to severe acute pain in adults, 18 years of age and older.

ACTION/KINETICS
Action
A centrally-acting narcotic analgesic thought to act through mu-opioid agonist activity and the inhibition of norepinephrine reuptake. Analgesia can be antagonized by selective mu-opioid antagonists (e.g., naloxone).

Pharmacokinetics
Mean absolute bioavailability: 32% due to extensive first-pass metabolism. **Maximum serum levels:** 1.25 hr. AUC and C_{max} are increased after a high-fat, high-calorie breakfast, although the drug can be given with or without food. Metabolized extensively in the liver, mainly by phase 2 conjugation but also by CYP2C9, CYP2C19, and CYP2D6. Unchanged drug and metabolites excreted in the urine. **t½:** 4 hr. **Plasma protein binding:** About 20%.

CONTRAINDICATIONS
Uses in severe hepatic or renal impairment. Use with significant respiratory depression or acute/severe bronchial asthma or hypercapnia in unmonitored settings or the absence of resuscitative equipment. Use in paralytic ileus or in those who are receiving MAOIs or who have taken them within the last 14 days (due to potential additive effects on norepinephrine levels, which may cause adverse CV effects). Use in those who may be susceptible to the effects of increased cerebrospinal fluid pressure (e.g., evidence of head injury and increased intracranial pressure). Use during and immediately prior to labor and delivery. Lactation.

SPECIAL CONCERNS
- **Has an abuse potential similar to hydromorphone. Can be abused and cause tolerance and dependence.**
- **Intracranial pressure may be markedly exaggerated in the presence of head injury or other intracranial lesions.**
- **Increased risk of respiratory depression in the elderly, debilitated, and in those suffering from hypoxia, hypercapnia, or upper airway obstruction.**
- **Use with caution in those with a history of seizures, with moderate hepatic impairment, or in biliary tract disease (including acute pancreatitis).**
- **Consider starting the elderly at a lower dose.**
- **Safety and efficacy not determined in children less than 18 years of age.**

SIDE EFFECTS
Most Common
N&V, dizziness, somnolence, constipation, pruritus.

CNS: Dizziness, somnolence, headache, tremor, lethargy, insomnia, confusion, abnormal dreams, anxiety, irritability, feeling drunk, hypoesthesia, paresthesia, disturbed attention, sedation, dysarthria, depressed level of consciousness, impaired memory, ataxia, presyncope, syncope, abnormal coordination, ***seizure***, euphoria, disorientation, restlessness, agitation, nervousness, abnormal thinking. **GI:** N&V, constipation, dry mouth, dyspepsia, abdominal discomfort, impaired gastric emptying. **CV:** Increased or decreased HR, decreased BP. **Respiratory:** Nasopharyngitis, URTI, decreased oxygen saturation, cough, dyspnea, res-

T

piratory depression (especially in the elderly). **GU:** UTI, urinary hesitation, pollakiuria. **Musculoskeletal:** Arthralgia, involuntary muscle contractions, sensation of heaviness. **Dermatologic:** Pruritus, hyperhidrosis, rash, hot flash, urticaria. **Ophthalmic:** Visual disturbance. **Body as a whole:** Fatigue, feeling hot, edema. **Miscellaneous:** Decreased appetite, drug withdrawal syndrome, hypersensitivity.

OVERDOSE MANAGEMENT

Symptoms: Symptoms are similar to other centrally-acting analgesics, including miosis, vomiting, CV collapse, varying degrees of CNS depression up to ***coma, seizures***, respiratory depression up to ***respiratory arrest***. *Treatment:* Re-establish a patent airway and institute assisted or controlled ventilation. Supportive treatment (oxygen, vasopressor) can be used to manage circulatory shock and pulmonary edema. Cardiac arrest or arrhythmias may require cardiac massage or defibrillation.

DRUG INTERACTIONS

CNS depressants (e.g., alcohol, analgesics, general anesthetics, phenothiazines, tranquilizers, sedatives, hypnotics) / Additive CNS depression → respiratory depression, hypotension, profound sedation, coma, death; if combined therapy is contemplated, reduce dose of one or both agents

MAOIs / Possible serotonin syndrome, including symptoms of agitation, hallucinations, coma, tachycardia, labile BP, hyperthermia, hyperreflexia, incoordination, N&V, diarrhea

Selective serotonin reuptake inhibitors / Possible serotonin syndrome, including symptoms of agitation, hallucinations, coma, tachycardia, labile BP, hyperthermia, hyperreflexia, incoordination, N&V, diarrhea

Tricyclic antidepressants / Possible serotonin syndrome, including symptoms of agitation, hallucinations, coma, tachycardia, labile BP, hyperthermia, hyperreflexia, incoordination, N&V, diarrhea

Triptans (e.g., sumatriptan, zolmitriptan) / Possible serotonin syndrome, including symptoms of agitation, hallucinations, coma, tachycardia, labile BP, hyperthermia, hyperreflexia, incoordination, N&V, diarrhea

HOW SUPPLIED

Tablets, Extended-Release: 50 mg, 100 mg, 150 mg, 200 mg, 250 mg; ***Tablets, Immediate-Release:*** 50 mg, 75 mg, 100 mg.

DOSAGE

TABLETS, IMMEDIATE-RELEASE

Analgesic.

Individualize according to severity of pain, previous experience with similar drugs, and ability to monitor the client.

Adults, 18 years and older: 50 mg, 75 mg, or 100 mg q 4–6 hr depending on pain severity. On the first day of dosing, the second dose may be given as soon as 1 hr after the first dose, if adequate pain relief is not reached with the first dose. Daily doses greater than 700 mg on the first day and 600 mg on subsequent days have not been studied and are not recommended.

TABLETS, EXTENDED-RELEASE

Analgesia.

Adults, initial: 50 mg twice a day; **then,** titrate to an effective and tolerable dose from 100–250 mg twice a day, up to a maximum of 500 mg a day.

NURSING IMPLICATIONS

IMPLEMENTATION/ADMINISTRATION/STORAGE

1. May be given with or without food.
2. No dosage adjustment is needed for mild or moderate renal impairment (drug not studied in severe renal impairment) or in mild hepatic impairment. For those with moderate hepatic impairment, initiate at 50 mg with the interval between doses no less than q 8 hr (i.e., maximum of 3 doses in 24 hr). Reflect further treatment to maintain analgesia with acceptable tolerability.

ASSESSMENT

1. Note type, location, onset, and characteristics of symptoms. Use a rating scale to rate pain levels.
2. Assess BP and for respiratory depression especially with asthma, COPD, and CNS depression. Note any evidence of head injury; precludes therapy.
3. List drugs prescribed to ensure none interact unfavorably. Note any seizure disorder or evidence of seizures and report.
4. Assess bowel function and ensure laxatives ordered as well as fluids and bulk added to diet.

T

5. Determine any evidence of mental status changes, changes in VS, coordination, or increased GI symptoms.
6. Monitor for tolerance and dependence. Check for any renal/liver dysfunction and adjust dosage.

CLIENT/FAMILY TEACHING

1. Use exactly as directed at the onset of pain and in the dose prescribed. May take with milk or food to ↓ GI upset.
2. Tapentadol ER must be swallowed whole and taken one at a time. The ER tablets may release all of their contents at once if split, broken, chewed, crushed, or dissolved, resulting in a risk of fatal overdose.
3. Do not pre-soak, lick, or otherwise wet the tablet prior to placing it in the mouth. Take each tablet with enough water to ensure complete swallowing immediately after placing it in the mouth.
4. Tapentadol ER tablets are intended for oral use only and must not be administered by any other route. If abused by parenteral route, may result in serious or even fatal complications.
5. Do not perform activities that require mental alertness or coordination. Change positions slowly to avoid dizziness.
6. Increase intake of fluids and fiber to offset constipating effects; use therapy as ordered.
7. Do not stop suddenly with long-term use; drug dependence occurs. Withdrawal symptoms may occur upon abrupt discontinuation; symptoms include anxiety, sweating, insomnia, rigors, pain, nausea, tremors, diarrhea, upper respiratory symptoms, piloerection, and, rarely, hallucinations. Stop therapy and report any evidence of seizures (drug may precipitate).
8. Avoid alcohol and any other CNS depressants without approval.
9. Report any unusual or intolerable side effects, difficulty breathing, or loss of pain control.
10. Practice reliable contraception; report if pregnant. Do not nurse while on therapy.
11. Store away from bedside to prevent accidental overdose.
12. Keep all F/U to assess response and for adverse SE.

OUTCOMES/EVALUATE

Control of pain

Telaprevir

(tel-**A**-pre-vir)

Classification(s): Antiviral drug, direct acting

Pregnancy Category: X

RX: Incivek.

INDICATIONS/USES

Treatment of genotype 1 chronic hepatitis C in combination with peginterferon alfa and ribavirin in adults with compensated liver disease, including cirrhosis, who are treatment-naive or who have previously been treated with interferon-based therapy, including null responders, partial responders, and relapsers.

ACTION/KINETICS

Action

Telaprevir is a direct-acting antiviral drug against the hepatitis C virus. It inhibits the serine protease necessary for the proteolytic cleavage of the HCV encoded polyprotein into mature forms of certain proteins that are essential for viral replication.

Pharmacokinetics

Absorbed from the small intestine. **C_{max}:** 4–5 hr. AUC increases significantly when telaprevir is taken with a standard fat meal. Extensively metabolized in the liver mainly by CYP3A4; non-CYP-mediated metabolism also plays a role after multiple telaprevir doses. Excreted mainly (92%) in the feces. **t½, elimination at steady state:** 9–11 hr.

CONTRAINDICATIONS

Use not recommended in those with decompensated liver disease or with moderate or severe hepatic impairment (Child-Pugh B or C, score of 7 or higher). Use in women who are pregnant; men whose female partners are pregnant. Coadministration with alfuzosin, cisapride, ergot derivatives (e.g., dihydroergotamine, ergonovine, ergotamine, methylergonovine), HMG-CoA reductase inhibitors (e.g., atorvastatin, lovastatin, simvastatin), midazolam (oral), pimozide, rifampin, sildenafil (Revatio when used to treat pulmonary hypertension), St. John's wort, tadalafil (Adcirca when used to treat pulmonary hypertension), or triazolam. Lactation.

T

SPECIAL CONCERNS

- **Systemic hormonal contraceptives may not be as effective in women while taking telaprevir.**
- **Safety and efficacy not established in children.**

SIDE EFFECTS

Most Common

Fatigue, rash, pruritus, N&V, diarrhea, anemia, dysgeusia, anorectal discomfort, hemorrhoids.

Side effects presented are for telaprevir combined with peginterferon alfa and ribavirin. **CNS:** Dysgeusia. **GI:** N&V, diarrhea, hemorrhoids, anorectal discomfort, anal pruritus, rectal burning. **Hepatic:** Hepatitis. **Dermatologic:** Rash (possible with eosinophilia), bullous rash, rash with vesicles/ulcers, pruritus, ***Stevens-Johnson syndrome.*** **GU:** Nephritis. **Hematologic:** Anemia. **Body as a whole:** Fatigue, fever. **Miscellaneous:** Facial edema.

LABORATORY TEST CONSIDERATIONS

↑ Bilirubin, uric acid. ↓ Hemoglobin, total WBCs, absolute neutrophils, absolute lymphocytes, mean platelets.

OVERDOSE MANAGEMENT

Symptoms: N&V, headache, diarrhea, decreased appetite, dysgeusia. *Treatment:* No specific antidote is available. Provide general supportive care, including monitoring of vital signs and observation of the client's clinical status. Also, remove unabsorbed drug from the GI tract, employing clinical monitoring (i.e., obtain an ECG).

DRUG INTERACTIONS

Alfuzosin / ↑ Alfuzosin plasma levels → ↑ risk for hypotension or cardiac arrhythmias; coadministration contraindicated

Antiarrhythmic drugs (e.g., amiodarone, bepridil, flecainide, systemic lidocaine, propafenone, quinidine) / ↑ Antiarrhythmic drug plasma levels → ↑ risk for serious and/or life-threatening side effects; use together with caution and monitor

Antidepressants (e.g., desipramine, trazodone) / ↑ Desipramine and trazodone plasma levels → ↑ risk of side effects (e.g., hypotension, syncope); use together with caution and consider a lower antidepressant dose

Atazanavir/Ritonavir / ↓ Telaprevir steady-state exposure; ↑ atazanavir steady-state exposure; monitor

Benzodiazepines (e.g., alprazolam, midazolam, triazolam) / ↑ Benzodiazepine levels → prolonged or increased sedation or respiratory depression; coadministration of oral midazolam and triazolam contraindicated

Bosentan / ↑ Bosentan concentrations; coadminister with caution and monitor

Calcium channel blockers (e.g., amlodipine, diltiazem, felodipine, nicardipine, nifedipine, nisoldipine, verapamil) / ↑ Calcium channel blocker concentrations; use together with caution

Carbamazepine / ↓ Telaprevir concentrations → ↓ virologic response; possible ↑ carbamazepine levels; coadminister with caution

Cisapride / ↑ Risk of cardiac arrhythmias; coadministration contraindicated

Clarithromycin / ↑ Plasma levels of both clarithromycin and telaprevir; possible QT interval prolongation and torsades de pointes; coadminister with caution

Colchicine / ↑ Colchicine plasma levels; those with hepatic or renal impairment should not receive colchicine and telaprevir; a reduction in colchicine dosage or an interruption in colchicine treatment recommended in those with normal hepatic or renal function (See ***Implementation/Administration/Storage***)

Corticosteroids, inhaled (e.g., budesonide, fluticasone) / ↑ Steroid levels; coadministration not recommended

Corticosteroids, systemic (e.g., dexamethasone) / ↓ Telaprevir levels → ↓ virologic response; possible ↑ steroid levels; coadministration not recommended

Cyclosporine / Marked ↑ cyclosporine plasma levels; closely monitor cyclosporine blood levels

Darunavir/Ritonavir / Steady-state exposure to both darunavir and telaprevir ↓ → ↓ virologic response; coadministration not recommended

Digoxin / ↑ Digoxin levels; start digoxin therapy with lowest dose; monitor digoxin serum levels

Efavirenz / Steady-state exposure to both efavirenz and telaprevir ↓ → ↓ virologic response; monitor

Ergot derivatives (e.g., dihydroergotamine, ergonovine, ergotamine, methylergonovine) / ↑ Risk of ergot toxicity (e.g., peripheral vasospasm or ischemia); coadministration contraindicated

Erythromycin / ↑ Plasma levels of both erythromcyin and telaprevir; possible QT interval prolongation and torsades de pointes; coadminister with caution

Escitalopram / ↑ Escitalopram concentrations; monitor and adjust escitalopram dose if necessary
Fosamprenavir/Ritonavir / Steady-state exposure to both fosamprenavir and telaprevir ↓ → ↓ virologic response; coadministration not recommended
HMG-CoA reductase inhibitors (e.g., atorvastatin, lovastatin, simvastatin) / ↑ Risk of myopathy, including rhabdomyolysis; coadministration contraindicated
Hormonal contraceptives (e.g., ethinyl estradiol, norethindrone) / ↓ Ethinyl estradiol exposure → ↓ efficacy; use two effective methods of nonhormonal contraception during telaprevir treatment; monitor those using estrogens as hormone replacement therapy for signs of estrogen deficiency
Itraconazole / Possible ↑ telaprevir concentrations; possible ↑ itraconazole plasma levels; do not give >200 mg itraconazole; coadminister with caution
Ketoconazole / Possible ↑ telaprevir concentrations; possible ↑ ketoconazole plasma levels; do not give >200 mg ketoconazole; possible QT prolongation; coadminister with caution
Lopinavir/Ritonavir / Steady-state exposure to telaprevir ↓ → ↓ virologic response; coadministration not recommended
Methadone / ↓ Methadone plasma levels; no dose adjustment needed when initiating telaprevir; monitor
Phenobarbital / ↓ Telaprevir concentrations → ↓ virologic response; ↑ or ↓ phenobarbital levels; coadminister with caution
Phenytoin / ↓ Telaprevir concentrations → ↓ virologic response; ↑ or ↓ phenytoin levels; coadminister with caution
Pimozide / ↑ Pimozide plasma levels → ↑ risk of serious and/or life-threatening side effects, including cardiac arrhythmias; coadministration contraindicated
Posaconazole / Possible ↑ telaprevir concentrations; possible ↑ posaconazole levels; possible QT interval prolongation and torsades de pointes; coadminister with caution
Rifamycins (e.g., rifabutin, rifampin) / ↓ Telaprevir plasma levels → ↓ virologic response; ↑ rifabutin levels; coadministration of rifabutin/telaprevir not recommended; coadministration of rifampin/telaprevir contraindicated
Salmeterol / ↑ Salmeterol concentrations → ↑ risk of CV side effects, including QT prolongation, palpitations, and sinus tachycardia; coadministration not recommended
Sildenafil / ↑ Risk for visual abnormalities, hypotension, prolonged erection, and syncope when used to treat pulmonary arterial hypertension; coadministration contraindicated; if used for erectile dysfunction, do not exceed a single dose of 25 mg in 48 hr
Sirolimus / ↑ Sirolimus blood levels; closely monitor sirolimus blood levels
St. John's wort / ↓ Telaprevir plasma levels → ↓ virologic response; coadministration contraindicated
Tacrolimus / Marked ↑ tacrolimus plasma levels; possible prolongation of QT interval; closely monitor tacrolimus blood levels
Tadalafil / ↑ Risk for visual abnormalities, hypotension, prolonged erection, and syncope when used to treat pulmonary arterial hypertension; do not exceed 10 mg single dose within 72 hr when used for erectile dysfunction
Telithromycin / ↑ Plasma levels of both telithromycin and telaprevir; possible QT interval prolongation; coadminister with caution
Tenofovir disoproxil fumarate / ↑ Tenofovir exposure; monitor; discontinue if tenofovir toxicity develops
Vardenafil / Possible QT interval prolongation; do not exceed a single dose of 2.5 mg within 72 hr when used for erectile dysfunction
Voriconazole / Possible ↑ telaprevir concentrations; either ↑ or ↓ voriconazole levels; possible QT interval prolongation and torsades de pointes; avoid coadministration
Warfarin / ↑ or ↓ Warfarin concentrations; monitor INR and adjust warfarin dose if needed
Zolpidem / ↓ Zolpidem plasma levels; monitor; zolpidem dose titration recommended

HOW SUPPLIED

Tablets: 375 mg.

DOSAGE

TABLETS

Chronic hepatitis C.

Adults, usual: 750 mg three times a day (7–9 hours apart) in combination with both peginterferon alfa and ribavirin. To prevent treatment failure, do not reduce the dose or interrupt telaprevir therapy. *NOTE:* Telaprevir must not be given as monotherapy and must be used with both peginterferon alfa and ribavirin.

NURSING IMPLICATIONS

IMPLEMENTATION/ADMINISTRATION/STORAGE

1. Do not start telaprevir combination treatment unless the female client has a negative pregnancy test immediately prior to initiation of treatment. Pregnancy testing should occur monthly during telaprevir combination treatment and for 6 months after all treatment has ended.
2. If peginterferon alfa or ribavirin is discontinued for any reason, telaprevir must also be discontinued.
3. If a dose is missed within 4 hr of the time it is usually taken, the prescribed dose should be taken as soon as possible. If more than 4 hr have passed since the dose is usually taken, the missed dose should not be taken; the client should resume the usual schedule.
4. Telaprevir must not be reduced or restarted if discontinued because of rash. Treatment of rash with oral antihistamines and/or topical corticosteroids may provide symptomatic relief but efficacy has not been determined. Treatment of rash with systemic corticosteroids is not recommended.
5. Use the following dosage recommendations if using colchicine and telaprevir: For treatment of gout flares, give colchicine 0.6 mg for 1 dose, followed by colchicine 0.3 mg 1 hr later. Do not repeat for 3 days. For prophylaxis of gout flares, reduce the colchicine dose to 0.3 mg daily if the original regimen was 0.6 mg colchicine twice a day. If the original regimen was 0.6 mg once a day, reduce the dose to colchicine 0.3 mg once every other day. To treat Mediterranean fever, the maximum colchicine dose should be 0.6 mg daily given once or 0.3 mg twice a day.
6. A ribavirin pregnancy registry has been established to monitor maternal-fetal outcomes of pregnancies in female clients and female partners of male clients exposed to ribavirin during treatment and for 6 months following cessation of treatment. Report such cases by calling 1-800-593-2214.
7. Store from 15–30°C (59–86°F). Once the bottle is open, use within 28 days.

ASSESSMENT

1. Note disease onset, genotype 1, if previously treated with interferon and ribavirin and failed therapy, or untreated with compensated liver disease.
2. List drugs prescribed to ensure none interact.
3. Confirm not pregnant and advise partners of males taking therapy use reliable contraception due to effects on fetus. Perform pregnancy test monthly and for 6 months following therapy.
4. Monitor VS, HCV-RNA levels and CBC regularly. Assess LFTs; avoid with decompensated liver disease or with moderate or severe hepatic impairment.

CLIENT/FAMILY TEACHING

1. Administer with food containing about 20 grams of fat (not low fat) within 30 min prior to each dose. Examples of foods that could be taken with telaprevir include the following: a bagel with cream cheese, ½ cup nuts, 3 Tbsp peanut butter, 1 cup ice cream, 2 oz American or cheddar cheese, 2 oz potato chips, or ½ cup trail mix.
2. Take with peginterferon alpha and ribavirin as directed; do not take alone. The recommended duration of treatment is 12 weeks in combination with peginterferon alfa and ribavirin. HCV-RNA levels will be monitored at weeks 4 and 12 to determine combination treatment duration and assess for treatment futility.
3. Telaprevir combination treatment may cause rash. The rash can be severe and may be accompanied by fever and skin breakdown. Report any skin changes or itching promptly to provider. Do not stop telaprevir because of rash unless instructed by provider because it may increase the possibility of treatment failure.
4. May experience fatigue, headaches, nausea, and taste changes; report if persistent or bothersome.
5. Review risks and S&S as anemia and neutropenia; may be increased when administered with peginterferon alfa and ribavirin.
6. Females must use two forms of contraception during and for 6 months following therapy if using nonhormonal form. Additionally will require a pregnancy test monthly during therapy and for 6 months following therapy. If pregnancy occurs, contact the Ribavirin Pregnancy

T

Registry by calling 1-800-593-2214 for tracking pregnancy outcome effects. Males receiving therapy must use reliable contraception as should female partners of childbearing age due to teratogenic fetal effects. Examples of nonhormonal methods of contraception include the following: a male condom with spermicidal jelly, female condom with spermicidal jelly (a combination of a male condom and a female condom is not suitable), a diaphragm with spermicidal jelly, a cervical cap with spermicidal jelly, or an intrauterine device (IUD).

7. Keep all F/U to assess response, for labs to determine continuation of therapy, and adverse SE.

OUTCOMES/EVALUATE

- Inhibition of HCV replication
- Significant reduction of HCV-RNA

Telbivudine

(tel-**BIV**-yoo-deen)

Classification(s): Antiviral drug, nucleoside reverse transcriptase inhibitor

Pregnancy Category: B

RX: Tyzeka.

INDICATIONS/USES

Treatment of chronic hepatitis B in adults with evidence of viral replication and either evidence of persistent elevations in serum ALT or AST or histologically active disease.

ACTION/KINETICS

Action

Telbivudine is phosphorylated by cellular kinases to the active telbivudine triphosphate. The triphosphate inhibits hepatitis B virus DNA polymerase (reverse transcriptase) by competing with the natural substrate, thymidine 5-triphosphate. Incorporation of telbivudine 5-triphosphate into viral DNA causes DNA chain termination, resulting in inhibition of hepatitis B viral replication.

Pharmacokinetics

Steady-state peak plasma levels: 1–4 hr. **Steady state:** About 5–7 days. Absorption not affected by food. **t½, intracellular:** About 14 hr. Food does not affect absorption. **t½, terminal:** 40–49 hr. Eliminated primarily by renal excretion of unchanged drug. Cross-resistance has been observed among hepatitis B nucleoside analogs. Hemodialysis (up to 4 hr) reduces systemic telbivudine exposure by about 23%. **Plasma protein binding:** About 3.3%.

CONTRAINDICATIONS

Hypersensitivity to telbivudine or any component of the product. Lactation.

SPECIAL CONCERNS

(1) Lactic acidosis and severe hepatomegaly with steatosis, including fatal cases, have been reported with the use of nucleoside analogs alone or in combination with antiretrovirals. (2) Severe acute exacerbations of hepatitis B have been reported in clients who have discontinued anti-hepatitis B therapy, including telbivudine. Closely monitor hepatic function with clinical and laboratory follow-up for at least several months in clients who discontinue anti-hepatitis B therapy. If appropriate, resumption of antihepatitis B therapy may be warranted.

- Exacerbations of hepatitis B are possible in those who have discontinued anti-hepatitis B therapy.
- Use caution with dose selection in the elderly.
- Safety and efficacy not determined in liver transplant recipients.
- Safety and efficacy not determined in children.

SIDE EFFECTS

Most Common

URTI, abdominal pain, fatigue, malaise, headache, nasopharyngitis, cough, diarrhea/loose stools, flu/flu-like symptoms, N&V, post-procedural pain.

CNS: Fatigue, malaise, headache, dizziness, insomnia, hypesthesia, paresthesia. **GI:** Abdominal distention/pain (including upper pain), diarrhea/loose stools, gastritis, N&V, dyspepsia, exacerbation of hepatitis. **Musculoskeletal:** Fibromyalgia, arthralgia, back pain, myalgia, myopathy, myositis, muscle cramps, musculoskeletal chest pain, pain in extremity, tenderness, rhabdomyolysis. **Respiratory:** Cough, URTI, nasopharyngitis, pharyngolaryngeal pain. **Hematologic:** Neutropenia, thrombocytopenia. **Dermatologic:** Rash, pruritus. **Body as a whole:** Flu and flu-like symp-

T

toms, pyrexia, pain, peripheral neuropathy. **Miscellaneous:** Post-procedural pain, exacerbation of hepatitis B, ***lactic acidosis and severe hepatomegaly with steatosis.***

LABORATORY TEST CONSIDERATIONS

↑ CPK, creatine kinase, ALT (including ALT flares), AST, lipase, amylase, total bilirubin.

DRUG INTERACTIONS

Drugs that alter renal function / Alteration of telbivudine plasma levels R/T telbivudine excretion mainly by the kidney

Pegylated interferon alfa-2a / ↑ Risk of peripheral neuropathy occurrence and severity

HOW SUPPLIED

Oral Solution: 100 mg/5 mL; *Tablets:* 600 mg.

DOSAGE

ORAL SOLUTION; TABLETS

Chronic hepatitis B.

Adults and children, 16 years and older: 600 mg once daily, with or without food. Adjustment of dosage, as follows, is necessary in those with impaired renal function: **C_{CR} 30–49 mL/min:** 600 mg tablet once every 48 hr or 20 mL (200 mg) of the solution per day; **C_{CR} <30 mL/min, not requiring dialysis:** 600 mg tablet q 72 hr or 10 mL (100 mg) of the solution per day; **end-stage renal disease on hemodialysis:** 600 mg once q 96 hr. Administer telbivudine after hemodialysis.

NURSING IMPLICATIONS

IMPLEMENTATION/ADMINISTRATION/STORAGE

1. Optimal treatment duration not established.
2. To monitor fetal outcomes of pregnant women exposed to telbivudine, health care providers should register such clients in the antiretroviral pregnancy registry by calling 1-800-258-4263.
3. Store from 15–30°C (59–86°F). Use PO solution within 2 months after opening the bottle. Do not freeze.

ASSESSMENT

1. Note reasons for therapy, disease onset, contact, other agents trialed, outcome.
2. Note liver biopsy date/findings and disease stage.
3. List drugs prescribed to ensure none interact.
4. Assess for S&S of unexplained muscle pain, tenderness, or weakness.
5. If client stops anti-hepatitis B therapy, continue to monitor LFTs for at least several months.
6. Monitor VS, renal and LFTs; reduce dose with dysfunction. Assess for Hep A, lactic acidosis, and monitor renal function in the elderly and those taking drugs that may alter renal function.

CLIENT/FAMILY TEACHING

1. Take as directed with or without food to control progression of HBV. Check and review medication guide with each fill.
2. Practice reliable contraception; drug does not reduce risk of transmission of HBV to others through blood contamination or sexual contact.
3. May experience muscle aches/pain, fatigue, fever, abdominal pain, diarrhea, headaches; report if persistent and if unexplained muscle weakness, pain, burning sensations, or numbness/tingling in extremities is experienced.
4. Do not stop drug suddenly, may cause exacerbation of HBV. Deterioration of liver disease may occur in some cases if treatment discontinued.
5. For those on a low-sodium diet, telbivudine solution contains approximately 47 mg of sodium per 600 mg (30 mL) dose.
6. Keep all F/U to assess response, labs, and for adverse SE.

OUTCOMES/EVALUATE

- ↓ HBV viral load
- ↑ Virological suppression

Telithromycin

(tel-ith-roe-**MYE**-sin)

Classification(s): Antibiotic, ketolide

Pregnancy Category: C

RX: Ketek.

SEE ALSO ***ANTI-INFECTIVE DRUGS.***

T

INDICATIONS/USES

Mild to moderate community acquired pneumonia due to *S. pneumoniae* (including multidrug resistant *S. pneumoniae* isolates, including isolates known as penicillin-resistant *S. pneumoniae* and isolates resistant to two or more of the following: penicillin, second-generation cephalosporins, macrolides, tetracyclines, and trimethoprim/sulfamethoxazole), *H. influenzae, M. catarrhalis, Chlamydophila pneumoniae,* or *Mycoplasma pneumoniae.*

ACTION/KINETICS

Action

A ketolide antibiotic structurally related to the macrolide family of antibiotics. Telithromycin blocks protein synthesis by binding to domains II and V of 23S rRNA of the 50S ribosomal subunit. By binding at domain II, the drug retains activity against gram-positive cocci in the presence of resistance caused by methylases that alter the domain V binding site of telithromycin. May also inhibit the assembly of nascent ribosomal units.

Pharmacokinetics

Maximum plasma levels: About 1 hr. Absolute bioavailability of 57%. Rate and extent of absorption not affected by food. **t½, terminal:** 9.8 hr (after multiple doses). About 50% metabolized in the liver by CYP3A4 and 50% of metabolism is CYP450-independent. Excreted in the feces and urine. **Plasma protein binding:** About 60–70% (mainly albumin).

CONTRAINDICATIONS

History of hypersensitivity to telithromycin and/or any components of the product or any macrolide antibiotic. Coadministration with cisapride or pimozide. Use with congenital prolongation of the QTc interval, in those with uncorrected hypokalemia or hypomagnesemia, clinically significant bradycardia, and in those receiving Class IA (quinidine and procainamide) or Class III (dofetilide) antiarrhythmics. Use to treat less serious bacterial infections, such as bronchitis and sinusitis. Use in myasthenia gravis, previous history of hepatitis and/or jaundice associated with the use of telithromycin or any macrolide antibiotic.

SPECIAL CONCERNS

Telithromycin is contraindicated in clients with myasthenia gravis. There have been reports of fatal and life-threatening respiratory failure in clients with myasthenia gravis associated with the use of telithromycin.

- **Due to potential severe liver problems, use of the drug is restricted to treating pneumonia.**
- **The elderly may be more sensitive to the drug.**
- **Use with caution during lactation.**
- **Safety and efficacy not determined in children.**

SIDE EFFECTS

Most Common

Diarrhea, N&V, dizziness, headache, dysgeusia, loose stools.

GI: Diarrhea, N&V, dysgeusia, loose/watery stools, abdominal distention/pain, anorexia, constipation, dyspepsia, flatulence, gastritis, gastroenteritis, GI upset, glossitis, oral candidiasis, stomatitis, upper abdominal pain, dry mouth, pseudomembranous colitis, *Clostridium difficile*-associated diarrhea, pancreatitis. **Hepatic:** Hepatitis with or without jaundice, hepatic dysfunction including increased liver enzymes, hepatocellular and/or cholestatic hepatitis with or without jaundice, ***fatal liver toxicity***. **CNS:** Dizziness, headache, insomnia, anxiety, somnolence, vertigo, paresthesia, loss of consciousness. **CV:** Bradycardia, hypotension, atrial arrhythmias, prolongation of QTc interval (may lead to ventricular arrhythmias), palpitations. **Dermatologic:** Rash, increased sweating, eczema, erythema multiforme, flushing, pruritus, urticaria. **Hypersensitivity:** Facial edema, ***angioedema, anaphylaxis***. **Musculoskeletal:** Muscle cramps, exacerbation of myasthenia gravis (rare). **GU:** Vaginal candidiasis, vaginitis, fungal vaginosis. **Ophthalmic:** Blurred vision, diplopia, difficulty focusing. **Body as a whole:** Fatigue.

LABORATORY TEST CONSIDERATIONS

↑ AST, ALT, blood alkaline phosphatase, eosinophil count, platelets, blood bilirubin.

DRUG INTERACTIONS

Antiarrhythmic drugs (amiodarone, bretylium, disopyramide, dofetilide, procainamide, quinidine, sotalol) / ↑ Risk of life-threating cardiac arrhythmias, including torsades de pointes; do not use telithromycin with class 1A and class III antiarrhythmics

Buspirone / ↑ Telithromycin plasma levels → ↑ pharmacologic and toxicologic effects

Cabergoline / ↑ Telithromycin plasma levels → ↑ pharmacologic and toxicologic effects

Carbamazepine / ↓ Telithromycin C_{max} and AUC → subtherapeutic levels R/T induction of CYP3A4 metabolism; ↑ or prolongation of the therapeutic and/or side effects of carbamazepine
Cisapride / ↑ Cisapride plasma levels → significant ↑ in the QTc interval; do not use together
Colchicine / ↑ Colchicine levels (possible toxicity) R/T inhibition of CYP3A4
Cyclosporine / ↑ Cyclosporine serum levels → ↑ or prolongation of therapeutic and/or side effects
Digoxin / ↑ Digoxin peak and trough levels by 73% and 21% respectively; monitor digoxin levels
Ergot alkaloids / Possible severe peripheral vasospasm and dysesthesia; do not use together
Hexobarbital / ↑ Hexobarbital serum levels → ↑ or prolongation of therapeutic and/or side effects
HMG-CoA Reductase Inhibitors (atorvastatin, lovastatin, simvastatin) / ↑ C_{max} and AUC of HMG-CoA reductase inhibitors; do not use together
Itraconazole / ↑ Telithromycin C_{max} and AUC by 22% and 54% respectively
Ketoconazole / ↑ Telithromycin C_{max} and AUC by 51% and 95% respectively
Metoprolol / ↑ Metoprolol C_{max} and AUC by 38%; use together with caution
Midazolam / ↑ Midazolam AUC R/T inhibition of metabolism by CYP3A4
Oral contraceptives containing ethinyl estradiol/levonorgestrel / ↑ Levonorgestrel steady state AUC by 50%
Phenobarbital / ↓ Telithromycin C_{max} and AUC → subtherapeutic levels R/T induction of CYP3A4 metabolism
Phenytoin / ↓ Telithromycin C_{max} and AUC → subtherapeutic levels R/T induction of CYP3A4 metabolism; ↑ or prolongation of the therapeutic and/or side effects of phenytoin
Pimozide / ↑ Pimozide plasma levels; do not use together
Ranolazine / ↑ Telithromycin plasma levels → ↑ pharmacologic and toxicologic effects
Repaglinide / ↑ Telithromycin plasma levels → ↑ pharmacologic and toxicologic effects
Rifampin / ↓ Telithromycin C_{max} and AUC by 79% and 86% respectively → subtherapeutic levels; do not use together
Sirolimus / ↑ Sirolimus serum levels → ↑ or prolongation of therapeutic and/or side effects
Sotalol / ↑ Risk of life-threating cardiac arrhythmias, including torsades de pointes; do not use telithromycin with Class 1A and Class III antiarrhythmics; also, ↓ sotalol C_{max} and AUC by 35% and 20% respectively
Tacrolimus / ↑ Tacrolimus serum levels → ↑ or prolongation of therapeutic and/or side effects
Theophylline / ↑ Theophylline C_{max} and AUC → worsening of N&V; give 1 hr apart
Triazolam / Possible ↑ triazolam levels R/T inhibition of metabolism by CYP3A4
Verapamil / ↑ Risk of cardiotoxicity; monitor closely
Warfarin / ↑ Warfarin anticoagulant effect; hemorrhage has occurred; monitor PT and INR

HOW SUPPLIED

Tablets: 300 mg 400 mg.

DOSAGE

TABLETS

Community-acquired pneumonia.

Adults and adolescents over 18 years of age: 800 mg (2 × 400 mg) once daily for 7–10 days without regard to food. In the presence of severe renal failure (e.g., C_{CR} <30 mL/min), including those who need dialysis, reduce the dose to 600 mg once daily. In those undergoing hemodialysis, give after the dialysis sesson on dialysis days. In the presence of severe impaired renal function with coexisting impaired hepatic function, reduce the dose to 400 mg once a day.

NURSING IMPLICATIONS

IMPLEMENTATION/ADMINISTRATION/STORAGE

Store at 25°C (77°F); limited time storage permitted at 15–30°C (59–86°F) for excursions.

ASSESSMENT

1. Note reasons for therapy, S&S of infections, culture results. List drugs prescribed to ensure none interact. Avoid use with Class 1A (i.e., quinidine, procainamide) or Class III (i.e., dofetilide) antiarrhythmics. Stop statins (simvastatin, lovastatin, and atorvastatin) during the course of treatment.
2. Check ECG for any QT prolongation; precludes drug therapy.
3. Assess for any history/evidence of myasthenia gravis (fatal and life-threatening respiratory failure has occurred), family history of QT pro-

T

longation or arrhythmias, clinically significant bradycardia, or hypokalemia.

4. This drug belongs to a new class of antibiotics called ketolides, and is structurally similar to the macrolides. Has caused fatal liver failure in some clients; monitor carefully for S&S of hepatitis (anorexia, fatigue, jaundice, malaise, or nausea).
5. Monitor VS, ECG, electrolytes, renal and LFTs; assess for dysfunction and report.

CLIENT/FAMILY TEACHING

1. Drug is used to treat pneumonia, and should not be used to treat less serious bacterial infections, or be used with viral conditions. Take as directed with or without food. Complete entire prescription even if feeling better, to prevent drug-resistant organisms.
2. If visual difficulties are experienced (blurred/double vision, difficulty focusing) during therapy, avoid driving a motor vehicle, operating dangerous equipment, or performing hazardous activities; avoid quick changes to view distant and close objects to minimize these effects. Usually noted with first or second doses, but may recur. Report if persistent or interferes with daily activities.
3. Drug may cause ECG changes; stop drug and report fainting/dizziness or loss of consciousness, right upper quadrant abdominal pain, yellow discoloration of skin or eyes during therapy.
4. Keep all F/U to assess response, labs, and for adverse SE.

OUTCOMES/EVALUATE

Resolution of pneumonia

Telmisartan

(**tell**-mih-**SAR**-tan)

Classification(s): Antihypertensive, angiotensin II receptor blocker

Pregnancy Category: C (first trimester); **D** (second and third trimesters)

RX: Micardis.

SEE ALSO ***ANGIOTENSIN II RECEPTOR ANTAGONISTS*** AND ***ANTIHYPERTENSIVES***.

INDICATIONS/USES

(1) Hypertension alone or in combination with other antihypertensives. (2) Reduce the risk of MI, stroke, or death from CV causes in clients 55 years of age and older at high risk of developing major CV events who are unable to take angiotensin-converting enzyme inhibitors.

ACTION/KINETICS

Pharmacokinetics

Control of BP in blacks is less than in whites. Is from 42–58% bioavailable (depending on dose). **Time to maximum levels:** 30–60 min. **t½, terminal:** About 24 hr. Excreted mainly in the feces by way of the bile. **Plasma protein binding:** Over 99.5%.

CONTRAINDICATIONS

Concomitant use with an ACE inhibitor.

SPECIAL CONCERNS

■ **Use in pregnancy.** When used in pregnancy, drugs that act directly on the renin-angiotensin system can cause injury and even death to the developing fetus. When pregnancy is detected, discontinue telmisartan as soon as possible. ■

- Use with caution in impaired hepatic function or in biliary obstructive disorders.
- Clients on dialysis may develop orthostatic hypotension.

SIDE EFFECTS

Most Common

URTI, diarrhea, pain, sinusitis, dizziness, fatigue, N&V, abdominal pain, myalgia, cough, pharyngitis, UTI, flu-like symptoms.

GI: Diarrhea, dyspepsia, heartburn, N&V, abdominal pain. **CNS:** Dizziness, headache, fatigue, anxiety, nervousness, insomnia. **Musculoskeletal:** Pain, including back/neck pain; myalgia, arthralgia. **Respiratory:** URTI, sinusitis, cough, rhinitis, pharyngitis, influenza, bronchitis. **Miscellaneous:** Chest pain, UTI, peripheral edema, rash, tachycardia, hypertension, flu-like symptoms.

LABORATORY TEST CONSIDERATIONS

↑ Creatinine (in small number of clients). ↓ Hemoglobin.

T

OVERDOSE MANAGEMENT

Symptoms: Hypotension, dizziness, tachycardia, or bradycardia. *Treatment:* Supportive for hypotension.

DRUG INTERACTIONS

↑ Digoxin peak plasma and trough levels

HOW SUPPLIED

Tablets: 20 mg, 40 mg, 80 mg.

DOSAGE

TABLETS

Antihypertensive.

Individualize dose. **Adults, initial:** 40 mg/day. **Maintenance:** 20–80 mg/day. If additional BP reduction is desired beyond that achieved with 80 mg/day, add a diuretic.

Cardiovascular risk reduction.

Adults, age 55 and older: 80 mg once per day.

NURSING IMPLICATIONS

IMPLEMENTATION/ADMINISTRATION/STORAGE

1. May be taken with or without food.
2. Correct depletion of intravascular volume or begin therapy under close supervision.
3. Most of the antihypertensive effect occurs within 2 weeks with maximal reduction of BP within 4 weeks.
4. Clients on dialysis may develop orthostatic hypotension; monitor BP closely.
5. Begin treatment with a low dose and under close medical supervision in those with biliary obstructive disorders or hepatic insufficiency.
6. Store from 15–30°C (59–86°F). Do not remove tablets from blisters until just before use.

ASSESSMENT

1. Note onset, duration, and characteristics of disease, other agents trialed, outcome.
2. Symptomatic hypotension may occur in clients who are volume- or salt-depleted. Correct prior to using telmisartan, use a lower starting dose and monitor closely.
3. With renal dialysis may develop orthostatic hypotension; monitor BP closely.
4. Monitor VS, ECG, electrolytes, H&H, renal and LFTs. With hepatic or renal dysfunction, use cautiously.

CLIENT/FAMILY TEACHING

1. Take as directed at the same time daily with or without food.
2. Do not remove tablets from blisters until just before use.
3. Use caution; may experience dizziness R/T low BP. Change positions slowly and report if persistent or bothersome.
4. Regular exercise, low-salt diet, weight control, and life-style changes (i.e., no smoking, low alcohol, low-fat diet, low stress, adequate rest) contribute to enhanced BP control. Monitor/record BP and HR regularly.
5. Use effective contraception; report pregnancy as drug use during second and third trimesters is associated with fetal injury and morbidity. Report drop in urine output.
6. Keep all F/U to assess response, labs, and for adverse SE.

OUTCOMES/EVALUATE

↓ BP

Temazepam

(teh-**MAZ**-eh-pam)

Classification(s): Sedative-hypnotic, benzodiazepine

Pregnancy Category: X

RX: Restoril, **C-IV**

Rx: Apo-Temazepam, CO Temazepam, Gen-Temazepam, PMS-Temazepam, ratio-Temazepam.

SEE ALSO ***TRANQUILIZERS/ANTIMANIC DRUGS/HYPNOTICS***.

INDICATIONS/USES

Insomnia in clients unable to fall asleep, with frequent awakenings during the night, and/or early morning awakenings.

ACTION/KINETICS

Action

Benzodiazepine derivative. Believed to potentiate GABA neuronal inhibition. The hypnotic action involves GABA receptors located in the CNS. The drug decreases sleep latency, the number of awakenings, and the time spent in the awake stage. Disturbed nocturnal sleep may occur the first one or two nights following discontinuance of the drug. Prolonged administration is not recommended, because physical dependence and tolerance may develop. See also *Flurazepam.*

Pharmacokinetics

Peak blood levels: 1.2–1.6 hr. **t½:** 10–17 hr. **Steady-state plasma levels:** 382 ng/mL (2.5 hr after 30-mg dose). Accumulation of the drug is minimal following multiple dosage. Metabolized in the liver to inactive metabolites. **Plasma protein binding:** 98%.

CONTRAINDICATIONS

Pregnancy.

SPECIAL CONCERNS

- Use with caution in severely depressed clients.
- Use during lactation may cause sedation and feeding problems in the infant.
- Geriatric clients may be more sensitive to the effects of temazepam.

SIDE EFFECTS

Most Common

Drowsiness, dizziness, light-headedness, incoordination.

CNS: Drowsiness, dizziness, light-headedness, incoordination, lethargy, confusion, euphoria, weakness, ataxia, lack of concentration, hallucinations. In some clients, paradoxical excitement (less than 0.5%), including stimulation and hyperactivity, occurs. **GI:** Anorexia, diarrhea. **Miscellaneous:** Tremors, horizontal nystagmus, falling, palpitations. Rarely, ***blood dyscrasias.***

HOW SUPPLIED

Capsules: 7.5 mg, 15 mg, 22.5 mg, 30 mg.

DOSAGE

CAPSULES

Insomnia.

Individualize. **Adults, usual:** 15–30 mg at bedtime (7.5 mg may be sufficient for some to improve sleep latency). **In elderly or debilitated clients, initial:** 7.5–15 mg until individual response is determined.

NURSING IMPLICATIONS

Do not confuse temazepam with flurazepam (a benzodiazepine hypnotic) or terazosin (an antihypertensive). Do not confuse Restoril with Vistaril (nonbenzodiazepine anti-anxiety drug) or Risperdal (an antipsychotic).

IMPLEMENTATION/ADMINISTRATION/STORAGE

Store from 15–25°C (68–77°F) in a well-closed, light-resistant container.

ASSESSMENT

1. Note reasons for therapy, onset, duration, characteristics of S&S, other agents trialed, outcome.
2. Assess mental status, sleep patterns, diet, lifestyle, routines; identify factors/triggers contributing to insomnia.
3. Report any depression or suicide ideations, pregnancy, or addiction history.
4. With long-term use may cause dependence, monitor CBC, renal and LFTs.

CLIENT/FAMILY TEACHING

1. Take only as directed; do not increase dose. May take several days before effects evident. Take 15 to 30 min before desired sleep.
2. May cause daytime drowsiness. Avoid activities that require mental alertness until drug effects realized. May need to supervise to ensure no falls or overuse.
3. Avoid alcohol and CNS depressants; may increase CNS depression. Avoid tobacco; decreases drug's effect.
4. No daytime napping. May still have difficulty getting to sleep, but once asleep will have increased rest. Keep diary listing routines, exercise time (do at least 4 hr before bedtime), use of caffeine, chocolate, alcohol, medications taking, distractions in bedroom.
5. Review nonpharmacologic methods of sleep induction (i.e., white noise, warm milk, chamomile tea, soft music, dark room, no TV).
6. Practice reliable birth control; drug may cause fetal harm.
7. For short-term use only. Long-term use can cause dependence and withdrawal symptoms. After more than 3 weeks of continuous use, may experience rebound insomnia. Sleep may be disturbed for 1 or 2 nights following discontinuation of temazepam therapy.
8. Keep all F/U to assess response, labs, and for adverse SE.

T

OUTCOMES/EVALUATE

Improved sleeping patterns; ↓ awakenings

IV

Temsirolimus

(**TEM**-sir-**OH**-lih-mus)

Classification(s): Antineoplastic, protein-tyrosine kinase inhibitor

Pregnancy Category: D

RX: Torisel.

INDICATIONS/USES

Treatment of advanced renal cell carcinoma.

ACTION/KINETICS

Action

Temsirolimus binds to an intracellular protein (FKBP-12); this protein-drug complex inhibits the activity of the target that controls cell division.

Pharmacokinetics

CYP3A4 is the major isoenzyme responsible for temsirolimus metabolites. Sirolimus is an active metabolite of temsirolimus. Temsirolimus inhibits CYP2D6 and CYP3A4 isoenzymes. Excreted mainly in the feces (78%) with a small amount (4.6%) excreted in the urine. **t½, mean:** 17.3 hr for temsirolimus and 54.6 hr for sirolimus.

CONTRAINDICATIONS

Avoid concomitant use of strong CYP3A4 inhibitors (e.g., atazanavir, clarithromycin, indinavir, itraconazole, ketoconazole, nefazodone, nelfinavir, ritonavir, saquinavir, telithromycin, voriconazole). Avoid concomitant use of strong CYP3A4 inducers (e.g., carbamazepine, dexamethasone, phenobarbital, phenytoin, rifampin, rifabutin, rifampicin). Lactation.

SPECIAL CONCERNS

- **Avoid the use of live vaccines and close contact with those who have received live vaccines (e.g., intranasal influenza, measles, mumps, rubella, oral polio, Bacille Calmette-Guérin, yellow fever, varicella, and TY21a typhoid vaccines).**
- **Safety and efficacy not determined in children.**

SIDE EFFECTS

Most Common

Anorexia, asthenia, edema, mucositis, N&V, rash, dysgeusia, diarrhea, back pain, dyspnea, cough, pain, pyrexia.

CNS: Dysgeusia (includes taste loss/perversion), headache, insomnia, depression. **GI:** Mucositis (includes aphthous stomatitis, glossitis, mouth ulceration, stomatitis), N&V, anorexia, diarrhea, abdominal pain, constipation, ***fatal bowel perforation.*** **CV:** Hypertension, ***DVT, pulmonary embolism***, thrombophlebitis, ***intracerebral hemorrhage.*** **Dermatologic:** Rash (includes eczema, exfoliative dermatitis, maculopapular/pruritic/pustular/vesiculobullous rash), pruritus, nail disorder, dry skin, acne. **Musculoskeletal:** Back pain, arthralgia, myalgia, chest pain. **Respiratory:** Dyspnea, cough, epistaxis, pharyngitis, rhinitis, pneumonia, URTI, ***interstitial lung disease*** (rarely fatal). **Hematologic:** Anemia, leukopenia, lymphopenia, thrombocytopenia. **GU:** Cystitis, dysuria, hematuria, urinary frequency, UTI, renal failure. **Hypersensitivity:** Dyspnea, flushing, chest pain, angioneurotic edema-type reactions (in those receiving ACE inhibitors with temsirolimus), ***anaphylaxis.*** **Ophthalmic:** Conjunctivitis, lacrimation disorder. **Metabolic:** Hyperglycemia/glucose intolerance, hyperlipemia. **Body as a whole:** Asthenia, edema (includes facial/peripheral edema), pain, pyrexia, infections (includes abscess, bronchitis, cellulitis, herpes simplex/zoster), weight loss, chills, impaired wound healing.

LABORATORY TEST CONSIDERATIONS

↑ Alkaline phosphatase, AST, serum creatinine, glucose, total bilirubin, total cholesterol, triglycerides. ↓ Phosphorus, potassium, hemoglobin, leukocytes, lymphocytes, neutrophils, platelets. Hyperglycemia, hyperlipemia, hypertriglyceridemia, hypophosphatemia,

OVERDOSE MANAGEMENT

Symptoms: Serious side effects, including ***thrombosis, bowel perforation, interstitial lung disease***, and psychosis are increased with doses greater than 25 mg. *Treatment:* No specific treatment for temsirolimus IV overdose.

DRUG INTERACTIONS

Azole antifungals (fluconazole, itraconazole, ketoconazole, posaconazole, voriconazole) / ↑ Temsirolimus levels R/T inhibition of CYP3A4; monitor temsirolimus levels and adjust dose if needed
Clarithromycin / ↑ Temsirolimus levels R/T inhibition of CYP3A4; monitor temsirolimus levels and adjust dose if needed

T

Cyclosporine / ↑ Sirolimus (active metabolite of temsirolimus) levels → ↑ toxicity
Dexamethasone / ↓ Temsirolimus levels R/T induction of CYP3A4; if concomitant use necessary, consider ↑ temsirolimus dose to 50 mg/week
Diltiazem / ↑ Temsirolimus levels R/T inhibition of CYP3A4; monitor temsirolimus levels and adjust dose if needed; also, ↑ sirolimus (active metabolite of temsirolimus) levels → ↑ toxicity
Grapefruit juice / ↑ Plasma sirolimus (a major metabolite of temsirolimus) levels; do not use together
Hydantoins (e.g., phenytoin) / ↓ Temsirolimus levels R/T induction of CYP3A4; if concomitant use necessary, consider ↑ temsirolimus dose to 50 mg/week
Mycophenolate / ↑ Mycophenolic acid trough levels → ↑ risk of toxicity
Phenobarbital / ↓ Temsirolimus levels R/T induction of CYP3A4; monitor temsirolimus levels and adjust dose if needed
Protease inhibitors (e.g., atazanavir, indinavir, nelfinavir, ritonavir, saquinavir) / ↑ Temsirolimus levels R/T inhibition of CYP3A4; monitor temsirolimus levels and adjust dose if needed
Rifamycins (e.g., rifabutin, rifampin, rifapentine) / ↓ Temsirolimus levels R/T induction of CYP3A4; consider ↑ temsirolimus dose to 50 mg/week
H ***St. John's wort*** / ↓ Temsirolimus levels R/T induction of CYP3A4; do not use together
Sunitinib / Dose-limiting toxicity (e.g., grade 3/4 erythematous maculopapular rash, gout/cellulitis requiring hospitalization)
Tacrolimus / ↓ Tacrolimus trough levels due to sirolimus (active metabolite) → ↓ pharmacologic effect; frequently monitor tacrolimus trough levels and adjust dose if needed

HOW SUPPLIED

Injection Solution, Concentrate: 25 mg/mL.

DOSAGE

IV INFUSION

Advanced renal cell carcinoma.

Adults: 25 mg infused over a 30- to 60-minute period once a week. Continue treatment until disease progression or unacceptable toxicity occurs.

NURSING IMPLICATIONS

IMPLEMENTATION/ADMINISTRATION/STORAGE

1. **IV** Do not add undiluted temsirolimus injection to infusion solutions; will cause the drug to precipitate. Always combine temsirolimus injection with the diluent provided before adding to infusion solutions. It is recommended that after the diluent is added, the drug should be given in 0.9% NaCl injection.
2. Premedicate with prophylactic diphenhydramine, 25–50 mg IV (or similar antihistamine) about 30 min before the start of each infusion of temsirolimus.
3. If a hypersensitivity reaction occurs during temsirolimus infusion, stop infusion and observe client for at least 30–60 min. At the discretion of the HCP, treatment may be resumed with the administration of an H_1-receptor antagonist (e.g., diphenhydramine) if not given previously and/or an H_2-receptor antagonist (e.g., famotidine, 20 mg IV or ranitidine, 50 mg IV) approximately 30 min before restarting the temsirolimus infusion. The infusion may then be resumed at a slower rate (up to 60 min).
4. Interrupt dosage if the absolute neutrophil count is <1,000/mm^3, platelet count is <75,000/mm^3, or for National Cancer Institute Common Terminology Criteria for Adverse Events grade 3 or greater adverse reactions. Once toxicities have resolved to grade 2 or less, temsirolimus may be restarted with the dose reduced by 5 mg weekly to a dose no lower than 15 mg/week.
5. Avoid concomitant use of strong CYP3A4 inhibitors (see *Contraindications* and *Drug Interactions*). If concomitant use is necessary, consider reducing the temsirolimus dose to 12.5 mg/week. If the strong inhibitor is discontinued, a washout period of about 1 week should be allowed before adjusting the temsirolimus dose back to the dose used prior to starting the strong CYP3A4 inhibitor.
6. Avoid concomitant use of strong CYP3A4 inducers (See *Contraindications* and *Drug Interactions*). If concomitant use is necessary, consider increasing the dose of temsirolimus to 50 mg/week. If the strong inducer is discontinued, the temsirolimus dose should be returned to the dose used prior to starting the strong CYP3A4 inducers.

T

7. Store the final temsirolimus dilution for infusion in polypropylene or glass bottles or polypropylene or polyolefin plastic bags. If polyvinyl chloride bags are used, the plasticizer di-2-ethylhexylphthalate may be leached from these bags.
8. Protect temsirolimus from excessive room light and sunlight.
9. Store from 2–8°C (36–46°F). The 10 mg/mL diluent/solution mixture is stable for up to 24 hr at controlled room temperature.
10. COMPATIBILITY 0.9% NaCl.
11. INCOMPATIBILITY Avoid adding other drugs or nutrients to admixtures of temsirolimus.

ASSESSMENT

1. Note disease onset, radiographic findings, other therapies trialed/failed.
2. List drugs prescribed to ensure none interact.
3. Assess lungs, heart, and abdomen (bowel perforations) regularly to ensure no adverse side effects.
4. Assess for other conditions (i.e., brain tumor, infections/wounds, or recent surgery). CNS tumors and anticoagulant therapy may increase risk of life-threatening intracerebral bleeding.
5. Determine that premedication with IV antihistamine (e.g., diphenhydramine 25 to 50 mg) given 30 min prior to start of each temsirolimus dose.
6. May require starting or increasing dose of lipid-lowering agents.
7. Check for diabetes, hyperlipidemia, liver problems, bone marrow problems, low WBC/platelet levels, or a weakened immune system. Follow administration guidelines R/T adverse events or lowered ANC/platelet count.
8. Monitor VS, renal and LFTs, lipids, BS, and CBC.

CLIENT/FAMILY TEACHING

1. Administered IV for advanced kidney cancer. Will receive premedication with an antihistamine (Benadryl) 30 min prior to therapy to help prevent allergic reactions.
2. Do not eat grapefruit or drink grapefruit juice while receiving this drug.
3. Report any facial swelling, breathing difficulty, increased abdominal pain, blood in stools, S&S of infection (i.e., fever, sore throat, rash, or chills), excessive thirst or urinary frequency.
4. May be more susceptible to infections, abnormal wound healing, interstitial lung disease–a severe and possibly fatal reaction, bowel perforation, kidney failure, or elevated triglycerides/cholesterol during therapy (may require therapy to control).
5. Vaccinations may not be as effective during therapy; avoid live vaccines and close contact with those who recently received a live vaccine.
6. Men with partners of childbearing potential should use reliable contraception throughout treatment and for 3 months after the last dose. Women should avoid pregnancy during and for 3 months following therapy; may cause fetal damage.
7. May increase blood sugar; report if confused, drowsy, or thirsty. May also cause flushing, fast breathing, or fruit like breath odor; report if evident.
8. Keep all F/U for weekly therapy, labs and to evaluate tumor response.

OUTCOMES/EVALUATE

Inhibition of malignant cell proliferation

IV

Tenecteplase

(teh-**NECK**-teh-plays)

Classification(s): Thrombolytic, tissue plasminogen activator

Pregnancy Category: C

RX: TNKase.

INDICATIONS/USES

Reduce mortality due to acute myocardial infarction (AMI). Begin treatment as soon as possible after onset of MI symptoms.

ACTION/KINETICS

Action

A tissue plasminogen activator produced by recombinant DNA. It binds to fibrin and converts plasminogen to plasmin. In the presence of fibrin, tenecteplase conversion of plasminogen to plasmin is increased relative to conversion in the absence of fibrin. Following the drug there are decreases in circulating fibrinogen.

T

Pharmacokinetics

t½, initial disposition: 20–24 min; **terminal disposition:** 90–130 min. Metabolized in the liver.

CONTRAINDICATIONS

Because of an increased risk of bleeding, do not use in the following conditions: Active internal bleeding, history of CVA, within 2 months of intracranial or intraspinal surgery or trauma, intracranial neoplasm, arteriovenous malformation or aneurysm, known bleeding diathesis, severe uncontrolled hypertension. IM use.

SPECIAL CONCERNS

The following high-risk conditions warrant an assessment of the risk of therapy versus the anticipated benefits:

- Recent major surgery (e.g., CABG, OB delivery, organ biopsy).
- Previous puncture of noncompressible vessels.
- CV disease.
- Recent GI or GU bleeding.
- Recent trauma; hypertension (systolic BP equal to or greater than 180 mm Hg or diastolic BP equal to or greater than 110 mm Hg).
- High likelihood of left heart thrombus (e.g., mitral stenosis with atrial fibrillation).
- Acute pericarditis.
- Subacute bacterial endocarditis.
- Hemostatic defects (including those secondary to severe hepatic or renal disease).
- Severe hepatic dysfunction.
- Pregnancy.
- Diabetic hemorrhagic retinopathy or other hemorrhagic ophthalmic conditions.
- Septic thrombophlebitis or occluded AV cannula at seriously infected site.
- Advanced age.
- Clients receiving PO anticoagulants (e.g., warfarin sodium).
- Recent administration of GP IIb/IIIa inhibitors.
- Any other condition in which bleeding constitutes a significant hazard or would be particularly difficult to manage because of its location.
- Possible cholesterol embolization and arrhythmias associated with reperfusion.
- Use with caution in the elderly, weighing the benefits versus risks, including bleeding.
- Use with caution during lactation.
- Safety and efficacy not determined in children.

SIDE EFFECTS

Most Common

Bleeding is the most common side effect (see the following).

Bleeding. Most common side effect. Major bleeding includes GI tract, urinary tract, puncture site (including cardiac catheterization site), retroperitoneal, respiratory tract. Minor bleeding includes hematoma, urinary tract, puncture site (including cardiac catheterization site), pharyngeal, GI tract, and epistaxis. Bleeding can also be divided into two broad categories: (a) Internal bleeding, involving intracranial and retroperitoneal sites, or the GI, GU, or respiratory tracts; and, (b) superficial or surface bleeding, seen mainly at vascular puncture or access sites (e.g., venous cutdowns, arterial punctures) or sites of recent surgical intervention. **CV:** Cardiogenic shock, arrhythmias (e.g., sinus bradycardia, accelerated idioventricular rhythm, ventricular premature depolarization, ventricular tachycardia), AV block, ***heart failure, cardiac arrest***, recurrent myocardial ischemia, ***myocardial reinfarction/rupture, cardiac tamponade***, pericarditis, pericardial effusion, mitral regurgitation, thrombosis, embolism, electromechanical dissociation. **Miscellaneous:** Pulmonary edema, N&V, hypotension, fever, ***serious allergic or anaphylactic reactions (rare).***

LABORATORY TEST CONSIDERATIONS

Results of coagulation tests or measures of fibrinolytic activity may be unreliable; specific precautions must be taken to prevent in vitro artifacts. Degradation of fibrinogen in blood samples removed for analysis is possible.

DRUG INTERACTIONS

Heparin, vitamin K antagonists, aspirin, dipyridamole, and GP IIb/IIIa inhibitors may increase the risk of bleeding if given prior to, during, or after tenecteplase therapy.

HOW SUPPLIED

Injection, Lyophilized Powder for Solution: 50 mg.

T

DOSAGE

IV ONLY

Acute myocardial infarction (AMI).

Dose is based on client weight, but not to exceed 50 mg. Given as a single bolus dose over 5 sec. **Less than 60 kg:**

30 mg (6 mL); **60 kg to less than 70 kg:** 35 mg (7 mL); **70 kg to less than 80 kg:** 40 mg (8 mL); **80 kg to less than 90 kg:** 45 mg (9 mL); **90 kg and over:** 50 mg (10 mL). *NOTE:* If serious bleeding, not controlled by local pressure, occurs, discontinue immediately as well as concomitant heparin or antiplatelet drugs.

NURSING IMPLICATIONS

IMPLEMENTATION/ADMINISTRATION/STORAGE

1. IV Initiate treatment as soon as possible after onset of symptoms of MI.
2. Reconstitute and administer as follows:
   - Aseptically withdraw 10 mL sterile water from that supplied. Use the red hub cannula syringe filling device. Do not discard the shield assembly. Do *not* use bacteriostatic water for injection.
   - Inject entire contents of the syringe (10 mL) into the tenecteplase vial. Direct the stream into the powder. Slight foaming may occur; any large bubbles will dissipate if allowed to stand undisturbed for several minutes.
   - Swirl contents gently until completely dissolved. Do not shake. The reconstituted product is colorless to pale yellow and is transparent with a concentration of 5 mg/mL and pH of about 7.3.
   - Determine appropriate dose of tenecteplase and withdraw correct volume (in mL) from the reconstituted vial with the syringe. Discard any unused portion.
   - With correct dose in the syringe, stand the shield vertically on a flat surface with the green side down and passively recap the red hub cannula.
   - Remove the entire shield assembly, including the red hub cannula by twisting counter-clockwise. The shield assembly also contains the clear-ended blunt plastic cannula; retain for split septum IV access.
   - Administer as a single IV bolus over 5 sec.
3. Tenecteplase contains no preservatives; thus, reconstitute immediately before use.
4. Use an upper-extremity vessel that is accessible to manual compression if an arterial puncture becomes necessary during the first few hours following therapy. Apply pressure for 30 or more minutes, apply a pressure dressing, and check the puncture site frequently for evidence of bleeding.
5. Coronary thrombolysis may occur in arrhythmias associated with reperfusion. Arrhythmias include sinus bradycardia, accelerated idioventricular rhythm, ventricular premature depolarization, and ventricular tachycardia. Have antiarrhythmic therapy for bradycardia or ventricular irritability available when tenecteplase is administered.
6. Store lyophilized tenecteplase at controlled temperatures not to exceed 30°C (86°F) or under refrigeration at 2–8°C (36–46°F).
7. If reconstituted drug is not used immediately, refrigerate tenecteplase vial at 2–8°C (36–46°F) and use within 8 hr.
8. COMPATIBILITY 0.9% NaCl.
9. INCOMPATIBILITY If given in an IV line with dextrose, precipitation may occur. Flush dextrose-containing lines with a saline prior to and following single bolus administration of tenecteplase.

ASSESSMENT

1. Note reasons for therapy, identifying symptom onset and site of infarct.
2. Do not use with active internal bleeding, history of CVA, recent: intracranial bleed, spinal surgery, trauma, neoplasm, AV malformation, aneurysm, or uncontrolled HTN.
3. Assess for reperfusion arrhythmias after therapy, which may include accelerated idioventricular rhythm, sinus bradycardia of short duration, VT, and return of elevated ST segment to near baseline. Have antiarrhythmic therapy for bradycardia or ventricular irritability available when tenecteplase is administered.
4. Obtain baseline cardiac enzymes, weight, CBC, bleeding times, type, and crossmatch. Monitor for S&S active bleeding; stop heparin infusion and report.

CLIENT/FAMILY TEACHING

1. Review inherent benefits and risks of drug therapy. Maintain bed rest during therapy.
2. To be effective, the therapy should be instituted as soon as possible after symptom onset of AMI.
3. Report any adverse side effects (i.e., sudden severe headache or active bleeding) immediately.

T

4. Encourage family members or significant other to learn CPR.

OUTCOMES/EVALUATE

↓ Mortality with AMI

IV

Teniposide (VM-26)

(teh-**NIP**-oh-side)

Classification(s): Antineoplastic, miscellaneous

Pregnancy Category: D

RX: Vumon.

SEE ALSO ***ANTINEOPLASTIC AGENTS***.

INDICATIONS/USES

In combination with other antineoplastic agents for induction therapy in clients with refractory childhood acute lymphoblastic leukemia (ALL). *Investigational:* Adult acute lymphocytic leukemia; non-Hodgkin lymphoma.

ACTION/KINETICS

Action

Acts in the late S or early G_2 phase of the cell cycle, preventing cells from entering mitosis. Inhibits type II topoisomerase activity, resulting in both single- and double-stranded breaks in DNA and DNA: protein cross-links. Active against sublines of certain murine leukemias that have developed resistance to amsacrine, cisplatin, daunorubicin, doxorubicin, mitoxantrone, or vincristine.

Pharmacokinetics

Terminal t½: 5 hr. Metabolized in the liver and excreted mainly through the urine (4–12% unchanged) with small amounts excreted in the feces. **Plasma protein binding:** More than 99%.

CONTRAINDICATIONS

Hypersensitivity to teniposide, etoposide, or the polyoxylethylated castor oil present in teniposide products. Lactation.

SPECIAL CONCERNS

(1) Teniposide is a cytotoxic drug. Administer under the supervision of a qualified health care provider experienced in the use of cancer chemotherapeutic agents. Appropriate management of therapy and complications is possible only when adequate treatment facilities are readily available. (2) Severe myelosuppression with resulting infection or bleeding may occur. (3) Hypersensitivity reactions, including anaphylaxis-like symptoms, may occur with initial or repeated dosing. Epinephrine with or without corticosteroids and antihistamines, has been employed to alleviate hypersensitivity reaction symptoms.

- **Clients with both Down syndrome and leukemia may be especially sensitive to myelosuppressive chemotherapy; thus, reduce initial dosing.**
- **Use with caution in clients with impaired hepatic function.**
- **Contains benzyl alcohol associated with a fatal "gasping" syndrome in premature infants.**

SIDE EFFECTS

Most Common

Thombocytopenia, neutropenia, anemia, leukopenia, nonspecified myelosuppression, mucositis, N&V, diarrhea, infection.

Hematologic: ***Severe myelosuppression***, leukopenia, neutropenia, thrombocytopenia, anemia, nonspecified myelosuppression. **Hypersensitivity reactions:** ***Anaphylaxis*** manifested by chills, fever, ***bronchospasm***, dyspnea, facial flushing, hypertension or hypotension, tachycardia. **CV:** Hypotension. **GI:** Mucositis, N&V, diarrhea. **Dermatologic:** Alopecia (reversible), rash, hepatic dysfunction/toxicity, peripheral neurotoxicity, infection, bleeding, renal dysfunction, metabolic abnormalities.

OVERDOSE MANAGEMENT

Symptoms: Myelosuppression, hypotension, anaphylaxis. *Treatment:* Anaphylaxis or overdose:

- Treat anaphylaxis promptly with antihistamines, corticosteroids, epinephrine, IV fluids, and other supportive measures. If a client who manifested a hypersensitivity reaction must be retreated, undertake pretreatment with corticosteroids and antihistamines; carefully observe client during and after the infusion.
- If hypotension occurs, stop the infusion and give fluids. Undertake other supportive therapy as needed.
- Myelosuppression may be treated with supportive care, including blood products and antibiotics.

T

DRUG INTERACTIONS

Antiemetic drugs / Acute CNS depression and hypotension in clients receiving high doses of teniposide and pretreated with antiemetics
Methotrexate / ↑ Plasma clearance of methotrexate
Sodium salicylate / ↑ Teniposide effect R/T displacement from plasma protein binding sites
Sulfamethizole / ↑ Teniposide effect R/T displacement from plasma protein binding sites
Tolbutamide / ↑ Teniposide effect R/T displacement from plasma protein binding sites

HOW SUPPLIED

Injection Solution, Concentrate: 10 mg/mL.

DOSAGE

IV INFUSION

Regimen 1 for childhood acute lymphoblastic leukemia (ALL) clients refractory to cytarabine-containing regimens.

Teniposide, 165 mg/m², and cytarabine, 300 mg/m² IV twice weekly for 8–9 doses.

Regimen 2 for childhood acute lymphoblastic leukemia (ALL) refractory to vincristine/prednisone-containing regimens.

Teniposide, 250 mg/m², and vincristine, 1.5 mg/m², IV weekly for 4–8 weeks, and prednisone, 40 mg/m² orally for 28 days.

NOTE: Dosage adjustment may be needed for clients with significant renal or hepatic dysfunction.

NURSING IMPLICATIONS

IMPLEMENTATION/ADMINISTRATION/STORAGE

1. **IV** Give over 30–60 min or longer; do not give by rapid IV infusion, as hypotension may occur.
2. The IV catheter or needle must be in the proper position and functional prior to infusion. Improper administration may cause extravasation, resulting in local tissue necrosis or thrombophlebitis. Also, occlusion of central venous access devices has occurred during 24-hr infusion at concentrations of 0.1–0.2 mg/mL.
3. Dilute with either D5W or 0.9% NaCl injection to give a final concentration of 0.1, 0.2, 0.4, or 1 mg/mL.
4. Contact of undiluted teniposide with plastic equipment/devices used to prepare IV infusions may result in softening, cracking, and possible drug leakage. To prevent extraction of plasticizer DEHP, prepare and give solutions in non-DEHP-containing LVP containers, such as glass, or polyolefin plastic bags or containers. Avoid PVC containers. Stability and use times are identical in glass and plastic parenteral solution containers.
5. Lipid administration sets or low DEHP-containing nitroglycerin sets will keep exposure to DEHP at low levels, and can be used. Diluted solutions are chemically/physically compatible with the recommended IV administration sets and LVP containers for up to 24 hr at ambient room temperature and lighting conditions.
6. Use caution in handling and preparing the solution as skin reactions may occur with accidental exposure, and drug is cytotoxic. Use of gloves is recommended; if the solution comes in contact with the skin, wash immediately with soap and water. If the drug comes in contact with mucous membranes, flush thoroughly with water.
7. Give solutions containing 1 mg/mL within 4 hr of preparation to reduce the potential for precipitation. Refrigeration of solutions is not recommended.
8. Precipitation of teniposide may occur at the recommended concentrations, especially if the diluted solution is agitated more than recommended during preparation. Also, minimize storage time prior to administration; take care to avoid contact of the diluted solution with other drugs or fluids.
9. Not for use in premature infants; contains benzyl alcohol.
10. Solutions prepared in D5W injection or 0.9% NaCl injection at teniposide concentrations of 0.1, 0.2, or 0.4 mg/mL are stable at room temperature for up to 24 hr after preparation. Solutions prepared at a concentration of 1 mg/mL should be given within 4 hr of preparation in order to reduce the potential for precipitation.

11. Refrigeration of teniposide solutions is not recommended.
12. Unopened ampules are stable until the date indicated if stored at 2–8°C (36–46°F) in the original package (protected from light).
13. COMPATIBILITY D5W, 0.9% NaCl.
14. INCOMPATIBILITY Because of the potential for precipitation, compatibility with other drugs, infusion materials, or IV pumps cannot be ensured. Heparin solution can cause precipitation of teniposide; flush administration apparatus thoroughly with D5W or 0.9% NaCl injection before and after administration.

ASSESSMENT

1. Determine indications for therapy, previous agents trialed and combination therapy ordered. Note any sensitivity to product derivatives, especially polyoxylethylated castor oil. Product also contains benzyl alcohol.
2. Premedicate with antiemetics; observe for enhanced CNS effects. If S&S of anaphylaxis occur (chills, fever, tachycardia, chest pain, dyspnea, or altered BP), interrupt infusion and report. May use corticosteroids and antihistamines in these clients if retreatment considered.
3. Reduce dose with Down syndrome.
4. Monitor VS, CBC, uric acid, renal and LFTs; reduce dose with dysfunction. May cause granulocyte and platelet suppression. Withhold if BP <90 systolic and platelet count <50,000/mm^3 or ANC <500/mm^3; do not resume treatment until hematologic recovery is evident. Nadir: 14 days; recovery: 21 days.

CLIENT/FAMILY TEACHING

1. Drug is administered IV over 30–60 min and with other anticancer agents to treat leukemia.
2. Report promptly if fever, chills, rapid heartbeat, infusion site pain, or difficulty breathing occurs.
3. N&V and hair loss are frequent drug side effects.
4. Avoid those with infections and crowds to prevent any infections.
5. Drug will cause fetal harm; use reliable contraceptive measures during treatment.
6. Keep all F/U to assess response, labs, and for adverse SE.

OUTCOMES/EVALUATE

Remission with relapsed or refractory ALL

Tenofovir disoproxil fumarate (PMPA)

(teh-**NOFF**-oh-veer)

Classification(s): Antiviral, nucleoside reverse transcriptase inhibitor

Pregnancy Category: B

RX: Viread.

SEE ALSO ***ANTIVIRAL DRUGS***.

INDICATIONS/USES

(1) In combination with other antiretroviral drugs to treat HIV-1 infection in adults and children, 12 years and older. (2) Chronic hepatitis B in adults. *NOTE:* Because of the risk of development of HIV-1 resistance, only use tenofovir in HIV-1 and HBV coinfected individuals as part of an appropriate antiretroviral combination regimen.

ACTION/KINETICS

Action

Tenofovir disoproxil fumarate requires initial diester hydrolysis for conversion to tenofovir and subsequent phosphorylation to form tenofovir diphosphate. Tenofovir diphosphate inhibits HIV-1 reverse transcriptase activity and HBV polymerase by competing with the natural substrate deoxyadenosine 5'-triphosphate and after incorporation into DNA, by DNA chain termination.

Pharmacokinetics

Bioavailability is about 25% in fasted clients. **Maximum serum levels:** About 1 hr. High-fat meals increase the PO bioavailability with an increase in C_{max} of about 14% and AUC of about 40%. About 70–80% excreted unchanged in the urine by a combination of glomerular filtration and active tubular secretion. Impairment of renal or hepatic function affects the pharmacokinetics. **t½, terminal:** 17 hr. **Plasma protein binding:** <7.2%.

CONTRAINDICATIONS

Hypersensitivity to tenofovir or any component of the product. Use in pregnancy only if clearly needed. Use in combination with emtricitabine/

T

tenofovir or efavirenz/emtricitabine/tenofovir. Lactation.

SPECIAL CONCERNS

■ (1) **Lactic acidosis and severe hepatomegaly with steatosis.** Lactic acidosis and severe hepatomegaly with steatosis, including fatal cases, have been reported with the use of nucleoside analogs alone or in combination with other antiretrovirals. (2) **Post-treatment exacerbation of hepatitis.** Severe acute exacerbations of hepatitis have been reported in hepatits B virus (HBV)-infected clients who have discontinued anti-hepatitis B therapy, including tenofovir. Monitor hepatic function closely with both clinical and laboratory follow-up for at least several months in clients who discontinue anti-hepatitis B therapy, including tenofovir. If appropriate, resumption of anti-hepatitis B therapy may be warranted. ■

- A high rate of virologic failure and emergence of nucleoside reverse transcriptase inhibitor resistance may occur in clients receiving a regimen containing didanosine enteric-coated beadlets, lamivudine, and tenofovir.
- Use caution with dose selection in the elderly.
- Safety and efficacy not determined in children younger than 12 years of age.

SIDE EFFECTS

Most Common

Abdominal pain, N&V, insomnia, pruritus, dizziness, pyrexia, back pain, diarrhea, dizziness, fatigue, headache, nasopharyngitis, skin rash, asthenia, depression, pain.

GI: N&V, diarrhea, flatulence, abdominal pain, anorexia, dyspepsia, ***pancreatitis***. **Hepatic:** Hepatitis, exacerbation of hepatitis after treatment discontinued. **CNS:** Headache, depression, insomnia, dizziness, abnormal dreams, paresthesia, anxiety, peripheral neuropathy. **Dermatologic:** Rash, pruritus, maculopapular rash, urticaria, vesiculobullous rash, pustular rash, sweating. **GU:** Renal toxicity, renal insufficiency/failure, proximal tubulopathy, acute renal failure, acute tubular necrosis, Fanconi syndrome, interstitial nephritis (include acute), nephrogenic diabetes insipidus, polyuria. **Respiratory:** Nasopharyngitis, pneumonia, dyspnea, sinusitis, URTI. **Musculoskeletal:** Myalgia, arthralgia, back/chest pain, bone toxicity (decreased bone density), muscle weakness, myopathy, osteomalacia (associated with proximal renal tubulopathy), bone fractures, rhabdomyolysis. **Body as a whole:** Asthenia, fatigue, peripheral neuritis, neuropathy, pain, fever/pyrexia, weight loss, allergic reaction (including angioedema). **Miscellaneous:** ***Lactic acidosis, severe hepatomegaly with steatosis***, virologic failure, redistribution and accumulation of body fat (including breast enlargement, central obesity, cushingoid appearance, dorsocervical fat enlargement, facial wasting, peripheral wasting), lipodystrophy, immune reconstitution syndrome (inflammatory response to indolent or residual opportunistic infections, including cytomegalovirus, *Mycobacterium avium* infection, *Pneumocystis jirovecii* pneumonia, and tuberculosis).

LABORATORY TEST CONSIDERATIONS

↑ AST, ALT, GGT, creatine kinase, creatinine, triglycerides, serum amylase, urine/serum glucose, fasting cholesterol/triglycerides. ↓ Neutrophils, hemoglobin. Hypophosphatemia, proteinuria, hematuria.

OVERDOSE MANAGEMENT

Symptoms: There is limited clinical experience at doses higher than the therapeutic dose of 300 mg. *Treatment:* Monitor for evidence of toxicity and undertake standard supportive treatment. Tenofovir is removed by hemodialysis.

DRUG INTERACTIONS

Abacavir / ↑ Abacavir C_{max}; AUC unchanged
Acyclovir / ↑ Levels of tenofovir (or other renally excreted drugs) R/T competition for tubular secretion
Adefovir dipivoxil / ↑ Levels of tenofovir (or other renally excreted drugs) R/T competition for tubular secretion; coadministration contraindicated
Atazanavir / ↓ Atazanavir levels; possible loss or lack of response; ↑ tenofovir AUC and C_{max}; do not coadminister without the addition of ritonavir
Cidofovir / ↑ Levels of tenofovir (or other renally excreted drugs) R/T competition for tubular secretion; ↑ risk of nephrotoxicity
Didanosine (buffered formulation or enteric-coated) / ↑ Maximum concentration and AUC of didanosine → ↑ side effects, including pancreatitis, lactic acidosis, and neuropathy; reduce the didanosine dose to 250 mg in adults >60 kg; discontinue didanosine in those who develop side effects

Entecavir / ↑ Entecavir AUC
Ganciclovir / ↑ Levels of tenofovir or ganciclovir (or other renally excreted drugs) R/T competition for tubular secretion
Indinavir / ↑ Tenofovir C_{max}; ↓ indinavir C_{max}; AUC remained the same for both drugs
Lamivudine / ↓ Lamivudine C_{max}; AUC unchanged
Lopinavir/Ritonavir / ↑ Tenofovir C_{max}; monitor closely
Nephrotoxic drugs / ↑ Risk of nephrotoxicity; avoid tenofovir in those receiving nephrotoxic drugs
NSAIDs (e.g., ibuprofen) / Possible ↑ Tenofovir pharmacologic/toxic effects; coadminister with caution
Saquinavir/Ritonavir / ↑ Saquinavir AUC and C_{max}; not expected to be clinically relevant
Tacrolimus / ↑ Tenofovir C_{max}; monitor closely
Valacyclovir / ↑ Tenofavir levels (or other renally excreted drugs) R/T competition for tubular secretion
Valganciclovir / ↑ Tenofavir levels (or other renally excreted drugs) R/T competition for tubular secretion

HOW SUPPLIED

Tablets: 300 mg (equivalent to 245 mg tenofovir disoproxil).

DOSAGE

TABLETS

HIV-1 infection; chronic hepatitis B in adults.

Adults and children, 12 years and older and 25 kg or more: 300 mg once daily taken PO without regard to food. Adjust the dose as follows in adults with renal impairment: **C_{CR}, 30–49 mL/min:** 300 mg q 48 hr; **C_{CR}, 10–29 mL/min:** 300 q 72–96 hr; **hemodialysis clients:** 300 mg q 7 days or after a total of about 12 hr of dialysis assuming 3 hemodialysis sessions a week of about 4 hr duration. Administer following completion of dialysis. *NOTE:* No dosing recommendation is available for those with C_{CR} <10 mL/min.

NURSING IMPLICATIONS

IMPLEMENTATION/ADMINISTRATION/STORAGE

1. Only use tenofovir in HIV-1 and HBV coinfected clients as part of an appropriate antiretroviral combination regimen.
2. To monitor fetal outcomes of pregnant women exposed to tenofovir, an antiretroviral registry has been created. Health care providers are encouraged to register clients by calling 1-800-258-4263.
3. Store from 15–30°C (59–86°F).

ASSESSMENT

1. Note reasons for therapy, disease onset, other therapies trialed. List drugs prescribed to ensure none interact or are nephrotoxic.
2. Assess for evidence of liver/renal disease, hepatitis B infection, bone abnormalities, and acidosis. If drug stopped suddenly, may exacerbate HBV.
3. Check bone density with history of pathologic bone fracture or if risk for osteopenia.
4. Monitor CBC, viral loads, CD4 counts, (HIV/Hep B), phosphorus, renal and LFTs; anticipate reduced dosing interval with renal dysfunction. Assess for lactic acidosis and severe hepatomegaly with steatosis.

CLIENT/FAMILY TEACHING

1. Drug is to be combined with other antiviral agents. When taken with didanosine, take the tenofovir 2 hr before or 1 hr after didanosine administration.
2. Take once a day as prescribed with a meal to enhance drug bioavailability. Do not stop suddenly without provider approval; may cause severe exacerbation of HBV.
3. May experience changes in body fat, N&V, diarrhea, and gas; report if persistent and if any yellowing of skin or eyes, abdominal pain, muscle aches/pains; stop drug therapy.
4. If profound weakness or tiredness, unexpected stomach discomfort, fatty diarrhea, feeling cold, dizzy, or light-headed or slow or irregular heartbeat, stop drug and report.
5. With HIV-associated osteopenia or osteoporosis need to take calcium and vitamin D supplementation.
6. Avoid crowds and persons with infections and OTC agents without provider approval.
7. Drug is not a cure for HIV; opportunistic infections may continue. Practice reliable contra-

T

ception; to prevent infecting infants with HIV, do not breast-feed. If pregnant, enroll in antiretroviral registry by calling 1-800-258-4263.

8. Keep all F/U visits to assess response, labs, and adverse SE.

OUTCOMES/EVALUATE

- Control of progression of tenofovir susceptible HIV infection
- ↓ HBV and treatment

Terazosin

(ter-**AY**-zoh-sin)

Classification(s): Antihypertensive, alpha-1-adrenergic blocking drug

Pregnancy Category: C

RX: Hytrin.

✱ Rx: Apo-Terazosin, Novo-Terazosin, PMS-Tarazosin, ratio-Terazosin.

INDICATIONS/USES

(1) Hypertension, alone or in combination with other antihypertensive drugs. (2) Symptoms of benign prostatic hyperplasia. *Investigational:* Ureteral stones, symptomatic treatment of chronic abacterial prostatitis.

ACTION/KINETICS

Action

Blocks postsynaptic alpha-1-adrenergic receptors, leading to a dilation of both areterioles and veins, and ultimately, a reduction in BP. Both standing and supine BPs are lowered with no reflex tachycardia. Also relaxes smooth muscle of the prostate and bladder neck. Usefulness in BPH is due to alpha-1-receptor blockade, which relaxes the smooth muscle of the prostate and bladder neck and relieves pressure on the urethra.

Pharmacokinetics

Food delays T_{max}. **Peak levels:** About 1 hr. **Onset:** 15 min. **Peak plasma levels:** 1–2 hr. **t½:** About 12 hr. **Duration:** 24 hr. Excreted unchanged and as inactive metabolites in both the urine (40%) and feces (60%). Clearance is decreased in the elderly.

SPECIAL CONCERNS

- Geriatric clients may be more sensitive to the hypotensive and hypothermic effects of terazosin.
- Use with caution during lactation.
- Safety and efficacy not determined in children.

SIDE EFFECTS

Most Common

Asthenia, dizziness, headache, somnolence, flu symptoms, nasal congestion, pharyngitis/rhinitis.

First-dose effect: Marked postural hypotension and syncope. **CV:** Palpitations, tachycardia, postural hypotension, hypotension, syncope, ***arrhythmias***, chest pain, vasodilation, atrial fibrillation. **CNS:** Dizziness, headache, somnolence, drowsiness, nervousness, paresthesia, depression, anxiety, insomnia, vertigo. **Respiratory:** Nasal congestion, dyspnea, sinusitis, epistaxis, bronchitis, ***bronchospasm***, cold or flu symptoms, increased cough, pharyngitis, rhinitis. **GI:** Nausea, constipation, diarrhea, dyspepsia, dry mouth, vomiting, flatulence, abdominal discomfort or pain. **Musculoskeletal:** Asthenia, arthritis, arthralgia, myalgia, joint disorders, back pain, pain in extremities, neck and shoulder pain, muscle cramps. **GU:** Impotence, urinary frequency, UTI, priapism. **Dermatologic:** Pruritus, rash, sweating. **Ophthalmic:** Blurred/abnormal vision, amblyopia, conjunctivitis, intraoperative floppy iris syndrome. **Miscellaneous:** Peripheral edema, weight gain, chest pain, fever, gout, tinnitus, edema, facial edema, thrombocytopenia, allergic reactions including ***anaphylaxis***.

LABORATORY TEST CONSIDERATIONS

↓ H&H, WBCs, albumin, total cholesterol.

OVERDOSE MANAGEMENT

Symptoms: Hypotension, drowsiness, ***shock***. *Treatment:* Restore BP and HR. Client should be kept supine; vasopressors may be indicated. Volume expanders can be used to treat shock.

DRUG INTERACTIONS

Alcohol / ↑ Risk of hypotension; avoid alcohol use
Finasteride / ↑ Finasteride plasma levels
Verapamil / ↑ Verapamil AUC, C_{max}, C_{min}, and ↓ T_{max}

HOW SUPPLIED

Capsules: 1 mg, 2 mg, 5 mg, 10 mg; *Tablets:* 1 mg, 2 mg, 5 mg, 10 mg.

DOSAGE

CAPSULES; TABLETS

Hypertension.

Individualized, initial: 1 mg at bedtime (this dose is not to be exceeded to minimize the potential for severe hypotension); **then,** increase dose slowly to obtain desired response. **Range:** 1–5 mg/day; doses as high as 20 mg may be required in some clients. Doses greater than 20 mg daily do not provide further BP control.

Benign prostatic hyperplasia.

Initial: 1 mg/day at bedtime (do not exceed this dose in order to minimize severe hypotension); **then,** increase dose in a stepwise fashion to 2 mg, 5 mg, and then 10 mg once daily to improve symptoms and/or urinary flow rates. Doses greater than 20 mg daily have not been studied.

Adjunctive therapy for ureteral stones.

2–5 mg/day for up to 1 month or until expulsion.

NURSING IMPLICATIONS

Do not confuse terazosin with temazepam (a sedative-hypnotic).

IMPLEMENTATION/ADMINISTRATION/STORAGE

1. The initial dosing regimen must be carefully observed to minimize severe hypotension.
2. Monitor BP 2–3 hr after dosing and at end of dosing interval to ensure BP control maintained.
3. Consider an increase in dose or twice a day dosing if BP control is not maintained at 24-hr interval.
4. To prevent dizziness or fainting due to a drop in BP, take the initial dose at bedtime; the daily dose can be given in the morning.
5. If terazosin must be discontinued for more than a few days, reinstitute the initial dosing regimen if restarted.
6. Due to additive hypotensive effects, use caution when combined with other antihypertensive agents (especially calcium channel blockers).
7. When treating BPH, a minimum of 4–6 weeks of 10 mg/day may be needed to determine if a beneficial effect has occurred.
8. Store from 15–30°C (59–86°F); protect from light and moisture.

ASSESSMENT

1. Note onset, duration, characteristics of S&S, other agents trialed.
2. A gradual increase in dose until symptom control, i.e., 1 mg/day for 7 days, then 2 mg/day for 7 days, then 3 mg/day for 7 days, then 4 mg/day for 7 days, and then 5 mg/day, may assist to diminish adverse effects and enhance compliance, especially in the elderly.
3. Note PSA levels, family history of prostate cancer, results of digital rectal exam (DRE) to ensure no prostate cancer.
4. Obtain BP and monitor R/T syncope and orthostatic effects with first dose.
5. Monitor DRE, PSA, I&O, BP, weight, urodynamic studies/BPH score.

CLIENT/FAMILY TEACHING

1. Take initial dose at bedtime to minimize side effects. Do not stop abruptly or titration must restart.
2. Use caution when performing activities that require mental alertness until drug effects realized; may cause dizziness or drowsiness.
3. Do not drive or undertake hazardous tasks for 12 hr after the first dose and after increasing dose or reinstituting therapy.
4. Avoid symptoms of dizziness (drop in BP) by rising slowly from a sitting or lying position and waiting until symptoms subside.
5. Do not take within 2 hr of meds used for erectile dysfunction due to additive BP lowering effects.
6. Record BP, weight twice a week; report excessive weight gain, low BP, dizziness or extremity swelling.
7. Report if nighttime urinary frequency increases or does not improve after 2 months of therapy.
8. Avoid OTC cold, cough, and allergy meds without provider approval.
9. Keep all F/U to assess response, labs, DRE, and for adverse SE.

OUTCOMES/EVALUATE

- Improvement in BPH symptoms
- ↓ BP

Terbinafine hydrochloride

(ter-**BIN**-ah-feen)

Classification(s): Antifungal

Pregnancy Category: B

OTC: DesenexMax, Lamisil AT.

RX: Lamisil, Terbinex.

Rx: Apo-Terbinafine, CO Terbinafine, Gen-Terbinafine, PMS-Terbinafine, Sandoz Terbinafine.

INDICATIONS/USES

Topical use: (1) Interdigital tinea pedis (athlete's foot), tinea cruris (jock itch), or tinea corporis (ringworm) due to *Epidermophyton floccosum, Trichophyton mentagrophytes,* or *T. rubrum.* (2) Plantar tinea pedis. (3) Tinea versicolor due to *Malassezia furfur. Investigational:* Cutaneous candidiasis and tinea versicolor.

Rx, Oral use: (1) Tablets: Onychomycosis of the toenail or fingernail due to dermatophytes (tinea unguium). (2) Oral Granules: Tinea capitis in those 4 years of age and older.

ACTION/KINETICS

Action

Inhibits squalene epoxidase, thus blocking the biosynthesis of ergosterol, an essential component of fungal cell membranes. Results in ergosterol deficiency and a corresponding accumulation of squalene leading to fungal cell death.

Pharmacokinetics

Approximately 75% of cutaneously absorbed drug is excreted in the urine, mostly as metabolites. Well absorbed following PO administration, with bioavailability after first-pass metabolism being about 40%. **Peak plasma levels:** 1 mcg/mL within 2 hr. Food enhances absorption. Slowly excreted from adipose tissue and skin. Inhibits CYP2D6-mediated metabolism. Extensively metabolized by CYP2C9, CYP1A2, CYP3A4, CYP2C8, and CYP2C19; about 70% of the dose eliminated in the urine. Renal or hepatic disease decreases clearance from the body. **Plasma protein binding:** More than 99%.

T

CONTRAINDICATIONS

Hypersensitivity to terbinafine or any component of the product. Ophthalmic or intravaginal use. PO use in chronic or active liver disease or renal impairment (C_{CR} less than 50 mL/min). Lactation.

SPECIAL CONCERNS

■ Rare cases of hepatic failure, some leading to death or liver transplant, have occurred with terbinafine use for the treatment of onychomycosis in those with and without preexisting liver disease. In the majority of such cases, clients had serious underlying systemic conditions and an uncertain causal relationship with terbinafine. Terbinafine is not recommended for those with chronic or active liver disease. Before prescribing, assess preexisting liver disease. Hepatotoxicity may occur in those with and without pre-existing liver disease. Pretreatment serum ALT and AST tests are advised for all those before taking terbinafine. ■

Safety and efficacy of tablets not determined in children less than 12 years of age.

SIDE EFFECTS

Most Common

Following oral use in adults: Headache, rash, diarrhea, dyspepsia, pruritus, nausea, taste disturbance.
Following oral use in children: Cough, headache, nasopharyngitis, pyrexia, URTI, vomiting.
Following topical use: Irritation, burning, itching, dryness.

Following oral use. GI: Diarrhea, dyspepsia, abdominal pain (including upper), nausea, flatulence, vomiting, taste disturbance, toothache, ***severe and fatal liver failure.*** Rarely, symptomatic idiosyncratic hepatobiliary dysfunction (including cholestatic hepatitis). **CNS:** Headache. **Dermatologic:** Rash, pruritus, urticaria, acute generalized exanthematous pustulosis, precipitation and exacerbation of cutaneous and systemic lupus erythematosus, psoriaform eruptions or exacerbation of psoriasis, ***Stevens-Johnson syndrome, toxic epidermal necrolysis.*** **Respiratory:** Nasopharyngitis, cough, nasal congestion, rhinorrhea, URTI. **Musculoskeletal:** Arthralgia, myalgia. **Ophthalmic:** Changes in ocular lens and retina. **Hematologic:** Severe neutropenia, thrombocytopenia. **Body as a whole:** Malaise, fatigue, pyrexia, influenza, infections. **Miscellaneous:** Taste disturbances/loss, hair loss, allergic reactions (including angioedema, ***anaphylaxis***).

Following topical use. Dermatologic: Irritation, burning, itching, dryness.

LABORATORY TEST CONSIDERATIONS

Liver enzyme abnormalities that are two or more times the upper limit of the normal range. ↓ Absolute neutrophil counts.

DRUG INTERACTIONS

Antiarrhythmics class type 1C (e.g. , flecainide, propafenone) / Inhibition of CYP2D6 by terbinafine may result in need for careful monitoring and dose reduction of the antiarrhythmic
Beta-blockers / ↓ Metabolism of beta-blockers by CYP2D6; possible ↑ pharmacologic and toxic effects; dose reduction may be needed
Caffeine / ↓ Clearance of caffeine
Cimetidine / Terbinafine clearance is ↓ by one-third
Cyclosporine / ↑ Cyclosporine clearance
Dextromethorphan / ↑ Dextromethorphan levels R/T ↓ liver metabolism by CYP2D6; possible dose reduction of dextromethorphan
Fluconazole / Single dose of fluconazole and terbinafine → ↑ terbinafine AUC and C_{max}
MAOIs type B / ↓ Metabolism MAOIs, type B by CYP2D6; possible ↑ pharmacologic and toxic effects
Rifampin / ↑ Terbinafine clearance (100%)
Selective serotonin reuptake inhibitors (e.g., paroxetine, venlafaxine) / ↓ Metabolism of SSRIs by CYP2D6; possible ↑ pharmacologic and toxic effects; possible dosage adjustment of SSRI
Tricyclic antidepressants (e.g., amitriptyline, desipramine, nortriptyline) / ↓ Metabolism of tricyclic antidepressants by CYP2D6; possible ↑ pharmacologic and toxic effects; possible TCA dosage adjustment
Warfarin / Possible ↑ or ↓PT

HOW SUPPLIED

Cream (OTC): 1%; ***Gel (OTC):*** 1%; ***Granules (Rx):*** 125 mg/packet, 187.5 mg/packet; ***Spray (OTC):*** 1%; ***Tablets (Rx):*** 250 mg.

DOSAGE

CREAM; GEL

Interdigital tinea pedis.

Apply to cover the affected and immediately surrounding areas twice a day for 1 week.

Tinea cruris or tinea corporis.

Apply to cover the affected and immediately surrounding areas 1–2 times per day for 1 week.

GRANULES

Tinea capitis in those 4 years and older.

Weight, less than 25 kg: 125 mg/day; **weight, 25–35 kg:** 187.5 mg/day; **weight, over 35 kg:** 250 mg/day. Give once daily for 6 weeks.

SPRAY

Tinea pedis, Tinea versicolor.

Spray twice a day for 1 week.

Tinea corporis, Tinea cruris.

Spray once daily for 1 week.

TABLETS

Onychomycosis.

Fingernail(s): One 250 mg tablet/day for 6 weeks. *Toenail(s):* One 250 mg tablet/day for 12 weeks. The optimal clinical effect is observed several months after mycologic cure and cessation of treatment due to slow period for outgrowth of healthy nails.

NURSING IMPLICATIONS

Do not confuse Lamisil with Lamictil (an anticonvulsant), lamivudine (an antiviral), labetalol (an alpha-beta adrenergic blocker), or Lomotil (an antidiarrheal).

IMPLEMENTATION/ADMINISTRATION/STORAGE

1. Avoid contact of cream with eyes, nose, mouth, or other mucous membranes.
2. Avoid occlusive dressings.
3. For topical use, many clients treated for 1–2 weeks continue to improve during the 2–4 weeks after drug therapy has been completed. Do not consider clients therapeutic failures until they have been observed for a period of 2–4 weeks off therapy.
4. Store the cream between 5–30°C (41–86°F). Protect tablets from light; store below 25°C (77°F). Store granules from 15–30°C (59–86°F).

ASSESSMENT

1. Describe clinical presentation; note location, onset, duration, and characteristics of symptoms. Assess for any depressive symptoms.
2. If presentation unclear, use infected tissue scrapings to confirm diagnosis.
3. Note any changes in sense of taste or smell or skin reactions.

4. Monitor CBC, AST, and ALT; note any liver or renal dysfunction and avoid therapy if evident.

CLIENT/FAMILY TEACHING

1. Drug used to treat fungal infections in those with no liver or renal dysfunction.
2. Cream for topical dermatologic use only; review application method.
3. Wash hands before and after topical application. Use a clean towel and washcloth; avoid sharing.
4. Avoid contact of cream with mouth, nose, eyes, and other mucous membranes; do not cover treated areas with occlusive dressing.
5. Sprinkle granules onto a spoonful of pudding, mashed potato, or other soft non-acidic food; swallow the entire spoonful without chewing. Do not use applesauce or fruit-based foods. If 2 packets (250 mg) are required for each dose, the contents of both packets can be sprinkled on 1 or 2 spoonfuls of nonacidic food. To be taken once a day for 6 weeks. Dosage is based on child weight for fungal infection of the scalp, in children ages 4 years and older.
6. Take tablets with food to ensure maximal absorption.
7. Report symptoms of increased irritation or possible sensitization such as redness, itching, burning, blistering, swelling, oozing, or rash. Also report persistent nausea, vomiting, right upper abdominal pain, fatigue, anorexia, dark urine, yellowing of the skin or eyes.
8. Use for prescribed time; do not skip or double up on doses.
9. Continued improvement in skin condition and/or mycotic nails may be noted for 2-4 weeks after therapy. Takes up to 6 weeks for fingernails and 12 weeks for toenail treatment.
10. Avoid OTC agents without provider approval during therapy.
11. Keep all F/U visits to assess response, labs, and adverse SE.

OUTCOMES/EVALUATE

- Improvement in dermatologic condition
- Clearing/healing of mycotic nail beds
- Resolution of fungal infection of scalp

Terbutaline sulfate

(ter-**BYOU**-tah-leen)

Classification(s): Sympathomimetic, direct-acting

Pregnancy Category: C

SEE ALSO ***SYMPATHOMIMETIC DRUGS***.

INDICATIONS/USES

Prophylaxis and treatment of bronchospasm in clients 12 years and older with asthma and reversible bronchospasms associated with bronchitis and emphysema. *Investigational:* PO: Premature labor (poor documentation). SC: Asthma in children 12 years and younger, premature labor.

ACTION/KINETICS

Action

Specific beta-2 receptor stimulant, resulting in bronchodilation and relaxation of peripheral vasculature. Minimal beta-1 activity. Action resembles that of isoproterenol.

Pharmacokinetics

PO, Onset: 30 min; **maximum effect:** 2–3 hr; **duration:** 4–8 hr. **SC, Onset:** 5–15 min; **maximum effect:** 30 min–1 hr; **duration:** 1.5–4 hr.

CONTRAINDICATIONS

PO or SC use not recommended for use in children less than 12 years of age. PO for acute or maintenance tocolysis. Injections for tocolysis for more than 48–72 hr. Lactation.

SPECIAL CONCERNS

Prolonged tocolysis. Terbutaline has not been approved and should not be used for acute or maintenance tocolysis. In particular, do not use terbutaline for maintenance tocolysis in the outpatient or home setting. Serious adverse reactions, including death, have been reported after administration of terbutaline to pregnant women. In mothers, these adverse reactions include increased heart rate, transient hyperglycemia, hypokalemia, cardiac arrhythmias, pulmonary edema, and myocardial ischemia. Increased fetal heart rate and neonatal hypoglycemia may occur as a result of maternal administration.

Large IV doses may aggravate preexisting diabetes and ketoacidosis.

SIDE EFFECTS

Most Common

Palpitations, tremor, dizziness/vertigo, nervousness/tension, N&V, PVCs/arrhythmias, drowsiness, headache.

See *Sympathomimetic Drugs* for a complete list of possible side effects. Also, **GI:** Heartburn, GI distress/disorder, N&V, dry mouth. **CV:** PVCs (arrhythmias, missed beats), BP changes, hypertension, ECG changes (e.g., atrial premature beats, ventricular premature beats, ventricular extrasystoles, AV block, sinus pause, ST-T wave depression, T-wave inversion, sinus bradycardia, atrial escape beat with aberrant conduction), tachycardia, chest tightness/pain/discomfort, angina, vasodilation, palpitations. **CNS:** Stimulation, anxiety, dizziness, vertigo, drowsiness, hallucinations, headache, insomnia, paresthesia, shakiness, nervousness, somnolence, tension, tremor, weakness, ***seizures***. **Respiratory**: Wheezing, dyspnea, throat dryness/irritation, pharyngitis. **Dermatologic:** Flushing, sweating. **Body as a whole:** Weakness, asthenia, hypertonia. **Miscellaneous**: ***Hypersensitivity reactions*** (including vasculitis, angioedema, bronchospasm, rash, urticaria), bad taste or taste change, muscle cramps, pain at injection site, elevation in liver enzymes, aggravation of diabetes (IV use).

LABORATORY TEST CONSIDERATIONS

↑ Liver enzymes. Hypokalemia.

HOW SUPPLIED

Injection: 1 mg/mL; *Tablets:* 2.5 mg, 5 mg.

DOSAGE

TABLETS

Asthma/Bronchospasms.

Adults and children over 15 years: 5 mg 3 times per day q 6 hr during waking hours, not to exceed 15 mg q 24 hr. If disturbing side effects are observed, dose can be reduced to 2.5 mg 3 times per day without loss of beneficial effects. Anticipate use of other therapeutic measures if client fails to respond after second dose. **Children 12–15 years:** 2.5 mg 3 times per day, not to exceed 7.5 mg q 24 hr.

Asthma/Bronchospasm in children 12 years and younger (investigational).

Children, 12 years and younger, initial: 0.05 mg/kg per dose q 8 hr; may increase dose if needed, up to a maximum of 5 mg/day or 0.15 mg/kg per dose q 8 hr.

SC ONLY

Asthma/Bronchospasm.

Adults and children 12 years and older: 0.25 mg SC. May be repeated 1 time after 15–30 min if no significant clinical improvement is noted. If client does not respond to the second dose, undertake other measures. Do not exceed a dose of 0.5 mg over 4 hr.

Asthma/Bronchospasm in children 12 years and younger (investigational).

Children, 12 years and younger, usual: 0.01 mg/kg per dose q 20 min as for 3 doses; **then** give q 2–6 hr as needed. **Maximum:** 0.4 mg per dose.

Premature labor (investigational).

Adults, initial: 0.25 mg q 20 min–3 hr. Hold the dose if the pulse exceeds 120 beats/min. Dose can be continued for a maximum of 48 hr. There are safety concerns with this dose.

NURSING IMPLICATIONS

Do not confuse terbutaline with terbinafine (antifungal) or tolbutamide (an oral hypoglycemic).

IMPLEMENTATION/ADMINISTRATION/STORAGE

1. Do not use ampules for IV use.
2. Inject SC into the lateral deltoid area.
3. Discard unused portion after single client use.
4. Do not use if solution is discolored.
5. Do not use for more than 3 days to prevent premature birth.
6. Store tablets from 15–30°C (59–86°F) protected from light. Store the injection from 20–25°C (68–77°F); protect from light by storing in original container until use.

ASSESSMENT

1. List type, onset, characteristics of S&S. Note triggers, other agents trialed.
2. Auscultate and document lung assessments, CXR, and PFTs. Observe for evidence of drug tolerance and rebound bronchospasm as well

T

as significant CV effects (BP, HR, and ECG changes).

3. Do not use terbutaline for maintenance tocolysis in the outpatient setting. Serious adverse reactions, including death, have been reported after administration to pregnant women. These adverse reactions include increased heart rate, transient hyperglycemia, hypokalemia, cardiac arrhythmias, pulmonary edema, and MI. Increased fetal heart rate and neonatal hypoglycemia may also occur.
4. Note VS, K^+, and ECG. Monitor lung sounds and LFTs.

CLIENT/FAMILY TEACHING

1. Take oral medication with meals to minimize GI upset.
2. Review and demonstrate appropriate method for administration. Review use of spacer to administer therapy and peak flow meter to assess response to therapy.
3. May use analgesic to relieve headache; use deltoid area for injections and, if bronchospasm occurs with inhalation therapy, report immediately.
4. Increase fluid intake to help liquefy secretions.
5. Report if chest pain, dizziness or headache, palpitations, or persisting symptoms of asthma continue with therapy.
6. Keep all F/U to assess response, labs, and for adverse SE.

OUTCOMES/EVALUATE

- Improved airway exchange
- Inhibition of uterine contractions (UL)

Terconazole nitrate

(ter-**KON**-ah-zohl)

Classification(s): Antifungal

Pregnancy Category: C

RX: Terazol 3, Terazol 7, Zazole.

✤ **Rx:** Tero-Terconazole.

INDICATIONS/USES

Vulvovaginitis caused by *Candida.* Ineffective in infections due to *Trichomonas* or *Haemophilus vaginalis.*

ACTION/KINETICS

Action

May exert its antifungal activity by disrupting cell membrane permeability, leading to loss of essential intracellular materials. Also inhibits synthesis of triglycerides and phospholipids, as well as inhibiting oxidative and peroxidative enzyme activity. When used for *Candida,* terconazole inhibits transformation of blastospores into the invasive mycelial form.

SPECIAL CONCERNS

- Consider discontinuing breastfeeding or the drug.
- Safety and efficacy not established in children.

SIDE EFFECTS

Most Common

Headache, dysmenorrhea, pain of the female genitalia, abdominal pain, vulvovaginal burning/irritation.

GU: Vulvovaginal burning, irritation, or itching; dysmenorrhea, pain of the female genitalia. **Miscellaneous:** Headache, body pain, photosensitivity, abdominal pain, chills, fever.

HOW SUPPLIED

Vaginal Cream: 0.4%, 0.8%; *Vaginal Suppositories:* 80 mg.

DOSAGE

VAGINAL CREAM

Vulvovaginitis due to Candida.

One applicator full (5 grams) intravaginally, once daily at bedtime for 7 consecutive days for the 0.4% cream and for 3 consecutive days for the 0.8% cream.

VAGINAL SUPPOSITORIES

Vulvovaginitis due to Candida.

One 80-mg suppository once daily at bedtime for 3 consecutive days.

NURSING IMPLICATIONS

ASSESSMENT

1. Note indications for therapy, onset, and characteristics of S&S; identify other agents trialed and outcome.
2. Obtain a thorough nursing history because recurrent candidiasis may be caused by oral

contraceptives, antibiotics, or diabetes, whereas intractable candidiasis may be the result of undetected diabetes mellitus or reinfection.
3. Prior to a second course of therapy, the diagnosis should be confirmed to rule out other pathogens associated with vulvovaginitis. KOH smear and/or cultures may be indicated with lack of response.

CLIENT/FAMILY TEACHING

1. Review the appropriate method for administration and cleansing (the cream should be inserted high into the vagina using the applicator). After suppositories administered, remain lying down for 30 min. Avoid douches during therapy. Wash hands before and after administration. Wash applicator in warm soapy water and rinse well.
2. Discontinue use and report if any burning, irritation, fever, chills, or pain occurs.
3. May stain clothes; use sanitary napkins during therapy and change frequently because damp sanitary napkins may harbor infecting organisms.
4. Cleanse external genitalia and avoid use of douches, tampons, or other vaginal OTC products while using the medication.
5. To avoid reinfection, refrain from sexual intercourse. Advise partner to use a condom as medication may also irritate partner.
6. May interact with latex and weaken latex condoms and diaphragms. Avoid these for 72 hr after application of medication.
7. Use for prescribed time frame even if symptoms subside. Report if infection recurs as cause needs to be determined.
8. Effect not affected by menses. Thus, continue to use during menses to ensure a full course of therapy.
9. Keep all F/U to assess response, labs, and for adverse SE.

OUTCOMES/EVALUATE

Resolution of fungal infections; symptomatic improvement

Tesamorelin

(tes-a-moe-**REL**-in)

Classification(s): Growth hormone releasing factor

Pregnancy Category: X

RX: Egrifta.

INDICATIONS/USES

Reduction of excess abdominal fat in HIV-infected clients with lipodystrophy.

ACTION/KINETICS

Action

Tesamorelin is an analog of human growth hormone-releasing factor (GHRH). GHRH acts on the pituitary somatotroph cells to stimulate the synthesis and pulsatile release of endogenous growth hormone which is both anabolic and lipolytic. By being lipolytic, excess abdominal fat is reduced.

Pharmacokinetics

Absolute bioavailability after 2 mg SC is <4% when tested in healthy subjects. **T_{max}:** 0.15 hr. **t½, mean elimination:** 26 min in healthy subjects and 38 min in HIV-infected clients after SC use for 14 days.

CONTRAINDICATIONS

Known hypersensitivity to tesamorelin and/or mannitol. Disruption of the hypothalamic-pituitary axis due to hypophysectomy, hypopituitarism, pituitary tumor/surgery, head irradiation, or head trauma. Use in children with open epiphyses because excess growth hormone and IGF-1 may result in linear growth acceleration and excessive growth. Active malignancy (newly diagnosed or recurrent). Pregnancy. Lactation.

SPECIAL CONCERNS

- Several side effects are due to the effect of growth hormone.
- Safety and efficacy not determined in children.

SIDE EFFECTS

Most Common

Hypersensitivity (rash, urticaria), arthralgia, carpal tunnel syndrome, extremity pain, hyperglycemia, peripheral edema, injection site reactions (erythema, irritation, pain, pruritus, swelling, urticaria, hemorrhage).

CNS: Hypesthesia, paresthesia, depression, insomnia, peripheral neuropathy. **GI:** N&V, dyspepsia, upper abdominal pain. **CV:** Hypertension, palpitations. **Dermatologic:** Pruritus, rash, hot flush, night sweats, urticaria. **Musculoskeletal:**

T

Arthralgia, carpal tunnel syndrome, extremity pain, joint stiffness/swelling, muscle spasms/strain, musculoskeletal pain/stiffness, myalgia. **Metabolic:** Hyperglycemia, glucose intolerance, increased risk to develop diabetes. **Injection site reactions:** Erythema, irritation, pain, pruritus, rash, swelling, urticaria, hemorrhage. **Hypersensitivity:** Rash, urticaria, erythema, flushing, pruritus. **Body as a whole:** Peripheral edema, pain, chest pain, fluid retention. **Miscellaneous:** Immunogenicity. Increased mortality in those with acute critical illness due to complications following open heart surgery, abdominal surgery, multiple accidental trauma, or those with acute respiratory failure

LABORATORY TEST CONSIDERATIONS

↑ IGF, blood creatine phosphokinase, HbA_{1c}

DRUG INTERACTIONS

Cortisone acetate / ↓ Conversion to biologically active metabolites R/T inhibition of the enzyme required for conversion; possibly ↑ maintenance or stress doses

Prednisone / ↓ Conversion to biologically active metabolites R/T inhibition of the enzyme required for conversion; possibly ↑ maintenance or stress doses

Ritonavir / ↓ Ritonavir AUC and C_{max}; extent of decrease not likely to be clinically important

Simvastatin / ↓ Simvastatin absorption; extent of decrease not likely to be clinically important

HOW SUPPLIED

Injection, Lyophilized Powder for Solution: 1 mg.

DOSAGE

SC

Lipodystrophy in HIV-infected clients.

Adults: 2 mg once a day.

NURSING IMPLICATIONS

IMPLEMENTATION/ADMINISTRATION/STORAGE

1. To prepare for administration, place the 1½ inch 18-gauge needle with its protective cap in place onto the syringe. Insert 2.2 mL of sterile water into the tesamorelin vial. Push the plunger slowly on a slight angle so water goes down the inside of the vial instead of directly onto the powder (i.e., to avoid foaming). While keeping the syringe with the needle attached in the vial and the vial upright, roll the vial gently for 30 seconds, until the sterile water and tesamorelin powder are well mixed. Do not shake the vial. Remove all of the liquid inside the vial (i.e., 2.2 mL).
2. Administer SC in the abdomen immediately after reconstitution. Rotate injection sites to different areas of the abdomen. Do not inject into scar tissue, bruises, or the navel.
3. Discard the reconstituted solution if it is not used immediately. Do not freeze or refrigerate the reconstituted solution.
4. Store unreconstituted vials from 2–8°C (36–46°F). Store the diluent, syringes, and needles from 20–25°C (68–77°F). Protect from light. Keep in the original box until use.

ASSESSMENT

1. Note number of years with disease, clinical presentation, measurements of hips and abdomen, and confirmation that visceral adipose tissue is unresponsive to exercise.
2. Determine any evidence of active malignancy, head trauma, head radiation, hypopituitarism, or pituitary tumor/surgery history; may preclude drug therapy.
3. Monitor eye exams, BP, CBC, HbA1c, CPK; also monitor insulin-like growth factor 1 (IGF-1) levels closely. Evaluate glucose status prior to initiating therapy and regularly during therapy. Those with diabetes require more rigid monitoring. Data concerning abdominal circumference or adiposity by CT should be documented regularly.

CLIENT/FAMILY TEACHING

1. After instruction, administer SC once a day in the stomach (avoid scar tissues, bruised and navel areas) as directed. Used to reduce excess abdominal fat in those with HIV; contains growth hormone-releasing factor (GRF).
2. May notice injection-site reactions, including bruising, erythema, irritation, pain, and pruritus. To reduce the incidence of injection-site reactions, rotate site of injections. Never share needles or syringes; use appropriate containers to discard.
3. Therapy may cause symptoms consistent with fluid retention, including arthralgia, carpal tunnel syndrome, and edema; report if evident.

4. Practice reliable contraception; stop drug and notify provider if pregnancy occurs. Do not breast-feed during therapy.
5. Report immediately any generalized rash, hives, trouble breathing, chest pain, or swelling of throat.
6. For additional information about this drug, go to www.EGRIFTA.com or contact AXIS Center toll-free at 1-877-714-2947.
7. Keep all F/U visits to access response, labs, and for adverse SE.

OUTCOMES/EVALUATE

↓ Abdominal visceral fat by circumference measurement/CT evaluation

Testosterone buccal system

(tess-**TOSS**-ter-ohn)

Classification(s): Androgen, naturally-occurring

Pregnancy Category: X

RX: Striant.

Testosterone cypionate in oil

Pregnancy Category: X

RX: Depo-Testosterone, **C-III**

Testosterone enanthate in oil

Pregnancy Category: X

RX: Delatestryl, **C-III**

Testosterone gel/solution

Pregnancy Category: X

RX: AndroGel 1% and 1.62%, Axiron, Fortesta, Testim, **C-III**

Testosterone pellets

Pregnancy Category: X

RX: Testopel, **C-III**

Testosterone transdermal system

Pregnancy Category: X

RX: Androderm, **C-III**

INDICATIONS/USES

Parenteral: (1) Replacement therapy in males due to conditions associated with symptoms of deficiency or absence of endogenous testosterone. (2) Primary or acquired congenital hypogonadism: testicular failure due to cryptorchidism, bilateral torsion, orchitis, vanishing testis syndrome, or orchidectomy. (3) Congenital or acquired hypogonadotropic hypogonadism: idiopathic gonadotropin or LHRH deficiency, or pituitary-hypothalamic injury from tumors, trauma, or radiation. (4) Delayed puberty (use testosterone enanthate only). (5) Metastatic mammary cancer in females (use testosterone enanthate only) who are 1–5 years postmenopausal.

Buccal/Gel/Solution/Transdermal: (1) Congenital or acquired primary hypogonadism. (2) Congenital or acquired hypogonadotropic hypogonadism.

Pellets: (1) Congenital or acquired primary hypogonadism. (2) Congenital or acquired hypogonadotropic hypogonadism. (3) Stimulation of puberty in carefully selected males with clearly delayed puberty.

ACTION/KINETICS

Action

Testosterone, the primary male androgen, is produced naturally by the Leydig cells of the testes. In many tissues, the action of testosterone is due to the active metabolite, dihydrotestosterone, which binds to cytosol receptors. The steroid-receptor complex is transported to the nucleus where it initiates transcription and other cellular changes. Exogenous testosterone administration results in inhibition of endogenous testosterone release due to negative feedback of pituitary LH. Large doses of exogenous testosterone may suppress spermatogenesis through feedback inhibition of pituitary FSH.

Pharmacokinetics

Oral testosterone is metabolized in the gut and 44% is cleared by the liver in the first pass. Thus, the parenteral, transdermal, and gel forms are used. Testosterone esters (cypionate or enanthate) are slowly absorbed after IM use. The t½ of testosterone varies over a wide range (10–100 min). **t½, testosterone cypionate after IM:** 8 days. Following use of the transdermal product to nonscrotal

T

skin, there is continual absorption over 24 hr. **Peak levels after transdermal:** 2–4 hr. Ninety percent is excreted through the urine as metabolites and 6% is excreted through the feces. **Plasma protein binding:** About 98%.

CONTRAINDICATIONS

Hypersensitivity to the drug or any component of the product. Serious renal, hepatic, or cardiac disease due to edema formation. Known or suspected prostatic or breast carcinoma in males. Use in pregnancy (masculinization of female fetus) and lactation. Discontinue if hypercalcemia occurs. Use of testosterone cypionate interchangeably with testosterone propionate (due to differences in duration of action).

SPECIAL CONCERNS

(1) Virilization has been reported in children who were secondarily exposed to transdermal testosterone. (2) Children should avoid contact with unwashed or unclothed application sites in men using transdermal testosterone. (3) Advise clients to strictly adhere to recommended instructions for use.

- **Prolonged use of high doses is associated with development of potentially life-threatening peliosis hepatitis, hepatic neoplasms, cholestatic hepatitis, jaundice, and hepatocellular carcinoma.**
- **Use with caution in young males who have not completed their growth (because of premature epiphyseal closure).**
- **Androgens may cause virilization in females or precocious sexual development in males.**
- **Elderly may manifest an increased risk of prostatic hypertrophy or prostatic carcinoma.**
- **Androgen therapy occasionally seems to accelerate metastatic breast carcinoma in women.**
- **Use of the gel not evaluated in women.**
- **Testosterone products are not safe and effective to enhance athletic performance and have the potential for serious side effects.**
- **Use with caution in children and prescribed only by those aware of the side effects on bone maturation.**

SIDE EFFECTS

Most Common

When used systemically or by implant: Headache, anxiety, depression, generalized paresthesia, acne, hirsutism, nausea, cholestatic jaundice, libido increased/decreased.

When used transdermally: Pruritus, application site itching/erythema, headache, dizziness/vertigo, burn-like blister under system.

Hepatic: Liver toxicity is the most serious side effect. Jaundice, cholestasis, alterations in BSP retention, AST, and ALT. Rarely, ***hepatic necrosis, hepatocellular neoplasms***, peliosis hepatitis, acute intermittent porphyria in clients with this disease. **GI:** N&V, diarrhea, anorexia, symptoms of peptic ulcer, dry mouth, abdominal pain, GI bleeding, increased appetite, stomatitis. **CNS:** Headache, pain, memory loss, nervousness, depression, dizziness, vertigo, anxiety, increased or decreased libido, insomnia, excitation, paresthesias, sleep apnea syndrome, personality disorder, CNS stimulation, generalized paresthesia, emotional lability, amnesia, hostility, thinking abnormalities, ***CNS hemorrhage***, choreiform movements, habituation, confusion (toxic doses). **CV:** Edema with or without CHF, hypertension, tachycardia, ***stroke***, deep vein phlebitis, vasodilation. **GU:** Testicular atrophy with inhibition of testicular function (e.g., oligospermia), impotence, abnormal ejaculation, breast pain/tenderness, dysuria, UTI, prostatitis, impaired urination, frequent erections, scrotal cellulitis, BPH, rectal mucosal lesion over prostate, hematuria, bladder cancer, papilloma on scrotum, prostate/testes/penis disorder, pelvic pain, incontinence, epididymitis, irritable bladder, prepubertal phallic enlargement, gynecomastia, priapism or excessive sexual stimulation, urethral obstruction in those with benign prostatic hypertrophy, hypercalcemia in breast cancer. **Dermatologic:** For transdermal products application site: itching, erythema, discomfort, irritation, pruritus, burning sensation, rash, burn-like blister under the system. Acne, alopecia, male pattern baldness, hirsutism, injection site pain/inflammation, seborrhea, discolored hair, dry skin. **Musculoskeletal:** Myalgia, back pain, arthralgia, muscle cramps. **Electrolyte:** Retention of sodium, chloride, calcium, potassium, phosphates. **Metabolic:** Hyperglycemia, hyperlipidemia, hyponatremia, electrolyte imbalance, hypercholesterolemia. **Hematologic:** Suppression of clotting factors (II, V, VII, X), polycythemia, leukopenia. **Body as a whole:** Flu syndrome, asthenia, fatigue, chills, infection, accelerated growth, sweating, ***anaphylaxis (rare).*** **Miscellaneous:** Flushing, accidental injury, papillary dilation, bronchitis. Hypercalcemia, especially in immobilized clients or those with metastatic breast carcinoma. Virilization in women.

In females: Menstrual irregularities (including amenorrhea), virilization, clitoral enlargement, hirsutism, increased libido, baldness (male pattern), virilization of external genitalia of female fetus.

In males: Decreased ejaculatory volume, oligospermia (high doses), gynecomastia, increased frequency and duration of penile erections.

In children: Disturbances of growth, premature closure of epiphyses, precocious sexual development. Inflammation and pain at site of IM or SC injection.

NOTE: Side effects of the cypionate and enanthate products are not readily reversible due to the long duration of action of these dosage forms. The patch may cause itching, irritation, erythema, or discomfort on skin areas where applied (Androderm). Potentially, small amounts of testosterone may be transferred to a sex partner.

LABORATORY TEST CONSIDERATIONS

Altered thyroid function tests, including ↓ levels of throxine-binding globulin causing decreased total T_4 serum levels and ↑ resin uptake of T_3 and T_4. False + or ↑ BSP, alkaline phosphatase, bilirubin, cholesterol, and acid phosphatase (in women). Alteration of glucose tolerance tests.

DRUG INTERACTIONS

Anticoagulants, oral / ↑ Anticoagulant effect
Antidiabetic agents / Additive hypoglycemia
Barbiturates / ↓ Androgenic effect R/T ↑ breakdown by liver
Corticosteroids, ACTH / ↑ Chance of edema; use together cautiously
Insulin / In diabetics, ↓ blood glucose → ↓ insulin requirements
Propranolol / ↑ Propranolol clearance if used with testosterone cypionate
H ***Saw palmetto*** / Antiandrogenic effect may ↓ testosterone activity

HOW SUPPLIED

Testosterone buccal system: 30 mg.
Testosterone cypionate in oil: ***Injection:*** 100 mg/mL, 200 mg/mL.
Testosterone enanthate: ***Injection:*** 200 mg/mL.
Testosterone gel/solution: ***Gel:*** *AndroGel:* 1% (50 mg) in packets or metered pumps and 1.62% (20.25 mg) in metered–dose pumps. *Testim:* 1% (50 mg) in unit–dose tubes. *Fortesta:* 10 mg/0.5 gram in metered–dose pumps; ***Solution:*** *Axiron:* 30 mg/1.5 mL in metered–dose pumps.
Testosterone pellets: ***Pellets:*** 75 mg.
Testosterone transdermal system: ***Patch, Extended-Release:*** *Androderm:* 2.5 mg/24 hr, 5 mg/24 hr.

DOSAGE

Testosterone cypionate.

IM ONLY

Male hypogonadism, replacement therapy.

Individualize depending on age, gender, and diagnosis. Adjust dosage based on client response. **Usual:** 50–400 mg q 2–4 weeks.

Testosterone enanthate

IM ONLY

Male hypogonadism.

Individualize depending on age, gender, and diagnosis. Adjust dosage based on client response. **Usual:** 50–400 mg q 2–4 weeks.

Males with delayed puberty.

Various dosage regimens have been used. Take into consideration the chronological and skeletal ages, both for the initial dose and any dosage adjustment. **Usual:** 50–200 mg q 2–4 weeks for a limited duration (e.g., 4–6 months). Take x-rays at appropriate intervals to determine amount of bone maturation and skeletal development.

Palliation of inoperable mammary cancer in women.

Usual: 200–400 mg q 2–4 weeks.

TESTOSTERONE BUCCAL SYSTEM

Primary hypogonadism, hypogonadotropic hypogonadism.

Apply 1 buccal system (30 mg) to the gum region twice a day, morning and evening (i.e., about 12 hr apart).

TESTOSTERONE GEL

Primary hypogonadism (congenital or acquired), hypogonadotropic hypogonadism.

AndroGel, Testim (Topical Gel, 1%). Adults, initial: 5 grams (to deliver 50 mg testosterone) applied once a day (preferable in the morning) to a clean, dry, intact skin of the shoulders and/or

T

upper arms. AndroGel may also be applied to the abdomen. Measure serum testosterone levels 14 days after initiation of therapy to ensure proper dosing. If the serum testosterone level is below the normal range, or if the desired clinical response is not achieved, the dose may be increased from 5 grams to 7.5 grams of AndroGel or 5 to 10 grams of Testim. If the serum testosterone level consistently exceeds the normal range at a daily dose of 5 grams, discontinue therapy.

AndroGel (Topical Gel, 1.62%). Adults, initial: 40.5 mg (2 pump actuations) applied topically once a day in the morning to the shoulders and upper arms. The dose can be adjusted between a minimum of 20.25 mg of testosterone (1 pump actuation) and a maximum of 81 mg (4 pump actuations). To ensure proper dosing, titrate the dose based on the pre–dose testosterone level from a single blood draw at about 14 and 28 days after starting treatment or following dose adjustment. Thereafter, assess serum testosterone levels periodically.

Fortesta (Topical Gel, 10 mg/0.5 gram). Adults, initial: 40 mg (4 pump actuations) applied once daily to the thighs in the morning. To ensure proper dosing, titrate the dose based on the serum testosterone level from a single blood draw 2 hr after applying testosterone and at approximately 14 days and 35 days after starting treatment or following dose adjustment. Thereafter, assess testosterone levels periodically.

TESTOSTERONE PELLETS

Replacement therapy.

Usual: 150–450 mg SC q 3–6 months.

Delayed puberty.

Often a lower dose range is used than for replacement and for a limited time duration (e.g., 4–6 months). The number of pellets to be implanted for all uses depends on the minimum daily requirement of testosterone determined by a gradual reduction of the amount given parenterally. The usual ratio is to implant two 75 mg pellets for each 25 mg testosterone propionate required weekly. About one-third of the material is absorbed during the first month, one-fourth the second month, and one-sixth the third month.

TESTOSTERONE TRANSDERMAL SYSTEM

Replacement therapy (congenital or acquired primary hypogonadism, congenital or acquired hypogonadotropic hypogonadism).

Androderm: **Initial dose, usual:** One 5-mg system or two 2.5-mg systems applied nightly for 24 hr providing a total dose of 5 mg/day. The systems are applied to a clean, dry area of the skin on the back, abdomen, upper arms, or thighs. Do not apply to the scrotum. *NOTE:* For the nonvirilized client, dosing may be started with one 2.5 mg system applied nightly.

TESTOSTERONE SOLUTION

Primary hypogonadism, hypogonadotropic hypogonadism.

Axiron (30 mg/1.5 mL). Adults, initial: 60 mg (2 pump actuations) applied once daily. Measure serum testosterone after initial of therapy to ensure the desired levels (300–1,050 nanograms/dL are achieved. Adjust the dose based on the serum testosterone level from a single blood draw 2–8 hr after application and at least 14 days after starting treatment or following dose adjustment. If the measured serum testosterone level is below 300 ng/dL, the daily testosterone dose may be increased from 60 mg (2 pump actuations) to 90 mg (3 pump actuations) or from 90 mg to 120 mg (4 pump actuations). If the serum testosterone level exceeds 1,050 ng/dL, decrease the daily testosterone dose from 60 mg (2 pump actuations) to 30 mg (1 pump actuation). If the serum testosterone level consistently exceeds 1,050 ng/dL at the lowest daily dose of 30 mg (1 pump actuation), discontinue therapy.

NURSING IMPLICATIONS

Do not confuse testosterone with testolactone (antineoplastic drug).

IMPLEMENTATION/ADMINISTRATION/STORAGE

1. Dosage of testosterone varies depending on the age and diagnosis of the client. Dosage is adjusted depending on client response and side effects.
2. The following information is applicable to testosterone cypionate and/or testosterone enanthate:
   - Do not use testosterone enanthate interchangeably with testosterone cypionate R/T differences in duration of action.
   - Redissolve crystals of testosterone enanthate or cypionate by warming and shaking the vial.
   - If needle or syringe is wet, product may become cloudy; this does not affect potency.
   - Warm unopened vial in warm water to decrease the viscosity of the oil. Vigorously rotate vial to resuspend drug in the oil. A film may appear on the sides of the vial. When no more suspended particles are observed on the bottom or sides of the vial, the drug has been suspended appropriately. Administer deep into the muscle; give slowly.
   - Continue therapy for at least 2 months for satisfactory response and 5 months for objective response.
   - When used for delayed puberty, consider the chronological and skeletal ages when determining initial and subsequent doses. Use is for a limited time (e.g., 4–6 months).
3. The following information is applicable to testosterone buccal:
   - Place buccal product in a comfortable position just above the incisor tooth on either side of the mouth. With each application, rotate to alternate sides of the mouth.
   - After opening the packet, place the rounded side surface of the buccal system against the gum and hold firmly in place with a finger over the lip and against the product for 30 seconds to ensure adhesion. The system is designed to stay in place until removed.
   - If the buccal system fails to adhere to the gum or should fall out of position within 4 hr before the next dose, apply a new buccal system; it may remain in place until the time of the next regularly scheduled dosing.
   - Take care to avoid dislodging the buccal system and check to see that it is still in place following toothbrushing, use of mouthwash, or consumption of food/beverages.
   - Do not chew or swallow the buccal system.
   - To remove the system, gently slide it downwards from the gum toward the tooth to avoid scratching the gum.
   - Store from 20–25°C (68–77°F). Protect from light and moisture. Dispose buccal systems in a manner that prevents accidental application or ingestion by children or pets.
4. The following information is applicable to testosterone gel:
   - Do not apply gel to the genitals.
   - Check the package insert for the various gel/solution products for appropriate application procedures.
   - After applying the gel, wait 5–6 hr or more before showering or swimming.
   - Testosterone from the gel will be transferred from males to female partners. Washing the area of contact on the other person as soon as possible with soap and water will remove residual testosterone from the skin surface.
5. The following information is applicable to testosterone pellets:
   - Pellet implantation is much less flexible for dosage adjustment compared with PO or IM use. Use great care when estimating the amount of testosterone pellets needed. If complications arise where testosterone should be discontinued, the pellets would have to be removed surgically.
   - Pellets are fat soluble and are implanted SC. In most men, an area on the anterior abdominal wall is selected 1 inch medial to the anterior superior iliac spine, avoiding previous scars. An area on either buttocks may also be chosen so that implantation is made beneath the external gluteus muscle.
   - Clean the skin with an antiseptic product and then anesthetize with 2–3 mL of local anesthetic. Some health care providers use

T

an epinephrine solution to ensure minimal capillary bleeding.
- Store testosterone pellets in a cool place.

6. The following information is applicable to *Androderm* transdermal system:
   - Do not apply the Androderm patch to bony areas such as the shoulders or hips; it is *not* to be applied to the scrotum.
   - Sites of application should be rotated, with an interval of 7 days between applications to the same site. Areas should not be oily, damaged, or irritated.
   - The system does not have to be removed during sexual intercourse or while taking a shower or bath.
   - Apply Androderm immediately after opening the pouch and removing protective liner. Press the system firmly in place, making sure there is good contact with the skin, especially around the edges of the patch.
   - To ensure proper dosing, measure the morning serum testosterone concentration following system application the night before. If the serum level is outside the normal range, repeat sampling making sure of proper system adhesion, as well as proper application time. Confirmed serum levels outside the normal range may require increasing the daily dose to 7.5 mg or decreasing the dose to 2.5 mg.
   - Skin irritation may be treated with over-the-counter topical hydrocortisone cream applied after system removal. Also, applying a small amount of triamcinolone acetonide 0.1% cream to the skin under the central drug reservoir of the transdermal system reduces the incidence and severity of skin irritation and does not affect transdermal absorption of testosterone.
   - Store from 15–30°C (59–86°F).
7. For transdermal products, do not use damaged patches. Excessive heat or pressure can cause drug reservoir to burst. Discard systems safely to prevent accidental application or ingestion by children, pets, or others.
8. Due to variability in analytical values among various diagnostic labs, have testosterone levels analyzed at the same lab so results can be compared more easily.

ASSESSMENT

1. Note reasons for therapy, type, onset, characteristics of S&S, and form prescribed.
2. Assess for any cardiac, renal, or hepatic dysfunction. List neurologic status, BP, respirations, heart sounds, and GU function.
3. Note hair distribution and skin texture.
4. Monitor for signs of mental depression such as insomnia, lack of interest in personal appearance, and withdrawal from social contacts.
5. Auscultate lung sounds and note any JVD. Report edema, as sodium retention and edema can be easily treated with diuretics.
6. Assess for relaxation of the skeletal muscles and pain deep in the bones. The discomfort in the bones is caused by a honeycombing; often caused by increased calcium levels. Flank pain may be caused by kidney stones from excessively high serum calcium levels. Administer large amounts of fluids to prevent renal calculi. If hypercalcemia is the result of metastases, initiate other appropriate therapy.
7. With a child, monitor closely for growth retardation and development of precocious puberty. Use with caution as the effect on the CNS in developing children is still being explored.
   - Review therapy with parents; often intermittent to allow for periods of normal bone growth.
   - Regular x-rays to monitor bone maturation and effects on epiphyseal centers; obtain q 6 months.
   - Record height/weight regularly.
8. If female, report the signs of virilization, (except in those with gender disorder requesting such changes) such as deepening of the voice, hirsuitism, acne, menstrual irregularity, and clitoral enlargement. Usually only evident with doses exceeding 200–300 mg/month. Increased libido in females may be early sign of drug toxicity.
9. Check prescribed medications for any drugs that may interact unfavorably (i.e., anticoagulants, hypoglycemic agents, and mineralocorticoids).
10. If prescribed high doses, periodically check H&H for evidence of polycythemia.
11. Treatment with aplastic anemia has resulted in several cases of hepatocellular carcinoma.

12. Determine if pregnant. Monitor CBC, H&H, serum glucose, calcium, electrolytes, PSA, renal and LFTs. To ensure proper dosing, measure testosterone levels as indicated. May alter serum lipid levels enhancing susceptibility to arteriosclerotic heart disease in women; monitor thyroid and lipid panel.

CLIENT/FAMILY TEACHING

1. Review method for administration/application, dosage, frequency of administration, site preparation, and timing of application. (see *Implementation/Administration/Storage*).
2. Pellets are fat soluble and are implanted SC by provider usually in abdominal wall.
3. Apply patches or gel to clean, dry skin; Androderm to back, abdomen, upper arms or thighs. AndroGel to upper arm and shoulders and Fortesta to thighs.
4. Apply patch once daily at the same time each day; night application is preferred. To apply: open packet and remove patch immediately prior to application, then remove release liner to expose adhesive side of patch and apply to clean, dry skin area of back, abdomen, thigh, or upper arm using firm pressure with fingers or palm to ensure good contact with skin, especially at edges of the patch.
5. Do not apply patch to scrotum, penis, skin that is not normal (e.g., inflamed or irritated), over a bony area, or to skin that may experience prolonged pressure during sleep or sitting.
6. Discard used patches carefully in trash and prevent accidental contact/ingestion by children or pets.
7. Do not have to remove patch during intercourse or while showering, bathing, or swimming.
8. OTC hydrocortisone may relieve mild rash S&S; report if irritation persists or worsens.
9. Apply gel once daily in the morning after bathing or showering completed. Do not apply gel to scrotum, penis, abdomen, or skin that is inflamed or irritated.
10. Gel is flammable; do not use near fire or open flame.
11. If gel accidentally gets into eyes, rinse eyes with warm, clean water and report if eye irritation develops.
12. Do not swim or bathe within 2 hr of applying Testim or within 5 to 6 hr of applying AndroGel; may reduce effectiveness.
13. Wash application site thoroughly with soap and water to remove drug residue before any situation in which direct skin-to-skin contact is anticipated (sexual contact).
14. If unwashed clothing or unclothed skin (where gel has been applied) comes in contact with skin of another person, especially a pregnant or breastfeeding partner, wash the general area of contact thoroughly with soap and water ASAP.
15. Be aware that virilization has been reported in children who were secondarily exposed to transdermal testosterone. Ensure children avoid contact with unwashed or unclothed application sites in those using transdermal testosterone.
16. The buccal system should be placed in a comfortable position just above the incisor tooth on either side of the mouth. Rotate to alternate sides of the mouth with each application. To apply the buccal system, place the rounded side surface against the gum and hold firmly in place with a finger over the lip and against the product for 30 seconds to ensure adhesion. If the system fails to adhere properly to the gum or should fall off during the 12-hr dosing interval, remove the old system and apply a new one. If the system falls out of position within 4 hr before the next dose, apply a new system; it may remain in place until the time of the next regularly scheduled dosing. To remove the system, gently slide it downwards from the gum toward the tooth to avoid scratching the gum. Take care to avoid dislodging the buccal system and check to see if it is still in place after toothbrushing, use of mouthwash or consumption of food or beverages. Do not chew or swallow the buccal system. Inspect gum area where buccal system applied and report any abnormality (including gum tenderness or irritation).
17. Report any unusual incidents of bleeding/bruising. Androgens suppress clotting factors (II, V, VII, and X); polycythemia and leukopenia may occur.
18. If drug received via pellets, sloughing can occur; report.

T

19. In older males, urinary obstruction may occur as a result of enlarged prostate.
20. Parents of children receiving testosterone should record weight twice a week and height every 2–3 months. X-rays will be performed periodically on prepubertal children to assess effect on bone growth.
21. Women with metastatic breast cancer need lab tests of serum and urine calcium levels, alkaline phosphatase, and serum cholesterol. If the serum cholesterol level is high, the dosage of drug may need to be changed. Follow a low-cholesterol diet and see dietitian for further assistance with diet. Facial hair and acne in females are reversible once drug withdrawn.
22. Drug may cause irregularities in the menstrual cycle; in postmenopausal women may cause withdrawal bleeding.
23. Use reliable birth control during and for several weeks after therapy withdrawn. Report if pregnancy suspected; increased risk of fetal abnormalities with this drug.
24. Males should report breast swelling or sustained erections; may necessitate drug withdrawal (at least temporarily).
25. Report any tingling of the fingers and toes or loss of appetite.
26. Follow a diet high in calories, proteins, vitamins, minerals, and other nutrients. Restrict sodium to reduce extremity swelling. Perform regular daily exercise to maintain weight and muscle mass.
27. With diabetes, low blood sugar may occur. Report extreme variations as diet and/or dose of antidiabetic agents may require modification.
28. In females with gender disorder, monitor testosterone levels and assess CBC, thyroid, and lipid panels regularly.
29. Review potential for drug abuse. High doses of androgens for enhancement of athletic performance can result in serious irreversible side effects/permanent physical damage.
30. Report yellow skin, fatigue or RUQ pain, itching, or a change in the color/consistency of stools (liver dysfunction).
31. Any easy bruising, bleeding, S&S sore throat or fever should be reported to rule out polycythemia and leukopenia.
32. If acne is severe, report as may be necessary to change dose.
33. Keep all F/U visits to assess response, labs, and adverse SE.

OUTCOMES/EVALUATE

- Replacement therapy with control of S&S of androgen deficiency
- Ablation of ovaries in metastatic breast cancer
- Suppression of breast tumor size and spread
- Delayed puberty (stimulation)

Tetracycline hydrochloride

(teh-trah-**SYE**-kleen)

Classification(s): Antibiotic, tetracycline

Pregnancy Category: D

RX: Capsules: Sumycin 250 and 500. **Syrup:** Sumycin Syrup.

🍁 **Rx:** Apo-Tetra, Novo-Tetra, Nu-Tetra.

SEE ALSO ***TETRACYCLINES.***

INDICATIONS/USES

PO:

1. Gram-negative organisms, including *Haemophilus ducreyi* (chancroid), *Francisella tularensis* (tularemia), *Yersinia pestis* (plague), *Bartonella bacilliformis* (bartonellosis), *Campylobacter fetus, Vibrio cholerae* (cholera), *Brucella* species (in conjunction with streptomycin), *Calymmatobacterium granulomatis* (granuloma inguinale).
2. Infections caused by: *Rickettsiae* (Rocky Mountain spotted fever, typhus fever and the typhus group, Q fever, rickettsialpox, tick fevers); *Mycoplasma pneumoniae* (respiratory tract infections), *Chlamydia trachomatis* (lymphogranuloma venerum, trachoma, inclusion conjunctivitis, uncomplicated urethral, endocervical or rectal infections), *Chlamydia psittaci* (psittacosis), *Borellia* species (relapsing fever), *Ureaplasma urealyticum* (nongonoccal urethritis).
3. Following susceptibility testing (resistance has been noted) for the following: *Escherichia coli, Enterobacter aerogenes, Acinetobacter* species, *Haemophilus influenzae* (URTI), *Klebsiella* species (respiratory and UTI), *Streptococcus pneumoniae* (upper respiratory infections), *Streptococcus pyogenes, S. pneu-*

T

moniae, Mycoplasma pneumoniae, Klebsiella species (lower respiratory tract infections). *Staphylococcus aureus, S. pyogenes* (skin and skin structure infections), *Bacteroides* and *Shigella* species.

4. Alternative therapy for the following when penicillin is contraindicated: Uncomplicated gonorrhea due to *Neisseria gonorrhoeae,* syphilis due to *Treponema pallidum,* yaws due to *Treponema pertenue, Listeria monocytogenes,* anthrax due to *Bacillus anthracis,* Vincent's infection due to *Fusobacterium fusiforme,* actinomycosis due to *Actinomyces* species, *Clostridium* species.
5. Adjunct with amebicides for acute intestinal amebiasis.
6. Adjunct therapy for severe acne.
7. Part of combination therapy to eradicate *Helicobacter pylori* infections. Complete eradication is possible.

Investigational: Pleural sclerosing agent in malignant pleural effusions (administered by chest tube); in combination with gentamicin for *Vibrio vulnificus* infections due to wound infection after trauma or by eating contaminated seafood.

ACTION/KINETICS

Pharmacokinetics

From 60–80% absorbed. **Time to maximum levels:** 2–4 hr. **t½, serum:** 6–12 hr. From 20 to 55% excreted unchanged in urine. Always express dose as the hydrochloride salt. **Plasma protein binding:** 20–65%.

CONTRAINDICATIONS

Use of PO products for streptococcal disease unless organism has been shown to be susceptible. Tetracyclines are not the drugs of choice to treat any type of staphylococcal infections.

SIDE EFFECTS

Most Common

Anorexia, N&V, diarrhea, dizziness, headache, rashes.

See *Tetracyclines* for a complete list of possible side effects.

HOW SUPPLIED

Capsules: 250 mg, 500 mg; *Syrup:* 125 mg/5 mL.

DOSAGE

CAPSULES; SYRUP

Mild to moderate infections.

Adults, usual: 500 mg twice a day or 250 mg 4 times per day.

Severe infections.

Adult: 500 mg 4 times per day. **Children over 8 years:** 25–50 mg/kg/day in four equal doses.

Eradication of H. pylori.

The following regimens may be used: (1) Tetracycline, 500 mg 4 times per day for 2 weeks, plus metronidazole, 250 mg 4 times per day for 2 weeks, plus bismuth subsalicylate, 525 mg 4 times per day for 2 weeks, plus an H_2-receptor antagonist for 28 days. (2) Clarithromycin, 500 mg twice a day for 2 weeks, plus ranitidine bismuth citrate, 400 mg twice a day for 4 weeks, plus either metronidazole, 500 mg twice a day, or amoxicillin, 1 gram twice a day, or tetracycline, 500 mg twice a day for 2 weeks. (3) Tetracycline, 500 mg 4 times per day for 2 weeks, plus metronidazole, 500 mg 3 times per day for 2 weeks, plus bismuth subsalicylate, 525 mg 4 times per day for 2 weeks, plus either lansoprazole, 30 mg once daily or omeprazole, 20 mg once daily, for 2 weeks.

Brucellosis.

500 mg 4 times per day for 3 weeks with 1 gram streptomycin IM twice a day for first week and once daily the second week.

Syphilis.

Sumycin only: Total of 30–40 grams over 10–15 days. **All products except Sumycin:** Early (<1 year): 500 mg 4 times per day for 15 days; >1 year duration: 500 mg 4 times per day for 30 days.

Uncomplicated gonorrhea.

500 mg q 6 hr for 7 days.

Uncomplicated urethral, endocervical, or rectal infections in adults due to Chlamydia trachomatis.

500 mg 4 times per day for minimum of 7 days.

Severe acne, long-term therapy.

Initially, 1 gram/day in divided doses; **then,** 125–500 mg/day (long-term). Alternate-day for intermittent therapy may be adequate in some clients.

NURSING IMPLICATIONS

IMPLEMENTATION/ADMINISTRATION/STORAGE

1. Treat streptococcal infections for at least 10 days.
2. Decrease recommended doses and/or extend dosing intervals in those with renal impairment.
3. Food, some dairy products, and antacids containing Al, Ca^{++}, or Mg^{++} interfere with tetracycline absorption.
4. In renal impairment, decrease the dose or extend dosing intervals.
5. Under no circumstances should outdated tetracyclines be given; degradation products of tetracyclines are highly nephrotoxic and may cause a Fanconi-like syndrome.
6. Store products below 30°C (86°F) protected from light and excessive heat.

ASSESSMENT

1. Note reasons for therapy, type, onset, characteristics of S&S.
2. Monitor cultures, CBC, liver and renal function studies; anticipate reduced dose or dosing intervals with renal dysfunction.

CLIENT/FAMILY TEACHING

1. Take PO form 1 hr before or 2 hr after meals and 1 hr before bedtime with a full glass of water. Avoid dairy products, antacids, or iron preparations for 2–3 hr of ingestion; reduces drug effectiveness.
2. May cause dizziness, light-headedness, or feeling of a whirling motion; use caution performing activities that require mental alertness until tolerance determined.
3. May cause photosensitivity reaction; avoid exposure to sunlight and wear protective clothing and sunscreen when exposed.
4. Drug may cause increased yellow-brown discoloration and softening of teeth and bones. *Not* advised for children under 8 years old.
5. Use additional nonhormonal form of contraception to prevent pregnancy; tetracycline may make birth control pills less effective.
6. Check expiration date; degraded drug is very nephrotoxic and may cause kidney damage. Discard any unused tetracycline by the expiration date noted on the label.
7. Report any new onset diarrhea, severe headache, or visual disturbances.
8. Keep all F/U to assess response, labs, and for adverse SE.

OUTCOMES/EVALUATE

- Resolution of infection; symptomatic improvement
- ↓ Acne lesions

Thalidomide

(thah-**LID**-ah-myd)

Classification(s): Immunomodulator

Pregnancy Category: X

RX: Thalomid.

INDICATIONS/USES

(1) Acute treatment of moderate to severe erythema nodosum leprosum (ENL). Not indicated for monotherapy for ENL in the presence of moderate to severe neuritis. (2) Maintenance therapy for prevention and suppression of the cutaneous symptoms of erythema nodosum leprosum recurrence. (3) In combination with dexamethasone to treat newly diagnosed multiple myeloma. *Investigational:* Prostate cancer in combination with docetaxel; graft vs. host disease after bone marrow transplantation; refractory multiple myeloma; primary brain tumors; appetite stimulant for cachexia in advanced cancer; aphthous ulcers.

ACTION/KINETICS

Action

Immunomodulatory drug; mechanism of action not known. Possesses immunomodulatory, anti-inflammatory, and antiangiogenic properties. Drug may suppress excessive tumor necrosis factor-alpha (TNF-α) production and down-modulation of selected cell surface adhesion molecules involved in leukocyte migration. When used to treat multiple myeloma, there is an increase in the number of circulating natural killer cells and an increase in plasma levels of interleukin-2 and interferon-gamma (associated with cytotoxic activity).

T

Pharmacokinetics

Peak plasma levels: 2.9–5.7 hr. High-fat meals increase the time-to-peak plasma levels to about 6 hr. **t½, elimination:** 5–7 hr. Appears to undergo nonenzymatic hydrolysis in the plasma. Excreted in the urine. **Plasma protein binding:** Approximately 60%.

CONTRAINDICATIONS

Never to be used in pregnancy or in those who could become pregnant while taking the drug (even a single 50 mg dose can cause severe birth defects). Use in males unless the client meets several conditions (see package insert). Use during heterosexual sexual contact. Use as monotherapy for ENL in the presence of moderate to severe neuritis. Lactation.

SPECIAL CONCERNS

(1) If taken during pregnancy, thalidomide can cause severe birth defects or death to a fetus. Thalidomide should never be used by women who are pregnant or who could become pregnant while taking the drug. Even a single dose (one 50, 100, or 200 mg capsule) taken by a pregnant woman can cause severe birth defects. Because of this toxicity and in an effort to make the chance of fetal exposure as negligible as possible, thalidomide is approved for marketing only under a special restricted distribution program approved by the FDA. This program is called the "System for Thalidomide Education and Prescribing Safety" (S.T.E.P.S.) Under this restricted distribution program, only prescribers and pharmacists registered with the program are allowed to prescribe and dispense the product at 1 month intervals. In addition, clients must be advised of, agree to, and comply with the requirements of the S.T.E.P.S. program in order to receive the product. (2) **Prescribers:** Thalidomide is prescribed only by licensed prescribers who are registered in the S.T.E.P.S. program and understand the risk of teratogenicity of thalidomide if used during pregnancy. The following major human fetal abnormalities related to thalidomide given during pregnancy have been documented:

- Absence of bones, absence of limbs (amelia), congenital heart defects, external ear abnormalities (including anotia, micropinna, small or absent external auditory canals), eye abnormalities (anophthalmos, microphthalmos), facial palsy, hypoplasticity of the bones, and phocomelia (short limbs). Alimentary tract, urinary tract, and genital malformations have also been documented.
- Mortality at or shortly after birth has been reported at about 40%. Effective contraception must be used for at least 1 month before beginning thalidomide, during therapy, and for 1 month following discontinuation of therapy. Reliable contraception is indicated even where there has been a history of infertility, unless the client has had a hysterectomy or has been postmenopausal for at least 24 months. Two reliable forms of contraception must be used simultaneously unless continuous abstinence from heterosexual sexual intercourse is the chosen method. Refer women of childbearing potential to a qualified provider of contraceptive methods, if needed. Sexually mature women who have not undergone a hysterectomy or who have not been postmenopausal for at least 24 consecutive months (i.e., who have had menses at some time in the preceding 24 consecutive months) are considered to be women of childbearing potential. Before starting treatment, administer a pregnancy test (sensitivity at least 50 milliunits/mL) to women of childbearing potential. Perform the test within the 24 hours prior to beginning therapy. A prescription for thalidomide for a woman of childbearing potential must not be issued until a written report of a negative pregnancy test has been obtained by the prescriber. Once treatment has been started, test for pregnancy weekly during the first 4 weeks of use, then repeat pregnancy testing at 4 weeks in women with regular menstrual cycles. If menstrual cycles are irregular, test for pregnancy every 2 weeks. Perform pregnancy testing and counseling if a client misses her period or if there is any abnormality in menstrual bleeding. If pregnancy occurs during thalidomide treatment, discontinue the drug immediately. Report any suspected fetal exposure to

thalidomide to the FDA immediately via MedWatch at 1-800-FDA-1088 and also to the manufacturer. Refer the client to an obstetrician/gynecologist experienced in reproductive toxicity for further evaluation and counseling.

(3) **Men:** Because thalidomide is present in the semen of clients receiving the drug, males receiving thalidomide must always use a latex condom during any sexual contact with women of childbearing potential even if he has undergone a successful vasectomy. Thalidomide is contraindicated in sexually mature men unless the client meets ALL of the following conditions:

- He understands and can reliably carry out instructions.
- He is capable of complying with the mandatory contraceptive measures that are appropriate for men, client registration, and client survey as described in the S.T.E.P.S. program.
- He has received both oral and written warnings of the hazards of taking thalidomide and exposing a fetus to the drug.
- He has received both oral and written warnings of the risk of possible contraception failure and of the presence of thalidomide in semen. He has been instructed that he must always use a latex condom during any sexual contact with women of childbearing potential, even if he has undergone a successful vasectomy.
- He acknowledges, in writing, his understanding of these warnings and of the need to use a latex condom during any sexual contact with women of childbearing potential, even if he has undergone a successful vasectomy, when having sexual intercourse with women of childbearing potential. Sexually mature women who have not undergone a hysterectomy or who have not been postmenopausal for at least 24 consecutive months (i.e., who have had menses at some time in the preceding 24 consecutive months) are considered to be women of childbearing potential.
- If the client is between 12 and 18 years of age, his parents or legal guardian must have read this material and agreed to ensure compliance.

(4) **Women:** Thalidomide is contraindicated in women of childbearing potential unless alternative therapies are considered inappropriate and the client meets ALL of the following conditions (i.e., essentially she is unable to become pregnant while on thalidomide therapy):

- She understands and can reliably carry out instructions.
- She is capable of complying with the mandatory contraceptive measures, pregnancy testing, patient registration, and patient survey as described in the S.T.E.P.S. program.
- She has received both oral and written warnings of the hazards of taking thalidomide during pregnancy and of exposing a fetus to the drug.
- She has received both oral and written warnings of the risk of possible contraception failure and of the need to use two reliable forms of contraception simultaneously, unless continuous abstinence from reproductive heterosexual intercourse is the chosen method. Sexually mature women who have not undergone a hysterectomy or who have not been postmenopausal for at least 24 consecutive months (i.e., who have had menses at some time in the preceding 24 consecutive months) are considered to be women of childbearing potential.
- She acknowledges, in writing, her understanding of these warnings and of the need for using two reliable methods of contraception for 4 weeks prior to starting thalidomide therapy, during thalidomide therapy, and for 4 weeks after stopping thalidomide therapy.
- She has had a negative pregnancy test with a sensitivity of at least 50 milli-international units/mL, within the 24 hr prior to beginning therapy.
- If the client is between 12 and 18 years of age, her parent or legal guardian must have read this material and agreed to ensure compliance.

(5) **Venous thromboembolic effects:** The use of thalidomide in multiple myeloma results in an increased risk of venous thromboembolic events, such as deep venous thrombosis and

pulmonary embolus. This risk increases significantly when thalidomide is used in combination with standard chemotherapeutic agents, including dexamethasone. In one controlled trial, the rate of venous thromboembolic events was 22.5% in clients receiving thalidomide in combination with dexamethasone, compared with 4.9% in clients receiving dexamethasone alone. Clients and health care providers are advised to be observant for the signs and symptoms of thromboembolism. Instruct clients to seek medical care if they develop symptoms such as arm or leg swelling, chest pain, or shortness of breath. Preliminary data suggest that clients who are appropriate candidates may benefit from concurrent prophylactic anticoagulation or aspirin treatment.

- **Clients with Hansen's disease may have an increased bioavailability of thalidomide.**
- **Safety and efficacy not determined in children less than 12 years of age.**

SIDE EFFECTS

Most Common

Dizziness, somnolence, orthostatic hypotension, acne, rash/desquamation, maculopapular rash, hematuria, leukopenia, fever, headache, neuropathy, dry mouth, flatulence, peripheral edema, pharyngitis, sinusitis, infection, constipation, dsypnea, edema.

NOTE: Only the most common side effects and possible serious side effects are listed. Included are common and/or serious side effects noted when combined with dexamethasone. **GI:** Constipation, dry mouth, flatulence, diarrhea, nausea, oral moniliasis, tooth pain, abdominal pain, anorexia, dyspepsia, N&V. **CNS:** Drowsiness, somnolence, dizziness, confusion, tremor, vertigo, headache, anxiety, agitation, depression, light-headedness, insomnia, paresthesia, seizures (including ***generalized tonic-clonic***). **Neurologic:** Peripheral sensory/motor neuropathy (may be permanent). **CV:** Orthostatic hypotension, bradycardia (may require medical intervention), hyper-/hypotension, embolism. Increased incidence of pulmonary embolism, DVT, thrombophlebitis, or thrombosis. **Respiratory:** Pharyngitis, rhinitis, sinusitis, dyspnea, cough. **Hematologic:** Neutropenia, leukopenia. **Hypersensitivity:** Erythematous macular rash, fever, tachycardia, hypotension. **Dermatologic:** Photosensitivity, rash (maculopapular, exfoliative, purpuric, bullous), dermatitis, desquamation, fungal nail disorder, pruritus, ***Stevens-Johnson syndrome, toxic epidermal necrolysis.*** **Musculoskeletal:** Back/neck/bone pain, neck rigidity, muscle weakness, arthralgia, myalgia. **Body as a whole:** Peripheral edema, accidental injury, infection (with/without neutropenia), weight gain/loss, asthenia, chills, malaise, pain, fatigue, fever. **Miscellaneous:** ***Human teratogenicity.*** HIV viral load increase, hematuria, impotence, facial edema.

LABORATORY TEST CONSIDERATIONS

↑ Alkaline phosphatase, AST, bilibrubin. ↓ Hemoglobin, leukocytes, neutrophils, platelets. Hyperglycemia, hyper-/hypokalemia, hypocalcemia, hyponatremia.

DRUG INTERACTIONS

Alcohol / Enhanced sedative effects
Barbiturates / Enhanced sedative effects
Chlorpromazine / Enhanced sedative effects
Isoniazid / Enhanced symptoms of peripheral neuropathy
Metronidazole / Enhanced symptoms of peripheral neuropathy
Vincristine / Enhanced symptoms of peripheral neuropathy

HOW SUPPLIED

Capsules: 50 mg, 100 mg, 200 mg.

DOSAGE

CAPSULES

Cutaneous erythema nodosum leprosum (ENL), initial therapy.

Adults, initial: 100–300 mg once daily with water, preferably at bedtime and at least 1 hr after the evening meal. Clients weighing less than 50 kg should be started at the low end of the dose range. In those with severe cutaneous ENL or who have required higher doses previously, dosing may be started at doses up to 400 mg once daily at bedtime or in divided doses with water 1 hr after meals. Continue initial dosing until signs and symptoms of active reaction have been eliminated (usually at least 2 weeks). Following this, taper clients off medication in 50 mg decrements q 2 to 4 weeks.

T

Maintenance therapy for prevention and suppression of ENL recurrence.

Maintain the minimum dose (see initial therapy) necessary to control the reaction. Attempt tapering of medication q 3 to 6 months, in decrements of 50 mg q 2 to 4 weeks.

Multiple myeloma.

Thalidomide, 200 mg, once daily with water preferably at bedtime, and at least 1 hr after the evening meal *plus* dexamethasone, 40 mg daily given PO on days 1–4, 9–12, 17–20 every 28 days.

NURSING IMPLICATIONS

IMPLEMENTATION/ADMINISTRATION/STORAGE

1. The product is supplied only to pharmacists registered with the S.T.E.P.S. program. The drug is dispensed in no more than a 1-month supply and only on presentation of a new prescription written within the previous 14 days and client signature. Pharmacists are required to obtain a confirmation number for each prescription and record that number on the prescription.
2. Specific informed consent and compliance with the mandatory client registry and survey are required of all male and female clients prior to dispensing the drug. The drug must not be repackaged.
3. Cutaneous absorption or inhalation of the drug, especially from handling the capsules or being exposed to body fluids of a thalidomide-user is possible. Wash exposed areas with soap and water.
4. Continue dosing until signs and symptoms of active reaction have subsided (usually 2 weeks). Clients may then be tapered off medication in 50 mg decrements q 2–4 weeks.
5. In clients with moderate to severe neuritis associated with severe erythema nodosum leprosum reactions, corticosteroids may be given along with thalidomide. Steroid doses can be tapered and discontinued when the neuritis has improved.
6. Discontinue if a rash occurs. Do not resume therapy if the rash is exfoliative, purpuric, or bullous, or if Stevens-Johnson syndrome or toxic epidermal necrolysis is suspected.
7. Concomitant use with carbamazepine, griseofulvin, HIV-protease inhibitors, modafinil, penicillins, phenytoin, rifabutin, rifampin, or certain herbal supplements (e.g., St. John's wort) with hormonal contraceptive drugs may decrease effectiveness of contraception for up to 1 month after discontinuing these therapies. Women requiring treatment with one or more of these drugs must use two other effective or highly effective methods of contraception, or abstain from heterosexual contact while taking thalidomide.
8. Store from 15–30°C (59–86°F). Protect from light.

ASSESSMENT

1. Note indications for therapy, onset, characteristics of S&S, other agents trialed and outcome. With leprosy, note characteristics including number of painful skin nodules and any systemic manifestations (fever, neuritis, malaise). With multiple myeloma, note protein levels and steroid failures.
2. Obtain negative pregnancy test. Drug is teratogenic; even one dose taken during pregnancy can cause severe birth defects. Pregnancy tests will be performed weekly during the first month of therapy and then monthly thereafter with regular menses and every 2 weeks with irregular menses. Monitor CBC; assess for neutropenia.
3. Drug will only be dispensed under a restricted distribution program (S.T.E.P.S.) requiring written consent. With relapsed MM client must still sign consent and agree to required monitoring.
4. If HIV-seropositive, monitor viral load the first and third month of treatment and then every 3 months. Monitor for signs of neuropathy at monthly intervals for the first 3 months of therapy.
5. Monitor CBC, pregnancy test (females not menopausal), and with HIV-viral load.

CLIENT/FAMILY TEACHING

1. Take as prescribed and each dose with a full glass of water at least 1 h after meals. For single daily doses, take at bedtime at least 1 h after the evening meal.
2. May cause dizziness/drowsiness; avoid activities that require mental acuity. Avoid alcohol and CNS depressants.

T

3. Women of childbearing age must practice two methods of reliable birth control or abstain continuously from heterosexual intercourse. Males must always wear a latex condom when engaging in sexual intercourse with women of childbearing age, despite successful vasectomy. During therapy do not donate blood or sperm.
4. Report any numbness, tingling, pain, or burning in the hands or feet. Peripheral neuropathy may occur and may be irreversible.
5. Review increased risk of venous thromboembolic events, such as DVT and pulmonary embolus. Risk increases with coadministration of standard chemotherapeutic agents. Seek medical care if any S&S such as shortness of breath, chest pain, or arm or leg swelling occur. (May benefit from concomitant prophylactic anticoagulation or aspirin treatment).
6. Drug is continued until S&S of active reaction subsides (approximately 2 weeks). The dosage may then be tapered by provider every 2–4 weeks.
7. Drug will only be dispensed in a 1 month supply, and only upon presentation of a valid prescription written within past 14 days. Drug therapy requires informed consent and compliance with the mandatory patient registry (MD must call company with drug ID number) and survey prior to dispensing and clinical monitoring during therapy (S.T.E.P.S. [system for thalidomide education and prescribing safety program]).
8. Keep all F/U to assess response, labs, and for adverse SE.

OUTCOMES/EVALUATE

- Suppression of cutaneous manifestations with ENL
- Inhibition of malignant cell proliferation

IV

Theophylline

(thee-**OFF**-ih-lin)

Classification(s): Antiasthmatic, xanthine derivative

Pregnancy Category: C

RX: Capsules, Extended-Release or Timed-Release: Theo-24. **Elixir:** Elixophyllin. **Tablets, Controlled-Release (24-hr) or Extended-Release (12-hr):** Theochron.

✦ **Rx:** Apo-Theo LA.

INDICATIONS/USES

PO, Injection: Symptoms and reversible airflow obstruction associated with chronic asthma and other chronic lung diseases, including emphysema and chronic bronchitis. *NOTE:* An inhaled beta-2 selective agonist, alone or with a systemically administered corticosteroid, is the most effective treatment for acute exacerbations of reversible airway obstruction. If an inhaled or parenteral beta agonist is not available, a loading dose of an oral immediate-release theophylline can be used as a temporary measure. *Investigational:* Apnea in preterm infants. Reduce essential tremor. Improve pulmonary function and dyspnea in chronic obstructive pulmonary disease.

ACTION/KINETICS

Action

Theophylline stimulates the CNS, directly relaxes the smooth muscles of the bronchi (relieve bronchospasms) and pulmonary blood vessels, produces diuresis, inhibits uterine contractions, stimulates gastric acid secretion, and increases the rate and force of contraction of the heart. Although the exact mechanism is not known, theophyllines may alter the calcium levels of smooth muscle, blocking adenosine receptors, inhibiting the effect of prostaglandins on smooth muscle, and inhibiting the release of slow-reacting substance of anaphylaxis and histamine.

Pharmacokinetics

PO liquids and uncoated tablets well absorbed; **maximal plasma levels:** 2 hr. Enteric-coated tablets and some sustained release forms may be unreliably absorbed. Rectal absorption is slow and erratic. Food may alter bioavailability and absorption of some sustained-release products. **Time to peak serum levels, extended-release capsules and tablets:** 4–7 hr. **Therapeutic plasma levels:** 10–20 mcg/mL. **t½:** 3–15 hr in nonsmoking adults, 4–5 hr in adult heavy smokers, 1–9 hr in children, and 20–30 hr for premature neonates. An increased t½ may be seen in individuals with CHF, alcoholism, liver dysfunction, or respiratory infections. Because of great variations in the rate of absorption (due to dosage form, food, dose level) as well as its extremely narrow therapeutic

T

range, theophylline therapy is best monitored by determination of the serum levels. 85–90% metabolized in the liver to various metabolites, including the active 3-methylxanthine. Theophylline is metabolized partially to caffeine in the neonate. The premature neonate excretes 50% unchanged theophylline and may accumulate the caffeine metabolite. Excretion is through the kidneys (about 10% unchanged in adults). **Plasma protein binding:** About 40%.

CONTRAINDICATIONS

Hypersensitivity to any xanthine, peptic ulcer, seizure disorders (unless on medication), hypotension, CAD, angina pectoris. PO theophylline products to treat status epilepticus. Lactation (use during lactation may result in irritability, insomnia, and fretfulness in the infant).

SPECIAL CONCERNS

- **Elderly (especially males) may manifest an increased risk of toxicity.**
- **Use with caution in the presence of gastritis, alcoholism, acute cardiac diseases, CHF, hypoxemia, severe renal and hepatic disease, severe hypertension, severe myocardial damage, hyperthyroidism, glaucoma.**
- **Use with caution in premature infants due to the possible accumulation of caffeine.**
- **Xanthines are not usually tolerated by small children because of excessive CNS stimulation.**

SIDE EFFECTS

Most Common

N&V, diarrhea, headache, insomnia, irritability.

Side effects are uncommon at serum theophylline levels less than 20 mcg/mL. At levels greater than 20 mcg/mL, 75% of individuals experience side effects including N&V, diarrhea, irritability, insomnia, and headache. At levels of 35 mcg/mL or greater, individuals may manifest ***cardiac arrhythmias***, hypotension, tachycardia (>10 mcg/mL in newborns), hyperglycemia, ***seizures, brain damage, or death.*** **GI:** N&V, diarrhea, anorexia, epigastric pain, hematemesis, dyspepsia, rectal irritation/bleeding, gastroesophageal reflux/aspiration during sleep or while recumbent. **CNS:** Headache, restlessness, insomnia, irritability, fever, dizziness, light-headedness, vertigo, reflex hyperexcitability, ***seizures***, depression, speech abnormalities, alternating periods of mutism and hyperactivity, ***brain damage, death***. **CV:** Hypotension, ***life-threatening ventricular arrhythmias***, palpitations, tachycardia, ***peripheral vascular collapse***, extrasystoles, dysrhythmias, worsening of existing arrhythmias. **Musculoskeletal:** Muscle twitching. **Respiratory:** Worsening of airway obstruction, tachypnea, ***respiratory arrest***. **Renal:** Proteinuria, excretion of erythrocytes and renal tubular cells, dehydration due to diuresis, urinary retention (men with BPH). **Miscellaneous:** Fever, flushing, hyperglycemia, inappropriate antidiuretic hormone syndrome, leukocytosis, rash, alopecia.

LABORATORY TEST CONSIDERATIONS

↑ Plasma free fatty acids, bilirubin, urinary catecholamines, ESR. Interference with uric acid tests and tests for furosemide and probenecid.

OVERDOSE MANAGEMENT

Symptoms: Excessive doses may cause severe toxicity. The incidence of toxicity increases significantly at serum levels >20 mcg/mL. Symptoms include agitation, headache, nervousness, restlessness, irritability, insomnia, tachycardia, extrasystoles, anorexia, N&V, fasciculations, tachypnea, tonic-clonic seizures. The first signs of toxicity may be seizures, ventricular arrhythmias, or even death. Acute overdose may also cause hypokalemia, hypercalcemia, hyperglycemia, and decreased serum bicarbonate levels. Overdosage with sustained release products may cause a dramatic increase in serum theophylline levels 12 hr or more later than the increases that occur with other products.

Treatment:

- Have gastric lavage equipment, and cathartics available to treat overdose if the client is conscious and not having seizures. Otherwise a mechanical ventilator, oxygen, diazepam, and IV fluids may be necessary for the treatment of overdosage.
- For postseizure coma, maintain an airway and oxygenate the client. To remove the drug, perform only gastric lavage and give the cathartic and activated charcoal by a large-bore gastric lavage tube. Charcoal hemoperfusion may be necessary.
- Treat atrial arrhythmias with verapamil and treat ventricular arrhythmias with lidocaine or procainamide.
- Use IV fluids to treat acid-base imbalance, hypotension, and dehydration. Hypotension may also be treated with vasopressors.

T

- To treat hyperpyrexia, use a tepid water sponge bath or a hypothermic blanket.
- Treat apnea with artificial respiration.
- Monitor serum levels of theophylline until they fall below 20 mcg/mL as secondary rises of theophylline may occur, especially with sustained-release products.

DRUG INTERACTIONS

Alcohol / Addition to liquid formulations is not necessary for absorption and may be potentially harmful
Allopurinol / ↑ Theophylline levels
Aminoglutethimide / ↓ Theophylline levels
Barbiturates / ↓ Theophylline levels
Benzodiazepines / Sedative effect may be antagonized by theophylline; coadministration may be beneficial in reversing theophylline-induced sedation
Beta-adrenergic agonists / Additive effects
Beta-adrenergic blocking agents (nonselective) / ↑ Theophylline levels
Calcium channel blocking drugs / ↑ Theophylline levels
Carbamazepine / Either ↑ or ↓ theophylline levels
Charcoal / ↓ Theophylline levels
Cimetidine / ↑ Theophylline levels
Ciprofloxacin / ↑ Theophylline plasma levels; ↑ possibility of side effects
Corticosteroids / ↑ Theophylline levels
Digitalis / ↑ Digitalis toxicity
Disulfiram / ↑ Theophylline levels
Ephedrine / ↑ Theophylline levels
Erythromycin / ↑ Theophylline effect R/T ↓ liver metabolism
Ethacrynic acid / Either ↑ or ↓ theophylline levels
Fluoroquinolones / ↑ Theophylline plasma levels → toxicity R/T ↓ metabolism by CYP1A2
Fluvoxamine / ↑ Risk of theophylline toxicity; decrease the usual daily maintenance dose of theophylline dose by one-third
Furosemide / Either ↑ or ↓ theophylline levels
Halothane / ↑ Risk of catecholamine-induced cardiac arrhythmias
Interferon / ↑ Theophylline levels
Isoniazid / Either ↑ or ↓ theophylline levels
Ketamine / Seizures of the extensor type
Ketoconazole / ↓ Theophylline levels
Lithium / ↓ Lithium plasma levels R/T ↑ rate of excretion
Loop diuretics / Either ↑ or ↓ theophylline levels
Macrolide antibiotics / ↑ Theophylline levels
Marijuana (smoking) / ↓ Theophylline levels
Mexiletine / ↑ Theophylline levels
Muscle relaxants, nondepolarizing / Dose-dependent reversal of neuromuscular blockade
Oral contraceptives / ↑ Theophylline effect R/T ↓ liver metabolism
Phenytoin / ↓ Theophylline levels; also possible ↓ phenytoin levels
Propofol / ↓ Propofol sedative effect
Quinolones / ↑ Theophylline levels
Ranitidine / ↑ Theophylline plasma levels
Rifampin / ↓ Theophylline levels
Smoking / ↑ Metabolism (including secondhand smoke exposure) of theophylline R/T induction of CYP1A2 → ↓ $t^{1/2}$; monitor levels
H ***St. John's wort*** / Possible ↓ theophylline plasma levels R/T ↑ metabolism
Sulfinpyrazone / ↓ Theophylline levels
Sympathomimetics / ↓ Theophylline levels
Tetracyclines / ↑ Risk of theophylline toxicity
Thiabendazole / ↑ Theophylline levels
Thyroid hormones / ↓ Theophylline clearance in hypothyroid clients; ↑ theophylline clearance in hyperthyroid clients
Tobacco smoking / ↓ Theophylline effect R/T ↑ liver metabolism; consider dosage ↑
Troleandomycin / ↑ Theophylline effect R/T ↓ liver metabolism
Verapamil / ↑ Theophylline effect
Zafirlukast / Possible ↑ theophylline levels

HOW SUPPLIED

Capsules, Extended-Release (12-hr or 24-hr): 100 mg, 125 mg, 200 mg, 300 mg, 400 mg; **Elixir:** 80 mg/15 mL; **Injection Solution:** 0.8 mg/mL, 1.6 mg/mL, 2 mg/mL, 3.2 mg/mL, 4 mg/mL; **Tablets, Controlled-Release (24-hr) or Extended-Release (12-hr):** 100 mg, 200 mg, 300 mg, 400 mg, 450 mg, 600 mg.

DOSAGE

ELIXIR (ELIXOPHYLLIN)

Bronchodilator, infants less than 1 year of age.

Premature neonates, <24 days postnatal, initial: 1 mg/kg q 12 hr.

Premature neonates, 24 days postnatal and older, initial: 1.5 mg/kg q 12 hr.

Full-term infants, up to age 26 weeks, initial: Calculate dosage according to the following:

T

Total daily dose (mg) = ([0.2 × age in weeks] + 5) × kg body wt. Divide the dose into 3 equal amounts given at 8 hr intervals.

Full-term infants, 26 weeks of age and older, initial: Use preceding formula to calculate total daily dose (mg). Divide the dose into 4 equal amounts given at 6 hr intervals.

Final dosage, infants <1 year of age: Adjust dosage to maintain a peak steady-state serum theophylline level of 5 to 10 mcg/mL in neonates and 10 to 15 mcg/mL in older infants. Up to 5 days may be required to achieve steady state in a premature infant while only 2 to 3 days may be required in an infant 6 months of age without other risk factors for impaired clearance in the absence of a loading dose. If a serum theophylline level is obtained before steady state is reached, the maintenance dose should not be increased, even if the serum theophylline level is less than 10 mcg/mL.

CAPSULES, EXTENDED-RELEASE OR CONTROLLED-RELEASE; ELIXIR; TABLETS, EXTENDED-RELEASE OR CONTROLLED-RELEASE

Bronchodilator, children less than 45 kg without risk factors for impaired clearance.

Elixir (Elixophyllin). Children, 1 to 15 years of age. Starting dose: 12–14 mg/kg/day, up to a maximum of 300 mg/day divided q 4 to 6 hr. **After 3 days, if tolerated, increase dose to:** 16 mg/kg/day, up to a maximum of 400 mg/day divided q 4 to 6 hr. **After 3 more days, if tolerated and needed, increase dose to:** 20 mg/kg/day, up to a maximum of 600 mg/day divided q 4 to 6 hr.

Extended-Release Capsules. Children, 1 to 15 years of age. Starting dose: 12–14 mg/kg/day, up to a maximum of 300 mg/day divided q 8 to 12 hr. **After 3 days, if tolerated, increase dose to:** 16 mg/kg/day, up to 400 mg/day divided q 8 to 12 hr. **After 3 more days, if tolerated and needed, increase dose to:** 20 mg/kg/day, up to a maximum of 600 mg/day divided q 8 to 12 hr.

Extended-Release Tablets, including Theochron. Children, 6 to 15 years of age. Starting dose: 12–14 mg/kg/day, up to a maximum of 300 mg/day divided q 12 hr. **After 3 days, if tolerated, increase the dose to:** 16 mg/kg/day, up to a maximum of 400 mg/day divided q 12 hr. After 3 more days, if tolerated and needed, increase dose to: 20 mg/kg/day, up to a maximum of 600 mg/day divided q 12 hr.

Theo-24 (Extended-Release Capsules). Children, 12 to 15 years of age. Starting dose: 12–14 mg/kg, up to a maximum of 300 mg/day given once q 24 hr. **After 3 days, if tolerated, increase dose to:** 16 mg/kg/day, up to a maximum of 400 mg/day given once q 24 hr. **After 3 more days, if tolerated and needed, increase dose to:** 20 mg/kg/day, up to a maximum of 600 mg/day given once q 24 hr.

NOTE: Clients with a more rapid metabolism should receive a smaller dose more often to prevent breakthrough symptoms. A reliably absorbed slow-release formulation will decrease fluctuations and permit longer dosing intervals.

Bronchodilator, children greater than 45 kg, and adults without risk factors for impaired clearance.

Elixir (Elixophyllin). Starting dose: 300 mg/day divided q 6 to 8 hr. **After 3 days, if tolerated, increase dose to:** 400 mg/day divided q 6 to 8 hr. **After 3 more days, if tolerated and needed, increase dose to:** 600 mg/day divided q 6 to 8 hr.

Theophylline Extended-Release Capsules. Starting dose: 300 mg/day divided q 8 to 12 hr. **After 3 days, if tolerated, increase dose to:** 400 mg/day divided q 8 to 12 hr. **After 3 more days, if tolerated and needed, increase dose to:** 600 mg/day divided q 8 to 12 hr.

Theophylline Extended-Release Tablets (including Theochron). Starting dose: 300 mg/day divided q 12 hr. **After 3 days, if tolerated, increase dose to:** 400 mg/day divided q 12 hr. **After 3 more days, if tolerated and needed, increase dose to:** 600 mg/day divided q 12 hr.

Theo-24 (Extended-Release Capsules). Starting dose: 300 to 400 mg/day given once q 24 hr. **After 3 days, if tolerated, increase dose to:** 400 to 600 mg/day given once q 24 hr. **After 3 more days, if tolerated and needed:** Doses greater than 600 mg should be titrated according to blood levels.

NOTE: Clients with a more rapid metabolism should receive a smaller dose more often to prevent breakthrough symptoms. A reliably absorbed slow-release formulation will decrease fluctuations and permit longer dosing intervals.

Clients with risk factors for impaired clearance, clients older than 60 years of age, and clients not feasible to monitor serum theophylline levels.

Elixophyllin, Theophylline Extended-Release Capsules. Children, 1 to 15 years of age: Final theophylline dose should not exceed 16 mg/kg/day, up to a maximum of 400 mg/day. **Adolescents 16 years of age and older and adults, including elderly clients:** Final theophylline dose should not exceed 400 mg/day.

Theophylline Extended-Release Tablets, Theochron. Children, 6 to 15 years of age: Final theophylline dose should not exceed 16 mg/kg/day, up to a maximum of 400 mg/day. **Adolescents 16 years of age and older and adults, including elderly clients:** Final theophylline dose should not exceed 400 mg/day.

Theo-24 (Theophylline-Extended Release Capsules) Theophylline-Extended Release Tablets only. Children, 12 to 15 years of age: Final theophylline dose should not exceed 16 mg/kg/day, up to a maximum of 400 mg/day. **Adolescents 16 years of age and older and adults, including elderly clients:** Final theophylline dose should not exceed 400 mg/day.

ELIXIR

Neonatal apnea.

Loading dose: Using the equivalent of anhydrous theophylline administered by NGT, 5 mg/kg; **maintenance:** 2 mg/kg/day in 2–3 divided doses given by NGT.

ANHYDROUS THEOPHYLLINE

Acute symptoms requiring rapid theophyllinization in clients not receiving theophylline.

PO loading dose for all groups: 5 mg/kg. **Maintenance doses for various groups follow. Otherwise healthy nonsmoking adults:** 3 mg/kg q 8 hr; **older clients and those with cor pulmonale:** 2 mg/kg q 8 hr; **clients with CHF:** 1–2 mg/kg q 12 hr; **children, 1–9 years of age:** 4 mg/kg q 6 hr; **children, 9–16 years of age and young adult smokers:** 3 mg/kg q 6 hr.

Acute symptoms requiring rapid theophyllinization in clients receiving theophylline.

Each 0.5 mg/kg theophylline given as a loading dose will increase serum theophylline levels by about 1 mcg/mL. Ideally, defer the loading dose if a serum theophylline level can be obtained rapidly. If this is not possible, exercise clinical judgment. When there is sufficient respiratory distress to warrant a small risk, administer 2.5 mg/kg theophylline in a rapidly absorbed form that is likely to increase serum levels by about 5 mcg/mL. If the client is not experiencing theophylline toxicity, this approach is not likely to cause dangerous side effects.

IV

Reversible airflow obstruction.

Because of marked client differences in the rate of theophylline clearance, the dose needed to reach a serum theophylline level in the 10 to 20 mcg/mL range varies 4-fold among otherwise similar clients in the absence of factors known to alter theophylline clearance.

The loading dose is dependent on a number of factors. When given IV, the serum concentration obtained from an initial loading dose is related primarily to the volume of distribution. If a mean volume of distribution is about 0.5 L/kg (range of 0.3 to 0.7 L/kg), each mg/kg (ideal body weight) of theophylline administered as a loading dose over 30 min results in an average 2 mcg/mL increase in serum theophylline levels. When a loading dose becomes necessary in an individual who has already received theophylline, estimation of the serum level based upon the history is not reliable; an immediate serum level determination is indicated.

The following guidelines should be followed to determine theophylline infusion rates. **Initial theophylline infusion rates following an appropriate loading dose.** The following recommendations serve as the upper limit for dosage adjustments in order to decrease the risk of potentially serious side effects associated with unexpected large increases in serum theophylline levels. *NOTE:* To achieve a target level of 10 mcg/mL, use ideal body weight for obese clients. Lower initial doses may be required for those receiving other drugs that decrease theophylline clearance (see *Drug Interactions*).

Neonates, postnatal age 24 days or less: 1 mg/kg q 12 hr to achieve a target concentration of 7.5 mcg/mL for neonatal apnea; **postnatal age >24 days:** 1.5 mg/kg q 12 hr to achieve a target concentration of 7.5 mcg/mL. **Infants, 6 to 52 weeks:** mg/kg/hr = (0.008) (age in weeks) × 0.21.

Young children, 1 to 9 years of age: 0.8 mg/kg/hr. **Older children, 9 to 12 years of age:** 0.7 mg/kg/hr.

Adolescents (cigarette or marijuana smokers), 12 to 16 years of age: 0.7 mg/kg/hr.

Adolescents, nonsmokers, 12 to 16 years of age: 0.5 mg/kg/hr, not to exceed 900 mg/day, unless serum levels indicate the need for a larger dose.

Adults, otherwise healthy nonsmokers, 16 to 60 years of age: 0.4 mg/kg/hr, not to exceed 900 mg/day, unless serum levels indicate the need for a larger dose.

Elderly, >60 years of age: 0.3 mg/kg/hr, not to exceed 400 mg/day, unless serum levels indicate the need for a larger dose. The maximum infusion rate should not exceed 17 mg/hr, unless the client continues to be symptomatic and steady-state serum theophylline level is less than 10 mcg/mL.

Cardiac decompensation, cor pulmonale, impaired liver function, sepsis with multiorgan failure, or shock: 0.2 mg/kg/hr, not to exceed 400 mg/day, unless serum levels indicate the need for a larger dose. In these clients, do not exceed an initial infusion rate exceeding 17 mg/hr, unless serum levels can be monitored at 24-hr intervals. In these clients, 5 days may be needed before steady state is reached.

NURSING IMPLICATIONS

IMPLEMENTATION/ADMINISTRATION/STORAGE

1. Individualize dosage on the basis of peak serum theophylline concentration measurements to achieve a dose that will provide maximum potential benefit with minimal risk of side effects.
2. Calculate dosage based on lean body weight (theophylline does not distribute to body fat). Once stabilized on a dosage, serum levels tend to remain constant.
3. Extended-release products are intended for clients with relatively continuous or recurring symptoms who need to maintain therapeutic theophylline serum levels. They are not intended to treat an acute episode of bronchospasm associated with asthma, chronic bronchitis, or emphysema. These clients require an immediate-release or IV theophylline preparation (or other bronchodilators).

4. Adjust dose following serum theophylline determinations as follows when using **oral** products:
   - If serum theophylline is 5–10 mcg/mL and symptoms are not controlled but current dosage is tolerated, increase dose by about 25%. Recheck serum levels after 3 days for further dosage adjustment.
   - If serum theophylline is from 10 to 20 mcg/mL and symptoms are controlled and current dosage is tolerated, maintain dosage and recheck serum theophylline levels at 6–12 month intervals. If symptoms are not controlled and current dosage is tolerated, consider adding additional medications(s) to treatment regimen.
   - If serum theophylline level is from 20 to 25 mcg/mL, decrease dose by 10%, even if no adverse reactions are present. Recheck serum levels after 3 days to guide further dosage adjustment.
   - If serum theophylline is from 25 to 30 mcg/mL, skip the next dose and decrease subsequent doses at least 25%, even if no adverse reactions are present. Recheck serum levels after 3 days to guide further dosage adjustment. If symptomatic, consider whether overdose treatment is indicated.
   - If serum theophylline levels are >30 mcg/mL, skip next 2 doses and decrease subsequent doses by at least 50%, and recheck serum levels after 3 days to guide further dosage adjustment.
5. Maximum daily theophylline dose (where the serum level is not measured) based on age follows: **Children, 1–9 years:** 24 mg/kg/day; **children, 9–12 years:** 20 mg/kg/day; **children, 12–16 years:** 18 mg/kg/day; **children, >16 years:** 13 mg/kg/day.
6. Transient caffeine-like side effects and excessive serum levels in slow metabolizers can be avoided in most clients by starting with a sufficiently low dose and slowly increasing the dose. Make dose increases only if the previous dosage is well tolerated and at intervals of no less than 3 days to allow serum theophylline levels to reach the new steady state.
7. Review list of agents with which theophylline derivatives interact.
8. Monitor serum theophylline levels in chronic therapy, especially if the maximum maintenance doses are used or exceeded. Obtain the serum sample at the time of peak absorption (1–2 hr) after administration for immediate-release products and 5–9 hr after the morning dose for sustained-release products (as long as the client has not missed doses during the previous 48 hr).
9. Once-daily dosing using the 12-hour extended-release capsules and tablets may be appropriate for adult nonsmokers with appropriate total body clearance, as well as others with low dosage requirements. Consider once-daily dosing only after the client has been gradually and satisfactorily treated to therapeutic levels with every-12-hour dosing. The trough concentration following conversion to once-daily dosing may be lower (especially in high clearance clients) and the peak levels may be higher (especially in low clearance clients) than that obtained with every-12-hour dosing.
10. Clients who metabolize theophylline rapidly (e.g., younger clients, smokers, some non-smoking adults) and who have symptoms repeatedly at the end of a dosing interval will require either increased doses given once a day or preferably, are likely to be better controlled by twice-daily dosing. Those who require increased daily doses are more likely to experience relatively wide peak-tough differences and may be candidates for a twice-a-day dosing schedule using theophylline extended-release capsules (12- and 24-hour) or extended-release tablets (12-hour).
11. The extended-release tablets or capsules are not recommended for children less than age 6. Dosage for once-a-day products has not been established in children less than 12 years old.
12. Serum levels may vary significantly following brand interchange.
13. When converting from an immediate-release to an extended-release product, keep the total daily dose the same; only the dosing interval is adjusted.
14. Consult the package insert of each theophylline product to determine the specific administration guidelines as they differ from product to product.

15. Store the elixir, extended-release and controlled-release tablets, and 12-hr extended-release capsules from 15–30°C (59–86°F). Store 24-hr controlled-release capsules below 25°C (77°F).
16. IV Adjust dose following serum theophylline determinations as follows when using **IV** products:
   - If serum theophylline levels are <9.9 mcg/mL and symptoms are not controlled but current dosage is tolerated, increase infusion rate about 25%. Recheck serum levels after 12 hr in children and 24 hr in adults for further dosage adjustment.
   - If serum theophylline levels are 10 to 14.9 mcg/mL and symptoms are controlled and current dosage is tolerated, maintain the infusion rate and recheck serum levels at 24-hr intervals. If symptoms are not controlled and current dosage is tolerated, consider adding additional medication(s) to the treatment regimen.
   - If serum theophylline levels are 15 to 19.9 mcg/mL, consider a 10% decrease in the infusion rate to provide a greater margin of safety, even if current dosage is tolerated.
   - If serum theophylline levels are 20 to 24.9 mcg/mL, decrease the infusion rate by 25%, even if no side effects are present. Recheck serum levels after 12 hr in children and 24 hr in adults to guide further dosage adjustment.
   - If serum theophylline levels are 25 to 30 mcg/mL, stop the infusion for 12 hr in children and 24 hr in adults and decrease subsequent infusion rate at least 25%, even if no side effects are present. Recheck serum levels after 12 hr in children and 24 hr in adults to guide further dosage adjustment. If symptomatic, stop the infusion and consider whether overdose treatment is indicated.
   - If serum theophylline levels are >30 mcg/mL, stop the infusion and treat overdose as indicated. If theophylline is subsequently resumed, decrease the infusion rate by at least 50% and recheck serum levels after 12 hr in children and 24 hr in adults to guide further dosage adjustment.
17. Do not use flexible container in series connections as such use could result in air embolism due to residual air being drawn from the primary container before administration of the fluid from the secondary container is completed.
18. Use aseptic technique in preparing theophylline for IV administration.
19. Store the injection at 25°C (77°F); avoid excessive heat and protect from freezing.
20. COMPATIBILITY D5W.
21. INCOMPATIBILITY No additive should be made to theophylline and D5W injections.

ASSESSMENT

1. Note reasons for therapy, type, onset, characteristics of S&S. Assess for hypersensitivity to xanthine compounds. List experience with this class of drugs.
2. List any hypotension, CAD, angina, PUD, during lactation, or with seizure disorders; avoid drug or use very cautiously with these conditions.
3. Assess for cigarette/marijuana use; induces hepatic metabolism of drug and may require increase in dosage from 50–100%.
4. Follow dosing guidelines carefully. Dosage based on peak serum concentration measurements and on lean body weight. Start low and gradually increase to achieve desired response.
5. Check for diet habits, which can influence the excretion of theophylline.
6. Assess lung fields closely. Note characteristics of sputum and cough; assess CXR, ABGs, and PFTs. Observe for any evidence of seizures.
7. Check levels; obtain serum sample at time of peak absorption (1–2 hr after administration for immediate release and 5–9 hr after the morning dose or sustained-release products). The client must not have missed doses during the previous 48 hr and the dosing intervals must have been reasonably typical during this time.
8. Monitor VS, ECG, CBC, calcium, renal and LFTs, and theophylline levels.

CLIENT/FAMILY TEACHING

1. Drug works by relaxing muscles in the lungs and chest, and makes the lungs less sensitive to allergens and other causes of bronchospasm.
2. To avoid epigastric pain, take with a snack or with meals. Do not crush, dissolve, chew, or break slow-release forms of the drug.

3. May cause dizziness, assess effects before performing activities that require mental alertness. Report S&S of toxicity such as N&V, anorexia, insomnia, restlessness/irritability, hyperexcitability; will need drug levels and ECG to assess for arrhythmias.
4. Do not smoke; may aggravate underlying medical conditions as well as interfere with drug absorption. Attend smoking cessation program. Do not take any OTC cough, cold, or breathing preparations without provider approval.
5. Protect from acute exacerbations of illness by avoiding crowds, dressing warmly in cold weather, obtaining the pneumonia vaccine and seasonal flu shot, covering mouth and nose so cold air is not directly inhaled, staying in air conditioning during excessively hot and humid weather, maintaining proper diet and nutrition, exercising daily, and consuming adequate fluids.
6. Report S&S of infections, adverse drug effects, difficulty breathing, and significant peak flow readings.
7. Drug will not stop asthma attack once started. Always carry rescue medicine (e.g., bronchodilator inhaler) in case of asthma attack.
8. Avoid caffeine- and xanthine-containing beverages and foods (chocolate, coffee, tea, colas) and daily intake of charbroiled foods; increases drug side effects.
9. When secretions become thick and tacky, increase intake of fluids, as these thin secretions and assist in their removal. (Avoid milk/milk products.)
10. Learn to pace activity and avoid overexertion at all times.
11. Hold medication and report side effects or excessive CNS depression/stimulation in children and infants (unable to report side effects).
12. Use caution; children and elderly more sensitive to theophylline effects.
13. Practice reliable contraception; may be harmful to an unborn baby.
14. Identify local support groups that may assist in understanding and coping with chronic respiratory disease/dysfunction.
15. Keep all F/U to assess response, labs, and for adverse SE.

OUTCOMES/EVALUATE

- Improved airway exchange and breathing patterns; ↓ wheezing
- Therapeutic drug levels without toxicity or serious side effects
- Stimulation of respirations in the neonate

Thioguanine (6-TG, 6-Thioguanine)

(thigh-oh-**GWON**-een)

Classification(s): Antineoplastic, antimetabolite

Pregnancy Category: D

RX: Tabloid.

🍁 **Rx:** Lanvis.

SEE ALSO ***ANTINEOPLASTIC AGENTS***.

INDICATIONS/USES

For remission, induction, consolidation, and maintenance therapy of acute nonlymphocytic leukemias (usually in combination with other drugs such as cyclophosphamide, cytarabine, prednisone, vincristine). Not recommended for maintenance therapy or long-term continuous treatment due to the high risk of liver toxicity. *NOTE:* Although thioguanine is one of several drugs that have activity in treating the chronic phase of chronic myelogenous leukemia, busulfun is usually regarded as the preferred drug. *Investigational:* Second-line therapy for Crohn's disease and ulcerative colitis. Psoriasis.

ACTION/KINETICS

Action

Purine antagonist that is cell-cycle specific for the S phase of cell division. Converted to 6-thioguanylic acid, which in turn interferes with the synthesis of guanine nucleotides by competing with hypoxanthine and xanthine for the enzyme phosphoribosyltransferase (HGPRTase). Ultimately the synthesis of RNA and DNA is inhibited. Resistance to the drug may result from increased breakdown of 6-thioguanylic acid or loss of HGPRTase activity.

Pharmacokinetics

Partially absorbed (30%) from GI tract. **t½, plasma disappearance:** 80 min. Metabolized by the liver and excreted in the urine. More effective in children than in adults. Cross-resistance with mercaptopurine.

CONTRAINDICATIONS

Resistance to mercaptopurine or thioguanine; there is usually complete cross-resistance between the two. Use for maintenance or long-term continuous therapy due to the high risk of liver toxicity from vascular endothelial damage; liver toxicity is not always associated with elevated liver-enzyme concentrations (signs of portal hypertension may indicate toxicity). Lactation.

SPECIAL CONCERNS

■ Thioguanine is a potent drug. Do not use unless a diagnosis of acute nonlymphocytic leukemia has been adequately established and the responsible physician is knowledgeable in assessing response to chemotherapy. ■

Clients having an inherited deficiency of thiopurine methyltransferase are usually sensitive to the myelosuppressive effects of mercaptopurine.

SIDE EFFECTS

Most Common

Myelosuppression (pancytopenia, anemia, leukopenia, thrombocytopenia-or any combination thereof), hyperuricemia.

See *Antineoplastic Agents* for a complete list of possible side effects. **Hematologic:** Myelosuppression (pancytopenia, anemia, leukopenia, thrombocytopenia—or any combination thereof), ***hepatoxicity.*** **GI:** N&V, anorexia, stomatitis, ***intestinal necrosis and perforation. hepatotoxicity.*** **Miscellaneous:** Loss of vibration sense, unsteadiness of gait, hyperuricemia. Adults tend to show a more rapid fall in WBC count than children.

LABORATORY TEST CONSIDERATIONS

↑ Uric acid in blood and urine.

OVERDOSE MANAGEMENT

Symptoms: N&V, hypertension, malaise, and diaphoresis may be seen immediately, which may be followed by myelosuppression and azotemia. ***Severe hematologic toxicity.*** *Treatment:* Induce vomiting if client is seen immediately after an acute overdosage. Treat symptoms. Hematologic toxicity may be treated by platelet transfusions (for bleeding) and granulocyte transfusions. Antibiotics are indicated for sepsis.

DRUG INTERACTIONS

Busulfan / Chronic concomitant therapy → esophageal varices associated with abnormal LFTs and evidence of nodular regenerative hyperplasia
Mesalamine / Exacerbation of rapid bone marrow suppression in clients with thiopurine methyltransferase deficiency
Olsalazine / Exacerbation of rapid bone marrow suppression in clients with thiopurine methyltransferase deficiency
Sulfasalazine / Exacerbation of rapid bone marrow suppression in clients with thiopurine methyltransferase deficiency

HOW SUPPLIED

Tablets: 40 mg.

DOSAGE

TABLETS

Acute nonlymphocytic leukemias.

Individualized. Adults and pediatric, initial: 2 mg/kg/day (or 75–100 mg/m^2) given at one time. From 2 to 4 weeks may elapse before beneficial results become apparent. Compute dose to nearest multiple of 20 mg. If no response after 4 weeks, dosage may be increased to 3 mg/kg/day. Dosage of thioguanine does not have to be decreased during administration of allopurinol (to inhibit uric acid production).

NURSING IMPLICATIONS

IMPLEMENTATION/ADMINISTRATION/STORAGE

1. Some individuals have an inherited deficiency of thiopurine methyltransferase and who may be unusually sensitive to the myelosuppressive effects of thioguanine resulting in rapid bone marrow suppression. Substantial dosage reduction may be needed to avoid the development of life-threatening bone marrow suppression.
2. Store from 15–25°C (59–77°F).

ASSESSMENT

1. Note reasons for therapy, onset, characteristics of S&S; list other agents trialed, outcome.
2. Identify those experiencing loss of vibration sense and with unsteady gaits (may be unable to rely on canes); may require assistance.

T

3. Expect hyperuricemia after tumor lysis, which may be reduced with administration of allopurinol, by preventing purine breakdown and excessive uric acid formation.
4. Perform platelet counts weekly; discontinue drug if abnormally large fall in blood count is noted, indicating severe bone marrow depression.
5. Monitor CBC, uric acid, renal and LFTs. Obtain CBC weekly and LFTs monthly during course of therapy; may cause granulocyte and platelet suppression. Nadir: 10 days; recovery: 21 days.

CLIENT/FAMILY TEACHING

1. Take on an empty stomach for best results. Expect maintenance doses to be continued during remissions.
2. Increase fluid intake (2–3 L/day) to minimize uric acid (crystals) in blood and urine.
3. Withhold drug and report yellowing of skin, decreased urine output, diarrhea, S&S of anemia (fatigue, dyspnea), or extremity swelling.
4. Avoid crowds, vaccinia, and persons with infectious diseases. Any sore throat, fever, or flu-like symptoms as well as increased bruising/bleeding require immediate reporting.
5. Practice reliable contraception.
6. Keep all F/U to assess response, labs, and for adverse SE.

OUTCOMES/EVALUATE

- Suppression of malignant cell proliferation
- Hematologic evidence of leukemia remission

Tiagabine hydrochloride

(tye-**AG**-ah-been)

Classification(s): Anticonvulsant, miscellaneous

Pregnancy Category: C

RX: Gabatril.

SEE ALSO ***ANTICONVULSANTS***.

INDICATIONS/USES

Adjunctive therapy for partial seizures in adults and children at least 12 years of age. *Investigational:* Bipolar disorders; posttraumatic stress disorder in adults. Refractory seizures in children.

ACTION/KINETICS

Action

Mechanism not known but activity of GABA, an inhibitory neurotransmitter, may be enhanced. Drug may block uptake of GABA into presynaptic neurons, allowing more GABA to bind to post-synaptic cells. This prevents propagation of neural impulses that contribute to seizures due to GABA-ergic action.

Pharmacokinetics

Well absorbed after PO; absolute bioavailability is about 90%. **Peak plasma levels:** About 45 min when fasting. High-fat meals decrease rate but not extent of absorption. **Steady-state:** 2 days. Metabolized in liver mainly by CYP3A and possibly CYP1A2, CYP2D6, and CYP2C19. Excreted in urine and feces. **t½, elimination:** 7–9 hr. The systemic clearance in induced clients is about 60% greater, resulting in significantly lower plasma levels and a t½ elimination of 2–5 hr. Diurnal effect occurs with levels being lower in evening compared with morning. **Plasma protein binding:** 96%.

CONTRAINDICATIONS

Hypersensitivity to tiagabine or any component of the product. Use during lactation only if benefit clearly outweighs risks.

SPECIAL CONCERNS

- Do not discontinue abruptly due to the possibility of withdrawal seizures.
- Increased risk of suicidal behavior and ideation.
- New onset seizures and status epilepticus are possible in clients without epilepsy.
- Safety and efficacy not determined in children less than 12 years of age.

SIDE EFFECTS

Most Common

Dizziness/light-headedness, asthenia, somnolence, nausea, nervousness/irritability, tremor, abdominal pain, abnormal/difficulty with concentration/attention.

NOTE: Side effects with an incidence of at least 1% or those that are life–threatening are listed.

CNS: Asthenia, dizziness/lightheadedness, nervousness, difficulty with concentration/attention, abnormal gait, agitation, ataxia, confusion, depression, difficulty with memory, emotional lability, hostility, insomnia, speech/language problems,

T

nystagmus, paresthesia, somnolence, fatigue, speech disorder, tremor, twitching, headache, anxiety, incoordination, depersonalization, dysarthria, euphoria, hallucinations, hyperkinesia, hypertonia, hypesthesia, hypokinesia, hypotonia, migraine, myoclonus, paranoid reaction, personality disorder, decreased reflexes, stupor, vertigo, ***suicidal behavior***/ideation, ***withdrawal seizures***. **GI:** N&V, diarrhea, abdominal pain, increased appetite, mouth ulceration, constipation, anorexia, dry mouth, flatulence, dyspepsia, gastroenteritis, gingivitis, stomatitis. **CV:** Vasodilation, hypertension, palpitation, syncope, tachycardia. **Dermatologic:** Rash (may be serious), pruritus, ecchymosis, acne, alopecia, dry skin, sweating. **Musculoskeletal:** Myasthenia, chest/back/neck pain, myalgia, arthralgia. **Respiratory:** Pharyngitis, increased cough, rhinitis, sinusitis, bronchitis, dyspnea, epistaxis, pneumonia. **GU:** UTI, urinary frequency, dysmenorrhea, dysuria, metrorrhagia, urinary incontinence, vaginitis. **Ophthalmic:** Amblyopia, conjunctivitis, diplopia, abnormal vision. **Otic:** Ear pain, otitis media, tinnitus. **Body as a whole:** Unspecified pain, flu syndrome, infection, lymphadenopathy, edema, peripheral edema, weight gain/loss, allergic reaction, chills, malaise, generalized weakness, fever, ***sudden unexplained death***. **Miscellaneous:** Accidental injury, cyst. *NOTE:* There is a risk of new onset seizures and status epilepticus in clients without a history of epilepsy, especially when used for unapproved indications (e.g., bipolar disorder).

LABORATORY TEST CONSIDERATIONS

EEG abnormalities.

OVERDOSE MANAGEMENT

Symptoms: Somnolence, impaired consciousness, agitation, confusion, drowsiness, lethargy, speech difficulties, hostility, depression, weakness, myoclonus, seizures (including status epilepticus), coma, ataxia, spike wave stupor, tremors, disorientation, vomiting, temporary paralysis, respiratory depression. *Treatment:*

- There is no specific antidote.
- Increase elimination by gastric lavage.
- Maintain the airway.
- Use general supportive care, including monitoring of vital signs and observation of the clinical status.
- Dialysis is not likely to be beneficial.

DRUG INTERACTIONS

Bupropion / ↑ Risk of seizures R/T bupropion lowering seizure threshold; use together with caution or select alternative therapy
Carbamazepine / ↑ Tiagabine clearance (60%) due to ↑ metabolism
Gemfibrozil / ↑ Tiagabine toxicity, including confusion, seizures, coma; closely monitor and adjust tiagabine dose as needed
Highly protein-bound drugs / ↑ Possibility of an interaction with other highly protein-bound drugs → ↑ free fractions of either drug; monitor effects and adjust dose as needed
Phenobarbital / ↑ Tiagabine clearance (60%) due to ↑ metabolism
Phenytoin / ↑ Tiagabine clearance (60%) due to ↑ metabolism
Primidone / ↑ Tiagabine clearance (60%) due to ↑ metabolism
Tramadol / ↑ Risk of seizures R/T tramadol lowering seizure threshold; use together with caution or select alternative therapy
Valproate / Significant ↓ tiagabine binding → 40% ↑ free tiagabine; significance is unknown

HOW SUPPLIED

Tablets : 2 mg, 4 mg, 12 mg, 16 mg.

DOSAGE

TABLETS

Partial seizures in those taking enzyme-inducing antiepileptic drugs.

Adults and children over 18 years, initial: 4 mg once daily. **Week 2:** 8 mg/day in 2 divided doses; **Week 3:** 12 mg/day in 3 divided doses; **Week 4:** 16 mg/day in 2–4 divided doses; **Week 5:** 20–24 mg/day in 2–4 divided doses; **Week 6:** 24–32 mg/day in 2–4 divided doses; **usual adult maintenance dose:** 32–56 mg/day in 2–4 divided doses. **Children, 12 to 18 years, initial, week 1:** 4 mg once daily. The total daily dose may be increased by 4 mg at the beginning of week 2. Thereafter, the total daily dose may be increased by 4–8 mg at weekly intervals until a clinical effect is noted or up to 32 mg/day in 2–4 divided doses is reached. Dosages above 32 mg/day have been tolerated for a short period of time in a small number of children. *NOTE:* Consider dosage adjustment whenever a change in the client's enzyme–inducing status occurs as a result of the addition, discontinuation, or dose change of the enzyme–inducing agent.

Partial seizures in those not taking an enzyme-inducing antiepileptic drug.

Adults and children, 12 years and older: The estimated plasma levels in noninduced clients is more than two times that in those receiving enzyme-inducing drugs. Thus, use in noninduced clients requires lower doses of tiagabine and such clients also require a slower titration of tiagabine compared with that of induced clients.

Refractory seizures in children (investigational).

Children, 2 years and older, initial: 0.25 mg/kg/day divided 2 times/day for 4 weeks. Increase at 4 week intervals to 0.1, 1, and 1.5 mg/kg/day until an effective dose is reached. **Maximum dose:** 0.73 +/- 0.44 mg/kg/day in those receiving enzyme–inducing antiepileptic drugs and 0.61 +/- 0.32 mg/kg/day in those receiving non enzyme-inducing antiepileptic drugs.

NURSING IMPLICATIONS

Do not confuse tiagabine with tizanidine (skeletal muscle relaxant).

IMPLEMENTATION/ADMINISTRATION/STORAGE

1. It is not necessary to modify dose of concomitant anticonvulsant drugs, unless clinically indicated.
2. Those with impaired liver function may require reduced initial and maintenance doses and/or longer dosing intervals compared with those with normal hepatic function.
3. The following recommendations for dosing apply to all clients taking tiagabine:
   - Give orally and take with food.
   - Do not use a loading dose.
   - Do not use rapid dose escalation and/or large dose increments.
   - Consider dosage adjustment whenever a change in the client's enzyme-inducing system occurs (i.e., as a result of the addition, discontinuation, or dose change of the enzyme-inducing agent).
4. If a dose is missed at the scheduled time, do not increase the next dose to make up for the missed dose.
5. Do not abruptly discontinue tiagabine. Withdraw gradually to minimize the potential for increased seizure frequency, unless safety concerns require a more rapid withdrawal.
6. To monitor the effects of in utero exposure to tiagabine, pregnant clients taking the drug should enroll in the North American Antiepileptic Drug Pregnancy registry by calling 1-888-233-2334
7. Store from 20–25°C (68–77°F) protected from light and moisture.

ASSESSMENT

1. Note reasons for therapy, characteristics of seizures, other agents trialed, outcome.
2. List drugs prescribed to ensure none interact.
3. Assess mental status and psychological state including any evidence of depression. Observe closely for impaired concentration, speech or language problems, and confusion as well as somnolence and fatigue.
4. Monitor LFTs; decrease dosage or dosing intervals with dysfunction.

CLIENT/FAMILY TEACHING

1. Take with food as directed. Do not stop abruptly; may trigger seizures.
2. Avoid activities requiring mental alertness until drug effects realized; may cause dizziness, sleepiness, or confusion.
3. Report any increased frequency or loss of seizure control, rash, weakness, or visual disturbances. Any behavioral changes or suicide ideations require immediate reporting.
4. Avoid alcohol and any other CNS depressants.
5. Practice reliable contraception; do not breastfeed.
6. Keep all F/U to assess response, labs, and for adverse SE.

OUTCOMES/EVALUATE

Control of seizures

T

Ticagrelor

(tye-**KA**-grel-or)

Classification(s): Antiplatelet drug, aggregation inhibitor

Pregnancy Category: C

RX: Brilinta.

INDICATIONS/USES

To reduce the rate of thrombotic CV events in clients with acute coronary syndrome (unstable angina, non-ST elevation MI, or ST elevation MI). Ticagrelor reduces the rate of a combined end point of CV death, MI, or stroke compared with clopidogrel. In clients treated with percutaneous coronary intervention, the rate of stent thrombosis is reduced. *NOTE:* Percutaneous coronary intervention clients who have received a loading dose of clopidogrel may be started on ticagrelor.

ACTION/KINETICS

Action

Ticagrelor and its major metabolite (are equally potent) reversibly interact with the platelet $P2Y_{12}$ adenosine diphosphate receptor; this prevents signal transduction and platelet activation.

Pharmacokinetics

T_{max}: 1.5 hr (range: 1–4 hr). T_{max} for the formation of the major active metabolite is 2.5 hr (range: 1.5–5 hr). Absolute bioavailability is 30–42%. A high fat meal increases AUC 21%; C_{max} of the active metabolite decreased by 22%. CYP3A4 is the major enzyme responsible for metabolism to the active metabolite. Ticagrelor is excreted through both the feces (58%) and urine (26%); the active metabolite is excreted through the bile, **t½, mean, ticagrelor:** 7 hr; **active metabolite:** 9 hr. **Plasma protein binding:** >99% for both ticagrelor and the active metabolite.

CONTRAINDICATIONS

History of intracranial hemorrhage or active pathological bleeding (e.g., peptic ulcer, intracranial hemorrhage). Severe hepatic impairment. Lactation.

SPECIAL CONCERNS

■ **Bleeding risk.** (1) Ticagrelor, like other antiplatelet agents, can cause significant, sometimes fatal, bleeding. (2) Do not use ticagrelor in clients with active pathological bleeding or a history of intracranial hemorrhage. (3) Do not initiate therapy with ticagrelor in clients planning to undergo urgent coronary artery bypass graft surgery. When possible, discontinue ticagrelor at least 5 days prior to any surgery. (4) Suspect bleeding in any client who is hypotensive and has recently undergone coronary angiography, percutaneous coronary intervention, coronary artery bypass graft, or other surgical procedures in the setting of ticagrelor. (5) If possible, manage bleeding without discontinuing ticagrelor. Stopping ticagrelor increases the risk of subsequent CV events. (5) **Aspirin dose and ticagrelor effectiveness.** Maintenance doses of aspirin above 100 mg reduce the effectiveness of ticagrelor; avoid such doses. After any initial dose, use with aspirin 75 to 100 mg/day. ■

- **Carefully consider use in those with moderate hepatic impairment.**
- **Risk factors for bleeding include older age, a history of bleeding disorders, performance of percutaneous invasive procedures, and concomitant use of drugs that increase the risk of bleeding (e.g., anticoagulant and fibrinolytic therapy, higher doses of aspirin, long-term use of NSAIDs).**
- **Suspect bleeding in any client who is hypotensive and has recently undergone coronary angiography, percutaneous coronary intervention, coronary artery bypass graft, or other surgical procedures even if the client has no signs of bleeding.**
- **Severe hepatic impairment increases the risk of bleeding.**
- **Safety and efficacy not determined in children.**

SIDE EFFECTS

Most Common

Bleeding events, dyspnea, cough, atrial fibrillation, dizziness, headache, nausea.

CV: Bleeding events (both early and later); bleeding may be major and ***life-threatening, intracranial bleeding.*** Also, atrial fibrillation, chest pain, hyper-/hypotension, bradyarrhythmias (including ventricular pauses). **CNS:** Headache, dizziness. **GI:** Diarrhea, nausea. **Respiratory:** Dyspnea (includes exertional dyspnea, dyspnea at rest, nocturnal dyspnea, and paroxysmal nocturnal dyspnea), cough. **GU:** Gynecomastia in men. **Body as a whole:** Fatigue. **Miscellaneous:** Back pain, noncardiac chest pain.

LABORATORY TEST CONSIDERATIONS

↑ Serum uric acid, serum creatinine.

OVERDOSE MANAGEMENT

Symptoms: Bleeding (most common), N&V, diarrhea, ventricular pauses. *Treatment:* No known treatment to reverse the effects of ticagrelor; drug is not dialyzable. Follow local standard medical practice to treat overdose. If bleeding occurs, take appropriate supportive measures. Monitor ECGs.

DRUG INTERACTIONS

NOTE: Ticagrelor is metabolized mainly by the CYP3A enzyme system. Substances known to inhibit these enzymes may decrease metabolism or increase bioavailability of ticagrelor. Also, drugs known to induce these enzyme systems may result in increased metabolism of ticagrelor or decreased bioavailability. Monitoring of blood levels and appropriate dosage adjustment are essential when such drugs are used together.

Aspirin / Use with aspirin doses >100 mg ↓ ticagrelor efficacy; after any initial loading dose of aspirin, use with aspirin 75–100 mg a day

Atazanavir / ↑ Ticagrelor plasma levels → ↑ pharmacologic/toxic effects; avoid concomitant use

Carbamazepine / ↓ Ticagrelor plasma levels → ↓ pharmacologic effect; avoid concomitant use

Clarithromycin / ↑ Ticagrelor plasma levels → ↑ pharmacologic/toxic effects; avoid concomitant use

Dexamethasone / ↓ Ticagrelor plasma levels → ↓ pharmacologic effect; avoid concomitant use

Digoxin / Possible ↑ digoxin levels R/T inhibition of the P–gp transporter → ↑ risk of toxicity; monitor digoxin levels

Indinavir / ↑ Ticagrelor plasma levels → ↑ pharmacologic/toxic effects; avoid concomitant use

Itraconazole / ↑ Ticagrelor plasma levels → ↑ pharmacologic/toxic effects; avoid concomitant use

Ketoconazole / ↑ Ticagrelor plasma levels → ↑ pharmacologic/toxic effects; avoid concomitant use

Lovastatin / ↑ Lovastatin serum levels R/T inhibition of metabolism by CYP3A4; avoid lovastatin doses >40 mg

Nefazodone / ↑ Ticagrelor plasma levels → ↑ pharmacologic/toxic effects; avoid concomitant use

Nelfinavir / ↑ Ticagrelor plasma levels → ↑ pharmacologic/toxic effects; avoid concomitant use

NSAIDs (e.g., ibuprofen) / ↑ Risk of bleeding; if coadministration cannot be avoided, closely monitor for bleeding

Phenobarbital / ↓ Ticagrelor plasma levels → ↓ pharmacologic effect; avoid concomitant use

Phenytoin / ↓ Ticagrelor plasma levels → ↓ pharmacologic effect; avoid concomitant use

Rifampin / ↓ Ticagrelor plasma levels → ↓ pharmacologic effect; avoid concomitant use

Ritonavir / ↑ Ticagrelor plasma levels → ↑ pharmacologic/toxic effects; avoid concomitant use

Saquinavir / ↑ Ticagrelor plasma levels → ↑ pharmacologic/toxic effects; avoid concomitant use

Simvastatin / ↑ Simvastatin serum levels R/T inhibition of metabolism by CYP3A4; avoid simvastatin doses >40 mg

Telithromycin / ↑ Ticagrelor plasma levels → ↑ pharmacologic/toxic effects; avoid concomitant use

Voriconazole / ↑ Ticagrelor plasma levels → ↑ pharmacologic/toxic effects; avoid concomitant use

HOW SUPPLIED

Tablets: 90 mg.

DOSAGE

TABLETS

Acute coronary syndrome.

Adults, loading dose: 180 mg; **maintenance dose:** 90 mg twice a day. After the initial loading dose of aspirin (usually 325 mg), use ticagrelor with a daily maintenance dose of aspirin, 75–100 mg.

NURSING IMPLICATIONS

IMPLEMENTATION/ADMINISTRATION/STORAGE

1. If a dose is missed, the client should take one 90 mg tablet (i.e., their next dose) at its scheduled time.
2. When possible, discontinue ticagrelor 5 days prior to surgery.
3. Avoid interruption of ticagrelor treatment. If ticagrelor must be temporarily discontinued (e.g., to treat bleeding, for elective surgery), restart as soon as possible. Discontinuation will increase the risk of MI, stent thrombosis, and death.

4. Store from 15–30°C (59–86°F). Keep in original container; keep tablets dry.

ASSESSMENT

1. Document indications for therapy, clinical presentation, other agents trialed and outcome.
2. List drugs prescribed to ensure none interact.
3. Review ECG, angiography and other cardiac studies. Assess heart sounds and rhythm.
4. Identify risk factors for bleeding: increased age, history of bleeding disorders, invasive procedures, and use of medications (NSAIDs, ASA) that increase the risk of bleeding.
5. Ensure that drug is stopped 5 days before any surgery, especially bypass.
6. Monitor CBC, uric acid, renal and LFTs.

CLIENT/FAMILY TEACHING

1. Administer with or without food as directed. Continue to take low dose aspirin unless otherwise instructed.
2. Drug administered to reduce risk of adverse events (death and stroke), and provide prevention over time of heart attack or stroke.
3. May lead to increased risk of bleeding; report any excessive bruising or prolonged bleeding or blood evident in urine or stool.
4. Practice reliable contraception; report if pregnancy suspected.
5. Notify all providers of use of this drug before undergoing surgical or dental procedures, or adding other medications to regimen.
6. May experience SOB; report if unexpected or severe.
7. Keep all F/U to assess response, labs, cardiac diagnostic studies and adverse SE.

OUTCOMES/EVALUATE

- ↓ Mortality with ACS
- ↓ Thrombotic cardiovascular events (MI, stroke) with acute coronary syndrome (ACS)

Combination Drug

IV

Ticarcillin disodium and Clavulanate potassium

(tie-kar-**SILL**-in, klav-you-**LAN**-ate)

Classification(s): Antibiotic, penicillin

Pregnancy Category: B

RX: Timentin.

SEE ALSO ***PENICILLINS.***

INDICATIONS/USES

(1) Septicemia, including bacteremia, due to beta-lactamase producing strains of *Klebsiella* species, *Staphylococcus aureus, Escherichia coli,* and *Pseudomonas aeruginosa* (and other *Pseudomonas* species). (2) Lower respiratory tract infections due to beta-lactamase producing strains of *S. aureus, Haemophilus influenzae,* and *Klebsiella* sp. (3) Bone and joint infections due to beta-lactamase producing strains of *S. aureus.* (4) Skin and skin structure infections due to beta-lactamase producing strains of *S. aureus, Klebsiella* sp., and *E. coli.* (5) UTIs (complicated and uncomplicated) due to beta-lactamase producing strains of *E. coli, Klebsiella* sp., *P. aeruginosa* (and other *Pseudomonas* species), *Citrobacter* sp., *Enterobacter cloacae, Serratia marcescens,* and *S. aureus.* (6) Endometritis due to beta-lactamase producing strains of *Prevotella melaninogenicus, Enterobacter* sp. (including *E. cloacae), E. coli, Klebsiella pneumoniae, S. aureus,* and *Staphylococcus epidermidis.* (7) Peritonitis due to beta-lactamase producing strains of *E. coli, K. pneumoniae,* and *Bacteroides fragilis* group. *NOTE:* Mixed infections due to ticarcillin-susceptible organisms and beta-lactamase-producing organisms susceptible to ticarcillin/clavulanate should not require addition of another antibiotic.

CONTENT

Each vial of the Powder for Injection and the Injection Solution (per 100 mL) contains: Ticarcillin disodium, 3 grams, and clavulanate potassium, 0.1 gram.

ACTION/KINETICS

Action

Ticarcillin has an antibacterial spectrum similar to carbenicillin. Contains clavulanic acid, which protects the breakdown of ticarcillin by beta-lactamase enzymes, thus ensuring appropriate blood levels of ticarcillin.

Pharmacokinetics

Peak plasma levels, ticarcillin, IV: 15 min. **t½:** 70 min.

SPECIAL CONCERNS

- **To reduce development of drug-resistant bacteria, use ticarcillin/clavulanate only to prevent or** treat infections that are proven or strongly suspected to be caused by susceptible bacteria.

- Use with caution in clients with impaired renal function and those on restricted salt diets.

SIDE EFFECTS

Most Common

Hypersensitivity, N&V, gastritis, stomatitis, diarrhea, skin rashes.

See *Penicillins* for a complete list of possible side effects. Neurotoxicity and neuromuscular excitability, especially in clients with impaired renal function. **Hematologic:** Neutropenia, leukopenia, thrombocytopenia, anemia. **GI:** N&V, diarrhea, constipation, abdominal pain, stomatitis, anorexia. **Respiratory:** Dyspnea, coughing. **Dermatologic:** Alopecia, rash. **Body as a whole:** Fatigue, fever, headache, pain (body, back, skeletal), asthenia.

HOW SUPPLIED

See *Content*.

DOSAGE

IV INFUSION

Systemic infections and urinary tract infections.

Adults, 60 kg or more: 3.1 grams (containing 0.1 gram clavulanic acid) q 4–6 hr for 10–14 days. **Adults <60 kg:** 200–300 mg ticarcillin/kg/day in divided doses q 4–6 hr for 10–14 days.

Gynecologic infections.

Adults, 60 kg or more, moderate infections: 200 mg/kg/day in divided doses q 6 hr; **severe infections:** 300 mg/kg/day in divided doses q 4 hr. **Adults, less than 60 kg:** 200–300 mg/kg/day in divided doses q 4–6 hr.

Mild to moderate infections in children.

Children, 60 kg or more: 3.1 grams q 6 hr. **Children, less than 60 kg:** 200 mg/kg/day (dosed at 50 mg/kg/dose) q 6 hr.

Severe infections in children.

Children, 60 kg or more: 3.1 grams q 4 hr. **Children, less than 60 kg:** 300 mg/kg/day (dosed at 50 mg/kg/dose) q 4 hr.

NURSING IMPLICATIONS

IMPLEMENTATION/ADMINISTRATION/STORAGE

1. IV Dosage for a client must consider the site and severity of the infection, the susceptibility of the organism causing the infection, and the status of the client's host defense mechanism.
2. For renal insufficiency: **Initially,** loading dose of 3 grams ticarcillin and 0.1 gram clavulanic acid; **then,** dose based on C_{CR} as follows. **C_{CR} >60 mL/min:** 3.1 grams q 4 hr; **C_{CR} from 30–60 mL/min:** 2 grams q 4 hr; **C_{CR} from 10–30 mL/min:** 2 grams q 8 hr; **C_{CR} <10 mL/min:** 2 grams q 12 hr; **C_{CR} <10 mL/min with hepatic dysfunction:** 2 grams q 24 hr. **Clients on peritoneal dialysis:** 3.1 grams q 12 hr; **clients on hemodialysis:** 2 grams q 12 hr and 3.1 grams after each dialysis.
3. To attain the appropriate dilution for 3 grams ticarcillin and 0.1 gram clavulanic acid, dilute with 13 mL of either NaCl or sterile water for injection. Further dilutions can be undertaken with D5W, RL injection, or NaCl.
4. Administer over a 30-min period, either through a Y-type IV infusion or by direct infusion. If a Y-type set up is used, temporarily discontinue administering any other solution during the infusion of ticarcillin/clavulanate.
5. Do not use plastic containers in serious connections, as this can result in embolism due to residual air being drawn from the primary container before administration of the fluid from the secondary container is complete.
6. Continue treatment for at least 2 days after S&S of infection have disappeared. The usual duration is 10–14 days.
7. Dilutions with NaCl or RL injection may be stored at room temperature for 24 hr or refrigerated for 7 days. Dilutions with D5W are stable at room temperature for 12 hr or for 3 days if refrigerated.
8. If used with another anti-infective agent (e.g., an aminoglycoside), give each drug separately.
9. Check the package insert for preparation of ADD-Vantage vial, pharmacy bulk package, or preparation for administration.
10. COMPATIBILITY D5W, RL injection, or NaCl.

T

11. [INCOMPATIBILITY] Sodium bicarbonate; administer separately.

ASSESSMENT

1. Note type, onset, characteristics of S&S. Obtain cultures before starting therapy; note clinical presentation.
2. Monitor bleeding times, CBC, cultures, renal and LFTs. Reduce dose with liver or renal dysfunction.

CLIENT/FAMILY TEACHING

1. Drug is administered parenterally to treat serious infections.
2. Report any symptoms of bleeding abnormalities, such as small purple spots on skin, easy bruising, or frank bleeding.
3. Extremity swelling, weight gain, or difficulty breathing may be precipitated by drug's large sodium content; notify provider.
4. Review drug side effects that should be reported if evident, especially persistent diarrhea.
5. Keep all F/U to assess response, labs, and for adverse SE.

OUTCOMES/EVALUATE

Resolution of infection; symptomatic improvement

Ticlopidine hydrochloride

(tie-**KLOH**-pih-deen)

Classification(s): Antiplatelet drug

Pregnancy Category: B

RX: Ticlid.

✤ **Rx:** Apo-Ticlopidine, Gen-Ticloplidine, Nu-Ticlopidine, Sandoz Ticlopidine.

INDICATIONS/USES

(1) With aspirin to decrease the incidence of sub acute stent thrombosis in clients undergoing successful coronary stent implantation. (2) Reduce the risk of fatal or nonfatal thrombotic stroke in clients who have manifested precursors of stroke or who have had a completed thrombotic stroke. Due to the risk of neutropenia or agranulocytosis, reserve for clients who are intolerant to aspirin therapy or who have failed aspirin therapy. *Investigational:* Chronic arterial occlusion, coronary artery bypass grafts, intermittent claudication, open heart surgery, primary glomerulonephritis, subarachnoid hemorrhage, sickle cell disease, uremic clients with AV shunts or fistulas.

ACTION/KINETICS

Action

Irreversibly inhibits ADP-induced platelet-fibrinogen binding and subsequent platelet-platelet interactions. This results in inhibition of both platelet aggregation and release of platelet granule constituents, as well as prolongation of bleeding time.

Pharmacokinetics

Peak plasma levels: 2 hr. **Maximum platelet inhibition:** 8–11 days after 250 mg twice a day. **Steady-state plasma levels:** 14–21 days. **t½, elimination:** 4–5 days. After discontinuing therapy, bleeding time and other platelet function tests return to normal within 14 days. Rapidly absorbed; bioavailability is increased by food. Extensively metabolized by the liver with approximately 60% excreted through the kidneys; 23% is excreted in the feces (with one-third excreted unchanged). Clearance of the drug decreases with age. **Plasma protein binding:** 98%.

CONTRAINDICATIONS

Use in the presence of neutropenia and thrombocytopenia, hemostatic disorder, or active pathologic bleeding such as bleeding peptic ulcer or intracranial bleeding. Severe liver impairment. Lactation.

SPECIAL CONCERNS

(1) Can cause life-threatening hematological side effects, including neutropenia/agranulocytosis and thrombotic thrombocytopenic purpura. (2) Severe hematological side effects may occur within a few days of starting therapy. The incidence of thrombotic thrombocytopenic purpura peaks after about 3–4 weeks of therapy and neutropenia peaks at about 4–6 weeks with both declining thereafter. Only a few cases have been seen after more than 3 months of therapy. (3) Hematological side effects cannot be reliably predicted by any demographic or clinical characteristics. During the first 3 months of therapy, hematologically and clinically monitor those receiving ticlopidine for evidence of neutropenia or thrombotic thrombocytopenic purpura (TTP). Immediately discontinue if there is any evidence of neutropenia or TTP.

- Use with caution in clients with ulcers (i.e., where there is a propensity for bleeding).

T

- Consider reduced dosage in impaired renal function.
- Elderly may be more sensitive to drug effects.
- Safety and efficacy not established in children less than 18 years of age.

SIDE EFFECTS

Most Common

Diarrhea, N&V, dyspepsia, rash, GI pain, neutropenia, purpura, flatulence, pruritus, dizziness.

Hematologic: Neutropenia, ***agranulocytosis, thrombotic thrombocytopenia purpura***, thrombocytopenia, pancytopenia, immune thrombocytopenia, ***hemolytic anemia with reticulocytosis***. **GI:** Diarrhea, N&V, GI pain, dyspepsia, flatulence, anorexia, GI fullness, peptic ulcer. **Hepatic:** Hepatitis, cholestatic jaundice, hepatocellular jaundice, ***hepatic necrosis***. **Bleeding complications:** Ecchymosis, hematuria, epistaxis, conjunctival hemorrhage, ***GI bleeding***, perioperative bleeding, posttraumatic bleeding, ***intracerebral bleeding (rare)***. **Dermatologic:** Maculopapular or urticarial rash, pruritus, urticaria. Rarely, erythema multiforme, exfoliative dermatitis, ***Stevens-Johnson syndrome***. **CNS:** Dizziness, headache. **Neuromuscular:** Asthenia, SLE, peripheral neuropathy, arthropathy, myositis. **Miscellaneous:** Tinnitus, pain, allergic pneumonitis, vasculitis, nephrotic syndrome, renal failure, angioedema, hyponatremia, serum sickness.

LABORATORY TEST CONSIDERATIONS

↑ Alkaline phosphatase, ALT, AST, serum cholesterol, and triglycerides. Abnormal LFTs.

DRUG INTERACTIONS

Antacids / ↓ Ticlopidine plasma levels
Aspirin / ↑ Effect of aspirin on collagen-induced platelet aggregation
Bupropion / ↑ Bupropion AUC and peak plasma levels and ↓ bupropion clearance R/T inhibition of metabolism by CYP2B6
Carbamazepine / ↑ Carbamazepine plasma levels → toxicity
Cimetidine / ↓ Ticlopidine clearance R/T ↓ liver metabolism
Digoxin / Slight ↓ in digoxin plasma levels
H *Evening primrose oil* / Potential for ↑ antiplatelet effect
H *Feverfew* / Potential for ↑ antiplatelet effect
H *Garlic* / Potential for ↑ antiplatelet effect
H *Ginger* / Potential for ↑ antiplatelet effect
H *Ginkgo biloba* / Potential for ↑ antiplatelet effect
H *Ginseng* / Potential for ↑ antiplatelet effect
H *Grapeseed extract* / Potential for ↑ antiplatelet effect
Phenytoin / ↑ Phenytoin plasma levels → somnolence and lethargy
Theophylline / ↑ Theophylline plasma levels R/T ↓ clearance

HOW SUPPLIED

Tablets: 250 mg.

DOSAGE

TABLETS

Adjunct with aspirin to reduce subacute stent thrombosis; reduce risk of thrombotic stroke.

250 mg twice a day.

NURSING IMPLICATIONS

Do not confuse Ticlid with Tequin (a fluoroquinolone antibiotic).

IMPLEMENTATION/ADMINISTRATION/STORAGE

1. To increase bioavailability and decrease GI discomfort, take with food or just after eating.
2. If switched from an anticoagulant or fibrinolytic drug to ticlopidine, discontinue the former drug before initiation of ticlopidine therapy.
3. IV methylprednisolone (20 mg) may normalize prolonged bleeding times, usually within 2 hr.

ASSESSMENT

1. Note reasons for therapy; assess for liver disease, bleeding disorders, or ulcer disease. Ascertain if aspirin intolerance.
2. See increased use of clopidogrel due to less side effect profile and once-daily dosing advantage.
3. List baseline hematologic profile (e.g., CBC, PT, PTT, INR), renal and LFTs. Monitor CBC biweekly to screen for possibly fatal thrombotic thrombocytopenic purpura (↓ platelets and ↓ WBCs) or aplastic anemia.

CLIENT/FAMILY TEACHING

1. Take with food or after meals to minimize GI upset.

T

2. **It may take longer than usual to stop bleeding; report unusual bleeding as severe hematological side effects may occur.**
3. **Brush teeth with a soft-bristle tooth brush, use an electric razor for shaving, wear shoes when ambulating, use caution and avoid injury, as bleeding times may be prolonged.**
4. **During the first 3 months of therapy, low white blood count can occur, resulting in an increased risk of infection. Come for scheduled blood tests and report any symptoms of infection (e.g., fever, chills, sore throat).**
5. **Any severe or persistent diarrhea, SC bleeding, skin rashes, or evidence of cholestasis (e.g., yellow skin or sclera, dark urine, light-colored stools) should be reported.**
6. **Avoid OTC agents without provider approval.**
7. **Keep all F/U to assess response, labs, and adverse SE.**

OUTCOMES/EVALUATE

- **Prevention of a complete or recurrent cerebral thrombotic event**
- **↓ Thrombosis with aspirin after coronary stent placement**

IV

Tigecycline

(tye-gah-**SYE**-kleen)

Classification(s): Antibiotic, miscellaneous

Pregnancy Category: D

RX: Tygacil.

INDICATIONS/USES

Treatment of the following infections in clients 18 years and older:

1. Complicated skin and skin structure infections due to *Escherichia coli, Enterococcus faecalis* (vancomycin-susceptible isolates only), *Staphylococcus aureus* (methicillin-susceptible and methicillin-resistant isolates), *Streptococcus agalactiae, Streptococcus anginosus* group (includes *S. anginosus, S. intermedius,* and *S. constellatus), Streptococcus pyogenes, Enterobacter cloacae, Klebsiella pneumoniae,* and *Bacteroides fragilis.*
2. Complicated intraabdominal infections due to *Citrobacter freundii, E. cloacae, E. coli, Klebsiella oxytoca, Klebsiella pneumoniae, E. faecalis* (vancomycin-susceptible isolates only), *S. aureus* (methicillin-susceptible and methicillin-resistant isolates), *S. anginosus* group (includes *S. anginosus, S. intermedius,* and *S. constellatus*), *B. fragilis, Bacteroides thetaiotaomicron, Bacteroides uniformis, Bacteroides vulgatus, Clostridium perfringens,* and *Peptostreptococcus micros.*
3. Community-acquired pneumonia due to *Streptococcus pneumoniae* (penicillin-susceptible isolates), including cases with concurrent bacteremia; *Haemophilus influenzae* (beta-lactamase negative isolates), and *Legionella pneumophila. Investigational:* Hospital–acquired pneumonia.

ACTION/KINETICS

Action

Tigecycline is a glycylcycline that inhibits protein translation in bacteria by binding to the 30S ribosomal subunit and blocking entry of amino-acyl tRNA molecules into the A site of the ribosome. This prevents incorporation of amino acid residues into elongating peptide chains. The drug is structurally similar to tetracyclines and may have similar side effects. Considered to be bacteriostatic, although bactericidal activity demonstrated against isolates of *S. pneumoniae* and *L. pneumophila.*

Pharmacokinetics

Is not extensively metabolized. Excreted through both the feces (59%) and urine (33%). **$t\frac{1}{2}$:** 42.4 hr after multiple doses. Systemic clearance is reduced and $t\frac{1}{2}$ increased in moderate or severe hepatic impairment. **Plasma protein binding:** 71–89%.

CONTRAINDICATIONS

Hypersensitivity to tigecycline or any component of the product. Use during tooth development unless other drugs are not likely to be effective or are contraindicated. Use in children less than 18 years of age.

SPECIAL CONCERNS

- **To reduce the development of drug-resistant bacteria and maintain efficacy, only use tigecycline to treat infections that are proven or strongly suspected to be caused by susceptible bacteria.**
- **Use with caution in severe hepatic impairment, in those with known hypersensitivity to tetracycline class antibiotics, and during lactation.**

T

- Use during tooth development (last half of pregnancy, infancy, childhood until age 8 years), may cause permanent discoloration of the teeth (yellow-gray-brown).
- Use caution when considering use in clients with complicated intra-abdominal infections secondary to clinically apparent intestinal perforation due to the possibility of sepsis/septic shock.
- Tigecycline is structurally similar to tetracyclines; thus, it may have similar side effects (e.g., photosensitivity, pseudotumor cerebri, pancreatitis, anti-anabolic action, azotemia, acidosis, and hypophosphatemia).
- Elderly clients may show greater sensitivity.
- Safety and efficacy not determined in children less than 18 years of age.

SIDE EFFECTS

Most Common

N&V, hypertension, headache, diarrhea, anemia, thrombocytopenia, hypoproteinemia, abdominal pain, fever, infection, injection site reaction.

GI: N&V, diarrhea, abdominal pain, dyspepsia, constipation, pseudomembranous colitis, abnormal stools, anorexia, dry mouth, *Clostridium difficile*- associated diarrhea, intestinal perforation (in those with complicated intra-abdominal infections), ***acute pancreatitis***. **Hepatic:** Jaundice, hepatic cholestasis, significant hepatic dysfunction/ ***hepatic failure***. **CNS:** Headache, dizziness, insomnia, somnolence. **CV:** Hypertension, hypotension, phlebitis, bradycardia, tachycardia, thrombophlebitis, vasodilation. **Respiratory:** Increased cough, dyspnea, pulmonary physical finding. **GU:** Leukorrhea, vaginal moniliasis, vaginitis. **Hematologic:** Thrombocytopenia, anemia, leukocytosis, eosinophilia, increased INR, prolonged APPT, prolonged PT. **Injection site:** Edema, inflammation, pain, phlebitis. **Body as a whole:** Infections (abscess, wound infections), fever, abnormal healing, asthenia, pruritus, rash, hypersensitivity/allergic reactions (including ***anaphylaxis/anaphylactoid reactions***), chills, pain, infection, superinfection (including fungi), ***sepsis/ septic shock***. **Miscellaneous:** Abscess, back pain, peripheral edema, taste perversion, infusion-related serious reactions, ***increased all–cause mortality***.

LABORATORY TEST CONSIDERATIONS

↑ Alkaline phosphatase, amylase, BUN, lactic dehydrogenase, AST, ALT, creatinine, INR, total bilirubin. Hyper-/hypoglycemia, hypokalemia, hypoproteinemia, hypocalcemia, hyponatremia. Prolonged aPTT and PT.

OVERDOSE MANAGEMENT

Symptoms: Increased incidence of N&V. *Treatment:* No specific information available on treating overdosage. Is not removed in significant quantities by hemodialysis.

DRUG INTERACTIONS

Cyclosporine / ↑ Cyclosporine levels → ↑ risk of toxic effects; monitor closely and adjust cyclosporine dose as needed

Oral contraceptives / Possible ↓ oral contraceptive effectiveness; advise to use an additional nonhormonal contraceptive method

Warfarin / ↓ Clearance of R-warfarin and S-warfarin by 40% and 23%, and increase in C_{max} by 38% and 43%, and an increase in AUC by 68% and 29% respectively; monitor PT and adjust warfarin dose as needed

HOW SUPPLIED

Injection, Lyophilized Powder for Solution: 50 mg.

DOSAGE

IV INFUSION

Complicated skin/skin structure infections; complicated intraabdominal infections; community-acquired pneumonia in adults.

Adults, initial: 100 mg given over 30–60 min; **then** 50 mg q 12 hr over 30–60 min for 5–14 days for complicated intra-abdominal infections and complicated skin and skin structure infections and for 7–14 days for community-acquired bacterial pneumonia. Duration of therapy is dependent on the severity and site of the infection and the client's clinical and bacteriological progress. *NOTE:* In severe hepatic impairment (Child-Pugh class C), the initial dose is 100 mg, followed by a reduced maintenance dose of 25 mg q 12 hr.

Hospital-acquired pneumonia.

Adults: Loading dose of 100 mg IV, followed by 50 mg IV q 12 hr for 13–20 days.

T

NURSING IMPLICATIONS

IMPLEMENTATION/ADMINISTRATION/STORAGE

1. IV To prepare the injection, reconstitute each vial with 5.3 mL of 0.9% NaCl injection, D5W injection, or Ringer's lactate injection to achieve a concentration of 10 mg/mL. Gently swirl the vial until the drug dissolves. Immediately withdraw 5 mL of the reconstituted solution and add to 100 mL IV bag for infusion (for a 100 mg dose, reconstitute 2 vials; for a 50 mg dose, reconstitute 1 vial) over 30–60 min. The maximum concentration in the IV bag should be 1 mg/mL. The reconstituted solution should be yellow to orange in color; discard if the solution is not this color. Inspect visually for particulate matter and discoloration (green, black) prior to administration. May be stored in the IV bag at room temperature for up to 6 hr or refrigerated for up to 24 hr.
2. May be given IV through a dedicated line or through a Y-site. If the same IV line is used for sequential infusion of several drugs, flush the line before and after tigecycline infusion with either 0.9% NaCl injection or D5W.
3. Is compatible with the following drugs when used with NaCl 0.9% injection or D5W injection: Amikacin, dobutamine, dopamine, gentamicin, haloperidol, lidocaine, metoclopramide, morphine, norepinephrine, piperacillin/tazobactam (EDTA formulation), potassium chloride, propofol, ranitidine, Ringer's lactate, theophylline, and tobramycin.
4. Prior to reconstitution, store from 15–30°C (59–86°F). Once reconstituted, may be stored at room temperature for up to 24 hr (up to 6 hr in the vial and the remaining time in the IV bag). If mixed with 0.9% NaCl injection or D5W injection, may be stored refrigerated for up to 48 hr following immediate transfer of the reconstituted solution into the IV bag.
5. COMPATIBILITY D5W, 0.9% NaCl, RL.
6. INCOMPATIBILITY If IV line is used for sequential infusion of other drugs, flush IV line with 0.9% NaCl, D5W, or Ringer's lactate injection before and after infusion of tigecycline. Incompatible with amphotericin B, amphotericin B lipid complex, diazepam, esomeprazole, and omeprazole.

ASSESSMENT

1. Note reasons for therapy, onset, characteristics of S&S, culture results, clinical presentation, other agents trialed.
2. Assess for any known hypersensitivity to tetracycline class antibiotics.
3. Monitor CBC, renal and LFTs; reduce dose with liver dysfunction. Use caution with hepatic dysfunction, during lactation and during tooth development (last half of pregnancy, infancy, childhood until age 8 years) may cause permanent discoloration of the teeth (yellow-gray-brown).
4. Assess for superinfection. Monitor PT/INR if used with warfarin and monitor for worsening hepatic function in those who develop abnormal LFTs and evaluate risk of continuing therapy.

CLIENT/FAMILY TEACHING

1. Drug is administered intravenously every 12 hours and used to treat bacterial infections, not viral infections. It should be administered exactly as directed despite feeling better. Skipping doses or not completing the full course of therapy may (a) decrease the effectiveness of the immediate treatment and (b) increase the likelihood that bacteria will develop resistance and will not be treatable by tigecycline or other antibacterial drugs in the future.
2. Use nonhormonal form of birth control as drug may impair effectiveness of these during therapy; avoid pregnancy.
3. Report any adverse or unusual side effects including bruising/bleeding, lack of response or worsening of symptoms, pain and swelling at injection site, diarrhea, or vaginal infection, or severe N&V.
4. Keep all F/U to assess response, labs, and for adverse SE.

OUTCOMES/EVALUATE

Resolution of infection; negative culture results

Tiludronate disodium

(tye-**LOO**-droh-nayt)

Classification(s): Bone growth regulator, bisphosphonate

Pregnancy Category: C

RX: Skelid.

T

INDICATIONS/USES

Paget's disease (osteitis deformans) where the level of serum alkaline phosphatase is at least twice upper limit of normal, in those who are symptomatic, or who are at risk for future complications of disease. *Investigational:* Osteoporosis with spinal cord injury.

ACTION/KINETICS

Action

Inhibits activity of osteoclasts and decreases bone turnover. Does not interfere with bone mineralization.

Pharmacokinetics

Poorly absorbed from GI tract in presence of food. **Peak serum levels:** 2 hr. Not metabolized; excreted in urine. **t½:** About 150 hr.

CONTRAINDICATIONS

Not recommended for those with C_{CR} less than 30 mL/min.

SPECIAL CONCERNS

- **Use with caution during lactation and in those with dysphagia, symptomatic esophageal disease, gastritis, duodenitis, or ulcers.**
- **Safety and efficacy not determined in children.**

SIDE EFFECTS

Most Common

Pain, diarrhea, dyspepsia, N&V, back pain, rales/rhinitis, sinusitis, URTI, accidental injury, flu-like symptoms.

GI: Diarrhea, N&V, dyspepsia, flatulence, tooth disorder, abdominal pain, constipation, dry mouth, gastritis, anorexia. **CNS:** Headache, dizziness, paresthesia, vertigo, somnolence, anxiety, nervousness, insomnia. **CV:** Dependent edema, peripheral edema, hypertension, syncope. **Musculoskeletal:** Arthralgia, arthrosis, pathological fracture, involuntary muscle contractions, jaw osteonecrosis, musculoskeletal pain. **Respiratory:** Rhinitis, sinusitis, URTI, coughing, pharyngitis, bronchitis. **Dermatologic:** Rash, skin disorder, pruritus, increased sweating, ***Stevens-Johnson type syndrome (rare)***. **Ophthalmic:** Cataract, conjunctivitis, glaucoma. **Body as whole:** Pain, back/chest pain, accidental injury, flu-like symptoms, asthenia, syncope, fatigue, flushing. **Miscellaneous:** Hyperparathyroidism, vitamin D deficiency, UTI, infection.

OVERDOSE MANAGEMENT

Symptoms: Hypocalcemia. *Treatment:* Standard medical practice to manage renal insufficiency or hypocalcemia.

DRUG INTERACTIONS

Antacids, Al or Mg⁺⁺ / Antacids, taken 1 hr before, ↓ tiludronate bioavailability
Aspirin / Aspirin, taken 2 hr after, ↓ tiludronate bioavailability by 50%
Calcium supplements / ↓ Tiludronate bioavailability by 80% when taken at same time
Indomethacin / ↑ Tiludronate bioavailability by 2- to 4-fold

HOW SUPPLIED

Tablets: 240 mg (equivalent to 200 mg tiludronic acid).

DOSAGE

TABLETS

Paget's disease.

Adults: Single 400 mg/day dose of tiludronate (2–240 mg tiludronate disodium tablets) taken with 6 to 8 oz of plain water for period of only 3 months. Maintain adequate vitamin D and calcium intake.

Osteoporosis with spinal cord injury (investigational).

Adults: 200 or 400 mg/day for 3 months (insufficient documentation).

NURSING IMPLICATIONS

IMPLEMENTATION/ADMINISTRATION/STORAGE

1. **Following therapy, allow an interval of 3 months to assess response.**
2. **Data regarding retreatment are limited, although favorable improvement has been observed.**
3. **Store from 15–30°C (59–86°F).**

ASSESSMENT

1. **Note reasons for therapy, other agents trialed, outcome. List clinical presentation, subjective complaints, BMD.**
2. **Monitor electrolytes, mineral panel, calcium, alkaline phosphatase, renal and LFTs.**

CLIENT/FAMILY TEACHING

1. Take with 6 to 8 oz of plain water. Do not take within 2 hr of food. Beverages other than water, food, and some medications reduce absorption of tiludronate.
2. Do not lie down for at least 30 minutes after taking drug.
3. Take aluminum- or magnesium-containing antacids, if needed, at least two hours after taking tiludronate.
4. Avoid aspirin, indomethacin, or calcium or mineral supplements within 2 hr before or 2 hr after therapy
5. May experience nausea, diarrhea, and GI upset; report if severe.
6. Consume adequate vitamin D and calcium supplements; take calcium 2 hr before or after therapy.
7. Report any rashes, itching, hives, severe stomach pains, bloody or black tarry stools, flank, bone or severe joint pain, or N&V.
8. Keep all F/U to assess response, labs, and for adverse SE.

OUTCOMES/EVALUATE

Inhibition of Paget's disease progression; ↓ Bone reabsorption and calcium levels

Timolol maleate

(**TIE**-moh-lohl)

Classification(s): Beta-adrenergic blocking agent

Pregnancy Category: C

RX: Ophthalmic Gel Forming Solution: Timoptic-XE. **Ophthalmic Solution:** Betimol, Istalol, Timoptic. **Tablets:** Blocadren.

🍁 **Rx:** Apo-Timol, Apo-Timop, Gen-Timolol, PMS-Timolol, Sandoz Timolol.

SEE ALSO ***BETA-ADRENERGIC BLOCKING AGENTS***.

INDICATIONS/USES

Ophthalmic Gel-Forming Solution (Timoptic-XE): Reduce elevated IOP in open-angle glaucoma or ocular hypertension.

Ophthalmic solution (Betimol, Istalol, Timoptic): Lower IOP in chronic open-angle glaucoma, selected cases of secondary glaucoma, ocular hypertension, aphakic (no lens) clients with glaucoma.

Tablets (Blocadren): (1) Hypertension (alone or in combination with other antihypertensives, especially thiazide diuretics). (2) Reduce CV mortality and risk of reinfarction in clinically stable MI survivors. (3) Prophylaxis of migraine. *Investigational:* Ventricular arrhythmias and tachycardias, essential tremors.

ACTION/KINETICS

Action

Exerts both beta-1- and beta-2-adrenergic blocking activity. Has minimal sympathomimetic effects, direct myocardial depressant effects, or local anesthetic action. Does not cause pupillary constriction or night blindness. The mechanism of the protective effect in MI is not known.

Pharmacokinetics

Peak plasma levels: 1–2 hr. **t½:** 4 hr. Metabolized in the liver. Metabolites and unchanged drug excreted through the kidney. Also reduces both elevated and normal IOP, whether or not glaucoma is present; thought to act by reducing aqueous humor formation and/or by slightly increasing outflow of aqueous humor. Does not affect pupil size or visual acuity. For use in eye: **Onset:** 30 min. **Maximum effect:** 1–2 hr. **Duration:** 24 hr.

CONTRAINDICATIONS

Hypersensitivity to drug. Bronchial asthma or bronchospasm including severe COPD. Use of the ophthalmic solution in those with sinus bradycardia, second- or third-degree AV block or overt cardiac failure, cardiogenic shock.

SPECIAL CONCERNS

■ Exacerbation of ischemic heart disease following abrupt withdrawal. Hypersensitivity to catecholamines has been observed in clients withdrawn from beta-blocker therapy; exacerbation of angina and, in some cases, MI have occurred after abrupt discontinuation of such therapy. When discontinuing chronically administered timolol, particularly in clients with ischemic heart disease, gradually reduce the dosage over a period of 1-2 weeks and carefully monitor the client. If angina markedly worsens or acute coronary insufficiency develops, reinstitute timolol administration promptly, at least temporarily, and take other measures appropriate for the management of unstable angina. Warn clients against interruption of discontinuation of therapy without the physician's advice. Because coronary artery disease is common and may be unrecognized, it may be prudent not to discontinue timolol therapy abruptly, even in clients treated only for hypertension.

- **Use ophthalmic preparations with caution in clients for whom systemic beta-adrenergic blocking agents are contraindicated.**
- **Safe use in children not established.**

SIDE EFFECTS

Most Common

When used ophthalmically: Ocular irritation (including conjunctivitis), local hypersensitivity reactions.

When used systemically: Insomnia, malaise/fatigue, anxiety, nervousness, impotence, bradycardia, dizziness, cold hands/feet.

See *Beta-Adrenergic Blocking Agents* for a complete list of possible side effects. **Following use of ophthalmic product:** Ocular irritation (including conjunctivitis), blepharitis, keratitis, blepharoptosis, decreased corneal sensitivity, visual disturbances (including refractive changes), diplopia, ptosis, local hypersensitivity reactions, slight decrease in resting HR.

DRUG INTERACTIONS

When used ophthalmically, possible potentiation with systemically administered beta-adrenergic blocking agents.

HOW SUPPLIED

Ophthalmic Gel Forming Solution: 0.25%, 0.5%; ***Ophthalmic Solution:*** 0.25%, 0.5%; ***Tablets:*** 5 mg, 10 mg, 20 mg.

DOSAGE

Timoptic-XE 0.25% or 0.5%

OPHTHALMIC GEL FORMING SOLUTION

Glaucoma.

1 gtt once daily.

Betimol or Timoptic, each 0.25% or 0.5%

OPHTHALMIC SOLUTION

Glaucoma.

1 gtt of 0.25 or 0.50% solution in each eye twice a day. If the decrease in intraocular pressure is maintained, reduce dose to 1 gtt once a day.

Istalol Ophthalmic (0.5%)

OPHTHALMIC SOLUTION

Glaucoma.

Initial: 1 gtt per affected eye once daily in the morning. If this does not adequately control intraocular pressure, an agent other than another topical beta-adrenergic blocker should be added to the regimen.

Blocadren

TABLETS

Hypertension.

Initial: 10 mg twice a day alone or with a diuretic; **maintenance:** 20–40 mg/day (up to 60 mg/day in two doses may be required), depending on BP and HR. If dosage increase is necessary, wait 7 days.

MI prophylaxis in clients who have survived the acute phase.

10 mg twice a day.

Migraine prophylaxis.

Initially: 10 mg twice a day. **Maintenance:** 20 mg/day given as a single dose; total daily dose may be increased to 30 mg in divided doses or decreased to 10 mg, depending on the response and client tolerance. If a satisfactory response for migraine prophylaxis is not obtained within 6–8 weeks using the maximum daily dose, discontinue the drug.

Essential tremor.

10 mg/day.

NURSING IMPLICATIONS

Do not confuse timolol with atenolol, each of which is a beta-adrenergic blocking drug

IMPLEMENTATION/ADMINISTRATION/STORAGE

1. **When transferring from another antiglaucoma agent, continue old medication on day 1 of timolol therapy (1 gtt of 0.25% solution). Then, discontinue former therapy. Initiate with 0.25% solution. Increase to 0.50% solution if response is insufficient. Further dosage increases are ineffective.**
2. **When transferring from several antiglaucoma agents, individualize the dose. If one of the agents is a beta-adrenergic blocking agent,**

discontinue it before starting timolol. Dosage adjustments should involve one drug at a time at 1-week intervals. Continue the antiglaucoma drugs with the addition of timolol, 1 gtt of 0.25% solution twice a day (if response is inadequate, 1 gtt of 0.5% solution may be used twice a day). The following day, discontinue one of the other antiglaucoma agents while continuing the remaining agents or discontinue based on client response.

3. Before using the gel, invert the closed container and shake once before each use.
4. Administer other ophthalmics at least 10 min before the gel.
5. The ocular hypotensive effect has been maintained when switching clients from timolol solution given twice a day to the gel once daily.
6. Store tablets from 15–30°C (59–86°F); protect from light.

ASSESSMENT

1. Note reasons for therapy, onset, characteristic of S&S, intraocular pressure readings/BP. With headaches describe characteristics/triggers.
2. Monitor BP/HR, ECG, IOPs, renal and LFTs.

CLIENT/FAMILY TEACHING

1. Drug is used in different forms for different conditions.
2. Do not perform tasks such as driving or operating machinery until drug effects are realized; may cause dizziness or drowsiness.
3. When tablets used for long-term prophylaxis against MI, do not interrupt therapy; abrupt withdrawal may precipitate reinfarction.
4. With eye drops, wash hands; do not allow dropper to touch eye. Tilt head back, looking up, pull lower eyelid down and instill prescribed number of drops. Close eye for 1 to 2 min, apply gentle pressure to bridge of nose for 1 to 3 min. Do not rub eye or touch top of dropper/bottle to eye, fingers, or other surface. If more than 1 topical eye drug used, give at least 5 min apart administering the ointment last. May experience temporary stinging or burning; report if bothersome or if eye/eyelid inflammation noted. Regular intraocular measurements by an eye doctor are required because ocular hypertension may recur without any overt S&S.
5. Report any evidence of rash, dizziness, heart palpitations, SOB, edema, or depression. May cause increased sensitivity to cold; dress appropriate.
6. With diabetes, drug may mask S&S of hypoglycemia.
7. Keep log of FS, pulse, and BP for provider review.
8. Advise surgeon before any surgery that this drug is being used (even as eye drops); may want to stop drugs temporarily. Do not stop oral drug suddenly; dose is usually tapered off to prevent complications.
9. Continue lifestyle modifications (i.e., weight reduction, regular exercise, reduced intake of sodium and alcohol, and no smoking) in the overall goal of BP control.
10. Keep all F/U to assess response, labs, and for adverse SE.

OUTCOMES/EVALUATE

- ↓ BP
- Myocardial reinfarction prophylaxis
- Migraine prophylaxis
- ↓ Intraocular pressures

Tinidazole

(tye-**NI**-dah-zole)

Classification(s): Antiprotozoal, second generation

Pregnancy Category: C

RX: Tindamax.

INDICATIONS/USES

(1) Intestinal amebiasis and amebic liver abscess due to *Entamoeba histolytica* in adults and children over 3 years of age. Not indicated to treat asymptomatic cyst passage. (2) Giardiasis due to *Giardia duodenalis (Giardia lamblia)* in adults and children over 3 years of age. (3) Bacterial vaginosis (formerly referred to as *Haemophilus* vaginitis, *Gardnerella* vaginitis, nonspecific vaginitis, or anaerobic vaginosis) in nonpregnant women. Rule out other pathogens commonly associated with vulvovaginitis (i.e., *Trichomonas vaginalis, Chlamydia trachomatis, Neisseria gonorrhoeae, Candida albicans,* and *Herpes simplex* virus). (4) Trichomoniasis caused by *T. vaginalis*. Treat partners of infected clients simultaneously in order to prevent reinfection.

ACTION/KINETICS

Action

An antiprotozoal drug. The nitro group of tinidazole is reduced by *Trichomonas*. The free nitro group generated may be responsible for the antiprotozoal activity. The drug causes DNA base changes in bacterial cells and DNA strand breakage in mammalian cells. The mechanism against *Giardia* and *Entamoeba* is not known.

Pharmacokinetics

Rapidly and completely absorbed. **Time to maximum levels:** 1.6 hr. Administration with food delayed the maximum levels by about 2 hr along with a decrease of 10% in C_{max}. Steady state reached 2.5–3 days after multiple-day dosing. Distributed to virtually all tissues and body fluids; crosses the blood brain barrier. Metabolized in the liver, mainly by CYP3A4. **t½, elimination:** 13.2 hr; **t½, plasma:** 12–14 hr. Excreted in both the feces and urine. **Plasma protein binding:** 12%.

CONTRAINDICATIONS

Hypersensitivity to tinidazole, any component of the product, or other nitroimidazole derivatives. Use during the first trimester of pregnancy. Lactation (interrupt during therapy and for 3 days following the last dose).

SPECIAL CONCERNS

■ Carcinogenicity has been seen in mice and rats treated chronically with metronidazole, another nitroimidazole agent. Although such data have not been reported for tinidazole, the two drugs are structurally related and have similar biologic effects. Reserve its use only for the conditions for which it is indicated. ■

- Avoid unnecessary use.
- Use with caution in those with evidence of or history of blood dyscrasias, in those with impaired hepatic function, and in selecting doses for the elderly.
- Safety and efficacy not demonstrated in children except to treat giardiasis and amebiasis in children over 3 years of age.

SIDE EFFECTS

Most Common

N&V, anorexia, excessive thirst, salivation, metallic/bitter taste, constipation, diarrhea, headache, darkened urine, swollen/sore/discolored tongue.

CNS: Headache, dizziness, ***seizures***, transient peripheral neuropathy (including numbness and paresthesia), ataxia, drowsiness, giddiness, insomnia, vertigo, coma (rare), confusion, depression (rare). **GI:** Metallic/bitter taste, N&V, abdominal pain, dyspepsia, cramps, epigastric discomfort, anorexia, constipation, diarrhea, stomatitis, decreased appetite, swollen/sore/discolored tongue, oral candidiasis, excessive thirst, salivation, flatulence, furry tongue (rare). **CV:** Palpitations. **Musculoskeletal:** Arthralgias, arthritis, myalgias. **Respiratory:** Bronchospasm, dyspnea, URTI, pharyngitis (rare). **GU:** Darkened urine, increased vaginal discharge/odor, vaginal candidiasis, menorrhagia, painful urination, pelvic pain, renal UTI, urine abnormality, vulvovaginal discomfort. **Hematologic:** Transient leukopenia, transient neutropenia, reversible thrombocytopenia (rare). **Hypersensitivity:** Angioedema, burning sensation, dry mouth, fever, flushing, pruritus, rash, salivation, sweating, thirst, urticaria. **Body as a whole:** Weakness, fatigue, malaise. **Miscellaneous:** *Candida* overgrowth, hepatic abnormalities (including increased transaminase levels).

LABORATORY TEST CONSIDERATIONS

Possible interference (values of zero) with serum chemistry values, including AST, ALT, LDH, triglycerides, and hexokinase glucose.

DRUG INTERACTIONS

Alcohol / Possible abdominal cramps, N&V, headaches, and flushing; avoid alcoholic beverages during therapy and for 3 days after discontinuation
Anticoagulants / ↑ Warfarin and other coumarin anticoagulant effect → prolonged PT; adjust anticoagulant dose as needed
Cholestyramine / Possible ↓ tinidazole bioavailability; separate doses of cholestyramine and tinidazole
Cimetidine / ↑ Tinidazole t½ and ↓ clearance R/T inhibition of metabolism by CYP3A4
Cyclosporine / Possible ↑ cyclosporine levels; monitor for toxicity
Disulfiram / Possible psychotic reactions; do not give to clients who have taken disulfiram within the past 2 weeks
Fluorouracil / ↓ Fluorouracil clearance → toxicity; monitor for fluorouracil toxicity if they must be taken together
Fosphenytoin / ↑ Tinidazole elimination → ↓ plasma levels R/T ↑ CYP3A4 metabolism

T

Ketoconazole / ↑ Tinidazole $t_{1/2}$ and ↓ clearance R/T inhibition of metabolism by CYP3A4
Lithium / Possible ↑ serum lithium levels; monitor lithium and creatinine levels
Oxytetracycline / May antagonize the effect of tinidazole
Phenobarbital / ↑ Tinidazole elimination → ↓ plasma levels R/T ↑ CYP3A4 metabolism
Phenytoin / ↑ Tinidazole elimination → ↓ plasma levels R/T ↑ CYP3A4 metabolism; also ↑ $t_{1/2}$ and ↓ phenytoin clearance following IV phenytoin
Rifampin / ↑ Tinidazole elimination → ↓ plasma levels R/T ↑ CYP3A4 metabolism
Tacrolimus / Possible ↑ tacrolimus levels; monitor for toxicity

HOW SUPPLIED

Tablets: 250 mg, 500 mg.

DOSAGE

TABLETS

Intestinal amebiasis.

Adults: 2 grams/day for 3 days with food. **Children over 3 years:** 50 mg/kg/day (up to 2 grams/day) for 3 days with food.

Amebic liver abscess.

Adults: 2 grams/day for 3–5 days with food. **Children over 3 years:** 50 mg/kg/day (up to 2 grams) for 3–5 days with food.

Giardiasis.

Adults: 2 grams as a single dose with food. **Children over 3 years:** 50 mg/kg (up to 2 grams) as a single dose with food.

Bacterial vaginosis.

Women, nonpregnant: 2 grams once daily for 2 days with food or 1 gram once daily for 5 days with food. Use in pregnant clients has not been studied.

Trichomoniasis.

Adults, men and women: 2 grams as a single dose with food.

NURSING IMPLICATIONS

IMPLEMENTATION/ADMINISTRATION/STORAGE

1. Take with food to minimize incidence of epigastric distress and other GI side effects. Food does not affect bioavailability.
2. Because trichomoniasis is a sexually transmitted disease, treat sexual partners with the same dose and at the same time.
3. If tinidazole is given on a day when hemodialysis is performed, give an additional dose of the drug equivalent to one-half the recommended dose after the end of the hemodialysis.
4. An extemporaneous oral suspension may be compounded as follows: Grind 4 × 500 mg tablets to a fine powder using a mortar and pestle. Add about 10 mL of cherry syrup to the powder and mix until smooth. Transfer the suspension to a graduated amber container. Use several small rinses of cherry syrup to transfer any remaining drug in the mortar to the final suspension for a final volume of 30 mL. The suspension in cherry syrup is stable for 7 days at room temperature; shake well before using.
5. Store tablets from 15–30°C (59–86°F) and protect from light.

ASSESSMENT

1. Note reasons for therapy, onset, characteristics of S&S, other agents trialed, culture results. Identify source/causative agent.
2. List drugs prescribed to ensure none interact.
3. Assess for any history/evidence of nervous system diseases or blood dyscrasia.
4. Monitor CBC, renal and LFTs.

CLIENT/FAMILY TEACHING

1. Take tablets as directed with food to ↓ GI upset. A metallic taste may be evident; will resolve when therapy completed.
2. Report any adverse side effects, such as numbness in extremities, chest pain, SOB, dizziness, drowsiness, unusual bruising/bleeding, confusion, or symptoms of infection.
3. Avoid alcohol during and for three days following therapy.
4. Practice reliable contraception, and do not breast feed during therapy.
5. With STD, ensure partner is also treated at the same time.
6. Keep all F/U to assess response, labs, and for adverse SE.

OUTCOMES/EVALUATE

Resolution of infection

Tinzaparin sodium

(tin-**ZAH**-pah-rin)

Classification(s): Anticoagulant, low molecular weight heparin

Pregnancy Category: B

RX: Innohep.

SEE ALSO ***HEPARINS, LOW MOLECULAR WEIGHT***.

INDICATIONS/USES

Treat acute symptomatic deep vein thrombosis (DVT) with or without pulmonary embolism when given with warfarin sodium. *Investigational:* Prophylaxis of DVT (which may lead to pulmonary embolism) in clients undergoing moderate risk surgery, orthopedic surgery, hip fracture surgery, gynecologic surgery, or neurosurgery at risk for thromboembolic complications.

ACTION/KINETICS

Pharmacokinetics

Is 86.7% bioavailable. **Maximum plasma levels:** 0.25–0.87 international units/mL within 4 to 5 hr after a single SC dose of 4,500 international units. Metabolized in the liver. **t½:** 3–4 hr. Excreted mainly in the urine. Clearance is reduced in impaired renal function.

ADDITIONAL CONTRAINDICATIONS

Use in those with a history of heparin-induced thrombocytopenia (HIT). Sensitivity to heparin, sulfites, benzyl alcohol, or pork products. Mixing with other injections or infusions.

SPECIAL CONCERNS

(1) **Spinal/epidural hematomas.** Epidural or spinal hematomas may occur in clients who are anticoagulated or scheduled to be anticoagulated with low molecular weight heparins or heparinoids and are receiving neuraxial anesthesia or undergoing spinal puncture. These hematomas may result in long-term or permanent paralysis. Consider these risks when scheduling clients for spinal procedures. Factors that increase the risk of developing epidural or spinal hematomas in these clients include use of indwelling epidural catheters; concomitant use of drugs that affect hemostasis, such as NSAIDs, platelet inhibitors, or other anticoagulants; a history of traumatic or repeated epidural or spinal punctures; and a history of spinal deformity or spinal surgery. (2) Monitor clients frequently for signs and symptoms of neurological impairment. If neurological compromise is observed, immediate treatment is necessary. (3) Consider the benefits and risks before neuraxial intervention in clients anticoagulated or to be anticoagulated for thromboprophylaxis.

- **Use with caution in pregnancy and only if clearly needed since benzyl alcohol in the product may cross the placenta and cause a fatal "gasping syndrome" in premature neonates.**
- **Contains metabisulfate that may cause allergic reactions, including anaphylaxis and life-threatening asthmatic episodes in susceptible individuals.**
- **Use with extreme caution in the elderly with renal impairment.**
- **Use with caution during lactation.**
- **Safety and efficacy not determined in children.**

SIDE EFFECTS

Most Common

Injection site reactions, chest pain, bleeding, constipation, N&V, UTI, epistaxis, dyspnea, pulmonary embolism, back pain, pain, fever, headache.

CV: Bleeding, ***hemorrhage (fatal or nonfatal)***, hypo-/hypertension, tachycardia, angina pectoris, deep thrombophlebitis, deep leg thrombophlebitis, cardiac arrhythmias, ***MI, coronary thrombosis***, thromboembolism, peripheral ischemia, hemoptysis, ocular hemorrhage, anorectal/rectal bleeding, cerebral/intracranial bleeding, hemarthrosis, hemoptysis, wound hematoma, ***GI hemorrhage, hemopericardium, spinal/epidural hematomas***. **Hematologic:** Thrombocytopenia, anemia, hematoma, agranulocytosis, pancytopenia, granulocytopenia, thrombocythemia. **GI:** N&V, abdominal pain, diarrhea, constipation, flatulence, GI disorder, dyspepsia, cholestatic hepatitis, hematemesis, melena, retroperitoneal/intra-abdominal bleeding, cholestatic hepatitis. **CNS:** Headache, dizziness, insomnia, confusion. **GU:** Priapism, UTI, hematuria, urinary retention, dysuria, ***vaginal hemorrhage***. **Respiratory: *Pulmonary embolism***, dyspnea, epistaxis, pneumonia, respiratory disorder. **Dermatologic:** Rash, erythematous rash, maculopapular rash, pruritus, bullous eruption, vesiculobullous rash, skin disorder,

T

skin necrosis, epidermal necrolysis, ischemic necrosis, urticaria, ecchymosis, purpura, cellulitis, allergic purpura, ***Stevens-Johnson syndrome***. **Injection site:** Mild local irritation, pain, hematoma, ecchymosis, necrosis, abscess, bleeding, irritation, pain. **Hypersensitivity:** ***Anaphylaxis***, allergic reaction, urticaria, angioedema. **Body as a whole:** Fever, impaired healing, infection, dependent edema, abcess, acute febrile reaction. **Miscellaneous:** Back/chest pain, pain, rash, neonatal hypotonia, congenital anomaly, ***fetal death***/distress, fetal/neonatal cutis aplasia of the scalp, ischemic necrosis, necrosis, neoplasm.

ADDITIONAL DRUG INTERACTIONS

Anticoagulants, oral / ↑ Risk of bleeding
Dextran / ↑ Risk of bleeding
Thrombolytics / ↑ Risk of bleeding

HOW SUPPLIED

Injection: 20,000 anti-Factor Xa international units/mL.

DOSAGE

SC ONLY

Deep vein thrombosis with or without pulmonary embolism.

Adults: 175 anti-Factor IX units/kg once daily for 6 days or until client is adequately anticoagulated with warfarin (INR at least 2.0 for two consecutive days). Initiate warfarin when appropriate (usually 1–3 days after tinzaparin initiation).

Venous thromboembolism prophylaxis in general surgery or gynecologic surgery (investigational).

Adults: 3,500 units given SC once/day started preoperatively (general surgery) or just before surgery (gynecologic surgery). For high-risk clients, tinzaparin may be given for up to 28 days after hospital discharge.

NURSING IMPLICATIONS

IMPLEMENTATION/ADMINISTRATION/STORAGE

1. Check package insert for dosing for treatment by body weight. If client weight is not given in the package insert, the following equation can be used to calculate the volume (mL) of tinzaparin 175 anti-factor Xa units/kg SC: client weight (kg) × 0.00875 mL/kg = volume (mL) to be given SC
2. **Do not give IM or IV.**
3. To ensure withdrawal of the correct volume, use an appropriately calibrated syringe.
4. Inspect visually before administration to ensure there is no particulate matter or discoloration of the vial contents.
5. Position clients either supine or sitting and give by deep SC injection. Alternate injections between left and right anterolateral and left and right posterolateral abdominal wall. Vary the injection site daily. Introduce the entire length of the needle into a skin fold held between the thumb and forefinger; hold the skin fold throughout the injection. To minimize bruising, do not rub the injection site after completing the injection.
6. Dosage adjustments are not required for the elderly and those with renal impairment.
7. Store between 15–30°C (59–86°F).
8. Do not mix with other injections or infusions.

ASSESSMENT

1. Note reason for therapy, onset, and characteristics of S&S. Assess for any bleeding disorders or active major bleeding, HIT, or any hypersensitivity to heparin sulfite, benzyl alcohol, or pork products.
2. Use cautiously with history of recent GI ulcerations, diabetic retinopathy, hemorrhage, uncontrolled HTN, or bleeding diathesis.
3. Assess for S&S of neurological impairment when spinal anesthesia or tap conducted.
4. Confirm PE by segmental lung scan defect and/or DVT by ultrasound. Start SC tinzaparin treatment × 6 days; add coumadin on day 2 and titrate to an INR of 2–3.
5. Weigh client; calculate dose for client weight (kg × 0.00875 mL/kg = volume in mL to be administered SC).
6. Monitor PT, INR, platelet count, CBC, renal function and stool for occult blood.

CLIENT/FAMILY TEACHING

1. Review indications for therapy, self administration techniques, and importance of site rotation.
2. To administer, wash hands, lie down or sit, and give by SC injection after instruction. Alternate sites between the left and right anter-

T

olateral and left and right posterolateral abdominal wall. Vary injection site daily.
3. Insert whole length of needle into a skin fold held between the thumb and forefinger. Hold skin fold throughout the injection.
4. To minimize bruising, do not rub site after administering and avoid OTC agents such as NSAIDs or aspirin.
5. Use caution to prevent injury; avoid contact sports, excessive jostling and use soft-bristle toothbrush and electric razor to prevent bleeding.
6. Report any unusual bruising, bleeding, chest pain, acute SOB, itching, rash, or swelling.
7. Keep all F/U to assess response, labs, and for adverse SE.

OUTCOMES/EVALUATE
- Anticoagulation and prevention of complications R/T clot formation
- Resolution of DVT

Tioconazole

(tie-oh-**KON**-ah-zohl)

Classification(s): Antifungal

Pregnancy Category: C

OTC: Monistat 1, Vagistat-1.

INDICATIONS/USES
Vulvovaginal candidiasis, including moniliasis and vaginal yeast infections.

ACTION/KINETICS
Action
Antifungal activity thought to be due to alteration of the permeability of the cell membrane of the fungus, causing leakage of essential intracellular compounds.

Pharmacokinetics
The systemic absorption of the drug in nonpregnant clients is negligible.

CONTRAINDICATIONS
Use of a vaginal applicator during pregnancy may be contraindicated.

SPECIAL CONCERNS
Safety and efficacy not determined during lactation or in children.

SIDE EFFECTS
Most Common
Burning, itching, irritation, vaginal discharge.

GU: Burning, itching, irritation, vulvar edema and swelling, discharge, vaginal pain/swelling/redness, dysuria, dyspareunia, nocturia, difficult or burning urination, desquamation, dryness of vaginal secretions. **Miscellaneous:** Headache, abdominal pain/cramping, URTI.

HOW SUPPLIED
Vaginal Ointment: 6.5%.

DOSAGE

VAGINAL OINTMENT
Vulvovaginal candidiasis, including moniliasis and vaginal yeast infections.

Single dose of about 4.6 grams (one applicator full) intravaginally at bedtime.

NURSING IMPLICATIONS

ASSESSMENT
1. Note indications for therapy, onset, and characteristics of S&S; identify other agents trialed and outcome.
2. Obtain a thorough nursing and gynecologic history; carefully evaluate symptoms, clinical presentation, and sources of infection.
3. If unresponsive, confirm infection by KOH smears and/or cultures.

CLIENT/FAMILY TEACHING
1. Review appropriate method for administration. Found to be effective as a single-dose treatment for vulvovaginal candidiasis and used just prior to bedtime.
2. Open foil packet just prior to use; remove purple cap. Insert entire contents of applicator into the vagina. Discard applicator after use.
3. Report if burning, irritation, or pain occurs. Effectiveness is not altered by menstruation.
4. May stain clothes; use sanitary napkins during therapy and change frequently because damp sanitary napkins may harbor infecting organisms. Avoid tampons during therapy.
5. To avoid reinfection, refrain from sexual intercourse. Symptomatic improvement is usually seen within 3 days and complete relief within 7 days.

T

6. The ointment base in Vagistat-1 may interact with rubber or latex products (condoms or vaginal contraceptive diaphragms); avoid use of these products within 72 hours following treatment.
7. Keep all F/U to assess response, labs, and for adverse SE.

OUTCOMES/EVALUATE
Resolution of fungal infection; symptomatic improvement

Tiotropium bromide

(tee-oh-**TROE**-pee-um)

Classification(s): Anticholinergic

Pregnancy Category: C

RX: Spiriva.

INDICATIONS/USES
(1) Long-term, once daily, maintenance treatment of bronchospasm associated with COPD, including chronic bronchitis and emphysema. (2) Reduce exacerbations in COPD clients. *NOTE:* Not intended for initial treatment of acute episodes of bronchospasms (i.e., rescue therapy).

ACTION/KINETICS
Action
Long-acting antimuscarinic (anticholinergic). In the airways it inhibits muscarinic M_3 receptors at the smooth muscle, leading to bronchodilation.

Pharmacokinetics
Since the drug is inhaled, the majority is deposited in the GI tract and, to a lesser extent, the lungs (site of action), although the fraction reaching the lung is highly available. The portion metabolized is through the CYP2D6 and CYP3A4 enzyme systems. However, most is excreted unchanged through the urine. **t½, terminal:** 5–6 days. **Plasma protein binding:** 72%.

CONTRAINDICATIONS
History of hypersensitivity to atropine or its derivatives, including ipratropium. Use for initial treatment of acute episodes of bronchospasm (rescue therapy). Use with other anticholinergics (e.g., ipratropium).

SPECIAL CONCERNS
- As an anticholinergic, drug may worsen S&S of narrow-angle glaucoma, prostatic hyperplasia, or bladder-neck obstruction; use with caution in these conditions.
- Immediate hypersensitivity reactions, including angioedema, may result after administration.
- Use with caution with narrow-angle glaucoma and in those with urinary retention.
- Use with caution during lactation.
- Safety and efficacy not determined in children.

SIDE EFFECTS
Most Common
URTI, dry mouth, constipation, accidents, sinusitis, pharyngitis/rhinitis, abdominal pain, chest pain (non-specific), dependent edema, UTI, dyspepsia.

GI: Dry mouth, dyspepsia, abdominal pain, constipation, vomiting, gastroesophageal reflux, GI disorder, stomatitis (including ulcerative), gingivitis, dysphagia, intestinal obstruction (including paralytic ileus), oral candidiasis. **CNS:** Depression, dysphonia, paresthesia, headache, insomnia, dizziness. **Respiratory:** URTI, sinusitis, pharyngitis, rhinitis, epistaxis, coughing, laryngitis, paradoxical bronchospasm, oropharyngeal candidiasis, hoarseness, throat irritation. **CV:** Angina pectoris (including aggravated angina pectoris), tachycardia, atrial fibrillation, SVT, palpitations. **Musculoskeletal:** Arthritis, skeletal pain, arthralgia, myalgia, joint swelling. **GU:** UTI, dysuria, urinary retention. **Dermatologic:** Rash, pruritus, urticaria, dry skin, skin infection/ulcer. Irritation, glossitis, mouth ulceration, pharyngolaryngeal pain. **Hypersensitivity:** Angioedema, itching, rash, paradoxical bronchospasm. **Application site: Metabolic:** Dehydration, dependent edema. **Ophthalmic:** Blurred vision, glaucoma (new onset or worsening), cataract, increased intraocular pressure. **Body as a whole:** Accidents, infection, moniliasis, flu-like symptoms, allergic reaction, ***angioedema.*** **Miscellaneous:** Herpes zoster, chest pain (non-specific), leg pain.

NOTE: The incidence of dry mouth, constipation, and UTI increase with age.

OVERDOSE MANAGEMENT
Symptoms: High doses cause anticholinergic signs and symptoms. However, acute intoxication by

inadvertent PO ingestion is unlikely as the drug is not well absorbed systemically.

DRUG INTERACTIONS

Use of tiotropium with other anticholinergic-containing drugs (e.g., ipratropium) has not been studied; thus, concomitant use is not recommended.

HOW SUPPLIED

Capsules, Containing Powder for Inhalation: 18 mcg (as base).

DOSAGE

CAPSULES CONTAINING POWDER FOR INHALATION

Chronic-obstructive pulmonary disease (COPD), including to reduce exacerbations of COPD.

Two inhalations of the contents of 1 tiotropium capsule once daily using the *HandiHaler* inhalation device.

NURSING IMPLICATIONS

IMPLEMENTATION/ADMINISTRATION/STORAGE

1. To administer tiotropium bromide, use the following guidelines:
   - Immediately before using the tiotropium dose, peel back the aluminum foil using the tab until 1 capsule is fully visible. Peel back the foil only as far as the "STOP" line printed on the blister foil in order to prevent exposure of more than 1 capsule. Use the drug immediately after opening the package or its effectiveness may be reduced.
   - Open the dust cap of the *HandiHaler* by pulling it upwards; then open the mouthpiece.
   - Place the capsule in the center chamber. It does not matter which end of the capsule is placed in the chamber.
   - Firmly close the mouthpiece until a click is heard, leaving the dustcap open.
   - Hold the *HandiHaler* device with the mouthpiece upwards; press the piercing button in completely once and release. This makes holes in the capsule and allows the medication to be released.
   - Breathe out completely. Do not breathe into the mouthpiece at any time.
   - Raise the *HandiHaler* device to the mouth and close lips tightly around the mouthpiece.
   - Keep head in an upright position and breath in slowly and deeply but at a rate sufficient to hear the capsule vibrate. Breathe in until lungs are full and then hold breath as long as is comfortable. At the same time, take the *HandiHaler* device out of the mouth and resume normal breathing.
   - To ensure getting the entire dose, repeat this once again.
   - After finishing the daily dose of tiotropium, open the mouthpiece again. Tip out the used capsule and dispose of it. Close the mouthpiece and dust cap for storage.
2. Do not swallow capsules as the intended effects on the lung will not occur.
3. Tiotropium capsules containing powder for inhalation are to be inhaled using a special device; do not take orally.
4. Store capsules from 15–30°C (59–86°F). Do not expose to extreme temperatures or moisture. Do not store capsules in the *HandiHaler.*

ASSESSMENT

1. List reasons for therapy, characteristics of S&S, other agents trialed, outcome.
2. Note CXR, PFTs, lung sounds, other drugs prescribed, overall physical condition/clinical presentation.
3. Assess ECG for QT prolongation, renal dysfunction, inability to self administer drug. Check for BPH, narrow angle glaucoma, bladder neck obstruction; drug may aggravate these conditions.
4. Closely monitor clients with moderate to severe renal impairment (C_{CR} 50 mL/min or less).

CLIENT/FAMILY TEACHING

1. Drug is administered once a day using the *HandiHaler* to control bronchospasms with lung disease. It is not to be used for acute bronchospasms or breathing problems; use rescue medication in this event.
2. Capsules come in sealed blisters. Do not remove until ready to use. If an additional blister is accidently opened, and pill is exposed

to air, discard capsule; do not save for next day use.

3. The capsules are to be placed in the *HandiHaler and punctured;* do not swallow. Review *Patient's Instructions for Use* (contains pictures with step-by-step instruction) enclosed with medication to fully understand how to correctly administer capsules. The medication is being inhaled even if the dose is not tasted or felt. Do not use a spacer with this therapy.
4. To administer follow these guidelines:
   - Open the dust cap of the *HandiHaler* by pulling it upwards; then, open the mouthpiece.
   - Place the capsule in the center chamber. It does not matter which end of the capsule is placed in the chamber.
   - Firmly close the mouthpiece until a click is heard, leaving the dustcap open.
   - Hold the *HandiHaler* device with the mouthpiece upwards; press the piercing button in completely once and release. This makes holes in the capsule and allows the medication to be released.
   - Breathe out completely. Do not breathe into the mouthpiece at any time.
   - Raise the *HandiHaler* device to the mouth and close lips tightly around the mouthpiece.
   - Keep head in an upright position and breath in slowly and deeply, but at a rate sufficient to hear the capsule vibrate. Breathe in until lungs are full and then hold breath as long as is comfortable. At the same time, take the *HandiHaler* device out of the mouth and resume normal breathing.
   - To ensure getting the entire dose, repeat this once again.
   - After finishing the daily dose of tiotropium, open the mouthpiece again. Tip out the used capsule and dispose of it. Close the mouthpiece and dust cap for storage.
5. Do not use *HandiHaler* with any other capsules or drugs. Clean as directed (usually once a month) and as needed following instructions in the *Patient's Instructions* pamphlet.
6. When using *HandiHaler,* do not permit powder to enter the eyes; may cause pupillary dilatation, and blurred vision. Report any eye pain/discomfort, colored images, blurred vision or vision halos associated with red eyes. May indicate glaucoma and should be immediately assessed by eye doctor.
7. Chest pain, ↑ SOB, mental status changes, tremors, abdominal pain, or severe constipation require prompt reporting.
8. Keep all F/U to assess response, lung function, and for adverse SE.

OUTCOMES/EVALUATE

- Improved airway exchange
- Long-term control of bronchospasm with COPD, emphysema and chronic bronchitis.

Tipranavir

(tye-**PRAN**-ah-veer)

Classification(s): Antiviral, protease inhibitor

Pregnancy Category: C

RX: Aptivus.

SEE ALSO ***ANTIVIRAL DRUGS***.

INDICATIONS/USES

Given with ritonavir to treat HIV-1 infected adults and children, 2 years and older, with evidence of viral replication who are highly treatment-experienced or have HIV-1 strains resistant to multiple protease inhibitors.

ACTION/KINETICS

Action

Tipranavir is a nonpeptidic HIV-1 protease inhibitor that inhibits the virus-specific processing of the viral Gag and Gag-Pol polyproteins in HIV-1 infected cells, thus preventing formation of mature virions. Development of resistance is possible, as well as cross-resistance to other antiviral drugs.

Pharmacokinetics

Absorption is limited. **t½ for tipranavir/ritonavir (taken for longer than 2 weeks):** 5.5 hr (women) and 6 hr (men); **T_{max}**: 2.9 hr (women) and 3 hr (men). These differences do not warrant a dose adjustment. Bioavailability is increased with a high-fat meal. Tipranavir is metabolized in the liver by CYP3A4. Excreted mainly in the feces. **Plasma protein binding:** >99.9%.

CONTRAINDICATIONS

Known hypersensitivity to any of the components of the product. Moderate to severe hepatic insufficiency (Child-Pugh class B and C, respectively). Coadministration of tipranavir and ritonavir with drugs that are highly dependent on CYP3A for clearance and for which elevated plasma levels are associated with serious and/or life-threatening side effects; see *Drug Interactions* for drugs involved. Lactation.

SPECIAL CONCERNS

■ (1) **Hepatotoxicity.** Clinical hepatitis and hepatic decompensation, including some fatalities, have been reported. Extra vigilance is warranted in clients with chronic hepatitis B or hepatitis C coinfection, as these clients have an increased risk of hepatotoxicity. (2) **Intracranial hemorrhage.** Both fatal and nonfatal intracranial hemorrhage have been reported. ■

- **Must be given with ritonavir to exert its therapeutic effect; failure to coadminister correctly will result in insufficient tipranavir plasma levels to achieve the desired effect.**
- **Use with caution in the elderly, in those with known sulfonamide allergy, and in those with mild hepatic impairment.**
- **Use with caution in those who may be at risk of increased bleeding from trauma, surgery, or other medical conditions, or who are receiving medications known to increase the risk of bleeding (e.g., antiplatelet drugs, anticoagulants), or who are taking supplemental doses of vitamin E. Tipranavir inhibits platelet aggregation.**
- **There is the potential for resistance/cross-resistance among protease inhibitors.**
- **Risk-benefit not determined in children less than 2 years of age.**

SIDE EFFECTS

Most Common

Adults: Diarrhea, N&V, pyrexia, cough, headache, fatigue, bronchitis, depression, insomnia, rash, abdominal pain, asthenia.

Children: Pyrexia, cough, rash, N&V, diarrhea, epistaxis

NOTE: Side effects listed are those for concomitant use of tipranavir and ritonavir. **GI:** N&V, diarrhea, abdominal pain/distension, anorexia, dyspepsia, flatulence, GERD, ***pancreatitis.*** **Hepatic:** Hepatitis, cytolytic hepatitis, ***hepatic failure***, hepatic steatosis, hyperbilirubinemia, toxic hepatitis, ***hepatic decompensation, with possible fatal outcome.*** **CNS:** Headache, depression, insomnia, dizziness, peripheral neuropathy, sleep disorder, somnolence. **CV:** ***Intracranial hemorrhage (both fatal and nonfatal).*** **Dermatologic:** Urticarial rash, maculopapular rash, photosensitivity, acquired lipodystrophy, exanthema, lipoatrophy, lipohypertrophy, pruritus. **Respiratory:** Bronchitis, cough, dyspnea, epistaxis. **Musculoskeletal:** Muscle cramps, myalgia. **GU:** Impaired renal function, breast enlargement. **Metabolic:** New-onset diabetes mellitus, exacerbation of preexisting diabetes mellitus, hyperglycemia, diabetic ketoacidosis, decreased appetite, dehydration, weight loss, mitochondrial toxicity. **Hematologic:** Anemia, neutropenia, thrombocytopenia, hemophilia, including spontaneous skin hematomas and hemarthrosis in those with hemophilia type A and B. Inhibition of platelet aggregation. **Body as a whole:** Pyrexia, fatigue, asthenia, malaise, redistribution/accumulation of body fat (including central obesity, dorsocervical fat enlargement, peripheral/facial wasting, and cushingoid appearance), hypersensitivity, flu-like illness. **Miscellaneous:** Reactivation of herpes simplex and varicella zoster, immune reconstitution syndrome.

LABORATORY TEST CONSIDERATIONS

↑ ALT, AST, amylase, creatine phosphokinase, GGT, lipase, cholesterol, triglycerides. ↓ WBCs. Abnormal LFTs. Hypercholesterolemia, hyperlipidemia, hyperglycemia, hyperamylasemia.

OVERDOSE MANAGEMENT

Symptoms: See *Side Effects. Treatment:* There is no known antidote. Treatment should consist of general supportive measures, including monitoring of vital signs and observation of clinical status. If needed, elimination of unabsorbed tipranavir can be achieved by gastric lavage or activated charcoal. Dialysis is unlikely to be of benefit.

DRUG INTERACTIONS

Tipranavir given with ritonavir is an inhibitor of CYP3A and may increase plasma levels of drugs that are primarily metabolized by CYP3A. Thus, coadministration of tipranavir/ritonavir with drugs highly dependent on CYP3A for clearance, and for which increased plasma levels are associated with serious and/or life-threatening side effects, is contraindicated. Coadministration with other CYP3A substrates may require a dosage adjustment and monitoring.

Abacavir / Possible ↓ abacavir plasma levels
Al- and Mg-based antacids / ↓ Tipranavir absorption; consider separating dosing
Antiarrhythmics (e.g., amiodarone, bepridil, flecainide, propafenone, quinidine) / Coadministration is contraindicated R/T potential for cardiac arrhythmias secondary to ↑ antiarrhythmic plasma levels
Anticholinergic drugs (e.g., darifenacin, fesoterodine, solifenacin, tolterodine) / Possible ↑ anticholinergic plasma levels → ↑ pharmacologic/toxic effects; if coadministered do not exceed daily doses as follows: darifenacin, 7.5. mg; fesoterodine, 4 mg; solifenacin, 5 mg; tolterodine, 2 mg
Aripiprazole / ↑ Aripiprazole plasma levels →↑ pharmacologic/toxic effects; monitor and adjust aripiprazole dose as needed
Azole antifungals (e.g., fluconazole, itraconazole, ketoconazole, voriconazole) / Fluconazole may ↑ tipranavir levels; high doses of fluconazole, itraconazole, ketoconazole not recommended
Benzodiazepines (e.g., oral midazolam, triazolam) / Coadministration contraindicated R/T risk of prolonged or increased sedation or respiratory depression; if parenteral midazolam used, monitor for respiratory depression and/or prolonged sedation; adjust midazolam dose as needed
Calcium channel blockers (e.g., diltiazem, felodipine, nicardipine, nisoldipine, verapamil) / Caution warranted and clinical monitoring recommended
Carbamazepine / ↓ Tipranavir concentrations → ↓ efficacy; use together with caution
Cisapride / ↑ Risk of arrhythmias; concurrent use contraindicated
Clarithromycin / ↑ Levels of both clarithromycin and tipranavir; for those with C_{CR}, 30–60 mL/min, ↓ clarithromycin dose by 50%; for those with C_{CR}, < 30 mL/min, ↓ clarithromycin dose by 75%
Colchicine / ↑ Colchicine plasma levels → life-threatening/fatal colchicine toxicity; avoid coadministration in those with hepatic/renal impairment; in others, do not exceed 0.3 mg dose of colchicine twice a day; monitor carefully
Contraceptives, oral (estrogen-containing) / ↓ Ethinyl estradiol levels by 50%; use nonhormonal contraceptives; also, ↑ risk of rash
Delavirdine / ↑ Tipranavir plasma levels and pharmacologic effects; also, ↓ delavirdine plasma levels and pharmacologic effects; may need to ↓ tipranavir dose and ↑ delavirdine dose
Desipramine / ↑ Desipramine levels; reduce desipramine dosage and monitor
Didanosine / ↓ Tipranavir levels; separate dosing from tipranavir/ritonavir by at least 2 hr
Digoxin / ↑ Digoxin plasma levels and pharmacologic effects; monitor closely; digoxin dose reduction may be needed
Disulfiram / Tipranavir capsules contain alcohol → disulfiram-like reaction
Dronedarone / ↑ Dronedarone plasma levels → ↑ pharmacologic/toxic effects; avoid coadministration
Efavirenz / Possible ↓ tipranavir levels
Eplerenone / ↑ Eplerenone plasma levels →↑ pharmacologic/toxic effects; monitor closely and adjust eplerenone dose as needed
Ergot derivatives (e.g., dihydroergotamine, ergonovine, ergotamine, methylergonovine) / ↑ Risk of ergot toxicity (peripheral vasospasms and ischemia of the extremities); do not use together
Erlotinib / ↑ Erlotinib plasma levels → ↑ pharmacologic/toxic effects; monitor and adjust erlotinib dose as needed
Eszopiclone / ↑ Eszopiclone plasma levels → ↑ pharmacologic/toxic effects; monitor closely and consider reducing eszopiclone dose
Fluticasone / ↑ Fluticasone plasma levels → significant ↓ serum cortisol levels; combination not recommended unless potential benefit outweighs the risk of systemic corticosteroid side effects
HMG-CoA reductase inhibitors (e.g., atorvastatin, lovastatin, rosuvastatin, simvastatin) / ↑ Risk of myopathy, including rhabdomyolysis; do not use tipranavir with lovastatin or simvastatin, but if using atorvastatin or rosuvastatin, start with the lowest possible dose with careful monitoring
Hypoglycemic drugs (e.g., glimepiride, glipizide, glyburide, pioglitazone, repaglinide, tolbutamide) / Careful glucose monitoring recommended
Immunosuppressants (e.g., cyclosporine, sirolimus, tacrolimus) / Careful drug concentration monitoring recommended
Loperamide / ↓ Levels of both loperamide and tipranavir; monitor tipranavir levels and client response; adjust therapy if indicated
Maraviroc / ↑ Maraviroc plasma levels → ↑ pharmacologic/toxic effects; monitor and adjust maraviroc dose as needed

T

Metronidazole / Tipranavir capsules contain alcohol → disulfiram-like reaction
Nevirapine / ↓ Tipranavir levels → ↓ efficacy; monitor and adjust tipranavir dose as needed
Omeprazole / May need to ↑ omeprazole dose
Opioid analgesics (e.g., meperidine, methadone) / Possible ↓ meperidine and methadone levels; levels of normeperidine (metabolite) may be ↑ → ↑ risk for seizures. Do not use increased meperidine doses or use meperidine long-term. May need to ↑ methadone dosage
Oral contraceptives (estrogen-containing) / Possible ↓ ethinyl estradiol levels; use alternate contraceptive methods; also, ↑ risk of rash
Phenobarbital / ↓ Tipranavir plasma levels; use together with caution
Phenytoin / ↓ Tipranavir plasma levels; use together with caution
Phosphodiesterase type 5 inhibitors (e.g., sildenafil, tadalafil, vardenail) / Use together with caution. Do not exceed sildenafil, 25 mg within 48 hr; tadalafil, 10 mg q 72 hr; or vardenafil, 2.5 mg q 72 hr if taken with tipranavir
Pimozide / ↑ Potential for cardiac arrhythmias; do not use together
Protease inhibitors (e.g., amprenavir, iopinavir, saquinavir) / Possible ↓ protease inhibitor levels; do not use together
Protein-tyrosine kinase inhibitors (e.g., dasatinib, sorafenib, sunitinib) / ↑ Protein-tyrosine kinase inhibitor levels →↑ pharmacologic/toxic effects; monitor response and adjust kinase inhibitor dose as needed
Quetiapine / ↑ Quetiapine plasma levels → ↑ pharmacologic/toxic effects; monitor and adjust quetiapine dose as needed
Ranolazine / ↑ Ranolazine plasma levels → ↑ risk of dose-related prolongation of QTc interval, torsades de pointes-type arrhythmias and sudden death; do not use together
Rifabutin / Possible loss of virologic response and possible resistance to tipranavir; do not use together. Also, possible ↑ rifabutin levels; reduce rifabutin dose by 75% (e.g., 150 mg q other day)
Rifamycins (e.g., rifampin, rifabutin) / Possible loss of virologic response and resistance to tipranavir; do not use together
H ***St. John's wort*** / Loss of virologic response and possible resistance to tipranavir; do not use together
Selective serotonin reuptake inhibitors (e.g., fluoxetine, paroxetine, sertraline) / SSRI dose may need to be adjusted
Tenofovir / ↓ Levels of both drugs; monitor levels of both drugs and adjust therapy as needed
Trazodone / Possible ↑ trazodone levels; use together with caution; consider a lower trazodone dose
Valproic acid / ↓ Valproic acid plasma levels → ↓ efficacy; use together with caution
Vasopressin receptor antagonists (e.g., conivaptan, tolvaptan) / ↑ Vasopressin receptor antagonist levels → ↑ pharmacologic/toxic effects; do not use together
Warfarin / Monitor INR frequently
Zidovudine / ↓ Tipranavir levels; separate dosing by at least 2 hr

HOW SUPPLIED

Capsules: 250 mg; ***Oral Solution:*** 100 mg/mL.

DOSAGE

CAPSULES; ORAL SOLUTION

HIV-1 infection.

Adults: Tipranavir, 500 mg (2 × 250 mg capsules or 5 mL of the oral solution), coadministered with ritonavir, 200 mg, twice daily. **Children, 2–18 years of age, usual:** 14 mg/kg tipranavir with 6 mg/kg ritonavir both taken twice a day, not to exceed tipranavir, 500 mg given with ritonavir, 200 mg, twice a day. **Alternative dosing in children:** tipranavir, 375 mg/m^2 with ritonavir 150 mg/m^2 each given twice a day. For children who develop intolerance or toxicity and cannot continue with tipranavir, 14 mg/kg with ritonavir, 6 mg/kg, consider decreasing the dose to tipranavir, 12 mg/kg with ritonavir, 5 mg/kg (or tipranavir, 290 mg/m^2 with ritonavir, 115 mg/m^2) given twice a day (provided their virus is not resistant to multiple protease inhibitors).

NURSING IMPLICATIONS

IMPLEMENTATION/ADMINISTRATION/STORAGE

1. **Tipranavir and ritonavir can be taken with or without food.**

2. Bioavailability is increased with a high-fat meal.
3. Failure to administer tipranavir with ritonavir results in reduced plasma levels of tipranavir that will be insufficient to reach the desired antiviral effect; also, some drug interactions will be altered.
4. The oral solution contains vitamin E, 116 units/mL, which is higher than the reference daily intake of 30 units for adults and about 10 units for children.
5. Prior to opening the bottle, store tipranavir in the refrigerator from 2–8°C (36–46°F). After opening the bottle, capsules and oral solution may be stored from 15–30°C (59–86°F). Use capsules and oral solution within 60 days.

ASSESSMENT

1. Note disease onset, characteristics of S&S, other agents trialed, outcome. Assess viral replication, in those who are highly treatment-experienced or have HIV-1 strains resistant to multiple protease inhibitors.
2. List drugs prescribed to ensure none interact unfavorably. Many require a reduction in dose, or discontinuation to prevent reaction or loss of effect.
3. In those with chronic hepatitis B or C co-infection, monitor carefully for hepatotoxicity. LFTs should be performed prior to initiating therapy and frequently throughout the duration of treatment. Those with chronic hepatitis B or C co-infection or elevations in liver enzymes prior to treatment are at increased risk (approximately 2.5-fold) for developing further liver enzyme elevations or severe liver disease; increased testing is warranted.
4. Monitor I&O, VS, weight, CBC, CD4 counts, viral load, lipids, renal and LFTs. With moderate to severe liver disease, avoid drug use.

CLIENT/FAMILY TEACHING

1. Swallow tipranavir capsules whole; do not chew. Prior to opening bottle store in refrigerator. After opening, capsules may be stored at room temperature.
2. Drug must be co-administered with 200 mg ritonavir to ensure therapeutic effect. Failure to correctly co-administer tipranavir with ritonavir will result in reduced plasma levels of tipranavir, which will not be sufficient to achieve the desired antiviral effect.
3. Do not alter the dose or stop therapy without provider approval. If a dose is missed, may take the dose as soon as possible and then return to normal dosing schedule. If a dose is skipped, do not double the next dose.
4. This drug, co-administered with 200 mg of ritonavir, has been associated with severe liver disease and some deaths. Stop drug and report S&S of hepatitis, which include fatigue, malaise, nausea, yellow skin or eyes, loss of appetite, change in stools, abdominal tenderness.
5. With oral solution, do not take supplemental vitamin E because tipranavir oral solution exceeds the RDI for vitamin E.
6. May experience a mild to moderate rash including a flat or raised rash or sensitivity to the sun; report if persistent or bothersome. May also experience joint pain/stiffness, throat tightness, generalized itching, muscle aches, fever, redness, blisters, or peeling of the skin.
7. Women receiving estrogen-based hormonal contraceptives will require an additional or alternative contraceptive measure during therapy. Increased risk of rash when tipranavir is used with hormonal contraceptives. Practice reliable contraception; drug does not reduce the risk of transmitting HIV to others through sexual contact. To monitor maternal-fetal outcomes of pregnant women exposed to tipranavir, an antiretroviral pregnancy registry has been developed; register by calling 1-800-258-4263.
8. A redistribution or accumulation of body fat may occur; cause and long-term health effects unknown at this time.
9. Drug combination is not a cure for HIV infection; may continue to develop opportunistic infections and other complications associated with this disease. Sustained decreases in plasma HIV RNA have been associated with a reduced risk of progression to AIDS and death.
10. Avoid use of any other prescription, nonprescription medication, or herbal products, particularly St. John's wort; may cause significant adverse drug interactions.
11. The Patient Package Insert should be reviewed with each refill as it provides updated written information concerning this drug and therapy.

12. **Keep all F/U to assess response, labs, and for adverse SE.**

OUTCOMES/EVALUATE
- **↓ HIV RNA**
- **Control of HIV progression**

IV

Tirofiban hydrochloride

(ty-roh-**FYE**-ban)

Classification(s): Antiplatelet drug

Pregnancy Category: B

RX: Aggrastat.

INDICATIONS/USES

In combination with heparin for acute coronary syndrome (ACS), including those being treated medically and those undergoing PTCA or atherectomy. Tirofiban decreases the rate of combined endpoint of death, new MI, or refractory ischemia/repeat cardiac procedure.

ACTION/KINETICS

Action

Non-peptide antagonist of the platelet glycoprotein (GP) IIb/IIIa receptor, which is the major platelet surface receptor involved in platelet aggregation. Activation of the receptor leads to binding of fibrinogen and von Willebrand's factor to platelets, and thus aggregation. Tirofiban is a reversible antagonist of fibrinogen binding to the GP IIb/IIIa receptor, thus inhibiting platelet aggregation.

Pharmacokinetics

t½: About 2 hr. Cleared from the plasma mainly unchanged by renal excretion (65%) and feces (25%). Plasma clearance is lower in clients over 65 years of age and is significantly decreased in those with a C_{CR} less than 30 mL/min.

CONTRAINDICATIONS

Active internal bleeding or history of diathesis within the previous 30 days; history of intracranial hemorrhage, intracranial neoplasm, AV malformation, or aneurysm; history of thrombocytopenia following prior use of tirofiban; history of stroke within 30 days or any history of hemorrhagic stroke; major surgical procedure or severe physical trauma within the last month; history, findings, or symptoms suggestive of aortic dissection; severe hypertension (systolic BP greater than 180 mm Hg or diastolic BP greater than 110 mm Hg); concomitant use of another parenteral GP IIb/IIIa inhibitor; acute pericarditis.

SPECIAL CONCERNS

- **Use with caution in clients with a platelet count less than 150,000/mm³ in hemorrhagic retinopathy or with other drugs that affect hemostasis (e.g., warfarin).**
- **Elderly clients have a higher incidence of bleeding complications than younger clients.**
- **Safety not determined when used in combination with thrombolytic drugs.**
- **Safety and efficacy not established in children less than 18 years of age.**

SIDE EFFECTS

Most Common

Bleeding (see *Side Effects*), bradycardia, coronary artery dissection, pelvic pain, dizziness, leg pain.

CV: Bleeding, including ***intracranial bleeding, retroperitoneal bleeding, major GI and GU bleeding***. Female and elderly clients have a higher incidence of bleeding than male or younger clients. **Miscellaneous:** Nausea, fever, headache, bradycardia, ***coronary artery dissection***, dizziness, edema or swelling, leg/pelvic pain, vasovagal reaction, sweating.

LABORATORY TEST CONSIDERATIONS

↓ H&H, platelets. ↑ Urine and FOB.

OVERDOSE MANAGEMENT

Symptoms: Bleeding, including minor mucocutaneous bleeding events and minor bleeding at the site of cardiac catheterization. *Treatment:* Assess clinical condition. Adjust or cease infusion, as appropriate. Can be removed by hemodialysis.

DRUG INTERACTIONS

Aspirin / ↑ Bleeding
H *Evening primrose oil* / Potential for ↑ antiplatelet effect
H *Feverfew* / Potential for ↑ antiplatelet effect
H *Garlic* / Potential for ↑ antiplatelet effect
H *Ginger* / Potential for ↑ antiplatelet effect
H *Ginkgo biloba* / Potential for ↑ antiplatelet effect
H *Ginseng* / Potential for ↑ antiplatelet effect

T

H *Grapeseed extract* / Potential for ↑ antiplatelet effect
Heparin / ↑ Bleeding
Levothyroxine / ↑ Tirofiban clearance
Omeprazole / ↑ Tirofiban clearance

HOW SUPPLIED

Injection: 50 mcg/mL; *Injection Concentrate:* 250 mcg/mL.

DOSAGE

IV

Acute coronary syndrome.

Initial: 0.4 mcg/kg/min for 30 min; **then** 0.1 mcg/kg/min. Use half the usual rate in those with severe renal impairment. Consult the package insert for the guide to dosage adjustment by weight in clients with normal renal function and in those with severe renal impairment.

NURSING IMPLICATIONS

Sound alike: Do not confuse Aggrastat with Argatroban (anticoagulant) or Aggrenox (antiplatelet drug).

IMPLEMENTATION/ADMINISTRATION/STORAGE

1. **IV** May be given in the same IV line as heparin, dopamine, lidocaine, potassium chloride, and famotidine. Do not give in the same IV line as diazepam.
2. Tirofiban injection (250 mcg/mL) must be diluted to the same strength as tirofiban injection premixed (50 mcg/mL). One of three methods can be used to achieve a final concentration of 50 mcg/mL (mix well prior to use):
   - Withdraw and discard 100 mL from a 500 mL bag of either sterile 0.9% NaCl or D5W; replace this volume with 100 mL of tirofiban injection (i.e., from two 50 mL vials).
   - Withdraw and discard 50 mL from a 250 mL bag of either sterile 0.9% NaCl or D5W and replace this volume with 50 mL of tirofiban injection (i.e., from two 25-mL vials or one 50-mL vial).
   - Add the contents of a 25 mL vial to a 100 mL bag of sterile 0.9% NaCl or D5W.
3. Tirofiban injection premix comes in 500 mL *Intravia* containers with 0.9% NaCl and tirofiban, 50 mcg/mL. To open the *Intravia* container, remove the dust cover. The plastic may be opaque due to moisture absorption during sterilization; the opacity will decrease gradually. Check for leaks by firmly squeezing the inner bag. Lack of sterility may be suspected if leaks are found; discard the solution. Do not use unless the solution is clear and the seal is intact.
4. Do not add other drugs or remove tirofiban from the bag without a syringe.
5. Do not use plastic containers in series connections, as an air embolism can result by drawing air from the first container if it is empty.
6. Store both the premixed and concentrated injection from 15–30°C (59–86°F); do not freeze and protect from light.
7. Discard any unused solution 24 hr after start of the infusion.
8. COMPATIBILITY D5W, 0.9% NaCl.
9. INCOMPATIBILITY Administer separately.

ASSESSMENT

1. Note reasons for therapy, onset, characteristics of S&S.
2. List any history of intracranial hemorrhage, neoplasm, AV malformation, or aneurysm.
3. Avoid excessive handling, sticks and procedures to prevent increased bleeding and assess for any evidence of bleeding.
4. Monitor VS, H&H, platelets, PTT initially and 6 hr after loading infusions of tirofiban and heparin, and daily; monitor renal function studies, reduce dosage with dysfunction (C_{CR} <30 mL/min).

CLIENT/FAMILY TEACHING

1. Drug is used IV with heparin to reduce death and symptoms associated with heart vessel blockage.
2. May experience bleeding so all sites will be carefully assessed and blood work evaluated frequently. Report immediately if noted.
3. May experience dizziness; use caution. If smoking, ask for help to stop now.
4. Encourage family to learn CPR.

OUTCOMES/EVALUATE

Inhibition of platelet aggregation with ↓ refractory ischemia, MI, and death

T

Tizanidine hydrochloride

(tye-**ZAN**-ih-deen)

Classification(s): Skeletal muscle relaxant, centrally-acting

Pregnancy Category: C

RX: Zanaflex.

✱ **Rx:** Apo-Tizanidine, Gen-Tizanidine.

SEE ALSO ***SKELETAL MUSCLE RELAXANTS, CENTRALLY ACTING.***

INDICATIONS/USES

Acute and intermittent management of increased muscle tone associated with muscle spasticity. Reserve use for daily activities and times when relief of spasticity is most important.

ACTION/KINETICS

Action

Acts on central alpha$_2$-adrenergic receptors; reduces spasticity by increasing presynaptic inhibition of motor neurons possibly by reducing release of excitatory amino acids. Greatest effects are on polysynaptic pathways. Also may reduce postsynaptic excitatory transmitter activity, decrease the firing rate of noradrenergic locus ceruleas neurons, and inhibit synaptic transmission of nociceptive stimuli in the spinal pathways.

Pharmacokinetics

Absolute bioavailability is about 40% due to extensive first-pass metabolism by CYP1A2 in the liver. The fed or fasted state have significant effects on the pharmacokinetics. Tablets and capsules are bioequivalent to each other under fasted conditions, but not under fed conditions. **Peak effect:** 1–2 hr. **Duration:** 3–6 hr. **t½:** About 2.5 hr. Excreted in urine and feces. Elderly clear drug more slowly.

CONTRAINDICATIONS

Hypersensitivity to tizanidine or any component of the product. Use with other α_2-adrenergic agonists. Concomitant use with fluvoxamine or ciprofloxacin.

SPECIAL CONCERNS

- **Use with caution in the elderly and during lactation.**
- **Use with extreme caution or not at all in hepatic or renal insufficiency and in those with C_{CR} of 25 mL/min or less.**
- **Safety and efficacy have not been determined in children.**

SIDE EFFECTS

Most Common

Sedation/somnolence, dry mouth, asthenia, dizziness, hypotension, bradycardia, UTI, infection

NOTE: Side effects listed are those with a frequency of 0.1% or greater. **CV:** Hypotension, bradycardia, arrhythmia, postural hypotension, syncope, vasodilation. **CNS:** Somnolence, dizziness, dyskinesia, nervousness, speech disorder, anxiety, depression, paresthesia, abnormal dreams, abnormal thinking, agitation, ***convulsion***, depersonalization, dysautonomia, emotional lability, euphoria, migraine, neuralgia, paralysis, stupor, tremor, vertigo, hallucinations, psychotic-like symptoms. **GI:** Dry mouth, constipation, vomiting, abdominal pain, diarrhea, dyspepsia, cholelithiasis, dysphagia, fecal impaction, flatulence, ***GI hemorrhage***, hepatitis, melena, hepatotoxicity (N&V, jaundice, anorexia). **Respiratory:** Pharyngitis, rhinitis, bronchitis, pneumonia, sinusitis. **GU:** UTI, urinary frequency, cystitis, enlarged uterine fibroids, kidney calculus, menorrhagia, pyelonephritis, urinary retention, urinary urgency, vaginal moniliasis, vaginitis. **Dermatologic:** Rash, skin ulcer, sweating, acne, alopecia, dry skin, pruritus, urticaria. **Musculoskeletal:** Back/neck pain, myasthenia, arthralgia, arthritis, bursitis, pathological fracture. **Hematologic/Lymphatic:** Anemia, ecchymosis, leukocytosis, leukopenia. **Metabolic:** Edema, weight loss. **Ophthalmic:** Amblyopia, conjunctivitis, eye pain, glaucoma, optic neuritis, retinal hemorrhage, visual field defect. **Otic:** Deafness, ear pain, otitis media, tinnitus. **Body as a whole:** Asthenia (weakness, fatigue, and/or tiredness), infection, flu syndrome, fever, allergic reaction, malaise, moniliasis, sepsis, ***death***. **Miscellaneous:** Abscess, cellulitis.

LABORATORY TEST CONSIDERATIONS

↑ ALT, AST. Abnormal LFTs. Hypercholesterolemia, hyperlipemia, hypothyroidism, adrenal cortical insufficiency, hyperglycemia, hypokalemia, hyponatremia, hypoproteinemia.

T

OVERDOSE MANAGEMENT

Symptoms: Lethargy, somnolence, confusion, coma, depressed cardiac function (bradycardia, hypotension), respiratory depression. *Treatment:* Ensure an adequate airway. Monitor CV and respiratory systems. Symptoms usually resolve in 1–3 days.

DRUG INTERACTIONS

Acyclovir / ↑ Tizanidine plasma levels → toxicity R/T inhibition of CYP1A2; do not use together
Alcohol / ↑ Tizanidine side effects; additive CNS depressant effects
$Alpha_2$-adrenergic agonists / Additive hypotension; use together contraindicated
Antiarrhythmics (e.g., amiodarone, mexiletine, propafenone, verapamil) / ↑ Tizanidine plasma levels → toxicity R/T inhibition of CYP1A2; do not use together
Antihypertensives / Use together with caution
Cimetidine / ↑ Tizanidine plasma levels → toxicity R/T inhibition of CYP1A2; do not use together
Ciprofloxacin / ↑ Tizanidine AUC and peak levels R/T inhibition of metabolism by CYP1A2; possible clinically significant hypotension; do not use together
Famotidine / ↑ Tizanidine plasma levels → toxicity R/T inhibition of CYP1A2; do not use together
Fluoroquinolones (e.g., norfloxacin) / Certain fluoroquinolones may inhibit tizanidine metabolism by CYP1A2 → ↑ plasma levels and toxicity
Fluvoxamine / ↑ Tizanidine AUC and peak levels R/T inhibition of metabolism by CYP1A2 → clinically significant hypotension; use together contraindicated
Oral contraceptives / ↓ Tizanidine clearance; during titration ↓ individual doses
Ticlopidine / ↑ Tizanidine plasma levels → toxicity R/T inhibition of CYP1A2; do not use together
Zileuton / ↑ Tizanidine plasma levels → toxicity R/T inhibition of CYP1A2; do not use together

HOW SUPPLIED

Capsules: 2 mg, 4 mg, 6 mg; ***Tablets:*** 2 mg, 4 mg.

DOSAGE

CAPSULES; TABLETS

Muscle spasticity.

Initial: 4 mg; **then** increase dose gradually in 2 to 4 mg steps to optimum effect. Dose can be repeated at 6–8 hr intervals, to maximum of 3 doses/24 hr, not to exceed 36 mg/day. There is no experience with repeated, single, daytime doses greater than 12 mg or total daily doses of 36 mg or more.

NURSING IMPLICATIONS

IMPLEMENTATION/ADMINISTRATION/STORAGE

1. Food has complex effects on tizanidine pharmacokinetics that differ with the different formulations as follows:
   - Switching administration to the tablet between the fed or fasted state.
   - Switching administration of the capsule between the fed or fasted state.
   - Switching between the tablet and capsule in the fed state.
   - Switching between the intact capsule and sprinkling the contents of the capsule on applesauce. These changes may result in increased side effects or delayed/more rapid onset of action.
2. To minimize hypotension, titrate the dose. Also, clients moving from a supine to fixed, upright position may be at increased risk for hypotension and orthostatic effects.
3. If the drug must be discontinued, especially in those receiving high doses for long periods, decrease the dose slowly to minimize the risk of withdrawal and rebound hypertension, tachycardia, and hypertonia.
4. Store from 25–30°C (59–86°F). Dispense in a tight, light-resistant container with child-resistant closure.

ASSESSMENT

1. Note reasons for therapy, onset, characteristics of S&S, clinical presentation, other agents trialed, and outcome.
2. Assess ROM, pain level, erythema, swelling, muscle spasticity, DTRs, sensory findings, muscle tone, and gait.
3. Observe those with a CrCl less than 25 mL/min for onset or increase in severity of common adverse reactions (eg, dry mouth, dizziness or somnolence).
4. Monitor VS, CBC, renal and LFTs; reduce dose with dysfunction. Check LFTs at 1, 3, and 6 months and periodically thereafter during long-term therapy.

T

CLIENT/FAMILY TEACHING

1. Drug works by blocking nerve impulses to the brain. It's used to treat spasticity by temporarily relaxing muscle tone.
2. Take consistently with or without food. May open capsule and sprinkle contents on applesauce; consume immediately. Capsule contents sprinkled on applesauce are not bioequivalent to consuming intact capsule under fasting conditions. Do not switch between intact capsules and capsule content sprinkled on food unless provider directed.
3. Do not perform activities that require mental alertness; drug causes sedation. Rise slowly from a lying or sitting position; avoid sudden position changes to prevent sudden drop in BP. Hot tubs/showers or baths may make dizziness and light-headedness worse.
4. Report if hallucinations or delusions experienced.
5. Avoid alcohol and any other CNS depressants.
6. Report loss of effect, visual problems, ↓ ROM, or worsening of symptoms.
7. With prolonged therapy do not stop suddenly; taper over a 1–2 week period.
8. Use reliable contraception; oral contraceptives may inhibit drug clearance by 50%.
9. Keep all F/U to assess response, labs, for adverse SE.

OUTCOMES/EVALUATE

↓ Spasticity; ↑ muscle relaxation

IV

Tobramycin sulfate

(toe-brah-**MY**-sin)

Classification(s): Antibiotic, aminoglycoside

Pregnancy Category: D (B for ophthalmic use)

RX: Inhalation: TOBI. **Ophthalmic:** AKTob Ophthalmic Solution, Defy Ophthalmic Solution, Tobrex Ophthalmic Ointment or Solution. **Parenteral:** Tobramycin for Injection, Tobramycin in 0.9% Sodium Chloride.

✤ **Rx:** Sandoz Tobramycin.

SEE ALSO ***AMINOGLYCOSIDES***.

INDICATIONS/USES

Systemic:

1. Complicated and recurrent UTIs due to *Pseudomonas aeruginosa, Proteus, Escherichia coli, Klebsiella, Enterobacter, Serratia, Staphylococcus aureus, Citrobacter,* and *Providencia.*
2. Lower respiratory tract infections due to *P. aeruginosa, Klebsiella, Enterobacter, E. coli, Serratia,* and *S. aureus* (penicillinase- and non-penicillinase-producing).
3. Intra-abdominal infections (including peritonitis) due to *E. coli, Klebsiella,* and *Enterobacter.*
4. Septicemia in neonates, children, and adults due to *P. aeruginosa, E. coli,* and *Klebsiella.*
5. Skin, bone, and skin structure infections due to *P. aeruginosa, Proteus, E. coli, Klebsiella, Enterobacter,* and *S. aureus.*
6. Serious CNS infections, including meningitis. Can be used with penicillins or cephalosporins in serious infections when results of susceptibility testing are not yet known.

Inhalation: Management of lung infections *(P. aeruginosa)* in cystic fibrosis clients. Also improves lung function.

Ophthalmic: Treat external ocular infections (involving the conjunctiva, or cornea) due to *Staphylococcus, S. aureus, Streptococcus, S. pneumoniae,* beta-hemolytic streptococci, *Corynebacterium, E. coli, Haemophilus aegyptius, H. ducreyi, H. influenzae, H. parainfluenzae, Klebsiella pneumoniae, Neisseria, N. gonorrhoeae, Proteus, Acinetobacter calcoaceticus, Enterobacter, Enterobacter aerogenes, Serratia marcescens, Moraxella, Pseudomonas aeruginosa,* and *Vibrio.*

ACTION/KINETICS

Action

Similar to gentamicin and can be used concurrently with carbenicillin.

Pharmacokinetics

Therapeutic serum levels, IM: 4–8 mcg/mL. **t½:** 2–2.5 hr. **Toxic serum levels:** >12 mcg/mL (peak) and >2 mcg/mL (trough).

CONTRAINDICATIONS

Use with diuretics or nephrotoxic drugs. Ophthalmically to treat dendritic keratitis, vaccinia, varicella, fungal or mycobacterial eye infections, after removal of a corneal foreign body. Lactation.

SPECIAL CONCERNS

See Aminoglycosides.

T

- Use with caution in premature infants and neonates.
- Ophthalmic ointment may retard corneal epithelial healing.

SIDE EFFECTS

Most Common

After ophthalmic use: Transient irritation/burning/stinging, itching, inflammation.
After systemic use: N&V, redness/irritation at injection site, dizziness, tinnitus, fatigue, pale skin, weakness.

See *Aminoglycosides* for a complete list of possible side effects. **Ophthalmic use:** Transient irritation/burning/stinging, itching, inflammation, angioneurotic edema, urticaria, vesicular and maculopapular dermatitis. **Systemic use:** Neurotoxicity, both auditory and vestibular ototoxicity. Nephrotoxicity (reversible).

OVERDOSE MANAGEMENT

Symptoms: Ophthalmic Use: Edema, lid itching, punctuate keratitis, erythema, lacrimation. *Treatment:* Treat symptomatically.

ADDITIONAL DRUG INTERACTIONS

Carbenicillin / ↑ Tobramycin effect when used for ***Pseudomonas*** infections
Cidofovir / ↑ Risk of nephrotoxicity
Ticarcillin / ↑ Tobramycin effect when used for ***Pseudomonas*** infections

HOW SUPPLIED

Injection: 10 mg/mL, 40 mg/mL; ***Injection Solution:*** 0.8 mg/mL, 1.2 mg/mL, 60 mg/mL; ***Ophthalmic Ointment:*** 0.3% (3 mg/mL); ***Nebulizer Solution:*** 300 mg/5 mL; ***Ophthalmic Solution:*** 0.3% (3 mg/mL); ***Powder for Injection:*** 1.2 grams.

DOSAGE

IM; IV

Non-life-threatening serious infections.

Adults: 3 mg/kg/day in three equally divided doses q 8 hr. For cystic fibrosis, an initial dosing regimen of 10 mg/kg/day IV in 3–4 equally divided doses is recommended as a guide.

Life-threatening infections.

Up to 5 mg/kg/day in three or four equal doses. **Pediatric:** Either 2–2.5 mg/kg q 8 hr or 1.5–1.9 mg/kg q 6 hr; **neonates 1 week of age or less:** Up to 4 mg/kg/day in two equal doses q 12 hr.

Impaired renal function.

Initially: 1 mg/kg; **then,** maintenance dose calculated according to information supplied by manufacturer.

NEBULIZER SOLUTION

Pseudomonas aeruginosa *in cystic fibrosis.*

Dose using a nebulizer twice a day for 10–15 min in cycles of 28 days on and then 28 days off. See package insert for detailed instructions for administration.

OPHTHALMIC OINTMENT (0.3%)

Mild to moderate infections.

0.5 in ribbon into the affected eye(s) 2–3 times a day.

Severe infections.

0.5 in ribbon into the affected eye(s) q 3–4 hr until improvement, followed by reduced treatment prior to discontinuation.

OPHTHALMIC SOLUTION, (0.3%)

Mild to moderate infections.

Instill 1–2 gtt into the affected eye(s) q 4 hr.

Severe infections.

Instill 2 gtt into the eye(s) hourly until improvement; reduce treatment prior to discontinuation.

NURSING IMPLICATIONS

IMPLEMENTATION/ADMINISTRATION/STORAGE

1. Use the nebulizer solution as close as possible to q 12 hr, but not less than q 6 hr.
2. Do not mix TOBI with dornase alfa in the nebulizer.
3. Store ophthalmic products from 8–27°C (46–80°F).
4. IV Prepare IV solution by diluting drug with 50–100 mL of dextrose or saline solution; infuse over 30–60 min.
5. Use proportionately less diluent for children than for adults.
6. Discard solution of drug containing up to 1 mg/mL after 24 hr at room temperature.
7. Store drug at room temperature no longer than 2 years.
8. COMPATIBILITY 0.9% NaCl, D5W.

9. INCOMPATIBILITY Do not mix with other drugs for parenteral administration.

ASSESSMENT

1. Note reasons for therapy and method of administration, type, onset, characteristics of S&S, other agents trialed, outcome.
2. Assess for renal, auditory, and vestibular dysfunction during therapy.
3. Monitor cultures, CBC, renal and LFTs; reduce dose with dysfunction.

CLIENT/FAMILY TEACHING

1. Drink plenty of fluids (2–3 L/day) during parenteral drug therapy.
2. With eye drops, wash hands, do not allow dropper to touch eye. Tilt head back, looking up, pull lower eyelid down, and instill prescribed number of drops. Close eye for 1 to 2 min; apply gentle pressure to bridge of nose for 1 to 3 min. Do not rub eye or touch top of dropper/bottle to eye, fingers, or other surface. If more than 1 topical eye drug used, give at least 5 min apart administering the ointment last. May experience temporary stinging or burning; report if bothersome or if eye/eyelid inflammation noted. Avoid wearing contact lenses until infection is cleared and provider approves.
3. With inhalation therapy, take over a 10–15 min period using a hand-held nebulizer with a compressor. If on multiple therapies, take other therapies first followed by tobramycin.
4. Inhale while sitting or standing upright and breathing normally through the mouthpiece of the nebulizer to ensure adequate dispersion. Nose clips may help to breathe through the mouth. Therapy is usually a month on and then a month off. Follow guidelines for proper equipment cleaning and care.
5. Report unusual bruising/bleeding, bloody diarrhea, loss of hearing, lack of response, numbness, twitching, or seizures immediately.
6. Keep all F/U to assess response, labs, and for adverse SE.

OUTCOMES/EVALUATE

- Negative cultures; resolution of infection
- Therapeutic drug levels (peak: 4–8 mcg/mL; trough: <2 mcg/mL)

■ IV

Tocilizumab

(**toe**-si-**LIZ**-oo-mab)

Classification(s): Immunomodulator

Pregnancy Category: C

RX: Actemra.

INDICATIONS/USES

(1) Treatment of adults with moderately to severely active rheumatoid arthritis who have had an inadequate response to one or more tumor necrosis factor (TNF) antagonist therapies. (2) Inhibition and slowing of structural joint damage, improvement in physical function, and reaching major clinical response in adults with moderately to severely active rheumatoid arthritis when combined with methotrexate. (3) Juvenile rheumatoid arthritis in children 2 years of age and older. *NOTE:* May be used alone or concomitantly with methotrexate or other disease-modifying antirheumatic drugs.

ACTION/KINETICS

Action

Binds specifically to both soluble and membrane-bound IL-6 receptors and inhibits IL-6-mediated signaling through these receptors. IL-6 has been shown to be involved in diverse physiological processes such as T-cell activation, induction of immunoglobulin secretion, initiation of hepatic acute phase protein synthesis, and stimulation of hematopoietic precursor cell proliferation and differentiation. IL-6 is also produced by synovial and endothelial cells, leading to local production of IL-6 in joints affected by inflammatory processes as rheumatoid arthritis.

Pharmacokinetics

Following IV use, tocilizumab undergoes biphasic elimination from the circulation. The terminal $t^{1/2}$ is concentration dependent; **$t^{1/2}$, 4 mg/kg dose:** 11 days; **$t^{1/2}$, 8 mg/kg dose:** 13 days (both when the drug is given q 4 weeks at steady state). Possible increased metabolism by CYP enzymes due to higher levels stimulated by tocilizumab; effect on CYP enzymes may persist for several weeks after stopping tocilizumab therapy.

CONTRAINDICATIONS

Use with tumor necrosis factor antagonists, interleukin-1 receptor antagonists, anti-CD20 mono-

T

clonal antibodies, and selective costimulation modulators due to possible increase immunosuppression and increased risk of infection. Initiation of use in clients with an ANC below 2,000/mm^3, platelet count below 100,000/mm^3, or ALT or AST about 1.5 × ULN. Use in clients with active hepatic disease or hepatic impairment. Use of live vaccines concurrently with tocilizumab. Lactation.

SPECIAL CONCERNS

■ (1) Clients treated with tocilizumab are at increased risk for developing serious infections that may lead to hospitalization or death. Most clients who developed these infections were taking concomitant immunosuppressants such as methotrexate or corticosteroids. (2) If a serious infection develops, interrupt tocilizumab until the infection is controlled. (3) Reported infections include the following (a) active tuberculosis, which may present with pulmonary or extrapulmonary disease. Test clients for latent tuberculosis before tocilizumab use and during therapy. Initiate treatment for latent infection prior to tocilizumab use. (b) Invasive fungal infections, including candidiasis, aspergillosis, and pneumocystis. Clients with invasive fungal infections may present with disseminated, rather than localized disease. (c) Bacterial, viral, or other infections caused by opportunistic pathogens. (4) Carefully consider the risks and benefits of treatment with tocilizumab prior to initiating therapy in clients with chronic or recurrent infection. Closely monitor clients for the development of signs and symptoms of infection during and after treatment with tocilizumab, including the possible development of tuberculosis in clients who tested negative for latent tuberculosis infection prior to initiating therapy. ■

- **Use with caution in elderly clients.**
- **Use with caution in those with preexisting or recent-onset demyelinating disorders (e.g., multiple sclerosis, chronic inflammatory demyelinating polyneuropathy).**
- **Most clients who develop GI perforations were taking concomitant nonsteroidal anti-inflammatory drugs or methotrexate.**
- **Safety and efficacy not determined in children.**

SIDE EFFECTS

Most Common

Serious infections, headache, hypertension, increased ALT, nasopharyngitis, URTI.

CNS: Headache, dizziness. **GI:** Abdominal pain (upper), gastritis, mouth ulceration, ***GI perforation*** (including complications of diverticulitis, generalized purulent peritonitis, lower GI perforation, fistula, abscess). **Respiratory:** Nasopharyngitis, URTI, bronchitis. **Hematologic:** Neutropenia, thrombocytopenia. **Infections:** Bacterial, mycobacterial, invasive fungal, viral, protozoal, and other opportunistic infections. Serious infections, including bacterial arthritis, cellulitis, diverticulitis, gastroenteritis, herpes zoster, pneumonia, ***sepsis***, UTI. **Infusion reactions:** Hypertension, headache, skin reactions (pruritus, rash, urticaria). **Body as a whole:** Hypersensitivity reactions (including ***anaphylaxis***), malignancies, rash, viral reactivation, immunogenicity.

LABORATORY TEST CONSIDERATIONS

↑ ALT, AST, lipids (total cholesterol, LDL, HDL, triglycerides). Abnormal LFTs.

DRUG INTERACTIONS

Anti-CD20 monoclonal antibodies (e.g., rituximab) / Possible ↑ immunosuppression and ↑ risk of infection; avoid coadministration
Contraceptives, hormonal / ↓ Pharmacologic effect → ↑ risk of contraceptive failure; consider alternative nonhormonal contraceptives or an additional method of contraception
Cyclosporine / ↓ Cyclosporine pharmacologic effect; closely measure cyclosporine levels when starting/stopping tocilizumab; adjust cyclosporine dose as needed
Dextromethorphan / ↓ Dextromethorphan pharmacologic effect; monitor and adjust dextromethorphan dose as needed
HMG-CoA reductase inhibitors (e.g., lovastatin, simvastatin) / ↓ HMG-CoA reductase inhibitor pharmacologic effect; monitor when starting/stopping the reductase inhibitor and adjust dose as needed
IL-1 receptor antagonists (e.g., anakinra) / Possible ↑ immunosuppression and ↑ risk of infection; avoid coadministration
Immunosuppressants (e.g., corticosteroids, methotrexate) / ↑ Risk of infections and malignancy; monitor and adjust treatment as needed
Proton pump inhibitors (e.g., omeprazole) / ↓ Pharmacologic effect of proton pump inhibitor;

monitor and adjust proton pump inhibitor dose as needed
Selective costimulation modulators (e.g., abatacept) / Possible ↑ immunosuppression and ↑ risk of infection; avoid coadministration
Theophylline / ↓ Theophylline pharmacologic effect; closely measure theophylline levels when starting/stopping tocilizumab and adjust theophylline dose as needed
Tissue necrosis factor antagonists (e.g., infliximab) / Possible ↑ immunosuppression and ↑ risk of infection; avoid coadministration
Warfarin / ↓ Pharmacologic effect of warfarin; monitor coagulation parameters more closely when starting/stopping tocilizumab and adjust warfarin dose as needed

HOW SUPPLIED

Injection Solution, Concentrate: 20 mg/mL.

DOSAGE

IV DRIP INFUSION

Rheumatoid arthritis as monotherapy or combined with methotrexate.

Adults, usual: 4 mg/kg q 4 weeks as a 60-min, single IV drip infusion. **Maximum dose:** 800 mg/infusion. Dose may be increased to 8 mg/kg based on clinical response. If liver enzymes become elevated or neutropenia or thrombocytopenia occur, reduce the dose from 8 to 4 mg/kg. See also *Implementation/Administration/Storage.*

Juvenile rheumatoid arthritis.

Children, 2 years and older: 12 mg/kg q 2 weeks for those who weigh less than 30 kg and 8 mg q 2 weeks for those who weigh at least 30 kg.

NURSING IMPLICATIONS

IMPLEMENTATION/ADMINISTRATION/STORAGE

1. IV Interrupt use if a client develops a serious infection until the infection is controlled.
2. Adjust the dose as follows for **liver enzyme abnormalities**: (a) If liver enzymes are greater than 1 to 3 × ULN, modify dose concomitant disease modifying antirheumatic drugs if appropriate. For persistent increases in this range, decrease tocilizumab dose to 4 mg/kg or interrupt tocilizumab until ALT/AST have normalized. (b) If liver enzymes are greater than 3 to 5 × ULN, interrupt tocilizumab dosing until they are less than 3 × ULN and follow previous recommendations for greater than 1 to 3 × ULN. For persistent increases greater than 3 × ULN, discontinue tocilizumab. (c) If liver enzymes are greater than 5 × ULN, discontinue tocilizumab.
3. Adjust the dose as follows for **neutropenia**: (a) If ANC >1,000 cells/mm³, maintain dose. (b) If ANC is 500–1,000 cells/mm³, interrupt tocilizumab dosing. When ANC is >1,000 cells/mm³, resume tocilizumab at 4 mg/kg and increase to 8 mg/kg as clinically appropriate. (c) If ANC <500 cells/mm³, discontinue tocilizumab.
4. Adjust the dose as follows for **thrombocytopenia**: (a) If platelets are 50,000–100,000 cells/mm³, interrupt tocilizumab dosing. If platelet count is >100,000/mm³, resume tocilizumab at 4 mg/kg and increase to 8 mg/kg as clinically appropriate. (b) If platelet count is <50,000 cells/mm³, discontinue tocilizumab.
5. Dilute tocilizumab to 100 mL using aseptic technique. From a 100 mL infusion bag or bottle, withdraw a volume of 0.9% NaCl injection equal to the volume of the tocilizumab solution needed for the client. Slowly add tocilizumab from each vial into the infusion bag/bottle. Gently invert the bag to mix; avoid foaming.
6. Allow the fully diluted solution to reach room temperature before beginning the infusion. Give over 60 min with an infusion set. **Do not administer as an IV push or bolus.**
7. Fully diluted solutions are compatible with polypropylene, polyethylene, and polyvinyl chloride infusion bags and polypropylene, polyethylene, and glass infusion bottles.
8. Do not use any product remaining in the vials.
9. Refrigerate from 2–8°C (36–46°F); do not freeze. Protect vials from light by storing in the original container until time of use. The fully diluted solution may be stored in the refrigerator or at room temperature for up to 24 hr protected from light.
10. To monitor outcomes of pregnant women exposed to tocilizumab, health care providers are encouraged to register clients and preg-

nant women are encouraged to register themselves by calling 1-877-311-8972.

11. COMPATIBILITY 0.9% NaCl.
12. INCOMPATIBILITY Administer separately.

ASSESSMENT

1. Note reasons for therapy, onset, characteristics of S&S, clinical presentation and joint findings, ROM, pain level, other agents trialed (TNF agents), and outcome.
2. List other agents prescribed to ensure none interact.
3. Assess for any evidence of infection and ensure TB testing performed. Evaluate any abdominal pain as perforation has occurred.
4. Review risk for developing serious infections that may lead to hospitalization or death especially in those taking concomitant immunosuppressants.
5. Determine any conditions that may preclude therapy; multiple sclerosis, chronic inflammatory demyelinating polyneuropathy, hepatitis, or severe infections.
6. Assess for any evidence of allergic reaction during infusion.
7. Monitor VS, lipids, CBC and LFTs; adjust dose for dysfunction and follow dosing guidelines carefully.

CLIENT/FAMILY TEACHING

1. Drug is administered once every 4 weeks as an infusion over 1 hr. May be used separately or with other agents to control symptoms of RA.
2. Drug may make one more likely to get infections or make any infection that one may have worse. Immediately report any S&S of infection (e.g., fever, chills, cough, sore throat, rash, painful urination).
3. Serious infections including TB (tuberculosis) and infections caused by viruses, fungi, or bacteria may occur with this therapy; report immediately; may be fatal.
4. Avoid crowds, persons with infections, and any vaccinations during therapy.
5. Any abdominal pain or new onset GI symptoms should be reported due to risk of perforation.
6. Practice reliable contraception (hormonal contraceptive effects may be decreased). Report if pregnancy suspected and register by calling 1-877-311-8972 to monitor outcome.
7. Keep all F/U to assess response, labs, and adverse SE.

OUTCOMES/EVALUATE

- ↓ Joint swelling/pain; ↑ mobility
- ↓ Pain, discomfort, and deformities

Tolcapone

(**TOHL**-kah-pohn)

Classification(s): Antiparkinson drug

Pregnancy Category: C

RX: Tasmar.

INDICATIONS/USES

Adjunct to levodopa and carbidopa for idiopathic Parkinson's disease. Since hepatotoxicity from the drug may be fatal, reserve for Parkinson clients on levodopa/carbidopa with symptom fluctuations who are not satisfactorily responding.

ACTION/KINETICS

Action

Reversible inhibitor of catechol-O-methyltransferase (COMT), resulting in an increase in plasma levodopa. When given with levodopa/carbidopa, plasma levels of levodopa are more sustained, allowing for more constant dopaminergic stimulation of the brain. May also increase side effects of levodopa.

Pharmacokinetics

Rapidly absorbed from the GI tract; **peak levels:** 2 hr. Food given within 1 hr before or 2 hr after PO use decreases bioavailability by 10–20%. **t½, elimination:** 2–3 hr. Almost completely metabolized in the liver; excreted in the urine (60%) and feces (40%). **Plasma protein binding:** More than 99.9%.

CONTRAINDICATIONS

Use with a nonselective MAOI. In clients with liver disease, history of nontraumatic rhabdomyolysis or hyperpyrexia, confusion possibly related to the drug, and in those withdrawn from tolcapone due to hepatocellular injury.

SPECIAL CONCERNS

■ (1) Because of the risk of potentially fatal, acute fulminant liver failure, use tolcapone in those with parkinsonism on levodopa/carbidopa who are experiencing symptom fluctuation and are not responding satisfactorily to, or are not appropriate candidates for other therapies. (2) Because of the risk of liver injury, withdraw clients from tolcapone who fail to show substantial improvement within 3 weeks of initiation of therapy. (3) Do not initiate tolcapone if there is clinical evidence of liver disease or ALT or AST values are greater than twice ULN. Treat those with severe dyskinesia or dystonia with caution. (4) Those who develop evidence of hepatocellular injury and are withdrawn from the drug for any reason may be at increased risk for liver injury if tolcapone is reintroduced. Do not consider such clients for retreatment. (5) Advise a prescriber who elects to use tolcapone in face of the increased risk of liver injury to monitor clients for evidence of emergent liver injury. Instruct clients about the need for self-monitoring for classical signs of liver disease (e.g., clay-colored stools, jaundice) and nonspecific signs (e.g., fatigue, appetite loss, lethargy). (6) Although frequent lab monitoring for evidence of hepatocellular injury is essential, it is not clear that baseline and periodic monitoring of liver enzymes will prevent fulminant liver failure. However, it is believed that early detection of drug-induced hepatic injury with immediate withdrawal of the drug enhances likelihood for recovery. Clients with preexisting hepatic disease are more vulnerable to hepatotoxins; thus, following the liver monitoring program is recommended. (7) Perform appropriate tests to exclude presence of liver disease before starting tolcapone therapy. Determine baseline levels of ALT and AST every 2 weeks for the first year of therapy, every 4 weeks for the next 6 months, and every 8 weeks thereafter. Monitor liver enzymes before increasing the dose to 200 mg 3 times per day and reinitiate at the frequency above. (8) Discontinue tolcapone if ALT or AST exceeds the ULN or if clinical signs and symptoms suggest the onset of hepatic failure (e.g., persistent nausea, fatigue, lethargy, anorexia, jaundice, dark urine, pruritus, and right upper quadrant tenderness).

Use with caution in severe renal or hepatic impairment, in those with severe dystonia/dyskinesias, and during lactation.

SIDE EFFECTS

Most Common

Dyskinesia, sleep disorder, dystonia, excessive dreaming, somnolence, confusion, dizziness, headache, nausea, anorexia, diarrhea, muscle cramps, orthostatic complaints.

GI: N&V, anorexia, diarrhea, constipation, xerostomia, abdominal pain, dyspepsia, flatulence, ***acute fulminant liver failure.*** **CNS:** Hallucinations, dyskinesias, sleep disorder, dystonia, excessive dreaming, somnolence, confusion, dizziness, headache, syncope, loss of balance, hyperkinesia, paresthesia, hypokinesia, agitation, irritability, mental deficiency, hyperactivity, panic reaction, euphoria, hypertonia, sudden uncontrolled sedation. **CV:** Orthostatic hypotension, chest pain, hypotension, chest discomfort. **Respiratory:** URTI, dyspnea, sinus congestion. **Musculoskeletal:** Muscle cramps, stiffness, arthritis, neck pain. **GU:** Hematuria, UTIs, urine discoloration, micturition disorder, uterine tumor. **Dermatologic:** Increased sweating, dermal bleeding, skin tumor, alopecia. **Ophthalmic:** Cataract, eye inflammation. **Body as a whole:** Falling, fatigue, influenza, burning, malaise, fever, rhabdomyolysis. *NOTE:* Clients over 75 years of age may develop more hallucinations but less dystonia. Females may develop somnolence more frequently than males.

LABORATORY TEST CONSIDERATIONS

↑ AST, ALT.

OVERDOSE MANAGEMENT

Symptoms: Nausea, vomiting, dizziness, possibility of respiratory difficulties. *Treatment:* Hospitalization is advised. Give supportive care.

HOW SUPPLIED

Tablets: 100 mg, 200 mg.

DOSAGE

TABLETS

Adjunct for idiopathic parkinsonism.

Initial: 100 mg 3 times per day with/without food. Use 200 mg 3 times per day only if anticipated benefit is justified. Do **not** increase the dose to 200 mg 3 times per day in those with moderate to severe liver cirrhosis.

NURSING IMPLICATIONS

IMPLEMENTATION/ADMINISTRATION/STORAGE

1. Even though 200 mg 3 times per day is reasonably well tolerated, the prescriber may start with 100 mg 3 times per day due to the potential for increased dopaminergic side effects and the possibility of adjustment of the concomitant levodopa/carbidopa dose.
2. A suggested dosing regimen is to give the first dose of tolcapone on the day with the first dose of levodopa/carbidopa; subsequent doses of tolcapone can be given 6 to 12 hr later.
3. Reductions in the daily dose of levodopa may be required.
4. Tolcapone can be used with either the immediate- or sustained-release formulations of levodopa/carbidopa.

ASSESSMENT

1. Note reasons for therapy, characteristics/duration of Parkinson's symptoms, other agents trialed/failed.
2. List drugs currently prescribed to ensure none interact unfavorably.
3. Ensure client aware of potential for liver toxicity; record informed consent.
4. May cause severe hepatotoxicity. Do not use with clinical evidence of liver disease or if ALT or AST twice the ULN. When used, monitor LFTs q 2 weeks for the first year of therapy, then q 4 weeks for the next 6 months and then q 8 weeks thereafter. Stop drug with ↑ evidence of liver dysfunction or if no improvement in symptoms after 3–4 weeks of therapy.

CLIENT/FAMILY TEACHING

1. Take as directed with your levodopa/carbidopa. Drug increases the action of levodopa by decreasing its metabolism in the peripheral tissues. If taken without levodopa, there is no treatment benefit. May experience nausea initially; should subside.
2. Do not drive or perform activities requiring mental alertness until drug effects realized; may cause sedation.
3. Review risk of intense urges and the possibility of hallucinations. Have client review and sign Patient Acknowledgement of risks associated with tolcapone therapy.
4. Stop drug and report any evidence of liver dysfunction: fatigue, loss of appetite, lethargy, yellow skin discoloration, clay-colored stools, hallucinations or diarrhea and report tremors or repetitive movements.
5. Rise slowly from a sitting or lying position to prevent low BP effects. May experience nausea initially and an increase in involuntary repetitive movements; these should subside. Six weeks into therapy may experience diarrhea; report if persistent or severe. May discolor urine bright yellow.
6. Practice reliable birth control; do not breastfeed.
7. Keep all F/U to assess response, labs, and for adverse SE.

OUTCOMES/EVALUATE

Control of S&S Parkinson's disease

Tolmetin sodium

(**TOLL**-met-in)

Classification(s): Nonsteroidal anti-inflammatory drug

Pregnancy Category: C

SEE ALSO ***NONSTEROIDAL ANTI-INFLAMMATORY DRUGS***.

INDICATIONS/USES

1. Relief of the signs and symptoms of acute flares and long-term management of rheumatoid arthritis and osteoarthritis.
2. Juvenile rheumatoid arthritis.

Investigational: Sunburn.

ACTION/KINETICS

Pharmacokinetics

Peak plasma levels: 30–60 min. Bioavailability is affected by food or milk but not by acute or chronic use of magnesium and aluminum hydroxides. **t½:** 2–7 hr. **Therapeutic plasma levels:** 40 mcg/mL. **Onset, anti-inflammatory effect:** Within 1 week; **duration, anti-inflammatory effect:** 1–2 weeks. Inactivated in liver and excreted in urine. **Plasma protein binding:** More than 93%.

SPECIAL CONCERNS

■ (1) **Cardiovascular risk.** NSAIDs may cause an increased risk of serious CV thrombotic events, myocardial infarction, and stroke, which can be fatal. This risk may increase with duration of use. Clients with CV disease or risk factors for CV disease may be at greater risk. (2) Tolmetin sodium is contraindicated for the treatment of perioperative pain in the setting of coronary artery bypass graft. (3) **GI risk.** NSAIDs cause an increased risk of serious GI adverse effects, including bleeding, ulceration, and perforation of the stomach or intestines, which can be fatal. These events can occur at any time during use and without warning symptoms. Elderly clients are at greater risk for serious GI events.

- Use with caution during lactation.
- Safety and efficacy not determined in children less than 2 years of age.

SIDE EFFECTS

Most Common

Hypertension, headache, dizziness, asthenia/malaise, diarrhea, N&V, flatulence, abdominal/GI distress, peripheral edema, edema.

See *Nonsteroidal Anti-Inflammatory Drugs* for a complete list of possible side effects.

LABORATORY TEST CONSIDERATIONS

Tolmetin metabolites give a false + test for proteinuria using sulfosalicylic acid.

HOW SUPPLIED

Capsules: 400 mg; ***Tablets:*** 200 mg, 600 mg.

DOSAGE

CAPSULES; TABLETS

Rheumatoid arthritis, osteoarthritis.

Adults: 400 mg 3 times per day (including one dose on arising and one at bedtime); adjust dosage according to client response after 1–2 weeks. **Maintenance, rheumatoid arthritis:** 600–1,800 mg/day usually in 3 divided doses; **osteoarthritis,** 600–1,600 mg/day generally in 3 divided doses. Doses larger than 1,800 mg/day for rheumatoid arthritis and osteoarthritis are not recommended.

Juvenile rheumatoid arthritis.

Children, 2 years and older, initial: 20 mg/kg/day in 3–4 divided doses to start; **then,** 15–30 mg/kg/day when control has been achieved. Doses higher than 30 mg/kg/day are not recommended. Beneficial effects may not be observed for several days to a week.

NURSING IMPLICATIONS

IMPLEMENTATION/ADMINISTRATION/STORAGE

1. A response is expected in a few days to a week. Expect progressive improvement during succeeding weeks of therapy.
2. Closely monitor those with impaired renal function; they may require a lower dose.
3. If GI symptoms occur, can give with antacids (but not sodium bicarbonate).
4. Store from 15–30°C (59–86°F). Protect from light.

ASSESSMENT

1. List reasons for therapy; note joint pain/level, deformity, swelling, inflammation, and ROM.
2. Determine history of ulcers, heart disease, or cardiac failure. May cause an increased risk of serious CV thrombotic events, MI, and stroke.
3. This class of drugs has been associated with increased risk of heart attacks/stroke (those with CV disease or risk factors for CV disease may be at higher risk); monitor for S&S and advise client.
4. Monitor for GI bleeding, ulceration, and perforation of the stomach or intestines, which can be fatal. Elderly clients are at higher risk for serious GI events.
5. Obtain eye exam if visual disturbance noted.
6. Assess BP, CBC and renal function studies.

CLIENT/FAMILY TEACHING

1. Doses should be spaced so that one dose is taken in the morning on arising, one during the day, and one at bedtime. The dosage is based on the treatment condition and varies according to indications. Take as directed. It may take several weeks or more before effects are evident.
2. Avoid taking with food or milk or immediately after meal unless GI irritation occurs, then may administer with meals, milk, a full glass of water, or antacids. Never administer with sodium bicarbonate. The elderly are particularly susceptible to gastric irritation and should take with milk, meals, an antacid, or stomach protectant if prescribed.

T

3. Avoid activities that require mental alertness until drug effects realized; may cause drowsiness, dizziness, or blurred vision.
4. Report any unusual bruising or bleeding, weight gain, edema, fever, blood in urine/stool or increased joint pain.
5. Avoid alcohol, smoking, and any OTC medications without approval.
6. Use protective clothing and sunscreen if any prolonged sun exposure, to prevent photosensitivity reaction.
7. Keep all F/U to assess response, labs, and for adverse SE.

OUTCOMES/EVALUATE

↓ Joint pain and inflammation; ↑ mobility

Tolnaftate

(toll-**NAF**-tayt)

Classification(s): Antifungal

Pregnancy Category: C

OTC: Absorbine Athlete's Foot Cream, Absorbine Footcare, Aftate for Athlete's Foot, Aftate for Jock Itch, Genaspor, Lamisil AF Defense, Quinsana Plus, Tinactin, Tinactin for Jock Itch, Ting, Ting Aerosol Spray.

SEE ALSO ***ANTI-INFECTIVE DRUGS***.

INDICATIONS/USES

(1) Tinea pedis, tinea cruris, tinea corporis, and tinea versicolor. (2) Fungal infections of moist skin areas.

ACTION/KINETICS

Action

Exact mechanism not known; is thought to stunt mycelial growth causing a fungicidal effect.

CONTRAINDICATIONS

Scalp and nail infections. Avoid getting into eyes. Use in children less than 2 years of age.

SIDE EFFECTS

Most Common

Mild skin irritation.

Dermatologic: Sensitivity, mild skin irritation.

HOW SUPPLIED

Cream: 1%; ***Gel:*** 1%; ***Powder:*** 1%; ***Solution:*** 1%; ***Spray Aerosol:*** 1%; ***Spray Liquid:*** 1%; ***Spray Powder:*** 1%.

DOSAGE

TOPICAL: CREAM; GEL; POWDER; SOLUTION; SPRAY AEROSOL; SPRAY LIQUID; SPRAY POWDER

Tinea pedia, tinea cruris, tinea corporis, tinea versicolor; fungal infections of moist skin areas.

Apply twice a day for 2–3 weeks although treatment for 4–6 weeks may be necessary in some instances.

NURSING IMPLICATIONS

ASSESSMENT

1. Note reasons for therapy, location, onset, characteristics of S&S. Inspect source of infection and presentation as the choice of vehicle is important for effective therapy.
   - Powders are used in mild conditions as adjunctive therapy.
   - For primary therapy and prophylaxis, creams, liquids, or ointments are used, especially if area is moist.
   - Liquids and solutions are used if area is hairy.
2. Assess cultures; use concomitant therapy if bacterial or *Candida* infections also present.

CLIENT/FAMILY TEACHING

1. Skin should be thoroughly cleaned and dried before applying. Use care; do not rub medication into or near the eye. Wash hands before and after application.
2. Continue to use as directed, despite improvement of symptoms. Takes 2-6 weeks to clear infection; local relief of symptoms should be evident within the first 24-48 hr.
3. Do not cover with dressing unless directed.
4. With foot infection wear well-fitting, ventilated shoes; change shoes and socks at least daily.
5. Keep all F/U to assess response, labs, and for adverse SE.

OUTCOMES/EVALUATE

- Symptomatic relief; skin healing
- Eradication of fungal infection

Tolterodine tartrate

(tohl-**TER**-oh-deen)

Classification(s): Urinary tract drug, anticholinergic

Pregnancy Category: C

RX: Detrol, Detrol LA.

INDICATIONS/USES

Overactive bladder with symptoms of urinary frequency, urgency, or urge incontinence.

ACTION/KINETICS

Action

Acts as a competitive muscarinic receptor antagonist in the bladder to cause increased bladder control.

Pharmacokinetics

Absolute bioavailability is highly variable (10–74%). Rapidly absorbed with peak serum levels within 1–2 hr. Metabolized by CYP2D6 by first pass effect in the liver to the active 5-hydroxymethyl derivative, which has similar activity as tolterodine. About 7% of individuals are slow metabolizers. Food increases bioavailability. Excreted in the urine (77%) and feces (17%). Both renal and hepatic impairment will affect disposition of the drug. **Plasma protein binding:** Highly bound.

CONTRAINDICATIONS

Hypersensitivity to the drug or components of the product. Urinary retention, gastric retention, uncontrolled narrow-angle glaucoma, lactation.

SPECIAL CONCERNS

- **Use with caution in renal impairment, in bladder outflow obstruction, in GI obstructive disorders (e.g., pyloric stenosis), and in those being treated for narrow-angle glaucoma.**
- **Safety and efficacy not determined in children.**

SIDE EFFECTS

Most Common

Immediate-Release: Dry mouth, headache, constipation, vertigo/dizziness, abdominal pain, diarrhea, dyspepsia, fatigue.

Extended-Release: Dry mouth, headache, constipation, abdominal pain, somnolence, dyspepsia, xerophthalmia.

GI: Dry mouth, dyspepsia, constipation, abdominal pain, N&V, diarrhea, flatulence. **CNS:** Headache, vertigo, dizziness, somnolence, anxiety, paresthesia, nervousness. **Respiratory:** URTI, bronchitis, coughing, pharyngitis, rhinitis, sinusitis. **Dermatologic:** Rash, erythema, dry skin, pruritus. **GU:** UTI, dysuria, urinary frequency, urinary retention. **Ophthalmic:** Abnormalities with vision, including accommodation; xerophthalmia, dry eyes. **Musculoskeletal:** Arthralgia, back pain, chest pain. **Body as a whole:** Fatigue, flu-like symptoms, infection, fungal infection. **Miscellaneous:** Hypertension, weight gain, fall, chest pain, tachycardia, peripheral edema, ***anaphylactoid reactions.***

OVERDOSE MANAGEMENT

Symptoms: Significant anticholinergic symptoms. *Treatment:* Symptomatic. Monitor ECG.

DRUG INTERACTIONS

Clarithromycin / ↑ Tolterodine levels R/T ↓ liver metabolism by CYP3A4; do not give tolterodine >1 mg twice a day

Cyclosporine / ↑ Tolterodine levels R/T ↓ liver metabolism by CYP3A4; do not give tolterodine >1 mg twice a day

Erythromycin / ↑ Tolterodine levels R/T ↓ liver metabolism by CYP3A4; do not give tolterodine >1 mg twice a day

Fluoxetine / ↑ Tolterodine levels R/T inhibition of CYP2D6; no dosage adjustment needed

Itraconazole / ↑ Tolterodine levels R/T ↓ liver metabolism by CYP3A4; do not give tolterodine >1 mg twice a day

Ketoconazole / ↑ Tolterodine levels R/T ↓ liver metabolism by CYP3A4; do not give tolterodine >1 mg twice a day

Miconazole / ↑ Tolterodine levels R/T ↓ liver metabolism by CYP3A4; do not give tolterodine >1 mg twice a day

Omeprazole / ↑ Tolterodine peak levels R/T ↑ rate of drug release from the extended-release product from ↑ gastric pH

Vinblastine / ↑ Tolterodine levels R/T ↓ liver metabolism by CYP3A4; do not give tolterodine >1 mg twice a day

Warfarin / Prolonged INR values → possible bleeding

HOW SUPPLIED

Capsules, Extended-Release: 2 mg, 4 mg; ***Tablets, Immediate-Release:*** 1 mg, 2 mg.

DOSAGE

CAPSULES, EXTENDED-RELEASE

Overactive bladder.

4 mg once daily taken with liquids and swallowed whole. May lower dose to 2 mg daily based on response and tolerability. For those with significantly decreased hepatic or renal function or who are taking drugs that are inhibitors of CYP3A4, the recommended dose is 2 mg daily.

TABLETS, IMMEDIATE-RELEASE

Overactive bladder.

Initial: 2 mg twice a day. Dose may be lowered to 1 mg twice a day based on individual response and side effects. Adjust dose to 1 mg twice a day in those with significantly reduced hepatic function or who are currently taking drugs that are inhibitors of CYP3A4 (see *Drug Interactions*).

NURSING IMPLICATIONS

IMPLEMENTATION/ADMINISTRATION/STORAGE

1. Do not give more than 1 mg twice a day (immediate-release), or 2 mg a day (extended-release) to those with significantly impaired hepatic function.
2. Protect from light.

ASSESSMENT

1. Note reasons for therapy, onset, occurrence/triggers, frequency, characteristics of S&S. Describe daily bladder function (use a voiding diary) and r/o infections and stones.
2. List drugs currently prescribed to ensure none interact or alter dosage. Determine evidence of urinary/gastric retention, GI obstructive disorders, or glaucoma.
3. Monitor renal and LFTs; decrease dose with dysfunction.

CLIENT/FAMILY TEACHING

1. Take as directed with or without food at same time each day. Swallow ER capsule whole.
2. Drug is used to help reduce the frequency and urgency associated with urination. It is not for stress incontinence or UTI but is for treatment of an overactive bladder.
3. May experience dizziness/drowsiness, headache, blurred vision, dry mouth and light sensitivity; use caution and report if persistent. If eye pain, rapid heart rate, SOB, urinary retention, rash or hives appears notify provider.
4. Dry mouth symptoms may be relieved with sugar free candy/gum, ice/water, or saliva substitute.
5. Practice reliable contraception; not for use during pregnancy.
6. For user support number call 1-800-896-8596 to enroll and to receive free information/updates and 24-hr hotline access or www.detrolLA.com.
7. Avoid alcohol and OTC antihistamines.
8. Keep all F/U to assess response, labs, and adverse SE.

OUTCOMES/EVALUATE

↑ Bladder control with ↓ urinary frequency, urgency, or urge incontinence

---

Topiramate

(toh-**PYRE**-ah-mayt)

Classification(s): Anticonvulsant, miscellaneous

Pregnancy Category: C

RX: Topamax, Topiragen.

🍁 **Rx:** Apo-Topiramate, CO Topiramate, Gen-Topiramate, PMS-Topiramate, ratio-Topiramate, Sandoz Topiramate.

SEE ALSO ***ANTICONVULSANTS.***

INDICATIONS/USES

(1) Adjunct treatment for partial onset seizures in adults and children, 2–16 years. (2) Adjunct treatment for primary generalized tonic-clonic seizures in adults and children, 2–16 years old. (3) Adjunct treatment of seizures associated with Lennox-Gastaut syndrome in clients 2 years of age and older. (4) Monotherapy in clients 10 years and older to treat partial-onset or primary generalized tonic-clonic seizures. (5) Prophylaxis of migraine headaches in adults. Use in acute treatment of migraines has not been studied. *Investigational:* Alcohol and cocaine dependence, binge eating disorder, bulimia nervosa, cluster headaches, infantile spasms, adjunctive therapy for bipolar disorder, weight loss in obesity, smoking.

ACTION/KINETICS

Action

Precise mechanism not known. The following effects may contribute to the anticonvulsant activity. (1) Action potentials seen repetitively by sustained depolarization of neurons are blocked in a time-dependent manner, suggesting an effect to block sodium channels. (2) Increases the frequency at which GABA activates $GABA_A$ receptors, thus enhancing the ability of GABA to cause a flux of chloride ions into neurons (i.e., enhanced effect of the inhibitory transmitter, $GABA_A$). (3) Antagonizes the ability of kainate to activate the kainate/AMPA subtype of excitatory amino acid aspartate, thus reducing the excitatory effect. (4) Inhibits the carbonic anhydrase enzyme, particularly isozymes II and IV.

Pharmacokinetics

Rapidly absorbed; **peak plasma levels:** About 2 hr. Bioavailability is about 80%. **t½, elimination:** 21 hr. **Steady state:** About 4 days in those with normal renal function. Excreted mostly unchanged in the urine. Plasma levels may be increased in hepatic impairment. **Plasma protein binding:** 15–41%; the fraction bound decreases with increased concentrations.

CONTRAINDICATIONS

Lactation.

SPECIAL CONCERNS

- **Use with caution in impaired hepatic and renal function.**
- **Clients taking the drug, especially children, should be monitored for decreased sweating and hyperthermia, especially those exposed to elevated environmental temperatures and/or engaged in vigorous activity.**
- **There is an increased risk of suicidal behavior and ideation.**
- **Safety and efficacy have not been determined in children less than 2 years old for adjunctive therapy of partial onset seizures, primary generalized tonic-clonic seizures, or seizures associated with Lennox-Gastaut syndrome.**

SIDE EFFECTS

Most Common

Dizziness, paresthesia, ataxia, anxiety, confusion, nervousness, depression, fatigue, somnolence, insomnia, URTI, anorexia, rhinitis, abnormal vision, diplopia, nystagmus, tremor, nausea.

NOTE: Side effects with an incidence of 0.1% or greater or those that are life–threatening are listed. **CNS:** Psychomotor slowing, including difficulty with concentration and speech or language problems. Somnolence, fatigue, dizziness, nervousness, ataxia, nystagmus, paresthesia, nervousness, difficulty with memory/concentration, tremor, confusion, depression, abnormal coordination, agitation, mood problems, aggressive reaction, hypoesthesia, apathy, emotional lability, depersonalization, hypo-/hyperkinesia, hyporeflexia, vertigo, stupor, ***clonic/tonic seizures***, hyperkinesia, hypertonia, insomnia, personality disorder, impotence, hallucinations, euphoria, psychosis, decreased libido, ***suicide behavior and ideation/attempt***, hyporeflexia, neuropathy, migraine, apraxia, hyperesthesia, dyskinesia, hyperreflexia, dysphonia, scotoma, dystonia, coma, encephalopathy, upper motor neuron lesion, paranoid reaction, delusion, paranoia, delirium, abnormal dreaming, neuroses, abnormal gait, tremor, vertigo. **GI:** Nausea, dyspepsia, anorexia, abdominal pain, constipation, dry mouth, thirst, gingivitis, glossitis, halitosis, diarrhea, vomiting, fecal incontinence, flatulence, gastroenteritis, GI disorder, gum hyperplasia, hemorrhoids, increased appetite, tooth caries, stomatitis, dysphagia, melena, gastritis, esophagitis, increased saliva, hiccough, gastroesophageal reflux, tongue edema, esophagitis, gallbladder disorder, gingival bleeding, enlarged abdomen, hepatitis, ***pancreatitis, hepatic failure (including fatalities)***. **CV:** Palpitation, hyper-/hypotension, postural hypotension, AV block, bradycardia, bundle branch block, angina pectoris, ***DVT***, abnormal EEG, syncope, vasodilation, phlebitis. **Body as a whole:** Asthenia, flu-like symptoms, infection, viral infections, hot flashes, body odor, edema, rigors, fever, malaise, syncope, enlarged abdomen, hyperthermia (especially in children during vigorous activity or exposure to elevated environmental temperatures). **Respiratory:** URTI, pharyngitis, sinusitis, rhinitis, epistaxis, dyspnea, coughing, bronchitis, asthma, pneumonia, respiratory disorder, ***bronchospasm, pulmonary embolism***. **Dermatologic:** Acne, alopecia, dermatitis, nail disorder, folliculitis, dry skin, urticaria, skin discoloration, pallor, eczema, photosensitivity reaction, erythematous rash, flushing, seborrhea, decreased/increased sweating, abnormal hair texture, facial edema, pemphigus, erythema multiforme, ***Stevens-Johnson syndrome, toxic dermal necrolysis.*** **GU:** Breast pain, renal stone formation, dysmenorrhea, amenorrhea, menstrual disorder, hematuria, intermenstrual bleeding, leukorrhea, menorrhagia, vaginitis, UTI, micturition frequency, urinary incontinence, abnormal urine, dysuria, renal calculus, ejaculation disorder, breast discharge, urinary retention, renal pain, nocturia, albuminuria, polyuria, oliguria, kidney stones, renal tubular acidosis, prostatic disorder. **Musculoskeletal:** Arthralgia, muscle weakness, arthrosis, osteoporosis, myalgia, skeletal pain, leg cramps, involuntary muscle contractions, back/chest/leg pain. **Metabolic:** Increased/decreased weight, dehydration, xeropthalmia, metabolic acidosis, diabetes mellitus. **Hematologic:** Anemia, leukopenia, lymphadenopathy, eosinophilia, lymphopenia, granulocytopenia, lymphocytosis, thrombocytothemia, purpura, thrombocytopenia, hematoma. **Ophthalmic:** Diplopia, abnormal vision, eye pain, conjunctivitis, abnormal accommodation, photophobia, abnormal lacrimation, strabismus, color blindness, acute myopia, mydriasis, ptosis, xerothalmia, scotoma, visual field defect, acute myopia with secondary angle-closure glaucoma, nystagmus. **Miscellaneous:** Decreased hearing, taste perversion, tinnitus, taste loss, parosmia, goiter, basal cell carcinoma.

LABORATORY TEST CONSIDERATIONS

↑ AST, ALT, gamma-GT, alkaline phosphatase, creatinine. Hypokalemia, hyperglycemia, hyperlipidemia, hyperchloremia, hypernatremia, hypocholesterolemia, hyponatremia, hypophosphatemia.

OVERDOSE MANAGEMENT

Symptoms: Abdominal pain, abnormal coordination, agitation, blurred vision, convulsions, depression, diplopia, dizziness, drowsiness, hypotension, lethargy, impaired mentation, metabolic acidosis, speech disturbance, stupor. *Treatment:* Gastric lavage or induction of emesis if ingestion is recent. Activated charcoal. Supportive treatment. Hemodialysis.

T

DRUG INTERACTIONS

Alcohol / CNS depression; cognitive and neuropsychiatric side effects
Amitriptyline / ↑ Amytriptyline levels; adjust amitripytline dose
Anticholinergics / ↑ Risk of heat-related disorders
Carbamazepine / ↓ Topiramate levels by about 40% R/T ↑ metabolism
Carbonic anhydrase inhibitors / ↑ Risk of renal stone formation and heat-related disorders
CNS depressants / CNS depression; cognitive and neuropsychiatric side effects
Digoxin / ↓ Serum digoxin AUC; clinical relevance not established
Estrogens / ↓ Effect of estrogens R/T ↓ estradiol AUC and plasma levels; consider ↑ estrogen dose
Hydantoins / ↓ Topiramate levels R/T ↑ metabolism; also, ↑ phenytoin levels R/T ↓ metabolism
Hydrochlorothiazide / ↑ Topiramate C_{max} and AUC; adjust dose accordingly
Lamotrigine / ↑ Topiramate levels
Lithium / ↓ Lithium AUC and C_{max}
Metformin / ↓ Metformin plasma clearance → ↑ AUC and C_{max}
Oral contraceptives / ↓ Effect of OCs; consider an alternate method of contraception or ↑ estrogen dose
Phenytoin / ↓ Topiramate levels and ↑ phenytoin levels; possible dosage adjustment
Pioglitazone / ↓ Topiramate's active metabolites; monitor carefully; also, ↓ pioglitazone AUC
Risperidone / ↓ Risperidone levels by 25%; monitor closely
Valproic acid / ↓ Levels of both topiramate and valproic acid; possible hyperammonemia with or without encephalopathy

HOW SUPPLIED

Capsules, Sprinkle: 15 mg, 25 mg; ***Tablets:*** 25 mg, 50 mg, 100 mg, 200 mg; ***Tablets, Film-Coated:*** 25 mg, 50 mg, 100 mg, 200 mg.

DOSAGE

CAPSULES, SPRINKLE; TABLETS; TABLETS, FILM-COATED

Epilepsy, monotherapy.

Adults and children, 10 years and older: 400 mg/day in 2 divided doses. Achieve this dosage using the following titration schedule: **Week 1:** 25 mg in the morning and evening; **Week 2:** 50 mg in the morning and evening; **Week 3:** 75 mg in the morning and evening; **Week 4:** 100 mg in the morning and evening; **Week 5:** 150 mg in the morning and evening; **Week 6:** 200 mg in the morning and evening.

Epilepsy, adjunctive therapy: Partial seizures, primary generalized tonic-clonic seizures, Lennox-Gastaut syndrome.

Adults, 17 years and older, initial: 25–50 mg/day; **then,** titrate in increments of 25 to 50 mg/week until an effective daily dose is reached. The recommended total daily dose is 200–400 mg/day; doses greater than 1,600 mg/day have not been studied. **Children, 2–16 years:** Begin titration at 25 mg or less (based on a range of 1–3 mg/kg/day) nightly for the first week. Then increase dose at 1- or 2-week intervals by increments of 1–3 mg/kg/day (given in 2 divided doses) to reach optimal clinical response. The recommended total daily dose is 5–9 mg/kg/day in two divided doses.

Migraine prophylaxis.

Week 1, initial: 25 mg at night; **Week 2:** 25 mg in the morning and evening; **Week 3:** 25 mg in the morning and 50 mg in the evening; **Week 4:** 50 mg in the morning and evening. **Maintenance:** 100 mg/day in 2 doses.

NURSING IMPLICATIONS

Do not confuse Topamax with Toprol-XL (antihypertensive) or with Tegretol and Tegretol-XR (anticonvulsants).

IMPLEMENTATION/ADMINISTRATION/STORAGE

1. If C_{CR} is <70 mL/1.73 m^2, use one half of the usual adult dose. These clients will require a longer time to reach steady state at each dose.
2. Plasma levels may be increased in those with hepatic impairment.
3. The sprinkle capsule is bioequivalent to the tablet and thus may be substituted as therapeutically equivalent.
4. Addition of topiramate to phenytoin therapy may require adjustment of the phenytoin dose to achieve an optimal response. The addition or withdrawal of phenytoin and/or carbamazepine during therapy with topiramate may require adjustment of the topiramate dose.
5. If necessary, withdraw topiramate gradually to minimize the risk of increased seizure frequency.
6. A prolonged period of dialysis may result in topiramate levels too low to maintain antiseizure effect. To avoid rapid falls in topiramate plasma levels during hemodialysis, a supplemental topiramate dose may be required.
7. Store tablets from 15–30°C (59–86°F) in a tightly closed container. Store sprinkle capsules at 25°C (77°F) in a tightly closed container. Protect capsules and tablets from moisture.

ASSESSMENT

1. Note reasons for therapy; with seizures note age at onset, type, and characteristics, other agents trialed, outcome.
2. List drugs currently prescribed to ensure none interact or lose effectiveness; MAOIs may promote kidney stones.
3. Document baseline psychomotor and mental status; assess for psychomotor slowing, speech or expression problems, difficulty concentrating, depression, fatigue, or sleepiness.
4. Evaluate for acute myopia or secondary angle closure glaucoma (eye exam). Immediately discontinue drug if symptoms present.
5. Measure baseline serum bicarbonate and monitor periodically during treatment to assess for metabolic acidosis.
6. Monitor CBC, liver, and renal function studies; reduce dose with renal dysfunction.

CLIENT/FAMILY TEACHING

1. Take exactly as prescribed! Swallow tablet whole. Due to the bitter taste of the drug, do not break tablets. Can be taken without regard for meals. Do not stop drug abruptly due to risk of increased seizure frequency.
2. For sprinkle capsules, either swallow whole or carefully open capsule and sprinkle the entire contents on a small amount (teaspoon) of soft food. Swallow the drug/food mixture immediately. Do not chew and do not store for future use.
3. Distinguish if drug affects motor or mental capacity before driving or performing activities that require mental alertness; may cause dizziness, confusion, drowsiness, and altered concentration.

T

4. **Review list of side effects, noting those that require attention. Report any blurred vision or periorbital edema immediately. May cause increased weight loss; consider additional food intake as needed.**
5. **Increase fluid intake to decrease concentration; drug may precipitate renal stone formation by increasing urinary pH and reducing urinary citrate excretion.**
6. **Avoid strenuous activity in hot weather; decreased sweating and increased body temperature, especially in hot weather may cause dehydration.**
7. **If using for migraine prophylaxis, must take daily as prescribed to prevent headaches.**
8. **Avoid alcohol and other CNS depressants during therapy.**
9. **May cause sensitivity reaction with prolonged sun exposure; use protective clothing and sunscreen if exposure necessary.**
10. **Use reliable, nonhormonal form of birth control; drug may compromise efficacy of PO contraceptives and cause birth defects.**
11. **Do not stop suddenly; should be tapered off over several weeks.**
12. **Keep all F/U to assess response, labs, and adverse SE.**

OUTCOMES/EVALUATE

- Control of seizures
- Migraine prophylaxis

IV

Topotecan hydrochloride

(toh-poh-**TEE**-kan)

Classification(s): Antineoplastic, hormone

Pregnancy Category: D

RX: Hycamtin.

SEE ALSO ***ANTINEOPLASTIC AGENTS.***

INDICATIONS/USES

Capsules: Treat relapsed small cell lung cancer in those with a prior complete or partial response who are at least 45 days from the end of first-line chemotherapy. **Injection:** (1) Metastatic cancer of the ovary after failure of initial or subsequent chemotherapy. (2) Small cell lung cancer sensitive disease after failure of first-line chemotherapy. (3) In combination with cisplatin to treat stage IV-B, recurrent, or persistent carcinoma of the cervix, that is not amenable to curative therapy with surgery and/or radiation therapy. *Investigational:* In combination with paclitaxel to treat advanced non-small cell lung cancer.

ACTION/KINETICS

Action

An inhibitor of topoisomerase I. Topoisomerase I relieves torsional strain in DNA by causing reversible single-strand breaks. Topotecan binds to the topoisomerase I-DNA complex and prevents religation of single-strand breaks. Cytotoxicity thought to be caused by double-strand DNA damage produced during DNA synthesis when replication enzymes interact with the ternary complex formed by topotecan, topoisomerase I, and DNA.

Pharmacokinetics

Rapidly absorbed after PO administration; **peak plasma levels after PO:** 1–2 hr. Hydrolyzed to the active lactone form of the drug. Following a high-fat meal, the time to maximum plasma levels is delayed from 1.5 to 3 hr for topotecan lactone and from 3 to 4 hr for total topotecan. About 30% of the drug is excreted in the urine. **t½, terminal:** 2 to 3 hr. About 30% of a dose is excreted in the urine. **Plasma protein binding:** About 35%.

CONTRAINDICATIONS

Hypersensitivity to topotecan or any component of the product. Pregnancy, lactation. Severe bone marrow depression, including those with baseline neutrophil counts less than 1,500 cells/mm^3.

SPECIAL CONCERNS

Capsules: Administer topotecan only to clients with baseline neutrophil counts of 1,500 cells/mm^3 or more and a platelet count of 100,000 cells/mm^3 or more. In order to assess the occurrence of bone marrow suppression, monitor blood cell counts. **Injection:** (1) Administer under the supervision of a physician experienced in the use of cancer chemotherapeutic drugs. Appropriate management of complications is possible only when adequate diagnostic and treatment facilities are readily available. (2) Do not give topotecan to those with baseline neutrophil counts of less than 1,500 cells/mm^3. In order to monitor the occurrence of bone marrow suppression (primarily neutropenia) that may be severe and result in infection and death, perform frequent peripheral blood cell counts on all clients receiving topotecan.

- **The dose limiting toxicity is leukopenia.**
- **Diarrhea is more common in those 65 years of age and older.**
- **WBC decreases with increasing doses.**
- **Safety and efficacy not determined in children.**

SIDE EFFECTS

Most Common

Myelosuppression (see *Side Effects*), headache, total alopecia, N&V, diarrhea, constipation, abdominal pain, pyrexia, pain, coughing, dyspnea.

Hematologic: Bone marrow suppression, including neutropenia (grade 4: <500 cells/mm^3), thrombocytopenia (grade 4: <25,000 cells/mm^3), anemia (severe: grade 3/4), leukopenia (<3,000 cells/mm^3), hemoglobin <8 grams/dL), sepsis or fever/infection with grade 4 neutropenia, platelet or RBC infusions, ***severe bleeding in association with thrombocytopenia*** (rare). **GI:** N&V, abdominal pain (partially associated with neutropenic colitis), constipation, diarrhea (may be severe), intestinal obstruction, stomatitis, anorexia. **CNS:** Headache, pain, paresthesias, neuropathy. **Musculoskeletal:** Arthralgia, myalgia. **Respiratory:** Dyspnea, coughing, pharyngitis, pneumonia. **Dermatologic:** Total alopecia, rash, severe dermatitis, severe pruritus. **At injection site:** Erythema, bruising. **Hypersensitivity:** Rash, allergic manifestations, anaphylactoid reactions, angioedema, ***anaphylaxis.*** **Body as a whole:** Anorexia, fatigue, asthenia, malaise, fever, pain, severe bleeding (in association with thrombocytopenia), ***sepsis.*** **Miscellaneous:** Chest pain, ocular disturbances, ***death.***

LABORATORY TEST CONSIDERATIONS

↑ AST, ALT, bilirubin.

OVERDOSE MANAGEMENT

Symptoms: Hematologic toxicity. *Treatment:* Observe carefully for bone marrow suppression. Consider supportive measures, including prophylactic use of granulocyte colony-stimulating factor and/or antibiotic therapy.

DRUG INTERACTIONS

Cisplatin / More severe myelosuppression
Cyclosporine A / P-glycoprotein inhibitors → significant ↑ in topotecan exposure
Cytotoxic drugs / More severe myelosuppression
Filgrastim / Prolonged duration of neutropenia; do not initiate until 24 hr after completion of topotecan treatment
Ketoconazole / P-glycoprotein inhibitors → significant ↑ in topotecan exposure
Ritonavir / P-glycoprotein inhibitors → significant ↑ in topotecan exposure
Saquinavir / P-glycoprotein inhibitors → significant ↑ in topotecan exposure

HOW SUPPLIED

Capsules: 0.25 mg, 1 mg; ***Injection, Lyophilized Powder for Solution:*** 4 mg.

DOSAGE

CAPSULES

Relapsed small cell lung cancer.

2.3 mg/m^2 per day given once daily for 5 consecutive days; repeat q 21 days. Round the calculated PO daily dose to the nearest 0.25 mg and then use the minimum number of 0.25 and 1 mg capsules. Use the same number of capsules for each of the 5 dosing days. In those with moderately impaired renal function (C_{CR} 30–49 mL/min), adjust the dose to 1.8 mg/m^2 per day. Insufficient data are available to provide a dose for clients with severely impaired renal function.

IV INFUSION

Metastatic ovarian cancer, small cell lung cancer.

Adults: 1.5 mg/m^2 by IV infusion over 30 min daily for 5 consecutive days, starting on day 1 of a 21-day course of therapy. The median time to response in ovarian cancer is 9–12 weeks and the median time to response in small cell lung cancer is 5–7 weeks. In the absence of tumor progression, a minimum of four courses is recommended. If severe neutropenia occurs, reduce the dose to 1.25 mg/m^2 for subsequent courses. Reduce doses similarly if the platelet count falls below 25,000 cells/mm^3. Also, for severe neutropenia, filgrastim may be given following the sub-

T

sequent course and before dosage reduction starting from day 6 of the course (i.e., 24 hr after completion of topotecan administration). Reduce the dose to 0.75 mg/m² for clients with a C_{CR} of 20–39 mL/min. No dosage reduction is required if the C_{CR} is 40–60 mL/min.

Cervical cancer.

Topotecan, 0.75 mg/m² daily over 30 min on days 1, 2, and 3 followed by cisplatin, 50 mg/m² on day 1 repeated every 21 days (i.e., a 21-day course of therapy). If severe febrile neutropenia (<1,000 cells/mm³) occurs, reduce the dose of topotecan to 0.6 mg/m² for subsequent courses. Also, decrease the dose of topotecan to 0.6 mg/m² if the platelet count falls below 10,000/mm³. Alternatively, in the event of severe febrile neutropenia, filgrastim (granulocyte colony-stimulating factor; G-CSF) can be given following the subsequent course and before reducing the dose. Give G-CSF starting from day 4 of the course (i.e., 24 hr after completion of topotecan dosing regimen). If febrile neutropenia occurs despite the use of G-CSF, reduce the dose of topotecan to 0.45 mg/m² for subsequent courses. *NOTE:* See cisplatin for administration and hydration guidelines.

NURSING IMPLICATIONS

IMPLEMENTATION/ADMINISTRATION/STORAGE

1. Capsules may be taken with or without food.
2. Clients should not be treated with subsequent courses of PO therapy until neutrophils recover to >1,000 cells/mm³, platelets recover to >100,000 cells/mm³, and hemoglobin levels recover to 9 grams/dL or more (with transfusion if necessary).
3. Reduce the PO dose to 0.4 mg/m²/day for subsequent courses if severe neutropenia (neutrophils <500 cells/mm³ associated with fever or infection or lasting for 7 days or more). Doses should be similarly reduced if the platelet count falls to <25,000 cells/mm³.
4. Reduce the PO dose to 0.4 mg/m²/day for subsequent courses for clients who experience grade 3 or 4 diarrhea. Those with grade 2 diarrhea, may need to follow the same dose modification guidelines.
5. Store capsules from 15–30°C (59–86°F); protect from light.
6. IV To begin therapy, clients must have a baseline neutrophil count >1,500 cells/mm³, a platelet count >100,000 cells/mm³, and a hemoglobin level of 9 mg/dL or higher. Do not retreat until neutrophils are >1,000 cells/mm³, platelets are >100,000 cells/mm³, and hemoglobin levels are 9 mg/dL or greater.
7. For those with moderately impaired renal function (C_{CR}, 20–39 mL/min), give a dose of 0.75 mg/m².
8. Only initiate cisplatin with topotecan if serum creatinine is 1.5 mg/dL or less.
9. Reconstitute the 4 mg topotecan vial with 4 mL of sterile water for injection. This may then be further diluted either with 0.9% NaCl or D5W and administered over 30 min. Because there is no antibacterial preservative in the product, use the reconstituted product immediately.
10. Inadvertant extravasation may cause mild local reactions, including erythema and bruising.
11. Topotecan is a cytotoxic drug. Prepare under a vertical laminar flow hood while wearing gloves and protective clothing. If topotecan solution contacts the skin, wash immediately and thoroughly with soap and water. If the drug contacts mucous membranes, flush thoroughly with water.
12. Reconstituted vials diluted for infusion are stable at controlled room temperature and ambient lighting conditions when stored for 24 hr.
13. Store vials in their original carton, protected from light, at controlled room temperature of 20–25°C (68–77°F).
14. COMPATIBILITY D5W, 0.9% NaCl.
15. INCOMPATIBILITY Administer separately.

ASSESSMENT

1. Note reasons for therapy, (prior complete or partial response) other agents/therapies trialed, when administered (at least 45 days from the end of first-line chemotherapy).

2. Monitor CBC, renal and LFTs; reduce dose with C_{CR} of 20–39 mL/m^2. Ensure baseline neutrophil count above 1,500 cells/mm^3 and platelet count at 100,000/mm^3. Do not readminister until neutrophils are above 1,000 cells/mm^3, platelets are 100,000 cells/mm^3, and hemoglobin levels are at least 9 mg/dL. Drug causes bone marrow suppression, neutropenia, and anemia. Nadir: 15 days.

CLIENT/FAMILY TEACHING

1. Swallow capsules whole; do not chew, crush, or divide capsules. If vomiting occurs after taking the dose of topotecan, do not take a replacement dose.
2. If the capsule contents come in contact with the skin or mucous membranes, wash thoroughly with soap and water or wash the eyes immediately with gently flowing water for at least 15 min. Report if skin reaction or if drug gets into the eyes.
3. May cause weakness or fatigue; use caution when performing activities that require mental alertness.
4. Drug may be administered IV over 30 min to stop the growth of cancer cells.
5. Report any evidence of infection: sore throat, fever, chills, unusual bruising/bleeding.
6. Practice reliable contraception; avoid breastfeeding.
7. May experience hair loss during therapy; should regrow once therapy completed.
8. Keep all F/U to assess response, labs, and for adverse SE.

OUTCOMES/EVALUATE

Control of malignant cell proliferation in metastatic cancer

Toremifene citrate

(**TOR**-em-ih-feen)

Classification(s): Antineoplastic, hormone (antiestrogen)

Pregnancy Category: D

RX: Fareston.

SEE ALSO ***ANTINEOPLASTIC AGENTS***.

INDICATIONS/USES

Metastatic breast cancer in postmenopausal women with positive estrogen-receptor (ER) or ER unknown tumors. *Investigational:* Desmoid tumors.

ACTION/KINETICS

Action

Estrogen agonist/antagonist that binds to estrogen receptors and may cause estrogenic, antiestrogenic, or both effects, depending on duration of treatment, gender, and endpoint/target organ selected. Antitumor effect is likely due to antiestrogenic effect, i.e., competes for estrogen at receptor and blocks growth-stimulating effects of estrogen in the tumor. There are increases in the QTc interval and T wave changes due to toremifene and N–demethyltoremifene (metabolite).

Pharmacokinetics

Well absorbed from GI tract; absorption not affected by food. **Peak plasma levels:** 3 hr. Steady state levels reached in 4–6 weeks. **t½, distribution:** About 4 hr. **t½, elimination:** About 5 days. Extensively metabolized in liver by CYP3A4 to N–demethyltoremifene which is also antiestrogenic but with weak antitumor potency. Mainly excreted in feces. The elimination half-life is increased in both the elderly and in those with hepatic insufficiency. **Plasma protein binding:** >99.5%.

CONTRAINDICATIONS

Hypersensitivity to toremifene or any component of the product. Congenital/acquired QT prolongation. Use with history of thromboembolic disease or in pediatric clients. Uncorrected hypokalemia or hypomagnesemia. Lactation.

SPECIAL CONCERNS

QT prolongation. Toremifene has been shown to prolong the QTc interval in a dose- and concentration-manner. Prolongation of the QT interval can result in a type of ventricular tachycardia called torsades de pointes, which may result in syncope, seizure, and/or death. Toremifene should not be prescribed to clients with congenital/acquired QT prolongation, uncorrected hypokalemia, or uncorrected hypomagnesemia. Avoid drugs known to prolong the QT interval and strong CYP3A4 inhibitors.

T

- **Hypercalcemia and tumor flare in some breast cancer clients with bone metastases during first weeks of treatment.**
- **In general, do not give long–term to those with preexisting endometrial hyperplasia.**
- **Use with caution in CHF, hepatic impairment, and electrolyte abnormalities.**
- **There is no indication for use in children.**

SIDE EFFECTS

Most Common

Hot flashes, sweating, N&V, vaginal discharge/bleeding, dizziness, edema.

CV: ***Cardiac failure, MI, pulmonary embolism, CVA, QT prolongation***, angina pectoris, arrhythmia, ischemic attack, thrombophlebitis, thrombosis, TIA. **GI:** Constipation, N&V, anorexia, jaundice. **Hematologic:** Leukopenia, thrombocytopenia. **Dermatologic:** Hot flashes, sweating, skin discoloration, dermatitis, alopecia, pruritus. **CNS:** Dizziness, tremor, vertigo, ataxia, depression. **Musculoskeletal:** Arthritis. **Respiratory:** Dyspnea. **GU:** Vaginal discharge/bleeding. **Ophthalmic:** Cataracts, dry eyes, abnormal vision, abnormal visual fields, diplopia, corneal keratopathy, glaucoma, reversible corneal opacity. **Body as a whole:** Edema, asthenia, rigors, fatigue, lethargy. **Miscellaneous:** Dyspnea, paresis, hypercalcemia and tumor flare, hypercalcemia.

LABORATORY TEST CONSIDERATIONS

↑ AST, alkaline phosphatase, bilirubin. Hypercalcemia.

OVERDOSE MANAGEMENT

Symptoms: Vertigo, headache, dizziness. Possibly, hot flashes, vaginal bleeding, vertigo, dizziness, ataxia, nausea. *Treatment:* General supportive measures.

DRUG INTERACTIONS

An additive effect of toremifene with other drugs that prolong the QT interval cannot be excluded. the following drugs may prolong the QT interval and increase the risk of life–threatening cardiac arrhythmias, including torsades de pointes: Amiodarone, arsenic trioxide, bretylium, chlorpromazine, clarithromycin, disopyramide, dofetilide, dolasetron, droperidol, erythromycin, gatifloxacin, granisetron, halofantrine, haloperidol, ibutilide, levofloxacin, levomethadyl, mefloquine, mesoridazine, moxifloxacin, ofloxacin, ondansetron, pentamidine, pimozide, probucol, procainamide, quinidine, sotalol, sparfloxacin, thioridazine, venlafaxine, and ziprasidone.

Atazanavir / ↑ Toremifene plasma levels R/T inhibition of metabolism by CYP3A4 → ↑ pharmacologic/toxic effects; closely monitor for QT prolongation

Carbamazepine / ↓ Toremifene blood levels R/T ↑ liver breakdown; monitor response and adjust toremifene dose as needed

Clarithromycin / ↑ Toremifene plasma levels R/T inhibition of metabolism by CYP3A4 → ↑ pharmacologic/toxic effects; closely monitor for QT prolongation

Clonazepam / ↓ Toremifene blood levels R/T ↑ liver breakdown

Dexamethasone / ↓ Toremifene blood levels R/T ↑ liver breakdown; monitor response and adjust toremifene dose as needed

Indinavir / ↑ Toremifene plasma levels R/T inhibition of metabolism by CYP3A4 → ↑ pharmacologic/toxic effects; closely monitor for QT prolongation

Itraconazole / ↑ Toremifene plasma levels R/T inhibition of metabolism by CYP3A4 → ↑ pharmacologic/toxic effects; closely monitor for QT prolongation

Ketoconazole / ↑ Toremifene plasma levels R/T inhibition of metabolism by CYP3A4 → ↑ pharmacologic/toxic effects; closely monitor for QT prolongation

Nefazodone / ↑ Toremifene plasma levels R/T inhibition of metabolism by CYP3A4 → ↑ pharmacologic/toxic effects; closely monitor for QT prolongation

Nelfinavir / ↑ Toremifene plasma levels R/T inhibition of metabolism by CYP3A4 → ↑ pharmacologic/toxic effects; closely monitor for QT prolongation

Phenobarbital / ↓ Toremifene blood levels R/T ↑ liver breakdown; monitor response and adjust toremifene dose as needed

Phenytoin / ↓ Toremifene blood levels R/T ↑ liver breakdown; monitor response and adjust toremifene dose as needed; also, possible ↑ phenytoin levels R/T ↓ metabolism by CYP2D9 (monitor phenytoin levels)

Rifabutin/Rifampin / ↓ Toremifene blood levels R/T ↑ liver breakdown; monitor response and adjust toremifene dose as needed

T

Ritonavir / ↑ Toremifene plasma levels R/T inhibition of metabolism by CYP3A4 → ↑ pharmacologic/toxic effects; closely monitor for QT prolongation
Saquinavir / ↑ Toremifene plasma levels R/T inhibition of metabolism by CYP3A4 → ↑ pharmacologic/toxic effects; closely monitor for QT prolongation
H ***St. John's wort*** / ↓ Toremifene blood levels R/T ↑ liver breakdown; monitor response and adjust toremifene dose as needed
Telithromycin / ↑ Toremifene plasma levels R/T inhibition of metabolism by CYP3A4 → ↑ pharmacologic/toxic effects; closely monitor for QT prolongation
Thiazide diuretics (e.g., hydrochlorothiazide) / ↑ Risk of hypocalcemia; monitor serum calcium
Tolbutamide / ↑ Tolbutamide levels R/T inhibition of metabolism by CYP2D9; monitor tolbutamide levels
Voriconazole / ↑ Toremifene plasma levels R/T inhibition of metabolism by CYP3A4 → ↑ pharmacologic/toxic effects; closely monitor for QT prolongation
Warfarin / ↑ Warfarin levels R/T inhibition of metabolism by CYP2D9 → ↑ PT; monitor warfarin levels

HOW SUPPLIED

Tablets: 60 mg.

DOSAGE

TABLETS

Metastatic breast cancer.

Adults, usual: 60 mg once daily. Continue until disease progression is observed.

NURSING IMPLICATIONS

IMPLEMENTATION/ADMINISTRATION/STORAGE

1. Toremifene is considered a potential teratogen. Follow safe handling procedures when preparing, administering, or dispensing the drug.
2. Store from 15–30°C (59–86°F); protect from light and heat.

ASSESSMENT

1. Note reasons for therapy, characteristics of S&S, other agents trialed, outcome.
2. Determine any history of prolonged QT syndrome and check ECG. Prolongation of the QT interval can result in torsades de pointes, which may result in syncope, seizure, and/or death. List drugs prescribed.
3. List any history/evidence of thromboembolic disorders.
4. Monitor CBC, calcium, renal and LFTs.

CLIENT/FAMILY TEACHING

1. Used to treat metastatic breast cancer in postmenopausal women with estrogen-receptor positive or unknown tumors. Drug acts to block the growth-stimulating effects of estrogen in the tumor.
2. Take once daily as directed. May take with food to decrease GI upset; do not crush, break or chew enteric coated products. Avoid taking foods that inhibit CYP3A4, including grapefruit products; may increase toremifene concentrations.
3. Use caution and notify provider if prescribed potent CYP3A4 inhibitors or medications that prolong the QT interval, review effects of toremifene on QT interval.
4. Report any unusual vaginal bleeding, muscle/bone pain, visual changes, or calf pain/tenderness, SOB, or chest pain.
5. May experience "tumor flare," syndrome of diffuse musculoskeletal pain and erythema with increased size of tumor lesions that regress later; if accompanied by hypercalcemia, must discontinue drug.
6. Avoid OTC medications or herbal supplements (such as St. John's wort) with toremifene; can reduce concentrations of coadministered drugs.
7. Use reliable barrier birth control as drug may induce ovulation.
8. Hair loss may occur and regrowth may be of a different texture and color.
9. Keep all F/U to assess response, labs, and for adverse SE.

OUTCOMES/EVALUATE

Control of malignant cell proliferation

Torsemide

(**TOR**-seh-myd)

Classification(s): Diuretic, loop

Pregnancy Category: B

RX: Demadex.

SEE ALSO ***DIURETICS, LOOP.***

INDICATIONS/USES

(1) Edema associated with congestive heart failure, renal disease, or hepatic disease. (2) Edema associated with chronic renal failure. (3) Hypertension alone or with other antihypertensive drugs. (4) Hepatic cirrhosis.

ACTION/KINETICS

Pharmacokinetics

Onset, PO: Within 60 min. **Peak effect, PO:** 60–120 min. **Duration:** 6–8 hr. **t½:** 210 min. Metabolized by the liver and excreted through the urine. Food delays the time to peak effect by about 30 min, but the overall bioavailability and the diuretic activity are not affected.

CONTRAINDICATIONS

Lactation.

SPECIAL CONCERNS

■ Loop diuretics are potent drugs; excess amounts can lead to a profound diuresis with water and electrolyte depletion. Careful medical supervision is required and dosage must be individualized. ■

- **Clients sensitive to sulfonamides may show allergic reactions to torsemide.**
- **Safety and efficacy not determined in children.**

SIDE EFFECTS

Most Common

Excessive urination, headache, dizziness, asthenia, diarrhea, abnormal ECG, arthralgia, nausea, rhinitis, increased cough.

CNS: Headache, dizziness, asthenia, insomnia, nervousness, syncope. **GI:** Diarrhea, constipation, nausea, dyspepsia, edema, ***GI hemorrhage***, rectal bleeding. **CV:** ECG abnormality, chest pain, atrial fibrillation, hypotension, ***ventricular tachycardia***, shunt thrombosis. **Respiratory:** Rhinitis, increase in cough. **Musculoskeletal:** Arthralgia, myalgia. **Miscellaneous:** Sore throat, excessive urination, rash.

LABORATORY TEST CONSIDERATIONS

Hyperglycemia, hyperuricemia, hypokalemia, hypovolemia

HOW SUPPLIED

Tablets: 5 mg, 10 mg, 20 mg, 100 mg.

DOSAGE

TABLETS

Edema associated with congestive heart failure.

Adults, initial: 10 or 20 mg once daily. If the dose is inadequate, titrate the dose upward by approximately doubling until the desired diuretic response is reached.

Edema associate with chronic renal failure.

Adults, initial: 20 mg once daily. If the dose is inadequate, titrate the dose upward by approximately doubling until the desired diuretic response is reached.

Edema associated with hepatic cirrhosis.

Adults, initial: 5 or 10 mg once daily given with an aldosterone antagonist or a potassium-sparing diuretic. If the dose is inadequate, titrate the dose upward by approximately doubling until the desired diuretic response is reached.

Hypertension.

Adults, initial: 5 mg once daily. If this dose does not lead to an adequate decrease in BP within 4–6 weeks, the dose may be increased to 10 mg once daily. If the 10 mg dose is not adequate, an additional antihypertensive agent is added to the treatment regimen.

NURSING IMPLICATIONS

Do not confuse torsemide with furosemide (also a loop diuretic).

IMPLEMENTATION/ADMINISTRATION/STORAGE

1. **Doses greater than 200 mg for CHF or chronic renal failure and greater than 40 mg for hepatic cirrhosis have not been adequately studied.**
2. **To prevent hypokalemia and metabolic alkalosis, use an aldosterone antagonist or potassium-sparing drug.**
3. **In clients with decompensated CHF, a small fraction of any given dose is delivered to the intraluminal site of action due to reduced renal clearance. Thus, at any given dose there is less natriuresis in clients with CHF.**

T

4. May be given without regard to meals.
5. It is not necessary to adjust the dose for geriatric clients.
6. Store from 15–30°C (59–86°F).

ASSESSMENT

1. Note reasons for therapy, onset, characteristics of S&S. List agents trialed, outcome.
2. Assess pulmonary, renal, and CV systems. List sensitivity to sulfonamides.
3. Monitor VS, weight, I&O, blood sugar, uric acid, BUN, creatinine, calcium, magnesium and potassium; drug may increase blood sugar and uric acid levels.

CLIENT/FAMILY TEACHING

1. Take only as directed in the a.m. to prevent nighttime awakening to void. May take with food to decrease GI upset. Store in a cool dry place away from BR.
2. Drug may cause dizziness, lightheadedness, and fatigue; use caution. Rise slowly from a sitting or lying position to minimize low BP effects.
3. Consume potassium-rich foods daily (banana, cantaloupe, and potatoes) unless restricted. Notify provider if vomiting and diarrhea occur or if signs of excessive potassium loss (eg, cramps, muscle weakness, nausea, dizziness) are noted.
4. With hypertension, keep a BP log for provider review.
5. Report immediately any chest pain, increased SOB, ringing in the ears, or sudden weight gain with extremity swelling.
6. May experience blurred vision, yellowing of vision, or sensitivity to sunlight. Avoid prolonged sun exposure; use sunscreen/protective clothing to avoid photosensitivity reaction.
7. Keep all F/U to assess response, labs, and for adverse SE.

OUTCOMES/EVALUATE

↓ Edema; ↑ diuresis; ↓ BP

Tramadol hydrochloride

(**TRAM**-ah-dol)

Classification(s): Analgesic, centrally-acting

Pregnancy Category: C

RX: Rybix ODT, Ryzolt, Ultram, Ultram ER.

✱ **Rx:** Ralivia.

INDICATIONS/USES

Immediate-Release (IR): Management of moderate to moderately severe pain in adults. *Investigational:* Premature ejaculation, restless legs syndrome.

Extended-Release (ER): Moderate to moderately severe chronic pain in adults who require around-the-clock pain therapy for an extended period of time.

ACTION/KINETICS

Action

A centrally-acting analgesic not related chemically to opiates. Precise mechanism is not known. Two complementary mechanisms may be applicable: It may bind to mu-opioid receptors and inhibit reuptake of norepinephrine and serotonin. The analgesic effect is only partially antagonized by the antagonist naloxone. Causes significantly less respiratory depression than morphine. In contrast to morphine, tramadol does not cause release of histamine. Produces dependence of the mu-opioid type (i.e., like codeine); however, there is little evidence of abuse. Tolerance occurs but is relatively mild; the withdrawal syndrome is not as severe as with other opiates.

Pharmacokinetics

Rapidly absorbed after PO administration. Food does not affect the rate or extent of absorption. **Onset:** 1 hr. **Peak effect:** 2–3 hr. **Peak plasma levels:** 2 hr. **Duration:** 2 hr for tramadol and 3 hr for the M1 active metabolite. **t½, plasma:** 6.3 hr for tramadol and 7.4 hr for the M1 active metabolite. Extensively metabolized in the liver by CYP2D6 and CYP3A4. Excreted in the urine, with about 30% excreted unchanged and 60% as metabolites. The M1-metabolite is active.

CONTRAINDICATIONS

Hypersensitivity to tramadol. In acute intoxication with alcohol, hypnotics, centrally acting analgesics, opiates, or psychotropic drugs. Use in clients with past or present addiction or opiate dependence or in those with a prior history of allergy to codeine or opiates. Use for obstetric preoperative medication or for postdelivery analgesia in nursing mothers. Use in children less than 16

T

years of age, as safety and efficacy have not been determined.

SPECIAL CONCERNS

- **Use with great caution in those taking MAOIs, as tramadol inhibits norepinephrine and serotonin uptake.**
- **Dosage reduction recommended with impaired hepatic or renal function and in clients over 75 years of age.**
- **Use with caution in increased intracranial pressure or head injury, in epilepsy, or in clients with an increased risk for seizures, including head trauma, metabolic disorders, alcohol or drug withdrawal, use of certain drugs (e.g., SSRIs, tricyclic compounds, cyclobenzaprine, promethazine), and CNS infections.**
- **Seizures may occur in any client, especially if the dose is increased.**
- **Tramadol may complicate the assessment of acute abdominal conditions.**
- **Has abuse potential for some clients.**

SIDE EFFECTS

Most Common

Dizziness, headache, CNS stimulation, ataxia, sedation/somnolence, vertigo, itching/pruritus, constipation, nausea.

CNS: Dizziness, vertigo, headache, somnolence, ataxia, CNS stimulation, anxiety, confusion, incoordination, euphoria, nervousness, sleep disorders, ***seizures***, paresthesia, cognitive dysfunction, hallucinations, tremor, amnesia, concentration difficulty, abnormal gait, migraine, development of drug dependence, speech disorders, depression, increased risk of seizures. **GI:** Nausea, constipation, vomiting, dyspepsia, dry mouth, diarrhea, abdominal pain, anorexia, flatulence, GI bleeding, hepatitis, stomatitis, dysgeusia, ***liver failure***. **CV:** Vasodilation, syncope, orthostatic hypotension, hypertension, tachycardia, abnormal ECG, myocardial ischemia, palpitations, pulmonary edema/embolism. **Dermatologic:** Pruritus, sweating, rash, itching, urticaria, vesicles, ***Stevens-Johnson syndrome***, ***toxic epidermal necrolysis***. **Body as a whole:** Asthenia, malaise, allergic reaction, accidental injury, weight loss, ***suicidal tendency***. **GU:** Urinary retention/frequency, menopausal symptoms, dysuria, menstrual disorder. **Ophthalmic:** Miosis, visual disturbancers, cataracts. **Miscellaneous:** ***Anaphylaxis***, deafness, tinnitus, hypertonia, dyspnea, serotonin syndrome.

LABORATORY TEST CONSIDERATIONS

↑ Creatinine, liver enzymes. ↓ Hemoglobin. Proteinuria.

OVERDOSE MANAGEMENT

Symptoms: Extension of side effects, especially ***respiratory depression and seizures***. *Treatment:* Naloxone will reverse some, but not all, of the symptoms of overdose. General supportive treatment, with special attention to maintenance of adequate respiration. Diazepam or barbiturates may help if seizures occur. Hemodialysis is not helpful.

DRUG INTERACTIONS

Alcohol / ↑ Respiratory depression
Anesthetics, general / ↑ Respiratory depression
Carbamazepine / ↓ Tramadol effect R/T ↑ metabolism
CNS depressants / Additive CNS depression
Cyclobenzaprine / ↑ Risk of seizures
Digoxin / ↑ Risk (rare) of digoxin toxicity
MAOIs / ↑ Risk of seizures
Naloxone / ↑ Risk of seizures if naloxone used for tramadol overdose.
Promethazine / ↑ Risk of seizures
Quinidine / ↑ Levels of tramadol and ↓ levels of M1 R/T inhibition of metabolism
SSRIs / ↑ Risk of seizures and ↑ risk of serotonin syndrome
Tricyclic antidepressants / ↑ Risk of seizures
Warfarin ↑ PT and INR

HOW SUPPLIED

Tablets, Extended-Release: 100 mg, 200 mg, 300 mg; ***Tablets, Immediate-Release:*** 50 mg; ***Tablets, Orally Disintegrating:*** 50 mg.

DOSAGE

TABLETS, IMMEDIATE-RELEASE; TABLETS, ORALLY DISINTEGRATING

Management of pain.

Individualize dose based on lowest effective dose. **Adults, 17 years and older, those requiring rapid onset of analgesia:** 50–100 mg q 4–6 hr, as needed, but not to exceed 400 mg/day. **Moderate to moderately severe chronic pain, initial:** 25 mg/day in the morning and titrate in 25 mg increments as separate doses q 3 days to reach 100 mg/day (25 mg four times a day). Thereafter, increase the total daily dose by 50 mg as tolerated q 3 days to reach 200 mg/day (50 mg 4 times a day). After titration, give 50–100 mg q 4–6 hr as needed for pain relief, not to exceed 400 mg/day. For clients over 75 years of age, the recommended dose is no more than 300 mg/day in divided doses. In impaired renal function with a C_{CR} less than 30 mL/min, the dosing interval should be increased to 12 hr, with a maximum daily dose of 200 mg. The recommended dose for clients with cirrhosis is 50 mg q 12 hr. Dialysis clients can receive their regular dose on the day of dialysis.

Premature ejaculation (Investigational).

50 mg given 2 hr before sexual activity.

Restless legs syndrome (Investigational).

50–100 mg/day for up to 24 months.

TABLETS, EXTENDED-RELEASE

Long-term around-the-clock management of pain in adults.

Clients not currently on tramadol immediate-release products. Adults, 18 years and older, initial: 100 mg once daily; titrate up as needed in 100 mg increments q 5 days. Maximum dose: 300 mg/day. **Clients currently on tramadol immediate-release products. Adults, 18 years and older:** Calculate the 24-hour tramadol immediate-release dose to the next lowest 100 mg increment. The dose may subsequently be individualized according to client need. Because there is limited flexibility of dose selection with the extended-release product, some clients maintained on the immediate-release product may not be able to convert to the extended-release form. **Maximum daily dose of extended-release products:** 300 mg. Administer with great caution to clients 65 years of age and older. Do not use the dosage form in clients with a C_{CR} <30 mL/min or in severely impaired hepatic function (Child-Pugh, class C).

NURSING IMPLICATIONS

Do not confuse tramadol hydrochloride with trazodone hydrochloride (an antidepressant) or Toradol (NSAID). Also, do not confuse Ultram with Ultrase (pancreatic enzymes).

IMPLEMENTATION/ADMINISTRATION/STORAGE

Store from 15–30°C (59–86°F) in a tight container.

ASSESSMENT

1. List reasons for therapy, location, onset, triggers, characteristics of S&S. Use a pain-rating scale to rate pain. List drugs prescribed to ensure none interact.
2. Assess for head trauma, history of drug addiction, allergy to opiates or codeine, seizures; may increase the risk of convulsions.
3. Determine any emotional problems or depression may preclude drug use.
4. Monitor VS, I&O, renal and LFTs; reduce dose with dysfunction and if over 75 years old. Avoid ER formulation with impairment.

CLIENT/FAMILY TEACHING

1. Take only as directed. May be taken without regard to meals. Do not exceed doses of tramadol; do not share medications and store safely out of reach of child.
2. Extended-release tablets are for oral use only and should not be chewed, crushed, dissolved, or split; swallow whole with a sufficient quantity of liquid.
3. Orally disintegrating tablets contain phenylalanine.
4. Do not perform activities that require mental alertness; drug may cause drowsiness and impair mental or physical performance. Avoid alcohol; may intensify drug effects.
5. Do not stop suddenly with prolonged therapy; taper dose to avert withdrawal S&S.
6. Report lack of response. Review list of side effects (nausea, dizziness, somnolence, pruritus, and constipation) that one may experience, and report if persistent or intolerable.
7. Avoid alcohol and CNS depressants. Report if pregnant or any seizure activity.
8. May mask abdominal pathology and obscure intracranial pathology due to abnormal pupil contraction. Carry ID/list of drugs currently prescribed.
9. Keep all F/U to evaluate response and adverse SE.

T

OUTCOMES/EVALUATE
Desired pain control

Combination Drug

Tramadol hydrochloride and Acetaminophen

(**TRAM**-ah-dol, ah-**SEAT**-ah-**MIN**-oh-fen)

Classification(s): Narcotic/nonnarcotic analgesic combination drug

Pregnancy Category: C

RX: Ultracet.

SEE ALSO ***TRAMADOL HYDROCHLORIDE*** AND ***ACETAMINOPHEN***.

INDICATIONS/USES
Short-term use (5 days or less) for management of acute pain. *NOTE:* Onset of analgesia is less than 1 hr and faster than tramadol alone.

CONTENT
Each Ultracet tablet contains tramadol hydrochloride *(narcotic analgesic)*, 37.5 mg and acetaminophen (*nonnarcotic analgesic*), 325 mg.

ACTION/KINETICS
Action
Tramadol is a centrally-acting synthetic opioid analgesic. Its mechanism is not completely known but both tramadol and its active metabolite bind to μ-opioid receptors and they are weak inhibitors of norepinephrine and serotonin reuptake. Tramadol is only partially antagonized by naloxone. Acetaminophen may cause analgesia by inhibiting CNS prostaglandin synthesis, although it has no anti-inflammatory activity.

Pharmacokinetics
Tramadol. Rapidly absorbed after PO administration; absolute bioavailability is about 75%. Food does not affect the rate or extent of absorption. **Onset:** 1 hr. **Peak effect:** 2–3 hr. **Peak plasma levels:** 2 hr. **Duration:** 2 hr for tramadol and 3 hr for the M1 active metabolite. **t½, plasma:** 6.3 hr for tramadol and 7.4 hr for the M1 active metabolite. Extensively metabolized in the liver by CYP2D6 and CYP3A4. Excreted in the urine, with about 30% excreted unchanged and 60% as metabolites. Excretion is reduced in those with C_{CR} <30 mL/min.

Acetaminophen. Peak plasma levels: 30–120 min. **t½:** 2–3 hr. **Therapeutic serum levels** (analgesia): 5–20 mcg/mL. Metabolized in the liver and excreted in the urine as glucuronide and sulfate conjugates. However, an intermediate hydroxylated metabolite is hepatotoxic following large doses of acetaminophen. **Plasma protein binding:** About 20% of tramadol is bound to plasma proteins.

CONTRAINDICATIONS
Not recommended for those with hepatic impairment. Hypersensitivity to any component of the product or to opioids. Use in acute intoxication with alcohol, hypnotics, narcotics, centrally-acting analgesics, opioids, or psychotropic drugs (CNS and respiratory depression may worsen). Not recommended for use during labor and delivery unless potential benefits outweigh risks. Lactation.

SPECIAL CONCERNS
- **Seizures may occur in those taking tramadol within the recommended dosage range; seizure risk is increased with doses above the recommended range, in those with epilepsy or a history of seizures, and in those with a recognized risk of seizures (e.g., head trauma, metabolic disorders, alcohol and drug withdrawal).**
- **Use with caution in those at risk for respiratory depression, in those with increased intracranial pressure or head injury, and in the elderly.**
- **Safety and efficacy not determined in children.**

SIDE EFFECTS
Most Common
Constipation, somnolence, increased sweating, nausea, diarrhea, anorexia, dizziness, dry mouth, insomnia, pruritus, prostatic disorder.

See *Tramadol* and *Acetaminophen* for a complete list of possible side effects. **Hypersensitivity:** Serious (but rarely fatal) ***anaphylactoid*** reactions, often following the first dose. Also, pruritus, hives, ***bronchospasm, angioedema, toxic epidermal necrolysis, Stevens-Johnson syndrome.***

OVERDOSE MANAGEMENT
Symptoms: **Tramadol:** Respiratory depression, lethargy, coma, ***seizure, cardiac arrest, death.*** **Acetaminophen:** Hepatic centrilobular necrosis leading to ***hepatic failure and death***. Also, renal

tubular necrosis, hypoglycemia, and coagulation defects. Early symptoms include N&V, diaphoresis, and general malaise. *Treatment:*

- Maintain adequate ventilation (primary concern).
- Naloxone will reverse some, but not all, symptoms of tramadol overdose but the risk of seizures increases.
- Provide supportive measures.
- For acetaminophen: Initially, induction of emesis, gastric lavage, activated charcoal. Oral N-acetylcysteine is said to reduce or prevent hepatic damage by inactivating acetaminophen metabolites, which cause liver toxicity.

DRUG INTERACTIONS

Acetaminophen-containing products / ↑ Potential for acetaminophen hepatotoxicity; do not use together
Alcohol / Do not use together
Amitriptyline / Possible inhibition of tramadol metabolism R/T inhibition of CYP2D6
Carbamazepine / Significantly ↓ analgesic effect of tramadol R/T ↑ metabolism; ↑ seizure risk, do not use together
Fluoxetine / Possible inhibition of tramadol metabolism R/T inhibition of CYP2D6
MAOIs / ↑ Risk of seizures and serotonin syndrome; use together with great caution
Naloxone / ↑ Risk of seizures if given in tramadol overdose
Neuroleptics / ↑ Risk of seizures
Opioids (other than tramadol) / ↑ Risk of seizures
Paroxetine / Possible inhibition of tramadol metabolism R/T inhibition of CYP2D6
Quinidine / ↑ Levels of tramadol and ↓ levels of the active metabolite R/T inhibition of CYP2D6
Selective serotonin reuptake inhibitors / ↑ Risk of seizures and serotonin syndrome
Tricyclic antidepressants / ↑ Risk of seizures
Warfarin / Rarely, alterations of warfarin effects, including ↑ PT

HOW SUPPLIED

See *Content.*

DOSAGE

TABLETS

Management of acute pain.

Adults: 2 tablets q 4–6 hr, as needed for relief of pain, up to a maximum of 8 tablets per day for 5 or fewer days. In those with C_{CR} <30 mL/min, do not exceed 2 tablets q 12 hr.

NURSING IMPLICATIONS

IMPLEMENTATION/ADMINISTRATION/STORAGE

1. Do not exceed the recommended dose.
2. Tramadol may cause psychological and physical dependence of the morphine-type. Withdrawal symptoms may occur if Ultracet is discontinued abruptly.
3. Store from 15–30°C (59–86°F).

ASSESSMENT

1. List reasons for therapy, onset, characteristics of S&S, clinical presentation, other agents trialed/outcome. Rate pain level.
2. Assess for head trauma, history of seizures, alcohol disorder.
3. Note drugs prescribed to ensure none interact; serotonergic agents (including SSRIs, SNRIs, and triptans) increase risk of seizures or serotonin syndrome.
4. Ensure x-ray/CT/MRI performed to assess skeletal damage. Note ROM, carefully assess areas of pain and reduced function.
5. Monitor renal and LFTs; reduce dose with dysfunction.

CLIENT/FAMILY TEACHING

1. Drug is a combination medication used to relieve pain; take as directed.
2. Avoid activities that require mental alertness until drug effects realized.
3. Do not take alcohol or OTC agents during therapy.
4. Practice reliable contraception, report if pregnancy suspected.
5. Do not stop suddenly after long-term use; withdrawal symptoms (craving/tolerance) may occur, which include: anxiety, sweating, insomnia, pain, nausea, tremors, rigors, diarrhea, upper respiratory symptoms, and, rarely, hallucinations; report if evident.
6. Keep all F/U to assess response, labs, and for adverse SE.

OUTCOMES/EVALUATE

Relief of pain

T

Trandolapril

(tran-**DOHL**-ah-pril)

Classification(s): Antihypertensive, ACE inhibitor

Pregnancy Category: C (first trimester); **D** (second and third trimesters)

RX: Mavik.

SEE ALSO ***ANGIOTENSIN CONVERTING ENZYME (ACE) INHIBITORS***.

INDICATIONS/USES

(1) Hypertension, alone or in combination with other antihypertensives such as hydrochlorothiazide. (2) For stable clients who have left-ventricular systolic dysfunction or who are symptomatic from CHF within the first few days after an acute MI. (3) Heart failure after MI.

ACTION/KINETICS

Pharmacokinetics

Rapidly absorbed; food slows rate, but not amount absorbed. Metabolized in liver to active trandolaprilat. **Onset:** 2–4 hr. Bioavailability is about 10% (70% of trandolaprilat, the active metabolite). Food slows absorption. **Peak plasma levels, trandolapril:** 30–60 min; **trandolaprilat:** 4–10 hr. **t½, elimination, trandolapril:** About 6 hr; **t½, trandoprilat:** About 10 hr. **Peak effect:** 4–8 hr. **Duration:** 24 hr. About one-third trandolaprilat is excreted in urine and two-thirds in feces. **Plasma protein binding:** About 80%.

CONTRAINDICATIONS

In those with a history of angioedema with ACE inhibitors. Lactation.

SPECIAL CONCERNS

■ When used during the second and third trimesters of pregnancy, injury and even death can result in the developing fetus. When pregnancy is detected, discontinue as soon as possible. ■

Safety and efficacy not determined in children.

SIDE EFFECTS

Most Common

Hypotension, dizziness, dyspepsia, cough, asthenia, syncope, myalgia, gastritis, hypocalcemia, intermittent claudication.

See also *Angiotensin Converting Enzyme Inhibitors* for a complete list of possible side effects. **Hypersensitivity**: ***Angioedema***. **CNS**: Dizziness, headache, fatigue, insomnia, paresthesias, somnolence, drowsiness, vertigo, anxiety. **GI**: Diarrhea, dyspepsia, gastritis, abdominal pain/distention, vomiting, constipation, pancreatitis. **Hepatic: *Hepatic failure***, including cholestatic jaundice, ***fulminant hepatic necrosis, death***. **CV**: Hypotension (may be severe following the first dose), bradycardia, chest pain, palpitations, ***cardiogenic shock***, intermittent claudication, first degree AV block, ***stroke***. **Respiratory**: Cough (may be chronic), dyspnea, URTI, epistaxis, throat inflammation. **Dermatologic**: Photosensitivity, flushing, pemphigus/pemphigoid, pruritus, rash. **GU**: UTI, impotence, decreased libido. **Musculoskeletal:** Muscle cramps, myalgia. **Hematologic:** Neutropenia, thrombocytopenia. **Miscellaneous**: Syncope, asthenia, intermittent claudication, edema, extremity pain, gout.

LABORATORY TEST CONSIDERATIONS

Hyperkalemia, hypocalcemia. ↑ Serum uric acid, BUN, creatinine.

DRUG INTERACTIONS

Diuretics / Excessive hypotensive effects
Diuretics, potassium-sparing: ↑ Risk of hyperkalemia
Lithium / ↑ Risk of lithium toxicity

HOW SUPPLIED

Tablets: 1 mg, 2 mg, 4 mg.

DOSAGE

TABLETS

Hypertension.

Initial: 1 mg once daily in non-Black clients (2 mg once daily in Black clients) for those not receiving a diuretic. Adjust dosage according to response; usually, adjustments are made at intervals of 1 week. **Maintenance, usual:** 4 mg once daily (twice daily dosing may be needed in some). If BP is still not adequately controlled, diuretic may be added.

Heart failure post-myocardial infarction/Left ventricular dysfunction post-MI.

Initial: 1 mg/day. Then increase the dose, as tolerated, to a target dose of

4 mg/day. If 4 mg is not tolerated, continue with the highest tolerated dose. If C_{CR} is less than 30 mL/min or if there is hepatic cirrhosis, initial dose is 0.5 mg daily. Titrate dose to optimal response.

NURSING IMPLICATIONS

IMPLEMENTATION/ADMINISTRATION/STORAGE

1. If client is on a diuretic, discontinue 2 to 3 days prior to beginning therapy with trandolapril to reduce likelihood of hypotension. If diuretic cannot be discontinued, use an initial trandolapril dose of 0.5 mg. Titrate subsequent dosage.
2. Dosage adjustment may be necessary in those with impaired hepatic function.
3. Store tablets from 20–25°C (68–77°F).

ASSESSMENT

1. Note reasons for therapy, disease onset, other agents trialed, outcome.
2. Assess hydration status. List studies of wall motion in LV dysfunction after MI or symptomatic CHF.
3. Monitor BP, weight, ECG, cardiac status, CBC, electrolytes, renal and LFTs; reduce dose with dysfunction.

CLIENT/FAMILY TEACHING

1. Take as directed with/without food.
2. Change positions slowly to prevent sudden drop in BP. Assess drug response before pursuing activities that require mental alertness.
3. May experience cough, dizziness, and diarrhea; report if persistent. Report any S&S of infection (fever, sore throat) to R/O neutropenia.
4. Practice reliable contraception; stop drug and report if pregnancy suspected.
5. Continue lifestyle changes (i.e., regular exercise, smoking/alcohol cessation, low-fat, low-salt diet in overall goal of BP control). Keep BP log for provider review.
6. With heart failure, record weights; report gains >3 lb/day or 5 lb/week.
7. Keep all F/U to assess response, labs, and for adverse SE.

OUTCOMES/EVALUATE

- ↓ BP
- Control of heart failure/ventricular dysfunction after MI

IV

Trastuzumab

(traz-**TOO**-zah-mab)

Classification(s): Antineoplastic, miscellaneous

Pregnancy Category: D

RX: Herceptin.

SEE ALSO ***ANTINEOPLASTIC AGENTS***.

INDICATIONS/USES

(1) Adjuvant treatment of clients with human epidermal growth factor receptor 2 (HER2)-overexpressing, node-positive or node negative (estrogen receptor/progesterone receptor negative or with one high risk factor) breast cancer as part of a regimen including doxorubicin, cyclophosphamide, and either paclitaxel or docetaxel. Also combined with docetaxel and carboplatin or used as a single agent following multimodality anthracycline–based therapy. (2) As a single agent for treatment of HER2-overexpressing breast cancer in those who have received one or more chemothrapy regimens for metastatic disease. (3) In combination with paclitaxel for first line treatment of HER2-overexpressing metastatic breast cancer. (4) In combination with cisplatin and capecitabine or 5–fluorouracil to treat HER2-overexpressing metastatic gastric or gastroesophageal junction adenocarcinoma in those who have not received prior treatment for metastatic disease.

ACTION/KINETICS

Action

A recombinant DNA-derived humanized monoclonal antibody that selectively binds with high affinity to the extracellular domain of the HER2 protein. Results in inhibition of the proliferation of human tumor cells that overexpress HER2 and mediates antibody-dependent cellular cytotoxicity. The HER2 protein is overexpressed in 25 to 30% of primary breast cancers.

Pharmacokinetics

t½, following loading dose of 4 mg/kg and weekly dose of 2 mg/kg: Average of 5.8 days (range from 1 to 32 days). Mean serum trough levels of trastuzumab, when given with paclitaxel,

T

were elevated 1.5 fold compared to use in combination with anthracycline plus cyclophosphamide.

CONTRAINDICATIONS

Lactation during therapy and for six months after the last trastuzumab dose.

SPECIAL CONCERNS

(1) **Cardiomyopathy:** Trastuzumab can result in subclinical and clinical cardiac failure. The incidence and severity was highest in clients who received trastuzumab concurrently with anthracycline-containing chemotherapy regimens. (2) Evaluate left ventricular function in all clients prior to and during treatment with trastuzumab. Discontinue trastuzumab treatment in clients receiving adjuvant therapy and withhold trastuzumab treatment in clients with metastatic disease for a clinically significant decrease in left ventricular function. (3) **Infusion reactions and pulmonary toxicity.** Trastuzumab administration can result in serious and fatal infusion reactions and pulmonary toxicity. Symptoms usually occur during or within 24 hours of administration of trastuzumab. Interrupt trastuzumab infusion for clients experiencing dyspnea or clinically significant hypotension. Monitor clients until signs and symptoms resolve completely. Discontinue trastuzumab for anaphylaxis, angioedema, interstitial pneumonitis, or acute respiratory distress syndrome.

- **Advanced age may increase the incidence of cardiac dysfunction.**
- **Use with caution during pregnancy and in those with sensitivity to Chinese hamster ovary proteins.**
- **Increased risk for severe pulmonary side effects in those with symptomatic intrinsic pulmonary disease (e.g., asthma, COPD) or those with extensive tumor involvement of the lungs.**
- **Contains benzyl alcohol that has been associated with a fatal "gasping syndrome" in premature infants.**
- **Safety and efficacy not determined in children.**

SIDE EFFECTS

Most Common

Anemia, diarrhea, dysgeusia, dyspnea, fatigue, fever, headache, increased cough, infection, infusion reactions, mucosal inflammation, myalgia, N&V, nasopharyngitis, neutropenia, rash, stomatitis, thrombocytopenia, URTI, weight loss.

CV: Tachycardia, ***vascular thrombosis***, embolism, arrhythmias, pericardial effusion, ***heart arrest***, ***hemorrhage***, ***shock arrhythmia***, hyper–/hypotension, palpitations, syncope. Cardiomyopathy, including left ventricular dysfunction and CHF. Cardiac dysfunction, including ***disabling cardiac failure***, dyspnea, increased cough, paroxysmal nocturnal dyspnea, peripheral edema, S3 gallop, reduced left ventricular ejection fraction. **GI:** Diarrhea, constipation, anorexia, N&V, abdominal pain (including upper), dysgeusia, dyspepsia, dysphagia, gastroenteritis, hematemesis, ileus, intestinal obstruction, colitis, esophageal ulcer, stomatitis. **Hepatic:** Hepatitis, pancreatitis, ***hepatic failure***. **CNS:** Dizziness, insomnia, headache, paresthesia, peripheral neuritis, depression, neuropathy, convulsion, ataxia, confusion, manic reaction. **Respiratory:** Increased cough, dyspnea, epistaxis, pharyngitis, rhinitis, sinusitis, apnea, pneumothorax, asthma, hypoxia, laryngitis, interstitial pneumonitis, nasopharyngitis, pharyngolaryngeal pain, pulmonary hypertension, pulmonary infiltrates, pleural effusions, noncardiogenic pulmonary edema, pulmonary insufficiency, pneumonia, pulmonary fibrosis, URTI, ***extreme respiratory distress, acute respiratory distress syndrome***. **Dermatologic:** Rash, desquamation, acne, herpes simplex/zoster, skin ulceration, nail changes, hot flashes, pruritus. **Hematologic:** Anemia, leukopenia, pancytopenia, thrombocytopenia, acute leukemia, coagulation disorder, lymphangiitis, exacerbation of chemotherapy-induced neutropenia, exacerbation of chemotherapy-induced neutropenia, ***febrile neutropenia and infection (may be fatal)***. **Musculoskeletal:** Arthralgia, myalgia, back pain, bone pain/necrosis, pathological fractures, muscle spasms, myopathy. **GU:** Hydronephrosis, kidney failure/impairment, cervical cancer, hematuria, hemorrhagic cystitis, UTI, pyelonephritis, nephrotic syndrome with glomerulopathy (rare). **Metabolic:** Peripheral edema, edema, hypoglycemia, growth retardation, hypothyroidism, autoimmune thyroiditis, weight loss. **First-infusion-associated reaction:** Chills, fever, N&V, pain, rigors, bronchospasm, hypoxia, headache, dizziness, dyspnea, severe hyper-/hypotension, rash, asthenia. More serious reactions, occurring infrequently, include bronchospasm, hypoxia, severe hypotension, ***death***. **Hypersensitivi-**

ty reactions: ***Anaphylaxis***, urticaria, ***bronchospasm***, angioedema, hypotension, hypoxia, dyspnea, pulmonary infiltrates, pleural effusions, noncardiogenic pulmonary edema, ***acute respiratory distress syndrome. Reaction may be fatal.*** **Body as a whole:** Accidental injury, allergic reaction, asthenia, chills, fatigue, fever, flu syndrome, mucosal inflammation, pain, pyrexia, ***sudden death***. **Miscellaneous:** Increased incidence of infections, especially of the upper respiratory tract, skin, and urinary tract; cellulitis, ascites, hydrocephalus, radiation injury, deafness, amblyopia, immunogenicity, oligohydramnios.

LABORATORY TEST CONSIDERATIONS

Hypercalcemia, hypokalemia, hypomagnesemia, hyponatremia.

OVERDOSE MANAGEMENT

Symptoms: There is no experience with overdosage in humans. *Treatment:* Conventional hemodialysis and peritoneal dialysis are ineffective in removing trastuzumab.

DRUG INTERACTIONS

Anthracycline / ↑ Risk of symptomatic cardiac dysfunction; monitor closely
Doxorubicin / ↑ Risk of symptomatic cardiac dysfunction; monitor closely
Paclitaxel / ↑ Trastuzumab serum levels; monitor closely for cardiac dysfunction
Warfarin / Hypoprothrombinemia and ↑ risk of bleeding

HOW SUPPLIED

Injection, Lyophilized Powder for Solution: 440 mg.

DOSAGE

IV INFUSION

Metastatic breast cancer.

Initial: 4 mg/kg as an IV infusion given over 90 min alone or in combination with paclitaxel; **maintenance, given once a week:** 2 mg/kg weekly, infused over 30 min if initial dose was tolerated. Give until tumor progression occurs.

Adjuvant breast cancer treatment: During and following paclitaxel, docetaxel, or docetaxel/carboplatin.

Adults, initial: 4 mg/kg by IV infusion over 90 min. **then,** 2 mg/kg by IV infusion over 30 min once a week during chemotherapy for the first 12 weeks (paclitaxel or docetaxel) or 18 weeks (docetaxel/carboplatin). **Maintenance:** One week following the last dose of trastuzumab, administer trastuzumab, 60 mg/kg as an IV infusion over 30–60 min q 3 weeks. **Duration:** A total of 52 weeks of trastuzumab therapy.

Adjuvant breast cancer treatment: Following completion of multimodality anthracycline-based chemotherapy regimens.

Adults, initial: 8 mg/kg as an IV infusion over 90 min within 3 weeks following completion of multimodality anthracycline-based chemotherapy. **Maintenance:** 6 mg/kg as an IV infusion over 30–60 min q 3 weeks. **Duration:** A total of 52 weeks of trastuzumab therapy.

Metastatic gastric cancer.

Adults, initial: 8 mg/kg as an IV infusion over 90 min. **Maintenance:** 6 mg/kg as an IV infusion over 30–90 min q 3 weeks until disease progression.

NURSING IMPLICATIONS

IMPLEMENTATION/ADMINISTRATION/STORAGE

1. **IV** For adjuvant treatment of metastatic breast cancer, do not coadminister with doxorubicin and cyclophosphamide. Following completion of doxorubicin and cyclophosphamide, give trastuzumab weekly for 52 weeks. During the first 12 weeks, coadminister trastuzumab with paclitaxel.
2. Decrease the rate of infusion for mild or moderate infusion reactions. Interrupt the infusion in those with dyspnea or clinically significant hypotension. Consider permanent discontinuation for severe and life-threatening infusion reactions.
3. Withhold trastuzumab dosing for at least 4 weeks and repeat left ventricular ejection fraction (LVEF) assessment q 4 weeks if there is a 16% or more absolute decrease in LVEF from pretreatment values or if LVEF falls below institutional limits of normal and there is a 10% or more absolute decrease in LVEF from pretreatment values. Resume the drug if, within 4–8 weeks, the LVEF returns to normal limits

T

and the absolute decrease in baseline is 15% or less. Permanently discontinue the drug for a persistent (more than 8 weeks) LVEF decline or for suspension of dosing on more than 3 occasions for cardiomyopathy.

4. Reconstitute each 440 mg vial with 20 mL bacteriostatic water, 1.1% benzyl alcohol, as supplied. Using a sterile syringe, slowly inject 20 mL of the diluent into the vial containing the lyophilized cake of trastuzumab. Direct the stream of diluent into the lyophilized cake. Swirl the vial gently to aid reconstitution. Do not shake; slight foaming may occur. Allow the vial to stand undisturbed for about 5 min. The resulting solution contains 21 mg/mL.
5. For those with sensitivity to benzyl alcohol, reconstitute with sterile water rather than bacteriostatic water for injection.
6. After reconstitution, immediately label vial in the area marked "Do not use after" with the date 28 days from the reconstitution date.
7. Shaking the reconstituted solution or causing excessive foaming during the addition of diluent may cause problems with dissolution and the amount of trastuzumab that can be withdrawn from the vial.
8. Interrupt trastuzumab infusion in all clients experiencing dyspnea or significant hypotension; initiate medical therapy, that may include epinephrine, corticosteroids, diphenhydramine, bronchodilators, and oxygen. Monitor carefully until complete resolution of all signs and symptoms. Consider permanent discontinuation in all those with severe infusion reactions.
9. Determine dose needed based on an initial dose of 4 mg/kg or a maintenance dose of 2 mg/kg. Calculate the volume needed from the reconstituted vial; withdraw this amount and add it to an infusion bag containing 250 mL of 0.9% NaCl. Gently invert the bag to mix the solution. Do not use D5W solution. The reconstituted preparation is a colorless to pale yellow transparent solution.
10. Give as an IV infusion over 90 min. If the initial infusion is tolerated, subsequent doses may be given over 30 min for weekly doses, or over 30–90 min if given q 3 weeks. Do not give as an IV push or bolus. May give in outpatient setting.
11. Prior to reconstitution, vials are stable at 2–8°C (36–46°F). When reconstituted with bacteriostatic water for injection, as supplied, is stable for 28 days when stored at 2–8°C and may be preserved for multiple use. If reconstituted with unpreserved sterile water for injection, use immediately and discard any unused portion. Do not freeze reconstituted or diluted solutions.
12. Trastuzumab diluted in polyvinylchloride or polyethylene bags containing 0.9% NaCl for injection may be stored at 2–8°C (36–46°F) or at room temperature for 24 hr or less. Since this solution contains no effective preservative, refrigeration is recommended.
13. Pregnant women with breast cancer who are receiving trastuzumab are encouraged to enroll in MotHER-the Herceptin Pregnancy Registry by calling 1-800-690-6720.
14. COMPATIBILITY 0.9% NaCl.
15. INCOMPATIBILITY Do not mix or dilute with other drugs. Do not administer through an IV line containing dextrose.

ASSESSMENT

1. Note breast cancer onset/diagnosis, other therapies trialed, outcome. Determine if first-line therapy or second-or third-line therapy for tumors overexpressing the HER2 protein.
2. During infusion assess for fever, chills, and other infusion-associated symptoms (see *Side Effects*). Assess for pulmonary hypersensitivity reactions; ARDS, dyspnea, pulmonary infiltrates, hypoxia and report any S&S.
3. Share risks of therapy: cardiomyopathy, pulmonary toxicity, embryo fetal toxicity.
4. Assess cardiac function. Obtain ECG, echocardiogram and/or MUGA to evaluate left ventricular function (LVEF) every 3 weeks during and upon completion of therapy. If treatment withheld for left ventricular cardiac dysfunction, repeat at 4 week intervals. Measure LVEF every 6 months for at least 2 yr following completion of trastuzumab treatment as a component of adjuvant therapy.
5. Monitor CBC and assess for anemia and leukopenia. Assess HER2 protein.

CLIENT/FAMILY TEACHING

1. Drug is used in combination regimens to treat metastatic disease. It is administered as an IV infusion once a week. May be given in an outpatient setting.

2. **Acetaminophen may help with flu-like symptoms after infusion; may also experience diarrhea, anemia, and infections during therapy; report.**
3. **Immediately report any S&S of ventricular dysfunction and congestive heart failure (SOB, cough, swelling of extremities); may cause cardiac toxicity. Also report any persistent nausea, vomiting, diarrhea, or worsening general body weakness.**
4. **Avoid crowds, persons with infections, and live vaccines during therapy.**
5. **Practice reliable contraception during and for 6 months following therapy.**
6. **Keep all F/U visits to assess response, labs, and adverse SE.**

OUTCOMES/EVALUATE

Inhibition of malignant breast cells that overexpress HER2 protein

Trazodone hydrochloride

(**TRAYZ**-oh-dohn)

Classification(s): Antidepressant, miscellaneous

Pregnancy Category: C

RX: Oleptro.

🍁 **Rx:** Apo-Trazodone, Apo-Trazodone D, Gen-Trazodone, PMS-Trazodone, ratio-Trazodine.

INDICATIONS/USES

Adults: Depression (immediate-release) and major depressive disorder (extended-release). *Investigational:* Treat insomnia associated with antidepressant use, depression, and mood disorders. Prevention of migraine.

ACTION/KINETICS

Action

May inhibit serotonin uptake by brain cells, therefore increasing serotonin concentrations in the synapse. May also act as an antagonist at 5-HT-2A/2C serotonin receptors. Response usually occurs after 2 weeks (75% of clients), with the remainder responding after 2–4 weeks. Causes a high degree of sedation, moderate orthostatic hypotensive effects (due to antagonism of alpha-1 adrenergic receptors), and slight anticholinergic effects. Does not inhibit MAO and is also devoid of amphetamine-like effects

Pharmacokinetics

Well absorbed. **Peak plasma levels, immediate-release:** 1 hr (empty stomach) or 2 hr (when taken with food); **extended-release:** 9 hr. **t½, initial, immediate-release:** 3–6 hr; **final:** 5–9 hr. **t½, terminal, extended-release:** 10 hr. **Effective plasma levels:** 800–1,600 ng/mL. **Time to reach steady state:** 3–7 days. Three-fourths of those with a therapeutic effect respond by the end of the second week of therapy. Metabolized in liver by CYP3A4 and excreted mainly through the urine. **Plasma protein binding:** 89–95%.

CONTRAINDICATIONS

During the initial recovery period following MI. Concurrently with electroshock therapy.

SPECIAL CONCERNS

Suicidality and antidepressant drugs. Antidepressants increase the risk, compared with placebo, of suicidal thinking and behavior (suicidality) in children, adolescents, and young adults in short-term studies of major depressive disorder and other psychiatric disorders. Anyone considering the use of trazodone or any other antidepressant in a child, adolescent, or young adult must balance this risk with the clinical need. Short-term studies did not show an increase in the risk of suicidality with antidepressants compared with placebo in adults older than 24 years of age; there was a reduction in risk with antidepressants compared with placebo in adults 65 years of age and older. Depression and certain other psychiatric disorders are themselves associated with increases in the risk of suicide. Appropriately monitor clients of all ages who are started on antidepressant therapy, and observe them closely for clinical worsening, suicidality, or unusual changes in behavior. Advise families and caregivers of the need for close observation and communication with the prescriber. Trazodone is not approved for use in children.

- **Use with caution in geriatric clients; they are more prone to sedative and hypotensive effects and hyponatremia.**
- **Use with caution during lactation and in impaired renal or hepatic function.**

- Use with caution in cardiac disease due to possible cardiac arrhythmias.
- Safety and efficacy not established in children 18 years and younger.

SIDE EFFECTS

Most Common

Immediate-Release Tablets: Drowsiness, dizziness/lightheadedness, dry mouth, N&V, fatigue, headache, syncope, insomnia, hypotension, nervousness, tremors, abdominal/gastric disorder, constipation, decreased appetite, blurred vision, musculoskeletal aches/pain.

Extended-Release Tablets: Somnolence, sedation, headache, dry mouth, dizziness, nausea, fatigue, diarrhea, constipation, blurred vision, back pain.

Immediate-Release Tablets. CNS: Drowsiness, dizziness/light-headedness, nervousness, fatigue, headache, insomnia, tremors, confusion, anger/hostility, decreased concentration, disorientation, incoordination, head full (heavy), excitement, impaired memory, nightmares/vivid dreams, paresthesia, akathisia, hallucinations, delusions, hypomania, impaired speech, numbness, clinical worsening and ***suicide risk***. **GI:** Dry mouth, N&V, decreased appetite, abdominal/gastric disorder, diarrhea, constipation, bad taste in mouth, flatulence, hypersalivation, increased appetite. **CV:** Syncope, hypertension, hypotension, tachycardia, palpitations, ***prolongation of QT/QTc interval with torsades de pointes with sudden, unexplained death***. **Respiratory:** Nasal/sinus congestion, shortness of breath. **Dermatologic:** Skin condition, edema, sweating, clamminess. **GU:** Delayed urine flow, early menses, hematuria, impotence, increased urinary frequency, missed periods, retrograde ejaculation, decreased/increased libido. **Musculoskeletal:** Aches/pains, muscle twitches. **Serotonin syndrome/Neuroleptic malignant syndrome:** Agitation, hallucinations, coma, tachycardia, labile BP, hyperthermia, hyperreflexia, incoordination, N&V, diarrhea, muscle rigidity, autonomic instability with possible rapid fluctuation of vital signs, mental status changes. **Ophthalmic:** Blurred vision, eyes red/tired/itching. **Otic:** Tinnitus. **Body as a whole:** Malaise, weight gain/loss. **Miscellaneous:** Allergic reaction, anemia, chest pain.

Extended-Release Tablets. CNS: Somnolence/sedation, headache, dizziness, fatigue, agitation, confusional state, abnormal coordination, disorientation, impaired memory, migraine, paresthesia, tremor, amnesia, aphasia, hypesthesia, speech disorder, vertigo. **GI:** Dry mouth, nausea, diarrhea, constipation, dysgeusia, abdominal pain, vomiting, reflux esophagitis. **Dermatologic:** Night sweats, acne, flushing, hyperhidrosis. **GU:** Ejaculation disorders, decreased libido, erectile dysfunction, abnormal orgasm, micturition urgency, bladder pain, urinary incontinence. **Musculoskeletal:** Back pain, myalgia, muscle twitching, gait disturbance. **Ophthalmic:** Blurred vision, visual disturbances, dry eye, eye pain, photophobia. **Otic:** Hyperacusis, tinnitus. **Miscellaneous:** Dyspnea, edema, hypersensitivity, photosensitivity reaction.

NOTE: A large number of side effects were noted in postmarketing studies. Listed previously are the most common side effects noted.

LABORATORY TEST CONSIDERATIONS

Low WBC and neutrophil counts (not considered clinically significant). Hyponatremia.

OVERDOSE MANAGEMENT

Symptoms: CNS depression, including ***respiratory arrest, seizures***, ECG changes, hypotension, priapism, as well as an increase in the incidence and severity of side effects noted previously (vomiting and drowsiness are the most common). *Treatment:* Ensure an adequate airway, oxygenation, and ventilation. Monitor cardiac rhythm and vital signs. Provide general supportive and symptomatic treatment (especially hypotension and sedation). Emesis is not recommended. However, gastric lavage with a large orogastric tube with appropriate airway protection may be indicated. Administer activated charcoal. Forced diuresis may be useful to remove the drug from the body.

DRUG INTERACTIONS

NOTE: An additive effect of trazodone with other drugs that prolong the QT interval is possible. The following drugs may prolong the QT interval and increase the risk of life-threatening cardiac arrhythmias, including torsades de pointes: amiodarone, arsenic trioxide, bretylium, chlorpromazine, disopyramide, dofetilide, dolasetron, droperidol, mefloquine, mesoridazine, moxifloxacin, pentamidine, pimozide, procainamide, quinidine, sotalol, tacrolimus, thioridazine, and ziprasidone.

Alcohol / ↑ Depressant effects

Barbiturates / ↑ Depressant effects

T

Carbamazepine / ↑ Carbamazepine plasma levels → ↑ pharmacologic and toxic effects; possible ↓ plasma levels of trazodone and metabolites
CNS depressants / ↑ CNS depression
Delavirdine / Possible ↑ plasma trazodone levels → ↑ pharmacologic and toxic effects; give together with caution and consider a lower trazodone dose
Digoxin / ↑ Digoxin levels; monitor digoxin levels, and adjust dose as needed
Dopamine antagonists (e.g., metoclopramide) / ↑ Risk of serotonin syndrome, including irritability, increased muscle tone, shivering, myoclonus, and altered consciousness; if concurrent use cannot be avoided, start with a low trazodone dose and closely monitor
H ***Ginkgo biloba*** / ↑ Plasma trazodone levels → ↑ pharmacologic and toxic (e.g., sedation) effects; adjust trazodone dose as needed
Itraconazole / ↓ Trazodone clearance → ↑ peak plasma levels and t½ R/T ↓ metabolism by CYP3A4 → potential side effects
Ketoconazole / ↓ Trazodone clearance → ↑ peak plasma levels and t½ R/T ↓ metabolism by CYP3A4 → potential side effects
Macrolide antibiotics (e.g., clarithromycin) / Possible ↑ plasma trazodone levels; coadminister with caution
MAOIs (e.g., phenelzine) / Possible serious, sometimes fatal, reactions; do not give together or within 14 days of discontinuing either the MAOI or trazodone
Nefazodone / ↑ Risk of serotonin syndrome, including irritability, increased muscle tone, shivering, myoclonus, and altered consciousness; if concurrent use cannot be avoided, start with a low trazodone dose and closely monitor
NSAIDs / ↑ Risk of bleeding; monitor for bleeding
Phenothiazines / ↑ Trazodone plasma levels → ↑ pharmacologic and toxic effects (e.g., sedation); monitor and adjust trazodone dosage as needed
Phenytoin / ↑ Phenytoin levels; monitor phenytoin levels and adjust dose as needed
Propranolol / Additive hypotensive effects; monitor BP and adjust antihypertensive dose if needed
Protease inhibitors (e.g., indinavir, ritonavir) / ↑ Trazodone plasma levels → ↑ pharmacologic and toxic effects (e.g., sedation); monitor and adjust trazodone dose as needed
Salicylates (e.g., aspirin) / ↑ Risk of bleeding; use with caution and monitor for bleeding
Selective serotonin reuptake inhibitors (e.g., fluoxetine) / ↑ Risk of serotonin syndrome, including irritability, increased muscle tone, shivering, myoclonus, and altered consciousness; if concurrent use cannot be avoided, start with a low trazodone dose and closely monitor
Sodium oxybate / ↑ Sleep duration and CNS depression
Triptans (e.g., sumatriptan) / ↑ Risk of serotonin syndrome, including irritability, increased muscle tone, shivering, myoclonus, and altered consciousness; if concurrent use cannot be avoided, start with a low trazodone dose and closely monitor
Tryptophan / ↑ Risk of serotonin syndrome, including irritability, increased muscle tone, shivering, myoclonus, and altered consciousness; if concurrent use cannot be avoided, start with a low trazodone dose and closely monitor
Warfarin / Either ↑ or ↓ PT; monitor frequently

HOW SUPPLIED

Tablets (generic): 50 mg, 100 mg, 150 mg, 300 mg; ***Tablets, Extended-Release (Oleptro):*** 150 mg, 300 mg.

DOSAGE

TABLETS

Depression.

Adults and adolescents, initial: 150 mg/day in divided doses; **then** increase by 50 mg/day every 3–4 days to maximum of 400 mg/day in divided doses (outpatients). Inpatients may require up to, but not exceeding, 600 mg/day in divided doses. **Maintenance:** Once an adequate dose has been reached, the dose may be decreased gradually; then adjust depending on the therapeutic response. Use lowest effective dose. Therapy may be required for several months. **Geriatric clients:** 75 mg/day in divided doses; dose can then be increased, as needed and tolerated, at 3–4 day intervals. **Children, 6 years and older, initial (investigational):** 1.5–2 mg/kg/day divided 2–3 times per day, up to a maximum of 6 mg/kg divided 3 times/day. Gradually increase the dose q 3–4 days.

T

Insomnia ((Investigational).

Adults: 50–100 mg/day as monotherapy.

Prevention of migraine (Investigational).

Adults: 100 mg/day.

TABLETS, EXTENDED-RELEASE

Major depressive disorder in adults.

Adults, initial: 150 mg once a day. Increase by 75 mg/day q 3 days (i.e., start 225 mg on day 4 of therapy), up to a maximum of 375 mg/day. Once an adequate response has been reached, dose may be reduced gradually, with dosage adjustment, depending on the therapeutic response. Maintain on the lowest effective dose; periodically reassess to determine need for continued treatment. Is generally recommended to continue treatment for several months after an initial response.

NURSING IMPLICATIONS

Ⓢ Do not confuse trazodone hydrochloride with tramadol hydrochloride (an analgesic).

IMPLEMENTATION/ADMINISTRATION/STORAGE

1. Initiate dose at the lowest possible level; increase gradually.
2. Beneficial effects may be observed within 1 week with optimal effects seen within 2 weeks.
3. Store from 15–30°C (59–86°F).

ASSESSMENT

1. List reasons for therapy, onset, symptoms, clinical presentation, associated factors, other agents trialed. Note any history of recent MI.
2. List drugs prescribed to ensure none interact.
3. Review risk of bleeding, including life-threatening hemorrhages, when used with NSAIDs, aspirin, or other drugs that may affect coagulation or bleeding.
4. Monitor VS, ECG, CBC, renal and LFTs.

CLIENT/FAMILY TEACHING

1. Take the immediate-release product with food to enhance absorption and minimize dizziness and/or light-headedness. Take major portion of dose at bedtime to reduce daytime side effects. Take extended-release tablets in late evening, preferably at bedtime, on an empty stomach.
2. The extended-release tablet may be taken whole or given as a half tablet by breaking the tablet along the score line (extended-release properties are not affected).
3. Use caution when driving or when performing other hazardous tasks; may cause drowsiness/dizziness. Avoid alcohol and CNS depressants.
4. Report any chest pain, SOB, confusion, convulsions, unusual bleeding, impotence, prolonged or inappropriate penile erections.
5. Use sugarless gum or candies and frequent mouth rinses to diminish dry mouth effects.
6. Inform surgeon if elective surgery is planned, to minimize interaction with anesthetic agent.
7. Record weight, as appetite may increase with drug. If also taking antihypertensives or nitrates, may have additive hypotensive effect.
8. Encourage family to share responsibility for drug therapy to optimize treatment, prevent overdosage, and observe for any overt behavioral changes or suicidal cues. Clients taking antidepressants and emerging from deepest phases of depression are more prone to suicide.
9. May take 2–4 weeks for full drug effects to be realized. Report any evidence of suicidal thoughts or ideas. Do not stop suddenly with prolonged therapy.
10. Keep all F/U to assess response, labs, and for adverse SE.

OUTCOMES/EVALUATE

- ↓ Depression (e.g., improved sleeping/eating patterns, ↓ fatigue, and ↑ social interactions)
- Treatment of aggression, cocaine withdrawal, neurogenic pain, panic disorder (unlabeled use)

IV

Treprostinil sodium

(treh-**PROSS**-tih-nill)

Classification(s): Antiplatelet drug

Pregnancy Category: B

RX: Remodulin, Tyvaso.

INDICATIONS/USES

Remodulin: (1) As a continuous IV or SC infusion to reduce symptoms associated with exercise in pulmonary arterial hypertension with NYHA Class II through Class IV to diminish symptoms associated with exercise. (2) To diminish the rate of clinical deterioration in clients requiring transition from epoprostenol. **Tyvaso:** To increase walk distance in clients with WHO group I pulmonary arterial hypertension and NYHA class III symptoms. Treatment timing can be adjusted for planned activities.

ACTION/KINETICS

Action

Causes direct dilation of pulmonary and systemic arterial vascular beds and inhibition of platelet aggregation. Also causes a dose-related negative inotropic and lusitropic effect. No major effects on cardiac conduction observed.

Pharmacokinetics

Rapidly and completely absorbed after SC infusion. Absolute bioavailability is 100%. **Steady state levels:** 10 hr. SC and IV administration showed bioequivalence at steady state at a dose of 10 nanograms/kg/hr. Metabolized in the liver and excreted in the urine (79%) and feces (13%). **t½, terminal:** 2–4 hr. Clearance is significantly reduced in those with impaired hepatic function. **Plasma protein binding:** 91%.

CONTRAINDICATIONS

Known hypersensitivity to the drug or structurally-related compounds.

SPECIAL CONCERNS

- **Use with caution in renal or hepatic impairment, during lactation, and in the elderly.**
- **Safety and efficacy not determined in children.**

SIDE EFFECTS

Most Common

Infusion-site pain and reaction (bleeding/bruising, erythema, induration), rash.

Some adverse reactions noted may be due to the underlying disease (e.g., chest pain, dyspnea, fatigue, pallor, right ventricular heart failure). **At site of injection:** Infusion site pain and reaction (bleeding/bruising, erythema, induration), rash, problems with the infusion system, arm swelling, pain. **GI:** Nausea, diarrhea. **CNS:** Headache, dizziness, paresthesias. **CV:** Vasodilation, hypotension. **Dermatologic:** Rash (including macular or papular), pruritus, hematoma. **Miscellaneous:** Jaw pain, edema, cellulitis. *NOTE:* Side effects listed above are those that occurred following SC use; data are not available on side effects following IV use.

OVERDOSE MANAGEMENT

Symptoms: Extensions of pharmacological effects, including flushing, headache, hypotension, N&V, diarrhea. *Treatment:* Symptoms are usually self-limiting and are treated with reducing or withholding the drug.

DRUG INTERACTIONS

Anticoagulants / ↑ Risk of bleeding especially in clients maintained on anticoagulants
Antihypertensive drugs / Significant BP reduction
Diuretics / Significant BP reduction
Vasodilators / Significant BP reduction

HOW SUPPLIED

Remodulin: ***Injection Solution:*** 1 mg/mL, 2.5 mg/mL, 5 mg/mL, 10 mg/mL.
Tyvaso: ***Solution for Oral Inhalation:*** 0.6 mg/mL.

DOSAGE

Remodulin

CONTINUOUS SC OR IV INFUSION ONLY

Pulmonary arterial hypertension.

Initial: 1.25 nanograms/kg/min given by continuous SC infusion or via a central IV line. If this dose cannot be tolerated, reduce to 0.625 nanograms/kg/min. Increase the infusion rate in increments of no more than 1.25 nanograms/kg/min per week for the first 4 weeks and then no more than 2.5 nanograms/kg/min per week for the remaining duration of infusion, depending on the response. Doses above 40 nanograms/kg/hr have not been studied sufficiently. Avoid abrupt cessation of the infusion or sudden large reductions in dose as worsening of symptoms may occur. In clients with mild or moderate hepatic insufficiency, decrease the initial dose to 0.625 nanograms/kg/min and increase cautiously. *NOTE:* **Dosage is in units of nanograms (ng) per kg per unit of time.**

Transition from epoprostenol to treprostinil.

Initiate the infusion of trepostinil and increase it while simultaneously reduc-

T

ing the dose of IV epoprostenol. Undertake the transition in a hospital with constant observation. During the transition, initiate treprostinil at a dose of 10% of the current epoprostenol dose; escalate as the epoprostenol dose is decreased. Use the following transition dose changes:

- Step 1: Epoprostenol dose unchanged; give treprostinil at 10% of the starting epoprostenol dose.
- Step 2: 80% of the starting epoprostenol dose; give treprostinil at 30% of the starting epoprostenol dose.
- Step 3: 60% of the starting epoprostenol dose; give treprostinil at 50% of the starting epoprostenol dose.
- Step 4: 40% of the starting epoprostenol dose; give treprostinil at 70% of the starting epoprostenol dose.
- Step 5: 20% of the starting epoprostenol dose; give treprostinil at 90% of the starting epoprostenol dose.
- Step 6: 5% of the starting epoprostenol dose; give treprostinil at 110% of the starting epoprostenol dose.
- Step 7: No epoprostenol given; give treprostinil at 110% of the starting epoprostenol dose + additional 5–10% increments as needed.

Tyvaso

ORAL INHALATION

Pulmonary arterial hypertension (WHO Class I and NYHA Class III symptoms).

Three breaths of 0.6 mg/mL per treatment session 4 times per day. If 3 breaths are not tolerated, reduce to 1–2 breaths and subsequently increase to 3 breaths as tolerated; may increase up to 9 breaths per treatment session 4 times per day.

NURSING IMPLICATIONS

IMPLEMENTATION/ADMINISTRATION/STORAGE

1. Treprostinil should be used only by those experienced in the diagnosis and treatment of pulmonary arterial hypertension. Initiation of therapy must be in a setting with adequate personnel and equipment for physiological monitoring and emergency care.
2. Treprostinil must be used only with the treprostinil inhalation system.
3. Do not mix treprostinil with other medications in the Optineb-ir device.
4. Give injection form by continuous SC or IV infusion.
5. Can be given as supplied or diluted for IV infusion with sterile water for injection or 0.9% NaCl.
6. Use the following formula to calculate SC infusion rates: SC infusion rate (mL/hr) = Dose (ng/kg/min) × weight (kg) × (0.00006) divided by treprostinil vial strength (i.e., mg/mL). Check the package insert for sample calculations for SC or IV infusion and for instructions on preparation for administration.
7. A single reservoir syringe can be given up to 72 hr at 37°C (99°F). Do not use a single vial for more than 14 days after initial introduction into the vial.
8. Given by continuous SC infusion via a self-inserted SC catheter using an infusion pump designed for SC drug delivery.
9. To avoid interruptions in drug delivery, the client must have available a backup infusion pump and SC infusion sets.
10. To prevent worsening symptoms, avoid abrupt withdrawal or sudden large increases in dosage of the drug.
11. Increase the dose for lack of improvement in or worsening of symptoms; decrease the dose for excessive pharmacologic effects or unacceptable side effects (e.g., anxiety, N&V, headache, infusion-site reaction, restlessness).
12. Unopened vials are stable until the date indicated if stored from 15–25°C (59–77°F). Solutions as dilute as 0.004 mg/mL are stable at ambient temperature for up to 48 hr.
13. IV If used IV, the product must first be diluted with sterile water for injection or 0.9% NaCl injection.
14. COMPATIBILITY Sterile water, 0.9% NaCl.
15. INCOMPATIBILITY Administer separately.

ASSESSMENT

1. Note NYHA stage, symptom characteristics and clinical presentation. List other agents trialed and the outcome. Identify if transplant candidate.

2. Usually administered SC with pump and delivery system; if IV therapy indicated, note reasons.
3. With inhalation therapy, use treprostinil inhalation system (Optineb-ir device).
4. Transition from epoprostenol to treprostinil should be done in monitored setting; follow dosing guidelines carefully.
5. Any pulmonary infections should be monitored closely for any worsening of lung disease and loss of drug effect.
6. List cardiopulmonary assessment findings and catherization results and monitor. Monitor renal and LFTs; use cautiously with dysfunction.

CLIENT/FAMILY TEACHING

1. Drug lowers blood pressure in the pulmonary artery that leads from the heart to the lungs. It is generally administered as a continuous infusion through an SC catheter with an infusion pump for an extended period of time. Do not stop therapy suddenly; may cause worsening of symptoms.
2. Review proper administration techniques, catheter insertion, site care, reservoir (drug) loading and pump maintenance/alarms/care/disposal of used supplies. Refer to home infusion agency/provider for management/support/backup equipment.
3. If prescribed the inhalation form, use only with the treprostinil inhalation system.
4. Do not mix solution with other medications in the Optineb-ir inhalation device.
5. It is dosed in 4 separate, equally spaced treatment sessions per day during waking hours, about 4 hr apart. Report acute respiratory infections; may worsen disease and alter drug effect.
6. One ampule of treprostinil contains enough medication for all 4 inhalation treatment sessions in a single day. At the end of each day, the medicine cup and any remaining medication must be discarded. Avoid contact with skin/eyes; if medication comes in contact with the skin/eyes, rinse immediately with water.
7. After opening foil pouch, use within 7 days. Treprostinil is light sensitive; store unopened ampules in foil pouch.
8. Report any persistent headache, diarrhea, dizziness, N&V, anxiety/restlessness, and infusion site pain so dose can be adjusted to control these effects yet improve present functioning level/exercise tolerance. Immediately report any worsening of SOB, chest pain, fatigue, injection site pain/reaction, itching or rash.
9. Keep close contact and all F/U visits to assess response, dose requirements, labs and adverse SE. May eventually require conversion to IV therapy.

OUTCOMES/EVALUATE

- ↑ Exercise tolerance
- ↑ CO with pulmonary artery hypertension

Tretinoin (Retinoic acid, Vitamin A acid)

(**TRET**-ih-noyn)

Classification(s): Retinoid

Pregnancy Category: C (Topical products); **D** (Oral products)

RX: Capsules: Tretinoin. **Topical Cream, Gel**: Atralin, Avita, Renova, Retin-A, Retin-A Micro, Tretin-X.

✱ **Rx:** Rejuva-A, Stieva-A.

INDICATIONS/USES

Dermatologic (Cream/Gel): *Altinac, Atralin, Avita, Retin-A, Retin-A Micro:* Topical treatment of acne vulgaris. *Renova, 0.02% Cream:* Adjunct for mitigation of fine wrinkles in those who use comprehensive skin care and sun avoidance programs. *Renova, 0.05% Cream:* Adjunct for mitigation of fine wrinkles, mottled hyperpigmentation, and tactile roughness of facial skin for those who do not achieve palliation using comprehensive skin care and sun avoidance programs alone. *NOTE:* It is advisable to rest a client's skin until effects of keratolytic agents wear off before beginning tretinoin therapy.

Oral (Capsules): Induce remission in acute promyelocytic leukemia (APL). After induction therapy with tretinoin, give clients a standard consolidation or maintenance chemotherapy regimen for APL, unless contraindicated.

ACTION/KINETICS

Action

Topical tretinoin is believed to decrease microcomedone formation by decreasing the cohesiveness of follicular epithelial cells. Also believed to increase mitotic activity and increase turnover of follicular epithelial cells as well as decrease keratin synthesis. In APL clients, tretinoin produces an initial maturation of the primitive promyelocytes derived from the leukemic clone, followed by a repopulation of the bone marrow and peripheral blood by normal, polyclonal hematopoietic cells. The exact mechanism of action for APL is unknown.

Pharmacokinetics

After topical use, some systemic absorption occurs (approximately 5% is recovered in the urine). Absorption after PO use is enhanced when the drug is taken with food. **Time to peak levels after PO:** 1–2 hr. **Terminal elimination t½:** 0.5–2 hr in APL clients. Metabolized by the liver by P450 enzymes, with about two-thirds excreted in the urine and one-third in the feces. **Plasma protein binding:** More than 95% (mainly to albumin).

CONTRAINDICATIONS

Eczema, sunburn. Use if inherently sensitive to sunlight or if taking other drugs that increase sensitivity to sunlight. Use of Renova if client is also taking drugs known to be photosensitizers (e.g., fluoroquinolones, phenothiazines, sulfonamides, tetracyclines, thiazides). Those allergic to parabens (preservative in the gelatin capsules). Use of PO form during lactation. Use around the eyes, mouth, angles of the nose, and mucous membranes.

SPECIAL CONCERNS

■ **For Capsules.** (1) Clients with acute promyelocytic leukemia (APL) are at high risk in general and can have severe side effects to tretinoin. Therefore, administer only to clients with APL under the strict supervision of a physician who is experienced in the management of those with acute leukemia and in a facility with lab and supportive services sufficient to monitor drug tolerance and to protect and maintain a client compromised by drug toxicity, including respiratory compromise. Use of tretinoin requires the physician to assess that the possible benefit to the client outweighs the following adverse reactions to the therapy. (2) **Retinoic acid-APL syndrome.** About 25% of clients with APL treated with tretinoin experienced the retinoic acid-APL (RA-APL) syndrome, characterized by fever, dsypnea, acute respiratory distress, weight gain, radiographic pulmonary infiltrates, and pleural or pericardial effusions, edema, and hepatic, renal, and multiorgan failure. This syndrome occasionally has been accompanied by impaired myocardial contractility and episodic hypotension. The syndrome has been observed with or without concomitant leukocytosis. Endotracheal intubation and mechanical ventilation have been required in some cases due to progressive hypoxia; several clients have died due to multi-organ failure. The syndrome generally occurs during the first month of treatment, with some cases following the first dose. (3) The management of retinoic acid-APL syndrome has not been defined rigorously, but high-dose steroids given at the first suspicion of the RA-APL syndrome appear to reduce morbidity and mortality. At the first signs suggestive of the syndrome (e.g., unexplained fever, dyspnea and/or weight gain, abnormal chest auscultatory findings, or radiographic abnormalities), initiate high-dose steroids (e.g., dexamethasone, 10 mg IV q 12 hr for 3 days or until resolution of symptoms) immediately, irrespective of the leukocyte count. The majority of clients do not require termination of tretinoin therapy during treatment of the retinoic acid-APL syndrome. However, in cases of moderate and severe RA-APL syndrome, consider temporary interruption of tretinoin therapy. (4) **Leukocytosis.** During tretinoin treatment, approximately 40% of clients will develop rapidly evolving leukocytosis. Clients who present with a high WBC at diagnosis (e.g., more than 5×10^9/L) have an increased risk of a further rapid increase in WBC counts. Rapidly evolving leukocytosis is associated with a higher risk of life-threatening complications. (5) If signs and symptoms of retinoic acid-APL syndrome are present with leukocytosis, immediately initiate treatment with high-dose steroids. Some investigators routinely add chemotherapy to tretinoin treatment in the case of clients presenting with a WBC count more than 5×10^9/L or in the case of a rapid increase in WBC count for clients leukopenic at the start of treatment, and have reported a lower incidence of the RA-APL syndrome.

T

Consider adding full-dose chemotherapy (including an anthracycline if not contraindicated) to tretinoin therapy on day 1 or 2 for clients presenting with a WBC count of more than 5×10^9/L; immediately add for clients presenting with a WBC count of less than 5×10^9/L, if the WBC count reaches greater than or equal to 6×10^9/L by day 5, greater than or equal to 10 or more $\times 10^9$/L by day 10, or greater than or equal to 15×10^9/L by day 28. (6) **Teratogenic effects.** Pregnancy Category D. There is a high risk that a severely deformed infant will result if tretinoin is given during pregnancy. If, nonetheless, it is determined that tretinoin represents the best available treatment for a pregnant woman or a woman of childbearing potential, it must be ensured that the client has received full information and warnings of the risk to the fetus if she were to be pregnant and of the risk of possible contraceptive failure. Instruct the client to use two reliable forms of contraception simultaneously during therapy and for 1 month following discontinuation of therapy, and emphasize the need to use dual contraception, unless abstinence is the chosen method. (7) Within 1 week prior to starting tretinoin therapy, collect blood or urine from the client for a serum or urine pregnancy test with a sensitivity of at least 50 milli-international units. When possible, delay tretinoin therapy until a negative result from this test is obtained. When a delay is not possible, place the client on two reliable forms of contraception. Repeat pregnancy testing and contraceptive counseling monthly throughout period of tretinoin treatment.

- Use topical products with caution during lactation.
- Safety and efficacy not determined in children.
- Excessive sunlight and weather extremes (e.g., wind and cold) may be irritating.
- Use Avita and Renova with caution with concomitant topical medications, medicated or abrasive soaps, shampoos, cleansers, cosmetics with a strong drying effect, permanent wave solutions, electrolysis, hair depilatories or waxes, and products with high concentrations of alcohol, astringents, spices, or lime.
- Safety and efficacy of Renova not determined in children less than 18 years of age, in individuals over the age of 50 years, or in individuals with moderately or heavily pigmented skin.
- Use of the PO form has resulted in retinoic acid-APL syndrome, especially during the first month of treatment.
- The safety and efficacy of oral tretinoin at doses less than 45 mg/m^2/day have not been evaluated in children.

SIDE EFFECTS

Most Common

After PO use: Headache, fever, weakness, fatigue, arrhythmias, flushing, hypertension, phlebitis, dizziness, anxiety, paresthesia, depression, confusion, GI hemorrhage, abdominal pain, diarrhea, constipation, anorexia, dyspepsia, renal impairment, hemorrhage, disseminated intravascular coagulation, peripheral edema, edema, URTI, dyspnea, respiratory insufficiency, pleural effusion, earache, malaise, shivering, infections, pain, chest discomfort, myalgia.

After topical use: Dry skin, peeling, burning, stinging, erythema, pruritus.

Following topical use: Dermatologic: Red, edematous, crusted, or blistered skin; temporary hyperpigmentation or hypopigmentation, increased susceptibility to sunlight, erythema, peeling, stinging, pruritus, burning, dryness. Excessive application will cause redness, peeling, or discomfort with no increase in results.

Following oral use: Retinoic acid-APL syndrome: Fever, dyspnea, weight gain, radiographic pulmonary infiltrate, pleural or pericardial effusions, edema; hepatic, renal, and multiorgan failure. Occasional impaired myocardial contractility and episodic hypotension; possibility of concomitant leukocytosis. ***Progressive hypoxemia with possible fatal outcome.*** Respiratory symptoms, including upper respiratory tract disorders, respiratory insufficiency, pneumonia, rales, expiratory wheezing, lower respiratory tract disorders, bronchial asthma, acute respiratory distress, ***pulmonary or larynx edema***, unspecified pulmonary disease.

Pseudotumor cerebri (especially in children): Papilledema, headache, N&V, visual disturbances. **Typical retinoid toxicity (similar to ingestion of high doses of vitamin A):** Headache, fever, dryness of skin and mucous membranes, bone pain, N&V, rash, mucositis, pruritus, increased sweating, visual disturbances, ocular disorders, alopecia, skin changes, changed visual acuity, bone

T

inflammation, visual field defects. **Body as a whole:** Malaise, shivering, infections, peripheral edema, pain, chest discomfort, anorexia, myalgia, flank pain, pallor, acidosis, hypothermia, ascites. **GI:** ***GI hemorrhage***, abdominal pain, various GI disorders, diarrhea, constipation, dyspepsia, abdominal distension, hepatosplenomegaly, hepatitis, ulcer, unspecified liver disorders. **CV:** Arrhythmias, flushing, hypotension, hypertension, phlebitis, ***cardiac failure***, ***cardiac arrest***, ***stroke***, MI, enlarged heart, heart murmur, ischemia, myocarditis, pericarditis, pulmonary hypertension, secondary cardiomyopathy, thrombosis (venous or arterial) during the first month of treatment involving various sites (e.g., CVA, MI, renal infarct). **CNS:** Dizziness, paresthesias, anxiety, insomnia, depression, confusion, ***cerebral hemorrhage***, ***intracranial hypertension***, agitation, hallucinations, abnormal gait, agnosia, aphasia, asterixis, cerebellar edema, cerebellar disorders, ***convulsions***, ***coma***, CNS depression, dysarthria, encephalopathy, facial paralysis, hemiplegia, hyporeflexia, hypotaxia, no light reflex, neurologic reaction, spinal cord disorder, tremor, leg weakness, unconsciousness, dementia, forgetfulness, somnolence, slow speech. **GU:** Renal insufficiency, dysuria, acute renal failure, micturition frequency, renal tubular necrosis, enlarged prostate. **Respiratory:** Upper respiratory tract disorders, dyspnea, respiratory insufficiency, pleural effusion, expiratory wheezing, pneumonia, rales, lower respiratory tract disorders, pulmonary infiltration, bronchial asthma, larynx edema, pulmonary edema, unspecified pulmonary disease. **Dermatologic**: Cellulitis, pallor, genital ulceration, vasculitis (predominately involving the skin). **Hematologic:** ***Hemorrhage, disseminated intravascular coagulation***, lymph disorders, thrombocytosis. **Metabolic:** Peripheral edema, edema, weight increase/decrease, facial edema, fluid imbalance. **Otic:** Earache, feeling of fullness in the ears, hearing loss, unspecified auricular disorders, irreversible hearing loss. **Miscellaneous:** Erythema nodosum, basophilia, hyperhistaminemia, Sweet's syndrome, organomegaly, hypercalcemia, pancreatitis, myositis.

T

LABORATORY TEST CONSIDERATIONS

Abnormal LFTs. Hypercholesterolemia.

DRUG INTERACTIONS

Aminocaproic acid / Rarely, cases of fatal thrombotic complications
Aprotinin / Rarely, cases of fatal thrombotic complications
Benzoyl peroxide / Use with topical tretinoin may cause significant skin irritation
Fluoroquinolones / Possible ↑ phototoxicity
Ketoconazole / Significant ↑ in tretinoin mean plasma AUC if ketoconazole given 1 hr prior to tretinoin
Phenothiazines / Possible ↑ phototoxicity
Resorcinol / Use with topical tretinoin may cause significant skin irritation
Salicylic acid / Use with topical tretinoin may cause significant skin irritation
Sulfonamides / Possible ↑ phototoxicity
Sulfur / Use with topical tretinoin may cause significant skin irritation
Tetracyclines / ↑ Risk of pseudotumor cerebri and intracranial hypertension; also possible ↑ phototoxicity
Thiazides / Possible ↑ Phototoxicity
Tranexamic acid / Rarely, cases of fatal thrombotic complications
Vitamin A / Possible aggravation of symptoms of hypervitaminosis A

HOW SUPPLIED

Capsules: 10 mg; ***Cream:*** 0.02%, 0.025%, 0.0375%, 0.05%, 0.1%; ***Gel:*** 0.01%, 0.025%, 0.04%, 0.05%, 0.1%.

DOSAGE

CREAM; GEL

Acne vulgaris.

Apply lightly over the affected areas once daily at bedtime. Beneficial effects many not be seen for 2–6 weeks.

CREAM

Palliation for skin conditions.

Apply cream (0.02% or 0.05%) once daily at bedtime, using only enough to lightly cover the entire affected area. Up to 6 months of therapy may be needed before effects are seen.

CAPSULES

Acute promyelocytic leukemia.

Adults: 45 mg/m²/day given as two evenly divided doses. Given until complete remission is obtained. Discontinue 30 days after achieving complete remission or after 90 days of treatment, whichever comes first.

NURSING IMPLICATIONS

IMPLEMENTATION/ADMINISTRATION/STORAGE

1. If after initiation of tretinoin the presence of the t(15;17) translocation is not confirmed by cytogenetics and/or by polymerase chain reaction studies and the client has not responded to tretinoin, alternative therapy appropriate for acute myelogenous leukemia should be considered.
2. Apply the liquid carefully with the fingertip, cotton swab, or gauze pad only to affected areas.
3. Excessive amounts of the gel will cause a "pilling" effect, which minimizes the likelihood of overapplication.
4. Before applying Renova, wash the face gently with a mild soap and pat the skin dry, waiting 20–30 min before applying. When applied, take care to avoid contact with eyes, ears, nostrils, and mouth. Wash hands thoroughly immediately after applying tretinoin.
5. Do not freeze Renova cream.
6. Treatment with Renova for more than 24 weeks does not appear to increase improvement. The results of continued irritation of the skin for more than 48 weeks are not known.
7. Store capsules from 15–30°C (59–86°F); protect from light.

ASSESSMENT

1. Note reasons for therapy, onset, characteristics of S&S, clinical presentation, other agents trialed/outcome.
2. With acute promyelocytic leukemia (APL) monitor carefully during induction therapy for adverse effects. Assess for APL syndrome within 1 month of therapy: fever, dyspnea, weight gain, pulmonary infiltrates by x-ray, and pleural or pericardial effusions. May also be accompanied by impaired myocardial contractility and episodic hypotension.
3. With acne, thoroughly describe pretreatment skin condition; obtain photographs to compare with results of therapy.
4. Check if pregnant. Monitor CBC renal and LFTs closely.

CLIENT/FAMILY TEACHING

Topical:

1. Keep away from normal skin, mucous membranes, eyes, ears, mouth, nostrils, and nose angles.
2. Wash with mild soap and warm water and pat skin dry. Wait 20–30 min before applying tretinoin. Do not wash face for 1 hr or more after applying tretinoin. Wash hands thoroughly before and after applying tretinoin.
3. On application there will be a transitory feeling of warmth and stinging. May use nonmedicated cosmetics during therapy but remove before treatment. Avoid any additional self-treatment with antiacne products.
4. Do not apply another skin care product or cosmetic and do not wash face for at least 1 hr after applying tretinoin. Expect dryness and peeling of skin from the affected areas.
5. May be more sensitive to wind and cold. Do not apply to wind or sunburned skin or to open wounds. Avoid excessive exposure to sunlamps and to the sun. If exposed, use a sunscreen and protective clothing over affected areas.
6. Avoid alcohol-containing preparations such as shaving lotions and creams, perfumes, cosmetics with drying effects, skin cleansers, and medicated soaps.
7. Initially, lesions may worsen, caused by the effect of the drug on deep lesions that had been previously undetected. Report if lesions become severe; discontinue drug until skin integrity restored.
8. Improvement should be evident in 6 weeks, but therapy should be continued for at least 3 months.
9. Practice reliable birth control; may cause fetal harm.

Oral:

1. Drug will be administered until complete remission is obtained. It will be stopped 30 days after remission or after 90 days of therapy, whichever comes first. This does not replace standard maintenance chemotherapy for APL.
2. Take with food to enhance absorption. Follow a low-fat diet and exercise regularly to reduce drug-induced elevated triglyceride levels.
3. Use caution with activities requiring mental alertness, may cause dizziness or confusion.

T

4. **Avoid supplemental vitamin A or products containing vitamin A (e.g., multivitamins) during therapy.**
5. **Report immediately: fever, SOB, fatigue, weight gain, cough (radiographic pulmonary infiltrates, and pleural or pericardial effusions).**
6. **Do not donate blood while on this therapy; may be harmful to recipient.**
7. **Avoid pregnancy. Must use two reliable forms of contraception during, and for 1 month following therapy; may cause fetal harm.**
8. **Keep all F/U to assess response, labs, and for adverse SE.**

OUTCOMES/EVALUATE

- ↓ Size/number of acne eruptions
- Clearing of skin condition; symptomatic improvement
- Remission with APL

Triamcinolone acetonide

(try-am-**SIN**-oh-lohn)

Classification(s): Glucocorticoid

Pregnancy Category: C

RX: Dental Paste: Kenalog in Orabase. **Inhalation Aerosol**: Azmacort (Oral), Nasacort AQ (Intranasal). **Parenteral**: Kenalog-10 and -40, Triesence (Intravitreal Suspension), Trivaris (Intravitreal Gel). **Topical Lotion/Ointment**: Kenonel, Triacet, Trianex, Triderm. **Topical Spray**: Kenalog.

🍁 **Rx: Dental Paste:** : Oracort.

Triamcinolone hexacetonide

Pregnancy Category: C

RX: Aristospan Intra-Articular, Aristospan Intralesional.

SEE ALSO ***CORTICOSTEROIDS.***

ADDITIONAL USES

(1) Pulmonary emphysema accompanied by bronchospasm or bronchial edema. (2) Diffuse interstitial pulmonary fibrosis. (3) With diuretics to treat refractory CHF or cirrhosis of the liver with ascites. (4) Multiple sclerosis. (5) Inflammation following dental procedures.

Triamcinolone acetonide: (1) **PO inhalation:** Maintenance treatment of chronic asthma as prophylactic therapy (use Azmacort) in adults and children 6 years of age and older. For those who require systemic therapy and for whom adding triamcinolone may reduce or eliminate the need for systemic corticosteroids. (2) **Intranasal:** Seasonal and perennial allergic rhinitis in adults and children 2 years of age and older (use Nasacort AQ). (3) **Intravitreal injection:** Sympathetic ophthalmia, temporal arteritis, uveitis, and ocular inflammatory conditions unresponsive to topical corticosteroids. Also, visualization during vitrectomy (Triesence only). (4) **Intraarticular**: Short-term administration (to tide client over in acute episode or exacerbation) for acute gouty arthritis, acute/subacute bursitis, acute nonspecific tenosynovitis, epicondylitis, rheumatoid arthritis, synovitis of osteoarthritis. (5) **Intralesional:** Alopecia areata; discoid lupus erythematosus; keloids; localized hypertrophic, infiltrated, inflammatory lesions of granuloma annulare; lichen planus; lichen simplex chronicus; psoriatic plaques; necroblosis lipoidica diabeticorum (use Kenalog-10 injection only). (6) **Intramuscular:** See *Uses* under *Corticosteroids*. Use Kenalog-40 or Trivaris injections only.

Triamcinolone hexacetonide, Intralesional: (1) Alopecia areata. (2) Discoid lupus erythematosus. (3) Keloids. (4) Localized hypertrophic, infiltrated inflammatory lesions of granuloma annulare, lichen planus, lichen simplex chronicus (neurodermatitis), and psoriatic plaques. (5) Necrobiosis lipoidica diabeticorum. (6) Cystic tumors of an aponeurosis or tendon (ganglia). **Intra-articular:** Adjunctive therapy for short-term administration (i.e., to tide client over in an acute episode or exacerbation) in acute gouty arthritis, acute and subacute bursitis, acute nonspecific tenosynovitis, epicondylitis, rheumatoid arthritis, or synovitis of osteoarthritis.

ACTION/KINETICS

Action

The anti-inflammatory effect is due to inhibition of prostaglandin synthesis. The drug also inhibits accumulation of macrophages and leukocytes at sites of inflammation and inhibits phagocytosis and lysosomal enzyme release. More potent than prednisone. Intermediate-acting. Has no mineralocorticoid activity.

Pharmacokinetics

Onset: Several hours. **Duration:** One or more weeks. **t½:** Over 200 min. Metabolized by the liver. About 60% excreted in the feces and 40% in the urine. **t½, after intranasal use:** 3.1 hr.

ADDITIONAL CONTRAINDICATIONS

Use of intranasal products with active or quiescent tuberculosis infections in the respiratory tract, or in untreated fungal, bacterial, or systemic viral infections, or ocular herpes simplex. Use of the intravitreal product for systemic fungal infections.

SPECIAL CONCERNS

Azmacort Aerosol: Particular care is needed in clients who are transferred from systemically active corticosteroids to triamcinolone inhalation aerosol because deaths due to adrenal insufficiency have occurred in asthmatic clients during and after transfer from systemic corticosteroids to aerosolized steroids in recommended doses. After withdrawal from systemic corticosteroids, a number of months is usually required for recovery of hypothalamic-pituitary-adrenal (HPA) function. For some clients who have received large doses of oral steroids for long periods of time before therapy with triamcinolone is initiated, recovery may be delayed for 1 year or longer. During this period of HPA suppression, clients may exhibit signs and symptoms of adrenal insufficiency when exposed to trauma, surgery, or infections, particularly gastroenteritis or other conditions with acute electrolyte loss. Although triamcinolone may provide control of asthmatic symptoms during these episodes, in recommended doses it supplies only normal physiological amounts of corticosteroid systemically and does not provide the increased systemic steroid that is needed for coping with these emergencies. During periods of stress or severe asthmatic attack, clients who have been recently withdrawn from systemic corticosteroids should be instructed to resume systemic steroids (in large doses) immediately and to contact their physician for further instruction. Instruct these clients to carry a warning card indicating that they may need supplementary systemic steroids during periods of stress or a severe asthma attack.

- **Use during pregnancy only if benefits clearly outweigh risks.**
- **Use special caution with decreased renal function or renal disease. Dose must be highly individualized.**

ADDITIONAL SIDE EFFECTS

Most Common

After nasal/respiratory use: Burning/dryness of nasal passages, nasal/throat irritation, sneezing, epistaxis, cough, pharyngitis, pyrexia.
After parenteral use: N&V, acne, diarrhea, constipation, headache, heartburn, restlessness, insomnia, sweating.
After intra-articular, intrasynovial, intrabursal use: Transient flushing, dizziness, local depigmentation, local irritation.
See *Corticosteroids* for a complete list of possible side effects. Exacerbation of symptoms has also been reported. A marked increase in swelling and pain and further restricted joint movement may indicate septic arthritis. Intradermal injection may cause local vesicular ulceration and persistent scarring. Syncope and ***anaphylactoid reactions*** have been reported with triamcinolone regardless of route of administration.

After intranasal use: Burning/dryness of nasal passages, nasal/throat irritation, pyrexia, sneezing, headache, vomiting, asthma symptoms, epistaxis, cough, rhinitis, pharyngitis, sinusitis, otitis media, perforation of nasal septum (rare), infection (rare).

HOW SUPPLIED

Triamcinolone acetonide: ***Aerosol Suspension, Oral Inhalation (Azmacort):*** 75 mcg/actuation; ***Cream:*** 0.025%, 0.1%, 0.5%; ***Dental Paste:*** 0.1%; ***Injection, Suspension:*** 3 mg/mL, 10 mg/mL, 40 mg/mL; ***Intranasal, Spray Suspension (AllerNaze, Nasacort AQ):*** 50 mcg/actuation (AllerNaze), 55 mcg/actuation (Nasacort AQ); ***Intravitreal Gel Suspension Injection:*** 80 mg/mL; ***Intravitreal Suspension Injection:*** 40 mg/mL; ***Lotion:*** 0.025%, 0.1%; ***Ointment:*** 0.025%, 0.05%, 0.1%, 0.5%; ***Topical Spray:*** 0.147 mg/gram (to deliver 0.2 mg).
Triamcinolone hexacetonide: ***Injection:*** 5 mg/mL, 20 mg/mL.

DOSAGE

Triamcinolone acetonide

AEROSOL, ORAL (AZMACORT)

Maintenance treatment of chronic asthma.

Adults, usual: 2 inhalations (150 mcg) 3–4 times per day or 4 inhalations (300 mcg) twice a day, not to exceed 16 inhalations (1,200 mcg/day). High initial doses (1,200–1,600 mcg/day) may be needed in those with severe asthma. **Pediatric, 6–12 years:** 1–2 inhalations (75–50 mcg) 3–4 times per day or 2–4 inhalations (150–300 mcg) twice a day, not to exceed 900 mcg/day (i.e., 12 inhalations). Use in children less than 6 years of age has not been determined. Improvement is usually apparent within 1–2 weeks after starting therapy. *NOTE:* Titrate to the lowest effective dose once asthma stability has been achieved.

INTRANASAL SPRAY (NASACORT AQ)

Seasonal and perennial allergic rhinitis.

Nasacort AQ. Titrate to the minimum effective dose to reduce the possibility of side effects. **Adults and children over 12 years of age, initial and maximum dose:** 2 sprays (110 mcg) in each nostril once daily (total of 220 mcg once daily). When the maximum benefit has been reached, reduce the dose to 110 mcg/day (1 spray in each nostril once daily). For the elderly, start at the low end of the dosing range. **Children, 5–12 years of age, initial:** 1 spray (55 mcg) in each nostril (total of 110 mcg) once daily; maximum recommended dose is 220 mcg/day as 2 sprays in each nostril once daily. Once symptoms are controlled, children may be able to be maintained on 110 mcg/day (1 spray in each nostril once daily). **Children, 2–5 years of age, initial:** 1 spray (55 mcg) in each nostril (total of 110 mcg/day) once a day. Maximum dose is 110 mcg/day (1 spray in each nostril once daily). Not recommended for children less than 2 years of age.

IM ONLY (NOT FOR IV USE)

Kenalog-40 and Trivaris. Adults, initial: 60 mg injected deeply into the gluteal muscle. Dosage is usually adjusted within the range of 40–80 mg, depending upon client response and duration of relief. Some clients may be controlled on doses of 20 mg or less. In certain overwhelming, acute, life-threatening situations, administration in doses exceeding the usual doses may be justified, and may be in multiples of the PO doses. *NOTE:* Kenalog-10 is not approved for IM use. **Children, initial:** Range of initial dosage is 0.11–1.6 mg/kg/day in 3 or 4 divided doses (or, 3.2–48 mg/m^2 body surface area per day). Dose depends on the specific disease being treated.

Acute exacerbation of multiple sclerosis.

Adults: 160 mg/day for a week, followed by 64 mg every other day for 1 month.

Hay fever or pollen asthma.

Adults: A single injection of 40–100 mg may help clients with hay fever or pollen asthma who are not responding to other therapy. Remission of symptoms may last through the pollen season after a single injection.

INTRA-ARTICULAR; INTRABURSAL; TENDON SHEATHS

Acute gouty arthritis, acute/subacute bursitis, acute nonspecific tenosynovitis, epicondylitis, rheumatoid arthritis, synovitis of osteoarthritis.

Adults. Kenalog-10, initial: May vary from 2.5–5 mg for smaller joints and from 5–15 mg for larger joints, depending on the specific disease being treated. **Usual dose:** A single injection is often sufficient; however, several injections may be needed for adequate relief of symptoms. Single injections into several joints, up to 20 mg or more, have been given. **Children, initial:** May vary from 2.5–5 mg for smaller joints and from 5–15 mg for larger joints, depending on the specific disease being treated. **Usual dose:** A single local injection is usually sufficient; however, several injections may be necessary for adequate relief of symptoms. Single injections into several joints, up to 20 mg or more, have been given. For children, use only Kenalog-10.

Adults. Kenalog-40, initial: May vary from 2.5–5 mg for smaller joints and from 5–15 mg for larger joints, depending on the specific disease being treated. Doses up to 10 mg for smaller areas and up to 40 mg for larger areas have usually been sufficient. **Usual dose:** A single injection is often sufficient; however, several injections may be needed for adequate relief of symptoms. Single injections into several joints, up to 80 mg or more, have been given.

Adults. Trivaris, initial: May vary from 2.5–100 mg, depending on the specific disease to be treated. In certain overwhelming, acute, life-threatening situations, doses exceeding the usual dosages may be justified and may be in multiples of PO doses.

INTRALESIONAL

Adults and children. Use Kenalog-10 injection only. Dosage per injection depends on the specific disease and lesion being treated. Multiple sites separated by 1 centimeter or more may be injected. Injections can be repeated, if needed, at weekly or less frequent intervals. *NOTE:* The more volume injected, the greater the risk for systemic absorption and systemic side effects.

INTRAVITREAL INJECTION

Ophthalmic diseases.

Triesence. Adults and children, initial: 4 mg/0.1 mL (100 mcL of 40 mg/mL suspension) with subsequent dosage as needed throughout the treatment course. **Trivaris. Adults:** A single injection of 4 mg/0.05 mL (50 mcL of the 80 mg/mL suspension).

Visualization during vitrectomy.

Triesence only. Adults and children: 1–4 mg (25–100 mcL of the 40 mg/mL suspension) given intravitreally.

CREAM; LOTION; OINTMENT; PASTE (ALL STRENGTHS); TOPICAL AEROSOL

Apply sparingly to affected area 2–4 times per day and rub in lightly.

Triamcinolone hexacetonide

INTRA-ARTICULAR (NOT FOR IV USE)

Small joints (interphalangeal, metacarpophalangeal). Large joints (knee, hip, shoulder).

Adults, initial: Varies from 2–48 mg/day, depending on the disease being treated. However, in certain overwhelming, acute, life-threatening conditions, administration of dosages exceeding the usual dosages may be justified and may be in multiples of the PO dosages. The dose depends on the size of the joint to be injection, the degree of inflammation, and the amount of fluid present. The average dose is 2–20 mg (0.1–1 mL). **Small joints (e.g., interphalangeal, metacarpophalangeal):** 2–6 mg; **large joints (e.g., hip, knee, shoulder):** 10–20 mg. When the amount of synovial fluid is increased, aspiration may be undertaken before administering the drug. The usual frequency of injection into a single joint is every 3 or 4 weeks; to avoid possible joint destruction from repeated use of intra-articular corticosteroids, injections should be as infrequent as possible. **Children, initial:** Varies from 0.11–1.6 mg/kg/day in 3 or 4 divided doses (alternative: 3.2–48 mg/m^2 body surface area/day).

INTRALESIONAL; SUBLESIONAL

Dermatological diseases.

Adults, initial: 2–48 mg/day depending on the disease being treated. The average dose is up to 0.5 mg per square inch of affected skin given intralesionally or sublesionally. **Children, initial:** 0.11–1.6 mg/kg/day (depending on the condition being treated) divided into 3 or 4 doses (alternative: 3.2–48 mg/m^2 body surface area/day). In certain overwhelming, acute, life-threatening situations, use of doses exceeding the usual

T

dosages may be justified and may be in multiples of the PO dosages. Use the lowest possible dose to control the condition being treated. When reduction in dosage is possible, do so gradually. If after long-term therapy, the drug is to be discontinued, withdraw gradually rather than abruptly.

NURSING IMPLICATIONS

IMPLEMENTATION/ADMINISTRATION/STORAGE

1. Use the lowest possible dose to control the condition being treated. When decreasing dosage, do so gradually. In order to minimize the potential growth effects of corticosteroids, titrate children to the lowest effective dose.
2. A risk/benefit decision must be made for each client as to dose and duration of treatment, and as to whether daily or intermittent therapy should be employed.
3. **Azmacort.** (a) Initially, use aerosol concomitantly with a systemic steroid. After 1 week, initiate a gradual withdrawal of systemic steroid. Make next reduction after 1–2 weeks, depending on response. If symptoms of insufficiency occur, dose of systemic steroid can be increased temporarily. Also, dose of systemic steroid may need to be increased in times of stress or during a severe asthmatic attack. (b) For best results, store Azmacort canister at room temperature and shake well before use. Prior to the first use, prime with 2 actuations. The canister will remain primed for 3 days. If the canister is not used for more than 3 days, reprime with 1 actuation. Do not puncture and do not use or store near heat or open flame; exposure to temperatures greater than 48.8°C (120°F) may cause bursting. (c) After using Azmacort, rinse the mouth. After 240 actuations, the amount delivered per actuation may not be consistent; discard the unit.
4. **Nasacort AQ.** (a) Individualize to the minimum effective dose to reduce the chance of side effects. (b) Nasacort AQ is viscous at rest but a liquid when shaken. This allows the drug to stay in the nasal airways at the site of inflammation for up to 2 hr. Nasacort HFA contains hydrofluoroalkane as the propellant instead of chlorofluorocarbon.
5. Store Azmacort and Nasacort AQ from 20–25°C (68–77°F). Do not puncture canister or store or use near heat or open flames. Exposure to temperatures above 49°C (120°F) may cause bursting. Keep Azmacort canister at room temperature before use.
6. **Nasal Spray.** Triamcinolone acetonide nasal spray for allergic rhinitis may be effective as soon as 12 hr after initiation of therapy. Reevaluate if improvement is not seen within 2–3 weeks.
7. **Triesence.** To prepare Triesence for intravitreal injection, use strict aseptic technique. Shake the vial vigorously for 10 seconds before use to ensure a uniform suspension. Before withdrawal, inspect for clumping or granular appearance; if agglomerated, do not use. After withdrawal, inject without delay to prevent settling in the syringe. Avoid possible entering of a blood vessel or introducing organisms that can cause infection. Store from 4–25°C (39–77°F). Do not freeze and protect from light.
8. **Trivaris.** (a) If using Trivaris, always allow the prefilled glass syringe to sit at room temperature for at least 30 min before the procedure. Use each syringe only for a single treatment, although multiple injections may be required to reach the recommended dose. (b) Use a 27gauge, ½-inch needle. Prepare the proper volume to be injected by advancing the plunger to the single line marked on the prefilled glass syringe shaft. Hold the syringe and needle at an angle and express excess gel suspension over a sterile surface. The plunger is correctly positioned when white compound is no longer visible between the plunger and the fill line on the syringe. This will provide the recommended dose of 4 mg/0.05 mL. Always check the needle to ensure it is firmly attached to the syringe before injection is undertaken. (c) Keep Trivaris refrigerated from 2–8°C (36–46°F) until use. Do not freeze; protect from light.
9. **Triesence and Trivaris.** (a) Carry out the injection procedure under controlled aseptic conditions, which include use of sterile gloves, a sterile drape, and a sterile eyelid speculum (or equivalent). Give adequate anesthesia and a broad-spectrum microbicide prior to the injection. (b) Use each vial or syringe only for

T

the treatment of a single eye. If the contralateral eye requires treatment, use a new vial, sterile field/gloves/drapes/speculum. Change injection needles before administration to the other eye. (c) Avoid the possibility of entering a blood vessel or introducing organisms that can cause infection. Strict aseptic technique is mandatory.

10. **Kenalog-10 and -40.** (a) When using Kenalog-10 or -40 (triamcinolone acetonide) parenterally, strict aseptic technique is to be maintained. Shake the vial before using to ensure a uniform suspension. Prior to withdrawal inspect for agglomeration. Do not use if the product shows agglomeration. After withdrawal, inject without delay to prevent settling in the syringe. (b) Store Kenalog-10 and -40 injections from 20–25°C (68–77°F). Avoid freezing and protect from light. Do not autoclave as the product is sensitive to heat.
11. **Kenalog-10.** When used intralesionally (Kenalog-10 only), inject directly into the lesion (i.e., intradermally or SC). It is preferable to use a tuberculin syringe and a small bore needle (23 to 25 gauge). Ethyl chloride spray may be used to ease the discomfort of the injection.
12. **Triamcinolone acetonide, intra-articular.** If using an intra-articular injection, excess synovial fluid, if present, should be aspirated to aid in pain relief and to prevent undue dilation of the steroid. However, all fluid is not removed. Prior use of a local anesthetic may be desired. Avoid injecting the drug into tissues surrounding the site, because tissue atrophy may occur.
13. **Triamcinolone acetonide, tenosynovitis.** If used for acute nonspecific tenosynovitis, take care to inject triamcinolone into the tendon sheath rather than the tendon substance. Epicondylitis may be treated by infiltrating the drug into the area of greatest tenderness.
14. **Triamcinolone acetonide, IM.** For IM use, inject deep into the gluteal muscle. For adults a minimum needle length of 1.5 inches is recommended. In obese clients, a longer needle may be required. Use alternate sites for subsequent injections. Avoid injection into the deltoid area due to a higher incidence of local atrophy; use the gluteal area.
15. **Triamcinolone acetonide.** Do not use the acetonide products if they clump due to exposure to freezing temperatures.
16. **Triamcinolone hexacetonide, intra-articular.** (a) The intra-articular suspension may be mixed with lidocaine HCl, 1% or 2%, using the formulations that do not contain parabens (causes flocculation of the steroid). These dilutions will retain full potency for 1 week; exercise care to avoid contamination of the vial's contents; discard the dilutions after 7 days. (b) Do not inject into an infected area.
17. **Triamcinolone hexacetonide, intra-articular.** Store from 20–25°C (68–77°F). Do not freeze.
18. **Triamcinolone hexacetonide, intralesional.** (a) Strict aseptic technique is essential. Gently agitate the syringe to achieve a uniform suspension before use. A small bore needle (not smaller than 24 gauge) may be used. Topical ethyl chloride may be used locally before injection. Do not inject into an infected area. (b) Carefully consider the site of the injection and the volume of injection.
19. **Triamcinolone hexacetonide, intralesional.** (a) The intralesional suspension may be mixed with lidocaine HCl, 1% or 2%, using the formulations that do not contain parabens (causes flocculation of the steroid). These dilutions will retain full potency for 1 week; exercise care to avoid contamination of the vial's contents; discard the dilutions afer 7 days. (b) The 5 mg/mL intralesional suspension may also be diluted, if desired, with D5W, D10W, NaCl injection, or sterile water for injection. Determine the optimum dilution (i.e., 1:1, 1:2, 1:4) by the nature of the lesion, its size, the depth of injection, the volume needed, and location of the lesion. In general, perform more superficial injections with greater dilution. Certain conditions (e.g., keloids) require a less diluted suspension, such as 5 mg/mL, with variation in dose and dilution determined by the client's condition.
20. **Triamcinolone hexacetonide, Intralesional.** Store from 20–25°C (68–77°F). Do not freeze. The product is sensitive to heat; do not autoclave.

ASSESSMENT

1. Note reasons for therapy and form/method prescribed; type, onset, and characteristics of S&S, other agents trialed, outcome.

2. Drug comes in various forms and is indicated for a variety of conditions; assess carefully.
3. Assess area/condition requiring treatment and clinical presentation.
4. Following intraocular injection, monitor for elevation of IOP and endophthalmitis, and if therapy given for more than 6 weeks.
5. Monitor bone density with long-term therapy. Routinely monitor growth of children.
6. Review specific agent to determine dosing guidelines.
7. Monitor blood sugar, CBC, electrolytes, renal and LFTs.

CLIENT/FAMILY TEACHING

1. Take at the same time each day. Review reasons for therapy, method/frequency of administration. Assess mouth and report any evidence of oral lesions with inhaled therapy. With paste, press small dab (about ¼ inch) on the lesion until thin film develops. Report any new blistering or peeling.
2. Ingest a liberal amount of protein; with regular use may experience gradual weight loss, associated with anorexia, muscle wasting, and weakness. See dietitian for assistance in meal planning.
3. Lie down if feeling faint; report if episodes persist and interfere with daily activities.
4. Report evidence of abnormal bruising/bleeding, weight gain, swelling of extremities, or SOB.
5. Drug may suppress reactions to skin allergy testing. Do not stop suddenly with long-term therapy.
6. With topical therapy, wash hands and apply to clean, slightly moist skin. Report if area does not improve with therapy or if symptoms worsen.
7. With nasal spray or inhaler, review appropriate method of administration and proper care and storage of equipment. Always rinse mouth and equipment after use. If bronchodilator also prescribed, use this first and allow at least 1 min before repeat inhalations.
8. For Nasacort AQ, prime the nasal spray before use by pushing down on the actuator until a fine spray appears (5 pumps). If the pump has not been used for more than 14 days, the pump must be reprimed with 1 spray. For Nasacort HFA, the canister must be primed with three actuations prior to the first use or after 3 days of non-use.
9. Store Nasacort AQ at room temperature. Discard container when the labeled number of actuations has been used, even if the bottle is not completely empty.
10. For dental paste: press small dab (about ¼ inch) on lesion until thin film develops. Do not rub the paste into the lesion. Apply at bedtime if being used once daily and after meals if being used more than once daily. If any local reactions occur: burning, irritation, itching, new blistering or peeling or new sores, stop drug and report.
11. With prolonged therapy, do not stop suddenly. Report any S&S of adrenal insufficiency (e.g., abdominal, joint, or muscle pain; depression; dizziness; fatigue; hypotension; nausea). Report immediately any new onset of depression, as well as aggravation of existing depressive symptoms.
12. Keep all F/U to assess response, labs, and for adverse SE.

OUTCOMES/EVALUATE

- ↓ Immune and inflammatory responses in autoimmune disorders and allergic reactions
- Improved airway exchange
- Restoration of skin integrity
- Relief of pain/inflammation; improved joint mobility
- Control of S&S allergic rhinitis

Triamterene

(try-**AM**-ter-een)

Classification(s): Diuretic, potassium-sparing

Pregnancy Category: C (D if used in gestational hypertension)

RX: Dyrenium.

INDICATIONS/USES

(1) Edema due to CHF, hepatic cirrhosis, and the nephrotic syndrome. (2) Steroid-induced edema. (3) Edema due to secondary hyperaldosteronism. (4) Idiopathic edema. May be used alone or with other diuretics.

ACTION/KINETICS

Action

Acts directly on the distal tubule to inhibit reabsorption of sodium in exchange for potassium or hydrogen ions. It increases urinary pH and occasionally increases serum potassium; is a weak folic acid antagonist. Promotes increased diuresis when clients are resistant or only partially responsive to thiazides or other diuretics due to secondary hyperaldosteronism.

Pharmacokinetics

Rapidly absorbed; 30–70% bioavailability. **Onset:** 2–4 hr. **Peak plasma levels:** 3 hr. **Peak effect:** 6–8 hr. Maximum therapeutic effect may not be seen for several days. **Duration:** 12–16 hr. **t½:** 3 hr. Metabolized to hydroxytriamterene sulfate, which is also active. About 20% is excreted unchanged through the urine. **Plasma protein binding:** 50–67%.

CONTRAINDICATIONS

Hypersensitivity to the drug or any component of the product. Anuria. Severe or progressive kidney disease or dysfunction with the possible exception of nephrosis. Severe hepatic disease. Use in those with preexisting elevated serum potassium >5.5 mEq/L (e.g., in impaired renal function, in azotemia, or in those who develop hyperkalemia while on the drug). Use of dietary potassium supplements, potassium salts, or potassium-containing salt substitutes. Use in those receiving other potassium-sparing drugs such as spironolactone, amiloride hydrochloride, or other formulations containing triamterene. Lactation.

SPECIAL CONCERNS

Safety and efficacy not determined in children.

SIDE EFFECTS

Most Common

N&V, diarrhea, dry mouth, headache, dizziness, malaise.

Electrolyte: Hyperkalemia, electrolyte imbalance. **GI**: N&V (may also be indicative of electrolyte imbalance), diarrhea, dry mouth, jaundice. **CNS**: Dizziness, drowsiness, fatigue, malaise, weakness, headache. **Hematologic**: Megaloblastic anemia, thrombocytopenia. **Renal**: Azotemia, interstitial nephritis, renal stones. **Metabolic:** Hyperkalemia, hypokalemia. **Hypersensitivity:** Rash, photosensitivity, ***anaphylaxis***. **Miscellaneous**: Muscle cramps, hyperglycemia.

LABORATORY TEST CONSIDERATIONS

↑ Uric acid. Nitrogen retention. Liver enzyme abnormalities. Possible metabolic acidosis.

OVERDOSE MANAGEMENT

Symptoms: Electrolyte imbalance, especially hyperkalemia. Also, N&V, other GI disturbances, weakness, hypotension, reversible acute renal failure. *Treatment:* Immediately induce vomiting or perform gastric lavage. Evaluate electrolyte levels and fluid balance and treat if necessary. Dialysis may be beneficial.

DRUG INTERACTIONS

Amantadine / ↑ Amantadine toxic effects R/T ↓ renal excretion
Anesthetic drugs / Effect potentiated by triamterene
Angiotensin-converting enzyme inhibitors / Significant hyperkalemia
Antihypertensives / Effect potentiated by triamterene
Captopril / ↑ Risk of significant hyperkalemia
Chlorpropamide / ↑ Risk of severe hyponatremia
Cimetidine / ↑ Bioavailability and ↓ clearance of triamterene
Digitalis / Inhibited by triamterene
Indomethacin / ↑ Risk of nephrotoxicity and acute renal failure; use this combination only when clearly needed
Lithium / ↑ Chance of lithium toxicity R/T ↓ renal clearance
Potassium salts / Possible severe hyperkalemia → cardiac arrhythmias or cardiac arrest; do not use together
Preanesthetic drugs / Potentiated by triamterene
Skeletal muscle relaxants, nondepolarizing / Potentiated by triamterene
Spironolactone / Additive hyperkalemia

HOW SUPPLIED

Capsules: 50 mg, 100 mg.

DOSAGE

CAPSULES

Diuretic.

Titrate dosage to the individual needs of the client. **Adults, initial:** 100 mg twice a day after meals; **maximum dai-**

ly dose: 300 mg. Use a lower initial dose when combined with another diuretic or antihypertensive agent.

NURSING IMPLICATIONS

Ⓢ Do not confuse triamterene with trimipramine (antidepressant).

IMPLEMENTATION/ADMINISTRATION/STORAGE

1. Minimize nausea by giving the drug after meals.
2. Store from 15–30°C (59–86°F); protect from light.

ASSESSMENT

1. Note reasons for therapy, characteristics of S&S, clinical presentation, other agents trialed; list agents prescribed to ensure none interact.
2. Assess for alcoholism; megaloblastic anemia may occur because triamterene is a weak antagonist of folic acid.
3. Monitor BP, weight, ECG, CBC, BS, uric acid, electrolytes, I&O, and renal function.

CLIENT/FAMILY TEACHING

1. Take in the a.m. with food to minimize GI upset/nausea.
2. Drug may cause dizziness; assess response before performing activities that require alertness.
3. Persistent headaches, fever, rash, drowsiness, vomiting, restlessness, mental wandering, lethargy, and foul breath may be signs of uremia; report.
4. Avoid alcohol and OTC agents. Also avoid potassium supplements, salt substitutes that contain potassium, and foods high in potassium; drug is potassium-sparing.
5. Urine may appear pale fluorescent blue.
6. Avoid direct sunlight for prolonged periods; may cause a photosensitivity reaction. Use sunscreens, sunglasses, hat, long sleeves, and pants when exposed.
7. Keep all F/U to assess response, labs, and for adverse SE.

OUTCOMES/EVALUATE

↓ Edema; ↑ diuresis; ↓ BP

Combination Drug

Triamterene and Hydrochlorothiazide

(try-**AM**-teh-reen, hy-droh-**kloh**-roh-**THIGH**-ah-zyd)

Classification(s): Antihypertensive, combination drug

Pregnancy Category: C

RX: Dyazide, Maxzide, Maxzide-25 MG.

🍁 **Rx:** Apo-Triazide, Novo-Triamzide, Nu-Triazide.

SEE ALSO ***HYDROCHLOROTHIAZIDE*** AND ***TRIAMTERENE***.

INDICATIONS/USES

Hypertension or edema in clients who manifest hypokalemia on hydrochlorothiazide alone. In clients requiring a diuretic and in whom hypokalemia cannot be risked (i.e., clients with cardiac arrhythmias or those taking digitalis). Usually not the first line of therapy, except for clients in whom hypokalemia should be avoided.

CONTENT

Capsules: Hydrochlorothiazide (*thiazide diuretic*), 25 or 50 mg and triamterene, (*potassium-sparing diuretic*), 37.5, 50, or 100 mg. **Tablets:** Hydrochlorothiazide, 25 or 50 mg and triamterene, 37.5 or 75 mg. (In Canada the tablets contain 25 mg of hydrochlorothiazide and 50 mg triamterene.)

ACTION/KINETICS

Action

Triamterene acts directly on the distal tubule to promote the excretion of sodium, bicarbonate, chloride, and fluid. It increases urinary pH. Hydrochlorothiazide promotes the excretion of sodium and chloride, and thus water by the distal renal tubule. Also increases excretion of potassium and to a lesser extent bicarbonate. The antihypertensive effect is thought to be due to direct dilation of the areterioles, as well as to a reduction in the total fluid volume of the body and altered sodium balance.

Pharmacokinetics

Triamterene. Onset: 2–4 hr. **Peak effect:** 6–8 hr. **Duration:** 7–9 hr. **t½:** 3 hr. Metabolized to hydroxytriamterene sulfate, which is also active.

About 20% is excreted unchanged through the urine.

Hydrochlorothiazide. Onset: 2 hr. **Peak effect:** 4–6 hr. **Duration:** 6–12 hr. **t½:** 5.6–14.8 hr. Hydrochlorothiazide is not metabolized but is eliminated rapidly by the kidney.

CONTRAINDICATIONS

Clients receiving other potassium-sparing drugs such as amiloride and spironolactone. Use in anuria, acute or chronic renal insufficiency, significant renal impairment, preexisting elevated serum potassium.

SPECIAL CONCERNS

- **Geriatric clients may be more sensitive to the hypotensive and electrolyte effects of this combination; also, age-related decreases in renal function may require a decrease in dosage.**
- **Use with caution during lactation.**

SIDE EFFECTS

Most Common

N&V, headache, anorexia, GI upset, diarrhea, flatulence, dizziness, photosensitivity.

See Diuretics, Thiazides, and *Triamterene* for a complete list of possible side effects.

LABORATORY TEST CONSIDERATIONS

Triamterene may impart blue fluorescence to urine, interfering with fluorometric assays (e.g., lactic dehydrogenase, quinidine). ↑ BUN, creatinine. ↑ Serum uric acid in clients predisposed to gouty arthritis.

HOW SUPPLIED

See *Content*.

DOSAGE

CAPSULES

Hypertension or edema.

Adults: Triamterene/hydrochlorothiazide, 37.5 mg/25 mg: 1–2 capsules given once daily with monitoring of serum potassium and clinical effect. Triamterene/hydrochlorothiazide, 50 mg/25 mg: 1–2 capsules twice a day after meals. Some clients may be controlled using 1 capsule every day or every other day. No more than 4 capsules should be taken daily.

TABLETS

Hypertension or edema.

Adults: Triamterene/hydrochlorothiazide, 37.5 mg/25 mg: 1–2 tablets/day (determined by individual titration with the components). Or triamterene/hydrochlorothiazide: 75 mg/50 mg to 1 tablet daily.

NURSING IMPLICATIONS

IMPLEMENTATION/ADMINISTRATION/STORAGE

Monitor clients who are transferred from less bioavailable formulations of triamterene and hydrochlorothiazide for serum potassium levels following the transfer.

ASSESSMENT

1. Note reasons for therapy, other agents trialed; list agents prescribed to ensure none interact.
2. Assess for alcoholism; megaloblastic anemia may occur because triamterene is a weak antagonist of folic acid. Note any history of kidney stones.
3. Monitor BP, weight, ECG, CBC, BS, uric acid, electrolytes, I&O, renal and LFTs; reduce dose with dysfunction.

CLIENT/FAMILY TEACHING

1. Drug is used to lower BP and reduce swelling of extremities. Take in the a.m. with food to minimize GI upset/nausea and nighttime voiding.
2. Use care, drug may cause dizziness/drowsiness; change positions slowly to prevent sudden drop in BP. Report any adverse effects, including sore throat, rash, or fever (S&S of blood dyscrasia) or lack of effectiveness.
3. Persistent headaches, drowsiness, vomiting, restlessness, mental wandering, lethargy, and foul breath may be signs of uremia; report. Any decrease in urinary output, jaundice, muscle cramps, weakness, nausea, blurred vision, or dizziness warrant reporting.
4. Avoid alcohol and OTC agents. Also limit sodium intake and avoid potassium supplements, salt substitutes that contain potassium, and foods high in potassium; drug is potassium-sparing.
5. Urine may appear pale fluorescent blue. Consume 2–3 L/day of fluids to prevent dehydration.

T

6. Avoid direct sunlight for prolonged periods; may cause a photosensitivity reaction. Use sunscreens, sunglasses, hat, and long sleeves and pants when exposed.
7. To help control BP: maintain healthy diet and limit intake of caffeine, avoid alcohol, salt substitutes, or high Na and high K foods, perform regular exercise, maintain weight, and stop smoking.
8. Keep all F/U to assess response, labs, BP, and for adverse SE.

OUTCOMES/EVALUATE

- Control of hypertension
- Resolution of edema

Triazolam

(try-**AYZ**-oh-lam)

Classification(s): Sedative-hypnotic, benzodiazepine

Pregnancy Category: X

RX: Halcion, **C-IV**

Rx: Apo-Triazo, Gen-Triazolam.

SEE ALSO ***TRANQUILIZERS, ANTIMANIC DRUGS,*** AND ***HYPNOTICS.***

INDICATIONS/USES

(1) Insomnia (short-term management, not to exceed 1 month). (2) May be beneficial in preventing or treating transient insomnia from a sudden change in sleep schedule.

ACTION/KINETICS

Action

Decreases sleep latency, increases the duration of sleep, and decreases the number of awakenings.

Pharmacokinetics

Time to peak plasma levels: 0.5–2 hr. **t½:** 1.5–5.5 hr. Metabolized in liver; inactive metabolites excreted in the urine. **Plasma protein binding:** 90%.

CONTRAINDICATIONS

Use concomitantly with itraconazole, ketoconazole, nefaxodone. Lactation (may cause sedation and feeding problems in infants).

SPECIAL CONCERNS

- Elderly may be more sensitive to the effects of triazolam.
- Safety and efficacy not established in children under 18 years of age.

SIDE EFFECTS

Most Common

Drowsiness, headache, dizziness, nervousness, light-headedness, coordination disorders/ataxia, N&V.

See *Tranquilizers, Antimanic Drugs, and Hypnotics* for a complete list of possible side effects. **CNS:** Rebound insomnia, anterograde amnesia, headache, ataxia, decreased coordination, traveler's amnesia. Psychologic and physical dependence. **GI:** N&V.

DRUG INTERACTIONS

Azole antifungals / ↑ Triazolam effect R/T ↓ liver metabolism
Clarithromycin / ↑ Triazolam effect R/T ↓ liver metabolism
Erythromycin / ↑ Triazolam effect R/T ↓ liver metabolism
Grapefruit juice / ↑ Triazolam effect R/T ↓ liver metabolism
Modafinil / ↑ Triazolam mean AUC and mean peak plasma levels
Protease inhibitors / ↑ Triazolam effect R/T ↓ liver metabolism
SSRIs / ↑ Triazolam effect R/T ↓ liver metabolism

HOW SUPPLIED

Tablets: 0.125 mg, 0.25 mg.

DOSAGE

TABLETS

Insomnia.

Adults, initial: 0.25–0.5 mg before bedtime. **Geriatric or debilitated clients, initial:** 0.125 mg; **then,** depending on response, 0.125–0.25 mg before bedtime.

NURSING IMPLICATIONS

ASSESSMENT

1. Note reasons for therapy, onset, duration, characteristics of S&S. Assess mental status

and note behavioral manifestations or evidence/history of depression.
2. Evaluate sleep patterns; determine underlying cause of insomnia so that source may be removed. With simple insomnia, try nonpharmacologic interventions to induce sleep, such as soft music, guided imagery, no daytime napping, or progressive muscle relaxation.
3. Initiate safety precautions (i.e., side rails, supervised ambulation, frequent observations), especially with elderly and confused clients.
4. Assess for tolerance and for psychologic and physical dependence. Monitor closely for CNS toxic effects especially during prolonged therapy (longer than 2 weeks). Monitor CBC and LFTs.

CLIENT/FAMILY TEACHING

1. Take only as directed. Store away from bedside.
2. Use caution when driving or operating machinery until daytime sedative effects evaluated. May notice morning drowsiness or tiredness.
3. Drug is for short-term use only; may cause physical and psychological dependence. Try warm baths/milk, and other methods to induce sleep, such as white noise simulator, soft music, guided imagery, or progressive muscle relaxation, rather than become dependent on drugs for insomnia.
4. Avoid alcohol and CNS depressants. Report unusual side effects, including hallucinations, nightmares, depression, or periods of confusion.
5. Record sleep diary, noting all foods, drinks, drugs consumed, activities before bedtime for provider review.
6. Keep all F/U to assess response, tolerance and for adverse SE.

OUTCOMES/EVALUATE

Improved sleeping patterns; insomnia relief

Combination Drug

IV

Trimethoprim and Sulfamethoxazole

(try-**METH**-oh-prim, sul-fah-meh-**THOX**-ah-zohl)

Classification(s): Antibiotic, combination

Pregnancy Category: C

RX: Bactrim, Bactrim DS, Septra, Septra DS, Sulfatrim.

Rx: Apo-Sulfatrim, Apo-Sulfatrim DS, Apo-Sulfatrim Pediatric, Novo-Trimel, Novo-Trimel DS, Nu-Cotrimox, Septra Injection.

SEE ALSO ***SULFONAMIDES***.

INDICATIONS/USES

PO:

1. Acute exacerbations of chronic bronchitis in adults due to *Haemophilus influenzae* or *Streptococcus pneumoniae*.
2. Acute otitis media in children due to *H. influenzae* or *S. pneumoniae*.
3. Enteritis in adults and children due to *Shigella flexneri* or *Shigella sonnei*.
4. Prophylaxis and treatment of *Pneumocystis carinii* pneumonitis in children and adults.
5. UTIs in adults and children due to *Escherichia coli, Klebsiella,* and *Enterobacter* species, *Proteus mirabilis* and *vulgaris,* and *Morganella morganii.*
6. Traveler's diarrhea in adults due to *E. coli.*

Investigational: Acute and chronic bacterial prostatitis in adults. Cholera and salmonella-type infections and nocardiosis in adults due to *Vibrio cholerae, Salmonella* species, and *Nocardia* species. Prophylaxis of recurrent UTIs in women. Skin and soft-tissue infections in adults and children due to methicillin-sensitive *Staphylococcus aureus* or methicillin-resistant *S. aureus.*

IV:

1. Enteritis in adults due to *S. flexneri* or *S. sonnei.*
2. Treatment of *P. carinii* pneumonitis in adults.
3. Severe or complicated UTIs in adults and children due to *E. coli, Klebsiella* and *Enterobacter* species, *P. mirabilis* and *P. vulgaris,* and *M. morganii.*

Investigational: Skin and soft-tissue infections in children due to methicillin-sensitive *S. aureus* or methicillin-resistant *S. aureus.* Cholera and salmonella-type infections and nocardiosis in adults due to *Vibrio cholerae, Salmonella* species, and *Nocardia* species.

CONTENT

These products contain the antibacterial agents sulfamethoxazole and trimethoprim.

T

Concentrate for injection: Sulfamethoxazole, 80 mg, and trimethoprim, 16 mg/mL.

Oral Suspension: Sulfamethoxazole, 200 mg, and trimethoprim, 40 mg/5 mL.

Tablets: Sulfamethoxazole, 400 mg, and trimethoprim, 80 mg/tablet.

Tablets, Double Strength (DS): Sulfamethoxazole, 800 mg, and trimethoprim, 160 mg/tablet.

ACTION/KINETICS

Action

Sulfamethoxazole inhibits bacterial synthesis of dihydrofolic acid by competing with para-aminobenzoic acid. Trimethoprim blocks the production of tetrahydrofolic acid by inhibiting the enzyme dihydrofolate reductase. Thus, this combination blocks two consecutive steps in the bacterial biosynthesis of essential nucleic acids and proteins essential to many bacteria.

Pharmacokinetics

The combination is rapidly and completely absorbed after PO use. Widely distributed throughout the body. **Peak plasma levels, after PO:** 1–4 hr; **after IV:** 1–1.5 hr. **Steady-state:** After 3 days. Urine concentrations are considerably higher than serum levels. **Sulfamethoxazole, t½, after PO:** 10 hr; **after IV:** 12.8 hr. **Trimethoprim, t½, after PO:** 8–10 hr; **after IV:** 11.3 hr. t½s are increased significantly in those with severely impaired renal function. Sulfamethoxazole is metabolized to inactive compounds, whereas trimethoprim is metabolized only to a small extent. Both are excreted through the kidneys.

CONTRAINDICATIONS

Hypersensitivity to trimethoprim or sulfonamides. Infants under 2 months of age. Pregnancy and lactation. Documented megaloblastic anemia due to folate deficiency. Marked hepatic damage. Severe renal insufficiency when status of renal function cannot be monitored. Use to treat group A beta-hemolytic streptococci infections.

SPECIAL CONCERNS

- **Use with caution in impaired liver or kidney function or with possible folate deficiency.**
- **AIDS clients may not tolerate or respond to this product.**
- **Hematologic changes indicative of folic acid deficiency may occur in the elderly or in those with preexisting folic acid deficiency or kidney failure.**

SIDE EFFECTS

Most Common

N&V, anorexia, rash, urticaria.

GI: Glossitis, anorexia, stomatitis, N&V, emesis, abdominal pain, diarrhea, pseudomembranous enterocolitis, hepatitis (including cholestatic jaundice and ***fulminant hepatic necrosis***), ***pancreatitis***, *Clostridium difficile*-associated diarrhea. **CNS:** Headache, mental depression, ***seizures***, ataxia, hallucinations, vertigo, insomnia, apathy, nervousness, aseptic meningitis, peripheral neuritis. **Musculoskeletal:** Arthralgia, myalgia, rhabdomyolysis (mainly in AIDS clients). **Respiratory:** Pulmonary infiltrates, cough, SOB. **GU:** Renal failure, interstitial nephritis, toxic nephrosis with oliguria and anuria, crystalluria, nephrotoxicity in association with cyclosporine. **Hematologic:** ***Agranulocytosis, aplastic anemia***, hemolytic anemia, megaloblastic anemia, thrombocytopenia, leukopenia, neutropenia, hypoprothrombinemia, eosinophilia, methemoglobinemia. **Hypersensitivity:** Erythema multiforme, ***Stevens-Johnson syndrome***, generalized skin eruptions, rash, toxic epidermal necrolysis, urticaria, serum sickness-like syndrome, pruritus, exfoliative dermatitis, ***anaphylaxis***, conjunctival and scleral injection, photosensitivity, allergic myocarditis, angioedema, drug fever, chills, Henoch-Schonlein purpura, systemic lupus erythematosus, generalized allergic reactions, periarteritis nodosa. **Metabolic:** Hyperkalemia, hyponatremia, hypoglycemia. **At infusion site:** Local irritation and inflammation due to extravasation. **Body as a whole:** Fatigue, weakness. **Miscellaneous:** Tinnitus, diuresis, and hypoglycemia (rare).

LABORATORY TEST CONSIDERATIONS

↑ Serum transaminase, bilirubin, and creatinine; BUN. Crystalluria. The drugs may interfere with the Jaffe alkaline picrate reaction assay for creatinine, resulting in overestimation by about 10% in the range of normal values. Trimethoprim: Possible interference with a serum methotrexate assay as determined by the competitive binding protein technique when a bacterial dihydrofolate reductase is used as the binding protein (no interference if methotrexate is measured by radioimmunoassay).

OVERDOSE MANAGEMENT

Symptoms: **Acute:** Anorexia, colic, N&V, dizziness, headache, drowsiness, unconsciousness, pyrexia, hematuria, crystalluria, depression, confusion; blood dyscrasias and jaundice are late manifestations. **Chronic:** Bone marrow depression manifested as thrombocytopenia, leukopenia, or megaloblastic anemia. *Treatment:*

- Usual supportive measures.
- Perform gastric lavage or emesis.
- Force oral fluids and give IV fluids if urine output is low and renal function is normal.
- Acidifying the urine will increase renal elimination of trimethoprim.
- Monitor blood counts and appropriate blood chemistries, including electrolytes.
- If blood dyscrasias or jaundice occur, begin specific therapy, including leucovorin, 5–15 mg/day.
- Peritoneal dialysis is not effective, and hemodialysis is only moderately effective in eliminating these drugs.

DRUG INTERACTIONS

NOTE: An additive effect of trazodone with other drugs that prolong the QT interval is possible. The following drugs may prolong the QT interval and increase the risk of life-threatening cardiac arrhythmias, including torsades de pointes: Amiodarone, arsenic trioxide, bretylium, chlorpromazine, disopyramide, dofetilide, dolasetron, droperidol, mefloquine, mesoridazine, moxifloxacin, pentamidine, pimozide, procainamide, quinidine, sotalol, tacrolimus, thioridazine, and ziprasidone.
ACE inhibitors / Hyperkalemia with cardiac arrhythmias or cardiac arrest R/T ↓ potassium excretion; monitor serum potassium levels
Alcohol / Possible disulfiram-like reaction; avoid drinking alcohol and taking alcohol-containing medications
Cyclosporine / ↓ Cyclosporine effect; ↑ risk of nephrotoxicity; monitor cyclosporine blood/plasma levels and serum creatinine; monitor for evidence of graft rejection
Dapsone / ↑ Plasma levels of both drugs → ↑ effect of both dapsone and trimethoprim; closely monitor for sulfone toxicity (e.g., methemoglobinemia)
Digoxin / ↑ Plasma digoxin levels, especially in the elderly; monitor digoxin levels
Dofetilide / ↑ Plasma dofetilide levels → ↑ risk of ventricular arrhythmias, including torsades de pointes. Do not use together
Hydantoins (e.g., phenytoin) / ↑ Phenytoin plasma levels and prolonged $t^{1/2}$ → ↑ risk of pharmacologic/toxic effects; monitor phenytoin levels and observe for toxicity
Indomethacin / ↑ Plasma sulfamethoxazole levels → ↑ pharmacologic/toxic effects
Methenamine / Potential for formation of insoluble precipitates in urine; use together contraindicated
Methotrexate / ↑ Risk of methotrexate toxicity R/T displacement from plasma protein binding sites; also, ↑ risk of methotrexate-induced bone marrow suppression and megaloblastic anemia; monitor hematologic status
Procainamide / ↑ Plasma procainamide and N-acetylprocainamide levels → ↑ pharmacologic procainamide effects; monitor plasma levels
Pyrimethamine / ↑ Risk of megaloblastic anemia in those receiving more than 25 mg pyrimethamine/week; assess for hematologic and neurologic signs of megaloblastic anemia
Repaglinide / ↑ Plasma repaglinide levels → ↑ risk of hypoglycemia; monitor BG
Sulfonylureas / ↑ Risk of hypoglycemia; monitor BG
Thiazide diuretics / ↑ Risk of thrombocytopenia with purpura in geriatric clients; monitor platelet count; may need to discontinue one or both drugs
Thiazolidinediones (e.g., pioglitazone) / ↑ Plasma thiazolidinedione levels → ↑ risk of hypoglycemia and other side effects; monitor BG
Tretinoin / Augmentation of phototoxicity; do not use together
Tricyclic antidepressants (e.g., amitriptyline) / ↓ Effect of tricyclic antidepressants; monitor response
Vaccines, live / Possible ↓ effectiveness of live vaccines
Warfarin / ↑ PT; monitor anticoagulant parameters and adjust dose as needed

HOW SUPPLIED

See *Content.*

DOSAGE

DOUBLE-STRENGTH (DS) TABLETS; ORAL SUSPENSION; TABLETS

Adults: Acute exacerbations of chronic bronchitis, enteritis, UTIs.

Adults: Sulfamethoxazole, 800 mg, and trimethoprim, 160 mg (i.e., 1 DS tablet, 2 tablets, or 4 teaspoonfuls of suspension) q 12 hr for 14 days to treat ex-

T

acerbations of chronic bronchitis, q 12 hr for 5 days to treat enteritis, and q 12 hr for 10–14 days to treat UTIs.

Children: Acute otitis media, enteritis, and UTIs.

Children, 2 months of age and older: Sulfamethoxazole, 40 mg/kg/day, and trimethoprim, 8 mg/kg/day, in 2 divided doses q 12 hr for 10 days to treat acute otitis media and UTIs and q 12 hr for days to treat enteritis. The following is a dosage guideline: **Body weight, 10 kg:** 5 mL of the suspension; **20 kg:** 10 mL of the suspension or 1 tablet; **30 kg:** 15 mL of the suspension or 1½ tablets; and **40 kg:** 20 mL of the suspension, 2 tablets, or 1 double-strength tablet.

Prophylaxis of P. carinii *pneumonia.*

Adults: Sulfamethoxazole, 800 mg, and trimethoprim, 160 mg, q 24 hr. Alternatively (investigational): Sulfamethoxazole, 400 mg, and trimethoprim, 80 mg, q 24 hr or sulfamethoxazole, 800 mg, and trimethoprim, 160 mg, 3 times a week. **Children:** Sulfamethoxazole, 750 mg/m^2, and trimethoprim, 150 mg/m^2, each day given in equally divided doses twice a day, on 3 consecutive days per week. Do not exceed a total daily dose of sulfamethoxazole, 1,600 mg, and trimethoprim, 320 mg.

Treatment of P. carinii *pneumonia.*

Adults and children: Sulfamethoxazole, 75–100 mg/kg/day, and trimethoprim, 15–20 mg/kg/day, given in equally divided doses q 6 hr for 14–21 days.

Traveler's diarrhea.

Adults: Sulfamethoxazole, 800 mg, and trimethoprim, 160 mg (i.e., 1 DS tablets), q 12 hr for 5 days.

Prostatitis, acute and chronic bacterial (Investigational).

Adults: Sulfamethoxazole, 800 mg, and trimethoprim, 160 mg (i.e., 1 DS tablet), twice a day for up to 12 weeks.

Nocardiosis (Investigational).

Adults: 1 mg/kg/day (based on trimethoprim) in 2 to 4 divided doses for 3–4 weeks; **then** decrease dose to 10 mg/kg/day (based on trimethoprim) in 2 to 4 divided doses for 3–6 months.

Prevention of recurrent UTIs in women (investigational).

Adult women: Sulfamethoxazole, 200 mg/day, and trimethoprim, 40 mg/day, at bedtime given a minimum of 3 times/week or postcoitally.

Skin and soft-tissue infections (investigational).

Adults: Sulfamethoxazole, 800–1,600 mg, and trimethoprim, 160–320 mg, twice a day. **Children:** 8–12 mg/kg (based on trimethoprim) in equally divided doses q 12 hr.

IV INFUSION

Enteritis, severe or complicated UTIs.

Adults and children: 8–10 mg/kg/day (based on trimethoprim) in 2 to 4 divided doses q 6, 8, or 12 hr for 5 days for enteritis and for up to 14 days for severe UTIs. **Maximum dose:** 60 mL/day (based on trimethoprim).

Treatment of P. carinii *pneumonia.*

Adults and children: 15–20 mg/kg/day (based on trimethoprim) in 3 or 4 equally divided doses q 6–8 hr for up to 14 days. For severely ill clients who are receiving continuous venovenous hemodiafiltration, a dose up to 10 mg/kg IV q 12 hr may be necessary.

Skin and soft-tissue infections in children (Investigational).

Children: 8–12 mg/kg (based on trimethoprim) in equally divided doses q 6 hr.

Nocardiosis (Investigational).

Adults, initial: 15 mg/kg/day (based on trimethoprim) in 2 to 4 divided doses for 3–4 weeks; **then** decrease the dose to 10 mg/kg/day (based on trimethoprim) in 2 to 4 divided doses for 3–6 months.

NURSING IMPLICATIONS

IMPLEMENTATION/ADMINISTRATION/STORAGE

1. **For clients with impaired renal function the following dosage is recommended: C_{CR} of**

T

15–30 mL/min: One-half the usual regimen, and for C_{CR} less than 15 mL/min: Use is not recommended.

2. The following is an alternate dosing regimen for trimethoprim/sulfamethoxazole for both PO and IV use: If C_{CR} is 30–50 mL/min, the dose of trimethoprim is 5–7.5 mg/kg/dose q 8 hr. If C_{CR} is 10–29 mL/min, the dose of trimethoprim is 5–10 mg/kg/dose q 12 hr. If C_{CR} is <10 mL/min, if the client is on hemodialysis, or if the client is on peritoneal dialysis, use of trimethoprim is not recommended; however, if used, give a dose of trimethoprim of 5–10 mg/kg/dose q 24 hr. For continuous renal replacement therapy, a dose of trimethoprim of 5–7.5 mg/kg/dose q 8 hr can be used.
3. **IV** Dilute each 5 mL vial to 125 mL with D5W and use within 6 hr. If a dilution of 5 mL/100 mL D5W is desired, use within 4 hr. If the amount of fluid should be restricted, each 5 mL can be diluted up to 75 mL with D5W and used within 2 hr. Do not refrigerate the diluted solution.
4. Administer IV infusion over a 60–90 min period. Avoid rapid infusion or bolus injection. Do not give IM.
5. As an alternative to the dose recommended for clients on hemodialysis, a dose of 5–20 mg/kg (based on trimethoprim) IV 3 times/week may be used in adults (assuming the client is receiving standard intermittent hemodialysis 3 times/week and completes the full dialysis sessions). Also, as an alternative a dose of 2.5–5 mg/kg (based on trimethoprim) q 12 hr is recommended for clients receiving continuous venovenous hemofiltration, continuous venovenous hemodialysis, or continuous venovenous hemodiafiltration; this dose assumes ultrafiltration and dialysis flow rates of 1–2 L/hr.
6. If the diluted IV infusion is cloudy or precipitates after mixing, discard and prepare a new solution.
7. Store vials from 15–30°C (59–86°F). Do not refrigerate; protect from light. After initial entry into the multidose vial, use the remaining contents within 48 hr.
8. COMPATIBILITY D5W.
9. INCOMPATIBILITY Do not mix the IV infusion with any other drugs or solutions.

ASSESSMENT

1. Note reasons for therapy, onset, characteristics of S&S, other agents trialed and culture results.
2. Assess for megaloblastic anemia; drug inhibits its ability to produce folinic acid. Simultaneous administration of folic acid (6–8 mg/day) may prevent antifolate drug effects.
3. Determine any severe allergy or bronchial asthma, sulfite sensitivity or G6PD-deficiency conditions, malabsorption problems, seizures, or alcoholism; requires close monitoring. Discontinue at the first sign of skin rash or adverse reaction.
4. If infected with AIDS virus, may be intolerant to product.
5. Monitor VS, I&O, lung sounds, cultures, CBC, urinalysis, renal and LFTs; reduce dose with dysfunction.

CLIENT/FAMILY TEACHING

1. Take with a full glass of water as directed. Complete entire prescription and do not share.
2. Report any symptoms of fever, inflammation/swelling of veins/lymph glands, N&V, watery diarrhea, skin rash, joint pain/swelling, mental disturbances, or lack of response.
3. Consume 2.5–3 L of fluids/day to prevent crystalluria and dehydration.
4. May experience dizziness, use caution with activities that require mental alertness.
5. Avoid during pregnancy.
6. Avoid prolonged sun exposure; use protective clothing, sunglasses, and sunscreen if exposure necessary.
7. Keep all F/U to assess response and for adverse SE.

OUTCOMES/EVALUATE

- Resolution of infection
- *P. carinii* pneumonia prophylaxis

Triptorelin pamoate

(**TRIP**-toh-rel-in)

Classification(s): Antineoplastic, gonadotropin-releasing hormone analog

Pregnancy Category: X

RX: Trelstar.

SEE ALSO ***ANTINEOPLASTIC AGENTS***.

T

INDICATIONS/USES

Palliative treatment of advanced prostate cancer when orchiectomy or estrogen therapy are either not indicated or unacceptable. *Investigational:* Ovarian cancer, pancreatic carcinoma, endometriosis, hyperandrogenism, growth hormone deficiency, in vitro fertilization, uterine leiomyomata. In children to treat central precocious puberty.

ACTION/KINETICS

Action

A synthetic decapeptide agonist analog of luteinizing hormone releasing hormone (LHRH or GnRH). Potent inhibitor of gonadotropic secretion when given continuously. Initially, there is a transient surge in circulating LH, FSH, estradiol, and testosterone. However, after 2–4 weeks, a sustained decrease in LH and FSH secretion and marked reduction of testicular and ovarian steroidogenesis occurs. In men, levels of serum testosterone fall to those seen in surgically castrated men. Thus, tissues and functions that depend on testosterone for maintenance become quiescent. These effects are reversible upon discontinuing therapy.

Pharmacokinetics

IM injection of the depot formulation achieves plasma levels over a 1 month period. **Time to maximum levels:** 1–3 hr. Metabolism is unknown but probably involves hepatic microsomal enzymes. Eliminated by the liver and kidneys. Is distributed and eliminated by a 3-compartment model; **t½:** About 6 min, 45 min, and 3 hr. There is a 2- to 4-fold increase in AUC in clients with impaired renal function.

CONTRAINDICATIONS

Hypersensitivity to triptorelin, other components of the product, other GnRH agonists, or GnRH. Women who are or may become pregnant. Lactation.

SPECIAL CONCERNS

- **Initially, due to transient increase in serum testosterone levels, there may be worsening signs and symptoms of prostate cancer during the first few weeks of treatment.**
- **Rarely, pituitary apoplexy occurs (see *Side Effects* for symptoms); immediate medical attention is required.**
- **Safety and efficacy not determined in children.**

SIDE EFFECTS

Most Common

Hot flushes, hypertension, headache, nausea, impotence, dysuria, skeletal/leg pain, leg edema, injection site pain, pain.

Worsening of signs/symptoms of prostate cancer: Bone pain, neuropathy, hematuria, urethral or bladder outlet obstruction, spinal cord compression with weakness or paralysis of lower extremities.

Side effects listed are combined for the three dosage strengths. **CNS:** Headache, insomnia, dizziness, emotional lability. **GI:** N&V, diarrhea, abdominal pain, anorexia, constipation, dyspepsia, ***pituitary apoplexy*** (includes symptoms of sudden headache, vomiting, visual changes, ophthalmoplegia, altered mental status, CV collapse). **CV:** Hypertension. **GU:** Impotence, urinary retention, UTI, breast pain, decreased libido, dysuria, gynecomastia, erectile dysfunction, testicular atrophy. **Musculoskeletal:** Skeletal pain, leg cramps/pain, arthralgia, back pain, myalgia, chest pain, pain in extremity. **Respiratory:** Coughing, dyspnea, pharyngitis, bronchitis. **Dermatologic:** Hot flushes, pruritus, rash. **Hematologic:** Anemia. **Metabolic:** Dependent edema, leg edema, peripheral edema, diabetes mellitus/hyperglycemia. **Hypersensitivity:** Angioedema, allergic reactions, ***anaphylactic shock.*** **Injection site:** Pain, local reactions. **Ophthalmic:** Conjunctivitis, eye pain. **Body as a whole:** Fatigue, pain, asthenia, influenza.

LABORATORY TEST CONSIDERATIONS

Suppression of the pituitary-gonadal axis may cause misleading results of diagnostic tests. Abnormal LFTs.

Triptorelin 11.25 mg: ↑ Glucose, serum urea nitrogen, AST, ALT, alkaline phosphatase. ↓ Hemoglobin and RBCs.

Triptorelin 22.5 mg: ↑ Glucose, hepatic transaminases. ↓ Hemoglobin.

DRUG INTERACTIONS

Do not give hyperprolactinemic drugs together with triptorelin, since hyperprolactinemia reduces the number of pituitary GnRH receptors.

HOW SUPPLIED

Injection, Lyophilized Microgranules for Suspension: 3.75 mg, 11.25 mg, 22.5 mg.

DOSAGE

IM

Advanced prostate cancer.

Adults: 3.75 mg IM once q 4 weeks, 11.25 mg IM once q 12 weeks, or 22.5 mg IM once q 24 weeks.

Central precocious puberty in children (investigational).

Children: 3.75 mg IM monthly. Consider giving calcium supplements.

NURSING IMPLICATIONS

IMPLEMENTATION/ADMINISTRATION/STORAGE

1. Give IM immediately after reconstitution. Inject the suspension into either buttock. Alter IM injection site periodically.
2. Follow package insert for preparation for administration.
3. Discard if not used immediately after reconstitution.
4. Store from 20–25°C (68–77°F).
5. Reconstitute in sterile water. Do not use any diluent, other than sterile water, to reconstitute.

ASSESSMENT

1. Note symptom onset, PSA levels, biopsy/staging results, other therapies trialed, outcome.
2. Carefully assess those with metastatic vertebral lesions and/or with upper or lower urinary tract obstruction during the first few weeks of therapy.
3. Monitor PSA, alkaline phosphatase, calcium, cholesterol profile, testosterone levels, CBC, renal and LFTs. Monitor response to triptorelin by measuring serum levels of testosterone.

CLIENT/FAMILY TEACHING

1. Drug therapy of the depo product consists of monthly IM injections and the LA product is every 84 days. Must continue to prevent progression of disease.
2. Hot flashes may occur with drug therapy R/T chemical castration.
3. May initially experience worsening of symptoms and/or onset of new symptoms such as bone pain, urine blood/obstruction, and numbness/tingling during the first few weeks of therapy. Immediately report any weakness, numbness, itching/hives/rash, respiratory difficulty or impaired urination.
4. Keep all F/U to assess response, labs, and for adverse SE.
5. Identify local support groups that assist in coping with disease.

OUTCOMES/EVALUATE

↓ Prostate tumor size and spread

IV

Tubocurarine chloride

(too-boh-kyour-**AR**-een)

Classification(s): Neuromuscular blocking drug

Pregnancy Category: C

RX: Tubocurarine Cl.

SEE ALSO ***NEUROMUSCULAR BLOCKING AGENTS.***

INDICATIONS/USES

(1) Muscle relaxant during surgery or setting of fractures and dislocations. (2) Spasticity caused by injury to or disease of CNS. (3) Treat seizures electrically induced or induced by drugs. (4) Diagnosis of myasthenia gravis.

ACTION/KINETICS

Action

Cumulative effects may occur. Most likely of the nondepolarizing drugs to cause histamine release. Narrow margin between therapeutic dose and toxic dose.

Pharmacokinetics

Onset, IV: 1 min; **IM:** 15–25 min. **Time to peak effect, IV:** 2–5 min. **Duration, IV:** 20–90 min. **t½:** 1–3 hr. About 43% excreted unchanged in urine.

ADDITIONAL CONTRAINDICATIONS

Clients in whom release of histamine is hazardous.

SPECIAL CONCERNS

- Use with caution during pregnancy and lactation and in children.
- If repeated doses are used before delivery, the newborn may manifest decreased skeletal muscle activity.

T

- **Children up to 1 month of age may be more sensitive to the effects of tubocurarine.**
- **Use with extreme caution in clients with renal dysfunction, liver disease, or obstructive states.**

SIDE EFFECTS

Most Common

Skeletal muscle weakness, prolonged skeletal muscle relaxation, respiratory insufficiency/apnea, flushing, increased salivation.

See *Neuromuscular Blocking Agents* for a complete list of possible side effects. Also, **Allergic reactions:** Excessive histamine secretion and circulatory collapse.

OVERDOSE MANAGEMENT

Symptoms: Respiratory insufficiency. *Treatment:* Overdosage chiefly treated by artificial respiration, although neostigmine, atropine, and edrophonium chloride should also be on hand.

ADDITIONAL DRUG INTERACTIONS

Acetylcholine / Antagonizes effect of tubocurarine
Anticholinesterases / Antagonizes effect of tubocurarine
Calcium salts / ↑ Tubocurarine effect
Diazepam / ↑ Risk of malignant hyperthermia
Potassium / Antagonizes effect of tubocurarine
Propranolol / ↑ Tubocurarine effect
Quinine / ↑ Tubocurarine effect
Succinylcholine chloride / ↑ Relaxant effect of both drugs

HOW SUPPLIED

Injection: 3 mg (20 units/mL).

DOSAGE

IM; IV

Adjunct to surgical anesthesia.

Adults, IM, IV, initial: 6–9 mg (40–60 units); **then** 3–4.5 mg (20–30 units) in 3–5 min if needed. Supplemental doses of 3 mg (20 units) can be given for prolonged procedures. Dosage can be calculated on the basis of 1.1 units/kg. **Pediatric, up to 4 weeks of age, IV, initial:** 0.3 mg/kg; **then,** give subsequent doses in increments of 1/5–1/6 the initial dose. **Infants and children, IV:** 0.6 mg/kg.

Electroshock therapy.

Adults, IV: 0.165 mg/kg (1.1 units/kg) given over 30–90 sec. It is recommended that the initial dose be 3 mg less than the calculated total dose.

Diagnosis of myasthenia gravis.

Adults, IV: 0.004–0.033 mg/kg. A test dose should be given within 2–3 min with IV neostigmine, 1.5 mg, to minimize prolonged respiratory paralysis.

NURSING IMPLICATIONS

IMPLEMENTATION/ADMINISTRATION/STORAGE

1. **IV Give IV as a sustained injection over 1–1.5 min. May also be given IM.**
2. **Give in incremental doses until relaxation is reached.**
3. **Decrease the initial dose if the inhalation anesthetic used enhances the action of curariform drugs or with compromised renal function.**
4. **Review the drugs with which tubocurarine interacts.**
5. **Have neostigmine methylsulfate available as an antidote.**
6. **COMPATIBILITY D5W, 0.9% NaCl.**
7. **INCOMPATIBILITY Administer separately; incompatible with alkaline solutions and may form a precipitate when mixed (e.g., methohexital sodium or thiopental sodium).**

ASSESSMENT

1. **Note reasons for therapy (diagnostic or anesthetic), onset, characteristics of symptoms and clinical presentation.**
2. **Utilize a peripheral nerve stimulator (train of four) to assess neuromuscular response and recovery.**
3. **Record length of time receiving drug. Should only be used on a short-term basis and in a continuously monitored environment. May experience residual muscle weakness with prolonged therapy.**
4. **Client may be fully conscious and aware of surroundings and conversations.**
5. **Drug does not affect pain or anxiety; administer analgesics and antianxiety agents as needed.**
6. **Have neostigmine methylsulfate available as an antidote.**

7. Continually monitor VS, I&O, ECG, and lab studies. Drug can cause vagal stimulation resulting in bradycardia, hypotension, and cardiac arrhythmias.

CLIENT/FAMILY TEACHING

1. Drug used to control movement and permit procedures/treatments and will make you feel like you are paralyzed; sensation will return once drug is discontinued and wears off.
2. Will be unable to move or talk and a machine will do all breathing. This will be in a setting that permits continous monitoring; response assessed with a peripheral nerve stimulator.
3. Explain all procedures and exams as consciousness is not affected by therapy. Reassure will be medicated for pain and anxiety during therapy (will be able to see and hear). All functions will return once the medication is discontinued.
4. Report any adverse or unusual side effects once medication therapy completed.

OUTCOMES/EVALUATE

- Skeletal muscle relaxation
- Control of drug or electrically induced seizures
- Diagnosis of myasthenia gravis

U

Ustekinumab

(**US**-teh-**KIN**-yoo-mab)

Classification(s): Immunomodulator
Pregnancy Category: B
RX: Stelara.

INDICATIONS/USES

Treatment of adults (18 years and older) with moderate to severe plaque psoriasis who are candidates for phototherapy or systemic therapy.

ACTION/KINETICS

Action

Binds with high affinity and specificity to the p40 protein subunit used by both interleukin (IL)-12 and interleukin-23 cytokines. IL-12 and IL-23 are involved in inflammatory and immune responses, such as natural killer cell activation and CD4+ T-cell differentiation and activation. Ustekinumab disrupts IL-12 and IL-23 mediated signaling and cytokine cascade thus reducing inflammation.

Pharmacokinetics

Median time to reach T_{max}: 8.5 days. **Steady-state, after multiple doses:** 28 weeks. Metabolic pathway has not been studied but is expected to be degraded into small peptides and amino acids. t½ varies over a wide range (4.6 to 80 days).

CONTRAINDICATIONS

Use with any clinically important active infection, including active tuberculosis. Use of BCG vaccines during treatment or for 1 year prior or 1 year after ustekinumab treatment.

SPECIAL CONCERNS

- Safety of ustekinumab given with other immunosuppressive drugs or phototherapy not evaluated.
- Use caution when considering use of ustekinumab in those with a chronic infection or a history of recurrent infection. Those genetically deficient in IL-12/IL-23 are especially vulnerable to disseminated infections from mycobacteria (including nontuberculous, environmental mycobacteria), salmonella (including nontyphi-strains), and Bacillus Calmette-Guérin (BCG) vaccinations. Serious infections and fatal outcomes have been reported.
- Use caution when giving live vaccines to household contacts of clients receiving ustekinumab due to the potential for shedding from the household contact and transmission to the client.
- Use with caution during lactation.
- Safety and efficacy not determined in children.

SIDE EFFECTS

Most Common

Nasopharyngitis, URTI, headache, fatigue.

CNS: Headache, fatigue, depression. **GI:** Diarrhea. **Dermatologic:** Pruritus, cellulitis. **Musculoskeletal:** Back pain, myalgia. **Respiratory:** Nasopharyngitis, URTI, pharyngolaryngeal pain. **Injection site:** Erythema, bruising, hemorrhage, in-

U

duration, irritation, pain, pruritus, swelling. **Body as a whole:** Fatigue, cellulitis. **Miscellaneous:** Increased risk of infections and reactivation of latent infections (may be serious and include bacterial, fungal, and viral), malignancies (including nonmelanoma skin cancers, breast, colon, head and neck, kidney, prostate, and thyroid), immunogenicity.

LABORATORY TEST CONSIDERATIONS

Presence of ustekinumab in serum may interfere with the detection of anti-ustekinumab antibodies resulting in inconclusive results due to assay interference.

DRUG INTERACTIONS

Consider monitoring for therapeutic effect (e.g., warfarin) or drug concentration (e.g., cyclosporine) in those receiving concomitant CYP450 substrates, especially those with a narrow therapeutic index.

HOW SUPPLIED

Injection Solution: 45 mg/0.5 mL, 90 mg/1 mL.

DOSAGE

SC

Plaque psoriasis.

Adults, weight >100 kg, initial: 90 mg; **then** after 4 weeks, give 90 mg q 12 weeks (the 45 mg dose was also effective but the 90 mg dose resulted in greater efficacy). **Adults, weight 100 kg or less, initial:** 45 mg; **then** after 4 weeks, give 45 mg q 12 weeks.

NURSING IMPLICATIONS

IMPLEMENTATION/ADMINISTRATION/STORAGE

1. Administer using a 27-gauge, ½-inch needle at a different anatomic location (e.g., upper arms, gluteal regions, thighs, or any quadrant of the abdomen) than the previous injection. Do not give in areas where the skin is tender, bruised, erythematous, or indurated.
2. Do not shake. Store upright from 2–8°C (36–46°F). Keep in original carton until time of use to protect from light. Discard any unused portion.

ASSESSMENT

1. Note disease onset, clinical presentation, previous treatments (topical, phototherapy, parental) trialed. List any medical conditions that may preclude therapy.
2. Identify if failed to respond to traditional therapy or if have associated psoriatic arthritis. Biologics work by blocking interactions between certain immune system cells. Although they are derived from natural sources rather than chemical ones, they must be used with caution because they have strong effects on the immune system and may cause life-threatening infections
3. Do not initiate treatment with active infection; use caution in those with chronic infection or history of recurrent infection and assess carefully for S&S of infection.
4. Update immunizations prior to starting therapy. Caution to avoid those that have received live vaccines due to potential for shedding.
5. Evaluate for tuberculosis risk factors and latent tuberculosis; test prior to starting therapy.
6. Consider cessation of therapy when significant infections, hematologic or CNS side effects occur. Malignancy has been observed in some clients receiving this therapy.
7. Monitor VS, CBC, renal and LFTs.

CLIENT/FAMILY TEACHING

1. Given SC with 2 starter doses: one initially and one in 4 weeks; then maintenance doses are given every 12 weeks. It is a treatment that targets the body's immune system by inhibiting the action of two proteins that are involved in plaque psoriasis.
2. May experience URTI, headaches and tiredness; report if bothersome.
3. Avoid live vaccines while undergoing this therapy.
4. Drug may lower the ability of your immune system to fight infections. Report any evidence or history of infections to provider.
5. Practice reliable contraception, report if pregnancy suspected.
6. Review risk of malignancies while receiving drug.
7. Keep all F/U visits to assess response, labs, and for adverse SE.

OUTCOMES/EVALUATE

- ↓ Plaque thickness, scaling and redness
- Clearing of psoriatic lesions

V

Valacyclovir hydrochloride

(**val**-ah-**SIGH**-kloh-veer)

Classification(s): Antiviral

Pregnancy Category: B

RX: Valtrex.

SEE ALSO ***ANTIVIRAL DRUGS***.

INDICATIONS/USES

(1) Treatment or suppression of genital herpes in immunocompetent adults and for suppression of recurrent genital herpes in HIV-infected individuals. When used as suppressive therapy in immunocompetent clients with genital herpes, the risk of heterosexual transmission to susceptible partners is reduced. (2) Herpes zoster (shingles) in immunocompetent adults. (3) Treatment of herpes labialis (cold sores) in clients 12 years and older. (4) Treatment of chickenpox in immunocompetent children, 2 to less than 18 years of age. *Investigational:* Prophylaxis to prevent cytomegalovirus disease in those who have undergone stem-cell or renal transplantation from a seropositive donor; use in those with AIDS for CMV prophylaxis is not recommended due to trend of increasing deaths with its use in this group.

ACTION/KINETICS

Action

Rapidly converted to acyclovir, which has inhibitory activity against herpes simplex virus types 1 (HSV-1) and 2 (HSV-2) and varicella-zoster virus. Acts by inhibiting replication of viral DNA by competitive inhibition of viral DNA polymerase, incorporation and termination of the growing viral DNA chain, and inactivation of the viral DNA polymerase.

Pharmacokinetics

Rapidly absorbed after PO administration (absolute bioavailability is about 55%) and is rapidly and nearly completely converted to acyclovir and l-valine by first-pass intestinal or hepatic metabolism. **Time to peak levels:** Approximately 1.5 hr. **Peak plasma levels:** Less than 0.5 mcg/mL of valacyclovir at all doses. **t½, acyclovir, plasma:** 2.5–3.3 hr. Approximately 50% is excreted through the urine. **Plasma protein binding:** 13.5–17.9%.

CONTRAINDICATIONS

Hypersensitivity or intolerance to acyclovir or valacyclovir. Use in immunocompromised individuals. Use in AIDS clients due to increasing deaths associated with use in this population. Lactation.

SPECIAL CONCERNS

- **Use with caution in renal impairment or in those taking potentially nephrotoxic drugs.**
- **Thrombotic thrombocytopenic purpura or hemolytic uremic syndrome seen in some clients.**
- **Safety and efficacy not determined in the following disease states: Immunocompromised clients, other than for the suppression of genital herpes in HIV-infected clients; for suppression of recurrent genital herpes in those with advanced HIV disease (CD4 count less than 100 cells/mm^3); to treat genital herpes in HIV-infected clients; and, to treat disseminated herpes zoster.**
- **Dosage reduction may be necessary in geriatric clients depending on the renal status.**
- **Use with caution during lactation.**
- **Safety and efficacy not determined in prepubertal children**

SIDE EFFECTS

Most Common

Headache, N&V, dizziness, fatigue, abdominal pain, rash, dysmenorrhea, arthralgia, depression.

GI: N&V, diarrhea, constipation, abdominal pain, anorexia, hepatitis. **CNS:** Headache, dizziness, depression, aggressive behavior, agitation, coma, confusion, ataxia, decreased consciousness, encephalopathy, mania, psychosis, auditory and visual hallucinations, ***seizures***, tremors. **CV:** Hypertension, tachycardia, leukocytoclastic vasculitis. **Hematologic:** Leukopenia, thrombocytopenia, anemia, thrombotic thrombocytopenic purpura, hemolytic uremic syndrome, ***aplastic anemia***.

V

Respiratory: Nasopharyngitis, URTI. **Dermatologic:** Erythema multiforme, rashes including photosensitivity, alopecia. **Musculoskeletal:** Arthralgia, dysarthria. **GU:** Dysmenorrhea, precipitation of acyclovir in renal tubules resulting in acute renal failure and anuria. **Hypersensitivity:** Rash, urticaria, pruritus, dyspnea, angioedema, ***anaphylaxis***. **Body as a whole:** Asthenia, fatigue. **Miscellaneous:** Facial edema, visual abnormalities.

LABORATORY TEST CONSIDERATIONS

↑ Creatinine, AST, ALT, alkaline phosphatase. ↓ WBCs, hemoglobin, platelet counts. Liver enzyme abnormalities.

OVERDOSE MANAGEMENT

Symptoms: Precipitation of acyclovir in renal tubules if the solubility (2.5 mg/mL) is exceeded in the intratubular fluid. *Treatment:* Hemodialysis until renal function is restored. About 33% of acyclovir in the body is removed during a 4-hr hemodialysis session.

DRUG INTERACTIONS

Cimetidine / May ↑ AUC and peak plasma acyclovir levels; also, ↓ acyclovir renal clearance
Interferon / ↑ Or synergistic antiviral effects
Ketoconazole / ↑ Or synergistic antiviral effects
Probenecid / May ↑ AUC and peak plasma acyclovir levels; also, ↓ acyclovir renal clearance
Zidovudine / ↑ CNS effects (i.e., profound drowsiness and lethargy)

HOW SUPPLIED

Tablets: 500 mg, 1 gram.

DOSAGE

TABLETS

Genital herpes, initial episodes.

1 gram twice a day for 10 days. Begin therapy within 72 hr of signs and symptoms. *Dosage with renal impairment:* C_{CR}, 30–40 mL/min: No reduction in dosage; C_{CR}, 10–29 mL/min: 1 gram q 24 hr; C_{CR} <10 mL/min: 500 mg q 24 hr.

Genital herpes, recurrent episodes.

Adults: 500 mg q 12 hr for 3 days. *Dosage with renal impairment:* C_{CR}, 30–49 mL/min: No reduction in dose; C_{CR}, 10–29 mL/min: 500 mg q 24 hr; and, C_{CR}, <10 mL/min: 500 mg q 24 hr.

Suppression of genital herpes.

Adults: 1 gram once daily in those with a healthy immune system (500 mg once daily for those who have 9 or fewer recurrences per year). *Dosage with renal impairment:* C_{CR}, 20–49 mL/min: No reduction in dose; C_{CR}, 10–29 mL/min: 500 mg q 24 hr for those taking 1 gram/24 hr and 500 mg q 48 hr for those taking 500 mg/24 hr; C_{CR}, <10 mL/min: 500 mg q 24 hr for those taking 1 gram/24 hr and 500 mg q 48 hr for those taking 500 mg/24 hr.

Suppressive therapy in HIV-infected clients with CD4 cell count at least 100 cells/mm³.

500 mg twice a day for chronic suppressive therapy of recurrent genital herpes (500 mg once daily in those with a history of 9 or fewer recurrence per year). *Dosage for renal impairment:* C_{CR}, 20– 40 mL/min: No reduction in dose; C_{CR}, 10–29 mL/min: 500 mg q 24 hr; C_{CR}, <10 mL/min: 500 mg q 24 hr.

Herpes zoster (shingles).

Adults: 1 gram 3 times per day for 7 days. *Dosage with renal impairment:* C_{CR}, 30–49 mL/min: 1 gram q 12 hr; C_{CR}, 10–29 mL/min: 1 gram q 24 hr; and, C_{CR}, <10 mL/min: 500 mg q 24 hr.

Herpes labialis (cold sores).

Clients, 12 years and older: 2 grams twice a day for 1 day taken about 12 hr apart. Initiate therapy at the earliest symptoms. Therapy beyond one day does not provide additional beneficial effects. *Dosage with renal impairment:* C_{CR}, 30–49 mL/min: 2 × 1 gram doses taken about 12 hr apart; C_{CR}, 10–20 mL/min: 2 × 500 mg doses taken about 12 hr apart; C_{CR}, <10 mL/min: Single 500 mg dose.

Chickenpox in immunocompetent pediatric clients.

Children, 2 to <18 years of age: 20 mg/kg three times a day for 5 days, not to exceed 1 gram 3 times a day. Initiate treatment within 24 hr after onset of rash.

NURSING IMPLICATIONS

Do not confuse valacyclovir with valganciclovir (also an antiviral drug).

IMPLEMENTATION/ADMINISTRATION/STORAGE

1. Begin therapy as soon as possible after herpes zoster has been diagnosed. The drug is most effective when started within 48 hr after the onset of rash. For recurrent genital herpes, initiate at the first S&S of a flare.
2. Clients requiring hemodialysis should receive the recommended dose after hemodialysis.
3. Store from 15–25°C (59–77°F).

ASSESSMENT

1. List reasons for therapy, onset, location, characteristics of S&S and frequency of occurrence. With herpes zoster, note dermatone(s) location, characteristics of lesions; most effective if initiated within 48 hr of rash/symptoms.
2. With recurrent genital herpes, note extent of lesions; initiate at first S&S of outbreak.
3. List drugs prescribed to ensure none interact.
4. Assess VS; ensure client adequately hydrated.
5. Monitor CBC, renal function studies; reduce dose if C_{CR} <50 mL/min.

CLIENT/FAMILY TEACHING

1. Take exactly as prescribed; do not share medications, skip, or double up on doses. Complete entire course of therapy. May take without regard to meals; food may decrease GI upset.
2. For cold sores, start therapy at the first symptom of a cold sore (eg, tingling, itching, burning). Do not exceed 2 doses taken about 12 hr apart.
3. With recurrent genital herpes, start therapy at the first S&S or recurrence; may not work well if started >24 hr after S&S occur. Abstain from sexual contact during acute outbreaks to prevent infecting partner; use condoms during all other times.
4. Vesicles with chickenpox/zoster usually become red or pustular after 4 or 5 days and by the 7th to 10th day dry up and crust over. The acute phase is completed by approximately 3 weeks, when the scabs slough from the skin.
5. During acute stage of shingles/pox, cover area and avoid contact with immunocompromised individuals, pregnant women, or anyone else who has not had the chickenpox virus. If unsure may check titers.
6. Immunocompromised clients usually experience a more severe case and disease course usually doubles. In clients with AIDS, review high risk potential with this drug use.
7. Report pain and headaches so appropriate analgesics can be prescribed. May cause drowsiness or dizziness. Report persistent pain once lesions have healed (postherpetic neuralgia may last many months to years), or if there is any eye involvement.
8. Avoid any prolonged sun or UV exposure during therapy to prevent sensitivity reaction.
9. Keep all F/U to assess response, labs, and for adverse SE.

OUTCOMES/EVALUATE

- ↓ Duration/progression of herpes zoster outbreak with reduced healing time; symptomatic relief
- ↓ Pain, ↓ duration, ↓ intensity, ↓ frequency/transmission with genital herpes/cold sore outbreak
- Treatment of chicken pox in immunocompetent child

Valganciclovir hydrochloride

(**val**-gan-**SIGH**-kloh-veer)

Classification(s): Antiviral

Pregnancy Category: C

RX: Valcyte.

SEE ALSO ***ANTIVIRAL DRUGS***.

INDICATIONS/USES

(1) Cytomegalovirus (CMV) retinitis in adults with AIDS. (2) Prevention of CMV disease in kidney, heart, and kidney-pancreas transplant adult clients at high risk (Donor CMV seropositive/Recipient CMV seronegative [(D+/R-)]. (3) Prevention of CMV disease in kidney and heart transplant pediatric clients, 4 months to 16 years of age, at high risk.

ACTION/KINETICS

Action

Is a prodrug that is metabolized to ganciclovir by intestinal and hepatic esterases. In CMV-infected cells, ganciclovir is first phosphorylated to ganciclovir monophosphate and then further phosphorylated to ganciclovir triphosphate. The triphosphate inhibits viral DNA synthesis. Resistant viruses to ganciclovir occur after prolonged treatment with valganciclovir.

Pharmacokinetics

Well absorbed from the GI tract. No other metabolites than ganciclovir have been identified. Excreted by the kidney. **t½, terminal:** About 4 hr.

CONTRAINDICATIONS

Hypersensitivity to ganciclovir or valganciclovir or any component of the product. Use if the absolute neutrophil count is <500 cells/mm^3, the platelet count is <25,000/mm^3, or the hemoglobin is <8 grams/dL. Use in clients receiving hemodialysis or in liver transplant clients. Lactation.

SPECIAL CONCERNS

■ The clinical toxicity of valganciclovir, which is metabolized to ganciclovir, includes granulocytopenia, anemia, and thrombocytopenia. In animal studies, ganciclovir was carcinogenic, teratogenic, and caused aspermatogenesis. ■

- Use with caution in pre-existing cytopenias or in those who have received or are receiving myelosuppressive drugs or irradiation.
- Use care with dose selection in the elderly.
- Safety and efficacy not determined in children for prevention of CMV disease in liver transplant clients, solid organ transplants other than those indicated, solid organ transplant clients younger than 4 months of age, or for treatment of congenital CMV disease.

SIDE EFFECTS

Most Common

Anemia, constipation, cough, diarrhea, graft rejection, hypertension, N&V, neutropenia, pyrexia, thrombocytopenia, tremor, URTI.

See also *Ganciclovir*. Side effects listed are those either with a frequency of 5% or more or those that are serious/life-threatening. **Hematologic:** Granulocytopenia, anemia, thrombocytopenia, severe leukopenia, neutropenia, pancytopenia, bone marrow depression, ***aplastic anemia***. **GI:** Diarrhea, N&V, constipation, abdominal distention/pain, ascites, dyspepsia. **CNS:** Headache, insomnia, paresthesia, ***convulsions***, psychosis, hallucinations, confusion, agitation, tremors, depression, dizziness. **CV:** Hyper-/hypotension. **GU:** Acute renal failure in the elderly (with or without reduced renal function), in those receiving potentially nephrotoxic drugs, and in clients without adequate hydration; dysuria, renal impairment, UTI. **Respiratory:** Cough, URTI, dyspnea, pharyngitis, nasopharyngitis, pleural effusion, rhinorrhea. **Dermatologic:** Acne, dermatitis, pruritus. **Musculoskeletal:** Arthralgia, back/limb pain, muscle cramps. **Metabolic:** Decreased appetite, dehydration, edema, peripheral edema. **Body as a whole:** Pyrexia, fatigue, weakness, pain, peripheral neuropathy, local and systemic infections and ***sepsis***, ***potential life-threatening bleeding due to thrombocytopenia***, hypersensitivity. **Miscellaneous:** Graft rejection, increased wound drainage, postoperative complications/pain/wound infection, wound dehiscence.

NOTE: Anemia, nasopharyngitis, neutropenia, pyrexia, and URTI occurred more frequently in children than in adults.

LABORATORY TEST CONSIDERATIONS

↑ Serum creatinine. Abnormal hepatic function. Hyperglycemia, hyperkalemia, hypocalcemia, hypokalemia, hypomagnesemia, hypophosphatemia.

DRUG INTERACTIONS

Since valganciclovir is rapidly metabolized to ganciclovir, any drug interactions will be those for ganciclovir. Thus, see ***Ganciclovir***.

HOW SUPPLIED

Tablets: 450 mg (as base); ***Powder for Oral Solution:*** 50 mg/mL as the base (after reconstitution).

DOSAGE

ORAL SOLUTION; TABLETS

Cytomegalovirus (CMV) retinitis, active disease.

Adults, initial: 900 mg (2 × 450 mg tablets) twice a day for 21 days with food. **Maintenance:** Following induction or in those with inactive CMV retinitis, give 900 mg (2 × 450 mg tablets) once daily with food.

Prevention of CMV disease.

Adults: 900 mg (two 450 mg tablets) once daily with food starting within 10 days of transplantation until 100 days posttransplantation. For all uses, adjust the dose as follows in those with renal impairment: If C_{CR} is 40 to 59 mL/min, give 450 mg twice a day for the initial dose and 450 mg once daily for the maintenance dose; if C_{CR} is 25 to 39 mL/min, give 450 mg once daily for the initial dose and 450 mg q 2 days for the maintenance dose; if C_{CR} is 10 to 24 mL/min, give 450 mg q 2 days for the initial dose and 450 mg twice weekly for the maintenance dose; use not recommended in those with a C_{CR} <10 mL/min or those on hemodialysis.

Children, 4 months-16 years: Use the following equation:

Dose (mg) = 7 × BSA × C_{CR} (calculated using a modified Schwartz formula)

C_{CR} (mL/min/1.73 m^2) = K × body length or height (cm)/serum creatinine (mg/mL)

where K = 0.45 for clients up to 2 years of age, 0.55 for boys 2 to younger than 13 years and for girls 2 to 16 years of age, and 0.7 for boys 13 to 16 years of age.

The dose is given once daily starting within 10 days of transplantation and until 100 days posttransplantation. Round all calculated doses to the nearest 25 mg increment. If the calculated dose exceeds 900 mg, a maximum dose of 900 mg once daily should be given. Dosing in children with renal impairment can be done using the recommended equation because C_{CR} is a component in the calculation.

NURSING IMPLICATIONS

Do not confuse valganciclovir with valacyclovir (also an antiviral drug). Also, do not confuse Valcyte with Valtrex (valacyclovir hydrochloride, also an antiviral).

IMPLEMENTATION/ADMINISTRATION/STORAGE

1. Valganciclovir tablets cannot be substituted for ganciclovir tablets on a one-to-one basis.
2. Use caution in handling valganciclovir tablets. Do not break or crush tablets; is potential teratogen and carcinogen. Avoid direct contact of broken/crushed tablets with the skin or mucous membranes. If contact occurs, wash thoroughly with soap and water; rinse eyes thoroughly with plain water.
3. The oral solution is preferred for children, as it provides the ability to administer a dose calculated according to the formula provided under *Dosage*. However, tablets may be used if the calculated dose is within 10% of the available tablets strength of 450 mg.
4. Cytopenia may occur at any time during treatment and may increase with continued dosing. Cell counts usually begin to recover within 3 to 7 days after stopping the drug.
5. Store tablets from 15–30°C (59–86°F). Store the constituted solution from 2–8°C (36–46°F) for no longer than 49 days. Do not freeze.

ASSESSMENT

1. Note reasons for therapy, characteristics of S&S, other agents trialed, cultures, outcome. Assess orientation and mentation levels.
2. Determine CMV retinitis by indirect ophthalmoscopy.
3. Review history and assess carefully for pre-existing cytopenias (granulocytopenia, anemia, and thrombocytopenia) or if have received or are receiving myelosuppressive drugs or irradiation.
4. Drug is converted to ganciclovir, but drugs are not interchangeable
5. In animal studies, ganciclovir was carcinogenic, teratogenic, and caused aspermatogenesis.
6. Assess for any S&S or evidence of infection.
7. Monitor VS, cultures, CBC, hold and report if ANC is <500 cells/mm^3, the platelet count is <25,000/mm^3, or the hemoglobin is <8 grams/dL. Anticipate reduced dose with renal dysfunction, see *Dosage*.

CLIENT/FAMILY TEACHING

1. Take with food to maximize bioavailability. Drug is not a cure; it controls symptoms and progression of disease.

V

2. Follow directions carefully for induction and then maintenance dosing. Valganciclovir *cannot* be substituted for ganciclovir on a mg to mg basis.
3. If others must handle the tablets, use caution. Do not break or crush tablets, and do not handle broken tablets. If contact with skin or mucous membranes occurs, wash thoroughly with soapy water and rinse eyes well with plain water.
4. Do not perform activities requiring mental alertness until drug effects realized; may cause dizziness, seizures, altered balance, and confusion.
5. Drug is a potential teratogen and carcinogen. Practice barrier contraception during and for 90 days following therapy.
6. Advise men temporary or permanent infertility may be drug induced.
7. Report any abnormal bruising or bleeding; drug impairs clotting.
8. Avoid crowds and those with active infections; wash hands frequently to reduce chances of infection. Report any S&S of infection (e.g., fever, sore throat, cough, or painful urination).
9. See eye doctor q 4–6 weeks as scheduled.
10. Keep all F/U to assess response, labs, and for adverse SE.

OUTCOMES/EVALUATE

↓ Progression of CMV retinitis

■ IV ℭ

Valproic acid

(val-**PROH**-ick)

Classification(s): Anticonvulsant, miscellaneous

Pregnancy Category: D

RX: Depacon, Depakene, Stavzor.

🍁 **Rx:** Apo-Valproic Acid, Gen-Valproic, PMS-Valproic Acid, PMS-Valproic Acid E.C., ratio-Valproic, Sandoz Valproic.

Divalproex sodium

(die-val-**PROH**-ex)

Pregnancy Category: D

RX: Depakote, Depakote ER.

🍁 **Rx:** Apo-Divalproex, Epival, Epival ER, Novo-Divalproex, Nu-Divalproex.

SEE ALSO ***ANTICONVULSANTS***.

INDICATIONS/USES

PO or IV. (1) Alone or in combination with other anticonvulsants for treatment of complex partial seizures in adults and children 10 years of age and older that occur either in isolation or in association with other types of seizures. (2) Use as sole and adjunctive therapy to treat simple and complex absence seizures (petit mal). (3) As an adjunct in multiple seizure patterns that include absence seizures.

PO. (1) Divalproex sodium delayed-release and extended-release tablets used for the acute treatment of acute manic or mixed episodes with or without psychotic features associated with bipolar disorder. (2) Divalproex sodium or valproic acid delayed-release capsules or tablets and extended-release tablets for prophylaxis of migraine headaches in adults. (3) Stavzor delayed-release tablets to treat manic episodes associated with bipolar disorder, complex partial seizures, or migraine headaches.

ACTION/KINETICS

Action

The precise anticonvulsant action is unknown; may increase brain levels of the neurotransmitter GABA. Other possibilities include acting on postsynaptic receptor sites to mimic or enhance the inhibitory effect of GABA, inhibiting an enzyme that catabolizes GABA, affecting the potassium channel, or directly affecting membrane stability.

Pharmacokinetics

Absorption is more rapid with the syrup (sodium salt) than capsules. Rapidly dissociates to the valproic ion in the stomach. Rate of absorption of the ion may vary with the formulation (i.e., liquid, solid, or sprinkle), conditions of use (fasting, after food), and the method of administration (i.e., whether sprinkled on food or taken intact). **Peak levels, with syrup:** 15 min-2 hr. Equivalent PO doses of divalproex sodium and valproic acid deliver equivalent amounts of valproate ion to the system. **Peak serum levels, capsules and syrup:** 1–4 hr (delayed if the drug is taken with food); **peak serum levels, enteric-coated tablet (divalproex sodium):** 3–4 hr. **t½:** 5–20 hr, with the lower time usually seen in clients taking other anticonvulsant drugs (e.g., primidone, phenytoin, phenobarbital, carbamazepine). **t½, children less than 10 days:** 10–67 hr; **t½, children over 2 months:** 7–13 hr. **t½, cirrhosis or acute hepatitis:** Up to 18 hr. **Therapeutic serum levels:** 50–150 mcg/mL, although a good correlation has not been established between daily dose, serum level, and therapeutic effect. Metabolized in the liver and inactive metabolites are excreted in the urine; small amounts of valproic acid are excreted in the feces. **Plasma protein binding:** 80–94%.

CONTRAINDICATIONS

Liver disease or dysfunction. Known urea cycle disorders. Lactation.

SPECIAL CONCERNS

(1) **Hepatotoxicity.** Hepatic failure (may be fatal) has occurred. Children less than 2 years of age are at considerably increased risk of developing fatal hepatotoxicity, especially those on multiple anticonvulsants, those with congenital metabolic disorders, those with severe seizure disorders accompanied by mental retardation, and those with organic brain disease. Use valproic acid with extreme caution and as a sole agent in this group. Above this age group, experience in epilepsy has indicated that the incidence of fatal hepatotoxicity decreases considerably in progressively older groups. These incidents have usually occurred during the first 6 months of treatment. Serious or fatal heptotoxicity may be preceded by nonspecific symptoms such as anorexia, facial edema, lethargy, malaise, vomiting, and weakness. In clients with epilepsy, a loss of seizure control may also occur. Closely monitor clients for appearance of such symptoms. Perform LFTs prior to therapy and at frequent intervals thereafter, especially during the first 6 months of therapy. (2) Valproate can produce teratogenic effects such as neural tube defects (e.g., spina bifida). Accordingly, the use of valproate products in women of childbearing potential requires that the benefits of use be weighed against the risk of injury to the fetus. This is especially important when the treatment of a spontaneously reversible condition not ordinarily associated with permanent injury or death (e.g., migraine) is contemplated. An information sheet describing the teratogenic potential of valproate is available for clients. (3) **Pancreatitis.** Cases of life-threatening pancreatitis have been reported in both children and adults receiving valproate. Some cases have been described as hemorrhagic with a rapid progression from initial symptoms to death. Cases have been reported shortly after initial use as well as after several years of use. Warn clients and caregivers that abdominal pain, N&V, and/or anorexia can be symptoms of pancreatitis that require prompt medical evaluation. If pancreatitis is diagnosed, discontinue valproate. Initiate alternative treatment for the underlying medical condition as clinically indicated.

- Use lower doses in geriatric clients due to possible increased free, unbound valproic acid levels in the serum.
- Use with caution with a history of hepatic disease; at particular risk are users of multiple anticonvulsants, children, and those with metabolic disorders, severe seizure disorders accompanied by mental retardation, and organic brain disease.
- Increased risk of suicidal behavior and ideation.
- Children less than 2 years of age are at a considerably increased risk of developing fatal hepatotoxicity.
- Safety and efficacy of divalproex sodium not determined to treat acute mania in children less than 18 years of age and to treat migraine in children less than 16 years of age.
- Safety and efficacy of divalproex sodium ER tablets not established for the prophylaxis of migraines in children; also, safety and efficacy of divalproex sodium ER not determined in children less than 10 years to treat complex partial seizures, simple and complex absence seizures, and multiple seizure types (that include absence seizures).
- Use of valproate sodium injection in children less than 2 years of age not studied.

SIDE EFFECTS

Most Common

Asthenia, headache, somnolence, dizziness, tremor, insomnia, amnesia, nervousness, ataxia, N&V, dyspepsia, diarrhea, abdominal pain, anorexia, flu syndrome, infection, nystagmus, diplopia, amblyopia/blurred vision, thrombocytopenia, alopecia.

V

Side effects listed include all uses. CNS: Somnolence, insomnia, sedation, dizziness, tremor, ataxia, emotional lability, abnormal thinking, amnesia, euphoria, headache, hypesthesia, nervousness, paresthesia, insomnia, depression, hallucinations, anxiety, confusion, abnormal gait, hypertonia, hypokinesia, increased reflexes, tardive dyskinesia, incoordination, abnormal dreams, personality disorder, emotional upset, psychosis, aggression, hyperactivity, behavioral deterioration, depression, emotional upset, psychosis, hostility, tremor, vertigo, parkinsonism, agitation, catatonic reaction, confusion, dysarthria, speech disorder, ***suicidal behavior/ideation***, coma (alone or with phenobarbital—rare), encephalopathy with and without fever (rare), reversible cerebral atrophy, dementia, ***hyperammonemic encephalopathy*** with urea cycle disorders (including ornithine transcarbamylase deficiency). **GI:** N&V, abdominal pain, dyspepsia, anorexia (with weight loss), dry mouth, stomatitis, tooth disorder, GI disorder, constipation, increased appetite (with weight gain), flatulence, hematemesis, eructation, periodontal abscess, taste perversion, indigestion, fecal incontinence, gastroenteritis, glossitis, acute intermittent porphyria, ***acute pancreatitis***. **CV:** Hypertension, palpitation, tachycardia, bradycardia, vasodilation, postural hypotension, hypotension, cutaneous vasculitis. **Hematologic:** Thrombocytopenia, ecchymosis, petechia, bruising, hematoma formation, ***frank hemorrhage***, relative lymphocytosis, macrocytosis, hypofibrinogenemia, leukopenia, eosinophilia, anemia (including macrocytic with or without folate deficiency), bone marrow suppression, pancytopenia, ***aplastic anemia***, acute intermittent porphyria. **Respiratory:** Infection, flu syndrome, pharyngitis, dyspnea, bronchitis, rhinitis, epistaxis, pneumonia, sinusitis, increased cough. **Musculoskeletal:** Arthralgia, arthrosis, leg cramps, myalgia, myasthenia, twitching. **Dermatologic:** Dry skin, rash, pruritus, petechiae, transient hair loss, skin rash, ecchymosis, erythema multiforme, photosensitivity, generalized pruritus, alopecia, sweating, rash, discoid lupus erythematosus, furunculosis, maculopapular rash, seborrhea, ***Stevens-Johnson syndrome, toxic epidermal necrolysis (rare)***. **GU:** Amenorrhea, dysmenorrha, urinary frequency, urinary incontinence, vaginitis, irregular menses, secondary amenorrhea, breast enlargement, galactorrhea, dysuria, cystitis, metrorrhagia, vaginal hemorrhage, polycystic ovary disease (rare), enuresis, UTI. **Metabolic:** Hyperammonemia, hyponatremia, inappropriate ADH secretion, Fanconi syndrome (rare; seen mainly in children), decreased carnitine concentrations. **Ophthalmic:** Nystagmus, diplopia, asterixis, "spots before eyes," amblyopia/blurred vision, abnormal vision, conjunctivitis, dry eyes, eye pain. **Otic:** Tinnitus, deafness, otitis media, hearing loss (either reversible or irreversible), ear pain, ear disorder. **Body as a whole:** Asthenia, flu syndrome, infection, malaise, weakness, fever, hypothermia, chills, chills and fever, injection site inflammation/pain reaction, unspecified pain, peripheral edema, infection, viral infection, accidental injury, lupus erythematosis, bone pain, multiorgan hypersensitivity reactions (rare), ***anaphylaxis***. **Miscellaneous:** Hyperammonemia, back/chest pain, neck pain/rigidity, facial edema.

LABORATORY TEST CONSIDERATIONS

False + for ketonuria. ↑ AST, ALT, LDH, serum bilirubin, amylase. Altered thyroid or liver function tests. Possible false interpretation of the urine ketone test.

OVERDOSE MANAGEMENT

Symptoms: Motor restlessness, asterixis, visual hallucinations, somnolence, heart block, ***deep coma.*** *Treatment:* Perform gastric lavage if client is seen early enough (valproic acid is absorbed rapidly). Undertake general supportive measures making sure urinary output is maintained. Naloxone has been used to reverse the CNS depression (however, it could also reverse the anticonvulsant effect). Hemodialysis and hemoperfusion have been used with success.

DRUG INTERACTIONS

Alcohol / ↑ Incidence of CNS depression
Amitriptyline / ↑ Amitriptyline levels
Antacids (Al-Mg hydroxide, Al-Mg trisilicate, calcium carbonate) / ↑ Risk of valproic acid toxicity; monitor carefully
Barbiturates / ↓ Valproic acid hepatic metabolism; may need to ↓ barbiturate dose
Carbamazepine / Variable changes in carbamazepine levels with possible loss of seizure control
Charcoal / ↓ Valproic acid absorption from the GI tract
Chlorpromazine / ↓ Clearance and ↑ elimination t½ of valproic acid → ↑ pharmacologic effects

Cholestyramine / ↓ Valproic acid serum levels with possible loss of seizure control; give valproic acid at least 3 hr before cholestyramine
Cimetidine / ↓ Clearance and ↑ $t\frac{1}{2}$ of valproic acid → ↑ pharmacologic effects
Clonazepam / ↑ CNS depression R/T ↓ plasma protein binding and ↓ metabolism; coadministration may induce absence status in those with a history of absence seizures
CNS depressants / ↑ Incidence of CNS depression
Diazepam / ↑ Diazepam effect R/T ↓ plasma protein binding and ↓ metabolism
Erythromycin / ↑ Serum valproic acid levels → valproic acid toxicity
Ethosuximide / ↑ Ethosuximide effect R/T ↓ metabolism; ↓ valproic acid levels
Etoposide / ↑ Etoposide levels
Felbamate / ↑ Mean peak valproate levels
Lamotrigine / ↓ Valproic acid serum levels and ↑ lamotrigine serum levels; reduce dose of lamotrigine
Lorazepam / ↑ Lorazepam effect R/T ↓ plasma protein binding and ↓ metabolism
Nimodipine / ↑ Nimodipine levels
Nortriptyline / ↑ Nortriptyline levels
Olanzapine / ↑ Hepatic enzymes; monitor AST and ALT q 3–4 months during the first year of therapy
Paroxetine / ↑ Paroxetine levels
Phenobarbital / ↑ Phenobarbital effect R/T ↓ liver breakdown; possible double the clearance of valproate
Phenytoin / ↑ Phenytoin effect R/T ↓ liver breakdown; ↓ effect of valproic acid R/T ↑ metabolism
Primidone / ↑ Primidone effect R/T ↓ liver breakdown; ↓ effect of valproic acid R/T ↑ metabolism
Rifampin / ↑ Valproate oral clearance
Salicylates (aspirin) / ↑ Effect of valproic acid in children R/T ↓ plasma protein binding and ↓ metabolism; monitor serum levels
Tolbutamide / Possible ↑ unbound fraction of tolbutamide; relevance not known
Topiramate / Possible ↑ metabolism of both drugs; hyperammonemia with and without encephalopathy
Tricyclic antidepressants / ↑ TCA plasma levels and side effects
Warfarin sodium / ↑ Warfarin effect R/T ↓ plasma protein binding. Also, additive anticoagulant effect
Zidovudine / ↓ Clearance in HIV-seropositive clients

HOW SUPPLIED

Valproic acid: ***Capsules:*** 250 mg; ***Injection, Concentrate:*** 100 mg/mL (as sodium valproate); ***Syrup:*** 250 mg/5 mL (as sodium valproate); ***Tablets, Delayed-Release (Stavzor):*** 125 mg, 250 mg, 500 mg.
Divalproex sodium: ***Capsules, Sprinkle:*** 125 mg; ***Tablets, Delayed-Release:*** 125 mg, 250 mg, 500 mg; ***Tablets, Extended-Release:*** 250 mg, 500 mg.

DOSAGE

Divalproex sodium, Valproic acid

CAPSULES; CAPSULES, SPRINKLE; DELAYED-RELEASE AND EXTENDED-RELEASE TABLETS (DIVALPROEX); SYRUP (VALPROIC ACID)

Complex partial seizures, monotherapy.

Adults and children 10 years and older: 10–15 mg/kg/day for monotherapy. Increase by 5–10 mg/kg/week until seizures are controlled or side effects occur, up to a maximum of 60 mg/kg/day. If a satisfactory response has not been reached, measure plasma levels to determine whether they are in the usually accepted therapeutic range of 50 to 100 mcg/mL. The probability of thrombocytopenia increases significantly at total trough valproate plasma levels above 100 mcg/mL in women and 135 mcg/mL in men. When converting to monotherapy, initiate at 10–15 mg/kg/day. Increase the dose by 5–10 mg/kg/week to achieve the optimum clinical effect. Concomitant antiepileptic drug dosage can usually be reduced by approximately 25% every 2 weeks. This reduction may be started at initiation of valproic acid therapy or delayed by 1 to 2 weeks if there is a concern that seizures are likely to occur with a reduction. The speed and duration of withdrawal of the concomitant antiepileptic

V

drug can be highly variable; monitor clients closely during this period for increased seizure frequency.

Complex partial seizures, adjunctive therapy.

Adults and children 10 years and older: Valproic acid may be added to the client's regimen at a dose of 10–15 mg/kg/day. The dose may be increased by 5–10 mg/kg/week to achieve the optimum clinical response. Usually, the optimum response is seen at daily doses less than 60 mg/kg/day. If the total daily dose exceeds 250 mg, give in divided doses.

Simple and complex absence seizures.

Initial: 15 mg/kg/day, increasing at 1-week intervals by 5–10 mg/kg/day until seizures are controlled or side effects occur. Usual recommended dose is 60 mg/kg/day. If the total daily dose exceeds 250 mg, give in divided doses. Therapeutic valproate serum levels for most clients with absence seizures are from 50 to 100 mcg/mL.

Acute manic episodes in bipolar disorder (use divalproex sodium delayed- or extended-release tablets).

Initial, using extended-release tablets: 25 mg/kg/day given once daily; increase the dose as rapidly as possible to reach the lowest therapeutic dose that will control symptoms. A trough plasma level between 85 and 125 mcg/mL may be effective. Maximum recommended dose: 60 mg/kg/day. **Initial, using delayed-release tablets:** 250 mg 3 times per day; **then** increase dose as rapidly as possible to reach the lowest therapeutic dose that will control symptoms. A trough plasma level between 50 and 125 mcg/mL may be effective. Maximum levels usually reached within 14 days. The maximum dose is 60 mg/kg/day.

Migraine (use divalproex sodium delayed- or extended-release tablets).

Initial, using extended-release: 500 mg once daily for 1 week; **then** increase to 1,000 mg once daily. **Initial, using delayed-release:** 250 mg twice daily; some may benefit from doses up to 1,000 mg/day. *NOTE:* The ER tablets are not bioequivalent to the delayed-release tablets.

IV

Epilepsy.

Give as a 60 min infusion at 20 mg or less per min with the same frequency as PO products. Use of the injection for more than 14 days has not been studied. Switch to PO valproate products as soon as possible.

Stavzor

TABLETS, DELAYED-RELEASE

Manic episodes with bipolar disorder, complex partial seizures, migraine headaches.

Adults: 750 mg/day in divided doses.

NURSING IMPLICATIONS

Do not confuse Depakote ER (extended-release divalproex sodium) and Depakote Delayed-Release (also divalproex sodium).

IMPLEMENTATION/ADMINISTRATION/STORAGE

1. Divide daily dosage if it exceeds 250 mg/day.
2. Do not confuse Depakote ER, an extended-release divalproex sodium, with Depakote delayed-release. The two forms can not be substituted for each other. Depakote still requires dosing q 8–12 hr whereas Depakote ER is given once daily.
3. Convert from Depakote to Depakote ER as follows: In adults and children over 10 years of age receiving Depakote, Depakote ER can be given once daily using a dose 8–20% higher than the total daily dose of Depakote. For those whose Depakote total daily dose can not be directly converted to Depakote ER, the client's Depakote total daily dose may be increased to the next higher dosage before converting it to the appropriate daily dose of Depakote ER.
4. To minimize GI irritation, initiate at a lower dose, give with food, or use delayed-release (Depakote).
5. To minimize CNS depression, give at bedtime.
6. Do not administer valproic acid syrup to clients whose *sodium* intake must be restricted. Consult provider if a sodium-restricted client is unable to swallow capsules.

7. With valproic acid therapy, conversion to divalproex sodium can be undertaken at the same total daily dose and dosing schedule.
8. Reduce starting dose in geriatric clients, depending on response. Younger children will require larger maintenance doses, especially if receiving enzyme-inducing drugs.
9. Do not abruptly discontinue antiepileptic drugs in clients in whom the drug is given to prevent major seizures due to the strong possibility of precipitating status epilepticus with accompanying hypoxia that is life-threatening.
10. IV Give as a 60 min infusion (not more than 20 mg/min) with the same frequency as PO products. More rapid infusion increases frequency of side effects.
11. When switching from PO to IV, the total daily dose of valproate sodium injection should be equivalent to the total daily dose of PO product. Monitor closely if receiving doses near maximum recommended dose of 60 mg/kg/day. If total daily dose exceeds 250 mg, give in divided doses.
12. The equivalence between injectable and PO products at a steady state is valid in every 6-hr regimen. If given less frequently, trough levels may fall below those of a PO dosage form; closely monitor trough plasma levels.
13. Well tolerated if infused over 5–10 min at rates up to 3 mg/kg/min at doses up to 15 mg/kg.
14. IV use for more than 14 days has not been studied. Switch to PO valproate products as soon as feasible.
15. Injection is compatible and chemically stable with dextrose (5%) injection, 0.9% NaCl, and LR injection for at least 24 hr when stored in glass or polyvinyl chloride bags at controlled room temperature.
16. COMPATIBILITY D5W, 0.9% NaCl and LR.
17. INCOMPATIBILITY Administer separately.

ASSESSMENT

1. Note reasons for therapy, type, onset, symptom characteristics. List other agents trialed, outcome.
2. Identify type, frequency, duration of behaviors that warrant therapy with bipolar disorder; assess mental status and presenting behaviors.
3. With seizures, document characteristics of seizures, onset, aura, and associated findings.
4. With migraine headaches, note triggers, aggravating/alleviating symptoms, duration and frequency.
5. Monitor CBC, bleeding times, and LFTs due to increased potential for hepatoxicity and pancreatitis. Follow dosing guidelines carefully.

CLIENT/FAMILY TEACHING

1. Take with or after meals to minimize GI upset and at bedtime to minimize sedative effects. Delayed-release products may reduce irritating GI side effects. Do not chew tablets or capsules; swallow whole to prevent irritation of mouth and throat. Do not take antacids, dairy products, or carbonated drinks with drug; hastens dissolution. Do not confuse ER form with regular form. The syrup may contain a high-sodium content; avoid in those salt restricted. Do not mix syrup with carbonated beverages.
2. Sprinkle capsules may be swallowed whole or the capsule opened and the contents sprinkled on a small amount (teaspoonful) of applesauce or pudding. Swallow the mixture immediately; do not chew. Do not store for future use.
3. Take only as directed, and do not stop suddenly; may induce seizures. Report any loss of seizure control.
4. Do not drive or perform activities that require mental alertness until drug effects realized and seizure control verified; may cause dizziness/drowsiness.
5. Report any unexplained fever, sore throat, skin rash, tremors, vision problems, yellow skin discoloration, unusual bruising/bleeding; may cause liver toxicity. Abdominal pain, N&V, or anorexia can be symptoms of pancreatitis that require prompt medical evaluation.
6. With diabetes, drug may cause a false positive urine test for ketones. Report symptoms of ketoacidosis (dry mouth, thirst, dry flushed skin).
7. Avoid alcohol, any CNS depressants, or OTC products without approval.
8. Practice reliable contraception. Do not take if pregnant.
9. Keep all F/U to assess response, for labs (CBC, drug levels, serum glucose/acetone, ammonia, and LFTs), and for adverse SE.

OUTCOMES/EVALUATE

- Control of seizures

V

- Migraine headache prophylaxis
- Control of manic episodes
- Therapeutic drug levels (50–150 mcg/mL)

Valrubicin

(val-**ROO**-bih-sin)

Classification(s): Antineoplastic, antibiotic

Pregnancy Category: C

RX: Valstar.

SEE ALSO *ANTINEOPLASTIC AGENTS*.

INDICATIONS/USES

Intravesical therapy of BCG-refractory carcinoma in situ of the urinary bladder in clients for whom immediate cystectomy would be associated with unacceptable morbidity or mortality.

ACTION/KINETICS

Action

Related to doxorubicin. Inhibits incorporation of nucleosides into nucleic acids, causes extensive chromosome damage, and arrests cell cycle G_2. Although minimal metabolism occurs when instilled into the bladder, valrubicin metabolites interfere with normal DNA breaking-resealing action of DNA topoisomerase II. It penetrates the bladder wall.

Pharmacokinetics

Almost completely excreted by voiding the instillate. Total systemic exposure during and after intravesical administration is dependent on the condition of the bladder wall.

CONTRAINDICATIONS

Hypersensitivity to anthracyclines or Cremophor EL. Concurrent UTIs, small bladder capacity (i.e., unable to hold 75 mL instillation). Use in those with a perforated bladder or when the integrity of the bladder mucosa has been compromised. IM or IV use. Lactation.

SPECIAL CONCERNS

- Use with caution in severe irritable bladder symptoms.
- The drug induces complete response in only 1 in 5 clients with BCG-refractory CIS. Delaying cystectomy could lead to metastatic bladder cancer, which is fatal.
- Safety and efficacy not determined in children.

SIDE EFFECTS

Most Common

Urinary frequency/urgency/incontinence, dysuria, bladder spasm, hematuria, bladder pain, cystitis.

GU: Local bladder symptoms, urinary frequency/urgency/incontinence/retention, dysuria, urinary bladder spasm, hematuria, bladder pain, urinary cystitis, nocturia, local burning symptoms, urethral pain, pelvic pain, UTI, poor urine flow, urethritis. **GI:** Abdominal pain, N&V, diarrhea, flatulence, taste loss, tenesmus. **Metabolic:** Hyperglycemia, peripheral edema. **CNS:** Headache, dizziness. **Dermatologic:** Rash, pruritus, local skin irritation, skin ulceration/necrosis (from inadvertant paravenous extravasation). **Body as a whole:** Asthenia, malaise, fever, myalgia. **Miscellaneous:** Back/chest pain, anemia, vasodilation, pneumonia.

LABORATORY TEST CONSIDERATIONS

↑ NPN.

HOW SUPPLIED

Solution for Intravesical Instillation: 40 mg/mL.

DOSAGE

SOLUTION FOR INTRAVESICAL INSTILLATION

Bladder cancer.

Adults: 800 mg once a week for 6 weeks.

NURSING IMPLICATIONS

IMPLEMENTATION/ADMINISTRATION/STORAGE

1. Administer under the supervision of a health care provider experienced in the use of intravesical cancer chemotherapeutic agents.
2. Use aseptic techniques during administration to avoid introducing contaminants into the GU tract or traumatizing the urinary mucosa.
3. Delay use for 2 or more weeks after transurethral resection or fulguration. Do not give to clients with a perforated bladder or to those where the integrity of the bladder mucosa has been compromised.
4. Insert a urethral catheter under aseptic conditions, drain bladder, and instill 75 mL valrubicin (diluted) slowly via gravity flow for several minutes. Withdraw catheter and have client retain drug for 2 hr before voiding.

5. Maintain adequate hydration following treatment.
6. Cremophor EL, which contains the valrubicin, may leach a hepatotoxic plasticizer from PVC bags and IV tubing. Thus, prepare and store the drug in glass, polypropylene, or polyolefin containers and tubing.
7. Do not mix with other drugs.
8. For each instillation, warm four 5-mL vials to room temperature slowly (do not heat). Withdraw 20 mL from the 4 vials and dilute with 55 mL 0.9% NaCl injection.
9. Valrubicin solution is clear red. Inspect for particulate matter and discoloration.
10. Valrubicin diluted in 0.9% NaCl is stable for 12 hr at temperatures up to 25°C (77°F).
11. At temperatures less than 4°C (30°F), Cremophor EL may form a waxy precipitate. If this occurs, warm vial in the hand until the solution is clear. If particulate matter is still seen, do not use.
12. Store unopened vials at 2–8°C (36–46°F). Do not freeze or heat vials.

ASSESSMENT

1. Note onset, diagnosis/BCG failure, other therapies trialed and outcome.
2. Ensure client unable to undergo, or not a candidate for cystectomy.
3. Do not start for at least 2 weeks after transurethral resection and/or fulguration. Determine bladder status prior to instillation of valrubicin. If evidence of bladder perforation, delay administration until bladder integrity restored.
4. Monitor VS, for evidence of infection, I&O.
5. Document cystoscopy and biopsy results, bladder wall integrity, and urine cytology; monitor every 3 months.

CLIENT/FAMILY TEACHING

1. Drug induces complete response in only about 1 in 5 clients. Delaying cystectomy could lead to metastatic bladder cancer.
2. Drug is administered into the bladder by a catheter once a week for 6 weeks. The catheter is removed and the drug retained in the bladder for 2 hr; then may void.
3. For the first 24–48 hr following instillation, red-tinged urine is typical. Report prolonged blood-tinged urine, irritation, pain, or other adverse effects.
4. Consume adequate fluids during therapy (2–3 L/day).
5. Men are to refrain from sexual intercourse; use reliable contraception during therapy.
6. Keep all F/U; evaluation for recurrence of bladder cancer should be done every 3 months with a biopsy, cystoscopy, and urine cytology.

OUTCOMES/EVALUATE

Control of bladder cancer

Valsartan

(val-**SAR**-tan)

Classification(s): Antihypertensive, angiotensin II receptor blocker

Pregnancy Category: C (first trimester); **D** (second and third trimesters)

RX: Diovan.

SEE ALSO ***ANGIOTENSIN II RECEPTOR ANTAGONISTS*** AND ***ANTIHYPERTENSIVE AGENTS***.

INDICATIONS/USES

(1) Alone or in combination with other antihypertensives to treat hypertension in adults and children, 6–16 years of age. (2) Heart failure (NYHA class II to IV). (3) In clinically stable clients with left ventricular failure or left ventricular dysfunction following an MI; used to reduce CV mortality.

ACTION/KINETICS

Action

Selectively blocks the binding of angiotensin II to the AT_1 receptor in vascular smooth muscle, resulting in a decrease in BP. Angiotensin II is a pressor agent causing vasoconstriction, stimulation of the synthesis of and release of aldosterone, cardiac stimulation, and renal reabsorption of sodium. Also reduces left ventricular hypertrophy.

Pharmacokinetics

About 25% bioavailable. Food decreases absorption. **Peak plasma levels:** 2–4 hr. **t½:** 6 hr. Eliminated mostly unchanged in feces (83%) and urine (about 13%). **Plasma protein binding:** 95%.

SPECIAL CONCERNS

When used in pregnancy during the second and third trimesters, drugs that act directly on the renin-angiotensin system can cause injury and even death to the developing fetus.

V

When pregnancy is detected, discontinue valsartan as soon as possible. The use of drugs that act directly on the renin-angiotensin system during the second and third trimesters of pregnancy has been associated with fetal and neonatal injury, including hypotension, neonatal skull hypoplasia, anuria, reversible or irreversible renal failure, and death. Oligohydramnios has also been reported, presumably resulting from decreased fetal renal function; oligohydramnios in this setting has been associated with fetal limb contractures, craniofacial deformation, and hypoplastic lung development. Prematurity, intrauterine growth retardation, and patent ductus arteriosus have also been reported, although it is not clear whether these occurrences were due to exposure to the drug. ■

- **Use with caution in severe hepatic or renal impaired function.**
- **May increase the death rate in clients also taking beta-blockers and ACE inhibitors for CHF.**

SIDE EFFECTS

Most Common

Dizziness, anxiety, nervousness, abdominal pain, viral infection

CNS: Headache, dizziness, fatigue, anxiety, insomnia, nervousness, paresthesia, somnolence. **GI:** Abdominal pain, diarrhea, nausea, constipation, dry mouth, dyspepsia, flatulence. **Respiratory:** URTI, cough, rhinitis, sinusitis, pharyngitis, dyspnea. **Body as a whole:** Viral infection, edema, asthenia, allergic reaction, viral infection. **Musculoskeletal:** Arthralgia, back pain, muscle cramps, myalgia. **Dermatologic:** Pruritus, rash. **Miscellaneous:** Palpitations, vertigo, neutropenia, impotence.

LABORATORY TEST CONSIDERATIONS

↓ H&H. ↑ Serum potassium, liver enzymes, serum bilirubin.

DRUG INTERACTIONS

Atenolol / ↑ Antihypertensive effect; no effect on HR

Potassium-sparing diuretics (e.g., amiloride, spironolactone, triamterene) / ↑ Serum potassium; also, ↑ serum creatinine in heart failure clients

HOW SUPPLIED

Tablets: 40 mg, 80 mg, 160 mg, 320 mg.

DOSAGE

TABLETS

Hypertension.

Adults, initial: 80 or 160 mg once daily as monotherapy in clients who are not volume depleted. A higher dose may be used in those requiring greater reductions. **Dose range:** 80–320 mg once daily. If additional antihypertensive effect is needed, dose may be increased to 160 mg or 320 mg once daily or diuretic may be added (has greater effect when valsartan dose increases beyond 80 mg). **Children, 6–16 years of age, initial:** 1.3 mg/kg once daily, up to 40 mg total. Adjust dosage according to BP response. Doses higher than 2.7 mg/kg (up to 160 mg) once daily have not been studied in this age group.

Heart failure.

Adults, initial: 40 mg twice a day. Increase dose to 80 and 160 mg twice a day as tolerated. **Maximum daily dose:** 320 mg in divided doses. Consider dose reduction of concomitant diuretics. Concomitant use with both an ACE inhibitor and beta-blocker is not recommended.

Postmyocardial infarction.

Initial: 20 mg twice daily (may be started as early as 12 hr after an MI). Dose may be titrated upward within 7 days to 40 mg twice daily, with subsequent titrations to a target maintenance dose of 160 mg twice daily, as tolerated. May be given with other postmyocardial infarction treatment, including aspirin, beta-blockers, thrombolytics, and statins.

NURSING IMPLICATIONS

Do not confuse Diovan with Diovan HCT (valsartan plus hydrochlorothiazide).

IMPLEMENTATION/ADMINISTRATION/STORAGE

1. **Give on an empty stomach.**
2. **Antihypertensive effect is usually seen within 2 weeks with maximum reduction after 4 weeks.**

3. For those who cannot swallow a tablet, a suspension can be prepared noting that the exposure to valsartan is 1.6 times more with the suspension than with the tablet. To prepare the suspension, add 80 mL of Ora-Plus (oral suspending vehicle) to an amber glass bottle containing 8 valsartan, 80 mg tablets. Shake for a minimum of 2 minutes. Allow the suspension to stand for 1 hr, after which shake the suspension for a minimum of 1 additional minute. Add 80 mL of Ora-Sweet SF (oral sweetening vehicle) to the bottle, and shake the suspension for at least 10 seconds to disperse the ingredients. The product can be stored for either up to 30 days at room temperature or up to 75 days refrigerated. Shake the bottle well (for at least 10 seconds) before each use.
4. Store tablets between 15–30°C (59–86°F) in a tight container protected from moisture.

ASSESSMENT

1. Note reasons for therapy, disease onset, characteristics of S&S, other agents trialed, outcome. List drugs prescribed to ensure none interact.
2. Ensure client is well hydrated.
3. Assess renal function in heart failure or post-MI clients regularly.
4. Monitor BP, CBC, electrolytes, renal and LFTs; note dysfunction.

CLIENT/FAMILY TEACHING

1. May take with or without food (works better without) and with other prescribed BP medications.
2. Change positions slowly and avoid dehydration to prevent sudden drop in BP and dizziness.
3. Practice reliable contraception; report if pregnancy suspected—may cause fetal death. Do not take if pregnant.
4. Continue low-fat, low-sodium diet, regular exercise, weight loss, smoking/alcohol cessation, and stress reduction in goal of BP control. Avoid salt replacements that contain potassium.
5. May experience headaches, coughing, diarrhea, nausea, and joint aches; report if persistent.
6. Before taking OTC drugs, obtain medical advice as some OTC drugs may affect the action of valsartan.
7. Record BP and pulse for provider review.
8. Keep all F/U to assess response, labs, and for adverse SE.

OUTCOMES/EVALUATE

- ↓ BP
- ↓ Cardiovascular death and CHF related hospitalizations

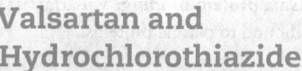

Combination Drug

Valsartan and Hydrochlorothiazide

(val-**SAR**-tan, **hy**-droh-klor-oh-**THIGH**-ah-zyd)

Classification(s): Antihypertensive combination drug

Pregnancy Category: C (first trimester); **D** (second and third trimesters)

RX: Diovan HCT.

SEE ALSO ***VALSARTAN*** AND ***HYDROCHLOROTHIAZIDE***.

INDICATIONS/USES

Treatment of hypertension. Not indicated for initial therapy.

CONTENT

Each Diovan HCT tablet contains the following amounts of valsartan (*angiotensin II receptor blocker*, listed first) and hydrochlorothiazide (*thiazide diuretic*): 80 mg/12.5 mg, 160 mg/12.5 mg, 160 mg/25 mg, 320 mg/12.5 mg, 320 mg/25 mg.

ACTION/KINETICS

Action

Valsartan selectively blocks the binding of angiotensin II to the AT_1 receptor in vascular smooth muscle, resulting in a decrease in BP. Angiotensin II is a pressor agent causing vasoconstriction, stimulation of the synthesis of and release of aldosterone, cardiac stimulation, and renal reabsorption of sodium. Also reduces left ventricular hypertrophy. Hydrochlorothiazide promotes the excretion of sodium and chloride, and thus water, by the distal renal tubule. Also increases excretion of potassium and to a lesser extent bicarbonate. The antihypertensive activity is thought to be due to direct dilation of the areterioles, as well as to a

V

reduction in the total fluid volume of the body and altered sodium balance.

Pharmacokinetics

Valsartan. About 25% bioavailable. Food decreases absorption. **Peak plasma levels:** 2–4 hr. **t½:** 6 hr. Eliminated mostly unchanged in feces (83%) and urine (about 13%). **Hydrochlorothiazide. Onset:** 2 hr. **Peak effect:** 4–6 hr. **Duration:** 6–12 hr. **t½:** 5.6–14.8 hr. Hydrochlorothiazide is not metabolized but is eliminated rapidly by the kidney. **Plasma protein binding:** Valsartan is about 95% bound to plasma proteins.

CONTRAINDICATIONS

Hypersensitivity to any component of the product. Use in those with anuria or hypersensitivity to other sulfonamide-derived drugs. Lactation.

SPECIAL CONCERNS

When used in pregnancy during the second and third trimesters, drugs that act directly on the renin-angiotensin system can cause injury and even death to the developing fetus. When pregnancy is detected, Diovan HCT should be discontinued as soon as possible.

- **Use with caution in those with impaired hepatic (including biliary obstructive disorders), or renal function or progressive liver disease (minor alterations of fluid and electrolyte balance may precipitate hepatic coma).**
- **Hypersensitivity reactions to hydrochlorothiazide may occur in clients with or without a history of allergy or bronchial asthma but are more likely in those with such a history.**
- **May increase the death rate in clients also taking beta-blockers and ACE inhibitors for CHF.**
- **Safety and efficacy have not been determined in children.**

SIDE EFFECTS

Most Common

Nasopharyngitis, headache, dizziness, orthostatic hypotension, hypokalemia.

See *Valsartan* and *Diuretics, Thiazides* for a complete list of possible side effects. **Miscellaneous:** Thiazides may exacerbate or activate systemic lupus erythematosus.

LABORATORY TEST CONSIDERATIONS

↑ Creatinine, BUN, liver enzymes. ↓ H&H.

OVERDOSE MANAGEMENT

Symptoms: Valsartan: Hypotension, tachycardia, bradycardia (if vagal stimulation occurs). Hydrochlorothiazide: Electrolyte depletion and dehydration. *Treatment:* Institute supportive treatment.

DRUG INTERACTIONS

See ***Valsartan*** and ***Diuretics, Thiazides***.

HOW SUPPLIED

See *Content.*

DOSAGE

TABLETS

Hypertension.

Adults: Clients whose BP is not controlled using valsartan alone can be switched to Diovan HCT (80/12.5 mg, 160/12.5 mg, or 320/12.5 mg) once daily. If BP remains uncontrolled after 3–4 weeks, increase the dose of valsartan or both components. Clients whose BP is inadequately controlled by hydrochlorothiazide, 25 mg daily or is controlled but experiences hypokalemia, may be switched to Diovan HCT (80/12.5 mg or 160/12.5 mg) once daily. If BP remains uncontrolled after 3–4 weeks, the dose may be increased up to a maximum of 320/25 mg. The maximal antihypertensive effect is reached in about 4 weeks after beginning therapy.

NURSING IMPLICATIONS

Do not confuse Diovan (valsartan alone) with Diovan HCT (valsartan and hydrochlorothiazide).

IMPLEMENTATION/ADMINISTRATION/STORAGE

1. **It is appropriate to begin combination therapy only after a client has failed to achieve the desired effect with monotherapy.**
2. **Diovan HCT can be given to clients with impaired renal function as long as the C_{CR} is >30 mL/min. In clients with more severe renal impairment, loop diuretics are preferred to thiazide diuretics.**
3. **No dosage adjustment is required in those with mild-to-moderate hepatic dysfunction.**
4. **May be given with other antihypertensive drugs.**

5. Store from 15–30°C (59–86°F) protected from moisture.

ASSESSMENT

1. Note reasons for therapy, disease onset, other agents trialed, outcome.
2. List drugs prescribed to ensure none interact.
3. Assess other medical conditions; ensure all stabilized. Dilutional hyponatremia may occur in edematous clients in hot weather; appropriate therapy is water restriction.
4. Hyperuricemia or frank gout may be precipitated in some receiving thiazide therapy.
5. In diabetics, dosage adjustments of insulin or oral hypoglycemic agents may be required. Hyperglycemia may occur with thiazide diuretics; latent diabetes mellitus may occur during thiazide therapy.
6. Thiazides have been shown to increase the urinary excretion of magnesium; may decrease urinary calcium excretion. Marked hypercalcemia may be evidence of hidden hyperparathyroidism. Thiazides should be discontinued before carrying out tests for parathyroid function.
7. Increases in cholesterol and triglyceride levels may be associated with thiazide therapy.
8. Monitor VS, renal and LFTs; ensure C_{CR} >30 mL/min. Use caution with impaired hepatic function or progressive liver disease; minor alterations of fluid and electrolyte balance may precipitate hepatic coma. Monitor electrolytes, Mg, and calcium.

CLIENT/FAMILY TEACHING

1. May take with or without food at the same time each day.
2. Use caution with activities that require mental alertness until drug effects realized; may experience dizziness. Change positions slowly to prevent sudden drop in BP (postural hypotension).
3. Ensure adequate fluid intake; especially during high activity, excessive sweating, nausea/vomiting, diarrhea, or in hot weather. May experience excessive drop in BP; record BP.
4. Report any unusual effects, changes in voiding patterns, swelling of the face, lips, or tongue, or lack of desired response. May experience headaches, coughing, diarrhea, nausea, and joint aches; report if persistent.
5. Continue low-fat, low-sodium diet, regular exercise, weight loss, smoking/alcohol cessation, and stress reduction in goal of BP control. Avoid salt replacements that contain potassium.
6. Avoid prolonged sun or UV exposure; may cause sensitivity reaction.
7. Practice reliable contraception; stop drug and report if pregnancy suspected.
8. Keep all F/U to assess response, labs, and for adverse SE.

OUTCOMES/EVALUATE

Desired BP control

IV

Vancomycin hydrochloride

(van-koh-**MY**-sin)

Classification(s): Antibiotic, miscellaneous

Pregnancy Category: C (**B** for capsules only)

RX: Vancocin.

SEE ALSO ***ANTI-INFECTIVE DRUGS***.

INDICATIONS/USES

PO: (1) Antibiotic-induced pseudomembranous colitis due to *Clostridium difficile.* (2) Enterocolitis due to *Staphylococcus aureus* (including methicillin-resistant strains).

IV: (1) Treatment of staphylococcal endocarditis. (2) Alone or in combination with aminoglycosides to treat endocarditis caused by *Streptococcus viridans* or *Streptococcus bovis.* Must combine with an aminoglycoside to treat endocarditis due to *Streptococcus faecalis.* (3) Treatment of diphtheroid endocarditis in combination with either rifampin, an aminoglycoside, or both in early-onset prosthetic valve endocarditis caused by *Staphylococcus epidermidis* or diphtheroids. (4) Certain parenteral products may be given PO for treatment of antibiotic-associated pseudomembranous colitis caused by *C. difficile* and for staphylococcal enterocolitis. Vancomycin is not effective PO for other types of infection. (5) Treatment of serious or severe infections due to susceptible strains of methicillin-resistant (beta-lactam resistant) staphylococci. It is indicated for those allergic to penicillin, those who cannot receive or who have failed to respond to other drugs (including penicillins or cephalosporins), and for infections due to vancomycin-susceptible organisms that are resistant to other antimicrobial drugs. Vancomycin is indicated for initial therapy when methicillin-resistant

V

staphylococci are suspected, but after susceptibility data are available, adjust therapy accordingly. (6) Efficacy has also been shown in infections due to staphylococci, including septicemia, bone infections, lower respiratory tract infections, and skin and skin structure infections.

ACTION/KINETICS

Action

Appears to bind to bacterial cell wall, arresting its synthesis and lysing the cytoplasmic membrane by a mechanism that is different from that of penicillins and cephalosporins. The drug also changes the permeability of the cytoplasmic membranes of bacteria, thus inhibiting RNA synthesis. Bactericidal for most organisms and bacteriostatic for enterococci. There is no cross resistance between vancomycin and other antibiotics.

Pharmacokinetics

Poorly absorbed from the GI tract. Diffuses in pleural, pericardial, ascetic, and synovial fluids after parenteral administration. **Peak plasma levels, IV:** 33 mcg/mL 5 min after 0.5 gram dosage. **t½, after PO:** 4–8 hr for adults and 2–3 hr for children; **t½, after IV:** 4–11 hr for adults and ranging from 2–3 hr in children to 6–10 hr for newborns. The half-life is increased markedly in the presence of renal impairment (240 hr has been noted). Primarily excreted in urine unchanged. Auditory and renal function tests are indicated before and during therapy.

CONTRAINDICATIONS

Hypersensitivity. Minor infections. Lactation.

SPECIAL CONCERNS

- **Use with extreme caution in the presence of impaired renal function or previous hearing loss.**
- **Geriatric clients are at a greater risk of developing ototoxicity. Use caution with dose selection.**
- **Those with inflammatory disorders of the intestinal mucosa may have significant systemic absorption of vancomycin, resulting in increased risk for development of side effects. The risk is greater if renal impairment is present.**
- **Safety and efficacy not determined of vancomycin administration by the intraperitoneal or intrathecal routes, although the drug has been used by the intraperitoneal route during continuous ambulatory peritoneal dialysis.**
- **Prescribing vancomycin without a proven or strongly suspected bacterial infection increases the risk of development of drug-resistant bacteria.**
- **Although used in children, safety and efficacy not determined. Coadministration of vancomycin and anesthetic agents has been associated with erythema and histamine-like flushing in children.**

SIDE EFFECTS

Most Common

Ototoxicity (including tinnitus), chills, coughing, drowsiness, anorexia, N&V, weakness, sore throat, fever.

GI: N&V, anorexia, pseudomembranous colitis, *C. difficile*-associated diarrhea. **CNS:** Vertigo, dizziness, drowsiness. **CV:** Exaggerated hypotension (due to rapid bolus administration), including ***shock and possibly cardiac arrest.*** **GU:** Renal failure (rare), interstitial nephritis (rare), ***nephrotoxicity*** (may lead to uremia). **Hematologic:** Eosinophilia, neutropenia (reversible). **Respiratory:** Wheezing, dyspnea, coughing, sore throat. **Dermatologic:** Urticaria, pruritus, macular rashes, exfoliative dermatitis, ***Stevens-Johnson syndrome, toxic epidermal necrolysis***, vasculitis (rare), drug rash with eosinophilia. **Hypersensitivity:** Dyspnea, "red man syndrome" ***(sudden and profound drop in BP*** with or without a maculopapular rash over the face, neck, upper chest, and extremities), hypotension, pain, muscle spasm of the chest/back, pruritus, urticaria, wheezing, drug fever, ***anaphylaxis***. **Otic:** Ototoxicity (may lead to deafness; deafness may progress after drug is discontinued), tinnitus. **At injection site:** Tissue irritation, including pain, tenderness, necrosis, thrombophlebitis. **Body as a whole:** Chills, fever, weakness, superinfection.

OVERDOSE MANAGEMENT

Treatment: Provide supportive care. Maintain glomerular filtration. Is poorly removed by dialysis. Hemofiltration and hemoperfusion with polysulfone resin increase vancomycin clearance.

DRUG INTERACTIONS

Aminoglycosides (e.g., gentamicin) / ↑ Risk of toxicity; monitor renal function and serum levels
Amphotericin B / ↑ Risk of toxicity; monitor renal function and serum levels
Anesthetics / ↑ Risk of erythema and histamine-like flushing in children; minimize by giving vancomycin as a 60 min infusion prior to induction of anesthesia

V

Bacitracin / ↑ Risk of toxicity; monitor renal function and serum levels
Cisplatin / ↑ Risk of toxicity; monitor renal function and serum levels
Indomethacin / Possible ↑ effects of vancomycin in neonates; monitor closely
Methotrexate / Possible ↑ methotrexate serum levels and markedly delayed methotrexate excretion; monitor and adjust methotrexate dose as needed
Muscle relaxants, nondepolarizing (e.g., vecuronium) / ↑ Neuromuscular blockade; do not use together
Nephrotoxic/Neurotoxic drugs / Carefully monitor with concurrent or sequential systemic or topical use
Polymyxin B / ↑ Risk of toxicity; monitor renal function and serum levels

HOW SUPPLIED

Capsules: 125 mg, 250 mg; ***Injection, Powder for Solution:*** 500 mg, 750 mg, 1 gram, 5 grams, 10 grams; ***Injection, Solution:*** 500 mg, 1 gram.

DOSAGE

CAPSULES

Pseudomembranous colitis, Staphylococcal enterocolitis.

Adults, usual: 0.5–2 grams/day in 3–4 divided doses for 7–10 days. **Children:** 40 mg/kg/day in 3–4 divided doses for 7–10 days, not to exceed 2 grams/day.

IV

Endocarditis.

Adults: 500 mg q 6 hr or 1 gram q 12 hr given at a rate of no more than 10 mg/min or over at least 60 min, whichever is longer. **Children, 1 month and older:** 10 mg/kg q 6 hr given over at least 60 min. **Infants, up to 1 month of age, initial:** 15 mg/kg for one dose; **then,** 10 mg/kg q 12 hr for neonates in the first week of life and q 8 hr thereafter up to 1 month of age. Give over 60 min. *NOTE:* In premature infants, vancomycin clearance decreases as postconceptional age decreases; thus, longer dosing intervals may be necessary in premature infants.

Pseudomembranous colitis, Staphylococcal enterocolitis.

Adults: 0.5–2 grams PO daily given in 3 or 4 divided doses for 7–10 days. **Children, usual:** 40 mg/kg/day given PO in 3 or 4 divided doses for 7–10 days, up to a maximum of 2 grams/day. See *Implementation/Administration/Storage* for use of IV products given PO.

Staphylococcal infections.

Adults: 2 grams IV divided as 500 mg q 6 hr or 1 gram q 12 hr given at a rate no faster than 10 mg/min or over at least 60 min, whichever is longer. **Children, 1 month and older:** 10 mg/kg per dose IV q 6 hr, given over at least 60 min. **Children, up to 1 month of age, initial:** 15 mg/kg, followed by 10 mg/kg q 12 hr for neonates in the first week of life and q 8 hr thereafter up to the age of 1 month. Give over 60 min. *NOTE:* In premature infants, vancomycin clearance decreases as postconceptional age decreases; thus, longer dosing intervals may be necessary in premature infants.

NURSING IMPLICATIONS

IMPLEMENTATION/ADMINISTRATION/STORAGE

1. Reduce dosage in renal disease; see package insert for procedure. In premature infants and the elderly greater dose reduction may be needed due to decreased renal function.
2. The parenteral form may be administered PO by diluting the 1-gram vial with 20 mL distilled or deionized water (each 5 mL contains about 250 mg vancomycin). Flavoring agents may be added to improve taste.
3. Store capsules from 15–30°C (59–86°F).
4. IV For IV use, reconstitute the 500 mg vial with 10 mL of sterile water for injection, the 750 mg vial with 15 mL of sterile water for injection, the 1 gram vial with 20 mL of sterile water for injection, the 5 gram pharmacy bulk package with 100 mL of sterile water for injection, or the 10 gram pharmacy bulk package with 95 mL of sterile water for injection. Reconstituted solutions of the 5 gram pharmacy bulk package contain 500 mg/10 mL and the reconstituted 10 gram pharmacy bulk package contain 1 gram/10 mL. Further dilution is required.
5. Reconstituted solutions must be diluted as follows: Those containing 500 mg vancomycin

V

must be diluted with at least 100 mL of diluent; those containing 750 mg vancomycin must be diluted with at least 150 mL of diluent, while reconstituted solutions containing 1 gram of vancomycin must be diluted with at least 200 mL diluent. Give the diluted dose by intermittent IV infusion of at least 60 min.

6. Thaw Galaxy containers at room temperature or under refrigeration; do not force thaw by immersion in a water bath or by microwave irradiation. Visually inspect for particulate matter and discoloration. Do not add supplementary medication. Store, before thawing, in a freezer capable of maintaining a temperature at or below –20°C (–4°F). Thawed solution in Galaxy containers are stable for 72 hr at room temperature or for 30 days stored under refrigeration. Do not refreeze thawed containers.
7. The initial dose should be 15 mg/kg even in those with mild to moderate renal insufficiency.
8. Intermittent infusion is the preferred route, but continuous IV drip may be used.
9. Avoid rapid IV administration, because this may result in hypotension, nausea, warmth, and generalized tingling. Administer over 60 min in concentrations of no more than 5 mg/mL and rates of no more than 10 mg/min in adults. For children, administer over at least 60 min.
10. Avoid extravasation during injections; may cause tissue necrosis.
11. Reduce risk of thrombophlebitis by rotating injection sites or adding additional diluent.
12. Aqueous solution is stable for 2 weeks.
13. Once rubber stopper is punctured, ampule should be refrigerated to maintain stability.
14. Store vials and pharmacy bulk packages from 20–25°C (68–77°F).
15. COMPATIBILITY D5W, D5/NSS, RL, D5/RL, Normosol-M/dextrose 5%, 0.9 % NaCl, and Isolyte E.
16. INCOMPATIBILITY Physically incompatible with beta-lactam antibiotics. Flush IV lines between administration of these antibiotics. Vancomycin solutions have a low pH and may cause physical instability of other compounds.

ASSESSMENT

1. Note reasons for therapy, type, onset, characteristics of S&S, culture results.
2. Assess renal and auditory functions (including 8th CN function). Monitor for hearing loss.
3. During IV administration, ensure that peak and trough drug levels are performed at the prescribed dosing interval, usually 30 min prior to scheduled IV dose (trough) and 1 hr following IV dose (peak) to accurately assess serum levels.
4. Report adverse drug effects, such as:
   - Ototoxicity, demonstrated by tinnitus, progressive hearing loss, dizziness, and/or nystagmus; may occur latently
   - Nephrotoxicity, demonstrated by albuminuria, hematuria, anuria, casts, edema, and uremia
5. Systemic infections require parenteral administration whereas pseudomembranous diarrhea *(C. difficile)* requires oral administration.
6. Monitor VS, weight, I&O, CBC, cultures, urinalysis, and renal function studies; reduce dose with renal dysfunction. Ensure adequate hydration.

CLIENT/FAMILY TEACHING

1. May be taken with or without food.
2. Complete entire course of drug therapy as prescribed, otherwise infection may recur. IV medication is given at regular intervals to maintain blood levels.
3. Report any fullness/ringing in ears, vertigo, or hearing loss.
4. Stay well hydrated during therapy.
5. Keep all F/U to assess response, labs, and for adverse SE.

OUTCOMES/EVALUATE

- Negative culture reports
- Relief of S&S R/T infection
- Therapeutic serum drug levels

Vardenafil hydrochloride

(var-**DE**-nah-fil)

Classification(s): Drug for erectile dysfunction

Pregnancy Category: B

RX: Levitra:, Staxyn:.

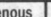

V

INDICATIONS/USES

Treatment of erectile dysfunction. *Investigational:* Raynaud phenomenon (film-coated tablets only).

ACTION/KINETICS

Action

During sexual stimulation, nitric oxide is released from nerve endings and endothelial cells in the corpus cavernosum of the penis. Nitric oxide activates the enzyme guanylate cyclase, causing an increased synthesis of cyclic guanosine monophosphate (cGMP) in the smooth muscle cells of the corpus cavernosum. The cGMP in turn causes smooth muscle relaxation, allowing increased blood flow to the penis, resulting in erection. Tissue levels of cGMP are regulated by both the rate of synthesis and degradation via phosphodiesterases (PDEs). The most abundant PDE in the human corpus cavernosum is the cGMP-specific phosphodiesterase type 5 (PDE5). Thus, inhibition of PDE5 enhances erectile function by increasing the amount of cGMP. Vardenafil is a selective inhibitor of PDE5.

Pharmacokinetics

Rapidly absorbed with a bioavailability of about 15%. **Maximum plasma levels:** 30–120 min after a single 20 mg dose. Food decreases C_{max} by 18–50%. **Onset:** About 20 min; **maximum effect:** 45–90 min. **Duration:** Less than 5 hr. Eliminated primarily by hepatic metabolism by CYP3A4 and to a minor extent by CYP2C isoforms. The major metabolite, M1, is active. **t½, terminal:** 4–5 hr for both vardenafil and the M1 metabolite. Excreted mainly in the feces (91–95%) with a small amount in the urine (2–6%). **Plasma protein binding:** About 95%.

CONTRAINDICATIONS

Regular or intermittent use with nitrates due to potentiation of hypotensive effects of nitrates. Known hypersensitivity to vardenafil or any component of the product. Use in clients with congenital QT prolongation and those taking Class 1A (quinidine, procainamide) or Class III (amiodarone, sotalol) antiarrhythmic drugs. Use of orally disintegrating tablets with potent or moderate CYP3A4 inhibitors, such as atazanavir, clarithromycin, erythromycin, indinavir, itraconazole, ketoconazole, and ritonavir. Use in unstable angina, hypotension, uncontrolled hypertension, recent history of stroke, life-threatening arrhythmia, MI (within the last 6 months), severe cardiac failure, severe hepatic impairment (Child-Pugh score from 10 to 15), end-stage renal disease requiring dialysis, known hereditary degenerative retinal disorders (including retinitis pigmentosa). Use of orally disintegrating tablets in those with moderate or severe hepatic impairment.

SPECIAL CONCERNS

- **Use with caution in clients with bleeding disorders or active peptic ulceration, in those with anatomical deformation (e.g., angulation, cavernosal fibrosis, Peyronie's disease) of the penis, or in those who have conditions that may predispose them to priapism (e.g., sickle cell anemia, multiple myeloma, leukemia).**
- **Use with caution when vardenafil is used concomitantly with alpha blockers due to the potential for an additive effect on BP leading to significant hypotension.**
- **Not known if vardenafil is excreted into human breast milk.**

SIDE EFFECTS

Most Common

Headache, dizziness, dyspepsia, nausea, diarrhea, rhinitis, sinusitis, accidental injury, back pain, flu syndrome, flushing, myalgia, rash, abnormal vision.

CNS: Headache, dizziness, hypertonia, hypesthesia, insomnia, paresthesia, somnolence, vertigo. **CV:** Hypo-/hypertension, ***MI, angina pectoris***, chest pain, ***myocardial ischemia***, palpitation, postural hypotension, syncope, tachycardia. **GI:** Dyspepsia, N&V, abdominal pain, diarrhea, dry mouth, dysphagia, esophagitis, gastritis, gastroesophageal reflux. **Musculoskeletal:** Arthralgia, back pain, myalgia, neck pain. **Respiratory:** Rhinitis, sinusitis, dyspnea, epistaxis, pharyngitis. **Dermatologic:** Flushing, photosensitivity reaction, pruritus, rash, sweating. **GU:** Abnormal ejaculation, priapism (including prolonged or painful erections). **Ophthalmic:** Abnormal/decreased/blurred vision, sudden vision loss (temporary or permanent), visual field defect, retinal vein occlusion, reduced visual acuity, chromatopsia, changes in color vision, conjunctivitis, dim vision, eye pain, glaucoma, photophobia, watery eyes, nonarteritic anterior ischemic optic neuropathy (rare). **Body as a whole:** Flu syndrome, asthenia, pain, facial edema, ***anaphylaxis (including laryngeal***

edema). **Miscellaneous:** Accidental injury, tinnitus.

LABORATORY TEST CONSIDERATIONS

↑ Creatine kinase, GGTP. Abnormal LFTs.

DRUG INTERACTIONS

Alcohol (substantial consumption) / ↓ BP, postural dizziness, and orthostatic hypotension
Alpha-adrenergic blockers / ↑ Risk of significant hypotension; use together with caution
Erythromycin / ↑ Vardenafil levels R/T ↓ metabolism by CYP3A4
Indinavir / ↑ Vardenafil levels R/T ↓ liver metabolism
Itraconazole / ↑ Vardenafil levels R/T ↓ liver metabolism by CYP3A4
Ketoconazole / ↑ Vardenafil levels R/T ↓ liver metabolism by CYP3A4
Nifedipine / Additional ↓ BP
Nitrates / Sudden, severe ↓ in BP → dizziness, syncope, heart attack, stroke; do not use together
Ritonavir / ↑ Vardenafil levels R/T ↓ liver metabolism

HOW SUPPLIED

Levitra. *Tablets:* 2.5 mg, 5 mg, 10 mg, 20 mg.
Staxyn. *Tablets, Orally Disintegrating:* 10 mg.

DOSAGE

TABLETS

Erectile dysfunction.

Adults, usual: 10 mg about 60 min before sexual activity. For film–coated tablets, the dose may be increased to 20 mg or decreased to 5 mg based on efficacy and side effects. Maximum recommended dose is 20 mg once a day. **Maximum dose, film–coated tablets:** 20 mg/dose once a day; **maximum dose, orally disintegrating tablets:** 10 mg/day. An initial dose of 5 mg should be considered in clients 65 years and older and in those with moderate hepatic impairment. Maximum dose for those with moderate hepatic impairment: 10 mg. Do not use orally disintegrating tablets in clients with moderate or severe hepatic impairment.

Raynaud's phenomenon (investigational).

10 mg twice a day for 2 weeks. *NOTE:* Safety concerns may limit use for this purpose.

NURSING IMPLICATIONS

Do not confuse vardenafil with varenicline (a smoking deterrent).

IMPLEMENTATION/ADMINISTRATION/STORAGE

1. The initial dose in those with moderate hepatic impairment (Child-Pugh score from 7 to 9) is 5 mg; the maximum dose in those with moderate hepatic impairment should not exceed 10 mg.
2. A single dose of 2.5 mg should not be exceeded in clients taking indinavir or ritonavir. No more than a single 2.5 mg dose should be taken in a 72-hr period in those taking ritonavir.
3. A dose of 2.5 mg daily should not be exceeded in those taking ketoconazole, 400 mg/day, or itraconazole, 400 mg/day. A dose of 5 mg daily should not be exceeded in those taking ketoconazole, 200 mg/day, itraconazole, 200 mg/day, or erythromycin.
4. In those stable on alpha-blockers, initiate vardenafil at a dose of 5 mg (2.5 mg when taken with certain CYP34A4 inhibitors).
5. Can be taken with or without food.
6. Staxyn 10 mg orally disintegrating tablet is not interchangeable with the 10 mg film-coated Levitra since Staxyn provides higher systemic exposure.
7. Sexual stimulation is required for a response to treatment.
8. Store from 15–30°C (59–86°F).

ASSESSMENT

1. Note onset and cause of erectile dysfunction, i.e., organic, psychogenic, or combined.
2. Assess cardiovascular status and obtain ECG. Clients using nitrates should not use this drug; should be nitrate free for 24 hr prior to use.
3. List drugs prescribed, as some may potentiate drug effects.
4. Ensure client aware of potential for visual changes/abnormalities.
5. Note any conditions that may predispose client to priapism, i.e., multiple myelomas, sickle cell anemia, or leukemia.

V

6. Assess for any anatomical deformation of penis (Peyronie's disease, angulation, or cavernosal fibrosis).
7. Monitor VS, renal and LFTs.

CLIENT/FAMILY TEACHING

1. May be taken with or without food.
2. Take only as directed 1 hr before anticipated act. Plan some form of sexual stimulation after ingestion to ensure desired erection obtained.
3. Staxyn tablet should be placed on the tongue, where it will disintegrate. Take without liquid immediately upon removal from the blister.
4. Report all medications currently prescribed to ensure none alter effects. Avoid nitrates and alpha-blocking drugs. Stop smoking; may inhibit drug effect.
5. Staxyn tablets contain phenylalanine; caution with phenylketonuria.
6. Practice safe sex; drug does not prevent disease transmission nor pregnancy.
7. May experience headache, flushing, upset stomach, stuffy nose, dizziness (from drop in BP) drowsiness, or abnormal vision (especially blue/green color discrimination); report any unusual, persistent or bothersome effects.
8. Do not use any other agent for erections with this therapy. Effects may be evident the day after therapy; assess before taking additional drug. Do not use more than once a day. Erections lasting more than 4 hr or painful erections lasting more than 6 hr require immediate ER care; penile damage may result.
9. Do not share medications or prescriptions due to potential for adverse interactions/effects. *Never* use this drug if currently taking nitrates in any form. May be fatal.
10. Keep all F/U to assess response, labs, and for adverse SE.

OUTCOMES/EVALUATE

Relief of erectile dysfunction; desired erection

Varenicline tartrate

(var-**EN**-ih-kline)

Classification(s): Smoking deterrent

Pregnancy Category: C

RX: Chantix.

INDICATIONS/USES

Aid to smoking cessation treatment.

ACTION/KINETICS

Action

Varenicline binds with high affinity and selectivity at alpha-4-beta-2 neuronal nicotinic acetylcholine receptors. The effectiveness in smoking cessation is thought to be due to the drug preventing nicotine from binding to alpha-4-beta-2 receptors. Thus, nicotine cannot stimulate the central nervous mesolimbic dopamine system, believed to be the neuronal mechanism underlying reinforcement and reward experienced by smoking.

Pharmacokinetics

Maximum plasma levels: 3–4 hr. **Steady state levels:** 4 days. Oral bioavailability is not affected by food. **t½, elimination:** 24 hr. Undergoes minimal metabolism with 92% excreted unchanged in the urine. **Plasma protein binding:** 20% or less.

CONTRAINDICATIONS

Use in children less than 18 years of age. Lactation.

SPECIAL CONCERNS

(1) Serious neuropsychiatric events, including, but not limited to, depression, suicidal ideation, suicide attempt, and completed suicide, have been reported in clients taking varenicline. Some reported cases may have been complicated by the symptoms of nicotine withdrawal in clients who stopped smoking. Depressed mood may be a symptom of nicotine withdrawal. Depression, rarely including suicidal ideation, has been reported in smokers undergoing a smoking cessation attempt without medication. However, some of these symptoms have occurred in clients taking varenicline who continued to smoke. (2) Observe all clients being treated with varenicline for neuropsychiatric symptoms, including changes in behavior, hostility, agitation, depressed mood, and suicide-related events, including ideation, behavior, and attempted suicide. These symptoms, as well as worsening of pre-existing psychiatric illness and completed suicide, have been reported in some clients attempting to quit smoking while taking varenicline in postmarketing experience. When symptoms were reported, most

were during varenicline treatment, but some were following discontinuation of varenicline therapy. (3) These events have occurred in clients with and without pre-existing psychiatric disease. Clients with serious psychiatric illness, such as schizophrenia, bipolar disorder, and major depressive disorder, did not participate in the pre-marketing studies of varenicline, and safety and efficacy of varenicline in these clients have not been established. (4) Advise clients and caregivers that the client needs to stop taking varenicline and contact a health care provider immediately if agitation, hostility, depressed mood, or changes in behavior or thinking that are not typical for the client are observed, or if the client develops suicidal ideation or suicidal behavior. In many postmarketing cases, resolution of symptoms after discontinuation of varenicline was reported, although in some cases the symptoms persisted; therefore, provide ongoing monitoring and supportive care until symptoms resolve. (5) Weigh the risks of varenicline against the benefits of its use. Varenicline has been demonstrated to increase the likelihood of abstinence from smoking for as long as 1 year compared with treatment with placebo. The health benefits of quitting smoking are immediate and substantial. ■

- **Due to decreased renal function in the elderly, use care in dose selection; consider monitoring renal function.**
- **Use with caution in impaired renal function; dosage adjustment is necessary.**
- **Potential for suicidal ideation and occasional suicidal behavior.**
- **Weigh the risks against the benefits of use of varenicline.**
- **Safety and efficacy not determined in children younger than 18 years of age.**

SIDE EFFECTS

Most Common

N&V, sleep disturbances, constipation, flatulence, abdominal pain, dyspepsia, headache, insomnia, abnormal dreams, dysgeusia, upper respiratory tract disorder, hypertension, hyperhidrosis, thirst.

CNS: Headache, insomnia, abnormal/frightening dreams, somnolence, lethargy, nightmares, sleep disorder, anxiety, panic, nervousness, tension, depression, mania, psychosis, attention disturbances, dizziness, emotional disorder, delusions, paranoia, irritability, restlessness, sensory disturbances, aggression, agitation, hostility, amnesia, disorientation, dissociation, decreased libido, migraine, mood swings, parosmia, psychomotor hyperactivity, restless legs syndrome, abnormal thinking, tremor, balance disorder, bradyphrenia, ***convulsions***, dysarthria, euphoria, facial palsy, hallucinations, mental impairment, multiple sclerosis, impaired psychomotor skills, psychotic disorder, homicidal ideation, ***suicidal behavior/ideation, completed suicide***. **GI:** N&V, flatulence, dysgeusia, abdominal pain, GERD, constipation, dyspepsia, dry mouth, diarrhea, gingivitis, dysphagia, enterocolitis, eructation, esophagitis, gastritis, ***GI hemorrhage***, mouth ulceration, gastric ulcer, intestinal obstruction, gallbladder disorder, ***acute pancreatitis***. **CV:** Hypertension, angina pectoris, arrhythmia, bradycardia, abnormal ECG, hypotension, ***MI***, palpitations, peripheral ischemia, syncope, tachycardia, ***thrombosis***, ventricular extrasystoles, acute coronary syndrome, atrial fibrillation, cardiac flutter, coronary artery disease, cor pulmonale, transient ischemic attack, ***CVA***. **Dermatological:** Rash, pruritus, hyperhidrosis, acne, dermatitis, dry skin, eczema, erythema, psoriasis, urticaria, photosensitivity reaction, hot flash, ***Stevens-Johnson syndrome, erythema multiforme***. **Respiratory:** Upper respiratory tract disorder, dyspnea, rhinorrhea, epistaxis, respiratory disorder, asthma, pleurisy, ***pulmonary embolism***. **GU:** Menstrual disorder, polyuria, erectile dysfunction, nephrolithiasis, nocturia, urethral syndrome, urine abnormality, sexual dysfunction, urinary retention, acute renal failure. **Musculoskeletal:** Arthralgia, back pain, muscle cramps, musculoskeletal pain, myalgia, arthritis, osteoporosis, myositis, chest pain. **Hypersensitivity:** ***Angioedema*** (swelling of the face, mouth, extremities, throat, larynx), ***respiratory compromise***. **Hematologic:** Anemia, lymphadenopathy, leukocytosis, splenomegaly, thrombocytopenia. **Metabolic:** Decreased/increased appetite, anorexia, increased weight, diabetes mellitus. **Ophthalmic:** Conjunctivitis, dry eye, eye irritation/pain, blurred vision, visual disturbance, acquired night blindness, transient blindness, subcapsular cataract, ocular vascular disorder, photophobia, vitreous floaters, nystagmus, visual field defect. **Otic:** Tinnitus, deafness, Ménière syndrome. **Body as a whole:**

Fatigue, malaise, asthenia, edema, flu-like illness, thirst, chills, pyrexia. **Miscellaneous:** Thyroid gland disorders, vertigo, chest discomfort, hypersensitivity, drug hypersensitivity.

LABORATORY TEST CONSIDERATIONS

Abnormal ECG, LFTs, urinalysis. ↑ Muscle enzymes. Hyperlipidemia, hypokalemia, hyperkalemia, hypoglycemia.

DRUG INTERACTIONS

Cimetidine / ↑ Varenicline exposure by 29% R/T ↓ renal clearance
Nicotine transdermal / ↑ Incidence of N&V, headache, dizziness, dyspepsia, and fatigue

HOW SUPPLIED

Tablets: 0.5 mg (as base), 1 mg (as base).

DOSAGE

TABLETS

Aid to smoking cessation.

Dosage titration beginning 1 week before the date to stop smoking, Days 1–3: 0.5 mg once a day; **days 4–7:** 0.5 mg twice a day. **Day 8 through end of treatment:** 1 mg twice a day. Treat clients for 12 weeks. Those who cannot tolerate the side effects may have the dose lowered temporarily or permanently. For those who have successfully stopped smoking at the end of 12 weeks, an additional course of 12 weeks is recommended to increase further the likelihood of long-term abstinence.

NURSING IMPLICATIONS

Do not confuse vareniciline with vardenafil (drug for erectile dysfunction).

IMPLEMENTATION/ADMINISTRATION/STORAGE

1. Clients who do not stop smoking during 12 weeks of initial therapy, or who relapse after treatment should be encouraged to make another attempt after identifying and addressing the factors that contributed to the failed attempt.
2. For clients with severe impaired renal function, the recommended initial dose is 0.5 mg once a day. Then titrate as needed to a maximum of 0.5 mg twice a day. For those with end-stage renal disease undergoing hemodialysis, a maximum dosage of 0.5 mg once a day may be given if well tolerated.
3. Smoking cessation may alter the pharmacokinetics or pharmacodynamics of certain drugs (e.g., insulin, theophylline, warfarin) for which an adjustment of dose may be necessary.
4. Store from 15–30°C (59–86°F).

ASSESSMENT

1. Note smoking history, other attempts to quit, activities that trigger desire to smoke.
2. List all drugs prescribed (e.g., theophylline, warfarin, insulin); drug may affect their actions/side effects. May require dosage adjustment.
3. Assess for any depression or psychiatric illness, note behavioral and clinical presentation; may preclude therapy.
4. Use with caution in the elderly; may be more sensitive to its effects.
5. Monitor renal and LFTs; reduce dose with renal dysfunction.

CLIENT/FAMILY TEACHING

1. Drug works in the brain to block the pleasurable effects of smoking. This helps to decrease desire to smoke.
2. Set a date to stop smoking. Start varenicline dosing 1 week before this date.
3. Take after eating and with a full glass of water (8 oz/240 mL).
4. If smoking still after quit date, continue to try to quit. If a dose is missed, do not take 2 doses at once.
5. May cause drowsiness or dizziness; may be worse with alcohol or certain medicines. Do not drive or perform activities that require mental alertness until drug effects realized.
6. Do not stop drug suddenly; may cause increased irritability or difficulty sleeping.
7. May experience nausea and insomnia; report if persistent as a dose reduction may be considered. May experience vivid, unusual, or strange dreams.
8. Report any depressed mood, agitation, changes in behavior, suicidal ideation; stop Chantix. Smoking cessation with or without treatment is associated with nicotine withdrawal S&S and the exacerbation of underlying psychiatric illness; use caution. Review provided educational materials and attend

V

counseling to support attempt to quit smoking.

9. Practice reliable contraception. Report if pregnancy suspected.
10. Keep all F/U to assess response and for adverse SE.

OUTCOMES/EVALUATE

- Smoking cessation
- Loss of desire to smoke

Vandetanib

(van-**DET**-a-nib)

Classification(s): Tyrosine kinase inhibitor.

Pregnancy Category: D

RX: Vandetanib.

INDICATIONS/USES

Treatment of symptomatic or progressive medullary thyroid cancer in those with unresectable locally advanced or metastatic disease.

ACTION/KINETICS

Action

Vandetanib inhibits endothelial cell migration, proliferation, and survival and new blood vessel formation in in vitro models of angiogenesis. Vandetanib also inhibits vascular endothelial growth factor-dependent cell survival. Also, the drug inhibits epidermal growth factor-stimulated receptor tyrosine kinase phosphorylation in tumor cells and endothelial cells and vascular endothelial growth factor-stimulated tyrosine kinase phosphorylation in endothelial cells. Vandetanib also caused sustained plasma concentration-dependent QT prolongation.

Pharmacokinetics

Absorption is slow. C_{max}: 4–10 hr. Metabolized mainly by CYP3A4. Unchanged drug is excreted in both the feces (44%) and urine (25%). **t½, median plasma:** 19 days.

CONTRAINDICATIONS

Congenital long QT syndrome. In those with moderate and severe (Child-Pugh Class B or C) hepatic impairment. Lactation.

SPECIAL CONCERNS

■ **QT prolongation, torsades de pointes, and sudden death.** Vandetanib can prolong the QT interval. Torsades de pointes and sudden death have been reported in clients receiving vandetanib. Do not use vandetanib in clients with hypocalcemia, hypokalemia, hypomagnesemia, or long QT syndrome. Hypocalcemia, hypokalemia, and/or hypomagnesemia must be corrected prior to vandetanib administration and should be periodically monitored. Avoid drugs known to prolong the QT interval. If a drug known to prolong the QT interval must be administered, more frequent electrocardiogram (ECG) monitoring is recommended. Given the half-life of 19 days, obtain ECGs to monitor the QT interval at baseline, at 2 to 4 and 8 to 12 weeks after starting treatment with vandetanib, and every 3 months thereafter. Following any dose reduction for QT prolongation or any dose interruptions more than 2 weeks, conduct QT assessment as previously described. Because of the 19-day half-life, adverse reactions, including a prolonged QT interval, may not resolve quickly. Monitor appropriately. Only health care providers and pharmacies certified with the restricted distribution program are able to prescribe and dispense vandetanib. ■

Safety and efficacy not determined in children.

SIDE EFFECTS

Most Common

Fatigue, headache, acne, rash, abdominal pain, decreased appetite, diarrhea, nausea, hypertension, decreased calcium and glucose, increased ALT.

CNS: Headache, depression, insomnia. **GI:** Abdominal pain, N&V, decreased appetite, diarrhea, colitis, dyspepsia, pancreatitis. **CV:** Hypertension, ECG QT prolonged, ***hypertensive crisis***, accelerated hypertension, bleeding events (***hemorrhage***), ischemic cerebrovascular events, ***cardiac failure with arrhythmia***. **Dermatologic:** Acne, rash, dermatitis acneiform, dry skin, photosensitivity reaction, pruritus, erythematous rash, generalized rash, macular rash, maculopapular rash, pruritic rash, exfoliative rash, dermatitis, dermatitis bullous, generalized erythema, eczema, ***Stevens-Johnson syndrome***, palmar–plantar erythrodysesthesia syndrome. **Respiratory:** Cough, nasopharyngitis,

respiratory failure/arrest, aspiration pneumonia, interstitial lung disease, pneumonitis. **Musculoskeletal:** Arthralgia. **Ophthalmic:** Blurred vision, corneal opacities, decreased visual acuity, halos. **Body as a whole:** Fatigue, asthenia, decreased weight, pyrexia, ***sepsis***. **Miscellaneous:** Hypothyroidism, reversible posterior leukoencephalopathy syndrome.

LABORATORY TEST CONSIDERATIONS

↑ ALT, creatinine, bilirubin. ↑ or ↓ Calcium, glucose, magnesium, potassium. ↓ WBCs, hemoglobin, neutrophils, platelets.

OVERDOSE MANAGEMENT

Symptoms: Increased severity of some side effects, including rash, diarrhea, and hypertension. Also, QT prolongation and torsades de pointes. Because of the 19-day half-life, side effects may not resolve quickly. *Treatment:* There is no specific treatment. Treat adverse effects symptomatically (especially severe diarrhea). Interrupt further doses of vandetanib. Do an ECG to determine QTc prolongation.

DRUG INTERACTIONS

An additive effect of vandetanib with other drugs that prolong the QT interval cannot be excluded. The following drugs may prolong the QT interval and increase the risk of life–threatening cardiac arrhythmias, including torsades de points: Amiodarone, arsenic trioxide, bretylium, chlorpromazine, cisapride, disopyramide, dofetilide, dolasetron, droperidol, gatifloxacin, halofantrine, levomethadyl, mefloquine, mesoridazine, moxifloxacin, pentamidine, pimozide, probucol, procainamide, quinidine, sotalol, sparfloxacin, thioridazine, and ziprasidone. Avoid coadministration.

Carbamazepine / ↓ Vandetanib plasma levels R/T induction of CYP3A4 → ↓ pharmacologic effect; avoid coadministration
Dexamethasone / ↓ Vandetanib plasma levels R/T induction of CYP3A4 → ↓ pharmacologic effect; avoid coadministration
Phenobarbital / ↓ Vandetanib plasma levels R/T induction of CYP3A4 → ↓ pharmacologic effect; avoid coadministration
Phenytoin / ↓ Vandetanib plasma levels R/T induction of CYP3A4 → ↓ pharmacologic effect; avoid coadministration
QT prolonging drugs (see list above) / ↑ Risk of life–threatening arrhythmias, including torsades de pointes; avoid coadministration; if coadministration is necessary, undertake more frequent ECG monitoring
Rifabutin, Rifampin, Rifapentine / ↓ Vandetanib plasma levels R/T induction of CYP3A4 → ↓ pharmacologic effect; avoid coadministration
H ***St. John's wort*** / ↓ Vandetanib plasma levels unpredictably; avoid coadministration

HOW SUPPLIED

Tablets: 100 mg, 300 mg.

DOSAGE

TABLETS

Medullary thyroid cancer.

Adults, usual: 300 mg/day.

NURSING IMPLICATIONS

IMPLEMENTATION/ADMINISTRATION/STORAGE

1. **In the event of QT interval corrected for heart rate, QTcF greater than 500 msec, interrupt dosing until QTcF returns to less than 450 msec; then resume at a reduced dose. For Common Terminology Criteria for Adverse Events grade 3 or greater toxicity, interrupt dosing until toxicity resolves or improves to grade 1 and then resume at a reduced dose. The 300 mg daily dose can be reduced to 200 mg and then to 100 mg for grade 3 or greater toxicities.**
2. **Avoid concomitant use of strong CYP3A4 inducers, including carbamazepine, dexamethasone, phenobarbital, phenytoin, rifampin, rifabutin, rifapentine, and St. John's wort.**
3. **If a dose is missed, the client should not take the missed dose if it is less than 12 hr before the next dose.**
4. **For those with moderate (C_{CR} 30–50 mL/min) to severe (C_{CR} <30 mL/min) renal impairment, reduce the starting dose to 200 mg.**
5. **If vandetanib tablets cannot be taken whole, they can be dispersed in a glass containing 60 mL of noncarbonated water and stirred for about 10 min until the tablet is dispersed (will not completely dissolve). No other liquids should be used. Swallow the dispersion immediately. Mix any residues in the glass with an additional 120 mL of noncarbonated**

V

water and swallow. The dispersion can also be given through a nasogastric or gastrostomy tube.

6. Vandetanib is a cytotoxic agent. Follow safe handling procedures when preparing, administering, or dispensing the drug.
7. Due to the risk of QT prolongation, torsades de pointes, and sudden death, vandetanib is available only through a restricted distribution program called the vandetanib risk evaluation and mitigation strategy (REMS) program. Only health care providers and pharmacies certified with the program are able to prescribe and dispense vandetanib. To enroll in the program call 1-800-817-2722 or visit http://www.vandetanibrems.com.
8. Store from 15–30°C (59–86°F).

ASSESSMENT

1. Document disease onset, other therapies trialed and that thyroid cancer is unresectable and locally advanced or has become metastatic.
2. Obtain ECG; drug can prolong QT interval and requires careful monitoring. List drugs prescribed and avoid concurrent use with any drugs that prolong QT interval.
3. Review risks associated with drug therapy: QT prolongation, interstitial lung disease, ischemic cerebrovascular events, heart failure, hemorrhage, severe skin reactions, diarrhea, hyperthyroidism, hypertension, reversible posterior leukoencephalopathy syndrome (RPLS). Due to possibility of death, this drug is only available through a restricted distribution program, called vandetanib REMS program.
4. Tablets should not be crushed. Direct contact of crushed tablets with the skin or mucous membranes should be avoided
5. Obtain ECG, VS, K^+, Ca^{++}, Mg^{++} and TSH prior to starting therapy, at 2-4 weeks and 8-12 weeks after starting treatment and every 3 months thereafter. Electrolytes and ECGs may require more frequent monitoring in the event of diarrhea. Monitor renal and LFTs, and reduce dose or stop therapy with dysfunction.

CLIENT/FAMILY TEACHING

1. Drug is used to treat thyroid cancer that cannot be removed by surgery or that has spread to other parts of the body. It takes a long time to get rid of this drug from your body and you may be at risk for side effects after you have stopped treatment.
2. May be taken with or without food. Do not crush the tablets. Direct contact of crushed tablets with the skin or mucous membranes should be avoided.
3. Frequent monitoring of your heart by an ECG and electrolytes will be performed. Vandetanib can prolong the QT interval in a concentration-dependent manner. Torsades de pointes, ventricular tachycardia, and sudden death have been reported.
4. Report any sudden onset or worsening of breathlessness, persistent cough, or fever immediately. Also contact provider if you experience seizures, headaches, visual disturbances, confusion, or difficulty thinking.
5. Avoid prolonged sun exposure and wear protective clothing and sunscreen if exposed. May be more susceptible to sunburn during and for 4 months following therapy. Notify provider if any rash develops.
6. May experience diarrhea with this therapy. Use standard antidiarrheal medications and report if diarrhea becomes persistent or severe.
7. Practice reliable contraception during and for 4 months following therapy. Do not breastfeed.
8. Keep all F/U to assess response, for labs/ECG, and for adverse SE.

OUTCOMES/EVALUATE

Inhibition of malignant cell proliferation with medullary thyroid cancer

IV

Vasopressin

(vay-so-**PRESS**-in)

Classification(s): Pituitary hormone

Pregnancy Category: C (Some recommend Pregnancy Category **B**)

RX: Pitressin Synthetic.

✱ **Rx:** Pressyn.

INDICATIONS/USES

(1) Neurogenic (central) diabetes insipidus (ineffective when diabetes insipidus is of renal origin-nephrogenic diabetes insipidus). (2) Prevention and treatment of postoperative abdominal disten-

tion. (3) Dispel interfering gas shadows in abdominal roentgenography. *Investigational:* Bleeding esophageal varices (IV or intra-arterial), pulseless cardiac arrest (IV or intraosseously), hemodynamic support of septic shock and vasodilatory shock due to systemic inflammatory response syndrome.

ACTION/KINETICS

Action

Released from the anterior pituitary gland; regulates water conservation by promoting reabsorption of water by increasing the permeability of the collecting ducts in the kidney. Depending on the concentration, the hormone acts directly on both V_1 and V_2 receptors. Also causes contraction of smooth muscle of the GI tract and all parts of the vascular system, especially the capillaries, small areterioles, and venules; has less effect on the small muscle of large veins. Also increases the smooth muscular activity of the bladder, GI tract, and uterus. The direct effect is not antagonized by adrenergic blockers or by vascular denervation.

Pharmacokinetics

Onset, IM, SC: variable; **duration,** 2–8 hr. **t½:** 10–20 min. **Effective plasma levels:** 4.5–6 microunits. Most is metabolized and rapidly destroyed by the kidneys and liver. About 5% excreted unchanged in the urine after 4 hr.

CONTRAINDICATIONS

Anaphylaxis or hypersensitivity to vasopressin or any component of the product. Vascular disease, especially when involving coronary arteries (may cause anginal pain with even small doses and possible MI with larger doses); angina pectoris. Chronic nephritis until reasonable blood nitrogen levels are attained.

SPECIAL CONCERNS

- **Increased risk of hyponatremia and water intoxication in pediatric/geriatric clients.**
- **Use caution during lactation and in the presence of asthma, epilepsy, migraine, CHF, or any condition in which rapid addition to extracellular water may produce a hazard for an already overburdened system.**
- **Use with extreme caution in CAD as even small doses may precipitate anginal pain and larger doses may cause an MI.**

SIDE EFFECTS

Most Common

Nausea, diarrhea, flatulence, pale-colored lips, stomach pain, headache, tremors, abdominal cramps, sweating.

GI: N&V, increased intestinal activity (e.g., belching, cramps, urge to defecate), diarrhea, abdominal cramps, flatulence. **CV:** Circumoral pallor, arrhythmias, decreased cardiac output, ***cardiac arrest***, angina, ***myocardial ischemia***, peripheral vasoconstriction, gangrene. **CNS:** Tremor, headache, vertigo, "pounding" in head. **Dermatologic:** Sweating, urticaria, skin blanching, pale-colored lips, cutaneous gangrene. **Respiratory:** Bronchial constriction. **Miscellaneous:** Tremor, ***allergic/hypersensitivity reactions, bronchoconstriction, anaphylaxis, water intoxication*** (drowsiness, listlessness, headache, ***coma, convulsions***). *NOTE:* Use of vasopressin may result in severe vasoconstriction and local tissue necrosis if extravasation occurs.

OVERDOSE MANAGEMENT

Symptoms: Water intoxication. *Treatment:* Withdraw vasopressin until polyuria occurs. If water intoxication is serious, administration of mannitol (i.e., an osmotic diuretic), hypertonic dextrose, or urea alone (or with furosemide) is indicated.

DRUG INTERACTIONS

Alcohol / May ↓ antidiuretic effect of vasopressin
Carbamazepine / May potentiate antidiuretic effect of vasopressin
Chlorpropamide / May potentiate antidiuretic effect of vasopressin
Clofibrate / May potentiate antidiuretic effect of vasopressin
Demeclocycline / May ↓ antidiuretic effect of vasopressin
Fludrocortisone / May potentiate antidiuretic effect of vasopressin
Ganglionic blocking drugs / May ↑ significantly sensitivity to pressor effects of vasopressin
Heparin / May ↓ antidiuretic effect of vasopressin
Lithium / May ↓ antidiuretic effect of vasopressin
Norepinephrine / May ↓ antidiuretic effect of vasopressin
Tricyclic antidepressants / May potentiate antidiuretic effect of vasopressin

HOW SUPPLIED

Injection Solution: 20 pressor units/mL.

V

DOSAGE

IM; INTRANASALLY; SC

Diabetes insipidus.

Adults: 5–10 units by injection 2–3 times per day as needed; **pediatric:** 2.5–10 units 3–4 times per day. When given intranasally by cotton pledgets, drops, or spray using the injection solution, the dosage and interval between doses must be determined individually for each client.

Postoperative abdominal distention.

Adults, initial: 5 units IM; **then,** may be increased to 10 units IM q 3–4 hr; **pediatric:** individualize the dose (usual: 2.5–5 units).

Abdominal roentgenography.

IM, SC: 2 injections of 10 units 2 hr and ½ hr, respectively, before x-rays are taken. Some recommend giving an enema before the first dose of vasopressin.

Esophageal varices.

Initial: 0.2 units/min IV or selective IA; **then,** 0.4 units/min if bleeding continues. The maximum recommended dose is 0.9 units/min.

Pulseless cardiac arrest.

1 dose of 40 units IV or intraosseously may replace either the first or second dose of epinephrine.

Hemodynamic support of septic shock and vasodilatory shock.

For refractory shock despite fluid resuscitation and conventional vasopressors, give at an infusion rate of 0.01 to 0.04 units/minute.

NURSING IMPLICATIONS

Do not confuse Pitressin (vasopressin) with Pitocin (oxytocin).

IMPLEMENTATION/ADMINISTRATION/STORAGE

1. It is desirable to give a dose not much larger than one just sufficient to cause the desired physiologic response. Excessive doses cause blanching of the skin, abdominal cramps, and nausea.
2. Administration of 1–2 glasses of water prior to use for diabetes insipidus will reduce side effects such as nausea, cramps, and skin blanching.
3. IV Store from 15–25°C (59–77°F).
4. COMPATIBILITY D5W, 0.9% NaCl.
5. INCOMPATIBILITY Administer separately.

ASSESSMENT

1. Note reasons for therapy, type, onset, characteristics of S&S.
2. Identify any vascular disease, especially involving the coronary arteries (e.g., hypertension, CHF, CAD) that may preclude therapy.
3. List any asthma, seizures, or migraine headaches. Assess closely for water intoxication to prevent seizures and coma.
4. Check skin turgor, mucous membranes, and presence of thirst to assess for dehydration.
5. Monitor BP and I&O; report any excessive BP elevation or lack of response characterized by a ↓ BP.
6. Record weight daily and assess for edema; report rapid gains.
7. Perform urine specific gravity, and report if <1.005 or >1.030. Determine urine osmolarity.
8. With abdominal distention, assess/document presence/characteristics of bowel sounds and passage of flatus/stool. An enema/rectal tube may facilitate expulsion of gas.
9. Injection solution may be used as nasal spray, in a dropper, or applied to cotton pledgets for topical administration.
10. Monitor VS, I&O, ECG, CBC, renal and LFTs.

CLIENT/FAMILY TEACHING

1. Lack of vasopressin causes your body to lose too much water.
2. Review appropriate method for administration/instillation. Rotate sites with SC injections. Take with 16 oz water to prevent N&V, skin blanching, and cramps.
3. With nasal therapy, insert tube into nasal cavity to administer drug. Follow provider guidelines for administration.
4. Avoid alcohol and OTC agents without approval.
5. Use caution and report any drowsiness, listlessness, and/or headache; restrict water intake.
6. Record weights, intake and output; urine output should decrease after use.
7. Keep all F/U to assess response, labs, and for adverse SE.

OUTCOMES/EVALUATE

- Prevention of dehydration: ↓ urinary output/osmolarity
- Control of intra-arterial bleeding
- ↓ Abdominal distention/discomfort; elimination of intestinal gas

IV

Vecuronium bromide

(veh-kyour-**OH**-nee-um)

Classification(s): Neuromuscular blocking drug, nondepolarizing

Pregnancy Category: C

RX: Norcuron.

SEE ALSO ***NEUROMUSCULAR BLOCKING AGENTS***.

INDICATIONS/USES

(1) Induce skeletal muscle relaxation during surgery or mechanical ventilation. (2) Facilitate ET intubation. (3) Adjunct to general anesthesia. *Investigational:* To treat electrically induced seizures or seizures induced by drugs.

ACTION/KINETICS

Action

Less likely than other agents to cause histamine release. Effects can be antagonized by anticholinesterase drugs.

Pharmacokinetics

Onset: 2.5–3 min; **peak effect:** 3–5 min; **duration:** 25–40 min using balanced anesthesia. About one-third more potent than pancuronium, but its duration of action is shorter at initial equipotent doses. No cumulative effects noted after repeated administration. **t½, elimination:** 65–75 min; a shortened half-life (35–40 min) has been noted in late pregnancy. Metabolized in liver and excreted through the kidneys and bile. Recovery may be doubled in clients with cirrhosis or cholestasis; renal failure does not affect recovery time. **Plasma protein binding:** 60–80%.

ADDITIONAL CONTRAINDICATIONS

Use in neonates, obesity. Sensitivity to bromides.

SPECIAL CONCERNS

Do not administer unless facilities for intubation, artificial respiration, oxygen therapy, and reversal agents are immediately available. Be prepared to assist or control respiration.

- Those from 7 weeks to 1 year of age are more sensitive to the effects of vecuronium, leading to a recovery time up to 1½ times that for adults.
- The dose for children aged 1–10 years of age must be individualized and may, in fact, require a somewhat higher initial dose and a slightly more frequent supplemental dosing schedule than adults.
- Those with myasthenia gravis or Eaton-Lambert syndrome may experience profound effects with small doses of vecuronium.
- Cardiovascular disease, old age, and edematous states result in increased volume of distribution and thus a delay in onset time-the dose should *not* be increased.

SIDE EFFECTS

Most Common

Skin flushing, itching, skeletal muscle weakness, wheezing, bronchial secretions, hives, increased HR, increased mean arterial pressure.

See *Neuromuscular Blocking Agents* for a complete list of possible side effects. Also, moderate to severe skeletal muscle weakness, which may require artificial respiration. ***Malignant hyperthermia.***

ADDITIONAL DRUG INTERACTIONS

Bacitracin / High IV or IP bacitracin doses → ↑ muscle relaxation
Sodium colistimethate / High IV or IP sodium colistimethate doses → ↑ muscle relaxation
Succinylcholine / ↑ Vecuronium effect
Tetracyclines / High IV or IP tetracycline doses → ↑ muscle relaxation

HOW SUPPLIED

Powder for Injection: 10 mg, 20 mg.

DOSAGE

IV

Intubation.

Adults and children over 10 years of age. 0.08–0.1 mg/kg.

For use after succinylcholine-assisted endotracheal intubation.

0.04–0.06 mg/kg for inhalation anesthesia and 0.05–0.06 mg/kg using balanced anesthesia. *NOTE:* For halothane anesthesia, doses of 0.15–0.28 mg/kg may be given without adverse effects.

For use during anesthesia with enflurane or isoflurane after steady state established.

0.06–0.085 mg/kg (about 15% less than the usual initial dose).

Supplemental use.

IV only: 0.01–0.015 mg/kg given 25–40 min following the initial dose; **then** given q 12–15 min as needed. **IV infusion:** Initiated after recovery from effects of initial IV dose of 0.08–0.1 mg/kg has started. **Initial:** 0.001 mcg; **then** adjust according to client response and requirements. Average infusion rate: 0.0008–0.0012 mg/kg/min (0.8–1.2 mcg/kg/min). After steady-state enflurane, isoflurane, and possibly halothane anesthesia has been established, reduce IV infusion by 25–60%.

NURSING IMPLICATIONS

Do not confuse vecuronium with rocuronium (another neuromuscular blocker). Also, do not confuse Norcuron with Natrecor (a cardiovascular drug).

IMPLEMENTATION/ADMINISTRATION/STORAGE

1. **IV Dosage must be individualized and depends on prior or concomitant use of anesthetics or succinylcholine.**
2. **Refrigerate after reconstitution. Use within 8 hr of reconstitution.**
3. **Have neostigmine, pyridostigmine, or edrophonium available to reverse vecuronium; atropine helps counteract muscarinic effects.**
4. **COMPATIBILITY Saline, D5W alone or with saline, RL solution, and sterile water for injection.**
5. **INCOMPATIBILITY Administer separately.**

ASSESSMENT

1. **Note reasons for therapy, anticipated time frame for use. Review conditions/drugs that antagonize and enhance neuromuscular blockade; assess for presence.**
2. **Provide ventilatory support. Monitor VS, ECG, and I&O. Can cause vagal stimulation, resulting in bradycardia, hypotension, and cardiac arrhythmias.**
3. **Use a peripheral nerve stimulator to determine neuromuscular blockade and muscle strength recovery. Anticholinesterase will reverse neuromuscular blockade but should not be used until some evidence of spontaneous recovery noted**
4. **Muscle fasciculations may cause soreness or injury after recovery. Give prescribed nondepolarizing agent and reassure that soreness is likely caused by unsynchronized contractions of adjacent muscle fibers just before onset of paralysis.**
5. **Monitor closely for any evidence of malignant hyperthermia, unresponsive tachycardia, jaw spasm, or lack of laryngeal relaxation. Stop infusion and report; temperature elevations are late S&S.**
6. **Drug should only be used on a short-term basis and in a continuously monitored environment.**
7. **Client is fully conscious and aware of surroundings and conversations. Drug does not affect pain or anxiety; give analgesics and antianxiety agents.**
8. **Position for comfort and so that the body is in proper alignment. Turn and perform mouth care and eye care frequently (protect eyes and instill liquid tears q 2 hr as blink reflex is suppressed).**
9. **Assess airway at frequent intervals. Have suction at the bedside.**
10. **Prolonged use, as in an ICU setting, may lead to skeletal muscle weakness and symptoms consistent with muscle disuse atrophy. This may complicate ventilator weaning; some may require extensive physical therapy.**
11. **Monitor ECG, VS, CBC, electrolytes, renal and LFTs, and lung assessments.**

CLIENT/FAMILY TEACHING

1. **Drug used to control movement and permit procedures/treatments and will make you feel like you are paralyzed; sensation will return once drug is discontinued and wears off. Procedures and activities will be explained at the time of performance.**
2. **Will be unable to move or talk, and a machine will do all breathing. This will be in a setting that permits continous monitoring; response assessed with a peripheral nerve stimulator.**

V

3. May have eyes patched; eye drops and patches used to protect corneas during prolonged therapy as blink reflex suppressed.
4. During therapy will be able to see and hear; medication will be given for pain and anxiety. All functions will return once the medication is discontinued.
5. Report any adverse or unusual side effects once medication therapy completed

OUTCOMES/EVALUATE

- Skeletal muscle relaxation
- Facilitation of intubation; tolerance of mechanical ventilation

Vemurafenib

(vem-you-**RAF**-e-nib)

Classification(s): Kinase inhibitor.

Pregnancy Category: D

RX: Zelboraf.

INDICATIONS/USES

Treatment of unresectable or metastatic melanoma with BRAF mutation as detected by a FDA-approved test.

ACTION/KINETICS

Action

Vemurafenib inhibits some mutated forms of BRAF serine-threonine kinase. Some mutations in the BRAF gene result in constitutively activated BRAF proteins, which can cause cell proliferation in the absence of growth factors that would normally be required for proliferation. Vemurafenib has antitumor effects in melanomas with mutated BRAF. Also, vemurafenib is associated with concentration-dependent QTc interval prolongation.

Pharmacokinetics

T_{max}, median: About 3 hr. Steady state is reached in about 15–22 days following dosing at 960 mg twice a day. About 94% of a dose is excreted in the feces and just 1% in the urine. **t½, elimination:** 57 hr. **Plasma protein binding:** >99%.

CONTRAINDICATIONS

Lactation.

SPECIAL CONCERNS

- Elderly clients older than 65 years may be more likely to experience side effects, including cutaneous squamous cell carcinoma, nausea, decreased appetite, peripheral edema, keratocanthoma, and atrial fibrillation.
- Use with caution in preexisting severe renal or hepatic impairment
- Safety and efficacy in children less than 18 years not established.

SIDE EFFECTS

Most Common

Alopecia, arthralgia, diarrhea, fatigue, headache, hyperkeratosis, N&V, photosensitivity reactions, pruritus, rash, skin papilloma, cutaneous squamous cell carcinoma,

CNS: Headache, dysgeusia, asthenia, dizziness, peripheral neuropathy, VIIth nerve paralysis. **GI:** N&V, diarrhea, constipation. **CV:** Atrial fibrillation, QT prolongation, vasculitis. **Dermatologic:** Alopecia, rash, photosensitivity reaction (mild to severe), cutaneous squamous cell carcinoma, hyperkeratosis, keratocanthoma, pruritus, skin papilloma, dry skin, seborrheic keratosis, sunburn, maculopapular rash, actinic keratosis, papular rash, basal cell carcinoma, erythema nodosum, folliculitis, keratosis pilaris, palmar–plantar erythrodysesthesia syndrome, ***Stevens-Johnson syndrome***. **Musculoskeletal:** Arthralgia, pain in extremity, myalgia, back pain, musculoskeletal pain, arthritis. **Respiratory:** Cough. **Metabolic/Nutritional:** Decreased appetite, decreased weight, peripheral edema. **Ophthalmic:** Retinal vein occlusion, uveitis. **Hypersensitivity:** ***Anaphylaxis***, generalized rash, erythema, hypotension. **Body as a whole:** Fatigue, pyrexia. **Miscellaneous:** New primary malignant melanoma. *NOTE:* Arthralgia, ↑ creatinine, photosensitivity and rash are seen more often in women whereas ↑ alkaline phosphatase and total bilirubin and keratocanthoma are seen more often in men.

LABORATORY TEST CONSIDERATIONS

↑ Creatinine, alkaline phosphatase, total bilirubin, ALT, AST, GGT.

OVERDOSE MANAGEMENT

Treatment: There is no specific antidote for vemurafenib overdose. Provide appropriate symptomatic treatment. Withhold vemurafenib and institute supportive care.

V

DRUG INTERACTIONS

An additive effect of vemurafenib with other drugs that prolong the QT interval cannot be excluded. The following drugs may prolong the QT interval and increase the risk of life–threatening cardiac arrhythmias, including torsades de pointes: Amiodarone, arsenic trioxide, bretylium, chlorpromazine, cisapride, disopyramide, dofetilide, dolasetron, droperidol, gatifloxacin, halofantrine, levomethadyl, mefloquine, mesoridazine, moxifloxacin, pentamidine, pimozide, probucol, procainamide, quinidine, sotalol, sparfloxacin, thioridazine, and ziprasidone.

Atazanavir / ↑ Vemurafenib plasma levels R/T inhibition of CYP3A4 metabolism → ↑ pharmacologic/toxic effects; use together with caution and monitor
Carbamazepine / ↓ Vemurafenib plasma levels R/T induction of CYP3A4 metabolism → ↓ therapeutic effect
Clarithromycin / ↑ Vemurafenib plasma levels R/T inhibition of CYP3A4 metabolism → ↑ pharmacologic/toxic effects; use together with caution and monitor
CYP1A2 substrates (e.g., caffeine) / ↑ Caffeine AUC 2.6 fold; use of vemurafenib with agents with a narrow therapeutic index that are metabolized by CYP1A2 is not recommended
CYP2D6 substrates (e.g., dextromethorphan) / ↑ Dextromethorphan C_{max} and AUC 36% and 47%, respectively; use of vemurafenib with agents with a narrow therapeutic index that are metabolized by CYP2D6 is not recommended
CYP3A4 substrates (e.g., midazolam) / ↓ Midazolam C_{max} and AUC 35% and 39% respectively; use of vemurafenib with agents with a narrow therapeutic index that are metabolized by CYP3A4 not recommended
Indinavir /↑ Vemurafenib plasma levels R/T inhibition of CYP3A4 metabolism → ↑ pharmacologic/toxic effects; use together with caution and monitor
Itraconazole / ↑ Vemurafenib plasma levels R/T inhibition of CYP3A4 metabolism → ↑ pharmacologic/toxic effects; use together with caution and monitor
Ketoconazole / ↑ Vemurafenib plasma levels R/T inhibition of CYP3A4 metabolism → ↑ pharmacologic/toxic effects; use together with caution and monitor
Nefazodone / ↑ Vemurafenib plasma levels R/T inhibition of CYP3A4 metabolism → ↑ pharmacologic/toxic effects; use together with caution and monitor
Nelfinavir / ↑ Vemurafenib plasma levels R/T inhibition of CYP3A4 metabolism → ↑ pharmacologic/toxic effects; use together with caution and monitor
Phenobarbital / ↓ Vemurafenib plasma levels R/T induction of CYP3A4 metabolism → ↓ therapeutic effect
Phenytoin / ↓ Vemurafenib plasma levels R/T induction of CYP3A4 metabolism → ↓ therapeutic effect
QT prolonging drugs (see list at beginning of this section) / ↑ Risk of life–threatening cardiac arrhythmias, including torsades de pointes; do not use together
Rifabutin, Rifampin, Rifapentine / ↓ Vemurafenib plasma levels R/T induction of CYP3A4 metabolism → ↓ therapeutic effect
Ritonavir / ↑ Vemurafenib plasma levels R/T inhibition of CYP3A4 metabolism → ↑ pharmacologic/toxic effects; use together with caution and monitor
Saquinavir / ↑ Vemurafenib plasma levels R/T inhibition of CYP3A4 metabolism → ↑ pharmacologic/toxic effects; use together with caution and monitor
Telithromycin / ↑ Vemurafenib plasma levels R/T inhibition of CYP3A4 metabolism → ↑ pharmacologic/toxic effects; use together with caution and monitor
Voriconazole / ↑ Vemurafenib plasma levels R/T inhibition of CYP3A4 metabolism → ↑ pharmacologic/toxic effects; use together with caution and monitor
Warfarin / ↑ AUC of S–warfarin (a CYP2C9 substrate); use together with caution and monitor INR frequently

HOW SUPPLIED

Tablets: 240 mg.

DOSAGE

TABLETS

Melanoma.

Adults, usual: 960 mg twice a day. The first dose should be taken in the morning and the second dose should be taken in the evening about 12 hr later.

V

Management of symptomatic side effects or prolongation of QTc may require dose reduction, treatment interruption, or treatment discontinuation. Dose modifications or interruptions are not recommended for cutaneous squamous cell carcinoma side effects.

NURSING IMPLICATIONS

IMPLEMENTATION/ADMINISTRATION/STORAGE

1. Treat clients with vemurafenib until disease progression or unacceptable toxicity occurs.
2. If a dose is missed, it can be taken up to 4 hr prior to the next dose to maintain the twice a day regimen. Do not take both doses at the same time.
3. Dose adjustments for adverse reactions graded by the Common Terminology Criteria for Adverse Events, v. 4.0 (CTC-AE):
   - (a) Grade 1 or Grade 2 (tolerable): Maintain vemurafenib dose of 960 mg twice a day.
   - (b) Grade 2 (intolerable) or grade 3, 1st appearance: Interrupt treatment until grade 0 to 1. Resume dosing at 720 mg twice a day.
   - (c) Grade 2 (intolerable) or grade 3, 2nd appearance: Interrupt treatment until grade 0 to 1. Resume dosing at 480 mg twice a day.
   - (d) Grade 2 (intolerable) or grade 3, 3rd appearance: Discontinue permanently.
   - (e) Grade 4, 1st appearance: Discontinue permanently or interrupt vemurafenib until grade 0 to 1. Resume dosing at 480 mg twice a day.
   - (f) Grade 4, 2nd appearance: Discontinue permanently.
4. Store from 15–30°C (59–86°F) in the original container with the lid tightly closed.

ASSESSMENT

1. Therapy is selectively indicated for clients with unresectable or metastatic melanoma with BRAF ^{V600E} mutation.
2. Treatment generally continues until disease progression or unacceptable toxicity occurs.
3. Drug can prolong QT interval and requires careful monitoring. List drugs prescribed and avoid concurrent use with any drugs that prolong QT interval. Monitor ECG as QT prolongation may require dose reduction, interruption or discontinuation.
4. Obtain a dermatologic evaluation prior to starting therapy and every 2 months while on therapy to assess for cutaneous squamous cell carcinoma (cuSCC). Any suspicious skin lesions should be excised, sent for dermatopathologic evaluation and treated as per standard protocol. Monitor skin condition for 6 months following discontinuation of therapy.
5. Routinely monitor patients for signs and symptoms of uveitis.
6. Review risks of therapy including development of new primary malignant melanoma, cuSCC, QT prolongation, hypersensitivity and photosensitivity reactions.
7. Confirmation of BRAF^{V600E} mutation-positive melanoma as detected by an FDA-approved test; is required for treatment with vemurafenib.
8. Obtain ECG and electrolytes (potassium, magnesium, calcium) before treatment and after dose modification. Monitor ECG 15 days after treatment initiation and then monthly during the first 3 months of therapy, and every 3 months thereafter or more often if clinically indicated. Monitor liver transaminases, alkaline phosphatase, and bilirubin before initiation of treatment and monthly during treatment, or as clinically indicated. Monitor renal and LFTs and reduce dose or stop therapy with dysfunction.

CLIENT/FAMILY TEACHING

1. Drug is used to treat a certain kind of melanoma that cannot be removed by surgery or that has spread to other parts of the body.
2. The first dose should be taken in the morning and the second dose should be taken in the evening approximately 12 hours later. Each dose can be taken with or without food.
3. Report any new warts, skin lesions that do not heal or bleed easily, and any changes in color or size of moles immediately. You may develop new melanoma lesions during therapy.
4. Frequent monitoring of your heart by an ECG and electrolytes will be performed. Vemurafenib can prolong the QT interval.
5. Report any eye pain, swelling, redness, or other vision changes and have regular eye exams performed.

V

6. May experience joint pain, rash, hair loss, fatigue, photosensitivity reactions, nausea, itching, and other skin growths; report if persistent or bothersome.
7. Avoid prolonged sun exposure and wear protective clothing and sunscreen if exposed. May be more susceptible to sunburn during and for 4 months following therapy. Notify provider if any rash develops.
8. Practice reliable contraception during and for 2 mo following therapy. Do not breast-feed.
9. Avoid OTC agents and any other prescribed agents without provider approval.
10. Keep all F/U to assess response, for labs/ECG, skin/eye exams, and for adverse SE.

OUTCOMES/EVALUATE

Inhibition of continued malignant cell proliferation with progressive BRAF mutation melanoma

Venlafaxine hydrochloride

(ven-lah-**FAX**-een)

Classification(s): Antidepressant, miscellaneous

Pregnancy Category: C (**D** during the second half of pregnancy)

RX: Effexor XR.

Rx: Novo-Venlafaxine XR.

INDICATIONS/USES

(1) Major depressive disorder. (2) Treatment of generalized anxiety disorder, as defined in DSM-IV. Use extended-release products only. (3) Treatment of social anxiety disorder (social phobia), as defined in DSM-IV. Use extended-release capsules and tablets only. (4) Adults with panic disorder, with or without agoraphobia as defined in DSM-IV. Use extended-release capsules only. *Investigational:* Hot flashes, autism, binge eating disorder, pain. Premenstrual dysphoric disorder. Posttraumatic stress disorder (after no response with a selective serotonin reuptake inhibitor for 8 weeks). Prevention of migraine in adults.

ACTION/KINETICS

Action

Not related chemically to any of the currently available antidepressants. Venlafaxine and the active metabolite, O-desmethylvenlafaxine, are potent inhibitors of the uptake of neuronal serotonin and norepinephrine in the CNS and a weak inhibitor of the uptake of dopamine. Has no anticholinergic, sedative, or orthostatic hypotensive effects.

Pharmacokinetics

Well absorbed (92%); absolute bioavailability is about 45%. Food does not affect the bioavailability. Metabolized in the liver by CYP2D6. Plasma levels of venlafaxine were higher in CYP2D6 poor metabolizers than extensive metabolizers. The major metabolite, O-desmethylvenlafaxine (ODV), is active. The drug and metabolite are eliminated through the urine (87%). **t½, venlafaxine:** 5 hr; **t½, ODV:** 11 hr. **Time to reach steady state:** 3 days. The half-life of the drug and metabolite are increased in clients with impaired liver or renal function. Food has no effect on the bioavailability of venlafaxine or the active metabolite.

CONTRAINDICATIONS

Hypersensitivity to venlafaxine or any components of the product. Use with a MAOI or within 14 days of discontinuation of a MAOI. Use of alcohol. Lactation.

SPECIAL CONCERNS

Suicidality and antidepressant drugs. Antidepressants increased the risk of suicidal thinking and behavior (suicidality) compared with placebo in short-term studies in children, adolescents, and young adults with major depressive disorder and other psychiatric disorders. Anyone considering the use of venlafaxine or any other antidepressant in a child, adolescent, or young adult must balance this risk with the clinical need. Short-term studies did not show an increased risk of suicidality with antidepressants compared with placebo in adults 24 years of age; there was a reduction in risk with antidepressants compared with placebo in adults 65 years of age and older. Depression and certain other psychiatric disorders are themselves associated with increases in the risk of suicide. Closely observe and appropriately monitor clients of all ages who are started on antidepressant therapy for clinical worsening, suicidality, or unusual changes in behavior. Advise families and caregivers of the need for close observation and communication with the prescriber. Venlafaxine is not approved for use in children.

- **Use with caution with impaired hepatic (e.g., cirrhosis) or renal (GFR = 10–70 mL/min) function, with a history of mania, and with diseases or conditions that could affect the hemodynamic responses or metabolism.**
- **Use with caution in clients with a history of seizures; also, in clients whose underlying medical condition might be compromised by increases in heart rate (i.e., hypothyroidism, heart failure, recent MI), especially those taking more than 200 mg/day of venlafaxine.**
- **Although possible for the elderly to be more sensitive, dosage adjustment is not necessary.**
- **Clinical worsening and suicide risk are possible in both adult and pediatric clients with major depressive disorder.**
- **Use for more than 4–6 weeks not evaluated.**
- **Safety and efficacy of the immediate-release or extended-release products not determined in children less than 18 years.**
- **Infants exposed to venlafaxine during the third trimester of pregnancy may develop complications requiring prolonged hospitalization, respiratory support, and tube feeding; carefully consider the potential risks and benefits of treatment and consider tapering the medication in the third trimester.**

SIDE EFFECTS

Most Common

N&V headache, somnolence, dizziness, insomnia, nervousness, anxiety, anorexia, blurred vision, tremor, constipation, asthenia, dry mouth, abnormal ejaculation/orgasm in men, impotence, sweating, abnormal dreams.

Side effects with an incidence of 0.1% or greater and life-threatening side effects are listed. **CNS:** Anxiety, headache, nervousness, insomnia, activation of mania or hypomania, ***seizures, suicide attempts/ideation***, dizziness, somnolence, tremors, twitching, abnormal dreams, hypertonia, paresthesia, decreased/increased libido, agitation, amnesia, confusion, abnormal thinking, depersonalization, worsening of depression, twitching, migraine, emotional lability, trismus, vertigo, apathy, ataxia, circumoral paresthesia, CNS stimulation, euphoria, hallucinations, hostility, hyperesthesia, hypesthesia, hyperkinesia, hyper-/hypotonia, incoordination, myoclonus, neuralgia, neuropathy, paranoid reaction, psychosis, psychotic depression, sleep disturbance, abnormal speech, stupor, akathisia, manic reactions, torticollis. **Serotonin syndrome:** Agitation, hallucinations, coma, tachycardia, labile BP, hyperthermia, hyperreflexia, incoordination, N&V, diarrhea, ***death***. **CV:** Sustained increase in BP (hypertension), vasodilation, tachycardia, increased pulse rate/heart rate, postural hypotension, palpitation, angina pectoris, extrasystoles, hypotension, arrhythmia, peripheral vascular disorder (mainly cold hands/feet), syncope, thrombophlebitis, peripheral edema, bradycardia, migraine. **GI:** Anorexia, N&V, dry mouth, constipation, diarrhea, dyspepsia, flatulence, abdominal pain, dysphagia, eructation, colitis, edema of tongue, esophagitis, gastroenteritis, gastritis, bruxism, glossitis, gingivitis, hemorrhoids, ***rectal hemorrhage***, melena, stomatitis, mouth ulceration, increased appetite, bruxism, GI ulcer, oral moniliasis, tongue edema. **Respiratory:** Bronchitis, increased cough, dyspnea, asthma, chest congestion, epistaxis, hyperventilation, laryngismus, laryngitis, pneumonia, voice alteration, pharyngitis, sinusitis, interstitial lung disease (rare), eosinophilic pneumonia (rare). **Dermatologic:** Acne, pruritus, rash, sweating, alopecia, brittle nails, contact dermatitis, dry skin, herpes simplex, herpes zoster, hot flashes, maculopapular rash, urticaria, eczema, psoriasis, skin hypertrophy. **Hematologic:** Ecchymosis, anemia, leukocytosis, leukopenia, lymphadenopathy, thrombocytopenia, thrombocythemia, abnormal WBCs. **Endocrine:** Hypothyroidism, hyperthyroidism, goiter, galactorrhea, thyroid nodule, thyroiditis. **Musculoskeletal:** Arthritis, arthralgia, arthrosis, bone pain/spurs, neck/chest/pelvic pain, bursitis, joint disorder, leg cramps, myasthenia, neck rigidity, tenosynovitis. **GU:** Urinary retention, abnormal ejaculation, impotence, urinary frequency, impaired urination, disturbed orgasm, menstrual disorder, anorgasmia (female), dysuria, hematuria, metrorrhagia, vaginitis, amenorrhea, kidney calculus, cystitis, leukorrhea, menorrhagia, nocturia, bladder pain, breast pain, kidney pain, pelvic pain, polyuria, prostatitis, enlarged prostate, prostate irritability, pyelonephritis, pyuria, urinary incontinence, urinary urgency, enlarged uterine fibroids, ***uterine hemorrhage, vaginal hemorrhage***, vaginitis, vaginal moniliasis. **Ophthalmic:** Blurred vision, mydriasis, abnormal accommodation, abnor-

V

mal vision, cataract, conjunctivitis, corneal lesion, diplopia, dry eyes, exophthalmos, eye pain, photophobia, subconjunctival hemorrhage, visual field defect. **Otic:** Tinnitus, ear pain, hyperacusis, otitis media. **Metabolic:** Weight gain/loss, dehydration, edema, diabetes mellitus, thirst, gout. **Body as a whole:** Asthenia, infection, chills, fever, trauma, yawning, accidental/intentional injury, malaise, enlarged abdomen, allergic reaction, cyst, facial edema, abnormal bleeding (especially ecchymosis), hangover effect, hernia, moniliasis, substernal chest pain, photosensitivity reaction. **Miscellaneous:** Taste perversion/loss, parosmia, hypoglycemic reaction, hemochromatosis, neuroleptic malignant syndrome, withdrawal syndrome. Possible changes in height of children.

LABORATORY TEST CONSIDERATIONS

↑ Alkaline phosphatase, creatinine, AST, ALT, serum cholesterol, serum triglycerides (fasting). Glycosuria, hyperglycemia, hyperlipemia, bilirubinemia, hyperuricemia, hypercholesterolemia, hypoglycemia, hypo-/hyperkalemia, hyponatremia, hypophosphatemia, hypoproteinemia, uremia, albuminuria.

OVERDOSE MANAGEMENT

Symptoms: Extensions of side effects, especially somnolence. Other symptoms include prolongation of QTc, mild sinus tachycardia, and ***seizures.*** Overdose occurs in combination with alcohol or other drugs. Symptoms include tachycardia, changes in level of consciousness (somnolence to coma), mydriasis, seizures, vomiting, prolongation of QT interval, bundle branch block, QRS prolongation, ventricular tachycardia, bradycardia, hypotension, liver necrosis, rhabdomyolysis, serotonin syndrome, vertigo, and death. *Treatment:* General supportive measures; treat symptoms. Ensure an adequate airway, oxygenation, and ventilation. Monitor cardiac rhythm and VS. Gastric lavage with a large bore orogastric tube with appropriate airway protection, if needed, may be helpful if performed soon after ingestion or in symptomatic clients. Administer activated charcoal. Induction of emesis is not recommended. Forced diuresis, dialysis, hemoperfusion, and exchange transfusion are unlikely to be beneficial.

DRUG INTERACTIONS

An additive effect of venlafaxine with other drugs that prolong the QT interval cannot be excluded. The following drugs may prolong the QT interval and increase the risk of life–threatening cardiac arrhythmias, including torsades de pointes: Amiodarone, arsenic trioxide, bretylium, chlorpromazine, cisapride, disopyramide, dofetilide, dolasetron, droperidol, mefloquine, mesoridazine, moxifloxacin, pentamidine, pimozide, procainamide, quinidine, sotalol, tacrolimus, thioridazine, and ziprasidone.

Aspirin / ↑ Risk of upper GI bleeding

Azole antifungals (e.g., itraconazole, ketoconazole) / ↑ Venlafaxine and O–desmethylvenlafaxine levels; adjust venlafaxine dose as needed

Bupropion / Possible serotonin syndrome; closely monitor. Also, paradoxical worsening of obsessive compulsive disorder

Cimetidine / ↓ First-pass metabolism of venlafaxine → ↓ oral clearance; use with caution in those with hypertension, impaired hepatic function, and in the elderly

Clozapine / Possible ↑ clozapine levels → side effects (including seizures); monitor and adjust clozapine dosage as needed when venlafaxine started or stopped

Cyproheptadine / ↓ Pharmacologic effects of venlafaxine; closely monitor

Dextromethorphan / ↑ Dextromethorphan plasma levels and toxicity; closely monitor

Fenfluramine / Possible serotonin syndrome R/T additive serotonergic effects; concurrent use not recommended

Haloperidol / ↑ Haloperidol serum AUC and C_{max}; monitor and adjust haloperidol dose as needed

Indinavir / ↓ Indinavir AUC and C_{max}; clinical significance unknown

Linezolid / ↑ Risk of serotonin syndrome (irritability, increased muscle tone, shivering, myoclonus, altered consciousness); monitor closely

Lithium / ↑ Lithium levels → neurotoxicity; also possible serotonin syndrome

MAOIs (e.g., phenelzine) / Serious and possibly fatal reaction, including hyperthermia, rigidity, myoclonus, autonomic instability with rapid changes in VS, extreme agitation, delirium, coma; concomitant use contraindicated.

Metoclopramide / ↑ Risk of serotonin syndrome (irritability, increased muscle tone, shivering, myoclonus, altered consciousness); monitor closely

Metoprolol / ↓ BP effects of metoprolol; clinical relevance not known
Methylene blue / ↑ Risk of CNS toxicity, including serotonin syndrome
Methylphenidate / Possible serotonin syndrome R/T additive effects; monitor closely
Metoclopramide / ↑ Risk of serotonin syndrome (irritability, increased muscle tone, shivering, myoclonus, altered consciousness); monitor closely
Metoprolol / ↓ Metoprolol BP lowering effect; use together with caution
Nefazodone / Possible serotonin syndrome R/T additive serotonergic effects; monitor closely
NSAIDs (e.g., ibuprofen, naproxen) / ↑ Risk of upper GI bleeding
Opioid analgesics (e.g., meperidine) / Possible serotonin syndrome R/T additive serotonergic effects; monitor closely
Propafenone / ↑ Levels of both propafenone and venlafaxine→ ↑ pharmacologic/toxic effects; monitor
Rasagiline / Possible serotonin syndrome R/T additive serotonergic effects; monitor closely
H ***Sour date nut*** /Possible serotonin syndrome R/T additive serotonergic effects; monitor closely
H ***St. John's wort*** / ↑ Risk of serotonin syndrome (irritability, increased muscle tone, shivering, myoclonus, altered consciousness); monitor closely
Selective norepinephrine reuptake inhibitors / ↑ Risk of serotonin syndrome (irritability, increased muscle tone, shivering, myoclonus, altered consciousness); monitor closely
Selective serotonin reuptake inhibitors (e.g., fluoxetine, paroxetine) / ↑ Risk of serotonin syndrome (irritability, increased muscle tone, shivering, myoclonus, altered consciousness); monitor closely
Sibutramine / ↑ Risk of serotonin syndrome (irritability, increased muscle tone, shivering, myoclonus, altered consciousness); monitor closely
Sympathomimetics (e.g., amphetamine) / ↑ Risk of serotonin syndrome (irritability, increased muscle tone, shivering, myoclonus, altered consciousness); monitor closely
Terbinafine / ↑ Venlafaxine plasma levels → ↑ pharmacologic/toxic effects; monitor and adjust venlafaxine dose if as needed
Tramadol / ↑ Risk of serotonin syndrome (irritability, increased muscle tone, shivering, myoclonus, altered consciousness); monitor closely
Trazodone / ↑ Risk of serotonin syndrome (irritability, increased muscle tone, shivering, myoclonus, altered consciousness); monitor closely
Tricyclic antidepressants (e.g., desipramine) / ↑ TCA levels → ↑ pharmacologic/toxic effects
Triptans (e.g., sumatriptan, zolmitriptan) / ↑ Risk of serotonin syndrome (irritability, increased muscle tone, shivering, myoclonus, altered consciousness); monitor closely
L-Tryptophan / Possible serotonin syndrome R/T additive or synergistic serotonergic effects; concomitant use not recommended
Warfarin / Possible ↑ PT, PTT, INR; monitor coagulation parameters when starting or stopping venlafaxine and adjust warfarin dose as needed

HOW SUPPLIED

Capsules, Extended-Release: 37.5 mg, 75 mg, 150 mg; ***Tablets, Extended-Release:*** 37.5 mg, 75 mg, 150 mg, 225 mg; ***Tablets, Immediate-Release:*** 25 mg, 37.5 mg, 50 mg, 75 mg, 100 mg.

DOSAGE

TABLETS, IMMEDIATE-RELEASE

Major depressive disorder.

Adults, initial: 75 mg/day given in 2 or 3 divided doses and taken with food. Depending on the response, the dose can be increased to the usual dose of 150–225 mg/day in divided doses. Make dosage increments up to 75 mg/day at intervals of 4 or more days. Severely depressed clients may require 375 mg/day in 3 divided doses. **Maintenance:** Periodically assess client to determine the need for maintenance treatment and the appropriate dose.

CAPSULES, EXTENDED-RELEASE; TABLETS, EXTENDED-RELEASE

Major depressive disorder.

Extended-Release Capsules/Tablets. Adults, initial: 75 mg as a single dose once daily in the morning or evening at about the same time each day. For some clients it may be desirable to start at 37.5 mg/day for 4–7 days to allow adjustment to the drug before increasing to 75 mg/day. Dose can be increased by

V

increments up to 75 mg no more often than every 4 days, to a maximum of 225 mg/day. **Maintenance:** 75–225 mg/day.

Generalized anxiety disorder.

Extended-Release Capsules, Adults, initial, usual: 75 mg/day as a single dose; if necessary, the dose may be increased to 225 mg/day. Increase in increments of up to 75 mg/day at intervals of not less than 4 days. To avoid overstimulation, some may need to start with 37.5 mg/day. Take on a daily basis, not on an as-needed basis. **Maintenance:** 75–225 (maximum) mg/day. Periodically reassess the need for continuing the medication.

Social anxiety disorder (social phobia).

Extended-Release Capsules/Tablets. Adults: 75 mg/day as a single dose.

Panic disorder.

Extended-Release Capsules, Adults, initial, usual: 37.5 mg per day for 7 days. Make dose increases in increments of up to 75 mg/day as needed at intervals of no less than 7 days. **Maintenance:** 75–225 mg/day. **Maximum dose:** 225 mg/day.

Hot flashes in otherwise healthy postmenopausal women (investigational).

Extended-Release formulation: 37.5–150 mg once a day, for up to 3 months. **Immediate-Release formulation:** 12.5 mg twice a day for 4 weeks.

NURSING IMPLICATIONS

IMPLEMENTATION/ADMINISTRATION/STORAGE

1. If switching from the immediate-release to extended-release, use the dosage form at the nearest equivalent dose. Individual dosage adjustments may be needed.
2. No dosage adjustment is recommended for the elderly based solely on age. Exercise caution, however.
3. Equal doses of venlafaxine ER tablets are bioequivalent to venlafaxine ER capsules when given under fed conditions.
4. In those with mild to moderate hepatic impairment, reduce the total daily dose by at least 50%; further dose reduction may be needed. In clients with cirrhosis, it may be necessary to reduce the dose more than 50%. Individualization of the dose may be needed in some.
5. In those with mild to moderate impaired renal function, reduce the total daily dose by 25–50% in those taking ER formulation and reduce the total daily dose by 25% in those taking immediate-release products. In those undergoing hemodialysis, reduce the total daily dose by 50% and withhold the dose until dialysis treatment is completed (4 hr).
6. When discontinuing after 1 week or more of therapy, taper dose to minimize risk of withdrawal syndrome. If drug has been taken for 6 weeks or more, taper dose gradually over a 2-week period.
7. At least 14 days should elapse between discontinuation of an MAOI and initiation of venlafaxine therapy; at least 7 days should elapse after stopping venlafaxine before starting an MAOI.
8. Take extended-release form in the morning or evening, but at the same time each day.
9. Abrupt discontinuation or dose reduction of venlafaxine (at various doses) may be associated with the appearance of new symptoms (frequency increased with increased dose level and with longer duration of treatment). Symptoms include agitation, anorexia, anxiety, confusion, impaired coordination, diarrhea, dizziness, dry mouth, dysphoric mood, fasciculation, fatigue, headaches, hypomania, insomnia, nausea, nervousness, nightmares, sensory disturbances (including shock-like electrical sensations), somnolence, sweating, tremor, vertigo, and vomiting. The dose should be decreased at a gradual rate.
10. Store extended-release capsules and immediate-release tablets from 20–25°C (68–77°F). Store extended-release tablets from 15–30°C (59–86°F).

ASSESSMENT

1. List reasons for therapy, onset, characteristics of S&S, mental status, any suicide ideations, clinical presentation. Note other agents trialed, outcome.
2. List agents prescribed to ensure none interact.
3. May cause sustained hypertension; monitor HR and BP regularly; assess ECG.

V

4. Prior to beginning treatment with an antidepressant, adequately screen clients with depressive symptoms to determine if they are at risk for bipolar disorder; may cause a mixed/manic episode.
5. Monitor VS, weight, CBC, lipid panel, renal and LFTs; reduce dose with hepatic/renal impairment.

CLIENT/FAMILY TEACHING

1. Give immediate-release tablets with food. Give extended-release capsules or tablets with food either in the morning or in the evening at about the same time each day.
2. Do not chew or crush extended-release tablets; swallow whole. The contents of the capsule may be sprinkled on applesauce and promptly consumed without chewing and followed with a glass of water to ensure complete swallowing of the pellets. Drug may impair appetite and induce weight loss; report if excessive.
3. Take only as directed; *do not* stop abruptly if used for 6 weeks or more-may cause withdrawal syndrome. Taper over a two week period.
4. Do not perform activities that require mental alertness until drug effects realized; may cause dizziness or drowsiness. Avoid alcohol and any unprescribed or OTC preparations.
5. Report any rash, hives, or other allergic manifestations immediately. May experience anxiety, palpitations, headaches, and constipation; report if persistent or intolerable.
6. Use reliable contraception. Notify provider if pregnant or intend to become pregnant while taking drug.
7. Avoid aspirin or aspirin-containing products, NSAIDs, Ginkgo biloba, or any other medication or herbal product that can affect coagulation (unless prescribed) because of increased risk of serious bleeding.
8. Any suicide ideations or abnormal behaviors should be reported. Due to the possibility of suicide, high-risk clients should be observed closely during initial therapy. Prescriptions should be written for the smallest quantity to reduce the risk of overdose. Family should supervise medication administration with severely depressed clients and report increased agitation, akathisia (psychomotor restlessness), anxiety, change in mood, change in personality, hostility or aggressiveness, impulsivity, insomnia, irritability, panic attacks, suicidal thoughts or behavior.
9. May take several weeks to notice any improvement in symptoms.
10. Keep all F/U to assess response, labs, BP/HR, and for adverse SE.

OUTCOMES/EVALUATE

- Improvement in symptoms of depression
- Control of anxiety/panic disorder

IV

Verapamil

(ver-**AP**-ah-mil)

Classification(s): Calcium channel blocker

Pregnancy Category: C

RX: Calan SR, Covera-HS, Isoptin SR, Verelan, Verelan PM.

🍁 **Rx:** Apo-Verap, Apo-Verap SR, Gen-Verapamil, Gen-Verapamil SR, Nu-Verap.

SEE ALSO ***CALCIUM CHANNEL BLOCKING AGENTS***.

INDICATIONS/USES

PO, Immediate-Release: (1) Angina pectoris due to coronary artery spasm (Prinzmetal's variant), chronic stable angina including angina due to increased effort, unstable angina (preinfarction, crescendo). (2) With digitalis to control rapid ventricular rate at rest and during stress in chronic atrial flutter or atrial fibrillation. (3) Prophylaxis of repetitive paroxysmal supraventricular tachycardia. (4) Essential hypertension. *Investigational:* Manic depression (alternate therapy), exercise-induced asthma, recumbent nocturnal leg cramps, cluster headaches.

PO, Extended-Release: (1) Essential hypertension (Covera-HS only). (2) Angina (Covera-HS only).

IV: (1) Paroxysmal supraventricular tachyarrhythmias. (2) Atrial flutter or fibrillation.

ACTION/KINETICS

Action

Slows AV conduction and prolongs effective refractory period. ↓ HR and ↑ PR interval. IV doses may slightly increase LV filling pressure. Moderately decreases myocardial contractility and peripheral vascular resistance. Worsening of heart

V

failure may result if verapamil is given to clients with moderate to severe cardiac dysfunction.

Pharmacokinetics

Onset, PO: 30 min; **IV:** 3–5 min. **Time to peak plasma levels (PO):** 1–2 hr (5–7 hr for extended-release). **t½, PO:** 4.5–12 hr with repetitive dosing; **IV, initial:** 4 min; **final:** 2–5 hr. **Therapeutic serum levels:** 0.08–0.3 mcg/mL. **Duration, PO:** 8–10 hr (24 hr for extended-release); **IV:** 10–20 min for hemodynamic effect and 2 hr for antiarrhythmic effect. Metabolized to norverapamil, which possesses 20% of the activity of verapamil. *NOTE:* Covera HS is designed to deliver verapamil in concert with the 24-hr circadian variations in BP. Verelan PM allows for bedtime dosing and incorporates a 4- to 5-hr delay in drug delivery so there are maximum plasma levels in the morning.

CONTRAINDICATIONS

Severe hypotension, second- or third-degree AV block, cardiogenic shock, severe CHF, sick sinus syndrome (unless client has artificial pacemaker), severe LV dysfunction. Cardiogenic shock and severe CHF unless secondary to SVT that can be treated with verapamil. Lactation. Use of verapamil, IV, with beta-adrenergic blocking agents (as both depress myocardial contractility and AV conduction). Ventricular tachycardia.

SPECIAL CONCERNS

- **Infants less than 6 months of age may not respond to verapamil.**
- **Use with caution in hypertrophic cardiomyopathy, impaired hepatic and renal function, and in the elderly.**

SIDE EFFECTS

Most Common

Infection, flu-like symptoms, URTI, rhinitis, nausea, dyspepsia, diarrhea, constipation, headache, fatigue/lethargy, dizziness, peripheral edema.

CV: CHF, bradycardia, ***AV block, asystole***, premature ventricular contractions and tachycardia (after IV use), peripheral and pulmonary edema, hypotension, syncope, palpitations, AV dissociation, ***MI, CVA***. **GI:** Nausea, constipation, abdominal discomfort or cramps, dyspepsia, diarrhea, dry mouth. **CNS:** Dizziness, headache, sleep disturbances, depression, amnesia, paranoia, psychoses, hallucinations, jitteriness, confusion, drowsiness, vertigo. IV verapamil may increase intracranial pressure in clients with supratentorial tumors at the time of induction of anesthesia. **Dermatologic:** Rash, dermatitis, alopecia, urticaria, pruritus, erythema multiforme, ***Stevens-Johnson syndrome***. **Respiratory:** URTI, rhinitis, nasal or chest congestion, dyspnea, SOB, wheezing. **Musculoskeletal:** Paresthesia, asthenia, muscle cramps or inflammation, decreased neuromuscular transmission in Duchenne's muscular dystrophy. **Body as a whole:** Infection, flu-like symptoms, sweating, flushing, fatigue, lethargy. **Miscellaneous:** Blurred vision, equilibrium disturbances, sexual difficulties, spotty menstruation, rotary nystagmus, gingival hyperplasia, polyuria, nocturia, gynecomastia, claudication, hyperkeratosis, purpura, petechiae, bruising, hematomas, tachyphylaxis.

LABORATORY TEST CONSIDERATIONS

↑ Alkaline phosphatase, transaminase.

OVERDOSE MANAGEMENT

Symptoms: Extension of side effects. *Treatment:* Beta-adrenergics, IV calcium, vasopressors, pacing, and resuscitation.

ADDITIONAL DRUG INTERACTIONS

Amiodarone / Possible cardiotoxicity with ↓ CO; monitor closely
Antihypertensive agents / Additive hypotensive effects
Antineoplastics / ↓ Verapamil absorption by several antineoplastics
Atorvastatin / ↑ Atorvastatin plasma levels
Barbiturates / ↓ Verapamil bioavailability
Buspirone / ↑ Buspirone effects
Calcium salts / ↓ Verapamil effect; can reverse clinical and toxic effects of verapamil
Carbamazepine / ↑ Carbamazepine effect R/T ↓ liver breakdown
Cimetidine / ↑ Verapamil bioavailability
Clarithromycin / Possible severe hypotension and bradycardia
Cyclosporine / ↑ Cyclosporine plasma levels → possible renal toxicity
Digoxin / ↑ Risk of digoxin toxicity R/T ↑ plasma levels
Disopyramide / Additive depressant effects on myocardial contractility and AV conduction
Dofetilide / ↑ Dofetilide plasma levels → ↑ risk of ventricular arrhythmias
Ethanol / Prolonged and ↑ ethanol effects
Etomidate / Anesthetic effect may be ↑ with prolonged respiratory depression and apnea

V

Fexofenadine / ↑ Fexofenadine peak plasma levels and AUC R/T ↑ bioavailability by inhibiting P-glycoprotein transport
Grapefruit juice / ↑ Verapamil plasma levels R/T ↓ liver metabolism
Imipramine / ↑ Imipramine serum levels
Lithium / ↓ Lithium levels; lithium toxicity also observed
Muscle relaxants, nondepolarizing / ↑ Neuromuscular blockade R/T verapamil effect on calcium channels
Prazosin / Acute hypotensive effect
Quinidine / Possibility of bradycardia, hypotension, AV block, VT, and pulmonary edema
Ranitidine / ↑ Verapamil bioavailability
Rifampin / ↓ Verapamil effect
Risperidone / Significant ↑ plasma risperidone levels R/T ↑ bioavailability through P-glycoprotein inhibition
Sirolimus / ↑ Sirolimus plasma levels
Smoking / ↓ Verapamil and norverapamil AUC and peak plasma levels R/T inhibition of CYP1A2
Sulfinpyrazone / ↑ Verapamil clearance
Tacrolimus / ↑ Tacrolimus plasma levels → ↑ toxicity
Theophylline / ↑ Theophylline effects
Vitamin D / ↓ Verapamil effects
Warfarin / Possible ↑ effect of either drug R/T ↓ plasma protein binding
NOTE: Since verapamil is significantly bound to plasma proteins, interaction with other drugs bound to plasma proteins may occur.

HOW SUPPLIED

Capsules, Extended-Release: 100 mg, 120 mg, 180 mg, 200 mg, 240 mg, 300 mg, 360 mg; *Injection:* 2.5 mg/mL; *Tablets, Extended-Release:* 120 mg, 180 mg, 240 mg; *Tablets, Immediate-Release:* 40 mg, 80 mg, 120 mg.

DOSAGE

TABLETS, IMMEDIATE-RELEASE

Angina at rest and chronic stable angina.

Individualized. Adults, initial: 80–120 mg 3 times per day (40 mg 3 times per day if client is sensitive to verapamil); **then** increase dose to total of 240–480 mg/day.

Arrhythmias.

Dosage range in digitalized clients with chronic atrial fibrillation: 240–320 mg/day in divided doses 3–4 times per day. Maximum effects will be noted during the first 48 hr of therapy.

Prophylaxis of paroxysmal supraventricular tachycardia.

240–480 mg/day in divided doses 3–4 times per day in nondigitalized clients. Maximum effects: During first 48 hr.

Essential hypertension.

Initial, when used alone: 80 mg 3 times per day. Doses up to 360–480 mg daily may be used. Effects are seen in the first week of therapy. In the elderly or in people of small stature, initial dose should be 40 mg 3 times per day.

Prophylaxis of migraine headache.

40–80 mg 3–4 times per day.

CAPSULES, EXTENDED-RELEASE (VERELAN, VERELAN PM); TABLETS, EXTENDED-RELEASE (CALAN SR, COVERA-HS, ISOPTIN SR)

Essential hypertension.

Calan SR or Isoptin SR, initial: 180 mg in the a.m. with food. If an adequate response is not reached, the dose may be increased as follows: 240 mg each morning, 180 mg each morning plus 180 mg each evening (or 240 mg each morning plus 120 mg each evening), or 240 mg q 12 hr. **Covera-HS, initial:** 180 mg at bedtime. If an adequate response is not reached, the dose can be increased as follows: 240 mg each evening, 360 mg each evening, or 480 mg each evening. **Verelan PM:** 200 mg/day at bedtime. Rarely, initial doses of 100 mg/day may be appropriate in those with an increased response to verapamil (e.g., impaired renal or hepatic function, elderly clients). If an adequate response is not reached, the dose can be increased as follows: 300 mg each evening or 400 mg each evening. **Verelan, initial:** 240 mg per day in the morning. Initial doses of 120 mg once daily in the morning; 120 mg per day may be warranted in those who have an increased response to verapamil. If an adequate response is

V

not reached with 120 mg per day, the dose may be increased as follows: 180 mg in the morning, 240 mg in the morning (usual dose), 360 mg in the morning, or 480 mg in the morning

SLOW IV

Supraventricular tachyarrhythmias.

Adults, initial: 5–10 mg (0.075–0.15 mg/kg) as an IV bolus given over 2 min (over 3 min in older clients); **then** 10 mg (0.15 mg/kg) 30 min later if response is not adequate. **Infants, up to 1 year:** 0.1–0.2 mg/kg (0.75–2 mg) given as an IV bolus over 2 min under continuous ECG monitoring; **1–15 years:** 0.1–0.3 mg/kg (2–5 mg, not to exceed 5 mg total dose) over 2 min. If response to initial dose is inadequate, it may be repeated after 30 min, but not more than a total of 10 mg should be given to clients from 1 to 15 years of age. **Elderly:** Give the dose over at least 3 min to minimize side effects.

NURSING IMPLICATIONS

Do not confuse Isoptin with Inotropin (a vasopressor), or Covera with Provera (a progestin).

IMPLEMENTATION/ADMINISTRATION/STORAGE

1. SR tablets (120 mg) may be useful for small stature and elderly clients who require less medication. The terms extended-release and sustained-released are sometimes used interchangeably.
2. Take SR tablets with food.
3. Verelan pellet-filled capsules may be carefully opened and the contents sprinkled on a spoonful of applesauce. Swallow applesauce immediately without chewing; follow with a glass of cool water to ensure complete swallowing of the pellets. Subdividing the contents of a capsule is not recommended.
4. Store capsules from 20–25°C (68–77°F); avoid excessive heat. Store tablets from 15–25°C (59–77°F).
5. IV Before administration, inspect ampules for particulate matter or discoloration.
6. Administer IV dosage under continuous ECG monitoring with resuscitation equipment readily available.
7. Give as slow IV bolus (5–10 mg) over 2 min (3 min to elderly clients) to minimize toxic effects.
8. Store ampules at 20–25°C (68–77°F); protect from light.
9. Always individualize dose in the elderly because the pharmacologic effects are more pronounced and more prolonged.
10. COMPATIBILITY Administer undiluted.
11. INCOMPATIBILITY Do not give verapamil in an infusion line containing 0.45% NaCl with $NaHCO_3$; a crystalline precipitate will form. Do not give by IV push in the same line used for nafcillin infusion, because a milky white precipitate will form. Do not mix with albumin, amphotericin B, hydralazine, trimethoprim/sulfamethoxazole, or dilute with sodium lactate in PVC bags. Verapamil will precipitate in any solution with a pH greater than 6.

ASSESSMENT

1. Note reasons for therapy, onset, characteristics of S&S. List agents trialed, outcome.
2. Review list of prescribed medications to ensure none interact.
3. During IV therapy, continuously monitor ECG (BP and PR interval) and administer with resuscitation equipment readily available.
4. Assess for conditions that preclude therapy: SSS, 2nd or 3rd degree AV block, hypotension, severe left ventricular dysfunction.
5. Use cautiously with decreased neuromuscular transmission; worsens myasthenia gravis. Also may ↑ ICP with supratentorial tumors at time of anesthesia induction.
6. Monitor VS; assess for bradycardia and hypotension, symptoms that may indicate overdosage. May lower BP to dangerously low levels if BP already low.
7. *Do not* administer concurrently with IV beta-adrenergic blocking agents.
8. Unless treating verapamil overdosage, withhold drugs that may elevate calcium levels.
9. Clients receiving concurrent digoxin therapy should be assessed for symptoms of toxicity and have digoxin levels checked periodically.
10. If disopyramide is to be used, do not administer for at least 48 hr before to 24 hr after verapamil dose.
11. Administer extended-release tablets with food to minimize fluctuations in serum levels.

12. Monitor VS, ECG, CBC, renal and LFTs; reduce dose with hepatic or renal impairment, compromised cardiac function, and in those prescribed beta-blockers.

CLIENT/FAMILY TEACHING

1. Verelan and Verelan PM capsules and the contents of the capsules should not be crushed or chewed. The capsules may be opened and the contents sprinkled on a tablespoon of applesauce. Swallow applesauce immediately without chewing, and follow by drinking a glass of cool water to ensure complete swallowing of the pellets.
2. Swallow verapamil ER tablets whole; do not crush or chew.
3. Calan SR and Isoptin SR may be split in half.
4. The medication in Covera-HS is released slowly through an outer shell that does not dissolve. May see the outer shell in stool as it passes from the body.
5. May cause dizziness and sudden drop in BP; use caution with activities that require mental alertness until drug effects realized.
6. Report irregular heartbeat, unusual bruising/bleeding, weight gain, ↑ SOB, swelling of hands or feet, or pronounced dizziness/hypotension.
7. Avoid alcohol, CNS depressants, and OTC agents without approval. Limit caffeine consumption.
8. Continue lifestyle modifications (low-fat and low-salt diet, decreased caloric and alcohol consumption, weight loss, no smoking, and regular exercise) in the overall goal of BP control.
9. Avoid prolonged sun exposure; use protection if exposed.
10. Ensure regular dental care and brush and floss teeth regularly.
11. Increase fluids and fiber in diet to prevent constipation. With higher doses constipation occurs more frequently. Report if bothersome, as psyllium (fiber) may be prescribed or, if severe, drug therapy may be changed.
12. Keep all F/U to assess response, labs, BP and HR log, and for adverse SE.

OUTCOMES/EVALUATE

- ↓ Frequency/severity of anginal attacks
- Control of BP
- Restoration of stable rhythm and rate
- Therapeutic drug levels (0.08–0.3 mcg/mL)

Vilazodone hydrochloride

(vil-**AZ**-oh-done)

Classification(s): Antidepressant, selective serotonin reuptake inhibitor.

Pregnancy Category: C

RX: Viibryd, Viibryd Patient Starter Kit.

INDICATIONS/USES

Treatment of major depressive disorder.

ACTION/KINETICS

Action

The mechanism is thought to be due to enhancement of serotonergic activity in the CNS through selective inhibition of serotonin reuptake.

Pharmacokinetics

Absolute bioavailability: 72%. C_{max}: 4–5 hr. Steady state reached in about 3 days. The AUC in the fasted state can be decreased by about 50% compared with the fed state and may result in decreased efficacy in some clients. Metabolized in the liver mainly by CYP3A4 with minor contributions from CYP2C29 and CYP2D6. **t½, terminal:** About 25 hr. **Plasma protein binding:** 96–99%.

CONTRAINDICATIONS

Use of alcohol. Severe hepatic impairment. Use with MAOIs or in those who have taken MAOIs within the preceding 14 days.

SPECIAL CONCERNS

Suicidality in children and adolescents. Antidepressants increased the risk compared with placebo of suicidal thinking and behavior (suicidality) in children, adolescents, and young adults in short-term studies of major depressive disorder (MDD) and other psychiatric disorders. Anyone considering the use of vilazodone or any other antidepressant in a child, adolescent, or young adult must balance this risk with the clinical need. Short-term studies did not show an increase in the risk of suicidality with antidepressants compared with placebo in adults older than 24 years of age; there was a reduction in risk with antidepressants compared with placebo in adults 65 years of age and older. Depres-

V

sion and certain other psychiatric disorders are themselves associated with increases in the risk of suicide. Clients of all ages who are started on antidepressant therapy should be monitored appropriately and observed closely for clinical worsening, suicidality, or any usual changes in behavior. Families and caregivers should be advised of the need for close observation and communication with the prescriber. Vilazodone is not approved for use in children.

- **Use during lactation only if the potential benefit outweighs the potential risk.**
- **Use during labor and delivery only if the potential benefit outweighs the potential risk.**
- **Safety and efficacy not determined in children.**

SIDE EFFECTS

Most Common

Diarrhea, N&V, insomnia.

CNS: Dizziness, somnolence, paresthesia, tremor, insomnia, abnormal dreams, decreased libido, restlessness, akathisia, restless legs syndrome, sedation, migraine, dysgeusia, panic attack, ***seizures***, activation of mania/hypomania. **GI:** Diarrhea, N&V, dry mouth, dyspepsia, flatulence, gastroenteritis. **CV:** Palpitations, abnormal bleeding, ventricular extrasystoles (rare). **Musculoskeletal:** Arthralgia. **GU:** Delayed ejaculation, erectile dysfunction, abnormal orgasm, anorgasmia, sexual dysfunction, pollakiuria. **Dermatologic:** Hyperhidrosis, night sweats. **Metabolic/Nutritional:** Increased/decreased appetite. **Ophthalmic:** Blurred vision, dry eye, cataracts. **Body as a whole:** Fatigue, feeling jittery/abnormal, serotonin syndrome, neuroleptic malignant like–syndrome.

LABORATORY TEST CONSIDERATIONS

Hyponatremia.

OVERDOSE MANAGEMENT

Symptoms: Serotonin syndrome, lethargy, restlessness, hallucinations, disorientation. *Treatment:* No known antidote. Provide supportive care. Ensure an adequate airway, oxygenation, and ventilation. Monitor cardiac rhythm and vital signs. If needed, gastric lavage with a large-bore orogastric tube with appropriate airway protection. Dialysis will likely not be effective due to the high percentage of the drug bound to plasma protein.

DRUG INTERACTIONS

Aspirin / ↑ Risk of bleeding
Buspirone / Possible serotonin syndrome
CYP3A4 inducers / Possible inadequate vilazodone concentrations → ↓ effectiveness
CYP3A4 strong/moderate inhibitors (e.g., ketoconazole) / ↑ Vilazodone plasma levels → ↑ pharmacologic/toxic effects
Monoamine oxidase inhibitors / Possible tremor, myoclonus, diaphoresis, N&V, flushing, dizziness, hyperthermia with features resembling neuroleptic malignant syndrome, seizures, rigidity, autonomic instability, mental status changes, including extreme agitation, delirium and coma; also possible serotonin syndrome
NSAIDs / ↑ Risk of bleeding
Selective norepinephrine reuptake inhibitors / Possible serotonin syndrome
Selective serotonin reuptake inhibitors (in addition to vilazodone) / Possible serotonin syndrome
Tramadol / Possible serotonin syndrome
Triptans / Possible serotonin syndrome
Tryptophan products / Possible serotonin syndrome
Warfarin / ↑ Risk of bleeding; monitor carefully

HOW SUPPLIED

Tablets: 10 mg, 20 mg, 40 mg. *NOTE:* Starter kit contains 7–10 mg tablets, 7–20 mg tablets, and 16–40 mg tablets.

DOSAGE

TABLETS

Major depressive disorder.

Adults, initial: Titrate dosage; start with an initial dose of 10 mg once a day for 7 days, followed by 20 mg once a day for an additional 7 days, and then an increase to 40 mg once a day. **Usual dose:** 40 mg once a day. Periodically assess to determine the need for maintenance treatment and the appropriate treatment dose.

NURSING IMPLICATIONS

IMPLEMENTATION/ADMINISTRATION/STORAGE

1. **Gradual dose reduction is recommended instead of abrupt discontinuation, whenever possible. Monitor for symptoms when discontinuing vilazodone. If intolerable symptoms**

occur following a dose reduction or upon discontinuation of treatment, consider resuming the previously prescribed dose and decreasing the dose at a more gradual rate.

2. At least 14 days must elapse between discontinuation of a MAOI and initiation of therapy with vilazodone. In addition, at least 14 days must be allowed after stopping vilazodone before starting an MAOI.
3. Reduce the dose to 20 mg when coadministered with strong CYP3A4 inhibitors.
4. No dose adjustment is needed on the basis of age, in those with mild to moderate hepatic impairment, or in those with mild, moderate, or severe renal impairment.
5. Store from 15–30°C (59–86°F).

ASSESSMENT

1. Note reasons for therapy, onset/characteristics of S&S, any events/triggers, and other agents trialed/outcome. Document behaviors and clinical presentation and screening; not for use with bipolar disorder.
2. List other drugs prescribed; ensure none interact. Avoid use within 14 days before or after MAOI use.
3. Assess for clinical worsening of depression, suicidality, or any other unusual changes in behavior.
4. If discontinued, decrease gradually to prevent discontinuation symptoms.
5. Use caution in those with seizure disorders; monitor the elderly, especially if on diuretics or volume depleted as they have exhibited clinically significant hyponatremia.
6. Monitor weight, ECG, VS, electrolytes, renal and LFTs.

CLIENT/FAMILY TEACHING

1. Take as directed, once daily, with food.
2. Use caution operating machines or cars until drug effects known. May impair judgment, thinking, or motor skills.
3. Avoid alcohol or other CNS depressants. Do not take aspirin or aspirin-containing products, NSAIDs, ginkgo biloba, or any other medication or herbal product that can affect coagulation. Risk for bleeding increases with this therapy.
4. Do not stop abruptly, discontinuation effects may occur when suddenly stopping vilazodone.
5. Advise that serotonin syndrome or Neuroleptic Malignant Syndrome (NMS)-like reactions may occur with use, especially with concomitant use of triptans, tramadol, tryptophan supplements, other serotonergic agents, or antipsychotic drugs; use caution.
6. Monitor and report any changes in behavior, mood swings, worsening of depression, or suicidal thoughts/behaviors immediately.
7. Report if S&S of allergic reaction occurs, such as rash, hives, swelling, or difficulty breathing.
8. Remind clients if they are treated with diuretics, or are otherwise volume depleted, or elderly, they have a greater risk of developing hyponatremia (low sodium).
9. Report pregnancy, intent to become pregnant, or breast-feeding to provider.
10. Keep all F/U to assess response, dose, labs, and for adverse SE.

OUTCOMES/EVALUATE

Relief/control of major depressive symptoms

IV

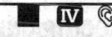

Vinblastine sulfate

(vin-**BLAS**-teen)

Classification(s): Antineoplastic, vinca alkaloid

Pregnancy Category: D

RX: Velban.

SEE ALSO ***ANTINEOPLASTIC AGENTS***.

INDICATIONS/USES

Palliative treatment of the following. **Frequently responsive malignancies.** (1) Palliative treatment of generalized Hodgkin's disease (stages III and IV, Ann Arbor modification of Rye staging system). (2) Lymphocytic lymphoma (nodular and diffuse, poorly and well differentiated). (3) Histiocytic lymphoma. (4) Advanced stages of mycosis fungoides. (5) Advanced testicular carcinoma. (6) Kaposi's sarcoma. (7) Letterer-Siwe disease (histiocytosis X). **Less frequently responsive malignancies.** (1) Choriocarcinoma resistant to other chemotherapy. (2) Breast cancer unresponsive to endocrine surgery and hormonal therapy.

Usually given in combination therapy. However, it has been used as a single agent to treat Hodgkin's disease and advanced testicular germinal-cell cancers (embryonal carcinoma, teratocar-

V

cinoma, choriocarcinoma), although combination therapy is more effective.

NOTE: Vinblastine enhances the effect of bleomycin if given 6–8 hr prior to giving bleomycin.

ACTION/KINETICS

Action

Believed to interfere with metabolic pathways of amino acids leading from glutamic acid to the citric acid cycle and urea. Also affects cell energy production needed for mitosis (affects growing cells in metaphase) and interferes with nucleic acid synthesis.

Pharmacokinetics

Rapidly cleared from plasma with extensive tissue binding but poor penetration to the brain. Also localizes in platelets and leukocyte fractions of whole blood. Almost completely metabolized in the liver after IV administration. **$t_{1/2}$, triphasic:** initial, 3.7 min; intermediate, 1.6 hr; final, 24.8 hr. Metabolites are excreted in the bile with smaller amounts in the urine. No cross-resistance with vincristine. **Plasma protein binding:** About 75%.

CONTRAINDICATIONS

Leukopenia, significant granulocytopenia (unless it is due to the disease being treated). Bacterial infections. Lactation.

SPECIAL CONCERNS

■ (1) It is extremely important that the needle be positioned properly in the vein before injected. If leakage into surrounding tissue occurs during IV administration of vinblastine sulfate, it may cause considerable irritation. Immediately discontinue the injection and introduce any remaining portion of the dose into another vein. Local injection of hyaluronidase and the application of moderate heat to the area of leakage will help disperse the drug and may minimize the discomfort and the possibility of cellulitis. (2) The drug is fatal if given intrathecally. It is for IV use only. ■

- **Intrathecal administration may cause death.**
- **Label syringes as follows: "Vinblastine Sulfate for Intravenous Use Only."**

SIDE EFFECTS

Most Common

Fatigue, alopecia, N&V, cough, fever, chills, infection, malaise, shortness of breath, easy bruising, lower back/side pain, painful/difficult urination.

See *Antineoplastic Agents* for a complete list of possible side effects. Toxicity is dose-related and more pronounced in clients over age 65 or in those suffering from cachexia (profound general ill health) or skin ulceration. **GI:** N&V, ileus, rectal bleeding, ***hemorrhagic enterocolitis***, vesiculation of the mouth, ***bleeding from a former ulcer***. **Dermatologic:** Total epilation, skin vesiculation. **Respiratory:** Acute SOB, ***severe bronchospasm***. **Neurologic:** Paresthesias, neuritis, mental depression, loss of deep tendon reflexes, ***seizures***. Extravasation may result in phlebitis and cellulitis with sloughing.

DRUG INTERACTIONS

Bleomycin sulfate and cisplatin / Combination of bleomycin, cisplatin, and vinblastine may produce signs of Raynaud's disease in clients with testicular cancer
Erythromycin / Severe myalgia, neutropenia, and constipation
Glutamic acid / Inhibits effect of vinblastine
Mitomycin C / Severe bronchospasm with SOB
Phenytoin / ↓ Effect of phenytoin due to ↓ plasma levels
Tryptophan / Inhibits effect of vinblastine

HOW SUPPLIED

Injection: 1 mg/mL; ***Powder for Injection:*** 10 mg.

DOSAGE

IV ONLY

All uses.

Individualized, using WBC count as guide. Administered once every 7 days. **Adults, initial:** 3.7 mg/m^2; **then,** after 7 days, graded doses of 5.5, 7.4, 9.25, and 11.1 mg/m^2 at intervals of 7 days (maximum dose should not exceed 18.5 mg/m^2). Usually the weekly dosage range is 5.5–7.7 mg/m^2. Do not increase the dose after the WBC count is reduced to about 3,000 cells/mm^3. **Children, initial:** 2.5 mg/m^2; **then,** after 7 days, graded doses of 3.75, 5.0, 6.25, and 7.5 mg/m^2 at intervals of 7 days (maximum dose should not exceed 12.5 mg/m^2). **Maintenance** doses are calculated based on WBC count-at least 4,000/mm^3. When the dose produces leukopenia of about 3,000 cells/mm^3, give a dose one increment smaller at

V

weekly intervals for maintenance. Even though 7 days have elapsed, do not give the next dose until the WBC count has returned to at least 4,000 cells/mm^3.

NURSING IMPLICATIONS

Do not confuse vinblastine with vincristine (another vinca alkaloid antineoplastic agent).

IMPLEMENTATION/ADMINISTRATION/STORAGE

1. IV Reconstitute the powder for injection under a laminar flow hood; add 10 mL of bacteriostatic NaCl, which is preserved with either benzyl alcohol or phenol for a final concentration of 1 mg/mL.
2. Inject into tubing of flowing IV infusion or directly into vein and administer over 1 min. To prevent cellulitis or phlebitis, secure the needles within the vein so that no solution extravasates. To further minimize extravasation, rinse syringe and needle with venous blood before withdrawal of the needles. Do not dilute the dose in large volumes of diluent (i.e., 100–250 mL) or give IV for prolonged periods of time (30 min or more) because this often causes vein irritation and increased risk of extravasation.
3. Assess peripheral IV site for patency to prevent extravasation, local irritation, and pain. If extravasation occurs, move infusion to another vein. Treat affected area with hyaluronidase injection and application of moderate heat to decrease local reaction.
4. Because of the increased risk of thrombosis, do not inject solution into an extremity in which circulation is impaired or potentially impaired by conditions, such as compressing or invading neoplasm, phlebitis, or varicosity.
5. If drug gets into the eye, immediately wash eye thoroughly with water to prevent irritation and ulceration.
6. After reconstitution and removal of a portion from the vial, the remainder may be stored in the refrigerator for 30 days. Unopened vials should be refrigerated at temperatures of 2–8°C (36–46°F).
7. COMPATIBILITY D5W or 0.9 % NaCl. Make solutions with either normal saline or 0.9% NaCl injection, each with or without a preservative.
8. INCOMPATIBILITY Do not reconstitute with solutions that raise or lower the pH from between 3.5 and 5.5. Administer separately.

ASSESSMENT

1. Note condition requiring treatment, other therapies trialed, biopsy, lab, and radiographic findings.
2. Take a thorough drug history; note reasons for therapy. List any neuropathies.
3. Administer antiemetic for N&V. Monitor I&O. Encourage fluid intake of 2–3 L/day. Assess infusion site closely; extravasation can cause severe local necrosis.
4. Observe for cyanosis and pallor of extremities and S&S of Raynaud's disease if also receiving bleomycin and severe bronchospasms if also receiving mitomycin.
5. Check for manifestations of neurotoxicity and report if evident; dosage may need to be adjusted. Monitor neurologic toxicity by checking reflexes and strength of hand grip.
6. Observe for S&S of gout; may use allopurinol empirically.
7. Do not increase dose after WBC count is reduced to about 3,000 cells/mm^3. When the dose causes such a degree of leukopenia, give a dose one increment smaller at weekly intervals for maintenance. Even though 7 days has elapsed, do not give the next dose until the WBC has returned to at least 4,000 cells/mm^3.
8. Monitor uric acid, renal function, and hematologic profiles. Drug may cause granulocyte and platelet suppression. Nadir: 10 days; recovery: 21 days.

CLIENT/FAMILY TEACHING

1. Drug is given by injection to interfere with the growth of cancer cells.
2. Report any signs of infection, fever, sore throat/mouth, unusual bruising/bleeding.
3. Avoid vaccinations and exposure to persons with infectious diseases during therapy
4. To prevent constipation, eat a high-fiber diet, increase intake of fluids, remain active, and take stool softeners as prescribed.
5. Wear protective clothing, sunglasses, and a sunscreen if exposure to sunlight is necessary.
6. Partial hair loss may occur; plan for cosmetic replacement.

V

7. Report any S&S of neurotoxicity: paresthesias, difficulty walking, and diminished reflexes; indication to discontinue drug therapy.
8. Practice barrier contraception.
9. Keep all F/U to assess response, labs, and for adverse SE.

OUTCOMES/EVALUATE

Control/regression of malignant process

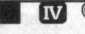

IV

Vincristine sulfate (VCR, LCR)

(vin-**KRIS**-teen)

Classification(s): Antineoplastic, vinca alkaloid

Pregnancy Category: D

RX: Oncovin, Vincasar PFS.

SEE ALSO ***ANTINEOPLASTIC AGENTS***.

INDICATIONS/USES

Frequently used in combination therapy. (1) ALL in children. (2) Hodgkin's and non-Hodgkin's lymphomas (lymphocytic, mixed-cell, histiocytic, undifferentiated, nodular, and diffuse). (3) Wilms' tumor, neuroblastoma, lymphosarcoma, rhabdomyosarcoma, reticulum cell sarcoma. *Investigational:* ITP; cancer of the breast, ovary, cervix, lung, colorectal area; malignant melanoma, osteosarcoma, multiple myeloma, ovarian germ cell tumors, mycosis fungoides, CLL, CML, Kaposi's sarcoma.

ACTION/KINETICS

Action

Inhibits mitosis at metaphase. The antineoplastic effect is due to interference with intracellular tubulin function by binding to microtubule and spindle proteins in the S phase.

Pharmacokinetics

After IV use, drug is distributed within 15–30 min to tissues. Poorly penetrates blood-brain barrier. **t½, triphasic:** initial, 5 min; intermediate, 2.3 hr; final, 85 hr. Approximately 80% is excreted in the feces and up to 20% in the urine. No cross-resistance with vinblastine.

CONTRAINDICATIONS

Use in demyelinating Charcot-Marie-Tooth syndrome or during radiation therapy. Lactation.

SPECIAL CONCERNS

(1) It is extremely important that the IV needle or catheter be properly positioned before injection. Leakage into surrounding tissue may cause considerable irritation. (2) Intrathecal use usually results in death. For IV use only.

Geriatric clients are more susceptible to the neurotoxic effects.

SIDE EFFECTS

Most Common

Fatigue, abdominal cramps, constipation, diarrhea, peripheral neuropathy, loss of fertility, alopecia, paralytic ileus, N&V, weight loss, rash, bloating.

See *Antineoplastic Agents* for a complete list of possible side effects. **Neurologic:** Paresthesias, depression of DTRs, foot drop, ***seizures***, difficulties in gait. **GI:** ***Intestinal necrosis or perforation***. Constipation, paralytic ileus. **Renal:** Inappropriate ADH secretion (polyuria or dysuria). Acute uric acid nephropathy. **Ophthalmic:** Blindness, ptosis, diplopia, photophobia. **Miscellaneous:** CNS leukemia, leukopenia or complicating infection, ***bronchospasm***, SOB. Less bone marrow depression than vinblastine. Significant tissue irritation if leakage occurs during IV use.

OVERDOSE MANAGEMENT

Symptoms: Exaggeration of side effects. *Treatment:*

- Treat side effects due to inappropriate secretion of ADH.
- Use an anticonvulsant (e.g., phenobarbital), if necessary.
- Prevent ileus by use of enemas, cathartics, or decompression of the GI tract.
- Monitor the CV system.
- Monitor blood counts daily to determine risk of infection and whether blood transfusions are necessary.
- Folinic acid, 100 mg IV q 3 hr for 24 hr and then q 6 hr for a minimum of 48 hr, may help with treating the symptoms of overdose.

DRUG INTERACTIONS

Antifungals, azole (including posaconazole) / ↑ Toxicity R/T inhibition of CYP3A4 and/or P-glycoprotein

L-Asparaginase / ↓ Vincristine renal clearance; give vincristine 12–14 hr before asparaginase

Calcium channel blocking drugs / ↑ Accumulation of vincristine in cells

Digoxin / ↓ Digoxin effect R/T ↓ plasma levels

Glutamic acid / Inhibits effect of vincristine

Itraconazole / ↑ Risk of neurotoxicity R/T ↓ vincristine metabolism

V

Methotrexate / Possible hypotension
Mitomycin C / Severe bronchospasm and acute SOB
Phenytoin / ↓ Phenytoin effect R/T ↓ plasma levels

HOW SUPPLIED

Injection: 1 mg/mL.

DOSAGE

IV ONLY (DIRECT, INFUSION)

Individualized for all uses with extreme care as overdose can be fatal.

Adults, usual, initial: 0.4–1.4 mg/m^2 (or 0.01–0.03 mg/kg) once a week; **children:** 1.5–2 mg/m^2 once a week. **Children <10 kg or with body surface area less than 1 m^2:** 0.05 mg/kg once a week. Hepatic insufficiency: If serum bilirubin is 1.5–3, administer 50% of the dose; if serum bilirubin is more than 3.1 or AST is more than 180, omit the dose.

NURSING IMPLICATIONS

Do not confuse vincristine with vinblastine (another vinca alkaloid antineoplastic agent).

IMPLEMENTATION/ADMINISTRATION/STORAGE

1. IV Dissolve powder in sterile water or isotonic saline injection to a concentration ranging from 0.01 to 1 mg/mL.
2. Inject either directly into a vein or into the tubing of a flowing IV infusion over a period of 1 min.
3. If extravasation occurs, move to another vein. Treat affected area with hyaluronidase injection (150 units/mL in 1 mL NaCl) and apply moderate heat to decrease local reaction.
4. Protect from light exposure.
5. Store in refrigerator. Dry powder is stable for 6 months. Solutions are stable for 2 weeks under refrigeration.
6. COMPATIBILITY NSS or D5W.
7. INCOMPATIBILITY Do not mix with any solution that alters the pH outside the range of 3.5–5.5. Administer separately.

ASSESSMENT

1. Note reasons for therapy, onset, characteristics of S&S, other agents trialed.
2. List neurologic assessment; monitor for early S&S of neurologic and neuromuscular side effects (e.g., sensory impairment, paresthesias) before neuritic pain and motor difficulties are apparent; neuromuscular manifestations are irreversible.
3. Premedicate and regularly administer antiemetic to control N&V.
4. Record I&O, weights, and assessment of nutritional/neurologic status.
5. Observe for S&S of gout. May add allopurinol empirically to prevent uric acid nephropathy.
6. Use laxatives and enemas to treat high colon impaction. Absence of bowel sounds is indicative of paralytic ileus; temporarily stop drug.
7. A 50% reduction in dose is recommended for those with a direct serum bilirubin more than 3 mg/dL.
8. Monitor CBC, uric acid, renal and LFTs. May cause granulocyte suppression. Nadir: 10 days; recovery: 21 days.

CLIENT/FAMILY TEACHING

1. Drug is administered IV to inhibit cancer cell progression.
2. Prevent constipation by increased intake of fluids (2–3 L/day), regular exercise, a high-fiber diet, and stool softeners as needed.
3. Report any S&S of neurotoxicity: paresthesias (numbness/tingling), difficulty walking, and diminished reflexes.
4. Avoid vaccinations and persons with infectious diseases.
5. Practice reliable contraception during and for 2 months following therapy.
6. Report any increased dyspnea, cough, fatigue, or unusual bruising or bleeding.
7. May cause hair loss; reversible when therapy stopped.
8. Avoid alcohol and OTC agents.
9. Keep all F/U to assess response, labs, and for adverse SE.

OUTCOMES/EVALUATE

Inhibition of malignant cell proliferation

IV

Vinorelbine tartrate

(vin-**OR**-el-been)

Classification(s): Antineoplastic, vinca alkaloid
Pregnancy Category: D
RX: Navelbine.

INDICATIONS/USES

Alone or in combination with cisplatin for first-line treatment of ambulatory clients with unresectable, advanced non-small cell lung cancer. In clients with Stage IV non-small cell lung cancer, can be used as a single agent or with cisplatin. In stage II non-small cell lung cancer, vinorelbine is not indicated for use with cisplatin. *Investigational:* Breast cancer, cisplatin-resistant ovarian carcinoma, and Hodgkin's disease.

ACTION/KINETICS

Action

Semisynthetic vinca alkaloid thought to act by inhibiting mitosis at metaphase through the drug's interaction with tubulin. Other possible actions may include interference with (a) amino acid, cyclic AMP, and glutathione metabolism, (b) calmodulin-dependent calcium transport ATPase activity, (c) cellular respiration, and (d) nucleic acid and lipid biosynthesis.

Pharmacokinetics

Following IV use, plasma levels decay in a triphasic manner. The initial rapid decline is due to distribution of the drug to peripheral compartments. The prolonged terminal phase is due to a slow efflux of the drug from peripheral compartments. **Terminal phase, t½:** Averages 27.7–43.6 hr. Metabolized by the liver and excreted through the urine and feces.

CONTRAINDICATIONS

Clients with pretreatment granulocyte counts less than 1,000 cells/mm^3. Lactation.

SPECIAL CONCERNS

■ (1) Give under the supervision of a physician experienced in the use of cancer chemotherapeutic agents. For IV use only; intrathecal use of other vinca alkaloids has been fatal. Label syringes containing this product: "Warning: Vinorelbine for IV use only. Fatal if given intrathecally." (2) Severe granulocytopenia, resulting in increased susceptibility to infection may occur. Granulocyte counts should be 1,000 or more cells/mm^3 prior to giving the drug. Adjust dosage according to CBC with differentials obtained on the day of treatment. (3) It is extremely important that the IV needle or catheter be properly positioned before injection. Improper administration of vinorelbine may result in extravasation causing local tissue necrosis or thrombophlebitis. ■

- Use with caution in clients with severe hepatic injury or impairment.
- Use with extreme caution in clients whose bone marrow reserve may have been compromised by chemotherapy or prior to irradiation; also, in those whose bone marrow function is recovering from the effects of previous chemotherapy.
- Elderly may be more sensitive to drug effects.
- Safety and efficacy not determined in children.

SIDE EFFECTS

Most Common

N&V, constipation, diarrhea, asthenia, injection site reactions/pain, peripheral neuropathy, alopecia, granulocytopenia, leukopenia, anemia.

Hematologic: Granulocytopenia (may require hospitalization), leukopenia, thrombocytopenia, anemia. **GI:** N&V, constipation (may be severe), diarrhea, paralytic ileus, anorexia, stomatitis, intestinal obstruction, ***necrosis, perforation***, dysphagia, mucositis. **CNS:** Mild to severe peripheral neuropathy including paresthesia and hypesthesia, loss of DTRs, headache. **CV:** Chest pain, especially in those with a history of CV disease or tumor within the chest; phlebitis, hyper-/hypotension, vasodilation, tachycardia, pulmonary edema. **Respiratory:** SOB (may be severe), dyspnea, interstitial pulmonary changes, pneumonia. **Dermatologic:** Alopecia, flushing, erythema, rash. **At injection site:** Vein discoloration, chemical phlebitis along the vein proximal to the site of injection, localized rash and urticaria, blister formation, skin sloughing. **Musculoskeletal:** Musculoskeletal aches and pains, back pain, jaw pain, myalgia, arthralgia. **Hypersensitivity:** Pruritus, urticaria, angioedema, ***anaphylaxis***. **Miscellaneous:** Asthenia, fatigue, hemorrhagic cystitis, SIADH secretion, vestibular and auditory deficits (especially when used with cisplatin), abdominal pain, pain in tumor-containing tissue, radiation recall events (e.g., dermatitis, esophagitis).

LABORATORY TEST CONSIDERATIONS

↑ Total bilirubin, AST. Transient elevations of liver enzymes.

OVERDOSE MANAGEMENT

Symptoms: Bone marrow suppression, peripheral neurotoxicity. *Treatment:* There is no known antidote for vinorelbine. For overdosage, begin general supportive measures together with appropriate blood transfusions and antibiotics, as necessary.

DRUG INTERACTIONS

Antifungals, azole (including posaconazole) / ↑ Toxicity R/T inhibition of CYP3A4 and/or P-glycoprotein
Cisplatin / ↑ Incidence of granulocytopenia
Mitomycin / Acute pulmonary reactions
Paclitaxel / Possible neuropathy when used together or sequentially

HOW SUPPLIED

Injection: 10 mg/mL.

DOSAGE

IV ONLY

Non-small-cell lung cancer.

Granulocytes (1,500 or more cells/mm^3) on the day of treatment: 30 mg/m^2 weekly given over 6–10 min into the side port of a free-flowing IV closest to the IV bag followed by flushing with at least 75–125 mL of the solution used to dilute the product. May also be given, at the same dose level, with cisplatin, 120 mg/m^2 on days 1 and 29 and then q 6 weeks. **Granulocytes (1,000–1,499 cells/mm^3) on the day of treatment:** 15 mg/m^2 weekly given over 6–10 min as described previously.

Breast cancer, Hodgkin's disease.

30 mg/m^2/week.

NURSING IMPLICATIONS

IMPLEMENTATION/ADMINISTRATION/STORAGE

1. **IV** During therapy, if clients have manifested fever or sepsis while granulocytopenic or had 2 consecutive weekly doses held due to granulocytopenia, give subsequent doses of vinorelbine as follows: 22.5 mg/m^2 for granulocytes equal to or >1,500 cells/mm^3 or 11.25 mg/m^2 for granulocytes from 1,000 to 1,499 cells/mm^3.
2. Ensure granulocyte counts are equal to or >1,000 cells/mm^3 prior to giving vinorelbine. Base dosage on granulocyte counts on the day of drug treatment.
3. If hyperbilirubinemia develops during treatment, adjust the dose of vinorelbine as follows: 30 mg/m^2 for a total bilirubin of 2 or less mg/dL, 15 mg/m^2 for a total bilirubin of 2.1–3 mg/dL, and 7.5 mg/m^2 for a total bilirubin >3 mg/dL.
4. Before any drug is given, properly position the needle or catheter, as leakage into surrounding tissue may cause considerable irritation, local tissue necrosis, or thrombophlebitis. If extravasation occurs, stop the injection immediately and give the remaining dose in another vein. Use institutional guidelines to treat extravasation.
5. Due to the toxicity of vinorelbine, wear gloves and use caution in handling/preparing the solution. If it comes in contact with skin or mucosa, wash the area immediately with soap and water. If the eye is affected, flush with water immediately.
6. Must be diluted in either a syringe or IV bag. If an IV bag is used, dilute the dose to a concentration between 0.5 and 2 mg/mL using one of the following solutions: D5W, 0.45% or 0.9% NaCl, D5W/0.45% NaCl, Ringer's, or RL injection. When dilution in a syringe is used, dilute the dose to a concentration between 1.5 and 3 mg/mL with D5W or 0.9% NaCl.
7. Diluted vinorelbine solutions may be used for up to 24 hr under normal room light when stored in polypropylene syringes or PVC bags at 5–30°C (41–96°F). Unopened vials are stable until the expiration date indicated if stored under refrigeration at 2–8°C (36–46°F). Protect unopened vials from light and do not freeze. Do not use if particulate matter present.
8. COMPATIBILITY D5W, 0.45% or 0.9% NaCl, D5/0.45% NaCl, Ringer's, or RL.
9. INCOMPATIBILITY Administer separately.

ASSESSMENT

1. Note reasons for therapy, other agents/therapies prescribed, when administered, outcome.
2. Drug may cause skin irritation with contact; avoid inhaling vapors.
3. Ensure IV catheter patent to prevent infiltration with resultant tissue necrosis.
4. List neurologic assessment; monitor for early S&S of neurologic and neuromuscular side effects.

V

5. Record VS, I&O, weights, and assessment of nutritional/neurologic status.
6. Observe for S&S of gout. May add allopurinol empirically to prevent uric acid nephropathy.
7. Monitor CBC, uric acid, renal, and LFTs. Reduce dose with impaired liver and hematologic function. Do not administer if granulocyte counts are not at least 1,000 cells/mm^3. Granulocyte nadir 7–10 days; recovery 7–14 days thereafter.

CLIENT/FAMILY TEACHING

1. Used IV to treat unresectable lung cancer.
2. Report any S&S of neurotoxicity: paresthesias (numbness/tingling), difficulty walking, and diminished reflexes.
3. Antiemetics will be given to prevent N&V; report if persistent. Ensure adequate fluid consumption.
4. Rinse mouth frequently and brush teeth often to prevent mouth sores; use unwaxed floss. Use multivitamin and nutritious diet to prevent weight loss.
5. Prevent constipation by increased intake of fluids (2–3 L/day), regular exercise, a high-fiber diet, and stool softeners as needed.
6. Report any fever or chills immediately; drug-induced granulocytopenia (reduction in WBC) makes one much more susceptible to infections.
7. Avoid crowds, persons with infectious diseases, and vaccinations during therapy.
8. May experience hair loss.
9. Practice reliable contraception during and for several months after therapy.
10. Keep all F/U to assess response, labs, and for adverse SE.

OUTCOMES/EVALUATE

Control of malignant cell proliferation.

IV

Voriconazole

(**vor**-ih-**KOH**-nah-zohl)

Classification(s): Antifungal

Pregnancy Category: D

RX: Vfend.

INDICATIONS/USES

(1) Invasive aspergillosis, usually due to *Aspergillus fumigatus.* (2) Serious fungal infections due to *Scedosporium apiospermum* (asexual form of *Pseudallescheria boydii*) and *Fusarium* species, including *Fusarium solani* in those intolerant of, or refractory to, other therapy. (3) Esophageal candidiasis. (4) Candidemia in those without low WBC counts (nonneutropenic clients) of the following: Disseminated infections in skin and infections in the abdomen, kidney, bladder wall, and wounds. *Investigational:* IV to treat catheter–related bloodstream infections in children.

ACTION/KINETICS

Action

Acts by inhibiting fungal cytochrome P450-mediated 14 alpha-lanosterol demethylation, which is an essential step in fungal ergosterol biosynthesis. Accumulation of 14 alpha-methyl sterols results in the loss of ergosterol in the fungal cell wall and is thought to be responsible for the antifungal activity.

Pharmacokinetics

Oral bioavailability is 96%, When the recommended PO loading dose regimen is given to healthy subjects, peak plasma levels close to steady state are reached within the first 24 hr of dosing. **Maximum plasma levels after IV:** 1–2 hr. High fat meals reduce both the C_{max} and AUC. Metabolized by hepatic cytochrome P450 enzymes CYP2C19 (major enzyme for metabolism of this drug), CYP2C9, and CYP3A4. Excreted mainly (>94%) in the urine. Terminal t½ is dose dependent and thus not useful in predicting accumulation or elimination of the drug. Fifteen to 20% of Asian populations are slow metabolizers compared with 3–5% of Caucasians and Blacks. **Plasma protein binding:** About 58%.

CONTRAINDICATIONS

Known hypersensitivity to the drug or product components or to other azoles. IV voriconazole in moderate or severe renal impairment unless benefit to risk justifies use. Use with CYP3A4 substrates (including cisapride, pimozide and quinidine), as increased plasma levels may cause QT prolongation and torsades de pointes (rare). Use with barbiturates (long-acting), carbamazepine, efavirenz, ergot alkaloids (ergotamine, dihydroergotamine), rifabutin, rifampin, ritonavir (400 mg q 12 hr), sirolimus and St. John's wort. Use in those with galactose intolerance, Lapp lactase deficiency, or glucose-galactose malabsorption. Lactation.

V

SPECIAL CONCERNS

- **Accumulation of the IV vehicle (sulfobutyl ether beta-cyclodextrin sodium) in those with moderate to severe renal dysfunction.**
- **Use with caution in clients with potential proarrhythmic conditions and in those hypersensitive to other azoles.**
- **Safety and efficacy not determined in children under 12 years of age.**

SIDE EFFECTS

Most Common

Abnormal pain, diarrhea, fever, headache, N&V, peripheral edema, rash, respiratory disorder, sepsis, visual disturbances.

Side effects listed are the more common or more serious. **Infusion reactions:** Flushing, fever, sweating, tachycardia, chest tightness, dyspnea, fainting, nausea, pruritus, rash. **Hematologic:** Thrombocytopenia, leukopenia, anemia, pancytopenia. **GI:** N&V, diarrhea, abdominal pain, dry mouth. **Hepatic:** Hepatitis, jaundice/cholestatic jaundice, abnormal LFTs; rarely, serious hepatic reactions, including clinical hepatitis, cholestasis, and ***fulminant hepatic failure***. **CNS:** Headache, hallucinations, dizziness. **Dermatologic:** Serious cutaneous reactions, including ***Stevens-Johnson syndrome and toxic epidermal necrolysis, erythema multiforme***, photosensitivity skin reaction (including squamous cell carcinoma of the skin and melanoma, especially with long-term use), rash, pruritus, maculopapular rash. **CV:** Tachycardia, hyper-/hypotension, vasodilation, prolongation of QT interval (rarely, ***torsades de pointes*** in seriously ill clients with multiple confounding risk factors), ***cardiac arrest***. **GU:** Abnormal kidney function, ***acute kidney failure*** (in severely ill clients often treated with nephrotoxic drugs as well). **Ophthalmic:** Visual disturbances, abnormal vision, color vision change, photophobia, chromatopsia, eye hemorrhage, optic neuritis, papilledema. **Body as a whole:** Fever, ***sepsis***, peripheral edema, chills. **Miscellaneous:** Respiratory disorders, chest pain.

LABORATORY TEST CONSIDERATIONS

↑ Alkaline phosphatase, hepatic enzymes, ALT, AST, creatinine, total bilirubin. Hypokalemia, hypomagnesemia, bilirubinemia.

DRUG INTERACTIONS

(1) Voriconazole is metabolized by CYP2C19, CYP2C9, and CYP3A4; thus, inhibitors or inducers of these three enzymes may increase or decrease voriconazole plasma levels. Also, voriconazole inhibits metabolic activity of these three enzymes; thus, there is the potential to increase plasma levels of other drugs metabolized by these CYP450 enzymes.
(2) An additive effect of voriconazole with other drugs that prolong the QT interval cannot be excluded. The following drugs may prolong the QT interval and and ↑ the risk of life–threatening cardiac arrhythmias, including torsades de pointes: Amiodarone, arsenic trioxide, bretylium, chlorpromazine, cisapride, disopyramide, dofetilide, dolasetron, droperidol, mefloquine, mesoridazine, moxifloxacin, pentamidine, pimozide, procainamide, quinidine, sotalol, tacrolimus, thioridazine, and ziprasidone.
Amprenavir / Metabolism of amprenavir may be inhibited; ↑ or ↓ metabolism of voriconazole
Aripiprazole / ↑ Aripiprazole plasma levels → ↑ pharmacologic/toxic effects; monitor and adjust aripiprazole dose as needed
Barbiturates (long-acting, including mephobarbital, phenobarbital) / Significant ↓ voriconazole levels R/T CYP450 induction; do not use together
Benzodiazepines (alprazolam, midazolam, triazolam) / ↑ Levels of benzodiazepines metabolized by CYP3A4; monitor for benzodiazepine side effects and adjust dose if necessary
Cabazitaxel / ↑ Cabazitaxel plasma levels → ↑ risk of pharmacologic/toxic effects; do not use together
Calcium channel blockers (e.g., felodipine) / Inhibition of metabolism of CCBs metabolized by CYP3A4 → ↑ plasma levels; monitor for CCB toxicity and adjust dose if necessary
Carbamazepine / Significant ↓ voriconazole levels R/T CYP450 induction; do not use together
Cimetidine / ↑ Voriconazole C_{max} and AUC; no dosage adjustment required
Clopidogrel / ↓ Clopidogrel plasma levels → ↓ pharmacologic effect; do not use together
Contraceptives, hormonal (e.g., containing ethinyl estradiol and norethindrone) / ↑ Plasma levels of both hormones; monitor for side effects related to contraceptive agent, as well as voriconazole
Cyclosporine / ↑ Cyclosporine C_{max} and AUC; reduce cyclosporine dose by 50%

V

Docetaxel / ↑ Docetaxel plasma levels → ↑ pharmacologic/toxic effects; do not give together; if coadministration cannot be avoided, ↓ docetaxel dose by 50% with close monitoring
Dronedarone / ↑ Dronedarone plasma levels → ↑ pharmacologic/toxic effects; coadministration contraindicated
Efavirenz / Significant ↓ voraconazole levels; significant ↑ efavirenz levels; if used together, ↑ voriconazole maintenance dose to 400 mg q 12 hr and ↓ efavirenz dosage to 300 mg q 24 hr
Ergot alkaloids (ergotamine, dihydroergotamine) / ↑ Ergot alkaloid plasma levels → possible ergotism; coadministration contraindicated
Erlotinib / ↑ Erlotinib plasma levels → ↑ risk of side effects; monitor; erlotinib dose ↓ may be needed
Erythromycin / ↑ Erythromycin plasma levels → ↑ risk of toxic effects, including sudden death due to cardiac causes; coadministration contraindicated
Everolimus / ↑ Everolimus plasma levels → ↑ pharmacologic/toxic effects; avoid coadministration; if coadministration necessary, monitor frequently for everolimus side effects; possibly ↓ everolimus dose
Fluconazole / ↑ Voriconazole C_{max} and AUC; coadministration not recommended; monitor closely if voriconazole given sequentially after fluconazole, especially within 24 hr of the last fluconazole dose
HMG-CoA reductase inhibitors (e.g., lovastatin) / Possible ↑ statin levels metabolized by CYP3A4 → ↑ risk of side effects, including rhabdomyolysis; consider dosage adjustment
Ixabepilone / ↑ Ixabepilone plasma levels → ↑ risk of pharmacologic/toxic effects; avoid coadministration; if coadministration necessary, ↓ ixabepilone dose may be needed
Maraviroc / ↑ Maraviroc plasma levels → ↑ risk of pharmacologic/toxic effects; ↓ maraviroc dose may be needed; coadministration contraindicated in those with severe renal impairment (C_{CR} <30 mL/min)
Methadone / ↑ Methadone levels → possible QT prolongation and other side effects, including respiratory depression; possibly reduce dose of methadone
Nelfinavir / Metabolism of nelfinavir may be inhibited; ↑ or ↓ metabolism of voriconazole
Nilotinib / ↑ Nilotinib plasma levels → ↑ pharmacologic/toxic effects; avoid coadministration; if coadministration necessary, interrupt nilotinib therapy
Nonnucleoside reverse transcriptase inhibitors (delavirdine, nevirapine) / Coadministration may ↑ or ↓ voriconazole metabolism; also, possible ↓ metabolism of nonnucleoside reverse transcriptase inhibitors; monitor for drug toxicity
NSAIDs (diclofenac, ibuprofen) / ↑ NSAID plasma levels; monitor frequently for toxicity; ↓ NSAID dosage may be needed
Omeprazole / ↑ Voriconazole AUC and C_{max}; ↑ omeprazole C_{max} and AUC; reduce dose of omeprazole by 50%
Opioid analgesics (alfentanil, fentanyl, oxycodone) / ↑ Opioid analgesic plasma levels; monitor for respiratory depression and other side effects; reduce opioid dose if needed
Phenytoin / ↓ Voriconazole C_{max} and AUC R/T ↑ CYP450 induction; ↑ phenytoin C_{max} and AUC up to 2 times; if phenytoin given with voriconazole, ↑ voriconazole PO dose from 200 to 400 mg q 12 hr (100 to 200 mg q 12 hr) in adults weighing <40 kg; for IV, ↑ voriconazole maintenance dose to 5 mg/kg q 12 hr
Pimozide / Metabolism of pimozide inhibited → possible QT prolongation and rarely torsades de pointes; do not use together
Prednisolone / ↑ Prednisolone C_{max} and AUC; no dosage adjustment needed
Quinidine / Metabolism of quinidine inhibited → possible QT prolongation and rarely torsades de pointes; do not use together
Rifabutin / Significant ↓ voriconazole levels; ↑ C_{max} and AUC of rifabutin by 3- or 4-fold; do not use together
Rifampin / Significant ↓ voriconazole levels; do not use together
Ritonavir (400 mg q 12 hr) / Significant ↓ voriconazole levels; do not use together
Romidepsin / ↑ Romidepsin plasma levels → ↑ pharmacologic/toxic effects, including QT prolongation; avoid coadministration
Saquinavir / Metabolism of saquinavir may be inhibited; ↑ or ↓ metabolism of voriconazole
Sirolimus / Significant ↑ sirolimus C_{max} and AUC; do not use together
St. John's wort / Multiple doses of St. John's wort + single dose of voriconazole → significant ↓ voriconazole AUC; do not use together
Sulfonamides / ↑ Sulfonamide levels; monitor for hypoglycemia

V

Sulfonylureas / ↑ Sulfonylurea levels; monitor for hypoglycemia; dosage adjustment of the sulfonylurea is recommended
Tacrolimus / Significant ↑ tacrolimus C_{max} and AUC; reduce the dose of tacrolimus to 33%; frequently monitor tacrolimus levels
Temsirolimus / ↑ Temsirolimus plasma levels → ↑ pharmacologic/toxic effects; avoid coadministration; if coadministration necessary, monitor frequently for temsirolimus side effects; possibly ↓ temsirolimus dose
Tyrosine kinase receptor inhibitors (dasatinib, lapatinib, pazopanib, sunitinib) / ↑ Tyrosine kinase receptor inhibitor plasma levels → ↑ pharmacologic/toxic effects; avoid coadministration
Vinca alkaloids (vinblastine, vincristine) ↑ Vinca alkaloid levels → neurotoxicity; consider dosage adjustment of the vinca alkaloid and monitor for toxicity
Warfarin / Significant ↑ maximum PT time; closely monitor; also, voriconazole may ↑ PT in clients receiving other coumarin anticoagulants
Zolpidem / ↑ Zolpidem plasma levels → ↑ pharmacologic/toxic effects; monitor frequently for zolpidem side effects; ↓ zolpidem dose may be needed

HOW SUPPLIED

Injection, Lyophilized Powder for Solution: 200 mg; ***Powder for Oral Suspension:*** 40 mg/mL (after reconstitution); ***Tablets:*** 50 mg, 200 mg.

DOSAGE

IV; ORAL SUSPENSION; TABLETS

Candidemia in nonneutropenic clients and other deep tissue Candida infections.

Adults and children 12 years and older, initial, IV loading dose: 6 mg/kg q 12 hr for the first 24 hr; **then** give an IV maintenance dose of 3–4 mg/kg q 12 hr or PO maintenance dose of 200 mg q 12 hr once the client can tolerate medication given PO. If clients are unable to tolerate 4 mg/kg IV, reduce the IV maintenance dose to 3 mg/kg q 12 hr. Treat clients for a minimum of 14 days after resolution of symptoms, or following the last positive culture, whichever is longer.

Invasive aspergillosis; scedosporiosis and fusariosis.

Adults and children 12 years and older, initial, IV loading dose: 6 mg/kg q 12 hr for the first 24 hr; **then** 4 mg/kg IV q 12 hr or 200 mg q 12 hr PO, once the client can tolerate PO medication. If clients are unable to tolerate 4 mg/kg IV, reduce the IV maintenance dose to 3 mg/kg q 12 hr.

ORAL SUSPENSION; TABLETS

Esophageal candidiasis.

Adults and children 12 years and older: 200 mg q 12 hr. **Maintenance:** 200 mg q 12 hr for clients weighing 40 kg or more; 100 mg q 12 hr for those weighing 40 kg or less. Treat clients for a minimum of 14 days and for at least 7 days following resolution of symptoms.

IV

Catheter-related bloodstream infection in children (investigational).

Children, 2 years and older: 6 mg/kg IV q 12 hr for 2 doses on day 1 (loading dose), followed by 4 mg/kg given IV q 12 hr.

NURSING IMPLICATIONS

IMPLEMENTATION/ADMINISTRATION/STORAGE

1. Use only the tablets in those with moderate to severe renal dysfunction as accumulation of the IV vehicle occurs. Only give IV if the benefit/risk to the client justifies IV administration.
2. The following recommendations for adults receiving continuous renal replacement therapy assumes ultrafiltration and dialysis flow rates of 1–2 liters/hr. Use a loading dose of 400 mg PO q 12hr for 2 doses; then, give a dose of 200 mg PO q 12hr for those receiving continuous venovenous hemofiltration, continuous venovenous hemodialysis, or continuous venovenous hemodiafiltration. For adults receiving intermittent hemodialysis, give 200 mg PO q 12 hr; this assumes the client is receiving standard intermittent hemodialysis 3 times per week and completes the full dialysis session.
3. In those with mild to moderate hepatic cirrhosis (Child-Pugh Class A and B), the standard loading dose can be used, but the mainte-

V

nance dose should be halved. Use not recommended in those with severe liver impairment.

4. Dosage adjustment: If client response is inadequate, the PO maintenance dose may be increased from 200 mg q 12 hr to 300 mg q 12 hr. For adult clients weighing 40 kg or less, the PO maintenance dose may be increased from 100 mg q 12 hr to 150 mg q 12 hr. If clients are unable to tolerate 300 mg PO q 12 hr, decrease the PO maintenance dose by 50 mg steps to a minimum of 200 mg q 12 hr (or 100 mg q 12 hr for clients weighing 40 kg or less).
5. To reconstitute the oral suspension, tap the bottle to release the powder. Add 46 mL of water to the bottle and shake vigorously for about 1 min. Remove the child-resistant cap and push the bottle adaptor into the neck of the bottle; replace the cap. The date of expiration of the reconstituted suspension should be written on the bottle label (shelf-life is 14 days at controlled room temperature).
6. Do not mix the suspension with any other medication or additional flavoring agent; do not dilute the suspension further with water or other vehicles.
7. Store the suspension from 2–8°C (36–46°F) before reconstitution. Store the reconstituted suspension and tablets from 15–30°C (59–86°F). Do not refrigerate or freeze the suspension. Discard any remaining suspension 14 days after reconstitution.
8. IV To reconstitute, add 19 mL of water for injection to obtain an extractable volume of 20 mL containing 10 mg/mL. Use a standard 20 mL (nonautomated) syringe to ensure the exact amount of 19 mL of water for injection is used. Discard the vial if a vacuum does not pull the diluent into the vial. Shake the vial until all of the powder is dissolved.
9. Must be infused over a maximum rate of 3 mg/kg/hr over 1–2 hr at a concentration of 5 mg/mL or less. Thus, the reconstituted solution must be further diluted as follows:
   - Calculate the volume of 10 mg/mL of concentrate required based on client weight (see package insert).
   - To allow the required volume of voriconazole to be added, withdraw and discard at least an equal amount of diluent from the infusion bag or bottle to be used. The volume of diluent remaining in the bag/bottle should be such that when 10 mg/mL of drug is added, the final concentration is not less than 0.5 mg/mL or more than 5 mg/mL.
   - Using an appropriate size syringe and aseptic technique, withdraw the required volume of 10 mg/mL voriconazole from the correct number of vials and add to the infusion bag/bottle. Discard partially used vials; do not use solutions that contain particles.
10. Store unreconstituted vials from 15–30°C (59–86°F). Use the reconstituted concentrate immediately. If not used immediately, do not store longer than 24 hr at 2–8°C (37–46°F). The injection solution is unpreserved and is for single use only. Discard any unused solution.
11. May be infused at the same time as TPN but must be infused in a separate line. If infused through a multiple-lumen catheter, TPN is administered using a different port from the one used for voriconazole.
12. COMPATIBILITY 0.9% NaCl, RL, D5/RL, D5/0.45% NaCl, D5W, D5W and 20 mEq KCl, 0.45% NaCl, and D5/NSS.
13. INCOMPATIBILITY Do *not* dilute with 4.2% sodium bicarbonate infusion, as the alkaline solution causes slight degradation of the drug after 24 hr at room temperature. Do not infuse voriconazole into the same line or cannula at the same time with other drug infusions, including parenteral nutrition. Also, do not give infusions of blood products or any electrolyte supplement at the same time as voriconazole.

ASSESSMENT

1. Note reasons for therapy, site, where contracted, characteristics of S&S, and fungal culture results.
2. List other agents prescribed to ensure none interact/compete.
3. During initial infusion, assess carefully for anaphylactoid-type reactions.
4. With prolonged therapy (>1 month), ensure that an eye exam for visual fields, acuity, and color perception is performed.
5. Monitor renal and LFTs carefully; reduce dose with dysfunction.

CLIENT/FAMILY TEACHING

1. Take tablets or oral suspension at least 1 hr before or 1 hr after a meal.
2. With oral suspension, shake for 10 sec before measuring dose. Use the oral dispenser supplied with the medication to measure.
3. Avoid activities that require mental alertness until drug effects realized; avoid driving or operating machinery if changes in vision noted. Do not drive at night, as drug may cause vision changes including blurred vision and light sensitivity.
4. Report any chills, fever, dark urine, N&V, rash, diarrhea, swelling of extremities, injection site reaction, visual disturbances, yellowing of skin/eyes.
5. Avoid prolonged sun exposure; photosensitivity reaction may occur. Use sunscreen and protective clothing if exposed.
6. Practice reliable contraception.
7. Drug is used for a prolonged period. Keep all F/U to assess response, labs, and for adverse SE.

OUTCOMES/EVALUATE

- Resolution of fungal infection
- Symptomatic improvement

Vorinostat

(voh-**RIN**-oh-stat)

Classification(s): Antineoplastic, histone deacetylase inhibitor

Pregnancy Category: D

RX: Zolinza.

SEE ALSO ***ANTINEOPLASTIC AGENTS.***

INDICATIONS/USES

Treat cutaneous manifestations of cutaneous T-cell lymphoma in those who have progressive, persistent, or recurrent disease on or following two systemic therapies.

ACTION/KINETICS

Action

Vorinostat inhibits activity of the enzymes histone deacetylases; these enzymes catalyze the removal of acetyl groups from the lysine residues of proteins, including histones. In some cancer cells there is an overexpression of histone deactylases or abnormal recruitment of histone acetylases causing hypoacetylation of histones. This leads to transcriptional activity of cancer cells. Vorinostat is believed to induce cell cycle arrest and/or apoptosis of some transformed cancer cells.

Pharmacokinetics

A high-fat meal modestly increases the extent of absorption but decreases the rate of absorption of the drug. Metabolized in the liver by glucuronidation and hydrolysis; liver microsomes are negligibly involved in the metabolism. Excreted in the urine; **t½, terminal:** 2 hr. **Plasma protein binding:** About 71%.

CONTRAINDICATIONS

Lactation.

SPECIAL CONCERNS

- Use with particular caution in those with congenital long QT syndrome or clients taking antiarrhythmics or other drugs that lead to QT prolongation.
- Do not rule out greater sensitivity of the elderly.
- Use with caution in impaired renal or hepatic function.
- Safety and efficacy not determined in children.

SIDE EFFECTS

Most Common

Anorexia, diarrhea, constipation, N&V, weight decrease, chills, fatigue, anemia, thrombocytopenia, dry mouth, dysgeusia, alopecia.

CNS: Fatigue, dizziness, headache, syncope, lethargy, spinal cord injury. **GI:** Diarrhea, N&V, dysgeusia, dry mouth, anorexia, constipation, decreased appetite, cholecystitis, ***GI hemorrhage***. **CV:** DVT, ischemic stroke, ***MI, pulmonary embolism.*** **Dermatologic:** Alopecia, pruritus, exfoliative dermatitis. **Hematologic:** Thombocytopenia, anemia, leukopenia, neutropenia. **Musculoskeletal:** Muscle spasms, chest pain. **Respiratory:** Cough, URTI, lobar pneumonia, ***pulmonary embolism***. **GU:** Pelvic-ureteric obstruction, ureteric obstruction. **Body as a whole:** Weight decrease, chills, peripheral edema, pyrexia, angioneurotic edema, asthenia, dehydration, infection, ***sepsis***, ***death of unknown cause***. **Miscellaneous:** Hyperglycemia, enterococcal infection, streptococcal bacteremia, T-cell lymphoma, squamous cell carcinoma.

V

LABORATORY TEST CONSIDERATIONS

↑ Serum glucose, serum creatinine. Proteinuria, hypokalemia, hyperglycemia.

DRUG INTERACTIONS

Valproic acid / Severe thrombocytopenia and GI bleeding; monitor platelet count every 2 weeks for the first 2 months

Warfarin / Prolongation of PT and INR; monitor carefully

HOW SUPPLIED

Capsules: 100 mg.

DOSAGE

CAPSULES

Cutaneous T-cell lymphoma.

Adults: 400 mg once daily with food. Continue treatment as long as there is no evidence of disease progression or unacceptable side effects. If intolerant to therapy, dose may be reduced to 300 mg once daily with food; the dose may be reduced further to 300 mg once daily with food for 5 consecutive days each week.

NURSING IMPLICATIONS

IMPLEMENTATION/ADMINISTRATION/STORAGE

1. Avoid direct contact of the powder in the capsules with the skin or mucous membranes. If contact occurs, wash thoroughly.
2. Store from 15–30°C (59–86°F).

ASSESSMENT

1. Note reasons for therapy, other systemic agents trialed with disease progression/recurrence.
2. Obtain ECG and monitor for QT prolongation during treatment.
3. List drugs prescribed. Assess for bleeding, pregnancy, severe N&V; may require antiemetics, fluids, or change in dosage.
4. Assess for conditions that may preclude therapy or require very close monitoring: DM, prolonged QT syndrome, blood clots, pregnancy.
5. Monitor CBC, platelets, chemistry, electrolytes, glucose, renal and LFTs every 2 weeks during first 2 months of therapy and monthly thereafter.

CLIENT/FAMILY TEACHING

1. Do not open or crush vorinostat capsules; if accidentally opened do not touch capsule or powder. Swallow capsule whole with food.
2. Consume at least eight 8-ounce glasses of water per day during therapy to prevent dehydration.
3. High glucose levels may occur; adjustment of diet and/or therapy for increased glucose may be required.
4. May experience N&V, diarrhea; report so antiemetics, antidiarrheals and fluid and electrolyte replacements may be prescribed.
5. Seek immediate medical attention if unusual bleeding occurs.
6. Report any sudden SOB or chest pain; may cause pulmonary embolus or DVT.
7. Practice reliable contraception; may cause fetal harm.
8. Keep all F/U to assess response, labs (every 2 weeks for the first 2 months of treatment then every month thereafter), and for adverse SE.

OUTCOMES/EVALUATE

Inhibition of progression of cutaneous T-cell lymphoma (CTCL)

W

■ IV ◎ 📷

Warfarin sodium

(**WAR**-far-in)

Classification(s): Anticoagulant, coumarin derivative

Pregnancy Category: X

RX: Coumadin, Jantoven.

🍁 **Rx:** Apo-Warfarin, Gen-Warfarin, Taro-Warfarin.

INDICATIONS/USES

PO or IV. (1) Prophylaxis and treatment of venous thrombosis and its extension. (2) Prophylaxis and treatment of the thromboembolic complications associated with atrial fibrillation and/or cardiac valve replacement. (3) Prophylaxis and treatment of pulmonary embolism. (4) Reduce the risk of death, recurrent MI, and thromboembolic events such as stroke or systemic embolization after MI.

ACTION/KINETICS

Action

Interferes with synthesis of vitamin-K dependent clotting factors resulting in depletion of clotting factors II, VII, IX, and X and the anticoagulant proteins C and S. Has no direct effect on an established thrombus, although therapy may prevent further extension of a formed clot as well as secondary thromboembolic problems.

Pharmacokinetics

Essentially completely absorbed from the GI tract, although food affects the rate (but not the extent) of absorption. Suitable for parenteral administration. **Peak concentrations:** 4 hr. The anticoagulant effect usually occurs within 24 hr after drug administration, but peak anticoagulant effect may be delayed 3–4 days. **Duration, after single dose:** 2–5 days. **t½:** 1–2.5 days. Metabolized in the liver by CYP-450 enzymes (including 2C9, 2C19, 2C8, 2C18, 1A2, and 3A4); inactive metabolites are excreted through the urine and feces. **t½, terminal:** 1 week but the effective half-life ranges from 20–60 hr. **Plasma protein binding:** Highly bound.

CONTRAINDICATIONS

Pregnancy. Hemorrhagic tendencies or blood dyscrasias; recent or contemplated surgery of the CNS, eye, or traumatic surgery resulting in large open surfaces; bleeding tendencies associated with active ulceration or overt bleeding of the GI, GU, or respiratory tracts; CV hemorrhage; aneurysms–cerebral, dissecting aorta; pericarditis and pericardial effusions, or bacterial endocarditis; threatened abortion, eclampsia and preeclampsia; inadequate laboratory facilities; unsupervised clients with senility, alcoholism, or psychosis or other lack of client cooperation; spinal puncture and other diagnostic or therapeutic procedures with potential for uncontrollable bleeding; major regional, lumbar block anesthesia, malignant hypertension; known hypersensitivity to warfarin or to any component of the product.

SPECIAL CONCERNS

Warfarin can cause major or fatal bleeding. Bleeding is more likely to occur during the starting period and with a higher dose (resulting in a higher INR). Risk factors for bleeding include high intensity of anticoagulation (INR of more than 4), 65 years of age and older, highly variable INRs, history of GI bleeding, hypertension, CV disease, serious heart disease, anemia, malignancy, trauma, renal function impairment, concomitant drugs, and long duration of warfarin therapy. Regular monitoring of INR should be performed on all treated clients. Those at high risk of bleeding may benefit from more frequent INR monitoring, careful dose adjustment to desired INR, and a shorter duration of therapy. Clients should be instructed about preventive measures to minimize risk of bleeding and to report immediately to health care provider signs and symptoms of bleeding.

- **Geriatric clients over age 60 are at an increased risk for bleeding, thromboembolic events, and atrial fibrillation.**
- **Anticoagulant use leads to increased risk with the following: Trauma, infection, renal insufficiency, sprue, vitamin K deficiency, severe to moderate hypertension, polycythemia vera, severe allergic disorders, vasculitis, indwelling catheters, severe diabetes, anaphylactic disorders, surgery or trauma resulting in large exposed raw surfaces.**
- **Use with caution in impaired hepatic and renal function.**
- **Use caution when herbal products are also taken, as there are many potential interactions.**
- **Carefully consider available alternatives to breastfeeding before undertaking the decision to breast-feed while on warfarin.**
- **Safety and efficacy not determined in children less than 18 years of age.**

SIDE EFFECTS

Most Common

Bleeding/hemorrhage (see the following possible symptoms).

CV: ***Hemorrhage*** is the main side effect and may occur from any tissue or organ. Symptoms of hemorrhage include headache, paralysis; pain in the joints, abdomen, or chest; difficulty in breathing or swallowing; SOB, unexplained swelling or shock. Angina syndrome, hypotension, syncope, vasculitis. Necrosis due to local thrombosis. Atheromatous plaque emboli or cholesterol microemboli leading to symptoms of purple toes syndrome; livedo reticularis; rash; gangrene; abrupt and intense pain in the leg, foot, or toes; foot ulcers; myalgia; penile gangrene; abdominal pain; flank or back pain; hematuria; renal function impairment; hypertension; cerebral ischemia, spinal cord infarction; pancreatitis; symptoms simulating polyarteritis. **CNS:** Dizziness, coma, headache, loss of consciousness, paresthesia (including feeling cold and chills). **GI:** N&V, diarrhea, sore mouth, mouth ulcers, anorexia, abdominal pain/cramping (including cramping, flatulence, bloating), paralytic ileus, taste perversion, intestinal obstruction (due to intramural or submucosal hemorrhage). **Hepatic:** Hepatitis, cholestatic hepatic injury, jaundice. **Dermatologic:** Rash, dermatitis (including bullous eruptions), exfoliative dermatitis, urticaria, pruritus, alopecia, necrosis or gangrene of the skin and other tissues (due to protein C deficiency). **GU:** Priapism, red-orange urine. **Respiratory:** Tracheal or tracheobronchial calcification (with long-term therapy), chest pain. **Hematologic:** Heparin-induced thrombocytopenia, leukopenia. **Body as a whole:** Hypersensitivity/allergic reactions, edema, fever, fatigue, lethargy, malaise, asthenia, pain, pallor, cold intolerance, hypersensitivity reactions (including ***anaphylaxis***).

LABORATORY TEST CONSIDERATIONS

False ↓ levels of serum theophylline determined by Schack and Waxler UV method (warfarin and dicumarol).

OVERDOSE MANAGEMENT

Symptoms: Early symptoms include melena, petechiae, microscopic hematuria, oozing from superficial injuries (e.g., nicks from shaving, excessive bruising, bleeding from gums after teeth brushing), excessive menstrual bleeding. *Treatment:* Discontinue therapy. Administer parenteral phytonadione (vitamin K_1), 5–25 mg parenterally. In emergency situations, 200–250 mL fresh frozen plasma or commercial factor IX complex. Fresh whole blood may be needed in clients unresponsive to phytonadione.

DRUG INTERACTIONS

Warfarin is responsible for more adverse drug interactions than any other group. Clients on anticoagulant therapy must be monitored carefully each time a drug is added or withdrawn. Monitoring usually involves determination of PT or INR. In general, a lengthened PT or INR means potentiation of the anticoagulant. Since potentiation may mean hemorrhages, a lengthened PT or INR warrants **reduction of the dosage of the anticoagulant.** However, the anticoagulant dosage must again be increased when the second drug is discontinued. A shortened PT or INR means inhibition of the anticoagulant and may require an increase in dosage.

Acetaminophen / ↑ Anticoagulant effect → ↑ risk of bleeding

Alcohol, ethyl / Chronic use ↓ warfarin effect R/T ↑ clearance; also, either ↑ or ↓ PT/INR responses

Allopurinol / ↑ Anticoagulant effect R/T ↓ warfarin hepatic metabolism

Aminoglutethimide / ↓ Warfarin effect R/T ↑ liver breakdown

Aminoglycoside antibiotics (oral) / ↑ Warfarin effect R/T interference with vitamin K

Aminosalicylic acid / ↑ Warfarin anticoagulant effect R/T effect on platelet function

Amiodarone / ↑ Anticoagulant effect R/T ↓ warfarin hepatic metabolism

Androgens / ↑ Anticoagulant effect → ↑ risk of bleeding

Anabolic steroids (e.g., danazol, oxandrolone, oxymethalone, stanozol) / ↑ Anticoagulant effect → ↑ risk of bleeding

Anticoagulants (e.g., argatroban, bivalirudin, dicumarol, lepirudin) / ↑ Anticoagulant effect → ↑ risk of bleeding

Antineoplastic drugs (e.g., capecitabine, cyclophosphamide, fluorouracil, gefitinib) / ↑ Anticoagulant effect → ↑ risk of bleeding

Aprepitant / ↓ Warfarin levels and INR R/T increased metabolism by CYP2C9

Ascorbic acid (high doses) / ↓ Warfarin effect by unknown mechanism

Aspirin / ↑ Risk of major bleeding; GI irritation

Atorvastatin / Either ↑ or ↓ PT/INR responses → ↑ or ↓ anticoagulant effect

H ***Avocado*** / Possible ↓ warfarin effect (↓ INR)

Azole antifungals (e.g., fluconazole, itraconazole, miconazole) / ↑ Anticoagulant effect R/T ↓ warfarin hepatic metabolism

Barbiturates / ↓ Warfarin effect R/T ↑ liver breakdown

Beta-adrenergic blockers / ↑ Anticoagulant effect → ↑ risk of bleeding
Bosentan / ↓ Warfarin effect R/T ↑ liver breakdown
H ***Bromelain*** / ↑ Tendency for bleeding
Carbamazepine / ↓ Warfarin effect R/T ↑ liver breakdown
Celecoxib / ↑ PT & INR; ↑ risk of upper GI hemorrhage in geriatric clients
Cephalosporins / ↑ Anticoagulant effect → ↑ risk of bleeding
Chenodiol / ↑ Anticoagulant effect → ↑ risk of bleeding
Chloral hydrate / Either ↑ or ↓ PT/INR responses → ↑ or ↓ anticoagulant effect
Chloramphenicol / ↑ Warfarin effect R/T ↓ liver breakdown
Chlordiazepoxide / ↓ Warfarin effect by unknown mechanism
Chlorpropamide / ↑ Anticoagulant effect → ↑ risk of bleeding
Cholestyramine / ↓ Anticoagulant effect R/T binding and ↓ absorption from GI tract
Cimetidine / ↑ Anticoagulant effect R/T ↓ warfarin hepatic metabolism; do not use together
H ***Cinchona bark*** / ↑ Anticoagulant effect
Clarithromycin / ↑ Anticoagulant effect R/T ↓ warfarin hepatic metabolism
Clofibrate / ↑ Anticoagulant effect → ↑ risk of bleeding
Clopidogrel / ↑ Risk of major bleeding
Clozapine / ↓ Warfarin effect by unknown mechanism
Contraceptives, oral / ↓ Anticoagulant effect R/T ↑ activity of certain clotting factors (VII and X); rarely, the opposite effect of ↑ risk of thromboembolism
Contrast media containing iodine / ↑ Warfarin effect by ↑ PT
Corticosteroids / ↑ Warfarin effect; also ↑ risk of GI bleeding R/T steroids ulcerogenic effect
H ***Cranberry*** / ↑ Warfarin effect R/T inhibition of cytochrome P450 isoenzymes
Cyclophosphamide / Either ↑ or ↓ PT/INR responses → ↑ or ↓ anticoagulant effect
Cyclosporine / ↓ Warfarin effect by unknown mechanism
H ***Danshen*** / Possible ↑ warfarin effects
Dextran / ↑ Anticoagulant effect → ↑ risk of bleeding
Dextrothyroxine / ↑ Anticoagulant effect → ↑ risk of bleeding
Diazoxide / ↑ Anticoagulant effect → ↑ risk of bleeding
Dicloxacillin / ↓ Warfarin effect R/T ↑ liver breakdown
Diflunisal / ↑ Anticoagulant effect and ↑ risk of bleeding R/T effect on platelet function and GI irritation
Dipyridamole / ↑ Risk of major bleeding
Disulfiram / ↑ Anticoagulant effect → ↑ risk of bleeding
H ***Dong quai*** / Potential for ↑ anticoagulant effects
Erythromycin / ↑ Warfarin effect R/T ↓ liver metabolism
Estrogens / ↓ Anticoagulant response by ↑ activity of certain clotting factors; rarely, the opposite effect of ↑ risk of thromboembolism
Etretinate / ↓ Warfarin effect R/T ↑ liver breakdown
H ***Evening primrose oil*** / Potential to ↓ platelet aggregation
Felbamate / ↑ Anticoagulant effect → ↑ risk of bleeding
Fenofibrate / ↑ Anticoagulant effect → ↑ risk of bleeding
H ***Feverfew*** / Potential to ↓ platelet aggregation
H ***Fish oil*** / ↑ Warfarin anticoagulant effect R/T interference with vitamin K
Fluconazole / ↑ Warfarin effect
Flutamide / ↑ Anticoagulant effect → ↑ risk of bleeding
H ***Garlic*** / Potential to ↓ platelet aggregation
Gatifloxacin / ↑ INR values
Gemfibrozil / ↑ Anticoagulant effect → ↑ risk of bleeding
H ***Ginger*** / Potential to ↓ platelet aggregation
H ***Ginkgo biloba*** / Potential to ↓ platelet aggregation; also, ginkgo biloba may ↑ warfarin metabolism
H ***Ginseng, panax*** / Potential to ↓ platelet aggregation
Glucagon / ↑ Anticoagulant effect → ↑ risk of bleeding
H ***Grapeseed extract*** / Potential to ↓ platelet aggregation
Griseofulvin / ↓ Warfarin effect by unknown mechanism
Halothane / ↑ Anticoagulant effect → ↑ risk of bleeding

Heparin / ↑ Anticoagulant effect → ↑ risk of bleeding
HMG-CoA reductase inhibitors (e.g., fluvastatin, lovastatin, simvastatin) / ↑ Anticoagulant effect R/T ↓ warfarin hepatic metabolism by CYP2C9; do not use together
Hydantoins / ↑ Warfarin effect; also, ↑ hydantoin serum levels
Hypoglycemics, oral / ↑ Warfarin effect R/T ↓ plasma protein binding; also, ↑ effect of sulfonylureas
Ifosfamide / ↑ Warfarin effect R/T ↓ liver breakdown and displacement from protein binding sites
Indomethacin / ↑ Warfarin effect R/T effect on platelet function; also, indomethacin is ulcerogenic → GI hemorrhage
Ifosfamide / ↑ Anticoagulant effect R/T ↓ warfarin hepatic metabolism; also, may displace warfarin from protein binding sites
Isoniazid / ↑ Anticoagulant effect → ↑ risk of bleeding
Isotretinoin / ↓ Warfarin effect by unknown mechanism
Itraconazole / Anticoagulant effect is enhanced
Ketoconazole / ↑ Warfarin effect
Leflunomide / ↑ Anticoagulant effect R/T ↓ warfarin hepatic metabolism
Levamisole / ↑ Anticoagulant effect → ↑ risk of bleeding
Loop diuretics / ↑ Warfarin effect by displacement from protein binding sites
Lovastatin / ↑ Warfarin effect R/T ↓ liver breakdown
Macrolide antibiotics (e.g., azithromycin, clarithromycin, erythromycin) / ↑ Anticoagulant effect R/T ↓ warfarin body clearance
Mefloquine / ↑ Warfarin effect by displacement from protein binding sites
Meprobamate / ↓ Warfarin effect by unknown mechanism
Mesalamine / ↓ Warfarin effect by unknown mechanism
Methimazole / Either ↑ or ↓ PT/INR responses → ↑ or ↓ anticoagulant effect
Methyldopa / ↑ Anticoagulant effect → ↑ risk of bleeding
Methylphenidate / ↑ Anticoagulant effect → ↑ risk of bleeding
Metronidazole / ↑ Anticoagulant effect R/T ↓ warfarin hepatic metabolism
Miconazole / ↑ Bleeding or bruising
Mineral oil / ↑ Hypoprothrombinemia by ↓ absorption of vitamin K from GI tract; also mineral oil may ↓ absorption of warfarin from GI tract
Mitotane / ↓ Warfarin effect R/T ↑ liver breakdown
Moricizine / Either ↑ or ↓ PT/INR responses → ↑ or ↓ anticoagulant effect
Nafcillin / ↓ Warfarin effect R/T ↑ liver breakdown
Nalidixic acid / ↑ Warfarin effect R/T displacement from protein binding sites
Neomycin / ↑ Warfarin anticoagulant effect R/T interference with vitamin K
Nevirapine / ↓ Warfarin effect R/T ↑ liver breakdown
NSAIDs / ↑ Warfarin effect; ↑ risk of bleeding R/T effects on platelet function and GI irritation; ↑ risk of upper GI hemorrhage in geriatric clients
Olsalazine / ↑ Warfarin anticoagulant effect R/T effect on platelet function
Omeprazole / ↑ Anticoagulant effect R/T ↓ warfarin hepatic metabolism
Orlistat / ↑ Anticoagulant effect → ↑ risk of bleeding
Oxandrolone / Large ↑ in INR; dose of warfarin may have to be greatly ↓
Penicillins, high IV doses (e.g., penicillin G, piperacillin, ticarcillin) / ↑ Warfarin effect → ↑ risk of bleeding R/T effects on platelet function
Pentoxifylline / ↑ Anticoagulant effect → ↑ risk of bleeding
Phenytoin / Either ↑ or ↓ PT/INR responses → ↑ or ↓ anticoagulant effect
Pravastatin / Either ↑ or ↓ PT/INR responses → ↑ or ↓ anticoagulant effect
Prednisone / Either ↑ or ↓ PT/INR responses → ↑ or ↓ anticoagulant effect
Primidone / ↓ Warfarin effect R/T ↑ liver breakdown
Propafenone / ↑ Anticoagulant effect R/T ↓ warfarin hepatic metabolism
Propoxyphene / ↑ Anticoagulant effect → ↑ risk of bleeding
Propylthiouracil / Either ↑ or ↓ PT/INR responses → ↑ or ↓ anticoagulant effect
Protease inhibitors (e.g., indinavir, ritonavir) / ↓ Warfarin effect by unknown mechanism
Proton pump inhibitors (e.g., esomeprazole, lansoprazole, omeprazole, pantoprazole, rabeprazole) /

W

↑ Anticoagulant effect R/T ↓ warfarin hepatic metabolism
Quinidine, quinine / ↑ Anticoagulant effect R/T ↓ warfarin hepatic metabolism
Quinolones (e.g., ciprofloxacin, levofloxacin, norfloxacin, ofloxacin) / ↑ Anticoagulant effect → ↑ risk of bleeding
Raloxifene / ↓ Warfarin effect by unknown mechanism
Ranitidine / Either ↑ or ↓ PT/INR responses → ↑ or ↓ anticoagulant effect
Ribavirin / ↓ Warfarin effect by unknown mechanism
Rifampin/Rifamycins / ↓ Anticoagulant effect R/T ↑ liver breakdown
Ropinirole / ↑ Anticoagulant effect → ↑ risk of bleeding
H ***St. John's wort*** / Possible ↓ warfarin plasma levels R/T ↑ metabolism
Salicylates / ↑ Warfarin effect and ↑ risk of bleeding R/T effect on platelet function and GI irritation
Selective serotonin reuptake inhibitors (e.g., fluoxetine, fluvoxamine, paroxetine, sertraline) / ↑ Anticoagulant effect → ↑ risk of bleeding
Sorafenib / ↑ INR
Spironolactone / ↓ Warfarin effect R/T hemoconcentration of clotting factors due to diuresis
Streptokinase / ↑ Warfarin effect
Sucralfate / ↓ Warfarin effect
Sulfamethoxazole and Trimethoprim / ↑ Warfarin effect R/T ↓ liver breakdown
Sulfinpyrazone / ↑ Anticoagulant effect R/T ↓ warfarin hepatic metabolism; do not use together
Sulfonamides / ↑ Anticoagulant effect R/T ↓ warfarin hepatic metabolism
Sulindac / ↑ Warfarin effect
Tamoxifen / ↑ Anticoagulant effect → ↑ risk of bleeding
Terbinafine / ↓ Warfarin effect R/T ↑ liver breakdown
Tetracyclines / ↑ Warfarin effect R/T interference with vitamin K
Thiazide diuretics / ↓ Warfarin effect R/T hemoconcentration of clotting factors due to diuresis
Thioamines / ↑ Warfarin effect
Thiopurines (e.g., azathioprine) / ↓ Warfarin effect R/T ↑ synthesis or activation of prothrombin
Thrombolytics (e.g., tissue plasminogen activator) / ↑ Anticoagulant effect → ↑ risk of bleeding
Thyroid hormones (including levothyroxine, liothyronine, liotrix) / ↑ Anticoagulant effect with ↑ risk of bleeding
Ticlopidine / ↑ Warfarin anticoagulant effect R/T effect on platelet function
Tolbutamide / ↑ Anticoagulant effect → ↑ risk of bleeding
Tolterodine / ↑ Anticoagulant effect → ↑ risk of bleeding
Tramadol / ↑ Anticoagulant effect → ↑ risk of bleeding
Trastuzumab / ↑ Anticoagulant effect → ↑ risk of bleeding
Trazodone / ↓ Warfarin effect by unknown mechanism
Trimethoprim/Sulfamethoxazole / ↑ Risk of bleeding
Urokinase / ↑ Warfarin effect
Valproate / ↑ Warfarin effect by displacement from protein binding sites
Vitamin A / Possible ↑ anticoagulant effect if using large doses of vitamin A
Vitamin C / Slightly prolonged PT
Vitamin E / ↑ Warfarin effect R/T interference with vitamin K
Vitamin K / ↓ Warfarin effect
Zafirlukast / ↑ Anticoagulant effect → ↑ risk of bleeding
Zileuton / ↑ Anticoagulant effect → ↑ risk of bleeding

HOW SUPPLIED

Powder for Injection, Lyophilized: 2 mg/mL when reconstituted; ***Tablets:*** 1 mg, 2 mg, 2.5 mg, 3 mg, 4 mg, 5 mg, 6 mg, 7.5 mg, 10 mg.

DOSAGE

IV; TABLETS

All uses.

Individualize based on PT/INR response. An INR of more than 4 probably does not provide additional therapeutic benefit in most clients and is associated with a higher risk of bleeding.

Adults, initial: 2–5 mg per day; **then** adjust dose based on prothrombin or INR determinations. A lower dose should be used in geriatric or debilitated clients or clients with genetic variations in CYP2C9 and VKORC1 enzymes. Dosage has not been established for children. **Maintenance:** 2–10 mg per day for most clients. Determine individual dose by PT response. Lower maintenance doses are recommended for elderly and/or debilitated clients and in those with a potential to show greater than expected PT/INR response to warfarin.

NURSING IMPLICATIONS

Sound Alike Drug: Do not confuse Coumadin with Cardura (doxazosin, antihypertensive) or with Avandia (rosiglitazone, an oral hypoglycemic).

IMPLEMENTATION/ADMINISTRATION/STORAGE

1. Frequent monitoring of PT/INR is recommended during the first week of therapy, during adjustment periods, and monthly thereafter.
2. The duration of therapy is individualized and should be continued until the danger of thrombosis and embolism has passed.
3. If a dose is missed, the dose should be taken as soon as possible on the same day. Doubling the daily dose to make up for the missed dose is not appropriate.
4. Do not change brands; may be differences in bioavailability.
5. The anticoagulant effect of warfarin is delayed. Thus, heparin is preferred initially for rapid anticoagulation. Conversion to warfarin may begin concomitantly with heparin therapy or may be delayed 3 to 6 days. To ensure anticoagulation, continue the full dose of heparin and overlap warfarin therapy with heparin for 4 to 5 days.
6. Levels of anticoagulation that are recommended for specific indications by the American College of Chest Physicians and the National Heart, Lung, and Blood Institute should be followed.
7. Asian clients may require lower initiation and maintenance doses of warfarin.
8. Impaired hepatic function can increase the response to warfarin through impaired synthesis of clotting factors and decreased warfarin metabolism.
9. Clients undergoing minor dental, dermatologic, or cataract removal should continue to receive warfarin.
10. Clients who require reversal of the anticoagulant effect of warfarin for an urgent procedure should be given low dose vitamin K, 2.5 to 5 mg IV or PO.
11. Protect from light; store at controlled room temperature. Dispense in tight, light-resistant container.
12. IV Give as slow bolus over 1–2 min into peripheral vein. Do not give IM.
13. To reconstitute for IV use: Add 2.7 mL sterile water for injection. Inspect for particulate matter and discoloration.
14. After reconstitution, injection stable for 4 hr at room temperature. There is no preservative; take care to ensure sterility of prepared solution.
15. Store injection from 15–30°C (59–86°F) protected from light. Do not refrigerate. Discard any unused portion.
16. COMPATIBILITY Sterile water.
17. INCOMPATIBILITY Administer separately. Vial is not for multiple use; discard unused solution.

ASSESSMENT

1. Note reasons for therapy, time-frame (i.e., DVT [initial] 6 months; recurrent/multiple DVT and heart valve replacement—lifetime); identify desired PT/INR range.
2. List drugs prescribed to ensure none interacts unfavorably by increasing or decreasing PT as a result of competition for protein binding at receptor sites.
3. Note any bleeding tendencies. Review PMH for conditions that may preclude therapy: PUD, chronic GI tract ulcerations, alcoholic, severe renal or liver dysfunction, endocardial infections.
4. Determine if pregnant. May cause fetal malformations and neonatal hemorrhage.
5. Some clients may be managed/discharged early on low molecular weight heparin injections and coumadin until desired INR obtained. Adjust oral anticoagulant weekly, especially if receiving one of the many drugs known to interact or compete with warfarin.
6. Have available vitamin K, FFP, or factor IX concentrate for warfarin overdoses.
7. With atrial fibrillation assess echocardiogram and ECG; monitor INR.
8. Review risk factors for adverse outcome, e.g., INR >4, over age 65 yr, highly variable INRs, history of GI bleeding, hypertension, cerebrovascular disease, serious heart disease, ane-

W

mia, malignancy, trauma, renal function impairment, long-term warfarin therapy.

9. Request written parameters noting the desired range for PT or INR, once anticoagulated (orally). It usually takes 36–48 hr for drug to reach steady state; therefore allow time to equilibrate. The INR is the PT ratio (test/control) obtained from human brain thromboplastin and is universally considered most accurate to calculate dosage.
10. Drug inhibits production of factors II, VII, IX, and X; onset in response is delayed because of degradation of clotting factors that have already been synthesized.
11. Sudden lumbar pain may indicate retroperitoneal hemorrhage.
12. GI dysfunction may indicate intestinal hemorrhage. Test for blood in urine and feces; check H&H to assess for abnormal bleeding.
13. Observe for "purple toes" syndrome related to inhibition of protein C and S. In those with deficiency of protein C/S anticoagulant response may increase risk of tissue necrosis.
14. Question about bleeding (gums, urine, stools, vomit, bruises). If urine discolored, determine cause, i.e., from drug therapy or hematuria. Indanedione-type anticoagulants turn alkaline urine a red-orange color; acidify urine or test for occult blood.
15. Monitor ECG, CBC, PT/PTT, INR, renal and LFTs.

CLIENT/FAMILY TEACHING

1. Take oral warfarin as prescribed and at the same time each day; must be compliant with therapy. Do not change brands of drug; may alter response. Avoid eating large amounts of grapefruit or drinking grapefruit or cranberry juice.
2. This drug does not dissolve clots but decreases the clotting ability of the blood and helps prevent the formation of harmful blood clots in the blood vessels and heart valves.
3. Avoid IM shots, activities/contact sports that may cause injury or cuts and bruises. Use a soft toothbrush, electric razor to shave, wear shoes, and use a night-light to avoid falls at night.
4. Report immediately unusual bruising/bleeding, dark brown or blood-tinged body secretions, injury or trauma, dizziness, abdominal pain or swelling, back pain, severe headaches, and joint swelling and pain.
5. If prescribed, may carry vitamin K for emergency use. (The usual dosage is 5–25 mg parenterally, to be used in the event of excessive bleeding.)
6. Foods high in vitamin K: asparagus, broccoli, cabbage, brussel sprouts, spinach, turnips, cheese, avocados, bananas, dried fruits, grapefruit, lima beans, nuts, oranges, peaches, potatoes, sunflower seeds, and tomatoes. Consistent intake of vitamin K foods should be done to ensure a stable INR as these may alter (lower) results.
7. Use reliable birth control. Menstruation may be prolonged and flow may be slightly increased. Report if excessive and unusual.
8. Skin eruptions may develop as an allergic reaction; report.
9. Avoid alcohol and OTC drugs. Check prior to taking any OTC drugs that have anticoagulant-type effects such as salicylates, NSAIDs, steroids, vitamin K, mineral preparations from health food stores, vitamins, herbals, herbal teas, alcohol. Check with provider to see if they intend continuation of baby aspirin. Should be done with AMI to prevent recurrence.
10. Wear identification and alert all providers of anticoagulant therapy.
11. Avoid smoking; increases dose requirements.
12. Identify social/economic situations that may alter compliance (lack of transportation for testing, inability to distinguish tablets or read directions); identify reliable resources.
13. Unusual hair loss and itching are common with the elderly; advise to report if intolerable or skin break down occurs.
14. Elderly are more prone to developing bleeding complications. Many elderly use multiple pharmacies and shop for value; stress the need to know what they are taking and why and to carry the name and dosage of ALL drugs prescribed. Do not skip a dose, as drug works for only 24 hr and must be readministered in order to be effective. Carry list of all meds/vitamins/herbals prescribed/consumed to all visits to provider/pharmacy.
15. Keep all F/U to assess response, regular labs, need for dosage changes. Once dose stabilized, PT/INR once monthly. Medication

W

should not be dispensed without confirmatory lab results.

OUTCOMES/EVALUATE

- PT within desired range (1.5–2 times the control)
- INR within desired range (2.0–3.0 with standard therapy; 2.5–4.0 with high-dose therapy)
- ↓ Risk of thromboembolism with prosthetic heart valves/AF
- Resolution/prophylaxis of DVT

Z

Zafirlukast

(zah-**FIR**-loo-kast)

Classification(s): Antiasthmatic, leukotriene receptor antagonist.

Pregnancy Category: B

RX: Accolate.

INDICATIONS/USES

Prophylaxis and chronic treatment of asthma in adults and children 5 years of age and older. *Investigational:* Chronic urticaria.

ACTION/KINETICS

Action

A selective and competitive antagonist of leukotriene receptors D_4 and E_4, which are components of slow-reacting substance of anaphylaxis. It is believed that cysteinyl leukotriene occupation of receptors causes asthma, including airway edema, smooth muscle constriction, and altered cellular activity associated with the inflammatory process. Zafirlukast inhibits bronchoconstriction caused by sulfur dioxide and cold air in clients with asthma. It also attenuates the early- and late-phase reaction in asthmatics caused by inhalation of antigens such as grass, cat dander, ragweed, and mixed antigens.

Pharmacokinetics

Rapidly absorbed after PO use; bioavailability may be decreased when taken with food. **Peak plasma levels:** 3 hr. **t½, terminal:** About 10 hr. Extensively metabolized in the liver by CYP2C9, with about 90% excreted in the feces and 10% in the urine. Clearance is reduced in clients with cirrhosis. Inhibits CYP2C9 and CYP3A4 isoenzymes. The C_{max} and AUC are increased in geriatric clients. **Plasma protein binding:** More than 99%.

CONTRAINDICATIONS

Hypersensitivity to zafirlukast or any component of the product. Use to terminate an acute asthma attack, including status asthmaticus. Lactation.

SPECIAL CONCERNS

- Clearance is reduced in clients 65 years of age and older.
- Safety and efficacy not determined in children less than 5 years of age.

SIDE EFFECTS

Most Common

Headache, N&V, diarrhea, abdominal pain, infection, asthenia, dizziness, fever.

GI: N&V, diarrhea, abdominal pain, dyspepsia. **CNS:** Headache, dizziness. **Hepatic:** Hepatic dysfunction, especially in women and girls. ***Hepatic failure***. Rarely, symptomatic hepatitis and hyperbilirubinemia. **Hypersensitivity:** Urticaria, angioedema, rashes (with and without blistering). **Hematologic:** Agranulocytosis, systemic eosinophilia with vasculitis consistent with Churg-Strauss syndrome. **Musculoskeletal:** Arthralgia, myalgia, back pain. **Body as a whole:** Asthenia, fever, bleeding, infection (especially in the elderly), generalized pain, bruising, edema. **Miscellaneous:** Accidental injury. *NOTE:* Headache and abdominal pain occurred frequently.

LABORATORY TEST CONSIDERATIONS

↑ ALT, liver enzymes (rare).

OVERDOSE MANAGEMENT

Symptoms: Rash, upset stomach. *Treatment:* Usual supportive measures, including removing unabsorbed drug from the GI tract and employing clinical monitoring.

DRUG INTERACTIONS

Use caution with coadministration of drugs known to metabolized by CYP2C9 and CYP3A4 since they are inhibited by zafirlukast.

Aspirin / ↑ Zafirlukast levels by about 45%
Erythromycin / ↓ Zafirlukast levels by about 40% R/T ↓ zafirlukast bioavailability
Theophylline (liquid product) / ↓ Mean plasma levels of zafirlukast by about 30%; no effect on plasma theophylline levels
Warfarin / Significant ↑ PT R/T inhibition of CYP2C9; closely monitor and adjust warfarin dose if needed

HOW SUPPLIED

Tablets: 10 mg, 20 mg.

DOSAGE

TABLETS

Asthma.

Adults and children aged 12 and older: 20 mg 2 times per day. **Children, 5–11 years:** 10 mg 2 times per day, even during symptom-free periods.

NURSING IMPLICATIONS

IMPLEMENTATION/ADMINISTRATION/STORAGE

Protect from light and moisture; store at controlled room temperatures of 20–25°C (68–77°F). Dispense in original air-tight container.

ASSESSMENT

1. Note reasons for therapy, onset, duration, characteristics of S&S and clinical presentation. List other agents trialed, outcome.
2. Note mental status and behavioral presentation and cardiopulmonary assessment findings. Document lung sounds, PFTS, and respiratory function.
3. Monitor labs, symptomatic complaints, and PFTs. Reinforce that drug is not for acute bronchospasm during asthma attack.
4. If liver dysfunction is suspected, discontinue therapy and perform LFTs immediately. If LFTs are consistent with hepatic dysfunction, do not resume therapy.

CLIENT/FAMILY TEACHING

1. Take 1 hr before or 2 hr after meals to prevent loss of bioavailability.
2. Take drug regularly during symptom-free periods. Do not increase or decrease dose without approval.
3. Drug is not appropriate for acute episodes of asthma. Continue all other antiasthma agents as prescribed.
4. Review peak flow meter use and set targets for intervention or additional therapy.
5. Avoid triggers (i.e., dust, chemicals, cigarette smoke, pollutants, pets, and perfumes).
6. Practice reliable birth control; do not breastfeed during therapy.
7. Keep all F/U to assess response and for adverse SE.

OUTCOMES/EVALUATE

Inhibition of bronchoconstriction; improved breathing patterns

Zalcitabine (Dideoxycytidine, ddC)

(zal-**SIGH**-tah-been)

Classification(s): Antiviral, nucleoside reverse transcriptase inhibitor

Pregnancy Category: C

SEE ALSO ***ANTIVIRAL DRUGS*** AND ***ANTI-INFECTIVE DRUGS***.

INDICATIONS/USES

In combination with antiretroviral drugs to treat HIV infection.

ACTION/KINETICS

Action

Converted in cells to the active metabolite, dideoxycytidine 5′-triphosphate (ddCTP), by cellular enzymes. ddCTP serves as an alternative substrate to deoxycytidine triphosphate for HIV-reverse transcriptase, thereby inhibiting the in vitro replication of HIV-1 and inhibiting viral DNA synthesis. The incorporation of ddCTP into the growing DNA chain leads to premature chain termination. ddCTP serves as a competitive inhibitor of the natural substrate for deoxycytidine triphosphate for the active site of the viral reverse transcriptase, which further inhibits viral DNA synthesis.

Pharmacokinetics

Food reduces the rate of absorption. Does not appear to undergo significant metabolism by the liver. **Elimination t½:** 1–3 hr. Approximately 70% of a PO dose is excreted through the kidneys and

10% in the feces. Prolonged elimination ($t^{1/2}$ up to 8.5 hr) is observed in clients with impaired renal function.

CONTRAINDICATIONS

Lactation.

SPECIAL CONCERNS

■ (1) Use has been associated with significant clinical side effects, some of which may be fatal. Zalcitabine can cause severe peripheral neuropathy; thus, use with extreme caution in those with pre-existing neuropathy. (2) May also cause pancreatitis (rare); immediately stop therapy in those who develop any symptoms suggestive of pancreatitis while using zalcitabine until this diagnosis is excluded. (3) Lactic acidosis and severe hepatomegaly with steatosis, including fatalities, have been reported with the use of antiretroviral nucleoside analogs alone or in combination, including zalcitabine. Also, rare cases of hepatic failure and death, possibly related to underlying hepatitis B and zalcitabine have been reported. ■

- **Use with extreme caution in clients with low CD_4 cell counts (<50/mm^3).**
- **Use with caution in clients with a history of pancreatitis or known risk factors for the development of pancreatitis.**
- **Clients with a C_{CR} less than 55 mL/min may be at a greater risk for toxicity due to decreased clearance.**
- **Clients may continue to develop opportunistic infections and other complications of HIV infection.**
- **Use with caution in moderate or severe peripheral neuropathy or with drugs that have the potential to cause peripheral neuropathy (see *Drug Interactions*).**
- **Possible severe peripheral neuropathy, pancreatitis (rare), hepatic failure (rare), lactic acidosis, and severe hepatomegaly with steatosis.**
- **Possible redistribution of accumulation of body fat.**
- **Use with caution in elderly.**
- **Safety and efficacy not determined in HIV-infected children less than 13 years of age.**

SIDE EFFECTS

Most Common

Peripheral neuropathy, abnormal hepatic function, fatigue, rash/pruritus/urticaria, convulsions, headache, abdominal pain, oral lesions/stomatitis, N&V, diarrhea, constipation, fever.

NOTE: The incidence of certain side effects is dependent on the duration of use and the dose of the drug. **Neurologic:** Peripheral neuropathy (may be severe) characterized by numbness and burning dysesthesia involving the distal extremities; this may be followed by sharp shooting pains or severe continuous burning pain if the drug is not withdrawn. The neuropathy may progress to severe pain requiring narcotic analgesics and may be irreversible. **GI:** ***Fatal pancreatitis, lactic acidosis and hepatomegaly with steatosis*** when given alone or with zidovudine. Esophageal ulcers, oral/esophageal ulcers, N&V, dysphagia, anorexia, abdominal pain, constipation, ulcerative stomatitis, aphthous stomatitis, diarrhea, dry mouth, dyspepsia, glossitis, ***rectal hemorrhage***, hemorrhoids, enlarged abdomen, gum disorders, flatulence, anorexia, tongue ulceration, dysphagia, eructation, gastritis, ***GI hemorrhage***, left quadrant pain, salivary gland enlargement, esophageal pain, esophagitis, rectal ulcers, melena, painful swallowing, mouth lesion, acute pharyngitis, abdominal bloating or cramps, anal/rectal pain, colitis, dental abscess, epigastric pain, gagging with pills, gingivitis, heartburn, ***hemorrhagic pancreatitis***, increased salivation, odynophagia, painful sore gums, rectal mass, sore tongue, sore throat, tongue disorder, toothache, unformed/loose stools. **Dermatologic:** Rash (including erythematous, maculopapular, follicular), pruritus, night sweats, dermatitis, skin lesions, acne, alopecia, bullous eruptions, increased sweating, urticaria, hot flashes, lip blister or lesions, carbuncle/furuncle, cellulitis, dry skin, dry rash desquamation, exfoliative dermatitis, finger inflammation, impetigo, infection, itchy rash, moniliasis, mucocutaneous/skin disorder, nail disorder, photosensitivity, skin fissure, skin ulcer. **CNS:** Headache, convulsions, dizziness, seizures, ataxia, abnormal coordination, Bell's palsy, dysphonia, hyperkinesia, hypokinesia, migraine, neuralgia, neuritis, stupor, aphasia, decreased neurologic function, disequilibrium, facial nerve palsy, focal motor seizures, memory loss, paralysis, speech disorder, ***status epilepticus***, tremor, vertigo, hypertonia, hand tremor, twitching, confusion, impaired concentration, insomnia, agitation, depersonalization, hallucinations, emotional lability, nervousness, anxiety, depression, euphoria, manic reaction, dementia, amnesia, somnolence, abnormal thinking, crying, loss of memory, decreased concentration/motivation/sexual desire, acute psychotic disorder, acute stress reaction, mood swings, paranoid states, ***suicide attempt.*** **Respiratory:** Coughing, dyspnea, respiratory distress, rales/rhonchi, nasal discharge, flu-like symptoms, cyanosis, acute nasopharyngitis, chest/sinus congestion, dry nasal mucosa, hemoptysis, sinus pain, sinusitis, wheezing. **Musculoskeletal:** Myalgia, arthralgia, arthritis, arthropathy, cold extremities, leg cramps, myositis, joint pain or inflammation, weakness in leg muscle, generalized muscle weakness, back pain, backache, bone aches and pains, bursitis, pain in extremities, joint swelling, muscle disorder/stiffness/cramps, arthrosis, myopathy, neck pain, rib pain, stiff neck. **Hepatic:** Exacerbation of hepatic dysfunction, especially in those with pre-existing liver disease or with a history of alcohol abuse. Abnormal hepatic function, hepatitis, jaundice, hepatocellular damage, severe hepatomegaly with steatosis, cholecystitis. **CV:** ***Cardiomyopathy***, CHF, abnormal cardiac movement arrhythmia, atrial fibrillation, ***cardiac failure***, cardiac dysrhythmias, heart racing, hypertension, palpitations, ***subarachnoid hemorrhage***, syncope, tachycardia, ventricular ectopy, epistaxis. **Hematologic:** Anemia, leukopenia, thrombocytopenia, alteration of absolute neutrophil count, granulocytosis, eosinophilia, neutropenia, hemoglobinemia, neutrophilia, platelet alteration, purpura, thrombus, unspecified hematologic toxicity, alteration of WBCs. **Hypersensitivity:** Urticaria, ***anaphylaxis*** (rare). **Endocrine:** Diabetes mellitus, gout, hot flashes, hypoglycemia, hyperglycemia, hypocalcemia, hypophosphatemia, hyper-/hyponatremia, hypomagnesemia, hyperkalemia, hypokalemia, hyperlipidemia, polydipsia. **GU:** Dysuria, toxic nephropathy, polyuria, renal calculi, ***acute renal failure***, hyperuricemia, increased frequency of micturition, abnormal renal function, renal cyst, albuminuria, bladder pain, genital lesion/ulcer, nocturia, painful/sore penis, penile edema, testicular swelling, urinary retention, vaginal itch/ulcer/pain, vaginal/cervix disorder. **Ophthalmic:** Abnormal vision, burning or itching eyes, xerophthalmia, eye pain or abnormality, blurred or decreased vision, eye inflammation/irritation, eye redness/hemorrhage, increased tears, mucopurulent conjunctivitis, photophobia, dry eyes, unequal sized pupils, yellow sclera. **Otic:** Ear pain/blockage, fluid in ears, hearing loss, tinnitus. **Body as a whole:** Fatigue, fever, rigors, chest pain or tightness, weight decrease, pain, malaise, asthenia, generalized edema, general debilitation, chills, difficulty moving, facial pain or swelling, flank pain, flushing, pelvic/groin pain. **Miscellaneous:** Lymphadenopathy, taste perversion, decreased taste, parosmia, lactic acidosis.

LABORATORY TEST CONSIDERATIONS

↑ ALT, AST, alkaline phosphatase, CPK, amylase, nonprotein nitrogen. Abnormal GGT, LDH, lactate dehydrogenase, triglycerides, lipase. Bilirubinemia. ↓ Hematocrit.

DRUG INTERACTIONS

The following drugs have the potential to cause peripheral neuropathy. **Concomitant use is not recommended.** Drugs include: Chloramphenicol, cisplatin, dapsone, didanosine, disulfiram, ethionamide, gold, hydralazine, iodoquinol, isoniazid, metronidazole, nitrofurantoin, phenytoin, ribavirin, vincristine. Drugs such as amphotericin, foscarnet, and aminoglycosides may increase the risk of peripheral neuropathy by interfering with the renal clearance of zalcitabine, thus increasing plasma levels.

Antacids (Mg/Al-containing) / ↓ Zalcitabine absorption
Cimetidine / ↓ Zalcitabine elimination by ↓ renal tubular secretion
Metoclopramide / ↓ Zalcitabine absorption
Pentamidine / ↑ Risk of fulminant pancreatitis
Probenecid / ↓ Zalcitabine elimination by ↓ renal tubular secretion

HOW SUPPLIED

Tablets: 0.375 mg, 0.75 mg.

DOSAGE

TABLETS

In combination with antiretroviral drugs (e.g., zidovudine) in advanced HIV infection.

Adults and children 13 years and older: 0.75 mg q 8 hr given at the same time with 200 mg zidovudine q 8 hr for a total daily dose of 2.25 mg zalcitabine and 600 mg zidovudine.

NURSING IMPLICATIONS

IMPLEMENTATION/ADMINISTRATION/STORAGE

1. Greater effect noted when new antiretroviral drugs are started at the same time as zalcitabine.

2. If C_{CR} is 10–40 mL/min, reduce dose to 0.75 mg/12 hr; if C_{CR} <10 mL/min, reduce dose to 0.75 mg/24 hr.
3. Dosage reduction not required for weights down to 30 kg.

ASSESSMENT

1. Note disease onset, clinical presentation, other agents trialed and outcome, and viral load/CD4 counts.
2. Assess abdomen, lactic acidosis, and hepatomegaly may be fatal.
3. Clients with a history of pancreatitis or elevated serum amylase should be followed closely while on zalcitabine therapy. Obtain baseline serum amylase and triglyceride levels with history of pancreatitis, increased amylase, those on parenteral nutrition, or those with a history of drug abuse.
4. Frequent monitoring of hematologic indices is recommended to detect serious anemia or granulocytopenia. In clients manifesting hematologic toxicity, decreases in hemoglobin may occur as early as 2–4 weeks after beginning therapy, whereas granulocytopenia may be seen after 6–8 weeks of therapy.
5. Assess for symptoms of peripheral neuropathy: pain, numbness, and tingling. If symptoms evident, drug may be reintroduced at 50% of the initial dose (i.e., 0.375 mg/8 hr) once all symptoms related to the peripheral neuropathy have improved to mild. Permanently discontinue the drug if severe discomfort due to peripheral neuropathy progresses for 1 week or longer.
6. Monitor CBC, CD_4 counts/viral loads, liver and renal function studies; adjust dose with renal dysfunction. Check for hepatitis A, B, and C; monitor closely.

CLIENT/FAMILY TEACHING

1. Take with or without food (with concurrently prescribed zidovudine, if appropriate) every 8 hr.
2. Drug is not a cure, may prolong life and helps to alleviate and manage the symptoms of HIV infections. May continue to develop opportunistic infections and other complications of HIV infection; remain under close medical supervision.
3. Use reliable contraceptive and practice safe sex.
4. Discontinue and report if symptoms of peripheral neuropathy occur, especially if they are bilateral and progress for more than 72 hr. Symptoms include numbness, tingling, or burning sensation, especially in the feet or tips of the toes. Peripheral neuropathy may continue to worsen despite interruption of therapy. If symptoms improve, drug may be reintroduced at a lower dose.
5. Schedule retinal exams q 6 months to assess for retinal depigmentation.
6. Identify local support groups that may assist client/family to understand and cope with this disease.
7. Keep all F/U to assess response, labs, and for adverse SE.

OUTCOMES/EVALUATE

Improved CD_4 cell counts, ↓ viral load, ↓ incidence of opportunistic infection, and improved survival rates in clients with advanced HIV infections

Zaleplon

(**ZAL**-leh-plon)

Classification(s): Sedative-hypnotic, nonbenzodiazepine

Pregnancy Category: C

RX: Sonata, **C-IV**

INDICATIONS/USES

Treat insomnia for up to 5 weeks.

ACTION/KINETICS

Action

Nonbenzodiazepine hypnotic. However, it interacts with the GABA-benzodiazepine receptor complex. It binds selectively to the brain omega-1 receptor located on the alpha subunit of $GABA_A$ receptor complex and potentiates t-butyl-bicyclophosphorothionate (TBPS) binding. Although it decreases the time to sleep, it does not increase total sleep time or decrease the number of awakenings. Decreased hangover effect.

Pharmacokinetics

Rapidly and almost completely absorbed. **Peak plasma levels:** 1 hr. Undergoes significant first-pass metabolism. A high-fat or heavy meal prolongs absorption. Extensively metabolized to inactive metabolites, which are excreted in the urine (70%) and feces (17%). **t½:** About 1 hr.

CONTRAINDICATIONS

Use with alcohol, severe hepatic impairment, or during lactation.

SPECIAL CONCERNS

- **Use with caution in diseases or conditions that could affect metabolism or hemodynamic responses, in clients with compromised respiratory function, or in clients showing signs or symptoms of depression.**
- **Abuse potential is similar to benzodiazepine and benzodiazepine-like hypnotics.**
- **Contains tartrazine (FD&C yellow #5), which may cause an allergic-type reaction, especially in those with aspirin hypersensitivity.**
- **May cause amnesia and dependence.**

SIDE EFFECTS

Most Common

Headache, myalgia, nausea, dyspepsia, eye pain, abdominal pain, asthenia, dysmenorrhea, fever, hyperacusis, vertigo, anorexia, abnormal vision, malaise, epistaxis.

Listed are side effects with an incidence of 0.1% or greater. **CNS:** Dizziness, amnesia, somnolence, anxiety, paresthesia, depersonalization, hypesthesia, tremor, hallucinations, vertigo, depression, hypertonia, nervousness, abnormal thinking/concentration, abnormal gait, agitation, apathy, ataxia, circumoral paresthesia, confusion, emotional lability, euphoria, hyperesthesia, hyperkinesia, hypotonia, incoordination, insomnia, decreased libido, neuralgia, nystagmus. **GI:** Nausea, dyspepsia, anorexia, colitis, constipation, dry mouth, eructation, esophagitis, flatulence, gastritis, gastroenteritis, gingivitis, glossitis, increased appetite, melena, mouth ulceration, rectal hemorrhage, stomatitis. **CV:** Migraine, angina pectoris, bundle branch block, hypertension, hypotension, palpitation, syncope, tachycardia, vasodilation, ventricular extrasystoles. **Dermatologic:** Pruritus, rash, acne, alopecia, contact dermatitis, dry skin, eczema, maculopapular rash, skin hypertrophy, sweating, urticaria, vesiculobullous rash. **GU:** Bladder/breast/kidney pain, cystitis, decreased urine stream, dysuria, hematuria, impotence, kidney calculus, menorrhagia, urinary frequency/incontinence/urgency, vaginitis, dysmenorrhea. **Respiratory:** Bronchitis, asthma, dyspnea, laryngitis, pneumonia, snoring, voice alteration. **Musculoskeletal:** Arthritis, arthrosis, bursitis, joint disorder (swelling, stiffness, pain), myasthenia, tenosynovitis. **Hematologic:** Anemia, ecchymosis, lymphadenopathy. **Metabolic:** Edema, gout, hypercholesterolemia, thirst, weight gain. **Ophthalmic:** Eye pain, abnormal vision, conjunctivitis, diplopia, dry eyes, photophobia, watery eyes. **Otic:** Ear pain, hyperacusis, tinnitus. **Body as a whole:** Headache, asthenia, myalgia, fever, malaise, chills, generalized edema. **Miscellaneous:** Abdominal pain, photosensitivity, peripheral edema, epistaxis, back pain, chest pain, substernal chest pain, face edema, hangover effect, neck rigidity, parosmia.

DRUG INTERACTIONS

Cimetidine / Significantly ↑ zaleplon levels
CNS depressants (anticonvulsants, antihistamines, ethanol) / Additive CNS depression
Rifampin / Significantly ↓ zaleplon levels

HOW SUPPLIED

Capsules: 5 mg, 10 mg.

DOSAGE

CAPSULES

Insomnia.

Adults, nonelderly: 10 mg for no more than 7–10 days. Consider 20 mg for the occasional client who does not benefit from the lower dose. Do not exceed a dose of 20 mg. **Mild to moderate hepatic impairment, elderly clients, or low-weight individuals:** 5 mg, not to exceed 10 mg.

NURSING IMPLICATIONS

ASSESSMENT

1. **Note reasons for insomnia, characteristics of S&S, contributing factors. Note drugs prescribed to ensure none interact; with cimetidine initially reduce zaleplon dose to 5 mg and assess response.**
2. **Assess sleep patterns, mental status, and identify any contributing factors eg. caffeine use, energy drinks, exercise before bedtime, medication usage.**
3. **List any depression, respiratory dysfunction, alcohol or drug dependence. Drug may cause**

dependence and amnesia and intensify depression symptoms.

4. Contains tartrazine (FD&C yellow #5); note any aspirin hypersensitivity. Monitor renal and LFTs; reduce dose with liver dysfunction.

CLIENT/FAMILY TEACHING

1. Due to its rapid onset, ingest immediately prior to going to bed or after going to bed and experiencing difficulty falling asleep. Store out of the reach of children.
2. Taking zaleplon with or immediately after a heavy, high-fat meal causes slower absorption leading to a reduced effect on sleep latency.
3. Do not engage in activities requiring mental alertness after ingesting drug and during the next day until drug effects realized. Avoid alcohol and CNS depressants.
4. May experience amnesia. Obtain at least 4 hr sleep after ingestion and before activity. If also taking cimetidine, take an initial lowered dose of 5 mg of zaleplon.
5. May experience withdrawal symptoms or worsening of insomnia with abrupt drug discontinuation especially with daily use for an extended period of time.
6. If behavioral changes or unusual thinking occur involving aggressiveness, confusion, loss of personal identity, agitation, hallucinations, increased depression or suicide ideations, report.
7. Identify triggers (caffeine, daytime naps) and alternative methods to induce sleep (i.e., soft music, warm milk, white noise simulator, etc).
8. Keep all F/U to assess response and for adverse SE.

OUTCOMES/EVALUATE

Relief of insomnia

Zanamivir

(zah-**NAM**-ih-vir)

Classification(s): Antiviral

Pregnancy Category: C

RX: Relenza.

INDICATIONS/USES

(1) Prophylaxis of influenza in adults and children at least 5 years of age. (2) Treatment of uncomplicated acute illness due to influenza virus A and B (limited) in adults and children 7 years and older who have been symptomatic for 2 or less days. *Investigational:* Chemoprophylaxis and treatment of H1N1 influenza A (swine flu) virus infection, including those with confirmed, probable, or suspected H1N1 influenza A and their close contacts. *NOTE:* There is no evidence that zanamivir is effective in any illness caused by agents other than influenza virus A and B.

ACTION/KINETICS

Action

Selectively inhibits influenza virus neuraminidase. The enzyme allows virus release from infected cells, prevents virus aggregation, and possibly decreases virus inactivation by respiratory mucus. Zanamivir may alter virus particle aggregation and release. There is the possibility of emergence of resistance. Does not prevent complications from bacterial infections.

Pharmacokinetics

About 4–17% is absorbed systemically. **Peak serum levels:** 17–142 ng/mL within 1–2 hr after a 10 mg dose. Readily excreted as unchanged drug in the urine. Unabsorbed drug is excreted in the feces. **t½, serum:** 2.5–5.1 hr after PO inhalation. **Plasma protein binding:** <10%.

CONTRAINDICATIONS

Hypersensitivity to zanamivir or any component of the product, including lactose (which contains milk proteins). Use in asthma or COPD.

SPECIAL CONCERNS

- Use with caution during lactation.
- Elderly may be more sensitive to the drug.
- Safety and efficacy not determined for preventing influenza in children younger than 5 years of age or in treating influenza in children less than 7 years of age, in clients with underlying chronic pulmonary disease, in those with high-risk underlying medical conditions (e.g., respiratory disease), or in those with severe renal insufficiency.
- Serious bacterial infections may begin with flu-like symptoms or may coexist with or occur as complications during the course of flu; zanamivir does not prevent such complications.
- Due to the potential for interference between live attenuated flu vaccine and zanamivir, do not give live attenuated influenza vaccine within 2 weeks before or 48 hr after administration of zanamivir unless medically indicated.

SIDE EFFECTS

Most Common

Dizziness, headache, N&V, diarrhea, bronchitis, cough, ENT infections, sinusitis

GI: Diarrhea, N&V, abdominal pain, anorexia, increased/decreased appetite. **Respiratory:** Nasal S&S, bronchitis, ***bronchospasm***, dyspnea, cough, sinusitis, ENT infections, ***ENT hemorrhages* in children**, asthma in children, throat/tonsil discomfort and pain in children, viral respiratory infections, nasal inflammation. **CNS:** Dizziness, headache, delirium, abnormal behavior, agitation, altered level of consciousness, anxiety, confusion, delusions, hallucinations, nightmares, ***seizures***. **CV:** Arrhythmias, syncope. **Hypersensitivity:** Oropharyngeal edema, serious skin rashes, ***anaphylaxis***. **Musculoskeletal:** Myalgia, arthralgia, muscle pain, articular rheumatism, musculoskeletal pain. **Dermatologic:** Facial edema, urticaria, rash, including serious cutaneous reactions. **Body as a whole:** Malaise, chills, fatigue, fever, allergic reactions (including oropharyngeal edema and serious skin rashes), serious bacterial infections with flu-like symptoms or as complications of flu.

LABORATORY TEST CONSIDERATIONS

↑ Liver enzymes, CPK. Lymphopenia, neutropenia.

HOW SUPPLIED

Power for Oral Inhalation, Blisters: 5 mg.

DOSAGE

POWDER FOR ORAL INHALATION (BLISTERS)

Prophylaxis of influenza: household setting.

Adults and children, 5 years and older: 10 mg inhaled once daily for 10 days. The 10 mg dose is obtained by 2 inhalations (one-5 mg blister/inhalation). Administer the dose about the same time each day. There are no data on the efficacy of prophylaxis in a household setting begun more than 1.5 days after the onset of signs and symptoms.

Prophylaxis of influenza: community outbreaks.

Adults and children, 12–16 years: 10 mg inhaled once daily for 28 days. The 10 mg dose is obtained by 2 inhalations (one-5 mg blister/inhalation). Administer the dose at about the same time each day. There are no data on the efficacy of prophylaxis in a community outbreak when started more than 5 days after the outbreak was identified. Safety and efficacy of prophylaxis have not been determined for longer than 28 days' duration.

Influenza treatment.

Adults and children over 7 years: 2 inhalations (one 5-mg blister/inhalation for a total dose of 10 mg) twice a day for 5 days. Two doses are taken on the first day of treatment whenever possible, provided there are 2 or more hr between doses. On subsequent days, doses are taken about 12 hr apart (i.e., morning and evening) at about the same time each day. Safety and efficacy of repeated treatment courses have not been studied.

Investigational: Prophylaxis of H1N1 influenza A (swine flu).

Adults and children 5 years and older: 10 mg (two 5-mg blisters) inhaled once a day for 10 days. Begin therapy within 7 days of exposure.

Investigational: Treatment of H1N1 influenza A (swine flu).

Adults and children 7 years and older: 10 mg (two 5-mg inhalations) twice a day for 5 days. Begin treatment within 2 days of onset of flu symptoms.

NURSING IMPLICATIONS

IMPLEMENTATION/ADMINISTRATION/STORAGE

1. The drug is given by oral inhalation only, using the Diskhaler provided.
2. Do not puncture the zanamivir blister until taking a dose using the Diskhaler.
3. For more information on use of zanamivir for prophylaxis and treatment of H1N1 influenza A, refer to the CDC guidelines at http://www.cdc.gov.
4. Store at from 15–30°C (59–86°F).

ASSESSMENT

1. Note reasons for therapy (prevention or treatment of influenza as dosing is different), onset, characteristics of S&S, contact with in-

fected individuals, any other medical conditions; note drug allergies.

2. Assess medical conditions, VS, clinical presentation, and history. Stop drug if bronchospasm or decline in peak flows evident. Not for use in those with asthma or COPD.
3. Assess carefully for neuropsychiatric events, especially in children.
4. Avoid live attenuated influenza vaccine administration within 2 weeks before or 48 hr after zanamivir dosing.
5. Monitor CBC, renal, LFTs, lung assessment findings. Note any renal dysfunction, as drug may be cumulative.

CLIENT/FAMILY TEACHING

1. Therapy is used to lessen the symptoms of influenza or to prevent the development of swine flu. To be given by oral inhalation only, using the Diskhaler provided. Review/demonstrate use of the delivery system.
2. Do not puncture any Relenza Rotadisk blister until taking a dose using the Diskhaler. Keep Diskhaler level and close lips around the mouth piece. Breathe in deep and steadily. Hold breath for a few seconds after inhaling to keep the drug in the lungs, then slowly release.
3. Continue treatment/therapy as prescribed despite feeling better. Take oral inhalations as directed at approximately the same time each day. Safety and efficacy of repeated treatment courses have not been evaluated.
4. If client is to use an inhaled bronchodilator at the same time as zanamivir, use the bronchodilator before taking zanamivir.
5. Does not reduce the risk of transmission of flu to others. Annual vaccination is still the primary means to prevent and control influenza and swine flu. Therapy may or may not improve symptoms and recovery time.
6. Clients with asthma or COPD may experience bronchospasm with zanamivir; weigh risk benefit ratio and have a fast-acting inhaled bronchodilator available. Stop zanamivir and contact provider immediately if worsening of respiratory symptoms or S&S of allergic reaction (i.e., hives, rash, swelling of throat).
7. An increased risk of confusion and unusual behavioral changes has been noted. The risk may be greater in children. Report symptoms of confusion or any other unusual behavioral changes.
8. Keep all F/U to assess response, labs, and for adverse SE.

OUTCOMES/EVALUATE

- ↓ Intensity/duration of S&S of influenza A and B or prophylaxis
- Prevention/treatment of confirmed, probable, or suspected H1N1 influenza A (swine flu) virus infection (unlabeled)

Ziconotide

(zye-**KOH**-noh-tide)

Classification(s): Analgesic

Pregnancy Category: C

RX: Prialt.

INDICATIONS/USES

Management of severe chronic pain in clients for whom intrathecal therapy is warranted and who are intolerant or refractory to other treatments (e.g., systemic analgesics, adjunctive therapies, or intrathecal morphine).

ACTION/KINETICS

Action

Ziconotide is a conopeptide that binds to N-type calcium channels located on the primary nociceptive (A-sigma and C) afferent nerves in the superficial layers of the dorsal horn of the spinal cord. The mechanism of action is not known, but it is believed the drug's binding blocks N-type calcium channels, which leads to a blockade of excitatory neurotransmitter release in the primary afferent nerve terminals resulting in analgesia. Ziconotide is not an opiate and will not prevent or relieve symptoms associated with opiate withdrawal.

Pharmacokinetics

The drug is administered intrathecally. Following passage from the CSF into the systemic circulation during continuous intrathecal administration, the drug is susceptible to proteolytic cleavage by various ubiquitous peptidases/proteases present in most organs (i.e., kidney, liver, lung, muscle). Thus, it is readily degraded to peptide fragments and free amino acids. **t½, terminal, from CSF:** 4.6 hr; **t½, plasma:** 1.3 hr.

CONTRAINDICATIONS

Hypersensitivity to ziconotide or any components of the product and in those with any other concomitant treatment or medical condition that would render intrathecal administration hazardous. Pre-existing history of psychosis with ziconotide. Presence of infection at the microinfusion injection site, uncontrolled bleeding diathesis, and spinal canal obstruction that impairs circulation of CSF. IV use of the product. Lactation.

SPECIAL CONCERNS

■ Severe psychiatric symptoms and neurological impairment may occur during treatment. Do not treat clients with a pre-existing history of psychosis with ziconotide. Monitor all clients frequently for evidence of cognitive impairment, hallucinations, or changes in mood or consciousness. In the event of serious neurological or psychiatric signs or symptoms, ziconotide therapy can be interrupted or discontinued abruptly without evidence of withdrawal effects. ■

Safety and efficacy not determined in children.

SIDE EFFECTS

Most Common

Dizziness, asthenia, somnolence, N&V, abnormal gait, ataxia, confusion, headache, hypertonia, impaired memory, diarrhea, anorexia, abnormal vision, pain.

CNS: Dizziness, somnolence, asthenia, confusion, ataxia, abnormal gait, headache, impaired memory, hyper-/hypotonia, anxiety, speech disorder, aphasia, dysesthesia, hallucinations, nervousness, paresthesia, vertigo, abnormal dreams, agitation, anxiety, aphasia, abnormal CSF, confusion, depression, difficulty concentrating, emotional lability, hostility, hyperesthesia, incoordination, insomnia, impaired memory, mental slowing, ***meningitis***, nervousness, neuralgia, paranoid reaction, decreased reflexes, speech disorder, stupor, abnormal thinking, tremor, twitching, vertigo, ***tonic-clonic seizures***, myoclonus, psychosis, ***suicidal ideations, suicide (rare)***. **GI:** N&V, diarrhea, anorexia, dry mouth, abdominal pain, constipation, dyspepsia, GI disorder. **CV:** Hyper-/hypotension, postural hypotension, syncope, tachycardia, vasodilation, atrial fibrillation, ***CVA***, abnormal ECG. **Respiratory:** Bronchitis, increased cough, dyspnea, lung disorder, pharyngitis, pneumonia, rhinitis, sinusitis, respiratory distress, ***fatal aspiration pneumonia (rare)***. **Dermatologic:** Cutaneous surgical complication, dry skin, pruritus, rash, skin disorder, sweating. **Musculoskeletal:** Arthralgia, arthritis, leg cramps, myalgia, myasthenia, myoclonus, rhabdomyolysis. **GU:** Urinary retention, dysuria, urinary incontinence, UTI, impaired urination, acute kidney failure. **Metabolic:** Dehydration, edema, peripheral edema, weight loss. **Ophthalmic:** Abnormal vision, nyastagmus, diplopia, photophobia. **Body as a whole**: Fever, pain, cellulitis, chills, fever, flu syndrome, infection, malaise, viral infection, ***sepsis***. **Miscellaneous:** Taste perversion, tinnitus, accidental injury, back pain, catheter complication, catheter-site pain, chest pain, neck pain/rigidity, pump-site complication, pump-site mass/pain.

LABORATORY TEST CONSIDERATIONS

↑ Creatinine phosphokinase.

OVERDOSE MANAGEMENT

Symptoms: Overdoses may occur because of pump programming errors or incorrect drug concentration preparations. Symptoms of overdose include ataxia, nystagmus, dizziness, stupor, unresponsiveness, spinal myoclonus, confusion, sedation, hypotension, word-finding difficulties, garbled speech, N&V. *Treatment:* There is no known antidote. Provide general medical supportive measures. Hospitalization may be necessary. The effects are not blocked by opioid antagonists. In the event of an inadvertent IV or epidural administration, hypotension could result; treat with a recumbent posture and BP support, as needed.

DRUG INTERACTIONS

CNS depressants / ↑ Incidence of CNS side effects, including confusion and dizziness

Opioids / Concomitant use with intrathecal opioids has not been studied; use together is not recommended

HOW SUPPLIED

Solution: 25 mcg/mL, 100 mcg/mL.

DOSAGE

INTRATHECAL

Management of severe chronic pain.

Initial: No more than 2.4 mcg/day (0.1 mcg/hr); titrate to client response. Adjust the dose of intrathecal administration according to the client's pain severity, their response to therapy, and the incidence of side effects. The effective dose is variable. The average dose level at the end of the 21-day titration used in clinical trials was 6.9 mcg/day (0.29 mcg/hr); maximum dose was 19.2 mcg/day (0.8 mcg/hr) on day 21.

Doses may be titrated upward by up to 2.4 mcg/day (0.1 mcg/hr) at intervals of no more than 2–3 times per week, up to a maximum of 19.2 mcg/day (0.8 mcg/hr) by day 21. Dose increases in increments of less than 2.4 mcg/day (0.1 mcg/hr) and increases in doses less frequently than 2–3 times per week may be used.

NURSING IMPLICATIONS

IMPLEMENTATION/ADMINISTRATION/STORAGE

1. The drug is used undiluted (20 mcg/mL in 20 mL vial) or diluted (100 mcg/mL in 1, 2, or 5 mL vials). Diluted drug is prepared with 0.9% NaCl injection using aseptic procedures to the desired concentration prior to placement in the microinfusion pump. The 100 mcg/mL formulation may be given undiluted once an appropriate dose has been established.
2. Saline solutions containing preservatives are not appropriate for intrathecal drug administration and are not to be used.
3. Refrigerate, but do not freeze, all ziconotide solutions after preparation and begin infusion within 24 hr.
4. Because of the lower incidence of serious side effects and discontinuation for side effects associated with a slower titration, use a faster titration schedule only if there is an urgent need for analgesic that outweighs the risk to the client's safety.
5. Ziconotide is intended for intrathecal delivery using a programmable implanted variable-rate microinfusion device or an external microinfusion device and catheter. Specific instructions and precautions for programming the microinfusion device and/or refilling the reservoir are available from the manufacturer's manual.
6. There is a higher incidence of confusion in elderly clients; dose selection for an elderly person should be cautious, starting at the low end of the dose range.
7. Refrigerate ziconotide during transit. Store from 2–8°C (36–46°F). Once diluted aseptically with saline, the drug may be stored from 2–8°C (36–46°F) for 24 hr. Protect from light. Discard any ziconotide solution if particulate matter or discoloration is observed; discard any unused portion remaining in the vial.

ASSESSMENT

1. Note reasons for therapy, onset, duration, characteristics and location of pain. Rate pain level; note other agents trialed/failed.
2. Review medical history to ensure no conditions that would preclude drug therapy (e.g., psychosis, severe depression, suicide attempts) and assess behavioral and clinical presentation.
3. This medication will not prevent withdrawal reactions from narcotics.
4. Medication should not be given into a vein (IV) or under the skin. It can cause fainting R/T severe hypotension if accidentally given into a vein. It is for intrathecal use only in those who have not responded to IV or intrathecal morphine, or other opioids for pain control.
5. Any fever, neck stiffness, N&V, altered mental status, assess for meningitis.
6. Assess client ability to perform steps to ensure safe administration. Set up a schedule for refilling pump. Check product visually for particles or discoloration.
7. Determine if using a narcotic (e.g., codeine, hydrocodone, morphine) regularly for more than a few weeks, or if it has been used in high doses; may be dependent on it. Suddenly stopping the narcotic will cause withdrawal reactions. When stopping extended, regular treatment with narcotics, gradually reducing the dosage will help prevent withdrawal reactions.
8. Monitor VS, renal and LFTs. May cause elevated CK levels, monitor for associated side effects.

CLIENT/FAMILY TEACHING

1. This is a pain reliever that works by blocking the nerves in the spinal cord that send pain signals. It decreases ongoing pain caused by cancer, AIDS, failed back surgery, multiple

sclerosis, neuropathy, and other causes that have not responded to other therapies.

2. This medication is injected into the spinal fluid (intrathecal) using a small pump. Treatment is usually started slowly and gradually increased to the dose that works best for you. To prevent infection, you will be taught how to handle the infusion pump, and learn proper care of the injection site. Call your provider/infusion nurse immediately if there is any sign of infection around the injection site (e.g., swelling, redness, tenderness). Must set up a schedule for refilling your pump. Before using, check this product visually for particles or discoloration. If either is present, do not use the liquid. Report any unusual soreness, worsening muscle pain, weakness and darkened urine, or if pain persists or worsens.
3. Do not engage in activities that require mental alertness or coordination while being treated with ziconotide.
4. Avoid alcohol and any other CNS depressant type drugs without provider approval.
5. Report any change in mental status (e.g., lethargy, confusion, disorientation, decreased alertness) or a change in mood, or perception (hallucinations, including unusual tactile sensations in the mouth) or symptoms of depression or suicidal thoughts. Also any nausea, vomiting, seizures, fever, headache, and/or stiff neck, which may be symptoms of developing meningitis require reporting.
6. Keep all F/U to assess response, labs, and for adverse SE.

OUTCOMES/EVALUATE

Relief of intractable pain

IV

Zidovudine (Azidothymidine, AZT)

(zye-**DOH**-vyou-deen, ah-**zee**-doh-**THIGH**-mih-deen)

Classification(s): Antiviral, nucleoside reverse transcriptase inhibitor

Pregnancy Category: C

RX: Retrovir.

✦ **Rx:** Apo-Zidovudine.

SEE ALSO ***ANTIVIRAL DRUGS*** AND ***ANTI-INFECTIVE DRUGS***.

INDICATIONS/USES

PO or IV: (1) Treatment of HIV-1 infection in combination with other antiretroviral drugs. (2) Prevention of maternal-fetal HIV-1 transmission. Indication is based on a dosing regimen that included three components: antepartum therapy of HIV-1 infected mothers, intrapartum therapy of HIV-1 infected mothers, and postpartum therapy of HIV-1 exposed infant. Used in combination with other antiretroviral drugs. Usually begin therapy between 14 and 34 weeks of gestation.

ACTION/KINETICS

Action

Zidovudine is phosphorylated intracellularly to the active 5'-triphosphate metabolite (zidovudine triphosphate). This metabolite inhibits reverse transcriptase via DNA chain termination after incorporation of the nucleotide analogue. Once incorporated, zidovudine triphosphate causes premature termination of the growth of the DNA chain. Zidovudine triphosphate is a weak inhibitor of the cellular DNA polymerases alpha and gamma and has been reported to be incorporated into the DNA of cells in culture.

Pharmacokinetics

Rapidly absorbed from the GI tract and is distributed to both plasma and CSF. Oral bioavailability is 64%. **Peak serum levels:** 0.5–1.5 hr. **t½:** Approximately 1 hr. **t½, elimination, fasting adults:** 0.5–3 hr. **t½, clients younger than 3 months of age:** 13 hr. In neonates 14 days of age or less, bioavailability is greater, total body clearance is slower, and half-life was longer than in pediatric clients over 14 days of age. Metabolized rapidly by the liver and excreted through the urine. **Plasma protein binding:** <38%.

CONTRAINDICATIONS

Allergy to zidovudine or components of the product. Lactation.

SPECIAL CONCERNS

(1) **Hematologic toxicity.** Zidovudine has been associated with hematologic toxicity, including neutropenia and severe anemia, particularly in clients with advanced HIV disease. (2) **Myopathy.** Prolonged zidovudine use has been associated with symptomatic myopathy. (3) **Lactic acidosis/severe hepatomegaly.** Lactic acidosis and severe hepatomegaly with

steatosis, including fatal cases, have been reported with the use of nucleoside analogs alone or in combination, including zidovudine and other antiretrovirals. Suspend treatment if clinical or laboratory findings suggestive of lactic acidosis or pronounced heptotoxicity occur. ■

- **Use with caution with bone marrow compromise evidenced by granulocyte count <1,000 cells/mm^3 or hemoglobin less than 9.5 grams/dL.**
- **Use caution with dose selection in the elderly.**
- **Not a cure for HIV; thus, clients may continue to acquire opportunistic infections and other illnesses associated with ARC or HIV.**
- **Not been shown to reduce the risk of HIV transmission to others through sexual contact or blood contamination.**

SIDE EFFECTS

Most Common

Headache, malaise, N&V, anorexia, constipation, asthenia, abdominal cramps/pain, arthralgia, chills, dyspepsia, fatigue, insomnia, musculoskeletal pain, myalgia, neuropathy.

Adults. Hematologic: Anemia (severe), neutropenia, granulocytopenia, thrombocytopenia, pure red cell aplasia, ***aplastic anemia***, hemolytic anemia, leukopenia, lymphadenopathy, pancytopenia with marrow hypoplasia. **Body as a whole:** Headache, asthenia, fever, fatigue, neuropathy, diaphoresis, malaise, body odor, chills, edema of the lip, flu-like syndrome, hyperalgesia, abdominal/chest/back pain. **GI:** N&V, GI pain, diarrhea, anorexia, dyspepsia, constipation, dysphagia, edema of the tongue, eructation, flatulence, bleeding gums, mouth ulcers, oral mucosa pigmentation, abdominal cramps/pain, ***rectal hemorrhage***. **Hepatic:** Hepatitis, ***hepatomegaly with steatosis***, jaundice, lactic acidosis, ***pancreatitis***. **CNS:** Somnolence, dizziness, paresthesia, insomnia, anxiety, confusion, emotional lability, depression, nervousness, vertigo, paresthesia, loss of mental acuity, mania, ***seizures***. **CV:** Vasodilation, syncope, vasculitis (rare), ***cardiomyopathy***. **Musculoskeletal:** Myalgia, myositis, arthralgia, tremor, twitch, muscle spasm, musculoskeletal pain, myopathy (with chronic use), myositis with pathological changes (similar to that produced by HIV disease), ***rhabdomyolysis***. **Respiratory:** Dyspnea, cough, epistaxis, rhinitis, pharyngitis, sinusitis, hoarseness. **Dermatologic:** Rash, pruritus, urticaria, acne, pigmentation changes of the skin and nails, sweating, ***Stevens-Johnson syndrome, toxic epidermal necrolysis***. **GU:** Dysuria, polyuria, urinary hesitancy/frequency, gynecomastia. **Ophthalmic:** Amblyopia, photophobia, macular edema. **Body as a whole:** Redistribution/accumulation of body fat including central obesity, dorsocervical fat enlargement, peripheral wasting, facial wasting, breast enlargement, and "cushingoid" appearance. **Miscellaneous:** Hearing loss, taste perversion, hypersensitivity reactions (including ***anaphylaxis***, angioedema, vasculitis), hyperbilirubinemia (rare), ***seizures***. Immune reconstitution syndrome, including an inflammatory response to indolent or residual opportunistic infections (such as *Mycobacterium avium*, cytomegalovirus, *Pneumocystis jirovecii* pneumonia, or tuberculosis).

Children. The following side effects have been observed in children, although any of the side effects reported for adults can also occur in children. **Body as a whole:** Granulocytopenia, anemia, fever, headache, phlebitis, bacteremia. **GI:** N&V, abdominal pain, diarrhea, weight loss, stomatitis, splenomegaly. **CNS:** Decreased reflexes, nervousness, irritability, insomnia, ***seizures***. **CV:** Abnormalities in ECG, left ventricular dilation, CHF, generalized edema, ***cardiomyopathy***, S_3 gallop. **GU:** Hematuria, viral cystitis

LABORATORY TEST CONSIDERATIONS

↑ ALT, AST, alkaline phosphatase, CPK, LDH, lipase, total amylase. Anemia, granulocytopenia, neutropenia, thrombocytopenia.

OVERDOSE MANAGEMENT

Symptoms: N&V. Transient hematologic changes. Headache, dizziness, drowsiness, confusion, lethargy. *Treatment:* Treat symptoms. Hemodialysis will enhance the excretion of the primary metabolite of zidovudine.

DRUG INTERACTIONS

Acyclovir / ↑ Risk of profound drowsiness and lethargy

Atovaquone / ↑ Zidovudine levels R/T inhibition of zidovudine glucuronidation

Bone marrow depressants / ↑ Zidovudine's hematologic toxicity

Cidofovir/Probenecid / Due to concomitant probenecid use to prevent cidofovir-induced nephrotoxicity, temporarily discontinue or decrease zidovudine dose by 50% on the day of cidofovir administration only
Cytotoxic drugs / ↑ Zidovudine's hematologic toxicity
Doxorubicin / Drugs antagonize each other; do not give together
Fluconazole / ↑ Zidovudine AUC; consider dose reduction in those with pronounced anemia or other severe side effects
Foscarnet / ↑ Risk of anemia
Ganciclovir / ↑ Plasma zidovudine levels → ↑ risk of hematologic toxicity; do not use together
Interferon alfa / ↑ Risk of hematologic toxicity
Interferon beta-1b / ↑ Risk of hematologic toxicity
Methadone / ↑ Zidovudine serum levels and AUC → ↑ risk of side effects
Nelfinavir/Ritonavir / ↓ Zidovudine AUC
Phenytoin / Levels of phenytoin may ↑, ↓, or remain unchanged; also, ↓ zidovudine excretion
Probenecid / ↓ Biotransformation or renal excretion of zidovudine → flu-like symptoms, including myalgia, malaise or fever, and maculopapular rash
Ribavirin / Possible antagonism of zidovudine against HIV; do not use together
Rifamycins / ↓ Zidovudine levels
Ritonavir / ↓ Zidovudine AUC
Stavudine/Ribavirin / Possible antagonism of zidovudine against HIV; do not use together
Valacyclovir / ↑ Risk of profound drowsiness and lethargy
Valganciclovir / ↑ Plasma zidovudine levels → ↑ risk of hematologic toxicity; do not use together
Valproic acid / ↑ Zidovudine AUC R/T ↓ glucuronidation
Vinblastine / ↑ Risk of cytotoxicity, nephrotoxicity, or hematologic toxicity
Vincristine / ↑ Risk of cytotoxicity, nephrotoxicity, or hematologic toxicity

HOW SUPPLIED

Capsules: 100 mg; ***Injection:*** 10 mg/mL; ***Syrup:*** 50 mg/5 mL; ***Tablets:*** 100 mg (water dispersible), 300 mg.

DOSAGE

CAPSULES; IV; SYRUP; TABLETS

Treatment of HIV infections.

Adults: 600 mg/day in divided doses in combination with other antiretroviral drugs. **Children, 4 weeks to younger than 18 years, 4 to <9 kg:** 24 mg/kg/day given as either 12 mg/kg twice a day or 8 mg/kg 3 times a day; **9 kg or greater to <30 kg:** 18 mg/kg/day given as 9 mg/kg twice a day or 6 mg/kg three times a day; **30 kg or greater:** 600 mg/day given as 300 mg twice a day or 200 mg 3 times a day. **Alternative dosing for children:** 480 mg/m^2/day in divided doses (either 240 mg/m^2 twice a day or 160 mg/m^2 3 times a day). *NOTE:* In some cases, the dose calculated by mg/kg will not be the same as that calculated by body surface area.

Prevent maternal-fetal HIV transmission (after week 14 of pregnancy).

Maternal dosing: 100 mg 5 times/day until the start of labor. During labor and delivery, zidovudine IV at 2 mg/kg over 1 hr followed by continuous IV infusion of 1 mg/kg/hr until clamping of the umbilical cord. **Infant dosing:** 2 mg/kg PO q 6 hr beginning within 12 hr after birth and continuing through 6 weeks of age. Infants unable to take the drug PO may be given zidovudine IV at 1.5 mg/kg, infused over 30 min q 6 hr.

NURSING IMPLICATIONS

Do not confuse Retrovir with ritonavir (also an antiviral drug) or Norvir (also an antiviral drug).

IMPLEMENTATION/ADMINISTRATION/STORAGE

1. The extent of absorption is equivalent for capsules, syrup, and tablets.
2. A 100-mg water dispersible tablet is available for individuals who can not swallow.
3. Dosage adjustment is recommended for clients with a C_{CR} <15 mL/min.
4. The recommended dose for those maintained on hemodialysis or peritoneal dialysis is 100 mg q 6–8 hr.
5. There are insufficient data to recommend dose adjustment in those with mild to moderate impaired hepatic function or liver cirrhosis.
6. Dose interruption until recovery may be required due to significant anemia (hemoglobin

less than 7.5 grams/dL or reduction of greater than 25% of baseline) and/or significant neutropenia (granulocyte count less than 750 cells/mm^3 or reduction of greater than 50% from baseline).

7. Lamivudine/zidovudine (Combivir) and abacavir/lamivudine/zidovudine (Trizivir) are combination products that contain zidovudine. Do not administer zidovudine concomitantly with either of these products.
8. Do not mix with blood products or protein solutions.
9. Zidovudine is considered a potential teratogen; thus, follow safe handling procedures when preparing, administering, or dispensing the drug.
10. Store from 15–30°C (59–77°F). Protect capsules from moisture.
11. IV Remove dose from 20-mL vial and dilute in D5W injection to a concentration not to exceed 4 mg/mL. Administer calculated dose IV at a constant rate over 1 hr.
12. After dilution, the solution is stable at room temperature for 24 hr and if refrigerated (2–8°C, 36–46°F) for 48 hr. To ensure safety from microbial contamination, give within 8 hr if stored at room temperature and 24 hr if refrigerated.
13. To monitor maternal-fetal outcomes of pregnant women exposed to zidovudine, register clients on the antiretroviral pregnancy registry by calling 1-800-258-4263.
14. COMPATIBILITY D5W or 0.9% NaCl.
15. INCOMPATIBILITY Administer separately.

ASSESSMENT

1. Note reasons for therapy, onset, other therapies trialed, baseline CD_4 counts, viral load.
2. Epoetin alfa recombinant may be administered with iron to stimulate RBC production. A blood transfusion may also be required.
3. Safety and effectiveness of chronic zidovudine therapy are not known, especially in those with a less advanced form of disease.
4. When used to prevent maternal-fetal transmission of HIV, zidovudine should be initiated in pregnant women between 14 and 24 weeks of gestation; also, IV zidovudine should be given during labor up until the cord is clamped, and newborn infants should receive zidovudine syrup. Infected mothers may not breast feed.
5. Monitor renal and LFTs. Initially monitor metabolic panel and CBC at least q 2 weeks. If lactic acidosis, anemia, or granulocytopenia severe, the dose must be adjusted or discontinued.

CLIENT/FAMILY TEACHING

1. Take with or without food q 4 hr ATC as ordered; sleep must be interrupted to take medication. Do not share and do not exceed the prescribed dose of zidovudine.
2. May cause drowsiness; use caution while driving or performing other tasks requiring mental alertness.
3. Report early S&S of anemia, e.g., SOB, weakness, lightheadedness, palpitations, and increased fatigue as well as muscle aches/pain (myopathy and myositis with pathological changes have been associated with prolonged use). Also report S&S of superinfections (e.g., furry tongue, mouth lesions, vaginal/rectal itching, rash).
4. Consume 2–3 L/day fluids to ensure adequate hydration. Maintain a record of weights and I&O.
5. Avoid acetaminophen and any other unprescribed drugs that may exacerbate the toxicity of zidovudine.
6. Drug is not a cure but helps to alleviate and manage symptoms of HIV infections and prolong life with continuous therapy. May continue to develop opportunistic infections and other complications due to AIDS or ARC.
7. The risk of transmission of HIV to others through blood or sexual contact is not reduced in individuals on zidovudine therapy. Practice safe sex and do not share needles.
8. With pregnancy, zidovudine therapy should start after the 14-week gestation period to help prevent the transmission from mother to infant. Once delivered, do not nurse infant.
9. Redistribution or accumulation of body fat may occur.
10. With HIV/hepatitis C virus confection, hepatic decomposition (some fatal) has occurred in those receiving combination antiretroviral therapy for HIV and interferon alfa with or without ribavirin.
11. Be aware, a rare but serious condition called lactic acidosis with liver enlargement can occur.

12. With accidental needlestick/occupational exposure, initiate therapy after incident for best outcome.
13. Identify local support groups that may assist one to understand/cope with this disease.
14. Keep all F/U to assess response, labs, and adverse SE.

OUTCOMES/EVALUATE

- Control of symptoms of HIV, AIDS, or ARC
- ↑ CD_4 counts; ↓ viral load; enhanced longevity
- ↓ Maternal fetal HIV transmission

Zileuton

(zye-**LOO**-ton)

Classification(s): Antiasthmatic, leukotriene receptor antagonist

Pregnancy Category: C

RX: Zyflo, Zyflo CR.

INDICATIONS/USES

Prophylaxis and chronic treatment of asthma in adults and children over 12 years of age.

ACTION/KINETICS

Action

Specific inhibitor of 5-lipoxygenase; thus, inhibits the formation of leukotrienes. Leukotrienes are substances that induce various biological effects including aggregation of neutrophils and monocytes, leukocyte adhesion, increase of neutrophil and eosinophil migration, increased capillary permeability, and contraction of smooth muscle. These effects of leukotrienes contribute to edema, secretion of mucus, inflammation, and bronchoconstriction in asthmatic clients. By inhibiting leukotriene formation, zileuton reduces bronchoconstriction due to cold air challenge in asthmatics.

Pharmacokinetics

Rapidly absorbed from the GI tract; **peak plasma levels:** 1.7 hr. Food affects the C_{max} of extended-release tablets but not immediate-release tablets. Metabolized in liver by CYP1A2, CYP2C9, and CYP3A4. Mainly excreted through the urine. **t½:** 2.5 hr (immediate-release) and 3.2 hr (extended-release). **Plasma protein binding:** 93%, primarily to albumin.

CONTRAINDICATIONS

Active liver disease or transaminase elevations greater than or equal to 3 times the ULN. Hypersensitivity (rash, eosinophilia) to any component of the product. Treatment of bronchoconstriction in acute asthma attacks, including status asthmaticus. Lactation.

SPECIAL CONCERNS

- Use with caution in clients who ingest large quantities of alcohol or who have a past history of liver disease.
- Women 65 years of age or older appear to have an increased risk of ALT elevations.
- Safety and efficacy not determined in children less than 12 years of age.

SIDE EFFECTS

Most Common

Extended-Release: Sinusitis, pharyngolaryngeal pain, nausea.

Extended-Release: GI: N&V, diarrhea, constipation, dyspepsia, flatulence, upper abdominal pain. **Hepatic:** Jaundice, hepatotoxicity, liver dysfunction, ***severe hepatic injury***. **CNS:** Headache, dizziness, sleep disorders, behavioral changes, insomnia, nervousness, somnolence. **Respiratory:** Sinusitis, pharyngolaryngeal pain, URTI. **Dermatologic:** Rash, pruritus. **Musculoskeletal:** Myalgia, arthralgia, chest pain, hypertonia, neck pain/rigidity. **GU:** UTI, vaginitis. **Ophthalmic:** Conjunctivitis. **Body as a whole:** Hypersensitivity, asthenia, fever, malaise, pain. **Miscellaneous:** Accidental injury, lymphadenopathy.

LABORATORY TEST CONSIDERATIONS

↑ LFTs, ALT. Low WBC count. Hyperbilirubinemia.

DRUG INTERACTIONS

CYP3A4 agents (calcium channel blockers, cyclosporine, ketoconazole) / Possible interaction; use caution and monitoring if coadministered with zileuton

Pimozide / ↑ Risk of life–threatening cardiac arrhythmias; coadministration contraindicated

Propranolol / ↑ Propranolol levels → ↑ effect; adjust propranolol dose as needed and monitor

Theophylline / ↑ Theophylline levels; ↓ theophylline dose by 50% and monitor theophylline levels

Warfarin / ↑ PT; adjust warfarin dose and monitor

HOW SUPPLIED

Tablets, Extended-Release: 600 mg; *Tablets, Immediate-Release:* 600 mg.

DOSAGE

TABLETS, EXTENDED-RELEASE

Symptomatic relief of asthma.

Adults and children, 12 years and older: 1,200 mg (two 600 mg tablets) twice daily, within 1 hr of morning and evening meals; **total daily dose:** 2,400 mg

TABLETS, IMMEDIATE-RELEASE

Symptomatic relief of asthma.

Adults and children, 12 years and older: One 600 mg tablet 4 times a day; total daily dose: 2,400 mg.

NURSING IMPLICATIONS

IMPLEMENTATION/ADMINISTRATION/STORAGE

1. Do not decrease dose or stop taking any other antiasthmatics when taking zileuton.
2. Dosage adjustment not necessary in those with renal dysfunction or those undergoing hemodialysis.
3. If a dose of the extended-release tablet is missed, take the next dose at the scheduled time; do not double the dose.
4. Store immediate-release and extended-release tablets from 20–25°C (68–77°F). Protect from light.

ASSESSMENT

1. Note onset, characteristics of S&S, and severity of disease. List triggers and currently prescribed therapy.
2. Screen for excessive alcohol use and any evidence of liver disease.
3. Document lung assessments, PFTs, peak flow readings, and CXR findings.
4. Monitor CBC, PFTs, and LFTs monthly × 3 months, then every 3 months during the first year of therapy.

CLIENT/FAMILY TEACHING

1. Take extended-release tablets within 1 hr of morning and evening meals; do not chew, cut, or crush tablets. Immediate-release tablets may be taken with meals and at bedtime.
2. Use caution, may cause dizziness; avoid hazardous activities until drug effects realized.
3. Continue to take other asthma medications as prescribed.
4. Drug will not reverse bronchospasm during acute asthma attack; use bronchodilators and other prescribed therapy. Seek care if symptoms are severe or peak flow readings indicate need. Use peak flow meter readings to monitor airway effectiveness and for medication increases.
5. Report immediately if experiencing RUQ pain, lethargy, itching, jaundice, fatigue, or flu-like symptoms (S&S of liver toxicity).
6. Review triggers (i.e., smoke, cold air, and exercise) that may cause increased hyperresponsiveness that can last up to a week. If more than the usual or maximum number of inhalations of short-acting bronchodilator treatment in a 24-hr period are required, notify provider.
7. Avoid alcohol and OTC agents without approval.
8. Report any overt behavioral changes or sleep disorders should they occur.
9. Keep all F/U to assess response, labs, adverse SE. Bring record of peak flow readings.

OUTCOMES/EVALUATE

Asthma prophylaxis; ↑ airway exchange.

Ziprasidone hydrochloride

(zigh-**PRAYZ**-oh-dohn)

Classification(s): Antipsychotic

Pregnancy Category: C

RX: Geodon.

INDICATIONS/USES

PO. (1) Treatment of schizophrenia. Due to the possibility of causing prolongation of the QT/QTc interval, other drugs should be considered first. (2) Acute manic or mixed episodes associated with bipolar disorder, with or without psychotic features. (3) As an adjunct to lithium or valproate for maintenance treatment of bipolar I disorder. *Investigational:* Autism, Tourette syndrome.

IM. Acute agitation in clients with schizophrenia for whom treatment with ziprasidone is appropriate and who need IM antipsychotic medication for rapid control of agitation.

ACTION/KINETICS

Action

Mechanism unknown. High affinity for dopamine D_2, D_3; serotonin 5–HT_{2A}, 5–HT_{2C}, 5–HT_{1A}, and 5–HT_{1D}; and alpha–1–adrenergic and moderate affinity for histamine H_1 receptors. Effect thought to be due to a combination of dopamine (D_2) and serotonin (5-HT_2) receptor antagonism. Causes moderate sedation, extrapyramidal symptoms, and orthostatic hypotension; low incidence of anticholinergic effects and weight gain.

Pharmacokinetics

Well absorbed; bioavailability is about 60% for PO product and 100% after IM administration. **Peak plasma levels:** 6–8 hr after PO and 1 hr after IM. Absorption increased up to 2-fold in the presence of food. Extensively metabolized in the liver by aldehyde oxidase, methylation, and oxidation by CYP3A4 and CYP1A2. About 20% excreted in the urine and 66% eliminated in the feces. **t½, terminal:** 7 hr after PO and 2–5 hr after IM administration. **Plasma protein binding:** More than 99%.

CONTRAINDICATIONS

Use with other drugs that prolong the QT interval, including class Ia and III antiarrhythmic drugs, chlorpromazine, dofetilide, dolasetron, droperidol, gatifloxacin, halofantrine, mefloquine, mesoridazine, moxifloxacin, pentamidine, pimozide, probucol, quinidine, sotalol, sparfloxacin, tacrolimus, or thioridazine. Do not use in clients with a known history of QT prolongation, with recent acute MI, with uncompensated heart failure, or cardiac arrhythmias. Lactation.

SPECIAL CONCERNS

Increased mortality in elderly clients with dementia-related psychosis. Elderly clients with dementia-related psychosis treated with atypical antipsychotic drugs are at an increased risk of death. Analysis of 17 placebo-treated trials (modal duration of 10 weeks), largely in clients taking atypical antipsychotic drugs revealed a risk of death in the drug-treated clients between 1.6 and 1.7 times that seen in placebo-treated clients. Over the course of a typical 10-week controlled trial, the rate of death in drug-treated clients was about 4.5%, compared with a rate of about 2.6% in the placebo group. Although causes of death were varied, most of the deaths appeared to be either cardiovascular (e.g., heart failure, sudden death) or infectious (e.g., pneumonia) in nature. Observational studies suggest that, similar to atypical antipsychotic drugs, treatment with conventional antipsychotic drugs may increase mortality. The extent to which the findings of increased mortality in observational studies may be attributed to the antipsychotic drug as opposed to some characteristic(s) of the clients is not clear. Ziprasidone is not approved for the treatment of clients with dementia-related psychosis.

- **Ziprasidone has a greater capacity to prolong the QT/QTc interval compared with other antipsychotic drugs. Prolongation of the QTc interval is associated with a torsades-de-pointes-type arrhythmia, which is a potentially fatal ventricular tachycardia. It is not known whether ziprasidone will cause torsades de pointes or increase the rate of sudden death.**
- **Use of antipsychotic drugs may cause tardive dyskinesia and/or neuroleptic malignant syndrome.**
- **Use with caution in those with a history of MI, ischemic heart disease, heart failure, or conduction abnormalities; in cerebrovascular disease; in conditions that predispose to hypotension; in those with a history of seizures or conditions that potentially lower the seizure threshold (e.g., Alzheimer's); in those with a history of glaucoma; in those at risk of aspiration pneumonia; or, in those with clinically significant prostatic hypertrophy, narrow-angle glaucoma, or a history of paralytic ileus.**
- **Use with caution in geriatric clients, as the drug may be excreted more slowly in this population (rate of death due to CV events or infections is higher in clients with dementia).**
- **Use IM ziprasidone with caution in those with renal impairment as the cyclodextrin excipient is excreted renally.**
- **Safety and efficacy not established in children.**

SIDE EFFECTS

Most Common

Akathisia, asthenia, drowsiness/sedation, extrapyramidal symptoms, headache, insomnia, rash, diarrhea, diverticulitis, dry mouth, dyspepsia, nausea, weight gain, increased cough, rhinitis, abnormal vision, accidental injury.

Mainly listed are side effects with an incidence of 1% or more or those that are life–threatening. **GI:** N&V, abdominal discomfort, constipation, dyspepsia, diarrhea, dry mouth, anorexia, diverticulitis, polydipsia, rectal hemorrhage, buccoglossal syndrome, ***pancreatitis***. **CNS:** Headache, agitation, drowsiness/sedation, insomnia, somnolence, ***suicide attempts***, akathisia, akinesia, amnesia, anxiety, ataxia, confusion, delirium, dizziness, dysarthria, dyskinesia, dystonia, extrapyramidal syndrome, hostility, hyperkinesia, hypertonia, hypotonia, hypesthesia, hypokinesia, incoordination, abnormal gait, neuropathy, tardive dyskinesia, migraine, neuropathy, paresthesia, personality disorder, speech disorder, tremor, vertigo, ***seizures***. **CV:** Orthostatic hypotension, hypertension, angina pectoris, premature atrial contractions, atrial fibrillation/flutter, bradycardia, tachycardia, QTc interval prolongation, ***sudden cardiac death, torsades de pointes***. **Respiratory:** Cold symptoms, URTI, rhinitis, increased cough, dyspnea, respiratory disorder. **Dermatologic:** Rash, urticaria, dermatitis, diaphoresis, fungal dermatitis, photosensitivity, rash. **Musculoskeletal:** Myalgia, rhabdomyolysis, choreoathetosis, cogwheel rigidity, flank pain. **GU:** Dysmenorrhea. **Metabolic:** Hyperglycemia, diabetes mellitus. **Ophthalmic:** Abnormal vision, diplopia, oculogyric crisis. **Body as a whole:** Asthenia, accidental injury/fall, chills, fever, hyperpyrexia, hypothermia, weight gain. **Miscellaneous:** Diabetes, facial edema, furunculosis, withdrawal syndrome, injection site pain.

LABORATORY TEST CONSIDERATIONS

↑ Prolactin.

OVERDOSE MANAGEMENT

Symptoms: Hypotension, ***circulatory collapse***, severe extrapyramidal symptoms. *Treatment:* Establish and maintain an airway and ensure adequate oxygenation and ventilation. Establish IV access. Undertake gastric lavage if necessary and consider activated charcoal with a laxative. Monitor CV status, including continuous ECG monitoring to detect possible arrhythmias. Treat hypotension and circulatory collapse with IV fluids (do not use epinephrine or dopamine). Give anticholinergic drugs to treat severe extrapyramidal symptoms.

DRUG INTERACTIONS

Antihypertensive drugs / Additive hypotension with certain antihypertensive drugs

Carbamazepine / ↓ Ziprasidone levels R/T ↑ liver metabolism

Centrally-acting drugs / Use caution due to CNS effects of ziprasidone

Dopamine agonists / Antagonism of agonist effect

Ketoconazole / ↑ Ziprasidone levels R/T inhibition of metabolism

Levodopa / Antagonism of levodopa effects

HOW SUPPLIED

Capsules: 20 mg, 40 mg, 60 mg, 80 mg; ***Injection, Lyophilized Powder for Solution:*** 20 mg/mL (as mesylate).

DOSAGE

CAPSULES

Schizophrenia.

Adults, initial: 20 mg twice a day with food. Adjust dose based on individual clinical status, up to 80 mg twice a day. If needed, adjust dose at intervals of 2 or more days, as steady state is reached in 1–3 days. To ensure use of the lowest effective dose, observe for several weeks for improvement before making upward dosage changes. **Maintenance:** Efficacy is maintained for 52 weeks or less at a dose of 20–80 mg (maximum) twice a day. The safety of doses above 100 mg twice a day has not been evaluated. Periodically assess to determine need for continued treatment.

Manic or mixed episodes associated with bipolar disorder (bipolar mania).

Adults: Day 1: 40 mg twice daily with food; **Day 2:** 60 or 80 mg twice daily; **then,** 40–80 mg twice daily, depending on client progress and tolerance. Continue the same dose on which the client was initially stabilized, within the range of 40–80 mg twice a day with food. Periodically assess to determine the need for maintenance treatment.

Autism (investigational).

Initial: 20 mg nightly, increased by 10–20 mg weekly in a twice-daily regimen. **Range:** 20–120 mg/day.

Tourette syndrome (investigational).

Initial: 10 mg twice a day, titrated to 30 mg 3 times a day over an 8-week period.

IM ONLY

Acute agitation in schizophrenia.

Adults: 10–20 mg IM, up to a maximum of 40 mg/day. Doses of 10 mg may be given q 2 hr and doses of 20 mg may be given q 4 hr, up to 40 mg/day. IM use for more than 3 consecutive days has not been evaluated. *NOTE:* If long-term therapy is needed, PO ziprasidone should replace IM administration as soon as possible.

NURSING IMPLICATIONS

IMPLEMENTATION/ADMINISTRATION/STORAGE

1. Do not coadminister both PO and IM forms.
2. Dosage changes are generally not required on the basis of age, gender, race, or renal or hepatic impairment.
3. If long-term ziprasidone therapy is indicated, the PO product should replace IM administration as soon as possible.
4. To reconstitute the injection for IM use, add 1.2 mL sterile water for injection and shake vigorously until the drug is dissolved. Each mL of reconstituted solution contains 20 mg ziprasidone. To administer a 10 mg dose, draw up 0.5 mL of the reconstituted solution and to give a 20 mg dose, draw up 1 mL of the reconstituted solution.
5. The product contains no preservative or bacteriostatic agent; thus, use aseptic technique in preparing final solution. Discard any unused portion.
6. Do not mix the reconstituted drug with any other drugs or solvents other than sterile water for injection.
7. Store capsules and the dry form of the injection at 15–30°C (59–86°F). Following reconstitution, injection can be stored, protected from light, for up to 24 hr from 15–30°C (59–86°F) or up to 7 days refrigerated at 2–8°C (36–46°F).

ASSESSMENT

1. Note disease onset, symptom characteristics, presenting behaviors, other agents trialed.
2. List drugs currently prescribed to ensure none interact unfavorably.
3. Note any history of CAD, abnormal QT interval, arrhythmias, CVA, Alzheimer's disease or seizures. If QTc interval >500 msec, do not give drug.
4. Hypokalemia and/or hypomagnesemia may increase the risk of QT prolongation and arrhythmias. Also monitor for S&S of diabetes mellitus.
5. Assess for tardive dyskinesia: involuntary body and facial movements and report as may be irreversible.
6. Not for use with the elderly with dementia-related psychosis due to increased risk of death.
7. Monitor VS, ECG, weight, BS, CBC, U/A, LFTs, electrolytes, and Mg^{++} levels. Those being considered for ziprasidone therapy who are at risk for significant electrolyte disturbances, especially hypokalemia, should have baseline serum K^{+} and Mg^{++} levels.

CLIENT/FAMILY TEACHING

1. Take as directed, twice a day with food. Do not stop suddenly; drug should be withdrawn slowly to prevent adverse side effects.
2. Continue regular psychotherapy sessions. Report any changes in behavior, loss of control, increased tremor, or evidence of seizures.
3. Avoid activities that require mental alertness until drug effects realized; dizziness and drowsiness may occur.
4. Change positions slowly to prevent drop in BP. Avoid hot baths/showers, hot tubs, as low BP may occur.
5. Do not perform strenuous activities in warm weather or high humidity; may suffer heat stroke.
6. Report any changes in mental status/personality or mood, dizziness, excessive drowsiness, fainting, high fever, weight gain, irregular/rapid pulse, muscle rigidity, involuntary body movements, palpitations, rash, seizures, or sweating.
7. Avoid OTC drugs and alcohol. Record BP regularly if on therapy for HTN.
8. Keep all F/U to assess response, labs, and for adverse SE.

OUTCOMES/EVALUATE

- Improved patterns of behavior with less agitation, less hyperactivity, and reality orientation
- Treatment of schizophrenia; bipolar disorder

Zoledronic acid

IV

(**ZOH**-leh-**dron**-ick)

Classification(s): Bone growth regulator, bisphosphonate

Pregnancy Category: D

RX: Reclast, Zometa.

INDICATIONS/USES

Reclast: (1)Treat Paget's disease of the bone in men and women who have elevations in serum alkaline phosphatase of 2 times or higher the upper limit of the age-specific normal reference range, or in those who are symptomatic, or those at risk for complications from their disease. Goal is to induce remission and normalize serum alkaline phosphatase. (2) Once-yearly dose to treat postmenopausal osteoporosis, including those who have recently had a low-trauma hip fracture; reduces the incidence of fractures. (3) Prevention of osteoporosis in postmenopausal women. (4) To increase bone mass in men with osteoporosis. (5) Prevention and treatment of glucocorticoid-induced osteoporosis in men and women who are initiating or continuing systemic glucocorticoids in a daily dosage equivalent to 7.5 mg or more of prednisone and who are expected to remain on glucocorticoids for at least 12 months.

Zometa: (1) Hypercalcemia of malignancy. (2) Multiple myeloma and those with documented bone metastases from solid tumors, in conjunction with standard antineoplastic therapy. Prostate cancer should have progressed after treatment with at least 1 hormonal therapy.

Investigational: (1) Osteopenia in androgen–deprived prostate cancer clients. (2) Osteopenia in estrogen–deprived breast cancer clients. (3) Prevention of post renal transplant bone loss (insufficient documentation).

ACTION/KINETICS

Action

Hyperactivity of osteoclasts causes excessive bone resorption in hypercalcemia of malignancy. Such hypercalcemia causes polyuria and GI disturbances with progressive dehydration and decreased glomerular filtration rate. Reducing excessive bone resorption and maintaining adequate fluid intake are essential to managing hypercalcemia of malignancy. Zoledronic acid acts to inhibit bone resorption perhaps by inhibiting osteoclastic activity and inducing osteoclast apoptosis. Zoledronic acid also blocks the osteoclastic resorption of mineralized bone and cartilage by binding to bone. It inhibits the increased osteoclastic activity and skeletal calcium release induced by various stimulatory factors released by tumors.

Pharmacokinetics

t½: 0.23 hr, 1.75 hr, and 167 hr for the distribution, elimination, and terminal elimination, respectively. Is primarily excreted through the urine unchanged.

CONTRAINDICATIONS

Hypersensitivity to zoledronic acid or other bisphosphonates. Hypocalcemia. Reclast is not recommended for use in those with severe renal impairment (C_{CR} <35 mL/min).

SPECIAL CONCERNS

- **Use with caution in aspirin-sensitive asthma.**
- **Safety and efficacy not determined in treating hypercalcemia associated with hyperparathyroidism or other non-tumor-related diseases.**
- **Use with caution during lactation and in the elderly.**
- **Safety and efficacy not determined in children.**

SIDE EFFECTS

Most Common

Anorexia, constipation, diarrhea, N&V, anemia, arthralgia, bone/skeletal pain, myalgia, dyspnea, edema/peripheral edema, fatigue, fever.

GU: ***Renal toxicity***, including deterioration of renal function and potential renal failure, UTI. **GI:** N&V, GI irritation/disorders, esophageal irritation, constipation, diarrhea, abdominal pain, anorexia, decreased appetite, dysphagia. **CNS:** Insomnia, anxiety, confusion, agitation, depression, dizziness, headache, hypesthesia, insomnia, paresthesia, somnolence. **CV:** Hypotension. **Hematologic:** Anemia, granulocytopenia, neutropenia, thrombocytopenia, pancytopenia. **Respiratory:** Dyspnea, coughing, pleural effusion, URTI. **Musculoskeletal:** Skeletal pain, myalgia, bone/joint/muscles pain, arthralgia, back pain, jaw osteonecrosis (in cancer clients). **GU:** Renal toxicity, acute renal failure, UTI. **Dermatologic:** Alopecia, dermatitis; rarely, rash, pruritus. **Ophthalmic:** Conjunctivitis. **Infusion site reaction:**

Redness, swelling. **Body as a whole:** Fever, fatigue, asthenia, rigors, ***progression of cancer***, flu-like syndrome (fever, chills, bone pain, arthralgias, myalgias), dehydration, edema/peripheral edema, chest pain, non-specific infection, dehydration, leg edema, mucositis, weight decreased, ***metastases***. **Miscellaneous:** Moniliasis, neoplasm.

LABORATORY TEST CONSIDERATIONS

↑ Creatinine. Hypocalcemia, hypokalemia, hypermagnesemia, hypomagnesemia, hypophosphatemia.

DRUG INTERACTIONS

Aminoglycosides / Possible additive effect to lower serum calcium levels for prolonged periods
Diuretics, loop / ↑ Risk of hypocalcemia

HOW SUPPLIED

Injection Solution (Reclast): 5 mg/100 mL; *Injection Solution, Concentrate (Zometa):* 4 mg/5 mL.

DOSAGE

Reclast

IV

The following recommended doses are for those with a C_{CR} of 35 mL/min or more.

Paget's disease of bone.

Adults, usual: 5 mg IV infusion given at a constant infusion rate over not less than 15 minutes. To reduce the risk of hypocalcemia, give clients elemental calcium 1,500 mg/day in divided doses (750 mg twice a day or 500 mg 3 times a day) and vitamin D 800 units/day, especially in the 2 weeks following zoledronic acid. Specific retreatment data are not available; however, retreatment may be considered in those who have relapsed, based on increases in serum alkaline phosphatase or in those who failed to achieve normalization of their serum alkaline phosphatase, or in those with symptoms.

Treatment of postmenopausal osteoporosis.

Adults, usual: 5 mg given once yearly as a 15-min IV infusion. Clients must be adequately supplemented with calcium and vitamin D if dietary intake is insufficient. An average of at least calcium 1,200 mg and vitamin D 800–1,000 units/day is recommended.

Prevention of osteoporosis in postmenopausal women.

Adults, usual: 5 mg by IV infusion once q 2 years over no less than 15 minutes. Clients must be adequately supplemented with calcium and vitamin D if dietary intake is insufficient. An average of at least calcium 1,200 mg and vitamin D 800–1,000 units/day is recommended.

Osteoporosis in men.

Adults, usual: A single 5 mg IV infusion once a year over no less than 15 minutes. Clients must be adequately supplemented with calcium and vitamin D if dietary intake is insufficient. An average of at least calcium 1,200 mg and vitamin D 800–1,000 units/day is recommended.

Glucocorticoid-induced osteoporosis.

Adults, usual: A single 5 mg IV infusion once a year given over no less than 15 minutes. Clients must be adequately supplemented with calcium and vitamin D if dietary intake is insufficient. An average of at least calcium 1,200 mg and vitamin D 800–1,000 units/day is recommended.

Zometa

IV ONLY

Hypercalcemia of malignancy.

Adults, usual: 4 mg as a single IV infusion given over at least 15 minutes. **Maximum recommended dose:** 4 mg if albumin-corrected serum calcium is greater than or equal to 12 mg/dL. Adequately hydrate clients prior to zoledronic acid administration. Consider retreatment if serum calcium does not return to normal or remain normal after initial treatment. Allow 7 days to elapse before retreatment.

Multiple myeloma and metastatic bone lesions from solid tumors.

Adults, usual: 4 mg infused over 15 min q 3 or 4 weeks if C_{CR} is higher than 60 mL/min. Optimal duration is not known. Give PO calcium supplement of 500 mg and a multiple vitamin containing 400 international units vitamin D per day.

NURSING IMPLICATIONS

IMPLEMENTATION/ADMINISTRATION/STORAGE

1. IV Clients must be appropriately hydrated prior to zoledronic acid administration. When used for hypercalcemia of malignancy, initiate vigorous saline hydration promptly and attempt to restore urine output to about 2 L/day throughout treatment. Avoid overhydration.
2. Administration of acetaminophen after zoledronic acid administration may decrease the incidence of acute-phase reaction symptoms.
3. When used for Paget's disease of the bone, infusion time must not be less than 15 min given over a constant infusion rate. Retreatment may be considered in those who have relapsed, based on increases in serum alkaline phosphatase, or in those who failed to achieve normalization of their serum alkaline phosphatase, or in clients with symptoms.
4. When used for hypercalcemia of malignancy, due to the risk of significant deterioration of renal function, do not exceed single doses of 4 mg of zoledronic acid with the duration of infusion no less than 15 minutes.
5. To reduce the risk of hypocalcemia, give all clients elemental calcium, 1,500 mg/day in divided doses (e.g., 750 mg twice a day or 500 mg 3 times per day) as well as vitamin D, 800 units/day, especially in the 2 weeks following drug administration.
6. Use the following dosage for Zometa in those with mild to moderate impaired renal function and who are being treated for multiple myeloma and bone metastases from solid tumors: If baseline C_{CR} is 50–60 mL/min, give 3.5 mg zoledronic acid; if baseline C_{CR} is 40–49 mL/min, give 3.3 mg zoledronic acid; if baseline C_{CR} is 30–39 mL/min, give 3 mg zoledronic acid. Dosage adjustments are not needed in treating clients with hypercalcemia of malignancy who have mild to moderate impaired renal function.
7. Reclast is contraindicated if C_{CR} is less than 35 mL/min.
8. Measure serum creatinine before each zoledronic acid dose; withhold treatment for renal deterioration. Use the following criteria in those who experience a decrease in renal function after zoledronic acid:
   - If the serum creatinine was normal prior to zoledronic acid and there is an increase of 0.5 mg/dL within 2 weeks of the next dose, withhold zoledronic acid until serum creatinine is at least within 10% of the baseline value.
   - If the serum creatinine is abnormal prior to zoledronic acid and there is an increase of 1.0 mg/dL within 2 weeks of the next dose, withhold zoledronic acid until serum creatinine is at least within 10% of the baseline value.
9. Preparation for administration of Zometa: Vials contain zoledronic acid concentrate allowing for the withdrawal of 5 mL of concentrate (equivalent to zoledronic acid 4 mg). Dilute this concentrate immediately in 100 mL of sterile NaCl 0.9% or D5W injection. To avoid inadvertant injection, do not store undiluted concentrate in a syringe. Give as a single IV infusion over no less than 15 min.
10. Store Reclast from 15–30°C (59–86°F). After opening, the solution is stable for 24 hr at 2–8°C (36–46°F). If refrigerated, allow solution to reach room temperature before administration.
11. Store Zometa from 15–30°C (59–86°F). If not used immediately after reconstitution, refrigerate. The total time between reconstitution, dilution, storage in the refrigerator, and the end of administration must not exceed 24 hr.
12. COMPATIBILITY D5W or 0.9% NaCl.
13. INCOMPATIBILITY Do not mix with calcium-containing solutions, such as lactated Ringer's. Administer separately.

ASSESSMENT

1. Note reasons for therapy, source of malignancy with cancer, clinical presentation, BMD, serum Ca^{++} levels, other agents/methods trialed.
2. Initiate vigorous NSS hydration to ensure urinary output is 2 L/day during treatment. Avoid diuretics until client is adequately hydrated.
3. Assess for kidney problems, any history of surgery to remove parathyroid glands or any in-

testinal surgery, or if unable to take calcium supplements.

4. Because of the possibility of osteonecrosis of the jaw in cancer clients, undertake a dental exam with appropriate preventive dentistry before beginning therapy (especially in those with risk factors such as cancer, chemotherapy, corticosteroids, or poor oral hygiene).
5. Note BMD with osteoporosis in postmenopausal women.
6. Monitor CBC, Ca^{++}, PO_4, Mg^{++}, electrolytes, and renal function. Ensure albumin corrected calcium level: (cCa, mg/dL = Ca + 0.8). Assess for renal failure and deficiency states, give calcium 1500 mg and vitamin D 800 international units daily.

CLIENT/FAMILY TEACHING

1. This drug is administered IV to reduce high calcium levels, which result from tumors that cause increased bone activity and skeletal calcium release, which cause your bones to weaken (Zometa). Also for postmenopausal osteoporosis (treatment/prevention and Paget's disease (Reclast).
2. Report adverse side effects or unusual response to therapy. Nausea, vomiting, diarrhea, constipation, pain/redness/swelling at the injection site, or flu-like symptoms (e.g., fever, chills, muscle/joint aches or pains) may occur. Immediately report any changes in urine output, rash, itching, dizziness, weakness, trouble breathing or swallowing, burning or painful urination, mental/mood changes (e.g., agitation, anxiety, confusion) and jaw pain, chest pain, SOB, swelling of the legs or mouth, eye or vision problems, persistent sore throat and fever, unusual bruising/bleeding.
3. Infusion-site reactions (e.g., hardness, pain, redness, swelling) may be treated with warm or cold packs and oral OTC analgesics (e.g., acetaminophen, ibuprofen); report if not responsive.
4. Maintain good oral hygiene; avoid invasive dental procedures (e.g., tooth extractions) during treatment with zoledronic acid.
5. Advise women of childbearing potential to use effective contraception during therapy.
6. Take oral calcium replacement of 1,500 mg and 800 international units of vitamin D daily.
7. Keep all F/U to assess response, labs, and for adverse SE.

OUTCOMES/EVALUATE

- ↓ Serum calcium levels in malignancy
- Inhibition of bone resorption (osteoporosis in postmenopausal women)
- Treatment of Paget's disease

Zolmitriptan

(zohl-mih-**TRIP**-tin)

Classification(s): Antimigraine drug

Pregnancy Category: C

RX: Zomig, Zomig ZMT.

INDICATIONS/USES

Treatment of acute migraine in adults with or without aura. Use only when there is clear diagnosis of migraine. *Investigational:* Migraines in adolescents.

ACTION/KINETICS

Action

Binds to serotonin 5-$HT_{1B/1D}$ receptors on intracranial blood vessels and in sensory nerves of trigeminal system. This results in cranial vessel constriction and inhibition of pro-inflammatory neuropeptide release.

Pharmacokinetics

Well absorbed after PO use. The PO forms are from 29–46% bioavailable, while the nasal form is 100% bioavailable. Orally disintegrating tablets may have a faster onset. **Time to onset of action:** 45 min (15 min for the nasal spray). **Peak plasma levels:** 1.5–3 hr. **t½, elimination:** About 3 hr (for zolmitriptan and active metabolite). Excreted in feces and urine. **Plasma protein binding:** About 25% bound to plasma proteins.

CONTRAINDICATIONS

Prophylaxis of migraine or management of hemiplegic or basilar migraine. Use in angina pectoris, history of MI, documented or silent ischemia, ischemic heart disease, coronary artery vasospasm (including Prinzmetal's variant angina), other significant underlying CV disease. Also use in uncontrolled hypertension, within 24 hr of treatment with another serotonin HT_1 agonist or an ergotamine-containing or ergot-type drug (e.g., dihydroergotamine, methysergide). Concurrent use with MAOI or within 2 weeks of discontinuing MAOI.

SPECIAL CONCERNS

- Use with caution in liver disease and during lactation.
- A significant increase in BP may occur with moderate-to-severe hepatic impairment.
- Safety and efficacy not determined for cluster headache.
- Safety for treating >3 headaches in a 30-day period using tablets or disintegrating tables not determined. Safety for treating >4 headaches in a 30-day period using the nasal spray not determined.
- Efficacy for migraine headaches not determined in children, 12–17 years old.

SIDE EFFECTS

Most Common

Warm/cold sensation, paresthesia, asthenia, dizziness, somnolence, chest tightness/pressure/heaviness, neck/throat/jaw pain, dry mouth, dyspepsia, nausea, pain.

GI: Dry mouth, dyspepsia, dysphagia, nausea, increased appetite, ***tongue edema***, esophagitis, gastroenteritis, abnormal liver function, thirst. **CV:** Palpitations, arrhythmias, hypertension, syncope. **Atypical sensations:** Hypesthesia, paresthesia, warm/cold sensation. **CNS:** Dizziness, somnolence, vertigo, agitation, anxiety, depression, emotional lability, insomnia. **Pain/pressure sensations:** Chest pain, tightness, pressure and/or heaviness. Pain, tightness, or heaviness in the neck, throat, or jaw. Heaviness, pressure, tightness other than in the chest or neck. **Musculoskeletal:** Myalgia, myasthenia, back pain, leg cramps, tenosynovitis. **Respiratory:** Bronchitis, ***bronchospasm***, epistaxis, hiccup, laryngitis, yawn. **Dermatologic:** Sweating, pruritus, rash, urticaria, ecchymosis, photosensitivity. **GU:** Hematuria, cystitis, polyuria, urinary frequency/urgency. **Body as a whole:** Asthenia, allergic reaction, chills, facial edema, edema, fever, malaise. **Miscellaneous:** Dry eye, eye pain, hyperacusis, ear pain, parosmia, tinnitus.

DRUG INTERACTIONS

Cimetidine / $t_{1/2}$ of zolmitriptan is doubled
Ergot-containing drugs / Prolonged vasospastic reactions
MAOIs / ↑ Zolmitriptan levels
Oral contraceptives / ↑ Zolmitriptan plasma levels
Selective serotonin reuptake inhibitors / Possible weakness, hyperreflexia, and incoordination
Sibutramine / Possible serotonin syndrome, including weakness, hyperreflexia, and incoordination

HOW SUPPLIED

Nasal Spray: 5 mg; *Tablets:* 2.5 mg, 5 mg; *Tablets, Oral Disintegrating:* 2.5 mg, 5 mg.

DOSAGE

NASAL SPRAY

Migraine headaches.

Give 1 dose of 5 mg. If headache returns, the dose may be repeated after 2 hr, not to exceed a maximum daily dose of 10 mg in any 24-hr period.

TABLETS

Migraine headaches.

Adults, initial: 2.5 mg or lower (break tablet in half). Dose of 5 mg may be required. If headache returns, repeat dose after 2 hr, not to exceed 10 mg in 24-hr period.

TABLETS, ORAL DISINTEGRATING

Migraine headaches.

Single dose of 2.5 mg. If headache returns, repeat dose after 2 hr, not to exceed 10 mg in 24-hr period.

NURSING IMPLICATIONS

IMPLEMENTATION/ADMINISTRATION/STORAGE

1. Use doses less than 2.5 mg in those with liver disease. Doses less than 2.5 mg may be obtained by manually breaking 2.5 mg tablet in half.
2. Safety of treating more than 3 headaches in a 30 day period has not been established.
3. Store nasal spray and tablets from 20–25°C (68–77°F); protect tablets from light and moisture.

ASSESSMENT

1. Note headache characteristics, including onset, frequency, type, duration of symptoms, triggers, and other agents trialed. Rate pain levels.
2. Assess neurologic exam, findings; review headache diary and note any triggers. Note mental status, N&V, vision changes/blurring,

tingling in extremities, and if precedes headache
3. Determine any cardiac problems or ischemic CV disease. Expect transient increases in BP.
4. Monitor BP, ECG, renal and LFTs; reduce dose with dysfunction.

CLIENT/FAMILY TEACHING

1. Take exactly as directed; strictly to relieve migraine headaches, not to prevent them. Do not exceed dosage or dosing intervals of 2 hr apart and total of 10 mg/24 hr. Take at the first symptom of migraine; attempt to identify triggers.
2. If using the orally disintegrating tablet, remove from the blister just prior to dosing. Place on the tongue where it will dissolve and be swallowed with saliva. Taking a liquid is not necessary. Do not break the orally disintegrating tablet.
3. Treating more than 4 headaches in a 30-day period with nasal spray (or 3 headaches in a 30-day period with tablets) has not been established; report if headaches are occurring more frequently.
4. Do not perform activities that require mental alertness until drug effects realized. May experience fatigue and dizziness.
5. Lying down in a dark room, avoiding light and noise may help diminish headache symptoms.
6. Report if chest pain, SOB, chest/throat tightness, wheezing, swelling of face occurs.
7. Practice reliable contraception; report if pregnancy suspected.
8. Avoid prolonged exposure to sunlight and wear protective clothing and sunscreen if exposed to prevent photosensitivity.
9. Keep all F/U to assess response, labs, and for adverse SE.

OUTCOMES/EVALUATE

Relief of migraine headache

Zolpidem tartrate

(**ZOL**-pih-dem)

Classification(s): Sedative-hypnotic, nonbenzodiazepine

Pregnancy Category: B (Immediate-Release); **C** (Extended-Release)

RX: Ambien, Ambien CR, Edluar, Tovalt ODT, Zolpimist, **C-IV**

INDICATIONS/USES

Oral Spray, Immediate-Release Tablets, Sublingual Tablets: Short-term treatment of insomnia (7–10 days of use). Re-evaluate if hypnotics are to be taken for more than 2–3 weeks.

Extended-Release/Orally Disintegrating Tablets: Treatment of insomnia characterized by difficulties with sleep onset and/or sleep maintenance.

ACTION/KINETICS

Action

May act by subunit modulation of the GABA receptor chloride channel macromolecular complex, resulting in sedative, anticonvulsant, anxiolytic, and myorelaxant properties. Although unrelated chemically to the benzodiazepines or barbiturates, it interacts with a GABA-benzodiazepine receptor complex and shares some of the pharmacologic effects of the benzodiazepines. Specifically, it binds to the omega-1 receptor preferentially. No evidence of residual next-day effects or rebound insomnia at usual doses; little evidence for memory impairment. Sleep time spent in stage 3 to 4 (deep sleep) was comparable to placebo with only inconsistent, minor changes in REM sleep at recommended doses.

Pharmacokinetics

Rapidly absorbed from the GI tract. **t½, elimination, immediate-release:** About 2.5 hr (increased in geriatric clients and those with impaired hepatic function). **t½, elimination, orally disintegrating:** 3.5 hr (nighttime dosing). **t½, elimination, extended-release:** 2.8 hr. Food decreases the bioavailability of zolpidem. Metabolized in the liver; inactive metabolites are excreted primarily through the urine. **Plasma protein binding:** 92.5%.

CONTRAINDICATIONS

Not recommended for use during lactation.

SPECIAL CONCERNS

- Use with caution and at reduced dosage with impaired renal or hepatic function, compromised respiratory function, and in clients with S&S of depression.

- **Impaired motor or cognitive performance after repeated use or unusual sensitivity to hypnotic drugs may be noted in geriatric or debilitated clients.**
- **Observe closely with any history of dependence on or abuse of drugs or alcohol as drug is habit-forming.**
- **Safety and efficacy not determined in children less than 18 years old.**

SIDE EFFECTS

Most Common

Immediate-Release/Oral Disintegrating: Dizziness, drowsiness, drugged feeling, headache, nausea, diarrhea, dyspepsia, myalgia, URTI.
Extended-Release: Headache, somnolence, dizziness, nausea, diarrhea, nasopharyngitis.

Listed are side effects with an incidence greater than 1%. **Immediate Release/Orally Disintegrating: CNS:** Headache, drowsiness, dizziness, depression, drugged feeling, lethargy, light-headedness, abnormal dreams, amnesia, anxiety, fatigue, nervousness, sleep disorder. **GI:** N&V, dyspepsia, dry mouth, diarrhea, constipation, abdominal pain, anorexia. **CV:** Palpitations. **GU:** UTI. **Musculoskeletal:** Myalgia, arthralgia, back pain. **Respiratory:** URTI, pharyngitis, rhinitis, sinusitis. **Miscellaneous:** Allergy, flu-like symptoms, chest pain, rash, infection, hypersensitivity reactions.

Extended-Release: CNS: Headache, somnolence, dizziness, hallucinations, disorientation, fatigue, memory disorders, depression, anxiety, apathy, balance disorder, depression, disturbed attention, hypoesthesia, psychomotor retardation, ataxia, binge eating, depersonalization, disinhibition, euphoria, mood swings, paresthesia, stress symptoms, tremor, ataxia, confusion, drowsiness, euphoria, insomnia, lethargy, vertigo, lightheadedness, burning sensation, postural dizziness. **GI:** N&V, constipation, abdominal discomfort/tenderness, abdominal pain, diarrhea, dyspepsia, hiccup, flatulence, frequent bowel movements, GERD, gastroenteritis. **CV:** Increased BP, palpitations. **GU:** Dysuria, vulvovaginal dryness, menorrhagia. **Dermatologic:** Rash, skin wrinkling, urticaria. **Musculoskeletal:** Back pain, myalgia, arthralgia, muscle cramps, neck pain/injury, involuntary muscle contractions. **Respiratory:** Throat irritation, dry throat, lower RTI, URTI, nasopharyngitis. **Ophthalmic:** Red eyes, visual disturbances, blurred vision, diplopia, altered visual depth perception. **Otic:** Vertigo, labyrinthitis, tinnitus, otitis externa. **Miscellaneous:** Asthenopia, appetite disorder, allergy, asthenia, increased body temperature, chest discomfort, contusion, pyrexia, flu, flu-like illness, hypersensitivity reactions.

Symptoms of withdrawal: Although there is no clear evidence of a withdrawal syndrome, the following symptoms were noted with zolpidem following placebo substitution: Fatigue, nausea, flushing, light-headedness, uncontrolled crying, emesis, stomach cramps, panic attack, nervousness, abdominal discomfort.

LABORATORY TEST CONSIDERATIONS

↑ ALT, AST, BUN. Hyperglycemia, hypercholesterolemia, hyperlipidemia, abnormal hepatic function.

OVERDOSE MANAGEMENT

Symptoms: Symptoms ranging from somnolence to light coma. Rarely, CV and respiratory compromise. *Treatment:* Gastric lavage if appropriate. General symptomatic and supportive measures. IV fluids as needed. Flumazenil may be effective in reversing CNS depression. Monitor hypotension and CNS depression and treat appropriately. Sedative drugs should not be used, even if excitation occurs. Zolpidem is not dialyzable.

DRUG INTERACTIONS

Alcohol / Additive effect on psychomotor performance
Azole antifungals (fluconazole, itraconazole, ketoconazole) / ↑ Zolpidem levels and therapeutic effects; monitor closely and adjust dose if necessary
Chlorpromazine / Additive ↓ alertness and psychomotor performance
CNS depressants / Additive CNS depression
Flumazenil / Reverses effect of zolpidem
Imipramine / ↓ Peak imipramine levels; additive decreased alertness
Rifamycins (e.g., rifampin) / ↓ Zolpidem levels and therapeutic effects; monitor closely and adjust dose if necessary
Ritonavir / Possible severe sedation and respiratory depression; do not use together
SSRIs / Shortened onset of zolpidem and ↑ effect

HOW SUPPLIED

Oral Spray: 5 mg, 10 mg; ***Tablets, Extended-Release:*** 6.25 mg, 12.5 mg; ***Tablets, Immediate-Re-***

lease: 5 mg, 10 mg; ***Tablets, Orally Disintegrating:*** 5 mg, 10 mg; ***Tablets, Sublingual:*** 5 mg, 10 mg.

DOSAGE

ORAL SPRAY; TABLETS, IMMEDIATE-RELEASE; TABLETS, ORALLY DISINTEGRATING; TABLETS, SUBLINGUAL

Hypnotic.

Adults, individualized, usual: 10 mg just before bedtime. In the elderly or in hepatic insufficiency, use an initial dose of 5 mg.

TABLETS, EXTENDED-RELEASE

Hypnotic.

Individualize dose. **Adults:** 12.5 mg just before bedtime. For elderly or debilitated clients, give 6.25 mg just before bedtime.

NURSING IMPLICATIONS

Do not confuse Ambien with Amen (a progestin).

IMPLEMENTATION/ADMINISTRATION/STORAGE

1. Limit therapy to 7–10 days. Reevaluate if the drug is required for more than 2–3 weeks.
2. Do not prescribe in quantities exceeding a 1-month supply.
3. Do not exceed 10 mg daily of the immediate-release or oral disintegrating tablets or 12.5 mg of the extended-release tablets.
4. Store the immediate-release and orally disintegrating tablets from 20–25°C (68–77°F) and the extended-release from 15–25°C (59–77°F).

ASSESSMENT

1. Note reasons for therapy, onset, characteristics S&S, triggers, other agents trialed and drugs prescribed to ensure none interact.
2. Assess for respiratory dysfunction (sleep apnea), pain, drug or alcohol dependence, and symptoms of depression.
3. Review sleep patterns (trouble falling/staying asleep, early a.m. awakenings) and lifestyle. Identify underlying cause(s) of insomnia (i.e., napping during the daytime, lack of exercise, ↑ stress, fear, loneliness, alcohol/caffeine/energy drink use, lack of routine).
4. Evaluate mental status, use lower dose in elderly/debilitated client; monitor for impaired motor/cognitive performance.
5. Monitor CBC, LFTs; reduce dose with dysfunction.

CLIENT/FAMILY TEACHING

1. Take only as directed. Tablets should be taken on an empty stomach with a full glass of water; oral spray should be taken just before going to bed. For faster sleep onset, do not administer with or immediately after a meal.
2. Do not take zolpidem unless planning to get 7 to 8 hr of sleep before being active again; less than 7 to 8 hr of sleep may result in daytime drowsiness, amnesia, or memory problems.
3. If using orally disintegrating tablets, open the blister pack and peel back the foil on the blister. Do not push the tablet through the foil. Remove the tablet and place it in the mouth where it will dissolve in seconds; then swallow with saliva. Can be taken with or without water. Do not chew, break, or split the tablet. Do not give with or immediately after a meal.
4. Swallow the extended-release tablets whole. Do not divide, crush, or chew the extended-release tablets.
5. With oral spray, prime by pressing down on pump 5 times. Press down completely on pump to deliver full dose (i.e., 5 mg). If 10 mg dose prescribed, then administer a second spray. Spray contents directly into mouth (colorless cherry-flavored solution). If oral spray is not used for 2 weeks, then prime again with 1 spray.
6. Do not perform any activities that require mental or physical alertness until drug effects realized. Evaluate response the following day to ensure that no residual effects are present
7. Avoid alcohol, caffeine, sodas, ice tea, energy drinks, chocolate after 4 p.m., and any unprescribed or OTC drugs.
8. Drug is for short-term use; keep a log and identify factors that may be contributing to insomnia. Review alternative methods for inducing sleep: relaxation techniques, daily early day exercise, soft music, no daytime napping, guided imagery, white noise, dietary changes, special effects simulator.
9. Those with depression are at a higher risk for suicide or intentional overdose. Advise family that these clients warrant closer observation

and limited prescriptions and to report any evidence of suicidal thoughts or aggressive behavior.
10. Keep out of reach of children, and store in a safe place away from bedside; drug has a high potential for abuse and withdrawal after 2 weeks of use.
11. Do not take if pregnant; use reliable contraception and report if suspected.
12. Review safety precautions with regard to falls, especially for elderly and debilitated clients.
13. May be habit forming; take only as prescribed.
14. Sleep may be disturbed for 1–2 nights following discontinuation of zolpidem therapy. If medication is discontinued after 2 or more weeks of nightly use, it will need to be slowly withdrawn.
15. Avoid alcohol and CNS depressants. Report any behaviors that are reportedly performed i.e. driving, preparing and eating meals without memory of event to provider.
16. Keep all F/U to assess response and for adverse SE.

OUTCOMES/EVALUATE

- Relief of insomnia
- ↓ Difficulty with sleep onset/maintenance

Zonisamide

(zoh-**NISS**-ah-myd)

Classification(s): Anticonvulsant, miscellaneous

Pregnancy Category: C

RX: Zonegran.

INDICATIONS/USES

Adjunctive therapy to treat partial seizures in adults with epilepsy.

ACTION/KINETICS

Action

Is a sulfonamide. Precise mechanism unknown. May block sodium channels and reduce voltage-dependent, transient inward currents (T-type Ca^{2+} currents), thus stabilizing neuronal membranes and suppressing neuronal hypersynchronization. May bind to the GABA/benzodiazepine receptor ionophore complex.

Pharmacokinetics

Peak plasma levels: 2–5 mcg/mL in 2–6 hr. Food delays time to maximum levels but does not affect bioavailability. Extensively binds to erythrocytes. Due to the long $t^{1/2}$, up to 2 weeks may be needed to achieve steady-state levels. **$t^{1/2}$, elimination:** About 63 hr from plasma and about 105 hr from erythrocytes. Excreted primarily in the urine as unchanged drug and the glucuronide metabolite (mediated by CYP3A4). **Plasma protein binding:** About 40%.

CONTRAINDICATIONS

Hypersensitivity to sulfonamides or zonisamide. Use in those with a glomerular filtration rate <50 mL/min. Lactation.

SPECIAL CONCERNS

- Hypersensitivity reactions are possible (zonisamide is a sulfonamide).
- Use with caution when coadministered with carbonic anhydrase inhibitors and drugs with anticholinergic activity.
- Use with caution in impaired hepatic or renal dysfunction.
- Use caution in dose selection in the elderly.
- Children seem to be at increased risk for zonisamide-associated oligohidrosis and hyperthermia.
- Increased risk of suicidal behavior and ideation.
- Abrupt withdrawal may precipitate increased seizure frequency or status epilepticus.
- Safety and efficacy not determined in children under 16 years of age.

SIDE EFFECTS

Most Common

Somnolence, anorexia, dizziness, headache, agitation/irritability, tiredness, nausea, diplopia, nystagmus, paresthesia, abdominal pain, dyspepsia, diarrhea, speech abnormalities, flu syndrome, rash, weight loss.

CNS-associated side effects are frequent. They can be classified as psychiatric symptoms (including depression and psychosis), psychomotor slowing (difficulty with concentration, speech, language), and somnolence or fatigue. Side effects listed are those with an incidence of 0.1% or more. **Hypersensitivity:** ***Stevens-Johnson syndrome, toxic epidermal necrolysis, fulminant hepatic necrosis, agranulocytosis, aplastic anemia.*** **CNS:** Somnolence, dizziness, headache, agitation, irritability, tiredness, ataxia, anxiety, confusion, depression, difficulty concentrating, difficulty with memory, speech/language problems, insomnia, mental slowing, paresthesia, nervousness, schizophrenia/schizophrenic behavior, tremor, convulsion, ***status epilepticus***, abnormal gait, hyperesthesia, incoordination, hypertonia, twitching, abnormal dreams, vertigo, decreased libido, neuropathy, hyperkinesia, movement disorder, incoordination, disarthria, hypotonia, peripheral neuritis, increased reflexes, euphoria, suicidal behavior/ideation. **GI:** Anorexia, nausea, abdominal pain, diarrhea, dry mouth, taste perversion, dyspepsia, constipation, vomiting, flatulence, gingivitis, gum hyperplasia, gastritis, gastroenteritis, stomatitis, cholelithiasis, glossitis, melena, rectal hemorrhage, ulcerative stomatitis, gastroduodenal ulcer, dysphagia, gum hemorrhage, ***pancreatitis***. **CV:** Palpitation, tachycardia, vascular insufficiency, ***CVA***, hypertension, hypotension, thrombophlebitis, syncope, bradycardia. **Respiratory:** Pharyngitis, increased cough, dyspnea, rhinitis. **Musculoskeletal:** Leg cramps, myalgia, myasthenia, arthralgia, arthritis. **Dermatologic:** Pruritus, maculopapular rash, acne, alopecia, dry skin, sweating, eczema, ecchymosis, urticaria, hirsutism, pustular rash, vesiculobullous rash, ***serious skin reactions (death possible)***. **GU:** Urinary frequency, dysuria, urinary incontinence, hematuria, kidney stones, impotence, urinary retention, urinary urgency, amenorrhea, polyuria, nocturia. **Hematologic:** Leukopenia, anemia, immunodeficiency, lymphadenopathy, ***aplastic anemia, agranulocytosis***. **Metabolic:** Peripheral edema, weight gain/loss, edema, thirst, dehydration. **Ophthalmic:** Diplopia, nystagmus, amblyopia, conjunctivitis, visual field defect, glaucoma, photophobia, iritis. **Otic:** Tinnitus, deafness. **Body as a whole:** Flu syndrome, accidental injury, asthenia, fatigue, malaise, allergic reaction. **Miscellaneous:** Difficulties in verbal expression, speech abnormalities, parosmia, chest pain, flank pain, facial edema, neck rigidity, ***unexplained death***. *NOTE:* Pediatric clients may get heat stroke, oligohydrosis, decreased sweating, and hyperthermia, especially in warm or hot weather.

LABORATORY TEST CONSIDERATIONS

↑ Serum creatinine, BUN, serum alkaline phosphatase, CPK.

OVERDOSE MANAGEMENT

Symptoms: CNS symptoms (see *Side Effects*). *Treatment:* Induce emesis or gastric lavage; protect the airway. Institute general supportive care, including frequent monitoring of vital signs. *NOTE:* Zonisamide has a long $t^{1/2}$.

DRUG INTERACTIONS

Carbamazepine / ↓ Zonisamide $t^{1/2}$ R/T ↑ liver metabolism

Phenobarbital / ↓ Zonisamide $t^{1/2}$ R/T ↑ liver metabolism

Phenytoin / ↓ Zonisamide $t^{1/2}$ R/T ↑ liver metabolism

Sulfonamides / Potentially fatal reactions, including Stevens-Johnson syndrome, toxic epidermal necrolysis, agranulocytosis, aplastic anemia, and other blood dyscrasias

Valproate / ↑ Zonisamide $t^{1/2}$ R/T ↓ liver metabolism

HOW SUPPLIED

Capsules: 25 mg, 50 mg, 100 mg.

DOSAGE

CAPSULES

Partial seizures.

Adults and those over 16 years of age: Individualize. **Initial:** 100 mg/day. May increase to 200 mg/day after 2 weeks. Additional increases to 300 and 400 mg/day may be made in 2 weeks or longer to achieve steady state. **Effective dose range:** 100–600 mg/day. Administer dosage once or twice daily except for the 100-mg dose

NURSING IMPLICATIONS

IMPLEMENTATION/ADMINISTRATION/STORAGE

Store from 15–30°C (59–86°F) in a dry place protected from light.

ASSESSMENT

1. Note type, onset, characteristics and frequency of seizures, other agents trialed, outcome. List other drugs prescribed to ensure none interact.
2. Note any sulfonamide allergy/use.
3. Assess behavioral presentation; note any evidence/history of depression/suicide idea-

tions. Note any skin rash; may require interruption of therapy.

4. Monitor VS, CBC, $NaHCO_3$, renal and LFTs; anticipate reduced dose with dysfunction.

CLIENT/FAMILY TEACHING

1. Take capsules once or twice a day as directed. May take with or without food, but should swallow capsules whole.
2. May cause drowsiness; do not perfom tasks that require alertness until drug effects realized and able to determine if drug affects performance.
3. Increase fluid intake (8 glasses of water/day) to reduce kidney stone risk. Report increased back or abdominal pain or any blood in urine. Stop drug and report immediately if a rash occurs or seizures worsen.
4. During the summer or hot weather, monitor temperature especially in children under age 17 as abnormally decreased sweating may occur, resulting in severe dehydration and heatstroke. Report if child taking zonisamide is not sweating as usual with or without a fever.
5. Any new onset fever, sore throat, easy bruising, oral ulcers, lack of sweating with fever or severe muscle pain and/or weakness require reporting.
6. Practice reliable birth control. Report if pregnancy suspected/anticipated or if breastfeeding, as drug should be avoided.
7. Abrupt withdrawal may precipitate increased seizure frequency or status epilepticus. Gradually reduce dose and report any loss of seizure control.
8. Report any mood or behavioral changes, increased depression, suicide ideations, aggressiveness or increased anger issues immediately.
9. Keep all F/U to assess response, labs, and adverse SE.

OUTCOMES/EVALUATE

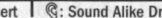

Control of seizures

Classifications

Chapter 2

Therapeutic Drug Classifications

Refer to the 2013 Delmar Nurse's Handbook website for additional drugs. Note that some drugs have recently been withdrawn from the market; consult www.fda.gov for more information.

ALKYLATING AGENTS

SEE ALSO THE FOLLOWING INDIVIDUAL ENTRIES:

Busulfan
Carboplatin
Carmustine
Chlorambucil
Cisplatin
Dacarbazine
Ifosfamide
Lomustine
Mesna

ACTION/KINETICS

Action

Alkylating agents donate an alkyl group (carbonium ion) to biologically important macromolecules, such as DNA. The molecule is inactivated, bringing *cell division* to a halt. This cytotoxic activity affects replication of cancerous cells and other cells, especially in rapidly proliferating tissues, such as the bone marrow, intestinal epithelium, and hair follicles. The toxic effects are usually cell-cycle nonspecific and become apparent when the cell enters the S phase and cell division is blocked at the G_2 phase (premitotic phase), resulting in cells having a double complement of DNA. Resistance of cancer cells to alkylating agents usually develops slowly and gradually. Resistance seems to be the sum total of several minor adaptations, including decreased permeability of the cells, increased production of noncancer receptors (nucleophilic substances), and increased efficiency of the DNA repair system.

NURSING IMPLICATIONS

ASSESSMENT

1. Note physical presentation, reasons for therapy, other agents trialed, outcome; ensure client is well hydrated. Restrict within 4 weeks after full XRT or chemotherapy to prevent critical bone marrow depression.
2. Monitor during therapy for adverse side effects; report. Assess IV catheter carefully to ensure patency and no extravasation.
3. Review VS, CBC, uric acid, renal and LFTs.

CLIENT/FAMILY TEACHING

1. Note reasons for therapy, anticipated results, frequency of dosing, and what to expect.
2. Review list of side effects (i.e., N&V, loss of appetite, fatigue), and identify ways to cope (i.e., small frequent meals, dividing dose, and consuming 8–10 glasses of fluid/day).
3. If infertility is a possible side effect, suggest clients who are considering families have eggs/sperm harvested prior to therapy. Drug may cause birth defects; use reliable contraception.
4. Practice good oral hygiene and complete dental work prior to starting therapy, or wait until after therapy when blood counts are stabilized.
5. Report unusual side effects, unusual bleeding/bruising, fever, chills, sore throat, cough, SOB, yellowing of skin/eyes, flank or stomach pain, changes in bladder/bowel function.
6. Avoid those with infections; drugs may cause immunosuppression and make one more susceptible to infections.
7. Review increased risk of secondary malignancies in clients treated with alkylating agents to ensure benefits outweigh risks.
8. Keep all F/U to assess response, labs, and adverse SE.

OUTCOMES/EVALUATE

Clinical/radiographic evidence of tumor regression and disease stabilization

Classifications

ALPHA-1-ADRENERGIC BLOCKING AGENTS ■

SEE ALSO THE FOLLOWING INDIVIDUAL ENTRIES:

Alfuzosin hydrochloride
Doxazosin mesylate
Prazosin hydrochloride
Tamsulosin hydrochloride
Terazosin

INDICATIONS/USES

(1) Hypertension, alone or in combination with diuretics or beta-adrenergic blocking agents. (2) Doxazocin, terazosin, and tamulosin are used to treat BPH. *Investigational:* Prazosin is used for refractory CHF, management of Raynaud's vasospasm, and to treat BPH. Doxazosin, along with digoxin and diuretics, is used to treat CHF.

ACTION/KINETICS

Action

Selectively blocks postsynaptic alpha-1-adrenergic receptors. Results in dilation of both areterioles and veins leading to a decrease in supine and standing BP. Diastolic BP is affected the most. Prazosin and terazosin do not produce reflex tachycardia. Terazosin also relaxes smooth muscle in the bladder neck and prostate, making it useful to treat BPH. Have many undesirable effects, which, although not toxic, limit their use. Always start treatment at low doses and increase gradually.

CONTRAINDICATIONS

Hypersensitivity to these drugs (i.e., quinazolines).

SPECIAL CONCERNS

- **The first few doses may cause postural hypotension and syncope with sudden loss of consciousness.**
- **Use with caution in lactation, with impaired hepatic function, or if receiving drugs known to influence hepatic metabolism.**
- **Safety and efficacy not established in children.**

SIDE EFFECTS

The following side effects are common to alpha-1-adrenergic blockers. See individual drugs as well. **CV:** Marked hypotension and/or syncope with sudden loss of consciousness (first-dose effect), palpitations, postural hypotension, hypotension, tachycardia, chest pain, arrhythmia. **GI:** N&V, dry mouth, diarrhea, constipation, abdominal discomfort/pain, flatulence. **CNS:** Dizziness, depression, decreased libido, sexual dysfunction, nervousness, paresthesia, somnolence, anxiety, insomnia, asthenia, drowsiness. **Musculoskeletal:** Pain in the shoulder, neck, or back; gout, arthritis, joint pain, arthralgia. **Respiratory:** Dyspnea, nasal congestion, sinusitis, bronchitis, ***bronchospasm***, cold symptoms, epistaxis, increased cough, flu symptoms, pharyngitis, rhinitis. **Ophthalmic:** Blurred vision, abnormal vision, reddened sclera, conjunctivitis, intraoperative floppy iris syndrome during phacoemulsification cataract surgery. **GU:** Impotence, urinary frequency, incontinence, priapism. **Miscellaneous:** Tinnitus, vertigo, pruritus, sweating, alopecia, lichen planus, headache, edema, weight gain, facial edema, fever.

OVERDOSE MANAGEMENT

Symptoms: Extension of the side effects, especially on BP.

Treatment: Keep supine to restore BP and normalize heart rate. Shock may be treated with volume expanders or vasopressors; support renal function.

DRUG INTERACTIONS

Ethanol / ↑ Risk of hypotension; advise clients to avoid alcohol
Clonidine / ↓ Antihypertensive effect of clonidine

LABORATORY TEST CONSIDERATIONS

↑ Urinary VMA.

DOSAGE

See individual agents.

NURSING IMPLICATIONS

IMPLEMENTATION/ADMINISTRATION/STORAGE

Take the first dose of prazosin and terazosin at bedtime to prevent dizziness.

ASSESSMENT

1. **Note reasons for therapy, characteristics of S&S, clinical presentation, other agents trialed, outcome.**
2. **Assess for heart or lung disease; note drugs currently prescribed. Some may cause vasospasm with Prinzmetal or vasospastic angina. If history of PUD, use drug cautiously.**
3. **Monitor electrolytes, ECG, VS. Base titration on standing BP R/T postural effects.**

4. Use cautiously in older clients; may fall R/T orthostatic hypotension. They may tolerate a slower, more gradual increase in dosage (i.e., terazosin 1 mg/day for 5 days followed by 2 mg/day for 5 days, etc., until desired response).

CLIENT/FAMILY TEACHING

1. May take with milk/meals to minimize GI upset. Do not stop abruptly; with terazosin, will have to re-titrate up to effective dosage if therapy stopped/interrupted. These drugs (alpha-1 blockers) relax the muscles of the bladder neck and prostate which allows easier urination. They work by keeping the hormone norepinephrine (noradrenaline) from tightening the muscles in the walls of smaller arteries and veins. Blocking that effect causes the vessels to remain open and relaxed. This improves blood flow and lowers blood pressure.
2. Take terazosin at bedtime especially first dose, to minimize fainting and low BP effects. Do not drive or perform hazardous tasks for 12–24 hr after first dose, after increasing dose, or following an interruption of dosage. Avoid low BP symptoms by rising slowly from a sitting or lying position and waiting until symptoms subside.
3. Finasteride and dutasteride (5-Alpha Reductase inhibitors) lower levels of hormones produced by the prostate, reducing the size of the prostate gland which helps increase urine flow rate, and decrease symptoms of BPH. It may take 3 to 6 months before you notice much improvement in your symptoms.
4. Record BP and weight. Report any weight gain or extremity swelling; without a diuretic, may experience retention of salt/water due to vessel dilation.
5. Dizziness, fatigue, headache, and palpitations may occur as well as transient apprehension, fear/anxiety. Report if persistent so dosage may be adjusted.
6. Report as indicated for DRE and PSA to ensure prostate lesion free.
7. Avoid alcohol, excess caffeine, and OTC agents (especially cold remedies).
8. Excessive exercise/heat exposure, prolonged standing, and alcohol may intensify side effects.
9. Review lifestyle changes needed for BP control (i.e., dietary restrictions of fat and sodium, weight reduction, regular physical exercise, decreased use of alcohol, stress reduction, and smoking cessation).
10. For BPH control: no fluid intake 4 hr before bedtime, empty bladder before going to sleep, avoid caffeine and alcohol in the evening.
11. Keep all F/U to assess response, labs, and adverse SE.

OUTCOMES/EVALUATE

- ↓ BP
- ↓ Nocturia, urgency/frequency
- Improved stream with BPH
- ↓ Nightmares (UL)

AMINOGLYCOSIDES

SEE ALSO THE FOLLOWING INDIVIDUAL ENTRIES:

Amikacin sulfate
Gentamicin sulfate
Neomycin sulfate
Tobramycin sulfate

INDICATIONS/USES

These are powerful antibiotics that induce serious side effects; **do not use for minor infections.** (1) Gram-negative bacteria causing bone and joint infections, septicemia (including neonatal sepsis), skin and soft tissue infections (including those from burns), respiratory tract infections, postoperative infections, intra-abdominal infections (including peritonitis), UTIs. (2) In combination with clindamycin for mixed aerobic-anaerobic infections. Also, see individual drugs.

Used for gram-positive bacteria only when other less toxic drugs are either ineffective or contraindicated. Use in CNS *Pseudomonas* infections such as meningitis or ventriculitis is questionable.

ACTION/KINETICS

Action

Broad-spectrum antibiotics believed to inhibit protein synthesis by binding irreversibly to ribosomes (30S subunit), thereby interfering with an initiation complex between messenger RNA and the 30S subunit. This leads to production of nonfunctional proteins; polyribosomes are split apart and are unable to synthesize protein. Usually bactericidal due to disruption of the bacterial cytoplasmic membrane.

Pharmacokinetics
Poorly absorbed from the GI tract; usually administered parenterally (exceptions: some enteric infections of the GI tract and prior to surgery). Also absorbed from the peritoneum, bronchial tree, wounds, denuded skin, and joints. Distributed in the extracellular fluid. Crosses the placental barrier, but not the blood-brain barrier. Penetration of the CSF is increased when the meninges are inflamed.

Rapidly absorbed after IM injection. **Peak plasma levels, after IM:** Usually ½–2 hr. Measurable levels persist for 8–12 hr after a single administration. **t½:** 2–3 hr (increases sharply in impaired kidney function). Ranges of t½ from 24 to 110 hr have been observed. Excreted mainly unchanged in urine. Resistance develops slowly.

CONTRAINDICATIONS
Hypersensitivity to aminoglycosides, long-term therapy (except streptomycin for tuberculosis).

SPECIAL CONCERNS
(1) Aminoglycosides cause significant nephrotoxicity or ototoxicity. They are excreted primarily by glomerular filtration; thus, serum half-life will be prolonged and significant accumulation will occur in clients with impaired renal function. Toxicity may develop even with conventional doses, especially in those with prerenal azotemia or impaired renal function. (2) Neurotoxicity, manifested as both auditory and vestibular ototoxicity can occur with any aminoglycoside. Auditory changes are irreversible, usually bilateral, and may be partial or total. The risk of hearing loss increases with the degree of exposure to either high peak or high trough serum levels and continues to progress after drug withdrawal. The risk is greater in clients with renal impairment and with preexisting hearing loss. High frequency deafness usually occurs first and can be detected by audiometric testing. When possible, obtain serial audiograms. There may be no clinical symptoms to warn of developing cochlear damage. Tinnitus or vertigo may occur and are evidence of vestibular injury. Other symptoms of neurotoxicity may include numbness, skin tingling, muscle twitching, and convulsions. Total or partial irreversible bilateral deafness may occur after drug discontinuation. (3) Vestibular toxicity is more predominant with gentamicin and streptomycin; auditory toxicity is more common with kanamycin, amikacin, and netilmicin. Tobramycin affects both functions equally. Relative ototoxicity is streptomycin = kanamycin >amikacin = gentamicin = tobramycin >netilmicin. Kanamycin, amikacin, and streptomycin appear in this relative comparison based on high dose (kanamycin, amikacin) and antituberculosis (streptomycin) therapy. (4) Renal toxicity is characterized by decreased creatinine clearance, cells or casts in the urine, decreased urine specific gravity, oliguria, proteinuria or evidence of nitrogen retention (increasing BUN, NPN, or serum creatinine). Renal damage is usually reversible. The relative nephrotoxicity of aminoglycosides is kanamycin = amikacin = gentamicin = netilmicin >tobramycin > streptomycin. (5) Closely observe all clients treated with aminoglycosides. Monitoring renal and eighth cranial nerve function at onset of therapy is essential for those with known or suspected renal impairment and in those whose renal function is initially normal, but who develop signs of renal dysfunction. (6) Evidence of renal impairment or ototoxicity requires drug discontinuation or appropriate dosage adjustments. When possible, monitor drug serum levels. Avoid concomitant use with other ototoxic, neurotoxic, or nephrotoxic drugs. Other factors that may increase risk of toxicity are dehydration and advanced age.

- **Safe use in pregnancy and during lactation not established.**
- **Assess premature infants, neonates, and older clients closely; they are particularly sensitive to toxic effects.**
- **Considerable cross-allergenicity occurs among the aminoglycosides.**

SIDE EFFECTS
Ototoxicity: Both auditory and vestibular damage have been noted. Increased risk with poor renal function and in the elderly. Auditory symptoms include tinnitus and hearing impairment, while vestibular symptoms include dizziness, nystagmus, vertigo, and ataxia. **Renal Impairment:** Characterized by cylindruria, oliguria, proteinuria, azotemia, hematuria, increase/decrease in frequency of urination; increased BUN, NPN, or creatinine;

and increased thirst. **Neurotoxicity:** Neuromuscular blockade, headache, tremor, lethargy, paresthesia, peripheral neuritis (numbness, tingling, or burning of face/mouth), arachnoiditis, encephalopathy, acute OBS. CNS depression, characterized by stupor, flaccidity, and rarely, ***coma, and respiratory depression in infants.*** Optic neuritis with blurred/loss of vision. **GI:** N&V, diarrhea, increased salivation, anorexia, weight loss. **Allergic:** Rash, urticaria, pruritus, burning, fever, stomatitis, eosinophilia. Rarely, ***agranulocytosis and anaphylaxis.*** Cross-allergy among aminoglycosides has been observed. **Miscellaneous:** Joint pain, ***laryngeal edema, pulmonary fibrosis***, superinfection.

OVERDOSE MANAGEMENT

Symptoms: Extension of side effects.

Treatment: Undertake hemodialysis (preferred) or peritoneal dialysis. N-acetylcysteine, 600 mg twice a day, lowers the incidence of gentamicin-(and perhaps other aminoglycosides) induced ototoxicity.

DRUG INTERACTIONS

Bumetanide / ↑ Risk of ototoxicity
Capreomycin / ↑ Muscle relaxation
Cephalosporins / ↑ Risk of renal toxicity
Ciprofloxacin HCl / Additive antibacterial activity
Cisplatin / Additive renal toxicity
Colistimethate / ↑ Muscle relaxation
Digoxin / Possible ↑ or ↓ effect
Ethacrynic acid / ↑ Risk of ototoxicity
Foscarnet / ↑ Risk of nephrotoxicity
Furosemide / ↑ Risk of ototoxicity
Methoxyflurane / ↑ Risk of renal toxicity
Penicillins / ↓ Effect of aminoglycosides
Polymyxins / ↑ Muscle relaxation
Skeletal muscle relaxants (surgical) / ↑ Muscle relaxation
Vancomycin / Additive ototoxicity and renal toxicity
Vitamin A / ↓ Effect R/T ↓ absorption from GI tract

LABORATORY TEST CONSIDERATIONS

↑ BUN, BSP retention, creatinine, AST, ALT, bilirubin. ↓ Cholesterol values.

DOSAGE

See individual drugs.

NURSING IMPLICATIONS

IMPLEMENTATION/ADMINISTRATION/STORAGE

1. Check expiration date.
2. Warn if drug being administered stings or causes a burning sensation.
3. During IM administration:
   - Inject deep into muscle mass to minimize transient pain.
   - Use a Z-track method for thin, elderly clients.
   - Rotate/document injection sites.
4. With IV administration:
   - Dilute with compatible solution.
   - Infuse at the rate ordered to prevent excessive serum concentrations.
5. Administer for only 7–10 days. Avoid repeating course of therapy unless serious infection present that does not respond to other antibiotics.
6. Administer ATC to maintain therapeutic drug levels.

ASSESSMENT

1. Note reasons for therapy, other agents trialed, characteristics of S&S. Assess clinical presentation and for presence/source(s) of infection. Monitor and document fever, culture/lab reports, wound characteristics (i.e., color, odor, drainage, temperature), and symptoms.
2. Assess for allergies; note any history of sensitivity to anti-infectives.
3. List drugs prescribed to ensure none interact/potentiate adverse effects.
4. Weigh/calculate BMI to ensure correct dosage. For peak drug level determinations, when applicable, draw blood 1 hr after IM injection and 30 to 60 min after IV infusion in non-heparinized tube. For trough levels, draw just before next dose due. Ensure adequate hydration to prevent renal tubule irritation.
5. Some formulations may contain sodium metabisulfite (may cause allergic-type reactions e.g., anaphylactic symptoms and life-threatening or less severe asthmatic episodes in some susceptible individuals).
6. Monitor VS and I&O; increase fluids to prevent renal tubule irritation. Monitor drug levels (e.g., amikacin levels >30 mcg/mL are considered toxic).

7. With vestibular dysfunction protect by supervised ambulation and side rails; note (potential for) fall hazard.
8. Assess for ototoxicity with pretreatment audiograms. Hearing loss is a dose-related side effect of drug therapy most commonly associated with amikacin, kanamycin, neomycin, or paromomycin. Tinnitus, dizziness, and loss of balance are also signs of vestibular injury and more commonly seen with gentamicin and streptomycin. Deafness may occur several weeks after discontinuing drug.
9. Do not administer concurrently or sequentially with a topical or systemic nephrotoxic or ototoxic drug (e.g., potent diuretics such as ethacrynic acid or furosemide) unless provider designates benefits outweigh risks.
10. Observe for neuromuscular blockade with muscular weakness leading to apnea, when administered with a muscle relaxant, after anesthesia, or too rapidly during IV infusion. Have calcium gluconate or neostigmine available to reverse blockade.
11. With IM injections select large muscle mass such as gluteal or midlateral thigh and administer deep to prevent tissue damage. May use ice to relieve pain at injection site.
12. Note cells or casts in the urine, oliguria, proteinuria, lowered specific gravity, increasing BUN/creatinine, all of which indicate altered renal function. Obtain/monitor VS, U/A, C&S, renal and LFTs, auditory, and vestibular function; assess for nephrotoxity.

CLIENT/FAMILY TEACHING

1. Review goals of therapy and prescribed method of administration. Infuse as prescribed, ATC, until prescription is completed when utilizing home infusion therapy.
2. Follow a well-balanced diet and consume at least 2–3 L/day of fluids. If N&V or loss of appetite occur, try small frequent meals and frequent mouth care.
3. Report S&S of superinfection (black, furry tongue; loose, foul-smelling stools; vaginal itching).
4. Report lack of response after 3 days of therapy, alterations in hearing, vision, and/or ambulation. Use safety measures to prevent injury.
5. Keep all F/U to assess response, labs/cultures, and adverse SE.

OUTCOMES/EVALUATE

- Negative culture reports
- Resolution of infection with ↓ WBCs, ↓ fever, symptomatic improvement

AMPHETAMINES AND DERIVATIVES ■

SEE ALSO THE FOLLOWING INDIVIDUAL ENTRIES:

Amphetamine mixtures
Dexmethylphenidate hydrochloride
Dextroamphetamine sulfate
Lisdexamfetamine dimesylate
Methylphenidate hydrochloride

INDICATIONS/USES

See individual drugs. Uses include: (1) To improve wakefulness in those with excessive daytime sleepiness associated with narcolepsy. (2) As part of a total treatment program for attention deficit disorder with hyperactivity in children 3–16 years of age. *Investigational:* Dextroamphetamine for treatment of cocaine dependence and to treat autism.

ACTION/KINETICS

Action

Thought to act on the cerebral cortex and reticular activating system (including the medullary, respiratory, and vasomotor centers) by releasing norepinephrine from central adrenergic neurons. High doses cause release of dopamine from the mesolimbic system. The stimulatory effect on the CNS causes an increase in motor activity and mental alertness, a mood-elevating effect, a slight euphoric effect, and an anorexigenic effect. The anorexigenic effect is thought to be produced by direct stimulation of the satiety center in the lateral hypothalamic feeding center of the brain.

Peripheral effects are mediated by alpha- and beta-adrenergic receptors and include increases in both systolic and diastolic BP, respiratory stimulation, and weak bronchodilator activity. Large doses may cause cardiac arrhythmias.

Psychic stimulation is often followed by a rebound effect manifested as fatigue. Tolerance will develop to all drugs of this class. There is a relatively wide margin of safety between the therapeutic and toxic doses of amphetamines. However, both acute and chronic toxicity can occur.

Pharmacokinetics

Readily absorbed from the GI tract and distributed throughout most tissues, with the highest concentrations in the brain and CSF. **Duration of anorexia (PO):** 3–6 hr. Metabolized in liver and excreted by kidneys. Excreted slowly (5–7 days); cumulative effects may occur with continued administration.

CONTRAINDICATIONS

Hyperthyroidism, advanced arteriosclerosis, moderate to severe hypertension, symptomatic CV disease, narrow-angle glaucoma, angina pectoris, CV disease, and individuals with hypersensitivity to these drugs. Use in emotionally unstable persons susceptible to drug abuse, in those with a history of drug abuse, and in agitated states. Use of methamphetamine to combat fatigue or replace rest in normal people. Psychotic children. Lactation. During or within 14 days of MAO inhibitor use (hypertensive crisis may occur). Use not recommended in children less than 3 years of age for attention deficit disorder with hyperactivity. Use not recommended for weight control.

SPECIAL CONCERNS

(1) Amphetamines have a high potential for abuse. Use in weight reduction programs only when alternative therapy has been ineffective. Administration for prolonged periods may lead to drug dependence and must be avoided. Pay particular attention to the possibility of individuals obtaining amphetamines for nontherapeutic use or distribution to others. Prescribe or dispense sparingly. (2) There is an increased risk of cardiovascular effects and adverse psychiatric symptoms. There are reports of sudden death in clients with underlying heart disease or serious heart defects and cases of stroke and MI. Clients with a history of heart disease, depression, or psychosis should not receive these medications.

- Use with caution in clients suffering from hyperexcitability states; in elderly, debilitated, or asthenic clients; and in clients with psychopathic personality traits or a history of homicidal or suicidal tendencies.
- Prescribe with caution for clients with even mild hypertension.
- Amphetamines have been significantly abused leading to tolerance, extreme psychological dependence, and severe social disability. Clients may increase the dosage to many times that recommended.
- Amphetamines may exacerbate symptoms of behavior disturbance and thought disorder in psychotic children, and they may exacerbate motor and phonic tics and Tourette's syndrome.

SIDE EFFECTS

CNS: Overstimulation, restlessness, dizziness, insomnia, dyskinesia, euphoria, dysphoria, tremor, headache, changes in libido, psychotic episodes at usual doses (rare). Rarely, psychoses. In children, manifestation of vocal and motor tics and Tourette's syndrome. **GI:** N&V, cramps, diarrhea, dry mouth, constipation, metallic taste, anorexia. **CV:** Arrhythmias, palpitations, dyspnea, pulmonary hypertension, peripheral hyper-/hypotension, precordial pain, fainting, tachycardia, increased BP, reflex decrease in HR, cardiomyopathy after chronic use. **Dermatologic:** Symptoms of allergy including rash, urticaria, erythema, burning. Pallor. **GU:** Urinary frequency, dysuria. **Ophthalmologic:** Blurred vision, mydriasis. **Hematologic:** ***Agranulocytosis***, leukopenia. **Endocrine:** Menstrual irregularities, gynecomastia, impotence, changes in libido. **Miscellaneous:** Alopecia, increased motor activity, fever, sweating, chills, muscle/chest pain, weight loss, urticaria, impotence. Long-term use results in psychic dependence, as well as high degree of tolerance. Growth inhibition in children after long-term use. *NOTE:* Abrupt cessation following prolonged high doses results in extreme fatigue, mental depression, and changes on the sleep EEG.

OVERDOSE MANAGEMENT

Symptoms of Acute Overdose (Toxicity): Restlessness, irritability, insomnia, tremor, hyperreflexia, rhabdomyolysis, rapid respiration, ***hyperpyrexia***, assaultiveness, hallucinations, panic states, sweating, mydriasis, flushing, hyperactivity, confusion, hyper-/hypotension, extrasystoles, tachypnea, fever, delirium, self-injury, arrhythmias, ***seizures, coma, circulatory collapse, death. Death usually results from CV collapse or convulsions.***

Symptoms of Chronic Toxicity: Chronic use/abuse is characterized by emotional lability, loss of appetite, severe dermatoses, hyperactivity, insomnia, irritability, somnolence, mental impairment, occupational deterioration, a tendency to withdraw from social contact, teeth grinding, continuous chewing, and ulcers of the tongue and lips. Prolonged use of high doses can elicit symptoms of paranoid schizophrenia, including auditory and visual hallucinations and paranoid ideation.

Treatment of Acute Toxicity (Overdosage):

- Symptomatic treatment. After oral ingestion, induce emesis or perform gastric lavage, followed by use of activated charcoal. Acidification of the urine increases the rate of excretion. Give fluids until urine flow is 3–6 mL/kg/hr; furosemide or mannitol may be beneficial.
- Maintain adequate circulation and respiration.
- Treat CNS stimulation with chlorpromazine. Reduce stimuli and maintain in a quiet, dim environment. Treat clients who have ingested an overdose of long-acting products for toxicity until all symptoms of overdosage have disappeared.
- IV phentolamine may be used for hypertension, whereas hypotension may be reversed by IV fluids and possibly vasopressors (used with caution).

DRUG INTERACTIONS

Acetazolamide / ↑ Amphetamine effect by ↑ renal tubular reabsorption
Ammonium chloride / ↓ Amphetamine effect by ↑ renal tubular excretion
Anesthetics, general / ↑ Risk of cardiac arrhythmias
Antihypertensives / ↓ Effect
Ascorbic acid / ↓ Amphetamine effect by ↓ renal tubular reabsorption
Furazolidone / ↑ Toxicity of anorexiants R/T MAO activity of Furazolidone
Guanethidine / ↓ Guanethidine effect by displacement from its site of action
Haloperidol / ↓ Amphetamine effect by ↓ drug uptake at its site of action
Insulin / Altered requirements
MAOIs / All peripheral, metabolic, cardiac, and central amphetamine effects are potentiated for up to 2 weeks after termination of MAOI therapy (symptoms include hypertensive crisis with possible intracranial hemorrhage, hyperthermia, convulsions, coma); death may occur. ↓ Amphetamine effect by ↓ drug uptake into its site of action
Methyldopa / ↓ Hypotensive effect by ↑ sympathomimetic activity
Phenothiazines / ↓ Amphetamine effect by ↓ drug uptake at its site of action
SSRIs / ↑ Sensitivity to amphetamines; possible serotonin syndrome; if given together, monitor for increased S&S of CNS effects.
Sodium bicarbonate / ↑ Amphetamine effect by ↑ renal tubular reabsorption
Thiazide diuretics / ↑ Amphetamine effect by ↑ renal tubular reabsorption
Tricyclic antidepressants / ↓ Amphetamine effects

LABORATORY TEST CONSIDERATIONS

↑ BUN and creatinine (both transient and reversible). ↑ Liver enzymes, plasma corticosteroids, serum bilirubin, uric acid, blood glucose. Small ↑ serum potassium. Urinary steroid determinations may be altered.

DOSAGE

See individual drugs. Administer at the lowest effective dose and individualize dosage. Many compounds are timed-release preparations.

NURSING IMPLICATIONS

IMPLEMENTATION/ADMINISTRATION/STORAGE

1. Extended-release amphetamine mixture products are indicated for children 6 years and older.
2. Use a small initial dose; then increase gradually as necessary. Use lowest effective dose.
3. Unless otherwise ordered, give last dose of day at least 6 hr before bedtime.
4. When used for ADD in children, interrupt therapy on occasion to determine necessity for continued therapy.

ASSESSMENT

1. Note reasons for therapy, clinical presentation, characteristics of S&S, other agents trialed, outcome. List all drugs currently taking.
2. Assess for conditions that would preclude using drugs in this category, i.e., ASHD, HTN, hyperthyroidism, DM, glaucoma. Note age and if debilitated.
3. If agitated or complains of sleeplessness, reduce dosage of drug. If somnolent or appears mentally or physically impaired, stop the drug. Observe for signs of psychologic dependence and drug tolerance.

4. If receiving MAOIs or received them 7–14 days before amphetamine therapy, assess for hypertensive crisis. Monitor and report fever, marked sweating, excitation, delirium, tremors, or twitching; pad side rails and have suction available.
5. Under the Controlled Substances Act; follow appropriate policy for dispensing/handling to restrict availability and discourage abuse.
6. Monitor VS, ECG. Assess for arrhythmias, tachycardia, or hypertension. CV changes with psychotic syndrome may indicate toxicity
7. Monitor electrolytes, ECG, need for continued therapy, weight/height to assess for growth inhibition, VS, and CBC.

CLIENT/FAMILY TEACHING

1. Take only as prescribed, 1 hr before meals and last dose 6 hr before bedtime to ensure adequate rest. Do not share medications. Report S&S of tolerance. Abrupt withdrawal may cause adverse symptoms.
2. Report any changes in attention span and ability to concentrate. May cause a false sense of euphoria and well being and mask extreme fatigue. These may impair judgment and ability to perform potentially hazardous tasks, such as operating a machine or an automobile. Using amphetamines to treat fatigue is inappropriate because rebound effects may be severe.
3. Seek medical assistance if experiencing extreme fatigue and depression once drug is discontinued. Periodic "drug holidays" may be ordered to assess progress and prevent dependence.
4. Avoid OTC agents and ingesting large amounts of caffeine in any form. Read labels for the presence of caffeine since this contributes to CV side effects.
5. Manage dry mouth by frequent rinsing, chewing sugarless gum, or sucking sugarless hard candies.
6. Store safely out of child's reach.
7. Keep all F/U to assess response, labs, and adverse SE.

OUTCOMES/EVALUATE

- ↑ Attention span/concentration
- ↓ Episodes of narcolepsy

ANGIOTENSIN II RECEPTOR ANTAGONISTS

SEE ALSO THE FOLLOWING INDIVIDUAL ENTRIES:

Candesartan cilexetil
Eprosartan mesylate
Irbesartan
Losartan potassium
Olmesartan medoxomil
Telmisartan
Valsartan

INDICATIONS/USES

(1) Hypertension, alone or in combination with other antihypertensive drugs. (2) Nephropathy in type II diabetes mellitus (irbesartan and losartan). (3) Heart failure (NYHA classes II to IV) in those intolerant to ACE inhibitors (valsartan). (4) Reduce risk of stroke in those with hypertension and left ventricular hypertrophy (losartan). *Investigational:* Congestive heart failure. Can be combined with ACE inhibitors to reduce morbidity and mortality in clients with moderate to severe CHF.

ACTION/KINETICS

Action

Angiotensin II, a potent vasoconstrictor, is the primary vasoactive hormone of the renin-angiotensin system; it is involved in the pathophysiology of hypertension. Angiotensin II increases systemic vascular resistance, causes sodium and water retention, and leads to increased HR and vasoconstriction. The angiotensin II receptor antagonists competitively block the angiotensin AT_1 receptor located in vascular smooth muscle and the adrenal glands, thus blocking the vasoconstrictor and aldosterone-secreting effects of angiotensin II. Thus, BP is reduced. No significant effects on HR with minimal orthostatic hypotension and no significant effect on potassium levels. Does not inhibit angiotensin converting enzyme (ACE).

CONTRAINDICATIONS

Hypersensitivity to any component of the products. Lactation.

SPECIAL CONCERNS

When used during the second and third trimesters of pregnancy, drugs that act directly on the renin-angiotensin system can cause injury and even death to the developing fetus. When pregnancy is detected, discontinue angiotensin II receptor antagonists as soon as possible. ■

- Symptomatic hypotension may occur in those who are intravascularly volume-depleted.
- Fetal and neonatal morbidity and death are possible if given to pregnant women.
- Safety and efficacy not determined in children less than 18 years of age.

DOSAGE

See individual drugs.

NURSING IMPLICATIONS

ASSESSMENT

1. Note reasons for therapy, characteristics of S&S, PMH, other agents trialed, outcome.
2. Ensure adequate hydration to prevent severe hypotensive episode.
3. Not for use during pregnancy or lactation. Observe infants exposed in utero for hypotension, oliguria, fetal defects, and ↑ K^+.
4. Assess for allergic reactions, i.e., rash, fever, itching, angioedema.
5. Monitor VS, ECG, CBC, electrolytes, and renal function; reduce dose with dysfunction.

CLIENT/FAMILY TEACHING

1. Take only as directed, usually once daily. May take with or without food.
2. Advise surgeon that ARB is prescribed; blockage of renin-angiotensin system following surgery may be problematic.
3. Avoid activities that cause reduction in fluid volume, i.e., excessive perspiration, vomiting, diarrhea, dehydration; may cause low BP.
4. Dizziness may occur; avoid activities that require mental alertness until drug effects realized. Change positions slowly to prevent sudden drop in BP.
5. Continue regular exercise, weight loss, dietary restrictions, including low salt; stop tobacco/alcohol; lifestyle changes needed to lower BP.
6. Practice reliable contraception. Stop drug and report if pregnancy suspected; do not nurse infant.
7. Record BP regularly at different times of day for provider review.
8. Keep all F/U to assess response, labs, and for adverse SE.

OUTCOMES/EVALUATE

- Control of BP
- Stabilization of CHF
- Renal stabilization

ANGIOTENSIN-CONVERTING ENZYME (ACE) INHIBITORS ■

SEE ALSO THE FOLLOWING INDIVIDUAL ENTRIES:

Benazepril hydrochloride
Captopril
Enalapril maleate
Fosinopril sodium
Lisinopril
Quinapril hydrochloride
Ramipril
Trandolapril

GENERAL STATEMENT

The following are guidelines on the evaluation and management of chronic heart failure. The guidelines stress the early diagnosis of heart failure, marked by four stages:

1. Stage A: High-risk clients with no structural heart disease or symptoms.
2. Stage B: Structural heart disease without signs or symptoms.
3. Stage C: Structural heart disease with prior or current symptoms.
4. Stage D: Refractory heart failure requiring specialized interventions.

These stages complement, but do not replace, the New York Heart Association functional classification for heart failure.

Treatment guidelines for the various stages follow:

1. Stage A: Prevention through treatment of identifiable risk factors for heart failure, including hypertension, diabetes, and atherosclerotic disease. The guidelines recommend the use of ACE inhibitors for preventing heart failure in stage A clients with atherosclerotic vascular disease, diabetes, or hypertension. As an alternate, angiotensin II receptor blockers are recommended.
2. Stage B: Clients with a history of MI and/or reduced left ventricular ejection fraction should be treated with an ACE inhibitor and a beta blocker. Angiotensin II receptor blockers are recommended for those intolerant of ACE inhibitors. Beta blockers recom-

mended are bisoprolol, carvedilol, or sustained-release metoprolol succinate (Toprol XL).

3. Stage C: For clients with reduced left ventricular ejection fraction, an aldosterone antagonist (e.g., spironolactone, eplerenone) is recommended in carefully selected clients with either moderate or severe heart failure or left ventricular dysfunction early after MI, has been added as a class I recommendation. Monitor potassium to avoid hyperkalemia.
4. Stage D: Use of a left ventricular assist device as a permanent "destination" therapy should be considered for select clients. Intermittent infusion of positive inotropes is not recommended; continuous infusions of these drugs should be considered only as palliation in end-stage clients.

Therapeutic considerations include the following guidelines:

- All symptomatic clients should be receiving, at a minimum, both an ACE inhibitor and a beta-blocker (unless contraindicated).
- The dose of ACE inhibitor should be titrated to levels found effective in clinical trials.
- The dose of beta-blocker should be started low and titrated gradually to avoid worsening of symptoms.
- Those receiving an aldosterone antagonist should be monitored closely for hyperkalemia, which is usually precipitated by renal impairment or concomitant use of potassium supplements, NSAIDs, COX-2 inhibitors, or high doses of ACE inhibitors.
- Clients should not be prescribed drugs that worsen heart failure, such as antiarrhythmic drugs (other than amiodarone and dofetilide), nondihydropyridine calcium-channel blockers, NSAIDs, and thiazolidinediones.

INDICATIONS/USES

See individual drugs. Uses include, but are not limited to: (1) Hypertension, alone or in combination with other antihypertensive agents (especially thiazide diuretics). Can be used as initial therapy either alone or in combination with thiazide diuretics. (2) CHF, often in combination with diuretics and/or digitalis. Use captopril, enalapril, fosinopril, lisinopril, or quinapril. (3) In stable clients who are symptomatic from CHF within the first few days after an acute MI (use ramipril or trandolapril). (4) Asymptomatic left ventricular dysfunction (enalapril). (5) Diabetic nephropathy (captopril). (6) Improve survival following MI in clinically stable clients with left ventricular dysfunction (ejection fraction of 40% or less) and to reduce incidence of overt heart failure and subsequent hospitalizations (captopril). (7) Reduction of risk of MI, stroke, and death from CV causes (ramipril). (8) Improve survival in hemodynamically stable clients within 24 hr of acute MI (lisinopril). (9) Use in stable clients with evidence of left ventricular systolic dysfunction (trandolapril).

ACTION/KINETICS

Action

Believed to act by suppressing the renin-angiotensin-aldosterone system. Renin, synthesized by the kidneys, produces angiotensin I, an inactive decapeptide derived from plasma globulin substrate. Angiotensin I is converted to angiotensin II by ACE. Angiotensin II is a potent vasoconstrictor that also stimulates secretion of aldosterone from the adrenal cortex, resulting in sodium and fluid retention. The ACE inhibitors prevent the conversion of angiotensin I to angiotensin II. This results in a decrease in plasma angiotensin II and subsequently a decrease in peripheral resistance and decreased aldosterone secretion (leading to fluid loss) and therefore a decrease in BP. There may be either no change or an increase in CO. Several weeks of therapy may be required to achieve the maximum effect to reduce BP. Standing and supine BPs are lowered to about the same extent. ACE inhibitors are also antihypertensive in low renin hypertensive clients. ACE inhibitors are additive with thiazide diuretics in lowering blood pressure; however, beta-blockers and captopril have less than additive effects when used with ACE inhibitors.

CONTRAINDICATIONS

Hypersensitivity to the products or a history of angioedema due to previous treatment with an ACE inhibitor. Use of enalapril, enalaprilat, or lisinopril in clients with hereditary or idiopathic angioedema. Use of most ACE inhibitors during lactation.

Classifications

SPECIAL CONCERNS

■ **Pregnancy.** When used in pregnancy during the second and third trimesters, ACE inhibitors can result in injury to and even death in the developing fetus. When pregnancy is detected, discontinue the ACE inhibitor as soon as possible. ■

- ACE inhibitors may also cause congenital malformations (atrial and ventricular septal defects, patent ductus arteriosus, spina bifida, microcephaly, renal dysplasia) when present during the first trimester of pregnancy.
- May cause a profound drop in BP following the first dose; initiate therapy under close medical supervision.
- Use with caution in renal disease (especially renal artery stenosis), as increases in BUN and serum creatinine have occurred.
- Use with caution in clients with aortic stenosis due to possible decreased coronary perfusion following vasodilator use.
- It is possible that clients taking an ACE inhibitor and high-dose aspirin (325 mg/day) will have a higher mortality rate than those taking an ACE inhibitor alone or an ACE inhibitor plus low-dose aspirin (less than 160 mg/day).
- Most are used with caution during lactation, if at all.
- Geriatric clients may show a greater sensitivity to the hypotensive effects of ACE inhibitors, although these drugs may preserve or improve renal function and reverse LV hypertrophy.
- Compliance in taking the medication and inadequate dosage are problems with ACE inhibitors.
- For most ACE inhibitors, safety and efficacy not determined in children.

SIDE EFFECTS

See individual entries. Side effects common to most ACE inhibitors include the following. **GI:** Abdominal pain, N&V, diarrhea, constipation, dry mouth, dyspepsia, hepatitis, pancreatitis. **CNS:** Sleep disturbances, insomnia, headache, dizziness, nervousness, paresthesias, depression, somnolence, drowsiness, vertigo. **CV:** Hypotension (especially following the first dose or in those volume- or salt-depleted), palpitations, angina pectoris, ***MI, CVA, cardiac arrest***, orthostatic hypotension, chest pain, tachycardia. **Dermatologic:** Diaphoresis, sweating, flushing, pemphigus/pemiphigoid, pruritus, rash, urticaria. **Hepatic:** Rarely, cholestatic jaundice progressing to ***hepatic necrosis and death.*** **Respiratory:** Chronic cough, dyspnea, URTI. **Body as a whole:** Fatigue, malaise, asthenia, fever, photosensitivity. **Miscellaneous:** Impotence, syncope, asthenia, anemia, tinnitus. ***Angioedema*** of the face, lips, tongue, glottis, larynx, extremities, and mucous membranes. ***Anaphylaxis.***

OVERDOSE MANAGEMENT

Symptoms: Hypotension is the most common.

Treatment: Supportive measures. The treatment of choice to restore BP is volume expansion with an IV infusion of NSS. Certain of the ACE inhibitors (captopril, enalaprilat, lisinopril, trandolaprilat) may be removed by hemodialysis.

DRUG INTERACTIONS

Aldosterone inhibitors (e.g., eplerenone) / ↑ Risk of serious hyperkalemia → cardiac arrhythmias or arrest; monitor serum potassium periodically

Aliskiren / ↑ Risk of hyperkalemia; closely monitor potassium levels

Allopurinol / ↑ Risk of hypersensitivity reactions

Anesthetics / ↑ Risk of hypotension if used with anesthetics that also cause hypotension

Angiotensin II receptor antagonists (e.g., telmisartan) / ↑ Risk of renal dysfunction; coadministration not recommended

Antacids / Possible ↓ bioavailability of ACE inhibitors

Capsaicin / May cause or worsen cough associated with ACE inhibitor use

Cyclosporine / ↑ Risk of hyperkalemia; monitor serum potassium frequently

Digoxin / ↑ or ↓ Digoxin levels; monitor levels; also, possible ↓ effect of loop diuretics and inhibition of angiotensin II production by ACE inhibitors

Diuretics / Possible excess ↓ BP especially in those with intravascular volume depletion

Gold salts / ↑ Risk of nitroid reaction (e.g., facial flushing, hypotension, N&V); monitor

Hypoglycemic drugs / Possible ↑ hypoglycemia

Indomethacin / ↓ Hypotensive effects of ACE inhibitors, especially in low renin or volume-dependent hypertensive clients

Insulin / Possible ↑ hypoglycemia

Lithium / ↑ Serum lithium levels → ↑ risk of toxicity

Classifications

Loop diuretics / ↓ Effect of loop diuretics; possible inhibition of angiotensin II production by the ACE inhibitor
NSAIDs / ↓ Hypotensive effect of ACE inhibitors
Phenothiazines / ↑ Effect of ACE inhibitors
Potassium-sparing diuretics / ↑ Potassium levels; use together with caution and monitor potassium levels
Potassium supplements / ↑ Potassium levels; use together with caution and monitor potassium levels
Salicylates / Possible ↓ hypotensive effect of ACE inhibitor; consider ↑ dose of ACE inhibitor or stop salicylate if BP control or renal function deteriorates
Thiazide diuretics / Additive effect to ↓ BP
Trimethoprim / ↑ Risk of serious hyperkalemia → cardiac arrhythmias and death; closely monitor serum potassium

LABORATORY TEST CONSIDERATIONS

↑ BUN and creatinine (both transient and reversible). ↑ Liver enzymes, serum bilirubin, uric acid, blood glucose. Small ↑ serum potassium.

DOSAGE

See individual drugs.

NURSING IMPLICATIONS

IMPLEMENTATION/ADMINISTRATION/STORAGE

Do not interrupt or discontinue ACE inhibitor therapy without consulting provider.

ASSESSMENT

1. List reasons for therapy, onset, characteristics of S&S. Note any previous therapy with ACE inhibitors or antihypertensive agents and outcome.
2. Monitor VS (BP-both arms while lying, standing, and sitting). With heart failure, list stage of disease and functional classification. With MI note date and cath reports; with ventricular dysfunction note ejection fraction.
3. Document hereditary angioedema (especially if caused by a deficiency of C1 esterase inhibitor). Report evidence of angioedema (swelling of face, lips, extremities, tongue, mucous membranes, glottis, or larynx) especially after first dose (but may also see delayed response). Relieve S&S with antihistamines. If involves laryngeal edema, observe for airway obstruction. *Stop* drug; use epinephrine (1:1,000 SC).
4. Those hypovolemic due to diuretics, GI fluid loss, or salt restriction may exhibit severe hypotension after initial doses; supervise ambulation until drug response evident.
5. Assess for neutropenia (especially with captopril); precludes drug therapy.
6. If undergoing surgery or general anesthesia with drugs that cause hypotension, ACE inhibitors will block angiotensin II formation; correct hypotension with volume expansion.
7. List risk factors and medical problems. Identify lifestyle changes needed to achieve and maintain lowered BP. Assess motivation and ensure that a trial of "good behavior" with dietary modifications and regular exercise for 3 months has been done unless BP stage >2 and/or proteinuria with diabetes.
8. Monitor VS, I&O, weight, electrolytes, CBC, renal and LFTs; check urine for protein if negative on urinalysis; check for microalbuminuria especially in diabetics.

CLIENT/FAMILY TEACHING

1. Take 1 hr before or 2 hr after meals and only as directed. Drugs control but do not cure hypertension; take as prescribed despite feeling better and do not stop abruptly.
2. Review prescribed dietary guidelines; avoid potassium or salt substitutes containing potassium.
3. Do not perform activities that require mental alertness until drug effects realized; initially may cause dizziness, fainting, or lightheadedness. Rise slowly from a lying position and dangle feet before standing; avoid sudden position changes to minimize low BP effects.
4. Take and record BP readings at various times during the day to share with provider.
5. Practice reliable contraception; report if pregnancy suspected. Do not nurse.
6. Report adverse side effects such as: nonproductive, persistent, cough, sore throat, fever, swelling of hands/feet, irregular heartbeat, chest pains, difficulty breathing, or hoarseness, excessive perspiration, dehydration, vomiting, and diarrhea, itching, joint pain, fever, or skin rash, swelling or weight gain of more than 3 lb/day or 5 lb/week.

Classifications

7. **With diabetes (with/without hypertension), ACE inhibitors have been shown to reduce proteinuria and renal protection.**
8. **Avoid excessive amounts of caffeine (e.g., tea, coffee, cola) and OTC agents, especially cold remedies.**
9. **NSAIDs and aspirin may impair the BP lowering effects of ACE inhibitors; antacids may decrease bioavailability. Advise surgeon that ACE is being taken.**
10. **Avoid activities that may lead to a reduction in fluid volume, i.e., excessive perspiration, vomiting, diarrhea, dehydration may all cause drop in BP.**
11. **Regular exercise, proper diet, weight loss, stress management, and adequate rest in conjunction with medications are needed in the overall management of high BP. Additional interventions such as stopping alcohol/tobacco products, and decreased salt intake may assist in BP control.**
12. **Keep all F/U to assess response, labs, and adverse SE.**

OUTCOMES/EVALUATE

- ↓ BP; ↓ Morbidity post-AMI
- Improvement in S&S of CHF
- ↓ Proteinuria/renal damage

ANTIANGINAL DRUGS-NITRATES/NITRITES

SEE ALSO BETA-ADRENERGIC BLOCKING AGENTS, CALCIUM CHANNEL BLOCKING DRUGS, AND THE FOLLOWING INDIVIDUAL ENTRIES:

Isosorbide dinitrate
Isosorbide mononitrate
Nitroglycerin IV
Nitroglycerin sublingual
Nitroglycerin sustained release capsules
Nitroglycerin topical ointment
Nitroglycerin transdermal system
Nitroglycerin translingual spray

INDICATIONS/USES

(1) Treatment and prophylaxis of acute angina pectoris (use sublingual, transmucosal, or translingual nitroglycerin). (2) First-line therapy for unstable angina. (3) Prophylaxis of chronic angina pectoris (topical, transdermal, translingual, transmucosal), or oral sustained-release nitroglycerin; isosorbide dinitrate and mononitrate. (4) IV nitroglycerin is used to decrease BP in surgical procedures resulting in hypertension, as well as an adjunct in treating hypertension or CHF associated with MI. *Investigational:* Nitroglycerin ointment has been used as an adjunct in treating Raynaud's disease. Also, isosorbide dinitrate with prostaglandin E_1 for peripheral vascular disease. Sublingual and topical nitroglycerin and oral nitrates have been used to decrease cardiac workload in clients with acute MI and in CHF.

ACTION/KINETICS

Action

Nitrates relax vascular smooth muscle by stimulating production of intracellular cyclic guanosine monophosphate. Dilation of postcapillary vessels decreases venous return to the heart due to pooling of blood; thus, LV end-diastolic pressure (preload) is reduced. Relaxation of areterioles results in a decreased systemic vascular resistance and arterial pressure (afterload). The oxygen requirements of the myocardium are reduced and there is more efficient redistribution of blood flow through collateral channels in myocardial tissue. Diastolic, systolic, and mean BP are decreased. Also, elevated central venous and pulmonary capillary wedge pressures, pulmonary vascular resistance, and systemic vascular resistance are reduced. Reflex tachycardia may occur due to the overall decrease in BP. Cardiac index may increase, decrease, or remain the same; those with elevated left ventricular filling pressure and systemic vascular resistance values with a depressed cardiac index are likely to see improvement of the cardiac index.

Pharmacokinetics

The onset and duration depend on the product and route of administration (sublingual, topical, transdermal, parenteral, oral, and buccal). **Onset:** 1 to 3 min for IV, sublingual, translingual, and transmucosal nitroglycerin or sublingual isosorbide dinitrate; 20 to 60 min for sustained-release, topical, and transdermal nitroglycerin or oral isosorbide dinitrate or mononitrate; and up to 4 hr for sustained-release isosorbide dinitrate. **Duration of action:** 3 to 5 min for IV nitroglycerin; 30 to 60 min for sublingual or translingual nitroglycerin; several hours for transmucosal, sustained-release, or topical nitroglycerin and all isosorbide dinitrate products; and up to 24 hr for transdermal nitroglycerin.

CONTRAINDICATIONS

Sensitivity to nitrites, which may result in severe hypotensive reactions, MI, or tolerance to nitrites. Severe anemia, cerebral hemorrhage, recent head trauma, postural hypotension, closed angle glaucoma, impaired hepatic function, hypertrophic cardiomyopathy, hypotension, recent MI. PO dosage forms should not be used in clients with GI hypermotility or with malabsorption syndrome. IV nitroglycerin should not be used in clients with hypotension, uncorrected hypovolemia, inadequate cerebral circulation, constrictive pericarditis, increased ICP, or pericardial tamponade.

SPECIAL CONCERNS

- **Use with caution during lactation and in glaucoma.**
- **Tolerance to the antianginal and vascular effects may occur.**
- **Safety and efficacy not determined during lactation and in children.**

SIDE EFFECTS

Systemic. CNS: Headaches (most common) which may be severe and persistent, restlessness, dizziness, weakness, apprehension, vertigo, anxiety, insomnia, confusion, nightmares, hypoesthesia, hypokinesia, dyscoordination. **CV:** Postural hypotension (common) with or without paradoxical bradycardia and increased angina, tachycardia, palpitations, syncope, rebound hypertension, crescendo angina, retrosternal discomfort, ***CV collapse***, atrial fibrillation, PVCs, ***arrhythmias***. **GI:** N&V, dyspepsia, diarrhea, dry mouth, abdominal pain, involuntary passing of feces and urine, tenesmus, tooth disorder. **Dermatologic:** Crusty skin lesions, pruritus, rash, exfoliative dermatitis, cutaneous vasodilation with flushing. **GU:** Urinary frequency, impotence, dysuria. **Respiratory:** URTI, bronchitis, pneumonia. **Allergic:** Itching, wheezing, tracheobronchitis. **Miscellaneous:** Perspiration, muscle twitching, methemoglobinemia, cold sweating, blurred vision, diplopia, ***hemolytic anemia***, arthralgia, edema, malaise, neck stiffness, increased appetite, rigors.

Topical. Peripheral edema, contact dermatitis: Tolerance can occur following chronic use. Nitrites convert hemoglobin to methemoglobin, which impairs the oxygen-carrying capacity of the blood, resulting in ***anemic hypoxia***. This interaction is dangerous in clients with preexisting anemia.

OVERDOSE MANAGEMENT

Symptoms (Toxicity): Severe toxicity is rarely encountered with therapeutic use. Symptoms include hypotension, flushing, tachycardia, headache, palpitations, vertigo, perspiring skin followed by cold and cyanotic skin, visual disturbances, syncope, nausea, dizziness, diaphoresis, initial hyperpnea, dyspnea and slow breathing, slow pulse, ***heart block***, vomiting with the possibility of bloody diarrhea and colic, anorexia, and increased ICP with symptoms of confusion, moderate fever, and paralysis. Tissue hypoxia (due to methemoglobinemia) may result in ***cyanosis, metabolic acidosis, coma, seizures, and death due to CV collapse.***

Treatment (Toxicity):

- Induction of emesis or gastric lavage followed by activated charcoal (nitrates are usually rapidly absorbed from the stomach). Gastric lavage may be used if the drug has been recently ingested.
- Maintain in a recumbent shock position and keep warm. Give oxygen and artificial respiration if required.
- Monitor methemoglobin levels.
- Elevate legs and administer IV fluids to treat severe hypotension and reflex tachycardia. Phenylephrine or methoxamine may also be helpful.
- Do not use epinephrine and similar drugs as they are ineffective in reversing severe hypotension.

DRUG INTERACTIONS

Acetylcholine / Effects ↓ when used with nitrates
Alcohol, ethyl / Hypotension and CV collapse R/T vasodilator effect of both agents
Antihypertensive drugs / Additive hypotension
Aspirin / ↑ Levels and effects of nitrates
Beta-adrenergic blocking drugs / Additive hypotension
Calcium channel blocking drugs / Additive hypotension, including significant orthostatic hypotension
Dihydroergotamine / ↑ Effect R/T ↑ bioavailability or antagonism → ↓ antianginal effects
Heparin / Possible ↓ effect
Narcotics / Additive hypotensive effect
Phenothiazines / Additive hypotension

Classifications

Sympathomimetics / ↓ Effect of nitrates; also, nitrates may ↓ effect of sympathomimetics → hypotension

LABORATORY TEST CONSIDERATIONS

↑ Urinary catecholamines. False negative ↓ in serum cholesterol.

DOSAGE

See individual agents.

NURSING IMPLICATIONS

IMPLEMENTATION/ADMINISTRATION/STORAGE

Store tablets and capsules tightly closed in their original container. Avoid exposure to air, heat, and moisture.

ASSESSMENT

1. Note onset, location, intensity, duration, extent, and any precipitating factors (i.e., activity, stress) surrounding anginal pain. Rate pain levels.
2. List any sensitivity to nitrites.
3. If history of anemia, administer with extreme caution.
4. Nitrates are contraindicated with elevated intracranial pressure and use of certain drugs for erectile dysfunction.
5. Assess experience with self-administered medications; note if SL tablets ordered for bedside.
6. While hospitalized, record when consumed so effectiveness can be determined and usage monitored: (a) frequency given; (b) duration and intensity of pain (use a pain-rating scale; rate pain initially and 5 min after administration), and if relief is partial or complete; (c) time it takes for relief to occur; (d) side effects, or ECG changes
7. Assess for sensitivity to hypotensive effects (N&V, pallor, restlessness, and CV collapse). Monitor VS and for hypotension when on additional drugs; adjust as needed. Supervise activities/ambulation until drug effects realized.
8. Check for S&S of tolerance that occur following chronic use but may begin several days after starting treatment; manifested by absence of response to the usual dose. (Nitrites may be discontinued temporarily until tolerance is lost, and then reinstituted. During interim, other vasodilators may be used.) Managed by 12 hr nitrate rest.
9. Observe for N&V, drowsiness, headache, or visual disturbances with long-term therapy (may require a change in drug). Note change in activity and response to drug therapy. Determine if less discomfort experienced when performing regular activity
10. Note any changes in ECG or elevated cardiac markers, results of echocardiogram, stress test, and/or catheterization.

CLIENT/FAMILY TEACHING

1. Take oral nitrates on an empty stomach with a glass of water. Drug decreases myocardial oxygen demand and reduces workload of the heart.
2. To prevent sudden drop in BP, use inhalation products or take SL tablets while sitting or lying down. Make position changes slowly and rise only after dangling feet for several minutes. The elderly should sit or lie down when taking NTG; may become dizzy and fall.
3. Monitor BP and pulse and keep record for provider review. Some drugs may lower heart rate (calcium channel/beta blockers), and BP.
4. Avoid changing from one brand to another due to differences in effectiveness between different companies.
5. Always carry SL tablets for use in aborting an attack. Check expiration date; replace when needed or every 6 months. A burning sensation under the tongue attests to drug potency. Carry SL tablets in a *glass* bottle, tightly capped. Keep in original container as heat, moisture, and air cause deterioration. Do not use plastic containers; drug deteriorates in plastic; avoid child-proof caps as tablets must be accessed quickly.
6. If pain is not relieved in 5 min by first SL tablet, may take up to 2 more tablets at 5-min intervals. If pain has not subsided 5 min after third tablet, client should be taken to the emergency room; *do not* drive; call 911.
7. Identify and take SL tablets 5–15 min prior to any situation likely to cause pain (e.g., climbing stairs, sexual intercourse, exposure to cold weather). Record attacks; report any increase in the frequency/intensity of attacks and loss of NTG effectiveness. Schedule frequent rest

periods, pace activities, and avoid stressful situations. Use acetaminophen for headaches.

8. Follow instructions on how to apply topical nitroglycerin. Remove at bedtime and apply upon arising; a nitrate-free period of 8 hr may reduce/prevent nitrate tolerance.
9. Avoid alcohol; nitrite syncope, a severe shock-like state, may occur. Inhalation products are flammable; do not use under situations where they might ignite.
10. Do not smoke. Review risks and lifestyle changes necessary to prevent further CAD (i.e., weight control, dietary changes, ↓ salt intake, modified regular exercise program, BP control, DM control, no alcohol/tobacco, and stress reduction).
11. Have family or significant other learn CPR; survival rate is greatly increased when CPR is initiated immediately. Carry ID with prescribed drugs. Know what you are taking and why.
12. Keep all F/U to assess response, labs, and for adverse SE.

OUTCOMES/EVALUATE

- ↓ Myocardial oxygen requirements; ↑ activity tolerance
- Improved myocardial perfusion
- Relief of pain/coronary artery spasm

ANTIARRHYTHMIC DRUGS

SEE ALSO THE FOLLOWING INDIVIDUAL ENTRIES:

Amiodarone hydrochloride
Calcium Channel Blocking Agents
Digoxin
Diltiazem hydrochloride
Dofetilide
Flecainide acetate
Lidocaine hydrochloride
Phenytoin
Phenytoin sodium
Procainamide hydrochloride
Propafenone hydrochloride
Propranolol hydrochloride
Quinidine gluconate
Quinidine sulfate
Verapamil

GENERAL STATEMENT

Examples of cardiac arrhythmias are *premature ventricular beats, ventricular tachycardia, atrial flutter, atrial fibrillation, ventricular fibrillation,* and *atrioventricular heart block.* The various antiarrhythmic drugs are classified according to both their mechanism of action and their effects on the action potential of cardiac cells. Importantly, one drug in a particular class may be more effective and safer in an individual client. The antiarrhythmic drugs are classified as follows:

1. Class I. Decrease the rate of entry of sodium during cardiac membrane depolarization, decrease the rate of rise of phase O of the cardiac membrane action potential, prolong the effective refractory period of fast-response fibers, and require that a more negative membrane potential be reached before the membrane becomes excitable (and thus can propagate to other membranes). Class I drugs are further listed in subgroups (according to their effects on action potential duration) as follows:
   - Class IA: Depress phase O and prolong the duration of the action potential. Examples: Disopyramide, procainamide, and quinidine.
   - Class IB: Slightly depress phase O and are thought to shorten the action potential. Examples: Lidocaine, mexiletine, phenytoin, and tocainide.
   - Class IC: Slight effect on repolarization but marked depression of phase O of the action potential. Significant slowing of conduction. Examples: Flecainide, and propafenone. *NOTE:* Moricizine is classified as a Class I agent but it has characteristics of agents in groups IA, B, and C.
2. Class II. Competitively block beta-adrenergic receptors and depress phase 4 depolarization. Examples: Acebutolol, esmolol, and propranolol.
3. Class III. Prolong the duration of the membrane action potential (relative refractory period) without changing the phase of depolarization or the resting membrane potential. Examples: Amiodarone, bretylium, dofetilide, ibutilide, and sotalol.
4. Class IV. Depresses phase 4 depolarization and lengthens phases 1 and 2 of repolarization. Example: Verapamil.

Adenosine and digoxin are also used to treat arrhythmias. Adenosine slows conduction time through the AV node and can interrupt the reentry pathways through the AV node. Digoxin causes a decrease in maximal diastolic potential and duration of the action potential; it also increases the slope of phase 4 depolarization.

SPECIAL CONCERNS

- **Monitor serum levels of antiarrhythmic drugs since some drugs can cause toxic side effects that can be confused with the purpose for which the drug is used. For example, toxicity from quinidine can result in cardiac arrhythmias.**
- **Antiarrhythmic drugs may cause new or worsening of arrhythmias, ranging from an increase in frequency of PVCs to severe ventricular tachycardia, ventricular fibrillation, or tachycardia that is more sustained and rapid. Such situations (called proarrhythmic effect) may make it difficult to distinguish the proarrhythmic effect from the underlying rhythm disorder.**

DRUG INTERACTIONS

H ***Aloe*** / Chronic aloe use → ↑ serum potassium loss causing ↑ effect of antiarrhythmics

H ***Buckthorn bark/berry*** / Chronic buckthorn use → ↑ serum potassium loss causing ↑ effect of antiarrhythmics

H ***Cascara sagrada bark*** / Chronic cascara use → ↑ serum potassium loss causing ↑ effect of antiarrhythmics

H ***Rhubarb root*** / Chronic rhubarb use → ↑ serum potassium loss causing ↑ effect of antiarrhythmics

H ***Senna pod/leaf*** / Chronic senna use → ↑ serum potassium loss causing ↑ effect of antiarrhythmics

NURSING IMPLICATIONS

ASSESSMENT

1. **Note reasons for therapy, drug sensitivity, any previous experiences with these drugs. Assess extent of palpitations, fluttering sensations, chest pains, fainting episodes, or missed beats, prolonged QT; obtain ECG/rhythm strips showing arrhythmia.**
2. **Assess heart sounds, VS, and EF. Use cardiac monitor if administering drugs by IV route; monitor for rhythm changes.**
3. **Monitor BP and pulse. A HR <60 bpm or >120 bpm should be avoided. Obtain written parameters for BP and pulse limits.**
4. **Assess lifestyle related to cigarettes and caffeine use, illicit drug use, alcohol consumption, and lack of regular exercise. Certain foods, emotional stress, and other environmental factors may also trigger arrhythmias; identify and eliminate before instituting drugs.**
5. **Monitor BS, lytes, lipid panel, drug levels, renal and LFTs. Ensure serum pH, electrolytes, pO_2 and/or O_2 sats are WNL. Review EPS, stress test/catherization results, and/or Holter findings.**

CLIENT/FAMILY TEACHING

1. **Drugs work by controlling the irregular heart beats so the heart can pump more efficiently. Take as ordered. If dose is missed, do not double up.**
2. **Avoid activities that require mental alertness until drug effects realized.**
3. **Follow recommended dietary guidelines, avoiding/limiting salt, and fluids as directed.**
4. **Avoid OTC products. Eliminate caffeine, cigarettes, salt, and alcohol; these substances alter drug absorption and may precipitate arrhythmias or cause fluid retention with certain agents.**
5. **Record BP and pulse for provider review; identify specific levels to hold drug, i.e., HR <60 or BP <90/60.**
6. **Report concerns/fears or problems R/T sexual activity and side effects of drug therapy. Always carry list of prescribed medications and condition being treated.**
7. **Family/significant other should learn CPR and how to use a defibrillator; survival rates are greatly increased when CPR is initiated immediately.**
8. **Keep all F/U to assess response, labs, and for adverse SE.**

OUTCOMES/EVALUATE

- **ECG evidence of arrhythmia control; restoration of stable cardiac rhythm**
- **Serum drug concentrations within therapeutic range.**

ANTICONVULSANTS ■

SEE ALSO THE FOLLOWING INDIVIDUAL ENTRIES:

Carbamazepine
Clobazam
Clonazepam
Clorazepate dipotassium
Diazepam

Ethosuximide
Ezogabine
Felbamate
Fosphenytoin sodium
Gabapentin
Lacosamide
Lamotrigine
Levetiracetam
Oxcarbazepine
Phenobarbital
Phenobarbital sodium
Phenytoin
Phenytoin sodium extended
Phenytoin sodium parenteral
Primidone
Rufinamide
Tiagabine hydrochloride
Topiramate
Valproic acid/Divalproex sodium
Vigabatrin
Zonisamide

GENERAL STATEMENT

Therapeutic agents cannot cure convulsive disorders, but do control seizures without impairing the normal functions of the CNS. This is often accomplished by selective depression of hyperactive areas of the brain responsible for the convulsions. Therefore, these drugs are taken at all times (prophylactically) to prevent the occurrence of the seizures. There are several different types of epileptic disorders; consult the International Classification of Epileptic Seizures. No single drug can control all types of epilepsy; thus, accurate diagnosis is important. Drugs effective against one type of epilepsy may not be effective against another. Therapy begins with a small dose of the drug, which is continuously increased until either the seizures disappear or drug toxicity occurs. Monotherapy is preferred, but if a certain drug decreases the frequency of seizures but does not completely prevent them, another drug can be added to the dosage regimen and administered concomitantly with the first. Failure of therapy most often results from the administration of doses too small to have a therapeutic effect or from failure to use two or more drugs together. With appropriate diagnosis and selection of drugs, four out of five cases of epilepsy can be controlled adequately, but it may take the provider some time to find the best drug or combination of drugs with which to treat the client.

INDICATIONS/USES

See individual drugs. Use is specific to the drug or drug class.

ACTION/KINETICS

See individual drugs.

SPECIAL CONCERNS

Many anticonvulsants can significantly lower bone mineral density at fracture-relevant sites; consider use of calcium/vitamin D supplements.

SIDE EFFECTS

See individual drugs. Drugs that are used to treat seizure disorders increase the risk of suicidal behavior and ideation.

DOSAGE

Dosage is highly individualized. However, trauma or emotional stress may necessitate an increase in drug dosage requirements (e.g., if the client requires surgery and starts having seizures). For details, see individual agents.

NURSING IMPLICATIONS

IMPLEMENTATION/ADMINISTRATION/STORAGE

1. Shake oral suspensions thoroughly before pouring to ensure uniform mixing.
2. Drug therapy must be individualized according to client needs.
3. Do not discontinue abruptly unless provider approved. To avoid severe, prolonged convulsions, withdraw over a period of days or weeks.
4. If there is reason to substitute one anticonvulsant drug for another, withdraw the first drug at the same time the dosage of the second drug is being increased.
5. Be prepared, in case of acute oral toxicity, to assist with inducing emesis (provided the client is not comatose) and with gastric lavage, along with other supportive measures such as administration of fluids and oxygen.

ASSESSMENT

1. List reasons for therapy, onset, characteristics of S&S, clinical presentation, others agents used and outcome. Check medical history for hypersensitivity to anticonvulsant drugs. Note derivatives to avoid.

2. Assess mental status: orientation to time and place, affect, reflexes, and VS. Check skin, eyes, and mucous membranes.
3. Note seizure classification (partial or generalized); frequency/severity noting location, duration, consciousness, type, frequency and any precipitating factors, i.e., presence of aura, other characteristics. Note EEG, CT/MRI results, and any surgical approaches.
4. Check to see if pregnant; may cause fetal abnormalities.
5. With IV administration, monitor closely for respiratory depression and CV collapse. Note any evidence of CNS side effects, such as blurred/dimmed vision, slurred speech, nystagmus, or confusion; supervise ambulation until resolved.
6. Observe for muscle twitching, loss of muscle tone, episodes of bizarre behavior, subsequent amnesia.
7. With phenytoin, check Ca^{++} level; contributes to bone demineralization, which can result in osteomalacia in adults and rickets in children. Risk increases with inactivity. May require calcium replacement with vitamin D and periodic dexa scan for BMD.
8. Administer vitamin K to pregnant women 1 month before delivery to prevent postpartum hemorrhage/bleeding in the newborn and mother.
9. Determine why receiving therapy and when. If not physiologic and no seizures for over 2 years with prophylactic therapy, may consider gradual drug discontinuation after EEG documents lack of irritable foci.
10. Monitor CBC, glucose, electrolytes, uric acid, urinalysis, renal and LFTs.

CLIENT/FAMILY TEACHING

1. Take drug as prescribed. Do not increase, decrease, or discontinue without approval; seizures may result. Lessen GI distress by taking with large amounts of fluids or with food. Increase fluid intake and include fruit and other foods with roughage and bulk in the diet.
2. Avoid driving. Many states require certification that one is seizure free for 6 months or more before license granted. May initially cause a decrease in mental alertness, drowsiness, headache, dizziness, and incoordination. CNS symptoms are dose-related and should subside with continued therapy; avoid hazardous tasks until symptoms resolve.
3. Dosage may change if undergoing physical trauma or emotional distress. Avoid alcohol and any other CNS depressants.
4. Calcium and vitamin D may be prescribed to prevent hypocalcemia (400 IU vitamin D and 600 mg Ca^{++} daily); folic acid may prevent megaloblastic anemia.
5. Regular oral hygiene is important. With loose gums, intensify oral hygiene, routinely use dental floss, soft toothbrush, massage gums, and get regular dental exams.
6. If slurred speech develops, try to consciously talk slower to avoid the problem. Avoid situations/exposures that result in fever and low sugar and sodium levels; may lower seizure threshold.
7. Report if rash, fever, severe headaches, pain/swelling of mouth, nose, and urinary tract, or balanitis (inflammation of the glans penis) occur; S&S of hypersensitivity; requires change in drug.
8. Report sore throat, easy bruising/bleeding, or nosebleeds: S&S of hematologic toxicity. Jaundice, dark urine, appetite loss, and abdominal pain may indicate liver toxicity. To detect hepatitis, hepatocellular degeneration, and fatal hepatocellular necrosis obtain labs for LFTs, as ordered.
9. Practice reliable birth control; may harm fetus. If nursing, observe infant for signs of toxicity.
10. Carry ID with the type of seizures and prescribed therapy. Family should learn CPR and how to protect client during a seizure.
11. Identify support groups (Epilepsy Foundation; Brain Injury Association National Help Line: 1-800-444-6443 and website: http://www.biausa.org) that may assist with understanding and coping with these disorders.
12. Keep all F/U to assess response, labs, and for adverse SE.

OUTCOMES/EVALUATE

- ↓ Frequency of seizures; improved seizure control
- Serum drug levels within desired range

ANTIDEPRESSANTS, TRICYCLIC ■

SEE ALSO THE FOLLOWING INDIVIDUAL ENTRIES:

Amitriptyline hydrochloride

Amoxapine*
Desipramine hydrochloride
Doxepin hydrochloride
Imipramine hydrochloride*
Imipramine pamoate*
Nortriptyline hydrochloride

Drugs marked with an * are available to view in the 2013 Nurse's Drug Handbook Website at www.cengage.com/community/nursesdrughandbook.

GENERAL STATEMENT

Drugs with antidepressant effects include the tricyclic antidepressants (TCAs); tetracyclic agents (i.e., maprotiline, mirtazapine); selective serotonin reuptake inhibitors (SSRIs) (i.e., citalopram, escitalopram, fluoxetine, fluvoxamine, paroxetine, sertraline); serotonin and norepinephrine reuptake inhibitors (i.e., desvenlafaxine, duloxetine, venlafaxine); and monoamine oxidase inhibitors (MAOIs) (i.e., isocarboxazid, phenelzine, tranylcypromine).

INDICATIONS/USES

(1) Endogenous and reactive depressions. (2) Drugs with significant sedative effects may be useful in depression associated with anxiety and sleep disturbances. The selective serotonin reuptake inhibitors are the most widely used antidepressants. See also individual drugs, as some are used for other purposes (e.g., enuresis, obsessive-compulsive disorder).

ACTION/KINETICS

Action

It is believed antidepressant drugs cause adaptive changes in the serotonin and norepinephrine receptor systems, resulting in changes in the sensitivities of both presynaptic and postsynaptic receptor sites. These effects may increase the sensitivity of postsynaptic alpha-1 adrenergic and serotonin receptors and decrease the sensitivity of presynaptic receptor sites. The overall effect is a reregulation of the abnormal receptor neurotransmitter relationship. The tricyclic antidepressants are chemically related to the phenothiazines; thus, they exhibit many of the same pharmacologic effects (e.g., anticholinergic, antiserotonin, sedative, antihistaminic, and hypotensive). The TCAs are less effective for depressed clients in the presence of organic brain damage or schizophrenia. Also, they can induce mania; note when given to clients with manic-depressive psychoses. *NOTE:* Genotyping may be able to predict response to antidepressants.

Pharmacokinetics

Well absorbed from the GI tract; significant first-pass effect. **Peak plasma levels:** 2–4 hr; the association between plasma levels and therapeutic effect has not been defined adequately. All have a long serum half-life. Up to 4 to 6 days may be required to reach steady plasma levels and maximum therapeutic effects may not be noted for 2 to 4 weeks. Because of the long half-life, single daily dosage may suffice. More than 90% bound to plasma protein. Partially metabolized in the liver; some are metabolized to active compounds. Excreted primarily in the urine.

CONTRAINDICATIONS

Severely impaired liver function. Use during acute recovery phase from MI. Concomitant use with MAOIs (See *Implementation/Administration/Storage*). Generally, not recommended for those less than 12 years of age.

SPECIAL CONCERNS

(1) Antidepressants increased the risk of suicidal thinking and behavior (suicidality) in short-term studies in children and young adults with major depressive disorder and other psychiatric disorders. Anyone considering the use of antidepressants in a child or young adult must balance this risk with the clinical need. Clients who are started on therapy should be observed closely for clinical worsening, suicidality, or unusual changes in behavior. Families and caregivers should be advised of the need for close observation and communication with the prescriber. (2) Short-term placebo-controlled trials of nine antidepressant drugs in children and adolescents with major depressive disorder, obsessive-compulsive disorder, or other psychiatric disorders revealed a greater risk of adverse reactions during the first few months of treatment. The average risk of such reactions in clients receiving antidepressants was 4%, twice the placebo risk of 2%. No suicides occurred in these trials.

- **Use of antidepressants in children, adolescents, and young adults may also be associated with suicidality; this group should be monitored care-**

fully if they are taking antidepressants to treat depression.

- **Use with caution during lactation and with epilepsy (seizure threshold is lowered), CV diseases (possibility of conduction defects, arrhythmias, CHF, sinus tachycardia, MI, strokes, tachycardia), glaucoma, BPH, suicidal tendencies, a history of urinary retention, and the elderly.**
- **Use during pregnancy only when benefits clearly outweigh risks.**
- **Geriatric clients may be more sensitive to the anticholinergic and sedative side effects.**
- **Electroconvulsive therapy may increase the hazards of therapy.**
- **Cross sensitivity may occur among clomipramine, desipramine, imipramine, nortriptyline, and trimipramine. Also, there may be cross sensitivity between doxepin and amoxapine.**

SIDE EFFECTS

Most frequent side effects are sedation and atropine-like reactions. **CNS:** Agitation, akathisia, EEG pattern alterations, ataxia, anxiety, coma, confusion, disorientation, disturbed concentration, dizziness, drowsiness, dysarthria, exacerbation of psychosis, excitement, excessive appetite, extrapyramidal symptoms (including tardive dyskinesia), fatigue, hallucinations, delusions, headache, hyperthermia, hypomania, incoordination, insomnia, mania, nervousness, neuroleptic malignant syndrome, numbness, panic, nightmares, paresthesias of extremities, peripheral neuropathy, tremors, seizures, restlessness, weakness, tingling. **Anticholinergic:** Dry mouth, blurred vision, increased IOP, disturbed accommodation, mydriasis, constipation, paralytic ileus, urinary retention, delayed micturition, urinary tract dilation, hyperpyrexia. **GI:** N&V, abdominal pain or cramps, anorexia, aphthous stomatitis, constipation, diarrhea, epigastric distress, black tongue, dysphagia, increased pancreatic enzymes, flatulence, indigestion, GI disorder, parotid swelling, stomatitis, taste disturbance, peculiar taste, ulcerative stomatitis, hepatitis (rare), jaundice. **CV:** Arrhythmias, ECG changes, flushing, change in AV conduction, ***heart block, stroke, sudden death***, hot flushes, hypertension, hypotension, orthostatic hypotension, palpitations, CHF, PVCs, syncope, tachycardia. **Dermatologic:** Skin rashes, urticaria, flushing, pruritus, petechiae, photosensitivity, edema. **GU:** Testicular swelling and gynecomastia in males, increase or decrease in libido, impotence, menstrual irregularities and galactorrhea in females, breast enlargement, impotence, painful ejaculation, nocturia, urinary frequency. **Hematologic:** Agranulocytosis, aplastic anemia, leukopenia, thrombocytopenia, purpura, eosinophilia. **Hypersensitivity:** Drug fever, edema (generalized or of face/tongue), itching, petechiae, photosensitivity, pruritus, rash, urticaria, vasculitis. **Metabolic:** Increase or decrease in blood sugar, inappropriate ADH secretion. **Miscellaneous:** Sweating, alopecia, fever, hyperthermia, proneness to falling, weight gain or loss, nasal congestion, abnormal lacrimation, tinnitus, chills, worsening of asthma.

High dosage increases the frequency of seizures in epileptic clients and may cause epileptiform attacks in normal subjects.

OVERDOSE MANAGEMENT

Symptoms: CNS symptoms include agitation, confusion, hallucinations, hyperactive reflexes, choreoathetosis, ***seizures, coma.*** Anticholinergic symptoms include dilated pupils, dry mouth, flushing, and ***hyperpyrexia.*** CV toxicity includes depressed myocardial contractility, decreased HR, decreased coronary blood flow, tachycardia, intraventricular block, ***complete AV block, re-entry ventricular arrhythmias, PVCs, ventricular tachycardia or fibrillation, sudden cardiac arrest***, hypotension, pulmonary edema.

Treatment: Admit client to hospital and monitor ECG closely for 3 to 5 days.

- Empty stomach in alert clients by inducing vomiting followed by gastric lavage and charcoal administration **after insertion of cuffed ET tube.** Maintain respiration and avoid the use of respiratory stimulants.
- Normal or half-normal saline to prevent water intoxication.
- To reverse the CV effects (e.g., hypotension and cardiac dysrhythmias), give hypertonic sodium bicarbonate. The usual dose is 0.52 mEq/kg by IV bolus followed by IV infusion to maintain the blood at pH 7.5. If hypotension is not reversed by bicarbonate, vasopressors (e.g., dopamine) and fluid expansion may be needed. If the cardiac dysrhythmias do not respond to bicarbonate, lidocaine or phenytoin may be used.
- Isoproterenol may be effective in controlling bradyarrhythmias and torsades de pointes ventricular tachycardia. Use propranolol,

0.1 mg/kg IV (up to 0.25 mg by IV bolus), to treat life-threatening ventricular arrhythmias in children.

- Treat shock and metabolic acidosis with IV fluids, oxygen, bicarbonate, and corticosteroids.
- Control hyperpyrexia by external means (ice pack, cool baths, spongings).
- To reduce possibility of convulsions, minimize external stimulation. If necessary, use diazepam or phenytoin to control convulsions. Avoid barbiturates if MAOIs have been used recently.

DRUG INTERACTIONS

Acetazolamide / ↑ Effect of tricyclics by ↑ renal tubular reabsorption
Alcohol, ethyl / Concomitant use may lead to ↑ GI complications and ↓ performance on motor skill tests; death has been reported
Ammonium chloride / ↓ Effect of tricyclics by ↓ renal tubular reabsorption
Anticholinergic drugs / Additive anticholinergic side effects
Anticoagulants, oral / ↑ Hypoprothrombinemia R/T ↓ liver breakdown
Anticonvulsants / TCAs may ↑ incidence of epileptic seizures
Antihistamines / Additive anticholinergic side effects
Ascorbic acid / ↓ TCA effects by ↓ renal tubular drug reabsorption
Barbiturates / Additive depressant effects; also, may ↑ liver breakdown of antidepressants
H ***Belladonna leaf/root*** / Additive anticholinergic effects
Benzodiazepines / TCAs ↑ effect of benzodiazepines
Beta-adrenergic blocking agents / TCAs ↓ effect of the blocking agents
Carbamazepine / ↓ Serum TCA levels; ↑ serum carbamazepine levels → ↑ pharmacologic/toxic effects
Charcoal / ↓ Absorption of TCAs → ↓ effectiveness (or toxicity)
Chlordiazepoxide / Concomitant use may cause additive sedative effects and/or additive atropine-like side effects
Cimetidine / ↑ Effect of TCAs (especially serious anticholinergic symptoms) R/T ↓ liver breakdown
Clonidine / Dangerous ↑ BP and hypertensive crisis
Diazepam / Concomitant use may cause additive sedative effects and/or additive atropine-like side effects
Dicumarol / TCAs may ↑ the t½ of dicumarol → ↑ anticoagulation effects
Disulfiram / ↑ Levels of TCAs; also, possibility of acute organic brain syndrome
Ephedrine / TCAs ↓ effects of ephedrine by preventing uptake at its site of action
Estrogens / Depending on the dose, estrogens may ↑ or ↓ the effects of TCAs
H ***Evening primrose oil*** / May worsen temporal lobe epilepsy or schizophrenia when taken with TCAs
Fluoxetine / ↑ Pharmacologic and toxic effects of TCAs (effect may persist for several weeks after fluoxetine discontinued)
Furazolidone / Toxic psychoses possible
Grepafloxacin / ↑ Risk of life-threatening cardiac arrhythmias, including torsade de pointes
Guanethidine / TCAs ↓ antihypertensive effect of guanethidine by preventing uptake at its site of action
Haloperidol / ↑ TCA effects R/T ↓ liver breakdown
H ***Henbane leaf*** / ↑ Anticholinergic effects
Histamine H-2 antagonists / ↑ Serum TCA levels
H ***Kava Kava*** / Additive effects
Levodopa / ↓ Effect of levodopa R/T ↓ absorption
MAOIs / Concomitant use may result in hyperpyretic crisis, excitation, hyperthermia, delirium, tremors, DIC, severe convulsions, coma, flushing, confusion, tachycardia, tachypnea, headache, mydriasis, and death although combinations have been used successfully
Meperidine / TCAs enhance narcotic-induced respiratory depression; also, additive anticholinergic side effects
Methyldopa / TCAs may block hypotensive effects of methyldopa
Methylphenidate / ↑ TCA effects R/T ↓ liver breakdown
Narcotic analgesics / TCAs enhance narcotic-induced respiratory depression; also, additive anticholinergic effects
Oral contraceptives / ↑ TCA plasma levels R/T ↓ liver breakdown
Oxazepam / Concomitant use may cause additive sedative effects and/or atropine-like side effects

Phenothiazines / Additive anticholinergic side effects; also, phenothiazines ↑ TCA effects R/T ↓ liver breakdown
Procainamide / Additive cardiac effects
Quinidine / Additive cardiac effects
Quinolone antibiotics / ↑ Risk of life-threatening cardiac arrhythmias, including torsade de pointes
Rifamycins / ↓ Serum TCA levels
H ***Scopolia root*** / ↑ TCA effects
SSRIs / ↑ Pharmacologic/toxic effects of TCAs; symptoms may persist for at least 5 weeks
Sodium bicarbonate / ↑ TCA effects by ↑ renal tubular drug reabsorption
Sparfloxacin / ↑ Risk of life-threatening cardiac arrhythmias, including torsades de pointes
Sympathomimetics / Potentiation of sympathomimetic effects → hypertension or cardiac arrhythmias
Tobacco (smoking) / ↓ Serum TCA levels R/T ↑ liver breakdown
Thyroid preparations / Mutually potentiating effects observed
Valproic acid / ↑ Plasma TCA levels → ↑ side effects
Vasodilators / Additive hypotensive effect

LABORATORY TEST CONSIDERATIONS

↑ Alkaline phosphatase, transaminase, prolactin, bilirubin; ↑ or ↓ blood glucose. False + or ↑ urinary catecholamines. Altered LFTs.

DOSAGE

See individual drugs. Dosage levels vary greatly in effectiveness from one client to another; therefore, carefully individualize dosage regimens.

NURSING IMPLICATIONS

IMPLEMENTATION/ADMINISTRATION/STORAGE

1. In adolescents, the elderly, and outpatients, use lower initial dosage than in adults; gradually increase dose as needed.
2. Individualize dose according to age, weight, physical, mental condition, and response to the therapy. Clients show the largest relative improvement during the first weeks of treatment.
3. For maintenance therapy, a single daily dose may suffice.
4. Dose usually administered at bedtime, so any anticholinergic and/or sedative effects will not impact ADL.
5. To reduce incidence of sedation and anticholinergic effects, start with small doses and then gradually increase to desired dosage levels.
6. Although tricyclic and MAOI combined use is usually contraindicated due to serious side effects, such combinations may offer significant advantages to those refractory to more conservative therapy. In conservative doses, with observance of MAOI dietary restrictions, and under close medical observation, combined therapy has been safe. Otherwise, at least 14 days (although some say 7 to 10 days) should elapse between MAOI discontinuation and tricyclic administration.

ASSESSMENT

1. Note reasons for therapy, behavioral manifestations, clinical presentation, symptom onset, and causative factors. Identify if receiving electroshock therapy; hazardous combination.
2. Monitor mental status. Assess for dysphoric mood, suicide ideations, and excessive appetite/weight changes. Note sleep disturbances, lethargy, apathy, physical hygiene, impaired thought processes, or lack of responses.
3. List drugs currently prescribed; some that may intensify depressive reactions include antihypertensives (i.e., methyldopa, beta blockers), antiparkinsonism, hormones, steroids, anticancer agents, and antituberculins (cycloserine) as well as barbiturates and alcohol.
4. Note S&S of allergic response, i.e., rash, alopecia, and eosinophilia. Sore throat, fever, easy bruising, unusual bleeding, presence of petechiae or purpura may be S&S of blood dyscrasias. Check for evidence of agranulocytosis, especially among elderly women and during the second month of therapy.
5. Assess for adverse endocrine disturbances such as increased/decreased libido, gynecomastia, testicular swelling, and impotence. With hyperthyroidism, assess for arrhythmias precipitated by TCAs. May alter blood sugar levels and require adjustment of hypoglycemic agent.
6. Report symptoms of cholestatic jaundice and biliary tract obstruction such as high fever, yellowing of the skin, mucous membranes and sclera, pruritus, and upper abdominal pain.

7. Discontinue TCAs several days prior to surgery; may adversely affect BP. Withdraw therapy slowly to avoid any withdrawal symptoms.
8. Assess for epileptiform seizures precipitated by the drug.
9. Note eye exam; report visual changes, headaches, halos, eye pain, dilated pupils, or nausea. May need to change, especially with glaucoma.
10. Monitor I&O; report abdominal distention, urinary retention, and absence of bowel sounds (i.e., paralytic ileus).
11. Differentiate type of depression based on diagnostic features related to reactive, major depressive, or bipolar affective disorders. Review symptoms to determine if affective, somatic, psychomotor, or psychological.
12. Monitor CBC, renal and LFTs. Record ECG, assess heart sounds, note any CAD, and evaluate neurologic functioning. Assess for tachycardia and increase in anginal attacks; may precede MI or stroke.

CLIENT/FAMILY TEACHING

1. Take sedating medications at bedtime to minimize daytime sedation; take those that cause insomnia in the a.m. or upon arising.
2. Use caution when performing tasks requiring mental alertness or physical coordination; may cause drowsiness or incoordination. Rise slowly from a lying position; do not remain standing in one place for any length of time. If feeling faint, lie down to minimize low BP effects. Determine best time to take.
3. GI complaints of anorexia, N&V, epigastric distress, diarrhea, blackened tongue, or a peculiar taste require a dosage adjustment. Take with or immediately following meals to reduce gastric irritation.
4. Increase oral hygiene, take frequent sips of water, suck on hard candy, or chew sugarless gum to maintain a moist mouth. A high-fiber diet, increased fluid intake, exercise, and stool softeners may prevent constipation. May affect carbohydrate metabolism; an adjustment of diabetes agent and diet may be indicated.
5. Avoid prolonged sun exposure, use sunscreen and protection if exposure necessary, may cause changes in skin pigmentation and skin burning.
6. May alter libido or reproductive function. Practice reliable birth control; report if pregnancy suspected. May consider sperm/egg harvesting prior to starting therapy.
7. Report alterations in perceptions, i.e., hallucinations, blurred vision, excessive stimulations. Watch those recovering from depression for suicidal tendencies; remove firearms/weapons from the home.
8. May take 4–6 weeks to realize a maximum clinical response; stay on treatment regimen. Will see provider more often the first 2–3 weeks; prescriptions will be for only small amounts to ensure compliance and to prevent an overdose; excess consumption can be lethal. Obtain number to call for help.
9. Do not stop abruptly, may experience withdrawal S&S. Avoid other drugs and alcohol during and for 2 weeks following TCA therapy.
10. Review when and how to take medications, reportable side effects, and importance of regular participation in psychotherapy programs (when indicated) to assist in goal attainment.
11. Keep all F/U to assess response, labs, and adverse SE.

OUTCOMES/EVALUATE

- Understand/accept illness, importance of counselling, drug therapy/medical supervision
- ↓ Depression evidenced by improved appetite, renewed interest in outside activities, ↑ socialization, improved sleeping patterns, ↑ energy
- ↓ Anxiety; improved coping skills

ANTIDIABETIC AGENTS: HYPOGLYCEMIC AGENTS

SEE ALSO ANTIDIABETIC AGENTS: INSULINS AND THE FOLLOWING INDIVIDUAL ENTRIES:

Acarbose
Exenatide
Glimepiride
Glipizide
Glyburide
Linagliptin
Liraglutide*
Metformin hydrochloride
Miglitol
Nateglinide
Pioglitazone hydrochloride
Pramlintide acetate
Repaglinide
Rosiglitazone maleate
Saxagliptin hydrochloride

Sitagliptin phosphate*

Drugs marked with an * are available to view in the 2013 Nurse's Drug Handbook Website at www.cengage.com/community/nursesdrughandbook.

GENERAL STATEMENT

The American Diabetes Association has developed standards for treating clients with diabetes. If followed, these standards will enable clients to decrease their blood glucose levels closer to normal; this will reduce the risk of complications, including blindness, kidney disease, heart disease, and amputations. The goals of these standards include establishing specific targets for control of blood glucose (usually between 80 and 120 mg/dL upon waking up and before meals, 160 mg/dL 2 hr afer a meal, and between 100 and 140 mg/dL at bedtime) and increased emphasis on educating clients for self-management of their disease. Targets for BP and lipid levels are also provided. If the guidelines are followed, it is estimated that the risk of development or progression of retinopathy, nephropathy, and neuropathy can be reduced by 50–75% in clients with insulin-dependent (type 1) diabetes. The guidelines suggest the following treatment modalities:

- Frequent monitoring of blood glucose.
- Regular exercise.
- Close attention to meal planning; consult a registered dietitian.
- For type 1 diabetics, either continuous SC insulin infusion or multiple daily insulin injections; for type 2 diabetics, consider insulin administration in certain situations, although dietary modification, exercise, and weight reduction are the cornerstone of treatment.
- Instruction in the prevention and treatment of hypoglycemia and other complications (both acute and chronic) of diabetes.
- Development of a process for ongoing support and continuing education for the client.
- Routine assessment of treatment goals.
- Control of BP.

INDICATIONS/USES

(1) Non-insulin-dependent diabetes mellitus (type 2) that does not respond to diet management and exercise alone. (2) Concurrent use of insulin and an oral hypoglycemic for type 2 diabetics who are difficult to control with diet and sulfonylurea therapy alone. One method used is the BIDS system: bedtime insulin (usually NPH) with daytime (morning only or morning and evening) oral hypoglycemic.Guidelines for oral hypoglycemic therapy include onset of diabetes generally in clients over 40 years of age (but is being noted more in children who are overweight and inactive, with poor dietary habits), duration of diabetes less than 5 years, absence of ketoacidosis, client is obese or has normal body weight, fasting serum glucose of 200 mg/dL or less, elevated glucose tolerance test, normal or high C-peptide, and hepatic and renal function is normal.

ACTION/KINETICS

Action

Sulfonylureas are classified as either first or second generation. *Generation* refers to structural changes in the basic molecule. Second-generation oral hypoglycemic drugs are more lipophilic and, as such, have greater hypoglycemic potency. Also, second-generation drugs are bound to plasma protein by covalent bonds, whereas first-generation drugs are bound to plasma protein by ionic bonds. The implication is that the second-generation drugs are potentially less susceptible to displacement from plasma protein by drugs such as salicylates and oral anticoagulants. First generation sulfonylureas include acetohexamide, chlorpropamide, tolazamide, and tolbutamide and are not widely used any longer. Second generation sulfonylureas include glipizide, glyburide, and glimepiride. In addition, there are several other classes of oral hypoglycemic drugs including (a) alpha-glucosidase inhibitors (e.g., acarbose, miglitol); (b) amylin analog (e.g., pramlintide acetate); (c) incretin mimetic agents (e.g., exenatide); (d) dipeptidyl peptidase-4 inhibitors (e.g., linagliptin, saxagliptin, sitagliptin); (e) biguanide (e.g., metformin); (f) meglitinides (e.g., nateglinide, repaglinide); (g) thiazolidinediones (e.g., pioglitazone, rosiglitazone). (h) glucagon-like peptide 1 (GLP-1) receptor agonist (e.g., liraglutide). These various classes act in a variety of ways (see below). *NOTE:* There are several combination products containing two oral hypoglycemic drugs (one of which is usually metformin) that act by different mechanisms (e.g., glyburide/metformin, glipizide/metformin, rosiglitazone/metformin).

The oral hypoglycemics act in one of the following ways: (1) Bind to plasma membranes of functional beta cells in the pancreas, causing a decrease in potassium permeability and membrane depolarization. This leads to an increase in intracellular calcium and subsequent release from insulin-containing secretory granules. The sulfonylureas enhance beta-cell response rather than change the sensitivity of beta-cells to glucose. To be effective, the client must have some ability for endogenous insulin production. (Examples are exenatide, glimepiride, glipizide, glyburide.) (2) Competitive, reversible inhibition of pancreatic alpha-amylase and membrane-bound intestinal alpha-glucosidase hydrolase enzymes, causing delayed glucose absorption (results in smaller increases in blood glucose following meals). Examples include acarbose and miglitol. (3) Acting as an amylinomimetic agent (i.e., affecting rate of postprandial glucose appearance), modulates gastric emptying, prevents postprandial rise in plasma glucagon, and causes satiety, which leads to decreased caloric intake and potential weight loss (example is pramlintide acetate). (4) Incretin mimetic agent that mimics the enhancement of glucose-dependent insulin secretion (example is exenatide). (5) Inhibitor of dipeptidyl peptidase-4 that results in slowing inactivation of incretin hormones, leading to increases in insulin release and decreasing circulating glucagon levels. Examples include saxagliptin and sitagliptin. (6) Decrease hepatic glucose production, decrease intestinal absorption of glucose, and improve insulin sensitivity by increasing peripheral glucose uptake and utilization (i.e., metformin). (7) Stimulate release of insulin from the pancreas (examples include nateglinide and repaglinide). (8) Decrease insulin resistance in the periphery and liver, resulting in increased insulin-dependent glucose disposal and decreased hepatic glucose output. These drugs are not insulin secretagogues. Examples include pioglitazone and rosiglitazone.

Differences in oral hypoglycemic drugs are mainly in their pharmacokinetic properties and duration of action.

CONTRAINDICATIONS

Stress before and during surgery, ketosis, severe trauma, fever, infections, pregnancy, diabetes complicated by recurrent episodes of ketoacidosis or coma; juvenile, growth-onset, insulin-dependent, or brittle diabetes; impaired endocrine, renal, or liver function. Use in diabetics who can be controlled by diet alone. Relapse may occur with the sulfonylureas in undernourished clients. Long-acting products in geriatric clients.

SPECIAL CONCERNS

- **Use with caution in debilitated and malnourished clients, during lactation since hypoglycemia may occur in the infant, and in those with impaired renal or hepatic function.**
- **Elderly may be more sensitive to oral hypoglycemics and hypoglycemia may be more difficult to recognize in these clients.**
- **Use of sulfonylureas has been associated with an increased risk of CV mortality compared to treatment with either diet alone or diet plus insulin.**
- **There may be loss of blood glucose control if the client experiences stress such as infection, fever, surgery, or trauma or develops syndrome X (insulin resistance or metabolic syndrome).**
- **Safety and efficacy not established in children.**

SIDE EFFECTS

Hypoglycemia is the most common side effect. **GI:** Nausea, heartburn, epigastric fullness, diarrhea, GI pain, constipation, dyspepsia, gastralgia, vomiting, proctocolitis, hunger, flatulence. **CNS:** Fatigue, dizziness, drowsiness, nervousness, asthenia, insomnia, tremor, anxiety, depression, chills, hypesthesia, hypertonia, somnolence, confusion, abnormal gait, decreased libido, migraine, anorexia, myalgia, arthralgia, weakness, paresthesia, vertigo, malaise, headache, confusion, abnormal gait, pain. **Hepatic:** Cholestatic jaundice, aggravation of hepatic porphyria, hepatitis. **CV:** Arrhythmia, hypertension, vasculitis. **Dermatologic:** Skin rashes, urticaria, erythema multiforme, pruritus, eczema, photophobia, morbilliform/maculopapular eruptions, allergic skin rash, exfoliative dermatitis, sweating, lichenoid reactions, porphyria cutanea tardia. **GU:** Polyuria, dysuria. **Respiratory:** Pharyngitis, dyspnea. **Hematologic:** Thrombocytopenia, leukopenia, ***agranulocytosis, aplastic/hemolytic anemia***, pancytopenia, eosinophilia. **Endocrine:** Inappropriate secretion of ADH resulting in excessive water retention, hyponatremia, low serum/high urine osmolality. **CV:** Arrhythmia, flushing, hypertension, vasculitis. **Ophthalmic:** Eye pain, blurred vision, conjunctivitis, retinal hemorrhage. **Miscellaneous:** Tinnitus, disulfiram-like reaction if taken with alcohol, rhinitis, polyuria, trace blood in stool, thirst, edema, leg cramps, syncope, resistance to drug action develops in a small percentage of clients.

OVERDOSE MANAGEMENT

Symptoms: Hypoglycemia. The following symptoms of hypoglycemia are listed in their general order of appearance: Tingling of lips and tongue, hunger, nausea, decreased cerebral function (lethargy, yawning, confusion, agitation, nervousness), increased sympathetic activity (tachycardia, sweating, tremor), seizures, stupor, coma.

Treatment: Mild hypoglycemia is treated with PO glucose and adjusting the dose of the drug or meal patterns. Severe hypoglycemia requires hospitalization. Concentrated (50%) dextrose is given by rapid IV and is followed by continuous infusion of 10% dextrose at a rate that will maintain blood glucose above 100 mg/dL. Client should be monitored for at least 24–48 hr, as hypoglycemia may recur (clients with chlorpropamide toxicity should be monitored for 3–5 days due to the long duration of action of this drug).

DRUG INTERACTIONS

Alcohol / Possible Antabuse-like syndrome, especially flushing of face and SOB. Also, ↓ effect of oral hypoglycemic R/T to ↑ liver breakdown
Androgens/anabolic steroids / ↑ Hypoglycemic effect
Anticoagulants, oral / ↑ Oral hypoglycemic effects by ↓ liver breakdown and ↓ plasma protein binding
Azole antifungals ↑ Oral hypoglycemic effect
Beta-adrenergic blocking agents / ↓ Hypoglycemic effect; also, symptoms of hypoglycemia may be masked
H ***Bilberry*** / Possible potentiation of antidiabetic agents
Calcium channel blockers / ↓ Hypoglycemic effect
Charcoal / ↓ Hypoglycemic effect R/T ↓ GI tract absorption
Chloramphenicol / ↑ Effect R/T ↓ liver breakdown and ↓ renal excretion
Cholestyramine / ↓ Hypoglycemic effect
Clarithromycin / Possible severe hypoglycemia in clients with moderately impaired renal function after taking sulfonylureas
Clofibrate / ↑ Hypoglycemic effect R/T ↓ plasma protein binding
Corticosteroids / ↓ Hypoglycemic effect
Diazoxide / ↓ Effects of both drugs
Digitalis glycosides / Possibly ↑ Digitalis serum levels
Estrogens / ↓ Hypoglycemic effect
Fenfluramine / ↑ Hypoglycemic effect
Fluconazole / ↑ Hypoglycemic effect
Gatifloxacin / Possible severe and persistent hypoglycemia refractory to IV dextrose after taking gatifloxacin
Gemfibrozil / ↑ Hypoglycemic effect
H ***Ginseng*** / ↑ Hypoglycemic effect
Histamine H_2 antagonists / ↑ Hypoglycemic effect R/T ↓ liver breakdown
Hydantoins / ↓ Effect of sulfonylureas R/T ↓ insulin release
Isoniazid / ↓ Hypoglycemic effect
Itraconazole / Possible hypoglycemia; monitor BG
Magnesium salts / ↑ Hypoglycemic effect
MAOIs / ↑ Hypoglycemic effect R/T ↓ liver breakdown
Methyldopa / ↑ Hypoglycemic effect R/T ↓ liver breakdown
Niacin,Nicotinic acid / ↓ Hypoglycemic effect
NSAIDs / ↑ Hypoglycemic effect of oral antidiabetics
Oral contraceptives / ↓ Hypoglycemic effect
Phenothiazines / ↓ Hypoglycemic effect
Probenecid / ↑ Hypoglycemic effect
Rifampin / ↓ Effect of sulfonylureas R/T ↑ liver breakdown
Salicylates / ↑ Effect of oral hypoglycemics by ↓ plasma protein binding
Sulfinpyrazone / ↑ Hypoglycemic effect
Sulfonamides / ↑ Effect of oral hypoglycemics by ↓ plasma protein binding and ↓ liver breakdown
Sympathomimetics / ↓ Hypoglycemic effect
Thiazides / ↓ Hypoglycemic effect
Thyroid products / ↓ Hypoglycemic effect
Tricyclic antidepressants / ↑ Hypoglycemic effect
Urinary acidifiers / ↑ Hypoglycemic effect R/T ↓ renal excretion
Urinary alkalinizers / ↓ Hypoglycemic effect R/T ↑ renal excretion

LABORATORY TEST CONSIDERATIONS

↑ BUN, serum creatinine, AST, LDH, alkaline phosphatase. Elevated LFTs. Hyponatremia.

DOSAGE

PO. See individual preparations. Adjust dosage according to needs of client. Exercise, weight loss, and diet are of primary importance in the control of diabetes.

NURSING IMPLICATIONS

IMPLEMENTATION/ADMINISTRATION/STORAGE

1. To decrease the incidence of gastric upset, take PO drugs with food.
2. If ketonuria, acidosis, increased glycosuria, or serious side effects occur, withdraw the medication.
3. Transfer from insulin:
   - If receiving 20 units or less of insulin daily, initiate oral hypoglycemic therapy and discontinue insulin abruptly.
   - For clients receiving 20–40 units of insulin daily, initiate oral hypoglycemic therapy and reduce insulin dose by 25–50%. Discontinue insulin gradually, using the absence of glucose in the urine as a guide. With glyburide, insulin may be discontinued abruptly.
   - For clients receiving more than 40 units of insulin daily, initiate PO therapy and reduce insulin by 20%. Discontinue insulin gradually, using glucose in the urine or finger sticks as a guide. It may be advisable to hospitalize clients on such high doses of insulin while they are being transferred to oral hypoglycemic agents.
4. Transfer from one oral hypoglycemic agent to another:
   - Except for chlorpropamide, no transition period is necessary. When transferring from chlorpropamide, use caution for 1–2 weeks due to the long chlorpropamide half-life.
   - Mild symptoms of hyperglycemia may appear during the transfer period. Perform finger sticks and test urine for ketones regularly (1–3 times daily) during the transfer period. Positive results must be reported.
5. Be prepared to treat if client develops severe hypoglycemia.
6. Review prescribed drugs to ensure none interact.
7. Type 2 diabetics who do not respond to the sulfonylureas are said to be *primary failures.* Responses to the sulfonylureas during the initial months of therapy followed by failure to respond are referred to as *secondary failures.* A Glucophage trial or combination therapy with insulin and/or up to three oral agents may be useful in these clients.

ASSESSMENT

1. Obtain a thorough nursing history. Assess mental functions to determine if able to understand the complexities of the monitoring and adjustment of medications, when and how to take prescribed agents, and impact on lifestyle.
2. If unsure of type of diabetes, may differentiate I and II with C-Peptide levels. C-peptide indicates endogenous insulin production. If not present, then total beta-cell failure has occurred, suggesting type 1 diabetes. Many younger children who are obese and inactive are developing type 2 diabetes at a very early age.
3. Note any previous experience with sulfonylureas and the outcome. Determine metformin and/or thiazolidinedione trial and the outcome; elderly do better with a slower metformin titration (i.e., increase dose weekly or increase by a half tablet instead of a whole tablet).
4. Document any stress. Clients about to undergo surgical procedures, who have suffered severe trauma, who have a fever and infection, or who are pregnant should generally not be placed on oral hypoglycemic agents.
5. Diabetics benefit from ACE and ASA therapy. Assess for metabolic syndrome or insulin resistance, i.e., obesity, HTN, ASHD, dyslipidemia, hyperinsulinemia and type 2 diabetes.
6. The underlying defect that causes type 2 diabetes is insulin resistance. Those with type 2 diabetes have an underlying genetic predisposition toward insulin resistance. Three factors that cause insulin resistance to worsen and lead to diabetes: getting older, gaining weight, and becoming more sedentary.
7. Routinely review eye and foot exams and labs for evidence of problems or loss of blood sugar control.
8. Monitor VS, ECG, lipid panel, electrolytes, CBC, HbA1c, and urine for microalbumin.

CLIENT/FAMILY TEACHING

1. Type 2 diabetes is a disease of metabolic dysfunction related to excessive weight gain, eating the wrong foods, insulin resistance, and physical inactivity. This disease may be reversed with weight loss, exercise, and changes in eating/lifestyle; identify goals.

2. Record blood sugar (and if directed, urine for ketones) at different times during the day and night for provider review. (Urine testing is not an accurate reflection of true serum glucose levels and should not be used to modify treatment.)
3. With hypoglycemic episodes, check finger stick at the time of the reaction. If BS <80 mg/dL drink 4 oz of juice (fast-acting CHO), followed by a longer acting CHO (approximately 10 grams) such as half a meat sandwich or 3–4 peanut butter crackers, and recheck finger stick in 15 min. If glucose is <100, repeat the process, i.e., juice and a CHO and another finger stick. Report frequency.
4. Medication helps to control high BS but does not cure diabetes; therapy is usually long term. Must adhere to prescribed diet if drug is to be effective; most secondary failures are due to poor dietary compliance; see dietitian as needed. Regular exercise (20–40 min 6 days per week), diet (men: 1,800–2,000 calories; women: 1,200–1,500 calories to maintain wt), weight control/loss are imperative.
5. Review list of high glycemic foods to avoid e.g., white and wheat bread, white potatoes, white sugar, cold cereals (except for bran), and white rice. Fiber helps to slow down how food is broken down, consume 25 grams per day.
6. Therapies that target insulin resistance (e.g., thiazolidinediones) and suppress hepatic gluconeogenesis (e.g., biguanide) provide the most benefit and are the preferred agents in early type 2 diabetes. Sulfonylureas are also useful in type 2 diabetes if the former two agents are not sufficient to control, blood glucose levels.
7. Insulin may be necessary if complications occur or sugar not well controlled. Review administration of insulin and how to rotate sites. Do not change brands of insulin or syringes. Review equipment use, methods of storage, and how to discard used syringes.
8. Report illness or if unusual itching, skin rash, jaundice, dark urine, fever, sore throat, nausea/vomiting, or diarrhea occurs.
9. With thyroid scans, advise lab that sulfonylureas interfere with the uptake of radioactive iodine.
10. Avoid alcohol; a disulfiram reaction may occur. Do not take any OTC agents without approval.
11. Need close medical supervision for the first 6 weeks and periodic lab tests until control attained; oral agents may cause blood dyscrasias, acidosis, or liver dysfunction.
12. Carry ID, a list of prescribed drugs, juice, and hard candy (such as Lifesavers need 6–8) or glucose tablets (chew 3) as source of fast-acting CHO. Avoid chocolate, as fat in chocolate may prevent rapid correction of blood sugar.
13. Keep all F/U to assess response, labs, and for adverse SE.

OUTCOMES/EVALUATE

- Knowledge/control of diabetes; adherence to exercise/drug/diet therapy
- ↓ Hypo-/hyperglycemic episodes
- HbA1c within desired range <8
- Prevention of target organ damage

ANTIDIABETIC AGENTS: INSULINS ■

SEE ALSO ANTIDIABETIC AGENTS: HYPOGLYCEMIC AGENTS AND THE FOLLOWING INDIVIDUAL ENTRIES:

Insulin aspart
Insulin detemir
Insulin glargine
Insulin glulisine
Insulin injection (Regular insulin)
Insulin injection concentrated
Insulin lispro injection
Isophane insulin suspension (NPH)
Isophane insulin suspension/Insulin injection 70/30, 50/50

GENERAL STATEMENT

Insulin preparations with different times of onset, peak activity, and duration of action have been developed. Such products are prepared by precipitating insulin in the presence of zinc chloride to form zinc insulin crystals. Based on these modifications, insulin products are classified as fast-acting, intermediate-acting, and long-acting. These preparations permit the provider to select the preparation best suited to the lifestyle of the client.

Rapid-Acting Insulins
1. Insulin aspart
2. Insulin glulisine
3. Insulin injection (Regular insulin)
4. Insulin lispro injection

Intermediate-Acting Insulins
1. Isophane insulin suspension (NPH)

Long-Acting Insulin
1. Insulin detemir
2. Insulin glargine

NOTE: Insulin preparations with various times of onset and duration of action are often mixed to obtain optimum control in diabetic clients.

INDICATIONS/USES
Human insulins are being used almost exclusively.
1. Replacement therapy in type 1 diabetes.
2. Diabetic ketoacidosis or diabetic coma (use regular insulin).
3. Type 2 diabetes when other measures have failed (e.g., diet, exercise, weight reduction), blood sugars are significantly elevated, or with surgery, trauma, infection, fever, endocrine dysfunction, pregnancy, gangrene, Raynaud's disease, kidney or liver dysfunction.
4. Glucose and regular insulin to treat hyperkalemia.
5. Insulin and oral hypoglycemic drugs have been used in type 2 diabetics who are difficult to control with diet and PO therapy alone.
6. Single component and human insulins for cases of local insulin allergy, immunologic insulin resistance, injection-site lipodystrophy, temporary insulin use (e.g., surgery, acute stress type 2 diabetes, gestational diabetes), and newly diagnosed diabetics.

ACTION/KINETICS
Action
Following combination with insulin receptors on cell plasma membranes, insulin facilitates the transport of glucose into cardiac and skeletal muscle and adipose tissue. It also increases synthesis of glycogen in the liver. Insulin stimulates protein synthesis and lipogenesis and inhibits lipolysis and release of free fatty acids from fat cells. This latter effect prevents or reverses the ketoacidosis sometimes observed in the type 1 diabetic. Insulin also causes intracellular shifts in magnesium and potassium.

Pharmacokinetics
Since insulin is a protein, it is destroyed in the GI tract. Thus, it must be administered SC so that it is readily absorbed into the bloodstream and distributed throughout the extracellular fluid. Metabolized mainly by the liver.

Diet
The dietary control of diabetes is as important as medication with appropriate drugs. The role of the nurse and dietitian in teaching the client how to eat properly cannot be underestimated. They must teach the client how to calculate exchange values of various foods. Food lists and food-exchange values published by the American Diabetes Association and the American Dietetic Association are valuable teaching aids. Diabetic clients should adhere to a regular meal schedule. The frequency of meals and the overall caloric intake vary with the type of drug taken and individual client needs. Close attention to meal frequency and meal planning is imperative, and a registered dietitian should be consulted. Diabetic children may be on a less restricted diet, adjusting the insulin dosage according to blood and urine glucose readings. Children with negative urine glucose tend to become hypoglycemic rapidly with exercise or decrease in appetite, and many providers allow for glucose spilling.

CONTRAINDICATIONS
Hypersensitivity to insulin. During episodes of hypoglycemia in clients sensitive to any component of the product.

SPECIAL CONCERNS
- **Pregnant diabetic clients often manifest decreased insulin requirements during the first half of pregnancy and increased requirements during the latter half.**
- **Inadequate or excessive insulin treatment of diabetic mothers inhibits milk production.**
- **Insulin is considered a high-alert medication in that it can cause injury when misused. Thus, it requires special handling to ensure safe use. Many products have similar names which may lead to errors related to confusion between Lente and Lantus insulins, Humulin and Humalog insulins, and between premixed products. Use ex-**

treme caution when selecting insulin to ensure the correct product will be used.

SIDE EFFECTS

Hypoglycemia: Due to insulin overdose, delayed or decreased food intake, too much exercise in relationship to insulin dose, or when transferring from one preparation to another. Even carefully controlled clients occasionally develop signs of insulin overdosage characterized by one or more of the following: Hunger, weakness, fatigue, nervousness, pallor or flushing, profuse sweating, headache, palpitations, numbness of mouth, tingling in the fingers, tremors, blurred and double vision, hypothermia, excess yawning, mental confusion, incoordination, tachycardia, loss of sensitivity, and loss of consciousness. Level of awareness is markedly diminished after an attack. Symptoms of hypoglycemia may mimic those of psychic disturbances. Severe prolonged hypoglycemia may cause brain damage, and in the elderly, may mimic stroke. **Allergic:** Urticaria, angioedema, lymphadenopathy, bullae, anaphylaxis. Occurs mostly following intermittent insulin therapy or IV administration of large doses to insulin-resistant clients. Antihistamines or corticosteroids may be used to treat these symptoms. **At site of injection:** Swelling, stinging, redness, itching, warmth. These symptoms often disappear with continued use. Lipoatrophy or lipodystrophy of subcutaneous fat tissue (minimize by rotating site of injection). **Insulin resistance:** Usual cause is obesity. Acute resistance may occur following infections, trauma, surgery, emotional disturbances, or other endocrine disorders. **Ophthalmic:** Blurred vision, transient presbyopia. Occurs mainly during initiation of therapy or in clients who have been uncontrolled for a long period of time.

Hypokalemia: Hyperglycemic rebound (Somogyi effect): Usually in clients who receive chronic overdosage.

DIFFERENTIATION BETWEEN HYPERGLYCEMIA (DIABETIC COMA) AND HYPOGLYCEMIC REACTION (INSULIN SHOCK)

Coma in diabetes may be caused by uncontrolled diabetes (high sugar content in blood or urine, ketoacidosis) or by too much insulin (insulin shock, hypoglycemia). Hyperglycemia is usually precipitated by the client's failure to take insulin. Hypoglycemia is often precipitated by the client's unpredictable response, excess exertion, stress due to illness or surgery, errors in calculating dosage, or failure to eat.

TREATMENT OF HYPERGLYCEMIA (DIABETIC COMA OR SEVERE ACIDOSIS)

Administer 30–60 units of regular insulin. This is followed by doses of 20 units or more q 30 min. To avoid a hypoglycemic state, 1 gram dextrose is administered for each unit of insulin given. Treatment is often supplemented by electrolytes and fluids. Urine/blood samples are collected for analysis, and VS are monitored regularly.

TREATMENT OF HYPOGLYCEMIA (INSULIN SHOCK)

Mild hypoglycemia can be relieved by PO administration of CHO such as orange juice, hard candy, or glucose tablets. If comatose, adults may be given 10–30 mL of 50% dextrose solution IV; children should receive 0.5–1 mL/kg of 50% dextrose solution. Epinephrine, hydrocortisone, or glucagon may be used in severe cases to cause an increase in blood glucose.

DRUG INTERACTIONS

ACE Inhibitors / ↑ Hypoglycemic effect of insulin
Acetazolamide / ↓ Hypoglycemic effect of insulin
AIDS antiviral drugs / ↓ Hypoglycemic effect of insulin
Albuterol / ↓ Hypoglycemic effect of insulin
Alcohol, ethyl / ↑ Hypoglycemia → low blood sugar and shock
Anabolic steroids / ↑ Hypoglycemic effect of insulin
Antidiabetics, oral / ↑ Hypoglycemic effect of insulin
Asparaginase / ↓ Hypoglycemic effect of insulin
Beta-adrenergic blocking agents / ↑ Hypoglycemic effect of insulin
Calcitonin / ↓ Hypoglycemic effect of insulin
Calcium / ↑ Hypoglycemic effect of insulin
Chloroquine / ↑ Hypoglycemic effect of insulin
Chlorthalidone / ↓ Hypoglycemic effect of antidiabetics
Clofibrate / ↑ Hypoglycemic effect of insulin
Clonidine / ↑ Hypoglycemic effect of insulin
Clozapine / ↓ Hypoglycemic effect of insulin
Contraceptives, oral / ↑ Dosage of antidiabetic R/T impairment of glucose tolerance; ↓ Hypoglycemic effect of insulin

Classifications

Corticosteroids / ↓ Effect of insulin R/T corticosteroid-induced hyperglycemia
Cyclophosphamide / ↓ Hypoglycemic effect of insulin
Danazol / ↓ Hypoglycemic effect of insulin
Dextrothyroxine / ↓ Effect of insulin R/T dextrothyroxine-induced hyperglycemia
Diazoxide / Diazoxide-induced hyperglycemia → ↓ diabetic control
Digitalis glycosides / Use with caution, as insulin affects serum potassium levels
Diltiazem / ↓ Hypoglycemic effect of insulin
Disopyramide / ↑ Hypoglycemic effect of insulin
Diuretics / ↓ Hypoglycemic effect of insulin
Dobutamine / ↓ Hypoglycemic effect of insulin
Epinephrine / ↓ Effect of insulin due to epinephrine-induced hyperglycemia
Estrogens / ↓ Effect of insulin due to impairment of glucose tolerance
Ethacrynic acid / ↓ Hypoglycemic effect of insulin
Fenfluramine / Additive hypoglycemic effects
Fibrates / ↑ Hypoglycemic effect of insulin
Fluoxetine / ↑ Hypoglycemic effect of insulin
Furosemide / ↓ Hypoglycemic effect of antidiabetics
H ***Ginseng*** / Possible additive hypoglycemic effects
Glucagon / Glucagon-induced hyperglycemia → ↓ effect of antidiabetics
Guanethidine / ↑ Hypoglycemic effect of insulin
Isoniazid / ↓ Hypoglycemic effect of insulin
Lithium carbonate / ↑ or ↓ Hypoglycemic effect of insulin
MAOIs / MAO inhibitors ↑ and prolong hypoglycemic effect of antidiabetics
Mebendazole / ↑ Hypoglycemic effect of insulin
Morphine sulfate / ↓ Hypoglycemic effect of insulin
Niacin / ↓ Hypoglycemic effect of insulin
Nicotine / ↓ Hypoglycemic effect of insulin
Octreotide / ↑ Hypoglycemic effect of insulin
Olanzapine / ↓ Hypoglycemic effect of insulin
Oxytetracycline / ↑ Effect of insulin
Pentamidine / ↑ Hypoglycemic effect of insulin; may be followed by hyperglycemia
Pentoxifylline / ↑ Hypoglycemic effect of insulin
Phenothiazines /↓ Hypoglycemic effect of insulin R/T phenothiazine-induced hyperglycemia
Phenytoin / Phenytoin-induced hyperglycemia → ↓ diabetic control
Propoxyphene / ↑ Hypoglycemic effect of insulin
Propranolol / Inhibits rebound of blood glucose after insulin-induced hypoglycemia
Protease inhibitors / ↓ Hypoglycemic effect of insulin
H ***Psyllium seed/ Blonde psyllium seed husk*** / Possible need to ↓ insulin dose
Pyridoxine / ↑ Hypoglycemic effect of insulin
Salicylates / ↑ Hypoglycemic effect of insulin
Somatropin / ↓ Hypoglycemic effect of insulin
Smoking / ↑ Insulin requirements in heavy smokers R/T ↓ SC insulin absorption; smoking may release endogenous substances that cause insulin resistance
Sulfinpyrazone / ↑ Hypoglycemic effect of insulin
Sulfonamides / ↑ Hypoglycemic effect of insulin
Terbutaline / ↓ Hypoglycemic effect of insulin
Tetracyclines / ↑ Hypoglycemic effect of insulin
Thiazide diuretics / ↓ Hypoglycemic effect of antidiabetics
Thyroid preparations / ↓ Effect of antidiabetic due to thyroid-induced hyperglycemia
Triamterene / ↓ Hypoglycemic effect of antidiabetic.

LABORATORY TEST CONSIDERATIONS

Hypoglycemia, hypokalemia. Alters liver function tests and thyroid function tests. False + Coombs' test, ↑ serum protein. ↓ Serum amino acids, calcium, cholesterol, and urine amino acids.

DOSAGE

Dosage highly individualized. Usually administered SC. Insulin injection (regular insulin) is the **only** preparation that may be administered IV. Give IV only for clients with severe ketoacidosis or diabetic coma. Dosage for insulin is always expressed in USP units. **Adults and children, usual dose:** 0.5–1 unit/kg/day. Dosage is established and monitored by blood glucose (often using glucose monitoring machines in the home), urine glucose, and acetone tests. Furthermore, since requirements may change with time, dosage must be checked at regular intervals. It may be advisable to hospitalize some clients while their daily insulin and caloric requirements are being established. The main goal is to control the blood sugar and send the client home to fine tune, as generally the home environment is more reliable for determining drug requirements.

In elderly clients, initial dosing, dosing increments, and maintenance dosing should be conservative to avoid hypoglycemic reactions, which may be difficult to recognize in the elderly.

In pregnancy, insulin requirements may increase suddenly during the last trimester. After delivery, requirements may suddenly drop to pre pregnancy levels. To prevent the development of hypoglycemia, insulin is often discontinued on the day of delivery and glucose is administered IV.

The various insulin preparations can be mixed to obtain the combination best suited for the individual client. However, mixing must be done according to the directions received from the physician/provider and/or pharmacist.

NURSING IMPLICATIONS

Also includes general applications for all clients with diabetes controlled by medication (whether it be insulin or an oral hypoglycemic agent).

IMPLEMENTATION/ADMINISTRATION/STORAGE

1. Read product information and any important notes inserted into the insulin package.
2. Color has been added to insulin packages to differentiate between products and prevent dispensing errors.
3. Lactating women may require adjustments in insulin dose and diet.
4. Discard open vials not used for several weeks or whose expiration date has passed.
5. Refrigerate stock supply of insulin but avoid freezing. Freezing destroys the manner in which insulin is suspended in the formulation.
6. Store vial in a cool place, avoiding extremes of temperature or exposure to sunlight.
7. Use the following guidelines with respect to mixing the various insulins:
   - Regular insulin may be mixed with NPH insulin. However, to avoid transfer of the longer-acting insulin into the regular insulin vial, withdraw regular insulin into the syringe first.
   - Give a mixture of regular insulin with NPH insulin within 15 min of mixing due to binding of regular insulin by excess zinc in the longer-acting preparations.
   - When used in an insulin infusion pump, insulin may be mixed in any proportion with either 0.9% NaCl injection or water for injection. Due to stability changes, use such mixtures within 24 hr of their preparation. Buffered insulin is usually the form prescribed and utilized in pumps.
8. Change insulins cautiously and under medical supervision. Changes in purity, strength, brand, type, or species source may require dosage adjustment.
9. Store compatible insulin mixtures for no longer than 1 month at room temperature or 3 months at 2–8°C (36–46°F); bacterial contamination may occur.
10. To ensure a constant amount of precipitate in each dose, invert the vial several times to mix before withdrawing the material. Avoid vigorous shaking and frothing of the material.
11. Discard any vial in which the precipitate is clumped or granular in appearance or which has formed a solid deposit of particles on the side of the vial.
12. To prevent dosage error, do not alter the order of mixing insulins or change the model or brand of syringe or needle.
13. Administer at a 90° angle with a 28- or 29-gauge needle. Syringes come in 0.3 mL (30 units), 0.5 mL (50 units) and 1 mL (100 units) sizes. Get the smallest syringe with the smallest needles to enhance dosage validity (e.g., if client is prescribed <30 units of insulin, advise to obtain the 0.3 mL syringe).
14. Provide an automatic injector for clients fearful of injections.
15. Assist visually impaired clients to obtain information and devices for self-administration by consulting their local diabetes association or by writing to the American Diabetes Association, 149 Madison Avenue, New York, NY 10016 (1-800-DIABETES or 1-800-342-2383), for their buyer's guide, which lists numerous products for diabetics. Clients may also contact The Lighthouse, Inc., 800 Second Avenue, New York, NY 10017 for additional information on visual impairments.
16. Lipoatrophy may occur. This may appear as mild dimpling of the skin or as deep pits in young girls and women and lipodystrophy appearing in well-developed muscle on the ante-

rior and lateral thighs of young boys and men. To prevent, rotate injection sites.

- Make a chart indicating the injection sites.
- Allow 3–4 cm between sites.
- Do not inject in the same site for at least 1–2 weeks.
- Avoid injecting within 1 cm around the umbilicus, because of the high vascularity in this area.
- Avoid injections around the waistline, because of the sensitive nerve supply to this area and the potential for fabric irritation.
- Use insulin at room temperature to prevent lipodystrophy.

17. Rotation of injection sites may lead to differences in blood levels of insulin. The abdomen is considered the best site due to constant insulin peak times with better gradual absorption. Apply gentle pressure after injection, but do not massage since this may alter rate of absorption.
18. If insulin has been refrigerated, allow it to remain at room temperature for at least 1 hr before using.
19. If breakfast is delayed for lab tests, check for dosage adjustment.

ASSESSMENT

1. Obtain thorough history and physical exam. Note any first-degree relatives with disease; there's a genetic predisposition.
2. There are several autoimmune diseases associated with type 1 diabetes. Celiac disease is the most common, but also Graves' disease, hypothyroidism, adrenal insufficiency, and pernicious anemia are related.
3. Specific autoantibodies to islet cells, insulin, and glutamic acid decarboxylase help identify those with autoimmune type 1 diabetes. Antibodies to glutamic acid decarboxylase 65 (GAD65) considered to be the most specific antibodies. Islet cell antibodies (ICA) are also present in the serum of patients with type 1 diabetes. Insulin autoantibodies can also be ordered but must be done before the client has any exposure to exogenous insulin
4. Assess for S&S of hyperglycemia: thirst, polydipsia, polyuria, drowsiness, blurred vision, loss of appetite, fruity odor to the breath, and flushed dry skin.
5. Assess for S&S of hypoglycemia: drowsiness, chills, confusion, anxiety, cold sweats, cool pale skin, excessive hunger, nausea, headache, irritability, shakiness, rapid pulse, and unusual weakness or tiredness.
6. For a *hyperglycemic reaction:*
   - Have regular insulin available.
   - Obtain BS or finger stick.
   - Monitor after giving insulin for further signs of hyperglycemia such as SOB, facial flushing, air hunger, and acetone breath.
7. Assess for S&S of *hypoglycemia,* such as easy fatigue, hunger, headache, cold, clamminess, drowsiness, nausea, lassitude, and tremulousness. Most likely to occur before meals, during or after exercise, and at insulin peak action times (i.e., 3 a.m. with evening dosing).
   - Weakness, sweating, tremors, and/or nervousness may occur later.
   - Excessive restlessness and profuse sweating at night.
   - Obtain BS or finger stick; promptly give 4 oz of juice and a CHO, if conscious.
   - If conscious and taking long-acting insulin, also give a slowly digestible CHO, such as bread with corn syrup or honey. Give additional CHO such as crackers and milk for the next 2 hr.
   - If unconscious, apply honey or Karo syrup to the buccal membrane or give glucagon.
   - If hospitalized, minimally responsive, or unconscious, give 10–20% IV dextrose solution.
8. A Somogyi effect is often mistaken as client not following the prescribed therapy. This occurs when hypoglycemia triggers the release of epinephrine and glucocorticoids, which stimulates glycogenesis and results in a higher a.m. BS level. Reduction in bedtime insulin dosage is necessary to stabilize. If treated for hypoglycemia, check 3 a.m. BS; if normal and then BS rises between 3 a.m. and 7 a.m., this is related to growth hormone release-termed the Dawn Phenomenon. To control, give long-acting insulin at bedtime instead of at dinnertime.
9. Juveniles with type 1 diabetes demand closer attention and observation for infection or emotional disturbances and hypoglycemia. They are more susceptible to insulin shock and have a more limited response to glucagon. Determine if managed with intensive or con-

ventional insulin therapy; adjust for hypoglycemia unawareness (when client passes out due to loss of catecholamine response). Assess for insulin pump placement for better control of sugars and lifestyle.

10. For the newly diagnosed elderly client, start insulin doses low and gradually increase.
11. The usual dose of NPH insulin is 0.8–1.5 units/kg; give two-thirds of dose in a.m. and one-third of dose in p.m. If using regular insulin, try 1:2 in a.m. and 1:1 in p.m. with NPH.
12. Identify BS goals, i.e., young child 80–150 mg/dL premeal and 100–150 mg/dL at bedtime; adolescent 70–150 mg/dL premeal and 100–150 mg/dL at bedtime; adult 70–150 mg/dL premeal and 100–150 mg/dL at bedtime. Adjust as symptoms and condition dictate.
13. Assess psychologic state, including disease acceptance, readiness to learn, support system, evidence of depression, or need for additional counseling.
14. During physical exam assess DTRs; check extremities (use monofilament) to assess sensation and for evidence of neuropathy. Review proper foot care with each visit.
15. Consider ACE therapy to prevent/preserve renal function and inhibit organ damage and baby aspirin for cardio-protection.
16. Assess injection sites, plot growth and weight every 3–4 months.
17. Schedule yearly eye exams if >12 years old or if client has had the disease for >5 years.
18. Monitor VS, weights, electrolytes, lipid profile, thyroid studies, BS, phosphate, Mg^{++}, CBC, HbA1c, and urinalysis. Assess for microalbuminuria. Monitor glucose levels carefully, especially in the elderly and those with hepatic or renal impairment.

CLIENT/FAMILY TEACHING

1. Medications assist to control diabetes but do not cure it. Type 1 diabetes is usually early onset when the pancreas makes little or no insulin; individuals with type 1 diabetes must take insulin injections or they will die. Type 2 diabetes is usually later onset and the pancreas still makes insulin, but the body cannot use it (termed insulin resistance); individuals with type 2 diabetes can use either oral hypoglycemic agents or insulin to lower their blood sugar or a combination of different oral agents to help them utilize their own insulin better.
2. The stomach destroys insulin, so it must be injected into fat under skin.
3. In type 1 diabetics, urine ketones indicate that there is not enough insulin to get the body's sugar into the cells, so it is burning body fat as an alternative and producing ketones as waste products; may lead to ketoacidosis, a life-threatening condition. May test urine for ketones with a "dip-and-read" product when:
   - Finger sticks >240 mg/dL
   - Pregnant
   - Experiencing severe stress
   - Vomiting or sick to stomach
   - Sick with flu/cold or virus infection
   - Experiencing symptoms of hyperglycemia (unusual fatigue, vision difficulty, increased thirst and/or hunger, polydipsia, unusually tired or sleepy, stomach pain, increased nausea, fruity odor to breath, rapid respirations, weight loss without altering food intake or activity patterns)
4. Perform finger sticks to monitor glucose levels. Review instructions for technique, calibration, operation, and device maintenance. Bring in periodically to double check machine accuracy and to review data bank to ensure values coincide with client log. Some general principles may be followed:
   - Rotate sites.
   - Cleanse area with soap and water or alcohol prior to stabbing.
   - Use a lancet and lancet device to access sample.
   - Stab finger outside, by nail, where the capillaries are abundant and let a bead of blood form.
   - Wipe off with a cotton ball.
   - Let blood bead reform and apply to the test strip.
   - Use proper test strips for designated machine; check expiration date.
   - Follow specific guidelines for the device in use.
   - When battery change occurs, reset machine date.
5. Regimens are specific to the individual, based on age, severity of diabetes, weight, any other

medical problems they have, as well as the philosophy of the health care team.

6. If not planning to eat, then do not take antihypoglycemic agents. Take 70/30 or regular insulin 30–40 min before a meal, Novolog 5–15 min before a meal. Administer at a 90° angle with a 28- or 29-gauge needle. Syringes come in 0.3 mL (30-units), 0.5 mL (50-units), and 1 mL (100-units) sizes. Purchase the smallest syringe with the smallest needles to enhance dosage validity (e.g., if prescribed less than 30 units of insulin, obtain the 0.3 mL syringe). May also be administered by pens or pumps. Although not recommended, may reuse disposable insulin syringes; based on comfort and perceived dullness. Review cleaning procedures to ensure adequately cleaned.
7. Use a chart to document and rotate injection sites to avoid lipohypertrophy of injection sites (lumps from scar tissue after many injections). Avoid these areas due to unreliable absorption. Warm refrigerated/cold insulin to room temperature and then roll between your palms to prevent lipodystrophy from injecting cold insulin.
8. For self-injection, wash hands, may brace the arm against a hard surface such as the wall or a chair.
   - Cleanse the area thoroughly with soap and water or alcohol and allow to dry. Then, depending on the condition of the skin, either pinch between the thumb and forefinger of one hand, or spread the skin using the thumb and fingers of one hand.
   - Insert into the subcutaneous tissue and aspirate to be sure needle is not in a blood vessel.
   - Inject insulin and withdraw the needle.
9. Review use and care of equipment, proper storage and disposal of needles and syringes, and provision and storage of drug.
10. *Always* check expiration dates; have an extra vial and equipment on hand for traveling, away from home, or when detained or hospitalized.
11. Have regular insulin for emergency use.
12. Must balance food, insulin, and exercise. Exercise increases the utilization of CHO and increases CHO needs. Have snacks available; 5–8 Lifesavers, 4 oz. juice, or glucose tabs (3) to counteract hypoglycemia.
13. Adhere to prescribed diet, weight control, and ingestion of food relative to the peak action of insulin being used. Record weekly weights; reduce intake of animal fats and salt; select a variety of foods to meet starch and sugar, protein, and fat requirements (usual recommendation, CHO 50%; protein 20%; fat 30%). Consume the kinds of fiber that help lower BS and fat levels (breads, cereals, and crackers made from whole grains, such as rye, bran, and brown rice, fresh vegetables and fruits, dried beans, and peas), low cholesterol and polyunsaturated and monosaturated fats.
14. Confer with dietitian for assistance in shopping, food selection/exchanges, diet, and meal planning. Consume premeal snacks in the a.m., midday, and at bedtime.
15. If ill and a meal is omitted because of fever, nausea, or vomiting, replace solid foods that contain starch and sugar, such as bread and fruit, with liquids that contain sugar (fruit juice, regular sodas) and follow designated sliding scale for "sick days." Do not omit insulin or hypoglycemic agents unless instructed. Perform finger sticks q 4 hr, and with type 1, also test urine for ketones; report if moderate or high.
16. Blurred vision may occur at beginning of insulin therapy; should subside in 6–8 weeks. The effect is caused by fluctuation of blood glucose levels, which produce osmotic changes in the lens of the eye and within the ocular fluids. If does not clear up in 8 weeks, consult eye doctor.
17. May experience allergic responses: Itching, redness, swelling, stinging, or warmth may occur at the injection site and usually disappears after a few weeks of therapy. Report, as purified or human insulins are used for local allergy and lipohypertrophy at injection site.
18. Failure to take insulin will result in ketoacidosis. Adjust insulin based on BS and guidelines for insulin administration during sick days. Identify soft foods and liquids to consume for sick days (i.e., regular soda, apple juice, clear broth, cream soups, puddings, applesauce, freezer pop, ice cream).
19. If ill, notify provider. To prevent coma, maintain adequate hydration by drinking 1 cup or more of noncaloric fluids such as coffee, tea, water, or broth every hour. Test finger sticks

and urine more. Identify when to go to the emergency room.

20. If there is no insulin/equipment to administer, decrease food intake by one-third and drink plenty of noncaloric fluids. Obtain supplies as soon as possible and return to prescribed diet and insulin dosage.
21. Follow good hygienic practices to prevent infection. Bathe daily with mild soap and lukewarm water. Use lotion to prevent skin dryness. Avoid injury from punctures. Avoid scratches; wear gloves when working with the hands. Always protect feet and wear shoes. Use sunscreen and protective clothing to avoid sunburn, and dress appropriately for the weather; prevent frostbite.
22. Establish a daily routine of checking and caring for the feet (use a mirror if unable to bend over). Wear comfortable shoes (leather or canvas) and stockings (no garters or elastic tops), and do exercises. Clip toenails (straight across); do not undertake any self-treatment for ingrown toenails, corns, warts, or calluses. Do not use any heat treatments, hot water bottles, or heating pads, and do not smoke, as this decreases blood flow to the feet. Obtain annual foot screen and periodic foot care as needed.
23. Hyperglycemia compounds the risk for tooth and gum problems; brush after meals, floss, and see dentist regularly.
24. Diabetes can damage the small blood vessels to the eye; obtain dilated eye exams. Eye damage has no symptoms in the early, treatable stage. Report blurred or double vision, narrowed visual fields, increased difficulty seeing in dim light, pressure or pain in the eye, or seeing dark spots.
25. May experience decreased sensation in feet, legs, and hands (neuropathy); use care when handling hot or cold items, wear shoes and socks to protect feet, and dress appropriately for the weather.
26. Carry ID noting "diabetic" and list of medications, who to notify, and what to do if unable to respond.
27. Avoid alcohol; causes hypoglycemia. Excessive intake may require a reduction of insulin; also causes a disulfiram-type reaction with oral hypoglycemic agents and increases peripheral neuropathy.
28. Carry all medications, syringes, glucagon, and blood testing equipment in carry-on luggage when traveling. Always carry diabetes ID. Keep to the usual meal and time, exercise, and medication routines as closely as possible. Carry food and fast-acting CHO in the event meals are delayed. Request medications for vomiting/diarrhea and plan ahead for mealtimes when crossing two or more time zones. Protect insulin and test strips from extremes in heat or cold (keeping between 15–30°C or 59–86°F).
29. Use only the insulin prescribed; check for correct origin (human or pork), brand name (Lispro, Humulin, etc.), and type (Regular, Lente, NPH, etc.).
30. Check vials before each dose is taken. Regular and Buffered Regular insulin (for pumps) should be clear and colorless, whereas other forms may be cloudy except for the newer long acting form.
31. Two kinds of insulin can be mixed in the same syringe:
    - Regular insulin can be mixed with any other insulin.
    - Do not mix the fast-acting lispro with other agents
    - A single form of insulin in a syringe can be stable for weeks or a month.
    - Except for the commercially prepared mixtures, mixtures of insulin are not stable and should be administered within 5 min of preparation.
    - When mixed, regular (unmodified) insulin should always be drawn up in the syringe first.
32. Impotence may be caused by damaged nerves and reduced blood flow related to diabetes; see urologist to find cause and best treatment.
33. Silent heart attacks may occur. Identify risk factors and alter lifestyle to prevent CAD (i.e., regular exercise, low-fat, low-salt, low-cholesterol diet, no tobacco or alcohol, stress/weight reduction, and BP and cholesterol LDL control).
34. Identify local diabetic educator and support groups to assist in understanding and coping with this disease. The American Diabetes Association (1-800-342-2383 and email: AskADA@diabetes.org) and local diabetes support

groups offer additional information and support.

35. Keep all F/U to assess response, labs, and for adverse SE.

OUTCOMES/EVALUATE

- Understanding/acceptance of DM
- Positive lifestyle changes to control blood sugars
- BS, renal and LFTs WNL; HbA1c <8
- Healthy skin at injection sites
- Prevent target organ damage

ANTIEMETICS

SEE ALSO THE FOLLOWING INDIVIDUAL ENTRIES:

Aprepitant
Dimenhydrinate
Diphenhydramine hydrochloride
Fosaprepitant dimeglumine
Granisetron hydrochloride
Meclizine hydrochloride
Ondansetron hydrochloride
Palonosetron hydrochloride
Prochlorperazine
Prochlorperazine edisylate
Prochlorperazine maleate
Scopolamine hydrobromide

GENERAL STATEMENT

Nausea and vomiting can be caused by a variety of conditions, such as infections, drugs, radiation, motion, organic disease, or psychologic factors. The underlying cause of the symptoms must be elicited before emesis is corrected. Many drugs used for other conditions, such as antidopaminergics (e.g., chlorpromazine, perphenazine, prochlorperazine, promethazine), anticholinergics (buclizine, cyclizine, dimenhydrinate, meclizine) and scopolamine have antiemetic properties. However, CNS depression may limit their use as antiemetics.

DRUG INTERACTIONS

Because of their antiemetic and antinauseant activity, the antiemetics may mask overdosage caused by other drugs.

DOSAGE

See individual drugs.

NURSING IMPLICATIONS

ASSESSMENT

1. Determine if nausea is an unusual occurrence or a recurring phenomenon; establish onset, duration, and associated factors such as vertigo, chemotherapy, or illness. Note past use of antiemetics and response.
2. Evaluate physiologic mechanism triggering N&V. Generally, if centrally mediated to the CTZ, would see nausea without vomiting, whereas if the vomiting center were triggered directly, then may see retching with vomiting.
3. Assess for other effects; antiemetics may mask signs of underlying pathology or overdosage of other drugs. Ensure no intestinal obstruction, drug overdose, or increased ICP. Monitor I&O; observe for dehydration. Offer liquids and advance to regular foods as tolerated.
4. With prolonged activity, monitor for electrolyte disturbance and replace as needed.

CLIENT/FAMILY TEACHING

1. Take exactly as directed. Drug may cause dizziness/drowsiness; avoid driving or other hazardous tasks until drug effects evaluated.
2. Practice measures to decrease nausea when possible, such as ice chips, sips of water, non-greasy foods, removal of irritating stimuli (odors or materials), and frequent mouth rinsing with water and oral hygiene. Advance diet only as tolerated.
3. Dangle legs before standing; rise slowly to prevent symptoms of low BP. Consume adequate fluids to prevent dehydration.
4. Avoid alcohol and any other unprescribed CNS depressants.
5. Keep all F/U to assess response, labs, and for adverse SE.

OUTCOMES/EVALUATE

- Control of N&V; prevention of dehydration/electrolyte imbalance
- Improved nutritional status with weight gain/ ↑ caloric intake

Classifications

ANTIHISTAMINES (H_1 BLOCKERS) ■

SEE ALSO THE FOLLOWING INDIVIDUAL ENTRIES:

FIRST GENERATION:
Chlorpheniramine maleate
Diphenhydramine hydrochloride
Meclizine hydrochloride
Promethazine hydrochloride

SECOND GENERATION:
Cetirizine hydrochloride
Desloratadine
Fexofenadine hydrochloride
Levocetirizine
Loratidine

OPHTHALMIC ANTIHISTAMINES:
Olopatadine hydrochloride*

Drugs marked with an * are available to view in the 2013 Nurse's Drug Handbook Website at www.cengage.com/community/nursesdrughandbook.

INDICATIONS/USES

PO: (1) Vasomotor, perennial, or seasonal allergic rhinitis and allergic conjunctivitis. Ophthalmic antihistamines may also be used. (2) Angioedema, urticarial transfusion reactions, urticaria, pruritus. (3) Atopic dermatitis, contact dermatitis, pruritus ani, pruritus vulvae, insect bites. (4) Sneezing and rhinorrhea due to the common cold. (5) Anaphylactic reactions. (6) Parkinsonism, drug-induced extrapyramidal reactions. (7) Vertigo. (8) Prophylaxis and treatment of motion sickness, including N&V. (9) Nighttime sleep aid.

Parenteral: (1) Relief of allergic reactions due to blood or plasma. (2) Adjunct to epinephrine in treating anaphylaxis. (3) Uncomplicated allergic conditions when PO therapy is not possible.

ACTION/KINETICS

Action

Compete with histamine at H_1 histamine receptors (reversible competitive inhibition), thus preventing or reversing the effects of histamine. First-generation antihistamines bind to central and peripheral H_1 receptors and can cause CNS depression or stimulation. Second-generation antihistamines are selective for peripheral H_1 receptors and cause less sedation. Antihistamines do not prevent the release of histamine, antibody production, or antigen-antibody interactions. Antihistamines prevent or reduce increased capillary permeability (i.e., decrease edema, itching) and bronchospasms. Allergic reactions unrelated to histamine release are not affected by antihistamines. Certain of the first-generation antihistamines also have anticholinergic, antiemetic, antipruritic, or antiserotonin effects. Clients unresponsive to a certain antihistamine may regain sensitivity by switching to a different antihistamine. From a chemical point of view, the antihistamines can be divided into the following classes.

FIRST GENERATION:

1. **Alkylamines.** Among the most potent antihistamines. Minimal sedation, moderate anticholinergic effects, and no antiemetic effects. Paradoxical excitation may also occur. Examples: Brompheniramine, chlorpheniramine, dexchlorpheniramine.
2. **Ethanolamine Derivatives.** Moderate to high sedative, anticholinergic, and antiemetic effects. Low incidence of GI side effects. Examples: Clemastine, diphenhydramine.
3. **Phenothiazines.** High antihistaminic, sedative, and anticholinergic effects; very high antiemetic effect. Example: Promethazine.
4. **Piperazine.** High antihistaminic, sedative, and antiemetic effects; moderate anticholinergic effects. Example: Hydroxyzine.
5. **Piperidines.** Moderate antihistaminic and anticholinergic effects; low to moderate sedation; no antiemetic effects. Examples: Azatadine, cyproheptadine, phenindamine.

SECOND GENERATION:

1. **Phthalazinone.** High antihistaminic effect; low to no sedative and anticholinergic effects; no antiemetic effect. Example: Azelastine.
2. **Piperazine.** Moderate to high antihistaminic effect; low to no sedation or anticholinergic effects; no antiemetic activity. Examples: Cetirizine, levocetirizine.
3. **Piperidines.** Moderate to high antihistaminic activity; low to no sedation and anticholinergic activity; no antiemetic action. Examples: Desloratadine, fexofenadine, loratidine.

Pharmacokinetics

The kinetics of most first-generation antihistamines are similar. **Onset:** 15–30 min; **peak:** 1–2 hr; **duration:** 4–6 hr (piperidines have a longer duration). Many antihistamines are available as timed-release preparations. Most first-generation antihistamines are metabolized by the liver and excreted in the urine. The pharmacokinetics of the second-generation antihistamines vary; consult individual drugs.

CONTRAINDICATIONS

First-generation antihistamines.

Hypersensitivity to the drug. Pregnancy or possibility thereof (some agents), lactation, premature and newborn infants, use with MAOIs. The phenothiazine-type antihistamines are contraindicated in CNS depression from any cause, bone marrow depression, jaundice, dehydrated or acutely ill children, and in comatose clients. Use to treat lower respiratory tract symptoms such as asthma, emphysema, chronic bronchitis (due to anticholinergic effects that may thicken secretions and impair expectoration). **Second-generation antihistamines.** Hypersensitivity to specific or chemically-related antihistamines.

SPECIAL CONCERNS

- **Antihistamines have varying degrees of atropine-like effects; use with caution in those with a predisposition to urinary retention, history of bronchial asthma, increased intraocular pressure, hyperthyroidism, CV disease, or hypertension.**
- **Also, use with caution in clients with convulsive disorders, respiratory disease, narrow-angle glaucoma, stenosing peptic ulcer, pyloroduodenal obstruction, symptomatic prostatic hypertrophy, bladder neck obstruction.**
- **Use phenothiazine antihistamines with caution in clients with CV disease, liver dysfunction, narrow-angle glaucoma, prostatic hypertrophy, stenosing peptic ulcer, pyloroduodenal obstruction, and bladder-neck obstruction.**
- **May diminish mental alertness in children and may occasionally cause excitation; larger doses may cause hallucinations, convulsions, and death in infants and children.**
- **Many recommend that antihistamines not be used in children less than 6 years of age while others set the minimum age for use of antihistamines as 2 years of age. Studies are continuing.**
- **Use in geriatric clients may result in dizziness, excessive sedation, syncope, toxic confusional states, and hypotension.**

SIDE EFFECTS

Systemic. CNS: Sedation ranging from mild drowsiness to deep sleep. Dizziness, incoordination, faintness, fatigue, confusion, lassitude, restlessness, excitation, nervousness, tremor, ***tonic-clonic seizures***, headache, irritability, insomnia, euphoria, paresthesias, oculogyric crisis, torticollis, catatonic-like states, hallucinations, disorientation, tongue protrusion (usually with IV use or overdosage), disturbing dreams, nightmares, pseudoschizophrenia, weakness, diplopia, vertigo, hysteria, neuritis, paradoxical excitation, epileptiform seizures in clients with focal lesions. Extrapyramidal reactions include opisthotonos, dystonia, akathisia, dyskinesia, and parkinsonism. **CV:** Postural hypotension, palpitations, bradycardia, tachycardia, reflex tachycardia, extrasystoles, increased or decreased BP, ECG changes (including blunting of T waves and prolongation of the Q-T interval), ***cardiac arrest***. **GI:** Epigastric distress, anorexia, increased appetite and weight gain, N&V, diarrhea, constipation, change in bowel habits, stomatitis. **GU:** Urinary frequency, dysuria, urinary retention, gynecomastia, inhibition of ejaculation, decreased libido, impotence, early menses, induction of lactation. **Hematologic:** Hypoplastic anemia, ***aplastic anemia, hemolytic anemia***, thrombocytopenia, leukopenia, pancytopenia, ***agranulocytosis***, thrombocytopenic purpura. **Respiratory:** Thickening of bronchial secretions, wheezing, nasal stuffiness, chest tightness, sore throat, ***respiratory depression;*** dry mouth, nose, and throat. **Ophthalmic:** Blurred vision, diplopia. **Miscellaneous:** Tinnitus, photosensitivity, hypersensitivity reactions, acute labyrinthitis, obstructive jaundice, erythema, high or prolonged glucose tolerance curves, glycosuria, elevated spinal fluid proteins, increased plasma cholesterol, increased perspiration, chills; tingling, heaviness, and weakness of the hands.

Topical. Prolonged use may result in local irritation and allergic contact dermatitis.

Nasal Spray. Glossitis, ulcerative and aphthous stomatitis, bitter taste, epistaxis, paroxysmal sneezing, rhinitis, conjunctivitis, eye abnormality, eye pain, nasal burning, taste loss, watery eyes, temporomandibular dislocation.

Classifications

OVERDOSE MANAGEMENT

Symptoms (Acute Toxicity): Although antihistamines have a wide therapeutic range, overdosage can nevertheless be fatal. Children are particularly susceptible. Early toxic effects may be seen within 30–120 min and include drowsiness, dizziness, blurred vision, tinnitus, ataxia, and hypotension. Symptoms range from CNS depression (sedation, ***coma***, decreased mental alertness) to ***CV collapse*** and CNS stimulation (insomnia, hallucinations, tremors, or ***seizures***). Also, ***profound hypotension, respiratory depression, coma, and death*** may occur. Anticholinergic effects include flushing, dry mouth, hypotension, fever, ***hyperthermia*** (especially in children), and fixed, dilated pupils. Body temperature may be as high as 107°F. In children, symptoms include hallucinations, toxic psychosis, delirum tremens, ataxia, incoordination, muscle twitching, excitement, athetosis, ***hyperthermia, seizures***, and hyperreflexia followed by postictal depression and ***cardiorespiratory arrest.***

Treatment:

- Treat symptoms and provide supportive care.
- Administer a slurry of activated charcoal and a cathartic. Gastric lavage within 3 hr after ingestion and even later if large amounts were taken.
- Hypotension can be treated with a vasopressor such as norepinephrine, dopamine, or phenylephrine (do not use epinephrine).
- For convulsions, use only short-acting depressants (e.g., diazepam). IV physostigmine can be used to treat centrally-mediated convulsions.
- Ice packs and a cool sponge bath are effective in reducing fever in children.
- Take precautions to protect against aspiration, especially in infants and children.
- Severe cases of overdose can be treated by hemoperfusion.

DRUG INTERACTIONS

Alcohol, ethyl / See CNS depressants

Antidepressants, tricyclic / Additive anticholinergic side effects

CNS depressants, antianxiety agents, barbiturates, narcotics, phenothiazines, procarbazine, sedative-hypnotics / Potentiation or addition of CNS depressant effects. Concomitant use may lead to drowsiness, lethargy, stupor, respiratory depression, coma, and possibly death

H ***Henbane leaf*** / Enhanced anticholinergic effects

Heparin / Antihistamines may ↓ the anticoagulant effects

MAOIs / Intensification and prolongation of anticholinergic and sedative side effects; use with phenothiazine antihistamine → hypotension and extrapyramidal reactions

SEE ALSO ***DRUG INTERACTIONS*** FOR ***PHENOTHIAZINES***

LABORATORY TEST CONSIDERATIONS

Discontinue antihistamines 4 days before skin testing to avoid false negative result.

DOSAGE

Usually PO

Parenteral administration is seldom used because of irritating nature of drugs. Topical usage is also limited because antihistamines often cause hypersensitivity reactions. When given for motion sickness, antihistamines are usually given 30–60 min before anticipated travel. See individual drugs.

NURSING IMPLICATIONS

IMPLEMENTATION/ADMINISTRATION/STORAGE

1. **Inject IM preparations deep into the muscle; irritating to tissues.**
2. **Swallow sustained-release preparations whole. May break scored tablets before swallowing. If difficulty swallowing capsules, may open and put contents into soft food for ingestion.**
3. **Do not apply topical preparations to raw, blistered, or oozing areas of the skin.**
4. **Do not apply to the eyes, around the genitalia, or to mucous membranes.**

ASSESSMENT

1. **List type, onset, characteristics of symptoms; note triggers. Stop antihistamines 2–4 days prior to skin testing to avoid false negative results.**
2. **Note any drug sensitivity; identify known allergens and all medications prescribed.**
3. **Monitor VS, I&O, CV status, lung sounds/status and characteristics of secretions. Determine any urinary retention, frequency, or pain.**
4. **Assess for any conditions that warrant close supervision or may preclude therapy: glaucoma (narrow angle), ulcers, BPH, heart dis-**

ease, HTN, seizures, pregnancy, hyperthyroidism.

5. Describe extent and characteristics of any rash, if present. Monitor CBC with long-term therapy; hemolytic anemia may rarely occur.

CLIENT/FAMILY TEACHING

1. Take before or at the onset of symptoms; cannot reverse reactions but may prevent them. Oral products may cause gastric irritation; administer with meals, milk, or a snack.
2. Do not drive or operate equipment until drug effects realized or drowsiness wears off. Sedative effects may disappear after several days or may not occur at all.
3. For motion sickness, take 30–60 min before travel time.
4. Report sore throat, fever, unexplained bruising, bleeding, or petechiae; may cause blood dyscrasias.
5. May cause sensitivity to sun or ultraviolet light; avoid long exposures, use sunscreen, sunglasses, and protective clothing when exposed.
6. Severe CNS depression is a symptom of overdosage. Report dizziness or weakness; avoid other CNS depressants.
7. Reduce symptoms of dry mouth by frequent rinsing with warm water, good oral hygiene, and sugarless gum or candies. Avoid overuse of mouthwash, as it may destroy normal flora and worsen dryness.
8. Ensure adequate hydration. If bronchial secretions are thick, increase fluids, and humidify air to decrease secretion viscosity; avoid milk temporarily. If problems with urination, void prior to taking the drug.
9. Exercise regularly; consume 2 L fluids/day and fruits, fruit juices, and dietary fiber to prevent constipation. Use stool softeners as needed.
10. Recurrent reactions may be referred to an allergist. Protect self from exposure, avoid triggers, and create an allergen-free living area.
11. Antihistamines raise BP, use with high BP only if medically supervised. Avoid alcohol or OTC agents without approval.
12. Children may manifest excitation rather than sedation. Clinical effectiveness may diminish with continued usage; switching to another class may restore drug effectiveness.
13. To ensure accurate skin testing, stop agent 4 days prior to testing.
14. Family/significant other should learn CPR; survival is greatly increased when CPR is initiated immediately.
15. Keep all F/U to assess response, labs, and for adverse SE.

OUTCOMES/EVALUATE

- ↓ Frequency/intensity of allergic manifestations; ↓ itching/swelling
- Prevention of motion sickness
- Effective nighttime sedation

ANTIHYPERLIPIDEMIC AGENTS-HMG-COA REDUCTASE INHIBITORS

SEE ALSO THE FOLLOWING INDIVIDUAL ENTRIES:

Atorvastatin calcium
Fluvastatin sodium
Lovastatin
Pitavastatin
Pravastatin sodium
Rosuvastatin calcium
Simvastatin

GENERAL STATEMENT

The National Cholesterol Education Program (NCEP) Expert Panel on Detection, Evaluation, and Treatment of High Blood Cholesterol in Adults has developed guidelines for the treatment of high cholesterol and LDL in adults. High-risk clients are defined as those with a greater than 20% risk for cardiovascular heart disease in the next 10 years. Cardiovascular heart disease includes a history of MI, unstable and stable angina, angioplasty, cardiac bypass surgery, or evidence of clinically significant myocardial ischemia. Risk factors include cigarette smoking, hypertension, low high-density lipoprotein cholesterol (HDL-C) less than 40 mg/dL, family history of premature cardiovascular heart disease and gender (men more than 45 years of age; women greater than 55 years of age). Moderately high-risk clients have two or more risk factors and a 10–20% risk for cardiovascular heart disease in the next 10 years. A client with moderate risk also has two or more risk factors, but the 10-year cardiovascular heart disease risk is less than 10%. A low-risk person has

0–1 risk factor with a 10-year cardiovascular heart disease risk at less than 10%.

The following are the NCEP's guidelines for LDL-C goals and cutpoints for therapeutic lifestyle changes and drug therapy in different risk categories:

1. CHD or CHD risk equivalents: 10-year risk >20%: LDL-goal is <100 mg/dL). LDL level at which to initiate therapeutic lifestyle changes: 100 mg/dL or greater. LDL level at which to consider drug therapy: 130 or greater mg/dL (100 to 129 drug optional).
2. CHD or CHD risk equivalents: 2 or more risk factors (10-year risk 20% or less). LDL-C goal: <130 mg/dL. LDL level at which to initiate therapeutic lifestyle changes: 130 mg/dL or more. LDL level at which to consider drug therapy: 10-year risk 10–20%: 130 mg/dL or more; 10-year risk <10%: 160 mg/dL or more.
3. CHD or CHD risk equivalents: 0 to 1 risk factor (almost all people with 0 to 1 risk factor have a 10-year risk 10% or less). LDL-C goal: <160 mg/dL. LDL level at which to initiate therapeutic lifestyle changes: 160 mg/dL or more. LDL level at which to consider drug therapy: 190 mg/dL or more (160 to 189: LDL-lowering drug optional).

The NCEP classification of cholesterol levels in children with a familial history of hypercholesterolemia or premature cardiovascular disease is as follows:

1. Acceptable level: Total-C: <170 mg/dL; LDL-C: <110 mg/dL.
2. Borderline: Total-C: 170 to 199 mg/dL; LDL-C: 110 to 129 mg/dL.
3. High: Total-C: 200 mg/dL or more; LDL-C: 130 mg/dL or more.

The goals for treatment are as follows:

1. For high-risk clients with LDL-C >100 mg/dL, an LDL-lowering drug is indicated along with therapeutic lifestyle changes. The threshold for LDL-lowering therapy has been lowered from >130 mg/dL, with drug therapy now optional for LDL-C levels between 100–129 mg/dL. Also, in high-risk clients with a pretreatment LDL-C of >100 mg/dL, initiation of an LDL-lowering drug to reach a treatment goal of <70 mg/dL is considered as an evidence-based therapeutic option.
2. For high-risk clients with high triglycerides or low LDL-C, it is recommended adding a fibrate or nicotinic acid to an LDL-lowering drug regimen. When triglycerides are >200 mg/dL, non-HDL-C is a secondary target of therapy, with a goal of 30 mg/dL higher than the previously identified LDL-C goal.
3. For moderately-high risk clients, an LDL-C treatment goal of <130 mg/dL is still recommended. However, a treatment goal of LDL <100 mg/dL is considered an evidence-based therapeutic option. If the LDL is >130 mg/dL, therapeutic lifestyle changes should be started. If the LDL level remains >130 mg/dL after implementation of therapeutic lifestyle changes, initiation of LDL-lowering drug therapy should be considered to achieve and sustain an LDL-C goal of <130 mg/dL. For those with an LDL level between 100–129 mg/dL, at baseline or after therapeutic lifestyle change implementation, beginning LDL-lowering drug therapy to reach an LDL level of <100 mg/ dL is a therapeutic option.
4. For clients at moderately high or high risk, LDL-lowering drug therapy, if used, should achieve at least a 30–40% reduction in LDL-C levels. Therapeutic lifestyle changes should also be started, regardless of the clients' LDL level, if the client has lifestyle related risk factors, such as obesity, physical inactivity, elevated triglycerides, low LDL, or metabolic syndrome.

INDICATIONS/USES

See individual drugs. Uses include: (1) Heterozygous familial hypercholesterolemia in adolescents. (2) Homozygous familial hyperlipidemia. (3) Hypertriglyceridemia, including Fredrickson type IV. Not indicated in such clients with low or normal LDL, despite elevated total cholesterol. (4) Mixed dyslipidemia, including Fredrickson types IIa and IIb. (5) Primary dysbetalipoproteinemia, including Fredrickson type III. (6) Primary hypercholesterolemia, including heterozygous familial and nonfamilial hypercholesterolemia. (7) Primary prevention of coronary events. (8) Secondary prevention of CV events. *Investigational:* Treatment of osteoporosis. Lower risk of developing type 2 diabetes and stroke when taken to reduce cholesterol. Lower cholesterol in women.

ACTION/KINETICS

Action

The HMG-CoA reductase inhibitors competitively inhibit HMG-CoA reductase; this enzyme catalyzes the early rate-limiting step in the synthesis of cholesterol. HMG-CoA reductase inhibitors increase HDL cholesterol and decrease LDL cholesterol, total cholesterol, apolipoprotein B, VLDL cholesterol, and plasma triglycerides. The mechanism to lower LDL cholesterol may be due to both a decrease in VLDL cholesterol levels and induction of the LDL receptor, leading to reduced production or increased catabolism of LDL cholesterol. The maximum therapeutic response is seen in 4–6 weeks. Statins may help prevent infections in clients with diabetes. Statins cause a significant reduction in CV events.

CONTRAINDICATIONS

Hypersensitivity to any component of the product. Active liver disease or unexplained persistent elevated liver function tests. Pregnancy, lactation. Use in children.

SPECIAL CONCERNS

- **Use with caution in those who ingest large quantities of alcohol or who have a history of liver disease.**
- **Rhabdomyolysis with acute renal failure secondary to myoglobinuria may occur with statins; fatalities are rare, however. Factors that may predispose a client to myopathy include age 65 years and older, inadequately treated or uncontrolled hypothyroidism, and renal insufficiency. The risk of myopathy/rhabdomyolysis is dose related. The risk also increases when statins are given with other drugs that inhibit their metabolism (e.g., cyclosporine, erythromycin, azole antifungals) or with drugs that can cause myopathy when given alone (e.g., fibrates, lipid-lowering doses of niacin).**
- **May cause photosensitivity.**
- **Safety and efficacy not established for atorvastatin, lovastatin, and simvastatin immediate-release products in prepubertal clients and children less than 18 years of age. Also, safety and efficacy not established for pravastatin in children younger than 8 years of age and for lovastatin ER, pitavastatin, and rosuvastatin in children.**

SIDE EFFECTS

The following side effects have been reported for HMG-CoA reductase inhibitors. Also see individual drugs. **GI:** N&V, diarrhea, constipation, abdominal cramps or pain, flatulence, dyspepsia, heartburn. Anorexia, cheilitis, colitis, duodenal ulcer, dysphagia, enteritis, eructation, esophagitis, gastritis, glossitis, gum hemorrhage, ***hemorrhage***, increased appetite, melena, pancreatitis, periodontal abscess, rectal mouth ulceration, stomach ulcer, stomatitis, tenesmus, ulcerative stomach. **Hepatic:** Biliary pain, cholestatic jaundice, cirrhosis, fatty changes in the liver, ***fulminant hepatic necrosis***, hepatitis (including chronic active hepatitis), hepatoma, increases in hepatic transaminases. **CNS:** Headache, dizziness, dysfunction of certain cranial nerves (e.g., alteration of taste, facial paresis, impairment of extraocular movement), tremor, vertigo, memory loss, paresthesia, anxiety, insomnia, depression, mental decline, aggressive behavior, ***suicide attempts***. Abnormal dreams, emotional lability, hyperkinesia, hypertonia, hypesthesia, incoordination, migraine, peripheral nerve palsy, peripheral neuropathy, psychic disturbances, somnolence, torticollis. **CV:** Cardiac chest pain, angina pectoris, arrhythmia, palpitations, phlebitis, postural hypotension, syncope, vasodilation. **Dermatologic:** Acne, rash, alopecia, contact dermatitis, eczema, seborrhea, skin ulcer, pruritus, sweating, urticaria, skin nodules/discoloration, dryness of skin/mucous membranes, changes in hair/nails. **Musculoskeletal:** Localized pain, bursitis, myalgia, muscle cramps or pain, myopathy, rhabdomyolysis, arthralgia, myasthenia, myopathy, myositis, pathological fracture, neck rigidity/pain, pelvic pain. **Respiratory:** URI, rhinitis, cough, asthma, dyspnea, epistaxis, pneumonia. **GU:** Abnormal ejaculation, albuminuria, breast enlargement, cystitis, dysuria, epididymitis, erectile dysfunction, fibrocystic breast, gynecomastia, hematuria, impotence, kidney calculus, loss of libido, metrorrhagia, nocturia, nephritis, renal failure, urinary frequency, incontinence, urinary retention/urgency, vaginal or uterine hemorrhage. **Hematologic:** Anemia, ecchymosis, lymphadenopathy, petechiae, thrombocytopenia. **Metabolic:** Diabetes mellitus, gout, hyperglycemia, hypoglycemia, weight gain. **Ophthalmic:** Progression of cataracts (lens opacities), baseline lenticular opacities, ophthalmoplegia, amblyopia, dry eyes, eye hemorrhage, glaucoma. **Otic:** Deafness, tinnitus.

Hypersensitivity: ***Anaphylaxis***, ***angioedema***, vasculitis, purpura, thrombocytopenia, leukopenia, ***hemolytic anemia***, lupus erythematosus-like syndrome, polymyalgia rheumatica, positive ANA, ESR increase, arthritis, arthralgia, eosinophilia, urticaria, photosensitivity, fever, chills, flushing, malaise, dyspnea, ***toxic dermal necrolysis***, ***Stevens-Johnson syndrome***. **Body as a whole:** Fatigue, influenza, edema, fever, malaise, generalized edema, photosensitivity reaction. **Miscellaneous:** Parosmia, taste loss/perversion, facial edema.

DRUG INTERACTIONS

See also individual drugs. ***NOTE***: Drugs that are inhibitors of P450 enzymes (especially CYP3A4) increase serum levels of several HMG-CoA reductase inhibitors.

Amiodarone / ↑ Levels of HMG-CoA inhibitors R/T ↓ metabolism → ↑ risk of rhabdomyolysis

Antifungals, Azole(e.g., itraconazole, ketoconazole) / ↑ Levels of HMG-CoA inhibitors R/T ↓ metabolism; may ↑ risk of rhabdomyolysis; do not use itraconazole with HMG-CoA inhibitors

Clarithromycin / ↑ Levels of HMG-CoA inhibitors R/T ↓ metabolism → ↑ risk of rhabdomyolysis

Clopidogrel / ↓ Clopidogrel effects on platelet function with atorvastatin or simvastatin

Colchicine / ↑ Risk of myopathy or rhabdomyolysis; if coadministration cannot be avoided, use together with caution and monitor

Cyclosporine / ↑ Risk of severe myopathy or rhabdomyolysis; if coadministration cannot be avoided, consider ↓ the dose of the HMG-CoA inhibitor and monitor closely

Digoxin / Slight ↑ in digoxin levels

Diltiazem / ↑ Levels of HMG-CoA inhibitors R/T ↓ metabolism → ↑ risk of rhabdomyolysis

Erythromycin / ↑ Risk of severe myopathy or rhabdomyolysis R/T ↓ metabolism of the statin

Fenofibrate / ↑ Risk of severe myopathy or rhabdomyolysis; if coadministration cannot be avoided, consider ↓ the dose of the HMG-CoA inhibitor

Gemfibrozil / ↑ Risk of severe myopathy or rhabdomyolysis; if coadministration can not be avoided, consider ↓ the dose of the HMG-CoA inhibitor

Grapefruit juice / Possible ↑ AUC, C_{max}, and elimination t½ of certain HMG-CoA reductase inhibitors → ↑ risk of rhabdomyolysis

Itraconazole / ↑ Levels of HMG-CoA inhibitors

Nefazodone / ↑ Levels of HMG-CoA inhibitors R/T ↓ CYP3A4 metabolism → ↑ risk of rhabdomyolysis

Niacin, Nicotinic acid / ↑ Risk of severe myopathy or rhabdomyolysis with niacin doses of 1 gram/day or more; if coadministration cannot be avoided, consider ↓ the dose of the HMG-CoA inhibitor

Propranolol / ↓ Antihyperlipidemic activity

Protease inhibitors / ↑ Levels of certain HMG-CoA inhibitors R/T ↓ metabolism → ↑ risk of myopathy

Verapamil / ↑ Levels of HMG-CoA inhibitors R/T ↓ metabolism → ↑ risk of rhabdomyolysis

Warfarin / ↑ Anticoagulant effect of warfarin

LABORATORY TEST CONSIDERATIONS

↑ AST, ALT, CPK, alkaline phosphatase, bilirubin, GGT. Abnormal thyroid and LFTs.

DOSAGE

See individual drugs.

NURSING IMPLICATIONS

IMPLEMENTATION/ADMINISTRATION/STORAGE

1. Lovastatin should be taken with meals; fluvastatin, pravastatin, and simavastatin may be taken without regard to meals.
2. Step-down therapy (e.g., pravastatin) may decrease medication effectiveness.

ASSESSMENT

1. Identify reasons for therapy, risk factors, other agents trialed, outcome.
2. Review lifestyle, risk factors, attempts to control with diet, exercise, and weight reduction. Also review PMH, FH, ROS, and physical exam.
3. Note any alcohol abuse or liver disease. Monitor LFTs as recommended. Transaminase levels 3 times normal may precipitate severe hepatic toxicity. If CK elevated, assess renal function as rhabdomyolysis with myoglobinuria could cause renal shutdown. Stop drug therapy and clearly mark chart and advise client not to take again.
4. Note nutritional analysis by dietitian; assess cholesterol profile (HDL, LDL, cholesterol, and triglycerides) after 3–6 months of exercise and diet therapy if risk factors do not require immediate drug therapy. With diabetes and

coronary heart disease, a more aggressive drug approach should be instituted in addition to diet therapy with goals of reducing LDL way below 100.

CLIENT/FAMILY TEACHING

1. Take only as directed. Drug is used to lower cholesterol levels and stabilize plaques in order to prevent heart attacks and progression of CAD as well as control coronary risk factors.
2. Report any pain in skeletal muscles or unexplained muscle pain, tenderness, or weakness promptly, especially with fever or malaise. Stop drug with any major trauma, surgery, or serious illness.
3. May cause photosensitivity; avoid prolonged sun or UV light exposure. Use sunscreens, sunglasses, and protective clothing when exposed.
4. Continue lifestyle modifications that include low-fat, low-cholesterol, and low-sodium diets, weight reduction with obese clients, smoking cessation, reduction of alcohol consumption, and regular aerobic exercise in the overall goal of cholesterol reduction.
5. Avoid OTC agents. May use Niaspan (SR form of niacin) with careful monitoring. Use a fibrate cautiously; lower statin dose is used and LFTs monitored.
6. Keep all F/U to assess response, labs, and for adverse SE.

OUTCOMES/EVALUATE

- ↓ LDL, triglycerides, and total cholesterol levels; ↓ risk of placque rupture and death

ANTIHYPERTENSIVE AGENTS

SEE ALSO THE FOLLOWING DRUG CLASSES AND INDIVIDUAL DRUGS:

Alpha-1-Adrenergic Blocking Agents
Alfuzosin hydrochloride
Doxazosin mesylate
Prazosin hydrochloride
Tamsulosin hydrochloride
Terazosin

Angiotensin-II Receptor Blockers
Azilsartan medoxomil
Candesartan cilexetil
Eprosartan mesylate
Irbesartan
Losartan potassium
Olmesartan medoxomil
Telmisartan
Valsartan

Angiotensin-Converting Enzyme Inhibitors
Benazepril hydrochloride
Captopril
Enalapril maleate
Fosinopril sodium
Lisinopril
Quinapril hydrochloride
Ramipril
Trandolapril

Beta-Adrenergic Blocking Agents
Atenolol
Betaxolol hydrochloride
Bisoprolol fumarate
Metoprolol succinate
Metoprolol tartrate
Nadolol
Nebivolol
Penbutolol sulfate
Propranolol hydrochloride
Timolol maleate

Calcium Channel Blocking Agents
Amlodipine
Clevidipine
Diltiazem hydrochloride
Felodipine
Isradipine
Nicardipine hydrochloride
Nifedipine
Nimodipine
Nisoldipine*
Verapamil

Centrally-Acting Agents
Methyldopa
Methyldopate hydrochloride

Combination Drugs Used for Hypertension
Amlodipine/Benazepril hydrochloride
Bisoprolol fumarate/Hydrochlorothiazide
Irbesartan/Hydrochlorothiazide
Lisinopril/Hydrochlorothiazide
Losartan potassium/Hydrochlorothiazide
Olmesartan medoxomil/Hydrochlorothiazide
Triamterene/Hydrochlorothiazide
Valsartan/Hydrochlorothiazide

Miscellaneous Agents
Aliskiren
Bosentan
Carvedilol
Epoprostenol sodium*
Minoxidil, oral*

Drugs marked with an * are available to view in the 2013 Nurse's Drug Handbook Website at www.cengage.com/community/nursesdrughandbook.

GENERAL STATEMENT

The Seventh Report of the Joint National Committee on Prevention, Detection, Evaluation and Treatment of High Blood Pressure classifies BP for adults aged 18 and over as follows: **Normal** as <120/<80 mm Hg, **Prehypertension** as 120–139/80–89 mm Hg, **Stage 1 Hypertension** as 140–159/90–99 mm Hg, and **Stage 2 Hypertension** as > or equal to 160/> or equal to 100 mm Hg. Drug therapy is recommended depending on the BP and whether certain risk factors (e.g., smoking, dyslipidemia, diabetes, age, gender, target organ damage, clinical CV disease) are present. Lifestyle modification is an important component of treating hypertension, including weight reduction, diet, reduction of sodium intake, aerobic physical exercise, cessation of smoking, and moderate alcohol intake. The risk of cardiovascular disease begins to increase when either the SPB exceeds 115 mm Hg or the DBP is greater than 75 mm Hg. Beyond 115/75 the risk of CV disease doubles with each advance of 20/10 mm Hg. In clients over 50 years of age, SBPs greater than 140 mm Hg are more important determinants of CV disease than are elevated DBPs. Generally speaking, the primary agents for initial monotherapy of Stage 1 hypertension to treat uncomplicated hypertension are thiazide diuretics; one may also consider ACE inhibitors, angiotensin receptor blockers, calcium channel blockers, and beta-adrenergic blocking agents. It should be noted that diet, exercise, and other life modifications are often sufficient to prevent or reduce hypertension. To treat Stage 2 hypertension, two drug combinations should be considered, i.e., usually a thiazide diuretic and an ACE inhibitor, or angiotensin receptor blocker, or a beta blocker, or a calcium channel blocker.

Various studies have shown that two or more antihypertensive drugs may be required for clients to reach their treatment goals. Such combinations may be beneficial to improve BP lowering efficacy, to obtain BP goals earlier, and to reduce major adverse CV events.

DRUG INTERACTIONS

See Individual Drugs

H ***Black cohosh*** / May potentiate antihypertensive drugs

H ***Garlic*** / May potentiate antihypertensive drugs

H ***Hawthorn*** / Cardioactive, hypotensive, and coronary vasodilator action of hawthorn may affect antihypertensive effect; monitor.

DOSAGE

See individual drugs.

NURSING IMPLICATIONS

ASSESSMENT

1. Note reasons for therapy, other agents trialed, family history of hypertension, stroke, CVD, CHD, MI, dyslipidemia, diabetes.
2. Assess baseline pulse rate and BP before starting antihypertensive therapy. To ensure accuracy of baseline readings, take BP in both (bared and supported) arms (lying, standing, and sitting) 2 min apart (30 min after last cigarette or caffeine consumption) at least three times during one visit, and on two subsequent visits. Document BMI (body mass index), height, weight and risk factors.
3. Ascertain lifestyle modifications (weight reduction, ↓ alcohol intake, regular exercise, reduced sodium/fat intake, stress reduction, and smoking cessation) needed to achieve lowered BP. Offer a trial following these modifications, and reassess in 3 months before starting therapy unless BP is in severe range or >2 risk factors.
4. Note funduscopic and neurologic exam findings. Assess for thyroid enlargement and presence of target organ damage. If difficult to control, assess for renal artery stenosis or secondary causes of HTN, and refer for 24 hr ambulatory BP monitoring.
5. Monitor ECG, electrolytes, CBC, uric acid, urinalysis, lipid panel, LFTs; always check for proteinuria.

Classifications

CLIENT/FAMILY TEACHING

1. Drugs control but do not cure hypertension. Take medications despite feeling fine and do not stop abruptly; may cause rebound hypertension. Drugs only provide protection/control of BP for the day in which they are taken. They must be taken daily as prescribed to ensure control. If dose missed, do not double up or take two doses close together.
2. Avoid activities that require mental alertness until drug effects realized.
3. Weakness, dizziness, and fainting may occur with rapid changes of position from lying to standing (postural hypotension). Rise slowly from a lying or sitting position and dangle legs for several minutes before standing to minimize low BP effects. Exercising in hot weather may worsen these effects. Do not become dehydrated.
4. There are generally no S&S of high blood pressure. When S&S become evident is when organ damage has already occurred. Keep a record of BP readings at different times during the day and evening to share with provider.
5. Adhere to a low-sodium, low-fat diet; see dietitian as needed for education, meal planning, and food selections. Avoid excessive amounts of caffeine (tea, coffee, chocolate, or colas).
6. Report any swelling in hands or feet, sudden weight gain, increased SOB, chest pain, or changes in urination, i.e., pain, frequency, or reduced amounts. Have yearly eye exams to detect early retinal changes from ↑ BP.
7. Avoid agents that may lower BP (e.g., alcohol, barbiturates, CNS depressants) or that could elevate BP (e.g., OTC cold remedies, oral contraceptives, steroids, NSAIDs [ibuprofen, naproxen], appetite suppressants, tricyclic antidepressants, MAOIs). Sympathomimetic amines in products used to treat asthma, colds, and allergies must be used with extreme caution
8. Report if sexual dysfunction occurs as medication can usually be changed to minimize symptoms or other options for sexual dysfunction explored.
9. Identify holistic interventions/lifestyle modifications necessary for BP control: dietary restrictions of fat and sodium (2–3 grams/day), weight reduction, ↓ alcohol (i.e., less than 24 oz beer or less than 8 oz of wine or less than 2 oz of 100-proof whiskey per day), tobacco cessation, ↑ physical activity, regular exercise programs, proper rest, and methods to reduce and deal with stress and how to incorporate into lifestyle.
10. Keep all F/U to assess response, labs, and adverse SE; bring log of BP and HR for provider review.

OUTCOMES/EVALUATE

- Understanding of disease/compliance with prescribed therapy
- ↓ BP (SBP <130 and DBP <80 mm Hg)
- Control/prevent target organ damage, stroke, MI, and/or death

ANTI-INFECTIVE DRUGS

SEE ALSO THE FOLLOWING INDIVIDUAL DRUGS AND DRUG CLASSES:

Aminoglycosides
Antiviral drugs
Bacitracin
Butenafine hydrochloride
Ceftaroline fosamil monoacetate
Cephalosporins
Chloramphenicol
Daptomycin
Doripenem*
Erythromycins
Fidaxomicin
Fluoroquinolones
Imipenem-Cilastatin sodium
Macrolides
Penicillins
Pentamidine isethionate
Pyrantel pamoate
Quinupristin/Dalfopristin
Sulfonamides
Telavancin hydrochloride*
Telithromycin
Tetracyclines
Tigecycline
Vancomycin hydrochloride

Drugs marked with an * are available to view in the 2013 Nurse's Drug Handbook Website at www.cengage.com/community/nursesdrughandbook.

GENERAL STATEMENT

The following general guidelines apply to the use of most anti-infective drugs:

1. Anti-infective drugs can be divided into those that are *bacteriostatic,* that is, arrest the multiplication and further development of the infectious agent, or *bactericidal,* that is, kill and thus eradicate all living microorganisms. Both time of administration and length of therapy may be affected by this difference.
2. Some anti-infectives halt the growth of or eradicate many different microorganisms and are termed *broad-spectrum antibiotics.* Others affect only certain specific organisms and are termed *narrow-spectrum antibiotics.*
3. Some of the anti-infectives elicit a hypersensitivity reaction in some persons. Penicillins cause more severe and more frequent hypersensitivity reactions than any other drug.
4. Because of differences in susceptibility of infectious agents to anti-infectives, the sensitivity of the microorganism to the drug ordered should be determined before treatment is initiated. Several sensitivity tests are commonly used for this purpose.
5. Certain anti-infective agents have marked side effects, some of the more serious of which are neurotoxicity, including ototoxicity, and nephrotoxicity. Care must be taken not to administer two anti-infectives with similar side effects concomitantly, or to administer these drugs to clients in whom the side effects might be damaging (e.g., a nephrotoxic drug to a client suffering from kidney disease). The choice of anti-infective also depends on its distribution in the body (i.e., whether it passes the blood-brain barrier).
6. Anti-infective drugs can also eradicate the normal intestinal flora necessary for proper digestion, synthesis of vitamin K, and control of fungi that may gain access to the GI tract (superinfection).

INDICATIONS/USES

See individual drugs. Anti–infective drugs are used systemically as well as locally (i.e., dermatologic, ophthalmic, otic, vaginal). The choice of the anti-infective depends on the nature of the illness to be treated, the sensitivity of the infecting agent, and the client's previous experience with the drug. Hypersensitivity and allergic reactions may preclude the use of the agent of choice. Labeling advises providers to prescribe antibiotics only to treat infections thought to be caused by bacteria or viruses and to counsel clients on the proper use of these drugs.

ACTION/KINETICS

Action

The mechanism of action of the anti-infectives varies. The following modes of action have been identified* Note the considerable overlap among these mechanisms:

1. Inhibition of synthesis of or activation of enzymes that disrupt bacterial cell walls leading to loss of viability and possibly cell lysis (e.g., penicillins, cephalosporins, cycloserine, bacitracin, vancomycin, miconazole, ketoconazole, clotrimazole).
2. Direct effect on the microbial cell membrane to affect permeability and leading to leakage of intracellular components (e.g., polymyxin, colistimethate, nystatin, amphotericin).
3. Effect on the function of 30S and 50S bacterial ribosomes to cause a reversible inhibition of protein synthesis (e.g., chloramphenicol, tetracyclines, erythromycin, clindamycin).
4. Bind to the 30S ribosomal subunit that alters protein synthesis and leads to cell death (e.g., aminoglycosides).
5. Effect on bacterial nucleic acid metabolism, which inhibits DNA-dependent RNA polymerase (e.g., rifampin) or inhibition of gyrase (e.g., fluoroquinolones).
6. Antimetabolites that block essential enzymes of folate metabolism.
7. Antiviral drugs that halt viral replication. Classes include (a) nucleic acid analogs such as acyclovir or gancyclovir that selectively inhibit viral DNA polymerase; (b) nucleic acid analogs such as lamivudine or zidovudine, that inhibit reverse transcriptase; (c) nonnucleoside reverse transcriptase inhibitors, such as efavirenz or nevirapine; and,

* Chemotherapy of Antimicrobial Diseases. In *Goodman and Gilman's The Pharmacological Basis of Therapeutics,* 11th ed. Edited by Brunton, Laurence, Lazo, John, and Parker, Keith. New York, McGraw-Hill, 2006.

(d) inhibitors of HIV protease or influenza neuraminidase.

CONTRAINDICATIONS

Hypersensitivity or allergies to the drug.

SIDE EFFECTS

The antibiotics and anti-infective agents have few direct toxic effects. Kidney and liver damage, deafness, and blood dyscrasias are occasionally observed.

The following undesirable manifestations, however, occur frequently: (1) Suppression of the normal flora of the body, which in turn keeps certain pathogenic microorganisms, such as *Candida albicans, Proteus,* or *Pseudomonas,* from causing infections. If the flora is altered, superinfections (monilial vaginitis, enteritis, UTIs), which necessitate the discontinuation of therapy or the use of other antibiotics, can result. (2) Incomplete eradication of an infectious organism. Casual use of anti-infectives favors the emergence of *resistant* strains insensitive to a particular drug. To minimize the chances for the development of resistant strains, anti-infectives are usually given at specified doses for a prescribed length of time after acute symptoms have subsided.

OVERDOSE MANAGEMENT

Treatment: Discontinue the drug and treat symptomatically. Supportive measures should be instituted as needed. Hemodialysis may be used although its effectiveness is questionable, depending on the drug and the status of the client (i.e., more effective in impaired renal function).

LABORATORY TEST CONSIDERATIONS

The bacteriologic sensitivity of the infectious organism to the anti-infective (especially the antibiotic) should be tested by the lab before initiation of therapy and during treatment.

DOSAGE

See individual drugs.

NURSING IMPLICATIONS

GENERAL NURSING CONSIDERATIONS FOR ALL ANTI-INFECTIVES

IMPLEMENTATION/ADMINISTRATION/STORAGE

1. Check expiration date.
2. Store according to recommended storage method.
3. Mark date and time of reconstitution, your initials, and the solution strength. Mark expiration date; store under appropriate conditions.
4. Complete infusion (or as ordered) before the drug loses potency; check drug info.

ASSESSMENT

1. Note onset, characteristics of S&S, clinical presentation, location, source of infection (if known), and culture results.
2. List any unusual reaction/sensitivity with any anti-infectives (usually penicillin). Note any previous experience with agent and outcome.
3. Conspicuously mark allergy: in red on the chart, medication record, ID band, care plan, pharmacy record, computerized record, and bed. Note if observed or reported by client.
4. Monitor VS, I&O; ensure adequate hydration. Assess for hives, rashes, or difficulty breathing, which may indicate a hypersensitivity or allergic response.
5. If drug mainly excreted by the kidneys, reduce dose with renal dysfunction. Nephrotoxic drugs are usually contraindicated with renal dysfunction because toxic drug levels are rapidly attained.
6. Verify orders when two or more anti-infectives are ordered for the same client, especially if they have similar side effects, such as nephro/neurotoxicity. Electronic entry prevents confusion.
7. Assess for superinfections, particularly of fungal origin, characterized by black furred tongue, nausea, and/or diarrhea.
8. Protect during hospitalization while immunocompromised by:
   - Limiting exposure to persons suffering from an active infectious process
   - Rotating IV site q 72–96 hr; changing IV tubing q 48 hr
   - Providing/emphasizing good hygiene
   - Washing hands carefully before and after contact with client
   - Screening visitors and having them wash hands before contact
9. Schedule administration throughout 24-hr period to maintain therapeutic drug levels. Administration schedule is determined by the drug half-life ($t^{1/2}$), severity of infection, evidence of organ dysfunction, and client's need

for sleep. Assess drug levels (peak and trough) to determine dosing and to assess adequacy of levels. Observe for mental status changes.

10. Obtain cultures before administering empiric therapy. Use correct procedure for obtaining, storing, and transporting specimens. Monitor VS, cultures, CBC, renal and LFTs.

CLIENT/FAMILY TEACHING

1. Take at prescribed intervals even if feeling better. Indentify ways to ensure proper dosing and complete therapy.
2. Use only under supervision. Do not share with friends or family members.
3. Prevent infection recurrence by completing entire prescription, despite feeling well. This ensures that the organism is eradicated and diminishes the emergence of drug-resistant bacterial strains. Incomplete therapy and indiscriminate use may render client unresponsive to the antibiotic with the next infection.
4. Report any unusual bruising or bleeding, e.g., bleeding gums, blood in stool, urine, or other secretions; S&S of allergic reactions, including rash, fever, itching, and hives or superinfections such as pain, swelling, redness, drainage, perineal itching, diarrhea, rash/sore throat or rash/joint pain/swelling as in serum sickness, or a change in S&S.
5. Report adverse side effects, lack of response, excessive diarrhea, or worsening of condition after 48–72 hr of therapy.
6. Take antipyretics as prescribed ATC for fever reduction as needed. Discard any unused drug after therapy completed.
7. Keep all F/U to assess response, labs, and for adverse SE.

OUTCOMES/EVALUATE

- Prevention/resolution of infection
- ↓ Fever, WBCs; ↑ appetite
- Negative culture reports
- Therapeutic serum drug levels

ANTINEOPLASTIC AGENTS ■

SEE ALSO THE FOLLOWING INDIVIDUAL ENTRIES:

Abiraterone acetate
Aldesleukin
Alemtuzumab
Altretamine*
Amifostine
Anastrozole
Asparaginase
Azacitidine
BCG Intravesical
Bendamustine hydrochloride
Bevacizumab
Bicalutamide
Bleomycin sulfate
Bortezomib
Brentuximab vedotin
Busulfan
Cabazitaxel
Capecitabine
Carboplatin
Carmustine
Cetuximab
Chlorambucil
Cinacalcet hydrochloride*
Cisplatin
Clofarabine
Crizotinib
Dacarbazine
Dasatinib
Daunorubicin citrate liposomal
Daunorubicin hydrochloride
Decitabine
Denileukin diftitox
Docetaxel
Doxorubicin hydrochloride conventional
Doxorubicin hydrochloride liposomal
Epirubicin hydrochloride
Eribulin mesylate
Erlotinib
Everolimus
Exemestane
Floxuridine
Fludarabine phosphate
Fluorouracil
Flutamide
Gefitinib
Gemcitabine hydrochloride
Goserelin acetate
Ibritumomab tiuxetan
Idarubicin hydrochloride
Ifosfamide
Imatinib mesylate
Interferon alfa-2b recombinant
Interferon alfa-n3
Ipilimumab

Irinotecan hydrochloride
Ixabepilone
Letrozole
Leuprolide acetate
Lomustine
Medroxyprogesterone acetate
Megestrol acetate
Mercaptopurine
Mesna
Methotrexate
Methotrexate sodium
Mitomycin
Nilutamide
Ofatumumab
Oxaliplatin
Paclitaxel
Panitumumab
Pazopanib hydrochloride
Pegaspargase
Pemetrexed
Pralatrexate
Procarbazine hydrochloride
Rituximab
Romidepsin
Sorafenib
Sunitinib maleate
Tamoxifen citrate
Temozolomide*
Temsirolimus
Teniposide
Thioguanine
Topotecan hydrochloride
Toremifene citrate
Trastuzumab
Triptorelin pamoate
Valrubicin
Vandetanib
Vemurafenib
Vinblastine sulfate
Vincristine sulfate
Vinorelbine tartrate
Vorinostat

Drugs marked with an * are available to view in the 2013 Nurse's Drug Handbook Website at www.cengage.com/community/nursesdrughandbook.

GENERAL STATEMENT

The choice of the chemotherapeutic agent(s) depends both on the cell type of the tumor and on its site of growth. All antineoplastic agents are cytotoxic (i.e., cell poisons) and therefore interfere with normal as well as neoplastic cells. However, neoplastic cells are more active and multiply more rapidly than normal cells and are thus more affected by the antineoplastic agents. Normal, rapidly growing tissue cells, such as those of the bone marrow, the GI mucosal epithelium, and hair follicles, are particularly susceptible to antineoplastic agents. The margin between the dose of antineoplastic drug needed to destroy the neoplastic cells and that needed to cause bone marrow damage, for example, is narrow. Since WBCs or platelets show the effect of an overdose more rapidly than do erythrocytes, the platelet and WBC counts are often used as a guide to dosage. If a blood or marrow test indicates a precipitous fall in the WBC or platelet count, the antineoplastic agent may have to be discontinued or the dosage modified significantly. Drugs are frequently withheld when the WBC count falls below 2,000/mm^3 and the platelet count falls below 100,000/mm^3. With the advent of granulocyte colony-stimulating factors, providers may now utilize this to support large dosing on an aggressive cancer, thus preventing postponement of therapy until recovery of the client's hematologic parameters. Sometimes the effect of the antineoplastic drugs on the bone marrow is cumulative, with the depression of WBCs and platelets occurring weeks or months after initiation of therapy.

GI tract toxicity is manifested by development of oral ulcers, intestinal bleeding, nausea, vomiting, loss of appetite, and diarrhea. Finally, alopecia often results from antineoplastic drug therapy.

INDICATIONS/USES

See individual drugs. Most of the drugs discussed in this section are used exclusively for neoplastic disease. A few are used on an experimental basis for some of the rheumatic diseases.

ACTION/KINETICS

Action

During division, cells go through a number of stages during which they may be susceptible to various chemotherapeutic agents (see *Action/Kinetics* of various drugs).

CONTRAINDICATIONS

Hypersensitivity to drug. Some antineoplastic agents may be contraindicated for up to 4 weeks after radiation therapy or chemotherapy with similar drugs. During first trimester of pregnancy.

Classifications

SPECIAL CONCERNS

- Use with caution, and at reduced dosages, in clients with preexisting bone marrow depression, malignant infiltration of bone marrow or kidney, liver dysfunction, or previous recent chemotherapy usage.
- Safe use during pregnancy not established.

SIDE EFFECTS

Bone marrow depression (leukopenia, thrombocytopenia, ***agranulocytosis***, anemia) is the major danger of antineoplastic therapy. ***Bone marrow depression can sometimes be irreversible.*** *It is mandatory that the client have frequent total blood counts and periodic bone marrow examinations. Precipitous falls must be reported to a physician.* **Other side effects include: GI:** N&V (may be severe), anorexia, diarrhea (may be hemorrhagic), stomatitis, mucositis, enteritis, abdominal cramps, intestinal ulcers. **Hepatic:** Hepatic toxicity including jaundice and changes in liver enzymes. **Dermatologic:** Dermatitis, erythema, various dermatoses including maculopapular rash, alopecia (reversible), pruritus, staining of vein path with some drugs, urticaria, cheilosis. **Immunologic:** Immunosuppression with increased susceptibility to viral, bacterial, or fungal infections. **CNS:** Depression, lethargy, confusion, dizziness, headache, fatigue, malaise, fever, weakness. **GU:** ***Acute renal failure***, reproductive abnormalities including amenorrhea and azoospermia. *NOTE:* Alkylating agents, in particular, may be both carcinogenic and mutagenic.

DOSAGE

See individual drugs.

NURSING IMPLICATIONS

GENERAL NURSING CONSIDERATIONS FOR ANTINEOPLASTIC AGENTS

IMPLEMENTATION/ADMINISTRATION/STORAGE

1. Antineoplastic drugs should be prepared only by trained personnel; avoid if pregnant.
2. Cytotoxic exposure may be through inhalation, ingestion, and absorption during preparation; prepare under a laminar flow (biologic) hood.
   - If not available, prepare in a separate room in a work area away from cooling or heating vents and away from other people. Cover work table area with a disposable plastic liner.
   - Use latex gloves (if not allergic) to protect the skin when reconstituting; do not use gloves made of PVC since these are permeable to some cytotoxic drugs. Good handwashing before and after preparation is essential. Prevent drug contact with skin or mucous membranes; document occurrence and wash area immediately with copious amounts of water.
   - Wear disposable, non permeable gown with closed front and knit cuffs completely covering wrists.
   - Wear goggles. Should material enter eyes, wash well with isotonic saline eyewash (or water if isotonic saline is unavailable) and consult ophthalmologist.
3. Start infusion with a solution not containing the chemotherapy drug. Avoid dorsum of the hand, wrist, or antecubital fossa as infusion site.
4. Use disposable Luer-loc fittings, protected needles, syringes, and connectors.
   - If drug is to be reconstituted from a vial, vent the vial at the beginning of the procedure. Venting lowers internal pressure and reduces risk of spilling/spraying (aerosolization) solution when needle is withdrawn.
   - Use sterile alcohol wipe around needle and vial top when withdrawing drug and when expelling air.
5. Wipe external surfaces of syringes and bottles once prepared. Place all disposable equipment in a separate plastic bag specifically marked for incineration.
6. Wear latex gloves when disposing of vomitus, urine, or feces.
7. Record all exposure times during preparation, administration, cleanup, and spills. Follow appropriate institutional guidelines governing exposures allowed, extravasation, spills, and periodic lab determinations.

ASSESSMENT

1. Note indications for therapy, onset, location, staging and type and length of infusion/therapy, other agents trialed, other options explored, outcome.
2. Assess infusion sites for evidence of infection, infiltration, or adverse reactions.

3. Assess client/family understanding of: illness, as well as risks of therapy, desire for treatment, importance of living will, and emotional support needs.
4. Monitor CBC, renal and LFTs carefully. Assess I&O, VS, skin integrity/color, and for evidence of bruising/bleeding, infection, fever, changes in bowel or urinary patterns, and mentation changes.

OUTCOMES/EVALUATE

- Understanding of illness, therapy options, drug side effects, and goals of therapy and desire for treatment
- Intolerance to therapy evidenced by tumor growth, acute renal failure, and liver/lung/cardiac toxicities
- N&V, pain, anorexia, or diarrhea may indicate inadequate levels of appropriate prescribed agents to control
- Presence and extent of psychologic depression, lethargy, or other mental status changes requiring therapy/intervention
- Prevention of adverse drug side effects
- Control of pain/fear
- Control/inhibition of malignant cell proliferation
- Hair regrowth
- Desired cure/remission

NURSING CONSIDERATIONS DURING INITIATION OF CHEMOTHERAPY

ASSESSMENT

1. Identify condition requiring therapy (onset, location, type, staging and S&S) and any previous radiation, surgery, or chemotherapy treatments.
2. Note any hypersensitivity to drugs or foods.
3. Determine nutritional status; note height, weight, and VS; doses are based on BSA (m^2) calculations (square root of Ht × Wt divided by 3,600).
4. Perform physical exam noting all findings and any deficiency. Examine carefully for abnormalities/problems including oral cavity, VS, Wt, and skin integrity.
5. Assess pathology reports, radiographic, MRI/CT, and other confirmatory studies. Share or interpret/clarify for client as requested.
6. Note prescribed route of administration: oral, IV, IM, or directly at the tumor site (intracavity, intrapleural, intrathecal, intravesical, intraperitoneal, intra-arterial, or topical).
7. Depending on the route, length of therapy, frequency of access, venous integrity, and client preference, determine need/location/type of access device.
8. Rate pain using a pain rating scale. Assess pain control regimen to ensure pain is well controlled.
9. Premedicate (antiemetic, antihistamine, and/or anti-inflammatory) 30–60 min before therapy and as needed.
10. Assess emotional status; evaluate need for antidepressant therapy and support groups.
11. Monitor bone marrow function (CBC with differential), platelets, liver and renal function.

INTERVENTIONS

1. Monitor VS, I&O. Report any pain, redness, or edema near injection site during or after treatment. If extravasation occurs, stop infusion and follow institutional protocol for minimizing effects. General guidelines for managing an extravasation include:
   - Document/report.
   - Aspirate drug through cannula with small syringe (tuberculin size).
   - Administer antidote as indicated.
   - Remove catheter/needle and apply ice (heat if vinca alkaloids).
   - Assess closely until site is healed.
2. Chart antineoplastic drugs on the medication administration record (MAR), electronic record, and according to the established protocol. Record therapy on the MAR:
   - Day 1: first day of the first dose.
   - Number each day after that in sequence, even though may not receive drug daily.
   - Indicate when nadir (the time of most severe physiologic depression) is likely to occur so that possible complications, such as infection and bleeding, can be anticipated and treated early; note recovery time.
   - When repeating drug regimen, first day of therapy is charted as day 1.
3. Establish interventions to promote client adherence. Keep informed and interpret complicated terminology/therapy/test results, treat symptoms, support client/family, and help distinguish/understand unconventional emotions/anger.
4. Identify references, information centers, websites, and support groups to assist in coping

with illness, understanding complex therapy, and emotional upset within the family unit.

5. Case management during therapy and assist client/family in navigating through diagnosis, to completion of therapy.

CLIENT/FAMILY TEACHING

1. Encourage to comply with all aspects of the therapeutic regimen to ensure success.
2. Practice reliable contraception. Determine if egg/sperm harvesting is indicated in young persons desiring a family.
3. Review information/literature R/T condition requiring treatment. The American Cancer Society provides many free booklets on cancers, chemotherapy, and how to deal with the side effects of treatments. Go to the library, internet, local cancer society, and provider with unanswered questions. May also call 1-800-4-CANCER, the Cancer Information Service at the National Cancer Institute (at http://www.cancer.gov/), or access other sites through the Internet or library.
4. Assist client to attain resource for second opinion if so desired.
5. Review drug side effects that may occur and a means for coping with disease and adverse effects.
6. Identify community support groups that offer assistance and support during chemotherapy treatments.
7. Identify who to call to report adverse side effects or to request clarification of instructions.
8. When antineoplastic agents are prepared and administered in the home, advise families how to dispose of urine, feces, vomitus, and equipment and how to handle spills and associated side effects.
9. Keep all F/U to assess response, labs, and for adverse SE.

NURSING CONSIDERATIONS FOR BONE MARROW DEPRESSION (MYELOSUPPRESSION)

LEUKOPENIA

ASSESSMENT

1. Assess for granulocytopenia or decreased WBCs (normal values: 5,000–10,000/mm^3).
2. Review differential (normal values: neutrophils 60–70%, lymphocytes 25–30%, monocytes 2–6%, eosinophils 1–3%, basophils 0.25–0.5%).
3. Note any sudden sharp drop in WBC count or a reduction below 2,000/mm^3; may require a dosage reduction, withdrawal of drug, protective isolation, and a granulocyte colony stimulating factor.
4. Determine nadir (time the blood count reaches its lowest point after chemotherapy) for prescribed agent (generally 7–14 days); assists to predict, monitor, and respond to effects of bone marrow depression.
5. Report fever above 38°C (100°F); limited resistance to infection due to leukopenia and immunosuppression. Assess for early S&S of infection: check oral cavity for sores/ulcerated areas and urine for odor or particulate matter. With reduced/absent granulocytes, local abscesses do not form with pus; infection becomes systemic.
6. Increased weakness or fatigue may indicate anemia or electrolyte imbalance. Fatigue is a significant side effect of therapy. With cytobines, e.g., interferon, fatigue may be overwhelming.

INTERVENTIONS

1. *Prevent infection* by using strict medical asepsis and frequent handwashing.
2. Provide frequent, meticulous, physical hygiene; maintain clean environment.
3. Cleanse and dry rectal area after each bowel movement. Apply ointment if irritated; use Tucks and/or Nupercainal for discomfort.
4. Use a gentle antiseptic to wash if tendency for skin eruptions.
5. Provide mouth care q 4–6 hr; otherwise mucosal deterioration occurs. Avoid lemon or glycerin; these tend to reduce saliva production and change pH of the mouth.
6. If WBC falls below 1,500–2,000/mm^3, may protect with:
   - Private room; explain reasons
   - Universal precautions; use gloves, masks, and gowns
   - Avoid indwelling urinary catheters
   - Frequent handwashing
   - Limit articles brought into room
   - Provide private bathroom or bedside commode
   - Minimize traffic in and out of room
   - Screen visitors for infection before they enter room; limit visitations

- Avoid exposure to dust, sprays, contaminated medical equipment
- Avoid deodorants; blocks sebaceous gland secretion
- Keep fresh fruits, vegetables, cut flowers, and any source of stagnant water (water pitcher, humidifiers, flower vases) away from client
- Review/stress kitchen hygiene and food safety at home
- Dogs, cats, birds, and other pets may carry infection; avoid contact
- Assess orders for granulocyte colony-stimulating factors and ensure availability

7. Prevent nosocomial infections from invasive procedures by:
   - Washing hands before and after any contact
   - Frequent assessment of skin integrity and all catheter sites
   - Cleansing skin with antiseptic before procedure
   - Changing IV tubing q 24 hr
   - Changing IV site q 48 hr, if no implanted device or other designated catheter for long-term use
   - Practice strict asepsis with all contacts, treatments and dressing changes
   - Keeping out of hospital if possible and managed at home

THROMBOCYTOPENIA

ASSESSMENT

1. Obtain platelet count (normal values: 150,000–400,000/mm^3). If below 50,000/mm^3, monitor closely.
2. Inspect skin for petechiae/bruising; assess all orifices for bleeding.
3. May hemorrhage spontaneously; transfuse if platelets <20,000.

INTERVENTIONS

1. Minimize SC or IM injections; apply pressure for 3–5 min to prevent leakage or hematoma.
2. Do not apply BP cuff or other tourniquet for excessive periods.
3. Avoid rectal temps and constipation; test all urine, GI secretions, and stool for occult blood.
4. Use safety precautions to avoid falls. Avoid unnecessary jostling or moving.
5. *Control bleeding* with:
   - Epistaxis: pinch nose for 10 min and apply pressure to upper lip to stop; in severe cases, small sponges saturated with neosynephrine ¼ % gently inserted into nare, or nasal packing, may be needed.
   - Transfusions, monitor VS before and 15 min after transfusion started and after completed. Assess for histo-incompatibility, indicated by chills, fever, and urticaria. Stop transfusion, provide supportive care, and follow appropriate institutional protocol for transfusion reaction.
6. Advise client to *prevent bleeding* by:
   - Not picking or forcefully blowing their nose
   - Avoiding contact sports and any activities that may cause injury
   - Reporting any severe frontal headaches
   - Using an electric razor for shaving rather than a blade
   - Using a soft-bristled toothbrush or massaging gums with fingers or a cotton ball and avoiding dental floss to limit irritation
   - Avoiding rectal irritation by contact with enemas, suppositories, or thermometers
   - Using a water-based lubricant before intercourse
   - Consuming plenty of fluids, increasing activity, and taking stool softeners to prevent constipation
   - Rearranging furniture so that area for ambulation is unimpeded and also to prevent bumping into furniture at night when getting out of bed to go to the bathroom
   - Having a nightlight to permit visualization during the night
   - Wearing shoes or slippers when ambulating

ANEMIA

ASSESSMENT

1. Assess for pallor, lethargy, dizziness, ↑ SOB, ↑ fatigue, ↓ BP or tilting.
2. Monitor CBC, reticulocyte count, MCV, and hemoglobin (normal values: men, 13.5–18.0 g/dL blood; women, 11.5–15.5 g/dL blood), and hematocrit (normal values: men, 40–52%; women, 35–46%), and iron panel.

INTERVENTIONS

1. *Minimize anemia* by:
   - Providing nutritious tolerable diet
   - Taking vitamins/iron supplements

2. *Assist with treatment of anemia* by:
   - Administering diet high in iron
   - Giving vitamins with minerals
   - Administering erythropoietin (Procrit) to stimulate RBC production
   - Administering blood transfusions
   - Spacing/scheduling activities to permit frequent rest periods
   - Positioning to facilitate ventilation; teaching breathing/relaxation techniques and administering oxygen
   - Controlling room temperature for comfort. Providing emotional support
   - Setting attainable goals with client and assisting them to attain these goals

NURSING CONSIDERATIONS FOR GI TOXICITY

NAUSEA AND VOMITING; ANOREXIA

ASSESSMENT

1. N&V may be due to either a CNS effect on the CTZ or direct irritation to the GI tract. With radiation therapy, N&V may be attributed to the accumulation of toxic waste products of cell destruction and localized damage to the lining of the throat, stomach, and intestine.
2. Anticipatory N&V is a conditioned response of unknown origin prior to chemotherapy which does respond to premedication.
3. Determine if refusing food or fluids or experiencing anorexia.
4. Monitor nutritional status and weights.
5. Examine the frequency, character, and amount of vomitus. List antiemetics prescribed and results.

INTERVENTIONS

1. *To prevent N&V:*
   - Antiemetics 30–60 min before or just after drug therapy
   - Therapy on empty stomach, with meals, or at bedtime
   - Antiemetic suppository
   - Ice chips at onset of nausea
   - Avoid carbonated beverages
   - Ingest dry carbohydrates such as toast/dry crackers before any activity
   - Wait for N&V to pass before serving food
   - Small, nutritious snacks; plan meal schedules to coincide with best tolerance time
   - Cold foods and salads with little cooking aroma to minimize N&V
   - Nourishing foods client likes
   - Consume a high-protein diet
   - Freeze and serve dietary supplements like ice cream; ↑ palatability
   - Avoid foods with overpowering aroma
   - Chew foods well
   - Good oral hygiene before and after meals (try 1 tsp baking soda in a glass of warm water for rinsing mouth)
   - Eat favorite foods.
   - Eat meals with others, preferably at a table. Sharing encourages eating.
   - Have client identify what works for them and what triggers symptoms
2. Antiemetics that have different actions/pharmacokinetics may be administered concurrently in an effort to control severe N&V.
3. *To treat N&V:*
   - Administer antiemetic(s). Report all vomiting; may require a change in therapy or dose or need for electrolyte correction.
   - Give other medications after meals.
   - Offer simple foods: rice, toast, noodles, bananas, scrambled eggs, mashed potatoes, custards, ice cream.
   - Offer salty foods (pretzels, crackers).
   - Avoid solid and liquid foods at the same meal.
   - Eliminate any room odors; avoiding malodorous foods (e.g., cabbage, sauerkraut, etc.).
   - Keep as comfortable, clean, and free from odor as possible.
   - Try another or concurrent antiemetic agents.
   - Correct electrolytes; provide hyperalimentation p.r.n.
   - Screen visitors/calls until client ready
   - Let client identify what appeals to them and what triggers symptoms.
4. *For anorexia:*
   - Provide small, frequent meals q 2 or 3 hr on schedule
   - Maximize caloric intake by offering nutrient-dense snacks and drinks (yogurt, cheese and crackers, peanut butter and jelly sandwiches, cereal, dried fruit, fruit nectar, and instant breakfast drink mixes)
   - Make nutrient-dense supplements with whole milk

- Suggest a walk or activity before eating to boost appetite
- Concentrate on obtaining favorite foods after identification
- Megace may stimulate appetite with certain forms of cancer while GI/colon cancers may require marinol therapy.

5. *To increase caloric intake and protein consumption:*
   - Add high-calorie foods such as mayonnaise, butter, and gravy to foods
   - Use whole milk in puddings, cream soups, custards
   - Make double-strength milk – add powdered milk to whole milk for gravies, hot cereals, mashed potatoes, eggs, casseroles, baked things, etc.
   - Add whipped cream to frosting and desserts
   - Offer milkshakes, nectar, and eggnog when thirsty
   - Offer peanut butter on crackers, bagels with cream cheese, trail mix, and nuts and seeds for snacks
   - Cut up meats and cheeses and add to salads, soups, scrambled eggs, etc.

BOWEL DYSFUNCTION (DIARRHEA/ ABDOMINAL CRAMPING)

ASSESSMENT

1. Note frequency and severity of cramping caused by hypermotility.
2. Document frequency, color, consistency, and amount of diarrhea; indicates tissue destruction. C&S stool.
3. Assess for dehydration and acidosis indicating electrolyte imbalance; monitor I&O and skin integrity on buttocks.
4. Encourage client to participate in care and identify what triggers symptoms and what helps

INTERVENTIONS

1. *To prevent diarrhea/abdominal cramping:*
   - Provide small, frequent meals on a schedule
   - Identify factors that aggravate/increase incidence
   - Use constipating foods, i.e., hard cheeses
2. *To treat diarrhea:*
   - Administer antidiarrheal and narcotic agent (i.e., codeine, tincture of opium, Imodium, or Lomotil). Report S&S, as a change in therapy or electrolyte correction may be needed.
   - Increase fluids/avoid dehydration
   - Provide foods to correct sodium and potassium losses, e.g., bananas, potatoes, fish and meat, apricot nectar, tomato juice, and sports drinks with "electrolytes," of Pedialyte
   - Avoid high-fiber foods that contain "insoluble fiber," such as wheat bran, brown rice, popcorn
   - Administer bulk-forming agents (i.e., Metamucil)
   - Offer "soluble-fiber" foods, i.e., white rice, oatmeal, applesauce, mashed potatoes, and pears
   - Avoid fried/greasy foods
   - Avoid excessive sweets; may aggravate diarrhea due to sorbitol, found in many gums and candies
   - Use aluminum-containing antacids
   - Avoid gas-forming foods, such as broccoli, corn, onion, garlic, lentils, and kidney beans
   - Avoid dairy products during acute episodes; consider lactose-free products or Lact-Aid, which facilitates digestion of lactose
   - Restrict intake to rest the bowel if necessary
   - Provide good skin care, especially to perianal area to prevent skin breakdown. Apply A&D ointment for perianal tenderness. Change gown and bed linens frequently; use special mattresses, frequent position changes, and room deodorizers as needed.
3. *To prevent constipation:*
   - Provide a high-fiber diet
   - Give stool softeners and bulk-forming agents
   - Increase fluid intake
   - Increase activity levels
   - Monitor frequency, consistency, and amount of stool
4. *To prevent obstruction:*
   - Aggressively manage constipation using lactose, sennosides, and softeners
   - Assess for early S&S such as abdominal pain, N&V, and diminished or absent bowel sounds

- Keep NPO, using NG suction to relieve before referring for surgical intervention.

STOMATITIS (MUCOSAL ULCERATION)

ASSESSMENT

1. Assess for mouth dryness, erythema, soreness, painful swallowing, and white patchy areas of oral mucosa.
2. Symptom onset usually 5 days to 2 weeks after starting therapy; assess regularly.

INTERVENTIONS

1. *To prevent stomatitis:*
   - Assess oral cavity 3 times/day and report bleeding gums or burning sensation when acid liquids such as fruit juice are ingested
   - Set up a regular schedule for oral preventive care
   - Provide good mouth care
   - Apply lubricant (Vaseline) to lips 3 times/day
2. *To treat stomatitis:*
   - Provide regular oral care
   - Apply topical viscous anesthetic, such as benzocaine 20%, or a swish and gargle anesthetic such as dyclonine hydrochloride 0.5%, or a swish, swallow/discard agent such as lidocaine 2% (Xylocaine), before meals or as needed to anesthetize oral mucosa. May swallow lidocaine after swishing it around oral cavity but encourage to expectorate it.
   - Puncture a vitamin E capsule and apply to painful lesions to promote healing
   - Offer "Magic Mouthwash," which consists of 4 grams (approx. 1/8 teaspoon) baking soda, 30 mL viscous Xylocaine, 30 mL Benadryl elixir, and 30 mL Maalox (optional) in 1 L NSS; swish and spit out q 1–2 hr as needed
   - Provide allopurinol mouthwash for fluorouracil-related stomatitis; or try sucking ice chips 1/2 hr before and during treatment
   - Offer small, frequent meals of bland foods at medium temperatures
   - Administer nystatin solution or clotrimazole troches orally for fungal infections
3. Administer medications (antifungals, antivirals) to prevent general infections.
4. Systemic antifungals may be required. If no relief investigate alternative therapies, i.e, Neupogen, etc. Do NOT let client continue to suffer as this is very painful and impairs recovery.

NURSING CONSIDERATIONS FOR NEUROTOXICITY

ASSESSMENT

1. Identify agents causing or having the potential to cause neurotoxic effects; further administration once symptoms have become prominent may be life threatening/non-reversible.
2. Involve neurology and client; report symptoms of minor neuropathies, i.e., tingling in hands and feet; loss of deep tendon reflexes. Use a tuning fork or monofilament to measure progressive loss of sensation. Report serious neuropathies, i.e., weakness of hands, ataxia, loss of coordination, foot drop, wrist drop, or paralytic ileus and hold therapy until evaluation completed.

INTERVENTIONS

1. *To prevent functional loss due to neurotoxicity:*
   - Identify neuropathies early so drug regimen can be adjusted/changed
   - Practice/teach seizure precautions
2. *To treat neuropathies:*
   - Use safety measures with functional losses
   - Maintain good body alignment by frequent and anatomically correct repositioning; ROM exercises.
   - Provide stool softeners/laxatives as needed
   - Identify causative agent and stop
   - Administer agents to help control pain
   - Use aids to prevent injury/falls i.e., cane, walker
   - Wear shoes to prevent injury, puncture, burn
   - Adjust water temperatures, wear protection when handling hot pots, bowls etc.

NURSING CONSIDERATIONS FOR OTOTOXICITY

ASSESSMENT

1. Assess for hearing difficulties before initiating therapy and monitor periodically during therapy.
2. Identify prescribed agents that may contribute to loss.

INTERVENTIONS

1. Report tinnitus or new onset hearing impairment.
2. Perform audiometry testing p.r.n. during therapy.

NURSING CONSIDERATIONS FOR HEPATOTOXICITY

ASSESSMENT

1. Assess for liver involvement, i.e., abdominal pain, high fever, diarrhea, and yellowing of skin/sclera. Screen for other sources of liver destruction, i.e., alcohol ingestion, heavy acetaminophen use, hepatitis B or C.
2. Identify prescribed agents that may contribute to liver dysfunction or medication combinations that may predispose one to progressive liver failure. Monitor LFTs regularly during therapy.
3. Obtain/assess the following LFTs:
   - Total serum bilirubin (normal values: 0.1–1.0 mg/dL); elevations may indicate liver disease or increased rate of RBC hemolysis.
   - AST (normal: 8–33 units/L). Elevations indicative of changes in liver, skeletal muscles, lungs, pancreas, and heart. Hepatitis produces striking elevations in the AST.
   - ALT (normal: 8–20 units/L). Elevations may precede hepatic necrosis.
   - LDH (normal: 70–250 units/L). Elevations may indicate hepatitis, pulmonary infarction, and CHF.

INTERVENTIONS

1. Prevent further hepatotoxicity by reporting LFT elevations and signs of liver involvement so drug regimen can be adjusted/changed.
2. Assist with treatment for hepatotoxicity by providing supportive nursing care for pain, fever, diarrhea, and jaundice associated symptoms.
3. Educate client on mechanism of disease and how to protect self from progressive liver destruction (i.e., avoid alcohol, high doses of acetaminophen, avoid OTC agents without provider approval).

NURSING CONSIDERATIONS FOR RENAL TOXICITY

ASSESSMENT

1. Report stomach pain, swelling of feet or lower legs, shakiness, reduced output, unusual body movements, or stomatitis.
2. Assess the following renal function tests:
   - Protein (normal urine: negative)
   - BUN (normal: 5–20 mg/dL)
   - Serum uric acid (normal: men, 3.5–7.0 mg/dL; women, 2.4–6.0 mg/dL)
   - C_{CR} (normal: women, 0.8–1.7 grams/24 hr; men, 1.0–1.9 grams/24 hr)
   - Quantitative uric acid (normal: 250–750 mg/day)

INTERVENTIONS

1. Monitor I&O. Test pH and alkalinize urine as indicated.
2. Consult nephrology for additional recommendations.
3. Monitor and control BP. Educate client concerning disease and how to protect self from progressive renal destruction, i.e., avoid elevated BP/BS, avoid OTC agents without provider approval.
4. Limit hyperuricemia with extra fluids to speed excretion of uric acid and to decrease hazard of crystal and urate stone formation. Administer uricosuric agents (i.e., probenecid) or antigout agents (i.e., allopurinol, colchicine) to lower uric acid levels.

NURSING CONSIDERATIONS FOR IMMUNOSUPPRESSION

ASSESSMENT

1. Assess for the presence of fever, chills, muscle aches, rigors, or sore throat.
2. Note changes in CBC (↓ WBC), skin integrity, urine changes, sputum production, drainage or other S&S R/T infections.

INTERVENTIONS

1. *To treat immunosuppression*:
   - Prevent infection as noted under bone marrow depression
   - Delay active immunization for several months after therapy is completed; may experience a hypo- or hyperactive response
   - Avoid contact with children who have recently taken the oral polio vaccine or are visibly sick
   - Avoid live vaccinia including zostrix
   - Avoid crowds and persons with known infections
   - Practice universal precautions
   - May be administered granulocyte colony-stimulating factor to boost immune system

2. Educate client to early S&S of infection and importance of early reporting. Regular frequent hand washing.
3. Review food safety (e.g., storage, handling, washing, cooking meats thoroughly, avoiding raw eggs) and stress importance of kitchen hygiene when preparing meals at home.
4. Have client identify food preparations at home and how to adjust to ensure safety.

NURSING CONSIDERATIONS FOR GU ALTERATIONS

ASSESSMENT

1. Assess for altered GU function. Most S&S, such as amenorrhea, cease after medication is discontinued.
2. Review risks; sterility may be a permanent result of therapy. Identify those that may be candidates for egg/sperm harvesting prior to therapy if pregnancy/child desired later.
3. Determine baseline function, assess regularly during therapy.

CLIENT/FAMILY TEACHING

1. Certain drugs may render individuals sterile. Advise that egg/sperm harvesting may be performed prior to therapy to accommodate future pregnancies/desired offspring.
2. To prevent fetal abnormalities/death, client and partner should use reliable contraceptive measures to avoid pregnancy, both during and for several months as directed after therapy.
3. Report any change in elimination patterns, new onset incontinence, pregnancy, or sexual dysfunction.
4. Keep regularly scheduled preventative appointments to evaluate function and to assess any adverse side effects.

NURSING CONSIDERATIONS FOR ALOPECIA

CLIENT/FAMILY TEACHING

1. Hair loss is a normal occurrence during chemotherapy. Treatment disrupts the mitotic activity of the hair follicle which weakens the hair shaft, causing it to break off. This includes all hair, i.e., eyebrows, body, and pubic hair.
2. Alopecia (hair loss) may occur within 2–3 weeks after the initial treatment. Assist to understand, be prepared for, and expect this as normal with chemotherapy. People respond differently; some may lose hair with a certain agent, others may not.
3. Hair usually will grow back but may be of a different texture or color. It should start to grow in again about 8 weeks after therapy is completed.
4. If receiving more than 4,500 rad to the cranium, hair loss may be permanent.
5. *To manage hair loss:*
   - Have client discuss their feelings/needs related to hair loss
   - Shop for a wig before hair loss begins
   - Wear a bandana or hat to cover head, and take special care to protect the bare head from sun exposure
   - Shave head, if hair starts to fall out in large clumps, and use a wig or scarf until scalp hair regrows
   - Wear a night cap at bedtime so hair that falls out during the night will be collected in one place and not all over the bed in the morning.
   - Attend support groups to share feelings related to changes in self-image and identify with others undergoing same
   - Report any loss of skin integrity or adverse effects

NURSING CONSIDERATIONS FOR ALTERATIONS IN SKIN

ASSESSMENT

1. Document skin color, turgor and integrity. Slight changes in skin color may occur during therapy.
2. Skin destruction R/T XRT requires aggressive treatment and care to prevent infection, pain, and further skin breakdown. Steroid therapy and topical creams may assist to reduce skin desquamation, scarring and disfigurement.
3. Identify additional stress that may contribute to skin changes, i.e. sun over-exposure, chemical contact dermatitis, systemic drug reactions.

INTERVENTIONS

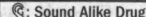

1. Maintain cleanliness of skin through bathing with oilated soaps in tepid water and frequent linen changes.
2. Prevent dryness and replenish skin moisture with regular application of emollient lotions and humidified air. Ensure adequate fluid and nutritional intake

Classifications

3. **Prevent excessive exposure to sun or artificial ultraviolet light; use sunscreen and protective clothing when exposed.**
4. **Use a special mattress or bed to redistribute weight on bony prominences and to minimize pressure and friction on pressure points. Establish and document a schedule for repositioning, massaging, and assessing skin condition.**
5. **If using wheelchair have special seat cushion to off set wt. and encourage to change positions frequently and to lie on belly on occasion to redistribute weight for a period of time.**
6. **With itching, attempt to stop scratching as this may impair skin integrity. Use antihistamines, corticosteroids, nonirritating moisturizers, and cool/ice compresses as needed.**
7. **Use analgesics to control pain as needed.**
8. **Refer for assistance with makeup application to enhance self esteem and if needed plastic surgery once therapy completed.**

OUTCOMES/EVALUATE

- **Inhibition of malignant cell proliferation**
- **Preservation of nerve function and hearing**
- **Knowledge of reproductive options**
- **Organ preservation**
- **Freedom from long term effects R/T adverse drug effects**
- **Self esteem intact**
- **Desired cure**

ANTIPARKINSON AGENTS

SEE ALSO THE FOLLOWING INDIVIDUAL ENTRIES:

Amantadine hydrochloride
Apomorphine hydrochloride
Benztropine mesylate
Carbidopa
Carbidopa/Levodopa
Diphenhydramine hydrochloride
Entacapone
Levodopa
Pramipexole
Rasagiline
Ropinirole hydrochloride
Tolcapone

GENERAL STATEMENT

Parkinson's disease is a progressive disorder of the nervous system, affecting mostly people over the age of 50. Parkinsonism is a frequent side effect of certain antipsychotic drugs, including prochlorperazine and chlorpromazine. Drug-induced symptoms usually disappear when the responsible agent is discontinued. The cause of Parkinson's disease is unknown; however, it is associated with a depletion of the neurotransmitter dopamine in the nervous system. Treatment focuses on administration of dopaminergic agents and/or anticholinergic drugs. Administration of levodopa-the precursor of dopamine-relieves symptoms in 75–80% of the clients. Most of the newer antiparkinsonian drugs must be given with levodopa. Anticholinergic agents also have a beneficial effect by reducing tremors and rigidity and improving mobility, muscular coordination, and motor performance. They are often administered together with levodopa. Certain antihistamines, notably diphenhydramine (Benadryl), are also useful in the treatment of parkinsonism. Clients suffering from Parkinson's disease need emotional support and encouragement because the debilitating nature of the disorder often causes depression. Comprehensive treatment also includes physical therapy.

SPECIAL CONCERNS

Clients taking dopamine agonists for parkinsonism may experience narcoleptic-sleep attacks.

DOSAGE

See individual drugs.

NURSING IMPLICATIONS

See *Nursing Implications* for individual drugs.

ASSESSMENT

1. **Note onset, characteristics of S&S, clinical presentation/impairment, PMH, family history of PD, disease progression, other agents/procedures trialed, and outcome.**
2. **List drugs prescribed. Determine if S&S are drug induced i.e., Haldol, phenothiazines) or are vascular forms (i.e., stroke induced), or atypical forms (i.e., multiple system atrophy, corticobasal degeneration and progressive supranuclear palsy). These forms can be differentiated from classic PD by different brain scans, blood tests and/or a thorough review**

of the history by a movement disorder specialist.

3. Monitor VS, I&O, and mental status. Assess for depression, affect, mood, behavioral changes, and suicide ideations.
4. Identify involvement in exercise, diet, PT/OT, and support groups; stress importance of these to improve mobility, flexibility, balance, range of motion and for preventing many of the disease's secondary symptoms such as depression and constipation.
5. Determine if surgical candidate for deep brain stimulation (DBS); most effective for those who experience disabling tremors, wearing-off spells and drug-induced dyskinesias.

CLIENT/FAMILY TEACHING

1. Parkinson's disease is a movement disorder that occurs when a group of cells in the substantia nigra (area of brain) begin to malfunction and die. These cells produce a chemical called dopamine which is a neurotransmitter (chemical messenger) that sends information to the parts of the brain that control movement and coordination. When dopamine-producing cells begin to die and the amount of dopamine produced in the brain decreases then these messages are sent/delivered more slowly thus leaving one incapable of initiating and controlling movements in a normal way.
2. It is thought that a combination of genetic and environmental factors contribute to this disease.
3. Drug therapy is aimed at restoring normal balances of cholinergic and dopaminergic influences in the brain (basal ganglia) to control tremor and permit desired activity.
4. Take only as prescribed; some agents have many adverse side effects. Taking with food may help to minimize GI upset. If stopped abruptly may induce parkinsonian crisis.
5. Close neurologic follow-up is imperative; some drugs may lose effectiveness and changes or additional therapy may be needed. Deep brain stimulation (DBS) involves the implantation of a battery-operated neurotransmitter under the collarbone to a wire which is placed through a small hole in the skull. The electrode tip is implanted in the target brain center. Electrical impulses are sent from the neurotransmitter up along the wire to the brain. These impulses interfere with and block the electrical signals that cause tremors and other symptoms of this disease. Subthalamic Nucleus DBS addresses not only tremors but also rigidity, slowness of movement, stiffness, and walking allowing a decrease in medications.
6. Avoid activities that require mental alertness and coordination until drug effects realized. Use caution to prevent falls and injury.
7. May use ice chips, fluids or sugarless candy/gum to relieve dry mouth symptoms. Increase fluids and fiber in diet, and activity to prevent constipation.
8. Talking systems, beeping watches, PDA's and multi-alarm timers will help remind you when you need to take certain meds before wearing off and loss of function occur.
9. Have client identify impact of disease on lifestyle and identify ways to reduce impact and manage symptoms.
10. For more information and updates refer to the Parkinson's disease foundation website http://www.pdf.org/.
11. Keep all F/U to assess response, labs, and for adverse SE.

OUTCOMES/EVALUATE

- ↓ Drooling, ↓ rigidity, ↓ tremors, ↓ slow movements
- Improved gait, posture, speech, balance and coordination

ANTIPSYCHOTIC AGENTS, PHENOTHIAZINES ■

SEE ALSO THE FOLLOWING INDIVIDUAL ENTRIES:

Chlorpromazine hydrochloride*
Perphenazine*
Prochlorperazine
Prochlorperazine edisylate
Prochlorperazine maleate

Drugs marked with an * are available to view in the 2013 Nurse's Drug Handbook Website at www.cengage.com/community/nursesdrughandbook.

GENERAL STATEMENT

Antipsychotic drugs do not cure mental illness, but they calm the intractable client, relieve the despondency of the severely depressed, activate the immobile and withdrawn, and make some clients more accessible to psychotherapy.

Most phenothiazines induce some sedation, especially during the initial phase of the treatment. Medicated clients can, however, be easily roused. In this manner, the phenothiazines differ markedly from the narcotic analgesics and sedative hypnotics. However, phenothiazines potentiate the analgesic properties of opiates and prolong the action of CNS depressant drugs. These drugs also cause sedation, decrease spontaneous motor activity, and may lower BP.

According to their detailed chemical structure, the phenothiazines belong to three subgroups:

1. **Aliphatic compounds.** Moderate to high sedative, anticholinergic, and orthostatic hypotensive effects. Moderate extrapyramidal symptoms. Often the first choice for clients in acute excitatory states. Examples: Chlorpromazine, promazine, triflupromazine.
2. **Piperazine compounds.** Act most selectively on the subcortical sites. Low to moderate sedative effects; low anticholinergic and orthostatic hypotensive effects; high incidence of extrapyramidal symptoms. Greatest antiemetic effects because they specifically depress the CTZ of the vomiting center. Examples: Fluphenazine, perphenazine, prochlorperazine, trifluoperazine.
3. **Piperidine compounds.** Low incidence of extrapyramidal effects; high sedative and anticholinergic effects; low to moderate orthostatic hypotensive effect. Examples: Mesoridazine, thioridazine.

INDICATIONS/USES

See also individual drugs.

(1) Psychoses, especially if excessive psychomotor activity manifested. Involutional, toxic, or senile psychoses. Used in combination with MAO inhibitors in depressed clients manifesting anxiety, agitation, or panic (use with caution). (2) With lithium in acute manic phase of manic-depressive illness. (3) As an adjunct in alcohol withdrawal to reduce anxiety, tension, depression, nausea, and/or vomiting. (4) For severe behavioral problems in children, manifested by hyperexcitable and/or combative behavior; also, for short-term use in hyperactive children who exhibit excess motor activity and conduct disorders. (5) Prophylaxis and control of severe N&V due to cancer chemotherapy, radiation therapy, postoperatively. Intractable hiccoughs, intermittent porphyria, tetanus (as adjunct). (6) As preoperative and/or postoperative medications. (7) Some phenothiazines are antipruritics. *NOTE:* Many phenothiazines are no longer used or used less frequently due to the availablity of newer, less toxic, and more effective drugs.

ACTION/KINETICS

Action

It has been postulated that excess amounts of dopamine in certain areas of the CNS cause psychoses. Phenothiazines are thought to act by blocking postsynaptic mesolimbic dopamine receptors, leading to a reduction in psychotic symptoms. Phenothiazines block both D_1 and D_2 dopamine receptors. The antiemetic effects are thought to be due to inhibition or blockade of dopamine (D_2) receptors in the chemoreceptor trigger zone in the medulla, as well as by peripheral blockade of the vagus nerve in the GI tract. Relief of anxiety is manifested as a result of an indirect decrease in arousal and increased filtering of internal stimuli to the brain stem reticular system. Alpha-adrenergic blockade produces sedation. Phenothiazines also raise pain threshold and produce amnesia due to suppression of sensory impulses. In addition, these drugs produce anticholinergic and antihistaminic effects and depress the release of hypothalamic and hypophyseal hormones. Peripheral effects include anticholinergic and alpha-adrenergic blocking properties.

Pharmacokinetics

Peak plasma levels: 2–4 hr after PO administration. Widely distributed throughout the body. **t ½(average):** 10–20 hr. Most metabolized in the liver and excreted by the kidney.

CONTRAINDICATIONS

Severe CNS depression, coma, clients with subcortical brain damage, bone marrow depression, lactation. In clients with a history of seizures and in those on anticonvulsant drugs. Geriatric or debilitated clients, hepatic or renal disease, CV disorders, glaucoma, prostatic hypertrophy. Contraindicated in children with chickenpox, CNS infections, measles, gastroenteritis, dehydration due to increased risk of extrapyramidal symptoms.

SPECIAL CONCERNS

- **Use with caution in clients exposed to extreme heat or cold and in those with asthma, emphysema, or acute respiratory tract infections.**

- **Certain phenothiazines (e.g., mesoridazine and thioridazine) may cause sudden cardiac death due to drug-prolonged QTc intervals.**
- **Use during pregnancy only when benefits outweigh risks.**
- **Children may be more sensitive to the neuromuscular or extrapyramidal effects (especially dystonias); those especially at risk include children with chickenpox, CNS infections, measles, dehydration, or gastroenteritis. Thus, generally, phenothiazines are not recommended for use in children less than 12 years of age.**
- **Geriatric clients often manifest higher plasma levels due to decreases in lean body mass, total body water, and albumin and an increase in total body fat. Also, geriatric clients may be more likely to manifest orthostatic hypotension, anticholinergic effects, sedative effects, and extrapyramidal side effects. Also, geriatric clients may have an increased risk of death.**

SIDE EFFECTS

CNS: Depression, drowsiness, dizziness, lethargy, fatigue. Extrapyramidal effects, Parkinson-like symptoms including shuffling gait or tic-like movements of head and face, tardive dyskinesia, akathisia, dystonia. ***Seizures***, especially in clients with a history thereof. ***Neuroleptic malignant syndrome (rare).*** **CV:** Orthostatic hypotension, increase or decrease in BP, tachycardia, fainting. **GI:** Dry mouth, anorexia, constipation, paralytic ileus, diarrhea. **Endocrine:** Breast engorgement, galactorrhea, gynecomastia, increased appetite, weight gain, hyper-/hypoglycemia, glycosuria. Delayed ejaculation, increased or decreased libido. **GU:** Menstrual irregularities, loss of bladder control, urinary difficulty. **Dermatologic:** Photosensitivity, pruritus, erythema, eczema, exfoliative dermatitis, pigment changes in skin (long-term use of high doses). **Hematologic:** ***Aplastic anemia***, leukopenia, ***agranulocytosis***, eosinophilia, thrombocytopenia. **Ophthalmic:** Deposition of fine particulate matter in lens and cornea leading to blurred vision, changes in vision. **Respiratory:** ***Laryngospasm, bronchospasm, laryngeal edema***, breathing difficulties. **Miscellaneous:** Fever, muscle stiffness, decreased sweating, muscle spasm of face, neck, or back; obstructive jaundice, nasal congestion, pale skin, mydriasis, systemic lupus-like syndrome. *Tardive dyskinesia* has been observed with all classes of antipsychotic drugs, although the precise cause is not known. The syndrome is most commonly seen in older clients, especially women, and in individuals with organic brain syndrome. It is often aggravated or precipitated by the sudden discontinuance of antipsychotic drugs and may persist indefinitely after the drug is discontinued. Early signs of tardive dyskinesia include fine vermicular movements of the tongue and grimacing or tic-like movements of the head and neck. Although there is no known cure for the syndrome, it may not progress if the dosage of the drug is slowly reduced. Also, a few drug-free days may unmask the symptoms of tardive dyskinesia and help in early diagnosis.

OVERDOSE MANAGEMENT

Symptoms: CNS depression including deep sleep and ***coma***, hypotension, extrapyramidal symptoms, agitation, restlessness, seizures, hypothermia, ***hyperthermia***, autonomic symptoms, ***cardiac arrhythmias***, ECG changes.

Treatment: Emetics are not to be used as they are of little value and may cause a dystonic reaction of the head or neck that may result in aspiration of vomitus.

- Hypotension: Volume replacement; norepinephrine or phenylephrine may be used (do not use epinephrine).
- Ventricular arrhythmias: Phenytoin, 1 mg/kg IV, not to exceed 50 mg/min; may be repeated q 5 min up to 10 mg/kg.
- Seizures or hyperactivity: Diazepam or pentobarbital.
- Extrapyramidal symptoms: Antiparkinsonian drugs, diphenhydramine, barbiturates.

DRUG INTERACTIONS

Alcohol, ethyl / Potentiation or addition of CNS depressant effects. Concomitant use may lead to drowsiness, lethargy, stupor, respiratory collapse, coma, or death
Aluminum salts (antacids) / ↓ Absorption from GI tract
Amphetamine / ↓ Drug effect by ↓ drug uptake to the action site
Anesthetics, general / See ***Alcohol***
Antacids, oral / ↓ Effect of phenothiazines R/T ↓ GI tract absorption
Antianxiety drugs / See ***Alcohol***
Anticholinergic drugs / Additive anticholinergic side effects and/or ↓ antipsychotic effect
Antidepressants, tricyclic / Additive anticholinergic side effects; also, ↑ TCA serum levels

Barbiturate anesthetics / ↑ Chance of tremor, involuntary muscle activity, and hypotension
Barbiturates / See ***Alcohol;*** also, barbiturates may ↓ effect R/T ↑ liver breakdown
Bromocriptine / Phenothiazines ↓ effect
Charcoal / ↓ Effect of phenothiazines R/T ↓ GI tract absorption
CNS depressants / See ***Alcohol;*** also, ↓ effect of phenothiazines R/T ↑ liver breakdown
Colistimethate / Additive respiratory depression
Diazoxide / Additive hyperglycemic effect
H ***Evening primrose oil*** / May worsen temporal lobe epilepsy or schizophrenia when used with phenothiazines
H ***Ginseng*** / Do not use with antipsychotics
Guanethidine / ↓ Drug effect by ↓ drug uptake at action site
H ***Henbane leaf*** / Additive anticholinergic effects
Hydantoins / ↑ Risk of hydantoin toxicity
Lithium carbonate / ↑ Risk of extrapyramidal symptoms, disorientation, or unconsciousness
MAO inhibitors / ↑ Effect of phenothiazines R/T ↓ liver breakdown
Meperidine / ↑ Risk of hypotension and sedation
Metrizamide / ↑ Risk of seizures during subarachnoid administration of metrizamide
H ***Milk thistle*** / Helps prevent liver damage from phenothiazines
Narcotics / See ***Alcohol***
Phenytoin / ↑ or ↓ Serum levels of phenytoin
Pimozide / Additive effect on QT interval; do not use together
Propranolol / ↑ Plasma levels of both drugs
Sedative-hypnotics, nonbarbiturate / See ***Alcohol***

LABORATORY TEST CONSIDERATIONS

False-positive: Bile (urine dipstick), ferric chloride, pregnancy tests, urinary porphobilinogen, urinary steroids, urobilinogen (urine dipstick). *False-negative*: Inorganic phosphorus, urinary steroids. *Caused by pharmacologic effects:* ↑ Alkaline phosphatase, bilirubin, serum transaminases, serum cholesterol, urinary catecholamines. ↓ Glucose tolerance, serum uric acid, 5-HIAA, FSH, growth hormone, LH, vanillylmandelic acid.

DOSAGE

See individual drugs. Effective over a wide dosage range. Dosage is usually increased gradually over 7 days to minimize side effects until the minimal effective dose is attained.

Dosage is increased more gradually in elderly or debilitated clients because they are more susceptible to the effects and side effects of drugs. After symptoms are controlled, dosage is gradually reduced to maintenance levels. It is usually desirable to keep chronically ill clients on maintenance levels indefinitely. Medication, especially in clients on high dosages, should not be discontinued abruptly.

NURSING IMPLICATIONS

IMPLEMENTATION/ADMINISTRATION/STORAGE

1. **Do not interchange brands of PO form of drug or suppositories; may differ in bioavailability.**
2. **To lessen injection pain, dilute commercially available injectable solutions in saline or local anesthetic. When administering IM, inject drug deeply into the muscle. Massage area of injection site after IM administration to reduce pain.**
3. **IV Do not use pink or markedly discolored solutions. When preparing or administering parenteral solutions, nurse and client should avoid contact of drug with skin, eyes, and clothing to prevent contact dermatitis.**
4. **Do not mix antipsychotic drugs with other drugs in the same syringe. Order a specific flow rate when administering parenteral solutions. Prevent extravasation of the IV solution.**
5. **Store solutions in a cool dry place in amber-colored containers.**

ASSESSMENT

1. **Take a complete medical and drug history; note any drug hypersensitivity or genetic predisposition. (These agents are referred to as neuroleptics in Europe.)**
2. **Assess for any history of asthma, emphysema, or seizures; this class of drugs may lower seizure threshold. Use caution in the elderly.**
3. **Note reasons for therapy. Assess baseline mental status, noting mood, behavior, reflexes, gait, coordination, sleeping problems, clinical presentation, and any reported depression.**
4. **These drugs are generally used less frequently due to the availablity of newer, less toxic, and more effective drugs.**
5. **If administering to children, note extent of hyperexcitability. Assess child for chickenpox,**

measles or other illness that may preclude drug therapy.

6. Monitor VS; assess BP in both arms in a reclining position, standing position, and sitting position, 2 min apart.
7. If administered IV, monitor flow rate and BP. Keep recumbent for at least 1 hr after IV completed, then slowly elevate HOB and observe for tachycardia, faintness, or dizziness; supervise ambulation.
8. If hospitalized, ensure that drug has been swallowed. May give a liquid preparation to permit better control over drug taking and to improve compliance.
9. Measure I&O; report abdominal distention and urinary retention. May need to reduce dosage, add antispasmodic, or change therapy.
10. Note any changes in carbohydrate metabolism (e.g., glycosuria, weight loss, polyphagia, increased appetite, or excessive weight gain); may require a change in diet/drug therapy and can be significant in those with diabetes.
11. Some may develop a hypersensitivity reaction with fever, asthma, laryngeal edema, angioneurotic edema, and anaphylactic reaction. *Stop* medication, notify provider, and treat symptomatically.
12. The antiemetic effects of phenothiazines may mask other pathology such as toxicity to other drugs, intestinal obstruction, or brain lesions; assess carefully.
13. If receiving barbiturates to relieve anxiety, reduce barbiturate dose. If administered as an anticonvulsant, do not reduce dosage.
14. Discontinue drug gradually to minimize severe GI disturbances or tardive dyskinesia. With evidence of EPS, such as akathisia, pseudoparkinsonism or tardive dyskinesia, notify provider. May require antiparkinsonian agent or discontinuation of therapy.
15. Encourage client to actively participate in goal setting and ways to attain.
16. Monitor hematologic profile, liver and renal function studies, urinalysis, ECG, and ocular findings.

CLIENT/FAMILY TEACHING

1. There are many different types of psychotic disorders. They comprise serious illnesses that affect the mind by altering one's ability to think clearly, make good judgments, respond emotionally, communicate effectively, understand reality and behave appropriately. When these symptoms are severe, one has difficulty staying in touch with reality and often is unable to meet the ordinary demands of daily life. It is extremely important to take the prescribed medications in order to better function in society and to decrease the mental and physical toll on those who care for and about these clients.
2. May take meds with food or milk to minimize GI upset. Take as directed; may be weeks or months before the full effects will be noticed; do not stop taking abruptly. Abrupt cessation of high doses of phenothiazines can cause N&V, tremors, sensations of warmth and cold, sweating, tachycardia, headache, and insomnia.
3. Avoid driving a car or operating heavy machinery or engaging in any activities that require mental alertness until drug effects realized; consult provider prior to resuming.
4. Report distress when in a hot or cold room; may affect heat-regulating mechanism.
   - Provide extra blankets if cold.
   - Bathe in tepid water if too warm.
   - Do *NOT* use heating pads or hot water bottles if feeling cold.
   - Avoid hot tubs, hot baths/showers; low BP may occur from vasodilation.
5. Report if excessively active or depressed. Spasms of face, neck, back, or tongue may be treated with antihistamines, or drug discontinuation.
6. Report S&S of blood dyscrasias: ↑ body temperature, weakness, easy bruising, or sore throat. May cause menstrual irregularity and false positive pregnancy tests; may develop engorged breasts and begin lactating. Keep accurate record of periods and report if pregnant.
7. Take slow, deep breaths if respiratory S&S occur; may depress cough reflex.
8. Males may experience decreased libido and develop breast enlargement. Report so drug can be adjusted.
9. May develop photosensitivity reactions; wear protective clothing, sunglasses, sunscreen, and avoid sunbathing or prolonged sun exposure.

10. Drug may discolor the urine pink or reddish brown. With long-term therapy may develop a yellow-brown skin reaction that may turn grayish purple.
11. Long-term therapy may affect vision; schedule regular eye exams. Report blurred vision and avoid driving.
12. Report evidence of early (cholestatic) jaundice, such as high fever, upper abdominal pain, nausea, diarrhea, itching, and rash. Withhold drug and report if yellowing of the sclera, skin, or mucous membranes occurs; may indicate biliary obstruction.
13. To prevent dry mouth, rinse mouth frequently, increase fluid intake, chew sugarless gum/hard candies. Increase fluids and bulk in diet to minimize constipation; may need laxatives. Report any urinary retention or persistent constipation. If administered to a child, note any reactions, especially if dehydrated or has an acute infection making child more susceptible to side effects.
14. Rise slowly from a lying or sitting position; dangle legs before standing to avoid low BP symptoms. Avoid alcohol, OTC drugs, and any other CNS depressants without approval.
15. With the elderly, be particularly observant for symptoms of tardive dyskinesia. May exhibit puffing of the cheeks or tongue; may develop chewing movements and involuntary movements of the tongue, head, extremities, and body.
16. Keep all F/U to assess response, labs, and for adverse SE. Continue regular case management and counselling sessions as prescribed and assist client to modify goals to fit desired lifestyle.

OUTCOMES/EVALUATE

- ↓ Excitable, withdrawn, agitated, or paranoid behaviors
- Orientation to time and place, and an understanding of illness
- Adherence to prescribed drug regimen

ANTIVIRAL DRUGS

SEE ALSO THE FOLLOWING INDIVIDUAL ENTRIES:

Antiviral, Antiherpes
Acyclovir
Famciclovir
Valacyclovir hydrochloride

Antiviral, Antiretroviral Fusion Inhibitor
Enfuvirtide

Antiviral, General
Adefovir dipivoxil
Amantadine hydrochloride
Cidofovir
Foscarnet sodium
Ganciclovir sodium
Oseltamivir phosphate
Penciclovir
Ribavirin
Rimantadine hydrochloride
Valganciclovir hydrochloride
Zanamivir

Antiviral, Integrase Inhibitor
Raltegravir potassium

Antiviral, Nonnucleoside Reverse Transcriptase Inhibitor
Delavirdine mesylate
Efavirenz
Etravirine
Nevirapine
Rilpivirine hydrochloride

Antiviral, Nucleoside Reverse Transcriptase Inhibitor
Abacavir sulfate
Didanosine
Emtricitabine
Lamivudine
Lamivudine/Zidovudine
Stavudine
Zalcitabine
Zidovudine

Antiviral, Nucleotide Analog Reverse Transcriptase Inhibitor
Tenofovir disoproxil fumarate

Antiviral, Protease Inhibitor
Atazanavir sulfate
Darunavir ethanolate
Fosamprenavir calcium
Indinavir sulfate
Nelfinavir mesylate
Ritonavir
Saquinavir mesylate
Tipranavir

Antiviral, Integrase Inhibitor
Raltegravir potassium

INDICATIONS/USES

HIV infection. Guidelines suggest five different combinations as initial therapy: (1) one protease inhibitor plus two nucleoside reverse transcriptase inhibitors; (2) two nucleoside reverse transcriptase inhibitors and a nonnucleoside reverse transcriptase inhibitor; (3) two protease inhibitors with or without nucleoside reverse transcriptase inhibitors; (4) a nucleoside reverse transcriptase inhibitor, a nonnucleoside reverse transcriptase inhibitor, and a protease inhibitor; or, (5) three nucleoside reverse transcriptase inhibitors.

ACTION/KINETICS

Action

To maintain their growth and reproduce, viruses must enter living cells. Thus, it is difficult to find a drug that is specific for the virus and that does not interfere with the function of the host cell. However, there are enzymes and replicative mechanisms that are unique to viruses and an increasing number of drugs with specific antiviral activity have been developed. The antiviral drugs currently marketed act by one of the following mechanisms:

1. Inhibition of enzymes required for DNA synthesis. Example: Idoxuridine.
2. Inhibition of viral nucleic acid synthesis by interacting directly with herpes virus DNA polymerase or HIV reverse transcriptase. Example: Foscarnet.
3. Inhibition of viral DNA or protein synthesis. Examples: Acyclovir, cidofovir, famciclovir, ganciclovir, penciclovir, trifluridine, valacyclovir, vidarabine.
4. Prevent penetration of the virus into cells by inhibiting uncoating of the RNA virus. Examples: Amantadine, rimantadine.
5. Protease inhibitors resulting in release of immature, noninfectious viral particles. Examples: Indinavir, nelfinavir, ritonavir, saquinavir.
6. Reverse transcriptase inhibitors (nucleoside and non-nucleoside) resulting in inhibition of replication of the virus. Examples of nucleoside inhibitors: Abacavir, didanosine, lamivudine, stavudine, zalcitabine, zidovudine. Examples of non-nucleoside inhibitors: Efavirenz, delavirdine, nevirapine.

It is often necessary to combine two antiviral drugs that have the same or different mechanisms of action in order to treat HIV infections and to minimize development of resistant viruses.

DOSAGE

See individual drugs. Many antiviral drugs are used in combination therapy to treat HIV disease.

NURSING IMPLICATIONS

ASSESSMENT

1. Note reasons for therapy, type/onset of S&S, exposure characteristics, and other agents trialed.
2. Identify clinical presentation, mental status and any underlying medical conditions that may preclude drug therapy.
3. List other agents prescribed to ensure none interact unfavorably. Assess support systems and client adherence potential as well as need for case management.
4. Determine need for antiemetic and antidiarrheal to control any adverse side effects.
5. Monitor CBC, renal and LFTs; also viral loads/T cells as indicated. Adjust dosage with renal dysfunction.

CLIENT/FAMILY TEACHING

1. Review method and frequency for drug administration. Stress importance of adherence to multidrug regimens and how to take exactly as directed even if feeling better; do not share medications.
2. Identify specific measures to decrease/halt disease spread. Continuous therapy without interruption has been shown to prolong life.
3. Maintain adequate nutrition; consume 2–3 L/day of fluids to prevent crystalluria.
4. Report any rashes or unusual drug side effects or if symptoms do not improve or worsen after specified time frame.
5. Practice reliable contraception as directed.
6. Assist client to set realistic, attainable goals that promote healthy, desirable lifestyle.
7. Close medical supervision/follow-up required during therapy. Keep all F/U to assess response, labs, and for adverse SE.

OUTCOMES/EVALUATE

- Prophylaxis of viral infections
- Reduction in length and severity of symptoms of viral infections
- ↓ Resistant viruses
- Increased recovery with HIV/Hep B, C infections

BETA-ADRENERGIC BLOCKING AGENTS

SEE ALSO ALPHA-1-ADRENERGIC BLOCKING AGENTS AND THE FOLLOWING INDIVIDUAL AGENTS:

Atenolol
Betaxolol hydrochloride
Bisoprolol fumarate
Esmolol hydrochloride
Levobunolol hydrochloride
Metoprolol succinate
Metoprolol tartrate
Nadolol
Penbutolol sulfate
Propranolol hydrochloride
Sotalol hydrochloride
Timolol maleate

INDICATIONS/USES

See individual drugs. Depending on the drug uses include, but are not limited to (1) Hypertension. (2) Angina pectoris. (3) MI. Are important in clients who have survived a first MI. (4) Migraine. (5) Part of the standard therapy for CHF. (6) May increase survival if taken prior to coronary artery bypass surgery. (7) Increase survival and decrease exacerbations in COPD. *NOTE:* See *Angiotensin Converting Enzyme (ACE) Inhibitors* for guidelines for the evaluation and management of chronic heart failure.

ACTION/KINETICS

Action

Combine reversibly with beta-adrenergic receptors to block the response to sympathetic nerve impulses, circulating catecholamines, or adrenergic drugs. Beta-adrenergic receptors are classified as beta-1 (predominantly in the cardiac muscle) and beta-2 (mainly in the bronchi and vascular musculature). Blockade of beta-1 receptors decreases HR, myocardial contractility, and CO; in addition, AV conduction is slowed. These effects lead to a decrease in BP, as well as a reversal of cardiac arrhythmias. Blockade of beta-2 receptors increases airway resistance in the bronchioles and inhibits the vasodilating effects of catecholamines on peripheral blood vessels. The various beta-blocking agents differ in their ability to block beta-1 and beta-2 receptors (see individual drugs); also, certain of these agents have intrinsic sympathomimetic action. Certain of these drugs (betaxolol, carteolol, levobunolol, metipranolol, and timolol) and used for glaucoma; act by reducing production of aqueous humor; metipranolol and timolol may also increase outflow of aqueous humor. Drugs have little or no effect on the pupil size or on accommodation.

CONTRAINDICATIONS

Sinus bradycardia, second- and third-degree AV block, cardiogenic shock, CHF unless secondary to tachyarrhythmia treatable with beta blockers, overt cardiac failure. Most are contraindicated in chronic bronchitis, bronchial asthma or history thereof, bronchospasm, emphysema, severe COPD.

SPECIAL CONCERNS

- **Use with caution in diabetes, thyrotoxicosis, cerebrovascular insufficiency, and impaired hepatic and renal function.**
- **Withdrawing beta blockers before major surgery is controversial.**
- **Safe use during pregnancy and lactation and in children has not been established.**
- **May be absorbed systemically when used for glaucoma; thus, there is the potential for an additive effect with beta blockers used systemically.**
- **Certain of the products for use in glaucoma contain sulfites, which may result in an allergic reaction.**
- **See individual agents for additional *Special Concerns*.**

SIDE EFFECTS

CV: Bradycardia, hypotension (especially following IV use), CHF, cold extremities, claudication, worsening of angina, strokes, edema, syncope, arrhythmias, chest pain, peripheral ischemia, flushing, SOB, sinoatrial block, pulmonary edema, vasodilation, increased HR, palpitations, conduction disturbances, ***first-, second-, and third-degree heart block***, worsening of AV block, ***thrombosis of renal or mesenteric arteries***, precipitation/worsening of Raynaud's phenomenon. Sudden withdrawal of large doses may cause angina, hypertensive reaction in those with pheochromocytoma, ***ventricular tachycardia***, ***fatal MI***, ***sudden death***, or ***circulatory collapse***. **GI:** N&V, gastric/epigastric pain, flatulence, gastritis, constipation, diarrhea, colon problems, dry mouth, heartburn, appetite disorder, anorexia, bloating, abdominal discomfort/pain, mesenteric arterial thrombosis, ischemic colitis, retroperitoneal fibrosis, hepatomegaly, dyspepsia, taste distortion, GI disorder, increased appetite, mouth ulceration, rectal disorders, dysphagia, abnormal taste, abdominal distension, taste perversion/abnormalities, digestive tract disorders, indigestion, salivation. **Hepatic:** Hepatomegaly, acute pancreatitis, elevated liver enzymes, acute hepatitis with jaundice, liver damage (especially with chronic use of phenobarbital). **Respiratory:** ***Bronchospasm***, dyspnea, cough, bronchial obstruction, rales, wheeziness, nasal stuffiness, pharyngitis, rhonchi, ***laryngospasm with respiratory distress***, asthma, rhinitis, sinusitis, pulmonary problem, upper respiratory tract problem, cold symptoms, flu symptoms, bronchitis, lung disorder, cough, epistaxis, pneumonia, tracheobronchitis. **CNS:** Dizziness, fatigue, lethargy, vivid dreams, depression, hallucinations, delirium, psychoses, paresthesias, insomnia, nervousness, nightmares, headache, vertigo, disorientation of time/place, hypo-/hyperesthesia, decreased concentration, short-term memory loss, change in behavior, emotional lability, slurred speech, lightheadedness. In the elderly, paranoia, disorientation, and combativeness have occurred, speech disorder. **Hematologic:** ***Agranulocytosis***, thrombocytopenia, nonthrombocytopenic or thrombocytopenic purpura, bleeding, eosinophilia, leukopenia, pulmonary emboli, hyperlipidemia, anemia, leukocytosis, lymphoadenopathy, purpura. **Allergic:** Respiratory distress, rash, pharyngitis, photosensitivity reaction, erythematous rash, fever combined with aching and sore throat, angioedema, ***laryngospasm***, ***anaphylaxis***. **Dermatologic:** Pruritus, rashes, increased skin pigmentation/irritation, sweating, dry skin, alopecia, psoriasis (reversible), pemphigoid rash. **Musculoskeletal:** Joint pain, arthralgia, muscle cramps/pain, back/neck pain, arthritis, twitching/tremor, localized pain, extremity pain, myalgia, pain, shoulder pain, joint disorder, arthropathy, tendonitis, chest pain, muscle cramps, midcapsular pain. **GU:** Sexual dysfunction, impotence, decrease libido, dysuria, nocturia, pollakiuria, urinary retention/frequency, UTI, cystitis, renal colic, GU disorder, renal failure, micturition disorder, oliguria, proteinuria, abnormal renal function, renal pain, menstrual disorders, prostatitis, breast pain, breast fibroadenosis. **Endocrine:** Hyper-/hypoglycemia, unstable diabetes, gout, acidosis, hypercholesterolemia, hyper-/hypokalemia, hyperlipemia, hyperuricemia. **Ophthalmic:** Visual disturbances, eye irritation, dry/burning eyes, blurred vision, conjunctivitis, ocular pain/pressure, abnormal lacrimation, ptosis, eye disorder, abnormal vision, blepharitis, ocular hemorrhage, iritis, cataract, scotoma, diplopia. **Otic:** Earache, tinnitus, labyrinth disorder, deafness. **Body as a whole:** Lupus syndrome/lupus-like reaction, Peyronie's disease, rigors, asthenia, malaise, infection, fever, cold sensation, ***death***. **Miscellaneous:** Facial swelling, weight gain/loss, decreased exercise tolerance, injury, thirst, increase symptoms of myasthenia gravis.

When used ophthalmically: Keratitis, blepharoptosis, diplopia, ptosis, and visual disturbances including refractive changes. **Systemic effects due to ophthalmic beta-1 and beta-2 blockers:** Headache, depression, arrhythmia, heart block, CVA, syncope, CHF, palpitation, cerebral ischemia, nausea, localized and generalized rash, ***bronchospasm*** (especially in those with preexisting bronchospastic disease), ***respiratory failure***, masked symptoms of hypoglycemia in IDDM, keratitis, visual disturbances (including refractive changes), blepharoptosis, ptosis, diplopia.

OVERDOSE MANAGEMENT

Symptoms: **CV:** Bradycardia, hypotension, low-output cardiac failure, cardiogenic shock, asystole, tachycardia (from partial agonists), prolonged QT interval (from sotalol), prolonged QRS complex (from membrane-stabilizing agents), ventricular dysrhythmias (from membrane-stabilizing agents), hypertension, ***AV block***. **CNS:** ***Seizures***, ***coma***, depressed level of consciousness. **GI:** Mesenteric ischemia, esophageal spasms. **Respiratory:** ***Apnea***, cyanosis, respiratory depression, ***bronchospasms***. **GU:** Renal failure. **Metabolic:** Hyperkalemia, hypoglycemia.

Treatment:

- Perform evaluation of airway, breathing, and circulation.
- To improve blood supply to the brain, place client in a supine position and raise the legs.
- Measure blood glucose and serum potassium. Monitor BP and ECG continuously.
- Provide general supportive treatment including artificial respiration. Give activated charcoal and perform gastric lavage in all clients who present within 1–2 hr after ingestion. In those who ingest sustained-release products, consider

whole bowel irrigation with polyethylene glycol solution.

- *Hypoglycemia:* IV glucagon.
- *Seizures:* Give IV diazepam or phenytoin; barbiturates are ineffective.
- *Excessive bradycardia:* If hypotensive, give atropine, 0.6 mg; if no response, give q 3 min for a total of 2–3 mg. Cautious administration of isoproterenol may be tried. Also, glucagon, 5–10 mg rapidly over 30 sec, followed by continuous IV infusion of 5 mg/hr may reverse bradycardia. Transvenous cardiac pacing may be needed for refractory cases.
- *Cardiac failure:* Digitalis, diuretic, and oxygen; if failure is refractory, IV aminophylline or glucagon may be helpful.
- *Hypotension:* Place client in Trendelenburg position. IV fluids unless pulmonary edema is present; also vasopressors such as norepinephrine (may be drug of choice), dobutamine, dopamine with monitoring of BP. If refractory, glucagon may be helpful. In intractable cardiogenic shock, intra-aortic balloon insertion may be required.
- *Premature ventricular contractions:* Lidocaine or phenytoin. Disopyramide, quinidine, and procainamide should be avoided as they depress myocardial function further.
- *Bronchospasms:* Give a beta-2-adrenergic agonist, epinephrine, or theophylline.
- *Heart block, second or third degree:* Isoproterenol or transvenous cardiac pacing.

DRUG INTERACTIONS

Aluminum salts / ↓ Bioavailability of certain beta-blockers → ↓ effect
Ampicillin / ↓ Bioavailability of certain beta-blockers → ↓ effect
Anesthetics, general / Additive depression of myocardium
Anticholinergic agents / Counteract bradycardia produced by beta-adrenergic blockers
Antihypertensives / Additive hypotensive effect
Barbiturates / ↓ Bioavailability of certain beta-blockers → ↓ effect
Benzodiazepines / ↑ Effect of certain benzodiazepines by lipophilic beta-blockers
Calcium channel blockers / ↑ Effect of certain beta-blockers
Calcium salts / ↓ Bioavailability of certain beta-blockers → ↓ effect
Chlorpromazine / Additive beta-adrenergic blocking action
Cholestyramine / ↓ Bioavailability of certain beta-blockers → ↓ effect
Cimetidine / ↑ Effect of beta blockers R/T ↓ liver breakdown
Clonidine / Paradoxical hypertension; also, ↑ severity of rebound hypertension
Colestipol / ↓ Bioavailability of certain beta-blockers → ↓ effect
Diphenhydramine / ↑ Plasma levels and CV effects of certain beta-blockers R/T ↓ metabolism
Disopyramide / ↑ Effect of both drugs
Epinephrine / Beta blockers prevent beta-adrenergic action of epinephrine but not alpha-adrenergic action → ↑ SBP/DBP and ↓ HR
Ergot alkaloids / ↑ Risk of peripheral ischemia R/T ergot alkaloid-mediated vasoconstriction and peripheral effects of beta-blockers
Flecainide / Possible ↑ bioavailability of either drug → ↑ effects
Furosemide / ↑ Beta-adrenergic blockade
Haloperidol / ↑ Risk of hypotensive episodes
Hydralazine / ↑ Effect of both beta-blockers and hydralazine
Indomethacin / ↓ Effect of beta blockers possibly due to inhibition of prostaglandin synthesis
Insulin / Beta blockers ↑ hypoglycemic effect of insulin
Lidocaine / ↑ Drug effect R/T ↓ liver breakdown
Methyldopa / Possible ↑ BP to alpha-adrenergic effect
Muscle relaxants, nondepolarizing / Beta-blockers may potentiate, counteract, or have no effect on action of nondepolarizing muscle relaxants
NSAIDs / ↓ Effect of beta blockers, possibly R/T inhibition of prostaglandin synthesis
Ophthalmic beta blockers / Additive systemic beta-blocking effects if used with oral beta blockers
Oral contraceptives / ↑ Effect of beta blockers R/T ↓ liver breakdown
Phenformin / ↑ Hypoglycemia
Phenobarbital / ↓ Effect of beta blockers R/T ↑ liver breakdown
Phenothiazines / ↑ Effect of both drugs
Phenytoin / Additive depression of myocardium; also ↓ effect of beta blockers R/T ↑ liver breakdown
Prazosin / ↑ First-dose effect of prazosin (acute postural hypotension)

Propafenone / ↑ Plasma levels of certain beta-blockers R/T ↓ liver metabolism
Quinidine / ↑ Plasma levels of beta-blockers in extensive metabolizers → ↑ effects
Quinolone antibiotics / ↑ Bioavailability of beta-blockers metabolized by the cytochrome P450 system
Rifampin / ↓ Effect of beta blockers due to ↑ breakdown by liver
Ritodrine / Beta blockers ↓ effect of ritodrine
Salicylates / ↓ Effect of beta blockers, possibly R/T inhibition of prostaglandin synthesis
SSRIs / Possible excessive beta-blockade R/T ↓ metabolism
Smoking / ↓ Antihypertensive and heart rate effects possibly R/T nicotine-mediated sympathetic activation; smokers may need ↑ dosages
Succinylcholine / Beta blockers ↑ effects of succinylcholine
Sulfonylureas / ↓ Effect of sulfonylureas
Sympathomimetics / Reverse effects of beta blockers
Theophylline / Beta blockers reverse the effect of theophylline; also, beta blockers ↓ renal drug clearance
Thioamines / ↑ Effects of beta-blockers
Thyroid hormones / Effects of certain beta-blockers may be ↓ when hypothyroid client is converted to euthyroid state
Tubocurarine / Beta blockers ↑ effects of tubocurarine
Verapamil / Possible side effects since both drugs ↓ myocardial contractility or AV conduction; bradycardia and asystole when beta blockers are used ophthalmically

LABORATORY TEST CONSIDERATIONS

↓ Serum glucose.

DOSAGE

See individual drugs.

NURSING IMPLICATIONS

IMPLEMENTATION/ADMINISTRATION/STORAGE

1. Sudden cessation of beta blockers may precipitate or worsen angina.
2. Lowering of intraocular pressure (IOP) may take a few weeks to stabilize when using betaxolol or timolol.
3. Due to diurnal variations in IOP, the response to twice a day therapy is best assessed by measuring IOP at different times during the day.
4. If IOP is not controlled using beta blockers, add additional drugs to the regimen, including pilocarpine, dipivefrin, or systemic carbonic anhydrase inhibitors.

ASSESSMENT

1. Note reasons for therapy, symptom characteristics, other agents trialed. List any history of depression; assess mental status. Review drugs currently prescribed to ensure none interact.
2. Check for any history of asthma, diabetes, or impaired renal function. With asthma, avoid nonselective beta antagonists due to beta-2 receptor blockade which may lead to increased airway resistance. With heart failure, weigh regularly, and with diabetes assess for hypoglycemia.
3. Monitor HR and BP; obtain written parameters for holding (e.g., for SBP <90 or HR <60).
4. When assessing respirations note rate and quality; may cause dyspnea and bronchospasm.
5. Monitor I&O and daily weights. Observe for increasing dyspnea, coughing, difficulty breathing, Wt gain, chest pain, fatigue, or edema; symptoms of CHF, may require digitalization, diuretics, and/or drug discontinuation.
6. Complaints of cold S&S, easy fatigue, or feeling lightheaded may require a drug change as well as impotence.
7. With diabetics watch for S&S of hypoglycemia, such as hypotension or tachycardia; S&S may be masked.
8. During IV administration, monitor ECG (may slow AV conduction and increase PR interval) and activities closely until drug effects evident.
9. Determine HR and BP in both arms lying, sitting, and standing. Monitor ECG, glucose, CBC, electrolytes, renal and LFTs. Note MUGA, echocardiogram, and/or stress test results.

CLIENT/FAMILY TEACHING

1. When prescribed for BP control, drug helps control BP but does not cure it. Must continue to take despite feeling better. With heart attack, drug is prescribed to prevent remodeling

of the heart and to decrease sudden death after heart attack.
2. Record BP and pulse immediately prior to first dose each day and record so medication can be adjusted. Review instructions for when to call provider, i.e., if HR <60 beats/min or SBP <90 mm Hg or as specified by provider.
3. Review lifestyle changes for BP control: regular exercise, weight loss, low-fat and reduced-calorie diet, decreased salt and alcohol intake, smoking cessation, and relaxation techniques.
4. Always consult provider before interrupting therapy; stopping abruptly may cause chest pain, heart attack, or ↑ BP. A 2-week taper is generally used.
5. May cause blurred vision, dizziness, or drowsiness; avoid activities that require mental alertness until drug effects realized.
6. Rise from a sitting or lying position slowly and dangle legs before standing to avoid S&S of sudden drop in BP. Elastic support hose may help decrease symptoms.
7. Dress warmly during cold weather. Diminished blood supply to extremities may cause cold sensitivity; check extremities for warmth.
8. Avoid excessive intake of alcohol, coffee, tea, or cola. Avoid OTC agents without approval.
9. If diabetic, monitor FS and report S&S of low sugar <60. With heart failure, check weight daily and report unusual weight gain (>2 lb per day or 5 lb per week), increased SOB, or chest pain.
10. Report any asthma-like symptoms, cough, or nasal stuffiness; may be symptoms of heart failure. Report any new-onset depression or marked fatigue.
11. Set realistic, attainable goals to ensure successful disease management.
12. Keep all F/U to assess response, labs, and for adverse SE.

OUTCOMES/EVALUATE

- ↓ BP; ↓ IOP; ↓ Remodeling
- ↓ Frequency/severity of anginal attacks; improved exercise tolerance
- ↓ Anxiety levels; ↓ tremors
- Migraine prophylaxis

CALCIUM CHANNEL BLOCKING AGENTS

SEE ALSO THE FOLLOWING INDIVIDUAL ENTRIES:

Amlodipine
Clevidipine butyrate*
Diltiazem hydrochloride
Felodipine
Isradipine
Nicardipine hydrochloride
Nifedipine
Nimodipine*
Nisoldipine*
Verapamil

Drugs marked with an * are available to view in the 2013 Nurse's Drug Handbook Website at www.cengage.com/community/nursesdrughandbook.

INDICATIONS/USES

See individual drugs. Uses include, but are not limited to: (1) Angina pectoris (chronic stable, unstable, vasospastic). (2) Hypertension. (3) Subarachnoid hemorrhage. (4) Atrial fibrillation/flutter. (5) Paroxysmal supraventricular tachycardia. *Investigational:* (1) Prevention of migraine headaches (diltiazem, verapamil). (2) Pulmonary hypertension (amlodipine, diltiazem, felodipine, nifedipine). (3) Raynaud's phenomenon (amlodipine, diltiazem, felodipine, isradipine, nifedipine). (4) Preterm labor (nifedipine). (5) Hypertrophic cardiomyopathy (verapamil).

ACTION/KINETICS

Action

For contraction of cardiac and smooth muscle to occur, extracellular calcium must move into the cell through openings called *calcium channels.* The calcium channel blocking agents (also called *slow channel blockers* or *calcium antagonists*) inhibit the influx of calcium through the cell membrane, resulting in a depression of automaticity and conduction velocity in both smooth and cardiac muscle. This leads to a depression of contraction in these tissues. Drugs in this class have different degrees of selectivity on vascular smooth muscle, myocardium, and conduction and pacemaker tissues. In the myocardium, these drugs dilate coronary vessels in both normal and ischemic tissues and inhibit spasms of coronary arteries. They also decrease total peripheral resistance, thus reducing energy and oxygen requirements of the heart. Also effective against certain cardiac arrhythmias by slowing AV conduction and prolonging repolarization. In addition, they depress the amplitude, rate of depolarization, and conduction in atria.

Classifications

CONTRAINDICATIONS

Sick sinus syndrome, second- or third-degree AV block (except with a functioning pacemaker). Use of bepridil, diltiazem, or verapamil for hypotension (<90 mm Hg systolic pressure). Lactation.

SPECIAL CONCERNS

- **Abrupt withdrawal may result in increased frequency and duration of chest pain.**
- **Hypertensive clients treated with calcium channel blockers have a higher risk of heart attack than clients treated with diuretics or beta-adrenergic blockers.**
- **May also be an increased risk of heart attacks in diabetics (only nisoldipine studied).**
- **Safety and efficacy of diltiazem, felodipine, and isradipine not established in children.**

SIDE EFFECTS

Side effects vary from one calcium channel blocker to another; refer to individual drugs.

OVERDOSE MANAGEMENT

Symptoms: Nausea, weakness, drowsiness, dizziness, slurred speech, confusion, marked and prolonged hypotension, bradycardia, junctional rhythms, ***second- or third-degree block.***

Treatment:

- Treatment is supportive. Monitor cardiac and respiratory function.
- If client is seen soon after ingestion, emetics or gastric lavage should be considered followed by cathartics.
- *Hypotension:* IV calcium, dopamine, isoproterenol, metaraminol, norepinephrine. Also, provide IV fluids. Place client in Trendelenburg position.
- *Ventricular tachycardia (caused by antegrade conduction in flutter/fibrillation with W-P-W or L-G-L syndromes):* IV procainamide or lidocaine; also, cardioversion may be necessary. Also, provide slow-drip IV fluids.
- *Bradycardia, asystole, AV block:* IV atropine sulfate (0.6–1 mg), calcium chloride, isoproterenol, norepinephrine; also, cardiac pacing may be indicated. Provide slow-drip IV fluids.

DRUG INTERACTIONS

Anesthetics / Potentiation of cardiac effects and vascular dilation associated with anesthetics; possible severe hypotension

Beta-adrenergic blocking agents / Beta blockers may cause depression of myocardial contractility and AV conduction

Cimetidine / ↑ Effect of CCBs R/T ↓ first-pass metabolism

Clarithromycin / ↑ Risk of hypotension or shock; may require hospitalization

H ***Dong quai*** / Possible additive effect

Erythromycin / ↑ Risk of hypotension or shock; may require hospitalization

Fentanyl / Severe hypotension or ↑ fluid volume requirements

Ginger / May alter CCBs effect R/T ↑ calcium uptake by heart muscle

Grapefruit juice / ↑ Serum levels of most calcium channel blockers

Itraconazole / Edema when used with amlodipine or nifedipine

Ranitidine / ↑ Effect of CCBs R/T ↓ first-pass metabolism

DOSAGE

See individual drugs.

NURSING IMPLICATIONS

ASSESSMENT

1. **Note reasons for therapy, onset, characteristics of S&S. List other agents used and outcome. Note any experience with these agents and the response. List drugs prescribed to ensure none interact.**
2. **Assess CV and mental status. These drugs cause peripheral vasodilation. Any excessive hypotensive response and increased HR may precipitate angina. Record VS, weight, ECG and BP in both arms while lying, sitting, and standing. Assess for CHF (weight gain, peripheral edema, dyspnea, crackles, jugular vein distention).**
3. **Monitor ECG, BS, electrolytes, I&O, renal and LFTs.**

CLIENT/FAMILY TEACHING

1. **These agents block the entry of calcium into the muscle cells of the heart and the arteries. Calcium causes the heart to contract and the arteries to narrow so by blocking entry, it decreases contraction of the heart and dilates (widens) the arteries.**
2. **Take with meals to ↓ GI upset. Do not stop therapy suddenly.**

3. **Do not perform activities that require mental alertness until drug effects realized. Report adverse effects such as dizziness, vertigo, unusual flushing, facial warmth, edema, nausea, constipation. Toxic drug effects are swelling of the hands or feet, pronounced dizziness, chest pain accompanied by sweating, SOB, or severe headaches.**
4. **If dizziness occurs (drop in BP), change positions slowly, especially when standing from a lying position. Sit down immediately if lightheadedness occurs. Move slowly from a lying to a sitting or standing position.**
5. **Avoid long periods of standing, excessive heat, hot showers or baths, and ingestion of alcohol; may worsen drop in BP.**
6. **Determine goals of therapy (e.g., ↓ DBP by 10 mm Hg, ↓ HR by 20 beats/min). Record pulse and BP at least twice a week as well as weights; review instructions regarding when to hold medications and notify provider.**
7. **Review lifestyle changes for BP control (i.e., regular exercise, weight loss, low-fat, low-cholesterol, reduced-calorie diet, decreased salt and alcohol consumption, smoking cessation, and stress reduction), and ways to incorporate these changes.**
8. **Keep all F/U to assess response, labs, and for adverse SE.**

OUTCOMES/EVALUATE

- Control of BP; ↓ HR
- ↓ Frequency/intensity of angina
- Stable cardiac rhythm
- Migraine headache prophylaxis

CALCIUM SALTS

SEE ALSO THE FOLLOWING INDIVIDUAL ENTRIES:

Calcium carbonate
Calcium chloride
Calcium gluconate

INDICATIONS/USES

IV: (1) Acute hypocalcemic tetany secondary to renal failure. (2) Hypoparathyroidism. (3) Premature delivery. (4) Maternal diabetes mellitus in infants. (5) Poisoning due to magnesium, oxalic acid, radiophosphorus, carbon tetrachloride, fluoride, phosphate, strontium, and radium. (6) Treat depletion of electrolytes. (7) During cardiac resuscitation when epinephrine or isoproterenol have not improved myocardial contraction (may also be given into the ventricular cavity for this purpose). (8) To reverse cardiotoxicity or hyperkalemia.

IM or IV: (1) Reduce spasms in renal, biliary, intestinal, or lead colic. (2) Relieve muscle cramps due to insect bites. (3) Decrease capillary permeability in various sensitivity reactions.

PO: (1) As a dietary supplement when calcium intake may be inadequate (including vitamin D deficiency, sprue, pregnancy, lactation, achlorhydria, chronic diarrhea, hypoparathyroidism, steatorrhea, menopause, renal failure, pancreatitis, hyperphosphatemia, alkalosis). (2) Osteoporosis, osteomalacia. (3) Chronic hypoparathyroidism. (4) Rickets. (5) Latent tetany. (6) Hypocalcemia secondary to use of anticonvulsant drugs. (7) Myasthenia gravis. (8) Eaton-Lambert syndrome. (9) Supplement for pregnant, postmenopausal, or nursing women. (10) Prophylactically for primary osteoporosis. *Investigational:* As an infusion to diagnose Zollinger-Ellison syndrome and medullary thyroid carcinoma. To antagonize neuromuscular blockade due to aminoglycosides.

ACTION/KINETICS

Action

Calcium is essential for maintaining normal function of nerves, muscles, the skeletal system, and permeability of cell membranes and capillaries. The normal serum calcium concentration is 9–10.4 mg/dL (4.5–5.2 mEq/L). Hypocalcemia is characterized by muscular fibrillation, twitching, skeletal muscle spasms, leg cramps, tetanic spasms, cardiac arrhythmias, smooth muscle hyperexcitability, mental depression, and anxiety states. Excessive, chronic hypocalcemia is characterized by brittle, defective nails, poor dentition, and brittle hair. Severe low-calcium tetany is best treated by IV administration of calcium gluconate. The hormone of the parathyroid gland is necessary for the regulation of the calcium level. Recommended daily allowances for men and women, age 19–24 years is 1,200 mg/day; and, for men and women, 25 years of age and older is 800 mg/day. Dietary reference intakes for men and women, 19–50 years of age is 1,000 mg/day; for men and women over 51 years of age is 1,200 mg/day; and, for pregnant and breastfeeding women is 1,000 mg/day.

Pharmacokinetics

Calcium is absorbed from the GI tract by passive diffusion and active transport. Calcium must be in a soluble, ionized form to be absorbed. Food increases calcium absorption. Vitamin D is required for absorption of calcium. Calcium enters the extracellular fluid and is rapidly incorporated into skeletal tissue. Calcium is excreted mainly through the feces (as much as 250–300 mg/day in healthy adults eating a regular diet).

CONTRAINDICATIONS

Digitalized clients, sarcoidosis, renal or cardiac disease, ventricular fibrillation. Cancer clients with bone metastases. Renal calculi, hypophosphatemia, hypercalcemia.

SPECIAL CONCERNS

- **Calcium requirements decrease in geriatric clients; thus, dose may have to be adjusted.**
- **Low levels of active vitamin D metabolites may impair calcium absorption in older clients.**
- **Use with caution in cor pulmonale, sarcoidosis, cardiac or renal disease, or in those receiving cardiac glycosides.**
- **May be irritating to the GI tract when given PO and may cause constipation.**
- **Some products contain phenylalanine.**

SIDE EFFECTS

Following PO use: GI irritation, constipation, renal calculi, mild (N&V, anorexia) or severe (confusion, delirium, stupor, coma) hypercalcemia.

Following IV use: Venous irritation, tingling sensation, feeling of oppression or heat, chalky taste. Rapid IV administration may result in vasodilation, decreased BP and HR, ***cardiac arrhythmias***, syncope, or ***cardiac arrest.***

Following IM use: Burning feeling, necrosis, tissue sloughing, cellulitis, soft tissue calcification. *NOTE:* If calcium is injected into the myocardium rather than into the ventricle, ***laceration of coronary arteries, cardiac tamponade, pneumothorax***, and ***ventricular fibrillation*** may occur.

Symptoms due to excess calcium (hypercalcemia): Lassitude, fatigue, GI symptoms (anorexia, N&V, abdominal pain, dry mouth, thirst), polyuria, depression of nervous and neuromuscular function (emotional disturbances, confusion, skeletal muscle weakness, and constipation), confusion, delirium, stupor, ***coma***, impairment of renal function (polyuria, polydipsia, and azotemia), renal calculi, arrhythmias, and bradycardia.

OVERDOSE MANAGEMENT

Symptoms: Systemic overloading from parenteral administration can result in an acute hypercalcemic syndrome with symptoms including markedly increased plasma calcium levels, lethargy, intractable N&V, weakness, ***coma***, and ***sudden death.***

Treatment: Discontinue therapy and lower serum calcium levels by giving an IV infusion of sodium chloride plus a potent diuretic such as furosemide. Consider hemodialysis.

DRUG INTERACTIONS

Atenolol / ↓ Drug effect R/T ↓ bioavailability and plasma levels
Corticosteroids / Interfere with absorption of calcium from GI tract
Digitalis / ↑ Digitalis arrhythmias and toxicity. Death has resulted from combination of digitalis and IV calcium salts
Iron salts / ↓ Absorption of iron from the GI tract; separate administration times if possible
H ***Lily-of-the-valley herb*** / ↑ Effectiveness and side effects of calcium
Milk / Excess of either may cause hypercalcemia, renal insufficiency with azotemia, alkalosis, and ocular lesions
Norfloxacin / ↓ Drug bioavailability
H ***Pheasant's eye herb*** / ↑ Effectiveness and side effects of calcium
Quinolones / ↓ GI absorption of quinolones (e.g., norfloxacin)
Sodium polystyrene sulfonate / Metabolic alkalosis and ↓ binding of resin to potassium with renal impairment
H ***Squill*** / ↑ Effectiveness and side effects of calcium
Tetracyclines / ↓ Tetracycline effect R/T ↓ GI tract absorption
Thiazide diuretics / Hypercalcemia R/T to thiazide-induced renal tubular reabsorption of calcium and bone release of calcium
Verapamil / Calcium antagonizes the effect of verapamil
Vitamin D / Enhances intestinal absorption of dietary calcium

DOSAGE

See individual agents. The usual daily dose as a dietary supplement is 500 mg to 2 grams,

2–4 times a day. Recommended doses for men older than 65 years of age and for post-menopausal women not taking estrogen replacement therapy is 1,500 mg/day

NURSING IMPLICATIONS

IMPLEMENTATION/ADMINISTRATION/STORAGE

The elemental calcium content of calcium salts is as follows: Calcium carbonate, 40% (20 mEq calcium/gram) and calcium gluconate, 9% (4.5 mEq calcium/gram).

ASSESSMENT

1. Perform a thorough nursing history, noting clinical presentation, indications for therapy and any precipitating causes. List drugs prescribed, especially if receiving digitalis products; drug may be contraindicated.
2. Identify any conditions that may preclude drug therapy, i.e., cancer, sarcoidosis, etc.
3. Assess for S&S of hypercalcemia, i.e., fatigue and CNS depression. With hypocalcemic tetany, protect client from injury.
4. Avoid giving at same time as iron, tetracycline, ciprofloxacin; wait 4 hrs when dosing with levothyroxine.
5. Note bone mineral density and fracture history.
6. Monitor calcium levels and renal function; assess for renal or parathyroid disease. Vitamin D facilitates absorption.

CLIENT/FAMILY TEACHING

1. General calcium requirements are best met by dietary sources (including milk in the diet) before menopause. Supplements should be taken with meals or milk and need vitamin D to facilitate absorption. Consult dietitian to assist with proper food selection and meal planning and preparation.
2. Multivitamin and mineral preparations are expensive and do not contain sufficient calcium to meet daily requirements. Usual prescribed replacement regimen:
   - Post-menopausal women: 1,000–1,500 mg
   - Pregnant or breast-feeding females: 1,200 mg
   - Adults and adolescents: 800–1200 mg
   - Children 1–10 years old: 500–800 mg
3. Do not use bone meal or dolomite as a source of calcium; they may contain lead.
4. Report adverse side effects, lack of desired response, and keep all F/U appointments to evaluate drug response and dosage adjustments to prevent hypercalcemia and hypercalciuria.

OUTCOMES/EVALUATE

- Resolution of hypocalcemia
- Relief of muscle cramps
- Osteoporosis prophylaxis
- Serum calcium levels within desired range (8.8–10.4 mg/dL)

CEPHALOSPORINS ■

SEE ALSO THE FOLLOWING INDIVIDUAL ENTRIES:

Cefaclor
Cefadroxil monohydrate
Cefdinir
Cefepime hydrochloride
Cefixime oral
Cefotaxime sodium
Cefoxitin sodium
Cefprozil
Ceftazidime
Ceftibuten
Ceftizoxime sodium
Ceftriaxone sodium
Cefuroxime axetil
Cefuroxime sodium
Cephalexin

GENERAL STATEMENT

Cephalosporins are broad-spectrum antibiotics classified as first-, second-, and third-generation drugs.

First-Generation Cephalosporins: Cefadroxil, cefazolin, cephalexin, cephapirin, cephradine.

Second-Generation Cephalosporins: Cefaclor, cefmetazole, cefonicid, cefotetan, cefoxitin, cefprozil, cefuroxime, and loracarbef.

Third-Generation Cephalosporins: Cefdinir, cefepime, cefixime, cefoperazone, cefotaxime, ceftazidime, ceftibuten, ceftizoxime, ceftriaxone.

The difference among generations is based on pharmacokinetics and antibacterial spectra. Generally, third-generation cephalosporins have more activity against gram-negative organisms and resistant organisms and less activity against gram-positive organisms than first-generation drugs. Third-generation cephalosporins are also stable against beta-lactamases. Cephalosporins can be destroyed by cephalosporinase.

INDICATIONS/USES

See individual drugs.

ACTION/KINETICS

Action

The cephalosporins interfere with a final step in the formation of the bacterial cell wall (inhibition of mucopeptide biosynthesis), resulting in unstable cell membranes that undergo lysis (same mechanism of actions as penicillins). Also, cell division and growth are inhibited. The cephalosporins are most effective against young, rapidly dividing organisms and are considered bactericidal.

Pharmacokinetics

Cephalosporins are widely distributed to most tissues and fluids. First- and second-generation drugs do not enter the CSF well but third-generation drugs enter inflamed meninges readily. Rapidly excreted by the kidneys.

CONTRAINDICATIONS

Hypersensitivity to cephalosporins or related antibiotics.

SPECIAL CONCERNS

- Safe use in pregnancy and lactation has not been established (pregnancy category: B).
- Use with caution in the presence of impaired renal or hepatic function, together with other nephrotoxic drugs, and in clients over 50 years of age.
- Perform C_{CR} on all clients with impaired renal function who receive cephalosporins.
- If hypersensitive to penicillin, may occasionally cross-react to cephalosporins.

SIDE EFFECTS

GI: N&V, diarrhea, constipation, abdominal cramps or pain, dyspepsia, glossitis, heartburn, sore mouth or tongue, dysgeusia, anorexia, flatulence, cholestasis, thirst, abdominal pain, oral candidiasis and moniliasis, flatulence, heartburn, gastritis, stomach cramps, eructation, melena, ***bleeding peptic ulcer***, ileus, gall bladder sludge, colitis (including pseudomembranous colitis). **Hepatic:** Hepatomegaly, hepatitis, jaundice, cholestasis, cholestatic jaundice, ***hepatic failure***. **CNS:** Headache, malaise, fatigue, vertigo, dizziness, lethargy, confusion, paresthesia, anxiety, hyperactivity, nervousness, insomnia, hypertonia, somnolence, precipitation of ***seizures*** (especially in clients with impaired renal function). **CV:** Hypotension, palpitations, chest pain, vasodilation, syncope. **Dermatologic:** Urticaria, diaphoresis, flushing, cutaneous moniliasis. **GU:** Pyuria, dysuria, vaginitis, vaginal discharge, genito-anal pruritus, genital candidiasis and moniliasis, reversible interstitial nephritis, hematuria, nephropathy, acute renal failure (rare). **Musculoskeletal:** Myalgia, arthralgia, rhabdomyolysis. **Respiratory:** Asthma, ***laryngeal edema***, dyspnea, interstitial pneumonitis, bronchitis, bronchospasm, pneumonia, ***respiratory failure***. **Hypersensitivity:** Urticaria, rashes (maculopapular, morbilliform, or erythematous), pruritus (including anal/genital areas), fever, chills, erythema, ***angioedema***, serum sickness, joint pain, exfoliative dermatitis, chest tightness, myalgia, erythema multiforme, edema, itching, numbness, chills, ***Stevens-Johnson syndrome, anaphylaxis.***

NOTE: Cross-allergy may be manifested between cephalosporins and penicillins. **Hematologic:** Leukopenia, leukocytosis, lymphocytosis, neutropenia (transient), eosinophilia, thrombocytopenia, thrombocythemia, ***agranulocytosis***, granulocytopenia, bone marrow depression, anemia, ***hemolytic anemia***, pancytopenia, decreased platelet function, ***aplastic anemia***, hypoprothrombinemia (may lead to bleeding), ***hemorrhage***, thrombocytosis (transient), lymphopenia, monocytosis. **Miscellaneous:** Superinfection including oral candidiasis and enterococcal infections, hypotension, sweating, flushing, dyspnea, interstitial pneumonitis.

NOTE: IV or IM use may result in local swelling, inflammation, cellulitis, paresthesia, burning, phlebitis, thrombophlebitis. IM use may also cause pain and induration, tenderness, increased temperature. Sterile abscesses have been observed following SC use. Nephrotoxicity (↑ BUN with and without ↑ serum creatinine) may occur in clients over 50 and in young children. Intrathecal use may result in hallucinations, nystagmus, or ***seizures.***

OVERDOSE MANAGEMENT

Symptoms: Parenteral use of large doses of cephalosporins may cause ***seizures***, especially in clients with impaired renal function.

Treatment: If seizures occur, discontinue the drug immediately and give anticonvulsant drugs. Hemodialysis may also be effective in cases of overwhelming overdosage.

DRUG INTERACTIONS

Alcohol / Antabuse-like reaction if used with cefazolin, cefmetazole, cefoperazone, or cefotetan
Aminoglycosides / ↑ Risk of renal toxicity with certain cephalosporins; monitor renal function closely
Antacids / ↓ Plasma levels of cefaclor, cefdinir, or cefpodoxime
Anticoagulants / ↑ Hypoprothrombinemic effects with cefazolin, cefmetazole, cefoperazone, or cefotetan
Colistimethate / ↑ Risk of renal toxicity; monitor renal function
Colistin / ↑ Risk of renal toxicity; monitor renal function
Ethacrynic acid / ↑ Risk of renal toxicity; monitor renal function
Furosemide / ↑ Risk of renal toxicity; monitor renal function
H_2 antagonists / ↓ Plasma levels of cefpodoxime or cefuroxime
Polymyxin B / ↑ Risk of renal toxicity; monitor renal function
Probenecid / ↑ Effect of cephalosporins by ↓ excretion by kidneys
Vancomycin / ↑ Risk of renal toxicity

LABORATORY TEST CONSIDERATIONS

↑ AST, ALT, total bilirubin, GGTP, LDH, alkaline phosphatase, neutrophil count (slight), PT (due to disturbances in vitamin K-dependent clotting function), platelets. ↓ H&H. False + for urinary glucose with Benedict's solution, Fehling's solution, or Clinitest tablets. False + Coombs' test and urinary 17-ketosteroids.

DOSAGE

See individual drugs.

NURSING IMPLICATIONS

IMPLEMENTATION/ADMINISTRATION/STORAGE

1. **IV** Parenteral solutions infused too rapidly may cause pain and irritation; dilute and infuse over 30 min unless otherwise indicated and assess site.
2. Continue therapy for at least 2–3 days after symptoms of infection have disappeared.
3. For group A beta-hemolytic streptococcal infections, continue therapy for at least 10 days to prevent the development of glomerulonephritis or rheumatic fever.

ASSESSMENT

1. Note reasons for therapy, physical presentation, S&S of infection, other agents trialed, outcome and culture results.
2. List allergy history. With hypersensitivity reactions to penicillin, assess for cross-sensitivity to cephalosporins.
3. The cephalosporins all have similar sounding and similarly spelled names. Use care when transcribing orders for administration and request clarification as needed.
4. Pseudomembranous colitis may occur. If diarrhea develops, report any fevers. Monitor VS, I&O, stool C&S, and electrolytes.
5. Those prescribed sodium salts of cephalosporins may have fluid retention; report if condition precludes this side effect.
6. If also prescribed other antibiotic give cephalosporins 1 hr before bacteriostatic antibiotics (erythromycins, tetracyclines and chloramphenicol) as these keep bacteria from growing by decreasing cephalosporin uptake by bacterial cell walls.
7. Persistent temperature elevations may be drug-induced fever.
8. Monitor VS, CBC, platelets, PT, BS, electrolytes, renal and LFTs. With renal impairment reduce dose; for dialysis clients, administer after treatment. May cause false positive Coombs' test.

CLIENT/FAMILY TEACHING

1. Oral medications should be taken on an empty stomach, but, if GI upset occurs, may be administered with meals. Take as directed and complete entire prescription despite feeling better.
2. Report any S&S that may necessitate drug withdrawal, such as vaginal itching/drainage, fever, or diarrhea. Immediately report any abnormal bleeding or bruising.
3. Yogurt or buttermilk (4 oz) may be prescribed daily for diarrhea related to intestinal superinfections (to restore intestinal flora); consult provider. Report signs of superinfection (black furry tongue, vaginal itching or discharge, and

Classifications

loose, foul-smelling stools). Nystatin may be ordered for secondary infections.

4. **May cause false positive Coombs' test. Would be of concern if being cross-matched for blood transfusions or in newborn where the mother used cephalosporins during pregnancy.**
5. **Avoid alcohol and alcohol-containing products during and for 3 days following completion of therapy, as a disulfiram-type reaction may occur.**
6. **Report adverse side effects, lack of response or inability to complete prescription. Keep all F/U to assess response, labs, and adverse SE.**

OUTCOMES/EVALUATE

- **Negative C&S reports**
- **Resolution of infection**
- **Symptomatic improvement, i.e., ↓ WBCs, ↓ fever, improved appetite, wound healing**

CHOLINERGIC BLOCKING AGENTS ■

SEE ALSO THE FOLLOWING INDIVIDUAL ENTRIES:

Atropine sulfate
Benztropine mesylate
Dicyclomine hydrochloride
Ipratropium bromide
Scopolamine hydrobromide
Scopolamine transdermal therapeutic system

INDICATIONS/USES

See individual drugs.

ACTION/KINETICS

Action

Cholinergic blocking agents prevent the neurotransmitter acetylcholine from combining with receptors on the postganglionic parasympathetic nerve terminal (muscarinic site). Effects include reduction of smooth muscle spasms, blockade of vagal impulses to the heart, decreased secretions (e.g., gastric, salivation, bronchial mucus, sweat glands), production of mydriasis and cycloplegia, and various CNS effects. In therapeutic doses, these drugs have little effect on transmission of nerve impulses across ganglia (nicotinic sites) or at the neuromuscular junction. Several anticholinergic drugs abolish or reduce the S&S of Parkinson's disease, such as tremors and rigidity, and result in some improvement in mobility, muscular coordination, and motor performance. These effects may be due to blockade of the effects of acetylcholine in the CNS.

CONTRAINDICATIONS

Glaucoma, adhesions between iris and lens of the eye, tachycardia, myocardial ischemia, unstable CV state in acute hemorrhage, partial obstruction of the GI and biliary tracts, prostatic hypertrophy, renal disease, myasthenia gravis, hepatic disease, paralytic ileus, pyloroduodenal stenosis, pyloric obstruction, intestinal atony, ulcerative colitis, obstructive uropathy. Cardiac clients, especially when there is danger of tachycardia; older persons suffering from atherosclerosis or mental impairment. Lactation.

SPECIAL CONCERNS

- **Use with caution in pregnancy.**
- **Infants and young children are more susceptible to the toxic side effects of anticholinergic drugs.**
- **Use in children when the ambient temperature is high may cause a rapid increase in body temperature due to suppression of sweat glands.**
- **Geriatric clients are particularly likely to manifest anticholinergic side effects and CNS effects, including agitation, confusion, drowsiness, excitement, glaucoma, and impaired memory.**
- **Use with caution in hyperthyroidism, CHF, cardiac arrhythmias, hypertension, Down syndrome, asthma, spastic paralysis, blonde individuals, allergies, and chronic lung disease.**

SIDE EFFECTS

These are desirable in some conditions and undesirable in others. Thus, the anticholinergics have an antisalivary effect that is useful in parkinsonism. This same effect is unpleasant when the drug is used for spastic conditions of the GI tract. Most side effects are dose-related and decrease when dosage decreases. **GI:** N&V, dry mouth, dysphagia, constipation, heartburn, change in taste perception, bloated feeling, paralytic ileus, epigastric distress, acute suppurative parotiditis, dilation of the colon, development of duodenal ulcer. **CNS:** Dizziness, drowsiness, nervousness, disorientation, headache, weakness, insomnia, fever (especially in children). Large doses may produce CNS stimulation including tremor and restlessness. **Anticholinergic psychoses:** Ataxia, euphoria, confusion, disorientation, loss of short-term memory, decreased anxiety, fatigue, insomnia, hallucinations, dysarthria, agitation. **CV:** Palpitations, tachycardia, hypotension, postural hypotension. **GU:** Urinary retention or hesitancy, dysuria, impotence. **Ophthalmic:** Blurred vision, dilated pupils, diplopia, increased intraocular tension, angle-closure glaucoma, photophobia, cycloplegia, precipitation of acute glaucoma. **Dermatologic:** Urticaria, skin rashes, other dermatoses. **Musculoskeletal:** Muscle weakness, muscle cramping. **Other:** ***Anaphylaxis***, flushing, decreased sweating, nasal congestion, numbness of fingers, suppression of glandular secretions including lactation. Heat prostration (fever and heat stroke) in presence of high environmental temperatures due to decreased sweating.

OVERDOSE MANAGEMENT

Symptoms (Belladonna Poisoning): Infants and children are especially susceptible to the toxic effects of atropine and scopolamine. Poisoning (dose-dependent) is characterized by the following symptoms: Dry mouth, burning sensation of the mouth, difficulty in swallowing and speaking, blurred vision, photophobia, dilated and sluggish pupils, rash, tachycardia, ***circulatory collapse, cardiac arrest***, increased respiration, ***increased body temperature*** (up to 109°F, 42.7°C), restlessness, irritability, confusion, anxiety, ataxia, hyperactivity, combativeness, toxic psychosis, anhidrosis, muscle incoordination, dilated pupils, hot dry skin, dry mucous membranes, dysphagia, foul-smelling breath, decreased bowel sounds, ***respiratory depression and paralysis***, tremors, ***seizures***, hallucinations, and ***death.***

Treatment (Belladonna Poisoning):

- Gastric lavage or induction of vomiting followed by activated charcoal. General supportive measures.
- Anticholinergic effects can be reversed by physostigmine (Eserine), 1–3 mg IV (effectiveness uncertain; thus use other agents if possible). Neostigmine methylsulfate, 0.5–2 mg IV, repeated as necessary.
- If there is excitation, diazepam, a short-acting barbiturate, IV sodium thiopental (2% solution), or chloral hydrate (100–200 mL of a 2% solution by rectal infusion) may be given.
- For fever, cool baths may be used. Keep client in a darkened room if photophobia is manifested.
- Artificial respiration should be instituted if there is paralysis of respiratory muscles.

DRUG INTERACTIONS

Amantadine / Additive anticholinergic side effects
Antacids / ↓ Absorption of anticholinergics from GI tract
Antidepressants, tricyclic / Additive anticholinergic side effects
Antihistamines / Additive anticholinergic side effects
Atenolol / Anticholinergics ↑ effects of atenolol
Benzodiazepines / Additive anticholinergic side effects
Corticosteroids / Additive ↑ intraocular pressure
Digoxin / ↑ Drug effect R/T ↑ GI tract absorption
Disopyramide / Potentiation of anticholinergic side effects
Guanethidine / Reversal of inhibition of gastric acid secretion caused by anticholinergics
Haloperidol / Possible worsening of schizophrenic symptoms, ↓ haloperidol serum levels, and development of tardive dyskinesia
Histamine / Reversal of inhibition of gastric acid secretion caused by anticholinergics
Levodopa / Possible ↓ drug effect R/T ↑ breakdown of levodopa in stomach (R/T delayed gastric emptying time)
MAO inhibitors / ↑ Effect of anticholinergics R/T ↓ liver breakdown
Meperidine / Additive anticholinergic side effects
Methylphenidate / Potentiation of anticholinergic side effects
Metoclopramide / Anticholinergics block action of metoclopramide
Nitrates, nitrites / Potentiation of anticholinergic side effects
Nitrofurantoin / ↑ Bioavailability of nitrofurantoin
Orphenadrine / Additive anticholinergic side effects
Phenothiazines / Additive anticholinergic side effects; also, ↓ phenothiazine effects
Primidone / Potentiation of anticholinergic side effects
Procainamide / Additive anticholinergic side effects
Quinidine / Additive anticholinergic side effects
Sympathomimetics / ↑ Bronchial relaxation
Thiazide diuretics / ↑ Bioavailability of thiazide diuretics
Thioxanthines / Potentiation of anticholinergic side effects

Classifications

DOSAGE

See individual drugs.

NURSING IMPLICATIONS

IMPLEMENTATION/ADMINISTRATION/STORAGE

Dosage is often small. To prevent overdosage, check dose and measure exactly.

ASSESSMENT

1. Note reasons for therapy and clinical presentation. Assess for asthma, glaucoma, or duodenal ulcer (precludes therapy).
2. List age; elderly clients, especially those with mental impairment or atherosclerosis, should not receive these drugs. Assess for constipation, urinary retention, and tolerance.
3. With eye therapy, determine any experience with these drugs and eye exam results. Document IOP; assess accommodation and pupillary response.
4. With GI therapy, document UGI and/or endoscopy findings.
5. With GU therapy, note PVR, cystoscopy and prostate exam results.
6. Drugs such as atropine may suppress thermoregulatory sweating; counsel client concerning activity (especially in hot weather) and appropriate clothing. Also, children and infants may exhibit "atropine fever."
7. Monitor VS and ECG. Assess for any hemodynamic changes and intraventricular conduction blocks. Note palpitations, renal disease, cardiac problems, or hepatic disease.

CLIENT/FAMILY TEACHING

1. May take with food or milk to ↓ GI upset. Do not stop suddenly.
2. Avoid activities that require mental alertness until drug effects realized.
3. Certain side effects are to be expected, such as dry mouth or blurred vision, and may have to be tolerated because of the overall beneficial effects of drug therapy. Report if persistent or bothersome; provider may reduce dose or temporarily stop drug.
4. With GI therapy, take early enough before a meal (at least 20 min) so that it will be effective when needed. Review printed information related to the prescribed diet; see dietitian for assistance in meal planning.
5. Gastric emptying times may be prolonged and intestinal transit time lengthened. Drug-induced intestinal paralysis is temporary and should resolve after 1–3 days of therapy.
6. With parkinsonism, do not withdraw abruptly. If the medication is changed, one drug should be withdrawn slowly and the other started in small doses.
7. Avoid prolonged heat exposure; may cause heat stroke.
8. May use ice, sips of fluids, or sugar free candy/gum to relieve dry mouth effects.
9. Avoid OTC cough and cold remedies with alcohol and antihistamines unless specifically directed by provider.
10. With eye administration review methods for instillation of drops or ointment and frequency. Wash hands and do not permit container to come in contact with eye tissue. Vision will be affected by the medications; temporary stinging and blurred vision will occur. Assess response and plan activities for safety. Night vision may be impaired. Photophobia, which may occur, can be relieved by wearing dark glasses.
11. Report any marked changes in vision, eye irritation, eye pain after instillation, or persistent headaches immediately.
12. With large doses, tears may diminish; may experience dry/sandy eyes that would benefit with liquid tears.
13. Report urinary retention; may be more pronounced in elderly men with BPH. Report if bladder distended; may need catheterization if no urine output >8 hr.
14. Consult with provider for medication adjustment if impotence occurs; may be drug-related.
15. Keep all F/U to assess response, labs, and for adverse SE.

OUTCOMES/EVALUATE

- Mydriasis and cycloplegia
- ↓ Heart rate
- ↓ Secretion production
- ↓ Tremors and rigidity

CORTICOSTEROIDS ■

SEE ALSO THE FOLLOWING INDIVIDUAL ENTRIES:

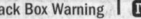

Beclomethasone dipropionate
Betamethasone

Betamethasone dipropionate
Betamethasone sodium phosphate and Betamethasone acetate
Betamethasone valerate
Budesonide
Ciclesonide
Cortisone acetate
Dexamethasone
Dexamethasone sodium phosphate
Flunisolide
Flunisolide hemihydrate
Fluticasone furoate
Fluticasone propionate
Hydrocortisone
Hydrocortisone acetate
Hydrocortisone butyrate
Hydrocortisone probutate
Hydrocortisone sodium succinate
Hydrocortisone valerate
Methylprednisolone
Methylprednisolone acetate
Methylprednisolone sodium succinate
Mometasone furoate
Mometasone furoate monohydrate
Prednisolone
Prednisolone acetate
Prednisolone sodium phosphate
Prednisolone tebutate
Prednisone
Triamcinolone
Triamcinolone acetonide
Triamcinolone hexacetonide

INDICATIONS/USES

When used for anti-inflammatory or immunosuppressant therapy, the corticosteroid should possess minimal mineralocorticoid activity. Therapy with glucocorticoids is not curative and in many situations should be considered as adjunctive rather than primary therapy. The following list is not inclusive but provides examples of the physiologic and pharmacologic uses of corticosteroids.

1. **Endocrine disorders.** Primary or secondary adrenal cortical insufficiency; cortisone or hydrocortisone are drugs of choice. For replacement therapy, drugs must possess both glucocorticoid and mineralocorticoid effects. Also, used for congenital adrenal hyperplasia, nonsuppurative thyroiditis, and hypercalcemia associated with cancer. Parenteral therapy is indicated for acute adrenal cortical insufficiency (cortisone or hydrocortisone are drugs of choice); preoperatively or in serious trauma or illness with known adrenal insufficiency or when adrenal cortical reserve is doubtful. Parenteral therapy is also used for shock unresponsive to conventional therapy if adrenal cortical insufficiency is suspected.
2. **Rheumatic disorders.** Adjunctive therapy for short-term use (acute episode or exacerbation) in rheumatoid arthritis (including juvenile), ankylosing spondylitis, acute and subacute bursitis, acute nonspecific tenosynovitis, acute gouty arthritis, psoriatic arthritis, post-traumatic osteoarthritis, synovitis of osteoarthritis, epicondylitis.
3. **Collagen diseases.** For exacerbation or maintenance therapy in selected cases of systemic lupus erythematosus, acute rheumatic carditis, or polymyositis.
4. **Allergic diseases.** Control of severe or incapacitating allergic conditions intractable to conventional treatment in serum sickness and drug hypersensitivity reactions. Parenteral therapy is indicated for urticarial transfusion reactions and acute noninfectious laryngeal edema (although epinephrine is the drug of choice).
5. **Respiratory diseases.** Prophylaxis and treatment of chronic bronchial asthma (including status asthmaticus), seasonal or perennial allergic rhinitis, symptomatic sarcoidosis, Loeffler's syndrome (not manageable by other means), berylliosis, fulminating or disseminated pulmonary tuberculosis (also use tuberculostatic drugs), aspiration pneumonitis. Regular use of inhaled steroids in children could be a life-saving treatment.
6. **Ocular diseases.** (a) Corneal injury from chemical, radiation, or thermal burns, or penetration of foreign bodies. (b) Steroid-responsive inflammatory conditions of the palpebral and bulbar conjunctiva, cornea, and anterior segment of the globe such as allergic conjunctivitis, acne rosacea, cyclitis, superficial punctate keratitis, herpes zoster keratitis, iritis, and selected infective conjunctivitis; noninfectious uveitis affecting the posterior segment of the eye; and postoperative inflammation following ocular surgery. (c) Seasonal allergic conjunctivitis.

7. **Otic diseases,** including inflammatory conditions of the external auditory meatus (e.g., allergic otitis externa and selected purulent and nonpurulent infective otitis externa). Dexamethasone sodium phosphate is most often used.
8. **Dermatologic diseases,** including angioedema or urticaria, contact dermatitis, atopic dermatitis, severe erythema multiforme (Stevens-Johnson syndrome), pemphigus, bullous dermatitis herpetiformis, mycosis fungoides, severe psoriasis, exfoliative or seborrheic dermatitis, acne rosacea.
9. **Diseases of the intestinal tract.** Used to carry the client over a critical period of the disease in ulcerative colitis, regional enteritis, and intractable sprue.
10. **Nervous system.** Acute exacerbations of multiple sclerosis.
11. **Malignancies.** Palliative management of leukemias and lymphomas in adults and acute leukemia in children.
12. **Edematous states.** To induce diuresis or remission of proteinuria in the nephrotic syndrome (without uremia) including that due to lupus erythematosus or of the idiopathic type.
13. **Hematologic diseases.** Acquired (autoimmune) hemolytic anemia, RBC anemia, idiopathic and secondary thrombocytopenic purpura in adults (IV only), congenital (erythroid) hypoplastic anemia.
14. **Intra-articular or soft tissue administration.** Short-term adjunctive therapy to carry the client over an acute episode in synovitis of osteoarthritis, rheumatoid arthritis, acute gouty arthritis, acute and subacute bursitis, epicondylitis, acute nonspecific tenosynovitis, post-traumatic osteoarthritis.
15. **Intralesional administration.** Keloids; hypertrophic, infiltrated, inflammatory lesions of lichen planus; psoriatic plaques, granuloma annulare, neurodermatitis, necrobiosis lipoidica diabeticorum, alopecia areata, discoid lupus erythematosus. Possibly effective in cystic tumors of an aponeurosis or tendon.
16. **Miscellaneous.** Tuberculosis meningitis with subarachnoid block or impending block when accompanied by appropriate tuberculostatic drugs; trichosis with neurologic or myocardial involvement.

Lotions are considered best for weeping eruptions, especially in areas subject to chafing (axilla, feet, and groin). Creams are suitable for most inflammations; ointments are preferred for dry, scaly lesions.

Investigational: Acute mountain sickness (dexamethasone), antiemetic (dexamethasone), bacterial meningitis (dexamethasone), bronchopulmonary dysplasia in preterm infants (dexamethasone), COPD (prednisone), diagnosis of depression (dexamethasone), Duchenne's muscular dystrophy (prednisone), Graves ophthalmopathy (prednisone), severe alcoholic hepatitis (methylprednisolone), hirsutism (dexamethasone), respiratory distress syndrome (prevention in premature infants using betamethasone; methylprednisolone is used in adults), septic shock (methylprednisolone), acute spinal cord injury (methylprednisolone), tuberculous pleurisy (prednisolone).

ACTION/KINETICS

Action

The hormones of the adrenal gland influence many metabolic pathways and all organ systems and are essential for survival. These processes include carbohydrate metabolism (e.g., glycogen deposition in the liver and conversion of glycogen to glucose), protein metabolism (e.g., gluconeogenesis, protein catabolism), fat metabolism (e.g., deposition of fatty tissue), and water and electrolyte balance (e.g., fluid retention, excretion of potassium, calcium, and phosphorus). According to their chemical structure and chief physiologic effect, the corticosteroids fall into two subgroups, which have considerable functional overlap. First are those, like cortisone and hydrocortisone, that mainly regulate the metabolic pathways involving protein, carbohydrate, and fat. This group is often referred to as *glucocorticoids.* In the second group are those, like aldosterone and desoxycorticosterone, that are more specifically involved in electrolyte and water balance. These are often referred to as *mineralocorticoids.* Hormones, such as cortisone and hydrocortisone, although classified as glucocorticoids, possess significant mineralocorticoid activity. Therapeutically, a distinction must be made between physiologic doses used for replacement therapy and pharmacologic doses used to treat inflammatory and other disease states.

The hormones have a marked anti-inflammatory effect because of their ability to inhibit prostaglandin synthesis. These agents also inhibit accumulation of macrophages and leukocytes at sites of inflammation, as well as inhibit phagocytosis and lysosomal enzyme release. They aid the organism in coping with various stressful situations (trauma, severe illness). The immunosuppressant effect is thought to be due to a reduction of the number of T lymphocytes, monocytes, and eosinophils. Corticosteroids also decrease binding of immunoglobulin to receptors on the cell surface and inhibit the synthesis and/or release of interleukins which, in turn, decrease T-lymphocyte blastogenesis and reduce the primary immune response.

Ocular corticosteroids are thought to act by induction of phospholipase A_2, inhibitory proteins, collectively called lipocortins. These proteins allegedly control the biosynthesis of potent mediators of inflammation, such as prostaglandins and leukotrienes by inhibiting the release of arachidonic acid, their common precursor. Arachidonic acid is released from membrane phospholipids by phospholipase A_2. Ocular corticosteroids may cause an increase in intraocular pressure.

CONTRAINDICATIONS

Suspected infection as these drugs may mask infections. Also peptic ulcer, psychoses, acute glomerulonephritis, herpes simplex infections of the eye, vaccinia or varicella, the exanthematous diseases, Cushing's syndrome, active tuberculosis, myasthenia gravis. Recent intestinal anastomoses, CHF or other cardiac disease, hypertension, systemic fungal infections, open-angle glaucoma. Also, hyperlipidemia, hyperthyroidism or hypothyroidism, osteoporosis, myasthenia gravis, tuberculosis, otitis media with effusion in children. Lactation (if high doses are used). Inhalation products to relieve acute bronchospasms. Topically in the eye for dendritic keratitis; fungal diseases of ocular structures; vaccinia, varicella and most other viral diseases of the cornea and conjunctiva; ocular tuberculosis; hypersensitivity; after uncomplicated removal of a superficial corneal foreign body; mycobacterial eye infection; acute, purulent, untreated eye infections that may be masked or enhanced by the presence of steroids. Topically in the ear in aural fungal infections and perforated eardrum. Topically in tuberculosis of the skin, herpes simplex, vaccinia, varicella, and infectious conditions in the absence of anti-infective agents. Inhalation products for relief of acute bronchospasms, primary treatment of status asthmaticus, or other acute episodes of asthma.

Ophthalmically to treat most viral diseases of the cornea and conjunctiva, including acute epithelial herpes simplex keratitis, vaccinia, and varicella; mycobacterial infections of the eye and fungal disease of ocular structures; tuberculosis of the eye; acute purulent untreated eye infections; known or suspected hypersensitivity to any of the components of products.

SPECIAL CONCERNS

(1) Deaths due to adrenal insufficiency have occurred in asthmatic clients during and after transfer from systemic corticosteroids to inhaled corticosteroids. After withdrawal from systemic corticosteroids, several months are needed for recovery of hypothalamic-pituitary-adrenal (HPA) function. During this time of HPA suppression, clients may exhibit symptoms of adrenal insufficiency when exposed to trauma, surgery, or infections (especially gastroenteritis or other conditions with acute electrolyte loss). Although inhaled glucocorticoids may control asthmatic symptoms during these episodes, they do not provide the necessary mineralocorticoids for the treatment of these emergencies. Clients previously maintained on 20 mg/day or more of prednisone (or equivalent) may be most susceptible, especially when their systemic corticosteroids have been almost completely withdrawn. (2) During periods of stress or a severe asthmatic attack, have clients who have been withdrawn from systemic corticosteroids resume them (in large doses) immediately; contact a physician. Have clients carry a warning card indicating that they may need supplementary systemic corticosteroids during such periods. To assess the risk of adrenal insufficiency in emergency situations, periodically perform routine adrenal cortical function tests, including measurement of early morning resting cortisol levels in all clients. An early morning resting cortisol level may be accepted as normal only if it falls at or near the normal mean level.

- **Use with caution in diabetes mellitus, hypertension, chronic nephritis, thrombophlebitis, convul-**

Classifications

sive disorders, infectious diseases, renal or hepatic insufficiency, pregnancy.

- Use of orally inhaled or intranasal products may inhibit the growth and development of children or adolescents, although this may only be temporary.
- Prolonged used of ophthalmic products may result in glaucoma, elevated intraocular pressure, optic nerve damage, defects in visual acuity and fields of vision, posterior subcapsular cataract formation or secondary ocular infections from pathogens liberated from ocular tissues.
- Ophthalmic products may retard corneal healing. The use of steroids following cataract surgery may delay healing and increase the incidence of bleb formation. Perforations of the cornea or sclera are possible.
- Benzalkonium chloride, a component of some ophthalmic products, may be absorbed by some soft contact lenses.
- Pediatric clients are at greater risk for developing cataracts, osteoporosis, avascular necrosis of the femoral heads, and glaucoma.
- Elderly are more likely to develop hypertension and osteoporosis (especially postmenopausal women).
- Use inhalation products with caution in children less than 6 years of age. Safety and efficacy of ophthalmic products not established in children.

SIDE EFFECTS

Small physiologic doses given as replacement therapy or short-term high-dosage therapy during emergencies rarely cause side effects. Prolonged therapy may cause a Cushing-like syndrome with atrophy of the adrenal cortex and subsequent adrenocortical insufficiency. A steroid withdrawal syndrome may occur following prolonged use; symptoms include anorexia, N&V, lethargy, headache, fever, joint pain, desquamation, myalgia, weight loss, hypotension.

SYSTEMIC USE

Fluid and electrolyte: Edema, hypokalemic alkalosis, hypokalemia, hypocalcemia, hypotension or shock-like reaction, hypertension, CHF. **Musculoskeletal:** Muscle wasting, muscle pain/weakness, osteoporosis, spontaneous fractures including vertebral compression fractures and fractures of long bones, tendon rupture, aseptic necrosis of femoral and humeral heads. **GI:** N&V, anorexia or increased appetite, diarrhea or constipation, abdominal distention, pancreatitis, gastric irritation, ulcerative esophagitis. Development or exacerbation of peptic ulcers with the possibility of perforation and hemorrhage; ***perforation of the small and large bowel***, especially in inflammatory bowel disease. **Endocrine:** Cushing's syndrome (e.g., central obesity, moon face, buffalo hump, enlargement of supraclavicular fat pads), amenorrhea, postmenopausal bleeding, menstrual irregularities, decreased glucose tolerance, hyperglycemia, glycosuria, increased insulin or sulfonylurea requirement in diabetics, development of diabetes mellitus, negative nitrogen balance due to protein catabolism, suppression of growth in children, secondary adrenocortical and pituitary unresponsiveness (especially during periods of stress). **CNS/Neurologic:** Headache, vertigo, insomnia, restlessness, increased motor activity, ischemic neuropathy, EEG abnormalities, ***seizures***, pseudotumor cerebri. Also, euphoria, mood swings, depression, anxiety, personality changes, psychoses. **CV:** Thromboembolism, thrombophlebitis, ECG changes (due to potassium deficiency), fat embolism, necrotizing angiitis, cardiac arrhythmias, ***myocardial rupture following recent MI***, syncopal episodes. **Dermatologic:** Impaired wound healing, skin atrophy and thinning, petechiae, ecchymoses, erythema, purpura, striae, hirsutism, urticaria, ***angioneurotic edema***, acneiform eruptions, allergic dermatitis, lupus erythematosus-like lesions, suppression of skin test reactions, perineal irritation. **Ophthalmic:** Glaucoma, posterior subcapsular cataracts, increased IOP, exophthalmos. **Miscellaneous:** Hypercholesterolemia, atherosclerosis, aggravation or masking of infections, leukocytosis, increased/decreased motility and number of spermatozoa. **In children:** Suppression of linear growth; reversible pseudobrain tumor syndrome characterized by papilledema, oculomotor or abducens nerve paralysis, visual loss, or headache.

PARENTERAL USE

Sterile abscesses, Charcot-like arthropathy, subcutaneous and cutaneous atrophy, burning or tingling (especially in the perineal area following IV use), scarring, inflammation, paresthesia, induration, hyper-/hypopigmentation, blindness when used intralesionally around the face and head (rare), transient or delayed pain or soreness, nystagmus, ataxia, muscle twitching, hiccoughs, ***anaphylaxis with or without circulatory collapse,***

cardiac arrest, bronchospasm, arachnoiditis after intrathecal use, foreign body granulomatous reactions.

INTRA-ARTICULAR USE

Postinjection flare, Charcot-like arthropathy, tendon rupture, skin atrophy, facial flushing, osteonecrosis. Due to reduction in inflammation and pain, clients may overuse the joint.

INTRASPINAL USE

Aseptic, bacterial, chemical, cryptococcal, or tubercular meningitis; adhesive arachnoiditis, conus medullaris syndrome.

OPHTHALMIC USE

Elevated intraocular pressure with possible development of glaucoma, optic nerve damage, and visual acuity and field defects; posterior subcapsular cataract formation; delayed wound healing; acute anterior uveitis; keratitis; conjunctivitis; corneal ulcers; mydriasis; conjunctival hyperemia; loss of accommodation; ptosis; perforation of the globe where there is thinning of the sclera. Rarely filtering blebs after cataract surgery. Transient stinging or burning upon installation, ocular irritation, foreign body sensation, visual disturbances (blurred vision). Development of secondary ocular infection (bacterial, viral, fungal). Allergic reactions, hypercorticoidism (rare), taste perversion.

TOPICAL USE

When used over large areas, when the skin is broken, or with occlusive dressings, may cause atrophy of the epidermis, drying of the skin, or atrophy of the dermal collagen. When used on the face, diffuse thinning and homogenization of the collagen, epidermal thinning, and striae formation. Occasionally, sensitization reaction may occur, which necessitates discontinuation of the drug.

INHALATION

In addition to systemic side effects, inhaled corticosteroids may cause hoarseness, oropharyngeal candidiasis, cough, dermatitis, thirst, and tongue hypertrophy.

OVERDOSE MANAGEMENT

Symptoms (Continued Use of Large Doses)-Cushing's Syndrome: Acne, hypertension, moonface, striae, hirsutism, central obesity, ecchymoses, myopathy, sexual dysfunction, osteoporosis, diabetes, hyperlipidemia, increased susceptibility to infection, peptic ulcer, electrolyte and fluid imbalance. Acute toxicity or death is rare.

Treatment of Chronic Overdose: Gradually taper the dose of the steroid and frequently monitor lab tests. During periods of stress, steroid supplementation is necessary. Dose should be reduced to the lowest one that will control the symptoms (or discontinue the steroid completely). Recovery of normal adrenal and pituitary function may take up to 9 months. Large, acute overdoses may be treated with gastric lavage, emesis, and general supportive measures.

DRUG INTERACTIONS

Acetaminophen / ↑ Risk of hepatotoxicity R/T ↑ rate of formation of hepatotoxic acetaminophen metabolite

Alcohol / ↑ Risk of GI ulceration or hemorrhage

H ***Aloe*** / Hypokalemia related to both drugs could potentiate the effect of digoxin

Amphotericin B / Corticosteroids ↑ K depletion caused by amphotericin B

Aminoglutethimide / ↓ Adrenal response to corticotropin

Anabolic steroids / ↑ Risk of edema

Antacids / ↓ Effect of corticosteroids R/T ↓ GI tract absorption

Antibiotics, broad-spectrum / Concomitant use may result in emergence of resistant strains, → severe infection

Anticholinergics / Combination ↑ IOP; aggravates glaucoma

Anticholinesterases / Anticholinesterase effects may be antagonized when used for myasthenia gravis

Anticoagulants, oral / ↓ Effect of anticoagulants by ↓ hypoprothrombinemia; also ↑ risk of hemorrhage R/T vascular effects of corticosteroids

Anticholinesterases / Corticosteroids may ↓ effect of anticholinesterases when used in myasthenia gravis

Antidiabetic agents / Hyperglycemic effect of corticosteroids may necessitate ↑ antidiabetic dose

Asparaginase / ↑ Hyperglycemic drug effect and the risk of neuropathy and disturbances in erythropoiesis

Barbiturates / ↓ Effect of corticosteroids R/T ↑ liver breakdown

Bumetanide / ↑ Potassium loss R/T potassium-losing properties of both drugs

Classifications

Carbonic anhydrase inhibitors / Corticosteroids ↑ K depletion caused by carbonic anhydrase inhibitors
Cholestyramine / ↓ Effect of corticosteroids R/T ↓ GI tract absorption
Colestipol / ↓ Effect of corticosteroids R/T ↓ GI tract absorption
Contraceptives, oral / Estrogen ↑ anti-inflammatory effect of hydrocortisone by ↓ liver breakdown
Cyclophosphamide / ↑ Effect of cyclophosphamide R/T ↓ liver breakdown
Cyclosporine / ↑ Effect of both drugs R/T ↓ liver breakdown
CYP 3A4 inhibitors (itraconazole, ketoconazole, miconazole, protease inhibitors) / ↑ Risk of serious side effects if used with budesonide or fluticasone
Digitalis glycosides / ↑ Chance of digitalis toxicity (arrhythmias) R/T hypokalemia
Ephedrine / ↓ Effect of corticosteroids R/T ↑ liver breakdown
Estrogens / ↑ Anti-inflammatory effect of hydrocortisone by ↓ liver breakdown
Ethacrynic acid / Enhanced potassium loss R/T potassium-losing properties of both drugs
Folic acid / Requirements may ↑
Furosemide / ↑ Potassium loss R/T potassium-losing properties of both drugs
H ***Ginseng*** / Possible additive effects; do not use together
Heparin / Ulcerogenic effects of corticosteroids may ↑ risk of hemorrhage
Hydantoins / ↑ Corticosteroid clearance → ↓ effects
Immunosuppressant drugs / ↑ Risk of infection
Indomethacin / ↑ Chance of GI ulceration
Insulin / Hyperglycemic effect of corticosteroids may necessitate ↑ antidiabetic dose
Isoniazid / ↓ Effect of isoniazid R/T ↑ liver breakdown and ↑ excretion
Ketoconazole / ↑ Corticosteroid availability and ↓ clearance → possible toxicity
H ***Licorice*** / ↑ Levels of corticosteroids
H ***Lily-of-the-valley*** / ↑ Effectiveness and side effects of chronic glucocorticoid therapy
Mexiletine / ↓ Effect of mexiletine R/T ↑ liver breakdown
Mitotane / ↓ Response of adrenal gland to corticotropin
Muscle relaxants, nondepolarizing / Effect of muscle relaxants may be ↑, ↓, or not changed
Neuromuscular blocking agents / ↑ Risk of prolonged respiratory depression or paralysis
NSAIDs / ↑ Risk of GI hemorrhage or ulceration
H ***Pheasant's eye herb*** / ↑ Effectivness and side effects of chronic glucocorticoid therapy
Phenobarbital / ↓ Effect of corticosteroids R/T ↑ liver breakdown
Phenytoin / ↓ Effect of corticosteroids R/T ↑ liver breakdown
Potassium supplements / ↓ Plasma levels of potassium
Potassium depleting drugs (e.g., diuretics) / Possible hypokalemia; monitor
Rifampin / ↓ Effect of corticosteroids R/T ↑ liver breakdown
Ritodrine / ↑ Risk of maternal edema
Salicylates / Both are ulcerogenic; also, corticosteroids may ↓ blood salicylate levels
Smoking / ↓ Response to inhaled corticosteroids in smokers
Somatrem, Somatropin / Glucocorticoids may inhibit effect of somatrem
H ***Squill*** / ↑ Effectiveness and side effects of chronic glucocorticoid therapy
Streptozocin / ↑ Risk of hyperglycemia
Tacrolimus / Higher tacrolimus doses needed for renal transplant clients also receiving corticosteroids
Theophyllines / Changes in effects of either drug may occur
Thiazide diuretics / ↑ Potassium loss R/T potassium-losing properties of both drugs
Tricyclic antidepressants / ↑ Risk of mental disturbances
Vitamin A / Topical vitamin A can reverse impaired wound healing in clients receiving corticosteroids

LABORATORY TEST CONSIDERATIONS

↑ Urine glucose, serum cholesterol, serum amylase. ↓ Serum potassium, triiodothyronine, serum uric acid. Alteration of electrolyte balance.

DOSAGE

See individual drugs. Corticosteroids are administered by a variety of routes.

NURSING IMPLICATIONS

IMPLEMENTATION/ADMINISTRATION/STORAGE

ORAL CORTICOSTEROIDS

1. **Administer PO forms of drug with food to minimize ulcerogenic effect. Discontinue gradually if used chronically.**

2. At frequent intervals, reduce the dose gradually to determine if symptoms of the disease can be effectively controlled by smaller drug dose.
3. When treating clients with conditions such as asthma, ulcerative colitis, and rheumatoid arthritis, corticosteroids, given every other day, provide the beneficial effect of the steroid while minimizing pituitary-adrenal suppression. With this therapy, twice the usual daily dose of an intermediate-acting steroid is given every other morning.
4. Local administration of corticosteroids is preferred over systemic therapy to minimize systemic side effects.
5. Use the lowest effective dose in children and monitor routinely to avoid reduced rate of growth.

TOPICAL CORTICOSTEROIDS

1. Cleanse area before applying the medication. Wash hands, wear gloves, apply sparingly, and rub gently into the area.
2. When prescribed, apply an occlusive dressing (not to be used if an infection is present) to promote hydration of the stratum corneum and increase the absorption of the medication. The following are two methods of applying an occlusive type dressing:
   - Apply a large amount of medication to the cleansed area. Cover with a thin, pliable, nonflammable plastic film, which is then sealed to the surrounding tissue with skin tape or held in place with gauze. Change the dressing q 3–4 days.
   - Apply a small amount of medication to the area and cover with a damp cloth. Then cover with a thin, pliable, nonflammable plastic film and seal to the surrounding tissue with tape, or hold in place with gauze. Change dressing twice a day.

ASSESSMENT

1. Note reasons for therapy, type, onset, characteristics of S&S; assess underlying cause: adrenal or non adrenal disorder and clinical presentation. Check for any allergic reactions to corticosteroids or tartrazine.
2. List medications taking; identify if any may interact with corticosteroids. These include antidiabetic agents, cardiac glycosides, oral contraceptives, anticoagulants, and drugs influenced by liver enzymes.
3. Assess mental status (i.e., mood, affect, aggression, behavioral changes, depression) and neurological function.
4. Monitor VS, I&O, and weight. Obtain CXR and PPD if therapy prolonged, assessing for infection. Note childhood illnesses and immunization status.
5. In conditions requiring long term therapy determine if other agents (e.g., methotrexate) can be used to spare long-term harmful steroid effects.
6. With trigger point injections, determine if oral trial effective in reducing pain levels before referral.
7. Monitor ECG, electrolytes, BS, urinalysis, renal and LFTs (usually see elevated BS and low K^+). If female, determine if pregnant.

INTERVENTIONS

TOPICAL CORTICOSTEROIDS

1. Note site of therapy e.g., size, color, location, depth, odor, swelling, drainage and nature of infection. Assess for local sensitivity reaction at site of application.
2. Absorption varies regionally with highest absorption in scrotal skin and lowest on the foot. Inflamed skin increases absorption severalfold. Better action has been noted with the ointment bases than with the lotion or cream vehicles.
3. Observe for S&S of infections since corticosteroids tend to mask. Avoid occlusive dressing when an infection is present. With large occlusive dressing, take temperatures q 4 hr. Report if elevated and remove the dressing.
4. Assess for evidence of systemic absorption. Protracted use of large quantities of potent topical corticosteroids to large BSAs may precipitate iatrogenic Cushing's syndrome. Symptoms may include edema and transient inhibition of pituitary-adrenal cortical function as manifested by muscular pain, lassitude, depression, hypotension, and weight loss.
5. Advise client when applying topical ointment, to wash hands and to wear gloves or to apply with a sterile applicator (e.g., tongue blade). Report redness, dilated blood vessels, purple discolorations, bruising, pustules, and depressed shiny, wrinkled skin. Prolonged use of potent topical corticosteroids may increase incidence of systemic side effects.

Classifications

ORAL CORTICOSTEROIDS

1. When first placed on corticosteroids, check BP twice a day until maintenance dose established.
2. Short-term oral therapy (e.g., 60 mg PO for 5 days) does not require divided doses or titration. With long-term therapy, monitor for symptoms of adrenal insufficiency, which include hypotension, confusion, restlessness, lethargy, weakness, N&V, anorexia, and weight loss; titrate dose to withdraw.
3. Evaluate for increased sodium and fluid retention. Monitor weight and observe for edema. If noted, adjust to low-sodium, high-potassium diet. Anticipate a small weight gain due to increased appetite, but sudden increases are probably due to edema. Edema occurs most frequently with cortisone or desoxycorticosterone acetate and less frequently with the synthetic agents.
4. Assess for SOB, distended neck veins, edema, and easy fatigue; S&S of CHF. Obtain CXR and ECG.
5. Monitor serum glucose, electrolytes, and platelet counts with long-term therapy. Report any unusual bleeding, bruising, presence of petechiae, symptoms of diabetes, and any other skin changes.
6. Assess muscles for weakness and wasting; signs of a negative nitrogen balance. Report changes in appearance, especially those resembling Cushing's syndrome (such as rounding of the face, hirsutism, presence of acne, and thinning of the hair and nails) so dosage can be adjusted.
7. With diabetes, may develop hyperglycemia necessitating a change in diet and insulin dosage.
8. Assess for signs of depression, lack of interest in personal appearance, insomnia or anorexia.
9. GI bleeding may occur; periodically test stools for occult blood and monitor hematologic profile. Discuss potential for menstrual difficulties and amenorrhea related to long-term therapy.
10. Observe for S&S of other illnesses; these drugs tend to mask their severity.

CLIENT/FAMILY TEACHING

1. Corticosteroids include both mineralocorticoids and glucocorticoids. Mineralocorticoids maintain salt and fluid balance in the body while glucocorticoids have metabolic and anti-inflammatory effects and are mediators of the stress response.
2. Take the oral medication with food in the early morning and report any symptoms of gastric distress. To prevent gastric irritation, may use antacids and eat frequent small meals. If the symptoms persist, diagnostic x-rays may be indicated. High doses of glucocorticoids stimulate the stomach to produce excess acid and pepsin and may cause peptic ulcers. Antacids 3–4 times per day may relieve epigastric distress. Report any unusual bruising/bleeding or dark stools.
3. Eat a diet high in protein to compensate for the loss due to protein breakdown from gluconeogenesis. Identify foods high in potassium and low in sodium to prevent electrolyte disturbances. Supplement diet with potassium-rich foods such as citrus juices, collard greens, or bananas. Read labels of canned or processed foods and consult dietician for assistance in selection and food preparation.
4. Obtain weight daily at the same time, wearing clothing of approximately the same weight, and using the same scales. Consistent weight gain may reflect fluid retention; initiate caloric management to prevent obesity.
5. Exercise daily and consume foods high in calcium to decrease possibility of osteoporosis (due to catabolic bone effects). Consume adequate protein, calcium, and vitamin D to minimize bone loss. On-going bone resorption with depressed bone formation is the cause of osteoporosis.
6. Report changes in mood or affect or insomnia. Take early in the day to mimic circadian rhythm and prevent insomnia. Avoid falls and accidents. Steroids may cause osteoporosis, which makes the bones more susceptible to fractures. Use a night light and a hand rail or other device for support and to prevent falls.
7. Corticosteroids can cause a loss of contraceptive action with oral contraceptives. Keep accurate menstrual records and consider alternative methods of birth control. May also have an adverse effect on sperm production and count. Weight gain, acne, and excess hair growth may occur.
8. With dosage reduction, flare-ups may occur caused by the reduction. Need to gradually

withdraw the medication when therapy has exceeded 7 consecutive days. This should proceed slowly so that the adrenal cortex will gradually be reactivated and take over the production of hormones. Sudden withdrawal may be life-threatening. Any sudden change will provoke symptoms of adrenal insufficiency.

9. With arthritis, do not overuse the joint once injected and painless. Permanent joint damage may result from overuse, because underlying pathology is still present.
10. With diabetes, monitor glucose levels frequently and report changes as insulin dose and diet may require adjustment.
11. Wounds may heal slowly because steroid therapy causes a delay in development of granulation tissue, increasing potential for infection. Observe any healing process for signs of infection and report any injury or postoperative separation of wound or suture line.
12. Delay any vaccinations, immunizations, or skin testing while receiving corticosteroid therapy because there is limited immune response. These drugs mask symptoms of infection and cause immunosuppression. Because antibody production is decreased by corticosteroids, clients are at risk for infection. Must maintain general hygiene and scrupulous cleanliness to avoid infection. Report if sore throat, cough, fever, malaise, or an injury that does not heal occurs. Avoid contact with persons with contagious diseases.
13. Clients on long-term eye therapy are prone to developing cataracts, exophthalmos, and increased IOP. Schedule routine eye exams and report any visual changes.
14. Avoid OTC medications, including aspirin and ibuprofen compounds, as well as alcohol, since these may aggravate gastric irritation and bleeding.
15. Check child's height and weight regularly and graph; growth suppression may occur with corticosteroid therapy; not prevented by growth hormone administration. Large doses of glucocorticoids in children may increase intracranial pressure (pseudotumor cerebri); report symptoms: vertigo, headache, and convulsions. These should disappear once therapy discontinued.
16. Carry ID, listing drugs and dosage, condition being treated, and who to contact in the event of an emergency. Periods of increased stress may require dosage increase temporarily.
17. Identify goals of therapy and ways to achieve desired outcomes.
18. Keep all F/U to assess response, labs, and for adverse SE.

OUTCOMES/EVALUATE

- Healing/clearing of dermatitis
- Chronic pain control
- Suppression of inflammatory/immune responses or disease manifestation in allergic reactions, autoimmune diseases, organ transplants
- Serum cortisol levels within desired range in adrenal deficiency states (8 a.m. level 110–520 nmol/L)

DIURETICS, LOOP

SEE ALSO DIURETICS, THIAZIDES, AND THE FOLLOWING INDIVIDUAL ENTRIES:

Bumetanide
Ethacrynate sodium
Ethacrynic acid
Furosemide
Torsemide

INDICATIONS/USES

See individual drugs.

ACTION/KINETICS

Action

Loop diuretics inhibit reabsorption of sodium and chloride in the proximal and distal tubules and the loop of Henle.

Pharmacokinetics

Metabolized in the liver and excreted primarily through the urine. Significantly bound to plasma protein.

CONTRAINDICATIONS

Hypersensitivity to loop diuretics or to sulfonylureas. In hepatic coma or severe electrolyte depletion (until condition improves or is corrected). Lactation.

SPECIAL CONCERNS

■ Loop diuretics are potent drugs; excess amounts can lead to a profound diuresis with water and electrolyte depletion. Careful medical supervision is required and dosage must be individualized.

- **Sudden alterations of electrolytes in hepatic cirrhosis and ascites may precipitate hepatic encephalopathy and coma.**
- **SLE may be activated or worsened.**
- **Ototoxicity is most common with rapid injection, in severe renal impairment, with doses several times the usual dose, and with concurrent use of other ototoxic drugs.**
- **The risk of hospitalization is doubled in geriatric clients who take diuretics and NSAIDs.**
- **Safety and efficacy of most loop diuretics not determined in children or infants.**

SIDE EFFECTS

See individual drugs. Excessive diuresis may cause dehydration with the possibility of ***circulatory collapse and vascular thrombosis or embolism.*** Ototoxicity including tinnitus, hearing impairment, deafness (usually reversible), and vertigo with a sense of fullness are possible. Electrolyte imbalance, especially in clients with restricted salt intake. Photosensitivity. Changes include hypokalemia, hypomagnesemia, and hypocalcemia.

OVERDOSE MANAGEMENT

Symptoms: Acute profound water loss, volume and electrolyte depletion, dehydration, decreased blood volume, and ***circulatory collapse with possibility of fascicular thrombosis and embolism.***

Treatment: Replace fluid and electrolyte loss. Carefully monitor urine and plasma electrolyte levels. Emesis and gastric lavage may be useful. Supportive measures may include oxygen or artificial respiration.

DRUG INTERACTIONS

Aminoglycosides / ↑ Ototoxicity with hearing loss
Anticoagulants / ↑ Drug activity
Chloral hydrate / Transient diaphoresis, hot flashes, hypertension, tachycardia, weakness and nausea
Cisplatin / Additive ototoxicity
Digitalis glycosides / ↑ Risk of arrhythmias R/T diuretic-induced electrolyte disturbances
Lithium / ↑ Plasma levels of lithium → toxicity
Muscle relaxants, nondepolarizing / Effect of muscle relaxants either ↑ or ↓, depending on diuretic dose
Nonsteroidal anti-inflammatory drugs / ↓ Effect of loop diuretics
Probenecid / ↓ Effect of loop diuretics
Salicylates / Diuretic effect may be ↓ with cirrhosis and ascites
Sulfonylureas / Loop diuretics may ↓ glucose tolerance
Theophyllines / Action of theophyllines may be ↑ or ↓
Thiamine / High doses of loop diuretics → thiamine deficiency
Thiazide diuretics / Additive effects with loop diuretics → profound diuresis and serious electrolyte abnormalities

DOSAGE

See individual drugs.

NURSING IMPLICATIONS

ASSESSMENT

1. **Note reasons for therapy. List other agents trialed and outcome. Identify sensitivity to sulfonamides; may exhibit cross-reactivity with furosemide.**
2. **Potent diuretic with site of action involving the loop of Henle in the kidneys. Increases elimination of sodium and chloride by primarily preventing reabsorption of sodium and chloride.**
3. **Assess auditory function carefully when large doses are anticipated or when used concurrently with other ototoxic agents. Ototoxicity is dose related and generally reversible.**
4. **Record VS, weights, I&O; keep bedpan or urinal within reach. Report absence/decrease in diuresis and note changes in lung sounds. Diuretics potentiate the effects of antihypertensive agents; monitor BP.**
5. **When ambulatory, check for edema in the extremities; if on bed rest, check for edema in the sacral area.**
6. **Monitor for serum electrolyte levels, pH, and the following *signs of electrolyte imbalance:***
    - ***Hyponatremia*** **(low-salt syndrome)-characterized by muscle weakness, leg cramps, dryness of mouth, dizziness, and GI upset.**
    - ***Hypernatremia*** **(excessive sodium retention)-characterized by CNS disturbances, i.e., confusion, loss of sensorium, stupor, and coma. ↓ Skin turgor and postural hypotension not as prominent as with combined sodium and water deficits.**

- *Water intoxication* (caused by defective water diuresis)-characterized by lethargy, confusion, stupor, and coma. Neuromuscular hyperexcitability with ↑ reflexes, muscular twitching, and convulsions if acute.
- *Metabolic acidosis*-characterized by weakness, headache, malaise, abdominal pain, and N&V. Hyperpnea occurs in severe metabolic acidosis. S&S of volume depletion: poor skin turgor, soft eyeballs, and dry tongue may be observed.
- *Metabolic alkalosis*-characterized by irritability, neuromuscular hyperexcitability, tetany if severe.
- ***Hypokalemia (potassium deficiency)***-characterized by muscular weakness, peristalsis failure, postural hypotension, respiratory embarrassment, and cardiac arrhythmias.
- ***Hyperkalemia (excess potassium)***-characterized by early signs of irritability, nausea, intestinal colic, and diarrhea; and by later signs of weakness, flaccid paralysis, dyspnea, dysphagia, and arrhythmias.

7. Hyper-/hypokalemia associated with diuretic therapy may potentiate the toxic effects of digitalis and precipitate arrhythmias.
8. With high doses monitor for hyperlipidemia and hyperuricemia; precipitating a gout attack. Assess for sore throat, skin rash, and yellowing of the skin or sclera; may be blood dyscrasias.
9. With liver dysfunction, assess for electrolyte imbalances, which could cause stupor, coma, and death.
10. If receiving EC potassium tablets, assess for abdominal pain, distention, or GI bleeding; can cause small bowel ulceration. Check stool for intact tablets.
11. May precipitate symptoms of diabetes with latent or mild diabetes. Test urine or perform finger sticks and monitor labs closely.
12. Monitor BP, weight, CBC, electrolytes, Mg^{++}, Ca^{++}, BS, uric acid, renal and LFTs; reduce dose with dysfunction.

CLIENT/FAMILY TEACHING

1. Take with food or milk to decrease GI upset. May cause frequent, copious voiding. Plan activities/travel; take in the a.m. to prevent sleep disruption.
2. These drugs help rid your body of sodium and water. They make your kidneys excrete more sodium in the urine which takes water with it from your blood. That decreases the amount of fluid going through your blood vessels, which reduces pressure on the walls of your arteries.
3. Include foods high in potassium, such as citrus, grape, cranberry, apple, pear, and apricot juices; bananas; meat, fish (salmon), melons, almonds, potatoes and spinach. This is preferable to taking potassium chloride supplements but potassium supplements are usually prescribed with non-potassium-sparing diuretics. Unless conditions such as gastric ulcer or diabetes exist, drink a large glass of orange juice daily. Consult dietitian as needed for assistance in selecting and preparing foods.
4. Weakness and/or dizziness may occur. Rise slowly from bed and sit down or lie down if evident. Use caution in driving a car or operating other hazardous machinery until drug effects apparent. The use of alcohol, standing for prolonged periods, and exercise in hot weather may enhance/lower BP.
5. Ensure adequate fluids; monitor BP and weight. Report excessive weight loss, loss of skin turgor or if dizziness, nausea, muscle weakness, cramps, SOB, chest, back, or leg pain, excessive weight gain, or tingling of the extremities occur.
6. Wear protective clothing, sunscreens, and sunglasses to prevent photosensitivity reactions. Avoid tanning booths and drink plenty of water when out in the sun to diminish dehydration potential. Avoid all OTC preparations without approval.
7. Keep all F/U to assess response, labs, and for adverse SE.

OUTCOMES/EVALUATE

- Symptomatic relief (↓ weight, ↓ swelling/edema, ↑ diuresis)
- Clinical improvement in S&S associated with CHF and renal failure
- ↓ BP

DIURETICS, THIAZIDES ■

SEE ALSO THE FOLLOWING INDIVIDUAL ENTRY:

Hydrochlorothiazide

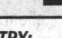

Classifications

INDICATIONS/USES

See individual drugs. (1) Edema due to CHF, nephrosis, nephritis, renal failure, PMS, hepatic cirrhosis, corticosteroid or estrogen therapy. (2) Hypertension. Hydrochlorothiazide is a component of a large number of combination drugs used to treat hypertension (*See Table 8*). (3) Premenstrual tension. *Investigational:* Thiazides are used alone or in combination with allopurinol (or amiloride) for prophylaxis of calcium nephrolithiasis. Nephrogenic diabetes insipidus.

ACTION/KINETICS

Action

Thiazides promote diuresis by decreasing the rate at which sodium and chloride are reabsorbed by the distal renal tubules of the kidney. By increasing the excretion of sodium and chloride, they force excretion of additional water. They also increase the excretion of potassium and, to a lesser extent, bicarbonate, as well as decrease the excretion of calcium and uric acid. Sodium and chloride are excreted in approximately equal amounts. Thiazides do not affect the glomerular filtration rate. Thiazides also have an antihypertensive effect which is attributed to direct dilation of the areterioles, as well as to a reduction in the total fluid volume of the body and altered sodium balance. The thiazide diuretics are related chemically to the sulfonamides. Although devoid of anti-infective activity, the thiazides can cause the same hypersensitivity reactions as the sulfonamides.

Pharmacokinetics

A large fraction is excreted unchanged in urine.

CONTRAINDICATIONS

Hypersensitivity to drug, anuria, renal decompensation. Impaired renal function and advanced hepatic cirrhosis. Do not use indiscriminately in clients with edema and toxemia of pregnancy, even though they may be therapeutically useful, because the thiazides may have adverse effects on the newborn (thrombocytopenia and jaundice).

SPECIAL CONCERNS

- **Geriatric clients may manifest an increased risk of hypotension and changes in electrolyte levels.**
- **The risk of hospitalization is doubled in geriatric clients who take diuretics and NSAIDs.**
- **Administer with caution to debilitated clients or to those with a history of hepatic coma or precoma, gout, diabetes mellitus, or during pregnancy and lactation.**
- **Particular care must be exercised when thiazides are administered concomitantly with drugs that also cause potassium loss, such as digitalis, corticosteroids, and some estrogens.**
- **Clients with advanced heart failure, renal disease, or hepatic cirrhosis are most likely to develop hypokalemia.**
- **May activate or worsen SLE.**

SIDE EFFECTS

The following side effects may be observed with most thiazides. See also individual drugs. **Electrolyte imbalance:** Hypokalemia (most frequent) characterized by cardiac arrhythmias. Hyponatremia characterized by weakness, lethargy, epigastric distress, N&V. Hypokalemic alkalosis. **GI:** Anorexia, epigastric distress or irritation, N&V, cramping, bloating, abdominal pain, diarrhea, constipation, jaundice, pancreatitis. **CNS:** Dizziness, lightheadedness, headache, vertigo, xanthopsia, paresthesias, weakness, insomnia, restlessness. **CV:** Orthostatic hypotension, MIs in elderly clients with advanced arteriosclerosis, especially if the client is also receiving therapy with other antihypertensive agents. **Hematologic:** ***Agranulocytosis, aplastic or hypoplastic anemia, hemolytic anemia***, leukopenia, thrombocytopenia. **Dermatologic:** Purpura, photosensitivity, dermatitis, rash, urticaria, necrotizing angiitis, vasculitis, cutaneous vasculitis. **Metabolic:** Neutropenia, hemolytic anemia. **Endocrine:** Hyperglycemia, glycosuria, hyperuricemia. **Miscellaneous:** Blurred vision, impotence, reduced libido, fever, muscle cramps, muscle spasm, respiratory distress.

OVERDOSE MANAGEMENT

Symptoms: Symptoms of plasma volume depletion, including orthostatic hypotension, dizziness, drowsiness, syncope, electrolyte abnormalities, hemoconcentration, hemodynamic changes. Signs of potassium depletion, including confusion, dizziness, muscle weakness, and GI disturbances. Also, N&V, GI irritation, GI hypermotility, CNS effects, cardiac abnormalities, ***seizures, hypotension, decreased respiration, and coma.***

Treatment:

- Induce emesis or perform gastric lavage followed by activated charcoal. Undertake measures to prevent aspiration.

- Electrolyte balance, hydration, respiration, CV, and renal function must be maintained. Cathartics should be avoided, as use may enhance fluid loss.
- Although GI effects are usually of short duration, treatment may be required.

DRUG INTERACTIONS

Allopurinol / ↑ Risk of hypersensitivity reactions to allopurinol
H ***Aloe*** / Hypokalemia as both drugs could potentiate effects of digoxin
Amphotericin B / Enhanced loss of electrolytes, especially potassium
Anesthetics / Thiazides may ↑ effects of anesthetics
Anticholinergic agents / ↑ Effect of thiazides R/T ↑ amount absorbed from GI tract
Anticoagulants, oral / Anticoagulant effects may be decreased
Antidiabetic agents / Thiazides antagonize hypoglycemic drug effects
Antigout agents / Thiazides may ↑ uric acid levels; thus, ↑ dose of antigout drug may be necessary
Antihypertensive agents / Thiazides potentiate drug effects
Antineoplastic agents / Thiazides may prolong drug-induced leukopenia
Calcium salts / Hypercalcemia R/T renal tubular reabsorption or bone release of calcium may be ↑ by exogenous calcium
Cholestyramine / ↓ Effect of thiazides R/T ↓ GI tract absorption
Colestipol / ↓ Effect of thiazides R/T ↓ GI tract absorption
Corticosteroids / Enhanced potassium loss R/T potassium-losing properties of both drugs
Diazoxide / Enhanced hypotensive effect. Also, ↑ hyperglycemic response
Digoxin / Thiazides produce ↑ K^+ and Mg^{++} loss with ↑ chance of digitalis-induced arrhythmias
Ethanol / Additive orthostatic hypotension
Fenfluramine / ↑ Antihypertensive effect of thiazides
Furosemide / Profound diuresis and electrolyte loss
Guanethidine / Additive hypotensive effect
Indomethacin / ↓ Effect of thiazides, possibly by inhibition of prostaglandins
Insulin / ↓ Effect R/T thiazide-induced hyperglycemia
H ***Licorice root*** / Potassium loss R/T thiazides and licorice → ↑ sensitivity to digitalis glycosides
Lithium / ↑ Risk of lithium toxicity R/T ↓ renal excretion; may be used together but monitored carefully
Loop diuretics / Additive effect to cause profound diuresis and serious electrolyte losses
Methenamine / ↓ Effect of thiazides R/T alkalinization of urine by methenamine
Methyldopa / ↑ Risk of hemolytic anemia (rare)
Muscle relaxants, nondepolarizing / ↑ Effect of muscle relaxants R/T hypokalemia
Norepinephrine / Thiazides ↓ arterial response to norepinephrine
Quinidine / ↑ Effect of quinidine R/T ↑ renal tubular reabsorption
Sulfonamides / ↑ Effect of thiazides R/T ↓ plasma protein binding
Sulfonylureas / ↓ Effect R/T thiazide-induced hyperglycemia
Tetracyclines / ↑ Risk of azotemia
Tubocurarine / ↑ Muscle relaxation and ↑ hypokalemia
Vasopressors (sympathomimetics) / Thiazides ↓ responsiveness of areterioles to vasopressors
Vitamin D / ↑ Effect of vitamin D R/T thiazide-induced hypercalcemia

LABORATORY TEST CONSIDERATIONS

Hypokalemia, hypercalcemia, hyponatremia, hypomagnesemia, hypochloremia, hypophosphatemia, hyperuricemia. ↑ BUN, creatinine, glucose in blood and urine. ↓ Serum PBI levels (no signs of thyroid disturbance). Initial ↑ total cholesterol, LDL cholesterol, and triglycerides.

DOSAGE

See individual drugs.

NURSING IMPLICATIONS

IMPLEMENTATION/ADMINISTRATION/STORAGE

1. **Clients resistant to one type of thiazide may respond to another.**
2. **Liquid potassium preparations are bitter. Administer with fruit juice or milk to enhance palatability.**
3. **To minimize electrolyte imbalance, thiazides may be taken every other day or on a 3- to 5-day basis for treatment of edema.**

Classifications

4. To prevent excess hypotension, reduce dose of other antihypertensive agents when beginning therapy.

ASSESSMENT

1. Note reasons for therapy and any previous use of these drugs. List any drug hypersensitivity.
2. Identify extent of edema; assess skin turgor, mucous membranes, extremities, and lung fields.
3. Determine presence of SLE; drug may worsen condition.
4. Works by inhibiting the reabsorption of sodium and chloride in the distal convoluted tubules in the kidneys.
5. Stop drug at least 48 hr before surgery. Thiazide inhibits pressor effects of epinephrine.
6. Potassium supplements should be given only when dietary measures are inadequate. If required, use liquid preparations to avoid ulcerations that may be produced by potassium salts in the solid dosage form. Exceptions include slow-K forms (potassium salt imbedded in a wax matrix) and micro-K forms (microencapsulated potassium salt).
7. Note any history of heart disease or gout; check uric acid levels. With cirrhosis, avoid K^+ depletion and hepatic encephalopathy.
8. Monitor BP, weight, CBC, uric acid, glucose, electrolytes, Ca^{++}, Mg^{++}, renal and LFTs.

CLIENT/FAMILY TEACHING

1. Take with food or milk if GI upset occurs. Consume in the morning so that major diuretic effect occurs before bedtime.
2. Eat a diet high in potassium. Include orange juice, bananas, citrus fruits, broccoli, spinach, tomato juice, cucumbers, beets, dried fruits, and apricots. Avoid large amounts of black licorice; may precipitate severe hypokalemia.
3. Rise slowly and dangle legs before standing to minimize low BP effects. Sit or lie down if feeling faint or dizzy. Record weight; report gains more than 2 lb/day or 5 lb/week and swelling of extremities.
4. With gout, avoid foods that precipitate attacks and continue antigout agents as prescribed. With diabetes, monitor finger sticks more frequently; may need adjustment of insulin or oral hypoglycemic agent.
5. Avoid alcohol; causes severe drop in BP. Do not take any other medication (including OTC drugs for asthma, cough and colds, hay fever, weight control) unless approved.
6. Report any severe weight loss/gain, muscle weakness, cramps, dizziness, or fatigue. Skin rashes may occur but severe symptoms R/T allergic reactions include acute SOB (pulmonary edema), abdominal pain (acute pancreatitis), easy bruising/bleeding (thrombocytopenia), yellowing of skin/eyes; itching (cholestatic jaundice); and pale, weak/dizzy (hemolytic anemia); report immediately.
7. Keep all F/U to assess response, labs, and adverse SE.

OUTCOMES/EVALUATE

- Control of hypertension; ↓ BP
- ↑ Urine output; ↓ edema; ↓ weight
- Normal electrolyte levels and fluid balance

ESTROGENS ■

SEE ALSO THE FOLLOWING INDIVIDUAL ENTRIES:

Esterified estrogens
Estradiol gel
Estradiol hemihydrate
Estradiol topical emulsion
Estradiol transdermal system
Estrogens conjugated, oral
Estrogens conjugated, parenteral
Estrogens conjugated, synthetic (A & B)
Estrogens conjugated, vaginal
Estropipate*
Oral Contraceptives

Drugs marked with an * are available to view in the 2013 Nurse's Drug Handbook Website at www.cengage.com/community/nursesdrughandbook.

INDICATIONS/USES

See individual drugs. Uses include, but are not limited to: (1) Hormone replacement therapy in postmenopausal women to relieve moderate to severe vasomotor symptoms and decrease the risk of osteoporosis. (2) Component of combination oral contraceptives and other forms for contraception. (3) Used vaginally for vulvar/vaginal atrophy (alternative therapies should be tried first), atrophic vaginitis, and treatment of moderate to severe vasomotor symptoms associated with menopause. (4) Less commonly used for palliative treatment of select breast or prostate cancer clients with advanced disease.

NOTE: Guidelines have been established for the routine use of combined estrogen and progestin hormone replacement therapy in women. Use of hormone replacement therapy carries both benefits and risks; overall risks are likely to exceed benefits. Thus, a D recommendation rating has been established for the routine use of combined estrogen and progestin in postmenopausal women and for the routine use of unopposed estrogen in postmenopausal women with hysterectomy for the prevention of chronic conditions.

Investigational: Turner syndrome (estrogen replicates the events of puberty).

ACTION/KINETICS

Action

The three primary estrogens in the human female are estradiol 17-β, estrone, and estriol, which are steroids. Estrogens combine with receptors in the cytoplasm of the cell, resulting in an increase in protein synthesis. For example, estrogens are required for development of secondary sex characteristics, development and maintenance of the female genital system, and breasts. They also produce effects in the pituitary and hypothalamus. In adult women, estrogens participate in bone maintenance by aiding the deposition of calcium in the protein matrix of bones. They increase elastic elements in the skin, tend to cause sodium and fluid retention, and produce an anabolic effect by enhancing the turnover of dietary nitrogen and other elements into protein. Furthermore, they tend to keep plasma cholesterol at relatively low levels.

Pharmacokinetics

Natural estrogens have a significant first-pass effect; thus, they are given parenterally. Synthetic derivatives can be given PO and are rapidly absorbed, distributed, and excreted. Estrogens are metabolized in the liver and excreted in urine (major portion) and feces. When given transdermally, the skin metabolizes estradiol only to a small extent.

CONTRAINDICATIONS

Known or suspected breast cancer, except in those clients being treated for metastatic disease. Cancer of the genital tract and other estrogen-dependent neoplasms. Undiagnosed abnormal genital bleeding. Active deep vein thrombosis or history of such. Active or recent (within the past year) arterial thromboembolic disease, including active thrombophlebitis, thrombosis, or thromboembolic disorders. History of thrombophlebitis, thrombosis, or thromboembolic disorders associated with previous estrogen use, except when used to treat breast or prostatic malignancy. Known or suspected pregnancy. Prolonged therapy in women who plan to become pregnant. Porphyria (estradiol vaginal tablets only). Use during lactation. May be contraindicated in clients with blood dyscrasias, hepatic disease, or thyroid dysfunction.

SPECIAL CONCERNS

(1) Estrogens have been reported to increase the risk of endometrial cancer in postmenopausal women exposed for more than 1 year. Incidence depends on duration of treatment and dose. When estrogens are used to treat menopausal symptoms, use the lowest dose and discontinue as soon as possible. When prolonged treatment is indicated, reassess the client at least semiannually by endometrial sampling to determine the need for continued therapy. (2) Close clinical surveillance of women taking estrogens is important. Adequate diagnostic measures, including endometrial sampling when indicated, should be undertaken to rule out malignancy in all cases of undiagnosed persistent or recurring abnormal vaginal bleeding. (3) There is no evidence that natural estrogens are more or less hazardous than synthetic estrogens at equiestrogenic doses. (4) Do not use estrogens during pregnancy as such use is associated with increased risk of congenital defects in the reproductive organs of the fetus and possibly other birth defects. There is no indication for estrogen therapy during pregnancy or during the immediate postpartum period. Estrogens are ineffective for the prevention and treatment of threatened or habitual abortion. Estrogens are not indicated for the prevention of postpartum breast engorgement. If estrogens are used during pregnancy, or if the client becomes pregnant while taking estrogens, inform her of the potential risks to the fetus. (5) Do not use estrogens with or without progestins for the prevention of CV disease. There is an increased risk of MI, stroke, invasive breast cancer, pulmonary emboli, and DVT in postmenopausal women during 5 years of treatment with conjugated equine estrogens (0.625 mg) combined with medroxyprogesterone acetate (2.5 mg) relative to placebo. Because of these risks, estrogens with or without

progestins should be prescribed at the lowest effective doses and for the shortest duration consistent with treatment goals and risks for the individual woman. (6) It has been reported that estrogens increase the risk of developing probable dementia in postmenopausal women 65 years or older during 4 years of treatment with conjugated estrogens plus medroxyprogesterone acetate compared with placebo. It is not known whether this is also true in younger postmenopausal women or women taking estrogen alone therapy. ■

- **Use with caution, if at all, in those with asthma, epilepsy, migraine, cardiac failure, renal insufficiency, diseases involving calcium or phosphorous metabolism, or a family history of mammary or genital tract cancer.**
- **Safety and efficacy not determined in children; use with caution in adolescents in whom bone growth is incomplete.**

SIDE EFFECTS

SYSTEMIC USE

Side effects to estrogens are dose dependent. **CV:** Potentially, the most serious side effects involve the CV system. ***Venous thromboembolism, deep and superficial venous thrombosis***, thrombophlebitis, ***MI, pulmonary embolism***, retinal thrombosis, ***mesenteric thrombosis, subarachnoid hemorrhage, postsurgical thromboembolism.*** Hypertension, edema, ***stroke***. **GI:** N&V, diarrhea, constipation, abdominal cramps/pain, dyspepsia, flatulence, gastritis, gastroenteritis, enlarged abdomen, hemorrhoids, bloating, cholestatic jaundice, colitis, ***acute pancreatitis***, changes in appetite, increased risk of gallbladder disease requiring surgery. **Dermatologic:** Most common are chloasma or melasma. Also, erythema multiforme, erythema nodosum, hemorrhagic eruptions, urticaria, dermatitis, photosensitivity, skin hypertrophy, loss of scalp hair, hirsutism, pruritus, rash, pruritus ani, acne. **Hepatic:** Cholestatic jaundice, aggravation of porphyria, benign (most common) or malignant liver tumors, including hepatic adenoma. **GU:** Breakthrough bleeding, spotting, changes in amount/duration of menstrual flow, amenorrhea during/after use, dysmenorrhea, UTI, leukorrhea, vaginitis, premenstrual-like syndrome, change in cervical eversion and degree of cervical secretion, cystitis-like syndrome, vaginal discomfort/pain, ***vaginal hemorrhage***, asymptomatic genital bacterial growth, hemolytic uremic syndrome, endometrial cystic hyperplasia, increased incidence of *Candida* vaginitis, genital moniliasis, cystitis, dysuria, frequent micturition, urethral disorder, vaginosis fungal, vaginal discharge, genital pruritus, urinary incontinence, endometrial hyperplasia, possible link between long-term use of estrogens after menopause and ovarian cancer, increase in size of pre-existing uterine leiomyomata. **CNS:** Mental depression, dizziness, changes in libido, chorea, insomnia, headache, sinus /tension headache, aggravation of migraine headaches, fatigue, nervousness, anxiety, emotional lability, mood disturbances, irritability, worsening of epilepsy, ***convulsions***. **Ocular:** Steepening of corneal curvature resulting in intolerance of contact lenses. Optic neuritis or retinal vascular thrombosis, resulting in sudden or gradual, partial or complete loss of vision, double vision, papilledema. **Respiratory:** URTI, sinusitis, rhinitis, bronchitis, pharyngitis, nasopharyngitis, cough, nasal congestion, pharyngolaryngeal pain, exacerbation of asthma. **Musculoskeletal:** Arthritis, arthralgia, skeletal pain. **Hematologic:** Increase in prothrombin and blood coagulation factors VII, VIII, IX, and X. Decrease in antithrombin III. **Local:** Pain at injection site, sterile abscesses, postinjection flare, redness/irritation at site of application of transdermal system. **Body as a whole:** Edema, reduced carbohydrate tolerance, pain, hypersensitivity reactions, flu-like symptoms, allergy, infection, accidental injury, asthenia, anemia, paresthesia, anaphylactoid/anaphylactic reactions (including urticaria and angioedema), fluid retention. **Miscellaneous:** Aggravation of porphyria, back pain, hot flushes, chest pain, leg edema, otitis media, toothache, tooth disorder, leg cramps, neck pain, neck rigidity, candidal infection, fungal infection, herpes simplex. Breast tenderness, enlargement, or secretions; galactorrhea, fibrocystic breast changes, breast cancer. Premature closure of epiphyses in children. Increased frequency of benign or malignant tumors of the cervix, uterus, vagina, and other organs. Increase or decrease in weight. Increased risk of congenital abnormalities. Hypercalcemia in clients with metastatic breast carcinoma. In males, estrogens may cause gynecomastia, loss of libido, decreased spermatogenesis, testicular atrophy, and feminization. Prolonged use of high doses may inhibit the function of the anterior pituitary. Estrogen therapy affects many laboratory tests.

VAGINAL USE

GU: Vaginal bleeding/discharge, endometrial withdrawal bleeding, serious bleeding in ovariectomized women with endometriosis. **Miscellaneous:** Breast tenderness.

DRUG INTERACTIONS

Anticoagulants, oral / ↓ Anticoagulant response by ↑ activity of certain clotting factors
Anticonvulsants / Estrogen-induced fluid retention may precipitate seizures. Also, contraceptive steroids ↑ drug effects by ↓ liver breakdown and ↓ plasma protein binding
Antidiabetic agents / Estrogens may impair glucose tolerance and thus change requirements for antidiabetic agent
Barbiturates / ↓ Effect of estrogen or changes in uterine bleeding profile by ↑ liver breakdown
H ***Black cohosh*** / May interfere with estrogen effects
Carbamazepine / ↓ Effect of estrogen or changes in uterine bleeding profile by ↑ liver breakdown
Corticosteroids / ↑ Pharmacologic/toxicologic effects of corticosteroids R/T inactivation of hepatic P450 enzyme
H ***Ginseng*** / Additive effects; avoid concomitant use
Grapefruit juice / Possible ↑ estrogen plasma levels
Hydantoins / Breakthrough bleeding, spotting, and pregnancy are possible; also, loss of seizure control R/T fluid retention
Itraconazole / ↑ Plasma estrogen levels → side effects
Ketoconazole / ↑ Plasma estrogen levels → side effects
Macrolide antibiotics / ↑ Plasma estrogen levels → side effects
Rifampin / ↓ Effect of estrogen or changes in uterine bleeding profile by ↑ liver breakdown
Ritonavir / ↑ Plasma estrogen levels → side effects
H ***Saw palmetto*** / ↓ Effect of hormones R/T antiestrogen effect
H ***St. John's wort*** / ↓ Effect of estrogen or changes in uterine bleeding profile by ↑ liver breakdown
Succinylcholine / Estrogens may ↑ drug effects
Thyroxine, thyroid hormone / Possible ↑ need for thyroxine, thyroid hormone
Topiramate / ↑ Estrogen metabolism → ↓ efficacy
Tricyclic antidepressants / Possible ↑ effects of both drugs (dose-dependent); possible ↑ incidence of toxic effects

LABORATORY TEST CONSIDERATIONS

Altered LFTs and thyroid function tests. False + urine glucose test. ↓ Serum cholesterol, total serum lipids, pregnanediol excretion, serum folate, antithrombin III, antifactor Xa. ↑ Serum triglyceride levels, thyroxine-binding globulin, sulfobromophthalein retention. ↑ PT, PTT, platelet aggregation time, platelet count, fibrinogen, plasminogen, norepinephrine-induced platelet aggregatability, and factors II, VII, IX, X, XI, VII-X complex, II-VII-X complex, and β-thromboglobulin. Impaired glucose tolerance, reduced response to metyrapone.

DOSAGE

PO, IM, SC, vaginal, topical, or by implantation. The dosage of estrogens is highly individualized and is aimed at the minimal effective amount.

NURSING IMPLICATIONS

IMPLEMENTATION/ADMINISTRATION/STORAGE

1. Most PO administered estrogens are metabolized rapidly and must be administered daily.
2. Parenterally administered estrogens are released more slowly from aqueous suspensions or oily solutions; give slowly and deeply.
3. To avoid continuous stimulation of reproductive tissue, cyclic therapy consisting of 3 weeks on and 1 week off is usually recommended for most uses.

ASSESSMENT

1. Note reasons for therapy, type/onset of symptoms. List other agents prescribed and outcome.
2. List history of thromboembolic problems as estrogens enhance blood coagulability; avoid use in smoker.
3. Assess mental status; note any history of depression, migraine headaches, or suicide attempts.
4. Identify any undiagnosed genital bleeding, liver disease, asthma, migraines, epilepsy, or cancer of the endometrium or breast (estrogen-dependent neoplasms), as these preclude drug therapy.
5. Monitor ECG, VS, BS, triglycerides, electrolytes, renal and LFTs.

CLIENT/FAMILY TEACHING

1. These are a group of hormones that primarily influence the female reproductive tract in sexual development, function (i.e., breast development, menstrual cycle) and maturation. In women, estrogens are produced mainly in the ovaries and in the placenta during pregnancy with smaller amounts produced by the adrenal glands. In men, small amounts are produced by the adrenal glands and testicles. Also, small amounts of estrone are made throughout the body in most tissues, especially fat and muscle. This is the major source of estrogen in women who have gone through menopause.
2. Taking oral agents with meals or a light snack will prevent gastric irritation and may eliminate nausea. Review the dose, form, and frequency of prescribed agent. With once-a-day therapy, taking at bedtime may eliminate problems. Nausea, bloating, abdominal cramping, changes in appetite, and vomiting may occur and usually disappear with continued therapy.
3. With cyclical therapy, take medications for 3 weeks and then omit for 1 week. Menstruation may then occur, but pregnancy will not because ovulation is suppressed. Keep a record of periods and problems, such as missed period, unusual vaginal bleeding, spotting, or irregularity. Report if pregnancy suspected.
4. Breast tenderness, enlargement, or secretion may occur. Perform BSE monthly (usually 2 weeks after menses) and report changes. Have mammogram and a breast exam performed by provider every year to help detect breast cancer as early as possible
5. Report immediately: leg pains, sudden onset of chest pain, dizziness, SOB, weakness of the arms or legs, or any numbness (S&S of thromboembolic problems).
6. Stop taking estrogen 4–6 weeks before any surgery or bed rest to decrease risk of blood clot development.
7. Report any alterations in mental attitude: depression or withdrawal, insomnia or anorexia, or a lack of attention to personal appearance.
8. Changes in the curvature of the cornea may make it difficult to wear contact lenses; consult ophthalmologist. Report any changes, such as hair loss or skin discoloration. Males may develop feminine characteristics or suffer from impotence; usually resolves once therapy completed.
9. May alter glucose tolerance. Monitor sugars and report increases; antidiabetic dose may need to be changed.
10. Insert suppositories high into the vault. Apply vaginal preparations at bedtime. Wear a sanitary napkin and avoid the use of tampons. Store suppositories in the refrigerator. Report if estrogen ointments cause systemic reactions.
11. If pregnant and planning to breast-feed, do not take estrogens. Consult provider for alternative forms of contraception; breast-feeding does not provide contraception.
12. *Do not smoke*. Attend formal smoking cessation programs.
13. Some potential risks, related to endometrial/breast cancer, have been associated with estrogen therapy. Close medical follow-up required.
14. Keep all F/U to assess response, labs, and for adverse SE.

OUTCOMES/EVALUATE

- Control of estrogen imbalance
- Effective contraceptive agent
- Relief of menopausal S&S
- Control of tumor size/spread in metastatic breast and prostate cancer

FLUOROQUINOLONES ■

SEE ALSO THE FOLLOWING INDIVIDUAL ENTRIES:

Ciprofloxacin hydrochloride
Gatifloxacin
Gemifloxacin mesylate
Levofloxacin
Moxifloxacin hydrochloride
Norfloxacin
Ofloxacin

INDICATIONS/USES

See individual drugs. Used for a large number of gram-positive and gram-negative infections.

ACTION/KINETICS

Action

Synthetic, broad-spectrum antibacterial agents. The fluorine molecule confers increased activity against gram-negative organisms as well as broadens the spectrum against gram-positive organisms. Are bactericidal agents by interfering with DNA gyrase and topoisomerase IV. DNA gyrase is an enzyme needed for the replication, transcription, and repair of bacterial DNA. Topoisomerase IV plays a key role in the partitioning of chromosomal DNA during bacterial cell division. Ciprofloxacin, levofloxacin, ofloxacin, and trovafloxacin may be given IV; all fluoroquinolones may be given PO.

Pharmacokinetics

Food may delay the absorption of ciprofloxacin, lomefloxacin, and norfloxacin.

CONTRAINDICATIONS

Hypersensitivity to the quinolone group of antibiotics, including cinoxacin and nalidixic acid. Tendinitis or tendon rupture associated with quinolone use. Clients receiving disopyramide and amiodarone or other drugs (e.g., quinidine, procainamide, sotalol) that prolong the QTc interval and which may cause torsade de pointes. Lactation. Use in children less than 18 years of age. Gatifloxacin with diabetes mellitus.

SPECIAL CONCERNS

- **Use lower doses in impaired renal function.**
- **May be differences in CNS toxicity between the various fluoroquinolones.**
- **Use may increase the risk of Achilles and other tendon inflammation and rupture.**
- **Several cause phototoxicity.**
- **May exacerbate the signs of myasthenia gravis and lead to life-threatening weakness of the respiratory muscles.**

SIDE EFFECTS

See individual drugs. The following side effects are common to each of the fluoroquinolone antibiotics. **GI:** N&V, diarrhea, abdominal pain or discomfort, dry or painful mouth, heartburn, dyspepsia, flatulence, constipation, pseudomembranous colitis. **CNS:** Headache, dizziness, malaise, lethargy, fatigue, drowsiness, somnolence, depression, insomnia, ***seizures***, paresthesia. **Dermatologic:** Rash, photosensitivity, pruritus (except for ciprofloxacin). **Hypersensitivity reactions:** Facial or ***pharyngeal edema***, dyspnea, urticaria, itching, tingling, loss of consciousness, ***CV collapse***. **Other:** Visual disturbances and ophthalmic abnormalities, hearing loss, superinfection, phototoxicity, eosinophilia, crystalluria, Achilles and other tendon inflammation and rupture. Fluoroquinolones, except norfloxacin, may also cause vaginitis, syncope, chills, and edema.

OVERDOSE MANAGEMENT

Symptoms: Extension of side effects.

Treatment: For acute overdose, vomiting should be induced or gastric lavage performed. The client should be carefully observed and, if necessary, symptomatic and supportive treatment given. Hydration should be maintained. Hemodialysis or peritoneal dialysis may help to remove ciprofloxacin but not other fluoroquinolones.

DRUG INTERACTIONS

Antacids / ↓ Serum fluoroquinolone levels R/T ↓ GI tract absorption
Anticoagulants / ↑ Anticoagulant effects
Cimetidine / ↓ Elimination of fluoroquinolones
Cyclosporine / ↑ Risk of nephrotoxicity
Didanosine / ↓ Serum fluoroquinolone levels R/T ↓ GI tract absorption due to Mg^{++} and aluminum buffers present in didanosine tablets
Iron salts / ↓ Serum fluoroquinolone levels R/T ↓ GI tract absorption
NSAIDs / ↑ Risk of CNS stimulation and seizures
Probenecid / ↑ Serum fluoroquinolone levels R/T ↓ renal clearance
Sucralfate / ↓ Serum fluoroquinolone levels R/T ↓ GI tract absorption
Theophylline / ↑ Theophylline plasma levels and ↑ drug toxicity R/T ↓ clearance
Zinc salts / ↓ Serum fluoroquinolone levels R/T ↓ GI tract absorption

LABORATORY TEST CONSIDERATIONS

↑ ALT, AST. False + opiate results in urinary assays. See also individual drugs.

DOSAGE

See individual drugs.

NURSING IMPLICATIONS

ASSESSMENT

1. **Note reasons for therapy, symptom characteristics, clinical presentation, and culture results. List any previous experiences with these antibiotics. Discontinue at first sign of rash or other allergic manifestations. Hypersensitivity reactions may occur latently.**

2. Assess soft tissue/extremity injury; note instability, pain, swelling, erythema, and discharge. Assess Achilles tendon for drug-induced injury.
3. If receiving anticoagulants and theophyllines, monitor closely; quinolones can cause increased drug levels with toxic drug effects (i.e., bleeding or seizures).
4. Monitor VS, I&O, CBC, cultures, renal and LFTs; reduce dose with renal dysfunction.

CLIENT/FAMILY TEACHING

1. Take only as directed. Avoid mineral supplements (i.e., iron or zinc) or antacids containing magnesium or aluminum simultaneously or 4 hr before or 2 hr after dosing with fluoroquinolones.
2. Do not perform hazardous tasks until drug effects realized; may experience dizziness, drowsiness, lightheadedness, or ↓alertness.
3. Report any bothersome symptoms; N&V and diarrhea are most frequently reported side effects. Symptoms of superinfection include furry tongue, vaginal or rectal itching, diarrhea.
4. Hypersensitivity reactions may occur, even after the first dose. Stop drug at first sign of skin rash or other allergic reaction.
5. Consume >2.5 L/day of fluids to ensure adequate hydration.
6. Wear protective clothing and sunscreens; avoid excessive sunlight or artificial UV light. Even brief exposure to sun can cause a severe sunburn or rash. Use a lip balm containing sun block and avoid the use of tanning beds, tanning booths, or sunlamps. Photosensitivity reactions may occur up to several weeks after stopping therapy.
7. Some fluoroquinolones may weaken the tendons in the shoulder, hand, or heel, making these fibrous bands of tissue more likely to tear. Stop drug and report any new onset tendon/extremity pain or inflammation as tendon rupture may occur.
8. Keep all F/U to assess response, labs, and for adverse SE.

OUTCOMES/EVALUATE

- Symptomatic improvement
- Resolution of infection (↓ WBCs, ↓ temperature, ↑ appetite)
- Negative culture reports

HEPARINS, LOW MOLECULAR WEIGHT ■

SEE ALSO THE FOLLOWING INDIVIDUAL ENTRIES:

Dalteparin sodium
Enoxaparin
Tinzaparin sodium

INDICATIONS/USES

See individual drugs. Uses include, but are not limited to: (1) Prophylaxis of DVT that may lead to pulmonary embolism. (2) Treatment of DVT with or without pulmonary embolism. (3) Prophylaxis of ischemic complications in unstable angina and non-Q-wave MI when given together with aspirin. (4) Prophylaxis of venous thromboembolism in cancer clients with central venous catheters. (5) Prophylaxis of venous thromboembolism in general surgery. (6) Prophylaxis of venous thromboembolism in gynecologic surgery.

ACTION/KINETICS

Action

As antithrombotic drugs they enhance the inhibition of Factor Xa and thrombin by binding to and accelerating antithrombin II activity. They potentiate the inhibition of Factor Xa preferentially; slightly affect thrombin and clotting time or activated partial thromboplastin time.

Pharmacokinetics

Primarily metabolized in the liver to lower molecular weight compounds with significantly less activity.

CONTRAINDICATIONS

Hypersensitivity to heparin, pork products, methylparaben, sulfites, or benzyl alcohol. Active major bleeding. Thrombocytopenia with positive in vitro tests for antiplatelet antibody in presence of a low molecular weight heparin. IM or IV use.

SPECIAL CONCERNS

■ (1) When spinal/epidural anesthesia or spinal puncture is used, those anticoagulated or scheduled to be anticoagulated with low molecular weight heparins or heparinoids to prevent thromboembolic complications are at risk of developing a spinal or epidural hematoma that can result in long-term or permanent paralysis. (2) The risk of these events is increased by the use of indwelling epidural catheters for administration of analgesia; the concomitant use of drugs affecting hemostasis, such as NSAIDs, platelet inhibitors, or other anticoagulants; a history of traumatic or repeated epidural or spinal puncture; or, a history of spinal deformity, spinal injury, or spinal surgery. (3) Frequently monitor clients for signs and symptoms of neurologic impairment. If neurological compromise noted, urgent treatment is necessary. (4) Consider the potential benefit versus risk before neuraxial intervention in clients anticoagulated or to be anticoagulated for thromboprophylaxis.

- **Use with extreme caution in clients with a history of heparin-induced thrombocytopenia.**
- **Use with extreme caution in clients with an increased risk of hemorrhage, including those with severe uncontrolled hypertension, bleeding diathesis, diabetic retinopathy, bacterial endocarditis, congenital or acquired bleeding disorders (including hepatic failure and amyloidosis), active ulceration and angiodysplastic GI disease, hemorrhagic stroke or shortly after brain, spinal, or ophthalmic surgery, or in those treated concomitantly with platelet inhibitors.**
- **Use with caution in severe liver or kidney disease.**
- **Use with caution during lactation.**
- **Safety and efficacy not determined in children.**

SIDE EFFECTS

See individual drugs. **Hemorrhagic side effects:** ***Clinically significant bleeding (fatal or nonfatal)*** from any tissue or organ, hemorrhage, injection site hematoma, wound hematoma. **Hemorrhagic complications:** Paralysis, paresthesia, headache, pain (chest, abdomen, joint, muscle, or other), dizziness, shortness of breath, difficulty breathing or swallowing, swelling, weakness, hypotension, ***shock, coma***. **Hepatic:** ↑ AST, ALT.

OVERDOSE MANAGEMENT

Symptoms: Hemorrhagic complications.

Treatment: Slow IV protamine sulfate (1%) at a dose of 1 mg for every 100 anti-Xa international units of dalteparin or 1 mg for every 1 mg of enoxaparin. A second infusion of protamine sulfate, 0.5 mg per 100 anti-Xa international units of dalteparin or per 1 mg of enoxaparin may be given if the aPTT measured 2–4 hr after the first infusion of protamine sulfate remains prolonged. Take care not to give an overdose of protamine.

DRUG INTERACTIONS

Aspirin / ↑ Risk of bleeding
H *Bromelain* / ↑ Risk of bleeding
Clopidogrel ↑ Risk of bleeding
Dextran / ↑ Risk of bleeding
Dipyridamole / ↑ Risk of bleeding
H *Feverfew* / Possible additive antiplatelet effect
H *Garlic* / Possible additive antiplatelet effect
H *Ginger* / Possible additive antiplatelet effect
Ketorolac tromethamine / ↑ Risk of bleeding
NSAIDs / ↑ Risk of bleeding
Sulfinpyrazone / ↑ Risk of bleeding
Thrombolytics / ↑ Risk of bleeding
Ticlopidine / ↑ Risk of bleeding

LABORATORY TEST CONSIDERATIONS

Asymptomatic ↑ AST, ALT.

DOSAGE

See individual drugs.

NURSING IMPLICATIONS

1. For SC administration only; do not give IM.
2. Low molecular weight heparins cannot be used interchangeably (i.e., unit for unit) with other low molecular weight heparins or unfractionated heparin.

ASSESSMENT

1. **Note reasons for therapy (prophylaxis/treatment), other agents trialed, outcome. Assess for any sensitivity to heparin, sulfite, methylparaben, or pork products.**
2. **Review list of special concerns that may preclude client receiving drugs. Those who received spinal anesthesia or taps require special monitoring to assess for neurologic S&S and spinal/epidural hematoma formation which may cause permanent paralysis.**
3. **List any evidence of active bleeding, bleeding disorders, or thrombocytopenia. Assess carefully for masked bleeding. Drug does not usually affect PT/PTT values; yet client may be hemorrhaging. Monitor VS, I&O, mental status, H&H, U/A, electrolytes, renal and LFTs; routinely check all potential bleeding sites. Any unexplained fall in BP or H/H should lead to a search for a bleeding site.**

CLIENT/FAMILY TEACHING

1. **Many clients are treated with low molecular weight heparins (LMWH) at home. Indications for therapy, self-administration techniques, length/frequency of therapy, and site rotation are important concerns. SC injection techniques and recognizing signs of complications are important. To minimize bruising, do not rub site after administering.**
2. **LMWHs are defined as heparin salts-produced by depolymerization of unfractionated heparin, rendering them smaller and more bioavailable than heparin. There is less binding to plasma proteins and less inactivation by platelet factor 4.**
3. **Due to LMWH predictable effects, they do not require the regular laboratory monitoring to ensure adequate anticoagulation and dose adjustment as does heparin.**
4. **Avoid aspirin, NSAIDs, and all OTC agents. Report any unusual effects, i.e., bruising, bleeding, chest pain, acute SOB, itching, rash, or swelling.**
5. **Keep all F/U to assess response, labs, and for adverse SE.**

OUTCOMES/EVALUATE

Thromboembolism/DVT/ischemic complication prophylaxis

HERBS ■

***SEE TABLE 1*.**

GENERAL STATEMENT

Herbs are medicinal plants, also called botanicals or phytomedicines. Herbal therapy is the use of plants or plant extracts for medicinal purposes (especially plants that are not part of the normal diet). Phytomedicines are medicinal products that contain plant material as their pharmacologically active component. They are often complex mixtures of compounds that generally do not exert a strong, immediate action. Consumers use herbal products as therapeutic agents for the treatment/cure of illness/disease symptoms and prophylactically to prevent disease and to maintain health and wellness.

Extracts are concentrated preparations of a liquid, powdered, or viscous consistency that are usually made from dried plant parts by maceration or percolation. Tincture is an alcoholic or hydroalcoholic solution prepared from botanicals. Plant juices are formed from the freshly harvested plant parts macerated in water and pressed. Herbal teas are potable infusions made from infusion (pour boiling water over the herb), decoction (cover herb with cold water and bring to a boil and simmer for 5–10 min), or cold maceration (place herb in tap water and let stand at room temperature for 6–8 hr).

Consumer use of herbs and medicinal products over the past two decades has risen dramatically. The World Health Organization has estimated that more than 70% of the world population use herbal medicine for some aspect of primary health care. In some Asian and African countries, 80% of the population relies on traditional medicine for primary health care. Up to 70% to 80% of the population in many developed countries have used some form of alternative or complementary alternative medicine, commonly known as CAM (e.g. acupuncture). The use of herbal treatments are the most popular form of traditional medicine, and are highly lucrative in the international marketplace generating billions of dollars in revenue. These agents are found in retail pharmacies, grocery stores, health food shops, corner markets, and other large outlet stores, as well as mail order and TV/Internet sales. Some major health insurance companies are including coverage for herbs under "alternative therapies" and many more are considering this coverage.

TABLE 1: Commonly Used Herbal Products

The following table presents some of the commonly used herbal products. It is not intended to be an extensive listing of information for each product. Rather, the table contains important information regarding use(s), dose, side effects, and other information. Importantly, labels for herbal products vary significantly in the quality and quantity of the information. Also, there is wide variation in plant part ingredients and recommended daily doses.

Name(s)	Use(s)	Dose	Contraindications	Side Effects	Other Information
Aloe juice/latex, Aloe gel	**PO::** *Juice/Latex*:: Laxative, cathartic. **Topical::** *Gel::* Promote burn or wound healing. Treat cold sores. Cosmetic products.	**Laxative::** 100–200 mg aloe, 50 mg extract, or 1–8 oz of the juice. **Topical::** Apply gel liberally.	PO in intestinal obstruction, Crohn's disease, ulcerative colitis, appendicitis, abdominal pain of unknown orign. Children under 12 years. Pregnancy, lactation.	Abdominal pain, cramps. Diarrhea with long-term use. Potassium loss, albuminura, hematuria, heart disturbances, weight loss, muscle weakness.	Do not use for more than 1-2 *weeks* without medical advice. Potassium loss can be increased by simultaneous use of corticosteroids, licorice, or thiazides. May interact with cardiac glycosides and antiarrhythmic drugs.
Bilberry fruit/leaf	**PO::** *Fruit::* Acute diarrhea. Improve visual acuity, including night vision. **Topical::** Mild for inflammation of the mouth and throat mucous membranes. *Leaf::* Diabetes, arthritis, gout, dermatitis, hemorrhoids, poor circulation, heart problems and prevention and treatment of GI, kidney, and urinary tract symptoms.	*Dried ripe berries::* 20–60 grams/day. *Decoction::* 5–10 grams in cold water; bring to boil and simmer 10 min; strain. *Extract::* 160 mg 2 times per day for retinopathy. **Topical::** Apply as a 10% concoction. *Leaf::* Drink as a tea:: 1–2 tsp. finely chopped dried leaf in 150 mL boiling water for 5–10 min; strain.	Chronic use of the leaf may cause anemia, jaundice, acute excitatory states, disturbance of muscle contraction.	Leaves contain high levels of chromium (may lower blood glucose). Avoid prolonged use of the tea. The leaf may interact with antidiabetic drugs and disulfiram.	
Cascara sagrada	**PO::** Most commonly as a laxative. Also for gallstones, liver ailments, and cancer. Used to make some sunscreens.	**Capsules, Syrup, Tablets::** 20–30 mg hydroxyanthracene derivatives/day, calculated as cascaroside A. *Fluid extract::* 2–5 mL 3 times per day. May also be used as a tea (2 grams finely chopped bark in 150 mL of boiling water for 5–10 min; strain).	Intestinal obstruction, Crohn's disease, colitis, appendicitis, abdominal pain of unknown origin, ulcers. Pregnancy. Lactation (may cause diarrhea).	Mild abdominal discomfort, colic, cramps. Chronic use:: Potassium depletion, albuminuria, hematuria, disturbed heart function, muscle weakness, finger clubbing, and cachexia. Improperly aged bark can cause severe vomiting.	Use with caution, if at all in children less than 2 years old. Potassium loss increased with concomitant use of corticosteroids, licorice, or thiazides. May interfere with absorption of some drugs due to reduced transit time through the GI tract. Increases side effects of cardiac glycosides (e.g., digoxin).

Name(s)	Use(s)	Dose	Contraindications	Side Effects	Other Information
Cat's Claw	**PO::** Diverticulitis, peptic ulcers, colitis, gastritis, hemorrhoids, parasites, leaky bowel syndrome. With zidovudine (AZT) for HIV positive clients.	**Capsules, Tablets::** 500–1,000 mg 1 to 3 times per day. *Tea::* Simmer 1 gram of root bark in 150 mL boiling water for 5–10 min; strain. Consume tea 3 times per day.	Pregnancy, lactation.	Diarrhea (high doses), hypotension. May contribute to unusual bruising or bleeding gums.	Use with caution if taking antihypertensives. Get up slowly to avoid dizziness. Avoid confusing cat's claw with devil's claw.
Chamomile, German Chamomile	**PO::** Flatulence, travel sickness, nasal mucous membrane inflammation, nervous diarrhea, restlessness, GI spasms, GI inflammatory disease, menstrual cramps. **Topical::** Hemorrhoids, mastitis, leg ulcers; inflammation of skin, anogenital, and mucous membranes, including the mouth and gums.	**PO::** 2–8 grams of the dried flower heads 3 times per day or 1 cup of tea 3 to 4 times per day. Prepare tea by steeping 3 grams of dried flower heads in 150 mL boiling water for 5–10 min; strain. *Liquid extract (1::1 in 45% alcohol)::* 1–4 mL 3 times per day. **Topical::** Prepared tea (4 tsp. of dried flower heads in 1.5 cups boiling water for 15 min); strain. **Ointment/ Gel (both 3 to 10%)::** For external use only.	Pregnancy (may be a teratogen). Lactation.	Highly concentrated tea can cause vomiting. Allergic reactions, including contact dermatitis, severe hypersensitivity reactions, and anaphylaxis. Can be irritating if used near the eyes. May exacerbate asthma.	Cautious use in those with allergies to ragweed, asters, chrysanthemums, or other members of the Asteraceae family. Use with benzodiazepines and other CNS depressants may cause additive effects. May interfere with anticoagulant therapy. Do not confuse with Roman chamomile.
Chondrotin sulfate	**PO::** Osteoarthritis. Ischemic heart disease, osteoporosis, hyperlipidemia. **IM::** Osteoarthritis. **Topical::** Dry eyes, as a viscoelastic agent in cataract surgery, medium for preservation of corneas used for transplantation. With other agents for osteoarthritis.	**PO::** 200–400 mg 2 to 3 times per day or 1,200 mg as a single daily dose for osteoarthritis. **IM::** 50–100 mg/day in 1 or 2 daily injections. Injection not available in the US.	Pregnancy, lactation. Use in those with clotting disorders.	**PO::** Epigastric pain, nausea, diarrhea, constipation, eyelid edema, lower limb edema, alopecia, estrasystoles. Allergic reactions. **Ophthalmic use::** Intraocular hypertension, discomfort, corneal edema after cataract surgery.	Possible increased risk of bleeding when used with antiplatelet or anticoagulant drugs. No evidence that use of chondroitin sulfate with glucosamine sulfate has a greater beneficial effect than either product alone.

Name(s)	Use(s)	Dose	Contraindications	Side Effects	Other Information
Comfrey	**Topical::** Ulcers, wounds and fractures. Above ground parts used for bruises and sprains. Gargle for gum disease and pharyngitis. **PO::** Tea for ulcers, excessive menstrual flow, diarrhea, bloody urine, persistent cough, rheumatism, pleuritis, bronchitis, cancer, angina.	**Topical::** Ointments and other external products made with 5 to 20% comfrey. Daily use should not exceed 100 mcg of the pyrrolizidine alkaloids. Apply externally only on unbroken skin.	Use of above ground parts during pregnancy and lactation.	Acute veno-occlusive disease, including symptoms of anorexia, lethargy, and a dull, dragging ache in the right upper abdomen with marked abdominal distention (may also be reduced urine output).	Use for no more than 10 days; maximum use is 4 to 6 weeks/year. Unsafe when the root or above ground parts are used PO due to potential for acute or chronic liver toxicity. Teas contain lesser levels of alkaloids but regular use can lead to toxicity. Dietary products are not required to list the amount of product; thus, all products used PO should be considered potentially dangerous.
Cranberry	**PO::** Prevention and treatment of urinary tract infections. As a urinary deodorizer for incontinent persons. Berries are used in foods, including juices, jelly, and sauce.	**PO, juice::** 3 oz (33% pure cranberry) daily for preventing UTIs and 12–32 oz daily to treat UTIs. **Capsules::** 6/day of dried cranberry powder (equivalent to 3 oz) juice. Or, 300 to 400 mg concentrated juice capsules 2 times per day.	Avoid using amounts greater than consumed in food during pregnancy and lactation.	No side effects. Consuming more than 3–4 L/day can cause diarrhea and other GI symptoms.	Might increase absorption of dietary vitamin B_{12} in clients taking proton pump inhibitors. Do not confuse with highbush cranberry.
Dong quai	**PO::** Root used for menstrual cramps, irregularity, retarded flow, weakness during menses, and menopausal symptoms. Treatment of skin pigmentation and psoriasis.	**PO, women::** 3 to 4 grams/day in divided doses with meals. Sometimes prepared as a tea. Dose of the extract is 1 mL (20 to 40 drops) 3 times per day.	Pregnancy due to uterine stimulant and relaxant effects. Lactation.	Severe photosensitivity and photodermatitis. Potentially carcinogenic and mutagenic.	Increased risk of bleeding if used with antiplatelet drugs or warfarin.

Name(s)	Use(s)	Dose	Contraindications	Side Effects	Other Information
Echinacea	**PO::** Treat or prevent colds and other upper respiratory tract infections. Also as an antiseptic, antiviral immune stimulant, UTIs, peripheral vasodilator, yeast infections. **Topical::** Skin wounds, chronic skin ulcers, psoriasis, herpes simplex.	**PO, tablets::** 500 mg 3 times per day on day 1; then, 250 mg 4 times per day for up to 10 days. For prophylaxis, take for 3 consecutive weeks and then not take for one week. **Juice::** 6–9 mL/day of juice from fresh above the ground parts for a maximum of 8 weeks. **Topical::** A semi-solid product containing at least 15% pressed juice of Echinacea purpura above ground parts.	Pregnancy and lactation. Use with tuberculosis, leukosis, collagenosis, multiple sclerosis, collagen disorders or other progressive systemic diseases due to potential for stimulating the autoimmune response. Use with AIDS, HIV infection, autoimmune disorders.	Allergic reactions, including acute asthma, urticaria, angioedema, and anaphylaxis. Fever, N&V. High doses may reduce male and female fertility.	Individuals sensitive to ragweed, marigolds, daisies, chrysanthemums, and many other herbs are more likely to experience an allergic reaction to echinacea. Use with caution in those with renal disease or who are immunocompromised. May interfere with immunosuppressant therapy. Clients with atopy are more likely to experience an allergic reaction. Induces CYP3A4; thus carefully monitor those receiving echinacea and CYP3A4 (as well as CYP1A2) substrates with a narrow therapeutic index. May interact with certain prescription medications; such drug-herb interactions are especially dangerous in elderly clients.
Evening primrose oil	**PO::** Premenstrual syndrome, hot flashes, mastalgia, endometriosis. Also, atopic eczema, psoriasis, acne, rheumatoid arthritis, Raynaud's phenomenon, multiple sclerosis, and Sjögren's syndrome.	**PO::** 3–4 grams/day for mastalgia; 2–4 grams/day for PMS. From 0.54–2.8 grams/day for rheumatoid arthritis. From 6–8 grams/day for atopic eczema. Children take 2–4 grams/day.	Pregnancy.	Indigestion, nausea, headache, soft stools, Large doses can cause loose stools and abdominal pain. May increase risk for pregnancy complications.	May worsen temporal lobe epilepsy or schizophrenia if used with phenothiazines or tricyclic antidepressants.
Feverfew	**PO::** Fever, headache, migraines, menstrual irregularities, stomach ache, N&V. **Topical::** Antiseptic, insecticide, toothache.	**PO::** 2.5 leaves/day for migraine prophylaxis (with or without food). The dose of freeze-dried leaf is 50–125 mg/day with or without food.	Pregnancy, lactation, and in children less than 2 years of age.	Mouth ulceration, tongue irritation, inflammation (with chewed leaves), abdominal pain, indigestion, diarrhea, N&V, flatulence. Post-feverfew syndrome:: Nervousness, tension headaches, insomnia, joint pain or stiffness, tiredness. **Topical::** Allergic contact dermatitis.	Allergic reactions can occur in those sensitive to ragweed, crysanthemums, daisies, marigolds, and many other herbs. May increase effect of anticoagulant and antiplatelet drugs. May decrease effectiveness of NSAIDs.

Name(s)	Use(s)	Dose	Contraindications	Side Effects	Other Information
Garlic	**PO::** Decrease BP, prevent coronary heart disease, prevent age-related vascular changes and atherosclerosis, reduce reinfarction, and mortality rate post-MI. Treat earaches and menstrual disorders. **Topical::** Oil is used for tinea pedis, tinea corporis, tinea cruris, and onychomycosis.	**PO::** 600–900 mg per day in 3 divided doses for hyperlipidemia and hypertension. Some use fresh garlic (1 clove or 4 grams/day). **Topical::** 0.4% cream and 0.6% gel for tinea infections.	PO use of large amounts during pregnancy and lactation (data vary). Topical use of large amounts.	Breath odor, mouth and GI burning or irritation, heartburn, flatulence, N&V, diarrhea. Possible changes in intestinal flora. Dermatitis when fresh garlic used topically.	Increased effects when used with warfarin (INR). Possible increased effects when used with aspirin, clopidogrel, enoxaparin, and others. Possible increased effects and toxicity when used with insulin or oral hypoglycemics. Can prolong bleeding time; discontinue 1–2 weeks before surgery. May interact with certain prescription medications; such drug-herb interactions are especially dangerous in elderly clients.
Ginger (African, Black, Cochin, Jamaica, Race)	**PO::** Motion sickness, colic, dyspepsia, flatulence, rheumatoid arthritis, post-surgical N&V, anorexa, URTI, cough, bronchitis. As a flavoring agent in foods/beverages. **Topical::** Juice used for thermal burns.	**PO::** 0.25–1 gram 3 times per day or 1 cup of tea (0.5–1 gram in 150 mL boiling water 5–10 min; strain) 3 times per day. Maximum daily dose:: 4 grams. For morning sickness:: 250 mg 4 times per day. Prevent post-operative N&V:: 1 gram powdered root 1 hr before induction of anesthesia. Antiemetic:: 2 grams freshly powdered root with water.	Use in those with gallstones until after medical evaluation.	Dermatitis in sensitive persons. CNS depression, cardiac arrhythmias, or hypoglycemia after high doses.	Use with herbs that have coumarin constituents or affect platelet aggregation thoretically increase the risk of bleeding. May enhance effect of barbiturates. May interfere with BP drug therapy or with diabetes therapy. May prevent cyclophosphamide-induced vomiting.

Name(s)	Use(s)	Dose	Contraindications	Side Effects	Other Information
Ginkgo biloba	*Leaf extract::* **PO::** Dementia syndromes or cerebral vascular insufficiency (memory loss, vertigo, dizziness, difficulty concentrating, mood disturbances, hearing disorders). Intermittent claudication. Reverse sexual dysfunction due to SSRI depressants. Cognitive disorders, attention deficit-hyperactivity disorder, premenstrual syndrome. Prevent acute mountain sickness. Various CV problems **Topical::** Wound dressings.	**PO::** Dementia syndromes or claudication:: 120–240 mg/day in 2 or 3 divided doses. Reverse sexual dysfunction due to SSRI's:: 60 mg 2 times per day, up to 240 mg 2 times per day. For vertigo or tinnitus disorders:: 120–160 mg/day in 2 or 3 divided doses. Prevent altitude sickness:: 160 mg 2 times per day.	Use in couples wishing to become pregnant.	Mild GI complaints, headache, dizziness, palpitations, allergic skin reactions. Large doses:: N&V, restlessness, diarrhea, weakness, lack of muscle tone. Bleeding disorders (rare). Possible seizures. Gingko pollen is strongly allergenic.	Increased risk of bleeding if used with anticoagulants or antiplatelet drugs. May increase BP if used with thiazide diuretics. May prevent cyclosporine-induced nephrotoxicity; however, may also increase bioavailability, AUC, and peak cyclosporine levels. Increased risk of bleeding if used with herbs that have coumarin constituents or affect platelet aggregation. Cross-reactivity possible with gingko fruit in those allergic to poison ivy, poison oak, poison sumac, mango rind, or cashew shell oil. May also interact with alprazolam, aspirin, haloperidol, ibuprofen, nifedipine, omeprazole, and trazodone. May interact with certain prescription medications; such drug-herb interactions are especially dangerous in elderly clients.
Ginseng, panaz	**PO::** General tonic to improve well-being and to stimulate immune function. To improve physical or athletic stamina, cognitive function, concentration, and work efficiency. To soothe irritated or inflamed tissues, as a diuretic, and an antidepressant. Improve psychological function in post-menopausal women.	**PO::** *Cut or powdered root::* 0.6–3 grams 1–3 times per day or 1 cup tea (3 grams of root in 150 mL of boiling water for 10–15 min or 1 ginseng tea bag usually containing 1,500 mg of the root) 1–3 times per day for 3–4 weeks. *Capsules::* 200–600 mg/day. Usual length of ingestion:: 3 weeks to 3 months. A panax-free period of 2 weeks is recommended between consecutive courses.	Use in cases of hemorrhage or thrombosis.	Insomnia, mastalgia, vaginal bleeding, tachycardia, mania, cerebral arteritis, Stevens-Johnson syndrome, edema, amenorrhea, decreased appetite, hyperpyrexia, pruritus, rose spots, hypotension, headache, vertigo, palpitations, euphoria, neonatal death. Diarrhea and allergic skin reactions after high doses. May prolong aPTT or PT. May reduce INR and PT in those treated with warfarin.	Use with herbs that affect platelet aggregation may increase the risk of bleeding. May interfere with effect of antipsychotic drugs. If used with digoxin, synergistic effects possible. No evidence of improved insulin sensitivity or beta–cell function in humans. May interfere with MAOI therapy. May potentiate the effects of stimulants, including caffeine in tea/coffee. Use with caution in cardiac disorders. Increased risk of hypoglycemia in diabetics. May interact with certain prescription medications; such drug-herb interactions are especially dangerous in elderly clients.

Name(s)	Use(s)	Dose	Contraindications	Side Effects	Other Information
Goldenseal	**PO::** Urinary tract infections, inflammation of vaginal and ureteral mucous membranes, hemorrhoids, gastritis, anorexia, peptic ulcers, colitis, postpartum hemorrhage, menorrhagia, dysmenorrhea, internal hemorrhage. **Topical::** Eczema, itching, acne, dandruff, ringworm, wounds.	**PO::** *Dried root or rhizome::* 0.5–1 gram 3 times per day. Prepare tea:: Simmer 0.5–1 gram in 150 mL boiling water for 5–10 min; strain. *Liquid extract::* 0.3–1 mL 3 times per day. *Tincture::* 2–4 mL 3 times per day **Topical::** Use as mouthwash 3–4 times per day; prepare by steeping 6 grams of dried herb in 150 mL boiling water for 5–10 min; strain and cool.	Use in infectious or inflammatory GI conditions and in newborns.	Prolonged PO use:: Digestive disorders, constipation, excitation, delirium (rare), hallucinations. Fresh plant may cause mucosal irritation. Use during pregnancy, lactation, or in newborns may cause kernicteris (may be fatal). Prolonged use:: Decrease B vitamin absorption. Increased bilirubin levels.	Enhanced therapeutic and adverse effects if used with herbs with sedative effects. May interfere with antacids, sucralfate, H_2 antagonists, and proton-pump inhibitors. May inhibit anticoagulant effects of heparin. Berberine in the herb may displace highly protein-bound drugs.
Grape seed extract (Muskat)	**PO::** Venous insufficiency, varicose veins, atherosclerosis, peripheral vascular disease, edema associated with injury or surgery, MI, cerebral infarction.	**PO::** *Extract as capsules/tablets::* 75–300 mg/day for 3 weeks; then, maintenance dose of 40–80 mg/day. For chronic venous insufficiency:: Extract procyanidin doses of 150–300 mg/day.	Pregnancy, lactation (avoid amounts greater than in food).	None reported.	May increase the effect of warfarin and the risk of bleeding.

Name(s)	Use(s)	Dose	Contraindications	Side Effects	Other Information
Green tea	**PO::** Stomach disorders, vomiting, diarrhea, headaches, diuretic, improve cognitive performance, Crohn's disease. Reduce risk of prostate cancer and colon cancer. Protect against heart disease, prevent kidney stones and dental caries. **Topical::** Wash to soothe sunburn, poultice for bags under the eyes, as a compress for headache or tired eyes, stop bleeding in tooth sockets.	**PO::** No reliable information; ranges between 1–10 cups daily. **Topical::** No typical dosage.	Use in infants, lactation. Use in those with gastric/duodenal ulcers.	GI upset and constipation. High doses:: Side effects due to caffeine (the active constituent). May induce cardiac arrhythmias in sensitive individuals.	Increased CNS stimulation when used with caffeine-containing products or ephedrine. Many possible drug interactions, including warfarin. Grapefruit juice can increase caffeine levels and increase risk of side effects. Milk may bind the antioxidants in tea and reduce beneficial effects. Possible prolonged bleeding time.
Hawthorn fruit, flower	**PO, Leaf::** Coronary circulation problems, improve perfusion of myocardium, chronic arrhythmias, hypotension. **Flower::** Improve heart function, coronary insufficiency, angina, cardiac neurasthenia, arrhythmias, cardiac asthma, sedation. **Topical, Leaf::** Poultice for boils, sores, ulcers.	Leaf used as a water extract, a water-alcohol extract, wine tea, and fresh juice. Dosage not available.	Use with cardiac glycoside-containing products (increased risk of toxicity). Pregnancy.	Nausea, GI complaints, fatigue, rash on hands, sweating, palpitations, headache, dizziness, sleeplessness, agitation, circulatory disturbances.	Additive effects when used with vasodilators or CNS depressants. May potentiate effects of digoxin (may need to decrease dose). May potentiate or interfere with conventional cardiovascular drug therapy. May interact with certain prescription medications; such drug-herb interactions are especially dangerous in elderly clients.
Kava	**PO::** Anxiety disorders, stress, insomnia, restlessness, epilepsy, psychosis, depression.	**PO::** *Extract::* 100 mg (70 mg kava-lactones) 3 times per day. For nervous anxiety, stress, restlessness:: 60–120 mg kava-lactones/day. *Tea::* 1 cup up to 3 times per day. To prepare tea:: Simmer 2–4 grams of the root in 150 mL boiling water for 5–10 min; strain.	Endogenous depression. Lactation.	**After PO::** GI complaints, headache, dizziness, enlarged pupils, disturbances of oculomotor equilibrium and accommodation, allergic skin reactions (rare). Mouth numbness if chewed. Drowsiness and impaired motor reflexes may affect ability to drive or operate machinery.	Possible additive effects if used with CNS depressants, including alcohol. Do not use more than 3 months without medical advice.

Name(s)	Use(s)	Dose	Contraindications	Side Effects	Other Information
Licorice (Glycyrrhiza, Licorice root)	**PO::** Inflammation of upper respiratory tract mucous membranes. Gastric and duodenal ulcers, bronchitis, chronic gastritis, colic, primary adrenocortical insufficiency, dry cough, arthritis, lupus, cholestatic liver disorders, hyperkalemia, hypotonia.	**PO::** *Powdered root::* 1–4 grams. *Tea::* 1 cup 3 times per day. To prepare tea:: Simmer 1–4 grams of powdered root in 150 mL boiling water for 5–10 min; strain.	Pregnancy, lactation. Use in diabetes, CHF, hypertension, cholestatic liver disorders, liver cirrhosis, hypokalemia, severe renal insufficiency, hypersensitivity to licorice.	Amenorrhea. High doses or chronic use:: Pseudoaldosteronism (hypertension, lethargy, headache, sodium/water retention, edema). Decrease serum testosterone and increase 17-hydroxyprogesterone:: May cause decreased libido and sexual dysfunction in men. Hypokalemia.	Increased risk of cardiac toxicity due to potassium depletion. Increased risk of bleeding if used with anticoagulants or antiplatelet drugs. Grapefruit juice may enhance mineralocorticoid activity. Increased potassium loss if used with thiazides. May interact with certain prescription medications; such drug-herb interactions are especially dangerous in elderly clients.
Melatonin	**PO::** Insomnia, especially to treat jet lag, sleep disorders, shift-work disorder. Many other uses.	**PO::** 0.3–5 mg at bedtime. For jet lag:: 5 mg at bedtime for one week beginning 3 days before the flight.	Pregnancy, lactation. Use with immunosuppressive drug therapy.	Headache, transient depressive symptoms, daytime fatigue, drowsiness, dizziness, abdominal cramps, reduced alterness, irritability. Worsen dysphoria in depressed clients.	Additive effects if used with CNS depressants. Do not drive or use machinery for 4–5 hr after taking melatonin. Use with caution in children.
Milk thistle (Lady's Thistle)	**PO::** *Fruit/Seeds::* Dyspeptic complaints, liver protectant, treat toxic liver damage due to chemicals, amanita mushroom poisoning, hepatic cirrhosis, chronic inflammatory liver disease, chronic hepatitis. *Above ground parts::* Treat and stimulate dysfunction of the liver and gallbladder. Jaundice, pleurisy, spleen diseases.	**PO::** *Fruit/Seeds::* 200–400 mg/day calculated as silibinin. Or, 12–15 grams of the dried fruit or seeds/day. *Above ground parts::* 1 cup of tea 2–3 times per day. Prepare tea by steeping 1/2 tsp. of the above grounds parts in 150 mL boiling water for 5–10 min; strain.	All parts of the plant during pregnancy and lactation.	*Fruit/Seeds::* Laxative effect. Mild allergic reactions.	All parts of the plant can cause an allergic reaction in those sensitive to ragweed, chrysanthemums, marigolds, daisies, and other herbs. May prevent liver damage due to cisplatin. Chemicals causing liver damage that may be treated with the herb include butyrophenones, phenytoin, phenothiazines, alcohol, acetaminophen, and halothane.

Name(s)	Use(s)	Dose	Contraindications	Side Effects	Other Information
Saw palmetto	**PO::** Benign prostatic hypertrophy. Mild diuretic, sedative, antiseptic, anti-inflammatory.	**PO::** For BPH:: 1–2 grams of whole berries or 320 mg of a lipophilic extract. Antiseptic, 1.5 mL. Tea:: 0.5–1 gram dried berry in 150 mL boiling water for 5–10 min; strain. Tea may not have sufficient levels of active ingredients.	Pregnancy, lactation.	Headache, stomach problems (rare), nausea, dizziness.	May interfere with oral contraceptive or hormone therapy. No significant effect on serum prostate-specific antigen (PSA) levels. Due to lack of proven efficacy, the FDA has banned all OTC products to treat BPH. May interact with certain prescription medications; such drug-herb interactions are especially dangerous in elderly clients.
Senna	**PO::** *Leaf, fruit::* Laxative for constipation, hemorrhoids, after anorectal surgery, to evacuate the GI tract to facilitate diagnostic tests.	**PO::** 15–30 mg hydroxyanthracene derivatives/day calculated as sennoside B. *Tea::* 1 cup in the a.m. or p.m. To make tea:: Steep 0.5–2 grams finely chopped leaf in warm, but not boiling water, for 10 min; strain. A cold water tea may have fewer GI side effects. To make a cold water tea:: Steep 0.5–2 grams finely chopped leaf in cold water for 10–12 hr; strain. *Liquid leaf extract::* 0.5–2 mL (frequency not specified).	Pregnancy, lactation. Use in those with abdominal pain, intestinal obstruction, acute intestinal inflammation, including Crohn's disease, ulcerative colitis, appendicitis, stomach inflammation, anal prolapse, hemorrhoids, undiagnosed abdominal pain. Use in those with dehydration, diarrhea, or loose stools.	Abdominal discomfort, colic, cramps. Chronic use:: Potassium deficiency, albuminuria, hematuria, "sluggish" colon, laxative-dependency syndrome. Possible senna-tea induced hepatitis (rare).	Loss of potassium may potentiate effect of cardiac glycosides, diuretics, and corticosteroids on heart function. Use with other stimulant laxatives increases the risk of potassium depletion.

Name(s)	Use(s)	Dose	Contraindications	Side Effects	Other Information
St. John's wort	**PO::** Depression, dysthymic disorder. Secondary symptoms due to depression, including fatigue, loss of appetite, insomnia, anxiety. OCD, migraine headache, neuralgia, diuretic, vitiligo, cancer. **Topical::** Treat bruises, abrasions, muscle pain, first degree burns, hemorrhoids, anti-inflammatory.	**PO::** For depression:: 300 mg 3 times per day of extract standardized to 0.3% hypericin. OCD:: 450 mg twice a day of extract standardized to 0.3% hypericin. *Crude drug::* 2–4 grams of above ground parts/day. *Liquid extract::* 2–4 mL/day. *Tincture::* 2–4 mL/day.	Pregnancy, lactation. Use with MAOIs, SSRIs, and tricyclic antidepressants due to potentiation of effects.	Insomnia, vivid dreams, anxiety, agitation, irritability, GI discomfort, fatigue, dry mouth, dizziness, N˘CC PT/INR in clients treated with warfarin, headache, delayed hypersensitivity, paresthesias. Also, hypomania or mania in depressed clients. Photosensitivity. Possible withdrawal symptoms similar to those seen with other antidepressants.	Questionable efficacy in treating depression. Large number of potential drug interactions (amtriptyline, atorvastatin, cyclosporine, fexofenadine, digoxin, midazolam, nifedipine, simvastatin, tacrolimus). Large doses with tyramine-containing foods may cause a hypertensive crisis. Can decrease results if used with warfarin. May cause breakthrough bleeding and irregular menstrual bleeding if used with oral contraceptives. Induces CYP3A4; ↓ serum imatinib levels. May interact with certain prescription medications; such drug-herb interactions are especially dangerous in elderly clients.
Valerian	**PO::** Insomnia, anxiety, stress, depression, epilepsy.	**PO::** 1 cup of tea several times per day. To prepare:: Steep 2–3 grams of the root in 150 mL boiling water for 5–10 min; strain. Maximum dose of root/day:: 15 grams. *Tincture::* 1–3 mL once to several times per day. *Extract::* 400–900 mg up to 2 hr before bedtime for up to 14 days.	Pregnancy, lactation.	Headache, excitability, cardiac disturbances, insomnia, uneasiness. Morning drowsiness; possible impaired alertness and information processing.	Warn clients not to drive or operate machinery after taking valerian. Additive effect when taken with other CNS depressants, including alcohol. Do not confuse with Valium.

Name(s)	Use(s)	Dose	Contraindications	Side Effects	Other Information
Yohimbe	**PO::** Impotence, aphrodisiac, exhaustion, angina, hypertension, diabetic neuropathy, postural hypotension.	Available in 5.4 mg tablets as a prescription drug with no FDA approval. Products are labeled with a standardized 15 mg yohimbine content.	Pregnancy, lactation. Use in angina, BPH, diabetes, depression, hypertension, hypotension, kidney or liver disease, prostate inflammation. Use with alpha-2 adrenergic blockers or phenothiazines due to possible increased alpha-adrenergic blockade.	Excitation, tremor, insomnia, anxiety, hypertension, tachycardia, N&V, salivation, irritability, fluid retention, Psychosis in people predisposed to it.	Use with caffeine, ephedra, MAOIs, sympathomimetics, tyramine-containing foods, or vasopressors may cause a hypertensive crisis. May interfere with antihypertensive drugs or antidiabetics. May interact with certain prescription medications; such drug-herb interactions are especially dangerous in elderly clients.

Herbs are regulated as Dietary Supplements under the Dietary Supplement Health and Education Act of 1994 (DSHEA). The WHO collaborates with member states to promote the safe use of traditional medicine in health care. More than 100 countries have established regulations for herbal medicines. Counterfeit, poor quality, or adulterated herbal products in the international market pose serious client safety threats. Depending on the country, a single herbal product could be defined as either a food, a dietary supplement, or an herbal medicine. There are no national standards, policies, or regulations that currently control this market.

Always ask about herbs, vitamins, teas or other remedies that the client may be using for a problem or to maintain health/wellness. Clients generally do not consider these significant or as medicines and often fail to mention them during a drug history. Many of these have the potential to interact or interfere with traditional drug therapies prescribed by the provider. Thus the importance of doing a careful drug history documenting all OTC therapies consumed (medication reconciliation). Herbals are not regulated by the FDA; they do not test or authorize any supplement. These may contain a variety of agents and some have been found not to contain any of the agent it portrays. Natural does not mean that it is safe.

Agents approved by the APhA (American Pharmacists Association) or U.S.P. which indicates the manufacturer followed standards established by the U.S. Pharmacopoeia should be those that the consumer purchases to ensure some degree of product reliability.

HISTAMINE H_2 ANTAGONISTS

SEE ALSO THE FOLLOWING INDIVIDUAL ENTRIES:

Cimetidine
Famotidine
Nizatidine
Ranitidine hydrochloride

INDICATIONS/USES

See individual drugs. Uses include: **Rx.** (1) Short-term treatment of benign gastric ulcer. Maintenance therapy after healing of acute ulcer (ranitidine). (2) Short-term treatment of active duodenal ulcer and maintenance therapy after the healing of the active ulcer. (3) GERD, including erosive or ulcerative disease diagnosed by endoscopy. (4) Prevention of upper GI bleeding in critically ill clients (IV cimetidine only). (5) Pathological hypersecretory conditions (except nizatidine), including Zollinger-Ellison syndrome, systemic mastocytosis, multiple endocrine adenomas. (6) As part of combination therapy to treat *Helicobacter pylori*- associated duodenal ulcer and maintenance therapy after healing of the active ulcer. (7) Prevent aspiration pneumonitis. (8) IV to prevent paclitaxel hypersensitivity (except nizatidine). (9) Prevent stress ulcers. (10) IV to reduce incidence of GI hemorrhage associated with stress-related ulcers (except nizatidine). (11) Suppress gastric acid secretion perioperatively. (12) In combination with histamine H_1 antagonists to treat certain types of urticaria.

OTC. (1) Relief of heartburn associated with acid indigestion and sour stomach. (2) Prevention of heartburn associated with acid indigestion and sour stomach due to certain foods and beverages.

ACTION/KINETICS

Action

Histamine H_2 antagonists are competitive blockers of histamine. As such they inhibit all phases of gastric acid secretion including that caused by histamine, gastrin, and muscarinic agents. Both fasting and nocturnal acid secretion are inhibited. In addition, the volume and hydrogen ion concentration of gastric juice are decreased. These drugs provide rapid symptomatic relief and accelerate ulcer healing when used with antibiotics for *Helicobacter pylori.* Cimetidine, famotidine, and ranitidine have no effect on gastric emptying; cimetidine and famotidine have no effect on lower esophageal pressure. Fasting or postprandial serum gastrin is not affected by famotidine, nizatidine, or ranitidine. Cimetidine is known to affect the cytochrome P450 drug metabolizing system for other drugs. Ranitidine also affects the P450 enzyme system, but its effect on elimination of other drugs is not significant. Famotidine and nizatidine do not affect the P450 enzyme system.

CONTRAINDICATIONS

Hypersensitivity. Use of cimetidine, famotidine, and nizatidine during lactation.

SPECIAL CONCERNS

- **Use with caution in impaired hepatic and renal function.**

Classifications

- Symptomatic response to these drugs does not preclude gastric malignancy.
- Elderly blacks have a greater risk of cognitive impairment if they have used these drugs for 2 or more years.
- Use ranitidine with caution during lactation.
- Safety and efficacy not established in children. Do not use cimetidine in children less than 16 years of age unless benefits outweigh risks.
- Is an increased risk of hip fractures especially with higher doses and long duration of use.

SIDE EFFECTS

The following side effects are common to all or most of the H_2-histamine antagonists. See individual drugs for complete listing. **GI:** N&V, abdominal discomfort, diarrhea, constipation, hepatocellular effects. **CNS:** Headache, fatigue, somnolence, dizziness, confusion, hallucinations, insomnia. **Dermatologic:** Rash, urticaria, pruritus, alopecia (rare), erythema multiforme (rare). **Hematologic:** Rarely, thrombocytopenia, agranulocytosis, granulocytopenia. **Other:** Gynecomastia, impotence, loss of libido, arthralgia, bronchospasm, transient pain at injection site, cardiac arrhythmias following rapid IV use (rare), arthralgia (rare), hypersensitivity reactions (bronchospasm, rash, eosinophilia, ***laryngeal edema, rarely anaphylaxis***).

OVERDOSE MANAGEMENT

Symptoms: No experience is available for deliberate overdose.

Treatment: Induce vomiting or perform gastric lavage to remove any unabsorbed drug. Monitor the client and undertake supportive therapy.

DRUG INTERACTIONS

See individual drugs.

Cephalosporins / Possible ↓ availability of certain cephalosporins (e.g., cefpodoxime, cefuroxime, cephalexin)

Ethanol / Possible ↑ ethanol plasma levels

Itraconazole / ↓ Itraconazole plasma levels due to changes in gastric pH

Ketoconazole / ↑ Gastric pH may inhibit ketoconazole absorption.

DOSAGE

See individual drugs.

NURSING IMPLICATIONS

IMPLEMENTATION/ADMINISTRATION/STORAGE

Dosage may need to be reduced in impaired renal function.

ASSESSMENT

1. Note onset, duration, intensity, other associated S&S, and previous treatments. Assess frequency of reflux occurrences. Chronic treatment usually initiated after two to three recurrences.
2. Perform CNS assessment noting level of orientation and monitor.
3. Check results of radiographic/endoscopic procedures; document *H. pylori* results and if/when treated.
4. For those unresponsive to maximum lifestyle and medical therapy evaluate if candidate for Implant to treat GERD (LINX Reflux Management System).
5. Monitor CBC, renal and LFTs; reduce dose with renal dysfunction. Determine gastric pH; maintain >5.

CLIENT/FAMILY TEACHING

1. May take without regard to meals; food prolongs drug effect and may help ↓ nausea, diarrhea and/or abdominal pain. Stagger doses of antacids, i.e., 1 hr before or 1 hr after cimetidine or ranitidine. Take as prescribed; do not stop if pain subsides or if "feeling better" as drug is necessary to inhibit gastric acid secretion so ulcer can heal.
2. Do not chew, break or crush SR tabs. If unable to swallow may open and sprinkle on applesauce or yogurt but must be swallowed immediately.
3. These agents reduce the secretion of gastric acid and are usually prescribed for 4–8 weeks initially to control symptoms and promote ulcer healing.
4. Avoid activities that require mental alertness until drug effects realized. Report any confusion or disorientation immediately. Any blood-tinged emesis or dark tarry stools as well as dizziness or rash, bruising, fatigue, and malaise, require immediate reporting. Avoid alcohol, caffeine, aspirin-containing products (cough and cold products), and foods that may cause GI irritation, i.e., harsh spices, black pepper.

Classifications

5. Do not take maximum dose of OTC products for more than 2 weeks without medical supervision. Prolonged use may contribute to depletion of intrinsic factor, necessary for vitamin B_{12} absorption especially in those >50 y.o.
6. Stop 24–72 hr before skin testing begins; may cause false negative response in tests with allergen extracts. May cause painful swelling of breast tissue and impotence, report as these are reversible.
7. Smoking may interfere with drug's action. Stop smoking and do not smoke after last dose of day.
8. Review GERD instructions, i.e., ↑ HOB, avoid lying down for at least 2 hr after eating, and dietary restrictions.
9. Report for all scheduled follow-up studies; a response to these agents does not preclude gastric malignancy.
10. Keep all F/U to assess response, labs, and for adverse SE.

OUTCOMES/EVALUATE

- Duodenal ulcer healing
- ↓ Gastric irritation/bleeding
- ↓ Abdominal pain/discomfort
- Gastric pH >5

LAXATIVES

SEE ALSO THE FOLLOWING INDIVIDUAL ENTRIES:

Docusate calcium
Docusate sodium
Psyllium hydrophilic muciloid

INDICATIONS/USES

See individual agents. (1) Short-term treatment of constipation. (2) Prophylaxis in clients who should not strain during defecation, i.e., following anorectal surgery or after MI (use fecal softeners or lubricant laxatives). (3) Evacuate the colon for rectal and bowel examinations (certain lubricant, saline, and stimulant laxatives). (4) In conjunction with surgery. (5) With anthelmintic therapy. (6) With chronic opioid therapy. *NOTE:* The underlying cause of constipation should be determined since a marked change in bowel habits may be a symptom of a pathologic condition.

ACTION/KINETICS

Action

Laxatives act locally, either by stimulating the smooth muscles of the bowel or by changing the bulk or consistency of the stools. Laxatives can be divided into seven categories.

1. *Stimulant laxatives:* Substances that directly stimulate the smooth muscles of the bowel to increase contractions. Also alter water and electrolyte secretion. Examples: Bisacodyl, cascara, casanthranol, and senna.
2. *Saline laxatives:* Substances that cause water retention, and therefore, increased intraluminal pressure of the intestine. Also cause cholecystokinin release. Examples: Magnesium salts and sodium phosphates.
3. *Bulk-forming laxatives:* Nondigestible substances that increase the bulk of the stools, thereby stimulating peristalsis; they form an emollient gel. Examples: Methylcellulose, polycarbophil, and psyllium.
4. *Emollient:* Agents that soften hardened feces and facilitate their passage through the lower intestine. Examples: Mineral oil.
5. *Fecal softener:* Facilitates admixture of fat and water to soften the stool. Example: Docusate.
6. *Hyperosmotic:* Glycerin causes local irritation and has a hyperosmotic action. Lactulose has an osmotic effect causing fluid retention in the colon, lowering the pH and increasing colonic peristalsis.
7. *Miscellaneous:* Castor oil has a direct action on the intestinal mucosa or nerve plexus; it alters water and electrolyte secretion.

CONTRAINDICATIONS

Severe abdominal pain or N&V that *might* be caused by appendicitis, enteritis, ulcerative colitis, diverticulitis, intestinal obstruction, fecal impaction, undiagnosed abdominal pain. Laxative use in these conditions may cause rupture of the abdomen or intestinal hemorrhage. Undiagnosed abdominal pain. Children under the age of 2.

SIDE EFFECTS

GI: Excess activity of the colon resulting in nausea, diarrhea, griping, or vomiting. Perianal irritation, bloating, flatulence. **Electrolyte balance:** Dehydration, disturbance of the electrolyte balance. **Miscellaneous:** Dizziness, fainting, weakness, sweating, palpitations.

Bulk laxatives: Obstruction in the esophagus, stomach, small intestine, or rectum.

Stimulant laxatives: Chronic abuse may lead to malfunctioning colon.

Mineral oil: Large doses may cause anal seepage resulting in itching, irritation, hemorrhoids, and perianal discomfort.

Chronic use of laxatives may cause laxative dependency and result in chronic constipation and other intestinal disorders because the client may start to depend on the psychologic effect and physical stimulus of the drug rather than on the body's own natural reflexes.

DRUG INTERACTIONS

Anticoagulants, oral / ↓ Absorption of vitamin K from GI tract induced by laxatives may ↑ effects of anticoagulants and result in bleeding
Digitalis / Cathartics may ↓ absorption of digitalis
Tetracyclines / Laxatives containing aluminum, Ca^{++}, or Mg^{++} may ↓ effect of tetracyclines R/T ↓ GI tract absorption

DOSAGE

See individual drugs.

NURSING IMPLICATIONS

IMPLEMENTATION/ADMINISTRATION/STORAGE

1. When administering a laxative, note the length of time it takes for the laxative to take effect and give it so that the result of the laxative will not interfere with the client's rest or digestion and absorption of nutrients.
2. Administer liquid laxatives at an agreeable temperature.
3. If laxative is administered in a liquid, select one palatable to client.
4. If ordered to prepare for a diagnostic exam, check directions carefully to ensure accurate administration.

ASSESSMENT

1. Note reasons for therapy, length of use and underlying causes; identify type/category taking and effectiveness. Determine stool characteristics and frequency. Client's definition of constipation may determine if, in fact, constipation exists.
2. With abdominal pain and discomfort, note location, triggers, and type of discomfort. Palpate for abnormalities and review patterns of elimination. R/O other intestinal disorders/obstruction where laxatives should not be used.
3. Note age, state of health, activity level, and general nutritional status. Identify recent lifestyle changes that may contribute to problem. Note any special restriction or limitation due to illness; may include fluid/sodium restrictions.
4. List other drugs that may contribute to constipation (i.e., diuretics, anticholinergics, antihistamines, antidepressants, narcotic analgesics, iron products, and some antihypertensive agents, especially verapamil).

CLIENT/FAMILY TEACHING

1. Take only as directed. Have a regular schedule for defecation; keep record of bowel function and response to all laxatives taken. Laxatives reduce the amount of time other drugs remain in the intestine and may diminish effectiveness.
2. If taken as preparation for a diagnostic study, review instructions. If unable to read, find someone to review directions to ensure an accurate test.
3. Review techniques that facilitate elimination; sitting with legs slightly elevated and leaning forward to increase abdominal pressure often encourages elimination. If ill at home, consider a commode at the bedside. This will promote better bowel function by encouraging client to move about and ensure privacy.
4. Bowel tone will be lost with long-term use of laxatives; reinforce that bowel movements do not have to occur daily. Use diet to achieve same purpose; two or three prunes a day are preferable to laxatives. Frequent use of any type of enemas may cause damage to the rectum and small bowel as well as inhibit bowel tone and may cause electrolyte abnormalities.
5. Review importance of diet high in fiber foods (and juices such as prune) and daily exercise in maintaining proper bowel function. Include bulk foods and sufficient fluids in diet to enhance elimination. Increase water consumption at least 6–8 8 oz glasses per day. Consult dietitian for assistance in meal planning/preparation and food selections.
6. If pregnant, consult with provider before taking any laxatives to treat constipation. Nursing mothers should avoid laxatives unless prescribed as many are excreted in breast milk and can cause infant diarrhea.

7. **Daily exercise will enhance regular elimination.**
8. **Report N&V, abdominal pain or if constipation persists because there could be a physiologic problem that requires attention.**
9. **Keep all F/U to assess response and for adverse SE.**

OUTCOMES/EVALUATE

- Relief of constipation; evacuation of a soft, formed stool
- Effective colon preparation for diagnostic procedures (no stool in bowel)

NARCOTIC ANALGESICS

SEE ALSO THE FOLLOWING INDIVIDUAL ENTRIES:

Alfentanil hydrochloride
Buprenorphine hydrochloride
Butorphanol tartrate
Codeine sulfate
Fentanyl citrate
Fentanyl transdermal system
Hydrocodone bitartrate and Acetaminophen
Hydromorphone hydrochloride
Meperidine hydrochloride
Methadone hydrochloride
Morphine sulfate
Oxycodone hydrochloride
Oxycodone hydrochloride and Acetaminophen
Remifentanil hydrochloride
Tapentadol hydrochloride
Tramadol hydrochloride
Tramadol hydrochloride and Acetaminophen

INDICATIONS/USES

See individual drugs. Uses include: (1) Treat pain due to various causes (e.g., MI, carcinoma, surgery, burns, postpartum). (2) Preanesthetic medication. (3) Adjunct to anesthesia. (4) Acute vascular occlusion. (5) Diarrhea. (6) Antitussive.

ACTION/KINETICS

Action

Narcotic analgesics are classified as agonists, mixed agonist-antagonists, or partial agonists depending on their activity at opiate receptors. The narcotic analgesics attach to specific receptors located in the CNS (cortex, brain stem, and spinal cord) resulting in various CNS effects. The mechanism is believed to involve decreased permeability of the cell membrane to sodium, which results in diminished transmission of pain impulses. Five categories of opioid receptors have been identified: mu, kappa, sigma, delta, and epsilon. Narcotic analgesics are believed to exert their activity at mu, kappa, and sigma receptors. Mu receptors are thought to mediate supraspinal analgesia, euphoria, and respiratory and physical depression. Pentazocine-like spinal analgesia, miosis, and sedation are mediated by kappa receptors while sigma receptors mediate dysphoria and hallucinations, as well as respiratory and vasomotor stimulation (caused by drugs with antagonist activity). In addition to an alteration of pain perception (analgesia), the drugs, especially at higher doses, induce euphoria, drowsiness, changes in mood, mental clouding, and deep sleep.

The narcotic analgesics also produce a large number of secondary pharmacologic effects. These include: (1) Depressed tidal volume and respiratory rate due to decreased sensitivity of the respiratory center to carbon dioxide. Death by overdosage is almost always the result of respiratory arrest. (2) Nausea and emesis due to direct stimulation of the CTZ. (3) Depression of the cough reflex by a direct effect on the medullary cough center. (4) Orthostatic hypotension and fainting due to peripheral vasodilation (when client stands), reduced peripheral resistance, and inhibition of baroreceptors. Little effect on BP when the client is in a supine position. (5) Pruritus, flushing, and red eyes due to histamine release. (6) Decrease in gastric motility leading to prolonged gastric emptying time and possible esophageal reflux. (7) In the small intestine decrease in biliary, pancreatic, and intestinal secretions causing delays in digestion of food. Increase in resting tone and periodic spasms occur. (8) Decreased propulsive peristalsis in the large intestine with an increase in tone to spasm. Causes severe constipation. (9) Constriction of the sphincter of Oddi causing epigastric distress or biliary colic. (10) Increased smooth muscle tone in the urinary tract can cause spasms with urinary urgency and difficulty with urination. (11) Pupillary constriction caused by certain narcotic analgesics is a sign of use/dependence. See also individual agents.

CONTRAINDICATIONS

Asthma, emphysema, kyphoscoliosis, severe obesity, convulsive states as in epilepsy, delirium tremens, tetanus and strychnine poisoning, diabetic acidosis, myxedema, Addison's disease, hepatic cirrhosis, and children under 6 months.

SPECIAL CONCERNS

- **Use with caution in clients with head injury or after head surgery because of morphine's capacity to elevate ICP and mask the pupillary response.**
- **Use with caution in the elderly, in the debilitated, in young children, in individuals with increased ICP, in obstetrics, and with clients in shock or during acute alcoholic intoxication.**
- **Use morphine with extreme caution in pulmonary heart disease (cor pulmonale). Deaths following ordinary therapeutic doses have been reported.**
- **Use cautiously in prostatic hypertrophy, because it may precipitate acute urinary retention.**
- **Use cautiously with reduced blood volume, such as in hemorrhaging clients who are more susceptible to the hypotensive effects of morphine.**
- **Since the drugs depress the respiratory center, give early in labor, at least 2 hr before delivery, to reduce the danger of respiratory depression in the newborn.**
- **When given before surgery, give at least 1–2 hr preoperatively so that the danger of maximum depression of respiratory function will have passed before anesthesia is initiated.**
- **These drugs may need to be withheld prior to diagnostic procedures so that the physician can use pain to locate dysfunction.**
- **Rapid IV injection increases the likelihood of respiratory depression, hypotension, apnea, circulatory collapse, cardiac arrest, and anaphylactoid reactions.**

SIDE EFFECTS

See individual drugs. The following side effects are common to most narcotic analgesics. **Respiratory:** ***Respiratory depression***, ***apnea***. **CNS:** Dizziness, lightheadedness, sedation, lethargy, headache, euphoria, mental clouding, fainting. Idiosyncratic effects including excitement, restlessness, tremors, delirium, insomnia. **GI:** N&V, vomiting, constipation, increased pressure in biliary tract, dry mouth, anorexia. **CV:** Flushing, changes in HR and BP, circulatory collapse. **Allergic:** Skin rashes including pruritus and urticaria. Sweating, ***laryngospasm***, edema. **Miscellaneous:** Urinary retention, oliguria, reduced libido, changes in body temperature. Narcotics cross the placental barrier and depress respiration of the fetus or newborn.

DEPENDENCE AND TOLERANCE

All drugs of this group are addictive. Psychologic and physical dependence and tolerance develop even when clients use clinical doses. Tolerance is characterized by the fact that the client requires shorter periods of time between doses or larger doses for relief of pain. Tolerance usually develops faster when the narcotic analgesic is administered regularly and when the dose is large.

OVERDOSE MANAGEMENT

Symptoms (Acute Toxicity): Severe toxicity is characterized by ***profound respiratory depression, apnea, deep sleep, stupor or coma, circulatory collapse, seizures, cardiopulmonary arrest, and death.*** Less severe toxicity results in symptoms including CNS depression, miosis, and respiratory depression. Serious overdosage is characterized by respiratory depression, extreme somnolence progressing to stupor or coma, constricted pupils, skeletal muscle flaccidity, and cold and clammy skin. Hypotension, bradycardia, hypothermia, pulmonary edema, pneumonia, shock occur in 40% or less of clients. The respiratory rate may be as low as 2–4 breaths/min. The client may be cyanotic. Urine output is decreased, the skin feels clammy, and body temperature decreases. If death occurs, it almost always results from ***respiratory depression.***

Symptoms (Chronic Toxicity): The problem of chronic dependence on narcotics occurs not only as a result of "street" use but is often found among those who have easy access to narcotics (physicians, nurses, pharmacists). All the principal narcotic analgesics (morphine, opium, heroin, codeine, meperidine, and others) have, at times, been used for nontherapeutic purposes. The nurse must be aware of the problem and be able to recognize signs of chronic dependence. These are constricted pupils, GI effects (constipation), skin infections, needle scars, abscesses, and itching, especially on the anterior surfaces of the body, where the client may inject the drug.

Withdrawal signs appear after drug is withheld for 4–12 hr. They are characterized by intense craving for the drug, insomnia, yawning, sneezing, vomiting, diarrhea, tremors, sweating, mental depression, muscular aches and pains, chills, and anxiety. Although the symptoms of narcotic withdrawal are uncomfortable, they are rarely life-threatening. This is in contrast to the withdrawal syndrome from depressants, where the life of the individual may be endangered because of the possibility of tonic-clonic seizures.

Treatment (Acute Overdose): Initial treatment is aimed at combating progressive respiratory depression by maintaining a patent airway and by artificial respiration. Gastric lavage and induced emesis are indicated in case of oral poisoning. Administer a narcotic antagonist (e.g., naloxone [Narcan], 0.4 mg IV), to reverse acute overdosage. The duration of respiratory depression may be longer than the duration of the opioid antagonist; thus, repeated administration of the antagonist may be necessary. Do not give a narcotic antagonist in the absence of clinically significant respiratory or CV depression. Note that administration of a narcotic antagonist to an opioid-tolerant person will precipitate a withdrawal syndrome. Respiratory stimulants (e.g., caffeine) should not be used to treat depression from the narcotic overdosage.

DRUG INTERACTIONS

Alcohol, ethyl / Potentiation or addition of CNS depressant effects; concomitant use may lead to drowsiness, lethargy, stupor, respiratory collapse, coma, or death
Anesthetics, general / See ***Alcohol***
Antianxiety drugs / See ***Alcohol***
Anticholinergics / ↑ Risk of urinary retention and/or severe constipation which may lead to paralytic ileus
Antidepressants, tricyclic / ↑ Narcotic-induced respiratory depression
Antihistamines / See ***Alcohol***
Barbiturates / See ***Alcohol***
Cimetidine / ↑ CNS toxicity (e.g., disorientation, confusion, respiratory depression, apnea, seizures)
CNS depressants/See ***Alcohol***
MAOIs / Possible potentiation of either MAOI (excitation, hypertension) or narcotic (hypotension, coma) effects; death has resulted
Methotrimeprazine / Potentiation of CNS depression
Narcotic analgesics, mixed agonist/antagonists (buprenorphine, butorphanol, nalbuphine, pentazocine) / May precipitate withdrawal symptoms in dependent clients
Phenothiazines / Analgesic effect of narcotics may be potentiated; however, there is an ↑ incidence of side effects
Sedative-hypnotics, nonbarbiturate / See ***Alcohol***
Skeletal muscle relaxants (surgical) / ↑ Respiratory depression/muscle relaxation

LABORATORY TEST CONSIDERATIONS

Altered liver function tests. False + or ↑ urinary glucose test (Benedict's). ↑ Plasma amylase or lipase.

DOSAGE

See individual drugs.

NURSING IMPLICATIONS

IMPLEMENTATION/ADMINISTRATION/STORAGE

1. **Review list of drugs prescribed and with which opioids interact and effects seen.**
2. **Request orders be rewritten at timed intervals as required for continued administration.**
3. **Record amount of opioid used on the controlled inventory sheet, noting drug, date, time, dose, and to whom, or if the drug was wasted; include appropriate witness as necessary, addressing all requirements for documentation.**
4. **Some states dispense prescription pads that must be used when ordering controlled substances.**
5. **IV Give by very slow IV injection, preferably as a diluted solution, with the client lying down. Do not give IV unless a narcotic antagonist and facilities for assisted or controlled respiration are available.**

ASSESSMENT

1. **Note reasons for therapy, type, onset, location, characteristics of symptoms; differentiate acute versus chronic syndromes and pain levels. Note prior experience with opioids and any adverse reactions.**
2. **Identify cause and document amount of pain or discomfort, intensity, duration, frequency of occurrence, and what therapy/drug was effective in the past. Use a pain rating scale (e.g., 0–10) to assess pain quantitatively so clients can accurately describe their level of pain and measure effectiveness of therapy.**
3. **Identify clinical conditions that may precipitate pain syndromes, i.e., cancer, neuropathic, postherpetic neuralgia, or musculoskeletal injury. Document amount of time elapsed between doses for relief from recurring pain. Note precipitating factors as well as the im-**

pact of the pain on the client's ability to function and perform ADLs.

4. Obtain baseline VS; generally, if the respiratory rate <12/min or the SBP <90 mm Hg, an opioid should not be administered unless there is ventilatory support or specific written guidelines, with parameters for administration. Note weight, age, and general body size. Too large a dosage for the client's weight and age can result in serious consequences.
5. Note asthma or other conditions that alter respirations. Determine if pregnant. Opioids cross the placental barrier and depress fetal respirations.
6. Explore source of pain; use nonopioid analgesics when possible. Coadministration (as with NSAIDs) may increase analgesic effects and permit lower opioid doses. Determine need for pain management referrals. Administer when needed; *prolonging administration until the maximum amount of pain experienced reduces drugs' effectiveness.*
7. Determine when to use supportive measures, such as relaxation techniques, repositioning, alternative therapies, and reassurance to assist in relieving pain.
8. Monitor VS and mental status. During parenteral therapy:
   - Monitor for ↓ respirations.
   - Opioids depress cough reflex. Turn q 2 hr; cough and deep breathe to prevent atelectasis. Splinting incisions and painful areas may assist in compliance. Administer opioid at least 30–60 min prior to activities or painful procedures.
   - Monitor for hypotension.
   - Report if HR below 50 beats/min in the adult or 110 beats/min in infant.
   - Observe for decrease in BP, deep sleep, or constricted pupils.
   - Assess during meals to prevent choking and aspiration.
   - Monitor closely when administered as sedation for a procedure.
   - Note effects on mental status. One who has experienced pain, fear, or anxiety may become euphoric and excited. Note dizziness, drowsiness, pupil reactions, or hallucinations.
9. Report if N&V occurs; may need an antiemetic or change in therapy. A snack or milk may decrease gastric irritation and lessen nausea when taken orally.
10. Monitor bowel function; opioids, especially morphine, can have a depressant effect on the GI tract and may promote constipation. Increase fluid intake to 2.5–3 L/day; consume fruit juices, fruits, and fiber. Increase level and frequency of exercise. Use stool softeners as needed.
11. Opioids may cause urinary retention. Monitor I&O; palpate abdomen for distention; empty bladder q 3–4 hr. Question about difficulty voiding, pain in the bladder area, sensation of not fully emptying the bladder, dysuria, or any unusual odors.
12. Monitor mental status. If bedridden, use side supports and safety measures; assist with ambulation, bathroom, and transfers to prevent falls. Note difficulty with vision. Check pupillary response to light; report if pupils remain constricted.
13. Reassure that flushing and a feeling of warmth may occur with therapeutic doses. May perspire profusely; be prepared to bathe; change clothes and linens frequently.
14. Assess for evidence of tolerance and addiction with ATC therapy. With terminal diseases and chronic debilitating pain, dependence on drug therapy is not a consideration, whereas *adequate pain control is of the utmost concern.*
15. Monitor CBC, electrolytes, renal and LFTs. Assess for dependence, drug-seeking behaviors, over use/consumption of prescription and identify those on long-term therapy so opioid agreement can be completed. Periodic drug testing may support proper use.

CLIENT/FAMILY TEACHING

1. Chronic pain is a multifaceted and complex syndrome, which adversely affects one's physical, emotional, socioeconomic, and spiritual foundations. It has been shown that identification of pain problems and adequate pain control are imperative in restoring a sense of well-being.
2. Oral drug formulations of extended-release, controlled-release, or sustained-release products are not made to be chewed, crushed, or dissolved.
3. One may never be totally pain free. The intent of therapy is to lower the pain level to one in

which activities can be performed R/T daily care, and those that are of interest and concern to the client including holding down a job and going to work every day; not to encourage one to sleep throughout the day. Education concerning chronic pain and its many facets will be reviewed to better prepare one for this chronic disease state.

4. Drug may become habit-forming; alternative methods for pain control will be explored and utilized. With chronic debilitating pain, addiction is not a concern whereas functionality is of concern. Take as prescribed before the pain becomes too severe. During prolonged usage, do not stop abruptly; withdrawal symptoms may occur. Providers may expect clients to sign opioid agreements for not only client education but for protection from liability and misuse issues.
5. Can cause drowsiness and dizziness especially initially and with dose adjustments; use caution when operating a motor vehicle or performing other tasks that require mental alertness. Rise slowly from a lying to sitting position and dangle before standing, to minimize orthostatic effects.
6. Determine extent of relief achieved with each dosage (e.g., pain level decreased from a level 5 to a level 2, 20 min after administration of medication). Keep a record of opioid use for breakthrough pain so that maintenance dose can be reviewed and adjusted.
7. Identify goals and techniques to enhance pain relief such as relaxation techniques, ice/heat applications, splinting incision, massage, supporting painful areas, and taking medication before strenuous activities and before pain becomes severe.
8. Do not take OTC agents without approval. Many contain small amounts of alcohol and some may interact unfavorably with the prescribed drug. Avoid alcohol in any form.
9. For fecal impaction, use preventive actions, such as increased fluid intake, increased use of fruit and fruit juices, fiber, and a stool softener.
10. Store all drugs in a safe place, out of the reach of children and away from the bedside to prevent accidental overdosage. When used as sedation for outpatient procedures, someone must accompany client. Expect a recovery period (to assess for adverse effects) up to several hours before release.
11. Identify appropriate support groups for assistance with understanding, accepting, and managing chronic pain. Seek locale of regional pain management center for nonresponders with chronic pain syndromes.
12. For those with terminal diseases, identify local support groups to provide contact with those experiencing similar symptoms and treatments and local hospice program.
13. For the elderly, blood levels of opioid may be higher, resulting in longer periods of pain relief. Assess physical parameters and client complaints carefully before readministering opioid for short-term pain control on the prescribed as-needed frequency.
14. Keep all F/U to assess response, labs, adverse SE, and refills through prescriptions.

OUTCOMES/EVALUATE

- Control of pain without altered hemodynamics or impaired level of consciousness
- Reduction in pain level on pain rating scale
- Ability to perform ADLs and desired activities that are of client importance
- Absence of acute toxicity, tolerance, or addiction, during short-term therapy

NARCOTIC ANTAGONISTS

SEE ALSO THE FOLLOWING INDIVIDUAL ENTRIES:

Naloxone hydrochloride
Naltrexone

ACTION/KINETICS

Action

Narcotic antagonists competitively block the action of narcotic analgesics by displacing previously given narcotics from their receptor sites or by preventing narcotics from attaching to the opiate receptors, thereby preventing access by the analgesic. Not effective in reversing the respiratory depression induced by barbiturates, anesthetics, or other nonnarcotic agents. These drugs almost immediately induce withdrawal symptoms in narcotic addicts and are sometimes used to unmask dependence.

DOSAGE

See individual drugs.

Classifications

NURSING IMPLICATIONS

ASSESSMENT

1. Note reasons for therapy, when and what agents consumed, and expected time frame for action. Determine etiology of respiratory depression. Narcotic antagonists do not relieve the toxicity of nonnarcotic CNS depressants.
2. Identify agent being reversed. If opioid is long acting or sustained release, repeated doses will be required in order to continue to counteract drug effects. Monitor VS and respirations closely after duration of action of antagonist; additional doses may be necessary.
3. Observe for symptoms of airway obstruction; if comatose, turn frequently and position on side to prevent aspiration. Maintain a safe, protective environment. Use side rails, supervise ambulation, and use soft supports as needed.
4. Observe for appearance of withdrawal symptoms characterized by restlessness, crying out due to sudden loss of pain control, lacrimation, rhinorrhea, yawning, perspiration, vomiting, diarrhea, sweating, writhing, anxiety, pain, chills, and an intense craving for the drug. If used to diagnose opioid use or dependence, observe for initial dilation of the pupils, followed by constriction.
5. Anticipate readministration of smaller doses of opioid (once depressant symptoms reversed) with terminal pain and conditions that warrant narcotic pain management.
6. Assess/monitor LOC, mental status, clinical presentation, and VS.

CLIENT/FAMILY TEACHING

Drug is used to reverse the effects of too much opioid. It may need to be readministered in order to attain this effect of increasing level of consciousness and reversing respiratory depression.

OUTCOMES/EVALUATE

- Reversal of toxic opioid analgesia evidenced by ↑ level of consciousness and improved breathing patterns
- Confirmation of opioid dependence

NEUROMUSCULAR BLOCKING AGENTS ■

SEE ALSO THE FOLLOWING INDIVIDUAL ENTRIES:

Atracurium besylate*
Cisatracurium besylate
Pancuronium bromide
Rocuronium bromide
Succinylcholine chloride
Tubocurarine chloride
Vecuronium bromide

Drugs marked with an * are available to view in the 2013 Nurse's Drug Handbook Website at www.cengage.com/community/nursesdrughandbook.

INDICATIONS/USES

See individual agents. Uses include, but are not limited to: (1) Adjunct to general anesthesia to cause muscle relaxation. (2) Reduce the intensity of skeletal muscle contractions in either drug-induced or electrically-induced convulsions. (3) Assist in the management of mechanical ventilation.

ACTION/KINETICS

Action

These drugs are categorized as competitive (nondepolarizing) and depolarizing agents, both of which act peripherally. Competitive agents include all of the above listed drugs *except* succinylcholine. They compete with acetylcholine for the receptor site in the muscle cells. The depolarizing agent-succinylcholine-initially excites skeletal muscle and then prevents the muscle from contracting by prolonging the time during which the receptors at the end plate cannot respond to acetylcholine (depolarization during refractory time). The muscle paralysis caused by the neuromuscular blocking agents is sequential in the following order: heaviness of eyelids, difficulty in swallowing/talking, diplopia, progressive weakening of extremities and neck, followed by relaxation of the trunk and spine. The diaphragm (respiratory paralysis) is affected last. They do not affect consciousness, and their use, in the absence of adequate levels of general anesthesia, may be frightening to the client. There is a narrow margin of safety between a therapeutically effective dose causing muscle relaxation and a toxic dose causing respiratory paralysis. **The neuromuscular blocking agents are always administered initially by a trained provider.** The nurse must be prepared to maintain and monitor respiration until the effect of the drug subsides.

Pharmacokinetics

After IV infusion, flaccid paralysis occurs within a few minutes with maximum effects within about

6 min. Maximal effects last 35–60 min and effective muscle paralysis may last for 25–90 min with complete recovery taking several hours.

CONTRAINDICATIONS

Allergy or hypersensitivity to any of these drugs.

SPECIAL CONCERNS

- **Use with caution in myasthenia gravis; renal, hepatic, endocrine, or pulmonary impairment; respiratory depression; during lactation; and in elderly, pediatric, or debilitated clients.**
- **Action may be altered in clients by electrolyte imbalances (especially hyperkalemia), some carcinomas, body temperature, dehydration, renal disease, and in those taking digitalis.**

SIDE EFFECTS

See also individual agents. ***Respiratory paralysis. Severe and prolonged muscle relaxation*.** **CV:** Cardiac arrhythmias, bradycardia, hypotension, cardiac arrest. These side effects are more frequent in neonates and premature infants. **GI:** Excessive salivation during light anesthesia. **Miscellaneous:** ***Bronchospasms*, *hyperthermia***, hypersensitivity (rare).

OVERDOSE MANAGEMENT

Symptoms: Decreased respiratory reserve, extended skeletal muscle weakness, prolonged apnea, low tidal volume, sudden release of histamine, ***CV collapse.***

Treatment: There are no known antidotes.

- Use a peripheral nerve stimulator to monitor and assess client's response to the neuromuscular blocking medication.
- Have anticholinesterase drugs, such as edrophonium, pyridostigmine, or neostigmine available to counteract respiratory depression due to paralysis of skeletal muscles. These drugs decrease the body's breakdown of acetylcholine. To minimize the muscarinic cholinergic side effects, give atropine.
- Correct BP, electrolyte imbalance, or circulating blood volume by fluid and electrolyte therapy. Vasopressors can be used to correct hypotension due to ganglionic blockade.

DRUG INTERACTIONS

The following drug interactions are for nondepolarizing skeletal muscle relaxants. See also succinylcholine.

Aminoglycoside antibiotics / Additive muscle relaxation, including prolonged respiratory depression
Amphotericin B / ↑ Muscle relaxation
Anesthetics, inhalation / Additive muscle relaxation
Carbamazepine / ↓ Duration or effect of muscle relaxants
Clindamycin / Additive muscle relaxation, including prolonged respiratory depression
Colistin / ↑ Muscle relaxation
Corticosteroids / ↓ Effect of muscle relaxants
Furosemide / ↑ or ↓ Effect of skeletal muscle relaxants (may be dose-related)
Hydantoins / ↓ Duration or effect of muscle relaxants
Ketamine / ↑ Muscle relaxation, including prolonged respiratory depression
Lincomycin / ↑ Muscle relaxation, including prolonged respiratory depression
Lithium / ↑ Recovery time of muscle relaxants → prolonged respiratory depression
Magnesium salts / ↑ Muscle relaxation, with prolonged respiratory depression
Methotrimeprazine / ↑ Muscle relaxation
Narcotic analgesics / ↑ Respiratory depression and ↑ muscle relaxation
Nitrates / ↑ Muscle relaxation, including prolonged respiratory depression
Phenothiazines / ↑ Muscle relaxation
Piperacillin / ↑ Muscle relaxation, including prolonged respiratory depression
Polymyxin B / ↑ Muscle relaxation
Procainamide / ↑ Muscle relaxation
Procaine / ↑ Muscle relaxation by ↓ plasma protein binding
Quinidine / ↑ Muscle relaxation
Ranitidine / Significant ↓ effect of muscle relaxants
Theophyllines / Reversal of effects of muscle relaxant (dose-dependent)
Thiazide diuretics / ↑ Muscle relaxation due to hypokalemia
Verapamil / ↑ Muscle relaxation, with prolonged respiratory depression

DOSAGE

See individual drugs.

NURSING IMPLICATIONS

ASSESSMENT

1. **Note reasons for therapy, desired outcome, and anticipated length of use.**

2. List other drugs receiving. Clients requiring neuromuscular blocking agents are often receiving other drugs that may prolong response to neuromuscular blocking agent.
3. Question client concerning changes in vision, ability to chew or move the fingers. Note age and condition; elderly and debilitated clients should not receive drugs in this category.
4. Note initial selective paralysis in the following sequence: levator muscles of the eyelids, mastication muscles, limb muscles, abdominal muscles, glottis muscles, intercostal muscles, and the diaphragm muscles; neuromuscular recovery occurs in the reverse order.
5. Administer in a closely monitored environment and generally only when client is intubated. Neuromuscular blocking agents are generally used in the ICU setting for three reasons: (a) to eliminate spontaneous breathing and promote mechanical ventilation (i.e., eliminate urge to fight the vent. (b) Cause a pharmacologic restraint so clients do not harm themselves. (c) To decrease oxygen consumption.
6. Prevent overdosage during infusions by frequent evaluations with a peripheral nerve stimulator (train-of-four) to document antagonism of neuromuscular blockade and recovery of muscle function and strength.
7. Whenever a paralytic agent is used, the Train of Four (TOF) is the test used to measure the degree of neuromuscular blockade. Do a baseline measurement before paralytic agent is started to determine what current is necessary to obtain twitch. Generally 20 mA may be enough. Complete and document until TOF to 2/4.
8. Instructions for use of Train of Four:
   - Explain to client exactly what you are doing, that it will not hurt, and why you are performing this test
   - Once instructed: Attach 2 electrodes along the course of the ulnar nerve. (Temporal may be used.)
   - Connect the lead to the peripheral nerve stimulator by inserting the jacks into the Proximal (red) and Distal (black) output jacks. Connect the other end to the client electrodes.
   - Turn stimulator on. Select the current necessary (usually 20) for that client to twitch when the stimuli is applied.
   - Press TOF once. It will deliver a train of four pulses where each is 0.5 seconds apart. Do NOT use the other buttons on the stimulator!
   - Count the number of twitches the client had out of four (0/4, 1/4, 2/4, 3/4, 4/4.) Adjust the medication as ordered. Goal is 1/4 to 2/4 twitches.
9. Perform frequent neurovascular assessments. Prolonged use of neuromuscular blocking agents may cause profound weakness and paralysis; may precipitate an acute myopathy.
10. Monitor VS frequently and pulmonary status continuously. Cardiac monitor and ventilator alarms should be set and checked frequently. Observe for excessive bronchial secretions or respiratory wheezing; suction to maintain patent airway.
11. Consciousness and pain thresholds are not affected by neuromuscular blocking agents; clients can still hear, feel, and see while receiving these agents. Avoid discussions that should not be overheard. Explain all contacts, injections, therapies, and procedures. Adequate anxiolytic therapy and analgesics should be administered for pain and/or fear with procedures and situations requiring this therapy.
12. Clients requiring prolonged ventilatory therapy should be adequately sedated with analgesics and benzodiazepines. Anxiety levels may be very high, but client cannot communicate this. Observe for drug interactions that may potentiate muscular relaxation and prove fatal.
13. Administer eye drops and patches to protect corneas during prolonged therapy; explain why this is done (i.e., blink reflex suppressed). Avoid corticosteroids during prolonged neuromuscular blockade unless benefits far outweigh the risks.
14. Perform frequent passive range-of-motion to prevent loss of function and contractures with prolonged therapy. Assess skin condition and turn frequently to prevent prolonged pressure on any one area as client unable to feel and thus unable to communicate discomfort.
15. Monitor CBC, electrolytes, CXR, ECG, renal and LFTs.

CLIENT/FAMILY TEACHING

1. Drug is used to paralyze functions so that procedures or controlled ventilation can occur.

2. Client will be constantly monitored and cared for. Medication will be administered for pain and anxiety as needed.
3. Client will regain the ability to move and talk once therapy is discontinued.

OUTCOMES/EVALUATE

- Skeletal muscle paralysis (pharmacologic restraint)
- Insertion of ET tube/tolerance of mechanical ventilation
- ↓ Oxygen consumption

NONSTEROIDAL ANTI-INFLAMMATORY DRUGS ■

SEE ALSO THE FOLLOWING INDIVIDUAL ENTRIES:

Celecoxib
Diclofenac potassium
Diclofenac sodium
Diflunisal
Etodolac
Fenoprofen calcium
Ibuprofen
Ibuprofen lysine
Indomethacin
Indomethacin sodium trihydrate
Ketoprofen
Ketorolac tromethamine
Meloxicam
Nabumetone*
Naproxen
Naproxen sodium
Oxaprozin
Oxaprozin potassium
Piroxicam
Sulindac
Tolmetin sodium

Drugs marked with an * are available to view in the 2013 Nurse's Drug Handbook Website at www.cengage.com/community/nursesdrughandbook.

INDICATIONS/USES

See individual drugs. **Systemic.** Uses include, but are not limited to: (1) Inflammatory disease, including rheumatoid arthritis, osteoarthritis, ankylosing spondylitis, gout, and other musculoskeletal diseases. (2) Nonrheumatic inflammatory conditions, including bursitis, acute painful shoulder, synovitis, tendinitis, or tenosynovitis. (3) Mild to moderate pain including episiotomy pain, strains and sprains, post extraction dental pain. (4) Primary dysmenorrhea. *Investigational:* Reduce risk of prostate cancer. Reduce risk of Alzheimer's disease (high doses).

Ophthalmic. (1) Ophthalmically to inhibit intraoperative miosis. (2) Postoperative inflammation and the reduction of ocular pain after cataract surgery. (3) Ocular itching due to seasonal allergic conjunctivitis. (4) Photophobia in those undergoing corneal refractive surgery. *Investigational:* Topical treatment of cystoid macular edema after cataract surgery.

ACTION/KINETICS

Action

The anti-inflammatory effect is likely due to inhibition of the enzyme cyclooxygenase (COX). There are two COX isoenzymes-COX-1 and COX-2. Depending on the NSAID, either COX-1 or COX-2 or both enzymes may be inhibited. Inhibition of cyclooxygenase results in decreased prostaglandin synthesis. Effective in reducing joint swelling, pain, and morning stiffness, as well as in increasing mobility in individuals with inflammatory disease. They do not alter the course of the disease, however. Their anti-inflammatory activity is comparable to that of aspirin. The analgesic activity is due, in part, to relief of inflammation. Other mechanisms that contribute to the anti-inflammatory effect include reduction of superoxide radicals, induction of apoptosis, inhibition of adhesion molecule expression, decrease of nitric oxide synthase, decrease of proinflammatory cytokine levels, modification of lymphocyte activity, and alteration of cellular membrane functions. Rheumatoid factor production may also be inhibited. The antipyretic action occurs by decreasing prostaglandin synthesis in the hypothalamus, resulting in an increase in peripheral blood flow and heat loss as well as promoting sweating. NSAIDs also inhibit miosis induced by prostaglandins during the course of cataract surgery; thus, these drugs are useful for a number of ophthalmic inflammatory conditions.

Pharmacokinetics

The NSAIDs differ from one another with respect to their rate of absorption, length of action, anti-inflammatory activity, and effect on the GI mucosa. Most are rapidly and completely absorbed from the GI tract; food delays the rate, but not the total amount, of drug absorbed. These drugs are metabolized in the kidney and are excreted through the urine, mainly as metabolites.

CONTRAINDICATIONS

Most for children under 14 years of age. Lactation. Individuals in whom aspirin, NSAIDs, or iodides have caused hypersensitivity, including acute asthma, rhinitis, urticaria, nasal polyps, bronchospasm, angioedema or other symptoms of allergy or anaphylaxis. Use in hepatic porphyria. Instillation of ophthalmic products while wearing contact lenses.

SPECIAL CONCERNS

- **Clients intolerant to one of the NSAIDs may be intolerant to others in this group.**
- **Use with caution in clients with a history of GI disease, reduced renal function, in geriatric clients, in clients with intrinsic coagulation defects or those on anticoagulant therapy, in compromised cardiac function, in hypertension, in conditions predisposing to fluid retention, and in the presence of existing controlled infection.**
- **The risk of hospitalization is doubled in geriatric clients taking NSAIDs and diuretics.**
- **Regular use of NSAIDs may hamper aspirin's prevention of first heart attacks; the risk of MI may be increased in new and current users of NSAIDs.**
- **The safety and efficacy of most NSAIDs have not been determined in children or in functional class IV rheumatoid arthritis (i.e., clients incapacitated, bedridden, or confined to a wheelchair).**
- **Use during pregnancy increases the risk of pulmonary hypertension in newborns.**
- **Products must carry a warning about the possibility of stomach bleeding in clients who consume three or more alcoholic drinks per day.**
- **Use with caution in individuals who have shown sensitivity to aspirin or phenylacetic acid derivatives.**
- **There is the potential for stomach bleeding in the following groups: Persons over age 60, those who have had prior ulcers or bleeding, persons who take a blood thinner, those taking more than one product containing an NSAID, and those taking a NSAID longer than prescribed.**
- **There is an increased risk for corneal adverse effects that may be sight-threatening if topical NSAIDs are used in clients with complicated ocular surgeries, corneal denervation, corneal epithelial defects, diabetes mellitus, dry eye syndrome, rheumatoid arthritis, or repeat ocular surgeries within a short period of time.**

SIDE EFFECTS

GI (most common): Peptic or duodenal ulceration and GI bleeding, intestinal ulceration with obstruction and stenosis, reactivation of preexisting ulcers. Heartburn, dyspepsia, N&V, anorexia, diarrhea, constipation, increased or decreased appetite, indigestion, stomatitis, epigastric pain, abdominal cramps or pain, gastroenteritis, paralytic ileus, salivation, dry mouth, glossitis, pyrosis, icterus, rectal irritation, gingival ulcer, occult blood in stool, hematemesis, gastritis, proctitis, eructation, sore or dry mucous membranes, ulcerative colitis, rectal bleeding, melena, ***perforation and hemorrhage of esophagus, stomach, duodenum, small or large intestine***. **CNS:** Dizziness, drowsiness, vertigo, headaches, nervousness, migraine, anxiety, mental confusion, aggravation of parkinsonism and epilepsy, lightheadedness, paresthesia, peripheral neuropathy, akathisia, excitation, tremor, ***seizures***, myalgia, asthenia, malaise, insomnia, fatigue, drowsiness, confusion, emotional lability, depression, inability to concentrate, psychoses, hallucinations, depersonalization, amnesia, ***coma***, syncope, aseptic meningitis. **CV:** CHF, hypo-/hypertension, arrhythmias, peripheral edema and fluid retention, vasodilation, exacerbation of angiitis, palpitations, tachycardia, chest pain, sinus bradycardia, peripheral vascular disease, peripheral edema. **Respiratory:** ***Bronchospasm, laryngeal edema***, rhinitis, dyspnea, pharyngitis, hemoptysis, SOB, eosinophilic pneumonitis. **Hematologic:** Bone marrow depression, neutropenia, leukopenia, pancytopenia, eosinophilia, thrombocytopenia, granulocytopenia, ***agranulocytosis, aplastic anemia, hemolytic anemia***, decreased H&H, anemia, hypercoagulability, epistaxis. **Ophthalmic:** Amblyopia, visual disturbances, corneal deposits, retinal hemorrhage, scotomata, retinal pigmentation changes or degeneration, blurred vision, photophobia, diplopia, iritis, loss of color vision (reversible), optic neuritis, cataracts, swollen, dry, or irritated eyes. **Dermatologic:** Pruritus, skin eruptions, sweating, erythema, eczema, hyperpigmentation, ecchymoses, petechiae, rashes, urticaria, purpura, onycholysis, vesiculobullous eruptions, cutaneous vasculitis, ***toxic epidermal necrolysis, angioneurotic edema***, erythema nodosum, ***Stevens-Johnson syndrome***, exfoliative dermatitis, photosensitivity, alopecia, skin irritation, peeling, erythema multiforme, desquamation, skin discoloration. **GU:** Menometrorrhagia, menorrhagia, impotence, menstrual disorders, hematuria, cystitis, azotemia, nocturia, proteinuria, UTIs, polyuria, dysuria, urinary frequency, oliguria, pyuria, anuria, renal insufficiency, nephrosis, nephrotic syndrome, glomerular/interstitial nephritis, urinary casts, acute renal failure in clients with impaired renal function, renal papillary necrosis. **Metabolic:** Hyper-/hypoglycemia, glycosuria, hyperkalemia, hyponatremia, diabetes mellitus. **Other:** Tinnitus, hearing loss/disturbances, ear pain, deafness, metallic or bitter taste in mouth, thirst, chills, fever, flushing, jaundice, sweating, breast changes, gynecomastia, muscle cramps, dyspnea, involuntary muscle movements, muscle weakness, facial edema, pain, serum sickness, aseptic meningitis, hypersensitivity reactions including asthma, acute respiratory distress, ***shock-like syndrome, angioedema***, angiitis, dyspnea, ***anaphylaxis***.

Following ophthalmic use: Transient burning and stinging upon installation, ocular irritation, keratitis, increased bleeding of ocular tissues following ocular surgery.

OVERDOSE MANAGEMENT

Symptoms: CNS symptoms include dizziness, drowsiness, mental confusion, lethargy, disorientation, intense headache, paresthesia, and ***seizures.*** GI symptoms include N&V, gastric irritation, and abdominal pain. Miscellaneous symptoms include tinnitus, sweating, blurred vision, increased serum creatinine and BUN, and acute renal failure.

Treatment: There are no antidotes; treatment includes general supportive measures. Since the drugs are acidic, it may be beneficial to alkalinize the urine and induce diuresis to hasten excretion.

DRUG INTERACTIONS

ACE inhibitors / Possible ↓ antihypertensive effect of ACE inhibitors
Acetaminophen / ↑ Risk of hypertension in women
Aminoglycosides / ↑ Aminoglycoside levels in premature infants due to ↓ glomerular filtration rate
Anticoagulants / Concomitant use results in ↑ PT
Aspirin / ↓ Effect of NSAIDs R/T ↓ blood levels; also, ↑ risk of adverse GI effects
Beta-adrenergic blocking agents / ↓ Antihypertensive effects R/T NSAID inhibition of prostaglandin synthesis, thus allowing unopposed pressor systems to potentiate hypertension
Bisphosphonates / ↑ Risk of gastric ulceration
Cholestyramine / ↓ GI absorption of NSAIDs → ↓ effect
Cimetidine / ↑ or ↓ Plasma levels of NSAIDs
Cyclosporine / ↑ Risk of nephrotoxicity of both drugs
Diuretics / ↓ Diuretic effects
H ***Gingko biloba*** / Additive effect on platelet aggregation → ↑ risk of bleeding
H ***Ginseng*** / Avoid concomitant use or monitor carefully
Lithium / ↑ Serum lithium levels
Loop diuretics / ↓ Drug effects
Methotrexate / ↑ Risk of methotrexate toxicity (i.e., bone marrow suppression, nephrotoxicity, stomatitis)
Phenobarbital / ↓ Effect of NSAIDs R/T ↑ liver breakdown
Phenytoin / ↑ Phenytoin pharmacologic and toxic effects R/T ↓ plasma protein binding
Probenecid / ↑ Levels and possibly toxicity of NSAIDs
Salicylates / Plasma levels of NSAIDs may be ↓; also, ↑ risk of GI side effects
SSRIs / ↑ Risk of significant GI side effects; do not use together
Sulfonamides / ↑ Drug effects R/T ↓ plasma protein binding
Sulfonylureas / ↑ Drug effects R/T ↓ plasma protein binding
Warfarin / ↑ Risk of upper GI hemorrhage

DOSAGE

See individual drugs.

NURSING IMPLICATIONS

IMPLEMENTATION/ADMINISTRATION/STORAGE

1. **Do not take alcohol or aspirin together with NSAIDs. If GI upset occurs, take with food, milk, or antacids.**
2. **NSAIDs may have an additive analgesic effect when administered with narcotic analgesics, thus permitting lower narcotic dosages.**
3. **Clients who do not respond clinically to one NSAID may respond to another.**
4. **Use of ophthalmic products more than 24 hr prior to surgery or beyond 14 days postsurgery**

may increase the risk for the incidence and severity of corneal side effects.

5. Topical NSAID products may slow or delay healing.

ASSESSMENT

1. Note reasons for therapy, onset, location, intensity, characteristics, and type of pain/swelling experienced. Rate pain level. Assess joint mobility/stability and ROM. Note other agents trialed and outcome.
2. Review indications and dosage prescribed. For anti-inflammatory effects, high doses are required whereas analgesia and pain relief may be achieved with much lower dosages. Metastatic bone pain responds effectively to NSAIDs but not as well to opiods.
3. Note allergic responses to aspirin or other anti-inflammatory agents. Asthma or nasal polyps may be exacerbated by NSAIDs. Children under age 14 generally should not receive drugs in this category.
4. Determine history of ulcers, heart disease, or cardiac failure. May cause an increased risk of serious CV thrombotic events, MI, and stroke. Risk increased with longer use and with heart disease.
5. Explain that the major effect of all NSAIDs is to decrease the synthesis of prostaglandins. This is achieved by reversibly inhibiting cyclooxygenase (COX), an enzyme that catalyzes the formation of prostaglandins and thromboxanes from arachidonic acid (the precursor). This is in contrast to salicylates, which irreversibly bind to COX and inhibit production for the entire life of the cell. Prostaglandins enhance the inflammatory response and renal blood flow, and offer cytoprotection of GI mucosa.
6. Make sure that client understands importance of not self medicating or taking other agents in this class of drug at the same time without provider approval.
7. Monitor VS, H&H, stool for occult blood, CBC, renal and LFTs; reduce dose with renal dysfunction. These drugs cause platelet inhibition that is reversible in 24–48 hr, whereas aspirin requires 4–5 days to reverse antiplatelet effects. COX-1 NSAIDs may inhibit the cardioprotective effects of aspirin. Separate dosing intervals.

CLIENT/FAMILY TEACHING

1. Take oral NSAIDs with a full glass of water or milk, with meals, or with a prescribed antacid and remain upright 30 min following administration to reduce gastric irritation or ulcer formation. Regular intake of drug needed to sustain anti-inflammatory effects. If not obtained, another NSAID may provide desired response.
2. Consume 2–3 L/day of water. Report any changes in stool consistency or symptoms of GI irritation. Sustained GI effects may require stomach protectant.
3. With topical use do not exceed dose and do not apply to skin that is not intact; stop therapy and report if rash occurs.
4. Use caution in operating machinery or in driving a car until drug effects realized; may cause dizziness or drowsiness.
5. Avoid alcohol, aspirin, and any other OTC preparations; may cause GI bleeding. Report any episodes of bleeding, chest pain, SOB, eye symptoms, ringing in ears, skin rashes, bruising, weight gain, swelling of limbs, decreased urine output, fever, or increased joint pain.
6. Record weights periodically and report any significant changes. NSAIDs cause sodium and water retention; avoid with CHF.
7. Diabetics need to be aware of the lowered blood sugar effect of NSAIDs on hypoglycemic agents. Dosage adjustments may be required.
8. Notify all providers of medications being taken to avoid unfavorable drug interactions.
9. Review risks associated with this class of drugs.
10. Keep all F/U to assess response, labs, and for adverse SE.

OUTCOMES/EVALUATE

- ↑ Joint mobility and ROM
- ↓ Discomfort/pain and swelling
- Improved pain scores

ORAL CONTRACEPTIVES: ESTROGEN-PROGESTERONE COMBINATIONS ■

SEE TABLE 2.

GENERAL STATEMENT

There are three types of combination (i.e., both an estrogen and progestin in each tablet) oral contraceptives: (1) **monophasic:** contains the same amount of estrogen and progestin in each tablet; (2) **biphasic:** usually contains the same amount of estrogen in each tablet, but the progestin content is lower for the first part of the cycle and higher for the last part of the cycle. Certain of the 28–day products (Beyez and Safyral) also contain levomefolate calcium along with the estrogen and progestin. The purpose of levomefolate calcium is to raise folate levels. (3) **triphasic:** the estrogen content may be the same or may vary throughout the medication cycle; the progestin content may be the same or varies, depending on the part of the cycle. Also, some products have a three month supply of tablets in the packet. The purpose of the biphasic and triphasic products is to provide hormones in a manner similar to that occurring physiologically. This is said to decrease breakthrough bleeding during the medication cycle. (4) **Four phases:** This product contains varying amounts of estrogen and progestin but in four different phases to be taken over a 26–day period (plus two inert tablets). The other type of oral contraceptive is the progestin-only ("mini-pill") product, which contains a small amount of norethindrone in each tablet. Also available is an emergency contraceptive (Ella, Next Choice, Plan B, Plan B-One Step). These products are intended to be used after unprotected intercourse or known or suspected contraceptive failure. These products are available over-the-counter for women 17 years and older and by prescription for younger women.

INDICATIONS/USES

(1) Prevention of pregnancy. (2) Prevent pregnancy after unprotected intercourse or a known or suspected contraceptive failure (Plan B-One Step only). (3) Moderate acne vulgaris in females aged 15 and older who have no contraindications to oral contraceptive therapy, have reached menarche, desire contraception, and who are unresponsive to topical antiacne drugs (Estrostep and Ortho Tri-Cyclen only).

ACTION/KINETICS

Combination oral contraceptives. Act by inhibiting ovulation due to an inhibition (through negative-feedback mechanism) of LH and FSH, which are required for development of ova. These products also alter the cervical mucus so that it is not conducive to sperm penetration and render the endometrium less suitable for implantation of the blastocyst should fertilization occur. The estrogen used in combination oral contraceptives is either ethinyl estradiol or mestranol. Ethinyl estradiol is rapidly absorbed; **peak levels:** 2 hr. Mestranol is demethylated to ethinyl estradiol in the liver. **t½:** 6–20 hr. Several different progestins are used in combination oral contraceptives: Desogestrel, drospirenone, ethynodiol diacetate, levonorgestrel, norethindrone, norethindrone acetate, norgestimate, or norgestrel. Terminal t½'s for progestins vary over a wide range.

Progestin-only oral contraceptives. These products inhibit ovulation in about 50% of users. However, these products also alter the cervical mucus, render the endometrium unsuitable for implantation, lower midcycle LH and FSH peaks, and slow the movement of the ovum through the fallopian tubes. These products contain norethindrone. This method of contraception is less reliable than combination therapy.

NOTE: Although oral contraceptives may be associated with serious side effects, a number of noncontraceptive health benefits have been confirmed. These include increased regularity of the menstrual cycle, decreased incidence of dysmenorrhea, decreased blood loss, decreased incidence of functional ovarian cysts and ectopic pregnancies, and decreased incidence of diseases such as fibroadenomas, fibrocystic disease, acute pelvic inflammatory disease, endometrial cancer, and ovarian cancer. OC use has also been associated with a reduction in colorectal cancer and positive effects on bone mineral density.

CONTRAINDICATIONS

Thrombophlebitis, history of deep-vein thrombophlebitis, thromboembolic disorders, cerebral vascular disease, CAD, MI, current or past angina, known or suspected breast cancer or estrogen-dependent neoplasm, endometrial carcinoma, hepatic adenoma or carcinoma, undiagnosed abnormal genital bleeding, known or suspected pregnancy, cholestatic jaundice of pregnancy, jaundice with prior tablet use, acute liver disease. Smoking. Use before menarche.

Combination oral contraceptives may interfere with lactation, decreasing the quantity and quality of breast milk. Also, a small amount of steroids is excreted in breast milk. If possible, defer use of oral contraceptive products until the infant has been weaned,

TABLE 2 Hormone Contraceptive Preparations Available in the United States

TRADE NAME	ESTROGEN	PROGESTIN
	MONOPHASIC	
Alesse (28-Day)	Ethinyl estradiol (20 mcg)	Levonorgestrel (0.1 mg)
Altavera (28-Day)	Ethinyl estradiol (30 mcg)	Levonorgestrel (0.15 mg)
Amethia (91-Day)	Ethinyl estradiol (30 mcg in first 84 tablets followed by 7 tablets containing 10 mcg)	Levonorgestrel (0.15 mg in 84 tablets)
Apri (28-Day)	Ethinyl estradiol (30 mcg)	Desogestrel (0.15 mg)
Aviane (28-Day)	Ethinyl estradiol (20 mcg)	Levonorgestrel (0.1 mg)
Azurette (28-Day)	Ethinyl estradiol (20 mcg in first 21 tablets, 2 inert tablets, 5 with only ethinyl estradiol, 10 mcg)	Desogestrel (0.15 mg in first 21 tablets)
Balziva (28-Day)	Ethinyl estradiol (35 mcg)	Norethindrone (0.4 mg)
Beyez (28-Day)	Ethinyl estradiol (20 mcg) (also contains levomefolate calcium to raise folate levels)	Drospirenone (3 mg)
Brevicon (28-Day)	Ethinyl estradiol (35 mcg)	Norethindrone (0.5 mg)
Camrese (91-Day)	Ethinyl estradiol (30 mcg in first 84 tablets followed by 7 tablets containing 10 mcg)	Levonorgestrel (0.15 mg in 84 tablets)
Cryselle (21- and 28-Day)	Ethinyl estradiol (30 mcg)	Norgestrel (0.3 mg)
Desogen (28-Day)	Ethinyl estradiol (30 mcg)	Desogestrel (0.15 mg)
Emoquette (28-Day)	Ethinyl estradiol (30 mcg)	Desogestrel (0.15 mg)
Ethinyl estradiol/Norethindrone Chewable Tablet	Ethinyl estradiol (25 mcg) (24-Days of estrogen/progestin plus 4 days of iron)	Norethindrone (0.8 mg)
Femcon Fe (28-Day) Chewable Tablets	Ethinyl estradiol (35 mcg)	Norethindrone (0.4 mg)
Gianvi (24-Day)	Ethinyl estradiol (0.2 mg)	Drospirenone (3 mg)
Jolessa (1 hormone-containing tablet/day for 84 days followed by one inert tablet/day for 7 days)	Ethinyl estradiol (30 mcg)	Levonorgestrel (0.15 mg)
Junel 21 Day 1/20	Ethinyl estradiol (20 mcg)	Norethindrone acetate (1 mg)
Junel 21 Day 1.5/30	Ethinyl estradiol (30 mcg)	Norethindrone acetate (1.5 mg)
Junel Fe 1/20 (28-Day)	Ethinyl estradiol (20 mcg)	Norethindrone (1 mg)
Junel Fe 1.5/30 (28-Day)	Ethinyl estradiol (30 mcg)	Norethindrone (1.5 mg)
Kariva* (28-Day)	Ethinyl estradiol (20 mcg and 10 mcg)	Desogestrel (0.15 mg)
Kelnor 1/35 (28-Day)	Ethinyl estradiol (35 mcg)	Ethynodiol diacetate (1 mg)
Lessina (21- and 28-Day)	Ethinyl estradiol (20 mcg)	Levonorgestrel (0.1 mg)
Levora (28-Day)	Ethinyl estradiol (30 mcg)	Levonorgestrel (0.15 mg)
Lo-Estrin Fe	Ethinyl estradiol (10 mcg) (First 24 contain both estrogen and progestin; next 2 contain only estogen; last 2 contain iron)	Norethindrone (1 mg)

TRADE NAME	ESTROGEN	PROGESTIN
	MONOPHASIC	
Loestrin 21 1/20	Ethinyl estradiol (20 mcg)	Norethindrone acetate (1 mg)
Loestrin 21 1.5/30	Ethinyl estradiol (30 mcg)	Norethindrone acetate (1.5 mg)
Loestrin 24 Fe (28-Day:: four iron-containing tablets)	Ethinyl estradiol (20 mcg)	Norethindrone acetate (1 mg)
Loestrin Fe 1/20 (28-Day)	Ethinyl estradiol (20 mcg)	Norethindrone acetate (1 mg)
Loestrin Fe 1.5/30 (28-Day)	Ethinyl estradiol (30 mcg)	Norethindrone acetate (1.5 mg)
Loryna (28-Day)	Ethinyl estradiol (20 mcg)	Drospirenone (3 mg)
LoSeasonique	Ethinyl estradiol, (20 mcg in 84 tablets followed by 10 mcg in 7 tablets)	Levonorgestrel (0.1 mg in 84 tablets; none in 7 tablets)
Low-Ogestrel (28-Day)	Ethinyl estradiol (30 mcg)	Norgestrel (0.3 mg)
Lutera (28-Day)	Ethinyl estradiol (20 mcg)	Levonorgestrel (0.1 mg)
Lybrel (28 tablets/pack; 1 hormone-containing tablet everyday without any tablet-free interval)	Ethinyl estradiol (20 mcg)	Levonorgestrel (90 mcg)
Microgestin Fe 1/20 (28-Day)	Ethinyl estradiol (20 mcg)	Norethindrone acetate (1 mg)
Microgestin Fe 1.5/30 (28-Day)	Ethinyl estradiol (30 mcg)	Norethindrone acetate (1.5 mg)
Mircette* (28-Day)	Ethinyl estradiol (20 mcg and 10 mcg)	Desogestrel (0.15 mg)
Modicon (28-Day)	Ethinyl estradiol (35 mcg)	Norethindrone (0.5 mg)
Necon 0.5/35 (21- and 28-Day)	Ethinyl estradiol (35 mcg)	Norethindrone (0.5 mg)
Necon 1/35 (21- and 28-Day)	Ethinyl estradiol (35 mcg)	Norethindrone (1 mg)
Necon 1/50 (21- and 28-Day)	Mestranol (50 mcg)	Norethindrone (1 mg)
Nordette 28 (28-Day)	Ethinyl estradiol (30 mcg)	Levonorgestrel (0.15 mg)
Norinyl 1 + 35 (28-Day)	Ethinyl estradiol (35 mcg)	Norethindrone (1 mg)
Norinyl 1 + 50 (28-Day)	Mestranol (50 mcg)	Norethindrone (1 mg)
Nortrel 0.5/35 (21- and 28-Day)	Ethinyl estradiol (35 mcg)	Norethindrone (0.5 mg)
Nortrel 1/35 (21- and 28-Day)	Ethinyl estradiol (35 mcg)	Norethindrone (1 mg)
Ocella (28-Day)	Ethinyl estradiol (30 mcg)	Drospirenone (3 mg)
Ogestrel 0.5/50 (28-Day)	Ethinyl estradiol (50 mcg)	Norgestrel (0.5 mg)
Orsythia (28-Day)	Ethinyl estradiol (20 mcg)	Levonorgestrel (0.1 mg)
Ortho-Cept (28-Day)	Ethinyl estradiol (30 mcg)	Desogestrel (0.15 mg)
Ortho-Cyclen (28-Day)	Ethinyl estradiol (35 mcg)	Norgestimate (0.25 mg)
Ortho-Novum 1/35 (28-Day)	Ethinyl estradiol (35 mcg)	Norethindrone (1 mg)
Ortho Novum 1/50 (28-Day)	Mestranol (50 mcg)	Norethindrone (1 mg)
Ovcon-35 (28-Day)	Ethinyl estradiol (35 mcg)	Norethindrone (0.4 mg)
Ovcon-50 (28-Day)	Ethinyl estradiol (50 mcg)	Norethindrone (1 mg)
Ovral (21- and 28-Day)	Ethinyl estradiol (50 mcg)	Norgestrel (0.5 mg)

TRADE NAME	ESTROGEN	PROGESTIN
	MONOPHASIC	
Portia (21- and 28-Day)	Ethinyl estradiol (30 mcg)	Levonorgestrel (0.15 mg)
Previfem (28-Day)	Ethinyl estradiol (35 mcg)	Norgestimate (0.25 mg)
Quasense (1 hormone-containing tablet/day for 84 days followed by one inert tablet/day for 7 days)	Ethinyl estradiol (30 mcg)	Levonortestrol (0.15 mg)
Reclipsen (28-Day)	Ethinyl estradiol (30 mcg)	Desogestrel (0.15 mg)
Safyral (28-Day)	Ethinyl estradiol (30 mcg) (Also contains levomefolate calcium to raise folate levels)	Drospirenone (3 mg)
Seasonale*	Ethinyl estradiol (30 mcg)	Levonorgestrel (0.15 mg)
Solia (28-Day)	Ethinyl estradiol (30 mcg)	Desogestrel (0.15 mg)
Sprintec (28-Day)	Ethinyl estradiol (35 mcg)	Norgestimate (0.25 mg)
Sronyx (28-Day)	Ethinyl estradiol (20 mcg)	Levonorgestrol (0.1 mg)
Syeda (28-Day) °	Ethinyl estradiol (30 mcg)	Drospirenone (3 mg)
Yasmin (28-Day)	Ethinyl estradiol (30 mcg)	Drospirenone (3 mg)
YAZ (1-hormone-containing tablet for 24 days followed by 1 inert tablet/day for 4 days)	Ethinyl estradiol (20 mcg)	Drospirenone (3 mg)
Zarah (28-Day)	Ethinyl estradiol (30 mcg)	Drospirenone (3 mg)
Zenchent (28-Day)	Ethinyl estradiol (35 mcg)	Norethindrone (0.4 mg)
Zovia 1/35 E (21- and 28-Day)	Ethinyl estradiol (35 mcg)	Ethynodiol diacetate (1 mg)
Zovia 1/50 E (21- and 28-Day)	Ethinyl estradiol (50 mcg)	Ethynodiol diacetate (1 mg)
	BIPHASIC	
Necon 10/11 (28-Day)	Ethinyl estradiol (35 mcg in each tablet)	Norethindrone (10 tablets of 0.5 mg followed by 11 tablets of 1 mg)
Ortho-Novum 10/11 (28-Day)	Ethinyl estradiol (35 mcg in each tablet)	Norethindrone (10 tablets of 0.5 mg followed by 11 tablets of 1 mg)
Seasonique*	Ethinyl estradiol (30 mcg in 84 tablets followed by 10 mcg in 7 tablets)	Levonorgestrel (0.15 mg in 84 tablets; none in 7 tablets)
	TRIPHASIC	
Aranelle (28-Day)	Ethinyl estradiol (35 mcg in each tablet for 21 days)	Norethindrone (0.5 mg the first 7 days, 1 mg the next 9 days, and 0.5 mg the last 5 days)
Caziant	Ethinyl estradiol (25 mcg in each tablet for 21 days)	Desogestrel (0.1 mg the first 7 days, 0.125 mg the next 7 days, and 0.15 mg the last 7 days)
Cesia (28-Day)	Ethinyl estradiol (25 mcg in each tablet for 21 days)	Desogestrel (0.1 mg the first 7 days, 0.125 mg the next 7 days, and 0.15 the last 7 days)

TRADE NAME	ESTROGEN	PROGESTIN
	TRIPHASIC	
Cyclessa (28-Day)	Ethinyl estradiol (25 mcg in each tablet for 21 days)	Desogestrel (0.1 mg the first 7 days, 0.125 mg the next 7 days, and 0.15 mg the last 7 days)
Enpresse (28-Day)	Ethinyl estradiol (30 mcg the first 6 days, 40 mcg the next 5 days, and 30 mcg the last 10 days)	Levonorgestrel (0.05 mg the first 6 days, 0.075 mg the next 5 days, and 0.125 mg the last 10 days)
Estrostep Fe (28-Day)	Ethinyl estradiol (20 mcg the first 5 days, 30 mcg the next 7 days, and 35 mcg the last 9 days)	Norethindrone (1 mg in each tablet)
Leena (28-Day)	Ethinyl estradiol (35 mcg in each tablet for 21 days)	Norethindrone (0.5 mg the first 7 days, 1 mg the next 9 days, and 0.5 mg the last 5 days)
Necon 7/7/7 (28-Day)	Ethinyl estradiol (35 mcg in each tablet for 21 days)	Norethindrone (0.5 mg the first 7 days, 0.75 mg the next 7 days, and 1 mg the last 7 days)
Ortho-Novum 7/7/7 (28-Day)	Ethinyl estradiol (35 mcg in each tablet for 21 days)	Norethindrone (0.5 mg the first 7 days, 0.75 mg the next 7 days, and 1 mg the last 7 days)
Ortho Tri-Cyclen (28-Day)	Ethinyl estradiol (35 mcg in each tablet for 21 days)	Norgestimate (0.18 mg the first 7 days, 0.215 mg the next 7 days, and 0.25 mg the last 7 days)
Ortho Tri-Cyclen Lo (28-Day)	Ethinyl estradiol (25 mcg in each tablet for 21 days)	Norgestimate (0.18 mg the first 7 days, 0.215 mg the next 7 days, and 0.25 mg the last 7 days)
Tilia Fe (28-Day)	Ethinyl estradiol (20 mcg in each tablet for the first 5 days, and 30 mcg for the next 7 days, and 35 mcg for the last 9 days)	Norethindrone acetate (1 mg in each tablet)
TriNessa (28-Day)	Ethinyl estradiol (35 mcg in each tablet for 21 days)	Norgestimate (0.18 mg the first 7 days, 0.215 mg the next 7 days, and 0.25 mg the last 7 days)
Triphasil (21- and 28-Day)	Ethinyl estradiol (30 mcg the first 6 days, 40 mcg the next 5 days, and 30 mcg the last 10 days)	Levonorgestrel (0.05 mg the first 6 days, 0.075 mg the next 5 days, and 0.125 mg the last 10 days)
Trivora (28-Day)	Ethinyl estradiol (30 mcg the first 6 days, 40 mcg the next 5 days, and 30 mcg the last 10 days	Levonorgestrel (0.05 mg the first 6 days, 0.075 mg the next 5 days, and 0.125 mg the last 10 days)
Velivet (28-Day)	Ethinyl estradiol (25 mcg in each tablet for 21 days)	Desogestrel (0.1 mg the first 7 days, 0.125 mg the next 7 days, and 0.15 mg the last 7 days)
	FOUR PHASES	
Natazia	2 tablets containing estradiol valerate (3 mg); 5 tablets containing estradiol valerate (2 mg) and dienogest (2 mg); 17 tablets containing estradiol valerate (2 mg) and dienogest (2 mg); and 2 tablets containing estradiol valerate (2 mg), i.e., 26-day hormone cycle (plus 2 inert tablets)	

TRADE NAME	ESTROGEN	PROGESTIN
	CONTRACEPTIVE PATCH	
ClimaraPro	Estradiol (45 mcg)	Levonorgestrel (0.015 mg)
	PROGESTIN-ONLY PRODUCTS**	
Camila (28-Day)		Norethindrone (0.35 mg)
Errin (28-Day)		Norethindrone (0.35 mg)
Jolivette (28-Day)		Norethindrone (0.35 mg)
Nor-QD (28-Day)		Norethindrone (0.35 mg)
Nora-BE (28-Day)		Norethindrone (0.35 mg)
Ortho-Micronor		Norethindrone (0.35 mg)
	EMERGENCY CONTRACEPTIVES	
Ella	No estrogen	Ulipristal acetate (30 mg)
One tablet as soon as possible within 120 hr (5 days) of unprotected intercourse or a known or suspected contraceptive failure. Use before menarche is not indicated.		
Next Choice	No estrogen	Levonorgestrel (0.75 mg)
One tablet within 72 hr after unprotected intercourse with the second tablet taken 12 hr after the first dose. Available OTC for women 17 years and older with a government-issued identification and by Rx for younger women.		
Plan B	No estrogen	Levonorgestrel (0.75 mg)
One tablet within 72 hr after unprotected intercourse with the second tablet taken 12 hr after the first dose. Available OTC for women 17 years and older with a government-issued identification and by Rx for younger women.		
Plan B One-Step	No estrogen	Levonorgestrel (1.5 mg)
1 tablet as soon as possible within 72 hr of unprotected intercourse or a known or suspected contraceptive failure. Available OTC for women 17 years and older and by Rx for younger women.		

* See Administration for special dosage/administration information.

** All progestin-only products contain 28 tablets/pack.

*** Except where noted or for progestin-only products, 28-day products contain either 7 inert tablets or 7 iron-containing tablets.

NOTE: Yasmin may cause hyperkalemia in high-risk clients. Do not use in clients with conditions that predispose to hyperkalemia (e.g., renal insufficiency, hepatic dysfunction, adrenal insufficiency).

SPECIAL CONCERNS

■ Cigarette smoking increases the risk of cardiovascular side effects from use of oral contraceptives. This risk increases with age and with heavy smoking (15 or more cigarettes per day) and is marked in women over 35 years of age. Women who use OCs should not smoke. ■

- There is an increased risk of thromboembolism, stroke, MI, hypertension, hepatic neoplasia, and gallbladder disease. The risk of CV and circulatory disease in OC users is significantly increased in women 35 years and older with other risk factors (e.g., smoking, uncontrolled hypertension, hypercholesterolemia, obesity, diabetes).
- Use with caution in clients with a history of hypertension, preexisting renal disease, hypertension-related diseases during pregnancy, familial tendency to hypertension or its consequences, a history of excessive weight gain or fluid retention during the menstrual cycle; these individuals are more likely to develop elevated BP.
- Use with caution in clients with asthma, epilepsy, migraine, diabetes, metabolic bone disease, renal or cardiac disease, and a history of mental depression.
- Use with drugs (e.g., barbiturates, hydantoins, rifampin) that increase the hepatic metabolism of oral contraceptives may result in breakthrough bleeding and an increased risk of pregnancy. The risk of becoming pregnant may be increased in overweight women.
- Progestin-only products do not appear to have any adverse effects on breastfeeding performance or on the health, growth, or development of the infant.

SIDE EFFECTS

Oral contraceptives. The oral contraceptives have wide-ranging side effects. These are particularly important, since the drugs may be given for several years to healthy women. Many authorities have voiced concern about the long-term safety of these agents. Some advise discontinuing therapy after 18–24 months of continuous use. The majority of side effects of oral contraceptives are due to the estrogen component. **CV:** ***Mesenteric thrombosis, MI, thrombophlebitis, venous thrombosis with or without embolism, pulmonary embolism, coronary thrombosis, cerebral thrombosis, arterial thromboembolism, mesenteric thrombosis, thrombotic and hemorrhagic strokes, postsurgical thromboembolism, subarachnoid hemorrhage, cerebral hemorrhage***, elevated BP, hypertension. **CNS:** Onset or exacerbation of migraine headaches, depression, headaches, dizziness. **GI:** N&V, bloating, diarrhea, abdominal cramps. **Ophthalmic:** Optic neuritis, retinal thrombosis, steepening of the corneal curvature, contact lens intolerance. **Hepatic:** ***Benign and malignant hepatic adenomas, benign liver tumors***, focal nodular hyperplasia, ***hepatocellular carcinoma***, gallbladder disease, cholestatic jaundice, acute intermittent porphyria. **GU:** Breakthrough bleeding, spotting, amenorrhea during and after treatment, change in menstrual flow, change in cervical erosion and cervical secretions, ***invasive cervical cancer***, bleeding irregularities (more common with progestin-only products), vaginal candidiasis, ***ectopic pregnancies in contraceptive failures, increase in size of pre-existing uterine fibroids***, temporary infertility after discontinuation, breast tenderness, breast enlargement, breast secretion. **Dermatologic:** Melasma (may persist), allergic rash, hirsutism (rare). **Miscellaneous:** Photosensitivity, congenital anomalies, edema/fluid retention, increase or decrease in weight, decreased carbohydrate tolerance, increased incidence of cervical *Chlamydia trachomatis,* decrease in the quantity and quality of breast milk.

Emergency contraceptives. Abdominal pain/cramps, breast tenderness, diarrhea, dizziness, fatigue, headache, menstrual irregularities, N&V.

DRUG INTERACTIONS

Acetaminophen / ↓ Effect of acetaminophen R/T ↑ liver metabolism

Acitretin / Acitretin interferes with effect of progestin-only products

Anticoagulants, oral / ↓ Effect of anticoagulants by ↑ levels of certain clotting factors (however, an ↑ effect of anticoagulants has also been noted in some clients)

Antidepressants, tricyclic / ↑ Effect of antidepressants R/T ↓ liver metabolism

Atorvastatin / ↑ AUC of steroid hormones

Barbiturates / ↓ OC effectiveness R/T ↑ liver metabolism
Benzodiazepines / ↑ Effect of alprazolam, chlordiazepoxide, diazepam, and triazolam R/T ↓ in liver breakdown; ↓ effect of lorazepam, oxazepam, and temazepam R/T ↑ liver breakdown
Beta-adrenergic blockers / ↑ Effect of beta blockers R/T ↓ liver metabolism
H ***Black cohosh*** / Interferes with effect of oral contraceptives
Caffeine / ↑ Effect of caffeine R/T ↓ liver metabolism
Carbamazepine / ↓ Effect of OCs R/T ↑ liver metabolism
Corticosteroids / ↑ Effect of corticosteroids R/T ↓ liver metabolism
Cyclosporine / ↑ Risk of cyclosporine toxicity R/T ↓ liver metabolism; do not use together
Dexamethasone ↓ Effect of OCs R/T ↑ liver metabolism
Ethosuximide / ↓ Effect of OCs R/T ↑ liver metabolism
Felbamate / ↓ Effect of OCs R/T ↑ liver metabolism
Griseofulvin / ↓ Effect of OCs R/T altered steroid gut metabolism; also, ↓ OC effectiveness R/T ↑ liver metabolism
Hydantoins / ↓ OC effectiveness R/T ↑ liver metabolism; also, effect of hydantoins may be altered
Hypoglycemics / ↓ Effect of hypoglycemics R/T OC effect on carbohydrate metabolism
Insulin / OCs may ↑ insulin requirements
Lamotrigine / ↓ Lamotrigine plasma levels R/T ↑ liver metabolism; also, ↓ oral contraceptive hormone levels
Modafinil / ↓ OC effectiveness R/T ↑ liver metabolism
Nevirapine / ↓ Effect of OCs R/T ↑ liver metabolism
Oxcarbazepine / ↓ Effect of OCs R/T ↑ liver metabolism
Penicillins, oral / ↓ Effect of OCs R/T altered steroid gut metabolism
Phenobarbital / ↓ Effect of OCs R/T ↑ liver metabolism
Phenytoin / ↓ Effect of OCs R/T ↑ liver metabolism
Primidone / ↓ Effect of OCs R/T ↑ liver metabolism
Protease inhibitors / ↓ Effect of OCs R/T ↑ liver metabolism
Pyridoxine / Concomitant use may ↑ pyridoxine requirements
Rifabutin,Rifampin, Rifapentine / ↓ Effect of contraceptives R/T ↑ liver metabolism
Ritonavir / ↓ Effect of contraceptives R/T ↑ liver breakdown of ethinyl estradiol
H ***Saw palmetto*** / ↓ OCs effect R/T antiestrogenic activity
Selegiline / ↑ Selegiline plasma levels R/T ↓ metabolism
Smoking / Possible ↓ OC effectiveness R/T ↑ metabolism of hormones in OC's
H ***St. John's wort*** / ↑ Risk of breakthrough bleeding and contraceptive failure R/T ↑ liver metabolism of OC hormones
Tetracyclines / ↓ Effect of contraceptives R/T altered steroid gut metabolism
Theophyllines / ↑ Effect of theophyllines R/T ↓ liver breakdown
Topiramate / ↓ Effect of contraceptive R/T ↑ hepatic metabolism
Troleandomycin / ↑ Chance of jaundice
Valproic acid / Possible ↑ seizure frequency R/T ↑ metabolism of valproic acid
Warfarin / ↑ Risk of clotting

LABORATORY TEST CONSIDERATIONS

↑ Prothrombin, factors VII, VIII, IX, X; fibrinogen; norepinephrine-induced platelet aggregation; thyroid-binding globulin, leading to ↑ total thyroid hormone (as measured by protein bound iodine T_4, by column or radioimmunoassay); corticosteroid levels; triglycerides and phospholipids; aldosterone; amylase; gamma-glutamyltranspeptidase; iron-binding capacity; sex-hormone-binding globulins, leading to ↑ levels of total circulating sex steroids and corticoids; transferrin; prolactin; renin activity; vitamin A.

↓ Antithrombin III; free T_3 resin uptake; response to metyrapone test; folate; glucose tolerance; albumin; cholinesterase; haptoglobin; tissue plasminogen activator; zinc; vitamin B_{12}; sex-hormone-binding globulin.

Progestin-only products: ↓ Thyroxine due to ↓ thyroid-binding globulin. Some progestins may ↑ LDL and ↓ HDL.

Oral contraceptives may ↑ HDL and cholesterol, ↑ or ↓ LDL, and ↓ LDL/HDL ratio while triglycerides remain unchanged.

DOSAGE

TABLETS

Contraception.

See *Implementation/Administration/Storage.* For any specific combination, use the dosage regimen that contains the least amount of estrogen and progestin compatible with a low failure rate and the needs of the client. Start new clients on products containing 35 mcg or less of estrogen.

Emergency contraception.

Take one tablet as soon as possible but within 72 hr (Next Choice, Plan B, Plan B-One Step) of unprotected intercourse. For Next Choice and Plan B, take a second tablet 12 hr after the first dose. For Ella, take one tablet within 5 days of unprotected intercourse. Can be used any time during the menstrual cycle.

Acne vulgaris.

Estrostep or Ortho Tri-Cyclen: Take 1 hormone-containing tablet daily for 21 days followed by 1 inert tablet daily for 7 days. After 28 tablets have been taken, a new course is started the next day.

NURSING IMPLICATIONS

IMPLEMENTATION/ADMINISTRATION/STORAGE

1. For combination oral contraceptive products:
   - *Sunday start.* If the product is to be started on Sunday, the first tablet should be taken the Sunday following the beginning of menses; if menses begins on Sunday, the first tablet should be taken that day.
   - *21-Day regimen.* Count the first day of menstrual bleeding as Day 1. Take 1 tablet per day for 21 days. No tablets are taken for 7 days. Whether menstrual flow has stopped or not, a new 21-day course of therapy is started. This schedule is followed whether flow occurs as expected or whether spotting or breakthrough bleeding occurs during the cycle. Withdrawal flow will usually begin about 3 days after the last hormone-containing tablet is taken.
   - *28-Day regimen.* To eliminate the necessity to count the days between cycles, many products contain 7 inert or iron-containing tablets. Hormone-containing tablets are taken for the first 21 days followed by 7 days of inert or iron-containing tablets, i.e., a tablet is taken every day of the year.
   - *Biphasic and Triphasic products.* The biphasic and triphasic products have varying amounts of estrogen and/or progestin, depending on the stage of the cycle; the client should understand fully how these preparations are to be taken and which tablets are to be taken at various times during the medication cycle. Often tablets are different shapes and/or colors to help with compliance. The client should be instructed when to take the various colored tablets in each product.
   - *Four phases.* The product contains four phases with each phase containing either estrogen alone (phases 1 and 4) or estrogen plus progestin (phases 2 and 3) for a total of 26 hormone-containing tablets; the product also contains 2 inert tablets.
2. Certain combination oral contraceptive products consist of chewable tablets.
3. *Progestin-only products.* The first tablet is taken on the first day of menses; thereafter, 1 tablet is taken daily every day of the year with no interruption between tablet packs. If the client is >3 hr late or misses 1 or more tablets, she should take the missed tablet as soon as remembered; then, go back to taking the progestin-only product at the regular time. A back up method of contraception (e.g. condom, spermicide) should be used every time the woman has sexual intercourse for the next 48 hr.
4. Ovcon 35 (norethindrone/ethinyl estradiol) is available as a chewable, oral, spearmint-flavored contraceptive tablet. The tablet may also be swallowed whole. If chewed, the woman should drink a full glass of water immediately after to ensure the full dose reaches the stomach.
5. Four of the monophasic oral contraceptive products are taken differently than other products. They are:
   - Kariva or Mircette. Each product contains ethinyl estradiol and desogestrel. Take one 20-mcg ethinyl estradiol/0.15 mg desogestrel tablet per day for 21 days followed

by 1 inert tablet per day for 2 days and then one 10-mcg ethinyl estradiol tablet per day for 5 days.

- Seasonale (ethinyl estradiol and levonorgestrel). Take one hormone-containing tablet per day for 84 days followed by 7 days of inert tablets (i.e., a total of 91 days per cycle). The client then begins the next and all subsequent cycles without interruption. Although women have menstrual periods only 4 times per year, there are more instances of unplanned bleeding and spotting between menstrual cycles, especially in the first few cycles of use. Withdrawal bleeding should begin during the 7 days following discontinuation of hormone-containing tablets. For the first 7 days of the first cycle, the client should use a nonhormonal backup method of birth control.
- Seasonique or LoSeasonique are extended-cycle oral contraceptives containing ethinyl estradiol (30 mcg for Seasonique or 25 mcg for LoSeasonique) and levonorgestrel (0.15 mg for Seasonique and 0.1 mg for LoSeasonique) in the first 84 tablets and ethinyl estradiol (10 mcg for both Seasonique and LoSeasonique) in the last 7 tablets. The 91-day cycle results in 4 menstrual periods per year (which occurs when the client is taking the 7 tablets containing 10 mcg ethinyl estradiol). Take the first tablet in a package on the first Sunday after the period begins, even if bleeding is still occurring. If the period starts on Sunday, take the first tablet that day. Another form of birth control should be used for the first 7 days after beginning Seasonique. Take one tablet every day at the same time, without interruption. After taking the last tablet containing 10 mcg ethinyl estradiol (white tablet), the client starts a new pack the very next day; no days are to be skipped.

6. Do not confuse the monophasic oral contraceptives Yasmin and Yaz.
7. Take tablets at approximately the same time each day.
8. Spotting or breakthrough bleeding may occur for the first 1–2 cycles; report if it continues past this time.
9. Side effects seen during the first few cycles may be transient. If they continue, dosage adjustment may be required as many of the side effects are related to the potency of the estrogen or progestin in the product.
10. For the initial cycle, use an **additional** form of contraception the first week.
11. For emergency contraception:
    - If vomiting occurs within 1 hr of taking either dose of the medication, the provider should be contacted to discuss whether or not to repeat the dose or take an antinausea medication.
    - Emergency contraception tablets are not to be used for ongoing pregnancy protection and are not to be used as a routine form of contraception by women.
12. If it is necessary to switch from combination therapy to progestin-only therapy, take the first progestin-only tablet the day after the last hormone-containing combination therapy tablet is finished. None of the 7 inactive tablets are to be taken. Many women have irregular periods after switching to progestin-only tablets; this is normal and to be expected. If switching from progestin-only to combination therapy, take the first hormone-containing combination therapy tablet on the first day of menses, even if the progestin-only pack is not finished. If switching to another brand of progestin-only products, start the new brand any time.
13. Non-nursing mothers may begin oral contraceptive therapy at the first postpartum exam (i.e., 4–6 weeks), regardless of whether spontaneous menstruation has occurred. Nursing mothers should not take oral contraceptives until the infant is weaned. Start no earlier than 4–6 weeks after a midtrimester pregnancy termination. Immediate postpartum use increases the risk of thromboembolism.
14. If the woman is fully breast-feeding (i.e., not giving the baby any food or formula), start the client on progestin-only products 6 weeks after delivery. If partially breast-feeding (giving the baby some food or formula), the client should start taking progestin-only products 3 weeks after delivery.
15. In the nonlactating mother, Seasonale may be started no earlier than day 28 postpartum because of the increased risk of thromboembol-

ism. Advise the client to use a nonhormonal backup method for the first 7 days of tablet-taking. However, if intercourse has already occurred, consider the possibility of ovulation and conception prior to beginning the medication. Seasonale may be started immediately after a first-trimester abortion; if the client starts Seasonale immediately, additional contraceptive measures are not needed.

ASSESSMENT

1. Note annual physical/internal exams, mammograms, and Pap smears. List any previous experience with these agents and results.
2. Report any family history of breast or uterine cancer or any existing medical condition that may preclude this drug therapy; assess smoking history.
3. Identify any abnormal vaginal bleeding. Assess contraceptive needs, and check to ensure not pregnant.
4. Explain that hormones (synthetic) that mimic natural estrogens and/or progesterone's attempt to "trick" the female reproductive system. They accomplish this by providing constant levels of these hormones in the blood and thus suppressing the release of follicle stimulating hormone (FSH) and leutinizing hormone (LH). FSH suppression inhibits the maturation of the egg in the ovary, while LH inhibits the release of the egg from the ovary. With a constant level of estrogen and progestin in the body, the endometrium will not be able to thicken sufficiently in order for the egg to attach.
5. A thick, opaque mucus is produced as a result of circulating progestins which prevents sperm from passing through and it also causes changes in the fallopian tubes that can impede the movement of the egg towards the uterus.
6. A combination of estrogen and progestin may interfere with the muscle contraction in the tubes and uterus thus interfering with implantation, all of which contribute to preventing pregnancy.
7. Reinforce that in no way do these hormones provide any protection against sexually transmitted diseases and protection must be used with each encounter.

CLIENT/FAMILY TEACHING

1. Take tablets or apply patches exactly as prescribed to prevent pregnancy. Take oral contraceptives with food. However, avoid taking with grapefruit juice.
2. If you vomit within 1 hr of taking Plan B for emergency contraception, contact your provider to determine whether or not to repeat that dose or take an antinauseant.
3. There is little likelihood that ovulation will occur if only 1 tablet is missed; however, the possibility of spotting or bleeding is increased. The possibility of ovulation occurring increases with each successive day that scheduled hormone-containing tablets are missed. The following guidelines can be followed for missed tablets:
   - If 1 combination therapy tablet is missed, take as soon as remembered or take 2 tablets the next day. As an alternative, take 1 tablet, discard the other missed tablet, and continue as scheduled. Use another form of contraception until menses.
   - If 2 combination therapy tablets are missed consecutively, take 2 tablets as soon as remembered with the next tablet at the usual time; or, take 2 tablets daily for the next 2 days and then resume the regular schedule. Use an additional form of contraception for the remainder of the cycle. If 2 hormone-containing tablets are missed in a row in the third week and the client is on a Sunday start regimen, take 1 tablet every day until Sunday. On Sunday, the rest of the pack is discarded and a new pack of tablets started that same day. If 2 hormone-containing tablets are missed in a row in the third week and the client is a Day 1 starter, discard the rest of the pack and a new pack is started on that day. Menses may not occur during this month; this is expected. If menses does not occur 2 months in a row, contact the provider as pregnancy is possible.
   - If 3 combination therapy tablets are missed consecutively and the client is a Sunday starter, she should keep taking 1 tablet per day until Sunday. On Sunday, the rest of the pack is discarded and a new pack started that same day. If the client is a Day 1 starter, the rest of the pack is dis-

carded and a new pack is started that same day. Menses may not occur during this month; this is expected. If menses does not occur 2 months in a row, contact the provider as pregnancy is possible. Pregnancy may occur during the 7 days after tablets are missed; thus, use another method of birth control as a back-up for those 7 days.

- If the client is more than 3 hr late or misses 1 or more progestin-only tablets, she should take the missed tablet as soon as remembered. Then, take tablets at the regular time. A back-up contraception method must be used every time she has intercourse for the 48 hr following the late or missed tablet. Report any missed menstrual periods. If two consecutive periods are missed, discontinue therapy until pregnancy ruled out.

4. Report pain in the legs or chest, respiratory distress, unexplained cough, severe headaches, dizziness, blurred vision, or partial loss of sight; stop therapy and notify provider immediately.
5. Oral contraceptives decrease the viscosity of cervical mucus, increasing the susceptibility to vaginal infections that are difficult to treat; regular careful hygienic practice is essential.
6. Report if persistent nausea, swelling, and skin eruptions develop and last beyond the four cycles; a dose adjustment or different combination may be needed.
7. Any changes in thought processes, depression, or fatigue should be reported; preparations with less progesterone may be needed.
8. Androgenic effects, such as weight gain, increased oiliness of the skin, acne, or ↑ hairiness may require a change in medication or dosage.
9. Do not take longer than 18 months without medical consultation. Report for yearly Pap smear testing, and physical examination; perform regular BSE (1 week after or 2 weeks before menstrual cycle) and report any changes/findings.
10. Practice another form of contraception if receiving ampicillin, anticonvulsants, rifampin, or tetracycline. These may cause intermittent bleeding and interactions could result in pregnancy.
11. Contraceptives interfere with the elimination of caffeine. Limit caffeine consumption to prevent insomnia, irritability, tremors, and cardiac irregularities.
12. If breast-feeding infant, another form of contraception should be used until lactation is well established.
13. **Do not smoke.** Attend formal smoking cessation program.
14. Avoid prolonged or excessive exposure to direct or artificial sunlight.
15. Oral contraceptives do not provide any protection against STDs; use appropriate barrier protection with intercourse.
16. Some potential risks, related to endometrial/breast cancer, have been associated with estrogen therapy. Close medical follow-up required.
17. Identify goals of therapy and best way to attain.
18. Keep all F/U to assess response, labs, and for adverse SE.

OUTCOMES/EVALUATE

- Desired contraception
- ↓ Severity of endometriosis
- Menstrual regularity
- ↓ Blood loss (hypermenorrhea) with hormone imbalances
- Emergency contraception with various products

PENICILLINS ■

SEE ALSO THE FOLLOWING INDIVIDUAL ENTRIES:

Amoxicillin
Amoxicillin and Potassium clavulanate
Ampicillin oral
Ampicillin sodium, parenteral
Ampicillin sodium/Sulbactam sodium
Penicillin G aqueous
Penicillin G benzathine and Penicillin G procaine
Penicillin G benzathine, intramuscular
Penicillin G procaine, intramuscular
Penicillin V potassium
Piperacillin sodium and Tazobactam sodium
Ticarcillin disodium and Clavulanate potassium

GENERAL STATEMENT

Penicillins may be classified as: (1) Natural: Penicillin G, Penicillin V. (2) Aminopenicillins: Amoxicillin, Amoxicillin/potassium clavulanate, Ampicillin, Ampicillin/sulbactam, Bacampicillin.

(3) Penicillinase-resistant: Cloxacillin, Dicloxacillin, Nafcillin, Oxacillin. (4) Extended spectrum: Carbenicillin, Mezlocillin, Piperacillin/Tazobactam sodium, Ticarcillin/Potassium clavulanate.

INDICATIONS/USES

See individual drugs. Effective against a variety of gram-positive, gram-negative, and anaerobic organisms.

ACTION/KINETICS

Action

The bactericidal action of penicillins depends on their ability to bind penicillin-binding proteins (PBP-1 and PBP-3) in the cytoplasmic membranes of bacteria, thus inhibiting cell wall synthesis. Some penicillins act by acylation of membrane-bound transpeptidase enzymes, thereby preventing cross-linkage of peptidoglycan chains, which are necessary for bacterial cell wall strength and rigidity. Cell division and growth are inhibited and often lysis and elongation of susceptible bacteria occur. Penicillin is most effective against young, rapidly dividing organisms and has little effect on mature resting cells. Depending on the concentration of the drug at the site of infection and the susceptibility of the infectious microorganism, penicillin is either bacteriostatic or bactericidal.

Pharmacokinetics

Penicillins are distributed throughout most of the body and pass the placental barrier. They also pass into synovial, pleural, pericardial, peritoneal, ascitic, and spinal fluids. Although normal meninges and the eyes are relatively impermeable to penicillins, they are better absorbed by inflamed meninges and eyes. **Peak serum levels, after PO:** 1 hr. **t½:** 30–110 min; protein binding: 20–98% (see individual agents). Excreted largely unchanged by the urine as a result of glomerular filtration and active tubular secretion.

CONTRAINDICATIONS

Hypersensitivity to penicillins, imipenem, beta-lactamase inhibitors, and cephalosporins. PO use of penicillins during the acute stages of empyema, bacteremia, pneumonia, meningitis, pericarditis, and purulent or septic arthritis. Use with a history of amoxicillin/clavulanate-associated cholestatic jaundice or hepatic dysfunction. Lactation.

SPECIAL CONCERNS

- **Use of penicillins during lactation may lead to sensitization, diarrhea, candidiasis, and skin rash in the infant.**
- **Use with caution in clients with a history of asthma, hay fever, or urticaria.**
- **Clients with cystic fibrosis have a higher incidence of side effects with broad-spectrum penicillins.**
- **Safety and efficacy of carbenicillin, piperacillin, and the beta-lactamase inhibitor/penicillin combinations (e.g., amoxicillin/potassium clavulanate, ticarcillin/potassium clavulanate) have not been determined in children less than age 12.**
- **The incidence of resistant strains of staphylococci to penicillinase-resistant penicillins is increasing.**
- **Use of prolonged therapy may lead to superinfection (i.e., bacterial or fungal overgrowth of nonsusceptible organisms).**
- **Cystic fibrosis clients have a higher incidence of side effects if given extended spectrum penicillins.**

SIDE EFFECTS

Penicillins are potent sensitizing agents; it is estimated that up to 10% of the U.S. population is allergic to the antibiotic. Hypersensitivity reactions are reported to be on the increase in pediatric populations. Sensitivity reactions may be immediate (within 20 min) or delayed (as long as several days or weeks after initiation of therapy).**Allergic:** Skin rashes (including maculopapular and exanthematous), exfoliative dermatitis, erythema multiforme (rarely, ***Stevens-Johnson syndrome***), hives, pruritus, wheezing, ***anaphylaxis***, fever, eosinophilia, hypersensitivity myocarditis, ***angioedema***, serum sickness, ***laryngeal edema, laryngospasm, prostration, angioneurotic edema, bronchospasm***, hypotension, ***vascular collapse, death***. **GI:** Diarrhea (may be severe), abdominal cramps or pain, N&V, bloating, flatulence, increased thirst, bitter/unpleasant taste, glossitis, gastritis, stomatitis, dry mouth, sore mouth/tongue, furry tongue, black "hairy" tongue, bloody diarrhea, rectal bleeding, enterocolitis, pseudomembranous colitis. **CNS:** Dizziness, insomnia, hyperactivity, fatigue, prolonged muscle relaxation. Neurotoxicity including lethargy, neuromuscular irritability, ***seizures***, hallucinations following large IV doses (especially in clients

Classifications

with renal failure). **Hematologic:** Thrombocytopenia, leukopenia, ***agranulocytosis***, anemia, thrombocytopenic purpura, ***hemolytic anemia***, granulocytopenia, neutropenia, bone marrow depression. **Renal:** Oliguria, hematuria, hyaline casts, proteinuria, pyuria (all symptoms of interstitial nephritis), nephropathy. Electrolyte imbalance following IV use. **Miscellaneous:** Hepatotoxicity (cholestatic jaundice), superinfection, swelling of face and ankles, anorexia, hyperthermia, transient hepatitis, vaginitis, itchy eyes. IM injection may cause pain and induration at the injection site, ecchymosis, and hematomas. IV use may cause vein irritation, deep vein thrombosis, and thrombophlebitis.

OVERDOSE MANAGEMENT

Symptoms: Neuromuscular hyperexcitability, ***convulsive seizures.*** Massive IV doses may cause agitation, asterixis, hallucinations, confusion, stupor, multifocal myoclonus, ***seizures***, coma, hyperkalemia, and encephalopathy.

Treatment (Severe Allergic or Anaphylactic Reactions): Administer epinephrine (0.3–0.5 mL of a 1:1,000 solution SC or IM, or 0.2–0.3 mL diluted in 10 mL saline, given slowly by IV). Corticosteroids should be on hand. In those instances where penicillin is the drug of choice, the physician may decide to use it even though the client is allergic, adding a medication to the regimen to control the allergic response.

DRUG INTERACTIONS

Aminoglycosides / Penicillins ↓ effect of aminoglycosides, although they are used together
Antacids / ↓ Effect of penicillins R/T ↓ GI tract absorption
Antibiotics (chloramphenicol, erythromycins, tetracyclines) / ↓ Effect of penicillins, although synergism has also been seen
Anticoagulants / ↑ Bleeding risk by prolonging bleeding time if used with parenteral penicillins
Aspirin / ↑ Effect of penicillins by ↓ plasma protein binding
Chloramphenicol / Either ↑ or ↓ effects
Erythromycins / Either ↑ or ↓ effects
Heparin / ↑ Risk of bleeding following parenteral penicillins
Oral contraceptives / ↓ Effect of OCs
Probenecid / ↑ Effect of penicillins by ↓ excretion
Tetracyclines / ↓ Effect of penicillins

LABORATORY TEST CONSIDERATIONS

↓ Hematocrit, hemoglobin, WBC lymphocytes, serum potassium, albumin, total proteins, uric acid. ↑ Basophils, lymphocytes, monocytes, platelets, serum alkaline phosphatase, serum sodium. ↑ AST, ALT, bilirubin, LDH following semisynthetic penicillins.

DOSAGE

See individual drugs. Penicillins are available in a variety of dosage forms for PO, parenteral, inhalation, and intrathecal administration. PO doses must be higher than IM or SC doses because a large fraction of penicillin given PO may be destroyed in the stomach.

NURSING IMPLICATIONS

IMPLEMENTATION/ADMINISTRATION/STORAGE

1. **IM and IV administration of penicillin causes a great deal of local irritation; thus, inject slowly.**
2. **IM injections are made deeply into the gluteal muscle. IV injections are usually diluted with a compatible IV infusion solution.**

ASSESSMENT

1. **Note reasons for therapy, onset, location, symptom characteristics, clinical presentation, other agents trialed/outcome, culture results.**
2. **Assess for allergic reactions; if reaction occurs, stop drug immediately. Allergic reactions are more likely to occur with a history of asthma, hay fever, urticaria, or allergy to cephalosporins.**
3. **Penicillins were the first antibiotics discovered as natural products from the mold *Penicillium*. They produce their bactericidal effects by inhibition of bacterial cell wall synthesis.**
4. **Detain in an ambulatory care site for at least 20 min after administering to assess for anaphylaxis. Approximately 300–500 people die each year from penicillin-induced anaphylaxis. In these individuals, the beta-lactam ring binds to serum proteins, initiating an IgE-mediated inflammatory response. There is a 10% cross reactivity with cephalosporins.**
5. **Long-acting types of penicillin are for IM use only; may cause emboli, CNS/cardiac pathol-**

Classifications

LABORATORY TEST CONSIDERATIONS

↑ AST, ALT, alkaline phosphatase, bilirubin.

DOSAGE

See individual drugs.

NURSING IMPLICATIONS

IMPLEMENTATION/ADMINISTRATION/STORAGE

1. Take with meals.
2. Antacids may be used with proton pump inhibitors.

ASSESSMENT

1. Note reasons for therapy, characteristics of S&S, other agents trialed. List drugs prescribed to ensure none interact or require acidity for metabolism.
2. Record abdominal assessments, x-ray (UGI, US, barium enema), CT/MRI, or endoscopic findings and *H. pylori* results.
3. Check BMD and for evidence of osteoporosis with long-term therapy.
4. Ensure those with MI hx and prescribed clopidogrel are aware that PPIs may block the effectiveness of clopidogrel and not reduce risk of another MI.
5. Identify what may be contributing to symptoms, i.e., tomato-based dishes, peppermint, consumption of alcohol and tobacco, lying down after eating, wearing tight waisted pants, Barrett's, *H. pylori* infection, etc. Determine if pregnant.
6. Assess LFTs; may reduce dose of some to every 4 days with dysfunction to prevent drug accumulations. Monitor CBC PRN.

CLIENT/FAMILY TEACHING

1. Take as directed with meals. Swallow tablets whole; do not open, crush, chew, or split tablets.
2. Do not perform activities that require mental alertness until drug effects realized. Report unusual bleeding, acid reflux, abdominal pain, severe lightheadedness/diarrhea, rash, worsening of symptoms or lack of effectiveness. Review drug-associated side effects; report if diarrhea persists.
3. Avoid alcohol, NSAIDs, and salicylates; may increase GI upset. Report any changes in urinary elimination, pain or discomfort.
4. Follow prescribed diet and activities to control S&S of GERD. Drug should be withdrawn once condition cleared/resolved and new eating behaviors and lifestyle changes in effect.
5. Long-term use significantly increases the risk of osteoporosis related fractures.
6. Generally these drugs are for short-term use only as they inhibit total gastric acid secretion. Side effects of prolonged therapy and suppression of acid secretion alter bacterial colonization and lead to hypochlorhydria and hypergastrinemia which may cause an increased risk for gastric tumors.
7. Keep all F/U to assess response, labs, and for adverse SE.

OUTCOMES/EVALUATE

- ↓ Intraesophageal acid exposure
- Promotion of ulcer/esophageal tissue healing; relief of pain
- ↓ Gastric acid production

SELECTIVE SEROTONIN REUPTAKE INHIBITORS

SEE ALSO THE FOLLOWING INDIVIDUAL ENTRIES:

Citalopram hydrobromide
Escitalopram oxalate
Fluoxetine hydrochloride
Fluvoxamine maleate
Paroxetine hydrochloride
Paroxetine mesylate
Sertraline hydrochloride

INDICATIONS/USES

See individual entries. Depending on the drug, uses include: (1) Depression. (2) Obsessive-compulsive disorder. (3) Panic disorder. (4) Bulimia nervosa. (5) Generalized anxiety disorder. (6) Premenstrual dysphoric disorder. (7) Posttraumatic stress disorder. (8) Social anxiety disorder. *Investigational:* Enuresis.

ACTION/KINETICS

Action

Antidepressant effect probably due to inhibition of CNS neuronal reuptake of serotonin and to a lesser extent to norepinephrine and dopamine neuronal reuptake. Not related chemically to tricyclic, tetracyclic, or other antidepressants. Slight to no anticholinergic, sedative, or orthostatic hypotensive effects.

Classifications

Pharmacokinetics

All are extensively metabolized by the liver. The mean maximum plasma levels are higher in geriatric clients and the elimination half-life is delayed in these clients.

CONTRAINDICATIONS

Hypersensitivity to any SSRI or any components of the products. Use in combination with an MAOI or within 14 days of stopping an MAOI. Lactation.

SPECIAL CONCERNS

■ Antidepressants increased the risk of suicidal thinking and behavior (suicidality) in short-term studies in children, adolescents, and young adults with major depressive disorder and other psychiatric disorders. Anyone considering the use of an SSRI or any other antidepressant in a child, adolescent, or young adult must balance this risk with the clinical need. Clients who are started on therapy should be observed closely for clinical worsening, suicidality, or unusual changes in behavior. Families and caregivers should be advised of the need for close observation and communication with the prescriber. Some SSRIs are not approved for use in pediatric clients. Studies have shown a greater risk of adverse reactions representing suicidal thinking or behavior during the first few months of treatment in those receiving antidepressants. The average risk of such reactions in those receiving antidepressants is 4%, twice the placebo risk of 2%. No suicides occurred in these trials. ■

- **Use with caution in clients with severe hepatic impairment.**
- **Use during pregnancy only if clearly needed; possible neonatal withdrawal and/or seizures may occur when therapy is used during pregnancy.**
- **Efficacy has not been determined for long-term use in OCD, panic disorder, or bulimia.**
- **SSRIs may be associated with an increased risk of fractures in those 50 years and older.**
- **Safety and efficacy not determined in children less than 18 years of age, other than pediatric clients with OCD and the use of fluoxetine in major depressive disorder.**

SIDE EFFECTS

See individual drugs. The following side effects (listed alphabetically) have been observed with several of the selective serotonin reuptake inhibitors (SSRIs): **CNS:** Abnormal dreams, abnormal thinking, agitation, akathisia, amnesia, anxiety, apathy, confusion, depersonalization, depression, dizziness, emotional lability, headache, hypertonia, hypoesthesia, hypo- or hyperkinesia, impaired concentration, insomnia, libido decrease, myoclonus, nervousness, paresthesia, somnolence, suicide ideation/attempts, tremor, vertigo. **CV:** Chest pain, hypertension, palpitations, postural hypotension, syncope, tachycardia, vasodilation, gestational hypertension and preeclampsia. **GI:** Abdominal pain, anorexia, constipation, diarrhea, dry mouth, dyspepsia, dysphagia, flatulence, gastroenteritis, increased appetite, nausea, tooth disorder/caries, vomiting. **Dermatologic:** Acne, pruritus, rash, sweating (excessive). **GU:** Abnormal ejaculation, anorgasmia, impotence, sexual dysfunction, urinary frequency, UTI, urination disorder/retention. **Musculoskeletal:** Arthralgia, myalgia, myasthenia, myopathy. **Respiratory:** Bronchitis, cough, dyspnea, rhinitis, sinusitis, yawn. **Body as a whole:** Accidental injury/trauma, allergic reaction, asthenia, chills, edema, fever, flu syndrome, malaise, weight gain or loss. **Miscellaneous:** Hyponatremia, taste perversion, tinnitus, vision (blurred/abnormal/disturbed).

DRUG INTERACTIONS

See individual drugs. The following drug interactions are possible with any of the SSRIs.

Alcohol / Possible increased impairment of mental and motor skills; do not use together
Aspirin / ↑ Risk of GI bleeding
Benzodiazepines / Possible ↓ clearance of benzodiazepines metabolized by hepatic oxidation (e.g., alprazolam, fluoxetine, fluvoxamine)
Beta adrenergic blockers / Certain SSRIs may ↓ metabolism of certain beta blockers
Coumarin anticoagulants / ↑ Risk of hospitalization for nongastrointestinal tract bleeding
Lithium / Possible ↓ serotonergic effects of SSRIs
L-Tryptophan / Both central (headache, sweating, dizziness, agitation, restlessness) and peripheral (GI distress, N&V) toxicity is possible
MAOIs / Serious (and possibly fatal) reactions, including hyperthermia, rigidity, myoclonus, autonomic instability, mental status changes

Metoclopramide / Possible serotonin syndrome (e.g., CNS irritability, shivering, myoclonus, altered consciousness), especially if used with sertraline
NSAIDs / ↑ Risk of GI bleeding and significant other GI side effects; do not use together
H ***St. John's wort*** / Possible mild serotonin syndrome
Sibutramine / Possible serotonin syndrome (e.g., CNS irritability, shivering, myoclonus, altered consciousness)
Sumatriptan / Weakness, hyperreflexia, incoordination
Sympathomimetics / ↑ Sympathomimetic effects and ↑ risk of serotonin syndrome
Tramadol / Possible serotonin syndrome (e.g., CNS irritability, shivering, myoclonus, altered consciousness)
Tricyclic antidepressants / Possible ↑ TCA plasma levels
Warfarin / Altered anticoagulant effects

DOSAGE

See individual drugs.

NURSING IMPLICATIONS

IMPLEMENTATION/ADMINISTRATION/STORAGE

Clients show the largest relative improvement during the first weeks of treatment.

ASSESSMENT

1. Note reasons for therapy, behavioral manifestations, symptom onset/characteristics, and contributing factors. List other drugs prescribed to ensure none interact; note agents trialed and outcome.
2. Differentiate type of depression based on diagnostic features related to reactive, major depressive, or bipolar affective disorders. Assess for dysphoric mood, suicidal ideations, and excessive appetite/weight changes. Include behavioral health review.
3. Note sleep disturbances, lethargy, apathy, impaired thought processes, or lack of response.
4. If over age 50 assess BMD and for fracture potential.
5. Carefully monitor adults and children, especially at the beginning of treatment, for worsening depression or emerging suicidal ideation.
6. A major depressive episode may be the initial symptom of bipolar disorder. Prior to initiating treatment with an antidepressant, adequately screen clients with depressive symptoms to determine if they are at risk for bipolar disorder.
7. Monitor ECG, CBC, renal and LFTs; use caution with liver dysfunction.

CLIENT/FAMILY TEACHING

1. May take with or without food as directed. Avoid other unprescribed or OTC agents and alcohol during therapy.
2. Use caution when performing tasks requiring mental alertness or physical coordination until drug effects realized. May cause drop in BP. Rise slowly from a lying or sitting position to minimize effects.
3. Increase oral hygiene, take frequent sips of water, suck on hard candy, or chew sugarless gum to maintain a moist mouth. A high-fiber diet, increased fluid intake, exercise, and stool softeners may prevent constipation.
4. May alter libido and sexual function. Practice reliable birth control; report if pregnancy suspected.
5. Report any alterations in perceptions, i.e., hallucinations, blurred vision, or excessive stimulations. Watch those recovering from depression for suicidal tendencies; remove firearms from the home and encourage support group therapy.
6. May take up to 4 weeks to notice any change in emotional state; stay on the treatment regimen. Will see provider more often the first 2–3 months; prescriptions will be for a small dosage to start and to prevent adverse side effects. Obtain number from provider to call for help or report adverse effects.
7. Do not stop abruptly at higher dosages; may experience withdrawal S&S. Review when and how to take medications, reportable side effects, especially rash or S&S of liver dysfunction (yellow skin, RUQ abdominal pain, itching, fatigue and change in stool color) and importance of regular participation in psychotherapy programs as prescribed.
8. SSRIs may be associated with an increased risk of fractures in those 50 years and older.
9. Report increased agitation/irritability, unusual behavioral changes, or suicide thoughts.

Classifications

10. Keep all F/U to assess response, labs, and for adverse SE.

OUTCOMES/EVALUATE

- **Understand illness and need for counselling, drug therapy/medical supervision**
- **↓ Depression evidenced by improved appetite, renewed interest in outside activities, ↑ socialization, improved sleeping patterns, ↑ energy**
- **↓ Anxiety; improved coping skills**

SEROTONIN 5-HT$_1$ RECEPTOR AGONISTS (ANTIMIGRAINE DRUGS) ■

SEE ALSO THE FOLLOWING INDIVIDUAL ENTRIES:

Almotriptan maleate
Eletriptan hydrobromide
Frovatriptan succinate
Naratriptan hydrochloride
Rizatriptan benzoate
Sumatriptan succinate
Zolmitriptan

INDICATIONS/USES

See individual drugs. Uses include: (1) Acute treatment of migraine with or without aura. Use only when a clear diagnosis of migraine has been determined. Drugs are not intended to prevent or reduce the number of migraine attacks. (2) Acute treatment of cluster headache episodes (sumatriptan injection only).

ACTION/KINETICS

Action

These drugs are selective 5-HT$_1$ receptor agonists. This receptor is present on human basilar arteries and in the vasculature of the dura mater. It is believed that symptoms of migraine are due to local cranial vasodilation or to the release of vasoactive and proinflammatory peptides from sensory nerve endings in an activated trigeminal system. Depending on the drug, the selective 5-HT$_1$ agonists have a high affinity for and combine with 5-HT$_{1B}$, 5-HT$_{1D}$, or 5-HT$_{1F}$ receptors on the extracerebral, intracranial blood vessels that become dilated during a migraine attack. Activation of the receptors causes cranial vessel vasoconstriction, inhibition of neuropeptide release, and reduced transmission in trigeminal pain pathways.

CONTRAINDICATIONS

IV use of injectable products (due to possibility of coronary vasospasm). Use in ischemic bowel disease, angina pectoris, history of MI, strokes, TIAs, documented silent ischemia, Prinzmetal's variant angina, in those with signs and symptoms of ischemic heart disease or coronary artery vasospasm, coronary artery disease (or in presence of risk factors for CAD), uncontrolled hypertension. Concurrent use (or within 24 hr of use) of ergotamine-containing products, dihydroergotamine, methysergide; also, MAOI therapy (or within 2 weeks of discontinuing an MAOI). Within 24 hr of another 5-HT$_1$ agonist. Use to manage hemiplegic or basilar migraine.

SPECIAL CONCERNS

- **Increased risk of myocardial ischemia or MI and other adverse cardiac events, including life-threatening disturbances of cardiac rhythm and death, cerebral hemorrhage, subarachnoid hemorrhage, stroke, coronary artery vasospasm, peripheral vascular ischemia, colonic ischemia with abdominal pain, bloody diarrhea, and significant increases in BP.**
- **Use with caution during lactation and in those with diseases that may alter the absorption, metabolism, or excretion of drugs.**
- **Safety and efficacy not determined in children.**

SIDE EFFECTS

See individual drugs. Most common side effects include paresthesia, asthenia, nausea, dizziness, fatigue, pain, somnolence, warm sensation, dry mouth, headache, flushing, hot or cold sensation, chest pain, and chest, jaw, or neck tightness or heaviness. More serious side effects follow: **CV:** ***Acute MI, life-threatening disturbances of cardiac rhythm***, and ***death*** within a few hours following use. ***Cerebral hemorrhage, subarachnoid hemorrhage, stroke, myocardial ischemia.*** Vasospastic reactions, including coronary artery vasospasm; peripheral vascular ischemia, colonic ischemia with abdominal pain and bloody diarrhea, hypertension, ***hypertensive crisis***. **Respiratory:** Nasal and throat irritation, burning, numbness, paresthesia, discharge, pain, soreness (all after using nasal spray). **Hypersensitivity:** ***Severe anaphylaxis/anaphylactoid reactions***. **Miscellaneous:** Chest, jaw, or neck tightness; pain, tightness, pressure, or heaviness over the precordium. Photosensitivity, long-term ophthalmic effects.

OVERDOSE MANAGEMENT

Symptoms: Hypertension and other more serious CV symptoms.

Treatment: There are no specific antidotes. Consider gastric lavage followed by activated charcoal in clients with suspected overdose. Begin standard supportive measures. If chest pain or other symptoms of angina are present, perform ECG monitoring for evidence of ischemia. Continue monitoring clients after an overdose for at least 10–20 hr depending on the drug.

DRUG INTERACTIONS

Ergot alkaloids / ↑ Risk of vasospastic reactions; do not use within 24 hr of each other
MAOIs / Do not use 5-HT_1 agonists within 2 weeks following discontinuation of an MAOI
SSRIs / Possible weakness, hyperreflexia, incoordination
Serotonin 5-HT_1 agonists / ↑ Risk of vasospastic reactions when two 5-HT_1 agonists are given within 24 hr of each other; use together is contraindicated
Sibutramine / Possible "serotonin syndrome," including symptoms of CNS irritability, motor weakness, shivering, myoclonus, and altered consciousness

DOSAGE

See individual drugs.

NURSING IMPLICATIONS

IMPLEMENTATION/ADMINISTRATION/STORAGE

1. Take a single PO dose with fluids as soon as symptoms of migraine appear. A second dose may be taken if symptoms return, but no sooner than 2 or 4 hours (depending on the drug) following the first dose.
2. If there is no response to the first dose, do not take a second dose without consulting provider.

ASSESSMENT

1. Note reasons for therapy, family history, characteristics of S&S; ensure not hemiplegic or basilar type of migraine headaches. List other drugs prescribed to ensure none interact and other agents trialed/outcome.
2. Review neurologic exam and CT/MRI results. A clear diagnosis of migraine should be made; the drug should not be given for headaches due to other neurologic events.
3. Assess for any CAD, CABG, uncontrolled HTN, circulation problems, IBD, or history of CVA/TIAs. With increased CAD risk factors give first dose in the office and assess client for adverse effects or have men undergo a stress test and women a thallium stress test.
4. Review headache diary and assess for triggers or agents that may cause headaches, i.e., tetracycline, niacin, nitrates, magnesium sulfate, red wines, Nutrasweet, caffeine, conjugated estrogens, etc.
5. Review ECG, renal and LFTs; evaluate for dysfunction. Monitor VS; expect transient increases in BP.

CLIENT/FAMILY TEACHING

1. Take exactly as directed; strictly for migraine headaches. Do not exceed dosage or dosing intervals, do not share medications with others regardless of symptoms; do not use for other types of headaches.
2. Use caution if driving or performing activities that require mental alertness; may cause dizziness or drowsiness. Report any chest pain, SOB, chest tightness, or wheezing.
3. Drug acts to shrink swollen blood vessels surrounding the brain that cause migraine headaches. Keep a headache diary and identify factors/foods/events that surround migraine headaches. Continue other remedies (i.e., noise reduction, reduced lighting, and bed rest) that assist to control S&S. Avoid known triggers, i.e., chocolate, cheese, citrus fruit, caffeine, alcohol, missing sleep/meals.
4. Review package insert and do not use with other similar headache medications.
5. Practice reliable contraception; report if pregnancy suspected.
6. Store away from heat, light, and moisture; store in a safe place. Report any unusual side effects, intolerance, or lack of response.
7. Keep all F/U to assess response, labs, and for adverse SE.

OUTCOMES/EVALUATE

Termination of migraine headaches

Classifications

SKELETAL MUSCLE RELAXANTS, CENTRALLY ACTING ■

SEE ALSO THE FOLLOWING INDIVIDUAL ENTRIES:

Baclofen
Cyclobenzaprine hydrochloride
Diazepam
Methocarbamol
Tizanidine hydrochloride

INDICATIONS/USES

See individual drugs. Uses include: (1) Musculoskeletal and neurologic disorders associated with muscle spasms, hyperreflexia, and hypertonia, including parkinsonism, tetanus, tension headaches, acute muscle spasms caused by trauma, and inflammation (e.g., low back syndrome, sprains, arthritis, bursitis). (2) Management of cerebral palsy and multiple sclerosis.

ACTION/KINETICS

Action

These drugs decrease muscle tone and involuntary movement. Many relieve anxiety and tension as well. Although the precise mechanism of action is unknown, most of these agents depress spinal polysynaptic reflexes. Their beneficial effects may also be attributable to their antianxiety activity. Several of the drugs in this group also manifest analgesic properties.

SIDE EFFECTS

See individual drugs.

OVERDOSE MANAGEMENT

Symptoms: Often extensions of the side effects. Stupor, ***coma, shock-like syndrome, respiratory depression***, loss of muscle tone, and impaired deep tendon reflexes may also occur.

Treatment: Symptomatic. Emesis or gastric lavage (followed by activated charcoal). If necessary, artificial respiration, oxygen administration, pressor agents, and IV fluids may be used. It may be possible to increase the rate of excretion of selected drugs by diuretics (including mannitol), peritoneal dialysis, or hemodialysis.

DRUG INTERACTIONS

CNS depressants (e.g., alcohol, barbiturates, sedatives and hypnotics, and antianxiety agents) / ↑ Sedative and respiratory depressant effects

H *Kava Kava* / Additive effects

DOSAGE

See individual drugs.

NURSING IMPLICATIONS

IMPLEMENTATION/ADMINISTRATION/STORAGE

1. If unable to swallow, crush tablets or empty capsules into a small amount of fruit juice.
2. If skeletal muscle relaxant is to be discontinued after long-term use, taper dose to prevent rebound spasticity, hallucinations, or other withdrawal symptoms.
3. Determine lowest dosage to treat symptoms.

ASSESSMENT

1. Note reasons for therapy, onset, and characteristics of S&S. List agents trialed/outcome.
2. Assess extent of musculoskeletal/neurologic disorders associated with muscle spasm. Note muscle tone, stiffness, pain, pain level, and extent of ROM.
3. Review baseline mental status. Note any seizures/history; may cause loss of seizure control.
4. Monitor BP q 4 hr. Supervise ambulation/transfers and ensure safe environment. If sedentary or immobilized, client is more prone to hypotension upon ambulation.
5. Assess level of mobility (ROM) and comfort (pain level) prior to and following drug administration. Check muscle responses and DTRs for evidence of drug overdose.
6. Monitor VS, renal and LFTs and urinary output; evaluate need for drugs to ↑ excretion rate.

CLIENT/FAMILY TEACHING

1. Take as directed with meals to reduce GI upset. If unable to swallow, crush tablets or empty capsules into a small amount of fruit juice.
2. These drugs may impair mental alertness; do not operate dangerous machinery or drive a car until drug effects realized. Avoid alcohol and any other CNS depressants. Antihistamines may cause an additive depressant effect.
3. Review additional therapies that may be prescribed for muscle spasm (heat, rest, exercise, physical therapy) and importance of adhering to prescribed regimen.

4. Increase fluids and bulk in diet to prevent constipation. Report if the urine becomes dark, the skin or sclera appears yellow, or skin itching develops.
5. Report persistent nausea, anorexia, or changes in taste perception, as nutritional state may become impaired.
6. Do not stop drug abruptly after prolonged use; may precipitate withdrawal symptoms, rebound spasticity, and hallucinations.
7. Report as scheduled for all lab and medical visits so therapy and symptoms can be evaluated and drug dosage/need assessed.

OUTCOMES/EVALUATE

- ↓ Muscle spasm and pain
- ↑ ROM with measurable improvement in muscle tone, mobility, and involuntary movements
- Relief of tension headaches

SULFONAMIDES ■

SEE ALSO THE FOLLOWING INDIVIDUAL ENTRIES:

Sulfacetamide sodium
Sulfadiazine
Sulfasalazine
Trimethoprim and Sulfamethoxazole

INDICATIONS/USES

PO, Parenteral. See individual drugs. Uses include, but are not limited to: (1) Urinary tract infections (e.g., pyelonephritis, cystitis, pyelitis). (2) Chancroid. (3) Meningitis caused by *Hemophilus influenzae,* meningococcal meningitis. (4) Rheumatic fever. (5) Nocardiosis. (6) Trachoma. (7) With pyrimethamine for toxoplasmosis. (8) With quinine sulfate and pyrimethamine for chloroquine-resistant *Plasmodium falciparum. (9)* With penicillin or erythromycin for otitis media due to *H. influenzae.* (10) Sexually transmitted diseases, including lymphogranuloma venereum and *Chlamydia trachomatis* infections.

Ophthalmic. (1) Conjunctivitis, corneal ulcer, and other superficial ocular infections due to susceptible organisms. (2) Adjunct to systemic sulfonamides to treat trachoma. (3) Inclusion conjunctivitis.

ACTION/KINETICS

Action

Structurally related to PABA and, as such, competitively inhibit the enzyme dihydropteroate synthetase, which is responsible for incorporating PABA into dihydrofolic acid. Thus, the synthesis of dihydrofolic acid is inhibited, resulting in a decrease in tetrahydrofolic acid, which is required for synthesis of DNA, purines, and thymidine. Are bacteriostatic.

Pharmacokinetics

Readily and completely absorbed from the GI tract. Distributed throughout all tissues, including the CSF, where concentrations attain 50–80% of those found in the blood. Metabolized in the liver and primarily excreted by the kidneys. Small amounts are found in the feces, bile, breast milk, and other secretions.

CONTRAINDICATIONS

Hypersensitivity to sulfonamides and chemically related drugs (e.g., thiazides, sulfonylureas, loop diuretics, carbonic anhydrase inhibitors, local anesthetics, PABA-containing sunscreens). Use in infants less than 2 years of age, except with pyrimethamine to treat congenital toxoplasmosis. Use at term during pregnancy. Use in infants less than 2 months of age who are nursing; use in premature infants with hyperbilirubinemia or G6PD deficiency. Group A beta-hemolytic streptococcal infections.

SPECIAL CONCERNS

- Use with caution, and in reduced dosage, in clients with impaired liver or renal function, intestinal or urinary tract obstructions, blood dyscrasias, allergies, asthma, and hereditary G6PD deficiency.
- The frequency of resistant organisms limits use as sole therapy to treat urinary tract infections.
- Use with caution if exposed to sunlight or ultraviolet light as photosensitivity may occur.
- Superinfection is a possibility.
- Use ophthalmic products with caution in clients with dry eye.
- Safety and efficacy of ophthalmic use in children not determined.

SIDE EFFECTS

Systemic. GI: N&V, diarrhea, abdominal pain, glossitis, stomatitis, anorexia, pseudomembranous enterocolitis, pancreatitis, hepatitis, ***hepatocellular necrosis*****. Allergic:** Rash, pruritus, photosensitivity, erythema nodosum or multiforme, generalized skin eruptions, ***Stevens-Johnson syndrome***, conjunctivitis, rhinitis, balanitis. Serum sickness,

Classifications

urticaria, pruritus, exfoliative dermatitis, ***anaphylaxis, toxic epidermal necrolysis*** with or without corneal damage, periorbital edema, conjunctival and scleral injection, allergic myocarditis, decreased pulmonary function with eosinophilia, disseminated lupus erythematosus, periarteritis nodosa, arteritis. **CNS:** Headaches, mental depression, ***seizures***, hallucinations, vertigo, insomnia, apathy, ataxia, drowsiness, restlessness. **Renal:** Crystalluria, toxic nephrosis with oliguria and anuria, elevated creatinine. **Respiratory:** Cough, shortness of breath, pulmonary infiltrates. **Hematologic:** ***Aplastic anemia***, leukopenia, neutropenia, ***agranulocytosis***, thrombocytopenia, hemolytic anemia, methemoglobinemia, purpura, hypoprothrombinemia. **Neurologic:** Peripheral neuropathy, polyneuritis, neuritis, optic neuritis. **Miscellaneous:** Jaundice, tinnitus, arthralgia, superinfection, hearing loss, drug fever, pyrexia, chills, lupus erythematosus phenomenon, transient myopia. By killing the intestinal flora, the sulfonamides also reduce the bacterial synthesis of vitamin K. This may result in ***hemorrhage.*** Administration of vitamin K to clients on long-term sulfonamide therapy is recommended. **Ophthalmic.** Headache, browache. Blurred vision, eye irritation, itching, transient epithelial keratitis, reactive hyperemia, conjunctival edema, burning and transient stinging. Rarely, ***Stevens-Johnson syndrome***, exfoliative dermatitis, ***toxic epidermal necrolysis***, photosensitivity, fever, skin rash, GI disturbances, and bone marrow depression.

OVERDOSE MANAGEMENT

Symptoms: N&V, anorexia, colic, dizziness, drowsiness, headache, unconsciousness, vertigo, toxic fever. More serious manifestations include ***acute hemolytic anemia, agranulocytosis***, acidosis, maculopapular dermatitis, hepatic jaundice, sensitivity reactions, toxic neuritis, ***death*** (several days after the first dose).

Treatment: Immediately discontinue the drug.

- Induce emesis or perform gastric lavage, especially if large doses were taken.
- To hasten excretion, alkalinize the urine and force fluids (if kidney function is normal). If there is renal blockage due to sulfonamide crystals, catheterization of the ureters may be needed.
- In the event of agranulocytosis, antibiotic therapy is needed to combat infection.
- To treat severe anemia or thrombocytopenia, blood or platelet transfusions are required.

DRUG INTERACTIONS

Anticoagulants, oral / ↑ Drug effects R/T ↓ plasma protein binding
Antidiabetics, oral / ↑ Hypoglycemic effect R/T ↓ plasma protein binding
Cyclosporine / ↓ Effect of cyclosporine and ↑ nephrotoxicity
Diuretics, thiazide / ↑ Risk of thrombocytopenia with purpura
Indomethacin / ↑ Effect of sulfonamides R/T ↓ plasma protein binding
Methenamine / ↑ Chance of sulfonamide crystalluria due to acid urine
Methotrexate / ↑ Risk of drug-induced bone marrow suppression
Phenytoin / ↑ Drug effect R/T ↓ liver breakdown
Probenecid / ↑ Effect of sulfonamides R/T ↓ plasma protein binding
Salicylates / ↑ Effect of sulfonamides R/T ↓ plasma protein binding
Silver products / Incompatible with ophthalmic products
Uricosuric agents / Potentiation of uricosuric action

LABORATORY TEST CONSIDERATIONS

False + or ↑ LFTs (amino acids, bilirubin, BSP), renal function (BUN, NPN, C_{CR}), blood counts, PT, Coombs' test. False + or ↑ urine glucose (copper reduction methods, such as Benedict's solution or Clinitest), protein, urobilinogen.

DOSAGE

See individual drugs.

NURSING IMPLICATIONS

IMPLEMENTATION/ADMINISTRATION/STORAGE

1. **Because sulfonamides are bacteriostatic, rather than bactericidal, a complete course of therapy is necessary to prevent immediate regrowth and development of resistance.**
2. **Do not use ophthalmic solutions if they have darkened or contain a precipitate.**
3. **Take care to avoid contamination of ophthalmic products.**

ASSESSMENT

1. Obtain a thorough nursing and drug history. List previous sulfonamide therapy/response.
2. Note reasons for therapy, onset, characteristics of S&S, culture results, other agents trialed, outcome.
3. Question concerning any conditions that may preclude drug therapy, i.e., intestinal problems, urinary tract obstructions, G6PD deficiency (may precipitate hemolysis), or allergies and explore further.
4. During drug therapy, assess for any of the following reactions that may require drug withdrawal:
   - Skin rashes, abdominal pain, anorexia, mouth irritation or tingling of extremities
   - Blood dyscrasias (characterized by sore throat, fever, pallor, purpura, jaundice, or weakness)
   - Serum sickness (characterized by eruptions of purpuric spots and swelling/pain in limbs and joints); onset 7–10 days after initiation of therapy
   - Early S&S of Stevens-Johnson syndrome (characterized by high fever, severe headaches, stomatitis, conjunctivitis, rhinitis, urethritis, and balanitis [inflammation of the tip of the penis])
   - Jaundice, indicating hepatic involvement; onset 3–5 days after initiation of therapy
   - Renal involvement (characterized by renal colic, oliguria, anuria, hematuria, and proteinuria)
   - Ecchymosis and hemorrhage (caused by decreased synthesis of vitamin K by intestinal bacteria)
   - Hemolytic anemia especially in the elderly
   - Behavioral changes or acute mental disturbances
5. Monitor I&O; ensure adequate fluid intake to prevent crystalluria. Check urinalysis for crystals. Minimum urine output should be 1.5 L/day. Test urine pH for excess acidity. Administration of a particularly insoluble sulfonamide may require urine alkalinization (i.e., $NaHCO_3$).
6. If administering long-acting sulfonamides, adequate fluid intake must be maintained for 24–48 hr after the drug has been discontinued.
7. Check if pregnant; drug may be harmful to developing fetus. Monitor VS, CBC, BS, bleeding times, cultures, renal and LFTs.

CLIENT/FAMILY TEACHING

1. Take on time and as prescribed despite feeling better. Take with 6–8 oz (180–240 mL) of water and maintain adequate fluid intake for 24–48 hr after therapy. May take with food if GI upset.
2. Do not perform activities that require mental alertness until drug effects realized.
3. May cause N&V and loss of appetite. Monitor I&O; consume >2.5 L/day of fluids.
4. May color urine orange-red or brown; not cause for alarm but report.
5. Test urine pH and report changes in acidity as additional drug therapy may be necessary. Avoid vitamin C; may make the urine more acidic and contribute to crystal formation.
6. If also taking anticoagulants, report increased bleeding tendencies.
7. Avoid prolonged exposure to sunlight; may cause a photosensitivity reaction. Wear protective clothing, sunglasses, and sunscreen.
8. Report any changes in vision or hearing. With ophthalmic use, report if no improvement in 5–7 days, if condition worsens, or if pain, redness, itching, or eye swelling occurs.
9. Vaginal intercourse should be avoided when using vaginal products.
10. Keep all F/U to assess response, labs, and for adverse SE.

OUTCOMES/EVALUATE

- Negative C&S results (note any organism resistance to sulfonamide)
- Resolution of infection; symptomatic improvement

SYMPATHOMIMETIC DRUGS

SEE ALSO THE FOLLOWING INDIVIDUAL ENTRIES:

Albuterol
Dobutamine hydrochloride
Dopamine hydrochloride
Epinephrine
Epinephrine hydrochloride
Formoterol fumarate
Pirbuterol acetate
Pseudoephedrine hydrochloride
Salmeterol xinafoate

Classifications

Terbutaline sulfate

INDICATIONS/USES

See individual drugs. Used mainly for relief of reversible bronchospasm associated with acute and chronic bronchial asthma, exercise–induced bronchospasm, and chronic COPD.

ACTION/KINETICS

Action

Adrenergic drugs act: (1) by mimicking the action of norepinephrine or epinephrine by combining with alpha and/or beta receptors (directly acting sympathomimetics) or (2) by causing or regulating the release of the natural neurohormones from their storage sites at the nerve terminals (indirectly acting sympathomimetics). Some drugs exhibit a combination of both effects. Adrenergic stimulation of receptors will manifest the following general effects:

- *Alpha-1-adrenergic:* / Vasoconstriction, decongestion, constriction of the pupil of the eye, contraction of splenic capsule, contraction of the trigone-sphincter muscle of the urinary bladder.
- *Alpha-2-adrenergic:* / Presynaptic to regulate amount of transmitter released; decrease tone, motility, and secretory activity of the GI tract (possibly involved in hypersecretory response also); decrease insulin secretion.
- *Beta-1-adrenergic:* / Myocardial contraction (inotropic), regulation of heartbeat (chronotropic), improved impulse conduction, ↑ lipolysis.
- *Beta-2-adrenergic:* / Peripheral vasodilation, bronchial dilation; ↓ tone, motility, and secretory activity of the GI tract; ↑ renin secretion, inhibition of uterine contractions.

Beta adrenergic drugs stimulate adenyl cyclase which catalyzes the formation of cyclic AMP from ATP. The formed cyclic AMP inhibits release of mediators from mast cells and basophils that cause hypersensitivity reactions. The increase in cyclic AMP leads to activation of protein kinase A, which inhibits phosphorylation of myosin and lowers intracellular ionic calcium levels causing smooth muscle relaxation.

CONTRAINDICATIONS

See individual drugs. Tachycardia due to arrhythmias; tachycardia or heart block caused by digitalis toxicity, angina, known hypersensitivity to sympathomimetics. Use of two or more beta-adrenergic bronchodilators simultaneously (potential additive effects). Use of bronchodilators with other sympathomimetic agents is not recommended.

SPECIAL CONCERNS

■ (1) Long-acting beta-2 agonists may increase the risk of asthma-related death. Data from a large placebo-controlled U.S. study that compared the safety of salmeterol or placebo added to usual asthma therapy showed an increase in asthma-related deaths in clients receiving salmeterol. This finding is considered a class effect of long-acting beta-2 agonists. All long-acting beta-2 agonists are contraindicated in clients with asthma without the use of a long-term asthma control medication. Currently available data are inadequate to determine whether current use of inhaled corticosteroids or other long-term asthma control drugs mitigates the increased risk of asthma related-death from long-acting beta-2 adrenergic agonists. (2) Once asthma control is achieved and maintained, assess the client at regular intervals and step down therapy (e.g., discontinue long-acting beta-2 agonist) if possible without loss of asthma control and maintain the client on a long-term asthma control medication, such as an inhaled corticosteroid. Do not use long-acting beta-2 agonists for clients whose asthma is adequately controlled on low- or medium-dose inhaled corticosteroids. (3) **Children and adolescents.** Available data from controlled clinical trials suggest that long-acting beta-2 agonists increase the risk of asthma-related hospitalization in children and adolescents. For children and adolescents with asthma, who require addition of a long-acting beta-2 agonist to an inhaled corticosteroid, a fixed-dose combination product containing both an inhaled corticosteroid and a long-acting beta-2 agonist should ordinarily be used to ensure adherence with both drugs. In cases where use of a separate long-term asthma control medication (e.g., inhaled corticosteroid) and along-acting beta-2 agonist is clinically indicated, appropriate steps must be taken to ensure adherence with both treatment components. If adherence cannot be ensured, a fixed-dose combination product containing both an inhaled corticosteroid and a long-acting beta-2 agonist is recommended.

- **Use with caution in hyperthyroidism, diabetes, prostatic hypertrophy, seizures, degenerative heart disease, especially in geriatric clients or those with asthma, emphysema, or psychoneuroses.**
- **Use with caution in clients with coronary insufficiency, CAD, ischemic heart disease, CHF, cardiac arrhythmias, hypertension, or history of stroke.**
- **Asthma clients who rely heavily on inhaled beta-2-agonist bronchodilators may increase their chances of death. Thus, use to "rescue" clients but do not prescribe for regular long-term use.**
- **Beta-2 agonists may inhibit uterine contractions.**
- **Long-acting beta-2 adrenergic agonists (e.g., formoterol, salmeterol) have been associated with an increased risk of severe asthma episodes and death.**
- **Paradoxical airway resistance with repeated excessive use of inhalation products is possible.**
- **Benzyl alcohol, contained in some products as a preservative, has been associated with a fatal "gasping" syndrome in premature infants.**
- **Lower doses may be required in the elderly due to increased sympathomimetic sensitivity.**

SIDE EFFECTS

See individual drugs; side effects common to most sympathomimetics are listed. **CV:** Tachycardia, arrhythmias, palpitations, BP changes, anginal pain, precordial pain, pallor, skipped beats, chest tightness, hypertension. **GI:** N&V, heartburn, anorexia, altered taste or bad taste, GI distress, dry mouth, diarrhea. **CNS:** Restlessness, anxiety, tension, insomnia, hyperkinesis, drowsiness, weakness, vertigo, irritability, dizziness, headache, tremors, general CNS stimulation, nervousness, shakiness, hyperactivity. **Respiratory:** Cough, dyspnea, dry throat, pharyngitis, ***paradoxical bronchospasm***, irritation, ***severe asthma episodes, including death***. **Miscellaneous:** Flushing, hypokalemia, sweating, ***allergic/hypersensitivity reactions***.

OVERDOSE MANAGEMENT

Symptoms:

Following inhalation: Exaggeration of side effects. **CV:** Anginal pain, hypertension, hypotension, tachycardia (rates may reach 200 beats/min), arrhythmias, palpitation, prolongation of the QTc interval, ***cardiac arrest***. **CNS:** Nervousness, headache, tremor, dizziness, insomnia, ***seizures***. **GI:** Dry mouth, nausea. **Musculoskeletal:** Muscle cramps. **Metabolic:** Hypokalemia, hyperglycemia. **Body as a whole:** Fatigue, malaise, metabolic acidosis.

Following systemic use: **CV:** Bradycardia, tachycardia, palpitations, extrasystoles, ***heart block***, elevated BP, chest pain, hypokalemia, transient arrhythmias, angina, hypo-//hypertension, significant drop in BP due to peripheral vasodilation. **CNS:** Anxiety, insomnia, tremor, delirium, drowsiness, headache, nervousness, ***convulsions, collapse***, and ***coma***. **GI:** N&V. **Metabolic:** Hypokalemia, hyperglycemia, increased insulin levels followed by rebound hypoglycemia. **Body as a whole:** Fever, chills, cold perspiration, sweating, mydriasis, and blanching of the skin.

Treatment: **For overdosage due to inhalation:** Discontinue the drug. Monitor BP and ECG. General supportive measures. Use metoprolol or atenolol cautiously as they may induce an asthmatic attack in clients with asthma. Dialysis is not appropriate.

For systemic overdosage: Discontinue drug or decrease dose. General supportive measures. Monitor BP, pulse, respiration, and ECG. Administer artificial respiration if respirations are shallow or cyanosis is present. For overdose due to PO agents, emesis, gastric lavage, or charcoal may be helpful. In severe cases, propranolol may be used but this may cause airway obstruction. Phentolamine may be given to block strong alpha-adrenergic effects. Vasopressors are contraindicated. In CV collapse, maintain BP. For hypertension, give phentolamine mesylate 5 mg, diluted in saline, may be given by slow IV or 100 mg PO may be used. Convulsions may be controlled by diazepam. Cool applications and dexamethasone, 1 mg/kg by slow IV, may control pyrexia.

DRUG INTERACTIONS

An additive effect of certain sympathomimetics (e.g., albuterol, formoterol, isoproterenol, salmeterol, terbutaline) with other drugs that prolong the QT interval is possible. The following drugs may prolong the QT interval and increase the risk of life-threatening cardiac arrhythmias, including torsade de pointes: amiodarone, arsenic trioxide, bretylium, chlorpromazine, cisapride, disopyramide, dofetilide, dolasetron, droperidol, mefloquine, mesoridazine, moxifloxacin, pentamidine,

pimozide, procainamide, quinidine, sotalol, tacrolimus, thioridazine, and ziprasidone.
Aminophylline / Enhanced toxicity (especially cardiotoxicity); also ↓ theophylline levels and potentiation of the hypokalemic effect of the sympathomimetic
Ammonium chloride / ↓ Effect of sympathomimetics R/T ↑ kidney excretion
Anesthetics / Halogenated anesthetics sensitize heart to adrenergics → cardiac arrhythmias
Anticholinergics / Concomitant use aggravates glaucoma
Antidiabetics / Hyperglycemic effect of epinephrine may necessitate ↑ dosage of insulin or oral hypoglycemic agents
Beta-adrenergic blocking agents / Inhibit adrenergic stimulation of the heart and bronchial tree; cause bronchial constriction; hypertension, asthma, not relieved by adrenergic agents
Bromocriptine / ↑ Risk of bromocriptine toxicity; if concurrent use cannot be avoided, monitor closely
Corticosteroids / Chronic use with sympathomimetics may result in or aggravate glaucoma; aerosols containing sympathomimetics and corticosteroids may be lethal in asthmatic children; also, potentiation of hypokalemic effect of the sympathomimetic
Digitalis glycosides / Combination may cause cardiac arrhythmias
Furazolidone / ↑ Effects of mixed-acting sympathomimetics (e.g., ephedrine)
Guanethidine / Direct-acting sympathomimetics ↑ drug effects, while indirect-acting sympathomimetics ↓ effects of guanethidine; also reversal of hypotensive drug effects
H ***Indian snakeroot*** / Initial significant ↑ BP
Linezolid / ↑ Effect of ephedrine (e.g., headache, hyperpyrexia, hypertension); minimal to no effect on direct-acting sympathomimetics
Lithium / ↓ Pressor effect of direct-acting sympathomimetics
MAOIs / All effects of sympathomimetics are potentiated; symptoms include hypertensive crisis with possible intracranial hemorrhage, hyperthermia, convulsions, coma; death may occur
Methyldopa / ↑ Pressor response
Methylphenidate / Potentiates pressor effect of sympathomimetics; combination hazardous in glaucoma
Oxytocics / ↑ Chance of severe hypertension
Phenothiazines / ↑ Risk of cardiac arrhythmias
Sodium bicarbonate / ↑ Effect of sympathomimetics R/T ↓ kidney excretion
Theophylline / Enhanced toxicity (especially cardiotoxicity); also ↓ theophylline levels and potentiation of the hypokalemic effect of the sympathomimetic
Thyroxine / Potentiation of pressor response of sympathomimetics
Tricyclic antidepressants / ↑ Effect of direct-acting sympathomimetics and ↓ effect of indirect-acting sympathomimetics

DOSAGE

See individual drugs.

NURSING IMPLICATIONS

IMPLEMENTATION/ADMINISTRATION/STORAGE

Discard colored solutions.

ASSESSMENT

1. Note reasons for therapy, contributing factors/triggers, clinical presentation, and desired response. Identify any sensitivity/previous use of adrenergic drugs/drugs in this class and outcome.
2. List history of CAD, tachycardia, endocrine disturbances, or respiratory tract problems.
3. Obtain baseline data regarding general physical condition, hemodynamic status including ECG, VS, labs, oxygen saturation, smoking history, work history with any exposure to chemicals/asbestos. Monitor PFTs and lab data including folate levels.

CLIENT/FAMILY TEACHING

1. Take exactly as directed. Do not increase dosage or take more frequently than prescribed. Consult provider if symptoms progress. Take early in the day to prevent insomnia.
2. Review prescribed drug therapy and potential side effects. Feelings/symptoms of fear or anxiety may be evident; these drugs mimic body's stress response. Avoid all OTC preparations.
3. Stop smoking to preserve current lung function. Attend formal smoking cessation classes.
4. Keep all F/U to assess response, labs, and for adverse SE.

Classifications

Special Nursing Considerations for Adrenergic Bronchodilators

ASSESSMENT

1. Obtain history and PE prior to starting therapy. Note any experience with this class of drugs.
2. Monitor VS; assess CV response. Evaluate cardiac function and note ejection fraction.
3. Observe effects on CNS; if pronounced, adjust dosage/frequency of administration.
4. With status asthmaticus and abnormal ABGs, continue to provide oxygen and ventilatory assistance even though the symptoms appear to be relieved by the bronchodilator. To prevent depression of respiratory effort, administer oxygen based on client's clinical symptoms and ABGs or O_2 saturations.
5. If three to five aerosol treatments of the same agent have been administered within the last 6–12 hr, with no relief, further evaluation is warranted. If dyspnea worsens after repeated excessive use of the inhaler, paradoxical airway resistance may occur. Be prepared to assist with alternative therapy and respiratory support.
6. Document lung assessment, ABGs (or O_2 saturation), and PFTs. Note characteristics of cough and sputum production.

CLIENT/FAMILY TEACHING

1. Review technique for use/care of inhalers and respiratory equipment. Rinsing of equipment and mouth after use is imperative to prevent oral fungal infections. Maintain record of peak flow readings and seek medical attention as directed.
2. To improve lung ventilation and reduce fatigue during eating, start inhalation therapy upon arising in the morning and before meals.
3. Regular, consistent use of the drug is essential for maximum benefit, but overuse can be life-threatening. If using inhaled medications and bronchodilators, use the bronchodilator first and wait 5 min before using the other medication.
4. A single aerosol treatment is usually enough to control an asthma attack. Overuse of adrenergic bronchodilators may result in reduced effectiveness, paradoxical reaction, and death from cardiac arrest. Consult provider if more than three (or prescribed number) aerosol treatments in a 24-hr period are required for relief.
5. With postural drainage, review how to cough productively and show family how to clap and vibrate the chest and position client to promote good respiratory hygiene.
6. Increased fluid intake will aid in liquefying secretions and removal. Consult provider if dizziness or chest pain occurs, or if there is no relief when the usual dose is used.
7. Avoid OTC preparations and any other unprescribed adrenergic medications.
8. **Stop smoking**; avoid crowds during "flu seasons," dress warmly in cold weather and cover mouth with scarf to filter cold air, receive the pneumonia vaccine and seasonal flu shot, and stay in air conditioning during hot, humid days to prevent exacerbations of illness. Identify triggers and practice avoidance.
9. Have family/significant other learn CPR.
10. Keep all F/U to assess response, labs, and for adverse SE.

OUTCOMES/EVALUATE

- Improved airway exchange with ↓ dyspnea/wheezing
- ↑ Exercise tolerance
- ↑ BP/cardiac output
- ↓ Nasal congestion

TETRACYCLINES

SEE ALSO THE FOLLOWING INDIVIDUAL ENTRIES:

Doxycycline calcium
Doxycycline hyclate
Doxycycline monohydrate
Tetracycline hydrochloride

INDICATIONS/USES

See individual drugs. Uses include: [linebrk/](1) Infections caused by *Rickettsiae* (Rocky Mountain spotted fever, typhus fever and the typhus group, Q fever, rickettsial pox, and tick fevers); *Mycoplasma pneumonia;* agents of psittacosis and ornithosis; agents of lymphogranuloma venereum and granuloma inguinale; *Borrelia recurrentis.*[linebrk/](2) Gram-negative infections caused by *Haemophilus ducreyi* (chancroid); *Yersinia pestis* (plague) and *Francisella tularensis* (tularemia). *Bartonella bacilliformis, Bacteroides* species, *Campylobacter fetus, Vibrio cholerae* (cholera), *Brucella* species (with streptomycin). [linebrk/](3) Infections due

Classifications

to *Chlamydia trachomatis* (lymphogranuloma venereum, trachoma, inclusion conjunctivitis, uncomplicated urethral, endocervical, or rectal infections), *Chlamydia psittaci* (psittacosis), *Borrelia* species (relapsing fever), *Ureaplasma urealyticum* (nongonococcal urethritis). [linebrk/](4) Infections caused by the following microorganisms when testing indicates appropriate susceptibility: *Escherichia coli, Enterobacter aerogenes, Shigella* species, *Acinetobacter calcoaceticus, H. influenzae* (respiratory infections), *Klebsiella* species (respiratory and urinary infections). *Streptococcus* species, including *S. pneumoniae. S. pyogenes* (skin and skin structure infections). *Mycoplasma pneumoniae,* and *Klebsiella* species (lower respiratory tract infections), *Staphylococcus aureus, Bacteroides,* and *Shigella* species. (*NOTE:* Up to 44% of *S. pyogenes* strains and 74% of *S. faecalis* strains are resistant to tetracyclines). [linebrk/](5) As part of combination therapy (e.g., with three or more of the following: Bismuth subsalicylate, metronidazole, omeprazole or lansoprazole, clarithromycin, amoxicillin, H_2-receptor antagonist) to provide symptomatic relief and accelerated ulcer healing for *Helicobacter pylori* eradication. [linebrk/](6) Treatment of trachoma, although the infectious agent is not always eliminated. [linebrk/](7) When penicillin is contraindicated, including infections caused by *Neisseria gonorrhoeae, Treponema pallidum,* and *T. pertenue* (syphilis and yaws). Also, *Listeria monocytogenes, Clostridium* species, *Bacillus anthracis, Fusobacterium fusiforme, Actinomycetes* species, *N. meningitis* (IV only). [linebrk/](8) Acute intestinal amebiasis due to *Entamoeba histolytica.*[linebrk/](9) PO in adults to treat uncomplicated urethral, endocervical, or rectal infections due to *Chlamydia trachomatis.*[linebrk/](10) PO as adjunctive therapy to treat severe acne (doxycycline, minocycline, tetracycline only). [linebrk/](11) PO with topical agents to treat inclusion conjunctivitis. [linebrk/](12) Anthrax, including inhalational anthrax (doxycycline only); used to reduce the incidence or progression of the disease following exposure to aerosolized *Bacillus anthracis.*[linebrk/](13) Prophylaxis of malaria due to *Plasmodium falciparum* (doxycycline only) in short-term travelers (less than 4 months) to areas with chloroquine and/or pyrimethamine-sulfadoxine resistant strains. [linebrk/](14) Treatment of asymptomatic meningococcal carriers of *N. meningitidis* (minocycline only).

NOTE: Do not use tetracyclines for streptococcal infections unless the organism has been shown to be susceptible. Tetracyclines are not the drugs of choice to treat any staphylococcal infection.

ACTION/KINETICS

Action

Tetracyclines inhibit protein synthesis by microorganisms by reversibly binding to the ribosomal 30S subunit, thereby interfering with protein synthesis. They block the binding of aminoacyl transfer RNA to the messenger RNA complex, thus inhibiting protein synthesis and thus cell growth. Cell wall synthesis is not inhibited. Are mostly bacteriostatic and are effective only against multiplying bacteria.

Pharmacokinetics

Adequately, but incompletely, absorbed from the GI tract. Well distributed throughout all tissues and fluids and diffuse through noninflamed meninges and the placental barrier (they enter fetal circulation and amniotic fluid). Are deposited in the fetal skeleton and calcifying teeth. **t½:** 7–18.6 hr (see individual agents); increased in the presence of renal impairment. They bind to serum protein (range: 20–93%; see individual agents). Concentrated in the liver in the bile; excreted mostly unchanged in the urine and feces. Excretion is significantly affected by renal function.

CONTRAINDICATIONS

Hypersensitivity. Use during tooth development stage (last trimester of pregnancy, neonatal period, during breastfeeding, and during childhood up to 8 years) because tetracyclines interfere with enamel formation and dental pigmentation. May be used in children under 8 years of age who have anthrax (including inhalational) only if other drugs are not likely to be effective or are contraindicated. Never administer intrathecally.

SPECIAL CONCERNS

- **Use with caution and at reduced dosage in clients with impaired kidney function.**
- **Avoid rapid IV administration due to possible thrombophlebitis.**

SIDE EFFECTS

See individual drugs. **GI:** Anorexia, N&V, diarrhea, glossitis, dysphagia, enterocolitis, inflammatory lesions (with monilial overgrowth) in the anogenital region, esophageal ulcerations, pancreatitis, dyspepsia, stomatitis, enamel hypoplasia, pseudomembranous colitis, esophagitis, bulky loose stools, sore throat, black hairy tongue, hoarseness. **CNS:** Dizziness, headache, bulging fontanel, pseudotumor cerebri, convulsions, hypesthesia, paresthesia, sedation, vertigo. **Dermatologic:** Maculopapular and erythematous rashes, photosensitivity, fixed drug eruptions, balanitis, erythema multiforme, ***Stevens-Johnson syndrome, toxic epidermal necrolysis***, skin and mucous membrane pigmentation, alopecia, erythema nodosum, hyperpigmentation of the nails, pruritus, vasculitis, exfoliative dermatitis (rare). **Hematologic:** Anemia, hemolytic anemia, thrombocytopenia, neutropenia, eosinophilia. **Hepatic:** Hepatic toxicity, hepatic cholestasis, ***hepatic failure***, hepatitis (rare). **Hypersensitivity:** Urticaria, angioneurotic edema, pericarditis, ***anaphylaxis***, anaphylactoid purpura, exacerbation of systemic lupus erythematosus, polyarthralgia, pulmonary infiltrates with eosinophilia. **Musculoskeletal:** Arthralgia, arthritis, bone discoloration, myalgia, joint stiffness, swelling. **GU:** Acute renal failure, interstitial nephritis, vulvovaginitis. **Respiratory:** Cough, dyspnea, bronchospasm, exacerbation of asthma. **Miscellaneous:** Brown-black microscopic discoloration of thyroid glands after prolonged therapy, tooth discoloration, lupus-like syndrome, fever, discolored secretions, tinnitus, decreased hearing, serum sickness-like syndrome. IV administration may cause thrombophlebitis. IM injections are painful and may cause induration at the injection site. Use of deteriorated tetracyclines may result in *Fanconi-like* syndrome characterized by N&V, acidosis, proteinuria, glycosuria, aminoaciduria, polydipsia, polyuria, hypokalemia.

OVERDOSE MANAGEMENT

Symptoms: The most common effects are dizziness and N&V.

Treatment: Discontinue the drug. Begin symptomatic treatment and supportive measures. Tetracyclines are not significantly removed by hemodialysis or peritoneal dialysis.

DRUG INTERACTIONS

Aluminum salts / ↓ Effect of tetracyclines R/T ↓ GI tract absorption
Antacids, oral / ↓ Effect of tetracyclines R/T ↓ GI tract absorption
Anticoagulants, oral / IV tetracyclines ↑ hypoprothrombinemia; also, ↑ action of PO anticoagulants R/T elimination of vitamin K-producing gut bacteria by tetracyclines
Bismuth salts / ↓ Effect of tetracyclines R/T ↓ GI tract absorption; give bismuth 2 hr after the tetracycline
H ***Bromelain*** / ↑ Plasma tetracycline levels
Bumetanide / ↑ Risk of kidney toxicity
Calcium salts / ↓ Effect of tetracyclines R/T ↓ GI tract absorption
Cholestyramine/Colestipol / ↓ or Delayed absorption of tetracyclines → ↓ plasma levels
Cimetidine / ↓ Effect of tetracyclines R/T ↓ GI tract absorption
Digoxin / ↑ Bioavailability of digoxin
Diuretics, thiazide / ↑ Risk of kidney toxicity
Ethacrynic acid / ↑ Risk of kidney toxicity
Furosemide / ↑ Risk of kidney toxicity
Insulin / Potentiation of ability of insulin to produce hypoglycemia; monitor BG closely and alter insulin regimen as needed
Iron preparations / ↓ Effect of tetracyclines R/T ↓ GI tract absorption
Isotretinoin / ↑ Incidence of pseudotumor cerebi; avoid concomitant use
Magnesium salts / ↓ Effect of tetracyclines R/T ↓ GI tract absorption
Methoxyflurane / ↑ Risk of kidney toxicity
Oral contraceptives / ↓ OC efficacy R/T interference with enterohepatic recirculation of certain contraceptive steroids by tetracyclines
Penicillins / Tetracyclines may interfere with the bactericidal activity of penicillins
Potassium citrate / ↑ Tetracycline excretion and ↓ serum levels
Sodium bicarbonate / ↓ Effect of tetracyclines R/T ↓ GI tract absorption
Sodium lactate / ↑ Tetracycline excretion and ↓ serum levels
Theophyllines / ↑ Incidence of theophylline side effects
Zinc salts / ↓ Effect of tetracyclines R/T ↓ GI tract absorption

LABORATORY TEST CONSIDERATIONS

False + or ↑ urinary catecholamines and urinary protein (degraded); ↑ coagulation time. False – or ↓ urinary urobilinogen, glucose tests (see *Nursing Implications*). Prolonged use or high doses may change liver function tests and WBC counts.

Classifications

DOSAGE

See individual drugs.

NURSING IMPLICATIONS

IMPLEMENTATION/ADMINISTRATION/STORAGE

1. Do not use outdated or deteriorated drugs, as a Fanconi-like syndrome may occur (see *Side Effects*).
2. Administer IM into large muscle mass to avoid extravasation into subcutaneous or fatty tissue.
3. Continue treatment for 24–48 hr after symptoms and fever subside. Treat all infections due to group A beta-hemolytic streptococci for 10 or more days.
4. **IV** Avoid rapid IV administration.
5. Prolonged IV use may cause thrombophlebitis.
6. Reserve IV use for situations where PO therapy is not indicated/tolerated. Institute PO therapy ASAP.

ASSESSMENT

1. Note reasons for therapy, onset, characteristics of S&S, clinical presentation, culture results. List other agents trialed and outcome.
2. Identify any drug allergens or sensitivity. IM form contains procaine HCl; assess for reactions.
3. Assess for colitis or other bowel problems. If pregnant, document trimester.
4. To prevent/treat pruritus ani, cleanse anal area with water several times a day and/or after each bowel movement. Observe for S&S of enterocolitis, such as diarrhea, pyrexia, abdominal distention, and scanty urine; may need to stop and try another antibiotic.
5. If GI disturbances occur, avoid antacids that contain calcium, magnesium, or aluminum. May take with a light meal or reduce dose, but increase administration frequency to reduce distress.
6. Assess with IV therapy for N&V, chills, fever, and hypertension resulting from too rapid administration or an excessively high dose; slow rate/report. Observe infant for bulging fontanel, which may be caused by a too rapid infusion rate.
7. Side effects such as sore throat, dysphagia, fever, dizziness, hoarseness, and inflammation of mucous membranes or candidal superinfections may occur. May cause onycholysis (loosening or detachment of the nail from the nail bed) or discoloration.
8. Monitor VS, weight, and I&O. Maintain adequate I&O as renal dysfunction may result in drug accumulation, leading to toxicity. With impaired renal function assess for increased BUN, acidosis, anorexia, N&V, weight loss, and dehydration; latent symptoms. Assess for altered level of consciousness or other CNS disturbances with impaired hepatic or renal function; may cause toxicity. Monitor CBC, BUN, creatinine, lytes, and cultures.

CLIENT/FAMILY TEACHING

1. Take on an empty stomach at least 1 hr before or 2 hr after meals. Withhold antacids, iron salts, dairy foods, and other foods high in calcium for at least 2 hr after PO administration. Do not take with milk, cheese, ice cream or yogurt. Take PO forms with plenty of fluids.
2. Zinc tablets or vitamin preparations containing zinc may interfere with drug absorption. Food sources high in zinc that should be avoided include oysters, fresh and raw; cooked lobster; dry oat flakes; steamed crabs; veal; and liver.
3. Avoid direct or artificial sunlight, which can cause a severe sunburn-like reaction; report if erythema occurs. Wear protective clothing, sunglasses, and sunscreen for up to 3 weeks following therapy.
4. Tetracyclines interfere with formation of tooth enamel and dental pigmentation from the third trimester of pregnancy through age 8.
5. Prevent/treat rectal itching by cleansing anal area with water several times a day and/or after each bowel movement.
6. Use alternative method of birth control, as drug may interfere with oral contraceptives; may also cause a vaginal infection.
7. Take only as directed and complete full prescription. Discard any unused capsules to prevent reaction from deteriorated drugs. Report loss of effectiveness or lack of response.
8. Keep all F/U to assess response, labs, and for adverse SE.

OUTCOMES/EVALUATE

- Resolution of infection (↓ temperature, ↓ WBCs, ↑ appetite)
- Symptomatic improvement
- Negative culture reports

THYROID DRUGS

SEE ALSO THE FOLLOWING INDIVIDUAL ENTRIES:

Levothyroxine sodium
Liothyronine sodium
Liotrix

INDICATIONS/USES

(1) Replacement or supplemental therapy in hypothyroidism due to all causes except transient hypothyroidism during the recovery phase of sub acute thyroiditis. (2) Treat or prevent euthyroid goiters, including thyroid nodules, subacute or chronic lymphocytic thyroiditis, multinodular goiter, and to manage thyroid cancer. (3) With antithyroid drugs for thyrotoxicosis (to prevent goiter or hypothyroidism). (4) Diagnostically to differentiate suspected hyperthyroidism from euthyroidism. (5) Myxedema coma and precoma. The treatment of choice for hypothyroidism is usually T_4 because of its consistent potency and its prolonged duration of action, although it does have a slow onset and its effects are cumulative over several weeks. *NOTE:* Exogenous thyroid hormone may cause regression of metastases from follicular and papillary thyroid carcinoma and is used as ancillary therapy in such conditions with radioactive iodine. Larger doses than those used for replacement therapy are needed.

ACTION/KINETICS

Action

The thyroid manufactures two active hormones: Thyroxine and triiodothyronine, both of which contain iodine. Synthetic derivatives include liothyronine (T_3), levothyroxine (T_4), and liotrix (a 4:1 mixture of T_4 and T_3). Thyroid hormones are released into the bloodstream where they are bound to protein. The mechanisms by which thyroid hormones exert their physiologic effect is not well understood. However, it is believed that most of the effects are exerted through control of DNA transcription and protein synthesis.

Thyroid hormones regulate growth by controlling protein synthesis and regulating energy metabolism by increasing the resting or basal metabolic rate. This increases respiratory rate, body temperature, CO_2, oxygen consumption, HR, blood volume, enzyme system activity, rate of fat, carbohydrate and protein metabolism, and growth and maturation. Excess thyroid hormone causes a decrease in TSH, and a lack of thyroid hormone causes an increase in the production and secretion of TSH. Normally, the ratio of T_4 to T_3 released from the thyroid gland is 20:1 with about 35% of T_4 being converted in the periphery (e.g., kidney, liver) to T_3.

Pharmacokinetics

PO administered T_4 absorption ranges from 40–80%; absorption is increased by fasting and decreased in malabsorption syndromes and by certain foods (e.g., soybean infant formula). Also, absorption may decrease with age and by certain drugs and foods. More than 99% of circulating hormone is bound to serum proteins, including thyroxine-binding globulin, thyroxine-binding prealbumin, and albumin. About 80% of T_3 comes from monodeiodination of T_4. Thyroid hormones are primarily excreted through the kidney, with about 20% eliminated in the feces. Urinary excretion of T_4 decreases with age.

CONTRAINDICATIONS

Uncorrected adrenal insufficiency, acute MI, hyperthyroidism, and untreated thyrotoxicosis. When hypothyroidism and adrenal insufficiency coexist unless treatment with adrenocortical steroids is initiated first. To treat obesity or infertility. Levothyroxine use in those with unrelated subclinical suppressed serum TSH with normal T_3 and T_4 levels and in acute MI.

SPECIAL CONCERNS

Drugs with thyroid hormone activity, alone or with other drugs, have been used for the treatment of obesity. In euthyroid clients, doses within the range of daily hormonal requirements are ineffective for weight reduction. Larger doses may produce serious or even life-threatening toxic effects, especially when given in association with sympathomimetic amines such as those used for their anorectic effects.

- **Geriatric clients and those with myxedema may be more sensitive to the usual adult dosage of these hormones.**
- **Use with extreme caution in the presence of angina pectoris, hypertension, and other CV diseases, renal insufficiency, and ischemic states.**
- **Use with caution during lactation and in clients with nontoxic diffuse goiter or nodular thyroid disease (i.e., to prevent thyrotoxicosis).**
- **Safety and efficacy not determined in children.**

Classifications

SIDE EFFECTS

Thyroid preparations have cumulative effects, and overdosage (e.g., symptoms of hyperthyroidism) may occur. **CV:** Arrhythmias, palpitations, angina, increased BP and pulse pressure, CHF, tachycardia, ***MI, cardiac arrest***, aggravation of CHF. **GI:** Abdominal cramps, diarrhea, N&V, appetite changes. **CNS:** Headache, nervousness, mental agitation, irritability, insomnia, tremors, hyperactivity, anxiety, emotional lability, seizures (rare). **Hypersensitivity:** Urticaria, pruritus, skin rash, flushing, angioedema, abdominal pain, N&V, diarrhea, fever, arthralgia, serum sickness, wheezing, allergic skin reactions (rare). **Miscellaneous:** Weight loss, hyperhidrosis, excessive warmth, irregular menses, heat intolerance, fatigue, fever, muscle weakness, dyspnea, hair loss, impaired fertility. Decreased bone density in pre- and postmenopausal women following long-term use of levothyroxine. *NOTE:* Pseudotumor cerebri and slipped capital femoral epiphysis seen in children receiving levothyroxine. Overtreatment may cause craniosynostosis in infants and premature closure of the epiphyses in children leading to compromised adult height.

OVERDOSE MANAGEMENT

Symptoms: Signs and symptoms of hyperthyroidism including headache, irritability, sweating, tachycardia, nervousness, increased bowel motility, palpitations, vomiting, psychosis, menstrual irregularities, ***seizures***, fever. Production or aggravation of angina or CHF, ***shock, arrhythmias, cardiac failure***.

Treatment: Reduce dose or temporarily discontinue therapy. Reinstitute therapy at a lower dosage.

DRUG INTERACTIONS

Amiodarone / ↓ T_3 levels
Antacids, Al- and Mg-containing / ↓ Thyroid absorption from the GI tract
Anticoagulants / ↑ Effect of anticoagulants by ↑ hypoprothrombinemia; monitor PT and INR
Antidepressants, tricyclic or tetracyclic / ↑ Therapeutic and toxic effects of both antidepressants and thyroid drugs
Antidiabetic agents / Hyperglycemic effect of thyroid preparations may necessitate ↑ in dose of both insulin or oral hypoglycemics
Beta-adrenergic blockers / ↓ Effect of beta blockers when the hypothyroid state is converted to the euthyroid state
Calcium salts / ↓ Thyroid absorption from the GI tract
Carbamazepine / ↑ Liver metabolism of levothyroxine → ↑ levothyroxine requirements
Cholestyramine / ↓ Effect of thyroid hormone R/T ↓ GI tract absorption
Colestipol / ↓ Effect of thyroid hormone R/T ↓ GI tract absorption
Corticosteroids / Thyroid preparations ↑ tissue demands for corticosteroids. Adrenal insufficiency must be corrected with corticosteroids before administering thyroid hormones. In clients already treated for adrenal insufficiency, dosage of corticosteroids must be increased when initiating therapy with thyroid drug
Digitalis compounds / ↓ Digitalis glycoside levels; ↓ therapeutic effects
Epinephrine / CV effects ↑ by thyroid preparations; ↑ risk of coronary insufficiency
Estrogens / May ↑ requirements for thyroid hormone
Growth hormone (somatrem, somatropin) / Excessive use of thyroid and growth hormone may accelerate epiphyseal closure
Iron salts / ↓ Absorption of thyroid from the GI tract
Ketamine / Concomitant use may result in severe hypertension and tachycardia
Levarterenol / CV effects ↑ by thyroid preparations; ↑ risk of coronary insufficiency
Oral contraceptives / May ↑ requirements for thyroid hormone
Phenobarbital / ↑ Liver metabolism of levothyroxine → ↑ levothyroxine requirements
Phenytoin / ↑ Liver metabolism of levothyroxine → ↑ levothyroxine requirements
Rifamycins / ↑ Liver metabolism of levothyroxine → ↑ levothyroxine requirements
Salicylates / Salicylates compete for thyroid-binding sites on protein
Simethicone / ↓ Thyroid absorption from the GI tract
Sodium polystyrene sulfonate / ↓ Thyroid absorption from the GI tract
H ***Soy*** / ↓ Absorption of supplemental thyroid hormones; space doses 2 hr apart
Sucralfate / ↓ Thyroid absorption from the GI tract

Theophylline / ↓ Theophylline clearance in hypothyroid; client is returned to normal when euthyroid state is reached

LABORATORY TEST CONSIDERATIONS

Alter thyroid function tests. ↑ PT. ↓ Serum cholesterol. A large number of drugs alter thyroid function tests.

DOSAGE

See individual hormone products.

NURSING IMPLICATIONS

IMPLEMENTATION/ADMINISTRATION/STORAGE

1. Initiate treatment with small doses that are gradually increased.
2. Check individual thyroid products for approximate dosage equivalents.
3. A child's dosage may be the same as the dosage for an adult.
4. Differences between brands of a drug mean that brand interchange is not recommended without consulting with provider or pharmacist. Use caution to prevent overdosage or relapse.
5. Store in a cool, dark place away from moisture and light.

ASSESSMENT

1. Perform a thorough history, documenting onset and characteristics of S&S and thyroid function tests (TFTs). Assess general physical condition (age, weight, disease severity/duration), and note angina, cardiac or other health problems.
2. Review all medications currently receiving to be sure none interacts with antithyroid drug, especially antidiabetic or anticoagulant therapy.
3. Assess clinical presentation noting S&S consistent with hypothyroidism (i.e., fatigue, lethargy, weight gain, puffy face and eyelids, large tongue, thyroid nodules, asymmetry, cold intolerance, hair loss, or cardiomegaly).
4. Note agent prescribed; thyroid extracts from hog or sheep do not have as predictable a response as the synthetic agents, may see more reactions. Animal derivatives are less stable and will degrade with exposure to moisture. Monitor thyroid function studies closely (for reduced T_3, T_4; ↑ radioimmunoassay of TSH).
5. Stop drug therapy 4 weeks before radioimmunoassay.
6. Observe for drug side effects; report complaints of headache, insomnia, and tremors. Note general response to therapy. Complaints of abdominal cramps, weight gain, edema, dyspnea, palpitations, angina, fatigue, or ↑ pallor may indicate cardiac problems.
7. Report any S&S or history of CAD. Monitor VS and cardiac rhythms; report if HR >100 bpm. Monitor weights. Observe for heat intolerance and excessive weight loss.
8. With anticoagulant therapy observe for purpura or ↑ bleeding. Monitor PT/PTT/INR closely; anticoagulant potentiated by thyroid preparations.
9. Obtain/monitor ECG, labs, TFTs, and assess need for radionuclide scanning.

CLIENT/FAMILY TEACHING

1. Drug must be taken only under medical supervision and must be taken for life. Take in a single morning dose, at the same time each day, to reduce the likelihood of insomnia.
2. Side effects may not appear for 4–6 weeks after the start of therapy or when dosage increased. Do not substitute or change brands without approval.
3. Record BP, pulse, and weight for review at each visit, to evaluate effectiveness of drug therapy. Any excessive weight loss, palpitations, leg cramps, nervousness, or insomnia requires immediate reporting, as dosage may be too high.
4. Carefully monitor child's growth and chart. Children may experience temporary hair loss.
5. With diabetes, thyroid preparations may require adjustment of insulin dosage. Monitor BS closely and report changes.
6. Certain foods, such as cabbage, turnips, pears, and peaches, are goitrogenic and may alter the requirements for thyroid hormone. Consult dietitian to discuss diet and assist with selecting foods according to increased energy demands resulting from the therapy. Thyroid hormones increase toxicity to iodine. Avoid foods high in iodine (dried kelp, iodized salt, saltwater fish/shellfish), multivitamins, dentifrices, and other nonprescription medications containing iodine.
7. Thyroid preparations potentiate the action of anticoagulants; if receiving anticoagulant ther-

apy, report excessive bleeding. Keep a record of menstrual cycles and report changes.
8. After several weeks of therapy, report if irritability, nervousness, and excitability occur; may indicate overdosage.
9. Keep all F/U to assess response, labs, and for adverse SE.

OUTCOMES/EVALUATE

- TFTs within desired range
- Normal metabolism evidenced by ↑ mental alertness, improvement in hair and skin condition, ↓ fatigue, ↓ panic attacks, normal growth/development, normal HR, regular bowel function

TRANQUILIZERS/ANTIMANIC DRUGS/ HYPNOTICS ■

SEE ALSO THE FOLLOWING INDIVIDUAL ENTRIES:

Alprazolam
Buspirone hydrochloride
Chlordiazepoxide
Clorazepate dipotassium
Diazepam
Eszopiclone
Hydroxyzine hydrochloride
Hydroxyzine pamoate
Lithium carbonate
Lithium citrate
Lorazepam
Midazolam hydrochloride
Ramelteon
Temazepam
Triazolam
Zaleplon
Zolpidem tartrate

INDICATIONS/USES

See individual drugs. Depending on the drug, used as antianxiety agents, hypnotics, anticonvulsants, and muscle relaxants. Many drugs also have special uses (see individual drugs).

ACTION/KINETICS

Action

Benzodiazepines are the major antianxiety agents. They are thought to affect the limbic system and reticular formation to reduce anxiety by increasing or facilitating the inhibitory neurotransmitter activity of GABA. Two benzodiazepine receptor subtypes have been identified in the brain-BZ_1 and BZ_2. Receptor subtype BZ_1 is believed to be associated with sleep mechanisms, whereas receptor subtype BZ_2 is associated with memory, motor, sensory, and cognitive function. When used for 3–4 weeks for sleep, certain benzodiazepines may cause REM rebound when discontinued. The benzodiazepines also possess varying degrees of anticonvulsant activity, skeletal muscle relaxation, and the ability to alleviate tension. The benzodiazepines generally have long half-lives (1–8 days); thus cumulative effects can occur. Several of the benzodiazepines are metabolized to active metabolites in the liver, which prolongs their duration of action.

Pharmacokinetics

Benzodiazepines are widely distributed throughout the body. Approximately 70–99% of an administered dose is bound to plasma protein. Metabolites of benzodiazepines are excreted through the kidneys. All tranquilizers have the ability to cause psychologic and physical dependence. Benzodiazepines have a wide margin of safety between therapeutic and toxic doses.

CONTRAINDICATIONS

Hypersensitivity, acute narrow-angle glaucoma, psychoses, primary depressive disorder, psychiatric disorders in which anxiety is not a significant symptom.

SPECIAL CONCERNS

- **Use with caution in impaired hepatic or renal function and in the geriatric or debilitated client.**
- **Use during lactation may cause sedation, weight loss, and possibly feeding difficulties in the infant.**
- **Geriatric clients may be more sensitive to the effects of benzodiazepines; symptoms may include oversedation, dizziness, confusion, or ataxia.**
- **Increased risk of hip fracture with benzodiazepine use in the elderly, especially during the first 2 weeks.**
- **When used for insomnia, rebound sleep disorders may occur following abrupt withdrawal of certain benzodiazepines.**

SIDE EFFECTS

CNS: Drowsiness, fatigue, confusion, ataxia, sedation, dizziness, vertigo, depression, apathy, lightheadedness, delirium, headache, lethargy, disorientation, hypoactivity, crying, anterograde amnesia, slurred speech, stupor, ***coma***, fainting, difficulty in concentration, euphoria, nervousness, irritability, akathisia, hypotonia, vivid dreams, "glassy-eyed," hysteria, ***suicide attempt***, psychosis. Paradoxical excitement manifested by anxiety, acute hyperexcitability, increased muscle spasticity, insomnia, hallucinations, sleep disturbances, rage, and stimulation. **GI:** Increased appetite, constipation, diarrhea, anorexia, N&V, weight gain or loss, dry mouth, bitter or metallic taste, increased salivation, coated tongue, sore gums, difficulty in swallowing, gastritis, fecal incontinence. **Respiratory:** ***Respiratory depression and sleep apnea***, especially in clients with compromised respiratory function. **Dermatologic:** Urticaria, rash, pruritus, alopecia, hirsutism, dermatitis, edema of ankles and face. **Endocrine:** Increased or decreased libido, gynecomastia, menstrual irregularities. **GU:** Difficulty in urination, urinary retention, incontinence, dysuria, enuresis. **CV:** Hypertension, hypotension, bradycardia, tachycardia, palpitations, edema, ***CV collapse***. **Hematologic:** Anemia, ***agranulocytosis***, leukopenia, eosinophilia, thrombocytopenia. **Ophthalmic:** Diplopia, conjunctivitis, nystagmus, blurred vision. **Miscellaneous:** Joint pain, lymphadenopathy, muscle cramps, paresthesia, dehydration, lupus-like symptoms, sweating, SOB, flushing, hiccoughs, fever, hepatic dysfunction. **Following IM use:** Redness, pain, burning. **Following IV use:** Thrombosis and phlebitis at site.

OVERDOSE MANAGEMENT

Symptoms: Severe drowsiness, confusion with reduced or absent reflexes, tremors, slurred speech, staggering, hypotension, SOB, labored breathing, ***respiratory depression***, impaired coordination, ***seizures***, weakness, slow HR, ***coma***. *NOTE:* Geriatric clients, debilitated clients, young children, and clients with liver disease are more sensitive to the CNS effects of benzodiazepines.

Treatment: Supportive therapy. In the event of an overdose of a benzodiazepine, have a benzodiazepine antagonist (flumazenil) readily available. Gastric lavage, provided that an ET tube with an inflated cuff is used to prevent aspiration of vomitus. Emesis only if drug ingestion was recent and client is fully conscious. Activated charcoal and saline cathartic may be given after emesis or lavage. Maintain adequate respiratory function. Reverse hypotension by IV fluids, norepinephrine, or metaraminol. **Do not** treat excitation with barbiturates.

DRUG INTERACTIONS

Alcohol / Potentiation or addition of CNS depressant effects; concomitant use may lead to drowsiness, lethargy, stupor, respiratory collapse, coma, or death
Anesthetics, general / See ***Alcohol***
Antacids / ↓ Rate of absorption of benzodiazepines
Antidepressants, tricyclic / Concomitant use with benzodiazepines may cause additive sedative effect and/or atropine-like side effects
Antihistamines / See ***Alcohol***
Barbiturates / See ***Alcohol***
Cimetidine / ↑ Effect of benzodiazepines R/T ↓ liver breakdown
CNS depressants / See ***Alcohol***
Digoxin / Benzodiazepines ↑ serum digoxin levels
Disulfiram / ↑ Effect of benzodiazepines by ↓ liver breakdown
Erythromycin / ↑ Effect of benzodiazepines by ↓ liver breakdown
Fluoxetine / ↑ Effect of benzodiazepines R/T ↓ liver breakdown
Grapefruit juice / ↑ Bioavailability of certain benzodiazepines (e.g., midazolam)
Isoniazid / ↑ Effect of benzodiazepines R/T ↓ liver breakdown
H ***Kava kava*** / Additive CNS depressant effect
Ketoconazole / ↑ Effect of benzodiazepines R/T ↓ liver breakdown
Levodopa / Effect may be ↓ by benzodiazepines
Metoprolol / ↑ Effect of benzodiazepines R/T ↓ liver breakdown
Narcotics / See ***Alcohol***
Neuromuscular blocking agents / Benzodiazepines may ↑, ↓, or have no effect on the action of neuromuscular blocking agents
Oral contraceptives / ↑ Effect of benzodiazepines R/T ↓ liver breakdown; or, ↑ rate of clearance of benzodiazepines that undergo glucuronidation (e.g., lorazepam, oxazepam)
Phenothiazines / See ***Alcohol***
Phenytoin / Concomitant use with benzodiazepines may cause ↑ effect of phenytoin R/T ↓ liver breakdown
Probenecid / ↑ Effect of selected benzodiazepines R/T ↓ liver breakdown
Propoxyphene / ↑ Effect of benzodiazepines R/T ↓ liver breakdown

Propranolol / ↑ Effect of benzodiazepines R/T ↓ liver breakdown
Ranitidine / May ↓ absorption of benzodiazepines from the GI tract
Rifampin / ↓ Effect of benzodiazepines R/T ↑ liver breakdown
Sedative-hypnotics, nonbarbiturate / See ***Alcohol***
Smoking / ↓ Benzodiazepine-induced sedation and drowsiness possibly R/T nicotine stimulation of the CNS
Theophyllines / ↓ Sedative effect of benzodiazepines
H ***Valerian*** / Additive CNS depressant effect
Valproic acid / ↑ Effect of benzodiazepines R/T ↓ liver breakdown

LABORATORY TEST CONSIDERATIONS

↑ AST, ALT, LDH, alkaline phosphatase.

DOSAGE

See individual drugs.

NURSING IMPLICATIONS

IMPLEMENTATION/ADMINISTRATION/STORAGE

1. Persistent drowsiness, ataxia, or visual disturbances may require dosage adjustment.
2. Lower dosage is usually indicated for older clients. For example, diazepam, 3 mg or more equivalents/day, increases the risk of hip fracture in the elderly.
3. GI effects are decreased when drugs are given with meals or shortly afterward.
4. Withdraw drugs gradually.

ASSESSMENT

1. Note reasons for therapy, onset of symptoms, behavioral manifestations/clinical presentation. Assess manner in which client responds to questions/problems. Identify any prior treatments, what was used, for how long, and the outcome.
2. List drugs currently prescribed to ensure none interact unfavorably. Check for any adverse reactions to this class of drugs. Review physical exam, reflexes, CNS findings and history for any contraindications to therapy.
3. Assess lifestyle and general level of health; note any situations that may contribute to these symptoms.
4. Administer the lowest possible effective dose, especially if elderly or debilitated. Note any symptoms consistent with overdosage.
5. Report complaints of sore throat (other than those caused by NG or ET tubes), fever, or weakness and assess for blood dyscrasias; check CBC.
6. Monitor BP before and after IV dose of antianxiety medication. Keep recumbent for 2–3 hr after IV. When hospitalized and given PO, remain until swallowed.
7. If client exhibits ataxia, or weakness or lack of coordination when ambulating, provide supervision/assistance. Use side rails once in bed and identify clients at risk for falls; utilize alarms to prevent falls.
8. Note any S&S of cholestatic jaundice: nausea, diarrhea, upper abdominal pain, or the presence of high fever or rash; check LFTs. Report if yellowing of sclera, skin, or mucous membranes evident (late sign of cholestatic jaundice and biliary tract obstruction); hold if overly sleepy/confused or becomes comatose.
9. With suicidal tendencies, anticipate drug will be prescribed in small doses/quantities. Report signs of increased depression immediately.
10. If history of alcoholism or if taking excessive quantities of drug, carefully supervise amount prescribed and dispensed. Note any evidence of physical or psychologic dependence. Assess for manifestations of ataxia, slurred speech, and vertigo (symptoms of chronic intoxication and that client may be exceeding dose).
11. Monitor VS, I&O, CBC, renal and LFTs; assess for blood dyscrasias or impaired function.

CLIENT/FAMILY TEACHING

1. Take most of daily dose at bedtime, with smaller doses during the waking hours to minimize mental/motor impairment. These drugs may reduce ability to handle potentially dangerous equipment, such as cars and machinery especially during the first 2 weeks of therapy; may decrease over time.
2. Rise slowly from a supine position and dangle legs over side of the bed before standing. If feeling faint sit/lie down immediately and lower the head. Allow extra time to prepare for daily activities; take precautions before arising, to reduce one source of anxiety and

stress. Identify/practice relaxation techniques that may assist in lowering anxiety levels.

3. Avoid alcohol while taking antianxiety agents. Alcohol potentiates the depressant effects of both the alcohol and the medication. Do not take any unprescribed or OTC medications without approval.
4. Do not stop taking drug suddenly. Any sudden withdrawal after prolonged therapy or after excessive use may cause a recurrence of the preexisting symptoms of anxiety. It may also cause a withdrawal syndrome, manifested by increased anxiety, anorexia, insomnia, vomiting, ataxia, muscle twitching, confusion, and hallucinations. May also develop seizures and convulsions.
5. These drugs are generally for short-term therapy; follow-up is imperative to evaluate response and the need for continued therapy. Report any adverse side effects and lack of response.
6. Avoid prolonged sun exposure and use protection if exposed. Do not overexert during hot weather, drink plenty of water, and remain cool; may cause heat stroke.
7. Attend appropriate counselling sessions as condition and length of therapy dictate.
8. Keep all F/U to assess response, labs, and for adverse SE.

OUTCOMES/EVALUATE

- ↓ Anxiety/tension episodes; ↑ coping ability
- ↓ Frequency/intensity of muscle spasms/tremor; seizure control
- Improved sleeping patterns
- Control of alcohol withdrawal symptoms

VACCINES

SEE TABLES 3, 4, AND 5.

GENERAL STATEMENT

Vaccines have played an important role in the health and life span of our population. They have been in use over 200 years, but since World War II, once the importance of disease prevention became evident, research into the area of vaccine development exploded.

More recently, the population has been exposed to the threat of biological warfare. This involves the use of a biologic microorganism in a bioterrorist attack. This may include radiation and dirty bombs, occupational health, food, and water security. Much discussion has been entertained as to how to deal with this threat, including mass immunizations and post-exposure prophylaxis. To this point, this question has not been resolved.

Additionally, the outbreak of swine flu, or the H1N1 virus, has taken forefront in our news. The H1N1 influenza virus has had a long history since first being identified in 1918 during what was termed the Spanish influenza pandemic, which infected one third of the world's population of 500 million people. Roughly 50 million people died during this viral outbreak. Not until the 1930s were the linked influenza viruses (now known as H1N1 viruses) isolated from pigs and then humans. In 1976, an outbreak of influenza occurred at Fort Dix in New Jersey and affected 200, some severely, with one death of a soldier who experienced feeling tired and weak and was dead the next day. Others during this outbreak were seriously ill. On March 18, 2009, the first illness (H1N1 influenza A) was reported in Mexico and continued to spread. By May 5, 2009, almost 600 more H1N1 influenza cases were confirmed in Mexico and 25 of these people died. Two children were diagnosed in April of 2009 in neighboring counties in southern California with swine influenza A (H1N1), and by April 26, 2009, the U.S. Department of Health and Human Services declared a national public health emergency involving H1N1 influenza A. People younger than 65 years of age are more severely affected by this disease. Those 18–64 years of age were most impacted by serious illness including hospitalizations, followed by people in the 0–17 years old age group. The CDC estimates that between 42 million and 86 million cases of H1N1 occurred between April 2009 and February 13, 2010, and between about 8,520 and 17,620 H1N1-related deaths occurred between April 2009 and February 13, 2010. The vaccine is the best way to protect against this virus. This is most important for people at higher risk of serious complications from H1N1, including those with certain health conditions, the very young, and those over age 65.

The annual 2010/2011 influenza vaccine incorporated the H1N1 vaccine. The fear of avian flu or the H5N1 influenza virus in migratory birds from Asia to Eastern Europe has raised the fear of a potential pandemic. WHO has recommended that the 2012-2013 vaccine viruses contain A/California/7/2009-like (2009H1N1), A/Victoria/361/2011-like (H3N2), and B/Wisconsin/1/2010-like (B/Yamagata lineage) viruses based on surveillance data and response to 2011-2012 trivalent seasonal vaccines.

Use of a vaccine (or actually contracting the disease) usually imparts a temporary or permanent resistance to an infectious disease. The human immune system has a memory. As the body is exposed to a disease-producing organism, the lymphocytes (immune cells) are activated and, by cell division, reproduce and attack the offending organism. Some of these lymphocytes remain in the body indefinitely with memory cells. Vaccines and toxoids promote the type of antibody production one would see if they had experienced the natural infection. This active immunization involves the direct administration of antigens to the host by intentionally exposing the immune system to a foreign infectious agent so it forms a memory of that agent. This causes the individual to produce the desired antibodies and cell-mediated immunity. These agents may consist of live attenuated agents or killed (inactivated) agents, or agents that alter the hosts' genetic structure. Immunizations confer resistance without actually producing disease.

Some vaccines are in short supply due to the push for immunization and are reserved for those individuals who have direct contact with the organism in the laboratory, military personnel deployed to an area with high risk for exposure to the organism, or other at risk individuals. Some organisms (anthrax) can be managed effectively with antibiotics in post-exposure prophylaxis. Passive immunization occurs when immunologic agents are administered. Immunoglobulins and antivenins only offer passive short-term immunity and are usually administered for a specific exposure.

There has been controversy surrounding some childhood vaccines. Some parents have claimed that their child was developing normally until they received their vaccinations. Many parents who have children with autism are attributing it to the thimerosal preservatives found in vaccines (influenza, DTP), which metabolizes into ethyl mercury.

The use of thimerosal has diminished since 1977, after recommendations by medical authorities, but trace amounts of thimerosal remain in many vaccines and in some vaccines, thimerosal has not yet been phased out despite recommendations. Some states have enacted laws banning the use of thimerosal in childhood vaccines. After review of the scientific literature, the Institute of Medicine (IOM) concluded that "the evidence favors rejection of a causal relationship between thimerosal-containing vaccines and autism." CDC supports the IOM conclusion.

Aggressive pediatric immunization programs have helped reduce preventable infections and death in children worldwide. Vaccines have contributed to the eradication of one of the most contagious and deadly diseases known to man, smallpox. Other diseases such as rubella, polio, chickenpox, measles, mumps, and typhoid are nowhere near as common as they were just 100 years ago. As long as a vast majority are vaccinated, it is much more difficult for a disease outbreak to occur, let alone spread. A recent publicized measles outbreak was related to lack of immunization. The other measles outbreaks have been related to international travel and imported. Polio, which is transmitted only between humans, has been targeted by an extensive campaign of eradication that has seen endemic polio restricted to only parts of four countries. Difficulty in reaching all children has caused the eradication date to be missed twice by 2006. This focus should continue and should be expanded to the adult population, many of whom have missed the natural infection and past immunizations. Some adults were never vaccinated as children. Also, some of the newer vaccines were not available when some adults were children. Immunity can begin to fade over time, so as we age, we become more susceptible to serious disease caused by common infections (e.g., flu, pneumococcus). A careful immunization history should be documented for every client, regardless of age. When in doubt or if disease/infection or immunization status is unknown, appropriate serologic evidence/titers may be drawn.

By 2010 27,500 cases of pertussis were reported and many more cases go unreported. Aggressive public health notices have advised that vaccinations of Tdap for pre-teens, teens, and adults occur, as protection from childhood vaccines fade over time. Pertussis outbreaks in hospitals and other clinical settings put infants and other patients at risk.

Shingles is caused by the varicella-zoster virus, the same virus that causes chickenpox. After an attack of chickenpox, the virus lies dormant in certain nerve tissue. As we age, the virus can reappear in the form of shingles. It is most common in people older than 50. Shingles is characterized by clusters of blisters that can cause severe pain that may last for weeks, months, or years. Zostavax is a live virus vaccine recently released that is given as a single injection under the skin (upper arm) to adults over age 50.

Vaccines remain one of the most powerful tools we have for disease prevention. Advances in biotechnology have ushered in a new era in vaccine development that holds even more promise for improving public health. Currently scientists are pursuing many promising new strategies in vaccine development and exploring novel ways to administer vaccines that may provide safer, more effective ways to fight disease. Table 3 lists some of the more common or currently discussed diseases, the general recommended schedule to confer immunization, and the length of immunity conferred. Table 4 outlines the active childhood immunization schedule, while Table 5 identifies an active Adult Immunization Schedule. For more information:

Academy of Pediatrics: http://www.aap.org

Centers for Disease Control and Prevention: http://www.cdc.gov

National Immunization Program: http://www.cdc.gov/vaccines

Infectious Diseases Society of America: http://www.idsociety.org

Immunization Action Coalition: http://www.immunize.org

National Network for Immunization Information (offers vaccination requirements by state): http://www.immunizationinfo.org

John Hopkins Center for Public Health Preparedness: http://jhsph.edu/preparedness

World Health Organization: http://www.who.int/en/

TABLE 3 Common Diseases, General Recommended Immunization Schedule, and Length of Immunity

Disease	Immunization Schedule	Length of Immunity
Anthrax	3 SC shots q 2 weeks followed by 3 additional SC shots given at 6, 12, and 18 months	1-year boosters (not available to public yet)
BCG vaccine (TB)	Adult/child >1 month:: 0.2–0.3 mL; child <1 month N˘cc dose by 50% following guidelines	TB post-exposure
Botulism	Pentavalent toxoid (types A,B,C,D,E) 0.5 mL SC (available from USAMRIID)	Post-exposure
Cholera	Two doses 1 week to 1 month apart (0.5 mL)	6 months
Diphtheria	Given as *DTaP; four doses at ages 2, 4, 6, and 15–18 months; booster at 4–6 years.	10 years
H1N1	0.25 mL, TIV age 6 months to 9 years (2 doses, 4 weeks apart); 0.5 mL over age 3	Lifetime
* Haemophilus influenzae (Hib)	Four doses at ages 2, 4, 6, and 15 months	Unknown (check titers)
*Hepatitis A	Initial dose with booster given at 6 months (2 doses, at least 6 months apart)	10 yrs
*Hepatitis B	Three doses:: At birth (or initial dose), 1 month later, and 6 months after second dose	Unknown (check titers)
Human Papillomavirus vaccine (HPV)	Three dose schedule with the second and third dose given 2 and 6 months after the first dose. Females age 11–12; as young as 9 years; catchup aged 13–26 years old if no previous vaccination or did not complete series: HPV4: males aged 9–26 years	Lifetime
*Influenza (flu)	One dose (or two doses of split virus if under 19 years, 4 weeks apart). All children 6–59 months; yearly	1 year
Measles	Given as *MMR at ages 12–15 months and 4–6 years	Lifetime
*Meningococcal meningitis	One dose (antibody response requires 5 days); 11 years for MCV4; 2 years for MPSV4; MCV4 at age 11–12 and at HS entry; antibiotic prophylaxis (rifampin 600 mg or 10 mg/kg q 12 hr for four doses should be given to all contacts per exposure)	?Lifetime; not consistently effective in those <2 years of age; booster may be needed
Mumps	Given as *MMR at ages 12–15 months and 4–6 years	Lifetime
Pertussis	Given as *DTaP; four doses at ages 2, 4, 6, and 15–18 months	10 years
*Pneumococcal (PCV)	One dose or 2 doses (0.5 mL)	Approx. 5–10 years
Poliovirus (OPV)	Four doses at ages 2, 4, and 6 months, then at age 4–6 years	Lifetime
* Poliovirus (IPV)	If all IPV or all OPV doses given before age 4, a fourth dose is necessary. If both given in the series, a total of four doses should be given and a fifth dose at ages 4–6.	Lifetime

(continues)

TABLE 3 Common Diseases, General Recommended Immunization Schedule, and Length of Immunity—*Continued*

Disease	Immunization Schedule	Length of Immunity
Rabies	Postexposure:: five doses on days 0, 3, 7, 14, and 28 with the rabies immune globulin; pre-exposure:: two doses 1 week apart, third dose 2–3 weeks later	Approx. 2 years
*Rotavirus (RV)	Given as three doses at ages 2, 4, and 6 months; do not start after age 12 weeks and do not give after age 32 weeks.	Unknown
Rubella	Given as *MMR at ages 12–15 months and 4–6 years	Lifetime
Smallpox	One dose; this vaccine available at CDC and local public health departments (critical in less than 4 days of exposure); vaccinia immune globulin in special cases, call USAMRIID	3–10 years
*Tetanus	Given initially as *DTaP; four doses at ages 2, 4, 6, and 15–18 months	Required every 10 years; 5 years if trauma
Typhoid	CPS vaccine (at-risk travelers)	IM 2 years; capsules 5 years
*Varicella vaccine	One dose (0.5 mL) age 12–15 months and a second dose (0.5 mL) at age 4–6 years	Unknown (check titers)
Varicella Zoster (shingles)	Zostavax (Zoster vaccine live)—SC—one dose	Lifetime
Yellow fever	One dose (>9 months old for at-risk travelers)	10 years

* Recommended immunizations

Centers for Disease Control and Prevention. Recommended immunization schedules, www.cdc.gov/vaccines

State Mandates on Immunization and Vaccine—Preventable Diseases www.immunize.org/laws

TABLE 4 Active Childhood Immunization Schedule

	First	Second	Third*	Fourth
DTaP	2 months	4 months	6 months	15–18 months
H1N1	6 months	4 weeks later		
Hepatitis A	2 doses between 12 and 23 months			
Hepatitus B	birth or initial dose	1 month after first dose	6 months or more after second dose	
Hib (*Haemophilus influenzae* type b)	2 months	4 months	6 months	12–15 months
Influenza	Yearly			
IPV (inactivated poliovirus vaccine)	2 months	4 months	6–18 months	4–6 years
MMR	12–18 months	4 years	-	-
OPV (oral poliovirus vaccine)	2 months	4 months	6 months	4–6 years
Pneumococcal, influenza	12–15 months At age 6 months and older—yearly			
Rotavirus	2 months	4 months	6 months	
Varicella	2 doses between 12–18 months; and 4–6 years			

Check with the CDC for catch up schedule: www.cdc.gov/vaccines

TABLE 5 Active Adult Immunization Schedule

HPV	3 doses for females through age 26
Influenza	Every year
Tetanus (Td/Tdap)	Tetanus booster every 10 years; with injury obtain one in 5 years; Tdap regardless of last Td
Pneumococcal	One dose after age 65
Varicella	2 doses (age 20 to >65)
Zostavax	One dose after age 60

VITAMINS

SEE TABLES 6, 7, AND 8.

GENERAL STATEMENT

Vitamins are essential, carbon-containing, noncaloric substances that are required for normal metabolism. They are organic compounds the body cannot produce but are produced by living materials such as plants and animals and they are generally obtained from the diet. They may also be referred to as nutrients. Vitamin D is synthesized in the body to a limited extent and Vitamin B_{12} is synthesized in the intestinal tract by bacterial flora.

Vitamins are essential for promoting growth, health, vitality, life, general well-being, and for the prevention and cure of many health problems and diseases. They are necessary for the metabolic processes responsible for transforming foods into tissue or energy. Vitamins are also involved in the formation and maintenance of blood cells, chemicals supporting the nervous system, hormones, and genetic materials. Vitamins do not provide energy because they contain no calories. Yet, some do help convert the calories in fats, carbohydrates, and proteins into usable body energy. Many misinformed people think vitamins can replace food. In fact, vitamins can not be assimilated without ingesting food. That is why they should be taken with a meal. Vitamins regulate metabolism, help convert fat and carbohydrates into energy, and assist in forming bone and tissue.

Disease states caused by severe nutritional deficiencies prompted the discovery of vitamins because scientists were able to reverse the signs and symptoms of these disease states with vitamins. Severe deficiencies include scurvy, rickets, pellagra, pernicious anemia, xerophthalmia, beriberi, osteomalacia, infantile hemolytic anemia, and hemorrhagic diseases of the newborn. Moderate vitamin deficiencies may also produce symptoms of impaired health.

Environmental factors and genetic predisposition may influence individual requirements for specific vitamins. Disease processes, growth, hormone balance, and drugs may also alter the dietary requirements and function of vitamins.

Many deficiency states can be traced to special circumstances such as pernicious anemia after gastrectomy; pellagra in corn-eating populations, and scurvy in the elderly subsisting on soft foods (e.g., eggs, bread, milk) while neglecting citrus fruits. Generally, although not common in the United States, vitamin deficiency usually involves multiple rather than single deficiencies and usually can be attributed to poor lifestyle choices and poor dietary habits with an inadequate intake of many nutrients, including all vitamins. Since vitamins are required in such small amounts, deficiencies are rare in industrialized nations. Vitamin toxicity/excess may occur and is more often the problem due to the ready availability of nutritional supplements.

There are two categories of vitamins: fat soluble and water soluble, depending on how the intestines absorb them. Fat soluble vitamins (A, D, E, and K) are found in the fat or oil of foods and require digestible fat and bile salts for absorption in the small intestine. The water-soluble vitamins, C and B complex (B-1, B-2, niacin, B-6, folic acid, B_{12}, pantothenic acid, and biotin) are found in the watery portion of foods and are well absorbed by the GI tract. They are easily lost through overcooking and do not require fat for absorption. Water soluble vitamins mix easily in the blood, are excreted by the kidneys, and only small amounts are stored in the tissues, so regular daily intake is essential. Fat soluble vitamins are stored in the body after binding to specific plasma globulins in fat parts of the body. In high doses they may accumulate in the body and cause adverse reactions.

Recommended Dietary Allowances (RDAs) are the recommended human vitamin and mineral intake requirements. These were developed by the Food and Nutrition Board, National Research Council of the National Academy of Sciences and have evolved over the past 50 years and are updated every 5 years. They are based on age, height, weight, and gender. These are only estimates of nutrient needs; each client and the surrounding factors warrant individualized evaluation when replacement is being considered. Pregnant and breast-feeding women, and children require more of some vitamins than most adults. The elderly seem more prone to deficiencies due to poor absorption during the aging process and due to decreased sun exposure, as their skin is not able to absorb enough to produce active forms of vitamin D. In fact, vitamin D deficiency is underdiagnosed and undertreated in our population today. Clients with impaired liver function should not

Classifications

take large amounts of fat soluble vitamins (i.e.; A, D, E, K) unless specifically prescribed due to the toxicity potential from cumulative effects.

The National Academy of Sciences Commission On Life Sciences has published the RDA for healthy people. RDAs are based on various kinds of evidence: 1) studies of subjects maintained on diets containing low or deficient levels of a nutrient, followed by correction of the deficit with measured amounts of the nutrient; 2) nutrient balance studies that measure nutrient status in relation to intake; 3) biochemical measurements of tissue saturation or adequacy of molecular function in relation to nutrient intake; 4) nutrient intakes of fully breastfed infants and of apparently healthy people from their food supply; 5) epidemiological observations of nutrient status in population in relation to intake; 6) in some cases, extrapolation of data from animal experiments. In practice there are only limited data on which estimates of nutrient requirements can be based. These are the elements that the advisory counsel has identified that has led their recommendations.

The HHS and USDA developed the Dietary Guidelines for Americans 2010. *Dietary Guidelines for Americans 2010* was released on January 13, 2011. The *Guidelines* must be issued at least every 5 years by law. (Public Law 101-445, Title III, 7 U.S.Code 301). This is available for view online at http://www.health.gov/dietaryguidelines/, and consist of six chapters with appendices and tables.

These guidelines emphasize:

- Balance calories with physical activity to manage weight.
- Consume more of certain foods and nutrients, such as fruits, vegetables, whole grains, fat-free and low-fat dairy products, and seafood.
- Consume fewer foods with sodium (salt), saturated fats, cholesterol, added sugars, and refined grains.

For women of childbearing age who may become pregnant: Eat foods high in heme-iron and/or consume iron-rich plant foods or iron-fortified foods with an enhancer of iron absorption, such as vitamin C-rich foods. Consume 400 micrograms of folic acid daily (foods, supplements). Additional recommendations for women who are pregnant or breast-feeding were addressed. Individuals age 50 and older are advised to consume foods fortified with vitamin B_{12}. The guidelines focus on building healthy eating patterns, and helping Americans make healthy choices.

NURSING IMPLICATIONS

ASSESSMENT

1. **Document indications for therapy, clinical presentation, and deficiency states. Have a full nutritional assessment done by a registered dietician as needed.**
2. **Determine client use and knowledge on the utilization of nutrients. Many overtake these agents and waste money on products of little use or that may even cause toxicity.**
3. **List agents prescribed to ensure none interact or impact vitamin absorption.**
4. **Identify if vegetarian. There is no vitamin B_{12} in any plant product. Also ↓ vitamin B_{12} absorption in the elderly. Use caution as folate administered to one deficient in vitamin B_{12} may result in subacute spine degeneration with paralysis.**
5. **With replacement, monitor levels as indicated to ensure requirements are met and levels are as desired (i.e., vitamin D test-25-OH).**
6. **Review *Dietary Guidelines for Americans 2010* with clients to ensure they have this information available for their review and understand updates and recommendations.**
7. **Assess metabolic panel and vitamin levels as indicated.**

CLIENT/FAMILY TEACHING

1. **Comply with dietary recommendations. The best source of vitamins is a well-balanced diet with foods from the basic food groups. Some require vitamin supplementation to replace those lost with continued drug use, certain conditions i.e. pregnancy, elderly, or certain disease states.**
2. **Take with food for best absorption and utilization.**

3. **Avoid self-medicating with vitamin supplements that exceed the RDA. Megadoses of vitamins (nutrients) for various medical conditions is unproven and may cause adverse side effects and toxicity. The fat soluble vitamins (A, D, E, & K) may accumulate and cause toxicity. At the least it will be a huge waste of money due to the fact that many vitamins in excess of body requirements are excreted.**
4. **Store away from heat in tight, light-resistant containers, out of childrens' reach. Regularly check for expiration dates and discard if expired.**
5. **Utilize reliable resources to expand knowledge of nutrient/vitamin use and always check with provider before adding to prescribed regimen. These should always be listed on medication lists and updated at each visit during medication reconciliation.**
6. **With deficiency states, keep all F/U to assess response, labs, and for any adverse SE.**

OUTCOMES/EVALUATE

- Prevention/decrease of symptoms of vitamin deficiencies
- Normal healthy functioning of body
- Prevention/cure of related health problems/diseases

TABLE 6 Common Vitamin Requirements For Adults

Vitamin	RDA	Physiologic Effects Essential for:
A (retinol, retinaldehyde, retonic acid)	Men: 5,000; Women: 4,000 international units	Growth and development; epithelial tissue maintenance; reproduction; prevents night blindness; stimulates production/activity of WBCs, takes part in remodeling bone
B complex::		Increasing intake of folic acid, vitamin B-6, and vitamin B-12 decreases homocysteine levels
B-1 (thiamine)	Male: 1.5 mg Female: 1.3 mg	Energy metabolism; normal nerve function
B-2 (riboflavin)	1.3–1.8 mg	Reactions in energy cycle that produce ATP; oxidation of amino acids and hydroxy acids; oxidation of purines
B-3 Niacin (nicotinic acid, nicotinamide)	14–20 mg	Synthesis of fatty acids and cholesterol; blocks FFA; conversion of phenylalanine to tyrosine
B-5 Pantothenic acid (calcium pantothenate, dexpanthenol)	5–10 mg	Synthesis of sterols, steroid hormones, porphyrins; synthesis and degradation of fatty acids; oxidative metabolism of carbohydrates, gluconeogenesis
B-6 (pyridoxine, pyridoxal, pyridoxamine)	2 mg	Amino acid metabolism; glycogenolysis, RBC/Hb synthesis; formation of neurotransmitters; formation of antibodies
Folacin (folic acid, pteroylglutamic acid)	400 mcg	DNA synthesis, formation of RBCs in bone marrow with cyanocobalamin; prevention of neural tube defects
B^{12} (cyanocobalamin, hydroxocobalamin, extrinsic factor)	3–6 mcg	DNA synthesis in bone marrow; RBC production with folacin; nerve tissue maintenance; prevents pernicious anemia
B-7 (Biotin)	300 mcg	Synthesis of fatty acids, generation of tricarboxylic acid cycle; formation of purines Coenzyme in CHO metabolism
C (ascorbic acid, ascorbate)	Men: 90 mg; Women: 75 mg; Extra 35 mg for smokers, alcoholics	Formation of collagen; conversion of cholesterol to bile acids; protects A and E and polyunsaturated fats from excessive oxidation; absorption and utilization of iron; converts folacin to folinic acid; some role in clotting, adrenocortical hormones, and resistance to cancer and infections; powerful antioxidant that can neutralize harmful free radicals
D (calcitriol, cholecalciferol, dihydrotachysterol, ergocalciferol, viosterol)	400 international units, or 10 mcg	Intestinal absorption and metabolism of calcium and phosphorus as well as renal reabsorption; release of calcium from bone and resorption
E (tocopherol, retinol)	Tocopherol: 22–33 international units; Retinol: 8–12 mcg (retinol equivalents)	May oppose destruction of Vitamin A and fats by oxygen fragments called free radicals; antioxidant; may affect production of prostaglandins which regulate a variety of body processes
K (menadione, phytonadione)	Men: 120 mcg; Women: 90 mcg	Formation of prothrombin and other clotting proteins by the liver; blood coagulation

TABLE 7 Vitamin Food Sources

Vitamin	Food Source
A (retinoic acid)	Eggs, liver, green leafy vegetables, milk, butter, colorful fruits and vegetables (carrots, tomatoes, sweet potatoes) some fish
B-1 (Thiamine)	Oatmeal, barley, rice bran, sunflower/sesame seeds
B-2 (Riboflavin)	Meat, liver, fish, green vegetables, milk products
B-3 (Niacin)	Pork, cereals (wheat, rye, corn), green vegetables, meat, fruits, legumes, milk, eggs, peanuts
B-6 (Pyridoxine)	Milk, cereals, meat, some vegetables, beans, fortified grains, banana, avocado
B_{12}	Liver, kidney, meat, dairy products, fortified cereals (vegetarians most at risk for deficiency)
C (Ascorbic acid)	Citrus fruits, juices, other fruits and vegetables, tomatoes, kiwi, broccoli, peppers, papaya
D	Cheese, eggs, fortified milk, butter, fish liver oils, fortified foods
E	Vegetable oils, widely available in a variety of foods, wheat germ, walnuts, almonds, sunflower seeds/oil, sweet potato, soybeans
K	Made by bacteria inside intestines; green leafy vegetables, cabbage, potatoes, cauliflower, liver, broccoli, lentils, chickpeas
Biotin (B-7)	Available in many food sources (almonds, peanuts, pecans, liver, cauliflower); made by intestinal bacteria
Folic Acid	Meats, kidney, liver, vegetables, beans, fortified cereals, fruits, dark green vegetables, asparagus, sweet potato, oranges
Panthothenic Acid (B-5)	Widely available in many different food sources (liver. kidney, chicken, turkey, eggs, salmon, vegetables)

Classifications

TABLE 8 Vitamin Deficiency States

Vitamin	Deficiency	Signs and Symptoms
A	Xerophthalmia	Progressive eye changes:: Night blindness to xerosis of conjunctiva and cornea with scarring
	Keratomalacia	Degeneration of epithelial cells with hardening and shrinking
B-1	Beriberi	Nerve damage, edema, CHF, Wernicke-Korsakoff syndrome
B-3 Niacin	Pellagra	Depression, anorexia, beefy red glossitis, cheilosis, dermatitis
B-6	Rare—usually seen with multiple B deficiencies	Fatigue, weight loss, weakness, irritability; headaches, insomnia, peripheral neuropathy, CHF, cardiomyopathy
B-7	Biotin deficiency	Hair loss, scaly red rash around eye, nose, mouth, and genital area; depression, lethargy, unusual facial fat distribution; numbness/tingling in extremities
B-12	Pernicious anemia	Macrocytic, megaloblastic anemia; progressive neuropathy R/T demyelination
C	Scurvy	Joint pain, growth retardation, anemia, poor wound healing with increased susceptibility to infection; petechial hemorrhages
D	Osteomalacia (adult), Rickets (child)	Demineralization of bones and teeth with bone pain and skeletal muscle deformities
E	Hemolytic anemia in low birth weight infants	Macrocytic anemia; increased hemolysis of RBCs and increased capillary fragility
K	Hemorrhagic disease in newborns	Increase tendency to hemorrhage

Appendix 1

Commonly Used Abbreviations and Symbols

A1C	hemoglobin A1C
ABG	arterial blood gas
ABI	ankle/brachial systolic pressure index
ACE	angiotensin-converting enzyme
ACLS	advanced cardiac life support
ACS	acute coronary syndrome
ACT	activated clotting time
ACTH	adrenocorticotropic hormone
ADA	adenosine deaminase
ADD	attention deficit disorder
ADE	adverse drug events
ADH	antidiuretic hormone
ADHD	attention deficit hyperactivity disorder
ADL	activities of daily living
ad lib	as desired, at pleasure
ADP	adenosine diphosphate
AF	atrial fibrillation
AFB	acid fast bacillus
AHF	antihemophilic factor
AIDS	acquired immune deficiency syndrome
AKA	above knee amputation
ALL	acute lymphocytic leukemia
ALS	amyotrophic lateral sclerosis
ALT	alanine aminotransferase
a.m., A.M.	morning
AMD	age-related macular degeneration
AMI	acute myocardial infarction
AML	acute myelogenous leukemia
AMP	adenosine monophosphate
ANA	antinuclear antibody
ANC	absolute neutrophil count
ANS	autonomic nervous system
APL	acute promyelocytic leukemia
aPTT	activated partial thromboplastin time
ARB	angiotensin receptor blocker
ARC	AIDS-related complex
ARDS	adult respiratory distress syndrome
ASA	aspirin (acetylsalicylic acid)
ASAP	as soon as possible
ASHD	arteriosclerotic heart disease
AST	aspartate aminotransferase
ATC	around the clock
ATP	adenosine triphosphate
ATU	antithrombin unit
AUC	area under the curve
AV	atrioventricular
AVB	abnormal vaginal bleeding, AV block
BBB	bundle branch block
BCG	Bacille Calmette-Guérin
BG	blood glucose
BIDS	bedtime insulin, daytime sulfonylurea
BK	below the knee
BKA	below knee amputation
BM	bowel movement
BMD	bone mineral density
BMI	body mass index
BMP	basic metabolic panel
BMR	basal metabolic rate
BMT	bone marrow transplant
BP	blood pressure
BPD	bronchopulmonary dysplasia
BPH	benign prostatic hypertrophy
bpm	beats per minute
BS	blood sugar, bowel sounds
BSA	body surface area
BSE	breast self-exam
BSP	Bromsulphalein
BUN	blood urea nitrogen
Bx	biopsy
C	Celsius/Centigrade
Ca	cancer, calcium
CABG	coronary artery bypass graft
CAD	coronary artery disease
CAP	community-acquired pneumonia
CAUTI	catheter associated urinary tract infections
CBC	complete blood count
CCB	calcium channel blockers
C_{CR}	creatinine clearance
CD_4	helper T4 lymphocyte cells
C&DB	cough and deep breathe
CDC	Centers for Disease Control and Prevention
CF	cystic fibrosis

CFU colony forming units
CHB complete heart block
CHD coronary heart disease
CHF congestive heart failure
CHO carbohydrate
CIS carcinoma in situ
CJD Creutzfeldt-Jakob disease
CK creatine kinase
CLL chronic lymphocytic leukemia
CLS capillary leak syndrome
cm centimeter
C_{max} maximum serum concentration
CML chronic myelocytic leukemia
CMV cytomegalovirus
CN cranial nerve
CNS central nervous system
CO cardiac output, carbon monoxide
CO_2 carbon dioxide
COLD chronic obstructive lung disease
COPD chronic obstructive pulmonary disease
CP cardiopulmonary
CPAP continuous positive airway pressure
CPB cardiopulmonary bypass
CPK creatine phosphokinase
CPR cardiopulmonary resuscitation
CRF/CRI chronic renal failure/chronic renal insufficiency
CRS cytokine release syndrome
C&S culture and sensitivity
CSF cerebrospinal fluid
CT computerized tomography
CTC common toxicity criteria (National Cancer Institute)
CTS carpal tunnel syndrome
CTZ chemoreceptor trigger zone
CV cardiovascular
CVA cerebrovascular accident
CVD cardiovascular disease
CVP central venous pressure
CXR chest x-ray
cysto cystoscopy
dATP deoxyadenosine triphosphate
DBP diastolic blood pressure
ddATP dideoxyadenosine triphosphate
DEA Drug Enforcement Agency
DEXA dual energy x-ray absorptiometry
DI diabetes insipidus
DIC disseminated intravascular coagulation
dL deciliter (one-tenth of a liter)
DM diabetes mellitus
DMARD disease-modifying antirheumatic drug
DNA deoxyribonucleic acid
DOA date of admission
DOB date of birth
DOE dyspnea on exertion
DPT diphtheria, pertussis, tetanus
dr. dram (0.0625 ounce)
DRE digital rectal examination
DSD dry sterile dressing
DSM-IV Diagnostic and Statistical Manual of Mental Disorders, Fourth Edition
DT delirium tremens
DTR deep tendon reflex
DVT deep vein thrombosis
Dx diagnosis
EC enteric-coated
ECB extracorporeal cardiopulmonary bypass
ECG electrocardiogram
ED erectile dysfunction
EDTA ethylenediaminetetra-acetic acid
EEG electroencephalogram
EENT eye, ear, nose, and throat
EF ejection fraction
e.g. for example
EMR electronic medical records
ENL erythema nodosum leprosum
ENT ear, nose, throat
EPS electrophysiologic studies, extrapyramidal symptoms
ER extended release
ERT estrogen replacement therapy
ESR erythrocyte sedimentation rate
ESRD end-stage renal disease
ET endotracheal
ETOH alcohol, ethanol
F Fahrenheit, fluoride
FBS fasting blood sugar
FDA Food and Drug Administration
FEV forced expiratory volume
FFP fresh frozen plasma
FOB fecal occult blood
FS finger stick
FSH follicle-stimulating hormone

F/U	follow-up
FUO	fever of unknown origin
FVC	forced vital capacity
fx	fracture
GABA	gamma-aminobutyric acid
G-CSF	granulocyte colony-stimulating factor
GERD	gastroesophageal reflux disease
GFR	glomerular filtration rate
GGT	gamma-glutamyl transferase
GGTP	gamma-glutamyl transpeptidase
GH	growth hormone
gi, GI	gastrointestinal
GnRH	gonadotropin-releasing hormone
GP	glycoprotein
G6PD	glucose-6-phosphate dehydrogenase
gtt	a drop, drops
GU	genitourinary
h, hr	hour
HA, HAL	hyperalimentation
HbA1c	glycosylated hemoglobin
HBV	hepatitis B virus
HCG, hCG	human chorionic gonadotropin
HCP	health care provider
HCT	hematocrit
HCV	hepatitis C virus
HDL	high density lipoprotein
HFN	high flow nebulizer
Hg	mercury
Hgb, Hct	hemoglobin, hematocrit
H&H	hemoglobin and hematocrit
HIT	heparin-induced thrombocytopenia
HIV	human immunodeficiency virus
HIV RNA	HIV virus
HLA	human leukocyte antigens
HJR	hepatojugular reflux
HMG-CoA	3-hydroxy-3-methyl-glutaryl-coenzyme A
HOB	head of bed
HPA	hypothalamic-pituitary-adrenal axis
HPG	hypothalamus-pituitary-gonadal axis
HR	heart rate
HRT	hormone replacement therapy
HSE	herpes simplex encephalitis
HSV	herpes simplex virus
ht	height
5-HT	5-hydroxytryptamine
HTN	hypertension
Hx	history
IA	intra-arterial
IBD	inflammatory bowel disease
IBS	irritable bowel syndrome
IBW	ideal body weight
ICP	intracranial pressure
ICU	intensive care unit
IDDM	insulin dependent diabetes mellitus
Ig	immunoglobulin
IGF	insulin-like growth factor
im, IM	intramuscular
IMV	intermittent mandatory ventilation
inh	inhalation
INR	international normalized ratio
I&O	intake and output
IOP	intraocular pressure
IP	intraperitoneal
IPPB	intermittent positive pressure breathing
IR	immediate release
ITP	idiopathic thrombocytopenia purpura
IUD	intrauterine device
iv, IV	intravenous
IVP	intravenous pyelogram
IVPB	IV piggyback, a secondary IV line
JVD	jugular venous distention
kg	kilogram (2.2 lb)
KVO	keep vein open
L	liter (1,000 mL), left
lab	laboratory
lb	pound
LBBB	left bundle branch block
LDH	lactic dehydrogenase
LDL	low density lipoprotein
LFTs	liver function tests
LHRH	luteinizing hormone-releasing hormone
LLQ	left lower quadrant
LOC	level of consciousness/loss of consciousness
LP	lumbar puncture
LUQ	left upper quadrant
LV	left ventricular
LVED	left ventricular end diastolic
LVEF	left ventricular ejection fraction
LVH	left ventricular hypertrophy

m^2	square meter
MAC	Mycobacterium avium complex
MAOI	monoamine oxidase inhibitor
MAP	mean arterial pressure
MAR	medication administration record
max	maximum
mcg	microgram
MCH	mean corpuscular hemoglobin
mCi	millicurie
mcL	microliter
MCV	mean corpuscular volume
MDI	metered-dose inhaler
MDRSP	multidrug resistant *Streptococcus pneumoniae*
MDS	myelodysplastic syndrome
meds	medications
mEq	milliequivalent
mg	milligram
MI	myocardial infarction
MIC	minimum inhibitory concentration
min	minute, minim
mL	milliliter
mm^3	cubic millimeter
MM	multiple myeloma
MME	mini mental exam
MMSE	mini mental state (status) examination
MRI	magnetic resonance imaging
MRSA	Methicillin-resistant *Staphylococcus aureus*
MS	multiple sclerosis, mitral stenosis
MTX	methotrexate
MUGA	multigated radionuclide angiography
NaCl	sodium chloride
NCI	National Cancer Institute
NG	nasogastric
NGT	nasogastric tube
NIDDM	non-insulin dependent diabetes mellitus
NHL	non-hodgkins lymphoma
NKA	no known allergies
NKDA	no known drug allergies
NMS	neuroleptic malignant syndrome
NPN	nonprotein nitrogen
NPO	nothing by mouth
NR	do not refill (e.g., a prescription)
NSCLC	non-small cell lung cancer
NSAID	nonsteroidal anti-inflammatory drug
NSR	normal sinus rhythm
NSS	normal saline solution
NTG	nitroglycerin
NYHA	New York Heart Association
N&V	nausea and vomiting
O_2	oxygen
OA	osteoarthritis
OBS	organic brain syndrome
OC	oral contraceptive
OCD	obsessive-compulsive disorder
OOB	out of bed
OR	operating room
O_2 sat	oxygen saturation
OTC	over the counter
oz	ounce
PA	pulmonary artery, physician assistant
PABA	para-aminobenzoic acid
PAC	premature atrial contraction
PACWP	pulmonary arterial capillary wedge pressure
PAF	paroxysmal atrial fibrillation
PAH	pulmonary artery hypertension
PBI	protein-bound iodine
p.c.	after meals
PCA	patient-controlled analgesia
PCI	percutaneous coronary intervention
PCN	penicillin
PCP	*Pneumocystis carinii* pneumonia
PCWP	pulmonary capillary wedge pressure
PDT	photodynamic therapy
PE	pulmonary embolus/embolism; physical exam
PEEP	positive end expiratory pressure
per	by, through
PFTs	pulmonary function tests
pH	hydrogen ion concentration
PID	pelvic inflammatory disease
PMH	past medical history
PMI	point of maximal intensity
PMS	premenstrual syndrome
PND	paroxysmal nocturnal dyspnea
p.o., PO	by mouth
PPD	purified protein derivative
PR	by rectum
PRN	when needed or necessary
PSA	prostatic specific antigen

PSVT paroxysmal supraventricular tachycardia
PT prothrombin time; physical therapy
PTCA percutaneous transluminal coronary angioplasty
PTH parathyroid hormone
PTSD post traumatic stress disorder
PTT partial thromboplastin time
PUD peptic ulcer disease
PUVA psoralen and ulraviolet A
PVC premature ventricular contraction; polyvinyl chloride
PVD peripheral vascular disease
PVR peripheral vascular resistance
q.h. every hour
q 2 hr every two hours
q 3 hr every three hours
q 4 hr every four hours
q 6 hr every six hours
q 8 hr every eight hours
RA right atrium; rheumatoid arthritis
RAIU radioactive iodine uptake
RBBB right bundle branch block
RBC red blood cell
RDA recommended daily allowance
REM rapid eye movement
RICE rest, ice, compression and elevation
RLQ right lower quadrant
RNA ribonucleic acid
R/O rule out
ROM range of motion
ROS review of systems
RRMS relapsing-remitting multiple sclerosis
RSV respiratory syncytial virus
R/T related to
RTC round the clock
RV right ventricular
RUQ right upper quadrant
Rx symbol for a prescription; treatment
SA sinoatrial; sustained-action
SAH subarachnoid hemorrhage
SARS severe acute respiratory syndrome
SBE subacute bacterial endocarditis
SBP systolic BP
SCC squamous cell carcinoma
SCI spinal cord injury
SCID severe combined immunodeficiency disease
SE side effects
SGGT serum gamma-glutamyl transpeptidase
SGOT serum glutamic-oxaloacetic transaminase
SGPT serum glutamic-pyruvic transaminase
S., Sig. mark on the label
SI sacroiliac
SIADH syndrome inappropriate antidiuretic hormone
SIMV synchronized intermittent mandatory ventilation
SL sublingual
SLE systemic lupus erythematosus
SOB shortness of breath
sol solution
sp. species
S/P status post
SR sustained release
SSNRI selective serotonin norepinephrine reuptake inhibitor
SSRI selective serotonin reuptake inhibitor
SSS sick sinus syndrome
S&S signs and symptoms
stat immediately
STD sexually transmitted disease
SV stroke volume
SVT supraventricular tachycardia
syr syrup
sz seizure
T temperature
t½ half-life
tab tablet
TB tuberculosis
TCA tricyclic antidepressant
TENS transcutaneous electric nerve stimulation
TFT thyroid function tests
TG triglycerides
THR total hip replacement
TIA transient ischemic attack
TIBC total iron binding capacity
TKR total knee replacement
T_{max} maximum threshold; time of maximum concentration
TNF tumor necrosis factor
TPN total parenteral nutrition
TSH thyroid stimulating hormone
tsp teaspoon

TURP	transurethral resection of the prostate
Tx	treatment
U/A	urinalysis
UGI	upper gastrointestinal
ULN	upper limit of normal
UO	urine output
URTI, URI	upper respiratory (tract) infection
US	ultrasound
USP	U. S. Pharmacopeia
UTI	urinary tract infection
UV	ultraviolet
UVB	ultraviolet B (portion of ultraviolet radiation spectrum)
VAD	venous access device
VF	ventricular fibrillation
VLDL	very low density lipoprotein
VMA	vanillylmandelic acid
V. O.	verbal order
VS	vital signs
VSZ	varicella
VT	ventricular tachycardia
WBC	white blood cell
WHO	World Health Organization
WNL	within normal limits
Wt	weight
XRT	radiation therapy
y.o.	years old
&	and
°	degree
>	greater than
<	less than
↑	increased, higher
↓	decreased, lower
–	negative, minus
/	per
%	percent
+	positive, plus
×	times, frequency

Please note that many abbreviations have double meanings or can be misread. It is better to write out the recommendations, especially when ordering specific procedures or specific directions for drug administration. See Appendix 2.

Appendix 2

Medication Errors: Importance of Reporting

Much news media coverage has been directed to the unnecessary loss of life due to medication errors, many of which were preventable. It is estimated that adverse drug reactions to prescription and over-the-counter medications kill at least 108,000 Americans and seriously injure an additional 2.3 million each year. One in 50 hospitalized patients experience a preventable adverse event. Staff must understand the potential for medication errors and the importance of the health care facility processes/procedures in place to prevent the errors. Encourage staff to report problems and make suggestions for improvements. Take the fear out of reporting errors by making the system non-punitive and removing the deterrent for not reporting errors. If errors go unreported, facilities have no means of correcting a situation that created the error. For a variety of reasons, some staff members have difficulty admitting their mistakes; however, they must be encouraged to report and participate in the correction of the process(es) that caused the error.

Some of the more common types of errors are:

- Drugs with similar sounding names
- Inappropriate abbreviations
- Poor handwriting; misplaced decimals and zeroes
- Confusion of metric and other dosing units and improper dosing
- Environmental factors such as noise, distractions, lighting, fatigue, workload
- Poor communication, interruptions/distractions
- Lack of complete patient data on allergies, medical conditions, and so forth
- Omissions

Last year, United States Pharmacopeia received more than 2,000 voluntary reports of medication reconciliation errors, and a 1999 Institute of Medicine report estimated that more than 7,000 deaths occur each year in hospitals alone due to medication errors. The Joint Commission's Sentinel Event Database also identifies medication errors as one of the most frequently occurring threats to patient safety. This Database reveals that 63% of the reported medication errors resulting in death or serious injury were due to breakdowns in communication, and approximately half of those would have been avoided through effective medication reconciliation. A 2005 patient safety goal was to initiate medication reconciliation at each facility and improve the safe use of high alert medications. This goal continues today.

The National Coordinating Council for Medication Error Reporting and Prevention (http://www.nccmerp.org) defines a medication error as "any preventable event that may cause or lead to inappropriate medication use or patient harm while the medication is in the control of the health care professional, patient, or consumer. Such events may be related to professional practice, health care products, procedures, and systems including prescribing; order communication; product labeling; packaging; and nomenclature; compounding; dispensing; distribution; administration; education; monitoring; and use."

The FDA maintains a site for reporting medication errors:
http://www.fda.gov/medwatch

The FDA began monitoring reports of medication errors in 1992. They reviewed reports that were sent to the FDA from the United States Pharmacopeia (USP) and the Institute for Safe Medication Practices (ISMP). The Med Watch reports were also reviewed. The Division of Medication Errors and Technical Support includes a medication error prevention program. This is staffed with pharmacists and support personnel who review the medication error reports sent to the USP-ISMP, Medication Errors Reporting Program (MERP), and Med Watch. Since many patient errors are related to medication errors, it is felt that if they share the knowledge gained, this information may lead to patient safety.

The FDA maintains other searchable safety databases related to medical devices, including: biologic products, recalls, drug shortages, vaccine safety, and dietary supplements. All reports are voluntary and without penalty. Forms are easily downloaded for completion or can be completed on line.

All medication error reports should be filed with the Institute for Safe Medication Practices at: http://www.ismp.org or 1-800-324-5723. Observed errors may be reported confidentially.

A searchable website for consumers is also available that you should share with your patients: http://www.safemedication.com

FDA's Medwatch Program and Online Reporting Forms (for serious adverse events reporting and safety information):
http://www.fda.gov/medwatch and http://www.fda.gov/medwatch/index.html
1-800-332-1088

Gain information and voluntarily report medication errors and/or fill out Form 3500, which you can download from the site, and return by mail or fax. You can also report the error by phone. This information allows the FDA to require labeling changes, withdraw a drug from market, and distribute safety information to other providers.

Center for Drug Evaluation and Research (FDA)
http://www.fda.gov/cder

This site offers highlights of new drugs, new safety information, drug safety, drugs recently approved, and generic and OTC products.

Initiatives to reduce medication error include improving medication systems through bar coding medications/patients (wrist bands), individual dose bins, and computer programs that screen for dosage problems, interactions, and allergies.

Another step is to provide additional warnings for certain medications with greater potential for harm, such as anticoagulants, potassium chloride, opiates, and insulin. Methods to prevent interruptions of health care providers administering medications are of utmost importance, as well as multi-professional team approaches. ISMP maintains a list of high-alert medications.

The Joint Commission approved a minimum list of dangerous abbreviations. The following abbreviations have been identified as those which promote medication errors and should no longer be used:

Eliminate	Use instead
U	unit
IU	international unit
qd	every day
qod	every other day
trailing zero	eliminate zero after a decimal point
lack of leading zero	write 0.X mg
MS	morphine sulfate
MSO_4	morphine sulfate
$MgSO_4$	magnesium sulfate

Other abbreviations that have been eliminated from the drug handbook for safety reasons include:

Eliminate	**Use instead**
b.i.d	twice a day
t.i.d	3 times per day
gm	gram

The Joint Commission also has a secondary list of suggested abbreviations to eliminate in the future:

Eliminate	**Use instead**
>	greater than
<	lesser than
@	at
cc	mL
µg	mcg or micrograms
Apothecary units	use metric units

Visit http://www.jointcommission.org for more information.

Health care professionals are urged to voluntarily report medication errors to the Institute for Safe Medication Practices (ISMP); phone: 1-800-324-5723. In addition, serious adverse events (including those resulting from medication errors) may be reported to the FDA MedWatch Program (1-800-FDA-1088).

Appendix 3

Controlled Substances in the United States and Canada

Controlled Substances Act—United States

The U.S. Federal Controlled Substances Act of 1970 placed drugs controlled by the Act into five categories or schedules based on their potential to cause psychologic and/or physical dependence as well as on their potential for abuse. The schedules are defined as follows:

Schedule I [C-I]: Includes substances for which there is a high abuse potential and no current approved medical use (e.g., heroin, marijuana, LSD, other hallucinogens, certain opiates and opium derivatives).

Schedule II [C-II]: Includes drugs that have a high ability to produce physical or psychologic dependence and for which there is a current approved or acceptable medical use (e.g. narcotics, certain CNS stimulants).

Schedule III [C-III]: Includes drugs for which there is less potential for abuse than drugs in Schedule II and for which there is a current approved medical use and moderate dependence liability. Certain drugs in this category are preparations containing limited quantities of codeine and nonbarbituate sedatives. Anabolic steroids are classified in Schedule III.

Schedule IV [C-IV]: Includes drugs for which there is less abuse potential than for Schedule III, for which there is a current approved medical use, and that have limited dependence liability (e.g., some sedatives, antianxiety drugs, nonnarcotic analgesics).

Schedule V [C-V]: Drugs in this category have limited abuse potential and consist mainly of preparations containing limited amounts of certain narcotic drugs for use as antitussives and antidiarrheals. Federal law provides that limited quantities of these drugs (e.g., codeine) may be bought without a prescription by an individual at least 18 years of age if allowed under state statutes. The product must be purchased from a pharmacist, who must keep appropriate records. However, state laws vary, and in many states such products require a prescription.

NOTE: Generally, prescriptions for Schedule II (high abuse potential) drugs cannot be transmitted over the phone and they cannot be refilled. Prescriptions for Schedule III, IV, and V drugs may be refilled up to five times within 6 months. Schedule II drugs are not necessarily "stronger" than drugs in Schedules III, IV, or V; Schedule II drugs are classified as such due to their high abuse potential. Drugs that are not controlled are indicated by an asterisk (*).

Controlled Substances—Canada

In Canada, there are eight schedules. They are:

I Some of the more common groups include opium derivatives and salts (e.g., codeine, morphine, hydrocodone, oxycodone, oxymorphone); coca derivatives and salts (e.g., cocaine); phenylpiperidines and derivatives and salts (e.g., difenoxin, diphenoxylate, pethidine); phenazepines and salts (e.g., ethoheptazine); amidones and salts (e.g., methadone); phenalkoxams and salts (e.g., dextropropoxyphene); morphinans and salts (e.g., buprenorphine, levorphanol); benzazocines and salts (e.g., pentazocine); phencyclidine and salts; and, fentanyls and salts (alfentanil, fentanyl, remifentanil, sufentanil). Note: The above list is not inclusive.

II Cannabis and derivatives (e.g., marijuana, cannabinol).

III Amphetamines, their salts and derivatives (e.g., amphetamine, benzphetamine). Also, methylphenidate, psilocin, psilocybin, mescaline.

IV Barbiturates and their salts and thiobarbiturates and salts. Also, anabolic steroids, benzodiazepines, chlorphentermine, diethylpropion, phendimetrazine, phentermine, butorphanol, nalbuphine, glutethimide, ethchlorvynol, maxindol, meprobamate, methyprylon.

V Phenylpropanolamine and propylhexedrine.

VI Ephedrine, ergotamine, LSD, pseudoephedrine.

VII Specific amounts of cannabis (3 kg), and cannabis resin (3 kg).

VIII Specific amounts of cannabis (30 g) and cannabis resin (1 g).

	Drug Schedule	
Drug	**United States**	**Canada**
Alfentanil	II	I
Alprazolam	IV	IV
Amobarbital sodium	II	IV
Amphetamine sulfate	II	III
Aprobarbital	III	IV
Benzphetamine HCl	III	III
Buprenorphine HCl	III	I
Butabarbital sodium	III	IV
Butorphanol tartrate	IV	IV
Chloral hydrate	IV	*
Chlordiazepoxide	IV	IV
Clonazepam	IV	IV
Clorazepate dipotassium	IV	IV
Cocaine	II	I
Codeine	II	I
Dexmethylphenidate HCl	II	Not available
Dextroamphetamine sulfate	II	III
Dextropropoxyphene		
Bulk	II	I
Dosage Forms	IV	I
Diazepam	IV	IV
Diethylpropion HCl	IV	IV
Difenoxin products	V	I
(0.5 mg/25 mcg atropine sulfate)		
Diphenoxylate products		
(2.5 mg/25 mcg atropine sulfate)	V	I

Appendix 3

Drug	Drug Schedule United States	Canada
Dronabinol	III	*
Estazolam	IV	IV
Ethchlorvynol	IV	IV
Fentanyl	II	I
Fluoxymesterone	III	IV
Flurazepam HCl	IV	IV
Glutethimide	II	IV
Halazepam	IV	IV
Hydrocodone	Not available alone (usually C-III in combination drugs)	I
Hydromorphone HCl	II	I
Ketamine	III	*
Levorphanol tartrate	II	I
Lorazepam	IV	IV
Mazindol	IV	IV
Meperidine HCl	II	I
Mephobarbital	IV	IV
Meprobamate	IV	IV
Methadone HCl	II	I
Methamphetamine HCl	II	III
Methandrostenolone	III	IV
Methylphenidate HCl	II	III
Methyltestosterone	III	IV
Midazolam	IV	IV
Modafinil	IV	*
Morphine sulfate	II	I
Nandrolone decanoate	III	IV
Opium	II	I
Opium products (100 mg/100 mL or grams)	V	I
Oxandrolone	III	IV
Oxazepam	IV	IV

(continues)

Drug	Drug Schedule United States	Canada
Oxycodone HCl	II	I
Oxymetholone	III	IV
Oxymorphone HCl	II	I
Paraldehyde	IV	*
Paregoric	III	I
Pemoline	IV	*
Pentazocine	IV	I
Pentobarbital sodium		
PO	II	IV
Rectal	III	IV
Phencyclidine	II	I
Phendimetrazine tartrate	III	IV
Phenobarbital	IV	IV
Phentermine HCl	IV	IV
Prazepam	IV	IV
Quazepam	IV	IV
Remifentanil HCl	II	–
Secobarbital sodium	II	IV
Sibutramine HCl	IV	–
Stanolone	III	IV
Stanozolol	III	IV
Sufentanil citrate	II	I
Tapentadol hydrochloride	II	–
Temazepam	IV	IV
Testosterone (all forms)	III	IV
Thiopental	III	IV
Triazolam	IV	IV
Zaleplon	IV	–
Zolpidem tartrate	IV	–

Appendix 4

Pregnancy Categories: FDA Assigned

The U.S. Food and Drug Administration's use-in-pregnancy rating system weighs the degree to which available information has ruled out risk to the fetus against the drug's potential benefit to the patient. The ratings, and their interpretation, are as follows:

Category	Interpetation
A	**CONTROLLED STUDIES SHOW NO RISK.** Adequate, well-controlled studies in pregnant women have failed to demonstrate a risk to the fetus in any trimester of pregnancy.
B	**NO EVIDENCE OF RISK IN HUMANS.** Either animal studies show risk but human findings do not, or if no adequate human studies have been done, animal findings are negative.
C	**RISK CANNOT BE RULED OUT.** Human studies are lacking, and animal studies are either positive for fetal risk or lacking. However, potential benefits may justify the potential risks.
D	**POSITIVE EVIDENCE OF RISK.** Investigational or post-marketing data show risk to the fetus. However, potential benefits may outweigh the potential risks. If needed in a life-threatening situation or serious disease, the drug may be acceptable if safer drugs cannot be used or are ineffective.
X	**CONTRAINDICATED IN PREGNANCY.** Studies in animals or humans, or investigational or post-marketing reports, have demonstrated positive evidence of fetal abnormalities or risk which clearly outweigh any possible benefit to the patient.

Appendix 5

Calculating Body Surface Area and Body Mass Index

Body Surface Area (BSA) Calculator

Use the following formulas to calculate the body surface area (BSA) for drug administration. These formulas replace the BSA Nomogram (Mosteller Formula).

BSA (metric) = $\sqrt{(\text{ht [cm]} \times \text{wt [kg]})/3600}$

BSA (English) = $\sqrt{(\text{ht [in]} \times \text{wt [lb]})/3131}$

Body Mass Index (BMI) Calculator

Calculate BMI to determine if overweight

1. Multiply weight in pounds by 703

2. Multiply height in inches times itself

3. Divide the first number by the second to give BMI

Example: Weight 190 lb and 5'5" (65") tall

1. 190 × 703 = 133,579

2. 65 × 65 = 4,225

3. 133,579 divided by 4,225 = 31.6

BMI is 31.6

- A BMI under 18.5 suggests underweight
- A BMI between 18.5 and 24.9 is considered a healthy weight
- A BMI between 25 and 29.9 indicates moderately overweight
- A BMI 30 or more indicates extremely obese

A precalculated BMI chart is available in most provider offices.

A precalculated BMI chart is available from the National Institutes of Health at: http://www.nhlbi.nih.gov/guidelines/obesity/bmi_tbl.htm

Appendix 6

Elements of a Prescription

To safely communicate the exact elements desired on a prescription, the following items should be addressed:

A. **The prescriber:** Name, address, phone number, and associated practice/specialty.

B. **The client:** Name, age/birthdate, address and any allergies of record.

C. **The prescription itself:** Name of the medication (generic); dosage form and quantity to be dispensed (e.g., number of tablets or capsules, 1 vial, 1 tube, volume of liquid); the strength of the medication (e.g., 125-mg tablets, 250 mg/5 mL, 80 mg/1 mL, 10%); and directions for use (e.g., 1 tablet PO 3 times per day; 2 gtt to each eye 4 times per day; 1 teaspoonful PO q 8 hr for 10 days; apply a thin film to lesions twice a day for 14 days).

D. **Other elements:** Date prescription is written, signature of the provider, number of refills; provider number: state license number and Drug Enforcement Agency (DEA) number (when applicable); and brand-product-only indication (when applicable).

To prevent misuse, many states require the use of tamper-resistant prescription pads. A typical prescription as follows:

A.

Julia Bryan, MSN, RN, CPNP
Pediatric Associates
1611 Kirkwood Highway
Wilmington, DE 19805
302-645-8261

Date: July 10, 20XX

B. **For: Kathryn Woods, Age 8**
27 East Parkway
Lewes, DE 19958

Rx **Amoxicillin susp. 250 mg/5 mL**
Disp. 150 mL
Sig: 1 teaspoon PO q 8 hr × 10 days

Refills: 0

Provider signature
Provider/State license number

Interpretation of prescription: The above prescription is written by Certified Pediatric Nurse Practitioner Julia Bryan for Kathryn Woods and is for amoxicillin suspension. The concentration desired is 250 mg/5 mL. The directions for taking the medication are 1 teaspoon (i.e., 5 mL) by mouth every 8 hr for 10 days. The prescriber wants 150 mL dispensed and no refills are allowed.

Appendix 7

Easy Formulas for IV Rate Calculation

To calculate the continuous drip rate for an IV infusion, the following information is necessary:

a. amount of solution to be infused
b. time for infusion to be administered
c. *drop factor (found in the tubing package)

$$\frac{\text{Total volume to be infused}}{\text{Total hours for infusion}} \times \frac{\text{*drop factor}}{60\ \text{min/hr}} = \text{gtt/min}$$

*if drop factor is:
60 gtt/min, then use 1 in the formula
10 gtt/min, then use $^1/_6$ in the formula
15 gtt/min, then use $^1/_4$ in the formula
20 gtt/min, then use $^1/_3$ in the formula

This gives you $\frac{\text{gtt}}{\text{min}}$

Example: Infuse 1,000 cc over 8 hr using tubing with a drop factor of 10 gtt/min.

$$\frac{1{,}000\ \text{mL}}{8\ \text{hr}} \times \frac{1}{6} = 20.8\ (21)\ \frac{\text{gtt}}{\text{min}}$$

Complete equation is:

$$\frac{1{,}000\ \text{mL}}{8\ \text{hr}} \times \frac{10\ \text{gtt/min}}{60\ \text{min/1 hr}} = \frac{1{,}000\ \text{mL}}{8\ \text{hr}} \times \frac{10\ \text{gtt}}{\text{mL}} \times \frac{1\ \text{hr}}{60\ \text{min}} = 21\ \frac{\text{gtt}}{\text{min}}$$

To get $\frac{\text{mL}}{\text{hr}}$ invert drop factor and multiply by $\frac{\text{gtt}}{\text{min}}$, or:

$$\frac{6}{1} \times 21\ \frac{\text{gtt}}{\text{min}} = 126\ \frac{\text{mL}}{\text{hr}}$$

When administering intermittent infusions, as with antibiotic therapy, use the following formula:

$$\text{Total volume to be infused} \div \frac{\text{minutes to administer}}{60\ \text{min/hr}} = \frac{\text{mL}}{\text{hr}}$$

Example: Administer 3 grams Zosyn in 100 mL of D5W over 45 min

$$100 \div \frac{45}{60}\ \text{(invert to multiply)}$$

or

$$100 \times \frac{60}{45} = 133.3\ (134)\ \frac{\text{mL}}{\text{hr}}$$

Appendix 8

List of Combination Drugs

NOTE: There are a significant number of combination drugs that are being reviewed and thus might be removed from the market. This is especially true for cough/cold products.

KEY: OTC: Available over-the-counter; Rx: Available by prescription only. sf: sugar free; C-II, C-III, C-IV: The schedule in which the product is controlled by the U.S. Federal Controlled Substances Act.

Accuretic Tablets (Rx): Quinapril HCl 10 mg + hydrochlorothiazide 12.5 mg; quinapril HCl 20 mg + hydrochlorothiazide 12.5 mg; quinapril HCl 20 mg + hydrochlorothiazide 25 mg

Actifed Cold and Allergy Tablets (OTC): Phenylephrine HCl 10 mg + chlorpheniramine maleate 4 mg

Actonel with Calcium Tablets (Rx): Risedronate 35 mg + calcium carbonate 1,250 mg

ActoPlus Met Tablets (Rx): Pioglitazone 15 mg + metformin HCl 500 mg; pioglitazone 15 mg + metformin HCl 850 mg

ActoPlus Met XR Tablets (Rx): Pioglitazone 15 mg + metformin HCl extended-release 1,000 mg; pioglitazone 30 mg + metformin HCl extended-release 1,000 mg

Advanced Formula Di-Gel Tablets (OTC): Calcium carbonate 280 mg + magnesium hydroxide 128 mg + simethicone 20 mg

Advicor Extended-Release Tablets (Rx): Lovastatin 20 mg + niacin extended-release 500 mg; lovastatin 20 mg + niacin extended-release 1,000 mg; lovastatin 40 mg + niacin extended-release 1,000 mg

Advil Allergy Sinus Tablets (OTC): Chlorpheniramine maleate 2 mg + ibuprofen 200 mg + pseudoephedrine HCl 30 mg

Advil Cold and Sinus Tablets (OTC): Ibuprofen 200 mg + pseudoephedrine HCl 30 mg

Advil Congestion Relief Tablets (OTC): Ibuprofen 200 mg + phenylephrine HCl 10 mg

Airacof Liquid (Rx, sf, C-V): Codeine phosphate 7.5 mg + diphenhydramine HCl 12.5 mg + phenylephrine HCl 7.54 mg/5 mL

Alavert Allergy and Sinus D-12 Hour Tablets (OTC): Loratidine 5 mg + pseudoephedrine HCl 120 mg

Aldactazide Tablets (Rx): Spironolactone 25 mg + hydrochlorothiazide 25 mg; spironolactone 50 mg + hydrochlorothiazide 50 mg

Aldex GS DM Tablets (Rx): Dextromethorphan HBr 15 mg + guaifenesin 190 mg + pseudoephedrine HCl 30 mg

Alenic Alka Tablets (OTC): Aluminum hydroxide 80 mg + magnesium trisilicate 20 mg

Aleve Cold and Sinus Tablets (OTC): Naproxen sodium 220 mg + pseudoephedrine HCl 120 mg

Aleve Sinus and Headache Tablets (OTC): Naproxen sodium 220 mg + pseudoephedrine HCl 120 mg

Alka-Seltzer Effervescent, Extra-Strength Tablets (OTC): Sodium bicarbonate 1,985 mg + aspirin 500 mg + citric acid 1,000 mg/tablet

Alka-Seltzer Gold Effervescent Tablets (OTC): Sodium bicarbonate 1,050 mg + citric acid 1,000 mg + potassium bicarbonate 344 mg/tablet

Alka-Seltzer Heartburn Relief Effervescent Tablets (OTC): Sodium bicarbonate 1,940 mg + citric acid 1,000 mg

Alka-Seltzer Lemon Lime Effervescent Tablets (OTC): Sodium bicarbonate 1,700 mg + citric acid 1,000 mg + aspirin 325 mg

Alka-Seltzer Plus Cold and Cough Liqui-Gels (OTC): Dextromethorphan HBr 10 mg + chlorpheniramine maleate 2 mg + phenylephrine HCl 5 mg + acetaminophen 325 mg

Alka-Seltzer Plus Cold Effervescent Tablets (OTC): Aspirin 325 mg + chlorpheniramine maleate 2 mg + phenylephrine HCl 7.8 mg

Alka-Seltzer Plus Cold Medicine Effervescent Tablets (OTC): Chlorpheniramine maleate 2 mg + phenylephrine HCl 5 mg + acetaminophen 250 mg

Alka-Seltzer Plus Cold Medicine Liqui-Gel Capsules (OTC): Chlorpheniramine maleate 2 mg + pseudoephedrine HCl 30 mg + acetaminophen 325 mg

Alka-Seltzer Plus Day and Night Cold Capsules (OTC): *Day:* Acetaminophen 325 mg + dextromethorphan HBr 10 mg + phenylephrine HCl 5 mg. *Night:* Acetaminophen 250 mg + dextromethorphan HBr 10 mg + doxylamine succinate 6.25 mg + phenylephrine HCl 5 mg

Alka-Seltzer Plus Day and Night Cold Effervescent Tablets (OTC): *Day:* Acetaminophen 250 mg + dextromethorphan HBr 10 mg + phenylephrine HCl 5 mg. *Night:* Acetaminophen 250 mg + dextromethorphan HBr 10 mg + doxylamine succinate 6.25 mg + phenylephrine HCl 5 mg

Alka-Seltzer Plus Day Cold Liquid (OTC): Dextromethorphan HBr 5 mg + phenylephrine HCl 2.5 mg + acetaminophen 162.5 mg/5 mL

Alka-Seltzer Plus Day Non-Drowsy Cold Capsules (OTC): Acetaminophen 325 mg + dextromethorphan HBr 10 mg + phenylephrine HCl 5 mg

Alka-Seltzer Plus Fast Crystal Packs Powder (OTC): Acetaminophen 650 mg + chlorpheniramine maleate 4 mg + phenylephrine HCl 10 mg/packet

Alka-Seltzer Plus Flu Effervescent Tablets (OTC): Aspirin 50 mg + chlorpheniramine maleate 2 mg + dextromethorphan HBr 15 mg

Alka-Seltzer Plus Mucus and Congestion Effervescent Tablets (OTC): Dextromethorphan HBr 10 mg + guaifenesin 200 mg

Alka-Seltzer Plus Mucus and Congestion Liquid-Filled Capsules (OTC): Dextromethorphan HBr 10 mg + guaifenesin 200 mg

Alka-Seltzer Plus Night Cold Liquid (OTC): Acetaminophen 162.5 + dextromethorphan HBr 5 mg + doxylamine succinate 3.125 mg + phenylephrine HCl 2.5 mg/5 mL

Alka-Seltzer Plus Night Cold Softgels (OTC): Acetaminophen 325 mg + dextromethorphan HBr 15 mg + doxylamine succinate 6.25 mg

Alka-Seltzer Plus Night-Time Cold Effervescent Tablets (OTC): Acetaminophen 250 mg + dextromethorphan HBr 10 mg + doxylamine succinate 6.25 mg + phenylephrine HCl 5 mg

Alka-Seltzer Plus Sinus Tablets (OTC): Acetaminophen 250 mg + phenylephrine HCl 5 mg

Alka-Seltzer Plus Sparkling Original Cold Formula Effervescent Tablets (OTC): Acetaminophen 250 mg + chlorpheniramine maleate 2 mg + phenylephrine HCl 5 mg

Allerest Maximum Strength Tablets (OTC): Chlorpheniramine maleate 2 mg + pseudoephedrine HCl 30 mg

Allerest PE Tablets (OTC): Phenylephrine HCl 10 mg + chlorpheniramine maleate 4 mg

Aludrox Suspension (OTC): Aluminum hydroxide 225 mg + magnesium hydroxide 200 mg + simethicone/5 mL

Ambifed CD Tablets (Rx, C-III): Codeine phosphate 10 mg + guaifenesin 400 mg + pseudoephedrine HCl 30 mg

Ambifed CDX Tablets (Rx, C-III): Codeine phosphate 20 mg + guaifenesin 400 mg + pseudoephedrine HCl 30 mg

Amturnide Tablets (Rx): Aliskiren 150 mg + amlodipine 5 mg + hydrochlorothiazide 12.5 mg; aliskiren 300 mg + amlodipine 5 mg + hydrochlorothiazide 12.5 mg; aliskiren 300 mg + amlodipine 5 mg + hydrochlorothiazide 25 mg; aliskiren 300 mg + amlodipine 10 mg + hydrochlorothiazide 12.5 mg; aliskiren 300mg + amlodipine 10 mg + hydrochlorothiazide 25 mg

Anacin Advanced Headache Tablets (OTC): Acetaminophen 250 mg + aspirin 250 mg + caffeine 65 mg

Anacin Caplets and Tablets (OTC): Aspirin 400 mg + caffeine 32 mg

Anacin Maximum Strength Tablets (OTC): Aspirin 500 mg + caffeine 32 mg

Anexia 5/500 Tablets (Rx, C-III): Hydrocodone bitartrate 5 mg + acetaminophen 500 mg

Anexia 7.5/650 Tablets (Rx, C-III): Hydrocodone bitartrate 7.5 mg + acetaminophen 650 mg

Anexia 10/660 Tablets (Rx, C-III): Hydrocodone bitartrate 10 mg + acetaminophen 660 mg

Angeliq Tablets (Rx): Drospirenone 0.5 mg + estradiol 1 mg

Antacid Suspension (OTC): Aluminum hydroxide 225 mg + magnesium hydroxide 200 mg/5 mL

Arthrotec 50 Tablets (Rx): Diclofenac sodium 50 mg + misoprostol 200 mcg

Arthrotec 100 Tablets (Rx): Declofenac sodium 100 mg + misoprostol 200 mcg

Aspirin Free Anacin PM Tablets (OTC): Diphenhydramine HCl 25 mg + acetaminophen 500 mg

Atacand HCT Tablets (Rx): Candesartan cilexetil 16 mg + hydrochlorothiazide 12.5 mg; candesartan cilexetil 32 mg + hydrochlorothiazide 12.5 mg; candesartan cilexetil 32 mg + hydrochlorothiazide 25 mg

Atripla Tablets (Rx): Efavirenz 600 mg + emtricitabine 200 mg + tenofovir disoproxil fumarate 300 mg

Avalide Tablets (Rx): Irbesartan 150 mg + hydrochlorothiazide 12.5 mg; irbesartan 300 mg + hydrochlorothiazide 12.5 mg; irbesartan 300 mg + hydrochlorothiazide 25 mg

Avandamet Tablets (Rx): Rosiglitazone 2 mg + metformin HCl 500 mg; rosiglitazone 2 mg + metformin HCl 1,000 mg; rosiglitazone 4 mg + metformin HCl 500 mg; rosiglitazone 4 mg + metformin HCl 1,000 mg

Avandaryl Tablets (Rx): Rosiglitazone 4 mg + glimepiride 1 mg; rosiglitazone 4 mg + glipepiride 2 mg; rosiglitazone 4 mg + glimepiride 4 mg, rosiglitazone 8 mg + glimepiride 2 mg; rosiglitazone 8 mg + glimepiride 4 mg

Azor Tablets (Rx): Amlodipine besylate 5 mg + olmesartan medoxomil 20 mg; amlodipine besylate 5 mg + olmesaratn medoxomil 40 mg; amlodipine besylate 10 mg + olmesartan medoxomil 20 mg; amlodipine besylate 10 mg + olmesartan medoxomil 40 mg

Back Pain-Off Tablets (OTC): Acetaminophen 250 mg + caffeine 50 mg + magnesium salicylate 250 mg

Bayer Plus Extra Strength (OTC): Aspirin 500 mg + calcium carbonate 250 mg

Bayer PM Extra Strength Aspirin Plus Sleep Aid Caplet (OTC): Aspirin 500 mg + diphenhydramine HCl 25 mg

Bayer Select Maximum Strength Night Time Pain Relief Tablets (OTC): Diphenhydramine HCl 25 mg + acetaminophen 500 mg

Benadryl Allergy and Cold Tablets (OTC): Diphenhydramine HCl 12.5 mg + phenylephrine HCl 5 mg + acetaminophen 325 mg

Benadryl Allergy and Sinus Headache Tablets (OTC): Diphenhydramine HCl 12.5 mg + phenylephrine HCl 5 mg + acetaminophen 325 mg

Benadryl Children's Allergy and Cold Fastmelt Tablets (OTC): Diphenhydramine HCl 12.5 mg + pseudoephedrine HCl 30 mg

Benadryl Severe Allergy and Sinus Headache Maximum Strength Tablets (OTC): Diphenhydramine HCl 25 mg + phenylephrine HCl 5 mg + acetaminophen 325 mg

Benadryl-D Allergy and Sinus Tablets (OTC): Diphenhydramine HCl 25 mg + phenylephrine HCl 10 mg

Benadryl-D Children's Allergy and Sinus Liquid (OTC, sf): Diphenhydramine HCl 12.5 mg + pseudoephedrine HCl 30 mg/5 mL

Benicar HCT Tablets (Rx): Olmesartan medoxomil 20 mg + hydrochlorothiazide 12.5 mg; olmesartan medoxomil 40 mg + hydrochlorothiazide 12.5 mg; olmesartan medoxomil 40 mg + hydrochlorothiazide 25 mg

Bio T Pres Liquid (Rx, sf): Dextromethorphan HBr 10 mg + guaifenesin 200 mg + phenylephrine HCl 5 mg/5 mL

Bio T Pres Pediatric Liquid (Rx, sf): Dextromethorphan HBr 5 mg + guaifenesin 75 mg + phenylephrine HCl 2.5 mg/5 mL

Bio-Tussi Pediatric Liquid (OTC, sf): Dextromethorphan HBr 5 mg + guaifenesin 75 mg + phenylephrine HCl 2.5 mg/5 mL

BioGtuss Liquid (Rx, sf): Dextromethorphan HBr 15 mg, guaifenesin 300 mg + phenylephrine HCl 10 mg/5 mL

Bromo Seltzer Effervescent Granules (OTC): Sodium bicarbonate 2,781 mg + acetaminophen 325 mg + citric acid 2,224 mg/dose

Bronkaid Dual Action Tablets (OTC): Ephedrine HCl 25 mg + guaifenesin 400 mg

Brotapp Liquid (OTC, sf): Brompheniramine maleate 1 mg + pseudoephedrine HCl 15 mg/5 mL

Bupap Tablets (Rx): Acetaminophen 650 mg + butalbital 50 mg

Butex Forte Capsules (Rx): Acetaminophen 650 mg + butalbital 50 mg

Caduet Tablets (Rx): Amlodipine besylate 2.5 mg + atorvastatin calcium 10 mg; amlodipine besylate 2.5 mg + atorvastatin calcium 20 mg; amlodipine besylate 2.5 mg + atorvastatin calcium 40 mg; amlodipine besylate 5 mg + atorvastatin calcium 10 mg; amlodipine besylate 5 mg + atorvastatin calcium 20 mg; amlodipine besylate 5 mg + atorvastatin calcium 40 mg; amlodipine besylate 5 mg + atorvastatin calcium 80 mg; amlodipine besylate 10 mg + atorvastatin calcium 10 mg; amlodipine besylate 10 mg + atorvastatin calcium 20 mg; amlodipine besylate 10 mg + atorvastatin calcium 40 mg; amlodipine besylate 10 mg + atorvastatin calcium 80 mg

Cafergot Tablets (Rx): Ergotamine tartrate 1 mg + caffeine 100 mg

Calcium 500 Chewable Tablets (OTC): Vitamin D 200 units + calcium 1,000 mg

Calcium 600 + D Tablets (OTC): Vitamin D 400 units + calcium 600 mg

Calcium Rich Rolaids Tablets (OTC): Calcium carbonate 412 mg + magnesium hydroxide 80 mg

Caltrate 600 + D Soft Chews (OTC): Calcium carbonate 600 mg + vitamin D3 400 units

Capacet Capsules (Rx): Acetaminophen 325 mg + butalbital 50 mg + caffeine 40 mg

Cardex Drops Concentrate (OTC): Chlorpheniramine maleate 1 mg + phenylephrine HCl 3.5 mg/mL

Cenhist Chewable Tablets (OTC): Brompheniramine maleate 6 mg + phenylephrine HCl 15 mg

Cepacol Ultra Sore Throat Plus Cough Lozenges (OTC): Dextromethorphan HBr 5 mg + benzocaine 7.5 mg

Citracal + D3 Maximum Tablets (OTC): Calcium 315 mg + vitamin D 250 units

Citrus Calcium + D Tablets (OTC): Vitamin D 200 units + calcium 200 mg; vitamin D 100 units + calcium 315 mg

Clarinex-D 24 Hour Tablets (Rx): Desloratidine 5 mg + pseudoephedrine HCl 240 mg

Claritin-D 12 Hour Tablets (OTC): Loratidine 5 mg + pseudoephedrine HCl 120 mg

Claritin-D 24 Hour Tablets (OTC): Loratidine 10 mg + pseudoephedrine HCl 240 mg

ClimaraPro Transdermal Patch (Rx): Estradiol 0.045 mg + levonorgestrel 0.015 mg/day

Clorpres Tablets (Rx): Clonidine HCl 0.1 mg + chlorthalidone 15 mg; clonidine HCl 0.2 mg + chlorthalidone 15 mg; clonidine HCl 0.3 mg + chlorthalidone 15 mg

CombiPatch Transdermal (Rx): Estradiol 0.05 mg + levonorgestrel 0.14 mg/day; estradiol 0.05 mg + levonorgestrel 0.25 mg

Combivir Tablets (Rx): Lamivudine 150 mg + zidovudine 300 mg

Complera Tablets: Emtricitabine 200 mg + rilpivirine 25 mg + tenofovir disoproxil fumarate 300 mg

Comtrex Maximum Strength Day and Night Flu Therapy Tablets – Day (OTC): Phenylephrine HCl 5 mg + acetaminophen 325 mg

Comtrex Maximum Strength Day and Night Severe Cold and Sinus Tablets – Night (OTC): Chlorpheniramine maleate 2 mg + phenylephrine HCl 5 mg + acetaminophen 325 mg

Comtrex Maximum Strength Non-Drowsy Cold and Cough Tablets (OTC): Dextromethorphan HBr 10 mg + phenylephrine HCl 5 mg + acetaminophen 325 mg

Concentrated Milk of Magnesia-Cascara Suspension (OTC): 15 mL equivalent to 30 mL milk of magnesia + aromatic cascara fluid extract 5 mL

Conex Cold & Allergy Solution (OTC): Dexbrompheniramine maleate 1 mg + pseudoephedrine HCl 30 mg/5 mL

Conex Cold & Allergy Tablets (OTC): Dexbrompheniramine maleate 2 mg + pseudoephedrine HCl 60 mg

Coricidin D Cold, Flu, and Sinus Tablets (OTC): Chlorpheniramine maleate 2 mg + phenylephrine HCl 5 mg + acetaminophen 325 mg

Coricidin HBP Cold and Flu Tablets (OTC): Chlorpheniramine maleate 2 mg + acetaminophen 325 mg

Coricidin HBP Cough and Cold Tablets (OTC): Chlorpheniramine maleate 4 mg + dextromethorphan HBr 30 mg

Coricidin HBP Maximum Strength Flu Tablets (OTC): Chlorpheniramine maleate 2 mg + dextromethorphan HBr 15 mg + acetaminophen 500 mg

Corvaryx H.S. Tablets (Rx): Esterified estrogens 0.625 mg + methyltestosterone 1.25 mg

Corzide Tablets 40/5 (Rx): Nadolol 40 mg + bendroflumethazide 5 mg

Corzide Tablets 80/5 (Rx): Nadolol 80 mg + bendroflumethazide 5 mg

Cough-X Oral Lozenges (OTC): Dextromethorphan HBr 5 mg + benzocaine 2 mg

Covaryx Tablets (Rx): Esterified estrogens 1.25 mg + methyltestosterone 2.5 mg

Deconamine Syrup (Rx): Chlorpheniramine maleate 2 mg + pseudoephedrine HCl 30 mg/5 mL

Deconomed SR Capsules (Rx): Chlorpheniramine maleate 8 mg + pseudoephedrine HCl 120 mg

Dexphen w/C Liquid (Rx, sf, C-V): Codeine phosphate 10 mg + dexchlorpheniramine maleate 1 mg + phenylephrine HCl 5 mg/5 mL

Di-Gel Liquid (OTC): Aluminum hydroxide 200 mg + simethicone 20 mg/5 mL

Dicel DM Chewable Tablets (OTC): Chlorpheniramine maleate 2 mg + dextromethorphan HBr 10 mg + pseudoephedrine HCl 30 mg

Difel-G Tablets (Rx): Diphylline 200 mg + guaifenesin 300 mg

Difil-G Forte Liquid (Rx): Diphylline 100 mg + guaifenesin 100 mg/5 mL

Dilex-G 200 Syrup (Rx, sf): Diphylline 100 mg + guaifenesin 200 mg/5 mL

Dilex-G 400 Tablets (Rx): Diphylline 200 mg + guaifenesin 400 mg

Dilex-G Syrup (Rx): Diphylline 100 mg + guaifenesin 100 mg/5 mL

Dimetane DX Liquid (Rx, sf): Brompheniramine maleate 2 mg + dextromethorphan HBr 10 mg + pseudoephedrine HCl 30 mg/5 mL

Dimetapp Children's Cold and Allergy Elixir (OTC): Phenylephrine HCl 2.5 mg + brompheniramine maleate 1 mg/5 mL

Dimetapp Long Acting Cough Plus Cold Syrup (OTC): Chlorpheniramine maleate 1 mg + dextromethorphan HBr 7.5 mg/5 mL

Diovan HCT Tablets (Rx): Valsartan 80 mg + hydrochlorothiazide 12.5 mg; valsartan 160 mg + hydrochlorothiazide 12.5 mg; valsartan 320 mg + hydrochlorothiazide 12.5 mg; valsartan 160 mg + hydrochlorothiazide 25 mg; valsartan 320 mg + hydrochlorothiazide 25 mg

DM/CPM/PE/GG Oral Syrup (Rx): Dextromethorphan HBr 15 mg + guiafenesin 100 mg + phenylephrine HCl 10 mg + chlorpheniramine maleate 2 mg/5 mL

DOK-Plus Syrup (OTC): Docusate sodium 60 mg + casanthranol 30 mg/15 mL

Dolgic Tablets (Rx): Acetaminophen 650 mg + butalbital 50 mg

Donatussin Drops (Rx): Phenylephrine HCl 1.5 mg + guaifenesin 20 mg/mL

Double Strength Gaviscon-2 Tablets (OTC): Aluminum hydroxide 160 mg + magnesium trisilicate 40 mg

Doxidan Capsules (OTC): Docusate sodium 100 mg + casanthranol 30 mg

Dristan Cold Multi-Symptom Formula Tablets (OTC): Chlorpheniramine maleate 2 mg + phenylephrine HCl 5 mg + acetaminophen 325 mg

Duac Topical Gel (Rx): Clindamycin 1% + benzoyl peroxide 5%

Duetact Tablets (Rx): Pioglitazone 30 mg + glimepiride 2 mg; pioglitazone 30 mg + glimepiride 4 mg

Duexis Tablets (Rx): Ibuprofen 800 mg + famotidine 26.6 mg

Dulera Inhalation Aerosol (Rx): Mometasone furoate 100 mcg + formoterol fumarate 5 mcg/actuation; mometasone furoate 200 mcg + formoterol fumarate 5 mcg/actuation

Duocet Tablets (Rx, C-III): Hydrocodone bitartrate 4 mg + acetaminophen 500 mg

Durabac Capsules (Rx): Acetaminophen 325 mg + caffeine 50 mg + phenyltoloxamine citrate 20 mg + salicylamide 250 mg

Duratuss A Tablets (Rx): Phenylephrine HCl 20 mg + guaifenesin 600 mg + acetaminophen 650 mg

Duratuss GP Tablets (Rx): Phenylephrine HCl 25 mg + guaifenesin 1,200 mg

Duratuss Tablets (Rx): Phenylephrine HCl 25 mg + guaifenesin 900 mg

Dyflex-G Tablets (Rx): Diphylline 200 mg + guaifenesin 200 mg

Dyphylline-GG Elixir (Rx): Diphylline 33.3 mg + guaifenesin 33.3 mg/5 mL

ED Bron GP Liquid (OTC, sf): Guaifenesin 100 mg + phenylephrine HCl 5 mg/5 mL

Ed ChlorPed D Solution Concentrate (OTC, sf): Chlorpheniramine maleate 2 mg + phenylephrine HCl 5 mg/mL

Ed-Bron G Liquid (Rx, sf): Theophylline 50 mg + guaifenesin 33.3 mg/5 mL

Embeda Capsules (Rx, C-II): Morphine sulfate 20 mg + naltrexone HCl 0.8 mg; morphine sulfate 30 mg + naltrexone HCl 1.2 mg; morphine sulfate 50 mg + naltrexone HCl 2 mg; morphine sulfate 60 mg + naltrexone HCl 2.4 mg; morphine sulfate 80 mg + naltrexone HCl 3.2 mg; morphine sulfate 100 mg + naltrexone HCl 4 mg

Empirin w/Codeine No. 3 Tablets (Rx, C-III): Codeine phosphate 30 mg + aspirin 325 mg

Empirin w/Codeine No. 4 Tablets (Rx, C-III): Codeine phosphate 60 mg + aspirin 325 mg

Endacon Oral Liquid (Rx, sf): Dextromethorphan HBr 20 mg + guiafenesin 100 mg + phenylephrine HCl 10 mg/5 mL

Endal CD Syrup (Rx, sf, C-V): Codeine phosphate 7.5 mg + chlorpheniramine maleate 2 mg + phenylephrine HCl 5 mg/5 mL

Endocet Tablets (Rx, C-II): Acetaminophen 325 mg + oxycodone HCl 5 mg; acetaminophen 325 mg + oxycodone HCl 7.5 mg; acetaminophen 500 mg + oxycodone HCl 7.5 mg; acetaminophen 325 mg + oxycodone HCl 10 mg; acetaminophen 650 mg + oxycodone HCl 10 mg

Entex LA Tablets (Rx): Phenylephrine HCl 30 mg + guaifenesin 800 mg (400 mg IR and 400 mg ER)

Entex Liquid (Rx, sf): Phenylephrine HCl 7.5 mg + guaifenesin 100 mg/5 mL

Entex LQ Liquid (OTC, sf): Guaifenesin 100 mg + phenylephrine HCl 10 mg/5 mL

Entex PSE Tablets (Rx): Pseudoephedrine HCl 120 mg + guaifenesin 600 mg

Epzicom Tablets (Rx): Abacavir 600 mg + lamivudine 300 mg

Equagesic Tablets (Rx, C-IV): Aspirin 325 mg + meprobamate 200 mg

Esgic Capsules (Rx): Acetaminophen 325 mg + caffeine 40 mg + butalbital 50 mg

Esgic Plus Capsules/Tablets (Rx): Acetaminophen 500 mg + caffeine 40 mg + butalbital 50 mg

Esocor P Oral Suspension (Rx): Chlorpheniramine maleate 4 mg + dextromethorphan HBr 30 mg + pseudoephedrine HCl 30 mg/5 mL

Estratest H.S. Tablets (Rx): Esterified estrogens 0.625 mg + methyltestosterone 1.25 mg

Estratest Tablets (Rx): Esterified estrogens 1.25 mg + methyltestosterone 2.5 mg

Etrafon A Tablets (Rx): Perphenazine 4 mg + amitriptyline 10 mg

Etrafon Forte Tablets (Rx): Perphenazine 4 mg + amitriptyline 25 mg

Etrafon Tablets (Rx): Perphenazine 2 mg + amitriptyline 25 mg

Excedrin Aspirin Free Caplets (OTC): Acetaminophen 500 mg + caffeine 65 mg

Excedrin Back and Body Extra Strength Caplets (OTC): Acetaminophen 250 mg + buffered aspirin 250 mg

Excedrin Extra Strength Caplets, Geltabs, Tablets (OTC): Acetaminophen 250 mg + aspirin 250 mg + caffeine 65 mg

Excedrin Migraine (OTC): Acetaminophen 250 mg + aspirin 250 mg + caffeine 65 mg

Excedrin P.M. Liquid (OTC): Diphenhydramine HCl 8.3 mg + acetaminophen 167 mg/5 mL; diphenhydramine HCl 50 mg + acetaminophen 1,000 mg/30 mL

Excedrin P.M. Liquigels (OTC): Diphenhydramine HCl 25 mg + acetaminophen 500 mg

Excedrin P.M. Tablets (OTC): Diphenhydramine citrate 38 mg + acetaminophen 500 mg

Excedrin Sinus Headache Tablets (OTC): Acetaminophen 325 mg + phenylephrine HCl 5 mg

Excedrin Tension Headache Caplets/Geltabs (OTC): Acetaminophen 500 mg + caffeine 65 mg

Exforge HCT Tablets (Rx): Amlodipine besylate 5 mg + valsartan 160 mg + hydrochlorothiazide 12.5 mg; amlodipine besylate 5 mg + valsartan 160 mg + hydrochlorothiazide 25 mg; amlodipine besylate 10 mg + valsartan 160 mg + hydrochlorothiazide 12.5 mg; amlodipine besylate 10 mg + valsartan 160 mg + hydrochlorothiazide 25 mg; amlodipine besylate 10 mg + valsasrtan 320 mg + hydrochlorothiazide 25 mg

Exforge Tablets (Rx): Amlodipine besylate 5mg + valsartan 160 mg; amlodipine besylate 5 mg + valsartan 320 mg; amlodipine besylate 10 mg + valsartan 160 mg; amlodipine besylate 10 mg + valsartan 320

Extra Action Cough Syrup (OTC): Dextromethorphan HBr 10 mg + guaifenesin 100 mg/5 mL

Extra Strength Doan's P.M. Tablets (OTC): Diphenhydramine 25 mg + magnesium salicylate 500 mg

Extra Strength Mintox Plus Liquid (OTC): Aluminum hydroxide 500 mg + magnesium hydroxide 450 mg + simethicone 40 mg/5 mL

Femhrt Tablets (Rx): Ethinyl estradiol 2.5 mcg + northindrone acetate 0.5 mg; ethinyl estradiol 5 mcg + norethindrone acetate 1 mg

Fioricet Tablets (Rx): Acetaminophen 325 mg + caffeine 40 mg + butalbital 50 mg

Fioricet w/Codeine Capsules (Rx, C-III): Codeine phosphate 30 mg + acetaminophen 325 mg + caffeine 40 mg + butalbital 50 mg

Fiorinal Capsules (Rx, C-III): Aspirin 325 mg + caffeine 40 mg + butalbital 50 mg

Fiorinal w/Codeine Capsules (Rx, C-III): Codeine phosphate 30 mg + aspirin 325 mg + caffeine 30 mg + butalbital 50 mg

Fosamax Plus D Tablets (Rx): Alendronate sodium 70 mg + cholecalciferol 70 mcg

Gaviscon Chewable Tablets (OTC): Aluminum hydroxide 80 mg + magnesium trisilicate 14.2 mg + sodium bicarbonate and magnesium

Gaviscon Extra Strength Antacid Tablets (OTC): Aluminum hydroxide 160 mg + magnesium carbonate 105 mg + sodium bicarbonate

Gaviscon Extra Strength Relief Formula Liquid (OTC): Aluminum hydroxide 254 mg + magnesium carabonate 237.5 mg/5 mL

Gaviscon Extra Strength Relief Formula Tablets (OTC): Aluminum hydroxide 160 mg + magnesium carbonate 105 mg

Gaviscon Liquid (OTC): Aluminum hydroxide 31.7 mg + magnesium carbonate 119.3 mg/5 mL

Gaviscon Tablets (OTC): Aluminum hydroxide 80 mg + magnesium trisilicate 20 mg

Gelusil Tablets (OTC): Aluminum hydroxide 200 mg + magnesium hydroxide 200 mg + simethicone 25 mg

Genasoft Plus Softgels (Capsules) (OTC): Docusate sodium 100 mg + casanthranol 30 mg

Gentex LA Tablets (Rx): Phenylephrine HCl 23.75 mg + guaifenesin 650 mg

Glucovance Tablets (Rx): Glyburide 1.25 mg + metformin HCl 250 mg; glyburide 2.5 mg + metformin HCl 500 mg; glyburide 5 mg + metformin HCl 500 mg

Haley's M-O Liquid (OTC): Magnesium hydroxide 900 mg (about) + mineral oil 3.75 mL/15 mL

Helidac (Rx): Bismuth subsalicylate chewable tablets, 262.4 mg + metronidazole tablets 250 mg + tetracycline capsules 500 mg

Hydrogesic Capsules (Rx, C-III): Hydrocodone bitartrate 5 mg + acetaminophen 500 mg

Hyzaar Tablets (Rx): Losartan potassium 50 mg + hydrochlorothiazide 12.5 mg; losartan potassium 100 mg + hydrochlorothiazide 12.5 mg; losartan potassium 100 mg + hydrochlorothiazide 25 mg

Ibudone Tablets (Rx, C-III): Hydrocodone bitartrate 5 mg + ibuprofen 200 mg; hydrocodone bitrartrate 10 mg + ibuprofen 200 mg

Iophen C-NR Liquid (Rx, C-V): Codeine phosphate 10 mg + guaifenesin 100 mg/5 mL

Iophen Dm-NR Liquid (Rx, C-V): Dextromethorphan HBr 10 mg + guaifenesin 100 mg/5 mL

Jalyn Capsules (Rx): Dutasteride 0.5 mg + tamsulosin HCl 0.4 mg

Janumet Tablets (Rx): Sitagliptin 50 mg + metformin HCl 500 mg; sitagliptin 50 mg + metformin HCl 1,000 mg

Jay-Phyl Syrup (Rx, sf): Diphylline 100 mg + guaifenesin 50 mg/5 mL

K-C Suspension (OTC): Kaolin 5.2 grams + pectin 260 mg + bismuth subcarbonate 260 mg/30 mL

Kaletra Oral Solution (Rx): Lopinavir 80 mg + ritonavir 20 mg/mL

Kaletra Tablets (Rx): Lopinavir 100 mg + ritonavir 25 mg; lopinavir 200 mg + ritonavir 50 mg

Kapectolin Suspension (OTC): Kaolin 90 grams + pectin 2 grams/30 mL

Kombiglyze XR Extended-Release Tablets (Rx): Saxagliptin 5 mg + metformin HCl 500 mg; saxagliptin 5 mg + metformin 1,000 mg; saxagliptin 2.5 mg + metformin 1,000 mg

Lexxel Extended-Release Tablets (Rx): Enalapril maleate 5 mg + felodipine 5 mg

Librax Capsules (Rx): Chlordiazepoxide 5 mg + clidinium bromide 2.5 mg

Limbitrol DS Tablets (Rx, C-IV): Chlordiazepoxide 10 mg + amitriptyline 25 mg

Liquibid D Tablets (Rx): Phenylephrine HCl 40 mg (ER) + guaifenesin 650 mg (250 mg IR + 400 mg ER)

Little Colds Decongestant Plus Cough Solution Concentrate (OTC): Dextromethorphan HBr 5 mg + phenylephrine HCl 2.5 mg/mL

LoHist Liquid (OTC, sf): Chlorpheniramine maleate 1 mg + phenylephrine HCl 2.5 mg/mL

LoHist PEB DM Liquid (OTC): Dextromethorphan HBr 20 mg + brompheniramine maleate 4 mg + phenylephrine HCl 10 mg/5 mL

LoHist PEB Liquid (OTC, sf): Brompheniramine maleate 4 mg + phenylephrine HCl 10 mg/5 mL

LoHist PSB Liquid (OTC, sf): Brompheniramine maleate 4 mg + pseudoephedrine HCl 20 mg/5 mL

Lopressor HCT 50/25 Tablets (Rx): Metoprolol tartrate 50 mg + hydrochlorothiazide 25 mg

Lopressor HCT 100/25 Tablets (Rx): Metoprolol tartrate 100 mg + hydrochlorothiazide 25 mg

Lopressor HCT 100/50 Tablets (Rx): Metoprolol tartrate 100 mg + hydrochlorothiazide 50 mg

Lorcet 10/650 Tablets (Rx, C-III): Hydrocodone bitartrate 10 mg + acetaminophen 650 mg

Lorcet Plus Tablets (Rx, C-III): Hydrocodone bitartrate 7.5 mg + acetaminophen 650 mg

Lortab 5/500 Tablets (Rx, C-III): Hydrocodone bitartrate 5 mg + acetaminophen 500 mg

Lortab 7.5/500 Tablets (Rx, C-III): Hydrocodone bitartrate 7.5 mg + acetaminophen 500 mg

Lortab 10/500 Tablets (Rx, C-III): Hydrocodone bitartrate 10 mg + acetaminophen 500 mg

Lortab Elixir (Rx, C-III): Hydrocodone bitartrate 2.5 mg + acetaminophen 167 mg/5 mL

Lortuss DM Liquid (Rx, sf): Dextromethorphan HBr 15 mg + doxylamine succinate 6.25 mg + pseudoephedrine HCl 30 mg/5 mL

Lortuss EX Suspension (Rx, sf, C-V): Codeine phosphate 10 mg + guaifenesin 100 mg + pseudoephedrine HCl 22.5 mg/5 mL

Lotensin HCT Tablets (Rx): Benazepril 10 mg + hydrochlorothiazide 12.5 mg; benazepril 20 mg + hydrochlorothiazide 12.5 mg; benazepril 20 mg + hydrochlorothiazide 25 mg;

Lotrel Capsules (Rx): Amlodipine 2.5 mg + benazepril HCl 10 mg; amlodipine 5 mg + benazepril HCl 10 mg; amlodipine 5 mg + benazepril HCl 20 mg; amlodipine 5 mg + benazepril HCl 40 mg; amlodipine 10 mg + benazepril HCl 20 mg; amlodipine 10 mg + benazepril HCl 40 mg

Lufyllin-GG Elixir (Rx): Diphylline 33.3 mg + guaifenesin 33.3 mg/5 mL

Maalox Advanced Maximum Strength Liquid (OTC): Aluminum hydroxide 400 mg + magnesium hydroxide 400 mg + simethicone 40 mg/5 mL

Maalox Advanced Regular Strength Liquid (OTC): Aluminum hydroxide 200 mg + magnesium hydroxide 200 mg + simethicone 20 mg/5 mL

Maalox Advanced Strength Chewable Tablets (OTC): Calcium carbonate 1,000 mg + simethicone 60 mg

Maalox Max Maximum Strength Chewable Tablets (OTC): Calcium carbonate 1,000 mg + simethicone 60 mg

Maalox Maximum Strength Multi-Symptom Liquid (OTC): Aluminum hydroxide 400 mg + magnesium hydroxide 400 mg + simethicone 40 mg/5 mL

Maalox Plus Antacid Junior Chewable Tablets (OTC): Calcium carbonate 400 mg + simethicone 24 mg

Maalox Regular Strength Liquid (OTC): Aluminum hydroxide 200 mg + magnesium hydroxide 200 mg + simethicone 20 mg/5 mL

Magaldrate Plus Suspension (OTC): Magaldrate 540 mg + simethicone 40 mg/5 mL

Malarone Pediatric Tablets (Rx): Atovaquone 62.5 mg + proguanil HCl 25 mg

Malarone Tablets (Rx): Atovaquone 250 mg + proguanil HCl 100 mg

Mapap Cold Formula Multi-Symptom Tablets (OTC): Acetaminophen 325 mg + dextromethorphan HBr 10 mg + phenylephrine HCl 5 mg

Mapap Sinus Congestion and Pain Maximum Strength Tablets (OTC): Acetaminophen 325 mg + phenylephrine 5 mg

Mapap Sinus Maximum Strength Tablets (OTC): Acetaminophen 500 mg + pseudoephedrine HCl 30 mg

Margesic Capsules (Rx): Acetaminophen 325 mg + caffeine 40 mg + butalbital 50 mg

Margesic H Capsules (Rx, C-III): Hydrocodone bitartrate 5 mg + acetaminophen 500 mg

Maxifed DM Liquid (Rx): Dextromethorphan HBr 10 mg + pseudoephedrine HCl 20 mg + guaifenesin 200 mg/5 mL

Maxifed DM Tablets (Rx): Dextromethorphan HBr 20 mg + pseudoephedrine HCl 40 mg + guaifenesin 400 mg

Maxifed DMX Tablets (Rx): Dextromethorphan HBr 20 mg + pseudoephedrine HCl 60 mg + guaifenesin 400 mg

Maxifed Tablets (Rx): Pseudoephedrine HCl 80 mg + guaifenesin 780 mg

Maxiphen DM Tablets (Rx): Dextromethorphan HBr 20 mg + phenylephrine HCl 10 mg + guaifenesin 400 mg

Maxiphen-G DM Extended-Release Tablets (Rx): Dextromethorphan HBr 30 mg + phenylephrine HCl 20 mg + guaifenesin 1,000 mg

Medi-First Extra Strength Pain Relief Tablets (OTC): Acetaminophen 110 mg + aspirin 162 mg + salicylamide 152 mg + caffeine 32.4 mg

Mesehist DM Liquid (Rx, sf): Chlorpheniramine maleate 4 mg + dextromethorphan HBr 15 mg + pseudoephedrine HCl 15 mg/4 mL

Metaglip Tablets (Rx): Glipizide 2.5 mg + metformin HCl 250 mg

Micardis HCT Tablets (Rx): Telmisartan 40 mg + hydrochlorothiazide 12.5 mg; telmisartan 80 mg + hydrochlorothiazide 12.5 mg; telmisartan 80 mg + hydrochlorothiazide 25 mg

Midol Maximum Strength Menstrual Caplets (OTC): Acetaminophen 500 mg + caffeine 60 mg + pyrilamine maleate 15 mg

Midol Maximum Strength PMS Caplets and Gelcaps (OTC): Acetaminophen 500 mg + pamabron 25 mg + pyrilamine maleate 15 mg

Midol Teen Maximum Strength Caplets (OTC): Acetaminophen 500 mg + pamabrom 25 mg

Mintox Plus Tablets (OTC): Aluminum hydroxide 200 mg + magnesium hydroxide 200 mg + simethicone 25 mg

Mintox Suspension (OTC): Aluminum hydroxide 225 mg + magnesium hydroxide 200 mg/5 mL

Mintox Tablets (OTC): Aluminum hydroxide 200 mg + magnesium hydroxide 200 mg

Moduretic Tablets (Rx): Amiloride 5 mg + hydrochlorothiazide 50 mg

Monopril-HCT Tablets (Rx): Fosinopril sodium 10 mg + hydrochlorothiazide 12.5 mg; fosinopril sodium 20 mg + hydrochlorothiazide 12.5 mg

Motrin Children's Cold Suspension (OTC): Ibuprofen 100 mg + pseudoephedrine HCl 15 mg/5 mL

Mucinex Cold for Kids Liquid (OTC): Phenylephrine HCl 2.5 mg + guaifenesin 100 mg/5 mL

Mucinex Cough for Kids Liquid (OTC): Dextromethorphin HBr 5 mg + guaifenesin/5 mL

Mucinex Cough Mini-Melts for Kids (OTC): Dextromethorphan HBr 5 mg + guaifenesin 100 mg

Mucinex D Maximum Strength Extended-Release Tablets (OTC): Guaifenesin 1,200 mg + pseudoephedrine HCl 120 mg

Mucinex D Tablets (OTC): Pseudoephedrine HCl 60 mg + guaifenesin 600 mg

Mucinex DM Extended-Release Tablets (OTC): Dextromethorphan HBr 30 mg + guaifenesin 600 mg

Mucinex DM Maximum Strength Extended-Release Tablets (OTC): Dextromethorphan HBr 60 mg + guaifenesin 1,200 mg

Mygel Suspension (OTC): Aluminum hydroxide 200 mg + simethicone 20 mg/5 mL

Mylagen Gelcaps (OTC): Calcium carbonate 311 mg + magnesium carbonate 232 mg

Mylagen II Liquid (OTC): Aluminum hydroxide 400 mg + magnesium hydroxide 400 mg + simethicone 40 mg/5 mL

Mylagen Liquid (OTC): Aluminum hydroxide 200 mg + simethicone 20 mg/5 mL

Mylanta Antacid Gelcaps (OTC): Magnesium hydroxide 125 mg + calcium carbonate 550 mg

Mylanta Extra Strength Liquid (OTC): Aluminum hydroxide 400 mg + magnesium hydroxide 400 mg + simethicone 40 mg/5 mL

Mylanta Gelcaps (OTC): Calcium carbonate 311 mg + magnesium carbonate 232 mg

Mylanta Liquid (OTC): Aluminum hydroxide 200 mg + magnesium hydroxide 200 mg + simethicone 20 mg/5 mL

Mylanta Maximum Strength Liquid (OTC): Aluminum hydroxide 400 mg + magnesium hydroxide 400 mg + simethicone 40 mg/5 mL

Mylanta Regular Strength Liquid (OTC): Aluminum hydroxide 200 mg + magnesium hydroxide 200 mg + simethicone 20 mg/5 mL

Mylanta Ultra Chewable Tablets (OTC): Magnesium hydroxide 300 mg + calcium carbonate 700 mg

Nasotuss Liquid (Rx, sf, C-V): Chlorcyclizine HCl 25 mg + codeine phosphate 10 mg + phenylephrine HCl 10 mg/5 mL

Nature's Remedy Tablets (OTC): Cascara sagrada 150 mg + aloe 100 mg

NeoTuss Oral Liquid (OTC, sf): Dextromethorphan HBr 30 mg + guiafenesin 200 mg/5 mL

Nighttime Pamprin Powder (OTC): Diphenhydramine HCl 50 mg + acetaminophen 650 mg/packet

NoHist LQ Liquid (OTC, sf): Phenylephrine HCl 10 mg + chlorpheniramine maleate 4 mg/5 mL

Norco 5/325 Tablets (Rx, C-III): Hydrocodone bitartrate 5 mg + acetaminophen 325 mg

Norco Tablets (Rx, C-III): Hydrocodone bitartrate 10 mg + acetaminophen 325 mg

Nortuss-NX Liquid (Rx, sf, C-V): Codeine phosphate 10 mg + chlorcyclizine HCl 9.375 mg/5 mL

Nortuss-NXD Liquid (Rx, sf, C-V): Codeine phosphate 10 mg + chlorcyclizine HCL 9.375 mg + pseudoephedrine HCl 30 mg/5 mL

Nuedexta Capsules (Rx): Dextromethorphan HBr 20 mg + quinidine sulfate 10 mg

Original Alka-Seltzer Effervescent Tablets (OTC): Sodium bicarbonate 1,700 mg + aspirin 325 mg + citric acid 1,000 mg + phenylalanine 9 mg/tablet; sodium bicarbonate 1,916 mg + aspirin 325 mg + citric acid 1,000 mg/tablet

OsCal Extra D Tablets (OTC): Vitamin D_3 500 units + calcium 500 mg

P Chlor DM Oral Drops (Rx, sf): Chlorpheniramine maleate 1 mg + dextromethorphan HBr 30 mg + phenylephrine HCl 3.5 mg/5 mL

Painaid Back Relief Tablets (OTC): Acetaminophen 250 mg + magnesium salicylate 250 mg

Pamprin Maximum Pain Relief Caplets (OTC): Magnesium salicylate 250 mg + pamabrom 25 mg

Pamprin Multi-Symptom Maximum Strength Caplets/Tablets (OTC): Pyrilamine maleate 15 mg + pamabrom 25 mg

PE/GG Oral Liquid (Rx): Guaifenesin 100 mg + phenylephrine HCl 7.5 mg/5 mL

PediaCare Children's NightRest Multi-Symptom Cold Liquid (OTC): Diphenhydramine HCl 12.5 mg + phenylephrine HCl 5 mg/5 mL

PediaCare Infant Decongestant and Cough (PE) Oral Drops (OTC, sf): Dextromethorphan HBr 3.125 mg + phenylephrine HCl 1.56 mg/mL

PediaCare Infant Decongestnat and Cough (PSE) Oral Drops (OTC): Dextromethorphan HBr 3.125 mg + pseudoephedrine HCl 9.375 mg/mL

Pepcid Complete Chewable Tablets (OTC): Famotidine 10 mg + calcium carbonate 800 mg + magnesium hydroxide 165 mg

Percocet Tablets (Rx, C-II): Oxycodone HCl 5 mg + acetaminophen 325 mg

Percodan Tablets (Rx, C-II): Oxycodone HCl 4.5 mg + oxycodone terephthalate 0.38 mg + aspirin 325 mg

Percogesic Extra Strength Tablets (OTC): Diphenhydramine HCl 12.5 mg + acetaminophen 500 mg

Percogesic Tablets (OTC): Acetaminophen 325 mg + diphenhydramine 12.5 mg

Percogesic Tablets (OTC): Phenyltoloxamine citrate 30 mg + acetaminophen 325 mg

Peri-Colace Capsules (OTC): Docusate sodium 100 mg + casanthranol 30 mg

Phrenilin c/Caffeine and Codeine (Rx, C-III): Acetaminophen 325 mg + codeine phosphate 30 mg + butalbital 50 mg + caffeine 40 mg

Phrenilin Forte Capsules: Acetaminophen 650 mg + butalbital 50 mg

Poly Hist DHC Liquid (Rx, sf, C-III): Dihydrocodeine bitartrate 7.5 mg + phenylephrine HCl 5 mg + pyrilamine maleate 7.5 mg/5 mL

Poly-Hist NC Liquid (Rx, sf, C-V): Codeine phosphate 10 mg + pseudoephedrine HCl 15 mg + triprolidine HCl 1.25 mg/5 mL

Poly-Tussin EX Oral Liquid (Rx, sf, C-III): Dihydrocodeine bitartrate 7.5 mg + guaifenesin 50 mg + phenylephrine HCl 7.5 mg/5 mL

Pram-HCA Rectal Cream (Rx): Hydrocortisone acetate 2.35% + pramoxine HCl 1%

Pramcort Topical Cream (Rx): Hydrocortisone acetate 1% + pramoxine HCl 1%

PrandiMet Tablets (Rx): Repaglinide 1 mg + metformin HCl 500 mg; repaglinide 2 mg + metformin HCl 500 mg

Prevpac (Rx): Amoxcillin capsules 500 mg + lansoprazole capsules 30 mg + clarithromycin tablets 500 mg/day

Primatene Asthma Tablets (OTC): Ephedrine HCl 12.5 mg + guaifenesin 200 mg

ProCort Rectal Cream (OTC): Hydrocortisone acetate 1.85% + pramoxine HCl 1.15%

Pylera Capsules (Rx): Bismuth subcitrate potassium 140 mg + metronidazole 125 mg + tetracycline 125 mg

Quadrapax Elixir (Rx, C-IV): Atropine sulfate 0.0194 mg + scopolamine HBr 0.0065 mg + hyoscyamine sulfate 0.1037 mg + phenobarbital 16.2 mg /5 mL

Quinaretic Tablets (Rx): Quinapril HCl 10 mg + hydrochlorothiazide 12.5 mg; quinapril HCl 20 mg + hydrochlorothiazide 12.5 mg; quinapril HCl 20 mg + hydrochlorothiazide 25 mg

Repan CF (Rx): Acetaminophen 650 mg + butalbital 50 mg

Reprexain Tablets (Rx, C-III): Hydrocodone bitartrate 2.5 mg + ibuprofen 200 mg; hydrocodone bitartrate 5 mg + ibuprofen 200 mg; hydrocodone bitartrate 10 mg + ibuprofen 200 mg

Rifamate (Rx): Rifampin 300 mg + isoniazid 150 mg

Rifater Tablets (Rx): Rifampin 120 mg + isoniazid 50 mg + pyrazinamide 300 mg

Riopan Plus Double Strength Suspension (OTC): Magaldrate 1,080 mg + simethicone 40 mg/5 mL

Riopan Plus Double Strength Tablets (OTC): Magaldrate 1, 080 mg + simethicone 20 mg

Riopan Plus Suspension (OTC): Magaldrate 540 mg + simethicone 40 mg/5 mL

Riopan Plus Tablets (OTC): Magaldrate 480 mg + simethicone 20 mg

Robafen DM Liquid (OTC): Dextromethorphan HBr 10 mg + guaifenesin 100 mg/5 mL

Robitussin Children's Cough & Cold CF Liquid (Rx): Dextromethorphan HBr 5 mg + guaifenesin 50 mg + phenylephrine HCl 2.5 mg/5 mL

Robitussin Cold, Cold and Congestion Tablets (OTC): Dextromethorphan HBr 10 mg + pseudoephedrine HCl 30 mg + guaifenesin 200 mg

Robitussin Cough and Cold D Liquid: Dextromethorphan HBr 15mg + pseudoephedrine HCl 30 mg + guaifenesin 200 mg/5 mL

Robitussin Cough and Congestion Liquid: Dextromethorphan HBr 10 mg + guaifenesin 200 mg/5 mL

Robitussin Cough Sugar-Free DM Liquid (OTC, sf): Dextromethorphan 10 mg + guaifenesin 100 mg/ 5 mL

Robitussin PE Head and Chest Congestion Liquid (OTC): Phenylephrine HCl 5 mg + guaifenesin 100 mg/ 5 mL

Robitussin Pediatric Cough and Cold Long-Acting Liquid (OTC): Chlorpheniramine maleate 1 mg + dextromethorphan HBr 7.5 mg/5 mL

Robitussin Pediatric Cough/Cold CF Drops (OTC): Dextromethorphan HBr 2 mg + phenylephrine HCl 1 mg + guaifenesin 40 mg/mL

Robitussin-DM Liquid (OTC): Dextromethorphan HBr 10 mg + guaifenesin 100 mg/5 mL

Rondex-DM Oral Drops (Rx, sf): Dextromethorphan HBr 3 mg + phenylephrine HCl 3.5 mg + chlorpheniramine maleate 1 mg /mL

Roxicet 5/500 Caplets (Rx, C-II): Oxycodone HCl 5 mg + acetaminophen 500 mg

Roxicet Oral Solution (Rx, C-II): Oxycodone HCl 5 mg + acetaminophen 325 mg/5 mL

Roxicet Tablets (Rx, C-II): Oxycodone HCl 5 mg + acetaminophen 325 mg

Roxilox Capsules (Rx, C-II): Oxycodone HCl 5 mg + acetaminophen 500 mg

Roxiprin Tablets (Rx, C-II): Oxycodone HCl 4.5 mg + oxycodone terephthalate 0.38 mg + aspirin 325 mg

Rulox Plus Tablets (OTC): Aluminum hydroxide 200 mg + magnesium hydroxide 200 mg + simethicone 25 mg

Rulox Suspension (OTC): Aluminum hydroxide 225 mg + magnesium hydroxide 200 mg/5 mL

Rynatan Pediatric Chewable Tablets (Rx): Chlorpheniramine maleate 4.5 mg + phenylephrine tannate 5 mg

Rynatan Pediatric Suspension (Rx); Chlorpheniramine maleate 4.5 mg + phenylephrine tannate 5 mg/5 mL

Rynatan Tablets (Rx): Chlorpheniramine maleate 9 mg + phenylephrine tannate 25 mg

Rynex PE (Rx, sf): Brompheniramine maleate 1 mg + phenylephrine HCl 2.5 mg/5 mL

Scot-Tussin DM Liquid (OTC, sf): Chlorpheniramine maleate 2 mg + dextromethorphan HBr 15 mg/5 mL

Scot-Tussin Original Clear 5-Action Cold and Allergy Formula Liquid (OTC, sf): Pheniramine maleate 13.3 mg + phenylephrine HCl 4.2 mg + caffeine citrate 25 mg + sodium citrate 83.3 mg + sodium salicylate 83.3 mg/5 mL

Scot-Tussin Original Clear 5-Action Cold and Allergy Formula Syrup (OTC): Pheniramine maleate 13.3 mg + phenylephrine HCl 4.2 mg + caffeine citrate 25 mg + sodium citrate 83.3 mg + sodium salicylate 83.3 mg/5 mL

Scot-Tussin Senior Clear Liquid (OTC, sf): Dextromethorphan HBr 15 mg + guaifenesin 225 mg/5 mL

Sedapap Tablets (Rx): Acetaminophen 650 mg + butalbital 50 mg

Senokot-S Tablets (OTC): Docusate sodium 50 mg + sennosides 8.6 mg

Sildec Oral Drops (Rx): Carbinoxamine maleate 1 mg + pseudoephedrine HCl 15 mg/mL

Sildec Syrup (Rx): Brompheniramine maleate 4 mg + pseudoephedrine HCl 45 mg/5 mL

Simcor Extended-Release Tablets (Rx): Simvastatin 20 mg + niacin extended-release 500 mg; simvastatin 20 mg + niacin extended-release 750 mg; simvastatin 20 mg + niacin extended-release 1,000 mg

Sine-Off Cough/Cold Tablets (OTC): Phenylephrine HCl 5 mg + dextromethorphan HBr 15 mg + guaifenesin 200 mg + acetaminophen 325 mg

Sine-Off Multi-Symptom Relief Tablets (OTC): Dextromethorphan HBr 15 mg + phenylephrine HCl 5 mg + acetaminophen 325 mg + guaifenesin 200 mg

Sine-Off Non-Drowsy Maximum Strength Tablets (OTC): Acetaminophen 325 mg + phenylephrine HCl 5 mg

Sine-Off Sinus/Cold Tablets (OTC): Chlorpheniramine maleate 2 mg + phenylephrine HCl 5 mg + acetaminophen 500 mg

Sinutab Non-Drying Capsules (OTC): Phenylephrine HCl 5 mg + guaifenesin 200 mg

Sinutab Sinus Maximum Strength Tablets (OTC): Acetaminophen 325 mg + phenylephrine HCl 5 mg

Sitrex PD Liquid (Rx, sf): Phenylephrine HCl 7.5 mg + guaifenesin 75 mg/5 mL

Sitrex Tablets (Rx): Phenylephrine HCl 20 mg + guaifenesin 1,200 mg

Sodol Compound (Rx): Carisoprodol 200 mg + aspirin 325 mg

Sominex Pain Relief Tablets (OTC): Diphenhydramine HCl 25 mg + acetaminophen 500 mg

Sonahist DM Solution Concentrate (Rx): Chlorpheniramine maleate 1 mg + dextromethorphan HBr 3 mg + phenylephrine HCl 2 mg/mL

Stagesic Capsules (Rx, C-III): Hydrocodone bitartrate 5 mg + acetaminophen 500 mg

Stalevo 50 Tablets (Rx): Carbidopa 12.5 mg + levodopa 50 mg + entacapone 200 mg

Stalevo 75 Tablets (Rx): Carbidopa 18.75 mg + levodopa 75 mg + entacapone 200 mg

Stalevo 100 Tablets (Rx): Carbidopa 25 mg + levodopa 100 mg + entacapone 200 mg

Stalevo 125 Tablets (Rx): Carbidopa 31.25 mg + levodopa 120 mg + entacapone 200 mg

Stalevo 150 Tablets (Rx): Carbidopa 37.5 mg + levodopa 150 mg + entacapone 200 mg

Stalevo 200 Tablets (Rx): Carbidopa 50 mg + levodopa 200 mg + entacapone 200 mg

Suboxone Sublingual Film (Rx, C-III): Buprenorphine 2 mg + naloxone 0.5 mg; buprenorphine 8 mg + naloxone 2 mg

Sudafed Children's Non-Drowsy Cold and Cough Liquid (OTC, sf): Dextromethorphan HBr 5 mg + pseudoephedrine HCl 15 mg/5 mL

Sudafed PE Day and Night Tablets (OTC): Phenylepherine HCl 10 mg (Day); Diphenhydramine HCl 25 mg + phenylephrine HCl 10 mg (Night)

Sudafed PE Multi-Symptom Cold and Cough Tablets (OTC): Dextromethorphan HBr 10 mg + phenylephrine HCl 5 mg + guaifenesin 100 mg + acetaminophen 325 mg

Sudafed PE Multi-Symptom Severe Cold Tablets (OTC): Diphenhydramine HCl 12.5 mg + phenylephrine HCl 5 mg + acetaminophen 325 mg

Sudafed PE Nighttime Cold Maximum Strength Tablets (OTC): Diphenhydramine HCl 25 mg + phenylephrine HCl 5 mg + acetaminophen 325 mg

Sudafed PE Nighttime Nasal Deongestant Tablets (OTC): Diphenhydramine HCl 25 mg + phenylephrine HCl 10 mg

Sudafed PE Non-Drying Sinus Caplets (OTC): Phenylephrine HCl 5 mg + guaifenesin 200 mg

Sudafed PE Sinus and Allergy Tablets (OTC): Phenylephrine HCl 10 mg + chlorpheniramine maleate 4 mg

Sudafed PE Sinus Headache Maximum Strength Tablets (OTC): Acetaminophen 325 mg + phenylephrine HCl 5 mg

SudoGest Sinus & Allergy Maximum Strength Liquid (OTC): Chlorpheniramine maleate 4 mg + pseudoephedrine HCl 60 mg

Symbicort Aerosol (Rx): Budesonide 80 mcg + formoterol fumarte 4.5 mcg/activation; budesonide 160 mcg + formoterol fumarate 4.5 mcg/activation

Symbyax Capsules (Rx): Olanzapine 3 mg + fluoxetine 25 mg; olanzapine 6 mg + fluoxetine 25 mg; olanzapine 6 mg + fluoxetine 50 mg; olanzapine 12 mg + fluoxetine 25 mg; olanzapine 12 mg + fluoxetine 50 mg

Synalgos-DC Capsules (Rx, C-III): Dihydrocodeine bitartrate 16 mg + aspirin 356.4 mg + caffeine 30 mg

T-Gesic Capsules (Rx, C-III): Hydrocodone bitartrate 5 mg + acetaminophen 500 mg

Tarka Tablets (Rx): Trandolapril 1 mg + verapamil HCl 240 mg; trandolapril 2 mg + verapamil HCl 180 mg; trandolapril 2 mg + verapamil HCl 240 mg; trandolapril 4 mg + verapamil HCl 240 mg

Tekamlo Tablets (Rx): Amlodipine besylate 5 mg + aliskiren 150 mg; amlodipine besylate 10 mg + aliskiren 150 mg; amlodipine besylate 5 mg + aliskiren 300 mg; amlodipine besylate 10 mg + aliskiren 300 mg

Tekturna HCT (Rx): Aliskiren 150 mg + hydrochlorothiazide 12.5 mg; aliskiren 150 mg + hydrochlorothiazide 25 mg; aliskiren 300 mg + hydrochlorothiazide 12.5 mg; aliskiren 300 mg + hydrochlorothiazide 25 mg

Tenoretic 100 Tablets (Rx): Atenolol 100 mg + chlorthalidone 25 mg

Tenoretic 50 Tablets (Rx): Atenolol 50 mg + chlorthalidone 25 mg

Teveten HCT Capsules (Rx): Eprosartan 600 mg + hydrochlorothiazide 12.5 mg; eprosartan 600 mg + hydrochlorothiazide 25 mg

Theraflu Caplets Nighttime Severe Cold Tablets (OTC): Acetaminophen 325 mg + chlorpheniramine maleate 2 mg + dextromethorphan HBr 10 mg

Theraflu Cold and Cough Powder (OTC): Dextromethorphan HBr 20 mg + pheniramine maleate 20 mg + phenylephrine HCl 20 mg/packet

Theraflu Cold and Sore Throat Powder (OTC): Pheniramine maleate 20 mg + phenylephrine HCl 10 mg + acetaminophen 325 mg/packet

Theraflu Daytime Severe Cold and Cough Packets (OTC): Acetaminophen 650 mg + dextromethorphan HBr 20 mg + phenylephrine HCl 10 mg/packet

Theraflu Daytime Severe Cold and Cough Tablets (OTC): Acetaminophen 325 mg+ dextromethorphan HBr 10 mg + phenylephrine HCl 5 mg

Theraflu Flu and Chest Congestion Powder (OTC): Acetaminophen 1,000 mg + guaifenesin 400 mg/packet

Theraflu Flu and Sore Throat Powder (OTC): Pheniramine maleate 20 mg + phenylephrine HCl 10 mg + acetaminophen 650 mg/packet

Theraflu Nighttime Severe Cough and Cold Powder (OTC): Acetaminophen 650 mg + diphenhydramine HCl 25 mg + phenylephrine HCl 10 mg/packet

Theraflu Sugar-Free Nighttime Severe Cough and Cold Powder (OTC, sf): Acetaminophen 650 mg + diphenhydramine HCl 25 mg + phenylephrine HCl 10 mg/packet

Theraflu Thinstrips Daytime Cough and Cold Strips (OTC): Dextromethorphan HBr 20 mg + phenylephrine HCl 10 mg/strip

Theraflu Thinstrips Nightime Cold and Cough Strips (OTC): Diphenhydramine HCl 25 mg + phenylephrine HCl 10 mg/strip

Theraflu Warming Relief Daytime Multi-Symptom Cold Tablets (OTC): Dextromethorphan HBr 10 mg + phenylephrine HCl 5 mg + acetaminophen 325 mg

Theraflu Warming Relief Flu & Sore Throat Liquid (OTC): Phenylephrine 1.67 mg + diphenhydramine HCl 4.165 mg + acetaminophen 108.3 mg/5 mL

Titralac Plus Liquid (OTC, sf): Calcium carbonate 500 mg + simethicone 20 mg/5 mL

Titralac Plus Tablets (OTC): Calcium carbonate 420 mg + simethicone 21 mg

TL-Hist CM Liquid (Rx, C-V): Chlorpheniramine maleate 2 mg + codeine phosphate 10 mg/5 mL

TobraDex ST Ophthalmic Suspension (Rx): Tobramycin 0.3% + dexamethasone 0.05%

Triaminic Chest and Nasal Congestion Liquid (OTC): Phenylephrine HCl 2.5 mg + guaifenesin 50 mg/5 mL

Triaminic Children's Thin Strips Day Time Cold and Cough Strips (OTC): Dextromethorphan HBr 5 mg + phenylephrine HCl 2.5 mg/strip

Triaminic Children's Thin Strips Night Time Cold and Cough Strips (OTC): Diphenhydramine HCl 12.5 mg + phenylephrine HCl 5 mg/strip

Triaminic Cold and Cough Thin Strips (OTC): Dextromethorphan HBr 5 mg + phenylephrine HCl 2.5 mg/strip

Triaminic Cold and Sore Throat Softchews (OTC): Dextromethorphan HBr 5 mg + acetaminophen 160 mg

Triaminic Cough and Runny Nose Chewable Tablets (OTC): Chlorpheniramine maleate 1 mg + dextromethorphan HBr 5 mg

Triaminic Daytime Cold and Cough Liquid (OTC): Dextromethorphan HBr 5 mg + phenylephrine HCl 2.5 mg/5 mL

Triaminic Flu, Cough and Fever Liquid (OTC): Chlorpheniramne maleate 1 mg + dextromethorphan HBr 7.5 mg + acetaminophen 160 mg

Triaminic Infant Decongestant Plus Cough Thin Strips (OTC): Phenylephrine HCl 1.25 mg + dextromethorphan 1.83 mg/strip

Triaminic-D Children's Syrup (OTC): Chlorpheniramine maleate 1mg + dextromethorphan HBr 7.5 mg + pseudoephedrine HCl 15 mg/5 mL

Tribenzor Tablets (Rx): Olmesartan medoxomil 20 mg + amlodipine 5 mg + hydrochlorothiazide 12.5 mg; olmesartan medoxomil 40 mg + amlodipine 5 mg + hydrochlorothiazide 12.5 mg; olmesartan medoxomil 40 mg + amlodipine 5 mg + hydrochlorothiazide 25 mg; olmesartan medoxomil 40 mg + amlodipine 10 mg + hydrochlorothiazide 12.5 mg; olmesartan medoxomil 40 mg + amlodipine 10 mg + hydrochlorothiazide 25 mg

Trigofen DM Liquid (Rx, sf): Chlorpheniramine maleate 1 mg + dextromethorphan HBr 3 mg + phenylephrine HCL 2 mg/5 mL

Trital DM (Rx, sf): Chlorpheniramine maleate 4 mg + dextromethorphan HBr 15 mg + phenylephrine HCl 10 mg/5 mL

Trizivir Tablets (Rx): Abacavir sulfate 300 mg + lamivudine 150 mg + zidovudine 300 mg

Truvada Tablets (Rx): Emtricitabine 200 mg + tenofovir disoproxil fumarate 300 mg

Tums Dual Action Chewable Tablets (OTC): Famotidine 10 mg + calcium carbonate 800 mg + magnesium hydroxide 165 mg

Tussbid Capsules (Rx): Phenylephrine HCl 15 mg + guaifenesin 400 mg

Tussbid PD Capsules (Rx): Phenylephrine HCl 7.5 mg + guaifenesin 200 mg

Twynsta Tablets (Rx): Telmisartan 40 mg + amlodipine 5 mg; telmisartan 40 mg + amlodipine 10 mg; telmisartan 80 mg + amlodipine 5 mg; telmisartan 80 mg + amlodipine 10 mg

Tylenol Allergy Multi-Symptom Gelcaps and Tablets (OTC): Chlorpheniramine maleate 2 mg + phenylephrine HCl 5 mg + acetaminophen 325 mg

Tylenol Allergy Multi-Symptom Nighttime Tablets (OTC): Diphenhydramine HCl 25 mg + phenylephrine HCl 5 mg + acetaminophen 325 mg

Tylenol Chest Congestion Liquid (OTC): Acetaminophen 166.67 mg + guaifenesin 66.67 mg/5 mL

Tylenol Chest Congestion Tablets (OTC): Acetaminophen 325 mg + guaifenesin 200 mg

Tylenol Children's Plus Flu Suspension (OTC): Acetaminophen 160 mg + chlorpheniramine maleate 1 mg + dextromethorphan HBr 5 mg + phenylephrine HCl 2.5 mg/5 mL

Tylenol Children's Plus Multi-Symptom Cold Suspension (OTC): Acetaminophen 160 mg + chlorpheniramine maleate 1 mg + dextromethorphan HBr 5 mg + phenylephrine HCl 2.5 mg/5 mL

Tylenol Cold Head Congestion Daytime Cool Burst Tablets (OTC): Dextromethorphan HBr 10 mg + phenylephrine HCl 5 mg + acetaminophen 325 mg

Tylenol Cold Head Congestion Nighttime Cool Burst Tablets (OTC): Dextromethorphan HBr 10 mg + chlorpheniramine maleate 2 mg + phenylephrine HCl 5 mg + acetaminophen 325 mg

Tylenol Cold Multi-Symptom Daytime Citrus Burst Liquid (OTC): Dextromethorphan HBr 3.33 mg + phenylephdrine HCl 1.67 mg + acetaminophen 108.33 mg/5 mL

Tylenol Cold Multi-Symptom Daytime Cool Burst Tablets (OTC): Dextromethorphan HBr 10 mg + phenylephrine HCl 5 mg + acetaminophen 325 mg

Tylenol Cold Multi-Symptom Daytime Gelcaps (OTC): Dextromethorphan HBr 10 mg + phenylephrine HCl 5 mg + acetaminophen 325 mg

Tylenol Cold Multi-Symptom Nighttime Cool Burst Liquid (OTC): Dextromethorphan HBr 3.33 mg + doxylamine succinate 2.08 mg + phenylephrine HCl 1.67 mg + acetaminophen 108.33 mg/5 mL

Tylenol Cold Multi-Symptom Nighttime Cool Burst Tablets (OTC): Dextromethorphan HBr 10 mg + chlorpheniramine maleate 2 mg + phenylephrine HCl 5 mg + acetaminophen 325 mg

Tylenol Cold Severe Congestion Tablets (OTC): Dextromethorphan HBr 15 mg + pseudoephedrine HCl 30 mg + guaifenesin 200 mg + acetaminophen 325 mg

Tylenol Cough and Sore Throat Daytime Liquid: Dextromethorphan HBr 5 mg + acetaminophen 166.7 mg/5 mL

Tylenol Infants' Drops Plus Cold (OTC): Acetaminophen 100 mg/mL + phenylephrine HCl 1.56 mg/mL

Tylenol Multi-Symptom Convenience Pack Tablets - Day (OTC): Chlorpheniramine maleate 2 mg + phenylephrine HCl 5 mg + acetaminophen 325 mg

Tylenol Multi-Symptom Convenience Pack Tablets – Night (OTC): Diphenhydramine HCl 25 mg + phenylephrine HCl 5 mg + acetaminophen 325 mg

Tylenol Multi-Symptom Menstrual Relief, Women's Tablets (OTC): Acetaminophen 500 mg + pamabrom 25 mg

Tylenol Plus Children's Cold Suspension (OTC): Chlorpheniramne maleate 1 mg + phenylephrine HCl 2.5 mg + acetaminophen 160 mg/5 mL

Tylenol Plus Children's Cough and Runny Nose Oral Suspension (OTC): Chlorpheniramine maleate 1 mg + dextromethorphan HBr 5 mg + acetaminophen 160 mg/5 mL

Tylenol Plus Children's Cough and Sore Throat Oral Suspension (OTC): Dextromethorphan HBr 5 mg + acetaminophen 160 mg/5 mL

Tylenol Plus Infants' Cold and Cough Concentrated Drops (OTC): Dextromethorphan HBr 3.125 mg + phenylephrine HCl 1.56 mg + acetaminophen 100 mg/mL

Tylenol PM Gelcaps/Tablets, Extra Strength (OTC): Diphenhydramine HCl 25 mg + acetaminophen 500 mg

Tylenol Severe Allergy Tablets (OTC): Diphenhydramine HCl 12.5 mg + acetaminophen 500 mg

Tylenol Sinus Congestion and Pain Nighttime Caplets (OTC): Phenylephrine HCl 5 mg + chlorpheniramine maleate 2 mg + acetaminophen 325 mg

Tylenol Sinus Congestion and Pain Severe Daytime Caplets (OTC): Phenylephrine HCl 5 mg + guaifenesin 200 mg + acetaminophen 325 mg

Tylenol Sinus Non-Drowsy Maximum Strength Gelcaps, Geltabs, and Tablets (OTC): Acetaminophen 325 mg + pseudoephedrine HCl 30 mg

Tylenol Sinus Severe Congestion Tablets (OTC): Pseudoephedrine HCl 30 mg + guaifenesin 200 mg + acetaminophen 325 mg

Tylenol Sore Throat Nighttime Liquid (OTC): Diphenhydramine HCl 8.3 mg + acetaminophen 166.6 mg/ 5 mL

Tylenol w/Codeine Elixir (Rx, C-V): Codeine phosphate 15 mg + acetaminophen 120 mg/5 mL

Tylenol w/Codeine No. 2 Tablets (Rx, C-III): Codeine phosphate 15 mg + acetaminophen 300 mg

Tylenol w/Codeine No. 3 Tablets (Rx, C-III): Codeine phosphate 30 mg + acetaminophen 300 mg

Tylenol w/Codeine No. 4 Tablets (Rx, C-III): Codeine phosphate 60 mg + acetaminophen 300 mg

Tylox Capsules (Rx, C-II): Oxycodone HCl 5 mg + acetaminophen 500 mg

Uniretic Tablets (Rx): Moexipril HCl 7.5 mg + hydrochlorothiazide 12.5 mg; moexipril HCl 15 mg + hydrochlorothiazide 12.5 mg; moexipril HCl 15 mg + hydrochlorothiazide 25 mg

Unisom with Pain Relief Tablets (OTC): Diphenhydramine HCl 50 mg + acetaminophen 650 mg

V-Cof Oral Suspension (Rx): Brompheniramine maleate 6 mg + carbetapentane citrate 25 mg + phenylephrine HCl 10 mg/5 mL

Valturna Tablets (Rx): Aliskiren 150 mg + valsartan 160 mg; aliskiren 300 mg + valsartan 320 mg

Vanex-HD Liquid (Rx, C-III): Hydrocodone bitartrate 1.7 mg + chlorpheniramine maleate 2 mg + phenylephrine HCl 5 mg/5 mL

Vaseretic Tablets (Rx): Enalapril maleate 5 mg + hydrochlorothiazide 12.5 mg; Enalapril maleate 10 mg + hydrochlorothiazide 25 mg

Vicks 44E Cough and Chest Congestion Relief Liquid (OTC): Dextromethorphan 6.67 mg + guaifenesin 66.7 mg/5 mL

Vicks Children's NyQuil Cold and Cough Relief Liquid (OTC): Chlorpheniramine maleate 0.67 mg + dextromethorphan HBr 5 mg/5 mL

Vicks DayQuil Multi-Symptom Cold/Flu Relief LiquiCaps (OTC): Dextromethorphan HBr 10 mg + phenylephrine HCl 5 mg + acetaminophen 325 mg

Vicks DayQuil Multi-Symptom Cold/Flu Relief Liquid (OTC): Dextromethorphan HBr 3.33 mg + phenylephrine HCl 1.67mg + acetaminophen 108.33 mg/5 mL

Vicks DayQuil Sinex Liquid-Filled Capsules (OTC): Acetaminophen 325 mg + phenylephrine HCl 5 mg

Vicks DayQuil Sinus Liqui-Caps (OTC): Acetaminophen 325 mg + phenylephrine 5 mg

Vicks Formula 44D Cough and Head Congestion Relief Liquid (OTC): Dextromethorphan HBr 6.67 mg + phenylephrine HCl 3.33 mg/5 mL

Vicks Formula 44E Pediatric Cough and Chest Congestion Relief Syrup (OTC): Dextromethorphan HBr 2.2 mg + guaifenesin 33.3 mg/5 mL

Vicks Formula 44M Cough, Cold and Flu Relief Liquid (OTC): Chlorpheniramine maleate 1 mg + dextromethorphan HBr 7.5 mg + acetaminophen 162.5 mg/5 mL

Vicks Formula 44M Pediatric Cough and Cold Relief Liquid (OTC): Chlorpheniramine maleate 0.67mg + dextromethorphan HBr 5 mg/5 mL

Vicks NyQuil Cough Syrup (OTC): Dextromethorphan HBr 5 mg + doxylamine succinate 2.08 mg/5 mL

Vicks NyQuil Multi-Symptom Cold/Flu Relief LiquiCaps (OTC): Dextromethorphan HBr 15 mg + doxylamine succinate 6.25 mg + acetaminophen 325 mg

Vicks NyQuil Multi-Symptom Cold/Flu Relief Liquid (OTC): Dextromethorphan HBr 5 mg + doxylamine succinate 2.08 mg + acetaminophen 166.67 mg/5 mL

Vicks NyQuil Sinex Liquid-Filled Capsules (OTC): Acetaminophen 325 mg + doxylamine succinate 6.25 mg + phenylephrine HCl 5 mg

Vicks NyQuil Sinus Liquid-Filled Capsules (OTC): Phenylephrine HCl 5 mg + doxylamine succinate 6.25 mg + acetaminophen 325 mg

Vicks Pediatric Formula 44M Cough and Cold Relief Liquid (OTC): Chlorpheniramine maleate 0.66 mg + dextromethorphan HBr 5 mg/5 mL

Vicoden ES Tablets (Rx, C-III): Hydrocodone bitartrate 7.5 mg + acetaminophen 750 mg

Vicoden HP Tablets (Rx, C-III): Hydrocodone bitartrate 10 mg + acetaminophen 660 mg

Vicoden Tablets (Rx, C-III): Hydrocodone bitartrate 5 mg + acetaminophen 500 mg

Vicoprofen Tablets (Rx, C-III): Hydrocodone bitartrate 7.5 mg + ibuprofen 200 mg

Vimovo Tablets (Rx): Naproxen 375 mg + esomeprazole 20 mg; naproxen 500 mg + esomeprazole 20 mg

Viravan-P Suspension (Rx): Pseudoephedrine HCl 30 mg + pyrilamine maleate 20 mg/5 mL

Vopac Tablets (Rx, C-III): Acetaminophen 650 mg + codeine phosphate 30 mg

Vytorin Tablets (Rx): Ezetimibe 10 mg + simvastatin 10 mg; ezetimibe 10 mg + simvastatin 20 mg; ezetimibe 10 mg + simvastatin 40 mg; ezetimibe 10 mg + simvastatin 80 mg

Xodol Tablets (Rx, C-III): Acetaminophen 300 mg + oxycodone bitartrate 5 mg; acetaminophen 300 mg + oxycodone bitartrate 7.5 mg; acetaminophen 300 mg + oxycodone bitartrate 10 mg

Xolox Tablets (Rx, C-II): Acetaminophen 500 mg + oxycodone HCl 2.5 mg

Z-Cof I Suspension (Rx): Dextromethorphan HBr 15 mg + guaifenesin 211 mg + pseudoephedrne HCl 30 mg/5 mL

Z-Tuss AC Liquid (Rx, sf, C-V): Chlorpheniramine maleate 2 mg + codeine phosphate 9 mg/ 5 mL

Z-Tuss E Liquid (Rx, sf, C-V): Codeine phosphate 9 mg + guaifenesin 200 mg + pseudoephedrine HCl 30 mg/5 mL

Zamicet Oral Solution (Rx, C-III): Acetaminophen 108.3 mg + hydrocodone bitartrate 3.3 mg/5 mL

Zebutal Capsules (Rx): Butalbital 50 mg + acetaminophen 500 mg + caffeine 40 mg

Zegerid Capsules (Rx): Omeprazole 40 mg + sodium bicarbonate 1,100 mg

Zegerid OTC Capsules (OTC): Omeprazole 20 mg + sodium bicarbonate 1,100 mg

Zegerid Powder for Oral Suspensin (Rx): Omeprazole 40 mg + sodium bicarbonate 1,680 mg

Zegerid Powder for Oral Suspension (OTC): Omeprazole 20 mg + sodium bicarbonate 1,680 mg;

Ziac Tablets (Rx): Bisoprolol fumarate 2.5 mg + hydrochlorothiazide 6.25 mg; bisoprolol fumarate 5 mg + hydrochlorothiazide 6.25 mg; bisoprolol fumarate 10 mg + hydrochlorothiazide 6.25 mg

ZoDen DM Drops (Rx, sf): Chlorpheniramine maleate 1 mg + dextromethorphan HBr 3 mg + phenylephrine HCl 1.5 mg/mL

Zydone Tablets (Rx, C-III): Hydrocodone bitartrate 5 mg + acetaminophen 400 mg; hydrocodone bitartrate 7.5 mg + acetaminophen 400 mg; hydrocodone bitartrate 10 mg + acetaminophen 400 mg

Zyrtec-D 12 Hour Tablets (Rx): Cetirizine HCl 5 mg (IR) + pseudoephedrine HCl 120 mg (ER)

Appendix 9

Drug/Food Interactions

A. DRUGS THAT SHOULD BE TAKEN WHILE FASTING

Alendronate
Ampicillin
Bethanechol (may experience N&V)
Bisacodyl
Captopril (take 1 hr before meals)
Ceftibuten (Cedax)
Cetirizine (Zyrtec)
Chloramphenicol
Cilostazol (Pletal)
Cyclosporine gel caps only (avoid fatty meals)
Demeclocycline (avoid high calcium foods/dairy products)
Dicloxacillin
Didanosine (Videx)
Digitalis preparations (not with high fiber foods)
Digoxin (avoid high fiber cereals and oatmeal)
Erythromycin base/estolate
Etidronate (Didronel)
Felodipine (Plendil)
Ferrous salts (not with tea, coffee, egg, cereals, fiber, or milk)
Fexofenadine
Flavoxate
Indinavir (Crixivan)
Ketoprofen (if GI distress occurs, may take with food)
Lansoprazole
Levodopa (not with high protein foods; meals delay absorption and peak plasma concentration; avoid caffeine)
Levothyroxine
Lomustine (empty stomach will reduce nausea)
Loracarbef (Lorabid)
Loratadine (Claritin)
Methotrexate (milk, cream, or yogurt may decrease absorption)
Methyldopa (not with high protein foods; meals delay absorption and peak plasma concentration; avoid caffeine)
Moexipril (Univasc)
Mycophenolate (Cellcept)
Nafcillin (inactivated by stomach acid; absorption variable with/without food)
Norfloxacin (milk, cream, or yogurt may decrease absorption)

Omeprazole
Oxacillin
Oxytetracycline (avoid dairy products and foods high in calcium)
Penicillamine (antacids, iron and food decreases absorption)
Perindopril (Aceon)
Phenytoin (if GI distress occurs, may take with food; food effect depends on preparation)
Propantheline
Repaglinide (Prandin)
Rifabutin (Mycobutin)
Rifampin
Riluzole (Rilutek)
Roxithromycin (take at least 15 min before or after meal)
Sotalol
Sucralfate
Sulfadiazine
Sulfamethoxazole-Trimethoprim (Bactrim)
Terbutaline sulfate
Tetracycline (avoid dairy products and foods high in calcium)
Theophylline (absorption of controlled release varies by preparation)
Thyroid hormone preparations (limit foods containing goitrogens)
Tolcapone (Tasmar)
Trientine (antacids, iron, and food reduces absorption)
Zafirlukast (Accolate)
Zalcitabine (Hivid)

B. DRUGS THAT SHOULD BE TAKEN WITH FOOD

Allopurinol (after meal)
Atovaquone (Mepron)
Augmentin
Aspirin
Amiodarone (Cordarone)
Baclofen (Lioresal)
Bromocriptine (Parlodel)
Buspirone
Carbamazepine (erratic absorption; Tegretol)
Carvedilol (Coreg)
Cefpodoxime (Vantin)
Chloroquine
Chlorothiazide
Cimetidine (Tagamet)
Clofazimine
Diclofenac (Voltaren)
Divalproex (Depakote)
Doxycyline

Felbamate (Felbatol)
Fenofibrate (TriCor)
Fiorinal
Fludrocortisone
Fenoprofen
Gemfibrozil
Glyburide (take with breakfast)
Griseofulvin (high fat meals)
Hydrocortisone
Hydroxychloroquine (Plaquenil)
Indomethacin
Iron products (take between meals, unless GI upset)
Isotretinoin
Itraconazole capsules
Ketorolac
Lithium
Mebendazole
Methenamine
Methylprednisolone
Metronidazole
Misoprostol (Cytotec)
Naltrexone
Naproxen
Nelfinavir (Viracept)
Niacin
Nifedipine (grapefruit juice increases bioavailability)
Nitrofurantoin
Olsalazine
Oxcarbazepine
Pentoxifylline
Pergolide
Perphenazine
Piroxicam
Potassium salts
Prednisone
Probucol (high fat meals)
Procainamide
Ritonavir (Norvir)
Salsalate
Saquinavir
Sevelamer (Renagel)
Spironolactone
Sulfasalazine

Sulfinpyrazone
Sulindac
Ticlopidine
Tolmetin
Trazodone
Troglitazone
Valproic acid
Verapamil SR (absorption varies by manufacturer; too rapid absorption may cause heart block)

C. CONSTIPATING AGENTS

Antacids (aluminum and calcium containing)
Anticholinergic drugs
Anticonvulsants
Antidepresssants
Antihistamines
Antiparkinsonian drugs
Antipsychotic drugs
Antispasmodics
Bisphosphonates
BP medications (calcium channel blockers)
Calcium supplements
Clonidine
Diuretics
Ganglionic blocking agents
Iron supplements
MAOIs
Muscle relaxants
Narcotics
NSAIDs
Octreotide
Opioids
Phenothiazines
Prostaglandin synthesis inhibitors
Tranquilizers
Tricyclic antidepressants

D. DIARRHEAL AGENTS

Adrenergic neuron blockers: guanethidine
Antacids (Mg^{++} containing); H_2 receptor antagonists (i.e., ranitidine); PPIs (i.e, omeprazole)
Antiarrhythmics (i.e., quinidine)
Antibiotics (especially broad spectrum agents)
Antidepressants (fluoxetine, sertraline)
Antihypertensives (beta blockers, ACE Inhibitors)
Anti-inflammatory drugs (NSAIDs, colchicine)

Antivirals
Chemotherapy agents
Cholinergic agonists and cholinesterase inhibitors
Colchicine
Corticosteroids (prednisone)
Digitalis
Glucophage (Metformin)
Laxative abuse
Lithium
Metoclopramide
Misoprostol
Mycophenolate (drugs to prevent organ transplant rejection)
NSAIDs
Olsalazine
Osmotic and stimulant laxatives (such as Ex-Lax, Ducolax, Correctol, Feen-a-Mint)
Radiation therapy
Theophylline (Theo-24)

E. TYRAMINE CONTAINING FOODS

Moderate amounts of tyramine:
Banana peel
Broad beans (fava)
Cheeses (all except cream cheese, ricotta, and cottage cheese)
Chianti, vermouth
Chocolate
Concentrated yeast extracts/Brewer's yeast
Fermented cabbage products: sauerkraut, kimchee
Hydrolyzed protein extracts for sauces, soups, gravies
Imitation cheese
Liquid and powdered protein supplements
Meat extracts
Nonalcoholic beers
Prepared meats (sausage, chopped liver, pate, salami, mortadella)
Raspberries
Some non-United States brands of beer
Yeast products

Significant amounts of tyramine:
Aged cheese
Aged or cured meats
Avocado
Bean curd
Cream from fresh pasteurized milk
Distilled spirits

Eggplant
Fruits (grapes, oranges, pineapple, plums, prunes, figs, raisins)
Peanuts, coconuts, Brazil nuts
Processed foods (Vegemite, sauerkraut, shrimp paste)
Red and white wines, port wines
Soy products (soy sauce, tofu, miso, teriyaki sauce)
Tap beer
Yogurt

F. FOODS CONTAINING GOITROGENS

Cruciferous vegetables:
Broccoli, brussel sprouts, cabbage, cauliflower, kale, rutabaga, mustard, turnips
Millet
Peaches
Peanuts
Radishes
Soy beans and soy-bean related foods (tofu)
Spinach
Strawberries

G. COUMARIN ANTICOAGULANTS AND DIETARY EFFECTS

Consumption of vitamin K-enriched foods may counteract the effects of anticoagulants since the drugs act through antagonism of vitamin K. Advise client on anticoagulants to maintain a steady, consistent intake of vitamin K-containing foods. The drug monograph for warfarin clearly lists these foods. Additionally, certain herbal teas (green tea, buckeye, horse chestnut, Woodruff, tonka beans, melitot) contain natural coumarins that can potentiate the effects of coumadin and should be avoided. Large amounts of avocado also potentiate the drug's effects. Green leafy vegetables: brussels sprouts, broccoli, spinach, kale, turnip greens, and other cruciferous vegetables increase the catabolism of warfarin thereby decreasing its anticoagulant activities. Caffeinated beverages (i.e., cola, coffee, tea, hot chocolate, chocolate milk) can affect therapy. Alcohol intake of more than three drinks per day can affect clotting times. Herbal supplements can also affect bleeding time: Coenzyme Q10 is structurally similar to vitamin K, feverfew, garlic, and ginseng. Avoid herbal medications while on warfarin therapy.

H. GENERAL DRUG CLASS RECOMMENDATIONS

ACE inhibitors: Take captopril and moexipril 1 hr before or 2 hr after meals; food decreases absorption. Avoid high potassium foods as ACE increases K^+.

Analgesic/Antipyretic: Take on an empty stomach as food may slow the absorption.

Antacids: Take 1 hr after or between meals. Avoid dairy foods as the protein in them can increase stomach acid.

Anti-anxiety agents: Caffeine may cause excitability, nervousness, and hyperactivity lessening the antianxiety drug effects.

Antibiotics: Penicillin generally should be taken on an empty stomach; may take with food if GI upset occurs. Do not mix with acidic foods: coffee, citrus fruits, and tomatoes; the acid interferes with absorption of penicillin, ampicillin, erythromycin and cloxacillin.

Anticoagulants: High vitamin K produces blood-clotting substance and may reduce drug effectiveness. Vitamin E >400 IU may prolong clotting time and increase bleeding risk.

Antidepressant drugs: May be taken with or without food.

Antifungals: Avoid taking with dairy products; avoid alcohol.

Antihistamines: Take on an empty stomach to increase effectiveness.

Bronchodilators with theophylline: High-fat meals may increase bioavailability while high-carbohydrate meals may decrease it. Food increases absorption of Theo-24 and Uniphyl which may cause increased N&V, headache, and irritability.

Cephalosporins: Take on an empty stomach 1 hr before or 2 hr after meals. May take with food if GI upset occurs.

Diuretics: Vary in interactions; some cause loss of potassium, calcium, and magnesium. Avoid salty food and natural black licorice as these increase K^+ and Mg^{++} losses. Large doses of vitamin D can elevate blood pressure.

H_2 blockers: May take with or without regard to food.

HMG-CoA reductase inhibitors: Take lovastatin with the evening meal to enhance absorption.

Laxatives: Avoid dairy foods as calcium can decrease absorption.

Macrolides: Take on an empty stomach 1 hr before or 2 hr after meals. May take with food for GI upset.

MAOIs: Have many dietary restrictions, so follow dietary guidelines as prescribed. Foods or alcoholic beverages containing tyramine may cause a fatal increase in BP.

Narcotic analgesics: Avoid alcohol as it may increase sedative effects.

Nitroimadazole (metronidazole): Avoid alcohol or food prepared with alcohol for at least 3 days after finishing the medicine. Alcohol may cause nausea, abdominal cramps, vomiting, headaches, and flushing.

NSAIDs: Take with food or milk to prevent irritation of the stomach.

Quinolones: Take on an empty stomach 1 hr before or 2 hr after meals. May take with food for GI upset but avoid calcium containing foods such as milk, yogurt, vitamins/minerals containing iron, and antacids because they decrease drug concentrations. Caffeine-containing products may lead to excitability and nervousness.

Sulfonamides: Take on an empty stomach 1 hr before or 2 hr after meals. May take with food if GI upset occurs.

Tetracyclines: Take on an empty stomach 1 hr before or 2 hr after meals. May take with food but avoid dairy products, antacids, and vitamins containing iron with tetracycline.

Appendix 10

Drugs Whose Effects Are Modified by Grapefruit Juice

Increasing numbers of drugs have been identified whose effects are modified by short-term or chronic use of grapefruit juice. The most frequent result is an increase in plasma levels of the drug, which may increase the risk and intensity of side effects. It is likely that the predominant mechanism for this effect is CYP3A4 isoenzyme inhibition by grapefruit. Another possibility, however is the effect of grapefruit juice on drugs whose absorption is highly dependent on the uptake drug transporter organic anion-transporting polypeptide (OATP1A2). Absorption of such drugs is decreased, leading to reduced plasma levels and therefore a decreased effect. It is also possible that other fruits (e.g., oranges, tangerines, apples) may also have an effect on this system.

The following is a representative list of drugs, including the mechanism, whose effects are modified by grapefruit juice.

Drug	Mechanism for Altered Effect
Albendazole	↑ Plasma albendazole levels and peak plasma concentration
Amiodarone	↑ Plasma amiodarone levels R/T inhibition of amiodarone metabolism
Amlodipine	↑ Plasma amlodipine levels R/T ↓ liver metabolism
Amprenavir	↓ Amprenavir peak levels and ↑ time to reach peak concentration
Artemether/Lumefantrine	Possible ↑ concentrations of artemether/lumefantrine → potentiation of QT R/T inhibition of CYP3A4
Atazanavir	↑ Atazanavir plasma levels → ↑ effect
Atorvastatin	↑ Plasma atorvastatin levels
Bexarotene	↑ Plasma bexarotene levels R/T ↓ liver metabolism
Budesonide	↑ Plasma budesonide levels
Buspirone	↑ AUC and peak plasma buspirone levels and time to reach peak levels
Calcium channel blockers	↑ Serum levels of calcium channel blockers
Carbamazepine	↑ Peak plasma carbamazepine levels
Cilostazol	↑ Plasma cilostazol levels R/T ↓ liver metabolism
Clarithromycin	↑ Clarithromycin plasma levels R/T ↓ metabolism; do not use together

Drug	Mechanism for Altered Effect
Cyclosporine	↑ Plasma cyclosporine levels R/T ↓ liver metabolism
Dextromethorphan	↑ Bioavailability of dextromethorphan
Digoxin	↑ Plasma digoxin levels
Dofetilide	Possible ↑ dofetilide plasma levels
Dronedarone	Avoid grapefruit juice
Ergot alkaloids	↑ Serum levels of ergotamine derivatives
Erythromycin	↑ Plasma erythromycin levels R/T ↓ metabolism in the small intestine
Estrogens	↑ Plasma levels of 17-beta estradiol/estrone combination
Etoposide	↓ Etoposide AUC and bioavailability
Everolimus	Significant ↑ exposure of everolimus; do not give together
Felodipine	↑ Plasma felodipine levels R/T ↓ liver metabolism
Fexofenadine	↓ Fexofenadine plasma levels R/T ↓ absorption by the drug transporter organic anion-transporting polypeptide
Fluvoxamine	↑ Fluvoxamine mean AUC and C_{max}
Fosamprenavir	See *Amprenavir*
HMG-CoA Reductase Inhibitors	Possible ↑ AUC, C_{max}, and elimination t½ of certain HMG-CoA reductase inhibitors → ↑ risk of rhabdomyolysis
Indinavir	Delay in indinavir absorption and time to reach peak plasma levels
Itraconzole	↓ Itraconzole bioavailability R/T inhibition of absorption
Ixabepilone	↑ Ixabepilone plasma levels
Lapatinib	↑ Lapatinib plasma levels
Losartan	↓ Liver metabolism to losartan's active form
Lovastatin	↑ Plasma lovastatin levels R/T ↓ liver metabolism
Lubasidone	Do not exceed a dose of 40 mg/day
Methylprednisolone	↑ Plasma methylprednisolone levels R/T ↓ liver metabolism
Midazolam	↑ PO midazolam plasma levels R/T ↓ liver metabolism
Mifepristone	↑ Plasma mifepristone levels R/T ↓ liver metabolism
Nicardipine	↑ Plasma nicardipine levels R/T ↓ liver metabolism

Drug	Mechanism for Altered Effect
Nifedipine	↑ Plasma nifedipine levels R/T ↓ liver metabolsim
Nilotinib	↑ Nilotinib plasma levels
Nisoldipine	↑ Plasma nisoldipine levels R/T ↓ liver metabolism
Pasugrel hydrochloride	↑ Pazopanib plasma levels → ↑ pharmacologic effects and ↑ risk of side effects; do not use together
Pimozide	↑ Pimozide plasma levels; possible QTc prolongation and increased risk of life-threatening cardiac arrhythmias. Do not use together.
Praziquantel	↑ Praziquantal AUC and C_{max}
Quinidine	↓ Quinidine absorption and ↓ quinidine metabolism to its major metabolite; effect on QTc interval delayed
Ranolazine	↑ Ranolazine levels and QTc prolongation R/T inhibition of metabolism by CYP3A; do not use together
Ritonavir	↑ Ritonavir plasma levels → ↑ pharmacologic effects
Romidepsin	↑ Romidepsin plasma levels R/T inhibition of metabolism by CYP3A4; use together with caution
Saquinavir	↑ Plasma saquinavir levels R/T ↓ liver metabolism
Saxagliptin	↑ Saxagliptin exposure; dosage adjustment not recommended
Scopolamine	↑ Scopolamine bioavailability and ↑ time to reach peak plasma levels
Sildenafil	↑ Plasma sildenafil levels R/T ↓ liver metabolism
Simvastatin	↑ Plasma simvastatin levels R/T ↓ liver metabolism
Sirolimus	↑ Plasma sirolimus levels R/T ↓ liver metabolism
Tacrolimus	↑ Tacrolimus blood trough levels in liver transplant clients R/T ↓ CYP3A metabolism
Temsirolimus	↑ Plasma sirolimus levels (sirolimus is a major metabolite of tensirolimus); do not use with grapefruit juice
Tolvaptan	↑ Tolvaptan levels 1.8-fold
Toremifene citrate	↑ Toremifene plasma levels → ↑ risk of side effects
Triazolam	↑ Plasma triazolam levels R/T ↓ liver metabolism
Verapamil	↑ Plasma verapamil levels R/T ↓ liver metabolism

Appendix 11

Drugs That Should Not Be Crushed

As a rule of thumb, any sustained-release or extended-release formulation should never be crushed. Instead, attempt to get a liquid formulation of the product so that it can be administered in that form. Coated products should also not be crushed. They were coated for a specific purpose, e.g., to prevent stomach irritation by the product, to prevent destruction of the product by stomach acid, to prevent an unwanted reaction, or to produce a prolonged or extended effect.

These are some of the drugs that should not be crushed:

Accutane
Aciphex
Actiq
Actonel
Adalat cc SR
Adderall XR
Advicor ER
Afrinol Repetab
Aggrenox
Allegra-D
Allerest capsule
Alprazolam ER
Altoprev
Ambien CR
Aminodur Duratab
Aptivus
Arthrotec
ASA E.C.
ASA Enseal
Augmentin XR
Avinza
Avodart
Azulfadine Entab
Betaphen-VK
Biaxin XL
Biscodyl EC
Boniva
Budeprion SR
Calan SR
Cardene SR
Cardizem LA, SR
Cardura XL
Ceclor CD
Ceftin
Cefuroxime
CellCept
Chlortrimeton SR
Choledyl SR
Cipro XR
Claritin-D
Colace
Colestid
Commit
Compazine Spansule
Concerta
Concerta SR
Covera-HS
Creon EC
Crixivan
Cymbalta
Cytovene
Depakote ER
Detrol LA
Dilacor XR
Ditropan XL
Divalproex XR
Drixoral tablet
Ducolax EC
DynaCirc CR
Ecotrin tablet
Effexor XR
E-Mycin tablet
Erythromycin EC
Evista

Feldene
Fentora
Feosol Spansule/Tablet
Ferro Grad-500 tablet/sequels
Flagyl ER
Flomax
Fosamax
Geocillin
Gleevec
Glipizide
Glucotrol XL
Glucophage XR
Imdur SR, LA
Inderal LA
Indocin SR
Innopran XL
Intelence
Isoptin SR
Isordil Tembids, Dinitrate
Isordil sublingual
Kadian
Kaon tablet
Kapidex
K-Dur, K-tab
Keppra XR
Ketek
Klor-Con
Lamictal XR
Lescol XL
Levbid SR
Lithobid SR
Luvox CR
Macrobid SR
Mestinon Timespans
Metadate CD, SR
Metoprolol ER
Motrin
MS Contin
Mucinex
Nexium
Niaspan
Nicotinic acid
Nifediac CC
Nifedipine ER
Nitroglycerin tablet
Nitrospan capsule
Norpace CR
OxyContin
Pancrease EC, MT
Paxil CR
Pentasa
Plendil SR
Prevacid
Prilosec SR
Procardia XL
Propecia
Proscar
Protonix
Prozac weekly
Ranexa
Razadyne ER
Renagel
Requip XL
Revlimid
Risperdal M-tab
Ritalin LA/SR
Rythmol SR
Seroquel XR
Sinemet CR
Slo-Niacin
Slow K tablet; Slow Mag, Slow Fe
Strattera
Sudafed SA capsule
Sular
Tasigna
Tegretol XR
Temodar
Tessalon Perles
Theobid Duracaps
Tiazac SR
Topamax
Toprol XL
Tracleer
Trental SR
Treximet
Tylenol ER

Ultram ER
Uniphyl SR
Uroxatral
Valcyte
Verapamil SR
Verelan PM
Videx EC
Voltaren EC/SR
Wellbutrin SR
Xanax SR
ZORprin
Zerit XR
Zolinza
Zomig ZMT
Zyban
Zyflo CR
Zyrtec-D

Appendix 12

National Patient Safety Goals (NPSG)

The purpose of the National Patient Safety Goals is to improve patient safety. The goals are developed to focus on problems in health care safety and how to solve them. Further information on the National Patient Safety Goals are located on the Joint Commission Website: www.jointcommission.org

Identify Patients Correctly

Goal 1: Improve the accuracy of patient identification

01.01.01. Use at least two patient identifiers when providing care, treatment, and services. This may include the patient's name and date of birth to ensure that each patient gets the correct medicine and treatment. (Hospital, Behavioral Health, Long-Term Care, Home Care)

01.03.01. Eliminate transfusion errors related to patient misidentification. (Hospital)

Improve Staff Communication

Goal 2: Improve the effectiveness of communication among caregivers

02.03.01. Report all critical results of tests and diagnostic procedures on a timely basis. Get important test results to the right staff person on time. (Hospital)

Use Medications Safely

Goal 3: Improve the safety of using medications

03.04.01. Before a procedure, label all medications, medication containers, i.e. medications in syringes, medicine cups, basins, and other solutions on and off the sterile field in perioperative and other procedural settings and in any area where medicines and supplies are set up. (Hospital)

03.05.01. Reduce the likelihood of patient harm associated with the use of anticoagulation therapy. (Hospital, Long-Term Care)

03.06.01. Maintain and communicate patient medication information.

Prevent Infection

Goal 7: Reduce the risk of health care-associated infections

07.01.01. Comply with either current Center for Disease Control hand hygiene guidelines or World Health Organization hand hygiene guidelines. Set goals for improving hand cleaning and use these goals to improve hand cleaning. (Hospital, Behavioral Health, Long-Term Care, Home Care)

07.03.01. Implement evidence-based practices to prevent health care-associated infections due to multidrug-resistant organisms in acute care hospitals. Use proven guideline to prevent infections that are difficult to treat. (Hospital)

07.04.01. Implement best practices or evidence-based guidelines to prevent central line-associated bloodstream infections. (Hospital)

07.05.01. Implement best practices/proven guidelines to prevent infection after surgery/surgical"… site. (Hospital)

07.06.01. Implement evidence-based practices to prevent indwelling catheter associated urinary tract infections (CAUTI).

Identify Patients at Risk for Suicide

(This requirement applies only to psychiatric hospitals and patients being treated for emotional or behavioral disorders in general hospitals.)

15.01.01. Identify patients at risk for suicide. Find out which patients are most likely to try and commit suicide. (Hospital, Behavioral Health). Identify at risk patients while under care and following discharge from health care organization.

Prevent Mistakes in Surgery

Universal Protocol (UP) for Preventing Wrong Site, Wrong Procedure, Wrong Person Surgery

01.01.01. Conduct a pre-procedure verification process. Make sure that the correct surgery is done on the correct patient and at the correct place on the patient's body. (Hospital)

01.02.01. Mark the procedure site. Mark the correct place on the patient's body where the surgery is to be done. (Hospital)

01.03.01. A time-out is performed before the procedure. Pause before the surgery/procedure to make sure that a mistake is not being made (time-out). (Hospital)

Appendix 13

Cultural Aspects of Medicine Therapy

As the diversity of the population increases, it has become clearer that health and medication administration practices should continually be reassessed. Culture and language are central to the process by which the health care provider tries to obtain information and learn from clients what their concerns, worries, and thoughts about their heath condition encompass. This enables the provider to be able to make appropriate assessments, diagnoses, treatment plans, medication selection, and identification of potential side effects. Both providers and clients are guided by their respective cultural norms. Providers may find difficulties in inducing changes in health-related behaviors that conflict with the typical cultural practices of these clients. Providers need to be able to assess the cultural differences in health beliefs and practices in the context of their individual social conditions to prevent confusing their individuality with national or other group stereotypes. Clinical care needs to be a private, yet, personalized situation where these clients can present their problems and complaints. The health care environment and interaction with front desk and other staff also influence the client's response to care. This is most important when there are language and cultural barriers in communication between providers and clients since accurate and honest communication between each is essential to the delivery of quality health services. Common approaches for dealing with communication problems include working with an interpreter, including bilingual family members for interpretation, and identifying those in the facility (employee, visitor, etc.) who are bilingual/bicultural.

Use an approach that is persuasive, but not confrontational or offensive. One can resolve conflict by developing trust, and understanding the social context helps. Elderly clients are especially sensitive about being corrected by younger individuals, so you may consider an older interpreter and one of the same gender as the client. Providers need to make sure that the information that they are giving to the client is understood, accepted, and applied as advised. This requires rewording or conversion of technical medical language into language that is culturally meaningful and that enhances the emotional support that the clients may need. Increased linguistic, racial, and cultural diversity of the population require increased sensitivity and culturally relevant approaches to disease control and health promotion. There is a sociomedical need to remove language and cultural barriers between providers and clients to reduce misunderstandings, inefficiencies, increase rapport with clients, and to prevent negative legal, ethical, and economic consequences. Clients need to be instructed on accessing timely, needed and appropriate health care. They may have a misunderstanding from culturally inappropriate and misleading translations such as verbal and gesture misinterpretation, physical distance and touching. They may experience distrust, fear of discrimination, of being stereotyped and misunderstood, and they may be burdened by unaffordable out of pocket costs.

There are medicine cultures within cultures: 1) Folk medicine: sacred, magic, and empirical (e.g., reading astrological signs, rituals, prayer, sacrifices, herbs, etc.) and the provider is referred to as: shaman or priest, spiritualist, herbalist, witch. 2) Popular medicine: horoscopes, cards, magic by "readers" and salespersons on interpersonal basis or using radio, TV, daily press, books, and magazines. This also includes advice by family, friends, coworkers, neighbors, and casual acquaintances (e.g., in subways, buses, sidewalks, waiting rooms, stores, salespersons, etc.). Popular medical practices include sharing prescriptions; taking patented medicines, injections, herbs, and controlled substances brought from abroad. 3) Biomedicine: science-based medical care. The client views the quality of care on the basis of his or her own values and preferences and these are guided and modified by his cultural orientation.

Cultural competence includes knowledge, attitudes, sensitivity, awareness, behaviors, and empathy. The provider must be knowledgeable and capable of managing the communication interplay between the culture and language of medical practice and the client's culturally-oriented health-related values, norms, beliefs and practices. Knowledge is the acquisition of accurate and unbiased information and understanding of the functioning norms, values, belief systems and the common understanding that prevails in one's community of service in relation to health and illness. Cultural awareness is the recognition that the ways of life, behaviors, meanings, and values of individuals are influenced by the social understandings within their communities or social groups. Cultural sensitivity is the ability to recognize similarities and differences in norms, standards of behavior, and conventions between, within and among populations and communities. Cultural sensitivity is expressed by the provider by empathy and respect for cultural differences. With increased diversification of the population, communication barriers have led to misinformation and misunderstandings that have contributed to increases in medical care errors, medication errors, lack of adherence, and lack of health improvement, thus indicating that providers need to reassess their communication skills in providing care.

There are public policies and professional guidelines to eliminate barriers between providers and clients. Among the federal laws and regulation is The Hill Burton Act of 1946 which requires meaningful access to health care as a condition of capital financing. It also requires that providers implement policies and procedures to document the conduct of periodic staff training, issue notices of the right of clients to translation and to oral language assistance, and take responsibility for monitoring these activities. Title VI of the Civil Rights Act of 1964 prohibits discrimination based on race, color, or national origin under any program or activity that receives federal aid. Under Medicare, Medicaid, and the Emergency Medical Treatment and Active Labor Act (EMTALA) guidelines for facilitating access to care have been issued. A variety of federal guidelines have been issued for services to persons of limited English proficiency. The Office of Minority Health (OMH) was established in 1986 to eliminate health disparities in racial and ethnic minority populations. According to the National Standards on Culturally and Linguistically Appropriate Services (CLAS) guidelines, staff members of a facility are expected to provide effective, understandable, and respectful care that is compatible with their clients' cultural health beliefs and practices and preferred language. There are numerous other national and state councils, medical societies, nursing associations and accreditation bodies that have also issued guidelines supporting the inclusion of cultural competence and language proficiency as tools for effective health care delivery services.

Appendix 14

Common Spanish Phrases and Terms Used in a Health Care Setting

Hello/Hi	Hola
Yes	Si
No	No
My name is	Me llamo
What can I do for you today?	¿Que puedo hacer yuo para usted hoy?
How are you feeling?	¿como se siente usted?
Do you take any medications?	¿Toma medicinas?
What are the names of the medications you are taking?	¿Cómo se llaman las medicinas que usted toma?
How old are you?	¿Cuantos anos tiene?
Are you allergic to anything?	¿Usted es alérgico a algo?
Do you have any medical problem?	¿Tiene usted algún problemamédico?
Are you having any pain?	¿Tiene usted aigu'n dolor?
Where is your pain located?	¿Dónde está su dolor localizado?
How long have you had it?	¿Cuán largo lo ha tenido usted?
Have you ever had this pain before?	¿Ha tenido jamás usted este dolor antes?
Are you pregnant?	¿Está embarazada?
How many months?	¿Cuántos meses?
Have you vomited?	¿Vomito?
Diarrhea	diarrea
Constipation	constipación
Have a cough?	¿Tiene una tos?
Have a fever?	¿Tiene una fiebre?
Please lie down	Acuestese, por favor
Relax	Rela'jese
What	Que
Where	Donde
When	Cuando
How long	Por cuanto tiempo
Please repeat	Repita, por favor
Insomnia	insomnia
Cold	frió

Cough	toser
Vision problem	problema de visión
Blurry vision	visión borrosa
Sore foot	dolorenel pie
Cannot urinate	no puede orinar
I have a pain in my stomach	Me duele mi estómago

Body Parts

Head	espuma
Eye	ojo
Nose	nariz
Ear	oído
Mouth	boca
Tongue	lengua
Teeth	diente
Shoulder	hombre
Back	enlomar
Arm	brazo
Hand	mano
Finger	dedo
Stomach	estómago
Leg	pierno
Knee	rodilla
Foot	pie
Toe	dedo del pie
Buttocks	nalgas
Genitals	genitals

Numbers

one	uno
two	dos
three	tres
four	cuatro
five	cinco
six	seis
seven	siete
eight	ocho
nine	nueve
ten	diez

twenty	veinte
thirty	treinta
forty	cuarenta
fifty	cincuenta
one hundred	Cien

Months

January	enero
February	febrero
March	marcha
April	abril
May	mayo
June	junio
July	julio
August	agosto
September	septiembre
October	octubre
November	noviembre
December	diciembre

Days of the Week

Monday	Lunes
Tuesday	Martes
Wednesday	Miercoles
Thursday	Jueves
Friday	Viernes
Saturday	Sabado
Sunday	Domingo

Colors

red	rojo
green	verde
blue	azul
black	negro
yellow	amarillo
brown	café
white	blanco
gray	gris

Miscellaneous

Right	diestro

Left	izquierda
Look up	ir aver
Look down	bajar los ojos
Turn	hacer girar
Sit down	sentarse
Stand up	poner a
Lie down	echarse

Appendix 15

Medication Reconciliation/Overdose/Misuse

Medication reconciliation is a process by which you obtain a complete and accurate list of the current medications from all sources that a patient is taking. This is performed at all points of contact by verifying the names and dosages of all medications to help reduce medication errors. It is done to prevent errors such as omission, duplications, dosing errors, or drug interactions. This process was developed to try and address the greater than 1.3 million adverse events, many related to medication.

Almost half of all medication errors occur at transition points such as transfer between units, upon admission and upon hospital discharge. One quarter of all medication errors occur in the outpatient setting. Medication errors account for at least 7,000 deaths yearly in the United States. More than 750,000 patients are injured because of medication errors yearly. Children are three times more at risk than adults for drug errors. Additionally, drug overdose rates have tripled over the past ten years.

Generally, verification can be accomplished by asking the patient to bring all the medications being taken to the visit so you can review them. Almost one-third of the time there is a difference between the medication orders and the information from the patient about what is actually being taken compared to what the medication label reads.

Hospitals have implemented medication reconciliation processes to collect and compare patient medication information. Hospitals may consider:

- Developing a list of patients' current medications
- Developing a list of medications that will be prescribed
- Comparing the two lists
- Making clinical decisions based on the comparison
- Communicating the new list to patients and caregivers

The list of current medications must include over-the-counter agents and herbals that the patient is consuming. It is much easier to generate and update the list on a computer-based operating system for patient orders, notes, and medications. This list is provided to patients so they can carry it to all providers and medical points of contact to ensure that the list is accurate, up-to-date, and followed by the patient.

The Joint Commission National Patient Safety Goals for 2011 included:

Goal 8 Accurately and completely reconcile medications across the continuum of care.

As of July 2011, this goal was incorporated into NPS6#3 "Improving the Safety of Using Medications." This occurred because there was no proven strategy for accomplishing medication reconciliation.

This goal requires that facilities "maintain and communicate accurate medication information" and compare the medication information the patient brought to the hospital with the medications ordered for the patient by the hospital in order to identify and resolve discrepancies.

Medication reconciliation should be performed at every care transition:

- On admission
- Before surgery
- After surgery

- With any inter-ward/floor transfer
- Any change in provider
- Upon discharge (facility or ED)
- At each visit
- With any change in therapy
- Changes in setting, service, provider, or level of care

A series of interventions, including medication reconciliation can successfully reduce the number of medication errors and patient deaths in this country.

If a form is developed to achieve this goal, the Medication Reconciliation Form should:

- List all of the medicines the patient is currently taking, including prescription and over-the-counter medications, such as aspirin, vitamins, and herbals (e.g., ginkgo, grape seed extract, ginseng, glucosamine, etc.).
- List medications that are taken only as needed, such as Advil, Tylenol, and nitroglycerin.
- Include the patient name and identifying information
- Document that you have reviewed the list of medications with the patient; that the patient understands the form will be updated to include future prescriptions ordered/taken; and that this form will be shared with all of the patient's providers and the pharmacist. They should alert the provider of any new prescriptions or OTC agents consumed.

Overdose/Misuse

Prescription painkiller overdoses killed 15,000 in the United States in 2008. In 2010, approximately 12 million Americans (1 in 20) admitted non-medical use of prescription painkillers. In 2009, 500,000 ER visits were attributed to abuse/misuse of prescription painkillers.

The United States government is developing programs to track this epidemic, educate health care providers, and develop programs and policies to prevent drug abuse/overdose while ensuring access to safe, effective pain treatment.

Many states are requiring that providers purchase prescription pads that are encrypted and cannot be reproduced, and developing electronic databases to track all prescriptions for painkillers in that state.

Health care providers can screen and monitor those they treat for substance abuse and mental health problems, prescribe only when other treatments have failed, prescribe only in small quantities and for the expected timeframe (length of anticipated therapy). Providers may perform random drug screens on those using long-term therapy, and continue to evaluate and educate patients in the safe use, storing, and disposal of prescription painkillers. Additionally, providers may use prescription drug monitoring programs (CPDUP) within the state to ensure proper use and distribution of painkillers, as well as tracking of all prescriptions issued.

IV Index

Boldface = generic drug name | CAPITALS = combination drugs

Index